Electroencephalography

Basic Principles, Clinical Applications, and Related Fields

FIFTH EDITION

Electroencephalography

Basic Principles, Clinical Applications, and Related Fields

FIFTH EDITION

ERNST NIEDERMEYER, M.D.

Consultant in Neurology
Sinai Hospital of Baltimore
Professor Emeritus of Neurology and Neurological Surgery
The Johns Hopkins University School of Medicine
Baltimore, Maryland

FERNANDO LOPES DA SILVA, M.D., PH.D.

Professor Emeritus
Swammerdam Institute for Life Sciences
University of Amsterdam
Amsterdam, The Netherlands

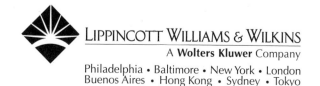

LIPPINCOTT WILLIAMS & WILKINS
A Wolters Kluwer Company

Philadelphia • Baltimore • New York • London
Buenos Aires • Hong Kong • Sydney • Tokyo

Acquisitions Editor: Anne M. Sydor
Developmental Editor: Lisa R. Kairis
Project Manager: Fran Gunning
Manufacturing Manager: Benjamin Rivera
Marketing Manager: Adam Glazer
Production Services: Print Matters, Inc.
Compositor: Compset, Inc.
Printer: Edwards Brothers

© 2005 by LIPPINCOTT WILLIAMS & WILKINS
530 Walnut Street
Philadelphia, PA 19106 USA
LWW.com

Printed in the USA

Library of Congress Cataloging-in-Publication Data

Electroencephalography : basic principles, clinical applications, and related
   fields / [edited by] Ernst Niedermeyer, Fernando Lopes da Silva.—5th ed.
      p. ; cm.
   Includes bibliographical references and index.
   ISBN 0-7817-5126-8
   1. Electroencephalography. I. Niedermeyer, Ernst, 1920– II. Lopes da
Silva, F.H., 1935–
   [DNLM: 1. Electroencephalography. 2. Central Nervous System
Diseases—diagnosis.
   WL 150 E384 2004]
   RC386.6.E43N54 2004
616.8'047547—dc22

                        2004056721

                        10 9 8 7 6 5 4 3 2 1

Preface to the First Edition

The history of clinical electroencephalography (EEG) has just passed the 50-year mark. The age of the pioneers was followed by the stage of expansion. What began in a few prestigious centers gradually became a tool of all academic medical institutions, and eventually of all major hospitals. In more recent years, EEG even invaded the private offices of practicing neurologists and other specialists interested in central nervous system (CNS) disease.

From this perspective, the history of clinical electroencephalography looks like the "via triumphalis" of a buoyantly dynamic new subspecialty. The elucidation of the electrophysiological processes underlying epileptic seizure disorders and a variety of other CNS dysfunctions was indeed a unique achievement made possible by the new method. The original intention of the founder of clinical EEG, Hans Berger, had been the exploration of mental and psychological processes, and even in this domain the yield has been substantial. Moreover, electroencephalographers have not confined themselves to the spontaneous wave patterns of the brain; forms of EEG data analysis with the aid of computers were introduced in order to demonstrate evoked and event-related potentials and to investigate the wealth of frequencies that constitute the EEG. In the search for the sources of EEG generation, the brain tissue became the target of exploration.

Depth electrodes became one of the most important tools of experimental neurophysiologists, who also investigated the single neuron using microelectrodes. The implantation of depth electrodes in the human brain has aided in the evaluation of chronic epileptics considered candidates for seizure surgery.

This impressive progress, however, has been counterbalanced by signs of pessimism, fatigue, and resignation. A certain malaise has inched its way into the hearts of thousands of electroencephalographers who have started to feel the grip of stagnation. Generation of EEG potentials has proved to be extremely complex and difficult to understand; the feeling of doing pragmatically useful work with an ill-understood method has been depressing to many workers in the field. The pragmatists have further suffered from the limitations of EEG as a method of localization of cerebral lesions. These feelings have been nourished by the phenomenal achievements of noninvasive radionuclear and radiological scanning methods; this progress of new methods in the field of structural diagnosis has been a matter of concern for many electroencephalographers. A more real danger, perhaps, is presented by the poorly trained colleagues who are tarnishing the image of EEG.

In reality, however, these challenges present a stimulus for the electrophysiological field. The function-oriented aspects of the neurological sciences will always be of paramount significance. The loss of function-oriented neurology would foreshadow the death of neurology. With all due respect for the structural aspects of lesions and tissue changes, neurology would be shallow and barren without awareness of the constant fluctuation of functional states in the CNS. Another important stimulus has been the establishment of standards of quality for electroencephalographers and EEG laboratories.

In these times of challenge, a review of the state of affairs in electroencephalography seems to be appropriate. Such thoughts have prompted the genesis of this large one-volume textbook which, by its mere size, sets itself apart from the group of smaller introductory textbooks and from the huge multivolume Handbook. The one-volume character of the book symbolizes the spirit of unity that should reign among clinical electroencephalographers, basic science researchers, and workers in the field of computerized data analysis.

One author can hardly undertake such a task alone. For this reason, we have reached out across the ocean for collaboration. It became clear, however, that a two-man effort would not suffice to cover the entire field in the relatively short working period of 2 years. We solicited for assistance and found a wonderful group of contributors in various special areas. Above all, coverage of the fields of neurophysiology and neuropharmacology have depended most heavily on the assistance of prestigious specialists.

Attempts at synthesis have not been the goal of this book. Instead the reader will find a more individualistic approach from which the personal basic philosophy of each author can be derived. No effort has been made to achieve strict standardization of symbols and terminology; as an example, frequencies are described in various terms (10 cps, 10/sec, 10 Hz, etc.). There is also some overlap between certain chapters; we feel that the reader will benefit from the presentation of a given topic as seen from two somewhat different viewpoints.

A piece of technical information might be worthwhile. Unless the filter setting is specifically indicated in the illustrations of EEG tracings, a time constant between 0.15 to 0.5 sec was used (above 0.4 sec when slow frequencies played a major role). The use of "muscle filters" was avoided.

We have tried to combine didactic and academic elements in this book. Hence, trainees as well as seasoned professionals in the field will, we hope, find what they are searching for. This dual approach does mean that some parts of the book require greater sophistication of the reader than do others.

Acknowledgments for invaluable help in this undertaking come from the depth of our hearts. Mr. Braxton Dallam Mitchell, President of Urban & Schwarzenberg in Baltimore,

Maryland, deserves the honor of having been the initiator of this book. His encouragement has been very much appreciated. Detlev Moos has coordinated the production of this book with care and efficiency; Suzanne Lohmeyer has copyedited and indexed it well; and Nan Tyler, Carola Sautter, and Victoria Doherty at the publisher's Baltimore office assisted with their experience. In the Johns Hopkins Hospital in Baltimore, Maryland, the technical staff of the laboratory deserves great praise: Mrs. Judy Nastalski, R. EEG T. and chief technologist, Mr. Eric DeShields, Mrs. Debbie Reichenbach, R. EEG T., Miss Sharon Vaughan, Mrs. Kathleen Daniecki, R. EEG T., Mrs. Cindy Haywood, and Miss Kim Rimel. How deeply the electroencephalographer depends on the quality of the recordings and the dedication of the technologists! Truly invaluable was the secretarial assistance of Mrs. Catherine Bonolis. The operation of the laboratory was further aided by the experience of Mrs. Marie Simpson. Important contributions came from Mr. Joe Dieter, who is responsible for the pictorial artwork, Mr. Ron Garret (lettering of tracings), and Mr. Zuhair Kareem and Mrs. Lillian Reich, the staff of Medical Photography.

Assistance and advice in the clinical EEG field was given most freely by Dr. Gisela Freund, Visiting Assistant Professor at the Johns Hopkins Hospital EEG Laboratory (1980/81), of the Department of Clinical Neurophysiology, Free University Berlin (Klinikum Westend). E.N.'s principal teacher in the field of electroencephalography, Dr. John R. Knott (presently of Boston, Massachusetts), and the great master of neurosurgery, epileptology, and neurophysiology, Dr. A. Earl Walker (presently of Albuquerque, New Mexico), deserve special gratitude.

Gratitude is expressed (by F.L.S.) to Professor Dr. W. Storm von Leeuwen, Dr. G. Wieneke, and Dr. K. Van Hulten (Utrecht University Hospital), Mr. N.J.I. Mars (Twente University of Technology), and Mr. A. Van Rotterdam (Institute of Medical Physics, Utrecht) for their advice and encouragement. The high professional competence of Mrs. Ada Van Schaik and Mr. Nico Haagen (Institute of Medical Physics, Utrecht) in their fields of secretarial work and art work was of invaluable help.

Heartfelt thanks are also expressed to the contributing authors of the book; they have naturally become a part of this undertaking. The response of these splendid co-workers was exemplary. Joseph J. Tecce and Lynn Cattanach, the authors of the article on contingent negative variation, substituted for a colleague who had to step down from his obligations at the last minute. They made possible the almost impossible when they declared their willingness to join the team of co-workers. To them, and to all the contributing authors of this volume, our deepest thanks.

ERNST NIEDERMEYER
FERNANDO LOPES DA SILVA
Spring 1981

Preface to the Fifth Edition

The inexorable flux of time has once again changed the electroencephalography (EEG) scene: a complex landscape with many outcroppings of the old classic electroencephalogram. Has it been a period of progress that separates us from the days of work on the fourth edition?

Digital EEG machines have made their triumphant entry into clinical as well as experimental laboratories. This change may not have materialized yet in less affluent countries where digital recording has remained unaffordable. Take heart, dear friends from those places: what your paper-written tracings show is, and will always be, a true electroencephalogram. It is not a question of modern vs. old-fashioned: The real question is the perennial dichotomy of good vs. poor EEG since deficient electrode attachment and uninspired interpretation spoil both paper-recorded and digital tracings.

And yet, with the advent of digital EEG something wonderfully new has arisen: the exploration of ultrafast and ultraslow EEG frequencies lies at our doorstep. It is up to you to make use of the new possibilities. In the enlarged EEG spectrum lies great promise for the clinical-epileptological EEGer and perhaps even greater prospects for the neurocognitive basic neuroscientist. The enlargement of our frequency range will give EEG a new completeness; therein lies the challenge of the ultraEEG—the EEG of the 21st century!

The exploration of what lies under scalp and skull has gained further importance. Classic forms of ultraEEG, the Franco-Swiss stereoelectroencephalography, subdural recording, and electrocorticography have become increasingly useful with this new wave of neurosurgical epilepsy treatment. Epilepsy centers with EEC-Video-Monitoring facilities have been mushrooming. Stimulation techniques have been tried and may still have to convince the doubters. Electrical and magnetic stimulation of the scalp have given us fascinating new vistas: this "stimulation from the top" has engendered powerful impetus for spinal monitoring during neurosurgical and orthopedic spinal procedures. The worlds of EEG and Magnetoencephalography appear to be closely intertwined and even involved in a competitive battle for the detection of epileptogenic foci. With all those similarities between EEG and MEG tracings, the gap between these two good neighborly fields should be bridged in the near future.

As before, much space is given in this book to the world of evoked and event-related potentials. These techniques explore CNS functions with remarkable efficacy. The role of the P 300 (and similar potentials) for psychological and psychiatric research has been steadily gaining strength.

This leads us to the part that used to be called "Psychophysiology" in earlier editions and is now appearing under the more timely heading of "Neurocognitive Functions." The relationship between brain and mind has remained shrouded in mystery like the Holy Grail at the legendary Montsalvat castle. Neurocognitive research has been flourishing over the past two decades; mostly with the use of neuroimaging methods while EEG and EP-related techniques have not abandoned the struggle for the highest prize. We may have to wait and think which features of cognitive functions can be analyzed neurophysiologically by way of ultraEEG/MEG whole-head recordings. This riddle might require philosophical expertise, and satisfactory answers may still lie years or decades ahead unless a phenomenal breakthrough occurs.

A plethora of new computer-assisted methods dedicated to the analysis of EEG/MEG signals has emerged from the research of mathematicians, physicists, and computer scientists allied with clinical neurophysiologists and is enriching our community with new tools to better understand the EEG. A glimpse into these new developments could not pass unnoticed in a new edition.

The writers of these lines express their profound gratitude to the publishers of this volume and, in particular, to Mr. Charley Mitchell and Ms. Lisa Kairis, who have been exuding the greatest encouragement for this undertaking. Next item: thanks for secretarial assistance. . . . Sorry, there was none. The years of retirement and emeritus status have drawbacks in this respect. But last, and certainly not least, we thank the host of coauthors, who have been wonderful. From them arose a spirit of enthusiasm that made our work much easier. Many, many thanks.

ERNST NIEDERMEYER
FERNANDO LOPES DA SILVA

Contents

Contributors

Franz Aichner, M.D.
Professor and Chief, Neurology
Landeskrankenhaus
Linz, Austria

Eckart O. Altenmüller, M.D.
Director and Chair
Institute of Music Physiology and Musicians' Medicine
University of Music and Drama
Hannover, Germany

Santiago Arroyo, M.D., Ph.D.
Medical Director
Department of CNS
EISAI Global Clinical Development
Ridgefield Park, NJ

Gerhard Bauer, M.D.
Professor
University Hospital for Neurology
Innsbruck, Austria

Richard Bauer, M.D.
University Hospital for Neurology
Pharmacological Institute
University of Innsbruck
Innsbruck, Austria

Aleksandar Beric, M.D., D.Sc.
Professor
Department of Neurology
New York University School of Medicine
Hospital for Joint Diseases
New York, NY

Warren T. Blume, M.D.
Professor, Neurology, Clinical Neurophysiology
University Hospital
London, Ontario, Canada

Richard P. Brenner, M.D.
Professor
Department of Neurology and Psychiatry
University of Pittsburgh School of Medicine
Director, EEG Laboratories
University of Pittsburgh Medical Center
Departments of Neurology and Psychiatry
Western Psychiatric Institute and Clinic
Pittsburgh, PA

Mitchell G. Brigell, Ph.D.
Associate Professor
Department of Neurology
Loyola University
Chicago, IL
Stritch School of Medicine
Maywood, IL

Roger J. Broughton, M.D., Ph.D.
Professor of Neurology
Department of Medicine
University of Ottawa Faculty of Medicine
Sleep Medicine Physician
Department of Medicine (Neurology)
Ottawa Hospital General Campus
Ottawa, Ontario, Canada

Peter Brown, M.D., F.R.C.P.
Professor
Sobell Department of Motor Neuroscience and Movement
    Disorders
Institute of Neurology
University College London
London, United Kingdom

Gastone G. Celesia, M.D.
Professor
Department of Neurology
Loyola University
Chicago, IL

Jan Claassen, M.D.
Research Fellow
Department of Neurology
Columbia University
The Presbyterian Hospital
New York, NY

Gabriel Curio, M.D., Ph.D.
Adjunct Professor
Department of Neurology
Campus Benjamin Franklin
Head
Neurophysics Group and Clinical Electroencephalography
Charité-University Medicine
Berlin, Germany

Gretchen L. Dike, M.D.
Department of Neurology
State University of Michigan
Lansing, MI

Günter Edlinger, M.Sc., Ph.D.
CEO
Department of Research and Development
g.tec Medical Engineering GmbH
Graz, Austria

Christian E. Elger, M.D., FRCP
Professor and Director
Department of Neurology (Epileptology)
University Hospital
Bonn, Germany

Mariella Fischer-Williams, M.D.
Milwaukee, WI

James D. Frost, Jr., M.D.
Professor
Departments of Neurology and Neuroscience
Baylor College of Medicine
Deputy Chief of Service
Department of Neurophysiology
The Methodist Hospital
Houston, TX

Christian Gerloff, M.D.
Center for Neurology
Neurologic University and Clinic
Tübingen, Germany

Pascal Grosse, Ph.D.
Department of Neurology
Humboldt University
Berlin, Germany

Hans-Christian Hansen, M.D.
Professor
Department of Neurology
University of Hamburg
Hamburg, Germany
Head
Departments of Neurology and Psychiatry
Friedrich-Ebert-Krankenhaus and Fachklinik Hahnknuell
Neumuenster, Germany

Riitta Hari, M.D., Ph.D.
Professor
Brain Research Unit, Low Temperature Laboratory
Helsinki University of Technology
Helsinki, Finland

Kai Kaila, Ph.D.
Professor
Department of Biological and Environmental Sciences
University of Helsinki
Helsinki, Finland

Anton Kamp
Biological Centre
University of Amsterdam
Amsterdam, The Netherlands

Gregory L. Krauss, M.D.
Professor
Department of Neurology
Director, Adult Epilepsy Clinic
The Johns Hopkins University School of Medicine
Baltimore, MD

Allan Krumholz, M.D.
Professor
Department of Neurology
University of Maryland School of Medicine
Baltimore, MD

Terrence D. Lagerlund, M.D.
Professor
Department of Neurology
The Mayo Clinic College of Medicine
Rochester, MN

Ronald P. Lesser, M.D.
Professor
Departments of Neurology and Neurosurgery
Zanvyl-Krieger Mind/Brain Institute
Johns Hopkins University
Baltimore, MD

Fernando Lopes da Silva, M.D., Ph.D.
Professor Emeritus
Swammerdam Institute for Life Sciences
University of Amsterdam
Amsterdam, The Netherlands

François Mauguière, M.D., Ph.D., D.Sc.
Professor
Department of Neurology
Claude Bernard Lyon I University
Faculty of Medicine Lyon-Nord
Chief Department of Functional Neurology and
    Epileptology
Neurological Hospital "Pierre Wertheimer"
Lyon, France

Janet M. Mullington, Ph.D.
Assistant Professor
Department of Neurology
Harvard Medical School
Department of Neurology
Beth Israel Deaconess Medical Center
Boston, MA

Thomas F. Münte, M.D.
Professor
Department of Neuropsychology
University of Magdeburg
Magdeburg, Germany

Sakkubai Naidu, M.D.
Professor
The Johns Hopkins University School of Medicine
Director
Clinical Neurogenetics
The Kennedy Krieger Institute
Baltimore, MD

Christa Neuper, Ph.D.
Senior Scientist
Department of Human–Computer Interfaces
University of Technology Graz
Associate Professor
Institute of Psychology
University of Graz
Graz, Austria

Ernst Niedermeyer, M.D.
Consultant in Neurology
Sinai Hospital of Baltimore
Professor Emeritus of Neurology and Neurological
    Surgery
The Johns Hopkins University School of Medicine
Baltimore, MD

Aurea Nogueira de Melo, M.D.
Professor of Pediatric Neurology
Department of Clinical Medicine
Federal University of Rio Grande do Norte
Hospital Universitário Onofre Lopes
Natal, Brazil

Marc R. Nuwer, M.D., Ph.D.
Professor, Clinical Neurophysiologist
Department of Neurology
UCLA School of Medicine
Department of Clinical Neurophysiology
UCLA Medical Center
Los Angeles, CA

James W. Packwood, Ph.D.
Clinical Neurophysiologist
Department of Neurology
UCLA School of Medicine
Department of Clinical Neurophysiology
UCLA Medical Center
Los Angeles, CA

Neal S. Peachey, M.D.
Assistant Professor
Department of Neurology
Loyola University-Chicago
Stritch School of Medicine
Maywood, IL
Hines VA Hospital
Hines, IL

Gert Pfurtscheller, Ph.D.
Professor
Department of Medical Informatics
Director
Institute of Biomedical Engineering
Graz University of Technology
Graz, Austria

Luis Felipe Quesney, M.D., Ph.D.
Center of Electroencephalography
Perez Modrego Medical Facility
Complutense University
Madrid, Spain

Manoj Raghavan, M.D., Ph.D.
Assistant Professor
Department of Neurology
Medical College of Wisconsin
Attending Physician
Department of Neurology
Froedtert Memorial Lutheran Hospital
Milwaukee, WI

Edward L. Reilly, M.D.
Professor
Residency Training Director
Department of Psychiatry
University of Texas Medical School
Department of Psychiatry
Harris County Psychiatric Clinic
Houston, TX

Erik Rumpl, M.D.
Professor
Chief, Department of Neurology
Landeskrankenhaus
Klagenfurt, Austria

Mark S. Scher, M.D.
Associate Professor
Case-Western Reserve University School of Medicine
Chief
Division of Pediatric Neurology
Rainbow Babies and Children's Hospital
Cleveland, OH

Frank W. Sharbrough, M.D.
Department of Neurology
The Mayo Clinic and Mayo Foundation
Rochester, MN

Joyce G. Small, M.D.
Professor Emerita
Department of Psychiatry
Indiana University School of Medicine
Larue D. Carter Memorial Hospital
Indianapolis, IN

Erwin-Josef Speckmann, M.D.
Professor
Institut fur Physiologie
Bereich Neurophysiologie
Westfälische Wilhelms-Universität
Muenster, Germany

Mircea Steriade, M.D., D.Sc.
Professor
Department of Physiology
Faculty of Medicine
Laval University
Quebec, Canada

Takeo Takahashi, M.D.
Director
Department of Neuropsychiatry
Yaotome Clinic
Sendai, Japan

Anne C. Van Cott, M.D.
Assistant Professor
Department of Neurology
University of Pittsburgh School of Medicine
Director
EEG Laboratory
Department of Neurology
VA Pittsburgh Health Care System
Pittsburgh, PA

Sampsa Vanhatalo, M.D., Ph.D.
Department of Neurophysiology
University Hospital of Helsinki
Helsinki, Finland

Ab van Rotterdam, Ph.D.
Senior Researcher (retired)
Radiobiological Laboratory
Radiobiological Institute TNO
Rijswijk, The Netherlands

Juha Voipio, Ph.D.
Professor
Department of Biological and Environmental Sciences
University of Helsinki
Helsinki, Finland

Albert Wauquier, Ph.D.
CEO
Dr. Drowsy, Inc.
Wichita, KS

W. Robert S. Webber, Ph.D.
Director of Programming
Epilepsy Monitoring Unit
The Johns Hopkins University School of Medicine
Baltimore, MD

Barbara F. Westmoreland, M.D.
Professor
Department of Neurology
The Mayo Medical School
Rochester, MN

Heinz Gregor Wieser, M.D.
Professor
Department of Epileptology and EEG
Neurology Clinic
Universitäts-Spital
Zurich, Switzerland

Gregory A. Worrell, M.D., Ph.D.
Associate Professor
Department of Neurology
Mayo Medical School
Consultant
The Mayo Clinic
Rochester, MN

Electroencephalography

Basic Principles, Clinical Applications, and Related Fields

FIFTH EDITION

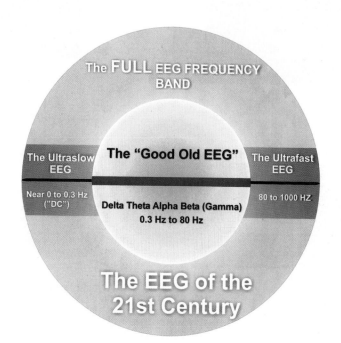

Figure 9.5

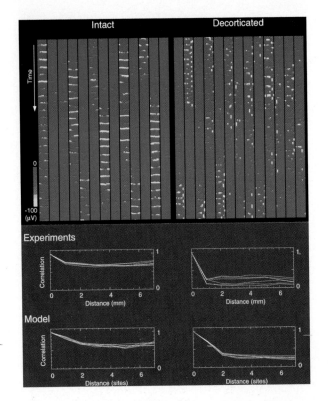

Figure 3.5

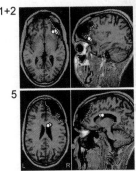

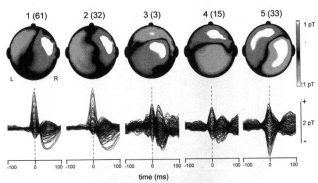

Figure 5.5

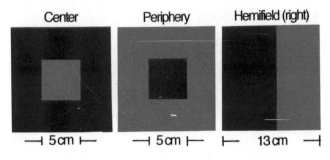

Figure 14.9

EEG premovement potentials

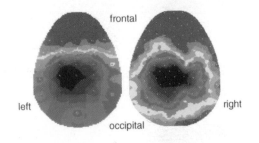

Figure 31.8

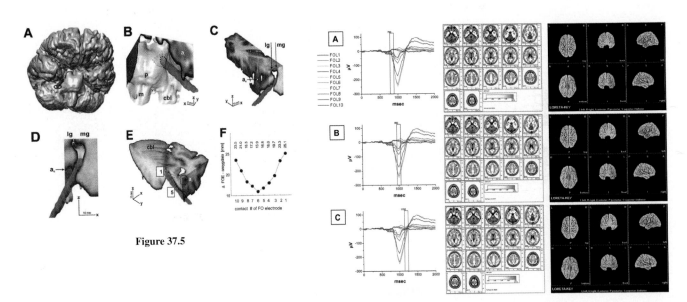

Figure 37.5

Figure 37.10

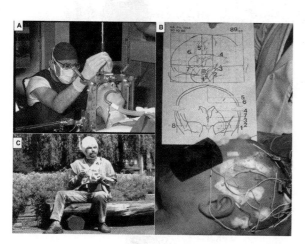

Figure 37.13

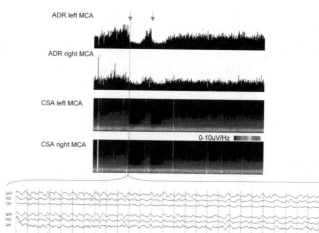

Figure 56.4

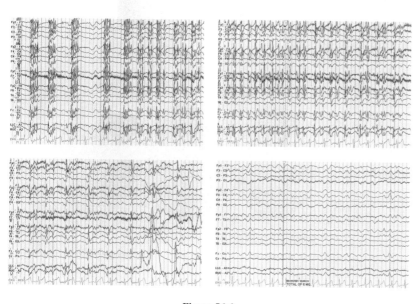

Figure 56.6

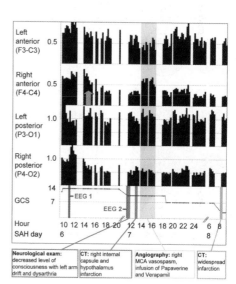

Figure 56.8a

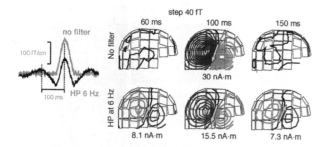

Figure 57.7

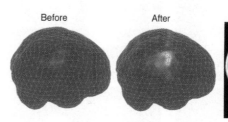

Figure 57.14

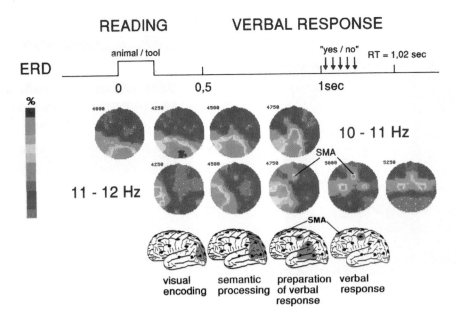

READING   **VERBAL RESPONSE**

ERD

animal / tool

"yes / no"   RT = 1,02 sec

0   0,5   1sec

%

10 - 11 Hz

SMA

11 - 12 Hz

SMA

visual encoding | semantic processing | preparation of verbal response | verbal response

Figure 58.17

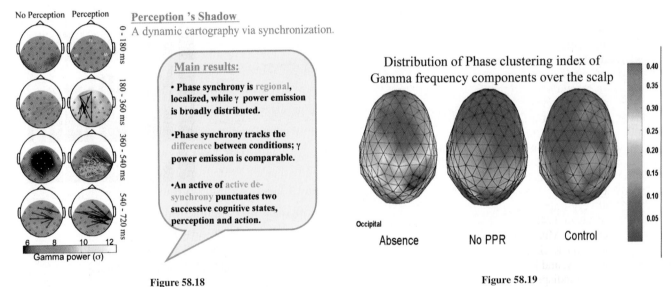

No Perception | Perception

0 - 180 ms
180 - 360 ms
360 - 540 ms
540 - 720 ms

6   8   10   12
Gamma power (σ)

Perception's Shadow
A dynamic cartography via synchronization.

Main results:

• Phase synchrony is regional, localized, while γ power emission is broadly distributed.

• Phase synchrony tracks the difference between conditions; γ power emission is comparable.

• An active of active de-synchrony punctuates two successive cognitive states, perception and action.

Figure 58.18

Distribution of Phase clustering index of Gamma frequency components over the scalp

0.40
0.35
0.30
0.25
0.20
0.15
0.10
0.05

Occipital

Absence   No PPR   Control

Figure 58.19

16 CHANNELS
uV 9.554
-1.641
EEG Systems Laboratory
Pjt17, Memory Move Locked Linked Ear 78 msec
A

27 CHANNELS
uV 10.78
-2.53
EEG Systems Laboratory
Pjt17, Memory Move Locked Linked Ear 78 msec
B

51 CHANNELS
uV 12.52
-5.868
EEG Systems Laboratory
Pjt17, Memory Move Locked Linked Ear 78 msec
C

LAPLACIAN DEBLURRING (51 CHANNELS)
uV/cm² 1.224
-0.964
EEG Systems Laboratory
Pjt17, No Memory Move Locked Laplacian 78,125 ms
D

Figure 59.12

MEG: distribution of sources per voxel

spindles

alpha

mu

max

min

Figure 59.13

1. Historical Aspects

Ernst Niedermeyer

Discovery of Electrical Phenomena

Thales from Miletos has been credited with the discovery of static electricity produced by friction (rubbing fur or glass with silk). He was one of the pre-Socratic "natural philosophers" of Greece (around 620–550 BC) and considered water the origin of all things. Thus, friction was recognized as the generator of a phenomenon that derived its name from the Greek work "electron," which stands for amber. This discovery fell into a dormant stage for more than two millennia.

Around 1600, William Gilbert began to study the electrical properties of various substances, and Otto von Guericke (1602–1686) invented the friction machine to create electrical fields. This machine eventually found its way into doctors' offices and even university hospitals. Its electrical field would make a patient's hair stand up, creating a strong impression on a psychologically gullible patient. These friction machines now ornament high school laboratories and technical museums. In the 17th and 18th centuries, the friction machine taught invaluable lessons on attraction and repulsion of charged bodies, on conductors and nonconductors, and on the rather questionable dualism of positive and negative electricity.

A new and very important piece of electrical equipment entered the scene in 1746 when the Leyden jar was introduced by Pieter van Musschenbroek (following the earlier work of Ewald von Kleist). This invention resulted in the storage of electricity, and its upshot, the condenser or capacitor, turned into an indispensable part of modern electronics. Benjamin Franklin's bold experiment caught electrical discharges of a thunderstorm in a Leyden jar.

What the friction machine could generate, the Leyden jar could store. Its sudden discharge was used in many experiments (O'Leary and Goldring, 1976).

The role of static electricity in medicine appeared to be forgotten for about 150 years and became resurrected with the introduction of the defibrillating cardioversion by William B. Kouwenhoven and his co-workers in the 1950s and 1960s; this approach may hold promises for cerebral applications (Niedermeyer, 2003a).

A serious scientific controversy developed in Italy between Luigi Galvani (1737–1798), professor at the University of Bologna, and Alessandro Volta (1745–1832) in the wake of Galvani's discovery of frog leg contractions within an electrical circuit and especially in the presence of a thunderstorm (1780). Volta doubted the biological nature of the contraction (animal electricity) and placed the emphasis on physics—on his "pile," the first battery (around 1800). This bimetallic pile was a generator capable of producing a steady flow of electricity. Volta's view more or less prevailed in this

hotly debated argument. The laws governing flowing electricity were soon discovered by Georg Ohm in 1827.

Nevertheless, Galvani's belief in "animal electricity" was not lost with other discarded false ideas. There still remained the nagging question of an active electrical contribution of animal muscle tissue.

Beginnings of Electrophysiology

The introduction of the galvanometer has been associated chiefly with the name of Nobili in Florence; this instrument was refined in 1858 by William Thompson (Lord Kelvin) in England (O'Leary and Goldring, 1976). These galvanometers would faithfully demonstrate continuous electrical currents and their variations in intensity but failed in the detection of instantaneous electrical phenomena.

Carlo Matteucci (1811–1868) in Bologna and Emil Du Bois-Reymond (1818–1896) in Berlin became the major proponents of an electrophysiologically based physiology of the nervous system. (The French name of Du Bois-Reymond indicates the Huguenot origin of this Prussian investigator.) Du Bois-Reymond coined the term *negative variation* for a phenomenon occurring during muscle contraction when the galvanometer indicated an unexpected decrease in current intensity (O'Leary and Goldring, 1976). This term was later resurrected in earliest electroencephalogram (EEG) research (Caton, 1875) and with the discovery of the "contingent negative variation" (Walter, 1964).

Hermann von Helmholtz (1821–1894) accurately measured the velocity of nerve conduction, which had been vastly overestimated up to that time. The electrodes used in physiological research were improved and made nonpolarizable (Du Bois-Reymond). The concept of "action current" was introduced by L. Hermann (1834–1919) and thus clarified Du Bois-Reymond's negative variations found during muscle contraction. Julius Bernstein (1839–1917) proposed a membrane theory of nerve tissue, which ultimately was elucidated as late as 1939 and the following years by A. L. Hodgkin and A. F. Huxley in England. Against this background of strongly evolving electrophysiology of the nervous system, the first observation of EEG-like electrical brain activity took place.

Caton: The First Attempt at the Electrical Activity of the Brain

Richard Caton (1842–1926) (Fig. 1.1) was a physician practicing in Liverpool who became deeply interested in electrophysiological phenomena and eventually received a grant from the British Medical Association to explore elec-

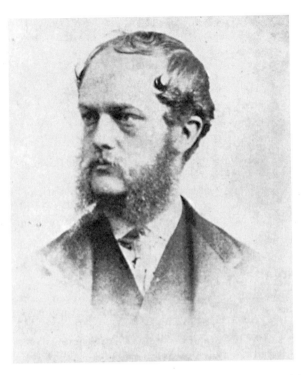

Figure 1.1.   Richard Caton at the time of his work on the electrical activity of the brain. (From Brazier, M.A.B. 1961. *A History of the Electrical Activity of the Brain. The First Half-Century.* London: Pitman, with permission from Macmillan.)

trical phenomena of the exposed cerebral hemispheres of rabbits and monkeys. According to Brazier (1961), Caton presented his findings to the association on August 24, 1875, and a very short report of 20 lines subsequently appeared in the *British Medical Journal*. A more detailed report was presented in the same journal in 1877 on experiments of more than 40 rabbits, cats, and monkeys, the rabbit having been principally employed.

Caton used a galvanometer. A beam of light was thrown on the mirror of the galvanometer and reflected on a large scale placed on the wall. With this type of visualization, Caton found that "feeble currents of varying direction pass through the multiplier when the electrodes are placed on two points of the external surface, or one electrode on the grey matter, and one on the surface of the skull." This sentence is regarded as indicating the birth of the electrophysiologram because one can assume that EEG phenomena made the needle move from one direction to the other. (The suffix "gram" naturally is out of place since "graphein" means "to write" and there was no written recording.) Even though artifacts could have played a major role, Caton deserves credit for the discovery of the fluctuating potentials that constitute the EEG.

Caton also described a few more interesting observations. He noted that the external surface of the gray matter was positive in relation to deep structures of the cerebrum. He also noted that the electric currents of the cerebrum appeared to have a relation to underlying function: "When any part of the grey matter is in a state of functional activity, its electric current usually exhibits negative variation." Thus,

Caton has also been credited with pioneer work on evoked potential. Furthermore, the difference in polarity found between cortical surface and deeper areas could be interpreted as the discovery of the "steady potential" ("DC potential"), but it might be wise to refrain from such statements that cannot be fully supported by the evidence. With regard to the fluctuations, Geddes (1987) pointed out that Caton's galvanometer had a very limited frequency response range from 0 to 6 Hz.

Caton found some measure of success and recognition with this work and held the chair of physiology at the University College of Liverpool from 1884 to 1891, when he resigned from this post. Later he became dean of the medical faculty and, in 1907, mayor (Lord Mayor) of Liverpool. The electrical activity of the brain did not occupy a predominant position in his further endeavors. Even though Caton became an EEG research dropout, his bold work will always remain a milestone in the history of the electrical activity of the brain. [More information on Caton's life and work is found in Mary Brazier's (1961) fine account.]

Eastern European Studies of Electrical Brain Activity

The time was ripe for further studies of electrical phenomena of the cerebrum. Concurrent with Caton's epochal work of 1875, physiologists of Eastern Europe began to demonstrate their independent observations and discoveries concerning the brain and its electrical activity. Another discovery of the 1870s had an incomparably greater impact on the neuroscientific world than Caton's demonstration of electrical activity of the brain. The capability of the human cerebral cortex to be electrically stimulated was discovered by G. Fritsch (1838–1927) and Julius Eduard Hitzig (1838–1907) in a joint study in 1870. According to O'Leary and Goldring (1976), an unusual observation had prompted Fritsch in his work: he had observed contralateral muscle contractions during dressing of an open brain wound in the Prussian-Danish War of 1864. The work of Fritsch and Hitzig was furthered by D. Ferrier and G. F. Yeo in 1880, who performed electrical stimulations of the cerebrum in apes and also in a patient who was operated on for a brain tumor. The repercussions of the stimulation studies were considerable since many investigators of that time held the view that the entire cerebrum is a homogeneous organ that harbors mental functions.

The response of the cortex to electrical stimulation probably was a special incentive for the study of its spontaneous electrical phenomena. This incentive was particularly strong in Eastern Europe, i.e., in laboratories of Russian and Polish universities. (In spite of the important historical ethnic and national differences, the fact cannot be ignored that most of Poland was part of the Czarist Russian Empire throughout the 19th century.)

Vasili Yakovlevich Danilevsky (1852–1939) was only 25 years old when he finished his thesis entitled "Investigations into the Physiology of the Brain" (Danilevsky, 1877), written at the University of Kharkov. This work was based on electrical stimulation as well as on spontaneous electrical activity in the brains of animals. Thus, Danilevsky walked in Caton's footsteps; in 1891, he gave full credit to Caton's priority. Mary Brazier (1961) comments on the disappointment of Danilevsky who saw his high hopes unfulfilled as far as the spontaneous electrical activity of the brain was concerned; he had expected better correlation with psychic and emotional processes. He remained deeply involved in brain physiology and published an extensive textbook of human physiology in 1915. He was not the only EEG researcher with shattered hopes in the field of psychophysiology.

The life and work of Adolf Beck (1863–1939) have been described in great detail by Brazier (1961). Beck worked in Kraków as well as in Lwow (the Polish province of Galicia, at that time a part of the Austrian-Hungarian monarchy). With nonpolarizable electrodes, Beck investigated the spontaneous electrical activity of the brain in rabbits and dogs. He observed the disappearance of rhythmical oscillations when the eyes were stimulated with light and thus became a forebear of Berger's discovery of alpha blocking. His work became widely known due to its publication in the *Central-blatt*.

To present a chronological account of the events, let us leave Eastern Europe for a moment, but not Vienna. In 1883, Ernst Fleischl von Marxow (1846–1891) deposited a sealed letter at the Imperial Academy of Sciences in Vienna that contained observations on cerebral electrical activity recorded over the visual cortex in various species of animals. He did not observe oscillatory activity. He claimed priority when Beck in 1890 published his data but was not aware of earlier work done by Caton and Danilevsky. The oddity of this episode is underscored by more recent historical accounts (Brazier, 1961; O'Leary and Goldring, 1976) that indicate that Fleischl von Marxow's work was not of first-rate quality. This does not detract from the renaissance-man versatility of this Austrian physiologist, who was well versed in linguistics (even Sanskrit), swimming, hunting, and mountain climbing.

Exciting new studies were being conducted in Eastern European universities. Napoleon Cybulski (1854–1919), who was Beck's teacher in Kraków and an internationally renowned leader in general physiology, presented experimental electroencephalographic studies in graphical form by using a galvanometer with a photographic attachment. He provided EEG evidence of an epileptic seizure in the dog caused by electrical stimulation.

Two Russian physiologists made further studies along these lines: Pavel Yurevich Kaufman (1877–1951) and Vladimir Vladimirovich Pravdich-Neminsky (1879–1952). Prior to the discussion of their work, a few words must be said about technological developments. The d'Arsonval galvanometer featured a mirror mounted on a movable coil; light focused on the mirror was deflected when a current passed the coil. The capillary electrometer was introduced by G. Lippmann and H. J. Marey [for further details, see O'Leary and Goldring (1976)]. Most important was the introduction by Willem Einthoven in 1903 of the string galvanometer, a very sensitive instrument that required photographic recording and became the standard instrumentation for electrocardiography at the turn of the century.

Kaufman's work and life are portrayed in Brazier's (1961) historical account. Kaufman expressed the view that an epileptic attack would have to be associated with abnor-

mal electrical discharges, and he studied the effects of cortical electrical stimulation. With World War I, he took the name of Rostoutsev and worked mainly at the University of Baku.

Pravdich-Neminsky began recording electrical brain activity of animals in 1912 with the string galvanometer. As Brazier (1961) has pointed out, his recordings, published in 1912, were the first pictorial demonstration of EEG and appeared two years earlier than Cybulski's tracings. Pravdich-Neminsky recorded the EEG from the brain, the dura, or the intact skull of the dog. He described a 12 to 14/sec rhythm under normal conditions and marked slowing under asphyxia. Furthermore, he coined the term *electrocerebrogram* (Fig. 1.2).

The achievements of the Eastern European neuroscientists during those 50 years preceding the outbreak of World War I fill us with awe and clearly demonstrate their special talent for electrophysiological neurophysiology. Limiting discussion to EEG history can show only the tip of the iceberg. To assess the true strength of their neuroscientific institutions, one must mention investigators in somewhat related electrophysiological areas. Ivan Michailovich Sechenov (1829–1905) appears to be founder of this powerful school of eminent neurophysiologists. He studied the electrical activity of the spinal cord and oblongata in the frog and was a predecessor of Pavlovian thought. Nikolai Yevgenevich Wedensky followed Sechenov as the chair and professor of physiology at St. Petersburg (known for the concept of Wedensky inhibition). Vladimir Efimovich Larionov, also working in St. Petersburg, conducted beautiful studies of the auditory cortex in the dog.

The greatest Russian neuroscientist was also the most eminent clinical neurologist of his country: Vladimir Mikhailovich Bechterev (also "Bekhterev") (1857–1927). He occupied the chair of psychiatry in St. Petersburg, which included the field of clinical neurology. He was a disciple of Du Bois-Reymond, Paul Emil Flechsig, and Wilhelm Wundt, and also worked at Charcot's clinic in Paris. The influence of Wundt prompted Bechterev's associative reflexology (I treasure his work "Allgemeine Grundlagen der Reflexologie des Menschen," Deuticke, Leipzig, 1926, even though I can hardly agree with his "objective study of personality"). He combined his clinical work and private practice with tireless psychophysiological methods. A photograph with one of his two assistants shows Bechterev wearing a thick winter coat in his institute in Leningrad, giving testimony to the icy cold in the unheated laboratory. "Functional anatomy of the brain, experimental psychology and clinical neurology were the three fields in which Bekhterev carved out a place for himself" (Yakovlev, 1953).

The Soviet regime had to choose between Bechterev and Ivan Petrovich Pavlov (1849–1936), a physiologist who had won the Nobel Prize in 1904 for his early work on conditioned reflexes. Pavlov was the choice, and the magic of conditioned reflex overshadowed all Soviet neurophysiology by highest decree (even though Pavlov himself was highly critical of the regime). The Pavlovian concept was closer to the ideology of dialectic materialism and this maxim with all its intolerant dogmatism outlasted Pavlov's death by two decades. This ideopolitically governed form of

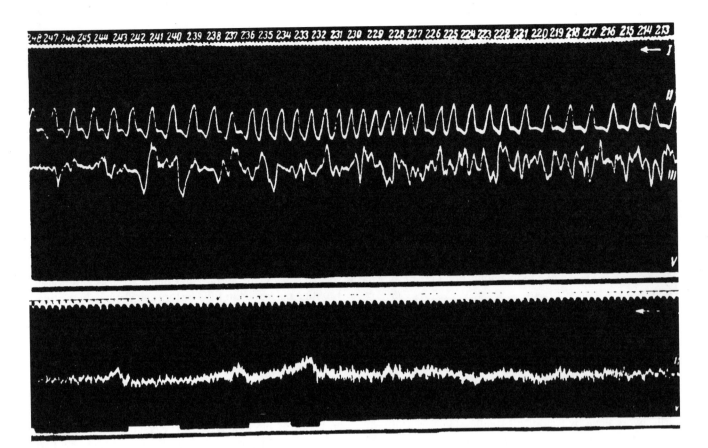

Figure 1.2. The first photographs to be published of electroencephalograms. In the upper record Neminsky shows (in the third trace) the brain potentials of a curarized dog with the pulsations from an artery in the brain recorded above them. In the lower record the sciatic nerve is being stimulated from time to time, and the decrease in activity noted by Neminsky can be seen. The record reads from right to left, line I being a time marker in fifths of a second, line III the galvanometer string, and line V the signal for stimulation. (From Pravdich-Neminsky, V.V. 1913. Ein Versuch der Registrierung der elektrischen Gehirnerscheinungen. *Zbl. Physiol.* 27:951–960, with permission from Dr. Mary Brazier and Macmillan.)

neuroscience stifled all progress of customary neurophysiology. The world leadership in EEG and related fields quickly crumbled, accompanied by a terrifying decline of a dogmatically governed neurophysiology.

Developments in Western and Central Europe

Electroencephalographic research was in a dormant state in Western and Central Europe while it was flourishing in Eastern European countries. This is quite amazing because neurophysiology in general was healthy and well outside Russia and her neighbors, but the ancestral lineage from Galvani to Du Bois-Reymond and Caton broke off and the neurophysiological field was watered by rivulets of different orientation. Thus, the work of Fleischl von Marxow lies like an erratic patch in the vast field.

The Western neurophysiologists followed attentively the work of their neuroanatomical confreres and the great controversy between network theories (the nerve cells forming a felt-like net) and the neuron theory (the neuron representing a unit). The net theory was supported by Joseph von Gerlach and by Camillo Golgi, the discoverer of the silver chromate staining method, but the neuron theory with its great principal proponent Santiago Ramón y Cajal (1852–1934) proved to be victorious in this struggle despite further attempts of new generations of "reticularist" believers in a continuous network of nerve cells.

In a similar manner, cerebral localizationists struggled against antilocalizationists. In Germany, Friedrich Leopold Goltz (1834–1902) removed the cerebral hemispheres in the "dog without cerebrum" living in a state of extreme lethargy and mental inertia (Goltz, 1888). H. Rothmann (1923) performed similar investigations. This type of research was aimed at the working of the cerebral hemispheres as a whole and de-emphasized aspects of cortical localization. As it was pointed out previously, the cerebral stimulation studies of Fritsch, Hitzig, Ferrier, and Yeo initiated a new era of interest in cortical localization.

In this period—the last third of the 19th and the dawning of the 20th century—the work of Charles Scott Sherrington (1857–1952), performed in Liverpool and Oxford, became most influential in the development of a modern Western type of reflexology. *The Integrative Action of the Nervous System* (Sherrington, 1906) was based on a series of lectures held at Yale University in 1904. The scope of this work reaches from reflexology to decerebrate rigidity, from motor cortex to sensory function, while the issue of mental function is being skirted with the modesty of a truly great neuroscientist. Inhibition is one of the great Sherringtonian discoveries. Even Ramón y Cajal's net of independent synaptically connected neurons stood solely in the service of neural excitation. (Incidentally, the term *synapse* was introduced by Sherrington.)

It is unfortunate that this greatest master of neurophysiology stood miles away from electrophysiological thought. His work was based chiefly on ablation techniques. He may hardly ever have given a thought to EEG methods even though he lived a full active life. His disciples—to name only Edward Liddell and Derek Ernest Denny-Brown—held similar views, while in Cambridge electrically oriented neurophysiology found its greatest proponent in Edgar Douglas Adrian (1889–1977), whom we discuss later in his relationship to Hans Berger's work.

Hans Berger and the Human Electroencephalogram

Hans Berger (1873–1941) (Fig. 1.3), the discoverer of the human EEG, was a neuropsychiatrist. What neuropsychiatry really meant in those years is poorly understood nowadays. Neurology and psychiatry formed one specialty, one discipline, in Germany, Austria, and a considerable number of other countries. Neuropsychiatric departments at university

hospitals and other institutions consisted of neurological and psychiatric floors; medical specialty training meant rotation from one discipline to the other, and a professor and head of department was supposed to master both domains. Pure neurology was just beginning to emerge as a special discipline in the German speaking countries [with the work of Wilhelm Erb (1840–1921), Max Nonne (1861–1959), and the incomparable Otfrid Foerster who, like Hans Berger, lived from 1873 to 1941].

Berger was not a leader, neither in neurology nor in psychiatry. Without his pioneering EEG work, his name would have been forgotten. Biographic sketches (especially Kolle, 1956) portray Berger as an extremely meticulous and conscientious person, somewhat aloof in his contact with his patients, a very strict and authoritarian department head, and an "anima candida" (a pure soul), a hard working professor without any interest in faculty schemes and diatribes. He hardly ever attended the annual meetings of the German neuropsychiatric society. His electroencephalographic work was carried out in a small and very primitive laboratory. His first scientific interest aimed at the cerebral circulation; plethysmographic methods were used in patients with skull defects. From 1902 to 1910, he studied the electrical activity of the cerebrum in the dog with a capillary electrometer after Lippmann, but the results were disappointing. Naturally, Berger was aware of the scanty pertinent literature from Caton to Cybulski and Pravdieh-Neminsky. His studies of the human EEG started in 1920; the introduction to Gloor's authoritative translation of Berger's work contains a plethora of interesting detail (Gloor, 1969).

Every electroencephalographer should be familiar with Berger's work, an undertaking that has been greatly facilitated by Gloor's English translation. It is true that the original German text is cumbersome and does not make easy reading, which is probably a reason for the very slow acceptance of Berger's work. Those 14 reports bear the same title: "On the Electroencephalogram of Man." Surely, a more attractive title would have helped somewhat. Berger's humanistic educational background becomes obvious in the rejection of the term *electrocerebrogram* of Pravdich-Neminsky for strictly linguistic reasons: the "ugly" mixture of Greek ("electro," "gram") and Latin ("cerebro") fragments. What Berger proposed in German was the term *Elektrenkephalogram* (Sic) since the root *enkephalo* from the Greek is linguistically more correct than *encephalo*.

Before Berger's work as such is brought into focus, we must discuss his electrophysiological instrumentation. He used a string galvanometer starting in 1910—first with the Einthoven type, later with the smaller Edelmann model, and after 1924 with the larger Edelmann model. In 1926, Berger started to use the more powerful Siemens double coil galvanometer (attaining a sensitivity of 130 µV/cm; Grass, 1984). With this instrument and the use of nonpolarizable pad electrodes, Berger recorded the human EEG tracings shown in his first report of 1929. The records were made on photographic paper with recordings from 1 to 3 minutes' duration. Berger used a bipolar recording technique with fronto-occipital leads for his one-channel EEG tracings along with simultaneous electrocardiogram (ECG) recording and a time marker. In 1932, he received an oscil-

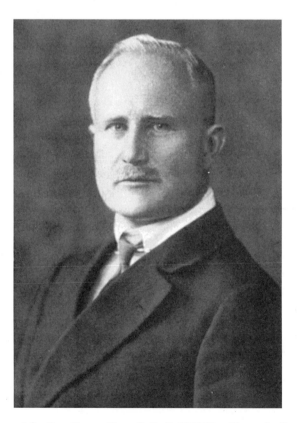

Figure 1.3. Hans Berger. (From Kolle K. 1956. Hans Berger. In *Gross Nervenärzte*, vol. 1, Ed. K. Kolle, pp. 1–6. Stuttgart: Thieme.)

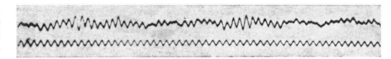

Figure 1.4. The first recorded electroencephalogram of a human. The lower line is a 10 cycles/sec sine wave for use as a time marker. The upper line is the recording from Berger's young son made in 1925. (From Berger, H. 1929. *Arch. Psychiat.* 87:527, with permission from Dr. Mary Brazier and Macmillan.)

lograph from Siemens but was unable to obtain further amplifiers with oscillographs in order to obtain multichannel recordings.

Studies of the human EEG began in 1924. Appointments were made for several patients with large skull bone defects (there was no scarcity of such patients in post-World War I Germany). On July 6, 1924, the small Edelmann string galvanometer showed oscillations presumably coming from the underlying brain. In 1925, Berger recognized that skull defects were not necessarily advantageous to obtaining a recording because of thickening of dura, postoperative adhesions, etc., and he found that recordings could be made just as well (or even better) through the intact skull and scalp. Between 1926 and 1929 Berger obtained good records with alpha waves; the double coil galvanometer was crucial for these observations. The data were often uncertain and, in 1928, Berger was beset with doubts concerning the authenticity of his observations (according to his diary entries, very impressively demonstrated by Jung, 1963).

The first report of 1929 features the alpha rhythm and the alpha blocking response (naturally along with a description of the smaller beta waves). Chlorinated silver needle electrodes, platinum wires, and zinc-plated steel needles were used in those years (Fig. 1.4). The bold first report of 1929 produced no "waves" until a confirming report came from Adrian in Cambridge (Adrian and Matthews, 1934). Throughout the 1930s, Berger's reports on the human EEG contained veritable gems: studies of fluctuation of consciousness, first EEG recordings of sleep (the first recording of spindles), the effect of hypoxia on the human brain, a variety of diffuse and localized brain disorders, and even an inkling of epileptic discharges. Eventually, Berger was invited to an international congress of psychologists in Paris in 1937 and to Bologna where the bicentennial of Galvani's birthday was celebrated (also 1937). His relationship to the Nazi regime was not good and Berger was most unceremoniously made a professor emeritus at earliest convenience, in 1938. This was indeed a hard blow to his plans for further electroencephalographic studies and, in the wake of a flu-like disease, he evidently developed a severe endogenous depression, which remained undiagnosed. He ended his life by suicide on June 1, 1941 at the age of 68. External factors may have contributed to his depression: in addition to his forced retirement at 65 (a few additional "years of honor" were granted to most retiring directors of university institutions), he also felt challenged by a group of independent EEG workers at the Institute of Brain Research at Berlin-Buch. This group was led by A. E. Kornmüller and produced excellent experimental EEG work, which is discussed later. Kornmüller might have had the better connections to the government institutions in Berlin, and the highly sensitive and often insecure Berger was afraid that his discovery was being taken away from him by his more aggressive colleagues in Berlin-Buch.

Berger was a very complex person and investigator. It was pointed out previously that he did not excel clinically, neither as psychiatrist nor as neurologist (even though he was very interested in cerebral localization and particularly in the localization of brain tumors). Berger also developed very unscientific ideas about the nature of the EEG, even though he was a meticulous scientist in his EEG work. The driving force in all his research work was the quest for the nature of the all-powerful force of mental energy ("*psychische Energie*"). An early personal experience convinced him that such a mental energy—even capable of transmitting thoughts and emotions from person to person—does exist. According to Berger's concept, influenced by the Danish physiologist Alfred Lehmann in 1901, mental energy is thought to be a partial product of metabolic energies (warmth and electricity being the other two products). This concept gives the EEG waves the eerie character of messengers within the mental activities, even as messengers from person to person.

Friedrich Rueckert (1788–1866), a great German poet of the Romantic period, was Berger's maternal grandfather. Behind the strict directorial facade of Berger was the gentle soul of a highly vulnerable man. It was the psychophysiologist Berger who searched for the correlate of mental energy and, on this voyage, he found the human electroencephalogram. It was one of those "Columbus syndromes": that a discovery is made as a by-product of a search for a different goal. Jung (1963) noted that Berger pursued his goal with the extremely powerful energy of a dilettante who had found a concept. Specialists like the excellent physiologist (and electrophysiologist) Wilhelm Biedermann in Jena were convinced that Berger's dilettantism would lead nowhere, but it was the dilettante and not the seasoned specialist who emerged victorious. Even though the EEG is not exactly what Berger assumed, his contribution was the greatest in the history of electroencephalography.

Berger's Contemporaries
The Berliner Group

The Institute of Brain Research (Hirnforschungs-Institut) in Berlin-Bush harbored a group of ambitious and energetic investigators in various neurosciences. Oskar Vogt (1870–1959), one of the great neuroanatomists and neuropathologists of his time and a remarkably independent thinker with a wide intellectual horizon, was the director of the institute. In 1936 he lost his "directorship for lifetime" when the Nazi government became aware of Vogt's activities at a similar institute in Moscow and his reluctance to get rid of Jewish co-workers (Hassler, 1959).

The Berliner Institute (a section of the Kaiser-Wilhelm Institutes) was composed of a variety of departments. In this context, the Department of Physiology under M. H. Fischer and the Department of Electrophysiology under A. E. Kornmüller must be singled out. These departments enjoyed the collaboration of an outstanding physicist and electronic engineer, J. F. Toennies (1902–1970), a personal friend of Oskar Vogt (both coming from the town of Husum in Holstein).

Toennies built the first ink-writing biological amplifier for the recording of brain potentials. While in New York as a fellow of the Rockefeller Foundation in 1932, he designed the differential amplifier—the still all-important principle of EEG amplification—but he shares this achievement with Brian Matthews, Adrian's ingenious co-worker whose work is discussed in the next section.

The collaboration with Toennies gave the Berlin group a much better tool for EEG research in comparison with Berger's instrumentation. Kornmüller quickly recognized the importance of recordings from a greater number of electrodes. His EEG studies in the human placed particular emphasis on the differences between given regions of the cerebrum ("*Hirnrindenfelder*") (Kornmüller, 1932, 1933, 1935, 1937). His studies of the clinical significance of EEG (Kornmüller, 1944) appear to be somewhat pale when compared with the importance of his earliest experimental EEG work carried out with Fischer and also with H. Löwenbach, who later came to the United States, where he became one of the earliest EEG pioneers. In those early studies, the EEG was obtained from the cortex of animals following poisoning with convulsive substances. This is the first EEG work focusing on epileptic manifestations and the first demonstration of epileptiform spikes (Fischer, 1933; Fischer and Löwenbach, 1934a,b; Kornmüller, 1935).

Oskar Vogt (his wife Cécile also being known as a great neuropathologist) developed a concept of strict cerebral compartmentalization in sharply separated areas. He showed indeed extremely impressive boundaries between healthy and diseased areas in the hippocampus (Vogt and Vogt, 1937) and conceived the cortex as divided into about 200 regions with precise demarcation from field to field. This concept became a powerful leitmotiv for Vogt's co-workers, and Kornmüller's EEG work clearly shows the marks of his authoritarian boss.

Richard Jung joined this group in 1937 when Vogt was already fired. (The tycoon Alfred Krupp provided the Vogts with a privately built institute in the Black Forest in his expression of personal gratitude. Decades earlier Vogt successfully treated an ailing Krupp—with hypnosis. Indeed, Vogt also used to be a master of this method!) Hugo Spatz replaced Vogt and considerably changed the goals of research. Toennies stayed with H. S. Gasser at the Rockefeller Institute in New York, where he constructed the first cathode follower to record from high-resistance electrodes. This was the birth of microelectrode recording, which developed into an enormously powerful scientific tool in the 1950s and 1960s.

Kornmüller's work declined after World War II, when he appeared to be obsessed with a totally unproven theory of glia as the generator of slow brain potentials. Jung, however, developed into one of the greatest electroneurophysiologists of his time.

Developments in Great Britain

Edgar Douglas Adrian (Baron of Cambridge and, as such, Lord Adrian) (1889–1977) was not only one of the greatest electrophysiological neurophysiologists of the 20th century; his name is also intimately associated with the discovery of the EEG because of his confirmation of Berger's observations (Adrian and Matthews, 1934). He showed his colleagues his own beautiful alpha rhythm and the blocking effect due to eye opening, but, alas, his great electronic wizard, Brian Matthews, apparently had a low-voltage EEG with no alpha rhythm. Due to some strange quirk, Adrian's recording from the head ganglion of a water beetle happened to be indistinguishable from Adrian's alpha rhythm and was blocked in the same manner, namely by light falling on the beetle's eyes. The Adrian-water beetle similarity and the Adrian-Matthews EEG dissimilarity must have been terribly confusing to the onlookers (also see Adrian, 1936).

Adrian was already a neurophysiologist of great prestige when he confirmed Berger's data. He had been credited with the demonstration of single sensory nerve fiber potential and the analysis of unit activity, which resulted in the Adrian-Bronk law (Adrian and Bronk, 1929). Incidentally, his collaborator Detlef Bronk became president of Johns Hopkins University in later years. Prior to Matthews, Keith Lucas had been Adrian's brilliant electronic engineer and experimental co-worker.

W. Grey Walter became the pioneer of clinical electroencephalography in England, and his discovery of foci of slow activity (delta waves, named by Walter) generated enormous clinical interest in the new method. Grey Walter, however, was a Ph.D., and this could have laid the foundation for the aversion of England's great neurologists toward the method of EEG, which in the following years was either ignored or left to Ph.D. electroencephalographers in the laboratory. We will find Grey Walter again in later decades; let it be said that he was one of the most brilliant minds in all neurosciences—an independent thinker, a powerful writer, quite often a man nearly consumed by the flame of his own brilliance. He founded a small but very effective school in Bristol at the Burden Institute.

Developments in France and Belgium

Thus far, France seems to be unduly neglected in this historical overview. It had its own proud neurophysiological schools in the 19th century, and the names of François Magendie (1783–1855) and, above all, Claude Bernard (1813–1878) belong in the pantheon of neuroscience.

A fine school of early electroencephalographers developed in Paris in the 1930s. A. Fessard at the Collège de France must be singled out as the most towering figure. Together with G. Durup, he also confirmed the results of Berger. Durup and Fessard even used EEG in the study of conditioned reflexes. Clinical electroencephalography started in France under the aegis of A. Baudouin and G. Fischgold. Fischgold had come from Rumania, developed into a leading clinical electroencephalographer, and—what an unusual combination—became a leader in neuroradiology. Baudouin was the key figure in the invitation of Berger to Paris in 1937.

Neighboring Belgium was the home of a giant in electrophysiological neurophysiology: Frederic Bremer (1892–1982) from the Université Libre of Brussels. Bremer quickly recognized the usefulness of EEG methods in the experimental investigation of the brain. He recognized the influence of afferent signals on the state of vigilance and compared his feline preparation called "*cerveau isolé*" (with midbrain transection) with the "*encéphale isolé*" resulting from transection at the boundary between the medulla oblongata and cervical cord. The former preparation would produce permanent coma; the latter would cause a variable state of vigilance, with waking and sleeping demonstrated on the EEG recording. In other words, trigeminal-sensory, auditory, visual, and probably also olfactory influences would help to keep the (artificially ventilated) *encéphale isolé* preparation in a waking-sleeping rhythm (Bremer, 1935).

The greatness of this investigator must be reemphasized, especially in today's era of short memory. Whoever reads his study entitled "Cerebral and Cerebellar Potentials" (Bremer, 1958) will roughly understand the dimensions of this neurophysiologist.

Developments in Other European Countries

Italy was one of the first countries where the EEG found fertile soil. Mario Gozzano, for many years professor of clinical neurology in Bologna (later in Rome), published his experiences with the new method as early as 1935. Gozzano personifies the (not too common) example of a leading neurologist assuming leadership in clinical electroencephalography (Mazza et al., 2002). All too often, eminent clinical neurologists spurned the new method.

A. Gemelli came from the diametrically opposite area of neurosciences. This great scholar was a monk, psychologist, philosopher, polyhistor, and president of the Catholic University in Milan. In 1937, he reported his first studies of the human EEG. Gemelli hence represents the psychological wing of EEG research, which subsequently spawned a number of outstanding Ph.D. electroencephalographers. (Others would come from the ranks of experimental neurophysiologists.)

The Austrian psychologist Hubert Rohracher falls into the Gemelli category. He held the chair of psychology for many years at the University of Vienna, but, in his early academic work, he fell under the spell of the alpha rhythm and even made a "pilgrimage" to Hans Berger in Jena (in the 1930s). His early EEG studies can be dated back to 1938.

America Enters the Scene

Around 1935, the center of gravity in the still modest bulk of EEG work started to shift from Europe to North America. Fascinating new reports came from the United States. European investigators started to travel across the Atlantic, and even Hans Berger was about to accept an invitation to the United States in 1939, when the beginning of World War II thwarted his plans.

In the pre-Berger development of experimental EEG studies, America had not played any role. Schwab (1951) reports that, in 1918, a medical student of Harvard Medical School, Donald McPherson, worked under the eminent physiologist Alexander Forbes. When McPherson placed two electrodes on the exposed brain of a cat and ran the output into a string galvanometer, he saw rhythmical 10/sec EEG activity. This finding was rejected as an artifact by Forbes. Was Forbes completely unaware of the work from Caton to Pravdich-Neminsky?

The rise of American EEG work to international fame is customarily associated with the work of Hallowell Davis, Frederic A. Gibbs, and Erna Gibbs at Harvard and also with Herbert Jasper's work at Brown University in Providence, Rhode Island. According to O'Leary and Goldring (1976), A. J. Derbyshire, a graduate student of Hallowell Davis, brought Berger's paper of 1929 to Davis's attention. Derbyshire, Pauline Davis, and H. N. Simpson then tried in vain to demonstrate their own alpha rhythms. There were finally shouts of joy when Hallowell Davis himself was found to have a good alpha rhythm. Otherwise, the first human EEG study in America would have been a negative one. This work was done in 1934, just before human EEG studies started to mushroom in the United States.

The EEG, however, had been used for animal experiments for some years in the United States, starting with Bartley and Newman (1930, 1931) and Bartley (1932), who produced EEG tracings in the dog. Howard Bartley did his work at Washington University in St. Louis, a place that had already developed into a hotbed of neurophysiology due to the magnificent work of Herbert S. Gasser, Joseph Erlanger, and George Bishop—a group that made excellent use of Braun's cathode ray oscilloscope (oscillograph) in the study of peripheral nerve potentials. This outstanding group was joined later by James L. O'Leary, a prominent neurophysiologist, electroencephalographer, and neurological clinician. Early experimental EEG work was done by Davis and Saul (1931), Travis and Dorsey (1931), Travis and Herren (1931), Bishop and Bartley (1932), Bartley (1932), and Gerard et al. (1933) (after Grass, 1984). The work of Ralph W. Gerard (1900–1974) is linked with the introduction of a concentric needle electrode for the stereotaxic exploration of the brain in experimental animals. Gerard joined forces (in 1934) with Franklin Offner, one of the leading electronic engineers in the development of EEG and related equipment.

American EEG work in the human started, as it was pointed out before, at Harvard in Boston (Hallowell and Pauline Davis, Frederic and Erna Gibbs, William G. Lennox), at Brown in Providence (Herbert H. Jasper), but also at the University of Iowa in Iowa City where Lee Travis worked, an experimental psychologist who became the founder of a powerful school (Herbert Jasper, Donald Lindsley, John R. Knott, and Charles Henry).

The great international breakthrough in clinical electroencephalography came in 1934 with studies of epileptic patients. Frederic Gibbs had come from Johns Hopkins University in Baltimore to join the Harvard group. He sought out William G. Lennox, who had already become a widely known epileptologist. It might be interesting to point out that Lennox had started studies of the cerebral circulation by measuring the O_2 and CO_2 content of the jugular veins (Lennox, 1930, 1931; Lennox and E. L. Gibbs, 1932). E. L. Gibbs was Erna L. Gibbs, originally the technical co-worker of Lennox but who became the wife of Frederic Gibbs and one of the world's first EEG technicians and the co-author of numerous papers. She had come to Boston as an immigrant from Germany. The pre-EEG work of Lennox and Gibbs on the cerebral blood flow was a milestone in this field. (One of the great present-day masters of cerebral blood flow, Louis Sokoloff from the National Institutes of Health, expressed to me in a personal communication his profound admiration for this pioneering work.) EEG simply exerted a greater degree of fascination to W. G. Lennox than did cerebral blood flow.

Twelve children with petit mal epilepsy were the clinical subjects for the petit mal epilepsy study of Gibbs and Davis (1935) and Gibbs et al. (1935, 1937). This work remains an evergreen in the entire EEG literature; hardly any EEG finding has left such an indelible impression as the association of petit mal absences and 3/sec spike-wave complexes. (Of course, it was found out later that spike waves could occur without petit mal.) While Berger was gripped by the rhythms, Frederic Gibbs came under the fascination of paroxysmal patterns such as spike waves. Shortly afterward, the EEG patterns of grand mal and psychomotor seizures were reported by the same team (Gibbs, Lennox, and Gibbs), but the stretches of fast spikes (in grand mal) and the rhythmical activity in 4/sec or 6/sec frequency (in psychomotor seizures) were no match in popularity for the 3/sec spike waves of petit mal.

The technical quality of the EEG tracings shown in these studies left much to be desired. Dr. and Mrs. Gibbs traveled to Germany in the summer of 1935, paid a visit to Hans Berger, spent some time at the Berlin-Buch Institute, and studied the "polyneurograph" instrument of Jan F. Toennies; they also saw the instrumentation of Matthews in England. Frederic Gibbs then contracted Albert Grass (then at the Massachusetts Institute of Technology) to build a three-channel preamplifier. In 1935, the Grass Model I went into use; it had three channels and an ink writer that recorded on rolls of paper (the folded paper not yet being in use).

The Gibbs-Gibbs-Lennox era of the 1930s proved to be perhaps the most exciting period in the history of EEG. In those years, EEG found the domain of greatest effectiveness: the realm of the epileptic seizure disorders. Epileptology can be divided historically into two periods: before and after the advent of EEG. Insights into the nature of the epileptic mechanisms deepened, not in a subtle manner but with a huge leap. What Fischer had started in 1931 with his experimental studies on picrotoxin and its effect on the cortical EEG in animals, the Gibbses and Lennox applied to human epileptology, and a wide door was flung open for the work of future decades. It is true that Berger in his seventh report (Berger, 1933) had shown a few examples of paroxysmal EEG discharges in a case of presumed petit mal attacks and also during a focal motor seizure in a patient with general paresis. These observations were just mentioned in passing and the opportunity of a major breakthrough was missed.

As to the other great pioneers of electroencephalography in North America, Hallowell and Pauline Davis produced fine work on the normal EEG and its variants. They were also among the earliest investigators of the human sleep EEG. In the domain of sleep, A. L. Loomis and his co-workers E. N. Harvey and G. A. Hobart were the first who methodically studied the human sleep EEG patterns and the

stages of sleep. This research was done off the academic track in Tuxedo Park, New Jersey (Loomis et al., 1935, their first study). The Davises eventually turned to audiology and moved to St. Louis. At Brown University in Providence, Rhode Island, Jasper studied the EEG of behavior disorders in children before he found his niche in basic and clinical epileptology at McGill University in Montreal in his epochal collaboration with Wilder Penfield (discussed later). Lee Travis gradually disappeared from the scene but his foremost disciples, John R. Knott and Charles E. Henry (Ph.D. electroencephalographers with strong clinical inclinations) were bound to assume a very important role in America's EEG work. Their ultimate skill and supreme dedication turned them into the "conscience of EEG," steering developments into the right direction and correcting the course when there was danger of going astray. D. Lindsley became one of the pioneers in the investigation of maturational EEG aspects; at the University of California at Los Angeles, he directed excellent neurophysiological EEG research.

This was the first wave of American EEG pioneers and their immediate disciples and followers. It is impossible for the historian to do justice to the second wave, which started before the great 1930s were over. There was Robert Schwab at Harvard and at the Massachusetts General Hospital in Boston, in whom the mastery of EEG was combined with great clinical neurological talents (especially in the field of myasthenia gravis, parkinsonism, and epilepsy). Across the Charles River, at the Massachusetts Institute of Technology, there was Warren McCulloch, a fiery genius like Grey Walter in Bristol and a profound thinker. His scope would range light years beyond the limits of EEG and neurophysiology. (One must read his *Embodiments of Mind* to fathom his greatness, even though one may be inclined to disagree in many points.) He and Grey Walter lived in the world of brain machines, but there was still a niche for a psyche (when one tries to read between the lines). Earlier at Northwestern University in Evanston, Illinois, outside Chicago, McCulloch had been involved with Dusser de Barenne in "neuronographic" work, an import from Utrecht, Netherlands; this work was based on topical strychnine poisoning of the cortex and exploration of transmitted spiking to other regions.

Clinical EEG research already started to conquer certain fields outside epileptology. Grey Walter's discovery of the delta focus (Walter, 1936) located over hemispheric brain tumors had opened the search for further relationships between brain lesions and focal EEG correlates; metabolic disturbances and especially hypoglycemia were explored with EEG. (The work of H. Hoagland and his co-workers dates back to 1937.)

When the 1930s ended, North America found itself in a leading position in the domain of EEG. By contrast, progress made in Europe was quite limited.

World War II and the 1940s

During World War II, from 1939 to 1945, research and clinical EEG activities were not flourishing, particularly not in Europe. There were some neurological units where the EEG was used in the localization of traumatic brain lesions and epileptogenic foci. After World War II, the gap between North America and Europe was bigger than ever before, and European EEG research found itself at a low point.

After the war, new activities started in England and France, while the situation in Germany looked desperate. W. Grey Walter with his associates V. J. Dovey and H. Shipton (a brilliant electronic engineer who later moved to Iowa City and then St. Louis) at the Burden Institute in Bristol discovered the paroxysmal response to flickering light at critical frequencies between 10 and 20/sec. Further work on epileptic photosensitivity immediately shifted from Bristol to Marseille, France, where a young and incredibly talented Henri Gastaut used this method, in combination with intravenous dosages of pentylenetetrazol, to determine the "*seuil épileptique*," i.e., the individual threshold for paroxysmal responses (Gastaut, 1949; Gastaut et al., 1948).

In 1947, the American EEG Society was founded and the First International EEG Congress was held in London; a second one followed in 1949 in Paris (in association with clinical neurology and other neurological disciplines). EEG activities in Germany were still minimal; Japan, however, gained attention by the work of K. Motokawa, a researcher of EEG rhythms. Switzerland started to develop its own profile; the neurophysiologist Marcel Monnier was instrumental in this regard. W. R. Hess, however, a Nobelist, had gained great prestige by the functional mapping of thalamus and hypothalamus with regard to autonomic responses to electrical stimulation.

The American scene was bustling with activities. Frederic A. Gibbs with his co-workers Erna Gibbs and B. Fuster from Uruguay produced another epochal study on the interictal anterior temporal spike or sharp wave discharge in the interseizure interval in patients with psychomotor seizures. This was an important step in the elucidation of temporal lobe epilepsy, a work with far-reaching consequences for the entire development of EEG laboratories and their routine work. It was found (Gibbs et al., 1948) that the anterior temporal discharges were often limited to the state of sleep. This observation meant that a tracing without a sleep portion could be insufficient, uninformative, and even misleading. Thus, EEG laboratories would include sleep in most (if not all) of their EEG evaluations. This required pasted electrodes (rather than rubber bands or caps), a much longer recording time, and a much smaller numerical output of recordings per technician (incidentally, an evolving profession, which is discussed later).

Transatlantic communication was poor at that time, and it was at this point when the routine work in American (or Canadian) EEG laboratories started to become more sophisticated than that of their European counterparts because of the inclusion of sleep.

Frederic Gibbs enjoyed enormous international prestige at that time as the world's leader in clinical electroencephalography. Nevertheless, his position at Harvard was much less prestigious; he held the academic rank of an instructor (below the professorial ranks), even though a visit to his laboratory was the goal of European colleagues (who could afford the trip). This disproportion drastically shows the negative attitude toward EEG in neurological departments (not universally, of course). Robert Schwab did not fare much better at Harvard in spite of his fine clinical-neurological talents.

Toward the end of the 1940s, Herbert H. Jasper turned into a strong competitor of Frederic Gibbs. Jasper had moved to the Neurological Institute of McGill University in Montreal, joining forces with Wilder Penfield, a neurosurgeon with a profound neuroscientific background. We discuss the rise of the Montreal group below (see Developments in the 1950s).

Two new developments started in the late 1940s. The EEG technique started to become invasive and, with the use of special depth electrodes, the exploration of deep intracerebral regions began. This is discussed below (see Developments in the 1950s). Automatic frequency analysis also started in the 1940s, but this development reached loftier heights in the 1960s.

A discussion of the 1940s would be incomplete without a brief glance at the work of the neurophysiologists. A large segment of neurophysiological work was dominated by the use of EEG. One of the most fascinating results of these researchers was the demonstration of thalamocortical relationships, thus far explored solely with anatomical methods (e.g., the study of the thalamus by A. Earl Walker in 1938, which propelled this young neuroscientist to great fame for decades to come). The work of Morison and Dempsey (1942) on the recruiting response had great impact on the neuroscientific world with the demonstration of cortical responses to relatively slow stimulation of the intralaminar structures of the thalamus in the cat. This work emphasized the role of the thalamus in the cortical electrogenesis and broke the ground for the concept of a "centrencephalic epilepsy," a concept promoted by Penfield and Jasper in Montreal (somewhat naively understood as a concept of the thalamic origin of primary generalized epilepsy).

Even greater was the impact of the work of Horace W. Magoun, who had studied the effects of descending and mostly inhibitory influences of the brainstem reticular formation during his work at Northwestern University. Together with G. Moruzzi (a fine neurophysiologist from Pisa, Italy, and investigator of basic epileptic mechanisms), Magoun subsequently studied the ascending system of the brainstem reticular formation (chiefly in the midbrain level) and the effect of high-frequency electrical stimulation, consisting of EEG desynchronization and behavioral arousal, on cortical function. Magoun, who had moved to the University of California at Los Angeles, subsequently investigated the effects of acute lesions made in the midbrain level reticular formation in cats. These cats remained in a comatose state with EEG slowing in spite of electrical brainstem stimulation because of the destruction of the all-important ascending portion of the brainstem reticular formation (Lindsley et al., 1949). It is no exaggeration when one describes the effect of these studies on the world of neuroscience as a "bombshell." For the ensuing 10 to 15 years, the association of consciousness with reticular formation and Magoun's name was so strong that it even had considerable influence on the Pavlovian dogmatism of the Eastern Bloc countries. Nowadays, however, even talented young neuroscientists react to Magoun's name with a blank expression—*sic transit gloria mundi!*

The reason for discussing this experimental work in a historical overview is to demonstrate the incredibly powerful role of EEG in the neurophysiology of the 1940s. This was a high water mark. Subsequently, experimental EEG work started to concentrate on single neurons while the "macro-EEG" gradually declined.

Developments in the 1950s

This is the last decade presented for historical analysis. Our story is gradually approaching the present, and a historical outline must shy away from events that comprise the last 30 years. It does not behoove the historian to place living and active colleagues into the focus of discussion (with few exceptions).

The 1950s was the decade when EEG became a household word. During the early stretch of the decade, almost every university (teaching) hospital had at least one EEG machine. At the end of the decade, EEG apparatuses had found their way into a large number of other hospitals and even into private practice. At university hospitals, central as well as departmental EEG laboratories emerged. The latter were usually limited to children or adults, and pediatric EEG units evolved (while specialized neonatological EEG units followed suit about 10 years later). Some psychiatric departments took particular pride in their clinical and research-oriented EEG work. It is absolutely true that psychiatry was always "nice" to the electroencephalographer. Psychiatry's domain was in need of organic or neurophysiological substrata of disorders and dysfunctions of psychiatric-psychological nature. What could the electroencephalographer give in return? It was very little, but the psychiatrists did not seem to mind. On the other hand, there was so much to give to neurology. At that time, it had become clear that the majority of diseases affecting the central nervous system (CNS) had more or less impressive EEG correlates, but the majority of neurologists remained either reserved or hostile to EEG. Neurosurgeons were interested as long as EEG could contribute to the determination of focal cerebral lesions (and before EEG became overpowered by noninvasive neuroimaging techniques). Some epilepsy-oriented neurosurgeons like W. Penfield or A. Earl Walker remained interested in EEG and its use in the depth of the cerebrum or on the cortex.

The epileptological EEG work of Herbert Jasper in collaboration with Wilder Penfield reached new heights, and Montreal reigned supreme as the place for neurosurgical treatment of focal epilepsies. Penfield was far more than a neurosurgeon. His operations for the removal of epileptogenic foci and, in a later phase, large portions of affected lobes were associated with electrical stimulation and a systematic study of the behavioral effects. At that time, local anesthesia was still widely used in neurosurgery. Jasper was chiefly a neuroscientist and not merely an electroencephalographer. The book entitled *Epilepsy and the Functional Anatomy of the Human Brain* (Penfield and Jasper, 1954) was a result of this fruitful collaboration.

Very controversial, however, was a concept of the primary generalized form of epilepsy characterized by generalized synchronous paroxysmal EEG discharges and exemplified by the 3/sec spike waves of petit-mal absences. Penfield and Jasper listed these epilepsies as "centrencephalic" with the concept of "center of the encephalon" (i.e., "thalamic midline structures") serving as the starting point of the bilateral discharges. Henri Gastaut from Marseille would follow the lead and so did many others, but Frederic Gibbs and a host of other electroencephalographers and neuroscientists became detractors of the centrencephalic concept. It wasn't until the late 1960s that it became clear that the centrencephalic concept stood on very shaky ground and was ripe for being dismantled. Montreal's own Pierre Gloor helped to do this in a cautious and diplomatic manner; others buried the centrencephalic concept more bluntly.

Frederic Gibbs had moved to the University of Illinois School of Medicine in Chicago (where full professorship was given to him instantly after Harvard had denied him any promotion for more than a decade). Chicago—especially the University of Chicago but also Northwestern University and the University of Illinois—had become a world leader in neurological sciences over the past 20 years. Percival Bailey, Paul Bucy, Roy Grinker, A. Earl Walker, Gerhardt Von Bonin, C. J. Herrick, Frederic Gibbs, and many others give testimony to the glory of neurological science in Chicago at the middle of that century. In the field of EEG, the Chicago group under the Gibbses and the Montreal group under Jasper and Gloor were strong rivals throughout the 1950s, especially with respect to leadership in epileptological electroencephalography. One of the greatest masters from the Chicago school, A. Earl Walker, came to Johns Hopkins in Baltimore in 1947, introducing depth EEG, electrocorticography, epilepsy surgery, and a scientifically oriented epileptology to his new place. Walker, who in 1972 had moved to the University of New Mexico and died in 1995, will always be remembered as one of the great scholars of neurosurgery and epileptology.

The 1950s saw a strong comeback of the Europeans. Henri Gastaut's intellectual brilliancy was hard to match. In Marseille, disciples of great stature flocked around him, especially Robert Naquet, Joseph Roger, and Annette Beaumanoir, to mention only the earliest nucleus of this group. At the great world centers of neurology, Salpêtrière Hospital in Paris and National Hospital, Queen Square, London, Antoine Remond and William Cobb, respectively, represented the EEG, but unfortunately too much in the shadow of the leading neurologists. Remond later turned into a protagonist of computerization of EEG data.

The star neurologists of both Queen Square and Salpêtrière lived in the world of classical neurology, which gave them so much satisfaction and happiness that one could hardly expect their openness for the world of brain potentials. The Queen Square guard appeared to be more detached from EEG than their Parisian confrères, perhaps due to the fact that Gastaut, the man from Marseille, came from the neurological ranks to achieve instant stardom with his EEG achievements. Probably no other famous neurologist has expressed his opinion about EEG more scathingly than Francis M. R. Walshe has done. He is the brilliant Queen Square star who apparently knew everything about neurology except EEG. To Sir Francis, the electrical activity of the brain was, "a bloodless dance of action potentials . . . hurrying to and fro of its molecules" (after Critchley, 1990). Let us assume, for everyone's benefit, that Sir Francis had meant it to be a joke.

Fine schools of EEG developed in the Netherlands with O. Magnus (son of a Nobel Prize winning physiologist) in Wassenaar and Storm van Leeuwen in Utrecht. In Switzerland, Rudolf Hess (also son of a Nobelist physiologist) created an important school of electroencephalographers at the Zurich University Hospital. Giuseppe Pampiglione, from Italy, initiated pediatric electroencephalography at the Hospital for Sick Children in London, concurrently with William Lennox's work at the Boston Children's Hospital.

These European centers of EEG activities had rather an international flavor with strong North American influence. This cannot be said about the evolving field of clinical EEG in West Germany, which was dominated by its prestigious leader Richard Jung in Freiburg. Jung's greatness pertained to experimental neurophysiology; he also had great interest in the clinical fields and even in philosophy. This renaissance man designed the outline for EEG training and the routine of the EEG laboratory—unfortunately not without shortcomings, which hamstrung the further development of clinical EEG in West Germany.

The 1950s also saw EEG sprouting into related fields. Depth electroencephalography with implanted intracerebral electrodes was used in the human for the first time by Meyers and Hayne (1948) and Knott et al. (1950) at the University of Iowa, Iowa City, and also by Hayne et al. (1949a) in Chicago. These short recordings served the study of EEG activity in the human basal ganglia and thalamus with regard to basal ganglia dyskinesias and epilepsy. In the following years, deep structures were also explored in patients with psychiatric disorders until doubt was cast upon the ethical basis of this invasive approach (see Chapter 36, "Depth Electroencephalography"). In the 1960s, depth EEG would find its true field in epileptic patients considered candidates for epilepsy surgery.

The origin of intraoperative electrocorticography dates back to Foerster and Altenburger (1935). How was it possible that Otfried Foerster, perhaps the greatest clinical neurologist ever and an amazing self-taught master of neurosurgery, failed to recognize the future potential of EEG? Did his mind work mainly in the world of Sherringtonian concepts? Most of the work in electrocorticography remains associated with the Montreal Neurological Institute and the names of Penfield and Jasper (also see Chapter 38, "Electrocorticography").

The related fields of EEG started to bloom in the 1950s. In a study entitled "A Summation Technique for Detecting Small Signals in a Large Irregular Background," George D. Dawson from the National Hospital, Queen Square, in London demonstrated evoked potentials to electrical stimulation of the ulnar nerve (Dawson, 1951). This required advanced analog technology. Thus, Dawson became the father of evoked potential studies, which developed into a major outcropping of electroencephalography, eventually constituting a field of its own. The ingenious superimposition method of Dawson was eventually superseded by the advent of computerized averaging methods in the 1960s.

Computational techniques of wave analysis started early in the history of EEG. First attempts were made by Hans

Berger (1932); he was assisted by the physicist Dietsch (1932), who applied Fourier analysis to short EEG sections. Further work in this field was produced by Grass and Gibbs (1938) and Knott and Gibbs (1939). At the Massachusetts Institute of Technology near Boston, Guillemin applied Fourier analysis to communication theory, and one of his students was Albert Grass who "could not wait to get the Gibbs interested" (Grass, 1984). The 1950s saw the early generation of automatic frequency analyzers approaching and eventually saw the end of these magnificent but mostly unused machines.

Eventually, the EEG branched out into the world of single neurons, and the microelectrode technique was introduced in the early 1950s. Microelectrodes can be made of metal such as tungsten with tips of 1 to 3 μm diameter; glass electrodes filled with electrolytes such as KCl have tips of 0.5 μm or even smaller. Because of their characteristics, microelectrodes reach very high impedance values (1–60 megohm), which render conventional EEG recording techniques unsuitable. The introduction of the cathode follower by Toennies created the technical prerequisite for single-cell recordings.

Extracellular microelectrode recording was used on a larger scale in the early 1950s (Jung et al., 1952; Li et al., 1952; Moruzzi, 1952). About 10 years later, extracellular microelectrode studies were even done intraoperatively in humans. Far more revolutionary was the introduction of the extremely laborious intracellular microelectrode technology (Brock et al., 1952, in the spinal cord; Phillips, 1961, in the cortex). This technique opened the gates to a new world of biochemical processes. These insights taught lessons in humility to the electrophysiological neurophysiologist. There was no doubt that the chemical changes were of primary significance, while the electrical phenomena were more or less by-products.

We cannot leave the 1950s without mentioning epochal developments in the field of sleep research. At the University of Chicago, N. Kleitman stood out as one of the world's leading investigators of the organization of sleep. This institution produced the first study of rapid eye movement (REM) sleep (Aserinsky and Kleitman, 1953), but it must be pointed out that Blake and Gerard (1937) described a "null stage" in the EEG of nocturnal sleep, thus indicating the desynchronization of EEG in REM sleep but without observation of the accompanying ocular, muscular, and other autonomic changes. William C. Dement continued the work of Kleitman and, following his move from Chicago to Stanford, became a world leader in the study of nocturnal sleep.

Sleep research gradually became based on polygraphic recording, and its share in the overall EEG research declined. This development led to a constantly widening gap between EEG and nocturnal sleep research (in the 1960s and the following decades).

The Rest of the Story

The last 30 years of the history of EEG and related fields can be gleaned directly from this book. The events of the 1960s, 1970s, and 1980s are just too close for us to see with the eyes of the historian. Nevertheless, modern trends are briefly discussed in this final section.

The development of clinical and experimental EEG work reached a high point around 1960 after 30 years of steady progress. There is no doubt that the 1960s slowed down the smooth progress. The interest of electroencephalographers in academic institutions tended to shift from the tracing, with all its waves and patterns, to automatic data analysis. Computerization was the direction—tendencies reaching back to Berger's coworker Dietsch (1932) but flourishing in the 1960s and 1970s. This development had many positive aspects. The names of Barlow, Brazier, Remond, Lopes da Silva, Bickford, Saltzberg, Dumermuth, Matousek, D. O. Walter, Cooper, Künkel, Lehmann, Gasser, Burch, Hjorth, Schenk, Matejcek, and Low should be mentioned in this context. In particular, Cooley and Tukey (1965) have been credited with the introduction of the fast Fourier transforms as the basis of power spectral analysis.

This work led us into a "brave new world" of EEG computerization and, as early as in 1967, we were told that customary EEG reading would soon be a thing of the past, replaced by a fully automatic EEG interpretation. The fears of many clinical electroencephalographers were unfounded; nobody became jobless, because such an automatization of EEG reading was fictional. It was found that EEG is far too complex for such automation. Its interpretation requires that wonderful computer that is located between the ears. One simply must consider that the methods of those years—frequency or time domain—were limited to an analysis of frequencies. Automatic spike detection had barely reached its earliest stage.

The electroencephalographer needed to be aware that all types of data computerization were nothing but the EEG in disguise—"an analog of an analog." Computerized frequency analysis was here to stay and to prove to be of enormous value not only in psychophysiological research but also in the assessment of neuropharmacological effects.

In the 1970s, the evoked potential technique progressed greatly. The introduction of the pattern changer in the visual evoked potential technique made this method highly reliable; the names of H. Speckrejse and R. Spehlmann ought to be mentioned in this context. In the field of auditory evoked potentials, the location of primary cortical discharge was elusive for many years, and the late vertex potential of limited clinical value. The introduction of the far field technique for the demonstration of the brainstem auditory evoked potentials (Jewell), however, proved to be extremely valuable. Analogous work in the field of somatosensory evoked potentials is associated with the names of Roger and Joan Cracco.

The 1960s and 1970s witnessed a regrettable alienation of EEG and epileptology, which had existed before in an almost perfect marriage. A sizable number of epileptologists lost interest in EEG. Was it early enthusiasm about the introduction of antiepileptic serum levels? Was the path to mastery of EEG becoming too laborious? This situation changed in the 1980s due to the rapidly increasing emphasis on EEG and related techniques in the presurgical workup of patients considered candidates for seizure surgery.

The 1970s and 1980s saw brilliant structural neuroimaging techniques emerging: computed tomography and magnetic resonance imaging. This seemed to knock out electroencephalography from the contributors to focal CNS diagnosis. Such a knockout blow, however, was also more apparent than real. The EEG, by its very nature, never was a structure-oriented test. Whether the patient has a hemispheric brain tumor, a vascular lesion, or a traumatic contusion, EEG can always demonstrate the degree of dysfunctional changes around the lesion (or secondary diffuse cerebral dysfunction). The sad story is that the neurologist of our day seems to lose interest in the realm of function and dysfunction. This development must be halted (and eventually will be).

Topical EEG diagnosis, however, has made a comeback of its own in the form of computerized brain mapping. This fascinating recent development is associated chiefly with the name of Frank Duffy. Again, it is the old EEG in new clothes: it can be understood only by an expert of the conventional EEG.

Starting in the late 1960s, a completely new development took place in the EEG exploration of the full-term and the premature newborn. The historical aspects of this development are found in Chapters 11 and 49.

This historical overview is not complete without a few words about the technicians (technologists) doing the EEG laboratory routine work. They had to place electrodes with greatest accuracy and to obtain a readable tracing, even under the most adverse conditions. They were considered the electroencephalographers' attendants for a long time, even though their work required considerable sophistication.

John R. Knott and Charles E. Henry invested incredible energy into the founding of the American Society of EEG (later Electroneurodiagnostic) Technologists, which came into being in 1962. Soon afterward, the first group of technicians underwent a stiff examination that made them registered EEG technologists. There have been similar developments in many other countries. This evolution has been helpful in giving EEG technologists the dignity they deserve, but this process is far from being completed. With every record we read, we must be thankful for the work of our technical staff and invest some of our energies in their continuous education and training, for the sake of better technical EEG quality and thus for the sake of our patients.

This historical overview remains a fragmented account because much remains untold in this story. However, it is hoped that the historical perspective this chapter brings to the reader will foster in our ranks insights that may help us avoid the mistakes of the past.

Epilogue: Thoughts About Present and Future

Clinical EEG

The role of clinical electroencephalography has been diminishing throughout the past 30 years except for epileptology, which has been using the tool of EEG video monitoring to its full extent. This produces an enormous accumulation of data and needs thorough analysis and interpretation—a highly time-consuming task that is often "farmed out" or subcontracted to outside readers of sometimes unacceptable EEG expertise. Presence, number or absence of spikes, and spike-related discharges are not the only criteria; full justice must be done to all EEG abnormalities of nonparoxysmal character, and this task is a lot more difficult. Such expensive long-term recordings should be either artfully interpreted or not done at all.

Acutely requested EEG on an emergency basis nowadays deals mainly with the question of "rule out status epilepticus" (Varelas et al., 2003). With presently widespread confusions concerning the limitations of nonconvulsive status epilepticus (see Chapter 27), the answer needs profound neurological-epileptological understanding. Cases of acute cerebral anoxia (post-cardiopulmonary arrest) may cause both convulsive as well as nonconvulsive pictures with massive paroxysmal EEG abnormalities but do not represent true status epilepticus (see Chapter 27).

Outside the confines of epileptic conditions, the EEG is full of information for the vast majority of neurological diseases. It is most regrettable that this rich source of information has been badly underused in most neurological teaching institutions and hospitals in general (Niedermeyer, 2003b).

The Basis of EEG

The cellular basis of EEG activity has been the topic of intensive studies of extracellular current flow and voltage-dependent intrinsic oscillations (see Buzsaki et al., 2003). Ongoing work on cortical and subcortical generators is found in Chapter 3 (also see Ebersole, 2003). This shows that the genesis of EEG is still a widely discussed issue.

EEG and Neurocognition

This area has become the perhaps most fascinating aspect of modern EEG interest (see Chapter 31). It is true that most of this type of research has been done with other tools such as functional magnetic resonance imaging, positron emission tomography (PET) scanning and single photon emission computed tomography (SPECT) (methods demonstrating regional blood flow and metabolic needs). With the extension of EEG into the ultrafast frequency ranges, a powerful upswing of EEG-oriented neurocognitive research in animals and humans can be expected. Neurocognition has assumed the position of the "Holy Grail" of all neuroscience, and EEG stands a great chance to become a principal contributor. After years of frantic efforts, it will be found that neuroscience can illuminate the "brain-mind barrier" only to a certain degree. For the time being, however, let us not disturb the glowing enthusiasm with Cassandra calls.

References

Major Historical Works

Brazier, M.A.B. 1961. *A History of the Electrical Activity of the Brain. The First Half-Century.* London: Pitman.
Critchley, M. 1990. *The Ventricle of Memory.* New York: Raven Press.
Gloor, P. 1969. *Hans Berger on the Electroencephalogram of Man.* Amsterdam: Elsevier.
Grass, A.M. 1984. The electroencephalographic heritage. Am. J. EEG Technol. 24:133–173.
Hassler, R. 1959. Cécile und Oskar Vogt. In *Grosse Nervenärzte,* vol. 2, Ed. K. Kolle, pp. 45–64. Stuttgart: Thieme.

Jung, R. 1963. Hans Berger und die Entdeckung des EEG nach seinen Tagebüchern und Protokollen. In *Jenenser EEG-Symposium: 30 Jahre Elektroenzephalographie,* Ed. R. Werner, pp. 20–53. Berlin: VEB Verlag Volk und Gesundheit.
Kolle, K. 1956. Hans Berger. In *Grosse Nervenärzte,* vol. 1, Ed. K. Kolle, pp. 1–6. Stuttgart: Thieme.
Mazza, S., Pavone, A., and Niedermeyer, E. 2002. Mario Gozzano: the work of an EEG pioneer. Clin. Electroencephalogr. 33:155–159.
Niedermeyer, E. 2003a. Benjamin Franklin and static electricity. Considerations of past, present, and future. Am. J. End. Technol. 43:26–29
O'Leary, J.L., and Goldring, S. 1976. *Science and Epilepsy.* New York: Raven Press.
Schwab, R.S. 1951. *Electroencephalography.* Philadelphia: WB Saunders.
Upton, M. 1960. *Electronics for Everyone.* New York: New American Library of World Literature (Signet Key Books).
Werner, R. 1963. Hans Berger zum Gedächtnis. In *Jenenser EEG-Symposium: 30 Jahre Elektroenzephalographie,* Ed. R. Werner, pp. 13–19. Berlin: VEB Verlag Volk und Gesundheit.

Work of Specially Mentioned EEG Pioneers

Adrian, E.D. 1936. The Berger rhythm in the monkey's brain. J. Physiol. 87:83P–84P.
Adrian, E.D., and Bronk, D.W. 1929. The frequency of discharge in reflex and voluntary contractions. J. Physiol. 67:119–151.
Adrian, E.D., and Matthews, B.H.C. 1934. The interpretation of potential waves in the cortex. J. Physiol. 81:440–471.
Aserinsky, W., and Kleitman, N. 1953. Regularly occurring episodes of eye motility and concomitant phenomena during sleep. Science 118:273–274.
Bartley, S.H. 1932. Analysis of cortical response to stimulation of the optic nerve. Amer. J. Physiol. 101:4P.
Bartley, S.H., and Newman, E.B. 1930. Recording cerebral action currents. Science 71:587.
Bartley, S.H., and Newman, E.B. 1931. Studies on the dog's cortex. Am. J. Physiol. 99:1–8.
Berger, H. 1929. Über das Elektrenkephalogramm des Menschen. 1st report. Arch. Psychiat. Nervenkr. 87:527–570.
Berger, H. 1932. Über das Elektrenkephalogramm des Menschen. 4th report. Arch. Psychiat. Nervenkr. 97:6–26.
Berger, H. 1933. Über das Elektrenkephalogramm des Menschen. 7th report. Arch. Psychiat. Nervenkr. 100:301–320.
Bishop, G.H., and Bartley, S.H. 1932. Electrical study of the cerebral cortex as compared to the action potential of excised nerve. Proc. Soc. Exp. Biol. (New York) 29:698–699.
Blake, K., and Gerard, R.W. 1937. Brain potentials during sleep. Am. J. Physiol. 119:692–703.
Bremer, F. 1935. Cerveau isolé et physiologie du sommeil. C. R. Soc. Biol. (Paris) 118:1235–1241.
Bremer, F. 1958. Cerebral and Cerebellar Potentials. Physiol. Rev. 38:357–388.
Brock, L.G., Coombs, J.S., and Eccles, J.C. 1952. The recordings of potentials from motor neurons with an intracellular electrode. J. Physiol. 117:431–460.
Buzsaki, G., Traub, R., and Pedley, T.A. 2003. The cellular basis of EEG activity. In *Current Practice of Clinical Electroencephalography,* 3rd ed., Eds. J.S. Ebersole and T.A. Pedley, pp. 1–11. Philadelphia: Lippincott Williams and Wilkins.
Caton, R. 1875. The electric currents of the brain. Br. Med. J. 2:278.
Cooley, J.W., and Tukey, J.W. 1965. An algorithm for the machine calculation of complex Fourier series. Math Comp. 19:267–301.
Danilevsky, V.D. 1877. Investigations into the Physiology of the Brain. Doctoral Thesis University Charkov (cited in Brazier, 1961).
Davis, H., and Saul, L.V. Action currents in the auditory tracts of the midbrain of the cat. Science 86:448–450.
Dawson, G.D. 1951. A summation technique for the detection of small signals in a large irregular background. J. Physiol. (London) 115:2P.
Dietsch, G. 1932. Fourier-Analyse von Elektrenkephalogrammen des Menschen. Pflugers Arch. Ges. Physiol. 230:106–112.
Ebersole, J.S. 2003. Cortical generators and EEG voltage fields. In *Current Practice of Clinical Electroencephalography,* 3rd ed., Eds. J.S. Ebersole and T.A. Pedley, pp. 12–31. Philadelphia: Lippincott Williams and Wilkins.

Fischer, M.H. 1933. Elektrobiologische Auswirkungen von Krampfgiften am Zentralnervensystem. Med. Klin. 29:15–19.

Fischer, M.H., and Löwenbach, H. 1934a. Aktionsströme des Zentralnervensystems unter der Einwirkung von Krampfgiften. 1. Mitteilung Strychnin und Pikrotoxin. Arch. Exp. Pathol. Pharmakol. 174:357–382.

Fischer, M.H., and Löwenbach, H. 1934b. Aktionsströme des Zentralnervensystems unter der Einwirkung von Krampfgiften. 2. Mitteilung: Cardiazol, Coffein und andere. Arch. Exp. Pathol. Pharmakol. 174:502–516.

Foerster, O., and Altenburger, H. 1935. Elektrobiologische Vorgänge an der mensehlichen Hirnrinde. D.Z. Nervenheilk. 135:277–288.

Gastaut, H. 1949. Effets des stimulations physiques sur l'E.E.G. de l'homme. Electroencephalogr. Clin. Neurophysiol. Suppl. No. 2:69–82.

Gastaut, H., Roger, J., Corriol, J.H., et al. 1948. Les formes expérimentales d l'épilepsie humaine. L'épilepsie induite par la stimulation lumineuse intermittente ou épilepsie photogénique. Rev. Neurol. (Paris) 80:161–183.

Geddes, L.A. 1987. What did Caton see? Electroencephalogr. Clin. Neurophysiol. 67:2–6.

Gerard, R.W., Marshall, W.H., and Saul, L.J. 1933. Cerebral action potentials. Proc. Soc. Exp. Biol. (New York) 30:1123–1125.

Gibbs, E.L., and Gibbs, F.A. 1947. Diagnostic and localizing value of electroencephalographic studies in sleep. Publ. Assoc. Res. Nerv. Ment. Dis. 26:366–376.

Gibbs, E.L., Fuster, B., and Gibbs, F.A. 1948. Peculiar low temporal localization of sleep-induced seizure discharges of psychomotor epilepsy. Arch. Neurol. Psychiatry (Chicago) 60:95–97.

Gibbs, F.A., and Davis, H. 1935. Changes in the human electroencephalogram associated with loss of consciousness. Am. J. Physiol. 113:49–50.

Gibbs, F.A., Davis, H., and Lennox, W.G. 1935. The electroencephalogram in epilepsy and in conditions of impaired consciousness. Arch. Neurol. Psychiatry (Chicago) 34:1133–1148.

Gibbs, F.A., Gibbs, E.L., and Lennox, W.G. 1937. Epilepsy paroxysmal cerebral dysrhythmia. Brain 60:377–388.

Goltz, F.L. 1888. Ueber die Verrichtungen des Groszhirns. Pflueger's Arch. Ges. Physiol. 42:419–467.

Grass, A.M., and Gibbs, F.A. 1938. A Fourier transform of the electroencephalogram. J. Neurophysiol. 1:521–526.

Hayne, R., Belinson, L., and Gibbs, F.A. 1949a. Electrical activity of subcortical areas in epilepsy. Electroencephalogr. Clin. Neurophysiol. 1:437–445.

Hayne, R., Meyers, R., and Knott, J.R. 1949b. Characteristics of electrical activity of human corpus striatum and neighboring structures. J. Neurophysiol. 12:185–195.

Hoagland, H., Rubin, M.A., and Cameron, D.F. 1937. The electroencephalogram of schizophrenics during insulin hypoglycemia and recovery. Am. J. Physiol. 120:559–570.

Jung, R., Baumgarten, R.V., and Baumgartner, G. 1952. Mikroableitungen von einzelnen Nervzellen im optischen Cortex der Katze. Die lich taktivierten B-Neurone. Arch. Psychiat. Z. Ges. Neurol. 189:521–539.

Knott, J.R., and Gibbs, F.A. 1939. A Fourier transform of the electroencephalogram from one to eighteen years. Psychol. Bull. 36:512–513.

Knott, J.R., Gibbs, F.A., and Henry, C.E. 1942. Fourier transforms of electroencephalogram during sleep. J. Exp. Psychol. 31:465–477.

Knott, J.R., Hayne, R.A., and Meyers, H.R. 1950. Physiology of sleep-wave characteristics and temporal relations of human electroencephalograms recorded from the thalamus, the corpus striatum and the surface of the scalp. Arch. Neurol. Psychiatry (Chicago) 63:526–527.

Kornmüller, A.E. 1932. Architektonische Lokalisation bioelektriseher Erscheinungen auf der Grosshirnrinde. 1. Mitteilung: Untersuchungen am Kaninchen bei Augenbelichtung. J. Psychol. Neurol. 44:447–459.

Kornmüller, A.E. 1933. Die Ableitung bioelektischer Effekte architektonischer Rindenfelder vom uneröffneten Schadel. J. Psychol. Neurol. 45:172–184.

Kornmüller, A.E. 1935. Der Mechanismus des epileptischen Anfalles auf Grund bioelektrischer Untersuchungen am Zentralnervensystem. Fortschr. Neurol. Psychiatry 7:391–400, 414–432.

Kornmüller, A.E. 1937. *Die Bioelektrischer Erseheinungen der Hirnrindenfelder.* Leipzig: Thieme.

Kornmüller, A.E. 1944. *Klinische Elektrenkephalographie.* Munich: Lehmann.

Kornmüller, A.E. 1947. *Die Elemente der Nervösen Tätigkeit.* Stuttgart: Thieme.

Lennox, W.G. 1930. The oxygen and carbon dioxide content of blood from the internal jugular and other veins. Arch. Intern. Med. 46:630–636.

Lennox, W.G. 1931. The cerebral circulation. Arch. Neurol. Psychiatry (Chicago) 26:719–724.

Lennox, W.G., and Gibbs, E.L. 1932. The blood flow in the brain and the leg of man, and the changes induced by alteration of blood gases. J. Clin. Invest. 1:1155–1177.

Li, C.L., Jasper, H.H., and McLennan, H. 1952. Décharge d'unités cellulaires en relation avec les oscillations électriques de l'écorce cérébrale. Rev. Neurol. (Paris) 87:149–151.

Liberson, W.T. 1937. Recherches sur les électroencéphalogramme transcraniens de l'homme. Travail Hum. 5:431–463.

Lindsley, D.B., Bowden, J.W., and Magoun, H.W. 1949. The effect of subcortical lesions upon the electroencephalogram. Am. Psychol. 4:233–234.

Loomis, A.L., Harvey, E.N., and Hobart, G.A. 1935. Potential rhythms of the cerebral cortex during sleep. Science 82:198–200.

Meyers, H.R., and Hayne, R. 1948. Electrical potentials of the corpus striatum and cortex in Parkinsonism and hemiballism. Trans. Am. Neurol. Assoc. 73:10–14.

Morison, R.S., and Dempsey, E.W. 1942. A study of thalamo-cortical relations. Am. J. Physiol. 135:281–292.

Moruzzi, G. 1952. L'attività dei neuroni corticali durante il sonne e durante la reazione elettroencefalografica di risveglio. Ricerca Sci. 22:1165–1173.

Moruzzi, G., and Magoun, H.W. 1949. Brain stem reticular format and activation of the EEG. Electroencephalogr. Clin. Neurophysiol. 1:455–473.

Niedermeyer, E. 2003b. The clinical relevance of EEG interpretation. Clin. Electroencephalogr. 34:93–98.

Penfield, W., and Jasper, H.H. 1954. *Epilepsy and the Functional Anatomy of the Human Brain.* Boston: Little, Brown.

Phillips, C.G. 1961. Some properties of pyramidal neurones of the motor cortex. In *The Nature of Sleep,* Eds. G.E.W. Wolstenholme and M. O'Conner, pp. 4–24. Boston: Little, Brown.

Rothmann, H. 1923. Zusammenfassender Bericht über den Rothmann'schen groszhirnlosen Hund nach klinischer und anatomischer Untersuchung. Z. Ges. Neurol. Psychiat. 87:247–313.

Sherrington, C.S. 1906. *Integrative Action of the Nervous System.* 1906. New Haven, CT: Yale University Press.

Travis, L.E., and Dorsey, J.M. 1932. Action current studies of simultaneously active disparate fields of the central nervous system of the rat. Arch. Neurol. Psychiat. 28:331–338.

Travis, L.E., and Herren, R.Y. 1931. The relation of electrical changes in the brain to reflex activity. J. Comp. Psychol. 12:23–29.

Travis, L.E., and Knott, J.R. 1936. Brain potential studies. I. Perseveration time to light. J. Psychol. 3:97–100.

Varelas, P.N., Spanaki, M.V., Hacein-Bey, L., et al. 2003. Emergent EEG. Neurology 61:702–704.

Vogt, C., and Vogt, O. 1937. *Sitz und Wesen der Krankheiten im Lichte der topistischen Hirnforschung und des Variierens der Tiere.* Leipzig: Barth.

Walter, W.G. 1936. The location of brain tumors by electroencephalogram. Proc. R. Soc. Med. 30:579–598.

Walter, W.G. 1964. Slow potential waves in the human brain associated with expectancy, attention and decision. Arch. Psychiat. Nervenkr. 206:309–322.

Walter, W.G., Dovey, V.J., and Shipton, H. 1946. Analysis of electrical responses of the human cortex to photic stimulation. Nature 158:540–541.

Walter, W.G., Cooper, R., Aldridge, V.J., et al. 1964. Contingent negative variation. An electric sign of sensorimotor association and expectancy in the human brain. Nature 203:380–384.

Yakovlev, P.I. 1953. Vladimir Mikhailovich Bekhterev (1857–1927). In *The Founders of Neurology,* Ed. W. Haymaker, pp. 244–247. Springfield, IL: Charles C Thomas.

2. Introduction to the Neurophysiological Basis of the EEG and DC Potentials[1]

Erwin-Josef Speckmann and Christian E. Elger

The clinical electroencephalographer correlates central nervous system (CNS) functions as well as dysfunctions and diseases with certain patterns of the electroencephalogram (EEG) on an empirical basis. Obviously, this method has been found valuable in clinical practice. Therefore, why should the clinical electroencephalographer study the basic elementary processes underlying the EEG? There is little doubt that the range of EEG interpretations can be much widened and misinterpretations avoided when the underlying elementary processes are also considered. This is true especially for convulsive disorders and cerebral metabolic disturbances. For example, an isoelectric EEG can be caused by selective pCO_2 increase while the brain is sufficiently supplied with O_2. On the other hand, in the presence of practically normal pCO_2 levels, cerebral hypoxia may be the cause. It will be pointed out below that the prognosis may be quite different in these two cases.

Elementary Processes of Extracellular Field Potential Generation

The basic mechanisms that give rise to potentials recorded outside the CNS elements will be described. Such extracellular potentials are generally known as field potentials (Speckmann and Caspers, 1979a).

In the course of this presentation, the morphology of generator structures is discussed briefly. Then, the electrical activity demonstrable with intracellular recordings from neurons and glia cells is described. On the basis of this information, the principles of the generation of extracellular field potentials are outlined and the various types of field potentials are characterized.

Generator Structures

The CNS essentially consists of nerve cells and glia cells. The arrangement of neurons usually shows a specific type of laminar character. Glia cells are located between neurons.

As shown in Fig. 2.1 several processes emerge from the nucleus-containing cellular soma (body) of the nerve cell. These processes can be divided into two types according to their function. Most of the processes are dendrites that branch off into numerous small ramifications. Every cell also has an axon that may split up into multiple collaterals. Such an axon provides contact with other nerve cells or with

other target organs. In the case of interneuronal connections, the contact consists of synapses that cover the dendrites, the soma, and the axon hillock in large numbers. Thus, nerve cells are usually covered with several thousand synapses (Palay and ChanPalay, 1977).

The glia cells are imbedded between nerve cell somata, dendrites, and axons. They usually have several processes that make contact with somata and processes of nerve cells; they may also make contact with vessels. This histological arrangement results in a cerebral extracellular space consisting of very narrow intercellular clefts (De Robertis and Carrea, 1965).

Neuronal Activity Recorded Intracellularly

Next, those essential potentials that can be demonstrated with intracellular recordings are characterized briefly. When the membrane of the nerve cell body is penetrated by a microelectrode, a potential of about 60 to 70 mV with negative polarity in the intracellular space can be recorded. This membrane potential is subject to various fluctuations that are elicited chiefly by synaptic activities. Their mechanisms are shown in greater detail in Fig. 2.2. As can be derived from this schematic illustration, the neuron from which the soma membrane potential is recorded has synaptic connections. The corresponding presynaptic structures are also explored with microelectrodes. If an action potential travels along the fiber, which ends in an excitatory synapse, an excitatory postsynaptic potential (EPSP) occurs in the following neuron (Fig. 2.2A). If two action potentials travel along the same fiber with a short interval, there will be a summation of EPSP triggering an action potential on the postsynaptic neuron after reaching the membrane threshold. If an action potential travels along a fiber ending in an inhibitory synapse, then hyperpolarization will occur, representing an inhibitory postsynaptic potential (IPSP) (Eccles, 1964; Hubbard et al., 1969; Shepherd, 1974).

Because of the time course of the various membrane potential fluctuations, the postsynaptic potentials are thought to contribute primarily to the generation of the extracellular field potentials in question (Creutzfeldt and Houchin, 1974; Hubbard et al., 1969; Speckmann and Caspers, 1979a; Speckmann et al., 1984). For this reason, the ionic mechanisms of these potentials are discussed in greater detail. The individual events of this process are presented with a magnified time base (see Fig. 2.4). With the elicitation of an EPSP, a net inflow of cations occurs across the subsynaptic membrane. This gives rise to depolarization of the subsynaptic

[1]This chapter was translated from German by E. Niedermeyer.

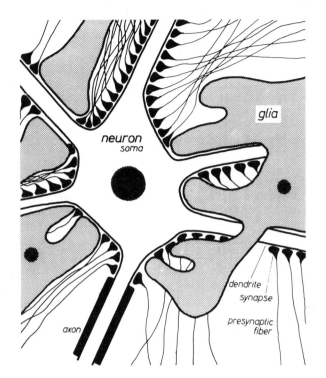

Figure 2.1. Schematic drawing of morphology and histology of neuronal and glial elements.

membrane. As shown in Fig. 2.2B, a potential gradient develops along the neuronal membrane in the intra- and extracellular space. Because of this potential gradient, cations move along the nerve cell membrane through the extracellular space in the direction of the subsynaptic region. An inversely directed flow takes place in the intracellular space. With the generation of an IPSP, there is an outflow of cations from the nerve cell and/or an inflow of anions into the nerve cell. These changes first increase the membrane potential at the subsynaptic membrane in comparison with the surrounding segments of the membrane. For this reason, a potential gradient develops along the nerve cell membrane, as in the case of the EPSP genesis. This potential gradient causes, in the extracellular space, a flow of cations from the subsynaptic region to the surrounding portions of the membrane. An inverse process develops in the intracellular space (Hubbard et al., 1969).

The ion fluxes in the extracellular space are of paramount significance in the generation of field potentials. Therefore, these processes are further discussed in the following chapters.

Glia Activity Recorded Intracellularly

In addition to the neurons, glial cells may also play a role in the generation of extracellular field potentials (Kuffler and Nicholls, 1966; Somjen and Trachtenberg, 1979). Therefore, the bioelectric properties of glial cells are summarized.

If a glia cell is penetrated with a microelectrode, a membrane potential can be recorded with a polarity similar to that of the nerve cells. The size of this membrane potential

approximates the potassium equilibrium potential and hence somewhat exceeds the membrane potential of nerve cells. In contrast to neurons, glial cells fail to show any action potentials, and there are also no postsynaptic potentials. Thus, in contrast to neurons, glial cells do not show characteristic potentials that distinguish them unmistakably from other cells. The glial membrane potential, however, is also not constant. An augmentation of the extracellular potassium concentration (potassium activity) causes depolarization of glial cells (Fig. 2.3A). Concentration changes of other ions cause only negligible alterations of the glial cell membrane potential. The glial cell is hence comparable to a potassium electrode (Kuffler and Nicholls, 1966; Kuffler et al., 1966).

The dependency of the glial membrane potential on the extracellular potassium concentration is the reason for a functional linkage with adjacent neuronal structures. Neuronal activity is associated with outflow of potassium ions.

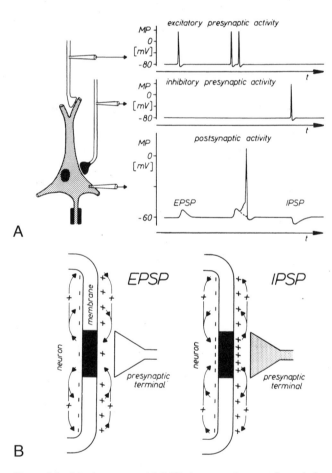

Figure 2.2. Membrane potential (MP) changes and current flows during synaptic activation. **A:** The MP of the postsynaptic neuron and the MP of the presynaptic fibers are recorded by means of intracellular microelectrodes. Action potentials in the excitatory and inhibitory presynaptic fiber lead to excitatory postsynaptic potential (EPSP) and inhibitory postsynaptic potential (IPSP), respectively, in the postsynaptic neuron. Two EPSPs sum up to a superthreshold potential, triggering an action potential in the postsynaptic neuron. **B:** During EPSP and IPSP, ionic current flows occur through as well as along the neuronal membrane, as shown by arrows. The density of + and − signs indicate the polarization of the subsynaptic (*dark area*) as well as that of the postsynaptic membrane during synaptic activation.

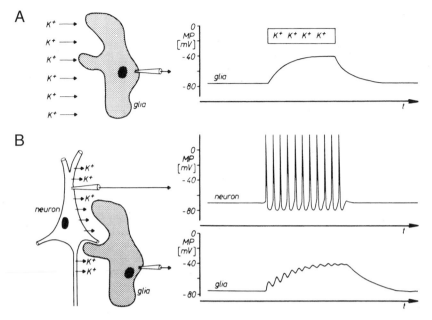

Figure 2.3. Membrane potential (MP) changes of glia cells induced by an increase in the extracellular K^+ concentration *(arrows in the schematic drawings)*. **A:** Potassium is applied extracellularly to the glia cell. **B:** The potassium concentration is increased due to an activation of a neighboring neuron. (From original tracings from Kuffler, S.W., Nicholls, J.G., and Orkand, R.K. 1966. Physiological properties of glial cells in the central nervous system of amphibia. *J. Neurophysiol.* 29:768–787.)

As shown schematically in Fig. 2.3B, repetitive firing of neurons gives rise to increased extracellular potassium concentration and hence to glial cell depolarization (Orkand et al., 1966; Speckmann, 1986). If the potassium concentration does not affect the entire glial cell membrane and remains increased only locally, then potential gradients build up along the glial cell, giving rise to intra- and extracellular current flows similar to the ones described in reference to neuronal synaptic transmissions (Fig. 2.4). Glial cells frequently have widespread processes and furthermore may have close connections with each other. For this reason, potential fields of considerable spatial extension may develop on the basis of the aforementioned mechanisms (Caspers et al., 1980, 1984; Somjen and Trachtenberg, 1979; Speckmann and Caspers, 1979a). In view of the above described functional interconnections, it is quite likely that in the gen-

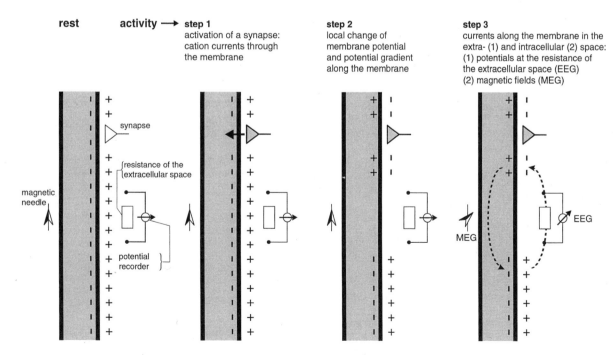

Figure 2.4. Basic mechanisms underlying generation of potentials (electroencephalogram; EEG) and of magnetic fields (magnetoencephalogram; MEG) in the extracellular space of central nervous system. The description is based on the assumption that an extended neuronal process, e.g., a dendrite, is locally depolarized by activation of an excitatory synapse.

esis of extracellular field potentials an amplifying effect can be attributed to the glial cells.

Generation of Extracellular Field Potentials

It has been shown in the preceding section that primary transmembranous currents generate secondary ionic currents along the cell membranes in the intra- and extracellular space. The portion of these currents that flows through the extracellular space is directly responsible for the generation of field potentials (Fig. 2.4). Particular significance must be ascribed to the synaptic processes as causing events for the field potentials in question, especially for their time course. In accordance with these statements, the generation of extracellular field potentials will be discussed as exemplified by extracellular fields accompanying synaptic activity (Caspers et al., l984; Hubbard et al., 1969; Rall, 1977; Speckmann et al., 1984). The discussion of these events will again make use of a very protracted time axis (Fig. 2.4). The explanation of the events is given in reference to the schematic view in Fig. 2.5. This figure shows a widely stretched neuronal element, with one end segment lying close to the surface of a central nervous structure. At both ends of this neuronal unit, the microelectrodes ME_1 and ME_2 are inserted. At the same time, the extracellular electrodes E_1 and E_2 are located at the surface and at the deeper end of the neuronal element. The potentials picked up from the intra- and extracellular electrodes are shown in the vicinity of each electrode. The potential recorded from the surface of the nervous structure is accentuated by *thicker lines*. Figure 2.5 shows active excitatory and inhibitory synapses, either close to the surface or located in the depth. As described elsewhere, the activation of an excitatory synapse leads to a net inward flow of cations. If this statement is applied to Fig. 2.5A1, then it becomes evident that the upper end of the neuronal element will be depolarized in comparison with other segments of the same cell. Accordingly, the synaptic current flow causes an EPSP at the microelectrode ME_1. This local depolarization then gives rise to further intra- and extracellular ionic currents along the nerve cell membrane. Because of the intracellular movements of positive charges, depolarization in the area of microelectrode ME_2 also takes place. This depolarization, however, is less steep and of smaller amplitude. At the superficially located extracellular electrode E_2, the inflow of positive charges into the neuronal element causes a negative field potential. The extracellular electrode E_2 is, metaphorically speaking, approached by positive charges so that a positive field potential will develop in this area. The point of reversal of the field potentials is localized between electrodes E_1 and E_2. The exact position of the point of reversal depends on the distribution of extracellular impedances.

Current flows of reversed direction (in reference to the recording electrodes) will occur if the active excitatory synapse is located at the deeper end of the neuronal element (Fig. 2.5A2). In this case, positive charges approach the superficially located electrode (E_1) (again speaking metaphorically) and remove themselves from the deeply located electrode (E_2). This arrangement of the active synaptic structures causes a positive field potential at the surface and a negative one at the deep electrode. The current flows accompanying the activation of inhibitory synapses located in deeper and in more superficial areas, respectively, are shown in Fig. 2.5B. As can be derived from this illustration, the activation of a deep inhibitory synapse (Fig. 2.5B1) produces a current flow that is largely similar to the one generated by the activation of a superficial excitatory synapse (Fig. 2.5A1). In the same manner, there are also similar current flows in the extracellular space when a superficial inhibitory synapse (Fig.

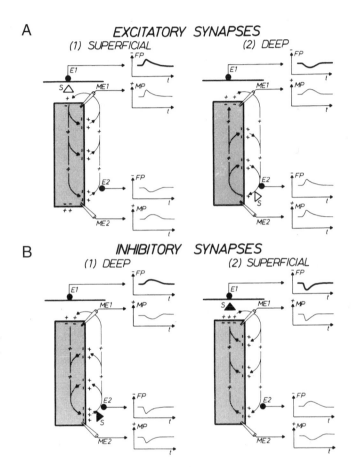

Figure 2.5. Membrane potential (MP) changes and field potentials (FPs) elicited by the activation of excitatory and inhibitory synapses in the central nervous system. The elementary processes are explained by means of a neuronal element *(hatched area)*, the one end of which contracts the surface of a structure in the central nervous system. The MP of the neuron element is recorded at both ends by the microelectrodes ME_1 and ME_2. The extracellular field is picked up at the surface of the neuronal structure by the electrode E_1, as well as in the vicinity of ME_2 by the electrode E_2. Active excitatory and inhibitory synapses are marked by *open triangles* and *black triangles* (S), respectively. **A1:** The inward current at S generates an EPSP that appears in the region of ME_1, as well as in that of ME_2. Because S is located superficially, the FP generated, due to the direction of the extracellular current flow *(arrows)*, is of negative polarity at the surface (E_1) and of positive polarity in the deeper recording (E_2). **A2:** The activation of a deep excitatory synapse elicits a current flow with inverse direction as compared with **A1**. Therefore, the extracellular FP consists in a positive deflection at the surface and in a negative one at the depth. **B1:** The outward current at S generates an IPSP in the region of ME_2, as well as in that of ME_1. Due to the direction of the extracellular current flow, the FP generated consists in a positive fluctuation in the depth (E_2) and in a negative one in the surface recording (E_1). **B2:** The current flow during the activation of a superficial inhibitory synapse is inverse as compared with **B1**. Therefore, the FP recorded from the surface consists of a positive fluctuation. Differences in the time course of the various potentials are caused by the electrical properties of the tissue.

2.5B2) or a deeply located excitatory synapse (Fig. 2.5A2) is activated. Accordingly, a negative field potential will develop at the surface of a central nervous structure (in the schematic view of Fig. 2.5) whenever a superficial excitatory or a more deeply located inhibitory synapse is activated. The corresponding principle applies to generation of the superficial field potentials of positive polarity.

Types of Field Potentials

The field potentials, whose generation has been described, can be subdivided into different types. If field potentials are recorded against an inactive reference point with an upper frequency limit of about 100 Hz, then two types of field potentials can be distinguished, depending on the time constant of the amplifying recording device. In the case of a time constant of 1 second or less, the extracellular field potentials correspond with that which is commonly known as the electroencephalogram (EEG). If the recording is carried out with an infinite time constant, i.e., with direct current (DC) amplifier, then slower potentials can also be picked up. Potentials recorded with this technique are generally known as DC potentials (Caspers, 1974; Caspers et al., 1984; Speckmann and Caspers, 1979a; Speckmann et al., 1984). Thus, DC potentials comprise slow as well as fast field potentials. The fast components correspond with the potential fluctuations of the EEG. Due to different time constants, however, the faster potential components may differ from each other as far as their time course is concerned when recordings are done either with conventional EEG amplifiers or with DC amplifiers.

Thus far, technical problems have made it difficult to carry out DC recordings from the scalp. Except for special areas of application, DC recordings are usually performed in animal experiments. DC potentials directly reflect the state of activity of central nervous cells and therefore contribute to the explanation of the mechanisms of genesis of cerebral field potentials (Caspers et al., 1980; Speckmann and Caspers, 1979b). For this reason, DC potentials will be discussed jointly with EEG waves.

For the sake of comparison, Fig. 2.6 shows the EEG and the DC potentials during convulsive activity, hypercapnia, and asphyxia. As shown in this illustration, a tonic-clonic convulsion is associated with a negative DC shift (Caspers and Speckmann, 1969; Caspers et al., 1980, 1984; Gumnit et al., 1970; Speckmann, 1986; Speckmann and Elger, 1984; Speckmann et al., 1984). Furthermore, it can be seen that the hypercapnia-induced disappearance of the EEG is associated with a monophasic positive DC shift. In the case of EEG extinction due to primary asphyxia, however, there are characteristic patterns of DC fluctuation. Hence, similar findings in the conventional EEG may be associated with different DC shifts.[2]

---

[2]What does the term *DC shift* mean? What is DC? Speaking from experience, many electroencephalographers have no clear concept regarding DC potentials or DC shifts. One cannot blame them because, for strange reasons, "DC" has two meanings in this context:

1. DC means direct current (and this is, of course, commonplace): a current without oscillations; a current derived from a battery source; a current maintained in one direction through a circuit. A more imperfect DC is

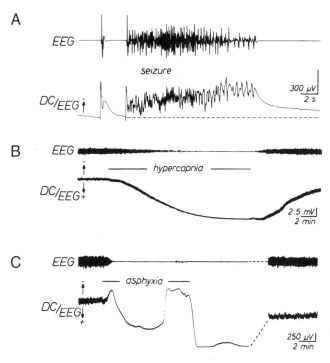

Figure 2.6. EEG (time constant: 1 second; upper frequency limit: 100 Hz) and DC/EEG recordings (DC recording: upper frequency limit, 100 Hz) during a generalized seizure induced by pentylenetetrazol (**A**), during hypercapnia (**B**), and during asphyxia (**C**). Original recordings were obtained from cats and rats. Note the different time scales.

Wave Generation

In the preceding sections, the generation of single field potentials was described. In this section, the principles of the generation of wavelike potential fluctuations are outlined. This is followed by the discussion of the laminar distribution of such potentials in the cerebral cortex.

Principal Mechanisms

To present the generation of wavelike potential fluctuations on the surface of a central nervous structure, a simple

---

produced by a rectifier, used to change alternating current (AC) into DC. For multilingual readers, DC is *courant continu* in French, *Gleichstrom* in German, and *corrente continuo* in Italian.

Electroneurophysiologically, DC shifts are ultraslow potentials, about as slow as 0.1 to 0.2/sec. This, however, is not true DC. Such slow activity is just a bit more "DC-like" since it does not show the faster "AC-like" activity. One simply has to live with this kind of misnomer.

2. DC also means direct coupling (and this is much less known). What coupling? The coupling between the stages of EEG amplification. Conventional EEG machines have stages coupled by capacitors. Now one has to remember that capacitors (a) reject DC and (b) determine the time constant. Even a very long time constant (several seconds duration) may not suffice for the recording of DC potentials. Direct coupling is a capacitor-free coupling between the stages of amplification and provides the optimal condition for DC recording. This is technically quite difficult in clinical conventional EEG recording but easier under experimental neurophysiological conditions in animals.

Hence, be aware of the dual significance of the term *DC* (also see the section Filters in Chapter 7). (This footnote added by Ernst Niedermeyer, editor.)

Figure 2.7. Principles of wave generation. The excitatory synapses of two afferent fibers contact the superficial dendritic arborization of two longitudinal neuronal elements. The afferent fiber activity is recorded by means of the intracellular electrodes E_1 and E_2, and the membrane potentials (MPs) of the dendritic elements are recorded by the electrodes E_3 and E_4. The field potential at the surface of the neuronal structure (cortex) is led by the electrode E_5. Synchronized groups of action potentials in the afferent fibers (E_1, E_2) generate wavelike EPSPs in the dendritic areas (E_3, E_4) and corresponding field potentials in the EEG and DC/EEG recording (E_5). Tonic activity in the afferent fibers results in a long-lasting EPSP with small fluctuations. During this period the EEG *(5b)* shows only a reduction in amplitude, whereas the DC/EEG recording *(5a)* reflects the depolarization of the neuronal elements as well.

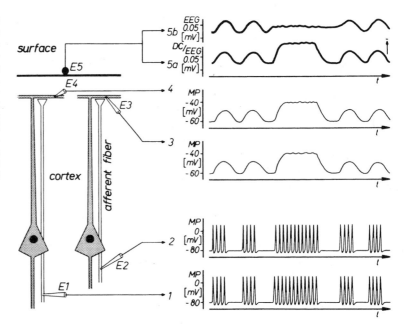

model as shown in Fig. 2.7 is used. This model consists of two extended pyramidal neurons of vertical orientation. Terminals of afferent fibers make contact with the superficial dendrites of both neurons via excitatory synapses. The bioelectrical activity of these structures is recorded with intracellular microelectrodes. The microelectrodes E_1 and E_2 are located in the ascending fibers and the microelectrodes E_3 and E_4 are in the superficial dendrites of the postsynaptic neurons. To pick up the extracellular field potentials, the electrode E_5 lies on the surface of the central nervous structure.

As shown in tracings 1 and 2, action potentials occur synchronously in the afferent fibers. There are grouped discharges that are temporarily supplanted by tonic activity. The ascending action potentials elicit individual EPSP in the upper dendrites of the neurons; these EPSPs are subsequently summated into major depolarizations in accordance with the discharge frequency. As shown in tracings 3 and 4, amplitude and duration of the depolarizations depend on the discharge pattern of the afferent fibers. The synaptic activity at the superficial structures gives rise to extracellular current flows resulting in superficial field potentials. With the use of DC recording techniques, the superficial field potentials reflect the potential fluctuations of the dendritic membrane. If, however, the superficial field potentials are recorded with a time constant of 1 second or less, then only the fast fluctuations of the superficial field potentials are demonstrable.

Thus far, the principles of genesis of EEG and DC waves have been shown in the schematic view of Fig. 2.7. Accordingly, the generation of physiological EEG waves may be explained as follows. If a grouped and synchronous influx takes place in afferent fiber systems toward the superficial generator structures, then EEG waves evolve that are of high amplitude and distinctly separated from each other. In case of a periodic sequence of the afferent bursts, the recording of the field potentials shows sinusoidal potential fluctuations. This mechanism has been presumed by several groups of investi-

gators as the principle of the generation of the alpha rhythm and slower periodic EEG waves. According to these workers, thalamocortical feedback loops are believed to play a significant role in the generation of the alpha rhythm (Andersen and Andersson, 1968; Speckmann and Caspers, 1979a).

If the afferent influx of impulses occurs at a high frequency for a longer period and/or synchronously, then negative field potentials with small fluctuations will result from the extracellular current flows. Accordingly, the EEG recording will pick up only waves of smaller amplitude and mostly higher frequency. In the DC recording, however, the prolonged depolarization of the superficial structures caused by the afferent high-frequency influx will express itself by a negative DC potential shift (Caspers, 1963; Goldring, 1974). There is a close correlation between the amplitude of the negative DC shift and average discharge frequency in the afferent fiber systems. This mechanism may apply principally to the generation of beta activity and other EEG waves of higher frequencies. A decrease of the amplitudes of the EEG waves can also occur when the afferent activity is diminished. In this case, however, the depression of EEG waves is accompanied by a positive DC shift (Caspers and Speckmann, 1974; also see Fig. 2.14).

Spatial Distribution Within the Cortex

The principles of generation of individual and wavelike field potentials at the surface of central nervous structures such as the cerebral cortex have been described. If the wavelike potential fluctuations are recorded not only from the cortical surface but also from different cortical layers, then it can be shown that potential fluctuations in the latter recordings may differ considerably from those at the surface. These differences imply polarity, frequency, and amplitude (Elger and Speckmann, 1983; Petsche et al., 1978; Speckmann and Caspers, 1979a). Such a recording from the cortex

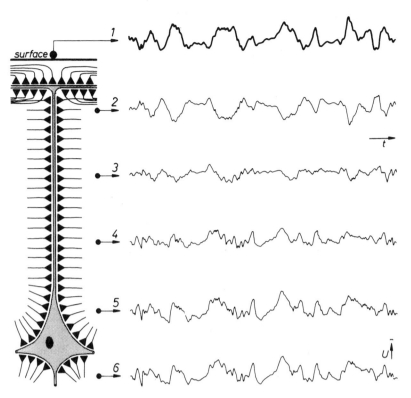

Figure 2.8. Surface *(1)* and laminar recordings *(2–6)* of EEG waves of the cortex. The schematic drawing symbolizes conical neuronal elements densely packed with synapses. (Drawings from original tracings obtained in experiments in the rat's motor cortex during pentobarbital anesthesia.)

of the rat is shown in Fig. 2.8. According to this illustration, field potentials reverse their polarity between electrode 1 (on the surface) and electrode 2 (located 300 μm beneath the cortical surface). Two and sometimes more of such phase reversals may be observed in deeper recording sites depending on the experimental conditions. The vertical distribution type of field potential will be discussed in greater detail in connection with the generation of cortical field potentials during convulsive activity.

In the course of the discussion of cerebral field potentials, it was pointed out that particular significance must be attributed to synaptic activity. A view of the laminar distribution of neurons in the cortex and the dense coverage of these unitary structures with synapses makes it clear that different patterns of potentials must necessarily occur in different layers when populations of synapses are activated in a different manner. This should be clarified by the schematic drawing in Fig. 2.8.

The difference of bioelectrical activity at cortical surface and in deeper cortical layers becomes very clear when voltage-sensitive dyes were used instead of field potential recordings (Köhling et al., 2000, 2002; Straub et al., 2003). With this technique neuronal activity can be seen, although the requirements for the generation of field potentials (see above) are not fulfilled.

Cortical Field Potentials During Epileptiform Activity

In the following subsections, the generation of cortical field potentials during convulsive activity is discussed. The first subsection deals with focal activity, and the second discusses generalized, tonic-clonic convulsive activity. For methodical reasons, we refer to data derived from experimental work in animals.

Focal Activity

If a convulsive substance such as penicillin is applied to the surface of the cerebral cortex, steep negative potentials of high amplitude can be picked up from the area of application after a short latency period. These discharges repeat themselves in stereotyped form and periodicity (Klee et al., 1982; Purpura et al., 1972; Speckmann, 1986) (Fig. 2.9A). If the membrane potential of a cortical neuron is simultaneously recorded with a microelectrode while a second microelectrode picks up the corresponding field potentials, then potential fluctuations occur as shown in Fig. 2.9B. It can be derived from this illustration that the monotonously recurrent negative field potentials are associated with equally stereotyped membrane potential fluctuations. These oscillations of the membrane commence with a steep depolarization that, having exceeded the membrane threshold, triggers a series of action potentials. This is followed by a plateau that, after 80 to 100 msec, changes into a steep repolarization, and frequently also into a hyperpolarization. These membrane potential fluctuations have proved to be characteristic in the epileptiform activity of individual neurons. They are generally known as paroxysmal depolarization shifts (PDSs) (Jasper et al., 1969; Speckmann, 1986).

Investigation of potential distribution within the cerebral cortex after the local application of penicillin yields a variety of findings. An appropriate model is shown in Fig. 2.10. In this experiment, recordings of interictal field potentials were

Figure 2.9. EEG (**A**) and membrane potential (MP) changes of a pyramidal tract neuron and extracellular field potential (FP) recorded in the vicinity of the impaled neuron (**B**) during focal interictal activity elicited by application of penicillin to the cortical surface (*hatched area* in **A**). Drawings of original tracings from experiments in the rat. The sweep speed in **B** is five times that in **A**. The recording sites are shown in the schematic drawings.

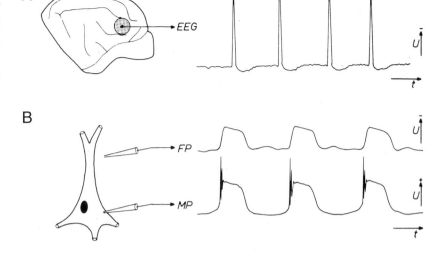

carried out from the cortical surface, from inside the cortex, and from the spinal cord. The spinal field potentials permit the observation of electrical activity descending from the cortex to the spinal cord. In Fig. 2.10A, negative field potentials are recorded from the cortical surface and from the two upper intracortical contacts after the application of penicillin together with penicillin-metabolizing enzyme penicillinase. There are, however, field potentials with predominantly positive components in the deeper contacts 4 through 6. If penicillin is applied to the surface without penicillinase, then negative field potential will also develop in deeper cortical layers. If it is assumed that the negative field potentials mirror the direct epileptiform activity of neuronal structures (Fig. 2.9), then it must also be assumed that deeper cortical elements are involved in convulsive activity shown in of Fig.

2.10B in contrast with Fig. 2.10A. This is further supported by the observation that neuronal activity descending to the spinal cord and producing characteristic spinal field potentials occurs only under the experimental conditions shown in Fig. 2.10B. If one compares the recordings in Fig. 2.10A and Fig. 2.10B, it becomes clear that, with a monotonous epileptiform potential at the cortical surface, the intracortical potential distribution and the occurrence of descending activity may differ considerably (Elger and Speckmann, 1980, 1983; Elger et al., 1981; also see Gumnit, 1974; Petsche et al., 1981; Speckmann and Elger, 1983; Wieser, 1983).

If penicillin is applied to deeper cortical laminae (Fig. 2.10C), then negative field potentials will be confined to that region. These potentials are consistently accompanied by descending activity to the spinal cord. Under these condi-

Figure 2.10. Cortical field potentials recorded at the surface (*1*) and from within the cortex (*2–6*) and spinal field potentials (*7*) during interictal activity. The interictal activity was elicited by penicillin. **A,B:** Potential distribution after surface application of the drug. In **A**, the spread of penicillin is limited by the use of penicillinase. **C:** Potential distribution after intracortical application of penicillin at recording point *4*. The areas directly involved in the epileptiform activity as indicated by negative field potentials are marked by hatching in the schematic drawings. Spinal field potentials are linked to the occurrence of negative field potentials in lamina V (**B** and **C**, *4*). Distance between the intracortical electrodes, 300 μm. (From original tracings from Elger, C.E., Speckmann, E.J., Caspers, H., et al. 1981. Focal interictal epileptiform discharges in the cortex of the rat: laminar restriction and its consequences for activity descending to the spinal cord. In *Physiology and Pharmacology of Epileptogenic Phenomena*, Eds. M.R. Klee, H.D. Lux, and E.J. Speckmann. New York: Raven Press.)

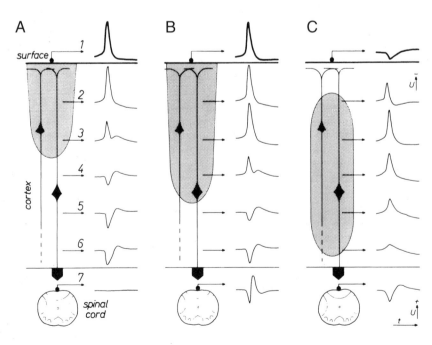

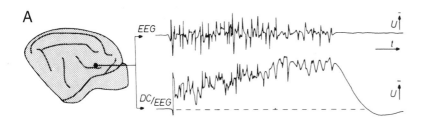

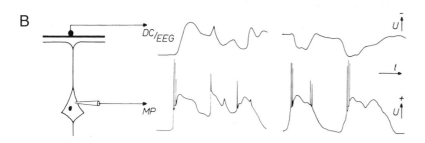

Figure 2.11. Simultaneous recordings of EEG and DC/EEG (**A**) and of DC/EEG and membrane potential (MP) of a pyramidal tract neuron (**B**) during generalized tonic-clonic seizures elicited by pentylenetetrazol. (Drawings after original tracings from experiments in the cat's motor cortex. The sweep speed in **B** is 10 times that in **A**.)

tions, there is frequently nothing but a positive potential fluctuation of minor amplitude at the cortical surface (Elger and Speckmann, 1983; Elger et al., 1981).

In summary, it can be derived from the described experimental models that, in focal convulsive activity limited to the cortex, the surface potential does not necessarily reflect the bioelectrical events in deeper cortical layers.

Generalized Tonic-Clonic Activity

Here, possible mechanisms involved in the generation of cortical field potentials during tonic-clonic convulsive activity are described. Again, data are based on experimental observations in animals. Tonic-clonic convulsive activity was triggered by repeated injections of pentylenetetrazol (also see Purpura et al., 1972; Speckmann, 1986).

Figure 2.11A shows a tonic-clonic convulsion recorded with a conventional EEG amplifier, as well as with a DC amplifier. There is a negative DC shift from the baseline during a convulsive seizure. This negative DC shift gradually recedes during the termination of the convulsions and frequently changes into a transient positive after shift (Caspers and Speckmann, 1969; Caspers et al., 1980, 1984; Gumnit, 1974; Speckmann, 1986; Speckmann and Caspers, 1979b; Speckmann and Elger, 1984).

When the membrane potential of a pyramidal tract neuron of lamina V is recorded during a convulsive seizure, it can be shown that under these conditions typical PDSs become manifest (Fig. 2.11B). If these PDSs are correlated with the potential fluctuations in the DC recording, it can be noticed that the PDS in pyramidal tract neurons are coupled at the beginning of the convulsive seizure with superficial negative potential fluctuations and at the end of the convulsive seizure with surface positive potential fluctuations (Fig. 2.11B) (Speckmann et al., 1978; Speckmann and Caspers, 1979a,b).

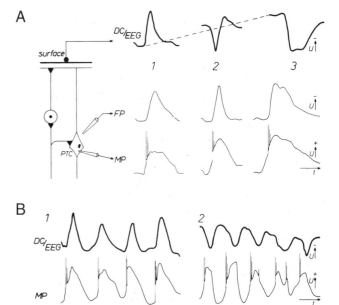

Figure 2.12. Single potential fluctuations at the cortical surface (DC/EEG) and concomitant membrane potential (MP) of a pyramidal tract cell (PTC) and field potentials (FP) in the PTC layer during generalized tonic-clonic seizures. The seizure activity was induced by pentylenetetrazol. **A:** The negative potential *(1)*, the positive-negative fluctuation *(2)*, and the positive potential *(3)* in the DC/EEG recording coincide with monophasic negative FP and stereotyped paroxysmal depolarization shift in the neuron. The negative DC shift occurring during the seizure is indicated by a *dashed line* in the upper row. Monophasic negative potentials in the DC/EEG recording occur with small and monophasic positive fluctuations along with a marked DC displacement. **B:** The relations between DC/EEG potentials and MP of PTC as described for A1 and A3 also hold true for trains of potentials *(1, 2)*. (From original tracings from Speckmann, E.J., Caspers, H., and Jansen, R.W.C. 1978. Laminar distribution of cortical field potentials in relation to neuronal field activities during seizure discharges. In *Architectonics of the Cerebral Cortex,* IBRO Monograph Series, vol. 3, Eds. M.A.B. Brazier and H. Petsche, pp. 191–209. New York: Raven Press.)

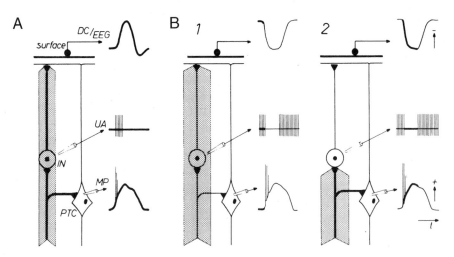

Figure 2.13. Flow charts of neuronal processes possibly responsible for the generation of DC/EEG waves of opposite polarity during a generalized tonic-clonic seizure. *Hatched arrows*, symbols for continuous asynchronous input to the cortex; *heavy lines*, symbols for phasic volleys giving rise to single convulsive discharges; PTC, pyramidal tract cell; IN, interneuron; MP, membrane potential; UA, extracellularly recorded unit activity. **A:** During a moderate asynchronous input to the cortex *(small hatched arrow)*, a burst of UA triggers a paroxysmal depolarization shift in a PTC. Simultaneously, it leads to a depolarization of superficial neuronal structures and therewith to a negative fluctuation in the DC/EEG recording at the cortical surface. **B:** With an increased asynchronous input to the cortex *(wide hatched arrow)*, the DC potential shifts to a more negative level than in **A** *(1)*. When in these conditions a phasic volley reaches the cortex, paroxysmal depolarization shifts are also triggered in PTC, whereas the enhanced asynchronous UA is interrupted mainly due to inactivation. The latter process results in a disfacilitation of the upper neuronal structures and therewith to a positive fluctuation of the superficial DC/EEG potential *(2)*. (From original tracings from Speckmann, E.J., Caspers, H., and Jansen, R.W.C. 1978. Laminar distribution of cortical fluid potentials in relation to neuronal field activities during seizure discharges. In *Architectonics of the Cerebral Cortex*. IBRO Monograph Series, vol. 3, Eds. M.A.B. Brazier and H. Petsche, pp. 191–209. New York: Raven Press.)

In addition to the field potentials of the cortical surface and the membrane potentials of the pyramidal tract cells, field potentials were also recorded in the fifth lamina. Under these conditions, it can be shown that every PDS is associated with a negative monophasic field potential in the depth (Fig. 20.12A). These stereotyped potential fluctuations in deep cortical layers correspond with field potentials at the cortical surface with either monophasic negative or positive (Fig. 2.12A1,3) or with polyphasic (Fig. 2.12A2) configurations. This statement does not merely apply to individual ictal potentials but is also true for prolonged trains of potentials during the convulsion. As Fig. 2.12B shows, paroxysmal depolarizations of pyramidal tract cells may be accompanied by a sequence of either negative or positive potentials on the cortical surface. If one correlates these various field potentials on the cortical surface with the slow DC shifts occurring during the convulsion (also see Fig. 2.12A), then it can be demonstrated that the surface-negative field potentials are associated primarily with a slight DC shift and that surface-positive field potentials will appear when the negative DC shift at the cortical surface reaches and exceeds a critical value (Speckmann and Caspers, 1979a,b; Speckmann et al., 1972, 1978).

These data are interpreted with flow charts in Fig. 2.13. The amplitude of the negative DC shift at the cortical surface depends greatly on the amount of the afferent influx of impulses to the generator structures in the superficial cortical laminae. This predominantly asynchronous afferent influx is symbolized by the width of hatched arrows in Fig. 2.13. Accordingly, the afferent influx in Fig. 2.13A is smaller than that in Fig. 2.13B. Therefore, there is a smaller DC shift in Fig. 2.13A and a prominent one in Fig. 2.13B. In

the case of Fig. 2.13A, a synchronized inflow of impulses from subcortical structures is assumed to reach the cortex (widened afferent fiber in schematic view). As a consequence, pyramidal tract cells will be stimulated to generate a PDS, and structures close to the surface will be depolarized through the mediation of interneurons. Accordingly, in such a constellation of excitatory processes, the paroxysmal depolarization in the depth will be coupled with a surface-negative field potential. With augmentation of the already existing afferent inflow of impulses, the interneurons involved will necessarily exhibit a heightened level of excitation (Fig. 2.13B). If an additional highly synchronized afferent influx of impulses takes place under these conditions, then further PDSs will be triggered in the pyramidal tract cells, but, in the interneurons, the previously existing high-frequency activity will be temporarily interrupted, chiefly due to inactivation. This causes a decline of the excitatory inflow of impulses to the superficial cortical structures. This disfacilitation gives rise to a positive field potential at the cortical surface. In this manner, a massive afferent inflow of impulses provides the basis for a correlation of positive epicortical field potentials with stereotyped paroxysmal depolarizations and monophasic negative field potentials in the depth (Speckmann et al., 1978; Speckmann and Caspers, 1979b).

Cortical Field Potentials During Gas Tension Changes in Tissue

This section deals with the alterations of epicortical field potentials and concomitant changes of the membrane potentials caused by deviations of the gas tension in brain tissue.

Such changes of the gas tension may occur when, for instance, the pulmonary and circulatory function is disturbed or when the local cerebral blood flow is inadequate.

First, the alterations of epicortical field potentials during selective hypercapnia are discussed; then, those associated with primary asphyxia are considered. It is shown that EEG changes may be similar under both conditions. The cortical DC potential, however, shows typical shifts that permit inferences concerning the cause of the accompanying EEG changes. The discussion of the effects of gas tension alterations on the bioelectrical activity of the CNS is based, again, on data derived from experimental work in animals.

Hypercapnia

If the CO_2 tension in the brain tissue is increased in a selective manner, typical reactions of the cortical field potentials as well as of the membrane potential and the postsynaptic potentials of individual neurons are found. These findings are shown in a summarized schematic view in Fig. 2.14.

The animal experiments on which Fig. 2.14 is based were carried out with the use of the so-called apnea technique. With this technique, interference of the effects of hypercapnia with simultaneous effects of hypoxia could be avoided. According to this technique, the experimental animal is ventilated for at least a half hour with pure oxygen. Thereafter, artificial ventilation is discontinued while the trachea of the animal remains connected with the O_2 reservoir. Under these conditions, the CO_2 tension progressively rises in the tissue for about 15 minutes without a concomitant fall of the oxygen tension below the baseline level.

With isolated increment of the CO_2 tension in the cerebral tissue by means of the apnea technique, the amplitude of the conventional EEG decreases progressively. This amplitude reduction affects first the waves of higher frequency and then those of lower frequency. Prior to the extinction of normal EEG activity, there is once again a phase characterized by high-frequency EEG activity in the range of 50 to 70 Hz (Caspers et al., 1979; Speckmann and Caspers, 1979a).

The extinction of the EEG is associated with a shift of the DC potential in a positive direction. If the CO_2 tension is then lowered again by reventilation, the EEG waves return in the original spectral composition after a short latency. At the same time, the positive DC shift resolves (Fig. 2.14). Experiments in animals have shown that, with reduction of the pCO_2, the EEG returns to normal activity even though the hypercapnia-induced suppression lasted for 1 hour or more. In these cases, a positive DC deflection of monophasic character was found to occur during the whole period of apnea (Caspers and Speckmann, 1974; Caspers et al., 1979; Speckmann and Caspers, 1974).

Under the aforementioned conditions, the recording of the membrane potential of a cortical nerve cell shows a hyperpolarization while the CO_2 tension is increased. Extensive experimental studies in animals have demonstrated that such a hyperpolarization is caused primarily by a reduction of the EPSP (Fig. 2.14; also see Speckmann and Caspers, 1974). Consideration of field potentials, of membrane potentials, and of EPSP shows that epicortical DC potentials reflect neuronal hyperpolarization. The disappearance of the EEG waves is presumed to be caused mainly by the reduction of postsynaptic activity.

Asphyxia

Primary asphyxia exemplified by respiratory arrest after air ventilation is associated with combined CNS effects of hypercapnia and hypoxia. The effects of gas tension changes on the field potentials and on the membrane potential of individual neurons are schematically shown in Fig. 2.15. In the corresponding animal experiments, the artificial ventilation with air was either temporarily (Fig. 2.15A) or persistently (Fig. 2.15B) interrupted.

With such an interruption of artificial ventilation with air, the conventional EEG waves disappear within less than 1 minute. This process is accompanied by a negative DC potential shift from the baseline, which has been characterized as *initial negativity* (1 in Fig. 2.15). While the EEG shows

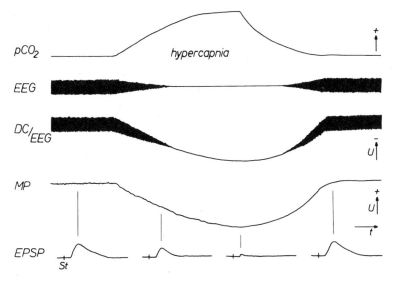

Figure 2.14. Effects of an isolated hypercapnia on epicortical field potentials (EEG, DC/EEG) and on membrane potential (MP). With increasing pCO_2, the EEG disappears even if the pO_2 is above normal levels. The disappearance of the EEG is associated with a positive DC shift and a hyperpolarization of most of the neurons. Simultaneously, the amplitudes of stimulus (St) evoked EPSP are markedly reduced. (From original tracings from Speckmann, E.J., and Caspers, H. 1974. The effect of O_2 and CO_2 tensions in the nervous tissue on neuronal activity and DC potentials. In *Handbook of Electroencephalography and Clinical Neurophysiology*, vol. 2, part C, Ed.-in-chief A. Remond, pp. 71–89. Amsterdam: Elsevier.)

Figure 2.15. Alterations of EEG, DC/EEG, and neuronal membrane potential (MP) during primary asphyxia. **A:** The abolition and the reappearance of EEG during a transient asphyxia goes in parallel with typical DC shifts: *(1)* initial negativity, *(2)* intermediate positivity, *(3)* reactive positivity. These DC fluctuations are accompanied by corresponding reactions of the MP. **B:** With continuing asphyxia, the EEG remains abolished and the intermediate positivity *(2)* turns over into a terminal negativity *(4)*. The latter DC negativity corresponds to a breakdown of neuronal membrane potential. (From original tracings from Speckmann, E.J., and Caspers, H. 1974. The effect of O_2 and CO_2 tensions in the nervous tissue on neuronal activity and DC potentials. In *Handbook of Electroencephalography and Clinical Neurophysiology,* vol. 2, part C, Ed.-in-chief A. Remond, pp. 71–89. Amsterdam: Elsevier.)

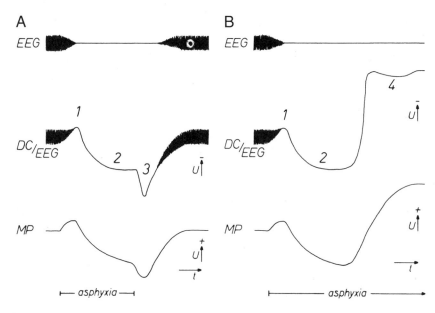

an isoelectric line in the further course of asphyxia, additional potential shifts are detectable with DC recording technique. The initial negativity is followed by a positive DC shift termed *intermediate positivity* (2 in Fig. 2.15). If reventilation is performed in this phase of asphyxia, an additional positive DC shift is observed, appropriately termed *reactive positivity* (3 in Fig. 2.15A). According to the analysis of the experimental work, the intermediate and the reactive types of positivity are due to an increase of CO_2 tension in the brain tissue. With the resolution of the reactive positivity, a restitution of the fast field potentials occurs that is also demonstrable with the conventional EEG. A comparison of the DC shifts and the alterations of the membrane potentials shows a parallelism of both events (Caspers and Speckmann, 1974; Caspers et al., 1979, 1980, 1984; Speckmann and Caspers, 1974, 1979a).

If the interruption of the artificial ventilation is continued for a longer period of time, then the intermediate positivity converts into the so-called terminal negativity (4 in Fig. 2.15B). This negative DC shift correlates with the breakdown of the neuronal membrane potential. The terminal effects are due to a critical lack of oxygen. The terminal negativity may be reversible for a substantial period of time under certain experimental conditions if the artificial ventilation is resumed and the reduction of the cerebral circulation is counteracted with circulation support measures (Speckmann and Caspers, 1974).

In summary, a comparison of EEG and DC potentials in selective hypercapnia and primary asphyxia shows that the recording of cortical field potentials with DC amplifiers provides a more accurate picture of the actual functional state of nerve cells.

References

Andersen, P., and Andersson, S.A. 1968. *Physiological Basis of the Alpha Rhythm.* New York: Meredith.

Caspers, H. 1963. Relations of steady potential shifts in the cortex to the wakefulness-sleep spectrum. In *Brain Function,* Ed., M.A.B. Brazier, pp. 177–213. Berkeley: University of California Press.

Caspers, H. (Ed.). 1974. DC potentials recorded directly from the cortex. In *Handbook of Electroencephalography and Clinical Neurophysiology,* vol. 10, part A, Ed.-in-chief A. Remond. Amsterdam: Elsevier.

Caspers, H., and Speckmann, E.J. 1969. DC potential shifts in paroxysmal states. In *Basic Mechanisms of the Epilepsies,* Eds. H. H. Jasper, A. A. Ward, Jr., and A. Pope, pp. 375–388. Boston: Little, Brown.

Caspers, H., and Speckmann, E.J. 1974. Cortical DC shifts associated with changes of gas tensions in blood and tissue. In *Handbook of Electroencephalography and Clinical Neurophysiology,* vol. 10, part A, Ed.-in-chief A. Remond, pp. 41–65. Amsterdam: Elsevier.

Caspers, H., Speckmann, E.J., and Lehmenkühler, A. 1979. Effects of CO_2 on cortical field potentials in relation to neuronal activity. In *Origin of Cerebral Field Potentials,* Eds. E.J. Speckmann and H. Caspers, pp. 151–163. Stuttgart: Thieme.

Caspers, H., Speckmann, E.J., and Lehmenkühler, A. 1980. Electrogenesis of cortical DC potentials. In *Motivation Factor and Sensory Processes of the Brain: Electrical Potentials, Behaviour and Clinical Use. Progress in Brain Research,* vol. 54, Eds. H.H. Kornhuber and L. Deecke, pp. 3–15. New York: Elsevier.

Caspers, H., Speckmann, E.J., and Lehmenkühler, A. 1984. Electrogenesis of slow potentials of the brain. In *Self-Regulation of the Brain and Behavior,* Eds. T. Elbert, B. Rockstroh, W. Lutzenberger, and N. Birbaumer, pp. 26–41. New York: Springer.

Creutzfeldt, O., and Houchin, J. 1974. Neuronal basis of EEG waves. In *Handbook of Electroencephalography and Clinical Neurophysiology,* vol. 2, part C, Ed.-in-chief A. Remond, pp. 5–55. Amsterdam: Elsevier.

De Robertis, E.D.P., and Carrea, R. (Eds.). 1964. *Biology of Neuroglia/ Progress in Brain Research,* vol. 15. New York: Elsevier.

Eccles, J.C. 1964. *The Physiology of Synapses.* Berlin: Springer.

Elger, C.E., and Speckmann, E.J. 1980. Focal interictal epileptiform discharges (FIED) in the epicortical EEG and their relations to spinal field potentials in the rat. Electroencephalogr. Clin. Neurophysiol. 48:447–460.

Elger, C.E., and Speckmann, E.J. 1983. Penicillin-induced epileptic foci in the motor cortex: vertical inhibition. Electroencephalogr. Clin. Neurophysiol. 56:604–622.

Elger, C.E., Speckmann, E.J., Caspers, H., et al. 1981. Focal interictal epileptiform discharges in the cortex of the rat: laminar restriction and its consequences for activity descending to the spinal cord. In *Physiology and Pharmacology of Epileptogenic Phenomena,* Eds. M.R. Klee, H.D. Lux, and E.J. Speckmann. New York: Raven Press.

Goldring, S. 1974. DC shifts released by direct and afferent stimulation. In *Handbook of Electroencephalography and Clinical Neurophysiology,* vol. 10, part A, Ed.-in-chief A. Remond, pp. 12–24. Amsterdam: Elsevier.

Gumnit, R. 1974. DC shifts accompanying seizure activity. In *Handbook of Electroencephalography and Clinical Neurophysiology,* vol. 10, part A, Ed.-in-chief A. Remond, pp. 66–77. Amsterdam: Elsevier.

Gumnit, R.J., Matsumoto, H., and Vasconetto, C. 1970. DC activity in the depth of an experimental epileptic focus. Electroencephalogr. Clin. Neurophysiol. 28:333–339.

Hubbard, J.I., Llinas, R., and Quastel, D.M.J. 1969. *Electrophysiological Analysis of Synaptic Transmission/Monographs of the Physiological Society.* London: Edward Arnold.

Jasper, H.H., Ward A.A., and Pope A. (Eds.). 1969. *Basic Mechanisms of the Epilepsies.* Boston: Little, Brown.

Klee, M.R., Lux, H.D., and Speckmann, E.J. (Eds.). 1982. *Physiology and Pharmacology of Epileptogenic Phenomena.* New York: Raven Press.

Köhling, R., Höhling, J.-M., Straub, H., et al. 2000. Optical monitoring of neuronal activity during spontaneous sharp waves in chronically epileptic human neocortical tissue. J. Neurophysiol. 84:2161–2165.

Köhling, R., Reinel, J., Vahrenhold, J. et al. 2002. Spatio-temporal patterns of neuronal activity: analysis of optical imaging data using geometric shape matching. J. Neurosci. Meth. 114:17–23.

Kuffler, S.W., and Nicholls, J.G. 1966. The physiology of neuroglial cells. Erg. Physiol. 57:1–90.

Kuffler, S.W., Nicholls, J.G., and Orkand, R.K. 1966. Physiological properties of glial cells in the central nervous system of amphibia. J. Neurophysiol. 29:768–787.

Orkand, R.K., Nicholls, J.G., and Kuffler, S.W. 1966. Effect of nerve impulses on the membrane potential of glial cells in the central nervous system of amphibia. J. Neurophysiol. 29:788–806.

Palay, S.L., and ChanPalay, V. 1977. General morphology of neurons and neuroglia. In *Handbook of Physiology/The Nervous System,* vol. 1, part 1, Ed. E.R. Kandel, pp. 5–37. Bethesda, MD: American Physiological Society.

Petsche, H., Muller-Paschinger, I.B., Pockberger, H., et al. 1978. Depth profiles of electrocortical activities and cortical architectonics. In *Architectonics of the Cerebral Cortex.* IBRO Monograph Series, vol. 3, Eds. M.A.B. Brazier and H. Petsche, pp. 257–280. New York: Raven Press.

Petsche, H., Pockberger, H., and Rappelsberger, P. 1981. Current source density studies of epileptic phenomena and the morphology of the rabbit's striate cortex. In *Physiology and Pharmacology of Epileptogenic Phenomena,* Eds. M.R. Klee, H.D. Lux, and E.J. Speckmann. New York: Raven Press.

Purpura, D.P., Penry, J.K., Tower, D.B., et al. (Eds.). 1972. *Experimental Models of Epilepsy.* New York: Raven Press.

Rall, W. 1977. Core conductor theory and cable properties of neurons. In *Handbook of Physiology/The Nervous System,* vol. 1, part 1, Ed. E.R. Kandel, pp. 39–97. Bethesda, MD: American Physiological Society.

Shepherd, G.M. 1974. *The Synaptic Organization of the Brain.* London: Oxford University Press.

Somjen, G.G., and Trachtenberg, M. 1979. Neuroglia as generator of extracellular current. In *Origin of Cerebral Field Potentials,* Eds. E.J. Speckmann and H. Caspers, pp. 21–32. Stuttgart: Thieme.

Speckmann, E.J. 1986. *Experimentelle Epilepsieforschung.* Darmstadt: Wissenschaftliche Buchgesellschaft.

Speckmann, E.J., and Caspers, H. 1974. The effect of O_2 and CO_2 tensions in the nervous tissue on neuronal activity and DC potentials. In *Handbook of Electroencephalography and Clinical Neurophysiology,* vol. 2, part C, Ed.-in-chief A. Remond, pp. 71–89. Amsterdam: Elsevier.

Speckmann, E.J., and Caspers, H. (Eds.). 1979a. *Origin of Cerebral Field Potentials.* Stuttgart: Thieme.

Speckmann, E.J., and Caspers, H. 1979b. Cortical field potentials in relation to neuronal activities in seizure conditions. In *Origin of Cerebral Field Potentials,* Eds. E.J. Speckmann and H. Caspers, pp. 205–213. Stuttgart: Thieme.

Speckmann, E.J., and Elger, C.E. (Eds.). 1983. *Epilepsy and Motor System.* Baltimore: Urban & Schwarzenberg.

Speckmann, E.J., and Elger, C.E. 1984. The neurophysiological basis of epileptic activity: a condensed overview. In *Epilepsy, Sleep, and Sleep Deprivation,* Eds. R. Degen and E. Niedermeyer, pp. 23–34. Amsterdam: Elsevier.

Speckmann, E.J., Caspers, H., and Janzen, R.W.C. 1972. Relations between cortical DC shifts and membrane potential changes of cortical neurons associated with seizure activity. In *Synchronization of EEG Activity in Epilepsies,* Eds. H. Petsche and M.A.B. Brazier, pp. 93–111. New York: Springer.

Speckmann, E.J., Caspers, H., and Janzen, R.W.C. 1978. Laminar distribution of cortical field potentials in relation to neuronal activities during seizure discharges. In *Architectonics of the Cerebral Cortex.* IBRO Monograph Series, vol. 3, Eds. M.A.B. Brazier and H. Petsche, pp. 191–209. New York: Raven Press.

Speckmann, E.J., Caspers, H., and Elger, C.E. 1984. Neuronal mechanisms underlying the generation of field potentials. In *Self-Regulation of the Brain and Behavior,* Eds. T. Elbert, B. Rockstroh, W. Lutzenberger, et al., pp. 9–25. New York: Springer.

Straub, H., Kuhnt, U., Höhling, J.-M., et al. 2003. Stimulus induced patterns of bioelectric activity in human neocortical tissue recorded by a voltage sensitive dye. Neuroscience 121:587–604.

Wieser, H.G. 1983. *Electroclinical Features of the Psychomotor Seizure. A Stereoencephalographic Study of Ictal Symptoms and Chronotopographical Seizure Patterns Including Clinical Effects of Intracerebral Stimulation.* Stuttgart: Gustav Fischer.

3. Cellular Substrates of Brain Rhythms

Mircea Steriade

The rhythms of the electroencephalogram (EEG) are defined as regularly recurring waveforms of similar shape and duration. They have been recognized since the beginnings of EEG recordings in humans and animals and some of them have been thoroughly described during the 1930s and 1940s. However, the detailed mechanisms of EEG rhythms could be analyzed only during the past four decades and especially since 1980. This was due to the advent of modern methods allowing the description of electroresponsive properties and ionic conductances of various types of individual cells as well as the network operations that account for the collective oscillations of large neuronal populations. This chapter discusses general notions about the cellular mechanisms of major EEG rhythms, with emphasis on the normal brain (as well as on the development from slow-wave sleep oscillations to paroxysmal episodes), and frames these oscillations within the behavioral context of various states of vigilance.

The neuronal substrates of some EEG rhythms have begun to be elucidated up to their most intimate aspects, while other types of oscillations are far from being understood at the single-cell and population level. We now know in much detail the intrinsic neuronal properties and network synchronization of spindle oscillation (7–14 Hz), characterizing the state of light sleep, that are generated in the thalamus and whose widespread synchronization is determined by corticothalamic projections. We also know the cellular mechanisms underlying the more recently described slow oscillation (generally 0.5–1 Hz) elaborated in the neocortex, reflected synaptically in the thalamus, and having the virtue of grouping other sleep rhythms (spindles and delta) as well as episodes of fast (beta/gamma) oscillations. The slow oscillation was originally described in intracellular recordings from anesthetized animals, but was also recognized in EEG and magnetoencephalography (MEG) during natural human sleep, and using extra- and intracellular recordings from neocortex during natural sleep of animals. We only begin to understand the sleep delta waves (1–4 Hz) at the level of single neurons and complex circuits, and we realize that the generic term *delta* comprises, in fact, at least two rhythms with different mechanisms and levels of genesis, within the thalamus or neocortex. The theta rhythm (4–7 Hz), produced in the hippocampus and occurring during different forms of arousal, especially in rodents, was intensively studied at the cellular level, but its precise mechanisms are still subject to controversies. We have still limited knowledge of various brain structures and neuronal types generating fast waves (20–60 Hz), so-called beta and gamma oscillations, which appear in a sustained manner during highly aroused and attentive states as well as in the dreaming state of rapid-eye-movement (REM) sleep. There is a continuous debate about

the significance of these fast rhythms, some arguing about their role in highly cognitive processes and consciousness, others challenging this hypothesis on the basis that the same rhythms also appear, discontinuously, during slow-wave sleep or deep anesthesia when consciousness is suspended. Finally, even though alpha waves, with frequencies largely overlapping those of spindling, have been described more than 60 years ago, we know little about the precise site(s) of production and virtually nothing about the underlying neuronal mechanism(s).

The order of sections in this chapter is not dictated by the frequencies of various rhythms, because waves ranging within a similar frequency range, such as alpha and spindling, are associated with quite opposite behavioral states (awareness and unconsciousness) and are probably generated at different brain levels (cerebral cortex and thalamus). Rather, I proceed from the synchronized EEG patterns of the sleepy thalamus and cerebral cortex (spindles, slow, and delta oscillations), and I describe the coalescence of these sleep rhythms within complex wave-sequences due to the corticothalamic volleys generated by the slow oscillation. Thus, although the description of the three distinct sleep oscillations is useful for didactic purposes, these rhythms are combined in the intact brain through reciprocal relations between the thalamus and cerebral cortex. I thereafter analyze the fast rhythms that accompany brain diffuse activation and focused attention, and discuss some modulatory systems that are essential for the shift from the closed brain during EEG-synchronized sleep to the open brain when information can be processed and analyzed. In sum, I will emphasize that the thalamus and cerebral cortex have to be considered as a unified oscillatory machine under the control of brainstem and forebrain modulatory systems.

Before entering the core of this chapter, devoted to the cellular substrates of brain rhythms, it is necessary to describe the major neuronal types and circuits that are implicated in the generation and synchronization of state-dependent oscillations.

Neuronal Types and Circuits Implicated in the Generation of Brain Rhythms

The major types of neurons implicated in the generation, synchronization, desynchronization, and activation of brain rhythms are located in the cerebral cortex, thalamus, and several generalized modulatory systems arising in the brainstem core, posterior hypothalamus, and basal forebrain. The morphological features and electrophysiological characteristics of these neurons have been investigated both *in vitro,* to elucidate the ionic nature of different conductances and classes of receptors, and *in vivo,* to shed light on neuronal features during the more or less rich synaptic activity in the intact brain and on their dependence on behavioral states. A comparison between *in vitro* and *in vivo* results concerning brain rhythms may be found in recent monographs (Steriade, 2001a, 2003). While all neuroscientists have to be informed about the analytical aspects of neuronal electrophysiology as described in slices maintained *in vitro,* some investigators prefer to benefit from collections of intact neurons in complex networks, as they operate in natural life. This is the main rationale for exploring the corticothalamic networks and their propensity for oscillatory activity in brains with preserved connectivity. One of the conclusions resulting from recent investigations is that synaptic activities within complex neuronal networks modulate, and often overwhelm, intrinsic neuronal properties. Intracellular analyses of neuronal types in the intact brain, especially in naturally alert preparations (Steriade et al., 2001), demonstrate that firing patterns ascribed to intrinsic neuronal properties display dramatic alterations during active behavioral states, due to changes in membrane potential and increased synaptic activity. The major neuronal types in the neocortex and thalamus, which are implicated in brain rhythms, are interconnected and they operate under the control of generalized modulatory systems (Fig. 3.1), a condition that cannot be explored in extremely reduced brain preparations.

Neuronal Types in Thalamus and Neocortex

At least three major types of neurons are involved in thalamocortical interactions: thalamic neurons with cortical projections (thalamocortical, TC); thalamic reticular (RE) neurons; and deeply lying cortical neurons, which project to these two types of thalamic neurons. There is a reciprocal circuit between excitatory (glutamatergic) neocortical and TC neurons and a recurrent inhibitory loop between TC neurons and RE neurons that use γ-aminobutyric acid (GABA) as neurotransmitter (Fig. 3.1). Local-circuit GABAergic thalamic interneurons are not often considered in this circuit, especially by investigators working on rodents, because, although local inhibitory interneurons constitute 25% to 30% of neurons in all thalamic nuclei of cats and primates, as well as in the dorsal lateral geniculate nucleus of rats, they are virtually absent in other nuclei of rodents (Steriade et al., 1997). It should be emphasized that 8% to 10% of GABAergic RE neurons project to local inhibitory thalamic interneurons (Liu et al., 1995), eventually leading to disinhibition of TC cells. This was shown by an increased incidence of inhibitory postsynaptic potentials (IPSPs) in TC neurons after excitotoxic lesions of RE perikarya (Steriade et al., 1985), as if local inhibitory interneurons were released from the inhibition arising in the RE nucleus. The connection between the two types of thalamic GABAergic cells, RE and local-circuit interneurons, was proposed to be

Figure 3.1. Neuronal loops in corticothalamic networks implicated in coherent oscillations and their control by brainstem cholinergic neurons. The top three neurons have been recorded and stained intracellularly in cats. The direction of their axons is indicated by *arrows. Insets* represent their responses to thalamic and cortical stimulation (*arrowheads* point to stimulus artifacts). The corticothalamic neuron (spikes truncated) from area 7 responded to thalamic stimulation of centrolateral intralaminar nucleus with antidromic *(a)* and orthodromic *(o)* action potentials (top superimposition, at a membrane potential of −55 mV). At more hyperpolarized levels (bottom superimposition, at −64 mV), the antidromic response failed but the orthodromic response survived as subthreshold excitatory postsynaptic potentials (EPSPs). The thalamic reticular γ-aminobutyric acid (GABA)ergic neuron (recorded from the rostrolateral district of the nucleus) responded to motor cortical stimulation with a high-frequency spike-burst, followed by a sequence of spindle waves on a depolarizing envelope (membrane potential, −68 mV). Spindle waves occur spontaneously, with a frequency of 7 to 14 Hz in animals (12–14 Hz in humans) during light sleep. In this case, spindles are elicited by cortical stimulation. The thalamocortical neuron (recorded from the ventrolateral nucleus) responded to motor cortex stimulation with a biphasic inhibitory postsynaptic potential (IPSP), leading to a low-threshold spike (LTS) and a sequence of hyperpolarizing spindle waves (membrane potential, −70 mV). For the sake of simplicity, local-circuit inhibitory neurons in cortex and thalamus are not illustrated. Shown below, the dual effects of brainstem cholinergic neurons, namely hyperpolarization of the thalamic reticular neuron and depolarization of the thalamocortical neuron. In this and similar figures, membrane potential is indicated at left. (Modified from Steriade, M. 2000. Corticothalamic resonance, states of vigilance, and mentation. *Neuroscience* 101: 243–276).

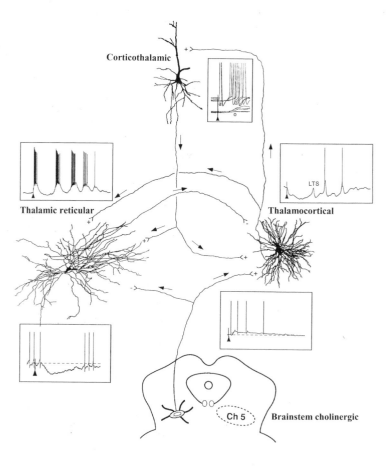

implicated in processes for focusing attention to relevant signals (Steriade, 1999).

The intrinsic electrophysiological properties of TC neurons recorded from different dorsal thalamic nuclei are similar. They consist mainly of a transient Ca^{2+} current (I_T) de-inactivated by hyperpolarization and underlying low-threshold spikes (LTSs) crowned by rebound spike-bursts (see TC neurons in Figs. 3.1 and 3.3); a hyperpolarization-activated cation current (I_H) that produces a depolarizing sag (see Fig. 3.20); high-voltage Ca^{2+} currents; a persistent Na^+ current ($I_{Na(p)}$); and different types of K^+ currents (reviewed in monographs by Steriade et al., 1990c, 1997). These intrinsic properties are important in the generation and synchronization of thalamic oscillations (Steriade and Llinás, 1988). A special class of TC neurons, recorded from the large-cell part of rostral intralaminar nuclei, with very fast conduction velocities (40–50 m/sec), generate unusually high-frequency (900–1,000 Hz), rhythmic (20–60 Hz) spike bursts at relatively depolarized levels; their LTSs have a shorter refractory phase (60–70 msec) than other TC neurons (150–200 msec), which allows them to rebound following each IPSP during sleep spindles (Steriade et al., 1993c).

The transient Ca^{2+} current that underlies the LTS is located in the soma and/or proximal dendrites of TC cells (Jahnsen and Llinás, 1984; Zhou et al., 1997), while it is located in distal dendrites of RE neurons (Contreras et al., 1993; Destexhe et al., 1996; Huguenard and Prince, 1992; Mulle et al., 1986). The spike bursts of RE neurons are much longer (30–80 msec, but up to 1 second when followed by a tonic tail) and have an *accelerando-decelerando* pattern, different from the short (5–15 msec) spike bursts with progressively increasing interspike intervals in TC neurons (Domich et al., 1986). The presence of spike bursts in presumed dendritic recordings from RE neurons and the graded nature of dendritic LTSs were revealed in intracellular recordings *in vivo* (Contreras et al., 1993). The highly excitable dendritic tree and the graded bursting behavior of RE neurons support their role as generators and synchronizers of spindle rhythmicity *in vivo* as well as the role of cortex in triggering sleep spindles by primarily acting on RE-cells' dendrites. A combined experimental and modeling study (Destexhe et al., 1996) showed that, in contrast to RE cells with intact dendritic arborizations in which there is a high density of low-threshold transient Ca^{2+} currents (I_{Ts}), RE cells in which most of the dendritic arborizations were removed have a much lower density of I_{Ts}; however, with a high density of I_{Ts} in distal dendrites, the spike-bursts showed *accelerando-decelerando* patterns, as is the case with RE neurons during natural slow-wave sleep (Steriade et al., 1986). It is likely that the very long (1.5–2 mm) dendrites of RE neurons are impaired when thalamic slices are prepared. This may explain some of the differences in results between *in vivo* and *in vitro* studies showing presence and absence, respectively, of spindle oscillations in the deafferented RE nucleus (see below).

In contrast to the relative homogeneity of either TC or RE neurons, there are several classes of neocortical neurons. Four cellular types are usually described (reviewed in Connors and Amitai, 1995; Connors and Gurnick, 1990; Steriade, 2001a,b, 2003): (1) Regular-spiking (RS) neurons constitute the majority of cortical neurons. They display trains of single spikes that adapt quickly or slowly to maintained stimulation. (2) Intrinsically bursting (IB) neurons generate clusters of action potentials, with clear spike inactivation, followed by hyperpolarization and neuronal silence. (3) Fast-rhythmic-bursting (FRB) neurons give rise to high-frequency (300–600 Hz) spike bursts recurring at fast rates (generally 30–50 Hz). (4) Fast-spiking (FS) neurons fire thin action potentials and sustain tonically very high firing rates without frequency adaptation.

Generally, RS, IB, and FRB neurons are pyramidal-shaped neurons, while FS firing patterns are conventionally regarded as defining local GABAergic cells. However, in addition to pyramidal-shaped FRB neurons, other neurons, with the same FRB firing patterns, are local-circuit, sparsely spiny interneurons (Steriade et al., 1998b). And some local inhibitory interneurons discharge like RS or bursting cells (Thomson et al., 1996).

The above classification in four neuronal types does not consider the role of cortical and thalamic synaptic activities in modifying the firing patterns resulting from intrinsic properties. Thus, IB neurons develop their firing pattern into that of RS neurons by depolarization (Steriade et al., 1993a; Timofeev et al., 2000; Wang and McCormick, 1993) or passing from slow-wave sleep to brain-activated states, waking or REM sleep (Steriade et al., 2001). Such a change explains why the proportion of IB neurons is so low (<5%) during natural brain alertness (Steriade et al., 2001). Also, FRB neurons change their firing pattern into that of FS neurons with depolarization (Steriade et al., 1998b), thus explaining the high proportion of FS-like discharge patterns during wakefulness (Steriade et al., 2001).

Therefore, the distinctions among cortical RS, IB, FS, and FRB neurons became much more subtle as we learned that one neuronal type may be transformed into another type, under certain physiological conditions.

Corticothalamic Circuits

Although all corticothalamic axons are glutamatergic (thus exerting excitatory actions on both RE and TC neurons), the effect of a natural or artificial corticofugal volley on TC neurons, which are the ultimate link for the transmission of information back to cortex, depends on the functional state of these neurons. During slow-wave sleep, when cortical activity is highly synchronized (Amzica and Steriade, 1995a; Steriade et al., 1993f) and TC neurons are in a state of hyperpolarization (Hirsch et al., 1983), the cortical influence is opposite on RE and TC neurons. Natural synchronous cortical volleys or electrical stimuli produce excitation and rhythmic spike bursts over a depolarizing envelope in RE neurons, whereas TC neurons simultaneously display rhythmic and prolonged IPSPs, followed by rebound excitations (Fig. 3.1). The cortically elicited IPSPs in TC neurons are bisynaptic as they are due to the prior excitation of GABAergic RE neurons. Pure signs of cortically evoked excitation in TC neurons may be seen only after removing the RE nucleus from this circuitry. These data suggest that the cortical projection to RE neurons is more powerful than the action it exerts on TC neurons. Indeed, the numbers of glutamate receptor subunits GluR4 are 3.7 times higher at corticothalamic synapses in RE neurons, compared to TC neurons, and the mean peak amplitude of corticothalamic excitatory postsynaptic currents (EPSCs) is about 2.5 higher in RE, than in TC, neurons (Golshani et al., 2001). These data are important because a series of natural phenomena, occurring especially in the sleeping brain as well as during abnormally synchronized events that characterize paroxysmal states, depend on the functional states of RE neurons, which have different consequences on TC neurons (Steriade, 2001c). The most potent effects on TC neurons are exerted by RE neurons when they fire prolonged, rhythmic, high-frequency spike bursts, which are the signature of these GABAergic neurons during slow-wave sleep, whereas the same neurons discharge tonically, in the single-spike mode, during waking and the state of sleep with rapid eye movements (Steriade et al., 1986). Thus, during slow-wave sleep, and even more so during some types of electrical seizures that develop from sleep patterns, the spike bursts fired by RE neurons induce greater postsynaptic inhibitory responses in TC neurons than those elicited by single spikes.

This sequence of events, from cortex to thalamus, first to RE neurons and then to TC neurons, underlies the coalescence of different sleep oscillatory types. Instead of simple rhythms, arising from simple circuits, as investigated in isolated thalamic or cortical slices maintained *in vitro,* the intact brains of animals and humans display complex wave sequences, comprising different types of low-frequency and high-frequency oscillations, which are produced by operations in interacting corticothalamic neuronal loops, under the control of generalized modulatory systems (Steriade, 2001a,b).

The above-mentioned results (Golshani et al., 2001) also shed light on controversial ideas about the initiation site (cortex or thalamus) and the processes implicated in the genesis of paroxysmal events consisting of spike-wave seizures, an electrographic pattern seen in experimental studies, which is similar to that observed in clinical absence (petit-mal) epileptic seizures. Experiments using multisite, extra- and intracellular recordings show that neocortical neurons become progressively entrained into the seizures that develop from slow-wave sleep oscillations, indicating that the buildup of these seizures obeys the rule of short-scale and long-scale synaptic circuits (Steriade and Amzica, 1994). During cortically generated spike-wave seizures, a majority of TC neurons are steadily hyperpolarized and display phasic IPSPs (Crunelli and Leresche, 2002; Pinault et al., 1998; Steriade and Contreras, 1995; Timofeev et al., 1998; reviewed in Steriade, 2003). These inhibitory potentials are mediated by RE neurons that faithfully follow each paroxysmal depolarizing shift of cortical neurons.

Besides these prevalent inhibitory projections from cortex to TC neurons, which are mediated through RE neurons during highly synchronized activities, excitatory cortical actions on TC neurons can also be revealed when RE neurons fire in the single-spike mode and their impact on TC neurons is less pronounced than when they fire long spike bursts.

Neuronal Types in Generalized Modulatory Systems

The neuromodulatory systems exert global actions by shifting the brain from one state of vigilance to another, and they also improve neuronal representations of behaviorally relevant stimuli in specific sensory systems. Activation is defined as a state of readiness in cerebral networks, a state of membrane polarization that brings neurons closer to firing threshold, thus ensuring safe synaptic transmission and quick responses to either external stimuli during waking or internal drives during REM sleep (Steriade, 1991). The resemblance between the brain-active states of waking and REM sleep results from data showing virtually identical EEG patterns in these two states, increased rates of spontaneous discharges as well as enhanced excitability to antidromic or orthodromic volleys in TC (Glenn and Steriade, 1982) and corticofugal (Steriade and Deschênes, 1974) neurons, and similar aspects of sensory-evoked field potentials in humans (Yamada et al., 1988). Only a few neuronal types, particularly the monoamine-containing neurons in the upper brainstem and posterior hypothalamus, are active in waking and silent during REM sleep (reviewed in Steriade and McCarley, 1990). This might account for the dissimilar mentation in waking and REM sleep, but the neuronal mechanisms underlying these psychological differences between logical thought in wakefulness and the hallucinatory state of dreaming have not yet been explored.

The intrinsic cellular properties of cholinergic mesopontine neurons, which project to the thalamus and depolarize TC neurons with increased input resistance (Curró Dossi et al., 1991), are characterized by a transient outward K^+ current (I_A) and high-threshold Ca^{2+} spikes. In adult animals, few neurons possess a low-threshold Ca^{2+} current (Kang and Kitai, 1990; Leonard and Llinás, 1990), whereas in young rats the majority of neurons displaying low-threshold spikes are cholinergic (Kamondi et al., 1992; Lübke et al., 1992). The fact that very few cholinergic neurons from mesopontine slices of adult animals display spike bursts is corroborated by *in vivo* studies of these neurons during natural states of vigilance showing that very short (<5 msec) interspike intervals, reflecting high-frequency spike bursts, represent only 2% to 4% of intervals during wakefulness and slow-wave sleep, and less than 7% of intervals during REM sleep (Steriade et al., 1990a). During REM sleep, spike bursts are related to the generation of ponto-geniculo-occipital (PGO) waves in one among several types of mesopontine cholinergic neurons (Steriade et al., 1990d). The high-threshold Ca^{2+}-mediated spike bursts are the slice equivalent of high-frequency (>500 Hz) spike bursts, occurring 20 to 40 msec before the thalamic PGO waves during REM sleep *in vivo,* and are preceded by a period of discharge acceleration suggesting their progressive depolarization (Steriade et al., 1990d).

Among other ascending activating systems, which are extrathalamic, the nucleus basalis (NB) provides the cholinergic innervation of the cerebral cortex. Studies of intrinsic properties and oscillations displayed by NB neurons showed that magnocellular NB neurons display rhythmic bursting activity mediated by a Ca^{2+}-dependent LTS (Khateb et al., 1992). A comparative study of cholinergic and noncholinergic NB neurons revealed that the former fire rhythmic spike bursts at low frequencies (<10 Hz) riding on LTSs and tonic firing (10–15 Hz) when depolarized. Noncholinergic neurons discharge in a unique mode, with clusters of spikes interspersed with rhythmic subthreshold membrane potential oscillations when depolarized from −55 mV (Alonso et al., 1996).

Sleep Spindles, Slow Sleep Oscillation, and Paroxysmal Developments

In this section I discuss the thalamically generated spindles (7–14 Hz), the cortically generated slow oscillation (<1 Hz), and the K complexes, because these major sleep landmarks are intimately related. I also discuss the neuronal plasticity and paroxysmal developments that occur as a consequence of sleep oscillations.

Generalities on Spindles

Classically, spindles have been regarded as the epitome of EEG synchronization during the early stage of quiescent sleep. This type of oscillation is defined by the association of two distinct rhythms: waxing and waning spindle waves at 7 to 14 Hz within sequences lasting for 1 to 2 seconds, and the periodic recurrence of spindle sequences with a slow rhythm, generally 0.2 to 0.5 Hz (*top part* in Fig. 3.2). The

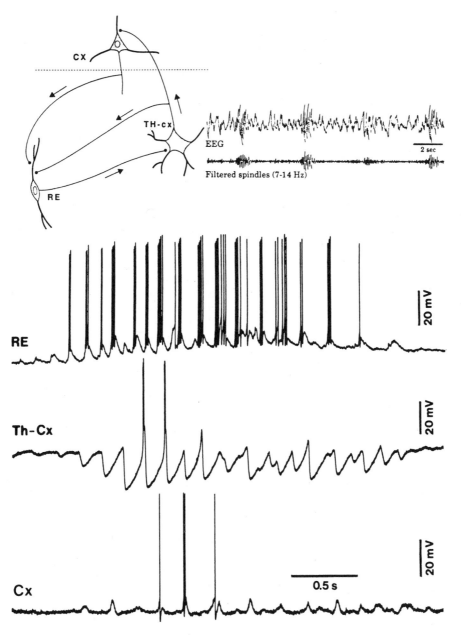

Figure 3.2. Spindle oscillations in reticular thalamic (RE), thalamocortical (Th-Cx, ventrolateral nucleus), and cortical (Cx, motor area) neurons. **Top:** Circuit of three neuronal types and two rhythms (7–14 Hz and 0.1–0.2 Hz) of spindle oscillations in cortical EEG. **Bottom:** Intracellular recordings in cats under barbiturate anesthesia. See text. (Modified from Steriade, M., and Deschênes, M. 1988. Intrathalamic and brainstem-thalamic networks involved in resting and alert states. In *Cellular Thalamic Mechanisms,* Eds. M. Bentivoglio and R. Spreafico, pp. 37–62. Amsterdam: Elsevier.)

slow rhythm of spindle sequences was described only two decades ago (Steriade and Deschênes, 1984) but, with the benefit of hindsight, it can be detected in earlier recordings of human's and cat's bioelectrical activity. While the rhythm of 7 to 14 Hz was intensively investigated and its cellular bases are largely known, the knowledge of intrinsic currents or synaptic actions that are implicated in the slower rhythm of 0.2 to 0.5 Hz is only at its beginnings.

Spindles are generated within the thalamus, but their shape and long-range synchronization is decisively influenced by the cerebral cortex. That spindles are produced within the thalamus was first demonstrated by Morison and Bassett (1945), who showed that such waves could still be recorded in the thalamus after total decortication and high brainstem transection. Thalamic spindles survive even more radical procedures, including the removal of the striatum and rhinencephalon (Villablanca, 1974). Although the intrinsic properties of individual thalamic cells play an important role in the patterning of sleep spindles (Steriade and Llinás, 1988), spindling is a network-generated oscillation in the recurrent inhibitory circuit including thalamic RE GABAergic cells, driven by TC neurons and projecting back to the latter (see *scheme* in Fig. 3.2).

Most of our knowledge on cellular bases of spindles derives from experimental studies in cat, the species of choice for the electrophysiological investigation of sleep spindles *in vivo,* and from *in vitro* studies in ferret's thalamic slices. The sleep cycle is similarly organized in human and cats; EEG spindles are similarly shaped in these species; and the RE nucleus, which plays a cardinal role in the generation of spindles, has similar ultrastructural features in cats and primates (see below). While cat's spindles are the electrographic landmark for the transition from wakefulness to sleep and are used as the main criterion for distinguishing the transition between these two behavioral states, stage 1 sleep is generally characterized in humans by the change from alpha waves to a mixed-frequency pattern of low-voltage waves, and spindles (in isolation or associated with sharp deflections termed K complexes) appear in the so-called stage 2 sleep. However, stage 1 sleep may or may not coincide with perceived sleep onset in humans, and many investigators recognize the clear-cut onset of sleep by the EEG correlates of stage 2, especially spindles and K complexes. Because spindles are generated in the thalamus and may primarily appear in discrete foci, it is also possible that neuronal processes associated with spindle oscillations are operating from the very onset of human sleep but are not visible at the usual inspection at the cortical surface, because of the absence of global thalamic synchronization during this initial stage.

Connectivity and Ultrastructure of the Thalamic Reticular Nucleus, the Spindle Pacemaker

The term *pacemaker* applied to RE nucleus is justified by experimental data showing that spindles are abolished in dorsal thalamic territories after disconnection from the RE nucleus (Steriade et al., 1985) and are preserved in the ros-

tral sector of the RE nucleus deafferented from thalamic inputs (Steriade et al., 1987; see details below).

The RE nucleus is a thin sheet of GABAergic neurons that covers the rostral, lateral, and ventral surfaces of the thalamus (Jones, 1985). Its major inputs arise in the thalamus, cerebral cortex, rostral part of the brainstem, and basal forebrain. The cortically projecting thalamic nuclei (constituting the dorsal thalamus) and cerebral cortex are structures that resonate within the spindle frequency and reinforce this oscillation. Distinctly, the brainstem and basal forebrain modulatory systems are mainly involved in inhibiting spindles through a variety of mechanisms that decouple the RE network, and thus they assist in promoting EEG activation patterns.

The output of RE neurons is mostly directed to the dorsal thalamus and, secondarily, to the rostral brainstem, but not to the cerebral cortex. The rule of RE projections backward to the dorsal thalamus has an important exception. In cat, the anterior thalamic nuclei (interposed in the limbic circuit between the hippocampus and the cingular cortex) and the lateral habenular nucleus do not receive inputs from RE neurons (Steriade et al., 1984; Velayos et al., 1989). This connectional feature has a physiological counterpart: spindling is absent in anterior thalamic nuclei (Paré et al., 1987), in the projection areas of the cingular cortex (Leung and Borst, 1987), as well as in habenular neurons (Wilcox et al., 1988). All these structures, devoid of RE afferences, but being part of circuits comprising the septum, hippocampus, and entorhinal cortex, display theta rhythmicity that globally characterizes the limbic system.

The neurons belonging to the RE nucleus are interconnected not only by means of their axons but also through their dendrites, which contain vesicles releasing GABA. The dendrodendritic contacts between RE neurons have been described in cats and primates (Asanuma, 1994; Deschênes et al., 1985; Williamson et al., 1994; Yen et al., 1985) but have not been generally found in rodents. As will be described below, the significance of dendrodendritic linkages is related to the possibility of synchronization of spindle oscillation within the pacemaking RE nucleus, with the consequent synchronization of the whole thalamus. Another way of synchronization could be realized by electrotonic coupling of RE neurons (Fuentealba et al., 2002; Landisman et al., 2002). Immunohistochemical results suggest the presence of a gap junction protein in a series of brain structures, including the RE nucleus (Nagy et al., 1988).

It is conventionally thought that the RE nucleus comprises a single type of cells. Intracellular staining of RE neurons revealed, however, two or three main types of RE elements on the basis of their shape, dendritic and axonal arborizations. One cellular type has axonal collaterals within the RE nucleus, while another seemingly does not (Spreafico et al., 1988, 1991). Electrophysiological data also indicate different types of intrinsic properties in RE neurons (Brunton and Charpak, 1997; Contreras et al., 1992; Llinás and Geijo-Barrientos, 1988).

The RE nucleus develops in ontogeny well before birth (Altman and Bayer, 1979). If considering the bulk of data on the RE role as a spindle pacemaker (see below), this early structural development would be conflicting with the common assumption that spindles appear quite late in ontogeny, as compared to other grapho-elements of the EEG (reviewed in Steriade et al., 1990c). However, in developmental studies, spindles have usually been recorded over the cortical surface, despite the fact that these waves are generated in the thalamus. When recording spindle oscillations in the thalamus of kittens, both rhythms (7–14 Hz and 0.1–0.2 Hz) have been found to appear as early as 6 to 7 hours after birth, but they are transferred to the cerebral cortex only beginning with the third to fourth days, and synchronous spindling in the thalamus and cerebral cortex occurs by the eighth to ninth days (Domich et al., 1987). This delay is probably due to the late development of thalamocortical axons and, especially, to the fact that the process of synaptogenesis continues for weeks after thalamocortical axons have entered the cortex (Wise et al., 1979).

Network Generation of Spindles

An early model of spindle generation postulated the existence of a recurrent inhibitory circuit between TC cells and local-circuit inhibitory cells within the limits of dorsal thalamic nuclei, the latter being driven by intranuclear axonal collaterals of TC cells and imposing IPSPs back onto TC cells that would fire postinhibitory rebound spike bursts at the offset of IPSPs (Andersen and Andersson, 1968). In that model, which had the merit of emphasizing the propensity of TC cells to produce an intrinsic rebound discharge after a period of inhibition, the corticothalamic feedback played no role in spindling.

In subsequent studies it was shown that (a) TC cells do not give rise to intranuclear axonal recurrent collaterals (Yen and Jones, 1983; Steriade and Deschênes, 1984); (b) local-circuit interneurons are not significantly implicated in spindle genesis since, after disconnection from RE nucleus, spindles are abolished in thalamic nuclei possessing a great number of local interneurons and prolonged, rhythmic IPSPs in TC cells are transformed into short and arrhythmic IPSPs; thus, the spindle-related IPSPs in TC cells are produced by the other class of inhibitory thalamic cells, GABAergic RE neurons (Steriade et al., 1985); (c) postinhibitory rebound spike bursts in TC cells are transferred to cortex where they elicit rhythmic EPSPs and occasional spike discharges in pyramidal neurons as well as other types of cortical cells (Fig. 3.2); and (d) the cerebral cortex potentiates and synchronizes thalamic spindles (Contreras et al., 1996a, 1997; Steriade et al., 1972). These data and the recent developments from *in vivo* and *in vitro* experiments are further discussed below.

The idea that spindles are generated in the RE nucleus stemmed from the patterns of spindle sequences recorded intracellularly in RE and TC neurons. Whereas spindles develop in RE cells as a slowly growing and decaying depolarization with superimposed spike barrages within the frequency of 7 to 14 Hz, TC cells simultaneously display 7 to 14 Hz IPSPs that occasionally lead to high-frequency (200–400 Hz) rebound spike bursts (Steriade and Deschênes, 1988) (Fig. 3.2). More recently, this result was obtained by means of dual simultaneous intracellular recordings from RE and TC cells *in vivo* (Timofeev and Steriade, 1996) and *in vitro* (Bal and McCormick, 1996). The spike bursts of TC cells are stigmatic events during sleep spindles (Steriade and Llinás, 1988). These bursts represent an intrinsic property of thalamic cells, due to a special conductance that is inactive at the resting membrane potential (around −55 to −60 mV) or at more depolarized levels, but becomes ready to be activated when the membrane potential is hyperpolarized by about 7 to 15 mV, which is the case of TC neurons during sleep with EEG synchronization (Fig. 3.3) (see above, Neuronal Types in Thalamus and Neocortex).

The various frequencies of spindles, which have often been interpreted as reflecting different types of oscillations, merely depend on various durations of the hyperpolarizations in TC neurons. Long duration (150–200 msec) hyperpolarizations, as during barbiturate anesthesia or deeply EEG-synchronized states, are associated with 7 Hz or even lower-frequency spindles, while relatively short hyperpolarizations (70–100 msec) result in spindles with higher frequencies (10–14 Hz). It can be postulated that lower-frequency spindles, which are recorded from some neocortical areas (especially in humans), are due to longer-duration hyperpolarizations of TC neurons in related dorsal thalamic nuclei.

Since the spindle oscillation is associated with a reciprocal (inverse) image in RE and TC neurons, we have hypothesized that the cyclic IPSPs in cortically projecting cells are produced by the rhythmic excitation of GABAergic RE neurons. Transections experiments and excitotoxic lesions of RE perikarya have indeed demonstrated that spindles and long-lasting IPSPs subserving them are abolished in cortically projecting thalamic territories deprived of RE connections (Steriade et al., 1985). To demonstrate that this loss was not due to traumatic events following the lesions, we took advantage of morphological data showing that cat's anterior thalamic cells are naturally devoid of RE afferents and showed that spindling is absent in anterior thalamic nuclei (see above). The absence of spindling in the anterior thalamic neurons, which have intrinsic properties similar to other thalamocortical neurons, emphasizes that *spindling is a synaptically generated oscillation in a circuit that necessarily includes the RE nucleus.*

However, the intrinsic properties of thalamic cells are quite important in shaping spindles. For example, the Ca^{2+}-dependent LTS is effective in inducing postinhibitory rebound bursts of thalamic cells transferred to the cerebral cortex. Without it, thalamic spindle waves would not be reflected on the cortical EEG. Another intrinsic property of thalamic cells is the voltage-dependent, noninactivating or very slowly inactivating, persistent sodium current, $I_{Na(p)}$ (Jahnsen and Llinás, 1984b). This current helps to generate postinhibitory rebound depolarizations. Indeed, after intracellular injections of quaternary derivatives of local anesthetics, which block $I_{Na(p)}$, spindles of TC cells are transformed into a single, long-lasting period of hyperpolarization (because it is unopposed by $I_{Na(p)}$) and rhythmic rebounds within the frequency range of spindles disappear (Mulle et al., 1985). Finally, the Ca^{2+}-dependent K^+ current,

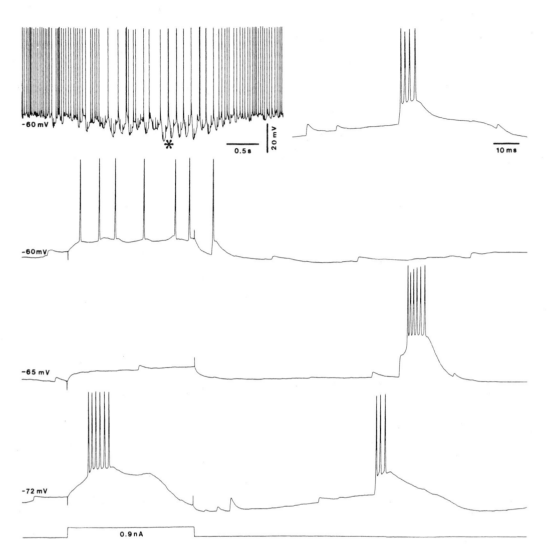

Figure 3.3. Two firing modes of thalamocortical cell. Intracellular recording in centrolateral intralaminar nucleus of cat under urethane anesthesia. **Top:** Trace of tonic firing at resting membrane potential (V_m −60 mV) and rhythmic (~8 Hz) high-frequency spike bursts during episode with spontaneous hyperpolarization. Burst indicated by *asterisk* is expanded at right. **Bottom:** Responses to depolarizing current pulses (identical parameters) at different V_m by applying direct current (DC) hyperpolarizing current. Note tonic firing at resting V_m (−60 mV), silent zone at −65 mV, and high-frequency burst at −72 mV. See also text. (From Steriade, M., unpublished data.)

$I_{K(Ca)}$, or some voltage-dependent K+ currents (Budde et al., 1992; McCormick, 1991) may prolong the long-lasting IPSPs generated in TC cells by RE neurons (Roy et al., 1984) and, thus, they assist in the production of the LTS and in inducing rebound bursts in TC cells.

The hypothesis that RE nucleus is the spindle pacemaker was finally strengthened by data showing that, after disconnection from its inputs (cerebral cortex, dorsal thalamus, and brainstem), the deafferented RE cells in the rostral pole of this nuclear complex continue to display both spindle rhythms (7–14 Hz and 0.2 Hz) and that spindle-related unit discharges are phase-locked with focal waves recorded by the same microelectrode (Steriade et al., 1987; Fig. 3.4). The spindle-related spike bursts of the isolated RE nucleus are in all respects identical to those of the RE neurons in the brain-intact animals (Domich et al., 1986; Steriade et al., 1986, 1987). Then, two major experimental requirements to sup-

port the idea of a spindle pacemaker (abolition of the oscillation in target structures disconnected from the pacemaker, and preservation of oscillation in the isolated rostral pole of RE nucleus) have been fulfilled.

It is then reasonable to propose that the deafferented RE cells support oscillations through an avalanche process within the dendrodendritic synaptic junctions of the RE nucleus. Hyperpolarization through dendrodendritic synapses of GABAergic RE cells would produce an LTS in the postsynaptic element (say *a*); Ca2+ entry in neuron *a* will be followed by GABA exocytosis and hyperpolarization of other dendrites, postsynaptic to those of cell's *a* dendrites; hyperpolarization in the latter elements would succeed in triggering an LTS. In this way, oscillations could spread to adjacent neurons and, ultimately, to large sectors of the RE nuclear complex. However, we have assumed that any excitatory drive impinging upon RE-cells' dendrites could start the

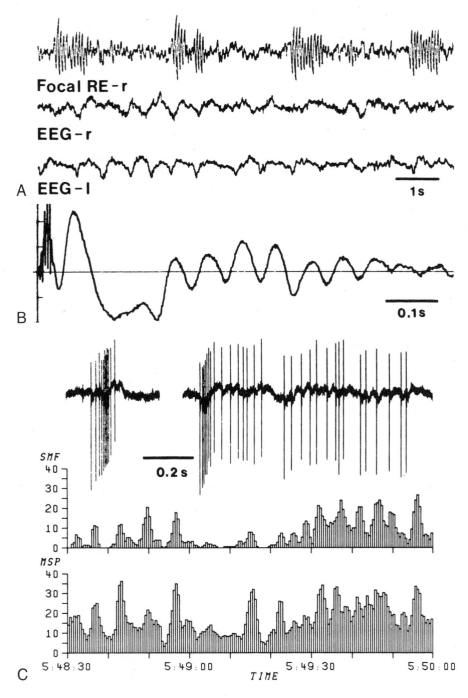

Figure 3.4. The deafferented thalamic reticular (RE) nucleus of cat generates spindle rhythmicity. For histology of transections that created an isolated island containing the rostral pole of the RE nucleus, see Figs. 1 and 2 in Steriade et al. (1987). **A:** Normal cyclic recurrence of spindle sequences in the rostral pole of the RE nucleus recorded by means of a microelectrode; absence of spindle rhythms (but persistence of delta waves) in cortical EEG recordings following thalamic transections. **B:** Oscillations within spindle frequency evoked in the rostral pole of the RE nucleus by stimulating (five-shock train) the white matter overlying the caudate nucleus (50 averaged traces). **C:** Slow rhythm of spindle sequences and related cell burst oscillations in the rostral pole of the RE nucleus deafferented by thalamic and corona radiata transections. Discharges of a single RE neuron were simultaneously recorded with focal spindle oscillations by the same microelectrode. Sequential mean frequency (SMF) of the neuron is depicted with the normalized amplitudes of focal waves filtered from spindle waves (MSP). Abscissa indicates real time. **Top:** Two (short and long) bursts from the same period. (Modified from Steriade, M., Domich, L., Oakson, G., et al. 1987. The deafferented reticular thalamic nucleus generates spindle rhythmicity. *J. Neurophysiol.* 57:260–273.).

process (Steriade et al., 1987). It is possible that the decreased firing rates of brainstem-thalamic cells at sleep onset (Steriade et al., 1982, 1990a) would induce hyperpolarization (through disfacilitation) in TC cells, with the consequence of burst discharges that, in turn, would excite RE-cells' dendrites and would set into motion the whole dendrodendritic inhibitory apparatus. The point should be stressed that, while TC-RE loops may assist in starting and developing spindles, the synchronization of the whole thalamus during spindling is possible only by invoking the widespread projections of RE neurons to the dorsal thalamus, because there is negligible, if any, crosstalk between dorsal

thalamic nuclei. Multisite recordings in the thalamus of anesthetized as well as naturally sleeping cats showed that distant and functionally different neurons beat synchronously during spindle sequences (Contreras et al., 1996a, 1997). Modeling studies of isolated RE neurons, with minimal or more realistic ionic models of RE cells (Bazhenov et al., 1999; Destexhe et al., 1994; Golomb et al., 1994; Wang and Rinzel, 1993), confirmed the idea that the deafferented RE nucleus generate spindles (Steriade et al., 1987). The modeling studies reached the conclusion that densely interconnected RE cells with GABA$_A$ and/or GABA$_B$ synapses are capable of spindle oscillations and that a modest

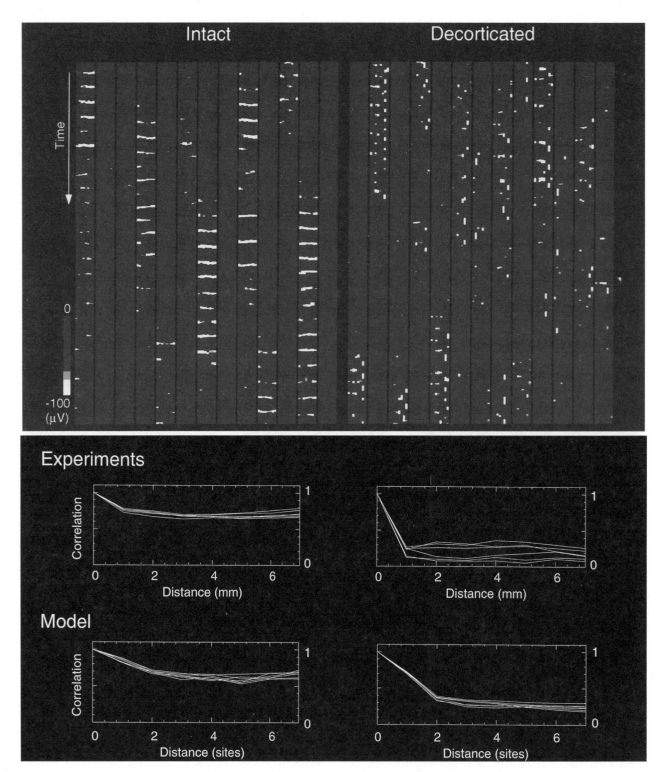

Figure 3.5. Control of spatiotemporal coherence of thalamic spindles by the cerebral cortex in cat. **Top panel:** Disruption of the spatiotemporal coherence of thalamic oscillation after removal of the neocortex. Spatiotemporal maps of electrical activity across the thalamus were constructed by plotting time (time runs from top to bottom in each column; *arrow* indicates 1 second), space (from left to right, the width of each column represents 8 mm in the anteroposterior axis of the thalamus), and local field potential (LFP) voltage [from *blue* to *yellow*, color represents the amplitude of the negative deflection of thalamic LFPs; the color scale ranged in ten steps from the baseline *(blue)* to −100 μV *(yellow)*]. Time was divided into frames, each representing a snapshot of 4 msec of thalamic activity. A total of 40 seconds is represented (9,880 frames). Each frame consisted of eight color spots, each corresponding to the LFP of one electrode from anterior to posterior (left to right in each column). **Middle column** (experiments): Decay of correlation with distance. Cross-correlations were computed for all possible pairs of thalamic sites, and the value at time zero from each correlation was represented as a function of the intersite distance for six different consecutive epochs of 20 seconds. Spatial correlation was calculated for thalamic recordings in the intact brain *(left)* and after removal of cortex *(right)*. **Bottom panel** (model): Decay of correlation with distance (in units of sites). Similar computation of cross-correlations as in the above panel from experiments, in the presence of cortex *(left)* and after decortication *(right)*. (Modified from Contreras, D., Destexhe, A., Sejnowski, T.J., et al. 1996. Control of spatiotemporal coherence of a thalamic oscillation by corticothalamic feedback. *Science* 274:771–774; and unpublished data of Destexhe, A., Contreras, D., Sejnowski, T.J., and Steriade, M.) (See Color Figure 3.5.)

excitation from input sources is effective in fully synchronizing the isolated RE network. The excitation may come from cortex and/or from TC cells.

Investigations in ferret visual thalamic slices maintained *in vitro,* containing the lateral geniculate and perigeniculate (caudal RE) nuclei, have analyzed the role of TC-RE interactions in spindle genesis and have specified the various receptors involved in the TC-to-RE excitation as well as in the GABA-mediated IPSPs imposed by RE onto TC neurons (Bal et al., 1995a,b; von Krosigk et al., 1993). The absence of spindles in the perigeniculate nucleus disconnected from the lateral geniculate nucleus (von Krosigk et al., 1993) may be explained by different factors in thalamic slices maintained *in vitro,* such as (a) a less intact and complete collection of RE cells (see note 13 in Steriade et al., 1993d), and (b) the absence of brainstem modulatory systems with depolarizing actions on RE neurons. Indeed, a modeling study (Destexhe et al., 1994b) has shown that network of isolated RE cells do not display spindle oscillatory behavior when no noradrenergic (NA)/serotonergic (5-HT) synapses are activated, but RE cells were brought to oscillation by activating 20% of the depolarizing NA/5-HT synapses.

The role of corticothalamic feedback in shaping, generation, and synchronization of spindles was demonstrated by (a) different shape and duration of spindles as a function of cortical stimulation (Contreras and Steriade, 1996) or by comparing thalamic spindles in intact-cortex and decorticated animals (Timofeev and Steriade, 1996); corticothalamic volleys produce brief and waning spindle sequences that lack the initial waxing component because these volleys succeed in entraining, right from the start, a great or the totality of thalamic cellular population implicated in spindle genesis; (b) eliciting spindles as response to cortical stimulation, even after contralateral cortical volleys to avoid antidromic activation of TC axons and collateral excitation of RE neurons (Steriade et al., 1972); (c) synchronizing RE cells, within spindle frequency, in response to cortical stimulation (Contreras and Steriade, 1996); and (d) synchronizing widespread thalamic territories to produce nearly simultaneous spindle sequences, since after decortication the coherence of spindles is much less organized (Contreras et al., 1996a, 1997) (Fig. 3.5). The propagation of spindles in thalamic slices (Kim et al., 1995) is likely due to the absence of corticothalamic projections and reduced background synaptic activity. The role of the cortical slow oscillation in grouping and synchronizing spindles is discussed below.

As TC neurons spend much of their sleep time during spindle-related IPSPs, there is a powerful inhibition of incoming messages in their route to the cerebral cortex. Recording field potentials evoked by stimulation of prethalamic axons (a method that permits the monitoring of the presynaptic deflection reflecting the magnitude of the afferent volley, together with the synaptically relayed, thalamically generated waves) revealed that the thalamus is the first station where afferent signals are completely blocked from the very onset of sleep. This obliteration of synaptic transmission in the thalamus leads to the deafferentation of the cerebral cortex, a prerequisite for the process of falling asleep (Steriade, 1984, 1991; Steriade et al., 1969). More re-

cently, our intracellular recordings from thalamic and cortical neurons have shown that, because of their hyperpolarization and increased membrane conductance during sleep spindles, TC cells do not transfer to cortex signals from prethalamic relay station, whereas the internal (corticocortical and corticothalamic) dialogue of the brain may be maintained during slow-wave sleep (Timofeev et al., 1996).

Augmenting Responses Within Spindle Frequencies and Neuronal Plasticity During Sleep

Repetitive (7–14 Hz) stimulation of dorsal thalamic nuclei evokes responses in projection cortical areas that increase in size during the pulse train (Fig. 3.6). This is the common way to mimic spindles in order to study the mechanisms of their waxing and waning pattern. Two types of incremental responses are known since their original description by Morison and Dempsey (1942): positive-negative waves at the cortical surface, also called *augmenting* response; and initially surface-negative waves, also termed *recruiting* responses. The different polarities of these two types of incremental responses reflect different projections of various thalamic nuclei to cortical layers. Most so-called specific dorsal thalamic nuclei preferentially project to midlayers III-IV of cortical areas, while some thalamic (for example, ventromedial and centrolateral) nuclei have prevalent projections to the superficial layer I. The surface-positivity (depth-negativity) of the augmenting response results from excitatory thalamocortical inputs, which create sinks in layers IV and supervening part of layer III, with current flow along the vertical core conductors represented by the apical dendrites of deeply lying, pyramidal-shaped neurons. The surface-negative (depth-positive) wave of recruiting responses results from direct depolarization of apical dendrites in layer I where recruiting-eliciting thalamic nuclei project. As to the negative component that follows the initially positive deflection in augmenting responses, it tends to be marked over wider cortical areas than the positive wave. This aspect is due to the fact that a series of specific thalamic nuclei, in addition to their prevalent projections to midlayers III to IV of restricted cortical regions, also project quite widely to layer I. The complexity of thalamocortical systems is such that a single cortical area receives afferents from multiple thalamic nuclei. This is the case, for example, of the cortical associational area 5, toward which the lateral posterior thalamic nucleus projects to layers III to IV and the ventral anterior thalamic nucleus projects to layer I. The result is an augmenting-type of response in cortical area 5 by stimulating lateral posterior nucleus, and a recruiting-type of response in the same cortical area by stimulating the ventral anterior nucleus (Steriade, 1978) (Fig. 3.6B).

However, most incremental potentials are mixed responses, with augmenting preceding the recruiting or vice versa (Spencer and Brookhart 1961), because of the multilaminar distribution of thalamic projections to cortex. For example, thalamocortical incremental responses evoked by rhythmic stimulation of rostral intralaminar nuclei (conventionally known as typically inducing recruiting responses) are of the

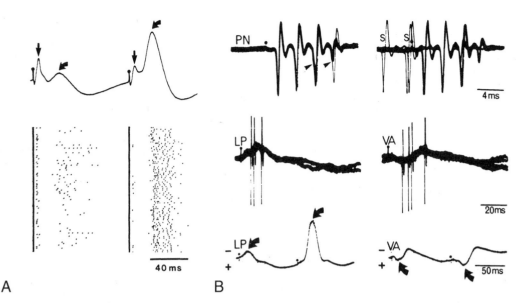

Figure 3.6. Augmenting and recruiting thalamocortical responses. **A:** Simultaneous recording of field potentials (50 averaged sweeps) and unit discharges (dot grams) at depth of 1 mm in cat anterior suprasylvian gyrus (area 5), evoked by two 0.1-second-delayed stimuli to the lateroposterior (LP) thalami nucleus; stimuli indicated by *dots* (field potential trace) and *vertical bars* (dot grams). Primary excitation indicated by *straight arrows,* and secondary excitation indicated by *oblique arrows.* The secondary depth-negative wave, associated with burst firing in the simultaneously recorded unit, is selectively augmented at second stimulus, whereas the primary excitation is simultaneously depressed. **B:** Augmenting and recruiting response patterns induced in the depth of cortical area 5 in the cat by stimulating LP thalamic nucleus projecting to middle cortical layers and ventroanterior (VA) thalamic nucleus projecting to the superficial layers. Chronically implanted, behaving preparations. **Top traces:** Thalamic-evoked field potentials and unit discharges are from a corticopontine neuron, as antidromically identified by stimulation of the pontine nuclei (PN); four-shock train at 370 Hz (only the artifact of the first shock is indicated by *dot*); break between initial segment and somadendritic spikes (third and fourth responses) or initial segment spike in isolation (fourth response) indicated by *arrowheads*; right superimposition shows collision of antidromic responses to the first shock by preceding spontaneous (S) discharges. **Middle traces:** Orthodromic discharges evoked in the same neuron by stimulating LP or VA thalamic nuclei. **Bottom traces:** Field potentials (50 averaged sweeps) evoked by stimulating LP or VA thalamic nuclei with two 100-msec-delayed shocks (unit discharges were cut off). Note augmenting (depth-negative) and recruiting (depth-positive) patterns of field responses to stimulation of LP and VA, respectively. (Modified from Steriade, M. 1978. Cortical long-axoned cells and putative interneurons during the sleep-waking cycle. *Behav. Brain Sci.* 1:465–514.)

recruiting type in one cortical area and of the augmenting type in another area of the same gyrus (because intralaminar nuclei project preferentially to layer I but also to deep layers); moreover, the latencies of both augmenting and recruiting responses evoked by thalamic intralaminar stimulation are equally short (<4 msec) (see Fig. 4 in Steriade et al. 1998c). Therefore, the distinction between augmenting and recruiting responses is no longer necessary. We can simply designate such responses as augmenting or incremental, describe their polarity, and keep in mind that thalamic neurons may project to middle, deep, and more superficial cortical layers.

The importance of augmenting responses is that they induce neuronal plasticity during as well as outlasting the stimulation period. As these incremental potentials are the experimental model of sleep spindles, they provide evidence that this major sleep oscillation may lead to potentiation of synaptic responsiveness. It was postulated that spindles as well as the slow sleep oscillation underlie the consolidation, during slow-wave sleep, of memory traces acquired during the state of wakefulness (Steriade et al., 1993b; Steriade and Timofeev, 2003). Work in humans is consistent with this hypothesis (Gais et al., 2000, 2002; Stickgold et al., 2000a,b).

In the thalamus of decorticated preparations, there are two forms of augmenting potentials (Steriade and Timofeev,

1997; Timofeev and Steriade, 1998). High-threshold responses to intrathalamic stimuli at ~10 Hz occur at a depolarized level of TC neurons, due to decremental responses in GABAergic RE neurons, the major source of inhibitory inputs to TC neurons. Prolonged and rhythmic thalamic stimulation eliciting high-threshold potentials leads to decreases in inhibitory responses of TC neurons and, consequently, to persistent and progressive increases in depolarizing synaptic responses (Fig. 3.7A). The neuronal mechanism of these responses depends on the activation of high-threshold Ca^{2+} currents (Hernández-Cruz and Pape, 1989; Kammermeir and Jones, 1997). By contrast, low-threshold responses develop with progressively increased IPSPs and postinhibitory rebound excitations in TC neurons (Fig. 3.7B1), produced by incremental responses of RE neurons (Fig. 3.7B2). Two essential mechanisms are needed for the generation of low-threshold augmenting responses: the transient T-current de-inactivated by membrane hyperpolarization and $GABA_B$-receptor–mediated inhibition of TC cells (Bazhenov et al., 1998a). Stimulation of prethalamic pathways does not induce augmenting responses because such volleys do not activate directly RE neurons (Bazhenov et al., 1998b).

In intact thalamocortical loops, dual intracellular recordings from TC and cortical neurons showed that aug-

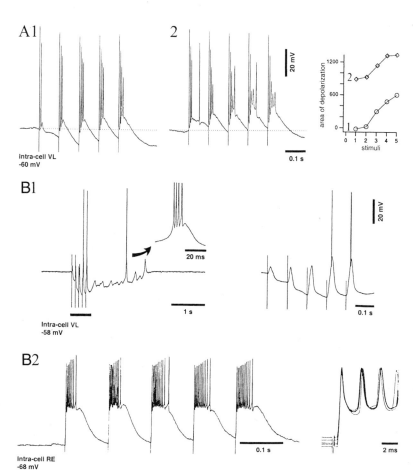

Figure 3.7. Two types of intrathalamic augmenting responses leading to neuronal plasticity. Unilaterally decorticated cats under ketamine-xylazine anesthesia. See the extent of decortication and callosal cut in Fig. 1 of the article by Steriade and Timofeev (1997). Intracellular recordings from thalamocortical (TC) in ventrolateral (VL) nucleus and thalamic reticular (RE) neurons. Stimulation in VL nucleus (pulse-trains of five stimuli at 10 Hz). **A:** Pulse trains at 10 Hz were delivered each 2 seconds. Responses of TC neuron to two pulse trains (*1* to *2*) are illustrated (*1* and *2* were separated by 18 seconds). Note that, with repetition of pulse trains, IPSPs elicited by the preceding stimuli were progressively reduced until their complete obliteration. The spike bursts contained more action potentials, with spike inactivation. The graph depicts the increased area of depolarization from the first to the fifth responses in each pulse train as well as from pulse trains *1* and *2*. The increase in the depolarization area was of about 500% from the first to the fifth response in pulse train *1* and 150% in the pulse train *2*. Also, the area of depolarization in the response to the second stimulus in the last pulse train *2* increased by about 800% compared to the already augmented response elicited by the second stimulus in pulse train *1*. **B1:** Low-threshold augmenting responses of TC neuron developing from progressive increase in IPSP-rebound sequences and followed by a self-sustained spindle. *Arrow* indicates expanded spike burst (action potentials truncated). The part marked by the *horizontal bar* and indicating augmenting responses is expanded at *right*. **B2:** Incremental responses RE neuron, accounting for the low-threshold-type of augmentation in TC neuron. (Modified from Steriade, M., and Timofeev, I. 1997. Short-term plasticity during intrathalamic augmenting responses in decorticated cats. *J. Neurosci.* 17:3778–3795; and Timofeev, I., and Steriade, M. 1998. Cellular mechanisms underlying intrathalamic augmenting responses of reticular and relay neurons. *J. Neurophysiol.* 79:2716–2729).

menting responses evoked by rhythmic thalamic stimulation at 10 Hz are characterized in cortical neurons by an increase in the secondary depolarization (Creutzfeldt et al., 1966; Purpura et al., 1964), at the expense of the primary EPSP (Steriade et al., 1998c) (Fig. 3.8A). The augmented secondary depolarizing component is quite sensitive to changes in the state of vigilance: it is selectively reduced or abolished by midbrain reticular stimulation and during naturally brain-activated states, such as arousal and REM sleep (Castro-Alamancos and Connors, 1996a; Steriade, 1970, 1981).

Are augmenting thalamocortical responses primarily due to events generated at the thalamic stimulated site (such as inhibitory potentials with subsequent rebound excitations transferred to the cerebral cortex), or do they reflect cortical events? That the cerebral cortex has the circuitry to elaborate such incremental responses in the absence of the thalamus was demonstrated by evoking augmenting responses to stimulation of white matter after lesions of the appropriate thalamic nuclei (Morin and Steriade, 1981), by antidromic activation of corticothalamic axons (Ferster and Lindström, 1986), and in isolated corti-

cal slabs *in vivo* (Timofeev et al., 2002a). The spatiotemporal features of augmenting responses have also been investigated in slices from motor cortex, and it was proposed that the initiation of these responses depends on the intrinsic properties and synaptic interconnections of deeply lying pyramidal cells (Castro-Alamancos and Connors, 1996b).

Dual intracellular recordings from TC and cortical neurons show that neuronal plasticity, in the form of self-sustained activity occurring within the same frequency range as that of evoked augmenting responses during the prior period of stimulation, is present in cortex despite the concomitant hyperpolarization and silence of TC neurons (Fig. 3.8B), which is due to the inhibitory pressure from thalamic RE neurons. This emphasizes that neuronal plasticity that follows augmenting potentials (Steriade et al., 1998c) as well as natural spindles (Timofeev et al., 2002a) has a cortical origin. Moreover, neuronal plasticity, with progressive membrane depolarization and increased synaptic responsiveness, is produced by intracortical volleys, through the callosal pathways, even in thalamectomized animals (Fig. 3.8C) (Steriade et al., 1993f).

Figure 3.8. Plasticity developing from augmenting responses in thalamocortical and intracortical neuronal networks. Intracellular recordings in cats under ketamine-xylazine (**A**), barbiturate (**B**), and urethane (**C**) anesthesia. **A:** Dual intracellular recording from the motor cortical (area 4) neuron and thalamocortical (TC) neuron in the ventrolateral (VL) nucleus. **Right:** Average of second and third responses in cortical and VL neurons. Note that the area of secondary depolarization in cortical neuron (*b*), which developed during augmentation (marked by *dots*), followed the rebound spike burst in TC neuron by ~3 msec. **B:** Self-sustained, postaugmenting oscillation in area 4 cortical neuron, simultaneous with persistent hyperpolarization in simultaneously recorded TC neuron. Dual intracellular recordings from thalamic ventrolateral (VL) nucleus and cortical area 4 neurons, in conjunction with field potential from the depth of area 4. Note persistent, spindle-like oscillation at the same frequency of augmenting responses in area 4, contrasting with a single low-threshold rebound and persistent hyperpolarization in the VL neuron. **C:** Changes in properties of the area 7 cortical neuron after repetitive callosal stimulation (10 Hz) of the homotopic point in the contralateral hemisphere. Ipsilateral thalamic lesion using kainic acid (see such lesions in Fig. 10A in Steriade et al., 1993b). Responses to pulse trains (each consisting of five stimuli at 10 Hz), repeated every 3 seconds, applied to contralateral area 7. The intracortical augmenting responses to the first and eighth pulse-trains are illustrated. Note depolarization by about 7 mV and increased number of action potentials within bursts after repetitive stimulation. (Modified from Steriade, M., Nuñez, A., and Amzica, F. 1993f. Intracellular analysis of relations between the slow (<1 Hz) neocortical oscillation and other sleep rhythms of the electroencephalogram. *J. Neurosci.* 13:3266–3283; and Steriade, M., Timofeev, I., Grenier, F., et al. 1998c. Role of thalamic and cortical neurons in augmenting responses: dual intracellular recordings *in vivo*. *J. Neurosci.* 18:6425–6443).

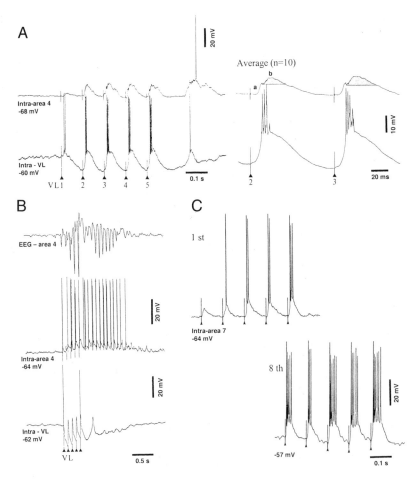

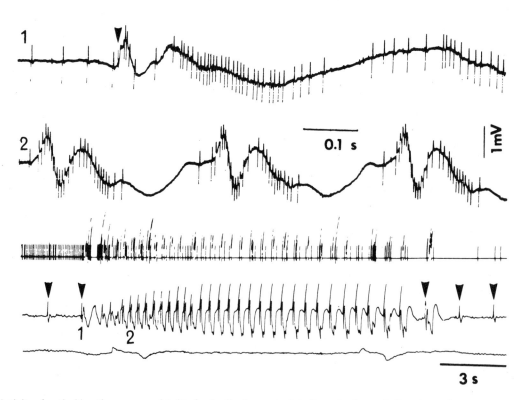

Figure 3.9. Activity of cortical bursting neurons related to focal epileptic spike-and-wave (SW) seizure in the behaving macaque monkey. Two oscilloscopic traces area shown; the numbers (*1* and *2*) indicate the corresponding parts in the ink-written recording depicted below. The three ink-written traces represent unit spikes, focal waves recorded by the same microelectrode in the motor (precentral) cortex, and eye movements. *Arrowheads* indicate single shocks to the ventrolateral thalamic nucleus. (Modified from Steriade, M. 1974. Interneuronal epileptic discharges related to spike-and-wave cortical seizures in behaving monkeys. *Electroencephalogr. Clin. Neurophysiol.* 37:247–263.)

Relations Between Sleep Spindles, Augmenting Potentials, and Self-Sustained Paroxysmal Events of the Spike-and-Wave Type

Several lines of evidence have suggested that the development of spike-and-wave (SW) complexes of the petit-mal epileptic type is related to the occurrence of spindles and/or related oscillations during the state of light sleep, and depends on resonant activities in the reciprocal thalamocorticothalamic loop: (a) SW activity increases during the spindle stage of EEG-synchronized sleep and is attenuated or blocked upon arousal (Kellaway, 1985). (b) In the feline generalized penicillin epilepsy model, spindles develop into bilaterally synchronous SW complexes and concomitant behavioral unresponsiveness, as in human petit-mal attacks (Gloor and Fariello, 1988). (c) Self-sustained SW cortical complexes at 2 to 3 Hz, lasting for 10 to 15 seconds, may follow thalamocortical (Steriade and Yossif, 1974) and corticothalamic (Steriade et al., 1976) augmenting responses in acutely prepared animals, or thalamic stimulation during behavioral drowsiness in primates (Steriade, 1974) (Fig. 3.9). (d) Stimulation of corticothalamic projections within the frequencies range of spindles may lead to self-sustained SW complexes in thalamic neurons (Steriade et al., 1976) (Fig. 3.10), similarly to the elicitation of cortical SW epileptic complexes following incremental thalamocortical responses.

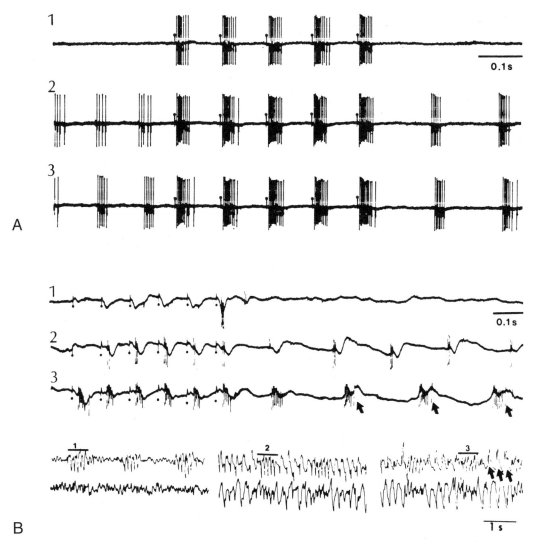

Figure 3.10. Cortically evoked responses in bursting thalamic neurons of cat lead to self-sustained spike-and-wave (SW) complexes. **A:** Ventrolateral cell was driven by motor cortex stimulation with five shocks at 10 Hz (in *1*), delivered every 2 seconds. Note the appearance of "spontaneous" bursts that resemble the evoked bursts at a late stage of stimulation (*2* and *3*). **B:** Effects of stimulation of the suprasylvian area 7 with trains of six shocks at 10 Hz (as in *1*) upon a bursting cell recorded from the lateroposterior (LP) nucleus. Beginning with the 12th shock train, the cell was regularly driven and displayed self-sustained rhythmic bursts at 5 Hz between cortical shock trains (in *2*). Self-sustained SW complexes appeared in *3* (28th shock train).

Bottom: The two ink-written traces represent focal waves in the LP nucleus, recorded by the same microelectrode used for unit recordings (*upper trace,* negativity upward), and EEG rhythms recorded from the surface of the suprasylvian gyrus *(bottom trace).* The numbers (*1–3*) on the EEG recordings correspond to the periods of stimulation depicted with the same numbers in the oscilloscope recordings. (Modified from Steriade, M. 1991. Alertness, quiet sleep, dreaming. In *Cerebral Cortex,* vol. 9, Eds. A. Peters and E.G. Jones, pp. 279–357. New York: Plenum; and Steriade, M., Oakson, G., and Diallo, A. 1976. Cortically elicited spike-wave afterdischarges in thalamic neurons. *Electroencephalogr. Clin. Neurophysiol.* 41:641–644.)

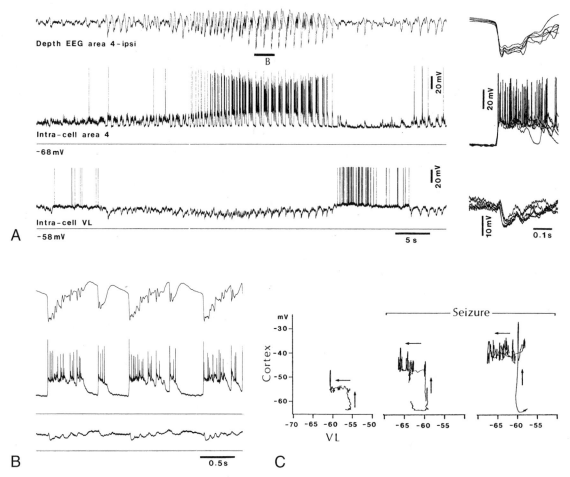

Figure 3.11. Dual intracellular recordings demonstrating hyperpolarization of thalamocortical (TC) cell in the ventrolateral (VL) nucleus during seizure depolarization and spike bursts in the area 4 cortical neuron. Cat under ketamine-xylazine anesthesia. **A:** Three traces depict simultaneous recording of depth-EEG from area 4, as well as intracellular activities of the area 4 cortical neuron and TC cell from the ipsilateral VL nucleus (below each intracellular trace, current monitor). The seizure was initiated by a series of EEG waves at about 0.9 Hz in the depth of area 4, continued with discharges at about 2 Hz, and ended with high-amplitude, periodic (0.9 Hz) EEG sequences consisting of wavelets at 14 Hz. All these periods were faithfully reflected in the intracellular activity of cortical neuron, whereas VL thalamic neuron displayed a tonic hyperpolarization throughout the seizure, with phasic sequences of IPSPs related to the large cortical paroxysmal depolarizations and spike bursts occurring at the end of the seizure. Note disinhibition of the VL cell after cessation of cortical seizure. At right, superimposition of six successive, expanded traces from the part indicated by *horizontal bar* (**B**) and continuing with subsequent three polyspike-wave complexes. Note spiky depth-negative EEG deflection associated with de-polarization of cortical cell and rhythmic IPSPs of VL thalamic neuron. Part marked by *B* is further depicted in the *bottom left panel*. **C:** Phase relations between simultaneously, intracellularly recorded area 4 cortical neuron and VL thalamic neuron are preserved during sleep and development of seizure activity. The three parts represent (from *left* to *right*): one period before seizure, during EEG sleep patterns; and two periods during early and late parts of the seizure. Phase plots of averaged membrane voltage of the area 4 cell (ordinate) against that of VL cell (abscissa). The development of seizure did not change the phase-relation between cells, but accentuated the amplitude of the elements constituting the normal (sleep) oscillatory behavior preceding the seizure. In essence, cortical depolarization *(upward arrows)* preceded the VL cell's hyperpolarization *(left-directed arrows)* in the three periods, although the amplitude of the membrane excursions were considerably enhanced during the seizure. (Modified from Steriade, M., and Contreras, D. 1995. Relations between cortical and thalamic cellular events during transition from sleep patterns to paroxysmal activity. *J. Neurosci.* 15:623–642; and unpublished data.)

The idea that the cerebral cortex may primarily generate SW seizures (Marcus et al., 1968a,b; Steriade, 1974) is also supported by the experiments of Gloor's group working with the penicillin model of such seizures (Avoli et al., 1983); however, since either the cortex or the thalamus may start the paroxysmal oscillatory behavior in the penicillin model, it was difficult to claim that one structure is exclusively playing the role of the prime mover in SW epilepsy. Recent data, using multisite recordings including dual intracellular recordings from cortex or from cortex and thalamus, strengthened the idea that the neocortex is preferentially implicated in the generation of seizures with SW complexes at 2 to 4 Hz or with poly-SW patterns interspersed with runs of fast EEG spikes at 10 to 20 Hz (Neckelmann et al., 1998; Steriade and Amzica, 1994; Steriade and Contreras, 1995; Steriade et al., 1998a). The results supporting this hypothesis basically consist of the fact that, with cortical and thalamic field potentials and cellular recordings, cortical processes are recruited well before any sign of thalamic entrainment.

Surprisingly, an important proportion (60% to 90% in different studies) of TC cells remained silent during cortically generated SW seizures, displaying a tonic hyperpolarization with phasic IPSPs in close time-relation with paroxysmal spike bursts in neocortical neurons (Fig. 3.11). This result, first obtained in cats (Steriade and Contreras, 1995) and subsequently confirmed in rats with genetically determined absence seizures (Crunelli and Leresche, 2002; Pinault et al., 1998), was explained by the fact that GABAergic RE neurons faithfully follow the spike bursts of cortical neurons and impose IPSPs onto TC cells, thus reinforcing through their exceedingly long spike bursts the hyperpolarization of TC cells before that the latter are able to burst. This was also demonstrated in computer network models of SW seizures (Lytton et al., 1997). Indeed, RE cells discharge spike bursts of about 40 to 50 msec during sleep (Domich et al., 1986; Steriade et al., 1986), but increase the duration of their spike bursts to 200 msec or more during SW seizures (Steriade and Contreras, 1995; Timofeev et al., 1998). Not only TC neurons are inhibited during cortically generated SW seizures, but also such seizures can be generated in cortex even after thalamectomy (Steriade and Contreras, 1998). Then, the minimal substrate for the generation of SW seizures is the neocortex. Nonetheless, the few numbers of TC neurons that, at an adequate level of membrane hyperpolarization, display postinhibitory spike bursts may reinforce and further synchronize cortical SW seizures.

What is the factor that accounts for the lowered frequency from around 10 Hz to about 3 Hz when spindling develops into SW epileptic discharges? An increased duration of inhibitory potentials is in keeping with Jasper's (1969) idea that "inhibitory rather than excitatory mechanisms play a leading role" (p. 435) in this form of epilepsy. Since the longest component of IPSPs in thalamic (Crunelli et al., 1988; Hirsch and Burnod, 1987; Paré et al., 1991) and cortical (Avoli, 1986) neurons is mediated by $GABA_B$ receptors linked with K^+ channels, and this phase is most susceptible to changes in state of vigilance (Curró Dossi et al., 1992b), the hypothesis of an increased duration of the potassium-dependent $GABA_B$-IPSP during

SW discharges was proposed in experimental (Liu et al., 1991) and computational (Destexhe, 1998) studies on thalamic and neocortical neurons. However, the "wave" component of SW complexes is *not* an active inhibitory (GABAergic) process, as shown by increased input resistance of cortical neurons during the wave (Neckelmann et al., 2000). Instead, the wave is due to disfacilitation combined with an increase in Ca^{2+}-dependent K^+ conductance, as shown by its reduction by 1,2-bis(2-aminophenoxy)etane-N,N,N,′N′-tetraacetic acid (BAPTA), as well as by the fact that long-lasting recordings with pipettes containing QX-314, a potent intracellular blocker of $GABA_B$ IPSPs, did not affect the generation of hyperpolarizing potentials related to the EEG wave component of SW seizures (Timofeev et al., 2003). The increase in $GABA_B$ IPSPs following blockade of $GABA_A$ receptors led to the slowing of the spindle rhythm (7–14 Hz) toward a slower oscillation (2–4 Hz) (Ralston and Ajmone-Marsan, 1956; von Krosigk et al., 1993), *but not to SW seizures* (Steriade and Contreras, 1998), as defined by paroxysmal episodes, in sharp contrast with the background activity, and with sudden arrest. On the other hand, the idea that the wave component is dependent on $GABA_A$-mediated IPSPs was refuted by showing that this component of SW complexes does not contain chloride-dependent inhibitory potentials (Timofeev et al., 2002b).

The Cortically Generated Slow Oscillation and Its Relations with Spindles and K-Complexes

A novel slow oscillation (less than 1 Hz) was first described in intracellular recordings from neocortical neurons in anesthetized animals and in EEG recordings from humans (Steriade et al., 1993e). It was subsequently found, with EEG and MEG recordings, during natural slow-wave sleep of animals (Steriade et al., 1996a) and humans (Achermann and Borbély, 1997; Amzica and Steriade, 1997a; Mölle et al., 2002; Massimini et al., 2003; Simon et al., 2000). The frequency of the slow oscillation depends on the anesthetic used and the behavioral state: it is mainly between 0.3 and 0.6 Hz under urethane anesthesia; between 0.6 and 0.9 Hz under ketamine-xylazine anesthesia; and between 0.7 and ~1 Hz during natural sleep. The best experimental condition under which single or dual simultaneous intracellular recordings can be made to investigate the mechanisms of the slow oscillation is the ketamine-xylazine anesthesia (Contreras and Steriade, 1995). Indeed, ketamine, a blocker of *N*-methyl-D-aspartate (NMDA) receptors, is placed among the most effective pharmacological tools in inducing slow-wave sleep patterns over the background of a wake state (Feinberg and Campbell, 1993). As to xylazine, an α_2-receptor agonist, it increases a K^+ conductance in a variety of central structures (see Nicoll et al., 1990). The similarity between the slow oscillation occurring in natural sleep and under ketamine-xylazine anesthesia was demonstrated in the same chronically implanted animal (Amzica and Steriade, 1997b).

It should be emphasized that the slow oscillation does not belong to the same category of brain rhythms as sleep

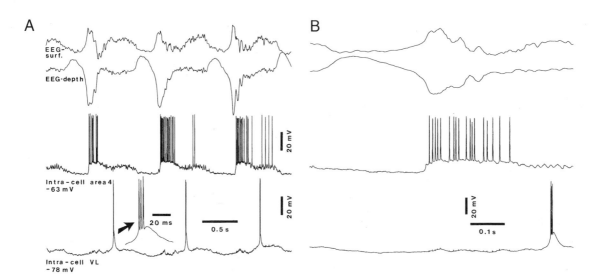

Figure 3.12. The slow oscillation (about 0.9 Hz) in dual simultaneous intracellular recordings from regular-spiking cell in cortical area 4 and thalamocortical cell in the ventrolateral nucleus. Cat under ketamine-xylazine anesthesia. *Arrow* in **A** points to a low-threshold spike-burst. An expanded cycle is shown in **B**. Note: *(a)* depth-positive (upward) EEG waves are associated with hyperpolarization of cortical and thalamic cells, whereas the sharp depth-negatives are associated with depolarization and action potentials in cortical cell, while the thalamic neuron display a rebound spike burst with a delay of 150 to 200 msec; *(b)* brief sequence of EEG spindles after the depth-negative (surface-positive) sharp deflection; and *(c)* fast depolarizing waves (40–50 Hz) in cortical neuron during the sustained depolarization. (Unpublished data of M. Steriade and D. Contreras.)

delta waves (see below, Two Types of Delta Waves Generated in the Thalamus and Cortex), nor is it similar to the "cyclic alternating pattern" recurring at 20 seconds or longer intervals (Terzano et al., 1988). The latter is associated with enhancement of muscle tone and heart rate, and was described as "arousal-related phasic events," whereas the slow oscillation is blocked during arousal in acute experiments as well as during natural awakening (Steriade et al., 1993a, 1996a).

The cortical nature of the slow oscillation was demonstrated by (a) its survival in the cerebral cortex after thalamectomy (Steriade et al., 1993f), and (b) its absence in the thalamus of decorticated animals (Timofeev and Steriade, 1996). The generation of the slow oscillation in neocortex was confirmed by its presence in cortical slices *in vitro* (Sanchez-Vives and McCormick, 2000) and in cortical slabs *in vivo* (Timofeev et al., 2000).

Intracellular analyses of the slow oscillation showed that cortical neurons throughout layers II to VI (with physiologically identified thalamic and/or callosal inputs, and with projections to the thalamus and/or homotopic points of the contralateral hemisphere) displayed a spontaneous oscillation recurring with periods of 1–1.5 to 5 seconds, depending on the anesthetic, and consisting of prolonged depolarizing and hyperpolarizing components (Fig. 3.12). The long-lasting depolarization of the slow oscillation consisted of EPSPs, fast prepotentials (FPPs), and fast IPSPs reflecting the action of synaptically coupled GABAergic local-circuit cortical cells (Steriade et al., 1993e). Data also indicated that the depolarizing com-

ponent is made up of both NMDA-mediated synaptic excitatory events and a voltage-dependent persistent sodium current, $I_{Na(p)}$. This was suggested by the suppression of the prolonged part of the depolarizing envelope by either administration of ketamine (NMDA blocker) or intracellular injection of QX-314 (a blocker of sodium currents), whereas the initial, short-lasting excitatory event of the depolarization was left intact (Steriade et al., 1993e). The long-lasting hyperpolarization, interrupting the depolarizing envelopes, is probably a combination of a $I_{K(Ca)}$ and disfacilitation in the corticothalamic network. Indeed, brain activation induced by stimulation of mesopontine cholinergic nuclei blocks the slow oscillation mainly through the suppression of the prolonged hyperpolarization, a muscarinic-mediated effect (Steriade et al., 1993a); it is known that activation of muscarinic receptors diminishes or suppresses the voltage- and calcium-dependent potassium current (McCormick and Williamson, 1989; Schwindt et al., 1989). As to the disfacilitation hypothesis, it is supported by measuring of the membrane input resistance (R_{in}) showing that R_{in} is highest during the long-lasting hyperpolarizing component of the slow oscillation (Contreras et al., 1996b). The disfacilitation is probably achieved by a progressive depletion of $[Ca^{2+}]_{out}$ during the depolarizing phase of the slow oscillation (Massimini and Amzica, 2001).

All major cellular classes in the cerebral cortex, as identified by electrophysiological characteristics and intracellular staining, display the slow oscillation: regular-spiking and intrinsically bursting cells, as well as local-circuit inhibitory basket cells (Contreras and Steriade, 1995; Steriade et al., 1993a,e). All these neuronal types exhibit similar relations with the EEG components of the slow oscillation: During the depth-positive EEG wave cortical neurons are hyperpolarized, whereas during the sharp depth-negative EEG deflection cortical neurons are depolarized (Fig. 3.12). The spectacular similarity between all types of cortical neurons and EEG waveforms raised the question of mechanisms underlying these synchronization processes. Dual intracellular recordings *in vivo* revealed that the overt synchronization of EEG patterns is associated with the simultaneous hyperpolarizations in cortical neurons (Fig. 3.13; Contreras and Steriade, 1995; Steriade et al., 1994). The intracortical synchronization of the slow oscillation was demonstrated by dual intracellular and field potential recordings from distant cortical foci, and by the disruption of synchronization after lidocaine injection between the two foci (Fig. 3.14; Amzica and Steriade, 1995b).

The neuronal synchronization also implicates thalamic neurons. Remarkably, RE thalamic cells (identified by their peculiar bursting pattern and cortically elicited spindle-like depolarizing oscillations), whose intrinsic electrophysiological properties are quite different from those of neocortical cells, exhibit patterns of the slow sponta-

neous oscillation, with prolonged depolarizations interrupted by prolonged hyperpolarizations, that are very similar to those of cortical neurons (Contreras and Steriade, 1995; Steriade et al., 1993b). The depolarizing component of the cortically generated slow oscillation is transmitted to RE thalamic neurons at which level it triggers rhythmic spike bursts and, consequently, is reflected in TC cells as rhythmic IPSPs leading to rebound spike bursts (Fig. 3.15), which are the basic mechanism for generation of sleep spindles. The slow oscillation was also recently described in thalamic slices maintained *in vitro* following activation of metabotropic glutamate receptor mGluR1a (Hughes et al., 2002). It is known that corticothalamic neurons use glutamate as neurotransmitter. The synchronous firing of neocortical neurons during the depolarizing component of the slow oscillation and the corticothalamic projections represent the mechanism that underlies the brief sequence of spindles that follows every cycle of the slow oscillation (Contreras and Steriade, 1995, 1996; Timofeev and Steriade, 1996). Our concept of a unified corticothalamic network, implying the coalescence of various sleep oscillations through the virtue of cortically generated slow oscillation to impinge on thalamic neurons and thus to group spindles within slow oscillation cycles (Contreras and Steriade, 1995; Steriade, 2001a,b; Steriade

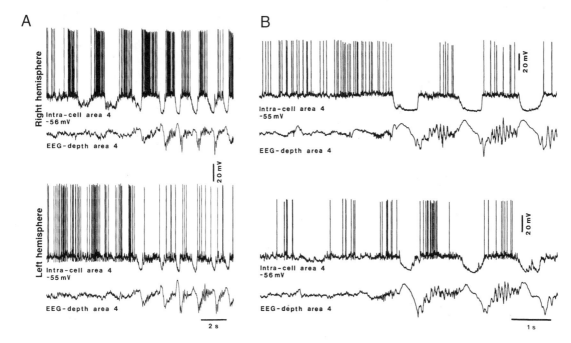

Figure 3.13. The synchronization of EEG is concomitant with simultaneous hyperpolarizations in neocortical neurons. Dual intracellular recordings from right and left areas 4. Two neuronal couples (**A** and **B**) are shown. **A:** While right area 4 neuron started to display low-amplitude, rhythmic hyperpolarizations, left area 4 neuron still displayed tonic firing, and the EEG showed an activated pattern; only when both cells simultaneously displayed large hyperpolarizations, was the EEG fully synchronized with the patterns of slow oscillation and brief spindle sequences. **B:** Simultaneous hyperpolarizations in the two neurons occurred suddenly. (Modified from Steriade, M., Contreras, D., and Amzica, F. 1994. Synchronized sleep oscillations and their paroxysmal developments. *Trends Neurosci.* 17:199–208; and Contreras, D., and Steriade, M. 1995. Cellular basis of EEG slow rhythms: a study of dynamic corticothalamic relationships. *J. Neurosci.* 15:604–622.)

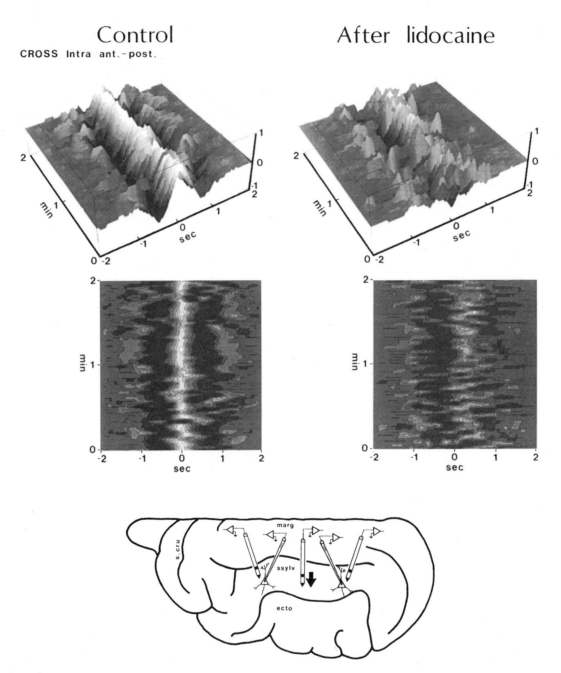

Figure 3.14. Disruption of synchronization of slow oscillation by intracortical disconnection of synaptic linkages. Dual intracellular recordings from the anterior and posterior parts of the suprasylvian gyrus in cat; lidocaine injection (40 μL, 20%) between the two micropipettes (see brain figurine). The synchrony and its disruption after lidocaine injections are represented by sequential field analyses. The control synchrony was char-acterized by well-aligned, high central peaks. After lidocaine injection, the previous pattern was replaced by a blurred sequence of lower peaks and lower valleys deviating from the central plane. (Modified from Amzica, F., and Steriade, M. 1995. Disconnection of intracortical synaptic linkages disrupts synchronization of a slow oscillation. *J. Neurosci.* 15:4658–4677.)

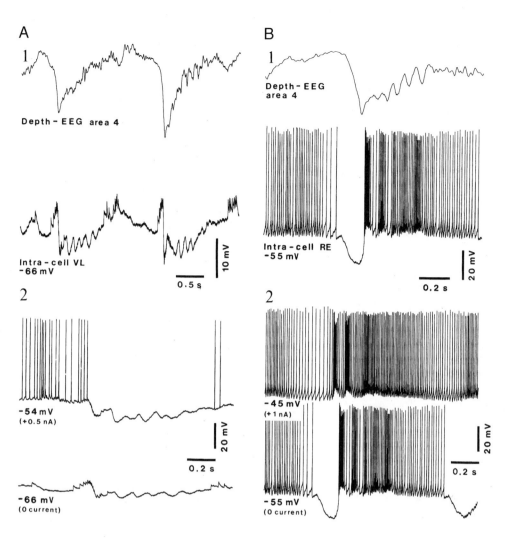

Figure 3.15. Effect of sharp cortico-thalamic volleys during the depolarizing phases of the slow sleep oscillation upon thalamocortical and thalamic reticular cells. Cat under ketamine-xylazine anesthesia. **A:** Depth-EEG from area 4 and intracellular recording from ventrolateral (VL) thalamocortical neuron. In *1*, two cycles of slow oscillation (0.5–0.6 Hz) at the resting membrane potential (−66 mV) of VL cell. Note brief sequence of spindle waves in EEG and corresponding IPSPs in VL cell following the sharp depth-EEG (depolarizing) component of the slow oscillation. In *2*, expanded traces to illustrate enhancement of spindle-related IPSPs with cell's depolarization. **B:** Depth-EEG from area 4 and intracellular recording from thalamic reticular (RE) neuron. In *1*, resting membrane potential (−55 mV). Note spindle-related spike bursts in association with EEG spindles that follow the hyperpolarizing phase of the slow oscillation. In *2*, expanded trace at the resting level and under depolarizing current. (Modified from Timofeev, I., and Steriade, M. 1996. Low-frequency rhythms in the thalamus of intact-cortex and decorticated cats. *J. Neurophysiol.* 76:4152–4168).

and Amzica, 1998), is supported by recent studies of human EEG during natural sleep (Mölle et al., 2002).

The resemblance between the pattern of slow oscillation during natural sleep and anesthesia concerns the two major components of this rhythm: the prolonged hyperpolarization during the depth-positive EEG wave is associated with silent firing, and the depolarizing component during the depth-negative EEG wave is accompanied by brisk firing that eventually leads to a sequence of spindle waves and to a depolarizing plateau associated with fast oscillations (Steriade et al., 1996a) (Fig. 3.16).

The sequence of grapho-elements consisting of an ample surface-positive transient followed by a slower, surface-negative component and, eventually, a few spindle waves is usually termed the K complex and is a reliable sign for stage 2 of human sleep, but surviving in all stages of quiet sleep (Loomis et al., 1938; Niedermeyer, 1993; Roth et al., 1956). This landmark of sleep was related with the slow oscillation in humans (Amzica and Steriade, 1997a) and its cellular substrates have been investigated in cats (Amzica and Steriade, 1997b). Briefly, (a) spectral analysis demonstrated the periodic recurrence of human K

complexes, with main peaks at 0.5 to 0.7 Hz; the other frequency bands in Fig. 3.17 are between 1 and 4 Hz (delta band, with several ill-defined peaks) and between 12 and 15 Hz for the spindling range; the decomposition of the signal into three digitally filtered channels (Fig. 3.17D) indicates that the S-lead reflects the slow oscillation, the Δ lead reflects the shape of the K complex, and the σ lead faithfully reflected the spindle activity of the original signal; (b) the laminar profile and intracellular substrates of the K complex during cat sleep or anesthesia revealed that the surface-recorded, positive K complexes reverse at a cortical depth of about 0.3 mm, and that the sharp depth-negative (surface-positive) wave of the K complex is associated with cells' depolarizations, eventually leading to a spindle sequence. These investigations indicate that the K complexes are the expression of the spontaneously occurring, cortically generated slow oscillation.

The depolarizing and hyperpolarizing phases of the cortical slow oscillation are also observed, with a different time course, in glial cells. Dual simultaneous intracellular recordings from neurons and adjacent glial cells were performed during sleep-like patterns produced by ketamine-

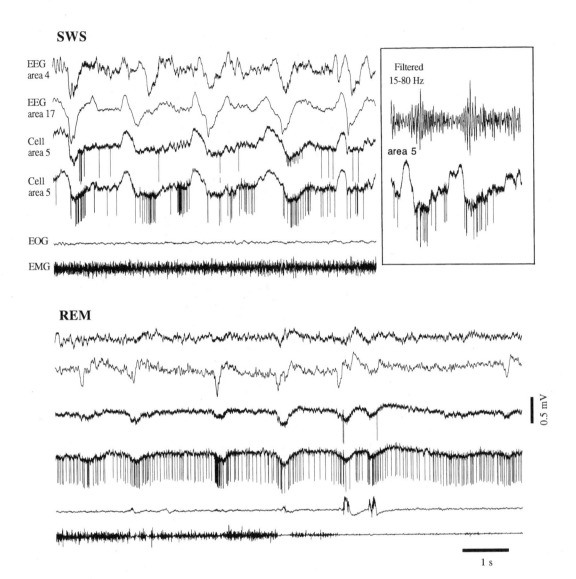

Figure 3.16. Patterns of slow oscillation during natural sleep are similar to those under ketamine-xylazine anesthesia. Selective reduction of fast rhythms during the inhibitory periods of the slow oscillation during natural sleep. Chronically implanted, naturally sleeping cat. SWS, slow-wave sleep. REM, rapid-eye-movement sleep. SWS is separated from REM by a nondepicted period of 34 seconds. Six traces represent: depth-EEG from motor (precruciate) area 4; depth-EEG from visual area 17; unit discharges and slow focal potentials from association area 5 in the anterior suprasylvian gyrus; and similar recording from an adjacent focus (2 mm apart) in area 5; electro-oculogram (EOG); and electromyogram (EMG). Right part in SWS panel shows reduction, up to disappearance, of fast rhythms (filtered 15–80 Hz) during the prolonged depth-positive wave of the slow oscillation that, in intracellular recordings, is associated with hyperpolarization of cortical and thalamic neurons. (Unpublished data by M. Steriade and F. Amzica; inset in SWS is adapted from Steriade, M., Amzica, F., and Contreras, D. 1996. Synchronization of fast (30–40 Hz) spontaneous cortical rhythms during brain activation. *J. Neurosci.* 16:392–417.)

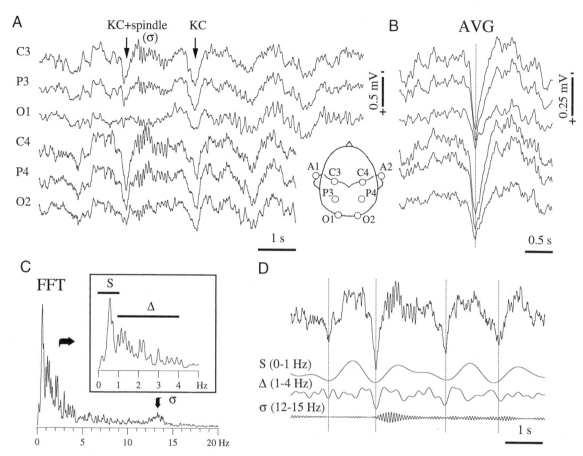

Figure 3.17. K-complex in human sleep. Scalp monopolar recordings with respect to the contralateral ear (see figurine). **A:** Short episode from a stage 3 period of sleep. The two *arrows* point to a K-complex (KC) followed by a spindle sequence (σ) and to a KC in isolation. The two KCs are embedded into a slow oscillation at about 0.6 Hz. Note the synchrony of KCs in all recorded sites and the diminution of their amplitudes in the occipital area. **B:** Average of 50 KCs aligned on the positive peak of the upper channel *(vertical dotted line)*. **C:** Power spectrum of the C3-lead for a period of 80 seconds of stable stage 3 activity containing the period depicted in **A**. The three frequency bands (S, Δ, and σ; further illustrated in **D**) are represented in the power spectrum. Moreover, the slow *(S)* activity displays a high peak, distinct from the onset of delta (Δ) activity (see inset). **D:** Frequency decomposition of the C3-lead *(upper trace)* into three frequency bands: slow *(S;* 0.1 Hz); delta (Δ; 1–4 Hz); and sigma (σ; 12–15 Hz). It is shown that the KC results from a combination of slow and delta waves. (Modified from Amzica, F., and Steriade, M. 1997. The K-complex: its slow (<1 Hz) rhythmicity and relation with delta waves. *Neurology* 49: 952–959.)

xylazine anesthesia to explore the possibility that glia may not only passively reflect, but also influence, the state of neuronal networks (Amzica and Steriade, 1998, 2000; Amzica et al., 2002). Simultaneous intracellular recordings of a neuron and a glial cell are illustrated in Fig. 3.18. The neuronal response to a cortical stimulus consists of an initial depolarization crowned by action potentials, an inhibitory potential, and a rebound excitation. The corresponding responses in the glia are a sluggish depolarizing slope, a further depolarization, and a negative wave, respectively. The fact that neuronal IPSP is reflected in the glia by a depolarizing potential may be explained by opening of Cl⁻ channels in glia by GABA_A action (Kettenmann and Schachner, 1985). During spontaneously occurring slow oscillation in anesthetized animals, the onset of the depolarizing phase in neurons is followed, after a lag of ~90 ms, by the depolarization of simultaneously recorded, adjacent (1–2 mm) glial cells (Fig. 3.18E) (Amzica and Neckelmann, 1999; Amzica and Steriade, 1998). Measurements of $[K^+]_{out}$ during the depolarizing phase of the slow oscillation indicate that glial cells phasically uptake part of the $[K^+]_{out}$ extruded by neurons (Amzica et al., 2002). Toward the end of the depolarizing phase, the glial membrane begins to repolarize before neurons. In view of the fact that the maximal glial depolarization is reached much later than the end of neuronal depolarization and that glial membrane potential returns to control value at the end of the slowly recurring oscillatory cycles, glial cells might control the pace of the oscillation through changes in $[K^+]_{out}$, which is known to modulate neuronal excitability. During the slow sleep oscillation, the $[K^+]_{out}$ amplitude reaches 1 to 2 mM, which when added to the physiological values of resting concentration, ~3 mM, may assist cortical neurons in oscillating between hyper- and hypoexcitability.

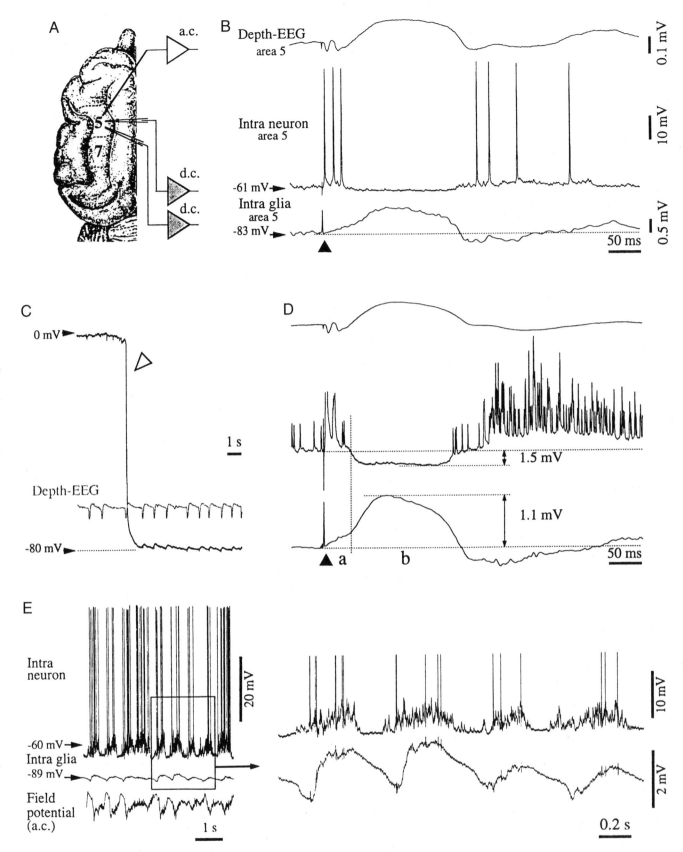

Figure 3.18. Responsiveness to cortical stimulus and spontaneously occurring slow oscillation in cortical neuron and glial cell. Dual simultaneous recordings in cat under ketamine-xylazine anesthesia. **A:** Top view of cat's brain with the localization of association areas 5 and 7 in the suprasylvian gyrus. **C:** Impalement of a glia cell is marked *(open arrowhead)* by a sudden voltage deflection from extracellular potential values (~0 mV) to −80 mV. Intraglial potentials (slow depolarizations) are reversed with respect to the extracellular ones. **D:** Dual intracellular (neuron and glia) and field potential recording in cortical area 5. Response to a single cortical stimulus *(black triangle)* delivered close to the field electrode. The recordings sites correspond to those indicated in **A**. See text for description of responses. Average of 25 responses evoked by cortical stimulation. The initial glial depolarization *(a)* is clearly separated from the following positive wave *(b)* by a change in the depolarizing slope. **E:** Slow oscillation in simultaneously recorded neuron and glial cell. (Modified from Amzica, F., and Steriade, M. 2000. Neuronal and glial membrane potentials during sleep and paroxysmal oscillations in the cortex. *J. Neurosci.* 20:6646–6665; and Amzica, F., and Neckelmann, D. 1999. Membrane capacitance of cortical neurons and glia during sleep oscillations and spike-wave seizures. *J. Neurophysiol.* 82:2731–2746.)

Two Types of Delta Waves Generated in the Thalamus and Cortex

As sleep deepens, the incidence of spindles diminishes and high-amplitude, slower EEG rhythms progressively develop. These waves are conventionally termed "delta," whence the term *delta sleep* applied to stages 3 to 4 of sleep in humans or to the later part of EEG-synchronized sleep in cats. A major task was to explore the cellular mechanisms that underlie the recently discovered slow oscillation (less than 1 Hz), described above, distinct from those that built up the conventional delta waves (1 to 4 Hz). Hereafter, the term *delta* will be conventionally used for oscillations within the frequency range of 1 to 4 Hz, and the term *slow* for waves below 1 Hz.

The difference between these two oscillatory types is emphasized because of their distinct origins and mechanisms (the slow oscillation emerges from network activity in the cerebral cortex, whereas at least one type of delta activity arises from the interplay between two intrinsic currents of thalamic cells) and because delta waves are grouped by the slow oscillation (Fig. 3.19; Steriade et al., 1993f). This underlines the fact that we deal with two different sleep oscillations. With the benefit of hindsight, one can see in previous EEG recordings cyclic groups of delta waves at 3 to 4 Hz recurring with a slow rhythm of 0.3 to 0.4 Hz in human sleep (Niedermeyer, 1993). Analyses of human sleep have also indicated the differences in dynamics between the slow and delta oscillations (Achermann and Borbély, 1997).

There are two types of delta activity. One is generated in the cortex, as it survives after thalamectomy, but its neuronal substrates have not yet been systematically investigated with intracellular recordings. The other originates in the thalamus, even after decortication, and its cellular mechanisms are quite well understood.

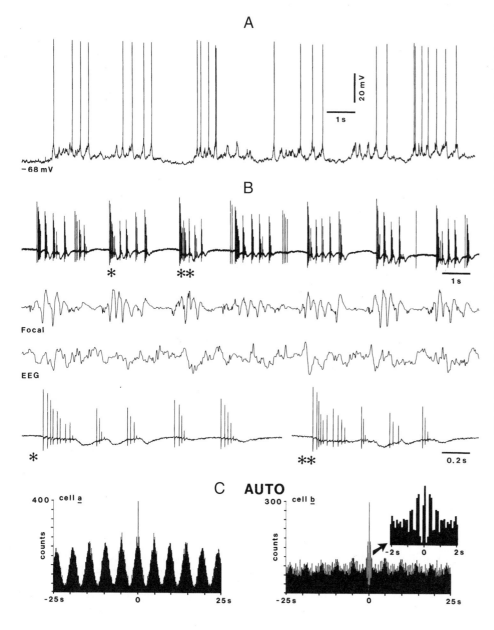

Figure 3.19. Grouping of delta waves by slow oscillation. Cats under urethane anesthesia. **A:** Intracellular recording of regular-spiking, corticothalamic cell in area 5, backfired from rostral intralaminar centrolateral (CL) and driven synaptically from lateroposterior (LP) nucleus. Note delta cellular oscillation (3–4 Hz) grouped within sequences recurring with a slow rhythm (0.3–0.4 Hz). **B:** Extracellular recording of bursting cell at a depth of 0.6 mm in area 7, convergently excited by LP and CL nuclei. Below the cellular trace, focal waves recorded through the same micropipette and gross EEG waves from the cortical surface are depicted. The sequence of spike-bursts marked by one and two *asterisks* are expanded below. Delta oscillations (3–4 Hz) are grouped by the slow oscillation (0.3–0.4 Hz). **C:** Slow and delta rhythms in two cells, recorded simultaneously, extracellularly (*a,* single-spike discharging; and *b,* bursting cell) from motor area 4 (depth 1.3 mm). Autocorrelograms show that both cells displayed the slow oscillation (0.2 Hz) and that cell *b* also oscillated in the delta frequency (2.5 Hz) within the slowly recurring sequences (see *arrow* and *inset*). (Modified from Steriade, M., Nuñez, A., and Amzica, F. 1993. Intracellular analysis of relations between the slow (<1 Hz) neocortical oscillation and other sleep rhythms of the electroencephalogram. *J. Neurosci.* 13:3266–3283.)

Early Studies

Until recently little, if anything, was known about the origin(s) and neuronal substrates of delta EEG waves. Their cortical origin was suggested on the basis that delta waves, at 1 to 2 Hz, survive on the EEG of athalamic cats (Villablanca, 1974). However, while "most of the thalamus was removed," in some animals the posterior parts were spared and "the rostral thalamus was only partially removed" (Villablanca, 1974, pp. 55–57). The thalamectomy by aspiration through the midline using a transcallosal approach to minimize direct cortical damage is heroic surgery and may leave intact important thalamic territories; even if only parts of the rostral intralaminar wing are spared, the widespread cortical projections of these nuclei may transfer to the cortex thalamically generated delta oscillations. In fact, thalamic recordings have shown the presence of focal delta waves even after cortical disconnection (see below).

As to the electrophysiological mechanisms, no intracellular data related to delta waves were available until the early 1990s. Stratigraphic studies (Calvet et al., 1964) and current source density analyses (Petsche et al., 1984) have indicated that delta waves result from vertically arranged dipoles between layers II to III and layer V. Extracellular recordings of cortical activity during pathological delta waves (as obtained by lesions of the subcortical white matter, the thalamus, or the mesencephalic reticular formation) have shown a relationship between the firing probability and the surface-positive (depth-negative) delta waves, whereas the depth-positive waves were associated with a diminution in discharge rates (Ball et al., 1977; see Fig. 1.21 in Steriade and Buzsáki, 1990). All these field-unit relationships might lead to the assumption that the depth-positive component of delta waves reflects the inhibition of pyramidal-shaped neurons by local-circuit cells. There are numerous types of GABAergic and/or peptidergic inhibitory interneurons in various cortical areas, such as large basket cells, small to medium-sized "chandelier" neurons, "spider" or "clutch" cells, and very small bipolar interneurons (e.g., Kisvárday et al., 1986, 1993; Somogyi et al., 1983, 1984; reviewed in Jones, 1987; Steriade et al., 1990e). GABAergic interneurons open chloride channels in pyramidal-type neurons and would then produce an extracellular current flow responsible for the depth-positivity of delta waves. Such a correlation would imply maximal firing of putative inhibitory interneurons during the depth-positive delta waves. However, this has not been found. It was then suggested (Steriade and Buzsáki, 1990; Steriade et al., 1990b) that, far from resulting exclusively from IPSPs, EEG delta waves are rather generated by summation of long-lasting afterhyperpolarizations (AHPs) produced by a variety of K+ currents in deeply lying pyramidal neurons.

Intracellular Analyses of the Thalamic Delta Rhythm

The role of TC neurons in the genesis of a clock-like, stereotyped delta (1–4 Hz) sleep oscillation, as well as the role of corticothalamic neurons in synchronizing thalamic delta waves and grouping them into sequences recurring within the frequency range of the slow oscillation, have recently been re-vealed by intracellular analyses. As is shown below, barbiturates induce an EEG picture with overwhelming spindle activity and they prevent the appearance of thalamic delta waves. Also, since it was necessary to block delta waves by setting into action brainstem-thalamic cholinergic systems (in order to mimic the behavioral state of arousal), barbiturates had to be avoided because, even in very small doses, they profoundly depress the cholinergic responses of TC and cortical neurons (Eysel et al., 1986; Krnjević, 1974).

Previous field potential and extracellular recordings have already indicated that (a) thalamic neurons display waves and unit discharges within delta (1–4 Hz) frequencies during EEG-synchronized sleep (McCarley et al., 1983; Steriade et al., 1971); (b) delta waves occur in RE thalamic nucleus even after disconnection from the cerebral cortex (Steriade et al., 1987); and (c) thalamic delta waves are suppressed during EEG-activation patterns induced by midbrain reticular stimulation (see Fig. 7 in Steriade et al., 1971). However, these observations did not elucidate the cellular mechanisms of thalamic delta waves.

That the thalamus is indeed implicated in the genesis of delta waves was demonstrated by a series of *in vitro* and *in vivo* studies that revealed that a clock-like oscillation within the delta frequency range is generated by the interplay of two intrinsic currents of thalamocortical cells. This intrinsic oscillation is potentiated and synchronized by network operations involving corticothalamic projections, with an intermediate link in the RE thalamic nucleus. *Whereas spindle oscillation is generated by synaptic interactions in the thalamic networks including RE nucleus, the thalamic delta oscillation is an intrinsic oscillation depending on two inward currents of TC cells.* Nonetheless, to be expressed at the macrophysiological level of the EEG, single cells should be united into neuronal ensembles by synchronizing devices that must have access to many dorsal thalamic nuclei. On an a priori ground, the only candidate for such a synchronization process is the RE thalamic nucleus that projects to widespread dorsal thalamic territories. Data related to the intrinsic electrophysiological properties of thalamic cells implicated in delta oscillation and to network synchronization of individual thalamic neurons are summarized below.

McCormick and Pape (1990a) found that a subpopulation of neurons recorded *in vitro* from the dorsal part of the lateral geniculate thalamic nucleus displayed rhythmic bursts of high-frequency spikes with an interburst frequency of 1 to 2 Hz. This oscillation results from the interplay between the transient calcium current I_T underlying the low-threshold spike (LTS) and a hyperpolarization-activated cation current (I_H). I_H is a noninactivating inward (anomalous) rectifier carried by Na+ and K+. The model proposed for the genesis of 1 to 2 Hz oscillation is depicted in Fig. 3.20A, from the work of McCormick and Pape (1990a), showing the proposed currents mediating the oscillation. At hyperpolarized levels of the membrane potential (V_m more negative than about −65 or −70 mV), I_H is activated and is expressed as a depolarizing sag of V_m toward rest. This depolarization activates the I_T (which was de-inactivated because of the membrane hyperpolarization), thus underlying an LTS that gives rise to a burst of high-frequency fast Na+ action potentials. The latter depolarization deactivates the I_H. Repolarization

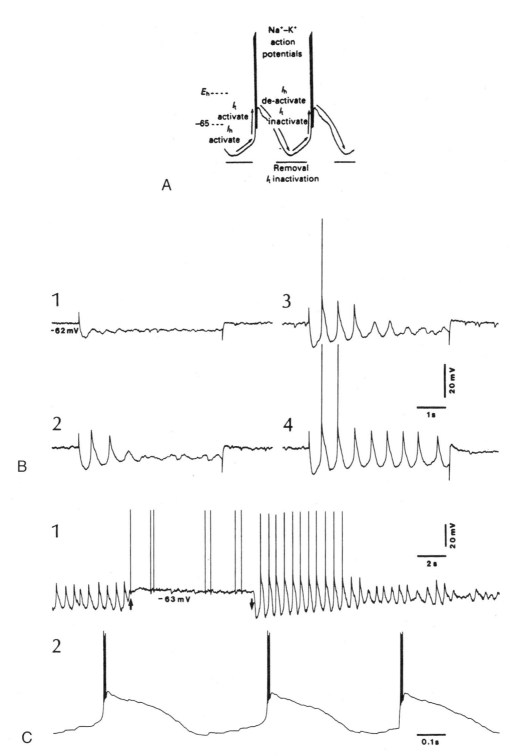

Figure 3.20. Delta oscillations in thalamocortical cells results from the interplay between two intrinsic currents, I_h and I_t. **A:** Proposed model for interaction between these intrinsic currents. Activation of the low-threshold calcium current, I_t, depolarizes the membrane toward threshold for a burst of sodium-dependent fast action potentials. The depolarization inactivates the portion of I_h that was active immediately before the calcium spike. Repolarization of the membrane due to I_t inactivation is followed by a hyperpolarizing overshoot, due to the reduced depolarizing effect of I_h. The hyperpolarization in turn deinactivates I_t and activates I_h, which depolarizes the membrane toward threshold for another calcium spike. **B:** Delta oscillation of cat ventral lateral thalamocortical cell triggered by hyperpolarizing current pulses (0.7 nA in *1,* 1 nA in *2,* 1.1 nA in *3,* and 1.2 nA in *4*). Note increasing number of cycles at a frequency of 1.6 Hz. **C:** Lateroposterior (LP) thalamocortical cell after decortication of areas projecting to LP nucleus. The cell oscillated spontaneously at 1.7 Hz. A 0.5-nA depolarizing current (between *arrows*) prevented the oscillation, and its removal set the cell back in the oscillatory mode. Three cycles after removal of depolarizing current in *1* are expanded in *2* to show high-frequency bursts crowning the low-threshold calcium spike. (**A** modified from McCormick, D.A., and Pape, H.-C. 1990a. Properties of a hyperpolarized-activated cation current and its role in rhythmic oscillation in thalamic relay neurons. *J. Physiol. (Lond.)* 431:291–318. **B** and **C** modified from Steriade, M., Curró Dossi, R., and Nuñez, A. 1991a. Network modulation of a slow intrinsic oscillation of cat thalamocortical neurons implicated in sleep delta waves; cortically induced synchronization and brainstem cholinergic suppression. *J. Neurosci.* 11:3200–3217.)

of the membrane is followed by a hyperpolarizing overshoot that, in turn, activates the I_H, which depolarizes the membrane toward another calcium-dependent LTS. The cycle is then repeatable. A similar rhythm was described *in vitro* by Leresche et al. (1991), and the two inward currents responsible for this oscillatory behavior have also been analyzed by Soltesz et al. (1991).

Our *in vivo* studies (Curró Dossi et al., 1992a; Nuñez et al., 1992b; Steriade et al., 1991a) have shown that antidromically identified TC cells recorded from a variety of sensory (lateral geniculate and ventral posterior), motor (ventral anterior and ventral lateral), associational (lateral posterior), and intralaminar (central lateral) thalamic nuclei display a delta rhythm induced by imposed hyperpolarization to values characteristic for late stages of EEG-synchronized sleep. The number of cycles in the elicited oscillation was correlated with the voltage deflection following the injection of hyperpolarizing current pulses (Fig. 3.20B). Moreover, *spontaneous* delta oscillation (without injecting current pulses) could be obtained by ablating the cortical areas projecting to the recorded thalamic nucleus. This deafferentation procedure removed the powerful depolarizing impingement from corticothalamic neurons and set thalamic cells at a more hyperpolarized V_m (around -70 mV) where delta oscillation is generated (Fig. 3.20C). The fact that rhythmic LTSs occurred in isolation (without super-imposed fast action potentials that could have synaptically engaged other elements in the thalamic and cortical networks) supported the idea that this oscillation is intrinsic.

Several other features characterize the intrinsic thalamic delta oscillation, as revealed in our *in vivo* experiments:

1. This oscillation is sensitive to barbiturates, even very low doses of short-acting barbiturates are effective in blocking it (Curró Dossi et al., 1992a). This effect is due to an increased conductance of TC cells produced by barbiturates, as already reported in *in vitro* experiments (Sykes and Thomson, 1989). The increased conductance prevents the interplay between the two inward currents responsible for the delta genesis. The sensitivity to barbiturates also explains why delta oscillation was not found in previous experiments on oscillatory properties of TC cells conducted under barbiturate anesthesia.

2. Delta oscillation is also blocked by spindle sequences, even those that occur in cerveau isolé preparations in the absence of barbiturates (Nuñez et al., 1992b) (Fig. 3.21A). The proposed mechanism of delta occlusion by spindles is the increased membrane conductance that is seen during and a few seconds after a spindle sequence (Fig. 3.21B). The hyperpolarization of TC cells outlasting the spindle sequence is ascribed to the long-lasting, tonic spike barrage of RE thalamic cells that follows the

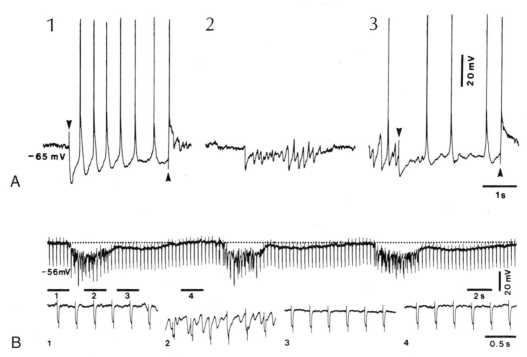

Figure 3.21. Incompatibility, at the single-cell level, between spindle and delta oscillations. Intracellular recordings of two (**A** and **B**) ventroanterior thalamocortical cells in cerveau isolé cats. **A:** *1,* hyperpolarizing current pulse (1.5 nA) generated delta oscillation at 2.5 Hz. *2,* spindle sequence occurring spontaneously. *3,* spindle sequence beginning before the hyperpolarizing current pulse (same parameters as in *1*) blocked delta oscillation. Note smaller voltage deflection evoked by hyperpolarizing current pulse during spindles. **B:** Change in membrane conductance during spindle sequences. Spontaneous spindle sequences show that, after the rhythmic IPSPs of spindles, the membrane potential remains hyperpolarized for 3 to 5 seconds. Short hyperpolarizing current pulses (0.8 nA) were injected to measure the membrane conductance. Epochs *1* to *4* are expanded below. Note increased conductance during spindles and, less marked, during the hyperpolarization following spindles, compared to control interspindle lulls. (Modified from Nuñez, A., Curró Dossi, R., Contreras, D., et al. 1992. Intracellular evidence for incompatibility between spindle and delta oscillations in thalamocortical neurons of cat. *Neuroscience* 48:75–85.)

spindle-related spike bursts in this GABAergic cell-type (Steriade et al., 1986). The increased membrane conductance during this prolonged hyperpolarization probably unbalances the interplay between I_H and I_T. This incompatibility between spindles and delta waves occurs at the singular cellular level. The presence of spindles at the EEG level (though they are greatly reduced) during late sleep stages when they may coexist with delta waves is due to the fact that some neuronal pools are still at the V_m where spindles are prevalent (see below, point *3*).

3. Spindles and delta oscillations appear at different V_m of TC cells. At the resting V_m (around -60 mV), thalamic cells display spontaneous or cortically elicited spindle oscillation, whereas at V_m more negative than -65 or -70 mV spindles progressively decrease in amplitude (due to the partial reversal of IPSPs that compose the cyclic hyperpolarizations in thalamocortical neurons) and the oscillations are within the delta frequency range (Fig. 3.22). Since delta oscillations, prevailing during late sleep stages, occur spontaneously or are triggered by cortical volleys at more negative V_m than spindles that characterize the early sleep stage, we have postulated a progressive hyperpolarization of thalamocortical cells

with the deepening of sleep with EEG synchronization (Steriade et al., 1991a). This is attributable to the progressive decrease in firing rates, during slow-wave sleep, of corticothalamic cells (Steriade, 1978) and thalamically projecting neurons located in the midbrain reticular formation (Steriade et al., 1982), mesopontine cholinergic nuclei (Steriade et al., 1990a), and monoaminergic nuclei (see details in Steriade and McCarley, 1990). The transmitters of all these neuronal types produce a depolarization of TC cells (McCormick and Prince, 1987, 1988; for review, see McCormick, 1990). That the partial removal of the depolarizing impingement exerted by corticothalamic cells is also effective in producing the V_m hyperpolarization required for setting thalamic neurons in the delta oscillatory mode (Curró Dossi et al., 1992a) is in keeping with Buzsáki's (1991) results, which showed that injections of NMDA blockers lead to a reduction in frequency of thalamic oscillations, from 8 to 2 Hz. It is known from human and animal studies that spindle and delta prevail during different sleep stages and that these two rhythms reciprocally oscillate within EEG-synchronized sleep (Lancel et al., 1992; Uchida et al., 1991). The intracellular data reported above provided

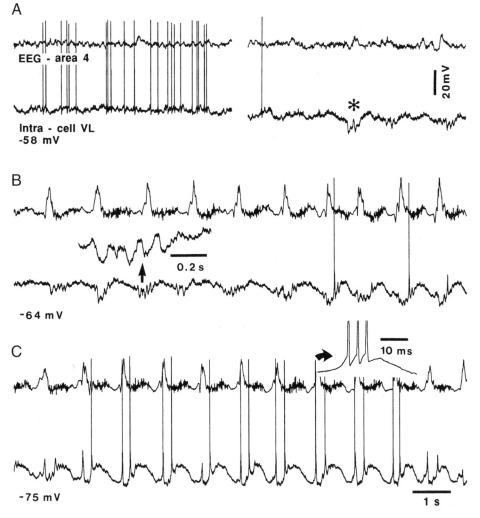

A
EEG - area 4
Intra - cell VL
-58 mV

20mV

*

B
0.2 s
-64 mV

C
10 ms
-75 mV
1 s

Figure 3.22. The dependency of transition from spindle to delta oscillation on the membrane potential of thalamocortical (TC) neurons in a cat under ketamine-xylazine anesthesia. Intracellular recording of a neuron from the ventral lateral nucleus, simultaneously with surface EEG from cortical area 4. **A:** *Left:* Tonic firing during activated EEG pattern; *right:* appearance of membrane potential oscillations in association with slight changes in EEG activity (*asterisk* marks the first hyperpolarizing sequence in association with the initial signs of EEG synchronization). **B:** Hyperpolarizing spindle oscillations (8–10 Hz) are grouped within sequences recurring with a slow rhythm (~0.8 Hz), in close time relation with the slow cortical EEG rhythm. One spindle sequence is expanded above *(arrow)*. **C:** A hyperpolarizing current step (-0.2 nA) transformed spindles into delta potentials (3 to 4 Hz), grouped by the same slow cortical rhythm (~0.8 Hz). One spike burst crowning the low-threshold spike is expanded above. (Modified from Steriade, M., Contreras, D., and Amzica, F. 1994. Synchronized sleep oscillations and their paroxysmal developments. *Trends Neurosci.* 17:199–208.)

the mechanisms accounting for this relative incompatibility between the two major sleep rhythms, mainly due to their differential voltage dependency.

4. Cortical volleys potentiate delta oscillation in thalamocortical cells (Steriade et al., 1991a). This synaptic action indicates that delta oscillation, resulting from the intrinsic properties of thalamic cells, is powerfully modulated by network operations. The facilitatory process is expressed by the transformation, as an effect of cortical stimulation, of subthreshold delta oscillation into rhythmic LTSs crowned by fast sodium action potentials. The LTSs may persist for 10 to 20 seconds as a self-sustained activity, after cessation of cortical volleys (Fig. 3.23A). Cortical stimuli also revive a hyperpolarization-activated

delta oscillation when it dampens after a few cycles (Fig. 3.23B). The question may arise as to how the corticothalamic activity is involved in maintaining a high level of activation in thalamic cells (since cortical ablation or functional disconnection leads to V_m hyperpolarization of thalamic cells and, consequently, delta oscillations; see point 3, above, while, on the other hand, it is also capable of potentiating delta oscillation formed by alternating LTS-AHP sequences on a background of increased hyperpolarization. The answer is that the influence of cortical cells on the thalamus varies with the behavioral state. Tonic, high-discharge firing rates of corticothalamic cells during waking (Steriade, 1978) exert a depolarizing impingement on thalamic cells through the release

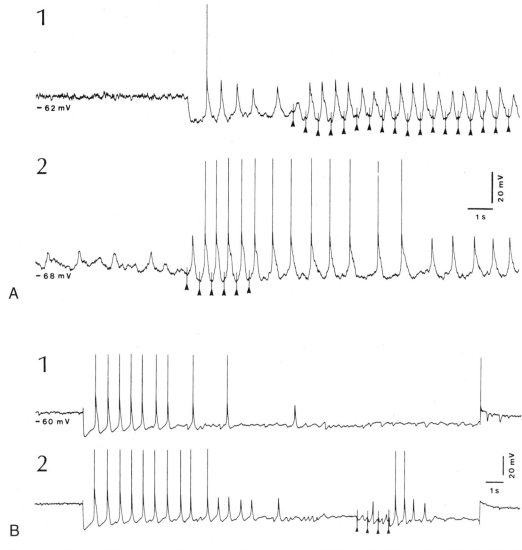

Figure 3.23. Cortical potentiation of thalamic delta oscillation. Intracellular recordings in cats under urethane anesthesia. **A:** Ventrolateral thalamocortical cell. *1,* hyperpolarization (0.8 nA) bringing the V_m from −62 to −78 mV induced a 2-Hz oscillation. When dampening of oscillation was imminent, cortical stimuli at 2 Hz evoked low-threshold spikes (LTSs). *2,* at V_m of −68 mV, a subthreshold oscillation appeared; six cortical stimuli (same parameters as in *1*) induced LTSs and, after cessation of stimuli, a self-sustained oscillation at 1 to 1.5 Hz ensued for 15 seconds. **B:** Another neuron, located in the centrolateral nucleus. Hyperpolarizing current pulses (duration, 22.5 seconds, 0.9 nA in *1*, 1 nA in *2*) elicited 1.4-Hz oscillation that dampened after 6 seconds *(1)* and 9 seconds *(2)*. Four shocks to the precruciate gyrus (*2, arrowheads* restarted the dampened oscillation, which thereafter continued in a self-sustained manner). (Modified from Steriade, M., Curró Dossi, R., and Nuñez, A. 1991a. Network modulation of a slow intrinsic oscillation of cat thalamocortical neurons implicated in sleep delta waves; cortically induced synchronization and brainstem cholinergic suppression. *J. Neurosci.* 11:3200–3217.)

of excitatory amino acids acting on non-NMDA, NMDA, as well as metabotropic glutamate receptors (McCormick and von Krosigk, 1992). Particularly, the prolonged excitation of thalamic relay cells resulting from the reduction of a "leak" potassium conductance through the activation of glutamatergic metabotropic receptors is capable of maintaining the activation patterns of TC cells, thus acting as a true descending activation system (McCormick and von Krosigk, 1992). Thus, the action of tonic, repetitive action potentials with depolar-

izing effects in the corticothalamic pathway prevents, during the alert state, the delta genesis since the interplay between I_H and I_T is critically dependent on membrane hyperpolarization. Removal of corticothalamic projections leads to hyperpolarization of their thalamic targets and greater propensity to delta oscillation (Curró Dossi et al., 1992a). Distinctly from the discharge patterns of corticothalamic cells during wakefulness, the same neurons have much lower rates during EEG-synchronized sleep and fire high-frequency bursts (Steriade, 1978) that

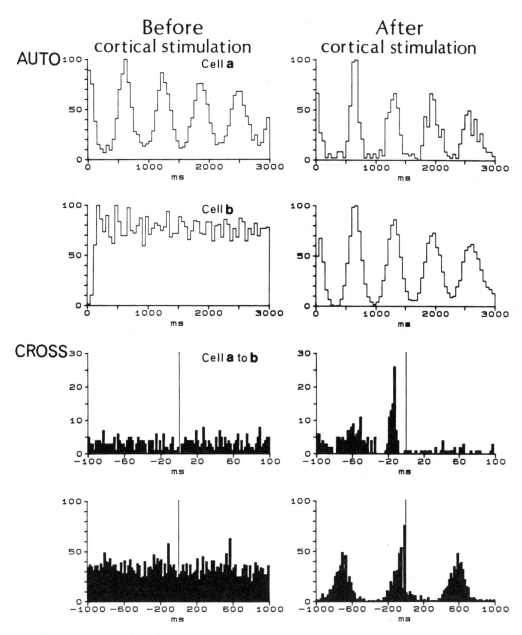

Figure 3.24. Auto- and cross-correlograms of two cells (*a* and *b*) recorded simultaneously in the ventrolateral thalamic nucleus of cat under urethane anesthesia. Four correlograms (before and after cortical stimulation) depict, from top to bottom, autocorrelogram of cell *a*, autocorrelogram of cell *b*, and the cross-correlogram of both cells (cell *b* is the reference cell) with two different bins (2 and 20 msec). Note, before cortical stimulation, delta (1.6-Hz) rhythm of cell *a*, flat contour (absence of rhythmicity) in cell *b*, and absence of coupling between these neurons.

After cortical stimulation, the background noise in cell *b* became rhythmic at the same frequency as cell *a* (1.6 Hz), and cross-correlograms show that cell *a* firing preceded cell *b* firing by about 10 to 20 msec. (Modified from Steriade, M., Curró Dossi, R., and Nuñez, A. 1991a. Network modulation of a slow intrinsic oscillation of cat thalamocortical neurons implicated in sleep delta waves; cortically induced synchronization and brainstem cholinergic suppression. *J. Neurosci.* 11:3200–3217.)

are more effective in phasically driving inhibitory RE and local-circuit thalamic cells. In turn, the latter induce IPSPs in thalamic relay neurons, thus creating the conditions for the appearance of the hyperpolarization-activated delta oscillation (Steriade et al., 1991a).

5. Lastly, corticothalamic volleys are capable of synchronizing delta-oscillating thalamic cells that were uncoupled prior to cortical stimuli (Steriade et al., 1991a) (Fig. 3.24). In this study, the cortically elicited synchronization of two or three simultaneously recorded neurons was obtained by using the same microelectrode. Thus, it was not possible to assess whether RE of local interneurons were responsible for the synaptic coupling between relay cells. (With the exception of lateral geniculate neurons, other TC cells do not have intranuclear recurrent axonal collaterals.) The role of the RE nucleus is suggested by the fact that the synchronizing process was elicited by stimulating a cortical (motor) area that is not directly related to the recorded (lateroposterior) thalamic nucleus. The only candidate for such a conjunction process is the RE nuclear complex. Many RE sectors (particularly the rostral pole and rostrolateral districts) are recipients of afferents from a variety of cortical areas and project to a variety of dorsal thalamic nuclei (Steriade et al., 1984). Extra- and intracellular recordings from various parts of the RE complex have indeed shown that RE cells discharge spike trains or high-frequency bursts within the frequency range of delta waves (Amzica et al., 1992; Steriade et al., 1993b).

Fast Rhythms (20–50 Hz) During Diffuse Arousal and Focused Attention

The brain substrate of EEG activation upon arousal has begun to be understood since the pioneering work of Moruzzi and Magoun (1949). They stimulated different foci of the brainstem reticular core in the deeply anesthetized (chloralosed) cat and elicited the transformation of high-voltage, low-frequency cortical EEG waves into low-voltage, fast rhythms, reminiscent of those occurring upon natural awakening. The cortical effect was thought to be mediated, at least in part, by the diffuse thalamic projecting system. Although this EEG response was obtained from many brainstem foci between the medulla and the mesencephalon (whence the notion of unspecific arousal systems), the most effective point was located in the rostral reticular core. Both the rostral brainstem reticular origin of at least one category of arousing neurons and their activating effects upon the cerebral cortex through a synaptic linkage in thalamic nuclei with widespread cortical projections have been supported by studies at the cellular level (Steriade and Glenn, 1982; Steriade et al., 1982).

The prevalent origin of arousal systems in the rostral reticular formation was also indicated by early transection experiments. Bremer's (1935) *cerveau isolé* (collicular-transected) cats were comatose and characterized by continuous EEG spindling. By contrast, the midpontine pretrigeminal preparation, realized by Moruzzi and his colleagues (Batini et al., 1958) by means of a transection only a few millimeters behind the collicular cut, displayed persistent EEG and ocular signs of alertness. The inescapable conclusion was that a small territory at the mesopontine junction, between the levels of collicular and midpontine transections, contains the neurons involved in the ascending activation of the thalamus and the cortex. During the past 15 years, two groups of cholinergic [pedunculopontine tegmental (PPT) and laterodorsal tegmental (LDT)] nuclei have been identified by using choline acetyltransferase (ChAT) immunohistochemistry. The projections to the thalamus of brainstem cholinergic cells were demonstrated by combining retrograde tracers with ChAT labeling (reviewed in Steriade and McCarley, 1990; Wainer and Mesulam, 1990). In addition to cholinergic nuclei, the brainstem territory at the mesopontine junction contains the noradrenaline-containing cells of the locus coeruleus and the serotonin (5-HT)-containing cells of the dorsal raphe nucleus. These monoaminergic aggregates have much less dense thalamic projections, but their axons directly innervate the cerebral cortex (reviewed in Saper, 1987). As will become clear in what follows, cholinergic neurons conjointly act with monoaminergic-containing cells to activate the thalamus and cortex during wakefulness. However, during REM sleep, characterized by brain excitability at least as high as that during arousal, only cholinergic neurons can account for forebrain activation, because locus coeruleus and dorsal raphe neurons are virtually silent (see Steriade and McCarley, 1990).

The "activation" response of Moruzzi and Magoun's (1949) experiments was, in fact, merely the suppression of spindles and slower EEG rhythms. The cellular mechanisms of this suppressing mechanism have recently been disclosed: (a) The blockage of spindle oscillations takes place at the very site of their genesis, the RE thalamic nucleus. Brainstem cholinergic neurons induce a hyperpolarization of RE cells by increasing a potassium conductance and, thus, they cut off the depolarizing envelope of spindle oscillations in RE neurons (Hu et al., 1989; McCormick and Prince, 1986). Other activating neuromodulators, 5-HT and NA, depolarize RE neurons (McCormick and Wang, 1991) and this action promotes single-spike activity of RE neurons, much the same as arousal. However, the combined effects of acetylcholine (ACh), 5-HT and NA, having quite different actions on the spindle pacemaking RE neurons, are far from being understood. (b) Thalamic delta waves are blocked by cholinergic (Steriade et al., 1991a) and monoaminergic (McCormick and Pape, 1990b) neurons, which exert depolarizing actions on their thalamic targets, and thus, bring them out of the voltage range where the intrinsic, clock-like delta oscillation is generated. Cortical delta waves are blocked by the cholinergic actions of nucleus basalis neurons (Buzsáki et al., 1988). The complex actions of modulatory cholinergic neurons on different types of thalamic and cortical cells are summarized in the cellular recordings and diagrams of Fig. 3.25.

At the time of Moruzzi and Magoun (1949), "activation" was thought to consist of negative events (suppression of EEG-synchronized waves), but no real sign of activated processes was observed, as their results mainly reported the flattening of the EEG following brainstem reticular formation. Only a decade later, evidence of increased excitability was provided. Cortical field potentials evoked by stimula-

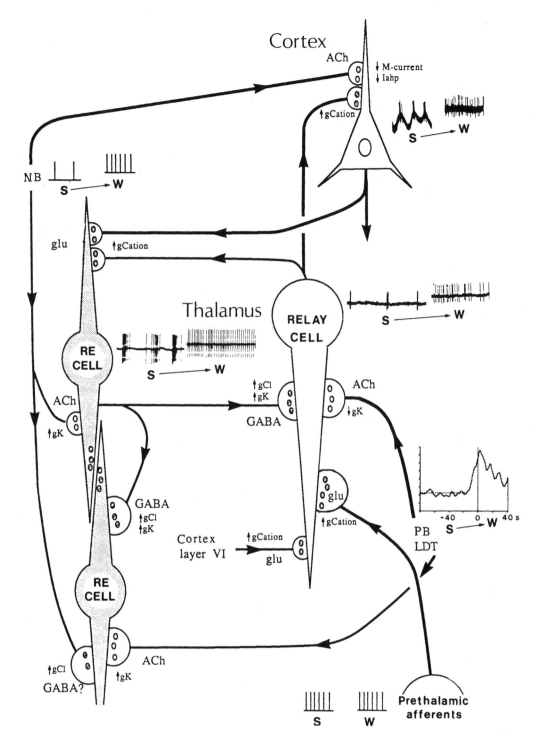

Figure 3.25. Schematic diagram of ascending cholinergic actions upon thalamocortical (relay) neurons, reticular thalamic (RE) GABAergic neurons, and pyramidal-shaped neurons of the cerebral cortex. Direction of axons is indicated by arrows. Acetylcholine (ACh) is released in the thalamus by peribrachial (PB) neurons of the pedunculopontine tegmental (PPT) nucleus and by laterodorsal tegmental (LDT) neurons. In the cortex, ACh is mostly released by nucleus basalis (NB) neurons. In relay and RE thalamic cells as well as in cortical pyramidal neurons, EEG-synchronized sleep (S) is characterized by rhythmic inhibitory periods and bursts of action potentials within the frequency range of spindle oscillations. These processes are associated with a decreased transfer function in thalamocortical cells. In cortical neurons, the activity evoked by prethalamic afferents is further reduced due to a relatively uninhibited M-current and slow afterhyperpolarizing current (I_{ahp}), which underlie spike frequency adaptation. Upon transition from S to waking (W), cholinergic PB/LDT neurons increase their rates of spontaneous firing, about 20 seconds before time 0 of W, taken as the most precocious change from EEG synchronization to desynchronization. An increased activity from S to W is also seen in NB neurons. Note that no change in firing rate from S to W is seen in neurons recorded from specific prethalamic relays. Increased activity of cholinergic PB/LDT and NB cells disrupts rhythm generation in the thalamus by depolarizing relay neurons, through a decrease in potassium conductance, g_K. As well, cortical pyramidal cells are activated through a decrease in M-current and I_{ahp}. There is, in addition, an excitatory action on cortical pyramidal cells by noncholinergic (glutamatergic) thalamocortical cells (increase in cationic permeability). Besides, the hyperpolarization of RE cells by cholinergic PB/LDT cells as well as by NB cholinergic and GABAergic cells underlies the blockage of spindle generation in the pacemaking RE neurons. Although PB/LDT cholinergic afferents hyperpolarize RE cells by an increase in g_K, these neurons are brought upon arousal toward single-spike firing, with increased discharge rates, because they are subject to excitatory influences from both relay and cortico-RE neurons using excitatory amino acids (glu). Schemes of changes in ionic conductances of thalamic and cortical neurons are modified from McCormick (1990) based on *in vitro* data of McCormick and Prince (1986, 1987). Data related to the S-W behavior of various types of depicted neurons are from chronic experiments on PB/LDT (Steriade et al., 1990a), RE thalamic (Steriade et al., 1986), and thalamocortical and cortical pyramidal cells (see details in Steriade et al., 1990c).

tion of prethalamic fibers (for example, the optic tract) were enhanced during midbrain reticular stimulation (Bremer and Stoupel, 1959; Dumont and Dell, 1960). In parallel studies, photically evoked field potentials recorded from the lateral geniculate thalamic nucleus were increased during brainstem reticular-induced arousal, without any sign of enhanced responses simultaneously recorded from the optic tract (Steriade and Demetrescu, 1960). Thus, the notion of activation was strengthened by data showing an increased synaptic excitability of both thalamic and cortical neurons during mesencephalic reticular stimulation.

The first demonstration that the EEG activated response to brainstem reticular stimulation is not only the blockage of spindles and slow waves, but also includes the appearance of peculiar fast rhythms characterizing arousal, belongs to Bremer and his colleagues (1960). They reported that a flattening of the cortical EEG is not the constant effect of brainstem stimulation. Instead, a clear-cut enhancement in amplitude of spontaneous rhythms and their regular acceleration to 40 to 45 Hz ("*accélération synchronisatrice*") appeared on the cortical EEG of the *encéphale isolé* (bulbospinal transected) preparation, simultaneously with the ocular syndrome of arousal.

Since then, a series of studies in various cortical areas have reported the presence of 20- to 40-Hz waves, during different conditions of increased alertness. The fast rhythm was observed in a canine subject in the occipital cortex while the dog paid intense attention to a visual stimulus (Lopes da Silva et al., 1970; Fig. 3.26A), during accurate performance of a conditioned response to a visual stimulus in monkey (Freeman and Van Dijk, 1988), during tasks requiring fine finger movements and focused attention in monkey motor cortical cells (Murthy and Fetz, 1992), during focused arousal prior to the performance of a complex task in humans (Sheer, 1984), and during behavioral immobility associated with an enhanced level of vigilance while the cat was watching a visible but unseizable mouse (Bouyer et al., 1987; Rougeul-Buser et al., 1983). Other studies have described stimulus-dependent oscillations at 25 to 45 Hz of the focal EEG and/or neuronal firing in the olfactory system (Freeman, 1975) and visual cortex (Eckhorn et al., 1988; Engel et al., 1990; Gray and Singer, 1989; Gray et al., 1989, 1990) (Fig. 3.26B). It was also reported that brainstem reticular stimulation selectively enhances the 80-Hz oscillatory waves composing the afterdischarge of the flash-evoked response in the visual cortex (Steriade et al., 1968) and facili-

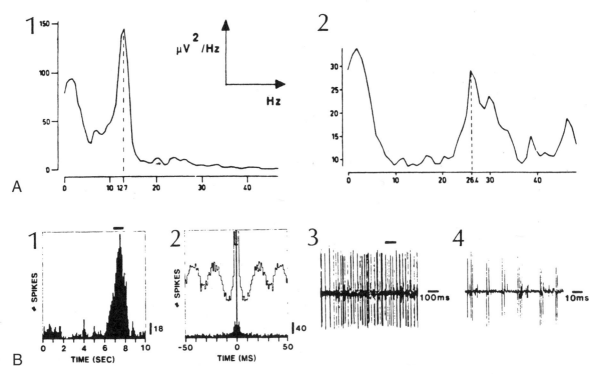

Figure 3.26. Induced beta (25–40 Hz) oscillations in visual cortex. **A:** Power spectra calculated from EEG signals recorded from the surface of the occipital cortex in the dog. The spectra in *1* were obtained while the awake animal kept its eye closed, and those in *2* when the animal paid intense attention to a visual object. Note that cortical activity had different dominant frequency components: alpha activity dominates in *1* and beta activity (peak around 26 Hz) dominates in *2*. **B:** The firing pattern of an oscillatory standard-complex cell of cat. *1,* poststimulus time-histogram of the neuronal spike train recorded over ten trials. The response is selective for the second direction of stimulus movements. *2,* autocorrelograms. *Filled bars* and *unfilled bars* display the correlograms computed for the first and second direction of stimulus movement, respectively. *3,* plot of the spike train recorded during a single presentation to the second direction of stimulus movement. *4,* high-resolution plot of the same data shown in *3.* (**A** modified from Lopes da Silva, F.H., Van Rotterdam, A., Storm van Leeuwen, W., et al. 1970. Dynamic characteristics of visual evoked potentials in the dog. II. Beta frequency selectivity in evoked potentials and background activity. *Electroencephalogr. Clin. Neurophysiol.* 29:260–268. **B** modified from Gray, C.M., Engel, A.K., König, P., et al. 1990. Stimulus-dependent neuronal oscillations in cat visual cortex: receptive field properties and feature dependence. *Eur. J. Neurosci.* 2:607–619.)

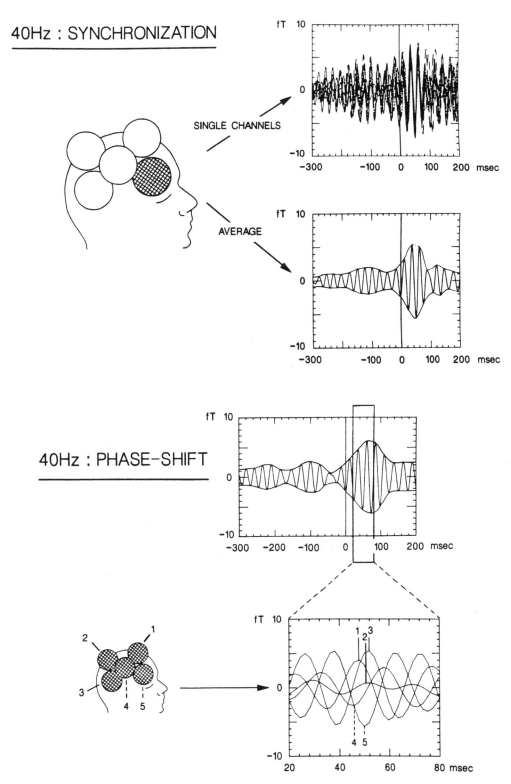

Figure 3.27. A 40-Hz rhythm in magnetoencephalographic recordings from awake humans. **Top:** Synchronization of 40-Hz oscillatory activity during auditory processing within seven single channels of one probe placed over lower frontal areas. The graph on the *top right* indicates a superimposition of 40-Hz activities, time locked to the stimulus onset, recorded from the seven channels. The graph on the *lower right* indicates an average of the seven individual channels, demonstrating synchronization over a large area (around 25 cm²). **Bottom:** Phase shift of 40-Hz oscillatory activity during auditory processing. The time period between 20 and 80 msec after the onset of the auditory stimuli is enlarged in the *lower panel*. The *lowest panel* shows the superimposition of averaged responses from all sensors in each of the five probe positions (hatched and numbered at *left*). Note the large, consistent phase shifts from region to region, indicating a continuous rostrocaudal phase shift over the hemisphere. (Modified from Llinás, R.R., and Ribary, U. 1992. Rostrocaudal scan in human brain: a global characteristic of the 40 Hz response during sensory input. In *Induced Rhythms in the Brain,* Eds. E. Basar and T. Bullock, pp. 147–154. Boston: Birkhauser.)

tates the coherency of 40-Hz responses in visual cortical neurons (Singer, 1990b). The possible significance of this rhythm resides in the fact that, in addition to the spatial mapping that allows a limited number of representations, a temporal component is brought about by synchronized oscillatory (around 40 Hz) responses across spatially separate cortical columns (Eckhorn et al., 1988; Gray et al., 1989). The conjunction of spatial and temporal factors is the basis of functionally coherent cell assemblies, distinguished by the phase and the frequency of their synchronous oscillatory activity (Singer, 1990a). The cell assemblies link spatially distributed elements and may be the bases for global and coherent properties of patterns, a prerequisite for scene segmentation and figure-ground distinction (Singer, 1990b). This "feature binding" and pattern recognition function was extended by data showing the role of 40-Hz oscillations in the mediation of higher-order motor functions (Murthy and Fetz, 1992). The issue of feature binding is controversial. Different opinions on this problem are exposed elsewhere (Shadlen and Movshon, 1999; Singer, 1999). This chapter does not discuss whether or not synchronized fast rhythms in distributed neuronal pools are needed for the representation of multiple facets of the external world into single percepts. Suffice it to say that fast rhythms are present and synchronized during states in which consciousness is suspended (see below).

The site(s) of origin, underlying intrinsic membrane properties, and network synchronization of the fast (generally termed: 40-Hz) rhythms have recently been investigated. The conclusion is that fast rhythms elicited by optimal sensory stimuli are only the tip of the iceberg, as these oscillations are present in the background (spontaneous) activity of the thalamus and cerebral cortex during cells' depolarization, not only during wakefulness when information processing is expected to occur, but also during deep anesthesia and natural slow-wave sleep (Steriade et al., 1991b, 1993c, 1996a,b). Magnetoencephalographic recordings in awake humans have revealed the presence of a 40-Hz oscillation over the entire cortical mantle, a phase-shift of oscillatory activity close to 12 msec between the rostral and caudal poles of the hemisphere, and a synchronization of this 40-Hz activity by presentation of auditory stimuli with random frequencies (Llinás and Ribary, 1992, 1993) (Fig. 3.27).

The origins and cellular mechanisms of fast rhythms are discussed below.

Site(s) of Origin

While the role played by cortical neurons in the genesis of the 40-Hz rhythm is generally accepted, the participation of resonant activities in thalamocortical circuits was denied in initial studies (Gray et al., 1989), in which it was assumed that geniculostriate cells do not usually display oscillatory responses within this frequency range. One of the arguments advanced by those authors against the mediation of 40-Hz rhythms by TC cells was that the collaterals of lateral geniculate neurons do not span sufficiently long distances to account for synchronized oscillations in columns of the visual cortex separated by up to 7 mm. Subsequent studies have demonstrated that 40-Hz rhythmic activities appear in intracellularly recorded, antidromically identified TC cells (Steriade et al.,

1991b, 1993c, 1996b). Other subcortical structures also have the intrinsic and network properties that could generate the fast rhythm not only at the single cell, but also at the population, level. The point is that the coherency between different various 40-Hz-generating brain levels can be accomplished both by different types of synaptic linkages within the cortex, thalamus, or other structures, and by reciprocal projections between distant brain structures (see below).

Intrinsic Membrane Properties and Network Synchronization

Llinás and collaborators (1991) have reported that the 40-Hz rhythm can be generated by intrinsic membrane properties of sparsely spinous interneurons recorded *in vitro* from layer 4 of guinea pig frontal cortex. It was found that these cells generate narrow-frequency (35–45 Hz) oscillations upon depolarization of the membrane potential and that these oscillations are generated by a voltage-dependent, persistent sodium current, with the involvement of a delayed rectifier. Similar voltage-dependent fast rhythms have been intracellularly recorded in identified callosal neurons (Nuñez et al., 1992a), a result that would explain the coherence of 40-Hz rhythm in cortical areas of both hemispheres. That some TC cells do also display the same oscillatory property is shown in Fig. 3.28 from *in vivo* experiments, depicting a special class of rostral intralaminar nucleus, projecting with high conduction velocities (40–50 m/sec) to association cortex (Steriade et al., 1991b). These TC cells discharged spike bursts at unusually high frequencies (900–1,000 Hz) that recurred within the frequency range of fast rhythms, around 40 Hz. Importantly, the intralaminar cells also discharged spike doublets or triplets, with the same exceedingly short interspike intervals, upon depolarization (Fig. 3.28), a feature that is consistent with their implications in fast oscillations during activated states associated with neuronal depolarizations, waking and REM sleep (Steriade et al., 1996a,b). Other neurons that generate intrinsic 40-Hz oscillatory waves upon cell depolarization include those of the amygdala nuclei (D. Paré, personal communication). The case of the amygdala is important in the light of its role in memory (Mishkin, 1982). Fast oscillations generated by these neurons could be transmitted through intraamygdaloid and distant connections to the cerebral cortex and the thalamus, and could thus contribute to the coherency of a series of forebrain structures in the consolidation of a memory trace (Llinás and Paré, 1991).

Further studies are required to elucidate the role of complex intrinsic properties of cortical neurons (Agmon and Connors, 1989; Berman et al., 1989; Chagnac-Amitai and Connors, 1989; Connors, 1984; Connors et al., 1982; McCormick et al., 1985; Schwindt et al., 1988a,b, 1989; Silva et al., 1991; Spain et al., 1991a,b; Stafstrom et al., 1985) in the genesis of fast (so-called 40 Hz) and related rhythms (Gray and McCormick, 1996; Gutfreund et al., 1995; Llinás et al., 1991; Nuñez et al., 1992; Steriade, 1997; Steriade et al., 1996a). Although some investigators emphasize the distinctness of some neuronal classes in displaying various types of discharge patterns and suppose that these patterns are invariant, other data show that the same neuron, either

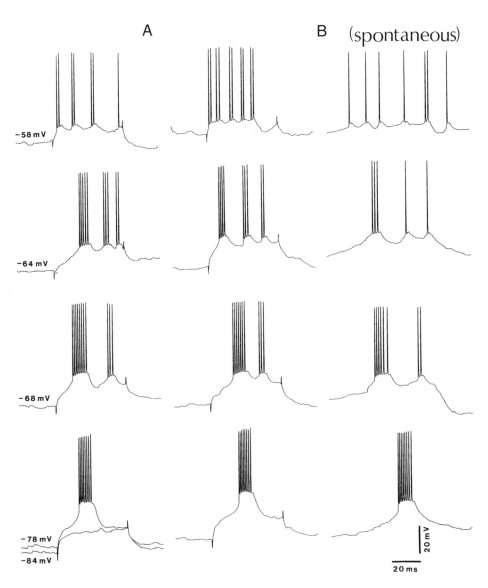

A   B (spontaneous)

Figure 3.28. Fast oscillatory patterns of neuron recorded from the dorsolateral part of the centrolateral (CL) intralaminar thalamic nucleus, characterized by exceedingly high-frequency (800–1000 Hz) spike bursts recurring rhythmically at 50 to 60 Hz. Intracellular recording in cat under barbiturate anesthesia. **A:** Activities triggered by depolarizing current pulses (+1.2 nA, 50 msec) at different levels of membrane potential (V_m, indicated at *left*). Two examples are illustrated for each V_m level. At *bottom*, presence of low-threshold spike (LTS) leading to high-frequency (800–1000 Hz) spike burst at −78 mVC and its absence at −84 mV. Note fast-recurring (50–60 Hz) spike doublets or spike triplets at relatively depolarized levels (−64 mV and −58 mV), a feature that is not seen in other types of thalamocortical neurons. **B:** Oscillatory patterns similar to those elicited by current injection occurred spontaneously at similar V_ms (from top to bottom, −58, −64, −68, and −78 mV). (Modified from Steriade, M., Curró Dossi, R., and Contreras, D. 1993. Electrophysiological properties of intralaminar thalamocortical cells discharging rhythmic (~40 Hz) spike-bursts at ~1000 Hz during waking and rapid eye movement sleep. *Neuroscience* 56:1–9.)

long-axoned (corticothalamic) or short-axoned, may change its firing elicited by depolarizing current pulses, from regular spiking to intrinsically bursting (or vice versa) and, furthermore, to fast spiking without spike frequency adaptation (Fig. 3.29; Steriade, 1997; Steriade et al., 1998b). Changes from one type of discharge to another have also been observed during the same depolarizing current pulse (Connors and Gutnick, 1990), during arousal elicited by stimulation of mesopontine cholinergic nuclei (Steriade et al., 1993a), and as an effect of activating neurotransmitters (Wang and McCormick, 1993).

Despite the fact that the fast oscillations (mainly 30–40 Hz) can be generated by the intrinsic properties of single cells, complex neuronal circuits are required for the synchronization of cellular ensembles so that the fast rhythm could be expressed in multiunit and EEG recordings. Several proposals have been made with respect to the synchronizing device(s) of this rhythm.

The intracortical circuits were emphasized since the initial works. Freeman (1975) postulated that the generation of

40- to 80-Hz activity in the olfactory bulb depends on feedback inhibitory circuits involving local-circuit GABAergic neurons acting on output elements, the mitral cells. Similarly, neocortical excitatory-inhibitory circuits have been thought to underlie the 40-Hz rhythm recorded in the visual cortex (Gray et al., 1990). *In vitro* studies of rat's somatosensory cortex have reported rhythmically synchronized activities around 37 Hz, generated by networks of intrinsically bursting pyramidal-shaped cells, in slices with reduced inhibition (Chagnac-Amitai and Connors, 1989). In that study, the short duration of oscillation suggested that a limited neuronal circuit, as in cortical slices, is inadequate to sustain oscillations for long periods. Data indicating synchronization of oscillations between striate and extrastriate cortices (Engel et al., 1991b) and a callosally mediated synchronization linking neurons recorded from areas 17 of both hemispheres (Engel et al., 1991b) were the basis for the hypothesis that the mechanism generating this oscillation are exclusively located at the cortical level. In support of the idea of an interhemispheric synchronization mediated by

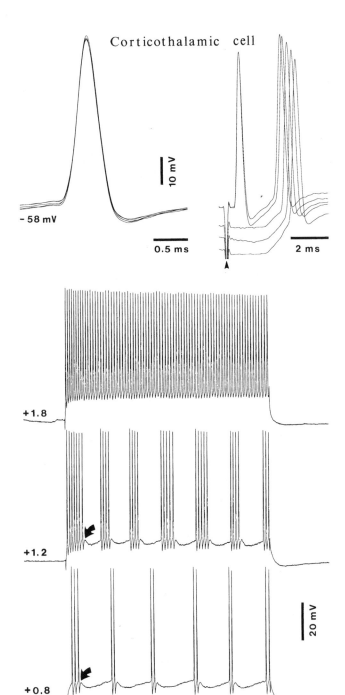

Corticothalamic cell

Figure 3.29. Continuum of discharge patterns elicited by depolarizing current pulses with different intensities. Intracellular recording (cat under ketamine-xylazine anesthesia) of corticothalamic neuron located in layer VI of cat suprasylvian area 7. **Top left:** Spontaneous action potentials had duration of 0.35 ms at half amplitude. **Top right:** Electrophysiological identification of thalamic projection and input: stimulus to thalamic lateral posterior nucleus *(arrowhead)* elicited antidromic activation (0.5 msec latency) and orthodromic spikes (2 msec latency). Five superimposed traces; the two top traces (at a V_m of -58 mV) depict both antidromic and synaptic responses, whereas antidromic spikes failed at more hyperpolarized levels. **Bottom:** Responses of the same neuron to 200-msec depolarizing current pulses of +1.8, +1.2, +0.8, and +0.5 nA. Note fast tonic firing (420 Hz) without spike frequency adaptation (+1.8 nA); spike bursts (intraburst frequency 400 Hz) recurring at 35 Hz (+1.2 nA); spike doublets or triplets (interspike intervals 2.5–3 msec) at 30 Hz (+0.8 nA); and passive response (+0.5 nA). *Oblique arrows* (+1.2 and +0.8) point to depolarizing afterpotentials. (Modified from Steriade, M. 1997. Synchronized activities of coupled oscillators in the cerebral cortex and thalamus at different levels of vigilance. *Cereb. Cortex* 7:583–604; and Steriade, M., Timofeev, I., Dürmüller, N., et al. 1998b. Dynamic properties of corticothalamic neurons and local cortical interneurons generating fast rhythmic (30–40 Hz) spike bursts. *J. Neurophysiol.* 79:483–490.)

tex to be essential for coordination of every movement (Murthy and Fetz, 1992). The fact that the stimulus-dependent 40-Hz oscillation occurs primarily in standard complex cells as opposed to complex and simple cells (Gray et al., 1990) may depend on connectivity features, differential receptive field responsiveness, or peculiar intrinsic properties.

Surprisingly, intracortical synchronization results in fast oscillations that do not show field reversal at any depth of the cortex (Steriade et al., 1996a). In those experiments, volume conduction was precluded because the negative field potentials of the fast oscillations were associated at all depths with neuronal firing and were not observable in the underlying white matter. The absence of depth reversal of fast oscillations was thought to be due to the fact that the current flow is mainly attributable to transmembrane components and less to internal longitudinal components. Vertically distributed currents are not completely ruled out, however, as current-source-density analyses show alternatively distributed microsinks and microsources (Steriade and Amzica, 1996). Thus, the lower intensity of vertical currents, compared with that of transmembrane currents, may explain the absence of potential reversal.

In addition to intracortical circuits, there is compelling evidence that subcortical structures (particularly the thalamus) are interposed in complex neuronal chains generating the 40-Hz rhythm. The hypothesis was proposed that corticothalamic projections drive RE thalamic neurons, thus leading to 40-Hz IPSP-rebound sequences in thalamic relay cells, which reenter the cortex (Llinás, 1990). If so, during the waking state when the 40-Hz rhythm is supposed to occur preferentially (see next section), the inhibitory input from RE thalamic neurons would sculpture the tonic firing of thalamocortical cells, and rhythmic spike trains would be transmitted back to the cortex. The resetting and transiently increased amplitude of fast oscillation in TC cells by short-lasting outward pulses suggests that short IPSPs originating in GABAergic neurons may reinforce fast oscillations (Pedroarena and Llinás, 1997). The relation between RE and

callosal projections, we were able to evoke 40-Hz oscillations upon depolarizing current pulses in cells recorded from the associational area 5 and antidromically identified as projecting to homotopic points in the contralateral cortex (Nuñez et al., 1992a). It was stressed that the 40-Hz oscillation is limited to a subpopulation of visual cortex neurons (Gray et al., 1990) and that it occurs too rarely in motor cor-

TC cells in this fast rhythm is not yet elucidated, especially because, at least in felines, RE cells have also access to thalamic inhibitory interneurons. This linkage would completely transform the simple inhibitory input from RE cells to TC neurons; disinhibition may even prevail (Steriade et al., 1985).

The fact is that TC cells do oscillate at 40 Hz, due to both intrinsic and extrinsic factors. Figure 3.30 demonstrates the coherence of fast oscillations between intracellularly re-corded TC cell and field potentials from the appropriate neo-cortical area. The presence of 40-Hz oscillatory neurons in the intralaminar central lateral nucleus (Steriade et al., 1991b, 1993c), which has widespread projections to the cerebral cortex (Jones, 1985) including the visual areas (Cunningham and LeVay, 1986), is important for the idea of thalamic conjunction and synchronization of distant cortical areas (Llinás and Ribary, 1993). It is also possible that the resonant thalamocorticothalamic circuits are only based on

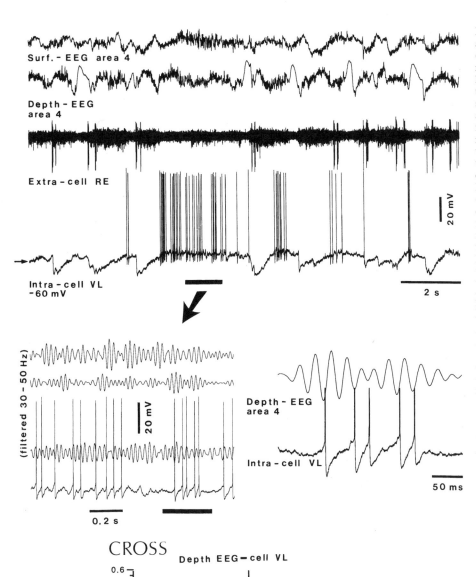

Figure 3.30. Episodes of tonic activation are associated with coherent fast rhythms (40 Hz) in cortical EEG and intracellularly recorded thalamocortical neuron. Cat under ketamine-xylazine anesthesia. **Top:** Four traces represent simultaneous recordings of surface and depth EEG from motor cortical area 4, extracellular discharges of neuron from the rostrolateral part of the thalamic reticular (RE) nucleus, and intracellular activity of thalamocortical neuron from ventrolateral (VL) nucleus. EEG, RE, and VL cells displayed a slow oscillation (0.7–0.8 Hz) during which the sharp depth-negative (excitatory) EEG waves led to IPSPs in VL cell, presumably generated by spike bursts in a cortically driven GABAergic RE neuron. Part marked by *horizontal bar*, taken from a short-lasting period of spontaneous EEG activation, is expanded below *(arrow)*, with EEG waves and field potentials from the RE nucleus filtered from 30 to 50 Hz; part marked by *horizontal bar* in this panel is further expanded at right to illustrate relations between action potentials of VL cell and depth-negative waves in cortical EEG at a frequency of 40 Hz. Cross-correlations (CROSS) between action potentials and depth-EEG shows clear-cut relation, with opposition of phase, between intracellularly recorded VL neuron and EEG waves. (Modified from Steriade, M., Contreras, D., Amzica, F., et al. 1996. Synchronization of fast (30–40 Hz) spontaneous oscillations in intrathalamic and corticothalamic networks. *J. Neurosci.* 16:392–417.)

direct excitatory projections, requiring just one interposed synapse in layer VI. Indeed, there is direct built-in frequency amplification in the corticothalamic pathway, as demonstrated by the fact that 30- to 50-Hz cortical volleys lead to a dramatic increase of EPSPs in target thalamocortical neurons (Lindström and Wróbel, 1990).

Potentiation by Arousing Cholinergic Systems

The hypothesis that 40-Hz oscillations reflect an increased level of alertness was tested by setting into action mesopontine cholinergic aggregates, the peribrachial (PB) area of the PPT nucleus and the LDT nucleus projecting to major thalamic nuclei. In addition, these nuclei project to the basal forebrain and, from there, they may influence the activity of the cerebral cortex. The cholinergic PB (PPT) and LDT cells, with identified thalamic projections, have been recorded in the behaving cat, and their activity was found to increase during waking and REM sleep, much above the lev-

els seen during EEG-synchronized sleep (Steriade et al., 1990a). This statistically significant increase in firing rates of PPT/LDT neurons took place 30 to 60 seconds in advance of the most precocious sign of EEG activation during the transition from slow-wave sleep to either arousal or REM sleep. Such a temporal correlation suggests that thalamically projecting cholinergic PPT/LDT neurons are causally involved in triggering and maintaining activation processes in thalamocortical systems.

There are two main effects of PPT or LDT stimulation upon thalamic function (Fig. 3.31): (a) Mesopontine cholinergic nuclei directly excite TC cells. This excitation has two components: a short-latency, short-duration depolarization mediated by nicotinic receptors and associated with an increase in membrane conductance; and a prolonged (in general 20-second, but up to 60-second) depolarization mediated by muscarinic receptors and associated with an increase in input resistance (Curró Dossi et al., 1991; see also Fig. 3.25. with *in vitro* data of ACh effects). The long-lasting muscarinic depolarization is the basis of the prolonged en-

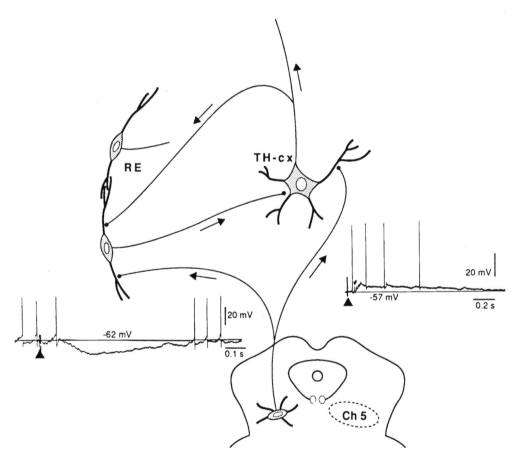

Figure 3.31.   Recurrent inhibitory loop of cat thalamocortical (TH-cx) and reticular thalamic (RE) neurons, and modulation of TH-cx and RE cells by mesopontine cholinergic afferents (only the Ch5 group of pedunculopontine tegmental neurons is depicted). In *insets*, Ch5 stimulation (brief pulse train, *arrowhead*) induces a depolarization of TH-cx neurons and a hyperpolarization of RE cells. The direct excitation of TH-cx cells is accompanied by their disinhibition (through inhibition of GABAergic RE cells). (Modified from Hu, B., Steriade, M., and Deschênes, M. 1989. The effects of brainstem peribrachial stimulation on perigeniculate neurons: the blockage of spindle waves. *Neuroscience* 31:1–12; Paré, D., Steriade, M., Deschênes, M., et al. 1990. Prolonged enhancement of anterior thalamic synaptic responsiveness by stimulation of a brainstem cholinergic group. *J. Neurosci.* 10:20–33; Steriade, M., Gloor, P., Llinás, R.R., et al. 1990b. Basic mechanisms of cerebral rhythmic activities. *Electroencephalogr. Clin. Neurophysiol.* 76:481–508.)

hancement in synaptic responsiveness of thalamic relay cells upon stimulation of mesopontine cholinergic cell aggregates (Paré et al., 1990). (b) The same cholinergic nuclei indirectly excite thalamocortical cells by inhibiting the RE cells through a hyperpolarization associated with increase in membrane conductance (Hu et al., 1989). Both these mechanisms are factors behind the increased firing rates and enhanced synaptic excitability of thalamocortical neurons, with consequently similar activated patterns in neocortical cells, during the states of wakefulness and REM sleep.

The above mechanisms of brainstem-thalamic cholinergic activation are also implicated in the potentiation of 40-Hz oscillations of TC neurons. Stimulation of the PB area in the PPT nucleus induces a twofold increase of cortical EEG waves around 40 Hz, a potentiating effect that is muscarinic-mediated as it was blocked by scopolamine (Steriade et al., 1991b, 1993a). Since mesopontine cholinergic nuclei project to the thalamus as well as through a more ventral path-

way to the basal forebrain, the latter structure was destroyed and the corpus callosum was cut in those experiments to provide evidence for the ipsilateral transmission of the facilitatory effect through the thalamus. The PPT-induced 40-Hz oscillation is associated in TC cells with a blockage of slow rhythms, due to a depolarization that sets these neurons out of the voltage range where delta waves are generated (Steriade et al., 1991a) (Fig. 3.32).

These data show that, far from serving only a resonant mechanism for reciprocally coupled groups in separate columns of the sensory and motor areas, the 40-Hz rhythm reflects a condition of diffusely increased vigilance of the brain (Steriade, 1993). The role of 40-Hz rhythm in motor cortical neurons during attentive behavior was demonstrated by Murthy and Fetz (1992). Further cellular studies are required to show the role of this fast rhythm in thalamic and cortical sensory processes involved in selective attention.

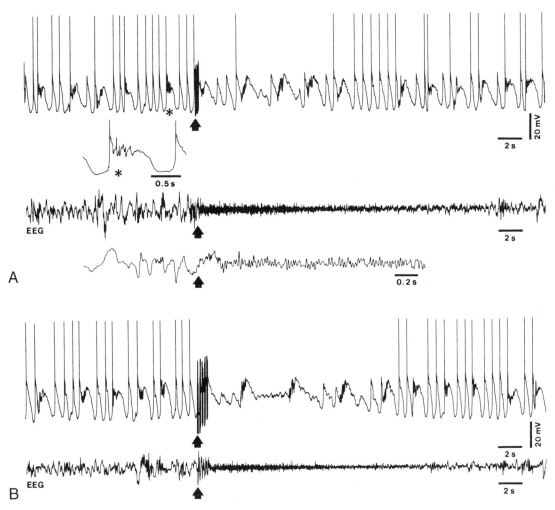

Figure 3.32. Intracellularly recorded delta oscillation in cat lateroposterior thalamocortical neuron, its suppression by mesopontine peribrachial (PB) stimulation (one and five pulse trains in **A** and **B**, respectively, indicated by *arrows*), and the appearance of 40-Hz oscillations. Below the top (intracellular) trace, cortical EEG (in **A**, an expanded epoch of EEG trace around the PB pulse train is also depicted to show the 40-Hz oscillation induced by PB stimulation). A sequence of fast depolarizing events in **A** *(asterisk)* is expanded and shown below. (Modified from Steriade, M., Curró Dossi, R., and Nuñez, A. 1991a. Network modulation of a slow intrinsic oscillation of cat thalamocortical neurons implicated in sleep delta waves: cortically induced synchronization and brainstem cholinergic suppression. *J. Neurosci.* 11:3200–3217.)

Theta Rhythm

Theta waves have been first described in the rabbit hippocampus during arousal elicited by sensory or brainstem reticular formation stimulation (Green and Arduini, 1954). This rhythm is usually considered within the frequency range of 4 to 7 Hz.

The cellular bases of theta waves have been intensively investigated in rodents (see below), but this rhythm is less evident in other mammals. In cats, the theta hippocampal activity is quite conspicuous during REM sleep, but occurs only exceptionally during wakefulness (Jouvet, 1965). It was also claimed that theta rhythm decreases in amplitude and regularity from rodents to other species and is poorly represented in primates (Crowne and Radcliffe, 1975; but see Stewart and Fox, 1991). As to humans, the presence of this rhythm was denied, even with deep electrodes inserted in the hippocampus (Brazier, 1968; Halgren et al., 1978, 1985). The normal theta activity, generally considered as poor or absent in primates, should not be confused with the so-called pathological theta waves, described as a slowing down of alpha activity, due to great reduction in cerebral blood flow (Ingvar et al., 1976), to metabolic encephalopathies (Saunders and Westmoreland, 1979), or occurring after disturbances in deep midline structures (Gloor, 1976).

Figure 3.33. Behavior-dependent macroscopic (EEG) states in the hippocampus and their intracellular correlates in the rat. **A:** Extracellular recordings from the CA1 stratum radiatum of the left *(l)* and right *(r)* hippocampus during the transition from exploration (walk) to being still (still). Note regular theta waves during waking and large, negative sharp waves (SPW) during immobility. Note also that SPWs are bilaterally synchronous. **B:** A single SPW with simultaneously recorded fast field oscillation from the CA1 pyramidal layer at a faster time scale. **C,D:** Intracellular correlates of field theta (**C**) and SPW (**D**) in CA1 pyramidal cells under urethane anesthesia. In **C**, extracellular and intracellular averages of theta (*n* = 80 to 200 repetitions) at three different polarization levels. Note that hyperpolarization leads to a reversal of intracellular theta *(dotted lines)* at chloride equilibrium potentials (details not shown). In **D**, a single ripple event (extra) showing the trigger pulse used for intracellular (intra) averaging of SPW events. Note that intracellular hyperpolarization reveals a strong depolarization force during the ripple. Intracellular traces are averages of 10 to 20 repetitions. (Modified from Buzsáki, G. 1996. The hippocampal-neocortical dialogue. *Cereb. Cortex* 6:81–92.)

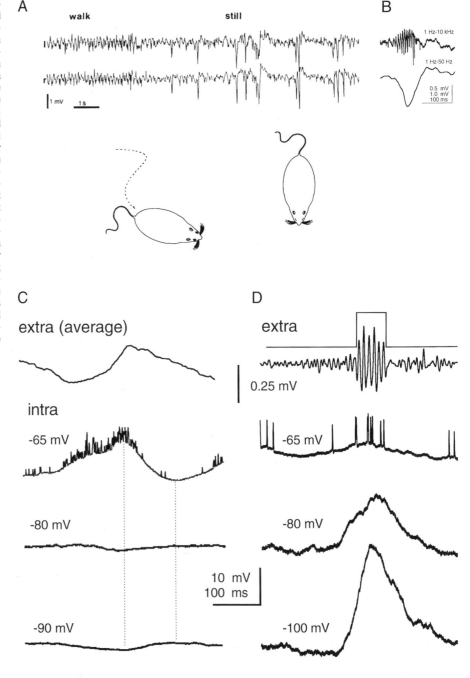

Because of the preponderance of theta waves in rodents, this section only briefly summarizes the origins and cellular mechanisms of theta waves in these species. The importance of theta rhythm transcends its relations with sensory processing and the control of different types of movements in rodents (Buzsáki, 1996; Grastyan et al., 1959; Vanderwolf and Leung, 1983) (Fig. 3.33). Indeed, the induction of long-term synaptic potentiation (LTP), a phenomenon involved in the beginnings of memory (Lynch, 1987), is optimal when the time interval between stimuli is about 0.2 seconds, which corresponds to the frequency band of hippocampal theta (Larson and Lynch, 1988; Larson et al., 1986; Pavlides et al., 1988). It was hypothesized (Larson and Lynch, 1988) that, at this frequency, the facilitation occurs because there is a suppression of IPSPs and a prolongation of the depolarization, resulting in an increased influx of calcium ions that would lead to an amplification of LTP.

Origins

Theta waves have been found in cortical limbic areas (such as hippocampus, entorhinal cortex, and cingular areas) where they are generally described as rhythmic slow activity (RSA) extending from 3–4 Hz to 10 Hz. The term *RSA* is used to avoid the term *theta rhythm*, which indicates a less broad frequency spectrum (4–7 Hz).

Some experimental results have suggested that the master structure controlling at least one type of theta activity is the septohippocampal cholinergic system, driven from the brainstem reticular core (Petsche et al., 1965). The rostral course of the ascending brainstem system triggering synchronized theta waves was traced by Vertes (1981, 1982) and the presence of theta-on cells in the caudal diencephalon was reported by Bland et al. (1995). Cellular recordings in the ventral part of the medial septum and the vertical branch of the diagonal band nucleus have shown that about half of these elements discharge in close time-relation with hippocampal RSA (Apostol and Creutzfeldt, 1974; Assaf and Miller, 1978; Gatzelu and Buño, 1982; Lamour et al., 1984). However, septal bursting cells are phase-locked with the hippocampal RSA even after fimbria cuts that interrupt the connections between septum and hippocampus (McLennan and Miller, 1976). On the other hand, lesions of the medial septum lead to the disappearance of hippocampal RSA (Petsche et al., 1962; Vinogradova et al., 1980). These data were at the basis of the claim that septum is the pacemaker of theta rhythm. Nonetheless, the local hippocampal circuits actively contribute to the genesis of theta waves as the application of the cholinergic agonist carbachol in hippocampal slices produces waves within the frequency range of theta (Konopacki et al., 1987).

Since atropine does not completely suppress theta activity, an additional (noncholinergic) system is believed to arise in the entorhinal cortex. Indeed, atropine totally eliminates hippocampal theta activity after entorhinal lesions (Vanderwolf and Leung, 1983). A dipole of RSA was found in the entorhinal cortex, with two amplitude maxima, one superficial in layer I-II and the other in layer III (Alonso and Garcia-Ausst, 1987a,b; Boejinga and Lopes da Silva, 1988; Mitchell and Ranck, 1980). Stellate cells in the layer II display intrinsic oscillations within the theta frequency (Alonso

and Llinás, 1989). The output from the entorhinal cortex activates the dentate granule cells and CA1 pyramids, regarded as main generators of hippocampal theta waves (Bland et al., 1980). The view that the most important inputs for the generation of theta activity are entorhinal afferents to the granule cells and CA1-CA3 pyramids (Buzsáki et al., 1983; Leung, 1984) is supported by experimental data showing that removal of the entorhinal input abolishes the large theta dipole in the hippocampal fissure (Ylinen et al., 1995). Another theta dipole is set up by inhibitory currents on pyramidal-cells' somata (Buzsáki et al., 1986; Soltesz and Deschênes, 1993) generated by hippocampal local-circuit inhibitory cells. Different dipoles have been found in restrained and freely moving animals (Bland et al., 1975; Green et al., 1960; Winston, 1974).

Cellular Mechanisms of Hippocampal Theta Waves

The discrepancies prevail over the agreements as to the cellular mechanisms underlying the genesis of the theta hippocampal theta waves. The first intracellular study showed that 85% of pyramidal cells impaled in CA1 and CA2 fields display oscillations of the membrane potentials that are synchronous with the field theta waves (Fujita and Sato, 1964). These authors considered the theta rhythm as mainly due to rhythmic EPSPs. The somatic hyperpolarizations were believed to result from the recurrent collateral activation of local-circuit inhibitory cells following the rhythmic discharges of pyramidal neurons driven by septal afferents. In addition to this recurrent inhibitory circuit, interneurons in the CA1 area are probably directly excited by septal inputs as well as by entorhinal inputs traveling in the perforant path (Buzsáki et al., 1983).

Whereas the prevalent view is that IPSPs are major events in CA1 pyramidal cells during RSA (Leung and Yim, 1983; Soltesz and Deschênes, 1993; see also Fig. 3.33C), Nuñez et al. (1987) claimed that RSA reflects excitatory postsynaptic potential (EPSPs) and presumably calcium-mediated slow spikes in CA1 and CA3 pyramids (Fig. 3.34). The majority of CA1 pyramidal cells undergo a sustained depolarization associated with a decrease in membrane conductance. Those authors concluded that the IPSPs do not play an essential role in the genesis of the focal theta waves. Thus, at the present time, there is not full agreement as to the PSPs and intrinsic currents involved in the different wave patterns of hippocampal RSA. Future studies should attempt simultaneous recordings from inhibitory interneurons and pyramidal cells to ascertain whether IPSPs contribute to the field theta activity. It was proposed that the sustained depolarization of pyramidal neurons during theta is due to a disinhibitory process due to a septum-induced suppression of tonic inhibition arising in hippocampal local-circuit inhibitory interneurons (Krnjević and Ropert, 1982; Krnjević et al., 1988).

Because the main origin of EEG waves should be searched in the synchronized PSPs and simultaneous intracellular recordings from a great number of neurons are impossible at this time, computer simulations have been used to produce oscillations similar to those observed in living

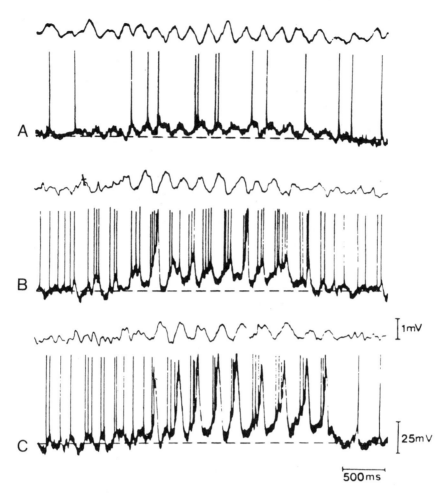

Figure 3.34. Theta rhythm generation. Hippocampal EEG *(upper trace)* and intracellular records of hippocampal pyramids *(lower trace)* in rats under urethane anesthesia. **A,B:** Two different CA1 pyramids. **C:** From CA3 pyramid. With theta waves, sustained depolarization above "resting" level *(broken lines)* are present in all cases. Smooth sine-like theta waves were recorded without (**A**), with occasional (**B**), or with continuously rhythmic (**C**) slow spikes. (Modified from Nuñez, A., Garcia-Ausst, E., and Buño, W. Jr. 1987. Intracellular theta rhythm generation in identified hippocampal pyramids. *Brain Res.* 416:289–300.)

animals. Traub and his colleagues (Miles et al., 1988; Traub et al., 1987, 1989; see also Pedley and Traub, 1990) have used models of the CA3 area with 200 to 20,000 pyramidal neurons as well as bursting and nonbursting inhibitory cells. Besides, they have endowed pyramidal neurons with slow inward currents to produce spontaneous spike bursts. Such a system displays a highly organized rhythmic activity at the population level, while individual elements show chaotic firing. These synchronized activities are similar to those seen experimentally.

Alpha Rhythm

This chapter ends with an account of what is presently known about the origin(s) of alpha rhythm occurring in the frequency range of 8 to 13 Hz. Although this is probably one of the few most important grapho-elements and its description dates back to Berger (1929), there is no knowledge about its cellular mechanisms because alpha waves have been mainly analyzed from scalp recordings in humans and laminar profiles of cortical field potentials in animals. For a description of different EEG patterns of alpha rhythms in the waking adult, see Niedermeyer (1987).

The temptation to understand the mechanisms of this rhythm at the cellular level by recording spindle oscillations under barbiturate anesthesia (Andersen and Andersson, 1968) is understandable, but alpha and spindle waves are quite different oscillations. Indeed, while the frequencies of these two rhythms may overlap, their origins and especially their behavioral context are dissimilar. Alpha waves are usually described as occurring during relaxed wakefulness. Some studies refer to them as a central timing mechanism regulating afferent and efferent signals (Sanford, 1971). The conventional wisdom that the occipital alpha rhythm is associated with reduced visual attention is challenged by the fact that the incidence of alpha waves increases during responses to visual stimuli or concentration on visual imagery (Mulholland, 1969) and the reports about augmentation of alpha activity during attention tasks (Creutzfeldt et al., 1969; Ray and Cole, 1985). Distinctly, spindle oscillations are associ-

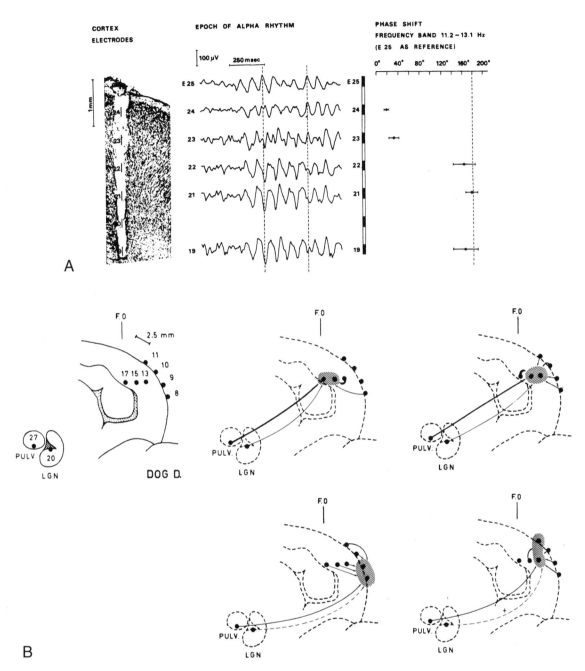

Figure 3.35. Alpha rhythm in dog. **A:** *Left,* photomicrograph of a section of the marginal gyrus (visual cortex). The electrode bundle consisted of seven wires with a bare tip of 0.15 mm. *Middle,* an epoch of alpha activity recorded simultaneously from six sites corresponding to those at *left,* against a common frontal cranial reference (negativity upward). Note that there is a polarity change between the most superficial sites (E25, 24) and the deepest sites (E22, 21, 19). *Right,* phase shift between the most superficial site (E25) and deeper lying sites computed by using spectral analysis based on the average of a number of epochs within the frequency band 11.2–13.1 Hz. The mean values of the phase shift and the corresponding standard deviations are indicated. **B:** Schematic view of the relationship between thalamic and cortical alpha activity. The *lines* indicate the amount of influence that a thalamic signal has on the coherence between a pair of cortical signals *(shaded area)* recorded during alpha activity. This was measured by partializing the intercortical coherence on the thalamic signals from the lateral geniculate nucleus (LGN) and pulvinar (PUL) or other cortical signals. Despite the fact that PUL has an influence on corticocortical domains of alpha activity, the intercortical factors play a significant role in the establishment of cortical domains of alpha activity. (Modified from Lopes da Silva, F.H., and Storm van Leeuwen, W. 1977. The cortical source of alpha activity. *Neurosci. Lett.* 6:237–241; and Lopes da Silva, F.H., Vos, J.E., Mooibroeck, J., et al. 1980. Relative contribution of intracortical and thalamo-cortical processes in the generation of alpha rhythms, revealed by partial coherence analysis. *Electroencephalogr. Clin Neurophysiol.* 50: 449–456).

ated with unconsciousness and with blockage of synaptic transmission through the thalamus from the very onset of sleep (Steriade et al., 1969; for review, see Steriade, 1991). Thus, the idea of an alpha-to-spindle continuum, or alpha viewed as an embryo of spindle oscillations, is untenable. As discussed below, not only the significance of spindle and alpha waves is different, but also their origins.

Lopes da Silva and his collaborators provided a series of experimental data toward the understanding of the origin of alpha rhythm in the dog. At variance with the thalamic origin of spindle oscillations, these authors suggested that alpha waves are mainly generated and spread within the cerebral cortex. Their data are as follows: (a) Alpha rhythms can be recorded from the visual cortex as well as from visual thalamic (lateral geniculate and pulvinar) nuclei (Lopes da Silva et al., 1973). (b) In the visual cortex, alpha waves are generated by an equivalent dipole layer centered at the level of the somata and basal dendrites of pyramidal neurons in layers IV and V (Lopes da Silva and Storm van Leeuwen, 1977) (Fig. 3.35A). (c) The coherence between alpha rhythms recorded in adjacent (~2 mm) foci of the visual cortex is larger than in any thalamocortical coherences measured in the same animal (Lopes da Silva and Storm van Leeuwen, 1978; Lopes da Silva et al., 1980) (Fig. 3.35B). These data led to the conclusion that a system of surface-parallel intracortical connections is mainly involved in the spread of alpha activity, while the influence of visual thalamic nuclei over the cerebral cortex is only moderate.

Final Remarks

The tendency of some investigators and practitioners to use the terms of various EEG rhythms by referring only to their frequency bands is misleading. Some points should be made: (a) EEG rhythms must be understood in the context of interconnected brain networks allowing synchronized activities of neuronal ensembles; (b) each rhythm should be placed within the context of distinct behavioral state; and (c) the knowledge of cellular mechanisms underlying various types of EEG oscillations is compelling. The last point is illustrated, for example, by the fact that various (slower and faster) types of spindle oscillations are easily understood on the basis of different durations of hyperpolarizations in TC cells, without calling for qualitatively different rhythmic activities.

Importantly, different sleep rhythms generated in neocortex and thalamus are coalesced due to the virtue of the cortically generated slow oscillation: during its depolarizing phase, all corticothalamic neurons fire synchronously, they drive thalamic reticular neurons, the pacemaker of spindles, thus each slowly oscillatory cycle also comprises a brief sequence of spindle waves (K complex). As well, the slow oscillation groups delta waves (Steriade and Amzica, 1998) and beta/gamma waves (Steriade et al., 1996a) because the latter are voltage (depolarization) dependent. This concept of a unified corticothalamic network that generates diverse types of brain rhythms grouped by the cortical slow oscillation (Steriade, 2001a,b) is supported by EEG studies in humans (Mölle et al., 2002).

The electrophysiologists interested in brain rhythmic activities perform analytical researches of central oscillations

by using intracellular recordings in *in vivo* preparations under various anesthetics or *in vitro* slices. Intracellular recordings of cortical cells in unanesthetized preparations are rarely used in relation with different behavioral conditions (but see Steriade et al., 2001; Timofeev et al., 2001); the difficulty to obtain stable recordings and to monitor the membrane potential in an animal with intense synaptic bombardment cannot be overemphasized. The *in vivo* studies on anesthetized animals and the *in vitro* works have provided the most reliable data on neuronal bases of EEG rhythms. This chapter is mainly built on their intracellular results. However, some anesthetics do not faithfully mimic the complex state of the EEG-synchronized sleep; for example, barbiturates induce overwhelming spindle oscillations that mask slower (0.1 to 4 Hz) rhythms. The ketamine-xylazine anesthesia is probably the best tool to obtain slow oscillations, in association with spindle waves, as well as fast rhythms during epochs associated with cells' depolarization. The *in vitro* techniques provide reliable data on intrinsic properties and ionic conductances of various cellular types. Of course, the very simplified circuitry in thin slices is far from the situation in the real nervous system, where a given structure displays a peculiar rhythm due to intrinsic membrane conductances and network properties, but also undergoes influences from a connected brain region exhibiting a different rhythmicity. Although brain slices represent a hypersimplified condition, some investigators use such terms as "spindles," "alpha," or "slow waves," only because of remote frequency similarities and despite the fact that the described rhythms have little to do with the patterns of bioelectrical activity in living animals. Future techniques will undoubtedly combine the opportunities provided by *in vitro* slices with the preserved connectivity of an intact brain.

References

Agmon, A., and Connors, B.W. 1989. Repetitive burst-firing in the deep layers of mouse somatosensory cortex. Neurosci. Lett. 99:137–141.

Alonso, A., and Garcia-Ausst, E. 1987a. Neuronal sources of theta rhythm in the entorhinal cortex of the rat. I. Laminar distribution of theta field potentials. Exp. Brain Res. 67:493–501.

Alonso, A., and Garcia-Ausst, E. 1987b. Neuronal sources of theta rhythm in the entorhinal cortex of the rat. II. Phase relations between unit discharges and theta field potentials. Exp. Brain Res. 67:502–509.

Alonso, A., and Llinás, R. 1989. Subthreshold theta-like rhythmicity in stellate cells of entorhinal cortex layer II. Nature 342:175–177.

Alonso, A., Khateb, A., Fort, P., et al. 1996. Differential oscillatory properties of cholinergic and noncholinergic nucleus basalis neurons in guinea pig brain slices. Eur. J. Neurosci. 8:169–182.

Altman, J., and Bayer, S.A. 1979. Development of the diencephalon in the rat. V. Thymidine-radiographic observations on internuclear and intranuclear gradients in the thalamus. J. Comp. Neurol. 188:473–500.

Amzica, F., and Neckelmann, D. 1999. Membrane capacitance of cortical neurons and glia during sleep oscillations and spike-wave seizures. J. Neurophysiol. 82:2731–2746.

Amzica, F., and Steriade, M. 1995a. Short- and long-range neuronal synchronization of the slow (<1 Hz) cortical oscillation. J. Neurophysiol. 73:20–39.

Amzica, F., and Steriade, M. 1995b. Disconnection of intracortical synaptic linkages disrupts synchronization of a slow oscillation. J. Neurosci. 15: 4658–4677.

Amzica, F., and Steriade, M. 1997a. The K-complex: its slow (<1 Hz) rhythmicity and relation with delta waves. Neurology 49:952–959.

Amzica, F., and Steriade, M. 1997b. Cellular substrates and laminar profile of sleep K-complex. Neuroscience 82:671–686.

Amzica, F., and Steriade, M. 1998. Electrophysiological correlates of sleep delta waves. Electroencephalogr. Clin. Neurophysiol. 107:69–83.

Amzica, F., and Steriade, M. 2000. Neuronal and glial membrane potentials during sleep and paroxysmal oscillations in the cortex. J. Neurosci. 20: 6646–6665.

Amzica, F., Nuñez, A., and Steriade, M. 1992. Delta frequency (1–4 Hz) oscillations of perigeniculate thalamic neurons and their modulation by light. Neuroscience 51:285–294.

Amzica, F., Neckelmann, D., and Steriade, M. 1997. Instrumental conditioning of fast (20- to 50-Hz) oscillations in corticothalamic networks. Proc. Natl. Acad. Sci. USA 94:1985–1989.

Amzica, F., Massimini, M., and Manfridi, A. 2002. Spatial buffering during slow and paroxysmal oscillations in cortical networks of glial cells in vivo. J. Neurosci. 22:1042–1053.

Andersen, P., and Andersson, S.A. 1968. *Physiological Basis of the Alpha Rhythm.* New York: Appleton-Century-Crofts.

Apostol, G., and Creutzfeldt, O.D. 1974. Cross-correlation between the activity of septal units and hippocampal EEG during arousal. Brain Res. 67:65–75.

Asanuma, C. 1994. GABAergic and pallidal terminals in the thalamic reticular nucleus of squirrel monkeys. Exp. Brain Res. 101:439–451.

Assaf, S.Y., and Miller, J.J. 1978. The role of the raphe serotonin system in the control of septal unit activity and hippocampal desynchronization. Neuroscience 3:539–550.

Avoli, M. 1986. Inhibitory potentials in neurons of the deep layers of the in vitro neocortical slices. Brain Res. 370:165–170.

Avoli, M., Gloor, P., Kostopoulos, G., et al. 1983. An analysis of penicillin-induced generalized spike and wave discharges using simultaneous recordings of cortical and thalamic single neurons. J. Neurophysiol. 50: 819–837.

Bal, T., and McCormick, D.A. 1996. What stops synchronized thalamocortical oscillations? Neuron 17:297–308.

Bal, T., von Krosigk, M., and McCormick, D.A. 1995a. Synaptic and membrane mechanisms underlying synchronized oscillations in the ferret lateral geniculate nucleus in vitro. J. Physiol. (Lond.) 483:641–663.

Bal, T., von Krosigk, M., and McCormick, D.A. 1995b. Role of the ferret perigeniculate nucleus in the generation of synchronized oscillations in vitro. J. Physiol. (Lond.) 483:665–685.

Ball, G.J., Gloor, P., and Schaul, N. 1977. The cortical electromicrophysiology of pathological delta waves in the electroencephalogram of cats. Electroencephalogr. Clin. Neurophysiol. 43:346–361.

Batini, C., Moruzzi, G., Palestini, M., et al. 1958. Persistent patterns of wakefulness in the pretrigeminal midpontine preparation. Science 128:30–32.

Bazhenov, M., Timofeev, I., Steriade, M., et al. 1998a. Cellular and network models for intrathalamic augmenting responses during 10-Hz stimulation. J. Neurophysiol. 79:2730–2748.

Bazhenov, M., Timofeev, I., Steriade, M., et al. 1998b. Computational models of thalamocortical augmenting responses. J. Neurosci. 18:6444–6465.

Bazhenov, M., Timofeev, I., Steriade, M., et al. 1999. Self-sustained rhythmic activity in the thalamic reticular nucleus mediated by depolarizing $GABA_A$ receptor potentials. Nat. Neurosci. 2:168–174.

Berger, H. 1929. Über das Elektoenkephalogramm des Menschen. Arch. Psychiatr. Nervenkr. 87:527–570.

Berman, N.J., Bush, P.C., and Douglas, R.J. 1989. Adaptation and bursting in neocortical neurons may be controlled by a single fast potassium conductance. Q. J. Exp. Physiol. 74:223–226.

Bland, B.H., Andersen, P., and Ganes, T. 1975. Two generators of hippocampal theta activity in rabbits. Brain Res. 94:199–218.

Bland, B.H., Andersen, P., Ganes, T., et al. 1980. Automated analysis of rhythmicity of physiologically identified hippocampal formation neurons. Exp. Brain Res. 38:205–219.

Bland, B.H., Konopacki, J., Kirk, I.J., et al. 1995. Discharge patterns of hippocampal theta-related cells in the caudal diencephalon of the urethan-anesthetized rat. J. Neurophysiol. 74:322–333.

Boejinga, P.H., and Lopes da Silva, F.H. 1988. Differential distribution of beta and theta EEG activity in the entorhinal cortex of the cat. Brain Res. 448:272–286.

Bouyer, J.J., Montaron, M.F., Vahnée, J.M., et al. 1987. Anatomical localization of cortical beta rhythm in cat. Neuroscience 22:863–869.

Brazier, M.A.B. 1968. Studies of the EEG activity of limbic structures in man. Electroencephalogr. Clin. Neurophysiol. 25:309–318.

Bremer, F. 1935. Cerveau "isolé" et physiologie du sommeil. C. R. Soc. Biol. (Paris) 118:1235–1241.

Bremer, F., and Stoupel, N. 1959. Facilitation et inhibition des potentiels évoqués corticaux dans l'éveil cérébral. Arch. Int. Physiol. 67:240–275.

Bremer, F., Stoupel, N., and Van Reeth, P.C. 1960. Nouvelles recherches sur la facilitation et l'inhibition des potentiels évoqués corticaux dans l'éveil réticulaire. Arch. Ital. Biol. 98:229–247.

Brunton, J., and Charpak, S. 1997. Heterogeneity of cell firing properties and opioid sensitivity in the thalamic reticular nucleus. Neuroscience 78:1671–1678.

Budde, T., Mager, R., and Pape, H.C. 1992. Different types of potassium outward current in relay neurons acutely isolated from the lateral geniculate nucleus. Eur. J. Neurosci. 4:708–722.

Buzsáki, G. 1991. The thalamic clock: emergent network properties. Neuroscience 41:351–364.

Buzsáki, G. 1996. The hippocampal-neocortical dialogue. Cereb. Cortex 6:81–92.

Buzsáki, G., Leung, L.S., and Vanderwolf, C.H. 1983. Cellular bases of hippocampal EEG in the behaving rat. Brain Res. 6:139–171.

Buzsáki, G., Czopf, J., Kondákor, I., et al. 1986. Laminar distribution of hippocampal rhythmic slow activity (RSA) in the behaving rat: current-source density analysis, effects of urethane and atropine. Brain Res. 365: 125–137.

Buzsáki, G., Bickford, R.G., Ponomareff, G., et al. 1988. Nucleus basalis and thalamic control of neocortical activity in the freely moving rat. J. Neurosci. 8:4007–4026.

Calvet, J., Calvet, M.C., and Scherrer, J. 1964. Etude stratigraphique corticale de l'activité EEG spontanée. Electroencephalogr. Clin. Neurophysiol. 17:109–125.

Castro-Alamancos, M.A., and Connors, B.W. 1996a. Spatiotemporal properties of short-term plasticity in sensorimotor thalamocortical pathways of the rat. J. Neurosci. 16:2767–2779.

Castro-Alamancos, M.A., and Connors, B.W. 1996b. Cellular mechanisms of the augmenting response: short-term plasticity in a thalamocortical pathway. J. Neurosci. 16:7742–7756.

Chagnac-Amitai, Y., and Connors, B.W. 1989. Synchronized excitation and inhibition driven by bursting neurons in neocortex. J. Neurophysiol. 62:1149–1162.

Connors, B.W. 1984. Initiation of synchronized neuronal bursting in neocortex. Nature 310:685–687.

Connors, B.W., and Amitai, Y. 1995. Functions of local circuits in neocortex: synchrony and laminae. In *The Cortical Neuron*, Eds. M.J. Gutnick and I. Mody, pp. 123–140. New York-Oxford: Oxford University Press.

Connors, B.W., and Gutnick, M.J. 1990. Intrinsic firing patterns of diverse neocortical neurons. Trends Neurosci. 13:99–104.

Connors, B.W., Gutnick, M.J., and Prince, D.A. 1982. Electrophysiological properties of neocortical neurons in vitro. J. Neurophysiol. 48:1302–1320.

Contreras, D., and Steriade, M. 1995. Cellular basis of EEG sleep rhythms: a study of dynamic corticothalamic relationships. J. Neurosci. 15:604–622.

Contreras, D., and Steriade, M. 1996. Spindle oscillation in cats: the role of corticothalamic feedback in a thalamically generated rhythm. J. Physiol. (Lond.) 490:159–179.

Contreras, D., Curró Dossi, R., and Steriade, M. 1992. Bursting and tonic discharges in two classes of reticular thalamic neurons. J. Neurophysiol. 68:973–977.

Contreras, D., Curró Dossi, R., and Steriade, M. 1993. Electrophysiological properties of cat reticular neurones in vivo. J. Physiol. (Lond.) 470: 273–294.

Contreras, D., Destexhe, A., Sejnowski, T.J., et al. 1996a. Control of spatiotemporal coherence of a thalamic oscillation by corticothalamic feedback. Science 274:771–774.

Contreras, D., Timofeev, I., and Steriade, M. 1996b. Mechanisms of long-lasting hyperpolarizations underlying slow sleep oscillations in cat corticothalamic networks. J. Physiol. (Lond.) 494:251–264.

Contreras, D., Destexhe, A., Sejnowski, T.J., et al. 1997. Spatiotemporal patterns of spindle oscillations in cortex and thalamus. J. Neurosci. 17:1179–1196.

Creutzfeldt, O.D., Watanabe, S., and Lux, H.D. 1966. Relations between EEG phenomena and potentials of single cells. I. Evoked responses after thalamic and epicortical stimulation. Electroencephalogr. Clin. Neurophysiol. 20:1–18.

Creutzfeldt, O., Grünvald, G., Simonova, O., et al. 1969. Changes of the basic rhythms of the EEG during the performance of mental and visuomotor tasks. In *Attention in Neurophysiology*. Eds. C.R. Evans and T.B. Mulholland, pp. 148–168. London: Butterworth.

Crowne, D.P., and Radcliffe, D.D. 1975. Some characteristics and functional relations of the electrical activity of the primate hippocampus and hypotheses of hippocampal function. In *The Hippocampus*. Eds. R.L. Isaacson and J.H. Pribram, pp. 185–203. New York: Plenum.

Crunelli, V., and Leresche, N. 2002. Childhood absence epilepsy: genes, channels, neurons and networks. Nat. Rev. Neurosci. 3:371–382.

Crunelli, V., Haby, M., Jassik-Gerschenfeld, D., et al. 1988. Cl⁻ and K⁺-dependent inhibitory postsynaptic potentials evoked by interneurons of the rat lateral geniculate nucleus. J. Physiol. (Lond.) 399:153–176.

Cunningham, E.T., and LeVay, S. 1986. Laminar and synaptic organization of the projection from the thalamic nucleus centralis to primary visual cortex in the cat. J. Comp. Neurol. 254:65–77.

Curró Dossi, R., Paré, D., and Steriade, M. 1991. Short-lasting nicotinic and long-lasting muscarinic depolarizing responses of thalamocortical neurons to stimulation of mesopontine cholinergic nuclei. J. Neurophysiol. 65:393–406.

Curró Dossi, R., Nuñez, A., and Steriade, M. 1992a. Electrophysiology of a slow (0.5–4 Hz) intrinsic oscillation of cat thalamocortical neurones in vivo. J. Physiol. (Lond.) 447:215–234.

Curró Dossi, R., Paré, D., and Steriade, M. 1992b. Various types of inhibitory postsynaptic potentials in anterior thalamic cells are differentially altered by stimulation of laterodorsal tegmental cholinergic nucleus. Neuroscience 47:279–289.

Deschênes, M., Paradis, M., Roy, J.P., et al. 1984. Electrophysiology of neurons of lateral thalamic nuclei in cat: resting properties and burst discharges. J. Neurophysiol. 51:1196–1219.

Deschênes, M., Madariaga-Domich, A., and Steriade, M. 1985. Dendrodendritic synapses in cat reticularis thalami nucleus, a structural basis for thalamic spindle synchronization. Brain Res. 334:169–171.

Destexhe, A. 1998. Spike-and-wave oscillations based on the properties of GABA_B receptors. J. Neurosci. 18:9099–9111.

Destexhe, A., Contreras, D., Sejnowski, T.J., et al. 1994a. A model of spindle rhythmicity in the isolated thalamic reticular nucleus. J. Neurophysiol. 72:803–818.

Destexhe, A., Contreras, D., Sejnowski, T.J., et al. 1994b. Modeling the control of reticular thalamic oscillations by neuromodulators. NeuroReport 5:2217–2220.

Destexhe, A., Contreras, D., Steriade, M., et al. 1996. In vivo, in vitro, and computational analysis of dendritic calcium currents in thalamic reticular neurons. J. Neurosci. 16:169–185.

Domich, L., Oakson, G., and Steriade, M. 1986. Thalamic burst patterns in the naturally sleeping cat: a comparison between cortically-projecting and reticularis neurones. J. Physiol. (Lond.) 379:429–450.

Domich, L., Oakson, G., Deschênes, M., et al. 1987. Thalamic and cortical spindles during early ontogenesis in kittens. Dev. Brain Res. 31:140–142.

Dumont, S., and Dell, P. 1960. Facilitation réticulaire des mécanismes visuels corticaux. Electrocephalogr. Clin. Neurophysiol. 12:769–796.

Eckhorn, R., Bauer, R., Jordan, W., et al. 1988. Coherent oscillations: a mechanism of feature linking in the visual cortex? Biol. Cybern. 60:121–130.

Engel, A.K., König, P., Gray, C.M., et al. 1990. Stimulus-dependent neuronal oscillations in cat visual cortex: inter-columnar interaction as determined by cross-correlation analysis. Eur. J. Neurosci. 2:588–606.

Engel, A.K., König, P., Kreiter, A.K., et al. 1991a. Interhemispheric synchronization of oscillatory neuronal responses in cat visual cortex. Science 252:1177–1179.

Engel, A.K., Kreiter, A.K., König, P., et al. 1991b. Synchronization of oscillatory neuronal responses between striate and extrastriate visual cortical areas of the cat. Proc. Natl. Acad. Sci. USA 88:6048–6052.

Eysel, U.T., Pape, H.C., and Van Schayck, R. 1986. Excitatory and differential disinhibitory actions of acetylcholine in the lateral geniculate nucleus of the cat. J. Physiol. (Lond.) 370:233–254.

Feinberg, I., and Campbell, I.G. 1993. Ketamine administration during waking increases delta EEG intensity in rat sleep. Neuropharmacology 9:41–48.

Ferster, D., and Lindström, S. 1986. Augmenting responses evoked in area 17 of the cat by intracortical axonal collaterals of corticogeniculate cells. J. Physiol. (Lond.) 367:217–232.

Freeman, W.J. 1975. *Mass Action in the Nervous System*. New York: Academic Press.

Freeman, W.J., and Van Dijk, B.W. 1988. Spatial patterns of visual cortical fast EEG during conditioned reflex in a rhesus monkey. Brain Res. 422:267–276.

Fuentealba, P., Crochet, S., Timofeev, I., et al. 2002. "Spikelets" in cat thalamic reticular nucleus in vivo. Soc. Neurosci. Abstr. 28:144.19.

Fujita, Y., and Sato, T. 1964. Intracellular records from hippocampal pyramidal cells in rabbit during theta rhythm activity. J. Neurophysiol. 27:1011–1025.

Gais, S., Plihal, W., Wagner, U., et al. 2000. Early sleep triggers memory for early visual discrimination skills. Nat. Neurosci. 3:1335–1339.

Gais, S., Mölle, M., Helms, K., et al. 2002. Learning-dependent increases in sleep density. J. Neurosci. 22:6830–6834.

Gatzelu, J.M., and Buño, W. 1982. Septo-hippocampal relationships during the EEG theta rhythm. Electroencephalogr. Clin. Neurophysiol. 54:375–387.

Glenn, L.L., and Steriade, M. 1982. Discharge rate and excitability of cortically projecting intralaminar thalamic neurons during waking and sleep states. J. Neurosci. 2:1287–1404.

Gloor, P. 1976. Generalized and widespread bilateral paroxysmal abnormalities. In *Handbook of Electroencephalography and Clinical Neurophysiology*, vol. 11, part B, Ed. A. Remond, pp. 11B52–11B87. Amsterdam: Elsevier.

Gloor, P., and Fariello, R.G. 1988. Generalized epilepsy: some of its cellular mechanisms differ from those of focal epilepsy. Trends Neurosci. 11:63–68.

Golomb, D., Wang, X.J., and Rinzel, J. 1994. Synchronization properties of spindle oscillations in a thalamic reticular nucleus. J. Neurophysiol. 72:1109–1126.

Golshani, P., Liu, X.B., and Jones, E.G. 2001. Differences in quantal amplitude reflect GluR4-subunit number at corticothalamic synapses on two populations of thalamic neurons. Proc. Natl. Acad. Sci. USA 98:4172–4177.

Grastyan, E., Lissak, K., Madarasz, I., et al. 1959. The hippocampal electrical activity during the development of conditioned reflexes. Electroencephalogr. Clin. Neurophysiol. 11:409–430.

Gray, C.M., and McCormick, D.A. 1996. Chattering cells: superficial pyramidal neurons contributing to the generation of synchronous oscillations in the visual cortex. Science 274:109–113.

Gray, C.M., and Singer, W. 1989. Stimulus-specific neuronal oscillations in orientation columns of cat visual cortex. Proc. Natl. Acad. Sci. USA 86:1698–1702.

Gray, C.M., König, P., Engel, A.K., et al. 1989. Stimulus-specific neuronal oscillations in cat visual cortex exhibit inter-columnar synchronization which reflects global stimulus properties. Nature 338:334–337.

Gray, C.M., Engel, A.K., König, P., et al. 1990. Stimulus-dependent neuronal oscillations in cat visual cortex: receptive field properties and feature dependence. Eur. J. Neurosci. 2:607–619.

Green, J.D., and Arduini, A. 1954. Hippocampal electrical activity in arousal. J. Neurophysiol. 17:533–557.

Green, J.D., Maxwell, D.S., Schindler, W.J., et al. 1960. Rabbit EEG "theta" rhythm: its anatomical source and relation to activity in single neurons. J. Neurophysiol. 23: 403–420.

Gutfreund, Y., Yarom, Y., and Segev, I. 1995. Subthreshold oscillations and resonant frequency in guinea-pig cortical neurons: physiology and modelling. J. Physiol. (Lond.) 483:621–640.

Halgren, E., Bab, T.L., and Crandall, P.H. 1978. Human hippocampal formation EEG desynchronizes during attentiveness and movement. Electroencephalogr. Clin. Neurophysiol. 44:778–781.

Halgren, E., Smith, M.E., and Stapleton, J.M. 1985. Hippocampal field potentials evoked by repeated vs nonrepeated words. In *Electrical Activity of the Archicortex*. Eds. G. Buzsáki and C.H. Vanderwolf, pp. 67–81. Budapest: Akademiai Kiadó.

Hernández-Cruz, A., and Pape, H.C. 1989. Identification of two calcium currents in acutely dissociated neurons from the rat lateral geniculate nucleus. J. Neurophysiol. 61:1270–1283.

Hirsch, J.C., and Burnod, Y. 1987. A synaptically evoked late hyperpolarization in the rat dorsolateral geniculate neurons in vitro. Neuroscience 23:457–468.

Hirsch, J.C., Fourment, A., and Marc, M.E. 1983. Sleep-related variations of membrane potential in the lateral geniculate body relay neurons of the cat. Brain Res. 259:308–312.

Hu, B., Steriade, M., and Deschênes, M. 1989. The effects of brainstem peribrachial stimulation on reticular thalamic neurons: the blockage of spindle waves. Neuroscience 31:1–12.

Hughes, S.W., Cope, D.W., Blethyn, K.L., et al. 2002. Cellular mechanisms of the slow (<1 Hz) oscillation in thalamocortical neurons in vitro. Neuron 33:947–958.

Huguenard, J.R., and Prince, D.A. 1992. A novel T-type current underlies prolonged Ca^{2+}-dependent burst firing in GABAergic neurons of rat thalamic reticular nucleus. J. Neurosci. 12:3804–3817.

Ingvar, D.H., Sjölund, B., and Ardo, A. 1976. Correlation between ECG frequency, cerebral oxygen uptake and blood flow. Electroencephalogr. Clin. Neurophysiol. 41:268–276.

Jahnsen, H., and Llinás, R. 1984a. Electrophysiological properties of guinea-pig thalamic neurones: an in vitro study. J. Physiol. (Lond.) 349: 205–226.

Jahnsen, H., and Llinás, R. 1984b. Ionic basis for the electroresponsiveness and oscillatory properties of guinea-pig thalamic neurones in vitro. J. Physiol. (Lond.) 349:227–247.

Jasper, H.H. 1969. Mechanisms of propagation: extracellular studies. In *Basic Mechanisms of the Epilepsies,* Eds. H.H. Jasper et al., pp. 421–438. Boston: Little, Brown.

Jones, E.G. 1985. *The Thalamus.* New York: Plenum.

Jones, E.G. 1987. GABA-peptide neurons of the primate cerebral cortex. J. Mind Behav. 8:519–536.

Jouvet, M. 1965. Paradoxical sleep—a study of its nature and mechanisms. In *Progress in Brain Research, vol. 18, Sleep Mechanisms,* Eds. K. Akert, C. Bally, and J.P. Schadé, pp. 20–57. Amsterdam: Elsevier.

Kammermeier, P.J., and Jones, S.W. 1997. High-voltage-activated calcium currents in neurons acutely isolated from the ventrobasal nucleus of the rat thalamus. J. Neurophysiol. 77:465–475.

Kamondi, A., Williams, J.A., Hutcheon, B., et al. 1992. Membrane properties of mesopontine cholinergic neurons studied with the whole-cell patch-clamp technique: implications for behavioral state control. J. Neurophysiol. 68:1359–1372.

Kang, Y., and Kitai, S.T. 1990. Electrophysiological properties of pedunculopontine neurons and their postsynaptic responses following stimulation of substantia nigra reticulata. Brain Res. 535:79–95.

Kellaway, P. 1985. Sleep and epilepsy. Epilepsia 26 (suppl. 1):15–30.

Kettenmann, H., and Schachner, M. 1985. Pharmacological properties of γ-aminobutyric acid-, glutamate-, and aspartate-induced depolarizations in cultured astrocytes. J. Neurosci. 5:3295–3301.

Khateb, A., Mühlethaler, M., Alonso, A., et al. 1992. Cholinergic nucleus basalis neurons display the capacity for rhythmic bursting activity mediated by low-threshold calcium spikes. Neuroscience 51:489–494.

Kim, U., Bal, T., and McCormick, D.A. 1995. Spindle waves are propagating synchronized oscillations in the ferret LGN in vitro. J. Neurophysiol. 74:1301–1323.

Kisvárday, Z.F., Cowey, A., and Somogyi, P. 1983. Synaptic relationships of a type of GABA-immunoreactive neuron (clutch cell), spiny stellate cells and lateral geniculate nucleus afferents in layer IVC of the monkey striate cortex. Neuroscience 19:741–761.

Kisvárday, Z.F., Beaulieu, C., and Eysel, U.T. 1993 Network of GABAergic large basket cells in cat visual cortex (area 18): implication for lateral disinhibition. J. Comp. Neurol. 327:398–415.

Konopacki, J., Bland, B.H., MacIvar, M., et al. 1987. Cholinergic theta rhythm in transected hippocampal slices: independent CA1 and dentate generators. Brain Res. 436:21–22.

Krnjević, K. 1974. Chemical nature of synaptic transmission in vertebrates. Physiol. Rev. 54:418–540.

Krnjević, K., and Ropert, N. 1982. Electrophysiological and pharmacological characteristics of facilitation of hippocampal population spikes by stimulation of the medial septum. Neuroscience 7:2165–2183.

Krnjević, K., Ropert, N., and Caullo, J. 1988. Septohippocampal disinhibition. Brain Res. 438:182–192.

Lamour, Y., Dutar, P., and Caullo, J. 1984. Septo-hippocampal and other medial septum-diagonal band neurons: electrophysiological and pharmacological properties. Brain Res. 309:227–239.

Lancel, M., van Riezen, H., and Glatt, A. 1992. The time course of sigma activity and slow-wave activity during NREMS in cortical and thalamic EEG of the cat during baseline and after 12 hours of wakefulness. Brain Res. 596:285–295.

Landisman, C.E., Long, M.A., Beierlein, M., et al. 2002. Electrical synapses in the thalamic reticular nucleus. J. Neurosci. 22:1002–1009.

Larson, J., and Lynch, G. 1986. Role of N-methyl-D aspartate receptors in the induction of synaptic potentiation by burst stimulation patterned after the hippocampal theta rhythm. Brain Res. 441:111–118.

Larson, J., Wong, D., and Lynch, G. 1986. Patterned stimulation at the theta frequency is optimal for the induction of hippocampal long-term potentiation. Brain Res. 368:347–350.

Leonard, C.S., and Llinás, R.R. 1990. Electrophysiology of mammalian pedunculopontine and laterodorsal tegmental neurons *in vitro*: implications for the control of REM sleep. In *Brain Cholinergic Systems,* Eds. M. Steriade and D. Biesold, pp. 205–223. Oxford: Oxford University Press.

Leresche, N., Lightowler, S., Soltesz, I., et al. 1991. Low-frequency oscillatory activities intrinsic to rat and cat thalamocortical cells. J. Physiol. (Lond.) 441:155–174.

Leung, L.S. 1984. Model of gradual phase shift of theta rhythm in the rat. J. Neurophysiol. 52:1051–1065.

Leung, L.S., and Borst, J.G.G. 1987. Electrical activity of the cingulate cortex. I. Generating mechanisms and relations to behavior. Brain Res. 407:68–80.

Leung, L.W.S., and Yim, C.Y. 1986. Intracellular records of theta rhythm in hippocampal CA1 cells of the rat. Brain Res. 367:323–327.

Lindström, S., and Wróbel, A. 1990. Frequency dependent corticofugal excitation of principal cells in the cat's dorsal lateral geniculate nucleus. Exp. Brain Res. 79:313–318.

Liu, Z., Vergnes, M., Depaulis, A., et al. 1991. Evidence for a critical role of GABAergic transmission within the thalamus in the genesis and control of absence seizures in the rat. Brain Res. 545:1–7.

Liu, X.B., Warren, R.A., and Jones, E.G. 1995. Synaptic distribution of afferents from reticular nucleus in ventroposterior nucleus of cat thalamus. J. Comp. Neurol. 352:187–202.

Llinás, R.R. 1988. The intrinsic electrophysiological properties of mammalian neurons: insights into central nervous function. Science 242: 1654–1664.

Llinás, R.R. 1990. Intrinsic electrical properties of mammalian neurons and CNS function. In *Fidia Research Foundation Neuroscience Award Lectures,* pp. 175–194. New York: Raven Press.

Llinás, R.R., and Geijo-Barrientos, E. 1988. *In vitro* studies of mammalian thalamic and reticularis thalami neurons. In *Cellular Thalamic Mechanisms,* Eds. M. Bentivoglio and R. Spreafico, pp. 23–33. Amsterdam: Elsevier.

Llinás, R., and Paré, D. 1991. On dreaming and wakefulness. Neuroscience 44:521–535.

Llinás, R., and Ribary, U. 1992. Rostrocaudal scan in human brain: a global characteristic for the 40 Hz response during sensory input. In *Induced Rhythms in the Brain,* Eds. E. Basar, and T. Bullock, pp. 147–154. Boston: Birkhauser.

Llinás, R., and Ribary, U. 1993. Coherent 40-Hz oscillation characterizes dream state in humans. Proc. Natl. Acad. Sci. USA 90:2078–2081.

Llinás, R., and Yarom, Y. 1981a. Electrophysiology of mammalian inferior olivary neurones in vitro. Different types of voltage-dependent ionic conductances. J. Physiol. (Lond.) 315:549–567.

Llinás, R., and Yarom, Y. 1981b. Properties and distribution of ionic conductances generating electroresponsiveness of mammalian inferior olivary neurones in vitro. J. Physiol. (Lond.) 315:569–584.

Llinás, R., Grace, A.A., and Yarom, Y. 1991. In vitro neurons in mammalian cortical layer 4 exhibit intrinsic oscillatory activity in the 10- to 50-Hz frequency range. Proc. Natl. Acad. Sci. USA 88:897–901.

Loomis, A.L., Harvey, N., and Hobart, G.A. 1938. Distribution of disturbance patterns in the human electroencephalogram, with special reference to sleep. J. Neurophysiol. 1:413–430.

Lopes da Silva, F.H., and Storm van Leeuwen, W. 1977. The cortical source of alpha rhythm. Neurosci. Lett. 6:237–241.

Lopes da Silva, F.H., and Storm van Leeuwen, W. 1978. The cortical alpha rhythm in dog: depth and surface profile of phase. In *Architecture of the Cerebral Cortex,* IBRO monograph series vol. 3, Eds. M.A.B. Brazier and H. Petsche, pp. 319–333. New York: Raven Press.

Lopes da Silva, F.H., Van Rotterdam A., Storm van Leeuwen, W., et al. 1970. Dynamic characteristics of visual evoked potentials in the dog. II. Beta frequency selectivity in evoked potentials and background activity. Electroencephalogr. Clin. Neurophysiol. 29:260–268.

Lopes da Silva, F.H., Van Lierop, T.H.M.T., Schrijer, C.F.M., et al. 1973. Organization of thalamic and cortical alpha rhythm: spectra and coherences. Electroencephalogr. Clin. Neurophysiol. 35:627–639.

Lopes da Silva, F.H., Vos, J.E., Mooibroeck, J., et al. 1980. Relative contribution of intracortical and thalamo-cortical processes in the generation of alpha rhythms, revealed by partial coherence analysis. Electroencephalogr. Clin. Neurophysiol. 50:449–456.

Lübke, J.I., Greene, R.W., Semba, K., et al. 1992. Serotonin hyperpolarizes cholinergic low-threshold burst neurons in the rat laterodorsal tegmental nucleus in vitro. Proc. Natl. Acad. Sci. USA 89:743–747.

Lynch, G. 1987. *Synapses, Circuits, and the Beginnings of Memory.* Cambridge, MA: MIT Press.

Lytton, W.W., and Sejnowski, T.J. 1991. Simulations of cortical pyramidal neurons synchronized by inhibitory interneurons. J. Neurophysiol. 66:1159–1179.

Lytton, W.W., Contreras, D., Destexhe, A., et al. 1997. Dynamic interactions determine partial thalamic quiescence in a computer network model of spike-wave seizures. J. Neurophysiol. 77:1679–1696.

Marcus, E.W., Watson, C.W., and Simon, S.A. 1968a. An experimental model of some varieties of petit mal epilepsy. Electrical-behavioral correlations of acute bilateral epileptogenic foci in cerebral cortex. Epilepsia 9:233–248.

Marcus, E.M., Watson, C.W., and Simon, S.A. 1968b. Behavioral correlates of acute bilateral symmetrical epileptogenic foci in monkey cerebral cortex. Brain Res. 9:370–373.

Massimini, M., and Amzica, F. 2001. Extracellular calcium fluctuations and intracellular potentials in the cortex during the slow sleep oscillation. J. Neurophysiol. 85:1346–1350.

Massimini, M., Rosanova, M., and Mariotti, M. 2003. EEG slow (~1 Hz) waves are associated with nonstationarity of thalamo-cortical sensory processing in the sleeping human. J. Neurophysiol. 89:1205–1213.

McCarley, R.W., Benoit, O., and Barrionuevo, G. 1983. Lateral geniculate nucleus unitary discharge in sleep and waking: state- and rate-specific aspects. J. Neurophysiol. 50:798–818.

McCormick, D.A. 1990. Cellular mechanisms of cholinergic control of neocortical and thalamic neuronal excitability. In *Brain Cholinergic Systems,* Eds. M. Steriade and D. Biesold, pp. 236–264. Oxford-New York: Oxford University Press.

McCormick, D.A. 1991. Functional properties of a slowly inactivating potassium current I_{As} in guinea pig dorsal lateral geniculate relay neurons. J. Neurophysiol. 66:1176–1189.

McCormick, D.A., and von Krosigk, M. 1992. Corticothalamic activation modulates thalamic firing through activation of glutamate metabotropic receptors. Proc. Natl. Acad. Sci. USA 89:2774–2778.

McCormick, D.A., and Pape, H.C. 1990a. Properties of a hyperpolarization-activated cation current and its role in rhythmic oscillation in thalamic relay neurones. J. Physiol. (Lond.) 431:291–318.

McCormick, D.A., and Pape, H.C. 1990b. Noradrenergic and serotonergic modulation of a hyperpolarization-activated cation current in thalamic relay cells. J. Physiol. (Lond.) 431:319–342.

McCormick, D.A., and Prince, D.A. 1986. Acetylcholine induces burst firing in thalamic reticular neurones by activating a K+ conductance. Nature 319:147–165.

McCormick, D.A., and Prince, D.A. 1987. Actions of acetylcholine in the guinea pig and cat medial and lateral geniculate nuclei, in vitro. J. Physiol. (Lond.) 392:147–165.

McCormick, D.A., and Prince, D.A. 1988. Noradrenergic modulation of firing pattern in guinea pig and cat thalamic neurons, in vitro. J. Neurophysiol. 59:978–996.

McCormick, D.A., and Wang, Z. 1991. Serotonin and noradrenaline excite GABAergic neurones of the guinea-pig and cat nucleus reticularis thalami. J. Physiol. (Lond.) 442:235–255.

McCormick, D.A., and Williamson, A. 1989. Convergence and divergence of neurotransmitter action in human cerebral cortex. Proc. Natl. Acad. Sci. USA 86:8098–8102.

McCormick, D.A., Connors, B.W., Lighthall, J.W., et al. 1985. Comparative electrophysiology of pyramidal and sparsely spiny stellate neurons of the neocortex. J. Neurophysiol. 54:782–806.

McLennan, H., and Miller, J.J. 1976. Frequency-related inhibitory mechanisms controlling rhythmical activity in the septal area. J. Physiol. (Lond.) 254:827–841.

Miles, R., Traub, R.D., and Wong, R.K.S. 1988. Spread of synchronous firing in longitudinal slices from the CA3 region of the hippocampus. J. Neurophysiol. 60:1281–1496.

Mishkin, M. 1982. A memory system in the monkey. Philos. Trans. R. Soc. Lond. B Biol. Sci. 298:85–95.

Mitchell, S., and Ranck, J.B., Jr. 1980. Generation of theta rhythm in medial entorhinal cortex of freely moving rats. Brain Res. 189:49–66.

Mölle, M., Marshall, L., Gais, S., et al. 2002. Grouping of spindle activity during slow oscillations in human non-REM sleep. J. Neurosci. 22:10941–10947.

Morin, D., and Steriade, M. 1981. Development from primary to augmenting responses in primary somatosensory cortex. Brain Res. 205:49–66.

Morison, R.S., and Bassett, D.L. 1945. Electrical activity of the thalamus and basal ganglia in decorticate cats. J. Neurophysiol. 8:309–314.

Morison, R.S., and Dempsey, E.W. 1942. A study of thalamocortical relations. Am. J. Physiol. 135:281–292.

Moruzzi, G., and Magoun, H.W. 1949. Brain stem reticular formation and activation of the EEG. Electroencephalogr. Clin. Neurophysiol. 1:455–473.

Mulholland, T. 1969. The concept of attention and the electroencephalographic alpha rhythm. In *Attention in Neurophysiology,* Eds. C.R. Evans and T.B. Mulholland, pp. 100–127. London: Butterworth.

Mulle, C., Steriade, M., and Deschênes, M. 1985. The effects of QX-314 on thalamic neurons. Brain Res. 333:350–354.

Mulle, C., Madariaga, A., and Deschênes, M. 1986. Morphology and electrophysiological properties of reticularis thalami neurons in cat: in vivo study of a thalamic pacemaker. J. Neurosci. 6:2134–2145.

Murthy, V.N., and Fetz, E.E. 1992. Coherent 25- to 35-Hz oscillations in the sensorimotor cortex of awake behaving monkeys. Proc. Natl. Acad. Sci. USA 89:5670–5674.

Nagy, J.I., Yamamoto, T., Shiosaka, S., et al. 1988. Immunohistochemical localization of gap junction protein in rat CNS: a preliminary account. In *Gap Junction,* Eds. E.L. Hertzberg and R.G. Johnson, pp. 375–389. New York: Alan R. Liss.

Necklemann, D., Amzica, F., and Steriade, M. 1998. Spike-wave complexes and fast components of cortically generated seizures. III. Synchronizing mechanisms. J. Neurophysiol. 80:1480–1494.

Necklemann, D., Amzica, F., and Steriade, M. 2000. Changes in neuronal conductance during different components of cortically generated spike-wave seizures. Neuroscience 96:475–485.

Nicoll, R.A., Malenka R.C., and Kauer, J.A. 1990. Functional comparison of neurotransmitter receptor subtypes in mammalian central nervous system. Physiol. Rev. 70:513–565.

Niedermeyer, E. 1987. The normal EEG of the waking adult. In *Electroencephalography,* 2nd ed., Eds. E. Niedermeyer and F. Lopes da Silva, pp. 99–117. Baltimore-Munich: Urban & Schwarzenberg.

Niedermeyer, E. 1993. Sleep and EEG. In *Electroencephalography,* 3rd ed., Eds. E. Niedermeyer and F. Lopes da Silva, pp. 153–166. Baltimore: Williams & Wilkins.

Nuñez, A., Garcia-Austt, E., and Buño, W., Jr. 1987. Intracellular theta rhythm generation in identified hippocampal pyramids. Brain Res. 416:289–300.

Nuñez, A., Amzica, F., and Steriade, M. 1992a. Voltage-dependent fast (20–40 Hz) oscillations in long-axoned neocortical neurons. Neuroscience 51:7–10.

Nuñez, A., Curró Dossi, R., Contreras, D., et al. 1992b. Intracellular evidence for incompatibility between spindle and delta oscillations in thalamocortical neurons of cat. Neuroscience 48:75–85.

Paré, D., Steriade, M., Deschênes, M., et al. 1987. Physiological properties of anterior thalamic nuclei, a group devoid of inputs from the reticular thalamic nucleus. J. Neurophysiol. 57:1669–1685.

Paré, D., Steriade, M., Deschênes, M., et al. 1990. Prolonged enhancement of anterior thalamic synaptic responsiveness by stimulation of a brainstem cholinergic group. J. Neurosci. 10:20–33.

Paré, D., Curró Dossi, R., and Steriade, M. 1991. Three types of inhibitory postsynaptic potentials generated by interneurons in the anterior thalamic complex of cat. J. Neurophysiol. 66:1190–1204.

Pavlides, C., Greenstein, Y.J., Goudman, M., et al. 1988. Long-term potentiation in the dentate gyrus is induced preferentially on the positive phase of the theta-rhythm. Brain Res. 439:383–387.

Pedley, T.A., and Traub, R.D. 1990. Physiological basis of EEG. In *Current Practice of Clinical Electroencephalography,* 2nd ed., Eds. D.D. Daly and T.A. Pedley, pp. 107–137. New York: Raven Press.

Pedroarena, C., and Llinás, R. 1997. Dendritic calcium conductances generate high-frequency oscillation in thalamocortical neurons. Proc. Natl. Acad. Sci. USA 94:724–728.

Petsche, H., Stumpf, C., and Gogolak, G. 1962. The significance of the rabbit's septum as a relay station between the midbrain and the hippocampus. The control of hippocampus arousal activity by septum cells. Electroencephalogr. Clin. Neurophysiol. 14:202–211.

Petsche, H., Gogolak, G., and van Zwieten, P.A. 1965. Rhythmicity of septal cell discharges at various levels of reticular excitation. Electroencephalogr. Clin. Neurophysiol. 19:25–33.

Petsche, H., Pockeberger, H., and Rappelsberger, P. 1984. On the search for the sources of the electroencephalogram. Neuroscience 11:1–27.

Pinault, D., Leresche, N., Charpier, S., et al. 1998. Intracellular recordings in thalamic neurones during spontaneous spike and wave discharges in rats with absence epilepsy. J. Physiol. (Lond.) 509:449–456.

Purpura, D.P., Shofer, R.J., and Musgrave, F.S. 1964. Cortical intracellular potentials during augmenting and recruiting responses. II. Patterns of synaptic activities in pyramidal and non-pyramidal tract neurons. J. Neurophysiol. 27:133–151.

Ralston, B., and Ajmone-Marsan, C. 1956. Thalamic control of certain normal and abnormal cortical rhythms. Electroencephalogr. Clin. Neurophysiol. 8:559–582.

Ray, W.J., and Cole, H.W. 1985. EEG alpha activity reflects attentional demands and beta activity reflects emotional and cognitive processes. Science 228:750–752.

Roth, M., Shaw, J., and Green, J. 1956. The form, voltage distribution and physiological significance of the K-complex. Electroencephalogr. Clin. Neurophysiol. 8:385–402.

Rougeul-Buser, A., Bouyer, J.J., Montaron, M.F., et al. 1983. Patterns of activities in the ventrobasal thalamus and somatic cortex SI during behavioral immobility in the awake cat: focal waking rhythms. Exp. Brain Res. (Suppl.) 7:69–87.

Roy, J.P., Clercq, M., Steriade, M., et al. 1984. Electrophysiology of neurons of the lateral thalamic nuclei in cat: mechanisms of long-lasting hyperpolarizations. J. Neurophysiol. 51:1220–1235.

Sanchez-Vives, M.V., and McCormick, D.A. 2000. Cellular and network mechanisms of rhythmic recurrent activity in neocortex. Nat. Neurosci. 3:1027–1034.

Sanford, A.J. 1971. A periodic basis for perception and action. In *Biological Rhythms and Human Perception,* Ed., W.P. Colquhoun, pp. 179–209. New York: Academic Press.

Saper, C.B. 1987. Diffuse cortical projection systems: anatomical organization and role in cortical function. In *Handbook of Physiology. The Nervous System,* vol. V, part 1, Eds. V.B. Mountcastle and F. Plum, pp. 169–210. Bethesda: American Physiological Society.

Saunders, M.G., and Westmoreland, B.F. 1979. The EEG in evaluation of disorders affecting the brain diffusely. In *Current Practice of Clinical Electroencephalography,* Eds. D.W. Klass and D.D. Daly, pp. 343–379. New York: Raven Press.

Schwindt, P.C., Spain, W.J., Foehring, R.C., et al. 1988a. Multiple potassium conductances and their functions in neurons from cat sensorimotor cortex *in vitro.* J. Neurophysiol. 59:424–449.

Schwindt, P.C., Spain, W.J., Foehring, R.C., et al. 1988b. Slow conductances in neurons from cat sensorimotor cortex in vitro and their role in slow excitability changes. J. Neurophysiol. 59:450–467.

Schwindt, P.C., Spain, W.J., and Crill, W.E. 1989. Long-lasting reduction of excitability by a sodium-dependent potassium current in cat neocortical neurons. J. Neurophysiol. 61:233–244.

Shadlen, M.N., and Movshon, J.A. 1999. Synchrony unbound: a critical evaluation of the temporal binding problem. Neuron 24:67–77.

Sheer, D. 1984. Focused arousal, 40 Hz, and dysfunction. In *Selfregulation of the Brain and Behavior,* Ed. T. Ebert, pp. 64–84. Berlin: Springer.

Silva, L.R., Amitai, Y., and Connors, B.W. 1991. Intrinsic oscillations of neocortex generated by layer 5 pyramidal neurons. Science 251:432–435.

Simon, N.R., Mandshanden, I., and Lopes da Silva, F.H. 2000. A MEG study of sleep. Brain Res. 860:64–76.

Singer, W. 1990a. Search for coherence: a basic principle of cortical self-organization. Concepts Neurosci. 1:1–26.

Singer, W. 1990b. Role of acetylcholine in use-dependent plasticity of the visual cortex. In *Brain Cholinergic Systems.* Eds. M. Steriade and D. Biesold, pp. 314–336. Oxford: Oxford University Press.

Singer, W. 1999. Neuronal synchrony: a versatile code for the definition of relations? Neuron 24:49–65.

Soltesz, I., and Deschênes, M. 1993. Low- and high-frequency membrane potential oscillations during theta activity in CA1 and CA3 pyramidal neurons of the rat hippocampus under ketamine-xylazine anesthesia. J. Neurophysiol. 70:97–116.

Soltesz, I., Lightowler, S., Leresche, N., et al. 1991. Two inward currents and the transformation of low-frequency oscillations of rat and cat thalamocortical cells. J. Physiol. (Lond.) 441:175–197.

Somogyi, P., Kisvárday, Z.F., Martin, K.A.C., et al. 1983. Synaptic connections of morphologically identified and physiologically characterized large basket cells in the striate cortex of cat. Neuroscience 10:261–294.

Somogyi, P., Hodgson, A.J., Smith, A.D., et al. 1984. Different populations of GABAergic neurons in the visual cortex and hippocampus of cat contain somatostatin- or cholecystokinin-immunoreactive material. J. Neurosci. 4:2590–2603.

Spain, W.J., Schwindt, P.C., and Crill, W.E. 1991a. Two transient potassium currents in layer V pyramidal neurones from cat sensorimotor cortex. J. Physiol. (Lond.) 434:591–607.

Spain, W.J., Schwindt, P.C., and Crill, W.E. 1991b. Postinhibitory excitation and inhibition in layer V pyramidal neurones from cat sensorimotor cortex. J. Physiol. (Lond.) 434:609–626.

Spencer, W.A., and Brookhart, J.M. 1961. Electrical patterns of augmenting and recruiting waves in the depths of the sensorimotor cortex of cat. J. Neurophysiol. 24:26–49.

Spreafico, R., De Curtis, M., Frassoni, C., et al. 1988. Electrophysiological characteristics of morphologically identified reticular thalamic neurons from rat slices. Neuroscience 27:629–638.

Spreafico, R., Battaglia, G., and Frassoni, C. 1991. The reticular thalamic nucleus (RTN) of the rat: cytoarchitectural, Golgi, immunocytochemical, and horseradish peroxidase study. J. Comp. Neurol. 304:478–490.

Stafstrom, C.E., Schwindt, P.C., Chubb, M.C., et al. 1985. Properties of persistent sodium conductance and calcium conductance of layer V neurons from cat sensorimotor cortex in vitro. J. Physiol. (Lond.) 53:163–170.

Steriade, M. 1970. Ascending control of thalamic and cortical responsiveness. Int. Rev. Neurobiol. 12:87–144.

Steriade, M. 1974. Interneuronal epileptic discharges related to spike-and-wave cortical seizures in behaving monkeys. Electroencephalogr. Clin. Neurophysiol. 37:247–263.

Steriade, M. 1978. Cortical long-axoned cells and putative interneurons during the sleep-waking cycle. Behav. Brain Sci. 3:465–514.

Steriade, M. 1981. Mechanisms underlying cortical activation: neuronal organization and properties of the midbrain reticular core and intralaminar thalamic nuclei. In *Brain Mechanisms and Perceptual Awareness,* Eds. O. Pompeiano and C. Ajmone-Marsan, pp. 327–377. New York: Raven Press.

Steriade, M. 1984. The excitatory-inhibitory response sequence of thalamic and neocortical cells: state-related changes and regulatory systems. In *Dynamic Aspects of Neocortical Function,* Eds. G.M. Edelman, W.E. Gall, and W.M. Cowan, pp. 107–157. New York: Wiley-Interscience.

Steriade, M. 1990. Spindling, incremental thalamocortical responses, and spike-wave epilepsy. In *Generalized Epilepsy,* Eds. M. Avoli, P. Gloor, G. Kostopoulos, and R. Naquet, pp. 161–180. Boston: Birkhäuser.

Steriade, M. 1991. Alertness, quiet sleep, dreaming. In *Cerebral Cortex,* vol. 9, Eds. A. Peters and E.G. Jones, pp. 279–357. New York: Plenum.

Steriade, M. 1993. Central core modulation of spontaneous oscillations and sensory transmission in thalamocortical systems. Curr. Opin. Neurobiol. 3:619–625.

Steriade, M. 1997. Synchronized activities of coupled oscillators in the cerebral cortex and thalamus at different levels of vigilance. Cereb. Cortex 7:583–604.

Steriade, M. 1999. Coherent oscillations and short-term plasticity in corticothalamic networks. Trends Neurosci. 22:337–345.

Steriade, M. 2000. Corticothalamic resonance, states of vigilance, and mentation. Neuroscience 101:243–276.

Steriade, M. 2001a. *The Intact and Sliced Brain.* Cambridge (MA): MIT Press.

Steriade, M. 2001b. Impact of network activities on neuronal properties in corticothalamic systems. J. Neurophysiol. 86:1–39.

Steriade, M. 2001c. The GABAergic reticular nucleus: a preferential target of corticothalamic projections. Proc. Natl. Acad. Sci. USA 98:3625–3627.

Steriade, M. 2003. *Neuronal Substrates of Sleep and Epilepsy.* Cambridge (UK): Cambridge University Press.

Steriade, M., and Amzica, F. 1994. Dynamic coupling among neocortical neurons during evoked and spontaneous spike-wave seizure activity. J. Neurophysiol. 72:2051–2069.

Steriade, M., and Amzica, F. 1996. Intracortical and corticothalamic coherency of fast spontaneous oscillations. Proc. Natl. Acad. Sci. USA 93:2533–2538.

Steriade, M., and Amzica, F. 1998. Coalescence of sleep rhythms and their chronology in corticothalamic networks. Sleep Res. Online 1:1–10.

Steriade, M., and Buzsáki, G. 1990. Parallel activation of thalamic and cortical neurons by brainstem and basal forebrain cholinergic systems. In *Brain Cholinergic Systems,* Eds. M. Steriade and D. Biesold, pp. 3–62. Oxford-New York: Oxford University Press.

Steriade, M., and Contreras, D. 1995. Relations between cortical and thalamic cellular events during transition from sleep patterns to paroxysmal activity. J. Neurosci. 15:623–642.

Steriade, M., and Contreras, D. 1998. Spike-wave complexes and fast runs of cortically generated seizures. I. Role of neocortex and thalamus. J. Neurophysiol. 80:1439–1455.

Steriade, M., and Demetrescu, M. 1960. Unspecific systems of inhibition and facilitation of potentials evoked by intermittent light. J. Neurophysiol. 23:602–617.

Steriade, M., and Deschênes, M. 1974. Inhibitory processes and interneuronal apparatus in motor cortex during sleep and waking. II. Recurrent and afferent inhibition of pyramidal tract neurons. J. Neurophysiol. 37:1093–1113.

Steriade, M., and Deschênes, M. 1984. The thalamus as a neuronal oscillator. Brain Res. Rev. 8:1–63.

Steriade, M., and Deschênes, M. 1988. Intrathalamic and brainstem-thalamic networks involved in resting and alert states. In *Cellular Thalamic Mechanisms,* Eds. M. Bentivoglio and R. Spreafico, pp. 51–76. Amsterdam: Elsevier.

Steriade, M., and Glenn, L.L. 1982. Neocortical and caudate projections of intralaminar thalamic neurons and their synaptic excitation from the midbrain reticular core. J. Neurophysiol. 48:352–371.

Steriade, M., and Llinás, R. 1988. The functional states of the thalamus and the associated neuronal interplay. Physiol. Rev. 68:649–742.

Steriade, M., and McCarley, R.W. 1990. *Brainstem Control of Wakefulness and Sleep.* New York: Plenum Press.

Steriade, M., and Timofeev, I. 1996. Intrathalamic mechanisms of short-term plasticity processes during incremental responses. Soc. Neurosci. Abstr. 22:2030.

Steriade, M., and Timofeev, I. 1997. Short-term plasticity during intrathalamic augmenting responses in decorticated cats. J. Neurosci. 17:3778–3795.

Steriade, M., and Timofeev, I. 2003. Neuronal plasticity in thalamocortical networks during sleep and waking oscillations. Neuron 37:563–576.

Steriade, M., and Yossif, G. 1974. Spike-and-wave afterdischarges in cortical somatosensory neurons of cat. Electroencephalogr. Clin. Neurophysiol. 37:633–648.

Steriade, M., Belekhova, M., and Apostol, V. 1968. Reticular potentiation of cortical flash-evoked afterdischarge. Brain Res. 11:276–280.

Steriade, M., Iosif, G., and Apostol, V. 1969. Responsiveness of thalamic and cortical motor relays during arousal and various stages of sleep. J. Neurophysiol. 32:251–265.

Steriade, M., Apostol, V., and Oakson, G. 1971. Control of unitary activities in cerebellothalamic pathway during wakefulness and synchronized sleep. J. Neurophysiol. 34:384–413.

Steriade, M., Wyzinski, P., and Apostol, V. 1972. Corticofugal projections governing rhythmic thalamic activity. In *Corticothalamic Projections and Sensorimotor Activities,* Eds. T.L. Frigyesi, E. Rinvik, and M.D. Yahr, pp. 221–272. New York: Raven Press.

Steriade, M., Oakson, G., and Diallo, A. 1976. Cortically elicited spike-wave afterdischarges in thalamic neurons. Electroencephalogr. Clin. Neurophysiol. 41:641–644.

Steriade, M., Oakson, G., and Ropert, N. 1982. Firing rates and patterns of midbrain reticular neurons during steady and transitional states of the sleep-waking cycle. Exp. Brain Res. 46:37–51.

Steriade, M., Parent, A., and Hada, J. 1984. Thalamic projections of nucleus reticularis thalami: a study using retrograde transport of horseradish peroxidase and double fluorescent tracers. J. Comp. Neurol. 229:531–547.

Steriade, M., Deschênes, M., Domich, L., et al. 1985. Abolition of spindle oscillations in thalamic neurons disconnected from nucleus reticularis thalami. J. Neurophysiol. 54:1473–1497.

Steriade, M., Domich, L., and Oakson, G. 1986. Reticularis thalamic neurons revisited: activity changes during shifts in states of vigilance. J. Neurosci. 6:68–81.

Steriade, M., Domich, L., Oakson, G., et al. 1987. The deafferented reticularis thalami nucleus generates spindle rhythmicity. J. Neurophysiol. 57:260–273.

Steriade, M., Datta, S., Paré, D., et al. 1990a. Neuronal activities in brainstem cholinergic nuclei related to tonic activation processes in thalamocortical systems. J. Neurosci. 10:2541–2559.

Steriade, M., Gloor, P., Llinás, R.R., et al. 1990b. Basic mechanisms of cerebral rhythmic activities. Electroencephalogr. Clin. Neurophysiol. 76:481–508.

Steriade, M., Jones, E.G., and Llinás, R.R. 1990c. *Thalamic Oscillations and Signaling.* New York: Wiley-Interscience.

Steriade, M., Paré, D., Datta, S., et al. 1990d. Different cellular types in mesopontine cholinergic nuclei related to ponto-geniculo-occipital waves. J. Neurosci. 10:2560–2579.

Steriade, M., Paré, D., Hu, B., et al. 1990e *The Visual Thalamocortical System and its Modulation by the Brain Stem Core,* vol. 10 in Sensory Physiology, pp. 1–124. Berlin: Springer.

Steriade, M., Curró Dossi, R., and Nuñez, A. 1991a. Network modulation of a slow intrinsic oscillation of cat thalamocortical neurons implicated in sleep delta waves: cortical potentiation and brainstem cholinergic suppression. J. Neurosci. 11:3200–3217.

Steriade, M., Curró Dossi, R., Paré, D., et al. 1991b. Fast oscillations (20–40 Hz) in thalamocortical systems and their potentiation by mesopontine cholinergic nuclei in the cat. Proc. Natl. Acad. Sci. USA 88: 4396–4400.

Steriade, M., Amzica, F., and Nuñez, A. 1993a. Cholinergic and noradrenergic modulation of the slow (~0.3 Hz) oscillation in neocortical cells. J. Neurophysiol. 70:1385–1400.

Steriade, M., Contreras, D., Curró Dossi, R., et al. 1993b. The slow (<1 Hz) oscillation in reticular thalamic and thalamocortical neurons: scenario of sleep rhythm generation in interacting thalamic and neocortical networks. J. Neurosci. 13:3284–3299.

Steriade, M., Curró Dossi, R., and Contreras, D. 1993c. Electrophysiological properties of intralaminar thalamocortical cells discharging rhythmic (~40 Hz) spike-bursts at ~1000 Hz during waking and rapid eye movement sleep. Neuroscience 56:1–9.

Steriade, M., McCormick, D.A., and Sejnowski, T.J. 1993d. Thalamocortical oscillations in the sleeping and aroused brain. Science 262:679–685.

Steriade, M., Nuñez, A., and Amzica, F. 1993e. A novel slow (<1 Hz) oscillation of neocortical neurons in vivo: depolarizing and hyperpolarizing components. J. Neurosci. 13:3252–3265.

Steriade, M., Nuñez, A., and Amzica, F. 1993f. Intracellular analysis of relations between the slow (<1 Hz) neocortical oscillation and other sleep rhythms of the electroencephalogram. J. Neurosci. 13:3266–3283.

Steriade, M., Contreras, D., and Amzica, F. 1994. Synchronized sleep oscillations and their paroxysmal developments. Trends Neurosci. 17:199–208.

Steriade, M., Amzica, F., and Contreras, D. 1996a. Synchronization of fast (30–40 Hz) spontaneous cortical rhythms during brain activation. J. Neurosci. 16:392–417.

Steriade, M., Contreras, D., Amzica, F., et al. 1996b. Synchronization of fast (30–40 Hz) spontaneous oscillations in intrathalamic and thalamocortical networks. J. Neurosci. 16:2788–2808.

Steriade, M., Jones, E.G., and McCormick, D.A. 1997. *Thalamus* (vol. 1, Organisation and Function). Oxford: Elsevier.

Steriade, M., Amzica, F., Neckelmann, D., and Timofeev, I. 1998a. Spike-wave complexes and fast runs of cortically generated seizures. II. Extra- and intracellular patterns. J. Neurophysiol. 80:1456–1479.

Steriade, M., Timofeev, I., Dürmüller, N., et al. 1998b. Dynamic properties of corticothalamic neurons and local cortical interneurons generating fast rhythmic (30–40 Hz) spike bursts. J. Neurophysiol. 79:483–490.

Steriade, M., Timofeev, I., Grenier, F., et al. 1998c. Role of thalamic and cortical neurons in augmenting responses: dual intracellular recordings in vivo. J. Neurosci. 18: 6425–6443.

Steriade, M., Timofeev, I., and Grenier, F. 2001. Natural waking and sleep states: a view from inside neocortical neurons. J. Neurophysiol. 85: 1969–1985.

Stewart, M., and Fox, S.E. 1991. Hippocampal theta activity in monkeys. Brain Res. 538:59–63.

Stickgold, R., James, L., and Hobson, J.A. 2000a. Visual discrimination learning requires sleep after training. Nat. Neurosci. 3:1237–1238.

Stickgold, R., Whitbee, D., Schirmer, B., et al. 2000b. Visual discrimination improvement. A multi-step process occurring during sleep. J. Cogn. Neurosci. 12:246–254.

Sykes, T.C.F., and Thomson, A.M. 1989. Sodium pentobarbitone enhances responses of thalamic relay neurones to GABA in rat brain slices. Br. J. Pharmacol. 97:1059–1066.

Terzano, M.G., Parrino, L., and Spaggiari, M.C. 1988. The cyclic alternating pattern sequences in the dynamic organization of sleep. Electroencephalogr. Clin. Neurophysiol. 69:437–447.

Thomson, A.M., West, D.C., Hahn, J., et al. 1996. Single axon IPSPs elicited in pyramidal cells by three classes of interneurons in slices of rat neocortex. J. Physiol. (Lond.) 496:81–102.

Timofeev, I., and Steriade, M. 1996. Low-frequency rhythms in the thalamus of intact-cortex and decorticated cats. J. Neurophysiol. 76:4152–4168.

Timofeev, I., and Steriade, M. 1998. Cellular mechanisms underlying intrathalamic augmenting responses of reticular and relay neurons. J. Neurophysiol. 79:2716–2729.

Timofeev, I., Contreras, D., and Steriade, M. 1996. Synaptic responsiveness of cortical and thalamic neurones during various phases of slow sleep oscillation in cat. J. Physiol. (Lond.) 494:265–278.

Timofeev, I., Grenier, F., and Steriade, M. 1998. Spike-wave complexes and fast runs of cortically generated seizures. IV. Paroxysmal fast runs in cortical and thalamic neurons. J. Neurophysiol. 80:1495–1513.

Timofeev, I., Grenier, F., Bazhenov, M., et al. 2000. Origin of slow oscillations in deafferented cortical slabs. Cereb. Cortex 10:1185–1199.

Timofeev, I., Grenier, F., Bazhenov, M., et al. 2002a. Short- and medium-term plasticity associated with augmenting responses in cortical slabs and spindles in intact cortex of cats in vivo. J. Physiol. (Lond.) 542:583–598.

Timofeev, I., Grenier, F., and Steriade, M. 2002b. The role of chloride-dependent inhibition and the activity of fast-spiking neurons during cortical spike-wave electrographic seizures. Neuroscience 14:1115–1132.

Timofeev, I., Grenier, F., and Steriade, M. 2003. Contribution of intrinsic neuronal factors in the generation of cortically generated electrographic seizures. Submitted.

Traub, R.D., Miles, R., Wong, R.K.S., et al. 1987. Models of synchronized hippocampal bursts in the presence of inhibition. II. Ongoing spontaneous population events. J. Neurophysiol. 58:752–764.

Traub, R.D., Miles, R., and Wong, R.K.S. 1989. Model of the origin of rhythmic population oscillations in the hippocampal slice. Science 243:1319–1325.

Uchida, S., Maloney, T., March, J.D., et al. 1991. Sigma (12–15 Hz) and delta (0.3–3.0 Hz) EEG oscillate reciprocally within NREM sleep. Brain Res. Bull. 27:93–96.

Vanderwolf, C.H., and Leung, L.W.S. 1983. Hippocampal rhythmic activity: a brief history and the effects of entorhinal lesions and phencyclidine. In *Neurobiology of the Hippocampus*, Ed., W. Seifert, pp. 275–302. New York: Academic Press.

Velayos, J.L., Jimenez-Castellanos, J., Jr., and Reinoso-Suárez, F. 1989. Topographical organization of the projections from the reticular thalamic nucleus to the intralaminar and medial thalamic nuclei in the cat. J. Comp. Neurol. 279:457–469.

Vertes, R.P. 1971. An analysis of ascending brain stem systems involved in hippocampal synchronization and desynchronization. J. Neurophysiol. 46:1140–1159.

Vertes, R.P. 1982. Brain stem generation of the hippocampal EEG. Prog. Neurobiol. 19:159–186.

Villablanca, J. 1974. Role of the thalamus in sleep control: sleep-wakefulness studies in chronic diencephalic and athalamic cats. In *Basic Sleep Mechanisms*, Eds. O. Petre-Quadens and J. Schlag, pp. 51–81. New York: Academic Press.

Vinogradova, O.S., Brazhnik, E.S., Karanov, A.N., et al. 1980. Analysis of neuronal activity in rabbit's septum with various conditions of deafferentation. Brain Res. 187:354–368.

Von Krosigk, M., Bal, T., and McCormick, D.A. 1993. Cellular mechanisms of a synchronized oscillation in the thalamus. Science 261:361–364.

Wainer, B.H., and Mesulam, M.-M. 1990. Ascending cholinergic pathways in the rat brain. In *Brain Cholinergic Systems*, Eds. M. Steriade and D. Biesold, pp. 65–119. Oxford: Oxford University Press.

Wang, X.J., and Rinzel, J. 1993. Spindle rhythmicity in the reticularis thalamic nucleus: synchronization among inhibitory neurons. Neuroscience 53:899–904.

Wilcox, K.S., Gutnick, M.J., and Cristoph, G.R. 1988. Electrophysiological properties of neurons in the lateral habenula nucleus: an *in vitro* study. J. Neurophysiol. 59:212–225.

Winson, J. 1974. Patterns of hippocampal theta rhythm in the freely moving rat. Electroencephalogr. Clin. Neurophysiol. 36:212–225.

Wise, S.P., Fleshman, J.W., Jr., and Jones, E.G. 1979. Maturation of pyramidal cell form in relation to developing afferent and efferent connections of rat somatic sensory cortex. Neuroscience 4:1275–1297.

Yamada, T., Kameyama, S., Fuchigami, Z., et al. 1988. Changes of short latency somatosensory evoked potential in sleep. Electroencephalogr. Clin. Neurophysiol. 70:126–136.

Yen, C.T., and Jones, E.G. 1983. Intracellular staining of physiologically identified neurons and axons in the somatosensory thalamus of the cat. Brain Res. 280:148–154.

Yen, C.T., Conley, M., Hendry, S.H.C., et al. 1985. The morphology of physiologically identified GABAergic neurons in the somatic sensory part of the thalami reticular nucleus in the cat. J. Neurosci. 5:2254–2268.

Ylinen, A., Soltesz, I., Bragin, A., et al. G. 1995. Intracellular correlates of theta rhythm in hippocampal pyramidal cells, granule cells and basket cell. Hippocampus 5:78–90.

Zhou, Q., Godwin, D.W., O'Malley, D.M., et al. 1997. Visualization of calcium influx through channels that shape the burst and tonic firing modes of thalamic relay cells. J. Neurophysiol. 77:2816–2825.

4. Dynamics of EEGs as Signals of Neuronal Populations: Models and Theoretical Considerations

Fernando Lopes da Silva

In Chapters 2 and 3 the neurophysiological basis of the electroencephalogram (EEG) was discussed with special emphasis on the phenomena at the cellular level. In Chapter 5 the biophysical aspects of the generation of EEG phenomena are considered mainly in terms of volume conduction, but the dynamic properties of EEG patterns are only briefly mentioned. These dynamic properties, however, are essential for understanding EEG phenomena. In this chapter, EEG signals are considered as the result of the dynamic behavior of neuronal populations as revealed by model studies. According to this perspective, it is necessary to integrate experimental and theoretical results. The latter must be obtained using models of neuronal networks and corresponding computer simulations. The mathematical treatment of such models has been avoided here; the interested reader is referred to a number of other publications that are cited for their thorough mathematical treatment of these areas.

The fundamental assumption on which the following discussion is based is that EEG signals reflect the dynamics of electrical activity in populations of neurons. A property of such populations that is of essential importance for the generation of EEG signals is the capacity of the neurons to work in synchrony. This depends on the connectivity between the neurons that form a network. The classic terminology of Freeman (1975) provides a useful systematization. Populations of neurons with mutual interactions are called KI sets; the interactions may be excitatory (KIe) or inhibitory (KIi). Groups of two interacting populations of neurons are called KII sets; they are formed by an interaction of a KIe set with a KIt set. Further, KIII sets formed by the interaction between two KII sets can be defined. A number of such KIII sets constitute a neural mass that may occupy a few square millimeters of cortical surface or a few cubic millimeters of nuclear volume in the brainstem or spinal cord. Typically, a neural mass consists of approximately 10^4 to 10^7 neurons. An example of a KIII set is given in a symbolic way in Fig. 4.1. An essential feature of such a basic module is the existence of multiple feedback loops. Such a set of neurons can produce oscillatory phenomena as revealed in EEG signals. The main parameters that characterize the dynamic behavior of the set are (a) the synaptic time constants; (b) the length constants, which define the distance of the interactions between different neurons; and (c) the gain factors, i.e., the strength of interactions, whether by way of chemical synapses or electrical couplings.

There are both inhibitory and excitatory feedback loops. The terms *negative feedback* and *positive feedback* are often used in a rather loose way to characterize the interactions between neuron populations. However, the sign of feedback is defined in an exact way by comparing the overall gain modulus of the system with feedback (closed loop gain: $|Y_o(j\omega)|$) and without feedback (open loop gain: $|Y_1(j\omega)|$). The feedback is said to be negative if $|Y_o(j\omega)| < |Y_1(j\omega)|$ and positive in the opposite case (Hammond, 1958). The exact sign of feedback in the interaction between neuron populations is in most cases not known. It therefore seems preferable to use the terms *excitatory* and *inhibitory feedback* to define the main synaptic type of interaction between neuron populations. This will be considered from the reference point of the "main" population, which usually is the population that receives the input from another source and/or sends its output to another structure.

In this chapter, models of the generation of characteristic types of EEGs, including the spatial spread of rhythmic activity over the cortex, and nonlinear dynamics as a new approach for understanding EEG phenomena are presented.

Models of EEG Generation

The processes of generation of EEG signals in a large number of neurons forming a neural mass are complex. Therefore, it is useful to use both analytic and synthetic approaches to understand such processes. It is essential to use both approaches in a dialectic way. The experimental data, obtained through histological or physiological analytic methods, must be put together just as pieces of a puzzle are assembled. However, knowledge of most neurophysiological systems is still rather limited. Very often the relationship between the different pieces is still unclear. It is at this level that a synthetic approach may be helpful. The point is then to put together the available data in such a way as to form the most likely pattern. In this way, a model of a neurophysiological system can be constructed. Such a model can help to advance knowledge of the system in two respects. First, it provides the possibility for testing the influence of different types of inputs upon the output of the system or of changing some of the properties of the constituting elements; in this way the model helps to systematize understanding of the system's behavior and to clarify individuals' thoughts. Second, it allows the formulation of hypotheses concerning new

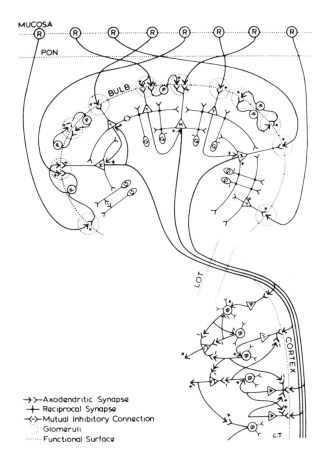

→>—Axodendritic Synapse
—+— Reciprocal Synapse
—<>—Mutual Inhibitory Connection
  ○ Glomeruli
.... Functional Surface

Figure 4.1. Diagram of the neuronal populations of the olfactory system according to Freeman (1975). (Abbreviations as in Fig. 4.2.)

elementary properties, relationships, and overall behavior; it may thus predict new properties of the system, raise new questions, and suggest new experiments to explore these hypotheses. In this way, the dialectic interplay between experimentation and theory can become reality. As Harmon (1964) stated long ago, it is in suggesting functional relationships between the activity of single neurons and the behavior of groups of neurons that theoretical neurophysiology may be most potent.

With these general objectives in mind, this chapter considers a few models of the generation of EEG phenomena that have been most elaborated in the past decades. These are (a) a model describing the generation of the EEG of olfactory areas of the brain as proposed extensively by Freeman (1975) and elaborated later (Freeman, 1979, 1986); (b) a model of the alpha rhythm of the thalamus and cortex as proposed by Lopes da Silva et al. (1974, 1976) and elaborated in more detail by Van Rotterdam et al. (1982), and later by Wright and Liley (1996) and by Nunez (1995); (c) a series of models of the membrane and synaptic properties of thalamic cells and circuits responsible for the generation of 7- to 14-Hz spindle rhythmicity that occurs at the onset and in the light stages of sleep, based on the experimental findings of Steriade and colleagues (Golomb and Rinzel 1993, 1994; Golomb et al. 1994, 1996; Wang 1994; Wang and

Rinzel 1992, 1993; Wang et al. 1991, 1995); (d) a model of the bistable behavior of a neuronal network, where abrupt transitions occur between two states: normal and paroxysmal (Suffczynski et al., 2000, 2004); (e) a model of the generation of epileptiform transients proposed by Wendling et al. (2002), and by Traub (1982), Traub and Wong (1983b), Traub et al. (1984, 2002), and Traub and Miles (1991); (f) a model of gamma rhythms developed by Traub et al. (1996) with realistic simulations of synapses (Jefferys et al., 1996a,b; Traub et al. 1996, 2002; Whittington and Traub, 2003).

Model of Olfactory Area EEG

First, it is useful to consider the structure of the main areas of interest: the olfactory bulb (OB) and the prepyriform cortex (PC) (Fig. 4.1). The axons of the primary olfactory nerve (PON) terminate in the glomeruli (gl) at the superficial layer of the bulb, where the PON axons make synaptic contacts with periglomerular neurons (P) and the dendrites of mitral (M) and tufted (T) cells (Freeman, 1972; Pinching and Powell, 1971; Reese and Shepherd, 1972). The output of this layer is fed to the layer of the M and T cells. These two types of neurons project into the underlying layer formed by granule cells (G). The output of the bulb is constituted by axons of the M cells that form the lateral olfactory tract (LOT). These axons terminate, among other areas, on the superficial pyramidal neurons (A) of the PC. The latter make synaptic contacts with the basket cells (B) and with deeper-lying pyramidal neurons (C). The axons of these last neurons constitute the output of the PC and project to several structures of the basal forebrain.

A scheme of the proposed interactions is shown in Fig. 4.2. In this scheme, the different types of neurons are represented as lumped systems because they are considered to have, on average, similar properties and reciprocal connections within the population. Freeman's basic methodology of study of those neural masses has been initially to follow a linear systems analysis approach. For linear analysis to be justifiable, the system under consideration must obey the superposition principle, which states that when the input is multiplied by a constant, k, the system's response must be multiplied by the same constant. It has been shown by Freeman (1972) that, within determined limits of input amplitude, the responses of the olfactory system's neural masses do in fact obey the principle of superposition. This fundamental property is not unique within the central nervous system. It has also been shown to hold, with some constraints, in the case of other types of sensory evoked potentials, as for example in the visual system, by Van der Tweel (1961), Spekreijse and van der Tweel (1970), Lopes da Silva et al. (1970), and Regan (1968). According to this approach, the output signal of the neural mass is a holistic event; it is a field potential the amplitude of which is proportional to the input. In conjunction with the field potentials, poststimulus time histograms of action potentials generated by single neurons may be recorded and analyzed in a similar fashion.

The main neuronal populations of these structures that are of importance for an understanding of the generation of the olfactory EEG can be summarized as follows: in the bulb, the mitral and tufted cell (MT) population, which is excitatory, and the granule cell population, which is inhibitory; in the

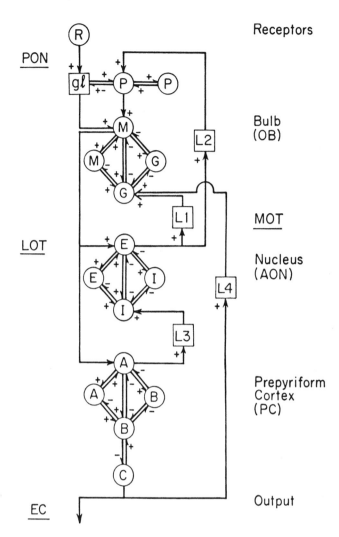

Figure 4.2. Lumped circuit diagram of the sets of neurons in the olfactory bulb (OB), the anterior olfactory nucleus (AON), and the prepyriform cortex (PC). PON, primary olfactory nerve; LOT, lateral olfactory tract; EC, external capsule; R, receptors of the nasal mucosa; gl, glomeruli; P, periglomerular neuron; M, mitral neuron; G, granule cell; E, superficial pyramidal cells of AON; I, inhibitory neuron; A, superficial pyramidal neuron; B, short local interneuron; C, deep pyramidal neuron; +, excitation; −, inhibition; L, latency. (Adapted from Freeman, W.J. 1986. Analytic techniques used in the search for the physiological basis of the EEG. In *Handbook of Electroencephalography and Clinical Neurophysiology*, vol. 1: *Methods of Analysis of Brain Electrical and Magnetic Signals*, Eds. A. Gevins and A. Remond. Amsterdam: Elsevier.)

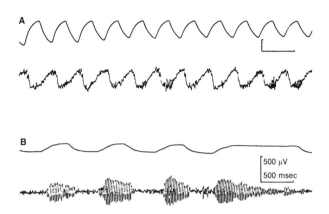

Figure 4.3. **A:** *Upper trace* shows respiration of a waking rabbit measured using a pneumograph; *lower trace* represents an EEG signal from the olfactory bulb (OB) in which the surface-negative wave peaks after each inhalation. **B:** *Upper trace* shows the air flow through the nose of an anesthetized cat; *lower trace* shows the EEG from the OB where the low frequencies have been filtered out. Note that each burst occurs with air inflow. (Adapted from Freeman, W.J. 1986. Analytic techniques used in the search for the physiological basis of the EEG. In *Handbook of Electroencephalography and Clinical Neurophysiology*, vol. 1: *Methods of Analysis of Brain Electrical and Magnetic Signals*, Eds. A. Gevins and A. Remond. Amsterdam: Elsevier.)

PC, the surface pyramidal population, which is excitatory, and the basket cell population, which is inhibitory. The interaction between the MT and the granule neuron populations forms an inhibitory feedback loop. The interaction between the surface pyramidal and the basket cell populations in the PC also forms an inhibitory feedback loop.

As can be seen in Fig. 4.2, there are also mutual excitatory interactions between M or T neurons in the bulb and between pyramidal A neurons in the PC, as well as mutual inhibitory interactions between granule cells in the bulb and basket cells in the PC. Excitation of the MT cells by PON inputs leads to excitation of the granule (G) neurons and to feed-

back inhibition of the MT neurons. In consequence, the G neurons are disexcited and the MT neurons are disinhibited. In this way, the MT neurons may become excited again, and the whole process may continue in an oscillatory mode. The basic oscillation is at 40 Hz in cat and 60 to 80 Hz in rabbit (Freeman, 1972) (Fig. 4.3). A similar type of inhibitory feedback loop occurs in the PC, and the EEG of this cortical structure resembles that of the OB in frequency content. In this model and similar ones, the action potentials are converted into graded currents at the somadendritic synapses causing the postsynaptic potentials. In a first approximation, these postsynaptic potentials may be considered to sum at the soma. At the trigger zone, the axon hillock, these potentials are transformed into spike trains depending on a threshold.

The postsynaptic potentials may be considered as the wave (W) mode of operation of the neural set; the action potentials represent the pulse (P) mode. This is, of course, a simplification of processes taking place at the membrane, but at the level of generalization at which EEG models are constructed, these are the main features that must be considered. The sensitivity of the threshold process in the bulb and cortex is controlled by centrifugal influences that originate in the forebrain and brainstem, among others from the locus coeruleus (Gray et al., 1984). The conversion between the postsynaptic potential (W mode) and the pulse rate (P mode) may be given in terms of the sigmoid curves shown in Fig. 4.4 for a single neuron and for the population or ensemble. The wave-pulse conversion can be considered as a static sigmoidal nonlinearity at the single neuron level. However, over small signal ranges this relation may be assumed to be linearized, and therefore it may be represented by a simple coefficient.

To simulate the local dynamics of the EEG, delays due to synaptic and conduction processes may be accounted for by

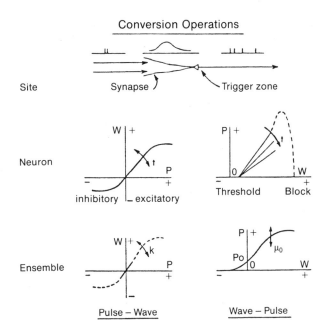

Figure 4.4. Conversion operations between the wave mode (W) and the pulse mode (P) for a neuron and an ensemble of neurons. At the neuronal level both operations are time-varying (t); the P-W conversion is nonlinear; the W-P conversion is linear between threshold and cathodal block. At the ensemble level, the P-W conversion is restricted to a small linear range and W-P conversion is static and nonlinear. The derivative of this curve defines the gain; this may change (μ_o) depending on arousal level. The P-W conversion can vary to represent synaptic changes occurring with learning. (Adapted from Freeman, W.J. 1983. Dynamics of image formation by nerve cell assemblies. In *Synergetics of the Brain,* Eds. E. Basar, H. Flohr, H. Haken, et al., pp. 102–121. Berlin: Springer-Verlag.)

a stage of integration. Along these lines, the dynamics of these structures may be represented by a mathematical model consisting of coupled differential equations that incorporate static nonlinear functions (for a mathematical treatment see Freeman, 1975, 1986, 2000). The main input to the populations of the OB comes from the olfactory mucosa and is modulated by the respiration rate (Fig. 4.3). A study of the behavior of the KII set described above shows that this set has multiple stable states. Two are of particular interest because they represent the most common situations. The first is a quasi-equilibrium state that is maintained by a steady input of low intensity; the second is the so-called carrier state (Freeman, 1986), characterized by a limit cycle with quasi-sinusoidal EEG activity at 40 Hz (cat) or 60 to 80 Hz (rabbit) that occurs during inspiration. This nonlinear oscillation represents a limit cycle because the feedback gain is displaced to the excitatory side of the resting value (Fig. 4.4) with an increase in pulse input (either of sensory origin or depending on arousal level) that may drive the KII set out of the equilibrium state. Certain drugs such as carbachol or picrotoxin can induce a limit cycle state of long duration (Freeman, 1986). Freeman's more recent interpretation of the EEG of these brain structures reveals that the KII set during a specific olfactory input is characterized by a limit cycle attractor that has a unique spatial amplitude pattern of the sinusoidal waves over the surface of the bulb. A later section shall consider the relevance of nonlinear dynamics

such as the theory of deterministic chaos for understanding EEG generation. Here it is sufficient to observe that the EEG signals simulated by the set of nonlinear coupled differential equations that describe the KII set approximate the experimentally recorded EEGs as shown in Fig. 4.5.

Alpha Rhythm Models: Spatial and Temporal Characteristics

A current view in neurophysiology is that the origin of certain rhythmic electrical activity seen in the EEG, such as that characteristic of some thalamic nuclei and cortical areas after administration of a barbiturate (Andersen and Andersson, 1968; Andersen et al., 1967) and possibly also that occurring spontaneously, such as sleep spindles and alpha rhythms (Steriade et al., 1990a,b) is to be found in populations of neurons characterized by the interaction between excitatory and inhibitory neuronal populations. Different types of models have been developed to account for the generation of EEG rhythmic activities within the alpha fre-

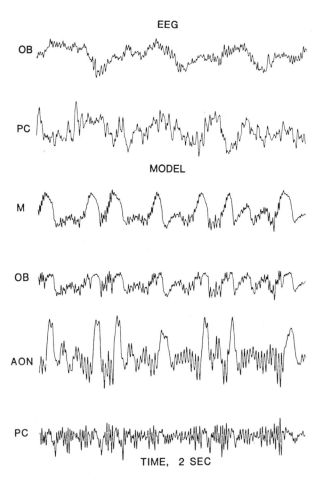

Figure 4.5. Examples of EEGs recorded from the OB and PC of a rat at rest and of signals generated by the model for several neuronal sets (OB, AON, and PC) and for the bulbar unit activity. (Adapted from Freeman, W.J. 1986. Analytic techniques used in the search for the physiological basis of the EEG. In *Handbook of Electroencephalography and Clinical Neurophysiology,* vol. 1: *Methods of Analysis of Brain Electrical and Magnetic Signals,* Eds. A. Gevins and A. Remond. Amsterdam: Elsevier.)

quency range. Some of these models operate at the microscopic level of the single neuron or the small local network (e.g., by Destexhe and colleagues, 1994, 1996), others at the macroscopic level with the aim of accounting for global properties of EEG signals recorded from the scalp (not limited to alpha rhythms) (e.g., by Nunez, 1995). Recently attempts have been made to combine the local and the global levels within a synthetic theoretical framework, among others by Nunez who developed a thoughtful "marriage of local and global theories" (Chapter 11 in Nunez 1995). A particular interesting discussion of this issue is the paper of Wright and Liley (1996) followed by a wide-open peer commentary.

Simplified Distributed and Lumped Alpha Models

At the cellular level, an important issue that has been repeatedly discussed in studies of the mechanisms underlying EEG rhythmic activities is the question of whether such rhythms are caused by single cells with pacemaker properties. A significant advance in this discussion was achieved when it was demonstrated by Jahnsen and Llinás (1984a,b) that some types of thalamic neurons display oscillatory behavior *in vitro*, even after blockage of synaptic transmission. Most neurons studied in this way tend to generate oscillations in the frequency range of 6 to 10 Hz. These intrinsic oscillatory properties of some neurons are most likely of importance in shaping the rhythmic behavior of the networks to which they belong. However, these properties may not be sufficient to account for the network rhythmic behavior. One main argument supports this statement: the disconnection of cortically projecting thalamic cells from their inputs, which arise in the reticular nucleus of the thalamus, abolishes spindles in thalamocortical relay (TCR) neurons (Steriade et al., 1985). However, single TCR neurons may preserve their intrinsic membrane oscillatory properties *in vitro* (Jahnsen and Llinás (1984a,b). Interestingly, the capacity of both TCR-RE circuits and the isolated reticular nucleus (RE), *in vivo*, to generate spindle oscillations contrasts with the fact that the RE nucleus isolated *in vitro* does not show spontaneous oscillations (Avanzini et al., 1989; Bal et al., 1995a,b; Huguenard and Prince, 1994; Von Krosigk et al., 1993; Warren et al., 1994). This is likely because the input conditions of the RE neurons *in vitro* are different from the situation *in vivo* because the neurons lack neuromodulation influences, including cholinergic, noradrenergic, and serotoninergic inputs. In modeling studies, the influence of neuromodulators on RE neurons membrane potential was simulated (Destexhe et al., 1994), namely noradrenaline and serotonin, by blocking leak K+ currents and thus depolarizing the RE neurons to the same level as observed *in vivo*. These studies showed that waxing-waning oscillations could occur in the RE network, similar to those seen *in vivo*. This finding provides clear evidence that the oscillatory behavior of these neuronal populations of RE neurons depends on specific levels of the neuronal membrane potential that is affected by several inputs, both at short- and long-range. Among the latter, the neuromodulatory inputs arising from the raphe nucleus (serotoninergic), the locus coeruleus (noradrenergic), as well as glutamatergic projections form forebrain areas are particularly important. Among the former it is interesting to note that gap junctions have been shown to exist between

RE nucleus (Landisman et al., 2002) and thus may also participate in the modulation of their oscillatory properties.

To understand how oscillations may be generated in thalamic nuclei, we must consider the basic structure of these neuronal networks. In the thalamic relay nuclei where this type of rhythmic activity can be recorded, namely the relay nuclei of the thalamus, three main types of neurons can be distinguished: the thalamocortical relay (TCR) neurons, whose axons project to the cortex; the reticular nucleus (RE) neurons that contribute to the inhibitory feedback control of the former; and the local, intrinsic, neurons. The RE forms a thin sheet of neurons that surround the anterior and lateral side of the thalamus and interact synaptically with the TCR neurons. The axons of the RE cells have as main target the TCR cells. Their dendrites make synaptic contacts with the axons of the TCR cells. Thus the TCR and the RE neurons are interconnected by means of a feedback loop as schematically shown in Fig. 4.6. Both the RE and the local-circuit neurons contain γ-aminobutyric acid (GABA) as transmitter. This implies that the feedback of the RE on the TCR neurons is GABAergic and thus inhibitory. The RE neurons receive fast GABA$_A$ mediated inhibitory postsynaptic potentials (IPSPs) from neighboring RE neurons; in this way these neurons form a chain of cells interconnected by in-

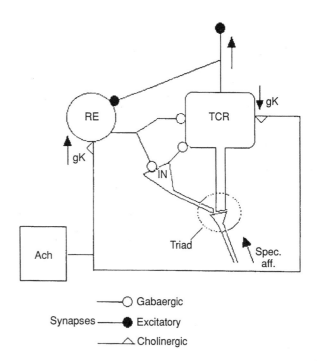

Figure 4.6. Simplified scheme of a thalamic neural network where the main features are presented. The thalamocortical relay (TCR), the reticular thalamic (RE), and the local-circuit interneurons (IN) are indicated, along with projections from a cholinergic population (ACh). The synaptic triad formed by the dendrites of TCR and IN neurons with the specific afferent (spec. aff.) fibers is also indicated. Three types of synapse are shown: excitatory, γ-aminobutyric acid (GABA)ergic (inhibitory) and cholinergic. The effect of the latter on RE neurons is assumed to be an increase in potassium conductance (g$_k$), whereas on the TCR neurons the effect is the opposite. (From Lopes da Silva, F.H. 1991. Neural mechanisms underlying brain waves: from neural membranes to networks. Electroencephalogr. Clin. Neurophysiol. 79:81–93, with permission.)

hibitory synapses. In addition they receive fast glutamatergic (AMPA type) excitatory postsynaptic potential (EPSPs) from TCR neurons. In turn the TCR neurons receive both fast $GABA_A$ and slow $GABA_B$ IPSPs from RE neurons (Bal et al., 1995a,b). In a thalamic nucleus, a number of feedback circuits can be distinguished between TCR and RE neurons.

In the context of this discussion, it is important to note that the TCR neurons can work essentially according to two distinct modes: either (a) as relay cells that simply depolarize and can produce single spikes in response to an adequate input volley, or (b) as oscillatory cells producing bursts of high-frequency spikes that are repeated in a rhythmic fashion. The resting membrane potential of a TCR neuron determines whether such a neuron will be active in the relay or in the oscillatory mode. To understand this question, it is necessary to take into account the intrinsic membrane properties of these cells, namely their main ionic conductances and the corresponding dynamics. It should be noted that these properties became known mainly due to microphysiological investigations in thalamic slices, *in vitro*, and in isolated brain preparations by the groups of Llinás and collaborators (Jahnsen and Llinás, 1984a,b). For a comprehensive account of these membrane properties, the reader is referred to the original publications and to the excellent reviews by Steriade and Llinás (1988), Steriade et al. (1990a,b), McCormick (1992), McCormick and Bal (1994), Destexhe et al. (1996), Destexhe and Sejnowski (2003), and to Chapter 3

A basic question is whether the different types of oscillations can be found *in vitro* in the absence of external inputs, since this would give support to the idea that these thalamic cells may support pacemaker rhythmic activity. Jahnsen and Llinás (1984a) provided an initial answer to this question, by showing that the oscillatory activity at about 10 Hz may be observed in the absence of external drive *in vitro*. However, we must also consider what is the contribution of the feedback circuits between TCR and RE neurons to the generation of EEG oscillations *in vivo*.

In this context the most direct experimental evidence pertains to the generation of spindle oscillations occurring during the early stages of sleep. Spindles appear in the EEG of most mammals as oscillations with a frequency in the range from 7 to 14 Hz, which form bursts lasting for 1.5 to 2 seconds that recur periodically with an irregular periodicity of about 5 to 10 seconds. This type of spindle can also be seen in animals under barbiturate anesthesia. It was shown by Steriade et al. (1985) that no thalamic nucleus is capable of generating spindle oscillations after disconnection from the RE nucleus. Therefore, the existence of feedback circuits including the RE nucleus is necessary for spindling to occur under normal conditions *in vivo*.

In conclusion, under the normal conditions of an intact brain, both synaptic interactions and input signals play an essential role in setting the conditions necessary for oscillatory behavior to occur. The frequency of this oscillation depends on the intrinsic membrane properties on the membrane potential of the individual neurons, and on the strength of the synaptic interactions.

A simplified model has been proposed (Lopes da Silva et al., 1974, 1976) that incorporates the limited physiological and histological data available at that time; these assumptions were sufficient to explain the generation of the alpha rhythm, i.e., the EEG stochastic signal that lies in the frequency range of 8 to 13 Hz. This appears mainly at eye closure and can be recorded best from the posterior regions of the scalp in humans. A similar type of activity has also been recorded at the visual cortex and some thalamic nuclei in dogs (Lopes da Silva et al., 1973) and cats (Chatile et al., 1992; Lanoir, 1972). The model in its most simple form consists of a set of simulated neurons, thalamocortical relay (TCR) cells, and interneurons (INs). The latter may be assumed to be the RE cells shown in Fig. 4.6, although the IN cells shown in this figure may have a complementary effect. For simplicity in the model, the cells providing feedback are denoted, in the following, as INs. In contrast with the lumped models, some examples of which have been given for the olfactory system, this model is a distributed one in the sense that each neuron is modeled individually; it occupies a specific position within a matrix of neurons. Such a distributed

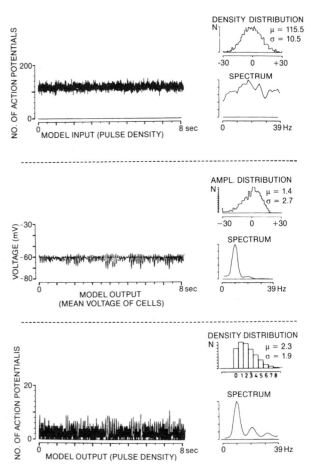

Figure 4.7. Results obtained with the distributed model of alpha rhythm. **Upper panel:** Input density of the input to all TCR neurons. **Middle panel:** Wave mode summed membrane potentials of all TCR neurons. **Lower panel:** Pulse mode: impulse density of all TCR neurons. *Right:* The amplitude distributions and the power spectra of the three signals are shown. Note the apparent waxing and waning of the simulated alpha rhythm and the dominant alpha rhythm with a second harmonic. (Adapted from Lopes da Silva, F.H., Hoeks, A., Smits, H., et al. 1974. Model of brain rhythmic activity. Kybernetik 15:27–37.)

model offers some special possibilities for theoretical studies that are not easily available in lumped models.

Without entering into great detail about the alpha rhythm distributed model, it is of interest to point out some of its characteristics. First, the structure of the distributed model initially used (Lopes da Silva et al., 1974) consisted of 144 TCR neurons and 36 INs; the 32 TCR neurons that surrounded one IN were responsible for its excitation, while each IN was responsible for the inhibition of the 12 TCRs around it. The excitation and inhibition were represented by time functions that were an approximation of the waveforms of EPSPs and IPSPs, respectively. The matrix of neurons should be viewed as lying at the surface of a torus. Furthermore, each neuron fired whenever the membrane potential exceeded a simple threshold; a short refractory period then followed. A basic characteristic of this model was that the input received by each TCR neuron was in the form of a series of pulses (action potentials) that had a Poisson distribution; the inputs to the individual TCR neurons were uncorrelated. The model's output signal was the sum of the membrane potential fluctuations of all TCR neurons. This output signal simulated the general spectral properties of an alpha rhythm. This result is illustrated in Figs. 4.7 to 4.9.

In the distributed model, it is also easy to investigate the result of changing the range of excitatory and inhibitory influence of, respectively, TCRs and INs. In the case of Fig. 4.7, there were 12 TCR neurons that were inhibited by one IN. This is the common situation; the effects of reducing this number to four and of increasing it to 21 are shown in Figs. 4.8 and 4.9. Reduction of the inhibitory area of influence of an IN results in a decrease of the spectral peak amplitude (alpha frequency) and an increase in bandwidth; an increase in the inhibitory area has the opposite effects. These are some of the phenomena that can be studied using a distrib-

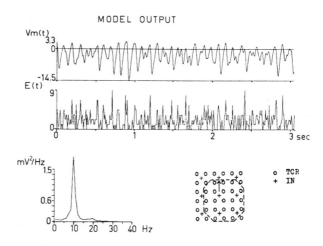

Figure 4.9. Similar to Fig. 4.8 but for a model with a larger inhibitory area. Here 1 IN inhibits 21 TCR neurons. Note that the intensity of the alpha peak is larger and the bandwidth is smaller in comparison with the model shown in Fig. 4.8. (Adapted from Lopes da Silva, F.H., van Rotterdam, A., Barts, P., et al. 1976. Models of neuronal populations: the basic mechanisms of rhythmicity. In *Perspectives of Brain Research*, Eds. M.A. Corner and D.F. Swaab. Prog. Brain Res. 45:281–308.)

uted neuronal model of rhythmic activity. However, this type of model has one main disadvantage: it is difficult to treat analytically. Therefore, it was necessary to develop a lumped model that would take into account the main characteristics of the distributed model. A lumped model of the same type as those of Freeman, previously described, permits a more general treatment of the activity of neuronal populations.

The development of the lumped model in analytical terms included the step of translating the properties of the discrete matrix of neurons into a system such as that depicted in Fig. 4.10. Essentially, the neural mass (here thalamic nucleus), the EEG of which is of interest, forms a KII set, which is constituted by the interaction of an excitatory (M) and an inhibitory (INIF) population (KIe and KIi sets). In addition, the scheme of Fig. 4.10 shows a second KIe (INEF) set that provides excitatory feedback and an additional KIe set that may receive a direct input (P(t)) from a source situated outside the neural mass and in this way lead to feed-forward inhibition. To obtain an analytic simplification of the distributed model, it is also useful to consider the general model of Wilson and Cowan (1972), who have formulated a set of equations that describe the overall activity (not specifically the EEG) in a cartel of excitatory and inhibitory neurons having a large number of interconnections. In this model, it is assumed that all types of interactions are possible, not only between excitatory and inhibitory neurons, but also within the same population.

Zetterberg (1973) has made use of this formulation to simplify the distributed model of alpha rhythm. Considering the simplified block diagram of Fig. 4.11, where the EPSPs and IPSPs are represented by $h_e(t)$ and $h_i(t)$, respectively, and the sigmoid wave pulse transfer functions are represented by $f_E(V)$ and $f_i(V)$, expressions for the transfer function of the simulated neuronal set can be obtained (for the

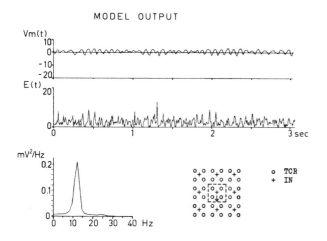

Figure 4.8. Output signals of the distributed alpha model: Vm(t) represents the summed membrane potentials of all TCR neurons and E(t) represents the impulse density of the same neurons. The power spectrum of Vm(t) is shown on the left below. In this case, a smaller inhibitory area than in the case of Fig. 4.9 has been simulated. Here one interneuron (IN) inhibits only four TCR neurons. (Adapted from Lopes da Silva, F.H., van Rotterdam, A., Barts, P., et al. 1976. Models of neuronal populations: the basic mechanisms of rhythmicity. In *Perspectives of Brain Research*, Eds. M.A. Corner and D.F. Swaab. Prog. Brain Res. 45:281–308.)

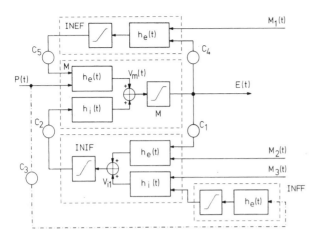

Figure 4.10. Block diagram of the lumped model for rhythmic activity with a possibility of modulation of inhibitory feedback and excitatory feedback. The cartel consists of four populations. M, main cells with input and output impulse density, respectively P(t) and E(t), and membrane potential, $V_m(t)$; spike generation nonlinearity sigmoid function. INIF, inhibitory population with membrane potential $V_{il}(t)$ and modulating inputs: excitatory by means of $M_1(t)$ and inhibitory by means of $M_2(t)$, spike generation with sigmoid. INFF, excitatory population driven by the main input P(t) inhibiting the inhibitory population INIF; INEF, excitatory population feeding back on to the main population, spike generation sigmoid. The interconnectivity constants giving the number of cells of one population projecting to one cell of the other population are C_1 and C_2 for the inhibitory feedback and C_4 and C_5 for the excitatory feedback. C_3 represents the number of cells of the INFF population excited by one input fiber (feed-forward). (Adapted from Lopes da Sila, F.H., van Rotterdam, A., Barts, P., et al. 1976. Models of neuronal populations: the basic mechanisms of rhythmicity. In *Perspectives of Brain Research*. Eds. M.A. Corner and D.F. Swaab. Prog. Brain Res. 45:281–308.)

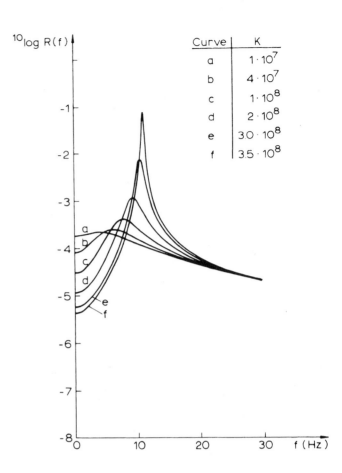

Curve	K
a	$1 \cdot 10^7$
b	$4 \cdot 10^7$
c	$1 \cdot 10^8$
d	$2 \cdot 10^8$
e	$30 \cdot 10^8$
f	$35 \cdot 10^8$

Figure 4.12. Power spectra of the output of the lumped alpha rhythm model shown in Fig. 4.11 for different values of the feedback gain (K), which is mainly determined by the coupling constants representing the synaptic interactions within the neuronal set. As the synaptic interactions become stronger and K increases, the spectrum acquires a clear selectivity at the alpha frequency. (Adapted from Lopes da Silva, F.H., Hocks, A., Smits, H., et al. 1974. Model of brain rhythmic activity. Kybernetik 15: 27–37.)

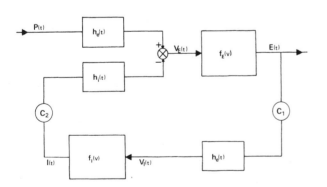

Figure 4.11. Block diagram of the lumped model for rhythmic activity of simplified alpha rhythm model. The thalamocortical relay (TCR) neurons are represented by two linear systems having impulse responses simulating an EPSP ($h_e(t)$) and an IPSP ($h_i(t)$), respectively, together with the static nonlinearity ($f_E(V)$) representing the spike-generating process. The interneurons (IN cells) are represented by one linear system ($h_e(t)$) and a nonlinearity ($f_I(V)$). C_1 represents the number of INs to which one TCR neuron projects; C_2 represents the number of TCRs to which one IN projects. (From Lopes da Silva, F.H., Hoeks, A., Smits, H., et al. 1974. Model of brain rhythmic activity. Kybernetik 15:27–37, with permission.)

mathematical treatment, see Lopes da Silva et al., 1976). One of the outputs of such a neuronal set represents the EEG signal of the population, assuming that the latter is determined by the somadendritic membrane potential of the main cells. The corresponding spectrum is shown in Fig. 4.12 for different values of K, which represents a measure of the gain factor of the neuronal set. The spectrum R(f) indeed shows a peak around 10 Hz, as was expected. The bandwidth and the peak frequency both depend on the coefficient K. Up to a point, a larger K will cause an increase in the frequency of the rhythmic activity, but too large a K will cause instability. K is also proportional to the derivatives $1/a_{el}$ and $1/a_{il}$ of the sigmoid functions in their working point, which in turn is determined by the mean input pulse density P(t). The peak frequency will increase and the bandwidth will decrease with an increase of the coupling constants, C_2 and C_1, i.e., with an increase in synaptic interactions within the neuronal cartel.

The linear analysis of the preceding section gives only a first approximation to the spectral characteristics of the

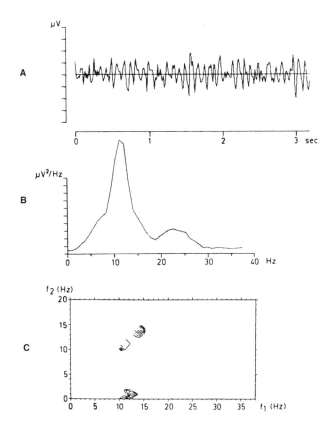

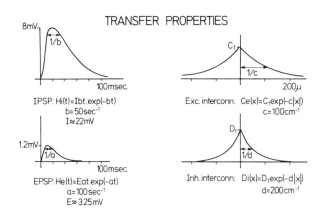

Figure 4.14. Transfer properties of the spatially distributed model or neuronal chain. *Left:* The time courses of the simulated IPSP and EPSP are shown with the corresponding equations. *Right:* The spatial connectivity functions are shown. Ce(x) and Di(x) describe the homogeneous interconnectivity functions for the excitatory and the inhibitory connections, which depend only on distance x. The values of the characteristic lengths correspond to $1/c$ and $1/d$. The numerical values of c and d in the figure are only indicative. (Adapted from Van Rotterdam, A., Lopes da Silva, F.H., Van den Ende, J., et al. 1982. A model of the spatial-temporal characteristics of the alpha rhythm. Bull. Math Biol. 44(2):283–305.)

Figure 4.13. An epoch of alpha rhythm (**A**) experimentally recorded from the visual cortex of the dog (technique as used in Lopes da Silva et al., 1973). The power spectrum (**B**) and the bicoherence (**C**) were obtained by ensemble averaging. Note the peak in the power spectrum at about 10 Hz and the smaller peak at the second harmonic frequency, which are related to each other as the bicoherence shows. **A:** Experimentally recorded alpha rhythm (arbitrary scale). **B:** Power spectrum (arbitrary scale). **C:** Bicoherence limits 99% at 0.119, 95% at 0.096, five lines from 0.18 until 0.26. (Adapted from Lopes da Silva, F.H., van Rotterdam, A., Barts, P., et al. 1976. Models of neuronal populations: the basic mechanisms of rhythmicity. In *Perspectives of Brain Research,* Eds. M.A. Corner and D.F. Swaab. Prog. Brain Res. 45:281–308.)

alpha rhythm, both experimentally measured and simulated. The spectrum of the experimentally measured alpha rhythm also presents a clear component at the second harmonic of the peak frequency (Fig. 4.13). It can be demonstrated by means of bispectral analysis that this component is indeed a second harmonic of the peak frequency. This fact implies that static nonlinear properties of the network have also to be taken into account.

The spatial properties of alpha rhythms are less well understood, although it has been found experimentally that, in the visual cortex of the dog, small cortical areas appear to act as "epicenters" from which alpha rhythm activity "spreads" in different directions (Lopes da Silva and Storm van Leeuwen, 1978). The spreading has been measured in terms of phase differences in rhythmic components at different locations on the cortical surface.

One hypothesis is that the propagation of alpha activity depends on spatial properties of the cortical neuronal net-

works; the strength of inhibition is a function of distance depending on the length of interneuronal connections. This hypothesis has been realized by way of a "spatially distributed model" of neurons and interneurons (Van Rotterdam et al., 1982), which is an extension of the lumped parameter model described by Lopes da Silva et al. (1974). In this spatially distributed model, it is assumed that two populations of neurons (main cells and local interneurons) are arranged in a one-dimensional row and are interconnected by means of recurrent collaterals and inhibitory fibers. Such a neuronal chain is assumed to have the following properties: (a) the transfer function of input-output spike densities are second-order linear functions with a longer time constant for inhibition than for excitation; (b) the interconnectivity properties are homogeneous in space, i.e., the strength of inhibition is only a function of distance between the interconnected neurons; and (c) the strength of interconnectivity decreases exponentially as a function of distance, as shown in Fig. 4.14.

To simulate alpha activity as a function of both space and time, the lumped model must be extended in such a way that it can account for spatial properties. This can be done as follows: the spatially distributed model consists of a chain of neurons and interneurons interconnected by means of spatially distributed excitatory collaterals and inhibitory fibers from the interneurons. The interconnections are described by Ce(k,l), denoting the number of excitatory synapses from the kth main cell projecting on the lth interneuron, and Ci(k,l), denoting the number of inhibitory synapses from the kth interneuron on the lth main cell. Figure 4.15 shows a schematic drawing of such a neuronal chain, where T_k is the kth main cell and I_k is the kth local interneuron. The main cells receive input along afferent fibers from outside the chain. Figure 4.16 shows the corresponding block diagram. The time-dependent behavior of the membrane potential

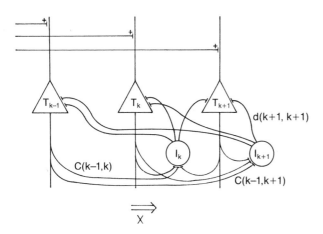

Figure 4.15. Schematic drawing of a section of the spatially distributed model (neuronal chain). For explanation see text. (Adapted from Van Rotterdam, A., Lopes da Silva, F.H., Van den Ende, J., et al. 1982. A model of the spatial-temporal characteristics of the alpha rhythm. Bull. Math. Biol. 44(2):283–305.)

U(k,t) of the kth cell is determined by the transfer functions he(t) and hi(t) of the lumped model. NI_e and NI_i denote the static nonlinearities that relate membrane potentials to impulse densities of main cells and interneurons, respectively. These static nonlinearities are assumed to have the same characteristics as $f_e(V_e)$ and $f_i(V_i)$ in the lumped model and hence can be approximated as linear gain factors in the neuronal chain. Finally, P(k,t) denotes the input impulse density on the main cell k.

To study propagation properties in the neuronal chain, various approaches can be used. In the first place, the expression describing the spatial and temporal characteristics of the model may be written as a linear inhomogeneous par-

tial differential equation, which is a rather complicated type of wave equation. By assuming a wave packet existing over a restricted length somewhere in the neuronal chain at some instant of time, one can try to determine group velocity and dispersion properties. Alternatively, the neuronal chain may be conceived as a two-dimensional linear system with a specified transfer function relating the input p(x,t) to the output u(x,t). The response to an arbitrary input can then be obtained in the time domain by means of a two-dimensional convolution or in the two-dimensional frequency domain by multiplication of the spectra of the transfer function and the input function (see mathematical treatment of Van Rotterdam et al., 1982).

It is reasonable to assume that, in order to simulate alpha rhythm conditions, the neuronal chain must be excited randomly in space as well as in time. Due to the linear character of the model, however, a simple local harmonic excitation of the chain already reveals the propagation properties of the neuronal chain.

If the neuronal chain is locally excited at $x = 0$ with a harmonic component of frequency ω_0, the model response with the same time characteristics has a local component at $x = 0$ and two components that spread in two directions along the chain. The amplitudes of these components decay exponentially proportional to $\exp[-\text{Re}\{k_i(\omega_0)\}|x|]$ and the phase shifts that reflect the propagation properties of the harmonic component equal $\exp[-\text{Im}\{k_i(\omega_0)\}|x|]$ radians when measured at a distance x in relation to $x = 0$. Both phase shift and decay are thus dependent on the frequency of excitation.

The results of the evaluation of the roots of the equation describing the output of the chain as a function of space and time (Van Rotterdam et al., 1982) show that the rhythmic components existing in the chain in the alpha band are less damped than the components outside the alpha band. Furthermore, it follows that the damping in the alpha band is mainly determined by the interconnectivity function with the largest characteristic length.

The model just described schematically has characteristics that are in qualitative agreement with experimental data on alpha rhythmic activity obtained from the visual cortex of dog (Lopes da Silva and Storm van Leeuwen, 1978). This can be examined in relation first to coherence analysis and second to experimental phase measurements:

1. Coherence analysis of EEG signals recorded from chronically implanted subdural electrodes lying directly on the marginal gyrus revealed a higher correlation between EEG components in the alpha band than between components outside that band (Lopes da Silva et al., 1980a,b). These experimental data support the conclusion from the model study that alpha rhythms are the least damped in the chain.

2. Phase shifts at the alpha frequency (around 12 Hz) measured on the marginal gyrus in four dogs reflected phase velocities that were about 30 cm/sec (Lopes da Silva and Storm van Leeuwen, 1978). Using the model, the characteristic length corresponding to this phase velocity and frequency was computed. The order of magnitude of the characteristic lengths 1/c and 1/d of the connectivity functions Ce(x) and Di(x) (Fig. 4.14) were estimated and

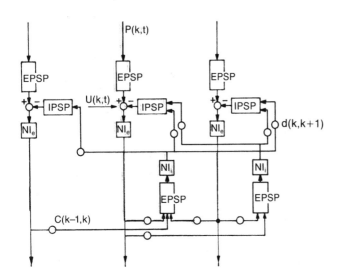

Figure 4.16. Block diagram of a section of the neuronal chain model showing the main excitatory and inhibitory interconnections as explained in text. (Adapted from Van Rotterdam, A., Lopes da Silva, F.H., Van den Ende, J., et al. 1982. A model of the spatial-temporal characteristics of the alpha rhythm. Bull. Math. Biol. 44(2):283–305.)

found to be within the range of 160 to 330 μm. The characteristic lengths correspond to the distance at which the influence of a neuron on a neighbor is reduced to 37% of the starting value and not to the whole length of the interconnecting fibers. The figures that were calculated using the model are in the same range as the dimensions of the basic cortical space module, which is considered to be a vertical cylinder of 200/300 μm diameter (Braitenberg, 1977; Chow and Leimann, 1970; Szentagothai, 1978a,b). Different systems of intracortical fibers, which involve much larger distances than the diameter of a column (at least distances one order of magnitude larger) assure the interconnectivity of several columns. One of these systems consists of tangential intracortical collaterals of the pyramidal cells. These may spread over distances of about 3 mm; they form the "pyramid collateral spread module" (Szentagothai, 1978b). Another system consists of long surface parallel terminal axons that may extend over distances of about 6 to 8 mm; this forms the "surface parallel intracortical system" (Szentagothai, 1978b). These systems of overlapping intracortical connections will lead to the establishment of cooperative action between large populations of cortical neurons and thus to the appearance of dynamic patterns over the cortex (Katchalsky et al., 1974). In addition to the corticocortical systems described above, one must also take into consideration the role of local interneurons; Tombol (1978) described, among others, basket cells in the cat cortex with vertical axons branching horizontally over 500 to 1,000 μm, with terminals surrounding and making contact with pyramidal cell somata; these basket cells are probably inhibitory interneurons. The collaterals belonging to the pyramid collateral spread module system of Szentagothai, which is most likely excitatory, and the axons of the inhibitory interneurons can be identified as the excitatory collaterals and the inhibitory fibers modeled in the model neuronal chain; because this system of interconnections ranges over distance in the order of magnitude of hundreds of micrometers, the estimated characteristic lengths computed from the experimentally measured alpha rhythm frequency and phase velocity with the help of the neuronal chain model are in agreement with neuroanatomical data.

Finally, note that the neuronal chain can be easily generalized to a neuronal network extending in two or three dimensions.

A more general approach that accounts for the generation of alpha rhythms and its spread in the cortex, has been proposed more recently by Liley and collaborators (Liley, 1997; Liley et al., 1999, 2002), who consider the cortex as an excitable spatial continuum of reciprocally connected excitatory and inhibitory neurons interacting by way of short-range (intracortical) and long-range (corticocortical) connections. An essential feature of this general model is that IPSPs are described by third-order differential equations, since according to these authors lower orders were not able to support widespread activity in the alpha band. This theoretical approach showed that the strength and form of synaptic interactions between inhibitory interneurons constitute the most

relevant determinants of the frequency and damping of alpha band oscillations. This feature derives from the assumption that local inhibitory-inhibitory loop delays are longer than the corresponding local and long-range excitatory-excitatory loop delays. This theory has been presented in the form of a set of nonlinear differential equations that can be solved by numerical methods, but most important predictions of the theory can be obtained by a simplified set of linear equations. In this way the input to the cortex can be assumed to be indistinguishable from band-limited white noise, while the cortex operates as a noise filter that passes preferentially frequencies around 8 to 13 Hz. The filter can be described by a transfer function, the properties of which are determined by the both the physiological state and the anatomical structure of the cortex.

Models of Oscillations at the Single Cell and Local Network Levels

In the last decades, important advances were obtained with respect to the physiology of single cells of the thalamus and to their patterns of interaction at the level of local networks, including the corresponding intrinsic membrane and synaptic properties. Interesting models incorporating these properties were proposed, among others by Wang (1994), Wang et al. (1995), Golomb et al. (1994, 1996), Destexhe et al. (1996), and have been reviewed extensively by Destexhe and Sejnowski (2003). These models are mainly based on the experimental results of Steriade and colleagues (e.g., Contreras and Steriade, 1996) and also of McCormick and collaborators (e.g., Bal et al., 1995a,b). The latter results were obtained in the ferret slice preparation that facilitates carrying out controlled experiments, although under circumstances that differ from the conditions in the intact brain. Nevertheless, in these slices it was possible to show (Bal et al., 1995a,b) the occurrence of spindles with main frequency between 5 and 9 Hz, during which the RE neurons tend to fire synchronously with almost every cycle of local rhythmic spindle. In contrast, TCR neurons tend to fire bursts also phase-locked to the local rhythm, but not at every cycle since they may skip one, two, or even more cycles. The modulation of this activity by blocking $GABA_A$ receptors results in a decrease of the main frequency to 2 to 4 Hz, whereas the rhythmic pattern is hardly changed by blocking $GABA_B$ receptors. In addition, the spindle bursts appear to propagate in the slice, as traveling fronts, at a velocity of about 1 mm/s.

As indicated above, the RE and the TCR neurons can exhibit oscillations of the membrane potential, that depend strongly on the state of the potassium leak conductance of the cells (g_{kl}). In the model of Golomb et al. (1996) both RE and TCR neurons are at rest, i.e., they do not display oscillatory behavior, for too small or too large values of g_{kl}, and they oscillate at intermediary levels. In this model the TCR neurons elicit EPSPs on RE neurons by way of glutamatergic (AMPA) synapses, whereas RE neurons elicit both $GABA_A$ and $GABA_B$ mediated IPSPs on TCR neurons. Due to the existence of a low-voltage activated Ca current (T current) the TCR neurons can elicit a rebound burst after a hyperpolarization due to the GABA-ergic IPSP, whether or not

A Synaptic Conductances

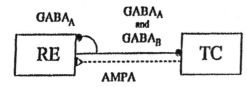

B One-Dimensional Architecture

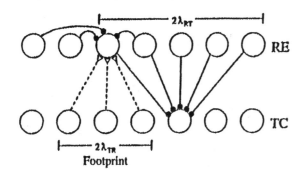

C Footprint Shapes

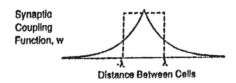

Figure 4.17. Synaptic architecture of the model of Golomb et al. (1996). **A:** Reticular neurons (RE) receive thalamocortical (TC) excitation via glutamatergic (AMPA) synapses and intra-RE inhibition via $GABA_A$ and $GABA_B$ synapses from other RE cells. **B:** This model has a one-dimensional architecture. The RE-to-TC coupling strength decays with distance. The typical decay length RT is called the synaptic footprint length. The same applies to the TC-to-RE coupling (TR), and to the RE-to-RE coupling (RR). **C:** A typical footprint shape of the synaptic coupling with distance; the decay length (either TR or RT or RR) is the distance for which the synaptic coupling reaches 1/e of its maximal value. (Adapted from Golomb, D., Wang, X.J., and Rinzel, J. 1996. Propagation of spindle waves in a thalamic slice model. J. Neurophysiol. 75:750–769.)

associated with a Ca-dependent K current [afterhyperpolarization (AHP) current]. In the model simulations if the neurons were not in intrinsic oscillatory mode, the network would be quiescent. However, the introduction of a few oscillating TCR neurons was sufficient to recruit the other neurons into a rhythmic spindle. The oscillation was critically dependent on the existence of a cationic current activated by hyperpolarization, the I_h or "sag" current, in these neurons (Wang, 1994).

Using this model it was possible to investigate the patterns of propagation of the oscillations throughout the network. The neurons in the network were connected by synaptic couplings, the strength of which decays with spatial distance, as shown in Fig. 4.17. An oscillation started typically at a focal site and propagated as a wavefront that re-

cruited successively more neurons into the oscillatory mode. The I_h current modulated the occurrence of these oscillations: a reduction of I_h led to sustained oscillations, whereas an up-regulation of I_h elicited refractoriness of the neurons, leading to extinction of the oscillations. In this model, the responses of the neuronal network to different stimulus patterns were not reported, although this is most important to understand the behavior of the network of the intact brain under physiological conditions.

Models of Epileptiform Activity

Here we consider those models by means of which one attempts to explain how EEG phenomena characteristic of epileptiform seizures may emerge from the normal ongoing activity. Most theoretical studies have addressed in general terms the question of how oscillations may take place in a network of neurons, assuming that such oscillations are akin to seizure activity. A general way to investigate this problem using a model of such a network is to analyze the trajectories in the phase plane whose coordinates are the potential and its first derivative. A nonlinear system that goes into stable oscillation even after the input stimulus has ceased will produce a closed trajectory in the phase plane; such a closed trajectory is called a limit cycle. Working from the model initially described by Lopes da Silva et al. (1974, 1976), Zetterberg et al. (1978) have shown that a slightly modified model may generate limit cycle oscillations that can simulate some forms of epileptogenic activity recorded from the cortex. Freeman noted that his KII model was not initially designed to simulate epileptiform activity. However, by using a different nonlinear gain curve, Babloyantz and Kaczmarek (1979) have generated limit cycle oscillations that are thought to resemble epileptiform activity. In such models, however, a more or less precise fit between simulated and recorded EEG activity was not attempted. More recently, models that attempt a precise waveform fit have been introduced. Such a model was proposed by Traub (1982) and Traub and Wong (1983a) and is based on experimental data at the cellular level concerning the membrane mechanisms responsible for epileptogenesis (Traub and Wong, 1983b) together with the properties of synaptic interactions in hippocampal neurons.

Cellular and Network Models of Epileptiform Activity

Observations at the cellular level obtained in the hippocampal slice preparation have yielded a number of new facts concerning the origin of an epileptogenic focus. It has been shown that pyramidal cells of the hippocampus (cornus ammonis or CA3) have active membrane regions, the so-called soma and dendritic hot spots that have voltage-dependent ion conductances (g) for Na^+, K^+, and Ca^{2+} and a calcium-activated K conductance; furthermore, a voltage-dependent inactivation of gK and a partial inactivation of gCa by the cytosolic accumulation of Ca^{2+} ions has been assumed (Traub, 1982). Incorporating all these properties, Traub (1982) has made a compartmental model by means of which spontaneous bursts in CA3 cells can be generated, as shown in Fig. 4.18. Using these elementary cellular components (Traub and Wong, 1982), Traub et al. (1984) constructed a network of CA3 neurons interconnected by

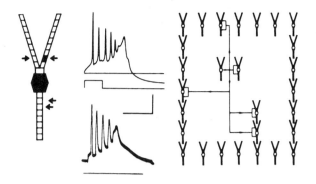

Figure 4.18. Simulation of a bursting neuron showing an epileptiform discharge. Each simulated neuron had a number of compartments and ion conductances, as explained in the text. The intracellular burst model is shown above a recorded burst. The network contains 100 neurons interconnected in a random synaptic network. Vertical calibration, 25 mV by 25 msec (model) and 40 msec (experimental). (Adapted from Traub, R.D., and Wong, R.K.S. 1982. Cellular mechanism of neuronal synchronization in epilepsy. Science 216:745–747.)

excitatory synaptic connections. The generation of epileptiform transients induced by the administration of antagonists of the neurotransmitter GABA was the first problem considered. The conditions for the production of a chain reaction of excitation that spreads over the whole network were found using the simulations. The most important of these conditions was that the excitatory interconnectivity should be sufficiently dense and the synaptic interactions of sufficient strength. A good fit between simulated and experimentally recorded epileptiform transients was obtained, as shown in Fig. 4.18. A second problem analyzed was how sustained afterdischarges can be produced in such a model. It was found that for the occurrence of repetitive afterdischarges, some form of pacing inhibitory process was needed. This was accomplished by introducing two additions in the model: (a) a slow voltage-dependent K+ conductance (M current), and (b) an axonal refractoriness that causes intermittent conduction from one to the next depolarized cell, located at the axonal initial segment, at branch points, or at presynaptic terminals.

Furthermore, a number of loops allowing reentrant paths within the neuronal population are of importance for the maintenance of a series of afterdischarges. Using this kind of models, in a series of studies Traub and collaborators (1996, 1999) investigated the role of a number of factors in inducing epileptiform oscillations similar to those observed in brain slices, *in vitro*, namely synaptic mediated activation of *N*-methyl-D-aspartate (NMDA) dendritic synapses, and intrinsic voltage-dependent conductances. The possible importance of the firing of ectopic presynaptic action potentials in eliciting the synchronization of neurons during epileptiform seizure-like activity was suggested (Traub et al., 1996). Another factor that may contribute to epileptiform activity has been put forward on the basis of models and *in vitro* physiological studies of Traub's group (2002): gap junctions located between the axons of principal hippocampal neurons would play a role in the generation of very fast (about 200 Hz) oscillations. These model simula-

tions have allowed making the prediction that action potentials can cross from axon to axon via gap junctions. Axonal network oscillations would, in turn, induce oscillatory activity in larger neuronal networks, by a variety of mechanisms, and could underlie *in vivo* ripples (to approximately 200 Hz in hippocampal EEG), to drive gamma (30-70 Hz) oscillations that appear in the presence of carbachol, and to initiate certain types of ictal discharges.

In addition model studies have also addressed the possibility that changes in extracellular ionic concentrations (increase of K+ and/or decrease of Ca2+) may be important for the generation of epileptiform seizure activity. Somjen and collaborators (Kager et al., 2000, 2001, 2002) used computer models to better understand how transmembrane ionic and water movements may affect neuronal excitability, and observed that the model produced epileptiform afterdischarges if during stimulation interstitial K+ concentration was sufficiently enhanced so that the persistent Na+ (slowly inactivating) current was activated. In order for firing of a neuron to be maintained after the end of a stimulus, the $[K^+_o]/[K^+_i]$ ratio had to be sufficiently large to maintain the neuronal membrane depolarized so that the inward currents could persist, which activated a series of action potentials. In the course of time the persistent Na+ current was inactivated and the ion pumps, associated with the buffering of K+ ions by glia cells, restored the normal levels of K+ extracellular concentration. These model studies strongly suggest that the elevation of extracellular K+ is not the initial stimulus for a seizure, but it may cause the transition from interictal to ictal discharges (Borck and Jefferys, 1999). The initial stimulus starting the seizure may require synaptic interactions among a population of interconnected neurons.

In contrast with the models described above, which are directed to the simulation of epileptiform activity as seen at the cellular level, especially in *in vitro* preparations, the model study of Wendling et al. (2000) focuses on high-frequency EEG activities (gamma band) that constitute one of the most characteristic EEG patterns in focal seizures of human epilepsy, especially those that have an epileptogenic zone in the hippocampus and associated limbic cortical areas (Allen et al., 1992; Bragin et al., 1999). This model starts from the hypothesis that networks of inhibitory interneurons with different properties are essential for the generation of gamma frequency oscillations (White et al., 2000). This lumped model includes different kinds of neuronal populations, in particular two kinds of GABAergic neurons: GABA_A fast and GABA_A slow populations, where the former cause IPSPs with short time constants on the soma of pyramidal neurons, while the latter cause IPSPs with slow time constants on the dendrites of these neurons. Furthermore as demonstrated experimentally by Banks et al. (2000), both classes interact: GABA_A slow cells inhibit not only pyramidal cells but also GABA_A fast interneurons. The model is based on the important experimental observation that a nonuniform alteration of GABAergic inhibition underlies the generation of epileptiform activity in hippocampus and associated areas of the limbic brain, namely a reduced dendritic inhibition and increased somatic inhibition (Cossart et al., 2001). The simulations show that strikingly realistic activities are produced by the model when

Figure 4.19. A: A real depth-EEG signal recorded in human hippocampus at the beginning of a partial temporal lobe seizure with intracerebral electrodes (SEEG). Four phases (a-1 to a-4) are distinguished according to the pseudo-stationary nature of the activities reflected by the signal: normal background activity (a-1), discharge of rhythmic spikes (a-2), low-voltage rapid discharge (a-3), and high amplitude quasi-sinusoidal slowing down activity (a-4). The normalized power spectral density (PSD) shows that part of the activity corresponding to phase a-3 belongs to the gamma band (55 to 60 Hz). **B:** A candidate path on the activity map, for a value of excitation (A = 5) and different values of slow (B) and fast (G) inhibition, showing the transitions between different types of activity observed in the real signal (type 1 → type 3 → type 4 → type 6). **C:** Slow and fast inhibitory synaptic gain profiles defined by the candidate path and used in the model to simulate a time-series signal with transitions in dynamics. **D:** Simulated EEG signal obtained with the model when the synaptic gains vary as a function of time and PSDs computed on the four periods of 10 seconds (b-1 to b-4). (Adapted from Wendling, F., Bartolomei, F., Bellanger, J.J., et al. 2002. Epileptic fast activity can be explained by a model of impaired GABAergic dendritic inhibition. Eur. J. Neurosci. 15(9):1499–1508.)

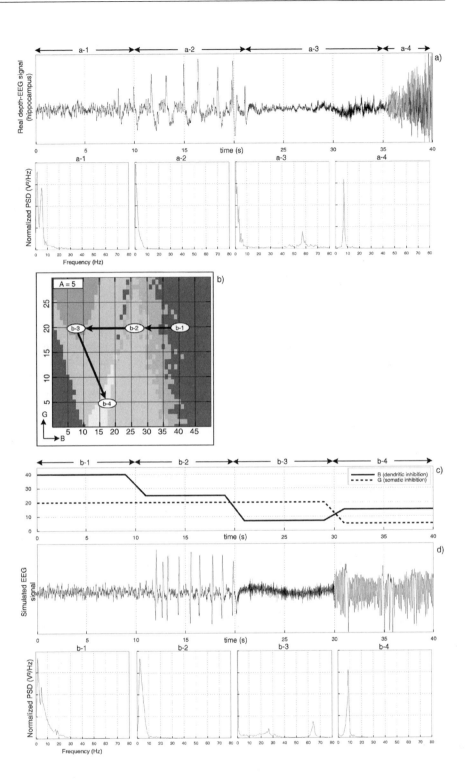

compared to real EEG signals recorded with intracerebral electrodes in patients with temporal lobe epilepsy. They show, further, that the transition between interictal and fast ictal activity is explained, in the model, by the impairment of dendritic inhibition (Fig. 4.19).

In general we may state that a variety of changes at the cellular level may lead to the occurrence of epileptiform seizure activity. In fact there is no unique process that can account for the generation of epileptiform activity.

Models of Thalamic Spike-and-Wave Seizures

Thalamic neurons can display different modes of activity including rhythmic bursting that are akin to spike-and-wave discharges characteristic of generalized epilepsies. In this respect the single neuron model of a thalamic relay neuron of Wang (1994), which shows both 10- and 3-Hz bursting dynamical modes, is particularly instructive. This model demonstrates clearly how distinct oscillatory modes depend on different balances of sets of ion currents. In this model the emergence of 3-Hz bursts, which resemble the 3-Hz oscillations seen in generalized epilepsies, depends on the value of the hyperpolarization-activated cationic current, I_h, the so-called sag current, although the T-type Ca current also plays an important role. According to this model the 10-Hz oscillatory mode is maintained, at the level of a single neuron, by the dynamics of the low-voltage activated Ca current, I_T. Under normal conditions the neuronal membrane does not hyperpolarize sufficiently to activate the I_h current.

Indeed if the neuronal membrane would be deeply hyperpolarized, it would stay in such a condition in case only I_T would be active, because the latter current is not sufficient to overcome a strong hyperpolarization. However, the presence of I_h allows the neuron to escape this strong hyperpolarized state. Thus the transition between the 10- and the 3-Hz modes depends on the level of hyperpolarization. This single neuron model is completely deterministic and it may display "strange attractors" typical of a chaotic dynamic state.

A model of a thalamic neuronal network that is closer to the reality of epileptic discharges than the single neuron model described above was developed to account for spike-and-wave (SW) seizures at the level of a neuronal population. The basic physiological phenomenon simulated was the finding that during SW discharges the RE neurons discharge with long spike bursts riding on a depolarization, whereas the TCR neurons are either entrained into the seizure oscillation or are quiescent (Lytton et al., 1997). The spatial model of these neuronal populations predicts that in a center of seizure activity there will be intense RE activity and TCR quiescence, and that this focus will be surrounded by an area where the TCR neurons will be less hyperpolarized such that low-threshold oscillatory spikes will occur. This surrounding area will be the forefront of a wave of propagating seizure activity. The model shows that the complex nonlinear dynamics of the neuronal network depends critically on the low-voltage activated (LVA) Ca-current I_T. In this context it is interesting to note that in the genetic model of absence epilepsy GAERS (Genetic Absence Epilepsy Rats of Strasbourg), the presence of a significantly enhanced LVA current in thalamic neurons was demonstrated by Tsakiridou et al., 1995. It is also noteworthy that drugs, like ethosuximide, that depress I_T should suppress seizure initiation. It should be noted, however, that more recent studies showed that ethosuximide acts also on the noninactivating Na^+ current and on a Ca^{2+}-activated K^+ current (Leresche et al., 1998). The level of hyperpolarization of TCR cells, which appears to be a crucial determinant of the dynamic behavior of the neuronal population, depends on synaptic mechanisms. The model of Destexhe et al. (1996) goes further than previous models and shows that the transition from 9–11 Hz to 3 Hz oscillations appears to depend on $GABA_B$ synapses. Relatively weak RE activity would mainly elicit $GABA_A$ responses, whereas stronger activity would recruit $GABA_B$ synapses and this would cause the quiescent

mode of the TCR neurons. Indeed, $GABA_B$ presynaptic inhibition is conspicuous between RE neurons, such that an enhancement of the latter would result in a decrease of intra-RE inhibition and, thus in an increase of inhibition of TCR neurons (quiescent state). Thus GABAergic drugs would aggravate the tendency for seizure oscillations to occur.

The models discussed above have given insight into some basic neuronal mechanisms of SW discharges, but do not address specifically the most essential issue of this type of epileptic activity—that a given thalamocortical loop can display both kinds of activity without specific adjustments of parameters being expressly made. Indeed the essence of epilepsy is that a patient displays (long) periods of normal EEG activity (i.e., nonepileptiform) intermingled with epileptiform paroxysmal activity only occasionally. Thus, it is essential to understand the mechanisms responsible for *transitions* from normal activity to paroxysmal SW discharges. This aspect of the dynamical process responsible for epilepsy was addressed in a computational model of absence epilepsy (Suffczynski et al., *submitted*). In this model the behavior of populations of interacting neurons integrating neuronal and network properties was simulated, as a more extended and elaborated version of a previous model of the alpha rhythm (Suffczynski et al., 1999). This approach facilitated investigating system *dynamics* at the macroscopic level, that is, at the level where electric brain signals such as local field potentials or EEG are recorded. The model may exhibit two qualitatively different types of behavior, such as seen in experimental animals with genetically determined absence-like seizure (WAG/Rij rats and GAERS animals). The output signal may display a waxing and waning "spindle-like" oscillation having a spectrum with a peak at approximately 11 Hz or a high amplitude "seizure-like" oscillation at a frequency around 9 Hz, as seen in these rats during absence seizures (Fig. 4.20). The former behavior corresponds to the normal ongoing activity, while the latter corresponds to the paroxysmal epileptiform activity. Thus, for a set of neuronal parameters, the model is in a "bistable regime" where it may generate both normal and paroxysmal oscillations and spontaneous transitions between these two types of behavior. This model facilitated making a number of important predictions that can be tested experimentally, both in animals and in humans: (a) The transitions between the normal and the paroxysmal states can emerge spontaneously and are not induced necessarily by any parameter changes. (b) Probabilities of transitions between normal neuronal activity and paroxysmal oscillations depend on a number of model parameters; therefore, these probabilities can be controlled in a nonunique way; in more general terms these probabilities may be described by gamma distributions, of which the exponential distribution is a special case. Interestingly, exponential shape of histograms of durations of ictal events has also been found in other types of human epilepsy. (c) Paroxysmal oscillations can be annihilated by a well-timed pulse, such that, under given conditions, this kind of seizures may be aborted. The model facilitates investigating these conditions such that the possibility of aborting seizures may be tested experimentally.

Simulation example

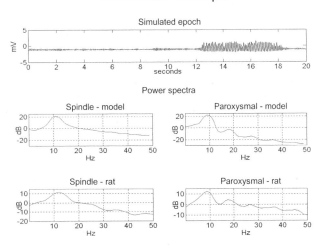

Figure 4.20. **Upper panel:** 20 seconds of a simulation with the occurrence of a spontaneous paroxysmal episode. **Middle panel:** Normal activity and a paroxysmal episode in an extended time scale. **Lower panel:** Average power spectra of signals simulated by the model and recorded from a WAG/Rij rat with absence seizures. *Left-hand side:* The spectra of normal activity. *Right-hand side:* The spectra of paroxysmal activity. (Adapted from Suffczynski, P., Kalitzin, S., and Lopes da Silva, F.H. 2004. Dynamics of non-convulsive epileptic phenomena modeled by a bistable neuronal network. *Submitted.*)

Relevance of Nonlinear Dynamic Systems for EEG Generation

The models of neuronal networks just introduced possess nonlinear wave-pulse functions. In a number of studies of such networks, a simplification has been introduced; it was assumed that this nonlinear characteristic could be approximated by a linearized version, at least under those conditions in which the input signals are limited to a small range of amplitude. However, such simplification is not necessary, and it may lead one to ignore essential nonlinear properties of the system, such as the generation of higher harmonics (Fig. 4.13). Indeed, it is possible to account for the behavior of neuronal networks assuming that these networks can be described by a number of coupled nonlinear differential equations as a function of time and space. In general, such a set of nonlinear differential equations may be considered to provide the basis for understanding the generation of all types of EEG activity.

A number of investigators, such as Freeman (1986) and Babloyantz (1985), started to explore the possibilities given by the modern mathematical field of research of nonlinear dynamic systems in order to obtain a better understanding of EEG phenomena. A relevant aspect for this discussion is that all nonlinear dynamic systems with more than two degrees of freedom can display unpredictable behavior over long time scales; in other words, they can display what mathematicians call chaotic behavior (Schuster, 1984). Such systems can have multiple stable states governed by "equilibrium," "limit cycle," or "chaotic" ("strange") attractors. Whether the system will find itself in one or another stable state depends on the input conditions and on the system's parameters.

These mathematical notions can be illustrated using the example of the KIII set defined by Freeman (1986). Such a set of neurons (Fig. 4.2) may have a least four equilibrium states. There is a rest state, in which the nonlinear pulse-wave function is set to zero and corresponds to the state during deep anesthesia. Another is a state in which a near-sinusoidal limit cycle occurs, such as is produced in the olfactory bulb and cortex by drugs and by hyperthermia (Freeman, 1975). Still another state is characterized by recurrent limit cycle behavior in which the olfactory bulb depends on the level of the normal respiratory rhythm (Fig. 4.3). If slightly structurally changed, a KIII set can be led to another state in which chaotic activity is generated. In such a case, the output consists of long stretches, or bursts, with unpredictable amplitudes and phases that resemble the fluctuations of the EEG at rest. A similar behavior can be obtained by giving a low-level random noise input to the KII set. This fact illustrates a general question with which one is faced when modeling the EEG: Is the ongoing EEG a manifestation of a chaotic attractor or of an equilibrium state under random perturbation? The mathematical techniques with which to characterize chaotic behavior of nonlinear dynamic systems and to differentiate it from random activity are described in detail in a number of specialized publications (Grassberger and Procaccia, 1983; Grassberger et al., 1991; Ott, 1993; Rapp et al., 1993; Schuster, 1984). Furthermore, the problems involved in applying these mathematical tools of nonlinear dynamical analysis to EEG signals are discussed in a number of publications (Basar, 1990; Casdagli et al., 1997; Elbert et al., 1994; Jansen, 1991; Pijn et al., 1991; Theiler and Rapp, 1996; Varela et al., 2001).

In general, one can state that it has been difficult to find unambiguous evidence for the existence of nonlinear determinism in EEG signals except for those recorded during epileptic seizures. The latter observations have led to the concept that a given neuronal network may present essentially different modes of activity, i.e., it may display different dynamics, depending on specific conditions. For some values of control parameters, a neuronal network may change its dynamical mode of activity; for example, instead of a random noisy state, a limit cycle or even a chaotic attractor may occur. Under these circumstances we say that a bifurcation has taken place. Thus a bifurcation represents a qualitative change and depends on a set of control parameters that define the operating regimen of the system. We hypothesized (Lopes da Silva et al., 2003) that the main difference between a normal and an epileptic brain is that the operating regimen of a neuronal network in the epileptic brain is much closer to a bifurcation point than in the normal brain, leading to a low-dimensional chaotic mode of behavior. This means that compared to the normal brain, where the operating regimen is situated far from such a bifurcation point, in an epileptic neuronal network the distance between operating and bifurcation points is so small that the system may easily switch from a stable equilibrium to a chaotic attractor, even in response to a very weak stimulus. The latter may pass undetected. Accordingly, in the case of epilepsy the basic question is which factors are responsible for the change in the operating point of the involved neuronal networks (Lopes da Silva and Pijn, 1995). It should be added that this nonlinear dynamical behavior, which we formulate here at the macroscopic level, has also been identified at the neuronal level, since near the transition from subthreshold to bursting oscillations in thalamic neurons an apparently chaotic oscillation was observed. This was made evident in the model studies of Wang (1994; et al., 1995).

Models of EEG Generation Involving Cortical and Subcortical Areas

The models presented in the previous section describe only a rather small number of EEG phenomena. There are many EEG patterns that have not yet been modeled in terms of sets of neuronal networks. Moreover, most models have been limited to simulations of the behavior of local neural networks. This chapter has already considered a model that involved a KIII set including networks of different areas. However, several EEG phenomena have started to be analyzed in these terms. For example, sleep EEG patterns are known in some detail in terms of cellular processes in a number of brainstem and cortical regions (Steriade, 1981; Steriade et al., 1993a,b; see also Chapter 3), and a model describing many essential features of slow wave sleep and activated states in the thalamocortical system as well as the transition between them was recently described (Bazhenov et al., 2002). Specific models that address the question of how pathological slow oscillations (Ball et al., 1977) may be generated have not yet been developed. It is to be expected that efforts in this direction will lead to a better understanding of such EEG phenomena by combining physiological data at the cellular level with mathematical modeling.

Another important theoretical aspect of the generation of EEG phenomena is the question of relating the temporal and spatial aspects of such phenomena. Most models are concerned with local networks, but not with the question of the coupling between relatively distant sets of neurons (for example, between the thalamus and the cortex). However, a model aimed at analyzing such a problem concerning the spatial organization of alpha rhythms has been introduced by Lopes da Silva et al. (1980a,b). A number of experimental studies of alpha rhythm in the dog have revealed that intracortical coherences are in general larger than any thalamocortical coherence measured in the same animal. This led investigators to question the amount of influence of thalamic sources on the large intracortical coherences. This amounts to choosing between two models: either thalamocortical relations are determined by point-to-point projections or each thalamic population may project to several cortical areas. Using partial coherence analysis (Lopes da Silva et al., 1980b), it has been shown that a model based on point-to-point projections cannot be accepted to explain the organization of thalamocortical alpha rhythms. Furthermore, it was found that there are widespread influences of populations of the dorsal thalamus on intracortical coherences. Notwithstanding these influences, the residual intracortical coherences were so large that other factors must be assumed to explain this intracortical coherent activity; these factors may have as an anatomical substrate inter- and intra-

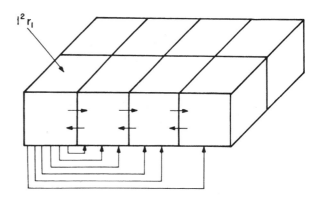

Figure 4.21. Representation of a cortical surface divided into volume elements that are interconnected by intracortical and other association fibers. (Adapted from Nunez, P.L. 1981. *Electric Field of the Brain.* New York: Oxford University Press.)

cortical systems of fibers responsible for the spatial distribution of alpha rhythms within the cortex. Indeed, if such systems did not exist, investigators would be left with a patchy nonoverlapping assembly of cortical modules with little intracortical coherence; it would be almost impossible in such a case to record an EEG at a relatively large distance from the cortex.

A similar problem has been mathematically elaborated by Nunez (1981), who developed a model, also based on the existence of interconnections between different cortical modules, to account for the global wave pattern of the EEG at the scalp (Fig. 4.21). In this way, Nunez takes into account that traveling EEG waves may coalesce to form standing waves because, he assumes, the cortex forms a closed surface. In his view, there is a fixed relationship between the nondimensional temporal and spatial frequency of EEG given by the dispersion relation. This relation relates the temporal frequency with the characteristic velocity of propagation of activity in associative cortical fibers and the so-called wave number.

Nunez (1989) discusses the theory proposed by Lopes da Silva et al. (1980b) and Van Rotterdam et al. (1982), which he calls the "local theory" of the electrocorticogram, in connection with his "global theory," which predicts traveling and standing waves with wavelengths up to the cortical circumference having phase velocities in the 10 m/sec range. According to the local theory, alpha activity spreads away from multiple epicenters with a preferred wave number range for alpha activity and with phase velocities of 30 to 120 cm/sec sec^{-1}. It is likely that a combined local/global theory is needed. Indeed, as Nunez points out (1989, 1995), the simultaneous existence of both short and long wavelength phenomena in the same frequency range can occur. Some EEG phenomena may be dominated by short-range intracortical interactions, while others are dominated by long-range corticocortical interactions. The human scalp EEG results probably from both types of activity. In the combined local-global theory of Nunez (1995), the input to the cortex consists of the modulating afferent input from subcortical areas and inputs from other cortical regions, whether distant or neighboring, through corticocortical fibers (Fig. 4.21). In this model, it is assumed that the local networks include inhibitory and excitatory feedback circuits, whereas the global corticocortical interactions are excitatory. Nunez and collaborators (Nunez, 2000; Nunez et al., 2001) proposed a theoretical framework supporting experimental measures of dynamic properties of human EEG. According to this model both globally coherent and locally dominated behavior can occur within the alpha band, depending on narrow band frequency, spatial measurement scale, and brain state. At the same time, alpha and theta phase locking between cortical regions during certain behavioral states can occur.

Models of Cortical Beta/Gamma Rhythms

In the cortex fast rhythms have been identified, both in the EEG and at the level of single neuronal activity, that are usually called beta or gamma rhythms, depending on frequency range. It has been found experimentally that fast frequency rhythms (33–45 Hz) occurring in the frontoparietal areas may occupy a restricted cortical area in the awake cat (Montaron et al., 1982). These thalamocortical beta rhythms are characteristic of attentive immobility. Beta rhythms with a different frequency (about 28 Hz) have been shown to be rather localized to occipital areas in dogs engaged in a visual discrimination task (Lopes da Silva et al., 1970). Particularly in the visual cortex, oscillations in the gamma frequency range (>30 Hz) at the single neuronal level (Gray et al., 1988) have been recorded (reviewed in Singer and Gray, 1995). In this way, synchronization occurs between neurons that represent related features of an object that should be integrated for the generation of a coherent visual percept. Furthermore, it was shown that neurons in other areas of the cerebral cortex may also synchronize their activity with those of the visual cortex, remarkably without time lags; this synchrony was particularly strong between areas subserving related functions (Roelfsema et al., 1997).

A large number of studies have demonstrated the existence of high-frequency rhythmic activities in the human EEG under different circumstances, particularly in relation with motor and cognitive functions (Freeman et al., 2003; Howard et al., 2003; Pfurtscheller et al., 2003; Sederberg et al., 2003). A review of clinically relevant beta rhythms is given in Chapter 9 and of the influence of drugs on these EEG activities in Chapter 34. Model studies of these EEG fast rhythms have been scarce. The demonstration of these high-frequency activities in animals, particularly in the hippocampus and associated areas, has inspired a number of model studies that try to account for the generation of these activities, integrating experimental observations and computer simulations. Such a model to account for the occurrence of fast oscillations in a neuronal network was proposed by Traub et al. (1996) and Jefferys et al. (1996a,b). The model consists of a chain of interconnected excitatory pyramidal and inhibitory interneurons. According to this model, when the excitatory drive on the interneurons reaches a level sufficient to induce pairs of action potentials at short intervals ("spike doublets") the network generates oscillations in the gamma frequency range on a millisecond

time scale from one end of the chain to the other. It should be noted, however, that neuronal oscillations in a similar frequency range have been found in other areas of the brain, mainly in olfactory bulb and cortex (Boeijinga and Lopes da Silva, 1988; Freeman, 1975, 1979; Kay et al., 1996), but also in the hippocampus and other limbic areas (for review, see Leung, 1992). These rhythmic activities have been modeled by means of cortical neuronal networks with recurrent inhibitory connections, and it was shown that such models, with the relevant physiological parameters, are capable of accounting for the 20- to 50-Hz gamma rhythms (see discussion on this topic by Freeman, 1996; Leung, 1996; and Jefferys et al., 1996a,b).

Based on experimental observations in brain slice preparations of the hippocampus or the neocortex, *in vitro*, where oscillations are induced by electrical stimulation and/or by exogenous drug application, a series of models was created as reviewed by Whittington et al. (2000). These models demonstrate that fast gamma rhythms can be generated by the mechanism of mutual inhibition in populations of interconnected inhibitory interneurons, which can be studied independently by pharmacological manipulations. In spite of the artificial conditions of these experiments, these physiological data have led to interesting theoretical generalizations (Whittington and Traub, 2003), as for instance the possible role of electrical coupling via gap junctions in the generation of very fast oscillations both under normal and epileptic conditions (Perez Velasquez and Carlen, 2000; Traub et al., 2001).

Recently, a generalized model that accounts for changes in rhythmic activities with behavioral state, from the slower alpha to the faster gamma and beta as arousal increases, was proposed (Pinto et al., 2003). This model is especially interesting because the same set of underlying intrinsic and network mechanisms appears to be responsible for the transitions between the rhythm types and between their synchronization properties. The effects of neuromodulation on ionic conductances were investigated in a cortical circuit model, consisting of synaptically coupled excitatory and inhibitory neurons that support rhythmic activity in the alpha, beta, and gamma ranges. It was shown that the effects of neuromodulation on ionic conductances are, by themselves, sufficient to induce transitions between synchronous gamma and beta rhythms and asynchronous alpha rhythms.

It should be noted that despite extensive search, no evidence was found by Menon et al. (1996) for globally correlated activity in the human EEG, either in narrow (i.e., 35–45 Hz) or broad (i.e., 20–50 Hz) frequency bands. Instead, spatially and temporally intermittent synchronization was observed between pairs of electrodes in 1-cm^2 regions with high variability. The distribution of correlation coefficients differed substantially from background levels at interelectrode distances of 1 cm and 1.4 cm but not 2 cm or more. These findings suggest that the surface diameters of domains of spatially correlated activity within the gamma band in human EEG are limited to less than 2 cm. Thus, if such gamma band spatial patterns exist in the human brain, no existing technology would be capable of measuring them at the scalp, and subdural electrode arrays for cortical surface recording would have to have spacings under 5 mm. This means that on the cortex there are well-characterized spatial domains of rhythmic activities that do not spread all over the cortical surface.

Conclusion

The complexity of EEG phenomena calls for the use of mathematical models and computer simulations in order to understand the underlying processes of generation. In the last few years, a number of problems in electroencephalography have been tackled in this way. Such theoretical studies are justified if they are combined with experimental investigations. In this way, one may not only obtain new insights about the generation of EEG patterns, but also formulate hypotheses to be tested under experimental conditions.

In the course of the last decades, a shift of attention from models describing the behavior of local neuronal networks in the temporal domain toward models that take into account the spatial properties of complex networks has occurred. Furthermore, an evolution can be seen in the techniques used. In the early phase, the approach was based mainly on the use of linear systems analysis, but more recently new mathematical tools for the analysis of nonlinear dynamic systems have been introduced in this domain of theoretical neurophysiology. Moreover, the availability of powerful computer tools opens new possibilities for modeling both complex membrane phenomena and network properties. The analysis of the dynamics of such networks is a challenge for the theoretical neurophysiologist interested in understanding EEG phenomena.

References

Allen, P.J., Fish, D.R., and Smith, S.J. 1992. Very high-frequency rhythmic activity during SEEG suppression in frontal lobe epilepsy. Electroencephalogr. Clin. Neurophysiol. 82(2):155–162.

Andersen, P., and Andersson, S.A. 1968. *Physiological Basis of Alpha Rhythm*. New York: Appleton-Century-Crofts.

Andersen, P., Andersson, S.A., and Lomo, T. 1967. Nature of thalamocortical relations during spontaneous barbiturate spindle activity. J. Physiol. 192:283–307.

Avanzini, G., de Curtis, M., Panzica, F., et al. 1989. Intrinsic properties of nucleus reticularis thalami neurons of the rat studied in vitro. J. Physiol. 416:111–122.

Babloyantz, A. 1985. Strange attractors in the dynamics of brain activity. In *Complex Systems Operational Approaches,* Ed. H. Haken, pp. 116–123. Berlin: Springer-Verlag.

Babloyantz, A., and Kaczmarek, L.K. 1979. Self-organization in biological systems with multiple cellular contacts. Bull. Math. Biol. 41:193–201.

Bal, T., von Krosigk, M., and McCormick, D.A. 1995a. Synaptic and membrane mechanisms underlying synchronized oscillations in the ferret LGNd in vitro. J. Physiol. (Lond.) 483:641–663.

Bal, T., von Krosigk, M., and McCormick, D.A. 1995b. Role of the ferret perigeniculate nucleus in the generation of synchronized oscillations in vitro. J. Physiol. (Lond.) 483:665–685.

Ball, G.J., Gloor, R., and Schaul, N. 1977. The cortical electromicrophysiology of pathological delta waves in the electroencephalogram of cats. Electroencephalogr. Clin. Neurophysiol. 43:346–361.

Banks, M.I., White, J.A., and Pearce, R.A. 2000. Interactions between distinct GABA(A) circuits in hippocampus. Neuron. 25(2):449–457.

Basar, E. 1990. Chaotic dynamics and resonance phenomena in brain function: progress, perspectives, and thoughts. In *Chaos in Brain Function,* Eds. E. Basar and T.H. Bullock, pp. 1–31. Berlin: Springer.

Bazhenov, M., Timofeev, I., Steriade, M., et al. 2002. Model of thalamocortical slow-wave sleep oscillations and transitions to activated states. J. Neurosci. 22(19):8691–8704.

Boeijinga, P.H., and Lopes da Silva, F.H. 1988. Differential distribution of beta and theta EEG activity in the entorhinal cortex of the cat. Brain Res. 448:272–286.

Borck, C., and Jefferys, J.G.R. 1999. Seizure-like events in disinhibited ventral slices of adult rat hippocampus. J. Neurophysiol. 82: 2130–2142.

Bragin, A., Engel, J. Jr., Wilson, C.L., et al. 1999. Hippocampal and entorhinal cortex high-frequency oscillations (100–500 Hz) in human epileptic brain and in kainic acid-treated rats with chronic seizures. Epilepsia, 40(2):127–137.

Braitenberg, V. 1977. *On the Texture of Brains.* New York: Springer-Verlag.

Casdagli, M.C., Iasemidis, L.O., Savit, R.S., et al. 1997. Nonlinearity in invasive EEG recordings from patients with temporal lobe epilepsy. Electroencephalogr. Clin. Neurophysiol. 102:98–105.

Chatile, M., Milleret, C., Buser, P., et al. 1992. A 10 Hz "alpha-like" rhythm in the visual cortex of the waking cat. Electroencephalogr. Clin. Neurophysiol. 83:217–230.

Chow, K.L., and Leimann, A.L. 1970. Aspects of the structural and functional organization of the neocortex. Neurosci. Res. Prog. Bull. 8(2): 157–183.

Contreras, D., and Steriade, M. 1996. Spindle oscillation in cats: the role of corticothalamic feedback in a thalamically generated rhythm. J. Physiol. (Lond.) 490:159–179.

Cossart, R., Dinocourt, C., Hirsch, J.C., et al. 2001. Dendritic but not somatic GABAergic inhibition is decreased in experimental epilepsy. Nat. Neurosci. 4(1):52–62.

Destexhe, A., Contreras, D., Sejnowski, T.J., et al. 1994. Modeling the control of reticular thalamic oscillations by neuromodulators. Neuroreport 5:2217–2220.

Destexhe, A., Bal, T., McCormick, D.A., et al. 1996. Ionic mechanisms underlying synchronized oscillations and propagating waves in a model of ferret thalamic slices. J. Neurophysiol. 76:2049–2070.

Destexhe, A., Sejnowski, T.J. 2003. Interactions between membrane conductances underlying thalamocortical slow-wave oscillations. Physiol. Rev. 83(4):1401–1453.

Elbert, T., Ray, W.J., Kowalik, J.E., et al. 1994. Chaos and physiology: deterministic chaos in excitable cell assemblies. Physiol. Rev. 74:1–47.

Freeman, W.J. 1972. Linear analysis of the dynamics of neural masses. Annu. Rev. Biophys. Bioeng. 1:225–256.

Freeman, W.J. 1975. *Mass Action in the Nervous System.* New York: Academic Press.

Freeman, W.J. 1979. Nonlinear dynamics of paleocortex manifested in the olfactory EEG. Biol. Cybern. 35:21–34.

Freeman, W.J. 1983. Dynamics of image formation by nerve cell assemblies. In *Synergetics of the Brain,* Eds. E. Basar, H. Flohr, H. Haken, et al., pp. 102–121. Berlin: Springer-Verlag.

Freeman, W.J. 1986. Analytic techniques used in the search for the physiological basis of the EEG. In *Handbook of Electroencephalography and Clinical Neurophysiology,* vol. 1: *Methods of Analysis of Brain Electrical and Magnetic Signals,* Eds. A. Gevins and A. Remond. Amsterdam. Elsevier.

Freeman, W.J. 1996. Feedback models of gamma rhythms (letter to editor). Trends Neurosci. 19:468.

Freeman, W.J. 2000. A proposed name for aperiodic brain activity: stochastic chaos. Neural. Netw. 13(1):11–13.

Freeman, W.J., Burke, B.C., and Holmes, M.D. 2003. Aperiodic phase resetting in scalp EEG of beta-gamma oscillations by state transitions at alpha-theta rates. Hum. Brain Mapp. 19(4):248–272.

Golomb, D., and Rinzel, J. 1993. Dynamics of globally coupled inhibitory neurons with heterogeneity. Physiol. Rev. E 48:4810–4814.

Golomb, D., and Rinzel, J. 1994. Clustering in globally coupled inhibitory neurons. Physica D 72:259–282.

Golomb, D., Wang, X.J., and Rinzel, J. 1994. Synchronization properties of spindle oscillations in a thalamic reticular nucleus model. J. Neurophysiol. 72:1109–1126.

Golomb, D., Wang, X.J., and Rinzel, J. 1996. Propagation of spindle waves in a thalamic slice model. J. Neurophysiol. 75:750–769.

Grassberger, P., and Procaccia, I. 1983. Measuring the strangeness of strange attractors. Physica 9D:189–208.

Grassberger, P., Schreiber, T., and Schaffrath, C. 1991. Chaos. Int. J. Bifurc. 1:521–547.

Gray, C.M., Freeman, W.J., and Skinner, J.E. 1984. Associative changes in the spatial amplitude patterns of rabbit olfactory EEG are norepinephrine dependent. Neurosci. Abstr. 10(36,2):121.

Gray, C., Konig, P., Engel, A., et al. 1988. Oscillatory responses in cat visual cortex exhibit intercolumnar synchronization which reflects global stimulus properties. Nature 338:334–337.

Hammond, P.H. 1958. *Feedback Theory and Its Applications.* London: English University Press.

Harmon, L.D. 1964. Problems in neural modeling. In *Neural Theory and Modeling, Proceedings of the 1962 OGAI Symposium,* Ed. R.F. Reiss. Stanford, CA: Stanford University Press.

Howard, M.W., Rizzuto, D.S., Caplan, J.B., et al. 2003. Gamma oscillations correlate with working memory load in humans. Cerebral Cortex 13: 1369–1374.

Huguenard, J.R., and Prince, D.A. 1994. Intrathalamic rhythmicity studied in vitro: nominal T-current modulations causes robust anti-oscillatory effects, J. Neurosci. 14:5485–5502.

Jahnsen, H., and Llinás, R. 1984a. Electrophysiological properties of guinea-pig thalamic neurones: an in vitro study. J. Physiol. (Lond.) 349: 205–226.

Jahnsen, H., and Llinás, R. 1984b. Ionic basis for the electro-responsiveness and oscillatory properties of guinea-pig thalamic neurons in vitro. J. Physiol. (Lond.) 349:227–247.

Jansen, B.H. 1991. Is it and so what? A critical review of EEG chaos. In *Measuring Chaos in the Human Brain,* Eds. D.W. Duke and W.S. Pritchard, pp. 49–82. Singapore: World Scientific.

Jefferys, J.G.R., Traub, R.D., and Whittington, M.A. 1996a. Neuronal networks for induced "40 Hz" rhythms. Trends Neurosci. 19:202–208.

Jefferys, J.G.R., Traub, R.D., and Whittington, M.A. 1996b. Reply. Trends Neurosci. 19:469–470.

Kager, H., Wadman, W.J., Somjen, G.G. 2000. Simulated seizures and spreading depression in a neuron model incorporating interstitial space and ion concentrations. J. Neurophysiol. 84(1):495–512.

Kager, H., Wadman, W.J., Somjen, G.G. 2000. Conditions for the triggering of spreading depression studied with computer simulations. J. Neurophysiol. 88(5):2700–2712.

Katchalsky, A.K., Rowland, V., and Blumenthal, R. 1974. Dynamic patterns of brain cell assemblies. Neurosci. Res. Prog. Bull. 12(1):1–187.

Kay, L.M., Lancaster, L.R., and Freeman, W.J. 1996. Reafference and attractors in the olfactory system during odor recognition. Int. J. Neural. Syst. 7:489–495.

Landisman, C.E., Long, M.A., Beierlein, M., et al. 2002. Electrical synapses in the thalamic reticular nucleus. J. Neurosci. 22:1002–1009.

Lanoir, J. 1972. Étude électrocorticographique de la veille et du sommeil chez le chat, organisation du cycle nycthéméral, rôle du thalamus. Thesis Doctor of Science, Centre Régional de recherche et de documentation Pédagogiques, Marseille, France.

Leresche, N., Parri, H.R., Erdemli, G., et al. 1998. On the action of the anti-absence drug ethosuximide in the rat and cat thalamus. J. Neurosci. 18(13):4842–4853.

Leung, L.S. 1996. Recurrent inhibition model of hippocampal CA in vivo (letter to editor). Trends Neurosci. 19:468–469.

Liley, D.T.J. 1997. A continuum model of the mammalian alpha rhythm. In *Spatiotemporal Models in Biological and Artificial Systems,* Eds. F. Lopes da Silva, J.C. Cadusch, and L. Borges de Almeida, pp. 89–96. Amsterdam: IOS Press

Liley, D.T.J., Cadusch, P.C., and Wright, J.J. 1999. A continuum theory of electro-cortical activity. Neurocomputing 26–27:795–800.

Liley, D.T.J., Cadusch, P.J., and Dafilis, M.P. 2002. A spatially continuous mean field theory of electrocortical activity. Network. Comp. Neural. Sys. 13:67–113.

Lopes da Silva, F.H. 1991. Neural mechanisms underlying brain waves: from neural membranes to networks. Electroencephalogr. Clin. Neurophysiol. 79:81–93.

Lopes da Silva, F.H., and Storm van Leeuwen, W. 1978. The cortical alpha rhythm in dog: The depth and surface profile of phase. In *Architectonics of the Cerebral Cortex,* Eds. M.A.B. Brazier and H. Petsche, pp. 319–333. New York: Raven Press.

Lopes da Silva, F.H., van Rotterdam, A., Storm van Leeuwen, W., et al. 1970. Dynamic characteristics of visual EP's in the dog. II. Beta frequency selectivity in evoked potentials and background activity. Electroencephalogr. Clin. Neurophysiol. 29:260–268.

Lopes da Silva, F.H., van Lierop, T.H.M.T., Schrijer, C.F., et al. 1973. Organization of the thalamic and cortical alpha rhythms: spectra and coherences. Electroencephalogr. Clin. Neurophysiol. 35:627–639.

Lopes da Silva, F.H., Hoeks, A., Smits, H., et al. 1974. Model of brain rhythmic activity. Kybernetik 15:27–37.

Lopes da Silva, F.H., van Rotterdam, A., Barts, P., et al. 1976. Models of neuronal populations: the basic mechanisms of rhythmicity. In *Perspectives of Brain Research,* Eds. M.A. Corner and D.F. Swaab. Prog. Brain Res. 45:281–308.

Lopes da Silva, F.H., Vos, J.E., Mooibroek, J., et al. 1980a. Partial coherence analysis of thalamic and cortical alpha rhythms in dog—a contribution towards a general model of the cortical organization of rhythmic activity. In *Rhythmic EEG Activities and Cortical Functioning,* Eds. G. Pfurtscheller et al., pp. 33–59. Amsterdam: Elsevier.

Lopes da Silva, F.H., Vos, J.E., Mooibroek, J., et al. 1980b. Relative contributions of intracortical and thalamocortical processes in the generation of alpha rhythms, revealed by partial coherence analysis. Electroencephalogr. Clin. Neurophysiol. 50:449–456.

Lopes da Silva, F.H., and Pijn, J.P. 1995. Epilepsy: network models of generation. In *The Handbook of Brain Theory and Neural Networks,* Ed. M.A. Arbib, pp. 367–369. Cambridge, MA: A Bradford Book, MIT Press.

Lopes da Silva, F., Blanes, W., Kalitzin, S.N., et al. 2003. Dynamical diseases of brain systems: different routes to epileptic seizures. IEEE Trans. Bio-Med. Eng. 50:540–549.

Lytton, W.W., Confreras, D., Desteche, A., et al. 1997. Dynamic interactions determine partial thalamic quiescence in a computer network model of spoke-and-wave seizures. J. Neurophysiol. 77:1676–1696.

McCormick, D.A. 1992. Neurotransmitter actions in the thalamus and cerebral cortex and their role in neuromodulation of thalamocortical activity. Prog. Neurobiol. 39:337–388.

McCormick, D.A., and Bal, T. 1994. Sensory gating mechanisms of the thalamus. Curr. Opin. Neurobiol. 4:550–556.

Menon, V., Freeman, W.J., Cutillo, B.A., et al. 1996. Spatio-temporal correlations in human gamma band electrocorticograms. Electroencephalogr. Clin. Neurophysiol. 98:89–102.

Montaron, M.F., Bouyer, J.J., Rougeul, A., et al. 1982. Ventral mesencephalic tegmentum (VMT) controls electrocortical beta rhythms and associated alternative behavior in the cat. Behav. Brain Res. 6:129–145.

Nunez, P.L. 1981. *Electric Field of the Brain.* New York: Oxford University Press.

Nunez, P.L. 1989. Generation of human EEG by a combination of long and short range neocortical interactions. Brain Topogr. 1:199–215.

Nunez, P.L. (Ed.) 1995. *Neocortical Dynamics and Human EEG Rhythms.* New York: Oxford University Press.

Nunez, P.L. 2000. Toward a quantitative description of large-scale neocortical dynamic function and EEG. Behav. Brain Sci. 23(3):371–398; discussion 399–437.

Nunez, P.L., Wingeier, B.M., and Silberstein, R.B. 2001. Spatial-temporal structures of human alpha rhythms: theory, microcurrent sources, multiscale measurements, and global binding of local networks. Hum. Brain Mapp. 13:125–164.

Ott, E. 1993. *Chaos in Dynamical Systems.* New York: Cambridge University Press.

Perez Velasquez, J.L.P., and Carlen, P. 2000. Gap junctions, synchrony and seizures. Trends Neurosci. 23:68–74.

Pfurtscheller, G., Graimann, B., Huggins, J.E., et al. 2003. Spatiotemporal patterns of beta desynchronization and gamma synchronization in corticographic data during self-paced movement. Clin. Neurophysiol. 114(7):1226–1236.

Pijn, J.P., Velis, D.N., and Lopes da Silva, F.H. 1991. Chaos or noise in EEG signals: dependence on state and brain site. Electroencephalogr. Clin. Neurophysiol. 79:371–381.

Pinching, A.J., and Powell, T.P.S. 1971. The neuron types of the glomerular layer of the olfactory bulb. J. Cell. Sci. 9:305–345.

Pinto, D.J., Jones, S.R., Kaper, T.J., et al. 2003. Analysis of state-dependent transitions in frequency and long-distance coordination in a model oscillatory cortical circuit. J. Comput. Neurosci. 15(2):283–298.

Rapp, P.E., Albano, A.M., Schmah, T.I., et al. 1993. Filtered noise can mimic low-dimensional chaos. Phys. Rev. E. 47:2289–2297.

Reese, T.S., and Shepherd, G.M. 1972. Dendrodendritic synapses in the central nervous system. In *Structure and Function of Synapses,* Eds. G.D. Pappas and D.P. Purpura, pp. 121–136. New York: Raven Press.

Regan, D.A. 1968. A high frequency mechanism which underlies visual evoked potentials. Electroencephalogr. Clin. Neurophysiol. 25:231–237.

Roelfsema, P.R., Engel, A.K., Koenig, P., et al. 1997. Visuomotor integration is associated with zero timelag synchronization among cortical areas. Nature 385:157–161.

Schuster, H.G. 1984. *Deterministic Chaos.* Weinheim: PhysikVerlag.

Sederberg, P.B., Kahana, M.J., Howard, M.W., et al. 2003. Theta and gamma oscillations during encoding predict subsequent recall. J. Neurosci. 23:10809–10814.

Singer, W., and Gray, C.H. 1995. Visual feature integration and the temporal correlation hypothesis. Annu. Rev. Neurosci. 18:555–586.

Spekreijse, H., and van der Tweel, L.H. 1970. System analysis of linear and nonlinear processes in electrophysiology of the visual system. In *Introduction to Biocybernetics,* Eds. M. Clynes, F.E. Yates, and J.H. Milsum. New York: John Wiley.

Steriade, M. 1981. Mechanisms underlying cortical activation: neuronal organization and properties of the midbrain reticular core and intralaminar thalamic nuclei. In *Brain Mechanisms and Perceptual Awareness,* Eds. O. Pompeiano and C. Ajmone-Marsan, pp. 327–377. New York: Raven Press.

Steriade, M., and Llinás, R.R. 1988. The functional states of the thalamus and the associated neuronal interplay. Physiol. Rev. 68:649–742.

Steriade, M., Deschènes, M., Domich, L., et al. 1985. Abolition of spindle oscillations in thalamic neurons disconnected from nucleus reticularis thalami. J. Neurophysiol. 54:1473–1497.

Steriade, M., Jones, E.G., and Llinás, R.R. 1990a. *Thalamic Oscillations and Signaling.* Neuroscience Institute Publications. New York: John Wiley & Sons.

Steriade, M., Gloor, P., Llinás, R.R., et al. 1990b. Report of the IFCN committee on basic mechanisms. Electroencephalogr. Clin. Neurophysiol. 76:481–509.

Steriade, M., Nunez, A., and Amzica, F. 1993a. A novel slow (<1 Hz) oscillation of neocortical neurons in vivo: depolarizing and hyperpolarizing components. J. Neurosci. 13:3252–3265.

Steriade, M., Nunez, A., and Amzica, F. 1993b. Intracellular analysis of relations between the slow (<1 Hz) neocortical oscillation and other sleep rhythms of the electroencephalogram. Neuroscience 13:3266–3283.

Suffczynski, P., Pijn, J.P.M., Pfurtscheller, G., et al. 1999. Event-related dynamics of alpha band rhythms: a neuronal network model of focal ERD/surround ERS. In *Event Related Desynchronization, Handbook of Electroencephalography and Clinical Neurophysiology,* Revised Series vol. 6, Eds. G. Pfurtscheller and F. Lopes da Silva, pp. 67–85. Amsterdam: Elsevier Science.

Suffczynski, P., Kalitzin, S., Pfurtscheller, G., et al. 2001. Computational model of thalamo-cortical networks: dynamical control of alpha rhythms in relation to focal attention. Int. J. Psychophysiol. 43(1):25–40.

Suffczynski, P., Kalitzin, S., and Lopes da Silva, F.H. 2004. Dynamics of non-convulsive epileptic phenomena modeled by a bistable neuronal network. 126(2):467–484.

Szentagothai, J. 1978a. Specificity versus (quasi) randomness in cortical connectivity. In *Architectonics of the Cortex,* Eds. M.A.B. Brazier and H. Petsche, pp. 77–97. New York: Raven Press.

Szentagothai, J. 1978b. The local neuronal apparatus of the cerebral cortex. In *Cerebral Correlates of Conscious Experience,* Inserm Symposium no. 6, Eds. P. Buser and A. Rougeaul-Buser, pp. 131–138. Amsterdam: Elsevier.

Theiler, J., and Rapp, P.E. 1996. Reexamination of the evidence for low-dimensional nonlinear structure in the human electroencephalogram. Electroencephalogr. Clin. Neurophysiol. 99:213–222.

Tombol, T. 1978. Comparative data on the Golgi architecture of interneurons of different conical areas in cat and rabbit. In *Architectonics of the Cerebral Cortex,* Eds. M.A.B. Brazier and H. Petsche, pp. 59–76. New York: Raven Press.

Traub, R.D. 1982. Simulation of intrinsic bursting in CA3 hippocampal neurons. Neuroscience 7:1233–1242.

Traub, R.D., and Miles, R. 1991. *Neuronal Networks of the Hippocampus.* Cambridge: Cambridge University Press.

Traub, R.D., and Wong, R.K.S. 1982. Cellular mechanism of neuronal synchronization in epilepsy. Science 216:745–747.

Traub, R.D., and Wong, R.K.S. 1983a. Synchronized burst discharge in disinhibited hippocampal slice. II. Model of cellular mechanism. J. Neurophysiol. 49:442–458.

Traub, R.D., and Wong, R.K.S. 1983b. Synaptic mechanisms underlying interictal spike initiation in a hippocampal network. Neurology 33: 258–266.

Traub, R.D., Knowles, W.D., Miles, R., et al. 1984. Synchronized afterdischarges in the hippocampus: simulation studies of the cellular mechanism. Neuroscience 12:1191–1200.

Traub, R.D., Whitington, M.A., Colling, S.B., et al. 1996. Analysis of gamma rhythms in the rat hippocampus in vitro and in vivo. J. Physiol. (Lond.) 493:471–484.

Traub, R.D., Jefferys, J.G., Whittington, M.A. 1999. Functionally relevant and functionally disruptive (epileptic) synchronized oscillations in brain slices. Adv. Neurol. 79:709–724.

Traub, R.D., Whittington, M.A., Buhl, E.H., et al. 2001. A possible role for gap junctions in generation of very fast EEG oscillations preceding the onset of, and perhaps initiating, seizures. Epilepsia 42:153–170.

Traub, R.D., Draguhn, A., Whittington, M.A., et al. 2002. Axonal gap junctions between principal neurons: a novel source of network oscillations, and perhaps epileptogenesis. Rev. Neurosci. 13(1):1–30.

Tsakiridou, E., Bertollini, L., de Curtis, M., et al. 1995. Selective increase in T-type calcium conductance of reticular thalamic neurons in a rat model of absence epilepsy. J. Neurosci. 15:3310–3317.

Van der Tweel, L.H. 1961. Some problems in vision regarded with respect to linearity and frequency response. Ann. N.Y. Acad. Sci. 89:829–856.

Van Rotterdam, A., Lopes da Silva, F.H., Van den Ende, J., et al. 1982. A model of the spatial-temporal characteristics of the alpha rhythm. Bull. Math. Biol. 44(2):283–305.

Varela, F., Lachaux, J.P., Rodriguez, E., Martinerie, J. 2001. The brainweb: phase synchronization and large-scale integration. Nat. Rev. Neurosci. 2(4):229–239.

Von Krosigk, M., Bal, T., and McCormick, D.A. 1993. Cellular mechanisms of a synchronized oscillation in the thalamus. Science 261:361–364.

Wang, X.J. 1994. Multiple dynamical modes of thalamic relay neurons: rhythmic bursting and intermittent phase-locking. Neuroscience 59:21–31.

Wang, X.J., and Rinzel, J. 1992. Alternating and synchronous rhythms in reciprocally inhibitory model neurons. Neural Comp. 4:84–97.

Wang, X.J., and Rinzel, J. 1993. Spindle rhythmicity in the reticularis thalami nucleus: synchronization among mutually inhibitory neurons. Neuroscience 53:899–904.

Wang, X.J., Rinzel, J., and Rogawski, M.A. 1991. A model of the T-type calcium current and the low threshold spike in thalamic neurons. J. Neurophysiol. 66:839–850.

Wang, X.J., Golomb, D., and Rinzel, J. 1995. Emergent spindle oscillations and intermittent burst firing in a thalamic model: specific neuronal mechanisms. Proc. Natl. Acad. Sci. USA 92:5577–5581.

Warren, R.A., Agmon, A., and Jones, E.G. 1994. Oscillatory synaptic interactions between ventroposterior and reticular neurons in mouse thalamus in vitro. J. Neurophysiol. 72:1993–2003.

Wendling, F., Bartolomei, F., Bellanger, J.J., et al. 2002. Epileptic fast activity can be explained by a model of impaired GABAergic dendritic inhibition. Eur. J. Neurosci. 15(9):1499–1508.

White, J.A., Banks, M.I., Pearce, R.A., et al. 2000, Networks of interneurons with fast and slow gamma-aminobutyric acid type A (GABA-A) kinetics provide substrate for mixed gamma-theta rhythm. Proc. Nat. Acad. Sci. USA 97:8128–8133.

Whittington, M.A., Traub, R.D., Kopell, N., et al. 2000. Inhibition-based rhythms: experimental and mathematical observations on network dynamics. Int. J. Psychophysiol. 38(3):315–336.

Whittington, M., and Traub, R.D. 2003. Inhibitory interneurons and network oscillations in vitro. Trends Neurosci. 26(12):676–682.

Wilson, H.R., and Cowan, J.D. 1972. Excitatory and inhibitory interaction in localized populations of model neurons. Biophys. J. 12:1–23.

Wright, J.J., and Liley, D.T.J. 1996. Dynamics of the brain at global and microscopic scales: neural networks and the EEG. Behav. Brain Sci. 19: 285–320.

Zetterberg, L.H. 1973. Stochastic activity in a population of neurons—A system analysis approach. Rep. Inst. Med. Physics, TNO, Utrecht 1:53.

Zetterberg, L.H., Kristiansson, L., and Mossberg, K. 1978. Performance of a model for a local neuron population. Biol. Cybern. 31:15–26.

5. Biophysical Aspects of EEG and Magnetoencephalogram Generation

Fernando Lopes da Silva and Ab Van Rotterdam

The electrical activity of the brain consists of ionic currents generated by biochemical sources at the cellular level. These ionic currents cause electric and magnetic fields that can be measured in the brain and surrounding tissues. The behavior of these fields can be predicted because they obey physical laws. This chapter is an introduction to the biophysical aspects of the generation of electroencephalogram (EEG) signals. It is convenient to consider the generation of EEG signals in biophysical terms because this is the exact way to determine the potential distribution at the scalp given a set of intracerebral current sources, i.e., the so-called forward problem of electroencephalography. An understanding of this problem is necessary to discuss the inverse problem that constitutes the main concern of clinical electroencephalography, which is to determine the intracerebral sources given a measured potential distribution at the scalp. The inverse problem has no unique solution, as shown long ago by Helmholtz (1855); therefore, it is essential to understand the forward problem so that constraints of the inverse problem may be well examined.

This chapter treats the biophysical basis of the generation of EEG potentials nonmathematically so that the general reader may follow it more easily; in the theoretical appendix, a mathematical treatment of the biophysical aspects is provided.

Space-Dependent Properties

The electrical potential at a point in the brain in principle can be computed if the microscopic cellular sources are known. In expression 5.8 of the Appendix, the field potential is given as a function of intracerebral current sources; in expression 5.10, it is given in terms of the membrane potential.

In general terms, the field potential of a population of neurons equals the sum of the field potentials of the individual neurons. To understand EEG phenomena, the activity of populations of neurons must always be considered. EEG phenomena can be measured only at a considerable distance from the source if the responsible neurons are regularly arranged and activated in a more or less synchronous way. A typical regular arrangement is the palisade, in which the neurons are distributed with the main axes of the dendritic trees parallel to each other and perpendicular to the cortical surface. When in such a population (for example, the pyramidal neurons of layer IV and V of the cortex) the neurons are more or less simultaneously activated by way of synapses lying at the proximal dendrites, extracellular currents will flow; their longitudinal components (i.e., parallel to the main axes of the neurons) will add, whereas their transverse components will tend to cancel out. The result is a laminar current along the main axes of the neurons. The net membrane current that results from the activation at the level of the synapse can be either a positive or a negative ionic current directed to the inside of the cell. Because there is no accumulation of charge anywhere in the medium (see also Appendix, expression 5.1), the injected current at the synaptic level is compensated by other currents flowing in the medium, as shown in Fig. 5.1. At the level of the synapse and in the case of an excitatory postsynaptic potential (EPSP), the synaptic current is carried by positive ions; in the case of an inhibitory postsynaptic potential (IPSP), the corresponding current is carried by negative ions. Because the direction of a current is defined by the direction along which the positive charge is transported, the ionic current is directed to the intracellular medium with an EPSP; with an IPSP, it is directed to the extracellular medium. Therefore, at the level of the synapse, there is an active sink in the case of a positive ionic current (EPSP) or an active source in the case of a negative ionic current (IPSP). The extracellular potential at the sink is negative; at the source, it is positive, as can be seen from expression 5.8. Along the cell and at a distance from the synaptic level, there exists a distributed passive source in the case of an EPSP or a distributed passive sink in the case of an IPSP.

In addition to postsynaptic potentials, other relatively slow variations of membrane potential, such as those associated with depolarizing or hyperpolarizing after potentials and dendritic events as calcium action potentials, may also be the sources of extracellularly measurable potentials.

At a macroscopic level, it may therefore be stated that the potential field generated by a synchronously activated palisade of neurons behaves like that of a dipole layer. This is no more than a rough model of reality. It may also be considered that an active sink (for instance, at the level of the cell somata in the cortex) is flanked by two passive sources, one lying more superficially and the other deeper than the sink; in such a case, the potential field should behave more like a quadrupole layer. This is, however, an unnecessary complication because in general the two sides of the quadrupole are rather asymmetrical; one is usually dominant. This is to be expected because it can be seen from histological sections of the cortex that there is a clear asymmetry of the pyramidal cells along a direction perpendicular to the cortex. These cells present a morphological polarization in the vertical direction because they are characterized by a rather long vertically directed apical dendrite that ramifies in the most

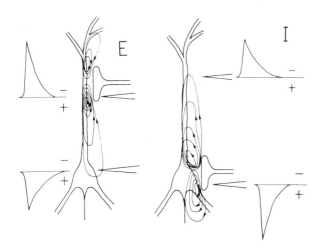

Figure 5.1. Current flow patterns in and around an idealized neuron owing to synaptic activation. *E,* current flow caused by activation of a synapse at the level of the apical dendrite resulting in depolarization of the membrane and flow of a net positive current. This current causes a sink at the site of the synapse. The extracellularly measured excitatory postsynaptic potential (EPSP) is drawn at the *left*; it has a negative polarity at the level of the synapse. At the soma there exists a distributed passive source resulting in an extracellular potential of positive polarity. *I,* current flow caused by activation of a synapse at the level of the soma resulting in hyperpolarization of the membrane and flow of a net negative current. This results in an active source at the level of the soma and passive sinks at the basal and distal dendrites. The extracellularly measured inhibitory postsynaptic potentials (IPSPs) at the soma and dendritic level are drawn. Note that an inhibition at the soma generates about the same extracellular potential field as an excitation at the apical or distal dendrites.

superficial layers of the cortex and by basal dendrites distributed around the soma; the axon runs vertically downward to the white matter. For the sake of simplicity, it therefore may be assumed that most potential fields generated in palisades of neurons can be mimicked by simple dipole layers. Lorente de No (1947) named this type of potential field the "open field" (Fig. 5.2C), in contrast to those fields generated by neurons with dendritic arborizations radially distributed about the soma; according to his description, these would generate "closed fields" as shown in Fig. 5.2A,B. In the latter case, the configuration of the radially oriented neurons is such that each neuron may be considered as generating a central source (or sink, depending on the type of synaptic activity) surrounded by spherically distributed sinks (or sources). The field potential in this case is equivalent to that of a distribution of radially oriented dipoles at the surface of a sphere. It can be seen intuitively that, under these circumstances, not only the tangential but also the radial components of current cancel each other; this can also be proved by the volume conduction theory (Fig. 5.3) (Klee and Rall, 1977).

Postsynaptic potentials in neuronal populations with an appropriate spatial organization can be sources of field potentials that can be measured at a distance and therefore are also sources of EEG signals. Can such other types of membrane potentials as action potentials also contribute to those EEG signals? This is not generally the case, for two reasons (see also Appendix). First, the membrane potential variation

caused by an action potential generates a field that is equivalent to that of a single dipole perpendicular to the membrane because the piece of membrane that is depolarized at any instant of time is small. In contrast, that of an electrotonically conducted postsynaptic potential extends, at any moment of time, over a larger portion of the membrane; thus it generates a field that corresponds rather to that of a dipole layer with dipoles perpendicular to the membrane surface. The latter attenuates with distance less rapidly than the former, as can be seen by comparing expressions 5.12 and 5.15 of the Appendix; this is illustrated in Fig. 5.10B and has also been discussed by Humphrey (1968). The second reason that they do not contribute to EEG signals is that action poten-

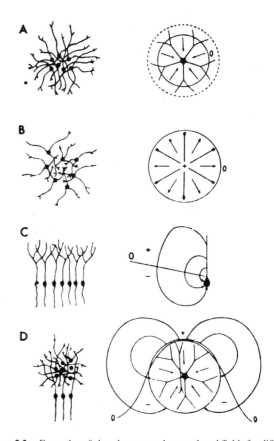

Figure 5.2. Examples of closed, open, and open-closed fields for different types of neuron pools in the central nervous system. *Left:* The populations are drawn. *Right:* Neurons representing the simultaneously activated pools are shown together with the arrows representing the lines of flow of current at the instant when the impulses have evaded the cell bodies. The zero isopotential lines (0) are also indicated. **A:** Oculomotor nucleus represented schematically by only one neuron with dendrites oriented radially outward. The isopotential lines are *circles*; the currents flow entirely within the nucleus, resulting in closed field (all points outside the nucleus remain at zero potential). **B:** Superior olive represented by neurons each having a single dendrite oriented radially inward. The currents result in a closed field. **C:** Accessory olive represented by only one neuron with a single long dendrite. The arrangement of sources and sinks in this structure permits the spread of current in the volume of the brain and thus results in an open field. **D:** Two structures mixed together, generating an open-closed field. (Modified from Lorente de No. 1947. Action potential of the motoneurons of the hypoglossus nucleus. J. Cell. Comp. Physiol. 29:207–287; Hubbard, J.I., Llinas, R., and Quastel, D.M.J. 1969. *Electrophysiological Analysis of Synaptic Transmission.* London: Edward Arnold Ltd.)

NEURON POPULATION POTENTIALS

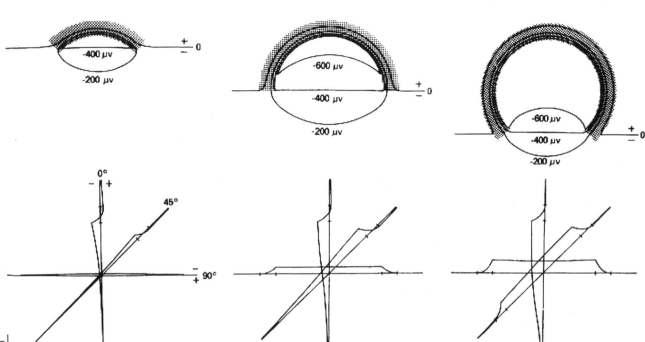

Figure 5.3. Equipotential plots and depth profiles for open cortices. Intersection of base lines of the depth profiles is at the center of the sphere. Tick marks represent the region of cells. Note that the 90-degree profile of the hemisphere and 45-degree profiles of the cap and punctured sphere run along the open edge of the cortex. (Adapted from Klee, M., and Rall, W. 1977. Computed potentials of cortically arranged populations of neurons. J. Neurophysiol. 40:647–666.)

tials, owing to their short duration (1–2 msec), tend to overlap much less than do postsynaptic potentials (EPSP and IPSP), which last longer (≈ 10–250 msec). In those cases in which action potentials do occur simultaneously (for example, when a group of fibers is excited by a short stimulus), the field of an action potential may also be recorded at relatively large distances in the form of what is generally called a compound action potential. The strength of the neuronal sources has been estimated (Hämäläinen et al., 1993) and shown to be in the order of 100 nA·mm^{-2}.

In summary, enough evidence exists to state that the EEG on the scalp is mainly caused by synchronously occurring postsynaptic potentials (De Munck et al., 1992).

Time-Dependent Properties

We have emphasized above the importance of synchrony of neuronal activity for the generation of EEG signals. We consider here the factors that cause this synchrony. The main factor is of a structural nature. Neuronal masses are, in general, organized as combinations of interlocked excitatory and inhibitory populations (Freeman, 1975; Katchalsky et al., 1974; Lopes da Silva et al., 1974, 1976; Wilson and Cowan, 1973); the interlocking takes place by way of recurrent collaterals forming different types of synapses that pos-

sibly include dendrodendritic synapses and even gap junctions (Schmitt et al., 1976).

These neural masses act as macroscopic sources of EEG signals. For example, in the case of the generation of alpha rhythms, it has been shown that such a macroscopic source is located within the cortex and behaves like a dipole layer directed perpendicularly to the cortical surface (Lopes da Silva and Storm van Leeuwen, 1978). The dynamic properties of alpha rhythms, such as their frequency, depend on the parameters of the neuronal populations, such as feedback gains, strength of connections, time properties of synaptic potentials, and nonlinear properties (i.e., thresholds and saturation).

Does this rhythmic activity propagate along the cortex or form a standing field? It has been shown experimentally (Lopes da Silva and Storm van Leeuwen, 1978) that, in the visual cortex of the dog, small cortical areas appear to act as "epicenters" from which alpha rhythm activity "spreads" in different directions. The existence of this type of spread has been concluded on the basis of phase differences in rhythmic components measured at different locations on the cortical surface. It has been shown in a model study (Van Rotterdam et al., 1982) that a neuronal chain, where the model neurons are interconnected by means of recurrent collaterals and interneurons such that the connectivity functions are homogeneous and their strength decays as an exponential function of distance, shows propagation of electrical activities characterized by frequencies in the alpha band with a velocity c in the order of magnitude of 0.3 $msec^{-1}$, which is in the range of experimental results. The dynamics of the activity of neuronal populations are treated in more detail in Chapter 4.

The propagation of electric activity in the cortex may result in the interesting phenomenon of time dilation, i.e., an EEG transient recorded at the cortex will seem to be of shorter duration than the transient recorded simultaneously at the scalp. This has been shown to occur in relation to epileptiform spikes (Lopes da Silva and van Hulten, 1978). The phenomenon of time dilation is due to the fact that a moving dipole seen from a distance can be observed over a longer time than when seen from nearby. The physical basis for this phenomenon is accounted for in the Appendix (expression 5.18).

Influence of Inhomogeneities

It has been assumed that the brain could be considered an infinite homogeneous medium, but in reality this is not the case. The field potentials are influenced not only by the geometry of the neuronal populations and the electrical properties of individual neurons but also by the existence of regions with different conductivities in the head, i.e., by the presence of inhomogeneities. For an interpretation of field potentials measured at the scalp, therefore, it is important to take into consideration the layers lying around the brain: the cerebrospinal fluid (CSF), the skull, and the scalp. These layers account, at least in part, for the attenuation of EEG signals measured at the scalp as compared to those recorded at the underlying cortical surface. This can be formulated in mathematical terms, as in the Appendix (expression 5.19).

To compute the potential distribution at the surface of the scalp caused by a dipole placed within the brain, it is necessary to compute the potential distribution at the surface of the different shells (that is, to solve the boundary value problem). This can be done by solving the Poisson equation (see equation 5.7) in polar coordinates as done in the Appendix. Already in the 1970s, the influence on the EEG of the specific electrical properties of the tissues surrounding the brain was recognized (Hosek et al., 1978; Kavanagh et al., 1978; Schneider, 1972, 1974; Witwer et al., 1972). The systematic study of Ary et al. (1981) led to the proposal of a method that would correct for the errors introduced by variations in skull and scalp thickness. Initially, the models of the head volume conductor consisted of concentric spheres, usually three to account for the brain, skull, and scalp; in some models a fourth layer was included representing the CSF. In the classic models, the three main concentric spheres typically had radii of 90, 83, and 78 mm. The values of the conductivities of the three layers commonly used were proposed by Geddes and Baker (1967): for the brain 0.33, for the skull 0.0042, and for the scalp also 0.33 $S \cdot m^{-1}$; in case the CSF was included, it had a conductivity of 1.0 $S \cdot m^{-1}$. Recently more precise estimates of these conductivities were obtained by way of measurements *in vivo*, using an electric impedance tomography (EIT) method combined with a realistic model of the head (Ferree et al., 2000;

Gonçalves et al., 2000, 2003). The results of the study of Gonçalves et al. (2003) showed that the ratio between the conductivities of the skull and the brain lies between 20 to 50 (for 6 subjects) rather than the traditionally assumed value of 80. The average values found in this investigation are the following: brain: 0.33 $S \cdot m^{-1}$; skull: 0.0081 $S \cdot m^{-1}$. It is also important to note that the variance of the estimates decreased by half when a realistic model was used, in comparison with a spherical model. However, a factor of 2.4 was found between the subjects with the extreme values of the ratio of conductivities. This implies that these values should be estimated for each individual to increase the reliability of the estimated conductivities.

In addition, it is known that the conductivity of the various tissues is not homogeneous. The conductivity of the skull varies with its thickness and bone structure. Law et al. (1993) showed that there is an inverse relation between skull resistivity and thickness. Cuffin (1993) and Eshel et al. (1995) investigated the effects of varying the conductivity of the skull; the former determined that the effect of local variations in skull and scalp thickness was slightly larger on the EEG than on the magnetoencephalogram (MEG), while the latter showed a correlation between interhemispheric asymmetry in skull thickness and the amplitude of the scalp EEG. The very thorough studies of Haueisen (1996; Haueisen et al., 1995) on the influence of various combinations of conductivities on both the EEG and MEG, showed that the scalp EEG is most influenced by the conductivities of the skull and the scalp, while the MEG was most influenced by the conductivities of the brain tissue and the CSF. We should note that the conductivity of the tissues of the head can also present anisotropy. Indeed, it is known that in brain tissue, the conductivity measured in a direction parallel to a fiber tract can be ten times larger that in the perpendicular direction (Nicholson, 1965). It is, however, difficult to integrate this finding in global models of the whole head, since fiber tracts are organized in a most complex way within the anatomical constraints of the folds of the brain. Nevertheless, De Munck (1989), using a model consisting of five concentric shells, solved the forward problem in an analytic form for the case in which the skull and the cortex had anisotropic properties. The effects of the anisotropic conductivity of the skull were determined by Bertrand et al. (1992) and by van den Broek (1997). The latter showed that the anisotropy of the skull causes the smearing out of the distribution of the EEG over the scalp, whereas the normal component of the MEG is not affected.

In addition, it is relevant to emphasize that the skull does not have a homogeneous surface, due to both the existence of regions with different thickness and the occipital opening and the eye sockets (Yan et al., 1991). The existence of holes in the skull, for example due to surgical interventions, influences also the distribution of the EEG over the scalp as demonstrated by Bertrand et al. (1992). In general, the localization of the dipoles is then shifted toward the hole.

Realistic Models of the Head and Numerical Methods

In the past, most solutions of the forward problem assumed that the head could be reasonably approximated by a spherical model with three or four shells. However, the geometry of this volume conductor is clearly not spherical. Therefore, since the late 1980s, realistically shaped models were gradually introduced and applied (Hämäläinen and Sarvas, 1989; He et al., 1987; Meijs et al., 1988a,b; Yvert et al., 1995). This was made possible by the advances in magnetic resonance imaging (MRI) that allow making realistic estimates of the three-dimensional geometry of the brain and surrounding tissues (Wieringa and Peters, 1993). To solve the forward problem in a realistic shaped volume of the head, it is necessary to apply numerical methods. This involves decomposing the volume conductor in a mesh consisting of a relatively large number of discrete elements. The accuracy of the method increases with the number of these elements, and, of course, is inverse proportional to their size, but the computational effort increases also accordingly. The most commonly used methods to compute the EEG potential distributions are the boundary element method (De Munck and Peters, 1991; Ferguson et al., 1994; Meijs et al., 1989), which is appropriate to the case where the volume conductor is assumed to be isotropic and piecewise homogeneous, and the volume element methods, which are needed in case the assumptions of isotropy and piecewise homogeneity do not hold. Examples of the latter are the finite-volume method (Eshel et al., 1995), the finite-difference and the finite-element methods (for details see reviews by van Uitert, Weinstein and Johnson, 2003). These methods are powerful, but they need reliable information about the structure of the brain and surrounding tissues, obtained from MRI scans, and of the corresponding conductivities, to be applied in a sensible way. They are particularly suited to calculate the influence of specific inhomogeneities such as the influence of the cerebral ventricles filled with CSF (van den Broek, 1997) and anisotropic conductivities (Haueisen, 1996).

In a number of studies, the advantage of using realistic models in comparison with spherical models has been demonstrated; differences in dipole reconstructions using EEG data were reported to reach 20 mm (Cuffin, 1996; Roth et al., 1993). Relatively smaller differences were obtained with MEG data, in the order of 4 mm (Menninghaus et al., 1994). This implies that the necessity of using realistic models, particularly those accommodating inhomogeneous volumes, is stronger for EEG than for MEG recordings. In the latter case, most calculations are based on the boundary-element method.

The Inverse Problem: Approaches to Estimate Solutions

The introduction stated that the problem of calculating the intracerebral sources of the potentials measured at the scalp, i.e., the so-called inverse problem of electroencephalography, has no unique solution. This means that different combinations of intracerebral sources can result in the same potential distribution at the scalp. Another problem in this respect is that the EEG is a differential measure; i.e., one measures potential differences between two points and there is no ideal reference point. The only way to tackle this problem is to make specific assumptions about the intracerebral sources that are assumed to cause a given EEG potential distribution and to make a model of the conductive media lying between the sources and the recording electrodes. This implies that first a particular type of forward problem is solved; thereafter, the theoretical scalp potentials obtained in this way are compared with those recorded experimentally. It should be noted that, on the one hand, a satisfactory comparison does not necessarily imply that the assumed sources are those really responsible for the measured EEG potentials. On the other hand, however, a bad comparison must lead to the conclusion that the assumptions are not correct either with respect to the sources or to the model, or both.

The numerical procedures by means of which the measured EEG/MEG distribution over the scalp is compared with that computed using the forward approach are not trivial. Usually one expresses the difference between the real and the simulated distributions as a summed squared difference. The question is to find a minimum of this function, which can be accomplished by several algorithms. The mostly used of this is that of Marquardt (1963). In the last decades many solutions of the inverse problem have been proposed, starting from the pioneer work of Schneider and Gerin (1970), Schneider (1972, 1974), Smith et al. (1973), Henderson et al. (1975), and many others as reviewed by Scherg (1990, 1992) and Stok (1986).

According to this approach, the intracerebral source is assumed to be an equivalent current dipole localized within the brain. Here we consider, in general terms, those aspects of the inverse problem that are common to EEG and MEG. The aim of the inverse procedure is to obtain an equivalent source, which in general is a dipole, determined by six parameters. This solution is called the *equivalent dipole* (ED), which must be considered a mathematical abstraction. It represents the theoretical dipole, which generates a potential (or magnetic field) distribution at the surface of the outer shell, that is the closest in the least square sense, to the measured distribution at the scalp. It should be emphasized that the estimation of an equivalent dipole located within the brain gives only a rough estimate of the center of gravity of the cortical area active at a given moment. For example in the case of the dipole layer shown in Fig. 5.3 the corresponding equivalent dipole would be located much deeper than the surface where the individual dipolar sources are placed.

Assuming that the activity of each cortical macro-column would be described by an equivalent current dipole, one would need several thousand to account for an EEG or MEG scalp distribution. The number of sensors, however, is much smaller, in the order of a maximum of 128 for the EEG and 300 for the MEG. Thus the problem of estimating brain sources of EEG or MEG data is underdetermined. Regularization methods have been proposed to help solving this major difficulty.

For solving the inverse problem, the method of the least-squares source estimation has been applied both to the activity measured at a single moment in time or within a time interval (Scherg and Von Cramon, 1985; Wood, 1982). In this context a convenient approach, proposed by De Munck (1989, 1990), is to split the set of parameters of the ED into linear and nonlinear parameters. This procedure consists schematically of the following steps: first, the time functions that describe the change of the source as function of time must be estimated for a given position and orientation of the

ED; second, the orientations must be found given the dipole time functions and position. These two steps must be performed alternatively a number of times until the best dipole orientation and time functions are found for given dipole positions. Thereafter, the nonlinear position parameters must be updated and the process repeated until a best fit is obtained. This procedure starts from the assumption that the position and orientation of the initial dipole are known, i.e., it is based on the stationary dipole model proposed by Scherg and Von Cramon (1985), although it is not constrained to the initial choice.

If a reasonable assumption on the initial position and orientation cannot be made, one may use the alternative approach of estimating EDs for a number of successive time samples of a given potential, or magnetic, distribution (so-called moving dipole approach) as done by Stok (1986) and Stok et al. (1990) and may others. In this way a series of EDs is obtained, as shown in Fig. 5.4. Those EDs that have about the same position and orientation can be clustered and the clustered dipoles can be averaged. If desired, these average ED clusters can be used as seed points for the procedure of de Munck as described above (Lopes da Silva and Spekreijse, 1991).

We should note that, in practice, if the distribution of the EEG potential or of the MEG field over the scalp is relatively simple, a single ED may be an appropriate model. Of course, one needs all available a priori information to speed up the so-

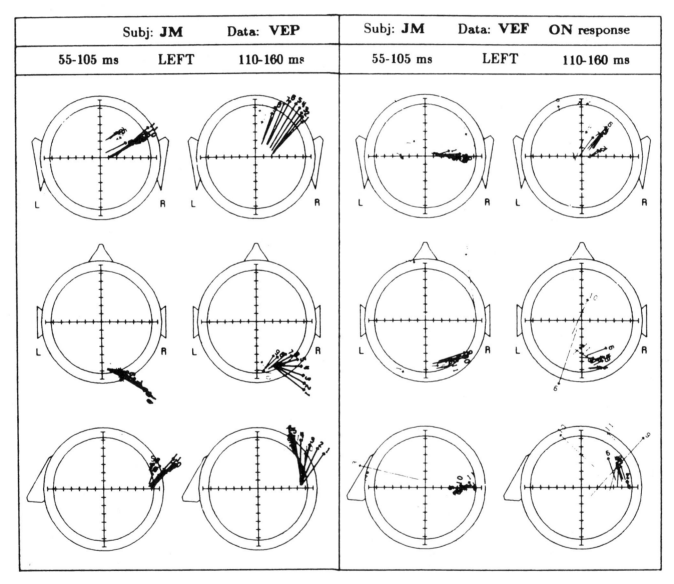

Figure 5.4. Projection of equivalent dipoles (EDs) based on visual evoked potentials (VEPs) *(left)* and visual evoked fields (VEFs) *(right)* during the on-response of subject JM, to the appearance of a checkerboard presented to the left half-visual field. Each ED is shown in three projection planes, namely occipital *(top)*, horizontal *(middle)*, and sagittal *(bottom)*. An *arrow* indicates the direction and length of the projection of the dipole and the starting point indicates the dipole location. Each *arrow* is identified by a small number that runs from 1 to 11. A group of *arrows* represents an interval of 50 msec, in steps of 5 msec, spanning the time interval of 55 to 160 msec after start of the stimulus. Scale: one division indicates 10 mm for the position and $6.7 \cdot 10^{-9}$ A · m, for the components. Each dipole is plotted with a line width corresponding to the measure of fit χ^2: thick for $\chi < 0.1$, medium for $0.1 < \chi < 0.2$, thin for $0.2 < \chi < 0.4$, very thin for $\chi \geq 0.4$. (Modified from Stok, C.J., Spekreijse, H.J., Peters, M.J., et al. 1990. A comparative EEG/MEG equivalent dipole study of the pattern onset visual response. New trends and advanced techniques in clinical neurophysiology. EEG Suppl. 41:34–50.)

lution and to give it high reliability. For instance, if it is to be expected that a given activity occurs simultaneously in both hemispheres in areas well defined anatomically, it is advisable to start by assuming two symmetrical dipoles at the appropriate sites (Scherg, 1992). An increase in the number of dipoles can easily lead to rather complex and ambiguous interpretations. Validation of equivalent dipole models can be obtained in retrospect by relating the solutions obtained to independent physiological or anatomical information. An example of an anatomical-physiological validation is the case of the dipolar sources of alpha, mu rhythms, and sleep spindles (Manshanden et al., 2002) that are distributed on brain areas as expected on the basis of animal and human physiological observations. An example of anatomical-pathological validation is given by the distribution of sources of epileptiform transients in patients with cortical lesions visible in MRIs (Fig. 5.5), where

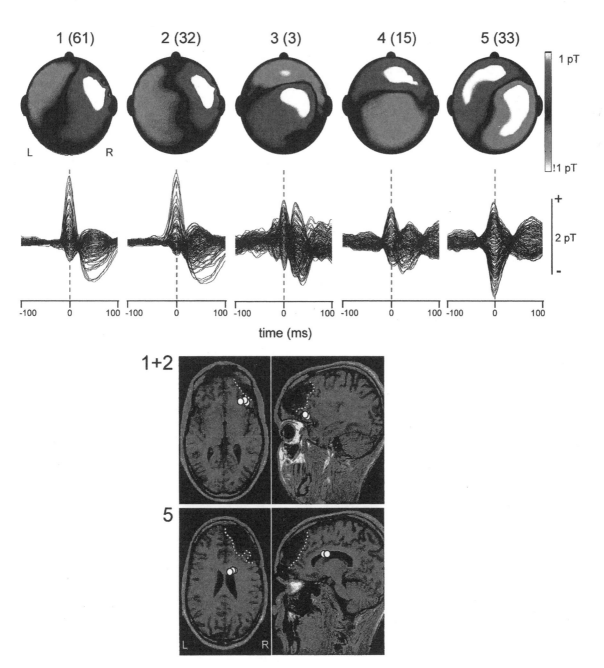

Figure 5.5. **Top:** Channel overlays and topographic maps of the average magnetic fields for the five spike clusters in patient C. The field maps represent the magnetic field distribution at the time of the marker, indicated in the channel overlays by the *dashed vertical red line*. Above each map the cluster number and, within brackets, the number of spikes it contains. **Bottom:** Position of equivalent dipoles. In the top axial and sagittal magnetic resonance imaging (MRI) slices the dipoles fitted to the average magnetoencephalogram (MEG) spike of clusters 1 and 2, combined. In the bottom slices are the dipole locations for cluster 5. For clusters 3 and 4 equivalent dipole sources with less than 10% residual error were not found. The boundary of the structural lesion in the right frontal lobe for this patient is marked by *dotted lines*. (Adapted from Van't Ent, D., Manshanden, I., Ossenblok, P., et al. 2003. Spike cluster analysis in neocortical localization related epilepsy yields clinically significant equivalent source localization results in magnetoencephalogram [MEG]. Clin. Neurophysiol. 114(10): 1948–1962.) (See Color Figure 5.5.)

the main epileptiform sources are located around the lesions (Schwartz et al., 2003; van't Ent et al., 2003).

A number of alternative methods have been developed to circumvent the obvious limitations of the equivalent dipole approach. One of these consists in applying spatial filtering to the data so that signals from a given location may be privileged with respect to the rest. This is the so-called linearly constrained minimum variance beam forming (Baillet et al., 2001) that has been applied in practice with some interesting results (Gross et al., 2001). Related methods are the synthetic aperture magnetometry (SAM) method introduced by Robinson and Vrba (1999), and the parametric mapping method applied by Dale et al. (2000). In addition, methods have been proposed to obtain estimates of multiple dipoles with little a priori information, such as the multiple signal classification (MUSIC) algorithm (Mosher and Leahy 1999; Mosher et al., 1992, 1999). A number of laboratories have pursued this issue by creating new algorithms based on the assumption that the sources are at fixed locations within the brain, namely at a given node of the triangular tessellation of the cortical surface as extracted from the subject's MRI. In this way the inverse solution is simplified to finding the linear parameters of the sources. Nevertheless, this problem is still underdetermined. The methods used to solve this problem use different forms of regularization parameters (Baillet and Garnero, 1992). In this way particular forms of inverse solutions can be obtained: minimum norm (MN) (Hämäläinen and Ilmoniemi, 1984, 1994; Wang et al., 1992, 1993), weighted resolution optimization (WROP) method of Grave de Peralta Menendez et al. (1997), and the low-resolution brain electromagnetic tomography (LORETA). The latter was proposed by Pascual-Marqui et al. (1994) and uses the discrete spatial Laplacian operator for regularization. This method yields a very smooth inverse solution (Pascual-Marqui et al., 2002).

In any case, dipole models provide less ambiguous solutions than the more sophisticated methods described above, since they are based on simpler assumptions. Nonetheless they yield images that are less attractive than the latter methods. In any case dipolar methods are only meaningful if the scalp field has approximately focal character.

Alternatively, the scalp EEG may be described using the surface Laplacian that estimates the local normal component of the current through the skull (Law et al., 1993) and can be computed by applying either a local or a global approach. According to the former (Hjorth, 1975; Le and Gevins, 1993; Le et al., 1994) the surface Laplacian is computed locally using a subset of neighboring sensors for differentiation. According to the global approach (Babiloni et al., 1997; Law et al., 1993; Nunez, 1981), an interpolation function is first applied to the measurements obtained over the

whole head and the differentiation is applied afterward. The relationship between the surface Laplacian and the cortical potential distribution is only simple in case of homogeneous skull and scalp layers. Zanow (1997) compared, in a computer simulation study, the performance of the surface Laplacian and a linear estimation approach with dipoles having free moment orientations, the so-called cortical potential reconstruction based on linear estimation (Fig. 5.6). Compared to the surface Laplacian method, the latter linear estimation method provided a more accurate cortical image of the sources (for a comprehensive review of these methodologies, see Knösche, 1997). Another alternative method consists in reconstructing the potential distribution on the inner boundary of the skull by the method of spatial deconvolution (Le and Gevins, 1993).

Currently a number of groups are attempting to solve the problem of the inherent ambiguity of the EEG/MEG inverse solutions by combining functional MRI (fMRI) data with EEG/MEG data, but these approaches are still in development (Dale et al., 2000). A problem is that the time course of the fMRI signal, i.e., the blood-oxygen-level dependent (BOLD) signal, differs from the corresponding local neurophysiological signals, since it is delayed with respect to the latter. Nonetheless, Logothetis and Wandell (2004) examined the relation between local field potentials (LFPs or local EEG), single- and multiunit activity (MUA) and high spatiotemporal fMRI responses recorded simultaneously in monkey visual cortex, and were able to demonstrate that only the LFP signal was significantly correlated with the hemodynamic response. Furthermore, the LFPs had the largest magnitude signal, and linear systems analysis showed that the LFPs were better than the MUAs at predicting the fMRI responses. These results provide a sound basis to develop appropriate methods to integrate EEG/MEG and fMRI data. Recently, Devor et al. (2003) reported the results of a systematic study in rat somatosensory cortex, to characterize the relationship between changes in blood oxygen content and the neural spiking and synaptic activity, showing that there is a nonlinear relationship between electrophysiological measures of neuronal activity and the hemodynamic response.

The Magnetoencephalogram (MEG)

As discussed above, the ionic currents originating from biochemical sources at the cellular level in the central nervous system generate not only electric fields but also magnetic fields.

Until Cohen's (1968) work, magnetic fields could not be detected owing to the extremely low strength of the MEG and the absence of sufficiently sensitive transducers. The magnetic field of the brain has a strength in the order of

Figure 5.6. The EEG *(top row)*, the brain potential reconstructed by means of linear estimation with minimum norm constraint *(center row)*, and the surface Laplacian maps *(bottom row)* of the deviant tones responses to a mismatch negativity experiment are shown at two latencies: at 140 msec *(left column)* and 180 msec *(right column)* after stimulus onset. Results were computed with the ASA (Advanced Source Analysis) software package. (Adapted from Zanow, F. 1997. Realistically shaped models of the head and their application to EEG and MEG, p. 144. Ph.D. thesis, University of Twente, Enschedé.)

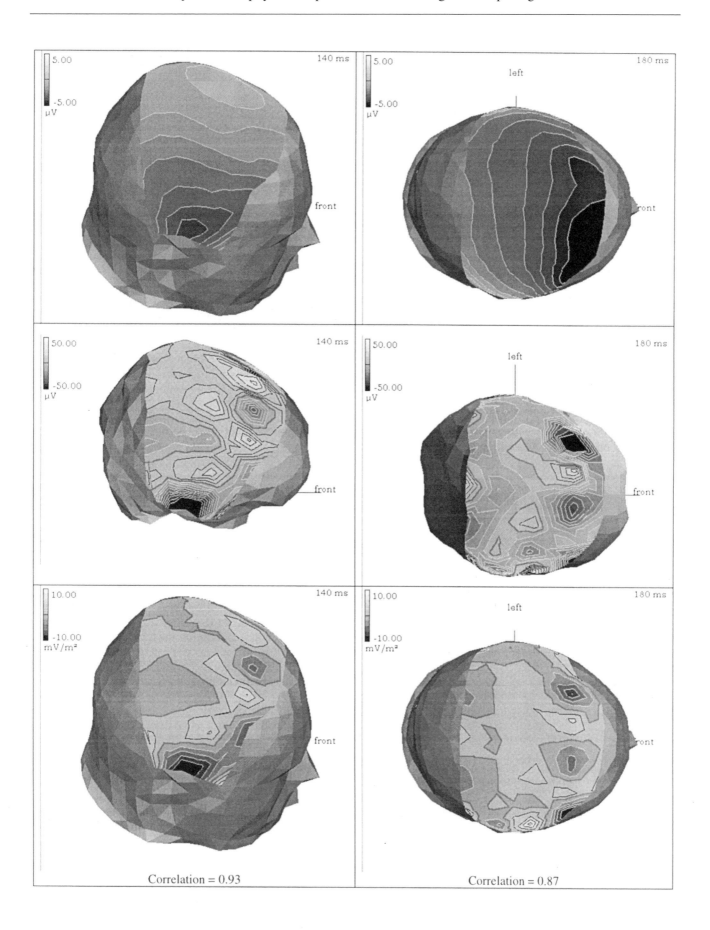

magnitude of 10^{-8} gauss (G) or, in meter-kilogram-second (mks) units, of 10^{-12} Weber m^{-2} or tesla (Wm^{-2} or T) (Reite et al., 1976), whereas the earth magnetic field has a strength in the order of magnitude of 0.5 G (Geselowitz, 1979). However, with the introduction of the superconducting quantum interference device (SQUID) magnetometer, based on a superconducting effect at liquid helium temperature, sensitivities in the order of magnitude of 10^{-10} G have been obtained (Reite et al., 1976).

The earth magnetic field and the urban magnetic noise fields (10^{-4} to 10^{-3} G) can be practically removed while recording the MEG by using the gradiometer technique. This is based on the fact that the disturbing fields are almost constant over large distances, whereas the MEG falls off rapidly with distance. This is done by subtracting the induced potentials in two coils placed close to each other; in this way, the earth and urban noise magnetic fields are suppressed. The magnetic field in stationary conditions obeys Ampere's laws and can be derived from the microscopic sources at the cellular level, as shown in the Appendix (from expression 5.22 onward). Whereas the electrical potential reflects the strength and localization of the current sources, the magnetic field reflects not only these properties but also the direction of the current densities. This can be seen in the Appendix by comparing expression 5.29 for the magnetic quantities with expression 5.8 for the electric potential. Whether the information about the direction of current densities in the brain may be derived from the MEG depends on the practical possibility of recording the magnetic fields in three directions. In general we may state that the EEG reflects mainly the volume or extracellular currents, whereas the MEG is more sensitive to the primary intracellular currents. There are very few experimental studies where magnetic and electric fields have been measured along with elementary electrophysiological properties of simple brain preparations. The recent study of Murakami et al. (2002) validates the assumption indicated above. This study examined whether evoked magnetic fields and intra- and extracellular potentials from longitudinal CA3 slices of guinea pig can be interpreted within a single theoretical framework that incorporates ligand- and voltage-sensitive conductances in the dendrites and soma of the pyramidal cells. The intracellular potentials in this validated model reveal that the spikes and slow waves of the magnetic fields are generated in or near the soma and apical dendrites, respectively.

In the section on the influence of inhomogeneities we have seen that, to explain the EEG, we must assume the existence of shells with different conductivities. The existence of these shells affects the electric potential in two ways: it causes an attenuation of the potential, and it introduces equivalent dipole layers at the boundaries of the inhomogeneities as shown in expression 5.19. However, the brain and surrounding tissues behave as a medium with constant magnetic permeability μ. Therefore, the magnetic field, in contrast to the electric field, is not influenced by those layers; it is nevertheless also affected by the induced dipole layers existing at the boundaries of the inhomogeneities in conductivity, as shown in the Appendix (expression 5.30).

Other properties of the MEG that should be mentioned are the following. Neither electrodes nor a reference point

are necessary for recording the MEG; the transducers for the MEG need not touch the scalp, because the magnetic field does not disappear where conductivity σ is zero (free space). From expression 5.29 it can be seen that the vector potential has the same direction as the intracerebral current density. Because the magnetic field is perpendicular to the vector potential, we can conclude that current dipoles directed perpendicularly to the surface of the skull result in magnetic fields tangential to the surface of the head and, vice versa, tangential current dipoles result in magnetic fields perpendicular to the skull.

Research on MEG has advanced considerably in recent years (see Chapter 57, "Magnetoencephalography as a Tool of Clinical Neurophysiology"). Both practical and theoretical aspects of magnetoencephalography have been elucidated, as summarized by Cohen and Cuffin (1983), Okada (1983), Cuffin (1985), Modena et al. (1982), Hari and Ilmoniemi (1986), Hämäläinen (1992), and Lewine and Orrison (1995). Some theoretical aspects of general interest will be mentioned here. Although EEG and MEG reflect in essence the same elementary phenomena, in practice the two types of measurement differ in a number of aspects.

First, the EEG is a relative measurement; it always needs a reference electrode. The magnetic field measurement does not need a reference point.

Second, the MEG is a measure of the magnetic fields perpendicular to the skull, which are caused by tangential current dipoles. The radial component of the current dipole does not generate a magnetic field outside a sphere-shaped volume conductor, and thus does not contribute to the MEG. By contrast, the EEG is a measure of both components. This means that the MEG reveals tangential current dipoles in a clear way, which in the EEG may be obscured by radial sources. The main intracortical dipolar current sources are perpendicular to the cortical surface (Fig. 5.1). Therefore, Cohen and Cuffin (1983), have pointed out that the MEG mainly measures the cortical current dipoles lying in the sulci and not on the convexity of the gyri. Thus, the former causes mainly tangential dipoles to the skull surface, whereas the latter produces mainly radial dipoles.

Third, the map representing the distribution of the magnetic field at the surface of the head caused by a tangential current dipole is rotated by 90 degrees to the corresponding EEG potential map as shown in Fig. 5.7. This means that to localize a dipole-like source in the x and y directions, both MEG and EEG should be used (Cohen and Cuffin, 1983), but it cannot be stated that one type of measurement is better than the other. Differences in localization of sources with both methods may be determined mainly by the direction along which the measurements were made.

Fourth, the EEG represents a sum of the potentials caused by primary and secondary sources or volume currents. In the Appendix, it is shown that the media of the head (brain, CSF, skull, and scalp) have different conductivities; thus, secondary sources of electric (expression 5.19) and magnetic fields (expression 5.30) are introduced. It is often stated, however, that the MEG is not affected by these volume currents (Cohen and Cuffin, 1983; Okada, 1983). It is still debatable how much these secondary sources contribute to the EEG and MEG under the conditions in which these

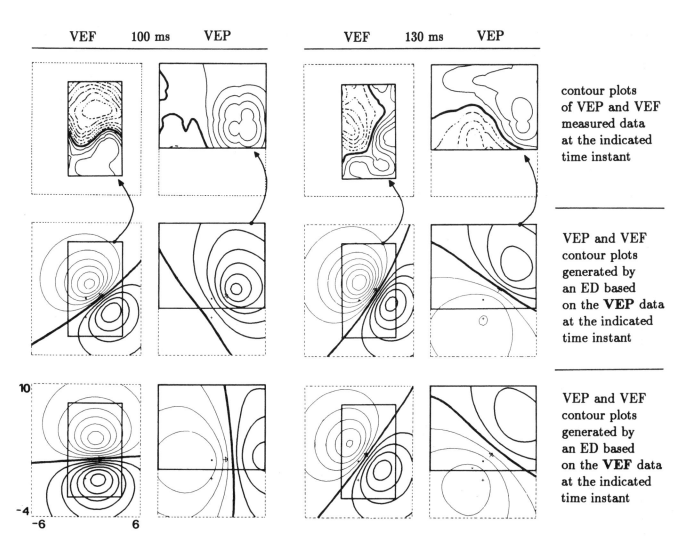

Figure 5.7. Examples of measured and computed maps corresponding to two time samples of a visual evoked potential (VEP) and magnetic field (VEF). The stimulus was the appearance of a checkerboard pattern as described in Stok (1986) and Stok et al. (1990). *Top row:* Measured VEF and VEP contour plots for two instants of time during the on-response: 100 and 130 msec. *Middle row:* Simulated VEF and VEP contour plots that correspond to the EDs that were estimated from the measured VEP distributions. *Bottom row:* The simulated contour plots that correspond to the VEF-based EDs. The *dashed rectangles* indicate the simulation area of 12 × 14 cm². Measures are in centimeters and with respect to the inion. In the contour plots of measured data, negativity is indicated by *dashed lines* and in the contour plots of simulated data by *thin lines*. The *thick lines* indicate the zero level. Note that these plots present theoretical and experimental examples of the three main differences that can be expected between EEG and MEG contour plots. (Modified from Stok, C.J., Spekreijse, H.J., Peters, M.J., et al. 1990. A comparative EEG/MEG equivalent dipole study of the pattern onset visual response. New trends and advanced techniques in clinical neurophysiology. EEG Suppl. 41:34–50.)

signals are experimentally measured. Plonsey (1982) pointed out that both the electric and magnetic fields are affected by secondary sources. Van Rotterdam (1986), using a model of a volume conductor represented by a lattice including inhomogeneities, showed that the magnetic field changes significantly in respect to the case of the homogeneous volume conductor under the influence of inhomogeneities in conductivity. In certain cases of spherical symmetry, however, the magnetic field distribution due to a current dipole is independent of spherically symmetrical variations in resistivity of the volume conductor (Nunez, 1986). Whether this will hold true for a real head is questionable.

Nevertheless, Cohen and Cuffin (1983) assume that the MEG would not be influenced by the volume currents and that this would explain why the MEG pattern is more focal, or tighter, than the corresponding EEG potential distribution. It appears that still tighter MEG patterns may be obtained by using transducers composed of a number of magnetic field-sensing coils in an array. Recent technological advances have made the practical use of multiple sensing coils for magnetic measurements over the head possible (Ricci et al., 1985).

Fifth, there are differences between MEG and EEG measurements regarding the representation of some types of non-dipolar sources, as discussed in detail by Cuffin (1985). Different types of sources give different results. For side-by-side line sources, forming a dipole layer, the EEG gives a more accurate representation of the actual sources than does the MEG; the reverse is true for in-line sources, i.e., a series of dipoles aligned along the same direction. However, it should be added that both EEG and MEG solutions of the inverse problems for the side-by-side and in-line sources lie deeper in the head and have a larger amplitude than the actual sources. In particular, the sources that are in the form of lines that are more than 2 cm long give different results when measured using EEG or MEG; the MEG solutions are deeper for the side-by-side sources, and EEG solutions are deeper for the in-line sources. These differences may be helpful in identifying the type of such sources in the brain (Cuffin, 1985).

Sixth, MEG and EEG appear to differ in their capability of localizing a current dipole source given a set of observations corrupted by noise. A single current dipole can be represented by six parameters; three determine its position inside the head and three define its components. It has been shown by Stok et al. (1984) that the EEG gives better estimates of the three components of the current dipole than the MEG, based on observations to which noise was added. The latter, however, gives better estimates of the three position parameters. Moreover, the inverse procedure, for cases with bad signal-to-noise ratios, fails more often with EEG than with MEG data. The equivalent dipoles estimated by the inverse procedure using EEG and MEG data separately may be combined in order to obtain an average estimate. Alternatively, the equivalent dipole may be calculated directly by determining the dipole that provides the least squares fit to EEG and MEG simultaneously. It can be demonstrated that the latter procedure provides slightly better results than the combination of the two estimates into an average estimate. This reinforces the statement that the two types of measurement, MEG and EEG, indeed provide complementary information and should be combined whenever precise source localization is desired.

Seventh, spherical models of the head perform much better with MEG than with EEG data, because the former is less sensitive to the influence of volume currents, while these currents are affected appreciably by deviations from the ideal head. This means that inverse solutions based on MEG data may be simpler to obtain since spherical models may be more readily used in this case than with EEG measurements (Leahy et al. 1998). Nevertheless, volume currents may still affect the MEG as shown by Van Uitert et al. (2003). Certainly one of the benefits that has been obtained by the introduction of the MEG technique is that a considerable amount of research on brain activity by competent multidisciplinary groups has led to a renewed interest in the biophysical study of the electric and magnetic activity recorded from the scalp. This led to the development of more sophisticated models of the neuronal sources and of the volume conductor (Wiejzeiu, 1887). These developments have been of interest for obtaining a better understanding not only of the MEG but also of the EEG. Initially the experimental results obtained by the new technique have led to the thought that the MEG is superior to the EEG in locating brain sources (Hari and Ilmoniemi, 1986).

However, the question of whether the MEG offers real practical advantages over the EEG has been raised (Stok, 1986). Stok et al. (1990) made a systematic theoretical and experimental comparison of EEG and MEG and concluded that the MEG is not, in general, superior over the EEG, although the MEG localizes the equivalent sources slightly better than the EEG, but it estimates the dipole components slightly worse. Two general conclusions of these studies should be put in evidence: (a) when model assumptions are not violated, the MEG and EEG lead essentially to the same inferences about the source (excluding magnetically silent sources); and (b) when model assumptions are violated, the MEG and EEG respond, in general, in different ways such that a comparison of the results obtained with both methods may give clues regarding the kind of model violation present. Therefore, it is important to use both methods to obtain a higher reliability in functional localization studies (Dale and Sereno, 1993).

This question has been addressed directly by comparing MEG and EEG maps obtained in patients where dipoles were implanted, using indwelling intracranial electrodes that were placed for the diagnosis of an epileptogenic focus (Cohen et al., 1990; Cuffin, 1996). These authors concluded, from a limited number of experimental measurements, that the average errors of localization were 10 mm for the EEG and 8 mm for the MEG, and thus that the MEG was not superior to the EEG. Nevertheless, the main advantage of the MEG may be the fact that the MEG is not affected by radial sources and, in this way, the use of both MEG and EEG may complement each other and help to establish a better model of the source, when it cannot be described as being a simple dipole.

In conclusion, more research is needed where the two methods are directly compared using the same data.

Appendix:
The Mathematical Basis

Ab Van Rotterdam

The ionic currents in the brain cause electrical and magnetic fields obeying Maxwell's and Ohm's laws. These fields have a direction and magnitude; they must, therefore, be represented as vector functions. The electric field is given by $\vec{E}(\vec{r}, t)$ and the magnetic field by $\vec{H}(\vec{r}, t)$, because these vectors depend on location $\vec{r}$ and on time t. (Vector quantities are indicated by an arrow above the symbol.)

In brain and surrounding tissues, the material constants are approximately the following: conductivity, $\sigma \approx 10^{-1}$ Ω^{-1} m^{-1}; dielectric constant, $\epsilon \approx 10^{-9}$ Fm^{-1}; and magnetic permeability, $\mu \approx 10^{-6}$ Hm^{-1}. Do potential changes taking place in the brain at a frequency of, for example, 1 kHz cause propagated electromagnetic waves in the medium that may be detected after a certain time at a distant point such as the scalp? It can be proved (Plonsey, 1969) that, in a medium such as the brain with the material constants indicated above, the propagation velocity of the electromagnetic waves is of the order of 10^5 ms^{-1}, which implies that one need not be concerned with the propagation of electromagnetic waves caused by potential changes within the brain. This means that, in practical terms, the effects of those potential changes may be detected simultaneously at any point in the brain or surrounding tissues. This important statement leads to the conclusion that the currents caused by sources in the brain at any moment in time behave in a stationary way. This means that no charge is accumulated at any time in the brain (Rosenfalck, 1969).

Therefore, it can be stated that for the current density $\vec{J}$ ($\vec{r}$) or, for simplicity, $\vec{J}$, at any moment of time:

$$\mathrm{div}\,\vec{J} = \mathrm{O} \tag{5.1}$$

where the operation div $\vec{J}$ is called divergence of the vector $\vec{J}$; $\vec{J}$ is the current density in Am^{-2}. The operator div must be understood as indicating differentiation of a vector; expression 5.1 can also be written in another way that may help in understanding its meaning. Let us consider the expression for $\vec{J}$ for the case of an infinitesimally small cube with sides dx, dy, and dz (Fig. 5.8). It holds that

$$\mathrm{div}\,\vec{J}\,\mathrm{dxdydz} = \left(\frac{\delta J_x}{\delta_x \,\mathrm{dydz}}\right)\mathrm{dx} + \left(\frac{\delta J_{\hat{y}}}{\delta_y \,\mathrm{dxdz}}\right)\mathrm{dy} \tag{5.2}$$
$$+ \left(\frac{\delta J_z}{\delta_z}\,\mathrm{dxdy}\right)\mathrm{dz}$$

In this expression the factors between brackets, such as $(\delta J_x/\delta_x\,\mathrm{dydz})$, represent the rate of change of current through the surfaces dydz, dxdz, and dxdy. To account for the total change of current, it is necessary that those factors are multiplied by the sides of the cube dx, dy, and dz; then these products must be summed. Thus expression 5.2 represents the total change of current in the volume of the cube. When no net current flows into the cube (i.e., the current that goes into the volume comes out again), this total change must be zero, as indicated in expression 5.1. Thus we may state that the current is stationary. In the case of a stationary current, the electrical field $\vec{E}(\vec{r})$, or simply $\vec{E}$, is related to the electrical potential $V(\vec{r})$, or simply V, by the following expression:

$$\vec{E} = -\mathrm{grad}V \tag{5.3}$$

In this expression the operator gradient (grad) indicates differentiation of the scalar function V, of space and time (time is considered here to be fixed) in the following way:

$$\mathrm{grad}V = \left(\frac{\delta V}{\delta x},\frac{\delta V}{\delta y},\frac{\delta V}{\delta z}\right)^{\mathrm{T}} \tag{5.4}$$

where gradV is a vector quantity called the gradient of V.

In a conductive medium, Ohm's law is valid; i.e.:

$$\vec{J} = \vec{J}_i + \sigma\vec{E} \tag{5.5}$$

where $\vec{J}$, is the current density injected in the medium (for example, a transmembrane current density caused by synaptic activity in a neuron).

Taking the divergence of both sides of expression 5.5 and using expression 5.1, one may write:

$$\mathrm{div}\vec{E} = \frac{-\mathrm{div}\,\vec{J}_i}{\sigma} \tag{5.6}$$

Substituting $\vec{E}$ by $-\mathrm{grad}V$ according to expression 5.3, one can write an expression that is called the Poisson equation for the potential field owing to an injected current:

$$\mathrm{div}\,\mathrm{grad}V = \frac{\delta^2 V}{\delta x^2} + \frac{\delta^2 V}{\delta y^2} + \frac{\delta^2 V}{\delta z^2} = \frac{\mathrm{div}\,\vec{J}_i}{\sigma} \tag{5.7}$$

In case the medium where $\vec{r}_o$ is situated is assumed to be infinite, isotropic, and homogeneous, it can be proved that the solution of the Poisson equation is the following:

$$V(\vec{r}^o) = -\frac{1}{4\pi\sigma}\int_{\mathrm{vol}}\frac{\mathrm{div}\,\vec{J}_i}{R}\,\mathrm{d}^3\mathrm{r} \tag{5.8}$$

which gives the values of the potential at a point $\vec{r}_o$ in the volume conductor from injected current densities $\vec{J}_i$, at points $\vec{r}$, lying at a distance R from $\vec{r}_o$ ($R = |\vec{r} - \vec{r}_o|$); the integral represents the summation over all current sources within the volume; note that divergence of the vector $\vec{J}$, gives a scalar quantity.

Summarizing, it has been shown that the space-varying and the time-varying parts of the electrical variables can be separated; the time-varying part is the same everywhere in the medium owing to the large propagation velocity, and the space-varying part can be computed for every instant in time according to expression 5.8.

This general expression is not the only way to define $V(\vec{r}_o)$. Two other expressions (5.10 and 5.12) are given below. These are more convenient because they relate the extracellular potential field directly to membrane processes of the individual neurons in the brain. One of these expressions can be derived assuming that the neuronal membrane can be considered as equivalent to a double layer with an inner (intracellular) membrane potential V_m and an outer (extracellular) potential V. In these terms, $V(\vec{r}_o)$ is given by the following expressions:

$$V(\vec{r}_o) = -\frac{1}{4\pi\sigma}\int_s (\sigma_i V_m(\vec{r}) - \sigma_e(\vec{r}))\mathrm{grad}\left(\frac{1}{R}\right)\cdot\mathrm{d}\vec{O}(\vec{r}) \tag{5.9}$$

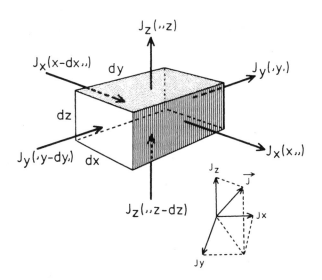

Figure 5.8. Cubic volume with sides dx, dy, and dz. Current density flowing in: J_z (x − dx, y − dy, z − dz); J_y (,y − dy) and J_z (,,z − dz) or $\vec{J}$ ($\vec{r}$ − d$\vec{r}$). Current densities flowing out: J_x (x,y,z); J_y (,y,) and J_z (,,z) or $\vec{J}$ ($\vec{r}$). When div $\vec{J}$ = 0, no charge is accumulated in volume dxdydz. *Inset:* Decomposition of current density vector $\vec{J}$ in components in x, y, and z direction as J_z, J_y, and J_x.

where σ_i is the intracellular and σ_e is the extracellular conductivity, and $d\vec{O}$ is pointing to the extracellular medium; the inner product grad $(1/R) \cdot d\vec{O}$ is called the solid angle $d\Omega(\vec{r} - \vec{r}_o)$ subtended by the surface element $d\vec{O}(\vec{r})$ on the membrane surface S and seen from the extracellular point $\vec{r}_o$. It must be emphasized that expression 5.8 takes the form of expression 5.9 only when the injected current densities $\vec{J}_i$ originate at the cell membrane as derived by Plonsey (1969). Expression 5.9 can be simplified to the following approximate expression, because $|\sigma_e V(\vec{r})| \ll |\sigma_i V_m(\vec{r})|$:

$$V(\vec{r}_o) \approx -\frac{\sigma_i}{4\pi\sigma_e} \int_s V_m(\vec{r}) d\Omega(\vec{r} - \vec{r}_o) \qquad (5.10)$$

The solid angle $d\Omega$ subtended by a membrane surface $d\vec{O}$ seen from a point $\vec{r}_o$ can be interpreted in a geometrical way, as shown in Fig. 5.9.

To understand the effect of the solid angle in a more practical way, it is useful to derive an explicit expression for $d\Omega$:

$$d\Omega(\vec{r} - \vec{r}_o) = \mathrm{grad}\left(\frac{1}{R}\right) \cdot d\vec{O}(\vec{r}) = \frac{\vec{R}}{R^3} \cdot d\vec{O}(\vec{r}) = \frac{\cos\theta}{R^2} d\vec{O}$$

$$(5.11)$$

where θ is the angle between $\vec{R}$ and $d\vec{O}$; it should be noted that $\vec{R}$ is the vector connecting the point $\vec{r}_o$ where V is measured and the point $\vec{r}$ where the dipole is located (see Fig. 5.8).

It should be noted in expression 5.9 that a change in membrane potential such as a depolarization in a small piece of membrane results in an intracellular potential V_m and an extracellular potential V. In this case, the membrane behaves like a current dipole consisting of a sink at the outside and a source at the inside. Thus, there is a jump in potential across the membrane. A current dipole, or simply a dipole, is defined by its strength and direction; it is represented by the vector $\vec{p}(\vec{r})$. In the example described above, the dipole is

oriented perpendicularly to the membrane surface $d\vec{O}$; thus, the dipole is represented as $p(\vec{r}) d\vec{O}$. According to the above, another expression for the potential $V(\vec{r}_o)$ caused by one dipole can be derived (Jackson, 1962):

$$V(\vec{r}_o) = \frac{p(\vec{r})}{4\pi\sigma} \mathrm{grad}\left(\frac{1}{R}\right) \cdot d\vec{O}(\vec{r})$$

or

$$V(\vec{r}_o) = \frac{p(\vec{r})\cos\theta}{4\pi\sigma R^2} d\vec{O} \qquad (5.12)$$

From expression 5.12 it can be concluded that in the case of a single dipole at the membrane, V decreases with the square of the distance R to the source and it is also proportional to $\cos\theta$; thus it is maximal when $\vec{R}$ is perpendicular to the surface $d\vec{O}$.

In many cases, the membrane depolarization (or hyperpolarization) does not remain limited to a small piece of membrane; rather, it spreads over a more or less extended membrane surface. In this way the equivalent current source cannot be accounted for in terms of a single dipole. One must, instead, assume that there exists a dipole layer at the membrane.

For a dipole layer located at the surface of the membrane, one must sum the effects of all individual dipoles; therefore, expression 5.12 becomes:

$$V(\vec{r}_o) = \frac{1}{4\pi\sigma} \int_s p(\vec{r}) \mathrm{grad}\left(\frac{1}{R}\right) \cdot d\vec{O}(\vec{r})$$

or

$$V(\vec{r}_o) = \frac{1}{4\pi\sigma} \int_s p(\vec{r}) d\Omega (\vec{r} - \vec{r}_o) \qquad (5.13)$$

From expression 5.13, it can be noted that, if p is constant over the closed membrane surface S, then $V(\vec{r}_o) = 0$, because the integral of the solid angle $d\Omega$ over an external closed surface is zero. Thus, to obtain a value of $V(\vec{r}_o)$ different from zero, p must vary over the membrane surface; in other words, the membrane potential must vary over the surface owing, for example, to local synaptic activity.

In this case, the attenuation of the potential in the volume conductor depends not only on distance R and angle θ, but also on the geometry of the dipole layer. For instance, for a dipole layer of constant strength with length l and height Δh located at x = 0 in the y-z plane (Fig. 5.10A) the potential field at a point $\vec{r}_o$ along the x axis will be given the following expression:

$$V(\vec{r}_o) = p \int_{y=-1/2}^{1/2} \int_{z=-\Delta h/2}^{\Delta h/2} \frac{r_o}{(r_0^2 + y^2 + z^2)^{3/2}} dyzy$$

$$(5.14)$$

For $r_o \gg \Delta h$ and $\Delta h \ll 1$, this can be estimated as follows:

$$V(\vec{r}_o) \approx \frac{p\Delta h}{r_o} \frac{1}{\{1 + (r_o/1)^2\}^{1/2}} \qquad (5.15)$$

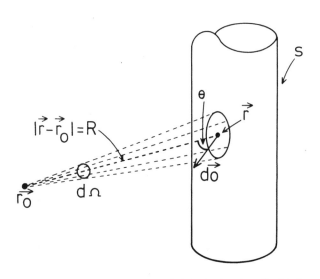

Figure 5.9. Solid angle subtended by infinitesimal surface dO with direction $d\vec{O}$ on membrane cylinder S seen from the extracellular point $\vec{r}_o$ lying at a distance $R = |\vec{r}_o - \vec{r}|$ from dO; the angle between the direction of the surface $d\vec{O}$ and $\vec{r}_o - \vec{r}$ is θ.

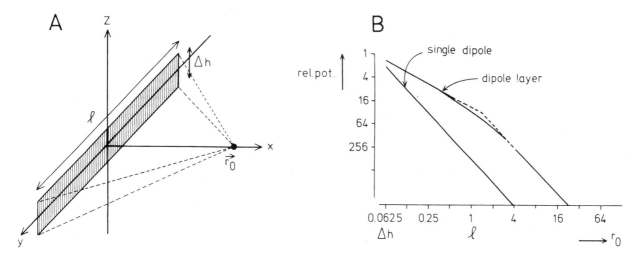

Figure 5.10. A: Dipole layer of length l and height Δh in the y-z plane seen from extracellular point $\vec{r}_o$ on the X axis. **B:** Attenuation (relative potential, rel. pot.) of extracellular potential as function of distance (r_o) in a log-log plot for the case of a single dipole and for the case of a dipole layer. Note that, in the latter case, two slopes can be distinguished, the decay of the potential with distance being more accentuated in the far field ($r_o > 1$). The arbitrary values of $\Delta h = 0.0625$ and l = 1 used in this model are indicated on the horizontal axis.

It can be seen that in the far field, $r_o \gg 1$, the potential tends to decay as in the case of the single dipole with r_o^2 where for short distances $\Delta h < r_o < 1$, the potential decays proportionally to distance r_o. In Fig. 5.10B, it can be seen that in the case of the dipole layer the attenuation has two slopes depending on the relation between r_o and 1, whereas in the case of a simple dipole there is only one slope.

Until now, the discussion has considered only the behavior of standing sources of EEG signals, i.e., sources that do not change in space. However, there is experimental evidence that leads one to assume that some macroscopic sources in the brain do propagate in space (Freeman, 1975; Lopes da Silva and Storm van Leeuwen, 1978; Nunez, 1981). This propagation of sources has a particular effect on the behavior of the potential field in time. This effect does not appear for standing sources where the time behavior of the field is the same as that of the sources.

In general terms, to allow for time-varying sources, expression 5.10 must be changed as follows:

$$V(\vec{r}_o, t) \approx -\frac{1}{4\pi\sigma_e} \int_S V_m(\vec{r}, t) d\Omega(\vec{r} - \vec{r}_o) \quad (5.16)$$

This effect can be illustrated by the following example (Fig. 5.11A). Let us assume a cell that can be simplified to an equivalent cylinder (Rall, 1962) oriented along the z axis where a membrane depolarization front propagate along the cylinder with an arbitrary velocity. In this case, we may write that the resulting potential $V(\vec{r}_o)$ is proportional to a time varying solid angle.

From expressions 5.11 and 5.16, the potential $V(\vec{r}_o,t)$ caused by a depolarization front along the cylinder is given by

$$V(\vec{r}_o, t) \approx \frac{\cos(\theta(t))}{|ct\vec{n}_z - \vec{r}_o|^2} dO \quad (5.17)$$

where $\vec{n}_z$ is the unit vector in the z direction. Note that the denominator in expression 5.17 represents the square of the distance R(t) between $\vec{r}_o$ and the time-varying location of the front.

At a point further away in the same direction, $\vec{r}_1 = \alpha\vec{r}_o$, V becomes:

$$V(\vec{r}_1, t) \approx \frac{1}{\alpha^2} V(\vec{r}_o, t/\alpha) \quad (5.18)$$

Therefore, the potential at a far location $\vec{r}_1$ is equal to the potential at location $\vec{r}_o$ attenuated in amplitude and in a more dilated time scale (Fig. 5.11B).

Influence of Inhomogeneities

Let us assume that the field potential $V(\vec{r}_o)$ generated by the activity of N neurons situated in a finite homogeneous medium containing M structures with different conductivities and bounded by surface S (outside the medium the conductivity is zero), can be expressed as follows (Van Rotterdam, 1978):

$$4\pi\sigma(\vec{r}_o)V(\vec{r}_o) = -\sigma_i \sum_{i=i}^N \int_{S_1} V_m^{(i)}(\vec{r}) d\Omega$$
$$+ \sigma_e \sum_{i=i}^N \int_{S_1} V(\vec{r}) d\Omega \quad (5.19)$$
$$+ \sum_{k=1}^M \int_{S_k} (\sigma_e - \sigma_k)V(\vec{r}) d\Omega$$
$$+ \sigma_e \int_S V(\vec{r}) d\Omega$$

in which S_1 represents the membrane surface that encloses the first neuron with membrane potential $V_m^{(i)}(\vec{r})$ and intracellular conductivity σ_i; the extracellular conductivity

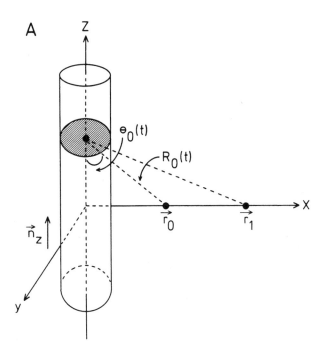

Figure 5.11. **A:** Membrane cylinder oriented along the Z axis in which a depolarization front propagates (with velocity c) along the Z direction, $\vec{r}_o$ and $\vec{r}_1$ are two extracellular points at which extracellular potentials are measured $\vec{r}_1 = \alpha\vec{r}_o$. Note that the potentials V at $\vec{r}_o$ and at $\vec{r}_1$ are different, because θ and R differ when seen from $\vec{r}_1$ instead or r_o. The changes in θ and R as a function of time depend on the propagation velocity c. **B:** Extracellular potentials V measured simultaneously at $\vec{r}_o$ and $\vec{r}_1$ (plot with arbitrary scales) showing time dilation.

is σ_e except in the regions bounded by the surfaces S_k, within these regions the conductivity is σ_k; $\sigma(\vec{r}_o)$ is the conductivity for the region where point $\vec{r}_o$ lies: $\sigma(\vec{r}_o) = \sigma_k$ if $\vec{r}_o$ is bounded by S_k and it is σ_e elsewhere, $d\Omega$ are the solid angles of surfaces pointing to the region with conductivity σ_e.

The second term on the right describes the influence that neurons have as inhomogeneities on the extracellular field; the third term describes the distorting influences of the M inhomogeneities, whereas the fourth term expresses the influence of the border of the medium.

Using expression 5.19, it is in principle possible to compute the EEG measured on the scalp and generated by N neurons.

In the following model, the brain and surrounding tissues are represented as a sphere with a number of shells within which a single dipole is situated. The potential field in and on the sphere is a solution of Poisson's equation obeying the following boundary conditions: the current densities normal to the surfaces of the shells are continuous and the tangential components of the electric field at the boundaries are also continuous.

Assuming radial symmetry, the solution for a radial dipole can be written as a Legendre series, in polar coordinates as follows (Jackson, 1962):

$$V(r, \phi, \theta) = \sum_{n=0}^{\infty} \{a_n r^{-(n+1)} + b_n r^n\} P_n^0(\cos\theta)$$

(5.20)

where $P_n^0(\cos\theta)$ is a Legendre polynomial of the nth order. For a tangential dipole, the solution is:

$$V(r, \phi, \theta) = \sum_{n=0}^{\infty} \{c_n r^{-(n+1)} + d_n r^n\} P_n^1(\cos\theta)\cos\phi$$

(5.21)

where $P_n^1(\cos\theta)$ is an associated Legendre polynomial.

The coefficients a_n, b_n, c_n, and d_n for all n in both cases should be evaluated on basis of the boundary conditions at the different boundaries and the fact that the source is a dipole (Hosek et al., 1978).

Magnetic Fields

In the stationary approximation of Maxwell's equations for the electromagnetic fields generated by microscopic sources at the cellular level, the behavior of the magnetic field $\vec{H}$ or the induction field $\vec{B} = \mu\vec{H}$ is governed by two experimental physical laws. These are Ampere's law in the stationary approximation:

$$\text{curl } \vec{H} = \vec{J}$$

(5.22)

and

$$\text{div } \vec{B} = 0$$

(5.23)

which expresses the experimental fact that magnetic monopoles do not exist. The term curl $\vec{H}$ is a differential operation called curl or rotation on a vector function; it is defined as follows:

$$\text{curl } \vec{H} = \left[\left(\frac{\partial H_y}{\partial z} - \frac{\partial H_z}{\partial y} \right) \cdot \left(\frac{\partial H_z}{\partial x} - \frac{\partial H_x}{\partial x} \right) \cdot \left(\frac{\partial H_x}{\partial y} - \frac{\partial H_y}{\partial x} \right) \right]^{\mathrm{T}} \tag{5.24}$$

For conservative or rotation-free fields, i.e., fields derivable from vector potentials (e.g., $\vec{E} = -\text{grad}V$), this differentiation results in a zero vector. However, for vector fields directed along a closed path (e.g., closed current density loops), the operation results in a vector field perpendicular to the original vector field. It can be proved that expression 5.23 is equivalent to the statement that $\vec{B}$ can be derived from a vector potential $\vec{A}$ as follows:

$$\vec{B} = \text{curl } \vec{A} \tag{5.25}$$

By substituting expression 5.25 in 5.22 and using the definition of $\vec{J}$ as a function of impressed current densities (expression 5), we obtain:

$$\frac{1}{\mu} \text{curl curl } \vec{A} = \vec{J}_i + \sigma\vec{E} \tag{5.26}$$

It can be shown that curl curl$\vec{A}$ = $-$div grad$\vec{A}$ + grad div$\vec{A}$, so that 5.26 becomes

$$\text{div grad}\vec{A} = -\mu\vec{J}_i + \text{grad div}\vec{A} - \mu\sigma\vec{E} \tag{5.27}$$

One can simplify expression 5.27 by making use of the ambiguity in the definition of $\vec{A}$ (Jackson, 1962) and choose $\vec{A}$ such that div$\vec{A} = -\mu\sigma V$; the two last terms of expression 5.27 then cancel out; expression 5.27 becomes the Poisson equation that for each separate component of $\vec{A}$ can be expressed as follows:

$$\text{div grad}\vec{A} = -\mu\vec{J}_i \tag{5.28}$$

In an infinite medium with constant μ and σ, the solution of equation 5.28 can be proved to be (Plonsey, 1969):

$$\vec{A}(\vec{r}_o) = \frac{\mu}{4\pi} \int_{\text{vol}} \frac{\vec{J}_i(\vec{r})}{R} \, d^3r \tag{5.29}$$

In this way, it can be seen that the magnetic vector potential $\vec{A}$ reflects the direction of the current densities $\vec{J}_i$. If there are inhomogeneities in conductivity, the expression becomes (Plonsey, 1972):

$$\vec{A}(\vec{r}_o) = \frac{\mu}{4\pi} \left[\int_{\text{vol}} \frac{\vec{J}_i(\vec{r})}{R} \, d^3r + \sum_k \int_{S_k} (\sigma_e - \sigma_k) \frac{V(\vec{r})}{R} \, d\vec{O}(\vec{r}) \right] \tag{5.30}$$

where S_k are surfaces enclosing regions with conductivity σ_k; elsewhere is the conductivity σ_e. The surfaces $d\vec{O}$ point to the region with conductivity σ_e; μ is assumed to be constant.

References

Ary, J.P., Klein, S.A., and Fender, D.H. 1981. Locations of sources of evoked scalp potentials; corrections for skull and scalp thicknesses. IEEE Trans. Biomed. Eng. 28:447–452.

Babiloni, F., Babiloni, C., Carducci, F., et al. 1997. A high resolution EEG method based on the correction of the surface Laplacian estimate for the subject's variable scalp thickness. Electroencephalogr. Clin. Neurophysiol. 103:486–492.

Baillet, S., and Garnero, L. 1997. A Baysenian approach to introducing anatamo-functional priors in the EEG/MEG inverse problem. IEEE Trans. Biomed. Eng. 44:374–385.

Baillet, S., Mosher, J.C., and Leahy, R.M. 2001. Electromagnetic brain mapping. IEEE Signal Processing Magazine, November, 14–30.

Bertrand, O., Thevenet, M., Perrin, F., et al. 1992. Effects of skull holes on the scalp potential distribution evaluated with a finite element model. Proceedings of the 14th International Conference of the IEEE Engineering in Medicine and Biology Society, Satellite Symposium on Neuroscience and Technology, November, Lyon, pp. 42–45.

Cohen, D. 1968. Magnetoencephalography. Evidence of magnetic fields produced by alpha rhythm current. Science 161:784–786.

Cohen, D., and Cuffin, B.N. 1983. Demonstration of useful differences between magnetoencephalogram and electroencephalogram. Electroencephalogr. Clin. Neurophysiol. 56:38–51.

Cohen, D., Cuffin, B.N., Yunokuchi, K., et al. 1990. MEG versus EEG localization test using implanted sources in the human brain. Ann. Neurol. 28:811–817.

Cuffin, B.N. 1985. A comparison of moving dipole inverse solutions using EEG's and MEG's. IEEE Trans. Biomed. Eng. 32:905–910.

Cuffin, B.N. 1993. Effects of local variations in skull and scalp thickness on EEG's and MEG's. IEEE Trans. Biomed. Eng. 40:42–48.

Cuffin, B.N. 1996. EEG localization accuracy improvements using realistically shaped head models. IEEE Trans. Biomed. Eng. 43:299–303.

Dale, A.M., and Sereno, M.I. 1993. Improving localization of cortical activity by combining EEG and MEG with MRI cortical surface reconstruction: a linear approach. J. Cogn. Neurosci. 5:162–176.

Dale, A.M., Liu, A.K., Fischl, B.R., et al. 2000. Dynamic statistical parameter mapping: combining fMRI and MEG for high resolution imaging of cortical activity. Neuron 26:55–67.

De Munck, J.C. 1989. A mathematical and physical interpretation of the electromagnetic field of the brain. Ph.D. thesis, University of Amsterdam, the Netherlands.

De Munck, J.C. 1990. The estimation of time varying dipoles on the basis of evoked potentials. Electroencephalogr. Clin. Neurophysiol. 77:156–160.

De Munck, J.C., and Peters, M.J. 1991. Mathematical aspects of biomagnetic modeling. 8th International Conference on Biomagnetism. Ed. M. Hoke, pp. 11–12. Munster: Excerpta Medica.

De Munck, J.C., Vijn, P.C.M., and Lopes da Silva, F.H. 1992. A Random dipole model for spontaneous brain activity. IEEE Trans. Biomed. Eng. 39:791–804.

Devor, A., Dunn, A.K., Andermann, M.L., et al. 2003. Coupling of total hemoglobin concentration, oxygenation, and neural activity in rat somatosensory cortex. Neuron 39(2):353–359.

Eshel, Y., Witman, S., Rosenfeld, M., et al. 1995. Correlation between skull thickness asymmetry and scalp potential estimated by a numerical model of the head. IEEE Trans. Biomed. Eng. 42:242–249.

Ferguson, A.S., Zhang, X., and Stroink, G. 1994. A complete linear discretization for calculating the magnetic field using the boundary element method. IEEE Trans. Biomed. Eng. 42:455–459.

Ferree, T.C., Eriksen, K.J., and Tucker, D.M. 2000. Regional head tissue conductivity estimation for improved EEG analysis. IEEE Trans. Biomed. Eng. 47:1584–1592.

Freeman, W.J. 1975. *Mass Action in the Nervous System.* New York: Academic Press.

Geddes, L.A., and Baker, L.E. 1967. The specific resistance of biological materials—a compendium of data for the biomedical engineer and physiologist. Med. Biol. Eng. 5:271–293.

Geselowitz, D.B. 1979. Magnetocardiography: an overview. IEEE Trans. Biomed. Eng. 26:497–504.

Gonçalves, S.I., de Munck, J.C., Heethaar, R.M., et al. 2000. The application of electrical impedance tomography to reduce systematic errors in the inverse EEG problem—a simulation study. Physiol. Meas. 21:379–393.

Gonçalves, S.I., de Munck, J.C., Verbunt, J.P.A., et al. 2003. In vivo measurement of the brain and skull resistivities using an EIT-based method and realistic models of the head. IEEE Trans. Biomed. Eng. 50:754–767.

Grave de Peralta Menendez, R., Hauk, O., Gonzalez Andino, S., et al. 1997. Linear inverse solutions with optimal resolution kernels applied to electromagnetic tomography. Hum. Brain Map. 5:454–467.

Gross, J., Kujala, J., Hämäläinen, M., et al. 2001. Dynamic imaging of coherent sources: studying neural interactions in the human brain. Proc. Natl. Acad. Sci. USA 98:694–699.

Hämäläinen, M.S. 1992. Magnetoencephalography: a tool for functional brain imaging. Brain Topogr. 5:95–103.

Hämäläinen, M.S., and Ilmoniemi, R.J. 1984. Interpreting measured magnetic fields of the brain: estimates of current distributions. Technical Report TKKFA559. Helsinki: University of Technology.

Hämäläinen, M.S., and Ilmoniemi, R.J. 1994. Interpreting magnetic fields of the brain: minimum norm estimates. Med. Biol. Eng. Comp. 32:35–42.

Hämäläinen, M.S., and Sarvas, J. 1989. Realistic conductivity geometry model of the human head for interpretation of neuromagnetic data. IEEE Trans. Biomed. Eng. 36(2):165–171.

Hämäläinen, M.S., Hari, R., Ilmoniemi, R., et al. 1993. Magnetoencephalography: theory, instrumentation and applications to the noninvasive study of human brain function. Rev. Med. Physics 65:413–497.

Hari, R., and Ilmoniemi, R. 1986. Cerebral magnetic fields. CRC Crit. Rev. Biomed. Eng. 14:93–126.

Haueisen, J. 1996. Methods of numerical field calculation for neuromagnetic source localization. Ph.D. thesis, Technische Universität Ilmenau, Shaker Verlag, Aachen.

Haueisen, J., Ramon, C., Czapski, P., et al. 1995. On the influence of volume currents and extended sources on neuromagnetic fields: a simulation study. Ann. Biomed. Eng. 23:728–739.

He, B., Musha, T., Okamoto, Y., et al. 1987. IEEE Trans. Biomed. Eng. 34:406–414.

Helmholtz, H. 1855. Ueber einige Gesetze der Verteilung elektrischer Ströme in Körperlichen Leitern mit Anwendung auf die thierischelektrischen Versuche. Prog. Ann. Physik. Chemie 89:211–233, 353–377.

Henderson, C.J., Buler, S.R., and Glass, A. 1975. The localization of equivalent dipoles of EEG sources by the application of electric field theory. Electroencephalogr. Clin. Neurophysiol. 39:117–130.

Hjorth, B. 1975. An online transformation of EEG scalp potentials into orthogonal source derivations. Electroencephalogr. Clin. Neurophysiol. 39: 526–530.

Hosek, R.S., Sances, A., Jodat, R.W., et al. 1978. The contributions of intracerebral currents to the EEG and evoked potentials. IEEE Trans. Biomed. Eng. 25:405–415.

Humphrey, D.R. 1968. Reanalysis of the antidromic cortical response. II. On the contribution of cell discharge and PSPs to the evoked potentials. Electroencephalogr. Clin. Neurophysiol. 25:421–442.

Jackson, J.D. 1962. *Classical Electrodynamics.* New York: John Wiley & Sons.

Katchalsky, A.K., Rowland, V., and Blumenthal, R. 1974. Dynamic patterns of brain cell assemblies. Neurosci. Res. Prog. Bull. 12/1.

Kavanagh, R.N., Darcey, T.M., Lehmann, D., et al. 1978. Evaluation of methods for three-dimensional localization of electrical sources in the human brain. IEEE Trans. Biomed. Eng. 25:421–429.

Klee, M., and Rall, W. 1977. Computed potentials of cortically arranged populations of neurons. J. Neurophysiol. 40:647–666.

Knösche, Th. 1997. Solutions of neuroelectromagnetic inverse problems an evaluation study. Ph.D. thesis, University of Twente, Enschedé.

Law, S.K., Nunez, P.L., and Wijesinghe, R.S. 1993. High-resolution EEG using spline generated surface Laplacians on spherical and ellipsoidal surfaces. IEEE Trans. Biomed. Eng. 40:145–153.

Le, J., and Gevins, A.S. 1993. Method to reduce blur distortion from EEGs using a realistic head model. IEEE Trans. Biomed. Eng. 40:517–528.

Le, J., Menon, V., and Gevins, A.S. 1994. Local estimate of surface Laplacian derivation on a realistically shaped scalp surface and its performance on noisy data. Electroencephalogr. Clin. Neurophysiol. 26:193–199.

Leahy, R.M., Mosher, J.C., Spencer, M.E., et al. 1998. A study of dipole localization accuracy for MEG and EEG using a human skull phantom. Electroencephalogr. Clin. Neurophysiol. 107:159–173.

Lewine, J.D., and Orrison, W. Jr. 1995. Magnetoencephalography and magnetic source imaging. In *Functional Brain Imaging,* pp. 369–417. St. Louis: Mosby Year Book.

Logothetis, N.K., Wandell, B.A. 2004. Interpreting the BOLD signal. Annu. Rev. Physiol. 66:735–769.

Lopes da Silva, F.H., and Spekreijse, H. 1991. Localization of brain sources of visually evoked responses: using single and multiple dipoles. An overview of different approaches. In *Event-Related Brain Research,* Eds. C.H.M. Brumia, G. Mulder, and M.N. Verbaten. EEG Suppl. 42:38–46. Amsterdam: Elsevier.

Lopes da Silva, F.H., and Storm van Leeuwen, W. 1978. The cortical alpha rhythm in dog: the depth and surface profile of phase. In *Architectonics of Cerebral Cortex,* Eds. M.A. Brazier and H. Petsche. New York: Raven Press.

Lopes da Silva, F.H., and van Hulten, K. 1978. Analyse quantitative de l'activite intercritique en E.E.G. et S.E.E.G. dans l'epilepsie. Rev. E.E.G. Neurophysiol. 8:198–204.

Lopes da Silva, F.H., Hoeks, A., Smits, A., et al. 1974. Model of brain rhythmic activity. Kybernetik 15:27–37.

Lopes da Silva, F.H., Van Rotterdam, A., Barts, P., et al. 1976. Models of neuronal populations. The basic mechanisms of rhythmicity. Prog. Brain Res. 45:281–308.

Lorente de No, R. 1947. Action potential of the motoneurons of the hypoglossus nucleus. J. Cell. Comp. Physiol. 29:207–287.

Manshanden, I., De Munck, J.C., Simon, N.R., et al. 2002. Source localization of MEG sleep spindles and the relation to sources of alpha band rhythms. Clin. Neurophysiol. 113(12):1937–1947.

Marquardt, D.W. 1963. An algorithm for least squares estimation of nonlinear parameters. J. Soc. Indust. Appl. Math. 11:431–441.

Meijs, J.W.H., Bosch, F.G.C., Peters, M.J., et al. 1987. On the magnetic field distribution generated by a dipolar current source situated in a realistically shaped compartment model of the head. Electroencephalogr. Clin. Neurophysiol. 66:286–298.

Meijs, J.W.H., Voorde, B.J. ten, Peters, M.J., et al. 1988a. The influence of various head models on EEGs and MEGs. In *Functional Brain Imaging,* Eds. G. Pfurtscheller and F.H. Lopes da Silva, pp. 31–45. Toronto: Hans Huber.

Meijs, J.W.H., Peters, M.J., Boom, H.B.K., et al. 1988b. Relative influence of model assumptions and measurement procedures in the analysis of the MEG. Med. Biol. Eng. Comput. 26:136–142.

Meijs, J.W.H., Weier, O.W., Peters, M.J., et al. 1989. On the numerical accuracy of the boundary element method. IEEE Trans. Biomed. Eng. 36:1038–1049.

Menninghaus, E., Lütkenhöner, B., and Gonzalez, S.L. 1994. Localization of a bipolar source in a skull phantom: realistic versus spherical model. IEEE Trans. Biomed. Eng. 41:986–989.

Modena, I., Ricci, G.B., Barbanera, S., et al. 1982. Biomagnetic measurements of spontaneous activity in epileptic patients. Electroencephalogr. Clin. Neurophysiol. 54:622–628.

Mosher, J.C., and Leahy, R.M. 1999. Source localization using recursively and projected (RAP) MUSIC. IEEE Trans. Signal Process. 47:332–340.

Mosher, J.C., Lewis, P.S., and Leahy, R.M. 1992. Multiple dipole modeling and localization from spatiotemporal MEG data. IEEE Trans. Biomed. Eng. 39:541–557.

Mosher, J.C., Baillet, S., and Leahy, R.M. 1999. EEG source localization using multiple signal classification approaches. J. Clin. Neurophysiol. 16:225–238.

Murakami, S., Zhang, T., Hirose, A., et al. 2002. Physiological origins of evoked magnetic fields and extracellular field potentials produced by guinea-pig CA3 hippocampal slices. J. Physiol. 544(pt 1):237–251.

Nicholson, P.W. 1965. Specific impedance of cerebral white matter. Exp. Neurol. 13:386–401.

Nunez, P.L. 1981. *Electrical Fields of the Brain.* New York: Oxford University Press.

Nunez, P.L. 1986. The brain's magnetic field: some effects of multiple sources on localization methods. Electroencephalogr. Clin. Neurophysiol. 63:75–85.

Okada, Y.C. 1983. Inferences concerning anatomy and physiology of the human brain based on its magnetic field. Il Nuovo Cimento 2D:379–409.

Pascual-Marqui, R.D., Michel, C.M., and Lehmann, D. 1994. Low resolution electromagnetic tomography: a new method for localizing electrical activity in the brain. Int. J. Psychophysiol. 18:49–65.

Pascual-Marqui, R.D., Esslen, M., Kochi, K., et al. 2002. Functional imaging with low-resolution brain electromagnetic tomography (LORETA): a review. Methods Find Exp. Clin. Pharmacol. 24(suppl C): 91–95.

Plonsey, R. 1969. *Bioelectric Phenomena.* New York: McGraw-Hill.

Plonsey, R. 1972. Capability and limitations of electrocardiography and magnetocardiography. IEEE Trans. Biomed. Eng. 19:239–244.

Plonsey, R. 1982. The nature of sources of bioelectric and biomagnetic fields. Biophys. J. 39:309–315.

Rall, W. 1962. Electrophysiology of a dendritic neuron model. Biophys. J. 2:145–167.

Reite, H., Zimmerman, J.E., Edrich, J., et al. 1976. The human magnetoencephalogram: some EEG and related correlations. Electroencephalogr. Clin. Neurophysiol. 40:59–66.

Ricci, G.B., Romani, G.L., Modena, I., et al. 1985. Multichannel neuromagnetic measurements in focal epilepsy. Electroencephalogr. Clin. Neurophysiol. 61:S34–S35.

Robinson, S.E., and Vrba, J. 1999. Functional brain imaging by synthetic aperture magnetometry (SAM). In *Recent Advances in Biomagnetism*, Eds. T. Yoshimoto, M. Kotani, S. Kuriki, et al., pp. 302–305. Sendai, Japan: Tohoku University Press.

Rosenfalck, R. 1969. Intra and extracellular potential fields of active nerve and muscle fibres. A physicomathematical analysis of different models. Acta Physiol. Scand. Suppl. 321:1–168.

Roth, B.J., Balish, M., Gorbach, A., et al. 1993. How well does a three-sphere model predict positions of dipoles in a realistically shaped head? Electroencephalogr. Clin. Neurophysiol. 87:175–184.

Scherg, M. 1990. Fundamentals of dipole source potential analysis. In *Auditory Evoked Magnetic Fields and Potentials,* Eds. F. Grandori, M. Hoke, and G.L. Romani, *Advances in Audiology,* vol. 6, pp. 40–69. Basal: S. Karger.

Scherg, M. 1992. Functional imaging and localization of electromagnetic activity. Brain Topogr. 5:103–111.

Scherg, M., and Von Cramon, D. 1985. Two bilateral sources of the late AEP as identified by a spatiotemporal dipole model. Electroencephalogr. Clin. Neurophysiol. 62:32–44.

Schmitt, F.O., Dev, P., Smith, B.H. 1976. Electronic processing of information by brain cells. Science 193:114–120.

Schneider, M.R. 1972. A multistage process for computing virtual dipolar sources of EEG discharges from surface information. IEEE Trans. Biomed. Eng. 19:1–12.

Schneider, M.R. 1974. Effect of inhomogeneities on surface signals coming from a cerebral current dipole source. IEEE Trans. Biomed. Eng. 21: 52–54.

Schneider, M.R., and Gerin, P. 1970. Une methode de localisation des dipoles cerebraux. Electroencephalogr. Clin. Neurophysiol. 28:68–78.

Schwartz, D.P., Badier, J.M., Vignal, J.P., et al. 2003. Non-supervised spatio-temporal analysis of interictal magnetic spikes: comparison with intracerebral recordings. Clin. Neurophysiol. 114(3):438–449.

Smith, D.B., Lell, M.E., Sideman, R.D., et al. 1973. Nasopharyngeal phase reversal of cerebral evoked potentials and theoretical dipole implications. Electroencephalogr. Clin. Neurophysiol. 34:654–658.

Stok, C.J. 1986. The inverse problem in EEG and MEG with application to visual evoked responses. Ph.D. thesis, University of Twente, The Netherlands.

Stok, C.J., Kouijzer, W.J.J., and Peters, M.J. 1984. Source localization based on EEG's and MEG's. Proceedings of the 5th Conference on Biomagnetics. Vancouver, Canada.

Stok, C.J., Spekreijse, H.J., Peters, M.J., et al. 1990. A comparative EEG/MEG equivalent dipole study of the pattern onset visual response. New trends and advanced techniques in clinical neurophysiology. EEG Suppl. 41:34–50.

Van den Broek, S.P. 1997. Volume conduction effects in EEG and MEG. Ph.D. thesis, University of Twente, Enschedé.

Van Oosterom, A. 1991. History and evolution of methods for solving the inverse problem. J. Clin. Neurophysiol. 8:371–380.

Van Rotterdam, A. 1978. A one-dimensional formalism for the computation of extracellular potentials: linear systems analysis applied to volume conduction. In *Progress Report No. PR6,* Eds. B. van Eijnsbergen and F.H. Lopes da Silva, pp. 115–122. Utrecht: Institute of Medical Physics TNO.

Van Rotterdam, A. 1986. Electric and magnetic fields of the brain: a systems analysis approach. Ph.D. Thesis, University of Amsterdam, The Netherlands.

Van Rotterdam, A., Lopes da Silva, F.H., van den Ende, J., et al. 1982. A model of the spatial-temporal characteristics of the alpha rhythm. Bull. Math. Biol. 44:283–305.

Van't Ent, D., Manshanden, I., Ossenblok, P., et al. 2003. Spike cluster analysis in neocortical localization related epilepsy yields clinically significant equivalent source localization results in magnetoencephalogram (MEG). Clin. Neurophysiol. 114(10):1948–1962.

Van Uitert, R., Weinstein, D., and Johnson, C. 2003. Volume currents in forward and inverse magnetoencephalographic simulations using realistic head models. Ann. Biomed. Eng. 31(1):21–31.

Wang, J.Z., Williamson, S.J., Kaufman, L. 1992. Magnetic source images determined by a lead-field analysis: the unique minimum-norm least-squares estimation. IEEE Trans. Biomed. Eng. 39(7):665–675.

Wang, J.Z. 1993. Minimum-norm least-squares estimation: magnetic source for a spherical model head. IEEE Trans. Biomed. Eng. 40(4):387–396

Wieringa, H.J., and Peters, M.J. 1993. Processing MRI data for electromagnetic source imaging. Med. Biol. Eng. Comput. 31:600–606.

Wilson, H.R., and Cowan, J.D. 1973. A mathematical theory of the functional dynamics of cortical and thalamic nervous tissue. Kybernetik 13:55–80.

Witwer, J.G., Tresek, G.J., and Jewett, D.L. 1972. The effect of media inhomogeneities upon intercranial electric fields. IEEE Trans. Biomed. Eng. 19:352–362.

Wood, C.C. 1982. Application of dipole localization methods to source identification in human evoked potentials. Ann. N.Y. Acad. Sci. 388: 139–155.

Yan, Y., Nunez, P.L., and Hart, R.T. 1991. Finite element model of the human head: scalp potentials due to dipole sources. Med. Biol. Eng. Comput. 29:475–481.

Yvert, B., Bertrand, O., Echallier, J.F., et al. 1995. Improved forward EEG calculations using local mesh refinement of realistic head geometries. Electroencephalogr. Clin. Neurophysiol. 95:381–392.

Zanow, F. 1997. Realistically shaped models of the head and their application to EEG and MEG. Ph.D. thesis, University of Twente, EnschedM.

6. Technological Basis of EEG Recording

Anton Kamp, Gert Pfurtscheller, Günter Edlinger, and Fernando Lopes da Silva

Electrodes and Interface Phenomena

The electrical contact between the input terminals of the recording apparatus and the tissue from which the electrical activities have to be recorded is made by means of electrodes. For recording of brain electrical activities, various types of electrodes are used; these are discussed in Chapter 7. The choice of electrode to be used depends on the location of the electrodes (on the scalp or within the brain) and on the behavioral situation in which the recordings take place. A basic property of any type of electrode is that there exists a metal/liquid junction in the electrical connection between tissue and apparatus. In the majority of electroencephalogram (EEG) examinations, scalp electrodes that are not in direct contact with the tissue are used; the indirect contact is established by an electrolyte bridge formed by an electrode jelly applied between the electrode and the skin. The electrochemical properties of the metal/liquid junction and the skin/electrolyte junction cause a steady electrical potential and an electrical impedance in the connection between tissue and apparatus. Both the electrode potential and the electrode impedance can restrict the performance of the recording system. Therefore, an analysis of these phenomena is necessary.

Direct Current (DC) Offset Voltage

When an electrode is placed in a conducting solution and no current is flowing, an electrical potential difference exists between the electrode and the bulk of the solution (Geddes and Baker, 1968). This electrode potential results from a difference between the electrical charge caused by the flow of ions from the metallic surface of the electrode into the solution and that caused by the flow of metallic ions from the solution into the metallic surface of the electrodes. An excess of charge in the solution causes the formation of an electrical double layer; in this way, an equilibrium is established. The value of the electrode potential is a function of the electrode material, the electrolyte composition, and the temperature. It may have values ranging from millivolts to volts. When scalp electrodes are used, depending on the electrolyte composition and the condition of the skin, a similar DC potential is generated at the skin/electrolyte junction.

These steady potentials generated at the electrodes, which cannot be eliminated, result in a DC offset voltage at the input of the EEG amplifier that can be large, as compared to the magnitude of the electrical activity recorded from the brain. Some electrode materials, such as stainless steel, exhibit a high resistance to DC current, which may cause a relatively high DC offset if amplifiers that draw input bias current are used. EEG amplifiers must be designed in such a way that their performance is not altered due to DC offset voltages or differences between offset voltages on the two inputs. A recommended maximum value for an acceptable DC voltage difference is ±0.3 V.

Blocking of the amplifier due to DC offset voltages when switching electrode montages can be prevented easily by means of antiblocking provisions.

Electrode Impedance

When a DC voltage is applied between electrodes placed in an electrolytic solution, the electrical double layers are disturbed and an electrical current flows. The magnitude of this current is dependent mainly on the transport of ions at the metal/electrolyte junction. The relation between voltage and current can be represented by a time-dependent electrode impedance; a simplified model is presented in Fig. 6.1. RD and CD signify the resistive and capacitive components of the transport mechanisms due to the electrical double layer. Rd and Cd represent the time-dependent, and thus frequency-dependent, diffusion impedance or Warburg impedance (Geddes, 1972). Rd and Cd are a function of $1/\sqrt{\omega}$. Req represents the electrolyte resistance, which in a practical situation involves the resistances of the body fluid, the skin, and the electrode jelly.

If the application of an external DC voltage to an electrode causes the flow of a steady current, the pathway formed by RD, Rd, and Cd is only resistive and the electrode is said to be nonpolarized, reversible, or inert. The AgAgCl electrode is an example of a reversible electrode that has a low resistance for DC and low frequency potentials. This type of electrode is commonly used for EEG recording. Many metal/electrolyte junctions do not have this property. In these cases, the current caused by a voltage step presents an initial transient onset but drops rapidly to a very small value. This can be explained (Fig. 6.1) by an initial impedance drop followed by an increase of the impedance component related to diffusion (Rd and Cd) to a large value of many megohms. This type of electrode is said to be polarized or nonreversible and cannot be used for the recording of DC potentials. The electrode impedance is determined to a large extent by the double layer capacitance CD. The value of CD is proportional to the size of the electrode surface. The metal used for electrodes cannot always be chosen on the basis of properties of the electrical impedance; other factors, such as toxicity, mechanical strength, or scalp irritation that may be caused by electrode application, may play a role and thus impose restrictions on the choice of the optimal electrode characteristics.

If scalp electrodes are used, the ultimate electrical impedance depends on the electrical resistance of the skin/electrolyte junction (Req in Fig. 6.1), which may have values

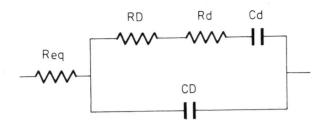

Figure 6.1. Simplified model of the impedance of a metal/electrolyte junction. Req, electrolyte resistance; RD and CD, electrical double-layer resistance and capacitance; Rd and Cd, time- and frequency-dependent diffusion impedance (Warburg impedance).

from kilo-ohms (Kohm) to hundreds of Kohm depending on the condition and preparation of the skin, the concentration of the electrode jelly, and the time elapsed after the application of the jelly (Almasi and Schmitt, 1970). To obtain an initial low resistance of reasonable stability, an electrode jelly with a high concentration of NaCl (5–10%) should be used in conjunction with a well-prepared skin from which the most superficial horny layer is scraped off.

Electrode Movement Artifacts

The motion of an electrode in relation to the scalp causes changes in the electrical double layer and thus alters the DC offset voltage; this causes an artifact in the EEG (Flasterstein, 1966). These artifacts can be reduced by using AgAgCl electrodes (Kahn, 1965), which, when properly prepared (Coles and Binnie, 1968) and handled with care, produce a relatively small and stable electrode potential (Cooper et al., 1969). A further improvement can be obtained by using electrodes in which the metallic surface is applied at some distance from the skin; in these cases, the electrically conducting connection between skin and metallic surface is made by means of an electrode/jelly bridge. This construction minimizes the effects of motion at the electrolyte/metal junction. Another source of movement artifacts, however, is the skin/electrolyte junction. The resistance and the DC potential generated at this junction may also change owing to motion; this may cause additional artifacts. This effect is felt more strongly if the amplifier draws a significant input current. Lowering the resistance at this junction by abrading the skin reduces this type of movement artifact.

The provisions that can be made to reduce electrode movement artifacts can be summarized as follows. Care should be taken that DC offset potentials and resistance in the pathway from skin to electrode surface are minimal; this implies a proper choice of electrodes and good skin preparation. The mechanical design of the electrodes and the way in which they are fixed to the scalp should provide minimal motion at both skin/electrolyte and electrolyte/metal junctions. To ensure relative mechanical stability of the electrode and the skin region in its vicinity, the mechanical load on the electrode should be kept as small as possible by using lightweight and flexible electrode leads.

Signal Attenuation and Accuracy of Measurements

Unwanted signal attenuation at the input of the amplifier is determined in general terms by the ratio of the electrode impedance and that of the EEG amplifier input stage. This interaction can be explained on the basis of the circuit given in Fig. 6.2, in which Z_{el_t} is the sum of the electrode impedances (with t representing time); Z_{cl_t} represents the impedance of the shunting capacitance of the cable connection between the electrodes and the amplifier; Z_{in} is the amplifier input impedance; and i_n and e_n represent, respectively, noise current and voltage sources inherent in the amplifier. In this way, a noise voltage e_{nt} at the amplifier input has to be taken into account. The signal attenuation is defined by the ratio between the amplifier input voltage e_{in} and the electrode open circuit voltage e_{sig}.

The ratio between e_{in} and e_{sig} is given by the expression:

$$e_{in}/e_{sig} = \frac{1}{1 + \dfrac{Z_{el_t}}{Z_{in}} + \dfrac{Z_{el_t}}{Z_{cl_t}}} \tag{6.1}$$

From this expression, it can be seen that e_{in} approximates e_{sig} if the total electrode impedance Z_{el_t} is sufficiently small as compared to the amplifier input impedance Z_{in} and the cable impedance Z_{el_t}. To obtain an attenuation as small as 0.99, the values of Z_{in} and Z_{cl_t} must be larger than 100 times Z_{el_t}. Because EEG scalp electrodes may easily have an electrical impedance of many Kohm, EEG amplifiers must have an input impedance of several megohms to prevent appreciable signal attenuation. This requirement becomes even more stringent if electrodes that, because of size and type of metal, have a relatively high impedance and/or a frequency-dependent impedance, are applied. Typical examples of such electrodes are sphenoidal electrodes and intracerebral electrodes. The cable capacitance may have a value of 0.001 µF or more; therefore, the shunting impedance Z_{cl_t} causes considerable attenuation at high frequencies if the electrodes have a relatively high impedance. This drawback has been overcome in certain EEG apparatus by locating the input amplifiers in the electrode terminal box. The signal attenuations for a number of stainless steel electrodes intended for intracerebral application that were measured using a certain

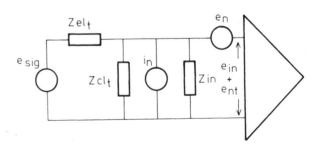

Figure 6.2. Simplified diagram of the input circuit of an EEG recording channel. Z_{elt}, total electrode impedance; Z_{clt} total cable impedance; Z_{in}, EEG amplifier input impedance; e_{sig}, EEG signal; i_n and e_n, noise current and noise voltage source inherent in input amplifier, respectively.

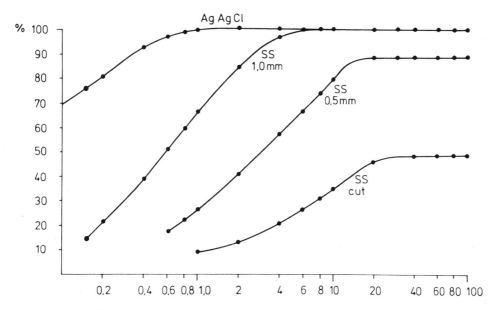

Figure 6.3. Example of the effect of the characteristics of different electrodes and amplifier input impedance on the recording sensitivity. The amplitudes recorded at various frequencies, using stainless steel wire electrodes ($\phi = 100$ μm) with different tip sizes, are compared to the amplitudes recorded with an AgAgCl electrode ($\phi = 500$ μm). Amplifier input impedance: 6 MΩ in parallel with a capacitor of 270 pF.

amplifier input impedance are represented in Fig. 6.3 by the decreases of the recording sensitivity.

The accuracy of measurement depends primarily on the magnitude of the noise voltage e_{nt}. This noise component e_{nt} is added to the amplifier input signal e_{in}. In this way, the accuracy of the measurement cannot be better than the magnitude of the noise. This accuracy can be expressed as the signal-to-noise ratio $S/N = e_{in}/e_{nt}$. The noise voltage source e_n is independent of the electrode/amplifier connection. The noise current source i_n, on the contrary, causes a current flow in the circuit $Z_{el_t}/Z_{cl_t}/Z_{in}$; thus the magnitude of the resulting noise voltage depends on the electrode impedance Z_{el_t}. Amplifiers having bipolar semiconductors (transistors) at the input stage have an appreciable noise current; the corresponding power spectrum decreases with frequency according to a 1/f law. The use of such amplifiers in conjunction with electrodes that have a relatively large impedance at low frequencies may result in significant alterations of the accuracy at the electrode/amplifier connection with decreasing frequency. For a general overview of patient-related and technical-related artifacts possibly disturbing and influencing EEG measurement, see Fig. 6.4.

Interference from External Electrical Sources

Mains power interference at the electrode/amplifier interface may introduce an artifact in EEG recordings. The effect of the electrodes on this frequency-encountered artifact can be explained on the basis of the circuit of Fig. 6.5.

Owing to capacitive coupling (C_{cm}) between the subject's body and power mains conductors in the environment, an alternating current i_{cm} flows via the subject's earth-electrode Z_{el_e} to earth. This current flow causes an alternating (AC) voltage e_{cm} ($e_{cm} = i_{cm} \cdot Z_{el_e}$) between the ground and the subject's body. In this way, both recording electrodes have an alternating potential with respect to the earth that is, at each moment, equal in amplitude and polarity. As regards the interference caused by this common mode AC electrode potential, the magnitude of the resultant AC potential differ-

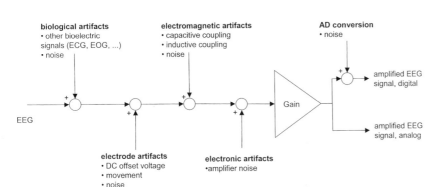

Figure 6.4. Biological and physical artifacts in EEG measurements. The brain activity can be superimposed by other biological signals such as electro-oculogram (EOG) artifacts, by electrode artifacts such as direct current (DC) offset voltages, by electromagnetic artifacts such as capacitive coupling from mains supply, and by electronic noise from the amplifier. The accuracy of the analog to digital converter is discussed in Chapter 42, Digital EEG.

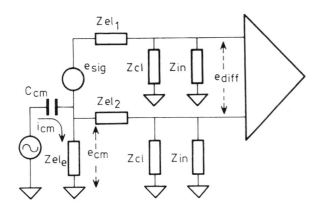

Figure 6.5. Schematic diagram representing the characteristics of an EEG amplifier input circuit in view of their effect on the reduction of mains interference.

ence e_{diff} at the amplifier input is of interest; e_{diff} should be small as compared with the amplitudes of the EEG signal e_{sig} being measured. If the two parallel impedances formed by the amplifier input impedances Z_{in} and the cable capacitance impedances Z_{cl} are assumed to be large as compared with the electrode impedances Z_{el_1} and Z_{el_2}, then e_{diff} can be approximated by:

$$e_{diff} \approx \frac{Z_{el_1} - Z_{el_2}}{Z_{cl}Z_{in}/(Z_{cl} + Z_{in})} e_{cm} \qquad (6.2)$$

From expression 6.2, it follows that in order to minimize e_{diff}, the difference between the two electrode impedances should be as small as possible. The impedance properties of the skin/electrolyte interface, however, may often result in impedance differences of several Kohm at mains frequency. Therefore, taking into account that the common mode voltage e_{cm} can easily have an amplitude of millivolts, the parallel impedance Z_{cl}, Z_{in} must be many Mohm in order to keep e_{diff} sufficiently small; Z_{in} should be in modern EEG apparatus at least 10 Mohm at mains frequency. A cable capacitance of 0.001 to 0.002 μF, which is realistic, corresponds at mains frequency to an impedance of a few Mohm. A cable capacitance of this order imposes a limitation on the obtainable reduction of mains interference; in certain circumstances additional provisions, such as electrostatic shielding of the patient, may be necessary.

An EEG apparatus with amplifier input stages located inside the electrode terminal box are to be favored in this respect, because in such apparatus mains interference is not affected by cable capacitance.

Interference from Magnetic Fields

Changing magnetic fields (e.g., from the alternating current of mains power supply or high-frequencey [HF] devices) induce also voltages e_{diff} in the electrode cables. The amplitudes of the induced voltages relate directly to the area A defined by the electrode cables and the strength and frequency f of the magnetic flux density B (expression 6.3).

$$e_{diff} = B * A * 2 * p * f \qquad (6.3)$$

The "magnetic-induced" artifacts cannot be suppressed by differential amplifiers. However, the induced voltages can be kept small if the area A is small, e.g., by twisting the electrode cables. With an amplitude for the magnetic flux density of 200 nT resulting from mains current, an induction area of 100 cm² and a mains frequency of 50 Hz, the induced voltage $e_{diff} = BA2\pi f$.

As the induced voltages depend on the frequency f of the magnetic flux density, the limiting values of the flux density amplitudes must be kept low for higher frequencies.

Interference from Electronic Amplifier Noise

The bioelectric signals are superimposed by electromagnetic influences (EMIs) and electronic noise. EMIs can be reduced, for example, by using shielded cables, but electronic noise cannot be eliminated. By using electronic amplifiers white noise (power spectral density is constant over frequency f) and pink noise (power spectral density is inversely proportional to frequency f) are superimposed to the EEG signals. The electronic noise depends on the layout of the amplifier, especially on the first amplification stage, and on the desired bandwidth or the amplifier. Typical electronic noise levels of commercial EEG amplifiers are in the range of 1 to 2 μV peak-to-peak for a bandwidth of 100 Hz and more than 4 μV peak-to-peak for a bandwidth of 3 kHz.

Principle of Amplification of EEG Signals

EEG recording concerns the measurement, amplification, and registration of differences between fluctuating electrical field potentials as a function of time. The fact that the potential differences fluctuate implies that the recorded signals have a certain bandwidth; this is a measure of the required frequency response of the recording system. For the majority of EEG examinations, a frequency response from 0.16 to 100 Hz is found to be adequate; however, if the investigation concerns very slowly varying potentials, a much lower frequency response down to DC might be required. A much higher frequency response (for example, up to 3,000 Hz) may also be required if brainstem auditory responses are studied. In most recording systems, signals within a certain frequency band can be discriminated in an optimal way.

An EEG recording should give a representation of the spatial distribution of the potentials over the scalp; therefore, different EEG signals must be simultaneously recorded from several electrodes. Usually, an EEG recording system is equipped with a number of identical recording channels, from 8, 16, 21 up to 256 or even more. The modern apparatus allows recording simultaneously from at least 21 standard electrode positions. In routine applications, a large number of electrodes are placed on the scalp. The recording system has the provision of selecting the desired combination of derivations. An EEG recording channel such as that shown in the block diagram of Fig. 6.6 is built from a series of elements, each of which has a specific function.

The input amplifier is connected to the recording electrodes; thus the actual measurement of the electrical field potentials is performed at this stage. Because the magnitude of common components of the potentials at the electrodes can be relatively large as compared to those components that

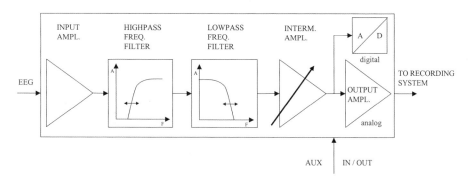

Figure 6.6. Block diagram of an EEG recording channel.

differ at both electrodes, the measuring principle of common mode rejection is used. This means that the input amplifier should be more sensitive in relation to the signal components that are different at the electrodes than to those components that are of equal amplitude and polarity (common mode). The discriminative power of the differential measurement is determined by the sensitivity of the input amplifier to common components in relation to the sensitivity to different components (discrimination factor).

An EEG recording channel is provided with adjustable high-pass (HP) and low-pass (LP) filters, by means of which the frequency response of the channel can be restricted to the frequency band of interest. The magnitudes of brain electrical activities can have values ranging from microvolts up to millivolts; they may differ considerably from one recording situation to another. Likewise, electrical activities simultaneously recorded from different pairs of electrodes can have significantly different magnitudes. To maintain an adequate input voltage (or current) for the output amplifier stage, an EEG recording channel is provided with adjustable gain, as illustrated in Fig. 6.6.

Two types of EEG amplifiers exist nowadays. The first type of amplifier provides the analog amplified EEG signal at the output, and the second type of amplifier provides the amplified EEG signal already digitally converted at the output.

The EEG signals are then transmitted via electrical or optical connections to the recording and/or processing devices.

The output amplifier delivers the voltage, current, or energy necessary for the registration system used.

Basic Characteristics of the EEG Apparatus

Input Circuit

The characteristics of the input amplifiers of the EEG apparatus are of great importance for accuracy of measurement. As discussed above, the discriminative power of the differential measurement performed at this stage depends to a large extent on the values of the amplifier input impedance as compared to those of the electrodes. This can be explained by considering the schematic diagram of the amplifier input circuit in Fig. 6.7. Z_{el_1}, Z_{el_2}, and Z_{el_e} represent, respectively, the impedances of the recording and the ground electrodes; ei_1 and ei_2 are the voltages at the two recording electrodes with respect to ground; e_{diff} represents the resul-

tant voltage difference at the amplifier input terminals. Two flows of current into the amplifier input circuit can be distinguished. One current, caused by e_{diff}, flows in the amplifier differential input impedance Z_{diff}; the other current, owing to the common mode component e_{cm} of ei_1 and ei_2, flows in the common mode input impedances Z_{cm}.

Assuming that $Z_{cm} \gg Z_{el_1}$, $Z_{cm} \gg Z_{el_2}$, and $Z_{diff} \gg (Z_{el_1} + Z_{el_2})$, the voltage difference e_{diff} at the amplifier input can be approximated by:

$$e_{diff} \approx \frac{ei_1}{1 + \dfrac{Z_{el_1} + Z_{el_2}}{Z_{diff}} + \dfrac{Z_{el_1}}{Z_{cm}}} - \frac{ei_2}{1 + \dfrac{Z_{el_1} + Z_{el_2}}{Z_{diff}} + \dfrac{Z_{el_2}}{Z_{cm}}} \quad (6.4)$$

From this expression, it can be seen that the values of the input impedances Z_{diff} and Z_{cm} as compared to the electrode impedances Z_{el_1}, and Z_{el_2} determine the accuracy of differential measurement at this stage. An accurate measurement of the voltage difference $ei_1 - ei_2$ requires that the two denominators in the expression approach unity; thus the sum of the impedance ratios $(Z_{el_1} + Z_{el_2})/Z_{diff}$ and Z_{ei}/Z_{cm} must be very small. If, for example, the electrode impedances have

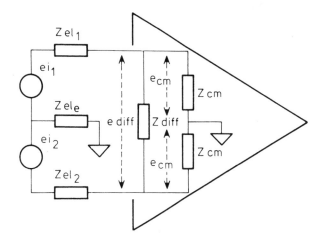

Figure 6.7. Input circuit of EEG differential amplifier input stage. Z_{el_1} and Z_{el_2}, impedances of recording electrodes; Z_{el_e}, impedance of ground electrode; Z_{diff}, differential input impedance; Z_{cm}, common mode input impedances; ei_1 and ei_2, electrical potentials between recording electrodes and around; e_{diff}, difference in potential between amplifier input terminals; e_{cm}, common mode potential between the two amplifier input terminals and ground.

values of about 10 Kohm, the input impedances Z_{diff} and Z_{cm} must have values of several Mohm in order to achieve an accuracy of at least 1%. An unbalance of the electrode impedances Z_{el_1} and Z_{el_2} results in unequal denominators in expression 6.4, and therefore imposes a further restriction on the accuracy of measurement. This is accentuated if ei_1 and ei_2 have relatively large common mode components; owing to this inequality, an additional unwanted voltage difference is caused at the amplifier input. The disadvantageous effect of electrode impedance unbalance will be much less if the relative contribution of Z_{ei}/Z_{cm} to the denominators of expression 6.4 is sufficiently small (e.g., $Z_{cm} \gg Z_{diff}$).

Balanced Amplifier

The measurement of the potential difference is performed by means of a balanced amplifier, also called a differential amplifier. The principle was reported by Offner (1937); a survey of application as an electroencephalograph amplifier was given by Parr and Walter (1943). Later information on semiconductor differential amplifiers was presented by Wu and Brandt (1969). The balanced amplifier is made up of a pair of amplifier circuits that are symmetrically connected with respect to ground and are balanced regarding the symmetrical active and passive components of the two circuits. The working principle will be explained on the basis of the diagram of Fig. 6.8, in which two identical active components (A1 and A2) are shown. Each has an output current that varies proportionally to the voltage (ei_1 and ei_2, respectively) between their inputs and ground. They have internal resistances R_1 and a common external resistor R_{cm} connected to ground.

The internal voltages across R_1 correspond, respectively, to the voltages e_{a1} and e_{a2}; the output voltages of the two circuits with respect to ground are, respectively $Z \cdot \dfrac{e_{a1}}{R_i}$ and $Z \cdot \dfrac{e_{a2}}{R_i}$. For this condition, it can be derived that a difference in voltage at the input $e_{diff} = ei_1 - ei_2$ results in an output

voltage difference $eo_{diff} = \dfrac{e_{diff}}{R_i} \cdot Z$, whereas common mode input voltages $e_{cm} = ei_1 = ei_2$ result in common mode output voltages $eo_{cm} = \dfrac{e_{cm}}{R_i + 2R_{cm}} \cdot Z$. Thus, the gain of the differential mode $G_{diff} = \dfrac{Z}{R_i}$, while the gain of the common mode $G_{cm} = \dfrac{Z}{R_i + 2R_{cm}}$. The discriminative power of a differential amplifier is determined by the ratio $\dfrac{G_{diff}}{G_{cm}} = \dfrac{R_i + 2R_{cm}}{R_i}$. This is called the discrimination factor F. To achieve a high value of F, the resistance R_{cm} must be large as compared to R_1. Therefore, an active constant current source is normally used for obtaining a very high resistance R_{cm} in the common pathway to ground. The ability of the amplifier to suppress common mode input signals, which is reflected by the common mode rejection ratio (CMRR), is closely related to the discrimination factor F. The specified CMRR of an EEG apparatus may have values from 10^3 (60 dB) to 10^4 (80 dB) or even 10^5 (100 dB). However, in many cases the specified CMRR does not represent the effective CMRR. The latter, as has been pointed out above, is dependent on the values of the differential amplifier input impedances as compared to the values of the other impedances in the amplifier input circuit. In some EEG apparatus, the recording electrodes are not directly connected to the input of the differential amplifier, but are connected by way of preamplifier stages that are located in the electrode terminal box. Such amplifiers usually have a high input impedance, whereas their output impedance is low; therefore, impedance transformation takes place before the electrode potentials are submitted to the differential amplifier stage. A very high value of the effective CMRR can be achieved by means of this provision if the preamplifier input impedances are sufficiently high. In this case, the CMRR is mainly affected by the possibility that the gains of the separate preamplifiers are not exactly equal.

Frequency Response and Time Constant

The bandwidth of a signal is defined by the frequency range within which the information of the signal is contained. If EEG signals are passed through a recording channel, information will be lost if the frequency response of the recording channel is narrower than the frequency range of the EEG signal. On the other hand, if the frequency range of the recording channel is wider than the bandwidth of the EEG signal, owing to noise, the recorded data will contain additional irrelevant information.

For the majority of EEG investigations, the frequency range of the recorded signal lies between 0.16 and 100 Hz. Thus, an EEG apparatus must provide recording within this frequency range without unacceptable amplitude distortion; in other words, it must have a flat frequency response within this range. In practice, a number of factors may impose restrictions on the frequency response used. Frequently, other biological electrical activities of cerebral or noncerebral origin or extraneous electrical activities such as interference potentials may be recorded simultaneously with the EEG

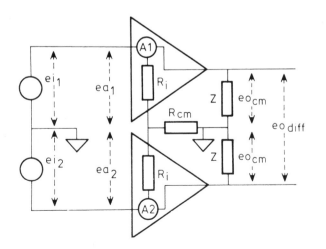

Figure 6.8. Schematic representation of the working principle of a balanced amplifier.

signals. In such circumstances, if the relevant EEG signals cover frequency ranges other than those of the unwanted activities, restriction of the frequency response of the recording channel may be indicated in order to improve the discrimination of the relevant EEG activities. Therefore, EEG recording channels are provided with an adjustable high-pass and low-pass frequency filter by means of which the frequency response of a channel can be chosen optimally for the recording conditions at hand. If, however, the frequency ranges of wanted and unwanted signals overlap, the ultimate selection of the frequency limits will always be a compromise.

Filter Characteristics, Amplitude, and Phase

Frequency selection filters can be characterized by the amplitude and phase of the output signal as a function of frequency in relation to the amplitude and phase of a sinusoidal input signal. This relation is graphically presented as the filter's frequency characteristic. Filter frequency characteristics are usually plotted with a logarithmic frequency scale, which provides equivalent resolution at low and high frequencies. In some cases, a normalized frequency scale is used. The amplitudes are usually presented relative to a reference output amplitude (amplitude at frequency with zero attenuation); the amplitude scale may be either linear (in percentages) or logarithmic (in decibels). The magnitude of the phase difference between input and output signals is given either in degrees or in radians (1 radian = 360°/2π).

Amplitude Characteristics

A high-pass filter has (within certain limits) a flat output amplitude down to a certain frequency; below this frequency the output amplitude gradually drops to zero (Fig. 6.9A). A low-pass filter, on the contrary, has a flat amplitude response up to a certain frequency (Fig. 6.9B). By cascading a high-pass and a low-pass filter (for example, the filters *A* and *B* of Fig. 6.9), a band-pass filter is formed (Fig. 6.9C). A filter

amplitude frequency characteristic is often represented by two parameters. First, there is the cutoff frequency, which corresponds with the frequency at which the output amplitude has dropped to 70.7% (3 dB) of the filter output amplitude at zero attenuation; second, there is the slope in decibels per octave, which is a measure of the maximum gradient of attenuation outside the pass-band. The filters shown in Fig. 6.9A,B have cutoff frequencies at 1.6 and 15 Hz, respectively, and have slopes of 6 dB/octave.

Phase Characteristics

Filters in commonly used EEG apparatus cause a phase difference as a function of frequency between the output and the input signal. This can be illustrated by the phase frequency characteristics of Fig. 6.9. Such a phase difference corresponds to a time displacement between input and output signals whereby the output signal is *leading* if the phase difference is positive and *lagging* if it is negative (Fig. 6.10).

In this way, it can be said that the negative phase of the high-pass filter of Fig. 6.9A corresponds to time lag, whereas the positive phase of the low-pass filter of Fig. 6.9B corresponds to time lead. The relation between frequency *f*, phase difference Φ, and the corresponding time τ is $\tau = \dfrac{\Phi}{f \cdot 360}$ if Φ is given in degrees, or $\tau = \dfrac{\Phi}{f \cdot 2\pi}$ if Φ is given in radians. Using this, it can be established that the time displacement introduced by the high-pass filter of Fig. 6.9A is strongly dependent on frequency, whereas in the low-pass filter of Fig. 6.9B the time displacement is reasonably frequency-independent in the frequency range of interest (f ≤ f_c) and is approximately 8 msec. Thus, if a complex signal, composed of several components at different frequencies, is passed through this high-pass filter, the original time relations between the several components will be modified, and the waveform of the output signal will be distorted as compared to the input signal. The low-pass filter will not cause such distortion, but there will be a time displacement of 8 msec between the input and output signal. The effect of low- and high-pass filtering on the EEG waveforms is shown in Fig. 6.11. Traces of the same input signal are shown

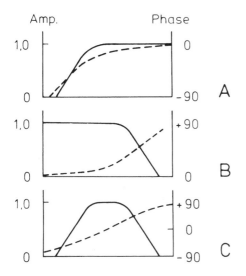

Figure 6.9. Frequency amplitude and frequency phase characteristics of a high-pass filter (**A**), a low-pass filter (**B**), and a band-pass filter (**C**), obtained by cascading the filters shown in **A** and **B**.

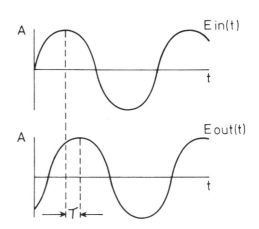

Figure 6.10. Time lag *T* between output signal $E_{out(t)}$ and harmonic input signal $E_{in(t)}$ owing to phase shift.

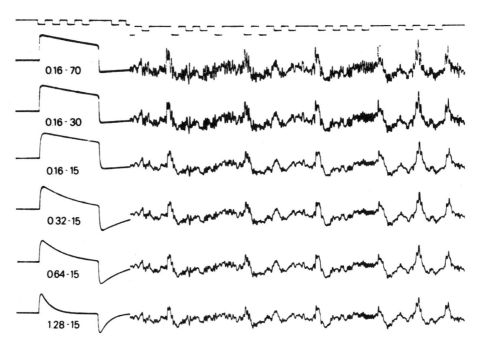

Figure 6.11. The same EEG signal recorded while using different positions of the high-pass and low-pass frequency filters. For each trace, the cutoff frequencies are given in hertz and the effect of the adjustment of the filter on the waveform of a square-wave input signal is also shown.

recorded while using various positions of the high- and low-pass filter selectors.

Time Constant

The simple capacitance resistor network shown in Fig. 6.12A is commonly used as a high-pass filter in an EEG apparatus and is usually specified by the time constant T = C · R of this first-order filter. If a DC voltage step $E_{in}(t)$ is applied to the input of this filter, the output voltage $E_{out}(t)$ will show an exponentially decaying wave form (Fig. 6.12B). The time constant T corresponds to the time elapsed between the presentation of the step voltage at t_o and the moment of time t_1, at which the output voltage has decayed to $\frac{1}{e} \cdot E_{in}$, where e = 2.7183, the base of the natural logarithm. The time constant is a measure for the behavior of the filter in the time domain. Information on the frequency response of the filter may, however, be more useful when considering EEG signals; this can be derived easily from the filter parameter *T*, because for this first-order filter the cutoff frequency is $f_e = \frac{1}{2\pi T}$, while the maximum slope is 6 dB/octave. For example, a time constant of 1 sec corresponds with a cutoff frequency (−3 dB point) of 0.16 Hz.

Sensitivity and Linearity

The sensitivity of a recording system is given by the relation between the magnitude of an input signal and that of the corresponding output signal. In practice, the sensitivity of an EEG recording system is expressed by the relation between the magnitude of an electrical potential at the input and the magnitude of the corresponding deflection on the paper rec-

ord; therefore, sensitivity is usually expressed in microvolts/mm or microvolts/cm. Given that a particular writing system has a certain dynamic range and resolution, the sensitivity of the recording system ultimately determines which range of input amplitudes will be represented with sufficient accuracy in the written data. In electroencephalography, the amplitudes of interest cover a range from a few microvolts up to millivolts; therefore, EEG recording systems are pro-

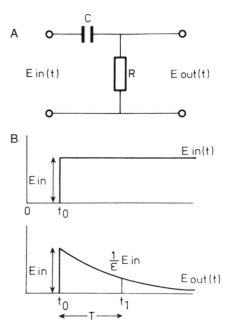

Figure 6.12.   A: First-order high-pass filter. **B:** The response $E_{out(t)}$ of this filter to an input voltage step $E_{in(t)}$. Time constant T = RC; R = resistance; C = capacitance.

vided with means for adjustment of recording sensitivity in accordance with any input amplitude range of interest. This adjustment is usually realized in a stepwise fashion; in this way, a range of fixed preadjusted sensitivities is available. Any continuous adjustment of sensitivity can only be realized by way of calibration of equalization procedures. Because the noise of a recording channel imposes a limitation on the ultimate accuracy of measurement, it is of little use to try to record a signal with an amplitude of the same order or less than that of the equivalent input noise of the recording channel. Accordingly, instrumental noise imposes a practical limitation on the upper side of the sensitivity range of an EEG recording channel.

The lowest sensitivity is chosen in such a way that EEG signals or other biological variables with the largest amplitudes that may occur can be recorded without distortion. To obtain a good representation of the distribution of electrical potentials over the scalp (topography), EEG recording in many instances is carried out using identical sensitivity for all recording channels. This can be achieved easily in practice because most EEG apparatus used in the clinical laboratory are equipped with a master sensitivity selector by means of which sensitivity adjustment of all recording channels can take place simultaneously. There are also provisions for sensitivity adjustment of the separate recording channels.

It is important in an EEG recording system that the similarity between the waveforms of the input and corresponding output signals be maintained. A recording system is said to be linear if, within the working amplitude range, the relation between input and output signals is constant; in other words, it is independent of the amplitudes of the recorded data, as exemplified in Fig. 6.13A for a triangular input signal. Within the usable amplitude range, a linear relationship, as demonstrated by the straight portion of line 1a, results in

a nondistorted output waveform (*solid curve*). Outside this amplitude range, owing to the finite recording span of the writing system, the output signal (*broken curve*) is clipped. The nonlinearity is represented by the sigmoid curve in Fig. 6.13A. In Fig. 6.13B, a nonlinear relationship, represented by line 1b, causes an output waveform that is distorted as compared to a triangular input signal. Nonlinear distortion, of course, causes a decrease of the accuracy of measurement. Considering that this form of distortion is, in most cases, amplitude-dependent, its amount is usually specified as a function of amplitude (for example, at full scale). In this way, the inaccuracy caused by distortion is given as a percentage of amplitude. Nonlinear distortion is not necessarily restricted to the written output of a recording system; it may also be specified in relation to electrical output signals used for storage and further analysis of EEG signals. Dissimilarities between the waveforms of the input and the corresponding output signals may also originate from the amplitude and the phase characteristic of the recording system. Because this form of distortion in principle is amplitude-independent, it is often referred to as linear distortion. The effect of the frequency characteristic on the relationship between input and output signals has already been discussed.

Signal Output and Input

Modern electroencephalographs are provided with extra output and input connections to be used in conjunction with auxiliary apparatus. The availability of output connections enables storage of EEG signals for off-line reproduction on the acquisition computer and/or enables on-line and even real-time data processing by a dedicated analyzer or a general computer. The input connections can be used in certain EEG studies for the simultaneous recording of other signals (see Chapter 47, Polygraphy) or to control the EEG apparatus, for example, for triggered recordings in evoked response studies. EEG apparatus are typically provided with sensitivity equalizers and shift controls for the electrical output signals. Such controls enable the output signals to be calibrated in terms of input voltage or in correspondence with the position of the recording sensitivity; in this way, the sensitivity of the output signal can be expressed in terms of input microvolts per output volts.

Electrical Safety

Electroencephalographs must meet the safety requirements for electrical equipment used in medical practice. These requirements particularly concern the electrical insulation of the part of the apparatus that conducts main current and the grounding of the equipment, which must provide an effective return path for the mains leakage current. From the point of view of electrical safety, the construction of the apparatus must ensure a sufficiently low value of earth leakage current under normal working conditions.

In certain special EEG recording conditions, i.e., during anesthesia monitoring or when recording from the critically ill, the patient often has to be in contact with other electrical equipment or grounded electrically conducting surfaces. Owing to ground loops and impedances in the return paths, fault currents may then flow easily from one instrument to

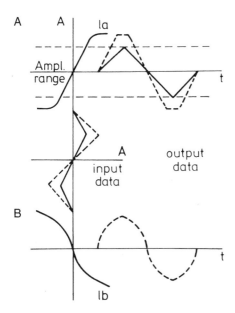

Figure 6.13. Example of nonlinear distortion owing to saturation outside the dynamic range of the recording system (**A**) and a nonlinear relationship between input and output signals (**B**).

another or to grounded surfaces. Effective protection of the patient can be obtained in such recording conditions if an EEG apparatus is used with an input system that effectively insulates the electroencephalograph from the other electrical equipment.

Connection of the signal inputs and outputs with auxiliary electrical equipment may result in a severe and hazardous deterioration of the safety conditions if the apparatus is not provided with protective electrical insulation of these connections. This particularly can occur if connections are made to equipment that does not meet the safety requirements for electromedical equipment. This usually applies to data acquisition and data storage equipment and to computerized data processing equipment constructed for general use.

Recently it became possible to record the EEG simultaneously with functional magnetic resonance imaging (fMRI). This provides a new dimension for the study of brain functions, both normal and pathological, but poses new technical problems. Most important is the problem of the subject's safety (risk of electrodes heating) (Lemieux et al., 1997), and the impairment of the EEG signal due to the static magnetic field and the gradients used for image acquisition. To avoid these problems it is important to use appropriate hardware and algorithms for artifact reduction (Allen et al., 1998; Goldman et al., 2000).

Safety conditions and the production and maintenance of medical equipment are regulated by mandatory regulations, and medical equipment must be approved by notified bodies for a dedicated use in patients/subjects. However, regulations for medical electrical equipment and standards vary for different countries. Therefore, it is important that the EEG apparatus has the appropriate approval (e.g., Communauté Européene [CE] mark, Food and Drug Administration clearance) for use in the hospital depending on the region. A base standard for the medical electrical equipment is given by IEC 60601–1 from the International Electrical Commission, which comprises the "General Requirements for Safety and Essential Performance." Based on this standard but with regional deviations and adaptions are the European standard EN 60601–1 or the United States standard UL-60601–1.

Testing of Systems

EEG recording systems must be tested regularly and, if necessary, be readjusted to ensure that their performance remains in accordance with the required specifications. Technical specifications and instructions for testing are usually provided by the manufacturer. Additionally, the recommendations on performance of EEG apparatuses formulated by the committee on EEG instrumentation of the International Federation of Societies for Electroencephalography and Clinical Neurophysiology (IFSECN) (Barlow et al., 1974; IFSECN Proceedings, 1978) can serve as a basis for carrying out performance tests. Because the calibration voltage is connected to the inputs of an EEG recorder, the functioning of an entire recording channel, from the input to the recorded output, can be checked easily and readily without extra instrumental provisions by making use of the calibration system of the apparatus. An inspection of the simultaneously recorded output signals corresponding to a known calibration signal in most instances provides a sufficient in-

dication of the improper performance of a channel. Most performance and maintenance tests can be carried out with relatively simple and inexpensive instruments, such as a multimeter of good precision for the measurement and adjustment of voltages and currents and a low-frequency signal generator covering at least the frequency range from 0.1 to 100 Hz. The latter should preferably be furnished with a calibrated attenuator, and it should also be provided with a battery power supply.

Calibration Systems and Recording Sensitivity

The recording sensitivity can be tested easily by using the manually operated calibration system. In this way, several calibration voltages can be applied at various recording sensitivities for testing and equalizing purposes. The method shown in Fig. 6.14 can be used to test both the calibration system and the recording sensitivity. The electrode montage selector is used to switch all channels to two arbitrary positions (A and B) of the electrode lead terminal box, which both are terminated with 100-Ω resistors. By means of the potentiometer (100 kΩ, 100 Ω), a 100-mV output signal of the low-frequency generator is attenuated to obtain a 100-μV input signal that can be used as a reference for testing the calibration voltage and for equalizing the recording sensitivities of the various recording channels. By varying the magnitude of the signal generator output voltage, the recording sensitivity also can be verified at other settings of the sensitivity control. When testing the calibration voltage and the recording sensitivity, the frequency of the signal generator must be adjusted in such a way that the frequency response of the recording system does not influence the accuracy of the measurement carried out.

The possibilities of using the calibration system for testing the linearity of the recording apparatus are rather restricted because the range of calibration voltages available in most EEG apparatuses does not permit an adequate determination of nonlinear distortion. For example, calibration voltages of 10, 20, 50, 100, and 200 μV applied at a recording sensitivity of 100 μV/cm do not permit an accurate representation of distortion owing to nonlinearities of the recording system. A better approach (Fig. 6.15) consists of applying an input signal $f(t)$ of constant amplitude with a second input signal $p(t)$ of a much lower frequency. Using the circuit of Fig. 6.16, this test condition can be obtained

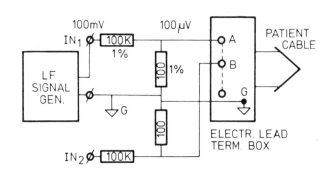

Figure 6.14. Electrical circuit for testing the sensitivity and the linearity of an EEG recording channel. For explanation, see text.

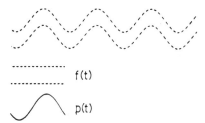

Figure 6.15. Signal for testing linearity. It is obtained by summation of a signal p(t) of low frequency (i.e., 0.5 Hz) and a signal f(t) of higher frequency (i.e., a square wave of 15 Hz; note that only the maxima and minima are shown). The amplitude of f(t) must remain constant in the entire working range of the writing system.

easily in the following way. The manually operated calibration signal (i.e., *f(t)* of Fig. 6.15) is applied in series with the electrode while recording; the low-frequency signal *p(t)* is obtained from the low-frequency signal generator. If the calibration system cannot be used in this manner, the test signal *f(t)* can be obtained from a second low-frequency generator that should be connected between ground (G) and INPUT 2 (IN$_2$, Fig. 6.14).

Frequency Response

The step function or square waveform produced by the calibration system can be used for testing and for adjusting the frequency response of the writing system. With the low-pass frequency filters set at maximum, this response should be in agreement with the manufacturer's specifications; otherwise, it should be adjusted in accordance with the procedure in the instruction manual. Under usual conditions, the response to a step function of square wave should have a small overshoot, which should be smaller than 5% of the amplitude of the recorded step response.

The calibration voltage step produced by the push of a single button can also be used for determining the time constant of a first-order high-pass filter. As has been pointed out, the time elapsed from the moment that the step function has been applied until the moment when the amplitude of the recorded wave form has decayed to 37% of its initial value corresponds to the time constant T of a high-pass filter

of first order having a cutoff frequency (-3 dB) fc = $1/2\pi$T. Thus, if a recording system is provided with first-order high-pass filters, the measurement of the time constants is a relatively easy procedure; in this way, a global check on whether the filters are in agreement with manufacturer's specifications can be carried out. Other detailed and precise information on high- and low-frequency responses of the recording system can be obtained by measuring the responses to sinusoidal input signals using a low-frequency signal generator as shown in Fig. 6.14. Applying sinusoidal input signals of constant amplitude, the recording sensitivity must be chosen such that the amplitudes of the corresponding recorded output signals can be measured with sufficient accuracy. In this way the output amplitude for different frequencies of the input can be measured and a frequency characteristic of the recording system can be obtained. To obtain complete information on the system's frequency responses, this procedure has to be carried out at various positions of the high- and low-pass filter frequency selectors.

Common Mode Rejection

A setup for testing the common mode rejection is shown in Fig. 6.16. Using the electrode montage selector, the two inputs of the channel of interest are connected to the arbitrary electrode positions A and B of the electrode lead terminal box, all other channel inputs are shorted and switched to ground. With switch S1 in position 1 and with a recording sensitivity of 100 µV/cm, a unit signal E_{i1} of 100 µV from a low-frequency generator should result in a recorded output signal having an amplitude corresponding to a deflection of 1 cm. Next, S1 is switched to position 2 and the signal amplitude is increased until again a 1-cm deflection is obtained at the output; this amplitude is given by E_{i2}. The ratio between E_{i2} and E_{i1} represents the CMRR. The same procedure with switch S2 open will produce a measure of the common mode rejection, taking into account an imbalance in electrode impedances. Because the common mode rejection is of importance for the reduction of mains interference, the measurement should also be carried out with the low-frequency generator put at mains frequency.

Interaction Between Channels

The amount of interaction between channels (crosstalk) can be determined by applying to each channel, one at a time while the other inputs are connected to ground, a 40-Hz input signal that should give, at a sensitivity of 100 µV/cm, a deflection in the output of 2 cm. The deflections in any of the other channels are then measured under these circumstances. Crosstalk can be expressed as the ratio between (a) the deflection measured in this manner and (b) the deflection recorded when the input signal of the same amplitude is applied to the same channel.

Digital EEG

The technological advances of the last few decades have led to a revolution in the techniques of EEG recording. This new technology can be called *digital EEG*. The basic principles of EEG recording techniques have not appreciably changed, but the forms of displaying EEG data have gained

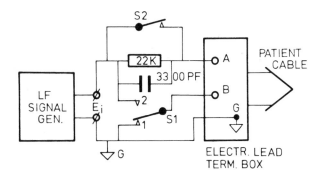

Figure 6.16. Electrical circuit for testing the common mode rejection of an EEG recording channel. For explanation, see text.

new dimensions with the possibilities offered by modern computer graphics (for a review, see Nuwer 1997). Furthermore, digital EEG permits one to manipulate EEG data in a flexible way and to combine different methods of analysis in time, frequency, and spatial domains. These new possibilities of digital EEG are presented in Chapter 41, Digital EEG.

References

Allen, P.J., Polizzi, G., Krakow, K., et al. 1998. Identification of EEG events in the MR scanner. The problem of pulse artifact and a method for its subtraction. NeuroImage 8:229–239.

Almasi, J.J., and Schmitt, O.H. 1970. Systematic and random variation of ECG electrode system impedance. Ann. N.Y. Acad. Sci. 46:509–519.

Barlow, J.S., Kamp, A., Morton, H.B., et al. 1974. EEG instrumentation standards: report of the committee on EEG instrumentation standards of the International Societies for Electroencephalography and Clinical Neurophysiology. Electroencephalogr. Clin. Neurophysiol. 37:539–553.

Coles, P.A., and Binnie, C.D. 1968. An alternative method of chloriding EEG electrodes. Proc. Electrophysiol. Technol. Assoc. 15:195–206.

Cooper, R., Osselton, J.W., and Shaw, J.C. 1969. *EEG Technology*. London: Butterworths.

Flasterstein, A.H. 1966. Voltage fluctuations of metal-electrolyte interfaces in electrophysiology. Med. Biol. Eng. 4:586.

Geddes, L.A. 1972. Interface design for bioelectrode system. IEEE Spectrum 9:41–47.

Geddes, L.A., and Baker, L.E. 1968. *Principles of Applied Biomedical Instrumentation*. New York: John Wiley.

Goldman, R.I., Stern, J.M., Engel J., Jr., et al. 2000. Acquiring simultaneous EEG and functional MRI. Clin. Neurophysiol. 111:1974–1980.

IFSECN Proceedings. 1978. EEG instrumentation standards. Electroencephalogr. Clin. Neurophysiol. 45:144.

Kahn, A. 1965. Monitor artifacts and streaming potentials in relation to biological electrodes. In *Digest of the 6th International Conference on Medical, Electrical, and Biological Engineering,* Tokyo, pp. 562–563.

Lemieux, L., Allen, P.J., Franconi, F., et al. 1997. Recording of EEG during fMRI experiments: patient safety. Magn. Reson. Med. 38:943–952.

Nuwer, M. 1997. Assessment of digital EEG, quantitative EEG, and EEG brain mapping: report of the American Academy of Neurology and the American Clinical Neurophysiology Society. Neurology 49:277–292.

Offner, F. 1937. Push-pull resistance coupled amplifiers. Rev. Sci. Int. 8:20–21.

Parr, G., and Walter, W.G. 1943. Amplifying and recording technique in electrobiology. J. Instn. Elect. Engrs. Part III 90:129–144.

Wu, C.C., and Brandt, R. 1969. Dual high gain differential amplifier. In *Designing with Linear Integrated Circuits*, Ed. J. Eimbinder, pp. 58–73. New York: John Wiley.

7. EEG Recording and Operation of the Apparatus

Edward L. Reilly

When the first edition of this book was published, this chapter stressed the importance of technical considerations in obtaining high-quality electroencephalogram (EEG) recordings. In the interval between the original and the current edition, there has been improvement in equipment, more integrated circuits, greater computerization, machine self-monitoring, machine automation, and less noisy electronics.

These changes can be great assets in attempting to produce a reliable diagnostic record, but as with many innovations, there can be a negative side. In the early EEG machines, a minor error in technique, whether a bad electrode or leaving some sort of electrical device such as a lamp in the room, created 60-cycle noise. Improved machinery is far more resistant to artifacts. In older machines, failure to plug the EEG cable to the jack box resulted in 60-cycle artifact of such severity that anyone in the room with the machine noticed it. An unplugged jack box in modern machines provides an extremely low voltage record that might be interpreted to represent extremely low voltage, but still plausible, brain activity if one was expecting severe damage to the central nervous system (CNS) of the patient or even electrocerebral silence.

In the office, such a record, of course, will be questioned and the error quickly picked up. But in an intensive care unit, where such an error is much more likely to happen, it may continue for minutes or longer before it is apparent and only after deliberate production of artifacts as a means of electrode verification.

Quality recordings continue to require the use of fail-safe techniques on the part of the technologist. In some instances, "smart" equipment is relied on but is run by less trained operators who have no troubleshooting skills. In reality, it may be necessary to have increasingly talented operators as we develop increasingly sophisticated equipment, if quality is to be maintained.

If one doubts the tendency to put less skilled operators with better equipment, one has only to go to the grocery store and compare the present-day cashier running a talking, adding, and subtracting register to the people who used to be hired to make change from their own calculations. In a few of the following subsections, specific points regarding the changing times will point out that the published guidelines for careful technology have become more critical, especially as related to evoked potentials or long-term ambulatory monitoring.

EEG Recording Electrode Placements

When EEG was first successfully carried out on humans by Hans Berger, electrodes were placed on the front and back of the head. Berger continued that method for a number of years and viewed what he saw as a measure of global cortical activity (Berger, 1929). It was discovered by others that, in fact, EEG activity varied in different locations on the head (Adrian and Matthews, 1934; Adrian and Yamagiwa, 1935).

By the mid-1930s, as the number of laboratories investigating EEG increased, there was a rapid proliferation of techniques and interpretations of the activity recorded. Multiple channels allowed investigators to record simultaneously from different scalp areas, and the presence of localized activity such as alpha rhythm and sleep spindles was discovered.

These observations were, in turn, followed by increased attempts to place electrodes at points where they might particularly enhance the observation of one or another type of activity (Gibbs and Gibbs, 1984). As awareness of pattern distribution improved and as new patterns were discovered, increased attempts were made to separate and discriminate between patterns and find electrode placements that would be most advantageous for demonstration of a particular pattern, such as sleep spindles, or demonstrate alpha activity not contaminated by the vertex activity. The observation that different types of activity occurred simultaneously encouraged the use of more electrodes for more channels of simultaneous recording. This was followed by attempts to place electrodes in a standardized manner so that a patient's record could be compared over time and different patients could be compared to each other. Initially, there was wide diversity from place to place in established methods and standard placements.

A committee of the International Federation of Societies for Electroencephalography and Clinical Neurophysiology recommended a specific system of electrode placement for use in all laboratories under standard conditions (Fig. 7.1) (Jasper, 1958). Their recommendation was the system now known as the International 10–20 system. Specific measurements from bony landmarks are used to determine the placement of electrodes. Many of the systems had done this earlier, but they generally used a specific standard interelectrode distance on every patient. The breakdown of such a system is apparent if the application of electrodes to a microcephalic patient is compared to application to a hydrocephalic patient using the same number of centimeters from landmark locations or between electrodes.

The International 10–20 system attempted to avoid both "eyeball" placement and unvarying distances by using specific anatomic landmarks from which the measurements

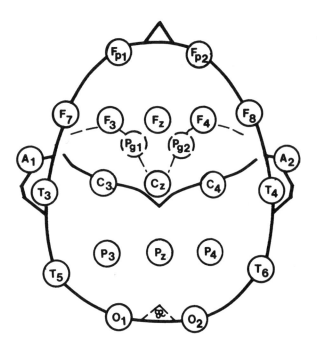

Figure 7.1. International 10–20 system placement and letter–number designation. Odd numbers on the *left*, even on the *right*, and Z, or zero, in the *midline*.

would be made and then using 10% or 20% of that specified distance as the electrode interval. Such electrode placement can be replicated consistently over time and can be replicated between laboratories. Although the measured distances change as the young individual grows, the basic placement remains much more consistent than is sometimes achieved without the use of measurements (i.e., on a properly measured head, a deviation of 1 cm is not necessary and should be corrected if it occurs). The consistency and replication over time may prove to have significant value, particularly in growing children and in longitudinal studies of evoked potential measurements. It is expected that this is more likely to be seen in the longer latency-evoked potential, in which near-field characteristics make placement more critical than in short latency far-field records.

The standard placement recommended by the American EEG Society for use in the International 10–20 system is for 21 electrodes. The system is designed to allow the use of additional electrodes with predictable and easily repeatable placement. The standard numbering system in the 10–20 system places odd-numbered electrodes on the left and even-numbered electrodes on the right, with the letter designating the anatomic area. As can be seen in Fig. 7.1, numbers are deliberately skipped so that the midline or zero electrodes are flanked by electrodes numbered 3 on the left and 4 on the right, allowing insertion of an electrode in the same anatomic designation numbered 1 or 2 if narrower spacing is wanted. Similarly, an electrode can be placed between the left frontal electrode (F3) and the left anterior temporal electrode (F7), which would be designated F5. As the diagram illustrates, the F7 electrode is really over the frontal lobe in a posterior and inferior position, and it is just

anterior to the temporal pole. It is clear that it is a sensitive electrode for temporal lobe activity. It has been suggested repeatedly that a still closer representation of temporal activity is desirable or at least might demonstrate maximum amplitude at points that are not currently positions for standard 10–20 system electrodes (Binnie et al., 1982). Greater specificity of temporal pole activity can be obtained with the use of specialized electrodes, but they are generally not necessary in standard recordings (see Chapter 36).

The American EEG Society, in 1991, added electrode placement nomenclature guidelines that designate specific locations and identification of 75 electrode positions along five anterior posterior planes lateral to the midline chain of 11 specific sites (Fig. 7.2). Similarly four coronal chains are anterior and four posterior to the chain of 13 electrode sites identifiable between the earlobe electrodes upthrough the midline C electrode (American EEG Society, 1994a-e).

The avoidance of a lockstep measurement system has been strongly advocated as one of the major advantages of the method now described as the anatomical placement of EEG electrodes (APEEGE) (Gibbs and Gibbs, 1984). Visual observation and application of electrodes without measurement, especially with distorted skulls, leads to individual decision making. These decisions may vary from test to test and observer to observer, so that one is less confident about whether a change in the EEG over time is due to a simple difference in electrode placement or to a change in the location of the activity being measured. Similarly, rules that require that an amplitude difference must be greater than 50% to be significant may be related more to common variation in electrode distances than to amplitude variation as an actual commonplace physiological feature.

The argument about the number of electrodes needed is based on many factors, including the montages used, the population routinely studied, the type of activity considered

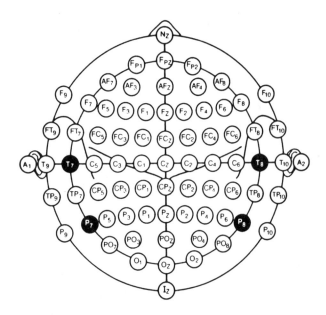

Figure 7.2. Modified combinatorial nomenclature. (Copyright 1990 American Electroencephalographic Society, with permission.)

important, the number of channels available, and the skills of the reader. Some systems are clearly more useful if one expects less skill and training for the technologist attempting to carry out the electrode application swiftly. Some of these combinations also allow more consistency throughout a recording, so the reader has a simpler task. Sometimes fewer electrodes are applied, as in infants, because it is believed that electrical activity is not recorded well from their heads because of small electrode distances; in fact, the voltage recorded on the heads of young children is not lower than in adults and in many cases is much higher. It is for this reason that the American EEG Society (1994b) guideline 2 noted that frequently a reduced sensitivity is needed to record from children. Similarly, the argument that fewer electrodes must be used in children because there is not room for the full 21 electrodes of the 10–20 system is spurious. As can be seen in Fig. 7.3, if collodion attachment of electrodes is used so that there is no smearing of the paste, the full 10–20 system can be applied. It provides very good reliability in heads with a circumference of as little as 23 cm. There is room for full electrode use on even smaller heads.

Some deviation from the International 10–20 system is seen in the research setting (Barrett et al., 1976; Halliday, 1978). Although the advantages sometimes apply to the test in question, issues of economy of time and lack of training of the technician are more often a factor than one would wish in attempting to find a common consistent method of applying electrodes.

Studies with magnetic resonance imaging (MRI) and computed tomography (CT) have demonstrated that the anatomical correlates of the scalp electrodes are imperfect (Myslobodsky et al., 1990) and the distortion may be more evident and lateralized in some sites such as the occipital region (Myslobodsky and Bar-Ziv, 1989).

Montage and Reasonable Use of Channels

The issue of montage and channels in a standard record is important because it has great bearing on the style of recording and the number of electrodes that are used. The term *montage* refers to the particular combination of electrodes examined at a particular point in time (Chatrian et al., 1974; Harner, 1977).

The montage is a tool used for a specific purpose; in most instances, multiple montages are more useful than single montages for long periods. It is probably useful to change the montage every 2 to 3 minutes unless there is clear indication to stay with the ongoing montage, e.g., when a procedure is expected to produce a specific change. The variation from baseline is important, and montage change is self-defeating for technologist and reader in such a case. In hyperventilation, the montage should be maintained for at least 1 minute before the procedure and at least 2 minutes after its completion for comparison. Another instance when montage variation should be done cautiously is in the midst of a seizure. Generally, here again one wants a consistent montage in order to follow the evolution of the seizure. For someone in seizure status who has continued to show the same activity for 5 or 10 minutes, it may become useful to vary the montage to get information about what is going on in other areas or from a different perspective. Endarterectomy, temperature, and anesthesia changes lend themselves to the single montage recording (Barlogie et al., 1979; Kaufman et al., 1977; Presbitero et al., 1980; Reilly et al., 1974, 1980).

Technologists and electroencephalographers use montages as one of the tools by which they record EEG activity. The montage is meant to carry out two simultaneous functions. One is to record from all areas of the scalp. The stan-

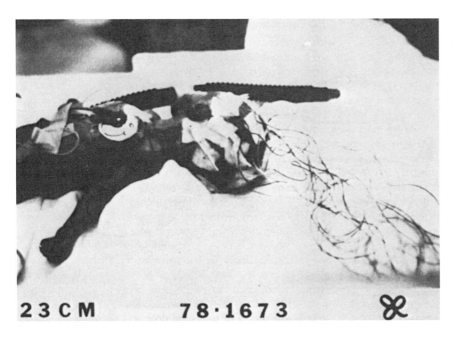

Figure 7.3. Collodion attachment of silver-disk electrodes (0.8 cm in diameter) on a premature infant with a head 23 cm in circumference.

23 CM   78·1673

dard montages and use of all the International 10–20 system electrodes accomplishes that goal. The second function is to record activity in such a manner that it is easily perceived by the reader. To some extent the various montages are used in an attempt to display more clearly activity that may, in fact, be present in several montages. The activity may be there but presented in a way not easily seen, unless some visual tricks are used to make it more evident for the reader. EEG, stored in memory and manipulated by computer at a later date, can be used to vary montages in different ways for a specific segment of data, but it is unlikely that the need for technician skill in changing for "cause" will decline.

There has long been debate within the EEG community as to the particular advantages or disadvantages of reference recording versus the scalp-to-scalp bipolar linkage. That debate, in turn, hinges on the quality of the technique involved in placing electrodes and on the type of abnormality being sought.

If one is mainly interested in a striking pattern, such as a spike-and-wave complex, then the display of such a pattern in a way that makes it stand out at a fairly large amplitude is desirable. For such a pattern, which is generally predominantly parasagittal, the use of the earlobe, whether ipsilateral or joined, is generally an excellent montage. If, on the other hand, the abnormality looked for is a fairly low-voltage limited pattern, perhaps involving only the midtemporal electrode and the reference electrode itself, there is great danger that the pattern can cancel out between the involved electrodes and not show up well. The use of reference electrodes also can lead to some rather complex situations in which there appears to be out-of-phase waveforms occurring both anteriorly and posteriorly (Garvin and Gibbs, 1971). In at least some instances, this phenomenon does not represent a physiological reversal of activity but the contaminated reference electrode effect on uninvolved electrodes (Reilly and Seward, 1980).

Reference Recording and Its Variants

The montages generally used in EEG are divided into two major categories. In one style of recording, the elec-

trodes in their various placements over the scalp are all referred to one single electrode, one common electrode on each side of the head, or the electrically combined activity from two or more electrodes (Fig. 7.4). When all electrodes are referred to a common electrode that, it is hoped, had little brain activity in it, it was convenient to call it "monopolar," but it is far better to recognize that such montages are reference and that it is virtually impossible to make either one of the electrodes in a pair so consistently neutral that the recording is indeed occurring in a monopolar fashion to a totally inactive reference electrode.

The value of a truly inactive electrode has always been evident, but the need is even greater with increased use of computed electrophysiological recording where subsequent display and analysis are quite vulnerable to reference influence.

A reference montage can be set up in two general ways. A common design for reference recording is to have alternating left and right electrodes so that comparable electrodes from each side are recorded next to each other. This sort of combination is particularly valuable when the major part of the abnormality is an asymmetry. Placing comparable electrodes next to each other allows for the observation and detection of subtle differences between the two sides. This is particularly useful if the activity observed might be acceptable if it were symmetrical in amplitude. Often waves are only abnormal because of an asymmetry. This situation is extremely common with activity observed in the temporal region, where one side demonstrates higher voltage and more persistent theta or delta activity than the other side. An asymmetry in the temporal region is frequently seen in drowsiness and light sleep at the time when there is a normally seen increase in amounts of theta and delta activity bilaterally. The asymmetry allows the reader to recognize existing abnormality, although some temporal differences have been reported in a number of normal or apparently normal individuals (Busse and Obrist, 1965; Drachman and Hughes, 1971; Kooi et al., 1964; Obrist and Busse, 1965; Obrist and Henry, 1958; Silverman et al., 1955; Yoshii, 1971). Interpretation of asymmetries will vary with the

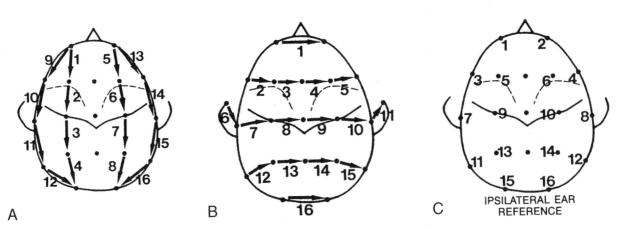

Figure 7.4.   A: A representation of bipolar (scalp-to-scalp) montage in a longitudinal or anteroposterior (AP) direction. This montage is designed for easy comparison of left-right differences in the parasagittal or temporal area, but a montage with strict left-to-right sequence of sets of four could provide the same information. **B:** This is a typical bipolar (scalp-to-scalp) montage in the transverse or coronal direction. **C:** This is a reference (monopolar) montage. This particular sequence is designed to allow a front-to-back sequencing of channels to provide anatomic continuity.

reader, but the visualization of the asymmetry, if it is present, depends on appropriate montages recorded at appropriate times. An asymmetry enhanced by drowsiness and maximal in the temporal regions may not be evident in longitudinal bipolar or ear reference records because of cancellation. Such an asymmetry is seen easily with coronal montages or reference montages using the vertex electrode (Morgan, 1968). These asymmetries will not be seen if the record is turned off while waiting for sleep or if the vertex electrode is considered contraindicated in sleep because of the vertex sharp transients. The latter is a striking large wave but not really an interpretive problem.

A sequential reference montage can be used to allow interhemisphere comparison if this is desirable. When it is useful, a montage might involve the left temporal electrodes with reference to the right ear, followed by the right temporal electrodes referenced to the left ear. Comparable electrodes from the two sides are further apart on the page, making comparison of very subtle differences more difficult, but the montage allows left-to-right comparison at any point in time at which the possible abnormalities appear. Such a "hemisphere sequence" is generally more valuable with bipolar montages than with reference, but it has its value with both types of recording.

One of the earliest and one of the staunchest advocates of monopolar recording was F. A. Gibbs (Gibbs and Gibbs, 1952, 1964). Some of the arguments for different electrode placement and the use of monopolar montages have been reviewed (Gibbs and Gibbs, 1984). In his various writings, Gibbs points out that many patterns are well delineated and were first seen on monopolar montages. These include sleep patterns, the 14/6 positive spike, and many of the specific seizure patterns. In contrast, Gibbs believes that bipolar montages number among their disadvantages the tendencies to (a) reduce voltages sometimes to the vanishing point and create complex waveforms, (b) make it difficult to recognize a "true" electrical sign, and (c) create out-of-phase relations that are hard to distinguish from true physiological out-of-phase voltages (Gibbs and Gibbs, 1964). False phase reversals are also created by involvement of the reference electrode and may be equally deceptive and require confirmation or elaboration by the use of bipolar techniques (Reilly and Seward, 1980).

One of the arguments for the theory that the earlobe electrode, or the two shorted together, makes a neutral reference is that it is, at times, relatively devoid of cortical activity. Unfortunately, one of the major sources of dysfunction and intermittent waves of high voltage is the temporal region, from which such activity is easily reflected in the earlobe electrode. In epileptics, temporal lobe abnormality may be present in as many as 70% of the patients; thus one or both earlobes can be "contaminated" in patients in whom the documentation and understanding of intermittent activity is quite important.

In an attempt to avoid the use of the earlobe electrodes in such patients, a balanced noncephalic electrode was developed by putting one electrode over the right sternoclavicular junction and another on the spine of the first thoracic vertebra. These electrodes are connected together through a 20,000-ohm variable resistor that can be changed in its resistance until the electrocardiogram is virtually canceled (Stephenson and Gibbs, 1949).

In a similar manner, many or all of the scalp electrodes were connected to a common reference lead of 1.5 megohm resistance (Goldman, 1949). Here again, the attempt is being made to average out the individual deviate voltages that may show up in only one or two electrodes. The average electrode concept works well unless there is some transient voltage that is either very high or involves a great many electrodes. In such a case, the transient voltage shows up with reverse polarity and much attenuated amplitude in a manner that may make it difficult to recognize. Of particular note is an eye blink artifact that very often gives a very high-voltage deflection in several electrodes. However, a transient, high-voltage abnormal waveform showing up in several electrodes simultaneously might be displaced in its apparent location and quite distorted in its actual amplitude. Various techniques to use electronics or computers to reconstitute signals in a more accurate way have been attempted (Hjorth, 1975, 1976, 1979; Ishiyama et al., 1982; Sorel and Ranwez, 1984).

Two of these methods are attempts to derive a more truly monopolar derivation (Ishiyama et al., 1982; Sorel and Ranwez, 1984). The latter article is also a good critique of some of the problems associated with bipolar recordings. Neoelectroencephalography (NEEG) is a recording with a true monopolar derivation that is derived by computer-reconstituted signals that use a reference electrode obtained from two electrodes on either side of the neck; the activity is subsequently subjected to Fourier analysis with continuous comparison of phase to determine whether or not the reference electrode is active. When it is determined that the reference electrode is active, it is automatically subtracted from the value of all other reference channels.

Source Derivation

From the early days of EEG, it has been recognized that the various combinations of electrodes represent an interplay of activity from surrounding areas and are particularly influenced by the two or more electrodes connected at any point in time. As noted above, a number of attempts have been made to reduce or eliminate the activity from one or two points so that the remaining observed discharge would become a truer reflection of the electrical activity at that particular point. A method of particular interest has been described by Hjorth (1975, 1976, 1979) with the intent of improving localization of focal activity from the scalp. This technique, which has been referred to as source derivation, has been examined not only for its potential use in EEG interpretation but for the examination of evoked potentials as well (Thickbroom et al., 1984). The technique replaces the visual estimation made by reviewing the various patterns from various combinations of electrodes with an on-line process designed to derive the source activity of each particular electrode (Hjorth, 1975). The method appears to enhance the activity that is unique to a particular electrode. It raises the possibility that one could make interpretations strictly using a single montage and review of the isolated activity from the various points involved in the EEG, rather than reviewing the various combinations, in order to make determinations about the origin of activity. In some particular clinical settings, such focal activity can be enhanced and made apparent when not seen with either bipolar or reference techniques, as has been demonstrated (Hjorth, 1976). Reviews of source derivation in clinical EEG in comparison to standard visual techniques indicated that abnormality detected by the source method but not conventional derivations actually occurred in only a small number of instances. The focal abnormalities, however, were often more pronounced with this technique (Wallin and Stalberg, 1980). There are still questions about the possibility of distortion with this technique, as with others (Gibbs and Gibbs, 1984). Subsequently, use of these techniques to look at visually evoked potentials also suggested that visually evoked potentials showed less spread to adjacent activities when examined by source derivation as well. Thus, the technique may have some localizing value for evoked potentials (Clement et al., 1985).

Nonreference Recording

In a further attempt to eliminate the influence of reference electrodes on the analyses of electrophysiological activity Lehmann et al. (1986) used vector diagram best fits to replicate an analysis without reference electrode or channel.

Some suggest that the closest technical fit to this may be the use of tied electrodes at the muscle free end of the mandible on each side rather than at the earlobe or mastoids (R. N. Harner, personal communication).

Bipolar Variants

In attempts to examine closely the symmetrical areas of the brain and to compare one side of the head with the other, there has been a tendency to use scalp-to-scalp linkages that are particularly useful in demonstrating a marked change in polarity in the so-called phase reversal. The latter phenomenon is greatly overrated and sometimes has been assumed to be evidence of an abnormality in itself. In fact, it is nothing but a tool to show the point of maximum deflection of one polarity or the other. Using bipolar scalp-to-scalp electrodes, it may be demonstrated in two electrode pairs over a common electrode (Fig. 7.5) or it may be seen only over three electrodes, with a middle pair of electrodes in fact canceling

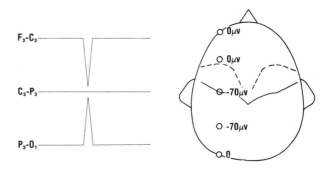

Figure 7.6. This is a classic phase reversal with equal surface negative activity in the C$_3$ and P$_3$ electrodes so that no deflection is seen in that channel, and the major deflections are seen between the uninvolved F$_3$ electrode and the heavily involved central electrode and between the heavily involved parietal electrode and the uninvolved occipital electrode.

out and the phase reversal only being seen if one looks at the electrode pair on either side of the two equally involved electrodes (Fig. 7.6). It is this latter phenomenon that causes some individuals so much difficulty with bipolar montages. If the reader is looking only for patterns (which are relatively rare) or an event in a single electrode, then this tendency for the focus to become low voltage and minimized in the most involved electrodes with bipolar techniques can be a source of confusion. If the phenomenon is recognized, looked for, and learned, it is a useful observation, but it requires the reader to use montages that put broader areas of the hemisphere close enough together to make the observation. Thus, when using bipolar linkage it is generally more desirable to place the channels for one hemisphere together on some part of a page where they can be compared to a similar sequence from the other hemisphere. Obviously, phase reversals and other phenomena can be seen if the left-right sequence of channels is being used, but it involves mastering a much larger part of the page while simultaneously separating the channels mentally into left and right side. For most readers, this is harder than looking at a hemisphere examined in toto and compared to the other hemisphere examined in toto.

The subject of montages over the years has shown a great deal of variability and a great many different strategies. Some assume that, once one has observed the activity from particular electrodes, one can extrapolate and deduce what any combination of electrodes would show. It certainly is the experience of most electroencephalographers that different montages may in fact make particular kinds of abnormalities more evident or more visible. An abnormality is not seen, perhaps, in other montages until a particular combination makes the activity optically more unmistakable, and in retrospect the existence of the abnormality in the montages where it was subtle and initially missed can be confirmed.

It is sometimes suggested that the montages must be presented in an unchanging consistent sequence or the reader will be slowed down or confused. On the contrary, it is probably more likely that activity will not be missed if the technologist is encouraged to change the sequence of montages or devise montages to enhance and more clearly demonstrate what the technologist sees in the record up to that time.

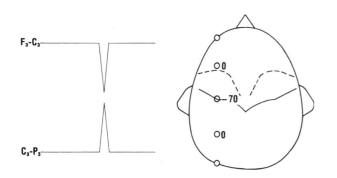

Figure 7.5. Classic surface negative phase reversal over the C$_3$ electrode which is 70 μV negative to both the F$_3$ and the P$_3$ electrode.

Montage selection is improved if the technologist has a good idea of the extent of the abnormal activity in question. This is the distribution or the field of abnormal activity. One attempts to find montages that have some of the electrodes in the field and some outside of the field. The importance of doing this relates to the way EEG amplifiers work. The amplifier does not measure the absolute electrical voltage under any one electrode but, rather, measures the difference in the electrical voltage from two electrodes connected to a particular amplifier. If two electrodes are demonstrating the same 100-μV delta wave and there is no activity in either electrode that is different from the other, connection of the two electrodes results in a flat line. In this instance, the flat line does not represent inactivity but shows that the activity is of equal potential (equipotential) in both electrodes (Chatrian et at., 1974). The term *isopotential* has been applied to this circumstance, but it implies to some the idea of no voltage. This is generally an error.

There is a general rule of thumb that higher voltages are seen as interelectrode distances increase. This is best seen as one records a bipolar montage and switches to a reference montage. The voltages appear to be much higher in the reference montage, and often it is necessary to decrease the sensitivity of the machine. It may be necessary to go back to higher amplification when returning to bipolar montages. It is clear that the voltage of brain activity is not changing.

This is a function of the montage change. The display of different voltages between the two montages is related to the fact that the bipolar anteroposterior (AP) chains of electrodes are close to each other, and the activity is similar in these relatively closely spaced electrodes. In most instances, there is a far greater difference between the voltage in the parasagittal electrodes and that from the earlobes. The latter may be inactive if truly neutral, but there is at least activity of a different voltage and frequency, which results in a higher voltage difference with the reference than the bipolar montages.

One may be attempting to work out the distribution of activity that is clearly abnormal. In this instance, a reference montage with electrodes from one hemisphere in sequence may be useful if the reference electrode is selected as one clearly out of the distribution of the abnormality (Binnie and Lloyd, 1970; Yoshii et al., 1966). This type of sequence is particularly useful with individuals who have focal epileptiform activity or those with a recognizable area of focal delta activity. This is easier to interpret if superimposed on a distinctly different background with a different frequency and voltage, so that the abnormal wave stands out and is recognizable simply when it appears and not just when it is compared to the other hemisphere.

The American EEG Society (1994d) has proposed that standard montages be used, not exclusively, but at least as part of every record. The recommendations are also based on the premise that the other minimal technical standards of EEG are being carried out. The montage recommendations are designed around the idea that at least eight channels are being used, and 16 or more channels are encouraged. It is assumed that the full 21 electrodes of the 10–20 system are being used.

The recommendations suggest that both bipolar and referential montages be used in a record. It is recommended that the electrode connections for each channel be indicated at the beginning of each montage, rather than using a cryptic number or letter as the only montage mark or attaching a copy of the montages on the front of a record. It is suggested that the bipolar connections should run in straight unbroken line with interelectrode distances equal. It is also recommended that over the course of a record, bipolar recordings be run both in the longitudinal direction (Fig. 7.4A) and the transverse direction (Fig. 7.4B). Referential recording should be done as well (Fig. 7.4C).

In accomplishing this, the guidelines suggest that when 16-channel or larger machines are used, at least one montage from each of the three classes will be needed. For 8- or 10-channel recordings, at least seven montages will be needed from the standardized list to meet the same requirements. Although it is still the belief in many laboratories that referential recordings alone or bipolar recordings alone are the only ones necessary, perhaps increased experience in laboratories using both will demonstrate to readers that in many instances it takes the combination to make clear which of at least two possibilities is correct when there is a particular asymmetry or unusual activity recorded.

Electrode Impedance

In the initial years of checking electrode attachments, it was common to measure resistance rather than impedance. Even now, when checking individual electrodes that are not attached to the patient's head, it is still sometimes simplest to take two electrodes, measure the resistance, and determine whether the resistance remains low when the two electrodes are slightly stretched. This has the advantage of picking up the "make-break" problem that is sometimes seen in an electrode that is conducting most of the time but is showing little intermittent breaks in conduction as the cable is moved. This is usually an electrode in which the inner wire is snapped but is not yet totally pulled apart. The stretching helps accentuate the break. Obviously, if this is done with excessive vigor, it may shorten the life of the electrode, which is costly and undesirable.

Once the electrode is attached, there can be discomfort and hazards in measuring electrode resistance (Seaba et al., 1973). As a result, it is useful to measure impedance rather than resistance once electrodes are attached to the patient (Seaba, 1985). To greatly minimize the hazards of measuring resistance, two major concerns can be cited: (a) the passage of current in the test may actually polarize or charge one of the electrodes, and the discharge of that electrode's potential buildup may show up in the record at some later point, looking like a plausible event from a focal source; (b) the other problem in measuring resistance through electrodes on the patient's head is that, if it is done with standard resistance meters rather than those specifically designed for patient use, it is likely that the current used is going to be felt by the patient with a sensation ranging from mild discomfort to clear pain.

Although resistance measurement depends predominantly on the material used for the electrode and on the ability of current to pass through the skin, the latter depends quite directly on the preparation of the skin before the electrode is attached. In contrast, impedance involves characteristics of resistance capacitance and inductance. As with resistance, electrode impedance is lower if the skin has been prepared by cleansing or rubbing to remove surface oil and superficial layers of the epidermis. Over the years, a wide array of materials, including acetone, alcohol, and even soapy water, have been used for this purpose. Now it is common to use materials that are themselves conducting electrolytes. The rubbing of the cleansing material requires some firmness, and one must be familiar with the material being rubbed in. A few of the currently available cleansing electrolyte materials have some abrasive substances embedded in the material. If such a cleanser with an abrasive is rubbed with the same enthusiasm and vigor as a cream without an abrasive, it is possible that there may actually be a break in the skin with some blood or later scab formation. This is undesirable. Often a small piece of gauze rubbed against the skin both carries the electrolyte material and has ridges sufficient to help remove the surface materials of the skin. The effect of the gauze can be enhanced by wrapping the piece of gauze around an eraser on the end of a pencil. The gauze can be held in place with a rubber band. The give under pressure on the soft eraser makes it less likely to injure the skin. Holding the pencil gives the technologist good control and a greater amount of pressure against the skin. A similar combination of both firmness and softness can be obtained with a cotton-tipped applicator. It remains imperative to look for the possibility of lack of similarity between impedance in different channels or changes in impedance over the course of the record. Such changes can result in record artifacts (Gordon, 1980). If skin preparation and electrode selection is done well, the impedance can be reduced below 3,000 ohm, and quite often 1,000-ohm impedance is reached without difficulty. An impedance over 5,000 ohm in any electrode should not be accepted as adequate (American EEG Society, 1994a; American Medical EEG Association, 1988).

It is important that impedance actually be measured. It cannot be assumed that routine attempts to reduce impedance and to apply the electrodes with reasonably consistent application will ensure low impedance. Failure to check impedance routinely leads to a variety of artifacts that can be interpreted as brain activity.

Even though the electrode has proper impedance at the beginning of the record, it can deteriorate during the recording. This point is given less recognition than is desirable. Technologists need to be encouraged to recheck impedance at regular intervals. Many machines have excellent methods of checking impedance in one channel or in all channels simultaneously. The output varies depending on the machine. Some instruments measure the difference in impedance between electrodes involved (lead imbalance); other machines measure total impedance of the two electrodes involved. The latter is preferable. It is essential that technologists and readers understand the method and implications of the method used for a particular machine. Whether the displayed output is the sum of the impedance of the involved electrodes or the difference between the impedance of each electrode must be understood by all those who work with the machine.

One often-neglected indicator of rising impedance is the development of a 60-cycle artifact from a particular electrode. This artifact is considered an unwanted interference in the recording, but there is a tendency for electrodes with rising impedance to show this and other artifacts. Such a development tells the technologist to test and fix an electrode before great difficulty develops. It can be of value if this is understood and if routine use of the 60-cycle notch filter is avoided.

Electrode Application

Once skin impedance has been appropriately lowered, the electrode can be attached to the skin in many ways. Attempts have been made to develop self-adhering or self-attaching electrodes. The needle electrode lies under the dermis and generally stays in place without additional means of holding it. It may fall out from its own weight, and it certainly falls out if the head is moved abruptly. Spring-loaded electrodes with flat surfaces or teeth are painful and not tolerated over the scalp, but a spring-loaded, flat, clip-type electrode on the earlobe can be used as the reference electrode. Most commonly, the conducting metal electrode is attached to the skin surface of the scalp, rather than embedded in the skin. Some relatively thick pastes with conducting properties are commercially available. A common method of attaching electrodes is to take an electrode and scoop up a ball of electrolyte paste; the electrode and paste are then firmly pressed onto the skin. The pressing of the electrode pushes the paste and electrode against the scalp. The paste folds around the edge of the electrode, and the attachment of the paste to the electrode is enhanced by pressing a cotton ball or a piece of gauze on top of the electrode and paste combination. This type of electrode is relatively easy to prepare, and good impedance recording can be obtained with it. One hazard of the method is spreading of the paste that makes electrode contact. The recording site is the size of the ball of paste on the scalp. If an unduly large amount of paste is used, the recording is from a much larger area than with the simple metal electrode. Masses of paste can spread as the head is moved and may touch each other and short out between electrodes. Also, the paste tends to dry. Contact becomes variable as the electrode becomes less consistently adherent. Such drying can occasionally be seen in less than 20 minutes but may not be seen in recordings extending well beyond 45 minutes. The smaller the amount of paste, the faster the drying, but large paste quantities increase the other problems described above.

To provide a more secure method of electrode attachment, collodion is applied to actually glue electrodes to the head. This can be done with a small ring of collodion at the edge of the electrode at the skin-electrode junction. More commonly, the collodion is used to soak a piece of gauze, which is then spread over the electrode and skin (Fig. 7.7A,B). This provides a large area with glue. Compressed air is used to speed the drying (Fig. 7.7C). It is critical for laboratories using this method to be aware that collodion, not flexible collodion, must be used. The latter is used more commonly in hospitals for dressings. In that situation, it is

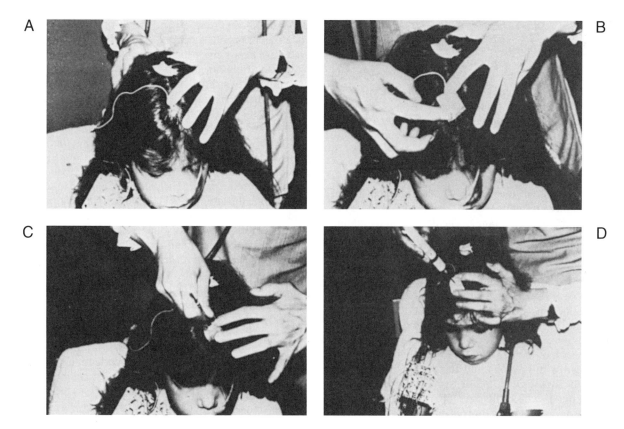

Figure 7.7.   **A:** The electrode is placed in the position on the head, which has been previously measured and has previously had the impedance lowered. **B:** A piece of gauze soaked with collodion is placed over the top of the electrode. **C:** Compressed air is sprayed on the collodion-soaked piece of gauze as the gauze is smoothed against the head. This causes rapid drying of the glue against the skin. A point in the compressed air applicator posi- tions the air in the center of the electrode and helps hold the electrode against the skin. **D:** A blunt-tipped needle that fits the hole in the electrode relatively tightly is passed through the hole in the gauze into the electrode and an electrolyte solution is added to fill the cup. This blunt metal tip can be used to scratch the skin and improve impedance if required.

not necessary to have the quick-drying characteristic needed for EEG application. The oil in flexible collodion makes adequate drying impossible. The electrolyte under the electrode can be scooped into the electrode before the electrode is glued in place. A more reliable method is to use electrodes that contain a hole (Fig. 7.8) so that the electrolyte can be added after the electrode is glued tightly on the head (Fig. 7.7D). Collodion-attached electrodes with a hole in the surface have the added advantage that they can be left in place for periods of up to 5 days without affecting the skin. Electrolyte can be added for each recording, and this allows re-recording to be carried out with greater ease and greater speed than if the electrodes are reapplied at each test. The electrolyte must not contain calcium if long-term contact is expected without skin effects. The collodion-attached electrodes as described here are probably the best for use in any short- or long-term recording session, whether those sessions take place over minutes or days. They are generally the best for surgical situations. This type of attachment appears to be the most reliable over hours, and it is generally much more feasible to gain access to an electrode and add more electrolyte solution through the hole in the electrode than it is to totally remove and reglue an electrode during surgery.

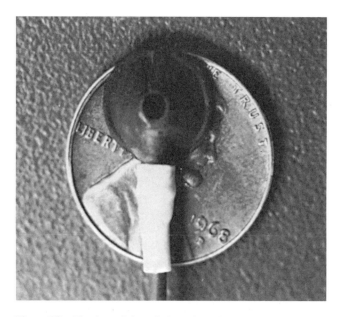

Figure 7.8.   The electrode has a hole so electrode paste can be added and skin can be reached to reduce impedance. The size of this 0.8-cm electrode is compared to the United States penny.

Calibration

The calibration signal simultaneously presents several bits of information. The calibration signal provides an assessment of the sensitivity of individual amplifiers. To be sure the machine is accurate, the technologist must be aware of the signal size expected, must provoke a signal of adequate size to measure, and must be able to measure the signal obtained (Fig. 7.9). In the illustration, three deflections have been obtained. One is a deflection in excess of the 12 mm from the baseline considered accurate and reliable on the particular machine used. The top calibration signal shows a distinct overshoot, which would not be included in the measurement even if this deflection were obtained within the adequate range. The deflection excluding the pen overshoot should be measured; this should be the appropriate deflection for input. If not, the amplifier should be adjusted. The lowest of the three calibrations in the illustration is so small that accurate measurement is difficult, if not impossible; it is best to try to arrive at calibration signals with deflections somewhere between 5 and 12 mm on most machines. With machines with narrow pen spacing, actual deflections cannot exceed 10 mm without exceeding the accurate arch of the pen. In Fig. 7.10, a page of calibrations is shown with the high and low linear filter settings marked on the sides. Only one or two square wave pulsations provoking the classically seen upward and then downward deflection of the alternating current (AC) are required. The tendency to recalibrate across the page for 10 or 20 seconds is unnecessary. The major use of the calibration signal is to provide a sample of the deflection, the rise time, the decay as modified by the low linear frequency setting or time constant, and a display of the sharpness of the square wave for some suggestion of the effect of the high-frequency filters.

The most critical part of calibration usage is that the deflections be carefully observed and measured in all channels at least once a day and preferably before the start of each record. The next most critical use of the calibration signal is as an assessment of pen alignment and time axis. Both of these are best seen if the calibration signal can be lined up with one of the time axis lines down the paper, as is seen in the initial upward deflection in Fig. 7.10. If a single pen is leading and pens both higher and lower on the paper than that particular pen are on the time axis line, the pen is misaligned and needs to be adjusted. If pen alignment has been adequately carried out, it is often found that the pens at the top of the page may be on the line; however, there is progressive deviation of the pens from the time axis line as one moves down the paper. The pens may lead or follow the line by the time the last channel is reached. This suggests that the paper is going through the machine crooked compared to the actual pen alignment. Readjustment of paper is sometimes difficult, but both pen and paper alignment are very important if the reader is to make an accurate assessment of onset of closely spaced events.

Two other types of calibration should be carried out. A low-voltage calibration such as a 5-μV input with a sensitivity of 7 or 7.5 μV/mm produces a very small deflection, less than 1 mm. The technologist and reader examine this to see if the onset of the wave is rounding or if there is absence of the deflection in one channel. The deflections are not measured, just examined. This is a very sensitive indicator when pen galvanometer difficulty begins. The ball bearings of the pen motor start to flatten, and the small signal is insufficient to make these flattened bearings move. The larger signal is sufficient to overcome that initial friction, and the large signal may show no apparent reduction in the deflection. The record will show loss of low-voltage signals, such as super-

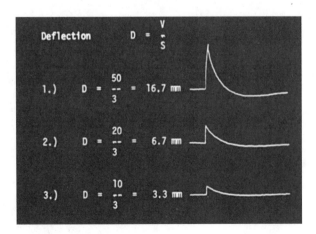

Figure 7.9. Calibration deflections in response to three signals but with a constant sensitivity. Only the center calibration has a deflection in a range where the pen is not exceeding its limits but is large enough for easy and accurate measurement.

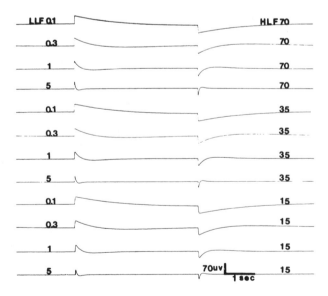

Figure 7.10. A series of deflections using a variety of low linear frequency settings (20% attenuation at the designated number) and a variety of high linear frequency settings (20% attenuation at the high-frequency number). The time axis marked on the paper lines up with the initial upward deflection.

imposed beta activity. Regular use of this small-voltage calibration signal is desirable to detect this potential problem at an early stage of development.

A "biological calibration" is essential. The "machine calibration" signal is internal to the machine; it gives no indication of the actual connection of the electrodes and does not actually involve the patient. The initial calibration signal tests only the machine, the amplifier, and the pen alignment. An additional calibration with the same two scalp-attached electrodes in all channels simultaneously demonstrates that all the amplifiers respond equally and correctly to a variety of frequencies and not just to a direct current (DC) signal. This tests the electrode cable and the patient's cerebral activity as well.

At the end of a recording, it is desirable to calibrate again, using all of the sensitivities and all of the filter settings used throughout the recording (American EEG Society, 1994a). In instances in which records of electrocerebral inactivity have been carried out, it is necessary to calibrate using a 2-μV calibration signal with the most sensitive amplification used in the recording. This is a demonstration of the deflection that would occur if this minimal level of EEG activity were recorded. The suggestion of using a 2-μV calibration signal is included in the minimum technical standards for EEG recordings of suspected cerebral death (American EEG Society, 1994c).

Filters

The use or misuse of filters provides one of the major sources of contention among electroencephalographers and technologists. The range of neurophysiological activity extends as high as 2,000 cycles/sec, as in the cerebellum. Slower frequencies of cortical origin extend down to one third of a cycle per second and probably to one quarter of a cycle per second. Still slower frequencies arise from the brain and are recorded under special circumstances, such as studies of the contingent negative variation (CNV) or studies of negative DC shifts prior to seizures. Slow brain frequencies are difficult to differentiate from the very slow potential changes that occur on the basis of sweat artifact or due to change in the galvanic skin response (GSR). Fortunately, study of evoked potentials brought the attention of neurophysiologists back to portions of the frequency band that had been ignored for a period of time. Some will argue for measuring the full range of provoked activity.

In general, one can assume that the greater the recorded frequency band, the greater the fidelity of reproduction of the actual activity. In theory, this is true, but recording a larger frequency band increases the amount of outside interference and noise in the signal. Filters are used to make a compromise between reduction of extraneous signals and preservation of as much as possible of the fidelity of the brain waves one particularly desires to observe. If the frequency band recorded for EEG is compared to that recorded for evoked potentials, a striking discrepancy in bands of value is apparent. In EEG there is little of value in the signal over 50 cycles/sec, whereas in recording short latency far-field evoked potentials, it is common to filter out frequencies under 100 or 150 cycles/sec but to continue recording

up to 3,000 or possibly 30,000 cycles/sec (Calloway et al., 1978; Cracco and Cracco, 1976; Stockard et al., 1979). One may insist on recording slow activity down to cycles/sec (direct current) but define it as acceptable to eliminate faster activity. In contrast, one may need to see all the fast activity but not care much about slower frequencies. In each case, one defines a frequency band. The component in equipment that eliminates unwanted frequencies and defines such limits is the filter. A filter range is the frequency that will appear without significant distortion at some determined level of accuracy. The question of significant distortion is answered variably for different kinds of studies.

For EEG activity, it is accepted that a frequency displayed at 70% or more of its actual voltage is acceptable. If the loss or attenuation to a particular frequency by the filter reduces the voltage more than 30% of its real value, the distortion is significant and puts the activity outside of the frequency band. This is an arbitrary number found acceptable by the EEG field and the various societies involved. Certainly, there is no reason why the societies cannot decide that 40% attenuation is acceptable or that 10% attenuation is too great. Electrocardiogram (ECG) equipment is allowed attenuation of only 10% or less within the defined frequency spectrum. Each industry or type of activity defines acceptable amounts of distortion at the limit of defined frequency bands.

The frequency band investigated in most detail by clinical neurophysiologists doing EEG has included frequencies under 50 cycles/sec. This limitation of the frequency leaves one with activity normally having the highest amplitude. Such frequencies were easier to record when equipment was less sensitive. The other reason for attention to slower frequencies (less than 100 cycles/sec) relates to limitation not of amplifiers, but of pens. Pens provide poor reproduction of activity over 100 cycles/sec. With the conventional pen and ink writing machine, there is little point in having an amplifier attempt to display activity faster than the pen will record.

One must consider what high-frequency and low-frequency activity is required in a particular record. A few of the most limiting filters overlap, but as a general rule filters used to influence low-frequency activity have no effect on the high-frequency waves. Those affecting the high-frequency activity do not do anything one way or the other to low-frequency waves. This is in contrast to manipulation of sensitivity or gain, which affects all frequencies recorded.

High-Frequency Filters

The filter that affects the high-frequency activity is described by several terms, including "high-frequency filter." Generally, a particular number is specified, such as high-frequency filter 70 or high-frequency filter 35. The designated number indicates which particular frequency has been reduced or attenuated in amplitude by the maximum attenuation allowed. The percentage attenuation cannot be taken for granted and is only know if the reader is familiar with the particular electroencephalograph machine used. In the United States, two common machines sold had different amounts of attenuation at the designated number. The Grass Instrument Company told the reader that the designated frequency would be attenuated 20% from its true amplitude.

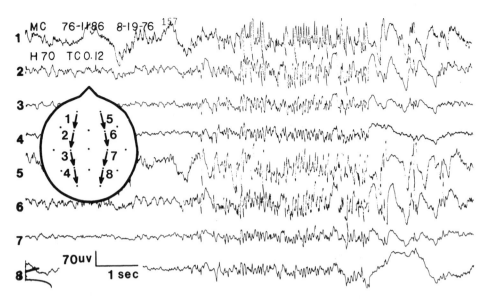

Figure 7.11. A sleeping patient demonstrates a train of multiple spikes blending into multiple spike and slow wave complexes. The individual spike is considerably faster than its repetition rate would suggest.

The Beckman Instrument Company told the reader that the attenuation at the designated number would be 30% or 3 dB. The latter degree of attenuation was the convention on machines some years ago, but flatter curves are now possible in modern amplifiers. With the many changes in companies and the variety of machines, the reader and technologist must find out the real effect on their particular machine.

A filter does not have a static or single level of attenuation at different frequencies. The high-frequency filter will affect the designated frequency by 20% or 30% and is expected to affect frequencies slower than the designated number at a progressively lesser degree (always less than the defined 20% or 30% attenuation) until there is no attenuation at all. In contrast, frequencies above the designated filter number will have progressively more than 20% or 30% attenuation, so that some higher frequencies may be attenuated to zero amplitude and be eliminated. The 1971 minimum standards of the American EEG Society originally recommended that 50 cycles/sec should not be attenuated by more than 50% of true amplitude. In the more recent versions of the standards (1994a-e), this recommendation has been changed. The 1994 standard suggested that 70 cycles/sec activity should not be attenuated by more than 30% of its true amplitude (attenuation of 3 dB).

Filter Issues in the Recording of Spikes

The upper frequency expected of spike discharges (those with a 20-msec base) is 50 cycles/sec, and the concern for this frequency is quite rational. For the individual interested in seizure disorders, the appropriate recording of high frequency may be of greatest concern. The filters on this end of the spectrum can be misused to provoke both underreading and overreading of the recording. Spikes by definition have a base of 20 to 70 msec, which ranges from 14.3 to 50 cycles/sec. Most recognize that spikes in the tonic phase of generalized seizure occur 13 to 20/sec, although Gibbs and

Gibbs (1952) report that they can repeat as fast as 40/sec. Observation clearly shows that these are often spikes with a base, indicating a faster frequency than the number seen in a second. The important concept is to recognize that a spike is defined by its base (Fig. 7.11). Readers are describing not the base, but the repetition rate. Thus, a 14 to 20/sec train of spikes may, in fact, consist of 40 to 50 cycles/sec spikes if each is measured individually (Fig. 7.12).

This is not merely an academic point. It is of clinical importance when considering the use of high-frequency filters. Fortunately, the term *muscle filter* has become less used, but some advocate the advantage of a rapid 30 cycles/sec "roll-off filter" to eliminate muscle faster than 30 cycles/sec. A high-frequency filter eliminates fast activity regardless of its origin. A 40 cycles/sec muscle potential and 40 cycles/sec spike appear the same to the filter and are attenuated and modified to the same degree by the filter. Both technologists and electroencephalographers need to develop understanding and familiarity with the filter curves for their machines.

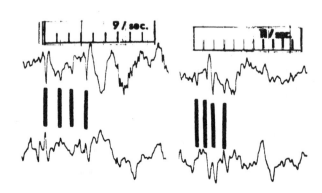

Figure 7.12. The frequency counter shows the repetition rate, but an uninvolved baseline exists between each spike.

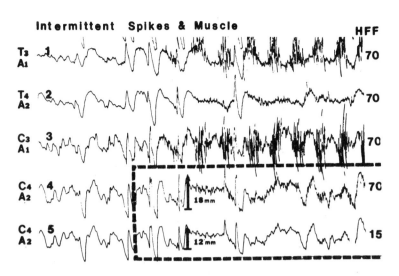

Intermittent Spikes & Muscle

Figure 7.13. The bottom two lines show the same spike and demonstrate the reduction in the amplitude and great modification of the spike pointedness of the wave as it occurs in channel 4 compared to its appearance in channel 5.

A 35 cycles/sec filter reduces 50 cycles/sec frequencies to only about 60% of their true amplitude. Some machines have 60 cycle "notch filters" that reduce 50 cycles/sec spikes 50% of their true amplitude. The 60-cycle filter and the high linear 35 cycles/sec filters have about equal effect on 40 cycles/sec activity, in that they both reduce it to about 60% of its original amplitude. The high linear filter 15, by definition, reduces 15 cycles/sec spikes by either 20% or 30% depending on the machine involved. It reduces spikes of 30 to 35 cycles/sec to less than two thirds of their true amplitude (Fig. 7.13).

It is critical that filters be used in such a way that they do not eliminate this wanted and desired spike activity. More specifically, the filters must not be used if a spike is to be clearly identified, because high-frequency filters also affect waveform. They round off the point crucial in the identification of a spike (Fig. 7.14). Once rounded off, it becomes difficult to separate a train of spikes from a high-voltage train

of beta waves. The reader who consistently berates the technologist for running records with excessive muscle artifact should be aware that technologists sensitized to use filters or to turn off the machine to avoid muscle activity will quite likely eliminate more than muscle artifact from records. This is antagonistic to the idea that seizure onset must be recorded. Seizures are preceded at times by multiple spikes. Spikes are easier to differentiate from muscle artifact with an open high-frequency filter than in a highly filtered and thus uninterpretable recording.

High-frequency filters are, in some instances, referred to as "low-pass filters," in that they pass low-frequency activity without affecting it. Thus their major influence is on the faster frequencies. This is certainly an accurate definition of their function, but there is more useful identification of their function when they are specified as high-frequency filters and the actual frequency they affect is specified.

Low-Frequency Filters

At the other end of the frequency band, there are low-frequency filters that are designated by numbers representing 20% or 30% attenuation at the particular frequency named. There are settings of low-frequency filter 1, low-frequency filter 0.1, or low-frequency filter 0.16, designating the frequency at which the expected attenuation occurs at the specified percent. The effect of a low-frequency filter is determined by the time constant involved. This feature in simpler, older amplifiers was determined by the combination of the resistance and capacitance in the amplifier. Resistance multiplied by capacitance equals the time constant in actual numbers. In more complex amplifiers, this ratio is not as linear as in the simpler circuits, but these components still are the features that determine the time constant. Time constant can be more operationally defined as the time it takes for a square wave deflection to drop 63% from its peak. That is the same as saying that time constant is the time it takes for a square wave signal deflection to drop within 37% of the original baseline. The technologist can make this measurement directly from the calibration signals that are, in fact, square wave deflections.

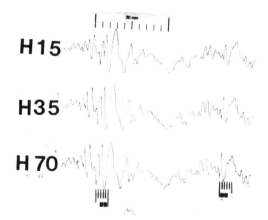

Figure 7.14. This close-up of the train of spikes and slow waves demonstrates a well-defined spike in the bottom line, but after filtering of the high-frequency activity, the point has been rounded off. It is less clear in the top channel that these waveforms could be defined unequivocally as spike discharges and not merely as high-voltage beta waves.

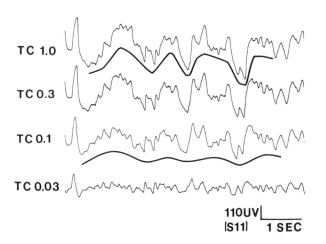

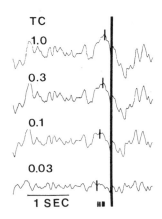

Figure 7.15. A series of shorter time constants measuring activity from the same two electrodes in each channel. UV, microvolts.

Figure 7.17. The same two electrodes with four different time constants demonstrate the apparent peak (marked to the left of the time axis bar). The peak seemingly occurs earlier with the short time constant, but in reality the pen is returning to baseline sooner with a progressively less accurate demonstration of the actual peak.

The terms *time constant* and *low linear frequency* are used interchangeably in considering the effect on slow activity, but the number is not the same where the terms are varied. A time constant of 1 second represents a low linear frequency filter of 0.1 or 0.16, depending on the machine involved. The time constant of 0.3 second may represent a low linear frequency filter of 0.5. It is critical to make the distinction that the same information can be conveyed using low linear frequency or time constant, but the number is not the same.

It has been stated that the time constant does not actually eliminate any of the slow frequencies, but only attenuates them. The effect, however, is that the reader finds the slow waves uninterpretable. Figure 7.15 demonstrates delta waves that are quite evident with longer time constants. The particular downward deflections of the delta components are evident even with the shortest time constant, but a reader is not apt to read or even see the slow activity at the shortest time constant, which is the equivalent of a low linear frequency 5 setting. In Fig. 7.16, it is observed that the delta waves on

the left and the right side of the illustration are attenuated to different degrees. This is because they are different frequencies of delta activity. The right-hand wave is slower and is attenuated more sharply. This reemphasizes the point that all frequencies below the designated frequency are *not* attenuated equally.

An additional effect of low linear frequency or time constant is to change the apparent peak of the observed slow wave. Figure 7.17 shows that the peak is closer to the vertical bar (time axis) with the longest time constant and appears to occur earlier with the shorter time constants. This effect is called "phase shift." Because the phase shift is dependent on the frequency of the wave attenuated, the degree of shift is different for each frequency and has the effect of modifying the relationship of waves to each other. This distorts relationships of different frequencies to each other. This is a major problem when the effect of the filter not only modifies the record but also modifies different components to a different degree, producing significant distortion.

The choice of the appropriate time constant can be critical in locating some asymmetrical discharges. It is general practice to start a record with the low linear frequency set at about 1, which suggests a time constant of 0.12 and 0.16 second. This is an appropriate time constant to use at the start of a record, but it is not the best; it is, in fact, a shorter time constant than is desirable in most records. At the start of a record, there is generally a good bit of patient movement; this relatively short time constant minimizes the artifact that is usually present in this part of the record. It should be routine to use a longer time constant; the 0.3- or 0.4-second time constant is appropriate in almost all records. When the patient is cooperative, it may be desirable to use even longer time constants. A time constant of 1 second, which approximates a low linear frequency of 0.1 cycle/sec, is useful. There is sometimes the feeling that, if an abnormality such as diffuse slowing is already evident in the record, nothing else needs to be done (Fig. 7.18). Readers and technologists both should be aware that records may have bilateral and relatively symmetrical 3 cycles/sec activity with

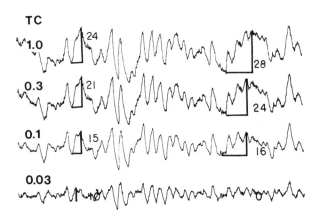

Figure 7.16. The same two electrodes are in all four channels but the time constants are different. It is observed that the slower delta wave on the *right* is attenuated more sharply than the faster delta wave on the *left*.

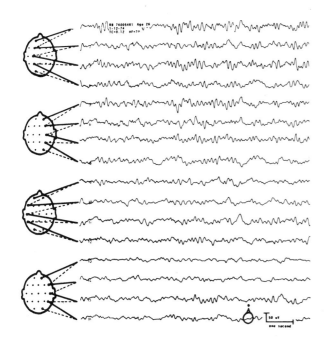

Figure 7.18. A record of a patient after a head injury. With a low linear frequency setting of 1, the record shows what appears to be reasonably symmetrical delta activity.

underlying lateralized 0.5 or 1 cycle/sec delta activity obscured unless a long time constant is used to allow the asymmetry to appear (Fig. 7.19). The search for subtle underlying asymmetries is of particular value in head trauma patients, who often have both diffuse slowing and focal changes. This is not the only etiology that shows this phenomenon; tumors may provoke similar dysfunction.

On occasion it is quite useful to deliberately eliminate much of the slow activity by use of the shortest time constant such as 0.03 or 0.35 second (Fig. 7.20). This attenuates most of the delta range activity. Some individuals believe that reducing the delta activity alone allows one to see faster frequencies more clearly. This may be more of a visual impression than a reality, because the faster frequencies, if observable at the particular sensitivity, are usually seen superimposed on the delta waves. The major value of reducing the delta activity is that it allows an increase in the sensitivity to a level that would be impossible without simultaneous attenuation of the delta waves. The mechanism of this effect is relatively simple, in that slower frequencies tend to be of higher voltage than faster frequencies. As a general rule, an

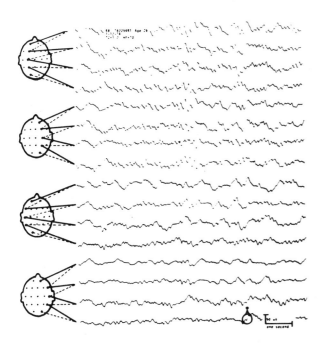

Figure 7.19. With the use of a time constant representing a low linear frequency of 0.1, there is very slow delta activity on the left anterior temporal midtemporal region, much more persistent than that observed in a comparable area on the right.

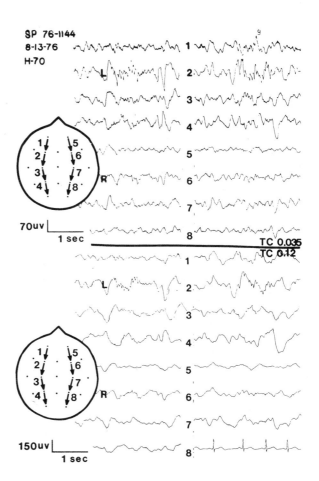

Figure 7.20. The *bottom portion* of the illustration is at S-15. Bilateral slow activity can be observed with some asymmetry, but the difference in the fast frequencies is only suggested. In the *upper portion* of the illustration, amplification was doubled after the removal of the delta components. The sleep spindles are quite visible and well defined, and the asymmetry is evident.

individual will demonstrate the lowest voltage for beta activity, somewhat higher voltage for alpha waves if they are present, higher voltages still for theta activity, and the highest voltage for delta waves. In some illnesses this sequence may be modified, but usually modification occurs only with relatively serious involvement; in the typical situation, the typical relationships are preserved. Because delta waves are generally of highest voltage, these peaks are likely to push the amplifier to its limit and require the use of a lower sensitivity. In Fig. 7.20, the sensitivity is 15 in the lower figure; the sleep spindles superimposed on the delta activity are visible but of quite low voltage, and their morphology is difficult to discern. The time constant was reduced to the low linear 5 setting, which means a time constant of 0.03 second. It was possible to increase the sensitivity to 7 μV/mm, which was not practical with the longer time constant. Now the hemispheric asymmetry and loss of spindles on the right compared to the left are more appreciable. An attempt to use sensitivity 7 without having reduced the time constant most likely would have resulted in amplifier and pen blocking and a barely readable record.

Sensitivity

The technologist has the ability to modify amplification in all channels of the EEG machine. Such changes can be different in each channel if this proves advisable, but this must be done with great caution.

Most EEG machines are linear, in that a specified number of microvolts deflects the pen 1 mm up to the point where the pen and/or the amplifier has reached its limit. Some older machines have compression amplifiers in which the sensitivity, in essence, decreases as the pen moves. The first millimeter from baseline might require 7 μV of electrical potential, but to move the pen from the 10th to the 11th mm from baseline might require 50 μV/mm. The virtue of this latter type of amplification is that there is less need for intervention by the technologist, and the pens are less likely to block even in the event of abrupt changes in voltage of EEG activity. The serious drawback of compression amplification is that clear and accurate measurement of each of the different types of activity is difficult.

There is no set guideline as to the amount of amplification desirable. Some electroencephalographers prefer to have sensitivity varied as little as possible. This lets one judge amplitude against a relatively constant baseline. Reading ability is limited by not using the full range of machine capability to display activity as clearly as possible. Another philosophy of amplification encourages the technologist to use the maximum amplification that can be employed at any time while avoiding consistent blocking of the pens or amplifiers and record distortion. Each change in sensitivity must be clearly and prominently marked on the EEG record so that the electroencephalographer can be aware of the voltage as the record continues. This latter approach allows for technically better recording of ongoing activity. The low-voltage record is further amplified; it becomes apparent whether or not the attenuation or low voltage involves all frequency bands or only the dominant frequency. Often the maneuver of increasing amplification can be critical in an asymmetrical record in determining whether the side with low voltage dominant activity is the better side in contrast to higher voltage slower frequencies or, in fact, is the more damaged side, because the loss of activity occurs in all bands and represents attenuation of voltage, as can commonly occur with vascular compromise and trauma.

The visual reader has the ability to see changes that involve a 0.5-mm deflection. Undoubtedly, there is individual variability, but the lower limit probably cannot be a greater visual sensitivity than 0.25 mm, because that is the width of the line drawn by an ink pen. If one assumes these estimates are reasonably accurate, a recording with a sensitivity of 7 μV/mm allows the reader to see changes of 3.5 μV when they occur, but not below that. Certainly, the reader of such a record would not see changes at the level of 1.75 μV, which is represented by only a 0.25-mm deflection. If this is kept in mind, the crucial importance of adequate sensitivity in particular circumstances, such as the recording of electrocerebral inactivity, becomes evident. The guidelines for minimal technical standards of EEG recording in suspected cerebral death (American EEG Society, 1994c) note that electrocerebral inactivity is defined as no activity over 2 μV. To have any chance to see 2-μV activity, the reader must have a sensitivity of 4 μV/mm. To display this activity, not just at the visual limit, but well above, would require a sensitivity of at least 2 μV/mm to make such change a readable 1 mm deflection. Present-day machines allow recordings of 1 μV/mm and 0.5 μV/mm sensitivity. These machines have a noise level of 2 μV/mm, but these are peak-to-peak extreme deflections. It is possible with experience to separate electrical noise from brain activity at levels of 1 and 1.5 μV. The argument is made that maximum amplification amplifies noise; this is quite correct. Discrimination between 1 μV noise and 1 μV cortical electrical activity is difficult but, at less than 2 μV/mm sensitivity, a distinction simply cannot be made. Increased sensitivity permits visualization of the activity but does not simplify the decision (Bennett et al., 1976). Some investigators contend that cortical activity at such low levels does not occur (Weiss et al., 1975), but there is reason to suspect that these lower levels of EEG activity have validity in determining ongoing brain function at the cortical level (Reilly et al., 1974, 1978, 1980).

Sensitivity, amplitude, voltage, deflection, and gain are all terms used as parameters with relationships that allow interchange if two of the three major features are known. The most useful formula is that voltage equals the pen deflection times the sensitivity ($V = D \times S$). One can calculate sensitivity (S), deflection (D), or voltage (V) if the other two are known. In every record, during calibration and patient recording, these relationships are used at least indirectly.

Sensitivity is defined as a ratio of input voltage to output pen deflection in an EEG channel (Chatrian et al., 1974). It is described as microvolts per millimeter (μV/mm). *Gain* is an older term and is the ratio of output signal voltage compared to input signal voltage (Chatrian et al., 1974). It is a multiplication factor. This is usable information in clinical EEG when instrument deflection can be converted to voltage. If input and output voltage are known, sensitivity can be determined. Voltage is the electric potential or potential difference between two points or, in EEG, between two electrodes. In EEG it is expressed in microvolts. *Deflection* is the vertical distance between two points, and the *amplitude* of a wave is the voltage of a wave measured peak to peak (Chatrian et al., 1974). Amplitude and voltage are essentially synonymous when indicated in measurements such as microvolts, but both are derived from deflection. The amplitude of a wave is sometimes described in millimeters, but this is incorrect even if commonly done. Amplitude is not the millimeter height of the wave but is the potential voltage that caused the pen to deflect that much. The relation established is that the amplitude is calculated by measuring the deflection, but it is not, in itself, deflection.

Use of Paper Drive Controls

An electroencephalograph displays patterns in a manner that becomes familiar to readers. The display can provide essentially the same information at a range of paper speeds, but the ease with which one makes determinations about the activity visually varies greatly depending on the paper speed used. Slow paper speed, such as 15 mm/sec, allows for economy of paper and economy of time in reviewing the record. This can be valuable if the activity recorded is carried out over a great length of time, as in surgery or sleep studies. Concentration of activity in a relatively small space may be quite adequate if the only changes of importance are activities that stand out from the ongoing activity because of some characteristic of the waveform. Very slow paper speed can be used to monitor repetitive episodes of high-voltage spike-and-wave discharge. Similarly, sudden drops in voltage, such as periods of attenuation or marked change in the frequency, may be evident at slow paper speeds.

Clinical laboratories in the United States and many other countries traditionally use a speed of 30 mm/sec. Clinical EEG machines are generally capable of running at half and twice this paper speed. A much wider range of frequencies is available for research machines. For some research applications, 25 mm/sec is as much of a standard as 30 mm/sec is for clinical use. This is particularly true with polygraph studies.

Slower Paper Speed

The paper speed that in some countries is considered slow (15 mm/sec) has been the conventional paper speed in other countries, particularly France. Comfort with one conventional speed over the other is, to a great extent, a matter of training and experience. Concern with the morphology and definition of very fast components such as spikes or with minimal asymmetries in the onset of spike discharges leads one to view 15 mm/sec paper speed less favorably. Particular interest in some of the slower components and in periods of attenuation or rhythmicity over longer periods of time makes slower speeds attractive. They have been particularly popular for studies of premature infants and records of neonatal sleep activity.

Possible subtle asymmetries of slow activity have been enhanced by changing from 30 to 15 mm/sec (Fig. 7.21). This maneuver does not change the amplitude of the wave in question, but it does change the ratio of amplitude to width and allows the reader to visualize asymmetries of slow activity that otherwise might not have been defined as clearly.

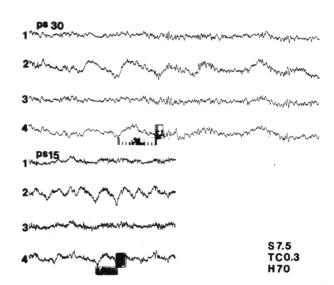

Figure 7.21. The *top four lines* show repetitive 1 cycle/sec delta activity. The *bottom four lines* show the same asymmetry; particularly in channel 2, the delta activity stands out and becomes more visible because of the change in its height/width ratio.

Faster Paper Speed

Increase in the paper speed will spread out various components. It is not infrequent for the technologist or reader to be concerned as to whether or not fast activity under observation is merely 60-cycle artifact or whether it represents muscle activity. The use of faster paper speed spreads fast frequencies out so that the metronome-like rhythmicity of 60-cycle artifact, versus the clear irregularity of the muscle activity defines the true origin.

Another important use of fast paper speed is the study of asymmetrical onset of seemingly synchronous activity. It is clinically important to distinguish secondary bilateral synchrony following onset from a lateralized focus from primary bilateral synchrony. When bilaterally synchronous epileptiform activity occurs, the onset may have hemispherical variation of 15 to 25 msec, but large (70–100 msec) differences suggest secondary bilateral synchrony (Tukel and Jasper, 1952).

Artifact

Artifacts fall into several major categories. The major class is machine and impedance artifact. The most common ones relate to problems with the electrode, such as the electrode itself being broken or improperly attached to the head. The next most common artifact in the machine category is the presence of 60-cycle artifact, either from nearby equipment or the very common ground loop. The latter often occurs when the patient has been grounded more than once and there is a difference between the grounds, causing 60-cycle artifact. Another source of 60-cycle artifact results when the ground electrode is shorted to one of the active electrodes. This is a particularly disconcerting artifact, in that the 60-cycle activity appears in many different channels. The chan-

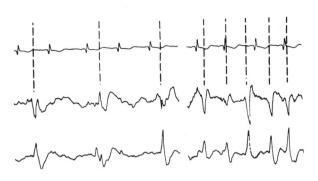

Figure 7.22. The *top line* represents the actual electrocardiogram (ECG), and the *bottom two lines* show relatively regular discharges that might be mistaken for repetitive EEG if the patient's own heart rate was not readily observable.

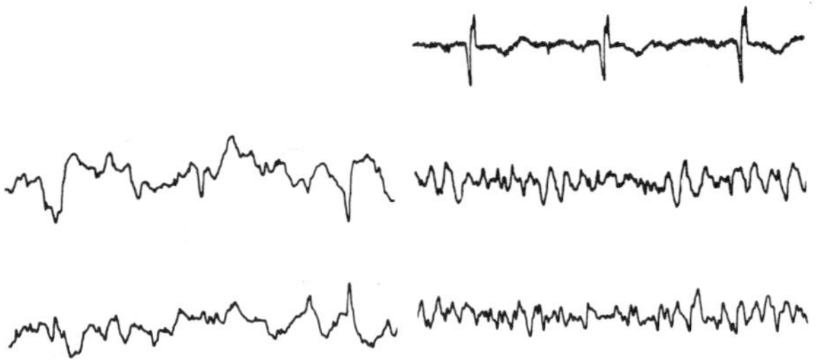

Figure 7.24. Cortical spike discharges have a great tendency to be sensitive to level of consciousness. The sharp activity on the left could have been cortical or occasional ECG complexes. Once the patient's level of consciousness is changed, as on the right, it is easy to make the discrimination, but the activity is no longer evident.

nels change from one montage to another. No matter how frequently one tries to correct individual scalp electrodes, the artifact continues. Testing the electrodes shows impedances that are adequate. It is only when the bridge between ground and scalp electrodes is removed and the area cleansed that the problem is eliminated.

The next major class of artifacts is physiological. There are a number of separate categories. The major and most common of the physiological artifacts are cardiac or oculographic in origin.

With cardiac artifacts, the most frequent and most troublesome is ECG artifact resulting from the QRS complex. This part of the ECG wave can have very rapid upward deflection resembling a sharp wave or spike in the EEG. The constant rhythm expected is not a sufficient discriminator (Fig. 7.22). The ECG complex is frequently intermittent even in a perfectly regular ECG; a particular ORS complex will be observed, then several complexes will be missed, and then another complex will be visible. This intermittent presentation complicates the distinction between ECG artifact and spikes. It is crucial to have an ECG monitor applied to every patient. A wrist lead is not necessary, and an EEG electrode on the shoulder referenced to the ear is adequate. If the monitor is attached, it can be initiated without changing the level of consciousness of the patient (Fig. 7.23). If it has to be added at the time the question arises, the addition

of the monitor may change the level of consciousness of the patient, and the questionable activity may no longer be present (Fig. 7.24). It remains uncertain whether the activity was ECG artifact or the arousal resulting in loss of the spike discharges.

Another cardiac-related artifact is pulsation artifact. This results from the blood pulsing through a vessel under an electrode. Recording ECG will demonstrate that this is time-locked to the pulsation artifact, which presents as a rhythmic slow wave. Touching the appropriate electrode demonstrates a pulsation. Slight movement of the electrode in whatever direction necessary to move it off the pulsating vessel is sufficient to eliminate the artifact. It is desirable to actually move this electrode; the artifact should not be allowed to continue through the record just because it is identified as pulsation artifact.

A less common cardiac-related artifact is the ballistocardiographic artifact, provoked by the rocking movement of the patient's entire body each time the heart beats. It is not due either to the ECG itself or to the blood vessel pulsation, but to actual movement of the head and body. This artifact is identified as time-locked to the heart by use of the ECG monitor. It can be eliminated by moving the patient's head or by putting a pillow under the patient's neck so that electrode movement against the bed is minimized.

Eye movement artifact is of most concern but easiest to document when it develops from vertical eye movement, in which it appears anteriorly and suggests the possibility of bilaterally synchronous delta waves. Proof of this type of eye movement artifact requires minimum expenditure of the technologist's time. Electrodes are placed under the center of the eye. (If the patient is looking straight ahead, the electrodes are under the pupil.) Referencing the frontal polar electrode to the ear and, in the next channel, referencing the ipsilateral under-eye lead to the ear will demonstrate in-phase waves between the two channels if the activity is coming from the frontal lobe (Fig. 7.25). Cortical activity has the same phase both above and below the eye. This montage will demonstrate out-of-phase waves if there is eye movement in the vertical plane (Matsuo et al., 1975). Outward phase reversal occurs, because the eye is a relative dipole with the anterior part (cornea) more positive than the poste-

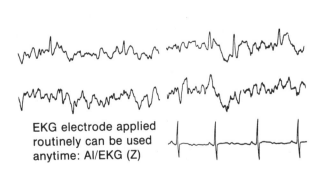

EKG electrode applied
routinely can be used
anytime: Al/EKG (Z)

Figure 7.23. On the *left*, two channels of EEG are seen with sharp waves that may be cardiac in origin. Addition of an ECG on the *right* demonstrates that this is not the case.

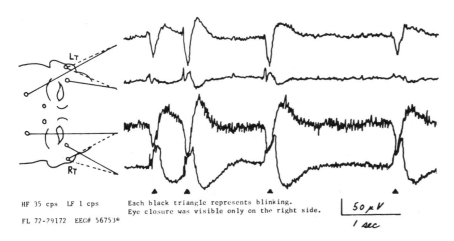

Figure 7.25. Simultaneous reference recording from above and below the eye gives out-of-phase responses to eye blink, but the synchronous delta activity of cortical origin would be in phase.

HF 35 cps   LF 1 cps

FL 72-79172   EEG# 56753*

Each black triangle represents blinking. Eye closure was visible only on the right side.

50 μV

1 sec

rior (retinal) portion, which is negative. With vertical movement, the cornea must move between the frontal polar electrode above the eye and the electrode below the eye. The electrode getting closer to the cornea becomes relatively positive; the electrode the cornea is moving away from becomes relatively negative. These electrodes are both input electrodes in their respective channels, and a phase reversal occurs.

In other instances, it is useful to record all eye movements. This requires electrode combinations that record lateral as well as vertical eye movements. One of the simplest methods of recording all eye movements is to connect an electrode at the lateral canthus of an eye to the frontal polar electrode ipsilateral to that eye. In the next channel, record from the other frontal polar electrode to the lateral canthus of the second eye. This montage does not distinguish between cortical activity and eye movement, but picks up eye movement deflections in any and all directions.

Troubleshooting

Identification and elimination of difficulties in a record relates to elements of recording discussed earlier in this section. Artifacts frequently are identifiable because of high voltage that is sufficient to cause the amplifiers to reach their limits and because they are frequently limited to a single electrode. Sudden voltage change with an almost instantaneous change from baseline to full voltage is uncharacteristic of true brain activity and alerts the reader to artifactual origin, but not the specific type of artifact occurring.

Troubleshooting requires consideration of the most common possibilities. It then involves a sequence of steps to eliminate the probable or possible causes. Because electrode application and electrode movement are the most common problems in EEG recording, the first step in eliminating a possible artifact is to check electrode impedance with the electrode test or lead imbalance features of the EEG machine. If there is high impedance, it is apparent that an electrode needs to be fixed. If there is not high impedance, it is possible that an intact electrode is making contact with the patient's pillow or is being touched or rubbed. Readjustment of the patient's position either by turning the head or placing

a pillow or towel roll under the patient's neck to lift *all* the electrodes into the air may become necessary. Sometimes it is necessary to move the jack box into which the electrodes are plugged. Simply moving the electrode cables as they go from the jack box to the patient's head can help. Touching the electrodes and verifying that they are attached tightly to the scalp is a valuable measure.

Computed Topographic Mapping and Analysis

The proliferation of recording systems that allow computation and display of electrophysiological activity in a display that uses the recorded activity to calculate and display the activity or its analyzed components continuously *between* the few points of actual data recorded has greatly increased the need for attention to almost all of the technical points related to records, including the number and consistent replacement of electrodes (Duffy et al., 1994).

Some of the procedures that at times are considered part of quantitative EEG are being used in more detailed analysis of the standard EEG activity. In some of these approaches to the standard EEG detection may include automated spike detection, using a dipole localization for artifact rejection (Flanagan et al., 2003), or multistage approach for automatic detection of epileptiform EEG (Liu et al., 2002).

Concluding Remarks

In recent years, there has been a tendency in some circles to devote more attention to the apparatus than to the actual operation of the machine and the recording of an EEG record or the evoked potential. As long as unpredictable episodic events continue to play a major role in the patient population generally seen in a clinical neurophysiology laboratory, it will remain necessary for attention to be given to the recording climate and to the skills of the people operating the machinery. This chapter presented a number of variations that cannot be incorporated into a standard record, but can be incorporated into the repertoire of the technologist recording the EEG, evoked potential, or operative record. If technologists are to become familiar with these various techniques and be able to use them in urgent situations, they must be given a degree of flexibility in recording so that they can try out these variations. The technologist, therefore, needs to be given latitude in routine situations and encouraged to try out different variations so that these tools can be used when a critical need arises.

If electrode integrity seems good, one is faced with the possibility that the artifact may in fact be related to the machine. It may be necessary to dial the same electrode combination into two amplifiers to see if they appear the same. Both amplifiers will show the artifact if it is from the electrode and/or jack box. If the waveform in the two channels differs, something is wrong with the amplifier. When an amplifier is seemingly disturbed, the settings of the sensitivity and filters in the individual amplifier should be reviewed. This is a common problem when, for some reason, two individual settings of an amplifier have been modified, making the response of the amplifier to the master control inoperative. Failure to return control to the master selector after a specific use is a common error.

References

Adrian, E.D., and Matthews, B.H.C. 1934. The interpretation of potential waves in cortex. J. Physiol. 81:440–471.

Adrian, E.D., and Yamagiwa, K. 1935. The origin of the Berger rhythm. Brain 58:323–351.

American EEG Society. 1994a. Guidelines (#1) in EEG. J. Clin. Neurophysiol. 11:2–5.

American EEG Society. 1994b. Guidelines (#2) in EEG. J. Clin. Neurophysiol. 11:6–9.

American EEG Society. 1994c. Guidelines (#3) in EEG. J. Clin. Neurophysiol. 11:10–13.

American EEG Society. 1994d. Guidelines (#7) in EEG. J. Clin. Neurophysiol. 11:30–36.

American EEG Society. 1994e. Guidelines (#13) in EEG. J. Clin. Neurophysiol. 11:111–113.

American Medical EEG Association. 1990. Electroencephalography Standards.

Barlogie, B., Corry, P.M., Yip, E., et al. 1979. Total-body hyperthermia with and without chemotherapy for advanced neoplasms. Cancer Res. 39:1481–1489.

Barrett, G., Blumhardt, L., Halliday, A.M., et al. 1976. A paradox in the lateralization of the visual evoked response. Nature 261:253–255.

Bennett, D.R., Hughes, J.R., Korein, J., et al. 1976. *An Atlas of EEG in Coma and Cerebral Death.* New York: Raven Press.

Berger, H., 1929. On the electroencephalogram of man. Arch. Psychiatr. Nervenkrankheiten. 87:527–570.

Binnie, C.D., and Lloyd, D.S.L. 1970. Letters to the editors. Common reference methods of derivation (response), Ed. J.W. Osseltron. Am. J. EEG Technol. 10:69–77.

Binnie, C.D., Dekker, E., Smit, A., et al. 1982. Practical consideration in the positioning of EEG electrodes. Electroencephalogr. Clin. Neurophysiol. 50:282–292.

Busse, E.W., and Obrist, W.D. 1965. Presenescent electroencephalographic changes in normal subjects. Gerontology 10:315–320.

Calloway, E., Tueting, P., and Coslow, S.H. 1978. *Event-Related Brain Potentials in Man.* New York: Academic Press.

Chatrian, G.E., Bergamini, L., Dondey, M., et al. 1974. A glossary of terms most commonly used by clinical electroencephalographers. Int. Fed. Soc. Electroencephalogr. Clin. Neurophysiol. 37:538–547.

Clement, R.A., Flanagan, J.G., and Harding, G.F. 1985. Source derivation of the visual evoked response to patten reversal stimulation. Electroencephalogr. Clin. Neurophysiol. 1:74–76.

Cracco, R.Q., and Cracco, J.B. 1976. Somatosensory evoked potential in man: far field potentials. Electroencephalogr. Clin. Neurophysiol. 41:460–466.

Drachman, D.A., and Hughes, J.R. 1971. Memory and hippocampal complexes. III. Aging and temporal EEG abnormalities. Neurology 2:1–14.

Duffy, F.H., Hughes, J.R., Miranda, F., et al. 1994. Status of quantitative EEG (QEEG) in clinical practice. Position Paper of the American Medical EEG Association on QEEG. Clin. Electroencephalogr. 25:VI–XXII.

Flanagan, D., Agarwal, R., Wang, Y.H., et al. 2003. Improvement in the performance of automated spike detection using dipole source features for artefact rejection. Electroencephalogr. Clin. Neurophysiol. 114(1): 38–49.

Garvin, J.S., and Gibbs, E.L. 1971. Focal frontal slow activity with physiological reversal of electrical sign in the occipital areas. Clin. Electroencephalogr. 2:218–223.

Gibbs, E.L., and Gibbs, T.J. 1984. Universal APEEGE (anatomical placement of EEG electrodes) system. Clin. EEG 15:1–21.

Gibbs, F.A., and Gibbs, E.L. 1952. *Atlas of Electroencephalography. Vol. 2, Methodology and Controls.* Reading, MA: Addison-Wesley.

Gibbs, F.A., and Gibbs, E.L. 1964. Exclusive monopolar recordings. Am. J. EEG Technol. 4:8–9.

Goldman, D. 1949. The use of a new type of "indifferent" electrode. Electroencephalogr. Clin. Neurophysiol. 1:523.

Gordon, M.R. 1980. Artifacts created by imbalanced electrode impedance. Am. J. EEG Technol. 20:149–160.

Halliday, A.M. 1978. Evoked potentials in neurological disorders. In *Event-related Brain Potentials in Man,* Eds. E. Calloway, P. Tueting, and S.H. Coslow, pp. 197–210. New York: Academic Press.

Harner, R.N. 1977. A recommendation for standard EEG montages. Am. J. EEG Technol. 17:105–114.

Hjorth, B. 1975. Technical contribution. An on-line transformation of EEG scalp potentials into orthogonal source derivations. Electroencephalogr. Clin. Neurophysiol. 39:526–530.

Hjorth, B. 1976. Localization of foci in the scalp field. In *Quantitiative Analytic Studies in Epilepsy,* Eds. P. Kellaway and I. Petersen. New York: Raven Press.

Hjorth, B. 1979. Multichannel EEG preprocessing. Analogue matrix operations in the study of local effects. Pharmakopsychiatr. Neuro-Psychopharmakol. 12:111–118.

Ishiyama, Y., Ebe, M., Homma, I., et al. 1982. Elimination of EGK artifacts from EEGs recorded with balanced noncephalic reference electrode method. Electroencephalogr. Clin. Neurophysiol. 53:662–665.

Jasper, H. 1958. Report of committee on methods of clinical exam in EEG. Electroencephalogr. Clin. Neurophysiol. 10:370–375.

Kaufman, H.H., Reilly, E.L., Porecha, H.P., et al. 1977. Cerebral ischemia during carotid endarterectomy with severe but reversible changes. Surg. Neurol. 7:195–198.

Kooi, K.A., Guevener, A.M., Tupper, J.C., et al. 1964. Electroencephalographic patterns of the temporal region in normal adults. Neurology 14:1029–1035.

Lehmann, D., Ozaki, H., and Pal, I. 1986. Averaging of spectral power and phase via vector diagram best fits without reference electrode or reference channel. Electroencephalogr. Clin. Neurophysiol. 64:350–363.

Liu, H.S., Zhang, T., and Yang, F.S. 2003. A multistage, multimethod approach for automatic detection and classification of epileptiform EEG. Electroencephalogr. IEEE Trans. Biomed. Eng. 49(12 patient 2):1557–1566.

Matsuo, F., Peters, J.F., and Reilly, E.L. 1975. Electrical phenomena associated with movements of the eyelid. Electroencephalogr. Clin. Neurophysiol. 38:507–511.

Morgan, P. 1968. Recording the temporal region spike. Am. J. EEG Technol. 8:7–22.

Myslobodsky, M.S., and Bar-Ziv, J. 1989. Location of occipital EEG electrodes verified by computer tomography. Electroencephalogr. Clin. Neurophysiol. 72:363–366.

Myslobodsky, M.S., Coppota, R., Bar-Ziv, J., et al. 1990. Adequacy of the International 10–20 electrode system for computed neurophysiologic topography. J. Clin. Neurophysiol. 7:507–518.

Obrist, W.P., and Busse, E.W. 1965. Application of electroencephalography in psychiatry. In *The Electroencephalogram in Old Age,* Ed. W. P. Wilson, pp. 185–205. Durham, NC: Duke University Press.

Obrist, W.P., and Henry, C.E. 1958. Electroencephalographic frequency analysis of aged psychiatric patients. Electroencephalogr. Clin. Neurophysiol. 10:621–632.

Presbitero, J.V., Ruiz, R.S., Rigor, B.M., Sr., et al. 1980. Intraocular pressure during influence and neuroplet anesthesia in adult patients undergoing ophthalmic surgery. Anesth. Analg. 59:50–54.

Reilly, E.L., and Seward, M.A. 1980. Reversal of electrical sign in the occipital area: physiological or montage artifact. Clin. Electroencephalogr. 11:57–66.

Reilly, E.L., Brumberg, J.A., and Doty, D.B. 1974. The effect of deep hypothermia and total circulatory arrest on the electroencephalogram in children. Electroencephalogr. Clin. Neurophysiol. 26:661–667.

Reilly, E.L., Kondo, C., Brunberg, J.A., et al. 1978. Visual evoked potentials during hypothermia and prolonged circulatory arrest. Electroencephalogr. Clin. Neurophysiol. 45:100–106.

Reilly, E.L., Barlogie, B., Seward, M.A., et al. 1980. Persistence of EEG activity with prolonged induced hyperthermic fever. Clin. Electroencephalogr. 11:22–27.

Seaba, P. 1985. *The Importance of Electrode Impedance. The Oxford Observer.* Clearwater, FL: Oxford Medilog. Inc.

Seaba, P., Reilly, E.L., and Peters, J.F. 1973. Patient discomfort related to measurement of electrode resistance. Am. J. EEG Technol. 13:7–12.

Silverman, A.J., Busse, E.W., and Barnes, R.H. 1955. Studies in the process of aging. Electroencephalographic findings in 400 elderly subjects. Electroencephalogr. Clin. Neurophysiol. 7:67–74.

Sorel, L., and Ranwez, R. 1984. Basis and use of a true monopolar derivation: the neo-electroencephalography (NEEG) Clin. Electroencephalogr. 2:71–82.

Stephenson, W., and Gibbs, F.A. 1949. Electroencephalograms recorded with non-cephalic electrodes as a reference. Electroencephalogr. Clin. Neurophysiol. 1:523.

Stockard, J.E., Stockard, J.J., Westmoreland, B.F., et al. 1979. Brainstem auditory-evoked responses. Arch. Neurol. 36:823–831.

Thickbroom, G.W., Mastaglia, F.L., Carroll, W.M., et al. 1984. Source derivation: application to topographic mapping of visual evoked potentials. Electroencephalogr. Clin. Neurophysiol. 59:279–285.

Tukel, K., and Jasper, H.H. 1952. The electroencephalogram in parasagittal lesions. Electroencephalogr. Clin. Neurophysiol. 4:481–494.

Wallin, G., and Stalberg, E. 1980. Source derivation in clinical routine EEG. Electroencephalogr. Clin. Neurophysiol. 50:282–292.

Weiss, M., Weiss, J., Cotton, J., et al. 1975. A study of the electroencephalogram during surgery with deep hypothermia and circulatory arrest in infants. J. Thorac. Cardiovasc. Surg. 70:316–329.

Yoshii, N. 1971. Electroencephalographic observation of apparently normal aged subjects. Tohoku J. Exp. Med. 103:202–215.

Yoshii, N., To, T.W., Murase, I., et al. 1966. A comparative study of average reference and routine monopolar ear lobe reference electrodes in EEG recording. Keio J. Med. 15:219–226.

8. The EEG Signal: Polarity and Field Determination

Ernst Niedermeyer

Every deflection of the electroencephalography (EEG) writing system indicates a change of voltage as well as a fluctuation of polarity, i.e., from negative to positive or vice versa. This raises the question of the nature of electrical positivity and negativity.

Positivity and negativity are seemingly confusing terms. Benjamin Franklin used these notions and based them on simple observations. When he rubbed a glass rod on silk, the glass was charged with one type of electricity; when he rubbed a stick of sealing wax on a cat's back, the sealing wax was charged with another type (Upton, 1960). It was then found that one kind of electricity would attract a pith ball and the other kind would repel it. This led to the rule that like charges of electricity repel each other, whereas unlike charges attract each other. Franklin also inferred that electric current flows from positive (+) to negative (−).

The basic rules of electrostatic induction (the basis of the aforementioned attraction and repulsion of charged objects) cannot explain the basic mechanisms of electricity. Insights into atomic structures have taught us that electricity consists of negatively charged particles called electrons. An electric current flows from an area of greater availability of electrons to an area of lesser availability of electrons. This latter area is then called positive because it contains a comparatively smaller amount of negatively charged electrons.

This principle of current flow is generally accepted in electrophysiological circles but stands in contrast to the view of electrotechnology in general (according to which current flows from positivity to negativity).

The assumption of two kinds of electricity was a fallacy. The question of negativity versus positivity is not a question of contrast, such as red versus green, or of different qualities; it is rather a question of quantity, of more versus less, of greater versus lesser availability of negatively charged electrons.

Constant changes of electron availability determine the pen movements of the EEG apparatus. As long as the EEG is composed of sinusoidal waves, the question of polarity (i.e., negativity versus positivity) is almost irrelevant. It usually suffices to determine the phase relationship (in phase versus out of phase) of such potentials over a given area.

Stretches of rhythmical EEG activity do not necessarily show sinusoidal character; one portion of each wave may be rounded and the other one sharp, as is the case in rolandic mu rhythm. Even more important is the polarity determination of single events, such as spikes or sharp waves. Such signals usually spread and form a field that can be plotted with appropriate EEG montages.

Pen Deflections and Polarity

The question of polarity and pen deflection has been discussed only sparingly in the comprehensive texts of EEG technology or clinical EEG. An excellent account of this subject has been given by Binnie et al. (1974) in their joint contribution to the *Handbook of Electroencephalography and Clinical Neurophysiology.* Earlier work in this field was done by Brazier (1949a,b), Magnus (1961), and, especially, Knott (1969), who has placed particular emphasis on correct interpretation of signal polarity. Niedermeyer (1978) discussed this problem following the principles laid down by Knott (1961, 1969). Richey and Namon (1976), Maulsby (1979), Tyner et al. (1983), Lesser et al. (1985), and Knott (1985) have also presented thorough discussions of this subject.

The formerly held concept that an upward pen deflection denoted negativity and a downward deflection denoted positivity is erroneous. This view ought to be laid to rest forever, because it ignores the complexity of a differential amplifier, with a dual input. There used to be input grids in vacuum tubes (hence the terms *grid 1* and *grid 2*), but modern transistors have a corresponding component called "base." We will refer to the dual input as "input 1" and "input 2."

Figure 8.1 shows inputs 1 and 2 of one given EEG channel. It shows on the left large clusters of negative charges at input 1 and a much smaller amount of negative charges at input 2; by comparison, input 2 is positive at this moment. Conversely, there is on the right a large negative charge at input 2 and a much smaller negative charge at input 1; this momentarily renders input 1 positive when compared with input 2.

The pen deflections in each of these circumstances are shown, and the rules of polarity can be readily derived:

Negativity of input 1: upward deflection.
Positivity of input 1: downward deflection.
Negativity of input 2: downward deflection.
Positivity of input 2: upward deflection.

To memorize this fundamental rule, it can be formulated as follows: negativity up, positivity down; correct for input 1, but input 2 reverses it!

Every commercially available EEG apparatus has been built according to this rule. However, there are some deviations from this rule in a number of apparatuses for computer-averaged evoked responses; some of these computer write-outs show upward deflections with positivity of input 1. This may be convenient in the case of the visual evoked response and its towering P 100 peak (positive and up), but

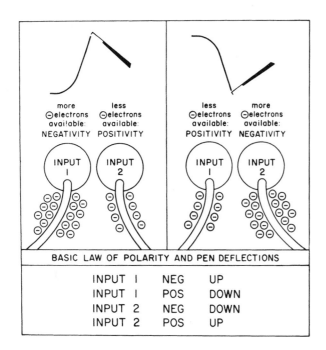

Figure 8.1. Inputs 1 and 2 of an EEG channel in schematic view.

it sadly reflects the lack of agreement among the branches of clinical electrophysiology.

The rules of polarity clearly indicate that a selected input for a certain channel (such as F_3–C_3) cannot be used inversely (C_3–F_3) without more or less confusing changes in a given montage. When F_3–C_3 is selected, the input from F_3 is connected with input 1 of the channel and C_3 is connected with input 2.

Examples of Signal Polarity and Field Analysis

Figure 8.2A shows a negative signal over C_4. This area alone is involved. In the second channel from the top (F_4–C_4), C_4 is connected with input 2; in the third channel from the top (C_4–P_4), it is connected with input 1. For this reason, channel 2 shows a downward deflection (negativity of input 2: down) and channel 3 shows an upward deflection

(negativity of input 1: up). This is a typical example of phase reversal in a bipolar montage.

In Fig. 8.2B, there is again a negative signal over C_4 with the same type of phase reversal, but F_4 and P_4 are also involved. In channel 1 (Fp_2–F_4), the pen goes down because of input 2 negativity. In channel 3 (P_4–O_2), the pen goes up because of input 1 negativity.

Figure 8.2C shows an example of a positive signal in C_4. In channel 2 (F_4–C_4), the pen moves up because of input 2 positivity and, in channel 3 (C_4–P_4), the pen moves down due to input 1 positivity. Figure 8.2D shows a positive signal over C_4 with spread into F_4 and P_4. In channel 1, F_4 is connected with input 2 and positivity causes an upward deflection; in channel 4, P_4 is connected with input 1, and positivity makes the pen move downward.

Figure 8.3 demonstrates more complicated examples of focal signals and their field distribution. In Fig. 8.3A, we are dealing with a negative signal in C_4 with spread into F_4 and P_4. The situation is almost the same as in Fig. 8.2B. Note, however, the differences of signal size. The small downward deflection in channel 2 shows that C_4 is only slightly more negative than F_4, while the gradient of negativity is much steeper between C_4 and P_4 (channel 3). From F_4, the gradient falls steeply to Fp_2, while the fall from P_4 and O_4 is not quite as steep, according to the size of the signal. The gradients can also be shown as slopes.

In Fig. 8.3B, there is a negative phase reversal between channels 1 and 3, whereas channel 2 shows equipotentiality. This means that two equally strong signals of the same polarity cancel out in this channel, because EEG signals are based on voltage differences and there is no difference in this case. In other words, the negative signal arises from a broad focus that comprises F_4 and C_4. The gradient falls from C_4 to P_4 (and eventually from P_4 to O_2). The focus is a "flat top" over F_4 and C_4, but an electrode interspersed between F_4 and C_4 might indicate the real focus.

In Fig. 8.3C, the flat top is further extended. Equipotentiality in channels 2 and 3 indicates that F_4, C_4, and P_4 represent the focus of the signal; the gradient falls toward Fp_2 and O_2.

Figure 8.3D shows a positive signal over C_4 with the typical positive phase reversal. The gradient falls gently to P_2 and a bit more steeply to F_4; there are steep gradients from F_4 to Fp_2 and from P_4 and O_2. Figure 8.3E shows a positive signal with a maximum in F_4 and C_4 and hence equipoten-

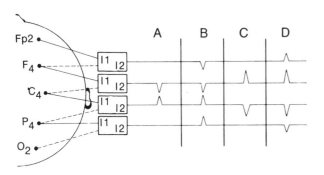

Figure 8.2. *I1*, input 1; *I2*, input 2.

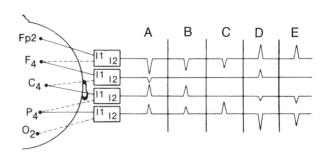

Figure 8.3. *I1*, input 1; *I2*, input 2. (From Niedermeyer, E. 1978. EEG Potentiale und Polarität. Die Bedeutung der Schreiberbewegungen in Hinblick auf Negativität und Positivität. *J. Electrophysiol. Tech.* 3:190–198.)

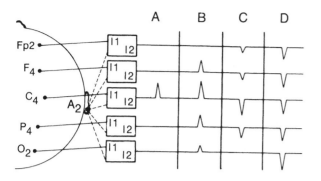

Figure 8.4. *I1*, input 1; *I2*, input 2.

tiality in channel 2. There is spread into Fp$_2$ as well as into P$_4$ and O$_2$.

Referential (unipolar) recording poses greater difficulties in the signal analysis; however, in most (but not all) cases, the peak area of the signal and its field distribution are interpretable. Figure 8.4A is suggestive of a negative signal in C$_4$, but other far-fetched explanations are also possible. Figure 8.4B shows a negative signal over C$_4$ with spread into F$_4$, P$_4$, and, to a very minor degree, O$_2$. In referential recordings, the size of the signal is of paramount significance; on the other hand, the interelectrode distance to the reference electrode must also be taken into account. Phase reversals materialize only when the reference (the ear in this case) itself is affected by the signal.

In Fig. 8.4C, a positive signal over C$_4$ with spread into F$_4$, P$_4$, and Fp$_2$ is the most plausible explanation, but there are also other possibilities, such as a negative signal in the ear electrode and strong involvement of O$_2$ (equipotentiality O$_2$–A$_2$). In Fig. 8.4D, a negative potential in the ear electrode A$_2$ is the most likely explanation, but no definite statement can be made in this case. There is no doubt that bipolar montages permit a better analysis of signal field distribution than do referential montages.

Figure 8.5 uses a temporal longitudinal montage in referential recording technique. Such a montage is more likely to show participation of the ear lead because of the vicinity of the temporal lobe. In Fig. 8.5A, a negative signal is most impressive in F$_8$. There is spread into Fp$_2$ and T$_4$. Interestingly,

T$_4$ could be more involved than Fp$_2$ despite the smaller signal deflection; the vicinity of T$_4$ to A$_2$ (hence a small interelectrode distance) must be considered. There is also slight spread into T$_6$.

Figure 8.5B looks confusing; every phase reversal in a referential array is indeed confusing. The plausible explanation is a negative signal in F$_8$ with spread into T$_4$, which is slightly more negative than A$_2$. Further spread goes into A$_2$, which also becomes negative. For this reason, A$_2$ is negative compared with Fp$_2$, T$_6$, and O$_2$; the input 2 negativity is particularly large in channel 4 (O$_2$–A$_2$) because of the large interelectrode distance. The possibility of slight involvement of Fp$_2$ cannot be ruled out.

Figure 8.5C shows almost the same situation, with a maximal negative signal in F$_8$. This time, however, there is an equal degree of spread into T$_4$ and A$_2$; this explains equipotentiality between these two electrodes (channel 3).

Further Comments

The foci shown in Figs. 8.2 through 8.5 are not necessarily the real foci. It is possible that a stronger signal in an electrode outside the small number of leads here demonstrated could be the real focus. To be more specific, a temporal longitudinal montage may show a signal with negative phase reversal in T$_4$. A parasagittal longitudinal montage may subsequently show a phase reversal in C$_4$. This indicates that T$_4$ and C$_4$ must be compared with each other. This is best done with a transversal (coronal) run, such as A$_1$–T$_3$, T$_3$–C$_3$, C$_3$–C$_z$, C$_z$–C$_4$, C$_4$–T$_4$, T$_4$–A$_2$. Presently, 16 or more channels are widely used and, with such apparatus, one montage often clarifies the issue.

Signal Polarity and the "Neoelectroencephalogram"

Comprehension of the principles of polarity facilitates the understanding of the method of "neoelectroencephalography" (Sorel and Ranwez, 1984). This method attempts to demonstrate "true monopolar derivations" with the use of a neck reference electrode. Phase angles and phase shifts are determined by means of a minicomputer. In fact, however, this interesting method is not revolutionary enough to warrant the prefix "neo."

The Dipole Concept and Polarity

The origin of EEG patterns has been thought to consist of numerous cerebral areas with opposite electrical poles that constantly fluctuate. This concept can be traced back to the work of Brazier (1949a,b); it will be discussed in greater detail in sections dealing with the origin of EEG potentials. More information can be derived from the work of Kooi (1971), Gloor (1971), Richey and Namon (1976), Maulsby (1979), and especially from the studies of Nunez (1981), and Gloor (1985).

The International Federation of Societies for Electroencephalography and Clinical Neurophysiology (IFSECN) published a glossary of EEG terms (Chatrian et al., 1974) in which a distinction is made between "instrumental phase reversal" and "true phase reversal." In this chapter, the term

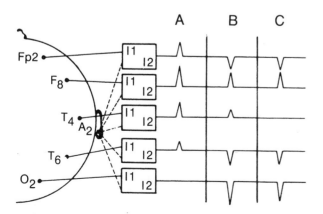

Figure 8.5. *I1*, input 1; *I2*, input 2.

Figure 8.6. Sleep tracing in a 7-month-old girl. The overall impression of the record was within normal limits of variability for age. The principal feature of this illustration is a train of sleep spindles with a sharp component that is normal at this age. In C_3, C_4, P_3, and P_4, the sharp component is negative. In Fp_1, Fp_2, F_7, F_8, F_3, and F_4, the sharp component is positive. The possibility of a large true dipole is worth discussion, although no convincing evidence can be provided for this hypothesis. Furthermore, the anterior spindle train with the positive sharp component lags somewhat behind the posterior spindles.

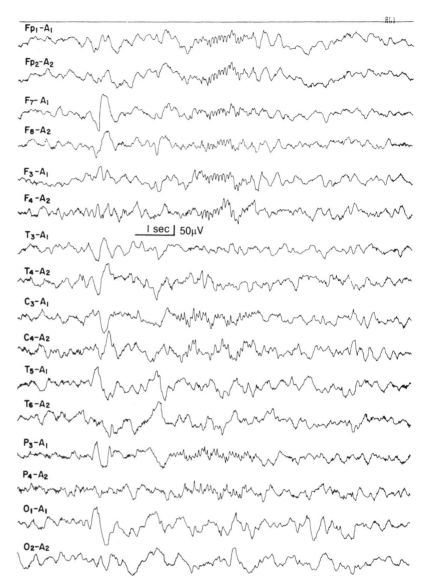

phase reversal is used only to mean "instrumental phase reversal"; it has been shown that, due to certain input characteristics of the apparatus, negativity and positivity may lead to well-defined pen deflections.

According to Chatrian et al. (1974), *true phase reversal* consists of "simultaneous pen deflection in opposite directions in two referential derivations using a suitable common reference electrode and displaying the same wave" (Fig. 8.6). According to these IFSECN committee members, "this phenomenon is rarely observed in scalp EEGs. When demonstrated beyond doubt in appropriate recording conditions, it indicates a 180° change in phase of an EEG wave between adjacent areas of the brain, on either side of a zero isopotential axis." Good examples of a dipole were found in the analysis of spike discharges from the lower rolandic region in children with benign rolandic epilepsy (Gregory and Wong, 1984). Further examples have been presented by Lesser et al. (1985).

It must be kept in mind that the dipole concept, although widely accepted, has not yet dispelled all uncertainties. Cases of true phase reversal as defined by IFSECN (1974) are indeed quite rare on the scalp, whereas depth and nasopharyngeal recordings often show phase reversals that could be explained according to the dipole concept as true phase reversals.

EEG-Electrogenesis, Micro-Dipoles, and EEG Signals

Thus far, the discussion has focused on the analysis of EEG signals based on the conventional EEG apparatus. This pragmatic approach must be understood and mastered by the clinical electroencephalographer, but it must be added that this is just the first step. The electrogenesis of EEG potentials and the current flow within myriad micro-dipoles are pivotal factors in a more refined analysis of EEG potentials.

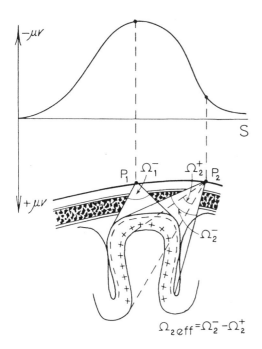

Figure 8.7. Potential distribution along line *S* on the scalp created by the synchronous activation of a curved portion of cortex that occupies the crown of a gyrus and its two sides forming the proximal walls of the two adjacent sulci. At P_1, the potential depends only on the solid angle Ω_1^-, since at this point an electrode "sees" only a portion of the negative side of the dipole layer. At P_2, an electrode sees the negative side of the portion of the dipole layer occupying the crown, the gyrus, and the wall of the proximal sulcus under the angle Ω_2^-; however, it also sees under the smaller angle Ω_2^+, the positive side of the portion of the dipole layer located in the wall of the distal sulcus. The potential at P_2 is therefore smaller than would be expected if only this were the angle determining the size of the potential at P_2 and is proportional to the effective solid angle Ω_{eff}, which equals the difference between Ω_2^- and Ω_2^+, the polarity being negative, since $\Omega_2^- > \Omega_2^+$. As is the case for a flat area of cortex oriented in parallel to the scalp, the potential profile is bell-shaped. (From Gloor, P. 1985. Neuronal generators and the problem of localization in electroencephalography: application of volume conductor theory to electroencephalography. *J. Clin. Neurophysiol.* 2:327–354.)

This has been pointed out in great detail by Gloor (1971, 1985). Figure 8.7 shows the EEG signal as the result of currents generated by a negative and a positive dipole layer. In Gloor's concept, the shape of the cortical garland with gyri and sulci is also taken into consideration (note the "solid angles"—Ω_1 and Ω_2).

Modern Biophysical Concepts

We are now facing an exciting new era of EEG signal analysis. New views have arisen from mapping techniques as well as from magnetoencephalographic concepts. Such views have been promoted by Burgess (1991), Van Oosterom (1991), Fender (1991), and Nunez and Pilgreen (1991). The monograph of Wong (1991) presents these views in a more comprehensive manner.

Figure 8.8 demonstrates different ways to map EEG signals. Wong (1991) explains this illustration (which is based on 21 electrodes) as follows: The potential field can be inspected using the simple contour line map (*middle*). This is

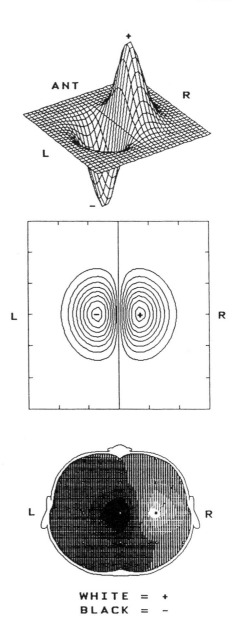

Figure 8.8. Different ways to map data. **Top:** Grid display. **Middle:** Contour map (vertex view). **Bottom:** Topographic map of head (same vertex view). For further explanation, see text. (From Wong, P.K.H. 1991. *Introduction to Brain Topography.* New York: Plenum.)

nothing more than a line drawing connecting locations (which may be real or interpolated from the 21 real values). These lines are the isopotential lines, and each is associated with a definite voltage value. In practice, it is inconvenient to display the actual number with each line, thus leading to possible confusion as to whether the isopotential lines represent a hill (positivity) or an abyss (negativity). A more refined remedy is to assign a different shading intensity to each isopotential line and to display the voltage-shading scale nearby. This is, of course, the now-familiar topographic display (Fig. 8.8, *bottom*).

As to the *top* of Fig. 8.8, Wong (1991) explains: "Grid displays can be looked upon as a set of rubber bands (isopotential lines) stretched across a frame (representing the head) parallel to each other in both directions. A positive voltage at a particular location would pull the rubber band up, while a negative voltage would push it down." Accordingly, the amount of travel is directly proportional to the voltage magnitude. The elasticity of the rubber bands smooths out any abrupt changes between electrodes. A similar mapping display method was described by Harris and Bickford (1968).

This new approach is eminently biophysical (whereas Gloor's approach is essentially neurophysiological). The biophysical approach places the stress on volume conduction of EEG signals. Propagation of EEG signals, however, does not solely depend on volume conduction. Jasper (1969) pointed out that propagation along conducting pathways represents the most important mechanism of signal spread (especially with regards to epileptiform signals).

Dipole theory has become fashionable in electroencephalography and there ought to be greater awareness of the serious limitations of this concept. This has been pointed out by Cooper et al. (1965) on the basis of their extensive depth EEG studies. A very critical attitude has been proposed by Niedermeyer (1996) in an analysis of dipole theory.

Acknowledgment

The author wishes to express his profound gratitude to Volker Milnik of Düren, Germany—one of the world's leading experts in this field.

References

Binnie, C.D., MacGillivray, B.B., and Osselton, J.W. 1974. Derivations and montages. In *Handbook of Electroencephalography and Clinical Neurophysiology,* vol. 3C, Ed. A. Remond, pp. 22–57. Amsterdam: Elsevier.

Brazier, M.A.B. 1949a. A study of the electrical fields at the surface of the head. Electroencephalogr. Clin. Neurophysiol. Suppl. 2:38–52.

Brazier, M.A.B. 1949b. The electrical fields at the surface of the head during sleep. Electroencephalogr. Clin. Neurophysiol. 1:195–204.

Burgess, R.C. 1991. Localization of neural generators (editorial). J. Clin. Neurophysiol. 8:369–370.

Chatrian, G.E., Bergamini, L., Dondey, M., et al. 1974. A glossary of terms most commonly used by clinical electroencephalographers. Electroencephalogr. Clin. Neurophysiol. 37:538–548.

Cooper, R., Winter, A.L., Crow, H.J., et al. 1965. Comparison of subcortical, cortical and scalp activity using chronic indwelling electrodes in man. Electroencephalogr. Clin. Neurophysiol. 18:217–228.

Fender, D.H. 1991. Models of the human brain and surrounding media: their influence on the reliability of source localization. J. Clin. Neurophysiol. 8:381–390.

Gloor, P. 1971. Volume theory and recording principles. Spike Wave (Special Issue) 2:1–48.

Gloor, P. 1985. Neuronal generators and the problem of localization in electroencephalography: application of volume conductor theory to electroencephalography. J. Clin. Neurophysiol. 2:327–354.

Gregory, D.L., and Wong, P.K. 1984. Topographical analysis of the centrotemporal discharges in benign rolandic epilepsy of childhood. Epilepsia 25:705–711.

Harris, J.A., and Bickford, R.G. 1968. Spatial display and parameter computation of the human epileptic spike focus by computer. Electroencephalogr. Clin. Neurophysiol. 24:281–282.

Jasper, H.H. 1969. Mechanisms of propagation: extracellular studies. In *Basic Mechanisms of the Epilepsies,* Eds. H.H. Jasper, A.A. Ward, Jr., and A. Pope, pp. 421–438. Boston: Little, Brown.

Knott, J.R. 1961. Concerning electrode arrays. Am. J. EEG Technol. 1:3–12.

Knott, J.R. 1969. Electrode montages revisited: how to tell up from down. Am. J. EEG Technol. 9:33–45.

Knott, J.R. 1985. Further thoughts on polarity, montages and localization. J. Clin. Neurophysiol. 2:63–75.

Kooi, K.A. 1971. *Fundamentals of Electroencephalography.* New York: Harper & Row.

Lesser, R.P., Lüders, H., Dinner, D.S., et al. 1985. An introduction to the basic concepts of polarity and localization. J. Clin. Neurophysiol. 2:46–61.

Magnus, O. 1961. On the technique of location by electroencephalography. In *Electroencephalography of Cerebral Tumours,* Eds. O. Magnus, W. Storm van Leeuwen, and W.A. Cobb, pp. 1–35. Amsterdam: Elsevier.

Maulsby, R.L. 1979. Basis for visual analysis: polarity convention, principles of localization and electrical fields. In *Current Practice of Clinical Electroencephalography,* Eds. D.W. Klass and D.D. Daly, pp. 27–36. New York: Raven Press.

Niedermeyer, E. 1978. EEG Potentiale und Polarität. Die Bedeutung der Schreiberbewegungen in Hinblick auf Negativität und Positivität. J. Electrophysiol. Tech. 3:190–198.

Niedermeyer, E. 1996. Dipole theory and the electroencephalogram. Clin. Electroencephalogr. 27:121–131.

Nunez, P.L. 1981. *Electrical Fields of the Brain.* New York-Oxford: Oxford University Press.

Nunez, P.L., and Pilgreen, K.L. 1991. The Spline-Laplacian in clinical neurophysiology: a method to improve EEG spatial resolution. J. Clin. Neurophysiol. 8:397–413.

Richey, E.T., and Namon, R. 1976. *EEG Instrumentation and Technology.* Springfield, IL: Charles C Thomas.

Sorel, L., and Ranwez, R. 1984. Basis and use of a true monopolar derivation: the neo-electroencephalography (N.E.E.G.). Clin. Electroencephalogr. 15:71–82.

Tyner, F.S., Knott, J.R., and Mayer, W.B., Jr. 1983. *Fundamentals of EEG Technology.* New York: Raven Press.

Upton, M. 1960. *Electronics for Everyone.* New York: New American Library of World Literature (Signet Key Books).

Van Oosterom, A. 1991. History and evolution of methods solving the inverse problem. J. Clin. Neurophysiol. 8:371–380.

Wong, P.K.H. 1991. *Introduction to Brain Topography.* New York: Plenum.

9. The Normal EEG of the Waking Adult

Ernst Niedermeyer

The presentation of the normal mature human electroencephalogram (EEG) and its basic features has a dual purpose. These are to promote knowledge of the boundaries between normality and abnormality in clinical EEG work and to enhance the understanding of the EEG as a phenomenon with important psychophysiological implications.

Both purposes are evident in Hans Berger's pioneering work, from the first report with its strong emphasis on psychophysiology and the discovery of the alpha rhythm (Berger, 1929) to his 14th report (Berger, 1938) of predominantly clinical interest. The question of how the EEG works remains to be answered by the experimental neurophysiologist. The nature of the normal EEG, how it reflects human behavior and mental functions, and the boundaries of normality are most legitimate guidelines for a chapter on the normal adult EEG.

EEG Frequencies

The EEG, as the continuous "roar" or "noise" of the brain, contains a fairly wide frequency spectrum, but it is not simply a hodgepodge of frequencies. Rhythmicity seems to create some law and order among waves of various lengths and amplitudes. The impression of prevailing rhythmicity and organization, however, is not a yardstick for the normality of an EEG. Pronounced rhythmicity may be a sign of abnormality, and a prima vista anarchic appearance does not necessarily imply abnormality. Reactivity may be the magic word in such cases; an EEG of mixed frequencies may be quite responsive to certain stimuli.

The *frequency range* of the EEG has a fuzzy lower and upper limit. There are ultraslow and ultrafast frequency components that play no significant role in the clinical EEG, with the exception of ultraslow activity in profound coma and near-terminal states. For these reasons, the frequency-response curve of an EEG apparatus concentrates on the clinically relevant frequency range, which is also the most important from the psychophysiological viewpoint. This range lies between 0.1/sec [or cycles per second (cps) or Hz] and 100/sec and, in a more restricted sense, between 0.3/sec and 70/sec. In the normal adult, the slow ranges (0.3–7/sec) and the very fast range (above 30/sec) are sparsely represented; medium (8–13/sec) and fast (14–30/sec) ranges predominate.

These frequencies are broken down into the following bands or ranges:

Delta below 3.5/sec (usually 0.1–3.5/sec)
Theta 4–7.5/sec
Alpha 8–13/sec
Beta 14–30/sec
Gamma above 30/sec (unlimited in upper range)

This is the "old-fashioned" breakdown of the EEG frequencies. The reader will find here and in several other chapters of this book discussions on ultraslow activity [below 0.1/sec to near 0 direct current (DC) potentials] and ultrafast activity (Curio, 2000a; also see Chapter 26). The exact width of the gamma range is still debated and may lie between 30 and 60/sec. There has been a proposal by Curio (2000b) for the following designations: omega range 60 to 120 Hz, rho range 120 to 500 Hz, and sigma range 500 to 1,000 Hz. This will need further clarifications. The reader will find below that the letters rho and sigma have been used for EEG phenomena occurring in sleep. Let us wait and see which of these terms will find general and lasting acceptance!

The sequence of these Greek letters is not logical and can be understood only in the historical view. The terms *alpha* and *beta* rhythm or waves were introduced by Berger (1929); the term *gamma* rhythm was subsequently used by Jasper and Andrews (1938) to designate frequencies above 30 or 35/sec; these were essentially 35 to 45/sec and superimposed on the occipital alpha rhythm (see Dutertre, 1977). This term was temporarily abandoned, and *gamma* frequencies became a part of the beta range.

The use of the term *gamma rhythm* or *gamma frequency range* has made an impressive comeback during the 1990s. The use of a *fast* beta range and a *very fast* gamma range might have been convenient for those who utilize frequency analysis with power spectra. Furthermore, modern EEG rhythm research in the 1990s has unearthed the all-but-forgotten term *gamma rhythm* (Basar, 1992; Bullock, 1992; Eckhorn et al., 1992; Gray et al., 1992). In this "new wave" of EEG rhythm research, rhythmic activities of the brain are conceived mainly as induced rather than as spontaneous rhythms.

The term *delta rhythm* was introduced by Walter (1936) to designate all frequencies below the alpha range. Walter himself, however, found a need to introduce a special designation for the 4 to 7.5/sec range and used the letter *theta*. He thus bypassed the Greek letters *epsilon, zeta,* and *eta*; he chose *theta* to stand for thalamus because he presumed a thalamic origin of these waves (also see Knott, 1976b).

The term *pi rhythm* has been used for the designation of posterior slow rhythms (3–4/sec) without harmonious relationship to the posterior alpha rhythm according to Dutertre (1977) who recommended the preferable (although certainly less precise) term *posterior slow rhythms*. Hardly anyone has used the term *pi rhythm* since the 1990s.

The term *phi rhythm* was suggested by D. Daly (according to Silbert et al., 1995) for the designation of monorhythmic posterior delta waves (less than 4/sec), distinct from the background and occurring within 2 sec of eye closure. This rhythm was also described by Belsh et al. (1983) as "posterior rhythmic slow activity after eye closure."

The term *occipital intermittent rhythmical delta activity (OIRDA)* (see Chapter 12) refers to a pattern of childhood that is usually found in epileptic patients (Gullapalli and Fountain, 2003). One may still wonder if the term *OIRDA* is really needed. On the other hand, FIRDA and TIRDA, for frontal and temporal rhythmical delta, are powerful and clinically informative patterns (see Chapters 12 and 27).

The alpha-like anterior temporal kappa rhythm (Laugier and Liberson, 1937) is a controversial pattern that is discussed later in this chapter. Kugler (1981) has been using the term *sigma activity* instead of *sleep spindles* and, furthermore, the term *sigma rhythm* for activity in the 11 to 15/sec range. The term *rho waves* was used for the activity known as POSTS (positive occipital sharp transients of sleep) (Kugler and Laub, 1971), but it has disappeared.

Other Greek letters have been proposed for the designation of distinct EEG activities. Mu rhythm and lambda waves are discussed in this chapter. The term *tau rhythm* is mentioned in Chapter 57, "Magnetoencephalography as a Tool of Clinical Neurophysiology," and it denotes a physiological alpha rhythm of the temporal region (in the author's opinion identical with the "third rhythm" discussed in this chapter). "Zeta wave" simply denotes a certain type of delta wave (rather than a rhythm) with some sharp configuration (Magnus and Van der Holst, 1987; Siepman et al., 2004).

Thus, 13 of the 23 letters of the Greek alphabet are being used in the EEG terminology, and this number could be even higher. In my opinion, it might be better to limit the Greek terms to the classical EEG frequency ranges retaining solely the letters *alpha, beta, gamma, delta,* and *theta.*

EEG Amplitudes

The EEG denotes voltage plotted against time. The voltage of the EEG signal determines its amplitude. The passage of the cortical EEG signal through leptomeninges, cerebrospinal fluid, dura mater, bone, galea, and scalp has a strongly attenuating effect on the original signal (Cooper et al., 1965); this is discussed in the section on the depth EEG. Corticographic discharges show amplitudes of 500–1.500 μ (0.5–1.5 mV) and several millivolts in prominent spiking. The amplitudes of the scalp EEG are markedly reduced and lie between 10 and 100 μV (in adults, more commonly between 10 and 50 μV).

The EEG amplitudes are measured from peak to peak. Precise determination of the voltage of each wave is unnecessary and should be discouraged as pseudoaccuracy; too many variables are involved (above all, the interelectrode distance and the type of montage, whether bipolar or referential recording). Electroencephalographers may indicate in their reports a certain amplitude range, such as "alpha rhythm from 20–30 μV," or, even better, limit themselves to statements such as "of medium voltage" or "of low to medium voltage."

A given frequency can be rendered abnormal by excessive voltage. This is true for all frequencies, and it is particularly important for the fast (beta) band. The problem of low voltage will be thoroughly discussed, because low amplitudes can indicate a life-threatening decline of cerebral voltage output, whereas the vast majority of low-voltage records are "desynchronized" (discussed later) and a variant of normalcy.

Alpha Rhythm
Definition

The International Federation of Societies for Electroencephalography and Clinical Neurophysiology (IFSECN) (committee chaired by G. E. Chatrian; see IFSECN, 1974) proposed the following definition of alpha rhythm:

> Rhythm at 8–13 Hz occurring during wakefulness over the posterior regions of the head, generally with higher voltage over the occipital areas. Amplitude is variable but is mostly below 50 μV in adults. Best seen with eyes closed and under conditions of physical relaxation and relative mental inactivity. Blocked or attenuated by attention, especially visual, and mental effort (IFSECN, 1974).

This committee also has pointed out that the term *alpha rhythm* must be restricted to rhythms fulfilling all of the above criteria. Rolandic mu rhythm may have the same frequency range, but its topography and reactivity are different (also see Markand, 1990).

Frequency

The chapter on EEG maturation shows the gradual frequency increase of a posterior basic rhythm that is detectable around the age of 4 months with a frequency of approximately 4/sec. This posterior basic rhythm shows a progressive frequency increase with average values of around 6/sec at age 12 months and 8/sec at age 3 years. At that time, the alpha frequency band is reached, and there is justification for the use of the term *alpha rhythm*. The frequency reaches a mean of about 10/sec at age 10 years. This is essentially the mean alpha frequency of adulthood; in other words, the progressive alpha rhythm acceleration usually ends around the age of 10 years, but the second decade of life (and to some degree also the third decade) features a constant decline of intermixed posterior slow activity that is usually present in considerable quantity at age 10.

The frequency of the alpha rhythm tends to decline in elderly individuals. This decline apparently reflects some degree of cerebral pathology, which is vascular or fibrillary degenerative, in most instances. Healthy and vigorous elderly people may show little or no alpha frequency decline, even in the ninth decade. An alpha rhythm with a consistent 8/sec frequency ought to be regarded as a mild abnormality.

The figure of 10.2 ± 0.9/sec has been indicated as the mean adult alpha frequency (Petersén and Eeg-Olofsson, 1971). An element of instability of the alpha frequency must be taken into consideration; according to Townsend et al. (1975), the alpha rhythm frequency can be stabilized by sinusoidally modulated light. Extreme upward gaze tends to facilitate the posterior alpha rhythm (Mulholland, 1969; Mulholland and Evans, 1965). Lateral eye deviations may have similar effects (Fenwick and Walker, 1969).

An alpha rhythm frequency shift to the faster portion of the band is not uncommon and is essentially within normal limits, as will be discussed later. The similarities between the frequencies of alpha rhythm and the physiological finger tremor have been discussed by Isokawa and Komisaruk (1983). Immediately after eye closure, the alpha frequency may be accelerated for a moment ("squeak effect," after Storm van Leeuwen and Bekkering, 1958).

Amplitude

Alpha rhythm amplitudes vary considerably from individual to individual and, in a given person, from moment to moment. The electroencephalographer, therefore, should look for stretches of optimal alpha output. A referential montage to the ipsilateral ear is usually most suitable for the determination of the alpha rhythm amplitude, but the interelectrode distances must always be considered. The maximum alpha voltage is usually over the occipital region as such, but a bipolar montage with a parasagittal array may obscure rather than reveal the true alpha maximum. The alpha amplitude may be quite small in the channels displaying P_3–O_1 and P_4–O_2 because of massive homophasic activity, which results in canceling out.

The alpha amplitudes tend to show constant waxing and waning. For this reason, trains of alpha waves show a typical spindle shape with a belly and a thin portion. However, the term *spindles* has been reserved for a classical pattern of sleep (see Chapter 10, "Sleep and EEG") and should not be used in this context.

Berger (1929) found alpha rhythm voltages of 15–20 μV; these are small values when one considers his fronto-occipital recording technique; their smallness was probably due to the instrument limitations of his Edelmann string galvanometer. According to Cobb (1963), the alpha rhythm voltage fluctuates between 0 and 40–50 μV in the individual record; values above 100 μV are uncommon in the adult, whereas maximums of 5–10 μV are frequently seen (Cobb, 1963). The work of Simon (also known as Simonova) and her co-workers has shed more light on this subject; Simonova et al. (1967) found amplitudes between 20 and 60 μV in 66% of their subjects; values below 20 μV were found in 28% and above 60 μV in 6% (also see Simon, 1977).

Higher alpha amplitudes are more likely to be found in association with slower alpha frequencies (Brazier and Finesinger, 1944; Wieneke et al., 1980). There is good evidence of a mild to moderate alpha amplitude asymmetry with higher voltage on the right (Cobb, 1963; Kellaway and Maulsby, 1966; Kiloh et al., 1972; Petersén and Eeg-Olofsson, 1971; Simon, 1977; Wieneke et al., 1980). This seems to indicate that the alpha rhythm is of greater amplitude over the nondominant hemisphere, but no convincing conclusion concerning handedness can be derived from this asymmetry (Petersén and Eeg-Olofsson, 1971). This physiological asymmetry has been confirmed by Matousek et al. (1981), who also found a reversal of this rule (i.e., higher voltage on the left occiput in patients with endogenous depression). Amplitude asymmetries must be demonstrated in both referential and bipolar montages from two or more posteriorly placed electrodes (such as parietal and posterior temporal) before it is considered significant (Markand, 1990).

There may be a fine line between physiological and truly abnormal alpha amplitude asymmetries.

Wave Morphology

The alpha rhythm is usually characterized by rounded or sinusoidal wave forms. However, a sizable minority of individuals have sharp alpha configuration. In such cases, the negative component appears to be sharp and the positive component appears to be rounded, similar to the wave morphology of rolandic mu rhythm.

The sharp configuration of posterior alpha waves is by no means an abnormality. It is a common finding, especially in young adults, adolescents, and older children. An admixture of beta waves is usually the cause of the sharp configuration; drug effects from sedatives or minor tranquilizers must sometimes be suspected in such cases. Unusual morphologies in childhood ("fused forms") are presented in Chapter 11, "Maturation of the EEG: Development of Waking and Sleep Patterns."

Spatial Distribution

The alpha rhythm is clearly a manifestation of the posterior half of the head and is usually found over occipital, parietal, and posterior temporal regions. This observation of Adrian and Matthews (1934) was doubted by Berger (1935), whose concept of alpha rhythm as a global cerebral rhythm was an erroneous conclusion from his fronto-occipital bipolar recording technique. The alpha rhythm may extend into central areas, the vertex, and also the midtemporal region. When the central region is strongly involved, the alpha rhythm must be distinguished from possibly coexisting rolandic mu rhythm. This is usually easily demonstrable with eye opening, blocking alpha rhythm but not blocking mu rhythm.

The alpha rhythm may occasionally extend slightly into the superior frontal leads (F_3, F_4). Extension into the frontopolar region (Fp_1, Fp_2) is practically unheard of. Apparent alpha rhythm in the frontopolar leads may be very prominent in referential (unipolar) montages if the referential ear electrode picks up the posterior alpha rhythm. This is particularly common when the mastoid region is used instead of the ear lobe (the mastoid being a preferred place with paste technique). Another source of confusion is eyelid flutter, with closed eyes giving rise to frontal artifacts in alpha frequency.

In depth electroencephalography and with occipital implants, posterior alpha rhythm can be demonstrated throughout the depth of the occipital lobe and even in the vicinity of the lateral geniculate body. According to Albe-Fessard (1975), alpha rhythm may be recorded from the medial pulvinar but not from the remaining thalamic nuclei in the human (also see Gücer et al., 1978). In the dog, Lopes da Silva et al. (1973a) demonstrated that alpha rhythm of the same peak frequency, bandwidth, and reactivity can be recorded from the visual cortex as well as from the visual thalamus (lateral geniculate body, pulvinar nuclei).

Further inferences on the alpha rhythm distribution can be made from the study of alpha rhythm generation. This topic is discussed later (also see Theories of Neurophysiological Basis of Mu Rhythm, below).

Reactivity

The posterior alpha rhythm is temporarily blocked by an influx of light (eye opening), other afferent stimuli, and mental activities. The degree of reactivity varies; the alpha rhythm may be completely blocked, suppressed, or attenuated with voltage reduction. The alpha blocking response to eye opening was discovered by Berger and described in his first report (1929) on the human EEG; it came as a great surprise for investigators who were searching for action potentials and hence would have expected enhancement of EEG voltage with influx of light (Fig. 9.1). Berger's own explanation was the concept of a zone of inhibition surrounding the area of excitation by the afferent stimulus (Berger, 1933a; also see Gloor, 1971).

It is noteworthy that in some subjects the alpha suppression is more pronounced than in others. These persons may have an alpha-free stretch of desynchronized and chiefly fast EEG activity for the duration of the eye opening, even in rather dim light. In others, the alpha blockage lasts for less than 1 second. According to Gibbs and Gibbs (1950) "after the eyes have been held open for a few minutes, low voltage alpha waves . . . usually reappear, unless the subject continues to look at something which holds his interest."

The amplitude ratio between eyes closed (well-developed alpha) and eyes open (beta of much smaller voltage) declines with advancing age (Könönen and Partanen, 1993).

Alpha attenuation due to auditory, tactile, and other somatosensory stimuli or heightened mental activity (such as solving difficult arithmetical problems) is usually less pronounced than the blocking effect with eye opening.

According to Niedermeyer et al. (1989), the blocking or attenuating effect of mental arithmetic on the posterior alpha rhythm is absent in most cases (Niedermeyer et al., 1989). In a study done in 1,280 patients (598 with normal EEG tracings, 682 with various degrees of EEG abnormality), alpha suppression or attenuation with calculation (serial sevens) was noted in only 21 (1.6%) of the patients. On the other hand, Berger (1931, 1932, 1933a,b, 1937) had shown fine examples of arithmetic-induced alpha blocking. We found, however, that even "serial seventeens" (100 minus 17, etc.) are mostly unassociated with any decrease of the posterior alpha rhythm. Does this mean that the venerable discoverer of the human EEG was all wrong as far as arithmetic-induced alpha blocking is concerned? Not at all. The arithmetical tasks given to his two teenage children, Klaus and Ilse, were just a lot more difficult: for Klaus (age 19) 23 × 43, and for Ilse (age 14) 196 ÷ 7. Difficulty of the task is not the only factor. Even simple arithmetic may cause alpha blocking if the subject shows great motivation trying to please the examiner. With a nonchalant approach, there is usually no alpha blocking.

No EEG is complete without certain reactivity tests. Although alpha rhythm disappears with the earliest approach of drowsiness, there are exceptional cases of persisting posterior alpha rhythm in profoundly comatose patients with pontine vascular lesions; their alpha rhythm shows no reactivity, even with strong nociceptive stimuli. According to Kiloh et al. (1972), "complete unresponsiveness of the alpha rhythm to visual stimuli is a rare and unequivocally abnormal finding."

Pfurtscheller (1990) conceives the stimulus-induced alpha blocking or attenuation as an "event-related EEG desynchronization." With the use of averaging techniques, he compared such desynchronizing effects with stimulus-induced evoked potentials and found different topographical patterns and time courses, presumably due to different underlying neuronal processes. This is just a small vignette of the "new wave" of alpha (and other EEG rhythms) research, which will be discussed in the further course of this chapter.

In albinism, misrouting of the optic nerve fibers with decussation anomaly is a frequent finding. Smith et al. (1998) have demonstrated that unilateral alpha activity to eye opening and closure can be found. In other words, there is right-sided alpha rhythm with left eye closed, left-sided alpha rhythm with right eye closed, and alpha blocking with closure of both eyes.

Alpha Rhythm and Vigilance

Alpha rhythm is the classical EEG correlate for a state of relaxed wakefulness best obtained with the eyes closed. A degree of higher alertness attenuates or suppresses the alpha rhythm, which is then supplanted by "desynchronized" low voltage fast activity.

The earliest stage of drowsiness is characterized by "alpha dropout" (Fig. 9.2). The trains of alpha waves become less and less continuous, and the last alpha fragments finally give way to a low-voltage pattern of mixed slow (mostly theta range) and fast frequencies. This type of alpha dropout is a hallmark of a normal adult EEG; in children and infants, various types of slow patterns appear (see Chapter

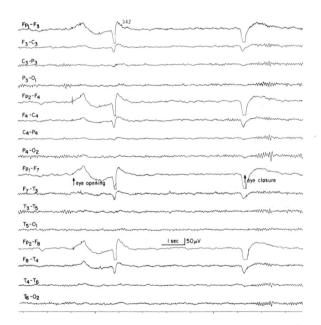

Figure 9.1. Normal record, in a patient age 27 years. Posterior 10–12/sec alpha rhythm. Good blocking response to eye opening and reactivation of alpha rhythm with eye closure. Note low-voltage fast activity and some return of alpha rhythm while eyes are kept open. Also note typical artifacts with eye opening, eye closure, and eye blink (caused by eye potential shifts).

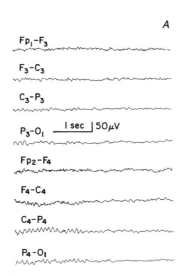

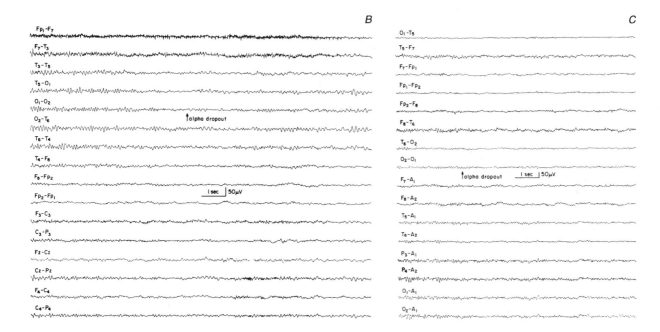

Figure 9.2. **A-C:** Three examples of alpha dropout at the earliest stage of drowsiness in normal adults. The close-up shows clearly the mixture of low-voltage fast and slow activity following alpha dropout. This is different from the low-voltage fast activity in the alpha blocking response to eye opening and heightened alertness.

11, "Maturation of the EEG: Development of Waking and Sleep Patterns"). In adults with some organic cerebral problems and in old age, a posterior alpha rhythm of normal appearance may be replaced by activity in the theta and delta range; a special pattern with rhythmical widespread (but mainly parietotemporal) 5 to 7/sec activity has been individualized recently by Westmoreland and Klass (1981), who consider this pattern "benign."

Interindividual Differences

When Adrian and Matthews demonstrated their own EEGs on May 12, 1934, at a meeting of the astonished members of the Physiological Society in Cambridge, England, it was found that Adrian's 10/sec alpha rhythm was quite impressive, whereas Matthews produced "no regular waves" (Adrian, 1971). Studies of further subjects showed that Adrian's alpha development was that of the majority,

whereas Matthews, the ingenious engineer and designer of Adrian's instrumentation, belonged to a minority of persons with little or no organized alpha rhythm.

Davis and Davis (1936) distinguished four types of records: (a) dominant alpha (found in 20% of healthy adults); (b) subdominant alpha (35%); (c) mixed alpha (20%); and (d) rare alpha (25%). Golla et al. (1943) distinguished three alpha types: M for minus or minimal, P for persistent, and R for responsive. The P type shows no real persistence of alpha, but has a very short blocking response to eye opening (also see Kiloh et al., 1972). Another type of alpha rhythm is the "monotonous high voltage alpha," which shows little or no waxing and waning of the amplitude (Kuhlo, 1976a).

These alpha traits are, to some degree, genetically transmitted (Davis and Davis, 1936; Lennox et al., 1945; Travis and Gottlober, 1936); marked similarities have been reported in identical twins. Here the question arises as to whether these alpha traits are EEG correlates of certain psychological personality traits. Such relationships were suggested by Lemere (1936), who related good alpha development with cyclothymic personalities and poor alpha development with schizothymic personalities (thus using the nomenclature of Kretschmer, 1931). Saul et al. (1937) found high alpha indices (i.e., a large quantity of alpha rhythm) in passive dependent people and low alpha indices in persons with a consistent drive to activity. This could not be confirmed by Lindsley (1938). An assumed correlation with extrovert and introvert personalities was not substantiated by the work of Henry and Knott (1941). Mental work given as tasks revealed a higher alpha percent time in introverts, according to Broadhurst and Glass (1969). Nowak and Marczynski (1981) studied the effects of anxiety traits and stress on the EEG; persons in the high-anxiety group showed stronger and more homogeneous alpha blocking responses, along with "paradoxical" alpha augmentation.

Earlier attempts at correlations between alpha rhythm and intelligence used to be futile or unconvincing (Berger, 1931, 1935, 1938; Gastaut, 1960; Henry, 1944; Kreezer, 1936; Shagass, 1946). More information is found in the handbook article of Knott (1976a). More sophisticated EEG technology appears to have shed more light on this topic. With the use of power spectral analysis, Gasser et al. (1983) found good correlations between alpha rhythm (plus other EEG criteria) and intelligence. Good memory performers are faster in retrieving information from memory and their alpha frequency tends to be higher by about 1/sec (Klimesch et al., 1996).

Intraindividual Differences

A person's EEG traits and alpha rhythm development must not be considered as permanent and unchangeable features like fingerprints. Every EEG tracing of some length gives testimony to a certain degree of variability, even within the state of relaxed vigilance. This is probably the effect of a large number of physiological and psychophysiological variables. To mention just one example, the waxing phase of alpha amplitudes has been related to the waning phase of afterimages (Jasper and Cruikshank, 1937). With advancing age, the alpha frequency tends to decrease (Fisch et al., 1990) but this is probably the effect of cerebral pathology occurring at old age.

Circadian studies of the EEG have been done sparingly (Frank, 1964; Scheich, 1969) and with inconclusive results (for further data, see Harding and Thompson, 1976). The *menstrual cycle* has been thought to influence the EEG and especially the alpha rhythm frequency. According to Dusser de Barenne and Gibbs (1942), a one-half cycle per second drop of the alpha frequency occurs for 1 to 2 days during the ovulation period and a similar decrease of 0.5/sec is also noted on the first day of menstrual flow. Lamb et al. (1953) found a maximum of alpha activity at the time of ovulation and a premenstrual increase of alpha frequency. Pitot and Gastaut (1954) reported alpha slowing (0.3–1/sec) immediately after ovulation and during menstruation. Later work was done with the use of frequency analysis (Harding, 1967;

Roubicek et al., 1968) and an integrator (Sugerman et al., 1970). Harding (1967) noted an activity increase in the alpha band during menstruation. Roubicek et al. (1968) observed increasing anterior theta activity at the time of menstruation. Harding and Thompson (1976) have summarized the work in this field as follows:

Preovulatory phase (days 5–14): Alpha frequency increased, amount of beta increased, photic driving reduced.

Postovulation or luteal phase (days 15–23): Alpha slower, amount of alpha increased, less beta and more theta activity, photic driving increased.

Premenstrual phase (days 23–28): Alpha frequency increased, amount of alpha reduced, more beta, less theta activity.

Menstrual phase (days 1–5): Alpha frequency slowed and amount increased, less beta, more theta activity.

According to Harding and Thompson (1976), no consistent changes have been found with the use of oral contraceptives. The study of Creutzfeldt et al. (1976) yielded slightly different results; there was a mild occipital alpha acceleration during the luteal phase (0.3/sec), along with slight decline of cognitive functions. These functions were significantly depressed in the group of women taking oral contraceptives (when compared with the group of women with spontaneous menstrual cycle). Small differences in the EEG of males and females have been reported by Veldhuizen et al. (1993).

Body temperature also modifies the alpha frequency; the alpha rhythm accelerates with increasing body temperature (Gundel, 1984). Therapeutic hyperthermia (up to 41°C) in cancer patients slows down the EEG to the delta range and depresses the overall EEG output (Dubois et al., 1980).

Alpha Conditioning and Alpha Feedback

The method of conditioning reflex formation was introduced in EEG research by Durup and Fessard (1935), who found that normally ineffective auditory stimuli when repeatedly presented in conjunction with visual stimuli were capable of producing alpha blocking. Similar observations had been made in passing by Berger (1930). Further work in this field was done by Cruikshank (1937), Jasper and Cruikshank (1937), Travis and Egan (1938), Knott and Henry (1941), and Jasper and Shagass (1941). Later studies were done by Visser (1961), Hofer and Hinkle (1964), Milstein (1965), and Torres (1968). Knott's (1976a) review of this topic is most illuminating.

Voluntary control of the alpha rhythm and the use of alpha feedback methods have been widely discussed topics since the late 1960s. This work was presumably prompted by the observation of well modulated alpha during meditation practiced by *yogis* (Anand et al., 1961; Bagchi and Wenger, 1958) or *zen buddhists* (Hirai, 1968, and Kasamatsu and Hirai, 1966, both articles cited in Gastaut, 1974). Nowlis and Kamiya (1970) and Brown (1970) associated alpha rhythm enhancement (on a "voluntary" basis) with a pleasant mood. Further work in this field was done by Wallace (1970), Wallace et al. (1971), and Banquet (1973), who studied states of *transcendental meditation.* Alpha amplitudes increased or decreased; in some subjects there were periods of low voltage theta activity. Knott (1976a) feels that such states are in essence periods of drowsiness and doubts the validity of the view that the high alpha state is a desirable condition. According to Stigsby et al. (1981), there is no consistent EEG pattern associated with successful or unsuccessful transcendental meditation. Gastaut (1974) has sharply criticized all forms of alpha cult. Hypnosis may induce states of relaxed wakefulness or lowered vigilance. The EEG simply reflects the level of vigilance (see Dongier et al., 1976). In the 1980s, the interest in alpha conditioning and alpha feedback started to decline.

Alpha Rhythm, Anxiety, and Emotional Tension

It has been pointed out that a relaxed waking state is the optimal condition for the posterior alpha rhythm. It is hence reasonable to assume that emotional tension attenuates or blocks the alpha rhythm. If this statement is correct, the EEG could serve as a tool for the assessment of emotional tension. This seems to hold true for the state of emotional tension in patients or subjects with pending litigation, after a head injury, or after other forms of physical damage (Scherzer, 1966). In such cases, the tension is, in essence, a state of expectancy pertaining to the outcome of an important test. In other states of tension and, especially, in psychotic individuals described as emotionally very tense, a well-developed alpha rhythm of average amplitude may be present. Catatonic schizophrenics in a state of extreme tension usually show low-voltage fast records.

Alpha Rhythm: Human Versus Animal

The posterior alpha rhythm shows considerable difference from species to species. The alpha frequency usually lies above 10/sec in primates, and the amplitude is surprisingly small in primates (recorded from dural electrodes). In the cat, an 8 to 13/sec rhythm was recorded from the most posterior part of the occipital cortex (Lanoir, 1972). Pampiglione (1963) demonstrated a fairly well developed posterior 6 to 8/sec rhythm in the dog at 1 year of age. This rhythm represents an equivalent of the human alpha rhythm (Storm van Leeuwen et al., 1967).

A 10/sec "alpha-like" rhythm in the visual cortex of the cat was reported by Chatila et al. (1992). Başar and Schürmann (1994) described evoked a alpha responses over the cat's visual cortex, evoked by visual stimuli. These data were obtained with extra- and intracranial recording.

Jurko and Andy (1967) compared the posterior alpha rhythm in three species of macaque monkeys. In rhesus (*Macaca mulatta*) and stumptail (*Rhesus speciosa*) monkeys, fairly well developed alpha rhythms, 10/sec and 12/sec, respectively, were recorded, whereas greater admixture of slow and fast frequencies was found in cynomolgus monkeys (*Macaca ira*). Caveness (1962) found an alpha average frequency of 9.8/sec in *Macaca mulatta.*

The closest resemblance to the human alpha is found in the dog (Storm van Leeuwen et al., 1963, 1967; also see Markand, 1990).

In this context, a study of Götze et al. (1959) on the EEG in healthy and diseased animals ought to be mentioned. This study deals with zoo monkeys and dogs. It is deplorable that collaboration between human electroencephalography and veterinary medicine has not intensified.

Alpha Rhythm and Its Generators

Alpha rhythm is of cortical origin, but the theory of a thalamic pacemaker function has frequently surfaced since the work of Berger (1933a), who presumed cortical genesis but thalamic governance of the alpha phenomenon. Bishop (1936) proposed the concept of corticothalamic reverberating circuits, and Andersen and Andersson (1968) are the proponents of a thalamic theory that is based on presumed similarities between human alpha rhythm and experimental barbiturate spindle activity in animals. According to this theory, the alpha rhythm is driven by presynaptic input to cortical neurons from the thalamic level (also see Andersen and Andersson, 1974; Frost, 1976). This concept has been challenged by Lopes da Silva et al. (1973a,b). Watanabe (1981) has postulated a "somewhat loose but stable oscillator system" subserving the generation of alpha rhythm.

Adrian and Yamagiwa (1935) regarded the alpha rhythm as cortical with maximal involvement of the visual area. Important new vistas were opened with the demonstration of some degree of interhemispheric asynchrony between alpha waves (Aird and Garoutte, 1958). It has been presumed that there is more than one alpha generator within the posterior regions of the cerebrum (Walter et al., 1966); this was further substantiated by depth EEG studies in the human (Perez-Boija et al., 1962). The technique of chronotopography has added further insight into the possibility of multiple sources of alpha generation (Remond, 1968). Further work on interhemispheric phase differences between alpha waves has been carried out with toposcopic analysis (Cooper and Mundy-Castle, 1960) and cross-correlation technique (Liske et al., 1967).

Posterior alpha generation and spread in posteroanterior direction (Walter et al., 1966) appears to be a fact. This concept, however, has been challenged by Inouye et al. (1983), who feel that alpha spread occurs in an anteroposterior direction in the dominant as well as in the nondominant hemisphere. These surprising views are based on the method of entropy analysis.

Our comprehension of alpha-rhythm genesis has not strikingly increased in the course of the 1980s and 1990s. It may be assumed that there are corticocortical and thalamocortical systems that interact in the generation of cortical alpha rhythms (Steriade et al., 1990). From the experimenter's as well as from the clinical EEGer's viewpoint, there is good reason to presume that alpha rhythm is most definitely a cortical phenomenon but there has been, thus far, no evidence of a synchronizing mechanism in cortical level.

The alpha rhythm caught the fancy of some of the most illustrious geniuses of the 20th century. In a book review of *Norbert Wiener, 1894–1964,* by P. R. Masani (Boston: Birkhauser, 1990), Barlow (1991) beautifully pointed out the alpha rhythm theories of Wiener and McCulloch and proceeded as follows:

In the next few years after 1953, Wiener evolved the concept of a stable component of the alpha rhythm (Wiener's interest in the EEG was essentially limited to the alpha rhythm) as a brain clock, to serve a gating function. (In *Cybernetics,* 1948), Wiener cites Pitts and McCulloch's 1947 idea of the alpha rhythm as a scanning rhythm; McCulloch, on the other hand, in one of the Macy Cybernetics Conference volumes, attributes the idea to Wiener's 1940 work on digital computer design.) Wiener added a mathematical basis, entailing nonlinear mutual entrainment (as an example of "self-organizing systems") a few years later (1958) and discussed the general concept at the 1963 Kershman Lecture (for which he had been suggested by John Hughes), under the title, "The Harmonic Analysis of Physiological Phenomena with Special Reference to Electroencephalography." Commentaries on Wiener's concept of the alpha rhythm as a brain clock, by Grey Walter and by this reviewer, can be found in *Survey of Cybernetics* (J. Rose [Ed.], 1969) and in Vol. 4 of *Collected Works* respectively.

If the alpha rhythm were to function as a brain clock, it would be a miserable time keeper. Virtually every EEG record with a well-formed posterior alpha rhythm shows minor or even more prominent fluctuations of its frequency. Such unrealistic alpha theories are simply not compatible with the clinical EEG practice (Niedermeyer, 1997).

An extracerebral artifact theory of alpha rhythm has been proposed by Lippold (1970, 1973), who has presumed that the alpha rhythm is caused by extraocular motor activity ("translational eye tremor modulating the position of the corneo-retinal potential"). There is little to substantiate this hypothesis. Some authors have taken pains to invalidate Lippold's theory; the work of Tait and Pavlovski (1978) has provided convincing evidence of its erroneous premises. Hess (1980) has further corroborated the cerebral genesis of alpha rhythm. The origin of the canine alpha was found in the cortex (phase reversal at laminae IV/V) (Lopes da Silva and Storm van Leeuwen, 1978; also see Steriade et al., 1990). Hogan and Fitzpatrick (1987) observed occipital alpha rhythm in the isolated canine brain after removal of mandible, orbit, and snout.

No neurophysiological or psychophysiological alpha rhythm theory has yet found general acceptance, and there are still uncertainties about the origin and psychophysiological significance of this remarkable phenomenon. And yet, our insights into the nature of the alpha rhythm (and other EEG rhythms) have been deepening. The ceaseless work of experimental neurophysiologists, psychoneurophysiologists, and neurotheoreticians has provided us with a better view of the nature of the alpha rhythm. Lopes da Silva (1991) has pointed out that "EEG signals can reflect functional states of neuronal networks." Accordingly, oscillatory mechanisms allow for changes between different behavioral modes. As in Wagnerian music, each oscillatory state may serve as a leitmotiv evoking different sets of mental associations and emotional states.

Rolandic (Central) Mu Rhythm

Rolandic (central) mu rhythm is in frequency and amplitude related to the posterior alpha rhythm, but its topography and physiological significance are quite different. Historically, the existence of a special central rhythm was presumed by Jasper and Andrews (1938) ("precentral alpha rhythm"), Maddocks et al. (1951) ("alphoid activity"), and Schütz and Müller (1951) ("high voltage rolandic alpha"). The features of mu rhythm were first described in detail by

Gastaut et al. (1952) and Gastaut (1952), who also included electrocorticographic tracings; these authors introduced the term *rhythme rolandique en arceau*. The epithet *en arceau* alludes to the arch-shaped wave morphology, which has also prompted the term *wicket rhythm* (Gastaut et al., 1954). Magnus (1954) used the term *central alpha* (see also Jasper and Andrews, 1938). Other terms are *arcade rhythm* (Van der Drift and Magnus, 1961), *comb rhythm* (Cobb, 1963), and *somatosensory alpha rhythm* (Kuhlman, 1978a).

Mu rhythm is not detectable in every mature subject; as will be discussed later, its prevalence is limited unless the "hidden" mu rhythm is visualized with special methods. Mu stands for motor; this rhythm is strongly related to functions of the motor cortex, but the contribution of the adjacent somatosensory cortex must not be ignored.

Mu rhythm and associated beta activity over the sensorimotor cortex have become a topic of special interest during the 1990s. As a matter of fact, mu rhythm as an interesting clinical EEG phenomenon has transcended into a powerful contributor to the understanding of motor activity in general. This development started with the work of Pfurtscheller on event-related desynchronization (ERD) (Pfurtscheller and Aranibar, 1978a,b)—a phenomenon briefly mentioned in our discussion of posterior alpha rhythm reactivity. The ERD pertains even more strongly to the rolandic mu rhythm (and furthermore to various cognitive tasks and their cortical EEG accompaniment) (Pfurtscheller, 1981, 1990, 1992; Pfurtscheller and Klimesch, 1992; Pfurtscheller and Neuper, 1992; Pfurtscheller et al., 1994). In other words, the ERD has become a new criterion for the assessment of cortical functioning, over the motor cortex but also over various cortical regions of strong afferent input related to neurocognitive activities. Further detail on the ERD is found in the work of Pfurtscheller and Lopes da Silva (1999a,b) and Chapter 51 of this book, also written by Pfurtscheller and Lopes da Silva.

Age and Prevalence

Central mu rhythm used to be considered scarce. The introduction of the International Electrode System (10–20 system) has contributed to a much greater awareness of this pattern. The C_3 and C_4 electrodes are located over the precentral gyrus in an optimal location for picking up central mu rhythm. Large material tested with a different electrode system showed a prevalence of only 3.2% (Klass and Bickford, 1957) and 2.9% (Schnell and Klass, 1966). This lies well below the figures found in other studies.

Gastaut et al. (1954) found mu rhythm in 10% of their adult patients; Beek (1958) observed this rhythm in 13% of a predominantly psychiatric patient population. In 500 essentially healthy young male adults, Gastaut et al. (1959a,b) found mu rhythm in 14.4%; the mu rhythm was often found in persons with certain psychopathic personality traits as evidenced by the Minnesota Multiphasic Personality Inventory (MMPI) test. Dongier and Dongier (1958) noted mu rhythm in 18% of a population of neurotic patients. Figures of 12% were reported by Picard et al. (1955) and Simonova et al. (1966).

In the patients of Niedermeyer and Koshino (1975), the prevalence of mu rhythm was 8.1% (182 of 2,248); broken down into age ranges, there were 9.0% between ages 0 and 10 years, 13.8% between 11 and 20 years, 8.4% between 21 and 40 years, and 4.5% above 41 years. These authors demonstrated rolandic mu rhythm in a 20-month-old child; this was thought to be an exceptionally early manifestation of mu rhythm. But was it really exceptionally early? Not when one considers the data of Stroganova et al. (1999), who demonstrated central mu rhythm (during a state of attention) in the tracing of an 8-month-old baby with a frequency of about 6 to 8.8/sec. The authors contend that mu rhythm tends to appear before the occipital alpha-equivalent because, unlike visual stimulation, somatosensory stimulation is present within the uterus.

Familial occurrence of mu rhythm has been reported by Koshino and Isaki (1986). With the use of frequency analysis, the prevalence of mu rhythm reaches values close to 100% (Schoppenhorst et al., 1980).

Wave Morphology, Frequency, and Spatial Distribution

Older synonyms such as *rhythme en arceau* or *wicket rhythm* pertain to the wave morphology; mu rhythm shows in most instances a sharp (or spiky) negative and a rounded positive phase. There are a few patterns with a monophasic spiky appearance. Posterior alpha rhythm may have a similar configuration: "wicket spikes" (Fig. 9.3) have a similar appearance. The same is true for 14 and 6/sec positive spikes, except for the spike positive and rounded negative compounded. (As to negativity and positivity, see Chapter 8, "The EEG Signal: Polarity and Field Determination.") All these patterns show a spatial distribution that is different from the mu rhythm or occurs at levels of vigilance that are usually incompatible with mu rhythm. The amplitudes are comparable to those of the posterior alpha rhythm (Fig. 9.3).

The most common frequency of the mu rhythm is 10/sec. Frequencies may lie below 9/sec and above 11/sec; a mu rhythm of less than 8/sec is probably a mild abnormality. Mu rhythm is often mixed with local activity around 20/sec (Fig. 9.4). According to Storm van Leeuwen et al. (1978), mu frequencies are slightly higher than alpha frequencies. The spatial distribution is essentially confined to the precentral-postcentral region; some spread into parietal leads is not uncommon. The C_3 and C_4 electrodes are mostly involved; occasionally, a vertex (C_z) maximum is noted. A special

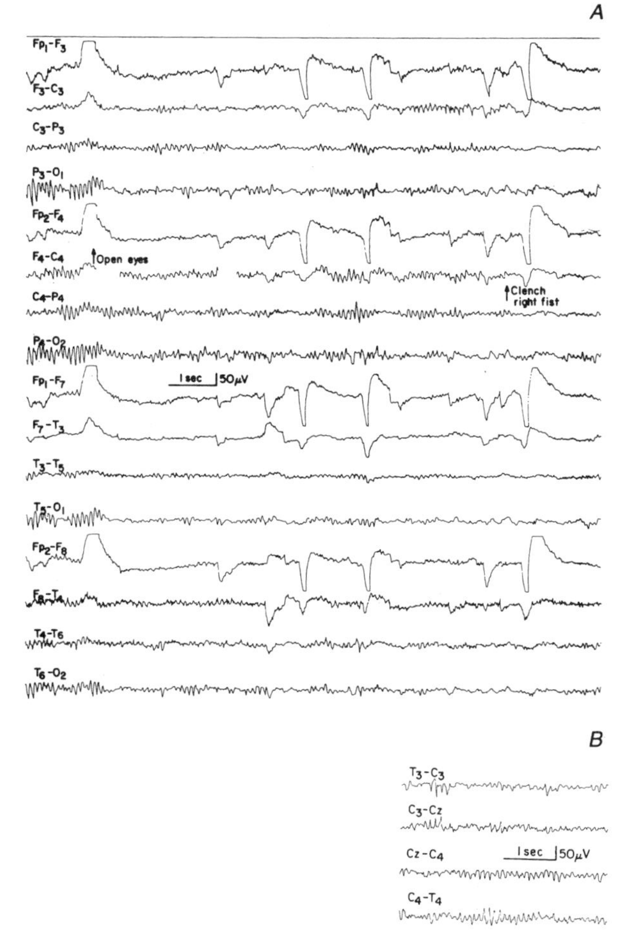

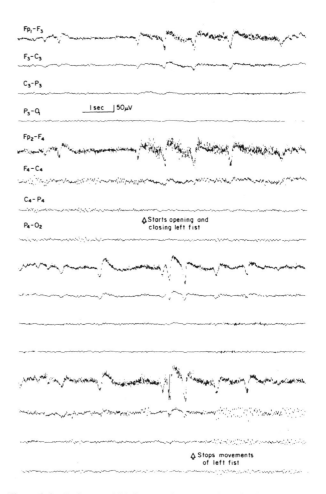

Figure 9.3. A: Rolandic mu rhythm, in a patient age 13 years. Stretches of central mu rhythm while eyes are kept open. These runs occur asynchronously on both sides and are blocked with clenching of right fist. Some posterior alpha rhythm persists after eye opening. Possible spread of mu rhythm into the parietal area makes differentiation of alpha and mu difficult in right parieto-occipital lead (eighth channel from the top). **B:** The close-up view of the same patient shows independent bilateral central mu rhythm.

Figure 9.4. Patient aged 51, 2 years after evacuation of a right-sided subdural hematoma. A right-sided central mu rhythm shows admixture of fast frequencies and spiky potentials. All components of this rhythm show a prominent and persistent blocking response to contralateral hand movements. (From Niedermeyer, E., and Koshino, Y. 1975. My-Rhythmus: Vorkommen und Klinische Bedeutung. *Z. EEG-EMG.* 6:69–78.)

vertex mu rhythm with special reactivity (lower limb) was described in aged patients by Farnarier et al. (1981). When recorded through bone defects, the mu rhythm is more widely distributed. According to Kuhlman (1978a), the maximum lies over the postcentral rather than the precentral cortex.

The alphoid (around 10/sec) and the fast (around 20/sec) component of the mu rhythm seem to be inseparably intermingled but, with more advanced technology, spatial separation is possible. According to Salmelin and Hari (1994a,b) the beta component arises from the motor cortex and the alphoid component from the sensory cortex. These magnetoencephalographic findings have been confirmed by Nashmi et al. (1994).

Mu rhythm usually occurs in short stretches. Persons with pronounced mu rhythm show long trains of mu rhythm.

In most persons with mu rhythm, this activity is bilateral but tends to shift from side to side. Coherence function studies have shown lack of bilateral coherence of mu rhythm in normal subjects (Storm van Leeuwen et al., 1978). Strictly unilateral mu rhythm must be scrutinized for the possibility of an ipsilateral rolandic disturbance as, for instance, an early stage of parasagittal meningioma, an arteriovenous malformation, or other types of neoplasm (Tannier et al., 1983). In such cases, even the possibility of a contralateral rolandic lesion must be taken into consideration (Gastaut, 1952; Hess, 1975; Kubicki et al., 1973). Above all, the possibility of a local cranial bone defect, surgical or traumatic, must be ruled out; a single burr hole in the rolandic region enables otherwise hidden mu rhythm to become manifest on the scalp (Fig. 9.4). Thus, mu rhythm represents at least a portion of rhythmical activity beneath bone defects ["breach rhythm," (Cobb et al., 1979)]; also see The "Third Rhythm" (Independent Temporal Alphoid Rhythm), below.

Reactivity

Mu rhythm is blocked by movements. These movements may be active (voluntary), passive, or reflexive (Chatrian, 1964, 1976a; Chatrian et al., 1959; Gastaut, 1952; Gastaut et al., 1952). The blocking effect is bilateral but more pronounced on the rolandic region contralateral to the site of movement; the effect appears prior to the onset of muscular contraction (Chatrian, 1976a; Chatrian et al., 1959; Gastaut, 1952; Gastaut et al., 1952; Klass and Bickford, 1957). According to Chatrian et at. (1959), there are delays of 50 msec to 7.5 seconds (average, 1.5 seconds) at the onset of the mu blocking effect after the initiation of the spontaneous flexion of the contralateral thumb, with the ipsilateral lagging behind the contralateral response. Gastaut et al. (1952) and Ciganek (1959) demonstrated a somatotopic distribution of the blocking effect (according to the functional anatomy of the rolandic cortex), but this observation could not be confirmed by Chatrian et al. (1959).

With the use of a gamma band (38–40/sec) frequency analysis focusing on the event-related synchronization (ERS) of the gamma component, Pfurtscheller et al. (1994) beautifully demonstrated the locus for right and left index finger movement, right toes, and the rather broad and bilateral area for tongue movements.

The mu blocking response is likely to be related to the conceptual design of the movement to be executed. Mere thoughts about performing movements and readiness to move block the mu rhythm (Chatrian, 1964, 1976a; Chatrian et al., 1959; Gastaut, 1952; Gastaut et al., 1952; Klass and Bickford, 1957). Mu blocking responses have also been demonstrated in persons with amputations of extremities; these mental activities concern movement of a phantom limb (Gastaut et al., 1965; Klass and Bickford, 1957).

Light tactile stimuli also produced a mu rhythm blocking effect that is most evident over the contralateral rolandic region (Chatrian, 1964, 1976a; Chatrian et al., 1959; Gastaut, 1952; Gastaut et al., 1952; Magnus, 1954). Kuhlman (1978a) has placed even greater emphasis on the sensory component and regards mu rhythm as the "idling" of the cortical sensory region, in analogy to the alpha rhythm as "idling" of the visual cortex and its vicinity. His work was carried out with power spectral analysis. This technique shows that central mu rhythm is a more common phenomenon than one would expect from the visual analysis of the scalp EEG (also see the power spectra study of Pfurtscheller and Aranibar, 1978a). These authors also showed simultaneous posterior alpha desynchronization (Pfurtscheller and Aranibar, 1978a,b). Coherence functions have also been used for the demonstration of rolandic mu rhythm (Schoppenhorst et al., 1980; Storm van Leeuwen et al., 1978).

It has been noted that rolandic mu rhythm is enhanced during intermittent photic stimulation (Brechet and Lecasble, 1965) and pattern vision (Koshino and Niedermeyer, 1975). The latter observation would contradict the basic law of mu rhythm as a rhythm of immobility; one is tempted to perceive the extraocular movements involved in pattern vision as a different ("extrarolandic") system in the motor organization.

Mu Rhythm, the (Slower) 20/Sec Beta and the (Faster) 40/Sec Beta (or Gamma) Components

The separation of the mu rhythm proper (around 10/sec) and the 20/sec beta component have been mentioned earlier. The 40/sec gamma component is not a spontaneous rhythm; rather, it constitutes the fast activity associated with the enhancement (event-related synchronization, ERS) of small preexisting activity with movement according to Pfurtscheller and his co-workers.

Cortical Rolandic Basis of Mu Rhythm

Jasper and Penfield (1949) found evidence of a strictly localized beta (around 20/sec) over the human motor cortex with electrocorticographic recording technique in the locally anesthetized patient. This rhythm could be blocked like mu rhythm with movement, especially contralateral movement, and also with thinking about the execution of movement. This rhythm is obviously the cortical equivalent of rolandic mu rhythm on the scalp. The mu waves on the scalp often show some notching or are imbedded in local fast activity, which is also blocked by movement. Gastaut (1952) confirmed the cortical precentral fast activity in electrocorticographic tracings. These data conflict with Kuhlman's (1978a) observation of a postcentral maximum of rolandic mu rhythm (scalp recordings with power spectral analysis). On the other hand, Graf et al. (1984) demonstrated precentral 8 to 10/sec mu rhythm in the electrocorticogram of an adult epileptic.

As mentioned earlier, mu rhythm around 10/sec on the scalp and cortical rolandic 20/sec activity appear to be harmonically related; such a relationship, however, does not exist between mu rhythm and rolandic beta activity on the scalp according to Pfurtscheller (1981) who used power spectral analysis. Quantitative EEG studies have also established a clean separating line between mu rhythm and posterior alpha rhythm (Van Huffelen et al., 1984).

A study of the functional significance of the mu rhythm from the human cortex was carried out with subdural electrodes by Arroyo et al. (1993). This work also showed the relationship of the cortical mu rhythm to the well-known somatotopic arrangement of the sensorimotor cortex.

Mu Rhythm-Like Activity in the Experimental Animal

A sensorimotor 7 to 14/sec rhythm has been demonstrated in quiet cats trained to obtain a reward (Chase and Harper, 1971; Sterman et al., 1969, 1970; Wyrwicka and Sterman, 1968). A similar rhythm of immobility was shown by Rougeul et al. (1972) in the cat; this is a 14/sec rhythm presumed to originate in the nucleus ventralis posterior of the thalamus (Bouyer et al., 1983).

Mu Rhythm Conditioning and Feedback Training

An impressive international study on mu rhythm and the phasic evolution of conditioning was presented by Gastaut et al. (1957). Mu rhythm feedback training has been used for various purposes, including the treatment of epileptic seizure disorders (Finley et al., 1975; Kuhlman, 1978b,c; Sterman et al., 1974). Roldan et al. (1981) observed the development of mu rhythm-like activity in the course of Hatha yoga exercises. This activity was called chi rhythm. It was believed to be a specific rolandic pattern of 11 to 17/sec waves and theta frequencies.

Evidence of More than One Type of Rolandic Mu Rhythm

This question has been raised by Covello et al. (1975), who feel that several entities of mu rhythm exist, even in one subject, and that their underlying physiological mechanisms may differ. Personal impressions lend some support to this idea. Earlier observations (Niedermeyer and Koshino, 1975) led to the conclusion that even the slightest degree of lessened vigilance (i.e., earliest drowsiness) was incompatible with mu rhythm; this view has been supported by Schoppenhorst et al. (1980). However, there have been some personal observations of patients demonstrating their best stretches of central mu rhythm in the light drowsy state after posterior alpha dropout. Yamada and Kooi (1975) even described mu rhythm in sleep [stages 1 and 2, as well as rapid-eye-movement (REM) sleep] in 20 individuals (19 patients with various complaints). The concept of Covello et al. (1975) is certainly in need of further study.

Mu Rhythm Status

The word *status* is not necessarily reserved for sustained epileptic activity (e.g., status migrainosus, status asthmaticus). Unusually sustained mu rhythm activity ("mu rhythm status") has been observed by Niedermeyer et al., 2004, in the setting of frontal lobe impairment and also in the absence of pathology (perhaps a side effect of levetiracetam).

Clinical Significance of Mu Rhythm

Rolandic mu rhythm as such is categorically within normal limits. In some cases, unusually spiky discharges may be present and even single spikes may stand out; such tracings are slightly abnormal. Children with benign rolandic epilepsy (see Chapter 27, "Epileptic Seizure Disorders") may gradually develop mu rhythm when rolandic spike activity subsides and the seizures appear to be under control. In such patients, grand mal or focal motor attack seizures may return later in adult life under unusual circumstances, such as severe stress with insomnia or infections. There are indeed a certain number of adults with rare grand mal attacks and normal EEG tracings featuring some central mu rhythm. This could be merely a coincidence, but there is reason to presume that mu rhythm may have a certain relationship to epileptic seizure disorders. Interestingly, in some children with benign rolandic epilepsy, cerebral spikes can be blocked by contralateral movements in the same manner as mu rhythm is blocked (Niedermeyer, 1972a,b). This response is not present in all children with rolandic spikes; this explains negative responses to motor activity reported by Isch-Treussard (1972).

Patients or control subjects with rolandic mu rhythm appear to be more prone to headaches than the average population (Schnell and Klass, 1966). Gastaut et al. (1954) and Bostem et al. (1964) emphasized relationships between mu rhythm and a variety of dysfunctions such as migraine, bronchial asthma, peptic ulcer eczema, tinnitus, arterial hypertension, and hyperthyroid states. Mu rhythm has been thought to be related to a low pain threshold (Niedermeyer et al., 1982).

According to Dongier and Dongier (1958), mu rhythm is common in patients with mild to moderate psychiatric disorders; it is associated with anxiety, aggressiveness, emotional instability, and psychosomatic disorders. Netchine et al. (1964) presented a psychodynamic theory of mu rhythm that is thought to be enhanced with repressed aggression and absent in patients with overt aggressiveness.

Relationships to other EEG patterns of marginal or mildly abnormal character have been pointed out (14 and 6/sec positive spikes, 6/sec spike waves; see Chapter 13). These patterns are often found in association with mild to moderate psychiatric disturbances and autonomic nervous system dysfunction.

Does this mean that rolandic mu rhythm—generally conceived as a physiological pattern—is, in reality, a mild abnormality? Let us reflect for a moment on the earlier statement that every healthy adolescent and adult harbors central mu rhythm when power spectra and coherence tests are utilized (see the aforementioned work of Schoppenhorst et al., 1980). Why then is mu rhythm evident in the conventional EEG in just a minority of persons? The answer is quite logical: their mu rhythm has to be more powerful than that of average persons in order to be picked up from the scalp. Thus, an individual with mu rhythm in the conventional EEG (and optimally placed electrodes) might already have a certain "excess" of mu rhythm. Such a presumed excess could be an indicator of local hyperexcitability. From here, the road could lead to autonomic (vegetative) dysfunctions, emotional dyscontrol and even to epileptic activities. Thus, life without a (conventionally recordable) mu rhythm could be easier than life with excessive mu rhythm activity.

In cases of strictly unilateral mu rhythm, a careful search for bone defects (bur holes) and/or local pathology is indicated. In the wake of ischemic hemiplegic insults, central mu rhythm may disappear or its reactivity may vanish (Pfurtscheller, 1986).

Theories of Neurophysiological Basis of Mu Rhythm

There are in essence three theories to be dealt with: (a) the hypothesis of "neuronal hyperexcitability" ("hyperexcitabilité neuronique"), either diffuse or locally restricted to the rolandic cortex (Beek, 1958; Gastaut, 1952; Gastaut et al., 1952; Van der Drift and Magnus, 1961); (b) the hypothesis of superficial cortical inhibition ("inhibition corticale superficielle"), comparable to aforementioned theories of "cortical idling"; this theory would explain the suppression of mu rhythm with motor activity (Bostem et al., 1964, 1965; Gastaut et al., 1964, 1965); and (c) the hypothesis of somatosensory "cortical idling," turning mu rhythm into an afference-dependent phenomenon (Kuhlman, 1978a).

In the discussion of central mu rhythm, simple mechanical factors must never be forgotten, not only the well-known facilitation of mu rhythm by local defects of bone, but even the possibility of an unusually thin scalp locally over the rolandic region.

Breach Rhythm (Rhythms Over Skull Defects)

The presence of cranial bone defects has considerable effect on the EEG frequency spectrum recorded from the overlying scalp. Fischgold et al. (1952) focused attention on this subject. In the following, this topic is discussed chiefly in connection with rolandic mu rhythm.

As has been pointed out, rolandic mu rhythm may become very prominent beneath a bone defect; this EEG pattern is naturally suppressed by motor activity. There is, however, a rhythmical activity in the 6 to 11/sec range that does not respond to movements and is found mainly over the midtemporal region (electrodes T_3 or T_4). This activity often shows spike character. The work of Cobb et al. (1979) has beautifully demonstrated the characteristics of this type of "breach rhythm" as a special entity among the EEG patterns. Bone replacement may or may not lead to some reduction of the midtemporal rhythm. Breach rhythm of the midtemporal variety is possibly an abnormal rhythm related to cerebral pathology; for this reason, its discussion in this chapter on the normal EEG may not be appropriate. In addition to surgical and traumatic skull lesions, an osteolytic skull metastasis can also give rise to local breach rhythm (Radhakrishnan et al., 1994).

The "Third Rhythm" (Independent Temporal Alphoid Rhythm)

Rhythmical activity in the alpha and upper theta range can be picked up from epidural electrodes over the midtem-poral region (Niedermeyer, 1990a-c, 1991, 1997). This rhythm is not detectable in the scalp EEG unless there is a local bone defect in the midtemporal region where it has been termed (together with coexisting central mu rhythm in the vicinity) "breach rhythm" by Cobb et al. (1979), who regarded the temporal activity as an abnormal rhythm.

There is now good reason to presume that the rhythmical temporal lobe activity, which is clearly independent from the posterior alpha and rolandic mu rhythm, constitutes a physiological rhythm.

The presence of such an independent temporal alpha rhythm has also been demonstrated with the use of magnetoencephalography in healthy adults by Hari (personal communication, 1990, 1991), who feels that this rhythm is strongly related to the cortical auditory function ("auditory alpha rhythm") (see Hari's Chapter 57, "Magnetoencephalography as a Tool of Clinical Neurophysiology"). Personal data (Niedermeyer, 1990a-c, 1991) do not provide good evidence for a relationship to auditory function. In some individuals, cognitive activities result in blocking responses of the third rhythm. It seems that the function of this rhythm is still debatable.

In the wake of the usual partial temporal lobectomy for the treatment of temporal lobe epilepsy, the third rhythm cannot be recorded despite the presence of surgical bone defects. Naturally, the auditory cortex remains preserved in this procedure. If the concept of an "auditory alpha rhythm" were correct, one would expect a particularly strong third rhythm after removal of overlying neocortical temporal lobe tissue. This is one more reason for disagreement with Hari's view.

Rhythmical activity in the alpha and upper theta range over the anterior temporal–midtemporal region in conventional scalp EEGs can be found in patients with cerebrovascular problems (Kendel and Koufen, 1970) and other types of temporal lobe changes but this abnormal rhythm can be differentiated from the physiological "third rhythm" (Niedermeyer, 1991).

Over the ensuing years, there has been almost no discussion concerning the nature of the third rhythm/tau rhythm. Bastiaansen et al. (1999) were unable to reach conclusions about these rhythms. Shinomiya et al. (1999) studied the third rhythm in eight patients with local bone defects. These authors carefully distinguished the third rhythm from the rhythmical form of temporal minor slow and sharp activity in cerebrovascular disorder.

Kappa Rhythm

This anterior temporal rhythm in alpha frequency was first reported by Laugier and Liberson (1937) and subsequently studied by Kennedy et al. (1948). Chatrian (1976b) has presented a lucid review of the literature on this phenomenon, which is unlikely to be an authentic cerebral rhythm. It is possibly an ocular artifact caused by discrete lateral oscillations of the eyeballs. Kappa rhythm has become all but forgotten and may be regarded as a nonissue in the field of EEG.

Beta Rhythms

The Greek letter *beta* stands for the frequency band above 13/sec. In customary EEG recording, frequencies above 70/sec are considerably attenuated due to filter effects. This establishes a natural upper limit of the beta band somewhere between 50 and 100/sec; otherwise, the upper limit of the beta band is open-ended. Faster chart speed or even special technical equipment is needed for studies of the fast frequency band. Any rhythmical EEG activity above 13/sec may be regarded as beta rhythm. Rhythmical beta activity is encountered chiefly over the frontal and central regions; it usually does not exceed 35/sec. A central beta rhythm is related to the rolandic mu rhythm and can be blocked by motor activity or tactile stimulation [see Rolandic (Central) Mu Rhythm, above]. The amplitude of beta activity seldom exceeds 30 μV. Beta activity may be locally enhanced over bone defects and shows considerable increase (in quantity and voltage) after the administration of barbiturates, some nonbarbituric sedatives, and minor tranquilizers. With very large amounts and high amplitudes of beta activity, abnormal proportions may be reached; in general, however, fast activity alone is seldom a cogent reason for calling a tracing abnormal.

Historically, the discovery of beta activity is closely linked to the first description of the alpha rhythm by Berger (1929). His first report on the human EEG of 1929 contains the following passage: "The electroencephalogram represents a continuous curve with continuous oscillations in which . . . one can distinguish larger first order waves with an average duration of 90 sigma (msec) and smaller second order waves of an average duration of 35 sigma (msec)" (after Gloor, 1971). In his second report, Berger (1930) pointed out: "For the sake of brevity I shall subsequently designate the waves of first order as alpha waves, the waves of second order as beta waves." Berger (1938) reversed earlier views and pointed out "that the beta waves and not the alpha waves of the EEG are the concomitant phenomena of mental activity." This concept is now provoking renewed interest.

As to differences between beta and gamma (around or above 40/sec) activity, the reader should return to the beginning of this chapter. The old term *gamma* for the designation of faster beta activity used to be all but forgotten until its resurrection around 1990.

Prevalence of Beta Activity

Beta activity is found in almost every healthy adult. Simon's (1977) statement that beta frequencies have been found in 22% of normal adults probably applies to more conspicuous forms of beta activity. Depth EEG studies and electrocorticograms show a remarkably large share of the beta band; such recordings have been obtained mostly in epileptics or in patients with neurological or psychiatric problems. Although obtained in patients and not in healthy persons, such depth records are quite informative concerning the spatial distribution of fast frequencies. Every scalp recording performed over a bone defect gives testimony to the wealth of cortical beta activity.

The prevalence of beta activity in the normal person can also be derived from various studies of normal volunteers (Brazier and Finesinger, 1944; Finley, 1944; Gallais et al., 1957; Gibbs et al., 1943; Mundy-Castle, 1951, 1953; Obrist, 1954; Picard et al., 1957; Roger and Bert, 1959; Vogel and Fujiya, 1969). The results of these studies have been re-

viewed by Kuhlo (1976b) in his thorough EEG handbook article on beta rhythms. Later work has been presented by Fortuin and Künkel (1983) and Kozelak and Pedley (1990).

The Gibbsian Approach: Distinction According to Beta Quantity

Gibbs and Gibbs (1950) distinguished two types of predominantly fast records. A moderate increase of fast activity was termed "F1" and a marked increase, "F2." Records of the F1 type were regarded as abnormal until the 40th year; F2 type records were regarded as abnormal at any age (Gibbs and Gibbs, 1950). Even an F3 type ("exceedingly fast") was introduced by Gibbs and Gibbs (1950).

Electroencephalographers have shown a more lenient philosophy toward fast tracings over the ensuing years. Beta activity must be particularly abundant in quantity and of rather high voltage to be termed abnormal. Even such fast records are categorically but slightly abnormal unless they occur in unresponsive patients, where such fast activity may represent a severe abnormality. This view is essentially congruent with the study of Drake (1984).

Further Attempts at a Differentiation of Beta Activities

Spatial Characteristics

In certain individuals, the posterior alpha rhythm is unusually fast and its frequency exceeds the upper limit of the alpha rhythm (13/sec). Such a 14 to 15/sec rhythm shows a good blocking response to eye opening and enhancement with eye closure; it may be considered a fast equivalent of the alpha rhythm. Gradual acceleration of the alpha frequency may be caused by hyperthyroidism (see Chapter 22, "Metabolic Central Nervous System Disorders," Fig. 22.9). Vogel and Götze (1962) separated the occipital 14 to 19/sec rhythm from the rest of beta activities, which were divided into frontocentral bursts of 20 to 30/sec waves and normal occipital alpha rhythm and diffuse beta activity generally mixed with alpha frequencies. Vogel (1962, 1966, 1970) subsequently divided the anterior beta activity into the 25 to 30/sec activity of the frontal region, occurring in brief trains, and the 20 to 25/sec activity of comparatively larger amplitudes occurring for variable periods.

Frontal runs of beta activity often exceed 30/sec and reach 35 to 40/sec when the patient is allowed to fall asleep. This activity may be found in unmedicated persons; sleep-inducing medication, which increases the activity in the 18 to 25/sec band, also augments activities in the faster beta range.

The region of fastest EEG frequencies and highest levels of cerebral blood flow (as well as oxygen and glucose uptake) is located in the frontocentral area. This observation has prompted the concept of "cerebral hyperfrontality" (Ingvar, 1987). This investigator has pointed out that (a) prefrontal activity constitutes an integral part of consciousness, and (b) abnormal prefrontal activity is accompanied by various forms of altered consciousness.

The physiological beta frequencies may be broken down as follows:

1. Frontal beta: fairly common, may be very fast, no relationship to physiological rhythm.

2. Central beta: partly but not generally the basis of rolandic mu rhythm often mixed with mu rhythm.
3. Posterior beta: often a fast alpha equivalent, reactive like alpha rhythm.
4. Diffuse beta: no linkage with any special physiological rhythm.

By contrast, "vertex beta" or "fast central midline rhythm" (Veilleux et al., 1988)—vertex activity in the 10 to 25/sec range—appears to be the expression of polyetiological focal abnormality in the frontocentral region.

Relationship to Personality Traits

Beta activity over the central region reportedly is absent in emotionally stable persons (Gallais et al., 1957; Picard et al., 1957; Remond and Lesèvre, 1957). Gastaut (1957) pointed out that the central fast rhythm and the closely related mu rhythm correlate with aggressive, domineering, and dynamic personality traits. Gastaut et al. (1960), however, felt that more detailed statistical analysis could not corroborate the aforementioned correlations.

In the older literature, fast activity was thought to be more common in patients with psychiatric problems (Finley, 1944). Cohn (1946) noted frontal beta activity (18–22/sec, 10–50 μV) in patients suffering from anxiety states. Gibbs and Gibbs (1950) reported a high incidence of very fast activity (above 30/sec) ("F3 type") in "dull psychopaths." Giannitrappani and Kayton (1974) demonstrated a prominent peak of 29/sec activity with the use of power spectral analysis in schizophrenic patients. A discussion of correlations between fast activity and neurological disorders would be inappropriate in a chapter dealing with the normal EEG. During the entire maturational period (including early adulthood), beta activity has been found to be relatively more prominent in females than in males (Matsuura et al., 1985).

Beta Activity and Drugs

This subject is discussed in Chapter 34, "EEG, Drug Effects, and Central Nervous System Poisoning."

Beta Activity at the Onset of Movements

Rhythmical 40/sec activity has been demonstrated over the left central region (C3 electrode) at the onset of self-paced voluntary right finger movements (Pfurtscheller and Neuper, 1992). With "event-related desynchronization" of local rhythmical activity around 10/sec in the movement-programming stage, a burst of 40/sec activity ("event-related synchronization") coincides with the initiation of movement. Naturally, the 40/sec activity had to be carefully separated from muscle potentials.

"Ultra-fast" EEG Activity

Interest in the ultrafast range from 80 to 1,000/sec has been surging over the past few years. The availability of digital EEG recording has flung open the gate to this new domain and it is just a matter of a few years and is going to stimulate new and very promising work. This range will provide us with new epileptological insights (Draguhn et al., 2000; Niedermeyer and Sherman, 2001a,b; Schiff et al., 2000) but also, above all, with a new understanding of corti-

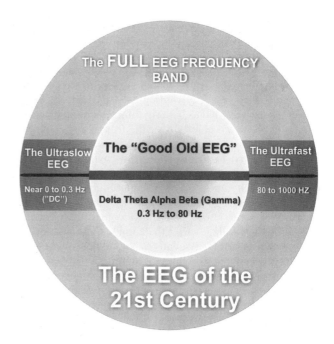

Figure 9.5.   The EEG of the 21st century. (See Color Figure 9.5.)

cal perception, motor activity, and, in particular, neurocognitive processes (Curio, 2000 a,b; Traub et al., 1999; Ziemann and Rothwell, 2000). A new chapter on ultrafast activity by Curio has been added to this volume (see Chapter 26).

Parallel with this new wave, there has been also renewed interest in ultraslow activity, from near zero (DC) up to 0.3/sec available nowadays. This range can improve focal epilepsy diagnosis (Vanhatalo et al., 2003, who have also contributed a new chapter to this volume; see Chapter 25). This range will also be fruitful for neurocognitive research and motor initiation not to leave aside sleep studies in prematurity (Vanhatalo et al., 2002).

Figure 9.5 illustrates these new research direction as the basis for the EEG of the 21st century. Interestingly, the very optimistic study on the future of EEG in assessing neurocognitive functions (Gevins, 1998) does not explicitly mention the possibilities provided by and enlarged frequency band but speaks of "fine-grain temporal resolution."

Very fast activity (beyond the conventional EEG range) has been found in cerebellar structures of animals, mostly in the range of 200 to 300/sec (Adrian, 1934; Bremer, 1958; Dow, 1938; Snider, 1950). Trabka (1963) found similar high EEG frequencies in the cerebrum of cats.

The Low-Voltage Record

A below-average voltage output is compatible with perfect central nervous system (CNS) functioning. In such individuals, the small amplitudes are the result of a lesser degree of synchronization of electrical activity in the neuronal level. Brainstem reticular formation systems strongly influence the degree of cortical neuronal synchronization; arousal mediated through the ascending mesodiencephalic reticular formation has a desynchronizing effect (Moruzzi and Magoun, 1949), whereas synchronizing effects are presumed to originate from the pontine portion of the ascending reticular formation (Magnes et al., 1961; Magni et al., 1959).

This type of brainstem regulation of the cortical EEG synchronization is likely to account for numerous fluctuations in the EEG amplitudes, especially those related to the level of vigilance. It is not clear whether these reticular effects account for a low-voltage EEG as a personal trait (with genetic determination, as will be pointed out later). Under pathological conditions, low-voltage tracings in vertebrobasilar artery insufficiency (to be discussed in Chapter 17) are probably due to some degree of pontine ischemia acting on the reticular formation. This could also be true for the frequently encountered low-voltage tracings of chronic alcoholics in advanced stages, with the possibility of early stages of pontine myelinolysis; this explanation, however, is but a working hypothesis (Lawson and Niedermeyer, 2002). True decline of the cerebral EEG voltage output (i.e., low-voltage activity independent of desynchronizing mechanisms) is a grave danger sign of a preterminal state unless it occurs for a few seconds only, as in certain syncopal attacks. It may also indicate diffuse chronic cortical degeneration (as described by Rosas et al., 2003).

Definition and Categories of Low-Voltage Records

The term *low-voltage EEG* has always proved to be quite flexible; it is in need of a strict definition. It was pointed out earlier in this chapter that precise figures concerning amplitudes are not truly accurate, because they depend on interelectrode distances and the montage; even an ear electrode may be slightly contaminated with EEG activity. The definition of Chatrian et al. (IFSECN, 1974) reads as follows:

> Low voltage record. A waking record characterized by activity of amplitudes not greater than 20 μV over all head regions. With appropriate instrumental sensitivities this activity can be shown to be composed primarily of beta, theta and, to a lesser degree, delta waves, with or without alpha activity, over the posterior areas.

This definition serves as a solid guideline. One could subdivide low-voltage records into two or three degrees; occasionally, one may see tracings in which 10 μV are not exceeded. Even such "very low voltage records" may be due to desynchronization and thus occur in a waking and alert patient or even in a control subject (Fig. 9.6). Low-voltage records are categorically within broad normal limits of variability and do not represent an abnormality unless the frequency spectrum shows abnormal local or diffuse slowing, asymmetries, or paroxysmal events. In a comatose patient, one must infer that the low voltage is due to true decline of cerebral activity and not merely caused by desynchronization. Such records must be regarded as extremely abnormal. This indicates that the record reader should depend on behavior observation (patient comatose, on respirator, etc.). On the other hand, the EEG as such reveals signs of telltale character for the experienced reader, such as presence or absence of eye blinks, types of artifacts, etc., even when he or she must read without any behavioral information.

The IFSECN (1974) definition does not elaborate on sleep and response to hyperventilation. It also omits the

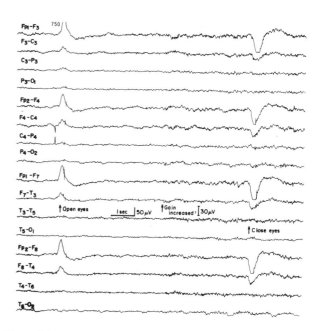

Figure 9.6. Low-voltage record with poor alpha organization, in a patient age 31 years. Note that recording was done with above-standard gain. Finer details demonstrable with further gain increase.

question of low-voltage alpha versus low-voltage fast records. One could add further categories of low-voltage records in the following manner:

1. Low-voltage fast record awake but voltage increase in non-REM sleep
   (a) with alpha improvement and voltage increase during hyperventilation (provided that the patient is cooperative in the test),
   (b) without alpha improvement and voltage increase during a well-performed hyperventilation;
2. Low-voltage fast record awake with persisting low voltage in non-REM sleep;
3. Low-voltage record awake with good alpha organization and voltage increase in sleep
   (a) with voltage increase during hyperventilation,
   (b) without voltage increase during hyperventilation;
4. Low-voltage record awake with good alpha organization and persisting low voltage in sleep.

The distinction between low voltage fast records and those with good alpha rhythm was suggested by Gastaut et al. (1957).

Prevalence and Electroclinical Correlations

Early studies of low-voltage tracings were carried out by Davis and Davis (1936), Jasper et al. (1939), and Finley (1944). Jasper et al. (1939) used the term *flat EEG*, which is not reserved for truly isoelectric records.

Gibbs et al. (1943) (also see Gibbs and Gibbs, 1950, 1964) found low-voltage fast records in 11.6% of 1,000 normal adult subjects. The study of Adams (1959) revealed a prevalence of 8% (in 427 normal individuals); the breakdown into age ranges is most important, because low-voltage tracings were found in 1% between ages 0 and 20 years, 7% between 20 and 39 years, and 11% between 40 and 69 years. Pine and Pine (1953) reported 7.25% low voltage records in 2,000 neurological and psychiatric patients between 17 and 70 years. Vogel and Götze (1959) found low-voltage tracings in 7.09% of 1,540 patients. In 7,000 patients including a large pediatric segment, only 3.6% were found to have a low-voltage tracing (Niedermeyer, 1963).

According to Gibbs and Gibbs (1950), the prevalence of low-voltage tracings increases sharply after age 13. This is congruent with the observations of Panzani and Turner (1952), Adams (1959), and Lucioni and Penati (1966). Low-voltage fast records in children below age 10 are suspect and clearly abnormal if neither hyperventilation nor non-REM sleep changes the low-voltage character of the tracing. In adults, persistence of low-voltage activity with hyperventilation and sleep is not categorically abnormal, although this lends more support to the presumption that such patients have an organic cerebral disorder. Chatrian (1976c) stressed the high incidence of low-voltage tracings in postconcussion syndrome and posttraumatic neurosis.

Posttraumatic records have been studied by Duensing (1948), Meyer-Mickeleit (1953), Vogel et al. (1961), Courjon (1962), Mifka and Scherzer (1962), Arfel et al. (1963), Lorenzoni (1963), and Scherzer (1966). Low-voltage records show a high incidence in posttraumatic patients, and "psychogenic alpha suppression" often accounts for the small amplitudes (Scherzer, 1966). Hyperventilation quickly leads to alpha development and voltage increase. Not all posttraumatic low-voltage records should be attributed to such psychological mechanisms of "posttraumatic neurosis" or "litigation neurosis"; there seems to be a niche for an organic posttraumatic syndrome with low-voltage EEG tracings (Chatrian, 1976c). Radermecker (1961) and Kugler (1964) have minimized the value of EEG as a method of "objectivation" of the patient's posttraumatic complaints.

Basal ganglia diseases show a somewhat higher incidence of low-voltage records. In the case of Huntington's chorea, however, progressive voltage decline could perhaps indicate "true" loss of cortical activity rather than desynchronization; a view supported by the work of Rosas et al. (2003). There has been some suggestion that endocrine and psychiatric disorders are associated with a greater incidence of low-voltage tracing (Adams, 1959).

There is some evidence that genetic factors play an important role in determining a low-voltage tracing in a healthy person (Vogel and Götze, 1959). This genetic predisposition, however, obviously does not manifest itself in infancy or childhood, a time when almost all low-voltage records bear the mark of abnormality. With adolescence (age 13, according to Gibbs and Gibbs [1950]), an unknown maturational change apparently starts to desynchronize the cortical EEG activity. Adams (1968) has contended that, in the presence of CNS pathology, the low-voltage fast character tends to change and the record shows local or diffuse slowing. The evolution of an epileptic seizure disorder is also likely to interfere with the previous low-voltage character of a tracing. The statement that the epileptic seizure disorders are very seldom associated with a low-voltage EEG (Adams, 1959) is certainly correct. However, a low-voltage record does not rule out an epileptic seizure disorder, even when one leaves aside the group of chronic alcoholics with withdrawal seizures and predominantly low-voltage tracings. This view has been supported by the work of Synek (1983).

According to this author's experience, two major groups of adult neurological patients are characterized by the frequent occurrence of low-voltage tracings: (a) patients with chronic vertebrobasilar artery insufficiency (even though this view has been criticized by Chatrian [1976c]), and (b) patients with chronic alcoholism (Krauss and Niedermeyer, 1991). Further discussion is found in Chapter 17, "Cerebrovascular Disorders and EEG," and Chapter 34, "EEG, Drug Effects, and CNS Poisoning."

Theta Rhythms

The term *theta* was introduced by Walter and Dovey (1944) and denotes the frequency range of 4 to 7/sec or 4 to 7.5/sec. This frequency band was a part of the delta range until Walter and Dovey felt that an intermediate band should be established. The term *theta* was chosen in order to allude to its presumed thalamic origin. The intermediate character of the theta band has been stressed in the German terminology *Zwischenwellen*, meaning intermediate waves. According to the international nomenclature, the theta band is the "frequency band from 4 to under 8 Hz" and the theta rhythm is the "rhythm with a frequency of 4 to under 8 Hz" (IFSECN, 1974).

Theta Activity in the Waking Adult

The normal adult waking record contains but a small amount of theta frequencies and no organized theta rhythm. Theta frequencies and theta rhythms, however, play an important role in infancy and childhood, as well as in states of drowsiness and sleep. The most important aspect is the maturational one; the reader will find more pertinent information in Chapter 11, "Maturation of the EEG: Development of Waking and Sleep Patterns." Larger contingents of theta activity in the waking adult are abnormal and are caused by various forms of pathology.

Studies of young adults such as army personnel and navy pilots have shown a sizable amount of theta activity (Gallais et al., 1957; Picard et al., 1957) because these slow frequencies tend to linger on through the third decade of life; the completely mature aspect of the human EEG cannot be expected before the age of 25 to 30 years.

On the basis of power spectra from normal adults, Rugg and Dickens (1982) presume that alpha and theta activity is generated by separate mechanisms.

Slow (theta and delta) EEG activity has been correlated with cholinergic activities and central cholinergic pathways (Steriade et al., 1990). The observation of slowing induced by the action of cholinergic substances on the ascending brainstem reticular formation dates back to Rinaldi and Himwich (1955). Further information is found in the overview of Riekkinen et al. (1991).

Hedonic Theta Rhythms

W. Grey Walter (1959) has associated theta activity with emotional processes, and thought that this activity might be a sign of "relative maturity of the mechanisms linking the cortex, the thalamus and the hypothalamus" (also see Knott, 1976b). He also attributed runs of theta waves to the emotional correlates of disappointment and frustration because of its appearance at the conclusion or interruption of a pleasurable stimulus. Similar views were expressed by Garsche (1956) and Lairy (1956). Maulsby (1971) presented a very impressive combined EEG and photographic demonstration of a 9-month-old girl and her EEG response to pleasurable stimuli; the most effective stimulus was being kissed by her mother. The response consisted of very pronounced rhythmical 4/sec activity of posterior accentuation, strongly spreading into central areas. This rhythm was different from the rhythmical 5 to 6/sec activity seen in this child's drowsy state. The 4/sec activity appeared to be pleasure-related rather than caused by the termination of a pleasurable stimulus. Similar rhythmical 4/sec activities were described by Kugler and Laub (1971) in children between the ages of 6 months and 6 years, elicited by watching puppets, moving objects, toys, and picture books ("puppet show theta rhythm"). Such hedonic EEG responses have not been observed in the adult EEG. According to Futagi et al. (1998), infantile theta rhythm associated with sucking, crying, gazing, and handling (including the hedonic type) is due to cortical activation driven by the limbic system.

From the Hedonic Theta Rhythm to EEG Findings During Sexual Activities

It may be interesting to note in this context that Mosovich and Tallaferro (1954) obtained EEG tracings from volunteers during coitus and masturbation. Further studies of human orgasm were carried out by Sem-Jacobsen (1968) and Heath (1972) with the use of depth electrodes in chronic psychiatric patients. Pre- and intraorgasmic paroxysmal discharges were reported by these authors (septal spiking; Heath, 1972), but the tracings of Heath show no special thalamic participation and no theta rhythm in the depth. A thorough EEG and polygraphic study of ejaculation and orgasm was carried out in young healthy males (Graber et al., 1985). The results turned out to be quite meager. "We have failed to demonstrate any significant and specific EEG changes during masturbation, ejaculation and the subjective experience of orgasm." This is probably a barren field for EEG research.

Other Physiological or Marginal Theta Rhythms

The 6 to 7/sec rhythm over the frontal midline is discussed in Chapter 11, "Maturation of the EEG: Development of Waking and Sleep Patterns." This rhythm usually disappears in adolescence. The theta activities described in children with primary generalized epilepsy and in their healthy siblings ("rhythmical monomorphic" 4 to 7/sec activity of parietal accentuation in children from 2 to 7 years) are discussed in Chapter 27, "Epileptic Seizure Disorders" and Chapter 11, "Maturation of the EEG: Development of Waking and Sleep Patterns."

With the use of a stress paradigm, Nowak and Marczynski (1981) produced in six of 24 healthy volunteers a rhythmical 5 to 6/sec theta response originating from either the occipital region or vertex during a state of maximal alertness.

A rhythmical 4/sec pattern occurring over the vertex solely in the waking state has been described as "4/sec vertex spindles" by Van Huffelen and Magnus (1973). This very rare pattern is likely to represent a mild abnormality. It is found mainly in adolescents with syncopal attacks and other signs of vasomotor instability. The use of the term *spindles* appears to be somewhat out of place when one considers the slow frequency and the occurrence in the waking state. Hence, Daoust-Roy (1989) proposed the term *4/sec vertex rhythm.*

Frontal Midline 6–7/Sec Theta Rhythm and Thinking

Rhythmical theta activity in the 6 to 7/sec range over the frontal midline region has been correlated with mental activities such as problem solving (Arellano and Schwab, 1950; Brazier and Casby, 1952; Ishihara and Yoshii, 1972; Mizuki, 1982, 1987; Mizuki et al., 1980, 1983). In personal studies of mental EEG activation, we were unable to produce this pattern (Niedermeyer et al., 1989); this indicates the technical difficulties in the demonstration of the task-related frontal theta rhythm.

Our inability to demonstrate frontal midline 6 to 7/sec activity as a response to mental tasks has been a nagging problem for the writer of this chapter. I asked Japanese and Chinese co-workers to solve mental tasks during EEG recordings (in hopes of finding a certain racial or cultural element specific to individuals from the Far East) with completely negative results. This vexing problem has been clarified by the work of Takahashi et al. (1997), who found that individuals with rhythmical frontal midline 6 to 7/sec activity in light drowsiness also had the same type of activity during mental tasks: "These two frontal theta rhythms closely resembled each other in frequency (94.6%) and distribution (83.8%)" (Takahashi et al., 1997). One wonders if these tasks become boring enough to produce light drowsiness rather than increased alertness (one is even tempted to utilize the old Pavlovian term *internal inhibition*, i.e., sleep induction in a certain repetitive experimental setting).

Macrosmatic mammals (rats, etc.) show a very powerful limbic and especially hippocampal rhythm from 3 to 12/sec (mainly 4 to 7/sec), which is further activated by arousal (Green and Arduini, 1954). An overview of limbic rhythmic theta activity has been presented by Lopes da Silva (1992).

Posterior Slow Activity

Posterior slow activities constitute a very important aspect of the EEG maturation in childhood, adolescence, and early adulthood (the third decade of life). All of these slow posterior activities in the theta and delta range are discussed in Chapter 11, "Maturation of the EEG: Development of Waking and Sleep Patterns." The mature adult waking record contains only traces of posterior slowing.

Lambda Waves
Definition and Historical Aspects

Lambda waves are "sharp transients occurring over the occipital region of the head of waking subjects during visual exploration. Mainly positive relative to other areas. Time-locked to saccadic eye movements. Amplitude varies, but is generally below 50 μV" (IFSECN, 1974).

This visually induced occipital activity was described by Y. Gastaut (1951); there was an earlier oral presentation by Evans (EEG Society in London, 1949). Subsequent EEG studies on lambda waves were presented by Cobb and Pampiglione (1952), Evans (1952, 1953), and Roth and Green (1953). A very extensive review of this subject is found in the handbook article of Chatrian (1976d).

Prevalence and Further Characteristics

Lambda waves are unmistakably present in some records and are not readily demonstrable in others. They are most prominent in waking patients intently viewing an illuminated visual field (Chatrian, 1976d). The prevalence essentially depends on the thoroughness of the EEG evaluation and the emphasis placed on the demonstration of this special phenomenon. According to Tsai and Liu (1965; quoted in Chatrian, 1976d), lambda waves are most frequent between ages 3 and 12 years (82.3%); their prevalence declines to 72% between 18 and 30 years and to 36.4% between ages 31 and 50 years.

Wave Morphology

Lambda waves have been described as biphasic or triphasic; the most prominent phase is positive. Their form has been described as triangular or saw-toothed shaped. The amplitude is usually below 20 μV and may exceed 50 μV in some persons. The overall duration of lambda waves lies between 200 and 300 msec. These waves repeat themselves, usually at intervals from 200 to 500 msec. Marton et al. (1982) have demonstrated the complexities of lambda waves; their predominant positive component is preceded and followed by a negative component.

Spatial Distribution

Lambda waves are most prominent in (or confined to) the occipital leads. Spread into parietal and posterotemporal areas is common and, in certain cases, the maximum may be found in areas adjacent to the occipital lobe (Evans, 1953; Roth and Green, 1953). Lambda activity is strictly bilateral synchronous. With the use of depth electrodes, Perez-Borja et al. (1962) demonstrated multiple foci of lambda waves, either in or near the calcarine region or more laterally in the occipital lobes.

Precipitating Factors

Voluntary scanning eye movements (exploratory saccades) play a very important role. It was found that most lambda waves follow an exploratory eye movement with a latency of 67 to 85 msec (mean, 78 msec) (Green, 1957). The preceding eye movement has been subsequently used as a trigger for computer techniques (Barlow, 1963, 1964; Barlow and Ciganek, 1969; Chatrian, 1964; Remond and Lesèvre, 1971; Remond et al., 1965; Scott and Bickford, 1967). Further interesting details on this subject are found in the handbook article of Chatrian (1976d) (Figs. 9.7 and 9.8).

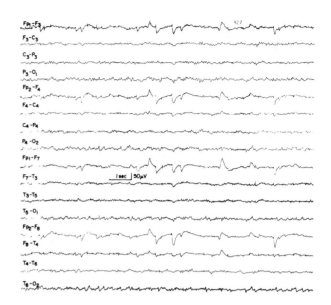

Figure 9.7. Occipital lambda waves while viewing pictures, in a patient age 15 years. Note ocular artifacts caused by scanning eye movements.

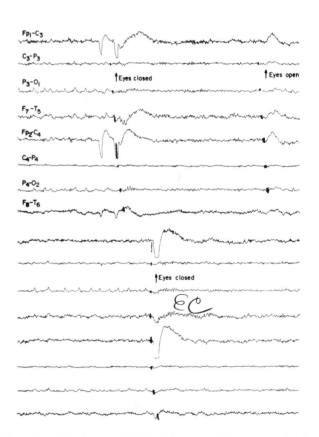

Figure 9.8. Prominent occipital lambda waves during eye opening. Patient, age 54 years, looking ahead in the dimly lit laboratory. There is no evidence of scanning ocular artifacts. Note instability and fast character of alpha rhythm (1–13/second and even faster). The *bottom part* shows continuation of the *upper part*.

Lambda waves are best found in brightly lit laboratories and cannot be elicited in darkness. The size of a given pattern and its distance and color are further variables. Binocular viewing of a picture may or may not produce larger lambda waves than monocular viewing (Bickford and Klass, 1964; Scott et al., 1967).

The role of psychological factors has also been pondered. Green (1954) felt that nervous tension would diminish lambda activity. Presentation of a new picture enhances lambda production (Chatrian, 1976d; Green, 1954). Lambda activity does not seem to be related to recognition of objects (Green, 1957). Hypnotic suggestion of a test picture failed to produce a lambda response (Scott et al., 1967).

Relationships to Alpha Rhythm and Visual Evoked Responses

There appears to be considerable independence between posterior alpha rhythm (with eyes closed) and lambda waves (with eyes open); no interaction or complementary action of these two activities has been found. Marked similarities between lambda waves and visual evoked responses have been reported by Remond et al. (1965) and Lesèvre (1967). Relationships between lambda waves and occipital photic driving were originally presumed by Y. Gastaut (1951) and Evans (1953) but could not be confirmed by Chatrian et al. (1960), Perez-Borja et al. (1962), and Scott et al. (1967).

Correlations with Neurological and Psychiatric Diseases

No such correlation has been demonstrated. There are also no correlations with certain personality traits.

Theories on the Basic Neurophysiological Mechanism

Lambda waves have been thought to be related to (a) visual evoked responses, (b) oculomotor-visual integration, (c) oculomotor potentials, or (d) arousal mechanisms. These theories have been thoroughly discussed by Chatrian (1976d).

Billings (1989) has proposed that there are two different occipital lambda waves in the human. The first one is the result of the release of peripheral visual inhibition during the braking phase of the primary saccade. This wave is transmitted via the faster conducting Y-type fibers of the optic nerve (subserving peripheral vision). The second wave is elicited by the return of normal central vision, during or slightly before the braking phase of the secondary corrective saccade. This wave is transmitted via the slower conducting X-type fibers of the optic nerve (subserving central vision). According to Billings, "lambda waves, long considered to be of rather trivial import by clinical electroencephalographers, are of considerable functional significance in the visual system."

Relationship to "Lambdoid" Activity or Positive Occipital Sharp Transients of Sleep (POSTS)

These occipital positive sharp discharges are discussed in the section on sleep. A relationship to lambda waves of the waking state appears to be quite obvious, but Chatrian (1976d) feels that the similarities between the patterns are only superficial.

Lambda Wave-Like Occipital Slow Discharges during Eye Blinks in Children

Large slow transients of a duration of 200 to 400 msec over the occipital region bisynchronously occurring after an eye blink with a latency of 100 to 200 msec have been described by Westmoreland and Sharbrough (1975). These waves were found mainly from ages 1 to 3 years. It has been thought that these discharges represent a variant of lambda waves. Pattern and picture scanning also produced these potentials.

EEG Rhythms: Are They Spontaneous or Induced?

The "new wave of EEG research" (initiated by Başar and Bullock) has emphasized the induced nature of EEG rhythms. The old adage of spontaneous EEG activity of either rhythmical or nonrhythmical character has been strongly challenged by the "new wave." This new line of research also has adopted a view in which there is hardly any gap left between EEG rhythms and evoked potentials.

In the old days of evoked potential work, it was shown that flash-evoked visual potentials are followed by a series of alphoid rhythmical waves (also called "ringing"). Thus, relationships between EEG rhythms and evoked potentials are not altogether new, though almost forgotten. Hence their revival in the 1990s must be warmly welcomed.

Imagine a jam-packed stadium with spectators watching an important ball game. There is noise—a gentle hum or single shouts or even tremendous outbursts of almost synchronously emitted vocal energies. Certainly, the most powerful activities are induced by the events on the field (analogy to "event-related potentials") but the constant hum cannot be attributed to any special outside event and may be called spontaneous. When, in less exciting phases of the game, the spectators' attention dwindles, then people start to talk to each other thus generating the hum that had prevailed when the crowd gathered prior to the game. It is reasonable to assume that, in periods of little action, cerebral neurons simply "talk to each other." Under the influence of synchronizing structures, this "hum" or "neuronal conversation" then turns into a spontaneous rhythm.

Concluding Remarks: Background Versus Foreground EEG Interpretation

This chapter presented the frequencies and patterns of the normal adult waking record. The reader may have searched in vain for a discussion of the background activity of the EEG. But what is background and what is foreground? This question touches problems of EEG interpretation that cannot be adequately taught in a textbook. The eye must be trained for the recognition of patterns that may be normal, abnormal-nonparoxysmal, or abnormal-paroxysmal. Above all, however, the interpreter must understand the gestalt of the record; this depends on a formidable number of variables. In this process of interpretation of EEG phenomena, the so-called background may have to be moved into the foreground and vice versa, depending on the momentary focus of emphasis.

This shows clearly where the limitations of an EEG textbook lie. There is simply no firm rule concerning the manner in which the record reader's eyes and brain have to operate in this process. There is simply no substitute for an adequate training period with regular joint reading sessions.

Every experienced electroencephalographer has his or her personal approach to EEG interpretation. This is also true for the manner in which the EEG report is written. Panel discussions on the EEG report and the proper way of writing reports consistently reveal striking differences among the panelists. Although standardization is an important goal in many areas of EEG technology, experienced electroencephalographers should not abandon a certain individualistic spirit, notwithstanding the fact that the eminent features of each tracing should be easily gleaned from the report. EEG reports should be sound and lucid, but the format does not have to be standardized. Why not? Because there is an element of science and an element of art in a good EEG interpretation; it is the latter that defies standardization.

References

Adams, A. 1959. Studies on flat electroencephalogram in man. Electroencephalogr. Clin. Neurophysiol. 11:34–41.

Adams, A. 1968. Frequenzanalyse des flachen EEG. Dtsch. Z. Nervenheilk. 193:57–72.

Adrian, E.D. 1934. Discharge frequency in cerebral and cerebellar cortex. J. Physiol. (Lond.) 83:32(abst).

Adrian, E.D. 1971. The discovery of Berger. In Handbook of Electroencephalography and Clinical Neurophysiology, vol. 1, Ed.-in-chief, A. Remond, pp. 5–10. Amsterdam: Elsevier.

Adrian, E.D., and Matthews, B.H.C. 1934. The Berger rhythm, potential changes from the occipital lobe in man. Brain 57:345–359.

Adrian, E.D., and Yamagiwa, K. 1935. The origin of the Berger rhythm. Brain 58:323–351.

Aird, R.B., and Garoutte, B. 1958. Studies on the "cerebral pacemaker." Neurology (Minneapolis) 8:581–589.

Albe-Fessard, D. 1975. Electrophysiological techniques used to differentiate thalamic nuclei. In Handbook of Electroencephalography and Clinical Neurophysiology, vol. 10B, Ed. A. Remond, pp. 46–58. Amsterdam: Elsevier.

Anand, B.K., China, G.S., and Singh, B. 1961. Some aspects of electroencephalographic studies in yogis. Electroencephalogr. Clin. Neurophysiol. 13:452–456.

Andersen, P., and Andersson, S.A. 1968. Physiological mechanisms of the alpha waves. In Clinical Electroencephalography of Children, Eds. P. Kellaway and I. Petersén, pp. 31–48. New York: Grune & Stratton.

Andersen, P., and Andersson, S.A. 1974. Thalamic origin of cortical rhythmic activity. In Handbook of Electroencephalography and Clinical Neurophysiology, vol. 2C, Ed. A. Remond, pp. 90–118. Amsterdam: Elsevier.

Arellano, A.P., and Schwab, R.S. 1950. Scalp and basal recording during mental activity. Proceed. 1st Internat. Congr. Psychiat., Paris.

Arfel, G., Fischgold, H., and Weiss, J. 1963. Le silence cérébral. In Problèmes de Base en Électroencéphalographie, Ed. H. Fischgold, pp. 118–152. Paris: Masson.

Arroyo, S., Lesser, R.P., Gordon, B., et al. 1993. Functional significance of the mu rhythm of human cortex: an electrophysiologic study with subdural electrodes. Electroencephalogr. Clin. Neurophysiol. 87:76–87.

Bagchi, B.K., and Wenger, M.A. 1958. Simultaneous EEG and other recordings during some yogi practices. Electroencephalogr. Clin. Neurophysiol. 10:193(abst).

Banquet, J.P. 1973. Comparative study on the EEG spectral analysis during sleep and yoga meditation. Proceed. 1st Europ. Cong. Sleep Res., Basel, pp. 389–394.

Barlow, J.S. 1963. Some statistical characteristics of electrocortical activity in relation to visual oculomotor tracking in man. Bol. Inst. Estud. Med. Biol. (Mex.) 21:497–518.

Barlow. J.S. 1964. Evoked responses in relation to visual perception and oculomotor reaction times in man. Ann. N.Y. Acad. Sci. 112:432–467.

Barlow, J.S. 1991. Book review (Norbert Wiener 1894–1964, P.R. Masani; Birkhauser, Boston, 1990).

Barlow, J.S., and Ciganek, L. 1969. Lambda responses in relation to visual evoked responses in man. Electroencephalogr. Clin. Neurophysiol. 26: 183–192.

Başar, E. 1992. Brain natural frequencies are causal factors for resonances and induced rhythms. In Induced Rhythms in the Brain, Eds. E. Başar and T.H. Bullock, pp. 425–467. Boston: Birkhäuser.

Başar, E., and Schürmann, M. 1994. Functional aspects of evoked alpha and theta responses in humans and cats. Biol. Cybern. 72:175–183.

Bastiaansen, M.C.M., Brunia, C.H.M., and Boecker, K.G.E. 1999. ERD as an index of anticipatory behavior. In Event-Related Desynchronization, Eds. G. Pfurtscheller and F.L. Lopes da Silva. Vol. 6 of Handbook of Electroencephalography and Clinical Neuropsychology, revised series, pp. 203–217. Amsterdam: Elsevier.

Beek, H. 1958. Age and the central rhythm "en arceau." Electroencephalogr. Clin. Neurophysiol. 10:356(abst).

Belsh, J.M., Chokroverty, S., and Barabas, G. 1983. Posterior rhythmic slow activity in EEG after eye closure. Electroencephalogr. Clin. Neurophysiol. 56:562–568.

Berger, H. 1929. Über das Elektrenkephalogramm des Menschen. Arch. Psychiat. Nervenkr. 87:527–570.

Berger, H. 1930. Über das Elektrenkephalogramm des Menschen. Zweite Mitteilung (2nd report). J. Psychol. Neurol. (Leipzig) 40:160–179.

Berger, H. 1931. Über das Elektrenkephalogramm des Menschen. Dritte Mitteilung (3rd report). Arch. Psychiat. Nervenkr. 94:16–60.

Berger, H. 1932. Über das Elektrenkephalogramm des Menschen. Vierte Mitteilung (4th report). Arch. Psychiat. Nervenkr. 97:6–26.

Berger, H. 1933a. Über das Elektrenkephalogramm des Menschen. Sechste Mitteilung (6th report). Arch. Psychiat. Nervenkr. 99:555–574.

Berger, H. 1933b. Über das Elektrenkephalogramm des Menschen. Siebente Mitteilung (7th report). Arch. Psychiat. Nervenkr. 100:301–320.

Berger, H. 1935. Über das Elektrenkephalogramm des Menschen. Zehnte Mitteilung (10th report). Arch Psychiat. Nervenkr. 103:444–454.

Berger, H. 1937. Über das Elektrenkephalogramm des Menschen. Zwölfte Mitteilung (12th report). Arch. Psychiat. Nervenkr. 106:165–187.

Berger, H. 1938. Über das Elektrenkephalogramm des Menschen. Vierzehnte Mitteilung (14th report). Arch. Psychiat. Nervenkr. 108:407–431.

Bickford, R.G., and Klass, D.W. 1964. Eye movements and the electroencephalogram. In The Oculomotor Systems, Ed. M.B. Bender, pp. 293–302. New York: Hoeber.

Billings, R.J. 1989. The origin of the occipital lambda wave in man. Electroencephalogr. Clin. Neurophysiol. 72:95–113.

Bishop, G.H. 1936. The interpretation of cortical potentials. Cold Spring Harb. Symp. Quant. Biol. 4:305–319.

Bostem, F., Dongier, M., Demaret, A., et al. 1964. Discussion à propos du rhythme mu. Rev. Neurol. (Paris). 111:335–337.

Bostem, F., Dongier, M., Demaret, A., et al. 1965. Discussion on mu rhythm. Electroencephalogr. Clin. Neurophysiol. 18:721(abst).

Bouyer, J.J., Tilquin, C., and Rougeul, A. 1983. Thalamic rhythms in cat during quiet wakefulness and immobility. Electroencephalogr. Clin. Neurophysiol. 55:180–187.

Brazier, M.A.B., and Casby, J.U. 1952. Crosscorrelation and autocorrelation studies of electroencephalographic potentials. Electroencephalogr. Clin. Neurophysiol. 4:201–211.

Brazier, M.A.B., and Finesinger, J.E. 1944. Characteristics of the normal electroencephalogram. I. A study of the occipital cortical potentials in 500 normal adults. J. Clin. Invest. 23:303–311.

Brechet, R., and Lecasble, R. 1965. Reactivity of mu rhythm to flicker. Electroencephalogr. Clin. Neurophysiol. 18:721–722.(abst).

Bremer, F. 1958. Cerebral and cerebellar potentials. Physiol. Rev. 38: 357–388.

Broadhurst, A., and Glass, A. 1969. Relationship of personality measures to the alpha rhythm of the electroencephalogram. Br. J. Psychiatry. 115: 199–204.

Brown, B.B. 1970. Recognition of aspects of consciousness through associations with EEG alpha activity represented by a light signal. Psychophysiology. 6:442–451.

Bullock, T.H. 1992. Introduction to induced rhythms: A widespread, heterogeneous class of oscillations. In Induced Rhythms in the Brain, Eds. E. Başar and T.H. Bullock, pp. 1–26. Boston: Birkhauser.

Caveness, W.F. 1962. Atlas of Electroencephalography in the Developing Monkey, Macaca mulatta. Reading, MA: Addison-Wesley.

Chase, M.H., and Harper, R.M. 1971. Somatomotor and visceromotor correlates of operantly conditioned 12–14/sec sensorimotor cortical activity. Electroencephalogr. Clin. Neurophysiol. 31:85–92.

Chatila, M., Milleret, C., Buser, P., et al. 1992. A 10 Hz "alpha-like" rhythm in the visual cortex of the waking cat. Electroencephalogr. Clin. Neurophysiol. 83:217–222.

Chatrian, G.E. 1964. Characteristics of unusual EEG patterns: Incidence, significance. Electroencephalogr. Clin. Neurophysiol. 17:471–472.

Chatrian, G.E. 1976a. The mu rhythms. In *Handbook of Electroencephalography and Clinical Neurophysiology,* vol. 6A, Ed. A. Remond, pp. 46–69. Amsterdam: Elsevier.

Chatrian, G.E. 1976b. The kappa rhythm. In *Handbook of Electroencephalography and Clinical Neurophysiology,* vol. 6A, Ed. A. Remond, pp. 104–114. Amsterdam: Elsevier.

Chatrian, G.E. 1976c. The low voltage EEG. In *Handbook of Electroencephalography and Clinical Neurophysiology,* vol. 6A, Ed. A. Remond, pp. 77–89. Amsterdam: Elsevier.

Chatrian, G.E. 1976d. The lambda waves. In *Handbook of Electroencephalography and Clinical Neurophysiology,* vol. 6A, Ed. A. Remond, pp. 123–149. Amsterdam: Elsevier.

Chatrian, G.E., Petersen, M.C., and Lazarte, J.A. 1959. The blocking of the rolandic wicket rhythm and some central changes related to movement. Electroencephalogr. Clin. Neurophysiol. 11:497–510.

Chatrian, G.E., Bickford, R.G., Petersen, M.C., et al. 1960. Lambda waves with depth electrodes in humans. In *Electrical Studies on the Unanesthetized Brain,* Eds. E.R. Ramey and D.S. O'Doherty, pp. 291–310. New York: Hoeber.

Ciganek, L. 1959. A contribution to the rolandic "arceau" rhythm. Electroencephalogr. Clin. Neurophysiol. 11:185–186.

Cobb, W.A. 1963. The normal adult EEG. In *Electroencephalography,* Eds. D. Hill and G. Parr, pp. 232–249. New York: Macmillan.

Cobb, W.A., and Pampiglione, G. 1952. Occipital sharp waves responsive to visual stimuli. Electroencephalogr. Clin. Neurophysiol. 4:110–111.

Cobb, W.A., Guiloff, R.J., and Cast, J. 1979. Breach rhythm: The EEG related to skull defects. Electroencephalogr. Clin. Neurophysiol. 47:251–271.

Cohn, R. 1946. The influence of emotions on the human electroencephalogram. J. Nerv. Ment. Dis. 104:351–357.

Cooper, R., and Mundy-Castle, A.C. 1960. Spatial and temporal analysis of the alpha rhythm: A toposcopic analysis. Electroencephalogr. Clin. Neurophysiol. 12:153–165.

Cooper, R., Winter, A.L., Crow, J.J., et al. 1965. Comparison of subcortical, cortical and scalp activity using indwelling electrodes in man. Electroencephalogr. Clin. Neurophysiol. 18:217–228.

Courjon, J. 1962. La place de l'électroencéphalographie en traumatologie cranienne. Cah. Méd. Lyon. 38:315–317.

Covello, A., DeBarros-Ferreira, M., and Lairy, G.C. 1975. Étude télémétrique des rhythmes centraux chez l'enfant. Electroencephalogr. Clin. Neurophysiol. 38:307–319.

Creutzfeldt, O.D., Arnold, P.M., Becker, D., et al. 1976. EEG changes during spontaneous and controlled menstrual cycles and their correlation with psychological performance. Electroencephalogr. Clin. Neurophysiol. 40:113–131.

Cruikshank, R.M. 1937. Human occipital brain potentials as affected by intensity-duration variables of visual stimulation. J. Exp. Psychol. 21:622–641.

Curio G. 2000a. Ain't no rhythm fast enough: EEG bands beyond beta. J. Clin. Neurophysiol. 17:339–340.

Curio G. 2000b. Linking 600-Hz "spike-like" EEG/MEG wavlets ("sigma bursts") to cellular substrates: concepts and caveats. J. Clin. Neurophysiol. 17:377–396.

Daoust-Roy, J. 1989. A waking 4 Hz vertex rhythm: 4 Cps vertex spindles revisited. Am. J. EEG Technol. 29:147–163.

Davis, H., and Davis, P.A. 1936. Active potentials of the brain in normal persons and in normal states of cerebral activity. Arch. Neurol. Psychiatr. (Chicago) 36:1214–1224.

Dongier, M., and Dongier, S. 1958. Quelques aspects de l'électroencéphalogramme des névroses. Évol. Psychiat. 1:1–18.

Dongier, M., McCallum, W.C., Torres, F., et al. 1976. Psychological and psychophysiological states. In *Handbook of Electroencephalography and Clinical Neurophysiology,* vol. 16A, Ed. A. Remond, pp. 195–256. Amsterdam: Elsevier.

Dow, R.S. 1938. The electrical activity of the cerebellum and its functional significance. J. Physiol. (Lond.) 94:67–86.

Draguhn A., Traub, R.D., Bibig, A., et al. 2000. Ripple (around 200-Hz) oscillations in temporal structures. J. Clin. Neurophysiol. 17:361–376.

Drake, M.E. 1984. Clinical correlates of very fast beta activity in the EEG. Clin. Electroencephalogr. 15:237–241.

Dubois, M., Sato, S., Lees, D.E., et al. 1980. Electroencephalographic changes during whole body hyperthermia in humans. Electroencephalogr. Clin. Neurophysiol. 50:486–495.

Duensing, F. 1948. Erfahrungen mit der Elektroenzephalographie bei Schädelschußverletzungen. Dtsch. A. Nervenheilk. 159:514–536.

Durup, G., and Fessard, A. 1935. À l'electroencephalogramme de l'homme. Ann. Psychol. 36:1–31.

Dusser de Barenner, D., and Gibbs, F. 1942. Variation in the electroencephalogram during the menstrual cycle. Am. J. Obstet. Gynecol. 44: 687–690.

Dutertre, F. 1977. Catalogue of the main EEG patterns. In *Handbook of Electroencephalography and Clinical Neurophysiology,* vol. 11A, Ed. A. Remond, pp. 40–79. Amsterdam: Elsevier.

Eckhorn, R., Schanze, T., Brosch, M., et al. 1992. Stimulus-specific synchronizations in cat visual cortex: Multiple microelectrode and correlation studies from several cortical areas. In *Induced Rhythms in the Brain,* Eds. E. Başar and T.H. Bullock, pp. 47–80. Boston: Birkhäuser.

Evans, C.C. 1952. Comments on "occipital sharp waves responsive to visual stimuli." Electroencephalogr. Clin. Neurophysiol. 4:111.

Evans, C.C. 1953. Spontaneous excitation of the visual cortex and association areas—lambda waves. Electroencephalogr. Clin. Neurophysiol. 5:69–74.

Farnarier, C., Mattei, J.P., and Naquet, R. 1981. The mu rhythm of the vertex and its reactivity: an infrequent observation. Electroencephalogr. Clin. Neurophysiol. 52:55P(abst).

Fenwick, B.B.C., and Walker, S. 1969. The effect of eye position on the alpha rhythm. In *Attention in Neurophysiology: An International Conference,* Eds. C.R. Evans and T.B. Mulholland, pp. 128–141. London: Butterworths.

Finley, K. 1944. On the occurrence of rapid frequency potential changes in the human electroencephalogram. Am. J. Psychiatry 101:194–200.

Finley, W.W., Smith, H.A., and Etherton, M.D. 1975. Reduction of seizures and normalization of EEG in a severe epileptic following sensorimotor biofeedback training. Biol. Psychol. 2:189–203.

Fisch, B.J., Lemos, M.S., and Hauser, W.A. 1990. Age-related changes in alpha rhythm frequency and reactivity. Electroencephalogr. Clin. Neurophysiol. 75:S45(abst).

Fischgold, H., Pertuiset, B., and Arfel-Capdeville, G. 1952. Quelques particularités électroencéphalographiques au niveau des brèches et des volets neurochirurgicaux. Rev. Neurol. (Paris). 86:126–132.

Fortuin, B., and Künkel, H. 1983. The beta-type EEG in adults. Electroencephalogr. Clin. Neurophysiol. 56:67P(abst).

Frank, G. 1964. Circadian periodicity in cerebral electrical output: relation to body temperature and stage of sleep-wakefulness cycles. Electroencephalogr. Clin. Neurophysiol. 17:712(abst).

Frost, J. 1976. Physiological bases of normal EEG rhythms. In *Handbook of Electroencephalography and Clinical Neurophysiology,* vol. 6A, Ed. A. Remond, pp. 150–160. Amsterdam: Elsevier.

Futagi, Y., Ishihara, T., Txuda, K., et al. 1998. Theta Rhythms Associated with sucking, Crying, Gazing, and Handling in Infants. Electroencephalogr. Clin. Neurophysiol. 106:392–399.

Gallais, P., Collomb, H., Milletto, G., et al. 1957. Confrontation entre les données de l'électroencéphalogramme et des examens psychologiques chez 522 sujets repartis en trois groupes differents. II. Confrontation des données de l'électroencéphalogramme et de l'examen psychologique chez 113 jeunes soldats. In *Conditionnement et Réactivité en Électroencéphalographie,* Eds. H. Fischgold and H. Gastaut. Electroencephalogr. Clin. Neurophysiol. Suppl. 6:294–303.

Garsche, R. 1956. Die Beta-Aktivität des Kindes. Z. Kinderheilk. 78: 441–457.

Gasser, T., Von Lucadou-Müller, I., Verleger, R., et al. 1983. Correlating EEG and IQ: A new look at an old problem using computerized EEG parameters. Electroencephalogr. Clin. Neurophysiol. 55:493–504.

Gastaut, H. 1952. Étude électrocorticographique de la réativité des rhythmes rolandiques. Rev. Neurol. (Paris) 87:176–182.

Gastaut, H. 1957. Confrontation entre les données de l'électroencéphalogramme et des examens psychologiques chez 522 sujets repartis en trois groupes differents. V. Conclusions d'ensemble. *In Conditionnement et Réactivité en Électroencéphalographie,* Eds. H. Fischgold and H. Gastaut. Electroencephalogr. Clin. Neurophysiol. Suppl. 6: 321–338.

Gastaut, H. 1960. Correlations between the electroencephalographic and the psychometric variables (M.M.P.I., Rosenzweig, intelligence tests). Electroencephalogr. Clin. Neurophysiol. 12:226–227.

Gastaut, H. 1974. Vom Berger-Rhythmus zum Alpha-Kult und zur Alpha-Kultur. Z. EEG-EMG. 5:189–199.

Gastaut, H., Terzian, H., and Gastaut, Y. 1952. Étude d'une activité électroencéphalographique méconnue: "Le rhythme rolandique en arceau." Marseille méd. 89:296–310.

Gastaut, H., Dongier, M., and Courtois, G. 1954. On the significance of "wicket rhythms" ("rhythmes en arceau") in psychosomatic medicine. Electroencephalogr. Clin. Neurophysiol. 6:687.

Gastaut, H., Jus, A., Jus, C., et al. 1957. Étude topographique des réactions électroencéphalographiques conditionées chez l'homme. Electroencephalogr. Clin. Neurophysiol. 9:1–34.

Gastaut, H., Bacher, F., Bert, J., et al. 1959a. Étude des corrélations entre les variables électroencéphalographiques et psychométriques (M.M.P.I., Rosenzweig). Rev. Neurol. (Paris). 101:376–384.

Gastaut, H., Dongier, S., and Dongier, M. 1959b. Electroencéphalographie et nevroses. Rev. Neurol. (Paris). 101:435–436.

Gastaut, H., Lee, M.C., and Laboureur, P. 1960. Comparative EEG and psychometric data for 825 French naval pilots and 511 control subjects of the same age. Aerospace Med. 31:547–552.

Gastaut, H., Broughton, R., Regis, H., et al. 1964. Quelques données nouvelles à propos due rhythme mu. Rev. Neurol. (Paris) 111:331–332.

Gastaut, H., Naquet, R., and Gastaut, Y. 1965. A study of the mu rhythm in subjects lacking one or more limbs. Electroencephalogr. Clin. Neurophysiol. 18:720–721.

Gastaut, Y. 1951. Un signe électroencéphalographique peu connu: les pointes occipitales survenant pendant l'ouverture des yeux. Rev. Neurol. (Paris) 84:640–643.

Gevins, A. 1998. The future of electroencephalography in assessing neurocognitive functioning. Electroencephalogr. Clin. Neurophysiol. 106: 165–172.

Giannitrappani, D., and Kayton, L. 1974. Schizophrenia and EEG spectral analysis. Electroencephalogr. Clin. Neurophysiol. 36:377–386.

Gibbs, F.A., and Gibbs, E.L. 1950. Atlas of Electroencephalography, vol. 1. Cambridge, MA: Addison-Wesley.

Gibbs, F.A., and Gibbs, E.L. 1964. Atlas of Electroencephalography, vol. 3. Reading, MA: Addison-Wesley.

Gibbs, F.A., Gibbs, E.L., and Lennox, W.G. 1943. Electroencephalographic classification of epileptic patients and control subjects. Arch. Neurol. Psychiat. (Chicago) 50:111–128.

Gloor, P. 1971. The work of Hans Berger. In Handbook of Electroencephalography and Clinical Neurophysiology, vol. 1A, Ed. A. Remond, pp. 11–24. Amsterdam: Elsevier.

Golla, F., Hutton, E.L., and Walter, W.G. 1943. The objective study of mental imagery. I. Physiological concomitance. Appendix on new method of electroencephalographic analysis. J. Ment. Sci. 89:216–223.

Götze, W., Kubicki, S., von Düring, et al. 1959. Über das EEG bei kranken und gesunden Tieren. Die Kleintier-Praxis. 4:97–103.

Graber, B., Rohrbaugh, J.W., Newlin, D.B., et al. 1985. EEG during masturbation and ejaculation. Arch. Sex. Behav. 14:492–503.

Graf, M., Niedermeyer, E., Schiemann, J., et al. 1984. Electrocorticography: Information derived from intra-operative recordings during seizure surgery. Clin. Electroencephalogr. 15:83–91.

Gray, C.M., Engel, A.K., König, P., et al. 1992. Mechanisms underlying the generation of neuronal oscillations in cat visual cortex. In Induced Rhythms in the Brain, Eds. E. Başar and T.H. Bullock, pp. 29–45. Boston: Birkhäuser.

Green, J.D., and Arduini, A.A. 1954. Hippocampal electrical activity in arousal. J. Neurophysiol. 17:533–557.

Green, J. 1954. Lambda waves in the EEG and their relation to some visual tasks. Proc. EPTA. 5(3).

Green, J. 1957. Some observations on lambda waves and peripheral stimulation. Electroencephalogr. Clin. Neurophysiol. 9:691–704.

Gücer, G., Niedermeyer, E., and Long, D.M. 1978. Thalamic recordings in patients with chronic pain. J. Neurol. (Berlin) 219:47–61.

Gullapalli, D., and Fountain, N. 2003. Clinical correlation occipital intermittent rhythmic delta activity. J. Clin. Neurophysiol. 20:35–41.

Gundel, A. 1984. The influence of body temperature on the waking EEG. Electroencephalogr. Clin. Neurophysiol. 57:33P(abst).

Harding, G.F.A. 1967. The use of automated low frequency analyzers in quantitative electroencephalography. Electroencephalogr. Clin. Neurophysiol. 23:487.

Harding, G.F.A., and Thompson, C.R.S. 1976. EEG rhythms and the internal milieu. In Handbook of Electroencephalography and Clinical Neurophysiology, vol. 6A, Ed. A. Remond, pp. 176–194. Amsterdam: Elsevier.

Heath, R.G. 1972. Pleasure and brain activity in man. Deep and surface electroencephalograms during orgasm. J. Nerv. Ment. Dis. 154:3–18.

Henry, C.E. 1944. Electroencephalograms of normal children. Monogr. Soc. Res. Child Dev., Nat. Res. Council, Washington, D.C. XI.

Henry, C.E., and Knott, J.R. 1941. A note on the relationship between personality and the alpha rhythm of the electroencephalogram. J. Exp. Psychol. 28:362–366.

Hess, R. 1975. Postoperative controls. In Handbook of Electroencephalography and Clinical Neurophysiology, vol. 14C, Ed. A. Remond, pp. 56–65. Amsterdam: Elsevier.

Hess, R. 1980. The origin of the alpha rhythm. Electroencephalogr. Clin. Neurophysiol. 49:110P

Hofer, M.A., and Hinkle, L.E., Jr. 1964. Conditioned alpha blocking and arousal: the effects of adrenaline administration. Electroencephalogr. Clin. Neurophysiol. 17:653–660.

Hogan, K., and Fitzpatrick, J. 1987. The cerebral origin of the alpha rhythm. Electroencephalogr. Clin. Neurophysiol. 69:79–81.

IFSECN. 1974. A glossary of terms commonly used by clinical electroencephalographers. Electroencephalogr. Clin. Neurophysiol. 37: 538–548.

Ingvar, D.H. 1987. The concept of "the cerebral hyperfrontality?" Electroencephalogr. Clin. Neurophysiol. 67:25P(abst).

Inouye, T., Shinosaki, K., and Yagasaki, A. 1983. The direction of spread of alpha activity over the scalp. Electroencephalogr. Clin. Neurophysiol. 55:290–300.

Isch-Treussard, C. 1972. Paroxysmal arched rhythms in the child. Electroencephalogr. Clin. Neurophysiol. 33:354(abst).

Ishihara, T., and Yoshii, N. 1972. Multivariate analytic study of EEG and mental activity in juvenile delinquents. Electroencephalogr. Clin. Neurophysiol. 33:71–80.

Isokawa, M., and Komisaruk, B.R. 1983. Convergence of finger tremor and EEG rhythm at the alpha frequency induced by rhythmical photic stimulation. Electroencephalogr. Clin. Neurophysiol. 55:580–585.

Jasper, H.H., and Andrews, H.L. 1938. Electroencephalography. III. Normal differentiation of occipital and precentral regions in man. Arch. Neurol. Psychiat. (Chicago) 39:96–115.

Jasper, H.H., and Cruikshank, R.M. 1937. Visual stimulation and the after-image as affecting the occipital alpha rhythm. J. Gen. Psychol. 17:29–48.

Jasper, H.H., and Penfield, W. 1949. Electrocorticograms in man: Effects of voluntary movement upon the electrical activity of the precentral gyrus. Arch. Psychiat. Nervenkr. 183:163–174.

Jasper, H.H., and Shagass, C. 1941. Conditioning of occipital alpha rhythm in man. J. Exp. Psychol. 28:377–388.

Jasper, H.H., Fitzpatrick, C.A., and Colomon, P. 1939. Analogies and opposites in schizophrenia and epilepsy. Am. J. Psychiatry 95:835–851.

Jurko, M.F., and Andy, O.J. 1967. Comparative EEG frequencies in rhesus, stumptail and cynomolgus monkeys. Electroencephalogr. Clin. Neurophysiol. 23:270–272.

Kellaway, P., and Maulsby, R.L. 1966. The Normative Electroencephalographic Data Reference Library, pp. 50–52. Final report. Houston: Baylor College of Medicine.

Kendel, K., and Koufen, H. 1970. EEG-Veränderungen bei zerebralen Gefäszinsulten des Hirnstamms. Dtsch. Z. Nervenheilk. 197:42–55.

Kennedy, J.L., Gottsdanker, R.M., Armington, J.C., et al. 1948. A new electroencephalogram associated with thinking. Science 108:527–529.

Kiloh, L.G., McComas, A.J., and Osselton, J.W. 1972. Clinical Electroencephalography, 3rd ed. London: Butterworths.

Klass, D., and Bickford, R.G. 1957. Observations on the rolandic arceau rhythm. Electroencephalogr. Clin. Neurophysiol. 9:570.

Klimesch, W., Doppelmayr, M., Schimke, H., et al. 1996. Alpha frequency, reaction time, and the speed of processing information. J. Clin. Neurophysiol. 13:511–518.

Knott, J.R. 1976a. The alpha rhythm. In Handbook of Electroencephalography and Clinical Neurophysiology, vol. 6A, Ed. A. Remond, pp. 7–29. Amsterdam: Elsevier.

Knott, J.R. 1976b. The theta rhythm. In Handbook of Electroencephalography and Clinical Neurophysiology, vol. 6A, Ed. A. Remond, pp. 69–77. Amsterdam: Elsevier.

Knott, J.R., and Henry, C.E. 1941. The conditioning of the blocking of the alpha rhythm in human electroencephalogram. J. Exp. Psychol. 28: 134–144.

Könönen, M., and Partanen, J.V. 1993. Blocking of EEG alpha activity during visual performance in healthy adults. A quantitative study. Electroencephalography 87:164–166.

Koshino, Y., and Isaki, K. 1986. Familial occurrence of the mu rhythm. Clin. Electroencephalogr. 17:44–50.

Koshino, Y., and Niedermeyer, E. 1975. Enhancement of rolandic mu rhythm by pattern vision. Electroencephalogr. Clin. Neurophysiol. 38: 535–538.

Kozelak, J.W., and Pedley, T.A. 1990. Beta and mu rhythms. J. Clin Neurophysiol. 7:191–207.

Krauss, G.L., and Niedermeyer, E. 1991. Electroencephalogram and seizures in chronic alcoholism. Electroencephalogr. Clin. Neurophysiol. 78:97–104.

Kreezer, G. 1936. Electrical potentials in the brain in certain types of mental deficiency. Arch. Neurol. Psychiatry (Chicago) 36:1206–1214.

Kretschmer, E. 1931. *Körperbau and Charakter.* Berlin: Springer.

Kubicki, S., Schoppenhorst, M., Sack, H.J., et al. 1973. Post-traumatischer mu wave Fokus: der Einfluß von Schlaf, Pharmaka und motorischer Aktivität. A. EEG-EMG. 4:203–209.

Kugler, J. 1964. *Electroencephalography in Hospital and General Consulting Practice.* Amsterdam: Elsevier.

Kugler, J. 1981. *Elektroenzephalographie in Klinik und Praxis,* 3rd ed. Stuttgart: Thieme.

Kugler, J., and Laub, M. 1971. "Puppet show" theta rhythm. Electroencephalogr. Clin. Neurophysiol. 31:532–533(abst).

Kuhlman, W.N. 1978a. Functional topography of the human mu rhythm. Electroencephalogr. Clin. Neurophysiol. 44:83–93.

Kuhlman, W.N. 1978b. EEG feedback training: enhancement of somatosensory cortical activity. Electroencephalogr. Clin. Neurophysiol. 45:290–294.

Kuhlman, W.N. 1978c. EEG feedback training of epileptic patients: clinical and electroencephalographic analysis. Electroencephalogr. Clin. Neurophysiol. 45:699–710.

Kuhlo, W. 1976a. The beta rhythms. In *Handbook of Electroencephalography and Clinical Neurophysiology,* vol. 6A, Ed. A. Remond, pp. 29–46. Amsterdam: Elsevier.

Kuhlo, W. 1976b. Slow posterior activities. In *Handbook of Electroencephalography and Clinical Neurophysiology,* vol. 6A, Ed. A. Remond, pp. 89–104. Amsterdam: Elsevier.

Lairy, G.C. 1956. Organisation de l'électroencéphalogramme normal et pathologique. Rev. Neurol. (Paris) 94:749–801.

Lamb, W., Ulett, G., Masters, W., et al. 1953. Premenstrual tension EEG, hormonal and psychiatric evaluation. Am. J. Psychiatry 109:840–848.

Lanoir, J. 1972. Étude électroencéphalographique de la veille et du sommeil chez le chat. Organisation du cycle nycthéméral. Rôle du thalamus. Thèse Doct. Sci. Marseille. Centre régional de recherche et de documentation pédagogique. Marseille, 520 pp.

Laugier, H., and Liberson, W.T. 1937. Contribution à l'étude de l'EEG humain. C.R. Soc. Biol. (Paris) 125:13–17.

Lawson, A.M., Niedermeyer, E. 2002. Central pontine myelinolysis: clinical and EEG considerations. Am. J. Electroneurol Diagn. Technol. 42:151–153.

Lemere, F. 1936. The significance of individual differences in the Berger rhythm. Brain 59:366–375.

Lennox, W.G., Gibbs, F.A., and Gibbs, E.L. 1945. The brain wave pattern, an hereditary trait. Evidence from 74 "normal" pairs of twins. J. Hered. 36:233–243.

Lesèvre, N. 1967. Étude des reponses moyennes récueillies sur la région postérieure du scalp chez l'homme au cours de l'exploration visuelle ("complexe lambda"). Psychol. Franç. 12:26–36.

Lindsley, D.B. 1938. Electrical potentials of the brain in children and adults. J. Gen. Psychol. 19:285–306.

Lippold, O.C.J. 1970. The origin of the alpha rhythm. Nature (Lond.) 226:616–618.

Lippold, O.C.J. 1973. *The Origin of the Alpha Rhythm.* Edinburgh: Churchill Livingstone.

Liske, E., Hughes, H.M., and Stowe, D.E. 1967. Cross-correlation of human alpha activity: normative data. Electroencephalogr. Clin. Neurophysiol. 22:429–436.

Lopes da Silva, F. 1991. Neural mechanisms underlying brain waves: From neural membranes to networks. Electroencephalogr. Clin. Neurophysiol. 79:81–93.

Lopes da Silva, F. 1992. The rhythmic slow activity (theta) of the limbic cortex: an oscillation in search of a function. In *Induced Rhythms in the Brain,* Eds. E. Başar and T.H. Bullock, pp. 83–102. Boston: Birkhäuser.

Lopes da Silva, F.H., and Storm van Leeuwen, W. 1978. The cortical alpha rhythm in dogs: the depth and surface profile of phase. In *Architectonics of Cerebral Cortex,* Eds. M.A. Brazier and H. Petsche. New York: Raven Press.

Lopes da Silva, F., Van Lierop, T.H.M.T., Schrijer, C.F., et al. 1973a. Organization of thalamic and cortical alpha rhythm: Spectra and coherences. Electroencephalogr. Clin. Neurophysiol. 35:627–640.

Lopes da Silva, F., Van Lierop, T.H.M.T., Schrijer, C.F., et al. 1973b. Essential differences between alpha rhythms and barbiturate spindles: spectra and thalamocortical coherences. Electroencephalogr. Clin. Neurophysiol. 35:641–645.

Lorenzoni, E. 1963. Der Wert des EEG beim Schädelhirntrauma. Wien. Med. Wschr. 42/43:787–789.

Lucioni, R., and Penati, G. 1966. Sulla frequencza e sul significato in psichiatria dei tracciati cosidetti piatti. Riv. Neurol. 36:200–208.

Maddocks, J.A., Hodge, R.S., and Rex, J. 1951. Observations on the occurrence of precentral activities at alpha frequencies. Electroencephalogr. Clin. Neurophysiol. 3:370(abst).

Magnes, J., Moruzzi, G., and Pompeiano, O. 1961. EEG-synchronizing structures in the lower brain stem. In *The Nature of Sleep,* Eds. G.I.W. Wolstenholme and M. O'Connor, pp. 57–78. London: Churchill Livingstone.

Magni, F., Moruzzi, G., Rossi, G.F., et al. 1959. EEG arousal following inactivation of the lower brain stem by selective injection of barbiturates into the cerebral circulation. Arch. Ital. Biol. 97:33–46.

Magnus, O. 1954. The cerebral alpha-rhythm ("rhythme en arceau"). Electroencephalogr. Clin. Neurophysiol. 6:349–350.

Magnus, O., and Van der Holst, M. 1987. Zeta waves: a special type of slow delta waves. Electroencephalogr. Clin. Neurophysiol. 67:140–146.

Markand, O.M. 1990. Alpha rhythms. J. Clin. Neurophysiol. 7:163–189.

Marton, M., Szirtes, J., Donauer, N., et al. 1982. Averaged lambda potentials in man and monkey. Electroencephalogr. Clin. Neurophysiol. 53:14P–15P(abst).

Matousek, M., Okawa, M., and Petersén. I. 1981. Inter-hemispheric differences in normals and in psychiatric patients with normal EEG. Electroencephalogr. Clin. Neurophysiol. 52:33P–34P(abst).

Matsuura, M., Yamamoto, K., Fukuzawa, H., et al. 1985. Age development and sex differences of various EEG elements in healthy children and adults. Quantification by a computerized wave form recognition method. Electroencephalogr. Clin. Neurophysiol. 60:394–406.

Maulsby, R.L. 1971. An illustration of emotionally evoked theta rhythm in infancy: hedonic hypersynchrony. Electroencephalogr. Clin. Neurophysiol. 31:157–165.

Meyer-Mickeleit, R.W. 1953. Das Elektrenzephalogramm nach gedeckten Kopfverletzungen Ein Beitrag zur Differentialdiagnose der Commotio und Contusio cerebri. Dtsch. Med. Wschr. 78:480–484.

Mifka, P., and Scherzer, E. 1962. Über die Wertigkeit des EEG im Spätstadium der Gehirnverletzung. Wien. Klin. Wschr. 74:573–576.

Milstein, V. 1965. Contingent alpha blocking: conditioning or sensitization. Electroencephalogr. Clin. Neurophysiol. 18:272–277.

Mizuki, Y. 1982. Frontal midline theta activity during performance of mental tasks. Electroencephalogr. Clin. Neurophysiol. 54:25P(abst).

Mizuki, Y. 1987. Frontal lobe: Mental functions and EEG. Am. J. EEG Technol. 27:91–101.

Mizuki, Y., Tanaka, O., Isozaki, H., et al. 1980. Periodic appearance of theta rhythm in the frontal midline during performance of a mental task. Electroencephalogr. Clin. Neurophysiol. 49:345–351.

Mizuki, Y., Takii, O., Nishijima, H., et al. 1983. The relationship between the appearance of frontal midline theta activity (Fm theta) and memory function. Electroencephalogr. Clin. Neurophysiol. 56:56P(abst).

Moruzzi, G., and Magoun, H.W. 1949. Brain stem reticular formation and activation of the EEG. Electroencephalogr. Clin. Neurophysiol. 1:455–473.

Mosovich, A., and Tallaferro, A. 1954. Studies of EEG and sex function at orgasm. Dis. Nerv. Syst. 15:218–220.

Mundy-Castle, A.C. 1951. Theta and beta rhythm in the electroencephalogram of normal adults. Electroencephalogr. Clin. Neurophysiol. 3:477–486.

Mundy-Castle, A.C. 1953. An analysis of central responses to photic stimulation in normal adults. Electroencephalogr. Clin. Neurophysiol. 5:1–22.

Mulholland, T. 1969. The concept of attention in the electroencephalographic rhythm. In *Attention in Neurophysiology: An International*

Conference, Eds. C.R. Evans and T. Mulholland, pp. 100–127. London: Butterworth.

Mulholland, T., and Evans, C.R. 1965. An unexpected artifact in the human electroencephalogram and the orienting of the eyes. Nature (Lond.) 207:36–37.

Nashmi, R., Mendonça, A.J., and MacKay, W.A. 1994. EEG rhythms of the sensorimotor region during hand movements. Electroencephalogr. Clin. Neurophysiol. 91:456–467.

Netchine, S., Harrison, A., Bergers, J., et al. 1964. Contribution à l'étude de la signification des rhythmes mu. Rev. Neurol. (Paris) 111:339–341.

Niedermeyer, E. 1963. Clinical correlates of flat or low voltage records. Electroencephalogr. Clin. Neurophysiol. 15:148(abst).

Niedermeyer, E. 1972a. *The Generalized Epilepsies.* Springfield, IL: Charles C Thomas.

Niedermeyer, E. 1972b. Focal and generalized seizure discharges in the electroencephalogram and their response to diazepam. Int. Med. Digest. 7:49–61.

Niedermeyer, E. 1990a. An independent alpha-like rhythm in the temporal region. Electroencephalogr. Clin. Neurophysiol. 75:S103(abst).

Niedermeyer, E. 1990b. Alpha-like rhythmical activity of the temporal lobe. Clin. Electroencephalogr. 21:210–224.

Niedermeyer, E. 1990c. Ein unabhängiger alpha-artiger Rhythmus über dem Temporallappen Das EEG-Labor. 12:165–173.

Niedermeyer, E. 1991. The "third rhythm": further observations. Clin. Electroencephalogr. 22:83–96.

Niedermeyer, E. 1997. Alpha rhythms as physiological and abnormal phenomena. Int. J. Psychophysiol. 26:31–49.

Niedermeyer, E., and Koshino, Y. 1975. My-Rhythmus: Vorkommen und klinische Bedeutung. Z. EEG-EMG. 6:69–78.

Niedermeyer, E., and Sherman, D.L. 2001a. Ultrafast frequencies: a new challenge for electroencephalography with remarks on ultraslow frequencies. Clin. Electroencephalogr. 32:119–121.

Niedermeyer, E., and Sherman, D.L. 2001b. Ultrafast EEG frequencies—not to be neglected in the future. Am. J. EEG Technol. 41:192–198.

Niedermeyer, E., Long, D.M., Hendler, N.H., et al. 1982. Chronic pain and mu rhythm. Electroencephalogr. Clin. Neurophysiol. 53:30P(abst).

Niedermeyer, E., Krauss, G.L., and Peyser, C.E. 1989. The electroencephalogram and mental activation. Clin. Electroencephalogr. 20:215–226.

Niedermeyer, E., Goldszmidt, A., and Ryan, D. 2004. "Mu rhythm status" and clinical correlates. Clin. Electroencephalogr. 35:215–218.

Nowak, S.M., and Marczynski, T.J. 1981. Trait anxiety is reflected in EEG alpha response to stress. Electroencephalogr. Clin. Neurophysiol. 52:175–191.

Nowlis, D., and Kamiya, J. 1970. The control of electroencephalographic alpha rhythms through auditory feedback and the associated mental activity. Psychophysiology 6:476–484.

Obrist, W.D. 1954. The electroencephalogram of normal aged adults. Electroencephalogr. Clin. Neurophysiol. 6:235–244.

Pampiglione, G. 1963. *Development of Cerebral Function in the Dog.* London: Butterworth.

Panzani, R., and Turner M. 1952. Étude électroencéphalographique de la maladie asthmatique. Correlations électroclinques-Hypothèses pathogéniques. Presse Méd. 3:1826–1828.

Perez-Borja, C., Chatrian, G.E., Tyce, F.A., et al. 1962. Electrographic patterns of the occipital lobes in man: a topographic study based on use of implanted electrodes. Electroencephalogr. Clin. Neurophysiol. 14:171–182.

Petersén, I., and Eeg-Olofsson, O. 1971. The development of the electroencephalogram in normal children from the age of 1 through 15 years. Nonparoxysmal activity. Neuropädiatrie 2:247–304.

Pfurtscheller, G. 1981. Central beta rhythms and sensorimotor activities in man. Electroencephalogr. Clin. Neurophysiol. 51:253–264.

Pfurtscheller, G. 1986. Rolandic mu rhythm and assessment of cerebral functions. Am. J. EEG Technol. 26:19–32.

Pfurtscheller, G. 1990. Event-related EEG desynchronization. Electroencephalogr. Clin. Neurophysiol. 75:S117(abst).

Pfurtscheller, G. 1992. Event-related synchronization (ERS): an electrophysiological correlate of cortical areas at rest. Electroencephalogr. Clin. Neurophysiol. 83:62–69.

Pfurtscheller, G., and Aranibar, A. 1978a. Occipital rhythm activity within the alpha band during conditioned externally paced movement. Electroencephalogr. Clin. Neurophysiol. 45:226–235.

Pfurtscheller, G., and Aranibar A. 1978b. Änderungen in der spontanen EEG-Aktivität vor Willkürbewegungen. Neue Wege bei der Untersuchung der zentralen mu-Aktivität. Z. EEG-EMG. 9:18–23.

Pfurtscheller, G., and Klimesch, W. 1992. Event-related synchronization and desynchronization of alpha and beta waves in a cognitive task. In *Induced Rhythms in the Brain,* Eds. E. Başar and T.H. Bullock, pp. 117–128. Boston: Birkhäuser.

Pfurtscheller, G., and Lopes da Silva, F.H. 1999a. Event-related EEG/MEG synchronization and desynchronization: basic principles. Clin. Neurophysiol. 110:1842–1857.

Pfurtscheller, G., and Lopes da Silva, F., eds. 1999b. Event-related desynchronization. *Handbook of Electroencephalography and Clinical Neurophysiology,* revised series, vol. 6. Amsterdam: Elsevier.

Pfurtscheller, G., and Neuper, C. 1992. Simultaneous EEG 10 Hz desynchronization and 40 Hz synchronization during finger movements. NeuroReport 3:1057–1060.

Pfurtscheller, G., Flotzinger, D., and Neuper, C. 1994. Differentiation between finger, toe and tongue movement in man based on 40 Hz EEG. Electroencephalogr. Clin. Neurophysiol. 90:456–460.

Picard, P., Laboureur, P., and Navranne, P. 1955. Examen électroencéphalographique de personnel navigeant. Méd. Aéronaut. 10:53–58.

Picard, P., Navaranne, P., Laboureur, P., et al. 1957. Confrontations des données de l'électroencéphalogramme et des examens psychologiques chez 522 sujets repartis en trois groupes differents. III. Confrontations des données de l'électroencéphalogramme et de l'examen psychologique chez 309 candidats pilotes a l'aéronautiques. In *Conditionnement et Réactivité en Électroencéphalographie,* Eds. H. Fischgold and H. Gastaut, pp. 304–314. Amsterdam: Elsevier.

Pine, I., and Pine, H.M. 1953. Clinical analysis of patients with low voltage EEG. J. Nerv. Ment. Dis. 117:191–198.

Pitot, M., and Gastaut, H. 1954. EEG changes during the menstrual cycle. Electroencephalogr. Clin. Neurophysiol. 6:162(abst).

Radermecker, J. 1961. La valeur médico-légale de l'électroencéphalographie dans les séquelles subjectives des traumas craneo-cérébraux fermés. Acta Neurol. Belg. 61:468–476.

Radhakrishnan, K., Silbert, P.L., and Klass, D.W. 1994. Breach activity related to an osteolytic skull metastasis. Am. J. EEG Technol. 34:1–5.

Remond, A. 1968. The importance of topographic data in EEG phenomena and an electric model to reproduce them. In *Advances in EEG Analysis,* Eds. D.O. Walter and M.A.B. Brazier, pp. 29–46. Amsterdam: Elsevier.

Remond, A., and Lesèvre, N. 1957. Remarques sur l'activité cérébrale des sujets normaux. La typologie électroencéphalographique dans ses rapports avec certains cactérs psychologiques. In *Conditionnement et Réactivité en Électroencéphalographie,* Eds. H. Fischgold and H. Gastaut, pp. 235–255. Amsterdam: Elsevier.

Remond, A., and Lesèvre, N. 1971. Étude de la fonction du regard par l'analyse des potentiels évoqués visuels (lumière, patterns complexes et mouvements des yeux). In *La Fonction du Regard,* Eds. A. Dubois Poulsen et al., pp. 127–175. Paris: Colloques de l'INSERM.

Remond, A., Lesèvre, N., and Torres, F. 1965. Étude chronotopographique de l'activité occipitale moyenne recueilli sur le scalp chez l'homme en rélation avec le déplacement du regard (complexe lambda). Rev. Neurol. (Paris) 113:193–226.

Riekkinen, P., Buzsaki, G., Riekkinen, P., Jr., et al. 1991. The cholinergic system and EEG slow waves. Electroencephalogr. Clin. Neurophysiol. 78:89–96.

Rinaldi, F., and Himwich, H.E. 1955. Cholinergic mechanisms involved in function of mesodiencephalic activating system. Arch. Neurol. Psychiatr. 73:396–402.

Roger, A., and Bert, J. 1959. Étude des corrélations entre les differents variables EEG. Rev. Neurol. (Paris) 101:334–360.

Roldan, E., Lepicovska, V., Dostalek, C., et al. 1981. Mu-like EEG rhythm generation in the course of Hatha-yogi exercises. Electroencephalogr. Clin. Neurophysiol. 52:13P(abst).

Rosas, H.D., Koroshetz, W.S., Chen, Y.I., et al. 2003. Evidence for more widespread cerebral pathology in early HD. Neurology 60:1615–1620.

Roth, M., and Green, J. 1953. The lambda wave as a normal physiological phenomenon in the human electroencephalogram. Nature (Lond.) 172:864–866.

Roubicek, J., Tachezy, R., and Matousek, M. 1968. Electrical activity of the brain during the menstrual cycle. Cs. Psychiatr. 64:90–94.

Rougeul, A., Letalle, A., and Corvisier, J. 1972. Activité rythmique du cortex somésthésique primaire en rélation avec l'immobilité chez le chat libre éveillé. Electroencephalogr. Clin. Neurophysiol. 33:23–39.

Rugg, M.D., and Dickens, A.M.J. 1982. Dissociation of alpha and theta activity as a function of verbal and visuospatial tasks. Electroencephalogr. Clin. Neurophysiol. 53:201–207.

Salmelin, R., and Hari, R. 1994a. Spatiotemporal characteristics of sensorimotor neuromagnetic rhythms related to thumb movement. Neuroscience 60:537–550.

Salmelin, R., and Hari, R. 1994b. Characterization of spontaneous MEG rhythms in healthy adults. Electroencephalogr. Clin. Neurophysiol. 91:237–248.

Saul, L.J., Davis, H., and Davis, P.A. 1937. Correlations between electroencephalograms and the psychological organization of the individual. Trans. Am. Neurol. Assoc. 63:167–169.

Scheich, H. 1969. Interval histograms and periodic diurnal changes of human alpha rhythm. Electroencephalogr. Clin. Neurophysiol. 26:442(abst).

Scherzer, E. 1966. Das flache EEG als bioelektrischer Ausdruck der Erwartungsspannung (psychogene Alphareduktion). Psychiatr. Neurol. (Basel) 152:207–212.

Schiff, S.J., Colella, D., Jacyna, G.M., et al. 2000. Brain chirps: spectrographic signatures of epileptic seizures. Electroencephalogr. Clin. Neurophysiol. 111:953–958.

Schnell, R.G., and Klass, D.W. 1966. Further observations on the rolandic arceau rhythm. Electroencephalogr. Clin. Neurophysiol. 20:95(abst).

Schoppenhorst, M., Brauer, F., Freund, G., et al. 1980. The significance of coherence estimates in determining cerebral alpha and mu activities. Electroencephalogr. Clin. Neurophysiol. 48:25–33.

Schütz, E., and Müller, H.W. 1951. Über ein neues Zeichen zentralnervöser Erregbarkeitssteigerung im Elektroenzephalogramm. Klin. Wochenschr. 29:22–23.

Scott, D.F., and Bickford, R.G. 1967. Electrophysiologic studies during scanning and passive eye movements in humans. Science 155:101–102.

Scott, D.F., Groethuysen, U.C., and Bickford, R.G. 1967. Lambda responses in the human electroencephalogram. Neurology (Minneapolis) 17:770–778.

Sem-Jacobsen, C.W. 1968. *Depth-Electrographic Stimulation of the Human Brain and Behavior.* Springfield, IL: Charles C Thomas.

Shagass, C. 1946. An attempt to correlate the occipital alpha frequency of the electroencephalogram with performance on a mental ability test. J. Exp. Psychol. 36:88–92.

Shinomiya, S., Fukenaga, T., and Nagata, K. 1999. Clinical aspects of the "third rhythm" of the temporal lobe. Clin. Electroencephalogr. 30:136–142.

Siepman, T.A.M., Cherian, P.J., and Visser, G.H. 2004. Zeta waves, an unusual EEG finding in structural brain lesions: Report of two patients. Am. J. END Technol. 44:24–29.

Silbert, P.L., Radhakrishnan, K., Johnson, J., et al. 1995. The significance of the phi rhythm. Electroencephalogr. Clin. Neurophysiol. 95:71–76.

Simon, O. (Simonova, O.) 1977. *Das Elektroenzephalogramm.* Munich: Urban & Schwarzenberg.

Simonova, O., Roth, B., and Stein, J. 1966. An EEG study of healthy subjects. Normal rhythms of the resting record. Electroencephalogr. Clin. Neurophysiol. 20:279(abst).

Simonova, O., Roth, B., and Stein, J. 1967. EEG studies of healthy population—normal rhythms of resting recording. Act. Unv. Carol. Med. (Praha) 13:543–551.

Smith, S.A., Wong, P.K.H., and Jan, J.E. 1998. Unilateral alpha activity: an electroencephalographic finding in albinism. J. Clin. Neurophysiol. 15:146–149.

Snider, R.S. 1950. Recent contributions to the anatomy and physiology of the cerebellum. Arch. Neurol. Psychiatry (Chicago) 64:196–219.

Steriade, M., Gloor, P., Llinas, R.R., et al. 1990. Basic mechanisms of cerebral rhythmical activities. Electroencephalogr. Clin. Neurophysiol. 76:481–508.

Sterman, M.B., Howe, R.C., and MacDonald, L. 1970. Facilitation of spindle-burst sleep by conditioning of electroencephalographic activity while awake. Science 167:1146–1148.

Sterman, M.B., MacDonald, L.R., and Stone, R.K. 1974. Biofeedback training of sensorimotor EEG in man and its effect on epilepsy. Epilepsia (New York) 15:395–416.

Sterman, M.B., Wyrwicka, W., and Roth, S.R. 1969. Electrophysiological correlates and neural substrates of alimentary behavior in the cat. In *Neural Regulation of Food and Water Intake,* Eds. J.P. Morgan and M. Wagner, Ann. N.Y. Acad. Sci. 157:723–739.

Stigsby, B., Rodenberg, J.C., and Moth, H.B. 1981. Electroencephalographic findings during mantra meditation (transcendental meditation). A controlled qualitative study of experienced meditators. Electroencephalogr. Clin. Neurophysiol. 51:434–442.

Storm van Leeuwen, W., and Bekkering, D.H. 1958. Some results obtained with the EEG spectrograph. Electroencephalogr. Clin. Neurophysiol. 10:563.

Storm van Leeuwen, W., Kamp, A., Kok, M.L., et al. 1963. Rélation entre l'activité électrique des certaines structures cérébrales et le comportement du chien. Rev. Neurol. (Paris) 109:258–259.

Storm van Leeuwen, W., Kamp, A., Kok, M.L., et al. 1967. Rélations entre les activités cérébrales du chien, son comportement et sa direction d'attention. Actual. Neurophysiol. (Paris) 7:167–186.

Storm van Leeuwen, W., Wieneke, G., Spoelstra, P., et al. 1978. Lack of bilateral coherence of mu-rhythm. Electroencephalogr. Clin. Neurophysiol. 44:140–146.

Stroganova, T.A., Orekhova, E.V., and Posikera, I.N. 1999. EEG alpha rhythm in infants. Clin. Neurophysiol. 110:997–1012.

Sugerman, A.A., Debruin, A.T., and Roth, C.W. 1970. Quantitative EEG change in the human menstrual cycle. Res. Commun. Chem. Pathol. Pharmacol. 1:526–534.

Synek, V.M. 1983. The low-voltage electroencephalogram. Clin. Electroencephalogr. 14:102–105.

Tait, G.A., and Pavlovski, R.P. 1978. Alpha and the eye. Electroencephalogr. Clin. Neurophysiol. 45:286–289.

Takahashi, N., Shinomiya, S., Mori, D., et al. 1997. Frontal midline theta rhythm in young healthy adults. Clin. Electroencephalogr. 28:49–54.

Tannier, C., Bentzinger, C., and Feuerstein, J. 1983. A case of a lesional unilateral mu rhythm: clinical and EEG evolution. Electroencephalogr. Clin. Neurophysiol. 56:21P(abst).

Torres, A.A. 1968. Sensitization and association in alpha blocking "conditioning." Electroencephalogr. Clin. Neurophysiol. 24:297–306.

Townsend, R.E., Lubin, A., and Naitoh, P. 1975. Stabilization of alpha frequency by sinusoidally modulated light. Electroencephalogr. Clin. Neurophysiol. 39:515–518.

Trabka, J. 1963. High frequency components in brain waves. Electroencephalogr. Clin. Neurophysiol. 14:453–464.

Traub, R.D., Jefferys, J.G.R., Whittington, M.A. 1999. *Fast oscillations in cortical circuits.* Cambridge, MA: MIT Press.

Travis, L.E., and Egan, J.P. 1938. Conditioning of the electrical response of the cortex. J. Exp. Psychol. 22:524–531.

Travis, L.E., and Gottlober, A.B. 1936. Do brain waves have individuality? Science 84:532–533.

Van der Drift, J.H., and Magnus, O. 1961. The EEG in cerebral ischemic lesions. Correlations with clinical and pathological findings. In *Cerebral Anoxia and the Electroencephalogram,* Eds. H. Gastaut and J.S. Meyer, pp. 180–196. Springfield, IL: Charles C Thomas.

Van Huffelen, A.C., and Magnus, O. 1973. 4 c/sec vertex spindles. Electroencephalogr. Clin. Neurophysiol. 34:543–546.

Van Huffelen, A., Poortvliet, D., and Van der Wulp, C. 1984. Quantitative electroencephalography in cerebral ischemia. Detection of abnormalities in "normal" EEGs. In *Brain Ischemia: Quantitative EEG and Imaging Techniques,* Eds. G. Pfurtscheller, J. Jonkman, and F.H. Lopes da Silva, pp. 3–28. Amsterdam: Elsevier.

Vanhatalo, S., Tallgren, P., Anderson, S., et al. 2002. DC-EEG recording discloses prominent very slow activity patterns in preterm infants. Clin. Neurophysiol. 113: 1822–1825.

Vanhatalo, S., Holmes, M.D., Tallgren, P., et al. 2003. Very slow EEG responses lateralize temporal lobe seizures. Neurology: 1098–1104.

Veilleux, M., Westmoreland, B.F., and Sharbrough, F.W. 1988. Fast central midline rhythm. Electroencephalogr. Clin. Neurophysiol. 69:91P–92P(abst).

Veldhuizen, R.J., Jonlman, E.J., and Poortvliet, D.C.J. 1993. Sex differences in age regression parameters of healthy adults—normative data and practical implications. Electroencephalogr. Clin. Neurophysiol. 86:377–384.

Visser, S.L. 1961. Correlations between the contingent alpha blocking, EEG characteristics and clinical diagnosis. Electroencephalogr. Clin. Neurophysiol. 13:438–446.

Vogel, F. 1962. Untersuchungen zur Genetik der Beta Wellen im EEG des Menschen. Dtsch. Z. Nervenheilk. 184:137–173.

Vogel, F. 1966. Zur genetischen Grundlage fronto-präzentraler Beta Wellen in EEG des Menschen. Hum. Genet. 2:227–237.

Vogel, F. 1970. The genetic basis of the normal human electroencephalogram (EEG). Hum. Genet. 10:91–114.

Vogel, F., and Fujiya, Y. 1969. The incidence of some inherited EEG variants in normal Japanese and German males. Hum. Genet. 7:38–42.

Vogel, F., and Götze, W. 1959. Familienuntersuchungen zur Genetik des normalen Elektroenzephalogramms. Dtsch. A. Nervenheilk. 178:668–700.

Vogel, F., and Götze, W. 1962. Statistische Betrachtungen über die Beta-Wellen im EEG des Menschen. Dtsch. Z. Nervenheilk. 184:112–136.

Vogel, F., Götze, W., and Kubicki, S. 1961. Der Wert von Familienuntersuchungen für die Beurteilung des Niederspannungs-EEG nach geschlossenen Schädeltrauma. Dtsch. A. Nervenheilk. 182:337–354.

Wallace, R.K. 1970. Physiological effects of transcendental meditation. Science 167:1751–1754.

Wallace, R.K., Benson, M., and Wilson, A.J. 1971. A wakeful hypometabolic physiologic state. Am. J. Physiol. 221:795–799.

Walter, D.O., Rhodes, J.M., Brown, D., et al. 1966. Comprehensive spectral analysis of human EEG generators in posterior cerebral areas. Electroencephalogr. Clin. Neurophysiol. 20:224–237.

Walter, W.G. 1936. The location of cerebral tumors by electroencephalography. Lancet 2:305–308.

Walter, W.G. 1959. Intrinsic rhythms of the brain. In *Handbook of Physiology,* Eds. J. Field, et al., Sec. 1, pp. 279–298. Washington, DC: American Physiological Society.

Walter, W.G., and Dovey, V.J. 1944. Electroencephalography in cases of sub-cortical tumour. J. Neurol. Neurosurg. Psychiatry 7:57–65.

Watanabe, S. 1981. Rhythmicity of EEG and stability of alpha rhythm. Electroencephalogr. Clin. Neurophysiol. 52:62P(abst).

Westmoreland, B., and Klass, O.W. 1981. A distinctive rhythmic EEG discharge of adults. Electroencephalogr. Clin. Neurophysiol. 51:186–191.

Westmoreland, B., and Sharbrough, F.W. 1975. Occipital slow waves associated with eye blinks in children. Electroencephalogr. Clin. Neurophysiol. 38:335(abst).

Wieneke, G.H., Deinema, C.H.A., Spoelstra, P., et al. 1980. Normative spectral data on alpha rhythm in male adults. Electroencephalogr. Clin. Neurophysiol. 49:636–645.

Wyrwicka, W., and Sterman, M.B. 1968. Instrumental conditioning of sensorimotor cortex EEG spindles in the waking cat. Physiol. Behav. 3:703–707.

Yamada, T., and Kooi, K.A. 1975. Level of consciousness and the mu rhythm. Clin. Electroencephalogr. 6:80–88.

Ziemann, U., and Rothwell, J.C. 2000. I-waves in motor cortex. J. Clin. Neurophysiol. 17:397–405.

10. Sleep and EEG

Ernst Niedermeyer

Sleep Recording in EEG and Special Sleep Laboratories

The chapter discusses the electroencephalogram (EEG) activity of sleeping healthy adults. This section is limited to sleep recordings obtained in the regular EEG laboratory. This type of sleep EEG recording has been done for about 60 years in many major laboratories to secure information not available in the usual waking-resting record with such activations as hyperventilation and intermittent photic stimulation. The purpose of these EEG sleep studies is to search for abnormalities that may be hidden in the waking state. The more this type of combined waking and sleep recording is carried out in the regular EEG laboratory, the greater will be the insight into the sleep patterns of normal individuals.

Nevertheless, the term *sleep EEG* may be somewhat presumptuous when one considers that only a short segment of sleep can be recorded under daytime recording circumstances. Furthermore, the recorded sleep is basically a nap, either spontaneous or induced by a sedative, and is thus different from nocturnal sleep. In the regular EEG laboratory, one can observe the process of falling asleep during the daytime. The ensuing sleep is relatively short and, for the most practical purposes, a duration of 10 to 30 minutes will suffice. The result is a tracing that shows the transition from the waking state to drowsiness and from drowsiness (stage 1) to light non-rapid-eye-movement (REM) sleep (stage 2). These stages of falling asleep and light sleep are usually the most informative stages for the electroencephalographer who is searching for clinically relevant abnormalities and especially for epileptic discharges not demonstrable in the waking state. In certain cases, deeper sleep (stage 3 or possible stage 4) may yield additional information; this may require a more prolonged sleep recording. REM stages usually emerge about 60 to 90 minutes after sleep onset; this is closer to 90 minutes in sedated sleep. This necessitates unusually prolonged recording and, in the hustle of a regular laboratory, blocks one of the recording units for an unduly long period.

Here the need for nocturnal sleep recording becomes obvious. There are now a growing number of specialized nocturnal sleep laboratories that offer 24-hour recordings of a given patient. These laboratories have concentrated on (a) nocturnal sleep research in healthy volunteers, (b) the exploration of the sequential nocturnal sleep phases in patients with sleep disorders, and (c) the study of poorly understood (and possible epileptic) attacks of strictly nocturnal occurrence.

Specialized sleep laboratories are polygraphically oriented and use EEG in combination with a variety of other physiological parameters. It is not unusual to find only two channels reserved for EEG recording. This polygraphic approach has made enormous progress over the past two decades; the required technology is the subject of a special section, and the clinical implications of modern polysomnography will be presented, with separate sections on newborns (Chapter 49) and on children and adults (Chapter 48).

The scoring of sleep stages (as it is being done in sleep laboratories) is essentially based on the rules laid down by Rechtschaffen and Kales (1968). These rules have been strongly criticized but no major changes have been introduced. The most consistent proponent of criticism have been Kubicki and his co-workers (Kubicki and Herrmann, 1996; Kubicki et al., 1986, 1987). Most of this criticism has been directed toward (a) lack of insufficient EEG information (limitation to central lead) and (b) misleading delta activity criteria resulting in erroneous scoring. This is particularly true with stage 1 and 2 segments occurring within REM sleep and falsely scored as REM sleep.

Practice and Technology of Sleep Recording in EEG Laboratory

The emphasis on sleep sections in routine laboratory work varies greatly and depends on the influence of major centers and schools. Most major American schools of EEG traditionally use sleep in routine EEG work to a great extent. Some laboratories try to attempt sleep in every or almost every patient at any age. In this author's laboratory, the proportion of sleep records was consistently around 60%. Debates about the usefulness of sleep can be heated; many electroencephalographers use sleep only as a method to obtain a tracing in uncooperative and otherwise unmanageable children. The informative value of short sleep recordings has been stressed by Gastaut et al. (1983, 1984) and Niedermeyer and Höller (1984).

There is no doubt that the overall information derived from a wakefulness record is greater and hence clinically more significant. There are, however, a number of conditions, especially in the domain of epileptic seizure disorders, in which sleep provides essential information. (This excludes the sleep disorders themselves, which ought to be evaluated in a specialized sleep laboratory.) For the sake of this important minority, sleep portions should be secured in most patients.

The drowsy state and light sleep (stage 2) are usually the most informative phases; for this reason, the sleep-onset portion with a length of 5 to 30 minutes in stage 2 sleep may be sufficient. In infants and children, a sleep section (nap recording) is almost a necessity, not simply because of easier management of the sleeping child but also because of the needed information. In infants and in small and preschool children, the EEG recording often cannot start until the child has fallen asleep. In these cases, great efforts must be made to secure a readable waking portion after awakening.

It can be understood readily that pad electrodes pressed against the scalp by caps or bands are counterproductive in a sleep laboratory. The slight discomfort caused by such electrodes is enough to keep the patient from falling asleep. For this reason, electrodes suitable for sleep recording ought to be fixed to the head by an adhesive.

In some laboratories, the technologist and the apparatus are placed in the same room where the patient lies. In the absence of video monitoring, this setup has advantages such as closer observation, especially in patients with clinical seizures, over the system of having patient and machine in separate rooms with a window permitting observation of the patient. With this latter setup, the technician can more effectively request help from colleagues or the medical director. Beds or carts are superior to reclining chairs.

Spontaneous Sleep, Sleep Deprivation, and Sedated Sleep

Spontaneous Sleep

Sleep without medication is undoubtedly preferable to sedated sleep. In an appropriately darkened room, many children and adults fall asleep quite readily. North American patterns of individual or family life often include watching late television shows, which incline some patients to be most willing to lie down and sleep during a daytime recording session. Outpatients from distant areas and those who have experienced strenuous travel in the early morning hours also are likely to sleep without medication.

Sleep Deprivation

Sleep deprivation prior to recording has been suggested over the past decade by a number of electroencephalographers. This method has been described by Bennett (1963), Bennett et al. (1964), Mattson et al. (1965), Oller-Daurella (1966), Pratt et al. (1968), Wittenbecker and Kubicki (1976), Rumpl et al. (1977), Deisenhammer and Klingler (1978), Degen (1980), Jovanovic (1991), Kubicki et al. (1991), and Klingler et al. (1991). It consists of sleep loss for 24 to 36 hours. Its goal is the detection of epileptic discharges that could be missed otherwise. According to the view of Pratt et al. (1968), a good deal of the activation of paroxysmal patterns may be ascribable to drowsiness and sleep as such, but some other factors specific for sleep deprivation have proved to be potent activators. In Pratt et al.'s research, activation of epileptic patterns was obtained in 41% of 114 patients.

Sleep deprivation may have drawbacks. Many individuals and especially children may be so fatigued that they fall asleep almost instantly in the laboratory with rapid evolution of stages 3 and 4; with the possible exception of temporal lobe epilepsy, these are much less informative electroencephalographically than stage 2. This is especially true in cases of generalized epilepsies (primary generalized epilepsy, Lennox-Gastaut syndrome) and benign focal spikes in children.

Naitoh and Dement (1976) have summarized the current status of sleep deprivation as follows:

1. One night of sleep loss is sufficient. Sleep loss can be performed at home with the help of a family member.
2. Anticonvulsant medication does not have to be discontinued.
3. Use sleep deprivation with other techniques of activation (see also Kubicki et al., 1991).
4. Patients must be kept awake during the test period.
5. Expect very few false-positive cases but many false-negative cases.
6. Sleep deprivation is a genuine activation method. Its efficacy in provoking abnormal EEG discharges is not due to drowsiness.

The insistence on keeping the patient awake during the recording may be debatable and its value should be thoroughly assessed. There is reason to presume that bilateral synchronous seizure discharges are triggered by short fluctuations of the level of awareness (light drowsiness followed by an arousing stimulus; see Niedermeyer, 1972); for this reason, the significance of short and minor drowsy periods should be emphasized rather than minimized.

As to the search for EEG abnormalities, a differentiation should be made between patients with primary generalized epilepsy and temporal lobe epilepsy. In the former, the strict routine suggested by Naitoh and Dement (1976) might be highly effective; these patients should by all means be kept awake during recording (also see Degen, 1980). In temporal lobe epilepsies, the ensuing deep sleep (stage 3) could be more informative.

Rodin et al. (1962) have extended the period of sleep loss in normal young volunteers to 120 hours of total sleep deprivation. There was evidence of frequent generalized bursts similar to those seen in primary generalized epilepsy. These changes, however, could not be confirmed by other investigators (Heinemann, 1966; Johnson, 1969; Jovanovic et al., 1971; Naitoh et al., 1969), who used sleep deprivation for periods as long as 264 hours. Welch and Stevens (1971) also feel that sleep deprivation does not activate the EEG of healthy subjects.

The suggestion of Gibbs and Gibbs (1964) to keep the patients awake until after midnight is helpful as a means to obtain sleep more readily the following morning in the laboratory. However, this widely used practice almost completely dilutes the basic principle of sleep deprivation. In practice, good sleep recordings in stage 2 are only slightly less informative than tracings obtained after sleep deprivation for 24 hours.

Sleep deprivation is a true activator, it is a specific stress imposed on the central nervous system (CNS) to activate otherwise hidden epileptic activity. Sleep recordings in general are done in a physiological state and should not be listed as activation. The sleep deprivation stress can be augmented by the effect of anticonvulsants with sedative effect (phenobarbital or primidone) against which the patient must fight. According to Klass and Fischer-Williams (1976), the benefits derived from sleep deprivation outweigh the risks of clinical seizures. These authors, however, point out that in

Table 10.1. Guidelines for sedation to obtain EEG sleep records

Recommended sedative: chloral hydrate (oral); chloral hydrate syrup U.S.P.
A. Adults and adolescents above 15 years
    Average weight (56–80 kg): 1.75–2.5 g
    Below average weight (40–55 kg): 1.25–2 g
    Above average weight (above 80 kg): 2.5–3.5 g
B. Children (5–14 years)
    1.0–2.0 g (depending on weight)
C. Infants and small children (4 months to 4 years)
    Below 1/2 year: 0.125–0.25 g
    1/2–1 year: 0.25–0.5 g (max. 0.75 g)
    1–4 years: 0.5–1.0 g (max 1.5 g if close to 4 years and above average weight)

Advantages of chloral hydrate: induced fast EEG activity less prominent than with barbiturates and rapidly metabolized.
Side effects (paradoxical excitation with irrational behavior) rare.

sleep-deprived persons photic stimulation requires greater caution. There is no doubt that emphasis being placed on sleep deprivation has clearly declined since the appearance of the second edition of this book in 1987.

Sedated Sleep

Whenever a sleep recording is desirable and cannot be obtained naturally, sedated sleep is dictated by necessity. The most important advice to a novice in this technique is patience; the patient must not be overpowered by strong and rapidly effective sedatives. Therefore, the intravenous and intramuscular routes must be avoided; with these the patient's sleep becomes very unnatural and contains elements of an early state of general anesthesia. The highly informative stages of drowsiness (stage 1) and light sleep (stage 2) are quickly passed, and the ensuing deep sleep yields very little information in most cases. Enormous amounts of fast activity may also obscure important details.

Orally or rectally administered sedatives act more gently and slowly. The ensuing sleep contains many or most features of spontaneous sleep. The author's personal experience is based on chloral hydrate and secobarbital (Seconal), but the former has proved to be preferable. The oral route is standard; rectal administration is usually confined to infants reluctant to take the medication by mouth. The dosages are shown in Table 10.1.

In special cases of temporal epilepsy there is still a place for the intravenous route and deep sleep. The use of ultra-short-acting barbiturates has been recommended by Kajtor et al. (1957); Wilder (1969) was particularly impressed with methohexital (Brevital). The effectiveness of these drugs lie in the fact that, in some cases of temporal lobe epilepsy, the anterior temporal spike focus becomes most active in stages 3 or 4.

Terminology of Sleep Stages

The Old Terminology

The first widely used terminology was proposed by Loomis et al. (1937, 1938). Stages of sleep were broken down as follows:

A	Awake, earliest drowsiness	Alpha
B_1	Light drowsiness	Alpha dropout
B_2	Deep drowsiness	Vertex waves
C	Light sleep	Spindles vertex waves, K complexes
D	Deep sleep	Much slowing, K complexes, some spindles
E	Very deep sleep	Much slowing, some K complexes

This classification reflects the state of knowledge prior to the discovery of REM sleep. The sleep investigators of the late 1930s, however, were not completely unaware of the existence of a rather unusual type of sleep, which they termed the "null stage" (Blake and Gerard, 1937). The occurrence of rapid eye movement and other physiological and psychological concomitants was not demonstrated by these investigators.

The Present Terminology

The discovery of human REM sleep has been attributed to Aserinsky and Kleitman (1953), who were able to demonstrate regularly recurrent periods of altered ocular motility during sleep. Further insight into the significance of the REM stages prompted a new terminology of sleep stages that emphasized the dichotomy of two basically different types of sleep: non-REM ("slow sleep") and REM sleep (also "paradoxical sleep" or "fast sleep").

This dualistic approach subsequently proved to be appropriate because of impressive differences of neurobiochemistry and neuronal circuitry (Dahlström and Fuxe, 1964; Jouvet, 1969, 1972; Jouvet and Delorme, 1965; Ungerstedt, 1971).

The presently used classification (essentially following that of Dement and Kleitman, 1957) divides sleep into the following stages:

1	Drowsiness	From alpha dropout to vertex waves
2	Light sleep	Spindles, vertex waves, K complexes
3	Deep sleep	Much slowing, K complexes, some spindles
4	Very deep sleep	Much slowing, some K complexes
REM	REM sleep	Desynchronization with faster frequencies

The transition from stage to stage may be somewhat imprecise, but in general, staging of sleep periods is not difficult for electroencephalographers who are used to reading records in both the waking state and sleep.

In the clinical EEG laboratory, most sleepers reach only stage 2, stage 3 is occasionally, and stage 4 seldom reached unless unusually long sleep recording time is allotted or in cases of profound tiredness after sleep loss. REM stages are seldom seen in the clinical laboratory except in infants, young children, and adults with sleep loss. Their occurrence at sleep onset may denote a primary sleep disorder (especially a narcolepsy-cataplexy complex), but REM sleep onset may also occur in patients with severely disturbed sleep due to central disturbances such as delirium tremens or in deep-seated cerebral pathology.

Reviews of the EEG characteristics (Erwin et al., 1984) and the neurobiochemical basis of sleep (Guilleminault and Baker, 1984) are warmly recommended sources of further information.

The "Microstructure" of Sleep: Cyclic Alternating Patterns

Sleep is not solely determined by macrostructural shifts of non-REM (NREM) and REM sleep stages. Evidence of a "microstructure" of sleep has been provided over the past 20 years. Transient activations phases ("phases transitoires") were reported by Schieber et al. (1971). "Cyclic alternating patterns" of sleep were observed by Terzano and his co-workers, first under severely abnormal conditions such as Creutzfeldt-Jakob disease (Terzano et al., 1981), later in normal individuals (Terzano and Parrino, 1987, 1991). Cyclic alternating patterns (CAPs) occur mainly in NREM sleep, are generally associated with transient lightening of sleep depth, and are independent of afferent stimuli, thus constituting modality-independent responses (Halász, 1988; Terzano and Parrino, 1991).

The cyclic alternating pattern consists of an A phase of enhancement of electrical activity and a subsequent B phase characterized by attenuation of EEG activity. Each phase lasts only between 2 and 60 seconds.

A somewhat different type of periodic activity of light sleep has been demonstrated by Evans (1992), who observed alternating periods of alpha and theta activity with a usual interval of about 16 seconds. This activity is thought to be related to intermittent arousing mechanisms involving cortex and brainstem activating systems (Evans, 1992). This study is also coupled with impressive thoughts about the failure of the physiological periodic activity in coma of either cortical and brainstem accentuation.

The State of Drowsiness

Early Drowsiness

The level of vigilance tends to fluctuate, and fleeting brief episodes of very light drowsiness are very common in waking records. Boredom, fatigue, and monotony may quickly induce such periods in a patient instructed to relax during the test. Drowsiness is a very interesting state from the electroencephalographer's viewpoint. It shows particularly marked age-determined changes; the "hypnagogic" rhythmical 4 to 6/sec theta activity of late infancy and early childhood represents a unique feature of that period of life (see Chapter 11, "Maturation of the EEG"). Later in childhood and, in many cases, in the declining years of life, the onset of drowsiness is characterized by greater amounts of slow activity mingling with the posterior alpha rhythm. An electroencephalographically defined drowsy state does not exist in the neonate and, in senility, abrupt transitions from wakefulness to light sleep are again quite common.

In the adult, the onset of drowsiness is characterized by gradual or brisk "alpha dropout." The alpha waves are replaced by low-voltage slow activity, mainly in the range of 2 to 7/sec. Very low voltage 15 to 25/sec activity may be

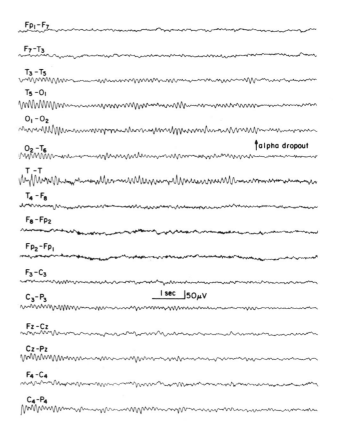

Figure 10.1. Alpha dropout with early drowsiness in normal adult.

mixed with the slowing (Fig. 10.1). Thus, the tracing appears to be desynchronized due to the general voltage decline. This state must be strictly separated from periods of enhanced alertness after eye opening or caused by mental or emotional stress (associated with alpha blocking). In enhanced alertness, there is also general desynchronization with low-voltage activity, but the slow frequency component is absent and beta frequency clearly predominates, mixed with some remnants of alpha. In patients with low-voltage fast waking records, the onset of early drowsiness may be quite poorly defined. Alpha dropout of early drowsiness and immediate slowing in adulthood is a suspect finding (Fig. 10.2).

Deepening of drowsiness is associated with enhancement of slow activity. Trains of 2 to 3/sec and 4 to 7/sec waves reach medium voltage and may become diffusely predominant. At this stage, arousing stimuli lead to immediate return of the posterior alpha rhythm, called "paradoxical alpha response" (Goldie and Green, 1960). These stretches of reactivated alpha rhythm are often characterized by higher amplitude than the individual's regular alpha rhythm. When alpha rhythm is reactivated in deep drowsiness or in non-REM sleep, the maximum is usually frontal rather that occipital ("short microarousals").

If a record is dominated by patterns of drowsiness and sleep and if waking states can be maintained for short periods only, then there is reason to presume that such a recording is not within normal limits. In such cases, there is

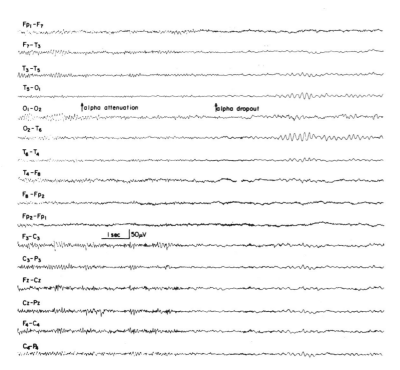

Figure 10.2. Early drowsiness in 56-year-old patient with dizziness and memory loss. Rhythmical 5–7/sec activity is noted over posterior regions very shortly after the disappearance of alpha waves. This rhythmical theta activity in earliest drowsiness is not categorically abnormal; however, incipient cerebrovascular disorder is suspected.

usually a large amount of diffuse slow (2–6/sec) activity preponderant during drowsiness and even in early drowsy states. In these individuals, the sequential structure of waking and sleeping is likely to be disturbed. Cerebrovascular and metabolic problems often account for such changes. Sleep deprivation must be ruled out in these cases, but in general healthy sleep-deprived adults are unlikely to exhibit excessive slowing in states of drowsiness.

A major study of the EEG in drowsiness has been presented by Santamaria and Chiappa (1987). Their work has placed special emphasis on changes in the alpha rhythm with occurrence of a centrofrontal alpha and temporal alpha (change in alpha distribution due to early drowsiness) as well as changes in alpha amplitude (diminution as well as increase).

These changes of alpha distribution in early drowsiness do not seem to be the rule. As Broughton and Hasan (1995) have pointed out, only a small portion of their subjects showed anterior diffusion of alpha rhythm (along with slowing by 0.5–1.5/sec) during drowsiness.

In light drowsiness, the P300 response (standard auditory paradigm) increases in latency and decreases in amplitude "but the counts of infrequent tones remained correct nevertheless" (Koshino et al., 1993). This important study shed some light on mental functioning in light drowsiness. On the other hand, EEG coherence studies show altered inter- and intrahemispheric EEG coherence in light drowsiness (Wada et al., 1996).

Deep Drowsiness

The hallmark of deep drowsiness is the appearance of *vertex waves*. These waves indicate an altered state of cerebral responsivity; vertex waves are secondary evoked potentials of several modalities, perhaps mostly auditory, that converge from their cortical projection areas in region underlying the vertex electrode. This region constitutes the posterior portion of the supplementary motor area of the frontal lobe along the interhemispheric fissure. The vertex waves represent an evoked event, like K complexes, discussed later (Fig. 10.3).

The term *vertex wave* was introduced by Liberson (1945). *On effect* (P.A. Davis, 1939), an earlier term, is no longer used. French authors have used the term *vertex spikes* ("pointes au vertex") (Bancaud et al., 1953; Gastaut, 1953). The catalogue of EEG patterns of the Handbook uses the term *vertex shark wave* (Dutertre, 1977). Other synonyms are *v waves* and *vertex sharp transients*. Surprisingly, Dutertre (1977) does not list the term *biparietal hump* (Gibbs and Gibbs, 1950) as a synonym of vertex waves and discusses this term among "slow waves." There is no doubt, however, that biparietal humps truly denote vertex waves. In the typical referential montages of Gibbs and Gibbs (1950, 1964), vertex waves appear most strikingly in parietal leads, because no midline and rolandic electrodes are placed.

The vertex wave is a compounded potential; a small spike discharge of positive polarity precedes the large following negative wave, which is almost always the most prominent feature of the discharge. Another small positive spiky discharge usually follows. The complexity of this potential reflects its neurophysiological character as an evoked potential. As a "secondary" evoked response, it is best compared with the vertex auditory evoked response that is maximal over the vertex (Kooi et al., 1971), despite the different views of Vaughan and Ritter (1970) (see discussion of Storm van Leeuwen, 1975). Its principal deflections are found in a latency range of 50 to 800 msec (Weitzman and Kremen, 1965). H. Davis et al. (1966) found a positive deflection P_1 at 50 to 60 msec, a negative N_1 at about 100 msec, a positive

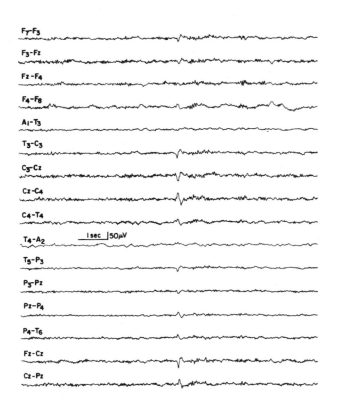

Figure 10.3. Vertex wave in deep drowsiness. Enhanced fast activity is due to medication (chloral hydrate).

P_2 at 170 to 200 msec, and a negative N_2 at about 300 msec. The authors feel that tactile vertex responses have slightly longer latency and show a more prominent P_1.

Vertex waves may occur as an isolated event; their large amplitude usually towers over the rest of the EEG activity. Quite frequently, salvos of repetitive vertex waves occur, firing at a range of about 1/sec or even somewhat faster.

Although the maximum of the vertex waves is almost invariably the vertex itself, their spread may reveal asymmetries that are fairly common in children. Pathology seldom selectively depresses the vertex wave, but such cases may occur (Niedermeyer and Pribram, 1966). Sharp boundaries must be drawn between vertex waves and rolandic spikes. Truly epileptogenic spikes may occur over the vertex. In practice, however, the differentiation between abnormal vertex spikes and the physiological vertex wave is not difficult, because the configuration of vertex spikes is more slender and more pointed (also see Kubicki et al., 1991). Vertex waves may become small and inconspicuous in aged individuals and are often poorly demonstrable in such persons.

Another important physiological potential of deep drowsiness is the positive occipital sharp transients of sleep (POSTS), which become apparent in deep drowsiness and persist during light sleep and deep sleep (Fig. 10.4).

This discharge was described first by Gibbs and Gibbs (1950) as "positive spike-like waves in occipital areas"; it was found most commonly in adolescents and young and middle-aged adults. Its prevalence declines after age 70 (Wright and Gilmore, 1984).

Similarities to occipital lambda waves were pointed out in several studies (Chatrian et al., 1960; Perez-Borja et al., 1962; Prior and Deacon, 1969; Roth et al., 1953), and the term *lambdoid* activity of drowsiness and sleep was used. Hess (1964) used the term *monophasic theta* in view of the predominant theta frequency of these chiefly rhythmical positive vents, whereas the term *occipital sharp waves of sleep* is found in the work of Arfel and Laurette (1973). Kugler and Laub (1971) used the term *lambda waves* during sleep and subsequently proposed the term *rho waves* (Kugler and Laub, 1973; Kugler, 1976). Vignaendra et al. (1974) studied the relationship of these potentials to the nocturnal sleep cycle, stressing their abundance in stage 2 and 3 sleep and scarcity or absence in REM sleep; these investigations also introduced the aforementioned term *positive occipital sharp transients of sleep* (POSTS).

These potentials are found in about 50% to 80% of a healthy adult population (49% according to Prior and Deacon, 1969; 79% according to Brenner et al., 1978). It is, therefore, quite difficult to attribute a special significance to this activity. A much lower figure (24%) and a striking preponderance of females were reported by Pristasova and Prochazka (1981).

Vignaendra et al. (1974) hypothesize that POSTS might represent a "playback" of information to the visual cortex in order to reexamine visual material collected during the day. A relationship of POSTS to dreaming (true dreams rather than hypnagogic imagery) in non-REM sleep (stage 2) was suggested by Niedermeyer and Lentz (1976), whereas Dement (1976) strongly emphasizes the lack of dreaming in this stage. According to Chatrian (1976), POSTS are unrelated to oculomotor activity as well as to visual imagery. In blind or severely amblyopic individuals, POSTS fail to materialize (Brenner et al., 1978)

The gamut of EEG patterns between earliest drowsiness and sleep onset was studied by Otto (1981). With the use of period analysis, eight different patterns were identified.

The observation of sleep spindles dates back to the work of Loomis et al. (1938). Gibbs and Gibbs (1950) have made remarkable contributions to the wave morphology of spindles. The first spindle trains show frequencies around 14/sec

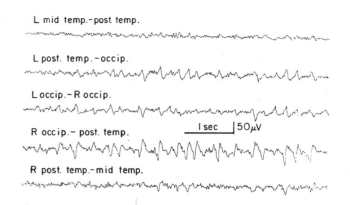

Figure 10.4. POSTS (positive occipital sharp transients of sleep) in a 34-year-old subject. (From Niedermeyer, E., and Lentz, W.J. 1976. Dreaming in non-REM sleep. *Waking and Sleeping* 1:49–59.)

(from 12.5 to 15.5/sec with a pronounced peak at exactly 14/sec, according to Gibbs and Gibbs). These investigators describe the spatial distribution of spindle trains as primarily central, but the use of midline electrodes shows a very definite maximum over the vertex. It is, therefore, worthwhile to include the vertex region in montages when it is anticipated that the patient will fall asleep.

Gibbs and Gibbs (1950) have separated the 14/sec spindle activity from the 12/sec and the 10/sec spindles (Fig. 10.5). The 12/sec spindle train appears a little later with deepening sleep although the patient is still in stage 2. These spindles range, according to Gibbs and Gibbs (1950), from 11 to 13.5/sec with a pronounced peak at 12/sec. Their spatial distribution is different; there is accentuation over frontal areas, with an impressive maximum over frontal midline. Gibbs and Gibbs stress bilaterally independent occurrence of 12/sec over frontal areas, but such asymmetries are not striking in the writer's opinion. Both types of spindles may be seen simultaneously in stage 2. With deepening sleep (at the transition from stage 2 to 3), an even slower type of spindle (around 10/sec) (Gibbs and Gibbs, 1950) is commonly seen; it is more widespread with a frontal maximum. These spindles are likely to be a forerunner of rhythmical activity in the 6 to 10/sec range, which is commonly found in stage 3. This type of activity should be differentiated from sleep spindles (Scheuler and Stinshoff, 1982).

In a 12-year-old patient of Reeves and Klass (1998), 14/sec spindles occurred on the left and asymmetric-shifting 12/sec spindles on the right where a frontal astrocytoma, grade 3 was found.

The ontogenetic evolution of sleep spindles in infancy and childhood is presented in Chapter 11, "Maturation of the EEG." Spindles are most impressive in childhood and adolescence; their voltage tends to become smaller throughout adulthood. In old age, spindles of low voltage are very common; this is probably not due to old age alone, but to vascular disorder as the faithful companion of old age. Sleep spindles share this decline of voltage with vertex and K complexes as age advances. Sleep spindles have been reported to be more frequent in women than in men (Gaillard et al., 1987); the same type of sex difference was also noticed in K complexes.

The physiological basis, nature, and significance of spindles are beyond the scope of this chapter. Briefly, Hess (1964) felt that spindles cannot be explained simply as "slowed beta activity." Spindles occur independently from faster, mostly 18 to 25/sec, activity and both patterns may be seen at the same time. Basic concepts of spindle activity have been discussed by Jankel and Niedermeyer (1985).

The *spatial distribution of spindles* indicates predominate frontal lobe involvement. The vertex regions, where spindles appear first, reflect activity from the most posterior portion of the supplementary motor region, or frontal lobe. This indicates a certain relationship to vertex waves (see above) and most K complexes (see below) recorded from the vertex region. Vertex waves as well as K complexes are often combined with spindle trains. There is evidence that vertex waves and K complexes are arousal responses, whereas the arousal-induced nature of spindles still requires convincing confirmation, despite the encouraging findings of Church et al. (1978) (also see Jankel and Niedermeyer, 1985).

In depth recordings with epileptic patients, sleep spindles tend to occur in deep frontal regions (from orbital cortex or from buried gyri of the inferior or middle frontal gyri) while the patient is drowsy and not yet asleep, according to scalp EEG evidence (Caderas et al., 1982; Jankel and Niedermeyer, 1985; Niedermeyer and Jankel, 1984; Niedermeyer et al., 1986; Zobniw, 1975).

With thalamic depth recordings in patients with states of chronic pain, independent thalamic (ventrobasal complex) spindles may appear in states of very light drowsiness (Gücer et al., 1978). These findings suggest the presence of multiple generator areas for spindles in humans.

Sleep spindles are probably found in most mammals (see Jankel and Niedermeyer, 1985). Unfortunately, the term *spindles* is used quite loosely in experimental neurophysiology. There has been a sizable bulk of literature dealing with spindles that, in reality, are trains of barbiturate-induced beta activity. Bremer (1958) suggested that barbiturate spindles are the animal counterpart of human alpha rhythm. Barbiturate spindles have been used as animal models for human alpha rhythm (Andersen and Andersson, 1968, 1974; Andersen and Eccles, 1962). It must not be forgotten that this work is based on drug-induced fast activity. Steriade et al. (1990) have strongly refuted the concept of Andersen and Andersson (1968, 1974). Based on experimental work in the cat, it is now presumed that the reticular thalamic nucleus of the thalamus generates

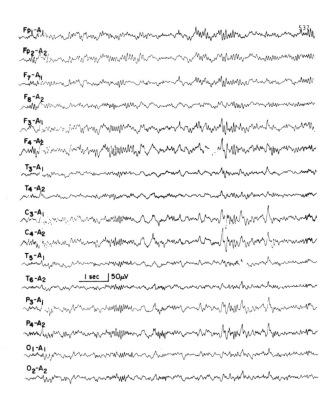

Figure 10.5. Light sleep (non-REM stage 2), in a patient age 31 years. Two categories of spindles are shown; spindles of 14–15/sec frequency dominate over centroparietal region, whereas less abundant spindles in the 12–13/sec range are found over frontal area.

spindle activity (Steriade and Deschênes, 1988; Steriade et al., 1990).

In very unusual cases, spindles may be present even in the waking state, although in attenuated form; this is true for occasional cases of "extreme spindles" (Gibbs and Gibbs, 1962); this pattern is discussed in Chapter 11, "Maturation of the EEG." Extremely rare are cases of typical (unmitigated) spindle activity—along with vertex waves and K complexes—in the presence of posterior alpha rhythm in a waking individual (Niedermeyer et al., 1979).

The term *limbic spindles* has been used by Reite (1975), who observed spindle-like bursts in beta frequency (around 20–50/sec) in nasopharyngeal leads and related this activity to respiration-linked trains of fast activity in the amygdala recorded in a variety of experimental animals (Delgado et al., 1970; Domino and Ueki, 1960; Reite et al., 1966). There has been convincing evidence that these spindles are artifacts due to mechanical vibration of nasopharyngeal electrodes (Engel et al., 1978; Niedermeyer et al., 1976) and sphenoidal electrodes (Engel et al., 1978) caused by snoring.

Vertex Waves

See the discussion under the heading of deep drowsiness.

K Complexes

K complexes make their appearance in stage 2 sleep and constitute an impressive response to arousing stimuli. These compounded potentials were first described by Loomis et al. (1938); the reason for calling them "K complexes" remains obscure (there have been reports that the naming was make on the spur of the moment without attaching any significance to the letter K). Others assume that "K" stands for "knocking" and the ensuing arousal activity in the EEG.

H. Davis et al. (1939) gave an excellent description of the single components of the K complex. As to the topographical distribution, the K complex shows a maximum over the vertex, but there are also K complexes with an indubitable maximum over the frontal midline. H. Davis et al. had already noted the existence of central and frontal K complexes, but these authors did not use midline electrodes. Brazier (1949) presumed two distinct generators; these were area 6, corresponding with the vertex, and area 9, corresponding with frontal midline. The distinction of these two types has some interesting epileptological implications that will be discussed in that context; unfortunately, modern descriptions and EEG glossaries have blurred the dividing lines. Dutertre (1977) stresses the vertex maximum only.

As to the wave morphology, the K complex consists of an initial sharp component, followed by a slow component that fuses with a superimposed fast component. The sharp component is biphasic and not seldom multiphasic. Its shape may closely resemble that of an isolated vertex wave, but in general the sharp component of the K complex shows greater complexity and greater variation from complex to complex. The sharp component was thoroughly investigated by Roth and Green (1956). The slow component is represented by a large slow wave that may exceed 1,000 msec in duration; its length and the degree of prominence greatly de-

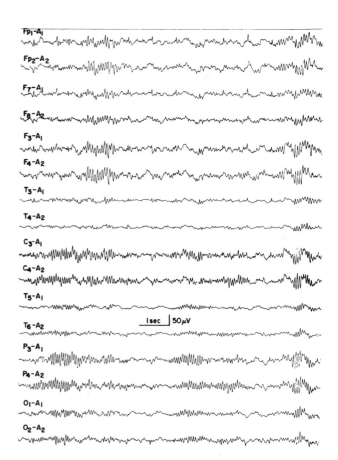

Figure 10.6. Light sleep (non-REM stage 2), in a patient age 40 years. Well-developed and rather widespread spindle activity, mostly in the range of 13–15/sec, most prominent in superior frontal, central, and parietal leads. Also note slow background activity.

pend on the filter setting. Shortening of the time constant all but suppresses the slow component. Superimposed on the slow component are 12 to 14/sec sleep spindles that represent the fast component. K complexes may follow each other in long stretches, but this is more common in deeper stages of sleep. In the recent catalogue of EEG signals in the Handbook, the K complex is described as having only a slow and a fast component; the initiating sharp component is equated with a vertex wave (Fig. 10.6).

The evoked nature of the K complex was clearly demonstrated by Niiyama et al. (1996) in healthy young adults. These authors confirmed N100–P200 components preceding the K complex (Ujszaszi and Halász, 1988; Weitzman and Kremen, 1965) and feel that even an apparently spontaneous K complex is, in reality, induced by an afferent stimulus.

The slow component of the K complex has been thought to be related to a cognitive process or information processing (Niiyama et al., 1995). This is a persuasive concept that is apt to explain the basic difference between afferent-arousing mechanisms of vertex waves and K complexes. The greater spread of the K complex into the frontal region would further bolster this concept.

Light Sleep (Stage 2)

General Considerations

The distinction between deep drowsiness and light sleep is imprecise and has necessarily been drawn in a somewhat arbitrary and artificial manner. In individuals with a well-developed drowsy state (i.e., in most children, adolescents, and adults), there is a very smooth transition from drowsiness to sleep. It is customary to regard the appearance of spindle trains in the 12 to 15/sec range as the signal of sleep onset. Not much can be gained by the observation of the patient. Even snoring may occur in what is deep drowsiness from the EEG viewpoint.

In EEG practice, montages ought to be suitable for the recognition of early sleep patterns. The first runs of spindles occur over the vertex with considerable spread into parietal and central leads. These areas should be well covered. A circular montage covering frontopolar, temporal, and occipital areas could miss the first minutes of stage 2 sleep. Referential linkages from the vertex and centroparietal areas to the ipsilateral ear are quite informative because of the wide interelectrode distance.

Once sleep has begun, the record shows a mixture of arousal-related patterns that truly deserve the often-overused term *background activity*. For the electroencephalographer, sleep would be a drab and dull affair if the picture were not enlivened by numerous arousal responses such as spindles, vertex waves, and K complexes. In addition, positive occipital transients of sleep are extremely common and may reflect some ongoing visual activities.

In sleep, the electrophysiological "roar" of the brain, which accounts for the alpha rhythm and a variety of other slow and fast activities, mellows and does not muffle event-related patterns to the same degree as in the waking state. Events expressing themselves as evoked potentials, such as the vertex wave, tower over the background activity, whereas the same events must be extracted by special averaging methods from the electroencephalographic "noise" of the brain in the waking state. In the more recent view of the "chaos theory," however, the EEG noise should not be regarded as an anarchic state (Röschke and Başar, 1990).

These are but a few words from the vantage point of the EEG laboratory. The polygraphic approach of nocturnal or 24-hour polysomnography is quite different and is presented in Chapter 48, "Polysomnograph." The polygraphic approach permits further insight into a variety of autonomically and neurobiochemically governed mechanisms. On the other hand, the polygraphic approach cannot do full justice to EEG details because of limitations of channels and data compression due to slow paper speed, so that the clinical electroencephalographer's insight into EEG sleep mechanisms retains its great value.

Slow and Fast Frequencies

Background activity shows considerable interindividual variation. *Slow frequencies* ranging from 0.75 to 4/sec are usually predominant; their voltage is high with a very prominent occipital peak in small children and gradually falls throughout adolescence and adulthood. The true amount of the slowest frequency components is not readily assessable because of limitations due to input capacitance and between-stages capacitance (determining the time constant and the low-frequency filtering). Very pronounced slowing, especially in frontal leads, is often due to perspiration artifacts, underscoring the need for air conditioning in areas with hot summer weather.

In adulthood, the voltage of the slow activity is moderate and may fall to the extent that the recording must be done with higher sensitivity in order to evaluate the background amplitudes.

Patients with low-voltage records in the waking state may also show below-average voltage while asleep. This is particularly true when the low-voltage awake tracing is likely to be related to organic cerebral problems affecting the synchronization of EEG activity, probably in the pontine level (see Magnes et al., 1961). Patients with vertebrobasilar artery insufficiency infrequently show such low-voltage patterns awake and asleep (Niedermeyer, 1963, 1972), and low-voltage patterns are also common in advanced cases of chronic alcoholism (Engel and Romano, 1959). On the other hand, the low-voltage waking records of tense and overly anxious patients (often noted in litigation cases) change to average voltage output in sleep.

Fast frequencies are commonly in the range of 15 to 30/sec, which lies clearly above the spindle frequency of 12 to 14/sec. This activity may occur even in unsedated patients with no history of chronic intake of sedatives. Some individuals show frequencies in the range of 28 to 40/sec, especially over frontal areas. Gibbs and Gibbs (1950) focused much attention on such fast patterns ("F_1, F_2, F_3 patterns") and consider very fast activity (above 30/sec) an abnormality.

These very fast waves occur in recurrent trains, mainly over anterior regions. In some individuals, this type of very fast activity could be drug-related, and one wonders if one is dealing with a 2:1 harmonic of the usual sedative-induced fast frequencies (customarily in the 18–25/sec range). Relationships to epileptic changes are not clearly demonstrable (Gibbs and Gibbs, 1964). Lorimer (1970) found a high prevalence of such fast patterns in a prison population. Kubicki et al. (1986, 1987) have emphasized the occurrence of "subvigil beta activity" during short arousal periods. With the use of the ultrafast frequency range (80–1,000 Hz, see Chapter 26), more light will be shed on the function of fast and ultrafast frequency during sleep.

According to human sleep studies of Marshall et al. (1994), a negative DC shift is associated with the transition from the waking state to sleep. Luthringer et al. (1995) reported a parallelism between slow wave activity and plasma renin levels in human sleep.

Sleep Spindles

Sleep spindles are also know as *sigma activity* or *sigma waves*. These latter terms were at first internationally encouraged, for instance by the International Federation of Societies for Electroencephalography and Clinical Neurophysiology (IFSECN) in 1961, but were discouraged in a later glossary from the same federation (IFSECN, 1974). In this glossary, spindles are defined as a "group of rhythmic waves characterized by progressively increasing, then gradually decreasing amplitude" (see also Dutertre, 1977).

This waxing and waning of amplitudes is exactly what the term *spindle* implies: a belly in the middle tapering off to the left and to the right. Unfortunately, experience teaches us time and again that this shape of spindle train is not the rule and may be rather uncommon. As a matter of fact a train of posterior alpha waves in the waking state may show better spindle shape than the average sleep spindles. Be this as it may, the fact remains that the term *sleep spindles* is in widespread use and should be retained in order to avoid confusion (Fig. 10.7).

The ontogenetic evaluation of the K complex has been pointed out in Chapter 11, "Maturation of the EEG." The K complex is largest in older children and in early adolescence; the sharp component is particularly impressive at that time. This again has certain epileptological implications that will not be discussed in this context. With advancing age, the K complex shows a decline of voltage and often degenerates into an insignificant slow potential with tiny superimposed spindle-like waves. A distinction between spontaneous and click-evoked K complexes was make by Halász et al. (1982), who investigated the relationship between these two types.

The K complex shows considerably interindividual variability. Paiva and Rosa (1991) distinguish six morphological types of K complexes, especially on the basis of variations in the negative component. These authors also found differences in the configuration of K complexes with regard to sleep stages 2, 3, and 4. Their study also confirmed the maximum of K-complex density in stage 2.

According to Weisz et al. (1995), the generation of K complexes is not controlled by the right hemisphere. Unilateral right-sided control of arousing mechanisms has been proposed by Heilman and Van den Abell (1979) following studies of unilateral spatial neglect (Heilman et al., 1978). In this condition, K complexes are present, whereas spindles are absent (Weisz et al., 1995). It might be interesting to note that both spindles and K complexes are absent in fatal thalamic degeneration with insomnia (Tinuper et al., 1989), a condition in which the anterior and the mediodorsal thalamic nuclei degenerate selectively.

Positive Occipital Transients of Sleep

These discharges remain quite active in stage 2 (see Deep Drowsiness, above).

Deep Sleep (Stage 3)

This stage is recorded much less often than stage 2 under routine EEG laboratory conditions. In this stage, the slow background activity moves into the foreground and dominates the picture. Delta frequencies in the 0.75 to 3/sec range are particularly prominent over the anterior regions. Rhythmical activity of lesser voltage and in the 5 to 9/sec range is quite common; these frequencies probably do not represent a slow spindle equivalent. Sleep spindles in the 10 to 12/sec and even in the 12 to 14/sec ranges are still present but gradually become less impressive; they seem to be "suffocated" by the luxuriant growth of high-voltage delta activity.

A close look at the anterior delta activity reveals interspersed sharp transients that may be just rudimentary. This indicates a certain relationship to K complexes, which seem to be present in unending sequences. Nevertheless, more typical isolated K complexes as response to arousing stimuli can also materialize, showing the typical three components and disrupting the general slow pattern (Fig. 10.8).

Anterior delta activity with interspersed minor sharp transients may form a pattern that has been described as "mitten pattern." This pattern has been amply discussed by Gibbs and Gibbs (1964), but there are older descriptions by Leemhuis and Stamps (1949), Lyketsos et al. (1953), Winfield and Sparer (1954), Halász and Kajtor (1962), and Gibbs and Gibbs (1963).

The authors have categorized the mitten patterns according to the shape and duration of the sharp component, which is called the "thumb section," while the slow component would represent the "hand section" of the mitten. In the A type (Gibbs and Gibbs, 1964), the thumb section has a duration of 1/8 to 1/9 sec; in the B type, the duration is from 1/10 to 1/12 sec. Slower thumb sections of 1/6th to 1/7th of a second have been called A-1 mittens. According to Gibbs and Gibbs (1964), A-1 mittens may be associated with deep and especially thalamic tumors in adults. The A mitten type is thought to be associated with parkinsonism and the B mitten type with psychosis (Gibbs and Gibbs, 1964).

These electroclinical correlations have not found wide acceptance. This may be because most EEG laboratories do not extend sleep into stage 3, in which mitten patterns thrive. The mitten shape also depends a good deal on referential (unipolar) recording techniques that place greater emphasis

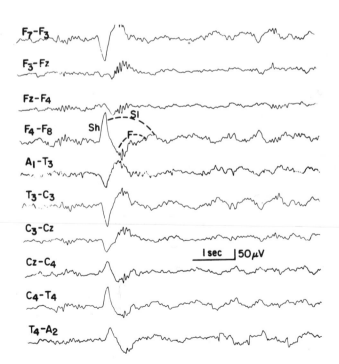

Figure 10.7. Close-up of a K complex, in a patient age 17 years. Note midline maximum (especially Cz: vertex) and the three principal components, the sharp, slow, and fast components.

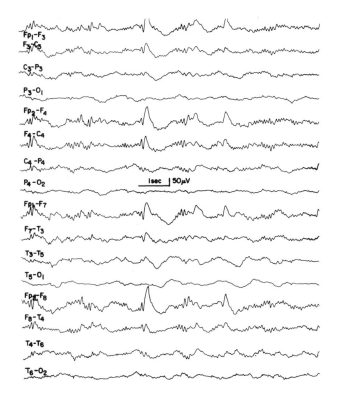

Figure 10.8. Deep sleep (non-REM stage 3), in a patient age 38 years. There is a greater amount of slow activity than in stage 2. Spindles are still abundant but less prominent than in stage 2. K complexes are noted over anterior areas, forming "mitten" patterns.

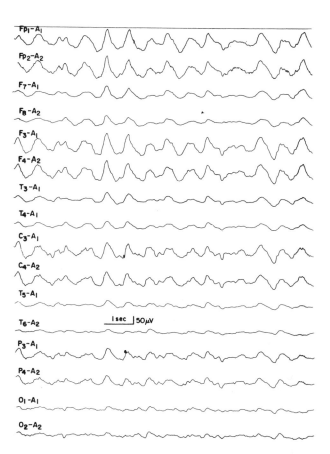

Figure 10.9. Very deep sleep (non-REM stage 4), in a patient age 41 years. Pronounced generalized 1.5–2/sec activity with frontal maximum and occasional traces of spindles.

on the mitten-like configuration. Of course, mitten patterns can also be demonstrated with bipolar montages, but then one must get used to slightly different shapes. The catalogue of EEG patterns (Dutertre, 1977) does not even mention the mitten pattern.

In a sizable number of healthy persons, there is an "alpha sleep pattern" that reaches its maximum in stage 3. This pattern was described first by Scheuler and Stinshoff (1982) and Scheuler et al. (1983); it is characterized by rhythmical 7 to 11/sec activity of frontal maximum, mostly intermingled with slow activity in the delta range. This pattern shows certain periodicities (Scheuler et al., 1990). The alpha sleep pattern must be differentiated from the alpha-delta sleep (Hauri and Hawkins, 1973; McNamara, 1993), a pattern associated with delta sleep deficit and often noted in patients with fibrositis (Moldofsky and Lue, 1980). By contrast, the alpha sleep pattern has been found to be associated with a stable sleep organization (Scheuler et al., 1988).

Very Deep Sleep (Stage 4)

Stage 4 is of rather little interest in the clinical EEG laboratory, although cases of temporal lobe epilepsy may occasionally withhold their spike activity until stages 3 and 4 are reached; this, however, is an exception rather than the rule.

In this stage, slow activity in the delta range becomes even more preponderant than in stage 3. Spindles become quite rare but are still detectable, sometimes only when slow frequencies are filtered out (Dement, 1976) (Fig. 10.9).

This stage of very deep sleep seems to have considerable endocrinological effect because the release of pituitary growth hormone is limited to stages 3 and 4 with a peak at stage 4 (Sassin et al., 1969). Arousal at this stage can be associated with manifestations of sleep disorders (somnambulism, nocturnal terror, or enuresis) in predisposed individuals (Gastaut and Broughton, 1964), and can produce marked confusion ("sleep drunkenness") in some patients. On the basis of coherence analysis, Banquet (1983) presumes that a transient partial interhemispheric disconnection occurs in stage 4.

REM Sleep (Stage REM)

REM sleep should be assessed with polygraphic methods; for this reason, this portion of sleep is discussed in Chapter 48, "Polysomnography." Under regular EEG laboratory conditions, the observation of REM sleep requires a long waiting period, because the first phase of REM does not appear before 60 to 90 minutes after sleep onset; sedation of the patient may even lengthen this period. A prolonged morning or afternoon recording may induce such REM stages, which are quite common in daytime naps (Salzarulo, 1971) provided that such naps are long enough.

Whenever the electroencephalographer must search specifically for REM periods (especially when no regional sleep laboratory with facilities for polysomnography is availability), stress must be laid on the use of two channels for electrooculography (two additional canthus electrodes, connected to the ears), one channel for cutaneous electromyography (submental region) and a thermocouple or strain gauge for pneumographic documentation.

In patients with a history of narcolepsy and additional attacks of cataplexy and/or sleep paralysis, REM sleep may occur at sleep onset (see Chapter 48, "Polysomnography"). Even with the regular EEG laboratory routine of short daytime sleep recordings, however, sleep-onset REM or a REM stage shortly after falling asleep may occur unexpectedly. Patients with severely disrupted sleep-waking cycles, in delirium tremens, or with deep-seated lesions or disturbances involving the brainstem may occasionally show early REM phases.

The REM stage EEG is of low-voltage activity, polyrhythmic, and similar to stage 1 (light drowsiness); periods of alpha waves, slightly slower than in wakefulness, or "sawtooth waves" in the 2 to 6/sec range appear in short bursts over frontal leads or vertex (Passouant, 1975). These sawtooth-like bursts may occur in conjunction with ocular movements (Schwartz, 1962). REM sleep also contains a good deal of alpha band activity, which is attenuated after REM sleep deprivation (Roth et al., 1999).

The sudden appearance of totally unexpected REM sleep in a routine EEG laboratory recording must not escape the electroencephalographer, even though the patient has no additional oculographic leads (Fig. 10.10) (also see Matsuo, 1981). The ocular potentials are mostly quite impressive and almost always give rise to marked eye movement artifacts in frontopolar and anterior temporal leads. Once familiarized with the tempo and shape of these discharges, the electroencephalographer will rarely miss REM states. Of course, the use of polygraphic documentation makes the task much easier. When a REM phase occurs directly at sleep onset, the transition from drowsiness to REM is not very pronounced in the EEG, whereas the change from deep non-REM sleep to REM is a very dramatic and unforgettable experience for every record reader.

Arousal from Sleep

In adolescents and adults, arousal from sleep is a quick process with almost immediate change from sleep into a waking pattern, usually with well-developed posterior alpha rhythm. One single K complex or a sequence of K complexes may mark the transition. Spectacular rhythmical theta activity during arousal from sleep in children is discussed in Chapter 11, "Maturation of the EEG."

Arousal is such a complex and multifaceted neurophysiological phenomenon that it cannot be discussed within the limitations of this chapter. The reader will certainly benefit from Steriade's chapter (see Chapter 3, "Cellular Substrates of Brain Rhythms").

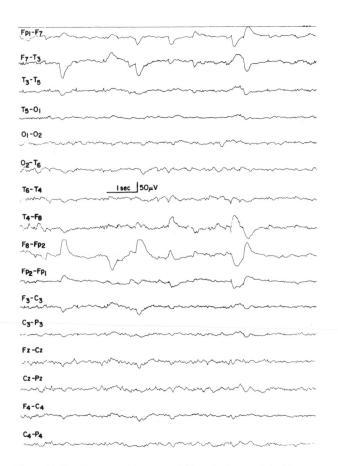

Figure 10.10. Unexpected sleep-onset REM episode, recorded without special ocular leads in a 26-year-old patient with brittle juvenile diabetes. Note ocular artifacts and general voltage attenuation with mixed frequencies.

References

Andersen, P., and Andersson, S.A. 1968. Physiological mechanisms of the alpha waves. In *Clinical Electroencephalography of Children*, Eds. P. Kellaway and I. Petersén, pp. 31–48. New York: Grune & Stratton (Stockholm: Almqvist and Wiksell).

Andersen, P., and Andersson, S.A. 1974. Thalamic origin of cortical rhythmic activity. In *Handbook of Electroencephalography and Clinical Neurophysiology,* vol. 2C, Ed.-in-chief, A. Remond, pp. 90–118. Amsterdam: Elsevier.

Andersen, P., and Eccles, J.C. 1962. Inhibitory phasing of neuronal discharge. Nature (Lond.) 196:645–647.

Arfel, G., and Laurette, G. 1973. Occipital sharp waves of sleep contrasted with lambda waves. Clin. Electroencephalogr. 4:16–32.

Aserinsky, E., and Kleitman, N. 1953. Regularly occurring episodes of eye mobility and concomitant phenomena during sleep. Science 118:273–274.

Bancaud, J., Bloch, V., and Paillard, J. 1953. Contribution E.E.G. à l'étude des potentiels évoqués chez l'homme au niveau de vertex. Rev. Neurol. (Paris) 89:399–418.

Banquet, J.P. 1983. Inter- and intrahemispheric relationships of the EEG activity during sleep in man. Electroencephalogr. Clin. Neurophysiol. 55: 51–59.

Bennett, D.R. 1963. Sleep deprivation and major motor convulsions. Neurology (Minneapolis) 13:953–958.

Bennett, D.R., Mattson, R.H., Ziter, F.A., et al. 1964. Sleep deprivation: neurological and electroencephalographic effects. Aerospace Med. 35: 888–890.

Blake, H., and Gerard, R.W. 1937. Brain potentials during sleep. Am. J. Physiol. 199:273–274.

Brazier, M.A.B. 1949. The electrical fields at the surface of the head during sleep. Electroencephalogr. Clin. Neurophysiol. 1:195–204.

Bremer, F. 1958. Cerebral and cerebellar potentials. Physiol. Rev. 38:357–388.

Brenner, R.P., Zauel, D.W., and Carlow, T.J. 1978. Positive occipital sharp transients of sleep in the blind. Neurology (Minneapolis) 28: 609–612.

Broughton, R., and Hasan, J. 1995. Quantitative topographic electroencephalographic mapping during drowsiness and sleep onset. J. Clin. Neurophysiol. 12:372–386.

Caderas, M., Niedermeyer, E., Uematsu, S., et al. 1982. Sleep spindles recorded from deep cerebral structures in man. Clin. Electroencephalogr. 13:216–225.

Chatrian, G.E. 1976. The lambda waves. In *Handbook of Electroencephalography and Clinical Neurophysiology,* vol. 6A, Ed.-in-chief, A. Remond, pp. 123–149. Amsterdam: Elsevier.

Chatrian, G.E., Bickford, R.G., Petersen, M.C., et al. 1960. Lambda waves with depth electrodes in humans. In *Electrical Studies in the Unanesthetized Brain,* Eds. E.R. Ramey and D.S. O'Doherty, pp. 291–310. New York: Hoeber.

Church, M.W., Johnson, L.C., and Seales, D.M. 1978. Evoked K complexes and cardiovascular responses to spindle-synchronous and spindle-asynchronous stimulus clicks during NREM sleep. Electroencephalogr. Clin. Neurophysiol. 45:443–453.

Dahlström, A., and Fuxe, K. 1964. Evidence for the existence of monoamino-containing neurons in the cerebral nervous system. I. Demonstration of monamines in the cell bodies of brain stem neuron. Acta Physiol. Scand. Suppl. 232:1–55.

Davis, H., Davis, P.A., Loomis, A.L., et al. 1939. Electrical reactions of human brain to auditory stimulation during sleep. J. Neurophysiol. 21: 500–514.

Davis, H., Mast, T., Yoshie, N., et al. 1966. The slow response of the human cortex to auditory stimuli. Electroencephalogr. Clin. Neurophysiol. 21: 105–113.

Davis, P.A. 1939. Effects of acoustic stimuli on the waking human brain. J. Neurophysiol. 2:494–499.

Degen, R. 1980. A study of the diagnostic value of waking and sleep EEGs after sleep deprivation in epileptic patients on anticonvulsive therapy. Electroencephalogr. Clin. Neurophysiol. 49:577–584.

Deisenhammer, E., and Klingler, D. 1978. Das Schlafentzug-EEG bei Kranken mit gesicherter und fraglicher Epilepsie sowie bei Kranken ohne epileptische Anfälle Z. EEG-EMG 9:38–42.

Delgado, J.M.R., Johnston, V.S., Wallace, J.D., et al. 1970. Operant conditioning of amygdala spindling in the free chimpanzee. Brain Res. 22: 347–362.

Dement, W.C. 1976. *Some Must Watch While Some Must Sleep.* San Francisco: San Francisco Book Co.

Dement, W., and Kleitman, N. 1957. Cyclic variations in EEG during sleep and their relation to eye movements, body motility and dreaming. Electroencephalogr. Clin. Neurophysiol. 9:673–690.

Domino, E.F., and Ueki, S. 1960. An analysis of the electric burst phenomenon in some rhinencephalic structures of the dog and monkey. Electroencephalogr. Clin. Neurophysiol. 12:635–648.

Dutertre, F. 1977. Catalogue of the main EEG patterns. In *Handbook of Electroencephalography and Clinical Neurophysiology,* vol. 11A, Ed.-in-chief, A. Remond, pp. 40–79. Amsterdam: Elsevier.

Engel, G.L., and Romano, J. 1959. Delirium, a syndrome of cerebral insufficiency. J. Chron. Dis. 9:260 (Quoted after Kiloh, L.G., McComas, A.J., and Osselton, J.W. 1972. *Clinical Electroencephalography.* London: Butterworth).

Engel, J., Jr., Jerrett, S., Niedermeyer, E., et al. 1978. "Limbic spindles." A re-appraisal. Electroencephalogr. Clin. Neurophysiol. 44:389–392.

Erwin, C.W., Somerville, E.R., and Radtke, R.A. 1984. A review of electroencephalographic features normal of sleep. Clin. Neurophysiol. 1: 253–274.

Evans, B.M. 1992. Periodic activity in cerebral arousal mechanisms—the relationship to sleep and brain damage. Electroencephalogr. Clin. Neurophysiol. 83:130–137.

Gaillard, J.-M., Baudat, J., and Blois, R. 1987. The effect of sex depressive state and minor tranquilizers on K potentials and spindles during sleep. Clin. Neurol. Neurosurg. 89:172–173.

Gastaut, H., and Broughton, R. 1964. A clinical and polygraphic study of episodic phenomena during sleep. In *Recent Advances in Biological Psychiatry,* vol. VII, Ed. J. Wortis, pp. 197–221. London: Plenum Press.

Gastaut, H., Gomez-Almanzar, M., and Taury, M. 1983. Der provozierte Mittagsschlaf: Eine einfache, erfolgreiche Methode zur Schlafaktivierung bie Epileptikern. Z. EEG-EMG 14:6–11.

Gastaut, H., Gomez-Almanzar, M., and Taury, M. 1984. The enforced nap: a simple effective method of inducing sleep activation in epileptics. In *Epilepsy, Sleep and Sleep Deprivation,* Eds. R. Degen and E. Niedermeyer, pp. 75–83. Amsterdam: Elsevier.

Gastaut, Y. 1953. Les pointes négatives évoquées sur le vertex: leur signification psychophysiologique et pathologique. Rev. Neurol. (Paris) 89: 382–389.

Gibbs, F.A., and Gibbs, F.A. 1962. Extreme spindles: correlation of electroencephalographic sleep pattern with mental retardation. Science 138: 1106–1107.

Gibbs, F.A., and Gibbs, E.L. 1950. *Atlas of Electroencephalography,* vol. 1. Cambridge, MA: Addison-Wesley.

Gibbs, F.A., and Gibbs, E.L. 1963. The mitten pattern: An electroencephalographic abnormality correlating with psychosis. J. Neuropsychiatry 5:6–13.

Gibbs, F.A., and Gibbs, E.L. 1964. *Atlas of Electroencephalography,* vol. 3. Reading, MA: Addison-Wesley.

Goldie, L., and Green, J.M. 1960. Paradoxical blocking and arousal in the drowsy state. Nature (Lond.) 187.

Gücer, G., Niedermeyer, E., and Long, D.M., 1978. Thalmic EEG recordings in patients with chronic pain. J. Neurol. (Berlin) 219:47–61.

Guilleminault, C., and Baker, T.L. 1984. Sleep and electroencephalography: points of interest and points of controversy. J. Clin. Neurophysiol. 1:275–291.

Halász, P. 1988. Information processing during sleep: introduction. In *Sleep 1986,* Eds. W.P. Koella, F. Obal, H. Schulz, et al., pp. 77–78. Stuttgart: Fischer.

Halász, P., and Kajtor, F. 1962. "Mittens"—a new form of electroencephalographic wave (Hungarian). Ideggyogy Szemle 15:46–57 (quoted after Gibbs, F.A., and Gibbs, E.L., 1964).

Halász, P., Pal, I., and Rajna, P. 1982. Relationship between spontaneous and evoked K complexes. Electroencephalogr. Clin. Neurophysiol. 53: 7P(abst).

Hauri, P., and Hawkins, D.R. 1973. Alpha delta sleep. Electroencephalogr. Clin. Neurophysiol. 34:233–237.

Heilman, K.M., and Van den Abell, T. 1979. Right hemisphere dominance for mediating cerebral activation (quoted after Weisz et al., 1995).

Heilman, K.M., Schwartz, H.D., and Watson, R.T. 1978. Hypoarousal in patients with neglect syndrome and indifference. Neurology 28:229–232.

Heinemann, L.G. 1966. Der Mehrtägige Schlafentzug in der experimentellen Psychoseforschung: Psychopathologie und EEG. Arch. Psychiatr. Nervenkr. 208:117–197.

Hess, R. 1964. The electroencephalogram in sleep. Electroencephalogr. Clin. Neurophysiol. 16:44–55.

IFSECN. 1974. A glossary of terms commonly used by clinical electroencephalographers. Electroencephalogr. Clin. Neurophysiol. 37:538–548.

Jankel, W.R., and Niedermeyer, E. 1985. Sleep spindles. J. Clin. Neurophysiol. 2:1–35.

Johnson, L.C. 1969. Psychological and physiological changes following total sleep deprivation. In *Sleep: Physiology and Pathology,* Ed. A. Kales, pp. 206–220. Philadelphia: JB Lippincott.

Jouvet, M. 1969. Biogenic amines and the states of sleep. Science 163:32–41.

Jouvet, M. 1972. Some monoaminergic mechanisms controlling sleep and waking. In *Brain and Human Behavior,* Eds. A.G. Karczmar and J.C. Eccles, pp. 131–161. New York: Springer.

Jouvet, M., and Delorme, F. 1965. Locus coeruleus et sommeil paradoxal. C.R. Soc. Biol. (Paris) 159:895–899.

Jovanovic, U.J. 1991. General considerations of sleep and sleep deprivation. In *Epilepsy, Sleep and Sleep Deprivation,* 2nd ed., Eds. R. Degen and E.A. Rodin, pp. 205–215. Amsterdam: Elsevier.

Jovanovic, U.J., Liebaldt, G.P., Mühl, M., et al. 1971. Schlafentzug und seine Begleiterscheinungen. Arch. Psychiatr. Nervenkr. 124:183–202.

Kajtor, F., Mullay, J., Farago, L., et al. 1957. Effect of barbiturate sleep on the electrical activity of the hippocampus of patients with temporal lobe epilepsy (a preliminary report). Electroencephalogr. Clin. Neurophysiol. 9:441–451.

Klass, D.W., and Fischer-Williams, M. 1976. Sensory stimulation, sleep and sleep deprivation. In *Handbook of Electroencephalography and Clinical Neurophysiology,* vol. 3D, Ed.-in-chief, A. Remond, pp. 5–73. Amsterdam: Elsevier.

Klingler, D., Tragner, H., and Deisenhammer, E. 1991. The nature of the influence of sleep deprivation on the EEG. In *Epilepsy, Sleep and Sleep*

Deprivation, 2nd ed., Eds. R. Degen and E.A. Rodin, pp. 231–233. Amsterdam: Elsevier.

Kooi, K.A., Tipton, A.C., and Marshall, R.E. 1971. Polarities and field configuration of the vertex components of the human auditory evoked response: a reinterpretation. Electroencephalogr. Clin. Neurophysiol. 31:166–169.

Koshino, Y., Nishio, M., Murata, T., et al. 1993. The influence of light drowsiness on the latency and amplitude of P300. Clin. Electroencephalogr. 24:110–113.

Kubicki, S., and Herrmann, W.M. 1996. The future of computer-assisted investigation of the polysomnogram: sleep-microstructure. J. Clin. Neurophysiol. 13:285–294.

Kubicki, St., Meyer, Ch., and Rohmel, J. 1986. Dies Schlafspindelperiodik. Z. EEG-EMG 17:55–61.

Kubicki, St., Höller, L., and Pastelak-Price, C. 1987. Subvigil beta activity: a study of fast EEG patterns in drowsiness. Am. J. EEG Technol. 27:15–31.

Kubicki, S., Scheuler, W., and Wittenbecher, H. 1991. Short-term sleep EEG recordings after partial sleep deprivation as a routine procedure to uncover epileptic phenomena: an evaluation of 719 EEG recordings. In *Epilepsy Sleep and Sleep Deprivation,* 2nd ed., Eds. R. Degen and E.A. Rodin, pp. 217–230. Amsterdam: Elsevier.

Kugler, J. 1976. Lambda waves and rho waves. Electroencephalogr. Clin. Neurophysiol. 40:193–194(abst).

Kugler, J., and Laub, M. 1971. Lambda waves during sleep. Electroencephalogr. Clin. Neurophysiol. 30:168(abst).

Kugler, J., and Laub, M. 1973. Lambdoid-Wellen (RHO-Wellen) in Schlaf. In *The Nature of Sleep,* Ed. U.J. Jovanovic, pp. 31–35. Stuttgart: Fischer.

Leemhuis, A.J., and Stamps, F. 1949. Mitten patterns in electroencephalogram of patients with Parkinsonism. Proc. Am. EEG Soc. Atlantic City, NJ.

Liberson, W.T. 1945. Functional electroencephalography in mental disorders. Dis. Nerv. Syst. 5:357–364.

Loomis, A.L., Harvey, E.N., and Hobart, G.A. 1937. Cerebral states during sleep as studied by human brain potentials. J. Exp. Psychol. 21:127–144.

Loomis, A.L., Harvey, E.N., and Hobart, G.A. 1938. Distribution of disturbance-patterns in the human electroencephalogram with special reference to sleep. J. Neurophysiol. 1:413–430.

Lorimer, F.M. 1970. Further clinical observations on exceedingly fast activity, a rare electroencephalographic abnormality. Clin. Electroencephalogr. 1:84–91.

Luthringer, R., Branderberger, G., Schaltenbrand, N., et al. 1995. Slow wave electroencephalic activity parallels renin oscillations during sleep in humans. Electroencephalogr. Clin. Neurophysiol. 95:318–322.

Lyketsos, G., Belinson, L., and Gibbs, F.A. 1953. Electroencephalograms of nonepileptic psychotic patients awake and asleep. Arch. Neurol. Psychiat. (Chicago) 69:707–712.

Magnes, J., Moruzzi, G., and Pompeiano, O. 1961. EEG-synchronizing structures in the lower brain stem. In *The Nature of Sleep,* Eds. G.E.W. Wolstenholme and M. O'Connor, pp. 57–78. London: Churchill.

Marshall, L., Molle, M., Schreiber, H., et al. 1994. Scalp recorded direct current potential shifts associated with the transition to sleep in man. Electroencephalogr. Clin. Neurophysiol. 91:346–352.

Matsuo, F. 1981. Recognition of REM sleep in standard EEG. Electroencephalogr. Clin. Neurophysiol. 52:490–493.

Mattson, R.H., Pratt, K.L., and Calverley, J.R. 1965. Electroencephalograms of epileptics following sleep deprivation. Arch. Neurol. (Chicago) 13:310–315.

McNamara, M.E. 1993. Alpha sleep: a mini review and update. Clin. Electroencephalogr. 24:192–193.

Moldofsky, H., and Lue, F.A. 1980. The relationship of alpha and delta EEG frequencies to pain and mood in "fibrositis" patients treated with chlorpromazine and I-tryptophan. Electroencephalogr. Clin. Neurophysiol. 50:71–80.

Naitoh, P., and Dement, W. 1976. Sleep deprivation in humans. In *Handbook of Electroencephalography and Clinical Neurophysiology,* vol. 7A, Ed.-in-chief, A. Remond, pp. 146–51. Amsterdam: Elsevier.

Naitoh, P., Kales, A., Kollar, E.J., et al. 1969. Electroencephalographic changes after prolonged deprivation of sleep. Electroencephalogr. Clin. Neurophysiol. 27:2–11.

Niedermeyer, E. 1963. The electroencephalogram and vertebrobasilar artery insufficiency. Neurology (Minneapolis) 13:412–422.

Niedermeyer, E. 1972. *The Generalized Epilepsies.* Springfield, IL: Charles C Thomas.

Niedermeyer, E., and Höller, L. 1984. Kurzschlaf im EEG-Eine Fundgrube sonst übersehener EEG-Abnormitäten. Z. EEG-EMG 15:57–66.

Niedermeyer, E., and Jankel, W.R. 1984. Falling asleep: depth EEG and thermographic observations. Electroencephalogr. Clin. Neurophysiol. 58:8P(abst).

Niedermeyer, E., and Lentz, W.J. 1976. Dreaming in non-REM sleep. Waking and Sleeping 1:49–51.

Niedermeyer, E., and Pribram, H.F.W. 1966. Unilateral suppression of vertex sharp waves in the sleep electroencephalogram (case report). Electroencephalogr. Clin. Neurophysiol. 20:401–404.

Niedermeyer, E., Schenk, G., Gücer, G., et al. 1976. "Limbic spindles." Facts or artifacts? Electroencephalogr. Clin. Neurophysiol. 41:201(abst).

Niedermeyer, E., Singer, H.S., Folstein, S.E., et al. 1979. Hypersomnia with simultaneous waking and sleep patterns in the electroencephalogram. A case report with neurotransmitter studies. J. Neurol. (Berlin) 221:1–13.

Niedermeyer, E., Jankel, W.R., and Uematsu, S. 1986. Falling asleep: Observations and thoughts. Am. J. EEG Technol. 26:166–175.

Niiyama, Y., Fushimi, M., Sekine, A., et al. 1995. K complex evoked in NREM sleep is accompanied by a slow negative potential related to cognitive process. Electroencephalogr. Clin. Neurophysiol. 95:27–33.

Niiyama, Y., Satoh, N., Kutsuzawa, O., et al. 1996. Electrophysiological evidence suggesting that sensory stimuli of unknown origin induce spontaneous K complex. Electroencephalogr. Clin. Neurophysiol. 98:394–400.

Oller-Daurella, L. 1966. La privation de sommeil comme méthode d'activation de l'EEG chez l'épileptique. Rev. Neurol. (Paris) 115:530–535.

Otto, E. 1981. Characteristics of EEG activity patterns occurring in the process of falling asleep. Electroencephalogr. Clin. Neurophysiol. 52:1P(abst).

Paiva, T., and Rosa, A. 1991. The K complex variability in normal subjects. In *Phasic Events and Organization of Sleep,* Eds. M.G. Terzano, P. Halász, and A.C. Declerck, pp. 167–187. New York: Raven Press.

Passouant, P. 1975. EEG and sleep. Electro-clinical semeiology. In *Handbook of Electroencephalography and Clinical Neurophysiology,* vol. 7A, Ed.-in-chief, A. Remond, pp. 3–11. Amsterdam: Elsevier.

Perez-Borja, C., Chatrian, G.E., Tyce, F.A., et al. 1962. Electrographic patterns of the occipital lobe in man: a topographic study based on use of implanted electrodes. Electroencephalogr. Clin. Neurophysiol. 14:171–182.

Pratt, K.L., Mattson, R.H., Weikers, N.J., et al. 1968. EEG activation of epileptics following sleep deprivation: a prospective study of 114 cases. Electroencephalogr. Clin. Neurophysiol. 24:11–15.

Prior, P.F., and Deacon, P.A. 1969. Spontaneous sleep in healthy subjects in long-term serial electroencephalograph readings. Electroencephalogr. Clin. Neurophysiol. 27:422–424.

Pristasova, E., and Prochazka, M. 1981. Bioccipital theta rhythmic and positive occipital sharp waves of sleep. Electroencephalogr. Clin. Neurophysiol. 52:1P–2P(abst).

Rechtschaffen, A., and Kales, A. 1968. A manual of standardized terminology, techniques, and scoring system for sleep stages of human subjects. University of California: Brain Information Service.

Reeves, A.L., and Klass, D.W. 1998. Frequency asymmetry of sleep spindles with focal pathology. Electroencephalogr. Clin. Neurophysiol. 106:84–86.

Reite, M. 1975. Non-invasive recording of limbic spindles in man. Electroencephalogr. Clin. Neurophysiol. 38:539–541.

Reite, M., Stephens, L., and Pegram, G.V. 1996. Uncal spindling in the chimpanzee. Brain Res. 3:393–395.

Rodin, E.A., Luby, E.D., and Gottlieb, S., Jr. 1962. The electroencephalogram during prolonged experimental sleep deprivation. Electroencephalogr. Clin. Neurophysiol. 14:544–551.

Röschke, J., and Başar, E. 1990. The EEG is not a simple noise: strange attractors in intracranial structures. In *Chaos in Brain Function,* Ed. E. Başar, pp. 49–62. Berlin: Springer.

Roth, C., Achermann, P., and Borbely, A.A. 1999. Alpha activity in the human REM sleep topography and effect of REM sleep deprivation. Clin. Neurophysiol. 110:632–635.

Roth, M., and Green, J. 1956. The form, voltage distribution and physiological significance of the K complex. Electroencephalogr. Clin. Neurophysiol. 8:385–402.

Roth, M., Shaw, J., and Green, J. 1953. The lambda wave as a normal physiological phenomenon in the human electroencephalogram. Nature (Lond.) 172:864–866.

Rumpl, E., Lorenzi, E., Bauer, G., et al. 1977. Zum diagnostischen Wert des EEG nach Schlafentzug. Z. EEG-EMG 8:205–209.

Salzarulo, P. 1971. Etude é'lectroencéphalographique et polygraphique du sommeil d'aprés-midi chez le sujet normal. Electroencephalogr. Clin. Neurophysiol. 30:399–407.

Santamaria, J., and Chiappa, K.H. 1987. *The EEG in Drowsiness.* New York: Demos.

Sassin, J., Parkee, D., Mace, J., et al. 1969. Human growth hormone release relation to slow-wave sleep and sleep-waking cycle. Science 165:513–515.

Scheuler, W., and Stinshoff, D. 1982. Das Alpha-Schlafmuster-eine kaum beachtete EEG-Variante. Z. EEG-EMG 13:34–41.

Scheuler, W., Stinshoff, D., and Kubicki, St. 1983. The alpha sleep pattern. Differentiation from other sleep patterns and effects of hypnotics. Neuropsychobiology 10:395–399.

Scheuler, W., Kubicki, St., Marquardt, J., et al. 1988. The alpha-sleep-pattern-quantitative analysis and functional aspects. In *Sleep 1986,* Eds. W.P. Koella, F. Obal, H. Schulz, et al. Stuttgart: Fischer.

Scheuler, W., Rappelsberger, P., Schmatz, F., et al. 1990. Periodicity analysis of sleep EEG in the second and minute ranges—example of application in different alpha activities in sleep. Electroencephalogr. Clin. Neurophysiol. 76:222–234.

Schieber, J.P., Muzet, A., and Ferrière, P.J.R. 1971. Les phases d'activation transitoire spontanées au cours du sommeil normal chez l'homme. Arch. Sci. Physiol. 25:443–464.

Schwartz, R.A. 1962. EEG et mouvements oculaires dans le sommeil de nuit. Electroencephalogr. Clin. Neurophysiol. 14:126–128.

Steriade, M., and Deschênes, M. 1988. Intrathalamic and brainstem-thalamic networks involved in resting and alert stages. In *Cellular Thalamic Mechanisms,* Eds. M. Bentivoglio and R. Spreafico, pp. 37–62. Amsterdam: Elsevier.

Steriade, M., Gloor, P., Llinas, R.R., et al. 1990. Basic mechanisms of cerebral rhythmic activities. Electroencephalogr. Clin. Neurophysiol. 76:481–508.

Storm van Leeuwen, W. 1975. Auditory evoked responses (AERs). *Handbook of Electroencephalography and Clinical Neurophysiology,* vol. 8A, Ed.-in-chief, A. Remond, pp. 71–85. Amsterdam: Elsevier.

Terzano, M.G., and Parrino, L. 1987. The phenomena of cyclic alternating pattern. Clin. Neurol. Neurosurg. 164–167.

Terzano, M.G., and Parrino, L. 1991. Functional relationship between micro- and macrostructure of sleep. In *Phasic Events and Dynamic Or-* *ganization of Sleep,* Eds. M.G. Terzano, P. Halász, and A.C. Declerck, pp. 101–119. New York: Raven Press.

Terzano, M.G., Mancia, D., Zacchetti, O., et al. 1981. The significance of cyclic EEG changes in Creutzfeldt-Jakob disease: prognostic value of their course in 9 patients. Ital. J. Neurol. Sci. 3:243–254.

Tinuper, P., Montagna, P., Medori, R., et al. 1998. The thalamus participates in the regulation of the sleep-waking cycle. A clinico-pathological study in fatal familial thalamic degeneration. Electroencephalogr. Clin. Neurophysiol. 73:117–123.

Ujszaszi, J., and Halász, P. 1988. Long latency evoked potential components in human slow wave sleep. Electroencephalogr. Clin. Neurophysiol. 69:516–522.

Ungerstedt, U. 1971. Stereotaxic mapping of the monoamine pathway in the rat brain. Acta Physiol. Scand. Suppl. 367:1–48.

Vaughan, H.G., Jr., and Ritter, W. 1970. The sources of auditory evoked responses recorded from the human head. Electroencephalogr. Clin. Neurophysiol. 28:360–367.

Vignaendra, V., Matthews, R.L., and Chatrian, G.E. 1974. Positive occipital sharp transients of sleep: relationships to nocturnal sleep cycle in man. Electroencephalogr. Clin. Neurophysiol. 37:239–246.

Wada, Y., Nanbu, Y., Koshino, Y., et al. 1996. Inter-and intrahemispheric EEG coherence during light drowsiness. Clin. Electroencephalogr. 27:24–88.

Weisz, J., Soroker, N., Oksenberg, A., et al. 1995. Effects of hemi-thalamic damage on K-complexes evoked by monaural stimuli during mid-afternoon sleep. Electroencephalogr. Clin. Neurophysiol. 94:148–150.

Weitzman, E.D., and Kremen, H. 1965. Auditory evoked responses during different stages of sleep in man. Electroencephalogr. Clin. Neurophysiol. 18:65–70.

Welch, L.K., and Stevens, J.B. 1971. Clinical value of the electroencephalogram following sleep deprivation. Aerospace Med. 42:349–351.

Wilder, B.J. 1969. Activation of epileptic foci in psychomotor epilepsy. Epilepsia (Amsterdam) 10:48(abstr.).

Winfield, D.L., and Sparer, P.J. 1954. The electroencephalogram in paralysis agitans. Dis. Nerv. Syst. 15:144–120.

Wittenbecker, H., and Kubicki, S. 1976. Statistische Auswertung von 719 Kurzschlafableitungen nach Schlafentzug. Z. EEG-EMC 8:205–209.

Wright, E.A., and Gilmore, R.L. 1984. Features of the geriatric EEG: age-dependent incidence of POSTS. Electroencephalogr. Clin. Neurophysiol. 58:49P(abst).

Zobniw, A.M., Yarworth, S., and Niedermeyer, E. 1975. Depth electroencephalography. J. Electrophysiol. Technol. 1:215–240.

11. Maturation of the EEG: Development of Waking and Sleep Patterns

Ernst Niedermeyer

General Principles

One of the first lessons the novice electroencephalographer must learn is the determination of brain potentials by two factors of paramount significance: level of vigilance and age. This chapter discusses the influence of age, and thus the ontogenetic evolution or maturation of the electroencephalogram (EEG).

The curve of human life, and life at all levels across the animal kingdom, is characterized by evolution, peak of maturity, and involution. However, there are basic differences between the ascending (evolutional) and descending (involutional) portions of the curve of life. Evolution proceeds along with maturation of neural tissues, the prerequisite of mental and intellectual growth.

The study of the *myelination of the brain* (Flechsig, 1920; Langworthy, 1930, 1933; Rorke and Riggs, 1969; Yakovlev and Lecours, 1967) has provided the structural basis of the maturation process in humans. Myelination, which is closely related to formation of lipids (Brante, 1949), seems to be the most important aspect in cerebral maturation, because this process accounts for the establishment of intercellular relationships that render the brain a functioning organ. Its biochemical composition has proved to be extremely complex (Norton, 1975a,b).

The declining curve of life is not determined by a reverse process such as "dematuration" (certainly not by demyelination), although the existence of a certain "wear out" of central nervous system (CNS) structures cannot be flatly denied. The predominant determining factor of CNS aging simply lies in a variety of pathological processes. The awareness of this basic difference between the ascending and the descending portions of life is of great significance in practical electroencephalography. Whereas the EEG of the years of maturation must be interpreted according to the rules of a statistical norm, the EEG evaluation of the aged individual must be guided by the ideal or optimal norm, because the optimal situation is absence of pathology, even in advanced age. With the application of a statistical norm, a mentally alert octogenarian with the frequency pattern of a normal middle-aged adult would have to be read as abnormal. This would be an absurdity.

Figure 11.1 demonstrates the maturational period, the peak of maturity, and the decline caused by pathology. The peak period of EEG maturation lies well into adulthood (after age 30), at a time when biological aging of body tissues has already started and physical capabilities or athletic performances have clearly passed their peak. This illustration, however, does not tell the whole truth. Cerebral maturation is not a smooth process of steady growth; one can observe certain quantum jumps in prematurity, as well as in infancy and childhood (Kellaway, 1957).

Historical Aspects

The first EEG studies in children were done by Berger (1932), who became aware of age-dependent changes. In his fifth report on the human EEG, he gave an account on his work with 17 children ranging in age from 8 days to 5 years. With the available equipment, a coil galvanometer, he was unable to demonstrate convincing EEG oscillations in newborns, although predominant delta activity was found at the age of 35 days. He related "the absence of the EEG in the first weeks of life" to Flechsig's (1920) demonstration of incomplete cortical myelination in the newborn.

Berger had to place the electrodes himself; this prompted some observations that have become commonplace for every EEG technician who deals with children: "a few children, however, screamed incessantly and became so restless that it was impossible to obtain the kind of continuous record necessary for interpretation." These problems have remained the same after more than 70 years of technical progress.

Over the ensuing years, further studies on the EEGs of normal and abnormal children have given testimony of increasing interest in this domain. Lindsley's (1936, 1939) longitudinal studies made significant contributions to EEG maturation. Further work was carried out by Bernhard (1939), Smith (1941), Henry (1944), Sureau et al. (1949), Gibbs and Gibbs (1950), Nekhorocheff (1950), Schütz et al. (1951), Kellaway and Fox (1952), and Garsche (1953). The use of spectral analysis has prompted further developmental EEG work (Benninger et al., 1984; Chavance and Samson-Dollfus, 1978; Colon et al., 1979; Corbin and Bickford, 1955; Dumermuth, 1968; Gibbs and Knott, 1949; Kasamatsu et al., 1964; Ohtahara, 1964; Samson-Dollfus and Goldberg, 1979; Walter, 1950). Gasser et al. (1983) studied the development of normal and mentally retarded children using factor analysis.

EEG neonatology has come of age as a special branch of developmental electroencephalography. The neonatal period in the premature and full-term newborn posed so many problems of a special electrophysiological nature, of EEG technology, and of interpretation that highly specialized investigators had to take over this burdensome task.

Earlier studies were made by Ellingson and Lindsley (1949), Arfel-Capdevielle (1950), Janzen et al. (1952), Mai and Schaper (1953), and Samson-Dollfus (1955). Full

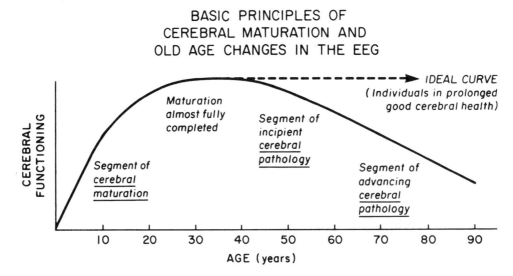

Figure 11.1.   Cerebral maturation (infancy, childhood, adolescence) versus cerebral pathology with regard to repercussions on the EEG.

recognition of EEG neonatology as a subspecialized field came with the deeper insights gained by a new approach, with or without computerized spectral analysis. The work of Dreyfus-Brisac (1964), as well as Dreyfus-Brisac and Monod (1964, 1975), occupies a special place; further major contributions have been made by Parmelee et al. (1968a,b), Prechtl et al. (1969), Engel (1975), Werner et al. (1977), Ellingson (1979), Lombroso (1979), and, with conservative recording technique, by Gibbs and Gibbs (1978). Further comprehensive work on the neonatal EEG (in atlas format) was presented by Stockard-Pope et al. (1992), Clancy et al. (1993), and De Weerd (1995). In a number of contributions to the premature and full-term neonatal EEG, Hughes and his coworkers investigated various important EEG patterns (Hughes, 1996; Hughes et al., 1983, 1987, 1990).

EEG evolution from infancy to adolescence in a large number of healthy juveniles has been the topic of extensive studies by Swedish authors (Eeg-Olofsson, 1971,a,b; Eeg-Olofsson et al., 1971; Petersén and Eeg-Olofsson, 1971; Petersén et al., 1975). This work has set standards for this branch of electroencephalography. In a remarkable study of 1,416 healthy subjects with an age range from 6 to 39 years, Matsuura et al. (1985) have investigated the development of various frequency ranges over the occipital, central, and frontopolar regions. These authors used automatic wave recognition methods. Gasser et al. (1988a,b) investigated the EEG development in children and adolescents with the use of frequency analysis and topographic demonstration.

EEG maturation in animals cannot be ignored. A study in the dog by Pampiglione (1963) and the work of Caveness (1962) in the rhesus monkey deserve special attention.

Premature Newborn

General Considerations

The EEG of the premature newborn reflects the immaturity of the fetal brain. These records may feature EEG activities that in mature adult life would be regarded as extremely abnormal or as heralding impending death. Suppression burst-like activity with long stretches of electrical silence may be normal in early stages of prematurity; discontinuity of the EEG activity is linked with striking asymmetries between both hemispheres. Somewhat later in the development, spikes or sharp waves loom impressively over the background of activity, but have to be interpreted as age-normal.

Difficulties in the assessment of EEG tracings of premature and full-term newborns cannot be overemphasized. The interpretation of these records is an awesome task which requires:

1. Adequate laboratory technique with the use of polygraphic parameters (oculogram, electromyelogram (EMG), pneumogram);
2. Familiarity with the characteristics of EEG phenomena through all stages of viable prematurity; and
3. Familiarity with the unusual correlates of the stages of vigilance, especially with rapid-eye-movement (REM) (active sleep) and non-REM (quiet sleep) phases, as well as mixed or intermediate sleep stages.

For this reason, the EEG of premature and full-term newborns will be presented in greater detail elsewhere in this book under special EEG methods, because mastery of polysomnographic techniques is a crucial prerequisite.

Significance of the Conceptional Age

The evaluation of the premature neonatal EEG is based on the conceptual age. The gestational age is calculated from the first day of the last menstrual period regardless of the date of birth. Gestational age plus age after birth equals the conceptional age.

Recordings Obtained from the Fetus

In a subject at a conceptional age of 3 months, Okamoto and Kirikae (1951) demonstrated slow activity (0.5–2/sec) with cortical electrodes. These tracings were obtained through cesarean section. Tharp (1990) reports that he saw those tracings and found considerable artifact overlay, which reduces the validity of these observations. Bergström (1969) studied the EEG of fetuses immediately after separation from the maternal circulation. He found primitive wave patterns of irregular frequency or intermittent complexes from the oral portion of the brainstem and from the hippocampus at a conceptional age of 17 weeks. According to this author, there is continuous EEG activity in the pontine level after 10 weeks of conceptional age.

EEG of Nonviable Fetuses before 24 Weeks of Conceptional Age

Rarely, EEG tracings can be secured in newborns with a life span of only a few hours. Engel (1964, 1975) recorded the EEG of a 19-week-old fetus (crown-rump length 14.8 cm). Initially, detectable activity in the 9 to 10/sec range (25 µV) flattened during the recording, while the newborn showed progressive bradycardia and gasping respiration.

Early Prematures: 24 to 27 Weeks

These premature newborns find themselves in an undifferentiated state of sleep that shows some characteristics of both "active" and "quiet" sleep. According to Dreyfus-Brisac and Monod (1975), before 28 weeks of conceptional age "the infant is active all the time but does not seem to be awake." These investigators pose the questions: "Does he really sleep? What is sleep at this age?" There are obviously no answers.

At this age, the EEG shows very slow (0.3–1/sec) waves of high voltage in bursts lasting 3 to 20 seconds (Dreyfus-Brisac and Monod, 1975). This activity is diffuse with occipital predominance. There are also short runs of rhythmical activity in the 8 to 14/sec range of moderate voltage (25–30 µV), mainly over the rolandic area (Dreyfus-Brisac and Monod, 1975). Rhythmical 4 to 5/sec activity may also occur superimposed on delta frequencies (Werner et al., 1977). The pattern is highly discontinuous and may alternate with stretches of general electrical quiescence of 2 to 3 minutes' duration (Dreyfus-Brisac and Monod, 1975; Engel, 1975). Bursts of activity usually occur simultaneously over both hemispheres.

An appraisal of the length of inactive (discontinuous) periods of EEG recordings was carried out by Benda et al. (1989). These investigators cast some doubt on earlier statements that periods of EEG inactivity of 2 to 3 minutes are within normal limits of variability. This may be true for some cases but, according to Benda et al. (1989), silent periods of more than 30 seconds carry a risk for nonsurvival, whereas short periods (less than 20 seconds) correlate with favorable outcome.

Benda et al. (1989) also showed that the use of phenobarbital (especially in premature infants with intraventricular hemorrhages) may affect the predictability of the EEG because of the fact that phenobarbital in large dosages induced or enhances burst-suppression activity.

The degree of EEG inactivity appears to be a better indicator for outcome than the severity of intraventricular hemorrhages (Benda et al., 1989; Clancy et al., 1984; Staudt et al., 1982; Watanabe et al., 1983).

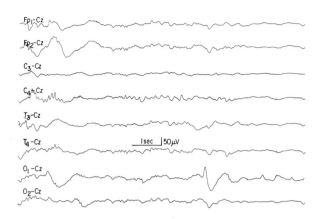

Figure 11.2. Conceptional age 29.5 weeks (gestational age 26 weeks, plus 3.5 weeks age after birth). Mixed slow and faster activity with rapid changes of voltage and an almost flat stretch. No definite EEG abnormalities.

Conceptional Age of 28 to 31 Weeks

The EEG remains discontinuous and no differentiation between waking and sleeping states can be made; there is also no basic difference between active and quiet sleep (Fig. 11.2). During stretches of EEG activity, delta activity (slower than 1/sec) may be quite prominent in all leads, frequently superimposed by short, low-voltage fast runs, mostly around 16/sec, known as "ripples of prematurity" (Engel, 1975) and also as "brushes" (Lombroso, 1979). Theta and alpha frequencies may be intermixed, and some inconspicuous sharp elements may be present. At age 31 weeks, bursts may be mixed with very pronounced sharp waves with temporal predominance (Werner et al., 1977). These premature babies usually have birth weights above 1,000 g. Hughes et al. (1983) studied periods of quiescence and activity in premature babies. Activity periods increased from 2% (at 24 weeks) to 80% (34 weeks). Periods of quiescence occurred in all premature infants up to the conceptual age of 32 weeks. Beautiful examples of brushes ("delta brushes") and so-called delta crests have been presented by Anderson et al. (1985).

Physiological rhythmical activity in the theta range has been described as "temporal, sawtooth waves" (Werner et al., 1977), "theta bursts" (Dreyfus-Brisac, 1979; Tharp, 1980) and "temporal sharp transients" or "bursts of sharp theta" (Lombroso, 1980, 1987). This pattern was extensively investigated by Hughes et al. (1987), who stressed the physiological character; absence or untimely disappearance of temporal theta activity was found to be a sign of abnormality. This pattern is most commonly in the 5 to 7/sec range and most prominent over the midtemporal region. Temporal theta maximizes at 29 to 31 weeks and then diminishes and disappears near term (Hughes et al., 1987) (Fig. 11.3).

Unlike the rhythmical theta activity of premature newborns, the sharp theta rhythm on the occipital areas of prematures (also known as STOP) shows an extremely early maximum at the conceptional age of 24 weeks and then gradually declines and is usually absent at full-term (Hughes et al., 1990) (Fig. 11.3). Vanhatalo et al. (2002)

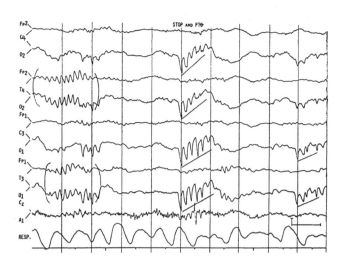

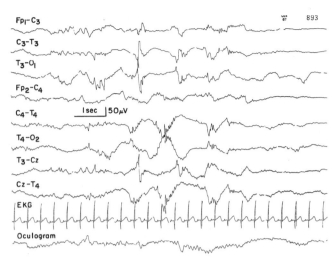

Figure 11.3. This illustration, taken from the work of J.R. Hughes, demonstrates sharp theta waves of prematurity, and *(underlined)* occipital sharp theta rhythm. The former is also known as "PT theta" and the latter as "STOP" ("sharp theta on the occipitals in prematures"). (Courtesy of Dr. J.R. Hughes and Clinical Electroencephalography.)

Figure 11.5. Age 11 days, born at 32 weeks' conceptional age. Seizures at birth, still occasional myoclonus. Note the impressive left midtemporal spikes. These spikes, however, are not abnormal at that age. Also note fast activity mixed with large slow waves ("delta brushes"), also a physiological pattern of this age. The baby is in "quiet" sleep. (Courtesy of *Handbook of Electroencephalography and Clinical Neurophysiology*, ed., J.A. Wada. Amsterdam: Elsevier, 1975.)

have strongly recommended the use of DC amplifiers, which are capable of demonstrating ultraslow EEG activity in stretches of nearly flat appearance with conventional recording technique.

Conceptional Age of 32 to 35 Weeks

This is the phase of beginning differentiation between wakefulness, active sleep, and quiet sleep. Slow activity, often with superimposed ripples around 16/sec, shows occipital predominance with a good deal of isosynchrony between both occipital areas. For this reason, running both occipital electrodes against each other may yield low-voltage slowing (Dreyfus-Brisac and Monod, 1975) (Fig. 11.4).

Portions of alternating and discontinuous activity with long flat stretches are noticeable in quiet sleep, whereas continuous irregular diffuse slowing with "ripples" is more

common in active sleep. Some oculographic activity of REM-like character is noted at this stage (Werner et al., 1977). Such continuous slow EEG activity, however, is also detectable in periods of wakefulness (Dreyfus-Brisac and Monod, 1975). At this conceptional age, single spikes may be quite prominent but do not constitute a categorical abnormality (Fig. 11.5).

Conceptional Age of 36 to 41 Weeks

Premature babies (36–38 weeks) show EEG features that can be seen in full-term newborns. Diffuse low-voltage patterns as well as diffuse slowing (mostly delta activity) with runs of 10 to 14/sec waves are common (Dreyfus-Brisac and Monod, 1975); typical ripples of prematurity decline and disappear (Monod et al., 1983).

For the first time, wakefulness and active and quiet sleep are correlated with three different EEG patterns. In quiet sleep, the recording shows discontinuous character during quiet sleep only. This pattern is well known as "tracé alternant." Bursts are of moderate to high voltage and of 1 to 10 seconds in duration, consisting of mixed slow, medium, and fast activity, often with intermingled spiky discharges. The "flat" periods between bursts are not truly flat, but show marked voltage depression with mixed frequencies; their duration ranges from 6 to 10 seconds (Werner et al., 1977). Oculographic activity is zero or inconspicuous; respiration is regular (Fig. 11.6). Moussalli-Salefranque et al. (1984) have clearly pointed out the important differences between a physiological tracé alternant and a seriously abnormal discontinuous EEG in full-term neonates. The term "tracé alternant" was introduced by Samson-Dollfus (1955), but the pattern as such was already known to several disciples of Fischgold (Pichot, 1953; presumably recognized by Fischgold himself—see Tharp, 1990). The periodicity of

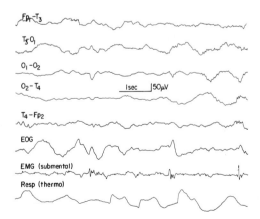

Figure 11.4. Conceptional age 34 weeks (gestational age 28 weeks, plus 6 weeks after birth). Note some REM-like oculographic activity and suggestions of "ripples" or "brushes" on the *right side* of this illustration.

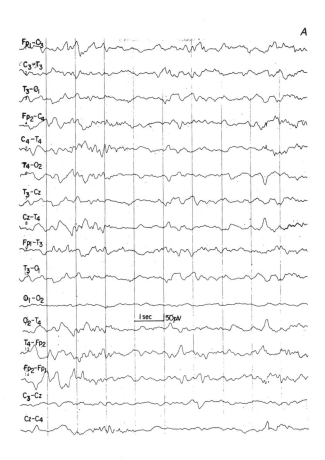

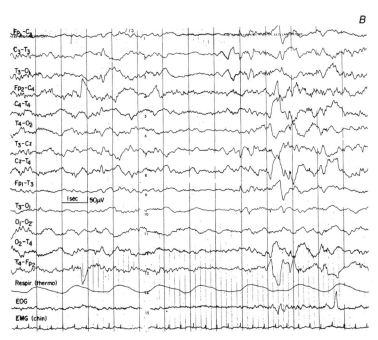

Figure 11.6. Tracé alternant in quiet (non-REM) sleep. **A:** Patient age 6 days, full-term. **B:** Patient age 1 month, full-term. The tracé alternant character is somewhat rudimentary; the low-voltage stretches are not very impressive. At this age, there is usually little or no evidence of tracé alternant.

stretches of greater and lesser EEG activity in the tracé alternant of quiet sleep was studied with the use of fast Fourier transforms; the results suggested a neuronal structure that functions as a clock, presumed to be located in the brainstem (Keidel et al., 1991).

Challamel et al. (1984) noticed periods of unilateral voltage depression in 3.13% of infants recorded in the neonatal period (conceptual age from 35 to 44 weeks); these asymmetries were shifting and occurred solely in quiet (non-REM) sleep. These infants suffered from a minor disease (not involving the CNS) and their outcome was excellent.

An EEG depression in sleeping full-term newborns was reported by O'Brien et al. (1987), who considered these stretches of depressed voltage "a benign variation." The voltage depression is frequently unilateral and may last from 30 seconds to 2 minutes. At the termination, there are bursts and stretches of "racé discontinue" (Challamel et al., 1984).

The emergence of different patterns for wakefulness and active and quiet sleep denotes a leap forward in the development of cerebral maturation that is not consistent with a smooth continuous process. Interhemispheric synchrony between homologous areas has markedly improved at full term (Ellingson et al., 1974; Joseph et al., 1976; Parmelee, 1969; Parmelee et al., 1969; Prechtl et al., 1974; Schulte et al., 1971; Varner et al., 1978). Cross-correlation coefficients have been found to be higher in neonatal active sleep than in quiet sleep (Varner et al., 1978). Coherence studies of normal newborns were carried out by Kuks et al. (1988). Scher et al. (1990) described a computer system for neonates that is capable of comparing behavioral and electrographic components of EEG sleep.

According to Passouant et al. (1965), the newborn's waking state represents 29% of the day. Sleep can be broken-down ("fast," REM) sleep. The intermediate forms with mixed traits of REM and non-REM sleep may exist (Fig. 11.7). Spontaneous arousal from sleep in the newborn invariably occurs in active (REM) sleep, according to Isch-Treussard et al. (1981).

In about one third of healthy full-term newborns, some rhythmical sharp activity is noted over the frontal midline and also over the vertex. This pattern has been described as "Fz theta/alpha bursts" (Hayakawa et al., 1987).

An extensive study of the benign nature of sharp activity of healthy preterm and full-term neonates was carried out by Scher et al. (1994a,b). On the other hand, Biagioni et al. (1996) discuss neonatal sharp activity under the heading of "abnormal EEG transients" and consider their prognostic significance rather ambivalent (the presumed underlying brain damage either remaining clinically silent or becoming evident in the further course).

This outline essentially describes the EEG activity of the full-term and near full-term neonate; far more detail on the neonatal EEG is found in Chapter 49, "Electroencephalography of the Newborn: Normal and Abnormal Features." The electroencephalographer who moves into the field of neonatal EEG evaluation must become familiar with the characteristics of the sleep stages at this age. In addition to the usual search for abnormal patterns, normal or abnormal sequential aspects of sleep stages must be taken into consideration.

The differentiation of sleep stages is rendered more difficult because of the smallness of the ocular potential in many cases at this age. For this reason, rapid eye movements may not give rise to the typical ocular artifacts in frontotemporal derivations. Even with special canthus electrodes, the ocular movements may be barely detectable, whereas direct observation will provide evidence for REM. These observations stress the importance of EMG and pneumogram. The reader will find a more detailed presentation of neonatological problems with more specific developmental, clinical, and electroencephalographic aspects in Chapter 49, "Electroencephalography of the Newborn: Normal and Abnormal Features."

Typical EEG Abnormalities in Prematurity and at Full Term

Discussion of abnormalities is out of place in a chapter discussing normal evolutional aspects. The author believes, however, that the electroencephalographer, confronted with the distinction between normalcy and abnormality, will appreciate a short discussion of abnormal neonatal tracings.

The distinction can be very difficult or even impossible. Engel (1975) puts it as follows: "It is difficult to describe the characteristics of an abnormal paroxysmal electrical discharge in detail because all individual graphoelements may occur independently in the EEG of normal neonates. In premature infants the differentiation between normal bursts and pathological paroxysms is even more difficult and sometimes arbitrary." The study of Lombroso (1979), based on quantification of certain EEG characteristics, has been very helpful in the detection of prognostically significant abnormalities. This has been confirmed by the work of Tharp et al. (1981).

Important distinctive characteristics of abnormal patterns in premature and full-term newborns can be listed as follows:

1. Marked asynchrony of bursts at a gestational age above 36 weeks.
2. Spike activity of prominent and consistent unilateral focal features in full-term and premature infants. Occa-

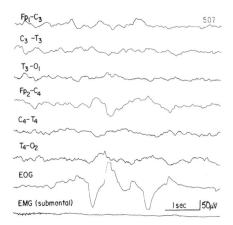

Figure 11.7. REM sleep, in a patient age 7 weeks, term. Note typical ocular artifact and depressed EMG activity.

sional sharp waves and spikes may occur even at week 41 in healthy babies, especially over the right midtemporal area, according to Karbowski and Nencka (1980) or with parietal predominance, after Statz and Dumermuth (1981).

3. The special case of large and often slow positive sharp waves in premature infants with intraventricular hemorrhages, chiefly over the rolandic area (Blume and Dreyfus-Brisac, 1982; Clancy and Tharp, 1984; Engel, 1975; Lombroso, 1982; Nowack and Janati, 1990; Tharp et al., 1981).
4. Repetitive ictal spiking with focal onset as a concomitant of neonatal convulsions, more common in full-term than in premature neonates.
5. Large prehypsarrhythmic disorganized patterns in full-term newborns with frequent short ictal episodes.
6. Flatness or near flatness, usually a sign of very severe cerebral involvement, such as acute herpes simplex encephalitis, massive asphyxia, severe cerebral malformation and especially hydrancephalic tissue destruction (Sternberg et al., 1984).
7. Stretches of rhythmical activity in alpha frequency. There is good evidence from the literature that this type of rhythmical activity represents camouflaged epileptic activity or reflects a CNS disturbance (Hrachovy and O'Donnell, 1999; Radvanyi-Bouvet, 1983; Staudt et al., 1983, 1984). In some cases, faster frequencies in the beta range may be found instead of rhythmical alpha activity (Radvanyi-Bouvet, 1983).
8. Excessive and burst-like theta activity (Hrachovy and O'Donnell, 1999).

Neonatal records of very low voltage are usually distinguishable from physiological low-voltage activity in newborns. This list includes only a few important abnormal patterns of the neonatal age.

To distinguish a normal tracé alternant from an abnormal suppression burst-like pattern:

1. Run the record long enough to find out if this alternating pattern is transient (tracé alternant) or constant (abnormal).
2. Distinguish between stretches of depressed voltage (in tracé alternant) and stretches of suppressed activity or near flatness (in abnormal suppression burst-like records).

The following might be helpful in the differentiation of tracé alternant and burst-suppression:

Tracé alternant: like MOUNTAINS AND HILLS.
Burst-suppression: like MOUNTAINS AND FLAT PLAINS.

Disappearance of Neonatal Patterns

The tracé alternant pattern as the EEG correlate of quiet sleep (non-REM sleep) is a common sight during the first 1 to 3 weeks of life in a full-term newborn, provided the record catches the baby in a quiet sleep episode. Active sleep (REM sleep) is more commonly encountered in the sleeping newborn (64% of sleeping time, according to Passouant et al., 1965). Tracé alternant portions disappear about

3 to 4 weeks after full-term birth (Dreyfus-Brisac and Curzi-Dascalova, 1975). Ellingson (1979), however, observed signs of tracé alternant up to the 47th day of life.

With the preponderance of active sleep (REM sleep), it is no surprise that the healthy full-term newborn shows active sleep at sleep onset. Quiet sleep onset is well established 1 month after full-term delivery (37 days, after Ellingson, 1979) and gradually emerges as the predominant type of sleep with the development of stages 2, 3, and 4.

Intervening diseases, even without affecting the CNS, may temporarily lead to a regression in the schedule of maturation. Hence the newborn may fall back into a prenatal pattern for the duration of the affliction.

With the disappearance of neonatal EEG characteristics and the emergence of patterns such as a posterior basic rhythm (the forerunner of alpha rhythm) and sleep spindles, the EEG starts to assume configurations that are more familiar to the electroencephalographer. At this point, the distinction between normalcy and abnormality starts to become easier.

Table 11.1 provides a condensed presentation of a number of EEG variables and their developmental aspects.

EEG in Infancy (2–12 Months)
General Considerations and Technical Aspects

The first 3 months of life are characterized by a gradual transition from neonatal to infantile EEG patterns. At the end of this period, the waking baby shows rhythmical posterior activity around 4/sec. This is a precursor of the posterior alpha rhythm and shows blocking effects with eye opening, although it is not quite as striking as later in life.

The waking infant is not an easy object for EEG studies. Babies tend to keep their eyes open, yet it is strongly recommended that stretches of waking record with eyes closed be obtained. Dreyfus and Curzi-Dascalova (1975) suggest a gentle passive occlusion of the eyes for short periods in order to demonstrate the posterior basic rhythm. Temporary use of a short time constant (0.1 sec) may be helpful to separate the posterior rhythm from movement artifacts. This rhythm may also be present in a crying baby (associated with forceful closure of eyes and concomitant frontal muscle artifacts), as well as in a quiet infant with open eyes. The baby usually closes the eyes as a sign of impending drowsiness.

In EEG laboratory practice, two basic philosophies characterize the approach to EEG recording in infancy. In the first, the recording is started in a sleeping baby. Spontaneous sleep is most desirable, and this goal can be achieved mainly when the recording is scheduled shortly after the baby has been fed. Otherwise, the baby will have to be sedated prior to recording (usually with chloral hydrate, 125–375 mg during the first 6 months of life, or secobarbital, 8–24 mg rectally or in a tasty fruit juice). The baby may be lying on a bed or in the mother's or the nurse's arms. This approach usually yields technically satisfactory sleep records, but it may be quite difficult to obtain a usable waking portion afterward. In a sedated infant, it is often impossible to secure a waking tracing. Using the second approach, the record routinely starts while the baby is awake. It is extremely difficult

Table 11.1.   A Condensed View of EEG Maturation

	Premature 27–27 Wk	Premature 28–31 Wk	Premature 32–35 Wk	Full-term Newborn 36–41 Wk
Continuity	Discontinuous, long flat stretches	Discontinuous	Continuous in waking state and REM sleep, discontinuous in non-REM sleep	Continuous except for tracé alternant in non-REM (quiet) sleep
Interhemispheric synchrony	Short bursts in synchrony	Mostly asynchronous activity	Partly synchronous, especially in occipital leads	Minor asynchronies still present
Differentiation of waking and sleeping	Undifferentiated	Undifferentiated	Waking distinguished from sleep early in the period, then differentiation of non-REM and REM sleep	Good
Posterior basic (alpha) rhythm	None	None	None	None
Slow activity (awake)	Very slow bursts, high voltage (state of vigilance undifferentiated)	Very slow activity predominant	Slow (delta) with occipital maximum	Slow (delta), mostly of moderate voltage
Temporal theta	Present and increasing	Prominent	Decreasing and disappearing	Disappearing or absent
Occipital theta	Prominent	Decreasing	Decreasing	Absent
Fast activity (awake)	Very little beta activity	Frequent ripples or brushes around 16/sec	Frequent ripples or brushes (16–20/sec)	Decreasing ripples, sparse fast activity
Low voltage	Long flat stretches	Flat stretches, mainly asynchronous	Low-voltage record suspect of serious cerebral pathology	Very low-voltage records are due to severe cerebral pathology; prognosis ominous
Hyperventilation	Not feasible	Not feasible	Not feasible	Not feasible
Intermittent photic stimulation	?	?	?	Driving response below 4 flashes/sec may occur, not easily elicited
Drowsiness	Undifferentiated	Undifferentiated	Undifferentiated	Undifferentiated
Tracé alternant	None	None	Present in non-REM (quiet) sleep	Present in non-REM (quiet) sleep
Spindles	None	None (but ripples present)	None (but ripples present)	None (but scanty ripples)
Vertex waves and K complexes	None	None	None	None
Positive occipital sharp transients of sleep	None	None	None	None
Slow and fast activity in sleep	Slow activity of high voltage, little slow activity (stage of vigilance undifferentiated)	Much slow activity, more irregular; little fast activity	Irregular slow activity of occipital predominance	Much delta and theta activity, continuous in REM sleep
REM sleep	Undifferentiated	Undifferentiated	Continuous slow activity; oculographically, REM present	Continuous slow activity, REM in EOG (more REM or "active" than non-REM sleep)
Rhythmical frontal theta activity (6–7/sec)	None	None	None	None
14 and 6/sec positive spikes	None	None	None	None
Psychomotor variant (marginal abnormality)	None	None	None	None
Sharp waves, spikes	Some intermixed sharp activity in bursts (normal)	Some intermixed sharp activity (normal)	Often prominent sharp waves or spikes (normal)	Some minor sharp transients (normal) (abnormal spikes more consistent and prominent)

Infancy 2–12 Mos	Early Childhood 12–36 Mos	Pre-school Age 3–5 Yrs	Older Children 6–12 Yrs	Adolescents 13–20 Yrs
Continuous	Continuous	Continuous	Continuous	Continuous
No significant asynchrony	No significant asynchrony	No significant asynchrony	No significant asynchrony	No significant asynchrony
Good	Good	Good	Good	Good
Starting at age 3–4 mos at 4/sec, reaching about 6/sec at 12 mos	Rising from 5–6/sec to 8/sec (seldom 9/sec)	Rising from 6–8/sec to 7–9/sec	Reaching 10/sec at age 10 yr	Averaging 10/sec
Considerable	Considerable	Marked admixture of posterior slow activity (to alpha rhythm)	Varying degree of posterior slow activity mixed with alpha	Posterior slow activity diminishing
None	None	None	None	None
None	None	None	None	None
Very moderate	Mostly moderate	Mostly moderate	Mostly moderate	Moderate, except for low voltage fast records
Uncommon, usually abnormal	Uncommon, usually abnormal	Uncommon, usually abnormal	Seldom as variant of normalcy	Occasionally and (at end of teenage period more often) as variant of normalcy
Not feasible	Mostly not feasible	Often marked delta response	Often marked delta response	Delta responses become less impressive
Improving driving to low flash rates after age 6 mos	Often good driving response to low flash rates	Often good driving response to low flash rates	Often good driving response, chiefly at medium flash rates (8–16/sec)	Often good driving response, chiefly at medium flash rates
Around age 6 mos, appearance of rhythmical theta	Marked "hypnagogic" rhythmical theta (4–6/sec)	Rhythmical theta gradually vanishing, other types of slow activity predominant	Gradual alpha dropout with increasing slow activity	Gradual alpha dropout with low-voltage stretches (mainly slow)
Disappears in 1st (seldom 2nd) mo	None	None	None	None
Appear after 2nd mo; 12–15/sec, sharp, shifting	In 2nd yr, sharp and shifting, then symmetrical with vertex maximum	Typical vertex maximum	Typical vertex maximum	Typical vertex maximum
Appear mainly at 5 mos, fairly large, blunt	Large, becoming more pointed	Large with an increasingly impressive sharp component	Large with a prominent sharp component	Not quite as large, sharp component not quite as prominent
None	Poorly defined	Poorly defined	Still poorly defined but gradually evolving	Often very well developed
Much diffuse 0.75–3/sec activity with posterior maximum; moderate fast activity	Marked posterior maximum of slow activity; often a good deal of fast activity	Predominant slowing but less prominent posterior maximum	Much diffuse slowing, slightly decreasing voltage	Much diffuse slowing with further attenuation of voltage
REM portion decreasing; mostly slow activity	Mostly slow, starting to become more desynchronized	Slow activity with some desynchronization	Less slowing and increasing desynchronization	Mature desynchronization
None	Seldom in 3rd yr of life	May occur, not very common	A bit more common	A bit more common, declining at end of period
None	Rare	May occur, not very common	Fairly common	Fairly common
None	None	Probably none	Uncommon	More common (although relatively rare)
Essential as abnormal phenomena	Spikes in seizure-free children, mainly occipital (mild abnormalities)	Spikes in seizure-free children, mainly occipital, also Rolandic (slight abnormalities)	Spikes in seizure-free children, mainly Rolandic (central-mid-temporal), slight to moderate abnormalities; physiological occipital spikes in congenitally blind children	Benign Rolandic spikes usually disappear before beginning of this period

to place electrodes under these circumstances; most infants resent this type of manipulation and their screaming can be very disruptive in a large laboratory.

Some EEG technologists have become extremely experienced in the art of handling a waking infant, and often succeed in obtaining both waking and spontaneous sleep records. Further information about the management of infants and children in North American EEG laboratories is found in the study of Leonberg (1984).

While the International Electrode System should be used for the electrode placement, the full set of 19 scalp and two ear reference electrodes does not have to be used. Ten electrodes are a bare minimum; 15 seems to be a reasonable number, with midline electrodes mandatory. The use of ocular leads, respiratory monitoring, and electrocardiogram (ECG) are helpful in the detection of artifacts, as well as in the assessment of sleep stages.

Many laboratories use rubber caps in small infant sizes; this technique is not conducive to sleep, and collodion is preferable. Whenever bentonite paste (recommended by Fois, 1961) or other types of paste are used, the possibility of rapid drying and thus deteriorating electrodes must be borne in mind with this technique; the electrode impedance values may remain particularly high, leaving aside the natural high impedance of the scalp in newborns and in early infancy. Needle electrodes are sometimes used in infants with good results. Excellent new types of paste are now used instead of bentonite.

EEG Characteristics in the Waking State

In early infancy (around age 2 months), irregular delta activity of 2 to 3.5/sec and medium to high voltage (50–100 μV) is widely preponderant (Dumermuth, 1972).

As mentioned above, rhythmical occipital 3 to 4/sec activity is often noted at the age of 3 to 4 months; this activity can be blocked by eye opening.

According to Dreyfus and Curzi-Dascalova (1975), this rhythm becomes more stable at age 5 months with acceleration to 5/sec. With further increase of frequency, an average frequency of 6 to 7/sec (occasionally 8/sec) is reached at age 12 months. The amplitudes range from 50 to 100 μV.

Some rhythmical rolandic activity of 5 to 8/sec may be present as early as age 3 months; its amplitude lies around 25 to 50 μV. This activity changes very little during the first year of life (Dreyfus and Curzi-Dascalova, 1975). These findings, obtained by visual analysis, have been bolstered and complemented by the use of power spectral analysis (Hagne, 1968; Hagne et al., 1972; Ohtahara, 1964).

EEG Characteristics in Drowsiness

Prior to the age of 5 to 8 months, the transition from the waking state to sleep is a gradual process characterized by progressive slowing into the delta frequency range. No specific drowsy state can be identified in the smooth progression of slow activity to the stage of sleep. Drowsiness becomes an indubitable entity between ages 6 and 8 months. This state is recognized by strong rhythmicity in the lower theta range, around 4/sec, with gradual acceleration to 5 and 6/sec over the ensuing months. The impressive theta rhythmicity is also known as "hypnagogic hypersynchrony" (Samson-Dollfus et al., 1981).

This drowsy pattern seems to develop from the posterior basic rhythm; such a development, however, might be more apparent than real. The transition from wakefulness to drowsiness is associated with a change of the distribution of amplitudes. The maximum or rhythmical theta activity moves into the centroparietal region where voltage values of 100 to 250 μV are quite common. Keep in mind that voltage values depend on the interelectrode distance and thus vary from montage to montage.

According to Dreyfus and Curzi-Dascalova (1975), the occipital rhythm may be somewhat slower than the diffusely predominant theta rhythm (possibly indicating a basic difference between two coexisting rhythmical theta patterns). In rare cases, the rhythmical theta activity of drowsiness may not materialize.

Sleep EEG and Non-REM Sleep

During the first 3 months of life, sleep may begin in a peculiar manner. Curzi-Dascalova et al. (1981) have shown that some infants fall asleep without eye closure, others with half-closed eyes, and others with brief alternating opening and closing of the eyes. The EEG and polygraphic data indicate sleep onset with active (REM) sleep in neonates and gradual evolution of sleep onset with quiet (non-REM) sleep during the ensuing weeks. The "slow" sleep of the infant is dominated by diffuse 0.75 to 3/sec activity with a maximum of amplitude (100–150 or 200 μV) over the occipital area. The amplitudes increase with deepening slow sleep. There are some intermixed theta, alpha, and beta frequencies of smaller amplitudes.

Spindles appear usually during the second month of life; occasionally, fragments of spindles may be observed somewhat earlier (Metcalf, 1969). The spindle frequency ranges from 12 to 15/sec, with 14/sec being the most commonly encountered frequency. Throughout infancy, spindles are maximal over central and parietal areas with shifting asymmetries. A clear-cut midline (vertex) maximum does not exist at this age. Spindles of infancy usually show a negative sharp component, whereas the positive component is rounded. The sharp spindle configuration (shown by Fois, 1961, and not specifically mentioned in earlier literature) is a typical hallmark of sleep in infancy. The comb-like shape of these runs may be erroneously interpreted as 14/sec positive spikes, but a careful analysis of polarity clearly shows negativity of the spiky components. The spatial distribution also is different; spindles are rolandic, 14/sec positive spikes of chiefly posterotemporal location. Finally, the 14/sec or 14 and 6/sec positive spike pattern is extremely rare before the age of 2 years and virtually nonexistent during the first year of life (Fig. 11.8).

According to Katsurada (1965), spindles may show sharp negative and positive phases after the age of 6 months; this type of spindle, however, is less common than those with a strictly negative sharp component.

The length of the spindle trains warrants some comment. These runs are of short duration and low voltage during the second month. With the third month, the amplitude increases and the duration of the runs becomes much longer (Lenard, 1970). The intervals between spindle trains become shorter, but the author cannot share the view that spindling is almost continuous between ages 2 and 6 months (Hagne et al.,

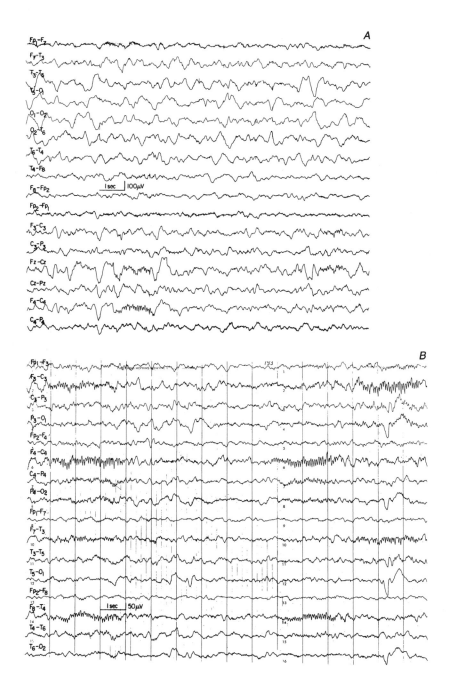

Figure 11.8. **A:** Patient age 10 months. Light non-REM sleep. Typical spindles of infancy, sharp and shifting. Normal posterior voltage maximum of slow activity (channels 3 to 7 from the top). **B:** Patient age 9 months. More prolonged trains of infantile spindles.

1972). Spindle bursts may reach a duration of 10 seconds, but there is a decline of the length of spindle runs in the second half of the first year, while the number of runs increases.

Dreyfus and Curzi-Dascalova (1975) have pointed out that complete absence of spindles at age 3 to 8 months represents a severe abnormality. This statement weighs heavily in view of the enormous material accumulated in the laboratory of these investigators; nevertheless, the electroencephalographer must use this dictum with great caution. The sleep record obtained must be sufficiently long in order "to give the baby a chance to produce spindles." At this age,

there is still a fair chance that the sleep recording is limited to REM sleep; this underscores the necessity of oculographic and pneumographic recording.

An excellent demonstration of the development of sleep spindles from age 10 weeks to 1 year was presented by Hughes (1996) (Fig. 11.9).

Vertex waves and *K complexes* are usually seen around the age of 5 months, although rudiments may be seen much earlier. Vertex waves may be quite large at age 5 to 6 months. At this age, K complexes are of considerable voltage, but the initiating sharp component is poorly developed

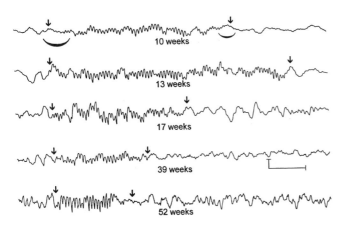

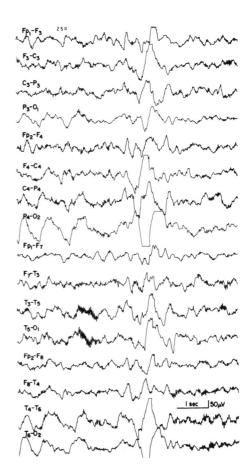

Figure 11.9. Sleep spindles at different ages. At 10 weeks note the very low amplitude at the beginning and end of the burst (underlined) with a duration of 5 seconds; at 13 weeks a long lasting spindle of 6.5 seconds; at 17 weeks, 3.5 seconds; at 39 weeks, 2 seconds; and 52 weeks, 1.5 seconds. Time (1 second) and voltage calibration (50 µV) are shown. Montage is bipolar linkage of the C_3-P_3 electrodes. *Arrows* designate the beginning and ending of typical spindles at the given age. (From Dr. John R. Hughes, 1996. Courtesy of the author and *Clinical Electroencephalography*.)

and somewhat "blunted" (Niedermeyer, 1972). In contrast, Metcalf et al. (1971) have stressed the comparatively low voltage of K complexes in infancy. These authors also noticed the appearance of K complexes in infants ages 5 to 6 months, but the complexes may be obscured by background activity (Figs. 11.10 and 11.11).

In infants in the first year of life, Ellingson et al. (1982) recorded brief apneic episodes ("respiratory pauses" lasting 3–10 sec) during sleep. These pauses are more common in REM sleep. All of these infants were clinically normal.

Figure 11.11. A K complex in a patient age 13 months; quite large with a blunted sharp component.

Sleep EEG and REM Sleep

The decrease of the REM sleep portion during the first year of life has been well established (Roffwarg et al., 1966; Stern et al., 1969); but the share of REM sleep activity is around 50% at birth, falling to 40% at 3 to 5 months and 30% between 12 and 24 months.

Dittrichova et al. (1972) and Dreyfus and Curzi-Dascalova (1975) reported the occurrence of sharp contoured occipital activity in the REM sleep of infants. This activity shows a frequency around 2/sec at 6 weeks and 2 to 4/sec at 12 to 16 weeks of age.

There is some intermixed delta and theta activity associated with the occipital sharp transients.

The REM sleep latency (time span from sleep onset to the first REM period) gradually lengthens in the course of the first year of life. The work of Schulz et al. (1983) has shown that the REM sleep latency underlies diurnal rhythmical changes, with the longest latencies between noon and 4 p.m. and the shortest between 4 a.m. and 8 a.m.

Reactivity and Evoked Responses

The evolution of evoked responses in newborns and infants will be discussed in Chapter 55, "Evoked Potentials in Infancy and Childhood."

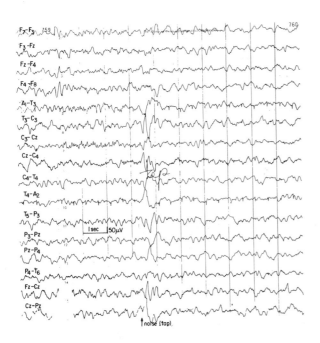

Figure 11.10. Patient age 9 months. Light non-REM sleep. A large vertex wave after auditory stimulus. The response is somewhat complex and resembles a K complex.

The blocking response of the posterior basic rhythm (obtained by passive eye closure, see above) is usually present at the age of 3 to 4 months. Similar rhythmical activity over the central region does not respond to eye opening (Dumermuth, 1972). A true rolandic mu rhythm cannot be identified during the first year of life, although forerunners of this activity are likely to be present. The author's earliest observation of unmistakable rolandic mu rhythm was made in a 20-month-old child (Niedermeyer and Koshino, 1975).

A photic driving response to flickering light may be obtained as early as 3 to 4 months after delivery; the responses are most prominent in the theta band (Hrbek et al., 1966; Vitova and Hrbek, 1972). There is probably no good evidence of occipital lambda wave activity during the first year of life.

EEG in Early Childhood (12–36 Months)

Waking Record

Readable waking records are not easily obtained in the second and third years of life. At this age, many little children resent being laid down in a supine position for electrode placement and recording and gradually become too heavy to be held comfortably in the nurse's or mother's arms. These children may successfully fight sleepiness and sleep and hence have to be sedated. For this reason, the waking portion is a postarousal tracing; it must be ascertained with great care that the child is truly awake. Some little children are so antagonistic to the procedure that they try to pull off their electrodes almost immediately after awakening.

The *posterior basic rhythm* is on the move from the upper theta to the lowest alpha range and is most commonly found between 6 to 7/sec during the second and 7 to 8/sec during the third year of life. The blocking response to eye opening intensifies; keep in mind that the degree of this response is considerably determined by darkness or brightness (more impressive response) of the recording room.

The evolution of the posterior basic rhythm and its gradual rise from the theta into the alpha frequency band has been the object of numerous studies (Bernhard, 1939; Gibbs and Knott, 1949; Henry, 1944; Kellaway and Fox, 1952; Lindsley, 1938, 1939; Smith 1937, 1938, 1941). Further studies were prompted by the use of spectral analysis (Corbin and Bickford, 1955; Dumermuth, 1968; Kasamatsu et al., 1964; Scheffner, 1968).

It can be gleaned from these studies that the posterior basic rhythm frequency is subject to considerable variation in the second and third year of life. According to Lindsley (1939), a frequency range from 5 to almost 10/sec can be observed in the second year, whereas the data of Eeg-Olofsson (1971a) show a surprisingly high mean frequency of 8/sec at this age.

Eye blinks are associated with a biphasic (negative-positive) potential of medium to high voltage in bilateral synchrony over occipital areas (Westmoreland and Stockard, 1977).

The amount of *fast activity* (Garsche, 1956) varies considerably. Unusually pronounced activity in the 18 to 25/sec range in unmedicated children may reach abnormal degrees in the waking state as well as in sleep; such records perhaps

suggest mild forms of cerebral palsy (Gibbs and Gibbs, 1964).

Frequencies slower than the posterior basic rhythm are practically always noted in the waking state at this age, mostly in the 2 to 5/sec range and widely scattered. The amount of this activity is also quite variable. Crying children may show increasing slowing due to a hyperventilation effect (Dumermuth, 1972).

The reactivity of the waking EEG becomes more prominent; the blocking response of the posterior basic rhythm is more clearly demonstrable than in the first year. Mu rhythm over the rolandic region may be identifiable in the second year of life (Niedermeyer and Koshino, 1975). The photic driving response to the strobe light remains accentuated in the low-frequency range.

Drowsiness

Generalized high-voltage (mostly 4–6/sec) theta activity of marked rhythmicity is the hallmark of the drowsy state in early childhood. This pattern is most pronounced in the central and parietal leads; it is less impressive over the temporal areas and sometimes least developed over the occipital region. The rhythmicity may assume quite monotonous character; the in-phase character of the ubiquitous pattern makes it tempting to theorize about an enormously extended generator area (Fig. 11.12). This pattern is widely known as "hypnagogic theta activity."

Gibbs and Gibbs (1950) paid special attention to a variant of the rhythmical theta activity of drowsiness. In a large number of small children, bursts of 4 to 5/sec activity may be present instead of the steady rhythmical theta activity. This pattern extends into the fourth year of life and shows mild paroxysmal activity without representing a true abnormality. Occasionally, small sharp or spiky discharges may be interspersed between the theta waves; the electroencephalographer must refrain from calling these discharges epileptic or spike-wave complexes. Unless indubitable spikes are detectable, the presence of such small spiky potentials is harmless and does not represent definite abnormality. The mature form of drowsy EEG activity with dropout of the posterior basic rhythm and general decline of the voltage output is quite common at this age.

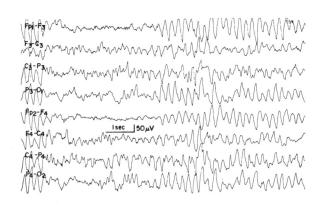

Figure 11.12. Patient age 3 years. Drowsiness. Rhythmical hypnagogic theta activity, 4–5/sec.

Figure 11.13. Patient age 9 months. Cerebral palsy, diplegic. Lack of posterior voltage maximum. Otherwise a normal record with sharp spindles of infancy.

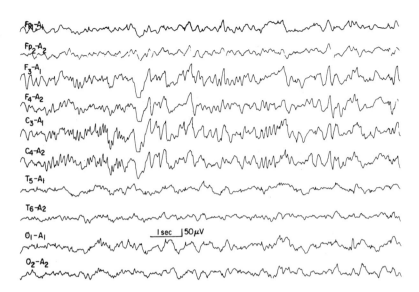

Sleep Record

The child falls into non-REM sleep and, with the usual length of a sleep recording in the EEG laboratory in daytime, REM stages are usually not observed. The hypnagogic theta hypersynchrony of drowsiness is supplanted by diffusely preponderant, irregular, high-voltage (1–3/sec and medium- to high-voltage 4–6/sec) activity. The maximum of amplitude is almost invariably found over the occipital area, where 0.75 to 2/sec waves may reach very high voltage (Fig. 11.8A). A different type of voltage distribution or even an anterior voltage maximum should warn the electroencephalographer; residual damage to the posterior regions is a good possibility, although none of the typical EEG abnormalities may be present (Fig. 11.13).

The varying degree of intermixed fast activity without premedication was mentioned earlier. *Spindle activity* in the 12 to 14/sec range is now found in a transitional stage; the shifting spindle runs over centroparietal areas with a negative spiky component are gradually replaced by symmetrical spindle activity with a maximum over vertex. A 14/sec spindle type appears first over the vertex; with deepening sleep (transition stage 2 to 3), spindles in the 12/sec range appear over frontal midline and upper frontal regions. Both types of spindles may be seen at the same time, but with the mentioned difference in spatial distribution.

Vertex waves, also known as "biparietal humps" (Gibbs and Gibbs, 1950), are quite prominent at this age; their amplitude is impressive, but their rise is not as abrupt and the configuration is not as sharp as in the ensuing period of life (age 4–12). This same is true for *K complexes,* which are abundantly noted in the stages of non-REM sleep.

Positive occipital sharp transients of sleep (occipital positive sharp activity, lambdoid activity) are absent or very poorly developed at this age.

REM sleep at this age is a rarely observed stage outside the specialized sleep laboratory; it starts to show signs of EEG desynchronization, but slow activity (mostly 2–5/sec, according to Cadilhac, 1975) is still preponderant (Fig. 11.14).

Unusual and Marginal Patterns in Sleep

Extreme spindles (Gibbs and Gibbs, 1962, 1964) represent an unusual variant of sleep spindle activity with high voltage, a wide frequency range (6–18/sec), and occasional paroxysmal traits. In a diminutive form, these spindles may even occur while the child is awake (coexisting with a posterior alpha rhythm) (Fig. 11.15).

According to Gibbs and Gibbs (1964), this pattern occurs in 0.05% of normal children, but the prevalence reaches 5% to 18% in children with mental retardation and/or cerebral palsy. This pattern is seen from age 1 to 12 years, with a peak at age 3; after age 12, the incidence falls to almost zero.

Following the original studies of Gibbs and Gibbs, there have been very few reports dealing with this pattern, which undoubtedly warrants greater attention. When clearly separable from typical spindle activity, extreme spindles might represent a mild abnormality.

The *fast spiky spindle variant* (Niedermeyer and Capute, 1967) is a very rare pattern (about one case in 2,000–3,000 EEGs of children). It consists of spindle-like activity in the range of 16 to 20/sec and may occur over a variety of areas (central, parietal, vertex, or midtemporal) in stage 2 or 3 of sleep. It is seen mainly in early childhood (around age 3) but also occurs in older children and adolescents. This discharge is usually seen in children with residual brain damage and probably indicates a mild abnormality.

The *14 and 6/sec positive spike discharge* is very uncommon before age 3 and will be discussed later.

Arousal from Sleep

Arousal from sleep is characterized by marked and prolonged activity of high-voltage 4 to 6/sec activity in all leads with some intermixed slower frequencies (Hess, 1964; Kellaway and Fox, 1952; Nekhorocheff, 1950). White and Tharp (1974) reported the observation of prolonged rhythmical sharp or spiky activity over the frontal areas in children between ages 2 and 12 years. According to these authors, this pattern was seen only in children with minimal cerebral dys-

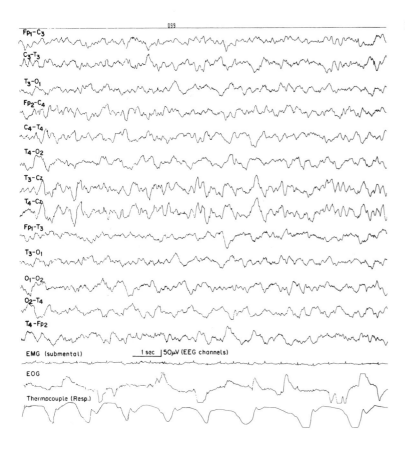

Figure 11.14. Patient age 22 months. REM sleep.

function. In the author's experience, this pattern has a very definite maximum over the frontal midline and is seen mainly from the second to the fourth year of life. Its mildly abnormal character is likely, but its clinical significance was thought to be debatable (Fig. 11.16).

Hughes has invalidated all doubts concerning the relationships of the "frontal arousal rhythm" to epileptic seizure

disorders. In a study of 50 cases (Hughes and Daaboul, 1999) epileptic seizures were present in 35 (70%) of the cases. Hughes (2003) also demonstrated a case in which the frontal arousal rhythm assumed ictal characteristics consisting of eyelid flutter and chewing.

Occurrence of Minor and Major Abnormalities in Early Childhood (Scarcity of Minor Abnormalities During the First 2 Years of Life)

When abnormalities are carefully and consistently graded as minimal, slight, moderate, marked, and severe, there is a statistically significant ($p < .001$) small number of minor (i.e., minimal, slight, and moderate) abnormalities prior to the age of 21 months. In other words, there is no real continuum of various forms of minor abnormalities between normal records on one side and markedly abnormal records on the other side (Niedermeyer and Yarworth, 1978). After the age of 21 months (approximately 2 years), minor abnormalities become much less scanty, and the aforementioned continuum of graded abnormalities is present.

One could theorize that there are but a limited number of EEG responses to cerebral impairment with lack of fine intermediate nuances of abnormality prior to the age of 21 months. It is, however, also possible that minor abnormalities are not so rare after all. The electroencephalographer may have to adopt new criteria of normalcy and abnormality for this early age. Recent progress in EEG neonatology has shown that classical signs of abnormality such as spikes, focal or diffuse slowing, or local voltage depression

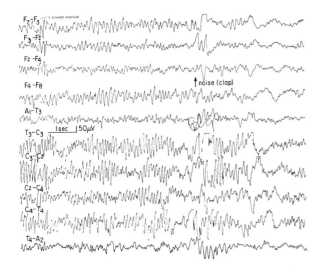

Figure 11.15. Patient age 22 months. Extreme spindles over central region; a somewhat slower type of spindles over frontal area.

Figure 11.16.   Patient age 16 months. Arousal from sleep. Pronounced rhythmical 6/sec activity with a sharp component, maximal over frontal midline.

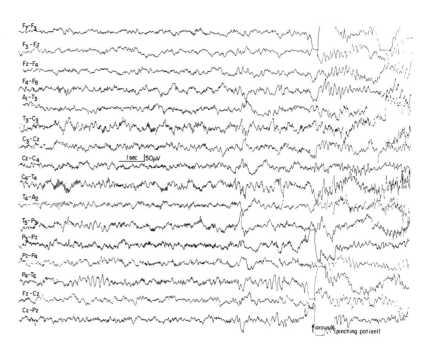

cannot serve as the only guideline; the sequences of sleep stages and their adequacy for the gestational age are important criteria for the newborn. It is possible that new valid criteria will evolve for infancy and early childhood; they might be, for instance, the voltage distribution of delta activity in sleep (lack of the posterior voltage maximum) (Slater and Torres, 1979; also see Fig. 11.13) or unorthodox features of sleep spindles. At this phase of ontogenetic evolution, there seems to be a period of limited eloquence of the EEG with a low yield for the referring clinician. From the data of Niedermeyer and Yarworth (1978), there is reason to presume that, with the presently used criteria, perinatal brain damage shows accompanying EEG abnormalities in the neonatal period, followed by a silent period with normal EEG findings yet ongoing clinical problems until the end of the second year of life, when EEG abnormalities tend to reappear.

Preschool Age EEG (3–5 Years)

Waking Record

At this age, it is much easier to obtain a waking record. With good handling by the technologist in the laboratory, many children prove to be quite cooperative. At age 3, the *posterior basic rhythm* has reached 8/sec and thus the alpha range. The alpha amplitude is almost always higher than in adolescence and adulthood. Leissner et al. (1970) have made attempts with ultrasound to correlate alpha voltage with thickness of the skull. The alpha voltage may reach 100 µV and tends to climb from age 3 to a peak at 8 or 9 years. Amplitudes are usually higher over the nondominant hemisphere (Petersén and Eeg-Olofsson, 1971).

The train of posterior alpha waves is frequently interrupted by intermingled slow waves, mostly in the range of 1.5 to 4/sec, extending from occipital into the posterior temporal and, less impressively, into the parietal regions. Alpha voltage, distribution, and admixture of slow activity create a picture that makes the tracing almost immediately identifiable as a record of childhood.

Posterior slowing may show a variety of forms. Most common is the irregularly interspersed type of slow activity. These slow waves are often preceded by a sharp contoured potential that blends together with the ensuing slow wave "slow fused transients" (Kellaway, 1957). The slowing is more often lateralized to the left hemisphere, according to Petersén and Eeg-Olofsson (1971); in the author's experience, however, lateralization to the right seems to be more common. Posterior slow activity can reach abnormal degrees, especially with towering amplitudes or abnormal rhythmicity such as prolonged trains of rhythmical slow waves. The differentiation of such abnormal forms from physiological posterior slow activity is usually not difficult.

In the *absence of posterior slow activity,* the posterior alpha rhythm in unbroken prolonged stretches assumes "mature" character. Eeg-Olofsson (1971b) and Petersén and Eeg-Olofsson (1971) list such tracings as "supernormal," which is a term comprehensible to every electroencephalographer, although it violates the rules of logical terminology. Such records suggest a hastened process of maturation, and a 5-year-old child may show the adult features of posterior alpha. Such an accelerated development (premature EEG maturation) may be associated with behavioral disturbances and subnormal intellectual development.

Anterior rhythmical 6 to 7/sec theta activity is not uncommonly found at preschool age but reaches its peak somewhat later. The clinical significance of this pattern is discussed in the next section.

Rolandic mu rhythm is clearly on the rise at this age before peaking early in the second decade of life.

At this age, *low-voltage records* with activity consistently below 25 to 30 µV are not seen as a variant of normalcy. Such tracings may be associated with states of cerebral palsy (Gibbs and Gibbs, 1964). *Excessively fast records* usually represent drug effect; otherwise, such records fall into the mildly to moderately abnormal range.

Activations

At the age of 4 years, children usually become very cooperative for *hyperventilation,* although one seldom finds a cooperative 3-year-old child. Four-year-olds seem to enjoy the test and are sometimes hard to stop.

Slow responses to hyperventilation can be very pronounced at this age and must be considered normal unless unequivocal epileptic discharges or marked asymmetries are found. Protracted slowing (either as rhythmical delta bursts or as continuous irregular delta-theta activity) after termination of hyperventilation usually indicates that the child continues overbreathing. In such cases, the effect of hypoglycemia must also be taken into consideration. (Check for last food intake; consider a rebound-type hypoglycemia after a breakfast consisting of carbohydrates.) Special studies in this field were done by Gibbs et al. (1943) and by Petersén and Eeg-Olofsson (1971).

The occipital driving response to *intermittent photic stimulation* is quite often slanted toward the lower part of the flicker frequency range; responses are most prominent below 8 flashes/sec (Petersén and Eeg-Olofsson, 1971). Paroxysmal responses to flicker (even in the normal child) are more likely to occur in school-age children.

Visser et al. (1982) investigated children at the age of 5 years with regard to their neurological condition at birth. EEG findings were found to be less significant than visual evoked potentials ("the more optimal the neurological condition at birth, the shorter the VEP peak latencies at the age of 5").

EEG Findings in Drowsiness

Past the age of 3 years, the aforementioned rhythmical high-voltage theta activity in the 4 to 6/sec range (hypnagogic theta) is bound to disappear; it is seldom seen in healthy children at age 6. Paroxysmal theta bursts are also on the decline. The admixture of posterior slow activity tends to increase in early drowsiness, and there is soon good evidence of enhanced delta and theta activity in all leads.

Anterior rhythmical 6 to 7/sec theta activity increases in early drowsiness but disappears in deep drowsiness. This pattern is more often encountered at school age and is discussed below.

The *14 and 6/sec positive spike discharge* manifests itself in deep drowsiness and vanishes in light sleep. This pattern is not too common at this age, and, for this reason, it will be discussed later.

Sleep EEG Records

The posterior maximum of diffusely predominant delta (1–3/sec) activity is not as pronounced as in infancy and early childhood. *Sleep spindles* have lost their sharp and bilaterally shifting feature of infancy and now show a well-defined maximum over the vertex. Frequencies around 14/sec are seen before more anterior spindles in the 10 to 12/sec range occur with deepening sleep.

Vertex waves and *K complexes* show a more prominent sharp component than in earlier years.

Positive occipital sharp transients of sleep (lambdoid activity) are absent or very poorly delineated at this age.

REM sleep is rarely recorded under regular laboratory conditions. The EEG shows little desynchronization at this age.

EEG in Older Children (6–12 Years)

General Considerations

At this age, one is usually dealing with fairly cooperative children, leaving aside marginal cases of hyperactivity or borderline intelligence. Complete records with a resting awake portion, hyperventilation, intermittent photic stimulation, and sleep are easily obtained.

This is a particularly well-explored age range because relatively large numbers of healthy children can be secured for such investigations from schools. The studies of Henry (1944), Gibbs and Knott (1949), Kellaway and Fox (1952), Gibbs and Gibbs (1964), and Netchine (1969) have dealt with in excess of 500 children. The most authoritative study in this field was carried out in Göteborg, Sweden, by Eeg-Olofsson (1971a) and Petersén and Eeg-Olofsson (1971) (also see Petersén et al., 1975). To secure a population of truly healthy children, a remarkable set of strict criteria was used, with the rejection of those with even minute signs of neurological, autonomic, and psychological dysfunction.

Waking Record

The *posterior alpha rhythm* gradually reaches a mean frequency of around 10/sec, which equals the mean frequency of the mature EEG of adulthood. This point is reached around the age of 10 years. In the work of Petersén and Eeg-Olofsson (1971), the mean value of 9/sec was reached at age 7 and 10/sec at 15 years. Interestingly, girls showed a statistically significant faster acceleration of the posterior alpha frequency than boys. These authors reported an increase of the alpha amplitude during early childhood until a peak was reached at age 6 to 9 years, with subsequent gradual decline. There was no sex difference. The alpha amplitude was determined by a bipolar occipitotemporal array, and a mean of 56 µV was found; such precise figures are completely dependent on the selection of electrodes and interelectrode distance.

The posterior alpha rhythm is usually of higher amplitude over the nondominant hemisphere and thus larger on the right side. According to Petersén and Eeg-Olofsson (1971), these asymmetries seldom exceed 20 µV. These authors were also unable to correlate alpha asymmetries with handedness.

Although the mature alpha frequency of 10/sec may be reached at age 10 or at least at age 15, there is still a considerable admixture of posterior slow activity interspersed between trains of alpha waves. The maturational process of the second decade of life is thus characterized by the gradual

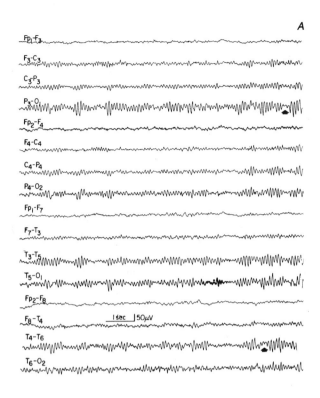

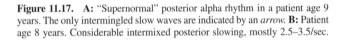

Figure 11.17. **A:** "Supernormal" posterior alpha rhythm in a patient age 9 years. The only intermingled slow waves are indicated by an *arrow.* **B:** Patient age 8 years. Considerable intermixed posterior slowing, mostly 2.5–3.5/sec. Slow waves often preceded by a sharp contoured large alpha wave (fused forms). Record is within normal limits of variability for age.

riddance of the intermixed posterior slow activity, excluding a few other minor changes in EEG evolution (Fig. 11.17).

Posterior slow activity is still quite prominent between age 6 and 12 years; "slow fused transients" (Kellaway et al., 1959) with sharp transients preceding single large slow waves are quite common. In addition to the common type of posterior slowing as randomly intermixed slow potentials, there are also other and more rhythmical forms of posterior slow activity.

Forms of *posterior slow activity* are broken down into arrhythmical and rhythmical slowing. This type of subdivision is also valid for adolescence and adulthood, although certain forms of posterior slowing are more common in children and others in adults. This subject has been extensively studied and discussed by Aird and Gastaut (1959); Gastaut et al. (1967); Petersén et al. (1975); and Kuhlo (1976).

In the age range from 6 to 12 years, the arrhythmical type of "slow, posterior waves found predominantly in youth" (Aird and Gastaut, 1959) is most commonly encountered. This pattern has been defined as consisting of waves in the delta and theta range, of variable form, lasting 0.35 to 0.5 second or longer without any consistent periodicity. Alpha waves are almost always intermingled or superimposed.

Among the rhythmical forms, the slow alpha variant represents a subharmonic of the alpha frequency (mostly 4 to 5/sec), often with intermixed alpha waves. In a neurologi-

cally normal 10-year-old girl, unilateral alpha subharmonics (left side, 4.5/sec) were noted (Attarian et al., 2001). Forms of pronounced rhythmical high-voltage 3 to 4/sec activity over occipital areas and adjacent regions are not uncommon at this age; these waves are often sharply contoured, and the moderately paroxysmal character of these slow runs places this activity into the mildly abnormal range. According to the extensive world of Kuhlo et al. (1969), the 4 to 5/sec rhythm, which is a special entity of posterior slowing, is not demonstrable during the first decade; it will be discussed later. Very rhythmical high voltage 3 to 4/sec waves may occur in prolonged runs in children with petit mal absences; this pattern is clearly abnormal and its significance is discussed in Chapter 27, "Epileptic Seizure Disorders."

In the discussion of the EEG frequencies in the initial part of Chapter 9, "The Normal EEG of the Waking Adult," other posterior slow rhythms were mentioned (including "pi" and "phi" rhythms) with little significance regarding the EEG maturation.

Fast activity usually does not play a major role at this age. According to Garsche (1956), beta frequencies are found in about 25% of the records, and there is little difference between younger and older children.

Rolandic mu rhythm is steadily on the rise until a peak reached between ages 11 and 15 years (Niedermeyer and

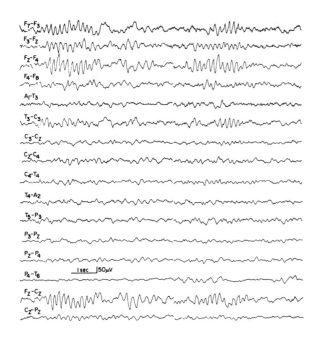

Figure 11.18. Rhythmical 6–7/sec activity over frontal midline and vicinity in a 12-year-old child.

Koshino, 1975). Occipital *lambda waves* are demonstrated more easily in older than in younger children but still lack the crisp and unmistakable contour of adulthood.

The prevalence of *anterior rhythmical 6 to 7/sec theta activity* picks up between ages 6 and 12 years before reaching a peak at age 13 to 15 (Palmer et al., 1976). These authors consider this pattern not an abnormality as such, but "of clinical interest because of its epileptological implications" (Fig. 11.18).

This view differs from the opinion of Petersén et al. (1975), who found a relatively high prevalence of anterior theta rhythm in healthy young individuals (21%). This figure is much larger than that of Palmer et al. (1976), who found up to 4%. Interestingly, Petersén et al. (1975) found a sex difference in the occurrence of this rhythm, with 24.9% in boys and 16.5% in girls.

More about the 6 to 7/sec theta rhythm and its presumed relationship to thinking is found in Chapter 9, "The Normal EEG of the Waking Adult."

A *4 to 6/sec theta rhythm* in children with predisposition to primary generalized epilepsy (spike-wave absences, etc.) has been described by Doose et al. (1968, 1972, 1973). This activity was seen mainly below age 8 years and was common in seizure-free siblings of children with petit mal absences. The predominantly centroparietal theta activity is considered abnormal (after careful differentiation from physiological activity and drowsiness).

Low-voltage records as a variant of normalcy are very rare at this age. Petersén and Eeg-Olofsson (1971) did not find a single case in their series. Schauseil-Zipf et al. (1984) reassessed the EEG at the age of 7 to 12 years in children who were regarded as "small-for-date" babies. Out of a total of 56 children, the EEG was normal in 36 and slightly to moderately abnormal in the remaining cases.

Activations

Hyperventilation shows particularly pronounced slowing of high voltage at this age. The slowing may start over posterior areas and gradually become diffuse with a frontal maximum; rhythmical slow activity usually ranges from 1.5 to 4/sec. A variety of responses has been reported by Daute et al. (1968) (with concomitant evaluation of pH and pCO_2 changes) and by Petersén and Eeg-Olofsson (1971). The normal character of the rhythmical and arrhythmical slow responses cannot be overemphasized (see Activations [Adolescents], below, for more details).

Intermittent photic stimulation shows a more mature type of occipital driving response, less prominent at low flash rates and more impressive in the medium range (6–16/sec). The work of Herrlin (1954), Doose et al. (1969), and Petersén and Eeg-Olofsson (1971) has been essential in the investigation of these responses. Further detailed information will be found in Chapters 15 and 28, "Brain Tumors and Other Space-Occupying Lesions" and "Nonepileptic Attacks," dealing with activation of the EEG and with epileptic seizure disorders.

Drowsiness

Drowsiness is characterized, at this age, by increasing theta and delta frequencies along with gradually fading posterior rhythmical alpha activity. The mature type of onset of drowsiness with gradual alpha dropout and mixed low-voltage slow and fast activity usually does not materialize in the first decade and slowly makes its appearance with early adolescence. On the other hand, the massive rhythmical theta activity of drowsiness (hypnagogic theta activity) seen in early childhood usually disappears around the age of 6 years.

Sleep

Under regular EEG laboratory conditions (leaving aside nocturnal or all-day sleep studies), non-REM sleep in its various stages is almost exclusively found unless the recording is prolonged to 1 hour or more.

Prior to the appearance of the first spindle trains, *vertex waves* are noted (transition from stage 1 to 2). These vertex waves are of remarkably high voltage and their sharp character may be poignant. These potentials are also known as "biparietal humps" because, in the montages of Gibbs and Gibbs (1950), there is a maximum over the parietal region, while neither vertex nor strictly central-rolandic electrodes are used (Fig. 11.19).

In school-age children, vertex waves may show moderate (seldom considerable) voltage asymmetries with asymmetrical spread into the vicinity. Under these circumstances, the physiological vertex activity may be confused with cerebral (rolandic) spikes; with greater experience, however, such errors can be avoided. The distinction between vertex waves and rolandic spikes, usually picked up by electrodes C_3 or C_4 over central areas, may occasionally arise from the vertex itself. When such a coexistence of vertex potentials exists, the physiological vertex waves are usually of longer duration and of somewhat higher voltage than the abnormal spikes (see also Chapter 13, Fig. 13.2).

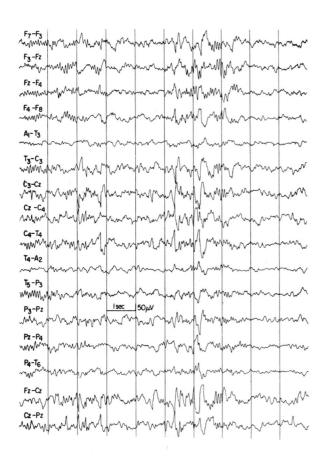

Figure 11.19. Patient age 10 years, non-REM sleep stage 2. Well-developed spindles, vertex waves, and K complexes.

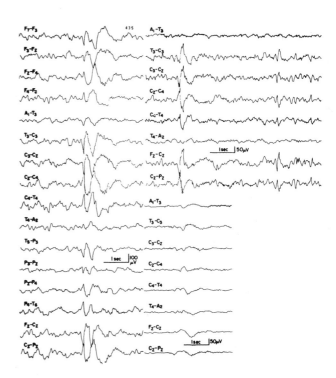

Figure 11.20. Evolutional and involutional phases of the K complex. *Left tracing,* patient age 5 years. Prominent initiating sharp component. *Upper right tracing,* patient age 8 years. Note very pronounced sharp component of K complex. *Far right,* a single vertex wave is shown. *Lower right,* patient age 47 years. K complex of moderate voltage; the initiating sharp component is markedly blunted. The slow component is inconspicuous; superimposed spindles are barely visible. This decline in the K complex suggests some cerebral pathology.

Prior to onset of stage 2 (light sleep), *positive occipital sharp transients of sleep* may already be noticeable. This pattern, however, is less common and less prominent in children than in adolescents and adults. A more detailed discussion is presented in the section dealing with the sleep EEG in general (see Sleep, below).

Sleep spindles show the features of maturity, with a well-defined vertex maximum. Its initial frequency of 14/sec or 12 to 14/sec may slow down to 10 to 12/sec with deepening sleep; the superior frontal electrodes (F_3, F_4) may show the spindles somewhat better than the central electrodes (C_3, C_4). The very maximum of spindle activity remains over the midline; a vertex maximum may or may not be replaced by a maximum over frontal midline (F_z) with deepening sleep (transition from stage 2 to 3). The spindle trains are usually shorter than 1 second. The waves are rounded; the physiological negative spiky spindle character has disappeared much earlier (age 2) (Fig. 11.19).

K complexes are often seen in association with spindles. The complex wave morphology of this pattern is extensively discussed in conjunction with sleep in general and again in Chapter 27, "Epileptic Seizure Disorders." K complexes and vertex waves represent fascinating responses to intrinsic or extrinsic stimuli; their neurophysiological substrate and clinical implications require more extensive discussion (Fig. 11.20).

REM sleep (rarely seen in a regular EEG laboratory) shows less slow activity and increasing desynchronization with mixed activities in the theta, alpha, and beta frequency range.

Arousal from sleep is characterized by an increasingly shorter transition from sleep to the waking state and decreasing length of high-voltage theta activity.

Patterns of Marginal and Possibly Abnormal Character in Drowsiness and Sleep

The 14 and 6/sec positive spike discharge is a common finding at this age. The sections on the sleep EEG and on abnormal (epileptic) patterns in the EEG discuss more extensively this type of activity, which was widely considered a genuine abnormality after the first report of Gibbs and Gibbs (1951). During the past 10 to 15 years, there has been accumulating evidence that this pattern is just marginally deviant but not categorically abnormal unless it appears in enormous abundance.

The *psychomotor variant* pattern (Gibbs et al., 1963; Gibbs and Gibbs, 1964) is predominantly seen in adolescents and young adults, but it is not uncommon in older children. It is usually associated with more serious behavioral or clinical problems, including occasional cases of proven epileptic seizure disorder; for this reason, one is inclined to regard this pattern as a mild abnormality. The wave morphology of this discharge is presented in other sections. The psychomotor variant occurs almost exclusively in very light drowsiness and disappears with deepening level of awareness.

EEG in Adolescents (13–20 Years)

General Considerations

The transition from the last years of childhood to puberty may be a major step in the biological and psychological development of the individual; EEG maturation, however, shows no dramatic changes in these years. In other words, there are no striking differences between the record of a healthy teenager and a healthy older child. Nevertheless, it is worthwhile to discuss these two age groups separately in view of a number of subtle changes.

Eeg-Olofsson (1971b) carried out a special study of the EEG development of normal adolescents and selected 185 persons from ages 16 to 21 years, according to the same strict principles by which these authors were guided in their aforementioned investigation of the childhood EEG. Earlier studies mostly dealt with mixed material comprising either adolescents and children (Brandt et al., 1961; Gibbs and Knott, 1949) or adolescents and adults (Lindsley, 1936, 1938; Matousek et al., 1967; Mundy-Castle, 1951, 1953; Picard, 1957; Roth et al., 1967; Selldén, 1964; Simonova et al., 1967; Vogel and Fujiya, 1969; Williams, 1941).

Waking Record

The *posterior alpha rhythm* shows a mean frequency around 10/sec; according to Petersén and Eeg-Olofsson (1971), the mean frequency lies at 10.2/sec in the male and 10.3/sec in the female. The entire alpha range, as reported by Petersén and Eeg-Olofsson, stretches from 8 to 12/sec; these authors observed a case of 8/sec alpha rhythm in a healthy 17-year-old boy (this would raise the suspicion of a minimal abnormality, in the opinion of some electroencephalographers). With the use of frequency analysis, Samson-Dollfus and Goldberg (1979) found mean alpha frequencies from 9.64 to 9.94/sec in subjects at age 15.

The posterior alpha rhythm is of moderately higher amplitude than in adulthood, but a slight decline from the height of alpha waves in childhood is noticeable. Alpha waves may show a negative sharp component (classically present in mu rhythm) that is due to a hidden or overt admixture of fast activity. Such sharp alpha waves are common in older children, adolescents, and young adults; this pattern is perfectly normal, a fact already stressed by Gibbs and Gibbs (1950). Amplitude asymmetries are practically the rule, and the voltage is usually somewhat higher on the right side but, according to Petersén and Eeg-Olofsson (1971), the difference seldom exceeds 20% of the greater amplitude.

The admixture of *posterior slow activity* constantly diminishes during the period of adolescence. In general, the amount of intermixed delta-theta activity (between alpha waves) lies around 10% to 15%; slightly or moderately higher figures are still acceptable as compatible with normalcy. Healthy adolescents' slow frequencies may show a wider distribution and their peak over the posterior regions is not quite as impressive as in older children. "Slow fused transients" (Kellaway et al., 1959) are not necessarily normal at this age.

A special form of posterior slow activity is the *posterior 4 to 5/sec rhythm* (Fig. 11.21), which probably constitutes a mild abnormality. This pattern is uncommon; probably one case was found in 1,000 or 2,000 tracings in the intake of a

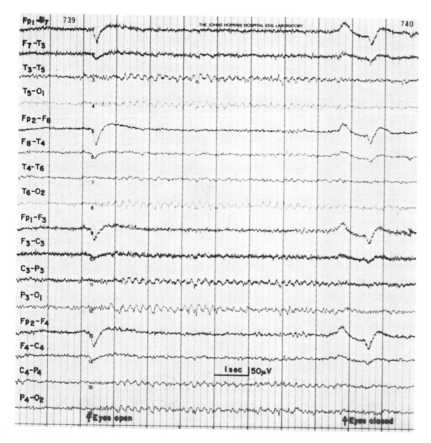

Figure 11.21. Patient age 21 years. An example of the 4–5/sec rhythm over the posterior region. Note that eye closure is followed by a few 12–13/sec alpha waves before a prominent posterior 4.5–5/sec rhythm emerges. This rhythm apparently vanishes shortly before eye opening. The record was otherwise normal. The patient was referred because of suspected psychogenic seizures.

large central EEG laboratory. The mean age at first examination was 24.15 years (Kuhlo et al., 1969), which indicates that this is a pattern of adolescence and young adulthood. Earlier descriptions of this type of activity were given by Nayrac and Beaussart (1956), Pitot and Gastaut (1956), Vallat and Lepetit (1957), Aird and Gastaut (1959), Vogel and Götze (1959), and Petersén and Sörbye (1962). More extensive investigations were subsequently carried out by Kuhlo (1967), Kuhlo et al. (1968, 1969), and Fröscher (1979). Acquired cerebral pathology (especially craniocerebral trauma), as well as genetic predisposition (Kuhlo et al., 1969), may play a determining role.

Another form of rhythmical posterior slow activity consists of *rhythmical 3 to 4/sec waves of high voltage over the occipital region* and its immediate vicinity. This pattern is brought on by eye closure after a latency period of 300 to 500 msec and lasts for about 1.5 to 3 seconds. This type of posterior slowing has been investigated by Belsh et al. (1983). These authors found this pattern only in children and adolescents from age 6 to 16 years. There is no doubt that this type of posterior rhythmical slowing represents a special entity. The rhythmical 3 to 4/sec waves exhibit a more or less obvious sharp component. This pattern occurs in children and juveniles with or without epileptic seizure disorder; one must agree with Belsh et al., who think that "such a discharge should not be interpreted as epileptiform activity." This pattern is also know as "phi rhythm" (Silbert et al., 1995).

Fast activity is more widely seen in adolescents than in older children. The maximum fast activity is most commonly found over the frontal areas. Well-defined and circumscript beta waves over the rolandic regions are seen, usually in conjunction with central mu rhythm.

The *rolandic mu rhythm* is fairly common in adolescents and gradually declines from a peak reached between ages 11 and 15 years (Niedermeyer and Koshino, 1975). *Occipital lambda waves* show their typical mature configuration. *Anterior rhythmical 6 to 7/sec theta activity* is gradually falling from its peak prevalence (age 13 to 15; see Fig. 11.21). A rare phenomenon is rhythmical 4/sec activity over the vertex ("*4/sec vertex spindles*") described by Van Huffelen and Magnus (1973); this occurs in the waking state only, mostly in adolescents, and especially in patients with vasomotor instability, such as syncope.

Low-voltage records, very rare in childhood, are more common in adolescents and may occur in about 5% of patients; these records are usually dominated by beta frequencies. This type of low-voltage fast record has been found more often in females (Mundy-Castle, 1951; Petersén and Eeg-Olofsson, 1971; Vogel and Fujiya, 1969; Vogel and Götze, 1962). Vogel (1962) investigated the role of predisposing genetic factors. In spite of hereditary predisposition, the fact remains that such low-voltage tracings do not manifest themselves until a certain age around puberty. In healthy adults, the prevalence of low-voltage records increases to 11.6% (Gibbs and Gibbs, 1950).

Activations

Hyperventilation does not yield spectacularly slow responses to the same extent as in children. Marked bilateral synchronous delta activity was found in 22% of the healthy adolescents studied by Petersén and Eeg-Olofsson (1971). It must be kept in mind, however, that hyperventilation is a poorly standardized procedure in which the intangibles of motivation and effort play a paramount role.

Intermittent photic stimulation shows essentially the mature type with a peak driving response in the medium and fast rate of flicker (mostly 6–20/sec). In adolescents, the predisposition to *paroxysmal flicker responses* must not be underrated; such responses of the photomyoclonic as well as of the photoconvulsive type (Bickford et al., 1952; also see Chapters 15 and 28, "Brain Tumors and Other Space-Occupying Lesions" and "Nonepileptic Attacks," dealing with activations and with epileptic seizure disorders, respectively) may occasionally occur in apparently healthy individuals. Further investigation of such persons sometimes unearths signs of mental, emotional, and autonomic nervous system instabilities.

Drowsiness

The transition from wakefulness to sleep (stage 1) shows, in general, the mature adult type with gradual alpha dropout and long stretches of a diffuse low-voltage pattern with mixed slow and fast activity. With deepening drowsiness, vertex waves appear, and positive occipital sharp transients of sleep may be present.

Sleep

In the commonly observed non-REM sleep onset tracings in regular EEG laboratories, there is little difference from the activity found in adults. The voltage of sleep spindles is somewhat greater than in adulthood, and this is also generally true for this amplitude of vertex waves and K complexes. Their sharp component is not quite as sharp as in older children. Positive occipital transients of sleep may be abundant in stage 2. REM sleep also shows the mature type in most cases. Arousal from sleep shows the mature type with very rapid transition from sleep patterns to waking activity.

Marginal Patterns

The *14 and 6/sec positive spike discharge* is not uncommon at this age. Incidence starts to show the first signs of decline; this is supported by the figures of Gibbs and Gibbs (1964) (15.8% at age 5–9, 20.8% at 10–14, and 1.65% at 15–19; there is marked further decline to 8.75% between ages 20 and 24 and 1.4% between 25 and 29). Similar data have been presented by Eeg-Olofsson (1971a). Deep drowsiness and light sleep facilitate this pattern, which is most prominent over the posterior temporal and occipital regions.

The *6/sec spike-wave complex* is occasionally seen in adolescents; Gibbs and Gibbs (1964) found this pattern in 2.8% of their 3,476 control subjects, a higher figure than at any other age. This pattern, however, already exceeds the boundaries of marginal activities and clearly belongs in the domain of mild to moderate abnormalities. It is discussed in Chapter 14 with epileptic seizure discharges.

The *psychomotor variant* pattern is much less common and reaches a slight peak at age 15 to 19 (0.4%), according to Gibbs and Gibbs (1964).

EEG in Young Adults (21–30 Years)

In subjects at the age when geniuses such as the composers Wolfgang Amadeus Mozart and Franz Schubert and the physicists and mathematicians Albert Einstein and Max Planck had reached the pinnacle of their creative work, the EEG often still shows lingering mild signs of immaturity.

These signs are limited to the posterior waking activity, which shows mild to moderate amounts of intermingled 1.5 to 3/sec and 4 to 7/sec waves that should not exceed medium voltage. This type of posterior slowing is normally not seen past age 30. Signs of psychological immaturity may or may not be present. As is true for the earlier segments of ontogenetic evolution, the EEG provides some insight into concepts of psychological immaturity but has failed to provide firm correlations.

Concluding Statements

This chapter provided a condensed description of the EEG maturation from birth through young adulthood. The basic rules of this process are not engraved in stone and must be viewed with a certain degree of flexibility. It is strongly recommended that terms such as *within broad (very broad) normal limits of variability for age* be used in mildly deviant but not definitely abnormal tracings, rather than making rigid distinctions between the "normal" and "abnormal" character of a given record.

The "clinician within ourselves" will demand statements concerning the clinical significance of mild deviations or definite abnormalities in the maturational process. The question has often been raised as to whether a child with above-average posterior slowing may show perceptive-cognitive deficits ("soft neurological signs") with possible reading and learning difficulties or the wide gamut of behavioral deviations (chiefly hyperkinetic behavior). The aforementioned marginal patterns, either within broad normal limits, such as the 14 and 6/sec positive spike discharge, or mildly abnormal, such as psychomotor variant and 6/sec spike-wave discharges, must be interpreted in a prudent and circumspect manner. In some cases, early jubilation over the discovery of such patterns and possible links between brain and psyche has done more harm than good to the field of electroencephalography.

It is also very difficult to make a firm and solidly founded statement as to whether deviations from the rules of EEG maturation (for instance, excessive posterior slowing at a given age) are simply a sign of immaturity or a sign of possible sustained structural insult to the brain.

References

Aird, R.B., and Gastaut, Y. 1959. Occipital and posterior electroencephalographic rhythm. Electroencephalogr. Clin. Neurophysiol. 11:637–656.

Anderson, C.M., Torres, F., and Faoro, A. 1985. The EEG of the early premature. Electroencephalogr. Clin. Neurophysiol. 60:95–105.

Arfel-Capdevielle, G. 1950. *Activité électrique cérébrale due nouveauné.* Thesis in Medicine, University of Paris.

Attarian, H.P., Pacquiao, P.A., and Erickson, S.M. 2001. Unilateral alpha subharmonics: a case report. Clin. Electroencephalogr. 32:32–35.

Belsh, J.M., Chokroverty, S., and Barabas, G. 1983. Posterior rhythmic slow activity in EEG after eye closure. Electroencephalogr. Clin. Neurophysiol. 56:562–568.

Benda, C.I., Engel, R.C.H., and Zhang, Y. 1989. Prolonged inactive phases during the discontinuous pattern of prematurity in the electroencephalogram of very-low-birthweight infants. Electroencephalogr. Clin. Neurophysiol. 72:189–197.

Benninger, C., Matthis, P., and Scheffner, D. 1984. EEG development of healthy boys and girls. Results from a longitudinal study. Electroencephalogr. Clin. Neurophysiol. 57:1–12.

Berger, H. 1932. Über das Elektroenzephalogramm des Menschen. 5. Mittlg. Arch. Psychiatr. Nervenkr. 98:231–254. [English translation: Gloor, P. 1969. Hans Berger. *On the Electroencephalogram of Man.* Amsterdam: Elsevier (see pp. 157–160).]

Bergström, R.M. 1969. Electrical parameters of the brain during ontogeny. In *Brain and Early Behavior.* Ed. R.J. Robinson, pp. 15–37. London: Academic Press.

Bernhard, C.G. 1939. Recherches sur la fréquence alpha de l'électroencéphalogramme chez l'enfant. Acta Psychiatr. (Kbh.) 14:223–231.

Biagioni, E., Boldrini, A., Bottone, U., et al. 1996. Prognostic value of abnormal EEG transients in preterm and full-term neonates. Electroencephalogr. Clin. Neurophysiol. 99:1–9.

Bickford, R.G., Sem-Jacobsen, C.W., White, P.C., et al. 1952. Some observations of the mechanisms of photic and photo-metrazol activation. Electroencephalogr. Clin. Neurophysiol. 4:275–282.

Blume, W.T., and Dreyfus-Brisac, C. 1982. Positive rolandic sharp waves in neonatal EEG: types and significance. Electroencephalogr. Clin. Neurophysiol. 53:277–282.

Brandt, H., Brandt, S., and Vollmund, K. 1961. EEG response to photic stimulation in 120 normal children. Epilepsia (Amsterdam) 2:313–317.

Brante, C. 1949. Studies on lipids in the nervous system. Acta Physiol. Scand. 18(suppl.):63.

Cadilhac, J. 1975. Ontogenesis and phylogenesis of sleep. In *Handbook of Electroencephalography and Clinical Neurophysiology,* Vol. 7A, Ed.-in-chief, A. Remond, Ed. P. Passouant, pp. 18–25. Amsterdam: Elsevier.

Caveness, W.F. 1962. *Atlas of EEG in the Developing Monkey (Macaca mulatta).* Reading, MA: Addison-Wesley.

Challamel, M.J., Isnard, H., Brunon, A.M., et al. 1984. Transient EEG asymmetry during quiet sleep. Electroencephalogr. Clin. Neurophysiol. 57:49P(abst).

Chavance, M., and Samson-Dollfus, D. 1978. Analyse spectrale de l'EEG de l'enfant normal entre 6 et 16 ans: Choix et validation des paramètres les plus informationnels. Electroencephalogr. Clin. Neurophysiol. 45:767–776.

Clancy, R.N., and Tharp, B.R. 1984. Positive rolandic sharp waves in the electroencephalograms of premature neonates with intraventricular hemorrhage. Electroencephalogr. Clin. Neurophysiol. 57:395–404.

Clancy, R.R., Tharp, B.R., and Enzman, D. 1984. EEG in premature infants with intraventricular hemorrhage. Neurology 34:583–590.

Clancy, R.R., Chung, H.J., and Temple, J.P. 1993. *Atlas of electroencephalography.* Vol. 1. *Neonatal Electroencephalography.* Amsterdam: Elsevier.

Colon, E.J., de Weerd, J.P.C., Notermans, S.L.H., et al. 1979. EEG spectra in children aged 8, 9, and 10 years. J. Neurol. 221:263–268.

Corbin, H.P.F., and Bickford, R.G. 1955. Studies of the electroencephalogram of normal children: comparison of visual and automatic frequency analysis. Electroencephalogr. Clin. Neurophysiol. 7:15–28.

Curzi-Dascalova, L., Monod, N., Guidasci, S., et al. 1981. Waking-sleeping transition in the newborn baby and in infants before the age of 3 months. Electroencephalogr. Clin. Neurophysiol. 52:57P(abst).

Daute, K.H., Frenzel, J., and Klust, E. 1968. Über den unspezifischen Hyperventilationseffekt im EEG des gesunden Kindes. I. Stärkegrad, Z. Kinderheilkd. 104:197–207.

De Weerd, A.W. 1995. *Atlas of EEG in the First Months of Life.* Amsterdam: Elsevier.

Dittrichova, J., Paul, K., and Pavlikova, E. 1972. Rapid eye movements in paradoxical sleep in infants. Neuropaediatrie 3:248–257.

Doose, H., Gerken, H., Horstmann, T., et al. 1968. Genetics of centrencephalic epilepsy in childhood. Epilepsia (Amsterdam) 9:107–115.

Doose, H., Gerken, H., Hien-Volpel, K.I.F., et al. 1969. Genetics of photosensitive epilepsy. Neuropaediatrie 1:56–73.

Doose, H., Gerken, H., Horstmann, T., et al. 1972. On the genetics of EEG anomalies in childhood. I. Abnormal theta rhythms. Neuropaediatrie 3:386–401.

Doose, H., Gerken, H., Horstmann, T., et al. 1973. Genetic factors in spike-wave absences. Epilepsia (Amsterdam) 14:57–75.

Dreyfus-Brisac, C. 1964. The electroencephalogram of the premature infant and full-term newborn. Normal and abnormal development of waking and sleeping patterns. In *Neurological and Electroencephalographic Correlative Studies in Infancy,* Eds. P. Kellaway and I. Petersén, pp. 186–207. New York: Grune & Stratton.

Dreyfus-Brisac, C. 1979. Neonatal electroencephalography. In *Reviews of Perinatal Medicine,* Eds. E.M. Scarpelli and V. Cosmi, pp. 379–483. New York: Raven Press.

Dreyfus, C., and Curzi-Dascalova, L. 1975. The EEG during the first year of life. In *Handbook of Electroencephalography and Clinical Neurophysiology,* vol. 6B, Ed.-in-chief, A. Remond, pp. 24–30. Amsterdam: Elsevier.

Dreyfus-Brisac, C., and Monod, N. 1964. Sleep of premature and full-term newborns. Polygraphic study. Proc. R. Soc. Med. 58:6–7.

Dreyfus-Brisac, C., and Monod, N. 1975. Electroencephalogram of full-term newborns and premature infants. In *Handbook of Electroencephalography and Clinical Neurophysiology,* vol. 6B, Ed.-in-chief, A. Remond, Ed. G.C. Lairy, pp. 6–23. Amsterdam: Elsevier.

Dumermuth, G. 1968. Variance spectra of electroencephalograms in twins. In *Clinical Electroencephalography in Children,* Eds. P. Kellaway and I. Petersén, pp. 119–154. New York: Grune & Stratton (Stockholm: Almqvist & Wiksell).

Dumermuth, G. 1972. *Elektroencephalographie im Kindesalter.* Stuttgart: Thieme.

Eeg-Olofsson, O. 1971a. The development of the EEG in normal children from age 1 to 15 years. The 14 and 6 Hz positive spike phenomenon. Neuropaediatrie 4:405–427.

Eeg-Olofsson, O. 1971b. The development of the electroencephalogram in normal adolescents from the age of 16 through 21 years. Neuropaediatrie 3:11–45.

Eeg-Olofsson, O., Petersén, I., and Selldén, U. 1971. The development of the electroencephalogram in normal children from the age of 1 through 15 years. Paroxysmal activity. Neuropaediatrie 2:375–404.

Ellingson, R.J. 1979. EEGs of premature and full-term newborns. In *Current Practice of Electroencephalography,* Eds. D.W. Klass and D.D. Daly, pp. 149–177. New York: Raven Press.

Ellingson, R.J., and Lindsley, D.B. 1949. Brain waves and cortical development in newborns and young infants. Am. Psychol. 4:248–249.

Ellingson, R.J., Dutch, S.J., and McIntire, M.S. 1974. EEGs of prematures: 3–8 year follow-up study. Dev. Psychobiol. 7:529–538.

Ellingson, R.J., Peters, J.F., and Nelson, B. 1982. Respiratory pauses and apnea during daytime sleep in normal infants during the first year of life: Longitudinal observations. Electroencephalogr. Clin. Neurophysiol. 53:48–59.

Engel, R. 1964. Abnormal electroencephalograms in the newborn period and their significance. Am. J. Ment. Deficiency 69:341–346.

Engel, R. 1975. *Abnormal Electroencephalograms in the Neonatal Period.* Springfield, IL: Charles C Thomas.

Flechsig, P. 1920. *Anatomie des menschlichen Gehirns und Rückenmarks auf myelogenetischer Grundlage.* Leipzig.

Fois, A. 1961. *The Electroencephalogram of the Normal Child.* Springfield, IL: Charles C Thomas.

Fröscher, W. 1979. Die okzipitale Grundrhythmusvariante und ihre Differentialdiagnose (4 ± 1/sec Grundrhythmusvariante). Z. EEG-EMG 10: 25–30.

Garsche, R. 1953. Grundzüge des normalen Elektroenzephalogramms im Kindesalter. Klin. Wochenschr. 31:118–123.

Garsche, R. 1956. Die Beta-Aktivität im EEG des Kindes. I. Mitteilung. Erscheinungsformen bei gesunden Kindern. Z. Kinderheilkd. 78:441–475.

Gasser, T., Mocks, J., and Bacher, P. 1983. Topographic factor analysis of the EEG with applications to development and mental retardation. Electroencephalogr. Clin. Neurophysiol. 55:445–463.

Gasser, T., Verleger, R., Bacher, P., et al. 1988a. Development of the EEG of school-age children and adolescents. I. Analysis of band power. Electroencephalogr. Clin. Neurophysiol. 69:91–99.

Gasser, T., Jennen-Steinmetz, C., Sroka, L., et al. 1988b. Development of the EEG of school-age children and adolescents. II. Topography. Electroencephalogr. Clin. Neurophysiol. 69:100–109.

Gastaut, H.J., Bostem, F., Waltrégny, A., et al. (Eds.). 1967. Les activités électriques cérébrales spontanées enregistrées sur la partie postérieure du scalp chez l'homme. In *Les Activités Électriques Cérébrales Spontanées et Évoquées chez l'Homme,* pp. 133–226. Paris: Gauthier-Villars.

Gibbs, E.L., and Gibbs, F.A. 1951. Electroencephalographic evidence of thalamic and hypothalamic epilepsy. Neurology (Minneapolis) 1:136–144.

Gibbs, E.L., and Gibbs, F.A. 1962. Extreme spindles: correlation of electroencephalographic sleep pattern with mental retardation. Science 138: 1106–1107.

Gibbs, F.A., and Gibbs, E.L. 1950. *Atlas of Electroencephalography,* Vol. 1. Cambridge, MA: Addison-Wesley.

Gibbs, F.A., and Gibbs, E.L. 1964. *Atlas of Electroencephalography,* Vol. 3. Reading, MA: Addison-Wesley.

Gibbs, F.A., and Gibbs, E.L. 1978. *Atlas of Electroencephalography,* Vol. 4. Reading, MA: Addison-Wesley.

Gibbs, F.A., and Knott, J.R. 1949. Growth of the electrical activity of the cortex. 1:223–229.

Gibbs, F.A., Gibbs, E.L., and Lennox, W.G. 1943. Electroencephalographic response to overventilation and its relation to age. J. Pediatr. 23:497–505.

Gibbs, F.A., Rich, C.L., and Gibbs, E.L. 1963. Psychomotor variant type of seizure discharge. Neurology 13:991–998.

Hagne, I. 1968. Development of waking EEG in normal infants during the first year of life. In *Clinical Electroencephalography of Children,* Eds. P. Kellaway and I. Petersén, pp. 97–118. New York: Grune & Stratton (Stockholm: Almqvist & Wiksell).

Hagne, I., Persson, J., Magnusson, R., et al. 1972. Spectral analysis via fast Fourier transform of waking EEG in normal infants. In *Automation of Clinical EEG,* Eds. P. Kellaway and I. Petersén, pp. 3–48. New York: Raven Press.

Hayakawa, F., Watanabe, K., Hakamada, S., et al. 1987. F_z theta/alpha bursts: a transient EEG pattern in healthy newborns. Electroencephalogr. Clin. Neurophysiol. 67:27–31.

Henry, C.E. 1944. Electroencephalograms of normal children. Monogr. Soc. Res. Child. Dev. National Research Council, Washington, D.C., XI, 71 pp.

Herrlin, K.M. 1954. EEG with photic stimulation: a study of children with manifest or suspended epilepsy. Electroencephalogr. Clin. Neurophysiol. 6:573–589.

Hess, R. 1964. The electroencephalogram in sleep. Electroencephalogr. Clin. Neurophysiol. 16:44–55.

Hrachovy, R.A., and O'Donnell, D.M. 1999. The significance of excessive rhythmic alpha and/or theta frequency activity in the EEG of the neonate. Clin. Neurophysiol. 110:438–444.

Hrbek, A., Vitova, Z., and Mares, P. 1966. Optic evoked potentials in children at different stimulation frequencies. Physiol. Bohemoslov. 15: 201–204.

Hughes, J.R. 1996. Development of sleep spindles in the first year of life. Clin. Electroencephalogr. 27:107–115.

Hughes, J.R. 2003. The frontal arousal rhythm (FAR) is an ictal pattern: a case report. Clin. Electroencephalogr. 34:13–14.

Hughes, J.R., and Daaboul, Y. 1999. The frontal arousal rhythm. Clin. Electroencephalogr. 34:13–14.

Hughes, J.R., Fino, J., and Gagnon, L. 1983. Periods of activity and quiescence in the premature EEG. Electroencephalogr. Clin. Neurophysiol. 56:23P(abst).

Hughes, J.R., Fino, J.J., and Hart, L.A. 1987. Premature temporal theta (PTth). Electroencephalogr. Clin. Neurophysiol. 67:7–15.

Hughes, J.R., Miller, J.K., Fino, J.J., et al. 1990. The sharp theta rhythm on the occipital area of prematures (STOP): a newly described waveform. Clin. Electroencephalogr. 21:77–87.

Isch-Treussard, C., Bapst-Reiter, J., and Kurtz, D. 1981. A study of spontaneous arousal in the newborn. Electroencephalogr. Clin. Neurophysiol. 52:57P(abst).

Janzen, R., Schroeder, C., and Heckel, H. 1952. Hirnbioelektrische Befunde bei Neugeborenen. Monatsschr. Kinderheilkd. 100:216–218.

Joseph, J.P., Lesèvre, N., and Dreyfus-Brisac, C. 1976. Spatiotemporal organization of EEG in premature infants and full-term newborns. Electroencephalogr. Clin. Neurophysiol. 40:153–168.

Karbowski, K., and Nencka, A. 1980. Right mid-temporal sharp EEG transients in healthy newborns. Electroencephalogr. Clin. Neurophysiol. 48: 461–469.

Kasamatsu, A., Hirai, T., Ando, N., et al. 1964. Development of EEG in normal infancy and childhood. Proc. Jpn. EEG Soc., pp. 23–25.

Katsurada, M.L. 1965. Electroencephalographic study of sleep in infants and young children. I. Development of spindle waves (in Japanese) Ann. Paediatr. Jpn. 2:391–394.

Keidel, M., Von Czettritz, G., Tirsch, W., et al. 1991. Periodic changes of amplitude in the EEG of premature infants. Electroencephalogr. Clin. Neurophysiol. 78:46P(abst).

Kellaway, P. 1957. Ontogenetic evolution of the electrical activity of the brain in man and animals. Fourth Int. Congr. Electroencephalogr. Clin. Neurophysiol. Acta Med. Belg., pp. 141–154.

Kellaway, P., and Fox, B.J. 1952. Electroencephalographic diagnosis of cerebral pathology in infants during sleep. I. Rationale, technique and the characteristics of normal sleep in infants. J. Pediatr. 41:262–287.

Kellaway, P., Crawley, J.W., and Kagawa, N. 1959. A specific electroencephalographic correlate of convulsive equivalent disorders in children. J. Pediatr. 55:582–592.

Kuhlo, W. 1967. Die 4–5/sec EEG-Grundrhythmusvariante im Schlaf und nach Contusio cerebri. Arch. Psychiatr. Nervenkr. 210:68–75.

Kuhlo, W. 1976. Slow posterior rhythms. In *Handbook of Electroencephalography and Clinical Neurophysiology,* Vol. 6A, Ed.-in-chief, A. Remond, pp. 89–104. Amsterdam: Elsevier.

Kuhlo, W., Heintel, H., Reichenmiller, H.E., et al. 1968. Familienuntersuchungen bei 4–5/sec Grundrhythmusvariante. Zentralbl. Gesamte Neurol. Psychiatr. 191:164(abst).

Kuhlo, W., Heintel, H., and Vogel, F. 1969. The 4–5/sec rhythm. Electroencephalogr. Clin. Neurophysiol. 26:613–618.

Kuks, J.B.M., Vos, J.E., and O'Brien, M.J. 1988. EEG coherence function for normal newborns in relation to their sleep state. Electroencephalogr. Clin. Neurophysiol. 69:295–302.

Langworthy, O.R. 1930. Medullated tracts in the brain of a seventh-month human fetus. Contr. Embryol. Carneg. Instr. 407, 120:37–51.

Langworthy, O.R. 1933. Development of behavior patterns and myelization of the nervous system in the human fetus and infant. Contr. Embryol. Carneg. Instr. 443, 139:1–57.

Leissner, P., Lindholm, L.E., and Petersén, I. 1970. Alpha amplitude dependency on skull thickness as measured by ultrasound technique. Electroencephalogr. Clin. Neurophysiol. 29:392–399.

Lenard, H.C. 1970. The development of sleep spindles during the first two years of life. Neuropaediatrie 1:264–276.

Leonberg, S.C. 1984. Management of infants and children for electroencephalography. Clin. Electroencephalogr. 15:202–207.

Lindsley, D.B. 1936. Brain potentials in children and adults. Science 84:354.

Lindsley, D.B. 1938. Electrical potentials of the brain in children and adults. J. Genet. Psychol. 19:285–306.

Lindsley, D.B. 1939. A longitudinal study of the alpha rhythm in normal children: frequency and amplitude standards. J. Genet. Psychol. 55:197–213.

Lombroso, C.T. 1979. Quantified electrographic scales on 10 preterm healthy newborns followed up to 40–43 weeks of conceptional age by serial polygraphic recordings. Electroencephalogr. Clin. Neurophysiol. 46:460–474.

Lombroso, C.T. 1980. Normal and abnormal EEGs in full-term neonates. In *Current Clinical Neurophysiology. Update on EEG and Evoked Potentials,* Ed. C.E. Henry, pp. 83–150. Amsterdam: Elsevier/North Holland.

Lombroso, C.T. 1982. Positive sharp waves in newborns: Observations on normals and on babies with proven pathologies. Electroencephalogr. Clin. Neurophysiol. 53:28P–29P(abst).

Lombroso, C.T. 1987. Neonatal electroencephalography. In *Electroencephalography,* 2nd ed., Eds. E. Niedermeyer and F. Lopes da Silva, pp. 725–762. Baltimore: Urban & Schwarzenberg.

Mai, H., and Schaper, G. 1953. Electroencephalographische Untersuchungen an Frühgeborenen. Ann. Paediatr. 180:345–365.

Matousek, M., Volavka, J., Roubicek, J., et al. 1967. EEG frequency analysis related to age in normal adults. Electroencephalogr. Clin. Neurophysiol. 23:162–167.

Matsuura, M., Yamamoto, K., Fukuzawa, H., et al. 1985. Age development and sex differences of various EEG elements in healthy children and adults. Quantification by a computerized wave form recognition method. Electroencephalogr. Clin. Neurophysiol. 60:394–406.

Metcalf, D.R. 1969. The effect of extrauterine experience on the ontogenesis of EEG sleep spindles. Psychosom. Med. 31:393–399.

Metcalf, D.R., Mondale, J., and Butler, F.K. 1971. Ontogenesis of spontaneous K complexes. Psychophysiology 8:340–347.

Monod, N., Curzi-Dacalova, L., and Vallecalle, M.H. 1983. Physiological fast EEG rhythms (brushes) in the premature and full-term newborn. Electroencephalogr. Clin. Neurophysiol. 56:66P(abst).

Moussalli-Salefranque, F., Mises, J., and Plouin, P. 1984. Values of discontinuous EEG in full-term neonates. Electroencephalogr. Clin. Neurophysiol. 57:50P(abst).

Mundy-Castle, A.C. 1951. Theta and beta rhythm in the electroencephalogram of normal adults. Electroencephalogr. Clin. Neurophysiol. 3:477–486.

Mundy-Castle, A.C. 1953. An analysis of central response to photic stimulation in normal adults. Electroencephalogr. Clin. Neurophysiol. 5:1–22.

Nayrac, P., and Beaussart, M. 1956. À propos des rhythmes à 2–4 c/s posterieurs chez les anciens traumatisés craniens. Rev. Neurol. (Paris) 94:849.

Nekhorocheff, M.I. 1950. L'électroencéphalogramme du sommeil chez l'enfant. Rev. Neurol. (Paris) 82:487–495.

Netchine, S. 1969. L'activité électrique cérébrale chez l'enfant 6 à 10 ans. In *Croissance de l'Enfant. Genèse de l'homme.* Paris: Presses Universitaires de France.

Niedermeyer, E. 1972. *The Generalized Epilepsies.* Springfield, IL: Charles C Thomas.

Niedermeyer, E., and Capute, A.J. 1967. A fast and spiky spindle variant in children with organic brain disease. Electroencephalogr. Clin. Neurophysiol. 23:67–73.

Niedermeyer, E., and Koshino, Y. 1975. My-Rhythmus: Vorkommen und klinische Bedeutung. Z. EEG-EMG 6:69–78.

Niedermeyer, E., and Yarworth, S. 1978. Scarcity of minor EEG abnormalities during the first two years of life. Electroencephalogr. 9:20–28.

Norton, W.T. 1975a. Myelin. In *Basic Neurochemistry,* Eds. R.W. Albers, C.J. Siegel, R. Katzman, et al. Boston: Little, Brown.

Norton, W.T. 1975b. Myelin: structure and biochemistry. In *The Nervous System,* Ed.-in-chief, D.B. Tower, pp. 467–481. New York: Raven Press.

Nowack, W.J., and Janati, A. 1990. Positive sharp waves in neonatal EEG. Am. J. EEG Technol. 30:211–222.

O'Brien, M.J., Lems, Y.L., and Prechtl, H.F.R. 1987. Transient flattenings in the EEG of newborns—a benign variation. Electroencephalogr. Clin. Neurophysiol. 67:16–26.

Ohtahara, S. 1964. Development of electroencephalogram during infancy and childhood. Proc. Jpn. EEG Soc., pp. 18–23.

Okamoto, Y., and Kirikae, T. 1951. EEG studies on brain of fetus of children of premature birth. Folia Psychiatr. Neurol. Jpn. 5:135–146.

Palmer, F.B., Yarworth, S., and Niedermeyer, E. 1976. Frontal midline theta rhythm. Electroencephalogr. Clin. Neurophysiol. 7:131–138.

Pampiglione, G. 1963. *Development of Cerebral Function in the Dog.* London: Butterworths.

Parmelee, A.H. 1969. EEG power spectral analysis of new-born infants' sleep states. Electroencephalogr. Clin. Neurophysiol. 27:690–691.

Parmelee, A.H., Akiyama, Y., Schultz, M.A., et al. The electroencephalogram in active and quiet sleep in infants. In *Clinical Electroencephalography in Children.* Eds. P. Kellaway and I. Petersén, pp. 77–88. New York: Grune & Stratton (Stockholm: Almqvist & Wiksell).

Parmelee, A.H., Schulte, F.J., Akiyama, Y., et al. 1968b. Maturation of EEG activity during sleep in premature infants. Electroencephalogr. Clin. Neurophysiol. 24:319–329.

Parmelee, A.H., Akiyama, Y., Schultz, M.A., et al. 1969. Analysis of the electroencephalogram of sleeping infants. Acta Nerv. Super. (Praha) 11:111–115.

Passouant, P., Cadilhac, J., and Delange, M. 1965. Le sommeil du nouveauné. Considérations sur la période de mouvements oculaires. Arch. Fr. Pediatr. 22:1087–1092.

Petersén, I., and Eeg-Olofsson, O. 1971. The development of the electroencephalogram in normal children from the age of 1 through 15 years. Neuropaediatrie 2:247–304.

Petersén, I., and Sörbye, R. 1962. Slow posterior rhythm in adults. Electroencephalogr. Clin. Neurophysiol. 14:161–170.

Petersén, I., Selldén, U., and Eeg-Olofsson, O. 1975. The evolution of the EEG in normal children and adolescents from 1 to 21 years. In *Handbook of Electroencephalography and Clinical Neurophysiology.* Vol. 6B, Ed.-in-chief, A. Remond, Ed. G.C. Lairy, pp. 31–68. Amsterdam: Elsevier.

Picard, P., Navarenne, P., Laboureur, R., et al. 1957. Confrontations des données de l'électroencéphalogramme et de l'examen psychologique chez 309 candidats pilotes a l'Aéronautique. Electroencephalogr. Clin. Neurophysiol. Suppl. 6:304–314.

Pichot, F. 1953. *Contribution a l'étude de l'électroencéphalogramme normal et pathologique du nouveau-né.* Thesis, Toulouse.

Pitot, M., and Gastaut, Y. 1956. Aspect électroencéphalographiques inhabituels des sequelles des traumatismes craniens. Il Les rhythmes postérieurs cycles-seconde. Rev. Neurol. (Paris) 94:189–191.

Prechtl, H.F.R., Weinmann, H., and Akiyama, Y. 1969. Organization of physiological parameters in normal and neurologically abnormal infants. Neuropaediatrie 1:101–129.

Prechtl, H.F.R., Vos, J.E., Akiyama, Y., et al. 1974. Neonatal EEG: age codes and coherence functions in relation to intrauterine growth and oestrogen levels. In *Ontogenesis of the Brain,* Vol. 2, Eds. L. Silek and S. Trojan, pp. 201–210. Praha: Universita Karlova.

Radvanyi-Bouvet, M.F. 1983. Pathological fast EEG rhythm (FR) in premature (PN) and full-term neonates (FTN). Electroencephalogr. Clin. Neurophysiol. 56:66P(abst).

Roffwarg, H.P., Muzio, J.N., and Dement, W.C. 1966. Ontogenetic development of the human sleep dream cycle. Science 152:604–619.

Rorke, L.B., and Riggs, H.E. 1969. *Myelination of the Brain in the Newborn.* Philadelphia: Lippincott.

Roth, B., Stein, J., and Simonova, O. 1967. Abnormal manifestations in resting EEG recordings of healthy persons. Acta Univ. Carol. Med. 13: 185–187.

Samson-Dollfus, D. 1955. L'EEG Prématuré jusqu' l'Age de 3 Mois et du Nouveau-né à Terme. Paris: Thesis in Medicine, Foulon.

Samson-Dollfus, D., and Goldberg, P. 1979. Electroencephalographic quantification by time domain analysis in normal 7–15 year old children. Electroencephalogr. Clin. Neurophysiol. 46:147–154.

Samson-Dollfus, D., Nogues, B., and Delagree, E. 1981. EEG recording during drowsiness in normal babies from 2 to 12 months of age. Electroencephalogr. Clin. Neurophysiol. 52:58P(abst).

Schauseil-Zipf, U., Hamm, W., and Mandl-Kramer, S. 1984. EEG findings in "small-for-date babies" at 7–12 years of age. Electroencephalogr. Clin. Neurophysiol. 57:33P–34P(abst).

Scheffner, D. 1968. Eine einfache Methode zur quantitativen Bestimmung langsamer Frequenzen im EEG von Kindern. Arch. Kinderheilkd. 177: 41–48.

Scher, M.S., Sun, M., Hatzilabrous, G.-M., et al. 1990. Computer analysis of EEG-sleep in the neonate: methodological considerations. J. Clin. Neurophysiol. 7:417–441.

Scher, M.S., Bova, J.M., Dokianakis, S.G., et al. 1994a. Positive temporal sharp waves on EEG recordings of healthy neonates: a benign pattern of dysmaturity in pre-term infants at post-conceptional term ages. Electroencephalogr. Clin. Neurophysiol. 90:173–178.

Scher, M.S., Bova, J.M., Dokianakis, S.G., et al. 1994b. Physiological significance of sharp wave transients on EEG recordings of healthy preterm and full-term neonates. Electroencephalogr. Clin. Neurophysiol. 90: 179–185.

Schulte, F.J., Hinze, G., and Schrempf, G. 1971. Maternal toxemia, fetal malnutrition and bioelectric brain activity in the newborn. Neuropaediatrie 2:439–460.

Schulz, H., Salzarulo, P., Fagioli, I., et al. 1983. REM latency: Development in the first year of life. Electroencephalogr. Clin. Neurophysiol. 56: 316–322.

Schütz, E., Müller, H.W., and Schönenberg, H. 1951. Über die Entwicklung zentralnervöser Rhythmen im Elektroenzephalogramm des Kindes. Z. Gesamte Exp. Med. 117:157–170.

Selldén, U. 1964. Electroencephalographic activation with Megimide in normal subjects. Acta Neurol. Scand. 40 (suppl. 12):30.

Silbert, P.L., Radhakrishnan, K., Johnson, J., et al. 1995. The significance of the phi rhythm. Electroencephalogr. Clin. Neurophysiol. 95:71–76.

Simonova, O., Roth, B., and Stein, J. 1967. EEG-studies of healthy population—normal rhythms of resting recording. Acta Univ. Carol. Med. 13:543–551.

Slater, G.E., and Torres, F. 1979. Frequency-amplitude gradient. A new parameter for interpreting pediatric sleep EEGs. Arch. Neurol. 36:465–470.

Smith, J.R. 1937. The electroencephalogram during infancy and childhood. Proc. Soc. Exp. Biol. Med. 36:384–386.

Smith, J.R. 1938. The electroencephalogram during normal infancy and childhood. II. The nature of the growth of the alpha waves. J. Genet. Psychol. 53:455–469.

Smith, J.R. 1941. The frequency growth of the human alpha rhythms during infancy and childhood. J. Psychol. 11:177–198.

Statz, A., and Dumermuth, G. 1981. Transient EEG patterns during sleep in healthy newborns. Electroencephalogr. Clin. Neurophysiol. 52:96P.

Staudt, F., Howieson, J., Benda, G.I., et al. 1982. EEG bei Neugeborenen mit intrakraniellen Blutungen: ein Vergleich mit klinischen Befunden und Ct-Scan. Z. EEG-EMG 13:143–148.

Staudt, F., Engel, R., and Coen, R.W. 1983. Rhythmische Alpha-Aktivität im EEG von Früh- und Neugeborenen. Z. EEG-EMG 14:22–27.

Staudt, F., Engel, R., and Coen, R.W. 1984. Rhythmical alpha activity in the EEG of premature and term infants. Electroencephalogr. Clin. Neurophysiol. 57:33P(abst).

Stern, E., Parmelee, A.H., Akiyama, Y., et al. 1969. Sleep cycle characteristics in infants. Pediatrics 43:65–70.

Sternberg, B., Frenkel, A.L., Plouin, P., et al. 1984. Aetiology of inactive EEG in the newborn. Electroencephalogr. Clin. Neurophysiol. 57:49P(abst).

Stockard-Pope, J.E., Werner, S.S., and Bickford, R.G. 1992. *Atlas of Neonatal Electroencephalography,* 2nd ed. New York: Raven Press.

Sureau, M., Fischgold, H., and Capdevielle, G. 1949. L'EEG du nouveauné normal de 0 à 36 heures. Rev. Neurol. (Paris) 81:543–545.

Tharp, B.R. 1980. Neonatal and pediatric electroencephalography. In *Electrodiagnosis in Clinical Neurology,* Ed. M.J. Aminoff, pp. 67–117. New York: Churchill Livingstone.

Tharp, B.R. 1990. Electrophysiological brain maturation in premature infants: an historical perspective. J. Clin. Neurophysiol. 7:302–314.

Tharp, B.R., Cukier, F., and Monod, N. 1981. The prognostic value of the electroencephalogram in premature infants. Electroencephalogr. Clin. Neurophysiol. 51:219–236.

Vallat, J.N., and Lepetit, J.M. 1957. Présentation de tracés de traumatismes craniens avec rhythmes postérieurs à quatre cycles-seconde. Notions sur les caractères évolutifs. Quelques réflexions à propos de l'expertise. Rev. Neurol. (Paris) 96:551–552.

Vanhatalo, S., Tallgren, P., Sainio, K., et al. 2002. DC-EEG Recording discloses prominent very slow activity patterns during sleep in preterm infants. Clin. Neurophysiol. 113:1822–1825.

Van Huffelen, A.C., and Magnus, O. 1973. 4c/sec vertex spindles. Electroencephalogr. Clin. Neurophysiol. 34:543–546.

Varner, J.L., Peters, J.F., and Ellingson, R.J. 1978. Interhemispheric synchrony in the EEG of full-term newborns. Electroencephalogr. Clin. Neurophysiol. 45:641–647.

Visser, S.L., Njiokiktjien, C.J., and De Rijke, W. 1982. Neurological condition at birth in relation to the electroencephalogram (EEG) and visual evoked potential (VEP) at the age of 5. Electroencephalogr. Clin. Neurophysiol. 54:458–464.

Vitova, Z., and Hrbek, A. 1972. Developmental study on the responsiveness of the human brain to flicker stimulation. Dev. Med. Chid. Neurol. 14:476–486.

Vogel, F. 1962. Ergänzende Untersuchungen zur Genetik des menschlichen Niederspannungs-EEG. Deutsch Z. Nervenheilk. 185:105–111.

Vogel, F., and Fujiya, Y. 1969. The incidence of some inherited EEG variants in normal Japanese and German mates. Hum. Genet. 7:38–42.

Vogel, F., and Götze, W. 1959. Familienuntersuchungen zur Genetik des normalen Elektroenzephalogramms. Deutsch Z. Nervenheilk. 178:668–700.

Vogel, F., and Götze, W. 1962. Statistische Betrachtungerüber über die Beta-Wellen im EEG des Menschen. Deutsch Z. Nervenheilk. 184:112–136.

Walter, W.G. 1950. Normal rhythms—their development, distribution and significance. In *Electroencephalography,* ed. 1, Eds. D. Hill and G. Parr, pp. 203–227. London: MacDonald.

Watanabe, K., Hakamada, S., Kuroyanagi, M.M., et al. 1983. Electroencephalographic study of intraventricular hemorrhage in preterm newborn. Neuropediatrics 14:225–230.

Werner, S.S., Stockard, J.E., and Bickford, R.G. 1977. *Atlas of Neonatal Electroencephalography.* New York: Raven Press.

Westmoreland, B.F., and Stockard, J.E. 1977. The EEG in infants and children: normal patterns. Am. J. EEG Technol. 17:187–206.

White, J.C., and Tharp, B.R. 1974. An arousal pattern in children with organic cerebral dysfunction. Electroencephalogr. Clin. Neurophysiol. 37:265–268.

Williams, D. 1941. The significance of an abnormal EEG. J. Neurol. Psychiatr. 4:257–268.

Yakovlev, P.I., and Lecours, A.R. 1967. Myelogenetic cycles of regional maturation of the brain. In *Symposium—Regional Development of the Brain in Early Life.* Oxford: Blackwell Scientific.

12. Nonspecific Abnormal EEG Patterns

Frank W. Sharbrough

Electroencephalogram (EEG) abnormalities can be divided into three descriptive categories: (a) distortion and disappearance of normal patterns, (b) appearance and increase of abnormal patterns, and (c) disappearance of all patterns. This description of EEG abnormalities can be further expanded by identifying their spatial extent (local or widespread, unilateral or bilateral) and their temporal persistence (brief and intermittent or prolonged and persistent). The intermittent abnormalities characterized by the sudden appearance and disappearance of a pattern are called "paroxysmal."

The above classification of EEG abnormalities is purely descriptive. In addition to descriptive categorization, EEG abnormalities can be subdivided on the basis of their usual clinical correlations. Most abnormal patterns, whether persistent or intermittent, are nonspecific because they are not associated with a specific pathological condition or etiology. However, some patterns usually occurring paroxysmally with distinctive waveforms (such as spike, spike and wave, sharp wave, seizure pattern, or periodic complexes) are specific in that they are frequently associated with specific pathophysiological reactions (such as epilepsy) or specific disease processes, such as subacute sclerosing panencephalitis (SSPE) or Jakob-Creutzfeldt disease. This chapter discusses the nonspecific abnormalities; later chapters discuss the specific abnormalities.

In spite of the fact that nonspecific abnormalities are not related to a specific pathophysiological reaction or a specific disease process, they nonetheless can be divided into three basic categories based on their usual association with different types of cerebral disturbances:

1. Widespread intermittent slow abnormalities, often associated with active (improving, worsening, or episodic) widespread brain dysfunction;
2. Bilateral persistent EEG findings, usually associated with impaired conscious cerebral responsivity; and
3. Focal persistent EEG findings, usually associated with focal cerebral disturbance.

The above divisions are based on the usual clinical correlates, but it is important to realize that these correlations are statistical and not absolute. The best intuitive grasp of the somewhat variable relationship between EEG abnormalities and clinical or other laboratory evidence of central nervous system (CNS) disturbance is obtained when the EEG is viewed as an extension of the neurological examination. When viewed from this perspective, the EEG studies electrical signs of neurological function, whereas the neurological examination studies physical signs. In any one patient, depending on the nature and location of the pathology, abnor-

malities may be found in both EEG and clinical examination, in only one examination, or in neither, just as abnormalities may be found in one, both, or neither of two subsets on the clinical examination, such as reflex and sensory examination. Furthermore, the results of both EEG and clinical evaluation may be normal, although the patient has anatomical abnormalities detectable by contrast studies or computed tomography (CT). The opposite also holds, in that both the EEG and clinical examination may show distinct abnormalities when radiographic studies are normal. An intelligent integration of the results of functional tests, such as the EEG and clinical examination, with radiographic tests that study anatomy, such as contrast studies or CT, requires an understanding of the value and limitation of each test, as well as the overall clinical field of neurology. With this conceptual background, this chapter discusses nonspecific EEG abnormalities based on the three general categories of clinical correlation.

Widespread Intermittent Slow Activity Often Associated with Active Widespread Brain Dysfunction

Description

Morphologically, this type of abnormality is characterized by intermittent commonly rhythmic slow activity often in the delta frequency range, thus accounting for its descriptive acronym, IRDA (intermittent rhythmic delta activity). When in the delta frequency range, it is often composed of runs of sinusoidal or saw-toothed waves with more rapid ascending than descending phases with mean frequencies close to 2.5 Hz (Cobb, 1976; Hess, 1975; Klass and Daly, 1979). The waves are relatively stereotyped in form and frequency and occur in short bursts (Figs. 12.1 and 12.2). This pattern, usually demonstrates reactivity; it is attenuated by alerting and eye opening and accentuated with eye closure, hyperventilation, or drowsiness [stage 1, non-rapid-eye-movement (REM) sleep]. With the onset of stage 2 and deeper levels of non-REM sleep, the abnormal IRDA disappears. However, in REM sleep the abnormal IRDA may again become apparent (Cobb, 1976; Hess, 1975; Klass and Daly, 1979; Scollo-Lavizzari, 1970).

Intermittent rhythmic delta activity is usually bilateral and widespread in distribution, with peak localization strongly influenced by age. In adults, the peak amplitude of the pattern is usually localized over the frontal area (Figs. 12.1 to 12.9) and especially over the frontopolar region (Zurek et al., 1985), thus giving rise to the acronym FIRDA (frontal IRDA), whereas in children the peak amplitude frequently develops over the occipital or posterior head regions

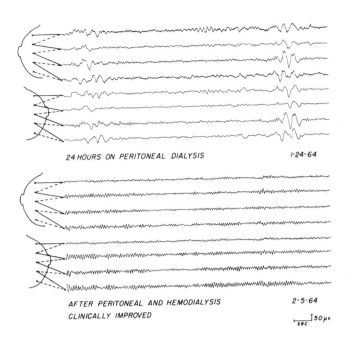

24 HOURS ON PERITONEAL DIALYSIS   1-24-64

AFTER PERITONEAL AND HEMODIALYSIS   2-5-64
CLINICALLY IMPROVED   ⌐────┐50μv.
                                         sec.

Figure 12.1. Widespread intermittent slow activity of the frontal intermittent rhythmic delta activity (FIRDA) type and disorganization of normal background activity resulting from uremic encephalography. The clinical and EEG manifestations resolved after peritoneal and hemodialysis.

(Figs. 12.10 to 12.12), resulting in the acronym OIRDA (occipital IRDA). This difference in location from adults to children is not related to difference in pathological processes, but simply reflects an age-determined variation in what is an otherwise similar, nonspecific reaction to a wide variety of changing pathological processes (Cobb, 1976; Daly, 1968; Hess, 1975; Klass and Daly, 1979).

Although the foregoing discussion concentrates on two of the more classical varieties of widespread intermittent slow activity using acronyms commonly applied to them (FIRDA or OIRDA), it has been clearly pointed out that other varieties of widespread intermittent slow activity made up of rhythmic theta or nonrhythmic delta exist and have essentially the same significance as the more classical forms with the rhythmic delta activity (Schaul et al., 1981a,b). Therefore, the subsequent comments regarding the more classical forms (FIRDA and OIRDA) also apply to these other varieties of widespread intermittent slow activity. In the German EEG literature, IRDA is also known as "parenrhythmia" (Penin, 1971).

Etiological Nonspecificity of IRDA

IRDA is not specific for a single etiology and can occur in response to systemic toxic or metabolic disturbances (Figs. 12.1 to 12.3) as well as to diffuse or focal intracranial diseases (Figs. 12.4 to 12.11). This may be due to diverse

Figure 12.2. Widespread intermittent slow (FIRDA type) disorganization of normal rhythms, and generalized persistent nonrhythmic delta activity (PNDA) associated with signs of disequilibrium, following hemodialysis.

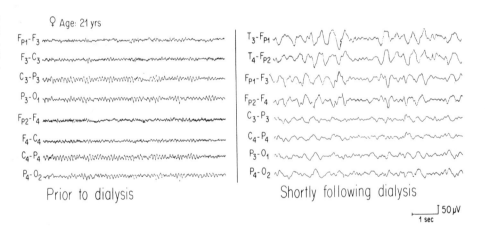

♀ Age: 21 yrs

Prior to dialysis   Shortly following dialysis

⌐────┐50 μV
1 sec

Figure 12.3. Widespread intermittent slow disorganization of normal rhythms (FIRDA), and generalized persistent nonrhythmic delta slowing (PNDA) produced by severe Dilantin intoxication.

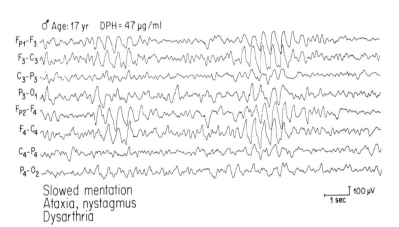

♂ Age: 17 yr   DPH = 47 μg/ml

Slowed mentation   ⌐────┐100 μV
Ataxia, nystagmus   1 sec
Dysarthria

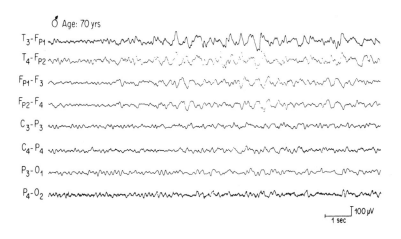

Figure 12.4. Widespread intermittent slow activity (FIRDA) and 7-Hz background activity associated with a senile dementia.

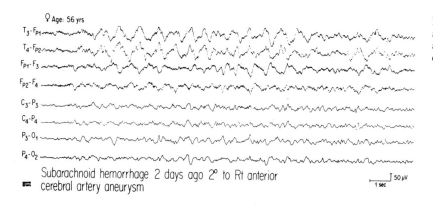

Figure 12.5. Widespread intermittent slow (FIRDA) activity and disorganization of the background 2 days after a subarachnoid hemorrhage from a right anterior cerebral artery aneurysm.

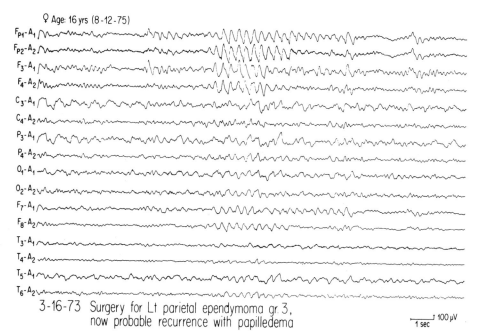

Figure 12.6. FIRDA and focal PNDA due to recurrent left parietal ependymoma. Some bursts of FIRDA predominate on the left side.

♀ Age: 13 Yr (9-18-73)

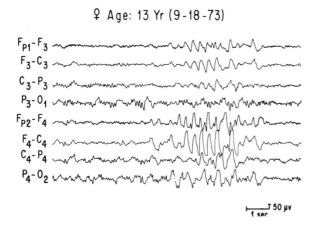

Figure 12.7. Widespread intermittent slow (FIRDA type) activity, maximum on the right, and focal disorganization of the background with persistent delta slowing (PNDA type), due to a right frontoparietal glioblastoma.

♀ Age: 36 yrs

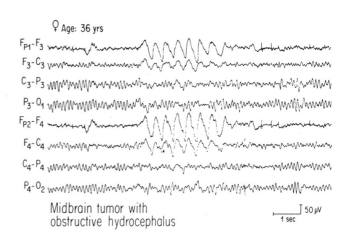

Midbrain tumor with obstructive hydrocephalus

Figure 12.9. Widespread intermittent slowing (FIRDA type) in a patient with midbrain tumor and symptomatic, obstructive hydrocephalus.

♀ Age: 16 yrs (11-10-72)

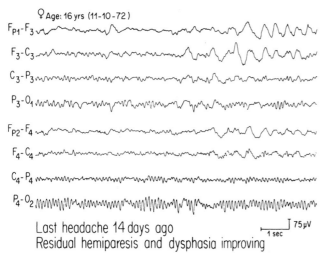

Last headache 14 days ago
Residual hemiparesis and dysphasia improving

Figure 12.8. Lateralized FIRDA, alpha asymmetry, and focal persistent delta slowing (PNDA type) associated with residual hemiparesis and dysphasia following a complicated migraine attack 14 days previously.

etiologies, such as infectious, inflammatory, degenerative, traumatic, vascular, or neoplastic disorders.

IRDA is also the nonspecific type of slowing that occurs in normal individuals in response to hyperventilation. In such cases, it should not be interpreted as an abnormality, but rather as the response of a normal CNS to the stress of an acutely changing pCO_2 (Fig. 12.12).

Nonlocalizing Nature of IRDA

Because IRDA may occur in response to systemic toxic or metabolic disturbances, diffuse intracranial pathology, or focal intracranial pathology, its localizing value obviously is limited. Even when it is due to a focal expanding lesion, the peak localization of the IRDA tends to be age-dependent [maximal frontal in adults (Figs. 12.1 to 12.9) and maximal posterior in children (Figs. 12.10 to 12.12)]. It is independent of the localization of the lesion, which may be at some distance, either in the supra- or infratentorial space, from the maximum expression of the IRDA. The recognition that IRDA is a non–localizing rhythm, even when associated with an intracranial lesion,

Figure 12.10. Widespread intermittent slowing [occipital intermittent rhythmic delta activity (OIRDA type)] in a 6-year-old patient with a right cerebellar astrocytoma and signs of increased intracranial pressure. Widespread intermittent slowing with a posterior maximum (OIRDA) is age-determined and not related to the location of the pathology.

♂ Age: 6 yrs

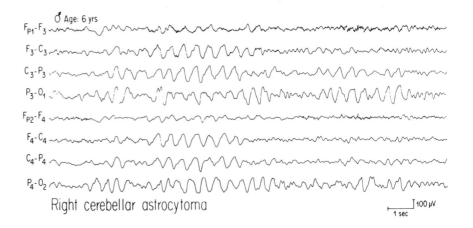

Right cerebellar astrocytoma

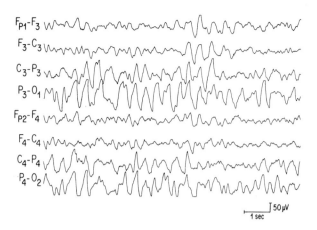

Figure 12.11. Widespread intermittent slowing (OIRDA type) and generalized PNDA associated with late infantile lipidosis.

led to its earlier designation as a "projected" or "distant" rhythm (Faure et al., 1951; Hess, 1975). Such a designation, however, can be misleading because it encourages the misconception that the IRDA, associated with a "distant" lesion, is morphologically distinct from IRDA due to diffuse intracranial disease or a systemic toxic or metabolic disturbance.

Although frequently bilateral, IRDA may occur predominantly unilaterally. Even when it occurs unilaterally in association with a lateralized supratentorial lesion, the lateralization of the IRDA, although usually ipsilateral (Figs. 12.6 to 12.8), may even be contralateral to the focal lesion (Fig. 12.12). Therefore, when IRDA is present, determining whether it is due to a focal lesion (and if so, the location of the focal lesion) is best based on persistent localizing signs, discussed later, and not on the morphology or even the laterality of IRDA.

TIRDA (temporal intermittent rhythmic delta activity) (Normand et al., 1995; Reither et al., 1989) is an "important

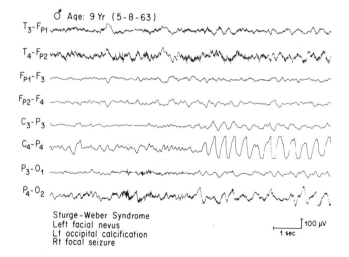

Figure 12.12. Lateralized OIRDA occurring as a normal response to hyperventilation in the intact right hemisphere; reduced on the left due to left occipital involvement with Sturge-Weber disease.

epileptogenic abnormality" (Normand et al., 1995), highly pathognomonic for temporal lobe epilepsy. These rhythmical unilateral delta trains indicate a focal lesion. Thus, TIRDA markedly differs from FIRDA and OIRDA (and their mainly global significance).

Mechanisms Responsible for IRDA

The mechanisms responsible for the genesis of IRDA are only partially understood. Earlier studies investigated the mechanism of IRDA-associated lesions producing increased intracranial pressure. It was recognized early that with benign intracranial hypertension (pseudotumor cerebri), IRDA was not present (Boddie et al., 1974; Hess, 1975; Klass and Daly, 1979; Sidell and Daly, 1961). However, in increased intracranial pressure with tumor or aqueductal stenosis, IRDA is frequently present. Based on this, earlier workers related the appearance of IRDA to increased transventricular pressure within the third ventricle tending to produce an acute or subacute dilatation of the third ventricle (Daly et al., 1953; Hess, 1975; Klass and Daly, 1979; Martinius et al., 1968). Some studies investigated the appearance of IRDA in diffuse encephalopathies with documented postmortem histopathological changes (Gloor et al., 1968). Based on these studies, it was concluded that the main correlate of IRDA was diffuse gray matter disease, both in cortical and subcortical locations. A later extension of this work (Schaul et al., 1981a) suggests that increased intracranial pressure alone, unless severe enough to produce secondary disturbance in cerebral circulation, does not produce IRDA, but rather IRDA appears only if the process responsible for the increased intracranial pressure also produces widespread brain dysfunction. Finally, any comprehensive theory about the origin of IRDA must not only take into account that IRDA is found in diverse systemic and intracranial processes, but also that IRDA is more likely to appear during the course of active fluctuating, progressing, or resolving widespread brain dysfunction and is less likely to be associated with chronic, stable brain dysfunction. Clinically, the earliest correlate of the appearance of IRDA, especially in an otherwise normal EEG, is a subtle, fluctuating impairment of attention and arousal (Schaul et al., 1981a). As the condition progresses, often leading to more persistent, bilateral abnormalities, frank alteration in consciousness appropriate to the degree of persistent, bilateral abnormalities usually appears.

In summary, IRDA is nonspecific in that it can be seen in association with a wide variety of pathological processes varying from systemic toxic or metabolic disturbances to focal intracranial lesions. Even when associated with a focal lesion, IRDA by itself is nonlocalizing. The common denominator in the wide variety of pathological processes producing IRDA is that, when such an abnormality appears, it is likely to be associated with the development of widespread brain dysfunction; the earliest clinical correlates are fluctuating levels of alertness and attention. With focal lesions, the mechanism may be sufficient distortion of the brain to produce secondary disturbances at both the subcortical and cortical levels. With primary intracranial encephalopathies, it appears to be due to widespread involvement of the gray matter at subcortical and cortical levels.

Bilateral Persistent EEG Findings, Usually Associated with Impaired Conscious Cerebral Responsivity

The relationship between different bilateral persistent EEG abnormalities and different states of impaired conscious cerebral responsivity is often confused in the literature. Articles frequently fail to identify which of several clearly distinct states is being considered. The origin of this confusion, as well as its possible solution, can be best appreciated by recognizing that the clinical evaluation of consciousness depends on the cooperative interaction of three closely related functions; at the risk of oversimplification, these can be identified and defined as follows.

Brainstem arousability: characterized by cyclic appearance of lid opening, blinking, and eye movement, which can occur whether or not consciousness is associated with this state. This minimal functional activity, without consciousness, requires only the upper brainstem and not cerebral cortical integrity, at least in the chronic states. Therefore, as defined, it may occur in the absence of cerebral consciousness. For example, the chronic vegetative state is a state of cerebral unconsciousness with preserved brainstem arousability.

Cerebral consciousness: characterized by cyclic awareness of self and environment that requires cerebral cortical integrity, as well as the integrity of subcortical structures down to and including those responsible for brainstem arousability as defined above. Because consciousness requires such a cooperative interaction of the cerebral cortex and the upper brainstem, consciousness does not occur in the absence of brainstem arousability. As a matter of fact, even the distorted consciousness of dreams during sleep occurs when there is considerable eye movement as evidence of upper brainstem activity, as is seen in REM sleep; furthermore, dreams occur in individuals capable of brainstem arousability. Sleep, by definition, is a nonwaking state with preserved brainstem arousability, in contrast to coma, which when most strictly defined consists of a nonwaking state with absent brainstem arousability.

Cerebral responsivity: characterized by purposeful motor responses to the external environment and, in its most differentiated forms, requires cerebral consciousness as well as a psychic desire to respond and an intact motor system capable of carrying out this intention.

Based on the foregoing definitions, three major neurological states can be identified with several subgroups under each of the major states. These can be identified and defined as follows.

States with conscious cerebral responsivity can be clinically divided into (a) those in which patients appear to have normal consciousness and (b) those in which consciousness is impaired. In the latter group, impaired consciousness is frequently designated as a *confused state* if impairment is relatively acute and likely reversible, whereas it is frequently designated as the demented state if impairment is chronic and frequently irreversible.

States with conscious cerebral unresponsivity can be divided into (a) those in which purposeful responsiveness is lost due to an organic paralysis either on a central or a peripheral basis producing the locked-in state and (b) those in which purposeful responsiveness is lost due to psychogenic factors producing a function unresponsiveness.

States with unconscious cerebral unresponsivity can be divided into (a) those in which brainstem arousability is maintained (the vegetative state) and (b) those in which brainstem arousability is lost (the strict definition of coma).

For a typical example of the type of confusion that may arise when the above conditions are not strictly defined, one has only to review the EEG literature concerning coma. Such a review shows that *coma* is frequently defined in any of three different ways; the reader is often left to infer from the context of the article which of the three different definitions the author is using for the word *coma*:

1. The strictest definition requires cerebral unconsciousness without brainstem arousability.
2. The looser definition requires only cerebral unconsciousness, either without brainstem arousability (strictly defined coma) or with brainstem arousability (the vegetative state).
3. The loosest definition requires only cerebral unresponsivity and thus includes unconscious states without brainstem arousability (strictly defined coma) and with brainstem arousability (the vegetative state), as well as conscious states with absent cerebral responsiveness because of paralysis (the locked-in state) or psychogenic reasons (psychogenic unresponsiveness).

This variability in the definition of coma explains in part why there has been such a discrepancy concerning the description of EEG findings in coma. This variable definition of coma introduces similar confusion into the neurological literature on irreversible coma; some authors use a strict definition of coma (Beecher, 1968; Chatrian, 1980), whereas others use a loose definition (Chatrian, 1980; Walker, 1977). In an attempt to avoid this type of confusion, EEG findings seen in association with impaired conscious purposeful responsiveness will be discussed separately for the three major states defined above.

States with Impaired Cerebral Responsivity: Description of EEG Findings Usually Associated with Impaired Consciousness

EEG findings in this category can usually be divided into (a) distortion and disappearance of normal patterns and (b) appearance and increase of abnormal patterns. Thus, the abnormalities seen in association with progressive impairment of consciousness include slowing of background frequency, such as slowing of the alpha rhythm in the posterior head region from the upper alpha frequency range into the theta frequency range (Figs. 12.13 and 12.14). The more anterior beta, especially the drug-induced type, may also slow from the upper beta range into the lower beta range and even into the upper alpha range as consciousness is progressively impaired. As the frequency of patterns seen in the normal patient drops out of the theta range into the delta range, usually the pattern begins to lose its rhythmicity and any recognizable resemblance to normal physiological patterns.

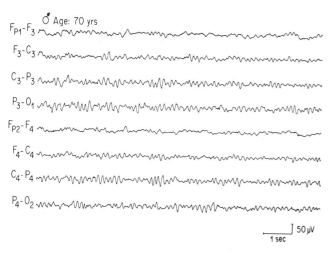

Figure 12.13. Slowing of occipital background rhythms into 7-Hz range with senile dementia.

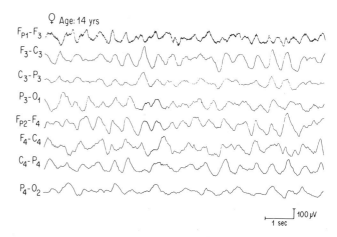

Figure 12.15. Frontally maximum persistent rhythmic delta slowing, as well as generalized persistent delta slowing (PNDA type), in a 14-year-old with encephalitis and bizarre behavior initially thought to be of functional origin.

Either concurrent with or following distortion and disappearance of recognizable patterns, it is common to see widespread, persistent nonrhythmic delta activity (PNDA) (Figs. 12.14 to 12.16). In addition to the above finding, especially with changing or evolving conditions, IRDA as discussed in the earlier sections may also appear (Figs. 12.4 and 12.5). As consciousness is progressively impaired (especially if acutely), the intermittent rhythmic delta activity may at times become relatively continuous in states with severely impaired consciousness (Fig. 12.15). The EEG findings discussed above in states with some elements of preserved purposeful responsiveness usually correlate at least roughly with the clinical estimate of impaired cerebral function based on impairment of consciousness.

States with Absent Cerebral Responsivity: Description of EEG Findings Usually Associated with Retained Consciousness

When purposeful responsiveness is absent, the clinical evaluation gives little insight into residual functional integrity at the cerebral hemispheric level, but usually reflects

only arousal function at the brainstem level and additional primitive reflex function at the brainstem and spinal cord level.

However, awareness may be maintained even in the absence of clinical signs of cerebral responsiveness, either due to organic paralysis (locked-in states) or psychogenic factors (functional unresponsiveness). In either case, the EEG is helpful in identifying patients who are likely to be conscious in spite of cerebral unresponsivity; these patients show normal patterns usually associated with conscious wakefulness, including a reactive alpha rhythm, at times an identifiable mu rhythm, and possible anterior beta activity (Fig. 12.17). Behavior non-REM sleep is associated with the usual spindles, as well as with slow wave components. However, REM sleep patterns may be lost or disturbed if the loss of purposeful responsiveness is due to a brainstem lesion (Chase et al., 1968; Chatrian, 1980; Markand, 1976;

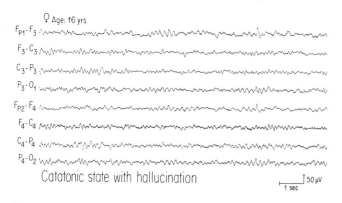

Figure 12.14. Slowing of background rhythms and low-voltage generalized persistent delta slowing (PNDA type) associated with lupus encephalopathy.

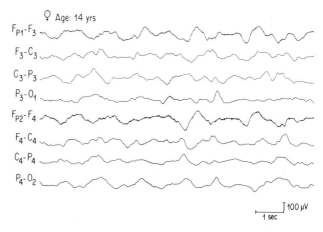

Figure 12.16. Generalized persistent delta slowing (PNDA type) and deteriorating EEG occurring in 14-year-old patient comatose 1 day after previous EEG (see Fig. 12-15).

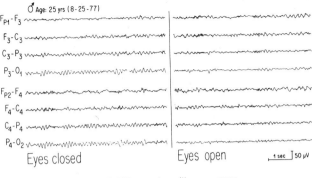

Eyes closed   Eyes open   1 sec ⌐50 μV

(1) Ocular bobbing and pupillary response
    to light
(2) Absent spontaneous respirations and calorics

Figure 12.17. Retained beta and reactive posterior alpha rhythm in a patient unresponsive with ocular bobbing due to a massive brainstem infarction secondary to complications of neck manipulation.

Westmoreland et al., 1975). In these cases, the distinction between functional and organic absence of purposeful responsiveness in spite of retained consciousness depends on clinical evidence suggesting the presence or absence of motor paralysis either on an upper or lower motor neuron basis.

States with Absent Cerebral Responsivity: Description of EEG Findings Usually Associated with Unconsciousness

With unconsciousness, all of the descriptive types of abnormalities noted above may occur. These include (a) distortion and disappearance of normal patterns, (b) appearance and increase of abnormal patterns, and (c) disappearance of all patterns.

Almost invariably, with the onset of unconsciousness the alpha rhythm commonly seen in the conscious state is lost. The anterior beta rhythm may persist in a recognizable form in unconscious patients, although its frequency tends to be slowed into the lower beta range and even into the alpha frequency range, as will be discussed later. In persistently unconscious patients, sleep-like patterns (spindles and vertex waves) may be seen when the patient is behaviorally quiescent (Fig. 12.18). These at times are referred to in the literature as "spindle coma," but in this context coma is defined loosely to include patients who are strictly comatose and unarousable and those who are arousable but vegetative (Bergamasco et al., 1968; Chatrian, 1980; Chatrian et al., 1963). In either case, the preservation of spindle patterns suggests a considerable degree of cerebral hemispheric functional integrity; not too surprisingly, this tends to be associated with a better prognosis (when all of the factors such as chronicity and etiology are equal) than other EEG patterns bearing no recognizable resemblance to normal physiological activity (Bergamasco et al., 1968; Chatrian, 1980).

Two alpha range patterns must be clearly distinguished from one another in patients without purposeful responsiveness. For the sake of contrasting these two patterns, the first is designated as the "conscious" alpha rhythm, because of its close if not perfect resemblance to the normal alpha rhythms seen in conscious, purposefully responsive subjects. The second is designated as the "unconscious" alpha pattern because of the more or less close resemblance of this pattern to that of alpha activity as seen in the unconscious state of anesthesia. The contrast and similarity between the conscious alpha rhythm and the unconscious alpha pattern (Fig.

Figure 12.18. Reactive spindle pattern in a patient comatose 2 days after cardiac arrest *(upper segment)*. Patient experienced a complete neurologic recovery with a normal follow-up EEG *(lower segment)*.

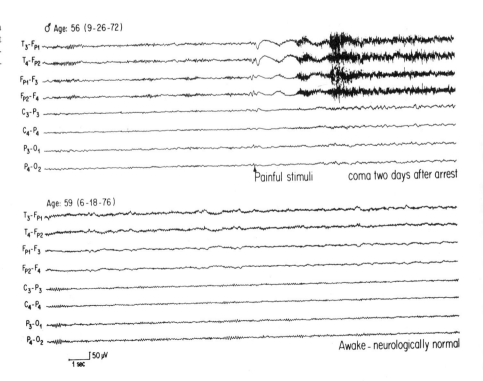

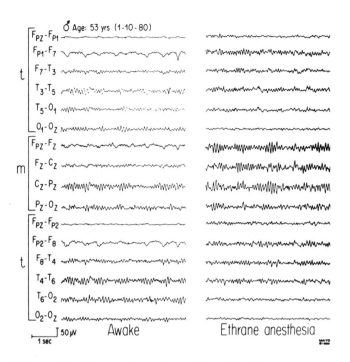

Figure 12.19. The normal posterior conscious alpha rhythm seen when a patient is awake is contrasted to the anterior unconscious alpha pattern seen under anesthesia (see text and Table 12.1 for further description).

Table 12.1. Conscious and Unconscious Alpha Patterns

	Normal Alpha Rhythm Conscious Alpha Pattern	Drug or Postarrest Unconscious Alpha Pattern
Temporal characteristics		
Frequency	Alpha	Alpha
Persistent	Persistent	Persistent
Spatial characteristics		
Peak	Posterior	Anterior
Boundary	Local	Widespread
Relational characteristics		
Relation to stimuli	Nonevoked, visually attenuated	Nonevoked, visually unattenuated

12.19) is outlined in Table 12.1 and can be summarized as follows. The conscious alpha rhythm has its peak located more posteriorly, with a local boundary, whereas the unconscious alpha pattern has its peak located anteriorly, with a widespread boundary. The frequency of both patterns by definition is usually in the alpha range, although with either the unconscious or conscious patterns the frequency may vary out of the alpha range into a faster (beta) frequency or a slower (theta) frequency. Both patterns are spontaneous rather than evoked and tend to occur in prolonged sequences. However, the conscious alpha rhythm is attenuated by eye opening, whereas the unconscious alpha pattern is unattenuated by eye opening. The unconscious pattern may be associated with other abnormal patterns, such as persistent irregular delta activity, but the conscious pattern may also be seen in association with persistent irregular delta activity. Therefore, the presence or absence of other abnormal patterns is not an absolute criterion for distinguishing the conscious from the unconscious alpha pattern.

Many of the patients with cerebral unresponsivity associated with the conscious alpha pattern on further examination may appear to be conscious with the absence of all or most purposeful responsiveness, due to either paralysis (locked-in state) (Figs. 12.17 and 12.20) or emotional factors (psychogenic unresponsiveness) (Chatrian, 1980; Grindal et al., 1977; Westmoreland et al., 1975). On the other hand, patients without purposeful responsiveness showing the unconscious alpha pattern usually do appear on closer examination to be truly unconscious (Figs. 12.19 and 12.20) (Grindal et al., 1977; Westmoreland et al., 1975). The possible mechanism for the latter unconscious alpha pattern, as well as its prognostic significance, is discussed in later sections.

As the EEG becomes more abnormal, there may be no patterns that resemble recognizable physiological activity. However, even if no recognizable physiological activity is maintained, higher voltage activity (usually greater than 50 mV) and reactivity (Fig. 12.21) tend to be of better prognostic significance than lower voltage patterns (less than 20 mV) and nonreactivity (Aoki and Lombroso, 1973) (Fig. 12.22).

The lower voltage patterns (less than 20 mV) may initially be intermittent (Brenner et al., 1975), but later become persis-

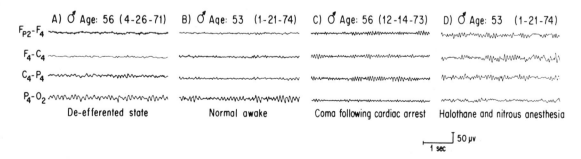

Figure 12.20. The alpha pattern in a patient locked-in due to brainstem infarction (**A**) appears to be a retention of the normal posterior (conscious) alpha rhythm seen in the normal awake individual (**B**). The posterior conscious alpha pattern, however, is clearly different from the anterior unconscious alpha pattern seen with postarrest unconsciousness (**C**) or with drug- or anesthetic-induced unconsciousness (**D**).

Figure 12.21. High-voltage PNDA and distorted FIRDA occurring as a response to stimulation in a comatose patient.

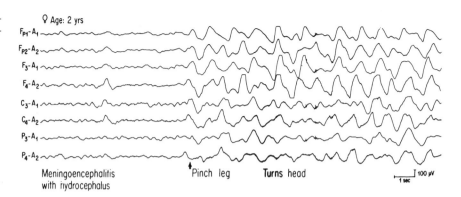

tent (Fig. 12.23). Obviously, the worst EEG finding is persistent electrocerebral inactivity (Figs. 12.22 to 12.24), defined for practical purposes as "no activity greater than 2 mV when using interelectrode distances of 10 cm or greater, a sensitivity of 2 mV/mm or greater, and other appropriate measures" (Guidelines in EEG, 1976; see also Chatrian, 1980).

All of the above patterns are quite nonspecific as far as etiology is concerned. However, there are specific EEG patterns that, when taken in context with the clinical picture, may suggest a specific etiology of impaired conscious purposeful responsiveness. These include such specific patterns as generalized spike and wave, making a diagnosis of confusion and stupor secondary to generalized seizure status. There are also periodic patterns that when taken in context with the clinical history may suggest a specific diagnosis such as Jakob-Creutzfeldt disease, SSPE, or herpes simplex encephalitis; there are other patterns as well that in an appropriate clinical setting suggest a particular etiology. However, these etiologically more specific patterns are discussed in later chapters. The nonspecific patterns described in the above section correlate more with severity of impaired cerebral hemispheric function rather than with etiology. The exact relationship of different EEG patterns and severity of cerebral functional impairment are discussed below (see Prognostic Significance of EEG Findings in an Unconscious Patient).

Limited Localizing Value

Most of the patterns mentioned above are widespread in distribution and give little information about localized path-

ology. Occasional exceptions to this general rule occur when there is marked attenuation of the abnormal pattern on the side of major intracranial pathology, such as a cerebral hemorrhage or massive subdural hematoma, which sometimes may not be clearly apparent based on clinical history (Fig. 12.25). Further, the combination of (a) an EEG showing relatively normal activity, (b) absent purposeful responsiveness, and (c) evidence of upper motor neuron involvement affecting all four extremities raises the real possibility of local brainstem disease (Fig. 12.17) versus a more widespread pathology (Chatrian, 1980). However, excluding these unusual situations, the patterns do not localize the disease to one particular area. Similar abnormalities may be seen with impaired consciousness due to cerebellar hemorrhage or to systemic toxic-metabolic conditions.

Prognostic Significance of EEG Findings in an Unconscious Patient

With the development of sophisticated capability for expensive, prolonged support of an unconscious life on one hand, and for lifesaving organ transplants on the other, it has become important to be able to make a reasonable prognosis concerning the chance that an unconscious patient, whether comatose or vegetative, has of regaining conscious life. For such predictions to be reasonably accurate, it is necessary to realize that a reliable prognosis requires the integration of three pieces of information. At the risk of oversimplification, these can be identified and defined as follows.

Figure 12.22. A,B: A 4-year-old demonstrates progressive decrease in EEG voltage associated with progressive clinical deterioration to cerebral death during the course of Reye's syndrome. **C:** A complete EEG satisfying the standard criteria showed no electrocerebral activity.

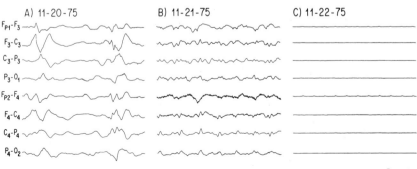

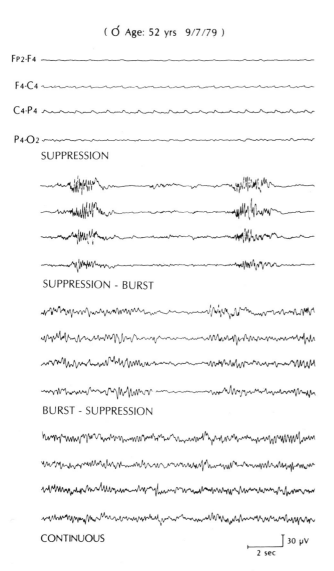

SUPPRESSION

SUPPRESSION - BURST

BURST - SUPPRESSION

CONTINUOUS   30 μV
                                            2 sec

Figure 12.23. Progressive EEG recovery after Pentothal given during hypothermia shows a progression from electrocerebral inactivity (first segment), to long suppression segments alternating with brief bursts (second segment), to prolonged rhythmic activity interrupted by brief attenuation (third segment), to the continuous unconscious alpha pattern (fourth segment). The reverse sequence of changes was more rapidly produced when the Pentothal was initially given.

Degree of Cerebral Functional Impairment

Unfortunately, in the absence of conscious purposeful responsiveness this cannot be adequately assessed based on the clinical examination alone. The clinical evaluation of impaired cerebral function depends entirely on the preservation of purposeful responsiveness. The absence of purposeful responsiveness effectively blocks clinical attempts to evaluate the degree of cerebral functional impairment; at times, it is clinically difficult to distinguish those cases in which there is little or no cerebral functional impairment with actual retention of consciousness from those in which there is the most severe cerebral functional impairment with total, or almost total, neuronal loss at the cerebral cortical level. Fortunately, even in such cases, the electroencepha-

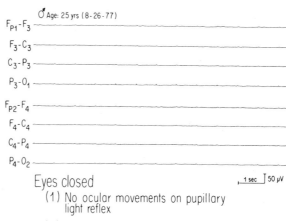

Eyes closed
(1) No ocular movements on pupillary light reflex
(2) Absent spontaneous respirations and calorics

Figure 12.24. No detectable cerebral activity at sensitivity 5 hours and short interelectrode distance 24 hours after cerebral death resulting from cardiovascular collapse consequent to brainstem infarction. (Notice detectable electrocardiogram in posterior derivation, indicating integrity of recording system. A full EEG following the accepted technical standards demonstrated no EEG activity.)

lographer continues to evaluate patterns of electrical activity at the cerebral cortical level. The EEG continues to give clues that help separate (a) those patients who are likely to be conscious in spite of absent purposeful responsiveness (Fig. 12.17), from (b) those who have severe impairment of cerebral hemispheric function to the degree of unconsciousness, nonetheless retaining a considerable amount of electrical activity (Figs. 12.16 and 12.18), from (c) those who are not only unconscious but who also have such extreme hemispheric functional impairment that they show no electrocerebral activity (Figs. 12.22 and 12.24). Therefore, in patients with absent purposeful responsiveness, the EEG becomes a most effective tool for evaluating whether the degree of cerebral functional impairment ranges from severe to extreme.

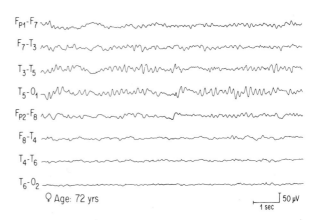

♀ Age: 72 yrs   50 μV
                                          1 sec

Figure 12.25. Right-sided attenuation of abnormal patterns correctly identifies the lateralization of an intracerebral hemorrhage resulting in flaccid, unresponsive coma without clinically localizing signs.

Chronicity and Evolution of Cerebral Functional Impairment

This is a very important factor in prognosis. Again, when purposeful responsiveness is absent, the clinical examination, which primarily looks at such functions as brainstem arousability and reflex activity at the brainstem and spinal cord level, may be misleading. This is because, in the absence of irreversible brainstem injury, prolonged survival usually is associated with recovery of brainstem function with return of brainstem arousability cycles and reflexes, even though patients may never recover enough cerebral hemispheric function to regain consciousness. In those cases, however, the EEG continues to give useful insights as to whether recovery is also simultaneously taking place at the cerebral level, even before clinical signs of conscious purposeful responsiveness return.

Potential Reversibility of Etiology

Obviously, this profoundly influences prognosis. Some conditions are relatively easily reversible, such as drug-induced coma in the absence of complicating cardiorespiratory impairment. Other conditions, such as postcardiorespiratory arrest, are much less readily reversible. Finally, there are conditions that not only are irreversible but tend to continually progress until death, including certain slow viral illnesses such as Jakob-Creutzfeldt disease and SSPE, as well as other progressive diseases.

Therefore, accurate prognosis is made difficult, because it depends on (a) the degree of cerebral functional impairment, (b) the chronicity and evolution of the impairment, and (c) the potential reversibility of the underlying etiology. A diagrammatic representation of how these three factors interact to influence the final prognosis for recovery of consciousness is presented in Table 12.2.

The influence of the severity of cerebral hemispheric functional impairment (as measured by EEG findings) on the ultimate prognosis for recovery of consciousness can be appreciated by recognizing that unconscious patients 24 hours after cardiac arrest with electrocerebral inactivity have no chance of recovering consciousness, whereas patients with retention of sleep spindles and good reactivity 24 hours after arrest (Fig. 12.18) have a reasonably good prog-

nosis of recovering their previous mental status barring additional superimposed complications.

An appreciation of the importance of chronicity can be achieved by recognizing that cerebral inactivity 3 minutes after cardiac arrest is quite compatible with good survival if resuscitation is initiated immediately, whereas electrocerebral inactivity persisting for 24 hours after resuscitation from cardiac arrest is not compatible with recovery of conscious life.

Finally, the important influence of the potential reversibility of the etiology upon the prognosis can be appreciated by recognizing that persistent electrocerebral inactivity for 24 hours during a drug coma without circulatory complications is compatible with complete recovery, in contrast to coma after cardiorespiratory arrest. Examples of EEG abnormalities of varying severity caused by etiology of varying degrees of reversibility (postencephalitic, posttraumatic, and postarrest unconsciousness) are reviewed in the following paragraphs.

The retention of recognizable sleep spindles in an unconscious patient is usually referred to in the literature as spindle coma (Klass and Daly, 1979). Here coma is defined loosely to cover the vegetative state as well as strict coma without brainstem arousability (Klass and Daly, 1979). However, in either case, the presence of spindles in coma is a good prognostic sign, regardless of whether it occurs in unconscious patients several days after cardiac arrest (Fig. 12.18) or in patients unconscious for several weeks with a nonprogressing condition such as a postencephalitic or posttraumatic state (Bergamasco et al., 1968; Chatrian et al., 1963; Klass and Daly, 1979; Scollo-Lavizzari, 1970). This does not mean that all unconscious patients with the spindle pattern recover; in such acutely ill patients, some may have irreversible brainstem injury or progressive disease or develop additional complications leading to additional irreversible injury or death.

The unconscious alpha pattern described in the previous section for the state of anesthesia not surprisingly is indistinguishable from that seen in drug overdose coma (Carroll and Mastaglia, 1979; Grindal et al., 1977), which clearly is nothing more than an unsupervised self-induced anesthetic state. However, an unconscious alpha pattern essentially identical to that seen in anesthesia and drug overdose coma be seen within several days after the onset of postarrest coma or even in a vegetative state (Grindal et al., 1977; Westmoreland et al., 1975).

Although the unconscious alpha pattern seen in anesthesia and drug-induced coma is quite similar to and at times indistinguishable from the unconscious alpha pattern seen in the postarrest state (Fig. 12.20), the ultimate prognosis is usually quite different. The cases of anesthesia and drug-induced coma progressively improve, with recovery of normal consciousness (Carroll and Mastaglia, 1979). Most of the postarrest cases either die in a subsequent arrest or survive for varying lengths of time in the vegetative state (Grindal et al., 1977; Westmoreland et al., 1975) (Fig. 12.22). The only postarrest cases that have recovered consciousness are those with arrests associated with electrocution (Grindal et al., 1977); it is possible that those cases involve a more reversible cause of the unconscious alpha pattern than is usually seen in arrest cases uncomplicated by electrocution.

Table 12.2. Prognosis for Recovery from Impaired Cerebral Function

(1) Functional impairment increases		
	(2) Chronicity without improvement increases	
		(3) Irreversibility of etiology increases

Increasingly poor prognosis for recovery of previous conscious cerebral life even if chronic, vegetative brainstem survival is possible.

However, any initial uncertainty about prognosis can be clarified by following the evolution of the unconscious alpha pattern with sequential EEG. In readily reversible drug- or anesthetic-induced patterns, there is a progressive improvement of the EEG with recovery of consciousness (Carroll and Mastaglia, 1979; Grindal et al., 1977). In post-arrest cases destined not to recover consciousness, the EEG deteriorates progressively, and usually there is a very low voltage, irregular, nonreactive pattern (Westmoreland et al., 1975) (Fig. 12.25).

If no recognizable physiological pattern can be detected, high voltage (greater than 50 mV) reactive abnormalities (Fig. 12.21) are generally a better prognostic sign than a persistently low voltage (less than 20 mV) nonreactive abnormality (Fig. 12.22), provided other factors such as chronicity and reversibility of etiology are equal (Aoki and Lombroso, 1973).

In an unconscious patient, low-voltage patterns of less than 20 mV represent a more severe abnormality and may alternate with higher voltage patterns producing first a picture of brief, intermittent suppression (Brenner et al., 1975), followed by more prolonged, intermittent suppression (Fig. 12.23). In more extreme cases, a low-voltage pattern may persist throughout; as the voltage of all activity persistently drops below detectable levels of 2 mV, the EEG stage of electrocerebral inactivity is reached (Chatrian, 1980) (Figs. 12.22 to 12.24). This latter pattern of electrocerebral inactivity is the worst of all EEG findings, indicating the most extreme state of cerebral hemispheric functional impairment. However, as mentioned above, even with this most extreme degree of impairment of cerebral hemispheric function, the prognosis not only depends on the absence of electrocerebral activity but also is strongly influenced by the reversibility of etiology. Such a pattern even if persistent for 24 hours is compatible with complete recovery of function if it is a drug-induced unconsciousness without cardiopulmonary complications. It is incompatible with recovery of consciousness if it is a postarrest unconsciousness (Chatrian, 1980).

Over the years, the laudable efforts of the EEG community to establish the criteria for electrocerebral inactivity (Chatrian, 1980; Guidelines for EEG, 1976) and its relationship to cerebral death have tended to obscure the following very important fact: Whether there is no electrocerebral activity above 2 mV or whether there is some activity between 2 and 5 mV does not materially alter the prognosis for recovery of consciousness provided that other factors such as chronicity and etiology are the same. The presence of some activity, however, does increase the likelihood that the patient's brainstem may have enough residual integrity to recover cycles of arousability, thus producing the vegetative state. This emphasizes the important point that, although chronic retention of some minimal electrocerebral activity due to some neuronal survival at the cerebral cortical level is not in itself adequate for the recovery of conscious life, it is usually associated with enough residual integrity at the brainstem level to allow for prolonged survival in the vegetative state if good, supportive medical care is given. In these cases, serious ethical and financial questions often arise. How long should these patients be supported with in-

tensive medical care? When intensive medical support is replaced by minimal supportive care of nutrition and hygiene, should antibiotics and other special medical treatment also be discontinued?

Mechanisms Responsible for EEG Findings in States with Cerebral Unresponsivity

When the absence of cerebral responsiveness is due to paralysis (the locked-in state) or a psychogenic cause (functional unresponsiveness), the patterns understandably appear to be simply a retention of a normal rhythm.

The presence of spindles and sleep-like activity in a persistently unconscious patient (whether unarousable and comatose or arousable but vegetative) most likely is related to the retention of enough physiological integrity of the cerebral cortex and subcortical regions so that generation of spindles is possible in spite of the absence of enough integrity of these structures to elaborate consciousness (Fig. 12.17). If this tentative interpretation is correct, it is not surprising, then, that many of these patients ultimately do well, because their unconsciousness is nonetheless associated with a considerable retention of functional integrity, giving them a reasonable chance for recovery, all other factors of chronicity and etiology being equal.

Widespread PNDA in association with impaired (Figs. 12.14 and 12.15) or absent (Fig. 12.16) consciousness is of less certain etiology. Evidence obtained from studies of encephalopathies producing widespread PNDA and associated with morphologically identifiable pathology at postmortem demonstrated that the pathology is primarily in the subcortical white matter (Gloor et al., 1968). At first glance, it is not obvious how such a theory would explain the appearance of irregular delta activity in the anesthetic state, where it seems more likely that the anesthesia exerts its effect at the synaptic level and not on the subcortical white matter. What appears to be an apparent discrepancy may be explicable based on the proposal (Gloor et al., 1977; Klass and Daly, 1979) that the primary pathology responsible for PNDA may be due to cortical deafferentation. If this is indeed the case, it would be possible to accomplish such cortical deafferentation either due to primary white matter disease or due to interference with synaptic input to the cortex directly by drugs or by metabolic means. However, the final answer to this question needs additional experimental investigation.

With the unconscious alpha pattern in anesthesia, there is fairly convincing evidence to suggest that it may be nothing more than a variant of the usual drug-induced beta rhythm that has been slowed into the alpha range with the onset of unconsciousness and anesthesia. In these cases, it is possible on the routine EEG to follow the first appearance of beta activity and then to see it become more widespread and slow in frequency as consciousness is lost (Fig. 12.26). Simultaneously with this, if present at the time of induction, the posterior waking alpha pattern tends to slow in frequency into the theta range before disappearing. This gives way to the unconscious alpha pattern mentioned above, which is itself likely to be a slowed variant of the drug-induced beta rhythms in the waking state. The relationship between these two patterns is further suggested by the fact that, with emer-

Figure 12.26. The EEG in a postarrest patient *(upper segments)* evolved from burst suppression, to the unconscious alpha pattern, to a low-voltage PNDA pattern 14 days after arrest with the patient remaining in the chronic vegetative state. In contrast, in a case of drug-induced coma *(lower segment)*, the EEG evolved from burst suppression, to the unconscious alpha pattern, to the normal conscious alpha rhythm 14 days later with complete neurological recovery.

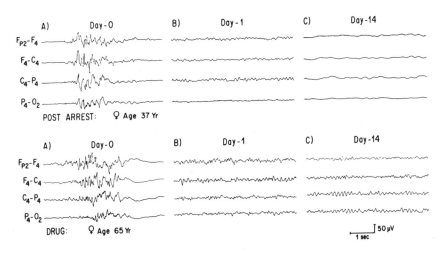

gence from anesthesia, the anterior unconscious alpha pattern increases in frequency into the beta range as the posterior alpha-range pattern reappears. This latter transition may be seen even before consciousness is verified by the patient's response to commands from the anesthesiologist.

Based on the above analogy, it seems quite reasonable to assume that the alpha pattern in drug-induced unconsciousness is, like the similar pattern under anesthesia, nothing more than a slowed variant of the drug-induced beta rhythm (Carroll and Mastaglia, 1979). The unconscious alpha pattern after arrest bears remarkable similarity, in terms of spatial and temporal characteristics and its lack of reactivity to visual stimuli, to the pattern seen in anesthesia or drug-induced unconsciousness (Carroll and Mastaglia, 1979; Grindal et al., 1977) (Figs. 12.20 and 12.27). Because of this close resemblance, it is tempting to postulate that both have similar mechanisms. However, since the basic mechanisms responsible for even the drug-induced beta rhythm are not known, and postarrest unconscious alpha pattern is often a transitional phenomenon that later disappears without recovery of consciousness (Westmoreland et al., 1975) (Fig. 12.26), further investigation of the basic mechanisms of all of these patterns will be necessary before anything more than the fact that they do have similar characteristics can be established. The similarity may make it impossible in an individual case to distinguish the pattern associated with a readily reversible stage of anesthesia from a transitional stage in severe postarrest brain injury, which will result in the vegetative state in cases with prolonged survival.

In summary, the above EEG findings in different stages of impaired, conscious, purposeful responsiveness are etiologically nonspecific, and the mechanisms responsible for their generation are only partially understood. However, in spite of these limitations, when the EEG findings are taken in context with other information concerning etiology and chronicity, they may be helpful in arriving more quickly at an accurate prognosis concerning the patient's chance of recovering his previous conscious life.

Focal Persistent EEG Findings Usually Associated with Focal Cerebral Disturbance

As was done in the preceding section on bilateral persistent EEG findings, focal persistent EEG abnormalities can

be divided into the following general descriptive types. These are (a) distortion and disappearance of normal patterns, (b) appearance and increase of abnormal patterns, and (c) disappearance of all patterns.

There is some overlap in the first two types of abnormalities, since abnormal rhythms may be related to the distortion of previously recognized normal rhythms. Disappearance of

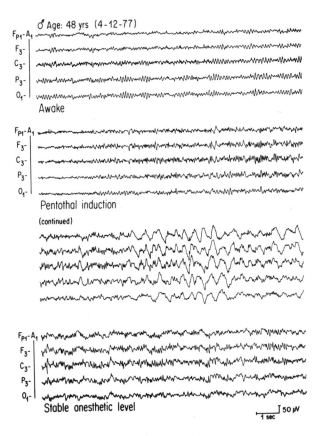

Figure 12.27. With Pentothal induction, the posterior conscious alpha rhythm *(upper segment)* disappears as 20-Hz beta appears and slows into the 14-Hz range *(second segment)*. This slowed beta pattern slows further into the alpha range, at first being intermixed with intermittent rhythmic slow *(third segment)* before developing into the stable unconscious alpha pattern of anesthesia *(fourth segment)*.

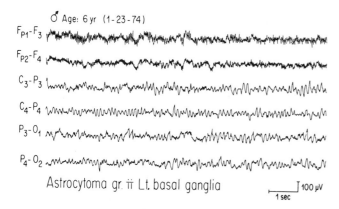

Astrocytoma gr. ﬁ Lt. basal ganglia

Figure 12.28. Higher amplitude beta activity ipsilateral to a left basoganglial astrocytoma.

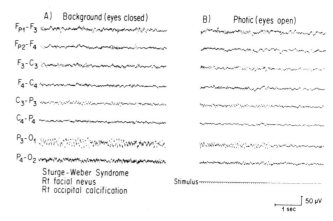

Sturge-Weber Syndrome
Rt facial nevus
Rt occipital calcification

Figure 12.30. Alpha activity, as well as photic driving, is reduced on the right in a patient with right occipital calcification with Sturge-Weber syndrome. The patient had infrequent focal seizures with a normal interictal neurological examination, including formal visual fields.

all rhythms in a focal area can seldom be seen at the cerebral cortex, although they may be detected with electrocorticography (Hess, 1975).

The focal distortion of normal rhythms may produce an asymmetry of amplitude, frequency, or reactivity of the rhythm. Amplitude asymmetries alone, unless extreme, are the least reliable finding. Amplitude may be increased (Fig. 12.28) or decreased (Figs. 12.29 and 12.30) on the side of focal abnormality. However, if there is focal slowing of physiological rhythms (for example, the alpha rhythm) by 1 Hz or more, this usually identifies reliably the side of focal abnormality, whether or not the amplitude of the rhythm is increased or decreased (Kooi et al., 1978). The unilateral loss of reactivity of a physiological rhythm, such as the loss of reactivity of the alpha rhythm to eye opening (Bancaud et al., 1955) or to mental alerting (Westmoreland and Klass, 1971) (Fig. 12.31) also reliably identifies the focal side of abnormality. Because of shifting asynchronies and asymmetries of the mu rhythm, the exact limits of normal asymmetry become more difficult to define; however, the asymmetrical

slowing of the central mu rhythm by 1 Hz or more, usually associated with an increase in amplitude, is a reliable sign of focal abnormality, often of a chronic nature (Cobb, 1976; Cobb and Muller, 1954). In addition to the waking rhythms discussed above, the normal activity of sleep-inducing spindles and vertex waves may be distorted or lost by a focal lesion in the appropriate distribution.

As normal rhythms are distorted, focal abnormalities may produce focal PNDA, one of the most reliable findings of a focal cerebral disturbance. The more persistent, the less reactive, and the more nonrhythmic and polymorphic such focal slowing, the more reliable an indicator it becomes for the presence of a focal cerebral disturbance (Cobb, 1976; Hess, 1975; Klass and Daly, 1979) (Figs. 12.32 to 12.36).

IRDA may be seen with a focal cerebral disturbance (Figs. 12.6 to 12.8) but, as mentioned earlier, it is both nonspecific, as far as etiology, and nonlocalizing. When present in association with a focal cerebral lesion, it usually implies

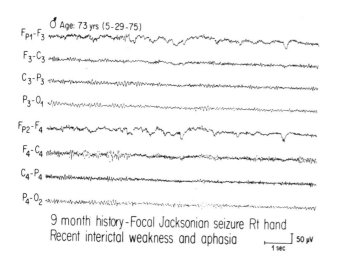

9 month history-Focal Jacksonian seizure Rt hand
Recent interictal weakness and aphasia

Figure 12.29. Lower amplitude beta activity ipsilateral to a left frontal astrocytoma.

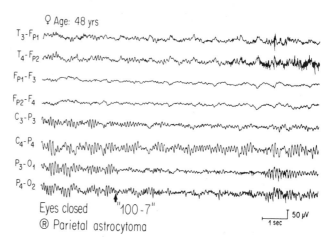

Eyes closed   "100-7"
Ⓡ Parietal astrocytoma

Figure 12.31. Reduced attenuation of alpha activity with mental alerting correctly identifies the hemisphere involved with a right parietal astrocytoma.

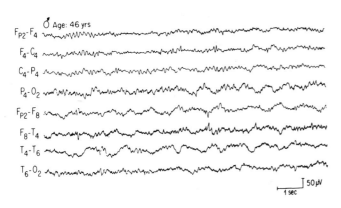

Figure 12.32. Focal PPDA and decreased background voltage on the side of a right temporal astrocytoma.

that the pathological process is beginning to produce an active widespread brain disturbance likely to be associated with clinical signs of an acute or subacute confusional episode or encephalopathy.

Focal epileptiform abnormality may occur in association with focal cerebral abnormalities, but because they have a relatively specific association with additional symptomatology such as epilepsy, they are not discussed here.

Etiological Nonspecificity

The above abnormalities do not reflect the underlying etiology but simply reflect that a pathophysiological process is present. Similar abnormalities may occur, whether they result from focal inflammation, trauma, vascular disease, brain tumor, or almost any other cause of focal cortical disturbance, including an asymmetrical onset of CNS degenerative diseases.

Figure 12.33. Focal persistent delta slowing (PNDA type) and reduced background activity on the side of a right subdural hematoma.

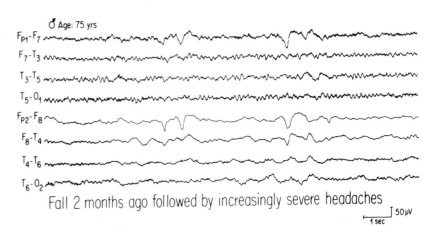

Figure 12.34. Focal persistent delta slowing (PNDA type) and reduced background voltage on the side of a left middle cerebral infarct occurring 2 days previously and associated with a residual dysphasia but a negative computed tomography (CT) scan.

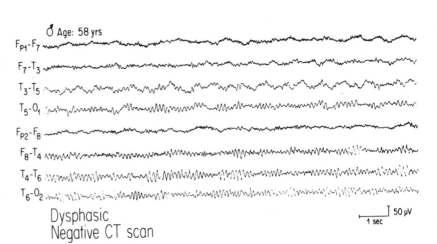

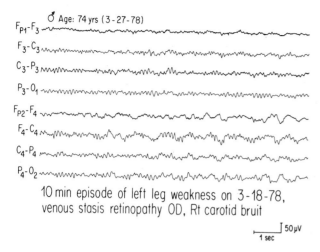

♂ Age: 74 yrs (3-27-78)

F_P1-F3
F3-C3
C3-P3
P3-O1
F_P2-F4
F4-C4
C4-P4
P4-O2

10 min episode of left leg weakness on 3-18-78, venous stasis retinopathy OD, Rt carotid bruit

50 μV
1 sec

Figure 12.35. Residual focal persistent delta slowing (PNDA type) 9 days after a right cerebral transient ischemic attack lasting 10 minutes. This patient had decreased retinal artery pressures and a carotid bruit on the right associated with an occluded right carotid.

Persistent Focal Abnormalities and Other Evidence of Focal Cerebral Disease

In general, no matter what the etiology, there is a rough correlation between the EEG evidence of focal cerebral disturbance and clinical as well as radiographic evidence of focal cerebral disturbance. However, in spite of this rough relationship, there are striking examples of lack of correlation in both directions. Some of this lack of correlation is understandable. For instance, a small infarct in the internal capsule is likely to be missed both by radiographic studies and EEG studies, in spite of the fact that its presence may be

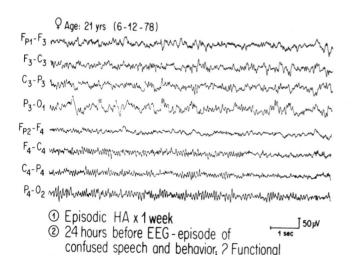

♀ Age: 21 yrs (6-12-78)

F_P1-F3
F3-C3
C3-P3
P3-O1
F_P2-F4
F4-C4
C4-P4
P4-O2

① Episodic HA x 1 week
② 24 hours before EEG - episode of confused speech and behavior; ? Functional
③ Asymptomatic during EEG

50 μV
1 sec

Figure 12.36. Focal persistent delta slowing (PNDA type) and reduced voltage of background activity in a patient now asymptomatic 24 hours after a left cerebral attack of complicated migraine. The CT scan was also negative.

readily detected by significant abnormalities on clinical examination. On the other hand, both the clinical examination and the EEG may be strikingly normal in spite of the fact that the CT scan shows evidence of a well-described cystic or calcified lesion in the silent area of the brain, which may have been present in a relatively nonprogressive form for a long period of time. Finally, the EEG may show major abnormalities in spite of a normal clinical examination with positive CT findings, provided the lesion is in a clinically silent area, such as one temporal or frontal lobe. With a transient ischemic attack, it is common for the clinical examination, the radiographic studies, and the EEG to be normal within attacks.

Nonetheless, in the author's experience, that small percentage of patients with transient ischemic attacks on a hemodynamic basis, rather than on the more common embolic basis, may retain a major EEG abnormality in spite of the fact that their CT scan is normal and their neurological examination has returned to normal after the transient attack (Fig. 12.35). The exact mechanism responsible for this is uncertain, but it is interesting to note that another apparent hemodynamic cause of transient neurological deficit in complicated migraine also may be associated with a marked residual EEG abnormality even when the neurological examination has returned to normal and even when the CT scan is normal (Fig. 12.36). Finally, it is not uncommon for the EEG to show clear-cut abnormalities and focal lesions without neurological deficit or CT abnormalities when there is an associated epileptogenic process.

Chronic widespread hemispheric disease, such as Sturge-Weber syndrome or infantile hemiplegia, characteristically produces widespread voltage attenuation over the abnormal hemisphere. In one study, this electrographic accompaniment was seen in every patient with Sturge-Weber disease even when there was no associated focal neurological deficit (Fig. 12.30). These asymmetries were noted even in young children prior to the development of the characteristic intracranial calcifications (Brenner and Sharbrough, 1976). Finally, local contusion or inflammatory disease may produce a dramatic and marked EEG change without CT accompaniment and with or without accompanying focal clinical deficit, depending on the location and intensity of the abnormality. However, even when the EEG picks up subclinical abnormalities not associated with roentgenographic changes, the abnormalities in general are quite nonspecific and require close correlation with the clinical history and other information before arriving at a specific diagnosis.

Focal EEG Findings and Skull Defects

Provided that there is no significant injury to the underlying generators, a skull defect produced by a craniotomy or a previous fracture can alter the voltage of the scalp-recorded potential in two different ways, depending on the orientation of the dipole axis of the generator to the bony defect. When the dipole axis of the generator is oriented perpendicular to the bony defect (as it is for underlying cortical neuronal generators), the skull defect usually increases the amplitude of the scalp-recorded potentials from

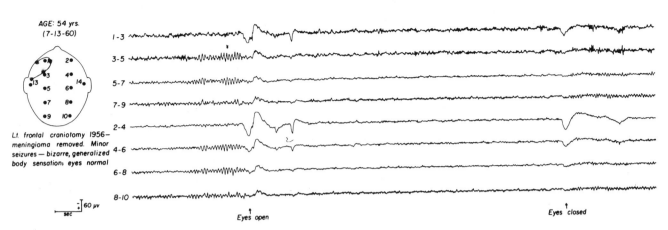

Figure 12.37. The voltage of beta activity is increased, whereas the voltage of eye blink and eye movement artifact is decreased on the side of a left-sided craniotomy. (See text for possible explanation of these phenomena.)

underlying generators. However, when the axis of the generator is parallel to the skull defect (as it is for the corneal-retinal potential of the eye underlying a frontal craniotomy), then the defect decreases the amplitude of the scalp-recorded potentials from the generator (Fig. 12.37). It is not intuitively clear why this same craniotomy has opposing effects on the amplitude of the scalp-recorded transmission from generators depending on whether the axis of the generator is oriented perpendicular or parallel to the skull defect. Mechanisms responsible for this phenomenon are discussed in a later section.

Because the axes of cerebral neuronal generators in the underlying cortex are consistently oriented at right angles to the overlying skull, a defect tends to increase their voltage recorded at scalp electrodes (Cobb et al., 1979). The tendency of the skull defect to increase such pickup may be offset injury (due to surgical intervention at the time of a craniotomy, due to trauma at the time of a skull fracture, or due to intrinsic pathology) to the underlying cerebral cortex, which tends to reduce the amplitude of the overlying scalp pickup. The net result as far as asymmetry of potentials from cerebral sources then depends on whether the depression of the cerebral cortical generators due to injury is great enough to offset the improved transmission due to the skull defect. This effect may change with time in any individual. For example, in the acute postoperative period after a temporal lobectomy, it is not uncommon to see lower amplitude background activity on the side of the craniotomy during the acute period of cerebral edema. However, in chronic follow-up recordings done months or years later, the amplitude of the background activity is often increased on the side of the craniotomy.

The complicated interaction of the above factors can be summarized as follows. The scalp-recorded potentials from cerebral cortical generators underlying a skull defect tend to be increased in amplitude unless acute or chronic injury has resulted in significant depression of underlying generator activity.

Mechanisms Responsible for EEG Findings Associated with Focal Cerebral Disturbance

In the absence of a clear-cut understanding of the mechanisms responsible for the generation of normal EEG activity, an accurate explanation of how focal cerebral disturbances result in distortion in the amplitude, frequency, and reactivity of normal scalp-recorded rhythms is not possible. However, in general, these distortions occur because focal abnormalities may alter the interconnections, number, frequency, synchrony, voltage output, and axis orientation of individual neuron generators, as well as the size and location and integrity of the cortical area containing the individual generators giving rise to the total signal ultimately detected on the scalp.

The theoretical origin of focal persistent nonrhythmic polymorphic delta activity has been touched on in the previous sections discussing generalized PNDA. In summary, there is general agreement among various researchers that focal pathology in the underlying white matter is commonly associated with PNDA (Gloor et al., 1977; Hess, 1975; Klass and Daly, 1979). In these cases, it is postulated that the white matter lesions produce PNDA by deafferenting the overlying cortex from its underlying white matter input. If so, this theory could also be extended to explain focal PNDA occurring postictally. Although it would not be reasonable to explain postictal focal PNDA on the basis of a primary white matter disturbance, it is reasonable to assume that the postictal state, either by exhaustion or inhibition, may functionally deafferent the cortex from its underlying white matter input. Finally, even if deafferentation of the cerebral cortex from its underlying white matter is the primary mechanism responsible for PNDA, whether focal or generalized, additional factors such as the acuteness or changing nature of the deafferentation would have to be postulated as additional important factors, inasmuch as PNDA is more commonly associated with acute, active disturbances and less commonly seen in chronic, stable disturbances (Kooi et al., 1978).

The mechanisms presumed to be responsible for bilateral IRDA have been discussed previously and are not reviewed here.

The cardiology literature discusses the theoretical explanation of why decreasing the resistance between a generator and an overlying surface may either increase or decrease the recorded surface voltage depending on whether the dipole axis of the generators is oriented perpendicularly (in which case the recorded surface voltage increases) or parallel (in which case the recorded surface voltage decreases) (Voukydis, 1974). This theoretical explanation is intricate and, at times, difficult to follow. However, a simple intuitive appreciation of the result may be grasped if one conceives of the scalp-recorded potential as being influenced by two competing circuits. One of the circuits, which includes the resistance of the skull perpendicular to and in series with the axis of the generator, transfers the generator signal to the scalp. The other circuit, which includes the skull resistance parallel to the dipole axis of the generator, shunts or diverts the generator signal from the scalp. This crude analogy predicts the observed changes resulting from the resistance decrease due to a frontal craniotomy. This decrease in resistance, which is in series with the dipole axis of neuronal generators, increases the transfer to the scalp recording electrodes. On the other hand, this decrease in resistance, which is in parallel to the dipole axis of the corneal-retinal potential, diverts and decreases the eye blink and eye movement potential being transferred to the scalp electrodes (Fig. 12.37).

As previously mentioned, the alteration of scalp-recorded EEG activity overlying a skull defect is influenced not only by the change in resistance due to the skull defect and the original characteristics of the underlying cortical generator, but also by injury to the cortical generator. In general, unless the injury is severe, the amplitude of normal and abnormal activity is likely to be increased by the effect of the craniotomy. Therefore, lower voltage patterns recorded over the side of the craniotomy suggest significant underlying cortical injury that may be temporary or permanent.

General Summaries and Conclusions

The nonspecific EEG abnormalities discussed in the preceding sections can be best thought of as electrical signs of cerebral dysfunction that may add new or confirmatory information about the patient's clinical condition. Although none of the findings in themselves are specific for a single etiology, taken in context with the clinical history they may be helpful in deciding between one of several possibilities (for example, functional versus organic), as well as in following the evolution of abnormality and giving prognostic information, especially in unconscious patients. In addition, EEG findings may suggest that additional studies and follow-up evaluation are needed. The nonspecific EEG findings were discussed under their usual clinical correlations, which are:

1. Widespread intermittent slow abnormalities, usually associated with active widespread brain dysfunction

2. Bilateral persistent abnormalities, usually associated with impaired conscious cerebral responsivity, and

3. Focal abnormalities, usually associated with focal cerebral disturbance.

Identification and categorization of these signs allows the EEG to be used as a dynamic tool to investigate function, especially if applied during the acute and evolving stages of various neurological conditions and if correlated with other available information. The specific EEG findings discussed in the following chapter are often helpful in giving additional insight into specific pathophysiologic reactions, such as epilepsy, or specific disease processes, such as SSPE or Jakob-Creutzfeldt.

References

Aoki, Y., and Lombroso, C. 1973. Prognostic value of electroencephalography in Reye's syndrome. Neurology (Minneapolis) 23:333–343.

Bancaud, J., Hécaen, H., and Lairy, G.C. 1955. Modifications de la réactivité E.E.G., troubles des fonctions symboliques et troubles confusionnels dans les lésions hémisphériques localisées. Electroencephalogr. Clin. Neurophysiol. 7:179.

Beecher, H.K. 1968. A definition of irreversible coma. Report of the Ad Hoc Committee of the Harvard Medical School to examine the definition of brain death. JAMA 205:337.

Bergamasco, B., Bergamini, L., Doriguzzi, T., et al. 1968. EEG sleep patterns as a prognostic criterion in post traumatic coma. Electroencephalogr. Clin. Neurophysiol. 24:374–377.

Boddie, H., Banna, M., and Bradley, W.G. 1974. "Benign" intracranial hypertension. Brain 97:313–326.

Brenner, R., and Sharbrough, F. 1976. Electroencephalographic evaluation in Sturge-Weber syndrome. Neurology 26:629–632.

Brenner, R., Schwartzman, R., and Richey, E. 1975. Prognostic significance of episodic low amplitude or relatively isoelectric EEG patterns. Dis. Nerv. Syst. 36:582.

Carroll, W., and Mastaglia, F. 1979. Alpha and beta coma in drug intoxication uncomplicated by cerebral hypoxia. Electroencephalogr. Clin. Neurophysiol. 46:95–105.

Chase, T., Moretti, L., and Prensky, A. 1968. Clinical and electroencephalographic manifestations of vascular lesions of the pons. Neurology 18:357.

Chatrian, G. 1980. Electrophysiologic evaluation of brain death: a critical appraisal. In *Electrodiagnosis in Clinical Neurology*, Ed. M. Aminoff. New York: Churchill Livingstone.

Chatrian, G., White, L. Jr., and Daly, D. 1963. Electroencephalographic patterns resembling those of sleep in certain comatose states after injuries to the head. Electroencephalogr. Clin. Neurophysiol. 15:272–280.

Cobb, W. (Ed.). 1976. Part B. EEG interpretation in clinical medicine. In *Handbook of Electroencephalography and Clinical Neurophysiology*, vol. 11, Ed.-in-chief, A. Remond. Amsterdam: Elsevier.

Cobb, W., and Muller, G. 1954. Parietal focal theta rhythm. Electroencephalogr. Clin. Neurophysiol. 6:455.

Cobb, W., Guiloff, R., and Cast, J. 1979. Breach rhythm: the EEG related to skull defects. Electroencephalogr. Clin. Neurophysiol. 47:251–271.

Daly, D. 1968. The effect of sleep upon the electroencephalogram in patients with brain tumors. Electroencephalogr. Clin. Neurophysiol. 25:521–529.

Daly, D., Whelan, J., Bickford, R., et al. 1953. The electroencephalogram in cases of tumors of the posterior fossa and third ventricle. Electroencephalogr. Clin. Neurophysiol. 5:203–216.

Faure, J., Drooglever-Fortuyn, J., Gastaut, H., et al. 1951. De la génèse et de la signification des rhythmes recueillis à distance dans les cas de tumeurs cérébrales. Electroencephalogr Clin. Neurophysiol. 3:429–434.

Gloor, P., Kalabay, O., and Giard, N. 1968. The electroencephalogram in diffuse encephalopathies: electroencephalographic correlates of grey and white matter lesions. Brain 91:779–802.

Gloor, P., Ball, G., and Schaul, N. 1977. Brain lesions that produce delta waves in the EEG. Neurology (Minneapolis) 27:326–333.

Grindal, A., Suter, C., and Martinez, A. 1977. Alpha-pattern coma: 24 cases with 9 survivors. Ann. Neurol. 1:371–377.

Guidelines in EEG No. 1. 1976. *Minimal Technical Standards for EEG Recording in Suspected Cerebral Death.* Willoughby, OH: American EEG Society.

Hess, R. (Ed.) 1975. Part C. Brain tumors and other space occupying processes. In *Handbook of Electroencephalography and Clinical Neurophysiology,* vol. 14, Ed.-in-chief, A. Remond. Amsterdam: Elsevier.

Klass, D., and Daly, D. (Eds.) 1979. *Current Practice of Clinical Electroencephalography,* 1st ed. New York: Raven Press.

Kooi, K., Tucker, R., and Marshall, R. 1978. *Fundamentals of Electroencephalography,* 2nd ed. Hagerstown, MD: Harper & Row.

Markand, O. 1976. Electroencephalogram in "locked-in" syndrome. Electroencephalogr. Clin. Neurophysiol. 40:529.

Martinius, J., Matthes, A., and Lombroso, C. 1968. Electroencephalographic features in posterior fossa tumors in children. Electroencephalogr. Clin. Neurophysiol. 25:128–139.

Normand, M.M., Wszolek, Z.K., and Lass, D.W. 1995. Temporal intermittent rhythmic delta activity in electroencephalograms. J. Clin. Neurophysiol. 12:280–284.

Penin, H. 1971. Das EEG der symptomatischen Psychosen. Nervenarzt 42:242.

Reither, J., Beaudry, M., and Leduc, C.P. 1989. Temporal intermittent rhythmic delta activity (TIRDA) and the diagnosis of complex partial epilepsy: sensitivity, specificity and predictive value. Can. J. Neurol. Sci. 16:398–401.

Schaul, N., Gloor, P., and Gotman, J. 1981a. The EEG in deep midline lesions. Neurology (New York) 31:157–167.

Schaul, N., Lueders, H., and Sachdev, K. 1981b. Generalized bilaterally synchronous bursts of slow waves in the EEG. Arch. Neurol. 38:690–692.

Scollo-Lavizzari, A. 1970. The effect of sleep on EEG abnormalities at a distance from the lesion: all night study of 30 cases. Eur. Neurol. 3:65–87.

Sidell, A., and Daly, D. 1961. The electroencephalogram in cases of benign intracranial hypertension. Neurology (Minneapolis) 11:413–417.

Voukydis, P. 1974. Effect of intracardiac blood on the electrocardiogram. N. Engl. J. Med. 291:612.

Walker, A.E. 1977. An appraisal of the criteria of cerebral death. A summary statement: a collaboration study. JAMA 237:982.

Westmoreland, B., and Klass, D. 1971. Asymmetrical attenuation of alpha activity with arithmetical attention. Electroencephalogr. Clin. Neurophysiol. 31:634–635(abst).

Westmoreland, B., Klass, D., Sharbrough, F., et al. 1975. Alpha coma: EEG, clinical, pathologic and etiologic correlations. Arch. Neurol. 32:713.

Zurek, R., Schiemann-Delgado, J., Froescher, W., et al. 1985. Frontal intermittent rhythmical delta activity and anterior bradyrhythmia. Clin. Electroencephalogr. 16:1–10.

13. Abnormal EEG Patterns: Epileptic and Paroxysmal

Ernst Niedermeyer

Electroencephalography has revolutionized the entire field of epileptology. This chapter discusses the role of the electroencephalogram (EEG) in the epilepsies, including electrical-clinical correlations in various epileptic conditions, and the semiology of the electrical signals that are contributory to the EEG diagnosis of epileptic phenomena in ictal states or in the interseizure interval.

The interictal paroxysmal phenomena is discussed first. These discharges represent the basic elements of more complex ictal patterns.

Principal Differences Between Interictal and Ictal Discharges

A distinction is made between ictal and interictal paroxysmal activity. This logical differentiation, however, is beset with great difficulties. It is sometimes difficult or even impossible to distinguish between ictal-clinical, ictal-subclinical, and interictal paroxysmal EEG activity, even with the use of neuropsychological tests. We must acknowledge the existence of a gray zone between interictal and ictal paroxysmal activities.

Sudden Change of Frequency

There are valid guidelines for the detection of true ictal events. The onset of a clinical seizure may be characterized by a sudden change of frequency. A new type of rhythm appears, hesitantly, then more distinctly; soon it boldly dominates the tracing. This rhythm may be in alpha frequency or it may be faster or slower; it clearly demonstrates a new element of the tracing, indicative of a completely new electrophysiological event. The abnormal rhythm may or may not show spiky character. It tends to become slower with increasing amplitudes and more distinct spiky phases of the rhythmical waves.

Sudden Loss of Voltage

Sudden "desynchronization" of electrical activity is found in *electrodecremental seizures*. The onset of these attacks may look almost flat locally and/or diffusely, but extremely fast very low voltage activity may gradually increase in voltage with decreasing frequencies. Ictal rhythmical activity may soon become preponderant, similar to that found in the sudden change of frequency. Arroyo et al. (1994) have stressed the role of the frontal lobes in electrodecremental seizures. Electrodecremental represents the most common EEG expression of infantile spasms occurring in the West syndrome (Kellaway, 1959; Ohtahara and Yamatogi, 1990).

Sudden Increase of Voltage

The classical example is the sudden steep rise of amplitude in a classical petit mal absence with 3/sec spike waves. There is hence considerable variability in the ictal EEG events. This has been quite discouraging for those concentrating on automatic devices for seizure detection. Even the eye of the experienced electroencephalographer may have difficulties in the determination of ictal episodes.

Ultraslow and Ultrafast Frequencies

These two aspects of paroxysmal activity are about to play an increasing role in the understanding of epileptiform EEG activity. For this reason, two new chapters have been added to this edition: Chapter 25 on infraslow activities by Vanhatalo et al. and Chapter 26 on ultrafast frequencies by Curio. In Chapter 27, on epileptic seizure disorders, there is also much emphasis being placed on those new "building blocks" of epileptic activity.

In the following discussion, the conventional approach is used with spikes and spike-related discharges as the centerpiece of paroxysmal EEG activity.

Problems of Terminology

Definitions of EEG events are indispensable, but they are also quite difficult to arrive at and are often unsatisfactory. Attempts to reassess the EEG terminology have been made from time to time; they often result in neologistic construction of terms that fail to receive general acceptance. The EEG terminology is filled with widely used, popular, and, alas, often quite sloppy and inaccurate terms. Nevertheless, most electroencephalographers know what is meant by such expressions in the professional jargon.

One could argue that the busy electroencephalographer will always be satisfied with the nomenclature he or she learned during the training period, whereas the academic thinkers among the electroencephalographers constantly strive for an unobjectionable and crystal-clear terminology free from linguistic flaws and capable of defining an EEG event from a variety of aspects. This view, however, is oversimplified. Academia sometimes has a vested interest in certain terms; it may bitterly resent new terms recommended by international committees.

A preliminary proposal by the International Federation of Societies for Electroencephalography and Clinical Neurophysiology (IFSECN, 1961) was followed by a definitive proposal (IFSECN, 1966) and a glossary of terms used by clinical electroencephalographers (IFSECN, 1974). The handbook catalogue of Dutertre (1977) exudes Cartesian lucidity and deserves admiration. Unfortunately, the definition of electrophysiological events can never do justice to all facets of the phenomenon. The question then arises as to whether we have to follow the new nomenclature rigidly. A negativistic attitude must be castigated, but pressure should not be put on the workers in the field to strictly adhere to the newly proposed terms. A consensus on the use of terms must come from within. Terms simply have to catch on.

As to epileptic discharges, there has been considerable disunity in the ranks of electroencephalographers. The term *epileptic discharge* has been attacked and condemned on the ground that such discharges may occur in the absence of clinical seizure manifestations or in individuals who have never had seizures. The same is true for the widely used term *seizure discharge*; even *paroxysmal discharge*, certainly a more cautious and unassuming term, has not found general acceptance.

Must electroencephalographers really become linguistic and philosophical hair splitters when we know very well what is meant? Assume that seizure discharges are "discharges that can be seen in seizures." In a less restrictive and more relaxed view, there is really nothing wrong with a term like *seizure discharges* as long as the reader of the reports knows that such terms should not be misconstrued.

Interictal Paroxysmal Patterns

Spike (Single or Random Spike)

According to IFSECN (1974), a spike is a transient, clearly distinguished from the background activity, with pointed peak at conventional paper speed and a duration from 20 to under 70 msec; the main component is generally negative. Amplitude is variable.

The distinction from the background activity is based on wave morphology and amplitude. In many cases, spikes stand out against the background because of their high voltage. If the voltage of spikes and background activity is approximately equal, the faster character (i.e., the shorter duration) of the spike is its distinctive feature. Is it possible that a spike of 50 msec duration and moderate amplitude may be embedded in 20/sec activity (50 msec wave duration), for instance in an epileptic with considerable drug-induced fast activity. Under these circumstances, the spike activity may be undetectable. In such a case, fast paper speed could demonstrate the morphological features of the spike (multiphasic and more pointed character with a dominant negative phase) in contrast with the more monotonous appearance of the fast waves.

Spikes have many characteristics in common and yet there are also remarkable inter- and intraindividual variations (Fig. 13.1) and inconsistencies between one spike and the next in the same lead (Kiloh et al., 1972). Spikes appear to be hypersynchronous events due to excessive simultaneous neuronal discharge. This view, however, is not congruent with the desynchronized (low-voltage) EEG aspect of "electrode-cremental seizures" or the electrode-incremental initiation of focal or generalized attacks. Definitions such as "epilepsy is paroxysmal hypersynchrony" (Roger et al.,

1949) may be correct on the neuronal level but partly incorrect from the viewpoint of the "macro-EEG."

Basic neurophysiologists have been cautioning against the casual use of terms such as *synchronization* and *desynchronization*. Low-voltage fast rhythms are not necessarily desynchronized and may be associated with enhancement and synchronization within intracortical networks (Steriade et al., 1996; see also Chapter 9, "The Normal EEG of the Waking Adult").

Processes on the neuronal level are presented in Chapters 2 and 3 and are also discussed in Chapter 27, on epileptic seizure disorders.

On the basis of long-term monitoring and computer analysis, Gotman (1984) has raised the question as to whether interictal spikes are in reality postictal. Gotman (1984) and Gotman and Marciani (1985) observed marked and prolonged increase of interictal spikes in a patient after a seizure (awake as well as asleep). Drug levels had little influence on the rate of spike activity, and there was no increase of spiking prior to a seizure.

The multiphasic character of a single spike warrants particular emphasis. A sequence of a minor positive, a major negative, and a second minor positive component (Fig. 13.1) is typical in most instances. A slow negative component may trail the spike discharge and often attain about the same amplitude as the negative main component of the spike. This trailing slow component of a single spike should not be regarded as evidence of a spike wave complex. Dutertre (1977) in his handbook catalogue shows examples of single spike wave complexes that one could just as well describe as compounded or multiphasic single spikes. From the vantage point of basic neurophysiology, there is some reason to presume that the trailing slow wave is caused by the same type of hyperpolarization demonstrated by Pollen et al. (1964) in the experimental analysis of the spike wave discharge.

The electroencephalographer very seldom finds single spikes on the scalp with predominant positive component (Matsuo and Knott, 1977; Maulsby, 1971). Positive single spikes are more common in electroencephalographic and

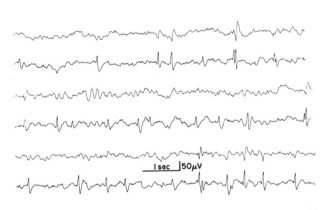

Figure 13.1. Various wave morphologies of spikes recorded from the same patient (age 6 years). Upper lead, T_3–T_5; lower lead, T_5–O_1. (First and second tracing from the top, continued in tracings 3 and 4, resp. 5 and 6.) Note multiphasic character of spikes with predominance of the negative phase (see Chapter 8, "The EEG Signal: Polarity and Field Determination") and occasional formation of double spikes.

depth recordings; on the scalp, predominant positivity of single spikes raises the question of defective superficial cortical laminae. Following surgery of cortical arteriovenous (AV) malformations or after traumatic laceration (Binnie et al., 1989), such positive spikes may be present occasionally. A special type of positive spiking over the vertex has been described by Bergen (1979) in a case that combined features of sphingolipidosis and mucopolysaccharidosis. [Also see the work of Engel et al. (1977) on the cherry red spot-myoclonus syndrome.] With dipole formation (especially in benign rolandic epilepsy), a positive spike discharge may be found in a moderate distance from the negative spike focus (Gregory and Wong, 1984; Wong and Gregory, 1988).

Spikes represent the basic element of paroxysmal activity in the EEG. A unitarian view that all spikes mean a hidden or overt paroxysmal event would be erroneous. The fine semiology of spikes is extremely important and the EEG interpreter ought to consider the following questions:

1. What is the precise wave morphology?
2. Where do the spikes occur?
3. What is the patient's age?
4. What is the state of awareness?
5. Is there any possibility of an artifact of similar appearance?
6. Is there any possibility of a physiological potential of similar appearance?

Discrepancies between spikes and behavioral epileptic events are not uncommon at all. This highly complex situation has been reinvestigated by Niedermeyer (1990).

Wave Morphology

The largest and most pronounced spikes are not necessarily associated with more serious epileptic seizure disorders. On the contrary, rolandic spikes in a child age 4 to 10 years are very prominent; however, the seizure disorder is usually quite benign or there may be no clinical seizures at all.

On the other hand, "small sharp spikes" are indeed marginal spike discharges and will be discussed separately. A very unusual type of rhythmically repetitive and yet interictal spike activity in two epileptic brothers was described by Bauer and Markoff (1970).

Spatial Distribution

In childhood, occipital spikes are, in general, the most benign spike discharges, with less than 50% having clinical seizures; rolandic central-midtemporal-parietal spikes are also quite benign, whereas frontal spikes or multifocal spikes are more epileptogenic.

Age

The significance of the age factor is enormous. From the spikes of an epileptic newborn to a seizure focus of old age, age-determined varieties of spikes can be distinguished.

Level of Awareness

Random spikes may occur at any state of waking-sleeping cycle and occur even in rapid-eye-movement (REM) sleep when bilateral synchronous bursts of spikes or spike waves are usually suppressed.

Repercussions on Perceptual Function

Shewmon and Erwin (1988a,b) investigated the impact of spikes located over the occipital region and its vicinity on visual perception and reaction time in three subjects with posterior spikes. Their work shows that the visuomotor reaction time was prolonged (or the response was absent) when the task was spike-locked. Furthermore, "spike-induced dysfunction was most pronounced when either response hand or visual field of stimulus was contralateral to the spike" (Shewmon and Erwin, 1988b). In a further study, Shewmon and Erwin (1988c) emphasized the significance of the trailing slow wave that follows a single spike discharge. The perceptive disturbance was particularly pronounced when the task was presented during the slow wave. These fascinating findings indicate that even single spikes of rapid duration may be capable of momentary impairment of the cortical visual function. This applies to visual tasks. During an ictal-subclinical episode of repetitive fast spiking over the occipital area and its neighborhood, correct mental arithmetic is possible (Niedermeyer et al., 1989).

Distinction from Similar Physiological Patterns

This differentiation is particularly important in the case of vertex sharp waves during deep drowsiness and stage 2 of light non-REM sleep. In childhood (after age 4), these waves may have a particularly spiky appearance and may be misinterpreted as paroxysmal spikes.

Physiological sharp or spiky vertex waves are usually quite easily distinguished from rolandic spikes in sleep (Fig. 13.2). Even in the more uncommon case of paroxysmal

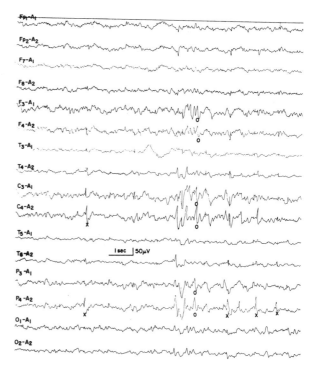

Figure 13.2. Coexistence of rolandic spikes and physiological vertex waves in light sleep (8-year-old boy, attacks of abdominal pain, no proven epileptic seizures). Right centroparietal spikes with occasional spread to the left are marked *X*; typical examples of a vertex wave are marked *O*.

spike discharges over the vertex, the differentiation from physiological vertex sharp waves is not difficult.

The physiological nature of the occipital lambda waves and "lambdoid" activity (positive occipital transients of sleep) must also be considered. The main component of this pattern is positive.

Distinction from Artifacts of Similar Appearance

This distinction depends on the electroencephalographer's experience and is usually an easy one.

The interpretation of the clinical significance of spikes can be extremely difficult and depends on the electroencephalographer's experience in the art of reading the EEG tracing and also on the clinical understanding of epileptological problems. Extensive personal laboratory experience is just as essential as scientific knowledge in interpreting the EEG.

Automatic Spike Detection

Since the pioneering work of Gotman et al. (1978) considerable controversy has arisen regarding computer-based automatic detection of spikes in the EEG. The pivotal question is "What should the computer imitate?" (Webber et al., 1993), and this question hinges on the precise definitions of spikes (Wilson et al., 1996): "A spike detected by any reader is a spike, a spike detected by the majority of readers is a spike, a spike detected by the weighted average of readers is a spike, etc." According to these authors, average spike attributes are calculated, and the resulting database can serve as a "gold standard" for testing computer algorithms or other readers. With the use of an "off-line" artificial neural network, attempts have been made at real-time detection of spikes (Webber et al., 1994).

Are Interictal Spikes Nothing but EEG Signals?

Our earlier view (found in this chapter in previous editions)—namely that single spikes are an EEG signal and nothing else—appears to be in need of some correction. This seems to be particularly true for "negative myoclonus" (ictally suppressed motor activity). Beautiful examples have been presented by Gambardella et al. (1997) and Werhahn and Noachtar (2000) (also see Fisch, 2003). A single spike may also cause changes in cerebral blood flow and increase of metabolic demands (Warach et al., 1996), demonstrated with the simultaneous use of EEG and functional magnetic resonance imaging (fMRI).

Even behavioral changes with impaired test performance may be associated with single interictal spikes (Aarts et al., 1984; Hughes, 1997). Further information is found in the work of Fisch (2003).

Sharp Waves

According to IFSECN (1974), a sharp wave is a transient, clearly distinguished from background activity, with pointed peak at conventional paper speeds and duration of 70 to 200 msec, i.e., more than approximately 1/14 to 1/5 sec. The main component is generally negative relative to the areas.

Jasper (1941) pointed out that the rising phase of the sharp wave is of the same order of magnitude as in spikes, but the descending phase is prolonged. The configuration

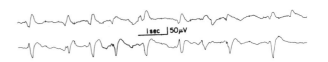

Figure 13.3. Recurrent sharp wave recorded from a 61-year-old patient. Upper lead, F_3–C_3; lower lead, C_3–P_3. A prominent negative phase is followed by a large and relatively slow trailing positive wave.

with a steeper ascending phase, however, is not always present. Examples of sharp waves are shown in Fig. 13.3.

A very unusual type of repetitive slow sharp wave activity has been reported in prematurely born infants with intraventricular hemorrhage; these discharges show predominantly positive polarity and are recorded mainly over the rolandic region (Cukier et al., 1974; Werner et al., 1977). The maximum of this activity is sometimes found over the vertex.

Spikes and sharp waves are neurophysiologically closely related phenomena; both of them are typical paroxysmal discharges and highly suggestive of an epileptic seizure disorder, although both phenomena may occur in patients without a history of seizure disorder.

Sharp waves are usually found as random focal discharges; most anterior temporal spikes are, in a strict sense, sharp waves. This is also true for most benign rolandic spikes of childhood. Sharp waves are more seldom found in generalized synchronous bursts where single spikes, spike waves, and polyspikes predominate.

It has been contemplated that sharp waves on the scalp correspond with spikes in the depth or on the cortex. Combined depth and scalp recording clearly refutes this view (Zobniw et al., 1975; see also Chapter 36, "Depth Electroencephalography"). One can detect spikes as well as sharp waves in depth recordings; a deep sharp wave usually corresponds with a sharp wave on the scalp if there is any corresponding scalp activity at all.

The long duration of a sharp wave permits better insight into the multiphasic character of this potential. A small preceding positive component may be very fast and qualify as a spike; even a small biphasic spike discharge may precede the much larger sharp wave. Some sharp waves even exceed the maximum length of 200 msec of the IFSECN definition (IFSECN, 1974) (Fig. 13.4), also named "slow sharp waves" (Ribeiro et al., 1999) or in cases of particularly long duration, "blunted sharp waves." Others become very complex. They consist of a constantly varying number of components; such compounded sharp waves may occur as the periodic discharges (periodic lateralized epileptiform discharges) of Chatrian et al. (1964).

It is certainly not incorrect to use the terms *spikes* and *sharp waves* synonymously when a local paroxysmal event is discussed, although purists of nomenclature would regard this as a breach of etiquette.

Polyspikes or Multiple Spikes

This discharge type represents a complex of spikes and may also be called polyspike complex. In modern terminology (IFSECN, 1974), the term *multiple spike complex* is preferred on the grounds of linguistic considerations, because

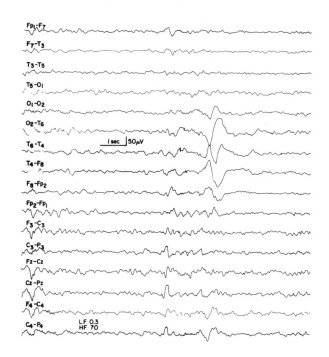

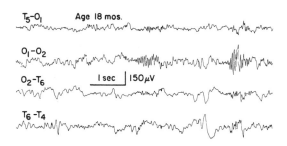

Figure 13.6. The differentiation between polyspikes and drug-induced fast activity may be difficult. The run of beta waves *(center)* certainly falls into the category of fast activity, but the more outstanding and burst-like run *(right)* is more likely to represent polyspike activity. A definitive statement depends on the impressions derived from the entire record.

Figure 13.4. An example of a very slow sharp wave (blunted sharp wave), maximal over T$_6$, obtained from a 6-year-old boy with craniocerebral trauma at age 4 followed by seizures.

"polyspikes" is an etymological hybrid. It has been defined as a complex paroxysmal EEG pattern with close association of two or more diphasic spikes occurring more or less rhythmically in bursts of variable duration, generally with large amplitudes (Dutertre, 1977) (Figs. 13.5 and 13.6).

Polyspike bursts are readily elicited by electrical stimulation of single depth leads, especially in limbic regions. On the scalp, however, polyspikes occur mostly as bilateral or generalized synchronous discharges. Exceptional focal polyspikes are occasionally encountered; these usually have a frontal maximum, except for occipital accentuation in hypsarrhythmia. Polyspikes and also polyspike-wave complexes are sometimes associated with concomitant myoclonus, especially in primary generalized epilepsy and in photosensitive individuals with this type of seizure disorder. Children with Lennox-Gastaut syndrome may also show association of polyspikes and myoclonus.

Runs of Rapid Spikes

This pattern has been described as "grand mal discharge" (Gibbs and Gibbs, 1952; Gibbs et al., 1935), "fast paroxysmal rhythms" (Jasper and Kershman, 1949), "rhythmic spikes" (Gastaut et al., 1966), and "generalized paroxysmal fast activity" (Brenner and Atkinson, 1982). It is seen only in sleep and occurs in older children, adolescents, and younger adults (Fig. 13.7). It consists of bursts of spike discharges at a rate from 10 to 25/sec, usually generalized but with a well-defined maximum over frontal regions; it may even be confined to the frontal leads. The voltage is in the medium to high range, often exceeding 100 or even 200 μV. The discharge rate is in most cases somewhat irregular. The bursts last for about 2 to 10 seconds; bursts of more than 5-second duration are usually associated with tonic seizures and thus represent an ictal pattern.

The obvious misnomer "grand mal discharges" is based on certain similarities with the ictal EEG of a grand mal seizure. In a patient population with grand mal seizures, runs of rapid spikes as an interictal pattern are a very rare finding. This has been confirmed by the data of Chayasirisobhon et al. (1984). The inappropriateness of the term *grand mal discharge* was stressed by Rodin et al. (1976), who thought that this pattern occurred in patients with primary generalized epilepsy who suffered from more than one type of seizure and especially from akinetic seizures. As already noted by Gastaut et al. (1966), this discharge is very typical in patients with Lennox-Gastaut syndrome; it is hardly ever found outside this clinical entity (Niedermeyer, 1969, 1972, 1974). It may be found in very rare instances of posttraumatic epilepsy with EEG traits of the Lennox-Gastaut syndrome (Niedermeyer et al., 1970). Brenner and Atkinson (1982), however, insist that runs of rapid spikes ("generalized paroxysmal fast activity") may be found outside the Lennox-Gastaut syndrome. In my experience, runs of rapid spikes may occur in all "imitators" of the Lennox-Gastaut syndrome (Niedermeyer, 1988).

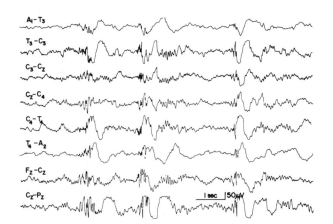

Figure 13.5. Polyspikes in light non-rapid-eye-movement (REM) sleep, especially over central region, associated with K complexes. (With permission of the AMA *Archives of Neurology.*)

Figure 13.7. A run of rapid spikes in a 19-year-old epileptic patient (Lennox-Gastaut syndrome). Note anterior maximum of the discharge. A few slow spike wave complexes are also seen (right temporo-occipital region).

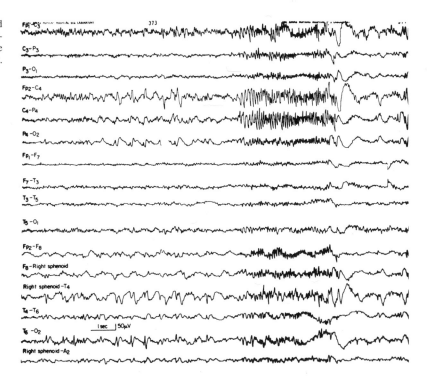

We know little about the neurophysiological underpinnings of this pattern. It is clearly a frontal lobe discharge, and the associated tonic seizures are probably arising from the premotor and supplementary motor portions of the frontal lobes. There could be certain similarities to the decremental seizure patterns, which also originate most commonly from the frontal lobe (Arroyo et al., 1994).

Unfortunately, those electroencephalographers who never use sleep portions in routine records will never see this fascinating pattern, which is definitely in need of further basic research.

Spike Wave Complex (Classical 3/Sec)

Classical 3/sec spike wave complexes are widely known even outside the community of electroencephalographers. It is officially termed *spike and slow wave complex* (IFSECN, 1974); this term comprises all types of spike wave complexes, which are listed separately because of markedly differing associated clinical-epileptological conditions. The official definition (IFSECN, 1974) is quite simple: "A pattern consisting of a spike followed by a slow wave." Older terms such as *spike-and-dome complex, wave-and-spike complex,* and *dart-and-dome complex* are seldom used these days and should be discouraged. The abridged term *3/sec spike wave* is certainly acceptable, because the omitted word *complex* is automatically implied.

Spike wave complexes of the classical variety (3/sec) have been described as the EEG pattern of petit mal absences (Gibbs et al., 1935). Since that time, the 3/sec spike wave discharge has been equated with petit mal epilepsy. Regrettable mistakes have occurred due to lack of communication between electroencephalographers and clinicians who initiated treatment with anticonvulsants specific for petit mal due to the use of the term *3/sec spike wave complexes* alone. The term *petit mal discharge* (Gibbs and Gibbs, 1952) has reinforced this type of reflex thinking. Fortunately, electroencephalographers and epileptologists have always cautioned against the misinterpretation of the term *petit mal discharges*; this should be interpreted as "discharges that occur in petit mal absences but also in other conditions." The work of Silverman (1954), Clark and Knott (1955), and Lundervold et al. (1959) has clearly shown that the spike wave discharge as an interictal event correlates with the occurrence of petit mal absences only in moderate percentage of patients (16% according to Clark and Knott).

The 3/sec spike wave discharge is a worthwhile subject for more detailed discussion. As to *wave morphology,* there is good evidence that the spike wave complex is not simply an association of a spike and a slow wave, although the above-mentioned definition is justifiable as a simplification. The spike wave complex contains hidden components that can be seen even with simple visual analysis at 30 mm/sec chart speed; special recording methods will reveal these extra components much better. Gastaut and Hunter (1950). Cohn (1954) and Weir (1965) have elucidated the components of this pattern. Most important is a spike of positive polarity during the descending portion of the slow wave (Weir, 1965), becoming evident as notching under usual recording conditions.

On the basis of experimental studies of cortical faradization, Jung and Toennies (1950) stressed the inhibitory character of the slow wave following a spike discharge ("Bremswelle"). Experimentally induced spike wave-like activity in cats, elicited by electrical stimulation of thalamic intralaminar structures, was studied with intracellular cortical microelectrodes (Pollen, 1964; Pollen et al., 1964; Weir and Sie, 1966). According to Pollen (1964), all components of the spike wave complex were the "consequence of post-synaptic activity." This author points out that "the initial positivity which may precede a negative spike (depending upon the intensity of the stimulation) results from depolarization of middle and deep lying neurons, whereas the surface negative spike is the result of EPSP [excitatory postsynaptic potential] generation primarily upon apical dendrites of vertically oriented pyramidal type neurons." According to Pollen (1964), the long surface negative wave is generated by inhibitory postsynaptic potentials (IPSPs) predominantly on or near the soma of similar pyramidal cells. Thus, the slow wave indeed appears to be related to inhibitory impulses.

From this vantage point, the spike wave discharge apparently represents an alternating succession of excitation and inhibition. The clinical ictal activities are thus constantly curbed by intervening inhibitory impulses that prevent the attack from progressing into massive downward discharges with motor effects (polyspikes with massive myoclonus) or to a full-blown grand mal attack. For this reason, motor manifestations of ictal episodes characterized by spike waves are almost always inconspicuous or modest. Furthermore, spike wave bursts rarely proceed into grand mal convulsions; such rare exceptions have been demonstrated by Halász (1972) and Niedermeyer (1976).

The distinction between classical (3/sec), slow (2–2.5/sec), and fast (4/sec) spike wave complexes and the smaller 6/sec spike wave discharge is justified on the basis of different clinical-epileptological correlates of each spike wave type; it is not an example of electroencephalographic hair splitting. The classical 3/sec spike wave discharge is most typical and most pronounced in children with petit mal absences. Clinical absences are usually present when the burst lasts for longer than 5 sec. Thus, shorter bursts are usually subclinical, but numerous psychophysiological attempts have been made to demonstrate certain fluctuations of level of awareness even in apparently subclinical spike wave bursts. This is discussed in greater detail in Chapter 27, "Epileptic Seizure Disorders." The classical spike wave

complex is, in most cases, easily activated by hyperventilation, whereas the slow and the fast forms of this discharge show little or no enhancement.

A classical 3/sec spike wave burst does not run exactly at a rate of 3/sec. The complexes are faster at the onset of the burst (mostly around 4/sec), then slow down to 3.5 and 3/sec for the main portion, and eventually slow to 2.5/sec at the end of the burst. During a burst, the spike discharges become gradually smaller, often shrinking to insignificance (Fig. 13.8) as in drowsiness and sleep.

The *spatial distribution* of the bursts is very typical; the maximum almost always lies over the frontal midline region, whereas a minimum is found over temporal and occipital areas. It is deplorable that somewhat different findings obtained by Dondey (1983) are based on EEG recordings in which no midline electrodes were used. Hence the data of the author do not invalidate the concept of a frontal midline maximum, which has been confirmed by Rodin and Ancheta (1987) with the use of brain mapping technique. The understanding of this distribution type is highly conducive to a better comprehension of the underlying mechanisms; this is pointed out in Chapter 27. Almost all spike wave bursts are bilateral synchronous or generalized synchronous; the synchrony, however, is not perfect (Cohn, 1954; Gotman, 1981). The age of distribution lies mainly in the range from 4 to 16 years.

The work of Lemieux and Blume (1983) has shed more light on the spatial distribution of the spike-wave complex on the basis of computer analysis. According to these authors, field distribution of spikes differed from that of the ensuing slow waves. Spikes "arose in one frontal region and propagated to the homologous part of the other frontal region with a peak-to-peak interval less than 15 msec. Less commonly, spikes first moved anteriorly within the initiating frontal region before contralateral propagation occurred." By contrast, negative slow waves were more diffuse, more symmetrical in evolution, and more posteriorly centered than the spikes.

The onset of the spike component in one frontal lobe is congruent with the earlier findings of Cohn (1954) and

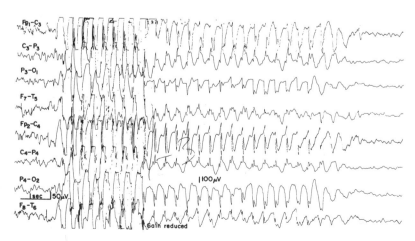

Figure 13.8. Petit mal absence with generalized synchronous spike wave complexes. The enormous amplitude of the discharges necessitates considerable lowering of the gain. The frontal voltage maximum is evident. Note gradual decline of the spike component at the end of attack, along with slight slow down of the frequency to about 2.5/sec.

Lüders et al. (1980), who noted asynchronies ranging from 5 to 20 msec. The frontal lobe is a large structure and subdivisions are necessary. Onset of spike-wave activity (and, in particular, of the spike component) over the frontal midline means in reality that a frontal portion in the immediate vicinity of the interhemispheric fissure is the origin of the discharge; this area belongs to the supplementary motor zone.

As to the neuropsychological correlates of subclinical generalized spike-wave bursts and clinical absences with spike-waves, see Chapter 27 (section on petit mal absences). In this context, it should be pointed out that the impact of apparently subclinical 3/sec spike-wave bursts might be stronger than one would expect from routine clinical observation. With its maximum over the frontal midline (frontal lobe close to interhemispheric fissure), there might be some impact on prefrontal lobe functions and, in particular, on the working memory. This concept of working memory, introduced by Baddeley (1986) and enormously refined by Fuster (1995, 1996), implies a system of constant perceptory afferences to the prefrontal dorsolateral region whence motor impulses emanate, resulting in readiness (set) for motor action. This system could be blocked for a moment by a few (even by a single) spike-waves and interfere with the working memory. In a clinical 3/sec spike-wave absence, blocking of the working memory might be the most likely explanation for the mild disturbance of consciousness and its immediate full recovery with the termination of the attack (Niedermeyer, 1997). No "true disturbance of consciousness"—epileptic or nonepileptic—can recover immediately. In other words, the function of working memory is simply suspended for the duration of the spike-waves.

Due to the uniqueness of primary generalized epilepsy with 3/sec spike-waves in the human (Niedermeyer, 1996), animal models for this response have great limitations. The arrest reaction of the monkey (Walker and Morello, 1967) produced by alumina cream injection into the fronto-orbital cortex has some resemblance to the human absence epilepsy; this cannot be said about the sudden freeze of motility noted in the cat stimulation of the cat's mesial anterior thalamus (Hunter and Jasper, 1949); there is no spike-wave activity associated with this type of arrest reaction.

According to Sperling and Skolnick (1995), there is a general decrease of cerebral blood flow (133 xenon method) during human generalized spike-wave activity, which, however, is less pronounced in frontal regions than in the parietal lobes. Transcranial magnetic stimulation of the motor cortex in patients with primary generalized epilepsy and 3/sec spike-waves produced motor evoked potentials of significantly reduced size when the cortical stimulus was time-locked to the slow wave component of the spike-wave complex (but slightly reduced or unchanged when the stimulus was time-locked with the spike) (Gianelli et al., 1994). This underscores the special inhibitory character of the slow wave component, which has been known since the work of Jung and Toennies (1950).

Spike Wave Complex (Slow 1–2.5/Sec)

After the demonstration of the 3/sec spike wave complex and its relationship to the petit mal absence (Gibbs et al., 1935), the Gibbses and William G. Lennox were struck by

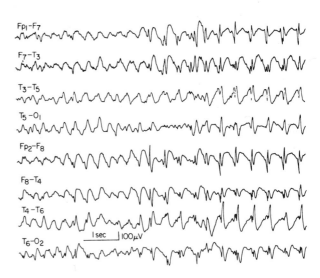

Figure 13.9. Generalized slow spike wave complexes (mostly around 2/sec) in a child with severe epileptic seizure disorder (Lennox-Gastaut syndrome).

the occurrence of slow spike-wave complexes in a much different type of patients with seizures other than the petit mal absence. The classical 3/sec spike wave complex was termed *petit mal discharge*. Consequently, the slow spike wave complex was termed *petit mal variant discharge*. This term was used first by Gibbs et al. (1939). In that study, hypoglycemia was induced in order to demonstrate an increase of classical 3/sec spike wave activity in the hypoglycemic state; an increase of slow spike wave activity, however, was not elicited with this activation method when used in appropriate patients.

The *wave morphology* of this pattern varies considerably. In the majority of the cases, the complex consists of a rather slow spike (according to the definition, a sharp wave, lasting 70 msec or longer) and a slow wave. In a sizable number of cases, true spikes (60 msec or less duration) are followed by a slow wave (Fig. 13.9).

The *spatial distribution* is, in most instances, quite similar to that of the 3/sec spike wave complex. In the vast majority of the cases, the bursts are bilateral or generalized synchronous (with imperfect synchrony, as discussed in Chapter 27); a frontal midline maximum is the rule in these discharges. Lateralization or occasional focal occurrence is sometimes observed, usually in children with severe residual brain damage in certain areas where parenchymatous destruction abolishes the spike-wave discharge.

Generalized slow spike wave discharges are often quite prolonged. In some children or adolescents, the entire sleep portion (light and moderately deep non-REM sleep) consists of unabated generalized slow spike wave activity. The diagnosis of an "electrical status epilepticus" may or may not be justified in such cases; there are usually no behavioral or polygraphic characteristics to suggest an ongoing ictal event.

In some cases, the slow spike-wave activity is found only in non-REM sleep; the author remembers a child in whom the waking state and light to deep non-REM sleep revealed perfectly normal findings, whereas the drowsy portion was characterized by prolonged generalized slow spike-wave activity.

Although the classical 3/sec spike wave complex is seldom seen before the age of 4 and almost never before 3.5 years, its slow counterpart appears much earlier, sometimes before the age of 6 months. At this early age, the frontal maximum may not be readily demonstrable.

The *clinical correlates* are discussed in Chapter 27. The slow spike wave complex is almost always associated with a severe and often uncontrollable type of childhood epilepsy (seldom with onset between ages 11 and 20 years) called Lennox-Gastaut syndrome (Gastaut et al., 1966; Gibbs et al., 1939; Lennox, 1960; Niedermeyer, 1969, 1974). Most of these children show a variety of minor attacks and evidence of mental retardation.

Thus, the distinction between slow (1–2.5/sec) and classical (3/sec) spike waves is of great clinical significance. One has to keep in mind, however, that many children or adolescents with slow spike waves also show series of 3/sec or even 4/sec spike wave complexes; the presence of these spike wave types is obviously of no significance in such cases and what counts is the slow type. On the other hand, patients with classical 3/sec spike wave complexes and a usually benign type of epileptic seizure disorder almost never show slow spike waves except when a 3/sec or 4/sec spike wave burst may slow down to 2.5/sec at the end. The reader will find further information in Chapter 27.

Spike Wave Complex (Fast 4/Sec, 4–5/Sec)

This pattern is closely related to the classical 3/sec spike wave complex; both discharge types are most commonly lumped together. A differentiation, however, is justified on clinical grounds.

Gastaut (1968) deserves credit for an outline of the distinctive features between the 3/sec and the 4/sec (or 4–5/sec) spike wave discharge. According to his investigations, the fast spike wave burst is usually of shorter duration (1–3 sec), it occurs in patients older than 15 years, the bursts are always subclinical, and the associated seizure disorder is usually characterized by myoclonic jerking, grand mal attacks, or a combination of both seizure types, whereas petit mal absences are quite uncommon. Paroxysmal flicker responses are common in such patients. A positive family history of epileptic seizures disorder is frequently found in this group of patients.

The 4/sec spike wave discharge is spatially distributed in the same manner as the 3/sec spike wave discharge; the frontal midline maximum is quite prominent (see Chapter 27).

The 6/Sec Spike Wave Complex (Wave and Spike Phantom, Miniature Spike and Wave)

This is a marginal paroxysmal pattern, described by Gibbs and Gibbs (1952) as follows: "The spike in this pattern has a strong positive component but the entire wave complex looks in general like a miniature reproduction of the 3 per second spike and wave of petit mal." In view of the positive component of the spike, Silverman (1967) has stressed similarities to the 6/sec component of the 14 and 6/sec positive spike discharge; he also observed transition from the former to the latter with deepening drowsiness. Marshall (1955) introduced the term *wave and spike phantom*, which has found but limited acceptance.

The clinical correlates of 6/sec spike wave complex have been elucidated by Thomas (1957), Gibbs and Gibbs (1964), Hughes et al. (1965), and Thomas and Klass (1968). It is usually a pattern of adulthood but may also occur in adolescents and children. About 50% to 60% of the patients suffer from indubitable epileptic seizures (mostly grand mal); the remainder show a history of syncopal attacks, posttraumatic states, or (as emphasized by Small, 1970) psychiatric problems.

The 6/sec spike wave complex is an uncommon but not rare pattern (about 0.5–1% in a central EEG laboratory).

The discharge may be recorded in waking state, drowsiness, and light non-REM sleep; light drowsiness appears to be the optimal recording condition (Fig. 13.10).

Investigations regarding the *spatial distribution* of this pattern have led to an important dichotomy. Hecker et al. (1979) pointed out that a distinction must be made between frontal accentuation and occipital accentuation. We are evidently dealing with two different types of discharge; the frontal type is most commonly associated with epileptic seizure disorders and sometimes found in combination with other paroxysmal discharge types. The occipital types are found predominantly in patients with no evidence of epilep-

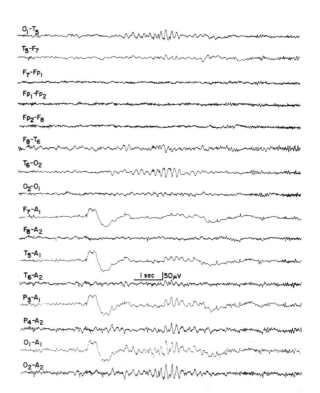

Figure 13.10. A short run of 6/sec spike waves, posterior type, recorded in a 52-year-old woman with a history of head injury 2 years earlier and subsequent headache, dizziness, and memory loss. There was computed tomography (CT) scan evidence of cortical atrophy.

tic seizure disorder. This distinction can be wholeheartedly endorsed on the basis of the writer's personal experience.

In a study of 839 patients with 6/sec spike wave complexes, Hughes (1980) placed particular emphasis on the distinction between frontal and occipital maximum. He summarized the principal features of both forms by the acronyms WHAM and FOLD:

W:	waking record	F:	females
H:	high in amplitude	O:	occipital
A:	anterior	L:	low in amplitude
M:	males	D:	drowsy record

An interesting sidelight of this observation is the uneven sex distribution, which is rather unique; no other EEG abnormalities show any gender preference.

According to Hughes (1991), patients with anterior 6/sec spike waves are more likely to have epileptic seizures, and those with posterior discharges tend to have neuroautonomic disturbances. Personal observations are not in agreement with this statement.

Kocher et al. (1975) were struck by the occurrence of 6/sec spike-wave complexes in the abstinence or withdrawal phase of drug-dependent individuals. Tharp (1966) produced the discharge by intravenous diphenhydramine (50 mg) in normal subjects. Hecker et al. (1979) found that the occipital form of the 6/sec spike wave complex is often related to drug dependence (hypoanalgesics, barbiturates) and withdrawal. All this underscores the need for a distinction of the two forms. Thus, the frontal form will have to be regarded as a truly epilepsy-related paroxysmal pattern, whereas the occipital form finds itself on the fringe of paroxysmal discharge types.

Benign EEG Variants and Patterns

The just-mentioned 6/sec spike-wave discharge has been listed under the heading of "benign EEG variants and patterns," which include patterns with "epileptiform morphology." According to Westmoreland (1990), the 6/sec spike-wave discharge has not been proved to be a reliable indicator of seizures (also see Klass and Westmoreland, 1985; Thomas and Klass, 1968). Other patterns listed under the heading of benign patterns are small sharp spikes, 14 and 6/sec positive spikes, wicket spikes, and the psychomotor variant pattern (discussed below).

According to Westmoreland, these patterns "have an epileptiform appearance but are considered normal or benign variants of EEG activity or activity of uncertain significance." These patterns may occur in healthy individuals, but there is no doubt that a variety of abnormalities (of pathologies of all kinds) can be harbored in a person who is able to function normally (Niedermeyer, 1987, 1988a). In this writer's opinion, it is false to interpret these patterns simply as normal (with the exception of the "14 and 6" discharge, which means normalcy in most instances). The other patterns are associated with potential epileptogenicity, which, in the case of the 6/sec spike-wave discharge, may reach 50% to 60%. They may also be forerunners of classical epileptiform discharges. I am in agreement with Westmoreland (1990) when she writes that "critical evaluation of the various types of EEG activity is important."

Rudimentary Spike Wave Complex ("Pseudo Petit Mal Discharge")

Gibbs and Gibbs (1964) described a paroxysmal discharge that consists of generalized or nearly generalized high-voltage 3 to 4/sec waves "with a poorly developed spike in the positive trough between the slow waves, occurring in drowsiness only." According to Gibbs and Gibbs, this pattern is most prominent over parietal areas. It is found only in infancy and early childhood when marked hypnagogic rhythmical theta activity is paramount in the drowsy state. In some of these children, the theta activity occurs in generalized bursts rather than in prolonged stretches; such bursts, sometimes as slow as 3 to 4/sec, may contain small spike elements that could justify a term like *rudimentary spike waves*. The Gibbsian term *pseudo petit mal discharge* could be conducive to an equation of spike wave and petit mal; this term has never caught on, and there is even some question as to whether this pattern should be considered to be a special paroxysmal discharge type.

One can agree with Gibbs and Gibbs (1964) that this pattern denotes a mild abnormality; transition into a classical or other spike wave pattern does not occur. It has been shown that a history of febrile illness is very often found in children with rudimentary spike waves; a history of febrile convulsions is also quite common in such children (Gibbs and Gibbs, 1964).

Small Sharp Spikes

This pattern has been delineated by Gibbs and Gibbs (1952, 1964). It is the most inconspicuous paroxysmal discharge and hence is easily overlooked. (Only the occipital type of the 6/sec spike wave complex is equally small and unimpressive.) The main negative and positive components are of about equally spiky character (Fig. 13.11). The discharge is fairly widespread and is seen chiefly over temporal and frontal areas, either shifting from side to side or synchronously firing. The pattern is almost exclusively found in drowsiness and/or light non-REM sleep. It is essentially a pattern of adulthood with a peak between ages 30 to 60 years; occurrence in adolescence and old age is somewhat less common. It is virtually absent in the first 10 years of life. This pattern is also known as benign epileptiform transients of sleep (BETS).

In our personal experience (Koshino and Niedermeyer, 1975), a prevalence of 1.36% was found with a peak of 2.9% between ages 30 and 40. In this study, two thirds (67.4%) of the patients had a history of epileptic seizures; this underscores the paroxysmal character of the discharge. Small sharp spikes sometimes are precursors of typical anterior temporal spikes or sharp waves, which, in such patients, simply occur somewhat later in drowsiness or sleep. This association was also noted by Gibbs and Gibbs (1964). In a depth EEG study by Westmoreland et al. (1979), an extensive generator area of small sharp spikes was found.

Among nonepileptics, the discharges may occur in patients with cerebrovascular disorder, syncopal attacks, and psychiatric problems. Small (1970) and Small et al. (1975) have placed special emphasis on the occurrence of this spike discharge in a psychiatric population and especially in patients with manic-depressive illness.

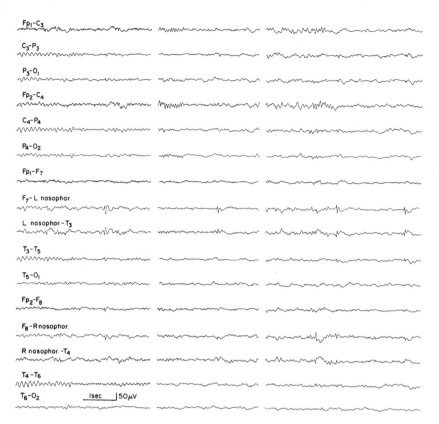

Figure 13.11. Small sharp spikes (51-year-old patient). Note the subtle character and moderate voltage of the discharge; also note its predominance in the left nasopharyngeal lead. There is evidence of spread into T_3, as well as into the right nasopharyngeal lead. The *left section* was recorded in the waking state (transition to earliest drowsiness); the *middle* and *right sections* were recorded in sleep. (Reproduced with permission from *Clinical Electroencephalography*.)

It is interesting to note that Gibbs and Gibbs (1964) found a rather high prevalence of small sharp spikes in presumed normal adult control subjects, reading 7.9% in the range from 40 to 49 years. Reiher and Klass (1968), Lebel et al. (1977), White et al. (1977), Klass and Westmoreland (1985), and Gutrecht (1989) have stressed the nonspecific nature of this pattern and do not regard its occurrence as an abnormality. By contrast, Low et al. (1984) as well as Hughes and Gruener (1984) have pointed out that small sharp spikes are not a normal or meaningless pattern. The data of these authors clearly show that this pattern indicates "a moderate degree of epileptogenicity" (Hughes and Gruener, 1984). This has been strongly confirmed by Saito et al. (1987) and also by Molaie et al. (1989). This is another indication of the inherent epileptogenic potentialities in so-called benign patterns.

Needle-Like Occipital Spikes of the Blind

Spike discharges of a particularly fast and needle-like character develop over the occipital region in most congenitally blind children (Gibbs and Gibbs, 1981; Gibbs et al., 1968; Lairy et al., 1964). These spikes are completely innocuous, unrelated to epileptic seizure disorder, and probably due to a state of functional deafferentation (Cannon and Rosenblueth, 1949). The discharges disappear during childhood or adolescence. The experimental basis of visual deafferentation spikes, however, is controversial (Kellaway et al., 1955).

Congenitally blind children with a history of *retrolental fibroplasia* often show evidence of accompanying cerebral impairment. Such children may show abundant and widespread but chiefly occipital spike activity; concomitant clinical epileptic seizures are fairly common in this condition (Gibbs and Gibbs, 1964; Gibbs et al., 1955). This type of spike activity must be differentiated from transient occipital spiking in nonepileptic congenitally blind children.

The 14 and 6/Sec Positive Spike Discharge (Fourteen and Six Positive Bursts)

Under the heading of "Fourteen and Six Hz Positive Bursts," this discharge has been defined as follows (IF-SECN, 1974). "Bursts of arch shaped waves at 13–17 Hz and/or 5–7 Hz, most commonly at 14 and/or 6 Hz, seen generally over the posterior temporal and adjacent areas of one or both sides of the head during sleep. The sharp peaks of its component are positive with respect to other regions." It is also pointed out in this definition that the amplitudes are generally below 75 μV, that the pattern is best demonstrated by referential recording using contralateral ear lobes or other remote reference leads, and that the clinical significance is controversial.

This excellent definition leaves nothing to be desired unless one would like to argue the use of "Hz," since one is not dealing with cycles per second at conventional paper speeds but with a certain rhythmical discharge rate of spikes. The synonymous term *ctenoids* was introduced by Lombroso et al. (1966) with regard to the comb-like shape. Contrary to Dutertre's (1977) statement, "mitten" is not a synonymous term.

The 14 and the six component may be observed independently. According to Gibbs and Gibbs (1964), the six com-

Figure 13.12. Various examples of 14/sec and 6/sec positive spikes *(underlined)*. Note posterior predominance for this pattern and shifting asymmetrics. Also note the sometimes blurred distinction between the 14 and 6 component, due to notch formation. The recording was obtained from a 12-year-old patient; montages to ipsilateral ear.

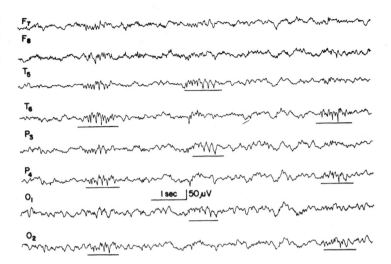

ponent prevails in early childhood and adulthood, while the 14 component is more prominent in older children and adolescents. Hughes (1960, 1965) emphasized the harmonic character of the major frequencies and preferred the term *14 and 7/sec positive spikes* (Fig. 13.12).

This pattern was described first by Gibbs and Gibbs (1951) and regarded as "evidence of thalamic and hypothalamic epilepsy." The following 15 years produced exciting correlations to autonomic nervous system dysfunctions and behavioral disorders (Gibbs and Gibbs, 1963; Henry, 1963; Hughes et al., 1961; Kellaway et al., 1959; Millen and White, 1954; Niedermeyer and Knott, 1961; Poser and Ziegler, 1958; Refsum et al., 1960; Schwade and Geiger, 1953; Shimoda, 1961; Stephenson, 1951; Walter et al., 1960). Enthusiasm flagged when it became clear that this pattern is too often found in healthy individuals (Lombroso et al., 1966; Long and Johnson, 1967). Little (1965) even presumed that this pattern "is more likely to be a sign of health than of disease."

The "14 and 6 pattern" may be confined to the regions lying beneath a skull defect (Beydoun and Drury, 1992) and hence could denote a "hidden pattern" that is not detectable from the scalp unless it reaches major proportions.

The pattern occurs most commonly in children after age 4 and adolescents and declines in adulthood; Gibbs and Gibbs (1964, 1978) recorded the 14 and 6 activity even in infants. Its occurrence in the waking state is exceptional; deep drowsiness and very light non-REM sleep are usually the ideal states for the documentation of the pattern, although deep sleep might be more conducive in very young children (Gibbs and Gibbs, 1964). Yürüker and Menzi (1971) elicited the 14 and 6 pattern with auditory stimuli presented in light sleep. Okada et al. (1990) noted 14 and 6/sec positive spikes in association with simultaneous negative spikes over the frontal area (suggestive of dipole formation).

Little is known about origin and neurophysiological discharge demonstrated in depth recordings at the thalamic as well as the basal ganglia level (Niedermeyer et al., 1967); the discharge was also repeatedly recorded in the amygdaloid complex.

The prevalence of the pattern used to be high in children, adolescents, and young adults, and increases with the recorded length of sleep. Much of the controversy about this pattern has arisen from differences of recording techniques and the use of routine sleep tracings and, in particular, the length of the sleep portion. The prevalence used to range from 10% to 30% at the age of 10 to 25 years, depending on type of patient. There has been good evidence of a marked—if not dramatic—decrease of the prevalence of "14 and 6" discharge according to Gibbs (1990). This author has pointed out the paralleling curve of the incidence of measles cases, but no strong inferences can be made from these similarities. Thus, the decline of the "14 and 6" observations remains an enigma.

Children with attacks of abdominal pain, older children with severe nonmigrainous headaches, children with certain forms of mental retardation, and adolescent or young adult aggressive sociopathic individuals have been presumed to show the 14 and 6/sec positive spike pattern more often than other patients and normal control subjects, but this is still shrouded in doubt and controversy. Proven cases of epileptic seizure disorder very seldom show 14 and 6/sec positive spikes as the only significant finding.

The author's laboratory reports records with 14 and 6 and no other abnormality as within broad normal limits of variability unless the pattern is extremely frequent and pronounced; then it is regarded as minimally abnormal. It appears to be a marginal pattern of no or very little epileptological significance.

The demonstration of 14 and 6/sec positive spikes in advanced states of metabolic encephalopathies, especially in hepatic coma (Silverman, 1964), is an interesting exception. For completely unknown reasons, this essentially innocuous discharge may appear when slow activity becomes extremely pronounced in such patients. A similar observation was reported by Ford and Freeman (1982). Drury (1989) reported 121 children with hepatic coma and mostly in association with Reye's syndrome. Seven of these children showed 14 and 6/sec positive spikes, occurring in an almost periodic manner, in four children activated by stimulation.

In all these cases, there was a background of severe EEG abnormality. Repeat tracings failed to show any 14 and 6 discharges (with one exception). The "14 and 6" pattern may also occur as a transient toxic effect of diphenhydramine hydrochloride (Benadryl).

Psychomotor Variant (Rhythmical Temporal Theta Bursts, Rhythmic Midtemporal Discharges)

This pattern is widely known as "psychomotor variant discharge" (Gibbs and Gibbs, 1952, 1964) because of certain similarities to rhythmical ictal activity occurring in psychomotor seizures (temporal lobe seizures, complex partial seizures). This term has been discouraged by IFSECN (1974), which recommended the term *rhythmical theta bursts of drowsiness*. The term *rhythmic midtemporal discharge* of Lipman and Hughes (1969) is also widely used.

The pattern consists of long runs of rhythmical activity in the range of 5 to 6.5/sec with a maximum over the midtemporal region, often with considerable spread into posterior temporal, anterior temporal, and occipital areas. The theta activity shows a well-defined negative sharp component (Fig. 13.13) that apparently stresses the paroxysmal character of the discharge. These trains of sharp theta waves may occur in a unilateral, bilateral shifting, or synchronous distribution type. The duration of a single run usually exceeds 10 seconds and may reach 1 minute or more. Very often, the first run is noted in early drowsiness; in deep drowsiness and light sleep, the pattern tends to disappear. According to Egli et al. (1978), patients with rhythmical theta bursts show shortened periods of REM sleep and also, to a lesser degree, of slow sleep in nocturnal sleep studies at the expense of log drowsy periods with the rhythmic theta pattern. Hughes (2001) has emphasized that the rhythmic midtemporal discharge is not limited by the drowsy state and may be very active in wakefulness. By no means should it be regarded as a normal drowsy pattern.

The pattern occurs mainly in younger or middle-aged adults; it is also seen in adolescents and children. It is a rare pattern; Egli et al. (1978) found a prevalence of 0.1% in a large laboratory.

The clinical significance is not clear. Despite its strongly paroxysmal appearance, its epileptogenic properties seem to be very low; most patients have no history of clinical seizures, although Lipman and Hughes (1969) found seizures in 36% of their patients. Personality disorders and some autonomic nervous system dysfunctions are common in patients with this pattern (Garvin, 1968; Gibbs and Gibbs, 1964; Lipman and Hughes, 1969). This view is shared by Eeg-Olofsson and Petersén (1982; cited in Boutros et al., 1986), who also studied the genetic transmission of this pattern and wondered about possible autosomal dominant inheritance. In the author's personal experience, this discharge represents a mild abnormality and we report such records as minimally or slightly abnormal if no other deviations are found.

Subclinical Rhythmic EEG Discharge of Adults (SREDA)

This pattern was originally described by Naquet et al. (1961) as a "paroxysmal discharge of the temporo-parieto-occipital junction," facilitated or triggered by temporary hypoxic conditions. In spite of certain paroxysmal features and its rhythmical sharp character, the possibility of an epileptic (ictal) event has been strongly de-emphasized. Herranz and Lopez (1984) have described this pattern as "subclinical paroxysmal activity" in 31 patients and stressed its rarity; it has an incidence of 0.02% to 0.045%.

Westmoreland and Klass (1981, 1997), and Miller et al. (1985) deserve particular credit for the elucidation of this discharge type. These authors disagree with the view of Naquet et al. (1961) concerning the major role of cerebrovascular insufficiency and hypoxia, although the average age of their patients was 61 years. The term "SREDA" has been proposed by Miller et al. (1985).

This pattern occurs mainly in the waking state or in light drowsiness. The onset may be fairly abrupt with widespread sharp rhythmical theta (4–7/sec) and occasionally with delta activity. In other cases, the onset is gradual with a few single sharp discharges that increasingly develop rhythmical character, first at delta, then at theta frequency. As to the spatial

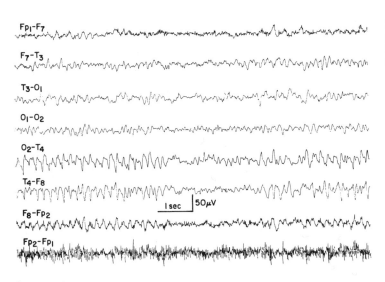

Figure 13.13. Psychomotor variant discharge of the right midtemporal region (T_4). Tracing was obtained from a 21-year-old woman. The record had low-voltage character; this necessitated the use of high gain.

distribution, a maximum of this discharge is usually found over the centroparietal region and especially over the vertex. Hyperventilation may induce this pattern.

In a "revisitation" of the SREDA pattern, O'Brien et al. (1998) analyzed this pattern in seven recent patients and only one of them showed evidence of cerebrovascular disorder.

Temporal Minor Sharp Transients of Old Age and Wicket Spikes

See Chapter 17, "Cerebrovascular Disorders and EEG."

Ictal Paroxysmal Patterns

Ictal EEG patterns may be a prolongation of a well-defined interictal pattern that becomes ictal by virtue of its long duration (this augmenting impact on neuronal function) or completely different from preceding interictal discharges. A typical example of the former case is the petit mal absences with short 3/sec spike wave bursts as interictal and prolonged 3/sec spike wave bursts as ictal phenomena. The emergence of a completely different ictal pattern is exemplified by partial forms of seizures (for instance, by cases of temporal lobe epilepsy with typical anterior temporal sharp waves in the interval and the sudden appearance of completely different patterns during a seizure).

Ictal patterns may be clinical, with the typical motor and behavioral changes of a seizure of whatever category or subclinical with no demonstrable motor or behavioral changes. In such clinically silent ictal episodes, neuropsychological studies may demonstrate some changes.

The following discussion of the ictal EEG patterns is cursory. A more detailed presentation is found in Chapter 27, "Epileptic Seizure Disorders." Special studies and atlases on epileptic seizures and their EEG correlates have been presented by Gibbs and Gibbs (1952), Ajmone Marsan and Ralston (1957), Gastaut and Broughton (1972), Karbowski (1975, 1985), and Oller-Daurella and Oller-Ferrer-Vidal (1977). The atlas of Oller-Daurella and Oller-Ferrer-Vidal is unique because of the beautiful cinematographic demonstration of clinical and EEG features. Further work on ictal EEG patterns was presented by Ralston (1958), Ralston and Papatheodorou (1960), Anziska and Cracco (1977), Geiger and Harner (1978), and Blume et al. (1983, 1984).

Grand Mal (Tonic-Clonic Seizures)

The ictal EEG is invariably obscured by muscle artifact; it is demonstrable only in patients treated with curare or other strong muscle relaxants with artificial respiration. Fast rhythmic spikes are present in all leads, with some accentuation in upper frontal leads. This fast spike activity characterizes the tonic stage and becomes discontinuous in the clonic stage. Rhythmic slow waves alternate with bursts of polyspikes synchronously with clonic jerks (polyspikes) and brief relaxation (slow bursts). A period of postictal electrical silence is usually fairly brief; a phase of very irregular slow activity follows during the ensuing minutes (see Chapter 27).

Petit Mal Absences

Typified by the generalized synchronous 3/sec spike wave complex occurring in more prolonged bursts, petit mal absences were discussed above (see Interictal Paroxysmal Patterns) and under petit mal absences in Chapter 27; also see discussion of 3/sec spike-wave in this chapter.

Psychomotor Seizures (Complex Partial Seizures, Temporal Lobe Seizures)

The ictal EEG patterns of these seizures are "as variable as the clinical features" (Gastaut and Broughton, 1972). The astounding variability of the ictal patterns is impressively demonstrated in the atlas of Oller-Daurella and Oller-Ferrer-Vidal (1977); also see Chapter 27.

In early work of Gibbs et al. (1936, 1937), the ictal EEG activity of psychomotor seizures was described as a special type of seizure discharge characterized by bursts of serrated slow waves, flat-topped 4/sec waves, and high voltage 6/sec waves ("seizure discharge of the psychomotor type"). Much greater complexities of the ictal patterns were stressed by Gastaut and Vigouroux (1958) and Klass (1975). In about 5% of the cases, a complex partial seizure may occur without any recordable ictal EEG activity (Gastaut and Broughton, 1972).

Focal Motor and Other Focal Seizures (Partial Seizures with Simple Symptomatology)

Cortical focal (partial) seizures are expected to be associated with a local discharge consisting of a sequence of repetitive spikes over the area contralateral to the motor or sensory (visual, auditory) clinical manifestations. This is correct in a large number of cases but does not pertain to all cases. According to Gastaut and Broughton (1972), there is no demonstrable ictal EEG discharge in about 30% of the cases. This is particularly true for circumscript motor rolandic attacks; ictal discharges arising from the precentral gyrus may be quite subtle and inconspicuous or not demonstrable at all in the EEG (Gibbs and Gibbs, 1952).

In cases with a well-documented EEG correlate of the seizure, the attack is often initiated by local desynchronization, i.e., very fast and very low voltage spiky activity, which gradually rises in amplitude with diminishing frequency (Geiger and Harner, 1978).

Myoclonic Seizures

Myoclonus is a very complex phenomenon; a considerable number of disorders with myoclonus do not fall into the epileptic category (Niedermeyer et al., 1979). Epileptic myoclonus is classically characterized by concomitant polyspikes or polyspike wave discharges in the EEG, of bilateral or generalized synchronous character, usually with maximum over the frontal regions. Further details are found in Chapter 27. A review of myoclonus and its relationship to epilepsy has been presented by Hallett (1985).

Tonic Seizures

The relationship between tonic seizures and massive fast spike activity was discussed above (see Interictal Paroxysmal Patterns and Runs of Rapid Spikes). This pattern is the typical correlate of tonic attacks occurring in patients with the Lennox-Gastaut syndrome.

Some tonic seizures are characterized by simple flattening or desynchronization of all activity during the attack (Gastaut and Broughton, 1972). These authors also describe rhythmical activity around 10/sec and a very rare diffuse slow wave pattern (mainly delta frequency) as EEG concomitants of tonic seizures.

Atonic Seizures

These seizures are customarily divided into a short form, such as simple drop attack, lasting only seconds, and a longer form, lasting minutes and described as "inhibitory." The EEG shows a few polyspike waves or spike waves of generalized distribution followed by large slow waves (short forms). More rhythmical spike activity around 10/sec and intermixed slow activity in all leads constitute the EEG correlate of the longer lasting attacks; rhythmical slow spike wave activity (1.5–2/sec) may also occur (Gastaut and Broughton, 1972; Oller-Daurella and Oller-Ferrer-Vidal, 1977). Suppression of the frontal premotor output might cause atonia and falls.

Akinetic Seizures

These attacks are characterized by arrest of all motion, which, however, is not caused by sudden loss of tone as in atonic seizure. The patients, usually children, are in an absence-like state; the EEG correlate is a slow (mostly 1–2/sec) spike-wave discharge, generalized synchronous and often with clocklike rhythmicity. This type of seizure is rather poorly understood and, in recent years, the use of this term has been discouraged.

Jackknife Seizures (Salaam Attacks)

The EEG correlates of this common type of seizure in children with hypsarrhythmia (infantile spasms, West syndrome) are divided into (a) sudden generalized flattening desynchronization, (b) rapid spike discharges of high voltage in all leads, and (c) no ictal alteration of the ongoing EEG activity (Kellaway, 1959; Gastaut and Broughton, 1972).

Periodic or Quasiperiodic Discharges

These rhythmically (or nearly rhythmically or "quasi-rhythmically") recurring discharges or patterns are of paroxysmal character, but they are usually not associated with epileptic seizure disorders characterized by chronically recurrent seizures. Periodic discharges or periodic activities are most commonly an important EEG feature of a severe ongoing central nervous system (CNS) disease with certain paroxysmal or even overt epileptogenic properties. They are hence disease-suggestive and sometimes virtually disease-specific, rather than suggestive of epileptic seizure disorders in general. A review of periodic activities was presented by Gaches (1971), as well as by Bauer and Pieber (1974).

The periodic character of these patterns in the presence of severe CNS involvement remains enigmatic; such rhythmi-

cal firing is markedly different from the predominantly random character of interictal seizure discharges (spikes, sharp wave, etc.). There is no satisfactory model to explain the periodicity of the discharges.

Periodic discharges are always of large amplitude, mostly in the range of 100 to 300 μV. These may be simple sharp waves, but of a duration that usually exceeds 150 msec. Other periodic discharges are compounded and polymorphic. Periodic discharges may be focal, widely scattered, or generalized synchronous. A fine tabulated review of periodic discharges has been presented by Spehlmann (1981).

Periodic Complexes in Subacute Sclerosing Panencephalitis (SSPE)

Features of this disease and the electroclinical correlations are presented in greater detail in Chapter 16, "The EEG in Cerebral Inflammatory Processes." The periodic complexes dominate the second state of this disease; this is a prolonged phase in which the clinical diagnosis is usually made.

The SSPE discharge has become exceptionally rare due to its relationship with measles and the excellent preventive effect of measles immunization. This type of complex discharge almost never occurs in other clinical conditions and is hence almost disease-specific. It is a very reliable and highly contributory diagnostic finding in this disease. These discharges were first mentioned by Balthazar (1944) and extensively described by Radermecker (1949, 1956) and Cobb and Hill (1950). The discharges show a duration from 0.5 to 3 seconds and are formed by two or more waves with mean amplitude of 500 μV (100–1,000 μV) (Rabending and Radermecker, 1977). In some cases, the voltage may even reach 1,400 μV (Kiloh et al., 1972).

The enormous height of this discharge may impress the inexperienced as a movement artifact; this idea is supported by frequent associated motor events such as myoclonus or sudden loss of tone.

The periodicity becomes manifest as the disease progresses; in its earlier stages, which are usually dominated by diffuse 1 to 3/sec activity of fairly rhythmical character, the compounded discharge may be aperiodic. Sometimes, the periodic discharge is present in the earliest stage of the disease and may persist to the fatal outcome; more often, this pattern disappears in the terminal or third stage. Vitrai et al. (1980) investigated the SSPE complex with the use of time functions of the auto- and cross-correlation coefficients.

The elements of the discharge are variable; a giant slow wave is usually mixed with several sharp waves. The discharge is generalized, with a maximum over the frontocentral areas and vertex. The frequency of the complexes ranges from 4 to 16/min (Rabending and Radermecker, 1977). The discharge is more impressive in the waking state (Fig. 13.14).

Accompanying myoclonus is fairly synchronous with the discharge; the motor activity may precede or trail the discharge in a range of 200 to 800 msec (Celesia, 1973); this author showed minor interhemispheric asynchronies (15 msec) and an earlier appearance in parieto-occipital areas than in frontocentral areas, where the discharge shows its most impressive voltage.

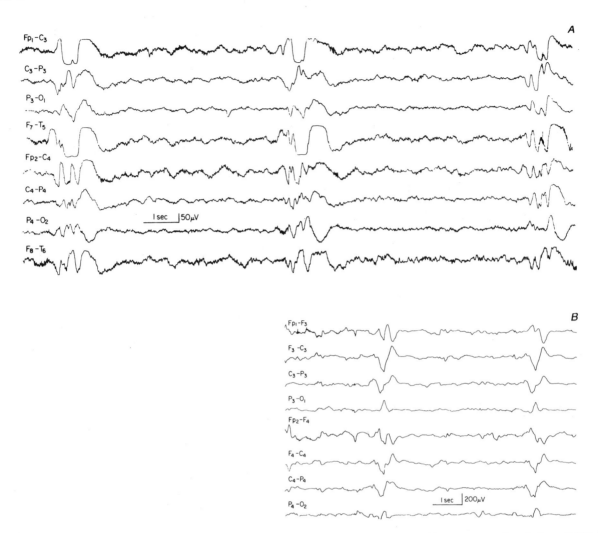

Figure 13.14.   Periodic discharges in subacute sclerosing panencephalitis (SSPE). **A:** At an earlier state with some preservation of other activities. **B:** At a more advanced state (recorded from two different patients, ages 8 and 9 years).

The background activity between the complexes is quite variable. The background may be normal with posterior alpha rhythm; however, this is exceptional; severely disordered background activity is most commonly found. Slow activity prevails and numerous spikes are sometimes recorded, especially over anterior areas. Spike-wave complexes may also be present; even clinical petit mal absences with classical 3/sec spike wave complexes have been observed (Broughton et al., 1973). A case of acute fulminant SSPE with only 2 months' duration was reported by Gökcil et al. (1998); the EEG showed very pronounced discharges.

Periodic discharges mimicking SSPE have been reported by Giovanardi Rossi et al. (1982) in children with myoclonic juvenile epilepsy of nonprogressive character. These discharges, however, were confined to ictal episodes. Most unusual is the observation of Prier et al. (1992): convincing periodic complexes of the aforementioned type in an indubitable case of multiple sclerosis (age 15 years).

The origin of the periodic SSPE discharge is controversial. Radermecker and Poser (1960) have proposed a deep thalamic or mesencephalic-reticular origin; this view has been supported by Cobb (1966, 1968), who performed depth EEG recordings, and by Lombroso (1968), who studied direct current (DC) potential changes during the periodic discharge. Other authors favor the idea of a cortical origin (Bogacz et al., 1959; Lesse et al., 1958; Storm van Leeuwen, 1964).

In an autopsy-confirmed case of SSPE, Martinovic (1986) demonstrated periodically occurring generalized high-voltage bursts firing at a rate of 11 to 13/sec with a spiky contour. There was a repetition interval of 27 to 28 seconds. This most unusual pattern was gradually replaced by the conventional type of periodic discharges.

Periodic Complexes in Herpes Simplex Encephalitis

In this extremely severe but not invariably fatal necrotizing encephalitis, slow repetitive spikes have been noted by Radermecker (1956). These observations were subsequently confirmed by Millar and Coey (1959), Perier et al. (1961),

Carmon et al. (1965), Rawls et al. (1966), Adams and Jennett (1967), Upton and Gumpert (1970), Gaches and Arfel (1972), Elian (1975), Kugler et al. (1976), and Cobb (1979). The discharge was also found in experimental disease inoculated rabbits by Gupta and Seth (1973).

In an earlier stage, local mostly unilateral temporal polymorphic delta waves are the most striking feature, but soon large sharp waves emerge over the most affected region. These discharges usually fire at intervals from 2 to 4 seconds. The discharge may be quite slow and exceed 1,000 msec; consider that a sharp wave is defined as having a duration from 70 to 150 msec. The amplitudes are in the range from 100 to about 500 μV. Similar periodic sharp discharges have been demonstrated in neonatal herpes simplex encephalitis (Fineyre, 1979). In the course of the disease, the originally regional discharge tends to become generalized synchronous; asynchronous bilateral discharges may also occur. Predominantly occipital localization of the periodic discharges have been reported by Bergey et al. (1982).

In contrast with the complexes found in SSPE, the periodic discharge of herpes simplex encephalitis is of short periodicity, with the greatest intervals of 4 seconds or less; according to Gaches (1971), this criterion is always met in the herpes simplex discharge. In some cases, the periodic discharge can be detected only when almost daily repeat records are carried out. This explains the fact that periodic discharges are not reported in all cases of herpes simplex encephalitis.

Periodic Discharges in Creutzfeldt-Jakob Disease

The clinical and neuropathological features of this subacute disease were established by the work of Creutzfeldt (1920), Jakob (1921), and Kirschbaum (1924, 1968). A very similar syndrome known as spongiform encephalopathy (Jones and Nevin, 1954) and a special variant described by Heidenhain (1929) were eventually found to be the same disease. Although originally presumed to be a degenerative CNS disorder, a slow virus was eventually demonstrated as the causative agent (C.J. Gibbs and Gajdusek, 1969; C.J. Gibbs et al., 1968). These investigators transmitted this virus to the chimpanzee with intracerebral inoculation and produced a similar invariably fatal disease. It is interesting to note that chimpanzees with the full clinical picture of Creutzfeldt-Jakob disease showed prominent delta activity in their EEG but neither spikes nor periodic discharges (Niedermeyer et al., 1972).

The periodic discharge consists of a sharp wave or a sharp triphasic complex of 100 to 300 msec duration with a repetition rate of 0.5 to 2/sec or intervals of 500 to 2,000 msec. The discharges occur against a severely disordered background of activity, mostly in generalized synchrony. Some cases show unilateral onset with discharges over one hemisphere or lateralized to one hemisphere for several days or weeks (Drury and Beydoun, 1996). According to Tariska et al. (1985), the periodic discharges may even remain unilateral in the course of the disease.

The periodic activity usually shows a maximum over the anterior region except for the Heidenhain form, which has a posterior maximum (Fig. 13.15); in this special form, cortical blindness is a common feature. In sleep, the periodic dis-

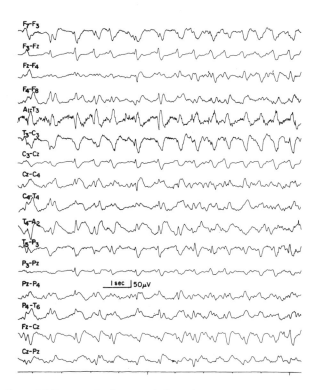

Figure 13.15. Periodic discharges in Creutzfeldt-Jakob disease. Note mild lateralization of the recurrent sharp waves to the left. The 68-year-old patient was demented, with psychotic features; there were long tract signs, fasciculation, and frequent myoclonus. Myoclonic jerking did not alter the tracing.

charges tend to disappear. The absence of periodic discharges after 10 weeks of illness militates against Creutzfeldt-Jakob disease (Chiappa and Young, 1978). EEG studies of Chiofalo et al. (1980) are based on the observation of 27 cases. The differential diagnosis of the combined clinical and electroencephalographic picture of this disease is quite complex (Poole, 1980).

Myoclonus is a typical clinical feature of this disease. The periodic patterns may or may not be associated with myoclonus (Niedermeyer et al., 1979).

In addition to periodic discharges, cyclic changes may also occur, and the periodic activity may get temporarily replaced by diffuse slow activity in the delta and theta range (Terzano et al., 1981).

The periodic EEG discharge of Creutzfeldt-Jakob disease may be caused by other conditions in rare instances. In Chapter 22, "Metabolic Central Nervous System Disorders," hypothyroidism is mentioned as a treatable cause of this pattern.

It has to be emphasized that the periodic discharges of Creutzfeldt-Jakob disease (a) do not occur in every case of this disease (even with numerous repeat-recordings) (Bortone et al., 1994) and (b) may occasionally be found in other disorders.

Periodic Lateralized Epileptiform Discharges (PLED)

In the wake of earlier work (Alajouanine et al., 1955; Barolin et al., 1962; Chatrian, 1961; Fischer-Williams, 1963;

LeBeau and Dondey, 1959; Pagni et al., 1960), Chatrian et al. (1964) gave an extensive account of periodic lateralized or focal discharge that may occur in a variety of acute neurological conditions. This pattern is most often associated with acute cerebral infarctions but may also occur in neoplastic and inflammatory pathology. Periodic discharges occurring in herpes simplex encephalitis are discussed earlier in this chapter. PLED activity, however, may also occur in other types of encephalitis—among others, in infectious mononucleosis encephalitis, according to Aminoff et al. (1982). As to acute vascular pathology, watershed-type infarctions are the most common structural substratum in patients with PLED. This pattern is also briefly discussed in Chapter 17, "Cerebrovascular Disorders and EEG." Markand and Daly (1971), Dauben and Adams (1974), and Bauer et al. (1981) presented further important work on this pattern, which also plays a major role in experimental cerebral embolism (Naquet and Vigouroux, 1972).

PLED may be simple and large sharp waves or complex (compounded) discharges with mixed spiky and slower elements. The amplitudes usually lie around 100 to 300 μV, but occasionally may be much higher. The firing rate may be as fast as 3/sec or as slow as 12/min (Chatrian et al., 1964) (Fig. 13.16).

The discharge is found over the maximally involved area, and the local background activity is almost always severely disordered. The mechanism of this form of infarction is discussed in Chapter 17. The focal maximum is customarily located over the boundary zone between middle and posterior cerebral arteries and thus over the posterior temporal region and its immediate vicinity. Watershed infarctions are seldom found between the territories of middle and anterior cerebral arteries, with a maximum of PLED activity over the superofrontal region.

The term *PLED* implies lateralization. It is possible, however, that PLED activity is generated independently over both hemispheres. De la Paz and Brenner (1982) have investigated the bilateral type of PLED referred to as "BIPLED" (also "bi-PLED"). Although strokes were found to be the leading cause in the PLED group, CNS infection and epileptic seizure disorders predominated in the group with BIPLED. Bilateral-synchronous (generalized-synchronous) periodic activity should not be listed as BIPLED in view of the original definition of Chatrian et al. (1964). This distinction, however, is not generally observed (see the report of Schear, 1984). Filley et al. (1984) have broken down their large material of PLED into typical and "indeterminate" discharges. The term *cerebral bigeminy* has been used by Aldrich and Pugh (1984) for bilaterally independent PLED activity. Even TRI-PLEDs, arising from three different areas, have been reported (left frontal,

left posterotemporal, and right posterotemporal) in an 85-year-old patient with renal encephalopathy (Hughes et al., 1998).

PLEDs are often associated with simultaneous focal motor twitching in contralateral face or fingers, hand, arm, leg, foot, etc. This underscores the paroxysmal character of the pattern. It is usually a temporary pattern that changes into other abnormalities within 1 to 2 days. Patients with PLED are in most cases acutely ill and often show a history of a variety of mixed problems, such as cerebral arteriosclerosis plus renal insufficiency or chronic alcoholism or diabetes mellitus. With all this emphasis on the vascular genesis of this pattern, the possibility of an underlying neoplasm must not be ignored.

Patients with PLED are commonly older adults; this pattern occasionally occurs in young adults and children (PeBenito and Cracco, 1979). Andriola (1982) noted PLED as well as BIPLED in 12 children with various types of acute CNS disease; those with bilateral activity (BIPLED) expired in the acute state. Ritaccio and March (1993) reported the association of BIPLEDs with complex partial status epilepticus. Silbert et al. (1996) described another variant of PLEDs with independent ipsilateral periodic lateralized discharges. A clinical curiosity appeared to be the observation of Chabolla et al. (1996): a young man suffering from multiple sclerosis (MS) with exacerbations ushered in by complex partial status epilepticus associated with an enhancing right frontal MRI lesion and PLEDs in the EEG. Another report on PLEDs in MS (right temporal PLEDs and MRI lesion) has been presented by Gandelman-Marton et al. (2003).

A very thoughtful study of PLEDs deserves special attention: a critical review of Pohlmann-Eden et al. (1996). These authors consider PLEDs as "an EEG signature of a dynamic pathophysiological state in which unstable neurobiological processes create an ictal-interictal continuum, with the nature of the underlying neuronal injury, the patient's preexisting propensity to have seizures, and the co-existence of any acute metabolic derangements all contributing to whether seizures occur or not." Pohlmann-Eden et al. have strongly reemphasized the dominant etiological role of strokes in the generation of PLEDs. From the evidence of functional neuroimaging studies, these authors feel that PLEDs "might reflect a key pattern for focal hyperexcitability in the penumbra zone of ischemic stroke."

A nonlateralized variant of PLEDs are periodic epileptiform discharges occurring in the midline (PEDIM), as cited by Westmoreland et al. (1997). These midline discharges are also presumed to arise from watershed areas: anterior and middle, middle, and posterior cerebral arteries.

Figure 13.16. **A:** Periodic lateralized epileptiform discharge (PLED) in a 70-year-old patient, widespread over left hemisphere with left midtemporal maximum. Note poorly developed background of activity. Cerebrovascular accident associated with twitching of right arm. Patient lethargic and obtunded. **B:** PLED over right central-midtemporal region, sometimes also involving the right parietal area. Note well-preserved physiological activities of waking and light drowsiness. Also note the complex and multiphasic character of the discharge. Patient is 68 years old with cerebrovascular disease with right centroparietal low-density area in CT scan (infarction).

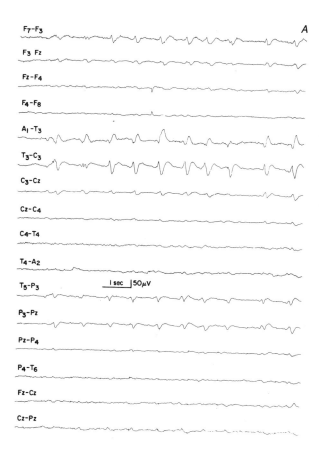

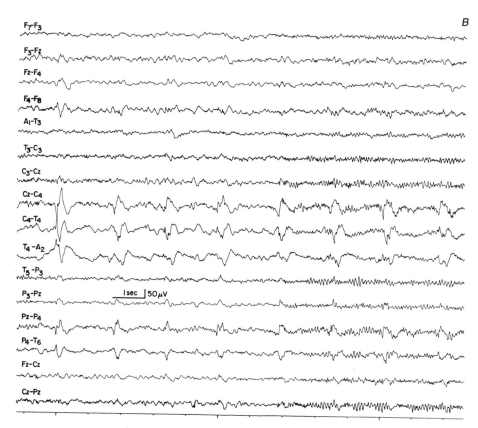

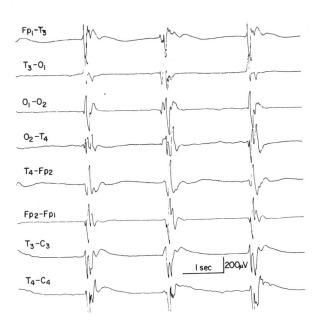

Figure 13.17. Comatose patient (acute cerebral anoxia), age 57. Constantly repetitive compounded spike discharges against a virtually flat background of activity. These discharges were associated with occasional generalized myoclonus.

Periodic Discharges in Acute Cerebral Anoxia

Repetitive simple or compounded sharp waves in generalized synchrony may occur against a flat (or at least seemingly flat) background of activity in patients with acute cerebral anoxia. Myoclonus is often found in association with this type of activity (Butenuth and Kubicki, 1971; Madison and Niedermeyer, 1970; Takahashi et al., 1993). In most cases, these discharges are probably aborted bursts in a suppression burst pattern. True periodic discharges, however, may also occur (Fig. 13.17). The reader will find more pertinent information in Chapter 23, "Cerebral Anoxia: Clinical Aspects."

Periodic Discharges of Other Etiologies

Periodic discharges may occasionally occur in other conditions, but such observations are rare. The presence of such discharges, whether regional or generalized, merely underscores the severity of the basic conditions. Figure 13-18 demonstrates periodic discharges over the right posterior quadrant in a 15-year-old girl with a history of Dandy-Walker syndrome, numerous shunt operations, and infections of the shunted area. These problems are compounded by a severe epileptic seizure disorder. These rhythmical discharges also show the tempo of propagation over the right posterior quadrant of the cerebrum (see legend).

Spikes and Other Paroxysmal Discharges in Healthy Nonepileptic Persons

The occurrence of focal or generalized paroxysmal discharges in apparently healthy individuals is a puzzling and even annoying finding that requires some discussion. These findings may be quickly termed as false positives, but the EEG abnormalities are real and their irrelevance in view of the individual's good health is more apparent than real. Such spikes are testimony of certain cerebral dysfunctions that may or may not become manifest in the further course of events. These findings do not discredit the method of electroencephalography, which, after artifacts are ruled out, can show only facts. These disturbing facts are in need of a reasonable interpretation. Let us contemplate the indubitable fact that a complete medical evaluation will yield certain physical shortcomings and organic abnormalities in almost every healthy individual; even acne pimples are cutaneous lesions and hence abnormalities. What the electroencephalographer needs in such cases is a commonsense philosophy as a basis for a wise interpretation. General medicine is full of examples of seemingly irrelevant and yet unmistakably present abnormalities that the prudent, seasoned physician will integrate into a holistic view of the individual. Seen from this angle, electroencephalography does not differ from the rest of medicine.

The EEG evaluation of comparatively large healthy populations usually shows a certain percentage of abnormalities. The work of Thorner (1942) showed paroxysmal discharges in 0.3% of 1,100 flying cadets; Gibbs et al. (1943)

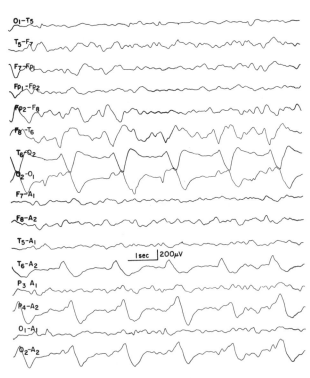

Figure 13.18. Waking record of a 15-year-old girl with Dandy-Walker syndrome in combination with a brainstem lipoma. The patient suffers from a severe epileptic seizure disorder; she had been treated with numerous shunt operations. Against a diffuse background of disorganized slow activity, a periodic discharge of "blunted" sharp character is very prominent over the right posterior quadrant. Both bipolar and unipolar derivations show a focal origin in the right posterotemporal lead (T_6) with prominent spread into right occipital (O_2) and right parietal (P_4) regions. This spread is so slow that the traveling character of the periodic discharges can be gleaned from bipolar and referential derivations.

found epileptic abnormalities in 0.9% of normal adult controls, whereas Harty et al. (1942) observed such abnormalities in 3% of candidates for medical service. "Larval epileptic disturbances" were noted in 9% of healthy controls by Williams (1944). The tumult of World War II was apparently conducive to such large-scale studies, which have become more scarce over the past decades.

A study of 682 Air Force applicants showed paroxysmal changes in 2.6%; about one fourth were focal and the rest were of nonfocal character (Buchthal and Lennox, 1953). Further studies of this kind were carried out in commercial flying personnel (Dell and Dell, 1958), candidates for commercial airplane pilot training (Blanc et al., 1964), and air cadets (O'Connor, 1964). Some studies concentrated on the classical 3/sec spike wave pattern, which was found in 0.2% of 3,070 normal controls (Gibbs et al., 1943) and 2.7% in the subjects of Hill (1952). Spike wave complexes were found in 0.9% to 1.5% of the groups studied by Dell and Dell (1958), in 1% of the subjects of Blanc et al. (1964), and in 0.5% of O'Connor's subjects (1964). No spike wave complexes were found in the normative study carried out for the National Aeronautics and Space Administration by Baylor University in Houston, Texas (Baylor University, 1966). Bennett (1967) evaluated the EEG of military and civil flying personnel (1,332 persons) and found spike wave discharges in only 0.6%. Gibbs and Gibbs (1964) found 6/sec spike waves in 1.3% to 2.0% of 3,476 adults, peaking in the range from 20 to 24 years, but was unable to detect any focal spikes or sharp waves. Focal sharp activity was reported in 1% of the material of Blanc et al. (1964). The reports of Lennox-Buchthal et al. (1959) and Kitamura and Asakura (1958) show a relatively high incidence of spikes (6.4 and 4%, respectively).

Zivin and Ajmone Marsan (1968) and Chatrian (1976) have contemplated the clinical significance of spikes in healthy persons. Above all, the interpretation must take into consideration age. In childhood, the occurrence of central-midtemporal (also parietal) spikes is associated with overt seizures in only 50% to 70% of the cases; this pertains mainly to the age from 3 to 12 years. In occipital spikes (mainly age 3–5 years), the epileptogenicity is even lower. Major studies on this subject based on large healthy populations were performed by Nekhorocheff (1950), Kellaway and Fox (1952), Brandt and Brandt (1955), Corbin and Bickford (1955), Trojaborg (1966), Eeg-Olofsson et al. (1971), and Cavazzuti et al. (1980). In general, "benign" focal spikes (such as seen in benign rolandic epilepsy) outnumber generalized synchronous bursts of spikes or spike waves by a slight to considerable margin. Cavazzuti et al. obtained EEG recordings of 3,726 children from 6 to 13 years of age without evidence of seizure or neurological deficits. Paroxysmal discharges were found in 131 cases (3.52%). Generalized, mainly polyspike, wave discharges were found in 41 cases, midtemporal spikes in 50, centroparietal spikes in 27, occipital spikes in two, and bilateral (midtemporal or parietal) spikes in 11 children. Change of spike localization occurred in but a few subjects; shifts from focal to generalized spiking and vice versa were also rare. The work of Cavazzuti et al. is particularly important because it includes follow-up periods of up to 9 years. In most children, the abnormalities disappeared, usually during ele-

mentary school age or in early adolescence. Only seven children developed clinical epileptic seizures; five had generalized discharges, one had midtemporal, and one had centroparietal spikes. In two subjects there was evidence of epileptic seizures in the family, while six children had siblings with spikes, either generalized or rolandic.

Both generalized synchronous (spike-wave, polyspike-wave) and rolandic (centroparieto-midtemporal) spikes in nonepileptic children suggest a *genetic predisposition* if no neurological deficit and no history of insult to the CNS are present. In children with a history of cerebral palsy and with no seizures but prominent spiking, the spike activity may herald future epileptic seizures (Gibbs and Gibbs, 1964). Even in perfectly healthy children with spikes, the possibility of future seizures cannot be completely ruled out, although the chances are slim.

In healthy children and especially in healthy adults with spikes, emphasis must be places on certain personality disorders that are not incompatible with normal functioning. Psychological and mild psychiatric deviations include poor impulse control, proneness to hysterical conversion reactions, and schizoid manifestations. In such individuals, the presence of a cerebral dysfunction with paroxysmal EEG changes may hamper the natural process of psychological maturation. In some of these cases, head injuries or infections of moderate severity might have prompted or facilitated the EEG changes as well as the psychological deviations.

The high incidence of anterior temporal-midtemporal sharp transients in older patients with some degree of cerebrovascular disorder is discussed in Chapters 17, "Cerebrovascular Disorders and EEG," and 27, "Epileptic Seizure Disorders." These patients may even have overt sharp waves; others show small sharp spikes. Unless there is evidence of epileptic seizures, these discharges indicate only some degree of temporal lobe dysfunction, often compatible with good health.

This section must be capped by a strong plea to clinicians to refrain from rash and ill-advised statements that a seizure-free person has epilepsy and must be treated because of spikes in the EEG. These persons need further medical attention, and repeat EEG should be done at reasonable intervals, such as every 2 years in a child or adolescent and every 5 years in an adult. Anticonvulsive treatment is not needed, but should not necessarily be denied to extremely apprehensive, introspective, and hypochondria-prone individuals. This author, too, has to refrain from rash verdicts; recent insights may indicate the use of antiepileptics in some seizure-free patients with spikes.

Concluding Remarks

Paroxysmal discharges in the EEG are indicators of deviant neuronal behavior that may or may not amount to clinical epileptic seizures. Solid experience in clinical EEG and familiarity with the multitude of epileptic seizure disorders are the indispensable prerequisites for a truthful and clinically useful interpretation of paroxysmal EEG events. The extensive chapter on EEG and epileptology, Chapter 27, provides the reader with further information on this subject.

Moreover, the reader will derive much benefit from the thoughtful review of interictal spike discharges by Hughes (1989). Considerations of the clinical relevance of paroxysmal discharges in general (Niedermeyer, 1990) reassess strength and limitations of EEG information in epileptic seizure disorders.

References

Aarts, J.H.P., Binnie, C.D., Smit, A.M., et al. 1984. Selective cognitive impairment during focal and generalized epileptiform EEG activity. Brain 107:293–308.

Adams, J.H., and Jennett, W.B. 1967. Acute necrotizing encephalitis: a problem in diagnosis. J. Neurol. Neurosurg. Psychiatr. 30:248–260.

Ajmone Marsan, C., and Ralston, B.L. 1957. *The Epileptic Seizures.* Springfield, IL: Charles C Thomas.

Alajouanine, T., Lecasble, R., and Remond, A. 1955. Eléments graphiques paroxystiques lents de survénue périodiques. Corrélations electrocliniquis. Rev. Neurol. (Paris) 93:477–478.

Aldrich, M.S., and Pugh, J.E. 1984. Cerebral bigeminy: alternating periodic epileptiform discharges. Electroencephalogr. Clin. Neurophysiol. 58:35P (abst).

Aminoff, M.J., Greenberg, D.A., and Wiekle, D.J. 1982. Periodic EEG complexes in infectious mononucleosis encephalitis. Electroencephalogr. Clin. Neurophysiol. 53:28P(abst).

Andriola, M. 1982. PLEDS and bi-PLEDS in children. Electroencephalogr. Clin. Neurophysiol. 53:88P(abst).

Anziska, B., and Cracco, R. 1977. Changes in frequency and amplitude in electrographic seizure discharges. Clin. Electroencephalogr. 8:206–210.

Arroyo, S., Lesser, R.P., Fisher, R.S., et al. 1994. Clinical and electroencephalographic evidence for sites of origin of seizures with diffuse electrodecremental pattern. Epilepsia 35:974–987.

Baddeley, A.D. 1986. *Working Memory.* Oxford: University Press.

Balthazar, K. 1944. Zur Kenntnis der Panencephalitis nodosa (Pette). Arch. Psychiatr. Nervenkr. 117:666.

Barolin, G., Scherzer, E., Naquet, R., et al. 1962. Étude électro-clinique des états de mal épileptiques survenants chez les apoplectiques. Rev. Neurol. (Paris) 107:242–243.

Bauer, G., and Markoff, R. 1970. Familienuntersuchungen bei einem seltenen paroxysmalen Muster. Z. EEG-EMG 1:19–26.

Bauer, G., and Pieber, R. 1974. Über periodische Komplexe im EEG. Z. EEG-EMG 5:75–86.

Bauer, G., Aichner, F., and Hengl, W. 1981. Der diagnostische Wert periodisch lateralisierter Komplexe im EEG. Z. EEG-EMG 12:135–141.

Baylor University College of Medicine and the Methodist Hospital. 1966. *The Normative Electroencephalographic Data Reference Library. Final Report.* Washington, DC: National Aeronautics and Space Administration.

Bennett, D.R. 1967. Spike-wave complexes in "normal" flying personnel. Aerospace Med. 38:1276–1282.

Bergen, D. 1979. A unique EEG pattern in mucolipidosis. Electroencephalogr. Clin. Neurophysiol. 46:80.

Bergey, G.K., Coyle, P.K., Krumholz, A., et al. 1982. Herpes simplex encephalitis with occipital localization. Arch. Neurol. (Chicago) 39:312–313.

Beydoun, A., and Drury, I. 1992. Unilateral 14 and 6 Hz positive bursts. Electroencephalogr. Clin. Neurophysiol. 82:310–312.

Binnie, C.D., Polkey, C.E., and Spencer, S. 1989. Positive spikes over a cortical laceration. Electroencephalogr. Clin. Neurophysiol. 72:106P(abst).

Blanc, C., Lafontaine, E., and Laplane, R. 1964. Les activités EEG paroxystiques généralisées ou focales chez les adultes non comitiaux: Études évolutive correlations longitudinales. Rev. Neurol. (Paris) 111:362–369.

Blume W.T., Lemieux, J.F., and Young, G.B. 1983. EEG morphology of early stage epileptic seizures. Electroencephalogr. Clin. Neurophysiol. 56:25P(abst).

Blume, W.T., Young, G.B., and Lemieux, J.F. 1984. EEG morphology of partial epileptic seizures. Electroencephalogr. Clin. Neurophysiol. 57: 295–302.

Bogacz, J., Castells, C., San Julian, J., et al. 1959. Nonepidemic progressive subacute encephalitis (type Van Bogaert). II. Serial EEG abnormalities and deep electrography. Acta Neurol. Lat.-Am. 5:158–183.

Bortone, E., Bettoni, L., Giorgi, C., et al. 1994. Reliability of EEG in the diagnosis of Creutzfeldt-Jakob disease. Electroencephalogr. Clin. Neurophysiol. 90:323–330.

Boutros, N.N., Hughes, J.R., and Weiler, M. 1986. Psychiatric correlates of the rhythmic mid-temporal discharges and the 6/sec spike and wave complexes. Biol. Psychiatr. 21:94–99.

Brandt, S., and Brandt, H. 1955. The electroencephalographic patterns in young healthy children from 0 to five years of life. Acta Psychiatr. Scand. 30:77–89.

Brenner, R.P., and Atkinson, R. 1982. Generalized paroxysmal fast activity: electroencephalographic and clinical features. Ann. Neurol. 11:386–390.

Broughton, R., Nelson, R., Gloor, P., et al. 1973. Petit mal epilepsy evolving to subacute sclerosing panencephalitis. In *Evolution and Prognosis of Epilepsies.* Eds. E. Lugaresi, P. Pazzaglia, and C.A. Tassinari, pp. 63–72. Bologna: Gaggi.

Buchthal, F., and Lennox, M. 1953. The EEG effect of Metrazol and photic stimulation in 682 normal subjects. Electroencephalogr. Clin. Neurophysiol. 5:545–558.

Butenuth, J., and Kubicki, St. 1971. Über die prognostische Bedeutung bestimmter Formen der Myoklonien und korrespondierender EEG-Muster nach Hypoxien. Z. EEG-EMG 2:78–83.

Cannon, W.B., and Rosenblueth, A. 1949. *The Supersensitivity of Denervated Structures: A Law of Denervation.* New York: Macmillan.

Carmon, A., Behar, A., and Beller, A. 1965. Acute necrotizing encephalitis presenting clinically as a space-occupying lesion. A clinico-pathological study of six cases. J. Neurol. Sci. 2:328–343.

Cavazzuti, G.B., Cappella, L., and Nalin, A. 1980. Longitudinal study of epileptiform EEG patterns in normal children. Epilepsia (New York) 21:43–55.

Celesia, G.G. 1973. Pathophysiology of periodic EEG complexes in subacute sclerosing panencephalitis (SSPE). Electroencephalogr. Clin. Neurophysiol. 35:293–300.

Chabolla, D.R., Moore, J.L., and Westmoreland, B.F. 1996. Periodic lateralized epileptiform discharges in multiple sclerosis. Electroencephalogr. Clin. Neurophysiol. 98:5–8.

Chatrian, G.E. 1961. EEG pattern: pseudo-rhythmic recurrent sharp waves. Its relationship to local cerebral anoxia and hypoxia. Electroencephalogr. Clin. Neurophysiol. 13:144(abst).

Chatrian, G.E. 1976. Paroxysmal pattern in "normal" subjects. In *Handbook of Electroencephalography and Clinical Neurophysiology.* vol. 6A, Ed.-in-chief, A. Remond, pp. 114–123. Amsterdam: Elsevier.

Chatrian, G.E., Shaw, C.M., and Leffman, H. 1964. The significance of periodic epileptiform discharges in EEG: an electrographic, clinical and pathological study. Electroencephalogr. Clin. Neurophysiol. 17: 177–193.

Chayasirisobhon, S., Cullis, P., Sack, R., et al. 1984. Grand mal discharge. Clin. Electroencephalogr. 15:155–158.

Chiappa, K., and Young, R. 1978. The EEG as a definitive diagnostic tool early in the course of Creutzfeldt-Jakob disease. Electroencephalogr. Clin. Neurophysiol. 45:26(abst).

Chiofalo, N., Fuentes, A., and Galvez, S. 1980. Serial EEG findings in 27 cases of Creutzfeldt-Jakob disease. Arch. Neurol. (Chicago) 37:143–145.

Clark, E.C., and Knott, J.R. 1955. Paroxysmal wave and spike activity and diagnostic sub-classification. Electroencephalogr. Clin. Neurophysiol. 7:161–164.

Cobb, W.A. 1966. The periodic events of subacute sclerosing leucoencephalitis. Electroencephalogr. Clin. Neurophysiol. 21:278–294.

Cobb, W.A. 1968. Depth recording in subacute sclerosing leucoencephalitis. In *Clinical Electroencephalography of Children.* Eds. P. Kellaway and I. Petersén, pp. 275–286. New York: Grune & Stratton (Stockholm: Almquist and Wiksell).

Cobb, W.A. 1979. Evidence on the periodic mechanism in herpes simplex encephalitis. Electroencephalogr. Clin. Neurophysiol. 46:345–350.

Cobb, W.A., and Hill, D. 1950. Electroencephalogram in subacute progressive encephalitis. Brain 73:392–404.

Cohn, R. 1954. Spike-dome complex in the human electroencephalogram. Arch. Neurol. Psychiatr. (Chicago) 71:699–706.

Corbin, H.P.F., and Bickford, R.G. 1955. Studies of the electroencephalogram of normal children: comparison of visual and automatic frequency analysis. Electroencephalogr. Clin. Neurophysiol. 7:15–28.

Creutzfeldt, H.G. 1920. Über eine eigenartige herdförmige Erkrankung des Zentralnervensystems. Z. Ges. Neurol. Psychiatr. 57:1. (Quoted after Kirschbaum, W.R., 1968.)

Cukier, F., André, N., Monod, N., et al. 1974. EEG contribution to diagnosing intraventricular haemorrhage in premature infants. Electroencephalogr. Clin. Neurophysiol. 36:840(abst).

Dauben, R.D., and Adams, A.H. 1974. Periodic lateralized epileptiform discharges in EEG. A review with special attention to etiology and recurrence. Clin. Electroencephalogr. 8:116–124.

De la Paz, D., and Brenner, R.P. 1982. Bilateral independent periodic lateralized epileptiform discharges—clinical significance. Electroencephalogr. Clin. Neurophysiol. 53:27P(abst).

Dell, A.R., and Dell, M.B. 1958. L'électroencéphalogramme systématique du personnel navigant. Étude préliminaire portant sur 1056 cas. Méd. Aéro. 13:33–47.

Dondey, M. 1983. Transverse topographical analysis of petit mal discharges: diagnostical and pathogenic implications. Electroencephalogr. Clin. Neurophysiol. 55:361–371.

Drury, I. 1989. 14- and 6-Hz positive bursts in diverse encephalopathies of childhood. Electroencephalogr. Clin. Neurophysiol. 72:12P(abst).

Drury, I., and Beydoun, A. 1996. Evolution of periodic complexes in Creutzfeldt-Jakob disease. Am. J. EEG Technol. 36:230–234.

Dutertre, F. 1977. Catalogue of the main EEG patterns. In *Handbook of Electroencephalography and Clinical Neurophysiology,* vol. 11A, Ed.-in-chief, A. Remond, pp. 40–79. Amsterdam: Elsevier.

Eeg-Olofsson, O., Petersén, I., and Selldén, U. 1971. The development of the electroencephalogram in normal children from the age of 1 through 15 years. Paroxysmal activity. Neuropaediatrie 2:375–404.

Egli, M., Hess, R., and Kuritzke, G. 1978. Die Bedeutung der "rhythmic mid-temporal discharges." Z. EEG-EMG 9:74–85.

Elian, M. 1975. Herpes simplex virus encephalitis and EEG. J. Electrophysiol. Technol. 1:161–170.

Engel, J., Jr., Rapin, I., and Giblin, D.R. 1977. Electrophysiological studies in two patients with cherry red spot-myoclonus syndrome. Epilepsia (New York) 18:73–87.

Filley, C.M., Kelly, M.A., Hwang, P.A.L.S., et al. 1984. An analysis of typical and "indeterminate" PLEDs. Electroencephalogr. Clin. Neurophysiol. 58:32P(abst).

Fineyre, R. 1979. Periodic discharge of unusually slow character in neonatal status epilepticus caused by necrotizing encephalitis (herpes simplex). Electroencephalogr. Clin. Neurophysiol. 46:80(abst).

Fisch, B.J. 2003. Interictal epileptiform activity: diagnostic and behavioral implications. J. Clin. Neurophysiol. 20:155–162.

Fischer-Williams, M. 1963. Burst-suppression activity as an indication of undercut cortex. Electroencephalogr. Clin. Neurophysiol. 15:723–724 (abst).

Ford, R.G., and Freeman, A.M. 1982. Positive spike bursts in a comatose adult. Electroencephalogr. Clin. Neurophysiol. 53:29P(abst).

Fuster, J.M. 1995. Memory and planning. In *Epilepsy and the Functional Anatomy of the Frontal Lobe,* Eds. H.H. Jasper, S. Riggio, and P.S. Patricia Goldman-Rakic, pp. 9–19. New York: Raven Press.

Fuster, J.M. 1996. *Memory in the Cerebral Cortex.* Cambridge, Mass: MIT Press.

Gaches, J. 1971. Les activitiés périodiques en EEG. Rev. EEG Neurophysiol. 1:9–33.

Gaches, J., and Arfel, G. 1972. Certitude et suspicions d'encéphalites herpétiques. Aspects électroencéphalographiques. Encéphale 61:510–549.

Gambardella, A., Aguglia, U., Oliveri, R.I., et al. 1997. Negative myoclonic status due to antiepileptic drug tapering: report of three cases. Epilepsia 38:819–823.

Gandelman-Marton, R., Rabey, J.M., and Flechter, S. 2003. Periodic lateralized epileptiform discharges in multiple sclerosis: a case report. J. Clin. Neurophysiol. 20:117–121.

Garvin, J.S. 1968. Psychomotor variant pattern. Dis. Nerv. Syst. 29:59–76.

Gastaut, H. 1968. Clinical and electroencephalographic correlates of generalized spike and wave bursts occurring spontaneously in man. Epilepsia (Amsterdam) 9:179–184.

Gastaut, H., and Broughton, R. 1972. *Epileptic Seizures.* Springfield, IL: Charles C Thomas.

Gastaut, H., and Hunter, J. 1950. An experimental study of the mechanism of photic activation in idiopathic epilepsy. Electroencephalogr. Clin. Neurophysiol. 2:263–287.

Gastaut, H., and Vigouroux, M. 1958. Electro-clinical correlations in 500 cases of psychomotor seizures. In *Temporal Lobe Epilepsy,* Eds. M. Baldwin, and P. Bailey, pp. 118–128. Springfield, IL: Charles C Thomas.

Gastaut, H., Roger, J., Soulayrol, R., et al. 1966. Childhood epileptic encephalopathy with diffuse slow spike-waves (otherwise known as "petit mal variant") or Lennox syndrome. Epilepsia (Amsterdam) 7:139–179.

Geiger, L.R., and Harner, R.N. 1978. EEG patterns at the time of focal seizure onset. Arch. Neurol. (Chicago) 35:276–286.

Gianelli, M., Cantello, R., Civardi, C., et al. 1994. Idiopathic generalized epilepsy: magnetic stimulation of motor cortex time-locked and unlocked to 3-Hz spike-and-wave discharges. Epilepsia 35:53–60.

Gibbs, C.J., Jr., and Gajdusek, D.C. 1969. Infection as the etiology of spongiform encephalopathy (Creutzfeldt-Jakob disease). Science 165:1023–1025.

Gibbs, C.J., Jr., Gajdusek, D.C., Asher, D.M., et al. 1968. Creutzfeldt-Jakob disease (spongiform encephalopathy): transmission to the chimpanzee. Science 161:388–389.

Gibbs, E.L., and Gibbs, F.A. 1951. Electroencephalographic evidence of thalamic and hypothalamic epilepsy. Neurology (Minneapolis) 1:136–144.

Gibbs, E.L., and Gibbs, F.A. 1981. Das Elektroenzephalogramm bei congenitaler Anophthalmie. Z. EEG-EMG 12:171–173.

Gibbs, E.L., Fois, A., and Gibbs, F.A. 1955. The electroencephalogram in retrolental fibroplasia. N. Engl. J. Med. 253:1102–1106.

Gibbs, F.A. 1990. An epidemiological note? Clin. Electroencephalogr. 21:112–118.

Gibbs, F.A., and Gibbs, E.L. 1952. *Atlas of Electroencephalography,* vol. 2. Cambridge, MA: Addison-Wesley.

Gibbs, F.A., and Gibbs, E.L. 1963. Fourteen and six per second positive spikes. Electroencephalogr. Clin. Neurophysiol. 15:353–358.

Gibbs, F.A., and Gibbs, E.L. 1964. *Atlas of Electroencephalography,* vol. 3. Reading, MA: Addison-Wesley.

Gibbs, F.A., and Gibbs, E.L. 1978. *Atlas of Electroencephalography,* vol. 4. Menlo Park, CA: Addison-Wesley.

Gibbs, F.A., Davis, H., and Lennox, W.G. 1935. The electroencephalogram in epilepsy and in conditions of impaired consciousness. Arch. Neurol. Psychiatr. (Chicago) 34:1133–1148.

Gibbs, F.A., Lennox, W.G., and Gibbs, E.L. 1936. The electro-encephalogram in diagnosis and localization of epileptic seizures. Arch. Neurol. Psychiatr. (Chicago) 36:1225–1235.

Gibbs, F.A., Gibbs, E.L., and Lennox, W.G. 1937. Epilepsy, a paroxysmal cerebral dysrhythmia. Brain 60:377–388.

Gibbs, F.A., Gibbs, E.L., and Lennox, W.G. 1939. The influence of blood sugar level on the wave and spike formation in petit mal epilepsy. Arch. Neurol. Psychiatr. (Chicago) 50:111–128.

Gibbs, F.A., Gibbs, E.L., and Lennox, W.G. 1943. Electroencephalographic classification of epileptic patients and control subjects. Arch. Neurol. Psychiatr. 50:111–128.

Gibbs, F.A., Gibbs, E.L., and Gibbs, T.J. 1968. Relation between specific types of occipital dysrhythmia and visual defects. Johns Hopkins Bull. 122:343–349.

Giovanardi Rossi, P., Gobbi, G., Moschen, R., et al. 1982. Subacute sclerosing panencephalitis-like EEG pattern and periodic myoclonic seizures: two case reports. Electroencephalogr. Clin. 54:3P(abst).

Gökcil, Z., Odabasi, Z., Aksu, A., et al. 1998. Acute fulminant SSPE: clinical and EEG features. Clin. Electroencephalogr. 29:43–48.

Gotman, J. 1981. Interhemispheric relations during bilateral spike-and-wave activity. Epilepsia (New York) 22:453–466.

Gotman, J. 1984. Could interictal epileptic spikes actually be postictal epileptic spikes? Electroencephalogr. Clin. Neurophysiol. 58:9P(abst).

Gotman, J., and Marciani, M.G. 1985. Electroencephalographic spiking activity, drug levels and seizure occurrence in epileptic patients. Ann. Neurol. 17:597–603.

Gotman, J., Gloor, P., and Schaul, N. 1978. Comparison of traditional reading of the EEG and automatic recognition of interictal epileptic activity. Electroencephalogr. Clin. Neurophysiol. 44:48–60.

Gregory, D.L., and Wong, P.K. 1984. Topographical analysis of the centrotemporal discharges in benign rolandic epilepsy of childhood. Epilepsia (New York) 25:705–711.

Gupta, P.C., and Seth, P. 1973. Periodic complexes in herpes simplex encephalitis. A clinical and experimental study. Electroencephalogr. Clin. Neurophysiol. 35:67–74.

Gutrecht, J.A. 1989. Clinical implications of benign epileptiform transients of sleep. Electroencephalogr. Clin. Neurophysiol. 72:486–490.

Halász, P. 1972. The generalized epileptic spike-wave mechanism and the sleep-wakefulness system. Acta. Physiol. Acad. Scient. Hungar. 42:293–314.

Hallett, M. 1985. Myoclonus: Relation to epilepsy. Epilepsia (New York) 26(suppl. 1):567–577.

Harty, J.E., Gibbs, E.G., and Gibbs, F.A. 1942. Electroencephalographic study of two hundred and seventy-five candidates for military service. War Med. (Chicago) 2:923–930.

Hecker, A., Kocher, R., Ladewig, D., et al. 1979. Das Minatur-Spike-Wave-Muster. Das EEG Labor 1:51–56.

Heidenhain, A. 1929. Klinische und anatomische Untersuchungen einer eignartiger organische Erkrankung des Zentralnervensystems im Praesenium. Z. Ges. Neurol. Psychiatr. 118:49–111.

Henry, E.E. 1963. Positive spike discharges in the EEG and behavior abnormality. In EEG and Behavior, Ed. G.E. Glaser, pp. 315–344. New York: Basic Books.

Herranz, F., and Lopez, S. 1984. Subclinical paroxysmal rhythmic activity. Electroencephalogr. Clin. Neurophysiol. 4:419–442.

Hill, D. 1952. EEG in episodic psychotic and psychopathic behaviour. A classification of data. Electroencephalogr. Clin. Neurophysiol. 4:419–442.

Hughes, J.R. 1960. The 14 and 7 per second positive spikes—a reappraisal following a frequency count. Electroencephalogr. Clin. Neurophysiol. 12:495–496.

Hughes, J.R. 1965. A review of the positive spike phenomenon. In Application of Electroencephalography in Psychiatry, Ed. W.P. Wilson, pp. 54–101. Durham: Duke University Press.

Hughes, J.R. 1980. Two forms of the 6/sec spike and wave complex. Electroencephalogr. Clin. Neurophysiol. 48:535–550.

Hughes, J.R. 1989. The significance of the interictal spike discharges. A review. J. Clin. Neurophysiol. 6:207–226.

Hughes, J.R. 1991. Changes in the annual incidence of the 6/sec spike and wave pattern. Clin. Electroencephalogr. 22:71–74.

Hughes, J.R. 1997. The significance of interictal spike discharge: a review. Clin. Electroencephalogr. 28:60(abst).

Hughes, J.R. 2001. The continuous rhythmic mid-temporal discharge. Clin. Electroencephalogr. 32:10–13.

Hughes, J.R., and Gruener, GT. 1984. Small sharp spikes revisited: further data on this controversial pattern. Electroencephalogr. Clin. Neurophysiol. 15:208–213.

Hughes, J.R., Gianturco, D., and Stein, W. 1961. Electro-clinical correlations in the positive spike phenomenon. Electroencephalogr. Clin. Neurophysiol. 13:599.

Hughes, J.R., Schlagenhauff, R.E., and Magoss, M. 1965. Electro-clinical correlations in the six per second spike and wave complex. Electroencephalogr. Clin. Neurophysiol. 18:71–77.

Hughes, J.R., Taber, J., and Uppal, H. 1998. TRI-PLEDs: a case report. Clin. Electroencephalogr. 29:106–108.

Hunter, J., and Jasper, H.H. 1949. Effects of thalamic stimulation in unanesthetized animals. Electroencephalogr. Clin. Neurophysiol. 1:303–324.

IFSECN, 1961. Preliminary proposal for an EEG terminology by the terminology committee of the International Federation for Electroencephalography and Clinical Neurophysiology. Electroencephalogr. Clin. Neurophysiol. 13:646–650.

IFSECN, 1966. Proposal for an EEG terminology committee of the International Federation for Electroencephalography and Clinical Neurophysiology. Electroencephalogr. Clin. Neurophysiol. 30:306–310.

IFSECN, 1974. A glossary of terms commonly used by clinical electroencephalographers. Electroencephalogr. Clin. Neurophysiol. 37:538–548.

Jakob, A. 1921. Über eigenartige Erkrankungen des Zentralnervensystems mit bemerkenswerten anatomischen Befunden (spastische Pseudosklerose, Encephalomyelopathie mit disseminierten Degenerationsbeschwerden). Deutsch Z. Nervenheilk. 70:132. (Quoted after Kirschbaum, W.R. 1968.)

Jasper, H.H. 1941. Epilepsy. In Epilepsy and Cerebral Localization, Eds. W. Penfield and T.C. Erickson, pp. 380–454. Springfield, IL: Charles C Thomas.

Jasper, H.H., and Kershman, J. 1949. Classification of the E.E.G. in epilepsy. Electroencephalogr. Clin. Neurophysiol. (suppl. 2):123–131.

Jones, D.P., and Nevin, S. 1954. Rapidly progressive cerebral degeneration (subacute vascular encephalopathy) with mental disorder, focal disturbances and myoclonic epilepsy. J. Neurol. Neurosurg. Psychiatr. 17:148–159.

Jung, R., and Toennies, F. 1950. Über Entstehung und Erhaltung von Krampfentladungen. Die Vorgänge im Reizort und die Krampffähigkeit des Gehirns. Arch. Psychiatr. Nervenkr. 1985:701–735.

Karbowski, K. 1975. Das Elekroenzephalogramm im epileptischen Anfall. Bern: Huber.

Karbowski, K. 1985. Epileptische Anfälle. Berlin: Springer.

Kellaway, P. 1959. Neurologic status of patients with hypsarrhythmia. In Molecules and Health, Ed. F.A. Gibbs, pp. 134–149. Philadelphia: JB Lippincott.

Kellaway, P., and Fox, B.J. 1952. Electroencephalographic diagnosis of cerebral pathology in infants during sleep. I. Rationale, technique and the characteristics of normal sleep in infants. J. Pediatr. 41:262–287.

Kellaway, P., Bloxsom, A., and MacGregor, M. 1955. Occipital spike foci associated with retrolental fibroplasia and other forms of retinal loss in children. Electroencephalogr. Clin. Neurophysiol. 7:469–470.

Kellaway, P., Crawley, J.W., and Kagawa, N. 1959. A specific electroencephalographic correlate of convulsive equivalent disorders in children. J. Pediatr. 55:582–592.

Kiloh, L.G., McComas, A.J., and Osselton, J.W. 1972. Clinical Electroencephalography, 3rd ed. London: Butterworth.

Kirschbaum, W.R. 1924. Zwei eigenartige Erkrankungen des Zentralnervensystems nach Art der spastischen Pseudosklerose (Jakob). Z. Ges. Neurol. Psychiatr. 92:157. (Quoted after Kirschbaum, W.R. 1968.)

Kirschbaum, W.R. 1968. Jakob-Creutzfeldt's Disease. New York: American Elsevier.

Kitamura, K., and Asakura, T. 1958. Clinical significance of spikes and sharp waves in EEG. Electroencephalogr. Clin. Neurophysiol. (suppl. 12):16.

Klass, D.W. 1975. Electroencephalographic complications in complex partial seizures. In Complex Partial Seizures and Their Treatment, Eds. J.K. Penry and D.D. Daly, pp. 113–140. New York: Raven Press.

Klass, D.W., and Westmoreland, B.F. 1985. Nonepileptogenic epileptiform electroencephalographic activity. Ann. Neurol. 18:627–635.

Kocher, R., Scollo-Lavizzari, G., and Ladewig, D. 1975. Miniature-spike-wave-Muster: Elektroencephalographisches Korrelat in der Abstinenzphase bei Medikamentenabhängigkeit. Z. EEG-EMG 6:78–82.

Koshino, Y., and Niedermeyer, E. 1975. The clinical significance of small sharp spikes in the electroencephalogram. Clin. Electroencephalogr. 6:131–140.

Kugler, J., Marltin, J.J., Radermecker, R.J., et al. 1976. Periodische Komplexe im EEG bei nekrotisierender Herpes-Enzephalitis. Z. EEG-EMG 7:63–71.

Lairy, G.C., Harrison, A., and Leger, E.M. 1964. Foyers EEG biocciptaux asynchrones de pointes chez l'enfant mal voyant et aveugle d'âge scolaire. Rev. Neurol. (Paris) 111:351–353.

LeBeau, F.E., and Dondey, M. 1959. Importance diagnostique de certaines activités électroencéphalographiques latéralisées périodiques ou à tendance périodique au cours des abscès de cerveau. Electroencephalogr. Clin. Neurophysiol. 11:43–58.

Lebel, M., Reiher, J., and Klass, D. 1977. Small sharp spikes (SSS). Reassessment of electroencephalographic and clinical significance. Electroencephalogr. Clin. Neurophysiol. 43:463(abst).

Lemieux, J.F., and Blume, W.T. 1983. Topographical evolution of the spike-wave complexes. Electroencephalogr. Clin. Neurophysiol. 56:30P (abst).

Lennox, W.G. 1960. Epilepsy and Related Disorders, vol. 1. Boston: Little, Brown.

Lennox-Buchthal, M., Buchthal, F., and Rosenfalck, P. 1959. Correlation of electroencephalographic findings with crash rate of military jet pilots. Epilepsia (Amsterdam) 1:366–373.

Lesse, S., Hoefer, P.F.A., and Austin, J.H. 1958. The electroencephalogram in diffuse encephalopathies. Arch. Neurol. Psychiatr. (Chicago) 79:359–375.

Lipman, I.L., and Hughes, J.R. 1969. Rhythmic mid-temporal discharges. An electroclinical study. Electroencephalogr. Clin. Neurophysiol. 27:43–47.

Little, S.C. 1965. A general analysis of the fourteen and six per second dysrhythmia. Proc. 6th International Congress Electroenceph. Clin. Neurophysiol., Vienna, pp. 313–315. Vienna: Wiener Med. Akad.

Lombroso, C.T. 1968. Remarks on the EEG and movement disorder in SSPE. Neurology (Minneapolis) 18:69–75.

Lombroso, C.T., Schwarts, I.H., Clark, D.M., et al. 1966. Ctenoids in healthy youth. Controlled study of 14 and 6-per-second positive spiking. Neurology (Minneapolis) 16:1152–1158.

Long, M.T., and Johnson, L.C. 1967. Fourteen and six positive spikes in nonpatient population. Neurology (Minneapolis) 17:316(abst).

Low, M.D., Henrikson, K., Lamont, D., et al. 1984. The relationship of small sharp spikes to seizures. Electroencephalogr. Clin. Neurophysiol. 58:11P(abst).

Lüders, H., Daube, J., Johnson, R., et al. 1980. Computer analysis of generalized spike-and-wave complexes. Epilepsia (New York) 21:183(abst).

Lundervold, A., Henriksen, G.F., and Fegersten, L. 1959. The spike wave complex. A clinical correlation. Electroencephalogr. Clin. Neurophysiol. 11:13–22.

Madison, D.S., and Niedermeyer, E. 1970. Epileptic seizures resulting from acute cerebral anoxia. J. Neurol. Neurosurg. Psychiatr. 33:381–386.

Markand, O.N., and Daly, D.D. 1971. Pseudoperiodic lateralized paroxysmal discharges in the electroencephalogram. Neurology (Minneapolis) 21:975–981.

Marshall, C. 1955. Some clinical correlates of the wave and spike phantom. Electroencephalogr. Clin. Neurophysiol. 7:633–636.

Martinovic, Z. 1986. Periodic generalized bursts of fast waves in subacute sclerosing panencephalitis. Electroencephalogr. Clin. Neurophysiol. 63:236–238.

Matsuo, F., and Knott, J.R. 1977. Focal positive spikes in electroencephalography. Electroencephalogr. Clin. Neurophysiol. 42:15–25.

Maulsby, R.L. 1971. Some guidelines for assessment of spikes and sharp waves in EEG tracings. Am. J. EEG Technol. 11:3–16.

Millar, J.H.D., and Coey, A. 1959. The EEG in necrotizing encephalitis. Electroencephalogr. Clin. Neurophysiol. 11:582–585.

Millen, F.J., and White, B. 1954. Fourteen and six per second positive spike activity in children. Neurology (Minneapolis) 4:541–549.

Miller, C.R., Westmoreland, B.F., and Klass, D.W. 1985. Subclinical rhythmic EEG discharge of adults (SREDA): further observations. Am. J. EEG Technol. 25:217–224.

Molaie, M., Santana, H.B., and Cavanaugh, W.A. 1989. Benign epileptiform transients of sleep (BETS) revisited. Electroencephalogr. Clin. Neurophysiol. 72:19P(abst).

Naquet, R., and Vigouroux, R.A. 1972. The EEG in relation to pathology in simple cerebral ischaemia. In Handbook of Electroencephalography and Clinical Neurophysiology, vol. 14A, Ed.-in-chief, A. Remond, pp. 38–44. Amsterdam: Elsevier.

Naquet, R., Louard, C., Rhodes, J., et al. 1961. À propos de certaines décharges paroxystiques du carrefour temporo-pariéto-occipital: leur activation par l'hypoxie. Rev. Neurol. (Paris) 105:203–207.

Nekhorocheff, M.I. 1950. La stimulation lumineuse intermittante chez l'enfant normal. Rev. Neurol. (Paris) 83:601–602.

Niedermeyer, E. 1969. The Lennox-Gastaut syndrome: a severe type of childhood epilepsy. D.Z. Nervenheilk. 195:263–283.

Niedermeyer, E. 1972. The Generalized Epilepsies. Springfield, IL: Charles C Thomas.

Niedermeyer, E. 1974. Compendium of the Epilepsies. Springfield, IL: Charles C Thomas.

Niedermeyer, E. 1976. Immediate transition from a petit mal absence into a grand mal seizure. Eur. Neurol (Basel) 14:11–16.

Niedermeyer, E. 1987. Controversial EEG patterns and their significance. Editorial. Am. J. EEG Technol. 27:129–132.

Niedermeyer, E. 1988a. Widersprüchlich beurteilte EEG-Tätigkeiten und ihre Bedeutung. EEG-Labor 10:3–7.

Niedermeyer, E. 1988b. The electroencephalogram in the differential diagnosis of the Lennox-Gastaut syndrome. In The Lennox-Gastaut Syndrome, Eds. E. Niedermeyer and R. Degen, pp. 177–220. New York: Alan R. Liss.

Niedermeyer, E. 1990. Clinical relevance of EEG signals in epilepsies. In Handbook of Electroencephalography and Clinical Neurophysiology, revised series, vol. 4, Eds. J.A. Wada and R.J. Ellingson, pp. 237–261. Amsterdam: Elsevier.

Niedermeyer, E. 1996. Primary (idiopathic) generalized epilepsy. Clin. Electroencephalogr. 27:1–21.

Niedermeyer, E. 1997. Frontal lobe functions and dysfunctions. Presented at Symposium, Lima (Peru).

Niedermeyer, E., and Knott, J.R. 1961. Über die Bedeutung der 14 and 6/sec-positiven Spitzen im EEG. Arch. Psychiatr. Nervenkrankh. 202:266–280.

Niedermeyer, E., Ray, C.D., and Walker, A.E. 1967. Depth studies in a patient with fourteen and six per second positive spikes. Electroencephalogr. Clin. Neurophysiol. 22:86–89.

Niedermeyer, E., Walker, A.E., and Burton, C. 1970. The slow spike-wave complex as a correlate of frontal and fronto-temporal posttraumatic epilepsy. Eur. Neurol. (Basel) 3:330–346.

Niedermeyer, E., Gibbs, C.B., Jr., Marsh, R., et al. 1972. EEG studies in subacute and degenerative neurological diseases experimentally produced in ferrets and chimpanzees. Electroencephalogr. Clin. Neurophysiol. 33:351–352(abst).

Niedermeyer, E., Fineyre, R., Riley T., et al. 1979. Myoclonus and the electroencephalogram. A review. Clin. Electroencephalogr. 10:75–95.

Niedermeyer, E., Krauss, G.L., and Pacer, C.E. 1989. The electroencephalogram and mental activation. Clin. Electroencephalogr. 20:215–227.

O'Brien, T.J., Sharbrough, F.W., Westmoreland, B.F., et al. 1998. Subclinical rhythmic electrographic discharges of adults (SREDA) revisited: a study using digital EEG analysis. J. Clin. Neurophysiol. 15:493–501.

O'Connor, P. 1964. Analysis of 500 routine EEGs of R.A.F. aircrew cadets. Electroencephalogr. Clin. Neurophysiol. 17:341(abst).

Ohtahara, S., and Yamatogi, Y. 1990. Evolution of seizures and EEG abnormalities in childhood onset epilepsy. In Handbook of Electroencephalography and Clinical Neurophysiology, revised series, vol. 4, Eds. J.A. Wada and R.J. Ellington, pp. 457–477. Amsterdam: Elsevier.

Okada, S., Kato, T., Miyashita, K., et al. 1990. 14 and 6 Hz positive spikes: relationship with a negative spiky phase in the frontal area. Electroencephalogr. Clin. Neurophysiol. 75:S108(abst).

Oller-Daurella, L., and Oller-Ferrer-Vidal, L. 1977. Atlas de Crisis Epilepticas. Geigy Division Farmaceut.

Pagni, C.A., Vitale, A., and Cassinari, V. 1960. Su alcuni casi di tracciati caratterizzati da elementi parassistici a ricorrenza ritmica periodica o pseudoperiodica. Riv. Neurol. 30:580–591.

PeBenito, R., and Cracco, J.B. 1979. Periodic lateralized epileptiform discharges in children. Ann. Neurol. 6:47–50.

Perier, O., Parmentier, B., Brihaye, J., et al. 1961. A case of inclusion body necrotizing encephalitis. In Encephalitides, Eds. L. Van Bogaert et al., pp. 235–242. Amsterdam: Elsevier.

Pohlmann-Eden, B., Hoch, D.B., Cochius, J.I., et al. 1996. Periodic lateralized epileptiform discharges—a critical review. J. Clin. Neurophysiol. 13:519–530.

Pollen, D.A. 1964. Intracellular studies of cortical neurons during thalamic induced wave and spike. Electroencephalogr. Clin. Neurophysiol. 17:398–406.

Pollen, D.A., Reid, K.H., and Perol, P. 1964. Micro-electrode studies of experimental wave and spike in the cat. Electroencephalogr. Clin. Neurophysiol. 17:57–67.

Poole, E.W. 1980. Jakob-Creutzfeldt disease. Patients who might have had this. Electroencephalogr. Clin. Neurophysiol. 49:89P.

Poser, C.M., and Ziegler, D.K. 1958. Clinical significance of 14 and 6 per second positive spike complexes. Neurology (Minneapolis) 8:903–912.

Prier, S., Benoit, C., and Cambier, J. 1992. Bilateral periodic stereo-typed EEG complexes in multiple sclerosis. Clin. Neurophysiol. 22 (suppl. 1–1992):107s(abst).

Rabending, G., and Radermecker, F.J. 1977. Subacute sclerosing panencephalitis (SSPE). In Handbook of Electroencephalography and Clinical Neurophysiology, vol. 15A, Ed.-in-chief, A. Remond, pp. 28–35. Amsterdam: Elsevier.

Radermecker, F.J. 1949. Aspects électroencéphalographiques dans trois cas d'encéphalite subaigue. Acta Neurol. Psychiatr. Belg. 49:222–232.

Radermecker, F.J. 1956. Systématique et électroencéphalographie des encéphalites et encéphalopathies. Amsterdam: Elsevier (Electroencephalogr. Clin. Neurophysiol., Suppl. 5).

Radermecker, F.J., and Poser, C.M. 1960. The significance of repetitive paroxysmal electroencephalographic patterns. Their specificity in subacute sclerosing leukoencephalitis. World Neurol. 1:422–433.

Ralston, B.L. 1958. The mechanism of transitions of interictal spiking foci into ictal seizure discharges. Electroencephalogr. Clin. Neurophysiol. 10:217–232.

Ralston, B.L., and Papatheodorou, C.A. 1960. The mechanisms of transition of interictal spiking foci into ictal seizure discharges. Part II. Observations in man. Electroencephalogr. Clin. Neurophysiol. 12:297–304.

Rawls, W.E., Dyck, P.J., Klass, D.W., et al. 1966. Encephalitis associated with herpes simplex virus. Ann. Intern. Med. 64:104–115.

Refsum, S., Presthus, J., Skulstad, A.A., et al. 1960. Clinical correlates of the 14 and 6 per second positive spikes. An electroencephalographic and clinical study. Acta Psychiatr. Scand. 35:330–344.

Reiher, J., and Klass, D.W. 1968. Two common EEG patterns of doubtful clinical significance. Med. Clin. North Am. 52:933–940.

Ribeiro, M., Niedermyer, E., and Hertz, S. 1999. Slow sharp waves. Clin. Electroencephalogr. 30:114–117.

Ritaccio, A.L., and March, G. 1993. The significance of BIPLEDs in complex partial status epilepticus. Am. J. EEG Technol. 33:27–34.

Rodin, E., and Ancheta, O. 1987. Cerebral electrical fields during petit mal absences. Electroencephalogr. Clin. Neurophysiol. 66:457–466.

Rodin, E., Smid, N., and Mason, K. 1976. The grand mal pattern of Gibbs, Gibbs and Lennox. Electroencephalogr. Clin. Neurophysiol. 40:401–406.

Roger, H., Cornil, L., and Paillas, J.E. 1949. *Les épilepsies.* Paris: Flammarion.

Saito, F., Fukushima, Y., and Kubota, S. 1987. Small sharp spikes: possible relationship to epilepsy. Clin. Electroencephalogr. 18:144–119.

Schear, H.E. 1984. Periodic EEG activity. Clin. Electroencephalogr. 15:32–39.

Schwade, E.D., and Geiger, S.G. 1953. Matricide with electroencephalographic evidence of thalamic or hypothalamic disorder. Dis. Nerv. Syst. 14:18–20.

Shewmon, D.A., and Erwin, R.J. 1988a. The effect of focal interictal spikes on perception and reaction time. I. General considerations. Electroencephalogr. Clin. Neurophysiol. 69:319–337.

Shewmon, D.A., and Erwin R.J. 1988b. The effect of focal interictal spikes on perception and reaction time. II. Neuroanatomic specificity. Electroencephalogr. Clin. Neurophysiol. 69:338–352.

Shewmon, D.A., and Erwin, R.J. 1988c. Focal spike-induced cerebral dysfunction is related to the after-coming slow wave. Ann. Neurol. 23:131–137.

Shimoda, Y. 1961. The clinical and electroencephalographic study of the primary diencephalic epilepsy or epilepsy of brain stem. Acta Neurovegetat. (Vienna) 23:181–191.

Silbert, P.L., Radhakrishnan, K., Sharbrough, F.W., et al. 1996. Ipsilateral independent periodic lateralized epileptiform discharges. Electroencephalogr. Clin. Neurophysiol. 98:223–226.

Silverman, D. 1954. Clinical correlates of the spike-wave complex. Electroencephalogr. Clin. Neurophysiol. 6:663–669.

Silverman, D. 1964. Fourteen and six per second positive spike pattern in a patient with hepatic coma. Electroencephalogr. Clin. Neurophysiol. 16:395–398.

Silverman, D. 1967. Phantom spike-wave and the fourteen and six per second positive spike pattern: a consideration of their relationship. Electroencephalogr. Clin. Neurophysiol. 23:203–217.

Small, J.G. 1970. Small sharp spikes in a psychiatric population. Arch. Gen. Psychiatr. 22:277–284.

Small, J.G., Small, I.F., Milstein, V., et al. 1975. Familial associations with EEG variants in manic depressive disease. Arch. Gen. Psychiatr. 32:43–48.

Spehlmann, R. 1981. *EEG Primer.* Amsterdam: Elsevier.

Sperling, M.R., and Skolnick, B.E. 1995. Cerebral blood flow during spike-wave discharges. Epilepsia 36:156–163.

Stephenson, W.A. 1951. Intracranial neoplasm associated with fourteen and six per second positive spikes. Neurology (Minneapolis) 1:372–376.

Steriade, M., Amzica, F., and Contreras, D. 1996. Synchronization of fast (30–40 Hz) spontaneous cortical rhythms during brain attention. J. Neurosci. 16:392–417.

Storm van Leeuwen, W. 1964. Electroencephalographical and neurophysiological aspects of subacute sclerosing leuco-encephalitis. Psychiatr. Neurol. Neurochir. (Amsterdam) 67:312–322.

Takahashi, M., Kubota, F., Nishi, Y., et al. 1993. Persistent synchronous periodic discharges caused by anoxic encephalopathy due to cardiopulmonary arrest. Clin. Electroencephalogr. 24:166–172.

Tariska, P., Gereby, G., and Majtenyi, K. 1985. The clinical significance of periodic lateralized epileptiform discharges (PLEDs). Electroencephalogr. Clin. Neurophysiol. 61:11P–12P(abst).

Terzano, M.G., Mancia, D., Calzetti, S., et al. 1981. Diagnostic value of EEG periodic discharges and cyclic changes in Creutzfeldt-Jakob disease. Electroencephalogr. Clin. Neurophysiol. 52:52P(abst).

Tharp, B.R. 1966. The 6-per-second spike and wave complex. Arch. Neurol. (Chicago) 15:533–537.

Thomas, J.E. 1957. A rare electroencephalographic pattern: the six-per-second spike and wave discharge. Neurology (Minneapolis) 7:438–442.

Thomas, J.E., and Klass, D.W. 1968. Six-per-second spike and wave pattern in the electroencephalogram: a reappraisal of clinical significance. Neurology (Minneapolis) 18:587–593.

Thorner, M.W. 1942. *Procurement of Electroencephalograph Tracings in 1000 Flying Cadets for Evaluating the Gibbs Technique in Relation to Flying Ability.* USAD School of Aviation Medical Research Report, No. 7–1.

Trojaborg, W. 1966. Focal spike discharges in children. Acta Paediatr. Scand. (Suppl.) 168:1–13.

Upton, A., and Gumpert, J. 1970. Electroencephalography in diagnosis of herpes simplex encephalitis. Lancet 1:650–652.

Vitrai, J., Czobor, P., Marosfi, S., et al. 1980. A study of periodicity and structure of EEG complexes in a case of SSPE. Electroencephalogr. Clin. Neurophysiol. 50:11–18.

Walker, A., and Morello, G. 1967. Experimental petit mal. Trans. Am. Neurol. Assoc. 57–61.

Walter, R.D., Colbert, E.G., Koegler, R.R., et al. 1960. A controlled study of the fourteen-and-six-per-second EEG pattern. Arch. Gen. Psychiatr. 2:559–566.

Warach, S., Ives, J.R., Schlaug, G., et al. 1996. EEG-triggered echo-planar functional MRI in epilepsy. Neurology 47:89–93.

Webber, W.R.S., Litt, B., Lesser, R.P., et al. 1993. Automatic spike detection: what should the computer imitate? Electroencephalogr. Clin. Neurophysiol. 87:364–373.

Webber, W.R.S., Litt, B., Wilson, K., et al. 1994. Practical detection of epileptiform discharges (Eds) in the EEG using an artificial neural network: a comparison of raw and parameterized EEG data. Electroencephalogr. Clin. Neurophysiol. 91:194–204.

Weir, B. 1965. The morphology of the spike-wave complex. Electroencephalogr. Clin. Neurophysiol. 19:284–290.

Weir, B., and Sie, P.G. 1966. Extracellular unit activity in cat during the spike-wave complex. Epilepsia (Amsterdam) 7:30–43.

Werhahn, K.J., and Noachtar, S. 2000. Epileptic negative myoclonus. In *Epileptic Seizures: Pathophysiology and Clinical Semiology*, Eds. H.O. Lueders and S. Noachtar, pp. 473–483. New York: Churchill Livingstone.

Werner, S.S., Stockard, J.E., and Bickford, R.G. 1977. *Atlas of Neonatal Electroencephalography.* New York: Raven Press.

Westmoreland, B.F. 1990. Benign EEG variants and patterns of uncertain clinical significance. In *Current Practice of Clinical Electroencephalography*, 2nd ed., Eds. D.D. Daly and T.A. Pedley, pp. 243–252. New York: Raven Press.

Westmoreland, B.F., and Klass, D.W. 1981. A distinctive rhythmic EEG discharge of adults. Electroencephalogr. Clin. Neurophysiol. 51:186–191.

Westmoreland, B.F., and Klass, D.W. 1997. Unusual variants of subclinical rhythmic electrographic discharge of adults (SREDA). Electroencephalogr. Clin. Neurophysiol. 102:1–4.

Westmoreland, B.F., Reiher, J., and Klass, D.W. 1979. Recording small sharp spikes with depth electroencephalography. Epilepsia (New York) 20:599–612.

Westmoreland, B.F., Frere, R.C., and Klass, D.W., 1997. Periodic epileptiform discharges in the midline. J. Clin. Neurophysiol. 14:495–498.

White, J.C., Langston, J.W., and Pedley, T.A. 1977. Benign epileptiform transients of sleep: clarification of the small sharp spike controversy. Neurology 27:1061–1068.

Williams, D. 1944. The nature of transient outbursts in the electroencephalogram of epileptics. Brain 67:10–37.

Wilson, S.B., Harner, R.N., Duffy, F.H., et al. 1996. Spike detection. I. Correlation and reliability of human experts. Electroencephalogr. Clin. Neurophysiol. 98:186–198.

Wong, P.K.H., and Gregory, D. 1988. Dipole fields in rolandic discharges. Am. J. EEG Technol. 28:243–250.

Yürüker, N., and Menzi, W. 1971. 14 and 6/s positive-Spikes im Schlaf nach akustischem Reiz. Z. EEG-EMG 2:121–124.

Zivin, L., and Ajmone Marsan, C. 1968. Incidence and prognostic significance of "epileptiform" activity in the EEG of nonepileptic subjects. Brain 91:751–777.

Zobniw, A.M., Yaworth, S., and Niedermeyer, E. 1975. Depth electroencephalography. J. Electrophysiol. Technol. 2:215–240.

14. Activation Methods

Takeo Takahashi

Various methods—such as hyperventilation, intermittent photic stimulation, or sleep—may be used to enhance preexisting abnormalities and induce abnormal findings in an otherwise normal electroencephalogram (EEG). Such methods are known as activation procedures. This chapter discusses common activation methods as well as methods that are less frequently carried out in EEG laboratories. Sleep-induced, sleep-deprived, and especially psychotropic drug-induced effects are not discussed here; they are covered in other chapters.

Hyperventilation

Precipitation of seizures by hyperventilation (HV) (Foerster, 1924) was known prior to discovery of human EEG. Therefore, EEG activation by HV has been widely used in almost all clinical EEG laboratories since its introduction. Nims et al. (1940) elucidated particular provocative efficacy of generalized-synchronous paroxysmal discharges and of absence seizures by this test. This method consists of deep and regular respiration at a rate of about 20/min for a period of 2 to 4 minutes. In adults, such HV will cause air exchange of 20 to 50 L/min and a drop in partial pressure of carbon dioxide (Pco_2) in the range of 4 to 7 mL% (Morrice, 1956). The characteristic EEG response to HV, most prominent in children, consists of a fluctuating increase of bilaterally synchronous slow activity and slowing of alpha and beta rhythms. In normal adults, although the slowing is generally not marked, there are wide differences among individuals.

With regard to the underlying mechanism of HV's provocation of slowing and seizure discharges, Gibbs et al. (1943) suggested that diffuse slowing is caused by inadequate compensatory vasoconstriction of the cerebrum in response to systemic hypocapnia. According to Gotoh et al. (1965), diffuse slowing is considered to be the direct result of cerebral ischemic anoxia resulting from hypocapnic cerebral vasoconstriction. Yamatani et al. (1994), measuring cerebral blood flow in the right carotid artery during HV, reported that decreased Pco_2 and cerebral blood flow were the fundamental factors causing EEG slowing. Fisch and So (2003) summarized the physiological basis of the EEG response to HV as the following: alteration of Pco_2, rather than pH or partial pressure of oxygen (Po_2), is the most important factor in producing EEG response to HV, whereas the most obvious and dramatic physiological effect of HV is decreased cerebral blood flow. Sherwin (1984) attributed the diffuse slowing to synchronous activity in the nonspecific thalamo-cortical projecting systems, which become more active in hypocapnia. Patel and Maulsby (1987) raised the possibility that hypocapnia induced by HV decreased activity in mesencephalic reticular formation, which then caused EEG slow-

ing, just as drowsiness and sleep produce EEG slowing. Similar mechanisms to those described above are considered to be important for provoking paroxysmal discharges (Niedermeyer, 1972b); hyperexcitability of neurons may be induced by respiratory alkalosis (Esquivel et al., 1991). However, the change from the pure delta response to the appearance of intermixed spikes and clear-cut spike-wave discharges remains obscure. Interestingly, it has been reported that intravenous administration of diazepam prevented HV-induced spike patterns, though it failed to attenuate the delta response (Niedermeyer, 1972a).

The magnitude of HV response depends upon a number of factors (Bostem, 1976). First, vigorous exchange of air can enhance activation effects. For the purpose of routine examination with HV, however, it is suggested that the rate of breathing be as close as possible to that of the resting rhythm (15–20 breaths/min) (Bostem, 1976). Second, age is an important factor. Slow waves appear much more abruptly, are more pronounced, and persist longer in children than in adults. The degree and abruptness of the response are related directly to age (Ziegler et al., 1975). The most dramatic EEG responses to HV usually occur between the ages of 8 and 12 years (Petersen and Eeg-Olofsson, 1971). According to Gibbs et al. (1943), in children between 3 and 5 years of age, 97% of epilepsy patients and 70% of normal subjects showed diffuse slowing with HV; after 20 years of age, more than 40% of epilepsy patients showed diffuse slowing, whereas it was seen in less than 10% of normal subjects. The areas most affected by HV in children are occipitotemporal regions (Kellaway, 1979). Delta waves tend to appear initially in the posterior regions and spread forward in the younger age group, whereas they tend to appear in the frontal regions and spread backward in the older age group (Bickford, 1979). Third, blood glucose level is also important in determining the degree of HV response. In adults, a low blood glucose level (less than 80 mg/dL) tends to enhance appearance of slow waves; a high level (more than 120 mg/dL) tends to inhibit or prevent such an effect (Davis and Wallace, 1942). Delta waves induced by HV can occasionally be the first indication of pathological hypoglycemia secondary to an islet cell tumor in a patient referred for an EEG (Bickford, 1979). Fourth, an erect position as compared to a reclining position enhances the effect of HV; EEG slowing occurs earlier and with greater intensity. This is thought to be a result of relative cerebral anoxia (Billinger and Frank, 1969). Diffuse slowing induced by HV usually disappears rapidly after ceasing HV; it may persist up to 30 seconds in normal adults.

Aside from diffuse slowing, HV may induce diffuse sharp waves or spike-wave discharges of epileptogenic significance; it is particularly effective in eliciting bilaterally synchronous spike-wave discharges in a patient with generalized epilepsies. Dalby (1969) found that patients with absence seizures were more sensitive to HV than patients with nonabsence seizures, with the incidence of spike-wave paroxysms being 50% in the former and 25% in the latter. During HV, not only absence seizures, but also complex partial seizures, are induced in epilepsy patients. In general, latent abnormalities are likely to be activated by HV. Slow wave foci associated with localized lesions may also be aggravated; abnormalities in temporal regions are more prone to accentuation than those elsewhere (Kiloh et al., 1972). Miley and Forster (1977) reported that vigorous HV of longer duration induced abnormal discharges with or without clinical seizures in 11% of epilepsy patients with complex partial seizures.

Unusually prolonged post-HV high-voltage slowing may be seen in patients with syncopal attacks of various etiologies (Engel, 1984). Buildup of slow waves after the end of HV ("re-buildup") may be a diagnostic finding in children with moyamoya disease (Kodama et al., 1979). In a study that addressed three cases of moyamoya disease, Kameyama et al. (1986) reported that this EEG re-buildup was noted about 5 minutes after HV cessation; moreover, corresponding decreases in cerebral blood flow and Po_2 were documented with it. Such a post-HV hypoxia 5 minutes after cessation of HV was also found in a study of nine normal adult subjects (Achenbach-Ng et al., 1994).

The American EEG Society Guidelines (AEEGS) Committee (1994) proposed the following minimum technical requirements: HV should be used routinely unless other medically justifiable reasons (e.g., a recent intracranial hemorrhage, significant cardiopulmonary disease, sickle cell disease or trait, or patient inability or unwillingness to cooperate) contraindicate it. It should be performed for a minimum of 3 minutes with continued recording for at least 1 minute after cessation of overbreathing. At times, HV must be performed for a longer period in order to obtain adequate EEG activation.

Intermittent Photic Stimulation

The effect of intermittent photic stimulation (IPS) on the human EEG was first studied by Adrian and Matthews (1934). They used sinusoidal IPS derived from a constant light source in front of which a disc with cutout sectors was rotated. After this earliest report, similar instruments were used for more than a decade (Bickford et al., 1953). Walter et al. (1946) were the first to report activation of paroxysmal discharges by IPS with an electronic strobe light. After this pioneering work, the method of IPS using a strobe light became popular (Kasteleijn-Nolst Trenité, 1998). The strobe lamp is placed at a distance of 20 to 30 cm in front of the subject's eyes. IPS is commonly presented through closed eyelids, but it can be administered with the eyes open. Details of IPS use in routine examination vary greatly between EEG laboratories. The following protocol is suggested by Bickford (1979): flashes at frequencies of 1, 3, 6, 9, 10, 15, 20, and 30 Hz each are given in trains of 5-second duration with eyes open and closed in a room with reduced illumination. It is sometimes advantageous to have patients open and close their eyes during the stimulation. In a standardization of screening methods for photosensitivity (Kasteleijn-Nolst Trenité et al., 1999), the following IPS frequencies are used: 1, 2, 3, 4, 6, 8, 10, 12, 14, 16, 18, 20, 60, 50, 40, 30, and 25 Hz (Fisch and So, 2003). The three main EEG changes induced by IPS are explained below.

Photic Driving Response

This is a physiological response consisting of rhythmic activity elicited over the posterior regions of the head by IPS frequencies of about 5 to 30 Hz. The term *photic driving response* (PDR) should be limited to activity time-locked to the stimulus and of a frequency identical or harmonically related to the stimulus frequency (Chatrian et al., 1974).

As a rule, PDR is found over posterior regions. In infants, PDR can be elicited a few hours after birth (Ellingson, 1960), but PDR remains relatively small up to about 6 years of age (Walter and Walter, 1951). In older children, PDR becomes much larger, particularly at low frequencies (Kiloh et al., 1972). The amplitude of PDR is usually higher in children than in adults and again tends to increase in elderly people. Regardless of age, however, an exaggerated PDR to low flash frequencies (0.5-3 Hz) usually signifies acute or subacute neuronal dysfunction (Kooi et al., 1978); examples include MELAS (mitochondrial myopathy, encephalopathy, lactic acidosis, and stroke-like episodes) (Fisch and So, 2003) and the late infantile form of ceroid lipofuscinosis (Pampiglione and Harden, 1977; Pinsard et al., 1978).

According to Fisch and So (2003), large positive occipital sharp-transients of sleep (POSTS) and lambda waves in response to scanning a complex pattern are predictive of a prominent PDR. Destructive cortical lesions may cause unilateral PDR depression, whereas irritative lesions, such as those associated with epileptic scars, may produce increased PDR on the side of the lesion (Bickford, 1979). Interpretation suggesting abnormal PDR should be made carefully because a minor and inconsistent asymmetry of PDR is infrequently seen even in normal subjects; Coull and Pedley (1978) claim that an asymmetry in amplitude only, in the absence of other EEG changes, should not be viewed as abnormal. Very low voltage or absence of PDR are of little diagnostic significance because some normal persons are not responsive to IPS (Kooi et al., 1978). According to Chiba et al. (1982), diffuse PDR could be observed in 25% of the patients who were receiving hemodialysis treatment.

It has been reported that PDR elicited by 5 Hz IPS with eyes closed is similar to that elicited by a red (saturated long-wave-length red) 5 Hz flicker stimulation, whereas PDR elicited by 5 Hz IPS with eyes open is similar to that elicited by a 5 Hz flickering dot pattern (Takahashi and Tsukahara, 1979). In that case, decreased luminance, such as 20 cd/m², was used. [This luminosity is very low compared to that of a stroboscopic IPS; e.g., Grass photostimulator (intensity 8): 3,939 cd/m² (Harding and Jeavons, 1994).] Furthermore, using a 5-Hz red flicker stimulation and, to a greater extent, a 5-Hz flickering dot pattern provided by a visual stimulator (Tsukahara and Takahashi, 1973), high-amplitude PDR over 50 µV was elicited more frequently. Such an excitatory effect of a dot pattern or other similar patterns on PDR (Tsukahara and Takahashi, 1979) can be

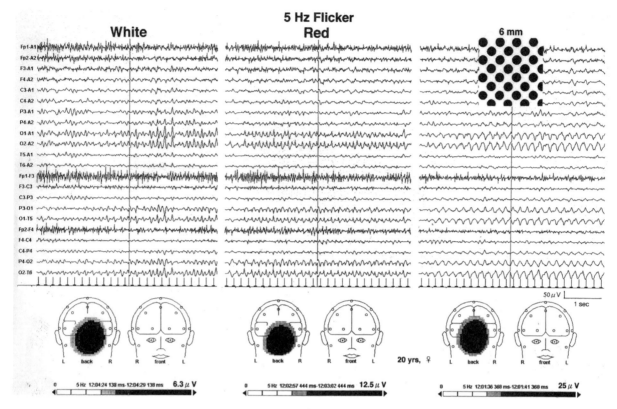

Figure 14.1. EEG changes in response to 5 Hz white-flicker, red-flicker, and flickering dot-pattern (6 mm in diameter) stimuli to the full-field (30 × 30 degrees) in a 20-year-old woman with occipital lobe epilepsy. Stimulus was provided by use of a square-type strobe-filter method (Takahashi, 2002); luminance was maintained at 20 candela (cd)/m². *Lower tracings* show mapping analysis of photic driving responses (PDRs) elicited by each flicker stimulation.

demonstrated easily by placing the pattern on the strobe light when IPS is given to the subject with eyes open (Takahashi, 1993a).

Studies of PDR utilizing 5-Hz red flicker and 5-Hz flickering dot pattern (6 mm in diameter) stimuli by means of visual stimulators (Tsukahara and Takahashi, 1973; Takahashi et al., 1980) yielded the following results (Takahashi, 1993a). High-amplitude PDR is more frequently elicited using either a red flicker stimulation or a flickering dot pattern stimulation, irrespective of diagnostic group, than a white flicker stimulation with equal luminance, such as 20 cd/m². High-amplitude PDRs elicited by flickering dot pattern and red flicker stimuli in adult patients suggest the presence of an occipital lobe disturbance. Incidence of high-amplitude PDR elicited by a flickering dot pattern stimulation in adult patients is 2.4 times higher in female patients than in male patients. A study of PDR in adult psychiatric outpatients showed that PDR amplitudes increased significantly with patient age (Takahashi et al., 1988). Figure 14.1 depicts EEG changes in response to 5-Hz flicker stimuli in a young patient with occipital lobe epilepsy: stimuli using white and red light elicited 5 and 10 Hz PDRs, whereas those by dot pattern [6 mm in diameter; 0.5 cycles/degree (c/deg)] elicited 5-Hz high-amplitude PDRs. Stimuli using dot patterns (0.5 mm: 4.9 c/deg; 1 mm: 2.1 c/deg; 2 mm: 1.5 c/deg; 4 mm: 0.8 c/deg) also showed a similar finding as that

shown in Fig. 14.1. As for high-amplitude PDRs observed in elderly individuals, they tend to be elicited by stimuli using moderate (2 mm in diameter) to large dot patterns (4 and 6 mm in diameter) as demonstrated in Fig. 14.2. Namely, when dot patterns with lower spatial frequencies are employed, high-amplitude PDR tends to be elicited in elderly patients (Takahashi, 1999), whereas its incidence increases in younger patients by use of dot patterns with higher spatial frequencies.

These PDRs elicited by visual stimuli not only to the full-field, but also to the center, periphery, and each hemifield (regional visual stimulation) provide us with useful clinical information (Takahashi, 1993b). Figure 14.3 shows results of 5-Hz fundamental PDRs elicited by regional visual stimulation in a total of 54 adult psychiatric outpatients, from whom patients with epilepsy and cerebral vascular disorders were excluded. We made a power spectral analysis on occipital PDRs elicited by a 5-Hz flickering dot-pattern (6 mm in diameter: 0.5 c/deg) stimulation to the center (11 × 11 degrees), periphery (11 × 11 degrees to 57 × 57 degrees), full-field (57 × 57 degrees), and each hemifield with luminance maintained at 10 cd/m². The average PDR amplitude in response to regional flickering dot-pattern stimuli in 28 patients aged over 45 years was higher than the average PDR amplitude in 26 patients aged 20 to 44 years. Amplitudes of PDRs elicited by stimuli to the periphery and lower hemi-

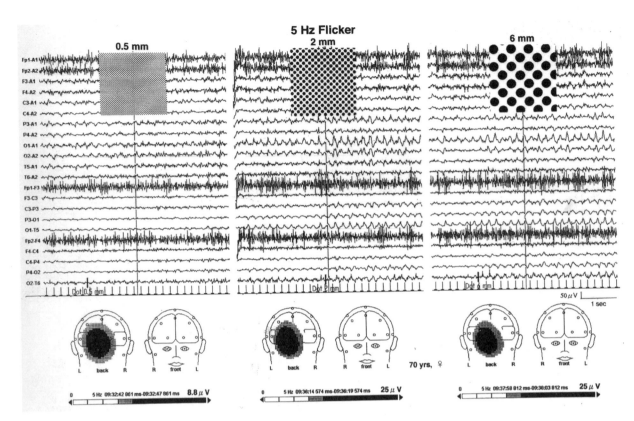

Figure 14.2. EEG changes in response to 5 Hz flickering dot-pattern (0.5, 2, and 6 mm in diameter) stimuli to the full-field (30 × 30 degrees) in a 70-year-old woman with benign paroxysmal positional vertigo. Stimulus was provided by use of a square-type strobe-filter method (Takahashi, 2002); luminance was maintained at 20 cd/m². *Lower tracings* show mapping analysis of PDRs elicited by each flickering dot-pattern stimulation.

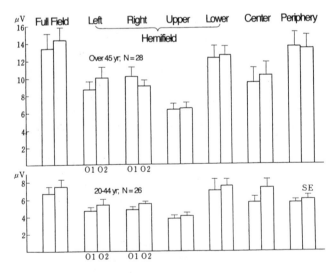

Figure 14.3. Photic driving response (PDR) elicited by regional visual stimuli in 54 adult psychiatric outpatients. We used an SLS-5100 visual stimulator (Nihon Kohden). Power spectral analysis was made on the record for 5 seconds after each 2-second stimulation. Power spectra are 5, 10, 15, 20, and 25 Hz PDRs; only that of 5 Hz fundamental PDR, which was the greatest, is shown in this figure. The root of each power is expressed for convenience to indicate amplitude. (Modified from Takahashi, T. 1993b. EEG activation by visual stimuli. In *The Newest Clinical Electroencephalography*, Eds. M. Sato and H. Matsuoka, pp. 323–344. Tokyo: Asakura Shoten.)

field were similar to those elicited by a stimulus to the full field. Regarding PDRs elicited by lateral hemifield stimuli, contralateral PDRs were slightly higher than ipsilateral ones, but their difference was not statistically significant. Particular efficiency in eliciting higher PDR by lower hemifield stimulation compared with other hemifield stimuli might be a result of its selective stimulus to the visual cortex, which is located closely beneath electrodes 01 and 02.

A power spectral analysis of PDRs elicited by the above visual stimuli may be used as a new tool for evaluation of drugs influencing the brain (Takahashi, 1999). Other clinical usefulness of this EEG examination is reported in the following discussion. In a patient with amblyopia, a distinct difference of PDRs evoked by stimulation of 5-Hz flickering dot-pattern to each eye was obtained (Takahashi et al., 1981); PDRs evoked by hemifield 5-Hz flickering dot-pattern stimuli enabled EEG diagnosis of a parietal lobe metastatic brain tumor in a patient who had suffered from breast cancer (Takahashi and Tomioka, 1985).

Photomyoclonic Response (Photomyogenic Response)

This is a response to IPS characterized by appearance of brief repetitive muscle spikes over anterior regions of the head. These often increase gradually in amplitude as stimulation continues and cease promptly when the stimulus is withdrawn. The response is associated frequently with eyelid flutter, a vertical oscillation of the eyelids and eyeballs; sometimes it is associated with discrete jerking, mostly involving musculature of the face and head (Chatrian et al., 1974).

Principal features of this response were first described by Gastaut and Rémond (1949) and Bickford et al. (1952), who introduced the term *photomyoclonic response* (PMR), which differs from photoparoxysmal response. Occasionally, a PMR can be seen with a photoparoxysmal response. The most effective triggering IPS frequency lies between 12 and 18 Hz (Niedermeyer et al., 1979). The PMR tends to appear in conjunction with muscular tension. The PMR occurs less often in children than in adults. Gastaut et al. (1958) reported that PMR was found in 0.3% of normal subjects, 3% of patients with epilepsy, 13% of patients with brainstem lesions, and 17% of patients with psychiatric disorders. The incidence of PMR in other studies (Kooi et al., 1960; Melsen, 1959; Reilly and Peters, 1973; Small, 1971), however, was lower than in that of Gastaut et al., ranging from 0.1% to 0.8%. The PMR is considered to be a nonspecific finding that is not significant for elimination diagnosis of a seizure disorder (Newmark and Penry, 1979). The PMR is enhanced in early stages of alcohol withdrawal in chronic alcoholics (Victor, 1970) or after sudden withdrawal from barbiturates and related sedatives (Wikler and Essig, 1970).

Photoparoxysmal Response (Photoconvulsive Response)

This is a response to IPS characterized by spike-and-wave and multiple spike-and-wave complexes that are bilaterally synchronous, symmetrical, and generalized and which may outlast the stimulus by a few seconds. There may be associated impairment of consciousness and brisk jerks involving musculature of the whole body, most predominantly that of the upper extremities and head (Chatrian et al., 1974). Newmark and Penry (1979) state that generalized slow activity and posterior spikes are not accepted universally as a *photoparoxysmal response* (PPR), but the significance of these discharges increases if they continue after stimulation is discontinued.

Although PPRs in photosensitive epilepsy patients are elicited by a broad range of IPS frequencies from 1 to 65 Hz (Harding and Harding, 1999), the most epileptogenic frequencies are within the range of 15 to 18 Hz (Topalkara et al., 1998). PPR is most frequently induced by 15-Hz IPS with eyes closed and 20-Hz IPS when the eyes are open (Klass and Fischer-Williams, 1976). When IPS is given with eyes open, careful attention to eye movement and position is needed because a directional change from central to lateral gaze diminishes the effect of IPS in evoking PPR. This effect is greater than the diminution effect with monocular IPS stimulation as compared with binocular IPS stimulation in eliciting PPR (Jeavons and Harding, 1975). Regarding levels of ambient light, with high-intensity IPS, the effects of normal ambient lighting may be negligible (Van Egmond et al., 1980). During IPS, the PPR may be induced by eye closure, especially immediately after eye closure (Panayiotopoulos, 1974). Patients with PPR are less sensitive to IPS when

asleep (Hishikawa et al., 1967; Sato et al., 1975). Generalized PPR may be most pronounced in the frontal, central, or occipital regions. Hishikawa et al. (1967) classified generalized PPR in photosensitive epilepsy patients into PPR that appear first in the occipital area and PPR that occur simultaneously over all areas or appear earlier over anterior regions. In the former group, an augmented visual evoked response could be obtained. Generalized PPR in children are usually rhythmic and higher in amplitude than those seen in adults. Occipital spikes as a sole response to IPS may not be indicative of epilepsy (Maheshwari and Jeavons, 1975). Unilateral occipital spikes are rarely induced by IPS. These patients, as opposed to patients with generalized PPR, often have a history of a local posterior lesion, mostly traumatic. Very rarely, frontal spikes can be provoked by IPS (Takahashi, 1982).

Jeavons (1969) found a PPR in 2.8% of the patients referred for EEG examination, a figure similar to that of Gastaut et al. (1958). The patients, whose seizures are induced by visual stimuli such as viewing a visual pattern, television (Wilkins et al., 1979), or eye closure, are particularly sensitive to IPS and tend to demonstrate PPR. Gastaut et al. reported that the PPR is almost entirely confined to patients with primary subcortical epilepsy and that it occurs in 40% of cases with absence seizures and in 20% of cases with generalized tonic-clonic seizures (GTCS). According to Stevens (1962), PPR occurred in 53% of that study's patients with nonfocal seizures, but in only 3% of that study's patients with focal seizures. A similar view has also been expressed by Niedermeyer (1972b), who states that generalized PPR are more highly associated with primary generalized epilepsy than with incompletely generalized or focal spikes. On the other hand, Guerrini et al. (1995) proposed a concept called idiopathic photosensitive occipital lobe epilepsy based on detailed analysis of ten patients with recurrent episodes of visually induced occipital seizures; all seizures were stimulus (mostly television and computer screen) related and began with elementary visual symptoms, followed in most patients by a slow clustering of cephalic pain, epigastric discomfort, and vomiting, with either normal or only mildly impaired responsiveness: All of them showed PPR of types 1 to 4 (see below). The ictal events that may accompany PPR are predominantly absence seizures, GTCS, and myoclonic jerks, especially of the eyelids or arms (Kasteleijn-Nolst Trenité et al., 1987). Gambardella et al. (1996) reported a 17-year-old girl with pure photosensitive epilepsy who showed photic-induced epileptic negative myoclonus (PPR was accompanied by loss of postural tone in both arms). They claim that negative myoclonus should be included among the ictal phenomena accompanying PPR.

Some studies have suggested that presence of PPR may be a familial trait (Doose et al., 1969; Jeavons and Harding, 1975; Takahashi, 1976a). Doose et al. (1969) reported that PPR may be regarded as a symptom of susceptibility to convulsions of the centrencephalic type. In a genetic study of photosensitive epilepsy, Waltz et al. (1992) classified PPR into four types: type 1, spikes with occipital rhythm; type 2, parieto-occipital spikes with a biphasic slow wave; type 3, parieto-occipital spikes with a biphasic slow wave and spread to the frontal region; type 4, generalized spikes and waves or polyspikes and waves. They found that type 4 occurred more often both in probands with epilepsy and their siblings than the respective controls, suggesting that coincidence of photosensitivity will appear as higher if only type 4 is considered to be indicative of photosensitivity. Photosensitivity is age-dependent, being highest in late childhood and early adolescence; it is more common in females (Doose et al., 1969). According to a prospective nationwide study made in Great Britain (Quirk et al., 1995a), the annual incidence of cases of epilepsy with type 4 PPR on their first EEG was approximately 2% of all new cases of epilepsy. When restricted to the age range of 17 to 19 years, the annual incidence rose to approximately 10% of all new cases of epilepsy presented in this age range. Analyzing generalized PPRs found in 128 chronic epilepsy patients, De Graaf et al. (1995) reported that there was a significantly higher occurrence in white persons (2.7%, 72 of 2,657) as compared with black persons (0.1%, 1 of 848) and subjects of mixed race (0.9%, 55 of 5,958), concluding that genetic rather than environmental factors influence generalized PPR.

For epileptic seizures triggered by television, photosensitivity remains the most common single mechanism (Harding and Jeavons, 1994). Since the first description of space invader epilepsy by Rushton (1981), patients with seizures triggered by electronic screen games (ESGs) such as video, console, and computer games have been reported (Kasteleijn-

Nolst Trenité et al., 2002; Takahashi, 2002). A nationwide study made in Great Britain (Quirk et al., 1995b) during 6-month periods identified 118 patients who had a first seizure while playing ESGs when they were 7 to 19 years old. Of 118 patients, 46 and 25 had definite and probable causal relationships, respectively; 47 patients had no such relationship. Within that age group, the annual incidence of first seizure triggered by playing ESGs (71 patients altogether) was estimated to be 1.5/100,000, representing approximately 3% of all new patients with epilepsy in this age range. Of 71 patients, 46 showed type 4 PPR, whereas 25 showed types 1 to 3 PPR. Although photosensitivity is thought to play the most important role in engendering ESG-induced seizures, other circumstances, acting either singly or in combination, should be taken into consideration (Binnie et al., 1994). Examples include (1) seizure precipitation by specific cognitive activities, decision making, hand movements, etc.; (2) seizure precipitation by nonspecific emotional factors relating to the subjects' engagement in games, such as anxiety or excitement; (3) lowering of the seizure threshold by fatigue or sleep deprivation; and (4) chance occurrence of a spontaneous seizure in a person with epilepsy while playing ESGs. Figure 14.4 illustrates generalized paroxysmal discharges elicited by a video game and generalized PPRs elicited by flickering visual stimuli in a 13-year-old boy who had an ESG-induced GTCS.

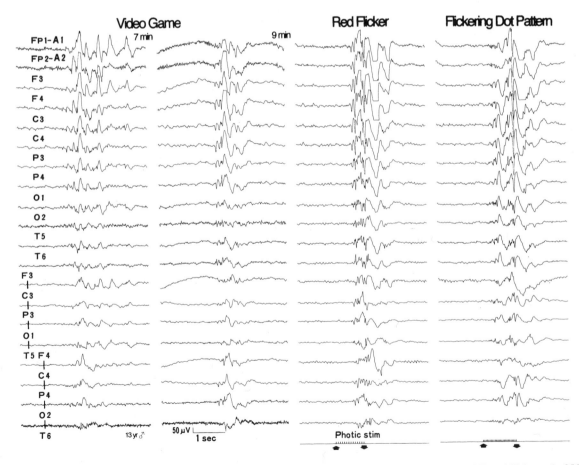

Figure 14.4.   Generalized paroxysmal discharges elicited by a video game (Super Tetris 2 + Bombliss) and generalized photoparoxysmal response (PPRs) elicited by flickering stimuli in a 13-year-old photosensitive epilepsy patient. We used a 12-inch television placed 1 m in front of the patient. Full-field (30 × 30 degrees) stimuli of a 15 Hz red flicker and a 25 Hz flickering 1.5 c/deg dot pattern provided by use of square type strobe-filter method elicited type 4 PPR. Luminance maintained at 20 cd/m². This EEG was recorded under drug-free conditions.

Occurrence of a PPR in an otherwise seizure-free individual is uncommon; these patients tend to have attacks of headache or psychological problems, such as personality disorder with hysterical reactions or an anxiety state (Niedermeyer et al., 1979). Incidence of PPR in nonepileptic, apparently normal subjects is estimated at probably less than 2% (Newmark and Penry, 1979). Reilly and Peters (1973) claim that the following criteria are useful for determining whether or not the patients are epileptic: prolonged PPR (outlasting the stimulus) suggests probable epilepsy (90%), whereas self-limited discharge is not diagnostic.

Especially in adults without previous seizures and without a family history of seizures, PPR usually suggests a toxic, metabolic, or drug withdrawal state (Kooi et al., 1978; Solomon and Fine, 1960; Victor and Brausch, 1967; Wikler and Essig, 1970). Symmetrical posterior high-amplitude spikes can be evoked at slow IPS rates in patients with diffuse encephalopathies, such as progressive myoclonic epilepsy or Creutzfeldt-Jakob disease (Coull and Pedley, 1978; Gastaut, 1969; Lee and Blair, 1973).

Several conditions are known to alter PPR. As described above, PPR is often associated with eye closure and is most likely to occur immediately after eye closure. This effect may also result from movement of the eyelids or of the eyes themselves. In addition, eye closure may produce activation by suddenly eliminating the visual pattern and by causing the field of vision to become red-hued (Bickford and Klass, 1969; Takahashi and Tsukahara, 1975). When stimuli are presented with the eyes open, a patterned field of vision (or flickering geometric pattern) has been found to be more effective than a homogeneous field (or white-light flicker) in eliciting PPR (Jeavons et al., 1972; Panayiotopoulos, 1974; Takahashi and Tsukahara, 1980). In addition, saturated long-wave-length red (red) facilitates induction of PPR (Takahashi and Tsukahara, 1976, 1992). An EEG activation by use of red flicker and flickering geometric pattern stimuli, which were given only in "eyes-open" conditions, revealed a higher rate of PPR provocation than by ordinary stroboscopic IPS (Takahashi et al., 1980). [In the former method, an SLS-5100 visual stimulator (Takahashi, 1993a) was employed and luminance maintained at 20 cd/m². Additional studies (Takahashi, 1989, 1994) have disclosed that elicited PPRs were found in 18% of epilepsy patients, suggesting that incidence of photosensitivity in epilepsy patients is 3.6 times higher than that of the commonly accepted 5% reported by Binnie and Jeavons (1992). Figure 14.5 shows a circular type strobe-filter (Takahashi, 2000, 2002), which is a simple device that is capable of inducing similar activation effects to the SLS-5100 visual stimulator. Using strobe-filters, visual stimuli (red flicker and flickering geometric pattern, luminance kept at 30 cd/m²) are easily presented to patients. Their stimulus luminance is far less intense than that of a stroboscopic IPS. In addition to examining photosensitivity with an ordinary strobe, such low luminance visual stimuli may be required for precise examination of photosensitive epilepsy patients.

Along with PPR, another term in use is *photoepileptiform response* (PER). This response is elicited by photic stimulation. According to their topography, they are divided into the following three categories (Fisch and So, 2003): 1, anterior dominant or generalized (bisynchronous and approximately symmetrical); 2, occipital dominant (bisynchronous and approximately symmetrical); and 3, occipital dominant and localized (unilateral or strongly lateralized). The category 1 PPR is one form of PER and is most closely associated with epilepsy.

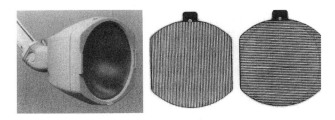

Figure 14.5. A flash lamp and a circular type strobe-filter. Luminance of direct stroboscopic intermittent photic stimulation (IPS) by use of LS-706A (Nihon Kohden), as shown in the *left tracing*, is 3,939 cd/m². Inserting a vertical grating pattern *(middle tracing)* along the filter holder on the front of the flash lamp as shown in the *left tracing* greatly reduces luminosity to 30 cd/m². Five strobe-filters are available (Nihon Kohden): red, dot pattern, vertical grating, horizontal grating *(right tracing)*, and white. Luminance of each strobe-filter is 30 cd/m² and spatial frequency of each pattern filter is 2 c/deg. Using this filter, the weakest possible stimuli of red flicker and pattern flicker ought to be used, taking great care not to induce clinical seizures in photosensitive individuals; one might, for example, start stimuli from lower flicker frequencies and terminate examinations when PPR appear (Takahashi, 2002).

Other Forms of Sensory Stimulation
Visual Stimulation

Various visual stimuli other than IPS may provoke PERs. The simple maneuver of eye closure induces posterior slow-wave transients, especially in children (Takahashi, 1976c; Westmoreland and Sharbrough, 1975) and may also provoke paroxysmal discharges (Gastaut and Tassinari, 1966; Green, 1968). Paroxysmal discharges similar to PPR seen in photosensitive epilepsy patients may even be induced by slow closure of the eyelids (Darby et al., 1980a). In the act of eye closure carried out in a lighted room, lights off and homogeneous visual field (Ganzfeld) (Forster, 1977; Gumnit et al., 1965; Takahashi, 1976b) are considered to play significant roles as visual stimuli in producing paroxysmal discharges. In fact, posterior sharp waves or spikes can be seen occasionally after or at the onset of IPS; these are called off-response and on-response, respectively (Colon et al., 1979; Jeavons and Harding, 1975). Spike-wave discharges associated with seizures can rarely be induced by a single-flash light stimulus (Bickford and Klass, 1969). Paroxysmal discharges may be evoked by red light alone (Forster, 1977; Takahashi and Tsukahara, 1972; Takahashi, 2002). Darkness may also induce paroxysmal discharges (Lugaresi et al., 1984; Panayiotopoulos, 1979). Similar paroxysmal discharges produced by Ganzfeld and total darkness have been reported by Panayiotopoulos (1994, 1998), who called it fixation-off-sensitivity (FOS); this unpatterned vision can be obtained either through +10 spherical lenses or through underwater goggles covered with semitransparent paper. He claims that FOS is suspected if EEG abnormalities appear and persist as long as the eyes remain closed and disappear when the eyes are opened. In such cases, EEG abnormalities

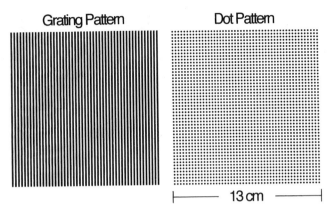

Figure 14.6. Geometric patterns used for square-type strobe-filter method. Each pattern was presented 30 cm before the eyes, resulting in its spatial frequency at 2 c/deg; pattern contrast is 0.98.

of FOS can be elicited by elimination of central vision and fixation; FOS is related to eyes-closed, not eye-closure EEG abnormalities. According to Panayiotopoulos (1994, 1998), the incidence of FOS-related EEG abnormalities appears to be as frequent as that of PPR in children younger than 12 years of age; FOS is probably more frequently associated with benign childhood epilepsy with occipital paroxysms than with any other epileptic condition.

Pattern, Pattern Flicker, and Red Flicker Stimulation

Geometric patterns often provoke paroxysmal discharges in epilepsy patients, particularly in photosensitive ones (Bickford and Klass, 1962; Binnie and Wilkins, 1998; Chatrian et al., 1970; Darby et al., 1980b; Klass, 2000). The patterns that are most effective for activation consist of closely spaced lines or dots with sharply contrasting interfaces that are arranged geometrically (Klass and Fischer-Williams, 1976). According to Wilkins et al. (1980), to induce paroxysmal discharges, patterns (black and white stripes of equal width and spacing) must have a spatial frequency between 1 and 4 c/deg. Line patterns are more epileptogenic than dot patterns (Fig. 14.6). Oscillation of a grating pattern greatly

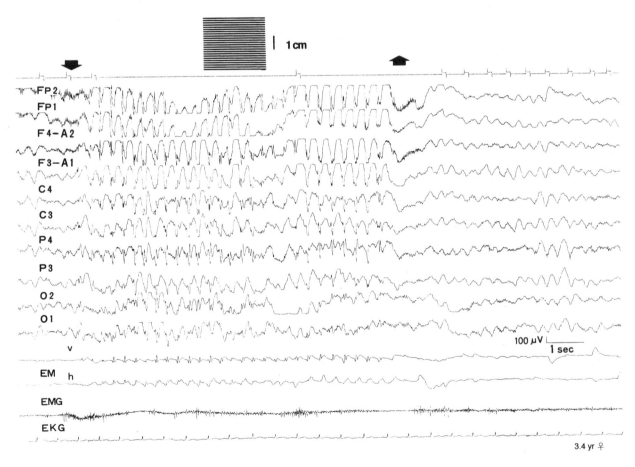

Figure 14.7. Generalized 3-Hz spike-and-wave complex elicited by a horizontal 2.1 c/deg grating pattern stimulation in a 3.4-year-old girl with severe myoclonic epilepsy in infancy. Vertical and horizontal eye movements, electromyogram (EMG) of the left hand, and electrocardiogram (ECG) were recorded simultaneously. *Downward* and *upward arrows* indicate the beginning and the end of a grating pattern stimulation, respectively.

In accordance with occurrence of a generalized paroxysmal discharge, regular button pressing shown at the *top* became absent, suggesting that she had an absence seizure. (Modified from Takahashi, T., and Sasaki, M. 1971. Pattern sensitivity: its activation method and clinical EEG findings. Rinsho Nohha (Osaka) 13:727–732.)

enhanced provocation of paroxysmal discharges; gratings oscillating in a direction orthogonal to the lines were the most effective, and the optimum oscillation frequency was in the range of 15 to 20 Hz (Binnie et al., 1985).

Figure 14.7 is an example of 3-Hz spike-and-wave complexes associated with an absence seizure induced by viewing a grating pattern in a 3.4-year-old girl with severe myoclonic epilepsy in infancy (Takahashi and Sasaki, 1971). This patient was very sensitive to vertical, horizontal, and oblique stripes with a wide range of spatial frequencies. She was also sensitive to dot patterns, but slightly less so than to stripes. Interestingly, this girl repeatedly stared at those patterns as if she were enjoying the absence seizures. A dot pattern, however, more frequently evokes lambda waves and rhythmic posterior slow activity than a grate pattern (Takahashi, 1974a). Lambda waves are more frequently evoked in subjects who show good photic driving responses, especially to low-frequency IPS. Photosensitive epilepsy patients are also often sensitive to pattern viewing, with an incidence of 5% (Bickford and Klass, 1969), 22% (Takahashi and Tsukahara, 1980), or 72% (Stefansson et al., 1977). Paroxysmal discharges induced by viewing usually arise from the occipital area, suggesting that they may arise primarily in an epileptogenic visual cortex (Chatrian et al., 1970; Takahashi and Tsukahara, 1975; Wilkins et al., 1980). Geometric pattern stimulus occasionally induces fast activity (beta rhythm) (Takahashi, 1999). Pattern viewing may also enhance mu rhythm (Koshino and Niedermeyer, 1975).

It has been reported that photosensitive epilepsy patients are particularly sensitive to full-field visual stimuli of a red flicker and flickering geometric pattern, when a decreased luminance, such as 10 to 20 cd/m^2, is used as a stimulating light source (Takahashi, 1989). Figure 14.8 illustrates EEG changes in response to stroboscopic IPS, red flicker, and flickering dot pattern stimuli in a photosensitive epilepsy patient. Particular emphasis ought to be given to the finding that IPS to eyes open was ineffective, whereas red flicker and flickering dot pattern stimuli elicited generalized PPRs, suggesting that stroboscopic IPS to eyes open, with luminance of 3,939 cd/m^2, is too strong to elicit PPR in this patient (Takahashi et al., 1999). In addition to hemifield (Soso et al., 1980; Takahashi, 1983, 1984, 1994; Wilkins et al., 1981) and quadrant-field (Takahashi, 1996) stimuli, visual stimulation to the center and periphery by use of the above stimuli can also yield useful information to further

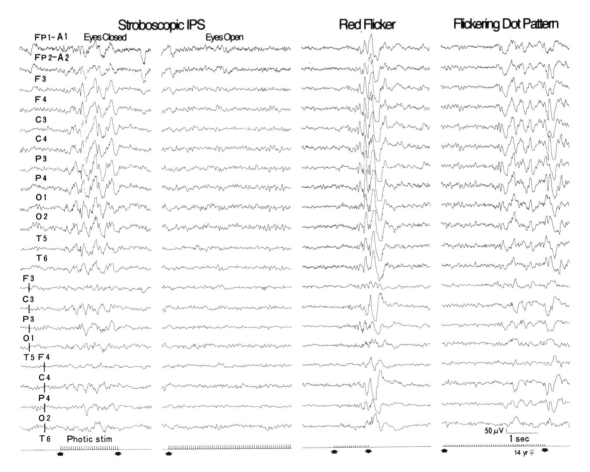

Figure 14.8. EEG changes in response to stroboscopic IPS, red flicker, and flickering dot pattern stimuli in a 14-year-old girl with photosensitive epilepsy. By use of Grass PS33-plus photic stimulator (intensity at 8), 15 Hz IPS was given 30 cm above the eye. Using the strobe-filter method, 15 Hz red flicker and 15 Hz flickering 2 c/deg dot pattern stimuli to the full-field (25 × 25 degrees) were given from 30 cm before the eye; luminance maintained at 20 cd/m^2.

Square Type Strobe-Filter

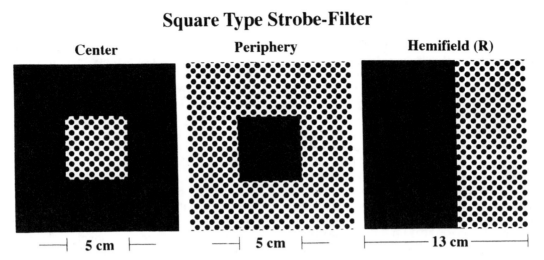

Figure 14.9. Dot pattern plastic filters used for regional flickering dot pattern stimuli by use of square-type strobe-filter method. Diameter of a single dot is 4 mm (0.8 c/deg), and luminance maintains at 20 cd/m². (See Color Figure 14.9.)

elucidate PPR (Takahashi, 1994). As an example, Fig. 14.9 shows filters used to provide a flickering dot pattern stimulation to the center, periphery, and hemifield by the square type strobe-filter method (Takahashi, 1999, 2002); similar field-size filters are used in red flicker stimuli. Figure 14.10 demonstrates EEG changes in response to such regional visual stimuli in the same patient shown in Fig. 14.8. A red flicker stimulation to the center promptly elicited generalized PPR as shown in the left tracing. That to the periphery, however, was less effective. Lateral hemifield stimuli elicited generalized PPR (equal PPR), but upper and lower hemifield ones were ineffective in this patient. In terms of PPR etiology, equal PPRs as shown in Fig. 14.10 are thought to be related to genetic factors, whereas an unequal PPR, in which either left or right hemifield stimulation elicits a PPR, is indicative of acquired cerebral disturbance, such as head trauma (Takahashi, 1994).

Regarding provocation of generalized PPR by visual stimuli to the center and periphery, a red flicker stimulation to the center is more effective than that to the periphery, indicating that macular stimulation plays a central role in it. In eliciting PPR by flickering dot pattern stimulation to the full field, a dot pattern with higher spatial frequency, such as 2.1 to 1.5 c/deg, shows the most significant efficacy; flicker frequencies must be between 20 and 15 Hz in that condition (Takahashi and Tsukahara, 1998). Flickering dot pattern stimulation to the center too, when a higher frequency dot pattern (2.1–4.9 c/deg) is used, elicits generalized PPR similar to that induced by red flicker stimulation to the center (Takahashi and Tsukahara, 2000), whereas that to the periphery by use of 0.5 c/deg dot pattern elicits generalized PPR with apparent local onset from posterior regions (Takahashi, 1994). Therefore, photosensitive epilepsy patients who are sensitive to red flicker and flickering dot pattern stimuli are thought to have hyperexcitable areas not only in the striate cortex, but also in the parastriate cortices. Local PPR in the striate cortex elicited by red flicker stimulation

would immediately transmit to the nonspecific diffuse projection system. This could engender generalized PPR with their simultaneous occurrence over all areas, as distinguished from those elicited by flickering dot pattern stimulation. In the latter, initial local PPR would seem to originate in the striate cortex as well as in the parastriate cortices. These might produce different generalized PPR, preceded by spikes over the posterior regions.

Of 18 photosensitive patients sensitive to red flicker stimulation (Takahashi et al., 1999), all cases were sensitive to at least one of the flickering geometric pattern stimuli. Although this finding suggests that common neuronal pathways are involved in PPR induction by red flicker and flickering geometric pattern stimuli, two different visual cortical pathways, namely the parvocellular (P) and the magnocellular (M) systems, are presumed to severally play a part in the following (Takahashi, 2002; Takahashi and Tsukahara, 1997): the P system deals with color, and V4 plays a central role for perception of both shape and color (Zeki, 1993). In human subjects, the region of the lingual and fusiform gyri has been identified as the color center (Allison et al., 1993; Lueck et al., 1989). Regarding reversing patterns, Harding and Jeavons (1994) maintain that they are dealing with transient phenomena and that perhaps the M system provides critical transmission that is similar to the mechanism of pattern sensitivity. This understanding may also hold true for flickering geometric pattern stimulation (Takahashi, 1999). From findings obtained by regional visual stimulation technique, however, the following view appears to be most likely: generalized PPRs elicited by red flicker and high spatial frequency pattern flicker stimuli to the center are mediated by the P system, whereas those elicited by low spatial frequency pattern flicker stimulation to the periphery are mediated by the M system (Takahashi, 2002).

The above knowledge obtained from EEG diagnosis by low-luminance visual stimuli provides us important clues

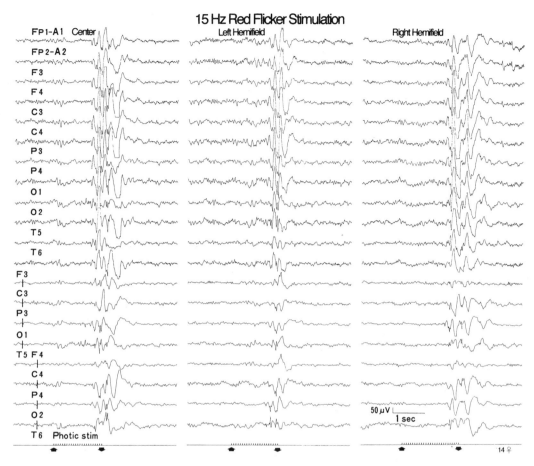

Figure 14.10.   Generalized PPRs elicited by regional red flicker stimuli in a 14-year-old girl with photosensitive epilepsy (the same patient shown in Fig. 14.8).

for detailed understanding particularly of seizures induced by stimulative screen images observed through use of TV, video systems, computer, etc. (Takahashi, 2002).

Auditory Stimulation

When compared with visual stimuli, activation of paroxysmal discharges by auditory stimuli is extremely rare. Being either transient or continuous, paroxysmal discharges provoked by auditory stimuli have been found mainly over temporal areas (Arellano et al., 1950; Gastaut et al., 1954; Peet et al., 1952; Takahashi, 1974b; Vigouroux et al., 1954). Pure tones have been shown by Arellano et al. (1950) to activate paroxysmal discharges in a psychomotor epilepsy patient. Prechtl (1959) reported that repetitive clicks caused aggravation of preexisting temporal lobe abnormalities in 37% of a large group of mixed cases. Stevens (1962) found the activating mechanism in 4.5% of temporal lobe epilepsy patients. These findings suggest that an epileptic disturbance in the primary auditory area of superior temporal gyrus (Heschl's gyrus) may chiefly be responsible for auditory stimuli that give rise to such paroxysmal discharges. On the other hand, Kiloh et al. (1972) showed that unilateral central sharp waves could be evoked by random taps. When generalized paroxysmal discharges appear to be induced by audi-

tory stimulation in drowsiness and sleep, special care in interpretation is needed because arousal secondary to auditory stimuli, not auditory stimulus per se, may play a role in triggering paroxysmal discharges.

Hearing-induced seizures are precipitated by hearing more or less specific music (Wieser et al., 1997), voices, and other sounds. According to Rosenow and Lüders (2000a), those patients usually have automotor seizures or generalized tonic-clonic seizures and temporal lobe epilepsy; the pathogenesis of auditory-induced seizures most probably involves activation of temporal auditory areas.

Somatosensory Stimulation

When areas of the primary sensorimotor cortex become hyperexcitable as a result of disease, contralateral afferent stimuli may trigger focal spikes and partial seizures. Along with tactile stimulation (De Marco and Negrin, 1973; De Marco and Tassinari, 1981; Deonna, 1998; Vignal et al., 1998), local stimuli by cold wind, rubbing, vibration, and stretching a muscle appear to rarely provoke spikes and seizures as reviewed by Takahashi (1999). Tapping anywhere about the upper torso or head produces myoclonic movements associated with diffuse spike-wave discharges in some young idiopathic epilepsy patients who are sensitive to afferent stimuli (Kooi et al., 1978). Focal areas that are sensitive to these stimuli are the finger, arm, shoulder, chest, face, head, and feet. In one patient, partial elementary seizures were evoked by tooth brushing (Holmes et al., 1982). O'Brien et al. (1996) reported a 23-year-old female complex epilepsy patient with seizures precipitated exclusively by tooth brushing and in whom structural and functional imaging demonstrated a right posterior frontal focus. Using tactile stimulation comprising tapping of the palmar tips of the fingers or toes, Langill and Wong (2003) investigated 304 patients with rolandic discharges. In this stimulus condition, right-hand tapping, for instance, would elicit discharges over the left central region, whereas tapping of either foot would elicit discharges at the vertex. Such tactile-enhanced discharges constituted 38.2%; they were regarded as benign, age-related phenomena.

Reviewing published cases of somatosensory reflex epilepsy, Servit (1962) stated that seizures are provoked by stimulation of the trigeminal somatosensory region in the majority of patients (over 80%). Exaggerated responses in such patients can be obtained by electrical stimulation of peripheral nerves. The amplitude of somatosensory evoked potentials (SEPs) to median nerve electrical stimulation is markedly enlarged (giant SEPs) in most patients with cortical myoclonus of various etiology (Berkovic et al., 1991; Dawson, 1947; Halliday, 1967; Shibasaki et al., 1985; Sutton and Mayer, 1974).

Mima et al. (1997) studied proprioception-related SEPs with passive flexion movement of the middle finger at the proximal interphalangeal joint in seven cortical myoclonus patients who had associated giant SEPs. In three of the seven patients, the proprioception-related SEPs were also enlarged. Therefore, the authors concluded that hyperexcitability of the sensorimotor cortex in cortical myoclonus is modality-specific; cortical excitability is exaggerated to both cutaneous and deep receptor inputs in some patients, but only to cutaneous input in others. Figure 14.11 shows an example of unilateral central-parietal spikes evoked by electrical stimulation of the contralateral median nerve in a patient with benign childhood epilepsy with centrotemporal spike.

Plasmati et al. (1992) found increased incidence of giant SEPs (38%) in 44 benign epilepsy with rolandic spikes (BERS) patients. According to their further study (Plasmati et al., 2000), which investigated 54 BERS patients and 61 age-matched control subjects, short latencies were normal in all BERS patients, whereas the amplitude of middle latency was increased in a significant percentage of children with BERS. Giant responses occurred in 25.9% of BERS patients and in 4.9% of normal subjects. This phenomenon was presumed to depend on physiologic, functional cortical hyperexcitability related to maturation processes. They state that the giant responses clearly differ from those observed in myoclonic epilepsies and are likely to be generated in different neuronal pools in the sensorimotor cortex. The similar distribution of these giant middle latency SEPs with tactile evoked EEG spikes suggests a common generator for these responses. Electrical stimulation of the median nerve on routine EEG examination evoked central-parietal spikes in 3% of patients; all of them were epilepsy patients, the majority of whom showed PPR as well (Takahashi, 1974b). In a case reported by Goldie and Green (1959), seizures elicited by rubbing the face could also be precipitated just by thinking about rubbing the face or by hypnotic suggestion of cutaneous stroking. Van Cott et al. (1996) reported four adult patients with stimulus-sensitive seizures and myoclonus following severe hypoxic-ischemic injury; their EEGs showed bursts of generalized spike and polyspike activity following tactile stimulation associated with clinical seizures.

Other Sensory Stimuli

Regarding EEG activation by olfactory stimulation, very few data exist. Stevens (1962) tested 61 epileptics with gross olfactory stimulation. The stimuli consisted of a strong

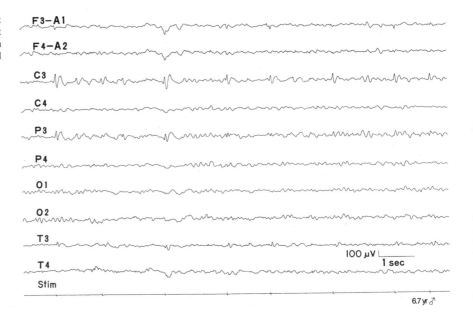

Figure 14.11. Electrical stimulation of right median nerve evoked spikes, maximal over left central-parietal areas, in a 6-year-old boy with benign childhood epilepsy with centrotemporal spike.

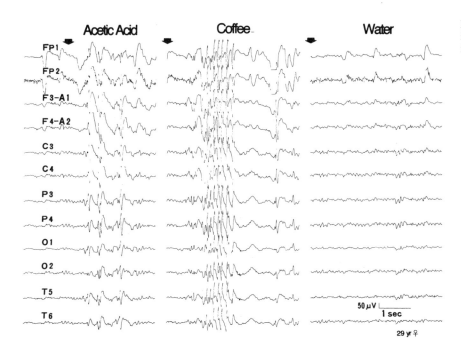

Figure 14.12. EEG responses to odorous stimuli in a 29-year-old woman with epilepsy with generalized tonic-clonic seizures (GTCSs) on awakening.

perfume (Tabu) and a malodorous H_2S compound. Sixteen out of 61 temporal lobe epilepsy patients demonstrated exaggerated spiking during or immediately after exposure to perfumed air. We also demonstrated EEG changes in response to olfactory stimuli in an adult epilepsy patient (Takahashi, 1982); generalized paroxysmal discharges were induced by ether and acetic acid. Figure 14.12 shows another example of odor sensitivity in a patient with GTCS seizures on awakening; olfactory stimuli with acetic acid and coffee elicited generalized paroxysmal discharges. In distinction to other modalities of sensory stimuli, repeated olfactory stimuli tend to quickly become ineffective. On EEG activation, olfactory stimuli using vanilla, coffee, etc., may be desirable because ammonia and similar pungent substances stimulate the trigeminal nerve.

Very little is known about the influence of vestibular stimulation on the EEG. Behrman and Wyke (1958) reported that bilateral 6-Hz activity arising from the temporal area could be evoked by caloric stimulation. Focal EEG changes were produced by rotational stimulation in 9 of 15 epileptics tested (Munter et al., 1964); in four patients, bilateral 2- to 7-Hz activity arose from the temporoparietal regions. Karbowski (1989) performed caloric stimulations in 62 epilepsy patients (irrigation for 15 seconds with 100 mL water at 27°C and at 44°C). In 22 cases, an increase in, or the appearance of, EEG abnormalities was detected. In two further cases epileptic seizures were triggered.

Multisensorial and Vegetative Sensory Stimuli

More than 600 patients with hot water epilepsy have been reported worldwide; more than 90% of them are from southern India (Acharya and Kotagal, 2000). The following factors are presumed to be involved in its pathophysiology: (a) high temperature, (b) direct contact of skin with water, (c) body part in contact with water, (d) mode of bathing. Generalized epileptiform abnormalities were found in 15% to 22%

of patients (Mani et al., 1975). Other reports have described both diffuse and focal abnormalities, predominantly in the temporal lobes. Ictal EEG abnormalities in ten patients include rhythmic left temporo-occipital spikes (Acharya and Kotagal, 2000; Lisovoski et al., 1992).

Seizures induced by eating (eating seizures) are rare. Rémillard et al. (1989, 1998) proposed two main clinical syndromes of eating seizures, differentiating temporolimbic from extralimbic, usually suprasylvian, seizure onset on clinical, radiologic, and EEG evidence. In addition, there was a subgroup of patients activated by certain tastes, such as sweets (Rémillard et al., 1989). They argued that the occurrence of eating seizures may be related to the excitation of a critical mass of epileptogenic cortex by various afferent stimuli, citing roles of the following: taste, mastication, gastric distension, somatosensory or proprioceptive input, and subcortical structures (Rémillard et al., 1998).

Seizures of "abdominal epilepsy" have reportedly been induced by vegetative sensory stimuli, such as enemas and injection of Prostigmin (Gastaut and Tassinari, 1966); such EEGs are characterized by appearance of generalized spike-wave complexes, occasionally associated with temporal and hemispheric foci.

Unexpected Startling Stimuli

One may rarely encounter patients with startle epilepsy (Alajouanine and Gastaut, 1955; Deonna, 1998; Vignal et al., 1998). Startle-induced seizures are focal or generalized tonic or atonic seizures, not always associated with loss of consciousness (Rosenow and Lüders, 2000b). Unexpected startling, mostly loud noises, and other unexpected somatosensory stimuli, such as sudden movements, are common precipitating factors; very rarely, visual stimuli are capable of startling. Those EEGs are usually accompanied by a temporary desynchronization followed by a generalized or focal seizure pattern (Gastaut and Tassinari, 1966). The interictal awake EEG shows frontal, central, or multifocal epileptiform discharges in the majority of patients (Aguglia et al., 1984; Manford et al., 1996; Saenz-Lope et al., 1984). Based on studies by animal models and clinical observations (Bancaud et al., 1975; Rosenow and Lüders, 2000b), startle epilepsy has been classified as "proprioceptive epilepsy" (Loiseau and Duché, 1989).

Transcranial Magnetic Stimulation

Hufnagel et al. (1990) used the method of transcranial magnetic stimulation (TMS) to induce paroxysmal discharge; positive findings were obtained in 12 of 13 patients. Schuler et al. (1993) statistically compared activation effects of paroxysmal discharge with those by TMS and HV in ten patients with drug-resistant partial epilepsy. TMS caused an activation of the focal paroxysmal discharges only in three patients, whereas HV produced it in six cases; TMS even caused significant reduction of paroxysmal discharge in two patients. These results led them to conclude that TMS was not better than HV. To contrast to low-frequency (<1 Hz) TMS studies, Tassinari et al. (2003) reported results obtained by high-frequency (>1 Hz) TMS (repetitive TMS; rTMS) in more than 60 epilepsy patients; rTMS-induced seizures were found in two of ten patients with progressive myoclonic epilepsy and in one of four patients with epilepsia partialis continua.

Other Forms of Activation

Eye Movements

Blinking is known to evoke spike-wave discharges (Green, 1966; Vignaendra et al., 1976). Nadkarni et al. (1994) reported that a 6-year-old boy's blinking triggered central midtemporal spikes (CMTSs) occurring reflexively, following the blinks by 100 to 200 msec. These blink-triggered CMTSs appeared almost exclusively while the patient was awake; it was inferred that the blinking while awake was associated with spikes resulting from abnormal and excessive excitatory interconnections between the precentral frontal areas and the epileptogenic zone of the rolandic cortex. In one patient, seizures were triggered by blinking when beginning to speak (Terzano et al., 1983). The phi rhythm (referring to posterior rhythmic slow waves occurring after eye closure) is an unusual age-related phenomenon seen mostly in young patients. According to Silbert et al. (1995), who defined it as a minimum of three consecutive monomorphic posterior delta waves occurring within 2 seconds of eye closure on at least two occasions, the phi rhythm has no significance for diagnosis of structural cerebral lesions or epilepsy. In epilepsy patients with this rhythm, however, the seizure disorder is more likely to be generalized than partial. In epilepsy patients, spike-wave discharges can also be induced not only by closing eyes (Gastaut and Tassinari, 1966; Green, 1966, 1968; Lewis, 1972; Robinson, 1939; Tieber, 1972), but also by opening of the eyes (Takahashi, 1976c) and performing conjugate eye movements (Shanzer et al., 1965; Takahashi, 1976c; Takahashi and Tsukahara, 1975). However, closing eyes is the most common effective technique (Takahashi, 1976c).

Paroxysmal discharges can also be provoked by voluntary eye closure and even by opening the eyes in darkness (Forster, 1977; Green, 1966; Lewis, 1972; Takahashi and Tsukahara, 1975; Vignaendra et al., 1976), indicating that spike-wave discharges may be evoked without the influence of visual stimuli. Generalized and focal paroxysmal discharges induced by such eye movements are usually maximal over the frontal areas (Takahashi and Tsukahara, 1975). Sensory afferents arising from contraction of the orbicularis oculi muscle (Vignaendra et al., 1976) and proprioceptive impulses from the ocular muscles (Shanzer et al., 1965) are thought to play a role in the mechanism of provocation of seizure discharges by closing eyes and by conjugate eye movements. In such epilepsy patients, similar paroxysmal

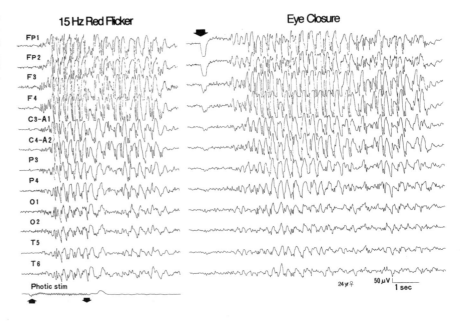

Figure 14.13. Generalized paroxysmal discharges induced by a 15-Hz red flicker stimulation and eye closure in a dark room in a 24-year-old woman with photosensitive epilepsy. A red flicker stimulus was provided by a visual stimulator (Tsukahara and Takahashi, 1973); luminance maintained at 20 cd/m².

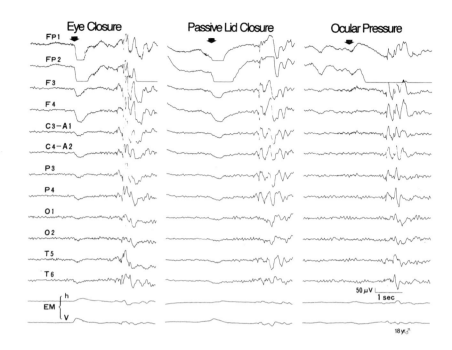

Figure 14.14. Generalized paroxysmal discharges induced by eye closure, passive lid closure, and ocular pressure in an 18-year-old man with photosensitive epilepsy. Simultaneous recordings of horizontal and vertical eye movements are shown *(bottom)*.

discharges to those described above may also be induced by ocular pressure (Robinson, 1939) or passive lid-closure in darkness (Toma et al., 1975). In an epilepsy patient, right occipital spikes and complex partial seizures could be induced by convergence (Vignaendra and Lim, 1978).

The above findings are most often seen in photosensitive epilepsy patients (Newmark and Penry, 1979). Figure 14.13 is an example of generalized spike-wave discharges with an anterior maximum induced by eye closure in darkness in comparison with that induced by a red flicker stimulation in a photosensitive epilepsy patient. Figure 14.14 shows another example of generalized spike-wave discharges induced by eye closure in darkness in a photosensitive epilepsy patient; similar spike-wave discharges were also induced by passive lid-closure and ocular pressure in darkness.

Limb and Trunk Movements

Just as the rolandic mu rhythm is blocked by contralateral movements, suppression of central spikes is also commonly observed with contralateral motor activities, such as clenching of the fist (Niedermeyer, 1972a). Alternatively, active or passive movements of the limbs may provoke focal motor seizures and focal paroxysmal discharges in a rare reflex epilepsy patient (Arseni et al., 1967). Forster (1977) reported a patient who had clonic seizures of the right hand; seizures invariably occurred with the use of the right hand, such as with writing or finger tapping, even occurring when the patient imagined movement of the hand. Rarely, seizure occurred with use of the left hand. These seizures were associated with focal spikes over the left motor areas.

Movement after various periods of rest may also induce seizures, including tonic seizure and paroxysmal choreo-athetosis (Forster, 1977; Hudgins and Corbin, 1966; Lishman et al., 1962). In such patients, in addition to startle or suddenness, the motor movement itself and the propriocep-

tive feedback secondary to the movements are thought to be involved in precipitating seizures (Forster, 1977; Loiseau and Duché, 1989).

Neuropsychological EEG Activation

Reflex epilepsies are divided into a simple and a complex group according to the triggering mechanism. The former comprises seizure precipitation by simple sensory stimuli and by movements, whereas the latter involves complex mental processes, such as reading (Radhakrishnan et al., 1995; Wolf, 2000), and a variety of other cognitive tasks. Regarding seizures elicited by cognitive tasks, the term *praxis-induced seizures* (Goossens et al., 1990; Inoue et al., 1994) has recently become popular. All descriptions cited below have only recently been grouped together as praxis-induced seizures (Wolf, 2000): epilepsia arithmetices, drawing-induced seizures, chess and card epilepsy, seizures during card games and draughts, reflex epilepsy evoked by decision making or by specific psychic activity, seizures evoked by playing with Rubik's cube, seizures induced by thinking, and reflex epilepsy with response to games of chance, calculations, and spatial decisions.

By use of a method of neuropsychological EEG activation (NPA), Matsuoka et al. (2000) reported results obtained from 480 Japanese patients with different types of epilepsy. NPA tasks consist of reading, speaking, writing, written arithmetic calculation, mental arithmetic calculation, and spatial construction. The NPA tasks provoked epileptic discharges in 38 patients (7.9%) and were accompanied by myoclonic seizures in 15 patients, absence seizures in eight, and simple partial seizures in one. Among the cognitive tasks, mental activities mainly associated with the use of the hands, i.e., writing (68.4%), written calculation (55.3%), and spatial construction (63.2%), provoked the most discharges, followed by mental calculation (7.9%) and reading (5.3%). As for precipitating events, action-programming type activities were thought to be the most crucial in 32 out of the 38 patients (84.2%), followed by thinking type activities in four patients (10.5%). Regarding classification of epilepsies, seizure-precipitating mental activities were almost exclusively (in 36 out of the 38 patients) related to idiopathic generalized epilepsies (IGEs), and were rarely (in only two out of the 38 patients) related to temporal lobe epilepsy. In IGE patients, provocative effects of NPA were related to myoclonic seizures rather than absence or generalized tonic-clonic seizures. These results suggest that NPA is a useful tool for examining the relationship between cognitive function and epileptic seizures.

Shown in Fig. 14.15 are paroxysmal discharges induced by written arithmetic in a juvenile myoclonic epilepsy (JME) patient; the following new question (right tracing) provoked more intensified paroxysmal discharges than those by the first one (left tracing). The right tracing of Fig. 14.16 illustrates bilateral paroxysmal discharges elicited by the Uchida-Kraepelin test (continuous one-digit addition) in a JME patient who had recurrent myoclonic seizures during video games; he was nonphotosensitive (Takahashi et al., 1995). Those shown on the right appear to be similar to generalized paroxysmal discharges evoked by a video game (the left tracing), suggesting that seizures induced by video games are not caused by visual stimuli, but are instead produced by combined factors of hand movements and calculation, which would be an example of praxis.

During mental work requiring concentration of attention, some subjects show theta activity bursts in the frontal midline (Ishihara and Yoshii, 1972). However, magnetoencephalography analysis (Sasaki et al., 1996) disclosed that frontal midline theta burst activities elicited by similar tasks in fact distribute widely in the frontal cortices of both cerebral hemispheres. Therefore, the authors claim that an expression of frontal mental theta waves is more appropriate than that of "frontal midline theta" being recorded maximally at the frontal midline (Yamaguchi, 1981).

Emotional Changes

It has long been thought that certain emotional states may be influential either directly or indirectly in precipitating seizures (Guey et al., 1969; Temkin and Davis, 1984). Stevens (1959) used emotional activation of the EEG in 30 epilepsy patients, eight with GTCS, and 22 with complex partial seizures. Stimuli consisted of a stressful interview that elicited strong feelings of anger, sorrow, embarrassment, mirth, and pleasure. Two thirds of GTCS patients showed no abnormal changes, while three quarters of complex partial seizure patients had abnormal findings. Abnormal changes not observed in previous tracings were seen in nearly half of the complex partial seizure group, but in only one patient in the GTCS group. Similar emotional activation of EEG patterns has been reported by Small et al. (1964).

Hypoglycemia

Provocation of convulsive seizures and spike discharges by hypoglycemia, especially during insulin shock treatment

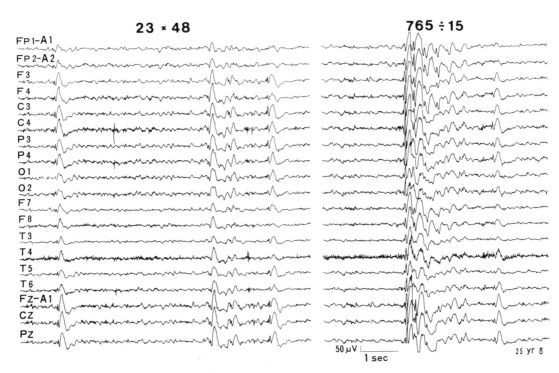

Figure 14.15. Generalized paroxysmal discharges induced by written arithmetic in a 25-year-old man with juvenile myoclonic epilepsy. The left paroxysmal discharge in the *left tracing* appeared 10 seconds after calculation was started. As shown in the *right tracing*, another question elicited intensified paroxysmal discharges that appeared 2 seconds after a calculation was started; simultaneous video-EEG monitoring revealed that myoclonic seizures of both arms were associated with it.

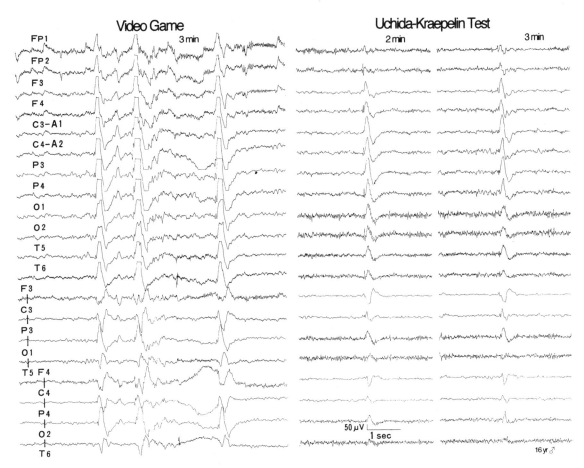

Figure 14.16. Paroxysmal discharges elicited by video game and Uchida-Kraepelin test in a 16-year-old boy with JME. The *left tracing* shows generalized paroxysmal discharges associated with myoclonic seizures of upper extremities; they occurred 3 minutes after the game (Puyo puyo) started. Uchida-Kraepelin test at 2 and 3 minutes elicited bilateral paroxysmal discharges associated with myoclonic seizures of both hands.

of schizophrenia (Sakel, 1935), has been well documented (Poire, 1969); spike-wave discharges are usually observed when the patient has "muscle twitches." Convulsions and EEG abnormalities also occur in patients with spontaneous episodes of hyperinsulinism secondary to islet-cell tumors of the pancreas; the same finding may be observed in rare patients with nonpancreatic tumors associated with hypoglycemia. Hypoglycemia of nonpancreatic origin (for example, ketogenic diet) occasionally facilitates generalized paroxysmal activity (Niedermeyer, 1972b). Therefore, EEG activation by fasting may be informative in generalized epilepsy patients if no paroxysmal discharges could be found on routine EEG examination. Attempts have also been made to induce paroxysmal activity through hypoglycemia produced by tolbutamide (Green, 1963; Mosowich, 1967). Hypoglycemic activation may also by a useful technique for predicting the presence of pathology in patients considered for anterior temporal lobectomy (Sperling, 1984).

Pharmacological Activation

Drugs

Alpha-chloralose or alpha-chloralose-scopolamine have occasionally been used for EEG activation in epilepsy pa-

tients with normal routine EEG (Bercel, 1953; Verdeaux et al., 1954). The adult patient was given a preparation consisting of scopolamine hydrobromide ½ mg and alpha chloralose 500 mg, in capsule form, by mouth (Bercel, 1953). Of 30 epilepsy patients, 22 showed activation efficacies. Intravenous tripelennamine (Pyribenzamine) is also known to activate focal or diffuse paroxysmal discharges (King and Weeks, 1965). In addition, it has been reported that intravenous administration of some antiparkinsonism agents, such as 1 mg of scopolamine hydrobromide (Vas et al., 1967a), 10 to 20 mg of procyclidine hydrochloride (Vas et al., 1967b), or 10 mg of methixene hydrochloride (Vas et al., 1967c), is capable of provoking focal paroxysmal discharges, especially in temporal lobe epilepsy patients. Intravenous alfentanil hydrochloride, which is a short-duration opioid analgesic, has been demonstrated to be effective in inducing temporal lobe spikes for intraoperative electrocorticographic and depth electrode recording (Cascino et al., 1993). These methods, however, have not been widely used.

Antiepileptic Drug Withdrawal Procedure for Long-Term Monitoring

Before epilepsy surgery, antiepileptic drug (AED) withdrawal in the video-EEG monitoring environment is currently being carried out for the purpose of increasing the probability of interictal and ictal abnormalities occurring during the record. The most important risk of AED withdrawal is the development of status epilepticus (Fagan and Lee, 1990; Simon, 1985). Such complications of AED withdrawal, however, can be prevented if patients are under the care of experienced staff (Fisch and So, 2003).

Metrazol and Megimide

Pentylenetetrazol (Metrazol) has been used therapeutically to induce convulsions in schizophrenia patients (von Meduna, 1935). Ziskind et al. (1946) demonstrated the value of Metrazol in triggering paroxysmal discharges. A series of similar studies followed: Kaufman et al. (1946), Ziskind and Bercel (1946), Cure et al. (1948), Jasper and Courtois (1953), and Bancaud (1976). The effectiveness of a given amount of Metrazol depends to a large extent on the rapidity of its injection as well as the total amount in relation to body weight (Jasper and Courtois, 1953). These authors recommended dilution of a 10% solution of Metrazol in normal saline so that 1 cc of the mixture contains 1 mg/kg of body weight. One milliliter is then given thereafter every 30 seconds.

Among epilepsy patients, those with bilaterally synchronous EEG disturbances were more sensitive than those with focal cortical seizures (Cure et al., 1948). On the other hand, Ajmone-Marsan and Ralston (1957) showed activation of various types of focal seizures by this method. They reported that the epileptogenic supplementary motor area appears to be very sensitive to Metrazol stimulation.

Gastaut (1950) described an activation method combined with Metrazol and IPS (see Takahashi, 1999). Gastaut pointed out that this test differentiates between epilepsies involving a subcortical diencephalic mechanism and those of cortical origin. A low threshold to IPS was found in idiopathic (absence seizure group in particular) and myoclonic epilepsies. Normal or elevated thresholds were found in the focal cortical group. Although this method was more sensitive than activation by Metrazol alone, a high incidence of low-threshold responses (5 mg/kg or less) in a number of other conditions such as schizophrenia and hysteria, and even normal subjects, has been observed.

Bemegride (Megimide) was first investigated as a barbiturate antagonist (Shulman et al., 1955). Megimide was then found to have a convulsant action similar to that of Metrazol (Delay et al., 1956; Drossopoulo et al., 1956).

Despite numerous studies, especially between 1946 and 1970 (Ajmone-Marsan, 2000), neither of the above tests is presently considered to be a satisfactory method for distinguishing between potential epileptic and nonepileptic individuals. Furthermore, the risk of failure in seizure control with resection of a focus that was localized by chemically (Megimide) induced seizures is two times higher than that with resection of a spontaneous seizure focus (Wieser et al., 1979). Therefore, drugs are no longer used to induce seizures for localization in epilepsy surgery (Fisch and So, 2003).

Reenactment of the Triggering Situation

When a fixed set of ambient circumstances is associated with convulsive or nonconvulsive paroxysmal attacks, reenactment of the situation, if possible, is desirable for reaching a diagnosis. Fariello et al. (1983) reported that reenactment determined the diagnosis in 30 of 32 patients with paroxysmal disorders. The authors claim that an appropriately executed reenactment should entail polygraphic recording of at least EEG, electrocardiogram, and respiration.

Concluding Remarks

The greater the number of different activation methods used in EEG evaluation of an epilepsy patient, the greater the chance of obtaining abnormal findings. From a practical point of view, however, desirable activations are those methods that can be carried out easily, in a short time, with affordable equipment, and without undesirable side effects for patients. Special methods of activation are needed in epilepsy patients for whom seizures tend to appear under certain conditions while awake.

Acknowledgments

The author wishes to thank Professor Y. Tsukahara for his discussions of the manuscript. The author is also very grateful to Mr. B.A. Fast for manuscript preparation assistance.

References

Acharya, J.N., and Kotagal, P. 2000. Activation of seizures by hot water. In *Epileptic Seizures: Pathophysiology and Clinical Semiology,* Eds. H.O. Lüders and S. Noachtar, pp. 615–627. New York: Churchill Livingstone.

Achenbach-Ng, J., Siao, T.C.P., Marvroudakis, N., et al. 1994. Effects of routine hyperventilation on PCO_2 and PO_2 in normal subjects: implications for EEG interpretations. J. Clin. Neurophysiol. 11:220–225.

Adrian, E.D., and Matthews, B.H.C. 1934. The Berger rhythm: potential changes from the occipital lobes in man. Brain 57:355–385.

AEEGS Guidelines Committee. 1994. Guideline one: minimum technical requirements for performing clinical electroencephalography. J. Clin. Neurophysiol. 11:4–5.

Aguglia, U., Tinuper, P., and Gastaut, H. 1984. Startle-induced epileptic seizures. Epilepsia 25:712–720.

Ajmone-Marsan, C. 2000. Pentylenetetrazol: historical notes and comments on its electroencephalographic activation properties. In *Epileptic Seizures: Pathophysiology and Clinical Semiology,* Eds. H.O. Lüders and S. Noachtar, pp. 563–569. New York: Churchill Livingstone.

Ajmone-Marsan, C., and Ralston, B.L. 1957. *The Epileptic Seizure:Its Functional Morphology and Diagnostic Significance.* Springfield, IL: Charles C Thomas.

Alajouanine, T., and Gastaut, H. 1955. La syncinésie-sursaut et l'épilepsie-sursaut è déclanchement sensorial ou sensitif inopiné. Les faits anatomocliniques (15 observations). Rev. Neurol. 93:29–41.

Allison, T., Begleiter, A., McCarthy, G., et al. 1993. Electrophysiological studies of color processing in human visual cortex. Electroencephalogr. Clin. Neurophysiol. 88:343–355.

Arellano, A.P., Schwab, R.S., and Casby, J.U. 1950. Sonic activation. Electroencephalogr. Clin. Neurophysiol. 2:215–217.

Arseni, C., Stoica, I., and Serbanescu, T. 1967. Electro-clinical investigations on the role of proprioceptive stimuli in the onset and arrest of convulsive epileptic paroxysms. Epilepsia 8:162–170.

Bancaud, J. 1976. EEG activation by Metrazol and Megimide in the diagnosis of epilepsy. In *Handbook of Electroencephalography and Clinical Neurophysiology,* Ed. A. Remond, pp. 105–120. Amsterdam: Elsevier.

Bancaud, J., Talairach, J., Lamarche, M., et al. 1975. Hypothèses neurophysiopathologiques sur l'épilepsie-sursault chez l'homme. Rev. Neurol. 131:559–571.

Behrman, S., and Wyke, B.D. 1958. Vestibulogenic seizures: a consideration of vertiginous seizures, with particular reference to convulsions produced by stimulation of labyrinthine receptors. Brain 81:529–541.

Bercel, N.A. 1953. Experience with a combination of scopolamine and alpha chloralose (S.A.C.) in activating normal EEG of epileptics. Electroencephalogr. Clin. Neurophysiol. 5:297–304.

Berkovic, S.F., So, N.K., and Andermann, F. 1991. Progressive myoclonus epilepsies: clinical and neurophysiological diagnosis. J. Clin. Neurophysiol. 8:261–274.

Bickford, R.G. 1979. Activation procedures and special electrodes. In *Current Practice of Clinical Electroencephalography,* Eds. D.W. Klass and D.D. Daly, pp. 269–305. New York: Raven Press.

Bickford, R.G., and Klass, D.W. 1962. Stimulus factors in the mechanism of television induced seizures. Trans. Am. Neurol. Assoc. 87:176–178.

Bickford, R.G., and Klass, D.W. 1969. Sensory precipitation and reflex mechanisms. In *Basic Mechanisms of the Epilepsies,* Eds. H.H. Jasper, A.A. Ward, and A. Pope, pp. 543–564. Boston: Little, Brown.

Bickford, R.G., Sem-Jacobsen, G.W., White, P.T., et al. 1952. Some observations on the mechanism of photic and photometrazol activation. Electroencephalogr. Clin. Neurophysiol. 4:275–282.

Bickford, R.G., Daly, D., and Keith, H.M. 1953. Convulsive effects of light stimulation in children. Am. J. Dis. Child. 86:170–183.

Billinger, T.W., and Frank, G.S. 1969. Effects of posture on EEG slowing during hyperventilation. Am. J. EEG Technol. 9:22–27.

Binnie, C.D., and Jeavons, P.M. 1992. Photosensitive epilepsies. In *Epileptic Syndromes in Infancy, Childhood and Adolescence,* 2nd ed., Eds. J. Roger, M. Bureau, C. Dravet, et al., pp. 299–305. London: John Libbey.

Binnie, C.D., and Wilkins, A.J. 1998. Visually induced seizures not caused by flicker (intermittent light stimulation). In *Reflex Epilepsies and Reflex Seizures: Advances in Neurology,* Vol. 75, Eds. B.G. Zifkin, F. Andermann, A. Beaumanoir, et al., pp. 123–138. Philadelphia: Lippincott-Raven.

Binnie, C.D., Findlay, J., and Wilkins, A.J. 1985. Mechanisms of epileptogenesis in photosensitive epilepsy implied by the effects of moving patterns. Electroencephalogr. Clin. Neurophysiol. 61:1–6.

Binnie, C.D., Harding, G.F.A., Richens, A., et al. 1994. Video games and epileptic seizures—a consensus statement. Seizure 3:245–246.

Bostem, F. 1976. Hyperventilation. In *Handbook of Electroencephalography and Clinical Neurophysiology,* vol. 3D, Ed. A. Remond, pp. 74–88. Amsterdam: Elsevier.

Cascino, G.D., So, E.L., Sharbrough, F.W., et al. 1993. Alfentanil-induced epileptiform activity in patients with partial epilepsy. J. Clin. Neurophysiol. 10:520–525.

Chatrian, G.E., Lettich, E., Miller, L.H., et al. 1970. Pattern-sensitive epilepsy. 1. An electrographic study of its mechanisms. Epilepsia 11:125–149.

Chatrian, G.E., Bergamini, L., Dondey, M., et al. 1974. A glossary of terms most commonly used by clinical electroencephalographers. Electroencephalogr. Clin. Neurophysiol. 37:538–548.

Chiba, T., Kitawaki, M., Aoki, Y., et al. 1982. Hemodialysis and electroencephalogram: through a long term observation. Rinsho Noha (Osaka) 24:195–201.

Colon, E.J., Vingerhoets, H.M., Notermans, S.L.H., et al. 1979. Off-response: its clinical incidence in very young children. Electroencephalogr. Clin. Neurophysiol. 46:601–604.

Coull, B.M., and Pedley, T.A. 1978. Intermittent photic stimulation: clinical usefulness of non-convulsive responses. Electroencephalogr. Clin. Neurophysiol. 44:353–363.

Cure, C., Rasmussen, T., and Jasper, H.H. 1948. Activation of seizures and electroencephalographic disturbances in epileptic and in control subjects with "Metrazol." Arch. Neurol. Psychiatry 59:691–717.

Dalby, M.A. 1969. Epilepsy and 3 per second spike and wave rhythms. Acta Neurol. Scand. 40(suppl.):1–183.

Darby, C.E., De Korte, R.A., Binnie, C.D., et al. 1980a. The self-induction of epileptic seizures by eye closure. Epilepsia 21:31–42.

Darby, C.E., Wilkins, A.J., Binnie, C.D., et al. 1980b. Routine testing for pattern sensitivity. J. Electrophysiol. Technol. 6:202–210.

Davis, H., and Wallace, W.M. 1942. Factors affecting changes produced in electroencephalograms by standardized hyperventilation. Arch. Neurol. Psychiatry. 47:606–625.

Dawson, G.D. 1947. Investigations on a patient subject to myoclonic seizures after sensory stimulation. J. Neurol. Neurosurg. Psychiatry 10:141–162.

De Graaf, A.S., Lombard, C.J., and Classen, D.A. 1995. Influence of ethnic and geographic factors on the classic photoparoxysmal response in the electroencephalogram of epilepsy patients. Epilepsia 36:219–223.

Delay, J., Schuller, E., Drossopoulo, G., et al. 1956. Un nouvel activant des électroencéphalogrammes: l'imide de l'acide éthyl-méthyl glutarique (NP 13), ou Mégimide. Rev. Neurol. 94:315–318.

De Marco, P., and Negrin, P. 1973. Parietal focal spikes evoked by contralateral tactile somatotopic stimulation in four non-epileptic subjects. Electroencephalogr. Clin. Neurophysiol. 34:308–312.

De Marco, P., and Tassinari, C.A. 1981. Extreme somatosensory evoked potential (ESEP): an EEG sign forecasting the possible occurrence of seizures in children. Epilepsia 22:569–575.

Deonna, T. 1998. Reflex seizures with somatosensory precipitation: clinical and electroencephalographic patterns and differential diagnosis, with emphasis on reflex myoclonic epilepsy of infancy. In *Reflex Epilepsies and Reflex Seizures: Advances in Neurology,* vol.75, Eds. B.G. Zifkin, F. Andermann, A. Beaumanoir, et al., pp. 193–206. Philadelphia: Lippincott-Raven.

Doose, H., Gerken, H., Hien-Volpel, K.F., et al. 1969. Genetics of photosensitive epilepsy. Neuropaediatrie 1:56–73.

Drossopoulo, G., Gastaut, H., Verdeaux, G., et al. 1956. Comparison of EEG "activation" by pentamethylenetetrazol (Metrazol) and bemegride (Megimide). Electroencephalogr. Clin. Neurophysiol. 8:710–711.

Ellingson, R.J. 1960. Cortical electrical responses to visual stimulation in the human infant. Electroencephalogr. Clin. Neurophysiol. 12:633–677.

Engel, J., Jr. 1984. A practical guide for routine EEG studies in epilepsy. J. Clin. Neurophysiol. 1:109–142.

Esquivel, E., Chaussai, M., Plouin, P., et al. 1991. Physical exercise and voluntary hyperventilation in childhood absence epilepsy. Electroencephalogr. Clin. Neurophysiol. 79:127–132.

Fagan, K., and Lee, S. 1990. Prolonged confusion following convulsion due to generalized nonconvulsive status epilepticus. Neurology 40:1689–1694.

Fariello, R.G., Booker, H.E., Chun, R.W.M., et al. 1983. Reenactment of the triggering situation for the diagnosis of epilepsy. Neurology 33:878–884.

Fisch, B.C., and So, E.L. 2003. Activation methods. In *Current Practice of Clinical Electroencephalography,* 3rd ed., Eds. J.S. Ebersole and T.A. Pedley, pp. 246–270. Philadelphia: Lippincott Williams & Wilkins.

Foerster, O. 1924. Hyperventilationsepilepsie. Zbl. Ges. Neurol. Psychiatr. 38:289–293.

Forster, F.M. 1977. *Reflex Epilepsy, Behavioral Therapy and Conditional Reflexes,* Springfield, IL: Charles C Thomas.

Gambardella, A., Aguglia, U., Oliveri, R.L., et al. 1996. Photic-induced epileptic negative myoclonus: a case report. Epilepsia 37:492–494.

Gastaut, H. 1950. Combined photic and Metrazol activation of the brain. Electroencephalogr. Clin. Neurophysiol. 2:249–261.

Gastaut, H. 1969. Introduction to the study of organic generalized epilepsies. In *The Physiopathogenesis of the Epilepsies,* Eds. H. Gastaut, H. Jasper, J. Bancaud, et al., pp. 147–157. Springfield, IL: Charles C Thomas.

Gastaut, H., and Rémond, A. 1949. L'activation de l'électroencéphalogramme dans les affections cérébrales non épileptogènes (vers une neurophysiolgie clinique). Rev. Neurol. 81:594–598.

Gastaut, H., and Tassinari, C.A. 1966. Triggering mechanisms in epilepsy: the electro-clinical point of view. Epilepsia 7:85–138.

Gastaut, H.J., Benoit, P.H., Vigouroux, M., et al. 1954. Potentiels évoqés par des stimuli auditifs sur la région temporale de certains épileptiques. Electroencephalogr. Clin. Neurophysiol. 6:557–564.

Gastaut, H., Trevisan, C., and Naquet, R. 1958. Diagnostic value of electroencephalographic abnormalities provoked by intermittent photic stimulation. Electroencephalogr. Clin. Neurophysiol. 10:194–195(abst).

Gibbs, F.A., Gibbs, E.L., and Lennox, W.G. 1943. Electroencephalographic response to overventilation and its relation to age. J. Pediatr. 23:497–505.

Goldie, L., and Green, J.N. 1959. A study of the psychological factors in a case of sensory reflex epilepsy. Brain 82:505–524.

Goossens, L.A.Z., Andermann, F., Andermann, E., et al. 1990. Reflex seizures induced by calculation, card or board games, and spatial tasks: a review of 25 patients and delineation of the epileptic syndrome. Neurology 40:1171–1176.

Gotoh, F., Meyer, J.S., and Takagi, Y. 1965. Cerebral effects of hyperventilation in man. Arch. Neurol. 12:410–423.

Green, J.B. 1963. The activation of electroencephalographic abnormalities by tolbutamide-induced hypoglycemia. Neurology 13:192–200.

Green, J.B. 1966. Self-induced seizures. Arch. Neurol. 15:579–586.

Green, J.B. 1968. Seizures on closing the eyes. Neurology 18:391–396.

Guerrini, R., Dravet, C., Genton, P., et al. 1995. Idiopathic photosensitive occipital lobe epilepsy. Epilepsia 36:883–891.

Guey, J., Bureau, M., Dravet, C., et al. 1969. A study of the rhythm of petit mal absences in children in relation to prevailing situations. The use of EEG telemetry during psychological examinations, school exercises and periods of inactivity. Epilepsia 10:441–451.

Gumnit, R.J., Niedermeyer, E., and Spreen, O. 1965. Seizure activity uniquely inhibited by patterned vision. Arch. Neurol. 13:363–368.

Halliday, A.M. 1967. The electrophysiological study of myoclonus in man. Brain 90:241–284.

Harding, G.F.A., and Jeavons, P.M. 1994. Photosensitive Epilepsy, new edition. London: MacKeith Press.

Harding, G.F.A., and Harding, P.F. 1999. Televised material and photosensitive epilepsy. Epilepsia 40 (suppl. 4):65–69.

Hishikawa, Y., Yamamoto, J., Furuya, E., et al. 1967. Photosensitive epilepsy: relationships between the visual evoked responses and the epileptiform discharges induced by intermittent photic stimulation. Electroencephalogr. Clin. Neurophysiol. 23:320–334.

Holmes, G.L., Blair, S., Eisenberg, E., et al. 1982. Tooth-brushing-induced epilepsy. Epilepsia 23:657–661.

Hudgins, R.L., and Corbin, K.B. 1966. An uncommon seizure disorder: familial paroxysmal choreoathetosis. Brain 89:199–204.

Hufnagel, A., Elger, C.E., Durwen, H.F., et al. 1990. Activation of the epileptic focus by transcranial magnetic stimulation of the human brain. Ann. Neurol. 27:49–60.

Inoue, Y., Seino, M., Kubota, H., et al. 1994. Epilepsy with praxis-induced seizures. In Epileptic Seizures and Syndromes, Ed. P. Wolf, pp. 81–92. London: John Libbey.

Ishihara, T., and Yoshii, N. 1972. Multivariate analytic study of EEG and mental activity in juvenile delinquents. Electroencephalogr. Clin. Neurophysiol. 33:71–80.

Jasper, H., and Courtois, G. 1953. A practical method for uniform activation with intravenous Metrazol. Electroencephalogr. Clin. Neurophysiol. 5: 443–444.

Jeavons, P.M. 1969. The use of photic stimulation in clinical electroencephalography. Proc. Electrophysiol. Technol. Assoc. 16:225–240.

Jeavons, P.M., and Harding, G.F.A. 1975. Photosensitive Epilepsy: A Review of the Literature and a Study of 460 Patients. London: Heinemann.

Jeavons, P.M., Harding, G.F.A., Panayiotopoulos, C.P., et al. 1972. The effect of geometric patterns combined with intermittent photic stimulation in photosensitive epilepsy. Electroencephalogr. Clin. Neurophysiol. 33: 221–224.

Kameyama, M., Shirane, R., Tsurumi, Y., et al. 1986. Evaluation of cerebral blood flow and metabolism in childhood moyamoya disease: an investigation into "re-build-up" on EEG by positron CT. Child. Nerv. Syst. 2:130–133.

Karbowski, K. 1989. Epileptic seizures induced by vestibular and auditory stimuli. In Reflex Seizures and Reflex Epilepsies, Eds. A. Beaumanoir, H. Gastaut, and R. Naquet, pp. 255–260. Geneva: Editions Médicine & Hygiène.

Kasteleijn-Nolst Trenité, D.G.A. 1998. Reflex seizures induced by intermittent light stimulation. In Reflex Epilepsies and Reflex Seizures: Advances in Neurology, vol. 75, Eds. B.G. Zifkin, F. Andermann, A. Beaumanoir, et al., pp. 99–121. Philadelphia: Lippincott-Raven.

Kasteleijn-Nolst Trenité, D.G.A., Binnie, C.D., and Meinardi, H. 1987. Photosensitive patients: symptoms and signs during intermittent photic stimulation and their relation to seizures in daily life. J. Neurol. Neurosurg. Psychiatry 560:1436–1549.

Kasteleijn-Nolst Trenité, D.G.A., Binnie, C.D., Harding, G.F.A., et al. 1999. Photic stimulation: standardization of screening methods. Epilepsia (suppl. 4) 40:75–79.

Kasteleijn-Nolst Trenité, D.G.A., Martins da Silva, A., Ricci, S., et al. 2002. Video games are exciting: a European study of video game-induced seizures and epilepsy. Epileptic Disord. 4:121–128.

Kaufman, I.C., Marshall, C., and Walker, A.E. 1946. Metrazol activated electroencephalography. Res. Publ. Ass. Nerv. Ment. Dis. 26:476–486.

Kellaway, P. 1979. An orderly approach to visual analysis: the parameters of the normal EEG in adults and children. In Current Practice of Clinical Electroencephalography, Eds. D.W. Klass and D.D. Daly, pp. 69–147. New York: Raven Press.

Kiloh, L.G., McComas, A.J., and Osselton, J.W. 1972. Clinical Electroencephalography, 3rd ed. London: Butterworths.

King, G., and Weeks, S.D. 1965. Pyribenzamine activation of the electroencephalogram. Electroencephalogr. Clin. Neurophysiol. 18:503–507.

Klass, D.W. 2000. Pattern activation of seizures. In Epileptic Seizures: Pathophysiology and Clinical Semiology, Eds. H.O. Lüders and S. Noachtar, pp. 598–608. New York: Churchill Livingstone.

Klass, D.W., and Fischer-Williams, M. 1976. Sensory stimulation, sleep and sleep deprivation. In Handbook of Electroencephalography and Clinical Neurophysiology, vol. 3D, Ed. A. Remond, pp. 5–73. Amsterdam: Elsevier.

Kodama, N., Aoki, Y., Hiraga, H., et al. 1979. Electroencephalographic findings in children with moyamoya disease. Arch. Neurol. 36:16–19.

Kooi, K., Thomas, M.H., and Mortenson, F.N. 1960. Photoconvulsive and photomyoclonic responses in adults: an appraisal of their clinical significance. Neurology 10:1051–1058.

Kooi, K.A., Tucker, P.R., and Marshall, R.E. 1978. Fundamentals of Electroencephalography, Hagerstown, MD: Harper & Row.

Koshino, Y., and Niedermeyer, E. 1975. Enhancement of rolandic mu-rhythm by pattern vision. Electroencephalogr. Clin. Neurophysiol. 38: 535–538.

Langill, L., and Wong, P.K.W. 2003. Tactile-evoked rolandic discharges: a benign finding? Epilepsia 44:221–227.

Lee, R.G., and Blair, R.D.G. 1973. Evolution of EEG and visual evoked response changes in Jakob-Creutzfeldt disease. Electroencephalogr. Clin. Neurophysiol. 35:133–142.

Lewis, J.A. 1972. Eye closure as a motor trigger for seizures. Neurology 22:1145–1150.

Lishman, W.A., Symonds, C.P., Whitty, C.W., et al. 1962. Seizures induced by movement. Brain 85:93–108.

Lisovoski, F., Prier, S., Koskas, P., et al. 1992. Hot-water epilepsy in an adult: ictal EEG, MRI and SPECT features. Seizure 1:203–206.

Loiseau, P., and Duché, B. 1989. Seizures induced by movement. In Reflex Seizures and Reflex Epilepsies, Eds. A. Beaumanoir, H. Gastaut, and R. Naquet, pp. 109–114. Geneva: Editions Médicine & Hygiène.

Lueck, C.J., Zeki, S., Friston, K.J., et al. 1989. The colour centre in the cerebral cortex of man. Nature 340:386–389.

Lugaresi, E., Cirignotta, F., and Montagna, P. 1984. Occipital lobe epilepsy with scotosensitive seizures: the role of central vision. Epilepsia 25: 115–120.

Maheshwari, M.C., and Jeavons, P.M. 1975. The clinical significance of occipital spikes as a sole response to intermittent photic stimulation. Electroencephalogr. Clin. Neurophysiol. 39:93–95.

Manford, M.R., Fish, D.R., and Shorvon, S.D. 1996. Startle provoked epileptic seizures: features in 19 patients. J. Neurol. Neurosurg. Psychiatry 61:151–156.

Mani, K.S., Mani, A.J., Ramesh, C.K. 1975. Hot-water epilepsy—a peculiar type of reflex epilepsy: clinical and EEG features in 108 cases. Trans. Am. Neurol. Assoc. 99:224–226.

Matsuoka, H., Takahashi, T., Sasaki, M., et al. 2000. Neuropsychological EEG activation in patients with epilepsy. Brain 123:318–330.

Melsen, S. 1959. The value of photic stimulation in the diagnosis of epilepsy. J. Nerv. Ment. Dis. 128:508–519.

Miley, C.E., and Forster, F.M. 1977. Activation of partial complex seizures by hyperventilation. Arch. Neurol. 34:371–373.

Mima, T., Terada, K., Ikeda, A., et al. 1997. Afferent mechanism of cortical myoclonus studied by proprioception-related SEPs. Electroencephalogr. Clin. Neurophysiol. 104:51–59.

Morrice, J.K.W. 1956. Slow wave production in the EEG, with reference to hyperpnoea, carbon dioxide and autonomic balance. Electroencephalogr. Clin. Neurophysiol. 8:49–72.

Mosowich, A. 1967. The role of oral hyperglycaemiants as activators in epilepsy. In Neurological Problems, Ed. J. Chorobski, pp. 117–130. Oxford: Pergamon.

Munter, M., Goetze, W., and Krokowski, G. 1964. Telemetrische EEG. Untersuchungen ratatorischer Vestibulatisreizung. Dtsch. Z. Nervenheilkd. 186:137–148.

Nadkarni, M.A., Postolache, V., Gold, A., et al. 1994. Central mid-temporal spikes triggered by blinking. Electroencephalogr. Clin. Neurophysiol. 90:36–39.

Newmark, M.E., and Penry, J.K. 1979. *Photosensitivity and Epilepsy: A Review.* New York: Raven Press.

Niedermeyer, E. 1972a. Focal and generalized seizure discharges in the electroencephalogram and their response to intravenous diazepam. Int. Med. Dig. 7:49–61.

Niedermeyer, E. 1972b. *The Generalized Epilepsies.* Springfield, IL: Charles C Thomas.

Niedermeyer, E., Fineyre, F., Riley, T., et al. 1979. Myoclonus and the electroencephalogram: a review. Clin. Electroencephalogr. 10:75–95.

Nims, L.F., Gibbs, E.L., Lennox, W.G., et al. 1940. Adjustment of acid-base balance of patients with petit mal epilepsy to overventilation. Arch. Neurol. Psychiatry 43:262–269.

O'Brien, T.J., Hogan, R.E., Sedal, L., et al. 1996. Tooth-brushing epilepsy: a report of a case with structural and functional imaging and electrophysiology demonstrating a right frontal focus. Epilepsia 37:694–697.

Pampiglione, G., and Harden, A. 1977. So-called neuronal ceroid lipofuscinosis: neurophysiological studies in 60 children. J. Neurol. Neurosurg. Psychiatry 40:323–330.

Panayiotopoulos, C.P. 1974. Effectiveness of photic stimulation on various eye-states in photosensitive epilepsy. J. Neurol. Sci. 23:165–173.

Panayiotopoulos, C.P. 1979. Conversion of photosensitive to scotosensitive epilepsy: report of a case. Neurology 29:1550–1554.

Panayiotopoulos, C.P. 1994. With comments and contributions from Binnie, C.D., and Takahashi, T. Fixation-off-sensitive epilepsies: clinical and EEG characteristics. In *Epileptic Seizures and Syndromes,* Ed. P. Wolf, pp. 55–66. London: John Libbey.

Panayiotopoulos, C.P. 1998. Fixation-off sensitive epilepsies: clinical and EEG characteristics. In *Reflex Epilepsies and Reflex Seizures: Advances in Neurology,* vol. 75, Eds. B.G. Zifkin, F. Andermann, A. Beaumanoir, et al., pp. 139–157. Philadelphia: Lippincott-Raven.

Patel, V.M., and Maulsby, R.L. 1987. How hyperventilation alters the EEG: a review of controversial viewpoints emphasizing neurophysiological mechanisms. J. Clin. Neurophysiol. 4:101–120.

Peet, R.M., Daly, D.D., and Bickoford, R.G. 1952. Some clinical and electroencephalographic responses to sound stimulation in epileptic patients. Trans. Am. Neurol. Assoc. 7:215–217.

Petersen, I., and Eeg-Olofsson, O. 1971. The development of the electroencephalogram in normal children from age 1 through 15 years—nonparoxysmal activity. Neuropaediatrie 2:247–304.

Pinsard, N., Livet, M.O., Saint-Jean, M. 1978. A case of cerebral lipidosis with an atypical presentation. Rev. Electroencephalogr. Neurophysiol. Clin. 8:175–179.

Plasmati, R., Michelucci, R., Forti, A., et al. 1992. The neurophysiological features of benign partial epilepsy with rolandic spikes. In *Benign Localized and Generalized Epilepsies of Early Childhood, Epilepsy Res. Suppl. 6,* Eds. R. Degan and F.E. Dreifuss, pp. 45–48. Amsterdam: Elsevier.

Plasmati, R., Pastorelli, F., and Tassinari, C.A. 2000. Giant midlatency somatosensory evoked potentials in benign epilepsy with rolandic spikes. In *Epileptic Seizures: Pathophysiology and Clinical Semiology,* Eds. H.O. Lüders and S. Noachtar, pp. 62–68. New York: Churchill Livingstone.

Poire, R. 1969. Hypoglycemic epilepsy: clinical, electrographic and biological study during induced hypoglycemia in man. In *The Physiopathogenesis of the Epilepsies,* Eds. H. Gastaut, H.H. Jasper, J. Bancaud, et al., pp. 75–110. Springfield, IL: Charles C Thomas.

Prechtl, H.F.R. 1959. Provocation of electroencephalographic changes in the temporal region by intermittent acoustic stimuli. Electroencephalogr. Clin. Neurophysiol. 11:511–519.

Quirk, J.A., Fish, D.R., Smith, S.J.M., et al. 1995a. Incidence of photosensitive epilepsy: a prospective national study. Electroencephalogr. Clin. Neurophysiol. 95:260–267.

Quirk, J.A., Fish, D.R., Smith, S.J.M., et al. 1995b. First seizures associated with playing electronic screen games: a community-based study in Great Britain. Ann. Neurol. 37:733–737.

Radhakrishnan, K., Silbert, P.L., and Klass, D.W. 1995. Reading epilepsy: an appraisal of 20 patients diagnosed at the Mayo Clinic, Rochester, Minnesota, between 1949 and 1989, and delineation of the epileptic syndrome. Brain 118:75–89.

Reilly, E.W., and Peters, J.F. 1973. Relationship of some varieties of electroencephalographic photosensitivity to clinical convulsive disorders. Neurology 23:1040–1057.

Rémillard, G.M., Andermann, F., Zifkin, B.G., et al. 1989. Eating epilepsy: a study of ten surgically treated patients suggests the presence of two separate syndromes. In *Reflex Seizures and Reflex Epilepsies,* Eds. A. Beaumanoir, H. Gastaut, R. Naquet, pp. 289–300. Geneva: Editions Médecine & Hygiéne.

Rémillard, G.M., Zifkin, B.G., and Andermann, F. 1998. Seizures induced by eating. In *Reflex Epilepsies and Reflex Seizures: Advances in Neurology,* vol. 75, Eds. B.G. Zifkin, F. Andermann, A. Beaumanoir, et al., pp. 227–240. Philadelphia: Lippincott-Raven.

Robinson, L.J. 1939. Induction of seizures by closing of the eyes, or by ocular pressure, in a patient with epilepsy. J. Nerv. Ment. Dis. 90:333–336.

Rosenow, F., and Lüders, H.O. 2000a. Hearing-induced seizures. In *Epileptic Seizures: Pathophysiology and Clinical Semiology,* Eds. H.O. Lüders and S. Noachtar, pp. 580–584. Philadelphia: Churchill Livingstone.

Rosenow, F., and Lüders, H.O. 2000b. Startle-induced seizures. In *Epileptic Seizures: Pathophysiology and Clinical Semiology,* Eds. H.O. Lüders and S. Noachtar, pp. 585–592. Philadelphia: Churchill Livingstone.

Rushton, D.N. 1981. Space invader epilepsy. Lancet 1:501.

Saenz-Lope, E., Herranz, F.J., and Masdeu, J.C. 1984. Startle epilepsy: a clinical study. Ann. Neurol. 16:78–81.

Sakel, M. 1935. *Neue Behandlugsmethode der Schizophrenie.* Wien: Moritz Perthes.

Sasaki, K., Tsujimoto, T., Nishikawa, S., et al. 1996. Frontal mental theta wave recorded simultaneously with magnetoencephalography and electroencephalography. Neurosci. Res. 26:79–81.

Sato, S., Dreifuss, F.E., and Penry, J.K. 1975. Photic sensitivity of children with absence seizures in slow wave sleep. Electroencephalogr. Clin. Neurophysiol. 39:479–489.

Schuler, P., Claus, D., and Stefan, H. 1993. Hyperventilation and transcranial magnetic stimulation: two methods of activation of epileptiform EEG activity in comparison. J. Clin. Neurophysiol. 10:111–115.

Servit, Z. 1962. The application of reflex theory in the interpretation of the clinical picture, genesis and treatment of epilepsy. Epilepsia 3:209–228.

Shanzer, S., Aprial, R., and Atkin, A. 1965. Seizures induced by eye deviation. Arch. Neurol. 13:621–626.

Sherwin, I. 1984. Hyperventilation: mode of action and application in electroencephalography. Am. J. EEG Technol. 24:201–211.

Shibasaki, H., Yamashita, Y., Neshige, R., et al. 1985. Pathogenesis of giant somatosensory evoked potentials in progressive myoclonic epilepsy. Brain 108:225–240.

Shulman, A., Shaw, F., Cass, N., et al. 1955. A new treatment of barbiturates intoxication. Br. Med. J. 1:1238–1244.

Silbert, P.L., Radhakrishnan, K., Johnson, J., et al. 1995. The significance of the phi rhythm. Electroencephalogr. Clin. Neurophysiol. 95:71–76.

Simon, R. 1985. Physiologic consequences of status epilepticus. Epilepsia 26(suppl. 1): S58–S66.

Small, J.G. 1971. Photoconvulsive and photomyoclonic responses in psychiatric patients. Electroencephalogr. Clin. Neurophysiol. 2:78–88.

Small, J.G., Stevens, J.R., and Milstein, V. 1964. Electroclinical correlates of emotional activation. J. Nerv. Ment. Dis. 138:146–155.

Solomon, S., and Fine, D. 1960. The precipitation of seizures by photic stimulation in a patient with hypoparathyroidism. J. Nerv. Ment. Dis. 130:253–260.

Soso, M.J., Lettich, E., and Belgum, J.H. 1980. Pattern-sensitive epilepsy. II. Effects of pattern orientation and hemifield stimulation. Epilepsia 21:313–323.

Sperling, M.R. 1984. Hypoglycemic activation of focal abnormalities in the EEG of patients considered for temporal lobectomy. Electroencephalogr. Clin. Neurophysiol. 58:506–512.

Stefansson, S.B., Darby, C.E., Wilkins, A.J., et al. 1977. Television epilepsy and pattern sensitivity. Br. Med. J. 2:88–90.

Stevens, J.R. 1959. Emotional activation of the electroencephalogram in patients with convulsive disorders. J. Nerv. Ment. Dis. 128:339–351.

Stevens, J.R. 1962. Control and peripheral factors in epileptic discharge: clinical studies. Arch. Neurol. 7:330–338.

Sutton, G.G., and Mayer, R.F. 1974. Focal reflex myoclonus. J. Neurol. Neurosurg. Psychiatry 37:207–217.

Takahashi, T. 1974a. Study of visual epilepsy. 4. Pattern activation and clinical EEG findings. Clin. Neurol. (Tokyo) 14:479–488.

Takahashi, T. 1974b. EEG responses to various stimuli. In *Atlas of Clinical EEG,* Eds. Y. Shimazono, K. Kitamura, and E. Otomo, pp. 157–193. Tokyo: Bunkodo.

Takahashi, T. 1976a. Photoconvulsive response and disposition. Folia Psychiatr. Neurol. Jpn. (Tokyo) 30:349–356.

Takahashi, T. 1976b. Influence on EEGs of gazing at a fixation point and of Ganzfeld. Brain Nerve (Tokyo) 28:95–103.

Takahashi, T. 1976c. EEG activation by movement of the eyelids and eyes. Rinsho Noha (Osaka) 18:334–344.

Takahashi, T. 1982. Activation methods. In *Electroencephalography: Basic Principles, Clinical Applications and Related Fields,* Eds. E. Niedermeyer and F. Lopes da Silva, pp. 179–195. Baltimore, Munich: Urban & Schwarzenberg.

Takahashi, T. 1983. Lateral hemifield flickering pattern stimulation in a patient with pattern-sensitive epilepsy. Epilepsia 24:548–556.

Takahashi, T. 1984. Hemifield red flicker stimulation in a patient with pattern-sensitive epilepsy. Epilepsia 25:223–228.

Takahashi, T. 1989. Techniques of intermittent photic stimulation and paroxysmal responses. Am. J. EEG Technol. 29:205–218.

Takahashi, T. 1993a. Activation methods. In *Electroencephalography: Basic Principles, Clinical Applications and Related Fields,* 3rd ed., Eds. E. Niedermeyer and F. Lopes da Silva, pp. 241–262. Baltimore: Williams & Wilkins.

Takahashi, T. 1993b. EEG activation by visual stimuli. In *The Newest Clinical Electroencephalography,* Eds. M. Sato and H. Matsuoka, pp. 323–344. Tokyo: Asakura Shoten.

Takahashi, T. 1994. Pathophysiological mechanisms of photosensitivity in IGEs. In *Idiopathic Generalized Epilepsies: Clinical, Experimental and Genetic Aspects,* Eds. A. Malafosse, P. Genton, E. Hirsch, et al., pp. 305–315. London: John Libbey.

Takahashi, T. 1996. Hemi- and quadrant-field visual stimuli in EEG diagnosis of photosensitive epilepsy. In *Recent Advances in Clinical Neurophysiology,* Eds. J. Kimura and H. Shibasaki, pp. 223–228. Amsterdam: Elsevier.

Takahashi, T. 1999. Activation methods. In *Electroencephalography: Basic Principles, Clinical Applications and Related Fields,* 4th ed., Eds. E. Niedermeyer and F. Lopes da Silva, pp. 261–284. Baltimore: Williams & Wilkins.

Takahashi, T. 2000. EEG diagnosis of photosensitive seizures and its preventive measures. Jpn. J. Clin. Neurophysiol. 28:236–245.

Takahashi T. 2002. *Photosensitive Epilepsy: EEG Diagnosis by Low-luminance Visual Stimuli and Preventive Measures.* Tokyo: IGAKU-SHOIN Publication Service.

Takahashi, T., and Sasaki, M. 1971. Pattern sensitivity: its activation method and clinical EEG findings. Rinsho Nohha (Osaka) 13:727–732.

Takahashi, T., and Tomioka, H. 1985. Photic driving evoked by hemi-field flickering dot pattern stimulation in a patient with brain tumor. Electroencephalogr. Clin. Neurophysiol. 61:381–384.

Takahashi, T., and Tsukahara, Y. 1972. EEG activation by red color. Igaku. No. Ayumi. (Tokyo) 83:25–26.

Takahashi, T., and Tsukahara, Y. 1975. Generalized paroxysmal discharges induced by visual stimuli and eye movements. Tohoku J. Exp. Med. (Sendai) 115:1–10.

Takahashi, T., and Tsukahara, Y. 1976. Influence of color on the photoconvulsive response. Electroencephalogr. Clin. Neurophysiol. 41:124–136.

Takahashi, T., and Tsukahara, Y. 1979. Influence of red light and pattern on photic driving. Tohoku J. Exp. Med. (Sendai) 127:45–52.

Takahashi, T., and Tsukahara, Y. 1980. Photoconvulsive response induced by use of "visual stimulator." Tohoku J. Exp. Med. (Sendai) 130:273–281.

Takahashi, T., and Tsukahara, Y. 1992. Usefulness of blue sunglasses in photosensitive epilepsy. Epilepsia 33:517–521.

Takahashi, T., and Tsukahara, Y. 1997. Photoparoxysmal response-evoked by regional visual stimuli in a photosensitive epilepsy patient. In *Pan-Pacific Conference on Brain Topography,* Eds. Y. Koga, K. Nagata, and K. Hirata, pp. 507–511. Amsterdam: Elsevier.

Takahashi, T., and Tsukahara, Y. 1998. Photoparoxysmal response elicited by flickering dot pattern stimulation and its optimal spatial frequency of provocation. Electroencephalogr. Clin. Neurophysiol. 106:40–43.

Takahashi, T., and Tsukahara, Y. 2000. Photoparoxysmal response elicited by flickering dot pattern stimulation to the center and periphery. Clin. Neurophysiol. 111:1968–1973.

Takahashi, T., Tsukahara, Y., and Kaneda, S. 1980. EEG activation by use of stroboscope and visual stimulator SLS-5100. Tohoku J. Exp. Med. (Sendai) 130:403–409.

Takahashi, T., Fukushi, S.M., and Suzuki, T. 1981. Diagnosis of amblyopia on the basis of the photic drivings evoked by flickering dot pattern. J. Sendai City Hosp. (Sendai) 2:21–26.

Takahashi, T., Kataoka K., and Tsukahara, Y. 1988. Power spectral analysis of photic driving elicited by flickering dot pattern and red flicker stimuli in adult psychiatric outpatients—with special reference to age and gender. Tohoku J. Exp. Med. (Sendai) 156:165–173.

Takahashi, Y., Shigematsu, H., Kubota, H., et al. 1995. Nonphotosensitive video game-induced partial seizures. Epilepsia 36:837–841.

Takahashi, T., Nakasato, N., Yokoyama, H., et al. 1999. Low-luminance visual stimuli compared with stroboscopic IPS in eliciting PPR in photosensitive patients. Epilepsia 40(suppl. 4):44–49.

Tassinari, C.A., Cincotta M., Zaccara G., et al. 2003. Transcranial magnetic stimulation and epilepsy. Clin. Neurophysiol. 114:777–798.

Temkin, N.R., and Davis, G.R. 1984. Stress as a risk factor for seizures among adults with epilepsy. Epilepsia 25:450–456.

Terzano, M.G., Parrino, L., Manzoni, G.C., et al. 1983. Seizures triggered by blinking when beginning to speak. Arch. Neurol. 40:103–106.

Tieber, E. 1972. Anfallmuster bei Augenschluss. Bericht über drei Fälle in einer Familie. Neuropaediatrie 3:305–312.

Toma, S., Mano, T., and Shiozawa, Z. 1975. Seizure discharges induced by eye closure. Clin. Neurol. (Tokyo) 15:340–346.

Topalkara, K., Alarcon, G., and Binnie, C.D. 1998. Effects of flash frequency and repetition of intermittent photic stimulation on photoparoxysmal responses. Seizure 7:249–255.

Tsukahara, Y., and Takahashi, T. 1973. Visual stimulator for EEG activation. Electroencephalogr. Clin. Neurophysiol. 35:333–335.

Tsukahara, Y., and Takahashi, T. 1979. Pattern-evoked high-amplitude photic driving in epileptic patients. In *Integrative Control Functions of the Brain,* vol. 2, Ed. M. Ito, pp. 90–92. Tokyo: Kodansha Scientific.

Van Cott, A.C., Blatt, I., and Brenner, R.P. 1966. Stimulus-sensitive seizures in postanoxic coma. Epilepsia 37:868–874.

Van Egmond, P., Binnie, C.D., and Veldhuizen, R. 1980. The effect of background illumination on sensitivity to intermittent photic stimulation. Electroencephalogr. Clin. Neurophysiol. 48:599–601.

Vas, C.J., Exley, K.A., and Parsonage, M.J. 1967a. An appraisal of hyoscine as an EEG activation agent. Electroencephalogr. Clin. Neurophysiol. 22:373–377.

Vas, C.J., Exley, K.A., and Parsonage, M.J. 1967b. Activation of the EEG by procyclidine hydrochloride in temporal lobe epilepsy. Epilepsia 8:241–251.

Vas, C.J., Exley, K.A., and Parsonage, M.J. 1967c. Methixene hydrochloride as an EEG activating agent. Epilepsia 8:252–259.

Verdeaux, G., Verdeaux, J., and Marty, R. 1954. L'activation des électroencéphalogrammes par le chloralose. Electroencephalogr. Clin. Neurophysiol. 6:19–28.

Victor, M. 1970. The role of alcohol in the production of seizures. In *Modern Problems of Pharmacopsychiatry—Epilepsy,* vol. 4, Ed. E. Niedermeyer, pp. 185–199. Basel: Karger.

Victor, M., and Brausch, C. 1967. The role of abstinence in the genesis of alcoholic epilepsy. Epilepsia 8:1–20.

Vignaendra, V., and Lim, C.L. 1978. Epileptic discharges triggered by eye convergence. Neurology 28:589–591.

Vignaendra, V., Ghee, L.H., Lee, L.C., et al. 1976. Epileptic discharges triggered by blinking and eye closure. Electroencephalogr. Clin. Neurophysiol. 40:491–498.

Vignal, J.-P., Biraben, A., Chauvel, P.Y., et al. 1998. Reflex partial seizures of sensorimotor cortex (including cortical reflex myoclonus and startle epilepsy). In *Reflex Epilepsies and Reflex Seizures: Advances in Neurology,* vol. 75, Eds. B.G. Zifkin, F. Andermann, A. Beaumanoir, et al., pp. 207–226. Philadelphia: Lippincott-Raven.

Vigouroux, M., Benoit, P., and Gastaut, H. 1954. Evoked potentials by auditory stimuli in the temporal region in an epileptic patient. Electroencephalogr. Clin. Neurophysiol. 6:163–164.

von Meduna, I. 1935. Versuch über die biologische Beeinflussung des Ablaufs der Schizophrenie. I. Campher und Cardiazol Krämpfe. Zbl. G. Neurol. Psychiat. 152:235–262.

Walter, V.J., and Walter, W.G. 1951. The effect of physical stimuli on the EEG. Electroencephalogr. Clin. Neurophysiol. 2 (suppl.):60–68.

Walter, W.G., Dovey, V.J., and Shipton, H. 1946. Analysis of the electrical response of the human cortex to photic stimulation. Nature (London) 158:540–541.

Waltz, S., Christen, H.-J., and Doose, H. 1992. The different patterns of photoparoxysmal response—a genetic study. Electroencephalogr. Clin. Neurophysiol. 83:138–145.

Westmoreland, B.F., and Sharbrough, F.W. 1975. Posterior slow wave transients associated with eye blinks in children. Am. J. EEG Technol. 15:14–19.

Wieser, H.G., Bancaud, J., Talairach, J., et al. 1979. Comparative value of spontaneous and chemically and electrically induced seizures in establishing the lateralization of temporal lobe seizures. Epilepsia 20:47–59.

Wieser, H.G., Hungerbueler, H., Siegel, A.M., et al. 1997. Musicogenic epilepsy: review of the literature and case report with ictal single photon emission computed tomography. Epilepsia 38:200–207.

Wikler, A., and Essig, C.F. 1970. Withdrawal seizures following chronic intoxication with barbiturates and other sedative drugs. In *Modern Problems of Pharmacopsychiatry—Epilepsy,* vol. 4, Ed. E. Niedermeyer, pp. 170–184. Basel: Karger.

Wilkins, A.J., Darby, C.E., Binnie, C.D., et al. 1979. Television epilepsy: the role of pattern. Electroencephalogr. Clin. Neurophysiol. 47:163–171.

Wilkins, A.J., Binnie, C.D., and Darby, C.E. 1980. Visually-induced seizures. Prog. Neurobiol. 15:85–117.

Wilkins, A.J., Binnie, C.D., and Darby, C.E. 1981. Interhemispheric differences in photosensitive epilepsy. I. Pattern sensitivity thresholds. Electroencephalogr. Clin. Neurophysiol. 52:461–468.

Wolf, P. 2000. Activation of seizures by reading and praxis. In *Epileptic Seizures: Pathophysiology and Clinical Semiology,* Eds. H.O. Lüders and S. Noachtar, pp. 609–614. New York: Churchill Livingstone.

Yamaguchi, Y. 1981. Frontal midline theta activity. In *Recent Advances in EEG and EMG Data Processing,* Eds. N. Yamaguchi and K. Fujisawa, pp. 391–396. Amsterdam: Elsevier.

Yamatani, M., Konishi, T., Murakami, M., et al. 1994. Hyperventilation activation on EEG recording in childhood. Epilepsia 35:1199–1203.

Zeki, S. 1993. *A Vision of the Brain.* Oxford: Blackwell Scientific.

Ziegler, D.K., Hassanein, R.S., and Dick, A.R. 1975. Effect of age and depth of hyperventilation on a quantitative electroencephalographic response. Clin. Electroencephalogr. 6:184–190.

Ziskind, E., and Bercel, N.A. 1946. Preconvulsive paroxysmal electroencephalographic changes after Metrazol injection. Res. Publ. Ass. Res. Nerv. Ment. Dis. 26:487–501.

Ziskind, E., Sjaardema, H., and Bercel, N.A. 1946. Minimal electroencephalographic response to Metrazol as a method for measuring the convulsive threshold for use in human beings. Science 104:462–463.

15. Brain Tumors and Other Space-Occupying Lesions

Mariella Fischer-Williams and Gretchen L. Dike

Alert physicians are wedded to change and are willing to forgo diagnostic tests when these are superseded by more reliable measures. With this reasoning, a chapter on the electroencephalogram (EEG) in brain tumors might be omitted. However, EEG stands the test of time because it monitors pathophysiological function as it fluctuates with time and is influenced by many factors. Therefore, the combination of magnetic resonance imaging (MRI) or computed tomography (CT) together with EEG gives the clinician a clearer anatomicophysiological picture than one or the other alone.

Cases in which an abnormal EEG is the first indication of a brain tumor continue to be noted. Thus, an abnormal EEG (Fig. 15.1) was the initial signal that a 28-year-old woman's headache, seemingly benign, required immediate investigation. In this case, the outpatient EEG showed right frontal 3- to 4-Hz waves; within 10 days the patient was admitted to the hospital, and 9 days later a right frontal astrocytoma was excised.

The EEG adds information on the functioning of the brain as a whole, either at the time of the initial diagnosis or during the long-term management of the patient. Abnormalities in EEG reflect general pathophysiological processes, raised intracranial pressure, cerebral anoxia or edema, and epileptogenesis but they show little specificity for a particular disorder (Binnie and Prior, 1994), which is why MRI or CT are also required.

EEG has adapted to the times. First, there is the technical change to digital EEG recording. Second, intraoperative neurophysiological monitoring, with intraoperative brain mapping, electrocorticography (ECoG), and magnetoencephalography have expanded the field. Depth electrodes may be indicated in specific cases (Fischer-Williams and Cooper, 1963); in this early report of 16 patients operated on for partial epilepsy, three of the patients had tumor. Now, information obtained from evoked potentials has, in many respects, revolutionized the subject (see below).

Although a thorough history and physical examination remain the basis for the evaluation of patients with a possible seizure disorder, EEG is a necessary extension for the neurological examination (Wyllie, 1996). However, MRI is now clearly the diagnostic tool par excellence for seizures in patients of all ages. Adjunctive tests such as ambulatory EEG, video/EEG, positron emission tomography (PET) or single photon emission computed tomography are indicated in specific circumstances (Wyllie, 1996), and functional MRI promises to give important information (Jack et al., 1994; Mueller et al., 1996).

Once a tumor has been diagnosed, and surgery planned, the addition of intraoperative neurophysiological monitoring is an important issue. Varieties of technique of ECoG and brain mapping are being used in many parts of the world, and the literature on this technique in the period 1994 through to mid-1997 is extensive. "Intra-operative neurophysiological monitoring is here to stay. . . . It is expected that such monitoring will become a routine part of all complex neurosurgical operations despite the current pressure to reduce the cost of health care" (Sekhar et al., 1995). On the other hand, "Intraoperative monitoring is not essential" (Malis, 1995). However, several recent detailed articles describe the usefulness of these measures, as discussed below.

Traditionally, the diagnosis and localization of brain tumors were based on morphological criteria. Anatomical details and topographical relations are now obtained by CT and MRI (Go et al., 1995). Mapping pathophysiological features by MRI at high spatial resolution may promise even greater detail (Degani et al., 1997). PET and magnetic resonance spectroscopy (MRS) also depict metabolic and blood flow aspects, and add information on the metabolism, structure, and pathophysiological relations of a tumor to the surrounding parenchyma. PET "provides measures of metabolism and substrate utilization in relatively large volumes (0.25 mL) of tissue in three dimensions, throughout the complete volume of the brain" (Therapeutics and Technology Assessment Subcommittee of the American Academy of Neurology, 1991). PET, because it gives information that is biochemical, "will typically show abnormalities prior to any change in the anatomy of the brain that might be identified with CT or MRI" (Therapeutics and Technology Assessment Subcommittee, 1991). Advances in the recording of function-related changes of the electromagnetic field may also at times give better definition of critical functional areas.

This chapter describes the characteristics of EEG in brain tumors, and analyzes the integration of MRI, CT, and EEG, and the valuable data on evoked potentials.

General Review of the EEG Abnormality in Gliomas, Meningiomas, and Metastatic Tumors

Gliomas, meningiomas, and metastatic tumors commonly cause the following abnormalities at the stage when the patient comes for definitive treatment with neurological symptoms and signs:

1. Polymorphic delta activity (PDA) or localized delta activity (LDA). These slow waves are usually localized to the side of the tumor, irregular in waveform (polymorphic) and continuous (Fig. 15.2).

Figure 15.1. EEG of a 28-year-old woman with headache and normal neurological examination, showing right frontal 3–5 Hz activity. Two weeks later, a right frontal astrocytoma was excised.

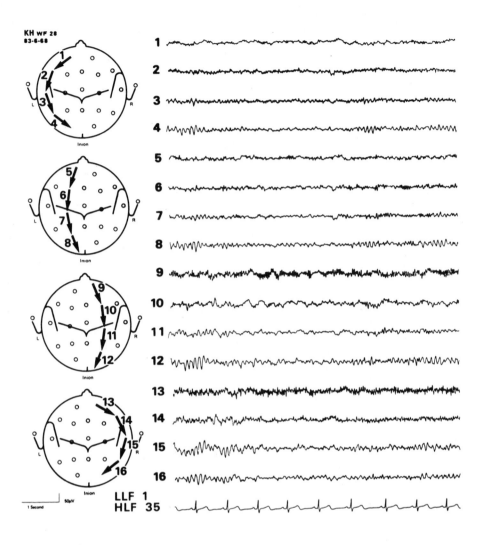

Figure 15.2. EEG of a 64-year-old man. Left temporal delta focus with suppression of background activity, left temporo-occipital. Craniotomy 11 days later showed left temporal glioblastoma.

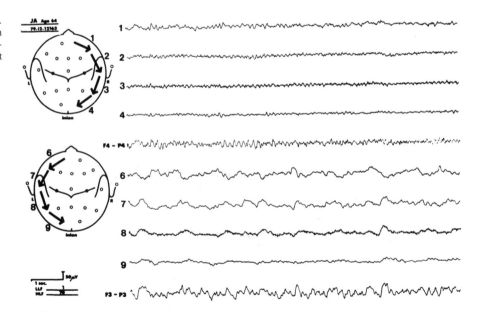

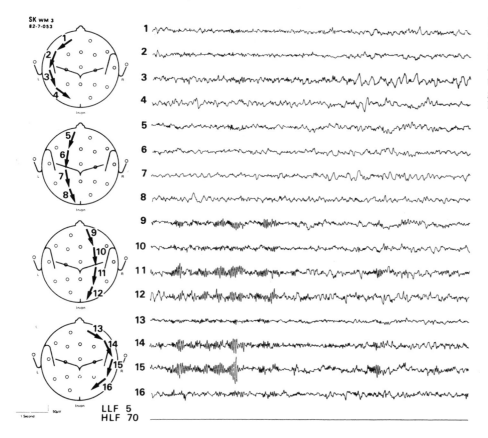

Figure 15.3. EEG of a 3-year-old child with a 10-day history of fever and cough, and 3 days of headache, vomiting, and irritability, but otherwise normal. Craniotomy 4 days after EEG showed large cystic astrocytoma grade 3 or papillary meningioma, a malignant variant of meningioma, left parietal.

2. Intermittent rhythmic delta activity (IRDA) or monorhythmic sinusoidal delta activity (MSDA).
3. Localized loss of activity over the area of tumor (Fig. 15.3). This is less commonly seen than localized delta activity, but when present it is a sure sign of the tumor site, whereas the delta activity with which it is usually associated may indicate the zone adjacent to the tumor.
4. Disturbance (usually slowing) of the alpha rhythm is commonly seen in posteriorly placed tumors.
5. Spikes, sharp waves, or spike-and-wave discharges may occur (Figs. 15.4 and 15.5). They appear only in those cases of tumor that provoke epilepsy and are uncommon even in these.

As an additional feature, periodic lateralized epileptiform discharges (PLED) may sometimes be recorded in tumor cases (Fig. 15.6). In a series of 282 patients showing typical PLED (Reyes and Jameson, 1979) tumor was present in 18% of the cases, as compared with "ischemia, i.e., occlusive disease, shock or cardiorespiratory arrest in 35%, and hemorrhage, post-cardiac surgery (presumably embolic) and post-partum (presumably cortical vein thrombosis) in 12%."

Regional Characteristics

Frontal Tumors

By the time the patient comes to surgery, the EEG is nearly always abnormal, and the abnormality is usually gross or well marked. Frontal lobe gliomas tend to cause local high-voltage delta discharges, sometimes over 100 μV. The discharges are often episodic, bifrontal, and regular in waveform [frontal IRDA (FIRDA)]. The background activity is sometimes well preserved. The abnormality may be only mild, but only rarely is the record within normal limits by the time the patient comes to surgery. This is more likely to occur in meningiomas and slow-growing astrocytomas grade 1.

Temporal Tumors

Most authors agree that temporal gliomas are the easiest to diagnose on the EEG because of the high percentage of cases showing polymorphic delta activity well localized over the tumor site (Fig. 15.2). In 89% of the cases, Fischer-Williams et al. (1962) noted that the abnormality remains unilateral; in one half of these the local delta activity is focal, and the phase reversal of the delta activity or focal sharp waves is a useful localizing sign. In over 90% of cases of temporal gliomas, the slow wave discharge is continuous (Fig. 15.2). Anterior temporal tumors are easier to diagnose than posterior temporal because of the more localized abnormality, particularly with fibrillary astrocytomas or oligodendrogliomas, and a sharp wave or spike or even a spike-and-wave complex may be observed.

Parietal Tumors

Parietal lobe gliomas are less easily diagnosed by the EEG than gliomas elsewhere. The delta discharge may be localized or generalized, but it nearly always remains ipsi-

Figure 15.4. EEG of the onset of a recorded seizure in a 79-year-old man with an astrocytoma of the right frontal lobe, diagnosed 3 months prior to recording.

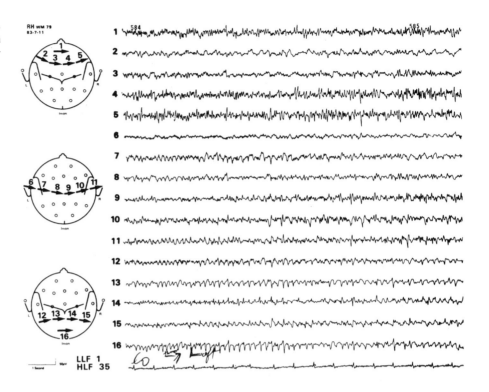

lateral. It tends to be continuous, irregular, and of only moderate voltage. The background activity is usually disturbed, particularly the alpha rhythm on both sides.

Occipital Tumors

The great majority of occipital gliomas produce focal changes; however, these abnormalities often extend into the parietal and temporal regions. Only occasionally do occipital meningiomas (mainly of the tentorium) cause focal changes. Alpha wave depression is very often found occipitally. As in parietal tumors the background record is either locally or generally impaired and in no case is alpha rhythm preserved.

Deep Tumors

These include tumors involving deep structures impinging on the lateral and third ventricle and its neighborhood, the hypothalamus, fornix, septum pellucidum, basal ganglia, internal capsule, optic nerves, and corpus callosum. Gliomas involving these deep structures characteristically cause episodic discharges. The component slow waves are usually monorhythmic, and this discharge is mainly bilateral. The

Figure 15.5. EEG of the end of the recorded seizure, lasting 55 seconds in a 79-year-old man with an astrocytoma of the right frontal lobe. The patient died 2 weeks after this EEG.

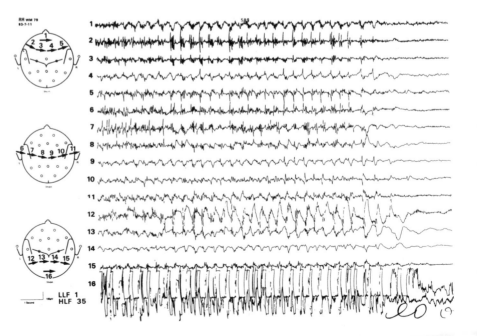

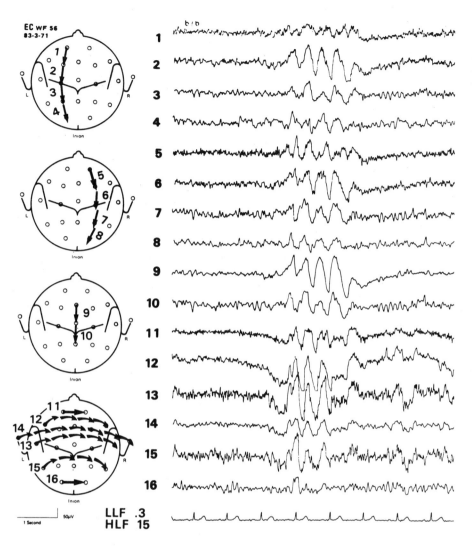

Figure 15.6. EEG of a 56-year-old woman showing paroxysmal discharges. At craniotomy 6 days after this EEG, an astrocytoma of the left parietal lobe was partially excised, followed by irradiation. She died exactly 1 year after this EEG.

LLF .3
HLF 15

---

typical EEG finding is IRDA. In no case is PDA found localized or focal.

Tumors of the Lateral Ventricles

These vary according to their tumor type. Intraventricular meningiomas are likely to show theta or delta activity in the temporal region. Intermittent theta or delta rhythms are usually confined to the tumor side.

Tumors of the Basal Ganglia

Tumors of the basal ganglia cause EEG changes similar to those of tumors associated with the lateral ventricles. Generalized changes with widespread theta activity may occur. IRDA may also occur, but in some cases the EEG remains normal.

Tumors of the Third Ventricle

Isolated tumors such as colloidal cysts or epidermoids are rare. Certain tumors such as craniopharyngiomas may encroach upon the third ventricle. A normal EEG is common in these patients, but there may be diffuse, frontal, or generalized EEG abnormalities. The EEG changes may largely depend on the nature of the underlying lesion and the rapidity

of the development of increased intraventricular pressure upon surrounding tissues. In general, the EEG findings of these midline tumors may be considered similar to those associated with tumors of the posterior fossa.

Tumors of the Sellar Region

The EEG in cases of intrasellar tumors nearly always show abnormalities in the temporal regions. All cases with increased intracranial pressure show general slowing of the EEG. The degree of compression of the hypothalamus seems important for EEG changes (Nauta et al., 1978).

Tumors of the Corpus Callosum

These tumors, together with cysts of the septum pellucidum, give rise to bilateral changes in about half the cases. Bilateral gliomas involving the corpus callosum (butterfly gliomas) invading the centrum ovale cause the same severe EEG abnormalities as do frontal tumors.

Posterior Fossa Tumors (Infratentorial Tumors)

It is this group that EEG is notoriously variable, and therefore MRI and CT are the diagnostic methods of choice. It is also in this group that evoked potentials can be diagnos-

Figure 15.7. EEG of a 56-year-old woman with right acoustic neuroma, removed at craniotomy 3 weeks later. The temporal delta discharges were bilateral or independent on the right or the left, but more frequent on the side opposite to the acoustic neuroma.

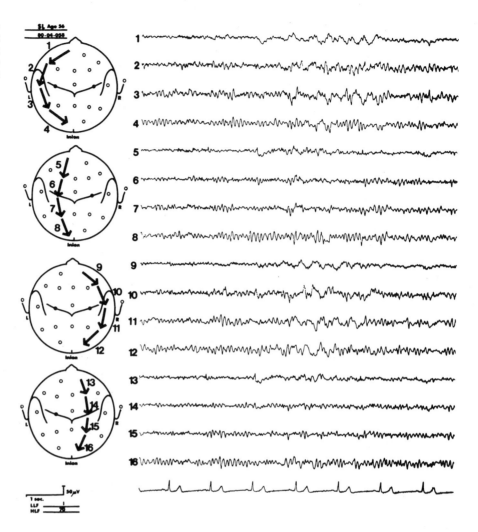

tically useful. The EEG abnormality may be gross, particularly in children, or the record may be normal. Abnormality is correlated with raised intracranial pressure or dilatation of the third ventricle. The main feature of posterior fossa gliomas is the bilateral appearance of the abnormality that can be mild or marked. Focal temporo-occipital delta activity may be present, particularly in young patients. However, a normal EEG does not preclude an infratentorial tumor.

Tumors of the Cerebellopontine Angle

In 10% to 15% of cases, there may be temporal or temporo-occipital abnormality, but the EEG abnormality may be on the side of the tumor, on the opposite side, or bilateral (Fig. 15.7). Of all brain tumors, the benign acoustic or trigeminal neurinomas at this site show the highest proportion of normal EEGs. Diagnosis is made with MRI and evoked potentials (see below).

Dysembryoplastic Neuroepithelial Tumor (DNT)

This tumor is a newly recognized brain mass lesion with distinctive pathological features and a favorable prognosis with surgery (Raymond et al., 1994). These authors describe the clinical, EEG, neuroimaging, and pathological features of 16 patients who underwent surgery. All but one of the patients had epilepsy. The mean age at seizure onset was 9.5 years (range: 1 week to 30 years) and at surgery 17 years (range: 7 months to 37 years). The mean verbal IQ was 94.6 (range 79–110) and performance IQ 105 (range 79–130). The EEG was abnormal in all cases reviewed (*n* = 13). Localized slow-wave activity was seen in 12 and interictal spiking in ten patients, being less extensive than or concordant with the lesion in three, and more extensive than or distant from the lesion in seven. X-ray CT was normal in three out of 11 patients. Calcification was seen on CT in four patients. MRI provided detailed anatomical information. The lesion was predominantly intracortical, although in six patients white matter was also involved. The lesion involved the temporal lobe in all but one patient where it was the cingulate gyrus. Postoperative follow-up ranged from 8 to 30 months (mean 16.2). Postoperatively, 12 patients were seizure-free and two had a more than 80% reduction in seizure frequency.

Correlation of EEG with Histological Type of Glioma

Excluding the tumors involving deep structures, the more slowly growing gliomas (oligodendrogliomas and fibrillary astrocytomas grade 1) can often be distinguished from the more rapidly growing astrocytomas grade 3 and 4 (glioblastoma multiforme). One case of oligodendroglioma was described with a 22-year history of focal jacksonian epileptic seizures (Aebi and Kraus-Ruppert, 1978). The EEG remained normal for many years. It appears that the longest duration recorded in the literature with a clinical history was over 29 years.

Comparison of EEG Features in Gliomas and Metastases

Several features have been noted to differentiate gliomas from metastases (Fischer-Williams et al., 1962). The overall abnormality is greater in gliomas than in metastases, being maximal in cases of glioblastoma.

Serial EEG Recording in Brain Tumors

Clinicians concerned with overall patient care and long-term management need to be aware of EEG progression. Many studies evaluate EEG evolution before and after treatment and are factors for prognosis and treatment (Fig. 15.8). In older patients vascular changes may occur after surgery, and the postoperative EEG frequently reflects a mixture of abnormality associated with the tumor and excision with additional ischemic changes.

Experimental Studies

The effects of malignant glioma on the EEG and on the seizure thresholds were investigated in experimental rodent gliomas using the epileptogenic drug pentylenetetrazole (PTZ) (Beaumont et al., 1996). Malignant gliomas were grown in adult Wistar rats. EEG (raw and spectrally analyzed) was recorded from the frontal and parietal regions. These studies confirmed that experimental gliomas alter not only the baseline EEG but also the EEG and behavioral response to PTZ. The authors discuss the reasons why glioma bearing rats have a raised seizure threshold, and a larger animal model might be helpful in the future, and useful in understanding the mechanism of epilepsy associated with tumors in humans.

Evoked Potentials in Brain Tumors

Evoked potentials (EPs) have brought a new dimension to the assessment of brain activity, giving information of dynamic change in specific pathways in response to sensory stimulation. A large variety of EPs, therefore, are recorded for the diagnosis and surgical treatment of brain tumors and will be described below.

The integration of MRI, CT, and EEG is noted in many areas, mainly in tumors causing epilepsy. In these cases, both structural and psychophysiological data are required.

Although surgery for epilepsy began more than a century ago (Horsley, 1886), it was not until the 1950s, when EEG was illuminating brain function, that surgery became more frequent (Jasper et al., 1951). Now, 50 years later, sophisticated data become integrated with video ictal viewing and the neurophysiological techniques noted above.

The percentage of tumors reported to be detected in patients with seizures varies depending on the type of popula-

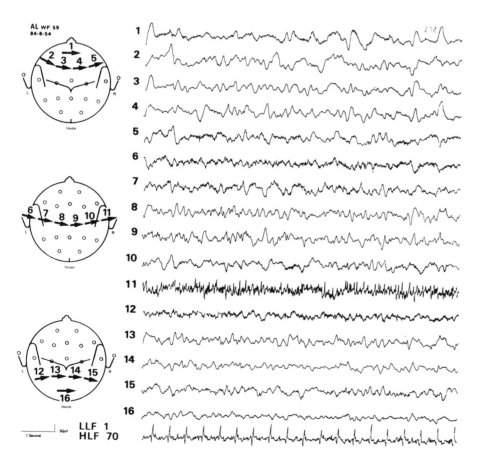

Figure 15.8. EEG of a 59-year-old woman recorded 4 months after subtotal removal of right temporal glioblastoma (grade 4 fibrillary astrocytoma). The generalized abnormality indicated poor prognosis and she deteriorated rapidly over the next month.

tion evaluated. In a series of 563 adults with "possible seizures" (Forsgren, 1996), the EEG, awake and/or asleep, was performed in 84% of the patients, CT in 80%, MRI in 58%, and PET in 57%. With these measures, the most common etiology for unprovoked seizures, after stroke, was brain tumor. Tumors were detected in 11% of these patients.

Shady et al. (1994) reported on 98 patients, aged 18 years or younger, with supratentorial astroglial neoplasms. The preoperative EEG accurately lateralized the tumor side in 88% of the cases, and localized to the correct lobe in 56%. However, authors in previous years stated that their EEG records showed more accurate detailed localization. For example, Goldensohn in 1980 showed that EEG was accurate in 68% of tumor cases, although this compared with 90% accuracy for CT.

In 1995, Montes et al. reported data for 18 children with complete excision of a cerebral lesion for epilepsy. Fifteen of these children had tumors. ECoG was done prior to and after resection. CT suggested that the lesions were indolent. MRI was better in differentiating neoplastic from developmental lesions. Interictal EEG showed epileptiform activity correlating with imaging in 54% of the children.

Surgical treatment of the epilepsies is fully documented in the comprehensive book edited by Engel (1993), and therefore overlaps some of the data given below.

Patients presenting with refractory partial epilepsy usually require extensive investigation. In a series of 20 such patients, (Boon et al., 1994), CT and/or MRI detected intracranial intraaxial structural lesions. The patients had presurgical neurological examination, video-scalp EEG monitoring with prolonged interictal and ictal recording, neuropsychological assessment, and PET. Intracranial EEG monitoring was performed in five patients in whom discrepancies among different tests were found. Interictal EEG showed focal epileptic activity in 85% and focal slowing in 30% of the patients. Lesions were mainly in the temporal lobe (55%), and most patients had complex partial seizures. Complete surgical removal of the lesions with free margins resulted in a more than 90% reduction of seizures without neurological deficit in 12 out of 13 patients.

In a retrospective study, Britton et al. (1994) described 51 consecutive patients who underwent operation for intractable partial epilepsy related to low-grade intracerebral neoplasm between 1984 and 1990. All patients had medically refractory partial seizures and a mass lesion identified by MRI. Lesionectomy was performed in 17 patients and 34 had lesion resection and corticectomy. Sixty-six percent of the patients were seizure-free and 88% experienced a significant reduction in seizure frequency. In 16 patients (31%) antiepileptic drugs were successfully stopped. The patients with complete tumor resection and no interictal epileptiform activity on postoperative EEG studies had the best operative outcome. This shows that in selected patients with tumor-related epilepsy, quality of life can improve with surgery.

Twenty-four patients with intractable epilepsy underwent surgery between 1969 and 1988 (Davies and Weeks, 1995). Localization was by noninvasive means using scalp EEG and CT. In 12 cases the focus was temporal and in eight frontal. Craniotomy was undertaken with intraoperative ECoG. There was a mass lesion in 12 cases, hippocampal sclerosis in two, and gliosis in six. The authors, after giving details of treatment and progress, conclude that where sufficient information exists to localize seizure activity by noninvasive means, invasive recording is not necessary. Intraoperative ECoG can prove useful to delineate the epileptogenic area in cases where there is a mass lesion, and the results can be rewarding.

Intraoperative brain mapping is a surgical adjunct during lesionectomy or epilepsy surgery in functional cortex. This procedure is typically performed at academic institutions by fellowship-trained neurosurgeons (Sartorius and Wright, 1997). However, the authors consider that most of the technology is straightforward and adaptable to the private practice setting.

In one study (Son et al., 1994), 12 patients operated on under local or general anesthesia for resection surgery of tumors diagnosed by neuroimaging underwent intraoperative recording (ECoG) and/or functional mapping by electrical stimulation or somatosensory evoked potential (SEPs) to identify the secondary epileptogenic area and/or functional area; two patients had meningiomas, five had astrocytomas, one had gangliocytoma, one had abscess, one had a small arteriovenous malformation (AVM), one had cysticercosis, and one had gliosis due to previous intracerebral hemorrhage from a middle cerebral artery aneurysm. Among these, additional corticectomy or anterior temporal lobectomy was performed in 11 patients. All the patients did well after surgery, without neurological deficits. The authors concluded that intraoperative recording and functional mapping of adjacent areas of the structural lesions of the brain are useful in surgery and can guide the extent of further resection.

In another study (Packer et al., 1994), cortical low-grade gliomas in childhood causing seizures were diagnosed by MRI and preoperative EEG studies. Sixty children with seizures and low-grade neoplasms were treated consecutively since 1981 by surgical resection without concomitant EEG monitoring or electrocortical mapping. After giving details of treatment and follow-up, the authors conclude that seizure control can be obtained 2 years after tumor surgery in the majority of children after extensive tumor resection without concomitant EEG monitoring or electrocortical mapping.

Under local anesthesia gliomas of the premotor and primary motor cortex can be surgically removed with minimal morbidity (Ebeling et al., 1995). However, since these neoplasms infiltrate toward the pyramidal tract and are frequently not well delineated from functional motor cortex, the long-term outcome is unfavorable. In such cases, to achieve further safe and radical surgery, intraoperative mapping and monitoring techniques are required. In Ebeling et al.'s series of 11 patients, five had recurrent tumor within 2 years of initial operation, and the authors therefore state that mapping and monitoring was required during this delicate surgery.

Zentner et al. (1996) state that functional topographic mapping, achieved by phase reversal of SEPs, allows precise localization of the central sulcus in surgery of the supplementary motor area (SMA). They operated with this technique on 28 patients for tumors (19 patients) or nontumors (nine patients). Seizures were the presenting symptom in 23 of these patients. Motor evoked potentials (MEP) monitoring, which was successfully performed in 13 of 15 cases during the resection procedure, showed no significant changes in any patient. This report is of interest for two main reasons: First, it shows that complete unilateral resection of the SMA could be done in 12 patients, without causing significant permanent deficits, although the SMA is known to control important functions such as initiation of motor activity or speech. Second, the report emphasizes that functional mapping and monitoring facilitates the exact delineation of the adequate resection plane along the precentral sulcus, and therefore allows this type of surgery. Postoperative MRI gave precise correlation of clinical and anatomical data.

A new method of intraoperative localization of the primary motor cortex was described by Maertens de Noordhout et al. (1996), based on the application of single anodal electric pulses to the brain surface. Primary motor areas could be localized in 18 out of 19 patients studied.

In 99 patients (Cedzich et al., 1996) with mass lesions in and around the central region, the central sulcus was localized during surgery with the use of SEP phase reversal. In 33 of these patients, the motor cortex was directly stimulated and electromyographic responses were recorded from the forearm flexor, thenar, and hypothenar muscles. An additional 25 patients, with subcortical lesions or lesions located directly at the pyramidal tract, were continuously monitored during surgery by MEPs. The central sulcus and the tumor could be localized exactly in all patients.

Thirty-four patients with tumoral parietal lobe epilepsy were treated surgically between 1934 and 1988 at the Montreal Neurological Institute (Salanova et al., 1995). Fifteen had right-sided and 16 left-sided resections. The remaining three patients had biopsies only. Follow-up ranging from 1 to 40 years (mean 12.3 years) was available for 28 patients. This review showed that parietal lobe tumors can be resected with good control of previously intractable seizures. The authors concluded that such an approach is preferable to postponing resection until the lesion enlarges.

In a study of 34 consecutive histologically confirmed supratentorial oligodendroglial brain tumors (15 oligoastrocytoma, 12 oligodendroglioma, and seven anaplastic oligodendroglioma), 25 patients presented with symptoms related to seizures (Whittle and Beaumont, 1995). The authors discuss management in detail. Twenty-four of the patients presenting with seizures underwent surgery (five stereotactic biopsy, five stereotactic guided resection, and 14 conventional craniotomy and resection) without intraoperative ECoG. Eighteen of the patients also had postoperative radiotherapy. Tumor resection and radiotherapy often facilitated control of seizures by anticonvulsants. Multiple clinicopathological and management variables require judgment.

Posterior Fossa Surgery

In 330 patients (Csecsei et al., 1995) with a space-occupying lesion of the posterior fossa, the blink (BR) and masseter (MR) reflexes and the brainstem auditory evoked response (BAER) and SEPs were recorded. With these techniques lesions within the brainstem could be differentiated from those outside the brainstem. The ipsilateral loss of BAER in cerebellopontine angle (CPA) tumors and the altered SEP in tumors within the brainstem were frequent, almost specific findings. Prolonged ipsi- and contralateral late BR responses and prolonged MR responses, a long so-

matosensory central conduction time of the SEP, and a prolonged wave III latency as well as a prolonged interpeak latency of the brainstem auditory evoked potential (BAEP) were not indicative but highly suspicious of a lesion within the brainstem. Prolonged early responses of the BR together with prolonged interpeak latencies of the BAEP were characteristic of CPA tumors (Csecsei et al., 1995).

However, in another study (Naessens et al., 1996) of 20 patients with CPA tumors the MRI was considered mandatory for diagnosis of small tumors because the auditory brain responses (ABR) lacked sensitivity in this group.

At a clinic for audiovestibular investigation, 237 patients were studied and 18 were found to have CPA tumors (Ferguson et al., 1996). The authors concluded that MRI scanning with gadolinium enhancement identifies virtually all tumors. Where MRI is available but waiting lists are long, the authors describe a strategy for using ABR to select priority referrals for MRI scanning.

Various ABR indices with true-positive and false-positive rates were studied to discriminate patients with brainstem lesions from those with cochlear lesions (Musiek and Lee, 1995). These characteristics are described and the authors conclude that there is a diagnostic advantage to using more than one ABR index in evaluating patients suspected of having brainstem involvement.

One case is described (Baran et al., 1995) in which significant ABR findings failed to document a large mass involving the low brainstem, but radiology and electronystagmometry (ENG) were valuable when there are vestibular symptoms and a lesion in the low brainstem.

Brainstem auditory evoked potentials (BAEPs) and blink reflexes (BRs) were obtained from 13 patients with CPA tumors (seven acoustic neurinoma, three meningioma, one neurinoma, one brainstem epidermoid tumor, and one AVM) (Nurlu et al., 1994). The main abnormality noted was in BAEPs generated by stimulating the ear ipsilateral to the lesion and also ipsilateral BRs obtained from ipsilateral stimulation of the supraorbital nerve.

Techniques of recording ABR are obviously of importance. In 40 patients with acoustic neuromas, Tanaka et al. (1996) reported that in six of these patients who had normal ABRs, valuable information was obtained when the click was given at high stimulus rates.

With MRI and BAER, small acoustic neuromas (less than 1 cm) can now be diagnosed. In one retrospective study of 70 patients (Dornhoffer et al., 1994) the BAER was abnormal in 65 (93%) on the basis of wave V latency prolongation and interaural latency differences.

Another retrospective study (Stanton and Cashman, 1996) mainly agrees with the above. In a series of 111 CPA tumor and 1,370 nontumor patients, individual ABR features were examined. The I-V measurement was best (sensitivity 82%, specificity 97%) but only for 44% of the population; I-III measurement (sensitivity 50%, specificity 96%) and III-V measurement (sensitivity 30%, specificity 07%) were worst. The authors describe different strategies for recording, corrected for hearing loss.

Brainstem Gliomas. Dorsally exophytic brainstem gliomas can be difficult to diagnose. In a series of 12 young children (Khatib et al., 1994) with median age of 3 years and

2 months, the tumors emanated from the pons, pontomedullary junction, or medulla. Eleven of the 12 patients had classic juvenile pilocytic astrocytomas, with signs of increased intracranial pressure and limited cranial nerve paresis. They had near-normal BAERs and the diagnosis was made by MRI with enhancement after gadolinium-diethylenetriamine pentaacetic acid (DTPA).

Both early BAEPs and middle latency auditory evoked potentials (MLAEPs) were recorded in nine patients suffering from a quadrigeminal plate tumor (Fischer et al., 1994). Technical details are fully reported in this article. The authors conclude that functional evaluation of the midbrain should not be limited to the recording of BAEPs, routinely performed for brainstem functional evaluation, but should also include recording of MLAEPs, although the technique is a little more delicate.

In another article (Eisner et al., 1995), full technical details are described for continuous electrophysiological monitoring of intrinsic brainstem motor function during surgery to remove space-occupying lesions in the fourth ventricle and brainstem. The authors' technique is analogous to that used during surgery in the CPA. Broadcasting electromyogram (EMG) responses through a loudspeaker gives the surgeon immediate feedback on the status of the motor nuclei being monitored in the fourth ventricle and brainstem. After this technique was used in 16 consecutive operations to remove cavernomas ($n = 9$), gliomas ($n = 4$), and other types of tumors ($n = 3$), surgical and neurological results showed the method to be reliable and simple to perform.

Neurophysiological localization of motor nuclei on the floor of the fourth ventricle by an "improved" method of brainstem mapping was described by Morota et al. (1995). The technique helped to locate intraoperatively the facial colliculus and the motor nuclei of cranial nerves IX/X and XII in 14 patients undergoing removal of brainstem tumors.

The motor nuclei of these cranial nerves are usually located relative to specific anatomical landmarks on the floor of the ventricle. These landmarks were not evident in most of the patients studied because of the distorting effects of the tumor. Mapping was performed before and after tumor resection. The authors consider that the technique is useful for locating cranial motor nuclei before tumor resection because it enables the surgeon to avoid damaging the nuclei when entering the brainstem. This is a mapping technique, not a continuous monitoring technique, during tumor resection.

BAEPs clearly enrich our physiological information. In one case operated on for an intrinsic tectal plate glioma (Bognar et al., 1994), BAEPs and middle latency potentials were recorded pre-, post-, and intraoperatively. At the end of surgery all waves were present with a marked delay in wave V and a slight delay of the Pa component. Remarkably, complete resection of the right inferior colliculus (IC) had no apparent auditory consequence. The pre- and postoperative tonal and vocal auditory tests were normal. The role of the IC hearing is discussed in this article.

Intraoperative neurophysiological monitoring of cranial nerve functions in surgery for microvascular decompression and tumors of the posterior fossa is important for minimizing the risk of permanent damage to the nerves (Broggi et al., 1995). These authors report that BAERs and the EMG

function of muscles innervated by trigeminal and facial muscles have been found useful in such cases.

Another technique is described for recording EEG and evoked-potential information directly from the cerebral hemispheres and brainstem (Stoeter et al., 1995). This is via an endovascular approach. Recordings were performed with polytef-insulated guidewires during interventional angiographies in 23 patients. All registrations were compared with simultaneous recordings from extracranial electrodes. This technique might help explore the electrical activity of deep cerebral structures that are otherwise accessible only by stereotactic puncture or electrode insertion.

The association between postoperative EEG abnormalities and persistent seizures after surgery for epilepsy as they relate to pathologic lesions was investigated (Berg and Spencer, 1995). Among 254 patients who underwent surgery for epilepsy between 1987 and 1991, there were 78 patients who had mesiotemporal sclerosis (MTS), and 47 who had low-grade brain tumors. Seizures persisted in 24% of the MTS group and in 27% of the tumor group. Epileptiform discharges and focal slowing were associated with seizure persistence in both groups, but to a significant extent only in the MTS group. Thus, the significance of the EEG after surgery for epilepsy is not fully understood.

Magnetoencephalography (MEG) may be used in a variety of ways. Cortical auditory function was evaluated (Nakasato et al., 1997) in 14 patients with temporal lobe tumors, using an MRI-linked whole-head MEG system. The authors describe the results in detail, which suggest that the MEG system can be used to evaluate cortical auditory function noninvasively before and after surgical treatment of temporal lobe tumors.

EEG Coherences in Patients with Brain Lesions

EEG coherence between pairs of combinations of the 10/20 system was studied (Harmony et al., 1994) in two groups: control subjects and patients with space-occupying lesions. Coherence was separately computed for the delta, theta, alpha, and beta bands. Comparisons between both groups showed highly significant differences in all bands. The authors concluded (what may have been self-evident) that with lesions disrupting cortex and adjacent white matter the coherence between this area and the remaining cortical areas is lower than normal, due to impairment of the fibers that connect the damaged area with the rest of the brain.

EEG in Brain Abscess

This disorder fortunately became rare in the countries reporting literature and therefore no new data concerning brain abscess are appearing in recent articles. The EEG abnormalities are sufficiently suggestive to permit the diagnosis of brain abscess. However, CT scanning undeniably furnishes high-quality reliable data, and Michel et al. (1979), compared the diagnostic value of CT and EEG in brain abscess.

Focal Signs

Large-amplitude delta activity has usually been observed, composed of particularly slow delta waves, less than 2 Hz. These are similar to but slower and more diffuse than in brain tumors. These findings are believed to be associated with diffuse edema.

Diffuse Abnormality

Most authors emphasize the difficulties in finding the EEG focus of a brain abscess. The tendency to diffusion of the slow delta rhythms over one or both hemispheres is greater with brain abscess than with any other space-occupying lesion. Such widespread abnormalities are even observed in cases of single well-circumscribed abscesses.

Intermittent Rhythmic Delta Activity

Bursts of monorhythmic delta waves predominantly over the frontal poles of one or both hemispheres have been described in cases of cerebellar abscess, but are more frequently found in cerebral abscess.

Evolution of EEG Changes in Intracranial Abscess

There is the same need for serial recordings after treatment in the acute phase as in brain tumors, particularly because of the high incidence of epilepsy after cerebral abscess. In a clinico-EEG study of 70 patients, Legg et al. (1973) noted that epilepsy developed in three fourths of their patients.

With modern methods of medical and surgical treatment, and in particular with prolonged prophylactic use of anticonvulsants in all patients after cerebral abscess, it is hoped that the incidence of seizures will be reduced.

EEG in Subdural Hematoma

Both in acute subdural hematoma, which is a neurosurgical emergency, and in chronic subdural hematoma, MRI or CT is the diagnostic method of choice. However, occasionally, the EEG may be the first procedure to indicate a subdural hematoma (Fig. 15.9) particularly in the EEG of a patient whose unconscious state is associated with alcohol in addition to concussion.

The EEG picture is subdural hematoma has been described as "the great imitator." The diversity of the EEG is associated with the fact that the clinical picture is protean; thus the pathology in neonates differs greatly from that in adults, and the stages of acute, subacute, and chronic subdural hematoma cover a wide range of pathology. A fluid or semifluid collection of blood may overlay the cerebral hemisphere on one side with a cystic hygroma on the other. In cases in which cerebral atrophy and cortical small vessel disease from chronic alcoholic encephalopathy existed prior to the injury that caused the subdural hematoma, brain function differs from that in cases of a young patient with a previously normal brain who suffers an acute injury with concussion and hematoma.

Acute Subdural Hematoma

In a series of 88 children under 2 years of age admitted for head injury (Der-Yang Cho et al., 1995), 23 patients were treated with medical or surgical methods for acute shaken/impact baby syndrome (SIBS) also known as the shaken baby syndrome (Ludwig and Warman, 1984). The diagnosis of acute SIBS depends on evidence of abuse in a child under 2 years of age; a history of shaking; symptoms of increasing intracranial pressure (ICP) including bulging fontanelle and coma; retinal hemorrhage by funduscopy; and CT or MRI evidence. The CT scan in this series showed an acute subdural hematoma in the interhemispheric, parasagittal, frontal, or occipital region with subarachnoid hemorrhage and brain swelling. Depending on the ICP measured, medical therapy was given. In ten children a decompressive craniotomy was performed, and a mean of 32 mL of subdural hematoma was removed. Ruptures of the bridging veins were found in four of these ten patients, which sup-

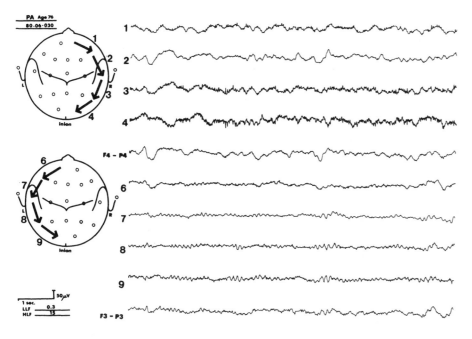

Figure 15.9. EEG of male, age 76, with continuous right hemisphere delta activity. At craniotomy on the day of EEG, a large subdural hematoma was evacuated from the right frontotemporoparietal region. A left temporofrontal hydroma was also removed.

ports the theory that rotational impact is a crucial factor for inducing SIBS (Aronyk, 1994), but all ten patients survived. Follow-up was done with CT or MRI, visual evoked potentials (VEPs), and auditory evoked potentials (AEPs). Hearing was better preserved in the operated patients than in the medically treated group. The authors concluded that with ICP more than 30 mm Hg patients are better treated with decompressive craniotomy. In some other reports of follow-up CT scans, massive brain swelling occurs, which develops into cerebral ischemia, infarction, or even necrosis.

Chronic Subdural Hematoma

The EEG is abnormal in about 90% of chronic subdural hematoma. The picture may resemble that recorded in glioblastoma or abscess, and the abnormalities are often bilateral. Accurate localization is variously reported and may be about 50%. Asymmetry of the alpha frequencies is helpful, with the maximum pathology being on the side of the slower alpha activity. However, the EEG may not show a local lesion, and therefore MRI or CT is indicated. Aoki (1990) described the clinical diagnosis and treatment of 30 cases of chronic subdural hematoma in infancy using CT technology.

The possibility of a subdural hematoma in the elderly should be considered, and should also be excluded when patients are being treated for alcohol withdrawal.

Experimental Subdural Hematoma

Studies on supratentorial subdural bleeding were carried out using a porcine model (Zwetnow et al., 1993). Blood from the abdominal aorta was led into a collapsed intracranial subdural rubber balloon. Bleeding caused an immediate rise in ICP. As a result the cerebral perfusion pressure decreased progressively, leading to an isoelectric EEG. Groups of the pigs received different treatment, and the authors noted that the beneficial effect of assisted ventilation on the course of subdural bleeding is multifactorial, involving both metabolic and mechanical mechanisms.

EEG and Evoked Potentials in Normal Pressure Hydrocephalus

The literature on EEG and EPs in normal pressure hydrocephalus (NPH) is limited. This is probably because NPH patients are a heterogeneous group with variable etiologies, and comparing findings in cases with mixed pathology may not be meaningful.

The EEG findings were described as nonspecific in 1985 by Peterson et al., reporting the surgical treatment in elderly patients at the Mayo Clinic.

Pattern-reversal VEPs in ten patients with hydrocephalus were analyses by Alani (1985) with 50 healthy volunteer controls. The response to whole- and half-field stimulation in four patients showed abnormalities consistent with optic nerve dysfunction. Two patients had asymmetrical responses to half-field stimulation, which suggested dysfunction of the visual pathways in the right hemisphere. The remaining four patients had normal responses. After surgical treatment of the hydrocephalus in four patients, there was marked improvement in two of three patients with preoperative abnormalities. This study suggests that VEPs may be useful in the follow-up of surgically treated hydrocephalic patients.

Quantitative EEG from the occipitoparietal region, gait, and psychometric tests were performed (Sand et al., 1994) in patients with idiopathic NPH before and after drainage of 40 mL of cerebrospinal fluid (CSF). The results were compared with those in demented controls. The EEG results were also analyzed for possible correlations with clinical, CSF dynamics, and psychometric variables. There were no significant differences between NPH patients and demented controls, either baseline EEG variables or in CSF tap-test-related change in EEG. The EEG response to the CSF tap test often did not exceed the day-to-day test-retest variability. EEG slowing (relative delta and theta power) correlated significantly with CSF outflow resistance. EEG band-power variables seemed to reflect some of the pathophysiology involved in idiopathic NPH, particularly increased resistance to CSF outflow. However, the practical value of the EEG method described in this article for the diagnosis and prognosis of NPH seems limited.

Central Nervous System (CNS) Oncological Complications

The CNS complications of systemic cancers include virtually every aspect of CNS pathology. Metabolic abnormalities due to the primary malignancy or the subsequent therapies are often unavoidable. Paraneoplastic entities are increasingly recognized, and with longer survival time, carcinomatous disease is more common. Aggressive approaches with bone marrow transplantation have contributed to the number of immunocompromised hosts at risk for various atypical CNS infections. Vascular disease and secondary coagulopathies remains a large problem. Metastatic lesions may occur literally anywhere on the neuraxis.

Despite great advances in the treatment of cancer, the age-adjusted mortality due to cancer in 1994 was 6% higher than the rate in 1970 (Bailar and Gornik, 1997). Although preventive measures and early detection have had some impact, CNS complications of malignancy remain common. Patients are surviving longer with their illness; hence, iatrogenic CNS complications of treatment are becoming a larger issue. In addition to new chemotherapeutic agents, entirely new modalities are becoming available. With new therapies and longer survival periods, new CNS complications are inevitable.

CNS Irradiation

In the 1980s the long-term CNS morbidity of survivors of pediatric malignancies who had received CNS radiation therapy (CRT) was recognized but not well understood. The role of EEG in assessing neurologic toxicity of CRT became clear when the later sequela of somnolence syndrome was fully described by Chien et al. in 1979. Somnolence syndrome is a transient encephalopathy seen in children 6 to 8 weeks after CRT in combination with high-dose methotrexate. In a prospective study with serial EEGs in 49 pediatric patients receiving CRT and varying chemotherapeutic regimens for acute lymphocytic leukemia (ALL), 29/49 (59%) developed somnolence syndrome. Of these children, 14 (48%) went on to have seizures and cognitive deficits. All 20 children who *did not* develop somnolence syndrome remained cognitively intact. The EEG pattern for somnolence syndrome patients was slow at the time of ALL diagnosis and showed a steady increase in background frequency until there was an abrupt slowing at the time they became encephalopathic. As their clinical status improved, the EEG returned to baseline, but the patients had significant long-term deficits. A retrospective study of patients at 2 to 18 years posttreatment showed 15% with mental defects, 25% with behavioral problems, and 49% with calcifications on brain CT (Danoff et al., 1980). Increased risk of somnolence syndrome was associated with younger age at time of treatment and higher CRT doses. The baseline EEG slowing was related primarily to the ALL and initially improved with treatment until toxicity of the CRT and chemotherapy caused somnolence syndrome (Chien et al., 1979).

Although somewhat controversial, P300 has been repeatedly used to monitor for CNS toxicity from CRT. The use of P300 for assessing cognitive function is limited due to poor specificity, but may be useful in such cases with a fairly high pretest probability of disease (Goodin, 1990). In comparing P300 values in ALL patients with and without a history of CRT, it was found that patients over 15 years old who had received CRT were especially inclined to have prolonged P300s. In another study, 33 survivors of childhood cancer were evaluated with P300, motor reaction time, and neuropsychiatric testing. Neuropsychiatric scores were decreased in those who had CRT and motor reaction time declined in the intrathecal (IT) chemotherapy group, but the most significant abnormalities occurred in the P300 values and neuropsychiatric evaluations of patients who had received CRT and high-dose chemotherapy. This suggested that slowing of cortical activity from white matter damage produces cognitive decline (Moore et al., 1992).

Although the toxicity of CRT has been described primarily in the pediatric population, there are notable effects in adults. Evaluation of serial EEG in adult monkeys exposed to whole-brain radiation revealed:

1. Decreased desynchronizing effect of photic stimulation on background rhythm
2. Decreased reception rate of rhythms of light flashes
3. Narrowed rhythm of light flashes frequency range
4. Increased reaction momentum

These changes were thought to be due to CRT-produced inhibition of cortical activity and impairment of sensory information processing (Legeza and Turlov, 1992). A prospective study of adults treated with IT chemotherapy and prophylactic CRT for leukemia and lymphoma showed only mild abnormalities with excess theta, slightly slowed alpha, and incomplete attenuation of alpha with visual attention. However, even these subtle changes were more prominent in younger adults, suggesting that they have lower thresholds for toxicity (Tucker et al., 1989).

Resection for single CNS metastasis has become the standard of care, but follow-up treatment with CRT in these cases remains controversial. Approximately 10% of 1-year survivors from CRT after metastatic resection develop ataxia, dementia, and urinary incontinence with cortical atrophy and white matter changes (Patchell, 1996). In a review of patients who had received whole-brain CRT, 12

of 12 patients developed these symptoms by 5 to 36 months without evidence of tumor recurrence (DeAngelis et al., 1989). Postmortem examination revealed radiation necrosis. Even isolated irradiation of the rhombencephalon has been associated with demyelinating plaques in the brainstem region directly involved at 2 to 3 months after treatment. Despite plaques evident at autopsy, no abnormalities have been seen in SEPs, brainstem auditory evoked potentials (BAERs), or visual evoked potentials (VERs). The demyelination is likely related to abnormal myelin turnover in the radiosensitive oligodendrocyte (Nightingale et al., 1984).

Chemotherapeutic Agents

Almost every antineoplastic agent used to date has been associated with some incidence of CNS toxicity. The focus here is on the role of EEG in evaluation of such toxicity. Tuxen and Hansen (1994) provide a more complete review.

Asparaginase. Asparaginase is an enzyme that catalyzes the hydrolysis of asparagine to L-aspartic acid and ammonia. It is used to treat leukemia and metastatic disease. Patients may develop lethargy, confusion, tremor, and personality changes associated with a nonspecific slowing of the background alpha and an elevation in the plasma ammonia. The severity of EEG abnormalities correlates better with the mental status than does the ammonia level (Moure et al., 1970).

Busulfan. Seizures during treatment with busulfan is common enough to warrant prophylactic treatment. Administration of phenytoin or benzodiazepines prevent most CNS toxicity. EEGs obtained in patients who have had seizures during busulfan therapy have revealed slowing and localized delta waves that resolve a few days after treatment is discontinued (Vassal et al., 1990).

Methotrexate. Many of the reported side effects of methotrexate (MTX) in the pediatric population occurred in the setting of CRT. In the past, higher MTX doses were typically used, had a devastating neurologic morbidity in survivors, and were associated with grossly abnormal EEGs even in patients who were left relatively intact (Meadows and Evans, 1976). A transient encephalopathy has also been reported in pediatrics after a single high dose of MTX with EEG PLEDs, suggesting functional deafferentation of cortical neurons (Kubo et al., 1992). Lasorella et al. (1993) looked at 25 patients who received IT MTX prophylactically for ALL and found CNS toxicity evident only in those who also had follow-up treatments after the intensive chemotherapy, implying chronicity of exposure or total dose is a contributing factor.

In adults high-dose MTX, with or without x-ray therapy, has been associated with a delayed necrotizing leukoencephalopathy (DNL). EEGs in these patients are typically diffusely slow. One patient with DNL was evaluated and found to have normal SEPs but an abnormal EEG showing (a) irregular slowing at 7 to 8 Hz alpha, (b) intermittent temporoparietal delta activity, and (c) complete lack of desynchronization to acoustic or painful stimuli. Postmortem pathology revealed loss of both thalamic and extrathalamic pathways to the internal capsule (Gutling et al., 1992). Possible mechanisms of injury include depression of cerebral glucose metabolism and alterations in blood-brain barrier function (Tuxen and Hansen, 1994).

Ifosfamide. Pratt et al. (1986) reviewed 50 pediatric patients with solid tumors receiving ifosfamide and mesna. Neurotoxicity including seizures, cranial nerve abnormalities, and cerebellar dysfunction occurred in 22%. Among the 50 patients, nonspecific EEG changes after ifosfamide treatment included development of a slowed background alpha rhythm, increased delta range activity, and triphasic waves. These changes were noted on the EEGs of patients with and without clinical neurotoxicity, and the severity of the EEG changes did not seem to predict the clinical situation. Patients with prior CNS disease, previous cisplatin use, and shorter infusion times may be at higher risk (Danesh et al., 1989; Pratt et al., 1989).

Ifosfamide in adults is associated with a 10% to 30% incidence of encephalopathy. EEGs show continuous, generalized, irregular slowing and sharp activity without a rhythmic or repetitive background. Both the EEG and the clinical encephalopathy improve with benzodiazepines (Simonian et al., 1993).

Cyclosporine. Cortical blindness has been described due to cyclosporine. Focal fronto-occipital slowing was noted on EEG.

Vinca Alkaloids. Transient focal neurological deficits may occur with cisplatin therapy (Berman and Mann, 1980; Cattaneo et al., 1988). Symptoms include cortical blindness, aphasia, focal seizures, and hemianopia. Associated features are neutropenic fevers, hypomagnesemia, mild renal impairment, and cumulative doses of at least 200 mg/m². EEGs with single and multiple spikes and slow waves or diffuse slowing have been reported. Imaging studies are normal and the symptoms generally resolve in 24 to 72 hours with supportive care only. Some patients with transient deficits have tolerated further cisplatin without difficulty (Gorman et al., 1989).

Cortical blindness that did not regress with cessation of treatment was reported in two patients given vindesine, another vinca alkaloid. Imaging studies were suggestive of ischemic events possibly due to a vasculitis (Heran et al., 1990). No EEG data were available on these individuals.

Fludarabine. Fludarabine is a purine nucleoside that has limited use, as doses high enough to produce clinical efficacy invariably produce severe CNS toxicity. Patients develop optic neuritis, cortical blindness, quadriparesis, and seizures often progressing to death (Warrell and Berman, 1986). EEGs have revealed severe slowing and irregular high-voltage rhythms (Chun et al., 1986).

Cytarabine. Cytarabine has been associated with cerebellar abnormalities related to Purkinje cell death. Somnolence and Broca's aphasia have also been reported with associated EEG slowing (Watson et al., 1985).

Paclitaxel (Taxol). Taxol is a novel antineoplastic agent that promotes microtubule polymerization and in animal models does not penetrate the blood-brain barrier. A transient encephalopathy has been noted after Taxol infusion and is associated with nonspecific theta activity. This encephalopathy is similar to that following high-dose MTX. Recurrence of symptoms with the subsequent doses has been reported (Perry and Warner, 1996).

Biological Response Modifiers

Interleukin-2 (IL-2). Immunomodulation with IL-2, a lymphokine, is used in human immunodeficiency virus (HIV) and various malignancies. IL-2 penetrates the blood-brain barrier with approximately 50% serum concentrations. At one institution, 8/1,500 patients who received parenteral IL-2 developed delirium with subsequent coma, ataxia, hemiparesis, seizures, and cortical syndromes, and displayed gray and white matter lesions on MRI. The pattern of lesions noted mirror those seen with cyclosporine toxicity, hypertensive encephalopathy, and eclampsia. Seven of the eight improved after the IL-2 was discontinued. Potential etiologies include a vasculopathy, direct IL-2 toxicity, and immune-mediated damage with induction of other cytokines. Frequently the EEG reflects the clinical focality much better than the MRI. EEGs were notable for focal right temporal PLEDs with a slow background, diffusely slow without focality, and FIRDA with left temporal slowing. It is important to recognize that these diverse EEG abnormalities can be related to the IL-2 and not a progression of the primary disease (Karp et al., 1996).

IL-2 may also produce neuropsychiatric problems. Pace et al. (1994) examined 20 patients before and after treatment using P300 and computer analysis of the EEG. Post-IL-2 changes included lengthened P300 and an increased percentage of EEG frequency in the delta and theta range, particularly frontally.

Delayed toxicity of intraventricular IL-2 has been associated with severe white matter abnormalities and a subcortical dementia (Meyers and Yung, 1993).

Interferons. Phase I clinical studies of interferon-α, which included serial EEGs, revealed progressive EEG changes that sequentially showed:

1. Slowing of the dominant alpha rhythm
2. Loss of attenuation of eye opening
3. Appearance of diffuse slow waves (theta then delta)
4. Decrease response of EEG to external stimuli
5. Prominent frontal intermittent delta bursts

However, these EEG changes also occurred in patients without clinical evidence of encephalopathy (Rohatiner et al., 1983). Patients with multiple myeloma who failed standard treatment developed confusion, somnolence and gait problems after alpha-interferon and their EEGs showed similar changes, but repeat EEGs reflected improving clinical status. Poor outcomes were common, but may reflect the severity of the underlying disease, as most patients had already failed traditional therapies (Suter et al., 1984).

Dose-related neuropsychiatric problems from interferon-α are more common than gross encephalopathy and are associated with diffuse slowing (Smedley et al., 1983). This can be significantly reduced with coadministration of steroids. In a prospective trial evaluating serial EEGs, 17/30 patients had CNS side effects that were apparent at the starting dose (Smedley et al., 1983). Five patients developed abnormal EEGs at the fourth dose and the EEG abnormalities were more severe at higher doses. EEG abnormalities were (a) diffuse slowing, (b) mild diffuse slowing with intermittent bursts of high-voltage slow waves, and (c) diffuse slowing with bifrontal focal rhythmic delta.

Intracerebral interferon-β has been used for brain tumors. In a prospective evaluation of patients who were to get interferon-β, EEG with computed spectral analysis (CSA) was found to be abnormal in 4/4 patients before treatment, likely reflecting tumor burden. No change was seen after treatment with interferon-β in the CSA EEG, but interestingly a decrease in percent EEG power predicted tumor recurrence before changes were visible on MRI (Knobler et al., 1988).

Local Sustained Release Chemotherapy

Administration of local chemotherapy into the tumor bed via a time-release wafer containing bischloroethylnitrosourea (BCNU) is available. Since this therapy has been used only in more aggressive tumors with minimal long-term survival, little is known of later sequelae. In the initial human trials, 41/100 (41%) of treatment patients versus 32/112 (29%) placebo patients had postoperative seizures (Brem et al., 1995a), and later studies evaluating safety showed 12/22 (55%) of patients with postoperative seizures (Brem et al., 1995b).

Gene Therapy

Gene therapy is still in its infancy and therefore its potential CNS complications have yet to be seen. With hundreds of human trials ongoing, CNS toxicity related to this intervention will soon become evident (Marcal and Grausy, 1997).

References

Aebi, M., and Kraus-Ruppert, R. 1978. Oligodendroglioma with twenty-two year history. J. Neurol. 219:139–144.

Alani, S.M. 1985. Pattern-reversal visual evoked potentials in patients with hydrocephalus. J. Neurosurg. 62:234–237.

Aoki, N. 1990. Chronic subdural hematoma in infancy. J. Neurosurg. 73:201–205.

Aronyk, K.E. 1994. Post-traumatic hematomas. In *Pediatric Neurosurgery*, 3rd ed., Eds. Cheek et al., pp. 279–296. Philadelphia: WB Saunders.

Bailar, J.C., and Gornik, H.L. 1997. Cancer undefeated. N. Engl. J. Med. 336:1569–1574.

Baran, J.A., Catherwood, K.P., and Musiek, F.E. 1995. "Negative" ABR findings in individual with large brainstem tumor: hit or miss? J. Am. Acad. Audiol. 6(3):211–216.

Beaumont, A., Clarke, M., and Whittle, I.R. 1996. The effects of malignant glioma on the EEG and seizure thresholds: an experimental study. Acta Neurochir. (Wien) 138:370–381.

Berg, P.S., and Spencer, S.S. 1995. EEG and seizure outcome after surgery. Epilepsia 36(3):236–240.

Berman, I.J., and Mann, M.P. 1980. Seizures and transient cortical blindness associated with cis-platinum diaminedichloride therapy in a thirty-year-old man. Cancer 45:764–766.

Binnie, C.D., and Prior, P.F. 1994. Electroencephalography. J. Neurol. Neurosurg. Psychiatry 57(11):1308–1319.

Bognar, L., Fischer, C., Turjman, F., et al. 1994. Tectal plate glioma. Part III: apparent lack of auditory consequences of unilateral inferior colliclar lesion due to localized glioma surgery. Acta Neurochir. 127(3–4):161–165.

Boon, P., Calliauw, L., DeReuck, J., et al. 1994. Clinical and neurophysiological correlations in patients with refractory partial epilepsy and intracranial structural lesions. Acta Neurochir. 128(1–4):68–83.

Brem, H., Ewend, M.G., Piantadosi, S., et al. 1995a. The safety on interstitial chemotherapy with BCNU-loaded polymer followed by radiation therapy in treatment of newly diagnosed malignant gliomas: phase I trial. J. Neurol. Oncol. 26:111–123.

Brem, H., Piantadosi, S., Berger, P.C., et al. 1995b. Placebo-controlled trial of safety and efficacy of intraoperative controlled delivery by biodegradable polymers of chemotherapy for recurrent gliomas. Lancet 345:1008–1012.

Britton, J.W., Cascino, G.D., Sharbrough, F.W., et al. 1994. Low-grade neoplasms and intractable partial epilepsy: efficacy of surgical treatment. Epilepsia 35(6):1130–1135.

Broggi, G., Scaiolo, V., Brock, S., et al. 1995. Neurophysiological monitoring of cranial nerves during posterior fossa surgery. Acta Neurochir. Suppl. 64:35–39.

Cattaneo, M.T., Filipazzi, V., Piazza, E., et al. 1988. Transient blindness and seizure associated with cisplatin therapy. J. Cancer Res. Clin. Oncol. 114:528–530.

Cedzich, C., Taniguchi, M., Schafer, S., et al. 1996. Somatosensory evoked potential phase reversal and direct motor cortex stimulation during surgery in and around the central region. Neurosurgery 38(5):962–970.

Chien, L.T., Aur, R.J.A., Stagner, S., et al. 1979. Long-term neurologic implications of somnolence syndrome in children with acute lymphocytic leukemia. Ann. Neurol. 8:273–277.

Chun, H.G., Leyland-Jones, B.R., Caryk, S.M., et al. 1986. Central nervous system toxicity of fludarabine phosphate. Cancer Treat. Rep. 70:1225–1228.

Csecsei, G.I., Klug, N., Szekely, G., Jr., et al. 1995. Multimodality electroneurophysiological findings in intra-axial and extra-axial lesions of the brain stem. Acta Neurochir. 137(1–2):48–53.

Danesh, M.M., De Giorgio, C.M., Beydoun, S.R., et al. 1989. Ifosfamide encephalopathy. Clin. Toxicol. 27:293–298.

Danoff, B.F., Cowchock, F.S., and Kramer, S. 1980. Assessment of the long term effects of primary radiation therapy for brain tumors in children. Radiat. Oncol. Biol. Phys. 6:1354–1355.

Davies, K.G., and Weeks, R.D. 1995. Results of cortical resection for intractable epilepsy using intra-operative corticography without chronic intracranial recording. Br. J. Neurosurg. 9(1):7–12.

DeAngelis, L.M., Delatte, J.Y., and Posner, J.B. 1989. Radiation-induced dementia in patients cured of brain metastasis. Neurology 39:789–796.

Degani, H., Gusis, V., Weinstein, D., et al. 1997. Mapping pathophysiological features of breast tumors by MRI at high spatial resolution. Nature Med. 3(7):780–783.

Der-Yang Cho, Yoeu-Chih Wang, and Chiang-Shiang Chi. 1995. Decompressive craniotomy for acute shaken/impact baby syndrome. Pediatr. Neurosurg. 23:192–198.

Dornhoffer, J.L., Helm, J., and Hoehmann, D.H. 1994. Presentation and diagnosis of small acoustic tumors. Otolaryngol. Head Neck Surg. 111(3 pt 1):232–235.

Ebeling, U., Fischer, M., and Kothbauer, K. 1995. Surgery of astrocytomas in the motor and premotor cortex under local anesthesia: report of 11 cases. Minim. Invasive Neurosurg. 38(2):51–59.

Eisner, W., Schmid, U.D., Reulen, H.J., et al. 1995. The mapping of continuous monitoring of the intrinsic motor nuclei during brain stem surgery. Neurosurgery 37(2):255–261.

Engel, J. (Ed.). 1993. *Surgical Treatment of the Epilepsies,* 2nd Ed. New York: Raven Press.

Ferguson, M.A., Smith, P.A., Lutman, M.E., et al. 1996. Efficiency of tests used to screen for cerebello-pontine angle tumors: a prospective study. Br. J. Audiol. 30(3):159–176.

Fischer, C., Bognar, L., Turjman, F., et al. 1994. Auditory early- and middle-latency evoked potentials in patients with quadrigeminal plate tumors. Neurosurgery 35(1):45–51.

Fischer-Williams, M., and Cooper, R.A. 1963. Depth recordings from the human brain in epilepsy. Electroencephalogr. Clin. Neurophysiol. 15:568–587.

Fischer-Williams, M., Last, S.L., Lyberi, G., et al. 1962. Clinico-EEG study of 128 gliomas and 50 intracranial metastatic tumors. Brain 85(1):1–46.

Forsgren, L., Bucht, G., Eriksson, S., et al. 1996. Incidence and clinical characterization of unprovoked seizures in adults: a prospective population-based study. Epilepsia 37(3):224–229.

Go, K.G., Kamman, R.L., Pruim, J., et al. 1995. On the principles underlying the diagnosis of brain tumors—a survey article. Acta Neurochir. 135(1–2):1–11.

Goldensohn, E.S. 1980. Evaluating focal intracranial lesions: complementary information between the EEG and CTT. Course given at annual meeting of the Academy of Neurology.

Goodin, D.S. 1990. Clinical utility of long latency "cognitive" event-related potentials (P3): the pros. Electroencephalogr. Clin. Neurophysiol. 76:2–5.

Gorman, D.J., Kefford, R., and Stuart-Harris, R. 1989. Focal encephalopathy after cisplatin therapy. Med. J. Aust. 150:399–401.

Gutling, E., Landis, T., and Kleihues, P. 1992. Akinetic mutism in bilateral necrotizing leukoencephalopathy after radiation and chemotherapy: electrophysiological and autopsy findings. J. Neurol. 239:125–128.

Harmony, T., Marosi, E., Fernandez, T., et al. 1994. EEG coherence in patients with brain lesions. Int. J. Neurosci. 74(1–4):203–226.

Heran, F., Defer, G., Brugieres, P., et al. 1990. Cortical blindness during chemotherapy: clinical, CT and MR correlations. J. Comput. Assist. Tomogr. 14:262–266.

Horsley, V.P. 1886. Brain surgery. Br. Med. J. 2:670–675.

Jack, C.R., Jr., Thompson, R.M., Butts, R.K., et al. 1994. Sensory motor cortex: correlation of presurgical mapping with functional MR imaging and invasive cortical mapping. Radiology 190(1):85–92.

Jasper, H., Pertuiset, B., and Flanigin, H. 1951. EEG and cortical electrograms in patients with temporal lobe seizures. Arch. Neurol. Psychiatry 65:272–290.

Karp, B.I., Yang, J.C., Khorsand, M., et al. 1996. Multiple cerebral lesions complicating therapy with interleukin-2. Neurology 47:417–424.

Khatib, Z.A., Heideman, R.L., Kovnar, E.H., et al. 1994. Predominance of pilocystic histology in dorsally exophytic brain stem tumors. Pediatr. Neurosurg. 20(1):2–10.

Knobler, R.L., Lublin, F.D., Streletz, L.J., et al. 1988. Intracerebral beta-interferon in brain tumor therapy. Ann. N.Y. Acad. Sci. 540:573–575.

Kubo, M., Azuma, E., Arai, S., et al. 1992. Transient encephalopathy following a single exposure of high-dose methotrexate in a child with acute lymphoblastic leukemia. Pediatr. Hematol. Oncol. 9:157–165.

Lasorella, A., Petrone, A., Colosimo, C., et al. 1993. High incidence of cerebral calcification associated with increased amount of intrathecal methotrexate in children with ALL. Proc. Annu. Meet. Am. Soc. Clin. Oncol. 12:A1065.

Legeza, V.I., and Turlov, I.S. 1992. [The effect of a high-intensity radiation exposure on the brain function of monkeys. The postradiation changes in the EEG response to rhythmic photostimulation.] Russian Radiobiol. 32: 98–107.

Legg, N.J., Gupta, P.C., and Scott, D.F. 1973. Epilepsy following cerebral abscess: a clinical and EEG study of 70 patients. Brain 96:259–268.

Ludwig, S., and Warman, M. 1984. Shaken baby syndrome: a review of 20 cases. Ann. Emerg. Med. 13:104–107.

Maertens de Noordhout, A., Born, J.D., Hans, P., et al. 1996. Intraoperative localization of the primary motor cortex using single electrical stimuli. J. Neurol. Neurosurg. Psychiatry 60(4):442–444.

Malis, L.I. 1995. Intra-operative monitoring is not essential (review). Clin. Neurosurg. 42:203–213.

Marcal, T., and Grausy, J.D. 1997. The TMC worldwide gene therapy enrollment report: end 1996. Hum. Gene Ther. 8:775–800.

Meadows, A.T., and Evans, A.E. 1976. Effects of chemotherapy on the central nervous system. Cancer 37:1079–1085.

Meyers, C.A., and Yung, W.K.A. 1993. Delayed neurotoxicity of intraventricular interleukin-2: a case report. J. Neurol. Oncol. 15:265–267.

Michel, F., Gastaut, J.L., and Bianchi, L. 1979. Electroencephalographic cranial computerized tomographic correlations in brain abscess. Electroencephalogr. Clin. Neurophysiol. 46:256–273.

Montes, J.L., Rosenblatt, B., Farmer, J.P., et al. 1995. Lesionectomy of MRI detected lesions in children with epilepsy. Pediatr. Neurosurg. 22(4):176–173.

Moore, B.D., Copeland, D.R., Ried, H., et al. 1992. Neurophysiological basis of cognitive deficits in long-term survivors of childhood cancer. Arch. Neurol. 49:809–817.

Morota, N., Deletis, V., Epstein, F.J., et al. 1995. Brain stem mapping: neurophysiological localization of motor nuclei on the floor of the fourth ventricle. Neurosurgery 37(5):922–930.

Moure, J.M.B., Whitecar, J.P., and Bodey, G.P. 1970. Electroencephalogram changes secondary to asparaginase. Arch. Neurol. 23:365–368.

Mueller, W.M., Yetkin, F.Z., Hammeke, T.A., et al. 1996. Functional magnetic resonance imaging mapping of the motor cortex in patients with cerebral tumors. Neurosurgery 39(3):515–520.

Musiek, F.E., and Lee, W.W. 1995. The auditory brain stem response in patients with brain stem or cochlear pathology. Ear Hear. 16(6):631–636.

Naessens, B., Gordts, F., Clement, P.A., et al. 1996. Re-evaluation of the ABR in the diagnosis of CPA tumors in the MRI-era. Acta Otorhinolaryngol. Belg. 50(2):99–102.

Nakasato, N., Kumabe, T., Kanno, A., et al. 1997. Neuromagnetic evaluation of cortical auditory function in patients with temporal lobe tumors. J. Neurosurg. 86(4):610–618.

Nauta, H.J.W., Contreras, F.L., Weiner, R.L., et al. 1987. Brain stem abscess managed with computer tomography guided stereotactic aspiration. Neurosurgery 20:476–480.

Nightingale, S., Schofield, I.S., and Dawes, P.J.D.K. 1984. Visual, cortical somatosensory and brainstem auditory evoked potentials following incidental irradiation of the rhombencephalon. J. Neurol. Neurosurg. Psychiatry 47:91–93.

Nurlu, G., Bavbek, M., Colak, A., et al. 1994. Brainstem auditory potential and blink reflexes in patients with pontocerebellar angle tumors. Neurosurg. Rev. 17(4):253–260.

Pace, A., Pietrangeli, A., Bove, L., et al. 1994. Neurotoxicity of antitumoral IL-2 therapy: evoked cognitive potentials and brain mapping. Ital. J. Neurol. Sci. 15:341–346.

Packer, R.J., Sutton, L.N., Patel, K.M., et al. 1994. Seizure control following tumor surgery for childhood cortical low-grade glioma. J. Neurosurg. 80(6):998–1003.

Patchell, R.A. 1996. The treatment of brain metastases. Cancer Invest. 14: 169–177.

Perry, J.R., and Warner, E.W. 1996. Transient encephalopathy after paclitaxel (Taxol) infusion. Neurology 46:1596–1599.

Peterson, R.C., Mokri, B., and Laws, E.R., Jr. 1985. Surgical treatment of idiopathic hydrocephalus in elderly patients. Neurology 35:307–311.

Pratt, C.B., Green, A.A., Horowitz, M.E., et al. 1986. Central nervous system toxicity following the treatment of pediatric patients with ifosfamide/mesna. J. Clin. Oncol. 4:1253–1261.

Pratt, C.B., Douglass, E.C., Etcubanas, E.L., et al. 1989. Ifosfamide in pediatric malignant solid tumors. Cancer Chemother. Pharmacol. 24:S24–27.

Raymond, A.A., Halpin, S.F., Alsanjari, N., et al. 1994. Dysembryoplastic neuroepithelial tumor. Features in 16 patients. Brain 117(pt 3):461–475.

Reyes, P., and Jameson, H.D. 1979. Clinical correlation of periodic lateralized epileptiform discharges in a general hospital. Electroencephalogr. Clin. Neurophysiol. 46:3P.

Rohatiner, A.X.S., Prior, P.F., Burton, A.C., et al. 1983. Central nervous system toxicity of interferon. Br. J. Cancer 47:419–422.

Salanova, V., Andermann, F., Rasmussen, T., et al. 1995. Tumoural parietal lobe epilepsy. Clinical manifestations and outcome in 34 patients treated between 1934 and 1988. Brain 118(pt 5):1289–1304.

Sand, T., Bovim, G., and Gimse, R. 1994. Quantitative electroencephalography in idiopathic normal pressure hydrocephalus: relationship to CSF outflow resistance and the CSF tap-test. Acta Neurol. Scand. 89:317– 322.

Sartorius, C.J., and Wright, G. 1997. Intraoperative brain mapping in a community setting—technical considerations. Surg. Neurol. 47(4):380–388.

Sekhar, L.N., Bejjani, G., Nora, P., et al. 1995. Neurophysiologic monitoring during cranial base surgery: is it necessary? Clin. Neurosurg. 42: 180–202.

Shady, J.A., Black, P.M., Kupsky, W.J., et al. 1994. Seizures in children with supratentorial astroglial neoplasms. Pediatr. Neurosurg. 21(1): 23–30.

Simonian, N.A., Gilliam, F.G., and Chiappa, K.H. 1993. Ifosfamide causes a diazepam-sensitive encephalopathy. Neurology 43:2700–2702.

Smedley, H., Katrak, M., Sikoa, K., et al. 1983. Neurological effects of recombinant human interferon. Br. Med. J. 286:262–264.

Son, E.I., Yi, S.D., Lee, S.W., et al. 1994. Surgery for seizure-related structural lesions of the brain with intraoperative acute recording (ECoG) and functional mapping. J. Korean Med. Sci. 9(5):409–413.

Stanton, S.G., and Cashman, M.Z. 1996. Auditory brainstem response. A comparison of different interpretation strategies for detection of cerebellopontine angle 1/4 tumors. Scand. Audiol. 23(2):109–120.

Stoeter, P., Dieterle, L., Meyer, A., et al. 1995. Intracranial electroencephalographic and evoked-potential recording form intravascular guide wires. AJNR 16(6):1214–1217.

Suter, C.C., Westmoreland, B.F., Sharbrough, F.W., et al. 1984. Electroencephalographic abnormalities in interferon encephalopathy: a preliminary report. Mayo Clin. Proc. 59:847–850.

Tanaka, H., Komatsuzaki, A., and Hentona, H. 1996. Usefulness of auditory brainstem responses at high stimulus rates in the diagnosis of acoustic neuroma. J. Otorhinolaryngol. Rel. Specialties 58(4): 224–228.

Therapeutics and Technology Assessment Subcommittee of the American Academy of Neurology. 1991. Assessment: positron emission tomography. Neurology 41:163–167.

Tucker, J., Prior, P.F., Green, C.R., et al. 1989. Minimal neuropsychological sequelae following prophylactic treatment of the central nervous system in adult leukemia and lymphoma. Br. J. Cancer 60:775–780.

Tuxen, M.K., and Hansen, S.W. 1994. Complications of treatment—neurotoxicity secondary to antineoplastic drugs. Cancer Treat. Rev. 20:191–214.

Vassal, G., Deroussent, A., Hartmann, O., et al. 1990. Dose-dependent neurotoxicity of high-dose busulfan in children: a clinical and pharmacologic study. Cancer Res. 50:6203–6207.

Warrell, R.P., and Berman, E. 1986. Phase I and II study of fludarabine phosphate in leukemia: therapeutic efficacy with delayed central nervous system toxicity. J. Clin. Oncol. 4:74–79.

Watson, P.R., Brubaker, L.H., and Yaghmai, F. 1985. Severe central nervous system toxicity from high-dose cytarabine: expressive aphasia after the second day of treatment. Cancer Treat. Rep. 69:313–314.

Whittle, I.R., and Beaumont, A. 1995. Seizures in patients with supratentorial oligodendroglial tumors. Clinicopathological features and management considerations. Acta Neurochir. 135(1–2):19–24.

Zentner, J., Hufnagel, A., Pechstein, U., et al. 1996. Functional results after resective procedures involving the supplementary motor areas. J. Neurosurg. 85(4):542–549.

Zwetnow, N.N., Orlin, J.R., Wu, W.H., et al. 1993. Studies on supratentorial subdural bleeding using a porcine model. Acta Neurochir. 121(1–2):58–67.

16. The EEG in Cerebral Inflammatory Processes

Barbara F. Westmoreland

Meningitis

The electroencephalogram (EEG) in meningitis shows various degrees of slow-wave abnormalities, depending on the type of meningitis and the degree of involvement of the central nervous system (CNS).

Moderate to severe diffuse slow-wave abnormalities are often present in *acute purulent meningitis*, and paroxysmal epileptiform activity may be present in those patients who have seizures (Kooi et al., 1978).

The electroencephalographic findings in *tuberculous meningitis* vary according to the location of the inflammatory process. In basal meningitis, the EEG may be normal and show only mild nonspecific slowing. When the inflammatory process involves the cortical meninges, moderate to severe slowing occurs (Fig. 16.1), depending on the degree of cortical involvement, the rate of progression of the disease process, the level of consciousness, the presence of metabolic or systemic factors, the pulmonary state of the patient, and the effects of medication (Radermecker, 1977). As with purulent meningitis, more severe slow-wave abnormalities are present in children, often with maximal slowing over the posterior head regions (Kiloh et al., 1972).

In *aseptic meningitis*, the EEG may be normal or show only mild slowing, and the EEG usually returns to normal within 1 to 2 weeks (Radermecker, 1977). The electroencephalographic findings may not necessarily correlate with the clinical severity of the inflammatory process or the development or degree of postinfectious sequelae (Radermecker, 1977).

Patients in whom meningoencephalitis develops in association with *infectious mononucleosis* may have mild to moderate, diffuse, or focal slow-wave abnormalities that may or may not coincide with the area of maximal neurological dysfunction (Schnell et al., 1966). On occasion, focal epileptiform abnormalities and, rarely, periodic slow-wave complexes have been observed in patients who experience seizures (Greenberg et al., 1982; Radermecker, 1977; Schnell et al., 1966).

The rate and degree of the improvement in the electroencephalographic abnormalities after treatment have some diagnostic and prognostic value (Radermecker, 1977). One of the characteristic features of *meningococcal meningitis* is the rapid improvement in the electroencephalographic findings, with the findings often returning to normal within 1 or 2 weeks after treatment (Turrell and Roseman, 1955). In other types of purulent meningitis and tuberculous meningitis, the electroencephalographic abnormalities often require several weeks to resolve (Kiloh et al., 1972; Kooi et al., 1978).

The EEG usually returns to normal in patients with uncomplicated meningitis (Kooi et al., 1978); however, persistent electroencephalographic abnormalities or evidence of deterioration in the EEG suggests an unfavorable course, the development of a complication such as an abscess or hydrocephalus, or the presence of residual brain damage (Kooi et al., 1978; Radermecker, 1977). Although the electroencephalographic findings are not essential for making the specific diagnosis of meningitis, the EEG and particularly serial recordings are helpful in following the course of the disease, detecting the development of complications or relapse, and indicating the presence of sequelae or residual brain damage (Radermecker, 1977) (Table 16.1).

Encephalitis

The electroencephalographic findings in encephalitis are similar to those in meningitis, although the abnormalities often are more severe; this may be a helpful point in the differential diagnosis.

The EEG is almost always abnormal during the *acute phase of encephalitis* (Kooi et al., 1978), with the most frequent finding being the presence of diffuse high-voltage, arrhythmic, and/or rhythmic delta slowing (Fig. 16.2, *top*). Diffuse polymorphic arrhythmic delta activity is more likely to occur when the white matter is involved, whereas paroxysmal, bisynchronous slow-wave activity is more likely to be present when the disease process involves the subcortical gray matter (Gloor et al., 1968). The degree of slowing depends on the severity of the infection, the amount of cerebral involvement, the level of consciousness, and other associated systemic or metabolic factors (Cobb, 1975; Kiloh et al., 1972; Scott, 1976). In general, the leukoencephalitides, which primarily involve the white matter and which are caused by the group B nonneurotropic viruses (measles, rubella, and variola) and the postvaccinal states, are associated with more severe electroencephalographic abnormalities than are those caused by the group A neurotropic viruses (mumps, St. Louis, and equine encephalitis with the exception of the severe Eastern form) (Gibbs et al., 1964; Kiloh et al., 1972). Children often show more severe electroencephalographic abnormalities than do adults. Epileptiform abnormalities also may be present, particularly if the patient is having seizures (Fig. 16.2, *bottom*).

Slow-wave abnormalities have also been observed during the *acute stages of uncomplicated childhood infections*, such as measles, mumps, rubella, chickenpox, and scarlet fever (Gibbs et al., 1959), in which there is no overt evidence of

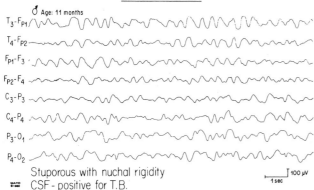

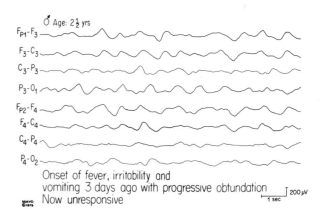

Figure 16.1. EEG showing generalized slowing in an 11-month-old boy with tuberculous meningitis.

nervous system involvement. The electroencephalographic abnormalities occur most frequently with measles infection (Gibbs et al., 1959), in which moderate to severe slow-wave abnormalities may be present as early as 1 to 4 days before the rash appears, reaching a maximum on the first day of the rash and then subsiding during the next 8 to 10 days (Pampiglione, 1964b). Transient slow-wave abnormalities also have been observed over the posterior head regions after measles vaccination (Pampiglione et al., 1971).

The electroencephalographic abnormalities usually diminish in association with clinical improvement, but on occasion the electroencephalographic changes lag behind the clinical findings. However, persistent or increased abnormalities, particularly if they are focal, are associated with an increased likelihood of brain damage or postencephalitic epilepsy. A return to a normal electroencephalographic pattern does not preclude residual brain damage (Kooi et al., 1978).

Congenital rubella encephalitis is associated with seizures and congenital malformations. The EEG abnormalities, which are usually apparent during the first month of life, consist of high-voltage slow waves and sharp-wave transients. The greatest percentage of abnormalities occur in patients who ultimately die or who have cataracts (Desmond et al., 1967; Dreyfus-Brisac and Ellingson, 1972). A lower incidence of abnormal EEGs is seen in patients with a hearing loss (Desmond et al., 1967).

Progressive rubella panencephalitis is an entity that consists of a delayed progressive neurological deterioration that occurs in the second decade of life in children who had congenital rubella (Vinken and Bruyn, 1978a; Wolinsky et al., 1976). The pathological findings are those of a subacute or chronic progressive panencephalitis. The EEG shows generalized slowing with intermittent slow waves. Periodic multiple spike complexes associated with myoclonic movements have been seen (Vinken and Bruyn, 1978a). Periodic high-voltage slow-wave complexes, occurring every 5 to 8 seconds and having features similar to those seen in subacute sclerosing panencephalitis, have also been seen but are not a constant finding (Vinken and Bruyn, 1978a; Wolinsky et al., 1976).

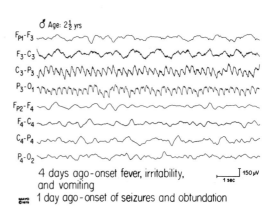

Figure 16.2. EEG of 2½-year-old boy with encephalitis. *Top,* generalized polymorphic delta activity; *bottom,* recorded seizure activity consisting of repetitive sharp waves over the left parietal and occipital head regions.

Congenital cytomegalovirus disease can cause severe damage to the developing CNS of fetuses and infants, resulting in various types of congenital defects, mental and motor retardation, and seizures (Dreyfus-Brisac and Ellingson, 1972). The EEG often shows significant abnormalities consisting of focal or generalized epileptiform discharges and diffuse or focal slow-wave abnormalities. Hypsarrhythmia, associated with infantile spasms, can also be seen (Dreyfus-Brisac and Ellingson, 1972). Cytomegalovirus disease can also occur in immunosuppressed patients, transplant recipients, and patients with AIDS; the EEG may show diffuse or focal abnormalities, depending on the involvement of the CNS.

The *enteroencephalitides* caused by coxsackievirus and enterocytopathogenic human orphan (ECHO) virus, which predominantly affect infants and young children, are accompanied by varying degrees of diffuse slow-wave abnormalities in the EEG (Radermecker, 1977).

Arthropod-borne viral encephalitides may be associated with changes in the EEG. In the mosquito-borne encephalitides, which include Western equine, Eastern equine, St. Louis, and Japanese encephalitis, variable slow-wave abnor-

Table 16.1.   EEG Abnormalities in Inflammatory Conditions

Condition	EEG Findings
Meningitis	
Acute purulent meningitis	Moderate to severe diffuse slow-wave abnormalities
Tuberculous meningitis	Mild to moderate slowing
Aseptic meningitis	Normal or mild slowing
Infectious mononucleosis	Mild to moderate slow-wave abnormalities; rarely epileptiform abnormalities
Encephalitis	
Acute encephalitis	Mild to severe slow-wave abnormalities; epileptiform abnormalities may also be present
Congenital rubella encephalitis	High-voltage slow waves and sharp waves
Progressive rubella encephalitis	Generalized slowing; on occasion spike discharges; rarely periodic slow-wave complexes
Congenital cytomegalovirus disease	Diffuse and focal slow-wave abnormalities; focal and generalized epileptiform abnormalities
California encephalitis	Varying degrees of diffuse slow-wave abnormalities
Coxsackie encephalitis	Varying degrees of diffuse slow-wave abnormalities
ECHO encephalitis	Varying degrees of diffuse slow-wave abnormalities
Western equine encephalitis	Varying degrees of diffuse slow-wave abnormalities
Eastern equine encephalitis	Varying degrees of diffuse slow-wave abnormalities
St. Louis encephalitis	Varying degrees of diffuse slow-wave abnormalities
Japanese encephalitis	Varying degrees of diffuse slow-wave abnormalities
West Nile encephalitis	Varying degrees of diffuse slow wave abnormalities
Tick-borne encephalitis	Varying degrees of diffuse slow-wave abnormalities
Rasmussen-Aguilar syndrome	Focal and generalized epileptiform abnormalities that migrate to different areas of the brain
Herpes simplex encephalitis	Periodic lateralized epileptiform discharges
Rabies	Widespread slowing
Rickettsial diseases	
Typhus	Diffuse or focal slow-wave abnormalities
Rocky Mountain spotted fever	Diffuse or focal slow-wave abnormalities
Tsutsugamushi fever	Diffuse or focal slow-wave abnormalities
Fungal diseases	
Histoplasmosis	Diffuse slow-wave abnormalities
Blastomycosis	Diffuse slow-wave abnormalities
Coccidioidomycosis	Diffuse slow-wave abnormalities
Cryptococcosis	Diffuse slow-wave abnormalities
Aspergillosis	Focal slow-wave abnormalities
Nocardiosis	Focal slow-wave abnormalities
Mucormycosis	Focal slow-wave abnormalities
Candidiasis	Focal slow-wave abnormalities
Prion diseases	
Creutzfeldt-Jakob disease	Generalized periodic sharp waves
Kuru	Slowing of the background
Subacute sclerosing panencephalitis	Generalized stereotyped periodic slow-wave complexes
Parasitosis	
Cysticercosis	Focal epileptiform and focal and generalized slow-wave abnormalities
Echinococcosis	Focal delta slowing and generalized slow-wave abnormalities
Toxoplasmosis	Infants: focal epileptiform abnormalities, hypsarrhythmia, delta slowing asymmetry Adults: normal or focal or generalized slow-wave abnormalities
African trypanosomiasis	Intermittent slow-wave bursts; abnormal sleep patterns
Malaria	Focal and generalized slowing
Filariasis	Normal or diffuse slow-wave abnormalities
Trichinosis	Diffuse slowing
Miscellaneous conditions	
Sydenham's chorea	Mild to moderate generalized slow-wave abnormalities; rhythmic slowing over posterior head regions
Reye's syndrome	Moderate to severe slow-wave abnormalities; epileptiform activity and seizure discharges
Neurosyphilis	Mild to moderate slowing
Neuro-Behçet's disease	Paroxysmal slow waves and generalized delta slowing
Multiple sclerosis	Normal or diffuse or focal slow-wave abnormalities
Hemiconvulsions, hemiplegia, epilepsy (HHE) syndrome	Unilateral epileptiform abnormalities and suppression of activity over affected hemisphere

malities can be seen in the EEG, which may or may not show a correlation with the clinical picture (Radermecker, 1977). Diffuse slow-wave abnormalities with at times more focal features and epileptiform activity may be seen in California encephalitis, and there is a fairly good correlation between the EEG and clinical findings, both during the acute stages of the disease and on follow-up examinations (Grabow et al., 1969; Radermecker, 1977).

The EEG in patients with meningitis and/or encephalitis secondary to West Nile virus has been described as showing generalized slowing that may be maximal over the frontal or temporal regions (Klein et al., 2002).

In *tick-borne encephalitis*, which includes Russian summer-spring encephalitis, Colorado tick fever, and the tick-borne encephalitis seen in Central and Eastern Europe, Scandinavia, and Finland, slow-wave abnormalities may be present prior to the onset of symptoms. The abnormalities do not necessarily correspond with the clinical symptoms and severity of the infection; slow-wave abnormalities, however, may continue to be present in those patients with postencephalitic symptoms and in some patients after the disease appears to have resolved (Hanzel, 1961; Lehtinen and Halonen, 1984; Radermecker, 1977).

EEG recordings have been done only rarely in patients with *rabies*. The recordings have been described as showing a depression or "extreme desynchronization" in one case and nonspecific findings in two other cases (Gastaut and Miletto, 1955; Radermecker, 1977). Prominent slowing with maximum over the vertex was noted in a case observed by Zschocke (1987). Diffuse slow-wave abnormalities similar to those seen in other postvaccinal states may be present after rabies vaccination (Radermecker, 1977).

Although abnormalities are usually not seen with pure spinal cord *poliomyelitis*, EEG abnormalities have been seen in polio, indicating a subclinical cerebral involvement (Radermecker, 1977).

The EEG recordings in the *rickettsial infections* (Eurasian typhus or spotted fever, Rocky Mountain spotted fever, and tsutsugamushi fever) range from normal to those showing diffuse or focal slow-wave abnormalities, with epileptiform activity present in those patients who develop seizures (Radermecker, 1977). The degree of EEG abnormality usually reflects the degree of encephalitic involvement.

Lyme disease, which is caused by a spirochete and is transmitted by a tick, may be accompanied by neurological symptoms and signs, including meningoencephalitis, cranial neuritis, and a radiculoneuritis (Pachner and Steere, 1985). Mild slowing has been seen in patients with encephalitic symptoms, and this has also been seen in some patients without evidence of encephalitis (Pachner and Steere, 1985).

Encephalitis or meningitis caused by *fungal diseases* (*histoplasmosis, blastomycosis, coccidioidomycosis,* and *cryptococcosis*) is associated with diffuse slow-wave abnormalities. These changes are similar to those produced by bacterial and viral agents. More focal EEG abnormalities may be present with focal cerebral involvement secondary to mycotic abscesses, granulomata, ischemia, vasculitis, thrombosis, hemorrhage, embolization, necrosis, or demyelination; these can be seen with *aspergillus, nocardiosis, mucormycosis,* and *candidiasis* (Radermecker, 1977). These complications are particularly likely to occur in compromised patients with altered immune states (Vinken and Bruyn, 1978b). As fungal infections tend to recur, the EEG may be helpful in following the clinical course of the patient and calling attention to a possible recurrence of the infection or the development of complications (Radermecker, 1977). The EEG may also be useful in monitoring the therapeutic and toxic effects of drugs (Radermecker, 1977).

As a rule, most of the different types of encephalitis do not give rise to specific types of EEG patterns. Instead, the EEG abnormalities are most often expressed as diffuse or focal slow-wave abnormalities, with the degree and extent of the slowing reflecting the intensity of parenchymal involvement (Radermecker, 1977).

Rasmussen's Encephalitis

Rasmussen's encephalitis is a chronic devastating disease occurring in children and young adults that predominantly affects one hemisphere and is characterized by progressive neurological and intellectual deterioration, hemiparesis, and recurrent episodes of intractable seizures (Aguilar and Rasmussen, 1960; Rasmussen and McCann, 1968). The seizures are variable; one type of seizure may be present at one time to be replaced by a different type of seizure occurring in a different location at another stage of the disease process. Epilepsia partialis continua is commonly seen in this entity (Andermann, 1991). The EEG shows various types of epileptiform and slow-wave abnormalities. The epileptiform abnormalities consist of focal, multifocal, unilateral, or bilaterally synchronous discharges (Andermann, 1991; Andrews, 1997), which can migrate or spread to different areas of the brain during the disease process (Fig. 16.3). Initially, the epileptiform activity is more prominent over the involved hemisphere. Later there is the development of bilateral epileptiform activity. As the disease progresses, the epileptiform activity becomes more frequent over the contralateral hemisphere and less frequent over the involved hemisphere (Andrews, 1977).

The pathological changes are consistent with a chronic encephalitis with perivascular inflammation, astrocytosis, lymphocytosis, gliosis, neuronal loss, and atrophy of the involved cerebral hemisphere (Andermann, 1991). There are areas of an active inflammatory process in some regions of the brain, while other regions show scarring or evidence of a "burned out" encephalitis (Rasmussen and McCann, 1968), which suggests that this may represent a chronic smoldering process that flares up intermittently, with an exacerbation of seizures and neurological and mental deficit (Andermann, 1991).

Investigators have reported the presence of an antibody to the GluR3 protein of the glutamate receptor in a subgroup of patients with Rasmussen's encephalitis and that rabbits immunized with the GluR3 antibody developed a syndrome similar to Rasmussen's encephalitis, which would suggest an immunopathological etiology (Andrews, 1996; Rogers, 1994).

There has also been a report of a cytomegalovirus genome found in some patients with Rasmussen's encephalitis, and the authors have suggested that the disease process could be

CHRONIC ENCEPHALITIS OF RASMUSSEN AND AGUILAR

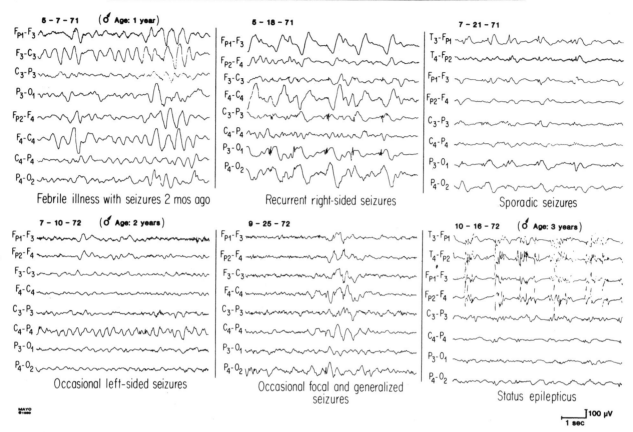

Figure 16.3. Serial EEG samples showing various types of electroencephalographic abnormalities in a patient with Rasmussen encephalitis; *upper left* segment shows generalized paroxysmal slow-wave abnormalities; *upper middle* shows focal spikes over the left posterior head region; *upper right* shows sharp waves over the left hemisphere; *lower left* shows rhythmic slowing and focal spikes in the right central-parietal derivation; *lower middle* shows spike and wave discharges maximal over the right hemisphere; *lower right* shows status epilepticus with repetitive generalized spike discharges, occurring maximally over the anterior head regions.

related to the persistence of the virus in the CNS (Jay et al., 1995; Power et al., 1990).

These findings suggest that Rasmussen's encephalitis is a chronic smoldering process that may be secondary to ongoing viral and/or immunological activity with an intermittent exacerbation of seizures and progressive neurological and mental deficit.

The interest in the possibility that immune mediated mechanisms may play a role in Rasmussen's encephalitis has led to a trial of immunosuppressive therapy, and there is a report in which the EEG findings, seizures, and clinical picture transiently improved in a few patients following plasmapheresis (Andrews, 1996). The EEG thus can be a helpful adjunct in following the course of patients undergoing various forms of therapy.

Herpes Simplex Encephalitis

The EEG often shows a characteristic pattern and temporal evolution (Kiloh et al., 1972) that can be of great value in making the diagnosis of herpes simplex encephalitis, especially when serial recordings are obtained (Upton and Gumpert, 1970). During the earlier stages of the disease process, the background activity is disorganized, and polymorphic delta activity develops in a focal or lateralized fashion, with a predominance over the involved temporal region; soon after this, focal or lateralized sharp- or slow-wave complexes appear, usually having a maximal expression over the involved temporal region (Ch'ien et al., 1977; Cobb, 1975; Gupta and Seth, 1973; Illis and Taylor, 1972; Kiloh et al., 1972; Radermecker, 1977; Rawls et al., 1966). These complexes rapidly evolve into a periodic pattern, with the sharp waves having a stereotyped appearance and recurring every 1 to 3 seconds (Fig. 16.4, *top*). The periodic pattern is usually seen between 2 and 5 days after the onset of the illness (Upton and Gumpert, 1970) but, on occasion, it has been observed up to 24 and 30 days after the onset of the illness (Elian, 1975; Illis and Taylor, 1972). If there is a bilateral involvement of the brain, bilateral periodic complexes may be present (Fig. 16.4, *bottom*), occurring synchronously or independently over the two hemispheres but often having a time-locked relationship with one another (Gaches and Arfel, 1972; Gupta and Seth, 1973; Illis and Taylor, 1972; Smith et al., 1975). Focal or lateralized electrographic seizure dis-

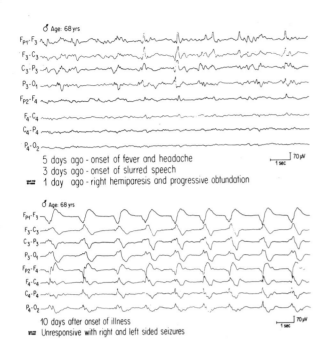

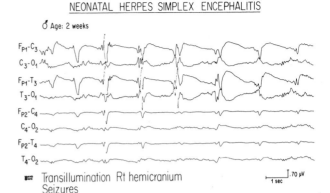

Figure 16.5. EEG of 2-week-old infant with neonatal herpes simplex encephalitis showing periodic discharges over the left hemisphere.

Figure 16.4. EEG of 68-year-old man with herpes simplex encephalitis. *Top*, periodic sharp waves over the left hemisphere; *bottom*, development of bilateral periodic complexes.

charges, consisting of repetitive sharp or slow waves or spike or polyspike bursts, may be present over the involved area or hemisphere. During this time, there is a transient obliteration of the periodic discharges on the side of the seizure discharges (Gaches and Arfel, 1972; Gupta and Seth, 1973; Smith et al., 1975). In the later stages of a fatal herpes simplex infection, the electrographic seizure discharges may occur in association with the periodic discharges without altering them. Additionally, during the later stages of the disease process, the periodic complexes often have a broader slow-wave appearance and a longer interburst interval. During the final stages of a fatal infection, the EEG assumes an almost isoelectric appearance.

In nonfatal herpes simplex encephalitis, the periodic complexes disappear as the disease process resolves; they are replaced by focal or lateralized slow-wave abnormalities or attenuation of activity over the involved area (Cobb, 1975; Kiloh et al., 1972). The resolution of the electroencephalographic abnormalities often lags behind the improvement in the clinical state (Illis and Taylor, 1972); the EEG frequently continues to show residual slow-wave abnormalities and focal epileptiform activity over the involved area.

As in adults, the presence of periodic complexes is a prominent feature in infants with herpes simplex encephalitis (Mizrahi and Tharp, 1982; Pettay et al., 1972; Sainio et al., 1983) (Fig. 16.5). The periodic activity consists of slow- or sharp-wave complexes that may occur in a focal or multifocal fashion or have a shifting emphasis from area to area (Mizrahi and Tharp, 1982; Pettay et al., 1972). The periodic waveforms are usually stereotyped in the same patient but

vary from patient to patient in morphological appearance. The periodic discharges may occur as intermittent paroxysms or persist throughout the recording without being altered by focal seizure discharges in other locations (Mizrahi and Tharp, 1982; Sainio et al., 1983). In the infants who survive, subsequent EEGs continue to show the presence of focal or multifocal epileptiform abnormalities and/or localized areas of attenuation overlying cystic areas of the brain (Smith et al., 1977). In infants who ultimately die, serial EEG recordings show a progression to a low-voltage or isoelectric tracing (Mizrahi and Tharp, 1982).

Although the findings in herpes simplex encephalitis are not pathognomonic for the disease, the presence of unilateral or bilateral periodic complexes in association with a febrile illness and a rapid evolution of neurological signs are strongly suggestive of herpes simplex encephalitis (Smith et al., 1975).

Acquired Immune Deficiency Syndrome (AIDS)

The human immunodeficiency virus (HIV) is a neurotropic virus involving both the nervous system and the immune system (Enzensberger et al., 1986; Klatzman et al., 1984; Levy and Bredesen, 1988; Nicholson, 1986). The most common CNS involvement consists of subacute encephalitis with dementia, also referred to as AIDS encephalopathy or the AIDS dementia complex (Levy and Bredesen, 1988; Snider et al., 1983). Various types of EEG abnormalities can be seen in patients with AIDS, including focal or generalized slowing, asymmetries, paroxysmal abnormalities, and/or epileptiform abnormalities (Bernad, 1991; Tinuper et al., 1990). These findings can occur as a result of primary infection by the AIDS virus or as a result of various opportunistic infections (candidiasis, cryptococcosis, toxoplasmosis, cytomegalovirus), neoplasms (primary CNS lymphoma, Kaposi's sarcoma), cerebrovascular complications, and/or the superimposed effects of more widespread systemic involvement (Levy and Bredesen, 1988).

Prion Diseases

Creutzfeldt-Jakob Disease

Creutzfeldt-Jakob disease is one of the prion diseases causing a diffuse disorder of the CNS that is now believed to be due to abnormal isoforms of the prion protein. The disease is characterized by progressive dementia, motor dysfunction, myoclonus, and a characteristic periodic electroencephalographic pattern that is valuable in making or confirming the diagnosis (Kiloh et al., 1972; May, 1968; Nevin et al., 1960).

The earliest electroencephalographic changes consist of a disorganization and decrease of normal background activity and the development of progressive slow-wave abnormalities (Burger et al., 1972). The slow-wave abnormalities are usually generalized, but at times they occur in a more focal or lateralized fashion. As the disease progresses, diphasic or triphasic slow-wave discharges appear. Initially, these discharges occur in a sporadic or intermittent fashion and may be asymmetric or predominate over one region (Burger et al., 1972), but eventually they evolve into the characteristic pattern, consisting of generalized and bisynchronous continuous periodic stereotyped sharp waves, recurring at intervals of 0.5 to 1 second and having a duration of 200 to 400 msec (Fig. 16.6) (Gloor, 1980; Jones and Nevin, 1954; Kiloh et al., 1972; May, 1968; Nevin et al., 1960; Radermecker, 1977). A majority of patients with Creutzfeldt-Jakob disease develops the characteristic EEG pattern by 12 weeks of the disease process (Levy, 1986). On a few occasions the discharges appear as periodic lateralized epileptiform discharges (PLEDs) before evolving into a bilateral pattern (Au et al., 1980). Myoclonic jerks often occur in association with the periodic sharp waves; however, there is not always a constant relationship between the myoclonic jerks and periodic sharp waves; one can occur without the other (Radermecker, 1977). This is particularly true during sleep or late in the course of the disease, when the myoclonic jerks decrease or disappear, but the periodic sharp waves persist (Burger et al., 1972; Jones and Nevin, 1954).

One characteristic feature of the periodic discharges in Creutzfeldt-Jakob disease is the reactivity of the sharp waves to alerting or afferent stimuli (Radermecker, 1977). Prior to the time when the periodic pattern has been established or when the sharp waves occur in a more intermittent or sporadic fashion, alerting the patient or arousing the patient out of sleep may bring out the periodic pattern (Cobb, 1975; F. W. Sharbrough, personal communication). When the periodic pattern is present, rhythmic photic, auditory, or somatosensory stimuli can pace or set the rhythm of the sharp waves if the frequency of the stimuli falls near the range of the frequency of the spontaneous periodic pattern. However, loud noises and certain types of drugs, such as diazepam and the barbiturates, can temporarily abolish the periodic sharp waves and myoclonic jerks (Elliott et al., 1974; Jones and Nevin, 1954; Nelson and Leffman, 1963; Radermecker, 1977).

As the disease progresses, the interburst interval increases and the amplitude of the periodic sharp waves decreases. In the final stages of the disease, the EEG becomes almost isoelectric, with intermittent bursts of sharp or slow waveforms that finally disappear in the terminal stages of the disease (Nevin et al., 1960).

In *Heidenhain's variant* of the disease, where there is a predominant involvement of the occipital head regions, the EEG often shows more focal abnormalities consisting of slowing and periodic complexes over the posterior head regions (Furlan et al., 1981). Some lateralization of the abnormalities may occur in the early stages, but the abnormalities usually become bilateral as the disease progresses. The periodic complexes may remain confined to the posterior head regions throughout the disease (Furlan et al., 1981), or they may become more widespread with a maximal amplitude over the posterior head regions.

On occasion Creutzfeldt-Jakob disease may progress rapidly, and the typical EEG abnormalities may evolve over a period of 1 to 3 weeks, and serial EEGs are helpful in making or confirming the diagnosis (Drury and Beydou, 1996; Levy et al., 1986). One should be aware, however, that some patients with Creutzfeldt-Jakob disease may not show the typical pattern of periodic sharp waves (Brown et al., 1984; Drury and Beydou, 1996; Tietjen and Drury, 1990).

The "mad cow" variant of Creutzfeldt-Jakob disease has been described as occurring at a younger age of onset than is typical for Creutzfeldt-Jakob disease and without the typical EEG changes of Creutzfeldt-Jakob disease (Will et al., 1996). The other atypical variants of Creutzfeldt-Jakob disease don't usually show the typical pattern of the generalized periodic sharp waves (Zerr et al., 2000).

Although the electroencephalographic findings are not pathognomonic for Creutzfeldt-Jakob disease, the presence of the periodic electroencephalographic pattern in association with the clinical findings of progressive dementia and myoclonus in an adult is a strong indication of Creutzfeldt-Jakob disease.

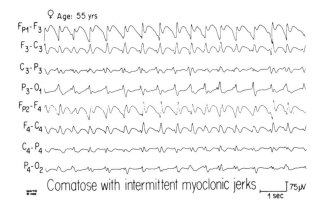

Figure 16.6. Typical EEG pattern of continuous bilaterally synchronous periodic sharp waves in 55-year-old woman with Creutzfeldt-Jakob disease.

Kuru

Kuru is a fatal cerebellar degenerative disease seen in the Fore people of New Guinea described by Gajdusek and Zigas (1957) and is now considered one of the variants of prion disease. Although the disease primarily involves the cerebellum, cerebral involvement occurs in the late stages as manifested by dementia and loss of emotional control. The EEG findings consist of slowing the alpha rhythm, an increase in theta activity, and, on occasion, delta slowing (Cobb et al., 1973). There has been no evidence for periodic or repetitive complexes (Cobb et al., 1973).

Subacute Sclerosing Panencephalitis

Subacute sclerosing panencephalitis (SSPE) is an inflammatory disease that occurs in children and adolescents; it is believed to be caused by the measles virus and is characterized by abnormal movements, a progressive intellectual deterioration, and a diagnostic electroencephalographic pattern. The characteristic electroencephalographic pattern was first described by Radermecker (1949) and Cobb and Hill (1950) and consists of high-voltage (300–1,500 mV) repetitive polyphasic and sharp- and slow-wave complexes ranging from 0.5 to 2 seconds in duration, usually recurring every 4 to 15 seconds (Cobb, 1966) (Fig. 16.7). On rare occasions, these complexes may occur at intervals ranging up to 1 to 5 minutes (Reiher et al., 1973; Westmoreland et al., 1977).

The periodic complexes may be present at any stage of the disease, but they usually are seen during the intermediate stages. Although the form and appearance of the periodic complexes are fairly constant and stereotyped in a single recording, the shape of the complexes varies in different patients and can change in the same patient at different stages of the disease process (Cobb, 1966; Kiloh et al., 1972). The complexes are usually generalized and bisynchronous, but at times they may be asymmetric, have a time lag from side to side or front to back (Cobb, 1966; Kooi et al., 1978), or occur in a more lateralized or focal fashion, particularly in the earlier stages of the disease. Initially, the complexes may occur at irregular intervals, but, once established, the complexes recur at regular intervals, although the repetition rate may vary during the course of the disease (Cobb, 1966;

Kiloh et al., 1972). Afferent stimuli do not usually affect the periodic complexes (Cobb, 1966; Radermecker, 1977); however, on rare occasions, the complexes can be evoked by external stimuli (Cobb, 1966; Westmoreland et al., 1979). This occurs when the complexes are present in an inconstant manner, either when they first make their appearance or toward the end of the period of remission (Cobb, 1966; Radermecker and Poser, 1960). Once the regular pattern of the complexes has been established, however, the complexes are no longer influenced by external stimuli (Radermecker and Poser, 1960). Drugs usually have little effect on the periodic complexes (Radermecker, 1977), although one report described the occurrence of periodic patterns after an intravenous injection of diazepam (Lombroso, 1968).

A prominent feature of SSPE is the stereotyped motor jerks or spasms occurring with the periodic complexes. The movements are often described as myoclonic jerks; however, they do not have the momentary lightning-quick nature of true myoclonus; instead, the movements consist of an initial "shock-like abruptness," followed by a momentary arrest of the movement, and then a gradual melting away to the position of rest (Metz et al., 1964). On less frequent occasions, the periodic complexes may be associated with an inhibitory phenomenon such as an arrest of movement, loss of tone, or drop attacks (Pampiglione, 1964a). The abnormal movements usually become evident at about the same time that the periodic complexes appear on the EEG; however, on occasion, and particularly in the early stages of the disease, the periodic complexes may be present without the associated motor movements (Cobb, 1966; Markand and Panszi, 1975). On the other hand, the presence of the motor jerks in the absence of the periodic complexes is uncommon (Cobb, 1966, 1975). The motor movements often disappear during sleep, despite a persistence of the periodic complexes. Certain drugs, such as diazepam, may reduce or abolish the motor movements without altering the electroencephalographic complexes.

The resting EEG may be relatively normal when the complexes first appear (Cobb, 1966; Kiloh et al., 1972). As

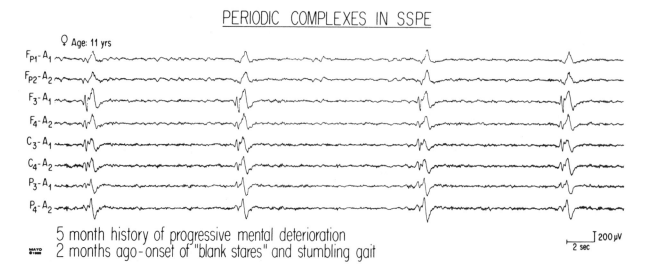

PERIODIC COMPLEXES IN SSPE

♀ Age: 11 yrs

5 month history of progressive mental deterioration
2 months ago-onset of "blank stares" and stumbling gait

200 μV
2 sec

Figure 16.7. Typical EEG pattern of periodic complexes in 11-year-old girl with subacute sclerosing panencephalitis (*SSPE*) (run at slow paper speed).

the disease evolves, however, the EEG shows various changes consisting of slowing and disorganization of the background, asymmetry of the background activity, or both. These changes are followed by an increase in the slow-wave abnormalities, usually occurring in a diffuse manner but at times having a focal or lateralized emphasis and coinciding with the area of maximal neurological involvement (Cobb, 1966; Radermecker, 1977). In the later stages of the disease, polymorphic delta activity or intermittent frontal dominant monorhythmic slow-wave activity may be present (Markand and Panszi, 1975). On occasion, there may be a transient flattening or attenuation of activity after the periodic complexes (Markand and Panszi, 1975; Radermecker, 1977). Various types of epileptiform discharges, spikes, sharp waves, or spike-and-wave complexes occurring in a focal or generalized fashion also may be present (Cobb, 1966; Markand and Panszi, 1975). Patients who have a remission or an improvement in the clinical state show a corresponding improvement on the EEG (Markand and Panszi, 1975).

The typical stages of sleep become less recognizable as the disease progresses, and identifiable sleep stages become limited to two main types: a low-voltage fast pattern with or without spindle activity and a high-voltage slow-wave pattern (Kooi et al., 1978; Radermecker, 1977). In the later stages of the disease, sleep spindles, V waves, and K complexes disappear and the electroencephalographic differentiation of the various stages of sleep is no longer possible (Petre-Quadens et al., 1968). The periodic complexes often persist during sleep, although their shape and frequency may be modified (Cobb, 1966). On rare occasions, periodic complexes may be activated or occur predominantly during the sleep recording (Westmoreland et al., 1977).

As the disease progresses, there may be a shortening in the interval between the complexes (Markand and Parisi, 1975; Wulff, 1982). In the final stages of the disease, there is often a reduction in amplitude and abundance of the electroencephalographic activity, and the recording may become almost isoelectric (Radermecker, 1977). In some instances, however, alpha activity may still be present shortly before death (Cobb, 1966; Markand and Panszi, 1975).

Although other entities may be associated with a periodic pattern, the stereotyped electroencephalographic complexes occurring in a regular and periodic fashion and having a constant relationship to motor movements make this pattern one of the most characteristic and specific of all electroencephalographic patterns (Cobb, 1966, 1975). Close attention to the EEG and clinical features aid in the diagnosis of SSPE and distinguish it from other types of encephalopathies or disease entities (Markand and Panszi, 1975).

Parasitosis

Cysticercosis is characterized by multifocal intracranial nodules and calcification secondary to parasitic cysts (Vinken and Bruyn, 1978b). The EEG shows focal epileptiform abnormalities and focal or diffuse slow-wave abnormalities depending on the site of the lesions and the degree of involvement of the brain (Radermecker, 1977; Vinken and Bruyn, 1978b).

Echinococcosis (*hydatidosis*) may present with cerebral hydatid cysts. More superficial cerebral cysts are associated with focal polymorphic delta slowing, while more deep-seated cysts are associated with unilateral or generalized monomorphic delta activity or paroxysmal slow-wave activity. Epileptiform activity may also be present but is less common (Radermecker, 1977).

Toxoplasmosis may present with focal or multifocal mass lesions, hemorrhagic lesions, metastatic granulomatosis, necrosis, meningoencephalitis, ependymitis, and hydrocephalus (Vinken and Bruyn, 1978b). Congenital toxoplasmosis has a particular affinity for the CNS and can cause severe damage to the fetus, resulting in mental and motor retardation, spasticity, visual difficulties, and seizures. The EEG is usually abnormal in infants with congenital toxoplasmosis and shows a variety of abnormalities consisting of delta slowing, attenuation of background activity, asymmetry, epileptiform abnormalities, and hypsarrhythmia (Dreyfus-Brisac and Ellingson, 1972; Radermecker, 1977).

The acquired form of toxoplasmosis seen in adults does not have the same affinity for the CNS as the congenital form, and the EEG shows less severe abnormalities or may be normal (Radermecker, 1977). Toxoplasmosis, however, is an important opportunistic pathogen in immunocompromised patients, transplant recipients, and patients with AIDS. It commonly involves the CNS, causing focal neurological deficits or a diffuse encephalopathy with corresponding abnormal EEGs.

In *African trypanosomiasis* (*sleeping sickness*) there is a disruption of the sleep-wake cycles with patients showing excessive drowsiness and sleepiness and sleep disturbances (Tapie et al., 1996). The waking EEG shows slowing of the background with bisynchronous slow-wave bursts that initially occur at 5- to 15-second intervals (Radermecker, 1977). As the disease progresses, the periodicity becomes more prominent. Later, the alpha activity disappears and the EEG shows a progressive attenuation of the background activity. Epileptiform activity may occur in the late stages of the disease and is often associated with seizures (Radermecker, 1977). Recordings during sleep show significant changes: (a) the various stages of sleep become less distinct as the typical markers of the various sleep stages, such as vertex waves and spindles, disappear, making it difficult to identify the various stages (Radermecker, 1977); (b) there is a telescoping of the various sleep stages; and (c) the more normal sequence of sleep stages is altered. Light sleep is interrupted by frequent arousals. Deep sleep (stage IV) is not always preceded by lighter stages and is also interrupted by frequent arousals. Low-amplitude theta and delta activity ranging from 3 to 7 seconds in duration may occur in a cyclic fashion during stage IV of sleep and may be associated with changes in cardiac and respiratory rhythms and tonic contractions of muscles. The drowsy state of the patient, coupled with the inability to enter sustained levels of deep sleep, produces a state of persistent hypersomnolence, i.e., "a true sleeping sickness" (Radermecker, 1977). With treatment, there is usually a rapid improvement in the EEG (Radermecker, 1977).

In *malaria*, minor changes may occur in the EEG in the absence of clinical CNS manifestations (Radermecker,

1977). With cerebral malaria in which the patient is co-matose, the EEG shows significant slow-wave abnormalities and, on occasion, spikes and sharp waves. In patients who recover, the EEG usually becomes normal; in patients with sequelae, the EEG may become normal or may continue to show a persistent abnormality (Radermecker, 1977).

In *filariasis*, the EEG may be normal or mildly abnormal in those patients with neuropsychiatric symptoms, but it is significantly abnormal in those with the encephalitic form (Radermecker, 1977; Vinken and Bruyn, 1978b). On occa-sion the EEG may become more abnormal when therapy causes lysis of the microfilarie (Radermecker, 1977).

Significant slowing can be seen in the EEG in the acute phase of meningoencephalitis caused by *trichinosis*; it may be disproportionate to the clinical symptoms. In the chronic phase, the EEG changes are usually less severe than the clin-ical symptoms (Perot et al., 1963; Radermecker, 1977).

Sydenham's Chorea

Sydenham's chorea is a movement disorder that occurs in patients with acute rheumatic fever. Sydenham's chorea oc-curs mainly in children and adolescents; it has been reported that more than half of the patients with Sydenham's chorea have abnormal electroencephalographic findings during the disease process (Johnson et al., 1964; Lavy et al., 1964). The electroencephalographic findings consist of slow-wave ab-normalities that vary from a mild slowing of the background to generalized delta slowing, with the degree of slowing being proportional to the severity of the movement disorder (Johnson et al., 1964; Kooi et al., 1978; Usher and Jasper, 1941). The slowing is usually diffuse but often has a maxi-mal expression over the posterior head regions (Fig. 16.8). In addition, brief trains of rhythmic 2- to 3-Hz bilaterally syn-chronous slow waves may be present over the posterior head

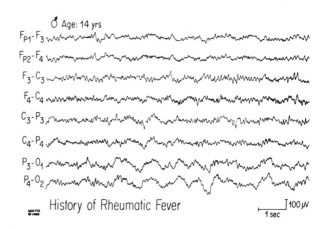

History of Rheumatic Fever

Figure 16.8. EEG of 14-year-old boy with Sydenham's chorea, showing slowing over the posterior head regions.

regions immediately after eye closure (Johnson et al., 1964). More lateralized slow-wave abnormalities may be present in hemichorea (Kooi et al., 1978). On rare occasions, epilepti-form abnormalities have been observed (Johnson et al., 1964). In general, the improvement on the EEG corresponds to the improvement in the clinical state, although on occasion the electroencephalographic abnormalities may lag behind the clinical state (Kooi et al., 1978; Lavy et al., 1964).

Reye's Disease

Reye's disease is a neurological disorder of children and adolescents that is characterized by a rapid, progressive en-cephalopathy and fatty infiltration of the viscera (Chaves-Carballo et al., 1975). The EEG shows various types of abnormalities that reflect the severity of the clinical state. In

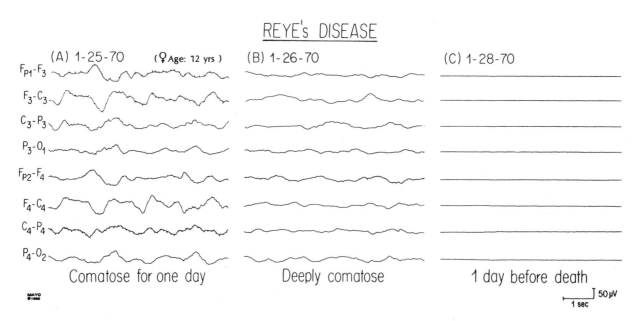

Figure 16.9. Serial electroencephalograms in 12-year-old girl with Reye's disease, showing generalized delta slowing (A), low amplitude slowing (B), and suppression of activity (C).

describing the prognostic value of the EEG in Reye's disease, Aoki and Lombroso (1973) observed that patients whose electroencephalograms showed mild to moderate degrees of theta and delta slowing often survived, whereas patients with severe EEG abnormalities consisting of very low-voltage delta slowing (Fig. 16.9) or a burst suppression pattern usually died. A third group of patients had an intermediate degree of abnormalities consisting of moderate- to high-voltage arrhythmic or semirhythmic delta slowing. Some of those patients survived and some died; serial recordings were helpful in determining whether the patient had a potential for improvement or would progress to an irreversible brain dysfunction.

Triphasic waves, which are seen in hepatic coma and hyperammonemia, are uncommon in Reye's disease (Aoki and Lombroso, 1973). Epileptiform abnormalities consisting of focal or multifocal sharp-wave discharges and electrographic seizure activity may be present, usually occurring in the later stages of the disease when the patient has deteriorated to a comatose state. It is not uncommon to see lack of clinical–electroencephalographic correlation (that is, seizures without an electroencephalographic abnormality or vice versa) (Aoki and Lombroso, 1973). This is usually a poor prognostic sign.

Neurosyphilis

The electroencephalographic findings in neurosyphilis vary, depending on the type, area, and degree of involvement of the nervous system, the stage of the disease, the rate of progression of the disease process, and the age of the patient (Arentsen and Voldby, 1952; Kiloh et al., 1972). Patients with tabes dorsalis or spinal cord disease usually show little or no electroencephalographic abnormality (Arentsen and Voldby, 1952). Patients with syphilis that involves the CNS, meningovascular syphilis, general paresis, or optic atrophy may show disorganization and slowing of the background, a monorhythmic theta pattern, or bursts of delta waves (Arentsen and Voldby, 1952; Kiloh et al., 1972; Kooi et al., 1978; Radermecker, 1977).

The slow-wave abnormalities often occur in a diffuse fashion, with the maximal emphasis over the anterior head regions (Arentsen and Voldby, 1952). At times, more focal slow-wave abnormalities and epileptiform discharges are present, particularly in patients with meningovascular syphilis (Kooi et al., 1978). In general, there is a relationship between the degree of electroencephalographic abnormalities and the degree of mental involvement, and the electroencephalographic pattern often becomes more abnormal as the disease progresses (Radermecker, 1977). Age also is a factor, in that younger patients tend to show a greater degree of abnormality than do older patients (Arentsen and Voldby, 1952).

After treatment, there is a decrease in the electroencephalographic abnormalities that parallels the clinical improvement. On occasion, some residual abnormalities may be present in patients with late inactive disease, and, conversely, neurological and psychological sequelae can be present despite a return to a normal electroencephalographic pattern (Radermecker, 1977).

In infants with *congenital syphilis*, the EEG may show slowing, asymmetry, focal or multifocal epileptiform abnormalities, or hypsarrhythmia (Dreyfus-Brisac and Ellingson, 1972).

Behçet's Disease

In *neuro-Behçet's disease* (uveomeningitis), the EEG usually shows some abnormality when pleocytosis of the spinal fluid is present (Vinken and Bruyn, 1978a). Paroxysmal slow-wave abnormalities and delta slowing are seen with more severe involvement of the CNS (Vinken and Bruyn, 1978a). Although the EEG abnormalities may not be related to the symptomatology, there is a correlation with the course of the disease, and progressive EEG abnormalities are seen in patients who show a deterioration (Vinken and Bruyn, 1978a).

Multiple Sclerosis

The incidence of electroencephalographic abnormalities in multiple sclerosis as reported in the literature varies from 20% to 50%, depending on the location of the CNS involvement, the stage of the disease, and the criteria used (Kiloh et al., 1972; Kooi et al., 1978; Lević, 1978). The electroencephalographic abnormalities, when present, usually consist of varying degrees of nonspecific slowing that may occur in a focal or diffuse manner. The abnormalities are more likely to be seen during periods of exacerbation and often resolve during periods of remission (Kooi et al., 1978). Patients with mental dysfunction may show moderate degrees of slow-wave abnormalities (Kooi et al., 1978) (Fig. 16.10). At times, focal electroencephalographic abnormalities may be present and show some correlation with the area of maximal cerebral involvement; more often, however, there is little correlation between the electroencephalographic findings and the clinical findings (Kiloh et al., 1972; Kooi et al., 1978; Lević, 1978). In rare instances, epileptiform abnormalities have been seen; however, in general, seizures are uncommon in patients with multiple sclerosis (Kiloh et al., 1972; Kooi et al., 1978). Periodic lateralized discharges have also been noted in patients with multiple sclerosis (Awerbuch and Verma, 1987; Chabolla et al., 1996).

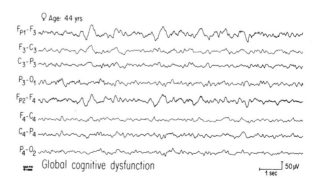

Figure 16.10. EEG showing generalized slowing in a 44-year-old woman with multiple sclerosis who has impaired mentation.

More useful than the EEG are the evoked potential studies in suggesting or confirming the presence of a demyelinating process affecting various areas of the nervous system (Kooi et al., 1978; Stockard and Sharbrough, 1980); this is discussed in more detail in the section on evoked potentials.

Prenatal Infections

Infections can affect the fetus at any stage of development. Infections that occur in the fetus during the first trimester cause congenital defects, developmental arrest, or organ malformations; those that occur near or at term produce effects similar to those seen with postnatal infections (Dreyfus-Brisac and Ellingson, 1972). The types of EEG abnormalities reflect the type and degree of CNS involvement rather than the specific type of infectious process. Sharp waves and high-voltage slow-wave activity are more likely to be seen with an encephalitic process. A low-voltage or almost flat tracing may be seen with hydranencephaly; a focal area of suppression can occur with porencephaly, and hypsarrhythmia can develop in any infant with a severe insult to the CNS (Dreyfus-Brisac and Ellingson, 1972). Although most infants with prenatal brain damage show some type of EEG abnormality, this may not be apparent at birth or may be present only during the sleep recording (Dreyfus-Brisac and Ellingson, 1972).

Neonatal Meningoencephalitis

In neonatal meningoencephalitis, the EEG is usually abnormal and shows the presence of focal or multifocal spikes or sharp waves, clinical and subclinical electrographic seizure discharges, theta or delta rhythms, or depression of activity (Dreyfus-Brisac and Ellingson, 1972). In infants who recover, the EEG shows a progressive improvement, although there may be a lag. In patients in whom the EEG remains abnormal, the infant either dies or is left with a residual deficit (Dreyfus-Brisac and Ellingson, 1972). Although the EEG findings are not specific for meningoencephalitis, as these types of findings can be seen with any severe insult to the neonatal CNS, serial recordings can be helpful in indicating the course of the disease, determining the severity of the cerebral damage, and predicting the development of sequelae (Dreyfus-Brisac and Ellingson, 1972).

Hemiconvulsions, Hemiplegia, and Epilepsy

In the *hemiconvulsions, hemiplegia, and epilepsy (HHE) syndrome*, the infant presents with a series of hemiconvulsions or with hemiconvulsive status during an acute febrile illness (Gastaut et al., 1959/1960). Following this, the patient is left with a flaccid hemiparesis that evolves into a spastic hemiplegia. Later the child has the onset of chronic epilepsy, most often arising from the temporal lobe (Gastaut et al., 1959/1960). The HHE syndrome may occur from birth up to 4 years of age but is most commonly seen between 6 months and 2 years of age. The EEG in the acute stages shows frequent or continuous spike or spike-and-wave dis-

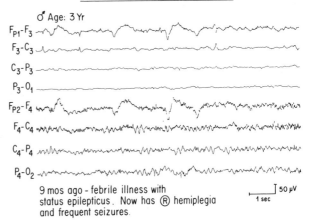

HEMICONVULSIONS, HEMIPLEGIA AND EPILEPSY (HHE) SYNDROME

♂ Age: 3 Yr

9 mos ago - febrile illness with status epilepticus. Now has ⓡ hemiplegia and frequent seizures.

50 µV
1 sec

Figure 16.11. EEG of a 3-year-old child with the HHE syndrome showing left frontal spikes and attenuation of the background activity over the left hemisphere.

charges over the involved side and may have some reflection to the contralateral side (Gastaut et al., 1959/1960). After the acute stages of seizures, there is a reduction in the activity over the involved side. In later recordings, there is a persistent attenuation of activity over the affected hemisphere, as well as the occurrence of focal or multifocal epileptiform discharges (Fig. 16.11). At times, bilateral discharges may be present, but with a decreased amplitude over the affected side (Gastaut et al., 1959/1960).

Brain Abscess

Brain abscesses may occur as a result of meningitis, septicemia, or septic emboli, or as an extension of an infectious process involving the ears, mastoids, and sinuses. In the early stages of an acute supratentorial abscess, the EEG may show diffuse slowing with a poorly defined focus. This pattern is more likely to occur with meningoencephalitis, if the patient is obtunded, and when the more focal abnormalities are obscured by generalized slow-wave abnormalities. Focal slowing becomes more apparent as the suppurative process becomes localized (Fig. 16.12); marked focal polymorphic delta slowing can develop overlying the site of the abscess, particularly if the lesion is located close to the surface of the brain. Focal attenuation or suppression of activity can also be seen (Pine et al., 1952). If there are multiple abscesses, multiple electroencephalographic foci may be present (Scott, 1976). More generalized, intermittent, or shifting bursts of rhythmic slow waves (that is, a projected rhythm) also may be present; these bursts may be seen with a disturbance of the frontal lobe (Michel et al., 1979) or as a secondary effect of the mass lesion on midline structures. On infrequent occasions, focal or lateralized periodic sharp- or slow-wave complexes (periodic lateralized epileptiform discharges) may be present over the involved area of the brain, probably reflecting a rapid expansion of the lesion (LeBeau and Dondey, 1959).

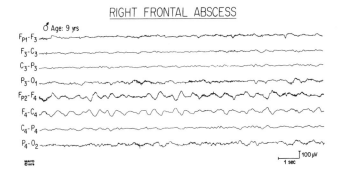

Figure 16.12. EEG showing focal delta slowing over the right frontal region in a 9-year-old boy with a right frontal abscess.

In general, the degree of electroencephalographic abnormalities reflects the severity of the inflammatory process. The electroencephalographic changes seen with an acute focal supratentorial abscess are often more pronounced than those seen with other focal cerebral lesions; this difference can be helpful in suggesting or confirming the presence of an abscess (Scott, 1976). It has been stated that between 90% and 95% of all patients with a supratentorial abscess will have some type of electroencephalographic abnormality (Scott, 1976), and that the EEG is helpful in localizing the site of the abscess in 70% (Kiloh et al., 1972).

Infratentorial abscesses produce less severe slow-wave abnormalities, and at times there may be little or no change on the EEG. When present, the slow-wave abnormalities usually consist of bilaterally synchronous or shifting groups of intermittent rhythmic slow waves (Kooi et al., 1978).

Chronic abscesses develop more slowly and insidiously and often without overt clinical signs of the infectious process. These are usually well-encapsulated abscesses that develop after the initial infection has been cured (Radermecker, 1977). A chronic abscess behaves like a progressive mass lesion and shows the same type of electroencephalographic findings as a tumor (that is, focal slow-wave abnormalities, asymmetry, or attenuation of the background activity), and, if there is increased intraventricular pressure, diffuse intermittent rhythmic slow-wave abnormalities. If the abscess develops very slowly, only minor or subtle electroencephalographic changes may be present.

After treatment, the slow-wave abnormalities improve; however, the EEG rarely returns to normal (Kooi et al., 1978). If surgical intervention is used, the postoperative EEGs show a rapid decrease in the degree of slow-wave abnormalities within the first few days after surgery; however, some slowing and asymmetry of activity often continues to be present over the surgical area. Epileptiform abnormalities are not very common in the acute stages of the abscess; however, about 75% of patients with cerebral abscesses subsequently suffer seizures (Legg et al., 1973; Scott, 1976), and those patients in whom the amount of epileptiform activity increases within the first 1 to 5 years have a greater tendency of developing subsequent seizures (Legg et al., 1973; Scott, 1976).

Subdural Empyema

An empyema is a localized focus of infection in the subdural space that usually develops from a local propagated infection and can spread easily, making it an even more serious infectious process than an abscess. The EEG in the early stages may show a poorly defined focus. Later, more distinct focal slow-wave abnormalities develop, together with focal epileptiform discharges, indicating an irritative cortical focus. As with a subdural hematoma, there is often an attenuation or suppression of background activity over the side of the empyema.

Thrombophlebitis

Thrombophlebitis of the dural veins can occur as a result of sepsis, a contiguous infection, or septic embolization. When this affects the superior lateral sinus, the patient often presents with a headache, seizures, paresis, and increased intracranial pressure (Radermecker, 1977). The EEG during the acute phases may show diffuse slowing with focal emphasis, bifrontal delta slowing, a reduction of the amplitude of the activity over the involved side, epileptiform abnormalities, or, at times, subclinical electrographic status (Lemmi and Little, 1960; Radermecker, 1977). Later EEGs show a residual asymmetry, persistent slow-wave abnormalities, and epileptiform activity (Lemmi and Little, 1960).

In thrombophlebitis of the lateral sinus, the EEG shows lateralized slowing and focal epileptiform abnormalities (Lemmi and Little, 1960; Radermecker, 1977).

Thrombosis of the superficial cortical veins often results in focal seizures and a focal neurological deficit, with the EEG showing focal slowing and epileptiform abnormalities over the involved area (Lemmi and Little, 1960; Radermecker, 1977).

Summary and Conclusions

Although the EEG shows a variety of patterns in association with various inflammatory processes, the EEG can help to (a) confirm and indicate the degree and extent of CNS involvement by the inflammatory process; (b) make the diagnosis of herpes simplex encephalitis, Creutzfeldt-Jakob disease, and SSPE when the characteristic electroencephalographic pattern of these diseases is present; (c) indicate the presence of a focal lesion; (d) monitor the course of the disease process; and (e) detect the development of complications or sequelae.

References

Aguilar, M.J., and Rasmussen, T. 1960. Role of encephalitis on the pathogenesis of epilepsy. Arch. Neurol. 2:663–676.

Andermann, F. 1991. *Chronic Encephalitis and Epilepsy. Rasmussen's Syndrome.* Toronto: Butterworth-Heinemann.

Andrews, P.I., Dichter, M.A., Berkovic, S.F., et al. 1996. Plasmapheresis in Rasmussen's encephalitis. Neurology 46:242–246.

Andrews, P.I., McNamara, J.O., and Lewis, D.V. 1997. Clinical and electroencephalographic correlates in Rasmussen's encephalitis. Epilepsia 38:189–194.

Aoki, Y., and Lombroso, C.T. 1973. Prognostic value of electroencephalography in Reye's syndrome. Neurology (Minneapolis) 23:333–343.

Arentsen, K., and Voldby, H. 1952. Electroencephalographic changes in neurosyphilis. Electroencephalogr. Clin. Neurophysiol. 4:331–337.

Au, W.J., Gabor, A.J., Vijayan, N., et al. 1980. Periodic lateralized epileptiform complexes (PLEDs) in Creutzfeldt-Jakob disease. Neurology 30: 611–618.

Awerbuch, G.I., and Verma, N.P. 1987. Periodic epileptiform discharges in a patient with definite multiple sclerosis. Clin. Electroencephalogr. 18: 38–40.

Bernad, P.G. 1991. The neurological and electroencephalographic changes in AIDS. Clin. Electroencephalogr. 22:65–70.

Brown, P., Rodgers-Johnson, P., Cathala, F., et al. 1984. Creutzfeldt-Jakob disease of long duration: Clinocopathological characteristics, transmissibility, and differential diagnosis. Ann. Neurol. 16:295–304.

Burger, L.J., Rowan, A.J., and Goldensohn, E.S. 1972. Creutzfeldt-Jakob disease. An electroencephalographic study. Arch. Neurol. 26:428–433.

Chabolla, D.R., Moore, J.L., and Westmoreland, B.F. 1996. Periodic lateralized epileptiform discharges in multiple sclerosis. Electroencephalogr. Clin. Neurophysiol. 98:5–8.

Chaves-Carballo, E., Gomez, M.R., and Sharbrough, F.W. 1975. Encephalopathy and fatty infiltration of the viscera (Reye-Johnson syndrome). A 17-year experience. Mayo Clin. Proc. 50:209–215.

Ch'ien, L.T., Boehm, R.M., Robinson, H., et al. 1977. Characteristic early electroencephalographic changes in herpes simplex encephalitis. Clinical and virologic studies. Arch. Neurol. 34:361–364.

Cobb, W. 1966. The periodic events of subacute sclerosing leucoencephalitis. Electroencephalogr. Clin. Neurophysiol. 21:278–294.

Cobb, W.A. 1975. Electroencephalographic changes in viral encephalitis. In Viral Diseases of the Central Nervous System, Ed. L.S. Illis, pp. 76–89, Baltimore: Williams & Wilkins.

Cobb, W., and Hill, D. 1950. Electroencephalogram in subacute progressive encephalitis. Brain 73:392–404.

Cobb, W.A., Hornabrook, R.W., and Sanders, S. 1973. The EEG of kuru. Electroencephalogr. Clin. Neurophysiol. 34:419–427.

Desmond, M.M., Wilson, G.S., Melnick, J.L., et al. 1967. Congenital rubella encephalitis: course and early sequelae. J. Pediatr. 71:311–331.

Dreyfus-Brisac, C., and Ellingson, R.J. 1972. Hereditary, congenital and perinatal diseases. In Handbook of Electroencephalography and Clinical Neurophysiology, vol. 15, part B, Ed.-in-chief, A. Remond. Amsterdam: Elsevier.

Drury, I., and Beydou, A. 1996. Evolution of periodic complexes in Creutzfeldt-Jakob disease. Am. J. End. Technol. 36:230–234.

Elian, M. 1975. Herpes simplex encephalitis. Prognosis and longterm follow-up. Arch. Neurol. 32:39–43.

Elliott, F., Gardner-Thorpe, C., Barwick, D.D., et al. 1974. Creutzfeldt-Jakob disease. Modification of clinical and electroencephalographic activity with methylphenidate and diazepam. J. Neurol. Neurosurg. Psychiatry 37:879–887.

Enzensberger, W., Helm, E.B., and Fischer, P.-A. 1986. EEG follow-up examinations in AIDS patients. Electroencephalogr. Clin. Neurophysiol. 63:28P(abst).

Furlan, A.J., Henry, C.E., Sweeney, P.J., et al. 1981. Focal EEG abnormalities in Heidenhain's variant of Creutzfeldt-Jakob disease. Arch. Neurol. 38:312–314.

Gaches, J., and Arfel, G. 1972. Certitude et suspicions d'encéphalites herpétiques. Aspects électroencéphalographiques. Encephale 61:510–549.

Gajdusek, D.C., and Zigas, V. 1957. Degenerative disease of the central nervous system in New Guinea. N. Engl. J. Med. 257:974–978.

Gastaut, H., and Miletto, G. 1955. Interprétation physiopathogénique de la rage furieuse. Rev. Neurol. (Paris) 92:1–25.

Gastaut, H., Poirier, F., Payan, H., et al. 1959/1960. H.H.E. Syndrome, hemiconvulsions, hemiplegia, epilepsy. Epilepsia 1:418–447.

Gibbs, F.A., Gibbs, E.L., Carpenter, P.R., et al. 1959. Electroencephalographic abnormality in "uncomplicated" childhood diseases. JAMA 171:1050–1055.

Gibbs, F.A., Gibbs, E.L., Spies, H.W., et al. 1964. Common types of childhood encephalitis. Electroencephalographic and clinical relationships. Arch. Neurol. 10:1–11.

Gloor, P. 1980. EEG characteristics in Creutzfeldt-Jakob disease. Arch. Neurol. 8:341.

Gloor, P., Kalabay, O., and Giard, N. 1968. The electroencephalogram in diffuse encephalopathies. Electroencephalographic correlates of grey and white matter lesions. Brain 91:779–802.

Grabow, J.D., Matthews, C.G., Chun, R.W.M., et al. 1969. The electroencephalogram and clinical sequelae of California arbovirus encephalitis. Neurology (Minneapolis) 19:394–404.

Greenberg, D.A., Weinkle, D.J., and Aminoff, M.J. 1982. Periodic EEG complexes in infectious mononucleosis encephalitis. J. Neurol. Neurosurg. Psychiatry 45:648–651.

Gupta, P.C., and Seth, P. 1973. Periodic complexes in herpes simplex encephalitis. A clinical and experimental study. Electroencephalogr. Clin. Neurophysiol. 35:67–74.

Hanzel, F. 1961. Aspects of tick encephalitis. In Encephalitides, Eds. L. Van Bogaert, J. Radermecker, J. Hazay, et al., pp. 661–670. Amsterdam: Elsevier.

Illis, L.S., and Taylor, F.M. 1972. The electroencephalogram in herpes-simplex encephalitis. Lancet 1:718–721.

Jay, V., Becker, L.E., Ostubo, H., et al. 1995. Chronic encephalitis and epilepsy (Rasmussen's encephalitis): detection of cytomegalovirus and herpes simplex virus 1 by the polymerase chain reaction and in situ hybridization. Neurology 45:108–117.

Johnson, D.A., Klass, D.W., and Millichap, J.G. 1964. Electroencephalogram in Sydenham's chorea. Arch. Neurol. 10:21–27.

Jones, D.P., and Nevin, S. 1954. Rapidly progressive cerebral degeneration (subacute vascular encephalopathy) with mental disorder, focal disturbances, and myoclonic epilepsy. J. Neurol. Neurosurg. Psychiatry 17: 148–159.

Kiloh, L.G., McComas, A.J., and Osselton, J.W. 1972. Clinical Electroencephalography, 3rd ed. London: Butterworths.

Klatzman, D., et al. 1984. Selective tropism of lymphadenopathy associated virus (LAV) for helper-inducer lymphocytes. Science 225:59–63.

Klein, C., Kimiagar, I., Pollak, L., et al. 2002. Neurological features of West Nile Virus infection during the 2000 outbreak in a regional hospital in Israel. J. Neurol. Sci. 200:63–66.

Kooi, K.A., Tucker, R.P., and Marshall, R.E. 1978. Fundamentals of Electroencephalography, 2nd ed. Hagerstown, MD: Harper & Row.

Lavy, S., Lavy, R., and Brand, A. 1964. Neurological and electroencephalographic abnormalities in rheumatic fever. Acta Neurol. Scand. 40:76–88.

LeBeau, J., and Dondey, M. 1959. Importance diagnostique de certaines activités électrecéphalographiques latéralisées, périodiques ou à tendance périodique au cours des abcès du cerveau. Electroencephalogr. Clin. Neurophysiol. 11:43–58.

Legg, N.J., Gupta, P.C., and Scott, D.F. 1973. Epilepsy following cerebral abscess. A clinical and EEG study of 70 patients. Brain 96:259–268.

Lehtinen, I., and Halonen, J.-P. 1984. EEG findings in tick borne encephalitis. J. Neurol. Neurosurg. Psychiatry 47:500–504.

Lemmi, H., and Little, S.C. 1960. Occlusion of intracranial venous structures. Arch. Neurol. 3:252–266.

Lević, Z.M. 1978. Electroencephalographic studies in multiple sclerosis. Specific changes in benign multiple sclerosis. Electroencephalogr. Clin. Neurophysiol. 44:471–478.

Levy, R.M., and Bredesen, D.E. 1988. Central nervous system dysfunction in acquired immunodeficiency syndrome. In AIDS and the Nervous System, Eds. M.L. Rosenblum et al., pp. 29–63. New York: Raven Press.

Levy, S.R., Chiappa, K.H., Burke, C.J., et al. 1986. Early evolution and incidence of electroencephalographic abnormalities in Creutzfeldt-Jakob disease. J. Clin. Neurophysiol. 3:1–21.

Lombroso, C.T. 1968. Remarks on the EEG and movement disorder in SSPE. Neurology (Minneapolis) 18:69–75.

Markand, O.N., and Panszi, J.G. 1975. The electroencephalogram in subacute sclerosing panencephalitis. Arch. Neurol. 32:719–726.

May, W.W. 1968. Creutzfeldt-Jakob disease. I. Survey of the literature and clinical diagnosis. Acta Neurol. Scand. 44:1–32.

Metz, H., Gregoriou, M., and Sandifer, P. 1964. Subacute sclerosing panencephalitis. A review of 17 cases with special reference to clinical diagnostic criteria. Arch. Dis. Child. 39:554–557.

Michel, B., Gastaut, J.L., and Bianchi, L. 1979. Electroencephalographic cranial computerized tomographic correlations in brain abscess. Electroencephalogr. Clin. Neurophysiol. 46:256–273.

Mizrahi, E.M., and Tharp, B.R. 1982. A characteristic EEG pattern in neonatal herpes simplex encephalitis. Neurology 32:1215–1220.

Nelson, J.R., and Leffman, H. 1963. The human diffusely projecting system. Evoked potentials and interactions. Arch. Neurol. 8:544–556.

Nevin, S., McMenemey, W.H., Behrman, S., et al. 1960. Subacute spongiform encephalopathy. A subacute form of encephalopathy attributable to vascular dysfunction (spongiform cerebral atrophy). Brain 83:519–564.

Nicholson, J., Gross, G., Callaway, C., et al. 1986. In vitro infection of human monocytes with human T-lymphotropic virus type III/lymphadenopathy associated virus (HTLV-III/LAV). J. Immunol. 137:323–329.

Pachner, A.R., and Steere, A.C. 1985. The triad of neurologic manifestations of Lyme disease: meningitis, cranial neuritis, and radiculoneuritis. Neurology 35:47–53.

Pampiglione, G. 1964a. Polymyographic studies of some involuntary movements in subacute sclerosing pan-encephalitis. Arch. Dis. Child. 39: 558–563.

Pampiglione, G. 1964b. Prodromal phase of measles. Some neurophysiological studies. Br. Med. J. 2:1296–1300.

Pampiglione, G., Griffith, A.H., and Bramwell, E.C. 1971. Transient cerebral changes after vaccination against measles. Lancet 2:5–8.

Perot, P., Lloyd-Smith, D., Libman, I., et al. 1963. Trichinosis encephalitis: a study of electroencephalographic and neuropsychiatric abnormalities. Neurology 13:477–485.

Petre-Quadens, O., Sfaello, Z., van Bogaert, L., et al. 1968. Sleep study in SSPE (first results). Neurology (Minneapolis) 18:60–68.

Pettay, O., Leinikki, P., Donner, M., et al. 1972. Herpes simplex virus infection in the newborn. Arch. Dis. Child. 47:97–103.

Pine, I., Atoynatan, T.H., and Margolis, G. 1952. The EEG findings in 18 patients with brain abscess: case reports and a review of the literature. Electroencephalogr. Clin. Neurophysiol. 4:165–179.

Power, C., Poland, S.D., Blume, W.T., et al. 1990. Cytomegalovirus and Rasmussen's encephalitis. Lancet 336:1282–1284.

Radermecker, F.J. (Ed.) 1977. *Infections and Inflammatory Reactions, Allergy and Allergic Reactions; Degenerative Diseases/Handbook of Electroencephalography and Clinical Neurophysiology*, vol. 15, part A. Ed.-in-chief, A. Remond. Amsterdam: Elsevier.

Radermecker, J. 1949. Aspects électroencéphalographiques dans trois cas d'encéphalite subaiguë. Acta Neurol. Psychiatr. Belg. 49:222–232.

Radermecker, J., and Poser, C.M. 1960. The significance of repetitive paroxysmal electroencephalographic patterns. Their specificity in subacute sclerosing leukoencephalitis. World Neurol. 1:422–431.

Rasmussen, T., and McCann, W. 1968. Clinical studies of patients with focal epilepsy due to "chronic encephalitis." Trans. Am. Neurol. Assoc. 93:89–94.

Rawls, W.E., Dyck, P.J., Klass, D.W., et al. 1966. Encephalitis associated with herpes simplex virus. Ann. Intern. Med. 64:104–115.

Reiher, J., Lapointe, L.R., and Lessard, L. 1973. Prolonged and variable intervals between EEG complexes in subacute inclusion body encephalitis. Can. Med. Assoc. J. 108:729–732.

Rogers, S.W., Andrews, P.I., Gahring, L.C., et al. 1994. Autoantibodies to glutamate receptor GluR3 in Rasmussen's encephalitis. Science 265: 648–651.

Sainio, K., Granstrom, M.L., Pettay, O., et al. 1983. EEG in neonatal herpes simplex encephalitis. Electroencephalogr. Clin. Neurophysiol. 56:556–561.

Schnell, R.G., Dyck, P.J., Bowie, E.J.W., et al. 1966. Infectious mononucleosis. Neurologic and EEG findings. Medicine 45:51–63.

Scott, D.F. 1960. *Understanding EEG. An Introduction to Electroencephalography.* London: Gerald Duckworth.

Smith, J.B., Westmoreland, B.F., Reagan, T.J., et al. 1975. A distinctive clinical EEG profile in herpes simplex encephalitis. Mayo Clin. Proc. 50:469–474.

Smith, J.B., Groover, R.V., Klass, D.W., et al. 1977. Multicystic cerebral degeneration in neonatal herpes simplex virus encephalitis. Am. J. Dis. Child. 131:568–572.

Snider, W.D., Simpson, D.M., Nielsen, S., et al. 1983. Neurological complications of acquired immune deficiency syndrome: analysis of 50 patients. Ann. Neurol. 14:403–418.

Stockard, J.J., and Sharbrough, F.W. 1980. Unique contributions of short-latency auditory and somatosensory evoked potentials to neurologic diagnosis. Prog. Clin. Neurophysiol. 7:231–263.

Tapie, P., Buguet, A., Tabaraud, F., et al. 1996. Electroencephalographic and polygraphic features of 24-hour recordings in sleeping sickness and healthy African subjects. J. Clin. Neurophysiol. 13:339–344.

Tietjen, G.E., and Drury, I. 1990. Familial Creutzfeldt-Jakob disease without periodic EEG activity. Ann. Neurol. 28:585–588.

Tinuper, P., de Carolis, P., Galeotti, M., et al. 1990. Electroencephalogram and HIV infection: a prospective study in 100 patients. Clin. Electroencephalogr. 21:3:145–150.

Turrell, R.C., and Roseman, E. 1955. Electroencephalographic studies of the encephalopathies. IV. Serial studies in meningococcic meningitis. Arch. Neurol. Psychiatr. 73:141–148.

Upton, A., and Gumpert, J. 1970. Electroencephalography in diagnosis of herpes-simplex encephalitis. Lancet 1:650–652.

Usher, S.J., and Jasper, H.H. 1941. The etiology of Sydenham's chorea. Electroencephalographic studies. Can. Med. Assoc. J. 44:365–371.

Vinken, P.J., and Bruyn, G.W. (Eds.) 1978a. *Infections of the Nervous System*, Part 2. Neurology, vol. 34. Amsterdam: North-Holland.

Vinken, P.J., and Bruyn, G.W. (Eds.) 1978b. *Infections of the Nervous System.* Part 3. Neurology, vol. 35. Amsterdam: North-Holland.

Westmoreland, B.F., Gomez, M.R., and Blume, W.T. 1977. Activation of periodic complexes of subacute sclerosing panencephalitis by sleep. Ann. Neurol. 1:185–187.

Westmoreland, B.F., Sharbrough, F.W., and Donat, J.R. 1979. Stimulus-induced EEG complexes and motor spasms in subacute sclerosing panencephalitis. Neurology (Minneapolis) 29:1154–1157.

Will, R.G., Ironside, J.W., Zeidler, M., et al. 1996. A new variant of Creutzfeldt-Jakob disease in the UK. Lancet 347:921–925.

Wolinsky, J.S., Berg, B.O., and Maitland, C.J. 1976. Progressive rubella panencephalitis. Arch. Neurol. 33:722–723.

Wulff, C.H. 1982. Subacute sclerosing panencephalitis: serial electroencephalographic recordings. J. Neurol. Neurosurg. Psychiatry 45:418–421.

Zerr, I., Schultz-Schaeffer, W.J., Giese, A., et al. 2000. Current clinical diagnosis in Creutzfeldt-Jakob disease: identification of uncommon variants. Ann. Neurol. 48:323–329.

Zschocke, S. 1987. EEG und Intensivüberwachung. Presented at EEG Course, German EEG Society, Munich, March 1987.

17. Cerebrovascular Disorders and EEG

Ernst Niedermeyer

Role of EEG in Diagnosis of Cerebrovascular Lesions

The electroencephalogram (EEG) has made a remarkable contribution to the diagnosis of cerebrovascular lesions. It occupies a favorable position when one considers that cerebrovascular accidents are acute catastrophic events that naturally have strong repercussions on the EEG. The tempo of evolution is an important factor; thus, acute vascular slow foci may be much more impressive than focal slowing caused by a slowly growing neoplasm. On the other hand, small deep vascular lesions are often too far distant from the cortex and may escape EEG detection, whereas deep vascular lesions in the brainstem and cerebellum reveal themselves only as secondary phenomena in the cerebral hemispheres. In an acute stroke, a massive and highly impressive EEG focus may be present before a computed tomography (CT) scan can demonstrate the lesion (Keilson et al., 1985). Magnetic resonance imaging (MRI) has been found to be even more precise and more informative than CT in the morphological evaluation of stroke; with this method, the lesion can be visualized within about 2 to 6 hours after the vascular accident, whereas CT scan demonstration usually requires 1 to 5 days before positive results are obtained. The EEG is an indicator of abnormal function; the function of the involved central nervous system (CNS) tissue breaks down before the structure shows its suffering. It has been shown experimentally (Gloor et al., 1977) as well as clinically with the use of CT scan (Gastaut et al., 1979) that edema alone does not account for delta activity in EEG. In the modern view, the factor of ischemic tolerance of the brain has been critically analyzed (Chen and Simon, 1997) along with the demonstration of a large number of biomolecular substances presumed to be involved in this complex process.

The role of EEG as an indicator of disturbed function (locally, regionally, or diffusely) in the event of a stroke has not always been duly appreciated. In an authoritative study on acute strokes, Hachinski and Norris (1980) have pointed out that "electroencephalography is not much help in the diagnosis of stroke, especially when CT scanning is available." Once again it must be stated that the evaluation of the degree and extension of cerebral dysfunction may be just as important as the demonstration of local or diffuse morphological changes. An experienced electroencephalographer with imagination might be able to provide valuable information about the regional and general functional (dysfunctional) state in a stroke. An imaginative approach to the EEG evaluation of strokes has been proposed by Velho-Groneberg (1986). Accordingly, the EEG reflects dynamic processes that occur in the wake of a stroke.

In addition to local or more diffuse slow activity, the EEG also shows a more or less serious decline of physiological patterns such as posterior alpha (basic) rhythm and intermixed slower or faster frequencies. Considerable localizing value has been ascribed to local depression of the background activity, while more extensive depression is regarded as somewhat less informative (Kok and Van der Drift, 1971; Van der Drift, 1972; Van der Drift and Kok, 1972). These authors believe that preservation of faster background activities, especially in subacute forms of middle cerebral artery ischemia, is indicative of considerable neuronal survival in the infarcted zone and hence indicative of a good prognosis.

The Changing Approach to Cerebrovascular Disasters in the 1990s

Reader, be lenient and understanding with regard to the presented literature, which may appear to be quite dated! Even now at the time of the fifth edition of this book in 2004, there has not been a lot of new EEG literature in this area. Not as far as acute stroke-like cerebrovascular problems are concerned. The stroke as the classical cerebrovascular catastrophe has become a domain of acute intensive care (critical care) neurology; diagnostic approaches have changed and, above all, therapeutic efforts have to be carried out with dramatic speed. In this acute situation, the new diagnostic approach emphasizes monitoring of cerebral, cardiovascular, and respiratory functions. Techniques of prolonged (continuous) EEG recording, often with the use of computerization of EEG data, have moved into the foreground and are described under the heading of such techniques.

We must not cut ourselves off from the historical development and, for this reason, a plethora of relatively old literature has not been eliminated.

Acute Cerebrovascular Accident

Acute cerebrovascular accident (CVA, apoplexy, or stroke) is essentially based on ischemic and hemorrhagic forms of pathology, rapidly leading to reversible and eventually irreversible hypoxia of the cerebral parenchyma. Ischemic damage has customarily been divided into local arterial thrombosis and embolic arterial obstruction. The result is a cerebral infarction (encephalomalacia) of the "white" type (nonhemorrhagic) or "red" type (hemorrhage due to reflux into the infarcted region as a secondary phenomenon). Cerebral hemorrhages are caused by the rupture of a diseased vessel.

This is a simple but outdated way of looking at the CVA. Modern clinical physiological cerebrovascular and neuropathological research has vastly improved our understanding of strokes and, for this reason, greater numbers of pathogenetic mechanisms have to be taken into consideration.

Arteriosclerosis (atherosclerosis) is not devoid of an inflammatory component (Lindsberg, 2000), but increased adhesion molecule expression has been found to be unassociated with symptomatic carotid disease (Nuotio et al., 2003). Table 17.1 (after Van der Drift, 1972) exemplifies this approach. Although a number of previously unknown mechanisms of CVA genesis have been added, no special emphasis is laid on the distinction between local arterial thrombosis and embolism, which are lumped together as "ischemia." Ischemic states usually pertain to the territory of the involved artery, but another mechanism has entered the picture. This is the concept of "extraterritorial ischemia," which gives rise to "watershed infarctions" ("boundary infarctions") along the borders of the major arterial territories, between middle, posterior, and anterior cerebral arteries.

This mechanism is based on a decline in the systemic circulation; this is a drop in blood pressure or cardiac output, usually combined with a diseased and plaque-ridden cerebral vasculature. It is a logical and convincing concept when it is assumed that boundary areas between the major cerebral arterial territories are most likely to suffer from ischemia. The work of Zülch and Behrend (1961) clearly demonstrates the distinction between the watershed type and the classical obstructive ischemic infarction.

Increasing emphasis has been placed on *transient ischemic attacks* over the past decade. These attacks precede more than 50% of cerebral arterial thrombosis (McHenry, 1978). These episodes consist of abrupt neurological (mostly hemiparetic or hemiparetic-dysphasic) deficits that resolve within minutes or hours. The attacks may involve either the internal carotid (middle cerebral artery), or the vertebrobasilar system. The sensorium is clear.

The delineation of *steal syndromes* has contributed further to the understanding of strokes and stroke-like deficits.

In the past, there has been considerable controversy about prevalence and incidence of the principal mechanisms of stroke. According to McHenry (1978), thrombosis of a cerebral artery accounts for more than 50% of all cases of stroke, followed by cerebral hemorrhage (25%) and embolism (5%). The remaining 20% is evenly divided into subarachnoid hemorrhage and subdural hematoma; these two mechanisms of intracranial bleeding, however, should be treated separately. In patients of ages 15 to 44 years, the most common causes are cardiac embolism, hematological disorder, and small vessel disease (lacunar disease) (Kittner et al., 1998).

Table 17.1. Pathogenic Mechanisms Involved in Cerebrovascular Accidents[a]

Primary Ischemia

I. Territorial ischemia (ischemia restricted to the area supplied by a cerebral artery): superficial flow area of the middle cerebral artery (MCA):
   A. Ischemia most marked in the distal (terminal) part of the flow area:
      1. Occlusion of the internal carotid artery (ICA);
      2. Incomplete occlusion or recanalization of the middle cerebral artery;
      3. Fall of blood pressure in addition to incomplete occlusion or small vessel disease;
      4. Decompensation of collateral circulation in old internal carotid artery occlusion.
      (In these cases there is a (collateral) circulation directly through the middle cerebral artery.)
   B. Ischemia most marked in the proximal part of the flow area (center of area of supply):
      1. Middle cerebral artery occlusion;
      2. Internal carotid occlusion with propagation of the thrombus in the middle cerebral artery.
      (In these cases there is a leptomeningeal collateral circulation.)
   C. Flow area of the anterior and posterior cerebral arteries
   D. Flow in deep arteries:
      1. Deep branches (rami striati) of the middle cerebral artery
      2. Rami perforantes
      3. Vertebrobasilar system
II. Extraterritorial ischemia-watershed infarction (Zülch and Behrend, 1969):
   A. Superficial border zones
   B. Deep border zones
III. Diffuse ischemia
IV. Venous thrombosis

Secondary Ischemia (Due to Cerebral Steal)

Extracerebral steal	Intracerebral steal
Subclavian steal	In cerebrovascular occlusion
Carotid steal	In arteriovenous malformation (AVM)
	In neoplasm

[a]With permission of Dr. J.H.A. Van der Drift and the North-Holland Publishing Company, Amsterdam.

EEG Correlates of Internal Carotid Artery Thrombosis

On the basis of anatomical studies, there is reason to presume that thrombotic arterial occlusions are found as often in the arterial trunks in the neck as in cerebral arteries (Alajouanine et al., 1961).

Thrombosis of the internal carotid artery is often heralded by clinical signs such as loss or diminution of the carotid pulsation in the neck, a bruit over the vessel in the neck, and decrease of retinal artery pressure evidenced by ophthalmodynamometry. Frontal headaches sometimes precede the CVA. The clinical symptomatology of the thrombosis depends greatly on the extension of the infarcted area. The entire territory may be softened, with subsequent massive cerebral edema, transtentorial herniation, and death. The other extreme is a clinically silent occlusion of the vessel. An entire gamut of pathological changes may be found between these two extremes, depending on the functioning of the collateral systems via the circle of Willis, subarachnoid (leptomeningeal) anastomoses, or ophthalmic artery. The diagnosis is made arteriographically; the CT scan and MRI can provide further information on the degree of concomitant edema.

In the presence of massive neurological deficits such as hemiplegia, with or without aphasia, the EEG shows pronounced delta activity over the affected hemisphere and especially over the frontocentrotemporal region. The delta activity may be very slow and is mostly of polymorphic character with superimposed theta and alpha frequencies. A temporal maximum of slow activity was stressed by Barré et al. (1950), Walkenhorst (1956), and Hass and Goldensohn (1959). Other investigators (Fuhrmann, 1953; Fuhrmann and Müller, 1954) noted ipsilateral voltage depression after carotid thrombosis, whereas Carreras et al. (1955) reported ipsilateral slowing followed by depression. Voltage depression may persist for some months over the affected hemisphere (Kooi, 1971). Runs of rhythmical intermittent delta waves may occur bilaterally over frontal areas (Kiloh et al., 1972). Initially preponderant mixed delta and theta activity over the affected hemisphere becomes more circumscript after 1 week, with prominent slowing over the temporal region (Corić et al., 1981).

The divergence of opinion on the role of voltage depression and slowing reflects the variety of parenchymatous involvement. Extremely slow activity over the affected hemisphere with decreasing amplitude and eventually poorly defined low-voltage activity indicates extremely extensive infarction. Clinically silent occlusion has no effect on the EEG.

Middle Cerebral Artery Thrombosis

The *acute form* of CVA caused by thrombotic occlusion of the middle cerebral artery may be quite similar to the acute internal carotid thrombosis as far as the hemiplegic or hemiplegic-aphasic neurological deficit is concerned. Confusion or semicoma is fairly common in the acute stage. Convulsive phenomena such as focal motor twitching contralaterally may be present but are more common in the special form of watershed ischemia (extraterritorial ischemia, to be discussed later). The cause and nature of the concomitant impairment of consciousness are not easily understood.

According to Van der Drift (1972) and Van der Drift and Kok (1972), the EEG is characterized by pronounced irregular and very slow delta activity ipsilaterally, of fairly high voltage, or fairly continuous character, and with frontotemporal maximum (temporal maximum according to Hubach and Struck, 1965). Traces of sharp activity may be present over the affected areas. There is marked depression of the background activity and, in severe strokes, transient global depression of EEG activity may be observed in all leads (Primavera et al., 1981). Frontal intermittent rhythmical delta runs may be seen in addition to the local and diffuse irregular (polymorphic) slowing. Strictly frontal polymorphic delta foci are not found in middle cerebral artery ischemia (Kok and Van der Drift, 1971) (Figs. 17.1 and 17.2). According to Kayser-Gatchalian and Neundörfer (1980), background abnormalities are of greater prognostic value than the focal slowing. Fairly good correlations between EEG

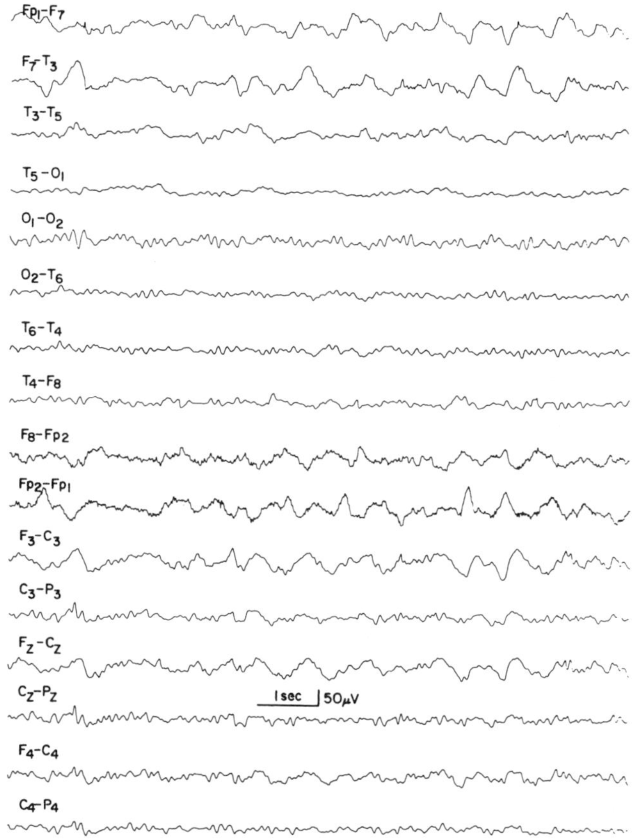

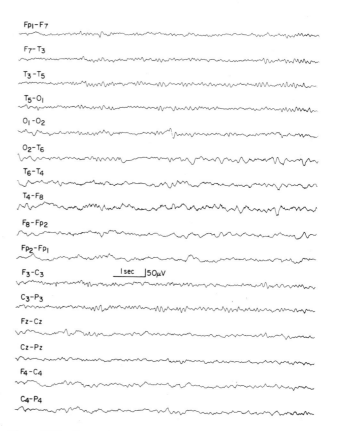

Figure 17.1. Age 57 years. Acute cerebrovascular accident (CVA) on the day before this record was obtained. There is marked left frontotemporal polymorphic delta activity. Also note alpha depression and loss of detail over left posterior quadrant. The right hemisphere and especially the right frontal area show some degree of delta activity.

Figure 17.2. Recent CVA (3 days earlier) due to right middle cerebral artery thrombosis and good computed tomography (CT) scan evidence of infarction in the corresponding territory. Acute left hemiplegia. Age 64 years. Patient awake; right-sided alpha diminished and a large zone of mixed 2–6/sec activity involving most of the right hemisphere.

findings in supratentorial strokes and cerebral circulation time data obtained with intravenously injected pertechnetate and a multidetector device have been reported by Tolonen and Ahonen (1983). The EEG faithfully reflects a variety of stroke complications and provides a valuable assessment of the patients condition (Velho-Groneberg, 1986). EEG slowing may spill over into the presumed healthy hemisphere. A study of computerized EEG findings and positron emission tomography in patients with infarctions of the middle cerebral artery showed surprising distant effects of some strokes: reduced cerebral blood flow and reduced metabolic rates in contralateral regions and even in the cerebellum (Nagata et al., 1989). These investigators also showed a fine correlation of EEG findings, cerebral blood flow, and metabolic rate except for the early stage of the stroke.

Preservation of background activity is a prognostically favorable sign. This is particularly true for the recovery from aphasia (Jabbari et al., 1979). In the wake of a hemiplegic stroke, augmentation of rolandic mu rhythm may develop over the affected side (Pfurtscheller, 1986). Such a mu rhythm may slow down into the 5 to 7/sec range.

In the ensuing period to recovery, a steady decline of the degree of slow activity parallels the clinical neurological improvement. A reversal of this process indicates complications. Full normalization may be present within 6 months. According to Christian (1975), ipsilateral spindle depression in sleep is the most persistent localizing sign. De Weerd et al. (1988) studied the recovery process with a quantified EEG method (neurometric analysis) and cerebral blood flow evaluation (xenon-133 inhalation). EEG and clinical data showed improvement that often was termed dramatic. A persistent neurological deficit was predicted by a low cerebral blood flow at the first measurement; such predictive statements could not be made from the initial EEG findings.

New methods of computer analysis in stroke patients have been introduced by Pfurtscheller and his co-workers (Pfurtscheller, 1993; also see Chapter 60, "Special Uses of EEG Computer Analysis in Clinical Environments"). Computed EEG topography in acute strokes was used by Jackel and Harner (1989) with very satisfactory results.

Luu et al. (2001) have advocated the use of EEG for continuous monitoring after an acute stroke for the sake of better understanding of the stroke pathology and its dynamic spatiotemporal changes. These authors feel that the use of spectral analysis derived from 64 or 128 channels is superior to the conventional EEG approach in stroke patients.

Negative shifts in the direct current (DC) potential were noted after permanent middle cerebral artery occlusions in Wistar rats. These DC shifts were associated with alkaline pH change in the ischemic penumbra (Back et al., 2000).

Ischemia (Thrombosis) in Deep Branches of the Middle Cerebral Artery

Occlusion of the rami striati, including lenticulo-optic and lenticulostriate perforating arteries, gives rise to marked contralateral hemiplegia due to the interruption of blood supply for the internal capsule. In these cases, the EEG may show little or no focal slowing; occasionally, demonstrable ipsilateral slowing is due to relative ischemia in superficial branches of the middle cerebral artery (Van der Drift, 1972).

Anterior Thalamic Infarction

Severe behavioral changes are found in association with infarction of the anterior thalamus (anterior thalamosubthalamic paramedian artery). The patients exhibit "palipsychism" (superimposition of mental activity normally processed sequentially) (Ghika-Schmid and Bogousslavsky, 2000). The symptomatology is prefrontal, presumably due to the strong connections between the dorsomedial thalamic nucleus and the prefrontal region.

Hemorrhage Involving Capsular Region (Middle Cerebral Artery Territory)

This form of stroke occurs mainly in hypertensive individuals; high blood pressure (BP) in combination with vascular disease (hyalinosis) may lead to a massive rupture. Occasionally, intracerebral hemorrhages are caused by aneurysms, arteriovenous malformations, or alteration of vessels inside a cerebral neoplasm. The most frequently involved vessel is the lenticulostriate artery, which is a small deep branch of the middle cerebral artery. Its nearness to the internal capsule explains the devastating effects on the motor outflow.

In hemorrhagic strokes, the patient appears to be more acutely ill than in a thrombotic CVA; there are usually no warning prodromal symptoms. The hemorrhage usually extends into the striatum and thalamus, prompting impairment of consciousness and even deep coma.

EEG changes, however, may be not quite as impressive as the clinical picture, probably due to the preservation of the cortical garland. Delta activity is present over the affected hemisphere (Hirose et al., 1981), maximally over the frontotemporal area, sometimes rhythmic and even sinusoidal (Kiloh et al., 1972) with intermittent runs, often of moderate voltage. There is more intermixed theta activity than in thrombosis. Involvement of the contralateral hemisphere is light to moderate; the posterior basic rhythm may be preserved or even enhanced unless the patient is unconscious. Sharp activity and frontal intermittent rhythmical delta runs play a very minor part. With lapse into coma, slowing becomes diffuse; the abnormalities become even more severe in the catastrophic event of hemorrhagic perforation into the lateral ventricle. A rapid fall of blood pressure, arterial vasospasm, and cerebral edema are further complications.

In view of such complicating factors, the distinction between capsular hemorrhage and middle cerebral artery thrombosis is practically impossible to make on EEG grounds, notwithstanding the fact that the uncomplicated hemorrhage shows less prominent slow activity.

The recovery phase shows a remarkable resolution of the initial abnormalities. One might assume that the process of recovery would be even faster than in comparable cases of thrombotic ischemia. Christian (1975), however, noticed focal EEG abnormalities 2 months after the insult in 85% of the patients with intracerebral hemorrhage and in 40% of those with thrombotic ischemia.

Can the EEG assist in making the distinction between infarction and hemorrhage? Lechner (1958) cast much doubt on such capabilities, but the work of Van der Drift (1972) seems to support a more optimistic view. The enormous clinical and pathological anatomical material of this author must be considered. The numbers of verified cases include 122 patients of subacute carotid-middle cerebral artery ischemia, 54 cases of lenticulostriate artery ischemia, 14 cases of anterior cerebral artery ischemia, and 75 cases of acute middle cerebral artery ischemia with edema.

With *computerized EEG data analysis,* Pfurtscheller et al. (1980) have shown asymmetries of the central mu rhythm with ipsilateral depression in the wake of the insult. This type of rolandic activity may be undetectable in the routine EEG. Van Huffelen et al. (1979, 1984) also used quantitative EEG data in the detection of abnormalities in acute unilateral cerebral ischemia. Sainio et al. (1983) have stressed the contribution of spectral analysis in acute strokes.

Thrombosis of the Anterior Cerebral Artery

Ischemic strokes involving the anterior cerebral artery are uncommon. Contralateral hemiplegia with predominant involvement of the leg is the most typical neurological deficit; confusion is frequently present, and profound coma may ensue. The degree of these signs and symptoms depends greatly on the extent of the infarcted area, which is determined by the functioning of collateral blood supply. Ipsilateral frontal delta activity is a typical EEG concomitant of this type of insult; the delta activity may be of rhythmical intermittent (although unilateral) character (Van der Drift and Kok, 1972).

Thrombosis of Perforating Arteries Arising from Anterior Cerebral Artery

These branches irrigate the greater part of the thalamus and the hypothalamus. According to Van der Drift (1972), this type of ischemia is not uncommon in the elderly after an acute drop in blood pressure. Dementia, grasp reflexes, and sphincter incontinence may ensue. The patients are confused and disoriented. The EEG is characterized by frontal intermittent rhythmical delta activity.

Motor Strokes Sparing the Leg

This is a fairly common situation (observed in 895 of a total of 3,901 stroke patients; De Freitas et al., 2000). According to these authors, this condition is usually due to more superficial infarcts caused by emboli from large-artery disease and atherosclerosis without stenosis. There are no good EEG data.

Thrombosis of the Posterior Cerebral Artery

This type of stroke leads to marked homonymous hemianopsia; contralateral sensory loss and a thalamic pain syndrome may be associated in a more extended ischemia. Delta activity is clearly accentuated over the ipsilateral parieto-occipital region (Georgiades et al., 1999).

Thrombosis of the External Geniculate Branch of the Posterior Cerebral Artery

This CVA gives rise to a typical thalamic lesion (Dejerine-Roussy syndrome), characterized by contralateral hemianesthesia with deep sensations being most severely damaged, hyperpathy (the basis of thalamic pain), mild limb ataxia, contralateral choreoathetoid movements, and mild temporary hemiparesis. The EEG may be unremarkable (Niedermeyer, 1957) or may show varying degrees of slow activity, which can be quite impressive in thalamic depth leads (Gücer et al., 1978).

With the use of somatosensory evoked potentials (SEP), Mauguiére and Desmedt (1988) were able to differentiate four subtypes of the Dejerine-Roussy syndrome:

1. No central pain, complete hemianesthesia and loss of cortical SEP on the affected side;
2. Central pain, severe hypoesthesia and loss of cortical SEP;
3. Central pain and hypoesthesia; cortical SEP present but reduced or delayed on the affected side;
4. Central pain with preserved touch and joint sensations and normal SEP.

In thalamic hemorrhages, there was evidence of delayed P3 event-related potentials (Onofrj et al., 1992).

Special Case of Cerebral Embolism as Cause of Thrombosis

All forms of cerebral embolism cause (and subsequent occlusions show) a variety of clinical and EEG changes. Lhermitte and his co-workers have demonstrated that a surprisingly large number of strokes believed to be thrombotic are due to embolism of cardiac origin (Lhermitte and Gautier, 1975; Lhermitte and Guiraud, 1968; Lhermitte et al., 1966).

Cerebral embolism that produces acute hemiplegic strokes may be lumped together with strokes due to local thrombosis (acute middle cerebral artery ischemia); in such cases, the constellation of clinical date and/or the autopsy will determine the true cause. Embolism of thrombotic material and gas and fat embolism may give rise to clinically and electroencephalographically similar pictures. In embolism, however, the extremely acute shock-like effect may trigger a chain of vasomotor responses in adjacent vascular territories. These responses either hasten the catastrophic events or resolve quickly so that recovery may evolve with unexpected speed.

Rasheva (1981) and Rasheva et al. (1981) noted clinical epileptic seizures in 10.1% and paroxysmal EEG discharges (spikes and sharp waves) in 57.1% of a large population (328 cases) with embolic stroke.

The importance of *cerebral gas embolism* during and after cardiac surgery is widely known. According to Naquet and Vigouroux (1972), gas embolism may produce EEG changes similar to those seen in watershed infarction, to be discussed in the following section. In *fat embolism,* Müller and Klingler (1965) reported marked delta-theta activity of frontotemporal accentuation. Similar findings were reported by Scherzer (1967).

In general, the EEG cannot effectively assist in the differentiation of thrombotic and thrombotic-embolic cerebral ischemia.

Experimental cerebral embolism lends itself to the study of immediate EEG effects. These are dramatic and instantaneous. In the rabbit, Hegedüs et al. (1985) demonstrated abrupt flattening of the affected hemisphere after embolization of the middle cerebral artery; there was even some volt-

Figure 17.3. Prompt flattening over the left hemisphere and some voltage decrease over right hemisphere (especially right frontal region) is noted after the experimental embolization of the left middle cerebral artery in the rabbit. (With permission from Dr. K. Hegedüs, Debrecen, and the editor-in-chief of *Journal of Neurology.*)

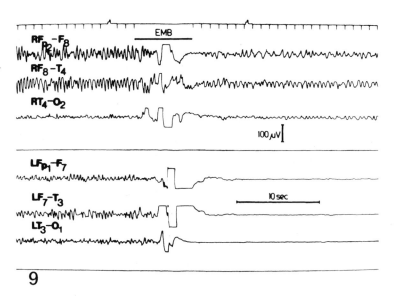

age decrease contralaterally (Fig. 17.3). This clearly shows that the effects of a major embolism extend beyond the involved arterial territory.

Watershed Ischemia

The pathophysiological mechanisms of watershed-type ischemias were discussed above. The discussion was essentially based on the physiological studies of Schneider (1950, 1961) and the clinical-pathological-anatomical observations of Adams and Van der Eecken (1953), Meyer (1953, 1958), Meyer et al. (1954), Alajouanine et al. (1957, 1959, 1961), Baker et al. (1963), Gastaut et al. (1971), and particularly on the work of Zülch (1953, 1971) and Zülch and Behrend (1961).

Acute watershed-type ischemia is found almost exclusively in old patients with a history of cerebral arteriosclerosis and chronic cardiovascular problems. A variety of illnesses may trigger the acute CVA. Acute infection, dehydration, uncontrolled diabetes mellitus, cardiovascular decompensation, severe anemia, recent craniocerebral trauma, extracerebral embolism, liver disease with portocaval encephalopathy, and severe arterial hypertension are events that can facilitate the occurrence of watershed ischemia (Naquet and Vigouroux, 1972).

Impairment of consciousness ranges from confusion to coma. A contralateral hemiparetic deficit is present; it is usually not as pronounced as in primary capsular ischemia or hemorrhage.

The EEG is slow (mixed delta-theta range) and severely disorganized; background activity is diffusely disordered. These changes are essentially diffuse with consistent lateralization to the affected hemisphere. Against this slow and disorganized background of rather moderate voltage, there are constantly repetitive large sharp waves or spikes, often compounded and consisting of several subcomponents and phases, usually over the posterotemporal-occipital-parietal region of the hemisphere that harbors the lesion. This periodic spike discharge is rhythmically or quasirhythmically repetitive at a rate of approximately 1/sec. The discharge

may become quite widespread, even reaching into the other hemisphere. Occasionally, the periodic spikes show a superior frontal maximum (see Fig. 13.16A,B in Chapter 13, "Abnormal EEG Patterns: Epileptic and Paroxysmal").

At this stage of repetitive spike activity, contralateral focal motor twitching (fingers or hand, face, abdomen, leg, foot, or toes) is the common accompaniment of the periodic spikes. The focal motor epileptic manifestations tend to linger on for hours or days; eventually, these twitches subside, although the general condition of the patient remains grave. Fatal outcome is very frequent. There has been some EEG literature on the periodic lateralized epileptiform discharges (PLEDs) (Chatrian et al., 1964). Such PLEDs often occur without accompanying motor activity. Further work on these discharges was presented by Alajouanine et al. (1955), Barolin et al. (1962), Markand and Daly (1971), and Pohlmann-Eden et al. (1996). These latter authors feel that PLEDs indicate focal hyperexcitability in the penumbra zone of an ischemic stroke. Multifocal epileptic seizures of partial character may also evolve in watershed ischemia, along with independent EEG foci (Matsuo, 1985). "Focal epileptic patterns" were reported in such cases by Berlit et al. (1988).

Deteriorating Strokes

Various complications may interfere with recovery from a cerebrovascular accident. The term *deteriorating stroke* has been used by Hachinski and Norris (1980) and includes progressively evolving strokes, recurrent strokes, and also spatially extending strokes. Their causes may be thrombotic, embolic, or hemorrhagic. Important pathogenic mechanisms include cerebral edema and the syndrome of inappropriate antidiuretic hormone (SIADH), which leads to reduction of cerebral sodium, potassium, and chloride content, altered brain energy metabolism, and neurotransmitter amino acid uptake (Hachinski and Norris, 1980). Cardiac factors, poststroke depression, and drug effects also may lead to poststroke deterioration. In evolving and deteriorating strokes, the ischemic penumbra plays a major role (Fisher and Garcia, 1996).

In deteriorating strokes, the EEG slowing tends to become more diffuse. It also may reflect drug effects (sedatives), but it is apt to remain notably unaltered in the case of poststroke depression.

Epileptic Seizures in Acute Stroke

The occurrence of epileptic seizures at the onset of a first-ever stroke underscores the severity of the lesion and in-hospital mortality is high, especially in aged persons with large hemorrhagic infarctions of a parietal lobe (Arboix et al., 1996).

Hemiplegic Migraine

Forms of acute hemiplegic migraine can mimic hemiplegic strokes. In some cases, the differential diagnosis is not easy, because migrainous vasospasm can lead to edema and infarction and thus to permanent cerebral parenchymatous damage (Schumacher and Wolff, 1941; Whitty, 1953). The EEG shows massive ipsilateral delta and theta activity (Bradshaw and Parsons, 1965; Heron, 1966; Heyck, 1956; Rosenbaum, 1960). More is found in Chapter 29, "The EEG in Patients with Migraine and Other Forms of Headache" (see Fig. 29.2).

Special Case of Acute Hemiplegia in Childhood

Acute hemiplegic episodes in infancy and childhood are not uncommon, but the literature has been rather scanty. The early work of Ford and Schaffer (1927; see also Ford, 1966) has been superseded by the extensive monograph of Isler (1969) based on 114 observations. This material is etiologically heterogeneous, with a predominance of infectious causes. Isler deserves much credit for the clarification of a clinical condition often believed to be of obscure origin. The EEG of childhood hemiplegias depends greatly on the underlying type of pathology.

Leukoaraiosis

Leukoaraiosis (Hachinski et al., 1987) "is a term used to describe radiological abnormalities in CT and MRI of the brain in elderly patients as bilateral areas of hypodensities in white matter of hemispheres" (Wiszniewska et al., 2000). This term comprises a number of cerebrovascular conditions and has no special EEG correlate.

Acute Cerebrovascular Accidents in Brainstem and Cerebellum

The preceding section dealt with vascular lesion within cerebral hemispheres including the capsular region and adjacent basal ganglia. Most of the above-described clinical-pathological conditions are characterized by contralateral hemiplegia.

Some conditions with different symptomatology, such as ischemia of the posterior cerebral artery and its external geniculate branch (giving rise to the thalamic pain syndrome) and the thalamohypothalamic manifestations caused by ischemia of the perforating branches arising from the anterior cerebral artery, have already been discussed.

This section deals with acute vascular syndromes in lower portions of the brain.

Thalamic Hemorrhage

Thalamic bleeding usually causes temporary loss of consciousness. Larger hemorrhages may give rise to ipsilateral delta activity. According to Jasper and Van Buren (1953), there is a reduction of alpha rhythm in the case of anteroventral thalamic damage. Alpha enhancement may be noted in patients with posterior thalamic lesions. Lack of sleep spindles has been reported (Hirose et al., 1981). Delayed P_3 responses were reported by Onofrj et al. (1992).

Basilar Artery Thrombosis

The thrombotic occlusion of the basilar artery is often preceded by warnings such as dizziness, vertigo, dysarthria, or cranial pareses (Siekert and Millikan, 1955). Hypertensive and diabetic individuals might be predisposed to this type of stroke. Most patients are over the age of 50.

The clinical picture and pathological substrata have been outlined in the work of Kubik and Adams (1946), Biemond (1951), French and Haines (1950), Silversides (1954), Siekert and Millikan (1955), Fang and Palmer (1956), Haugstedt (1956), Cravioto et al. (1958), and Loeb and Meyer (1965). There is marked variation depending on the tempo of development, whether abrupt or progressive over hours and days, and extent of the lesion. According to Plum and Posner (1966), about 50% of the patients are in coma from the onset of the thrombosis, and most of the rest are either confused or obtunded and delirious. Respiratory disturbances are very common; pupillary anomalies ranging from miosis (pontine) to mydriasis (in mesencephalic level) are almost always present (Plum and Posner, 1966). Cranial nerve involvement may be widespread. Long tract signs are very common, with quadriplegia and sometimes hemiplegia. Swallowing is severely impaired.

The *locked-in syndrome* consists of quadriplegia and paralysis of all cranial nerves except those that control vertical eye movements (Feldman, 1971; Nordgren et al., 1971; Patterson and Grabois, 1986; Plum and Posner, 1966). Basilar artery thrombosis is its most common cause; the lesions usually occupy the ventral pons. The patients are not in coma; the EEG is, in the majority of the cases, normal or only slightly abnormal (Bauer et al., 1979; Markand, 1976). Jacome and Morilla-Pastor (1990) describe a case of locked-in syndrome with a well-developed but unreactive posterior alpha rhythm. According to Gütling et al. (1996), three out of five patients with locked-in syndrome had no alpha reactivity of the EEG. A considerable number of cases of basilar thrombosis have been shown to be embolic in nature (Kubik and Adams, 1946).

In cases with *mesodiencephalic involvement,* bilateral slowing of the EEG has been observed (Abbott and Bautista, 1949; Kubik and Adams, 1946; Watson and Adams, 1951) (Fig. 17.4). Roger et al. (1954) pointed out that upper brainstem involvement is associated with slowing, whereas *lower (ponto-oblongata) pathology* is usually associated with diffuse low-voltage tracings. Further evidence of low-voltage activity was provided by the observation of acute cases with autopsy verification by Lundervold et al. (1956), Tucker (1958), and Paddison and Ferris (1961). Further work in this field was presented by Friedlander (1959), Birchfield et al.

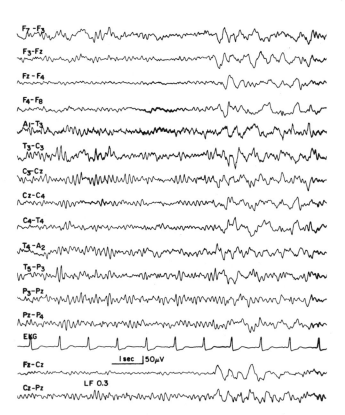

Figure 17.4.   Recent brainstem stroke in a 67-year-old patient. Thrombosis of basilar artery with midbrain infarction. Patient awake and in recovery. Note posterior 6–9/sec basic rhythm and a run of bilateral 1.5–4/sec waves with frontal maximum.

(1959), Potes et al. (1961), Kaada et al. (1961), Van der Drift and Magnus (1961), Chase et al. (1968), Kendel and Koufen (1970), and Ketz (1971).

From the EEG viewpoint, it is important to reflect on the significance of low-voltage tracings, which are very common in acute as well as in chronic lower brainstem disease. This will be discussed more extensively in the section on chronic vertebrobasilar artery insufficiency; such low-voltage tracings are not categorically abnormal.

Thrombosis of the basilar artery can also be caused secondarily by supratentorial space-occupying lesions via the *mechanisms of transtentorial herniation.* The work of Loeb (1962) has been particularly valuable in this field.

Thrombosis of the Vertebral Artery

This is the most common cause of lateral medullary infarction (Fisher et al., 1961). It may be the cause of typical or incomplete Wallenberg syndrome (Duffy and Jacobs, 1958). Thrombosis of the vertebral artery is usually associated with ill-defined low-voltage activity in the EEG.

Thrombosis of Branches of the Vertebral and Basilar Artery

Thrombotic occlusions of the paramedian, short circumferential, and long branches (posterior inferior cerebellar, anterior inferior cerebellar, superior cerebellar anterior) do not offer any interesting aspects from the EEG viewpoint. Poorly defined low-voltage activity is the most common finding.

Midbrain Hemorrhage

Mesencephalic bleeding without extension into the pons is most likely to give rise to Parinaud's syndrome; it is seldom fatal. The EEG often shows diffuse activity in the upper theta range (7/sec, according to Van der Drift and Kok, 1972).

Lower Brainstem Hemorrhage

These uncommon strokes almost always give rise to coma and respiratory anomalies (Plum and Posner, 1966), sometimes progressing to acute respiratory failure (Steegman, 1951). The pupils are usually very small. Quadriplegia is very common; bouts of decerebrate posturing also occur.

The EEG may show the striking finding of a well-preserved posterior alpha rhythm that cannot be blocked by various modalities of stimuli (Loeb and Poggio, 1953; Loeb et al., 1959; Neundörfer et al., 1974), but, in exceptional cases, the reactivity of the alpha rhythm may persist (Radermecker, 1967). Other patients show diffuse low-voltage tracings as seen in cases of lower brainstem infarction (see Basilar Artery Thrombosis, above).

Cerebellar Hemorrhage

Acute cerebellar hemorrhage rapidly leads to coma after a few minutes of headaches, dizziness, or vertigo. Cerebellar edema rapidly produces a pressure cone (tonsillar herniation) with fatal outcome. The rapidity of the evolution usually precludes EEG studies. A remarkable study of 22 cases was carried out by Rasheva et al. (1981); it demonstrated high-voltage delta activity, more over the contralateral cerebral hemisphere. In patients with cerebellar stroke, movement-related cortical potentials were found to be depressed (Gerloff et al., 1996).

Chronically Recurrent Minor Strokes (Transient Ischemic Attacks, Cerebrovascular Insufficiency, Intracerebral Steal Syndromes)

Concepts of basic mechanisms in recurrent minor strokes have undergone marked changes over the past 50 years. Many of these attacks used to be ascribed to forms of neurosyphilis (in some cases, rightly) before vasospasm was widely regarded as the cause of transient neurological deficits. Vasospasm, however, was scarcely demonstrable in the bulk of CVA-producing cerebrovascular disorders. Denny-Brown (1960) stressed the role of hemodynamic factors and introduced the widely used term *cerebrovascular insufficiency,* usually caused by stenosing plaques in combination with a fall in systemic blood pressure. In such cases of transient cerebrovascular insufficiency, however, the possibility of microembolisms due to material from ulcerated plaques cannot be ruled out. Therefore, the term *transient ischemic attacks* (TIAs) is generally preferred now (Alajouanine et al., 1960; Marshall, 1964).

Hemiparetic Transient Ischemic Attacks (Internal Carotid or Middle Cerebral Artery Insufficiency)

Recurrent attacks of transient hemiparesis with or without speech difficulties are of great clinical interest, not simply as a sign of incipient cerebrovascular disease, but especially as a possible forerunner of a progressive internal carotid artery thrombosis. The present possibility of successful surgical treatment by endarterectomy or a bypass in the neck region means that these attacks have to be taken very seriously; the use of cranial arteriography must not be delayed. These attacks may be associated with ipsilateral amaurosis fugax when the ophthalmic artery is affected.

The EEG very often is normal in patients referred because of a recent transient ischemic attack. During the attack, there may be ipsilateral minor slow (mostly theta range) and somewhat sharp activity. According to Van der Drift and Kok (1972) prominent ipsilateral delta activity over the temporal region indicates that the recovery will take longer than 24 hours, even though the alpha rhythm may be completely preserved. In general, the EEG does not allow a differentiation between a rather harmless temporary insufficiency state of the middle cerebral artery and the onset of a progressive and life-threatening internal carotid thrombosis. With the progression of the latter, the EEG will show marked gradual increase of ipsilateral and eventually diffuse delta and theta activity.

Transient states of subacute to chronic insufficiency of the middle cerebral artery have been described by Gastaut et al. (1959) and Bruens et al. (1960). These states were associated with ipsilateral slowing in the delta and theta range. A predominance of normal records was noted by Silva and Gross (1983), while abnormal findings prevailed in the material of Kogeorgos and Scott (1981).

In patients with occlusion or high-grade stenosis of the common or internal carotid artery and a history of strokes or TIAs, contralateral arm and/or leg movements may occur, precipitated by standing, walking, or neck hyperextension (Yanagihara et al., 1985). According to these authors, these movements are not of epileptic character, as evidenced by unremarkable EEG findings during the motions.

Multi-Infarct Dementia

This is the final product of chronically recurrent minor lacunar strokes. Diffuse EEG slowing is present in these cases, mostly at a moderate, and sometimes at a severe, degree.

The differential diagnosis from Alzheimer-type senile dementia is very important, but unfortunately the EEG does not offer reliable distinctive criteria. Elevated serum copper has been suggested as diagnostic of Alzheimer-type dementia, being not elevated in multi-infarct dementia (Squitti et al., 2003).

Insufficiency of Vertebrobasilar Artery System

Symptoms of vertebrobasilar artery insufficiency are quite common in patients over age 45. In mild forms, such transient states may recur over four decades without leading to massive thrombosis with brainstem infarction.

The most common symptoms and signs are dizziness and light-headedness, vertigo, suboccipital headache, blurring of vision, and syncope. Less common are bilateral amaurosis fugax, drop attacks (syncope with sudden fall), cranial nerve deficits (V to XII), cerebellar ataxia, and long tract signs. Vertigo/dizziness is also the preeminent symptom in bilateral intracranial vertebral artery disease (Shin et al., 1999).

This symptomatology has been outlined by Siekert and Millikan (1955), Loeb et al. (1961), Loeb and Meyer (1965), Marshall (1972), and Toole and Patel (1974). Arteriosclerotic changes and cervical spondylosis ("spondylitic vertebral artery compression," Sheehan et al., 1960) are the most important pathogenic factors. Extreme head movements such as backing a car or screwing in a light bulb can trigger symptoms of vascular insufficiency in the presence of spondylitic changes.

In spite of the clinical evidence, the demonstration of corresponding hemodynamic deficit proved to be very difficult. Trouillas et al. (1991) eventually demonstrated indubitable "nuclear hemodynamic vertebrobasilar insufficiency" with xenon-133 inhalation, corroborated with positron emission tomography scan using intravenous technetium-99m-labeled hexamethylpropylene amine oxime.

A more chronically protracted form of mild vertebrobasilar artery insufficiency with mixed neuropsychiatric symptomatology was delineated by Niedermeyer (1960).

The EEG contributes to the diagnosis to a limited extent. According to Niedermeyer (1963), the records may be:

1. Completely normal and unremarkable;
2. Within broad normal limits but consistently of diffuse low-voltage character;
3. Same as 2, plus very pronounced photic driving response to flicker with unusually prominent responses to single flashes and a very wide range of driving; also perhaps a driven eye blink response (blink reflex);
4. Same as 2 or 3, plus sporadic runs of left anterior temporal-midtemporal minor slow and sharp activity, mostly on the left side (with this combination, the record may have to be considered as minimally or slightly abnormal); or
5. Within normal limits but with unusually pronounced alpha voltage; there may or may not be an enhanced photic driving response to flicker (Figs. 17.5 to 17.8).

The low-voltage type of record may be of mildly disorganized fast type with little or no organized posterior alpha rhythm; more seldom, alpha rhythm of consistently low voltage may be quite stable with good response to eye opening. With hyperventilation (to be done with caution), the low-voltage character remains unchanged, in contrast with the alpha improvement in some emotionally tense patients with low-voltage records. In sleep, the voltage of spindles, vertex waves, and K complexes and the background activity remain below average.

Thus, the EEG can contribute to the diagnosis of vertebrobasilar artery insufficiency but is far from being diagnostic or even specific. The limitations of its diagnostic value have been stressed by Oller-Daurella (1974). There are various causes of the desynchronized low-voltage character of an EEG (discussed in Chapter 9, "The Normal EEG of the Waking Adult"). Temporal minor slow and sharp activity is

Figure 17.5. Age 57 years. Chronic vertebrobasilar artery insufficiency (suffering from vertigo and depression). The generally predominant low-voltage fast record shows a very prominent photic driving response to intermittent photic stimulation. There is some spread into adjacent areas.

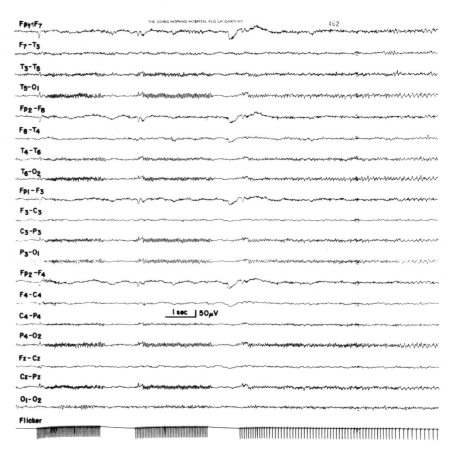

well known as a common pattern of old age, although its basis may be vascular or possibly hippocampic ischemia due to vertebrobasilar-posterior cerebral artery insufficiency (see below). The enhanced photic driving responses as such are absolutely nonspecific and probably caused by enhanced excitability of the mildly ischemic occipital cortex (Scheuler, 1983). The neurophysiological basis of the low-voltage character in vertebrobasilar artery insufficiency is obscure. Hypothetically, pontine ischemia could lead to a disturbance of the "synchronizing" pontine portion of the ascending brainstem reticular formation (described by Magnes et al., 1961) with subsequent impairment of cortical EEG synchronization. This explanation, however, is mere conjecture.

Recurrent Ictal States in Vertebrobasilar and Posterior Cerebral Artery Insufficiency

This is a rare condition; it is not discussed in EEG textbooks and is virtually unknown in the entire EEG literature. Such cases, however, are observed from time to time, and an understanding of the underlying disturbance can be very helpful. Naquet et al. (1961) has brought these cases into the open with strong de-emphasis on the epileptological facets. Further observations have been reported by Picornell et al. (1984).

These patients (most of them over age 50) may have mild attacks of dizziness, blurred vision, homonymous hemianopsia, or visual hallucinations. The EEG shows a status-like succession of ictal fast spike activity starting over the left or right occipital area with spread over the entire posterior quadrant and to the contralateral posterior regions. The attacks last about 30 to 90 seconds. The patients function fairly well despite the abundance of attacks. This condition may persist for days or even weeks without any significant consequences. Anticonvulsive medication is not needed and is probably of limited value. These patients are unlikely to have any other epileptic manifestations (Fig. 17.9). This recurrent pattern might be related to or even identical with the rhythmic and sharp contoured discharges described by Westmoreland and Klass (1981). These are also called subclinical rhythmic EEG discharge of adults (SREDA) by Miller et al. (1985).

Transient Global Amnesia

Transient states of severely impaired memory and confusion have been described by Bender (1956) as "episodes of confusion with amnesia" and by Fisher and Adams (1964) as "transient global amnesia." Further studies on this subject were presented by Jaffe and Bender (1966), Mumenthaler and Von Roll (1969), Steinmetz and Vroom (1972), Ganner (1974), Müller (1975), Kugler et al. (1975), Fogelholm et al. (1975), and on a larger scale by Mumenthaler et al. (1980), and Mumenthaler and Treig (1984).

The peak manifestation age lies around 50 to 60 years. The episodes last for several hours or a few days, and there is usually complete restitution of the massive retrograde am-

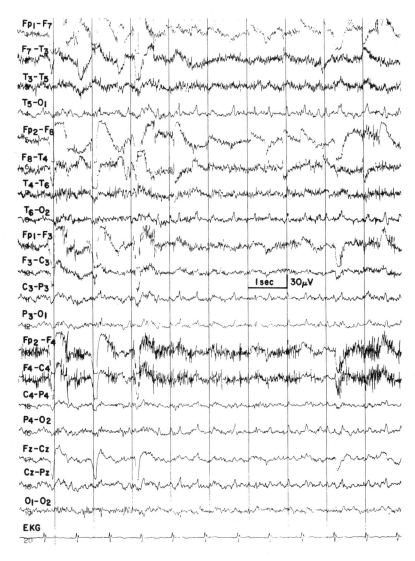

Figure 17.6. Same patient as in Fig. 17.5. Presentation of pictures evokes an unusually pronounced degree of occipital lambda wave activity. This and the enhanced photic driving response to flicker suggest heightened excitability of the central visual system.

nesia that dominates the clinical picture. The patients usually appear to be confused, but in some cases they act adequately during the entire episode; suddenly it dawns on them that they cannot recall any event during the amnestic period. The function of speech is preserved. There is some evidence of a cerebrovascular disorder in some of these patients: in others, however, the cause remains unclear. The most likely basis of global amnesia is a state of vertebrobasilar artery insufficiency associated with hippocampic ischemia; this view is supported by most authors. Fogelholm et al. (1975) assume an insufficiency of the anterior choroidal artery. A relationship to migraine has been stressed by Crowell et al. (1984).

The differential diagnosis depends heavily on the EEG. There is usually no major degree of slow activity; some minor slowing and also some rather unimpressive sharp and spiky transients may be recorded over the anterior temporal and midtemporal regions (Tharp, 1969). This author presumes a state of temporal lobe epilepsy caused by vertebrobasilar artery insufficiency. Petit mal absence status, which may also occur in the elderly, must be differentiated on the basis of the

EEG findings. The somewhat blurred boundary between vascular insufficiency states and prolonged epileptic manifestations in conditions such as status epilepticus, petit mal absence status, and psychomotor status is discussed further in Chapter 27, "Epileptic Seizure Disorders."

Most workers in the field agree that the EEG is normal in the interval and also during the attack in the majority of the cases. Normal records were obtained in 66% during the attack (Frank, 1981) and in practically 100% in the interval (Mumenthaler and Treig, 1984). By contrast, Logar et al. (1981) reported abnormal EEG findings in 18 out of 30 patients; the temporal region was most often involved. Most of their recordings were carried out during the interval.

According to Jacome (1989, 1990), who presented a review of the literature, transient global amnesia is a benign episodic disorder, rarely associated with structural lesion of the brain, but associated with isolated shorter memory loss with variable degrees of retrograde amnesia. This author feels that a vascular pathophysiological mechanism might underlie transient global amnesia, a mechanism similar to the one implicated in migraine. The EEG is believed to be

Figure 17.7. Same patient as in Figs. 17.5 and 17.6. In light drowsiness, the otherwise low-voltage activity is punctuated by stretches of medium 5–7/sec waves over the left anterior temporal-midtemporal region. This is a variant of "minor slow and sharp activity" usually found over the same region in early stages of cerebrovascular disorder.

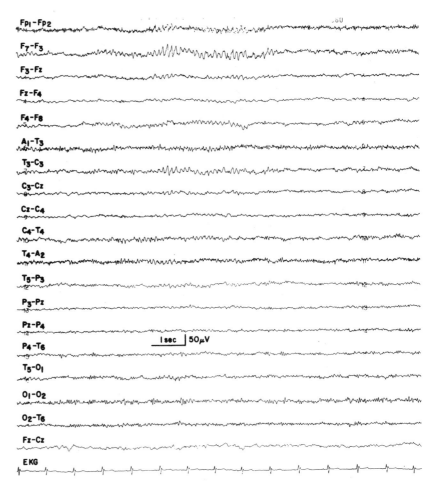

Figure 17.8. Age 53 years. Presumed chronic vertebrobasilar artery insufficiency in an early stage. The left portion of the figure shows unusually prominent and enhanced posterior alpha rhythm of above average voltage. The right portion shows a trace of left anterior temporal-midtemporal minor sharp and slow activity.

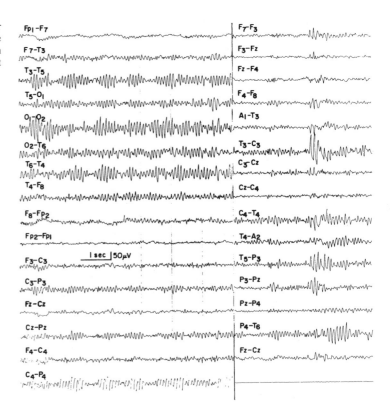

useful in discarding true or primary epileptic mechanisms and is normal in most cases. Secondary epileptic mechanisms may occur but are unusual. Treatment with antiepileptic drugs is not warranted and the recurrence rate is low.

In the wake of intravenous doses of diazepam, a special form of transient global amnesia may materialize. The EEG correlates have been investigated by Hynek et al. (1981) and show the expected increase of beta activity along with voltage reduction (desynchronization).

Intracerebral Steal Syndromes

The best known "steal" phenomenon is the *subclavian steal syndrome* (Toole, 1964), in which an occlusion of the left subclavian artery at its origin leads to a reversed blood flow in the left vertebral artery; this blood is siphoned into the left subclavian artery distal to the occlusion. The blood is hence derouted from its encephalic destination. An occlusion of the right innominate artery can lead to similar changes of the cerebral blood flow. EEG changes simply depend on the degree of the steal, which may produce minor or more prominent cerebral ischemia.

Steal syndromes also occur in a variety of intracranial conditions (Van der Drift and Kok, 1972). In an arteriovenous malformation, a redistribution of the circulating blood may lead to contralateral ischemia and to areas of EEG slowing on the structurally apparently (but not truly) uninvolved hemisphere.

EEG of Early Stages of Cerebrovascular Disorder

Local Slowing Over the Temporal Regions

With advancing age, local slowing over the temporal regions and especially in the anterior temporal and midtemporal areas is a very common finding. The slowing is usually quite subtle; brief trains of 3 to 8/sec waves are most often noted, but slow activity is often mixed with faster frequencies (mostly 9–14/sec). Mild to moderately sharp transients are very often intermingled. Instead of the mixed type of slow activity, one may observe rhythmical activity in the lower alpha range (7.5–9/sec), clearly separable from the posterior alpha rhythm (Kendel and Koufen, 1970). For unknown reasons, these temporal abnormalities are markedly lateralized to the left hemisphere in about 75% to 90%. Gibbs and Gibbs (1964) have described these patterns under the heading of "minimal temporal slow activity." Maynard and Hughes (1984) have stressed the rhythmical character of this pattern with the introduction of the term *bursts of rhythmical temporal theta.* However, this comprises only one aspect of minor temporal slow and sharp activity. Asokan et al. (1987) use the term *temporal minor slow and sharp activity.* The sharp component of this pattern needs further comment. It is sometimes hidden in the waking state but tends to appear in early drowsiness. In light non-rapid-eye-movement (NREM) sleep, the pattern may change to brief trains of

A

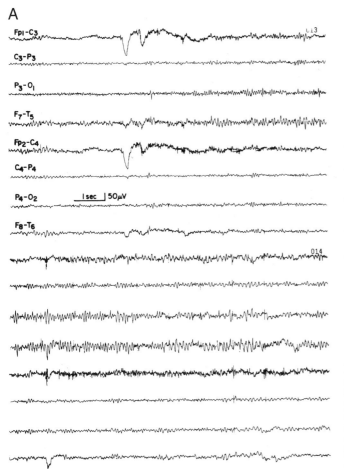

B

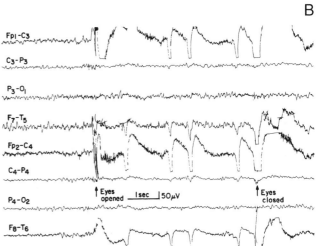

Figure 17.9. Age 67 years. Recent onset of right homonymous hemianopsia with hemianopic hallucinations. Presumed posterior cerebral artery insufficiency. **A:** Gradual buildup of rhythmical 12–15/sec activity over left posterior quadrant, slightly spreading to the right. *Lower portion* shows continuation of upper portion; there is gradual slowing of the rhythmical activity to 8–9/sec. **B:** Same patient, 10 seconds after the tracing in **A**. A posterior alpha rhythm in the 8–10/sec range has been restored; the blocking response to eye opening is poor on the left side and good on the right side.

rhythmical spiking over the anterior and midtemporal areas (discussed below under the heading of wicket spikes).

The occurrence of this pattern in normal middle aged and elderly population is high. In a study of 3,476 normal control subjects "minimal temporal slow activity" was encountered in 1.3% at ages 50 to 59 years and in 3.2% at above 60 years of age (Gibbs and Gibbs, 1964). Mundy-Castle (1962), Busse and Obrist (1963, 1965), Kooi et al. (1964), Otomo and Tsubaki (1966), Kazis et al. (1982), and Torres et al. (1983) demonstrated these changes in community volunteers with up to 30% to 40% showing evidence of temporal slowing. Similar data were reported in hospital populations (Revitch and Zallarski, 1969). In the mixed material (from birth to old age) of Asokan et al. (1987), the temporal changes ("minor slow and wharp activity") were found in 3.5%.

Is this pattern a sign of pathology? Is it associated with a particular cluster of clinical signs? According to Gibbs and Gibbs (1964), the activity is associated with nonspecific and often subjective complaints such as headache, dizziness, and mild signs of intellectual impairment. However, no significant differences between the memory function of normal elderly persons with and without temporal lobe foci were found (Drachman and Hughes, 1971; Obrist, 1971). There is usually no evidence of neurological deficit (Kooi et al., 1964). In some individuals, indubitable sharp waves and spikes replace the initially very minor sharp transients. These spikes and sharp waves are of remarkably low epileptogenicity, and most of these patients are completely seizure-free; caution is advised in order not to construe a case of temporal lobe epilepsy in the presence of symptoms such as dizziness, blurring of vision, and syncopes.

Decrease in cerebral blood flow has been suggested as the causative factor. Niedermeyer (1962, 1963) demonstrated minor temporal slow and sharp activity in a sizable number of patients with chronic vertebrobasilar artery insufficiency. In the study of Maynard and Hughes (1984), there is evidence that rhythmical temporal theta is associated with cerebrovascular disorder in the absence of major neurological disease. Visser et al. (1987) and Asokan et al. (1987) also support the view that this pattern is caused by cerebrovascular problems and not simply by old age. The possibility of hippocampal ischemia has been raised but there is no convincing evidence for this assumption. In spite of the established relation between EEG frequency and cerebral blood flow (Ingvar et al., 1976), there is no consensus regarding the best parameters for assessing ischemia. Based on quantified EEG data, the correlation is poorer for theta than for alpha and delta activity (Nagata et al., 1984).

Some reports stress a female predominance (Asokan et al., 1987; Hughes and Cayaffa, 1977), suggesting hormonal involvement. Sexual hormones influence cerebral excitability; estrogen increases and progestin decreases cortical excitability (Holmes and Donaldson, 1987). Receptors show a differential distribution throughout the brain modulated by the neuroendocrine climate (Pfaff and McEwen, 1983). The amygdala and hippocampus show only few progestin receptors, still further decreasing at menopause. In some patients and/or conditions, this reduction might become critical, especially in the presence of other factors, genetic or vascular. This may eventually induce subclinical EEG signs of local-

ized increased excitability or new late-onset generalized absence seizures in elderly women. These mechanisms are still speculative and need further research. There is no satisfactory mechanism to explain the vast preponderance of left temporal theta foci (Arenas et al., 1986).

A temporal lobe pattern of dysfunction has been noted on the basis of psychological assessment in persons with cognitive decline (Butters et al., 1996).

Unusual Patterns Associated with Drowsiness and Marginal Patterns of Sleep

Anterior Bradyrhythmia

Sequences of bilateral anterior slow activity in the delta range (mostly 1.5–2.5/sec) are sometimes noticed in the tracings of aging individuals. These trains of delta waves are fairly rhythmical but do not assume strictly monorhythmical character; their maximum clearly lies over the frontal areas with some spread into central and anterior temporal regions. Their duration varies between 2 and 10 seconds, and the voltage output may be considerable. The pattern has been termed "anterior bradyrhythmia" by Gibbs and Gibbs (1964). More recently, Katz and Horowitz (1983) have presented a study on "sleep onset" frontal intermittent rhythmical delta activity (FIRDA) in a normal geriatric population. These authors rightly distinguish sleep onset FIRDA from "true" FIRDA and point out that the former occurs in normal elderly persons, whereas the latter represents an abnormal condition. Unfortunately, Katz and Horowitz were not aware of the already existing term *anterior bradyrhythmia,* which certainly denotes the same phenomenon.

Prevalence and incidence of this pattern in a healthy elderly population are unknown. With a strict waking EEG routine, this pattern may be missed because it is most often seen in drowsiness or light sleep. This pattern is less rhythmical than frontal intermittent delta waves in patients with space-occupying lesions, a pattern of the waking state, subsiding in sleep. Further information on the distinction of anterior bradyrhythmia from FIRDA is found in the studies of Zurek et al. (1985) and Shiohama et al. (1993).

The pathological significance of this pattern is uncertain and the underlying mechanisms unknown. There is reason to presume that a mild arousing stimulus triggers the train of delta waves. The pattern is not consistently present and may reflect transient states of deterioration in the health of an elderly person, such as caused by infection, trauma, or minor stroke. Gibbs and Gibbs (1964) feel that vascular disease is the usual cause of this activity, although the reported symptom profiles are nonspecific.

Wicket Spikes

Wicket spikes (or wicket waves) consist of trains of monophasic arciform waveforms or single spike-like waveforms that resemble mu (wicket) activity. The wicket waves have a frequency of 6 to 11 Hz and range from 60 to 200 µV in amplitude (Reiher and Lebel, 1977). Wicket waves occur bilaterally or independently over the temporal regions or they may occur predominantly on one side, usually the left. When they occur as a simple waveform, they must be differentiated from a spike discharge. Wicket spikes are best seen during drowsiness and light sleep and tend to disappear with deepening sleep. Wicket spikes occur predominantly in adults usually older than 50 years; their clinical significance is rather minor but this pattern is not altogether irrelevant and could signal some degree of cerebrovascular problems. They are presented by some as a sleep variant of temporal minor slow and sharp activity (Asokan et al., 1987).

Subclinical Rhythmic Electrographic Discharge of Adults

The pattern consists of sharp-contoured or sinusoidal theta waveforms in the range of 5 to 7 Hz occurring in a widespread distribution with maximal expression over the parietotemporal regions. The pattern is usually bilateral, but it may be asymmetric, its duration ranges from seconds to minutes. The onset may be abrupt or the discharge may progressively build up; it may end abruptly or subside gradually.

It is an uncommon subclinical rhythmic pattern occurring in less than 0.5% of a general EEG laboratory population older than 50 years (Miller et al., 1985). It usually occurs during wakefulness or drowsiness but has been recorded during stage 2 NREM sleep. There is no correlation with a history of epileptic seizures. It was initially thought to be associated with vascular insufficiency by Naquet et al. (1965). Although the underlying mechanisms remain uncertain, it is probably a benign EEG pattern with little diagnostic significance (Westmoreland and Klass, 1981, 1997).

Arterial Hypertension and Chronic Progressive States of Cerebral Arteriosclerosis (Status Lacunaris)

Arterial Hypertension

In essential as well as in renal hypertension, the clinical symptomatology of nervous tension, brief periods of dizziness, vertigo, headache, and angiospastic retinal changes is usually unassociated with EEG abnormalities. Normal EEG findings in the vast majority of these cases have been reported by Bagchi et al. (1950), Jost et al. (1952), Obrist et al. (1961), and Gibbs and Gibbs (1964). In advanced stages of arterial hypertension, Krump (1953) found runs of frontal theta waves (5–7/sec). Christian (1975) observed episodes of critical hypertensive bouts (up to 280/150 mm Hg) without concomitant EEG changes. Böhm et al. (1967) noticed gradual slowing of the alpha frequency in advanced stages; Mitschke (1969) reported the development of focal or diffuse EEG abnormalities with the progression of the disease.

In old age, arterial hypertension as such has little or no effect on the EEG, whereas hypotension in arteriosclerotic individuals often gives rise to EEG changes, neurological deficits, and dementia (Harvald, 1958; Obrist et al., 1961; Turton, 1958).

With the use of induced arterial systemic hypertension during carotid endarterectomy, Bassi et al. (1984) noted normalization of preexisting focal EEG changes.

Hypertensive Encephalopathy

In this condition, severe arterial hypertension gives rise to cerebral edematous changes and hence to signs of intracra-

nial hypertension. Headache may reach an excruciating degree, especially in the morning, augmented by coughing and straining and sometimes accompanied by vomiting. Transient attacks of blindness may occur, and generalized as well as focal epileptic seizures may materialize. Papilledema with retinal arteriolar spasms and hemorrhages is common. The condition may progress into somnolence, delirium, stupor, and coma (Toole and Patel, 1974).

The EEG may show surprisingly little in this serious cerebral disorder. There is reason to presume that the neuronal oxygenation does not reach critically low values in spite of the fact that the cerebral blood flow is diminished in this condition (Heine, 1953). In the case of epileptic convulsions, EEG changes are usually limited to the period immediately before, during, and after the attacks. This is akin to the acute encephalopathy of eclampsia gravidarum, where EEG abnormalities are barely detectable in the preeclamptic state and are practically limited to the grand mal convulsions themselves.

However, there have been reports of very pronounced EEG abnormalities in hypertensive encephalopathy. Aguglia et al. (1984) described severe parieto-occipital changes with prominent paroxysmal features. After acute onset of hypertensive encephalopathy (blood pressure of 300/140 and age 70), Benna et al. (1984) observed generalized spikes and polyspikes followed by a slow wave. With gradual improvement of hypertension, the paroxysmal pattern lingered on. Figure 17-10 shows marked diffuse slowing in a patient with hypertensive encephalopathy.

There is also a form of hypertensive encephalopathy associated with moderate hypertension; it is also found in conjunction with renal insufficiency. It causes a reversible posterior leucoencephalopathy without infarction (Hickey et al., 1996).

Chronic Diffuse Cerebral Arteriosclerosis (Atherosclerosis) and Lacunar States

Milder forms of diffuse cerebral arteriosclerosis are characterized by memory impairment, dizziness, light-headedness, vertigo, blurring of vision, and suboccipital headache. This condition is usually based on the principal symptomatology of vertebrobasilar artery insufficiency (see above), in addition to more or less serious decline of memory functions. *Runs of mixed slow and medium frequency activity with intermingled sharp transients* occur over anterior temporal-midtemporal areas, in most cases on the left. This pattern has been well known since the earlier work of Strauss et al. (1952) and Busse et al. (1954). The work of Visser et al. (1987) and Asokan et al. (1987) has shed more light on this pattern and its relationship to cerebrovascular disorder in its early stages.

Advancing cerebral arteriosclerosis gradually leads to *slowing of the alpha rhythm* and to *diffuse slowing* with general increase of theta and delta frequencies. These abnormalities are quite common in elderly patients. Differentiation from neurofibrillary senile/presenile dementias may become impossible at this stage.

Sleep and arousal mechanism need some discussion. A routine sleep EEG of a patient with advanced diffuse cerebral arteriosclerosis shows *frequent brief catnap-like periods of*

Figure 17.10. Age 42 years. Hypertensive encephalopathy with epileptic seizures. Note diffuse slowing, which is briefly attenuated with a mental task.

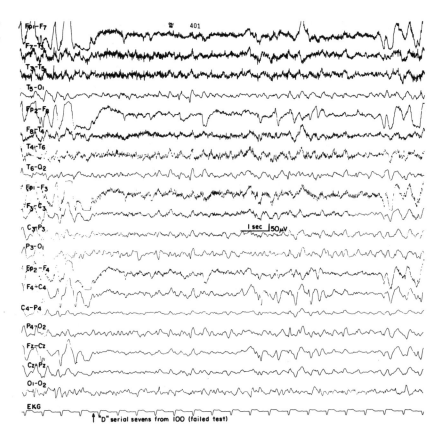

sleep. These episodes of light non-REM (stage 2) sleep show abrupt onset and abrupt termination; their duration may be less than 10 seconds. Drowsy states are virtually skipped, and a waking state with alpha rhythm and light sleep with spindles may be seen on the same page of the tracing. It could be hypothesized that this instability of the sleep-waking regulation is caused by ischemic states in the ascending brainstem reticular formation. The same disturbance may also account for nocturnal restlessness and agitation.

Lacunar states (status lacunaris) are determined by a special type of pathology that tends to evolve in elderly hypertensive arteriosclerotics. Multiple irregular cavities (0.5–15 mm in size) are found, chiefly in basal ganglia, pons, thalamus, and white matter, but not in the cerebral cortex (Toole and Patel, 1974). A minor stroke may result in altered cerebral vasoregulation, which increases the risk for further strokes (Novak et al., 2003).

The clinical symptomatology of lacunar states has been studied extensively by Fisher (1965, 1967, 1969), who described a variety of syndromes with marked bilateral white matter lacunar formation. According to Kappelle and Van Huffelen (1989), the EEG is quite useful in the assessment of recent lacunar infarctions; their impressions seem to be based on alpha/mu rhythm asymmetries and amplitude differences rather than on spectacular delta foci. A rather limited value of EEG in lacunar infarctions was reported by Labar et al. (1989a). States of *pseudobulbar palsy* occur with bilateral lower cranial nerve signs, dysarthria, dyspha-

gia, dementia, and reflex-like spells of crying. Patients with lacunar states may become very rigid with pseudo-parkinsonian features. The EEG is not contributory in these conditions; uncharacteristic low-voltage activity or diffuse slowing may be present.

Lacunar states often result in *multi-infarct dementia.* The EEG correlates have been investigated by Logar et al. (1983), who found a strong predominance of abnormal findings. Excessive slowing often exhibits focal features, in contrast to Alzheimer-type dementias.

In rare form of *subcortical arteriosclerotic encephalopathy (Binswanger's type)* (Burger et al., 1976; Olszewski, 1962), slow progression of mental deterioration is associated with aphasia, hemiparesis, sensory deficits, and visual field cuts. There is severe atheromatosis in small arteries of white matter and basal ganglia. In a pathologically confirmed case, White (1979) and Hacke et al. (1982) noted periodic discharges in the EEG over the chiefly involved hemisphere.

Epileptic seizure disorder with chronically recurrent attacks may be the consequence of advancing cerebrovascular disease. According to Fischer (1959), epileptic seizures requiring neuropsychiatric admission occur in 4% of patients with cerebrovascular disorders.

The role of the temporal lobe and Ammon's horn lesions has been stressed (Niedermeyer, 1958; Takahashi et al., 1965), with emphasis on left-sided foci. Clinically epileptogenic lesions seemingly evolve from milder temporal lobe disturbances, which so abundantly produce minor slow and sharp activity over the temporal lobe. The chronically recurrent seizure disorder of late onset must be separated from the acute convulsive states seen mainly in watershed ischemias.

Subarachnoid Hemorrhage (Intracranial Aneurysms, Arteriovenous Malformations, and Other Causes)

The extremely dramatic symptomatology of a subarachnoid hemorrhage with acute meningeal signs does not need special discussion. Cranial nerve deficits are quite common. In more severe cases, there is evidence of cerebral involvement with impairment of consciousness and, in about 10% to 20% of the cases, epileptic seizures.

The EEG shows diffuse changes, disorganization, disruption of the posterior alpha rhythm, and excessive slow activity. Occasionally, lateralization of slow activity may be indicative of the primarily involved hemisphere (Christian, 1975; Daly and Markand, 1990; Roseman et al., 1951). With total dependence on arteriographic demonstration of the causative lesion and partial dependence on refined CT scan methods, there is no practical need for an EEG in the search for the correct localization. The EEG, however, remains a valuable indicator of the general state of cerebral functioning (Labar et al., 1989b; Logar et al., 1982).

The patient's general condition seriously deteriorates when subarachnoid bleeding is followed by vasospasm. The pathogenesis of such widespread vasospasm is poorly understood (Echlin, 1965; Heros et al., 1983; Levitt, 1970). According to Kiloh et al. (1972), marked delta foci occur in areas of massive vasospasm. Such secondary lesions are sometimes associated with sharp activity (Van der Drift and Kok, 1972). Prolonged vasospasm and a decrease of cerebral blood flow may lead to dementia and diffuse cerebral atrophy. The area of massive vasospasm correlates with the area of local EEG slowing (Rumpl et al., 1977).

Ruptured bifurcation aneurysms (circle of Willis and vicinity) are the most common cause of subarachnoid hemorrhage. Margerison et al. (1970) carried out extensive EEG studies in 70 patients with ruptured aneurysms in a search for valid localizing signs.

Massive bleeding from a ruptured aneurysm into the cerebral parenchyma is prognostically ominous and can be fatal within less than 1 hour. The EEG pattern of intracerebral hematomas resulting from such bleeding was studied by Van der Drift (1972). Regional polymorphic delta activity was found to be more pronounced than in acute middle cerebral artery ischemia.

In survivors of subarachnoid hemorrhages from aneurysms, epileptic seizures have been found in 12.5% (Walton, 1953); marked EEG changes with spikes are also found (Kiloh et al., 1972). Scott and Cabral (1975) stressed the frequent occurrence of epileptic seizures following intracranial aneurysm surgery (clipping, wrapping).

Survivors of subarachnoid bleeding from an aneurysm of the anterior communicating artery sometimes develop severe personality changes and dementia. Their state of apathy and loss of drive is not associated with typical EEG changes.

Severe frontal and hypothalamic (deep perforating branches of anterior cerebral artery) lesions might account for this lamentable clinical picture.

Arteriovenous malformations or arteriovenous aneurysms are the cause of subarachnoid hemorrhages that are much less severe and life threatening than is bleeding from a ruptured aneurysm. These malformations may also give rise to focal or generalized epileptic seizures that usually start between ages 10 and 35.

The EEG of patients with arteriovenous malformations has been described as abnormal in all observed cases (Husby et al., 1953). The interpretation of the abnormalities is beset with difficulties, because a sizable number of cases may show an "erroneous" lateralization with slowing or sharp activity over the "wrong" hemisphere (Groethuysen et al., 1955; Mosmans and Jonkman, 1980; Walton, 1994; Yeh et al., 1990). As impractical as such findings may be, their pathophysiological substratum is not devoid of clinical interest, since the misleading lateralization is determined by intracerebral steal phenomena. In the writer's personal experience, even a very large arteriovenous malformation may be found without any EEG abnormality. This evidently indicates the lack of consistent hypoxic impairment of the cortical function.

Subarachnoid bleeding may occur without demonstrable cause. In some cases, the source of bleeding consists of aneurysmatic widening of a bacterially infected artery (arteritis leading to a "mycotic" aneurysm). Bacterial endocarditis is usually the cause of this type of vascular pathology. During treatment with endovascular embolization, EEG monitoring may detect clinical hazards (Paiva et al., 1995).

Intracranial Venous Thrombosis

In the era of antibiotic therapy, episodes of infectious intracranial venous thrombosis and thrombophlebitis have become rare. Complicated ear infections (transverse sinus) or facial carbuncles (cavernous sinus) occasionally cause such a progression of infectious material into the venous system of the cranial cavity. Complications of abortion are another cause; widespread cortical venous thrombosis may develop intrapartum. Reviews of the field have been presented by Garcin and Pestel (1949), Dubois (1956), Huhn (1957, 1969), and Carter (1972).

EEG changes in *cortical venous thrombosis intrapartum* can be very pronounced, with widespread prominent delta activity; these patients are not necessarily in a state of impaired consciousness but show marked changes of higher cortical functions, such as aphasia, mutism, or apraxia, and the course of ensuing recovery may be very slow (Fig. 17.11).

Literature on the EEG in cerebrovenous pathology is scanty. The work of Huhn (1957), Lemmi and Little (1960), Franco (1961), and Hubach and Struck (1965) has been particularly informative. Van der Drift and Kok (1972) demonstrated the underlying pathophysiological mechanisms as well as the correlations of EEG and venous pathology. Focal slowing and ictal epileptic activity have been reported (Griewing et al., 1991).

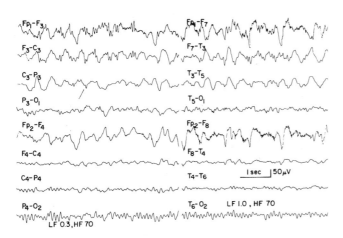

Figure 17.11. Age 20 years. Central nervous system (CNS) complication postabortion, probably due to cerebral venous thrombosis. The patient exhibited decorticate posturing and convulsions in the acute state. The EEG was done 3 weeks after the acute stage. The patient was quite alert during the recording, but there was marked global aphasia. Note lateralization of delta activity to left hemisphere; also note left-sided alpha depression and/or suppression.

Cerebrovascular Involvement in Connective Tissue Diseases

Systemic lupus erythematosus gives rise to neurological signs and symptoms in 25% to 35% of the patients (Aita, 1975). This is due to small patchy vessel involvement. Convulsions and psychotic episodes are the most common CNS changes. About 2% to 5% of the patients with lupus erythematosus develop cerebrovascular syndromes with occlusion and focal cerebral deficit (Aita, 1975).

The EEG in CNS complication of lupus erythematosus is determined by the severity of clinical neurological deficits and may range from normal to markedly abnormal findings of either focal or diffuse character.

EEG studies of systemic lupus erythematosus and other collagen or connective tissue diseases such as periarteritis nodosa, scleroderma, giant cell arteritis, or rheumatoid arthritis have been scanty (Krump, 1955; Stein and Stava, 1961; Taylor and Pacella, 1949; see also Gibbs and Gibbs, 1964). According to Finn et al. (1980), the EEG is useful in the early detection of this disease. Kogeorgos and Scott (1982) studied 74 cases; EEG abnormalities were present in 79%. Gottwald and Sturm (1984) reported abnormal records in 78% of 40 patients. The EEG abnormalities consist of focal or diffuse slowing, spikes or sharp waves of focal or multifocal character, and "dysrhythmic phenomena." Glanz et al. (1998) reported a history of seizures in 19.9% of patients with systemic lupus erythematosus (95 out of 478). These authors were struck by the lateralization of EEG abnormalities to the left hemisphere (79.6% to the left, 7.4% to the right, and 13% bilaterally). In another study, Glanz et al. (2001) confirmed the lateralization and stressed the left temporal maximum of the abnormalities. Interestingly, this distribution is not much different from that of the pattern known anterior temporal-midtemporal minor slow and sharp activity, which is so common in early stages of cerebrovascular disorder (see above).

In *Wegener's granulomatosis,* CNS involvement is less common than in lupus erythematosus. EEG abnormalities may occur; metabolic (renal) causes have to be ruled out (Molaie and Fariello, 1981). In *morphea* (localized scleroderma), epileptic seizures are fairly common (25%), and both epileptic and nonepileptic EEG abnormalities are three times as common as in age-matched control population (Hwang et al., 1981).

In *Sjögren's syndrome,* the CNS may be affected by an aseptic meningoencephalitis (Alexander and Alexander, 1983). Cognitive disturbances and dementia may also be caused by vasculitis, which is treatable with corticosteroids in high dosages (Caselli et al., 1991). These authors also found diffuse EEG abnormalities in a patient with vasculitis. In a personal observation, I saw a diffuse low-voltage record with sporadic anterior temporal spikes (mainly on the left), although there was no convincing evidence of epileptic seizures.

Other Types of Vascular Disease

In *thromboangiitis obliterans cerebri,* temporary focal delta activity may be found over areas of recent cortical damage, but these changes disappear quickly; the EEG is probably of little diagnostic value in this disease (Bernsmeier and Held, 1972). EEG findings are also regarded as noncontributory in patients with *moyamoya disease* (Nishimoto and Takeuchi, 1972). According to Aoki et al. (1977), a reappearance of the hyperventilation-induced buildup of slow activity approximately 20 to 60 seconds after the activation is a typical finding in moyamoya disease. This phenomenon has been studied more extensively by Ohyama et al. (1983). Hyperventilation may induce transient ischemic attacks along with limb shaking in *moyamoya* disease (Kim et al., 2003).

Granulomatous angiitis (Cravioto and Feigin, 1959; Kolodny et al., 1968) is a progressive and fatal disease. Prominent diffuse or local slowing of the EEG is a common finding.

In *sickle cell anemia,* neurological complications may occur occasionally. Impairment of consciousness, convulsions, and neurological deficits may prevail for several days or weeks. Marked EEG changes are noted (Hill et al., 1950; Gibbs and Gibbs, 1964). Focal slowing was found to be more impressive than the corresponding neurological symptomatology, with considerable attenuation of the EEG changes during sleep (Neidengard and Niedermeyer, 1975).

Neurological and electroencephalographic changes due to *blood diseases* are discussed under the headings of metabolic encephalopathies (in Chapter 22) and brain tumors in neuro-oncology (in Chapter 15). Briefly, intracerebral hematomas are not uncommon in hemophilia, thrombocytopenia, and leukemia. In such cases, marked focal or diffuse slowing is found in the EEG.

Cerebral Manifestations of Cardiac Diseases

Basic Considerations

Cardiac diseases and dysfunctions can impair the brain in various ways with a wide variety of pathological changes.

Only a part of the CNS lesions and disturbances caused by cardiac problems falls into the category of cerebrovascular disorder. Cerebrovascular phenomena such as arterial embolism are inseparably associated with bacterial infections such as cerebritis and brain abscess. In other cases, one is dealing with hypoxic-anoxic cerebral pathology, especially in complications of open heart surgery.

Congenital Heart Disease

Neurological disturbances are quite frequent in patients with congenital heart disease. According to Tyler and Clark (1957), neurological deficits occur in 25%, blackout spells in 12%, and convulsions in 6% of the cases. It is therefore no surprise that abnormal EEG tracings are fairly common in congenital heart disease (Beaussart et al., 1961; Bekény et al., 1963; Kalyanaraman et al., 1968; Lesny et al., 1961; Losev, 1958; Shev and Robinson, 1958, 1961).

Brain abscess is a well-known complication of congenital heart disease, especially in infancy and early childhood. Focal polymorphic delta activity is usually very prominent in these abscesses. This type of brain abscess is unassociated with endocarditis and dissemination of infected emboli. Diffuse cerebral hypoxia may give rise to impairment of consciousness and marked diffuse slowing in the EEG. Focal slowing may also occur. Such hypoxic lesion may gradually become epileptogenic (Kalyanaraman et al., 1968; Niedermeyer, 1972).

Cerebral hypoxia may develop in cyanotic as well as in noncyanotic forms of congenital heart disease, but it is more frequently found in the former.

Acquired Heart Disease

CNS complications of acute or subacute bacterial endocarditis are essentially infectious diseases and are discussed under that heading (in Chapter 16). In *cardiac decompensation,* a variety of causes and mechanisms eventually lead to cerebral hypoxia with slowing and terminal flattening of the EEG (Gibbs and Gibbs, 1964; Krump, 1958; Obrist and Bissell, 1955).

EEG abnormalities are common in *chronic bronchopneumopathy* with *cor pulmonale.* These changes may (Davidson and Jefferson, 1959) or may not parallel the degree of impaired consciousness (Goulon et al., 1961).

Paroxysmal tachycardia may be associated with transient EEG abnormalities (Subbotnik et al., 1955; Tucker and Yoe, 1956), especially when the attack leads to impairment of consciousness. Walsh et al. (1968) emphasized paroxysmal cerebral discharges in conjunction with *paroxysmal atrial tachycardia,* which was considered secondary to the cerebral events.

The *Adams-Stokes syndrome* is usually associated with a permanent heart block and a very slow pulse rate. The electroencephalographer is advised to use EEG monitoring throughout the recording. During the attack, slow activity appears after a few seconds of asystolia with progressive amplitude of delta waves (Broser, 1958) (see also Chapter 28, "Nonepileptic Attacks," Fig. 28.1).

References

Abbott, J.A., and Bautista, P.C. 1949. Electroencephalographic findings in various types of vascular accidents. Electroencephalogr. Clin. Neurophysiol. 1:252(abst).

Adams, R.D., and Van der Eecken, H.M. 1953. Vascular diseases of the brain. Ann. Reo. Med. 4:213–252.

Aguglia, U., Tinuper, P., Farnarier, G., et al. 1984. Electroencephalographic and anatomo-clinical evidences of posterior cerebral damage to hypertensive encephalopathy. Clin. Electroencephalogr. 15:53–60.

Aita, J.A. 1975. *Neurologic Manifestations of General Diseases.* Springfield, IL: Charles C Thomas.

Alajouanine, T., Lecasble, R., and Remond, A. 1955. Éléments graphiques paroxystiques lents de survénue périodiques. Corrélations électrocliniques. Rev. Neurol. (Paris) 93:477–478.

Alajouanine, T., Castaigne, P., and Lhermitte, F. 1957. Physiopathologie des accidents vasculaires cérébraux. In *La Thérapeutique des Affections Vasculaires Cérébrales.* Paris: Masson.

Alajouanine, T., Castaigne, P., Lhermitte, F., et al. 1959. Les obstructions bilatérales de la carotide interne. Sem. Hôp. Paris 35:1149–1160.

Alajouanine, T., Lhermitte, F., and Gautier, J.C. 1960. Transient cerebral ischemia in atherosclerosis. Neurology (Minneapolis) 10:906–914.

Alajouanine, T., Castaigne, P., Lhermitte, F., et al. 1961. Factors inducing ischemic cerebro-vascular accidents in arteriosclerosis. In *Cerebral Anoxia and the Electroencephalogram,* Eds. H. Gastaut and J.S. Meyer, pp. 172–179. Springfield, IL: Charles C Thomas.

Alexander, E.L., and Alexander, G.E. 1983. Aseptic meningoencephalitis in primary Sjögren syndrome. Neurology 33:593–598.

Aoki, Y., Hiraga, H., and Ichijo, S. 1977. EEG of moyamoya disease. Electroencephalogr. Clin. Neurophysiol. 43:490(abst).

Arboix, A., Comes, E., Massons, J., et al. 1996. Relevance of early seizures for in-hospital mortality in acute cerebrovascular disease. Neurology 47:1429–1435.

Arenas, A.M., Brenner, R.P., and Reynolds, C.F. 1986. Temporal slowing in the elderly revisited. Am. J. EEG Technol. 26:105–114.

Asokan, G., Pareja, J., and Niedermeyer, E. 1987. Temporal minor slow and sharp EEG activity and cerebrovascular disorder. Clin. Electroencephalogr. 18:201–210.

Back, T., Hoehn, M., Mies, G., et al. 2000. Penumbra tissue alkalosis in focal cerebral ischemia: relationship to energy metabolism in blood flow and steady potential. Ann. Neurol. 47:485–492.

Bagchi, B.K., Kooi, K.A., Hoobler, S.W., et al. 1950. Electroencephalographic findings in hypertension. I. Correlation with clinical status. Univ. Mich. Med. Bull. 16:92–103.

Baker, A.B., Dahl, E., and Sandler, S. 1963. Cerebrovascular disease. Etiologic factors in cerebral infarction. Neurology (Minneapolis) 13:445–454.

Barolin, C., Scherzer, E., Naquet, R., et al. 1962. Étude électroclinique des états de mal épileptiques survénant chez les apolectiques. Rev. Neurol. (Paris) 107:242–243.

Barré, J.A., Rohmer, F., and Isch, F. 1950. Étude électroencéphalographique des thromboses de la carotide interne. Rev. Neurol. (Paris) 82:568–571.

Bassi, P., Feller, S., and Sbrascini, S. 1984. Focal EEG changes normalized by induced arterial systemic hypertension during carotid endarterectomy. Electroencephalogr. Clin. Neurophysiol. 58:73P(abst).

Bauer, G., Gerstenbrand, F., and Rumpl, E. 1979. Varieties of the locked-in syndrome. J. Neurol. 221:77–92.

Beaussart, M., Dupuis, D., and Dupuis, R. 1961. Electroencephalographic studies of cyanotic congenital heart disease. In *Cerebral Anoxia and the Electroencephalogram,* Eds. H. Gastaut and J.S. Meyer. Springfield, IL: Charles C Thomas.

Bekény, G., Horányi, B., Péter, A., et al. 1963. Elektroenzephalographische Untersuchungen bei kongenitalen Herzfehlern. In *Jenenser EEG-Symposion,* 30 Jahre Elektroenzephalographie, pp. 194–200. Berlin: VER Verlag Volk und Gesundheit.

Bender, M.B. 1956. Syndrome of isolated episode of confusion with amnesia. J. Hillside Hosp. 5:212–215.

Benna, P., Bergamini, L., Tarenzi, L., et al. 1984. Hypertensive encephalopathy: association with unusual EEG changes. Electroencephalogr. Clin. Neurophysiol. 58:74P(abst).

Berlit, P., Bühler, B., and Krause, K.H. 1988. EEG findings in borderline infarcts. Electroencephalogr. Clin. Neurophysiol. 69:4P(abst).

Bernsmeier, A., and Held, K. 1972. Thromboangiitis obliterans cerebri. In *Handbook of Neurology,* vol. 11, Eds. P.J. Vinken and G.W. Bruyn, pp. 292–326; vol. 12, pp. 384–397; Amsterdam: North-Holland.

Biemond, A. 1951. Thrombosis of the basilar artery. Brain 74:300–317.

Birchfield, R.I., Heyman, A., and Wilson, W. 1959. An evaluation of electroencephalography in vertebral infarction and ischemia due to arteriosclerosis. Neurology (Minneapolis) 9:859–870.

Böhm, H., Trlica, J., and Veljacikova, N. 1967. The EEG in different phases of essential vascular hypertension. Electroencephalogr. Clin. Neurophysiol. 22:286–287(abst).

Bradshaw, P., and Parsons, M. 1965. Hemiplegic migraine: a clinical study. Q. J. Med. 34:65–85.

Broser, F. 1958. *Die cerebralen vegetativen Anfälle.* Berlin: Springer.

Bruens, J.H., Gastaut, H., and Giove, G. 1960. Electroencephalographic study of the signs of chronic vascular insufficiency of the Sylvian region in aged people. Electroencephalogr. Clin. Neurophysiol. 12:283–295.

Burger, P.C., Burch, J.G., and Kunze, U. 1976. Subcortical arteriosclerotic encephalopathy (Binswanger's disease). Stroke 7:626–631.

Busse, E.W., and Obrist, W.D. 1963. Significance of focal electroencephalographic changes in the elderly. Post Grad. Med. 34:179–182.

Busse, E.W., and Obrist, W.D. 1965. Pre-senescent electroencephalographic changes in normal subjects. J. Gerontol. 20:315–320.

Busse, E.W., Barnes, R.H., Silverman, A.J., et al. 1954. Studies of the process of aging: factors that influence the psyche of elderly persons. Am. J. Psychiatry 110:897–908.

Butters, M.A., Lopez, O.L., and Becker, J.T. 1996. Focal temporal lobe dysfunction in probable Alzheimer's disease predicts a slow rate of cognitive decline. Neurology 46:687–692.

Carreras, M., Angeleri, F., and Urbani, M. 1955. L'electtroencefalografia nelle diagnosi differenziali delle malattie cerebrovascolari occlusive. Riv. Neurobiol. 112:213–236.

Carter, A.B. 1972. Clinical aspects of infarction. In *Handbook of Neurology,* Eds. P.J. Vinken and G.W. Bruyn, pp. 292–326. Amsterdam: North-Holland.

Caselli, R.J., Scheithauer, B.W., Bowles, C.A., et al. 1991. The treatable dementia of Sjögren syndrome. Ann. Neurol. 30:98–101.

Chase, T.N., Moretti, L., and Prensky, E.L. 1968. Clinical and electroencephalographic manifestations of vascular lesions of the pons. Neurology (Minneapolis) 18:357–365.

Chatrian, G.E., Shaw, G.M., and Leffman, H. 1964. The significance of periodic lateralized epileptiform discharges: an electrographic, clinical and pathological study. Electroencephalogr. Clin. Neurophysiol. 17:177–193.

Chen, J., and Simon, R. 1997. Ischemic tolerance in the brain. Neurology 48:306–311.

Christian, W. 1975. *Klinische Elektroenzephalographie,* 2nd ed. Stuttgart: Thieme.

Corić, B., Mihajlović, M., Jagodic, D., et al. 1981. EEG correlates in carotid artery occlusion. Electroencephalogr. Clin. Neurophysiol. 52: 14P(abst).

Cravioto, H., and Feigin, I. 1959. Non-infectious granulomatous angiitis with a predilection for the nervous system. Neurology (Minneapolis) 9: 599–609.

Cravioto, H., Rey-Bellet, J., Prose, P., et al. 1958. Occlusions of the basilar artery. A clinical and pathological study. Neurology (Minneapolis) 8: 145–152.

Crowell, G.F., Stump, D.A., Biller, J., et al. 1984. The transient global amnesia-migraine connection. Arch. Neurol. 41:75–79.

Daly, D.D., and Markand, O.N. 1990. Focal brain lesions. In *Current Practice of Clinical Electroencephalography,* 2nd ed. Eds. D.D. Daly and T.A. Pedley, pp. 335–370. New York: Raven Press.

Davidson, L.A.G., and Jefferson, J.M. 1959. Electroencephalographic studies in respiratory failure. Br. Med. J. 2:296.

De Freitas, G.R., Devuyst, G., van Melle, G., et al. 2000. Motor strokes sparing the leg. Arch. Neurol. 57:513–518.

Denny-Brown, D. 1960. Recurrent cerebrovascular episodes. Arch. Neurol. 2:194–210.

De Weerd, A.W., Veldhuizen, R.J., Veering, M.M., et al. 1988. Recovery from cerebral ischaemia, EEG, cerebral blood flow and clinical symptomatology in the first three years after a stroke. Electroencephalogr. Clin. Neurophysiol. 70:107–204.

Drachman, D.A., and Hughes, J.R. 1971. Memory and the hippocampal complexes. III. Aging and temporal EEG abnormalities. Neurology 21: 1–14.

Dubois, J. 1956. Les thrombophlébites cérébrales post-partum. Gynecol. Obstet. 55:478.

Duffy, P., and Jacobs, G.B. 1958. Clinical and pathological findings in vertebral artery thrombosis. Neurology (Minneapolis) 8:862–869.

Echlin, F. 1965. EEG changes following spasms of the basilar and vertebral arteries produced by experimental subarachnoid hemorrhage. Electroencephalogr. Clin. Neurophysiol. 19:319(abst).

Fang, H.C.H., and Palmer, J.J. 1956. Vascular phenomena involving brain stem structures. Neurology (Minneapolis) 6:402–419.

Feldman, M.H. 1971. Physiological observations in a chronic case of "locked-in" syndrome. Neurology (Minneapolis) 21:459–478.

Finn, R., Kamaldeen, S., Moona, G., et al. 1980. The EEG in systemic lupus erythematosus. Electroencephalogr. Clin. Neurophysiol. 49:91P.

Fischer, H. 1959. Symptomatische Epilepsie bei cerebralen Gefäßprozessen. Arch. Psychiatr. Nervenkr. 199:296–310.

Fisher, C.M. 1965. Lacunes. Small, deep cerebral infarcts. Neurology (Minneapolis) 15:774–786.

Fisher, C.M. 1967. A lacunar stroke. The dysarthria-clumsy hand syndrome. Neurology (Minneapolis) 17:614–617.

Fisher, C.M. 1969. The arterial lesions underlying lacunes. Acta Neuropathol. (Berl.) 12:1.

Fisher, C.M., and Adams, R.D. 1964. Transient global amnesia. Acta Neurol. Scand. 40:Suppl. 9.

Fisher, C.M., Karnes, W.E., and Kubik, C.S. 1961. Lateral medullary infarction. The pattern of vascular occlusion. J. Neuropathol. Exp. Neurol. 20:323–379.

Fisher, M., and Garcia, J.H. 1996. Evolving stroke and the ischemic penumbra. Neurology 47:884–888.

Fogelholm, R., Kivalo, E., and Bergstrom, L. 1975. The transient global amnesia syndrome. An analysis of 35 cases. Eur. Neurol. 13:72–84.

Ford, F.R. 1966. *Diseases of the Nervous System in Infancy, Childhood and Adolescence.* Springfield, IL: Charles C Thomas.

Ford, F.R., and Schaffer, A.J. 1927. The etiology of infantile acquired hemiplegia. Arch. Neurol. Psychiatry 18:323–347.

Franco, P.J. 1961. Electroencephalography in venous disturbances of the brain. Rev. Neuro-Psiquiatr. 24:447–452.

Frank, G. 1981. *Amnestische Episoden.* Berlin: Springer.

French, L.A., and Haines, G.L. 1950. Unilateral vertebral artery ligation: report of a case ending fatally with basilar artery thrombosis. J. Neurosurg. 7:156–158.

Friedlander, W.J. 1959. Electroencephalographic changes in acute brain stem vascular lesions. Neurology (Minneapolis) 9:24–34.

Fuhrmann, W. 1953. Das EEG bei akuten Kreislaufstörungen des Gehirns. Verh. Dtsch. Ges. Neurol. Neurochir., Hamburg, 1952: see Zentralbl. Ges. Neurol. Psychiatr. 122:24–25.

Fuhrmann, W., and Müller, D. 1954. L'EEG nelle alterazioni circulatori acute del cervello. G. Psichiatr. Neuropatol. 82:1–14.

Ganner, H. 1974. Ictus amnesticus. In *Das Gedächtnis. Gedächtnisstörungen,* Eds. D. Fontanari, J. Kugler, and H. Lechner, pp. 73–80. Munich: Banaschewski.

Garcin, R., and Pestel, M. 1949. *Thrombophlébites Cérébrales.* Paris: Masson.

Gastaut, H., Bruens, J.H., Roger, J., et al. 1959. Étude électroencéphalographique des signes d'insuffisance circulatoire sylvienne chronique. Rev. Neurol. (Paris) 100:59–65.

Gastaut, H., Naquet, R., and Vigouroux, R.A. 1971. The vascular syndrome of the parieto-temporo-occipital "triangle." Based on 18 cases. In *Cerebral Circulation and Stroke,* Ed. K.J. Zülch, pp. 82–92. Heidelberg: Springer.

Gastaut, J.L., Michel, B., Sabet Hassan, S., et al. 1979. Electroencephalography in brain edema (127 cases of brain tumor investigated by cranial computerized tomography). Electroencephalogr. Clin. Neurophysiol. 46: 239–255.

Georgiades, A.L., Yamamoto, Y., Kwan, E.S., et al. 1999. Anatomy of sensory findings in patients with posterior cerebral artery territory infarction. Arch. Neurol. 56:835–838.

Gerloff, C., Altenmüller, E., and Dichgans, J. 1996. Disintegration and reorganization of cortical motor processing in two patients with cerebellar stroke. Electroencephalogr. Clin. Neurophysiol. 98:59–68.

Ghika-Schmid, F., and Bogousslavsky, J. 2000. The acute behavioral syndrome of anterior thalamic infarction: A prospective study of 12 cases. Ann. Neurol. 48:220–227.

Gibbs, F.A., and Gibbs, E.L. 1964. *Atlas of Electroencephalography,* vol. 3, 2nd ed. Reading, MA: Addison-Wesley.

Glanz, B.I., Schur, P.H., and Khoshbin, S. 1998. EEG abnormalities in systemic lupus erythematosus. Clin. Electroencephalogr. 29:128–131.

Glanz, B.I., Laoprasert, P., Schur, P.H., et al. 2001. Lateralized EEG findings in patients with neuropsychiatric manifestations of systemic lupus erythematosus. Clin. Electroencephalogr. 32:14–19.

Gloor, P., Ball, G., and Schaul, N. 1977. Brain lesions that produce delta waves in the EEG. Neurology (Minneapolis) 27:326–333.

Gottwald, W., and Sturm, U. 1984. EEG findings in lupus erythematosus. Electroencephalogr. Clin. Neurophysiol. 57:34P–35P.

Goulon, M., Picidalo, J.J., Christophe, M., et al. 1961. Clinical, electroencephalographic and biological correlations in 34 cases of chronic broncho-pneumopathy with asphyxia. In *Cerebral Anoxia and the Electroencephalogram.* Eds. H. Gastaut and J.S. Meyer, pp. 565–577. Springfield, IL: Charles C Thomas.

Griewing, B., Mertins, L., Lütcke, A., et al. 1991. Das Elektroenzephalogramm in der Verlaufsbeobachtung und Diagnostik von Thrombosen des Hirnnervensystems. EEG-Labor 13:103–117.

Groethuysen, U.C., Bickford, R.G., and Svien, H.J. 1955. The EEG in arteriovenous anomalies of the brain. Arch. Neurol. Psychiatry 74:506–513.

Gücer, G., Niedermeyer, E., and Long, D.M. 1978. Thalamic EEG recordings in patients with chronic pain. J. Neurol. (Berl.) 219:47–61.

Gütling, E., Isenmann, S., and Wichmann, W. 1996. Electrophysiology in the locked-in-syndrome. Neurology 46:1092–1101.

Hachinski, V., and Norris, J.W. 1980. The deteriorating stroke. Quoted by Hachinski, V., and Norris, J.W. 1985. *The Acute Stroke.* Philadelphia: Davis.

Hachinski, V.C., Potter, P., and Merskey, H. 1987. Leuko-araiosis. Arch. Neurol. 44:21–23.

Hacke, W., Kolmann, H.L., and Zeumer, H. 1982. Neurophysiologische Befunde bei der subkortikalen arteriosklerotischen Enzephalopathie (M. Binswanger). Z. EEG-EMG 13:121–128.

Harvald, B. 1958. EEG in old age. Acta Psychiatr. Scand. 33:193–196.

Hass, W.K., and Goldensohn, E.S. 1959. Clinical and electroencephalographic considerations in the diagnosis of carotid artery occlusion. Neurology (Minneapolis) 9:575–589.

Haugstedt, H. 1956. Occlusion of the basilar artery. Neurology (Minneapolis) 6:823–828.

Hegedüs, K., Fekete, I., Tury, F., et al. 1985. Experimental focal cerebral ischaemia in rabbits. J. Neurol. (Berl.) 232:223–230.

Heine, G. 1953. Vergleichende Untersuchung über Hirndurchblutungsgröße und Hirnstrombild beim Menschen. Verh. Dtsch. Ges. Kreislaufforsch. 19:196–210.

Heron, J.R. 1966. Migraine and cerebrovascular disease. Neurology (Minneapolis) 16:1097–1104.

Heros, R.C., Zervas, N.T., and Varsos, V. 1983. Cerebral vasospasm after subarachnoid hemorrhage: an update. Ann. Neurol. 14:599–608.

Heyck, H. 1956. *Neue Beiträge zur Klinik und Pathogenese der Migräne.* Stuttgart: Thieme.

Hickey, J., Chaves, C., Appignani, G., et al. 1996. A reversible posterior leukoencephalopathy syndrome. N. Engl. J. Med. 334:494–500.

Hill, F.S., Hughes, J.G., and Davis, B.C. 1950. Electroencephalographic findings in sickle cell anemia. Pediatrics 6:277–285.

Hirose, G., Saeki, M., Kosoegawa, H., et al. 1981. Delta waves in the EEGs of patients with intracerebral hemorrhage. Arch. Neurol. 38:170–175.

Holmes, G.L., and Donaldson, J.O. 1987. Effect of sexual hormones on the electroencephalogram and seizures. J. Clin. Neurophysiol. 4:1–22.

Hubach, H., and Struck, G. 1965. Zur Korrelation von EEG und pathomorphologischen Befunden cerebraler Gefäßprozesse. Arch. Psychiatr. Nervenkr. 206:641.

Hughes, J.R., and Cayaffa, J.J. 1977. The EEG in patients at different ages without organic cerebral disease. Electroencephalogr. Clin. Neurophysiol. 42:766–784.

Huhn, A. 1957. Die Hirnvenen- und Sinusthrombose Fortschr. Neurol. 25:440.

Huhn, A. 1969. Die venöse Abflußstörung. In *Die zerebralen/Durchblutungsstörungen des Erwachsenenalters,* Ed., J. Quandt, pp. 773–800. Berlin: VEB Verlag Volk und Gesundheit.

Husby, K., Norlen, G., and Petersen, Z. 1953. Electroencephalographic findings in intracranial arterial and arteriovenous aneurysms and subarachnoid hemorrhages. Acta Psychiatr. Scand. 28:387–400.

Hwang, P., Andermann, F., Metrakos, K., et al. 1981. The seizures of morphea. Electroencephalogr. Clin. Neurophysiol. 52:47P(abst).

Hynek, K., Cerny, M., and Posmurova, M. 1981. The EEG correlates of diazepam-induced amnesia. Electroencephalogr. Clin. Neurophysiol. 52:16P(abst).

Ingvar, D.H., Sjölund, B., and Ardo, A. 1976. Correlation between EEG frequency, cerebral oxygen uptake and blood flow. Electroencephalogr. Clin. Neurophysiol. 41:268–276.

Isler, W. 1969. *Akute Hemiplegien und Hemisyndrome im Kindesalter.* Stuttgart: Thieme.

Jabbari, B., Maulsby, R.L., Holtzapple, P.A., et al. 1979. Prognostic value of EEG in acute vascular aphasia: a long term clinical-EEG study of 53 patients. Clin. Electroencephalogr. 10:190–197.

Jackel, R.A., and Harner, R.N. 1989. Computed EEG topography in acute stroke. Neurophysiol. Clin. 19:185–197.

Jacome, D.E. 1989. EEG features in transient global amnesia. Clin. Electroencephalogr. 20:183–192.

Jacome, D.E. 1990. Transient global amnesia: clinical and EEG considerations. Am. J. EEG Technol. 30:195–209.

Jacome, D.E., and Morilla-Pastor, D. 1990. Unreactive EEG: pattern in locked-in syndrome. Clin. Electroencephalogr. 21:31–36.

Jaffe, R., and Bender, M.B. 1966. EEG studies in the syndrome of isolated episodes of confusion with amnesia "transient global amnesia." J. Neurol. Neurosurg. Psychiatry 29:472–474.

Jasper, H.H., and Van Buren, J. 1953. Interrelationship between cortex and subcortical structures: clinical electroencephalographic studies. Electroencephalogr. Clin. Neurophysiol. 4:168–188.

Jost, H., Ruimann, C.J., Hill, T.S., et al. 1952. Studies in hypertension. J. Nerv. Ment. Dis. 115:35–48, 152–162.

Kaada, B.R., Harknzark, W., and Stokke, O. 1961. Deep coma associated with desynchronization in EEG. Electroencephalogr. Clin. Neurophysiol. 13:785–798.

Kalyanaraman, K., Niedermeyer, E., Rowe, R., et al. 1968. The electroencephalogram in congenital heart disease. Arch. Neurol. (Chicago) 18:98–106.

Kappelle, L.J., and Van Huffelen, A.C. 1989. EEG assessment in patients with lacunar infarcts. Electroencephalogr. Clin. Neurophysiol. 73:54P (abst).

Katz, R.I., and Horowitz, G.R. 1983. Sleep-onset frontal rhythmic slowing in a normal geriatric population. Electroencephalogr. Clin. Neurophysiol. 56:27P.

Kayser-Gatchalian, M.C., and Neundörfer, B. 1980. The prognostic value of EEG in ischaemic cerebral insults. Electroencephalogr. Clin. Neurophysiol. 49:608–617.

Kazis, A., Karlovasitou, A., and Xafenias, D. 1982. Temporal slow activity of the EEG in old age. Arch. Psychiat. Nervenkr. 231:547–554.

Keilson, M.J., Miller, A.E., and Drexler, E.D. 1985. Early EEG and CTT scanning in stroke—a comparative study. Electroencephalogr. Clin. Neurophysiol. 61:21P(abst).

Kendel, K., and Koufen, H. 1970. EEG-Veränderungen bei cerebralen Gefäßinsulten des Hirnstamms. Dtsch. Z. Nervenheilkd. 197:42–55.

Ketz, E. 1971. Die Vertebro-Basilaris-Thrombose im konventionellen EEG. Z. EEG-EMG 2:36–43.

Kiloh, L.G., McComas, A.J., and Osselton, J.W. 1972. *Clinical Electroencephalography,* 3rd ed. London: Butterworths.

Kim, H.Y., Chung, C.S., Lee, J., et al. 2003. Hyperventilation-induced limb shaking TIA in Moyamoya disease. Neurology 60:137–139.

Kittner, J.J., Stern, B.J., Wozniak, M., et al. 1998. Cerebral infarctions in young adults. Neurology 50:1890–1894.

Kogeorgos, J., and Scott, D.F. 1981. EEG aspects of transient ischaemic attacks. Electroencephalogr. Clin. Neurophysiol. 52:103P(abst).

Kogeorgos, J., and Scott, D.F. 1982. Neuropsychiatric and EEG features in 74 cases of systemic lupus erythematosus with cerebral involvement. Electroencephalogr. Clin. Neurophysiol. 53:1P(abst).

Kok, N.K.D., and Van der Drift, J.H.A. 1971. The significance of the EEG for localization and prognosis of supratentorial ischemic disease. A clinical pathological study. Preliminary report. Rev. EEG Neurophysiol. 1:295–307.

Kolodny, E.H., Reibeiz, J.J., Caviness, V.S., et al. 1968. Granulomatous angiitis of the central nervous system. Arch. Neurol. 19:510–524.

Kooi, K.A. 1971. *Fundamentals of Electroencephalography.* New York: Harper & Row.

Kooi, K.A., Güvener, A.M., Tupper, C.J., et al. 1964. Electroencephalographic patterns of the temporal region in normal adults. Neurology 14:1029–1034.

Krump, J.E. 1953. Elektroenzephalographische Untersuchungen bei essentieller Hypertension. Verh. Dtsch. Ges. Kreislaufforsch. 19:200–209.

Krump, J.E. 1955. Modifications électroencéphalographiques des maladies du collagène. Rev. Neurol. (Paris) 92:593–607.

Krump, J.E. 1958. Die Lebenswandlung des Elektroenzephalogramms bei Herz-und Kreislaufkranken. Verh. Dtsch. Ges. Kreislaufforsch. 24:258–265.

Kubik, C.S., and Adams, R.D. 1946. Occlusion of the basilar artery—a clinical and pathological study. Brain 69:72–121.

Kugler, J., Doenicke, A., and Laub, M. 1975. Matabolisch verursachte amnestische Episoden. Muench. Med. Wochenschr. 117:1585–1592.

Labar, D.R., Petty, G.W., Fisch, B.Y., et al. 1989a. Electroencephalographic findings in lacunar infarctions. Electroencephalogr. Clin. Neurophysiol. 73:42P(abst).

Labar, D.R., Fisch, B.J., Fink, M.E., et al. 1989b. Quantitative EEG following subarachnoid hemorrhage: a comparison of methods. Electroencephalogr. Clin. Neurophysiol. 72:2P–3P(abst).

Lechner, H. 1958. Das EEG im vaskulären Geschehen. Wien. Klin. Wochenschr. 70:90–99.

Lemmi, H., and Little, S.C. 1960. Occlusion of intracranial venous structures. A consideration of the clinical and electroencephalographic findings. Arch. Neurol. 3:252–266.

Lesny, I., Bor, I., and Vlach, V. 1961. EEG changes in children suffering from congenital heart disease: influence of O_2 inhalation. Electroencephalogr. Clin. Neurophysiol. 13:173–179.

Levitt, P. 1970. The effects of subarachnoid blood on the electrocorticogram of the cat. Proc. Am. EEG Soc., Hans Berger Award Lecture, Washington, DC.

Lhermitte, F., and Gautier, J.C. 1975. Sites of cerebral arterial occlusions. In Modern Trends in Neurology, Ed. D. Williams, pp. 123–140. London: Butterworths.

Lhermitte, F., and Guiraud, B. 1968. Ischemic accidents in the middle cerebral artery. Arch. Neurol. 19:248.

Lhermitte, F., Gautier, J.C., and Derouesne, C. 1966. Anatomopathologie et physiopathologie des sténoses carotidiennes. Rev. Neurol. (Paris) 115:641.

Lindsberg, P.J. 2000. Clinical evidence of inflammation as a risk factor in ischemic stroke. In Inflammation and Stroke, Ed. G. Feuerstein, pp. 13–26. Basel: Birkhaeuser.

Loeb, C. 1962. Patologia del circolo sottotentoriale. Sist. Nerv. 14:213–323.

Loeb, C., and Meyer, J.S. 1965. Strokes Due to Vertebro-Basilar Disease. Springfield, IL: Charles C Thomas.

Loeb, C., and Poggio, G.F. 1953. Electroencephalogram in a case with pontomesencephalic haemorrhage. Electroencephalogr. Clin. Neurophysiol. 5:295–296.

Loeb, C., Rosadini, G., and Poggio, G.F. 1959. Electroencephalograms during coma. Neurology (Minneapolis) 9:610–618.

Loeb, C., Garello, L., and Pastorino, P. 1961. Aspetti clinici dell'insufficienza cerebrovascolare. Sist. Nerv. 13:334–351.

Logar, C., Ladurner, G., Enge, S., et al. 1981. Wert des EEG bei Patienten mit transitorischen globalen Amnesien. EEG-EMG 12:158–160.

Logar, C., Enge, S., Körner, E.M., et al. 1982. Zur klinischen Wertigkeit des EEG bei Subarachnoidalblutung. Z. EEG-EMG 13:68–72.

Logar, C., Enge, S., Ladurner, G., et al. 1983. Das EEG bei Multiinfarkten mit und ohne intellektuellen Abbau. Z. EEG-EMG 14:204–208.

Losev, J.E. 1958. Kocenke funkcionajnogo softojanija kory golovnogo mozga ditej a vrozdenymi serdca osnovanij elektroencefalograficeskich issledovanij. Vop. Okhrany Materin. Dets. 34:66–75 (cited in Lesny et al., 1961).

Lundervold, A., Hauge, T., and Löken, A.C. 1956. Unusual EEG in unconscious patients with brain stem atrophy. Electroencephalogr. Clin. Neurophysiol. 8:665–670.

Luu, P., Tucker, D.M., Englander, R., et al. 2001. Localizing acute stroke-related EEG changes. J Clin. Neurophysiol. 18:302–317.

Magnes, J., Monezzi, G., and Pompeiano, O. 1961. Electroencephalogram-synchronizing structures of the lower brain stem. In The Nature of Sleep, Eds. G.E.W. Wolstenholme and M. O'Connor, pp. 57–78. Boston: Little, Brown.

Magni, F., Moruzzi, G., Rossi, G., et al. 1959. EEG arousal following inactivation of the lower brain stem by selective injection of barbiturate into the vertebral circulation. Arch. Ital. Biol. 97:33–46.

Margerison, J.H., Binnie, C.D., and McCaul, I.R. 1970. Electroencephalographic signs employed in the location of ruptured intracranial arterial aneurysms. Electroencephalogr. Clin. Neurophysiol. 28:296–306.

Markand, O.N. 1976. Electroencephalogram in the "locked-in" syndrome. Electroencephalography 40:529–534.

Markand, O.N., and Daly, D.D. 1971. Pseudoperiodic lateralized paroxysmal discharges in the electroencephalogram. Neurology (Minneapolis) 21:975–981.

Marshall, J. 1964. The natural history of transient ischaemic cerebrovascular attacks. Q. J. Med. 33:309–324.

Marshall, J. 1972. A survey of occlusive disease of the vertebrobasilar arterial system. In Handbook of Neurology, vol. 12, Eds. P.J. Vinken and G.W. Bruyn, pp. 1–12. Amsterdam: North-Holland.

Matsuo, F. 1985. Multifocal epileptic seizures associated with acute cerebral ischemia. Electroencephalogr. Clin. Neurophysiol. 61:25P(abst).

Mauguière, F., and Desmedt, J.E. 1988. Thalamic pain syndrome of Déjérine-Roussy. Arch. Neurol. 45:1312–1320.

Maynard, S.D., and Hughes, J.R. 1984. A distinctive electrographic entity: bursts of rhythmical temporal theta. Clin. Electroencephalogr. 15:145–150.

McHenry, L.C., Jr. 1978. Cerebral Circulation and Stroke. St. Louis: Green.

Meyer, J.-E. 1953. Über die Lokalisation frühkindlicher Hirnschäden in arteiellen Grenzgebieten. Arch. Psychiatr. Nervenkr. 190:328–341.

Meyer, J.-E. 1958. Zur Lokalisation arteriosklerotischer Erweichungsherde in arteriellen Grenzgebieten des Gehirns. Arch. Psychiatr. Nervenkr. 196:421–432.

Meyer, J.S., Fang, H.C., and Denny-Brown, D. 1954. Polarographic studies of cerebral collateral circulation. Arch. Neurol. Psychiatry 72:296–312.

Miller, C.R., Westmoreland, B.F., and Klass, D.W. 1985. Subclinical rhythmic EEG discharge of adults (SREDA): further observations. Am. J. EEG Technol. 25:217–224.

Mitschke, H. 1969. EEG in arterial hypertension. Electroencephalogr. Clin. Neurophysiol. 27:660(abst).

Molaie, M., and Fariello, R.G. 1981. EEG detection of cerebral involvement in Wegener granulomatosis. Electroencephalogr. Clin. Neurophysiol. 51:37P(abst).

Mosmans, P.C.M., and Jonkman, E.V. 1980. The significance of the collateral vascular system of the brain in hunt and steal syndromes. Clin. Neurol. Neurosurg. 82:145–156.

Müller, D. 1975. Beitrag zur Kenntnis der amnestischen Episoden. Psychiatr. Neurol. Med. Psychol. 27:463–469.

Müller, H.R., and Klinger, M. 1965. The electroencephalogram in cerebral fat embolism. Electroencephalogr. Clin. Neurophysiol. 18:278–386.

Mumenthaler, M., and Von Roll, L. 1969. Amnestische Episoden. Analyse von 16 eigenen Beobachtungen. Schweiz. Med. Wochenschr. 99:133–139.

Mumenthaler, M., and Treig, T. 1984. Amnestische Episoden. Analyse von 111 eigenen Beobachtungen. Schweiz. Med. Wschr. 114:1163–1170.

Mumenthaler, M., Mumenthaler, M., and Meier, C. 1980. Amnestische Episoden. Analyse von 70 eigenen Beobachtungen, davon 63 mit Katamnese. In Status Psychomotoricus, Ed. K. Karbowski, pp. 117–137. Bern: Huber.

Mundy-Castle, A.C. 1962. Central excitability in the aged. In Medical and Clinical Aspects of Aging, Ed. M.T. Blumenthal, pp. 575–595. New York: Columbia University Press.

Nagata, K., Yunoki, K., Araki, G., et al. 1984. Topographic electroencephalographic study of ischemic attacks. Electroencephalogr. Clin. Neurophysiol. 58:291–301.

Nagata, K., Tagawa, K., Hiroi, S., et al. 1989. Electroencephalographic correlates of blood flow and oxygen metabolism provided by positron emission tomography in patients with cerebral infarctions. Electroencephalogr. 72:16–30.

Naquet, R., and Vigouroux, R.A. 1972. EEG in cerebral gas emboli from cardiac surgery. In Handbook of Electroencephalography and Clinical Neurophysiology, vol. 14A, Ed.-in-chief, A. Remond, pp. 38–44. Amsterdam: Elsevier.

Naquet, R., Louard, C., Rhodes, J., et al. 1961. À propos de certaines décharges paroxystiques du carrefour temporo-pariéto-occipital: leur activation par l'hypoxie. Rev. Neurol. (Paris) 105:203–207.

Naquet, R., Franck, G., and Vigouroux, R. 1965. Données nouvelles sur certaines décharges paroxystiques du carrefour pariéto-temporo-occipital rencontrées chez l'homme. Zentralbl. Neurochir. 25:153–180.

Neidengard, L., and Niedermeyer, E. 1975. The electroencephalogram in neurological complications of sickle cell anemia (SS-hemoglobinopathy). Clin. Electroencephalogr. 6:68–74.

Neundörfer, B.L., Meyer-Wahl, L., and Meyer, J.G. 1974. Alpha-EEG und Bewußlosigkeit. Ein kasuistischer Beitrag zur likaldiagnostischen Bedeutung des Alpha-EEG beim bewußtlosenPatienten. Z. EEG-EMG 5: 106–114.

Niedermeyer, E. 1957. Motorische Herdepilepsie bei Thalamus-Syndrome (Kasuistische Mitteilung zur Frage der "diencephalen Jackson-Epilepsie"). Wien Klin. Wochenschr. 69:702–705.

Niedermeyer, E. 1958. Über Epilepsie im höheren Lebensalter. Arch. Psychiatr. Nervenkr. 197:248–262.

Niedermeyer, E. 1960. Considérations au suject d'un syndrome (crises méniériformis, neurasthénia, désynchronisation du tracé EEG), probablement déterminé par une ischémie chronique bénigne dans le territoire de l'artère basilaire. Rev. Neurol. (Paris) 102:281–285.

Niedermeyer, E. 1962. EEG und Basilarinsuffizienz. Psychiatr. Neurol. (Basel) 144:212–244.

Niedermeyer, E. 1963. The electroencephalogram and vertebrobasilar artery insufficiency. Neurology (Minneapolis) 13:412–422.

Niedermeyer, E. 1972. The EEG in cardiac diseases. In *Handbook of Electroencephalography and Clinical Neurophysiology,* vol. 14A, Ed.-in-chief, A. Remond, pp. 65–67. Amsterdam: Elsevier.

Nishimoto, A., and Takeuchi, S. 1972. Moyamoya disease. Abnormal arterial networks in the cerebral basal region. In *Handbook of Neurology,* vol. 12, Eds. P.J. Vinken and G.W. Bruyn, pp. 352–383. Amsterdam: North-Holland.

Nordgren, R.E., Markesbery, W.R., Fukuda, K., et al. 1971. Seven cases of cerebromedullospinal disconnection: the "locked-in" syndrome. Neurology (Minneapolis) 21:1140–1148.

Novak, V., Chowthary, A., Farrar, B., et al. 2003. Altered cerebral vasoregulation in hypertension and stroke. Neurology 60:1657–1663.

Nuotio, K., Lindsberg, P.J., Carpén, O., et al. 2003. Adhesion molecule expression in symptomatic and asymptomatic carotid stenosis. Neurology 60:1890–1899.

Obrist, W.D. 1971. EEG and intellectual function in the aged. Proceed. Am. EEG Soc. Minneapolis, Sept. 1971.

Obrist, W.D., and Bissell, L.F. 1955. The electroencephalogram of aged patients with cardiac and cerebral vascular disease. J. Gerontol. 10: 315–330.

Obrist, W.D., Busse, E.W., and Henry, C. 1961. Relation of electroencephalogram to blood pressure in elderly persons. Neurology (Minneapolis) 11:151–158.

Ohyama, H., Niizuma, H., Kinjo, T., et al. 1983. Changes of EEG and tissue pCO$_2$ with hyperventilation in children with Moyamoya disease. Electroencephalogr. Clin. Neurophysiol. 56:55P(abst).

Oller-Daurella, L. 1974. El EEG de los sindromes vasculares vertebrobasilares. Rev. Infect. Med. 49:195–202.

Olszewski, J. 1962. Subcortical arteriosclerotic encephalopathy. World Neurol. 3:359–375.

Onofrj, M., Curatola, L., Malatesta, P., et al. 1992. Delayed P3 event-related potentials (ERPs) in thalamic hemorrhage. Electroencephalogr. Clin. Neurophysiol. 83:52–61.

Otomo, E., and Tsubaki, T. 1966. Electroencephalography in subjects sixty years and over. Electroencephalogr. Clin. Neurophysiol. 20:77–82.

Paddison, R.M., and Ferris, G.S. 1961. The electroencephalograms in cerebral vascular disease. Electroencephalogr. Clin. Neurophysiol. 13:99–110.

Paiva, T., Campos, J., Baeta, E., et al. 1995. EEG monitoring during endovascular embolization of cerebral arteriovenous malformations. Electroencephalogr. Clin. Neurophysiol. 95:3–13.

Patterson, J.R., and Grabois, M. 1986. Locked-in syndrome: a review of 139 cases. Stroke 17:758–764.

Pfaff, D.W., and McEwen, B.S. 1983. Action of estrogens and progestins on nerve cells. Science 219:808–814.

Pfurtscheller, G. 1986. Rolandic mu rhythms and assessment of cerebral functions. Am. J. EEG Technol. 26:19–32.

Pfurtscheller, G. 1993. Special uses of EEG computer analysis in clinical environments. In *Electroencephalography,* 3rd ed., Eds. E. Niedermeyer and F. Lopes da Silva, pp. 1125–1133. Baltimore: Williams & Wilkins.

Pfurtscheller, G., Wege, W., and Sager, W. 1980. Asymmetrien in der zentralen alpha-Aktivität (My-Rhythmus) unter Ruhe und Aktivitätsbedingungen bei zerebrovaskulären Erkrankungen. Z. EEG-EMG 11:63–71.

Pfurtscheller, G., Ladurner, G., Maresch, H., et al. 1984. Brain electrical activity mapping in normal and ischemic brain. In *Brain Ischemia—Quantitative EEG and Imaging Techniques,* Eds. G. Pfurtscheller, J. Jonkman, and F. Lopes da Silva, pp. 287–302. Amsterdam: Elsevier.

Picornell, I., Luengo, A., Mola, S., et al. 1984. EEG study of certain subclinical paroxysmal discharges recorded at the parieto-temporo-occipital crossing. Electroencephalogr. Clin. Neurophysiol. 57:69P(abst).

Plum, F., and Posner, J.B. 1966. *Diagnosis of Stupor and Coma.* Philadelphia: Davis.

Pohlmann-Eden, B., Hoch, D.B., Cochius, J.L., et al. 1996. Periodic lateralized epileptiform discharges: a critical review. J. Clin. Neurophysiol. 13:519–530.

Potes, J., McDowell, F., and Wells, C.E. 1961. Electroencephalogram in brain stem infarction. Arch. Neurol. 21:94(abst).

Primavera, A., Abbruzzese, M., and Siani, C. 1981. Transient depression of cerebral electrical activity in acute stroke. Electroencephalogr. Clin. Neurophysiol. 51:58P(abst).

Prior, P.F. 1973. *The EEG in Acute Cerebral Anoxia.* Amsterdam: Excerpta Medica.

Radermecker, J. 1967. Severe acute necrosis of the pons with long survival: electroclinical symptoms and absence of cerebral lesions. Electroencephalogr. Clin. Neurophysiol. 23:281–282(abst).

Rasheva, M. 1981. Epileptic seizures in the acute stage of embolic stroke. Electroencephalogr. Clin. Neurophysiol. 52:78P(abst).

Rasheva, M., Stamenov, E., Todorova, P., et al. 1981. Dynamics of electrical activity of the brain in cerebellar haemorrhage. Electroencephalogr. Clin. Neurophysiol. 52:78P(abst).

Reiher, J., and Lebel, M. 1977. Wicket spikes: Clinical correlates of a previously undescribed EEG pattern. Can. J. Neurol. Sci. 4:39–47.

Revitch, E., and Zallarski, Z. 1969. Slow anterior temporal foci in a mental hospital population. Behav. Neuropsychiatry 1:8–23.

Roger, J., Roger, A., and Gastaut, H. 1954. Electro-clinical correlation in 36 cases of vascular syndromes of brain stem. Electroencephalogr. Clin. Neurophysiol. 6:164(abst).

Roseman, E., Bloom, B.M., and Schmidt, R.P. 1951. The electroencephalogram in intracranial aneurysms. Neurology (Minneapolis) 1:25–38.

Rosenbaum, H.E. 1960. Familial hemiplegic migraine. Neurology (Minneapolis) 10:164–170.

Rumpl, E., Bauer, G., and Stampfel, G. 1977. Der Angiospasmus bei der Subarachnoidalblutung als wichtige Ursache für fokale Veränderungen im EEG Z. EEG-EMG 8:200–204.

Sainio, K., Stenberg, D., Kesimäki, I., et al. 1983. Visual and spectral EEG analysis in the evaluation of the outcome in patients with ischemic brain infarction. Electroencephalogr. Clin. Neurophysiol. 56:117–124.

Scherzer, E. 1967. EEG-Veränderungen bei zerebraler Fettembolie. Psychiatr. Neurol. 153:337.

Scheuler, W. 1983. Zur klinischen Bedeutung der gesteigerten Photostimulationsreaktion im Alpha-Frequenzbereich. Z. EEG-EMG 14:143–153.

Schneider, M. 1950. Die Physiologic der Hirndurchblutung. Dtsch. Z. Nervenheilkd. 162:113–119.

Schneider, M. 1961. Survival and revival of the brain in anoxia and ischemia. In *Cerebral Anoxia and the Electroencephalogram,* Eds. H. Gastaut and J.S. Meyer, pp. 134–143. Springfield, IL: Charles C Thomas.

Schumacher, G., and Wolff, H.G. 1941. Experimental studies on headache. Arch. Neurol. Psychiatry 45:199–214.

Scott, D.F., and Cabral, R. 1975. Development and prevention of seizures after neurosurgical procedures including ruptured cerebral aneurysms. Proc. Am. Epilepsy Soc., New York.

Sheehan, S., Bauer, R.B., and Meyer, J.S. 1960. Vertebral artery compression in cervical spondylosis. Arteriographic demonstration during life of vertebral artery insufficiency due to rotation and extension of the neck. Neurology (Minneapolis) 10:968–986.

Shev, E.E., and Robinson, S.J. 1958. Electroencephalographic findings associated with congenital heart disease. Preliminary report. Electroencephalogr. Clin. Neurophysiol. 10:253–258.

Shev, E.E., and Robinson, S.J. 1961. Electroencephalographic findings associated with congenital heart disease. In *Cerebral Anoxia and the Electroencephalogram,* Eds. H. Gastaut and J.S. Meyer, pp. 578–589. Springfield, IL: Charles C Thomas.

Shin, H.K., Yoo, H.M., Chang, H.M., et al. 1999. Bilateral intracranial vertebral artery disease in the New England Medical Center Posterior Circulation Registry. Arch Neurol 56:1353–1358.

Shiohama, N., Shinomiya, S., and Nagaoka, M. 1993. Clinical features of anterior bradyrhythmia. Clin. Encephalogr. 24:194–201.

Siekert, G., and Millikan, C. 1955. Studies in cerebrovascular disease. II. Some clinical aspects of thrombosis of the basilar artery. Mayo Clin. Proc. 30:93–100.

Silva, A., and Gross, P.T. 1983. Use of EEG in the evaluation of TIAs. Electroencephalogr. Clin. Neurophysiol. 56:13P(abst).

Silversides, J.L. 1954. Basilar artery stenosis and thrombosis. Proc. R. Soc. Med. 47:290–293.

Squitti, E., Pasqualetti, P., Casetta, E., et al. 2003. Elevation of serum copper levels discriminates Alzheimer's disease from vascular dementia. Neurology 660:2013–2014.

Steegman, A.T. 1951. Primary pontile hemorrhage. J. Nerv. Ment. Dis. 114: 35–65.

Stein, J., and Stava, Z. 1961. Electroencefalogram u sklerodermie. Czechoslov. Derm. 36:501–512 (cited in Gibbs, F.A., and Gibbs, E.L., 1964).

Steinmetz, E.F., and Vroom, F.Q. 1972. Transient global amnesia. Neurology (Minneapolis) 22:1193–1200.

Strauss, H., Ostow, M., and Greenstein, L.D. 1952. *Diagnostic Electroencephalography.* New York: Grune & Stratton.

Subbotnik, S.I., Feinberg, Y.S., and Spielberg, P.I. 1955. Electroencephalography in paroxysmal tachycardia. Electroencephalogr. Clin. Neurophysiol. 7:577–584.

Takahashi, T., Niedermeyer, E., and Knott, J.R. 1965. The EEG in older and younger adult groups with convulsive disorder. Epilepsia (Amsterdam) 6:24–32.

Taylor, R.M., and Pacella, B.C. 1949. Electroencephalograms in scleroderma. J. Nerv. Ment. Dis. 107:42–47.

Tharp, B.R. 1969. The electroencephalogram in transient global amnesia. Electroencephalogr. Clin. Neurophysiol. 26:96–99.

Tolonen, U., and Ahonen, A. 1983. Relationship between regional pertechnetate cerebral circulation time and EEG in patients with cerebral infarction. Electroencephalogr. Clin. Neurophysiol. 56:125–132.

Toole, J.F. 1964. Reversed vertebral artery flow and cerebral vascular insufficiency. Arch. Intern. Med. 61:159–162.

Toole, J.F., and Patel, A.N. 1974. *Cerebrovascular Disorders,* 2nd ed. New York: McGraw-Hill.

Torres, F., Faoro, A., Loewenson, R., et al. 1983. The electroencephalogram of elderly subjects revisited. Electroencephalogr. Clin. Neurophysiol. 56:391–398.

Trouillas, P., Nighogossian, N., and Philippon, B. 1991. Nuclear hemodynamic vertebrobasilar insufficiency. Arch. Neurol. 48:921–929.

Tucker, J.S. 1958. The electroencephalogram in brain stem vascular disease. Electroencephalogr. Clin. Neurophysiol. 10:405–416.

Tucker, J.S., and Yoe, R.H. 1956. Simultaneous EEG-EKG recording: Study of a case with complete heart block and ventricular tachycardia. Electroencephalogr. Clin. Neurophysiol. 8:129–132.

Turton, E.C. 1958. The EEG as a diagnostic and prognostic aid in the differentiation of organic disorders in patients over 60. J. Ment. Sci. 104: 461–465.

Tyler, H.R., and Clark, D.B. 1957. Incidence of neurological complications in congenital heart disease. Arch. Neurol. Psychiatry 77:17–22.

Van der Drift, J.H.A. 1972. The EEG in cerebro-vascular disease. In *Handbook of Clinical Neurology,* vol. 11, Eds. P.J. Vinken and G.W. Bruyn, pp. 267–291. Amsterdam: North-Holland.

Van der Drift, J.H.A., and Kok, N.K.D. 1972. The EEG in cerebrovascular disorders in relations to pathology. In *Handbook of Electroencephalography and Clinical Neurophysiology,* vol. 14A, Ed.-in-chief, A. Remond, pp. 12–30, 47–64. Amsterdam: Elsevier.

Van der Drift, J.H.A., and Magnus, O. 1961. The EEG in cerebral ischemic lesions. Correlations with clinical and pathological findings. In *Cerebral Anoxia and the Electroencephalogram,* Eds. H. Gastaut and J.S. Meyer, pp. 180–196. Springfield, IL: Charles C Thomas.

Van Huffelen, A.C., Poortvliet, D., Van der Wulp, C., et al. 1979. Quantitative EEG in cerebral ischemia: A. Parameters for the detection of abnormalities in "normal" EEGs in patients with acute unilateral cerebral ischemia (AU CI). In *Second European Congress of Clinical Neurophysiology,* Eds. H. Lechner and A. Aranibar, Int. Congress Series No. 506, pp. 25–26. Amsterdam-Oxford: Excerpta Medica.

Van Huffelen, A.C., Roelvink, N.C.A., and Van der Wulp, C.J.M. 1984. Quantitative EEG in cerebral ischemia. Electroencephalogr. Clin. Neurophysiol. 58:108P(abstr.).

Velho-Groneberg, P. 1986. The EEG: an important (and often underrated) tool in the diagnosis of stroke. Am. J. EEG Technol. 26:213–224.

Visser, S.L., Hooijer, C., Jonker, C., et al. 1987. Anterior temporal focal abnormalities in normal aged subjects, correlations with psychological and CT brain scan findings. Electroencephalogr. Clin. Neurophysiol. 66:1–7.

Walkenhorst, A. 1956. Gefäszabhängige Prozesse hinsichtlich ihrer Seitenlokalisation im Hirnstrombild. Nervenarzt 27:180–183.

Walsh, G., Masland, W., and Goldensohn, E.S. 1968. Paroxysmal cerebral discharge associated with atrial tachycardia. Electroencephalogr. Clin. Neurophysiol. 24:187(abst).

Walton, A. 1994. Pre- and postoperative findings in an arteriovenous aneurysm. A case study. Am. J. EEG Technol. 34:55–65.

Walton, J.N. 1953. The electroencephalographic sequelae of spontaneous subarachnoid haemorrhage. Electroencephalogr. Clin. Neurophysiol. 5: 41.

Watson, C.W., and Adams, R.D. 1951. The electroencephalogram in relation to consciousness and responsiveness in destructive lesions of the brain stem: a clinical pathology study of brain stem diseases, particularly basilar artery occlusion. Electroencephalogr. Clin. Neurophysiol. 3:371 (abst).

Westmoreland, B.F., and Klass, D.W. 1981. A distinctive rhythmic EEG discharge of adults. Electroencephalogr. Clin. Neurophysiol. 51:186–191.

Westmoreland, B.F., and Klass, D.W. 1997. Unusual variants of subclinical electrographic discharge of adults (SREDA). Electroencephalogr. Clin. Neurophysiol. 102:1–4.

White, J.C. 1979. Periodic EEG activity in subcortical arteriosclerotic encephalopathy (Binswanger's type). Arch. Neurol. 36:485–489.

Whitty, C.W.M. 1953. Familial hemiplegic migraine. J. Neurol. Neurosurg. Psychiatr. 16:172–177.

Wiszniewska, M., Devuyst, G., Bogousslavsky, J., et al. 2000. What is the significance of leukoaraiosis in patients with acute ischemic stroke. Arch. Neurol. 57:967–973.

Yanagihara, T., Piepgras, D.G., and Klass, D.W. 1985. Repetitive involuntary movements associated with episodic cerebral ischemia. Ann. Neurol. 18:244–250.

Yeh, H.S., Kashiwagi, S., Tew, J., et al. 1990. Surgical management of epilepsy with cerebral arteriovenous malformations. J. Neurosurg. 72: 216–223.

Zülch, K.J. 1953. Neue Befunde und Deutungen aus der Gefäszpathologie des Hirns und Rückenmarks. Zentralbl. Allg. Pathol. Anat. 90:402.

Zülch, K.J. 1971. Some basic patterns of collateral circulation of the cerebral arteries. In *Cerebral Circulation and Stroke,* Ed. K.J. Zülch, pp. 106–122. Berlin: Springer.

Zülch, K.J., and Behrend, R.C.H. 1961. The pathogenesis and topography of anoxia and ischemia of the brain in man. In *Cerebral Anoxia and the Electroencephalogram,* Eds. H. Gastaut and J.S. Meyer, pp. 144–163. Springfield, IL: Charles C Thomas.

Zurek, R., Schiemann-Delgado, J., Froescher, W., et al. 1985. Frontal intermittent rhythmical delta activity and anterior bradyrhythmia. Clin. Electroencephalogr. 16:1–10.

18. EEG and Dementia

Anne C. Van Cott and Richard P. Brenner

Dementia is a syndrome that consists of a decline in cognitive and intellectual abilities occurring in an awake and alert patient, which is severe enough to interfere significantly with work, usual social activities, or relationships with others (American Psychiatric Association, 1994). Areas affected may include memory, abstract thinking, judgment, cognitive function, and personality. Since the disorder occurs predominantly in the elderly, the prevalence of dementia will increase dramatically with the aging of the United States population (Corey-Bloom et al., 1995). Dementia is a symptom complex that can occur in over 70 disorders (Geldmacher and Whitehouse, 1997) and needs to be differentiated from other disorders that are common in the elderly, such as delirium and depression.

EEG Changes in Dementia

The EEG can be helpful in the evaluation of dementia for several reasons. It may confirm that an abnormality of cerebral function exists, particularly when the differential diagnosis is between a primary degenerative dementia, such as Alzheimer's disease (AD), and a psychiatric disorder, such as depression with cognitive impairment (depressive pseudodementia). In other patients, the EEG may indicate that a focal, rather than a diffuse, process is responsible for the dementia syndrome. Rarely, the EEG may suggest the presence of an unsuspected seizure disorder. In the appropriate clinical setting, an EEG pattern can be strongly supportive, but not pathognomonic of Creutzfeldt-Jakob disease (CJD) (Cambier et al., 2003; Levy et al., 1986; Steinhoff et al., 1996). Robinson et al. (1994) found the waking EEG helpful in the exclusion of AD and considered that its widespread availability, low cost, and high sensitivity support the use of EEG in the diagnosis of this disease.

Harner (1975) stated that in a patient with dementia, particularly early in the course of the illness, a normal or mildly abnormal EEG favors a primary degenerative disorder and argues against metabolic, toxic, or infectious etiologies. In contrast, with these treatable disorders, the EEG is usually more abnormal. The following clinical rule has been suggested: if the EEG looks much worse than the patient's mental state, there is a high probability that a treatable cause exists. On the other hand, if the EEG is normal or near normal while the degree of cognitive impairment is marked, either a cortical dementia, such as frontotemporal dementia, or a depressive pseudodementia is probable (Boutros and Struve, 2002; Cummings and Benson, 1992; Rosen, 1997). Obviously, there are exceptions; however, while the EEG is not diagnostic, it often provides clues that may help direct the investigation.

Classification of Dementia

In the past, dementias have been clinically classified based on the neurological signs and symptoms accompanying impaired memory. Although the differentiation between subcortical and cortical dementia profiles may be clinically useful, the separation has no firm basis on either clinical or neuropathological grounds (Whitehouse, 1986). The term *subcortical dementia* refers to individuals with dementia accompanied by psychomotor slowing, apathy, and depression. Subcortical dementias encompass Parkinson's disease (PD), progressive supranuclear palsy (PSP), and Huntington's disease (HD). In contrast, cortical dementia patients have more difficulties with language, perception, and praxis (Chui, 1989; Cummings and Benson, 1992). AD is the prototypical cortical dementia. Degenerative processes such as CJD and vascular dementia that present with varied clinical features have been classified as mixed cortical/subcortical dementias.

Although such a division is an oversimplification, it is useful when applied in the EEG laboratory since cortical and "mixed" dementias are more frequently associated with EEG abnormalities (Pedley and Miller, 1983; Verma et al., 1987). Although Pedley and Miller (1983) did not find consistent EEG differences between patients with cortical dementia (AD) and subcortical dementia, patients with subcortical dementia had a higher percentage of normal records. Verma et al. (1987) found that 14 of 15 (93%) patients with subcortical dementia had relatively normal EEGs as compared to only three of 15 (20%) patients with cortical dementia, matched for age, sex, and severity of dementia. The authors felt that these findings validated the classification of dementia into subcortical and cortical categories. Other electrophysiological studies, such as auditory long latency event-related potentials, have shown distinct changes in the early components of the response, supporting these subtypes of dementia (Goodin and Aminoff, 1986, 1987). Recognizing the limitations of this dichotomy, for purposes of discussion, this classification system is used in this chapter.

Cortical Dementia

Alzheimer's Disease

AD is the most common dementing illness, accounting for approximately 50% to 80% of individuals presenting with dementia. Typical features include an insidious onset, a progressive course, and involvement in multiple areas of cognition in a patient who is otherwise alert, healthy, and free of motoric or other neurological signs. The first symptoms characteristically are problems with difficulty in recent

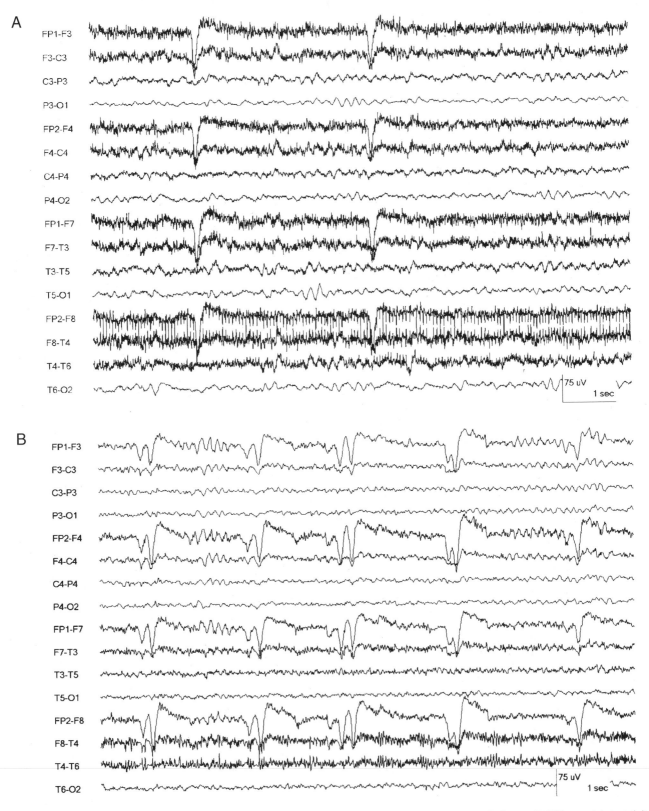

Figure 18.1.   **A:** There is diffuse slowing of background rhythms in this 83-year-old woman with Alzheimer's disease. **B:** Widespread theta activity, maximal anteriorly, in this 62-year-old man with Alzheimer's disease.

memory and remembering names; however, some patients begin primarily with language or visuospatial complaints (Katzman, 1986). There are criteria for the diagnosis of AD, which include the categories of possible, probable, and definite AD (McKhann et al., 1984).

EEG findings in AD, using conventional visual analysis (Fig. 18.1) may include a slowing of the dominant posterior rhythm, an increase in diffuse slow (delta and theta) activity, and/or generalized bursts of slow activity that are usually maximal anteriorly (Brenner et al., 1988; Liddell, 1958; Rae-Grant et al., 1987; Soininen et al., 1982), and a reduction in alpha (Gordon and Sim, 1967; Letemendia and Pampiglione, 1958) and/or beta activity (Weiner and Schuster, 1956; Letemendia and Pampiglione, 1958).

Although a number of early investigators emphasized the prominent EEG abnormalities in AD, the patients they studied usually had moderate to severe dementia. Clearly, with mild impairment, particularly early in the illness, the EEG can be normal. In some patients, although the dominant posterior rhythm is still within the alpha frequency (8-13 Hz), if previous EEGs are available it may be evident that the frequency has slowed. Prominent focal slowing is not a feature of the EEG in patients with AD. However, as in normal elderly subjects, occasional focal (temporal) slowing, consisting of delta and theta activity, may occur, particularly over the left side (Klass and Brenner, 1995; Obrist, 1976).

Epileptiform discharges are rare in AD (Thal et al., 1988). Triphasic waves (TWs) can occur in AD, although they are most often seen in metabolic disorders, particularly hepatic dysfunction. Muller and Kral (1967) described triphasic complexes, which were often sharp in appearance and maximal in the posterior head regions, in patients with severe dementia. Rae-Grant et al. (1987) found TWs in 15 of 268 (6%) EEG studies done in AD patients. The authors did not comment on the distribution of the TWs. These complexes were always associated with other severe EEG disturbances, such as excessive delta activity. Sundaram and Blume (1987) evaluated the clinical correlation and morphology of TWs in 63 consecutive patients and found that TWs were maximal anteriorly in the majority of AD patients. Further studies (Blatt and Brenner, 1996; Primavera and Traverso, 1990; Primavera et al., 1989) found the discharges usually maximal posteriorly (Fig. 18.2).

Generalized periodic patterns have been described in autopsy proven case reports of AD. Ehle and Johnson (1977) reported a 66-year-old man who presented with a subacute dementia and EEG changes resembling CJD. Watson (1979) reported a 55-year-old woman who had a rapidly progressive dementia, myoclonus, and periodic complexes. However, as Gloor (1980) indicated, these cases did not meet the definition of periodicity. Furthermore, generalized periodic patterns may occur in a variety of other illnesses that affect the elderly, such as toxic-metabolic disorders or following anoxia (Brenner and Schaul, 1990).

There is a good correlation between the severity of EEG abnormalities and cognitive impairment (Anderer et al., 1994; Brenner et al., 1988; Claus et al., 1999; Erkinjuntti et al., 1988; Hughes et al., 1989; Johannesson et al., 1979; Kaszniak et al., 1979; Knott et al., 1999; Kowalski et al., 2001; Liddell, 1958; Merskey et al., 1980; Obrist and Busse, 1965; Obrist et al., 1962; Roberts et al., 1978; Rae-Grant et al., 1987; Schreiter-Gasser et al., 1994; Soininen et al., 1982; Weiner and Schuster, 1956). Thus, the sensitivity of the EEG in discriminating AD patients from normal elderly

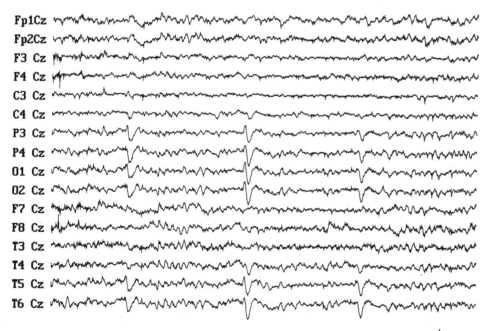

Figure 18.2. An 81-year old woman with Alzheimer's disease. Several triphasic waves, maximal posteriorly, are present. (From Blatt, I., and Brenner, R.P. 1996. Triphasic waves in a psychiatric population: a retrospective study. J Clin Neurophysiol 13:324–329. Philadelphia: Lippincott-Raven, with permission.)

100 µV

1 sec

individuals or, for example, from those with major depression, is dependent on the severity of the dementia.

In the hope of increasing the diagnostic value of EEG, interest has developed in computerized EEG spectral analysis, which provides more quantitative data than does conventional visual EEG analysis. Findings with quantitative EEG (qEEG) are similar to those reported with conventional EEG analysis. Numerous studies (Bennys et al., 2001; Brenner et al., 1986; Coben et al., 1983, 1985; Giaquinto and Nolfe, 1986; Knott et al., 1999; Miyauchi et al., 1994; Schreiter-Gasser et al., 1993; Visser et al., 1985) have shown a shift of the spectrum to slower frequencies, with an increase in theta activity and a decrease in beta activity, in patients with AD compared to normal elderly subjects. There is a correlation between spectral EEG measures, such as mean frequency and severity of dementia (Brenner et al., 1986; Canter et al., 1982; Duffy et al., 1984; Penttila et al., 1985; Rodriquez et al., 1999; Rosen, 1997; Sloan and Fenton, 1993; Streletz et al., 1990). In mild dementia, there is an increase in theta and a decrease in beta activity (Coben et al., 1983, 1985), whereas with greater severity of dementia there are also decreases in alpha and increases in delta activity (Coben et al., 1985; Elmstahl et al., 1994; Hier et al., 1991; Miyauchi et al., 1994; Penttila et al., 1985; Soininen and Partanen, 1988; Stigsby et al., 1981).

In a study comparing the diagnostic efficacy of computerized spectral versus visual EEG analysis in elderly normal and AD subjects, Brenner et al. (1988) found that spectral analysis afforded only modest advantages over visual EEG analysis in differentiating AD patients from elderly controls. Since the degree of spectral and visual EEG abnormalities correlated with the severity of dementia, both tests more often correctly classified those AD patients with lower Mini-Mental State Examination (MMSE) (Folstein et al., 1975) scores. Also, both tests identified primarily the same patients. The authors did not find the computer to be more sensitive than the eye in the identification of AD patients with mild impairment, and such patients, who are more difficult to diagnose clinically, may not be identified by EEG criteria. However, computerized spectral data was derived from only four channels, while 16 channels and a longer recording time were used for visual analysis. Schreiter-Gasser et al. (1994) found quantitative data, particularly absolute power of delta activity, to be the best predictor of degree of dementia. Both qEEG and visual EEG analysis were highly correlated with degree of dementia. Subsequently, Strijers et al. (1997) utilizing 19 channels for visual analysis and 12 channels for computerized data, which included both frequency analysis and coherence, indicated that the accuracy in identifying demented patients was comparable between visual analysis and qEEG. However, only a small number of AD patients (nine) were studied.

Currently, although both visual analysis of EEG and qEEG compare favorably to other imaging modalities, such as computed tomography (CT), magnetic resonance imaging (MRI), single photon emission computed tomography (SPECT), and positron emission tomography (PET), in the evaluation of dementia (Hegerl and Moller, 1997; Jonkman, 1997; Robinson et al., 1994), for mild degrees of dementia the specificity and sensitivity are limited. This may be im-

proved with further development of quantitative techniques and mathematical manipulations, such as discriminant analysis and artificial neural networks (Anderer et al., 1994; Besthorn et al., 1997; Musha et al., 2002; Petrosian et al., 2001; Pritchard et al., 1994). At present, the clinical usefulness of qEEG in dementia is limited, as most changes can be seen in routine EEG testing (Nuwer, 1997). Unlike Jonkman (1997), we do not believe that qEEG is the preferred study, and concur with Nuwer (1996) that qEEG should not be employed separately from routine EEG. Although qEEG may help probe brain function and connectivity in new ways (Holschneider and Leuchter, 1999), it remains a research tool, but as yet an unproven diagnostic tool for AD (Knott et al., 2001).

In addition to spectral analysis, qEEG studies have also evaluated coherence, which is a measure of the synchronizational neuronal activity between two cortical sites. Several studies have reported decreased alpha coherence in AD patients, suggesting fewer neuronal connections (Adler et al., 2003; Besthorn et al., 1994; Dunkin et al., 1995; Hogan et al., 2003; Knott et al., 2000). It has been proposed that the decreased alpha coherence may be related to an alteration of corticocortical connections (Locatelli et al., 1998).

There have been several longitudinal EEG studies of AD patients. Coben et al. (1985) found overall changes in power spectra (increases in delta and theta and decreases in beta, alpha, and mean frequency) over a 2.5-year period. Sloan and Fenton (1993) did not find significant power spectra changes in an 18-month follow-up of AD patients. Hooijer et al. (1990) found visual analysis to be better for showing a progression of slowing of the EEG in AD patients than power spectral analysis. However, with progression of disease, the conventional EEG does not invariably worsen in all AD patients (Rae-Grant et al., 1987).

What is the role of the EEG as a predictor of progression in dementia? Some studies (Berg et al., 1984; Forstl et al., 1996b), using spectral measures, did not find this test to be predictive of progression of dementia in AD patients, while others (Claus et al., 1998a) found slowing of the qEEG to be marker for rate of subsequent cognitive and functional decline in early AD, independent of demographic disease characteristics. Helkala et al. (1991), using both conventional visual EEG analysis and spectral measures, found that AD patients with an abnormal EEG at an early stage of the disease had a different pattern of cognitive decline than AD patients (matched for severity of dementia) with a normal EEG. Those with deteriorating EEGs during the initial 1-year follow-up subsequently showed a greater decline in praxic functions, as well as a tendency toward a higher frequency of extrapyramidal symptoms and a greater risk of institutionalization than AD patients with stable EEGs during the first year. Lopez et al. (1991) found more marked EEG abnormalities (conventional visual and spectral analysis) in AD patients with delusions and hallucinations compared to AD patients matched for severity of dementia, but without delusions and hallucinations. Patients with these psychotic symptoms had a more rapid rate of decline as measured by the MMSE (Folstein et al., 1975). In a subsequent study, Lopez et al. (1997) found both abnormal EEG and psychosis to be independent predictors of disease progression. Edwards-Lee et al. (2000) also reported greater qEEG abnormalities in AD patients with psychosis compared to those with similar cognitive impairment but without psychosis. Although several studies have suggested that qEEG may have prognostic relevance and be useful for clinical purposes such as predicting loss of activities of daily living, incontinence, and death (Claus et al., 1998b; Nobili et al., 1999; Rodriguez et al., 1996), the use EEG for prediction of survival in individual cases remains to be determined (Claus et al., 1998b).

Although the pathophysiological basis of AD is uncertain, a cholinergic deficit may be responsible for some of the symptoms (Cummings and Kaufer, 1996; Dringenberg, 2000; Lehtovirta et al., 2000). Anticholinergic drugs, such as scopolamine, can produce EEG slowing and behavioral changes, including confusion and memory impairment, in healthy volunteers (Sannita et al., 1987), whereas cholinergic drugs can transiently shift EEG spectral analysis into more normal patterns and improve memory and attention performances in AD patients (Adler and Brassen, 2001; Agnoli et al., 1983). Rodriquez et al. (2002) reported that long-term treatment with donepzil, an oral anticholinesterase, resulted in a lesser deterioration of the EEG in patients with mild to moderate AD compared to controls. Riekkinen et al. (1990, 1991) reviewed the role of the nucleus basalis of Meynert (a cholinergic nucleus located in the basal forebrain and a major source of cortically projecting cholinergic fibers) and choline acetyltransferase, and their relationship to EEG slowing and cognitive decline.

Dementia with Lewy Bodies

Dementia with Lewy bodies (DLB), a recently defined neurodegenerative disorder, is considered by some the second most common form of dementia in the elderly (Galvin, 2003). Patients with DLB typically have a more rapid rate of disease progression and respond differently to a variety of medications, making the accurate antemortem diagnosis an important clinical issue. In addition to progressive cognitive decline, the Consortium on Dementia with Lewy Bodies (CDLB) defines three major clinical criteria of DLB: visual hallucinations, fluctuating cognition, and spontaneous motor features of parkinsonism (McKeith et al., 1996). Pathologically, Lewy bodies are typically described as subcortical, but can also be located cortically again raising the issue of the "subcortical-cortical" classification of dementia.

Several reports have examined the validity of the CDLB criteria and have found them to be sensitive but not highly specific (McKeith, 2000; Verghese et al., 1999). Merdes et al. (2003) propose that concomitant AD tangle pathology alters the clinical phenotype of DLB, decreasing clinical diagnostic accuracy. EEG does not definitively distinguish DLB from other forms of dementia, and controversy exists in the literature regarding it diagnostic role in the evaluation and treatment of patients with DLB. Crystal et al. (1990) reported in their small series that EEGs were frequently abnormal, often early in the course of the illness. The abnormalities included background posterior slowing and frontally dominant burst of delta and theta activity, at a time of mild to moderate dementia. Recently, frontal intermittent rhythmic delta activity was found to be more common in patients with DLB (seven of ten) than in patients with AD (two of nine), despite a similar degree of cognitive impairment (Calzetti et al., 2002). In another study (Briel et al., 1999), standard EEG recordings from patients with autopsy-confirmed DLB and AD were compared. Greater slowing was found in the tracings of DLB patients, with the majority showing a loss of alpha activity and temporal lobe slow-wave transients. The temporal slow waves were reported to correlate with a clinical history of loss of consciousness. The authors proposed that temporal slow wave transients might be a useful diagnostic feature in DLB. Walker et al. (2000) examined EEG activity of patients with DLB or AD, and elderly controls. The authors reported that fluctuations in cognition and level of arousal correlated with rapid changes in background EEG frequency assessed quantitatively and proposed that EEG may play a role in diagnosis and treatment studies. Contradicting these reports, Barber et al. (2000) compared EEGs from patients who fulfilled the clinical criteria for DLB and "probable" AD. Patients with DLB had a shorter duration of their illness but were more severely demented as assessed by the MMSE. EEG slowing was present in both groups, consisting predominately of theta activity of 4 to 7 Hz. There was no statistically significant difference in the EEG findings between the two groups, although the authors reported a correlation between the severity of EEG slowing and the MMSE score. One autopsy-verified case of DLB had generalized periodic discharges resembling CJD (Yamamoto and Imai, 1988).

Frontotemporal Dementia

Frontotemporal lobar degeneration is the third most common cause of dementia. A consensus on clinical diagnostic criteria (Neary et al., 1998) defines three neurobehavioral syndromes including frontotemporal dementia (FTD), progressive nonfluent aphasia, and semantic dementia. FTD is a common cause of early-onset dementia (Ratnavalli et al., 2002). Typically considered a "focal" dementia, FTD is characterized by profound changes in affect and social conduct. Some familial cases of FTD are associated with mutations in the tau gene (Snowden et al., 2002). The conventional EEG in patients with FTD is characteristically normal. No focal or epileptiform abnormalities are present despite the neuropathological evidence of focal frontal and anterior temporal lobe degeneration. In fact, a normal conventional EEG despite clinical evidence of dementia is considered a supportive diagnostic feature in the diagnostic criteria of FTD (Neary et al., 1998).

Stigsby et al. (1981) compared EEG activity of autopsy-confirmed cases of AD and FTD (referred to as Pick's disease) and reported the EEG was normal in FTD. In a kinship study of family members, 11 patients had normal EEG activity while two were reported to have excessive frontoparietal theta activity with a preserved alpha rhythm (Groen and Endtz, 1982). Stigsby (1988) pointed out that EEG tracings in FTD may appear normal with visual analysis, but frequency analysis shows clear differences from a healthy control group. Yener et al. (1996) also suggested that qEEG might be helpful in distinguishing subjects with AD from those with FTD. Like visual analysis, qEEG studies have found EEG changes to be less severe in FTD patients than those with AD (Forstl et al., 1996a; Yener et al., 1996). This concept is supported again by a recent study that incorporated healthy controls (Lindau et al., 2003) and found that qEEG abnormalities of FTD patients were distinctly different, with an absence of slow activity and a decrease in fast activity, compared to AD patients.

Mixed Cortical/Subcortical Dementia

Creutzfeldt-Jakob Disease

Creutzfeldt-Jakob disease (CJD) is a human prion disease with four currently recognized clinicopathological forms (Knight and Will, 2003). The neuropathological characteristic of CJD is the abnormal accumulation of cellular prion protein (PrP) in the brain. Sporadic CJD is the most common form (annual incidence approximated at 1 per million) of the illness. The cause of the sporadic form is unknown. Clinically, sporadic CJD is characterized by a rapidly progressive dementia frequently associated with ataxia and myoclonus. Iatrogenic CJD, the result of accidental transmission of CJD during medical care, can be divided into central (e.g., neurosurgical instrument, dura mater grafts) and peripheral (e.g., human growth hormone) routes of transmission. While central transmission has clinical features similar to sporadic CJD, peripherally acquired CJD is characterized by a progressive cerebellar syndrome. Interest has recently focused on the appearance of a clinicopathological variant of CJD attributed to the transmission of bovine

spongiform encephalopathy from cattle to humans. Variant CJD, commonly called "mad cow disease," has a more protracted clinical course than sporadic CJD with additional psychiatric and painful sensory symptoms (Weihl and Roos, 1999). Genetic CJD, an autosomal dominantly inherited disease, is linked to mutations of the *PrP* gene and has a more protracted clinical course with heterogeneous clinical features. The recent recognition of the different types of CJD may explain some of the conflicting information with regard to EEG findings during the course of the illness.

The EEG often shows a characteristic periodic pattern in CJD (Fig. 18.3), but is not pathognomonic (Brenner and Schaul, 1990). However, in the clinical setting of rapid cognitive decline, ataxia, chorea, or myoclonus, the EEG can be suggestive of CJD. There are progressive EEG changes during the illness. Early in the course of the illness, the EEG may show diffuse slowing; during the second phase of CJD (usually within 3 months after onset) periodic sharp-wave complexes (PSWCs), most often triphasic or biphasic, occur approximately every second. The discharges are diffuse and generally symmetrical, but initially they may be asymmetric and occasionally lateralized (Au et al., 1980). Cambier et al. (2003) described eight CJD patients with lateralized periodic sharp waves in conjunction with focal cortical dysfunction, elevated 14-3-3 protein, and focal abnormalities of the cortical ribbon and deep gray matter on fluid-attenuated inversion recovery (FLAIR) MRI imaging. With progression of the disease, there is a decrease in the amplitude of the background activity. The periodic complexes often persist

Figure 18.3. Generalized periodic sharp triphasic waves, maximal anteriorly, in a 74-year-old woman with Creutzfeldt-Jakob disease.

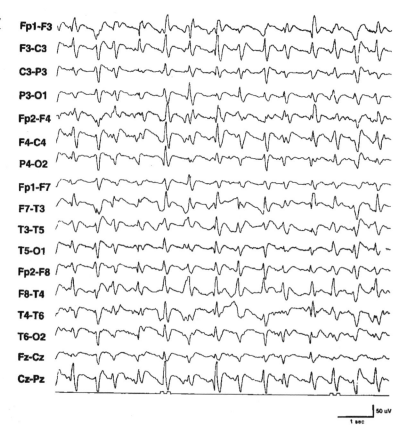

(Burger et al., 1972; Chiofalo et al., 1980), whereas the interval between complexes may lengthen (Lee and Blair, 1973).

The characteristic periodic pattern occurs in the majority (75% to 94%) of CJD patients (Aguglia et al., 1987; Brown et al., 1986; Burger et al., 1972; Chiofalo et al., 1980; Hansen et al., 1998; Masters et al., 1979; Steinhoff et al., 1996). Bortone et al. (1994) reported that all 15 patients in their study had PSWC at some point in their illness. In their literature review, Levy et al. (1986) noted that PSWCs were reported in 66 of 75 (88%) patients with CJD who had adequate EEG data during this initial 3-month period. Steinhoff et al. (1996), in a study of 29 patients (15 with neuropathologically confirmed CJD and 14 patients suspected of having CJD but in whom other diagnoses were established), assessed the accuracy and reliability of PSWC in CJD. They found the sensitivity and specificity of PSWC on EEG to be 67% and 86%, respectively. Levy et al. (1986) believe that the absence of PSWC in the EEG after 12 weeks of illness argues strongly against a diagnosis of CJD unless it is a rare subtype of long duration, which is less likely to show periodic complexes. Brown et al. (1986) concluded that although the presence of dementia, myoclonus, and periodic EEG activity may be lacking in as many as 25% of patients, the combined absence of involuntary movements and periodic EEG activity is highly unusual and makes the diagnosis of CJD unlikely. However, this does occur (Zochodne et al., 1988), particularly in familial cases (Tietjen and Drury, 1990).

Cerebrospinal fluid (CSF) analysis for 14-3-3 proteins has recently gained popularity as evidence for the diagnosis of CJD. 14-3-3 is a normal brain protein that is released into the spinal fluid in the setting of neuronal destruction (Knight and Will, 2003). Based on the reported high specificity and sensitivity for the diagnosis of CJD in patients with dementia (Hsich et al., 1996; Zerr et al., 1998), the 2001 American Academy of Neurology Guidelines recommend 14-3-3 protein CSF analysis for "confirming or rejecting the diagnosis of CJD in clinically appropriate circumstances." Recently, Huang et al. (2003) have disputed the sensitivity and specificity of 14-3-3 proteins and reported a finding of >10% false-positive cases based on clinical diagnosis; the main limitation of this study was lack of confirmation by tissue diagnosis. Zerr and colleagues (2000) analyzed the diagnostic value of both CSF 14-3-3 and EEG prospectively from pooled data of 805 cases of sporadic CJD and reported that both the sensitivity and specificity of 14-3-3 protein was higher than for PSWCs on EEG. Combining EEG and 14-3-3 data increased the sensitivity, but decreased the specificity of the diagnosis. Poser et al. (1999) performed a prospective follow-up of 364 suspected CJD patients and found that the presence of 14-3-3 protein in the CSF was superior to EEG and MRI in discriminating CJD from other rapidly progressive dementias.

As indicated, the periodic pattern present in CJD is not pathognomonic and can occur with reversible toxic encephalopathy due to baclofen (Hormes et al., 1988; Zak et al., 1994), ifosamide (Wengs et al., 1993), lithium (Smith and Kocen, 1988), and levodopa (Neufeld, 1992), for example. In addition, Isozumi et al. (1994) described a 50-year-old woman with subacute dementia, myoclonus, and periodic

complexes, initially thought to be due to CJD, who improved. The final diagnosis was a mitochondrial encephalopathy. Thomas and Borg (1994) reported a 40-year-old man who presented with a myoclonic encephalopathy and an EEG pattern suggestive of CJD. However, the patient, who had the acquired immunodeficiency syndrome (AIDS) dementia complex, improved following treatment and the EEG returned to normal.

Multi-Infarct Dementia

Vascular dementia (VaD) classically has an abrupt onset associated with stroke. Cognitive deficits are typically accompanied by focal neurological findings and supratentorial infarcts on neuroimaging studies. In contrast to AD, VaD patients may have early and severe impairment of executive function with less prominent memory problems (Roman, 2002). The National Institute of Neurological Disorders and Stroke, with the support of the AIREN (Association internationale pour la recherche et l'enseignement en neurosciences) (Roman, 2003), has established diagnostic criteria that emphasize not only clinical aspects of the illness and diagnostic testing, but also the heterogeneity of VaD syndromes. Both routine EEG and qEEG play a limited role in differentiating VaD from other dementia types. Not surprisingly, focal abnormalities, such as spikes, sharp waves, and slowing, are more common in patients with VaD than in patients with AD (Bucht et al., 1984; Harrison et al., 1979; Roberts et al., 1978; Soininen et al., 1982; Striano et al., 1981). The presence of focal abnormalities depends on the size and location of the infarcts; the more superficial and larger the infarcts, the more prominent the focal abnormalities. Small deep lacunar infarcts have relatively little effect on the EEG (Ettlin et al., 1989; Macdonell et al., 1988).

Spectral studies have compared AD and VaD. Erkinjuntti et al. (1988) compared AD patients to VaD patients in groups that were similar with regard to sex, age, education, and degree of dementia. Spectral analysis revealed a decline in the percentage of alpha power and a concomitant increase in theta and delta power relative to the degree of dementia for both groups. They found no significant group differences, while others have reported differences (d'Onofrio et al., 1996; Leuchter and Walter, 1989; Leuchter et al., 1987, 1992; Sloan and Fenton 1993).

Cerebral autosomal-dominant arteriopathy with subcortical infarcts and leukoencephalopathy (CADASIL) is a genetically determined early-onset VaD due to an arteriopathy (Hedera and Turner, 2002). A mutation in the *NOTCH-3* genes was identified as a cause of CADASIL (Joutel and Tournier-Lasserve, 1998). The clinical syndrome was first described in a large family with subcortical strokes and dementia (Tournier-Lasserve et al., 1993). Cerebral ischemia (not associated with stroke risk factors) is the most common manifestation of CADASIL, followed by cognitive decline. Typically cognitive deficits occur in the classic stepwise fashion associated with VaD, but many patients may present with progressive deterioration resembling a subcortical neurodegenerative dementia. Migraines with aura are common in CADASIL, having been reported in almost half of all patients (Hedra and Turner, 2002). Epilepsy, most often following strokes, had been reported in 2% to

10% of CADASIL patients. No specific EEG changes have been associated with CADASIL.

Subcortical Dementia

Parkinson's Disease

It is estimated that up to 40% of patients with Parkinson's disease (PD) develop dementia (Goldstein and Price, 2003). Typically the dementia is usually associated with long-standing disease, 5 to 10 years from PD onset, and may have characteristics similar to DLB. The EEG abnormalities reported in PD consist of nonspecific diffuse changes, such as slowing of background rhythms posteriorly and an increase in theta and delta activity (England et al., 1959; Sirakov and Mezan, 1963). Occipital slowing has been associated with dementia and the degree of motor disability in PD patients (Neufeld et al., 1988). Soikkeli et al. (1991) reported similar findings using spectral analysis, and Neufeld et al. (1994) found a nonsignificant but consistent trend of increased amplitude in the delta and theta range in the demented PD patients compared to nondemented PD subjects and normal controls. Rivastigmine, a cholinesterase inhibitor, produced a significant increase in relative alpha activity in demented parkinsonian patients. An increase in beta activity and a decrease in slower frequencies (delta and theta) were also observed; however, these were not statistically significant (Fogelson et al., 2003).

Progressive Supranuclear Palsy

Next to DLB, progressive supranuclear palsy (PSP) is the second most common "dementia with parkinsonism." PSP causes a dementia similar to that of PD in up to 75% of patients (Goldstein and Price, 2003). Su and Goldensohn (1973) found that the initial EEG was normal in eight of 12 (67%) patients with PSP. In cases where subsequent records were performed, EEG abnormalities consisted of background slowing and bursts of frontal intermittent rhythmic delta activity (FIRDA) with progression of the dementia. Fowler and Harrison (1986) compared the EEGs of 22 patients with PSP to 22 patients with a comparable (mild to moderate) degree of dementia due to AD. Twelve of 22 (55%) patients with PSP had normal EEGs. The most common abnormality was an excessive amount of theta activity. Similar nonspecific abnormalities were found in the comparable AD group. Like others (Gordon and Sim, 1967; Harner, 1975; Torres and Hutton, 1986), the authors felt that in AD severe EEG abnormalities are seen in the more advanced cases. Thus, Fowler and Harrison (1986) did not feel that PSP patients could be distinguished from mild to moderately demented AD patients on the basis of EEG findings. Montplaisir et al. (1997) compared qEEG in six patients with PSP to controls and found that PSP patients had slowing over the frontal lobes during wakefulness. In addition, abnormalities of sleep architecture were identified, including REM sleep abnormalities.

Huntington's Disease

Huntington's disease is an autosomal-dominant neurodegenerative disease caused by an expanded trinucleotide (CAG) repeat. Even in the absence of clinical symptoms, it is easily diagnosed with genetic testing. In the past, the EEG was felt to have potential value in diagnosing HD. Low-voltage (less than 10 µV) EEGs have been described in approximately 40% of cases of HD (Scott et al., 1972; Sishta et al., 1974). Because of the proposed rarity of this pattern in normal individuals, some investigators have felt that the EEG is particularly helpful in the diagnosis of this disease (Scott et al., 1972; Torres and Hutton, 1986). However, earlier research (Adams, 1959) reported low-voltage tracings in 10% of adults without neurological or psychiatric conditions. With respect to HD, Pedley and Miller (1983) did not feel that a low-voltage pattern is characteristic of the illness, at least in the early stages when the diagnosis was previously difficult to make. The EEG has not proven to be of predictive value in indicating which family members will eventually develop the disease (Chandler, 1966) and has no role with advances in genetic testing. Streletz et al. (1990), using computerized analysis, found increased theta and decreased alpha activity in patients with HD; quantitatively similar changes were found in patients with AD. Bylsma et al. (1994) used qEEG in 16 HD patients and found frontal and temporal abnormalities and decreased EEG amplitude that correlated with the severity of neurological impairment. Myoclonus is a rare phenomenon in HD, but has been reported is a few families, and is associated with cortical epileptiform discharges (Thompson et al., 1994; Vogel et al., 1991).

Normal Pressure Hydrocephalus

Normal pressure hydrocephalus (NPH) presents classically with gait apraxia, urinary urgency or incontinence, and mental status changes. NPH is considered a potentially reversible dementia since it is due to a structural change that can be surgically treated (Goldstein and Price, 2003). Relatively few EEG studies have been described in this disorder. Brown and Goldensohn (1973) reported 11 cases; six had normal EEGs. The remainder had a variety of changes usually with normal background rhythms. In only one patient was FIRDA present, and it occupied only a small portion of the record. Several reports revealed a higher incidence of abnormal EEG tracings in patients diagnosed with NPH (Greenberg et al., 1977; Petersen et al., 1985; Wood et al., 1974). Hashi et al. (1976) described that the majority of NPH patients studied (12/13) had abnormal EEG tracings; the most common pattern showed bihemispheric monorhythmic bursts of slowing. Four of five patients who underwent shunting procedures had significant improvement of their EEG postoperatively.

Human Immunodeficiency Virus-1 Encephalopathy

It is estimated that 15% to 20% of AIDS patients develop a progressive encephalopathy resulting in dementia. The clinical manifestations, neuroimaging studies, and pathological features of this entity, which are due to direct brain infection by the retrovirus, suggest predominantly subcortical involvement, at least initially (Navia et al., 1986). In patients with HIV encephalopathy, EEG findings are nonspecific, consisting of excessive generalized slowing (Gabuzda et al., 1988; Goodin et al., 1990; McArthur, 1987). Harden et al. (1993) described unusual low-amplitude slow and featureless EEG patterns in some severely demented AIDS patients who also had atrophy on CT scan. EEG abnormalities were not found to correlate with clinical and imaging criteria for early encephalopathy (Harrison et al. 1998). However, in the more advanced stages, EEG slowing has been reported to parallel neurological deterioration (Tinuper et al., 1990). With respect to asymptomatic HIV-1-infected individuals, some researchers reported that EEG abnormalities were the earliest indicator of subtle central nervous system (CNS) dysfunction and could potentially predict the development of neurological disease (Koralnik et al., 1990; Parisi et al., 1989) in patients. This has been refuted by the Multicenter AIDS Cohort Study (MACS), which found no difference in the incidence of EEG abnormalities in asymptomatic individuals compared to seronegative controls (Nuwer et al., 1992).

Other Disorders

Delirium

Delirium is characterized by an acute change in mental status and consciousness and affects 10% to 30% of hospitalized patients (Gleason 2003). Delirium is common in the elderly, and dementia is often a predisposing factor underlying delirium in this group (Beresin, 1988; Lipowski, 1989; Francis et al., 1990; Strub and Black, 1988). For example, Purdie et al. (1981) found that 44 of 100 consecutive admissions for undiagnosed acute confusional states had a chronic organic brain syndrome with a superimposed acute insult causing decompensation. There are clinical features that usually help in the differentiation of delirium from dementia, such as rapidity of onset, brief duration, and clouding of consciousness. However, the conditions often coexist.

The EEG is often helpful in indicating whether the delirium is due to (a) a diffuse encephalopathy; (b) a focal brain lesion; or (c) continued epileptic activity without motor manifestations, such as nonconvulsive status epilepticus. See Brenner (1991) and Klass and Brenner (1995) for a review of the role of the EEG in delirium.

Most often, patients with delirium have a toxic-metabolic encephalopathy. Generally, with progression of the encephalopathy, there is a diffuse slowing of background rhythms from alpha to theta, with delta activity becoming predominant when the patient is comatose. The EEG may also show FIRDA. Although a diffusely slow record indicates cerebral dysfunction, it is not specific for a single etiology. The degree of slowing usually parallels the degree of alteration of consciousness and indicates its severity; however, there are exceptions. Spectral analysis also indicates an association between spectral EEG changes and severity of cognitive deterioration in delirium (Jacobson and Jerrier, 2000). In one study, the percentage of delta and mean frequency correlated with the length of both delirium and hospitalization (Koponen et al., 1989). Similar findings were reported by Jacobson et al. (1993), who reported that the most abnormal conventional and qEEG results occurred in subjects with delirium coexisting with dementia.

Occasionally, patients with focal lesions appear to have a confusional state due to global impairment. For example, patients with Wernicke's aphasia may be mistaken for having a global rather than a focal deficit. Several types of EEG abnormalities may occur in patients with focal lesions including polymorphic delta activity, focal attenuation of activity, a decrease of faster frequencies over the affected side, and epileptiform abnormalities, such as periodic lateralized epileptiform discharges (PLEDs).

The EEG is extremely useful in the identification of nonconvulsive status epilepticus, particularly when the cause of this acute confusional state is not clinically apparent. There are two major categories of nonconvulsive status: generalized, often termed absence status; and complex partial status. In the former, the EEG shows more or less continuous generalized, bilaterally synchronous, symmetric epileptic activity, usually maximal anteriorly (Fig. 18.4). In complex partial status epilepticus, the EEG abnormalities usually are focal, most often affecting the temporal area, although they can become generalized. At times, however, these two conditions can be difficult to distinguish, even with ictal EEG recordings (Guberman et al., 1986; Tomson et al., 1986). Some feel that ictal confusion due to generalized nonconvulsive status epilepticus appearing for the first time in later life is a distinct entity (Ellis and Lee, 1978; Lee, 1985; Primavera et al., 1994; Schwartz and Scott, 1971). Some cases may represent drug toxicity (Wengs et al., 1993; Zak et al., 1994) or an uncommon complication of drug (benzodiazepine) withdrawal (Thomas et al., 1992, 1993).

In the differential diagnosis of delirium, psychiatric causes include schizophrenia, atypical psychoses, mood disorders, and hysteria (Beresin, 1988; Gleason, 2003; Lipowski, 1989), and drugs that produce acute psychological disturbances, particularly a heightened state of arousal (Engel and Romano, 1959). Most patients with delirium have a diffusely slow EEG, which is helpful in separating an organic from a functional, purely psychiatric, psychosis that may share features of delirium. In patients with psychiatric disorders, the EEG is generally normal or, when abnormal, does not usually show the degree or magnitude of slowing seen in a confused patient with an organic disorder (Bostwick and Philbrick, 2002; Strub and Black, 1988). However, the EEG may be of less value in the acutely fearful, agitated, and delirious patient, because it would not appear to be significant different from that in other agitated patients, such as those with schizophrenia or other functional psychoses (Pro and Wells, 1977). The effects of drug or electroshock treatments on the EEG may also blur the distinction between a psychiatric disorder and an organic encephalopathy.

The EEG has been cited as helpful in distinguishing delirium from dementia, often showing generalized bilateral slowing in delirium due to toxic-metabolic disorders (except in cases of withdrawal symptoms, where low-voltage fast activity is seen), and usually being normal or showing only mild slowing in dementia (Beresin, 1988; Jacobson and Jerrier, 2000). Engel and Romano (1959) felt that the EEG in dementia showed slowing less consistently when compared to delirium and that a significant proportion of mildly to moderately demented patients had normal or borderline EEGs. In a study to validate the distinction between delir-

Figure 18.4. Generalized nonconvulsive status epilepticus (absence status) in an 84-year-old woman with no previous history of seizures. (From Klass, D.W., and Brenner, R.P. 1995. Electroencephalography of the elderly. J Clin Neurophysiol 12:116–131. New York: Raven Press, with permission.)

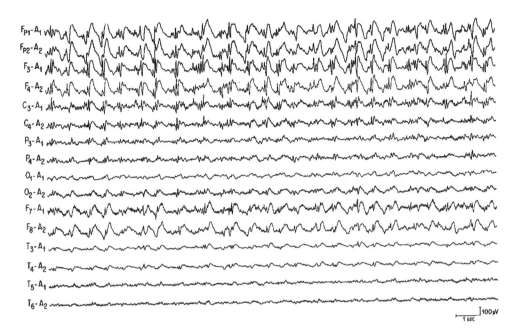

ium and dementia, Rabins and Folstein (1982) found that delirious patients, when compared to demented patients, were more likely to have a diffusely slow EEG. EEGs were abnormal in 87% of delirious patients and 89% of demented patients, but the percentage of abnormal EEGs that were diffusely slow differed between the two groups. Eighty-one percent of the delirious patients had such recordings, while 33% of the demented patients had diffusely slow EEGs. This difference was statistically significant ($p < .001$). Thus, the authors felt that the EEG findings supported the use of the EEG as an aid in diagnosing delirium. They concluded that in patients on acute medical inpatient units a diffusely slow EEG is more suggestive of delirium. However, diffusely slow records also occur in dementia, with the severity of the dementia being the important variable. Furthermore, delirium and dementia often coexist.

Depression

When present in depressed patients, EEG abnormalities detected by visual analysis are usually mild (Brenner et al., 1988). In an early study of aged psychiatric patients, Obrist and Henry (1958) found that the majority with an organic brain syndrome had diffuse slowing on the EEG, while most patients with functional disorders (including depression) had normal tracings. The clinical value of the EEG in the evaluation of depression often is to help exclude other disorders that may mimic an affective disorder (Small, 1983). In addition, the EEG can be helpful in distinguishing dementia from pseudodementia, which is frequently due to depression (Boutrous and Struve, 2002; Hegerl and Moller, 1997; Rosen, 1997). The EEG is more often abnormal in the former and normal in the latter (Ron, 1979; Wilson et al., 1977). However, the EEG in patients with dementia can also be normal, particularly in the early stages, while abnormal in patients with depression. Furthermore, some patients may have mixed symptoms.

Brenner et al. (1989) reported EEG findings in 33 elderly patients with mixed symptoms of depression and dementia followed longitudinally to confirm diagnosis. Two groups of patients—patients with dementia with depressive features, and patients with depressive pseudodementia—were defined. Also included for comparison were patients with probable AD without depressive features, patients with major depression without cognitive impairment, and healthy elderly controls. There were significant group differences on waking EEGs between those mixed patients who did well after treatment for depression (depressive pseudodementia) and those patients having dementia with secondary depression. The majority of patients with either dementia or dementia with secondary depression had abnormal EEGs, with approximately one third having moderate or severe abnormalities. In contrast, in patients with either depression or depressive pseudodementia, the EEG was usually normal or showed only mild abnormalities. Pozzi et al. (1995), using qEEG, reported differences in depressed patients with or without dementia, with delta activity increased posteriorly in AD patients compared to those with only depression.

Epilepsy and Dementia

Dementia can be due to a variety of causes (Geldmacher and Whitehouse, 1997). Although some authors (Walstra et al., 1996) report a low prevalence (1%) of "reversible" dementias in elderly patients evaluated at a memory clinic, the evaluation of an individual with dementia still includes a careful search for potentially treatable causes of cognitive impairment. In the adult epilepsy population, selective cognitive impairment and amnesia have been attributed to epileptiform activity (Aarts et al., 1984; Zeman et al., 1998). Of great interest with regard to dementia are case reports of patients who presented with progressive memory impairment in whom memory dysfunction was attributed to unrecognized seizures. Tatum and colleagues (1998) described five patients over the age of 67 who had complaints of memory loss with a waxing and waning pattern. All had initial nondiagnostic EEGs, but prolonged EEG monitoring documented seizure activity, four with electrographic seizure onset over the left temporal lobe. Three had resolution of memory deficits with antiepileptic drugs (AED) treatment. Hogh et al. (2002) reported three patients with progressive memory impairment and an initial diagnosis of AD who had abnormal EEGs (two with temporal epileptiform discharges, one with intermittent sharply contoured frontotemporal theta activity). All three had sustained and measurable improvement on cognitive testing following initiation of AED therapy. Since unrecognized seizures can produce memory deficits and be misdiagnosed as dementia, epilepsy should be considered in the differential diagnosis of dementia. In addition, patients with a diagnosis of dementia may also have epilepsy.

Seizures are now the third most frequently encountered neurological problem in the elderly population, preceded by stroke and dementia. One of the most commonly identified causes for epilepsy in the elderly individual is dementia (Hauser, 1992). Based on a review of the literature, dementia appears to be a risk factor for the development of epilepsy. There is conflicting data regarding the percentage of patients with dementia who develop unprovoked seizures, varying from 2.4% to 17% (Hauser, 1997; Hesdorffer et al., 1996; Mendez et al., 1994; Romanelli et al., 1990; Scheuer et al., 2000).

Making the diagnosis of epilepsy in elderly patients with dementia can be challenging since they may be poor historians, be unaware of their seizures, have had unwitnessed spells, or have concomitant medical problems that confound the clinical picture. The presence of interictal epileptiform discharges on EEG support the diagnosis of epilepsy, but is reported to be less frequent in older individuals (Ajmone-Marsan and Zivin, 1970). In a retrospective study, Drury and Beydoun (1998) reported that in patients with seizure onset after the age of 60, interictal epileptiform activity was present in only 26% of 70 patients (mean age of 70). Prolonged monitoring, either ambulatory or closed circuit television (CCTV) EEG, is a valuable diagnostic tool in establishing the correct epilepsy diagnosis in the elderly patient. Equally important, monitoring may identify patients with other treatable medical or psychiatric conditions who are receiving anticonvulsant medications for nonepileptic spells (Drury et al., 1999; Lancman et al., 1996). Although a potentially challenging procedure in an uncooperative patient, monitoring should be considered in demented patients with spells suspected of being seizures.

Summary

The EEG is often useful in the evaluation of dementia. It can aid in differentiating between a degenerative disorder, such as AD, and pseudodementia due to psychiatric illness. In patients with dementia, the EEG may indicate whether the process is focal or diffuse. It can also provide early evidence for CJD or suggest the possibility of a toxic-metabolic disorder. Finally, a previously unrecognized seizure disorder

may be discovered. However, the EEG does have limitations. The most common abnormality, diffuse slowing, is nonspecific and occurs in many different types of dementia, as well as in other disorders, such as delirium. Furthermore, EEG changes in dementia are usually related to severity of illness, particularly in AD, so that the EEG can be normal early in the course of the illness when the diagnosis is more difficult clinically. Perhaps future qEEG techniques will help in classification, monitoring, and prognostication of dementia.

References

Aarts, J.H., Binnie, C.D., Smit, A.M, et al. 1984. Selective cognitive impairment during focal and generalized epileptiform EEG activity. Brain 107:293–308.

Adams, A. 1959. Studies on flat electroencephalogram in man. Electroencephalogr. Clin. Neurophysiol. 11:34–41.

Adler, G., and Brassen, S. 2001. Short-term rivastigmine treatment reduces EEG slow-wave power in Alzheimer's patients. Neuropsychobiology 43:273–276.

Adler, G., Brassen, S., and Jajcevic, A. 2003. EEG coherence in Alzheimer's dementia. J. Neural Transm. 110:1051–1058.

Agnoli, A., Martucci, N., Manna, V., et al. 1983. Effect of cholinergic and anticholinergic drugs on short-term memory in Alzheimer's dementia: a neuropsychological and computerized electroencephalographic study. Clin. Neuropharmacol. 6:311–323.

Aguglia, U., Farnarier, G., Tinuper, P., et al. 1987. Subacute spongiform encephalopathy with periodic paroxysmal activities: clinical evolution and serial EEG findings in 20 cases. Clin. Electroencephalogr. 18:147–158.

Ajmone-Marsan, C., and Zivin, L.S. 1970. Factors related to the occurrence of typical paroxysmal abnormalities in the EEG records of epileptic patients. Epilepsia 11:361–381.

American Psychiatric Association, Committee on Nomenclature and Statistics. 1994. *Diagnostic and Statistical Manual of Mental Disorders: DSM-IV,* 4th ed. rev. Washington, DC: American Psychiatric Association.

Anderer, P., Saletu, B., Kloppel, B., et al. 1994. Discrimination between demented patients and normals based on topographic EEG slow wave activity: comparison between Z statistics, discriminant analysis and artificial neural network classifiers. Electroencephalogr. Clin. Neurophysiol. 91:108–117.

Au, W.J., Gabor, A.J., Viyan, N., et al. 1980. Periodic lateralized epileptiform complexes (PLEDS) in Creutzfeldt-Jakob disease. Neurology 30:611–617.

Barber, P.A., Varma, A.R., Lloyd, J.J., et al. 2000. The electroencephalogram in dementia with Lewy bodies. Acta Neurol. Scand. 101:53–56.

Bennys, K., Rondouin, G., Vergnes, C., et al. 2001. Diagnostic value of quantitative EEG in Alzheimer's disease. Neurophysiol. Clin. 31:153–160.

Beresin, E.V. 1988. Delirium in the elderly. J. Geriatr. Psychiatry Neurol. 1:127–143.

Berg, L., Danziger, W.L., Storandt, M., et al. 1984. Predictive features in mild senile dementia of the Alzheimer type. Neurology 34:563–569.

Besthorn, C., Forstl, H., Geiger-Kabisch, C., et al. 1994. EEG coherence in Alzheimer disease. Electroencephalogr. Clin. Neurophysiol. 90:242–245.

Besthorn, C., Zerfass, R., Geiger-Kabisch, C., et al. 1997. Discrimination of Alzheimer's disease and normal aging by EEG data. Electroencephalogr. Clin. Neurophysiol. 103:241–248.

Blatt, I., and Brenner, R.P. 1996. Triphasic waves in a psychiatric population: a retrospective study. J. Clin. Neurophysiol. 13:324–329.

Bortone, E., Bettoni, L., Giorgi, C., et al. 1994. Reliability of EEG in the diagnosis of Creutzfeldt-Jakob disease. Electroencephalogr. Clin. Neurophysiol. 90:323–330.

Bostwick, J.M., and Philbrick, K.L. 2002. The use of electroencephalography in psychiatry of the medically ill. Psychiatr. Clin. North Am. 25:17–25.

Boutros, N.N., and Struve, F. 2002. Electrophysiological assessment of neuropsychiatric disorders. Semin. Clin. Neuropsychiatry 7:30–41.

Brenner, R.P. 1991. Utility of electroencephalography in delirium: past views and current practice. Int. Psychogeriatr. 3:211–229.

Brenner, R.P., and Schaul, N. 1990. Periodic EEG patterns: classification, clinical correlation and pathophysiology. J. Clin. Neurophysiol. 7:249–267.

Brenner, R.P., Ulrich, R.F., Spiker, D.G., et al. 1986. Computerized EEG spectral analysis in elderly normal, demented and depressed subjects. Electroencephalogr. Clin. Neurophysiol. 64:483–492.

Brenner, R.P., Reynolds, C.F., and Ulrich, R.F. 1988. Diagnostic efficacy of computerized spectral versus visual EEG analysis in elderly normal, demented and depressed subjects. Electroencephalogr. Clin. Neurophysiol. 169:110–117.

Brenner, R.P., Reynolds, C.F., and Ulrich, R.F. 1989. EEG findings in depressive pseudodementia and dementia with secondary depression. Electroencephalogr. Clin. Neurophysiol. 72:298–304.

Briel, R.C., McKeith, I.G., Barker, W.A., et al. 1999. EEG findings in dementia with Lewy bodies and Alzheimer's disease. J. Neurol. Neurosurg. Psychiatry 66:401–403.

Brown, D.G., and Goldensohn, E.S. 1973. The electroencephalogram in normal pressure hydrocephalus. Arch. Neurol. 29:70–71.

Brown, P., Cathala, F., Castaigne, P., et al. 1986. Creutzfeldt-Jakob disease: clinical analysis of a consecutive series of 230 neuropathologically verified cases. Ann. Neurol. 20:597–602.

Bucht, G., Adolfsson, R., and Winblad, B. 1984. Dementia of the Alzheimer type and multi-infarct dementia. A clinical description and diagnostic problems. J. Am. Geriatr. Soc. 32:491–498.

Burger, L.J., Rowan, A.J., and Goldensohn, E.S. 1972. Creutzfeldt-Jakob disease: an electroencephalographic study. Arch. Neurol. 26:428–433.

Bylsma, F.W., Peyser, C.E., Folstein, S.E., et al. 1994. EEG power spectra in Huntington's disease: clinical and neuropsychological correlates. Neuropsychologia 32:137–150.

Calzetti, S., Bortone, E., Negrotti, A., et al. 2002. Frontal intermittent rhythmic delta activity (FIRDA) in patients with dementia with Lewy bodies: a diagnostic tool? Neurol. Sci. 23(suppl 2):S65–66.

Cambier, D.M., Kantarci, K., Worrell, G.A., et al. 2003. Lateralized and focal clinical, EEG, and FLAIR MRI abnormalities in Creutzfeldt-Jakob disease. Clin. Neurophysiol. 114:1724–1728.

Canter, N.L., Hallett, M., and Growdon, J.H. 1982. Lecithin does not affect EEG spectral analysis or P300 in Alzheimer disease. Neurology 32:1260–1266.

Chandler, J.H. 1966. EEG in prediction of Huntington's chorea. An eighteen-year follow-up. Electroencephalogr. Clin. Neurophysiol. 21:79–80.

Chiofalo, N., Fuentes, A., and Galvez, S. 1980. Serial EEG findings in 27 cases of Creutzfeldt-Jakob disease. Arch. Neurol. 37:143–145.

Chui, H.C. 1989. Dementia. A review emphasizing clinicopathologic correlation and brain-behavior relationships. Arch. Neurol. 48:806–814.

Claus, J.J., Kwa, V.I., Teunisse, S., et al. 1998a. Slowing on quantitative spectral EEG is a marker for rate of subsequent cognitive and functional decline in early Alzheimer disease. Alzheimer Dis. Assoc. Disord. 12:167–174.

Claus, J.J., Ongerboer de Visser, B.W., Walstra, G.J.M., et al. 1998b. Quantitative spectral electroencephalography in predicting survival in patients with early Alzheimer disease. Arch. Neurol. 55:1105–1111.

Claus, J.J., Strijers, R.L., Jonkman, E.J., et al. 1999. The diagnostic value of electroencephalography in mild senile Alzheimer's disease. Clin. Neurophysiol. 110:825–832.

Coben, L.A., Danziger, W., and Berg, L. 1983. Frequency analysis of the resting awake EEG in mild senile dementia of Alzheimer type. Electroencephalogr. Clin. Neurophysiol. 55:372–380.

Coben, L.A., Danziger, W., and Storandt, M. 1985. A longitudinal EEG study of mild senile dementia of Alzheimer type: changes at 1 year and at 2.5 years. Electroencephalogr. Clin. Neurophysiol. 61:101–112.

Corey-Bloom, J., Thal, L.J., Galasko, D., et al. 1995. Diagnosis and evaluation of dementia. Neurology 45:211–218.

Crystal, H.A., Dickson, D.W., Lizardi, J.E., et al. 1990. Antemortem diagnosis of diffuse Lewy body disease. Neurology 40:1523–1528.

Cummings, J.L., and Benson, F.D. 1992. Laboratory aids in the diagnosis of dementia. In *Dementia: A Clinical Approach*, pp. 345–364. Boston: Butterworth-Heinemann.

Cummings, J.L., and Kaufer, D. 1996. Neuropsychiatric aspects of Alzheimer's disease: the cholinergic hypothesis revisited. Neurology 47:876–883.

d'Onofrio, F., Salvia, S., Petretta, V., et al. 1996. Quantified-EEG in normal aging and dementias. Acta Neurol. Scand. 93:336–345.

Dringenberg, H.C. 2000. Alzheimer's disease: more than a "cholinergic disorder"—evidence that cholinergic-monoaminergic interactions contribute to EEG slowing and dementia. Behav. Brain Res. 115:235–249.

Drury, I., and Beydoun, A. 1998. Interictal epileptiform activity in elderly patients with epilepsy. Electroencephalogr. Clin. Neurophysiol. 106:369–373.

Drury, I., Selwa, L.M., Schuh, L.A., et al. 1999. Value of inpatient diagnostic CCTV-EEG monitoring in the elderly. Epilepsia 40:1100–1102.

Duffy, F.H., Albert, M.S., and McAnulty, G. 1984. Brain electrical activity in patients with presenile and senile dementia of the Alzheimer type. Ann. Neurol. 16:439–448.

Dunkin, J.J., Osato, S., and Leuchter, A.F. 1995. Relationships between EEG coherence and neuropsychological tests in dementia. Clin. Electroencephalogr. 26:47–59.

Edwards-Lee, T., Cook, I., Fairbanks, L., et al. 2000. Quantitative electroencephalographic correlates of psychosis in Alzheimer disease. Neuropsychiatry Neuropsychol. Behav. Neurol. 13:163–170.

Ehle, A.L., and Johnson, P.C. 1977. Rapidly evolving EEG changes in a case of Alzheimer disease. Ann. Neurol. 1:593–595.

Ellis, J.M., and Lee, S.I. 1978. Acute prolonged confusion in later life as an ictal state. Epilepsia 19:119–128.

Elmstahl, S., Rosen, I., and Gullberg, B. 1994. Quantitative EEG in elderly patients with Alzheimer's disease and healthy controls. Dementia 5:119–124.

Engel, G.L., and Romano, J. 1959. Delirium, a syndrome of cerebral insufficiency. J. Chronic Dis. 3:260–277.

England, A.C., Schwab, R.S., and Peterson, E. 1959. The electroencephalogram in Parkinson's syndrome. Electroencephalogr Clin. Neurophysiol. 11:723–731.

Erkinjuntti, T., Larsen, T., Sulkava, R., et al. 1988. EEG in the differential diagnosis between Alzheimer's disease and vascular dementia. Acta Neurol. Scand. 77:36–43.

Ettlin, T.M., Staehelin, H.B., Kischka, U., et al. 1989. Computed tomography, electroencephalography, and clinical features in the differential diagnosis of senile dementia. Arch. Neurol. 46:1217–1220.

Fogelson, N., Kogan, E., Korczyn, A.D., et al. 2003. Effects of rivastigmine on the quantitative EEG in demented Parkinsonian patients. Acta Neurol. Scand. 107:252–255.

Folstein, M.F., Folstein, S.E., and McHugh, P.R. 1975. "Mini-Mental State": a practical method for grading the cognitive state of patients for the clinician. J. Psychiatr. Res. 12:189–198.

Forstl, H., Besthorn, C., Hentschel, F., et al. 1996a. Frontal lobe degeneration and Alzheimer's disease: a controlled study on clinical findings, volumetric brain changes and quantitative electroencephalography data. Dementia 7:27–34.

Forstl, H., Sattel, H., Besthorn, C., et al. 1996b. Longitudinal cognitive, electroencephalographic and morphologic brain changes in ageing and Alzheimer's disease. Br J. Psychiatry 168:280–186.

Fowler, C.J., and Harrison, M.J.G. 1986. EEG changes in subcortical dementia: a study of 22 patients with Steel-Richardson-Olszewski (SRO) syndrome. Electroencephalogr. Clin. Neurophysiol. 64:301–303.

Francis, J., Martin, D., and Kapoor, W.N. 1990. A prospective study of delirium in hospitalized elderly. JAMA 263:1097–1101.

Gabuzda, D.H., Levy, S.R., and Chiappa, K.H. 1988. Electroencephalography in AIDS and AIDS-related complex. Clin. Electroencephalogr. 19:1–6.

Galvin, J.E. 2003. Dementia with Lewy bodies. Arch. Neurol. 60:1332–1335.

Geldmacher, D.S., and Whitehouse, P.J. 1997. Differential diagnosis of Alzheimer's disease. Neurology 48(suppl 6):S2–S9.

Giaquinto, S., and Nolfe, G. 1986. The EEG in the normal elderly: A contribution to the interpretation of aging and dementia. Electroencephalogr. Clin. Neurophysiol. 63:540–546.

Gleason, O.C. 2003. Delirium. Am. Fam. Physician 67:1027–1034.

Gloor, P. 1980. EEG characteristics in Creutzfeldt-Jakob disease. Ann. Neurol. 8:341.

Goldstein, M.A., and Price, B.H. 2003. Non-Alzheimer dementias. In *Office Practice on Neurology*, Eds. M.A. Samuels and S.K. Feske, pp. 873–886. Philadelphia: Churchill Livingstone.

Goodin, D.S., and Aminoff, M.J. 1986. Electrophysiological differences between subtypes of dementia. Brain 109:1103–1113.

Goodin, D.S., and Aminoff, M.J. 1987. Electrophysiological differences between demented and nondemented patients with Parkinson's disease. Ann. Neurol. 21:90–94.

Goodin, D.S., Aminoff, M.J., Chernoff, D.N., et al. 1990. Long latency event-related potentials in patients infected with human immunodeficiency virus. Ann. Neurol. 27:414–419.

Gordon, E.B., and Sim, M. 1967. The E.E.G. in presenile dementia. J. Neurol. Neurosurg. Psychiatry 30:285–291.

Greenberg, J.O., Shenkin, H.A., and Adam, R. 1977. Idiopathic normal pressure hydrocephalus—a report of 73 patients. J. Neurol. Neurosurg. Psychiatry 40:336–341.

Groen, J.J., and Endtz, L.J. 1982. Hereditary Pick's disease: second re-examination of the large family and discussion of other hereditary cases, with particular reference to electroencephalography, a computerized tomography. Brain 105:443–459.

Guberman, A., Cantu-Reyna, G., Stuss, D., et al. 1986. Nonconvulsive generalized status epilepticus: clinical features, neuropsychological testing, and long-term follow-up. Neurology 36:1284–1291.

Hansen, H.C., Zschocke, S., Sturenburg, H.J., et al. 1998. Clinical changes and EEG patterns preceding the onset of periodic sharp wave complexes in Creutzfeldt-Jakob disease. Acta Neurol. Scand. 97:99–106.

Harden, C.L., Daras, M., Tuchman, A.J., et al. 1993. Low amplitude EEGs in demented AIDS patients. Electroencephalogr. Clin. Neurophysiol. 87:54–56.

Harner, R.N. 1975. EEG evaluation of the patient with dementia. In *Psychiatric Aspects of Neurological Diseases,* vol. 1, Eds. F.D. Benson and D. Blummer, pp. 63–82. New York: Grune and Stratton.

Harrison, M.J.G., Thomas, C.J., DuBoulay, G.H., et al. 1979. Multi-infarct dementia. J. Neurol. Sci. 40:97–103.

Harrison, M.J., Newman, S.P., Hall-Craggs, M.A., et al. 1998. Evidence of CNS impairment in HIV infection: clinical, neuropsychological, EEG, and MRI/MRS study. J. Neurol. Neurosurg. Psychiatry 65:301–307.

Hashi, K., Nishimura, S., Kondo, A., et al. 1976. The EEG in normal pressure hydrocephalus. Acta Neurochir. (Wien) 33:23–35.

Hauser, W.A. 1992. Seizure disorders: the changes with age. Epilepsia 33(suppl 4):S6–14.

Hauser, W. 1997. Epidemiology of seizures and epilepsy in the elderly. In *Seizures and Epilepsy in the Elderly,* Ed. A. Rowan, pp. 7–18. Boston: Butterworth-Heinemann.

Hedera, P., and Turner, R.S. 2002. Inherited dementias. Neurol. Clin. 20:779–808.

Hegerl, U., and Moller, H.J. 1997. Electroencephalography as a diagnostic instrument in Alzheimer's disease: reviews and perspectives. Int. Psychogeriatr. 9:237–246.

Helkala, E.-L., Laulumaa, V., Soininen, H., et al. 1991. Different pattern of cognitive decline related to normal or deteriorating EEG in three-year follow-up study with patients of Alzheimer's disease. Neurology 41:528–532.

Hesdorffer, D.C., Hauser, W.A., Annegers, J.F., et al. 1996. Dementia and adult-onset unprovoked seizures. Neurology 46:727–730.

Hier, D.B., Mangone, C.A., Ganellen, R., et al. 1991. Quantitative measurement of delta activity in Alzheimer's disease. Clin. Electroencephalogr. 22:178–182.

Hogan, M.J., Swanwick, G.R., Kaiser, J., et al. 2003. Memory-related EEG power and coherence reductions in mild Alzheimer's disease. Int J. Psychophysiol. 49:147–163.

Hogh, P., Smith, S.J., Scahill, R.I., et al. 2002. Epilepsy presenting as AD: neuroimaging, electroclinical features, and response to treatment. Neurology 58:298–301.

Holschneider, D.P., and Leuchter, A.F. 1999. Clinical neurophysiology using electroencephalography in geriatric psychiatry: neurobiologic implications and clinical utility. J. Geriatr. Psychiatry Neurol. 12:150–164.

Hooijer, C., Jonker, C., Posthuma, J., et al. 1990. Reliability, validity and follow-up of the EEG in senile dementia: sequelae of sequential measurement. Electroencephalogr. Clin. Neurophysiol. 76:400–412.

Hormes, J.T., Benarroch, E.E., Rodriguez, M., et al. 1988. Periodic sharp waves in baclofen-induced encephalopathy. Arch. Neurol. 45:814–815.

Hsich, G., Kenney, K., Gibbs, C.J., et al. 1996. The 14-3-3 brain protein in cerebrospinal fluid as a marker for transmissible spongiform encephalopathies. N. Engl. J. Med. 335:924–930.

Huang, N., Marie, S.K., Livramento, J.A., et al. 2003. 14-3-3 protein in the CSF of patients with rapidly progressive dementia. Neurology 61:354–357.

Hughes, J.R., Shanmugham, S., Wetzel, L.C., et al. 1989. The relationship between EEG changes and cognitive functions in dementia: a study in a VA population. Clin. Electroencephalogr. 20:77–85.

Isozumi, K., Fukuuchi, Y., Tanaka, K., et al. 1994. A MELAS (mitochondrial myopathy, encephalopathy, lactic acidosis, and stroke-like episodes) mtDNA mutation that induces subacute dementia which mimics Creutzfeldt-Jakob disease. Intern. Med. 33:543–546.

Jacobson, S., and Jerrier, H. 2000. EEG in delirium. Semin. Clin. Neuropsychiatry 5:86–92.

Jacobson, S.A., Leuchter, A.F., and Walter, D.O. 1993. Conventional and quantitative EEG in the diagnosis of delirium among the elderly. J. Neurol. Neurosurg. Psychiatry 56:153–158.

Johannesson, G., Hagberg, B., Gustafson, L., et al. 1979. EEG and cognitive impairment in presenile dementia. Acta Neurol. Scand. 59:225–240.

Jonkman, E.J. 1997. The role of the electroencephalogram in the diagnosis of dementia of the Alzheimer type: an attempt at technology assessment. Neurophysiol. Clin. 27:211–219.

Joutel, A., and Tournier-Lasserve, E. 1998. Notch signalling pathway and human diseases. Semin. Cell Dev. Biol. 9:619–625.

Kasczniak, A.W., Garron, D.C., Fox, J.H., et al. 1979. Cerebral atrophy, EEG slowing, age, education, and cognitive functioning in suspected dementia. Neurology 29:1273–1279.

Katzman, R. 1986. Differential diagnosis of dementing illnesses. Neurol. Clin. 4:329–340.

Klass, D.W., and Brenner, R.P. 1995. Electroencephalography of the elderly. J. Clin. Neurophysiol. 12:116–131.

Knight, R., and Will, B. 2003. Prion disease. In *Neurological Disorders Course and Treatment,* 2nd ed., pp. 707–720. San Diego: Academic Press.

Knott, V., Mohr, E., Hache, N., et al. 1999. EEG and passive P300 in dementia of the Alzheimer type. Clin. Electroencephalogr. 30:64–72.

Knott, V., Mohr, E., Mahoney, C., et al. 2000. Electroencephalographic coherence in Alzheimer's disease: comparisons with a control group and population norms. J. Geriatr. Psychiatry Neurol. 13:1–8.

Knott, V., Mohr, E., Mahoney, C., et al. 2001. Quantitative electroencephalography in Alzheimer's disease: comparison with a control group, population norms and mental status. J. Psychiatry Neurosci. 26:106–116.

Koponen, H., Partanen, J., Paakkonen, A., et al. 1989. EEG spectral analysis in delirium. J. Neurol. Neurosurg. Psychiatry 52:980–985.

Koralnik, I.J., Beaumanoir, A., Hausler, R., et al. 1990. A controlled study of early neurologic abnormalities in men with asymptomatic human immunodeficiency virus infection. N. Engl. J. Med. 323:864–870.

Kowalski, J.W., Gawel, M., Pfeffer, A., et al. 2001. The diagnostic value of EEG in Alzheimer disease: correlation with the severity of mental impairment. J. Clin. Neurophysiol. 18:570–575.

Lancman, M.E., O'Donovan, C., Dinner, D., et al. 1996. Usefulness of prolonged video-EEG monitoring in the elderly. J. Neurol. Sci. 142(1–2):54–58.

Lee, R.G., and Blair, R.D.G. 1973. Evolution of EEG and visual evoked response changes in Jakob-Creutzfeldt disease. Electroencephalogr. Clin. Neurophysiol. 35:133–142.

Lee, S.I. 1985. Nonconvulsive status epilepticus: ictal confusion in later life. Arch. Neurol. 42:778–781.

Lehtovirta, M., Partanen, J., Kononen, M., et al. 2000. A longitudinal quantitative EEG study of Alzheimer's disease: relation to apolipoprotein E polymorphism. Dement. Geriatr. Cogn. Disord. 11:29–35.

Letemendia, F., and Pampiglione, G. 1958. Clinical and electroencephalographic observations in Alzheimer's disease. J. Neurol. Neurosurg. Psychiatry 21:167–172.

Leuchter, A.F., Newton, T.F., Cook, I.A., et al. 1992. Changes in brain functional connectivity in Alzheimer-type and multi-infarct dementia. Brain 115:1543–1561.

Leuchter, A.F., and Walter, D.O. 1989. Diagnosis and assessment of dementia using functional brain imaging. Int. Psychogeriatr. 1:63–71.

Leuchter, A.F., Spar, J.E., Walter, D.O., et al. 1987. Electroencephalographic spectra and coherence in the diagnosis of Alzheimer's-type and multi-infarct dementia. Arch. Gen. Psychiatry 44:993–998.

Levy, S.R., Chiappa, K.H., Burke, C.J., et al. 1986. Early evolution and incidence of electroencephalographic abnormalities in Creutzfeldt-Jakob disease. J. Clin. Neurophysiol. 3:1–21.

Liddell, D.W. 1958. Investigations of E.E.G. findings in presenile dementia. J. Neurol. Neurosurg. Psychiatry 21:173–176.

Lindau, M., Jelic, V., Johansson, S.E., et al. 2003. Quantitative EEG abnormalities and cognitive dysfunctions in frontotemporal dementia and Alzheimer's disease. Dement. Geriatr. Cogn. Disord. 15:106–114.

Lipowski, Z.J. 1989. Delirium in the elderly patient. N. Engl. J. Med. 320:578–582.

Locatelli, T., Cursi, M., Liberati, D., et al. 1998. EEG coherence in Alzheimer's disease. Electroencephalogr. Clin. Neurophysiol. 106:229–237.

Lopez, O.L., Becker, J.T., Brenner, R.P., et al. 1991. Alzheimer's disease with delusions and hallucinations: neuropsychological and electroencephalographic correlates. Neurology 41:906–912.

Lopez, O.L., Brenner, R.P., Becker, J.T., et al. 1997. EEG spectral abnormalities and psychosis as predictors of cognitive and functional decline in probable Alzheimer's disease. Neurology 48:1521–1525.

Macdonell, R.A.L., Donnan, G.A., Baldin, P.F., et al. 1988. The electroencephalogram and acute ischemic stroke. Arch. Neurol. 45:520–524.

Masters, C.L., Harris, J.O., Gajdusek, D.C., et al. 1979. Creutzfeldt-Jakob disease: patterns of worldwide occurrence and the significance of familial and sporadic clustering. Ann. Neurol. 5:177–188.

McArthur, J.C. 1987. Neurological manifestations of AIDS. Medicine 66:407–437.

McKeith, I.G. 2000. Clinical Lewy body syndromes. Ann. N.Y. Acad. Sci. 920:1–8.

McKeith, I.G., Galasko, D., Kosaka, K., et al. 1996. Consensus guidelines for the clinical and pathologic diagnosis of dementia with Lewy bodies (DLB): report of the consortium on DLB international workshop. Neurology 47:1113–1124.

McKhann, G., Drachman, D., Folstein, M., et al. 1984. Clinical diagnosis of Alzheimer's disease: report of the NINCDS-ADRDA work group under the auspices of the Department of Health and Human Services Task Force on Alzheimer's Disease. Neurology 34:939–944.

Mendez, M.F., Catanzaro, P., Doss, R.C., et al. 1994. Seizures in Alzheimer's disease: clinicopathologic study. J. Geriatr. Psychiatry Neurol. 7:230–233.

Merdes, A.R., Hansen, L.A., Jeste, D.V., et al. 2003. Influence of Alzheimer pathology on clinical diagnostic accuracy in dementia with Lewy bodies. Neurology 60:1586–1590.

Merskey, H., Ball, M.J., Blume, W.T., et al. 1980. Relationships between psychological measurements and cerebral organic changes in Alzheimer's disease. Can. J. Neurol. Sci. 7:45–49.

Miyauchi, T., Hagimoto, H., Ishii, M., et al. 1994. Quantitative EEG in patients with presenile and senile dementia of the Alzheimer type. Acta Neurol. Scand. 89:56–64.

Montplaisir, J., Petit, D., Decary, A., et al. 1997. Sleep and quantitative EEG in patients with progressive supranuclear palsy. Neurology 49:999–1003.

Muller, H.F., and Kral, V.A. 1967. The electroencephalogram in advanced senile dementia. J. Am. Geriatr. Soc. 15:415–426.

Musha, T., Asada, T., Yamashita, F., et al. 2002. A new EEG method for estimating cortical neuronal impairment that is sensitive to early stage Alzheimer's disease. Clin. Neurophysiol. 113:1052–1058.

Navia, B.A., Jordan, B.D., and Price, R.W. 1986. The AIDS dementia complex: I. Clinical features. Ann. Neurol. 19:517–524.

Neary, D., Snowden, J.S., Gustafson, L., et al.1998. Frontotemporal lobar degeneration: a consensus on clinical diagnostic criteria. Neurology 51:1546–1554.

Neufeld, M.Y. 1992. Periodic triphasic waves in levodopa-induced encephalopathy. Neurology 42:444–446.

Neufeld, M.Y., Inzelberg, R., Korczyn, A.D. 1988. EEG in demented and non-demented parkinsonian patients. Acta Neurol. Scand. 78:1–5.

Neufeld, M.Y., Blumen, S., Aitkin, I., et al. 1994. EEG frequency analysis in demented and nondemented parkinsonian patients. Dementia 5:23–28.

Nobili, F., Copello, F., Vitali, P., et al. 1999. Timing of disease progression by quantitative EEG in Alzheimer's patients. J. Clin. Neurophysiol. 16:566–573.

Nuwer, M.R. 1996. Quantitative EEG analysis in clinical settings. Brain Topogr. 8:201–208.

Nuwer, M. 1997. Assessment of digital EEG, quantitative EEG, and EEG brain mapping: report of the American Academy of Neurology and the American Clinical Neurophysiology Society. Neurology 49:277–292.

Nuwer, M.R., Miller, E.N., Visscher, B.R., et al. 1992. Asymptomatic HIV infection does not cause EEG abnormalities: results from the Multicenter AIDS Cohort Study (MACS). Neurology 42:1214–1219.

Obrist, W.D. 1976. Problems of aging. In Handbook of Electroencephalography and Clinical Neurophysiology, vol. 6, Ed. A. Remond. pp. 275–292. Amsterdam: Elsevier.

Obrist, W.D., and Busse, E.W. 1965. The electroencephalogram in old age. In Applications of Electroencephalography in Psychiatry, Ed. W.P. Wilson, pp. 185–205. Durham: Duke University Press.

Obrist, W.D., and Henry, C.F. 1958. Electroencephalographic findings in aged psychiatric patients. J. Nerv. Ment. Dis. 126:254–267.

Obrist, W.D., Busse, E.W., Eisdorfer, C., et al. 1962. Relation of the electroencephalogram to intellectual function in senescence. J. Gerontol. 17:197–206.

Parisi, A., Strosselli, M., Di Perri, G., et al. 1989. Electroencephalography in the early diagnosis of HIV-related subacute encephalitis: analysis of 185 patients. Clin. Electroencephalogr. 20:1–5.

Pedley, T.A., and Miller, J.A. 1983. Clinical neurophysiology of aging and dementia. In Advances in Neurology: The Dementias, vol. 38, Eds. R. Mayeux and W.G. Rosen, pp. 31–49. New York: Raven Press.

Penttila, M., Partanen, J.V., Soininen, H., et al. 1985. Quantitative analysis of occipital EEG in different stages of Alzheimer's disease. Electroencephalogr. Clin. Neurophysiol. 60:1–6.

Petersen, R.C., Mokri, B., and Laws, E.R., Jr. 1985. Surgical treatment of idiopathic hydrocephalus in elderly patients. Neurology 35:307–311.

Petrosian, A.A., Prokhorov, D.V., Lajara-Nanson, W., et al. 2001. Recurrent neural network-based approach for early recognition of Alzheimer's disease in EEG. Clin. Neurophysiol. 112:1378–1387.

Poser, S., Mollenhauer, B., Kraubeta, A., et al.1999. How to improve the clinical diagnosis of Creutzfeldt-Jakob disease. Brain 122:2345–2351.

Pozzi, D., Golimstock, A., Petracchi, M., et al. 1995. Biol. Psychiatry 38:677–683.

Primavera, A., and Traverso, F. 1990. Triphasic waves in Alzheimer's disease. Acta Neurol. Belg. 90:274–281.

Primavera, A., Traverso, F., and Perfumo, P. 1989. Triphasic waves in dementia syndromes. Riv. Neurol. 59:146–149.

Primavera, A., Giberti, L., Scotto, P., et al. 1994. Nonconvulsive status epilepticus as a cause of confusion in later life: a report of 5 cases. Neuropsychobiology 30:148–152.

Pritchard, W.S., Duke, D.W., Coburn, K.L., et al.1994. EEG-based, neural-net predictive classification of Alzheimer's disease versus control subjects is augmented by non-linear EEG measures. Electroencephalogr. Clin. Neurophysiol. 91:118–130.

Pro, J.D., and Wells, C.E. 1977. The use of the electroencephalogram in the diagnosis of delirium. Dis. Nerv. Syst. 38:804–808.

Purdie, F.R., Hareginin, B., and Rosen, P. 1981. Acute organic brain syndrome: review of 100 cases. Ann. Emerg. Med. 10:455–461.

Rabins, P.V., and Folstein, M.F. 1982. Delirium in dementia: diagnostic criteria and fatality rates. Br. J. Psychiatry 140:149–153.

Rae-Grant, A., Blume, W., Lau, C., et al. 1987. The electroencephalogram in Alzheimer-type dementia: a sequential study correlating the electroencephalogram with psychometric and quantitative pathologic data. Arch. Neurol. 44:50–54.

Ratnavalli, E., Brayne, C., Dawson, K., et al. 2002. The prevalence of frontotemporal dementia. Neurology 58:1615–1621.

Riekkinen, P.J., Riekkinen, P.J., Sr., Soininen, H., et al. 1990. Regulation of EEG delta activity by the cholinergic nucleus basalis. In Alzheimer's Disease. Epidemiology, Neuropathology, Neurochemistry, and Clinics, Eds. K. Maurer, P. Riederer, and H. Beckman, pp. 437–445. Berlin: Springer-Verlag.

Riekkinen, P., Buzsaki, G., Riekkinen, P., Jr., et al. 1991. The cholinergic system and EEG slow waves. Electroencephalogr. Clin. Neurophysiol. 78:89–96.

Roberts, M.A., McGeorge, A.P., and Caird, F.I. 1978. Electroencephalography and computerised tomography in vascular and non-vascular dementia in old age. J. Neurol. Neurosurg. Psychiatry 41:903–906.

Robinson, D.J., Merskey, H., Blume, W.T., et al. 1994. Electroencephalography as an aid in the exclusion of Alzheimer's disease. Arch Neurol. 51:280–284.

Rodriguez, G., Nobil, F., Arrigo, A., et al. 1996. Prognostic significance of quantitative electroencephalography in Alzheimer patients: preliminary observations. Electroencephalogr. Clin. Neurophysiol. 99:123–128.

Rodriguez, G., Copello, F., Vitali, P., et al. 1999. EEG spectral profile to stage Alzheimer's disease. Clin. Neurophysiol. 110:1831–1837.

Rodriguez, G., Vitali, P., De Leo, C., et al. 2002. Quantitative EEG changes in Alzheimer patients during long-term donepezil therapy. Neuropsychobiology 46:49–56.

Roman, G.C. 2002. Vascular dementia revisited: diagnosis, pathogenesis, treatment, and prevention. Med. Clin. North Am. 86:477–499.

Roman, G.C. 2003. Vascular dementia: distinguishing characteristics, treatment, and prevention. J. Am. Geriatr. Soc. 51(suppl 5):S296–304.

Romanelli, M.F., Morris, J.C., Ashkin, K., et al. 1990. Advanced Alzheimer's disease is a risk factor for late-onset seizures. Arch. Neurol. 47:847–850.

Ron, M.A., Toone, B.K., Garralda, M.E., et al. 1979. Diagnostic accuracy in presenile dementia. Br. J. Psychiatry 134:161–168.

Rosen, I. 1997. Electroencephalography as a diagnostic tool in dementia. Dement. Geriatr. Cogn. Disord. 8:110–116.

Sannita, W.G., Maggi, L., and Rosadini, G. 1987. Effects of scopolamine (0.25–0.75 mg i.m.) on the quantitative EEG and the neuropsychological status of healthy volunteers. Neuropsychobiology 17:199–205.

Scheuer, M.L., Lopez, O.L., Brenner, R.P., et al. 2000. Tonic-clonic seizures in patients with probable Alzheimer disease. Neurology 54 (suppl 3):A415.

Schreiter-Gasser, U., Gasser, T., and Ziegler, P. 1993. Quantitative EEG analysis in early onset Alzheimer's disease: a controlled study. Electroencephalogr. Clin. Neurophysiol. 86:15–22.

Schreiter-Gasser, U., Gasser, T., and Ziegler, P. 1994. Quantitative EEG analysis in early onset Alzheimer's disease: correlations with severity, clinical characteristics, visual EEG and CT. Electroencephalogr. Clin. Neurophysiol. 90:267–272.

Schwartz, M.S., and Scott, D.F. 1971. Isolated petit-mal status presenting de novo in middle age. Lancet 2:1399–1401.

Scott, D.F., Heathfield, K.W.G., Toone, B., et al. 1972. The EEG in Huntington's chorea: a clinical and neuropathological study. J. Neurol. Neurosurg. Psychiatry 35:97–102.

Sirakov, A.A., and Mezan, I.S. 1963. EEG findings in parkinsonism. Electroencephalogr. Clin. Neurophysiol. 15:321–322.

Sishta, S.K., Troupe, A., Marszalek, K.S., et al.1973. Huntington's chorea: an electroencephalographic and psychometric study. Electroencephalogr. Clin. Neurophysiol. 36:387–393.

Sloan, E.P., and Fenton, G.W. 1993. EEG power spectra and cognitive change in geriatric psychiatry: a longitudinal study. Electroencephalogr. Clin. Neurophysiol. 86:361–367.

Small, J.G. EEG in affective disorders. 1983. In *EEG and Evoked Potentials in Psychiatry and Behavioral Neurology,* Eds. J.R. Hughes and W.P. Wilson, pp. 41–54. Woburn: Butterworths.

Smith, S.J.M., and Kocen, R.S. 1988. A Creutzfeldt-Jakob like syndrome due to lithium toxicity. J. Neurol. Neurosurg. Psychiatry 51:120–123.

Snowden, J.S., Neary, D., and Mann, D.M. 2002. Frontotemporal dementia. Br. J. Psychiatry 180:140–143.

Soikkeli, R., Partanen, J., Soininen, H., et al. 1991. Slowing of EEG in Parkinson's disease. Electroencephalogr. Clin. Neurophysiol. 79:159–165.

Soininen, H., and Partanen, J.V. 1988. Quantitative EEG in the diagnosis and follow-up of Alzheimer's disease. In *The EEG of Mental Activities,* Eds. D. Giannitrapani and L. Murri, pp. 42–49. Basel: Karger.

Soininen, H., Partanen, V.J., Heilkala, E.-L., et al. 1982. EEG findings in senile dementia and normal aging. Acta Neurol. Scand. 65:59–70.

Steinhoff, B.J., Racker, S., Herrendorf, G., et al. 1996. Accuracy and reliability of periodic sharp wave complexes in Creutzfeldt-Jakob disease. Arch. Neurol. 53:162–166.

Stigsby, B. 1988. Dementias (Alzheimer's and Pick's disease): dysfunctional and structural changes. Am. J. EEG Technol. 28:83–97.

Stigsby, B., Johannesson, G., and Ingvar, D.H. 1981. Regional EEG analysis and regional cerebral blood flow in Alzheimer's and Pick's diseases. Electroencephalogr. Clin. Neurophysiol. 51:537–547.

Streletz, L.J., Reyes, P.F., Zalewska, M., et al. 1990. Computer analysis of EEG activity in dementia of the Alzheimer's type and Huntington's disease. Neurobiol. Aging 11:15–20.

Striano, S., Vacca, G., Bilo, L., et al. 1981. The electroencephalogram in dementia: differential diagnostic value in Alzheimer's disease: senile dementia and multi-infarct dementia. Acta Neurol. 36:727–734.

Strijers, R.L., Scheltens, P., Jonkman, E.J., et al. 1997. Diagnosing Alzheimer's disease in community-dwelling elderly: a comparison of EEG and MRI. Dement. Geriatr. Cogn. Disord. 8:198–202.

Strub, R.L., and Black, F.W. 1988. Acute confusional states (delirium). In *Neurobehavioral Disorders—A Clinical Approach,* pp. 107–139. Philadelphia: F.A. Davis.

Su, P.C., and Goldensohn, E.S. 1973. Progressive supranuclear palsy. Electroencephalographic studies. Arch. Neurol. 29:183–186.

Sundaram, M.B.M., and Blume, W.T. 1987. Triphasic waves: clinical correlates and morphology. Can. J. Neurol. Sci. 14:136–140.

Tatum, W.O.T., Ross, J., and Cole, A.J. 1998. Epileptic pseudodementia. Neurology 50:1472–1475.

Thal, L.J., Grundman, M., Klauber, M.R. 1988. Dementia: characteristics of a referral population and factors associated with progression. Neurology 38:1083–1090.

Thomas, P., and Borg, M. 1994. Reversible myoclonic encephalopathy revealing the AIDS-dementia complex. Electroencephalogr. Clin. Neurophysiol. 90:166–169.

Thomas, P., Beaumanoir, A., Genton, P., et al. 1992. "De novo" absence status of late onset: report of 11 cases. Neurology 42:104–110.

Thomas, P., Lebrun, C., and Chatel, M. 1993. De novo absence status epilepticus as a benzodiazepine withdrawal syndrome. Epilepsia 34:355–358.

Thompson, P.D., Bhatia, K.P., Brown, P., et al. 1994. Cortical myoclonus in Huntington's disease. Mov. Disord. 9:633–641.

Tietjen, G.E., and Drury, I. 1990. Familial Creutzfeldt-Jakob disease without periodic EEG activity. Ann. Neurol. 28:585–588.

Tinuper, P., de Carolis, P., Galeotti, M., et al. 1990. Electroencephalogram and HIV infection: a prospective study in 100 patients. Clin. Electroencephalogr. 21:145–150.

Tomson, T., Svanborg, E., and Wedlund, J. 1986. Nonconvulsive status epilepticus: high incidence of complex partial status. Epilepsia 27:276–285.

Torres, F., and Hutton, J.T. 1986. Clinical neurophysiology of dementia. Neurol. Clin. 4:369–386.

Tournier-Lasserve, E., Joutel, A., Melki, J., et al.1993. Cerebral autosomal dominant arteriopathy with subcortical infarcts and leukoencephalopathy maps to chromosome 19q12. Nat. Genet. 3:256–259.

Verghese, J., Crystal, H.A., Dickson, D.W., et al. 1999. Validity of clinical criteria for the diagnosis of dementia with Lewy bodies. Neurology 53:1974–1982.

Verma, N.P., Greiffenstein, M.F., Verma, N., et al. 1987. Electrophysiologic validation of two categories of dementias—cortical and subcortical. Clin. Electroencephalogr. 18:26–33.

Visser, S.L., Van Tilburg, W., Hooijer, C., et al. 1985. Visual evoked potentials (VEPs) in senile dementia (Alzheimer type) and in non-organic behavioural disorders in the elderly: comparison with EEG parameters. Electroencephalogr. Clin. Neurophysiol. 60:115–121.

Vogel, C.M., Drury, I., Terry, L.C., et al. 1991. Myoclonus in adult Huntington's disease. Ann. Neurol. 29:213–215.

Walker, M.P., Ayre, G.A., Cummings, J.L., et al. 2000. Quantifying fluctuation in dementia with Lewy bodies, Alzheimer's disease, and vascular dementia. Neurology 54:1616–1625.

Walstra, G.J., Teunisse, S., van Gool, W.A., et al. 1997. Reversible dementia in elderly patients referred to a memory clinic. J. Neurol. 244:17–22.

Watson, C.P. 1979. Clinical similarity of Alzheimer and Creutzfeldt-Jakob disease. Ann. Neurol. 6:368–369.

Weihl, C.C., and Roos, R.P. 1999. Creutzfeldt-Jakob disease, new variant Creutzfeldt-Jakob disease, and bovine spongiform encephalopathy. Neurol. Clin. 17:835–859.

Weiner, H., and Schuster, D.B. 1956. The electroencephalogram in dementia. Some preliminary observations and correlations. Electroencephalogr. Clin. Neurophysiol. 8:479–488.

Wengs, W.J., Talwar, D., and Bernard, J. 1993. Ifosfamide-induced nonconvulsive status epilepticus. Arch. Neurol. 50:1104–1105.

Whitehouse, P.J. 1986. The concept of subcortical and cortical dementia: another look. Ann. Neurol. 19:1–6.

Wilson, W.P., Musella, L., and Short, M.J. 1977. The electroencephalogram in dementia. In *Dementia,* Ed. C.E. Wells, pp. 205–221. Philadelphia: F.A. Davis.

Wood, J.H., Bartlet, D., James, A.E., Jr., et al. 1974. Normal-pressure hydrocephalus: diagnosis and patient selection for shunt surgery. Neurology 24:517–526.

Yamamoto, T., and Imai, T. 1988. A case of diffuse Lewy body and Alzheimer's disease with periodic synchronous discharges. J. Neuropathol. Exp. Neurol. 47:536–548.

Yener, G.G., Leuchter, A.F., Jenden, D., et al. 1996. Quantitative EEG in frontotemporal dementia. Clin. Electroencephalogr. 27:61–68.

Zak, R., Solomon, G., Petito, F., et al. 1994. Baclofen-induced generalized nonconvulsive status epilepticus. Ann. Neurol. 36:113–114.

Zeman, A.Z., Boniface, S.J., and Hodges, J.R. 1998. Transient epileptic amnesia: a description of the clinical and neuropsychological features in 10 cases and a review of the literature. J. Neurol. Neurosurg. Psychiatry 64:435–443.

Zerr, I., Bodemer, M., Gefeller, O., et al. 1998. Detection of 14-3-3 protein in the cerebrospinal fluid supports the diagnosis of Creutzfeldt-Jakob disease. Ann. Neurol. 43:32–40.

Zerr, I., Pocchiari, M., Collins, S., et al. 2000. Analysis of EEG and CSF 14-3-3 proteins as aids to the diagnosis of Creutzfeldt-Jakob disease. Neurology 55:811–815.

Zochodne, D.W., Young, G.B., McLachlan, R.S., et al. 1988. Creutzfeldt-Jakob disease without periodic sharp wave complexes: a clinical, electroencephalographic, and pathologic study. Neurology 38:1056–1060.

19. Degenerative Disorders of the Central Nervous System

Sukkubai Naidu and Ernst Niedermeyer

The term *degenerative central nervous system (CNS) disorders* is controversial; the nature of these diseases is quite heterogeneous. The complexity of the pathogenetic factors cannot be discussed in this short presentation. More detailed information can be found in the *Handbook of Clinical Neurology*, Volumes 10, 13, and 14 (1970 and 1972), as well as in the work of Rapin (1976), Adams and Lyon (1982), Dyken and Krawiecki (1983), Kolodny and Cable (1983), Nyhan and Sakati (1987), Desnick (1991), Chaves-Carballo (1992), and Moser (1992).

"True" degeneration of the CNS may occur as abiotrophic processes causing premature aging of certain neuronal structures, probably on a genetic basis. Presenile and senile dementias are typical examples of degenerative abiotrophic processes, but, for practical reasons, these disorders are presented separately under the heading of electroencephalography (EEG) and dementia.

Most so-called degenerative CNS disorders are caused by metabolic disturbances of chronically progressive character. In view of the chronic progression, these diseases should not be incorporated into the section of metabolic encephalopathies with predominantly acute or subacute course and rapid fluctuations.

In this context, we cannot do full justice to the neurobiochemical, pathophysiological, and pathogenetic considerations, as we concentrate on the EEG features. In this disease group, EEG abnormalities are extremely common and often quite pronounced. The degree of abnormality apparently depends on the type of affected neuronal systems, some of which might be electroencephalographically more eloquent than others.

The number of presumed degenerative CNS diseases and syndromes has already exceeded the 300 mark. Underlying biochemical aberrations are being rapidly elucidated. This makes it clear that this chapter must be confined to the better known and more important diseases and syndromes.

Over the past two decades, the association of neurodegenerative diseases with the dysfunction of organelles within the cellular structure has gained increasing importance. Lysosome, peroxisome, and mitochondria are such vulnerable organelles; their disorders have been recognized as the primary cause of various degenerative diseases. These new vistas have vastly changed the landscape by the establishment of new principles of classification.

Lysosomal Disorders

Tay-Sachs Disease

This disease belongs to a group of diseases that has been listed as "lysosomal disorders." In addition to Tay-Sachs disease, this group includes Batten's disease, GM1 gangliosidosis, cherry red spot myoclonus syndrome, and other forms of lipidosis.

Tay-Sachs disease in its classical form is clinically characterized by macular degeneration ("cherry red spot"), mental deterioration, epileptic seizures, blindness, and amyotrophy. It manifests itself in the first year of life. Neuropathologically, the disease is a GM2 gangliosidosis (Klenk, 1941) with ganglioside accumulation in nerve cells.

Myoclonus involves limbs and extremities and is easily triggered by auditory stimuli (Gastaut and Tassinari, 1966; Schneck, 1964). The EEG is normal in the early phase, but gradually shows high-voltage delta bursts with sharply contoured potentials; spike and sharp wave activity of widespread distribution may be noted (Cobb et al., 1952; Pampiglione and Lehovsky, 1968) with acoustically induced myoclonic seizures. During these attacks, the EEG may be flattened. Progressive decline of voltage output is common in the final stage (Fig. 19.1). The electroretinogram remains normal throughout the illness (Pampiglione and Harden, 1977).

Two variants of Tay-Sachs disease are known as *Sandhoff's disease* and *AB variant*. These are fairly rapidly progressive encephalopathies with cherry-red spot, myoclonic seizures, dementia, and fatal outcome after a short course.

There are also *juvenile forms* such as juvenile Tay-Sachs disease, juvenile Sandhoff's disease, ataxia variety, and a variety with lower motor neuron involvement. These forms are less aggressive than the infantile forms.

There is also an *adult-onset form* of Tay-Sachs disease. Epileptic seizures, dementia, and normal pressure hydrocephalus are the common features. Startle-induced myoclonus may occur, but (according to the authors' personal observation) the startle is unassociated with EEG changes, and the entire record may be within normal limits. There is even an *asymptomatic form* of adult-onset Tay-Sachs disease with typical biochemical changes in the absence of neurological and mental deficits.

A more recently established B1 variant of Tay-Sachs disease is found in childhood. It is characterized by ataxia, basal ganglia disorder, and seizures.

GM1 Gangliosidosis

This is a rare inborn error of metabolism due to a deficiency of β-galactosidase leading to accumulation of GM1 gangliosides. An infantile (type I) and a juvenile form (type II) are distinguished. Epileptic seizures may occur in both forms. The EEG, particularly around the age of 2 to 3 years, is characterized mainly by slowing with prominent rhythmi-

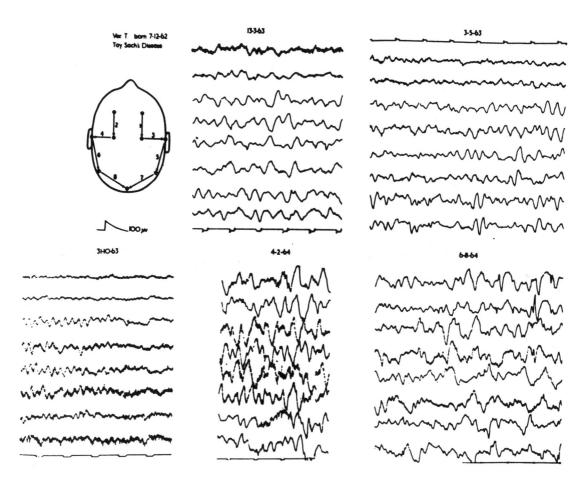

Figure 19.1.   Tay-Sachs disease. Gradual evolution of abnormalities (age 3, 5, 11, 14, and 18 months). (Courtesy of Dr. G. Pampiglione, London, England, with permission of Grune & Stratton, New York and London.)

cal 4 to 5/sec activity that is maximal over temporal areas (Harden et al., 1982).

Cherry Red Spot Myoclonus Syndrome

Sialidosis Type I

A syndrome of childhood featuring a macular cherry-red spot, progressive myoclonus, and easily controllable epileptic seizures has been described by Rapin et al. (1975). Dementia is notably absent. This disease has been tentatively classified as a mucolipidosis.

The EEG shows rhythmical spiking over the vertex, with positive polarity; this occurs against a poorly defined low-voltage background (Engel et al., 1977). These vertex spikes are enhanced in sleep; no slowing materialized in non-rapid-eye-movement (REM) sleep (Engel et al., 1977) (Fig. 19.2). Myoclonus is preceded by a time-locked EEG spike (Tobimatsu et al., 1983).

Exacerbation of myoclonus with cigarette smoking and the menstrual cycle has been reported (Steinman et al., 1980; Thomas et al., 1979).

Sialidosis Type II

This disorder is more progressive than type I (cherry red spot myoclonus syndrome). There is skeletal dysmorphism with dementia and punctuate cataracts. Myoclonic activity may be quite subtle and does not alter the EEG, which is of moderate voltage with mixed theta and beta frequencies. There are occasional generalized 4 to 6/sec paroxysms (Messenheimer et al., 1984).

Niemann-Pick's Disease

Niemann-Pick's disease is caused by accumulation of sphingomyelin due to deficiency of sphingomyelinase. At least four types (A to D) are distinguished. There are marked organomegalies. Neurological involvement may be present. EEG abnormalities are undetermined, but were rather mild in a personal observation of an adolescent. Some patients (types C and D) may present with cataplexy that responds to protriptyline (Kandt et al., 1982).

Gaucher's Disease

Gaucher's disease is a lipid storage disease with accumulation of glucocerebroside (a sphingolipid). Severe mental retardation may occur, and there are marked organomegalies.

Three types have been described. Type I is the chronic neuronopathic form of adult onset without central neurological defects. Type II begins in infancy (acute neuronopathic

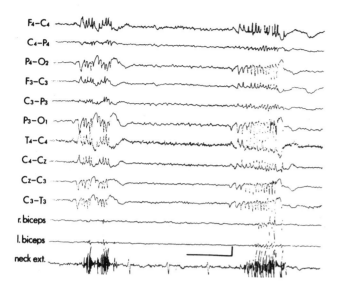

Figure 19.2. Vertex positive spikes in a 28-year-old patient with cherry red spot myoclonus disease. Note accompanying myoclonus in electromyogram (EMG) leads. The positive polarity of the vertex spikes can be derived from the phase reversal in Cz (see Chapter 6, "Technological Basis of EEG Recording"). (Courtesy of Dr. J. Engel, Jr., Los Angeles, California, with permission of Raven Press, New York.)

form), and type III begins later in life (subacute neuronopathic form). The CNS is affected in types II and III. These forms present with epileptic seizures, myoclonus, spasticity, ataxia, dementia, and cranial nerve deficits. Paroxysmal EEG abnormalities may occur in these forms prior to the onset of clinical seizures; EEG worsening parallels the deteriorating clinical course. According to Nishimura et al. (1980), EEG abnormalities are most prominent in type III and include polyspikes, rhythmical sharp waves (6–10/sec), and spike-wave discharges; these abnormalities are diffuse but most prominent over posterior areas. Paroxysmal flicker responses are common in type III. Interestingly, normal EEG tracings predominate in type II notwithstanding severe neurological deficits.

Farber's Disease (Farber's Lipogranulomatosis)

Farber's disease is an autosomal-recessive disorder caused by acid ceramidase deficiency. It begins in childhood and is associated with moderate to severe mental retardation. Infantile spasms may occur and, in milder cases, petit mal absence-like seizures with generalized spike waves may occur (Hodson et al., 1983). Most children show a progressive course with fatal outcome within 3 years.

Globoid Leukodystrophy (Krabbe's Disease, Diffuse Sclerosis)

Globoid leukodystrophy is caused by an autosomal-recessive deficiency of the enzyme that catalyzes the hydrolytic cleavage of the galactose moiety of galactocerebroside (ceramide galactose) (Suzuki and Suzuki, 1970; also see Brady, 1975). It is autosomal recessive, with onset around age 4 to 5 months with hyperirritability and episodic fever, then convulsions, blindness, deafness, and mental retarda-

tion. Incessant screaming is common. Tonic convulsion may be triggered by light or noise (Allen, 1964). A state of permanent rigidity dominates the terminal phase of the disease. In this stage, the EEG is almost flat in all leads. In earlier stages, hypsarrhythmia-like patterns may be present (Andrews et al., 1971; Suzuki and Suzuki, 1983; Williams et al., 1979).

Onset in late infancy, childhood, or adolescence has also been reported (Loonen et al., 1985). The EEG shows slowing and paroxysmal discharges, especially over frontotemporal regions. The gene and its multiple mutation have been identified.

Metachromatic Leukodystrophy

More common than other lipidoses, metachromatic leukodystrophy is caused by accumulation of a galactocerebroside (sulfatide) *in vitro*, corrected by crude arylsulfatase. Onset is in the second year of life with peripheral motor deficits (flaccidity of arms and legs), followed by mental retardation and especially by loss of speech. The occurrence of seizures in the classical as well as in the juvenile form has been reported by MacFaul et al. (1982).

EEG findings are comparatively mild and even normal except for the late stages (Pampiglione, 1968; also see Dumermuth, 1972). Animal models of this disease are now available for further studies of pathogenesis.

Fabry's Disease

Fabry's disease is an X-linked recessive disorder, chiefly found in males and due to accumulation of ceramide-trihexoside (ceramide-glucose-galactose-galactose). Onset is mainly in adolescence, with pain and a burning sensation in hands and feet, exacerbated by hot weather because of lack of sweating. There are corneal opacities, widespread arteriosclerosis, and renal damage. The latter may respond very well to dialysis, thus averting early death. EEG findings are unremarkable.

Mucolipidosis II (I Cell Disease)

This disease evolves in the first decade and leads to dysmorphism and mental retardation. It has to be differentiated from the complex of mucopolysaccharidosis. Mucolipidosis III has been termed "pseudo-Hurler" because of clinical similarities. According to Siegel et al. (1998), six out of ten patients with mucolipidosis type IV showed numerous spikes in the EEG, but only one of them had clinical seizures.

Schindler's Disease

This is a rare familial autosomal-recessive disorder based on α-*N*-acetyl-galactosaminidase deficiency (Van Diggelen et al., 1988).

There is a rapidly progressive cerebral impairment starting at age 9 to 12 months, resulting in cortical blindness, spasticity, myoclonus, and profound mental retardation.

The EEG shows diffuse and multifocal paroxysmal discharges and slowing, maximal over centroparieto-occipital regions. The evoked potentials of all modalities are delayed and of low amplitude.

Despite neuropathological similarities with infantile neuroaxonal dystrophy and Hallervorden-Spatz disease, the biochemical abnormality clearly differs from these two conditions.

Mucopolysaccharidosis

The autosomal-recessive, X-linked type I (Hurler syndrome, gargoylism) must be distinguished from type II (Hunter's syndrome), type III (Sanfilippo's syndrome), type IV (Morquio's syndrome), type V (Scheie's syndrome), and type VI (Maroteaux-Lamy syndrome). Various degrees of mental retardation occur in these subforms. Abnormal facial appearance (gargoylism), kyphosis, abdominal hernias, retarded bone growth, and some degree of hydrocephalus are more or less developed in these syndromes. Mucopolysaccharides are accumulated and also excreted in the urine; the liver and spleen are enlarged. EEG abnormalities seem to be congruent with the degree of CNS impairment (Gibbs and Gibbs, 1964), but no specific findings have been reported.

It has been established that type III (Sanfilippo) can be associated with frequent epileptic seizures and mental retardation.

Peroxisomal Disorders

Disorders resulting from dysfunction of the peroxisome have been recognized as a whole new class of degenerative diseases.

Adrenoleukodystrophy

This X-linked disorder occurs in boys (Schaumberg et al., 1974;1975), and the enzyme defect involves the metabolism of very long chain fatty acids alone (Moser, 1986). This disease is associated with cortical blindness, motor impairment, and hyperactivity.

There is pronounced high-voltage polymorphic delta activity in the EEG (Andriola, 1979) that chiefly affects the temporo-occipital areas (Battaglia et al., 1981; Mamoli et al., 1979) (Fig. 19.3).

Schilder disease (diffuse sclerosis) is characterized by extensive destruction of the occipital lobes. This disorder is now recognized as adrenoleukodystrophy.

Sudanophilic Leukodystrophy

This form is pathophysiologically unclear; little is known about EEG changes. Onset is mainly in late childhood; pendular nystagmus and head tremor may be in the foreground. Massive EEG showing with occasional ictal "tonic discharge" was reported by Rodière et al. (1979).

This disease appears to be closely related to (and sometimes identical with) adrenoleukodystrophy.

Zellweger's Syndrome

This cerebrohepatorenal syndrome is a recessive disorder that results from a lack of peroxisomes, causing accumulation of very long chain fatty acids, pipecolic acid and bile acid, and a deficiency of glycerolipids. Clinically, there are severe hypotonia (apparent at birth), epileptic seizures (first week of life), hepatomegaly, renal cysts, retinopathy, dysmorphic fea-

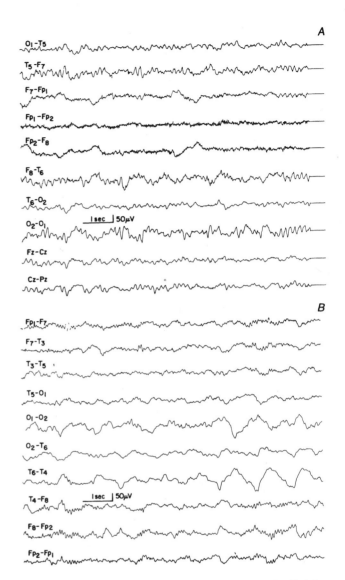

Figure 19.3. Adrenoleukodystrophy. Age 18 years. **A:** Awake. **B:** Asleep. Note persistent right occipitoposterotemporal slowing in waking state and sleep. Record slightly abnormal.

tures, and severe mental retardation (Moser, 1986). Bilateral spiking in the EEG, especially over temporal regions, has been reported (Volpe and Adams, 1972). There may be continuous spike and sharp-wave activity when the patient is both awake and asleep, with consistent accentuation over the vertex region (Govaerts et al., 1984). Very pronounced spiking over central areas was noted in a premature neonate with Zellweger syndrome (Panjan et al., 2001). Milder variants exist. Multiple mutations in genes involved in peroxisomal biogenesis or protein transport have been identified.

Mitochondrial Disorders

Kearns-Sayre Syndrome

This is a hereditary disorder characterized by progressive external ophthalmoplegia, retinal pigmentary degeneration, heart block, elevated serum lactate and pyruvate levels, and elevated cerebrospinal fluid (CSF) protein. The disorder begins in childhood; seizures may occur, but little is known about the EEG.

With the use of nerve conduction time evaluation and transcranial magnetic stimulation, Schubert et al. (1994) provided evidence of central and peripheral nervous system involvement.

MELAS Syndrome (Mitochondrial Myopathy, Encephalopathy, Lactic Acidosis, and Stroke)

The MELAS syndrome is characterized by attacks of classic migraine resulting in ischemia-encephalomalacia affecting mainly the occipital lobes (multiple strokes). Intractable epileptic seizures are associated with this syndrome. The disorder is found in children, adolescents, and adults; the course is progressive (Dvorkin et al., 1987).

The myopathic component of this syndrome often features ragged red fibers and is hence related to the syndrome of myoclonus with epilepsy and with ragged red fibers (MERRF) (Dvorkin et al., 1987).

The EEG shows slowing and spike or spike-wave activity of occipital accentuation, often unilateral; some cases do not feature any paroxysmal activity.

The EEG may also show periodic lateralized epileptiform discharges (PLEDs) over the chiefly affected occipital lobe (Bell, 1995).

MERRF Syndrome (Myoclonus with Epilepsy and with Ragged Red Fibers)

Cerebellar ataxia with dysmetria and intentional tremor is usually found at the onset in childhood or early adolescence; intentional tremor and action myoclonus may become inseparable. Major epileptic convulsions may be entirely absent, in contrast with essential hereditary myoclonus epilepsy. Dementia may or may not be present.

This condition may be associated with widespread myopathy that exhibits the features of "ragged red fiber myopathy"

described by Black et al. (1975). Figure 19.4 shows a tracing of such a patient. In this case, the family history was negative. On the other hand, familial cases also occur and have been reported in three generations by DeBarsy et al. (1969).

The EEG (according to personal impressions) shows more rhythmical and organized character than the tracings found in essential hereditary myoclonus epilepsy. Bursts of spikes are noted, often without relationship to clinical myoclonus (Fig. 19.4). Bergamasco et al. (1967) were struck by the total absence of REM sleep in 24-hour recordings and hypothesized that myoclonus might serve as an equivalent of REM sleep because the patient did not suffer from the REM sleep deficit. Depth EEG studies in eight patients were carried out by Tassinari et al. (1971).

Clinical features of MELAS and MERRF may occur in the same patients and both syndromes may become intertwined (Berkovic et al., 1988). Detailed electrophysiological studies of MERRF have been presented by So et al. (1988) and Becker et al. (1990), the latter study still referring to the older term *dyssynergia cerebellaris myoclonical Ramsay Hunt* (with emphasis being placed on the sensorimotor mechanisms involved in the genesis on myoclonus). A combination of MERRF syndrome and myoclonus epilepsy has been reported by Ohtsuka et al. (1993). The *Fukuhara syndrome* (Fukuhara et al., 1980) is now considered identical with the MERRF syndrome.

Leigh's Encephalomyelopathy (Leigh's Syndrome)

A rare and presumably inherited autosomal-recessive disease of infancy and earliest childhood, Leigh's encephalomyelopathy is characterized by impairment of consciousness, respiratory disturbances, and ataxia. The disease progresses fairly rapidly to a terminal state with ensuing death. Brainstem, cerebellum, and spinal cord are bilaterally affected with spongiform changes, microhemorrhages, and infarctions (Pincus, 1972). Little is known about EEG changes.

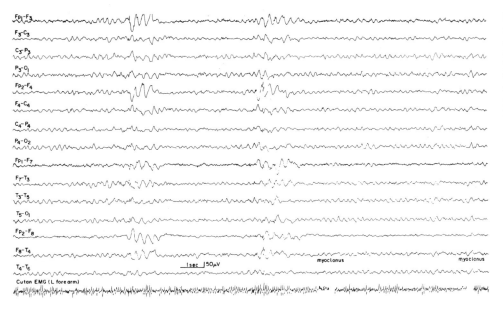

Figure 19.4. Progressive cerebellar degeneration with myoclonus, ataxia, dementia, and "ragged red fiber" myopathy. Age 19 years. There is slow basic rhythm at 5/sec, punctuated with generalized 2–3/sec bursts mixed with spikes. Clinical myoclonus is not associated with bursts in the EEG.

Inborn Disturbances of the Urea Cycle

Disturbances such as citrullinemia may result in extremely high serum ammonia levels and may be manifest in early infancy. The EEG is usually abnormal (personal observation). Mental retardation may be profound. Allan et al. (1958) reported two siblings with excessive excretion of argininosuccinic acid associated with mental retardation, generalized seizures, and ataxia. The EEG showed spikes and massive slowing.

The symptoms of urea cycle disturbances may be manifest in the neonatal and early infantile period as poor sucking, hypotonia, vomiting, irritability, lethargy, epileptic seizures, and coma. Onset in childhood is likely to present as recurrent ataxia, cyclic vomiting, behavioral disturbances, lethargy, and coma. In either condition, delay of therapy leads to severe brain damage or death (Batshaw, 1984).

Verma et al. (1984) documented severe EEG abnormalities (ornithine transcarbamylase deficiency and arginosuccinic acid synthase deficiency) in infants who developed seizures between the 4th and 36th day of life. The EEG showed multifocal spikes, spike waves, sharp waves, and slowing. Dietary protein restriction may lead to EEG normalization. Low-voltage slow activity with superimposed fast activity was found in infants with citrullinemia and seizures; spike activity was also noted against this background of mixed activity (Engel and Buist, 1985).

Severe EEG abnormalities with burst suppression were found in *acute neonatal citrullinemia* (Clancy and Chung, 1991). This rare inborn error of metabolism is due to deficient enzymatic activity of arginosuccinic acid synthetase.

Aminoacidurias

Phenylketonuria (PKU)

This well-known and rather widespread condition used to be found in 0.5% of the institutionalized mentally retarded population (Ford, 1966). Deficiency of liver phenylalanine hydroxylase results in the inability to metabolize phenylalanine normally. Screening of newborns with the ferric chloride test has led to early discovery and subsequent dietary treatment (Fig. 19.5).

Mental deficiency with markedly delayed milestones of psychomotor development is the outstanding feature. Behavioral changes include restlessness, viciousness, and aggressiveness. Convulsions are not uncommon, sometimes in the form of infantile spasms with hypsarrhythmia in the EEG (Low et al., 1957). According to Metcalf (1972), the EEG is unequivocally abnormal in 25%, mildly disturbed in 51%, and normal in 24%. Hypsarrhythmic findings in infancy are supplanted by irregular generalized spike wave-like bursts, mostly 3/sec, according to Dumermuth (1972). This author also contends that there is no correlation between degree of EEG changes, phenylalanine concentration in serum and CSF, and excretion of phenylpyruvic acid. Further EEG studies were done by Fois et al. (1955), Stadler (1961), Herrlin (1962), Fisch et al. (1965), Gross et al. (1981), Wasser et al. (1981), Behbehani (1985), and Pietz et al. (1987). De Giorgis et al. (1983) emphasized the high correlation of epileptiform abnormalities and elevated blood levels of phenylalanine, es-

pecially in the second and third months of life. Salomon et al. (1981) noted bursts of spikes and polyspikes as well as sharp theta activity during REM sleep in the new variant of PKU due to *dihydropteridin reductase deficiency*.

Lowe's Syndrome (Oculocerebrorenal Syndrome)

This condition is not yet fully understood; it is probably a sex-linked recessive disorder. There is excessive excretion of amino acids associated with impaired renal tubular function. The affected children show severe mental deficiency and hyperactivity. Vision is reduced due to hydrophthalmos and cataract. Signs of osteomalacia are present. Attacks of fever and dehydration are common. Intermittent ophthalmoplegia and pseudotumor cerebri may develop; hypoglycemia is noted in about 50% of the patients. The clinical course is unrelated to enzyme levels (Menkes, 1985) and may be prolonged or rapid, with death occurring within 1 month. The EEG is abnormal in most cases (Dumermuth, 1972; Illig et al., 1963), usually after the first year of life. Multifocal sharp wave activity may occur.

Maple Syrup Disease

This is a severely destructive condition due to defective metabolism of branched chain amino acids (leucine, isoleucine, valine) and blockage of decarboxylation. The neurological deficits are manifest at birth; there is rapid disappearance of the Moro reflex, then rigidity and intermittent states of decerebration with opisthotonos. EEG abnormalities may be nonspecific (Dancis et al., 1960) or markedly paroxysmal (Dent and Westall, 1961; Pampiglione, 1968).

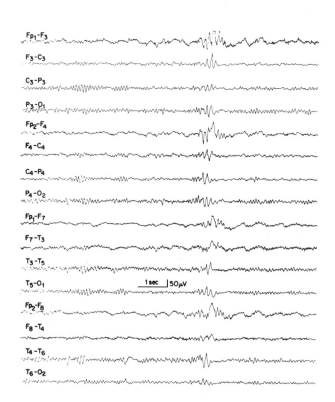

Figure 19.5. Phenylketonuria. Patient, age 28 years, normalized with dietary treatment. A brief generalized theta burst occurs after challenge diet.

Hartnup Disease

Hartnup disease is a very rare autosomal-recessive disorder arising from failed tubular absorption of a group of monoamino monocarboxylic acids (especially tryptophan), resulting in aminoaciduria with bountiful excretion of indolacetic acid and indican. The disease itself is episodic rather than chronically progressive, with skin rashes, diarrhea, cerebellar ataxia, and mental disturbance. EEG findings are unremarkable.

Homocystinuria

Homocystinuria is an autosomal-recessive condition. Methionine and homocystine excretion are elevated due to a defect in cystathionine synthase. The disorder is characterized by ectopia lentis, skeletal changes suggesting Marfan's syndrome, osteoporosis, and thrombotic lesions of arteries and veins (Carson and Neill, 1962; Gerritsen et al., 1962; Schimke et al., 1965). Intracranial arterial thrombosis may lead to severe neurological deficits. Mental retardation is common (two thirds of the cases). EEG changes are variable and sometimes quite pronounced, especially in children with epileptic seizures (based on personal observation).

Marfan Syndrome

Marfan syndrome shows some superficial similarities to the aforementioned syndrome of homocystinuria: osteoporosis, arachnodactylia, ectopia lentis, and vascular problems such as aneurysms and thrombotic lesions. Changes of fibrillin, however, distinguish Marfan syndrome from homocystinuria. EEG findings are unremarkable.

Genetic research has established the role of Marfan syndrome as a nosological entity.

Nonketotic Hyperglycinemia

This is an autosomal-recessive disorder of glycine metabolism that manifests itself in early infancy with intractable epileptic seizures, lethargy, severe psychomotor retardation, and early death (Nyhan, 1978). Serial EEG studies have shown burst-suppression patterns in the newborn period; in the further course, slowing along with multifocal spikes and polyspikes are the dominant features (Markand et al., 1982).

Treatment with large dosages of diazepam in combination with choline, sodium benzoate, and folic acid may improve the EEG and the seizure frequency without dramatic developmental gains (Matalon et al., 1983). More recently, dextromethorphan has also been used in the treatment (Hamosh et al., 1992).

Canavan's Disease

This is a rapidly progressive combined gray and white matter disease leading to spongiform changes. It has also been termed the Van Bogaert-Bertrand type of spongy degeneration. It is an autosomal-recessive disease that is more common among Jewish children.

The disease begins around age 3 months with rapid psychomotor regression, visual loss, optic atrophy, irritability, poor feeding, and hypotonia followed by spasticity. Megalencephaly occurs along with computed tomography (CT) scan evidence of white matter degeneration. Epileptic seizures occur in about half of the infants, with choreoathetosis in a few.

In spite of severe neuropathological changes, the EEG often remains normal (Buchanan and Davis, 1965; Kamoshita et al., 1968).

Canavan's disease used to be listed among progressive CNS diseases of unknown origin. The demonstration of *N*-acetyl-aspartic aciduria along with aspartoacylase deficiency, and the genetic defect in the aspartoacylase gene have shed more light on the nature of this disease.

Other Metabolic Diseases

Lesch-Nyhan Syndrome

This is a sex-linked disorder; it is confined to males and associated with hyperuricemia, mental retardation, spasticity, choreoathetosis, and self-mutilation (first reported by Catel and Schmidt, 1959). Reduced amounts of the enzyme hypoxanthine-guanine phosphoribosyltransferase (HGPRT) represent the underlying defect. The dopamine concentration is reduced in the basal ganglia. Basal ganglia-type dyskinesias begin around the age of 2 years. Seizures may occur but must not be confused with episodes of decerebrate posturing. Allopurinol or substitution of catecholamines does not improve neurological symptoms. Attempts at gene therapy are being made. The EEG may be normal or abnormal with excessive slowing (Kelley and Wyngaarden, 1983).

Glycogen Storage Diseases

Eight different types of glycogen storage disorders have been described. Those with neurological manifestations include type II (Pompe's disease), type V (McArdle's disease), and type VII (Tansi disease). All are autosomal-recessive disorders with muscular involvement; in type II, the heart is also affected. No specific EEG abnormalities have been reported (Howell and Williams, 1983).

Cerebrotendinous Xanthomatosis (CTX)

This recessively inherited lipid storage disease, described by Van Bogaert et al. (1937) as characterized by CNS involvement, cataracts, and xanthomata of Achilles and other tendons, is believed due to a hepatic enzyme abnormality. There is evidence of progressive dementia, ataxia, spastic quadriparesis, mild peripheral neuropathy, and epileptic seizures (Berginer et al., 1982). The EEG is characterized by slowing of the background activity, paroxysmal high-voltage delta bursts, spikes, sharp waves, and polyspikes. When treated with chenodeoxycholic acid, neurological progression may be arrested or reversed with improvement of CT scan and EEG; improvement of visual and brainstem auditory evoked potentials may also be noted (Pedley et al., 1985).

Pelizaeus-Merzbacher Disease

This is a rare form of leukodystrophy, pathophysiologically unclear and probably X-linked recessive. Nystagmus, head tremor, and ataxia usually dominate the clinical picture. The EEG is essentially unremarkable.

On the other hand, brainstem auditory (prolonged I–V interpeak interval) and visual evoked potentials [prolonged P1 (P100) latency] are diagnostically helpful. These tests, however, cannot identify unaffected carriers of the disease (Borkowski et al., 1991).

Biotinidase Deficiency

These patients suffer from reduced activity of biotinidase with a resultant inability to liberate bound biotin from holocarboxylases. The clinical symptomatology is characterized by epileptic seizures, ataxia, muscular hypotonia, deafness, developmental delay, skin rash, alopecia, metabolic acidosis, and organic aciduria (Wolf et al., 1983a,b). In some of the children, seizures may be the only presenting symptom (Wolf, 1983a,b, 1985). Little is known about the EEG findings. Treatment with biotin reverses most of the clinical symptoms.

Refsum's Disease

This disorder was first described by Refsum (1946); it is a rare autosomal-recessive disorder with the cardinal manifestations of retinitis pigmentosa, peripheral neuropathy, ataxia, deafness, anosmia, and ichthyosis. Exogenous phytanic acid accumulates due to reduced oxidation. Early treatment with a low phytanic acid diet and plasmapheresis arrests the progress of the disease.

No specific EEG changes have been described. The electroretinogram is often present but subnormal; the visual evoked responses have been described as normal.

Galactosemia

This autosomal-recessive disease chiefly affects the liver and the digestive system. It is caused by absence of galactose-1-phosphate uridyltransferase; galactose-1-phosphate concentration rises in cells. Mental retardation is common, but neurologic deficits are notably absent (Allen, 1964). Abnormal EEG tracings with excessive slowing have been observed.

Batten's Disease (Cerebromacular Degeneration, Neuronal Ceroid Lipofuscinosis)

This disease has been presumed to be due to the accumulation of ceroid and lipofuscin (Zeman and Dyken, 1969), but this view is still debatable. Its onset occurs in late infancy or childhood; loss of vision with macular degeneration

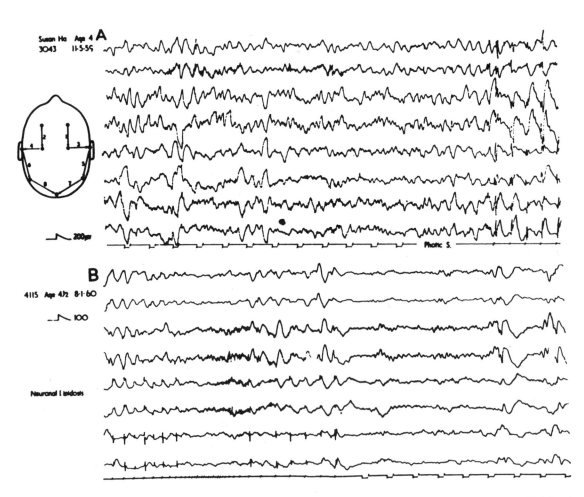

Figure 19.6. Lipidosis, probably Bielschowsky-Jansky form. Age 4 years (**A**) and 4.5 years (**B**). With photic stimulation, large driven posterior spikes. (From Pampiglione, G. 1968. In *Clinical Electroencephalography of Children*, Eds. P. Kellaway and I. Petersén. New York/London: Grune & Stratton.)

and optic nerve atrophy occurs, associated with decline of intellectual functions and epileptic seizures.

At present, many of the following disorders have been clarified metabolically as well as by genetic mutational analysis.

EEG abnormalities are already present in the early stage. Marked slowing develops; spike activity may be associated with brief generalized bursts; some children show marked posterior accentuation of slow activity. The electroretinogram is abolished in all forms of this disease (Pampiglione and Harden, 1977).

With low-frequency intermittent photic stimulation, large occipital spikes can be induced (Fig. 19.6) (Green, 1971; Pampiglione and Harden, 1973; Pampiglione and Lehovsky, 1968). According to Pampiglione and Harden (1977), Westmoreland and Sharbrough (1978), and Pinsard et al. (1979), the flicker-induced occipital spike response is seen only in the late infantile *Bielschowsky-Jansky form* and not in the juvenile or adult forms (*Spielmeyer-Vogt form, Batten form, Kufs form*) (Fig. 19.6).

A *variant of the Bielschowsky-Jansky form* was described in Finland (Sainio et al., 1982). The onset occurs around age 5 to 7 years with early failure of visual function. Flicker-driven spikes over posterior regions appeared in the EEG around age 7 to 8 years and disappeared after age 11 years. The record tends to flatten over the ensuing years.

Occasionally, the EEG may show slow spike-wave activity; this and the occurrence of atonic seizures may initially suggest the diagnosis of Lennox-Gastaut syndrome (Pinsard et al., 1979). This pattern is more common in the Spielmeyer-Vogt form (Pampiglione and Harden, 1977), but its occurrence in the Bielschowsky-Jansky form has also been noted (Rey-Pias and Morales Blanquez, 1972).

All of the above-mentioned subforms have undergone a change in nomenclature:

CNL 1: (CNL standing for lipofuscinosis neuronal): Infantile onset (Haltia, Santavuori, Hagberg variants).
CNL 2: Late infantile onset: Jansky-Bielschowsky.
CNL 3: Juvenile onset: Spielmeyer-Vogt.
CNL 4: Adult onset: Kufs.
CNL 5: Late infantile variant.

Metabolic Disturbances and Degeneration Affecting Chiefly the Basal Ganglia

Hallervorden-Spatz Disease

This is a somewhat controversial nosological entity. The original report described a sibship of 12, in which five sisters showed increasing dysarthria and dementia; brown discoloration of globus pallidus and substantial nigra were found at autopsy. Progressive rigidity of the extremities is usually associated with choreoathetoid movements; epileptic seizures and mental deterioration may occur (Hallervorden and Spatz, 1922; Meyer, 1966). The disease usually begins in childhood; death occurs in early adulthood.

According to Radermecker (1977), the EEG is severely marred by artifacts; some low-voltage slowing and fast activity has been observed in a few cases, whereas normal tracings were found in other patients.

Swaiman et al. (1983) reported two siblings with Hallervorden-Spatz disease who also demonstrated sea-blue histiocytes in the bone marrow and cytoplasmic inclusions in circulating lymphocytes, indicating extracerebral manifestations. One of them had clinical epileptic seizures. His EEG was characterized by bursts of generalized slow activity and sharp waves; there were also infrequent bilateral multifocal spikes, as well as excessive posterior slowing.

Infantile Neuroaxonal Dystrophy (Seitelberger's Disease)

This disease was first believed to be an infantile form of the Hallervorden-Spatz disease (Seitelberger, 1952), but it is now widely considered a unique disease entity (Cowen and Olmstead, 1963; Fadiloglu, 1971; Radermecker, 1977). After onset at the age of 1 year, there is mental deterioration, general hypotonia, and spasticity. Death ensues after several years. In the majority of the cases, the EEG findings were normal, but unusually large amounts of fast activity may occur, even reaching abnormal degrees (Radermecker, 1977; Radermecker and Dumon-Radermecker, 1972).

According to Ferriss et al. (1977), fast activity (chiefly in the 16–24/sec range) of high voltage is very typical of this disease; this view is shared by Mises et al. (1983), who regard the fast pattern as nearly disease specific. The fast activity shows no response to eye opening or closure. With hyperventilation or during breath-holding attacks, fast activity may be supplanted by diffuse slowing (Ferriss et al., 1977). Fast activity even persists in sleep, although some degree of slow activity may also be noted; K complexes are absent (Ferriss et al., 1977). The EEG changes develop in the third year of life.

Tonic spasms were studied with EEG-video analysis and found to be associated with irregular sharp and high-voltage slow wave complexes followed by desynchronization (Wakai et al., 1994).

Infantile neuroaxonal dystrophy and Hallervorden-Spatz disease show considerable similarities (Seitelberger, 1971). Cases of Hallervorden-Spatz disease with onset before age 10 years may be inseparable from infantile neuroaxonal dystrophy. Sensory evoked potentials reveal abnormalities in the "Hallervorden-Spatz neuroaxonal dystrophy complex" (Mutoh et al., 1990).

Paroxysmal Choreoathetosis

This is a rare and sometimes familial condition in which storms of choreoathetoid movements occur in seizure-like episodes, mostly triggered by active or passive movements. Stevens (1966) and Perez-Borja et al. (1967) have stressed the relationship to reflex epilepsy.

These attacks may start in the first year of life and continue into adulthood. Familial occurrence was reported by Mount and Reback (1940), who have been credited with the first description of this syndrome.

The EEG is normal in the interval and during the dyskinetic episodes (confirmed by a personal observation), although cases with epileptic discharges have also been noted (Perez-Borja et al., 1967). In Radermecker's opinion (1977), epileptic seizures are merely a complication of the disease.

Familial studies with EEG were presented by Pryles et al. (1952), Richards and Barnett (1968), and Rodin and Chayasirisobhon (1980). Jacome and Risko (1984) demonstrated large bilateral occipital spike discharges driven by low flicker frequencies in an elderly patient with a lifelong history of paroxysmal choreoathetosis.

Wilson's Disease (Hepatolenticular Degeneration)

Chronic hepatocerebral degeneration, the acquired form, is discussed in Chapter 22.

Wilson's disease is caused by copper retention and ceruloplasmin deficiency. Onset is in childhood or adolescence with tremor, rigidity, a very typical slow punctuated speech, and mask-like facial expression. Hepatic cirrhosis and the corneal Kayser-Fleischer ring are present.

The EEG has been reported frequently as normal or almost normal (Denny-Brown and Porter, 1951; Hornbostel, 1954; Strauss et al., 1952). Gibbs and Gibbs (1964) found normal tracings in the majority of the cases. Some cases may show pronounced slowing, even with spiky discharges (Heller and Kooi, 1962; Konovalov et al., 1957; Zhirmunskaya and Chukhrova, 1959). EEG abnormalities do not correlate with low ceruloplasmin levels (Heller and Kooi, 1962) or with ammonia level, even in the presence of triphasic waves (Asao and Oji, 1968). According to Hansotia et al. (1969), marked EEG abnormalities occur only in serious complications of the disease.

Liu et al. (1983) confirmed the nonspecific EEG changes of paroxysmal slow waves or sharp transients in 54.7% of cases; these did not correlate with copper or ceruloplasmin levels, age of onset, or duration of illness, but did correlate with severity of illness. EEG changes after BAL and penicillamine therapy followed a similar course. Asymptomatic siblings also had normal to mildly abnormal tracings similar to their diseased relatives. Sack et al. (1981) presented long-term EEG studies in 74 patients. In untreated patients, the record was normal in about 50%; the remaining patients showed either localized or diffuse slowing. With d-penicillamine treatment, slowing in the EEG decreased, most significantly during the first 2 years. According to Ferrari et al. (1981), sleep spindle activity is reduced in Wilson's disease and normalizes during treatment.

Parkinson's Syndrome

Parkinson's syndrome is discussed in Chapter 18, "EEG and Dementia."

Multiple System Atrophy

This rather modern term for an atypical Parkinson syndrome characterized by cerebellar and pyramidal signs (outweighing basal ganglia symptomatology) is based on older neuropathological studies of striatonigral, nigrostriatal, and cerebello-nigro-striatal degeneration (Adams et al., 1961, 1964). An overview of Ben-Shlomo et al. (1997) shows that there have been no EEG studies in this area.

Menkes' Disease (Kinky Hair Disease)

This sex-linked disorder of gray CNS matter, which affects only males, was first described by Menkes et al. (1962); association with low serum copper and ceruloplas-

min was demonstrated by Danks et al. (1972). There is also liver and brain copper accumulation due to poor intestinal absorption. A defective metallothionein has been considered the causative agent. The symptoms start in the neonatal period and consist of hypothermia, poor feeding, hypotonia, and epileptic seizures. The striking feature is the colorless, friable, and twisted hair. Cerebral vessels may be elongated and tortuous. According to Daish et al. (1978), early treatment increases copper and ceruloplasmin levels but does not prevent further CNS impairment.

The EEG shows multifocal abnormalities (White et al., 1993) and hypsarrhythmia; the electroretinogram is normal but the visual evoked potential is absent (Friedman et al., 1978). Other variants of this condition have been documented (McKusick, 1983).

Dystonia Musculorum Progressiva (Torsion Spasm)

Dystonia musculorum is a poorly understood disease that is characterized by massive twisting slow movements involving the extremities and the musculature of the trunk, neck, and face. Both familial and nonfamilial forms are observed; older children, adolescents, and young adults are most often affected. The EEG may be almost completely obscured by muscle artifacts; the readable portions are essentially within normal limits of variability. Nocturnal sleep studies have demonstrated an unusual wealth of spindles that attain relatively high voltage, a decrease of REM sleep, and generally poor quality of sleep (Jankel et al., 1983; Wein and Golubev, 1979).

Writer's cramp and similar occupational cramps are forms of dystonia. The work of Hamano et al. (1999) has shown that the primary disturbance might be prefrontal affecting the planning phase. In their study, the contingent negative variation showed lowered amplitudes between the first and second signal, selectively involving the cramp-affected hand movements.

Myoclonic Dystonia

This is a rare disorder characterized by myoclonus and rare dystonia; epileptic seizures may also occur. The EEG may show epileptiform changes (Obeso et al., 1983). A recently discovered hereditary form also showed EEG slowing (mainly temporal) and sporadic paroxysmal activity (Foncke et al., 2003).

Tourette Syndrome

This is an etiologically and pathogenetically obscure condition occurring mainly in children and adolescents. It is characterized by massive uncontrolled movements of face, trunk, and extremities. The patients often produce barking noises or may shout obscenities. In the absence of convincing organic findings (negative neuropathological and CT scan findings), this condition has often been thought to be basically psychiatric. No serious progression occurs in the course; there is a good response to haloperidol.

The EEG may be seriously marred by muscle and movement artifacts; the findings are mostly normal. EEG observations have been reported by Dolmierski and Klossovna (1958), Gajdosova et al. (1972), Sweet et al. (1973), Lucas and Rodin (1973), Bergen et al. (1980), and Marra et al. (1980). Marra et al. also observed a patient with additional generalized epileptic seizures and another patient with clonic movements contralateral to a spike focus. Krumholz et al. (1983) noted EEG abnormalities in 12.5% of the patients; these consisted of slowing of background, minor paroxysmal slow activity, and central spikes. A higher incidence of EEG abnormalities (29.2%) was reported by Barabas (1984) and Volkmar et al. (1984) (45%).

Obeso et al. (1981) studied the EEG during tics and voluntarily mimicked tics in patients with Tourette's syndrome. The voluntary jerk was preceded by a premovement negative potential of about 7 µV amplitude and commenced 500 msec prior to the electromyelographic (EMG) discharge. The spontaneous tic did not show this change. This was interpreted as a significant physiological difference between truly abnormal tics and voluntary movements in Tourette's syndrome. An exaggerated startle reflex has been demonstrated by Gironell et al. (2000).

Cerebellar Degenerations

Spinocerebellar Degeneration

In spinocerebellar degenerations (Friedreich's form, Pierre Marie's form), the EEG is usually normal (Liversedge and Emery, 1961; Thiébaut and Gruner, 1961). In Friedreich's form, the spinocerebellar symptomatology may be combined with epileptic seizures (Andermann et al., 1976; Davies, 1949; Gayral and Gayral, 1969; Newmark and Penry, 1980). Massive generalized slow spike-wave activity and the occurrence of typical minor motor seizures are indicative of a combination with the Lennox-Gastaut syndrome (personal observation) or with progressive myoclonus epilepsy (Smith et al., 1978). The EEG is normal in the Roussy-Levy syndrome (Biemond, 1954).

The spectrum of Friedreich ataxia has been reassessed and found to be broader than previously thought (Dürr et al., 1996). A special gene deficit has been demonstrated in Friedreich ataxia and other forms of spinocerebellar degeneration.

Olivopontocerebellar Atrophies

Olivopontocerebellar atrophy was originally regarded as a single nosological entity (Dejerine and Thomas, 1900). Duvoisin (1984) has attempted to reclassify a heterogeneous group of disorders on the basis of common clinical and morphological features such as ataxia and extrapyramidal signs associated with cerebellar or pontine atrophy, but with clearly distinct genetic and biochemical characteristics. The dominantly acquired variety includes the Menzel type, Schut's disease, and Joseph's disease with slow saccades, peripheral neuropathy, retinal degeneration, dementia, and extrapyramidal signs in conjunction with glycolipiduria. The sporadic or recessively inherited type includes the originally described form of Dejerine and Thomas, characterized by glutamate dehydrogenase deficiency, striatal degeneration, and autonomic nervous system failure.

The EEG has been described as normal or minimally abnormal (due to slowing) in forms with glutamate dehydrogenase deficiency; in these forms, sleep apnea may be demonstrable in sleep studies. Brainstem auditory evoked potentials have suggested cochlear nerve dysfunction due to the involvement of spiral ganglia and dorsal root ganglion cells; visual evoked potentials may also be abnormal (Duvoisin and Chokroverty, 1984). In other types of olivopontocerebellar atrophy, the EEG has been reported as normal (Wadia, 1984; Caplan, 1984).

Forms of Progressive Myoclonus Epilepsy

Myoclonus epilepsies of either progressive or benign character are degenerative CNS diseases with metabolic derangement and genetic predisposition. These myoclonic disorders—in severe forms associated with grand mal seizures, ataxia, and dementia—are neither common nor particularly rare; their epileptic features tend to be so prominent that a special presentation is justified.

Essential Hereditary Myoclonus Epilepsy

This group of degenerative CNS diseases is characterized by autosomal-recessive genetic transmission; there is massive myoclonus (symmetrical or asymmetrical), and major epileptic convulsions (grand mal) are more or less common. Cerebellar ataxia develops, and basal ganglia dyskinesias and a varying degree of dementia occur. Neuropathology shows widespread lesions in the cerebellum, brainstem, thalamus, and cortex. Forms of varying severity can be differentiated.

Lafora Disease

The form described by Lafora and Glueck (1911) shows the most rapid progression and tends to be fatal within 5 years. According to Roger (1965), this disease begins between 6 and 19 years of age (mean age, 11.5 years) and presents in 80% of the cases with seizures: clonic, tonic-clonic, and myoclonic. In addition, there are also focal seizures, especially of a visual character (Tinuper et al., 1983). The myoclonus is described as fragmentary and segmental rather than massive and is worsened by movements or intended movements. Mental deterioration may occur at an early stage or with some delay. Pyramidal signs, cerebellar ataxia, and basal ganglia dyskinesias gradually evolve.

The EEG may show a well-preserved alpha rhythm in the early state, punctuated by generalized bursts of spikes and polyspikes but with no organized spike waves. Subsequently, the EEG deteriorates and becomes highly disorganized (Gastaut, 1968; Grinker et al., 1938; Roger et al., 1965). Such a disorganized EEG (Fig. 19.7) shows irregular slow activity of medium to high voltage. Bursts of spikes may be bilateral-synchronous with a frontal maximum and often associated with myoclonus. There is also multifocal spiking. Needle-like spikes over frontal and temporal areas are myogenic and must be differentiated from authentic cerebral spikes. Myoclonus often occurs with any appreciable concomitant EEG burst. Photosensitivity (to intermittent photic stimulation) may occur in the early stage and persist; massive photoconvulsive responses can be temporarily blocked by small dosages of intravenous diazepam

Figure 19.7. Essential myoclonus epilepsy (Lafora-Unverricht-Lundborg). Unverricht form, age 17 years. Severe diffuse disorganization with abundant bilateral-frontal or generalized spiking. Extremely fast and needle-like spikes over anterior areas are probably myogenic; others are authentically cerebral. A body jerk barely alters the tracing.

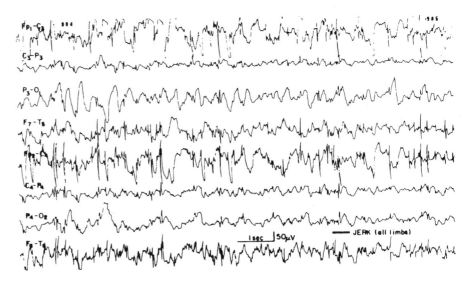

(Niedermeyer, 1970). The myoclonus as such can also be temporarily blocked by benzodiazepines (Barolin and Pateisky, 1969; Gastaut, 1968; Scharfetter and Schmoigl, 1968). Complete EEG disorganization characterizes the final stage of the disease.

Roger et al. (1965) have stressed the presence of spikes and polyspikes and the absence of spike wave and polyspike wave complexes. Other authors have noted massive polyspike wave activity (Barolin and Pateisky, 1969; Gambi et al., 1970; Hambert and Petersén, 1970; Riehl et al., 1967; Tükel and Caliskan, 1964; Yokoi et al., 1965). According to Tassinari et al. (1979), polyspike activity develops about 3 to 5 years after onset of disease. The EEG deterioration was also corroborated by Reese et al. (1993).

On the other hand, a gradual increase of spike-wave activity was reported in four members of a Palestinian family with Lafora disease (Yen et al., 1991).

Lafora disease is a recessive hereditary condition. Inclusion bodies (Lafora bodies) constitute a major feature of the neuropathological changes and can be demonstrated by cutaneous, muscular, and hepatic biopsies (Carpenter and Karpati, 1981). Death tends to occur after an average of 2 to 10 years following onset (Roger et al., 1992).

The Unverricht-Lundborg Type (Also Known as Baltic Type or Baltic Myoclonus Epilepsy)

This type was described relatively early by Unverricht (1891) in a patient living in Estonia and by Lundborg (1903, 1911) in southwestern parts of Sweden. Eldridge et al. (1983) recognized a similar root in both forms. The Baltic type used to be milder than the Lafora form, although (according to Eldridge et al.) phenytoin treatment might have worsened the character of the disease in recent decades. Nevertheless, cases of the Unverricht type may have a rather rapidly fatal course even in the absence of phenytoin treatment. There are significant similarities in clinical symptomatology with the Lafora form; neuropathologically, however, the absence of Lafora bodies in the Baltic form serves as a distinctive characteristic in the biopsy.

A thoroughly investigated *Finnish type of Baltic myoclonus epilepsy* has been delineated by Koskiniemi et al. (1974a). Inheritance is recessive; onset occurs between 8 and 13 years of age. Cerebellar ataxia is rapidly associated with seizures of the myoclonic and grand mal type; myoclonus may be segmental, fragmentary, or massive, and can be triggered by various stimuli and especially by movements. Pyramidal signs are found in 30% of the patients. Mental deterioration is rather slow, but the motor deterioration progresses so that the patients are bedridden about 5 to 10 years after onset. Death tends to occur after about 15 years. Appropriate anticonvulsive treatment can slow down the course of the disorder.

The EEG is characterized by gradually progressive slowing with generalized 3 to 5/sec spike-wave-like bursts of frontal accentuation (Fig. 19.8), whereas spike-wave complexes are alien to the EEG picture of Lafora disease. Paroxysmal flicker responses are the rule (Roger et al., 1992); there are generalized spikes and polyspikes with photic stimulation. According to Koskiniemi et al. (1974b), spikes, spike waves, polyspikes, and photosensitivity increase during the terminal stage. The EEG abnormalities and evoked potentials were studied with magnetoencephalographic technique by Karhu et al. (1994).

Our knowledge concerning the genetics of this disorder can be summarized as follows: the Unverricht-Lundborg type (also known as EMP 1) has been linked to the human chromosome 21q22.3; the gene encoding cystatin B was shown to be localized to this area (Pennacchio et al., 1996).

Nonprogressive Benign Myoclonus

For many decades, cases of widespread but nonprogressive myoclonus without other neurological deficits, without major convulsions, and without dementia were usually listed as *paramyoclonus multiplex* or *Friedreich's disease*—a condition described by Friedreich (1881). Familial forms with an autosomal mode of heredity have been reported by Hartung (1920) and Mahloudji and Pikielny (1967) (Hartung syndrome). The EEG findings are normal (Fig. 19.9).

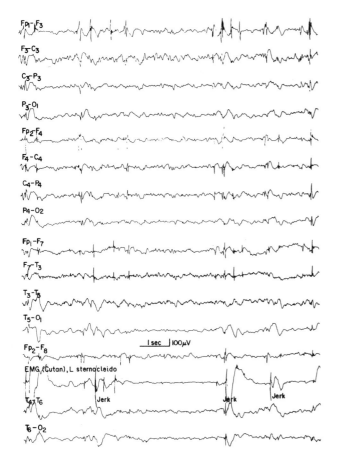

Figure 19.8. Essential myoclonus epilepsy. Unverricht form, age 23 years. There is evidence of spikes with concomitant muscle jerks and without any muscular accompaniment.

Other Progressive CNS Degenerations

Alper's Disease

This is a clinicopathological syndrome with initially normal development followed by psychomotor retardation with prominent myoclonic, focal, and generalized tonic-clonic convulsions. Epilepsia partialis continua may be the most impressive clinical manifestation. The EEG may show continuous anterior high-voltage 1 to 3/sec spike-wave-like activity regardless of ongoing focal motor seizures (Brick et al., 1984). These authors also found that paroxysmal EEG activity gradually diminishes and background activity slows, regardless of continuing focal epileptic seizures, in the terminal phase of the disease. Diffuse low-voltage activity also has been reported. Epilepsia partialis continua and grand mal status were observed by Walton (1996).

Alexander's Disease

This is a rare disease with combined gray and white matter involvement (Alexander, 1949). The onset occurs mainly in infancy, but juvenile and adult forms are known.

Children present with failure to thrive, psychomotor retardation, epileptic seizures, spasticity, and progressive macrocephaly. Peculiar eosinophilic hyaline bodies (Rosen-

thal fibers) are present below the pia and around blood vessel throughout the brain and spinal cord. Destructive white matter changes are most prominent in the frontal lobes.

No specific EEG changes are known; Friede (1964) reported a child with diffuse slowing and focal spikes.

CADASIL (Cerebral Autosomal-Dominant Arteriopathy with Subcortical Infarcts and Leukoencephalopathy)

This disorder is characterized by headaches, transient ischemic attacks, and strokes with onset during adulthood and progression leading to dementia and pseudobulbar palsy (Chabriat et al., 1995). It is a disease of the small- and medium-sized arteries, associated with mutation of the *Notch3* gene on chromosome 19 (Tournier-Lasserve et al., 1993) and delayed VEP 100 (Parisi et al., 2000).

Phacomatoses

Phacomatoses are congenital conditions of dominant inheritance with variable and widespread manifestations that often affect the CNS (Francois, 1972). According to Francois, the four cardinal features of phacomatosis are as follows:

1. Small spots or patches on skin or mucous membranes ("phakos," like "nevus," denotes birthmark).
2. Localized tumor-like hyperplastic formations of different types.

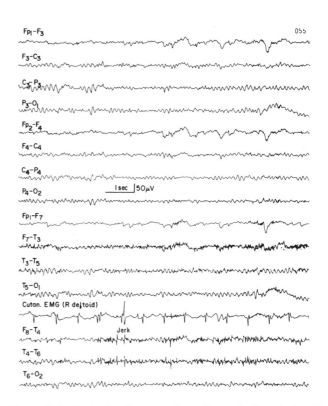

Figure 19.9. Benign hereditary myoclonus (Hartung's disease). Age 25 years. The alpha frequency (8–9/sec) is slower than average, but no definite abnormalities are present. A muscle jerk is unassociated with EEG events.

3. True tumors, arising from undifferentiated embryonic cells (benign or malignant).
4. Other congenital abnormalities (of the viscera, bones, etc.).

Tuberous Sclerosis

Tuberous sclerosis is practically always characterized by cutaneous lesions (adenoma sebaceum, shagreen plaques, depigmented areas), ophthalmological lesions ("phakoma," a retinal tumor, and other retinal changes), and CNS manifestations that are caused by cortical tuberosities and spongioblastic tumor formation in the cerebrum (Donegani et al., 1972). Epileptic seizures are extremely common and practically obligatory when the CNS is involved. In infancy, these attacks may present themselves as infantile spasms (Krauthammer, 1965). Grand mal as well as psychomotor and other partial types of seizures may occur. A neonatal form with onset of seizures in the newborn period has been described by Pohowalla and McIntyre (1984).

Mental retardation is not quite as common as the epileptic seizure disorder (Lagos and Gomez, 1967). Various neurological deficits may be present.

The EEG has been found to be abnormal in 87% of the cases (Lagos and Gomez, 1967); a similar figure was found by Dickerson and Hellman (1952). The EEG changes reflect the seizure disorder as well as the tumoral lesions (Fig. 19.10). Typical hypsarrhythmia is found in the presence of infantile spasms. In patients with cutaneous formations only, the EEG is normal (Harvald and Hauge, 1955).

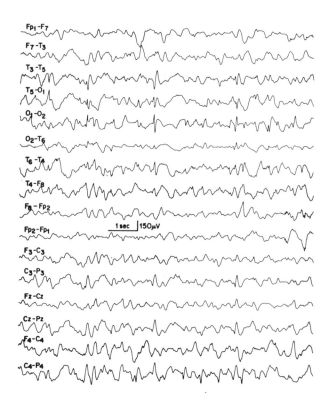

Figure 19.10. Tuberous sclerosis with frequent epileptic seizures. Age 2 years 8 months. There is massive diffuse slowing (patient lethargic, only 5 minutes after a major convulsion). Sporadic spikes occur mainly over left occipitoposterotemporal region.

Ganji and Hellman (1985) reported the EEG data of 60 patients (320 records) with tuberous sclerosis. Normal tracings were found in five patients (8.3%); diffuse slowing (84%) was the most common abnormality; slow spike-wave discharges were found in 42%, focal spikes in 16%, and multifocal spikes in 16%. Clinical seizures were noted in 58 patients (97%); in 80%, the seizures started in the first year of life. Generalized seizures (evidently grand mal) occurred in 44 patients, infantile spasms in 27, myoclonic attacks in 15, focal seizures in 15, and atonic-akinetic seizures in 15 patients. From the presence of slow spike-wave patterns and atonic-akinetic seizures, one can infer that, in some of the patients, a superimposed Lennox-Gastaut syndrome materializes.

Curatolo et al. (1988) reported congruence of EEG spike foci and MRI lesions in tuberous sclerosis. Genetic studies have shown two underlying gene defects, which do not break up the disease into different entities.

Neurofibromatosis (Von Recklinghausen's Disease)

This disease is characterized by multiple tumors arising from the peripheral nervous system, by abnormal cutaneous pigmentation, and by CNS tumors. Café-au-lait spots are usually the first clinical manifestation (Whitehouse, 1966), followed by the development of neurofibromatous changes. In type 2, bilateral acoustic neurinomas are common; multiple meningiomas and intraspinal tumors may also occur. The gene of type 1 has been mapped to chromosome 17 and type 2 to 22.

Epileptic seizures are not common in this disease. EEG tracings are either normal or slightly abnormal unless intracranial tumor growth or epileptic seizures dominate the picture.

Sturge-Weber Syndrome

This disease is clinically characterized (after Alexander, 1972) as follows:

1. Cutaneous vascular nevus (nevus flammeus or capillary nevus) affecting mainly the upper part of the face
2. Epileptic seizures in practically every case
3. Homonymous hemianopsia (majority of cases)
4. Gyriform intracranial calcifications becoming radiologically manifest after infancy
5. Glaucoma or buphthalmos
6. Some degree of mental retardation
7. Hemiparetic deficit with hemihypertrophy of body or face

Leptomeningeal angiomatosis is the most significant pathological substratum. The facial nevus is present at birth. The psychomotor development of the infant is normal until the first seizures occur; this often dramatically changes the course, and both neurological and mental deficits become apparent.

The seizures usually start around age 2. Because most lesions are located in the occipital-parietal region, the seizures may have a focal onset (scotomatous field defect).

The EEG shows local voltage depression of the area. In more advanced cases, the intravenous diazepam-induced beta response is absent over the affected region (Jansen et al., 2002). Spikes may be present, but according to personal observations, the abnormalities are not very impressive. Alexander and Norman (1960) and Alexander et al. (1962) presented electrocorticographic observations with sharply demarcated flattening over the angiomatous region surrounded by a zone of spiky activity. Occipital lobectomy usually leads to seizure control (Alexander and Norman, 1960). In severe cases with extensive pathology, early hemispherectomy (before age 1 year) may be helpful (Revol et al., 1988). More recently, aspirin has been used over long periods in order to prevent thrombosis; the results have been encouraging (Roach et al., 1985).

Further information on Sturge-Weber syndrome is found in Chapter 27, "Epileptic Seizure Disorders," in the section on occipital lobe epilepsy.

Incontinentia Pigmenti

This disorder is also known as Bloch-Sulzberger syndrome and may be listed in the group of phacomatoses. It is characterized by disturbed skin pigmentation, sometimes in association with ocular, dental, and cardiac anomalies. The CNS may be severely affected in some cases. In a personal observation, a young adult was profoundly mentally retarded and suffered from a very severe and recalcitrant epileptic seizure disorder with various types of major and minor seizures. The EEG was abnormal with almost constantly repetitive spikes against a grossly disordered background of activity.

Hypomelanosis (Ito)

This disease is associated with prominent epileptic seizure disorder (generalized tonic-clonic), mental retardation, language disability, autistic behavior, and hypotonia. Hypopigmented skin lesions show a linear pattern (Ruggieri et al., 1996).

Chromosomal Aberrations
Down Syndrome (Mongolism, Trisomy 21)

The clinical characteristics and the underlying chromosomal aberration are well known. There have been numerous EEG reports since Kreezer's first study (1939). Most of this work has been discussed by Ellingson et al. (1970).

According to Ellingson et al. (1970) and Ellingson (1972), EEG abnormalities occur in 20% to 30% of mongoloids and are more common in childhood than in adulthood. Epileptic seizures are less frequent in mongolism than in mental retardation due to other causes (Walter et al., 1955). Gibbs and Gibbs (1964) described bilateral spike-like activity over parietal areas in sleep records of mongoloid children and also noted widespread monorhythmic 4/sec waves (chiefly frontal and parietal) in the waking state. Prominent occipital high-voltage 1 to 2/sec waves with a sharp component in the terminal phase were also reported (Gibbs and Gibbs, 1964). These authors also stressed the scarcity of 14 and 6/sec positive spikes in Down syndrome. There are no correlations between EEG abnormalities and special clinical features. A maturational lag in the development of infantile sleep patterns has been reported by Ellingson et al. (1970). The features of Alzheimer's presenile dementia tend to develop early in the adult life of the Down syndrome patient. There have been reports about the combination of Down syndrome and infantile spasms (West syndrome) (Silva et al., 1996).

Longitudinal intrahemispheric and interhemispheric coherence studies showed some differences between children with Down syndrome and healthy controls (Schmid et al., 1992).

Progeria

This is an extremely rare condition, characterized by rapidly evolving precocious senility with onset in early infancy; death occurs usually before age 10 years and is caused by coronary disease. Autosomal-recessive inheritance is suspected (Gabr et al., 1960). EEG findings in two cases reported by Gibbs and Gibbs (1964) were normal; repeat studies in one case remained normal for the chronological age.

Hereditary Optic Nerve Atrophy (Leber's Disease)

This is probably a heterogeneous disease (McKusick, 1983) with an unclear genetic mode of transmission. Age of onset is variable, mostly around age 20 years. Rabache et al. (1960) reported EEG abnormalities in nine of 16 cases; slowing of the alpha frequency (7.5–8/sec) and frontotemporal bursts were found (Fig. 19.11). Some of these cases may be of mitochondrial origin.

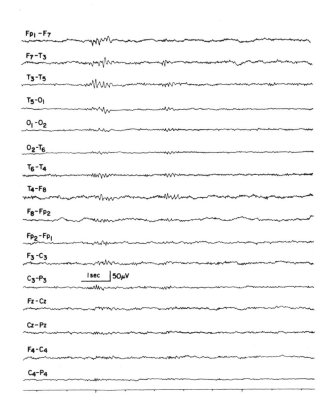

Figure 19.11. Leber's optic atrophy (bilateral). Patient, 49 years old, had recent syncope without convulsive movement. Computed tomography scan is normal. The EEG shows train of 7–10/sec waves with mildly sharp transients over temporal areas, more on the left. This same type of mild abnormality is commonly seen in early cerebrovascular disorder.

Myotonic Dystrophy

This well-known disease is not confined to the neuromuscular level. Autonomic and endocrine functions are disturbed, and there is evidence of mental change; cerebral atrophy is often demonstrable. This autosomal-dominant disorder may be diagnosed in early adulthood or adolescence (Schubert et al., 1980).

About 50% of the patients show EEG abnormalities consisting mainly of excessive slow activity (Lundervold et al., 1969). The EEG abnormalities may correlate with mental changes (Okuma et al., 1970). The alpha rhythm was found to be slower than average, monotonous, and of low voltage (Beijersbergen et al., 1980). An increase in theta frequencies was reported by Murri et al. (1990).

Congenital Muscular Dystrophy

This is an autosomal-recessive disease that affects *in utero* skeletal muscle as well as the CNS (Fukuyama, 1960). It is characterized by severe mental retardation, hypotonia, joint contractures, and epileptic seizures. According to Yoshioka et al. (1981), seizures occur in two thirds of the patients. The EEG is abnormal and demonstrates slowing, spikes, and sharp waves. The slowing corresponds with areas of cerebral atrophy.

Dystrophia Musculorum Progressiva (Duchenne's Disease)

Subnormal mental functioning has been noted frequently in this disease. A variety of EEG abnormalities, especially excessive slowing, have been reported (Paolozzi et al., 1965; Sirakov, 1965; Zellweger and Niedermeyer, 1965).

Other Chromosomal Aberrations

In *translocation 6q:14q*, hypsarrhythmic EEG patterns have been reported (Hattori et al., 1985). The *fragile X syndrome* is associated with mental retardation, macroorchidism, large ears, prominent jaw, and high-pitched jocular speech; the EEG is unremarkable (DeArce and Kearns, 1984).

The *Aicardi syndrome* with flexion spasms, chorioretinal abnormalities, and agenesis of the corpus callosum occurs solely in girls; this syndrome is now considered to be transmitted as an X-linked dominant gene that is lethal to boys. The EEG shows multifocal paroxysmal discharges and assumes burst-suppression-like features, but there is total asynchrony between the hemispheres (Fariello et al., 1977). These abnormalities are common in the first 6 months and are replaced by multiple epileptic foci. All sleep stages are severely altered.

The *Wolf-Hirschhorn syndrome* is an autosomal disorder caused by partial deletion of the short arm of chromosome 4. Clinically, there are myoclonic seizures (unilateral or generalized), followed by brief absences. EEG studies in four children with this syndrome showed impressive high-voltage spike-wave-like bursts (Sgró et al., 1995). This pattern is thought to be similar to that found in Angelman syndrome (Srgó et al., 1995).

There have been only very few EEG observation in cases of *trisomy D, trisomy E,* and *"maladie de cri du chat."*

Sex Chromosome Aberrations

The prevalence of EEG abnormalities in *Klinefelter's syndrome (XXY)* might be higher than in the average population; the reports are inconclusive (Dumermuth, 1961; Hambert and Frey, 1964; Nielsen and Pedersen, 1969). The alpha frequency seems to be below average; otherwise, no consistent EEG abnormalities have been shown.

In *Turner's syndrome (XO)*, poorly specified EEG abnormalities have been reported (see Ellingson, 1972).

In the *XYY syndrome*, mild EEG abnormalities are quite common (Borgoankar et al., 1968). Ellingson (1972) suspects that these abnormalities could be due partly to sampling prison and hospital populations.

Duchenne's type of muscular dystrophy (see above) would also fall into this category.

Further Degenerative Diseases of Unclear Origin

Rud Syndrome

This is a rare disorder; the main features are ichthyosis, epileptic seizures, mental retardation, neurosensory hearing loss, and hypogonadism. This disorder has been associated with steroid sulfatase deficiency in cultured skin fibroblasts (Andria et al., 1984). Both generalized and focal motor seizures have been reported. EEG abnormalities include slowing of the background activity with frontotemporal and midtemporal paroxysmal discharges as well as bilateral synchronous spike-wave activity; EEG abnormalities have also been noted in seizure-free patients (Maldonado et al., 1975; Marxmiller et al., 1985; York-Moore and Rundle, 1962).

Angelman Syndrome (Happy Puppet Syndrome)

This syndrome has been described in young children, adolescents, and adults (Angelman, 1965; Jay et al., 1991). These patients present with peculiar craniofacial features, tongue protrusion, paroxysmal laughter, and movements of puppet-like jerkiness. They also may suffer from optic nerve atrophy, cerebral atrophy, and frequent epileptic seizures. The etiology is unclear. A linkage to chromosome 15 has been demonstrated.

Pampiglione and Martinez (1983) observed "very large discharges" (facilitated with eye closure) up to the age of 8 years. Thereafter, the EEG tends to improve. This suggests an early developmental anomaly with limited progression. Ganji and Duncan (1989) noted two types of development with serial EEG tracings: one with arrest of electrical maturation at age 1 to 3 years, and another with signs of gradual improvement and EEG maturation. The cortical myoclonus found in Angelman syndrome was investigated in great detail by Guerrini et al. (1996). According to Valente et al. (2003), very abnormal EEG records are the rule in Angelman syndrome; the most common pattern, however, is diffuse delta activity of very high voltage with more or less prominent intermingled spiking, sometimes assuming slow spike-wave character.

Heller's Syndrome (Dementia Infantilis, Dementia Praecocissima)

This is a poorly delineated and etiologically obscure syndrome with certain schizophrenic traits and disturbed communicative and social behavior, starting at age 3 to 4 years and associated with speech deterioration or complete loss of language. True schizophrenic development and organic cerebral features appear to be almost inseparably intermingled.

The EEG is uncharacteristic and may be normal. Left frontal slowing was found in a right-handed older child with mutism but no intellectual defect (personal observation).

Rett Syndrome

This syndrome was described first by Rett (1966) and was subsequently confirmed by Hagberg et al. (1983); its underlying cause has remained undetermined in spite of a sizable bulk of investigations. The disease is confined to the female gender.

Following a period of normal development from birth to age 6 to 18 months, a progressive decline of psychomotor functions is associated with language impairment, loss of motor skills (even true apraxia), and very typical (and virtually diagnostic) stereotypic hand movements: wringing, washing, rubbing motions. Epileptic seizures occur in 75% to 80%. Grand mal, psychomotor (complex partial), and focal motor seizures have been reported.

The EEG is almost always abnormal. Spikes are a common finding and are most often noted over the central regions, especially in sleep (Niedermeyer et al., 1991). In some cases, central spikes can be blocked with passive hand movements (Niedermeyer and Naidu, 1990) (Fig. 19.12). On the other hand, Robertson et al. (1988) elicited central spikes and spike waves with contralateral tactile stimulation. Slow spike-wave complexes may also occur (Niedermeyer et al., 1986) along with signs of a concomitant Lennox-Gastaut syndrome (Olmos Gracia de Alba et al., 1987).

Prominent theta rhythms in the 4 to 6/sec range have been noted over vertex area and its vicinity (Niedermeyer et al., 1997).

With the progression of the disorder, epileptic seizures and EEG spikes tend to disappear: "later motor deterioration stage" (Hagberg and Witt-Engerström, 1986). In this stage (after age 10 years), the EEG most commonly shows diffuse slowing (Niedermeyer et al., 1986).

Abnormal breathing was observed by Lugaresi et al. (1985). According to Kerr et al. (1990), episodes of hyperventilation are associated with disappearance of delta activity. Sleep studies (Aldrich et al., 1990) show rather poorly defined spindles and K complexes. A distinction between true epileptic seizures and episodic disturbances of non-epileptic character in children with Rett syndrome was attempted by Glaze et al. (1998).

The smallness of the frontal lobe in Rett syndrome has been thought to be the cause of disinhibition of the motor cortex hence leading to uncontrolled motor activity (awake) and central spikes (mainly in sleep) (Niedermeyer et al., 1997).

Degenerative CNS Diseases with Autonomic Dysfunctions

Familial Dysautonomia (Riley-Day Disease)

This autosomal-recessive disorder occurs almost exclusively in children of Ashkenazic Jewish lineage. It is associated with severe progressive autonomic nervous system dysfunction; death in childhood or adolescence is the rule. Neuropathological studies have been surprisingly inconclusive. Postural hypotension, absence of tears, skin blotching, abnormal temperature control, and periodic vomiting are typical clinical signs. There is indifference to pain, areflexia, poor coordination, and dysarthria. Syncopal attacks are common; epileptic seizures or major convulsions also occur with or without fever.

Gibbs and Gibbs (1964) found predominantly normal EEG tracings. Niedermeyer et al. (1967) found abnormal records in every one of ten cases and reported excessive slowing as well as generalized bursts of slow activity with spikes and sharp waves (Fig. 19.13).

Idiopathic Orthostatic Hypotension (Shy-Drager Syndrome)

This is a sporadic and occasionally familial condition with pronounced orthostatic hypotension, based on degeneration of the intermediolateral column of the spinal cord and the dorsal vagal nuclei (Bannister and Oppenheimer, 1972; Chokroverty et al., 1969; Shy and Drager, 1960). There is

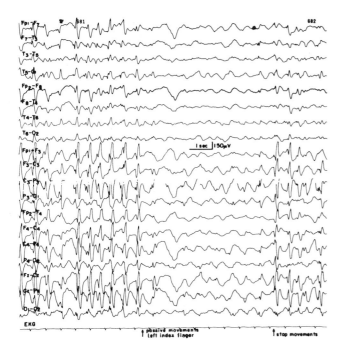

Figure 19.12. Age 11 years. Rett syndrome. EEG shows massive bilateral-synchronous spikes and slow spike waves, maximal over central areas and vertex, immediately and independently blocked with passive movements of left index finger. Also note immediate return of spikes and spike waves after cessation of movements. This portion was obtained in a state of lethargy-wakefulness.

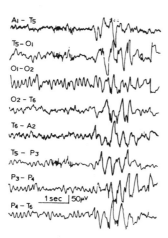

Figure 19.13. Riley-Day syndrome (familial dysautonomia). Age 11 years, no history of epileptic seizures. Note generalized burst with intermixed spikes. (With permission of Elsevier, Amsterdam.)

anhidrosis, impotence, dysuria, and absence of compensatory vasomotor reflexes. Parkinsonian features such as tremor, rigidity, and ataxia are often present.

The resting EEG is unremarkable. When recorded in orthostatic posture and after slight exertion, very prominent diffuse delta activity occurs, while the first signs of fainting are noticeable. The heart rate remains unchanged due to lack of compensatory mechanisms (Fig. 19.14). In contrast, patients with orthostatic dizziness and fainting due to vertebrobasilar artery insufficiency show no concomitant EEG changes.

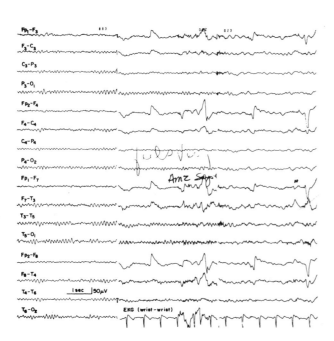

Figure 19.14. Shy-Drager syndrome in a 54-year-old man. The unactivated record was within normal limits of variability. *Left portion,* patient at rest; *center portion,* patient standing; he feels very dizzy but there is no significant EEG change; *right portion,* patient has started to move up and down a small stepladder consisting of two steps 25 cm apart. Note moderate diffuse EEG slowing without change of heart rate.

References

Adams, R.D., and Lyon, G. 1982. *Neurology of Hereditary Metabolic Diseases of Children.* New York: McGraw-Hill.

Adams, R.D., Van Bogaert, L., and Van der Eecken, H. 1961. Dégénerescences nigro-striées et cérébello-nigro-striées. Neurol. Psychiatr. (Basel) 142:219–259.

Adams, R.D., Van Bogaert, L., and Van der Eecken, H. 1964. Striatonigral degeneration. J. Neuropathol. Exp. Neurol. 23:584–608.

Aldrich, M.S., Garofalo, E.A., and Drury, I. 1990. Epileptiform abnormalities during sleep in Rett syndrome. Electroencephalogr. Clin. Neurophysiol. 75:365–370.

Alexander, G.L. 1972. Sturge-Weber syndrome. In *Handbook of Clinical Neurology,* vol. 22, Eds. P.J. Vinken and G.W. Bruyn, pp. 223–240. Amsterdam: North Holland.

Alexander, G.L., and Norman, R.M. 1960. *The Sturge-Weber Syndrome.* Bristol: John Wright & Sons.

Alexander, G.L., Cooper, R., and Crow, H.J. 1962. EEG, ECoG and oxygen availability in the cortex of a case of Sturge-Weber syndrome. Electroencephalogr. Clin. Neurophysiol. 14:284(abst).

Alexander, W.S. 1949. Progressive fibrinoid degeneration of fibrillary astrocytes associated with mental retardation in hydrocephalic infant. Brain 72:373–381.

Allan, J.D., Cusworth, D.C., Dent, C.E., et al. 1958. A disease, probably hereditary, characterized by severe mental deficiency and a constant gross abnormality of amino acid metabolism. Lancet 275:185.

Allen, N. 1964. Developmental and degenerative diseases of the brain. In *Pediatric Neurology,* Ed. T.W. Farmer, pp. 162–284. New York: Hoeber Medical Division, Harper & Row.

Andermann, E.D., Remillard, G.M., Goyer, C., et al. 1976. Genetic and family studies on Friedreich's ataxia. Can. J. Neurol. Sci. 3:287–301.

Andrews, J.M., Cancilla, P.A., Grippo, J., et al. 1971. Globoid cell leukodystrophy (Krabbe's disease): morphological and biochemical studies. Neurology 21:337–352.

Andria, G., Ballabio, G., Parenti, S., et al. 1984. Steroid sulphatase deficiency is present in patients with the syndrome "ichthyosis and male hypogonadism" and with "Rud syndrome." J. Inherited Metab. Dis. 7(suppl 2):159–160.

Andriola, M.R. 1979. The EEG in adrenoleucodystrophy (Schilder's disease). Electroencephalogr. Clin. Neurophysiol. 46:2P(abst).

Angelman, H. 1965. "Puppet" children: a report on three cases. Dev. Med. Child. Neurol. 7:681–688.

Asao, H., and Oji, K. 1968. *Hepatocerebral Degeneration.* Springfield, IL: Charles C Thomas.

Bannister, R., and Oppenheimer, D.R. 1972. Degenerative diseases of the nervous system associated with autonomic failure. Brain 95:457–474.

Barabas, G., Matthews, W.S., and Holowinsky, M. 1984. Electroencephalographic abnormalities in Tourette's syndrome. Ann. Neurol. 16:93–94.

Barolin, G.S., and Pateisky, K. 1969. Geschwister mit Myoklonuskörperchenkrankheit (Unverricht-Lundborg). Familien- und Lngschnittuntersuchung. Wien Z. Nervenheilk. 27:1–8.

Batshaw, M. 1984. *Hyperammonemia: Current Problems in Pediatrics.* Chicago: Year Book.

Battaglia, A., Harden, A., Pampiglione, G., et al. 1981. Neurophysiological studies in 14 patients with adrenoleucodystrophy. Electroencephalogr. Clin. Neurophysiol. 51:53P(abst).

Becker, W.J., Kunesch, E., and Freund, H.-J. 1990. Myoclonus and sensorimotor mechanisms in Ramsay-Hunt syndrome (RHS). Electroencephalogr. Clin. Neurophysiol. 75:S9(abst).

Behbehani, A.W. 1985. Termination of strict diet therapy in phenylketonuria. A study of EEG sleep patterns and computer spectral analysis. Neuropediatrics 16:92–97.

Beijersbergen, R.S.H.M., Kemp, A., and Storm van Leeuwen, W. 1980. EEG observations in dystrophia myotonica (Curschmann-Steinert). Electroencephalogr. Clin. Neurophysiol. 49:143–151.

Bell, A.J. 1995. MELAS syndrome: Overview and case study. Am. J. EEG Technol. 35:83–91.

Ben-Shlomo, Y., Wenning, G.K., Tison, F., et al. 1997. Survival of patients with pathologically proven multiple system atrophy: a meta-analysis. Neurology 48:384–393.

Bergamasco, B., Bergamini, L., and Mutani, R. 1967. Spontaneous sleep abnormalities in a case of dyssynergia cerebellaris myoclonica. Epilepsia (Amsterdam) 8:271–281.

Bergen, D., Tanner, C., and Wilson, R. 1980. The EEG in Gilles de la Tourette syndrome. Electroencephalogr. Clin. Neurophysiol. 49:23P (abst).

Berginer, V.M., Radwan, H., Korczyn, A.D., et al. 1982. EEG in cerebrotendonous xanthomatosis. Clin. Electroencephalogr. 13:89–96.

Berkovic, S.F., Andermann, F., Karpati, G., et al. 1988. The epileptic syndromes associated with mitochondrial disease. Electroencephalogr. Clin. Neurophysiol. 69:50P(abst).

Biemond, A. 1954. La forme radiculo-cordonale postérieure des dégénérescences spino-cérébelleuses. Rev. Neurol (Paris) 91:3–21.

Black, J.T., Judge, D., Demers, L., et al. 1975. Ragged red fibers. A biochemical and morphological study. J. Neurosci. 26:479–488.

Borgoankar, D.S., Murdoch, J.L., McKusick, V.A., et al. 1968. The YY syndrome. Lancet 2:461–462.

Borkowski, W.J., Jr., Marks, H.G., and Strivastava, R. 1991. BAERs and VERs in Pelizaeus-Merzbacher disease, patients and carriers. Electroencephalogr. Clin. Neurophysiol. 79:44P(abst).

Brady, R.O. 1975. Lipidoses. In *The Nervous System*, vol. 2, Ed.-in-chief, D.B. Tower, pp. 219–227. New York: Raven Press.

Brick, J.F., Westmoreland, B.F., and Gomez, M.R. 1984. The electroencephalogram in Alper's disease. Electroencephalogr. Clin. Neurophysiol. 58:31P(abst).

Buchanan, D.S., and Davis, R.L. 1965. Spongy degeneration of the nervous system: a report of four cases with a review of the literature. Neurology 15:207–222.

Caplan, L.R. 1984. Clinical features of sporadic (Déjérine-Thomas) olivopontocerebellar atrophies. In *Olivopontocerebellar Atrophies*, Eds. R.C. Duvoisin and A. Plataikas, pp. 217–224. New York: Raven Press.

Carpenter, S., and Karpati, G. 1981. Sweat gland duct cells in Lafora disease: diagnosis by skin biopsy. Neurology 31:1564–1568.

Carson, N.A., and Neill, D.W. 1962. Metabolic abnormalities detected in a survey of mentally backward individuals in Northern Ireland. Arch. Dis. Child. 37:509–513.

Catel, W., and Schmidt, J. 1959. Über eine familäre gichtische Diathese in Verbindung mit zerebralen und renalen Symptomen bei einem Kleinkind. Deutsch. Med. Wochenschr. 84:2145.

Chabriat, H., Vahedi, K., Iba-Zen, M.T., et al. 1995. Clinical spectrum of CADASIL: a study of 7 families' cerebral autosomal dominant arteriopathy with subcortical infarcts and leukoencephalopathy. Lancet 346: 934–939.

Chaves-Carballo, E. 1992. Detection of inherited neurometabolic diseases. Pediatr. Neurol. 39:801–820.

Chokroverty, S., Barron, K.D., Katz, F.H., et al. 1969. The syndrome of primary orthostatic hypotension. Brain 92:743–748.

Clancy, R.R., and Chung, H.J. 1991. EEG changes during recovery from acute severe neonatal citrullinemia. Electroencephalogr. Clin. Neurophysiol. 78:222–227.

Cobb, W., Martin, F., and Pampiglione, G. 1952. Cerebral lipidosis: electroencephalographic study. Brain 75:343–357.

Cowen, D., and Olmstead, D. 1963. Infantile neuro-axonal dystrophy. J. Neuropathol. Exp. Neurol. 22:175–236.

Curatolo, P., Cusmai, R., Trasatti, G., et al. 1988. Tuberous sclerosis relationships between the site of EEG spike foci and cortical lesions by MRI. Electroencephalogr. Clin. Neurophysiol. 70:16P(abst).

Daish, P., Wheeler, E.M., Roberts, P.F., et al. 1978. Menkes syndrome: report of a patient treated from 21 days of age with parenteral copper. Arch. Dis. Child. 53:956–958.

Dancis, J., Levitz, M., and Westall, R.G. 1960. Maple syrup urine disease. Branched-chain ketoaciduria. Pediatrics 25:72–79.

Danks, D.M., Campbell, P.E., Stevens, B.J., et al. 1972. Menkes kinky hair syndrome. An inherited defect in copper absorption with widespread effects. Pediatrics 50:188–201.

Davies, D.L. 1949. Psychiatric changes associated with Friedreich's ataxia. J. Neurol. Neurosurg. Psychiatr. 12:246–250.

DeArce, M.A., and Kearns, A. 1984. The fragile X syndrome: the patients and their chromosome. J. Med. Genet. 21:84–91.

DeBarsy, T., Myle, G., Troch, C., Matthys, R., et al. 1969. La dyssynergie cérébelleuse myoclonique (R. Hunt); affection autonomique ou variante du type dégéneratif de l'épilepsie myoclonie progressive (Unverricht-Lundborg): approche anatomo-clinique. J. Neurol. Sci. 8: 111–127.

De Giorgis, G.F., Antonozzi, I., Del Castello, P.G., et al. 1983. EEG as a possible tool in phenylketonuria. Electroencephalogr. Clin. Neurophysiol. 55:60–68.

Déjérine, J., and Thomas, A. 1900. L'atrophie olivo-ponto-cérébelleuse. Nouv. Iconograph. Salpêt. 13:330–370.

Denny-Brown, D., and Porter, H. 1951. The effect of BAL (2,3 mercaptopropanol) on hepato-lenticular degeneration (Wilson's disease). N. Engl. J. Med. 245:917–925.

Dent, C.E., and Westall, R.G. 1961. Studies in maple syrup urine disease. Arch. Dis. Child. 36:259–268.

Desnick, R.J. 1991. *Treatment of Genetic Diseases*. New York: Churchill Livingstone.

Dickerson, W.W., and Hellman, C.D. 1952. Electroencephalographic study of patients with tuberous sclerosis. Neurology (Minneapolis) 2: 248–254.

Dolmierski, R., and Klossovna, M. 1958. On the disease of Gilles de la Tourette (Polish). Neurol. Neurochir. Psychiatr. Polska 8:639–646.

Donegani, G., Grattarola, F.R., and Wildi, E. 1972. In *Handbook of Clinical Neurology*, vol. 14, Eds. P.J. Vinken and G.W. Bruyn, pp. 340–389. Amsterdam: North Holland.

Dumermuth, G. 1961. EEG Untersuchungen beim jugendlichen Klinefelter-Syndrome. Helvet. Paediatr. Acta 16:702–710.

Dumermuth, G. 1972. *Elektroencephalographie im Kindesalter*, 2nd ed. Stuttgart: Thieme.

Dürr, A., Cossee, M., Agid, Y., et al. 1996. Clinical and genetic abnormalities in patients with Friedreich's ataxia. N. Engl. J. Med. 335: 1175.

Duvoisin, R.C. 1984. An apology and introduction to the olivopontocerebellar atrophies. In *Olivopontocerebellar Atrophies*, Eds. R.C. Duvoisin and A. Plataikas, pp. 5–12. New York: Raven Press.

Duvoisin, R.C., and Chokroverty, S. 1984. Clinical expression of glutamate dehydrogenase deficiency. In *Olivopontocerebellar Atrophies*, Eds. R.C. Duvoisin and A. Plataikas, pp. 267–279. New York: Raven Press.

Dvorkin, G.S., Andermann, F., Carpenter, S., et al. 1987. Classical migraine, intractable epilepsy and multiple strokes: a syndrome related to mitochondrial encephalomyopathy. In *Migraine and Epilepsy*, Eds. F. Andermann and E. Lugaresi, pp. 203–232. Boston: Butterworths.

Dyken, P., and Krawiecki, N. 1983. Neurodegenerative diseases of infancy and childhood. Ann. Neurol. 13:351–364.

Eldridge, R., Iivananainen, M., Stern, R., et al. 1983. "Baltic myoclonus epilepsy": hereditary disorder of childhood made worse by phenytoin. Lancet 2:838–842.

Ellingson, R.J. 1972. EEG in disorders associated with chromosome anomalies. In *Handbook of Electroencephalography and Clinical Neurophysiology*, vol. 15, Ed.-in-chief, A. Remond, pp. 19–23. Amsterdam: Elsevier.

Ellingson, R.J., Menolascino, F.J., and Eisen, J.D. 1970. Clinical-EEG relationship in mongoloids confirmed by karyotype. Am. J. Ment. Defic. 74:645–650.

Engel, J., Jr., Rapin, I., and Giblin, D.R. 1977. Electrophysiological studies in two patients with cherry red spot-myoclonus syndrome. Epilepsia (New York) 18:73–87.

Engel, R.C., and Buist, N.R.M. 1985. The EEG of infants with citrullinemia. Dev. Med. Child. Neurol. 27:199–206.

Fadiloglu, S. 1971. Sur les formes infantiles familiales précoces de l'atrophie pigmentaire pallidoréticulée. Acta. Neurol. Belg. 71:392–406.

Fariello, R.G., Chun, R.W.M., Doro, J.M., et al. 1977. EEG recognition of Aicardi's syndrome. Arch. Neurol. (Chicago) 34:563–566.

Ferrari, E., Puca, F.M., Specchio, L.M., et al. 1981. Sleep spindles in Wilson's disease. Electroencephalogr. Clin. Neurophysiol. 51:59(abst).

Ferriss, G.S., Happel, L.T., and Duncan, M.C. 1977. Cerebral cortical isolation in infantile neuroaxonal dystrophy. Electroencephalogr. Clin. Neurophysiol. 43:168–182.

Fisch, R.O., Sines, L.K., Torres, F., et al. 1965. Studies on families of phenylketonurics: observations in intelligence and electroencephalographic changes. Am. J. Dis. Child. 109:427–431.

Fois, A., Rosenberg, C., and Gibbs, F.A. 1955. The electroencephalogram in phenylpyruvic oligophrenia. Electroencephalogr. Clin. Neurophysiol. 7:569–572.

Foncke, E.M.J., Klein, C., Koelman, T.M., et al. 2003. Hereditary myoclonus-dystonia associated with epilepsy. Neurology 60:1988–1990.

Ford, F.R. 1966. *Diseases of the Nervous System in Infancy, Childhood and Adolescence*, 5th ed. Springfield, IL: Charles C Thomas.

Francois, J. 1972. A general introduction to phacomatoses. In *Handbook of Clinical Neurology*, vol. 14, Eds. P.J. Vinken and G.W. Bruyn. Amsterdam: North Holland.

Friede, R.L. 1964. Alexander's disease. Arch. Neurol. (Chicago) 11:414–422.

Friedman, E., Harden, A., and Koivikko, M. 1978. Menkes' disease: Neurophysiological aspects. J. Neurol. Neurosurg. Psychiatry 41:505–510.

Friedreich, N. 1881. Neuropathologische Beobachtungen: Paramyoclonus multiplex. Virchow's Arch. Pathol. Anat. 86:421–430.

Fukuhara, N., Tokiguchi, S., Shirakawa, S., et al. 1980. Myoclonus epilepsy associated with ragged red fibers (mitochondrial abnormalities): disease entity or syndrome? Light and electron microscopic studies of two cases and review of the literature. J. Neurol. Sci. 47:117–133.

Fukuyama, T., Haruna, H., and Kawazura, M. 1960. A peculiar form of congenital progressive muscular dystrophy. Pediatr. Univ. Tokyo 4:5–8.

Gabr, M., Hashem, N., Hashem, M., et al. 1960. Progeria, a pathologic study. J. Pediatr. 57:70–77.

Gajdosova, D., Sramka, M., and Nadvornik, P. 1972. Pozorovanie u choroby Gilles de la Tourette (Some observations in Gilles de la Tourette's disease; Czechoslov.) Cesk. Neurol. Neurochir. 35:294–297.

Gambi, D., Ferro, F.M., and Mazza, S. 1970. Analysis of sleep in the progressive myoclonus epilepsy. Eur. Neurol. (Basel) 3:347–364.

Ganji, S., and Duncan, M.C. 1989. Angelman's (happy puppet) syndrome: clinical, CT scan and serial electroencephalographic study. Clin. Electroencephalogr. 20:128–140.

Ganji, S., and Hellman, C.D. 1985. Tuberous sclerosis: long-term follow-up and longitudinal electroencephalographic study. Clin. Electroencephalogr. 16:219–224.

Gastaut, H. 1968. Séméiologie des myoclonies et nosologie analytiue des syndromes myocloniques. Rev. Neurol. (Paris) 119:1–30.

Gastaut, H., and Tassinari, C.A. 1966. Triggering mechanisms in epilepsy. The electroclinical point of view. Epilepsia (Amsterdam) 7:85–128.

Gayral, J., and Gayral, L. 1969. Epilepsie et heredodegenerations spinocerebelleuses. J. Genet. Hum. 17:127–136.

Gerritsen, T., Vaughn, J.G., and Waisman, H.A. 1962. The identification of homocystinuria in the urine. Biochem. Biophys. Res. Commun. 9:493–496.

Gibbs, F.A., and Gibbs, E.L. 1964. *Atlas of Electroencephalography*, 2nd ed., vol. 3. Reading, MA: Addison-Wesley.

Gironell, A., Rodriguez-Fornells, A., Kulisevsky, J., et al. 2000. Abnormalities of the acoustic startle reflex and reaction time in Gilles de la Tourette syndrome. Clin. Neurophysiol. 111:1366–1371.

Glaze, D.G., Schultz, R.J., and Frost, J.D. 1998. Rett syndrome: characterization of seizures versus non-seizures. Electroencephalogr. Clin. Neurophysiol. 106:79–83.

Govaerts, L., Colon, E., and Monnens, L. 1984. Neurophysiological study of the cerebro-hepato-renal syndrome of Zellweger. Electroencephalogr. Clin. Neurophysiol. 58:108P(abst).

Green, J.B. 1971. Neurophysiological studies in Batten's disease. Dev. Med. Child Neurol. 13:477–498.

Grinker, R.R., Serota, H., and Stein, I. 1938. Myoclonic epilepsy. Arch. Neurol. Psychiatr. (Chicago) 40:968–980.

Gross, P.T., Berlow, S., Schuett, V.E., et al. 1981. EEG in phenylketonuria: attempt to establish clinical importance of EEG changes. Arch. Neurol. (Chicago) 38:122–126.

Guerrini, R., DeLorey, T.M., Bonanni, P., et al. 1996. Cortical myoclonus in Angelman syndrome. Ann. Neurol. 40:39–48.

Hagberg, B., and Witt-Engerström, T. 1986. Rett syndrome: a suggested staging system for describing impairment profile with increasing age toward adolescence. Am. J. Med. Genet. 24:47–59.

Hagberg, B., Aicardi, J., Dias, K., et al. 1983. A progressive syndrome of autism, dementia, ataxia, and loss of purposeful hand use in girls: Rett's syndrome. Ann. Neurol. 14:471–479.

Hallervorden, J., and Spatz, H. 1922. Eigenartige Erkrankung im extrapyramidalen System mit besonderer Beteiligung des Globus pallidus und der Substantia nigra. Ein Beitrag zu den Beziehungen zwischen diesen beiden Zentren. Z. Ges. Neurol. Psychiatr. 79:254–297.

Hamano, T., Katayama, M., Kubori, T., et al. 1999. Abnormal contingent negative variation in writer's cramp. Clin Neurophysiol. 110:508–515.

Hambert, G., and Frey, T.S. 1964. The electroencephalogram in the Klinefelter syndrome. Acta Psychiatr. Scand. 40:28–36.

Hambert, O., and Petersén, I. 1970. Clinical, electroencephalographical and neuropharmacological studies in syndromes of progressive myoclonus epilepsy. Acta. Neurol. Scand. 46:149–186.

Hamosh, A., McDonald, J.W., Valle, D., et al. 1992. Dextromethorphan and high-dose benzoate therapy for non-ketotic hyperglycinemia in an infant. J. Pediatr. 121:131–135.

Hansotia, P., Harris, R., and Kennedy, J. 1969. EEG changes in Wilson's disease. Electroencephalogr. Clin. Neurophysiol. 27:523–528.

Harden, A., Martinovic, Z., and Pampiglione, G. 1982. EEG/ERG/VEP studies in GM1 gangliosidosis. Electroencephalogr. Clin. Neurophysiol. 53:2P(abst).

Hartung, E. 1920. Zwei Fälle von Paramyoclonus multiplex mit Epilepsie. Zentralbl. Ges. Neurol. Psychiatr. 565:150–153.

Harvald, B., and Hauge, M. 1955. The electroencephalogram in patients with tuberous sclerosis. Electroencephalogr. Clin. Neurophysiol. 7:573–576.

Hattori, H., Hayashi, K., Okuno, T., et al. 1985. De nova reciprocal translocation t(6;14) (q27;q13.3) in a child with infantile spasms. Epilepsia (New York) 26:310–313.

Heller, G.L., and Kooi, K.A. 1962. The electroencephalogram in hepatolenticular degeneration (Wilson's disease). Electroencephalogr. Clin. Neurophysiol. 14:520–526.

Herrlin, K.M. 1962. A clinical and electroencephalographic study of a pair of monozygotic twins with phenylketonuria. Acta Paediatr. (Uppsala) 51:137–154.

Hodson, A.K., Lewis, D.V., and Coleman, R.A. 1983. Absence seizures in Farber's lipogranulomatosis. Electroencephalogr. Clin. Neurophysiol. 56:5P(abst).

Hornbostel, H. 1954. Neuere Erkenntnisse über das hepatolentikuläre Syndrom. Schweiz. Med. Wschr. 84:7–11.

Howell, R.R., and Williams, J. 1983. Glycogen storage diseases. In *The Metabolic Basis of Inherited Diseases*, Eds. J.B. Stanbury, J.B. Wyngaarden, D.S. Fredrickson, et al., pp. 141–166. New York: McGraw-Hill.

Illig, R., Dumermuth, G., and Prader, A. 1963. Das oculo-cerebrorenale Syndrom. Klinische, metabolische und elektroencephalographische Befunde bei 3 Fällen. Helv. Paediatr. Acta 18:173–202.

Jacome, D.E., and Risko, M. 1984. Photic-induced-driven PLEDs in paroxysmal dystonic choreoathetosis. Clin. Electroencephalogr. 15:151–154.

Jankel, W.R., Allen, R.P., Niedermeyer, E., et al. 1983. Polysomnographic findings in dystonia musculorum progressiva. Sleep 6:281–285.

Jansen, F.E., van Huffelen, A.C., Witkamp, Th.D., et al. 2002. Diazepam-enhanced activity in Sturge-Weber syndrome: its diagnostic significance in comparison with MRI. Clin. Neurophysiol. 113:1025–1029.

Jay, V., Becler, L.E., Chan, F.-W., et al. 1991. Puppet-like syndrome of Angelman: a pathologic and neurochemical study. Neurology 41:416–422.

Kamoshita, S., Rapin, I., Suzuki, K., et al. 1968. Spongy degeneration of the brain. Neurology 18:975–985.

Kandt, R.S., Emerson, R.G., Singer, H.S., et al. 1982. Cataplexy in variant forms of Niemann-Pick disease. Ann. Neurol. 12:284–288.

Karhu, J., Hari, R., Paetau, R., et al. 1994. Cortical reactivity in progressive myoclonus epilepsy. Electroencephalogr. Clin. Neurophysiol. 90:93–102.

Kelley, W.N., and Wyngaarden, J.B. 1983. Clinical syndromes associated with hypoxanthine guanine phosphoribosyl-transferase deficiency. In *The Metabolic Basis of Inherited Disease*, 5th ed., Eds. J.B. Stanbury, J.B. Wyngaarden, D.S. Fredrickson, et al., pp. 1115–1143. New York: McGraw-Hill.

Kerr, A., Southall, D., Amos, P., et al. 1990. Correlation of electroencephalogram, respiration and movement in the Rett syndrome. Brain Dev. 12:61–68.

Klenk, E. 1941. Über die Ganglioside des Gehirns bei der infantilen amaurotischen Idiotie vom Typus Tay-Sachs. Ber. Deutsch. Chem. Ges. 75:1632–1640.

Kolodny, E.H., and Cable, W.J.L. 1983. Inborn errors of metabolism. Ann. Neurol. 11:221–232.

Konovalov, N.V., Zhimunskaja, E.A., and Chukrova, V.A. 1957. Electricheskaia aktivonostmozga prihepato-lentikularnoi degenerasti. Zh. Neuropat. Psikhiat. 57:584–590.

Koskiniemi, M., Donner, M., Majuri, H., et al. 1974a. Progressive myoclonus epilepsy. A clinical and histopathological study. Acta Neurol. Scand. 50:307–332.

Koskiniemi, M., Toivakka, E., and Donner, M. 1974b. Progressive myoclonus epilepsy. Electroencephalographic findings. Acta Neurol. Scand. 50:333–359.

Krauthammer, W. 1965. EEG observations in children with tuberous sclerosis. Electroencephalogr. Clin. Neurophysiol. 21:201(abst).

Kreezer, G. 1939. Intelligence level and occipital alpha rhythm in the Mongolian type of mental deficiency. Am. J. Psychol. 52:503–532.

Krumholz, A., Singer, H.S., Niedermeyer, E., et al. 1983. Electrophysiological studies in Tourette's syndrome. Ann. Neurol. 14:638–641.

Lafora, G.R., and Glueck, B. 1911. Beitrag zur Histopathologie der myoklonischen Epilepsie. Z. Gesamte Neurol. Psychiatry 6:1–14.

Lagos, J.C., and Gomez, M.R. 1967. Tuberous sclerosis: re-appraisal of a clinical entity. Proc. Mayo Clin. 42:26–49.

Laura, A.E.M., Renier, W.O., Arts, W.F., et al. 1997. Evolution of epilepsy and EEG findings in Angelman syndrome. Epilepsia 38:195–199.

Liu, X.Q., Xu, J.Q., and Feng, Y.K. 1983. Wilson's disease. An electroencephalographic study. Chin. Med. J. 96:835–840.

Liversedge, L., and Emery, V. 1961. Electroencephalographic changes in cerebellar degenerative lesions. J. Neurol. Neurosurg. Psychiatry 24:326–330.

Loonen, M.C.B., Van Diggelen, O.P., Janse, H.C., et al. 1985. Late onset globoid cell leukodystrophy (Krabbe's disease): clinical and genetic delineation of two forms and their relation to the early infantile form. Neuropediatrics 16:137–142.

Low, N.L., Bosma, J.F., and Armstrong, M.D. 1957. Studies on phenylketonuria. VI. EEG studies in phenylketonuria. Arch. Neurol. Psychiatry (Chicago) 77:359–365.

Lucas, A.R., and Rodin, E.A. 1973. Electroencephalogram in Gilles de la Tourette's disease. Dis. Nerv. Syst. 37:85–89.

Lugaresi, E., Cirignotta, F., and Montagna, P. 1985. Abnormal breathing in the Rett syndrome. Brain Dev. 7:329–333.

Lundborg, H. 1903. *Die progressive Myoklonus-Epilepsie (Unverricht's Myoklonie)*. Uppsala: Almqvist.

Lundborg, H. 1911. *Medizinisch-biologische Familienforschung*. Jena: Fischer.

Lundervold, A., Refsum, S., and Jacobsen, W. 1969. The EEG in dystrophia myotonica. Eur. Neurol. (Basel) 2:279–284.

MacFaul, R., Cavanaugh, N., Lake, B.D., et al. 1982. Metachromatic leukodystrophy: review of 38 cases. Arch. Dis. Child. 57:168–175.

Mahloudji, M., and Pikielny, R.T. 1967. Hereditary essential myoclonus. Brain 90:669–674.

Maldonado, R.R., Tamayo, L., and Carnevale, A. 1975. Neuro-ichthyosis with hypogonadism (Rud's syndrome). Int. J. Dermatol. 5:347–352.

Mamoli, B., Graf, M., and Toifl, K. 1979. EEG pattern evoked potentials and nerve conduction velocity in a family with adrenoleucodystrophy. Electroencephalogr. Clin. Neurophysiol. 47:411–419.

Markand, O., Garg, B.P., and Brandt, I.K. 1982. Non-ketotic hyperglycinemia: electroencephalographic and evoked potential abnormalities. Neurology 32:151–156.

Marra, T.R., Reynolds, N.C., Jr., and Dahl, D.S. 1980. Tourette syndrome, an acquired encephalopathy? A report of two cases with epileptiform dysrhythmia. Clin. Electroencephalogr. 11:118–123.

Marxmiller, J., Trenkle, I., and Ashwal, S. 1985. Rud syndrome revisited: ichthyosis, mental retardation, epilepsy and hypogonadism. Dev. Med. Child Neurol. 27:335–343.

Matalon, R., Naidu, S., Hughes, J.R., et al. 1983. Nonketotic hyperglycinemia: treatment with diazepam—a competitor for glycine receptors. Pediatrics 71:581–584.

McKusick, V.A. 1983. *Mendelian Inheritance in Man*, 6th ed. Baltimore: Johns Hopkins.

Menkes, J.H. 1985. Metabolic diseases of the nervous system. In *Textbook of Child Neurology*, Ed. J.H. Menkes, pp. 1–122. Philadelphia: Lea & Febiger.

Menkes, J.H., Alter, M., Steigleder, G.K., et al. 1962. A sex-linked recessive disorder with retardation of growth, peculiar hair and focal cerebral and cerebellar degeneration. Pediatrics 29:764–779.

Messenheimer, J.A., Greenwood, R.S., Aylsworth, A.S., et al. 1984. Electrophysiological changes in sialidosis type 2. Electroencephalogr. Clin. Neurophysiol. 58:32P(abst).

Metcalf, D.R. 1972. EEG in inborn errors of metabolism. In *Handbook of Electroencephalography and Clinical Neurophysiology*, vol. 158, Ed.-in-chief, A. Remond, pp. 14–18. Amsterdam: Elsevier.

Meyer, A. 1966. The Hallervorden-Spatz syndrome. In *Greenfield's Neuropathology*, Eds. W. Blackwood, W.H. McMenemey, A. Meger, et al., pp. 412–414. Baltimore: Williams & Wilkins.

Mises, J., Moussalli-Salefranque, F., Hagenmuller, M.P., et al. 1983. Fast EEG rhythms in metabolic diseases of children. Electroencephalogr. Clin. Neurophysiol. 56:68P(abst).

Moser, H.W. 1986. Periorxisomal disorders [editorial]. J. Pediatr. 108:89–91.

Moser, H.W. 1992. Genetic and metabolic diseases: Mechanisms and potential for therapy. In *Diseases of the Nervous System, Clinical Neurobiology*, Eds. A.K. Asbury, G.M. McKhann, and W.I. McDonald, 2nd ed., vol. 1, pp. 670–680. Philadelphia: W.B. Saunders.

Mount, L.A., and Reback, S. 1940. Familial paroxysmal choreoathetosis. Arch. Neurol. Psychiatr. (Chicago) 44:841–847.

Murri, L., Massetani, R., Rossi, B., et al. 1990. Electrophysiological abnormalities in myotonic dystrophy. Electroencephalogr. Clin. Neurophysiol. 75:S101(abst).

Mutoh, K., Okuno, T., Ito, M., et al. 1990. Somatosensory evoked potentials in Hallervorden-Spatz-neuroaxonal-dystrophy complex with dorsal column involvement. Clin. Electroencephalogr. 21:58–66.

Newmark, M.E., and Penry, J.K. 1980. *Genetics of Epilepsy: A Review*. New York: Raven Press.

Niedermeyer, E. 1970. Intravenous diazepam and its anticonvulsive action. Johns Hopkins Med. J. 127:79–96.

Niedermeyer, E., and Naidu, S. 1990. Further EEG observations in children with Rett syndrome. Brain Dev. 12:53–54.

Niedermeyer, E., McKusick, V.A., Brunt, P., et al. 1967. The EEG in familial dysautonomia (Riley-Day syndrome). Electroencephalogr. Clin. Neurophysiol. 23:67–73.

Niedermeyer, E., Rett, A., Renner, H., et al. 1986. Rett syndrome and the electroencephalogram. Am. J. Med. Genet. 24:195–199.

Niedermeyer, E., Naidu, S., and Nogueira de Melo, A. 1991. The usefulness of electroencephalography in Rett syndrome. Am. J. EEG Technol. 31:27–37.

Niedermeyer, E., Naidu, S., and Plate, C. 1997. Unusual EEG theta rhythms over central region in Rett syndrome and considerations of underlying dysfunction. Clin. Electroencephalogr. 28:36–43.

Nielsen, J., and Pedersen, E. 1969. Electro-encephalographic findings in patients with Klinefelter's syndrome. Acta Neurol. Scand. 45:87–94.

Nishimura, R., Omos-Lau, N., Ajmone-Marsan, C., et al. 1980. Electroencephalographic findings in Gaucher's disease. Neurology 30:152–159.

Nyhan, W.L. 1978. Nonketotic hyperglycinemia. In *The Metabolic Basins of Inherited Diseases*, Eds. J.B. Stanbury, J.B. Wyngaarden, D.S. Fredrickson, et al., pp. 518–527. New York: McGraw-Hill.

Nyhan, W.L., and Sakati, N.O. 1987. *Diagnostic Recognition of Genetic Disease*. Philadelphia: Lea & Febiger.

Obeso, J.A., Rothwell, J.C., and Marsden, C.D. 1981. Simple tics in Gilles de la Tourette syndrome are not prefaced by a normal premovement EEG potential. J. Neurol. Neurosurg. Psychiatry 44:735–738.

Obeso, J.A., Rothwell, J.C., Lang, A.E., et al. 1983. Myoclonic dystonia. Neurology 33:825–830.

Ohtsuka, Y., Amano, R., Oka, E., et al. 1993. Myoclonus epilepsy with ragged-red fibers: a clinical and electrophysiological study on two sibling cases. J. Child Neurol. 8:366–372.

Okuma, T., Sarai, K., Ishino, H., et al. 1970. Myotonia dystrophica. Report of six cases in three families with special reference to the mental disorder and EEG. Brain Nerve (Tokyo) 22:77–85.

Olmos Garcia de Alba, G., Domingo Gamboa Marrufo, J., Rangifo Ramos, O., et al. 1987. Rett syndrome with Lennox-Gastaut pattern. Clin. Electroencephalogr. 18:187–190.

Pampiglione, G. 1968. Some inborn metabolic disorders affecting cerebral electrogenesis. In *Some Recent Advances in Inborn Errors of Metabolism*, Eds. K.S. Holt and V.P. Coffey, pp. 80–100. London: Livingstone.

Pampiglione, G., and Harden, A. 1973. Neurophysiological identification of a late infantile form of neuronal lipidosis. J. Neurol. Neurosurg. Psychiatry 36:68–74.

Pampiglione, G., and Harden, A. 1977. So-called neuronal ceroid lipofuscinosis. Neurophysiological studies in 60 children. J. Neurol. Neurosurg. Psychiatry 40:323–330.

Pampiglione, G., and Lehovsky, M. 1968. The evolution of EEG features in Tay-Sachs' disease and amaurotic family idiocy in 24 children. In *Clinical Electroencephalography in Children*, Eds. P. Kellaway and I. Petersen, pp. 287–306. New York: Grune & Stratton (Stockholm: Almqvist and Wiksell).

Pampiglione, G., and Martinez, A. 1983. Evolution of the Angelman syndrome. Follow-up of 3 new cases. Electroencephalogr. Clin. Neurophysiol. 56:72P(abst).

Panjan, D.P., Pečarič, N., and Neubauer, D. 2001. A case of Zellweger syndrome with extensive MRI abnormalities and unusual EEG findings. Clin. Electroencephalogr. 32:28–31.

Paolozzi, C., Rinaldi, F., and Buscaino, G.F. 1965. Changes with time of EEG abnormalities in muscular dystrophy. *Proceedings of the 6th International Congress of Electroencephalography and Clinical Neurophysiology*, pp. 285–287. Vienna: International League Against Epilepsy.

Parisi, V., Pierelli, F., Malandrini, A., et al. 2000. Visual electrophysiological responses in subjects with cerebral autosomal arteriopathy with subcortical infarcts and leukoencephalopathy (CADASIL). Clin. Neurophysiol. 111:1582–1588.

Pedley, T.A., Emerson, R.G., Warner, C.L., et al. 1985. Treatment of cerebrotendinous xanthomatosis with chenodeoxycholic acid. Ann. Neurol. 18:517–518.

Pennacchio, L.A., Lehesjoki, A.-E., Stone, N., et al. 1996. Mutations in the gene encoding cystatin B in progressive myoclonus epilepsy (EPM 1). Science 271:1731–1734.

Perez-Borja, C., Tassinari, A.C., and Swanson, A.G. 1967. Paroxysmal choreoathetosis and seizures induced by movement (reflex epilepsy). Epilepsia (Amsterdam) 8:260–270.

Pietz, J., Benninger, C., Schmidt, H., et al. 1987. EEG development in early treated phenylketonuria. Electroencephalogr. Clin. Neurophysiol. 66:73P(abst).

Pincus, J.H. 1972. Subacute necrotizing encephalomyopathy (Leigh's disease). Dev. Med. Child Neurol. 14:87–101.

Pinsard, N., Livet, M.O., and Saint-Jean, M. 1979. A case of cerebral lipidosis with an atypical presentation. Electroencephalogr. Clin. Neurophysiol. 46:38P(abst).

Pohowalla, P., and McIntyre, H.B. 1984. Neonatal tuberous sclerosis. Electroencephalogr. Clin. Neurophysiol. 58:37P.

Pryles, C., Livingston, S., and Ford, F. 1952. Familial paroxysmal choreoathetosis of Mount and Reback. Pediatrics 9:44–47.

Rabache, R., François, P., Asseman, R., et al. 1960. L'électroencéphalographie dans 16 cas de maladie de Leber. Rev. Neurol. (Paris) 102:360–361.

Radermecker, F.J. 1977. Degenerative disease of the nervous system. In *Handbook of Electroencephalography and Clinical Neurophysiology*, vol. 15A, Ed.-in-chief, A. Remond, pp. 162–191. Amsterdam: Elsevier.

Radermecker, F.J., and Dumon-Radermecker, M.A. 1972. À propos de EEG dans la dystrophie neuroaxonale et la maladie de Hallervorden-Spatz infantile. Rev. Electroencephalogr. Clin. Neurophysiol. 2:406–413.

Rapin, I. 1976. Progressive genetic-metabolic diseases of the central nervous system in children. Pediatric Annals II. Pediatr. Neurol. 56:313–316, 349.

Rapin, I., Katzman, R., and Engel, J., Jr. 1975. Cherry red spots and progressive myoclonus without dementia: a distinct syndrome with neuronal storage. Trans. Am. Neurol. Assoc. 100:39–42.

Reese, K., Toro, C., Malow, B., et al. 1993. Progression of the EEG in Lafora-Body disease. Am. J. EEG Technol. 33:229–235.

Refsum, S. 1946. Heredopathia atactica polyneuritiformis: a familial syndrome not hitherto described. Acta Psychiatr. Neurol. Scand. Suppl. 38:1–303.

Rett, A. 1966. *Über ein cerebral-atrophisches Syndrom bei Hyperammonaemie.* Vienna: Brüder Hollinek.

Revol, M., Lapras, C., Gilly, R., et al. 1988. Epilepsy and Sturge-Weber disease. Discussion of early hemispherectomy. Electroencephalogr. Clin. Neurophysiol. 70:10P(abst).

Rey-Pias, J.M., and Morales Blanquez, C. 1972. Lennox-Gastaut Syndrom bei amaurotischer Idiotie (Typ Jansky-Bielschowsky). EEG und Therapie in 2 Fällen. Z. EEG-EMG 3:161–166.

Richards, R.N., and Barnett, H.J.M. 1968. Paroxysmal dystonic choreoathetosis. A family study and review of the literature. Neurology (Minneapolis) 18:461–469.

Riehl, J.L., Lee, D.K., Andrews, J.M., et al. 1967. Electrophysiological and neuropharmacological studies in a patient with Unverricht-Lafora's disease. Neurology (Minneapolis) 17:502–511.

Roach, E.S., Riela, A.R., McLean, W.T., Jr., et al. 1985. Aspirin therapy for Sturge-Weber syndrome. Ann. Neurol. 18:387(abst).

Robertson, R., Langill, L., Wong, P.K.H., et al. 1988. Rett syndrome: EEG presentation. Electroencephalogr. Clin. Neurophysiol. 70:388–395.

Rodière, M., Georgescu, M., Alric, J., et al. 1979. The EEG and EMG findings in sudanophilic leucodystrophy. Electroencephalogr. Clin. Neurophysiol. 46:38P(abst).

Rodin, E., and Chayasirisobhon, S. 1980. Familial paroxysmal choreoathetosis. Electroencephalogr. Clin. Neurophysiol. 50:225P(abst).

Roger, J., Gastaut, H., Toga, M., et al. 1965. Epilepsie myoclonie progressive avec corps de Lafora (étude clinique, polygraphique et anatomique d'un cas). Rev. Neurol. (Paris) 112:50–61.

Roger, J., Soulayrol, R., Hassoun, J., et al. 1968. La dyssynergie cérébelleuse myoclonique (Maladie de Ramsay Hunt). Rev. Neurol. (Paris) 119:85–106.

Roger, J., Genton, P., Bureau, M., et al. 1992. Progressive myoclonus epilepsies in childhood and adolescence. In *Epileptic Syndromes in Infancy, Childhood and Adolescence*, 2nd ed., Eds. J. Roger, M. Bureau, F.E. Dreifuss, et al., pp. 381–400. London: Libbey.

Rolando, S. 1985. Rett syndrome: report of eight cases. Brain Dev. 7:290–296.

Ruggieri, M., Tigano, G., Mazzone, D., et al. 1996. Involvement of the white matter in hypomelanosis of Ito (incontinentia pigmenti achromiens). Neurology 46:485–492.

Sack, G., Lössner, J., and Bachmann, H. 1981. Long-term EEG investigations in 74 patients with Wilson's disease. Electroencephalogr. Clin. Neurophysiol. 52:18P(abst).

Sainio, K., Santavuori, P., and Renlund, M. 1982. EEG in Salla disease and in a variant of Jansky-Bielschowsky disease. Electroencephalogr. Clin. Neurophysiol. 54:48P(abst).

Salomon, F., Fagioli, I., Rey, F., et al. 1981. EEG sleep activity in a phenylketonuronic child of the "new variant" type before and after treatment with 5-HTP and 1-DOPA. Rev. Electroencephalogr. Clin. Neurophysiol. 7:212–217.

Scharfetter, C., and Schmoigl, S. 1968. Über das Syndrom der progressiven Myoklonus-Epilepsie nach Unverricht-Lundborg (Eine Verlaufsbeobachtung durch ein-einhalb Jahrzehnte). Schweiz. Arch. Neurol. Psychiatry 102:145–154.

Schaumburg, H.H., Powers, J.M., Suzuki, K., et al. 1974. Adrenoleucodystrophy (sex-linked Schilder disease). Inclusions in the cerebral nervous system. Arch. Neurol. (Chicago) 31:210–213.

Schaumburg, H.H., Powers, J.M., Raine, C.S., et al. 1975. Adrenoleucodystrophy. A clinical and pathological study of 17 cases. Arch. Neurol. (Chicago) 32:577–591.

Schimke, R.N., McKusick, V.A., Huang, T., et al. 1965. Homocystinuria. A study of 20 families with 38 affected members. JAMA 193:711–719.

Schmid, R.G., Tirsch, W.S., Rappelsberger, P., et al. 1992. Comparative coherence studies in healthy volunteers and Down's syndrome patients from childhood to adult age. Electroencephalogr. Clin. Neurol. 83:112–123.

Schneck, L. 1964. Clinical manifestations of Tay-Sachs disease. In *Tay-Sachs Disease*, Ed. B.W. Volk, pp. 16–30. New York: Grune & Stratton.

Schubert, M., Zierz, S., and Dengler, R. 1994. Central and peripheral nervous system conduction in mitochondrial myopathy with chronic progressive external ophthalmoplegia. Electroencephalogr. Clin. Neurophysiol. 90:304–312.

Schubert, T., Jerusalem, F., Martenet, A.-C., et al. 1980. Myotonic dystrophy. Early detection and genetic counseling. J. Neurol. (Berlin) 223:13–22.

Seitelberger, F. 1952. Eine unbekannte Form von Lipoidspeicherkrankheit des Gehirns. *Proc. First Internat. Congr. Neuropathol.* Rome, pp. 323–333. Turin: Rosenberg and Sellier.

Seitelberger, F. 1971. Neuropathological conditions related to neuroaxonal dystrophy. Acta Neuropathol. (Berlin) 5(suppl):17–29.

Sgró, V., Riva, E., Canevini, M.P., et al. 1995. 4p-syndrome: a chromosomal disorder associated with a particular EEG pattern. Epilepsia 36:1206–1214.

Shy, G.M., and Drager, G.A. 1960. A neurological syndrome associated with orthostatic hypotension. Arch. Neurol. (Chicago) 2:511–527.

Siegel, H., Frei, K., Greenfield, J., et al. 1998. Electroencephalographic findings in patients with mucolipidosis type IV. Electroencephalogr. Clin. Neurophysiol. 106:400–403.

Silva, M.L., Cieuta, C., Guerrini, R., et al. 1966. Early clinical and EEG features of infantile spasms in Down syndrome. Epilepsia 37:977–982.

Sirakov, A. 1965. EEG findings in progressive muscular dystrophy. *Proceedings of the 6th International Congress of Electroencephalography and Clinical Neurophysiology*, pp. 289–291. Vienna: Wien, Med. Akad.

Smith, N.J., Espir, M.L.E., and Matthews, W.B. 1978. Familial myoclonic epilepsy with ataxia and neuropathy with additional features of Friedreich's ataxia and peroneal muscle atrophy. Brain 101:461–472.

So, N., Kuzniecky, R., Berkovic, S., et al. 1988. Electrophysiological studies in myoclonus epilepsy with ragged-red fibers (MERRF). Electroencephalogr. Clin. Neurophysiol. 69:50P(abst).

Stadler, H. 1961. Über das EEG bei der Phenylketonurie. Ann. Paediatr. 197:429–451.

Steinman, L., Tharp, B.R., Dorfman, J., et al. 1980. Peripheral neuropathy in cherry red spot myoclonus syndrome (sialidosis type I). Ann. Neurol. 7:450.

Stevens, H. 1966. Paroxysmal choreoathetosis—a form of reflex epilepsy. Arch. Neurol. (Chicago) 14:415–420.

Strauss, H., Ostow, M., and Greenstein, L.D. 1952. *Diagnostic Electroencephalography.* New York: Grune & Stratton.

Suzuki, K., and Suzuki, Y. 1970. Globoid cell leukodystrophy (Krabbe's disease): deficiency of galactocerebroside beta-galactosidase. Proc. Natl. Acad. Sci. U.S.A. 66:302–309.

Suzuki, K., and Suzuki, Y. 1983. Galactosylceramide lipidoses: globoid cell leukodystrophy (Krabbe's disease). In *The Metabolic Basis of Inherited Diseases*, 5th ed., Eds. J.B. Stanbury, J.B. Wyngaarden, D.S. Fredrickson, et al., pp. 857–880. New York: McGraw-Hill.

Swaiman, K., Smith, S.A., Trock, G.L., et al. 1983. Sea blue histiocytes, lymphocytic cytosomes, movement disorder. 59Fe uptake in basal ganglia: Hallervorden-Spatz disease or ceroid storage disease with abnormal isotope scan? Neurology 33:301–305.

Sweet, R.D., Soloman, G.E., Wayne, H., et al. 1973. Neurological feature of Gilles de la Tourette's syndrome. J. Neurol. Neurosurg. Psychiatr. 36:1–9.

Tassinari, C.A., Roger, J., Regis, H., et al. 1971. Die myoklonische zerebelläre Dyssynergie nach Ramsay Hunt und Aktionsmyoklonie beim Lance-Adams-Syndrom. Z. EEG-EMG 2:86–91.

Tassinari, C.A., Bureau-Pallas, M., Dalla Bernardina, B., et al. 1979. Lafora disease. Electroencephalogr. Clin. Neurophysiol. 46:37P(abst).

Thiébaut, F., and Gruner, J.E. 1961. Hérédo-dégénérescence spinocérébelleuse. *Encyclopédie Medico-Chirurgicale, Neurologie,* vol. 2, 17082, pp. 1–9. Paris: Masson.

Thomas, P.K., Abrams, J.D., Swallow, D., et al. 1979. Sialidosis type I: cherry red spot myoclonus syndrome with sialidase deficiency and altered electrophoretic mobilities of some enzymes known to be glycoproteins. J. Neurol. Neurosurg. Psychiatry 42:873.

Tinuper, P., Aguglia, U., Pellissier, J.F., et al. 1983. Ictal visual phenomena in a case of Lafora disease proven by skin biopsy. Epilepsia (New York) 24:214–218.

Tobimatsu, S., Fukui, R., Shibasaki, H., et al. 1983. Electrophysiological studies in cherry red spot myoclonus syndrome. Electroencephalogr. Clin. Neurophysiol. 56:54P–55P(abst).

Tournier-Lasserve, E., Joutel, A., Melki, J., et al. 1993. Cerebral autosomal dominant arteriopathy with subcortical infarcts and leukoencephalopathy maps to chromosome 19 p20 Nat. Genet. 3:256–259.

Tükel, K., and Caliskan, A. 1964. A l'étude électroencéphalographique d'une famille dont deux membres sont atteints d'épilepsie myoclonique d'Unverricht-Lundborg. Rev. Neurol. (Paris) 110:231–246.

Unverricht, H. 1891. *Die Myoclonie.* Leipzig: Deuticke.

Valente, K.D., Andrade, J.Q., Grossmann, R.M., et al. 2003. Angelman syndrome: difficulties in EEG pattern recognition and possible misinterpretations. Epilepsia 44:1051–1063.

Van Bogaert, L., Scherer, H.F., and Epstein, L. 1937. *Une forme cérébrale de cholesterinose généralisée.* Paris: Masson.

Van Diggelen, O.P., Schindler, D., Willemsen, R., et al. 1988. Alpha-*N*-acetylgalactosaminidase deficiency, a new lysosomal storage disorder. J. Inherited Metab. Dis. 11:349–357.

Verma, N.P., Hart, Z.H., and Kooi, K.A. 1984. Electroencephalographic findings in urea-cycle disorders. Electroencephalogr. Clin. Neurophysiol. 57:105–112.

Vogel, F., Wendt, G., and Oepen, H. 1961. Das EEG und das Problem einer Frühdiagnose der Chorea Huntington. Deutsch. Z. Nervenheilk. 182:355–361.

Volkmar, F.R., Leekman, J.F., Detlor, J., et al. 1984. EEG abnormalities in Tourette's syndrome. J. Am. Acad. Child Psychiatry 23:352–353.

Volpe, J.J., and Adams, R.D. 1972. Cerebro-hepato-renal syndrome of Zellweger: an inherited disorder of neuronal migration. Acta Neuropath. (Berlin) 20:175–198.

Wadia, N.H. 1984. A variety of olivopontocerebellar atrophy distinguished by slow eye movements and peripheral neuropathy. In *Olivopontocerebellar Atrophies*, Eds. R.C. Duvoisin and A. Plataikas, pp. 149–177. New York: Raven Press.

Wakai, S., Asanuma, H., Hayasaka, H., et al. 1994. Ictal video-EEG analysis of infantile neuroaxonal dystrophy. Epilepsia 35:823–826.

Walter, R.D., Yeager, C.L., and Rubin, H.K. 1955. Mongolism and convulsive seizures. Arch. Neurol. Psychiatr. (Chicago) 74:559–563.

Walton, A. 1996. A case study of Alpers' disease in siblings. Am. J. EEG Technol. 36:18–27.

Wasser, S., Theile, H. Bergmann, L., et al. 1981. EEG studies on the termination of therapy in phenylketonuria. Electroencephalogr. Clin. Neurophysiol. 52:14P(abst).

Wein, A., and Golubev, V. 1979. Polygraphic analysis of sleep in dystonia musculorum progressiva. Waking and Sleeping 3:41–50.

Westmoreland, B.F., and Sharbrough, F.W. 1978. The EEG in cerebromacular degeneration. Electroencephalogr. Clin. Neurophysiol. 45:28P–29P(abst).

White, S.R., Reese, K., Sato, S., et al. 1993. Spectrum of EEG findings in Menkes disease. Electroencephalogr. Clin. Neurophysiol. 87:57–61.

Whitehouse, D. 1966. Diagnostic value of the café-au-lait spot in children. Arch. Dis. Child. 41:316–319.

Williams, R.S., Ferrante, R.J., and Caviness, V.S. 1979. The isolated human cortex. A Golgi analysis of Krabbe's disease. Arch. Neurol. (Chicago) 36:134–139.

Wolf, B., Grier, R.E., and Allen, R.J. 1983a. Phenotypic variation in biotinidase deficiency. J. Pediatr. 103:233–237.

Wolf, B., Grier, R.E., Allen, R.J., et al. 1983b. Biotinidase deficiency: the enzyme defect in late onset multiple carboxylase deficiency. Clin. Chim. Acta 131:272–281.

Wolf, B., Heard, G.S., Secor, et al. 1985. Biotinidase deficiency. Ann. N.Y. Acad. Sci. 447:252–262.

Yen, C.E., Beydoun, A., and Drury, I. 1991. Longitudinal EEG studies in a kindred with Lafora disease. Electroencephalogr. Clin. Neurophysiol. 78:14P(abst).

Yokoi, S., Kobori, H., and Yoshihara, H. 1965. Clinical and neuropathological studies of myoclonic epilepsy. Acta Neuropathol. (Berlin) 4:370–379.

York-Moore, M.E., and Rundle, A.T. 1962. Rud's syndrome. J. Ment. Defic. Res. 6:108–118.

Yoshioka, M., Okuno, T., Ito, M., et al. 1981. Congenital muscular atrophy (Fukuyama type): repeated CT studies in 19 children. Comput. Tomogr. 5:81–88.

Zellweger, H., and Niedermeyer, E. 1965. Central nervous system, manifestations of childhood muscular dystrophy. I. Psychometric and electroencephalographic findings. Ann. Paediatr. 205:25–42.

Zeman, W., and Dyken, P. 1969. Neuronal ceroid lipofuscinosis (Batten's disease), relationship to amaurotic idiocy. Pediatrics 44:570–582.

Zhirmunskaya, E.A., and Chukhrova, J.A. 1959. The electric activity of the brain in hepatolenticular degeneration. In *Proceedings of the First International Congress of Neurological Science,* vol. 3, Brussels, 1957, pp. 336–337. London: Pergamon Press.

20. The EEG in Infantile Brain Damage, Cerebral Palsy, and Minor Cerebral Dysfunctions of Childhood

Aurea Nogueira de Melo and Ernst Niedermeyer

This chapter discusses various forms of insult to the fetal, neonatal, or infantile brain. These forms of pathology lead to a wide variety of residual brain damage. The residual character separates them from degenerative central nervous system (CNS) diseases, in which progressive damage is caused by a neurobiochemical-metabolic process.

Dysplasias and malformations of the brain due to poorly defined causes are discussed in this chapter, along with structural damage caused by birth anoxia, trauma at birth or in infancy, severe infection, and vascular catastrophes. A final section on the syndrome of minimal cerebral dysfunction discusses a heterogeneous group of disturbances that has been presumed to represent a very mild form of residual infantile brain damage.

Severe Congenital Malformation of the Brain

Anencephaly

In these newborns, the entire cerebrum is absent; the brainstem is usually intact up to the midbrain level. The survival period is naturally very short. For this reason, electroencephalogram (EEG) studies are very scanty (André-Thomas and Fischgold, 1949; Bernstine and Borkowski, 1960; Cohadon et al., 1966). Some type of EEG activity is recordable from remainders of parenchyma, and the activity may not look strikingly abnormal.

Holoprosencephaly

Holoprosencephaly results from failure of segmentation and cleavage of the embryonic forebrain into paired symmetric cerebral hemispheres. The cerebrum remains holospheric and the primitive prosencephalic ventricle a single cavity.

Severe EEG abnormalities have been noted in this condition; isoelectric activity, voltage depression with loss of detail, slowing, and spike activity occur in accordance with localization of the malformation (Crawley and Proler, 1972). More extensive studies were done by De Myer and White (1964). An excellent review of EEG findings in children with holoprosencephaly (Clegg et al., 2002) stressed the following consistent abnormalities in this condition: hypersynchronous theta during waking state and sleep, hypersynchronous beta (asleep), episodic attenuation of cerebral activity, and a wide range of various epileptic discharges.

Hydranencephaly

Hydranencephaly is a devastating CNS malformation consisting of nearly complete absence of the cerebral hemispheres with intact meninges and skull, the resulting cavity being filled with cerebrospinal fluid (Hamby et al., 1950). It is generally accepted to be the result of a severe encephaloclastic event (probably vascular).

Electroencephalography has been useful in this condition (Hamby et al., 1950; Puech et al., 1947; Sutton et al., 1980).

Iinuma et al. (1989) have pointed out that the EEG is helpful in the differentiation of hydranencephaly from maximal hydrocephalus when computed tomography (CT) scan shows morphological similarities. The EEG tracings tend to be of very low voltage and featureless character; some regional slow or mixed activity may be present (Fig. 20.1). McAbee et al. (2000) reported two infants with prenatally acquired hydranencephaly with prolonged survival. Their EEG was read as isoelectric.

Lissencephaly

This is a rare developmental condition that is most commonly but not necessarily associated with agyria. In incomplete lissencephaly, the brain is pachygyric. Lissencephaly is the major anomaly of several familial syndromes but is also found as an isolated developmental defect (Dobyns et al., 1984, 1985). In most cases, there is microcephaly; the cortex is thick and its lamination altered (with four rather than six laminae). In type I lissencephaly (Dobyns et al., 1984), there are dysmorphic syndromes such as the Miller-Dieker and the Norman-Roberts syndrome; an anomaly of chromosome 17 is found in the former.

Type II was described by A. Earl Walker (1942); it is commonly associated with massive ventricular enlargement and cerebellar and ocular defects. This condition is strongly related to the Dandy-Walker malformation (Dobyns et al., 1985).

The EEG was studied by Dulac et al. (1984) and Gastaut et al. (1987). The authors stressed the occurrence of very high voltage with rapid frequencies (alpha and theta range), mixed with delta waves and infrequent spikes. Similar findings were reported by De Rijk-Van Andel et al. (1988) and Hodgkins (2000).

A rare case of cerebrocerebellar lissencephaly (Elia et al., 1995) was characterized by a "pseudohypsarrhythmic" pattern subsequently replaced by consistent rhythmical spikes and sharp waves, independently firing over frontal areas. In

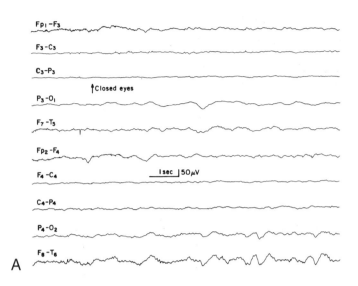

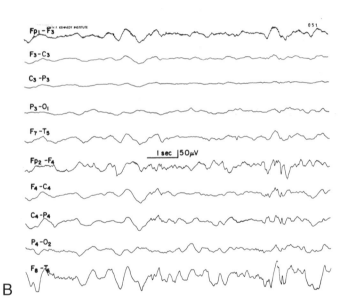

Figure 20.1. Age 10 months. Hydrancephaly (hydranencephaly). **A:** Waking state. An almost flat record at average gain over left hemisphere except for some temporo-occipital slowing. Over right hemisphere, the anterior portion is almost flat, while slowing is noted posteriorly. **B:** Sleep record. Marked voltage depression and loss of detail over left hemisphere. Disorganized slowing and suggestions of sharp transients on the right.

a personal observation (Fig. 20.2), there was also an unusually high-voltage output with pronounced slowing and prominent multifocal spikes and sharp waves; arousing stimuli would lead to desynchronization with rhythmical fast activity and irregular movements (but no startle).

Myelomeningocele

In this well-known malformation, the EEG is normal unless the cases are complicated by hydrocephalus with cerebral impairment (Dumermuth, 1972).

Abnormal Ventricles

Predominantly abnormal EEG findings have been reported in cases of *cavum septi pellucidi, cavum vergae* (Bergleiter and Fekas, 1964; Dumermuth, 1972; Larroche and Baudy, 1961), and *cisterna interventricularis.*

Porencephaly and Schizencephaly

Porencephaly consists of gross cystic defects in the cerebral hemispheres, either due to developmental (schizencephalic) disturbances or as the result of ischemic encephalomalacia. Congenital hemiplegia, bilateral hemiplegia, or tetraplegia are the most common neurological consequences.

EEG abnormalities are usually quite prominent with local slowing or spiking or with zones of featureless low-voltage activity. Smaller porencephalic cysts may be associated with normal records (Murphy and Garvin, 1947).

Pohowalla et al. (1984) described severe EEG changes in newborns with cystic brain disease. The EEG was characterized by suppressed background activity, focal or multifocal spikes, and sharp waves that correlated with the anatomical site of the cysts. The term *schizencephaly* (Yakovlev and Wadsworth, 1946) implies a cerebral cleft lined with gray matter. There is a "pial-ependymal seam" covering the cleft and reaching the ependymal lining of the ventricle. This feature is crucial in the differentiation of schizencephaly from other malformations (Barkovich and Kuzniecky, 1996). The extent of the schizencephalic aberration parallels the severity of motor and mental impairment is not congruent with the severity of epileptic seizure disorder (Granata et al., 1996). Interictal EEG recordings show normal background activity; there is slowing over the cleft region, and local spike activity may also be contralateral (Granata et al., 1996).

A 3-year-old girl with porencephaly and hydrocephaly was reported by Haginoya et al. (1999); her EEG was of focal-hypsarrhythmic character, but the tonic spasms were quite symmetrical. Dennis et al. (2000) described ten cases of unilateral and bilateral schizencephaly along with their EEG and imaging findings.

Agenesis of the Corpus Callosum

Agenesis of the corpus callosum is a cerebral defect that is being increasingly recognized due to the use of transfontanellar ultrasonography and CT scan. Among malformations, agenesis of the corpus callosum is the leading cause of mental retardation. This underscores the significance of EEG studies in this condition.

A variety of asymmetries in the EEG have been described in this condition (Fermaglich and O'Doherty, 1972; Goldensohn et al., 1941; Green and Russell, 1966). Many of these infants are clinically asymptomatic, and it is hence not surprising that Dumermuth (1972) found normal EEG records in 50% of the cases. Familial occurrence of this condition was discussed by Aichner et al. (1983).

On the other hand, severe CNS damage may occur in conjunction with callosal agenesis, and marked EEG abnormalities may be present. Hypsarrhythmic changes are common in infants with the Aicardi syndrome, which is discussed in Chapter 27, "Epileptic Seizure Disorders," and

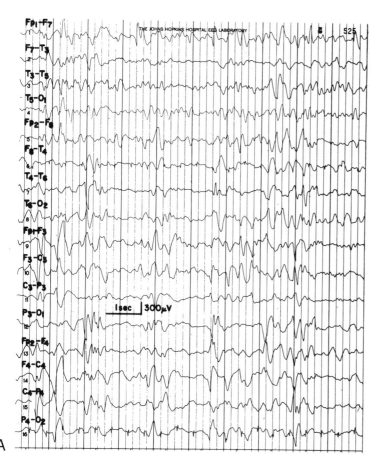

A

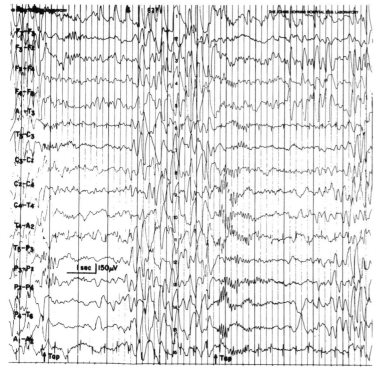

B

Figure 20.2. **A:** Age 15 months. Lissencephaly with profound mental retardation and severe epileptic seizure disorder (mostly tonic seizures). Sleep portion. Note the enormous voltage output and massive spike and sharp wave activity, more over right hemisphere. Some spindle activity is present on the left side (right portion of figure). There are some enigmatic phase reversals of sharp activity over left occipital and right frontopolar region. **B:** Same patient as in **A**. Arousing stimuli (taps) in sleep give rise to general desynchronization and also to spiky 14–18/sec runs. These responses were often associated with tonic posturing.

Chapter 19, "Degenerative Disorders of the Central Nervous System" (Fig. 20.3).

With the use of inter- and intrahemispheric coherence methods, Koeda et al. (1995) demonstrated a decrease of interhemispheric EEG coherence in acallosal children. These authors also noted lowered intrahemispheric coherence in the right hemisphere (compared to normals), suggesting reduced connectivity within right hemisphere (mainly in the beta band). These authors assume compensatory left hemisphere mechanisms.

Hemimegalencephaly

This condition denotes a rare brain malformation characterized by congenital hypertrophy of one cerebral hemisphere and ipsilateral ventriculomegaly (Bignami et al., 1969). The clinical signs include unilateral motor deficit (hemiplegia), mental retardation, and epilepsy.

Abnormal EEG findings have been reported by Tjiam et al. (1978), Dambska et al. (1984), Vigevano et al. (1984), King et al. (1985), and Ohtsuka et al. (1999). These authors reported "alpha-like" activity, triphasic complexes, and burst-suppression patterns.

Some authors have stressed the usefulness of EEG in hemimegalencephaly with regard to diagnosis and prognosis. "Alpha-like" activity was exhibited by patients with a somewhat more favorable outcome. These patients learned to walk and to talk. On the other hand, "triphasic complexes" seem to have a more severe prognostic significance.

Hwang et al. (1989) reported five cases of unilateral megalencephaly (age 11 days to 10 years). All of them had epileptic seizures (focal motor, complex partial; also infantile spasms and status epilepticus). The posterior basic rhythm was absent over the involved hemisphere. Spikes were multifocal and most prominent over frontal, temporal, and central areas. Periodic lateralized epileptiform discharges (PLEDs) were frequently found. Ictal events were electrocorticographically documented. Improvement of the seizure disorder occurred after hemidecortication. Epileptic negative myoclonus ("negative myoclonus"; see Chapter 27 under myoclonus) in a newborn with hemimegalencephaly and a constant nonreactive burst suppression pattern in the EEG was described by Guzzetta et al. (2002).

Hydrocephalus

Dilated ventricles, brain atrophy, and enlargement of the head are the hallmarks of infantile hydrocephalus. Its etiologies and pathogenic mechanisms are multifold and complex; a full discussion of them is beyond the scope of this chapter.

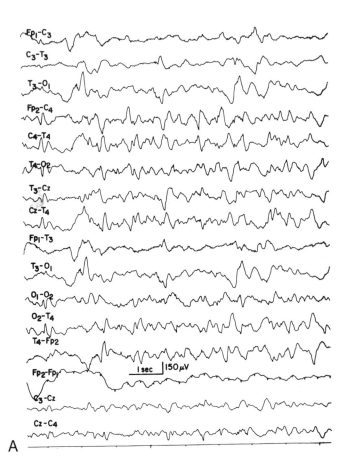

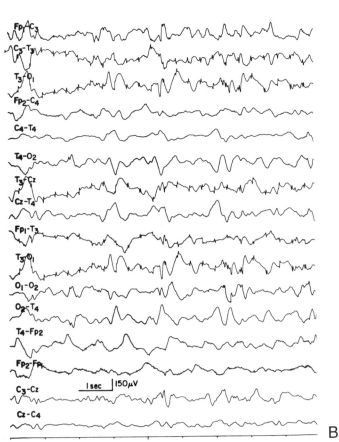

Figure 20.3.   Three-month-old girl with Aicardi's syndrome (full blown). **A:** Voltage depression and washed-out slow activity over left hemisphere. **B:** Somewhat later after a very brief stretch of widespread ictal subclinical activity, voltage depression and loss of detail have shifted to right hemisphere. Note high voltage output and a few spikes (not to be confused with electrocardiogram artifact in T_3).

The EEG is frequently abnormal; the abnormalities reflect the type and degree of damage to the cerebral parenchyma. Massive slowing and spiking may be present locally or diffusely, especially in postinfectious hydrocephalus in the wake of acute meningitis. A normal record was found in 20% (Dumermuth, 1958, 1972). Multiple spike foci and/or hypsarrhythmia were noted in one third of the patients (Dumermuth, 1958, 1972). Garvin and Gibbs (1975) have stressed the frequent occurrence of asynchronous sleep patterns (also see Watanabe et al., 1984).

Further observations were reported by Heppner and Lechner (1955), Fois et al. (1958), Bogacz and Rebollo (1962), and Pampiglione and Lawrence (1962). Laws and Niedermeyer (1970) found consistent abnormalities after shunt procedures, mostly over the hemisphere used for surgery. The possibility of a smoldering low-grade infection along the catheter was considered.

While hydrocephaly as such is not commonly recognized as a cause of epileptic seizure disorder, shunt treatment is frequently associated with seizures, especially in children (Bourgeois et al., 1999; Sato et al., 2001). Gelisse et al. (2003) reported EEG findings resembling benign epilepsy of childhood with centrotemporal spikes in two cases of shunted hydrocephalus.

Anomalies of the Cranium

Microcephaly

In microcephaly, an overall reduction of cranial capacity results in small skull size and small brain size. The cortex may be hyperplastic or may show patches of microgyria, macrogyria, or argyria. A variety of disorders may cause microcephaly.

These cortical changes are essentially the cause of EEG abnormalities of various degrees (Fois and Rosenberg, 1957; Fritzche and Fritzche, 1957). According to Dumermuth (1958, 1972), about two thirds of the cases show abnormal records.

Craniosynostosis

In this condition, premature fusion of cranial bones may occur independently of cerebral growth, resulting in compression of neural structures (Allen, 1964). The EEG serves as an indicator of cerebral impairment and is, according to Dumermuth (1958, 1972), very useful in the assessment of cerebral functioning prior to surgical intervention.

Brain Damage Caused by Prenatal Infections

Rubella Syndrome

Maternal rubella during the first trimester of pregnancy, especially during the first 4 weeks when the risk is almost 50%, leads to a variety of birth defects caused by the virus. Malformations of the eye, inner ear, and heart are common; the viral disease may linger on postnatally for several months, causing myocarditis, hepatitis, purpura, pneumonia, and encephalitis.

The EEG findings are inconsistent; even in the presence of severe CNS abnormalities, the EEG may be normal (Barnet, 1972). Polysomnography may reveal an abnormal sequence of sleep stages. Evoked response studies of all modalities are presumed to be helpful.

Other Causes of Prenatal Brain Damage

Transplacental infections with *cytomegalovirus* (leading to chorioretinitis, hepatosplenomegaly, hearing loss, microcephaly, mental retardation, and seizures), *syphilis* (leading to saddle nose, keratitis, meningovascular involvement, convulsions, deafness, and mental retardation), and *toxoplasmosis* (leading to chorioretinitis, hydrocephalus, intracerebral calcifications, seizures, and mental retardation) are the most widely known causes of fetal infection. EEG abnormalities may be quite pronounced, and even hypsarrhythmia has been reported in these three conditions (Barnet, 1972; Radermecker, 1960; Stern et al., 1969).

Fetal Alcohol Syndrome (FAS)

Fetal alcohol syndrome results from maternal alcohol consumption during pregnancy. The incidence in the United States is from 1:600 to 1:300 live births. The clinical manifestations include growth deficiencies, facial abnormalities, neurological disorder (microcephaly, hyperactivity, developmental delays, attention-deficit disorder, seizures, mental retardation), cardiac septal defects and minor joint and limb abnormalities. Kaneko et al. (1996), studying children with FAS, demonstrated that alpha activity was significantly reduced in the absence of slow activity. The left hemisphere was more seriously affected. These data suggest that the left hemisphere may be more vulnerable to prenatal alcohol exposure.

Cerebral Palsy

The term *cerebral palsy* encompasses various forms of infantile brain damage with prominent motor disturbances. The etiologies are multifold and often not clearly demonstrable. The type of cerebral palsy is determined by the preponderant type and distribution of motor deficit or dysfunction. The underlying pathological substratum varies considerably and makes it understandable that some clinicians individualize the forms of cerebral palsy (Ford, 1966).

Neither neuropathological nor etiological classifications are satisfactory. Even the logical distinction between mechanical trauma at birth and birth anoxia (asphyxia) "tends to obscure the complex interplay of the pathogenetic factors often involved" (Norman, 1966). According to this author, compression of arteries during such mechanical birth injury as distortion of the head may be facilitated by neonatal shock, itself an expression of anoxia. Clinical-neurological classifications, therefore, are generally preferred and will be used in this section.

Epileptic seizures are a frequent symptom of cerebral palsy; their occurrence and the question of the predictability of future seizures heighten the significance of EEG studies. There is good evidence that EEG abnormalities are more serious and more frequently noted in cerebral palsy cases with (rather than without) epileptic seizure disorder (Al-Sulaiman, 2001; Senebil et al., 2002).

Diplegic Forms

Diplegic forms are characterized by spastic paresis or paralysis with predominant involvement of the lower extremities, caused by venous stasis and bleeding (Schwartz, 1924, 1961) or by arterial compression (Earle et al., 1953; Lindenberg, 1955). These early lesions lead to lobar sclerosis with cortical changes such as ulegyria, microgyria, pachygyria, or disturbed cortical lamination. These conditions impinge strongly on the pyramidal motor outflow, thus causing a typical spastic deficit with marked spasticity of the legs and knock-knees or "scissoring" (genu valgum). Arm involvement is mostly limited to clumsiness. Various degrees of mental retardation are found in 31% of the children (Gibbs and Gibbs, 1964).

EEG studies are essentially based on the unrivaled work and material of Perlstein and Gibbs (1949), Perlstein et al. (1955), and Gibbs and Gibbs (1964).

Excessive slow and fast activity is quite common in children with the diplegic form of cerebral palsy. Predominant fast activity has been reported by Shinners et al. (1950), Gibbs and Gibbs (1964), and Dumermuth (1972). Normal records are most common in the first 2 years of life; typical abnormalities such as spikes, diffuse or focal slowing, or asymmetries tend to become more evident after the age of 2 years. It is hence worthwhile to focus attention on the absence of physiological patterns. This is particularly true for light non-rapid-eye-movement (REM) sleep (absence of spindles, vertex waves, K complexes); this and the general voltage depression in sleep has been emphasized by Gibbs and Gibbs (1964). In the first 2 years of life, slow activity in non-REM sleep shows a physiological voltage maximum over the occipital region. The absence of a posterior voltage maximum as a sign of early childhood brain damage, suspected by Niedermeyer and Yarworth (1978), has been unequivocally demonstrated by Slatter and Torres (1979). Other deviant findings in the sleep EEG were reported by Levy-Alcover et al. (1959).

Spike activity is very common and is present in about half of the cases of the diplegic form. Occipital spikes (below age 5) and midtemporal or cerebral spikes (above age 5) predominate among the paroxysmal discharges (Gibbs and Gibbs, 1964). According to these authors, spike activity is by far more common in children with seizures and is rare in seizure-free diplegic children. Gibbs and Gibbs (1964) also have stressed the value of spike activity in the EEG in predicting imminent clinical seizures; unfortunately, the predictive value is low below the age of 2 years. Further studies on spike foci were made by Skatvedt and Lundervold (1956) and Skatvedt (1958).

Severe forms of epileptic seizure disorder may develop in the presence of hypsarrhythmic patterns with infantile spasm or slow spike-wave activity with a variety of minor seizures, as in Lennox-Gastaut syndrome. These serious forms of childhood epilepsy, however, are more common in the hemiplegic form of cerebral palsy. The presence of the 14 and 6/sec positive spike discharge usually indicates a benign form of seizure disorder. This pattern probably does not correlate with the degree of mental retardation.

Quadriplegic Form

This form is closely related to the diplegic form and is distinguished from the latter by equally serious involvement of upper and lower extremities. The underlying lesion, therefore, is somewhat more extensive; basic characteristics are otherwise essentially the same.

According to Gibbs and Gibbs (1964), epileptic seizures are more common in the quadriplegic (59%) than in the diplegic form (31%). This is concurrent with a greater number of cases with spikes in the quadriplegic form. The incidence of low-voltage waking activity, low-voltage or absence of sleep spindles, and vertex waves is particularly high among quadriplegics, followed by diplegic patients; it is lowest in hemiplegic patients. Similar findings have been reported in the work of Gururaj et al. (2003).

Hemiplegic Form

The hemiplegic form of cerebral palsy is most commonly due to peri- and postnatal causes rather than to prenatal etiologies. Massive acute cerebrovascular accidents such as hemorrhage or thrombosis of major cerebral arteries are the most common substratum. Ensuing cystic formations, termed "false porencephaly" by Ford (1966), who distinguished this condition from true porencephalies, are common. Severe acute meningoencephalitis may also result in infantile hemiplegia.

The hemiplegic form is very common and, in the work of Gibbs and Gibbs (1964), was even more frequently found than the diplegic and quadriplegic forms combined. The prevalence of epileptic seizures is high [62.5% according to Gibbs and Gibbs (1964)]. Panteliadis et al. (2002) showed that the frequency of epilepsy in children with congenital hemiplegia is paralleled by the degree of EEG abnormalities (approaching 85% in patients with severe EEG abnormalities).

EEG abnormalities are found in the vast majority of these infants or children, and very severely disordered tracings are quite common. In cases of extensive porencephalic or pseudoporencephalic cysts, the EEG is usually depressed, featureless, or even almost flat over the involved hemisphere; small regions of less depressed EEG activity may be present. Those children with massive contralateral hemiplegia and usually intractable epileptic seizure disorders often benefit from hemispherectomy, which demonstrates enormous cystic degeneration. In such cases the destroyed cortex is usually unable to generate spike activity, which is understandable in view of the almost complete lack of voltage output, whereas epileptic discharges may be recorded over the presumed healthy hemisphere. The abnormalities persist in sleep, and pronounced spindle depression may be present on the affected side.

In many cases, marked high-voltage output with mixed slow activity and spikes is noted over the affected hemisphere; this was found in two thirds of the cases of Dumermuth (1972). This author also noted hypsarrhythmia and infantile spasms in 8% of the cases; this is regarded as prognostically unfavorable. About one fourth of the children with unilateral high-voltage slow and spiky activity have no clinical seizures.

After hemispherectomy, pronounced flattening is noted over the altered hemisphere, which is not totally removed;

gray masses remain in the basal ganglia and thalamic level. The persistence of these parenchymatous rests may explain the low-voltage activity encountered over the side of surgery; furthermore, potentials from the remaining hemisphere can be recorded through cerebrospinal fluid, skull, and scalp (Cobbs and Sears, 1960).

Bilateral (Double) Hemiplegic Form

In this form, lesions of the hemiplegic form are found in both hemispheres. As in the hemiplegias, the arms are more paretic than the legs (in contrast to the diplegic and quadriplegic forms), and pseudobulbar motor deficits are also common; the mental deficit is of high grade (Ford, 1966). This form is rare. The severity of the bilateral EEG abnormalities reflects the extent of the structural damage.

Choreoathetoid Form

About one fourth of all cases of cerebral palsy take this form. The underlying pathological substratum varies, and several types of brain damage may contribute to the choreoathetoid forms (also called the "extrapyramidal" or "basal ganglia" form). Forms such as status marmoratus and other basal ganglia pathology have been found to be caused by kernicterus, which is probably the most common etiology of this form. The motor control of these children or adolescents is often very severely impaired, whereas the mental deficit tends to be mild or nonexistent. In spite of the preponderance of subcortical damage, about 25% of those affected are epileptics.

The EEG is normal in about 30% to 50% of the cases. Focal spike activity is the most common abnormality; local or diffuse slowing and asymmetries are also common. Dumermuth (1972) has stressed the moderate degree of abnormality. Gibbs and Gibbs (1964) noticed that low-voltage activity in sleep with depression of spindles, vertex waves, and K complexes is common in spastic forms but uncommon in the choreoathetoid form. "Extreme spindles" (Gibbs and Gibbs, 1964; also see Chapter 11, "Maturation of the EEG: Development of Waking and Sleeping Patterns") have also been observed frequently in this form.

Hypotonic Form

This form is not generally recognized. It is essentially based on early cerebellar damage and must be carefully differentiated from infantile neuromuscular disorder ("floppy babies"). Normal EEG tracings were found in 57% of this group (Dumermuth, 1972).

Hypotonic-Dystonia Syndrome

A syndrome characterized by early-onset hypotonia and frequent episodes of paroxysmal dystonia was delineated by Andermann et al. (1994). EEG findings were either normal or mildly abnormal (without paroxysmal activity).

Mental Retardation

There is a fairly large literature on the EEG in mental retardation. There is no chapter devoted to mental retardation in this book because mental deficits are caused by a large number of distinct and ill-defined clinical conditions. Such conditions are found in Chapter 19, "Degenerative Disorders of the Central Nervous System," as well as in this chapter and in Chapter 27, "Epileptic Seizure Disorders."

New aspects of mental retardation have emerged of the last two decades, especially with regard to *fragile X syndrome,* which is found in approximately 1/1,250 males and 1/2,500 females. In addition to mental retardation, the fragile X syndrome is characterized by a distinctive facial appearance with large ears and long face, hypermobile joints, and macro-orchidism. The affected males exhibit fragility of the distal end of the chromosome. Epileptic seizures occur in 10% to 20% of these patients (Berry-Kravis, 2002) and focal seizures with centrotemporal spikes (similar to benign rolandic epilepsy) are the most common seizure manifestation (Berry-Kravis, 2002; Singh et al., 1999).

Other Causes of Early Brain Damage and Dysfunction

Malnutrition, parasitic infestation, and goiter represent factors that may cause cerebral impairment (Gallais et al., 1951). EEG findings in affected school children showed slowing in 27% and spike (sharp wave, spike-wave) activity in 6.6% (Levav et al., 1995).

Minimal Cerebral Dysfunction

This large group of behaviorally disturbed children can hardly be considered a nosological or clinical entity. A study of such patients is beset with terminological problems.

In general, the term *minimal cerebral dysfunction* has been used to describe a syndrome in children characterized by hyperkinetic behavior, short attention span, lability of mood, and various minor perceptual disturbances (MacKeith, 1963). The lack of gross neurological deficits sets it apart from the cerebral palsy complex, although it is possible that a continuum exists (Paine, 1962). The significance of an organic cerebral basis has been stressed by Birch (1964).

Electroencephalographers have shown interest in behaviorally disturbed children for some decades. Solomon et al. (1937, 1938) found a high incidence of EEG abnormalities in "childhood behavior disorder" and suggested an underlying cerebral component. This line of thinking was reinforced by the observation of favorable response to amphetamine sulfate in some of these children (Cutts and Jasper, 1939; Lindsley and Cutts, 1940; Lindsley and Henry, 1942). Other children responded favorably to diphenylhydantoin (Walker and Kirkpatrick, 1947).

On the basis of a very large population, Cohn (1958), Cohn and Nardini (1958), and Gervasio (1978) focused their attention on the significance of posterior slow activity in the waking record. Other investigators concentrated on 14 and 6/sec positive spike discharge, described first by Gibbs and Gibbs (1951) and interpreted by these authors as "evidence of thalamic and hypothalamic epilepsy." A relationship to childhood or juvenile behavior disorder was presumed by Schwade and Geiger (1956), Walter et al. (1960), Niedermeyer and Knott (1961), and Henry (1963), along with considerable de-emphasis on the epileptogenic character of the discharge. This was followed by a series of studies that have markedly lessened the clinical significance of the 14 and 6/sec positive spike discharge (Little, 1965; Lombroso et al., 1966; Metcalf, 1963).

It has become clear since the first review of this topic by Ellingson (1954) that it is exceedingly difficult to establish clinical-electrical correlation in this wide and heterogeneous field. A study by Capute et al. (1968) showed EEG abnormalities in precisely 50% of 106 children diagnosed as having minimal cerebral dysfunction; there was a variety of mild to moderate EEG abnormalities, while only eight patients had markedly abnormal records. The 14 and 6/sec positive spike pattern played a rather minor role among the abnormalities. In contrast, Klinkerfuss et al. (1965) found EEG abnormalities in 90%.

The complexity of this topic is highlighted by Satterfield and Schell's study (1984), which was a follow-up study from childhood into adolescence. It was found that hyperactive children with abnormal EEGs and abnormal auditory evoked potentials had a good outcome (for example, no police arrest in adolescence). On the other hand, hyperactive children with normal EEGs and normal evoked potential studies tended to be delinquent in adolescence.

Attention Deficit and Minimal Cerebral Dysfunction

The outdated term *minimal cerebral dysfunction* has been replaced by the now widely used term *attention-deficit hyperactivity disorder* (ADHD) (American Psychiatric Association, 1994). This is a very common disorder with a prevalence ranging from 5% to 7% of children. The onset lies around age 7 years; boys are about three to nine times more frequently affected than girls. The underlying cause has remained a mystery.

The EEG contribution to the understanding of ADHD has been fairly meager. Rather minor and nonspecific abnormalities were found in half of these patients (Capute et al., 1968). With the use of quantitative EEG, Grünewald-Zuberbier et al. (1975) found that children with ADHD showed higher alpha amplitudes and less beta activity; there was also a reduced response to arousing stimuli (and hence a deficient concentration of attention).

Richer et al. (2002) noted a higher prevalence of epileptiform abnormalities in ADHD (using hyperventilation and photic stimulation) in comparison with normal children. Hughes et al. (2000) found epileptiform discharges in 30.1% of 176 children with ADHD. Most abnormalities were located over temporal and occipital areas.

Other studies of ADHD placed special stress on frequency bands. According to Clarke et al., there are two distinct EEG clusters of children: (a) those with increased high-amplitude theta and deficiencies in the delta and beta band, and (b) those with increased slow waves and deficiencies in the fast range. These subtypes were found in boys (Clarke et al., 2002) and, with less variance in their EEG profile, in girls with ADHD (Clarke et al., 2003). Barry et al. (2003) placed their emphasis on elevated theta power and reduced alpha and beta power. Excessive beta activity was found primarily in the frontal regions (Clarke et al., 2001). This was thought to be related to frontal lobe functions such as self-regulation and inhibition control.

Cerebral blood flow studies in ADHD demonstrated hypoperfusion of the frontal region (Lou et al., 1984). Methylphenidate augmented frontal and decreased motor-sensory cortical perfusion (Lou et al., 1984).

These findings clearly support the concept of a frontal-motor cortex disconnection syndrome (Niedermeyer, 2001; Niedermeyer and Naidu, 1996). While there is no structural abnormality in ADHD, the frontal lobe is conceived as being "lazy" and thus not exerting the physiological inhibition on the motor cortex (an inhibitory function that loses significance in the course of adolescence and adulthood). This disinhibition would result in the enhanced urge to move. On the other hand, a "lazy" frontal lobe does not provide for the normal degree of general and selective attention (Niedermeyer and Naidu, 1996). Seen from this angle, the calming effect of the stimulant methylphenidate in ADHD is not paradoxical; on the contrary, this is a logical response of an activated frontal lobe capable of generating the normal degree of inhibition on the motor cortex. This concept was derived from preceding analogous observations made in Rett syndrome (a rare disorder; see Chapter 19, "Degenerative Disorders of the Central Nervous System"). The frontal lobe is of smaller size in Rett syndrome (Armstrong, 1995) and there is definite cerebral organicity found in Rett syndrome, while the ADHD is strictly based on CNS dysfunction rather than structural anomalies. Central EEG abnormalities in Rett syndrome (Niedermeyer et al., 1997) were instrumental in the development of the frontal-motor cortex disconnection concept, which can be transferred from an organically determined to a dysfunctional clinical syndrome.

The work of Steger et al. (2000) revealed subtle but specific visual-attentional, central, and premotor-frontal dysfunctions in ADHD. In this context, a beneficial response to methylphenidate in mania should be mentioned (Bschor et al., 2001). According to these authors, there seems to be a pattern of light drowsiness (alpha mixed with theta and beta) in the manic state. With 20 mg methylphenidate (Ritalin), the EEG showed a very regular alpha-EEG of wakefulness along with psychiatric normalization. Although this is just a single case, one could speculate that the manic state could be due to disinhibition caused by weakened frontal lobe functions in adulthood when motor hyperactivity is no longer a major problem.

Dyslexia and the EEG

Dyslexia is a complex and controversial topic. Dyslexia is not merely a delay in the ability to learn to read. It comprises problems of symbolic visual perception and cognition along with word usage, significance, meaning, pronunciation, spelling, and others.

Primary dyslexia is thought to be of a developmental nature, whereas secondary dyslexia is the result of early structural brain damage. Primary developmental dyslexia is more common in boys (at a ratio of about 2.5:1). In the absence of unequivocal neurological deficits, "soft neurological signs"—a term introduced by Schilder—have been reported in primary dyslexia (and also in children with minimal cerebral dysfunction/attention deficit disorder). These mild signs encompass clumsiness, mild incoordination, right-left confusion, failure to reproduce a geometrical shape from memory, and other cognitive dysfunctions. Critchley (1986), however, has emphasized the dexterity and excellent athletic skills of dyslexic children and found no signs of hyperactivity.

Earlier EEG studies showed larger numbers of EEG abnormalities in dyslexic children in comparison with normal controls. Hughes and Park (1968) found EEG abnormalities in 36% of their large dyslexic patient population. These investigators have pointed out that "the most common type of EEG abnormality was the 6–7/sec and 14/sec positive spike phenomenon seen in one half of the abnormal records. Excessive occipital slowing was seen in 27% of the abnormal cases." Hughes (1978) reported 45% of EEG abnormalities; this figure was derived from ten studies. Today, in hindsight, these abnormalities must be considered either marginal or perhaps as anomalies found "within broad normal limits of variability." Methodological weaknesses of EEG studies in dyslexic children were pointed out by Conners (1978).

Over the past two decades, EEG studies of dyslexia have been based mainly on computer analysis of EEG data. Fein et al. (1986) were unable to detect major differences between dyslexics and a control group with the use of power spectral analysis. Yingling et al. (1986) utilized the neurometric approach of John (1977), but even this highly sophisticated technique could not detect any special anomalies in dyslexics. It must be noted that, in computerized data analysis, only a limited number of EEG channels are analyzed in most cases. According to Byring et al. (1991), quantified EEG shows some temporoparieto-occipital abnormalities in children with spelling disabilities.

A study of fluent and dyslexic reading with magnetoencephalography showed no essential differences in the cortical sequential processing from left inferior occipitotemporal cortex to left superior temporal cortex (Salmelin et al., 2000); these authors emphasized that dyslexia is chiefly associated with phonological problems.

Dyslexia still remains a clinical, neuropsychological, and electroencephalographic problem and essentially an unresolved riddle.

References

Aichner, F., Vogl, G., Mayr, U., et al. 1983. Balkenmangel und Epilepsie bei zwei Brüdern. Z. EEG-EMG. 14:195–198.

Al-Sulaiman, A. 2001. Electroencephalographic findings in children with cerebral palsy: a study of 151 patients. Funct. Neurol. 16:325–328.

Allen, N. 1964. Developmental and degenerative diseases of the brain. In *Pediatric Neurology*, Ed. T.W. Farmer, pp. 162–284. New York: Hober Medical Division (Harper & Row).

American Psychiatric Association. 1994. *Diagnostic and Statistical Manual of Mental Disorders*, 4th ed. (DSM-IV). Washington, DC: APA.

Andermann, F., Ohtahara, S., Andermann, E., et al. 1994. Infantile hypotonia and paroxysmal dystonia: a variant of alternating hemiplegia of childhood? Mov. Disord. 9:227–229.

André-Thomas, and Fischgold, H. 1949. Étude électroencéphalographique d'un anencéphale. Ann. Méd. Psychol. 107:70–72.

Armstrong, D.D. 1995. The neuropathology of Rett syndrome—overview 1994. Neuropediatrics 26:100–104.

Barkovich, A.J., and Kuzniecky, R.L. 1996. Neuroimaging of focal malformations of cortical development. J. Clin. Neurophysiol. 13:481–494.

Barnet, A.B. 1972. Prenatal infections involving the brain. In *Handbook of Electroencephalography and Clinical Neurophysiology*, vol. 15B, Ed.-in-chief, A. Remond, pp. 27–32. Amsterdam: Elsevier.

Barry, R.J., Clarke, A.R., and Johnstone, S.J. 2003. A review of electrophysiology in attention-deficit/hyperactivity disorder: I. Quantitative and qualitative electroencephalography. Clin. Neurophysiol. 114: 171–183.

Bergleiter, R., and Fekas, L. 1964. Das Cavum septi pellucidi und Cavum vergae in Klinik und Röntgenbild. Fortschr. Neurol. Psychiatr. 32:361–399.

Bernstine, R.L., and Borkowski, W.T. 1960. Electroencephalographic studies in anencephalics. Am. J. Obstet. Gynecol. 80:1151–1153.

Berry-Kravis, E. 2002. Epilepsy in fragile X syndrome. Dev. Med. Child Neurol. 44:724–728.

Bignami, A., Palladini, G., and Zappella, M. 1969. Unilateral megalencephaly with nerve cell hypertrophy. An anatomical and quantitative histochemical study. Brain Res. 9:103–114.

Birch, H.G. 1964. The problem of "brain damage" in children. In *Brain Damage in Children*, Ed. H.G. Birds, pp. 3–12. Baltimore: Williams & Wilkins.

Bogacz, J., and Rebollo, M.A. 1962. Electroencephalographic abnormalities in non-tumor hydrocephalus. Electroencephalogr. Clin. Neurophysiol. 14:123–125.

Bourgeois, N., Sainte-Rose, C., Cinalli, G., et al. 1999. Epilepsy in children with shunted hydrocephalus. J. Neurosurg. 90:274–281.

Bschor, T., Mueller-Oerlinghausen, B., and Ulrich, G. 2001. Decreased level of EEG vigilance in acute mania as a possible predictor for a rapid effect of methylphenidate: a case study. Clin. Electroencephalogr. 32: 36–39.

Byring, R.F., Salmi, T.K., Sainio, K.O., et al. 1991. EEG in children with spelling disabilities. Electroencephalogr. Clin. Neurophysiol. 79:247–255.

Cantwell, D.P. 1983. Diagnostic validity of the hyperactive child (attention deficit disorder with hyperactivity) syndrome. Psychiatr. Dev. 3:277.

Capute, A.J., Niedermeyer, E., and Richardson. F. 1968. The electroencephalogram in children with minimal cerebral dysfunction. Pediatrics 41:1104–1114.

Clarke, A.R., Barry, R.J., McCarthy, R., et al. 2001. Excess beta activity in children with attention deficit/hyperactivity disorder: an atypical electrophysiological group. Psychiatr. Res. 103:205–218.

Clarke, A.R., Barry, R.J., McCarthy, R., et al. 2002. EEG evidence for a new conceptualisation of attention deficit-hyperactivity disorder. Clin. Neurophysiol. 113:1036–1044.

Clarke, A.R., Barry, R.J., McCarthy, R., et al. 2003. EEG activity in girls with attention–deficit/hyperactivity disorder. Clin. Neurophysiol. 114:319–328.

Clegg, N.J., Gerace, K.L., Sparagana, S.P., et al. 2002. Holoprosencephaly: a review. Am. J. EEG Technol. 42:59–72.

Cobbs, W., and Sears, T.A. 1960. A study of the transmission of potentials after hemispherectomy. Electroencephalogr. Clin. Neurophysiol. 12:371–383.

Cohadon, E., Leurzor, G., Vital, C., et al. 1966. Étude clinique, anatomique et électroencéphalographique d'un cas d' anencéphalie. Rev. Neuropsychiatr. Infant. 14:817–831.

Cohn, R. 1958. On the significance of bi-occipital slow wave activity in the electroencephalogram of children. Electroencephalogr. Clin. Neurophysiol. 10:766.

Cohn, R., and Nardini, J.E. 1958. The correlation of bilateral occipital slow activity in the human EEG with certain disorders of behavior. Am. J. Psychiatr. 115:44–54.

Conners, C.K. 1978. Clinical review of electroencephalographic and neurophysiological studies in dyslexia. In *Dyslexia: An Appraisal of Current Knowledge*, Eds. A.L. Benton and D. Pearl. New York: Oxford University Press.

Crawley, J.W., and Proler, M.L. 1972. Hydrocephalus and cerebral malformation. In *Handbook of Electroencephalography and Clinical Neurophysiology*, vol. 15B, Ed.-in-chief, A. Remond, pp. 24–26. Amsterdam: Elsevier.

Critchley, M. 1986. *The Citadel of the Senses*. New York: Raven Press.

Cutts, K.K., and Jasper, H.H. 1939. Effect of benzedrine sulfate and phenobarbital on behavior problem children with abnormal electroencephalogram. Arch. Neurol. Psychiatr. (Chicago) 41:1138–1145.

Dambska, M., Wisniewski, K., and Sher, J. 1984. An autopsy case of hemimegalencephaly. Brain Dev. 6:60–64.

De Myer, W., and White, P.T. 1964. EEG in holoprosencephaly (arrhinencephaly). Arch. Neurol. (Chicago) 11:507–520.

Dennis, D., Charell, J.F., Brun, M., et al. 2000. Schizencephaly: clinical and imaging features in 30 infantile cases. Brain Dev. 22:475–483.

De Rijk-Van Andel, J.F., Arts, W.F.M., and Deweerd, A.W. 1988. EEG in type I lissencephaly. Dev. Med. Child Neurol. 30:126–129.

Dobyns, W.B., Stratton, R.F., and Greenberg, F. 1984. Syndromes with lissencephaly. Am. J. Med. Genet. 18:509–526.

Dobyns, W.B., Kirkpatrick, J.B., Hittner, H.M., et al. 1985. Syndromes with lissencephaly. II: Walker-Warberg and cerebro-oculo-muscular syndromes and a new syndrome with type II lissencephaly. Am. J. Med. Genet. 22:157–195.

Dulac, O., Plouin, P., Perulli, L., et al. 1984. EEG aspect of agyria. Electroencephalogr. Clin. Neurophysiol. 57:51P(abst).

Dumermuth, G. 1958. Über die elektroenzephalographische Untersuchung dyskranieller Kinder (Mikro-und Makrocephalie, Kraniosynostose). Helvet. Padiatr. Acta. 13:618–635.

Dumermuth, G. 1972. Elektroenzephalographie im Kindesalter. Stuttgart: Thieme.

Earle, K.M., Baldwin, M., and Penfield, W. 1953. Incisural sclerosis and temporal lobe seizures produced by hippocampal herniation at birth. Arch. Neurol. Psychiat. 65:27–42.

Elia, M., Musemeci, S.A., Ferri, R., et al. 1995. Unusual EEG features in a child with cerebrocerebellar lissencephaly. Epilepsia 36(suppl 3):S78 (abst).

Ellingson, R.J. 1954. The incidence of EEG abnormality among patients with mental disorders of apparently non-organic origin: a critical review. Am. J. Psychiatry 111:263–275.

Fein, G., Yingling, C.D., Johnstone, J., et al. 1986. EEG spectra in dyslexic and control boys during resting condition. Electroencephalogr. Clin. Neurophysiol. 63:87–97.

Fermaglich, J., and O'Doherty, D.S. 1972. Agenesis of the corpus callosum: an electroencephalographic study. Epilepsia (Amsterdam) 13:345(abst).

Fois, A., and Rosenberg, C.M. 1957. The electroencephalogram in microcephaly. Neurology (Minneapolis) 7:703–704.

Fois, A., Gibbs, E.L., and Gibbs, F.A. 1958. Bilaterally independent sleep patterns in hydrocephalus. Arch. Neurol. Psychiatry (Chicago) 79:264–268.

Ford, F.R. 1966. Disease of the Nervous System in Infancy, Childhood and Adolescence, 5th ed. Springfield, IL: Charles C Thomas.

Fritzche, I., and Fritzche, H. 1957. Microcephaly and the electroencephalogram. Ann. Paediatr. (Basel) 188:45–53.

Gallais, P., Miletto, G., Corriol, J., et al. 1951. Introduction à l'étude d'EEG physiologogique du noir d'Afrique. Méd. Tropicale. 11:128–146.

Garvin, J.S., and Gibbs, F.A. 1975. Electroencephalogram in hydrocephalus. Clin. Electroencephalogr. 6:29–40.

Gastaut, H., Pinsard, N., Raybaud, Ch., et al. 1987. Lissencephaly (agyria-pachygyria): clinical findings and serial EEG studies. Dev. Med. Child Neurol. 29:167–180.

Gelisse, P., Corda, D., Raybaud, C., et al. 2003. Abnormal neuroimaging in patients with benign epilepsy with centrotemporal spikes. Epilepsia 44:372–378.

Gervasio, L. 1978. Clinical observations of posterior slow activity. Electroencephalogr. Clin. Neurophysiol. 45:2P(abst).

Gibbs, E.L., and Gibbs, F.A. 1951. Electroencephalographic evidence of thalamic and hypothalamic epilepsy. Neurology (Minneapolis) 1:136–144.

Gibbs, F.A., and Gibbs, E.L. 1964. Atlas of Electroencephalography, vol. 3. Reading, MA: Addison-Wesley.

Goldensohn, L.N., Clark, E.R., and Levine, R. 1941. Agenesis of the corpus callosum: report of a case with neuropsychiatric, psychologic, electroencephalographic and pneumoencephalographic studies. J. Nerv. Ment. Dis. 93:567–580.

Granata, T., Battaglia, G., D'Incerti, L., et al. 1996. Schizencephaly: neuroradiologic and epileptologic findings. Epilepsia 37:1185–1193.

Green, J.B., and Russell, D.J. 1966. Electroencephalographic asymmetry with midline cyst and deficient corpus callosum. Neurology (Minneapolis) 16:541–545.

Grünewald-Zuberbier, E., Grünewald, G., and Raschke, A. 1975. Hyperactive behavior and EEG arousal. Electroencephalogr. Clin. Neurophysiol. 38:149–159.

Gururaj, A.K., Sztriha, L., Bener, A., et al. 2003. Epilepsy in children with cerebral palsy seizure. Eur. J. Epilepsy 12:110–114.

Guzzetta, F., Battaglia, D., Lettori, D., et al. 2002. Epileptic negative myoclonus in a newborn with hemimegalencephaly. Epilepsia 43:1106–1109.

Haginoya, K., Kon, K., Tanaka, S., et al. 1999. The origin of hypsarrhythmia and tonic spasms in West syndrome: evidence from a case of porencephaly and hydrocephalus with focal hypsarrhythmia. Brain Dev. 21:129–131.

Hamby, W.S., Krauss, R., and Beswich, W.F. 1950. Hydranencephaly: clinical diagnosis. Presentation of seven cases. Pediatrics 6:371–383.

Henry, C.E. 1963. Positive spike discharges in the EEG and behavior abnormality. In EEG and Behavior, Ed. G.E. Glaser, pp. 315–344. New York: Basic Books.

Heppner, F., and Lechner, H. 1955. Die Bedeutung des EEG für die Diagnose des kindlichen Hydrocephalus. Zbl. Neurochir. 15:11–17.

Hodgkins, P.R., Kris, A., Boyd, S., et al. 2000. A study of EEG, electroretinogram, visual evoked potential and eye movement in classical lissencephaly. Dev. Med. Child Neurol. 42:28–52.

Hughes, J.R. 1978. Electroencephalographic and neurophysiological studies in dyslexia. In Dyslexia: An Appraisal of Current Knowledge, Eds. A.L. Benton and D. Pearl, pp. 205–240. New York: Oxford University Press.

Hughes, J.R., and Park, G.E. 1968. The EEG in dyslexia. In Clinical Electroencephalography in Children, Eds. P. Kellaway and I. Petersén, pp. 307–327. Stockholm: Almqvist and Wiksell.

Hughes, J.R., DeLeo, A.J., and Melyn, M.A. 2000. The electroencephalogram in attention deficit-hyperactivity disorder. Epilepsy Behav. 1:271–274.

Hwang, P.A., Shahar, E., Hoops, R., et al. 1989. The EEG of unilateral megalencephaly. Electroencephalogr. Clin. Neurophysiol. 72:13P–14P (abst).

Iinuma, K., Handa, I., Kojima, A., et al. 1989. Hydranencephaly and maximal hydrocephalus: usefulness of electrophysiological studies for their differentiation. J. Child Neurol. 4:114–117.

John, E.R., Karmel, B.Z., Corning, W.C., et al. 1977. Neurometrics. Science 196:1393–1410.

Kaneko, W.M., Phillips, E.R., Riley, E.P., et al. 1996. EEG findings in fetal alcohol syndrome and Down syndrome children. Electroencephalogr. Clin. Neurophysiol. 98:20–28.

King, M., Stephenson, J.B.P., Ziervogel, M., et al. 1985. Hemimegalencephaly. A case for hemispherectomy? Neuropediatrics 16:46–55.

Klinkerfuss, G.H., Lang, P.H., Weinberg, W.A., et al. 1965. Electroencephalographic abnormalities of children with hyperkinetic behavior. Neurology (Minneapolis) 15:883.

Koeda, T., Knyazeva, M., Nijokiktjien, C., et al. 1995. The EEG in acallosal children. Coherence values in the resting state: Left hemisphere compensatory mechanism? Electroencephalogr. Clin. Neurophysiol. 95:397–407.

Larroche, J.C., and Baudy, J. 1961. Cavum septi pellucidi, cavum Vergae, cavum veli interpositi. Cavités de la ligne médiane. Biol. Neonat. (Basel) 3:193–236.

Laws, E.R., Jr., and Niedermeyer, E. 1970. EEG findings in hydrocephalic patients with shunt procedures. Electroencephalogr. Clin. Neurophysiol. 29:325(abst).

Levav, M., Cruz, M.E., and Mirsky, A.F. 1995. EEG abnormalities, malnutrition, parasitism and goiter: a study of school children in Ecuador. Acta Paediatr. 84:197–202.

Levy-Alcover, N.A., Terris, A., and Tardieu, G. 1959. Étude électroencéphalographique des enfants atteints de séquelles motrices d'encéphalopathies infantiles sans comitialité. Rev. Neurol. (Paris) 100:382–391.

Lindenberg, R. 1955. Compression of brain arteries as pathogenetic factors for tissue necroses and their areas of predilection. J. Neuropath. Experim. Neurol. 14:223–243.

Lindsley, D.B., and Cutts, K.K. 1940. Electroencephalograms of constitutionally inferior and behavior problem children. Comparison of those of normal children and adults. Arch. Neurol. Psychiatry (Chicago) 44:1199–1209.

Lindsley, D.B., and Henry, C.E. 1942. The effects of drugs on behavior and electroencephalogram of children with behavior disorder. Psychosomat. Med. 4:140–149.

Little, S.C. 1965. A general analysis of the fourteen and six per second dysrhythmia. Proceedings of the 6th International Congress of Electroencephalography and Clinical Neurophysiology, Vienna, pp. 313–315. Vienna: Wiener Medizinische Akademie.

Lombroso, C.T., Schwartz, I.H., Clark, D.M., et al. 1966. Ctenoids in healthy youths. Controlled study of 14 and 6-per-second positive spiking. Neurology (Minneapolis) 16:1152–1158.

Lou, H.C., Henriksen, L., and Bruhn, P. 1984. Focal cerebral hypoperfusion in children with dysphasia and/or attention deficit disorder. Arch. Neurol. 41:825–829.

MacKeith, R.C. 1963. Defining the concept of "minimal brain damage." *Proceedings of the International Study Group, Oxford,* 1962, Little Club Clinic. Develop. Med. No. 10, pp. 1–9. National Spastics Society. London: Heinemann.

McAbee, G.N., Chan, A., and Erde, E.L. 2000. Prolonged survival with hydranencephaly: report of two patients with literature review. Pediatr. Neurol. 23:80–84.

Metcalf, D.R. 1963. Controlled studies of the incidence and significance of 6 and 14 per second positive spiking. Electroencephalogr. Clin. Neurophysiol. 15:161(abst).

Murphy, J.P., and Garvin, J.S. 1947. The electroencephalogram in porencephaly. Arch. Neurol. Psychiatry (Chicago) 58:436–446.

Niedermeyer, E. 2001. Frontal lobe disinhibition, Rett syndrome, and attention deficit hyperactivity disorder. Clin. Electroencephalogr. 32:20–23.

Niedermeyer, E., and Knott, J.R. 1961. Über die Bedeutung der 14 and 6/sec-positiven Spitzen im EEG. Arch. Psychiatr. Nervenkr. 206:266–280.

Niedermeyer, E., and Naidu, S. 1996. Rett syndrome, EEG and sensorimotor cortex. Proceed. World Congr. Rett Syndrome, Goeteborg.

Niedermeyer, E., and Yarworth, S. 1978. Scarcity of minor EEG abnormalities during the first two years of life. Clin. Electroencephalogr. 9:20–28.

Niedermeyer, E., Naidu, S., and Plate, C. 1997. Unusual EEG theta rhythms over central region in Rett syndrome and considerations of underlying mechanisms. Clin. Electroencephalogr. 28:36–43.

Norman, R. 1966. The pathogenesis of temporal lobe epilepsy. In *Biological Factors in Temporal Lobe Epilepsy. Clinics in Developmental Medicine No. 22.* Eds. C. Ounsted, J. Lindsay, and R. Norman. pp. 32–49. London: Heineman.

Ohtsuka, Y., Ohno, S., and Oka, E. 1999. Electroclinical characteristics of hemimegalencephaly. Pediatr. Neurol. 20:390–393.

Paine, R.S. 1962. Minimal chronic brain syndromes in children. Dev. Med. Child. Neurol. 4:21.

Pampiglione, G., and Lawrence, M. 1962. EEG and clinico-pathological observations in hydrocephalic children. Arch. Dis. Child 37:491–499.

Panteliadis, C., Jacobi, G., Covanis, A., et al. 2002. Epilepsy in children with congenital hemiplegia: correlation between clinical EEG and neuroimaging findings. Epileptic Disord. 4:251–255.

Perlstein, M.A., and Gibbs, F.A. 1949. Clinical significance of electroencephalography in cases of cerebral paralysis. Arch. Neurol. Psychiatry (Chicago) 62:682–685.

Perlstein, M.A., Gibbs, E.L., and Gibbs, F.A. 1955. The electroencephalogram in infantile cerebral palsy. Am. J. Phys. Med. 34:477–496.

Pohowalla, P., McIntyre, H.B., and Worthen, N. 1984. EEG in neonatal intracranial cysts. Electroencephalogr. Clin. Neurophysiol. 58:36P(abst).

Puech, P., Guilly, P., Fischgold, H., et al. 1947. Un cas d'anencéphalique hydrocéphalique. Étude électroencéphalographique. Rev. Neurol. (Paris) 79:117–124.

Radermecker, F.J. 1960. Das Elektroenzephalogramm bei den Encephalitiden und Encephalopathien des Kindesalters. Nervenarzt. 31:529–541.

Richer, L.P., Shevell, M.I., and Rosenblatt, B.R. 2002. Epileptiform abnormalities in children with attention-deficit-hyperactivity disorder. Pediatr. Neurol. 26:125–129.

Salmelin, R., Helenius, P., and Service, E. 2000. Neurophysiology of fluent and impaired reading: a magnetoencephalographic approach. J. Clin. Neurophysiol. 17:163–174.

Sato, O., Yamaguchi, T., Kittaka, M., et al. 2001. Hydrocephalus and epilepsy. Child Nerv. Syst. 17:76–86.

Satterfield, J.H., and Schell, A.M. 1984. Childhood brain function differences in delinquent and non-delinquent hyperactive boys. Electroencephalogr. Clin. Neurophysiol. 57:199–207.

Schwade, E.D., and Geiger, S.G. 1956. Abnormal electroencephalographic findings in severe behavior disorders. Dis. Nerv. Syst. 17:307–317.

Schwartz, P. 1924. Erkrankungen der Zentral-nervensystems nach traumatischer Geburtsschädigung. Z. ges. Neurol. Psychiat. 90:263–468.

Senebil, N., Sonnel, B., Aydin, O.F., et al. 2002. Epileptic and non-epileptic cerebral palsy: EEG and cranial imaging findings. Brain Dev. 24:166–169.

Shinners, B.M., Krauss, R.F., and Maddigan, C. 1950. High beta rhythm in children: its clinical significance. Electroencephalogr. Clin. Neurophysiol. 2:360.

Singh, R., Sutherland, G.R., and Manson, J. 1999. Partial seizures with focal epileptogenic electroencephalographic patterns in three related female patients with fragile-X syndrome. J. Child Neurol. 14:108–112.

Skatvedt, M. 1958. *Cerebral Palsy.* Oslo: University Press.

Skatvedt, M., and Lundervold, A. 1956. The significance of electroencephalographic spike foci in patients with cerebral palsy without epileptogenic seizures. Acta Paediat. (Uppsala) 45:440–443.

Slatter, G.A., and Torres, F. 1979. Frequency-amplitude gradient. A new parameter for interpreting pediatric sleep EEG. Arch. Neurol. (Chicago) 36:465–470.

Solomon, P., Jasper, H.H., and Bradley, C. 1937. Studies in behavior problem children. Arch. Neurol. Psychiatry (Chicago) 38:1350–1351.

Solomon, P., Bradley, C., and Jasper, H.H. 1938. Electroencephalographic analyses of behavior problem children. Am. J. Psychiatry 95:641–658.

Steger, J, Imhof, K., Steinhausen, H.C., et al. 2000. Brain mapping of bilateral interactions in attention deficit hyperactivity disorder and control boys. Clin. Neurophysiol. 111:1141–1156.

Stern, H., Elek, S.D., Booth, J.C., et al. 1969. Microbial causes of mental retardation. The role of prenatal infections with cytomegalovirus, rubella virus and toxoplasma. Lancet 2:443–448.

Sutton, L.N., Bruce, D.A., and Schut, L. 1980. Hydranencephaly versus maximal hydrocephalus. An important clinical distinction. Neurosurgery 6:35–38.

Tjiam, A.T., Stefanko, S., Schenk, V.W.D., et al. 1978. Infantile spasms associated with hemihypsarrhythmia and hemimegalencephaly. Dev. Med. Child Neurol. 20:779–798.

Vigevano, F., Aicardi, J., Lini, M., et al. 1984. La sindrome del nevo sebaceo lineare: presentazione di una casistica multicentrica. Boll. Lega Ital. Epilessia. 45/46:59–63.

Walker, A.E. 1942. Lissencephaly. Arch. Neurol. Psychiatry 48:13.

Walker, C.F., and Kirkpatrick, B.B. 1947. Dilantin treatment for behavior problems in children with abnormal electroencephalograms. Am. J. Psychiatry 103:484–492.

Walter, R.D., Colbert, E.G., Koegler, R.R., et al. 1960. A controlled study of the fourteen- and six-per-second EEG pattern. Arch. Neurol. (Chicago) 2:559–566.

Watanabe, K., Yamada, H., Hara, K., et al. 1984. Neurophysiological evaluation of newborns with congenital hydrocephalus. Clin. Electroencephalogr. 15:22–31.

Yakovlev, P.I., and Wadsworth, R.C. 1946. Schizencephalies. A study of the congenital clefts in the cerebral mantle. 1. Clefts with fused lips. J. Neuropathol. Exp. Neurol. 5:116–130.

Yingling, C.D., Galin, D., Fein, G., et al. 1986. Neurometrics does not detect "pure" dyslexics. Electroencephalogr. Clin. Neurophysiol. 43:426–430.

21. Craniocerebral Trauma

Erik Rumpl

A craniocerebral trauma raises the important question of the degree of cerebral disturbance. This question may be answered easily in cases of commotio cerebri or slight concussion of the brain; this is a reversible impairment of consciousness of brief duration with no clinical evidence of any gross structural change in the brain substance. The question of brain function becomes more important in cases of cerebral contusion after more severe injury with prolonged unconsciousness and signs of brainstem dysfunction. Brainstem damage may result from primary brainstem injury (Jellinger, 1967; Maciver et al., 1958) or from secondary brainstem lesion due to downward transtentorial herniation (Jefferson, 1952). It has been shown that brainstem injury does not exist in isolation; it is merely one aspect of diffuse brain damage (Mitchell and Adams, 1973).

The clinical parameter of the grade of disintegration of brain function and impairment of the brainstem is demonstrated by the development of an acute secondary midbrain and bulbar brain syndrome. The symptoms of the well-known rostrocaudal deterioration, first described by McNealy and Plum (1962) and Plum and Posner (1966) and modified by Gerstenbrand and Lücking (1970), allow a clear clinical statement about the depth of posttraumatic coma. In addition to the neurological examination, cranial computed tomography (CT) and magnetic resonance tomography (MRI) easily identify a space-occupying lesion and sometimes demonstrates the displacement of the brainstem (Osborn, 1977; Reich et al., 1993). These methods, however, fail to give any information about cerebral activity. Therefore, the electroencephalogram (EEG) is still important in the diagnosis of traumatic cerebral lesions, especially in the assessment of the degree of cortical activity, which shows reasonably good correlation with the depth of posttraumatic coma (Arfel, 1975; Bricolo and Turella, 1973; Chatrian et al., 1963; Rumpl et al., 1979; Silverman, 1963; Stone et al., 1988; Synek, 1990).

Chronic stages of craniocerebral trauma demonstrate a diminished electroencephalographic-neurological correlation (Jung, 1953; Lücking et al., 1977; Meyer-Mickeleit, 1953; Mifka and Scherzer, 1962b; Radermecker, 1964). However, there is an approximate correlation between the EEG and clinical improvement, especially in patients who have had systematic follow-up studies of EEG and clinical examination (Courjon and Scherzer, 1972; Jabbari et al., 1986; Koufen and Dichgans, 1978; Koufen and Hagel, 1987). Occasionally, the EEG may return to normal when neurological or psychiatric abnormalities persist, a disparity that indicates a bad prognosis (Lücking et al., 1977; Strnad and Strnadová, 1987; Walter et al., 1948; Williams, 1941b). By contrast, in some patients with normal clinical findings,

an abnormal EEG may be the forerunner of an intracranial complication such as posttraumatic epilepsy (Courjon and Scherzer, 1972).

Earlier EEG Work in Craniocerebral Trauma

Williams (1941a) studied a few patients after mild craniocerebral trauma and observed that normal records can be obtained within a few hours of injury. Further electroencephalographic studies in brain injuries were done by Dow et al. (1944), who included patients with more severe injuries and repeated studies during the recovery of the patients. Dawson et al. (1951) continued to observe patients and studied the evolution of abnormalities with repeated records. Extensive work in this field was done by Meyer-Mickeleit (1953), Schneider and Hubach (1962), Courjon and Scherzer (1972), and Koufen and Dichgans (1978).

The impairment of consciousness to any degree was usually found to be accompanied by an abnormal EEG (Dow et al., 1944; Dawson et al., 1951; Duensing, 1948; Meyer-Mickeleit, 1953; Scherzer, 1965; Schneider and Hubach, 1962). Most of these authors directed their attention to the frequency of the basic activity and to focal, general, or epileptic abnormalities, but no further distinction of the EEG pattern was made. High-voltage delta activity was regarded as the electroencephalographic correlate of coma, which in turn was considered an equivalent of deep sleep (Davis and Davis, 1939; Hill, 1950; Schwab, 1951). Further studies in coma (Fischgold and Mathis, 1959; Loeb, 1958; Mathis et al., 1957) made it clear that states of coma were associated with a variety of EEG patterns, often with the criteria of sleep (Chatrian et al., 1963; Naquet et al., 1967; Silverman, 1963). The manifestation of sleep patterns appeared to be of prognostic significance, supported by the results of overnight or prolonged EEG recordings (Bergamasco et al., 1968; Bricolo et al., 1968; Valente et al., 2002). The role of reactivity in the assessment of the depth of coma was first pointed out by Fischgold et al. (1955) and is an important prognostic indicator for good outcome (Fischer and Mutschler, 2002). In addition to these findings, asymmetry in reactivity was considered a reliable lateralizing sign (Courjon et al., 1971).

During the last decade, important reviews concerning posttraumatic comatose states have given detailed insight into the EEG in altered states of consciousness (Arfel, 1975; Chatrian, 1975; Vigouroux, 1975). Early and late changes of the EEG after craniocerebral trauma were discussed extensively by Courjon and Scherzer (1972) and Stockard et al. (1975).

Experimental Work

Williams and Denny-Brown (1941) found an immediate reduction in amplitude (sometimes approaching isoelectricity) in the EEG in cats subjected to experimental head concussion. After a short period of delta activity, the EEG returned to normal within a period of seconds to a few minutes. Dow et al. (1944) studied the physical factors responsible for the injury in humans. These factors appeared to be of the same order as those necessary to produce experimental concussion in animals (Denny-Brown and Russel, 1941). Interestingly, the threshold velocity that provoked concussion at the moment of impact in animals also marked the limit between the average velocity in patients with borderline and abnormal EEG (Dow et al., 1944). Other than this finding, pathological observations made in humans could not be convincingly duplicated in experimental studies. This might be due to the smaller mass of brain in animals and the restriction in impact techniques (Ommaya and Gennarelli, 1974; Ommaya et al., 1971). Even in standardized animal experiments, the analysis of the EEG did not provide adequate indices of injury severity, and there was no correlation found with the duration of coma (Ommaya et al., 1973).

Following the convulsive theory of slight concussion (Shaw, 2002) the energy imported to the brain may generate turbulent rotatory and other movements of the cerebral hemispheres provoking a convulsive disorder, which might present a mild form of cerebral concussion with a sudden short loss of consciousness, paralysis of reflex activity, and loss of memory (commotio cerebri). This theory may explain the observation that the EEG returns to normal within 24 hours in these cases.

Some closer correlations to EEG changes in comatose states in humans were found in other animal experiments producing localized destructive brain lesions or using local electrical stimulation. Local lesions in the white matter and in thalamic structures were immediately followed by the appearance of delta waves, which were accompanied by spindles in the case of thalamic lesions. Slow activity developed gradually in mesencephalic reticular formation lesions; it was absent in cortical lesions (Gloor et al., 1977). EEG changes similar to those seen in thalamic destructive lesions were found after stimulation of thalamic nuclei (Akert et al., 1952; Hunter and Jasper, 1949). Stimulation at the level of the mesencephalic reticulum induced behavior and EEG arousal in sleeping in otherwise intact animals, whereas destructive lesions at mesencephalic levels caused coma and EEG activity reminiscent of different types of sleep (Jouvet, 1961). All these mechanisms may be involved in posttraumatic comatose states as long as delta waves and spindles are generated by otherwise relatively normal cortical neurons.

EEG Changes in the Acute Stages of Posttraumatic Coma

Comatose posttraumatic states may be associated with a multitude of abnormal waveforms other than delta (Chatrian et al., 1963; Fischgold and Mathis, 1959; Mathis et al., 1957; Silverman, 1963). These abnormal waveforms, especially the different patterns of sleep, depend above all on the patient's level of consciousness (Chatrian, 1975). Therefore, a detailed neurological description of comatose patients is necessary to define coma (Fischer, 1969) in order to establish a sufficient correlation between different EEG changes and different stages of coma.

Classification of EEG

Different parameters have been used in the breakdown of EEG signs in comatose states (Arfel, 1975; Bricolo and Turella, 1973; Chatrian et al., 1963; Courjon and Scherzer, 1972; Fischgold and Mathis, 1959; Hockaday et al., 1965; Kubicki et al., 1970; Prior, 1973; Silverman, 1963). To increase the value of the EEG in posttraumatic coma, all these parameters were integrated and correlated with the stages of rostrocaudal deterioration (Rumpl et al., 1979).

The EEG abnormalities may be classified in five grades (Rumpl et al., 1979): grade 1, predominant alpha and little theta activity; grade 2, predominant theta and little delta activity; grade 3, predominant high-voltage rhythmic and arrhythmic delta and subdelta activity; grade 4, diffuse, mostly low-voltage delta and subdelta activity and low-voltage activity only recognizable with increased amplification (3.5 μV/mm); and grade 5, isoelectric record.

Other signs apart from these grades can also be noted in the EEG: (a) superimposed fast activity (6–18 c/sec localized over the frontal region or diffusely spread; (b) normal-looking sleep records; (c) diffuse slowing accompanied by "typical sleep potentials" (spindles, vertex sharp waves, K complexes); (d) diffuse slowing accompanied by altered "sleep potentials," listed under "atypical sleep potentials"; (e) spontaneously alternating EEG patterns with a rapid succession of low-voltage delta activity and high-voltage slow waves [this activity can be classified as delta bursts (0.5–2 seconds) and short (2–5 seconds) and long (more than 5 seconds in duration) runs of delta with frequencies of 0.5–4 c/sec]; (f) "lateralized signs" such as local slow activity ("local slowing"), unilateral predominant slow activity, unilateral low-voltage output, and unilateral depression of superimposed fast activity listed under the heading of "unilateral predominant slowing," asymmetries of "typical or atypical sleep potentials," and asymmetries of response to external stimuli; (g) four types of reaction to external stimuli: (1) appearance of widespread 1 to 7 c/sec activity, (2) blocking of slow activity, (3) appearance of alternating EEG patterns, and (4) appearance or disappearance of "typical or atypical sleep potentials"; and (h) epileptiform patterns: (1) focal or generalized runs of spikes and sharp spike waves, (2) periodic lateralized epileptiform discharges (PLEDs), and (3) triphasic waves.

Reactivity may be immediate or delayed. Delayed reactivity is a slow EEG response inducing a new pattern under the influence of repetitive stimulation (Arfel, 1975). Fischgold and Mathis (1959) emphasize the usefulness of auditory and painful stimuli in contrast to the insignificant effect of visual stimulation. In lighter stages of coma, stimulation may also provoke extracerebral changes such as muscle activity and respiratory artifacts.

Classification of Coma

Physiologically, the loss of consciousness implies that the patient has suffered widespread dysfunction of cerebral hemi-

Table 21.1. Clinical Signs in Posttraumatic Patients at the Different Stages of the Midbrain Syndrome (MBS) and Bulbar Brain Syndrome (BBS)[a]

	MBS 1	MBS 2	MBS 3	MBS 4	BBS 1	BBS 2
Spontaneous limb postures	Nonstereotyped movements in the arms and legs	Nonstereotyped movements in the arms Extension of the legs	Decorticate posturing	Decerebrate posturing	Flaccidity	Flaccidity
Motor response to pain	Nonstereotyped withdrawal of the limbs	Nonstereotyped withdrawal of the arms Extensor response of the legs	Decorticate response	Decerebrate response	Decerebrate response	No response
Eye position	Roving movements	Roving, more irregular movements	Immobile, straight ahead	Immobile, divergent	Immobile, divergent	Immobile, divergent
Pupil size and reaction	Normal Reacting	Normal small Reacting	Small Small range of contraction	Enlarged Small range of contraction	Large Unreacting	Large Unreacting
Respiration pattern	Normal	Cheyne-Stokes	Cheyne-Stokes Rapid regular hyperventilation	Regular hyperventilation	Ataxic	No respiration

[a]From Rumpl, E., Prugger, M., Bauer, G., et al. 1983. Incidence and prognostic value of spindles in post-traumatic coma. Electroencephalogr. Clin. Neurophysiol. 56:420–429.

spheres or the brainstem or both. When there is a diffuse swelling of the brain or bilateral hemispheric lesions, the cerebral hemispheres, the diencephalon, and the adjoining midbrain are displaced downward through the tentorial notch. In this case, the herniation through the tentorium is symmetrical (central tentorial herniation). If downward displacement continues, the contents of the posterior fossa will finally be pressed through the foramen magnum. This brain shift evokes a number of characteristic clinical signs that have been described by various authors (Gerstenbrand and Lücking, 1970; McNealy and Plum, 1962; Plum and Posner, 1966). The most prominent clinical signs of central herniation are listed in Table 21.1. According to Gerstenbrand and Lücking (1970) posttraumatic comatose states can be broken down into six stages, including four stages of midbrain syndrome (MBS) and two stages of bulbar brain syndrome (BBS). With regard to the terminology of Plum and Posner (1966), MBS 1 and MBS 2 correspond to the early diencephalic stage, MBS 3 to the late diencephalic stage, MBS 4 to the midbrain-upper pons stage, BBS 1 to the lower pontine-upper medullary stage, and BBS 2 to the medullary stage.

In cases with expanding lesions in the lateral middle fossa or temporal lobe, the medial edges of the uncus and hippocampal gyrus are commonly pushed toward the midline and over the free lateral edge of the tentorium, compressing the third cranial nerve (early uncal herniation). During uncal herniation, an unilateral dilated pupil is the most consistent finding (Plum and Posner, 1966). Other neurological signs may be present at this early stage and may provide hints concerning the original hemispheric lesion. Once the pupil dilates fully (late uncal herniation), the patients become comatose, and abnormal postures and motor responses evolve (Gerstenbrand and Rumpl, 1983; Plum and Posner, 1966). Eventually, with increasing intracranial pressure, lateralizing signs disappear and the patients show the clinical signs of MBS 4 or BBS 1.

Neurological signs different from this expected rostrocaudal deterioration may be found in cases of primary brainstem injury. Maciver et al. (1958) state that a primary brainstem lesion can be suspected if the neurological signs do not fit the classical stages of rostrocaudal deterioration (i.e., the relatively intact oculomotor functions are in contrast to decerebrate posturing and respiratory abnormalities). The CT scan is diagnostic and eliminates a supratentorial lesion causing secondary brainstem dysfunction. The MRI scan shows the extent of brainstem damage in the further course.

Relation of EEG Abnormalities to the Stage of Coma

The EEG patterns in the different stages of MBS and BBS are presented in Fig. 21.1. The significance of this observation is somewhat hampered by the fact that the figure presents EEG data obtained within 1 week after brain injury, thereby neglecting the special behavior of spindle activity (see Relation of EEG Abnormalities to Outcome, below). Nevertheless, the figure demonstrates well the principal relation of EEG to the stages of coma. There is a decrease in the number of different EEG patterns related to the stages of MBS and BBS, indicating the increase of intracranial pressure. Unfavorable prognosis is shown by the disappearance of "typical or atypical sleep potentials," alternating patterns, and loss of reactivity (Arfel, 1975; Bricolo et al., 1968; Chatrian et al., 1963; Courjon and Scherzer, 1972; Rumpl et al., 1979; Silverman, 1963). In accordance with the mildly diffuse cortical disturbance, the EEG is slightly or moderately abnormal in MBS 1.

Stimuli to diencephalic or rostromesencephalic structures (Bricolo, 1975) may induce delta bursts or short runs of delta waves. Local slow activity can be seen only in an otherwise mildly abnormal EEG, while increasing diffuse slowing may overwhelm local abnormalities (Hess, 1961). Borderline EEG patterns occur at MBS 1 but not in deeper

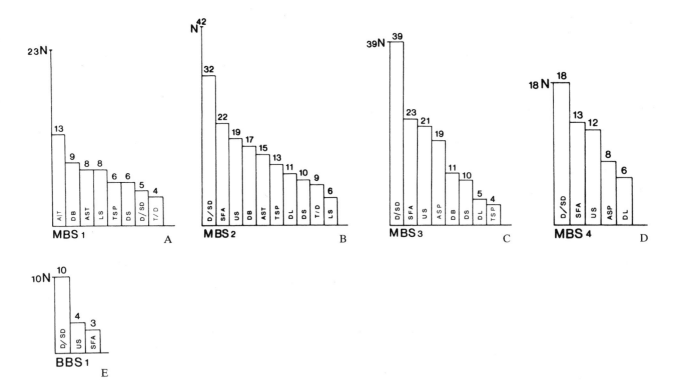

Figure 21.1. The EEG patterns at the different stages of acute traumatic secondary midbrain and bulbar brain syndrome. Note reduction in the variety of EEG patterns in the course of increasing rostrocaudal deterioration. At bulbar brain syndrome stage 2, the EEG is isoelectric. The records were listed under one or more of the following categories: A/T, predominant alpha and little theta activity; T/D, predominant theta and little delta activity; D/SD, predominant diffuse rhythmic and arrhythmic delta and subdelta activity; DB, delta bursts; DS, short runs of delta; DL, long runs of delta; TSP, typical sleep potentials; ASP, atypical sleep potentials; S, spindles; LS, local slowing; US, unilateral predominant slowing; SFA, superimposed fast activity; MBS, midbrain syndrome; BBS, bulbar brain syndrome; *N*, number of records. (From Rumpl, E. 1979. Elektro-neurologische Korrelationen in den frühen Phasen des posttraumatischen Komas. I. Das EEG in den verschiedenen Phasen des akuten traumatischen sekundären. Mittelhirn und Bulbärhirnsyndroms. Z. EEG-EMG 10:148–157; and Rumpl, E., Lorenzi, E., Hackl, J.M., et al. 1979. The EEG at different stages of acute secondary traumatic midbrain and bulbar brain syndromes. Electroencephalogr. Clin. Neurophysiol. 46:487–497, somewhat modified).

stages of MBS. In MBS 2, the amount of slow activity increases. This increasing abnormality may be due to a direct cortical disturbance (Hess, 1965) or to a more remote effect from deeper structures (Bricolo, 1975; Lücking, 1970). However, "sleep or sleep-like potentials" (see Figs. 21.6A and 21.7A) indicate a relatively intact cortex (Silverman, 1963). In MBS 2, the EEG shows the widest range of different EEG patterns. In MBS 3, a clear reduction in the number of EEG patterns is noted. A decrease of spontaneous alternating patterns and "sleep potentials" has been thought to indicate an increasing disturbance of the diencephalic and mesencephalic systems (Chatrian et al., 1963).

Increasing rostrocaudal deterioration is further characterized by the increased change of typical or atypical sleep potentials (Silverman, 1963) and the shift of superimposed fast activity, diffusely spread in lighter stages of MBS, to the frontal regions (Rumpl, 1979). The EEG patterns are still more simplified in MBS 4 and BBS 1. The absence, reduction, and deterioration of sleep potentials or alternating patterns are suggestive of marked damage at the diencephalic level (Bricolo et al., 1968; Naquet et al., 1967). The telencephalon (Arfel, 1975) must also be involved, considering the diffuse brain edema in advanced stages of MBS. In BBS 1, low-voltage delta and subdelta activity appears, followed

by low-voltage cerebral activity, often recognizable only with increased amplification. No electrical cerebral activity can be observed in patients with BBS 2 (Rumpl et al., 1979). Patients with an isoelectric EEG or an EEG with repeated isoelectric periods will die (Hutchinson et al., 1991). The high prognostic value of an EEG classification with a great number of different EEG patterns was supported by the development of an EEG score, which included many of these phenomena weighted according to their perceived prognostic value and scored as dichotomous variables—present or absent (Rae-Grant et al., 1991).

Unreactive alpha activity or "alpha-like" rhythms (Chokroverty, 1975) are not seen in patients in BBS 1 after supratentorial lesions causing secondary brainstem involvement. This pattern usually appears in polytraumatic patients at this stage, and thereby strongly suggests an additional hypoxic or anoxic cerebral lesion. The same suggestion can be made with theta-pattern coma, which was found to be a variant of alpha coma (Synek and Synek, 1984). Usually, both patterns are predictors of fatal outcome. Rhythmic coma in children especially in the alpha frequency range has generally a better prognosis than in adults (Horton et al., 1990).

Primary brainstem injuries may produce clinical symptoms that are hardly separable from symptoms of secondary brainstem injury caused by downward herniation. Although primary brainstem damage rarely exists in pure form (Mitchell and Adams, 1973), a primary brainstem lesion may be the principal cause of coma. In these cases, the EEG can be a helpful diagnostic tool. Patients in coma from caudally placed brainstem lesions may have nonreactive alpha activity even in an unresponsive decerebrate state (Chatrian et al., 1964a). Sleep spindles, vertex sharp waves, and K complexes suggest that the lesion is below the still intact thalamocortical system (Jasper and Van Buren, 1953). This suggestion has been confirmed by Steudel et al. (1979), who described brainstem lesions with evidence based on cranial CT and autopsy findings in all their decerebrate patients with spindles and/or alpha activity in the EEG. During the first week, these activities were replaced by delta waves, indicating that EEG patterns similar to the one seen in prolonged comatose states are rare (Chatrian, 1975; Rumpl, 1980).

The reaction to external stimuli further characterizes the depth of coma (Arfel, 1975; Courjon and Scherzer, 1975). In MBS 1, sensory stimulation may briefly block the slow activity; sleep, easily recognizable at this stage, may have a similar effect (Stockard et al., 1975). In further stages of MBS, reactivity consists of widespread delta activity, alternating patterns, and typical or atypical sleep potentials (see Fig. 21.13A). In BBS 1 and BBS 2, no reactivity can be observed.

Generalized burst suppression occurs in posttraumatic coma only when cerebral anoxia was sustained with the trauma (Rumpl, 1979; Stockard et al., 1975). Burst suppression activity due to an overdose of soporific drugs tends to produce uniform intersuppression activity, in contrast to the intersuppression activity in anoxic coma, in which delta waves and intermittent spikes are observed frequently (Stockard et al., 1975). This type of activity carries a poor prognosis because it indicates a diffuse anoxic encephalopathy that interferes with the original traumatic brain damage.

Metabolic derangements certainly have an important impact on coma and accompanying EEG abnormalities (Arfel, 1975; Goulon et al., 1959; Merill and Hampers, 1970; Naquet et al., 1967; Silverman, 1963; Wilson and Sieker, 1958). The number of metabolic disturbances is obviously higher in patients in deep stages of posttraumatic coma (Rumpl et al., 1979). Most of these patients suffer from multiple trauma including the liver, kidneys, and lungs. The combination of metabolic and traumatic encephalopathy carries the worst prognosis. The EEG changes due to metabolic disturbance interfere with the EEG changes because of the herniation itself, thus blurring the rules concerning the decrease of different EEG patterns with advancing deterioration. Further influences on the EEG are caused by the effects of sedative or anesthetic drugs frequently used in intensive care units.

Early electroencephalographic seizure activity is only seen in cases of severe craniocerebral trauma, in which patients may have clinical seizures shortly before or shortly after the discharges are found in the EEG (Fig. 21.2). Acute epileptic and paroxysmal EEG discharges may also accompany nonconvulsive (subclinical) seizures or status epilepticus in severe brain injuries. In cases of nonconvulsive seizures or status, a more severe clinical picture is simu-

lated. Seizures either are generalized from the start or more often are focal with subsequent generalization (Courjon and Scherzer, 1972). Focal seizure activity consists of runs of spikes and sharp waves and is more likely to occur in patients with underlying intracranial hematoma. The EEG is of considerable localizing value in these cases, and there has been only one reported case of focal seizure activity occurring contralateral to the posttraumatic hematoma (Courjon and Scherzer, 1972).

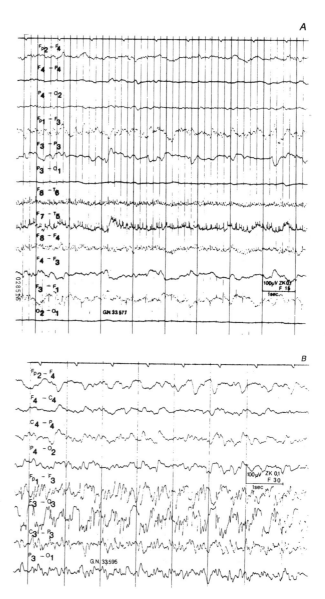

Figure 21.2. **A:** EEG from 32-year-old woman in midbrain syndrome stage 2 and with clinical signs of a left hemisphere lesion. No clinical evidence of epileptic fits. Unilateral predominant slowing in the left hemisphere. Sharp waves in left upper frontal region. **B:** EEG from the same patient in midbrain syndrome stage 1, one day after first recording. Right-sided clinical focal motor attacks. Continuous focal spikes in left upper frontal-central region. (From Rumpl, E. 1979. Elektro-neurologische Korrelationen in den frühen Phasen des posttraumatischen Komas. I. Das EEG in den verschiedenen Phasen des akuten traumatischen sekundären. Mittelhirn und Bulbärhirnsyndroms. Z. EEG-EMG 10:148–157.)

Usually, the appearance of the electroencephalographic seizure activity at these stages of coma carries a worse prognosis (Courjon and Scherzer, 1972) and is associated with a mortality that is about three times higher than in the absence of seizure activity (Stockard et al., 1975). Additionally, status epilepticus associated with generalized motor seizures may be the result of severe cerebral trauma. Death occurs in more than 50% of these cases within the first few days (Courjon and Scherzer, 1972). In children, posttraumatic status epilepticus is associated with a far less ominous prognosis than in adults (Grand, 1974). Isolated spikes and slow waves are rare after a recent injury (Kiloh and Osselton, 1966), but they may occur in severe cases. Although prognosis in cases with early seizures is generally bad, acute convulsions are a more serious complication in patients with brain tumor and metabolic encephalopathies (Bauer and Niedermeyer, 1979). Unfortunately, quantitative EEG has difficulties detecting spikes, brief seizures, burst suppression, PLEDs, triphasic waves, and intermittent theta and delta activity. Therefore, the use of serial standard EEG recordings at least three times a week is still required in intensive care patients (Jordan, 1993).

PLEDs are rare events in posttraumatic coma; they are usually seen in cases of subdural hematoma (Toyonaga et al., 1974). More frequent PLEDs are seen in patients with acute unilateral lesions of vascular origin (Chatrian et al., 1964b; Markand and Daly, 1971). Triphasic waves may also be produced by subdural hematoma, but they are more characteristic of metabolic disturbances (Bickford and Butt, 1955; Hall and Joffe, 1973), especially when no asymmetry can be detected.

The lateralizing signs in the EEG (other than epileptic discharges) demonstrate a close correlation to the lateralizing signs of the neurological examination (Fig. 21.3). In

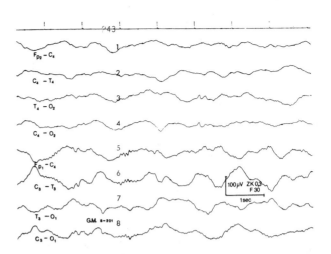

Figure 21.4. EEG from 42-year-old man in midbrain syndrome stage 3, one day after surgical evacuation of a right epidural hematoma. Unilateral slowing in right hemisphere and asymmetrical (and mildly atypical) spindles point to the original lesion.

MBS 4 and BBS 1, the neurological examination reveals no lateralizing signs at all. At these stages, the EEG gives a hint of local cerebral lesion. The localized signs in the EEG may accompany all local cerebral lesions including the three major types of hematoma—subdural, epidural, and intracerebral (Fig. 21.4). Asymmetry in reactivity (Courjon et al., 1971) is helpful to ascertain uncertain lateralizing signs in the acute stages of coma (see Chapter 26, Fig. 26.9); in prolonged comatose states, asymmetry often does not manifest itself unless the patient is stimulated (Stockard et al., 1975).

Relation of EEG Abnormalities to Outcome

According to Jennet and Bond (1975), patient outcome may be classified in four categories: death, severe disability, moderate disability, and good recovery. In the results presented here, the category of severe disability includes patients in an apallic (vegetative) state. Because there has been much doubt concerning the prognostic significance of spindle activity in posttraumatic coma, special attention was paid to spindle activity in a study based on 70 EEGs taken in the acute stage of coma (within the first 2 days after brain injury) and 63 EEGs recorded in a prolonged comatose state (days 3 through 12 after brain injury). The incidence of spindles, form of spindles, and asymmetries of spindle activity in the different outcome categories are listed in Table 21.2. (Rumpl et al., 1983).

In patients with good recovery, spindles are seen in all EEGs recorded during the acute stage of coma (100%). Atypical (8%) and asymmetrical spindles (12%) were rarely observed in these cases. In prolonged coma, spindles occurred in only 44% of patients with good outcome; there were atypical spindles in 11% and asymmetry in 25% of spindle EEGs. The EEGs of patients with moderate disability outcome showed spindles in 90% of all records during the acute stage of coma, but atypical spindles (33%) and asymmetry (33%) significantly increased. A remarkable increase of atypical spindles (50%) was seen in prolonged coma. The EEGs of patients who developed severe disability showed spindles in 61% of

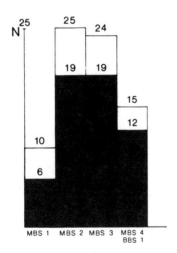

Figure 21.3. Correlation of lateralizing signs in the EEG with the neurological or postmortem examinations. *Dark columns* demonstrate corresponding neurological and EEG signs of lateralization in midbrain syndrome (MBS) stages 1, 2, and 3. In midbrain syndrome stage 4 and bulbar brain syndrome (BBS) stage 1 (listed in one column), results of the autopsy have to be used in some cases to determine lateralization. (From Rumpl, E., Lorenzi, E., Hackl, J.M., et al. 1979. The EEG at different stages of acute secondary traumatic midbrain and bulbar brain syndromes. Electroencephalogr. Clin. Neurophysiol. 46:487–497.)

Table 21.2. Incidence of Spindles, Form of Spindles, and Asymmetries of Spindle Activity in Different Outcome Categories[a]

Outcome Categories	Acute Coma (Total %)							Prolonged Coma (Total %)						
	N^b	Spindles		Atypical		Asymmetry Spindles		N	Spindles		Atypical		Asymmetry Spindles	
Good recovery	26	26	100	2	8	3	12	18	8	44	2	11	2	25
Moderate disability	10	9	90	3	33	3	33	7	4	57	2	50	1	25
Severe disability	18	11	61	5	45	7	63	21	5	24	5	100	2	40
Brain death	16	9	56	4	44	8	88	17	2	12	1	50	2	100
Total coma	70	64	91	14	22	24	33	63	19	30	10	53	7	37

[a]The percentages of atypical spindles and symmetry of spindles remarkably increase with worsening of outcome. Spindles are seen in most cases in acute coma within the first 2 days after injury but show clear reduction in prolonged coma (days 3 to 12 after injury) (from Rumpl, E., Prugger, M., Bauer, G., et al. 1983. Incidence and prognostic value of spindles in post-traumatic coma. Electroencephalogr. Clin. Neurophysiol. 56:420–429.)
[b]N, number of patients and EEGs.

all cases. Atypical spindles were found in 45%; asymmetry was found in 63% of spindle EEGs. Patients with prolonged coma and subsequent severe disability showed only atypical spindles, and the percentage of spindles decreased to 24%. Asymmetries were seen in 40%. Patients who suffered brain death within 2 weeks after trauma showed spindles in 56% in the acute stage of coma. Asymmetry of spindles was seen in 88% and atypical spindles were seen in 44% of spindle coma. In prolonged coma, spindles were seen in only two cases (12%), and both were asymmetrical.

From these findings, one can conclude that the observation of spindles largely depends on the time of the EEG recording. Variations of the timing of EEG recordings account for the incidence of spindles varying between 14% and 67% in different reports (Bergamasco et al., 1968; Steudel et al., 1979) and may also explain why the prognostic value of spindles was doubted (Hansotia et al., 1981; Hughes et al., 1976; Lorenzoni, 1975). Within 2 days after brain injury, the vast majority of EEGs showed spindles. Chatrian et al. (1963), Courjon et al. (1971), Steudel et al. (1979), and Hansotia et al. (1981) found spindle activities when their records were made within 2 days after trauma.

Vigouroux et al. (1964) and Courjon et al. (1971) observed the decrease of spindles in prolonged coma independent of the outcome. This observation was further corroborated by Bricolo et al. (1978), using compressed spectral array in long-term EEG monitoring. These authors found the disappearance of frequencies of the 12- to 14-c/sec range between days 3 and 5 after trauma to be one of their most striking results. On the third day after trauma, a change of sleep-like activity with spindles to a slow monotonous pattern was also observed in children. There was no influence of this change on the final outcome (Dusser et al., 1989). On the other hand a sleep organization close to normal based on 24-hour polysomnographic recordings in prolonged stages of posttraumatic coma was a reliable prognostic marker, both for survival and for functional recovery (Valente et al., 2002).

Good Outcome Category

Typical spindles and reactivity are seen in the majority of EEGs in acute coma, but spindles are clearly reduced in prolonged coma (Fig. 21.5). Reactivity of the alerting type is

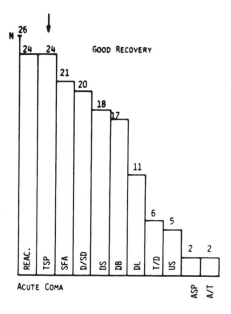

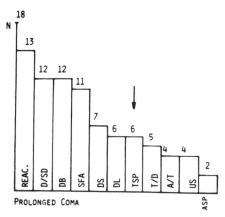

Figure 21.5. The EEG patterns in acute *(top)* and prolonged *(bottom)* coma in patients with good recovery. Typical spindles *(arrow)* are seen in the majority of EEGs in acute coma but are clearly reduced in prolonged coma. REAC, reactivity; other abbreviations as in Figure 21.1. (From Rumpl, E., Prugger, M., Bauer, G., et al. 1983. Incidence and prognostic value of spindles in post-traumatic coma. Electroencephalogr. Clin. Neurophysiol. 56:420–429.)

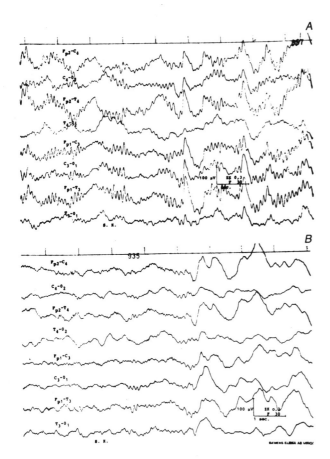

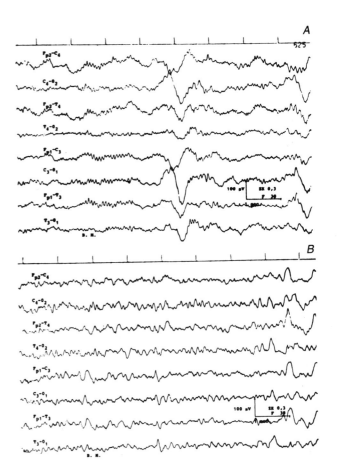

Figure 21.6. **A:** EEG from a 23-year-old man in acute coma due to secondary brainstem dysfunction (classical midbrain syndrome stage 2 without lateralization). Easily recognizable typical spindles, symmetrical over both hemispheres, accompanied by K complexes and diffuse slowing. Computed tomography (CT) scan: moderate brain edema with scattered contusional areas in left frontoparietal and right temporal regions. No signs of compression at tentorial level. Blood within the interhemispheric fissure. **B:** EEG from the same patient in prolonged coma. No spindles, superimposed fast activity, and change to high-voltage short and long delta runs (alternating pattern). No lateralizing signs in the EEG. Outcome: good recovery. (From Rumpl, E., Prugger, M., Bauer, G., et al. 1983. Incidence and prognostic value of spindles in post-traumatic coma. Electroencephalogr. Clin. Neurophysiol. 56:420–429.)

Figure 21.7. **A:** EEG from a 20-year-old man in acute coma due to primary brainstem injury. Neurological signs of atypical midbrain syndrome stage 4 (decerebrate posture). Typical spindles, delta bursts, and superimposed fast activity accompanied by diffuse slowing. CT scan: normal. **B:** EEG from the same patient in prolonged coma. Predominant alpha/theta activity, several delta waves, reactivity in form of blocking slow waves, and no lateralizing EEG signs. Characteristic EEG pattern for pontine lesions. Outcome: good recovery. (From Rumpl, E., Prugger, M., Bauer, G., et al. 1983. Incidence and prognostic value of spindles in post-traumatic coma. Electroencephalogr. Clin. Neurophysiol. 56:420–429.)

the most prominent response, but, in rare cases, reactivity of the blocking type or disappearance of spindles was the result of auditory or painful stimulation. The variety of the different EEG patterns is high and only slightly reduced in prolonged coma. Hence, these EEG patterns strongly correspond to the patterns found in MBS 2 (Fig. 21.1). Interestingly, eight patients showed decerebrate posture, leading to the classification of MBS 4. In contrast to these alarming neurological findings, the CT scan was normal or slightly abnormal in these cases. Therefore, a primary brainstem lesion was thought to be the principal cause of coma. Typical spindles were noted in patients with either primary or secondary brainstem lesions (Figs. 21.6 and 21.7).

Moderate Disability Outcome Category

The EEG patterns in acute and prolonged coma show a wide range of variability, similar to that seen in the good

outcome category (Fig. 21.8). Typical spindles are reduced in prolonged coma, but otherwise no significant change in other EEG patterns is seen.

Severe Disability Outcome Category

There is a decrease of spindles and reactivity and rarefaction of the number of EEG patterns in acute and prolonged coma (Fig. 21.9). No typical spindles are found in prolonged coma. These alterations in EEG patterns are similar not only to those found in MBS 3 and MBS 4 (Fig. 21.1), but also to those seen in the transitional stage to the apallic syndrome (see EEG Changes in Prolonged Comatose States and the Apallic Syndrome, below).

Brain Death Category

All EEG patterns already reduced in acute coma showed further reduction in prolonged coma (Fig. 21.10). Low-volt-

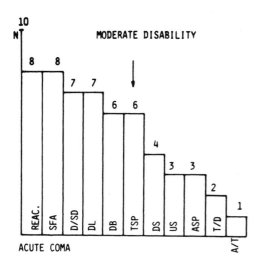

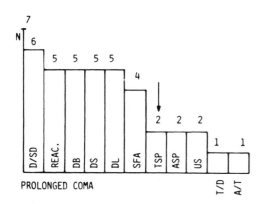

Figure 21.8. The EEG patterns in acute and prolonged coma in patients with moderate disability outcome. Typical spindles *(arrow)* are frequently seen in acute coma and show reduction in prolonged coma. No dramatic change in other EEG patterns between acute and prolonged coma. Reactivity is closely related to the capacity for spindling. Observations hampered by small number of patients. REAC, reactivity; other abbreviations as in Figure 21.1. (From Rumpl, E., Prugger, M., Bauer, G., et al. 1983. Incidence and prognostic value of spindles in post-traumatic coma. Electroencephalogr. Clin. Neurophysiol. 56:420–429.)

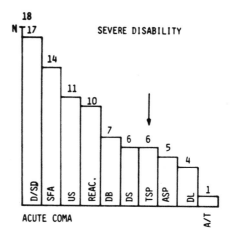

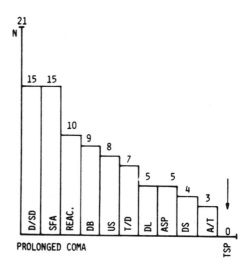

Figure 21.9. The EEG patterns of patients with severe disability outcome in acute and prolonged coma. Note the decrease of typical spindles *(arrow)* in acute coma and the total loss of typical spindles in prolonged coma. Also reactivity is less frequently seen in these cases. Note general decrease in the variety of EEG patterns. REAC, reactivity; other abbreviations as in Figure 21.1. (From Rumpl, E., Prugger, M., Bauer, G., et al. 1983. Incidence and prognostic value of spindles in post-traumatic coma. Electroencephalogr. Clin. Neurophysiol. 56:420–429.)

age output EEGs were seen in three cases in acute coma. In prolonged coma, the number of low-voltage output EEGs increased to seven, and isoelectric EEG was found in four cases. Reactivity was poor in acute and prolonged coma. Typical spindles were rarely seen; they were symmetrical only in one case. In rare cases, remnants of spindles were noted (Fig. 21.11). On the whole, these patterns correlate strongly with the findings in BBS 1 and BBS 2, respectively.

There is good reason to assume that spindle activity is of great prognostic value in acute coma (i.e., within 2 days after trauma). With worsening of outcome, there is a steady decrease of spindle activity accompanied by an increase of atypical spindles and asymmetry. In prolonged coma, spindles are less frequent; atypical forms and asymmetries correspond with the outcome, as in cases of acute coma. The overall incidence of spindles in the first 2 days of coma is

high (91%), but it shows a remarkable decrease of 30% in the following days. The brain's capacity for spindling is closely related to its capacity for EEG arousal; both are partially lost in late stages of MBS and BBS, as well as in prolonged coma. The disappearance of spindles in prolonged coma suggests that spindle activity cannot predict the outcome in prolonged coma. On the other hand, if spindle activity is present, asymmetry and distortion are of prognostic value. Atypical spindles and asymmetries significantly increase in patients with bad outcome. Generally, the decrease of spindles not only indicates the deepening of coma, but more frequently heralds the transition to a prolonged comatose state. In such a case, the loss of spindles is of less prognostic significance when other EEG signs of favorable outcome, such as reactivity, alternating patterns, high voltage, and symmetry of activities, remain unchanged.

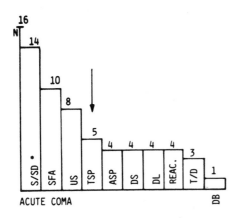

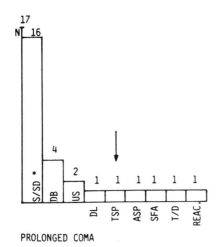

mary and secondary brainstem lesions are compared. One must consider, however, that cases of isolated primary brainstem injury are rare (Mitchell and Adams, 1973) and that the hemispheres are frequently also involved. This may be especially true in patients with bad outcome.

Although there is increasing doubt about the effect of barbiturate anesthesia in the treatment of intracranial hypertension, barbiturate anesthesia may be advisable in certain cases (Miller, 1979). This therapy profoundly alters the EEG activity. The EEG by itself is not sufficient to predict the level of barbiturate anesthesia under clinical conditions in which adjuvant medications are used (Myers et al., 1977). However, it is generally accepted that the appearance of burst-suppression activity points to a therapeutic plasma level of barbiturates (Newlon et al., 1983). There is no doubt that the EEG patterns mentioned above are widely suppressed by this ther-

Figure 21.10. The EEG patterns in patients who suffered brain death within 14 days after brain injury. In acute coma, typical spindles are rarely seen (symmetrical only in one case). In prolonged coma, typical but asymmetrical spindles are seen in one case only. There is similar decrease in reactivity and limited variety of EEG patterns. Columns of delta/subdelta activity include three low-voltage EEGs in acute coma and seven low-voltage EEGs and four isoelectric EEGs in prolonged coma. REAC, reactivity; other abbreviations as in Figure 21.1. (From Rumpl, E., Prugger, M., Bauer, G., et al. 1983. Incidence and prognostic value of spindles in post-traumatic coma. Electroencephalogr. Clin. Neurophysiol. 56:420–429.)

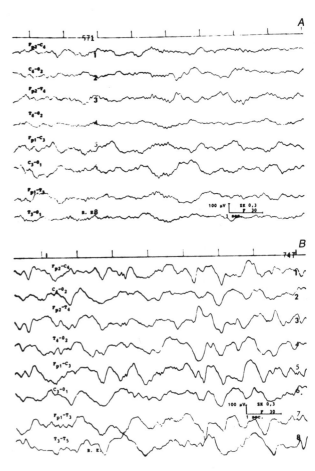

Figure 21.11. **A:** EEG from a 17-year-old girl in acute coma due to secondary brainstem involvement (classical midbrain syndrome stage 4). Typical (mildly abnormal) and asymmetrical spindles. Spindles are better seen on the *left*. Slight reduction in amplitudes of slow waves on the *right*. CT scan: areas of local brain contusions at basal ganglia level on both sides. Small hemorrhagic lesion in the posterior part of the left internal capsule. Signs of tentorial compression. Blood in the third ventricle. **B:** EEG from the same patient in prolonged coma. Atypical severely distorted spindles in the left frontal region. Spindles are hardly recognizable and can only be detected from knowledge of the previous EEG (**A**). Outcome: brain death. (From Rumpl, E., Prugger, M., Bauer, G., et al. 1983. Incidence and prognostic value of spindles in post-traumatic coma. Electroencephalogr. Clin. Neurophysiol. 56:420–429.)

There is no significant influence of small contusional areas in the CT scans on spindle activity (Rumpl et al., 1983). Larger hemispheric lesions are accompanied by increasing asymmetry of spindle activity. Furthermore, the neurological findings show close correlation with symmetry and form of spindles as well as with the results of CT scan. Exceptions are seen in cases of primary brainstem injury. Despite decerebrate posturing, many patients recover well (Chatrian et al., 1963; Rumpl et al., 1983); others die or survive in a state resembling a posttraumatic locked-in syndrome (Britt et al., 1977). In these cases, one might assume either reversible or irreversible impairment of the midbrain or brainstem, respectively, but undisturbed thalamocortical connections subserve well-formed spindle activity. On the other hand, there are no significant differences in spindle activity in the different outcome categories when cases of pri-

apy; consequently, any prognostic value of the EEG is lost. Therefore, obtaining early EEG recordings before treating with barbiturates is advocated. This also pertains to cases treated with large doses of other sedative drugs.

EEG Changes in Prolonged Comatose States and the Apallic Syndrome

In prolonged coma, neurological findings are similar to those seen at the acute stage; only small differences are observed (Overgaard et al., 1973). The EEG changes in this period have been described in detail elsewhere in this chapter. There are, however, more characteristic EEG patterns during the transitional stage from MBS to the traumatic apallic syndrome (Avenarius and Gerstenbrand, 1977). The clinical symptomatology of the transitional stage is not limited to patients with evolution into the full stage of an apallic (vegetative) syndrome, but also occurs in patients who recover with a marked organic brain syndrome characterized by various severe neurological signs of multilocal brain damage.

Classification of Prolonged Coma and the Apallic Syndrome

Transitional Stage to the Apallic Syndrome

During this prolonged evolution of a comatose state, the patients are still in deep coma with closed eyes. At the end of this stage, within 2 or 3 weeks, the survivors begin to open their eyes, initially for very short periods and after arousing stimuli. A steady increase of chewing, a decrease of decorticate or decerebrate rigidity, an increase of extrapyramidal symptoms, and normalization of the reflex eye movements can be observed. Patients react to painful or acoustic stimuli with varying degrees of extensor and flexor response in the limbs accompanied by an altered respiratory pattern. The most important and characteristic feature of this stage is the onset of overactivity of the sympathetic nervous system, leading to extensive tachycardia. This overactivity has been confirmed by the demonstration of high catecholamine plasma levels (mainly of norepinephrine) (Hörtnagl et al., 1980). This sequence of events may begin in stages 2 to 4 of MBS, but is most frequently seen in MBS 3 and 4 (Gerstenbrand et al., 1980).

Full Stage of the Apallic Syndrome

The term *apallic* is used for a clinical syndrome (Gerstenbrand, 1967) without any implication of a particular cerebral lesion. The patients lie with open eyes for longer periods, paying no attention to events around them. They seem to be awake, but not aware. They do not notice events around them. They may show no blink response to menace and react with abnormal movements only to painful stimulation. There are no emotional reactions. Chewing or teeth grinding occurs spontaneously or may be evoked by tactile perioral stimuli. The muscle tone is increased, and only fragments of coordinated movements can be observed. The sleep-waking rhythm seems to be controlled by exhaustion. In the waking state, the overactivity of the sympathetic nervous system continues; during sleep, a shift to a parasympathetic set of responses may be observed.

State of Stupor and Confusion

In less severe cases, the patients show prolonged symptoms of early MBS (usually MBS 1) and pass into a state of stupor and confusion. The patients are usually drowsy, lying in a flexed attitude. During the waking state, patients may be resistant to nursing care and examinations, disoriented, and sometimes noisy and violent. Neurological focal symptoms become more evident. Most of these patients need sedative drugs. This condition may last for days or even weeks and gradually passes. Symptoms of local brain damage may persist and may cause neurological and mental deficits of varying severity.

Relation of EEG Abnormalities to the Stages of Prolonged Coma and the Apallic Syndrome

The EEG patterns of patients in the transitional stage of the apallic syndrome are compared with an EEG recorded during the acute MBS 3 in Fig. 21.12. There is a clear decrease in the variety of EEG patterns, especially of sleep or sleep-like potentials and alternating patterns (Dolce and Kaemmerer, 1967; Rumpl, 1980). A complete loss of spindles is noted in these patients (Fig. 21.13). This evolution of the EEG patterns from waveforms of sleep into rather uniform, frequently high-voltage activity creates the impression of increasing rostrocaudal deterioration. This impression may be supported by the decrease of reactivity; there may be no reactivity to any mode of sensory stimulation (Stockard et al., 1975; Rumpl, 1980). A similar evolution of the EEG is seen in patients developing the transition stage from MBS 2. In contrast to the unfavorable outcome of patients with increasing intracranial pressure, the loss of the activities mentioned above does not carry a poorer prognosis when seen in

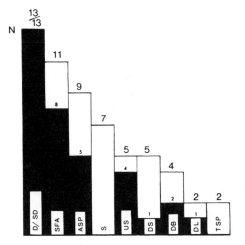

Figure 21.12. The EEG patterns of 13 patients in the transitional stage to the traumatic apallic syndrome evolving from midbrain syndrome Stage 3. *Dark columns* demonstrate the decrease of EEG patterns at the transition stage compared with the EEG patterns at the acute stage of midbrain syndrome *(white columns)*. Note the complete loss of spindles in these cases. Abbreviations as in Figure 21.1. (From Rumpl, E. 1980. Elektro-neurologische Korrelationen in den frühen Phasen des posttraumatischen Komas. II. Das EEG im Übergang zum, und im Vollbild des traumatischen apallischen Syndroms. Z. EEG-EMG 11:43–50.)

Figure 21.13.   A: EEG from 24-year-old woman in acute midbrain syndrome stage 3 without clinical signs of lateralization. After acoustic stimulus *(arrow)*, appearance of spindles followed by delta and subdelta activity of higher amplitude. Note symmetry of reaction. **B:** EEG from the same patient in the transition stage to the apallic syndrome, 4 days after first recording. Uniform delta and subdelta activity; loss of spindles. After acoustic stimulus *(arrow)*, long run of delta. Note symmetry of reaction.

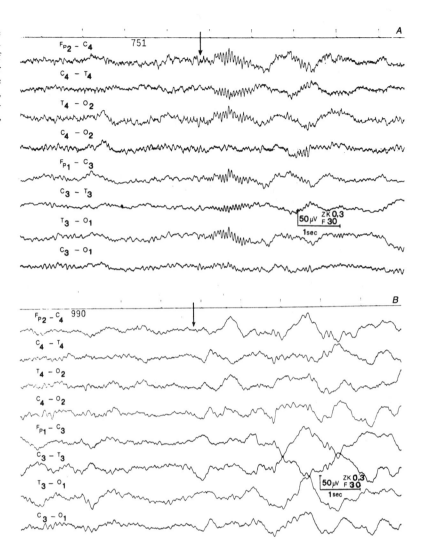

patients at the transition stage (Chatrian, 1975; Rumpl, 1980). Patients in MBS 4 show an already-simplified EEG pattern with only slight further changes at the transition stage. Loss of atypical sleep potentials may be observed, or reactivity may be abolished (Rumpl, 1980).

The variety of EEG patterns is also reduced in the full stage of the apallic syndrome, but this reduction is less marked than in the transitional stage. The variety of EEG patterns increases as soon as cyclic sleep and waking activity can be identified. This is associated with the spindles and long runs of delta (Fig. 21.14). On the other hand, the EEG of patients developing the full stage of the apallic syndrome from MBS 4 remains rather uniform and shows only a little difference between sleep and waking activities. Periods of fast activity of low voltage, along with eye closure, usually characterize sleep, whereas high-voltage slow waves indicate the waking state (Butenuth and Kubicki, 1975; Rumpl, 1980). Passouant et al. (1964), Cadilhac et al. (1966), Bergamasco et al. (1968), and Bricolo et al. (1968) found similar alternating periods of faster low-voltage activity and high-voltage slow waves during sleep in long-lasting nocturnal records. The appearance of EEG sleep patterns and circadian

EEG variations is a favorable prognostic sign (Bergamasco et al., 1968). Completely organized sleep patterns or increasing organization of nocturnal sleep in successive recordings indicates a more favorable outcome than the absence of such patterns. The occurrence of REM sleep is especially significant in this regard (Dolce and Kaemmerer, 1967). This finding may be supported by reports of the reappearance of slow-wave sleep with continued absence of the REM phase in patients who never regained consciousness after brainstem vascular accidents (Chase et al., 1968; Ferguson and Benett, 1974). In rare cases, positive sharp waves in the occipital regions are seen during sleep (Courjon and Scherzer, 1972).

In contrast to reports that suggest that sleep or sleep-like activities point to a favorable outcome, there is no evidence that sleep or sleep-like activity found at the full stage of the apallic syndrome months after the brain injury gives any information about further outcome (Rumpl et al., 1984). Patients with relatively well-developed sleep stages persisted clinically at the stage of an apallic syndrome or remained severely disabled (Fig. 21.15), whereas patients with severely altered sleep showed further recovery. However, the value

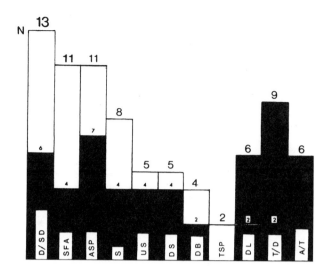

Figure 21.14. The EEG patterns of the same 13 patients as in Figure 21.12 at the full stage of the apallic syndrome *(dark columns)* compared with the EEG patterns at the acute stage of midbrain syndrome *(white columns)*. Note the general acceleration and the reappearance of spindles and altered sleep activities. Abbreviations as in Figure 21.1. (From Rumpl, E. 1980. Elektro-neurologische Korrelationen in den frühen Phasen des posttraumatischen Komas. II. Das EEG im Übergang zum, und im Vollbild des traumatischen apallischen Syndroms. Z. EEG-EMG 11:43–50.)

of long-term EEG recordings in these patients was hampered by the fact that given stages of sleep or wakefulness lasted no longer than a few seconds or minutes. This phenomenon appears to be rather characteristic for apallic patients (Butenuth and Kubicki, 1975; Rumpl et al., 1984). REM sleep was hardly separated from sleep stage 1; rapid eye movements appeared at any stage, even during synchronized sleep. Atypical and asymmetric spindle activity continued to be of prognostic significance by indicating a persistent structural hemispheric lesion. Generally, the prognostic value of long-lasting nocturnal EEG recordings is very limited in apallic or severely disabled patients if done months after the craniocerebral trauma.

The EEG patterns of patients in the state of stupor and confusion show a decrease in the variety of EEG patterns similar to the one seen in prolonged coma. However, sleep or sleep-like potentials are more frequently seen in these patients in diurnal examinations. Generalized theta with less delta activity is the predominating pattern at this stage; it is usually seen in waking periods and without further change after stimulation. The value of most records at this stage is hampered by the use of the sedative drugs needed to obtain technically satisfactory recordings. Drug-induced sleep activities might also indicate a favorable outcome in most of these patients, and asymmetries in sleep potentials might be of diagnostic significance in cases of chronic subdural hematoma.

The reaction to external stimulation is remarkably reduced in the transitional stage of the apallic syndrome. In most cases, no response can be observed (Rumpl, 1980; Stockard et al., 1975). Less frequently, a delayed reactivity characterized by long runs of delta is noted. No reactivity is seen in patients in the full stage of the apallic syndrome dur-

ing the waking state, whereas stimulation during sleep frequently induces long-lasting waking activity (Butenuth and Kubicki, 1975; Fischgold and Mathis, 1959).

Metabolic disturbances decrease in patients in prolonged comatose states (Arfel, 1975). Therefore, the EEG abnormalities are less influenced by metabolic factors than in the stages of MBS. Nevertheless, the influence of metabolic disturbances and drugs must be taken into consideration at these stages.

Epileptic discharges are not seen in patients in the transitional stage or full stage of the apallic syndrome (Lücking et al., 1977; Rumpl, 1980), but may occur in the state of stupor and confusion and during the remission stage from the apallic syndrome (Lücking et al., 1977).

Lateralized signs in the EEG are slightly reduced in prolonged comatose states, mainly due to the loss of asymmetrical typical or atypical sleep potentials. Asymmetry of reactivity is diagnostically helpful (Stockard et al., 1975).

Prognostic criteria can be derived from EEG findings only with great care and caution. A gradual increase in frequency from delta to faster activity points to a favorable index only for survival, not for recovery (Strnad and Strnadová, 1987). Improvement of EEG must be accompanied by clinical improvement to have any prognostic significance (Lücking et al., 1977; Strnad and Strnadová, 1987). An isoelectric EEG indicates loss of bioelectrical activity, to be discussed in Chapter 26, on coma and brain death. Patients who survive with an isoelectric EEG are classified as complete apallic syndromes by some authors (Biniek et al., 1989; Ingvar and Brun, 1972). In cases of very low-voltage EEG in repeated recordings, one can expect survival without hope of recovery as a social human being (Ingvar and Brun, 1972). In patients who develop the symptomatology of the apallic syndrome from MBS 4 accompanied by rather rarified EEG patterns, the prognosis for social recovery is also very poor (Gerstenbrand et al., 1980; Rumpl, 1980). The favorable clinical out-

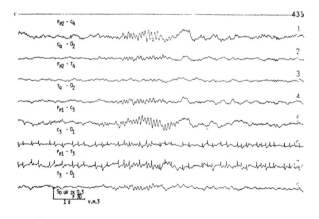

Figure 21.15. Nocturnal EEG from a 29-year-old woman at the full stage of an apallic (vegetative) syndrome. She has learned to move the left lower extremity on command but remains severely disabled. Typical spindles, K complexes during sleep, stage 2. Continuous myogenic spiking in left temporal region due to palatal myoclonus. (From Rumpl, E., Prugger, M., and Bauer, G. 1984. Zum prognostischen Wert elektroenzephalographischer Schlafbeobachtungen im traumatisch bedingten apallischen Syndrom. Neuropsychiatr. Clin. 3:219–232.)

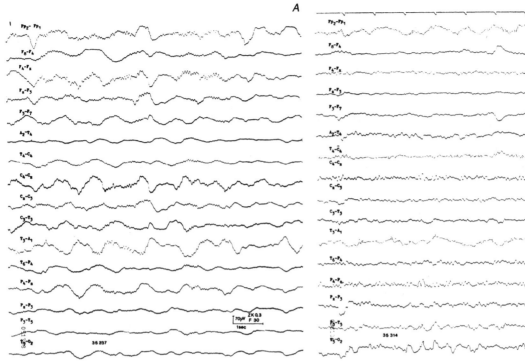

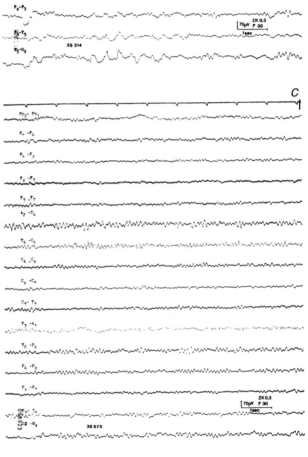

Figure 21.16.   A: EEG from 20-year-old woman with cerebral contusion, drowsiness, and clinical signs of left frontoparietal lesion. Delta and sub-delta activity, unilateral slowing, and suppression of altered spindles in the left hemisphere. **B:** EEG from the same patient, 1 day after first recording. Reappearance of reactive alpha activity, local slowing in left frontotem-poroparietal region. **C:** EEG from the same patient, 3 days after first recording. The EEG is nearly normal; intermittent slow waves in left temporal region. Full clinical recovery with the exception of headache, lack of concentration, and dizziness.

come of patients with organized sleep has been mentioned above. The persistence of sleep patterns or sleep-like activities at the transitional stage of the apallic syndrome might also indicate a favorable outcome, although the value of this observation is hampered by the very small number of cases studied (Bergamasco et al., 1977; Rumpl, 1980).

EEG Changes at Early Stages after Craniocerebral Trauma without Evidence of Brainstem Dysfunction

In mild or moderate head or brain injuries, there may be no or only mild disturbances of consciousness with no clinical signs of primary or secondary brainstem dysfunction. In general, the EEG recovery is fast in these patients, who fortunately form the vast majority of cases after craniocerebral trauma.

Relation of EEG Abnormalities to Mild or Moderate Stages of Cerebral Concussion

In cases of commotio cerebri (cerebral concussion with loss of consciousness) but with no impairment of consciousness at the time the records were taken, normal or borderline EEGs were found in the vast majority of cases within the first 24 hours (Dow et al., 1944; Scherzer, 1965; Williams, 1941a). No slowing of the alpha rhythm could be detected by Meyer-Mickeleit (1953) in these recordings. The slowing of alpha rhythm is usually considered to be the slightest degree of generalized disturbance after contusio cerebri (Meyer-Mickeleit, 1953) and may only be found with repeated EEG, because the significant slowing occurs in the alpha frequency range (Koufen and Dichgans, 1978).

The mildest disturbance of consciousness seen after craniocerebral trauma is drowsiness and hypersomnia, which are accompanied by the EEG findings of normal sleep (Stockard et al., 1975). There are usually generalized slowing of all frequencies and altered sleep patterns in patients with barely existent periods of wakefulness. Sensory stimulation will block the slowing and sleep. There may be gliding clinical and electroencephalographic transitions to the first stage of MBS. However, the change from abnormal EEG activity to a more normal pattern is fast in these cases (Fig. 21.16).

In contrast to the aforementioned fairly good correlation of EEG and clinical findings, there are many patients with head injury who show marked discrepancies between EEG patterns and clinical findings. A normal neurological status in a patient with no or little complaint may be accompanied by impressively abnormal EEGs (Figs. 21.17 and 21.18). Similar EEG findings may also be seen in patients with cerebral concussion without loss of consciousness but with a short or longer lasting alteration in mental status (Kelly and Rosenberg, 1997). The EEG would most likely detect cortical disease in acute cases with mild injury, even if the CT scan or MRI is normal. Very little is said in the literature about these cases, and only a few authors regard them as mild forms of concussion (Denny-Brown, 1961; Tönnis, 1956; Verjaal, 1972). In contrast, a normal EEG can be seen in patients with significant impairment in neuropsychological performance after mild traumatic brain injury within 24 hours and up to 6 weeks after injury (Voller et al., 1999).

Particularly pronounced discrepancies between electrical cortical activity and the clinical state may be found in children (Dumermuth, 1965; Lenard, 1965; Melin, 1949). Children may show high-amplitude generalized delta activity for weeks or months after a mild craniocerebral trauma and in the presence of normal consciousness (Stockard et al., 1975). Immaturity might enhance functional traumatic (postconcussion) disturbances and produce focal or generalized EEG abnormalities (Courjon and Scherzer, 1972). On the other hand, focal changes have been thought to be a significant sign of contusional brain damage (Christian, 1968).

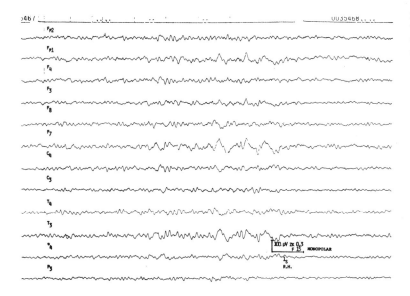

Figure 21.17. EEG from a 35-year-old man complaining of vertigo after mild cerebral contusion. At the time of EEG recording, normal neurological status and CT scan. Intermittent slow activity (theta and delta) in left frontotemporal region.

Figure 21.18. EEG from a 45-year-old woman after mild cerebral contusion without signs of brainstem impairment. Some complaints about vertigo. At the time of EEG recording, normal neurological and CT scan findings. Intermittent left temporal theta focus.

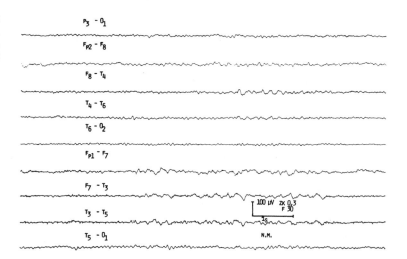

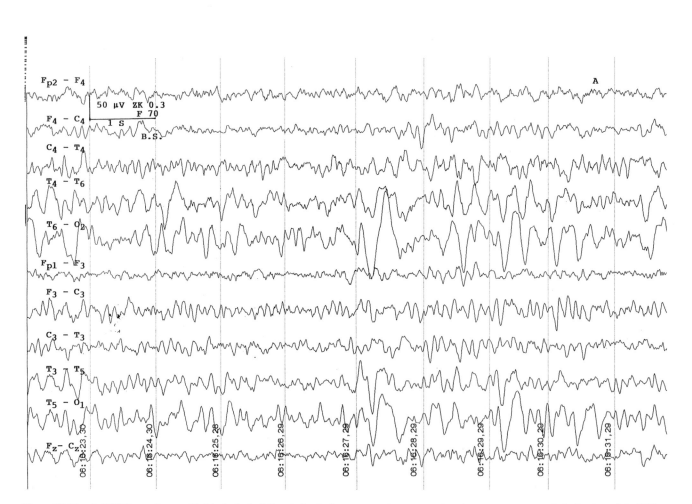

Figure 21.19. **A:** EEG from a 6-year-old girl who had a fall on the back of her head after an unexpected push while playing. She had a period of blurred vision, delayed answers to questions, disorientation, drowsiness, and stereotyped finger movements, which lasted about 1 hour. The CT and magnetic resonance imaging scans were normal. At the time of the EEG recording 2 days after the accident, the patient was alert with no neurological or mental deficit. The EEG showed high-voltage occipital delta activity intermingled with sharp transients.

The recovery of EEG abnormalities follows the same pattern as in adults (Koufen and Dichgans, 1977). In children with transient cortical blindness following mild head trauma, posterior slowing with subsequent fast normalization can be observed (Yamamoto and Bart, 1989).

Lateralized signs consist mainly of focal slow waves in the theta and delta range (Jung, 1953; Koufen and Dichgans, 1978; Meyer-Mickeleit, 1953; Scherzer, 1965), whereas the other cerebral regions show only minor changes (Hess, 1961). A close correlation with neurological deficits is seen within the first months (Jung, 1953; Meyer-Mickeleit, 1953; Mifka and Scherzer, 1962b; Radermecker, 1964).

Elderly persons may have pretraumatic EEG abnormalities, especially in the temporal regions, due to cerebrovascular insufficiency. The combination of traumatic and vascular factors makes it difficult to distinguish the EEG abnormalities caused by the cerebral contusion. There is particularly high mortality in elderly patients with early epileptic seizures (Vigouroux et al., 1966). The loss of reactivity may appear in light stages of coma, indicating a bad prognosis (Courjon and Scherzer, 1972).

Epileptic Discharges

The term *early epilepsy* should be confined to fits in the first week after injury (Jennett, 1969). Localized focal motor epilepsy is most common in the first week, whereas acute temporal lobe epilepsy with psychomotor or complex partial seizures is never found during this period. Courjon and Scherzer (1972) found generalized seizures in 50% of the cases, while the other 50% had focal attacks. These authors believe that there is a higher percentage of focal seizures because of secondary generalization and doubtful clinical observation. After 2 weeks, posttraumatic epilepsy in adults may have any type of epileptic manifestation, with the exception of petit mal attacks with generalized rhythmic synchronous 3/sec spike-and-wave activity in the EEG (Courjon and Revol, 1966). Although epilepsy during the first week recurred or persisted in less than one third of patients (the recurrence rate in the second week is over 70%), the risk for late epilepsy is significantly greater for patients with early fits than for those without (Jennett, 1969). A threefold increase in the incidence of both early and late seizures is seen in patients with depressed skull fractures when compared with injuries accompanied by nondepressed fractures (Stockard et al., 1975). Occipital status epilepticus is a rare event in posttraumatic blindness (Black et al., 1996). While cortical blindness in traumatic brain injured patients with no or minimal occipital pathology on CT or MRI scanning is generally transient (Fig. 21.19), occipital status epilepticus accompanied by occipital edema may lead to persistent visual deficit if not detected for early treatment.

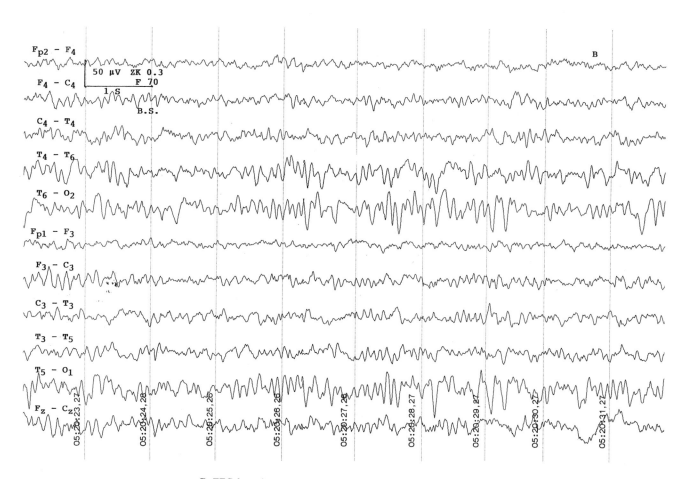

B: EEG from the same patient 3 days later within the range of normal.

Long runs of continuous activity of focal spikes or unilateral spike-wave discharges are the most common EEG pattern in early epilepsy (Courjon and Scherzer, 1972). In general, focal epileptiform patterns associated with diffuse EEG abnormalities suggest a greater probability of subsequent chronic epilepsy than does focal epileptiform activity in an otherwise normal EEG (Stockard et al., 1975). Using standard 24-hours recordings seizure activity can be seen after trauma in up to 35% of patients with mild or severe head-brain injury in the first weeks after trauma, but accompanying epileptic fits are rare (Kazibutowska et al., 1992). In cases of severe brain injury early electroencephalographic seizure activity might be seen in patients who will have clinical seizures shortly before or after the discharges are found in the EEG (Fig. 21.2).

Epileptiform activities are more frequently seen in children than in adults. These are isolated spikes or spike waves, sharp waves, and spike-wave complexes, localized or generalized. A single epileptic focus in the EEG after severe head trauma has the same favorable outcome as in benign focal epilepsy (Wohlrab et al., 1997). Generalized irregular spike-wave activity is occasionally seen (Stockard et al., 1975). The 14 and 6 positive spikes can be an abnormal finding after mild or severe head injury in children. This pattern may appear as a delayed reaction to mild injury, but may also be seen during recovery from severe injury (Gibbs and Gibbs, 1987). However the significance of 14 and 6 positive spikes is of less value, because it may also be seen in healthy children (Niedermeyer and Knott, 1961). All of these discharges can be observed within hours of the trauma (more commonly within days or weeks), and all are associated with a good prognosis.

EEG Changes at Late Stages After Craniocerebral Trauma

In late stages after craniocerebral trauma, clinical and EEG examination demonstrate diminished correlation, which further increases after a 3-month interval (Courjon and Scherzer, 1972; Jung, 1953; Meyer-Mickeleit, 1953; Mifka and Scherzer, 1962b). This lack of correlation may also occur in patients during recovery from an apallic syndrome (Lücking et al., 1977).

Clinical Classification

Recovery from the Apallic Syndrome

Although the symptomatology of the apallic syndrome is remarkably uniform, there are different degrees of telencephalic lesions, so that recovery is possible (Gerstenbrand, 1967). During the remission stage (Gerstenbrand, 1977), there is evidence of increasing reintegration of higher brain function. The onset is indicated by primitive emotional reactions in response to painful stimuli followed by optical fixation and displeasure reactions. The first voluntary movements are usually seen in the fingers. The patient starts to respond to simple orders. In patients who make a reasonable recovery, further stages of remission appear, marked by the symptomatology of the Klüver-Bucy syndrome, the Korsakoff syndrome, and, finally, the organic brain syndrome of varying severity. Symptoms of local brain lesions can now

be clearly determined. These lesions may be permanent, but in some cases the apallic syndrome is transient with complete recovery of the patient.

In mild and moderate brain injuries, the onset of the late stage can be clinically defined by the disappearance of disturbances of consciousness and confusion and by the stabilization of neurological deficits and psychic syndromes (Courjon and Scherzer, 1972). Usually, a gradual recovery is seen, but in some cases neurological and mental deficits may persist.

Posttraumatic Syndrome

According to Caveness (1966), this syndrome comprises headache, vertigo, dizziness, nervousness, irritability, impaired memory, disturbances of concentration, excessive fatigue, insomnia, and intolerance to alcohol. Practically, in 50% of the patients, the symptoms disappear within 2 weeks after mild injury, while in 25% the symptoms continue for months and sometimes years (Verjaal and Van't Hooft, 1975). However, it should be noted that most of the posttraumatic complaints do not appreciably differ from nontraumatic neurotic syndromes.

Relation of EEG Abnormalities to the Late Stages of Craniocerebral Trauma

EEG recovery from the full stage of the apallic syndrome is generally associated with an acceleration of EEG activity. Theta and (fewer) delta waves characterize the apallic syndrome months after the brain injury (Jellinger et al., 1963; Lücking et al., 1977). Recovery from this stage is characterized by the decline of theta and delta waves and reappearance of reactive alpha activity. Favorable outcome is associated with faster regression of theta waves and more progressive reinstitution of alpha activity (Jellinger et al., 1963; Pateisky et al., 1963). In a summary of their findings, Lücking et al. (1977) have been able to draw the following conclusions on the prognostic value of the EEG in the apallic syndrome: (a) Predominant theta and delta activity unchanged for several months points to a significant lesion of the hemispheres. (b) An early and progressive appearance of alpha activity in the absence of clinical improvement suggests slight cortical, but extensive subcortical, lesions. (c) Alpha frequency may show a gradual acceleration within years without further clinical improvement. (d) Focal symptoms become more marked after the decrease of general changes and may shift from side to side in cases of temporal foci. (e) Epileptic discharges may occur in patients with no evidence of epileptic fits, although patients with focal epileptic attacks may have no epileptic discharges in repeated EEGs.

EEG recovery of generalized abnormalities is characterized by a steady increase in frequency. After comatose states, generalized theta activity is one of the most constant features of the EEG recovery (Stockard et al., 1975) and may show further improvement with gradually evolving reactive alpha activity. After mild head injuries with cerebral contusion and slowing of the basic rhythm, follow-up EEGs are often characterized by a gradual increase of alpha frequency returning to normal within several weeks or months (Jung, 1953; Koufen and Dichgans, 1978; Meyer-Mickeleit, 1953; Scherzer, 1965). Six months after trauma, alpha slowing persists in only 4% of the cases (Koufen and Dichgans, 1978).

EEG recovery of lateralizing signs shows a characteristic evolution in uncomplicated cases. Unilateral slowing or a delta focus will gradually change into a theta focus or a focus of irregular waves of changing frequency. This focus may turn into the focal slowing of alpha rhythm in the parietal, posterior, and occipital regions with the slightest degree of local disturbance (Jung, 1953; Meyer-Mickeleit, 1953). This focal slowing usually disappears quickly and may sometimes be followed by focal reduction in amplitude (Courjon and Scherzer, 1972). The diagnostic value of such alpha asymmetries is doubtful, however, when one considers the frequent occurrence of such asymmetries in healthy persons (Radermecker, 1964). Another rare and transient local sign is focal activation of alpha rhythm (Duensing, 1948) characterized by a focal slowing and increase of alpha amplitude by eye closure; eye opening fails to block the activity.

In cases with traumatic psychosis (delirium, Korsakoff syndrome, changes of affect), EEG foci are demonstrated in 95% of cases, bilaterally in 70%. Normalization occurs within 3 months in 48%, with foci persisting more than 2 years in 22% mostly in patients with traumatic epilepsy. Focal signs initially consist of delta waves (85%) and finally of focal dysrhythmia (73%) with temporal localization increasing from 58% to 82% (Koufen and Hagel, 1987).

Even in the late posttraumatic stage, focal EEG abnormalities may show a close correlation with the clinical focal deficit (Koufen and Dichgans, 1978; Schneider and Hubach, 1962). After closed head injuries, focal EEG abnormalities tend to disappear within 6 months (Koufen and Dichgans, 1978) to 2 years (Meyer-Mickeleit, 1953) in the vast majority of cases. In contrast, Goetze (1953) found focal changes in 50% of his cases 20 years after an open craniocerebral trauma; Schneider and Hubach (1962) found focal changes in 40% of their patients with prolonged confusional states. Focal abnormalities decrease more slowly than generalized ones and may even be found some years after injury (Courjon and Scherzer, 1972). The area of the focal abnormality usually shrinks in size and may narrow down to a temporal or parieto-occipital focus (Courjon and Scherzer, 1972). In penetrating head injury, a close correlation between focal slowing and focal neurological deficit may be found even 12 to 16 years after injury (Jabbari et al., 1986). In open craniocerebral trauma, foci often persist over the area of penetration, and migration to posterior regions is unusual (Christian, 1968). In rare cases, the location of the focal abnormality may shift from one area to another (Dawson et al., 1951; Koufen and Dichgans, 1978). More frequently, the foci shift to the frontal rather than to the occipital region, but they may return to the original locus in both cases (Dawson et al., 1951).

Epileptic Discharges

Apart from early attacks, late epilepsy may develop within a month or two of the injury or may be delayed for many years. Early attacks will predispose to late ones (Jennett, 1969). A detailed discussion of posttraumatic epilepsy is presented in Chapter 27.

The EEG in the posttraumatic syndrome can neither prove nor rule out the existence of traumatic symptoms (Courjon, 1962; Kugler, 1966). Even pronounced EEG abnormalities are not necessarily associated with posttraumatic syndromes (Courjon and Scherzer, 1972). In contrast, a normal EEG cannot exclude severe cerebral damage.

EEG Changes in Whiplash Injuries, Cervical Fractures, and Dislocations

Whiplash injuries may be accomplished by EEG abnormalities; similarly, patients with cervical fractures and dislocations may demonstrate EEG changes even in the absence of loss of consciousness at the moment of the accident (Courjon and Scherzer, 1972). Torres and Shapiro (1961) found the incidence of generalized and focal EEG changes (focal spikes and focal slow waves) in a selected group of whiplash injury cases to be the same as in patients with closed head injury. An additional injury to the head was carefully excluded in their patients. On the average, their EEGs were done 6 months after the accident. Temporal lobe foci were more frequently seen in whiplash injury than in closed head trauma, but this did not prove to be statistically significant. Slow waves appeared to be accentuated over the posterior regions of the brain. In contrast to the EEG changes after closed head injuries, the EEG became increasingly abnormal in many of their cases when follow-up records were studied. Moreover, many cases showed marked fluctuations in the degree of abnormality suggesting a vascular mechanism for these changes.

The EEG changes might indeed be due to fluctuations in the blood supply from the vertebral arteries, which can be impaired by hyperextension of the neck (Kuhlendahl, 1964; Mifka and Scherzer, 1962a). Vertebral fractures with displacement of fragments may directly compress the vertebral arteries. Similar patterns in the EEG may appear in this case. There are also alternative explanations for the genesis of EEG abnormalities in the wake of neck injuries. The acceleration-deceleration as such may directly affect the cerebral parenchyma (Denny-Brown and Russel, 1941), or the rapid sequence of backward-forward movements of head and neck may cause traumatic lesions as the cerebrum strikes the inner table of the skull (Torres and Shapiro, 1961). Jacome (1987) found mostly normal EEG (and also 24-hour cassette recording) findings in 68 cases with whiplash injuries (and without accompanying head injury).

Compressed Spectral Array and Brain Mapping

Continuous EEG monitoring of patients in the first days following injury requires the use of computer-assisted (Fourier transform) analysis using compressed spectral analysis (CSA) or similar techniques. With this method the power spectra or specific EEG frequency bands may be monitored for the long term. The dominant frequencies, their distribution, and their amplitude may be better assessed with CSA than with conventional EEG (Stone et al., 1988). Two or four channels appear to be adequate to regain significant data regarding the outcome of patients (Bricolo et al., 1978; Cant and Shaw, 1984; Sironi et al., 1983; Steudel and Krüger, 1979). Unfavorable outcome was seen in patients with slow and monotonous CSA and in patients with significant interhemispheric amplitude asymmetry. Favorable outcome was frequently found in patients with changeable CSA, especially with sleep-like CSA (Bricolo et al., 1978; Sironi et al., 1983). Persistence or return of activity within the alpha or theta range pointed to good outcome in most cases (Cant and Shaw, 1984). Repeated studies of CSA showed an increase in the absolute and relative amplitudes of the alpha and theta ranges in patients who survived (Steudel and Krüger, 1979). Difficulties in interpretation may appear in patients in alpha or theta pattern coma, as well as in patients undergoing barbiturate therapy. Further difficulties are that CSA may fail to show paroxysmal patterns, such as spikes, brief seizures, burst suppression, PLEDs, triphasic waves, and intermittent theta and delta activity (Jordan, 1993).

Calculation of the theta/beta power ratios in patients with deep coma revealed long-lasting EEG reactions after standardized repetitive stimulation (Pfurtscheller et al., 1986). With this method EEG reaction may be elicited even in cases where other methods fail to evoke an EEG response—acute or delayed—at all. The theta/beta ratio decreased with recovery of cerebral functions. A bolus injection of 100 to 500 mg of thiopental evokes short-lasting beta stimulation in CSA. This response was of high prognostic significance since 84% of patients with this reaction survived (Klein et al., 1988).

In mild head trauma discriminating EEG power spectral analysis indicated three classes of variables that are attributable to mechanical head injury: (1) increased coherence and decreased phase in frontal and frontotemporal regions; (2) decreased power differences between anterior and posterior cortical regions; (3) reduced alpha power in posterior cortical regions (Thatcher et al., 1989). These authors speculate that these electrophysiological features are consistent with the mechanics of cerebral trauma and may explain persistent symptoms after mild trauma such as headache, dizziness, memory loss, short attention span, and reduced ability to process complex information. Subsequently, EEG measures of cerebral asymmetry such as EEG coherence and phase and amplitude symmetry were found to be best predictors of outcome also in patients with severe brain injury. EEG coherence and phase have been shown to reflect to some extent the magnitude of diffuse axonal injury (Thatcher et al., 1991).

Topographic brain mapping (TBM) can demonstrate subtle asymmetries and lateralization and localization effects more efficiently than standard EEG, when the recording is done properly from a technical standpoint (Hooshmand et al., 1989; Jerret and Corsak, 1988). In 135 patients after mild or moderate head injury, abnormal TBM was found in 56% of cases years after injury. The temporofrontal regions were involved in 65%, the temporo-occipital regions in 25%, and the parieto-occipital regions in 9% of patients. The most common type of abnormality was absolute voltage asymmetry. In contrast the standard EEG showed abnormalities in 30% of cases consisting mainly of mild, nonspecific generalized slowing (Hooshmand et al., 1989). TBM appears to provide better detection of low-amplitude slow activity not easily discernible by routine EEG (Jerrett and Corsak, 1988).

Head Injury in Sports

A generalized reduction in amplitude and slow irregular theta activity has been observed in boxers within 15 to 30 minutes after fighting, with a significant increase of these findings in boxers who had sustained a knockout blow (Busse and Silverman, 1952; Larsson et al., 1954; Pampus and Grote, 1956). Although the EEG might detect even slight degrees of cerebrovascular autoregulation disturbance, the method is not routinely used to avoid second impact syndrome in contact-sports head trauma (Kelly and Rosenberg, 1997; Saunders and Harbaugh, 1984). However, the method should be more sensitive than CT or MRI scanning.

In long-term observations Pampus and Grote (1954) found a correlation between the frequency of abnormal EEGs and the number of fights and, furthermore, a correlation between EEG abnormalities and short time intervals between fights. Repeated fights within a short period have particularly ill effects on the brain, and the extent and degree of EEG abnormalities increased after each fight (Courjon and Scherzer, 1972; Pampus and Grote, 1956). Usually the EEG of young boxers shows more serious changes than that of older ones. No severe abnormalities were found in amateur boxers either with many or few matches. There was a somewhat higher incidence of slight or moderate EEG deviations among boxers than among soccer players and track and field athletes. No neurophysiological variable was correlated to the number of bouts, number of lost fights, or length of boxing career. Also an abnormal EEG did not predict the degree of clinical impairment. EEG abnormalities showed no correlation to neurological findings or the number of bouts the fighter has waged (Roberts, 1969). In general, no signs of serious brain damage were found among amateur athletes (Haglund and Persson, 1990). On the other hand, a significantly increased incidence of focal theta activity was found in soccer players at the end of their careers, probably as the result of a cumulative effect due to repeated heading (Tysvaer et al., 1989). Slightly abnormal to abnormal EEGs were found in 35% of active and in 32% of former soccer players. Interestingly enough, there were fewer abnormal EEG changes among the typical "headers" than among the "nonheaders" (Tysvaer, 1992).

There is a chronic progressive traumatic encephalopathy in boxers, especially in those with a history of repeated knockout defeats. Critchley (1957) found a significant increase of EEG abnormalities in boxers who suffered from this encephalopathy, which is known as the *punch drunk state* (Martland, 1928) or *dementia pugilistica* (Millspaugh, 1937), in comparison to the EEG of more successful boxers. Critchley (1957), however, found no correlation between the degree of boxer's encephalopathy and the EEG. Similar conclusions were drawn by Mawdsley and Ferguson (1963) and Johnson (1969). The EEG may be useful in determining the severity of trauma after a fight, but it is a less sensitive indicator of boxer's encephalopathy during and beyond the active career. No correlation with clinical findings was established even with the use of psychometric tests (Johnson, 1969). As in EEG recovery after craniocerebral trauma of other origins, a normal EEG cannot exclude the existence or the development of encephalopathy.

Other sports, such as horseback riding, American football, and rugby, may carry a similar risk of repeated concussion. The number of injuries might be quite different from that of boxers, but some of them may be more severe than those usually occurring in the boxing ring. Temporal lobe epilepsy and persisting mental impairment was found in professional jockeys after repeated riding accidents (Forster et al., 1976).

Conclusion

There is a close correlation between clinical and electroencephalographic findings in acute posttraumatic comatose states. A declining number of observable EEG patterns may suggest increasing rostrocaudal deterioration and poor prognosis, as well as the development of a prolonged comatose state. An assessment of the EEG abnormalities without knowledge of the clinical symptoms is difficult in these stages. Metabolic disturbances and drugs may also influence the EEG patterns. Early epileptic discharges in the EEG are of prognostic significance if they appear prior to clinical seizures. In cases of primary brainstem damage, the EEG can help to differentiate these lesions from secondary brainstem involvement. In comatose states, follow-up EEG is necessary to determine the state of cortical activity and its evolution. Early EEG recordings are stressed in all cases of craniocerebral trauma because of increasing lack of correlation between clinical and EEG data in later stages. No conclusion can be drawn from a single EEG at a late stage as to the severity of the original trauma. A single record may only be useful in the case of epileptic manifestations. Serial tracings during acute and late stages accompanied by close clinical examinations will increase the value of the EEG in any case. Secondary deterioration of the EEG after a period of recovery suggests late intracranial complications, such as epilepsy, hematoma, hydrocephalus, abscess, and meningitis, or the development of a concomitant cerebral disease.

References

Akert, K., Koella, W.P., and Hess, R., Jr. 1952. Sleep produced by electrical stimulation of the thalamus. Am. J. Physiol. 168:260–267.

Arfel, G. 1975. Introduction to clinical and EEG studies in coma. In *Handbook of Electroencephalography and Neurophysiology*, vol. 12, Eds. A. Remond, R. Harner, and R. Naquet, pp. 5–23. Amsterdam: Elsevier.

Avenarius, H.J., and Gerstenbrand, F. 1977. The transition stage from midbrain syndrome to the traumatic apallic syndrome. In *The Apallic Syndrome*, Eds. G. Dalle Ore, F. Gerstenbrand, C.H. Lücking, et al., pp. 22–25. Berlin/Heidelberg/New York: Springer.

Bauer, G., and Niedermeyer, E. 1979. Acute convulsions. Clin. Electroencephalogr. 10:127–144.

Bergamasco, B., Bergamini, L., Doriguzzi, T., et al. 1968. EEG sleep patterns as a prognostic criterion in post-traumatic coma. Electroencephalogr. Clin. Neurophysiol. 24:374–377.

Bergamasco, B., Bergamini, L., Bricolo, A., et al. 1977. Studies on sleep during the apallic syndrome. In *The Apallic Syndrome,* Eds. G. Dalle Ore, F. Gerstenbrand, C.H. Lücking, et al., pp. 155–159. Berlin/Heidelberg/New York: Springer.

Bickford, R.G., and Butt, H.R. 1955. Hepatic coma: the electroencephalic pattern. J. Clin. Invest. 34:790–799.

Biniek, R., Ferbert, A., Rimpel, J., et al. 1989. The complete apallic syndrome—a case report. Intensive Care Med. 15:212–215.

Black, K., Obayan, A., Zafonte, R.D., Mann, N.R., Hammond, F.M., and Wood, D.L. 1996. Occipital status epilepticus: an unusual case of posttraumatic blindness. Neuro. Rehabilitation 7:219–221.

Bricolo, A. 1975. Neurosurgical exploration and neurological pathology as means for investigating human sleep semiology and mechanism. In *Experimental Study of Human Sleep: Methodological Problems,* Eds. G.C. Lairy and P. Salzarulo, pp. 55–82. Amsterdam: Elsevier.

Bricolo, A., and Turella, G. 1973. Electroencephalographic patterns of acute traumatic coma: diagnostic and prognostic value. J. Neurosurg. Sci. 17:278–285.

Bricolo, A., Gentilomo, A., Rosadini, G., et al. 1968. Akinetic mutism following cranio-cerebral trauma. Physiopathological considerations based on sleep studies. Acta Neurochir. (Wien) 18:68–77.

Bricolo, A., Turazzi, S., Faccioli, F., et al. 1978. Clinical application of compressed spectral array in long-term EEG monitoring of comatose patients. Electroencephalogr. Clin. Neurophysiol. 45:211–225.

Britt, R.H., Herrick, M.K., and Hamilton, R.D. 1977. Traumatic locked-in syndrome. Ann. Neurol. 1:590–592.

Busse, E.W., and Silverman, A.J. 1952. Electroencephalographic changes in professional boxers. JAMA. 149:1522–1525.

Butenuth, J., and Kubicki, S. 1975. Klinisch-elektroenzephalographische Schlafbeobachtungen im apallischen Syndrome. Z. EEG-EMG 6:185–188.

Cadilhac, J., El Kassabgui, M., and Passouant, P. 1966. La réorganisation du sommeil nocturne après les comas posttraumatiques. Rev. Neurol. 115:529(abst).

Cant, B.R., and Shaw, N.A. 1984. Monitoring by compressed spectral array in prolonged coma. Neurology 34:35–39.

Caveness, W.F. 1966. Posttraumatic sequelae. In *Head Injury, Conference Proceedings,* Eds. W.F. Caveness and A.E. Walker, pp. 209–219. Philadelphia/Toronto: Lippincott.

Chase, T.N., Moretti, L., and Prensky, A.L. 1968. Clinical and electroencephalographic manifestations of vascular lesions of the pons. Neurology (Minneapolis) 18:357–368.

Chatrian, G.E. 1975. Electrographic and behavioral signs of sleep in comatose states. In *Handbook of Electroencephalography and Clinical Neurophysiology*, vol. 12, Eds. A. Remond, R. Harner, and R. Naquet, pp. 63–77. Amsterdam: Elsevier.

Chatrian, G.E., White, J.R., and Daly, P. 1963. Electroencephalographic patterns resembling those of sleep in certain comatose states after injuries to the head. Electroencephalogr. Clin. Neurophysiol. 15:272–280.

Chatrian, G.E., Lowell, M.D., White, E., Jr., et al. 1964a. EEG pattern resembling wakefulness in unresponsive decerebrate state following traumatic brain stem infarct. Electroencephalogr. Clin. Neurophysiol. 16:285–289.

Chatrian, G.E., Shaw, C.M., and Leffman, H. 1964b. The significance of periodic lateralized epileptiform discharges in the EEG: an electroencephalographic, clinical and pathologic study. Electroencephalogr. Clin. Neurophysiol. 17:177–193.

Chokroverty, S. 1975. "Alpha-like" rhythms in electroencephalograms in coma after cardiac arrest. Neurology (Minneapolis) 25:655–663.

Christian, W. 1968. *Klinische Elektroenzephalographie. Lehrbuch und Atlas,* pp. 264–274. Stuttgart: Thieme.

Courjon, J. 1962. La place de l'électroencéphalographie en traumatologie crânienne. Cah. Méd. Lyon 38:315–317.

Courjon, J., and Revol, M. 1966. Traumatismes crâniens et épilepsie. Cah. Méd. Lyon 42:1343–1350.

Courjon, J., and Scherzer, E. 1972. Traumatic disorders. In *Handbook of Electroencephalography and Clinical Neurophysiology,* vol. 14, Eds. A. Remond, O. Magnus, and J. Courjon, pp. 8–95. Amsterdam: Elsevier.

Courjon, J., Naquet, R., Baurand, C., et al. 1971. Valeur diagnostique de l'E.E.G. dans les suites immédiates des traumatismes crâniens. Rev. EEG Neurophysiol. 1:133–150.

Critchley, M. 1957. Medical aspects of boxing, particularly from a neurological standpoint. Br. Med. J. 1:357–362.

Davis, P.A., and Davis, H. 1939. The electrical activity of the brain. Its relation to physiological states and to states of impaired consciousness. Res. Publ. Assoc. Res. Nerv. Ment. Dis. 19:50–80.

Dawson, E.E., Webster, J.E., and Gurdjian, E.S. 1951. Serial electroencephalography in acute head injuries. J. Neurosurg. 8:613–630.

Denny-Brown, D. 1961. Brain trauma and concussion. Arch. Neurol. 5:1–3.

Denny-Brown, D., and Russel, W.R. 1941. Experimental cerebral concussion. Brain 64:93–164.

Dolce, G., and Kaemmerer, E. 1967. Contribute anatomico-clinico ed elettroencefalografico all conoscenza della sindromi apallica. Studio dell evoluzione dell EEG da sonne in 5 casi. Sist. Nerv. 1:12–23.

Dow, R., Ulett, G., and Raaf, J. 1944. Electroencephalographic studies immediately following head injury. Am. J. Psychiatr. 101:174–183.

Duensing, F. 1948. Die Alphawellenaktivierung als Herdsymptom in Elektroencephalogramm. Nervenarzt 19:544–552.

Dumermuth, G. 1965. *Elektroencephalographie im Kindesalter*, pp. 262–266. Stuttgart: Thieme.

Dusser, A., Navelet, Y., Devictor, D., et al. 1989. Short- and long-term prognostic value of the electroencephalogram in children with severe head injury. Electroencephalogr. Clin. Neurophysiol. 73:85–93.

Ferguson, J.M., and Benett, D.R. 1974. Sleep in a patient with pontine infarction. Electroencephalogr. Clin. Neurophysiol. 36:210–211(abst).

Fischer, C.M. 1969. The neurological examination of the comatose patient. Acta Neurol. Scand. 36(suppl):45–56.

Fischer, C., and Mutschler, V. 2002. Traumatic brain injuries in adults: from coma to wakefulness. Neurophysiological data. Ann. Readapt. Med. Phys. 45:448–455.

Fischgold, H., and Mathis, P. 1959. *Obnubilations, comas et stupeurs, études électroencéphalographiques.* Electroencephalogr. Clin. Neurophysiol. 11(suppl):27–68.

Fischgold, H., Torrubia, H., Mathis, P., et al. 1955. Réaction EEG d'éveil (arousal) dans le coma. Corrélations cortico-cárdio-respiratoires. Presse Méd. 61:1231–1233.

Forster, J.B., Leiguarda, R., and Tilley, P.J.B. 1976. Brain damage in national hunt jockeys. Lancet 1:981–987.

Gerstenbrand, F. 1967. *Das traumatische apallische Syndrome.* Wien/New York: Springer.

Gerstenbrand, F. 1977. The symptomatology of the apallic syndrome. In *The Apallic Syndrome*, Eds. G. Dalle Ore, F. Gerstenbrand, C.H. Lücking, et al., pp. 14–21. Berlin/Heidelberg/New York: Springer.

Gerstenbrand, F., and Lücking, C.H. 1970. Die akuten traumatischen Hirnstammschäden. Arch. Psychiatr. Nervenkr. 213:264–281.

Gerstenbrand, F., and Rumpl, E. 1983. Das prolongierte Mittelhirnsyndrom traumatischer Genese. In *Hirnstamml sionen*, Ed. K.J. Neumrker, pp. 236–248. Leipzig: Hirzel.

Gerstenbrand, F., Rumpl, E., and Prugger, M. 1980. Die apallische Symptomatik. In *Neurotraumatologie, Derzeitige Schwerpunkte, 8. Internationales Symposium Erlangen 1979*, Ed. H.H. Wiek, pp. 235–239. Stuttgart: Thieme.

Gibbs, F.A., and Gibbs, E.L. 1987. Electroencephalographic study of head injury in childhood. Clin. Electroencephalogr. 18:10–11.

Gloor, P., Ball, G., and Schaul, N. 1977. Brain lesions that produce delta waves in the EEG. Neurology 27:326–333.

Goetze, W. 1953. Das Hirnstrombild bei offenen Hirnverletzungen. Mschr. Unfallheilk. 56:297–305.

Goulon, M., Pocidalo, J.J., Christophe, M., et al. 1959. Clinical, electroencephalographic and biological correlations in 34 cases of bronchopneumonia with asphyxia. In *Cerebral Anoxia and the Electroencephalogram*, Eds. H. Gastaut and J.S. Meyer, pp. 565–577. Springfield, IL: Charles C Thomas.

Grand, W. 1974. The significance of post-traumatic status epilepticus in childhood. J. Neurol. Neurosurg. Psychiatry 37:178–180.

Haglund, Y., and Persson, H.E. 1990. Does Swedish amateur boxing lead to chronic brain damage? 3. A retrospective clinical neurophysiological study. Acta Neurol. Scand. 82:353–360.

Hall, R.C., and Joffe, J.R. 1973. Hypomagnesemia: physical and psychiatric symptoms. JAMA. 244:1749–1751.

Hansotia, P., Gottschalk, P., Green, P., et al. 1981. Spindle coma: incidence, clinicopathologic correlates, and prognostic value. Neurology (Minneapolis) 31:83–87.

Hess, R. 1961. Significance of EEG signs for localization of cerebral tumours. Electroencephalogr. Clin. Neurophysiol. 19(suppl):75–110.

Hess, R. 1965. Sleep and sleep disturbances in the electroencephalogram. Prog. Brain Res. 18:127–139.

Hill, D. 1950. Psychiatry. In *Electroencephalography*, Eds. D. Hill and G. Parr, pp. 319–363. London: MacDonald.

Hockaday, J.M., Potts, F., Epstein, E., et al. 1965. EEG changes in acute cerebral anoxia from cardiac or respiratory arrest. Electroencephalogr. Clin. Neurophysiol. 18:575–586.

Hooshmand, H., Beckner, E., and Radfor, F. 1989. Technical and clinical aspects of topographic brain mapping. Clin. Electroencephalogr. 20:235–247.

Hörtnagl, H., Hammerle, A.F., Hackl, J.M., et al. 1980. The activity of the sympathetic nervous system in the course of severe head injury. Intensive Care. Med. 6:169–177.

Horton, E.J., Goldie, W.D., and Baram, T.Z. 1990. Rhythmic coma in children. J. Child Neurol. 5:242–247.

Hughes, J.R., Boshes, B., and Leestma, J. 1976. Electro-clinical and pathologic correlations in comatose patients. Clin. Electroencephalogr. 7: 13–30.

Hunter, J., and Jasper, H.H. 1949. Effects of thalamic stimulation in unanesthetized animals. Electroencephalogr. Clin. Neurophysiol. 1:305–324.

Hutchinson, D.O., Frith, R.W., Shaw, N.A., et al. 1991. A comparison between electroencephalography and somatosensory evoked potentials for outcome prediction following severe head injury. Electroencephalograph. Clin. Neurophysiol. 78:228–233.

Ingvar, D.H., and Brun, A. 1972. Das komplette apallische Syndrom. Arch. Psychiatr. Nervenheilkd. 215:219–239.

Jabbari, B., Vengrow, M.I., Salazar, A.M., et al. 1986. Clinical and radiological correlates of EEG in the late phase of head injury: a study of 515 Vietnam veterans. Electroencephalogr. Clin. Neurophysiol. 64: 285–293.

Jacome, D.E. 1987. EEG in whiplash: a reappraisal. Clin. Electroencephalogr. 18:41–45.

Jasper, H.H., and Van Buren, J. 1953. Interrelationships between cortex and subcortical structures. Clinical electroencephalographic studies. Electroencephalogr. Clin. Neurophysiol. 4(suppl):168–202.

Jefferson, M. 1952. Altered consciousness associated with brain stem lesions. Brain 75:55–67.

Jellinger, K. 1967. Häufigkeit und Pathogenese zentraler Hirnläsionen nach stumpfer Gewalteinwirkung auf den Schädel. Wien Z. Nervenheilkd. 25:223–249.

Jellinger, K., Gerstenbrand, F., and Pateisky, K. 1963. Die protrahierte Form der posttraumatischen Enzephalopathie. Nervenarzt. 34:145–163.

Jennett, W.B. 1969. Early traumatic epilepsy. Lancet 1:1023–1025.

Jennet, B., and Bond, M. 1975. Assessment of outcome after severe brain damage. Lancet 1:480–484.

Jerrett, S.A., and Corsak, J. 1988. Clinical utility of topographic EEG brain mapping. Clin. Electroencephalogr. 19:134–143.

Johnson, J. 1969. The EEG in the traumatic encephalopathy of boxers. Psychiatr. Clin. 2:204–211.

Jordan, K.G. 1993. Continuous EEG and evoked potential monitoring in the neuroscience intensive care unit. J. Clin. Neurophysiol. 10:445–475.

Jouvet, M. 1961. Telencephalic and rhombencephalic sleep in the cat. In *The Nature of Sleep*, Eds. G.E.W. Wolstenholme and M. O'Connor, pp. 188–208. Boston: Little, Brown.

Jung, R. 1953. Neurophysiologische Untersuchungsmethoden. In *Handbuch der Inneren Medizin V*, vol. 1, Eds. G. Bergmann, W. Frey, and H. Schwiegk, pp. 1286–1293. Berlin: Springer.

Kazibutowska, Z., Stelmach-Wawrzyczek, M., and Majchrzak, R. 1992. Results of prospective 24-hour EEG studies of patients after craniocerebral injuries. Neurol. Neurochir. Pol. 26:304–310.

Kelly, J.P., and Rosenberg, J.H. 1997. Diagnosis and management of concussion in sports. Neurology (Minneapolis) 48:575–580.

Kiloh, L.G., and Osselton, J.W. 1966. *Clinical Electroencephalography*, p. 125. London: Butterworths.

Klein, H.J., Rath, S.A., and Göppel, F. 1988. The use of EEG spectral analysis after thiopental bolus in the prognostic evaluation of comatose patients with brain injuries. Acta Neurochirurg. 42(suppl):31–34.

Koufen, H., and Dichgans, J. 1978. Häufigkeit und Ablauf von traumatischen EEG-Veränderungen und ihre klinischen Korrelationen. Fortschr. Neurol. Psychiatr. 46:165–177.

Koufen, H., and Hagel, K.H. 1987. Systematic EEG follow-up study of traumatic psychosis. Eur. Arch. Psychiatr. Neurol. Sci. 237:2–7.

Kubicki, S., Rieger, H., and Busse, G. 1970. EEG in fatal and near fatal poisoning with soporific drugs. I. Typical EEG patterns. Clin. Electroencephalogr. 1:5–13.

Kugler, J. 1966. *Elektroenzephalographie in Klinik und Praxis.* 2. Aufl., p. 203. Stuttgart: Thieme.

Kuhlendahl, K. 1964. Die neurologischen syndrome bei der Überstreckungsverletzung der Halswirbelsäule und dem sogenannten Schleudertrauma. M. Med. Wschr. 106:1025–1030.

Larsson, L.E., Melin, K.A., Nordström-Öhrberg, B.O., et al. 1954. Acute head injuries in boxers. Acta Psychiatr. Scand. 95(suppl):1–42.

Lenard, H.G. 1965. EEG-Veränderungen bei frischen Schädeltraumen im Kindesalter. Med. Wschr. 107:1820–1827.

Loeb, C. 1958. Electroencephalographic changes during the state of coma. Electroencephalogr. Clin. Neurophysiol. 10:589–606.

Lorenzoni, E. 1975. Das EEG im posttraumatischen Koma. Fortschr. Neurol. Psychiatr. 43:155–191.

Lücking, G.H. 1970. Sleep-like patterns and abnormal arousal reactions in brain stem lesions. Electroencephalogr. Clin. Neurophysiol. 28:214 (abst).

Lücking, G.H., Müllner, E., Pateisky, K., et al. 1977. Electroencephalographic findings in the apallic syndrome. In *The Apallic Syndrome,* Eds. G. Dalle Ore, F. Gerstenbrand, C.H. Lücking, et al., pp. 144–154. Berlin/Heidelberg/New York: Springer.

Maciver, J.N., Lassman, L.P., Thomas, C.W., et al. 1958. Treatment of severe head injuries. Lancet 2:544–550.

Markand, O.N., and Daly, D.D. 1971. Pseudoperiodic lateralized paroxysmal discharges in electroencephalogram. Neurology (Minneapolis) 21:975–981.

Martland, H.S. 1928. Punch drunk. JAMA. 91:1103–1107.

Mathis, P., Turrubia, H., and Fischgold, H. 1957. Réactivité, périodicité et corrélation cortico-cardio-respiratoire dans le coma. Electroencephalogr. Clin. Neurophysiol. 6(suppl):27–68.

Mawdsley, C., and Ferguson, F.R. 1963. Neurological disease in boxers. Lancet 2:795–801.

McNealy, D.E., and Plum, F. 1962. Brain stem dysfunction with supratentorial mass lesions. Arch. Neurol. 7:26–48.

Melin, K.A. 1949. Electroencephalography following head injuries in children. Acta Pediatr. (Uppsala) 75:152–174.

Merill, J.P., and Hampers, C.L. 1970. Uremia (part 1). N. Engl. J. Med. 289:953–961.

Meyer-Mickeleit, R.W. 1953. Das Elektroenzephalogramm nach gedeckten Kopfverletzungen. Dtsch. Med. Wschr. 1:480–484.

Mifka, P., and Scherzer, E. 1962a. Zur Pathogenese zerebraler Symptomatik bei Verletzungen der Halswirbelsäule. Münch. Med. Wschr. 10:1686–1690.

Mifka, P., and Scherzer, E. 1962b. Über die Wertigkeit des EEG im Spätstadium der Gehirnverletzung. Wien. Klin. Wschr. 74:573–576.

Miller, J.D. 1979. Barbiturates and raised intracranial pressure (editorial). Ann. Neurol. 6:189–193.

Millspaugh, J.A. 1937. Dementia puglistica (punch drunk). U.S. Nav. Med. Bull. 35:297–303.

Mitchell, D.E., and Adams, J.H. 1973. Primary focal impact damage to the brain stem in blunt injuries. Does it exist? Lancet 2:215–218.

Myers, R.R., Stockard, J.J., and Saidman, L.J. 1977. Monitoring of cerebral perfusion during anesthesia by time-compressed Fourier analysis of the electroencephalogram. Stroke 8:331–337.

Naquet, R., Vigouroux, R.P., Choux Bourand, C., et al. 1967. Étude électroencéphalographique des traumatismes craniens récents dans un service de ré-animation. Rev. Neurol. 117:512–513(abst).

Newlon, P.G., Greenberg, R.P., Enas, G.G., et al. 1983. Effects of therapeutic pentobarbital coma on multimodality evoked potentials recorded from severely head-injured patients. Neurosurgery 12:613–619.

Niedermeyer, E., and Knott, J. 1961. Über die Bedeutung der 14 and 6/sec positiven Spitzen in EEG. Arch. Psychiatr. Nervenkr. 202:266–280.

Ommaya, A.K., and Gennarelli, T.A. 1974. Cerebral concussion and traumatic unconsciousness. Brain 97:633–654.

Ommaya, A.K., Grupp, R.L., Jr., and Naumann, R.A. 1971. Coup and contre-coup: observations on the mechanics of visible brain injuries in the rhesus monkey. J. Neurosurg. 35:503–517.

Ommaya, A.K., Corrao, P.G., and Letcher, F. 1973. Head injury in the chimpanzee: Part I. Biodynamics of traumatic unconsciousness. J. Neurosurg. 39:152–166.

Osborn, A.G. 1977. Diagnosis of descending herniation by cranial computed tomography. Radiology 123:93–96.

Overgaard, J., Hvid-Hansen, O., Land, A.M., et al. 1973. Prognosis after head injury based on early clinical examination. Lancet 2:631–635.

Pampus, F., and Grote, W. 1956. Elektroencephalographische und klinische Befunde bei Boxern und ihre Bedeutung fr die Pathophysiologie der traumatishcen Hirnschädigung. Arch. Psychiatr. Nervenkr. 194:152–178.

Passouant, P., Cadilhac, J., Delange, M., et al. 1964. Différentes stades électriques et organization en cycle des comas posttraumatiques. Enrégistrement polygraphique de long durée. Rev. Neurol. 111:391(abst).

Pateisky, K., Gerstenbrand, F., and Jellinger, K. 1963. The EEG in the posttraumatic apallic syndrome. Electroencephalogr. Clin. Neurophysiol. 15:713(abst).

Pfurtscheller, G., Schwartz, G., and List, W. 1986. Long-lasting EEG reactions in comatose patients after repetitive stimulation. Electroencephalogr. Clin. Neurophysiol. 64:402–410.

Plum, F., and Posner, J.B. 1966. *Diagnosis of Stupor and Coma.* Philadelphia: F.A. Davis.

Prior, P.F. 1973. *The EEG in Acute Cerebral Anoxia,* pp. 43–46. Amsterdam: Excerpta Medica.

Radermecker, J. 1964. Das EEG bei gedeckten Hirnschäden und seine Beziehung zu den subjektiven Beschwerden. Med. Wschr. 106:1315–1322.

Rae-Grant, A.D., Barbour, P.J., and Reed, J. 1991. Development of a novel EEG rating scale for head injury using dichotomous variables. Electroencephalogr. Clin. Neurophysiol. 79:349–357.

Reich, J.B., Sierra, J., Camp, W., et al. 1993. Magnetic resonance imaging measurements and clinical changes accompanying transtentorial and foramen magnum brain herniation. Ann. Neurol. 34:748–749.

Roberts, A.H. 1969. *Brain Damage in Boxers.* London: Pitman Medical Scientific Publishing.

Rumpl, E. 1979. Elektro-neurologische Korrelationen in den frühen Phasen des posttraumatischen Komas. I. Das EEG in den verschiedenen Phasen des akuten traumatischen sekundären. Mittelhirn und Bulbärhirnsyndroms. Z. EEG-EMG 10:148–157.

Rumpl, E. 1980. Elektro-neurologische Korrelationen in den frühen Phasen des posttraumatischen Komas. II. Das EEG im Übergang zum, und im Vollbild des traumatischen apallischen Syndroms. Z. EEG-EMG 11:43–50.

Rumpl, E., Lorenzi, E., Hackl, J.M., et al. 1979. The EEG at different stages of acute secondary traumatic midbrain and bulbar brain syndromes. Electroencephalogr. Clin. Neurophysiol. 46:487–497.

Rumpl, E., Prugger, M., Bauer, G., et al. 1983. Incidence and prognostic value of spindles in post-traumatic coma. Electroencephalogr. Clin. Neurophysiol. 56:420–429.

Rumpl, E., Prugger, M., and Bauer, G. 1984. Zum prognostischen Wert elektroenzephalographischer Schlafbeobachtungen im traumatisch bedingten apallischen Syndrom. Neuropsychiatr. Clin. 3:219–232.

Saunders, R.L., and Harbaugh, R.E. 1984. The second impact in catastrophic contact sports head trauma. JAMA 252:538–539.

Scherzer, E. 1965. Wert der Elektroenzephalographie beim Schädel-trauma. Wien. Klin. Wschr. 77:543–547.

Schneider, E., and Hubach, H. 1962. Das EEG der traumatischen Psychosen. Dtsch. Z. Nervenheilkd. 183:600–627.

Schwab, R.S. 1951. *Electroencephalography in Clinical Practice*, p. 195. Philadelphia: Saunders.

Shaw, N.A. 2002. The neurophysiology of concussion. Prog. Neurobiol. 67:281–344.

Silverman, D. 1963. Retrospective study of EEG in coma. Electroencephalogr. Clin. Neurophysiol. 15:486–503.

Sironi, V.A., Ravagnati, L., Signorini, G., et al. 1983. Diagnostic and prognostic value of EEG compressed spectral analysis in posttraumatic coma. In *Advances in Neurotraumatology,* Eds. R. Vilani, J. Papo, M. Giovanelli, et al., pp. 328–330. Amsterdam: Excerpta Medica.

Steudel, W.I., and Krüger, J. 1979. Using the spectral analysis of the EEG for prognosis of severe brain injuries in the first post-traumatic week. Acta Neurochir. 28(suppl):40–42.

Steudel, W.I., Krüger, J., and Grau, H. 1979. Zur Alpha- und Spindel-Aktivitt bei komatsen Patienten nach einer Schdel-Hire-Verletzung unter besonderer Berücksichtigung der Computertomographie. Z. EEG-EMG 10:143–147.

Stockard, J.J., Bickford, R.G., and Aung, M.H. 1975. The electroencephalogram in traumatic brain injury. In *Handbook of Clinical Neurology,* vol. 23, Eds. P.J. Vinken and G.W. Bruyn, pp. 217–367. Amsterdam/Oxford: North-Holland.

Stone, J.L., Ghaly, R.F., and Hughes, J.R. 1988. Electroencephalography in acute head injury. J. Clin. Neurophysiol. 5:125–133.

Strnad, P., and Strnadová, V. 1987. Long-term follow-up EEG studies in patients with traumatic apallic syndrome. Eur. Neurol. 26:84–89.

Synek, V.M. 1990. Value of a revised EEG coma scale for prognosis after cerebral anoxia and diffuse head injury. Clin. Electroencephalogr. 21:25–30.

Synek, V.M., and Synek, B.J.L. 1984. Theta pattern coma, a variant of alpha pattern coma. Clin. Electroencephalogr. 15:116–121.

Thatcher, R.W., Walker, R.A., Gerson, I., et al. 1989. EEG discriminant analysis of mild head trauma. Electroencephalogr. Clin. Neurophysiol. 73:94–106.

Thatcher, R.W., Cantor, D.S., McAlaster, R., et al. 1991. Comprehensive predictions of outcome in closed head-injured patients. Ann. N.Y. Acad. Sci. 620:82–101.

Tönnis, A. 1956. Beobachtungen an frischen gedeckten Hirnschädigungen. In *Das Hirntrauma*, Ed. E. Rehwald, p. 772. Stuttgart: Thieme.

Torres, F., and Shapiro, S.K. 1961. Electroencephalograms in whiplash injury. Arch. Neurol. 5:28–35.

Toyonaga, K., Schlagenhauff, R.E., and Smith, B.H. 1974. Periodic lateralized epileptiform discharges in subdural hematoma. Case-reports and review in literature. Clin. Electroencephalogr. 5:113–118.

Tysvaer, A.T., Storli, O.V., and Bachen, N.I. 1989. Soccer injuries to the brain. A neurologic and electroencephalographic study of former players. Acta Neurol. Scand. 80:151–156.

Tysvaer, A.T. 1992. Head and neck injuries in soccer. Impact of minor trauma. Sports Med. 14:200–213.

Valente, M., Placidi, F., Oliveira, A.J., et al. Sleep organization pattern as a prognostic marker at the subacute stage of post-traumatic coma. 2002. Clin. Neurophysiol. 113: 1798–1805.

Verjaal, A. 1972. Trauma capitis. In *Neurologie vor de algemene praktijk*, Eds. R. van den Bergh and J.F. Folkerts, pp. 170–187. Brussels: Agon-Elsevier.

Verjaal, A., and Van't Hooft, F. 1975. Commotio and contusio cerebri (cerebral concussion). In *Handbook of Clinical Neurology*, vol. 23, Eds. P.J. Vinken and G.W. Bruyn, pp. 417–444. Amsterdam/Oxford: North-Holland.

Vigouroux, R.P. 1975. Between life and death. In *Handbook of Electroencephalography and Clinical Neurophysiology*, vol. 12, Eds. A. Remond, R. Harner, and R. Naquet, pp. 95–98. Amsterdam: Elsevier.

Vigouroux, R., Naquet, R., Baurand, C., et al. 1964. Évolution électroradio-clinique de comas graves prolongés post-traumatiques. Rev. Neurol. 110:72–81.

Vigouroux, R.P., Naquet, R., and Gastaut, H. 1966. Aspects particuliers de certaines manifestations épileptiques précoces lors de traumatismes crânio-cérébraux survénus chez des sujects âgés. Rev. Neurol. 115: 976–980.

Voller, B., Benke, T., Benedetto, K., et al. 1999. Neuropsychological, MRT and EEG findings after very mild traumatic brain injury. Brain Inj. 13: 821–827.

Walter, W., Hill, D., and Williams, D. 1948. Discussion of the electroencephalogram in organic cerebral disease. Proc. Soc. Med. Lond. 41:237–250.

Williams, D. 1941a. The electro-encephalogram in acute head injuries. J. Neurol. Psychiatry 4:107–130.

Williams, D. 1941b. The electroencephalogram in chronic posttraumatic states. J. Neurol. Psychiatry 4:131–146.

Williams, D., and Denny-Brown, D. 1941. Cerebral electrical changes in experimental concussion. Brain 64:223–238.

Wilson, W.P., and Sieker, H.L. 1958. A study of the factors responsible for changes in the electroencephalogram in chronic pulmonary insufficiency. Electroencephalogr. Clin. Neurophysiol. 10:89–96.

Wohlrab, G., Schmitt, B., and Botshauser, E. 1997. Benign focal epileptiform discharges in children after severe head trauma: prognostic value and clinical course. Epilepsia. 38:275–278.

Yamamoto, L.G., and Bart, R.T. 1989. Transient blindness following mild head trauma. Clin. Pediatr. 27:479–483.

22. Metabolic Central Nervous System Disorders

Ernst Niedermeyer

Introduction and Historical Remarks

A quick glance at neuronal electrogenesis tells us it is dependent on metabolic homeostasis. Nutritive and energy-providing metabolic systems represent the fuel for neuronal and glial structures; abnormalities in their composition may lead to pronounced clinical and electroencephalographic acute and subacute changes; these are usually reversible, but sometimes irreversible progression evolves.

Cerebral metabolic disturbances and/or electroencephalogram (EEG) changes due to blood alkalosis from hyperventilation and anoxia are presented elsewhere. This chapter deals mainly with alterations of the blood sugar level, failure of the hepatic and renal organ systems, states of electrolyte imbalance, changes due to endocrine disorders, and certain toxic-metabolic conditions. Some chronic metabolic disturbances such as inborn errors of metabolism are discussed under the heading of degenerative disorders.

Berger's (1937) observation of slow activity induced by hypoglycemia in schizophrenic patients treated with insulin marked the beginning of EEG studies in human metabolic disorders. Over the ensuing years, EEG studies in metabolic disorders remained somewhat in the background when compared with activity in the fields of epileptic seizure disorder and structural cerebral lesions. Most of the metabolic disorders belong to the domain of internal medicine, a field of understandably limited interest in EEG investigations.

Major progress was made when the work of Foley et al. (1950) and Bickford and Butt (1955) on hepatic coma showed very pronounced slowing and formation of triphasic waves. The contributions of Condon et al. (1954), Krump (1955), Thiébaut et al. (1958), Cadilhac et al. (1959), and Glaser (1960) have provided further important information on the EEG correlates of metabolic encephalopathies.

There has been persistent interest in the EEG of metabolic disorders; this is probably due to the discovery of renal encephalopathies after dialysis in chronic renal insufficiency and the availability of modern EEG monitoring techniques (MacGillivray, 1976).

Hypoglycemia

Cerebral functioning depends on an adequate supply of glucose. Hypoglycemia-induced EEG changes have been shown experimentally by Moruzzi (1938), Himwich et al. (1939), Gellhorn and Kessler (1942), and Davis (1943). It was found that the electrical activity of the cortex disappears earlier than that of deep structures. Level of awareness, blood sugar level, and EEG changes do not necessarily parallel

each other (Gellhorn and Kessler, 1942). Later work in the cat by Waltrégny (1969) placed special emphasis on hypoglycemic epileptic seizures. Creutzfeldt and Meisch (1963) studied the behavior of single neurons in hypoglycemia.

Early clinical EEG observations were reported by Berger (1937), Hoagland et al. (1937), Gibbs et al. (1940), Davis (1943), Engel et al. (1944), Weinland and Weinland (1949), Lafon et al. (1950), Gibbs and Murray (1954), Hetzel and Niedermeyer (1955), Shagass and Roswell (1954), and Regan and Browne-Mayers (1956). It was found that very low blood sugar levels were compatible with a normal EEG (Ziegler and Presthus, 1957) and also with wakefulness. Clinical observations had already shown that impairment of consciousness and disturbance of central nervous system (CNS) functions were dependent mainly on the rapid fall of the blood sugar level, rather than on absolute values (Von Braunmühl, 1947). Patients with insulin-dependent diabetes mellitus may be unaware of hypoglycemia; their nearly normal glycosylated hemoglobin levels result in normal cerebral glucose uptake and preserve cerebral metabolism (Boyle et al., 1995).

Most of the aforementioned work was based on administration of insulin for therapeutic purposes in schizophrenic patients (Sakel cure). During the 1960s, the decline of this type of treatment and the substitution of major tranquilizers dampened further investigations in the human, aside from major studies by Poiré et al. (1966) and Poiré (1969).

All of this work shows an extremely impressive degree of slowing in the EEG combined with epileptic activity that may be more or less prominent depending on individual propensities. Particularly impressive is the rapidity of the EEG normalization after stomach tube feeding or intravenous administration of glucose.

Spontaneous states of hypoglycemia (functional or neoplastic hyperinsulinism) may give rise to varying degrees of EEG change (Gastaut et al., 1969). In some of these patients, profound coma and/or major convulsions may occur; the EEG may be characterized by massive spiking (Hoefer et al., 1946). Even psychomotor (complex partial) seizures have been reported in a case of insulinoma (Scarpino et al., 1985).

With the use of long-term EEG, Lefebre et al. (1990) demonstrated a grand mal in the early morning hours, associated with a blood sugar level of 28 mg/dL. A hyperinsulinoma was diagnosed; surgery rendered the patient seizure-free.

Hyperglycemia

Hyperglycemic states are much less eloquent in the EEG than states of hypoglycemia. Gibbs et al. (1940) found mixed slow and fast frequencies and some intermingled spiking in patients with blood sugar levels exceeding 400 mg/100 mL. In advanced diabetic coma, however, very pronounced slowing may occur, and the record may become indistinguishable from a hypoglycemic state (Krump, 1955). According to Cadilhac et al. (1959), the EEG abnormalities may persist for several days despite effective treatment. Occasionally, epileptogenic lesions may result from comatose states (Engel et al., 1954), but such sequelae are more likely to be caused by the hypo- rather than the hyperglycemic state.

A distinction has to be made between ketotic and nonketotic hyperglycemia; the latter entity was described by DiBenedetto et al. (1965) and appears to be rich in neurological complications. Epileptic seizures of focal character are common in this condition (Daniel et al., 1969; Maccario et al., 1965; Vastola et al., 1967), as are, above all, focal motor seizures with rolandic EEG spike foci and contralateral clonic motions (Aquino and Gabor, 1980; Singh and Strobos, 1980). These seizures can be induced by movement (Gabor, 1974; Duncan et al., 1991). Occipital lobe seizures may be an initial manifestation (Harden et al., 1991) and can be triggered by lateral gaze (Duncan et al., 1991). The hyperglycemic states do not have to be nonketotic in order to cause focal seizures but, in such cases, a ketotic-nonacidotic situation is found (Daniel et al., 1969).

Liver Disease (Hepatic Encephalopathy)

Liver disease as such does not necessarily produce major EEG changes; even chronically confused and disoriented patients may show only moderate EEG abnormalities (Guggenheim et al., 1964; Penin, 1967); in other instances, very pronounced EEG slowing predominates. Absence or presence of prominent EEG changes obviously hinges on certain pathogenetic or pathophysiological mechanisms. For this reason, some discussion of the pathophysiological mechanisms and their clinical expression is needed.

A distinction must be made between the concept of *portal-systemic encephalopathies* (Sherlock et al., 1954) and *acute massive hepatic cellular failure.* Portal-systemic encephalopathies are based on portocaval anastomosis (Eck's fistula); protein loads from, for example, eating meat lead to hepatic coma. This condition is found in chronic cirrhosis of the liver with portal-systemic venous shunts. Complete acute breakdown of the liver results in hepatic encephalopathy with coma. Toxic (mainly nitrogenous) substances reach the brain in either case. In advanced states, the distinction between both pathophysiological mechanisms is impossible, and the neurological and EEG changes of a full-fledged hepatic coma become indistinguishable, regardless of the mechanism (MacGillivray, 1976).

Clinically, hepatic encephalopathy is ushered in by a decline of mental functioning. Apathy, euphoria, childishness, irritability, and impaired intellectual abilities are common. Constructional apraxia is an early sign (Summerskill et al., 1956), followed by slurred speech and lethargy. Asterixis is an early neurological sign and consists of recurrent sudden loss of muscle tone in the outstretched and dorsiflexed hand (Adams and Foley, 1949, 1953). Parkinsonian traits appear (Knell et al., 1974), and pyramidal signs may be present before hypo- and areflexia emerge in profound coma. The

level of consciousness decreased from confusion to lethargy, semicoma and stupor, coma, and deep coma with unresponsiveness. Five stages have been distinguished by Rumpl et al. (1979).

The *biochemical mechanisms* of hepatic encephalopathy are still controversial. The role of *hyperammonemia* has been strongly emphasized (Gabuzda, 1962, 1967; Gabuzda et al., 1952; McDermott and Adams, 1954; Sherlock et al., 1954; Summerskill et al., 1956). The role of an *abnormal glutamine metabolism* and the influence of α-*ketoglutaramate* has been stressed by Duffy et al. (1974). The importance of *false neurotransmitters* with decreased synthesis of brain *norepinephrine* has also been advocated (Fischer, 1974; Fischer and Baldessarini, 1971). The pathogenic mechanisms have been extensively reviewed by Fraser and Arieff (1985).

The *electroencephalographic changes* of hepatic encephalopathy have been well known since the studies of Foley et al. (1950) and Bickford and Butt (1955). The degree of slowing often parallels the level of blood ammonia; this was beautifully demonstrated by Kiloh et al. (1972). Posterior alpha rhythm may be preserved during the early stage of enhanced slowing (Foley et al., 1950). Sudden shifts between a normal alpha frequency (around 9–10/sec) and slow substitutes (around 5–7/sec or 6–8/sec) are common (Bickford and

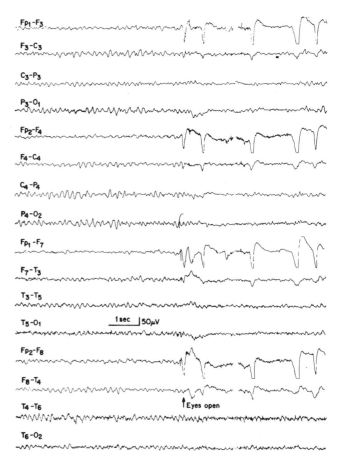

Figure 22.1. Hepatic encephalopathy in a 59-year-old patient. Good treatment response. Blocking response of posterior 5–6/sec basic rhythm. There are also some intermixed 8–10/sec alpha waves of lower voltage.

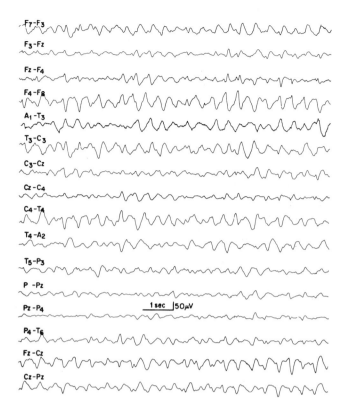

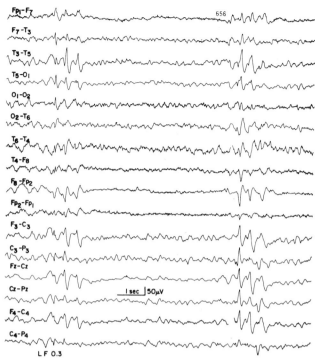

Figure 22.2. Hepatic encephalopathy in a 42-year-old patient. Predominant activity around 2.5/sec, most prominent over frontocentral regions. Note several triphasic waves, especially in channels 4 and 15 in the right portion of the illustration.

Figure 22.4. Triphasic waves of unusually paroxysmal configuration in a 59-year-old patient with hepatic encephalopathy and no history of seizures. Also note the distribution of the potentials and a posterior maximum of the triphasic waves; this is not altogether uncommon.

Butt, 1955; Friedlander, 1956; Laidlaw, 1959; Laidlaw et al., 1961; MacGillivray, 1976; Silverman, 1962) (Fig. 22.1).

Massive EEG slowing, with or without triphasic waves, may be found in the absence of coma and even in conjunction with positive responses to certain mental tasks (Niedermeyer et al., 1989), whereas constructional apraxia is an early sign and precursor of hepatic encephalopathy (Sherlock, 1957). The dynamics of cognitive brain dysfunctions are mirrored by event-related P300 potentials—even with a minor degree of dysfunction (Kügler et al., 1994). Even in the absence of encephalopathy, an abnormal Bereitschaftspotential and magnetic resonance imaging (MRI) pallidal signal may occur in cirrhotic patients (Kulisevsky et al., 1995).

Bickford and Butt (1955) introduced the term *triphasic waves*, which denotes slow waves (usually 1.5–3/sec) with an initiating sharp transient that sometimes may assume the character of a frank spike (Figs. 22.2 to 22.5). The wave morphology of this discharge was recognized earlier by Foley et al. (1950). Bickford and Butt (1955) felt that the triphasic wave complex was highly indicative, if not specific, in hepatic encephalopathy, and there is little doubt that this pattern is more commonly seen in this clinical context than in other usually metabolic cerebral disorders. Triphasic waves are found with deepening impairment of consciousness and sometimes even in patients who are fully awake. When such patients are allowed to fall asleep, normalization of the record takes place for the duration of sleep. Triphasic waves are replaced by further slowing of delta frequencies and general flattening in profound coma and impending death (Jones et al., 1967; Kennedy et al., 1973). In the state of profound coma, very slow delta activity occasionally may be mixed with trains of 14 and 6/sec positive spikes. In general, the incidence of triphasic waves in hepatic encephalopathy lies around 25% (Rumpl et al., 1979; Silverman, 1962; Simsarian and Harner, 1972).

Karnaze and Bickford (1984) reassessed the significance of triphasic waves. According to these authors, triphasic waves are highly characteristic but not pathognomonic for

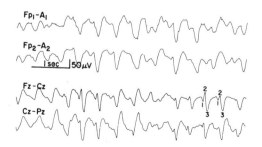

Figure 22.3. Examples of triphasic waves taken from two patients with hepatic encephalopathy. Note wave morphology. The numbers 1, 2, and 3 indicate the phase of the triphasic wave.

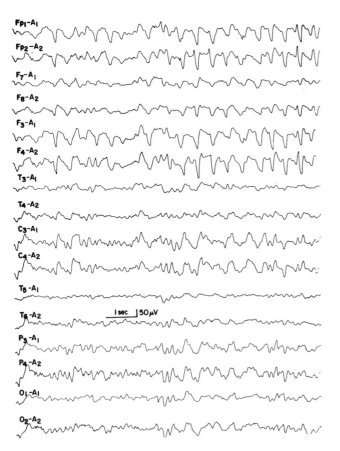

Figure 22.5. What looks like a classical example of triphasic waves in metabolic encephalopathy is, in reality, the EEG of a 37-year-old epileptic who had had three grand mal attacks over the past 2 days.

hepatic encephalopathy. A similar reevaluation of triphasic waves was carried out by Sundaram and Blume (1984).

The question of the clinical significance or specificity of triphasic waves is still engulfed in controversy. Fisch and Klass (1988) have reemphasized the diagnostic specificity of triphasic waves on the basis of their blind study of 56 tracings with triphasic wave patterns. On the other hand, Bahamon-Dussan et al. (1989) pointed out that triphasic waves occur most often in patients with metabolic encephalopathies, cannot be used to distinguish different diagnostic entities, and indicate a poor prognosis for survival. This pessimistic view is justified if (a) the patient is comatose or (b) the background EEG activity is severely disturbed. Aguglia et al. (1990) even underscored the occurrence of triphasic waves in nonmetabolic encephalopathies and brain lesions (stroke, craniopharyngioma, glioma in thalamic level, cortical and subcortical carcinomatosis of the cerebrum, Binswanger's subcortical encephalopathy). Triphasic waves are not uncommon in aged psychiatric patients treated with lithium (Blatt and Brenner, 1996).

Quantification of EEG data has been done by some authors (Cohn and Castell, 1969; Kennedy et al., 1973; Kurtz et al., 1972; Laidlaw, 1959; MacGillivray, 1969, 1976; Van de Rijt et al., 1984; Yaar et al., 1981). According to personal experience with power spectral analysis of four EEG chan-

nels, this method is not superior to visual analysis. A decline of slow delta activity (below 1/sec) along with increasing theta activity has been reported in liver cirrhosis with subclinical hepatic encephalopathy (Elena et al., 2002).

Despite the paroxysmal appearance of triphasic waves, clinically overt epileptic manifestations are not very common in hepatic encephalopathy and occur much less frequently than in renal encephalopathies (Bauer and Niedermeyer, 1979; Gastaut et al., 1969; Plum and Posner, 1966). Surprisingly, Adams and Foley (1953) found an approximately equal incidence of seizures in renal and hepatic failure. Similarities between triphasic waves and spike-wave complexes cannot be denied. The boundaries between spike waves and triphasic waves were discussed by Hughes (1990), Klass (1990), and Ghigo (1990). Ficker et al. (1997) demonstrated various forms of spikes, focal sharp waves, and generalized spike waves in patients with hepatic encephalopathy. These patients also had epileptic seizures and their outcome was poor.

The work of Sherlock (1971), Sherlock and Parbhov (1971), and Kennedy et al. (1973) and the review of MacGillivray (1976) underscore the very important role of the EEG in monitoring the course of the treatment as well as the prognostic aspects of hepatic encephalopathy. "Even small shifts (of 0.5/sec) . . . can be sensitive indicators of the beginning of a trend" (MacGillivray, 1976). The EEG has also proved to be very useful in blind evaluation of patients temporarily treated with calcium and arginine salts of ketoanalogues of branched chain amino acids (Riley et al., 1979; also see Pinelli et al., 1982).

The reason for the particular EEG sensitivity of hepatic encephalopathy is unclear; special features of the cerebral pathology, such as cerebral edema (Silverman, 1962), cerebellar involvement (Ware et al., 1971), and especially astrocytic changes (Cavanagh, 1974), may account for it.

Chronic hepatocerebral degeneration may lead to a variety of EEG changes. The *acquired form* (Victor, 1974; Victor et al., 1965) is neurologically characterized by dysarthria, ataxia, intention tremor, and choreoathetosis affecting chiefly the cranial musculature. This clinical entity is considered to occur much more frequently than the *familial form (Wilson's disease)* (Victor, 1974). The acquired form may develop in various chronic liver diseases and often leads to the above-described picture of hepatic encephalopathy. Such a development is less common in Wilson's disease.

With predominance of basal ganglia syndromes, little or moderate EEG change is present; even normal records are found (Victor et al., 1965). EEG findings in Wilson's disease usually consist of mild or moderate degrees of slowing (Hansotia et al., 1969). In the extensive material of Liu et al. (1983), 54.7% had abnormal tracings. Evoked potential studies in neurologically active cases of Wilson's disease are significantly abnormal, especially auditory brainstem and somatosensory potentials (Grimm et al., 1992).

Cerebral disturbances after liver transplant are not uncommon, caused by factors such as general anesthetics, impaired liver function, sepsis, or hypoxia (Lehmkuhl et al., 1988). The EEG may be used in the assessment of cerebral dysfunction. EEG findings (and especially quantified data) proved to be very useful in the prognostication of liver transplants (Epstein et al., 1992). Girier et al. (1989) investigated the EEG findings in *fulminant hepatic failure in children* and described the stages of progressive EEG deterioration. Inferences with regard to the need of a liver transplant can be made on the basis of the EEG findings.

Renal Disease (Renal Encephalopathy, Uremia)

Impressive EEG changes have been reported in acute as well as in chronic renal failure (Cadilhac, 1976; Cadilhac and Ribstein, 1961; Gloor et al., 1969; Hughes et al., 1950; Jacob et al., 1965; Klinger, 1954; Mises et al., 1968; Prill et al., 1969; Zysno, 1966).

In *acute uremia,* the neurological picture is characterized by agitation, confusion, tremor, fasciculations, myoclonus, coma, and occasional major convulsions (Cadilhac, 1976). There are various EEG abnormalities. Irregular low-voltage activity with slowing of the posterior basic rhythm and occasional theta bursts are noted; other cases show prolonged bursts of bilateral synchronous mixed slow and sharp activity or frank spikes.

Bilateral spike discharges may or may not be associated with widespread myoclonic jerking. Grand mal attacks and, exceptionally, focal (partial) seizures may materialize (Tyler, 1968). About one third of the patients with renal insufficiency develop epileptic seizures (Locke et al., 1961; Prill et al., 1969). Seizures are usually due to water–electrolyte imbalance (Glaser, 1974; Zuckermann and Glaser, 1972).

Epileptic discharges and overt clinical seizures may be prompted by hemodialysis and may occur either during or after the therapeutic procedure (Kennedy et al., 1963; Prill et al., 1969); even status epilepticus may develop (Prill et al., 1969). Convulsions may occur suddenly without preceding EEG changes (Cadilhac, 1976). The pathophysiological mechanisms of the acute dialysis syndrome with seizures (*dysequilibrium syndrome*) have been outlined by Prill et al. (1969) and Glaser (1974). In chronic dialysis treatment, the syndrome of *dialysis dementia* has been reported (Alfrey et al., 1972; Bercaw et al., 1984; Chokroverty and Gandhi, 1982; Hughes and Schreeder, 1981; Kogeorgos et al., 1982; Mahurkar et al., 1973; Stockard and Trauner, 1984). These patients develop, over months and years of dialysis treatment, signs such as confusion, dyspraxia, speech disturbances, memory loss, myoclonus, and psychotic behavior, mostly leading to coma and death. The EEG picture of dialysis dementia requires some clarification. This syndrome usually occurs in hemodialyzed patients, but it has also been reported in peritoneal dialysis (Smith et al., 1980). With glucose added to the hemodialysis fluid, postdialytic EEG worsening could be avoided (Bercaw et al., 1984). Nogues and Vecchierini-Blineau (1987) studied the EEG of 36 patients with renal insufficiency treated with hemodialysis. The EEG worsened after dialysis sessions in 22 cases.

In *chronic uremia,* EEG and mental function are usually stable thanks to prolonged dialysis treatment. Cadilhac (1976) has been impressed with the presence of signs suggestive of a chronic polyneuropathy. Occasional periods of deterioration may occur with seizures and diffuse delta and theta activity (Fig. 22.6) in the EEG. Hughes (1980) found the EEG changes correlated best with blood urea nitrogen

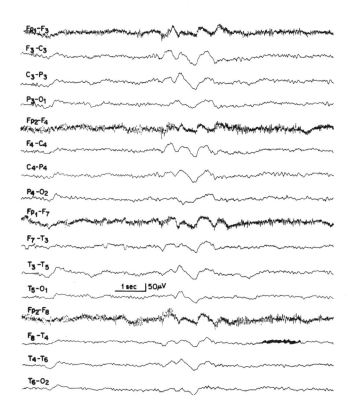

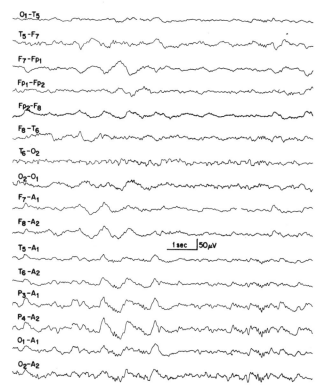

Figure 22.6. **Left:** Encephalopathy due to chronic renal failure (age 50 years). Note intermittent delta runs. **Right:** The same patient in sleep. Trains of delta waves with superimposed spindles, not exceeding the normal limits of variability. The tendency toward normalization in sleep is found in most forms of metabolic encephalopathy.

fluctuations. Generalized spike-wave-like bursts were noted in 8% to 9% of uremic patients (Hughes, 1984). Sensitivity to photic stimulations may be heightened (Tyler, 1965), and changes of the flicker response have been noted (Hamel et al., 1978). Sleep records of chronic uremic patients may show some abnormalities. Long bursts of high-voltage 12 to 13/sec waves with enhanced vertex sharp activity in drowsiness, lack of spindles (14/sec) in stage 2 sleep, and prolonged high-voltage slow bursts with awakening have been reported (Jacob et al., 1965). In rapid-eye-movement (REM) sleep, ocular movements are enhanced; they may even be continuous and associated with blinking and brief myoclonic motions. Nocturnal sleep studies show long periods of insomnia (Cadilhac, 1976). Brass (1980) has stressed the significance of EEG monitoring in terminal renal failure. In *children with renal failure*, diffuse slowing (Lehovsky et al., 1983) and generalized bursts of spikes or spike-wave-like activity (Stockard and Trauner, 1984) are commonly noted.

Patients with *renal transplant* sometimes develop CNS problems associated with EEG slowing. The mechanisms of this type of encephalopathy are very complex.

Eclampsia Gravidarum

Eclampsia gravidarum is a metabolic-toxic syndrome that is pathophysiologically poorly understood. Renal, cerebral, and hepatic functions are involved; grand mal attacks occur at the height of the disturbance intrapartum. Weiss and Dexter (1941) presumed that preeclampsia was an endothelia cell dysfunction giving rise to marked edema. Their speculation was supported by the findings of Belizan et al. (1991) (Ferris, 1991). On the other hand, Schobel et al. (1996) conceived preeclampsia as "a state of sympathetic overactivity" on the basis of sympathetic neurograms.

EEG documentation of the ictal and interictal state has been quite scanty (Guieu et al., 1976; Maltby and Rosenbaum, 1942; Pinto et al., 1981; Thomas et al., 1995; Torgard et al., 1965). In the acute stage of eclampsia, posterior alpha rhythm is seldom recorded; this is probably due to the preferential localization of the main process in the occipital lobes (Calloni et al., 1981). Occipital predominance of EEG abnormalities is congruent with clinical (cortical blindness; Grimes et al., 1980; Gurjinder et al., 1989) and MRI findings (Frederiksson et al., 1989).

According to Calloni et al. (1981, 1982), diffuse EEG slowing is a prominent finding in all cases. Thomas et al. (1995) noted focal and generalized spikes; these authors also stressed certain similarities between eclampsia and hypertensive encephalopathy. The eclamptic-toxemic state must be carefully differentiated from intrapartum cortical venous thrombosis.

Lips (1988) emphasized the EEG improvement in the treatment course of eclamptic patients. Brophy and Brophy (1991) reported rapid EEG normalization with intravenous pyridoxine treatment. Chronically lingering epileptic seizures as a consequence of eclampsia are exceptional ("posteclamptic epilepsy," Ledermair and Niedermeyer, 1956).

Hypocalcemia

Hypocalcemia, the closely related syndrome of hypoparathyroidism, and the clinical picture of tetany represent complex clinical entities that cannot be discussed in great detail. The extensive study of Alajouanine et al. (1958) and the concise handbook review of Kurtz (1976) are recommended to the reader with electroencephalographic interest.

Severe hypocalcemia is highly epileptogenic and produces marked EEG changes with slowing and generalized bursts of spikes (Fig. 22.7). It is evident that tetanic carpopedal spasms are very common in such patients, and it must be emphasized that these tetanic manifestations are essentially noncerebral. Glaser and Levy (1960) found a good correlation between hypocalcemic epileptic seizures and paroxysmal EEG abnormalities. On the other hand, no correlation was found among calcium serum level, onset of seizures, and EEG changes (Goldberg, 1959; Rohmer et al., 1959; Thiébaut et al., 1958). Experimentally, Corriol et al. (1969) found massive spike activity and tonic and grand mal epileptic seizures in dogs a few days after removal of the parathyroid gland; these animals also showed sensitivity to flickering light. Epileptic manifestations develop at calcium levels around 6.0 or 5.0 mg/100 mL in the human as well as in the experimental animals of Corriol et al. (1969).

The clinical syndromes of *normocalcemic tetany* and *neurogenic tetany* are often or predominantly associated with normal EEG records. *Neonatal hypocalcemia* produces acute epileptic seizures and severe transient EEG changes but no carpopedal spasms. *Rachitic tetany* (common infantile tetany) is associated with hypocalcemia, carpopedal spasms, laryngospasm, convulsions, and the clinical signs of rickets; the EEG changes are usually mild with no spike activity (Kurtz, 1976).

In *pseudohypoparathyroidism* with short stature, osteochondral dysplasia, short fourth finger, hypocalcemia, and tetany, the EEG is most often abnormal as in cases of hypocalcemia (Guberman and Jaworski, 1979; Swash and Rowan, 1972; Vignaendra et al., 1977). No significant EEG changes have been found in *pseudopseudohypoparathyroidism*.

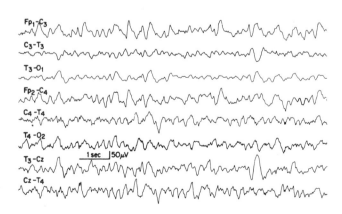

Figure 22.7. Hypocalcemia (Ca 5.2 mg/100 mL). Note marked diffuse slowing along with scattered sharp activity.

The EEG was found to be normal in five of six patients with *Fahr disease;* the remaining patient showed mild slowing (Devlesc Howard and Manyam, 1989).

Hyponatremia and Water Intoxication

Hyponatremia and acute water intoxication lead to severe EEG abnormalities with pronounced generalized slowing. Following earlier observations (Kiloh and Osselton, 1961; Saunders and Westmoreland, 1979), Zwang and Cohn (1981) reported a case of acute compulsive water intake resulting in a serum sodium of 116.4 mg/100 mL. There was papilledema and status epilepticus grand mal with diffuse 0.5 to 2/sec activity in the EEG. In spite of rapid normalization of the electrolytes, EEG recovery was slow. Okura et al. (1990) reported EEG slowing, spike waves, and status epilepticus in water intoxication.

Hypercalcemia

Hypercalcemic conditions may be due to hyperplasia or neoplasm of the parathyroids, excessive parathyroid activity caused by renal failure or skeletal decalcification, vitamin D intoxication, or a paraneoplastic state in cancers with bony metastases.

Neurological deficits and mental impairment are accompanied by EEG abnormalities consisting mainly of slowing of the basic rhythm and bursts of 1 to 2/sec waves (Allen et al., 1970; Lehrer and Levitt, 1960; Moore, 1967; Strickland et al., 1967; Swash and Rowan, 1972). According to Spatz et al. (1977), EEG changes appear when the serum calcium level reaches 13 mg/100 mL.

None of these authors reported the occurrence of spike activity. Huott et al. (1974), however, described a case of hypercalcemia with a calcium serum level of 16.6 mg/100 mL with acute development of a right homonymous hemianopsia, two grand mal attacks, and massive spike activity independently over the right and left occipital regions; this was due to prolonged ingestion of calcium tablets. A very similar observation of left occipital spiking in hypercalcemia at a level of 16 mg/100 mL was made by Barolin and Karbowski (1973). In addition to slow activity, triphasic waves may appear (Marchau, 1982).

Vitamin Deficiencies

Pyridoxin (vitamin B$_6$) deficiency on a nutritional basis has been recognized as a rare cause of severe and even fatal convulsions in neonates and infants (Coursin, 1954; Reilly et al., 1953). *Pyridoxin dependency* develops during fetal life as a genetic disorder and produces both intrauterine and postnatal seizures (Bejsovec et al., 1967; Hunt et al., 1954; Waldinger and Berg, 1968). The investigators of these syndromes reported massive generalized spike activity in the EEG (also see Glaser, 1976). Seizures and EEG changes respond quickly to administration of pyridoxin.

The pyridoxine response must include EEG improvement and stoppage of ongoing clinical seizures in order to be diagnostic of pyridoxine dependency. For more details, see Mikati et al. (1991).

Thiamine (vitamin B$_1$) deficiency may give rise to *Wernicke's encephalopathy* with or without Korsakoff's syndrome, associated with predominant oculomotor and cerebellar symptomatology (Victor et al., 1971). EEG changes range from mild to severe and, in general, parallel the severity of the neurological deficits (Dreyfus and Victor, 1961). Initial alpha slowing is gradually followed by the appearance of theta and delta frequencies (Frantzen, 1966) and, in severely ill patients, by diffuse sharp and slow wave complexes (Fournet and Lanternier, 1956). The administration of thiamine quickly improves the symptomatology of the Wernicke syndrome, but the resolution of the Korsakoff syndrome requires weeks or months.

Pellagra with the well-known "four D" symptomatology (dermatitis, diarrhea, depression, and dementia) produces diffuse EEG slowing (Srikantia et al., 1968; Vallat et al., 1962).

Vitamin B$_{12}$ deficiency (pernicious anemia) gives rise to spinal cord and peripheral nerve changes; in addition, the brain may also be affected with clinical evidence of mental changes such as confusion or delirium. Slow activity in the EEG may be quite pronounced (Diefenbach et al., 1953; Krump, 1955; Martinez-Barros et al., 1994; Samson et al., 1952; Walton et al., 1954); even temporal spike and sharp wave activity has been reported (Walton et al., 1954). A beautiful example of severe slowing and its response to therapy has been shown by Kiloh et al. (1972). Abnormal EEG findings have been found to be unrelated to the presence of myelopathy or neuropathy (Andersen and Stigsby, 1985).

Very pronounced epileptiform EEG abnormalities have been reported in the early-onset cobalamin C/D deficiency: an inborn error of intracellular cobalamin metabolism with high plasma levels of methylmalonic acid, homocystine, and homocysteine (Biancheri et al., 2002). The EEG demonstrates massive spikes of either focal or generalized character in the further course (childhood); the MRI shows diffuse loss of white matter. A variety of metabolic encephalopathies may occur in patients with *oncological problems* (Fig. 22.8).

Abnormal EEG findings with focal slowing and/or sharp-wave activity have been described in children and adolescents with *severe hemophilia.* These focal changes may not be associated with clinical neurological abnormalities (Lipinski and Weisser, 1987).

Endocrine Disorders

Adrenal Cortex

Adrenocortical insufficiency (Addison's disease) may be associated with pronounced delta and theta activity in the EEG, but such changes are found in serious cases only (Cloche et al., 1952; Dreyfus-Brisac and Mises, 1953; Engel and Margolin, 1942; Glaser, 1958; Hernandez-Peniche, 1953; Hoffman et al., 1942; Nishitani, 1962; Thiébaut et al., 1958). In milder forms, the EEG shows little or no abnormality. Cortisone can dramatically improve the clinical and electroencephalographic picture, and it has been suggested that the EEG abnormalities are caused mainly by the altered glucose metabolism. The EEG slowing reaches high

Figure 22.8. Metabolic encephalopathy. Hyperviscosity syndrome in a 52-year-old patient with multiple myeloma. The patient is awake, although somewhat lethargic; note fragments of a posterior basic rhythm.

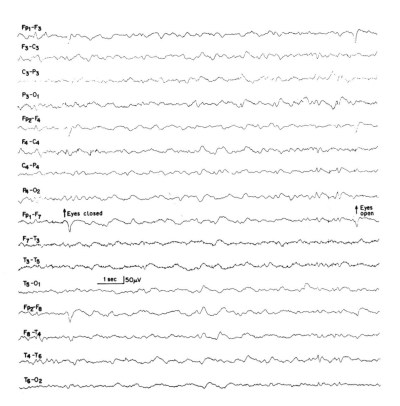

voltage in states of addisonian crisis. Addisonian states may be found in a variety of diseases (Oelkers, 1996). Adrenoleukodystrophy, a peroxisomal neurodegenerative disease (see Chapter 19, "Degenerative Disorders of the Central Nervous System"), may be dominated by addisonian symptoms.

In *adrenal cortical hyperfunction (Cushing's disease),* EEG abnormalities are less prominent than in addisonian states. Slow as well as fast frequencies may be excessively developed (Garcia-Austt et al., 1950; Glaser, 1953, 1958, 1976; Krankenhagen et al., 1970). No specific metabolic disturbance could be attributed to the EEG changes. Therapeutic dosages of adrenocorticotropic hormone (ACTH) or cortisone also produce mild to moderate EEG changes along with frequent mental changes and enhanced seizure susceptibility (Friedlander and Rottger, 1951; Pine et al., 1951). In adult epileptics with abnormal EEG tracings, the EEG changes are enhanced by intravenous cortisone (Glaser et al., 1955), in striking contrast to the beneficial effect of ACTH and cortisone in hypsarrhythmic infants.

Pituitary Gland

The EEG changes caused by advanced intrasellar tumors or craniopharyngiomas will not be discussed. Postpartum necrosis of the anterior lobe of the pituitary gland (*Sheehan's syndrome*) is the most common cause of severe hypopituitarism with pluriglandular insufficiency. The EEG shows massive diffuse theta and delta activity, especially in association with impaired consciousness (Christian, 1975; Cloche and Stuhl, 1959; Hughes and Summers, 1956;

Kennedy et al., 1955; Krump, 1955; Salmon, 1956; Storm van Leeuwen et al., 1957). These EEG abnormalities are most likely to reflect the secondary depression of the adrenocortical function.

Thyroid Gland

Hyperthyroidism is commonly associated with acceleration of alpha rhythm frequency. Such observations can be traced back to Rubin et al. (1937), Lindsley and Rubinstein (1937), Bertrand et al. (1938), and Ross and Schwab (1939) (Fig. 22.9). Enhancement of fast activity (15–30/sec) was reported by Gibbs and Gibbs (1941), Terracol et al. (1951), Vague et al. (1952, 1957), and Condon et al. (1954). Wilson et al. (1964) found the highest incidence of abnormalities in premenopausal females. These authors felt that "endocrinological factors other than the thyroid may play an important role in the production of EEG abnormalities in patients with hyperthyroidism." According to Vague et al. (1957), rolandic mu rhythm may be augmented by hyperthyroidism.

Paroxysmal bursts and clinical seizures such as grand mal (but also adversive and focal motor attacks) have been reported by Skanse and Nyman (1956), Korcyzn and Bechar (1976), and Jabbari and Huott (1980). Administration of thyroxin produces epileptic activity. Epileptic patients with thyroid dysfunction may respond poorly to anticonvulsants unless the endocrine problem is properly treated. The occurrence of anterior delta bursts was noted by Berlit and Rakicky (1991). Prominent EEG abnormalities have been noted in *thyrotoxic crisis with encephalopathy* prompted by

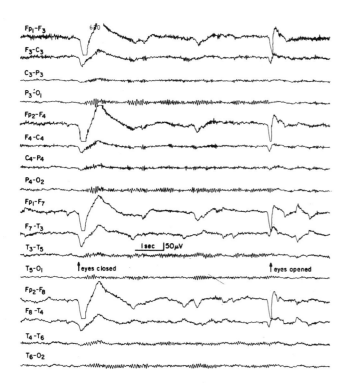

Figure 22.9. Hyperthyroidism in a 52-year-old woman. Note fast basic rhythm of 14–16/sec with good blocking effect. Somewhat faster activity over central regions does not show the blocking response.

severe infection, surgical intervention, and so forth. Cranial nerve signs, acute myeloencephalopathy, and choreic movements may occur. The EEG is dominated by marked slowing; fast activity may be superimposed (Cadilhac, 1976; Spatz et al., 1975). Van Zandycke et al. (1977) reported triphasic waves in two cases. Passouant et al. (1966) reported changes in the nocturnal EEG with difficulty in falling asleep and unduly lengthened REM periods (up to 40 or 50 minutes). Diffuse EEG abnormalities in *Hashimoto thyroiditis* have been described by Shaw et al. (1991) and also by Henchey et al. (1995).

Hypothyroidism reveals itself in a variety of clinical conditions such as congenital myxedema, cretinism, and myxedema in adulthood with complications such as myxedematous coma.

In *myxedematous infants,* a delay of the EEG development and especially of the sleep spindle development has been reported by Schultz et al. (1968). Excessive slowing and generally low voltage have been noted by Nieman (1961), Horstmann and Martinius (1964), and Harris et al. (1965). An excess of low-voltage slow activity has also been reported in *hypothyroid adult patients* (Ross and Schwab, 1939; Thiébaut et al., 1958); the alpha blocking response may be poor or even absent. The pathophysiology of *myxedematous coma* is poorly understood; epileptic seizures may precede the comatose state (Forester, 1963). Wackenheim (1955) reported predominant slow activity of low voltage in myxedematous coma. In this condition, triphasic

waves were noted by River and Zelig (1993). Wynn et al. (1989) found generalized periodic sharp wave discharges (mimicking Jakob-Creutzfeldt encephalopathy) in an elderly patient with hypothyroidism. The EEG normalized with thyroid treatment.

Other Hormonal Disturbances

The physiological influence of *estrogens* on the EEG has been demonstrated by some investigators. Mild to moderate slowing of the alpha frequency was found at the end of pregnancy (Gibbs and Reid, 1942) and 1 to 3 days prior to menstruation (Dusser de Barenne and Gibbs, 1942). Subtle changes caused by the influence of sexual hormones have been reported by Faure (1961). Margerison et al. (1964) observed some decrease in the low alpha frequency range in the premenstrual phase. Further information on this subject is found in Chapter 9, "The Normal EEG of the Waking Adult." These changes are practically negligible in clinical electroencephalographic work.

Shterev et al. (1981) studied the EEG of 46 patients with *Stein-Leventhal syndrome.* In spite of the absence of neurological signs or symptoms, 37 of these patients showed EEG abnormalities.

Pheochromocytomas give rise to extremely high blood pressure values; even in these critical states (with values of up to 280/170 mm Hg), the EEG may remain normal (Christian, 1975). Similar observations were made by Raab and Smithwick (1949).

Acute Porphyria

In acute porphyria, the EEG remains normal when the symptomatology is limited to abdominal pain and polyneuropathy. With the appearance of mental impairment and delirium, theta and delta frequencies become predominant (Goldberg, 1959; Kiloh and Nevin, 1950). Asymmetrical slowing and spike or sharp wave activity may also occur (Dow, 1961). Pronounced slowing is found in *central forms* of porphyria (Fig. 22.10).

In a case of acute intermittent porphyria and inappropriate antidiuretic hormone release, Ackermann and Scollo-Lavizzari (1982) found pronounced diffuse slowing followed by recovery.

Seizures are fairly common (up to 20%) in acute porphyria (Birchfield and Cowger, 1996; Bonkovsky and Schady, 1982; Bylesjö et al., 1996; Kaplan and Lewis, 1986), and their treatment causes great problems because of the well-known induction of porphyria with the use of antiepileptic medication (gabapentin considered to be an exception and thus the treatment of choice; Krauss et al., 1995).

Mixed-Type Encephalopathy

This polyetiological condition (Niedermeyer et al., 1999) stands apart from all of the well-defined metabolic encephalopathies. It is a quite common condition, mostly acute, characterized simply by change of mentation (confusion, delirium, etc.) with little or no neurological deficits but with indubitable diffuse EEG slowing. A variety of

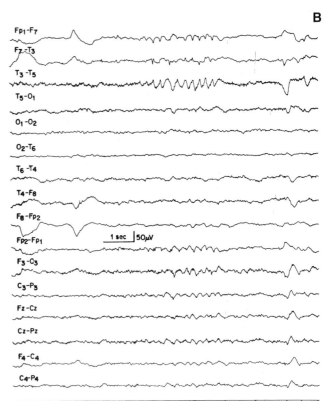

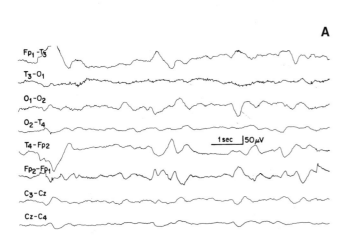

Figure 22.10. **A:** Cerebral form of acute intermittent porphyria in a 24-year-old woman. Slow mentation, personality change, and grand mal seizures. **B:** Same patient, improving although still somewhat lethargic. Note runs of rhythmical slowing over left frontotemporal region. This is an example of occasional focal characteristics in metabolic encephalopathies.

medical conditions (such as pneumonia or influenza in aged patients) and postsurgical conditions (excluding neurosurgical cases) play a major role in the genesis of mixed-type encephalopathy. The length of time of anesthesia augments the problem in postsurgical cases (thus introjecting a pharmacological element). Here is the usual sequence of events: concern about the patient's mental decline leads to neuroimaging, which yields normal findings; then comes the EEG request. These findings are always abnormal with moderate slowing (less than in the classical metabolic encephalopathies). Fortunately, the EEG reader can inform the clinician that this mixed type of encephalopathy usually carries a good prognosis. A special form of mixed-type encephalopathies occurs in 30% of severe burns; in these cases, however, the prognosis is guarded (Niedermeyer et al., 1999).

Chronic Respiratory (Pulmonary Insufficiency)

Chronic bronchial disease and pulmonary emphysema, along with right cardiac failure (*cor pulmonale*), may lead to a chronic encephalopathy clinically characterized by headache, papilledema, elevated cerebrospinal fluid pressure, and twitching of extremities (Austen et al., 1957; Conn et al., 1957; Glaser, 1960, 1976). The EEG shows considerable diffuse delta and theta activity; occasionally, anterior delta waves may show the configuration of triphasic waves. Appropriate treatment may quickly reverse these changes, but oxygen administration may be dangerous.

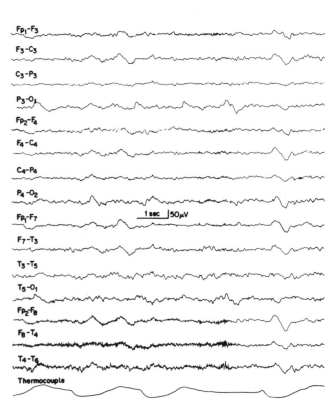

Figure 22.11. Abnormally slow and disorganized waking record in a patient (age 30 years) with pickwickian syndrome.

Chronic alveolar hypoventilation in conjunction with obesity gives rise to the *Pickwickian syndrome* with excessive somnolence (Gastaut et al., 1965, 1966; Jung and Kuhlo, 1965). Most of these patients also suffer from *sleep apnea,* especially from the obstructive type (see Chapter 48, "Polysomnography: Principles and Applications in Sleep and Arousal Disorders"). The routine EEG also shows abnormal amounts of diffuse slow activity (Fig. 22.11).

References

Ackermann, H.P., and Scollo-Lavizzari, G. 1982. EEG-Veränderungen bei einer Patientin mit akut intermittierender Porphyrie und einem Schwartz-Bartter-Syndrom (SIADH). Z. EEG-EMG 13:117–120.

Adams, R.D., and Foley, J.M. 1949. The neurological changes in the more common types of severe liver disease. Trans. Am. Neurol. Assoc. 74: 217–219.

Adams, R.D., and Foley, J.M. 1953. Neurological complications of liver disease. Publ. Assoc. Res. Neuro. Ment. Dis. 32:198–237.

Aguglia, U., Gambardella, A., Oliveri, R.L., et al. 1990. Nonmetabolic causes of triphasic waves: a reappraisal. Clin. Electroencephalogr. 21: 120–125.

Alajouanine, T., Contamin, F., and Cathala, H.P. 1958. *Le syndrome tétanie.* Paris: Baillère.

Alfrey, A.C., Mishell, J.M., Burks, J., et al. 1972. Syndrome of dyspraxia and multifocal seizures associated with chronic hemodialysis. Trans. Am. Soc. Artif. Intern. Organs 18:257–260.

Allen, M.E., Singer, F.R., and Melamed, D. 1970. Electroencephalographic abnormalities in hypercalcemia. Neurology (Minneapolis) 20:15–22.

Andersen, K., and Stigsby, B. 1985. Quantitative EEG analysis in patients with pernicious anemia. Electroencephalogr. Clin. Neurophysiol. 61: 33P(abst).

Aquino, A., and Gabor, A.J. 1980. Movement-induced seizures in nonketotic hyperglycemia. Neurology 30:600–604.

Austen, F.K., Carmichael, M.W., and Adams, R.D. 1957. Neurologic manifestations of chronic pulmonary insufficiency. N. Engl. J. Med. 257: 579–590.

Bahamon-Dussan, J.E., Celesia, G.G., and Grigg-Damberger, M.M. 1989. Prognostic significance of EEG triphasic waves in patients with altered states of consciousness. J. Clin. Neurophysiol. 6:313–319.

Barolin, G.S., and Karbowski, K. 1973. Okzipitale Krisen im "Grenzland der Epilepsie." Z. EEG-EMG 4:1–8.

Bauer, G., and Niedermeyer, E. 1979. Acute convulsions. Clin. Electroencephalogr. 10:127–144.

Bejsovec, M., Kulenda, Z., and Ponca, E. 1967. Familial intrauterine convulsions in pyridoxine dependency. Arch. Dis. Child. 42:201–207.

Belizan, J.M., Villar, J., Gonzalez, L., et al. 1991. Calcium supplementation to prevent hypertensive disorders of pregnancy. N. Engl. J. Med. 325: 1399–1405.

Bercaw, B.L., Ramirez, G., and Mathis, H. 1984. EEG changes in patients with chronic renal failure undergoing hemodialysis with and without glucose in the dialysis fluid. Electroencephalogr. Clin. Neurophysiol. 58: 31P(abst).

Berger, H. 1937. Das Elektrenkephalogramm des Menschen. 12 Mittlg. (12th report). Arch. Psychiatr. Nervenkr. 106:165–187.

Berlit, P., and Rakicky, J. 1991. The EEG in metabolic and endocrine encephalopathies. Clin. Neurophysiol. 78:36P(abst).

Bertrand, I., Delay, J., and Guillain, J. 1938. L'électroencéphalogramme dans le myxoedème. C. R. Soc. Biol. (Paris) 129:395–398.

Biancheri, R., Cerone, R., Rossi, A., et al. 2002. Early-onset cobalamin C/D deficiency: epilepsy and electroencephalographic features. Epilepsia 43: 616–622.

Bickford, R.G., and Butt, H.R. 1955. Hepatic coma: the electroencephalograph pattern. J. Clin. Invest. 34:790–799.

Birchfield, R.I., and Cowger, M.L. 1996. Acute intermittent porphyria with seizures. Am. J. Dis. Child. 112:561–565.

Blatt, I., and Brenner, R. 1996. Triphasic waves in a psychiatric population: a retrospective study. J. Clin. Neurophysiol. 13:324–329.

Bonkovsky, H.L., and Schady, W. 1982. Neurologic manifestations of acute porphyria. Semin. Liver Dis. 2:108–124.

Boyle, P.J., Kempers, S.F., O'Connor, A.M., et al. 1995. Brain glucose uptake and unawareness of hypoglycemia in patients with insulin-dependent diabetes mellitus. N. Engl. J. Med. 333:1726–1731.

Brass, N. 1980. Verlaufsuntersuchungen ber EEG-Veränderungen während Hämodialyse bei terminaler Niereninsuffizienz. Z. EEG-EMG 11: 51–57.

Brophy, E., and Brophy, M.H. 1991. Pyridoxal phosphate normalization of the EEG in eclampsia. Electroencephalogr. Clin. Neurophysiol. 79:36P (abst).

Bylesjö, I., Forsgren, L., Lithner, F., et al. 1996. Epidemiology and clinical characteristics of seizures in patients with acute intermittent porphyria. Epilepsia 37:230–235.

Cadilhac, J. 1976. The EEG in renal insufficiency. In *Handbook of Electroencephalography and Clinical Neurophysiology,* vol. 15C, Ed.-in-chief, A. Remond, pp. 351–369. Amsterdam: Elsevier.

Cadilhac, J., and Ribstein, M. 1961. The EEG in metabolic disorders. World Neurol. 2:296–308.

Cadilhac, J., Ribstein, M., and Jean, R. 1959. EEG et troubles métaboliques. Rev. Neurol. (Paris) 100:270–296.

Calloni, M.V., Porazzi, D., and Rovetta, P. 1981. Cerebral dysfunction in eclampsia: a longitudinal EEG study. Electroencephalogr. Clin. Neurophysiol. 51:79P(abst).

Calloni, M.V., Porazzi, D., and Rovetta, P. 1982. Further observations on focal onset of eclamptic seizures. Electroencephalogr. Clin. Neurophysiol. 54:1P(abst).

Cavanagh, J.B. 1974. Liver bypass and the glia. In *Brain Dysfunction in Metabolic Disorders,* Ed. F. Plum, pp. 313–335. New York: Raven Press.

Chokroverty, S., and Gandhi, V.K. 1982. EEG in patients with progressive dialytic encephalopathy and chronic renal failure on long-term hemodialysis. Electroencephalogr. Clin. Neurophysiol. 53:29P(abst).

Christian, W. 1975. *Klinische Elektroenzephalographie,* 2nd ed. Stuttgart: Thieme.

Cloche, R., and Stuhl, L. 1959. Aspects de l'EEG dans quelques cas d'insuffisance hypophysaire globale. Rev. Neurol. (Paris) 100:336.

Cloche, R., Azerad, E., and Stuhl, T. 1952. Les modifications de l'électroencéphalogramme dans l'insuffisance surrénale. Ann. Méd. 53:689–708.

Cohn, R., and Castell, D.O. 1969. The effect of acute hyperammonemia on the electroencephalogram. J. Lab. Clin. Med. 68:195–205.

Condon, J.V., Becka, D.R., and Gibbs, F.A. 1954. Electroencephalographic abnormalities in endocrine disease. N. Engl. J. Med. 251:638–641.

Conn, H.O., Dunn, J.P., Newman, H.A., et al. 1957. Pulmonary emphysema simulating brain tumor. Am. J. Med. 22:524–533.

Corriol, J., Papy, J., Rohner, J.J., et al. 1969. Electroclinical correlations established during tetanic manifestations induced by parathyroid removal in the dog. In *The Physiopathogenesis of the Epilepsies,* Eds. H. Gastaut, H.H. Jasper, J. Bancaud, et al., pp. 3128–3140. Springfield, IL: Charles C Thomas.

Coursin, D.B. 1954. Convulsive seizures in infants with pyridoxine deficient diet. JAMA 154:406–408.

Creutzfeldt, O.D., and Meisch, J.J. 1963. Changes of cortical neuron activity of EEG during hypoglycemia. In *The Physiological Basis of Mental Activity,* Ed. R. Hernandez-Peon, pp. 158–171. Amsterdam: Elsevier.

Daniel, J.C., Chokroverty, S., and Barron, K.D. 1969. Anacidotic hyperglycemia and focal seizures. Arch. Intern. Med. 124:701–706.

Davis, P.A. 1943. Effect on the electroencephalogram of changing blood sugar level. Arch. Neurol. Psychiatry (Chicago) 49:186–194.

Devlesc Howard, A.B., and Manyam, B.V. 1989. Electroencephalography in Fahr's disease. Electroencephalogr. Clin. Neurophysiol. 73: 68P(abst).

DiBenedetto, R.J., Crocco, J.A., and Soscia, J.L. 1965. Hyperglycemic nonketotic coma. Arch. Intern. Med. 116:74–82.

Diefenbach, W.C., Beyers, M.R., and Meyer, L.M. 1953. The electroencephalographic and psychologic changes in pernicious anemia. Acta Haematol. (Basel) 9:201–208.

Dow, R.S. 1961. The electroencephalographic findings in acute intermittent porphyria. Electroencephalogr. Clin. Neurophysiol. 13:425–437.

Dreyfus, P.M., and Victor, M. 1961. Effects of thiamine deficiency on the cerebral nervous system. Am. J. Clin. Nutr. 9:414–425.

Dreyfus-Brisac, D., and Mises, R. 1953. Étude EEG des 28 addisoniens. Electroencephalogr. Clin. Neurophysiol. 5:133–134.

Duffy, T.E., Vergara, F., and Plum, R. 1974. Alpha-ketoglutaramate in hepatic encephalopathy. In *Brain Dysfunction in Metabolic Disorders,* Ed. F. Plum, pp. 339–352. New York: Raven Press.

Duncan, M.B., Jabbari, B., and Rosenberg, M.L. 1991. Gaze-evoked visual seizures in nonketotic hyperglycemia. Electroencephalogr. Clin. Neurophysiol. 32:221–224.

Dusser de Barenne, D., and Gibbs, F.A. 1942. Variations in the electroencephalogram during the menstrual cycle. Am. J. Obstet. Gynecol. 44:687–690.

Elena, M., Fernandes, J., Romero, M., et al. 2002. Subclinical hepatic encephalopathy shows an important decrease of slow waves in the sleep EEG. Clin. Neurophysiol. 13:1370(abst).

Engel, G.L., and Margolin, S.G. 1942. Neuropsychiatric disturbance in internal disease: metabolic factors and electroencephalographic correlations. Arch. Intern. Med. 70:236–259.

Engel, G.L., Romano, J., Ferris, E.G., et al. 1944. A simple method of determining the frequency spectrum of the electroencephalograph. Observations on physiological variations in glucose, oxygen, posture and acid base balance on the normal electroencephalogram. Arch. Neurol. Psychiatr. (Chicago) 51:134–146.

Engel, R., Halberg, F., Tichy, F.Y., et al. 1954. Electrocerebral activity and epileptic attacks at various blood sugar levels. Acta Neuroveget. (Vienna) 9:147–167.

Epstein, C.M., Riether, A.M., Henderson, R.M., et al. 1992. EEG in liver transplantation: visual and computerized analysis. Electroencephalogr. Clin. Neurophysiol. 83:367–371.

Faure, J. 1961. L'activité électrique du cerveau. Influence des agents hormonaux et métaboliques. World Neurol. 2:879–894.

Ferris, T.F. 1991. Pregnancy, preeclampsia and the endothelial cell. N. Engl. J. Med. 325:1439–1440.

Ficker, D.M., Westmoreland, B.F., and Sharbrough, F.W. 1997. Epileptiform abnormalities in hepatic encephalopathy. J. Clin Neurophysiol. 14:230–234.

Fisch, B.J., and Klass, D.W. 1988. The diagnostic specificity of triphasic wave patterns. Electroencephalogr. Clin. Neurophysiol. 70:1–8.

Fischer, J.E. 1974. False neurotransmitters and hepatic coma. In *Brain Dysfunction in Metabolic Disorders,* Ed. F. Plum, pp. 353–373. New York: Raven Press.

Fischer, J.E., and Baldessarini, R.J. 1971. False neurotransmitters and hepatic failure. Lancet 2:75–79.

Foley, J.M., Watson, C.W., and Adams, R.D. 1950. Significance of the electroencephalographic changes in hepatic coma. Trans. Am. Neurol. Assoc. 75:161–165.

Forester, L.F. 1963. Coma in myxoedema. Arch. Intern. Med. 111:734–743.

Fournet, A., and Lanternier, M. 1956. Constatations électroencéphalographiques dans 17 cas d'encéphalopathie de Gayet-Wernicke. Rev. Neurol. (Paris) 94:644–645.

Frantzen, E. 1966. Wernicke's encephalopathy. Acta Neurol. Scand. 42:426–441.

Fraser, C.L., and Arieff, A.I. 1985. Hepatic encephalopathy. N. Engl. J. Med. 313:865–873.

Frederiksson, K., Lindvall, O., Ingemarsson, I., et al. 1989. Repeated cranial computed tomographic and magnetic resonance imaging scans in two cases of eclampsia. Stroke 20:547–553.

Friedlander, W.J. 1956. Electroencephalographic changes in hyperammonemia. Electroencephalogr. Clin. Neurophysiol. 8:513–516.

Friedlander, W.J., and Rottger, E. 1951. The effect of cortisone on the electroencephalogram. Electroencephalogr. Clin. Neurophysiol. 3:311–313.

Gabor, A.J. 1974. Focal seizures induced by movement without sensory feedback mechanisms. Electroencephalogr. Clin. Neurophysiol. 36:403–408.

Gabuzda, G.J. 1962. Hepatic coma: clinical considerations, pathogenesis and management. In *Advances in Internal Medicine,* vol. 311, Eds. W. Dock and I. Snapper. Chicago: Year Book.

Gabuzda, G.J. 1967. Ammonium metabolism and hepatic coma. Gastroenterology 53:806–810.

Gabuzda, G.J., Phillips, G.B., and Davidson, C.S. 1952. Reversible toxic manifestations in patients with cirrhosis of the liver given cation exchange resins. N. Engl. J. Med. 246:124–130.

Garcia-Austt, E., Torrents, E., and Mussio-Fournier, F. 1950. The electroencephalogram in Cushing's disease. Electroencephalogr. Clin. Neurophysiol. 2:103.

Gastaut, H., Tassinari, C.A., and Duron, B. 1965. Étude polygraphique des manifestations épisodiques (hypniques et respiratoires) diurnes et nocturnes du syndrome de Pickwick. Rev. Neurol. (Paris) 112:573–579.

Gastaut, H., Duron, B., Papy, J., et al. 1966. Étude polygraphique comparative du cycle nychtémérique chez les narcoleptiques, les pickwickiens, les obèses et les insuffisants respiratoires. Rev. Neurol. (Paris) 115:456–462.

Gastaut, H., Rohmer, F., Cossette, A., et al. 1969. Introduction to the study of functional generalized epilepsies. In *The Physiopathogenesis of the Epilepsies,* Eds. H. Gastaut, H.H. Jasper, J. Bancaud, et al., pp. 15–25. Springfield, IL: Charles C Thomas.

Gellhorn, E., and Kessler, M. 1942. The effect of hypoglycemia on the electroencephalogram at varying degrees of oxygenation of the blood. Am. J. Physiol. 136:1–6.

Ghigo, J. 1990. Principles in the differentiation of atypical spike-waves and triphasic waves: a technologist's view. Am. J. EEG Technol. 30:315–316.

Gibbs, F.A., and Gibbs, E.L. 1941. *Atlas of Electroencephalography,* 1st ed. Cambridge, MA: Addison-Wesley.

Gibbs, F.A., and Murray, E.L. 1954. Hypoglycemic convulsions. Electroencephalogr. Clin. Neurophysiol. 6:674.

Gibbs, F.A., and Reid, D.E. 1942. The EEG in pregnancy. Am. J. Obstet. Gynecol. 44:672–675.

Gibbs, F.A., Williams, D., and Gibbs, E.L. 1940. Modification of the cortical frequency spectrum by changes in CO_2, blood sugar and oxygen. J. Neurophysiol. 3:49–58.

Girier, B., Clouzeau, J., Navelet, Y., et al. 1989. Fulminant hepatic failure (FHF) in children. EEG prognosis. Electroencephalogr. Clin. Neurophysiol. 73:48P–49P(abst).

Glaser, G.H. 1953. Psychotic reactions induced by corticotropin (ACTH) and cortisone. Psychosomat. Med. 4:280–291.

Glaser, G.H. 1958. EEG activity and adrenal-cortical dysfunction. Electroencephalogr. Clin. Neurophysiol. 10:366.

Glaser, G.H. 1960. Metabolic encephalopathy in hepatic, renal and pulmonary disorders. Postgrad. Med. 27:611–619.

Glaser, G.H. 1974. Brain dysfunction in uremia. In *Brain Dysfunction in Metabolic Disorders,* Ed. F. Plum, pp. 3173–3197. New York: Raven Press.

Glaser, G.H. 1976. The EEG in certain metabolic disorders. In *Handbook of Electroencephalography and Clinical Neurophysiology,* vol. 315C, Ed.-in-chief, A. Remond, pp. 316–325. Amsterdam: Elsevier.

Glaser, G.H., and Levy, L.L. 1960. Seizures and idiopathic hypoparathyroidism. A clinical-electroencephalographic study. Epilepsia (Amsterdam) 1:454–465.

Glaser, G.H., Kornfeld, D.S., and Knight, R.P. 1955. Intravenous hydrocortisone, corticotropin and the electroencephalograms. Arch. Neurol. Psychiatr. (Chicago) 73:338–344.

Gloor, P., Jacob, J.C., Elwan, O.H., et al. 1969. The electroencephalogram in chronic renal failure. In *The Physiopathogenesis of the Epilepsies,* Eds. H. Gastaut, H.H. Jaspers, J. Bancaud, et al., pp. 3209–3236. Springfield, IL: Charles C Thomas.

Goldberg, A. 1959. Acute intermittent porphyria. A study of 50 cases. Q. J. Med. 28:183–202.

Goldberg, H.H. 1959. The electroencephalogram in hypocalcemic syndromes. Electroencephalogr. Clin. Neurophysiol. 11:398.

Grimes, D.A., Ekbladh, L.E., and McCartney, W.H. 1980. Cortical blindness in preeclampsia. J. Gynecol. Obstet. 17:601–603.

Grimm, G., Madl, C., Katzenschlager, R., et al. 1992. Detailed evaluation of evoked potentials in Wilson's disease. Electroencephalogr. Clin. Neurophysiol. 82:119–124.

Guberman, A., and Jaworski, Z.F.G. 1979. Pseudohyperparathyroidism and epilepsy. Diagnostic value of computerized cranial tomography. Epilepsia 20:541–553.

Guggenheim, P., Regli, F., Hafen, G., et al. 1964. Elektroenzephalographische Untersuchungen bei chronischen Lebererkrankungen vor und nach Belastung mit Morphin. Deutsch. Med. Wochenschr. 89:749.

Guieu, J.D., Milbled, G., and Pruvot, P. 1976. Unusual EEG events during a case of puerperal eclampsia. Electroencephalogr. Clin. Neurophysiol. 40:549(abst).

Gurjinder, P.S., Dhand, U.K., and Chopra, J.S. 1989. Balint's syndrome following eclampsia. Clin. Neurol. Neurosurg. 91:161–165.

Hamel, B., Bourne, J.R., Ward, J.W., et al. 1978. Quantitative assessment of photic driving in renal failure. Electroencephalogr. Clin. Neurophysiol. 45:719–730.

Hansotia, P., Harris, R., and Kennedy, J. 1969. EEG changes in Wilson's disease. Electroencephalogr. Clin. Neurophysiol. 27:523–528.

Harden, C.L., Rosenbaum, D.H., and Daras, M. 1991. Hyperglycemia presenting with occipital seizures. Epilepsia 32:215–220.

Harris, R., Della-Rovere, M.D., and Prior, P. 1965. Electroencephalographic studies in infants and children with hypothyroidism. Arch. Dis. Child. 40:612–617.

Henchey, R., Cibula, J., Helveston, W., et al. 1995. Electroencephalographic findings in Hashimoto's encephalopathy. Neurology 45:977–981.

Hernandez-Peniche, J. 1953. El electroencefalograma en la enfermedad de Addison. Rev. Invest. Clin. (Mexico City) 5:439–444.

Hetzel, H., and Niedermeyer, E. 1955. Der Gehirnhydrolysat-Weckeffekt im hypoglykaemischen Koma und sein hirnelektrisches Bild. Arch. Psychiatr. Nervenkr. 76:369–382.

Himwich, H.E., Frostig, J.P., Hoagland, H., et al. 1939. Clinical electroencephalographic and biochemical changes during insulin hypoglycemia. Proc. Soc. Exp. Biol. (New York) 40:401–402.

Hoagland, H., Cameron, D.E., and Rubin, M. A. 1937. The electroencephalogram of schizophrenics during insulin treatments. Am. J. Psychiatry 94:183–208.

Hoefer, P.F.A., Guttmann, S.A., and Sands, I.J. 1946. Convulsive states and coma in cases of islet cell adenoma of the pancreas. Am. J. Psychiatry 102:486–495.

Hoffman, W.C., Lewis, R.A., and Thorn, G.W. 1942. The electroencephalogram in Addison's disease. Bull. Johns Hopkins Hosp. 70:335–361.

Horstmann, W., and Martinius, J. 1964. Das Hirnstrombild der kindlichen Hypothyreose unter Hormontherapie. Arch. Kinderheilk. 170:56–60.

Hughes, J.G., Hill, F.S., and Davis, B.C. 1950. Electroencephalographic findings in acute nephritis. J. Pediatr. 36:451–459.

Hughes, J.R. 1980. Correlations between EEG and chemical changes in uremia. Electroencephalogr. Clin. Neurophysiol. 48:583–594.

Hughes, J.R. 1984. EEG in uremia. Am. J. EEG Technol. 24:1–10.

Hughes, J.R. 1990. Principles in the differentiation of atypical spike-waves and triphasic waves. Am. J. EEG Technol. 30:309–312.

Hughes, J.R., and Schreeder, M.T. 1981. EEG in dialysis encephalopathy. Electroencephalogr. Clin. Neurophysiol. 51:36P(abst).

Hughes, R.R., and Summers, Y.K. 1956. Changes in the electroencephalogram associated with hypopituitarism due to post-partum necrosis. Electroencephalogr. Clin. Neurophysiol. 8:87–96.

Hunt, A.D., Jr., Stokes, J., Jr., McCrory, W.W., et al. 1954. Pyridoxine dependency: Report of a case of intractable convulsions in an infant controlled by pyridoxine. Pediatrics 13:140–145.

Huott, A.D., Madison, D.S., and Niedermeyer, E. 1974. Occipital lobe epilepsy. A clinical and electroencephalographic study. Eur. Neurol. (Basel) 11:325–339.

Jabbari, B., and Huott, A.D. 1980. Seizures in thyrotoxicosis. Epilepsia (New York) 21:91–96.

Jacob, J.C., Gloor, P., Elwan, O.H., et al. 1965. Electroencephalographic changes in chronic renal failure. Neurology (Minneapolis) 15:419–429.

Jones, E.A., Clain, D., Clink, H.M., et al. 1967. Hepatic coma due to acute hepatic necrosis treated by exchange blood transfusion. Lancet 2:169–172.

Jung, R., and Kuhlo, W. 1965. Neurophysiological studies of abnormal night sleep in the Pickwickian syndrome. In *Sleep Mechanisms,* Eds. K. Akert, C. Bally, and J. Schade, pp. 140–159. Amsterdam: Elsevier.

Kaplan, P.W., and Lewis, D.V. 1986. Juvenile acute intermittent porphyria with hypercholesterolemia and epilepsy. A case report and review of the literature. J. Child Neurol. 1:38–45.

Karnaze, D.S., and Bickford, R.G. 1984. Triphasic waves: a reassessment of their significance. Electroencephalogr. Clin. Neurophysiol. 57:193–198.

Kennedy, A.C., Lintona, A.L., Luke, R.G., et al. 1963. Electroencephalographic changes during haemodialyses. Lancet 1:408–411.

Kennedy, J., Parbhoo, J.P., MacGillivray, B.B., et al. 1973. Effect of extracorporeal liver perfusion on the electroencephalogram of patients in coma due to acute liver failure. Q. J. Med. 42:549–561.

Kennedy, J.M., Thomson, A.P., and Whitfield, I.C. 1955. Coma and electroencephalographic changes in hypopituitarism. Lancet 2:907–908.

Kiloh, L.G., and Nevin, S. 1950. Acute porphyria with severe neurological changes. Proc. R. Soc. Med. 43:948.

Kiloh, L.G., and Osselton, J.W. 1961. *Clinical Electroencephalography.* London: Butterworth.

Kiloh, L.G., McComas, A.J., and Osselton, J.W. 1972. *Clinical Electroencephalography,* 3rd ed., London: Butterworth.

Klass, D.W. 1990. Principles in the differentiation of atypical spike-waves and triphasic waves. Am. J. EEG Technol. 60:313–314.

Klinger, M. 1954. EEG observations in uremia. Electroencephalogr. Clin. Neurophysiol. 6:519.

Knell, A.J., Davidson, A.R., Williams, R., et al. 1974. Dopamine and serotonin metabolism in hepatic encephalopathy. Br. Med. J. 1:549–551.

Kogeorgos, J., Marsh, F., Scholtz, K., et al. 1982. Dialysis dementia: neurophysiological and EEG aspects. Electroencephalogr. Clin. Neurophysiol. 53:2P(abst).

Korczyn, A.D., and Bechar, M. 1976. Convulsive fits in thyrotoxicosis. Epilepsia (New York) 17:33–34.

Krankenhagen, B., Penin, H., and Zeh, W. 1970. Prä- und postoperative Untersuchungen bei Patienten mit Cushing-Syndrom. Z. EEG-EMG 1:14–19.

Krauss, G.L., Simmons-O'Brien, E., and Campbell, M. 1995. Successful treatment of seizures in acute intermittent porphyria. Neurology 45:594–595.

Krump, J.E. 1955. Die Klinische Bedeutung des Elektroenzephalogrammes bei Vergiftungen, Endotoxikosen und Endokrinopathien. *Proceed. Deutsche Internisten-Tagung,* Leipzig. Berlin: VEB Verlag Volk und Gesundheit.

Kügler, C.F.A., Petter, J., Taghavy, A., et al. 1994. Dynamics of cognitive brain dysfunction in patients with chronic liver disease: an event-related P300 potential perspective. Electroencephalogr. Clin. Neurophysiol. 91:33–41.

Kulisevsky, J., Conill, J., Avila, A., et al. 1995. Abnormalities of the Bereitschaftspotential and MRI pallidal sign in non-encephalopathic cirrhotic patients. Electroencephalogr. Clin. Neurophysiol. 94:425–431.

Kurtz, D. 1976. The EEG in parathyroid dysfunction. In *Handbook of Electroencephalography and Clinical Neurophysiology,* vol. 15C, Ed.-in-chief, A. Remond, pp. 77–87. Amsterdam: Elsevier.

Kurtz, D., Zenglein, J.P., Imler, M., et al. 1972. Étude de sommeil nocturne au cours de l'encéphalopathie porto-cave. Electroencephalogr. Clin. Neurophysiol. 33:167–179.

Lafon, R., Passouant, P., Billet, M., et al. 1950. Étude électroencéphalographique du coma insulinique. Ann. Méd. Psychol. 2:251–254.

Laidlaw, J. 1959. The application in general medical conditions of a visual method of assessing and representing generalized electroencephalographic abnormalities. J. Neurol. Neurosurg. Psychiatr. 24:58–70.

Laidlaw, J., Read, A.E., and Sherlock, S. 1961. Morphine tolerance in hepatic cirrhosis. Gastroenterology 40:389–396.

Ledermair, O., and Niedermeyer, E. 1956. Posteklamptische Epilepsie. Geburtshilfe und Frauenheilk. 16:679–684.

Lefebre, Ch., Lefebre, B., and Skotzek, B. 1990. An unusual case of hyperinsulinoma with confusional states and tonic-clonic seizures diagnosed with the help of long-term video-EEG recording. Electroencephalogr. Clin. Neurophysiol. 75:S81(abst).

Lehmkuhl, P., Kaukemuller, J., Pohl, S., et al. 1988. EEG monitoring of intensive care patients after liver transplantation. Electroencephalogr. Clin. Neurophysiol. 69:17P(abst).

Lehovsky, M., Spicakova, V., and Jencikova, B. 1983. EEG findings in 24 children with renal failure. Electroencephalogr. Clin. Neurophysiol. 55:28P(abst).

Lehrer, G.M., and Levitt, M.F. 1960. Neuropsychiatric presentation of hypercalcemia. J. Mt. Sinai Hosp. 27:10–18.

Lindsley, D.B., and Rubenstein, B.B. 1937. Relationships between brain potentials and some other physiological variables. Proc. Soc. Exp. Biol. (New York) 35:558–563.

Lipinski, C.G., and Weisser, J. 1987. EEG findings in children and adolescents with severe hemophilia. Electroencephalogr. Clin. Neurophysiol. 66:70P(abst).

Lips, U. 1988. EEG changes in a standardized treatment of eclampsia. Electroencephalogr. Clin. Neurophysiol. 69:70P(abst).

Liu, X.Q., Xu, J.Q., and Feng, Y.K. 1983. Wilson's disease. An electroencephalographic study. Chin. Med. J. 96:835–840.

Locke, J., Merrill, J.P., and Tyler, H.R. 1961. Neurologic complications of uremia. Arch. Intern. Med. 108:519–530.

Maccario, M.J., Messis, C.P., and Vastola, E.F. 1965. Focal seizures as a manifestation of hyperglycemia without ketoacidosis. Neurology (Minneapolis) 15:195–206.

MacGillivray, B.B. 1969. An EEG monitor incorporating simple pattern recognition. J. Physiol. (London) 201:65–67.

MacGillivray, B.B. 1976. The EEG in liver disease. In *Handbook of Electroencephalography and Clinical Neurophysiology,* vol. 15C, Ed.-in-chief, A. Remond, pp. 26–50. Amsterdam: Elsevier.

Mahurkar, S.D., Dhar, S.K., Salta, R., et al. 1973. Dialysis demtia. Lancet 1:1412–1415.

Maltby, G.L., and Rosenbaum, M. 1942. Relation of cerebral dysrhythmia to eclampsia. Proc. Soc. Exp. Biol. (New York) 50:10–12.

Marchau, M.M.B. 1982. Das Elektroenzephalogramm bei Hyperkalzämie. Z. EEG-EMG 13:61–67.

Margerison, J., Anderson, W., Dawson, J., et al. 1964. Plasma sodium and the EEG during the menstrual cycle of normal human female. Electroencephalogr. Clin. Neurophysiol. 17:540–544.

Martinez-Barros, M., Ramos-Peek, J., Escobar-Izquierdo, A., et al. 1994. Clinical, electrophysiologic, and neuroimaging findings in Wernicke's syndrome. Clin. Electroencephalogr. 25:148–152.

McDermott, W.V., and Adams, R.D. 1954. Episodic stupor associated with an Eck fistula in the human with particular reference to the metabolism of ammonia. J. Clin. Invest. 33:1–9.

Mikati, M.A., Trevathan, E., Krishnamoorthy, K.S., et al. 1991. Pyridoxine-dependent epilepsy: EEG investigation and long-term follow-up. Electroencephalogr. Clin. Neurophysiol. 78:215–221.

Mises, J., Lerique-Koechlin, A., and Rimbot, A. 1968. The EEG during renal insufficiency. Electroencephalogr. Clin. Neurophysiol. 25:91(abst).

Moore, J.M.B. 1967. The electroencephalogram in hypercalcemia. Arch. Neurol. (Chicago) 17:34–51.

Moruzzi, G. 1938. Action de l'hypoglycémie insulinique sur l'activité spontanée et provoquée de l'écorce cérébrale. C. R. Soc. Biol. Paris 128:1181–1184.

Niedermeyer, E., Krauss, G.L., and Efron Peyser, C. 1989. The electroencephalogram and mental activation. Clin. Electroencephalogr. 20:215– 227.

Niedermeyer, E., Ribeiro, M., Hertz, S. 1999. Mixed-type encephalopathy: preliminary considerations. Clin. Electroencephalogr. 30:12–15.

Nieman, E.A. 1961. The electroencephalogram in congenital hypothyroidism. A study of 10 cases. J. Neurol. Neurosurg. Psychiatry 24:50–57.

Nishitani, H. 1962. Electroencephalogram in endocrine disease. II. Adrenal diseases. Jpn. Arch. Intern. Med. 9:413–418.

Nogues, B., and Vecchierini-Blineau, M.F. 1987. Electroencephalographic modifications induced by dialysis in patients with chronic renal insufficiency. Electroencephalogr. Clin. Neurophysiol. 67:66P(abst).

Oelkers, W. 1996. Adrenal insufficiency. N. Engl. J. Med. 335:1206–1211.

Okura, M., Nagamine, I., Okada, K., et al. 1990. EEG changes during and after water intoxication. Electroencephalogr. Clin. Neurophysiol. 75: S110(abst).

Passouant, P., Passouant-Fontaine, T., and Cadilhac, J. 1966. L'influence de l'hyperthyroidie sur le sommeil. Étude clinique et expérimentale. Rev. Neurol. (Paris) 115:335–366.

Penin, H. 1967. Über den diagnostischen Wert des Hirnstrombildes bei der hepatoportalen Encephalopathie. Zugleich ein klinisch-statistischer Beitrag zur Frage neurologischer und psychischer Veränderungen bei Leberzirrhosen und portocavaler Anastomosenoperation. Fortschr. Neurol. Psychiatr. 35:173.

Pine, I., Engel, F.L., and Schwartz, T.P. 1951. The electroencephalogram in ACTH and cortisone treated patients. Electroencephalogr. Clin. Neurophysiol. 3:301–310.

Pinelli, P., Scremin, S., Pistollato, G., et al. 1982. Therapy with selective amino acid infusion in patients with alcoholic cirrhosis: clinical and EEG study. Electroencephalogr. Clin. Neurophysiol. 54:4P(abst).

Pinto, F., Stefanini, M.C., Onofrj, M., et al. 1981. Prognostic value of the EEG in eclampsia. Electroencephalogr. Clin. Neurophysiol. 51:57P–58P (abst).

Plum, F., and Posner, J.B. 1966. *Diagnosis of Stupor and Coma.* Philadelphia: F.A. Davis.

Poiré, R. 1969. Hypoglycemic epilepsy: Clinical, electrographic and biological study during induced hypoglycemia in man. In *The Physiopathogenesis of the Epilepsies,* Eds. H. Gastaut, H.H. Jasper, J. Bancaud, and A. Waltrégny, pp. 75–110. Springfield, IL: Charles C Thomas.

Poiré, R., Feuillet, C., Stoianoff-Nenoff, S., et al. 1966. Étude clinique et électrographique des manifestations convulsives de la cure de Sakel. Ann. Méd. Psychol. 2:686–687.

Prill, A., Quellhorst, E., and Scheler, F. 1969. Epilepsy: clinical and electroencephalographic findings in patients with renal insufficiency. In *The Physiopathogenesis of the Epilepsies,* Eds. H. Gastaut, H.H. Jasper, J. Bancaud, et al., pp. 60–68. Springfield, IL: Charles C Thomas.

Raab, W., and Smithwick, R.H. 1949. Pheochromocytoma with hypothalamic manifestations and excessive hypermetabolism. J. Clin. Endocrinol. 9:782–790.

Regan, P.F., and Browne-Mayers, A.N. 1956. Electroencephalography: Frequency analysis and consciousness. A correlation during insulin-induced hypoglycemia. J. Nerv. Ment. Dis. 124:142–147.

Reilly, R.H., Killam, K.F., Jenney, E.H., et al. 1953. Convulsant effects of isoniazid. JAMA 152:1317–1321.

Riley, T., Fineyre, F., Maddrey, W.C., et al. 1979. EEG studies in hepatic encephalopathy. "Blind" EEG evaluation. Electroencephalogr. Clin. Neurophysiol. 46:9P(abst).

River, Y., and Zelig, O. 1993. Triphasic waves in myxedema coma. Clin. Electroencephalogr. 24:146–150.

Rohmer, F., Wackenheim, A., and Kurtz, D. 1959. L'EEG dans les syndromes endocriniens hypophysaires, thyroidiens, surrénaux et dans la tétanie de l'adulte. Rev. Neurol. (Paris) 100:297–314.

Ross, D.A., and Schwab, R.J. 1939. The cortical alpha rhythm in thyroid disorders. Endocrinology 25:75–79.

Rubin, M.A., Cohen, H.C., and Hoagland, H. 1937. The effect of artificially raised metabolic rate and the electroencephalogram of schizophrenic patients. Endocrinology 21:536–540.

Rumpl, E., Hackl, J.M., Gerstenbrand, F., et al. 1979. Zum EEG im Leberkoma. Z. EEG-EMG 10:88–94.

Salmon, H.A. 1956. Case of hypopituitary coma with serial electrocephalography. Br. Med. J. 1:1397–1399.

Samson, D.C., Swisher, J.N., Christian, R.M., et al. 1952. Cerebral metabolic disturbance and delirium in pernicious anemia: clinical and electroencephalographic studies. Arch. Intern. Med. 90:4–14.

Saunders, M.G., and Westmoreland, B.F. 1979. The EEG for evaluation of disorders affecting the brain diffusely. In *Current Practice of Clinical Electroencephalography,* Eds. D.W. Klass and D.D. Daly, pp. 343–379. New York: Raven Press.

Scarpino, O., Mauro, A.M., and Del Pesce, M. 1985. Partial complex seizures and insulinoma: a case report. Electroencephalogr. Clin. Neurophysiol. 61:90P(abst).

Schobel, H.P., Fischer, T., Heuszer, K., et al. 1996. Preeclampsia—a state of sympathetic overactivity. N. Engl. J. Med. 335:1480–1485.

Schultz, M.A., Schulte, F.J., Akiyama, Y., et al. 1968. Development of EEG sleep phenomena in hypothyroid infants. Electroencephalogr. Clin. Neurophysiol. 25:351–358.

Shagass, C., and Roswell, P.N. 1954. Serial electroencephalographic and clinical studies in a case of prolonged insulin coma. Arch. Neurol. Psychiatr. (Chicago) 72:705–711.

Shaw, P.J., Walls, T.J., Newman, M.B., et al. 1991. Hashimoto's encephalopathy: a steroid-responsive disorder associated with high antithyroid antibody titers—report of 5 cases. Neurology 41:228–233.

Sherlock, S. 1957. Altered consciousness in liver failure (hepatic precoma and coma). Proceed. First Internat. Congr. of Neurol. Sciences, Brussels, 1957. Les editions "Acta Medica Belgica." Brussels, 1957, pp. 115–133.

Sherlock, S. 1971. *Diseases of the Liver and Biliary System,* 4th ed. Oxford: Blackwell.

Sherlock, S., and Parbhov, S.P. 1971. The management of acute hepatic failure. Post. Grad. Med. J. 47:493–498.

Sherlock, S., Summerskill, W.H.J., White, L.P., et al. 1954. Portosystemic encephalopathy. Neurological complications of liver disease. Lancet 2: 453–457.

Shterev, A., Daskalov, D., and Dokumov, S. 1981. EEG investigation of women with Stein-Leventhal syndrome. Electroencephalogr. Clin. Neurophysiol. 52:79P(abst).

Silverman, D. 1962. Some observations on the EEG in hepatic coma. Electroencephalogr. Clin. Neurophysiol. 14:53–59.

Simsarian, J.P., and Harner, R.N. 1972. Diagnosis of metabolic encephalopathy: significance of triphasic waves in the electroencephalogram. Neurology (Minneapolis) 22:456.

Singh, B.M., and Strobos, R.J. 1980. Epilepsia partialis continua associated with nonketotic hyperglycemia: clinical and biochemical profile of 21 patients. Ann. Neurol. 8:155–160.

Skanse, B., and Nyman, G.E. 1956. Thyrotoxicosis as a cause of cerebral dysrhythmia and convulsive seizures. Acta Endocrinol. (Copenhagen) 22:246–263.

Smith, D.B., Lewis, J.A., Burks, J.S., et al. 1980. Dialysis encephalopathy in peritoneal dialysis. JAMA 244:365–366.

Spatz, R., Nagel, J., Kollmannsberger, A., et al. 1975. Das Elektroenzephalogramm bei der Hyperthyreose und im thyreotoxischen Koma. Z. EEG-EMG 6:14–18.

Spatz, R., Kugler, J., and Angstwurm, H. 1977. Zur Bedeutung elektorenzephalographischer Veränderungen beim Hyperkalzämie-Syndrom. Z. EEG-EMG 8:70–76.

Srikantia, S.G., Veeraghava-Reddy, M., and Krishnaswamy, K. 1968. Electroencephalographic patterns in pellagra. Electroencephalogr. Clin. Neurophysiol. 25:386–388.

Stockard, J.J., and Trauner, D.A. 1984. Distinctive EEG abnormalities in progressive renal encephalopathy of childhood: Similarity to those in progressive dialytic encephalopathy (PDE) of adults. Electroencephalogr. Clin. Neurophysiol. 57:60P(abst).

Storm van Leeuwen, W., Demanet, J., de Graeff, J., et al. 1957. Effects of therapy on electro-encephalographic abnormalities in hypopituitarism. Acta Med. Scand. 159:381.

Strickland, N.J., Bold, A.M., and Medd, W.E. 1967. Bronchial carcinoma with hypercalcemia simulating cerebral metastasis. Br. Med. J. 3:590–592.

Summerskill, W.H.J., Davidson, E.A., Sherlock, S., et al. 1956. The neuropsychiatric syndrome associated with hepatic cirrhosis and extensive portal circulation. Q. J. Med. 25:245.

Sundaram, M.B., and Blume, W.T. 1984. Triphasic waves revisited. Electroencephalogr. Clin. Neurophysiol. 58:51P(abst).

Swash, M., and Rowan, A.J. 1972. Electroencephalographic criteria of hypocalcemia and hypercalcemia. Arch. Neurol. (Chicago) 26:218–228.

Terracol, I., Passouant, P., Gesp, H., et al. 1951. Les anomalies EEG au cours de la maladie de Basedow. Presse Méd. 59:1316–1318.

Thiébaut, F., Rohmer, F., and Wackenheim, A. 1958. Contribution à l'étude électroencéphalographique des syndromes endocriniens. Electroencephalogr. Clin. Neurophysiol. 10:1–30.

Thomas, S.V., Somanathan, N., and Radhakumari, R. 1995. Interictal EEG changes in eclampsia. Electroencephalogr. Clin. Neurophysiol. 94:271–275.

Torgard et al. 1965. Quoted in Gastaut, H., Rohmer, F., Cossette, A., et al. 1969. Introduction to the study of functional generalized epilepsies. In *The Physiopathogenesis of the Epilepsies,* Eds. H. Gastaut, H.H. Jasper, J. Bancaud, et al., pp. 5–25. Springfield, IL: Charles C Thomas.

Tyler, H.R. 1965. Neurological complications of dialysis, transplantation and other forms of treatment in chronic uremia. Neurology (Minneapolis) 15:1081–1088.

Tyler, H.R. 1968. Neurologic disorders in renal failure. Am. J. Med. 44:734–748.

Vague, J., Gastaut, H., Favier, G., et al. 1952. Les données de l'électroencéphalographie en pathologie endocrinienne. Marseille Méd. 89:1–17.

Vague, J., Gastaut, H., Codaccioni, J.L., et al. 1957. L'électroencéphalographie des maladies thyroidiennes. Ann. Endocrinol. 18:996.

Vallat, J.N., Lepetit, J.M., Demarti, D., et al. 1962. Accidents neurologiques de la pellagra. Á propos d'une observation électroclinique. Presse Md. 70:625–626.

Van der Rijt, C.C.D., Schalm, S.W., De Groot, G.H., et al. 1984. Objective measurements of hepatic encephalopathy by means of automated EEG analysis. Electroencephalogr. Clin. Neurophysiol. 57:423–426.

Van Zandycke, M., Orban, L., and Van der Eecken, H. 1977. Ondes lentes triphasiques dans deux cas d'encéphalopathie thyréotoxique. Acta Neurol. Belg. 77:115–120.

Vastola, E.F., Maccario, M., and Homan, R. 1967. Activation of epileptogenic foci by hyperosmolality. Neurology 17:520–526.

Victor, M. 1974. Neurologic changes in liver disease. In *Brain Dysfunction in Metabolic Disorders,* Ed. F. Plum, pp. 1–12. New York: Raven Press.

Victor, M., Adams, R.D., and Cole, M. 1965. The acquired (non-Wilsonian) type of chronic hepatocerebral degeneration. Medicine (Baltimore) 44:345–396.

Victor, M., Adams, R.D., and Collins, G.H. 1971. The *Wernicke-Korsakoff Syndrome.* Philadelphia: F.A. Davis.

Vignaendra, V., Frank, A.O., and Lim, C.L. 1977. Absence status in a patient with hypocalcemia. Electroencephalogr. Clin. Neurophysiol. 43:429–433.

Von Braunmühl, A. 1947. *Insulinschock und Heilkrampf in der Psychiatrie.* Stuttgart: Wissenschaftliche Verlagsgesellschaft.

Wackenheim, A. 1955. Contribution à l'Étude Électroencéphalographique des Syndromes Endocriniens. Strasbourg: Thesis (Medicine).

Waldinger, C., and Berg, R.B. 1968. Signs of pyridoxine dependency manifest at birth in siblings. Pediatrics 32:161–168.

Walton, J.N., Kiloh, L.G., Osselton, J.W., et al. 1954. The electroencephalogram in pernicious anaemia and subacute combined degeneration of the cord. Electroencephalogr. Clin. Neurophysiol. 6:45–64.

Waltrégny, A. 1969. Epilepsy and insulinic hypoglycemia: an experimental study. In *The Physiopathogenesis of the Epilepsies,* Eds. H. Gastaut, H.H. Jasper, J. Bancaud, et al., pp. 111–214. Springfield, IL: Charles C Thomas.

Ware, A.J., D'Agostino, A.N., and Combes, B. 1971. Cerebral oedema: a major complication of massive hepatic necrosis. Gastroenterology 61:877–884.

Weinland, W.L., and Weinland, W. 1949. Über elektroencephalographische Beobachtungen beim Insulinschock. Arch. Psychiatr. Nervenkr. 18:34–44.

Weiss, S., and Dexter, L. 1941. *Preeclamptic and eclamptic toxemia in pregnancy.* Baltimore: Williams & Wilkins.

Wilson, W.P., Johnson, J.E., and Feist, F.W. 1964. Thyroid hormone and brain functions. Changes in photically elicited EEG responses following the administration of tri-iodo-thyronine to normal subjects. Electroencephalogr. Clin. Neurophysiol. 16:329–331.

Wynn, D., Lagerlund, T., Mokri, B., et al. 1989. Periodic complexes in hypothyroidism masquerading as Jakob-Creutzfeldt disease: a case report. Electroencephalogr. Clin. Neurophysiol. 72:31P(abst).

Yaar, I., Shapiro, M.B., and Pottala, E.W. 1981. An EEG power spectral analysis of dopaminergic mechanisms in patients with hepatic coma. Electroencephalogr. Clin. Neurophysiol. 51:31P(abst).

Ziegler, D.K., and Presthus, J. 1957. Normal electroencephalogram at deep levels of hypoglycemia. Electroencephalogr. Clin. Neurophysiol. 9:523–526.

Zuckermann, E.C., and Glaser, G.H. 1972. Urea-induced myoclonic seizures. An experimental study of mechanism and site of action. Arch. Neurol. (Chicago) 27:14–28.

Zwang, H.J., and Cohn, D. 1981. Electroencephalographic changes in acute water intoxication. Clin. Electroencephalogr. 12:35–40.

Zysno, E. 1966. EEG changes and electrolyte metabolism in uremia. Electroencephalogr. Clin. Neurophysiol. 20:755(abst).

23. Cerebral Anoxia

Franz Aichner and Gerhard Bauer

Basic Mechanisms

The brain is metabolically one of the most active of all the organs in the body. Cerebral oxygen consumption in normal conscious young persons is approximately 3.5 mL/100 g brain/min. The rate of oxygen consumption by an entire brain of average weight (1,400 g) amounts to 49 mL O_2/min in the basal state. The average man weighs 70 kg and consumes about 250 mL O_2/min in the basal state. Therefore, the brain alone, which represents only approximately 2% of total body weight, accounts for 20% of the resting total body oxygen consumption (Table 23.1) (Clarke and Sokoloff, 1994).

Oxygen is utilized in the brain almost entirely for the oxidation of carbohydrate (Sokoloff, 1960). The average critical level of oxygen tension in the brain below consciousness and the normal electroencephalogram (EEG) pattern are lost, lies between 15 and 20 mm Hg (Hossmann and Kleihus, 1973; Martin et al., 1994). The average rate of blood flow in the human brain amounts to 57 mL/100 g tissue/min corresponding to 800 mL/min or approximately 15% of total basal cardiac output for the entire brain (Table 23.1). Regulation of the cerebral blood flow (CBF) is achieved mainly by control of cerebral vessels. High $PaCO_2$, low PaO_2, and low pH tend to dilate the blood vessels and increase CBF. Changes in the opposite direction constrict the vessels and decrease blood flow.

Glucose is the only significant substrate for the brain energy metabolism. The O_2 consumption and CO_2 production are equivalent to a rate of glucose utilization of 26 mmol/100 g tissue/min. The glucose utilization actually measured amounts to 31 mmol/100 g/min. Excess glucose (5.5 mmol O_2/mmol glucose) is probably metabolized in part to lactate, pyruvate, and other intermediates of carbohydrate metabolism.

Because of the high rate of oxygen metabolism and the lack of tissue oxygen stores, interruption of oxygen delivery to the brain causes immediate cell dysfunction and rapidly leads to cell death. Oxygen delivery to the brain is calculated as the product of the oxygen content of arterial blood and the CBF. Inadequate oxygen delivery (hypoxia, anoxia) can result from inadequate CBF (ischemic hypoxia/ anoxia), inadequate partial pressure of oxygen in arterial blood (hypoxic hypoxia/anoxia), or inadequate oxygen-carrying capacity of arterial blood (anemic hypoxia/anoxia) (Auer and Benveniste, 1997).

The most common cause of brain hypoxia is ischemia or inadequate CBF. Reduction of CBF below 15 mL/min/100 g of tissue results in failure of electrical activity. Reduction to less than 10 mL/min/100 g of tissue results in loss of the transmembrane ionic gradient (Heiss and Rosner, 1983).

Cellular energy depletion appears to be a triggering event of the damaging biochemical process during ischemia. Biochemical events involved in reperfusion determining cell death are listed in Table 23.2. The molecular consequences of brain ischemia include changes in cell signaling (neurotransmitters, neuromodulators), in signal transduction (receptors, ion channels, second messengers, phosphorylation reactions), in metabolism (carbohydrate, protein, fatty acid, free radicals), and in gene regulation and expression (Benveniste et al., 1984; Pulsinelli and Cooper, 1994; Siesjö et al., 1995). Changes of neurochemical markers and their normalization could be monitored by intracerebral microdialysis in a patient during cardiac resuscitation (Bauer et al., 2004).

Delayed neuronal death refers to the neuronal degeneration occurring days after an episode of complete ischemia of short duration (Hori et al., 1991; Petito et al., 1987). Factors of these secondary deleterious processes are reperfusion injury (Hallenbeck and Dutka, 1990); neuronal hyperactivity in the postischemic period, possibly due to enhanced sensitivity of postischemic neurons to afferent stimuli; mitochondrial perturbations; as well as postischemic alterations in calcium, potassium, and glutamate homeostasis. The importance of delayed neuronal death lies in the implication that the postischemic period before the neurons have died represents, at least in theory, a therapeutic window (Auer and Benveniste, 1997). The above-described processes have to be distinguished from delayed ischemic neurodegeneration leading to cognitive impairments and parkinsonian-like syndromes after focal cerebral ischemia (Fujioka et al., 2003).

In global ischemia, blood supply to the entire brain is interrupted. Conditions causing anoxic–ischemic encephalopathy are myocardial infarction, cardiac arrest (CA), hemorrhage with shock and circulatory collapse, shock, suffocation from drowning, strangulation, aspiration of vomiting or blood, compression of the trachea, foreign body in the trachea, diseases paralyzing respiration muscles, and carbon monoxide poisoning. In focal ischemia, blood supply to a particular region of the brain is interrupted.

In patients who sustained a period of systemic hypotension or elevated intracranial pressure after brain injury, infarctions have been observed in the watershed or boundary zones of adjacent vascular territories. After short episodes neuronal damage may occur in selectively vulnerable regions of the brain. Administration of graded ischemic insults of 10-, 20-, and 30-minute duration has indicated a vulnerability in the following decreasing order: hippocampal regions (CA 1 > CA4 > CA3) > cerebellar Purkinje cells > cerebellar stellate and basket cells > striatum: small > large neurons > neocortical layers 3, 5, and 6 > layers 2 and 4 (Brierley, 1976). The basis of this selective vulnerability has

Table 23.1. Cerebral Blood Flow and Metabolic Rate in a Normal Young Adult Man

Function	Per 100 g of Brain Tissue	Per Whole Brain (1,400 g)
Cerebral blood flow (ml/min)	57	798
Cerebral O_2 consumption (ml/min)	3.5	49
Cerebral glucose utilization (mg/min)	5.5	77

(after Sokoloff, 1960)

Table 23.3. Hypoxic Thresholds for CNS Dysfunction

Simulated Altitude (ft)	F_1O_2 (%)	PaO_2 (Torr)	Neurological Status
Sea level	21	90	Normal
5,000	17	80	Impaired dark vision
8,000–10,000			Impaired short-term memory; difficulty learning complex tasks
	15–14	55–54	
15,000–20,000			Loss of judgment, euphoria, obtundation
	11–9	40–30	
>20,000	<9	<25	Coma

(after Pulsinelli and Cooper, 1994)

not been entirely determined, although many differences between vulnerable and less vulnerable cells might account for it (Lipton, 1999; Pulsinelli et al., 1982). In the most severe ischemic brain injury, tissue edema and elevated intracranial pressure stop CBF following resuscitation.

Hypoxia constitutes the lack of oxygen due to low oxygen tension in the inhaled air, such as may happen during a sojourn in thin air at high altitude, or result from depletion of oxygen stores during general anesthesia or diving excursions. Frequent causes are obstruction of airways, pulmonary edema, atelectasis, pneumonia, terminal emphysema, asthma, anaphylaxis, epiglottitis, croup, bronchiolitis, and apnea. With these conditions, the hypoxemia tends to be accompanied by hypercapnia as a result of insufficient removal of carbon dioxide. The condition is also called asphyxia (Go, 1991).

Pure hypoxic encephalopathy, uncomplicated by the effects of reduced CBF, occurs rarely in humans, since hypoxia induces cardiac arrhythmias, and systemic hypotension causes cerebral hypoperfusion. However, isolated hypoxic hypoxia is different from ischemic hypoxia with regard to pathophysiology and prognosis (Miyamoto and Auer, 2000).

Hypoxic thresholds for central nervous system (CNS) dysfunction are given in Table 23.3. At approximately 1,500 to 10,000 feet, which corresponds to $PaO_2 = 40$ to 30 torr, cognitive function becomes severely impaired with loss of judgment, delirium, and muscular incoordination. Acute hypoxia, equivalent to an altitude of 10,000 feet or above, which corresponds to $PaO_2 = 25$ to 20 torr, is associated with rapid loss of consciousness. The ultimate cause of hypoxic encephalopathy is a fall in the partial pressure of tissue oxygen to levels that no longer support mitochondrial respiration (Pulsinelli and Cooper, 1994).

Neurological Signs

The clinical course of anoxic–ischemic brain injury reflects more the rate of onset and severity than the precise nature of the insult (Heiss and Rosner, 1983). Asystole leads to loss of consciousness in 4 to 8 seconds in the upright position and after 12 to 15 seconds in the supine. EEG signs of syncopes are dealt with below (see also Chapter 28). If the CA lasts longer than 15 to 20 seconds, tonic posturing ensues. Cyanosis appears along with incontinence of both urine and feces. Pupils become unreactive and bilateral Babinski signs occur. In more chronic situations, the patient may gradually develop lethargy and confusion, followed by multifocal myoclonus, general rigidity, focal neurologic deficits, and finally coma (Table 23.4) (Binder and Gerstenbrand, 1986). Pro-

Table 23.2. Major Events in Brain Ischemia

Early changes (sec-min)
Release of free fatty acids
Ca^{2+} influx
Activation of lipolytic enzymes
Mitochondrial swelling
Increased NADH
Increased adenosine
Intermediate changes (<10 min)
Increased glycolysis
Decreased glucose, glycogen
Increased lactate
Decreased energy charge
Failure of Na, K-ATPase
Neurotransmitter release
Increased cyclic AMP
Late changes (>10 min)
Decreased protein synthesis
Increased proteolysis
Activation of lysosomal enzymes
Development of edema
Induction of heat shock proteins
Induction of c-*fos*
Induction of ornithine decarboxylase

(after Farooqui et al., 1994)

Table 23.4. Neurological Signs of Cerebral Anoxic Injury

Primary Phase	Secondary Phase
No pupillary light reaction	Normal pupil reaction
Preserved corneal reflex	Preserved corneal reflex
Inconstant oculocephalic reflex	Positive oculocephalic reflex
Inconstant vestibulocephalic reflex	
No motoric pattern	
Flaccid muscle tone	Extensor spasm, paratonic rigidity
Elevated tendon jerks	Rigidity
No spinal reflexes	Spasticity
No spasticity	Myoclonic jerks: ocular pharyngofacial diaphragmal trunk extremity

(after Binder and Gerstenbrand, 1986)

Table 23.5. Relationship between Level of Consciousness and Cerebral Metabolic Rate

Level of Consciousness	Cerebral Blood Flow (ml/100 g/min)	Cerebral O_2 Consumption (ml/100 g/min)
Mentally alert	54	3.3
Normal young men		
Mentally confused	48	2.8
Brain tumor		
Diabetic acidosis		
Insulin hypoglycemia		
Cerebral arteriosclerosis		
Comatose	57	2.0
Brain tumor		
Diabetic coma		
Insulin coma		
Anesthesia		

(after Sokoloff, 1969)

gressive reductions in the level of consciousness are paralleled by corresponding decreases in the cerebral metabolic rate (Tables 23.5 and 23.6) (Sokoloff, 1969).

Neurological syndromes following the acute anoxic insult may be classified into three categories: transient deficits after brief coma, persistent focal deficits after more prolonged coma (>12 hours), and global damage with no recovery. Patients with brief episodes of cerebral anoxia may tolerate circulatory arrest and recover rapidly and completely. Coma lasts only several hours. After severe and prolonged hypotension, focal or multiple infarcts, especially within the border zones of the cerebral circulation, may occur. Such patients remain in coma for more than 12 hours,

Table 23.6. Cerebral Blood Flow and Metabolic Rate in Humans with Various Disorders Affecting Mental State

Condition	Mental State	Cerebral Blood Flow (ml/100 g/min)	Cerebral O_2 Consumption (ml/100 g/min)
Normal	Alert	54	3.3
Increased intracranial pressure (brain tumor)	Coma	34	2.5
Insulin hypoglycemia			
Arterial glucose level			
74 mg/100 ml	Alert	58	3.4
19 mg/100 ml	Confused	61	2.6
8 mg/100 ml	Coma	63	1.9
Thiopental anesthesia	Coma	60	2.1
Postconvulsive state			
Before convulsion	Alert	58	3.7
After convulsion	Confused	37	3.1
Diabetes			
Acidosis	Confused	45	2.7
Coma	Coma	65	1.7
Hepatic insufficiency	Coma	33	1.7

(after Sokoloff, 1969)

and focal or multifocal neurological deficits are observed after regaining consciousness. Global CNS damage following cardiac arrest results in irreversible brain damage with widespread destruction of gray and white matter (Fig. 23.1) (Plum and Posner, 1982). Circulatory arrest produces irreversible brain injury after 4 minutes, whereas anoxia (with Pao_2 > 20 mm Hg) without ischemia lasting up to 40 minutes may still permit an excellent outcome. Recovering patients awake within the first 24 to 48 hours. Patients who do not awake within these time limits are in danger of dying or of surviving in a persistent vegetative state (Maiese and Caronna, 1988).

After prolonged episodes of hypotension, patients remain in coma for >12 hours, and posthypoxic syndromes develop: persistent coma or persistent vegetative state, dementia without or with extrapyramidal signs, personality changes, amnestic states, visual disorders, parkinsonism and choreoathetosis, seizures (Snyder et al., 1980b), as well as brainstem, cerebellar, and spinal cord disorders (Gorelick and Kelly, 1993).

Puzzling phenomenons are myoclonic jerks after an anoxic episode. They occur as myoclonic status in acute postanoxic coma (Bauer and Niedermeyer, 1979; Jumao-as and Brenner, 1990; Krumholz et al., 1988; Wijdicks et al., 1994; Young et al., 1990), even as selective stimulus-provoked myoclonus (Gatzonis et al., 2001; Niedermeyer et al., 1977), and as postanoxic intention myoclonus after regaining consciousness (Lance and Adams, 1963). The differentiation of these types of myoclonias is important with regard to etiology and prognosis. Whereas myoclonic jerks in a comatose state carry a grim prognosis (see below), postanoxic intention myoclonus mostly occurs after awakening from a hypoxic insult due to an asthmatic attack (Morris et al., 1998; Werhan et al., 1997). The movement disorder tends to improve with time (Werhan et al., 1997). 5-Hydroxytryptamine (5-HT) (serotonin) receptors seem to play a role in this type of posthypoxic myoclonus (Pappert et al., 1999).

Less severely affected patients are able to communicate on awakening and may have slight or moderate intellectual impairment. Personality and behavioral changes include irritability, verbal aggressiveness, violence, impulsiveness, moodiness, and depression. Hypomania has also been described. Amnesia associated with cerebral anoxia results from ischemic damage to the hippocampus or thalamus or failure of oxygen dependent neurotransmitter systems. Unlike alcoholic Korsakoff syndrome, amnestic patients after cerebral hypoxia are oriented and do not confabulate (Volpe and Hirst, 1983). Visual dysfunction may be due to ischemia to arterial border zones between the posterior and middle cerebral arteries. Visual motor behavior is impaired due to disconnection of the primary visual system and the centers subserving eye and limb movements. Optic ataxia, simultanagnosia, and ocular apraxia may occur (Balint syndrome). Movement disorders like dystonia, tremor, parkinsonism, and chorea may follow cerebral anoxia or ischemia (Bhatt et al., 1993; Hawker and Lang, 1990; Janavs and Aminoff, 1998; Li et al., 2000; Scott and Jankovic, 1996). Carbon monoxide exposure serves as a model for anoxia-associated parkinsonism (Brucher, 1985). Magnetic resonance imaging (MRI) shows abnormalities within the basal ganglia (Arbelaez et al., 1999).

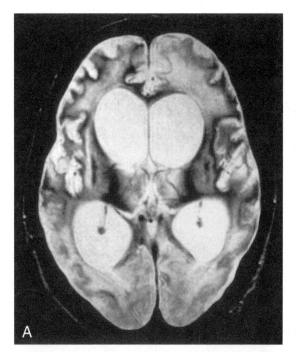
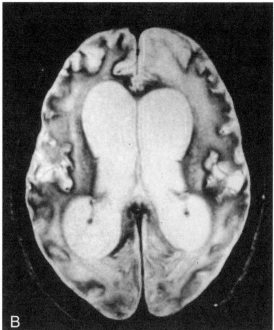
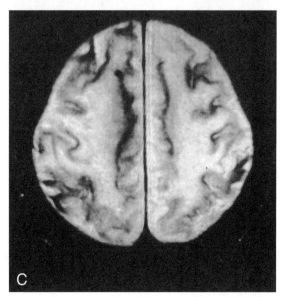

Figure 23.1.   A–C: A 45-year-old man in a vegetative state 42 days after cerebral anoxia due to cardiac arrest (CA). On magnetic resonance imaging (MRI), axial T2-weighted images showing severe ventricular enlargement, diffuse cortical and subcortical atrophy, as well as T2 prolongation in both cerebral hemispheres indicating severe diffuse encephalopathy.

In some patients, CA leads to necrosis of brainstem nuclei, with relative preservation of other CNS structures. Key neurological features include mutism, quadriplegia, preservation of vertical gaze, and ocular bobbing. Autonomic dysfunctions are observed. Brainstem signs include absence of oculocephalic response, absence of oculovestibular response, roving eye movements, persistent downward deviation of the eyes, and ocular bobbing. In severe anoxic injury, brainstem reflexes are absent (Ropper, 1981).

Autopsy and Neuroimaging Findings

Autopsy findings demonstrate ischemic cell changes in all types of anoxia (Brierley et al., 1973). The pattern of damage generally depends on the extent and duration of per-fusion failure. With severe global reduction of CBF, massive diffuse cortical necrosis occurs (Adams et al., 1966; Lindenberg, 1963). With partial perfusion failure, i.e., reduction in systemic blood pressure and CBF, lesions are confined to arterial boundary zones and the pattern corresponds to the "watershed" or "geographical" distribution (Brierley et al., 1973; Prior, 1973; Zülch and Behrend, 1961). In acute cases of massive anoxic brain damage, cerebral edema and consecutive transtentorial herniation are common complications (Lindenberg, 1963).

In an attempt to define the structural basis of the vegetative state, Adams et al. (2000) have undertaken a detailed neuropathological study of the brains of 49 patients who remained vegetative until death 1 month to 8 years after an acute brain insult. Of these, 14 patients had sustained some type of acute hypoxic-ischemic brain damage, in the neocortex in nine cases (64%) and focal damage in four (29%). The thalamus was abnormal in every case. One can conclude that the fundamental structural abnormality in patients in a vegetative state is subcortical and related to damage to the white matter of the cerebral hemispheres and/or the thalamus (Adams et al., 2000).

Early in the course of acute anoxic coma, computed tomography (CT) of the brain may exhibit no abnormalities. Later in the course, diffuse mass effects with effacement of cerebral sulci and cisterns, global decrease in the cortical gray matter density from edema, bilaterally low-density lesions of the basal ganglia, and decreased gray matter density in bilateral watershed distributions are seen (Kjos et al., 1983; Morimoto et al., 1993). In MRI series, the most frequently encountered types of hypoxic cerebral damage were watershed infarctions and bilateral selective neuronal necroses within the globus pallidus, putamen, caudate nuclei, thalamus, parahippocampal gyrus, hippocampus, cerebellum, and brainstem nuclei (Birbamer et al., 1991; Christophe et al., 2002; Sawada et al., 1990; Singhal et al., 2002; Takahashi et al., 1993). Roine et al. (1993) found CA associated with deep cerebral infarcts but not with leukoaraiosis. Early white matter injuries after an anoxic-ischemic insult have also been identified (Chalela et al., 2001). The sensitivity of MRI in the detection of ischemic hypoxic lesions is markedly superior to that of CT. The use of magnetic resonance spectroscopy (MRS), diffusion-weighted MRI, and positron emission tomography (PET) may identify viable brain tissue and allow on-line monitoring of therapeutic interventions. MRS is more sensitive than MRI in detecting hypoxic damage and is also diagnostic at a much earlier stage of the disease. In the instant early stage of hypoxia, pH, phosphocreatine and adenosine triphosphate (ATP) are diminished, whereas lactate is elevated. In the early stage of hypoxia N-acetyl-aspartate (NAA) is reduced and lactate may still be present over days and weeks (Felber et al., 1992; Martin et al., 1991).

In a PET study of brain glucose metabolism in patients with postanoxic syndrome, De Volder et al. (1990) demonstrated that brain anoxia can result in global brain hypometabolism. The extent of these abnormalities is related to the depth of coma, the location to arterial border zones such as parieto-occipital cortex, frontomesial area, striatum, and visual cortex. PET provides a useful index of residual brain tissue function after anoxia (De Volder et al., 1990). Using the 133 xenon blood flow technique, Beckstead et al. (1978) reported that CBF and cerebral metabolic rate for oxygen were severely reduced in patients at 2 to 6 hours after cardiac arrest. Cohan et al. (1989) found that patients regaining consciousness had relatively normal CBF before regaining consciousness, but those who died without regaining consciousness had increased CBF, which appeared within 24 hours after resuscitation. The increase in CBF might indicate the onset of irreversible brain damage (Cohan et al., 1989). PET documents a severe and irreversible damage of supratentorial cortical structures in postanoxic vegetative state. PET distinguishes functional alterations in vegetative state from those in non-rapid-eye-movement (REM) sleep and documents that patients in vegetative state are in a state

closely related to deep anesthesia (Rudolf, 2000; Schaafsma et al., 2003).

EEG Abnormalities

Basic Mechanisms of EEG Changes

Oxidative metabolism supplies the energy for the maintenance of the membrane potentials of nerve cells. Therefore, the EEG reflects disturbances of cerebral metabolism such as anoxia. Reduction of po_2 and increase of pco_2 frequently occur concomitantly. These biochemical changes exert reverse effects on most cortical and spinal nerve cells (Speckmann, 1970). With isolated lowering of po_2, the neuronal membrane potential declines and the discharge rate rises. By contrast, an increase in $pcoO_2$ leads to an increase in the membrane potential and to an inhibition of spontaneous activity. With further lowering of po_2, the membrane potential breaks down and electrical activity ceases.

Experimentally, lowering of O_2 leads to EEG changes consisting of progressive reduction in voltage accompanied by an increase in frequency (Meyer and Marx, 1972). With further lack of O_2, diffuse slowing and, finally, electrical silence occur. The sequence of electrophysiological disturbances underlying the response of the EEG to anoxia has been studied in detail (Martin et al., 1994). Neuronal death occurs as a result of increase of excitatory mechanisms mediated by glutamate. Before the final accumulation of glutamate, modest changes in membrane potential and intracellular and extracellular ion concentrations are connected with the EEG changes listed above.

The selective vulnerability of nerve cells can also be noted in electrical terms. Electrical activity disappears first in the most recently (phylogenetically) developed areas of the brain. Cortical electrical silence is accompanied by maximal activity recorded from brainstem structures (Naquet and Fernandez-Guardiola, 1959; Noell and Dombrowski, 1947; Sugar and Gerard, 1938; Ward and Wheatley, 1947).

EEG Changes During Arrest of Cerebral Circulation and with Syncope (see also Chapter 28)

The just-mentioned sequence of electrical events can clearly be demonstrated in complete cerebral ischemia due to cardiac arrest, excessive hypotension, or mechanical interruption of CBF (Dell et al., 1961; Fischer-Williams and Cooper, 1964; Gastaut and Fischer-Williams, 1957; Lavy and Stern, 1967; Meyer et al., 1967; Rohmer et al., 1952). During the first 3 to 6 seconds after arrest of circulation, no clinical or EEG signs can be observed. When the arrest lasts about 7 to 13 seconds, slow waves of increasing amplitude and decreasing frequency appear. If the arrest of circulation is prolonged, attenuation of activity and flattening of the EEG occur. Return of normal cerebral activity after restoration of circulation is attained in a reverse manner. Visser et al. (2001) have been able to monitor the EEG during implantation of an internal cardioverter defibrillator. The first spectral change after circulatory arrest was an increase in alpha power and a decrease in beta power. After 15 seconds alpha power started to decrease and the sequence of EEG changes followed the above-described pattern.

Syncope in a strictly linguistic sense means loss of consciousness accompanied by a drop to the floor. In clinical terms, it implies a cardiovascular etiology (see also Chapter 28), resulting in cerebral circulatory arrest (Mattle et al., 1995). Brenner (1997) gives an excellent review of the pathophysiology and EEG of this very common disorder. The EEG signs are essentially the same as mentioned above. It has to be noted that syncope of cardiovascular origin and epileptic seizures exhibit complex interactions, i.e., syncope can lead to seizures (Bergey et al., 1997; Emery, 1990) and seizures to syncope (Reeves et al., 1996). Furthermore, aura phenomena with syncope closely resemble epileptic auras (Benke et al., 1997; Lempert et al., 1994). Therefore, simultaneous electrocardiogram (ECG) is important when EEG is used in the evaluation of loss of consciousness (Pitney et al., 1994).

EEG Patterns in Prolonged Conditions After Anoxia

In the daily routine work of an EEG laboratory, records of prolonged conditions after hypoxia are much more common than those of acute CA. EEG changes are principally the same as with other comatose states and are described in detail in Chapter 24(AQ6), dealing with coma and brain death. This section gives some details specific for hypoxic coma states.

Diffuse Slowing

Diffuse slowing of varying degrees characterizes the less severe grades of diffuse postanoxic or hypoxic (Pampiglione, 1964; Prior, 1973; Silverman, 1975) and respiratory encephalopathies (Vazquez, 1979). Intermingled spindle activity resembling physiological sleep spindles was found in 64% of the patients (Hulihan and Syna, 1994). In cases with spindles, the EEG was more frequently changed by exogenous stimulation.

Frontal Intermittent Rhythmic Delta Activity (FIRDA)

This ubiquitous sign of initial defect in arousal consists of rhythmical trains of large delta waves over frontotemporal regions. With cerebral anoxia, this pattern seems to be characteristic of chronic diffuse ischemia (Van der Drift, 1972) or encephalopathies secondary to pulmonary insufficiency (Vazquez, 1979; Wilson and Sieker, 1958). Somewhat different from FIRDA are intermittent polymorphic delta activities over the anterior regions (anterior bradyrhythmia), which may occur in confusional states in the elderly. Although most probably related to some type of reduced CBF, compared with FIRDA anterior bradyrhythmia usually represents a transient and more benign EEG abnormality.

Continuous Spiking

Many records of patients in deep coma after CA are characterized by continuous diffuse spike or sharp-wave activity occasionally resembling triphasic waves (Calham and Ettinger, 1966; Silverman, 1975) (Fig. 23.2). Asymmetries in the paroxysmal activity may be observed, and transitions to periodic lateralized epileptiform discharges (PLEDs) (Fig. 23.3) or bilateral independent PLEDs (Bi-PLEDs) may occur (Suter, 1977). In advanced cases, stretches of near flatness interrupt the continuous spiking, suggesting a close relationship to the burst suppression pattern.

Periodic Spikes and Burst-Suppression Activity

Both patterns indicate coma with dissolution of cerebral functions down to the midbrain level (Bauer and Niedermeyer, 1979). Periodic phenomena are frequently encountered in severe posthypoxic coma and may occur with the suppression burst pattern (Fig. 23.3A), PLEDs (Fig. 23.3B), with single spikes and polyspikes and waves (Fig. 23.4) (Niedermeyer et al., 1999; Thömke et al., 2002). Suppression burst activity may occur in diversified forms and

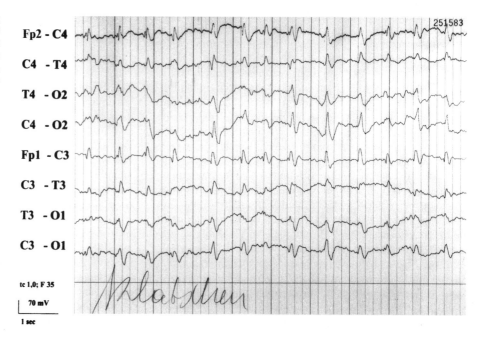

Figure 23.2. A 66-year-old man in a coma after CA. Died 9 days after the EEG was recorded. Periodic triphasic waves during the whole record. No change with exogenous stimuli (acoustic "Klatschen"). Note inconspicuous 60-Hz artifact in channel 1.

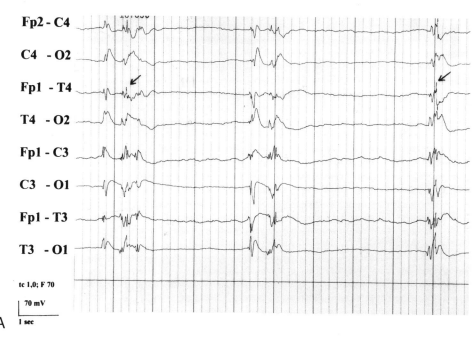

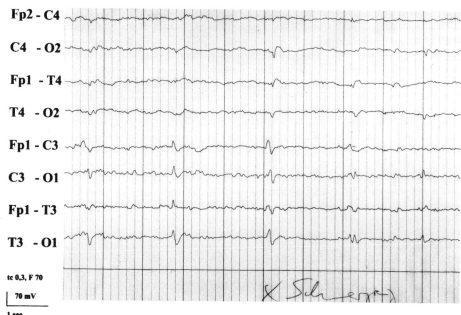

Figure 23.3. **A:** A 49-year-old man with residual epilepsy due to marked right frontal posttraumatic lesion. He had a seizure with consecutive anoxic episode of unknown duration. Comatose, on respirator. Suppression burst pattern. Myoclonic jerks time-locked to EEG bursts (see muscle artifacts indicated by *arrows*). **B:** Same patient; EEG was recorded 1 day later. Comatose, on respirator, no further jerks. Periodic transients more over the left hemisphere. Alpha frequencies in between the periodic transients. No change with noxious stimuli ("Schmerzreiz"). The EEG might be considered improved over that in **A**, but the patient died 1 month later due to a septic syndrome.

with a great variance in interburst intervals (Beydoun et al., 1991). Sinclair et al. (1999) subclassified burst suppression patterns in continuous and not continuous or incomplete (i.e., modified) types in neonatal hypoxic-ischemic encephalopathies. Transitions exist between suppression burst patterns, periodic and continuous spiking, as well as monorhythmical alpha and theta activities with sequential recordings or even within one given record (Thömke et al., 2002).

With EEGs exhibiting continuous spiking or periodic paroxysmal anomalies, a great number of involuntary movement abnormalities (see above) may be observed. Mostly, they consist of myoclonic jerks (Bauer and Niedermeyer,

1979), time-locked to the bursts (Figs. 23.3A and 23.4) or without a clear-cut correlation to EEG (Fig. 23.5). They might be stimulus sensitive (Niedermeyer et al., 1977; Van Cott et al., 1996) or unreactive to stimuli. Generalized tonic-clonic seizures, "erratic status" epilepticus (Bortone et al., 1992), and myoclonic status epilepticus (see above) may be seen (Fig. 23.4). The epileptic nature of myoclonic jerks without accompanying EEG spikes might be debatable. Furthermore, there are nonepileptic motor phenomena in hypoxic states with suppression burst EEG. Transient tonic eye opening is especially troublesome because it might give the impression of voluntary eye opening to inexperienced clinicians or relatives (Jordan et al., 1982; McCarty and Mar-

Figure 23.4. A 73-year-old man who is comatose after CA, on respirator. Continuous periodic polyspikes and waves every 2.5 seconds intermingled with muscle artifacts. In between the polyspikes and waves, rhythmic 1/sec spikes and waves without artifacts. Periodic polyspikes and waves were accompanied by myoclonic jerks (myoclonic status epilepticus).

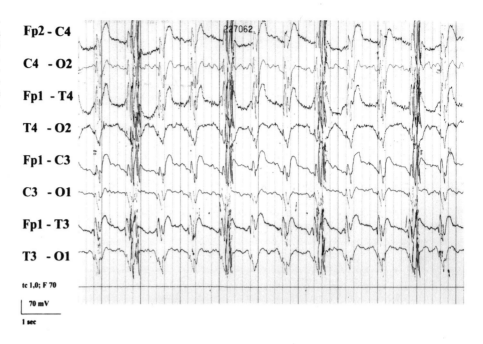

shall, 1981; Mori et al., 1983; Reeves et al., 1997). With deepening coma, epileptic and nonepileptic motor phenomena and also decerebrate posturing disappear. This must be regarded as a sign of further dissolution of brainstem functions, rather than improvement.

Monorhythmical Activities

Widespread rhythmical activities in the alpha or theta frequency are a puzzling phenomenon in severe coma (Hockaday et al., 1965; Kaplan et al., 1999; McKeown and Young, 1997; Prior, 1973; Silverman, 1975; Synek and Synek, 1984; Westmoreland et al., 1975). Alpha and theta rhythms might alternate in the same record (Thömke et al., 2002; Young et al., 1994) (Fig. 23.6) or represent a successor pattern to suppression burst activities with sequential records (Fig. 23.7). With anoxic coma, alpha or theta rhythms may occur monotonously over the anterior regions. No other frequencies are present. This specific type was termed complete alpha or theta coma (Berkhoff et al., 2000). Intermingled slow waves or some type of reactivity constitute the incomplete alpha/theta coma (Berkhoff et al., 2000). Alpha and theta coma demonstrate the difficulties of an EEG evaluation solely based on the frequency spectrum.

Figure 23.5. An 82-year-old man in a coma after CA due to myocardial infarction. Burst and prolonged burst with repetitive polyphasic transients. Myoclonic jerks (see artifacts in electrocardiogram channel) without a correlation to bursts. Exhibited prominent unreactive alpha frequencies 1 day later and died 2 days after admission. Channel 8 (T_3–O_1) out of working condition.

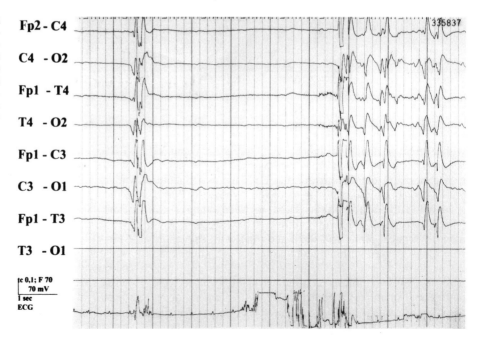

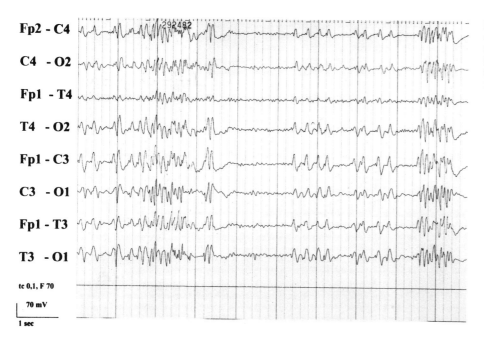

Figure 23.6. A 61-year-old man in a coma after CA. Comatose, on respirator, died the next day. Paroxysmal rhythmical activities of varying frequencies and intermittent periods with lowered amplitudes and 10–13/sec rhythmical activities.

Low-Voltage Output EEG and Electrocerebral Silence

These patterns indicate the breakdown of neuronal electrical activity due to irreversible depolarization of the membrane potential. It is not clear whether the reversible flattening during CA, the intermittent flat periods with the suppression burst pattern, and flattening immediately after some generalized seizures are likewise related to depolarization or to excessive hyperpolarization. Low-voltage output EEG is not to be mixed up with genetically determined low-voltage EEG (Steinlein et al., 1992) or records of anxious patients.

The Role of Evoked Potentials in the Diagnosis of Anoxic Coma

Evoked potentials (EPs) have advantages over EEG in the evaluation of comatose patients (Bettinger et al., 1992; Ganes and Lundar, 1988; Kotchoubey et al., 2001; Walser et al., 1985). With EP there is a possibility to study subcortical pathophysiology. Furthermore, sedative drugs frequently used in the intensive care unit (ICU) alter EEG activity but not short latency EP. Details about EP in coma may be found elsewhere in the book.

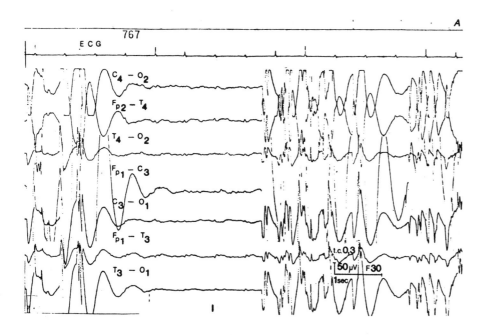

Figure 23.7. A: A 50-year-old woman in a hypoxic coma with impaired brainstem functions due to hanging in a suicide attempt. Patient had irregular muscular twitching in the face. Burst suppression-like pattern in EEG, recorded after administration of succinylcholinchloride i.v. Note the low voltage irregular mixed activity in between the bursts.

Figure 23.7. *(continued)* **B:** Record taken 3 days after that in **A**. Bulbar brain syndrome at neurological examination with completely dissolute brainstem functions. Rhythmical alpha activity during the whole record, maximal over frontotemporal regions (alpha coma). The patient died 3 days later.

Prognosis

The knowledge of the underlying etiology of the comatose state is essential for prognostication of outcome. Patients in traumatic coma recover somewhat better than those in nontraumatic coma. Patients with hypoxic-ischemic coma after CA have an intermediate prognosis between the metabolic and cerebrovascular groups. The success rate for initial resuscitation and ultimate survival from an out-of-hospital CA depends in part on the etiology of the event. Ventricular tachycardia carries a relatively good prognosis (67% survivors) followed by ventricular fibrillation (30%). Asystole and electromechanical dissociation have dismal outcome statistics. The most common causes of death during hospitalization after resuscitated CA are related to the severity of injury to the CNS. Anoxic encephalopathy and infections subsequent to prolonged respirator dependence account for 60% of deaths. Another 30% occur as a consequence of low cardiac output states, which fail to respond to interventions. Paradoxically, recurrent arrhythmias are the least common cause of death, accounting for only 10% of in-hospital deaths (Myerburg and Castellanos, 1991).

Selected studies suggest that the 40% to 50% of out-of-hospital cardiac arrest patients may be discharged alive from the hospital after resuscitation (Earnest et al., 1979; Longstreth et al., 1983; Snyder et al., 1980a). In the standard treatment group of a well-designed study, 20% were alive at 1 year at follow-up (Brain Resuscitation Clinical Trial I Study Group, 1986). In a second report of the same group, mortality was 83% at 6 months (Brain Resuscitation Clinical Trial II Study Group, 1991). Return to normal wakefulness and cognition ranges from 13% to 54%. Bassetti et al. (1996) reported the outcome in 60 patients comatose for more than 6 hours after a CA; 20% made a good recovery, and 80% died or remained in a vegetative state. A prospective investigation of out-of-hospital CA treated by early defibrillation in 200 patients yielded the following numbers: 145 (72%) patients survived to hospital admission, 74 (40%) have been neurologically intact at discharge, and 19 died after discharge. The mean length of follow-up was 4.8 ± 3.0 years (Bunch et al., 2003). In patients after in hospital CPR a range of 93–99% with good recovery is reported (Murphy and Murray, 1989).

Survival following immersion is dependent on short duration of the submersion and bystander-initiated cardiopulmonary resuscitation (CPR). Among survivors of near-drowned children, neurological injury is common. If one considers all survivors, neurological sequelae range from 0% to 30%. Patients arriving at the emergency department pulseless or with a Glasgow Coma Scale (GCS) score of 3 rarely survive. Among the survivors 60% to 100% exhibit neurological deficits (Allmann et al., 1986; Nichter and Everett, 1989).

The incidence of CA related to anesthesia has been studied in Australia (National Health and Medical Research Council, 1985–87), Canada (Cohen et al., 1986), the United Kingdom, the United States, and France (Tiret et al., 1986). The most common causes of CA and death related to anesthesia are listed on Table 23.7. The major risk factors are age (children and the elderly) and emergency surgery.

Clinical Outcome Predictors

All studies of coma prognosis are plagued by methodological problems. Outcome after CPR is determined by patient-dependent and resuscitation-dependent factors (Tables 23.8 and 23.9). Patient-dependent factors are intrinsic heart disease, other associated medical conditions, and the presenting cardiac rhythm (Grubb et al., 1995). Resuscitation-dependent factors are witnessed versus unwitnessed arrest, bystander–initiated CPR, and the duration of anoxia. The duration of anoxia, confirmed by the observation of a bystander, is a major determinant of brain damage. CPR reduces prehospital and overall mortality (Cummins et al., 1991; Mullie et al., 1989). A significant difference on dura-

Table 23.7. Causes of Cardiac Arrest Related to Anesthesia

Drug overdose
Inadequate ventilation/failed intubation
Acid aspiration
Airway obstruction
Anaphylaxis
Cardiac failure
Cardiogenic shock
Cerebral hypoxia
Halothane-related hepatic failure
Intravenous injection of local anesthetic
Malignant hyperpyrexia
Lack of experience/care/knowledge

Table 23.9. Laboratory Predictors after CPR

Parameter	Unfavorable Prognosis
1. Blood glucose on admission	>300 mg%
2. Serum lactate	Elevation
CSF lactate	Presence
Brain lactate (1 HMRS)	Presence
3. N-Acetyl-Aspartate (1 HMRS)	Reduction
4. Neuron specific enolase	>120 mg/ml

tion of anoxia has been described in patients with favorable and unfavorable outcome after CPR (mean, 4.1 minutes versus 8 minutes; Berek et al., 1995). However, the time of anoxia is often difficult to determine.

The duration of postanoxic coma is easier to determine. Bokonjic and Buchthal (1961) reported that 90% of patients in coma for less than 48 hours made a complete recovery. Bell and Hodgson (1974) stated that full recovery from coma of more than 3 days' duration is exceptional, and several observers have noted that persistence of unresponsive coma for 48 hours after CA was predictive of poor outcome. Permanent brain damage was extremely rare if the coma lasted less than 6 hours (Thomassen and Wernberg, 1979). Other authors found that approximately 80% of CA survivors regain consciousness within the first hour after CPR (Bates et al., 1977). In a prospective clinical study, Abramson and Safar (1986) have shown that 20% of patients who are unconscious 10 minutes after successful resuscitation recovered to a normal or near-normal condition after 1 year, while the remaining patients exhibited severely impaired brain function until death.

The prognostic significance of pupillary signs and motor responses to noxious stimuli has been investigated by various authors (Attia and Cook, 1998; Chen et al., 1996; Edgren et al., 1994; Levy et al., 1981, 1985;

Table 23.8. Clinical Predictors after Cardiopulmonary Resuscitation

Clinical Parameter	Poor Prognosis
1. Duration of anoxia	>8–10 minutes
Duration of CPR	>30 minutes
Duration of postanoxic coma	>72 hours
2. Pupillary light reaction	absent on day 3
Motor response to pain	absent on day 3
Brainstem reflexes	absent
3. Innsbruck coma scale (ICS) on admission	<2 (Death)
	<5
Glasgow coma scale (GCS) on day 3	<5
Glasgow-Pittsburgh coma scale (GPCS) on day 3	<22
The Longstreth awaking score coma scale (on admission)	<4
The Grubb prognostic scoring system	4–6
4. Seizures: myoclonic status epilepticus, presence of generalized status epilepticus	

Longstreth et al., 1983; Rothstein et al., 1991; Willoughby and Leach, 1974). Absence of motor responses on day 3 after CA together with unreactive pupils was followed by a persistent vegetative state in all patients (Edgren et al., 1994; Levy et al., 1981). The most predictive variable at the initial examination was the pupillary light reflex. None of 52 patients unreactive at the initial examination survived with a good outcome or moderate disability. Motor responses are considered the clinical sign with the second most important predictive power. According to Willoughby and Leach (1974) no response or merely stereotyped reflex responses 1 hour after CA indicate a generally poor prognosis. At 3 days, no motor response or flexor and extensor posturing was universally predictive of poor outcome. Nevertheless, analysis of individual patients showed that the absence of both pupillary light reaction and motor responses gave false-positive results in up to 7% and 5%, respectively. Further prognostic important signs were spontaneous eye movements, eye opening, and oculocephalic response (Levy et al., 1985).

Mullie et al. (1989) reported the predictive value of the GCS in the first 2 to 6 days of coma after out-of-hospital CA. The GCS, which had been initially developed for studies of head trauma, predicted outcome correctly in 80% of patients. Edgren et al. (1987) assessed the prognostic value of the Glasgow-Pittsburgh Coma Scale (GPCS) and an Uppsala modification. Forty-eight hours after CA these coma scales predicted good outcome correctly in 94% and 96%, respectively. In an international clinical multicenter trial, a total of 262 comatose CA survivors were followed for 1 year (Edgren et al., 1994). Poor outcome could be predicted immediately after reperfusion with an accuracy ranging from 52% to 84% for various signs and scores. Multivariate analysis identified lack of motor response to pain as the only independent predictor of poor outcome at a time later than 16 hours post-CA. Sandroni et al. (1995) compared the predictive values of evoked potentials and the GCS. The GCS showed a higher sensitivity and correlation with the Glasgow Outcome Scale than evoked potentials, but was associated with a high percentage of false-positive results, and its specificity was only 67%.

Grubb et al. (1995) reported on 346 consecutive cases of out-of-hospital cardiac arrest. There were associations between in-hospital mortality and prearrest variables, resuscitation variables, and factors measured during admission. A prognostic scoring system was developed based on three variables with the strongest independent relation with in-hospital mortality. Patients with a score of 4 to 6 points are unlikely to survive to discharge, whereas patients with a score of 0 points have an in-hospital mortality between 5% and 14%. Berek et al. (1997) studied 112 consecutive patients after out-of-hospital CA using the Innsbruck Coma Scale (ICS). Coma rating done initially by the mobile ICU at the time of arrival was not informative, whereas coma rating 20 to 30 minutes later predicted both favorable/nonfavorable outcome and survival/nonsurvival.

Myoclonic status epilepticus after CA has been considered an agonal phenomenon (Wijdicks et al., 1994). Several researchers agreed with the predictive value for poor outcome (Bauer and Niedermeyer, 1979; Krumholz et al., 1988; Young et al., 1990). According to Morris et al. (1998), myoclonic status is not necessarily an agonal event. However, the authors reported patients with Lance-Adams syndrome, a condition quite different from status myoclonicus in a comatose state.

Predictive Value of EEG

The predictive value of the EEG concerning outcome has been open to controversy (Allen, 1977; Attia and Cook, 1998; Plum and Posner, 1982). Therapeutic administration of muscle relaxants blurs neurological signs, and administration of sedatives blurs both neurological and EEG signs. No systematic testing of the modifying influences of sedatives has been reported. The accuracy of prognostic statements is greatest in records with very mild or very severe EEG abnormalities; the prognostic meaning of the intervening grades of abnormality is less certain (Chen et al., 1996; Hockaday et al., 1965; Prior, 1973; Rothstein et al., 1991; Silverman, 1975). EEG changes observed in the early phase after CA are of less prognostic significance than are those after 24 to 48 hours. Serial recordings are helpful (Chen et al., 1996; Pressler et al., 2001). Developments in either direction, either deterioration or progression toward normalization, allow corresponding statements. Fig. 23.3 presents an example of an exception to this rule. Several grading scales of EEG abnormalities have been developed (Scollo-Lavizzari and Bassetti, 1987; Synek, 1988, 1990). The overall accuracy of prognosis from EEG has been thought to be 80% to 90% (Hockaday et al., 1965; Prior, 1973). This figure might be improved further using long-term EEG recordings and data analysis (Geocadin et al., 2000; Morillo et al., 1983).

Malignant EEG patterns like burst-suppression pattern, periodic spiking, low-voltage output EEG, and electrocerebral silence are hard-core signs of poor outcome. Exceptions from this rule have repeatedly been reported. However, there are virtually no false pessimistic statements, if one differentiates between complete and incomplete alpha/theta coma (Berkhoff et al., 2000) and between real and modified burst suppression patterns (Sinclair et al., 1999) (see above). Especially the careful analysis of rhythmical alpha frequencies in coma and the diagnosis of complete alpha coma increase the certainty of prognostic statements (Bauer et al., 1982; Westmoreland et al., 1975).

Predictive Value of Evoked Potentials (for details see Chapter 56)

A meta-analysis of commonly encountered clinical and electrophysiological predictors of poor outcome in anoxic-ischemic coma, based on 33 studies with a total of more than 4,500 patients, revealed that absence of early cortical somatosensory evoked responses is the most discriminating predictor of poor outcome in patients with anoxic ischemic coma [0–2% for 95% confidence interval (CI) of pooled false-positive tests] (Zandbergen et al., 1998). A practical procedure in comatose patients after CA has been proposed (Zandbergen et al., 1998). Considerations regarding neurological outcome should be postponed until 72 hours after the onset of coma. After 72 hours, patients with either absent pupillary reflexes or motor response to pain no better than flexion will undergo somato-sensory evoked potential (SSEP) testing. In patients in whom early HSSEP responses are bilaterally absent after this procedure, only palliative care will be given.

Predictive Value of Neuroimaging

Brain swelling defined by the absence or compression of cerebral sulci, ventricles, and cisterns on CT was found in the early postresuscitation period, indicating a poor neurological outcome (Kjos et al., 1983). MRI is superior to CT, and MRS as well as diffusion imaging are even more sensitive than MRI in detecting hypoxic damage (Arbelaez et al., 1999; Christophe et al., 2002; Dubowitz et al., 1998; Singhal et al., 2002; Wijdicks et al., 2001). Furthermore, these methods are diagnostic at an earlier stage of the disease (Warach et al., 1995; Younkin, 1993). Martin et al. (1991) studied 31 P MRS in eight patients with severe postanoxic encephalopathy after CA. Mean brain pH was significantly more alkalotic when compared to age- and sex-matched normal controls. There was a marked metabolic heterogeneity, ranging from normal values to complete absence of high-energy phosphates with only inorganic phosphate remaining. These findings have also been observed in patients with brain death (Aichner et al., 1992). In the early and late stage of hypoxia 1 H MRS reveals reduced NAA and accumulation of lactate. Lactate intensity was correlated with lesion size, single photon emission computed tomography (SPECT) score, the Toronto Stroke Scale, and outcome index. NAA, by contrast, correlated with outcome index but not with lesion size, SPECT score, and the Toronto Stroke Scale (Graham et al., 1995). The severity of changes in MRS appears to correlate with clinical outcome. Lactate-negative patients recovered well or died of cardiac causes, whereas patients with elevated lactate level died or remained neurologically severely disabled (Berek et al., 1995).

Hexamethylpropyleneamine oximr (HMPAO)-SPECT studies of the brain after CA showed frontal hypoperfusion that tended to improve over time, but persisted in most patients. The relative size of the total perfusion defect improved in recovering patients. Patients with a total perfusion deficit size of more than 50% of the supratentorial brain remained comatose and died, but even large perfusion deficits up to 40% did not exclude the possibility of good recovery.

The occurrence or severity of frontal hypoperfusion did not predict either the recovery of consciousness or the outcome (Roine et al., 1991).

Predictive Value of Laboratory Parameters in Serum and Cerebrospinal Fluid

The prognostic significance of glycemia in the postresuscitation period could be demonstrated by various studies. Longstreth et al. (1983, 1984, 1986) suggested that the association between poor neurological recovery and high blood glucose level on admission after CA could be linked to prolonged CPR, leading to both higher levels of blood glucose and worse neurological outcome. The relation of high glycemia on admission and poor outcome after CPR was confirmed by Calle et al. (1989).

Elevated serum lactate revealed to be of prognostic importance in patients suffering from shock due to sepsis, trauma, CA, and other causes (Tuchschmidt and Mecher, 1994). Arterial lactate concentrations reflect the severity of the perfusion defect and correlate with outcome. Neuron-specific enolase (NSE) in blood and in cerebrospinal fluid (CSF) can be used as a prognostic parameter both in cerebrovascular diseases and hypoxic ischemic brain damage (Edgren et al., 1983; Karkela et al., 1992; Meynaar et al., 2003). NSE values exceeding 120 ng/mL during the first 5 days after hypoxia-ischemia point to an unfavorable outcome. In contrast, NSE concentrations below 35 ng/mL mostly indicate a good recovery. S-100 protein serves also as an early predictor and sensitive marker of hypoxic brain damage and outcome after cardiac arrest in humans (Böttiger et al., 2001; Hachimi-Idrissi et al., 2002).

Concluding Remarks on Prognostic Statements

In spite of enormous advances in modern emergency medicine, many patients with CA die. In cases of survival, problems of prognosis and morbidity are of great medical, ethical, and financial importance. Summarizing all the data, prognosis can be made with a great probability. On the other hand, with a given single patient an absolutely certain statement seems to be impossible. This perception carries important implications. Signs of poor outcome should not automatically lead to discontinuation of therapy, which may result in a self-fulfilling prophecy (Shewmon and De Giorgio, 1989). In every acute situation, optimal therapy should be continued until the course of treatment proves the poor outlook (Berek and Aichner, 1999).

References

Abramson, N.S., and Safar, P. 1986. Brain Resuscitation Clinical Trial I Study Group. Randomized clinical study of thiopental loading in comatose survivors of cardiac arrest. N. Engl J. Med. 314:397–403.

Adams, J.H., Brierley, J.B., Connor, R., et al. 1966. The effects of systemic hypotension upon the human brain. Clinical and neuropathological observations in 11 cases. Brain 89:235–268.

Adams, J.H., Graham, D.I., and Jennett, B. 2000. The neuropathology of the vegetative state after an acute brain insult. Brain 123:1327–1338.

Aichner, F., Felber, S., Birbamer, G., et al. 1992. Magnetic resonance: a noninvasive approach to metabolism, circulation, and morphology in human brain death. Ann. Neurol. 32:507–511.

Allen, N. 1977. Life or death of the brain after cardiac arrest. Neurology 27:805–806.

Allmann, F.D., Nelson, W.B., and Pacentini, G.A. 1986. Outcome of near drowning resuscitation in severe pediatric near drowning. Am. J. Dis. Child. 140:571–575.

Arbelaez, A., Castillo, M., and Mukherji, S.K. 1999. Diffusion-weighted MR imaging of global cerebral anoxia. AJNR 20:999–1007.

Attia, J., and Cook, D.J. 1998. Prognosis in anoxic and traumatic coma. Crit. Care Clin. 14:497–511.

Auer, R.N., and Benveniste, H. 1997. Hypoxia and related conditions. In *Greenfield's neuropathology*, Eds. D.I. Graham and P.L. Lantos, pp. 263–314. London: Edward Arnold.

Bassetti, C., Bomio, F., Mathis, H., et al. 1996. Early prognosis after cardiac arrest: a prospective clinical, electrophysiological, and biochemical study of 60 patients. J. Neurol. Neurosurg. Psychiatry 61:610–615.

Bates, D., Caronna, J.J., Cartlidge, N.E.F., et al. 1977. A prospective study of non-traumatic coma: methods and results in 310 patients. Ann. Neurol. 2:211–220.

Bauer, G., and Niedermeyer, E. 1979. Acute convulsions. Clin. Electroencephalogr. 10:127–144.

Bauer, G., Aichner, F., and Klingler, D. 1982. Aktivitäten im Alpha-Frequenzbereich und Koma. Z.EEEG-EMG 13:28–33.

Bauer, R., Gabl, M., Obwegeser, A., et al. 2004. Neurochemical monitoring using intracerebral microdialysis during cardiac resuscitation. Intensive Care Med. 30:159–161.

Beckstead, J.E., Tweed, W.A., Lee, J., et al. 1978. Cerebral blood flow and metabolism in man following cardiac arrest. Stroke 9:569–573.

Bell, J.A., and Hodgson, H.J.F. 1974. Coma after cardiac arrest. Brain 97:361–372.

Beltinger, A., Riffel, B., and Stöhr, M. 1992. Prognostischer Stellenwert des EEG im Vergleich zu evozierten Potentialen bei schwerer hypoxischer Hirnschädigung. Z. EEG-EMG 75–81.

Benke, Th., Hochleitner, M., and Bauer, G. 1997. Aura phenomena during syncope. Eur. Neurol. 37:28–32.

Benveniste, H., Drejer, J., Schousboe, A., et al. 1984. Elevation of the extracellular concentrations of glutamate and aspartate in rat hippocampus during transient cerebral ischemia monitored by intracerebral microdialysis. J. Neurochem. 43:1369–1374.

Berek, K., and Aichner, F. 1999. Prognosis of cerebral hypoxia after cardiac arrest. Curr. Opin. Crit. Care 5:211–215.

Berek, K., Lechleitner, P., Luef, G., et al. 1995. Early determination of neurological outcome after pre-hospital cardiopulmonary resuscitation. Stroke 26:543–549.

Berek, K., Schinnerl, A., Traweger, C., et al. 1997. The prognostic significance of coma rating, duration of anoxia and cardiopulmonary resuscitation in out-of-hospital cardiac arrest. J. Neurol. 244:556–561.

Bergey, G.K., Krumholz, A., and Fleming, C.P. 1997. Complex partial seizure provocation by vasovagal syncope: video-EEG and intracranial electrode documentation. Epilepsia 38:118–121.

Berkhoff, M., Donati, F., Bassetti, C. 2000. Postanoxic alpha (theta) coma: a reappraisal of its prognostic significance. Clin. Neurophysiol. 111:297–304.

Beydoun, A., Yen, C.E., and Drury, I. 1991. Variance of interburst intervals in burst suppression. Electroencephalogr. Clin. Neurophysiol. 79:435–439.

Bhatt, M.H., Obeso, J.A., and Marsden, C.D. 1993. Time course of post-anoxic akinetic-rigid and dystonic syndromes. Neurology 43:314–317.

Binder, H., and Gerstenbrand, F. 1986. Das anoxische Koma. Intensivbehandlung 1:84–90.

Birbamer, G., Aichner, F., Felber, S., et al. 1991. MRI of cerebral hypoxia. Neuroradiology 33(suppl):53–55.

Bokonjic, N., and Buchthal, F. 1961. Post anoxic unconsciousness as related to clinical and EEG recovery in stagnant anoxia and carbon monoxide poisoning. In *Cerebral Anoxia and Electroencephalogram*, Eds. J.S. Meyer and H. Gastaut, pp. 118–127. Springfield, IL: Charles C Thomas.

Bortone, E., Bettoni, G., Giorgi, C., et al. 1992. Adult postanoxic "erratic" status epilepticus. Epilepsia 33:1047–1050.

Böttiger, B.W., Möbes, S., Glätzer, R., et al. 2001. Astroglial protein S-100 is an early and sensitive marker of hypoxic brain damage and outcome after cardiac arrest in humans. Circulation 103:2694–2698.

Brain Resuscitation Trial I Study Group. 1986. Randomized clinical study of cardiopulmonary-cerebral resuscitation: thiopental loading in comatose survivors of cardiac arrest. N Eng J Med 314:397–403.

Brain Resuscitation Clinical Trial II Study Group. 1991. A randomized clinical trial of a calcium entry-blocker (lidoflazine) in the treatment of comatose survivors of cardiac arrest. N. Engl. J. Med. 324:1225–1231.

Brenner, R.P. 1997. Electroencephalography in syncope. J. Clin. Neurophysiol. 14:197–209.

Brierley, J. 1976. Cerebral hypoxia. In Greenfield's Neuropathology, Eds. W. Blackwood and J. Corsellis, pp. 43–85. London: Edward Arnold.

Brierley, J.B., Graham, D.H., Adams, J.H., et al. 1973. The threshold and neuropathology of cerebral "anoxic-ischemic" cell change. Arch. Neurol. 29:367–374.

Brucher, J.M. 1985. Leucoencephalopathie in anoxic-ischemic process. In Handbook of Clinical Neurology, Eds. P.J. Vinken, G.W. Bruyn, and H. Klawans, Vol. 47(3), Demyelinating Diseases, pp. 525–549. Amsterdam: Elsevier Science Publishers.

Bunch, T.J., White, R.D., Gersh, B.J., et al. 2003. Long-term outcomes of out-of-hospital cardiac arrest after successful early defibrillation. N. Engl. J. Med. 348:2626–2633.

Calham, C.L., and Ettinger, M.G. 1966. Unusual EEG in coma after cardiac arrest. Electroencephalogr. Clin. Neurophysiol. 21:385–388.

Calle, P.A., Buylaert, W.A., and Vanhaute, O.A., and the Cerebral Resuscitation Study Group. 1989. Glycemia in the post-resuscitation period. Resuscitation 17(suppl):181–188.

Chalela, J.A., Wolf, R.L., Maldjian, J.A., et al. 2001. MRI identification of early white matter injury in anoxic-ischemic encephalopathy. Neurology 56:481–485.

Chen, R., Bolton, C.F., and Young, B. 1996. Prediction of outcome in patients with anoxic coma: a clinical and electrophysiological study. Crit. Care Med. 24:672–678.

Christophe, C., Fonteyne, C., Ziereisen, F., et al. 2002. Value of MR imaging of the brain in children with hypoxic coma. AJNR 23:716–723.

Clarke, D.D., and Sokoloff, L. 1994. Circulation and energy metabolism of the brain. In Basic Neurochemistry: Molecular, Cellular, and Medical Aspects, 5th ed., Eds. G.J. Siegel, et al., pp. 645–680. New York: Raven Press.

Cohan, S.L., Mun, S.K., Petite, J., et al. 1989. Cerebral blood flow in humans following resuscitation from cardiac arrest. Stroke 20:761–765.

Cohen, M.M., Duncan, P.G., and Pope, W.D.P. 1986. A survey of 112,000 anesthetics at one teaching hospital (1975–83). Can. Anaesth. Soc. J. 33:22–33.

Cummins, R.O., Ornato, J.P., Thies, W.H., et al. 1991. Improving survival from sudden cardiac arrest: the "chain of survival" concept. Circulation 83:1832–1847.

Dell, P., Hugelin, A., and Bonvallet, M. 1961. Effects of hypoxia on the reticular and cortical diffuse systems. In Cerebral Anoxia and the Electroencephalogram, Eds. H. Gastaut and J.S. Meyer, pp. 46–58. Springfield, IL: Charles C Thomas.

De Volder, A.G., Goffinet, A.M., Bol, A., et al. 1990. Brain glucose metabolism in postanoxic syndrome. Arch. Neurol. 48:625–629.

Dubowitz, D.J., Bluml, St., Arcinue, E., et al. 1998. MR of hypoxic encephalopathy in children after near drowning: correlation with quantitative proton MR spectroscopy and clinical outcome. AJNR 19:1617–1627.

Earnest, M.P., Breckinridge, J.C., Yarnell, P.R., et al. 1979. Quality of survival after out-of-hospital cardiac arrest; predictive value of early neurologic evaluation. Neurology 29:56–60.

Edgren, E., Terent, A., Hedstrand, U., et al. 1983. Cerebrospinal fluid markers in relation to outcome in patients with global cerebral ischemia. Crit. Care Med. 11:4–6.

Edgren, E., Hedstrand, U., Nordin, M., et al. 1987. Prediction of outcome after cardiac arrest. Crit. Care Med. 15:820–825.

Edgren, E., Hedstrand, U., Kelsey, S., et al., and BRCT 1 Study Group. 1994. Assessment of neurological prognosis in comatose survivors of cardiac arrest. Lancet 343:1055–1059.

Emery, E. 1990. Status epilepticus secondary to breath-holding and pallid syncopal spells. Neurology 40:859.

Felber, S., Aichner, F., Sauter, R., et al. 1992. Combined MR-imaging and MR-spectroscopy of patients with acute stroke. Stroke 23:1106–1110.

Fischer-Williams, M., and Cooper, R.A. 1964. Some aspects of electroencephalographic changes during open heart surgery. Neurology (Minneapolis) 14:472.

Fujioka, M., Taoka, T., Matsuo, Y., et al. 2003. Magnetic resonance imaging shows delayed ischemic striatal neurodegeneration. Ann. Neurol. 54:732–747.

Ganes, T., and Lundar, T. 1988. EEG and evoked potentials in comatose patients with severe brain damage. EEG Clin. Neurophysiol. 69:6–13.

Gastaut, H., and Fischer-Williams, M. 1957. Electro-encephalographic study of syncope. Its differentiation from epilepsy. Lancet 2:1018–1025.

Gatzonis, S.D., Zournas, Ch., Michalopoulos, A., et al. 2001. Area-selective stimulus-provoked seizures in post-anoxic coma. Seizure 10:294–297.

Geocadin, R.G., Ghodara, R., Kimura, T., et al. 2000. A novel quantitative EEG injury measure of global ischemia. Clin. Neurophysiol. 111:1779–1787.

Go, K.G. 1991. Cerebral pathophysiology. Amsterdam: Elsevier.

Gorelick, P.B., and Kelly, M.A. 1993. Neurological complications of cardiac arrest. In Handbook of Clinical Neurology, Eds. C. G. Goetz et al., vol. 19(63), Systemic Diseases, part 1, pp. 205–230. Amsterdam, New York: Oxford North Holland Publishing Company.

Graham, G.D., Kalvach, P., Blamire, A.M., et al. 1995. Clinical correlates of proton magnetic resonance spectroscopy findings after acute cerebral infarction. Stroke 26:225–229.

Grubb, N.R., Elton, R.A., and Fox, K.A.A. 1995. In-hospital mortality after out-of-hospital cardiac arrest. Lancet 346:417–421.

Hachimi-Idrissi, S., Van der Auwera, M., Schiettecatte, J., et al. 2002. S-100 protein as early predictor of regaining consciousness after out of hospital cardiac arrest. Resuscitation 53:251–257.

Hallenbeck, J.M., and Dutka, A.J. 1990. Background review and current concepts of reperfusion injury. Arch. Neurol. 47:1245–1254.

Hawker, K., and Lang, A.E. 1990. Hypoxic-ischemic damage of the basal ganglia. Case reports and a review of the literature. Mov. Disord. 5:219–224.

Heiss, W.D., and Rosner, G. 1983. Functional recovery of cortical necrosis as related to degree and duration of ischemia. Ann. Neurol. 14:294–301.

Hockaday, J.M., Potts, F., Epstein, E., et al. 1965. EEG changes in acute cerebral anoxia from cardiac or respiratory arrest. Electroencephalogr. Clin. Neurophysiol. 18:575–586.

Hori, A., Hirose, G., Kataoka, S., et al. 1991. Delayed postanoxic encephalopathy after strangulation. Arch. Neurol. 48:871–874.

Hossmann, K.A., and Kleihus, P. 1973. Reversibility of ischemic brain damage. Arch. Neurol. 29:375–384.

Hulihan, J.F., and Syna, D.R. 1994. Electroencephalographic sleep patterns in postanoxic stupor and coma. Neurology 44:758–760.

Janavs, J.L., and Aminoff, M.J. 1998. Dystonia and chorea in acquired systemic disorders. J. Neurol. Neurochir. Psychiatry 65:436–445.

Jordan, J.E., Parrish, D., Cliett, J.B., et al. 1982. Suppression burst associated with eye opening. Arch. Neurol. 3:602.

Jumao-as, A., and Brenner, R.P. 1990. Myoclonic status epilepticus: a clinical and electroencephalographic study. Neurology 40:1199–1202.

Kaplan, P.W., Genoud, D., Ho, T.W., et al. 1999. Etiology, neurologic correlations, and prognosis in alpha coma. Clin. Neurophysiol. 110:205–213.

Karkela, J., Bock, K., Kaukinen, S., et al. 1992. Evaluation of hypoxic brain injury with spinal fluid enzymes, lactate, and pyruvate. Crit. Care Med. 20:378–386.

Kjos, B.O., Brant-Zawadzki, M., and Young, R.G. 1983. Early CT findings of global central nervous system hypoperfusion. AJNR 4:1043–1048.

Kotchoubey, B., Lang, S., Baales, R., et al. 2001. Brain potentials in human patients with extremely severe diffuse brain damage. Neurosci. Lett. 301:37–40.

Krumholz, A., Stern, B., and Heiss, H.D. 1988. Outcome from coma after cardiopulmonary resuscitation: relation to seizure and myoclonus. Neurology 38:401–405.

Lance, J.W., and Adams, R.D. 1963. The syndrome of intention or action myoclonus as a sequel to hypoxic encephalopathy. Brain 86:111–133.

Lavy, S., and Stern, S. 1967. Electroencephalographic changes following sudden cessation of artificial pacing in patients with heart block. Confin. Neurol. (Basel) 29:47.

Lempert, T., Bauer, M., and Schmidt, D. 1994. Syncope: a videometric analysis of 56 episodes of transient cerebral hypoxia. Ann. Neurol. 36:233–237.

Levy, D.E., Bates, D., Caronna, J.J., et al. 1981. Prognosis in nontraumatic coma. Ann. Intern. Med. 94:293–301.

Levy, D.E., Caronna, J.J., Singer, B.H., et al. 1985. Predicting outcome from hypoxic-ischemic coma. JAMA 253:1420–1426.

Li, J.Y., Lai, P.H., Chen, C.Y., et al. 2000. Postanoxic parkinsonism: clinical, radiologic, and pathologic correlation. Neurology 55:591–593.

Lindenberg, R. 1963. Patterns of CNS vulnerability in acute hypoxemia, including anesthesia accidents. In *Selective Vulnerability of the Brain in Hypoxaemia*, Eds. J.P. Schade and W.H. McMenemey, pp. 189–205. Philadelphia: Davis.

Lipton, P. 1999. Ischemic cell death in brain neurons. Physiol. Rev. 79:1431–1568.

Longstreth, W.T., Jr., and Inui, T.S. 1984. High blood glucose level on hospital admission and poor neurological recovery after cardiac arrest. Ann. Neurol. 15:59–63.

Longstreth, W.T., Jr., Diehr, P., and Inui, T.S. 1983. Prediction of awakening after out-of-hospital cardiac arrest. N. Engl. J. Med. 308:1378–1382.

Longstreth, W.T. Jr., Diehr, P., Cobb, L.A., et al. 1986. Neurologic outcome and blood glucose levels during out-of-hospital cardiopulmonary resuscitation. Neurology 36:1186–1191.

Maiese, K., and Caronna, J.J. 1988. Coma after cardiac arrest: clinical features, prognosis and management. In *Neurological and Neurosurgical Care*, Eds. A.H. Ropper and S.F. Kennedy, pp. 233–245. Rockville, MD: Aspen.

Martin, G.B., Paradis, N.A., Helpern, J.A., et al. 1991. Nuclear magnetic resonance spectroscopy study of human brain after cardiac resuscitation. Stroke 10:1–29.

Martin, R.L., Lloyd, H.G.E., and Cowan, A.L. 1994. The early events of oxygen and glucose deprivation: setting the scene for neuronal death. Trends Neurosci. 17:251–257.

Mattle, H.P., Nirkko, A.C., Baumgartner, R.W., et al. 1995. Transient cerebral circulatory arrest coincides with fainting in cough syncope. Neurology 45:498–501.

McCarty, G.E., and Marshall, D.W. 1981. Transient eyelid opening associated with postanoxic EEG suppression-burst pattern. Arch. Neurol. 38:754–756.

McKeown, M.J., and Young, G.B. 1997. Comparison between the alpha pattern in normal subjects and in alpha pattern coma. J. Clin. Neurophysiol. 14:414–418.

Meyer, J.S., and Marx, P.W. 1972. The pathogenesis of EEG changes during cerebral anoxia. In *Cardiac and Vascular Diseases/Handbook of Electroencephalography and Clinical Neurophysiology*, Eds. J.H.A. Van der Drift, vol. 14A, part A, pp. 5–11. Amsterdam: Elsevier.

Meyer, J.S., Sakamato, K., Akijama, M., et al. 1967. Monitoring cerebral blood flow, metabolism and EEG. Electroencephalogr. Clin. Neurophysiol. 23:497–508.

Meynaar, I.A., Straaten, H.M., van der Wetering, J., et al. 2003. Serum neuron-specific enolase predicts outcome in post-anoxic coma: a prospective cohort study. Intensive Care Med. 29:189–195.

Miyamoto, O., and Auer, R.N. 2000. Hypoxia, hyperoxia, ischemia, and brain necrosis. Neurology 54:362–371.

Mori, E., Yamadori, A., Tsuruta, H., et al. 1983. Transient eye opening with EEG suppression-burst pattern in postanoxic encephalopathy. Arch. Neurol. 40:189.

Morillo, L.E., Tullock, J.W., Gummit, R.J., et al. 1983. Compressed spectral array patterns following cardiopulmonary arrest. Arch. Neurol. 40:287–289.

Morimoto, Y., Kemmotsu, O., Kitami, K., et al. 1993. Acute brain swelling after out-of-hospital cardiac arrest: pathogenesis and outcome. Crit. Care Med. 21:104–110.

Morris, H.R., Howard, R.S., and Brown, P. 1998. Early myoclonic status and outcome after cardiorespiratory arrest. J. Neurol. Neurosurg. Psychiatry 64:267–268.

Mullie, A., Lewi, P., Van Hoeyweghen, R., and the Cerebral Resuscitation Study Group 1989. Pre-CPR conditions and the final outcome of CPR. Resuscitation 17 (suppl):11–21.

Murphy, D.J., and Murray, A.M. 1989. Outcome of cardiopulmonary resuscitation in the elderly. Ann. Intern. Med. 111:199–203.

Myerburg, R.J., and Castellanos, A. 1991. Cardiovascular collapse, cardiac arrest and sudden death. In *Harrison's Principles of Internal Medicine*, 12th ed., vol. 1, Eds. Wilson et al., pp. 237–242. New York: McGraw-Hill.

Naquet, R., and Fernandez-Guardiola, A. 1959. Effects of various types of anoxia on spontaneous and evoked cerebral activity in the cat. In *Cerebral Anoxia and the Electroencephalogram*, Eds., H. Gastaut and J.S. Meyer, pp. 72–88. Springfield, IL: Charles C Thomas.

National Health and Medical Research Council. 1985–87. Report on anesthetic related mortality in Australia.

Nichter, M.A., and Everett, P.B. 1989. Childhood near drowning: is cardiopulmonary resuscitation always indicated? Crit. Care Med. 17:993–998.

Niedermeyer, E., Bauer, G., Burnite, R., et al. 1977. Selective stimulus-sensitive myoclonus in acute cerebral anoxia—a case report. Arch. Neurol. 34:365–368.

Niedermeyer, E., Sherman, D.L., Geocadin, R.J., et al. 1999. The burst suppression electroencephalogram. Clin. Electroencephalogr. 30:99–105.

Noell, W.G., and Dombrowski, E.B. 1947. Cerebral localization and classification of convulsions produced by a severe oxygen lack. Project 497, Report 1. Randolph Field, TX: School of Aviation Medicine.

Pampiglione, G. 1964. Seizures after resuscitation. Elelectroencephalogr. Clin. Neurophysiol. 17:474.

Pappert, E.J., Goetz, C.G., Vu, T.Q., et al. 1999. Animal model of post-hypoxic myoclonus. Effects of serotonergic antagonists. Neurology 52:16–21.

Petito, C.H., Feldmann, E., Pulsinelli, W.A., et al. 1987. Delayed hippocampal damage in humans following cardiorespiratory arrest. Neurology 37:1281–1286.

Pitney, M.R., Beran, R.G., and Jones, A. 1994. A simultaneous electrocardiogram is important when electroencephalography is used in the evaluation of loss of consciousness. Electroencephalogr. Clin. Neurophysiol. 90:246–248.

Plum, F., and Posner, J.B. 1982. Prognosis in coma. In *The Diagnosis of Stupor and Coma*, Eds. F. Plum and J.B. Posner, pp. 329–348. Philadelphia: F.A. Davis.

Pressler, R.M., Boylan, G.B., Morton, M., et al. 2001. Early serial EEG in hypoxic ischaemic encephalopathy. Clin. Neurophysiol. 112:31–37.

Prior, P.F. 1973. *The EEG in Acute Cerebral Anoxia*. Amsterdam: Excerpta Medica.

Pulsinelli, W.A., and Cooper, A.J.L. 1994. Metabolic encephalopathies and coma. In *Basic Neurochemistry: Molecular, Cellular and Medical Aspects*, 5th ed., Eds. G.J. Siegel et al., pp. 841–857. New York: Raven Press.

Pulsinelli, W.A., Brierly, J.B., and Plum, F. 1982. Temporal profile on neurological damage in a model of transient forebrain ischemia. Ann. Neurol. 11:491–498.

Reeves, E.L., Nollet, K.E., Klass, D.W., et al. 1996. The ictal bradycardia syndrome. Epilepsia 37:983–987.

Reeves, E.L., Westmoreland, B.F., and Klass, D.W. 1997. Clinical accompaniments of the burst-suppression EEG pattern. J. Clin. Neurophysiol. 14:150–153.

Rohmer, F., Gastaut, Y., and Dell, M.B. 1952. L'EEG dans la pathologie vasculaire du cerveau. Rev. Neurol. 87:93–124.

Roine, R.O., Launes, J., Nikkinen, P., et al. 1991. Regional cerebral blood flow after human cardiac arrest. Arch. Neurol. 48:625–629.

Roine, R.O., Raininko, R., Erkinjuntti, T., et al. 1993. Magnetic resonance imaging findings associated with cardiac arrest. Stroke 24:1005–1014.

Ropper, A.H. 1981. Ocular dipping in anoxic coma. Arch. Neurol. 38:297–299.

Rothstein, T.L., Thomas, E.M., and Sumi, S.M. 1991. Predicting outcome in hypoxic-ischemic coma. A prospective clinical and electrophysiologic study. Electroencephalogr. Clin. Neurophysiol. 79:101–107.

Rudolf, J. 2000. Positron emission tomography in diagnosis and prognosis of postanoxic cerebral dysfunctions. Fortschr. Neurol. Psychiatr. 68:344–351.

Sandroni, C., Barelli, A., Piazza, O., et al. 1995. What is the best test to predict outcome after prolonged cardiac arrest? Eur. J. Emerg. Med. 2:33–37.

Sawada, H., Udaka, F., Seriu, N., et al. 1990. MRI demonstration of cortical laminar necrosis and delayed white matter injury in anoxic encephalopathy. Neuroradiology 32:319–321.

Scollo-Lavizzari, G., and Bassetti, C. 1987. Prognostic value of EEG in post-anoxic coma after cardiac arrest. Eur. Neurol. 26:161–170.

Scott, B.L., and Jankovic, J. 1996. Delayed-onset progressive movement disorders after static brain lesions. Neurology 46:68–74.

Schaafsma, A., de Jong, B.M., Bams, J.L., et al. 2003. Cerebral perfusion and metabolism in resuscitated patients with severe post-hypoxic encephalopathy. J. Neurol. Sci. 210:23.30.

Shwmon, D.A., and De Giorgio, C.M. 1989. Early prognosis in anoxic coma. Reliability and rationale. Neurol. Clin. 7:823–843.

Siesjö, B.K., Zhao, Q., Pahlmark, K., et al. 1995. Glutamate, calcium, and free radicals as mediators of ischemic brain damage. Ann. Thorac. Surg. 59:1316–1320.

Silverman, D. 1975. The electroencephalogram in anoxic coma. In *Altered States of Consciousness. Coma, Cerebral Death/Handbook of Electroencephalography and Clinical Neurophysiology,* Eds. R. Harner, and R. Naquet, vol. 12, pp. 81–94. Amsterdam: Elsevier.

Sinclair, D.B., Campbell, M., Byrne, P., et al. 1999. EEG and long-term outcome of term infants with neonatal hypoxic-ischemic encephalopathy. Clin. Neurophysiol. 110:655–659.

Singhal, A.B., Topcuoglu, M.A., and Koroshetz, W.J. 2002. Diffusion MRI in three types of anoxic encephalopathy. J. Neurol. Sci. 196:37–40.

Snyder, B.D., Loewenson, R.B., Gumnit, R.J., et al. 1980a. Neurologic prognosis after cardiac arrest: II. Level of consciousness. Neurology 30: 52–58.

Snyder, B.D., Loewenson, R.B., Gumnit, R.J., et al. 1980b. Neurological prognosis after cardiac arrest: III. Seizure activity. Neurology 30:1292–1297.

Sokoloff, L. 1960. The metabolism of the CNS in vivo. In *Handbook of Physiology–Neurophysiology,* vol. 3, Eds. J. Field, H.W. Magoun, and V.E. Hall, pp. 1843–1864. Washington, DC: American Physiological Society.

Sokoloff, L. 1969. Cerebral circulation and behavior in man strategy and findings. In *Psychochemical Research in Man,* Eds. A.J. Mandell and M.P. Mandell, pp. 237–252. New York: Academic.

Speckmann, E.J. 1970. Changes in neuronal activity in hypoxia and asphyxia. Electroencephalogr. Clin. Neurophysiol. 29:206(abst).

Steinlein, O., Anokhin, A., Yping, M., et al. 1992. Localization of a gene for the human low voltage EEG on 20q and genetic heterogeneity. Genomics 12:69–73.

Sugar, O., and Gerard, R.W. 1938. Anoxia and brain potentials. J. Neurophysiol. 1:558–572.

Suter, C. 1977. Brain death. MCV Q. 13(3):83–87.

Synek, V.M. 1988. EEG abnormality grades and subdivisions of prognostic importance in traumatic and anoxic coma in adults. Clin. Electroencephalogr. 19:160–166.

Synek, V.M. 1990. Value of a revised EEG coma scale for prognosis after cerebral anoxia and diffuse head injury. Clin. Electroencephalogr. 21:25–30.

Synek, V.M., and Synek, B.J.L. 1984. Theta pattern coma, a variant of alpha pattern coma. Clin. Electroencephalogr. 15:116–121.

Takahashi, S., Higano, S., Ishii, K., et al. 1993. Hypoxic brain damage: cortical laminar necrosis and delayed changes in white matter at sequential MR imaging. Radiology 189:449–456.

Thomassen, A., and Wernberg, M. 1979. Prevalence and prognostic significance of coma after cardiac arrest outside intensive care and coronary units. Acta Anaesth. Scand. 23:143–148.

Thömke, F., Brand, A., and Weilemann, S.L. 2002. The temporal dynamics of postanoxic burst-suppression EEG. J. Clin. Neurophysiol. 19:24–31.

Tiret, L., Desmonts, J.M., and Hatton, F. 1986. Complications associated with anesthesia. A prospective survey in France. Can. Anesth. Soc. J. 33: 336–341.

Tuchschmidt, J.A., and Mecher, C.E. 1994. Predictors of outcome from critical illness: shock and cardiopulmonary resuscitation. Crit. Care Clin. 10:179–195.

Van Cott, A.C., Blatt, I., and Brenner, R.P. 1996. Stimulus-sensitive seizures in postanoxic coma. Epilepsia 37:868–874.

Van der Drift, J.H.A. 1972. The EEG in cerebrovascular disease. In *Handbook of Clinical Neurology,* Eds. P.J. Vinken and G.W. Bruyn, vol. 11, pp. 267–291. Amsterdam-New York: North Holland.

Vazquez, J.O. 1979. Neurological manifestations of chronic respiratory diseases. In *Handbook of Clinical Neurology,* Eds. P.J. Vinken and G.W. Bruyn, vol. 38, pp. 285–307. Amsterdam: North Holland.

Visser, G.H., Wienecke, G.H., Van Huffelen, A.C., et al. 2001. The development of spectral EEG changes during short periods of circulatory arrest. J. Clin. Neurophysiol. 18:169–177.

Volpe, B.T., and Hirst, W. 1983. The characterization of an amnesic syndrome following hypoxic ischemic injury. Arch. Neurol. 40:436–440.

Walser, H., Mattle, H., Keller, H.M., et al. 1985. Early cortical median nerve somatosensory evoked potentials. Prognostic value in anoxic coma. Arch. Neurol. 42:32–38.

Warach, S., Gaa, J., and Siewert, B. 1995. Acute human stroke studied by whole brain echo planar diffusion weighted magnetic resonance imaging. Ann. Neurol. 37:231–241.

Ward, A.A., and Wheatley, F.R. 1947. Sodium cyanide. Sequence of changes of activity induced at various levels of the central nervous system. J. Neuropathol. Exp. Neurol. 6:292–294.

Werhan, K.J., Brown, P., Thompson, P.D., et al. 1997. The clinical features and prognosis of chronic posthypoxic myoclonus. Mov. Disord. 12:216–220.

Westmoreland, B.F., Klass, D.W., Sharbrough, F.M., et al. 1975. Alphacoma. Electroencephalographic, pathologic and etiologic correlations. Arch. Neurol. 32:713–718.

Wijdicks, E.F.M., Parisi, J.E., and Sharbrough, F.W. 1994. Prognostic value of myoclonic status in comatose survivors of cardiac arrest. Ann. Neurol. 35:239–243.

Wijdicks, E.F.M., Campeau, N.G., and Miller, G.M. 2001. MR imaging in comatose survivors of cardiac resuscitation. AJNR. 22:1561–1565.

Willoughby, J.O., and Leach, B.G. 1974. Relation of neurological findings after cardiac arrest to outcome. Br. Med. J. 3:437–439.

Wilson, W.P., and Sieker, H.O. 1958. A study of the factors responsible for changes in the electroencephalogram in chronic pulmonary insufficiency. Electroencephalogr. Clin. Neurophysiol. 10:89–96.

Young, G.B., Gilbert, J.J., and Zochodne, D.W. 1990. The significance of myoclonic status epilepticus in postanoxic coma. Neurology 40:1843–1848.

Young, G.B., Blume, W.T., Campbell, V.M., et al. 1994. Alpha, theta and alpha-theta coma: a clinical outcome study utilizing serial records. EEG Clin. Neurophysiol. 91:93–99.

Younkin, D.P. 1993. Magnetic resonance spectroscopy in hypoxic-ischemic encephalopathy. Clin. Invest. Med. 16:115–121.

Zandbergen, E.G.J., de Haan R.J., Stoutenbeek, C.P., et al. 1998. Systematic review of early prediction of poor outcome in anoxic-ischaemic coma. Lancet 352:1808–1812.

Zülch, K.J., and Behrend, R.C.H. 1961. The pathogenesis and topography of anoxia, hypoxia and ischemia of the brain in man. In *Cerebral Anoxia and the Electroencephalogram,* Eds. H. Gastaut and J.S. Meyer, pp. 144–163. Springfield, IL: Charles C Thomas.

24. Coma and Brain Death

Gerhard Bauer

Definition of Coma

The definition of coma rests on the definition of consciousness. Because consciousness evades any direct observation, there cannot be a scientific definition, although published books and papers on consciousness and its neuronal correlates have increased in number in the past decade (Baars, 1998; Block, 1996; Niedermeyer, 1999; Zeman, 2001). For medical purposes, a descriptive approach defines coma as unarousable unresponsiveness (Plum and Posner, 1966). Responses to stimuli are basic to the examination of comatose states. In cases of widespread paralysis, the behavioral pattern does not correlate with the presence or absence of consciousness. Therefore, coma detached from neurological signs remains an abstraction (Fischer, 1969). A medically meaningful description encompasses the whole range of neurological symptoms and electroencephalogram (EEG) signs.

From the clinical viewpoint, two main categories of consciousness are identifiable: the contents of consciousness and the global quality of vigilance (Cairns, 1952). The word *coma*, as it is used in this chapter, is limited to alterations of vigilance. This operational description allows a clear separation from profound disturbances of higher cortical functions, i.e., organic brain syndromes, dementia, and chronic vegetative states.

Pathophysiology of Coma

Neuronal structures necessary for the maintenance of normal consciousness are the cerebral cortex, the ascending reticular activating system, and the connecting fibers of both structures. The functional or lesional disturbance of the ascending reticular activating system plays a definite role in the alteration of global consciousness. Summarizing experimental works in animals (Batini et al., 1959; French and Magoun, 1952; Lindsley et al., 1949, 1950), Amytal injection experiments in humans (Alema et al., 1966), and clinicopathological observations (Chase et al., 1968; Halsey and Downie, 1966; Orthner, 1969; Rossi, 1964, 1965; Specht, 1964), it becomes clear that the part of the activating system sensitive for the maintenance of alertness lies in the pontomesencephalic tegmentum. Disturbances leading to coma must occupy both sides of the midline, be located at the pontomesencephalic junction, and be either acutely acquired or fairly large in extent (Plum, 1972). Recent neuroanatomical correlates suggest that structures in the upper pontine tegmentum may have a more important role (Parvizi and Damasio, 2003).

Coma with Supratentorial Lesions

Several different processes may involve the tegmental pontomesencephalic junction either directly or indirectly. Supratentorial lesions are unlikely to produce coma directly, provided the definition of coma excludes states of profoundly depressed cortical function. Furthermore, elevated intracranial pressure per se is not apt to cause coma. The crucial mechanism represents cerebral herniation, consequent compression of or traction upon the brainstem, and secondary vascular brainstem lesions. Uncal and central herniations have been differentiated (McNealy and Plum, 1962). Both mechanisms disrupt the mesodiencephalic arousal system that lies close to the level of the tentorial notch. This concept has been questioned on the basis of computed tomography (CT) (Ropper, 1986) and magnetic resonance imaging (MRI) (Ropper, 1993), which stress the importance of horizontal displacement. Descending transtentorial herniation could be visualized during life by MRI and can precede the appearance of neurological signs and symptoms (Feldmann et al., 1988; Reich et al., 1993; Wijdicks and Miller, 1997). Downward displacement of the midbrain can be suggested by midbrain kinking due to rotation of the cerebral hemisphere and rotation of the brainstem in the coronal plane. These parameters reflect upper brainstem dysfunction most closely (Inao et al., 1993). Leaving these anatomical details aside, secondary alterations on the brainstem play a crucial role in coma with supratentorial lesions.

Coma with Infratentorial Lesions

Infratentorial lesions cause coma in different ways. The lesions may destroy the paramedian pontomesencephalic reticular formation directly. Those conditions occur with vascular lesions (Facon et al., 1958; Ingvar et al., 1964; Jouvet, 1969; Nyberg-Hansen et al., 1978), especially with pontine hemorrhages (Dinsdale, 1964). The occurrence of direct and primary traumatic brainstem lesions has not been generally accepted. The existence of such lesions has been questioned (Adams et al., 1977; Mitchell and Adams, 1973), but, according to other investigators (Gerstenbrand and Lücking, 1970; Tsubokowa et al., 1980), there is reason to presume that such lesions occur in rare cases. With the introduction of MRI in the examination of brain-injured patients, evidence of primary brainstem lesions has become more convincing (Gentry et al., 1989) (Fig. 24.1), although lesions in the cerebral hemispheres with consecutive transtentorial herniations seem to be leading (Jenkins et al., 1986). In a prognostic view, diffuse axonal injuries, i.e.,

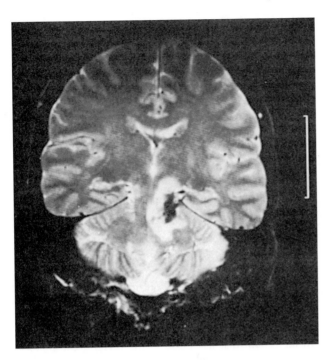

Figure 24.1. R.J., a 30-year-old man in a deep coma after a car accident. No coma grading possible because of immediate sedation for intubation. Magnetic resonance imaging (MRI) at the midbrain level (Cor. T2; TR = 2,400 msec; TE = 90 msec). Vast contusional region in the left upper brainstem representing an example of a primary traumatic brainstem lesion.

cephalic level. At some time during the disintegration, the neurological symptoms may resemble those observed with transtentorial herniations (Bauer and Niedermeyer, 1979), whereas an orderly progression in the rostral-caudal direction is never observed (Plum and Posner, 1966).

Differentiation of Coma from Other Conditions of Altered Responsiveness

Sleep

Several conditions of altered responsiveness must be distinguished from coma. Sleep denotes physiological loss of consciousness. Its differentiation from coma is based on arousability. Although coma resembles sleep in a popular sense, it is due not to disinhibition or stimulation of the sleep-inducing systems but to an organic or functional disturbance of the waking system (Jouvet, 1969). Nevertheless, in light coma, parts of the arousal system are still functioning and may be subject to modulations caused by the systems that serve sleep. From a clinico-encephalographic point of view, differentiation of initial stages of coma from physiological but exaggerated sleep due to prolonged sleep deprivation or states after intoxication with alcohol or central nervous system (CNS)-depressant drugs may be difficult. Because exact criteria have not been established, the clinician as well as the electroencephalographer depend on impressions based on personal experience.

shearing injuries of the cerebral white matter are of particular importance (Adams et al., 1991). Infratentorial processes located outside the brainstem lead to coma by pressure on the reticular formation either directly or by upward herniation through the tentorial notch. Downward herniation through the foramen magnum has no compressing effect on the tegmentum but leads to secondary anoxic changes.

Coma with Diffuse Brain Disturbances

Prolonged or chronic diffuse encephalopathies are associated with depressions of cortical activities but have preserved cycles of sleep and wakefulness. In acute and severe cases, coma is common and indicates a dysfunction of the arousal system. Two pathophysiological possibilities exist. First, the encephalopathy may lead to a diffuse brain edema with consecutive herniation (Lindenberg, 1963). The brain edema can also be demonstrated by CT of the brain (New and Scott, 1975; Ruggiero et al., 1977; Torack et al., 1976). Second, phylogenetically most recently developed structures of the brain are more susceptible to anoxic, metabolic, and toxic damages (Gastaut and Fischer-Williams, 1959; Himwich, 1951; Hoagland et al., 1939; Meyer et al., 1967; Naquet and Fernandez-Guardiola, 1959; Noell and Dombrowski, 1947; Richardson et al., 1959; Sugar and Gerard, 1938; Ward and Wheatley, 1947). This selective vulnerability can be demonstrated by MRI (Birbamer et al., 1991) (Fig. 24.2) and represents the basis for comatose conditions with disintegrated cerebral functions down to the mesen-

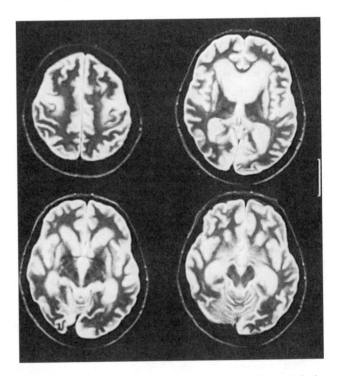

Figure 24.2. S.-T.C., a 26-year-old woman in a coma after resuscitation from cardiac arrest slipping into a chronic vegetative state. MRI of the brain (Ax. T2; TR = 2,400 msec; TE = 90 msec; 1.ST.; CP. Head; FUV = 27 cm). Cortical and subcortical atrophy, changes in the signal intensity in the basal ganglia and hippocampic gyri. Example of disturbed cerebral structures according to the selective vulnerability against hypoxia.

Locked-In Syndrome

A clearly defined and easily recognized condition is the locked-in syndrome (Plum and Posner, 1966). There is no alteration of consciousness. The patient is completely paralyzed except for vertical eye movements and is able to communicate complex ideas by blinking Morse code (Feldman, 1971). Synonyms are "pseudo-coma" and "de-efferented state." Lesions are located in the ventral part of the pons or, in rare cases, in the midbrain (Bauer et al., 1979; Chia, 1991; Dehaene and Dom, 1982; Hochmann et al., 1985; Karp and Hurtig, 1974; Meienberg et al., 1979; Uematsu et al., 1985) and bilateral internal capsules (Chia, 1984). Completely de-efferented states with acute inflammatory polyradiculitis have also been termed locked-in syndrome (Loeb et al., 1984) and may be differentiated from pontine transsection syndromes by accompanying neurological symptoms.

Akinetic Mutism

Akinetic mutism (Cairns et al., 1941) is somewhat less strictly defined. The patient is mute or speaks in fragments, and does not move spontaneously but moves secondary to exogenous stimuli. Communication is severely reduced but not abolished. The lesions spare the cortex but affect the thalamus, the basal ganglia, the posterior part of the third ventricle, and the gyrus cinguli bilaterally (Cairns, 1952; Jouvet, 1969). Transient mutism was also observed with posterior fossa surgery (Gelabert-González and Fernández-Villa, 2001). Immobility is considered to be caused by the failure of extrapyramidal coordination (Jouvet, 1969); in other words, this is an extrapyramidal locked-in syndrome.

Vegetative State

The most frequently encountered chronic condition of altered consciousness is "a syndrome in search of a name" (Jennet and Plum, 1972). The different faces of this syndrome have been called *apallic syndrome* (Gerstenbrand, 1967; Kretschmer, 1940), complete and incomplete apallic syndrome (Ingvar and Brun, 1972), prolonged coma (Vigouroux, 1975), and persistent vegetative state (Jennet and Plum, 1972). Absence of any clinical sign of cortical function combined with alternating periods of sleep and wakefulness are the essentials of this condition. The eyes are opened periodically, but there are no signs of appreciation of the environment. Accompanying prominent pyramidal signs allow a clear separation from akinetic mutism. Pathologically, no common pattern of lesion can be defined. Prognosis, EEG signs, and appropriate management rest on the strict or broadened definition of this condition (Levin et al., 1991; Molinari, 1991; Munsat et al., 1989; Spudis, 1991). Terminological and prognostic controversies have been cleared by the Multi-Society Task Force on Persistent Vegetative State (PVS) (1994a,b). Recently, a minimally conscious state (MCS) has been declared a separate clinical condition (Giacino et al., 2002). Questions remain about the boundaries to coma and vegetative state. Persons who are treating patients in a vegetative state always have to be very alert for some kind of environmental perception (Kassubek et al., 2003).

Coma Vigile

This term was used as a synonym for the apallic syndrome (Schiffter and Schliack, 1975), for distinct varieties of the apallic syndrome (Gerstenbrand, 1967; Kubicki and Haas, 1975), for locked-in syndrome (Ingvar and Brun, 1972), and for akinetic mutism (Jennet and Plum, 1972). The author refrains from further interpretations of this multifaceted term.

EEG Patterns in Coma

The EEG is an essential part of the neurological assessment of a comatose patient. Numerous EEG patterns have been observed that are not significant per se but are extremely helpful for diagnostic or prognostic statements in the context of neurological abnormalities.

Diffuse Slowing

Diffuse continuous slowing, either in the theta or delta range, is characteristic of a variety of comatose states regardless of etiology (Gibbs et al., 1937). Slowing of a reactive basic rhythm is not consistent with coma but suggests a diffuse brain syndrome or demented state. Gradual dissolution of the alpha rhythm and intermittently interspersed theta frequencies occur in the earliest phases of coma and mimic normal drowsiness.

Intermittent Delta Rhythms

Intermittent rhythmic and bilaterally synchronous delta activity is frequently seen in the initial phases of coma. The voltage is maximal over frontal regions in adults and over occipital regions in children (Cobb, 1957). This pattern has also been termed frontal intermittent rhythmic delta activity (FIRDA) (Daly, 1979) or occipital intermittent rhythmic delta activity (OIRDA). Intermittent delta rhythms occur with subcortical (Gloor, 1976), deep frontal (Arfel and Fischgold, 1961; Hess, 1961), and other supratentorial lesions (Hess, 1962). Furthermore, they can be observed in metabolic and hypoxic encephalopathies (Harner and Katz, 1975). The combination of a focal abnormality with intermittent delta rhythms is extremely suggestive of a supratentorial mass lesion with incipient herniation (Hess, 1962). With frontal lesions, the delta rhythms may be seen only over the opposite hemisphere. Polymorphous low-voltage slow activity indicates the affected frontal lobe. Paroxysmal delta rhythms in an otherwise normal EEG hint of a deep-seated lesion; these rhythms in combination with diffuse slowing suggest, above all, a metabolic encephalopathy. Although FIRDA is an unspecific EEG sign with regard to etiology and affected structures, its appearance is highly suggestive of early phases of coma and represents an initial sign of dysfunction of the arousal system (Schaul et al., 1981). In contrast to frontal and occipital rhythmic delta activities, temporal abnormalities (TIRDA; Reither et al., 1989) represent an important epileptogenic pattern (Normand et al., 1995).

EEG Patterns Usually Seen During Sleep

In some types of coma, EEG patterns were observed that otherwise are considered typical of sleep, i.e., sleep spindles (sigma waves) and K complexes (Chatrian et al., 1963; Hess, 1962; Jasper and Van Buren, 1953; Lücking, 1970; Silverman, 1963) (Fig. 24.1). These patterns have a cyclic appearance, suggesting that the comatose patient may be subject to the influences of the sleep-inducing systems (Bergamasco et al., 1968; Passouant et al., 1964). The gradual abolition of those organized phenomena with deepening coma might be due to increasing cortical dysfunction (Hess, 1965) or to direct involvement of brainstem mechanisms.

Alternating Pattern

In states with Cheyne-Stokes respiration, a cyclic alternation of low-voltage irregular activity and high-voltage slow waves can be recorded (Arfel, 1975a; Fischgold and Mathis, 1959; Romano and Engel, 1944). Phases with predominant high-voltage slow activity correlate with hyperventilation and increased pulse rate. Every stimulus applied during the low-voltage period leads to high-voltage slow activity. Thus, the patients seem to be more aroused during the slow-wave period. The cause of cyclic changes was suspected in a pacemaker function of the arousal system, temporarily released by depression of cortical inhibition influences (Evans, 1976). This pacemaker, however, could also be the respiration center itself, which roughly follows the chemical influences of blood gases.

Prolonged Bursts of Delta Waves and the Reactivity of EEG

Prolonged bursts of bilateral high-voltage delta activity have been described in a wide variety of intracranial conditions, mainly in patients with head injuries (Arfel, 1975a; Fischgold and Mathis, 1959; Kubicki et al., 1970; Li et al., 1952; Lücking, 1970; Schwartz and Scott, 1978). The high-voltage delta activity lasts for several seconds or often for minutes. Delta bursts occur either spontaneously or secondary to exogenous stimuli (Fig. 24.3) and have been considered to be some type of exaggerated K complex (Kubicki and Haas, 1975; Lücking, 1970; Silverman, 1963). The pattern is associated with greater muscle activity and restlessness, as well as attempts to communicate. A busy intensive care unit (ICU) may give continuous acoustic stimulation. The resultant activation pattern, consisting of large delta waves, gives the erroneous impression of deepening coma.

Systematic testing of reactions to stimuli is an essential part of an EEG examination in a comatose subject. Slow-wave responses to arousal are only one type, the alerting type. Another response consists of voltage reduction and filtering of remnants of the basic rhythm, the blocking type (Li et al., 1952). In deep coma, no response, even to repetitive stimulation, can be observed. There are further types of EEG changes secondary to exogenous stimuli, i.e., flattening of voltage without or with blocking of slow waves, filtering of delta waves combined with the occurrence of nonrhythmical frequencies in the alpha and theta range, and muscle artifacts without changes in the EEG.

Epileptiform Activities

Spikes and/or sharp waves are predominant in some comatose patients; this is frequently but not invariably associated with seizures. Generalized paroxysmal activities may occur continuously during the whole record, indicating a certain type of myoclonic status epilepticus (Lowenstein and Aminoff, 1992). In other cases, no visible motor phenomena may be present (Bauer and Niedermeyer, 1979; Lowenstein and Aminoff, 1992; Suter, 1974). In cases of unilateral continuous spiking (Fig. 24.4), the patient may not be truly unconscious, but aphasic or otherwise unable to react adequately. Periodic lateralized epileptiform discharges (PLEDs) (Chatrian et al., 1964a) are seen in coma, but 50% of patients show no alterations in vigilance. PLEDs occur mainly with acute convulsions in vascular structural lesions, but a wide variety of other conditions are also known to produce PLEDs (Bauer et al., 1981; Bauer and Pieber, 1974; Chatrian et al., 1964a; Kuroiwa and Celesia, 1980; Markand and Daly, 1971; Schwarz et al., 1973). Evidence that coma or confusional states accompanied by PLEDs represent a specific type of nonconvulsive status epilepticus (Terzano et al., 1986) comes from positron emission tomography (PET) studies (Handforth et al., 1994). However, in many cases intravenous antiepileptic drug treatment does not ameliorate either the clinical condition or the EEG changes.

Triphasic Waves

This pattern is generally considered fairly characteristic of a hepatic coma. Typical triphasic waves have been sepa-

Figure 24.3. B.M., a 17-year-old girl with secondary traumatic midbrain syndrome. Spindle activities and prolonged burst of delta waves secondary to hand clapping.

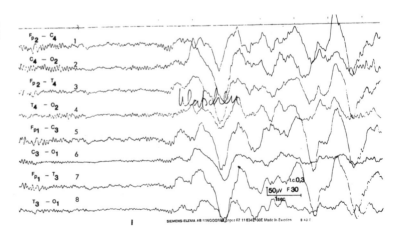

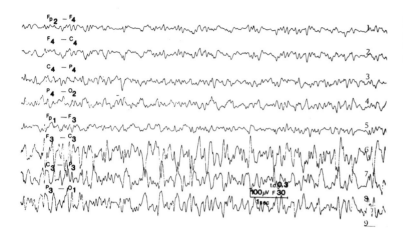

Figure 24.4. P.M., a 34-year-old woman in an unresponsive state after termination of status epilepticus due to relapse of a left temporal astrocytoma. Continuous left central spikes and sharp waves.

rated from atypical forms (Bickford and Butt, 1955; Reiher, 1970) (Fig. 24.5). The characteristics of the typical pattern consist of medium- to high-voltage triphasic waves, occurring in rhythmical trains at a rate of 1.5 to 2.5 cycles/sec, bilaterally synchronous and symmetrical over both hemispheres. An anterior-posterior time delay has been emphasized as an important criterion for the typical form but is rarely observed with referential or transverse montages (Simsarian and Harner, 1972). Furthermore, a gamut of transitions exists between typical and atypical forms. Hepatic coma with continuously occurring triphasic waves has been considered a type of status epilepticus nonconvulsivus (Yamamoto and Hosokawa, 1984; Yasuda et al., 1988). Triphasic waves were also seen in hypoxic states (Calham and Ettinger, 1966; Prior, 1973; Silverman, 1975), intoxication (Kubicki et al., 1970), other metabolic derangements (Harner and Katz, 1975; Madison and Niedermeyer, 1970), cases of subdural hematoma/brainstem infarction (Towsend and Drury, 1991), sepsis-associated encephalopathy (Young et al., 1992), and cerebral carcinomatosis (Miller et al., 1986). Furthermore, in a different clinical context, nearly continuously occurring sharp and slow waves with absence status of Lennox-Gastaut syndrome (Bauer et al., 1983) might also be confused with triphasic waves. Triphasic waves have also been observed with preserved consciousness in Alzheimer's disease, prion diseases, and unspecified demented states (Blatt and Brenner, 1996).

Suppression-Burst Activity

Many records of deeply comatose patients are characterized by a suppression-burst pattern: high-voltage bursts of slow waves with intermingled sharp transients or spikes occur against a depressed background or complete flatness. The bursts are quasi periodically repeated and frequently, but not invariably, accompanied by diffuse myoclonic jerks (Bauer and Niedermeyer, 1979; Butenuth and Kubicki, 1971; Madison and Niedermeyer, 1970; Pampiglione and Harden, 1968; Suter, 1974). The bursts and the accompanying jerks follow an endogenous repetition rate, which can be altered by exogenous stimuli in exceptional cases. According to the morphology, several types of burst-suppression activity might be differentiated. Remnants of cerebral activity in between the bursts frequently consist of nonreactive rhythmical activities in the alpha and theta ranges (Bauer et al., 1989; Zaret, 1985).

Periodic Spiking

Periodic spiking represents an EEG sign closely related to suppression-burst activity. Single or multiple spikes occur on a flat background activity (Fig. 24.6). The repetition rate is higher than with the burst-suppression pattern. Slow waves are less prominent or even lacking. Periodic spikes are likewise accompanied by myoclonic jerks (Bauer and

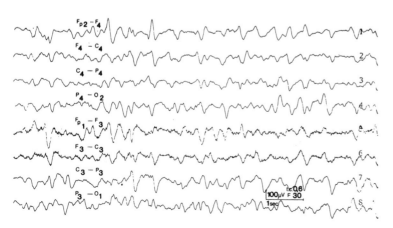

Figure 24.5. K.M., a 73-year-old woman in a confused state after seizures during dialysis treatment for chronic renal insufficiency. Diffuse slowing and atypical triphasic waves.

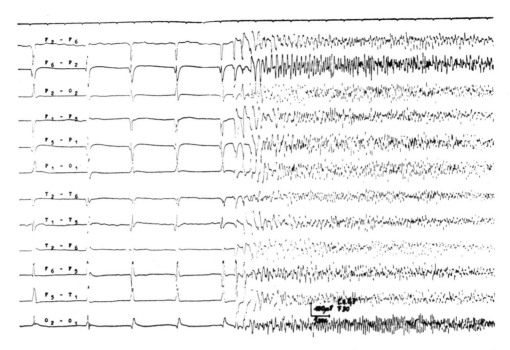

Figure 24.6.   W.H., 36-year-old man with secondary traumatic midbrain syndrome complicated by pneumococcal meningitis. Recording after application of intravenous succinylcholine chloride. Periodic spiking turning into generalized continuous spike activity.

Niedermeyer, 1979; Suter, 1974). No definite one-to-one relation to the spikes can be found.

Monorhythmical Activities

A striking phenomenon is normal-looking rhythmical activities in the alpha range in deep comatose states. This is encountered in unresponsive conditions after brainstem lesions (Chatrian et al., 1964b; Loeb and Poggio, 1953; Lundervold et al., 1956; Rohmer et al., 1965; Westmoreland et al., 1975) and in severe anoxic encephalopathies (Binnie et al., 1970; Chokroverty, 1975; Grindal and Suter, 1975; Sharbrough et al., 1975; Vignaendra et al., 1974; Westmoreland et al., 1975). These alpha frequencies are different from normal alpha rhythm in terms of spatial distribution and reactivity. They occur steadily throughout the whole record and are diffusely spread or accentuated over the anterior regions. There are no or minor fluctuations in amplitude, and there is definitely no reaction to any stimulus. "Alpha coma" has to be carefully separated from spindle-like activities (Bauer et al., 1982; Nogueria de Melo et al., 1990), from 10 to 18 cycles/sec rhythms due to intoxication (Kubicki et al., 1970; Okonek and Rieger, 1975; Sharbrough et al., 1975), from normal alpha rhythm in the locked-in syndrome, and from transient epileptic discharges (Fig. 24.7) (Karbowski, 1975; Staudt et al., 1983). The real alpha coma has been considered a temporary antemortem stage (Arfel, 1975a) following a burst-suppression pattern (Bauer et al., 1982; Westmoreland, 1975; Zaret, 1985). In this narrow definition, alpha pattern coma is thought to carry an unfavorable prognosis. This is also true for nonreactive alpha frequencies not ful-

Figure 24.7.   R.J., a 51-year-old woman in a metabolic coma accompanied by myoclonic jerks. Rhythmical activities occurring independently over both hemispheres. The changing frequencies and the mu-like shape suggest the epileptic nature of the rhythms.

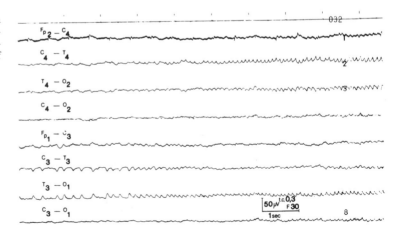

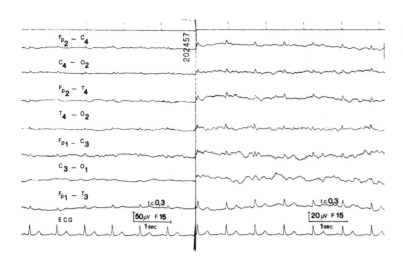

Figure 24.8. C.A., a 23-year-old man with secondary traumatic bulbar brain syndrome. Remnants of cerebral activity (low-voltage output EEG) becoming more visible with increased gain.

filling the rigid criteria of alpha pattern coma and for theta pattern coma (Synek and Synek, 1984). The invariable ominous significance has been doubted and cases of good recovery have been reported (Austin et al., 1988; Iragui and McCutchen, 1983; Synek and Glasgow, 1985; Tomassen and Kamphuisen, 1986; Young et al., 1994).

Low-Voltage Output EEG

This pattern is a precursor of electrocerebral silence. The term denotes remnants of cerebral activity of less than 20 µV (Fig. 24.8). Low-voltage records of conscious subjects should not be confused with severe and global depression of EEG activities (see Chapter 9).

Focal Abnormalities in Coma

Coma due to localized supratentorial lesions is likely to be associated with focal EEG signs. The lateralizing signs may become blurred and even abolished with deepening coma. They consist of localized or unilateral slowing, asymmetrical depression of slow or fast activities, especially of sleep spindles, and asymmetrical responses to exogenous stimuli. Prolonged delta bursts are depressed over the more affected hemisphere (Arfel, 1975a) (Fig. 24.9). The differentiation between consistent unilaterally accentuated slowing and asymmetrical alerting responses is crucial for correct lateralization in comatose states.

On the other hand, localized EEG abnormalities are not uncommon with diffuse encephalopathies (Bauer and Niedermeyer, 1979; Harner and Katz, 1975). The nonketotic hyperosmolar diabetic coma is particularly apt to produce focal neurological deficits, partial seizures, and corresponding EEG signs (Gerich et al., 1971; Harner and Katz, 1975; Maccario et al., 1965).

EEG and the Etiology of Coma

The EEG can never be specific for etiological entities. Nevertheless, electrical patterns observed in coma show several correlations with underlying disease. Because EEG changes in relation to etiology are discussed in other parts of this book, this section presents only a short outline.

EEG in Supratentorial Lesions

The EEG in supratentorial lesions that cause coma is nearly always markedly abnormal. Focal slowing indicates the site of the lesion, whereas diffuse slowing parallels the degree of herniation. Detailed electroclinical correlations in acute secondary midbrain syndromes are presented in Chapter 21, on EEG and trauma.

EEG in Infratentorial Lesions

Neurological signs and EEG abnormalities are frequently disproportional in coma due to infratentorial processes. In contrast with apparent comatose behavior, the EEG may look unexpectedly normal. This is especially true in brainstem infarcts with predominant alpha frequencies. In such instances, one should be aware of the possibility that the patient is not comatose but locked-in. There are a few observations of so-called total locked-in syndrome (Bauer et al., 1979; Dehaene et al., 1985). Such patients are totally immobile, including vertical eye movements. The reactive alpha

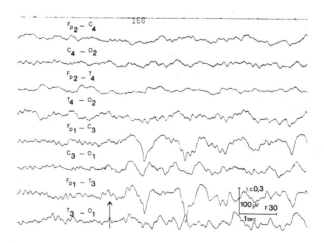

Figure 24.9. O.V., a 24-year-old woman in a coma after removal of a right-sided subdural hematoma. Depression of rhythmical 7 cycles/sec activity over the right hemisphere. With exogenous stimulation (*arrow*), burst of delta waves (alerting response), depressed over the right hemisphere.

rhythm represents the only clue that the patient is not comatose but rather totally locked-in.

EEG in Anoxic Coma

The number of patients in postanoxic coma has increased during the past decades due to modern advances in emergency treatment. Continuous triphasic wave-like seizure discharges, burst-suppression activity, periodic spiking, and monorhythmical alpha frequencies are typical EEG patterns. Clinical and EEG signs of status epilepticus, especially of myoclonic status epilepticus, are frequently present (Krumholz et al., 1988; Kuroiwa et al., 1982; Simon and Aminoff, 1986; Young et al., 1990). A more detailed description is presented in Chapter 23 on cerebral anoxia.

Infectious Diseases

EEG abnormalities in CNS infections show some characteristics (Radermecker, 1956). Diffuse slowing is exceptionally prominent; it is often rhythmical or quasiperiodic. Superimposed diffuse theta or alpha frequencies are scarce. Generalized periodic phenomena are highly suggestive for subacute sclerosing panencephalitis (Balthasar, 1944; Cobb and Hill, 1950; Martin et al., 1950; Radermecker and Macken, 1951) or Jakob-Creutzfeldt disease (Abbot, 1959; Amler and Bergner, 1967; Gloor et al., 1968; Lee and Blair, 1975); they occur also in diffuse encephalitides (Lesse et al., 1958; Storm van Leeuwen, 1964) and in various other conditions (Bauer and Pieber, 1974; Kuroiwa and Celesia, 1980; Kiloh et al., 1972). Lateralized periodic complexes in herpes simplex encephalitis are of great diagnostic importance (Illis and Taylor, 1972; Kugler et al., 1976; Lesse et al., 1958; Millar and Coey, 1959; Upton and Gumpert, 1970).

EEG in Metabolic Coma

The enormous complexity of pathophysiological mechanisms in metabolic coma stands in contrast to the lack of specificity of accompanying EEG signs. Diffuse slowing is always seen in metabolic coma. In cases of disproportionate degrees of coma and slowing, a metabolic cause is unlikely (Harner and Katz, 1975). Focal slowing does not exclude the diagnosis. Triphasic waves are suggestive of a metabolic disorder, especially of hepatic origin. The diagnostic significance of triphasic waves may have been overstressed, but it is still important when this pattern is encountered in an undiagnosed insidiously developing coma. With hepatic coma, spikes may also be encountered (Ficker et al., 1997). Uremia is frequently complicated by generalized tonic-clonic seizures and generalized polyspikes associated with diffuse slow activity. Photomyoclonic responses are not infrequent. Diffuse slowing may become exaggerated during or after dialysis with or without clinical signs of a disequilibrium syndrome. Paroxysmal bursts of slow waves and slowing of the basic rhythm were seen in all cases of the dialysis dementia syndrome (Burks et al., 1976; Chang Chui and Damasio, 1980; Garret et al., 1988). Modern advances in dialysis techniques made this complication an exceptional event.

Epileptic Conditions

Epileptic conditions lead to prolonged coma in convulsive status epilepticus, in postictal states with lingering subclinical paroxysmal activities (Bauer, 1975a), and in typical and atypical absence status (Bauer, 1975b; Brett, 1966; Niedermeyer and Khalifeh, 1965) and in other types of nonconclusive status epilepticus (Kaplan, 1996). In most instances, the EEG shows prominent seizure activity and is instrumental in the establishment of the correct diagnosis, although an EEG without spikes does not categorically exclude the epileptic nature of the altered state of consciousness. On the other hand, many comatose states are complicated by interspersed epileptic seizures. Coma with acute convulsions is accompanied by a markedly abnormal EEG, which in most instances is characterized by seizure discharges (Bauer and Niedermeyer, 1979).

EEG in Relation to the Depth of Coma

The EEG as a functional test should be closely related to the degree of impaired cerebral function. There are several reasons why this relation is far from being perfect. The main reason is found in local brainstem coma, which leaves the cortex and the EEG comparatively unaffected.

Attempts to classify coma into clinical stages are numerous. The most logical coma grading is based on an orderly sequence of neurological symptoms down the levels of the neuraxis in cases of transtentorial herniations (Cairns, 1952; Gerstenbrand and Lücking, 1970; McNealy and Plum, 1962; Plum and Posner, 1966). Different stages of a midbrain syndrome have been distinguished from a bulbar brain syndrome. Similar neurological symptoms have been observed in infectious diseases (Dodge and Swartz, 1965; Williams et al., 1964) and anoxic states (Bauer and Niedermeyer, 1979; Jellinger and Seitelberger, 1970). Several attempts have been made to introduce practical coma scales to enable neurologically untrained medical staff to get immediate information (Diringer and Edwards, 1997; Gerstenbrand et al., 1984; Rowley and Fielding, 1991; Sacco et al., 1990; Shakhnovich et al., 1980; Teasdale and Jennet, 1974). Pupillary responses serve as a reliable parameter, possibly superior even to brainstem evoked potentials and intracranial pressure monitoring (Krieger et al., 1993). Therefore, coma scales should include pupillary responses. Neurological coma grading becomes impossible with early sedation for therapeutic purposes and is confined to auxiliary tests. An International Federation of Societies for Electroencephalography and Clinical Neurophysiology (IFCN) committee recommended standards for electrophysiological monitoring in comatose and other unresponsive states (Chatrian et al., 1996).

Regardless of the etiology, the following information about the grade of *rostral-caudal deterioration* can be supported by EEG evidence in the following manner:

1. The degree and generalization of slowing is related to the level of unresponsiveness (Harner and Katz, 1975; Loeb, 1975a; Romano and Engel, 1944). The most important exception to this rule is prolonged bursts of delta waves secondary to exogenous stimuli. Furthermore, in children the degree of slowing is frequently disproportionate to the clinical state.
2. The effect of stimulation yields good information about the depth of coma. As one proceeds down the scale of coma, the blocking type of response is replaced by the

alerting type. Finally, the EEG becomes unreactive even to repeated stimulation (Arfel, 1975a; Fischgold and Mathis, 1959; Schwartz and Scott, 1978; Vigouroux et al., 1964). Motor responses without changes of EEG should not be regarded as a sign of cortical functions. They might be mediated by the lower brainstem or even by the spinal cord and can be present with cortical death and electrocerebral silence (ECS).

3. Potentials otherwise seen during sleep become progressively scarcer and finally disappear with deepening coma (Bergamini et al., 1966; Chatrian et al., 1963; Lücking, 1970; Rumpl et al., 1979; Silverman, 1963).

4. Patterns highly suggestive of a late midbrain or initial bulbar brain syndrome are (a) progressive voltage depression (Arfel, 1975a; Fischgold and Mathis, 1959; Vigouroux et al., 1964); (b) extreme slowing with extinction of superimposed fast activities (Fischgold and Mathis, 1959; Kubicki et al., 1960); (c) intermittent isoelectric periods; (d) periodic spiking or burst-suppression activity (Bauer and Niedermeyer, 1979; Fischgold and Mathis, 1959; Kubicki et al., 1960, 1970; Suter, 1974; Silverman, 1975); and (e) monorhythmic unreactive alpha and theta frequencies (Westmoreland et al., 1975; Synek and Synek, 1984).

Prognostic Criteria from EEG

The EEG is certainly of great prognostic value in comatose states (Celesia, 1999). Its significance is limited by the fact that the outcome is often not determined by the brain disturbance itself but by the underlying metabolic or cardiovascular problems. Furthermore, prognostic criteria do not apply if anesthetics or other CNS depressant drugs have been used. This fact has become especially important with the widespread use of sedative drugs in comatose states. In these patients, neurological and EEG examinations may be misleading, and valuable monitoring seems to be confined to evoked potentials (Ganes and Lundar, 1983; Hume and Cant, 1981; Hutchinson et al., 1991; Rumpl et al., 1983b). The barbiturate treatment of comatose states, however, has never been generally accepted (Cremer et al., 2001; Schwab et al., 1997), and its use has declined progressively (Brain Resuscitation Clinical Trial, 1986; Dearden, 1985).

In general, the prognostic significance of EEG patterns parallels their correlations to the grade of rostral-caudal deterioration. Prognostically favorable signs are reactions to exogenous stimuli (Arfel, 1975a; Evans and Bartlett, 1995; Gütling et al., 1995; Kubicki et al., 1970; Lücking, 1970) and normal-looking sleep potentials or sleep cycles (Arfel, 1975a; Bergamasco et al., 1968; Bergamini et al., 1966; Bricolo et al., 1967; Chatrian et al., 1963; Lücking, 1970; Rumpl et al., 1983a; Valente et al., 2002). Spindle coma indicates relative integrity of the cerebral hemispheres (Nogueira de Melo et al., 1990). Its prognostic significance depends on the underlying etiology (Kaplan et al., 2000). Best outcomes occurred when spindle coma was due to drugs, encephalopathy, or seizures. With posttraumatic coma, normal-looking sleep spindles carry a good prognosis. On the other hand, several posttraumatic cases exhibiting spindle coma have a poor outcome probably due to prominent primary or secondary brainstem lesions (Kaplan et al., 2000;

Rumpl et al., 1983a). The absence of spindles in anoxic coma was associated with poor outcome, whereas its presence did not indicate a favorable course (Hulihan and Syna, 1994). Improvement of EEG signs at serial recordings may represent the first indication of a favorable course. Fast activities over the anterior regions are considered a favorable sign in intoxication (Kubicki et al., 1970).

On the other hand, absence of reactivity has been judged an ominous sign (Arfel, 1975a; Li et al., 1952). With rostral-caudal deterioration, the number of patterns decreases (Rumpl et al., 1979). A very poor prognosis is indicated by monotonous, high-voltage 0.5- to 3-Hz activity without changes occurring spontaneously or secondary to exogenous stimuli (Dusser et al., 1989), by the burst-suppression pattern (Bauer and Niedermeyer, 1979; Bickford et al., 1965; Hockaday et al., 1965; Pampiglione, 1962a,b; Prior, 1973; Silverman, 1975), by generalized periodic phenomena (Binnie et al., 1970; Pampiglione, 1962a,b; Prior, 1973), by intermittent flattening, by monorhythmical alpha frequencies (Arfel, 1975a; Binnie et al., 1970; Prior, 1973; Westmoreland et al., 1975), and by a low-voltage output EEG (Bauer and Niedermeyer, 1979; Bickford et al., 1965; Binnie et al., 1970; Hockaday et al., 1965; Prior, 1973; Silverman, 1975). With intoxications, the aforementioned patterns are of less serious significance. Triphasic waves indicate a poor prognosis in liver diseases (MacGillivray, 1976) and also with intoxication (Kubicki et al., 1970). Paroxysmal abnormalities in coma represent an unfavorable sign (Binnie et al., 1970), except in posttraumatic coma (Bauer and Niedermeyer, 1979).

Brain Death
Definition

The entire problem of cerebral death is a by-product of improved medical care; it has become urgent because of the need for organs for transplantation surgery. There is nearly complete agreement that cerebral death determines the death of an individual (Saunders, 1975). Its definition is left to the medical profession and rests on an exact description of a syndrome that encompasses the clinical and EEG picture, etiological factors, and evolution (Loeb, 1975b).

Numerous terms are used for the same clinical entity: (a) aperceptive, areactive, apathic, and atonic syndrome (Jouvet, 1969); (b) brain death; (c) stage IV coma (Fischgold and Mathis, 1959); (d) coma dépassé (Mollaret and Goulon, 1959); (e) irreversible coma (Vigouroux, 1975); (f) cerebral death; (g) cerebral death syndrome; and (h) irreversible breakdown of cerebral functions (Gerstenbrand, 1973).

In recent times, a new, twofold discussion was started about brain death. Especially in Germany the equalization of brain death and individual death has been vigorously questioned calling transplantation surgeons "vivisectionists" (quoted by Simm, 1996). On the other hand, because of the chronic shortage of organs for transplantation, donorship was expanded to anencephalic infants (Arras and Shinnar, 1988; Peabody et al., 1989; Truog and Fletcher, 1989) and to non-heart-beating patients (Koostra et al., 1995). With these discussions a considerable factual and conceptual confusion arose. This confusion can easily be cleared by sticking to the long-established principles.

The equation of brain death with individual death is a matter of social agreement. There is no rational argument to doubt the criterion of brain death. Anencephalic infants might be considered donors provided brain death, including the brainstem, has been properly diagnosed. From a neurological point of view, there are two problems with non-heart-beating donors. No data exist about how long the heart beat has to be arrested until the brain is irreversibly out of any function. Category 3 patients, according to Koostra et al. (1995), are ICU patients dying from severe brain trauma with no chance for recovery but who do not meet the criterion of brain death. To harvest organs, medical support is withdrawn until cardiac arrest occurs. Ethically, this procedure can hardly be accepted. With the other categories of non-heart-beating donors, neurologists and electroencephalographers might not be involved in the decision-making process.

Pathophysiology

Whatever the cause of coma, a common final pathway can be assumed in all fatal cases. The crucial mechanism consists of elevation of intracranial pressure. If it approaches the systemic arterial pressure, EEG activity ceases, and arrest of intracerebral circulation occurs. This experimentally confirmed pathomechanism (Baldy-Moulinier and Frerebeau, 1969; Kramer and Tuyman, 1967) is also responsible for the development of brain death in human subjects. The findings at autopsy show a wide range of intensity, from light softening to total liquefaction ("respirator brain") (Loeb, 1975b). In cases of primary hemispheric lesions, signs of transtentorial or tonsillar herniations are almost always present. The intensity of pathological changes depends on the development of intracranial circulatory arrest. According to Lindenberg (1963), morphological changes occur with quickly developing brain edema ("morphotropic necrobiosis"), whereas no major changes are found if the intracranial circulatory arrest is preceded by a period of severe hypoxia of sufficient length ("morphostatic necrobiosis"). In cases of prolonged ventilatory support, a certain degree of reperfusion leads to later changes in brain death (Alvarez et al., 1988a; Schröder, 1983).

Neurological Signs

In the diagnosis of cerebral death, the first step is the demonstration of a brain death syndrome based on neurological examination. Neurological signs of cortical functions and brainstem activity must be absent. Pupils must be fixed even with a strong light stimulus. Peripheral third nerve injuries should be excluded. Oculovestibular responses must be absent (Buettner and Zee, 1989; Nayyar et al., 1987). No motor activity can be observed in the muscles innervated by cranial nerves. Muscle artifacts in EEG have been considered to be evidence of brainstem functions (Arfel, 1975b; Hirsch et al., 1970). In other cases, however, the recorded muscle activity was assumed to be due to hyperexcitability of the nerve membrane caused by artificial hyperventilation (Mayr et al., 1990). Spontaneous respiration must be absent; no respiration movements should be detectable after removal from the respirator. Testing for apnea is necessary to conform the neurological brain death syndrome. The practical procedure differs markedly within different centers (Earnest et al., 1986; Marks and Zisfein, 1990; Van Donselaar et al., 1986). Hypotension and other cardiovascular complications can pose a significant risk to patients undergoing apnea testing (Goudreau et al., 2000; Jeret and Benjamin, 1994). Apneic oxygenation can reduce the risk (Marks and Zisfein, 1990). A standardized procedure has been suggested for apnea testing (Wijdicks, 1995).

The Harvard criteria of brain death (Beecher, 1968) include the absence of spinal reflexes. This is not only overdemanding but plainly incorrect. After an initial phase of spinal shock due to a total brain infarct down to the level of C-1, many patients exhibit simple or complex spinal reflexes (Becker et al., 1970; Butenuth et al., 1975; Chang, 2002; Crenna et al., 1989; Gerstenbrand, 1973; Gros et al., 1969; Ivan, 1973; Schwartz and Vendrely, 1969; Vigouroux, 1975). Complex spinal reflexes such as the tonic plantar response, priapism, and tonic contractions of the cremaster, abdominal, and vaginal muscles can be regarded as a positive sign of brain death (Gerstenbrand, 1973) in the absence of brainstem and cortical functions.

Electrocerebral Silence (ECS)

An isoelectric EEG is confirmatory for the establishment of cerebral death (Beecher, 1968; Bennet et al., 1976; Hirsch et al., 1970; Penin and Käufer, 1969; Schwab et al., 1963; Silverman et al., 1969; Suter, 1977). It must be emphasized, however, that ECS per se does not mean cerebral death. Isoelectric EEG recordings have been found with the complete apallic syndrome (Ingvar and Brun, 1972), with intoxication and full recovery (Bennet et al., 1976; Bird and Plum, 1968; Haider et al., 1971; Mantz et al., 1971; Mellerio, 1969; Sament and Huott, 1969), with hypothermia (Prior, 1973; Williams and Spencer, 1958), and with transient decorticate states followed by varying degrees of recovery (Fischgold and Mathis, 1959). Since therapeutic hypothermia is not beneficial in the management of comatose states (Clifton et al., 2001; Harris et al., 2002), it has to be considered only in rare circumstances. Therefore, ECS can be taken as a sign of brain death only if neurological signs of cortical and brainstem functions are lacking, and intoxication and marked hypothermia can be excluded. A brain death syndrome at the neurological examination is based on brainstem death and does not exclude ongoing cortical activities reflected by EEG activity (Fig. 24.10) (Grigg et al., 1987; Ogata et al., 1988). To consider EEG activity with brainstem death as a pitfall of EEG in determining brain death, because brainstem death equals brain death, turns the logic upside down. Brainstem death does not mean brain death, defined as irreversible loss of functions of all parts of the brain. Ongoing EEG activity with isolated brainstem death proves this statement. In cases of primary brainstem lesions, the EEG is not only confirmatory but essential for correct diagnosis. The same is true for fulminant demyelinating polyradiculopathy resembling brainstem death (Drury et al., 1987; Marti-Masso et al., 1993; Stojkovic et al., 2001).

The relationship between brain death diagnosed on the basis of neurological and EEG examinations and respirator brain at autopsy has been reassessed (Leestma et al., 1984). Overly rigid criteria for the differentiation of ECS from the

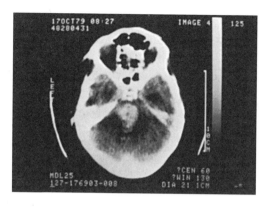
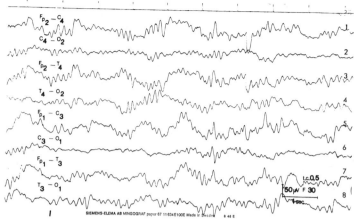

Figure 24.10. K.J., a 48-year-old man; computed tomography showed extensive hemorrhage in pontine level, EEG diffuse slowing with superimposed spindle-like 7–8 cycles/sec activities. This EEG was recorded after the diagnosis of a brain death syndrome at neurological examination.

very low voltage output EEG and excess noise have been criticized (Horikawa et al., 2003; Spudis et al., 1984). In spite of certain shortcomings, EEG has proved to of paramount importance in the evaluation of brain death. Shortcomings are of a technical nature, as are conceptual misunderstandings, such as with primary brainstem death and the overinterpretation of artifacts. However, real cerebral EEG waves exclude brain death by definition. To bypass these difficulties, several attempts have been made to redefine brain death and to confine it to brainstem death (Rothstein, 1993). The concept of whole-brain death delivers high diagnostic practicability and certainty and has achieved a high level of acceptance in Western society (Bernat, 1992). There is no urgent need to change it to brainstem death or neocortical death.

Technical Standards for the EEG Recording in Brain Death

The definition and reliability of ECS is based on the technical standards applied for its registration. Many records referred to as ECS show low-voltage output EEG or use insufficient technical standards.

Several national EEG societies have published recommendations for EEG recordings in suspected brain death (Bätz et al., 1994; Bennet et al., 1976; American Electroencephalographic Society, 1994; Hirsch et al., 1970; Silverman et al., 1970). These suggestions do not differ essentially among the national recommendations. They include the following:

1. A minimum of eight scalp electrodes and reference electrodes to cover the major brain areas;
2. Interelectrode impedances under 10,000 ohms but over 100 ohms;
3. Testing the integrity of the entire recording system;
4. Interelectrode distances of at least 10 cm to enlarge the amplitudes and to pick up electrical fields originating in deep structures;
5. Sensitivity increase up to 2 µV/mm during most of the recording to distinguish ECS from low-voltage output EEG;
6. Use of time constants of 0.3 to 0.4 second;
7. Use of monitoring techniques, with simultaneous ECG recording to be mandatory;
8. Testing EEG reactivity to exogenous stimuli;
9. Recording time of at least 30 minutes;
10. Recording to be made only by a qualified technologist.

The most important recommendation is the use of high instrument sensitivity along with the need for continuous recognition and elimination of artifacts. This is indeed a painstaking task in a busy ICU.

Practical Procedures in the Determination of Brain Death

There is an urgent need for a practical procedure to determine the earliest point of time for harvesting organs for transplantation surgery. The first step is the neurological examination demonstrating a brain death syndrome. Prerequisites for a safe neurological diagnosis are clinical or imaging evidence of an acute cerebral catastrophe that is compatible with the diagnosis, and the exclusion of confounding conditions like severe electrolyte imbalance, drug intoxication or poisoning, and hypothermia (Quality Standards Subcommittee of the American Academy of Neurology, 1995). The following steps in the procedure of brain death determination vary according to national recommendations (Beirat der Bundesärztekammer, 1997; Haupt and Rudolf, 1999; Quality Standards Subcommittee of the American Academy of Neurology, 1995; Schweizerische Akademie der Medizinischen Wissenschaften, 1996; Wijdicks, 2001). In general, three possibilities exist: (1) No confirmatory laboratory tests but an extended observation time of at least 12 hours and exclusion of a primary brainstem lesion. (2) Use of EEG as a confirmatory test and the demonstration of ECS. (3) Use of a so-called terminal pan-angiography as a confirmatory test and the demonstration of a nonfilling phenomenon. This method is potentially dangerous (Waugh and Sacharias, 1992). Legally, it needs a declaration of consent, obviously not possible in the condition under discussion. Examinations subject to patient's consent are considered illegal in unconscious patients, unless they are performed in order to help the patient. Therefore, many lawyers consider "terminal angiography" illegal. Furthermore, persistence of isolated flow in the internal carotid artery has been observed in brain death (Freitas et al., 2003). Transcranial Doppler examinations criteria for brain death have yet to be clarified (Jacobs et al., 2003).

If the EEG is chosen as a confirmatory laboratory test, the length of observation time until a second and final EEG should be recorded was under discussion for a long time. Silverman et al. (1970) demand 24 hours, Loeb (1975b) and Richter (1973) consider 12 hours a reasonable time, and Kugler et al. (1973) proposed 6 hours in cases with adequate observation of clinical and electrical signs during the time prior to the development of brain death. Nowadays, in diagnostically doubtless cases no further observation time is recommended (Beirat der Bundesärztekammer, 1997; Quality Standards Subcommittee of the American Academy of Neurology, 1995). In cases with diagnostic or technical uncertainties, repeated recordings are advised. The usefulness of EEG in the evaluation of brain death in children has been discussed (Alvarez et al., 1988b; Celesia, 1989; Moshé, 1989; Schneider, 1989; Shewmon, 1988). With optimal technical standards, similar criteria to those used in adults can be applied.

References

Abbot, J. 1959. The EEG in Jakob-Creutzfeldt's disease. Electroencephalogr. Clin. Neurophysiol. 11:184(abst).

Adams, J.H., Mitchell, D.E., Graham, D.I., et al. 1977. Diffuse brain damage of immediate impact type. Brain 100:489–502.

Adams, J.H., Graham, D.I., Genarelli, T.A., et al. 1991. Diffuse axonal injury in non-missile head injury. J. Neurol. Neurosurg. Psychiatry 54:481–483.

Alema, G., Perria, L., Rosadini, G., et al. 1966. Functional inactivation of the human brainstem related to the level of consciousness. J. Neurosurg. 24:629–639.

Alvarez, L.A., Lipton, R.B., Hirschfield, A., et al. 1988a. Brain death determination by angiography in the setting of a skull defect. Arch. Neurol. 45:225–227.

Alvarez, L.A., Moshé, S.L., Belman, A.L., et al. 1988b. EEG and brain death determination in children. Neurology 38:227–230.

American Electroencephalographic Society. 1994. Guideline Three: minimum technical standards for EEG recording in suspected cerebral death. J. Clin. Neurophysiol. 11:10–13.

Amler, G., and Bergner, M. 1967. Typisches EEG-Muster beim Creutzfeldt-Jakob-Syndrom unter Berücksichtigung diagnostischer und differntialdiagnostischer Gesichtspunkte. Psychiatr. Neurol. (Basel) 154:373–383.

Arfel, G. 1975a. Introduction to clinical and EEG studies in coma. In Altered States of Consciousness, Coma, Cerebral Death. Handbook of Electroencephalography and Clinical Neurophysiology, vol. 12, Eds. R. Harner and R. Naquet, pp. 5–23. Amsterdam: Elsevier.

Arfel, G. 1975b. Brain death—evidence contributed by laboratory studies other than surface EEGs. In Altered States of Consciousness, Coma, Cerebral Death. Handbook of Electroencephalography and Clinical Neurophysiology, vol. 12, Eds. R. Harner and R. Naquet, pp. 116–121. Amsterdam: Elsevier.

Arfel, G., and Fischgold, H. 1961. EEG signs in tumors of the brain. In Electroencephalography and Cerebral Tumors. Electroencephalogr. Clin. Neurophysiol. Suppl. 19:36–50.

Arras, J.D., and Shinnar, S. 1988. Anencephalic newborns as organ donors: a critique. JAMA 259:2284–2285.

Austin, E.J., Wilkus, R.J., and Longstreth, W.T. 1988. Etiology and prognosis of alpha coma. Neurology 38:773–777.

Baars, B.J. 1998. Metaphors of consciousness and attention in the brain. TINS 21:58–62

Baldy-Moulinier, M., and Frerebeau, P. 1969. Cerebral blood flow in cases of coma following severe head injury. In Cerebral Blood Flow, Eds. M. Brock et al., pp. 216–219. Berlin: Springer-Verlag.

Balthasar, K. 1944. Zur Kenntnis der Panencephalitis nodosa (Pette). Arch. Psychiatr. Nervenkr. 117:667.

Batini, C., Moruzzi, G., Palestini, J., et al. 1959. Effects of complete pontine transection on the sleep wakefulness rhythm: the mid-pontine pretrigeminal preparation. Arch. Ital. Biol. 97:1–12.

Bätz, B., Besser, R., Flemming, I., et al. 1994. Empfehlungen der Deutschen Gesellschaft für Klinische Neurophysiologie (Deutsche EEG-Gesellschaft) zur Bestimmung des Hirntodes. Z. EEG-EMG 25:163–166.

Bauer, G. 1975a. Der Wert von EEG-Kontrollen möglichst bald nach einem epileptischen Anfall. Z. EEG-EMG 6:125–130.

Bauer, G. 1975b. Psychische Veränderungen bei kontinuierlichen epileptischen Entladungen. Schweiz. Arch. Neurol. Neurochir. Psychiatr. 116:241–255.

Bauer, G., and Niedermeyer, E. 1979. Acute convulsions. Clin. Electroencephalogr. 10:127–144.

Bauer, G., and Pieber, R. 1974. Über periodische Komplexe im EEG. Z. EEG-EMG 5:75–86.

Bauer, G., Gerstenbrand, F., and Rumpl, E. 1979. Varieties of the locked-in syndrome. J. Neurol. 221:77–91.

Bauer, G., Aichner, F., and Hengl, W. 1981. Der diagnostische Wert periodischer lateralisierter Komplexe im EEG. Z. EEG-EMG 12:135–141.

Bauer, G., Aichner, F., and Klingler, D. 1982. Aktivitäten im Alphaequenzbereich und Koma. Z. EEG-EMG 13:28–33.

Bauer, G., Aichner, F., and Mayr, U. 1983. Status atypischer Absencen in Jugend- und Erwachsenenalter. Nervenarzt 54:100–105.

Bauer, G., Prugger, M., Bohr, K., et al. 1989. Relationship between the suppression burst pattern and rhythmical activities in the alpha and theta bands of EEG of comatose patients. Electroencephalogr. Clin. Neurophysiol. 76:72P.

Becker, D.J., Becker, D.P., Robert, C.M., Jr., et al. 1970. An evaluation of the definition of cerebral death. Neurology (Minneapolis) 20:459–462.

Beecher, H.K. 1968. A definition of irreversible coma: report of the ad hoc committee of the Harvard Medical School to examine the definition of brain death. JAMA 205:337–340.

Beirat der Bundesärztekammer. 1997. Kriterien des Hirntodes. Entscheidungshilfen zur Feststellung des Hirntodes. Buudesürtz-Kammer Köln.

Bennet, D.R., Hughes, J.R., Korein, J., et al. 1976. Atlas of Electroencephalography in Coma and Cerebral Death. New York: Raven Press.

Bergamasco, B., Bergamini, L., Doriguzzi, T., et al. 1968. EEG sleep patterns as a prognostic criterion in post-traumatic coma. Electroencephalogr. Clin. Neurophysiol. 24:374–377.

Bergamini, L., Bergamasco, B., Mombelli, A., et al. 1966. Autocorrelazione in sogetti in coma. Rev. Neurol. 36:233–236.

Bernat, J.L. 1992. Brain death occurs only with destruction of the cerebral hemispheres and the brain stem. Arch. Neurol. 49:569–570.

Bickford, R.G., and Butt, H.R. 1955. Hepatic coma: the electroencephalographic pattern. J. Clin. Invest. 34:790–799.

Bickford, R.G., Dawson, B., and Takeshita, H. 1965. EEG evidence of neurologic death. Electroencephalogr. Clin. Neurophysiol. 18:513.

Binnie, C.D., Prior, P.F., Lloyd, D.S.L., et al. 1970. Electroencephalographic prediction of fatal anoxic brain damage after resuscitation from cardiac arrest. Br. Med. J. 4:265–268.

Birbamer, G., Aichner, F., Felber, S., et al. 1991. MRI of cerebral hypoxia. Neuroradiology 33:53–55.

Bird, T.D., and Plum, F. 1968. Recovery from barbiturate overdose coma with a prolonged isoelectric electroencephalogram. Neurology (Minneapolis) 18:456–460.

Blatt, I., and Brenner, R.P. 1996. Triphasic waves in a psychiatric population: a retrospective study. J. Clin. Neurophysiol. 13:324–329.

Block, N. 1996. How can we find the neural correlate of consciousness? TINS 19:456–459.

Brain Resuscitation Clinical Trial I Study Group. 1986. Randomized clinical study of Thiopental loading in comatose survivors of cardiac arrest. N. Engl. J Med. 314:397–403.

Brett, E.M. 1966. Minor epileptic status. J. Neurol. Sci. 3:53–75.

Bricolo, A., Gentilomo, A., Roadini, G., et al. 1967. Long lasting post-traumatic unconsciousness. Acta Neurol. Scand. 19:512–532.

Buettner, U.W., and Zee, D.S. 1989. Vestibular testing in comatose patients. Arch. Neurol. 46:561–563.

Burks, J.S., Alfrey, A.C., Huddlestone, J., et al. 1976. A fatal encephalopathy in chronic haemodialysis patients. Lancet I:764–768.

Butenuth, J., and Kubicki, S. 1971.Über die prognostische Bedeutung bestimmter Formen der Myoklonien und korrespondierender EEG-Muster nach Hypoxien. Z. EEG-EMG 2:78–83.

Butenuth, J., Fuchs, E.C., Schiffter, R., et al. 1975. Klinische Kriterien zur Bestimmung der Komatiefe. Akt. Neurol. 2:81–102.

Cairns, H. 1952. Disturbances of consciousness with lesions of the brain stem and diencephalon. Brain 75:109–146.

Cairns, H., Oldfield, R.C., and Pennybacker, J.B. 1941. Akinetic mutism with an epidermoid cyst of the third ventricle. Brain 64:173–290.

Calham, C.L., and Ettinger, M.G. 1966. Unusual EEG in coma after cardiac arrest. Electroencephalogr. Clin. Neurophysiol. 21:385–388.

Celesia, G.G. 1989. Brain death in children: editorial comment. Electroencephalogr. Clin. Neurophysiol. 73:271.

Celesia, G.G. 1999. EEG and coma: is there a prognostic role for EEG? Editorial. Clin. Neurophysiol. 110:203–204.

Chang, G.Y. 2002. "Belly dancing" in coma. Eur. Neurol. 48:51.

Chang Chui, H., and Damasio, A.R. 1980. Progressive dialysis encephalopathy ("dialysis dementia"). J. Neurol. 222:145–157.

Chase, T.N.L., Moretti, L., and Prensky, A.L. 1968. Clinical and electroencephalographic manifestations of vascular lesions of the pons. Neurology (Minneapolis) 18:357–368.

Chatrian, G.E., White, L.E., and Daly, D. 1963. Electroencephalographic pattern resembling those of sleep in certain comatose states after injuries to the head. Electroencephalogr. Clin. Neurophysiol. 15:272–280.

Chatrian, G.E., Shaw, C.M., and Leffman, H. 1964a. The significance of periodic lateralized epileptiform discharges in EEG: an electrographic, clinical and pathological study. Electroencephalogr. Clin. Neurophysiol. 17:177–193.

Chatrian, G.E., White, L.E., and Shaw, C.-M. 1964b. EEG pattern resembling wakefulness in unresponsive decerebrate state following traumatic brain stem infarct. Electroencephalogr. Clin. Neurophysiol. 16:285–289.

Chatrian, G.-E., Bergamasco, B., Bricolo, A., et al. 1996. IFCN recommended standards for electrophysiologic monitoring in comatose and other unresponsive states. Report of an IFCN committee. Electroencephalogr. Clin. Neurophysiol. 99:103–122.

Chia, L.G. 1984. Locked-in state with bilateral internal capsule infarcts. Neurology 34:1365–1367.

Chia, L.G. 1991. Locked-in syndrome with bilateral ventral midbrain infarcts. Neurology 41:445–446.

Chokroverty, S. 1975. "Alpha-like" rhythms in electroencephalograms in coma after cardiac arrest. Neurology (Minneapolis) 25:655–663.

Clifton, G.L., Miller, E.R., Choi, S.C., et al. 2001. Lack of effect of induction of hypothermia after acute brain injury. N. Engl. J. Med. 344:556–563.

Cobb, W.A. 1957. Electroencephalographic abnormalities as signs of localized pathology. EEG abnormalities at a distance from the lesion. IVe Congrès International d'Électro-encéphalographie et de Neurophysiologie clinique. Acta Medica Belgica, Brussels, pp. 205–223.

Cobb, W.A., and Hill, D. 1950. Electroencephalogram in subacute progressive encephalitis. Brain 73:392–404.

Cremer, O.L., Moons, K.G.M., Bouman, E.A.C., et al. 2001. Long-term propofol infusion and cardiac failure in adult head-injured patients. Lancet 357:117–118.

Crenna, P., Conci, F., and Boselli, L. 1989. Changes in spinal reflex excitability in brain-dead humans. Electroencephalogr. Clin. Neurophysiol. 73:206–214.

Daly, D.D. 1979. Use of EEG for diagnosis and evaluation of epileptic seizures and nonepileptic episodic disorders. In *Current Practice of Clinical Electroencephalography,* Eds. D.D. Klass and D.D. Daly, pp. 221–268. New York: Raven Press.

Dearden, N.M. 1985. Ischaemic brain. Lancet 2:255–259.

Dehaene, J., and Dom, R. 1982. A mesencephalic locked-in syndrome. J. Neurol. 227:255–259.

Dehaene, J., Dom, R., Marchau, M., et al. 1985. Locked-in syndrome with bilateral ptosis: combination of bilateral horizontal pontine gaze paralysis and nuclear oculomotor nerve paralysis. J. Neurol. 232:366–367.

Dinsdale, H.B. 1964. Spontaneous hemorrhage in the posterior fossa. Arch. Neurol. 10:200–217.

Diringer, M.N., and Edwards, D.F. 1997. Does modification of the Innsbruck and the Glasgow coma scales improve their ability to predict functional outcome? Arch. Neurol. 54:606–611.

Dodge, P.R., and Swartz, M.N. 1965. Bacterial meningitis. II. Special neurologic problems, postmeningitis complications and clinico-pathological correlations. N. Engl. J. Med. 272:954–960.

Drury, I., Westmoreland, B.F., and Sharbrough, F.W. 1987. Fulminant demyelinating polyradiculoneuropathy resembling brain death. Electroencephalogr. Clin. Neurophysiol. 67:42–43.

Dusser, A., Nevelet, Y., Devictor, D., et al. 1989. Short- and long-term prognostic value of electroencephalogram in children with severe head injury. Electroencephalogr. Clin. Neurophysiol. 73:85–93.

Earnest, M.P., Beresford, H.R., and McIntyre, H.B. 1986. Testing for apnea in suspected brain death: methods used by 129 clinicians. Neurology 36:542–544.

Evans, B.M. 1976. Patterns of arousal in comatose patients. J. Neurol. Neurosurg. Psychiatry 39:392–402.

Evans, B.M., and Bartlett, J.R. 1995. Prediction of outcome in severe head injury based on recognition of sleep related activity in the polygraphic electroencephalogram. J. Neurol. Neurosurg. Psychiatry 59:17–25.

Facon, E., Steriade, M., and Wertheim, N. 1958. Hypersomnie prolongée engendrée par des lésions bilatérales due système activateur médial. Le syndrome thrombotique de la bifurcation du tronc basilaire. Rev. Neurol. 98:117–133.

Feldman, M.H. 1971. Physiological observations in a chronic case of "locked-in" syndrome. Neurology (Minneapolis) 21:459–478.

Feldmann, E., Gandy, S.E., Becker, R., et al. 1988. MRI demonstrates descending transtentorial herniation. Neurology 38:697–701.

Ficker, D.M., Westmoreland, B.F., and Sharbrough, F.W. 1997. Epileptiform abnormalities in hepatic encephalopathy. J. Clin. Neurophysiol. 14:230–234.

Fischer, C.M. 1969. The neurological examination of the comatose patient. Acta Neurol. Scand. 45(suppl 36):56.

Fischgold, H., and Mathis, P. 1959. Obnubilations, comas et stupeurs: Études électroencéphalographique. Electroencephalogr. Clin. Neurophysiol. (suppl 11). Paris: Masson.

Freitas, G.R., André, C., Bezerra M., et al. 2003. Persistence of isolated flow in the internal carotid artery in brain death. J. Neurol. Sci. 210:31–34.

French, J.D., and Magoun, H.W. 1952. Effects of chronic lesions in central cephalic brain stem of monkeys. Arch. Neurol. Psychiatry 68:591–604.

Ganes, T., and Lundar, T. 1983. The effect of Thiopentone on somatosensory evoked responses and EEG's in comatose patients. J. Neurol. Neurosurg. Psychiatry 46:509–514.

Garret, P.J., Mulcahy, D., Carmody, M., et al. 1988. Aluminium encephalopathy: clinical and immunological features. Q. J. Med. 69:775–783.

Gastaut, H., and Fischer-Williams, M. 1959. The physiopathology of epileptic seizures. In *Handbook of Physiology,* Eds. Y. Field et al., vol. 1, pp. 329–363. Washington: American Physiological Society.

Gelabert-González, M., and Fernández-Villa, J. 2001. Mutism after posterior fossa surgery. Review of the literature. Clin. Neurol. Neurosurg. 103:111–114.

Gentry, L.R., Godersky, J.C., and Thompson, B.H. 1989. Traumatic brain stem injury: MR imaging. Radiology 171:177–187.

Gerich, J.E., Martin, M.M., and Recan, L. 1971. Clinical and metabolic characteristic of hyperosmolar nonketotic coma. Diabetes 20:228–238.

Gerstenbrand, F. 1967 *Das Traumatische Apallische Syndrome.* Wien-New York: Springer-Verlag.

Gerstenbrand, F. 1973. Die klinische Symptomatik des irreversiblen Ausfalls der Hirnfunktionen (Das Vorstadium und die spinalen Reflexe). In *Die Bestimmung des Todeszeitpunktes,* Eds. W. Krösl and E. Scherzer, pp. 33–40. Wien: Maudrich.

Gerstenbrand, F., and Lücking, C.H. 1970. Die akuten traumatischen Hirnstammsträden. Arch. Psychiatr. Nervenkr. 213:264–281.

Gerstenbrand, F., Hackl, J.M., Mitterschifffthaler, G., et al. 1984. Die Innsbrucker Koma-Skala. Klinisches Koma-Monitoring. Intensivbehandlung 9:133–144.

Giacino, J.T., Ashwal, S., Childs, N., et al. 2002. The minimally conscious state. Neurology 58:349–353.

Gibbs, F.A., Gibbs, E.L., and Lennox, W.G. 1937. Effect on the electroencephalogram of certain drugs which influence nervous activity. Arch. Intern. Med. 60:154–166.

Gloor, P. 1976. Generalized and widespread bilateral paroxysmal activities. In *EEG Interpretation in Clinical Medicine. Handbook of Electroencephalography and Clinical Neurology,* vol. 11B, Ed. W. Cobb, pp. 52–87. Amsterdam: Elsevier.

Gloor, P., Kalabay, O., and Giard, N. 1968. The electroencephalogram in diffuse encephalopathies: electroencephalographic correlates of grey and white matter lesions. Brain 91:779–802.

Goudreau, J.L., Wijdicks, E.F.M., Emery, S.F. 2000. Complications during apnea testing in the determination of brain death: predisposing factors. Neurology 55:1045–1048.

Grigg, M.M., Kelly, M.A., Celesia, G.G., et al. 1987. Electroencephalographic activity after brain death. Arch. Neurol. 44:948–954.

Grindal, A.B., and Suter, C. 1975. "Alpha-pattern coma" in high voltage electrical injury. Electroencephalogr. Clin. Neurophysiol. 38:521–526.

Gros, C., Baldy-Moulinier, M., Gros-Massoubre, A., et al. 1969. L'avenir éloigné des comas traumatiques de l'enfant. Neuro-chirurgie 15:35–50.

Gütling, E., Gonser, A., Imhof, H-G., et al. 1995. EEG reactivity in the prognosis of severe head injury. Neurology 45:915–918.

Haider, I., Matthew, H., and Oswald, I. 1971. Electroencephalographic changes in acute poisoning. Electroencephalogr. Clin. Neurophysiol. 30: 23–31.

Halsey, J.H., and Downie, A.W. 1966. Decerebrate rigidity with preservation of consciousness. J. Neurol. Neurosurg. Psychiatry 29:350–354.

Handforth, A., Cheng, J.T., Mandelkern, M.A., et al. 1994. Markedly increased mesiotemporal lobe metabolism in a case with PLEDs: further evidence that PLEDs are a manifestation of partial status epilepticus. Epilepsia 35:876–881.

Harner, R.N., and Katz, R.I. 1975. Electroencephalography in metabolic coma. In Altered States of Consciousness, Coma, Cerebral Death. Handbook of Electroencephalography and Clinical Neurophysiology, vol. 12, Eds. R. Harner and R. Naquet, pp. 47–62. Amsterdam: Elsevier.

Harris, O.A., Colford, J.M., Good, M.C., et al. 2002. The role of hypothermia in the management of severe brain injury. Arch. Neurol. 59: 1077–1083.

Haupt, W.F., and Rudolf, J. 1999. European brain death codes: a comparison of national guidelines. J. Neurol. 246:432–437.

Hess, R. 1961. Significance of EEG signs for location of cerebral tumors. Electroencephalogr. Clin. Neurophysiol. Suppl. 19:75–110.

Hess, R. 1962. Die bioelektrischen Zeichen der cerebralen Massenverschiebung bei Hirntumoren. Schweiz. Med. Wschr. 92:1537–1542.

Hess, R. 1965. Sleep and sleep disturbances in the electroencephalogram. Prog. Brain Res. 18:127–139.

Himwich, H.E. 1951. Brain Metabolism and Cerebral Disorders. Baltimore: Williams & Wilkins.

Hirsch, H., Kubicki, S., Kugler, J., et al. 1970. Empfehlungen der Deutschen EEG-Gesellschaft zur Bestimmung der Todeszeit. Z. EEG-EMG 1:53–54.

Hoagland, H., Himwich, H.E., Campbell, E., et al. 1939. Effect of hypoglycemia and pentobarbital sodium on electrical activity of cerebral cortex and hypothalamus (dogs). J. Neurophysiol. 2:276–288.

Hochmann, M.S., Sowers, J.J., and Bruce-Gregorius, J. 1985. Syndrome of the mesencephalic artery: report of a case with CT and necropsy findings. J. Neurol. Neurosurg. Psychiatry 48:1179–1181.

Hockaday, J.M., Potts, F., Epstein, E., et al. 1965. EEG changes in acute cerebral anoxia from cardiac or respiratory arrest. Electroencephalogr. Clin. Neurophysiol. 18:575.

Horikawa, M., Harada, H., and Yarita, M. 2003. Detection limit in low-amplitude EEG measurement. J. Clin. Neurophysiol. 20:45–53.

Hulihan, J.F., and Syna, D.R. 1994. Electroencephalographic sleep patterns in post-anoxic stupor and coma. Neurology 44:758–760.

Hume, A.I., and Cant, B.R. 1981. Central somatosensory conduction after head injury. Ann. Neurol. 10:411–419.

Hutchinson, D.O., Frith, R.W., Shaw, N.A., et al. 1991. A comparison between electroencephalography and somatosensory evoked potentials for outcome predictions following severe head injury. Electroencephalogr. Clin. Neurophysiol. 78:228–233.

Illis, L.S., and Taylor, F.M. 1972. The electroencephalogram in Herpes-simplex encephalitis. Lancet 1:718–721.

Inao, S., Kuchiwaki, H., Kanaiwa, H., et al. 1993. Magnetic resonance imaging assessment of brainstem distortion associated with a supratentorial mass. J. Neurol. Neurosurg. Psychiatry 56:280–285.

Ingvar, D.H., and Brun, A. 1972. Das komplette apallische Syndrom. Arch. Psychiatr. Nervenkr. 215:219–239.

Ingvar, D.H., Haggendal, E., Nilsson, N.J., et al. 1964. Cerebral circulation and metabolism in a comatose patient. Arch. Neurol. 11:13–21.

Iragui, V.J., and McCutchen, Ch.B. 1983. Physiologic and prognostic significance of "alpha coma." J. Neurol. Neurosurg. Psychiatry 46:632–638.

Ivan, L.P. 1973. Spinal reflexes in cerebral death. Neurology (Minneapolis) 23:650–652.

Jacobs, B.S., Carhuapoma, J.C., and Castellanos, M. 2003. Editorial. Clarifying TCD criteria for brain death—are some arteries more equal than others? J. Neurol. Sci. 210:3–4.

Jasper, H.H., and Van Buren, J. 1953. Interrelationships between cortex and subcortical structures. Clinical electroencephalographic studies. Electroencephalogr. Clin. Neurophysiol. Suppl. 4:168–202.

Jellinger, K., and Seitelberger, F. 1970. Protracted post-traumatic encephalopathy: pathology, pathogenesis and clinical implications. J. Neurol. Sci. 10:51–94.

Jenkins, A., Teasdale, G., Hadley, M.D.M., et al. 1986. Brain lesions detected by magnetic resonance imaging in mild and severe head injuries. Lancet 1:445–446.

Jennet, B., and Plum, F. 1972. Persistent vegetative state after brain damage. A syndrome in search of a name. Lancet 1:734–737.

Jeret, J.S., and Benjamin, J.L. 1994. Risk of hypotension during apnea testing. Arch. Neurol. 51:595–599.

Jouvet, M. 1969. Coma and other disorders of consciousness. In Handbook of Clinical Neurology, vol. 3, Eds. P.J. Vinken and G.W. Bruyn, pp. 62–79. Amsterdam: North-Holland.

Kaplan, P.W. 1996. Nonconvulsive status epilepticus in the emergency room. Epilepsia 37:643–650.

Kaplan, P.W., Genoud, D., Ho, T.W., et al. 2000. Clinical correlates and prognosis in early spindle coma. Clin. Neurophysiol. 111:584–590.

Karbowski, K. 1975. Das Elektroencephalogramm im epileptischen Anfall. Bern: Hans Huber.

Karp, J.S., and Hurtig, H.I. 1974. "Locked-in" state with bilateral midbrain infarcts. Arch. Neurol. 30:176–178.

Kassubek, J., Juengling, F.D., Els, T., et al. 2003. Activation of a residual cortical network during painful stimulation in long-term postanoxic vegetative state: a 15O-H2O PET study. J. Neurol. Sci. 212:85–91.

Kiloh, C.G., Canas, A.J., and Osselton, J.W. 1972. Clinical Electroencephalography. London: Butterworths.

Koostra, G., Daemen, J.H.C., and Oomen, A.P.A. 1995. Categories of non-heart-beating donors. Transpl. Proc. 27:2893–2894.

Kramer, W., and Tuyman, J.A. 1967. Acute intracranial hypertension. An experimental investigation. Brain. Res. 686–705.

Kretschmer, E. 1940. Das apallische Syndrom. Z. Ges. Neurol. Psychiatr. 169:576–579.

Krieger, D., Adams, H.-P., Schwarz, St., et al. 1993. Prognostic and clinical relevance of pupillary responses, intracranial pressure monitoring, and brain stem auditory evoked potentials in comatose patients with supratentorial mass lesions. Crit. Care Med. 21:1944–1950.

Krumholz, A., Stern, B.J., and Weiss, H.D. 1988. Outcome from coma after cardiopulmonary resuscitation: relation to seizures and myoclonus. Neurology 38:401–405.

Kubicki, S., and Haas, J. 1975. Elektroklinische Korrelationen bei Komata unterschiedlicher Genese. Akt. Neurol. 2:103–112.

Kubicki, S., Just, O., and Trede, M. 1960. Die Bedeutung des EEG bei Herzoperationen in Hypothermie und extracorporaler Zirkulation. Anästhesist. 9:119–123.

Kubicki, S., Rieger, H., Busse, G., et al. 1970. Elektroenzephalographische Befunde bei schweren Schlafmittelvergiftungen. Z. EEG-EMG 1: 80–93.

Kugler, J., Angstwurm, H., Finsterer, U., et al. 1973. In Die Bestimmung des Todeszeitpunktes, Eds. W. Krösl and E. Scherzer, pp. 93–102. Wien: Maudrich.

Kugler, J., Martin, J.J., Radermecker, F.J., et al. 1976. Periodische Komplexe im EEG bei nekrotisierender Herpes-Enzephalitis. Z. EEG-EMG 7:63–71.

Kuroiwa, Y., and Celesia, G.G. 1980. Clinical significance of periodic EEG patterns. Arch. Neurol. 37:15–20.

Kuroiwa, Y., Celesia, G.G., and Chung, H.D. 1982. Periodic EEG discharges of the cerebral cortex in anoxic encephalopathy: a necropsy case report. J. Neurol. Neurosurg. Psychiatry 45:740–742.

Lee, R.G., and Blair, R.D.G. 1975. Evolution of EEG and visual evoked response changes in Jakob-Creutzfeldt disease. Electroencephalogr. Clin. Neurophysiol. 35:133–142.

Leestma, J.E., Hughes, J.R., and Diamond, E.R. 1984. Temporal correlates in brain death. Arch. Neurol. 41:147–152.

Lesse, S., Hoefer, P.F.A., and Austin, J.H. 1958. The electroencephalogram in diffuse encephalopathies. Arch. Neurol. Psychiatry. 79:359–375.

Levin, H.S., Saydjari, Ch., Eisenburg, H.M., et al. 1991. Vegetative state after closed-head injury. Arch. Neurol. 48:580–585.

Li, C.L., Jasper, H., and Henderson, L. 1952. The effect of arousal mechanisms of various forms of abnormality in the electroencephalogram. Electroencephalogr. Clin. Neurophysiol. 4:513–526.

Lindenberg, R. 1963. Patterns of CNS vulnerability in acute hypoxaemia, including anaesthesia accidents. In *Selective Vulnerability of the Brain in Hypoxaemia*, Eds. J.P. Schadé and W.H. McMenemy, pp. 189–205. Philadelphia: F.A. Davis.

Lindsley, D.B., Bowden, J.W., and Magoun, H.W. 1949. Effect upon the EEG of acute injury to the brain stem activating system. Electroencephalogr. Clin. Neurophysiol. 1:475–486.

Lindsley, D.B., Schreiner, L.H., and Magoun, H.W. 1950. Behavioral and EEG changes following chronic brain stem lesion in the cat. Electroencephalogr. Clin. Neurophysiol. 2:483–498.

Loeb, C. 1975a. Correlative EEG and clinico-pathological studies of patients in coma. In *Altered States of Consciousness, Coma, Cerebral Death,* vol. 11, Eds. R. Harner and R. Naquet, pp. 24–36. Amsterdam: Elsevier.

Loeb, C. 1975b. Pathology of cerebral death. In *Altered States of Consciousness, Coma, Cerebral Death,* vol. 11, Eds. R. Harner and R. Naquet, pp. 106–110. Amsterdam: Elsevier.

Loeb, C., and Poggio, G. 1953. Electroencephalograms in a case with ponto-mesencephalic haemorrhage. Electroencephalogr. Clin. Neurophysiol. 5:295–296.

Loeb, C., Mancardi, G.L., and Tabaton, M. 1984. Locked-in syndrome in acute inflammatory polyradiculoneuropathy. Eur. Neurol. 23:137–140.

Lowenstein, D.H., and Aminoff, M.J. 1992. Clinical and EEG features of status epilepticus in comatose patients. Neurology 42:100–104.

Lücking, C.H. 1970. Sleep-like patterns and abnormal arousal reactions in brain stem lesions. Electroencephalogr. Clin. Neurophysiol. 28:214(abst).

Lundervold, A., Hange, T., and Löken, A.C. 1956. Unusual EEG in unconscious patient with brain stem atrophy. Electroencephalogr. Clin. Neurophysiol. 8:665–670.

Maccario, M., Messis, C.P., and Vastola, E.F. 1965. Focal seizures as a manifestation of hyperglycemia without keto acidosis. Neurology (Minneapolis) 15:195–206.

MacGillivray. 1976. The EEG in liver disease. In *Metabolic, Endocrine and Toxic Diseases. Handbook of Electroencephalography and Clinical Neurophysiology,* vol. 15, Ed. D.D. Daly, pp. 26–50. Amsterdam: Elsevier.

Madison, D., and Niedermeyer, E. 1970. Epileptic seizures resulting from acute cerebral anoxia. J. Neurol. Neurosurg. Psychiatry 33:381–386.

Mantz, J.M., Tempe, J.D., Jager, A., et al. 1971. Silence électrique cérébral de 24 heurs au cours d'une intoxication massive par 10 g de Pentobarbital-Hémodialyse-Guérison. Presse Med. 79:1243–1246.

Markand, O.N., and Daly, D.D. 1971. Pseudoperiodic lateralized paroxysmal discharges in electroencephalogram. Neurology (Minneapolis) 21:975–981.

Marks, St.J., and Zisfein, J. 1990. Apneic oxygenation in apnea tests for brain death. A controlled trial. Arch. Neurol. 47:1066–1068.

Marti-Masso, J.F., Suarez, J., Lopez, de Munain, A., et al. 1993. Clinical signs of brain death simulated by Guillain-Barré syndrome. J. Neurol. Sci. 120:115–117.

Martin, F., Macken, J., and Hess, R. 1950. Sur une encéphalite subaigue, ayant les caractères de la leuco-encéphalite sclérosante, avec inclusions. Schweiz. Arch. Neurol. Psychiatr. 66:217–260.

Mayr, N., Zeitlhofer, J., Auff, E., et al. 1990. Die Bedeutung von EMG-Artefakten im isoelektrischen EEG. Z. EEG-EMG 21:56–58.

McNealy, D.E., and Plum, F. 1962. Brainstem dysfunction with supratentorial mass lesions. Arch. Neurol. 7:10–32.

Meienberg, O., Mumenthaler, M., and Karbowski, K. 1979. Quadriparesis and nuclear oculomotor palsy with total bilateral ptosis mimicking coma. Arch. Neurol. 36:708–710.

Mellerio, F. 1969. Problèmes posés par les aspects de silence cérébral électrique en toxicologie (à propos d'une intoxication aigue). Rev. Neurol. 120:481–482.

Meyer, J.S., Sakamoto, K., Akiyama, M., et al. 1967. Monitoring cerebral blood flow, metabolism and EEG. Electroencephalogr. Clin. Neurophysiol. 23:497–508.

Millar, J.H.D., and Coey, A. 1959. The EEG in necrotizing encephalitis. Electroencephalogr. Clin. Neurophysiol. 11:582–585.

Miller, J.W., Klass, D.W., Mokri, B., et al. 1986. Triphasic waves in cerebral carcinomatosis. Arch. Neurol. 43:1191–1193.

Mitchell, D.E., and Adams, J.M. 1973. Primary focal impact damage to the brainstem in blunt head injuries. Does it exist? Lancet II:215–218.

Molinari, G.F. 1991. Persistent vegetative state, do not resuscitate . . . and still more words doctors use. J. Neurol. Sci. 102:125–127.

Mollaret, P., and Goulon, M. 1959. Le coma dépassé. Rev. Neurol. 101:3–15.

Moshé, S. 1989. Usefulness of EEG in the evaluation of brain death in children: the pros. Electroencephalogr. Clin. Neurophysiol. 73:272–275.

Multi-Society Task Force on PVS. 1994a. Medical aspects of the persistent vegetative state (first of two parts). N. Engl. J. Med. 330:1499–1508.

Multi-Society Task Force on PVS. 1994b. Medical aspects of the persistent vegetative state (second of two parts). N. Engl. J. Med. 330:1572–1578.

Munsat, Th.L., Stuart, W.H., and Cranford, R.E. 1989. Guidelines on the vegetative state. Neurology 39:123–124.

Naquet, R., and Fernandez-Guardiola, A. 1959. Effects of various types of anoxia on spontaneous and evoked cerebral activity in the cat. In *Cerebral Anoxia and the Electroencephalogram,* Eds. H. Gastaut and J.S. Meyer, pp. 72–88. Springfield, IL: Charles C Thomas.

Nayyar, M., Strobos, R.J., Singh, B.M., et al. 1987. Caloric-induced nystagmus with isoelectric electroencephalogram. Ann. Neurol. 21:98–100.

New, P.F.J., and Scott, W.R. 1975. *Computerized Tomography of the Brain and Orbit.* Baltimore: Williams & Wilkins.

Niedermeyer, E. 1999. A concept of consciousness. Ital. J. Neurol. Sci. 20:7–15.

Niedermeyer, E., and Khalifeh, R. 1965. Petit mal status ("spike wave stupor"). Epilepsia 6:250–262.

Noell, W.G., and Dombrowski, E.B. 1947. Cerebral localization and classification of convulsions produced by a severe oxygen lack. Project 497, Report 1. Randolph Field. TX: School of Aviation Medicine.

Nogueira de Melo, A., Krauss, G.L., and Niedermeyer, E. 1990. Spindle coma: observations and thoughts. Clin. Electroencephalogr. 21:151–161.

Normand, M.M., Wszolek, Z.K., and Klass, D.W. 1995. Temporal intermittent rhythmic delta activity in electroencephalograms. J. Clin. Neurophysiol. 12:280–284.

Nyberg-Hansen, R., Loken, A.C., and Tenstad, O. 1978. Brainstem lesion with coma for five years following manipulation of the cervical spine. J. Neurol. 218:97–105.

Ogata, J., Imakita, M., Yutani, C., et al. 1988. Primary brainstem death: a clinic-pathological study. J. Neurol. Neurosurg. Psychiatry 51:646–650.

Okonek, S., and Rieger, H. 1975. EEG-Veränderungen bei Alkylphosphat-Vergiftungen. Z. EEG-EMG 6:19–27.

Orthner, H. 1969. Neuroanatomische Gesichtspunkte der Schlaf-Wach-Regulierung. In *Der Schlaf,* Ed. U. Jovanovic, pp. 49–84. München: Barth.

Pampiglione, G. 1962a. EEG studies after cardio-pulmonary resuscitation. Proc. R. Soc. Med. 55:653.

Pampiglione, G. 1962b. Resuscitation after cardiac arrest. Electroencephalogr. Clin. Neurophysiol. 14:294.

Pampiglione, G., and Harden, A. 1968. Resuscitation after cardio-vascular arrest. Prognostic evaluation and early electroencephalographic findings. Lancet 1:1261–1264.

Parvizi, J., and Damasio, R. 2003. Neuroanatomical correlates of brainstem coma. Brain 126:1524–1536.

Passouant, P., Cadilhac, J., Delange, M., et al. 1964. Différents stades électriques et organisation en cycles des comas post-traumatiques. Enrégistrage polygraphique de longue durée. Rev. Neurol. 111:391.

Peabody, J.L., Janet, R.E., and Ashwal, St. 1989. Experience with anencephalic infants as prospective organ donors. N. Engl. J. Med. 321:344–350.

Penin, H., and Käufer, C. (Eds.) 1969. *Der Hirntod.* Stuttgart: Thieme.

Plum, F. 1972. Organic disturbances of consciousness. In *Scientific Foundations of Neurology,* Eds. M. Critchley, J.L.O. O'Leary, and B. Jennet, pp. 193–201. Philadelphia: F.A. Davis.

Plum, F., and Posner, J.B. 1966. *The Diagnosis of Stupor and Coma.* Philadelphia: F.A. Davis.

Prior, P.F. 1973. *The EEG in Acute Cerebral Anoxia.* Amsterdam: Excerpta Medica.

Quality Standards Subcommittee of the American Academy of Neurology. 1995. Practice parameters for determining brain death in adults. Neurology 45:1012–1014.

Radermecker, J. 1956. Systématique et électroencéphalographie des encéphalites et encéphalopathies. Electroencephalogr. Clin. Neurophysiol. Suppl. 5.

Radermecker, J., and Macken, J. 1951. Aspects électroencéphalographiques et cliniques de la leucoencéphalite sclérosante subaigue. Rev. Neurol. 83:341.

Reich, J.B., Sierra, J., Camp, W., et al. 1993. Magnetic resonance imaging and clinical changes accompanying transtentorial and foramen magnum brain herniation. Ann. Neurol. 33:159–170.

Reiher, J. 1970. The electroencephalogram in the investigation of metabolic comas. Electroencephalogr. Clin. Neurophysiol. 28:104.

Reither, J., Braudry, M., and Leduc, C.P. 1984. Temporal intermittent delta activity (TIRDA) and the diagnosis of complex partial epilepsy: sensitivity, specificity, and predictive value. Can. J. Neurol. Pei.16:398–401.

Richardson, J.C., Chambers, R.A., and Heywood, P.M. 1959. Encephalopathies of anoxia and hypoglycemia. Arch. Neurol. 1:178–190.

Richter, H.R. 1973. Elektroencephalographie (EEG), Todeszeitbestimmung und der Tod als modernes Tabu. In *Die Bestimmung des Todeszeitpunktes,* Eds. W. Krösl and E. Scherzer, pp. 85–91. Wien: Maudrich.

Rohmer, R., Kurtz, D., and Kiffer, A. 1965. Étude critique de l'activité E.E.G. dan les syndromes vasculaires du tronc cérébral. Rev. Neurol. 113:278–284.

Romano, J., and Engel, G.L. 1944. Delirium. I: Electroencephalographic data. Arch. Neurol. Psychiatry 52:290–295.

Ropper, A.H. 1986. Lateral displacement of the brain and level of consciousness in patients with an acute hemispheral mass. N. Engl. J. Med. 314:953–958.

Ropper, A.H. 1993. Syndrome of transtentorial herniation: is vertical displacement necessary? J. Neurol. Neurosurg. Psychiatry 56:932–935.

Rossi, G.F. 1964. A hypothesis on the neural basis of consciousness. Considerations based upon some experimental work. Acta Neurochir. 12: 187–197.

Rossi, G.F. 1965. Some aspects of the functional organization of the brain stem: neurophysiological and neurosurgical observations. Copenhagen. III Int. Congr. Neurol. Surg. Excerpta Med., pp. 117–122.

Rothstein, T.L. 1993. Redefining brain death. Lancet 342:180.

Rowley, G., and Fielding, K. 1991. Reliability and accuracy of the Glasgow Coma Scale with experienced and unexperienced users. Lancet 337: 535–538.

Ruggiero, G., Sabattini, L., and Nuzzo, G. 1977. Computerized tomography and encephalography. Neuroradiology 13:45–48.

Rumpl, E., Lorenzi, E., Hackl, J.M., et al. 1979. The EEG at different stages of acute secondary traumatic midbrain and bulbar brain syndromes. Electroencephalogr. Clin. Neurophysiol. 46:487–497.

Rumpl, E., Prugger, M., Bauer, G., et al. 1983a. Incidence and prognostic value of spindles in posttraumatic coma. Electroencephalogr. Clin. Neurophysiol. 56:420–429.

Rumpl, E., Prugger, M., Gerstenbrand, F., et al. 1983b. Central somatosensory evoked potentials in posttraumatic coma. Electroencephalogr. Clin. Neurophysiol. 56:583–596.

Sacco, R.L., VanGool, R., Mohr, J.P., et al. 1990. Nontraumatic coma. Glasgow coma score and coma etiology as predictors of 2-week outcome. Arch. Neurol. 47:1181–1184.

Sament, S., and Huott, A.D. 1969. The EEG in acute barbiturate intoxication with particular reference to isoelectric EEGs. Electroencephalogr. Clin. Neurophysiol. 27:695.

Saunders, M.G. 1975. Medico-legal aspects of brain death. In *Altered States of Consciousness, Coma, Cerebral Death. Handbook of Electroencephalography and Clinical Neurophysiology,* vol. 11, Eds. R. Harner and R. Naquet, pp. 129–143. Amsterdam: Elsevier.

Schaul, N., Gloor, P., and Gotman, J. 1981. The EEG in deep midline lesions. Neurology (New York) 31:157–167.

Schiffter, R., and Schliack, H. 1975. Bewußtseinsverlust. Akt. Neurol. 2:69–72.

Schneider, S. 1989. Usefulness of EEG in the evaluation of brain death in children: the cons. Electroencephalogr. Clin. Neurophysiol. 73:276–278.

Schröder, R. 1983. Later changes in brain death. Signs of partial recirculation. Acta Neuropathol. (Berl.) 62:15–23.

Schwab, R.S., Potts, F., and Bonazzi, A. 1963. EEG as an aid in determining death in the presence of cardiac activity (ethical, legal and medical aspects). Electroencephalogr. Clin. Neurophysiol. 15:147–148.

Schwab, S., Spranger, M., Schwarz, S., et al. 1997. Barbiturate coma in severe hemispheric stroke: useful or obsolete? Neurology 48:1608–1613.

Schwartz, B., and Vendrely, E. 1969. Un des problèmes posés par le diagnostic du coma dépassé: EEG nul et diamètre pupillaire. Rev. Neurol. 121:319–323.

Schwartz, M.S., and Scott, D.F. 1978. Pathological stimulus-related slow wave arousal response in the EEG. Acta Neurol. Scand. 57:300–304.

Schwartz, M.S., Prior, P.F., and Scott, D.F. 1973. The occurrence and evolution in the EEG of a lateralized periodic phenomenon. Brain 96:613–622.

Schweizerische Akademie der Medizinischen Wissenschaften. 1996. Richtlinien zur Definition und Feststellung des Todes im Hinblick auf Organtransplantationen. Schweiz. Ärztezeitung 30:1773–1780.

Shakhnovich, A.R., Thomas, J.G., Duboca, S.D., et al. 1980. The prognosis of the outcome of comatose states. Resuscitation 8:243–255.

Sharbrough, F.W., Westmoreland, B.F., Reagan, T.J., et al. 1975. The significance of a transitional monorhythmic EEG pattern in patients after cardiopulmonary arrest. Neurology (Minneapolis) 27:384–385.

Shewmon, D.A. 1988. Commentary on guidelines for the determination of brain death in children. Ann. Neurol. 24:789–791.

Silverman, D. 1963. Retrospective study of the EEG in coma. Electroencephalogr. Clin. Neurophysiol. 15:486–503.

Silverman, D. 1975. The electroencephalogram in anoxic coma. In *Altered States of Consciousness, Coma, Cerebral Death. Handbook of Electroencephalography and Clinical Neurophysiology,* vol. 11, Eds. R. Harner and R. Naquet, pp. 81–94. Amsterdam: Elsevier.

Silverman, D., Saunders, M.G., Schwab, R.S., et al. 1969. Cerebral death and the electroencephalogram. JAMA 209:1505–1510.

Silverman, D., Masland, R.L., Saunders, M.G., et al. 1970. Irreversible coma associated with electrocerebral silence. Neurology (Minneapolis) 20:525–533.

Simm, M. 1996. Germany struggles with organ transplantation. Nature Med. 2:615.

Simon, R.P., and Aminoff, M.J. 1986. Electroencephalographic status epilepticus in fatal anoxic coma. Ann. Neurol. 20:351–355.

Simsarian, J.P., and Harner, R. 1972. Diagnosis of metabolic encephalopathy: Significance of triphasic waves in the electroencephalogram. Neurology (Minneapolis) 22:456.

Specht, F. 1964. Ponstumoren und Bewußtseinszustand. Arch. Psychiat. Z. Ges. Neurol. 20:323–344.

Spudis, E.V. 1991. The persistent vegetative state—1990. J. Neurol. Sci. 102:128–136.

Spudis, E.V., Penry, J.K., and Link, A.S. 1984. Paradoxical contributions of EEG during protracted dying. Arch. Neurol. 41:154–156.

Staudt, F., Engel, R.C., and Coen, R.W. 1983. Rhythmische Alpha-Aktivitäten im EEG von Früh- und Neugeborenen. Z. EEG-EMG 14:22–27.

Stojkovic, T., Verdin, M., Hurtevent, J.F., et al. 2001. Guillain-Barré syndrome resembling brainstem death in a patient with brain injury. J. Neurol. 248:430–432.

Storm van Leeuwen, W. 1964. Electroencephalographical and neurophysiological aspects of subacute sclerosing leucoencephalitis. Psychiatr. Neurol. Neurochir. (Amst.) 67:312–322.

Sugar, O., and Gerard, R.W. 1938. Anoxia and brain potentials. J. Neurophysiol. 1:558–572.

Suter, C. 1974. Clinical advances in the evaluation of deep coma. MCV Q. 10:152–162.

Suter, C. 1977. Brain death. MCV Q. 13:83–87.

Synek, V.M., and Glasgow, G.L. 1985. Recovery from alpha coma after decompression sickness complicated by spinal cord lesions at cervical and midthoracic levels. Electroencephalogr. Clin. Neurophysiol. 60:417–419.

Synek, V.M., and Synek, B.J.L. 1984. Theta pattern coma, a variant of alpha pattern coma. Clin. Electroencephalogr. 15:116–121.

Teasdale, G., and Jennet, B. 1974. Assessment of coma and impaired consciousness. A practical scale. Lancet 2:81–83.

Terzano, M.G., Parrino, L., Mazzuchi, A., et al. 1986. Confusional states with periodic lateralized epileptiform discharges (PLEDs): a peculiar epileptic syndrome in the elderly. Epilepsia 27:446–457.

Tomassen, W., and Kamphuisen, H.A.C. 1986. Alpha coma. J. Neurol. Sci. 76:1–11.

Torack, R.M., Alcala, H., Gado, M., et al. 1976. Correlative assay of computerized cranial tomography (CCT), water content and specific gravity in normal and pathological post mortem brain. J. Neuropathol. Exp. Neurol. 34:385–392.

Towsend, J.B., and Drury, J. 1991. Triphasic waves in coma from brainstem infarction. Eur. Neurol. 31:47–49.

Truog, R.D., and Fletcher, J.C. 1989. Anencephalic newborns. Can organs be transplanted before brain death? N. Engl. J. Med. 321:388–391.

Tsubokawa, T., Nishimoto, H., Yamamoto, T., et al. 1980. Assessment of brainstem damage by the auditory brainstem response in acute severe head injuries. J. Neurol. Neurosurg. Psychiatry 43:1005–1011.

Uematsu, D., Suematsu, M., Fukunchi, Y., et al. 1985. Midbrain locked-in state with oculomotor subnucleus lesion. J. Neurol. Neurosurg. Psychiatry 48:952–956.

Upton, A., and Gumpert, J. 1970. Electroencephalography in diagnosis of herpes-simplex encephalitis. Lancet 1:650–652.

Valente, M., Placidi, F., Oliveira, A.J., et al. 2002. Sleep organization pattern as a prognostic marker at the subacute stage of post-traumatic coma. Clin. Neurophysiol. 113:1798–1805.

Van Donselaar, C.A., Meerwaldt, J.D., and VanGijin, J. 1986. Apnea testing to confirm brain death in clinical practice. J. Neurol. Neurosurg. Psychiatry 49:1071–1073.

Vignaendra, V.M.B., Wilkus, R.J., Copass, M.K., et al. 1974. Electroencephalographic rhythms of alpha frequency in comatose patients after cardiopulmonary arrest. Neurology (Minneapolis) 24:582–588.

Vigouroux, R.P. 1975. Between life and death. In *Altered States of Consciousness, Coma, Cerebral Death. Handbook of Electroencephalography and Clinical Neurophysiology,* vol. 11, Eds. R. Harner and R. Naquet, pp. 95–99. Amsterdam: Elsevier.

Vigouroux, R., Naquet, R., Baurand, C., et al. 1964. Évolution electro-radioclinique de comas graves prolongés post traumatiques. Rev. Neurol. 110:72–80.

Ward, A.A., and Wheatley, F.R. 1947. Sodium cyanide. Sequence of changes of activity induced at various levels of the central nervous system. J. Neuropathol. Exp. Neurol. 6:292–294.

Waugh, J.R., and Sacharias, N. 1992. Arteriographic complications in the DSA era. Radiology 182:243–246.

Westmoreland, B.F., Klass, D.W., Sharbrough, F.W., et al. 1975. Alpha-coma. Electroencephalographic, clinical, pathologic and etiologic correlations. Arch. Neurol. 32:713–718.

Wijdicks, E.F.M. 1995. Determining brain death in adults. Neurology 45:1003–1011.

Wijdicks, E.F.M. 2001. The diagnosis of brain death. N. Engl. J. Med. 344:1215–1221.

Wijdicks, E.F.M., and Miller, G.M. 1997. MR imaging of progressive downward herniation of the diencephalon. Neurology 48:1456–1459.

Williams, C.P.S., Swanson, A.G., and Chapman, J.T. 1964. Brain swelling with acute purulent meningitis. Pediatrics 34:220–227.

Williams, G.R., and Spencer, F.C. 1958. The clinical use of hypothermia following cardiac arrest. Ann. Surg. 148:462.

Yamamoto, M., and Hosokawa, K. 1984. Triphasic spike-wave stupor in portal-systemic encephalopathy: a case report. J. Neurol. Neurosurg. Psychiatry 48:386–387.

Yasuda, Y., Akiguchi, I., and Kameyama, M. 1988. Prolonged disturbance of consciousness with periodic EEG discharges after fulminant hepatitis. J. Neurol. 235:318–320.

Young, G.B., Gilbert, J.J., and Zochodne, D.W. 1990. The significance of myoclonic status epilepticus in postanoxic coma. Neurology 40:1843–1948.

Young, G.B., Bolton, C.F., Archibald, Y.M., et al. 1992. The electroencephalogram in sepsis-associated encephalopathy. J. Clin. Neurophysiol. 9:145–152.

Young, G.B., Blume, W.T., Campbell, V.M., et al. 1994. Alpha, theta and alpha-theta coma: a clinical outcome study utilizing serial recordings. Electroencephalogr. Clin. Neurophysiol. 91:93–99.

Zaret, B.S. 1985. Prognostic and neurophysiological implications of concurrent burst suppression and alpha patterns in the EEG of postanoxic coma. Electroencephalogr. Clin. Neurophysiol. 61:199–209.

Zeman, A. 2001. Consciousness. Brain 124:1263–1289.

25. Infraslow EEG Activity

Sampsa Vanhatalo, Juha Voipio, and Kai Kaila

The conventional way of recording electroencephalogram (EEG) is about half a century old. The early pioneers were faced with the challenge to design routine EEG techniques that enabled recordings of the most salient features in the human EEG known at that time. A major obstacle was encountered in attempts to faithfully record slow events. Electrode drifts that produced artefactual slow signals tended to saturate the amplifier's dynamic range, and they also pushed the polygraph recorder pens out of scale. To circumvent these problems, the EEG amplifiers became furnished with an in-built high-pass filter. Hence, all kinds of slow signals, whether physiological or artefactual, were eliminated.

In practice, the technical compromise described above means that the conventional EEG has a poor low-frequency response, which results in attenuation and distortion of signals at <0.5 Hz. This is in sharp contrast with a wealth of data showing that the physiological frequency range of human EEG signals ranges from infraslow (0.01 Hz or even less, as discussed in this chapter) to ultrafast (up to several hundreds of Hz; see Chapter 26) frequencies. We will present several lines of evidence to demonstrate that, at the present stage of EEG technology, any trade-off in attempts to improve the stability of recordings at the expense of their frequency response has no solid scientific or technical basis. In fact, filtering off the lower end of the EEG spectrum by the standard high pass at around 0.5 Hz can lead to a situation where the most salient features of the EEG are effectively deleted. This kind of a massive loss of relevant data is clearly evident, for instance, in standard EEG recordings of the immature human brain, and during epileptic events.

Due to historical reasons, the terminology related to recording slow EEG events is somewhat confusing. The term *direct-current EEG* (DC EEG) has been widely used in older literature, to imply an ideal frequency response of the EEG with a minimum at 0 Hz. However, the term *DC* has at least two connotations, which are misleading. First, it is practically impossible to have a *by definition* 0-Hz response, since this would mean that slow EEG voltage shifts with a time constant of weeks, months, and even years could be recorded. Second, the use of the term *DC EEG* puts an a priori emphasis on the low-frequency part of the EEG spectrum, but, as we will show below, looking at low frequencies does not compromise any simultaneous analyses carried out at fast or even ultrafast frequencies. The results described here show that EEG responses, with a time course of several minutes to achieve their peak levels, can be easily recorded if attention is paid to trivial aspects of EEG electrode and amplifier design and characteristics (Bauer et al., 1989; Vanhatalo et al., 2003a–c; Voipio et al., 2003).

Hence, instead of the old DC-EEG nomenclature, we prefer using the term *full-band EEG* (FbEEG). This conveys the idea that the full, physiologically and clinically relevant EEG bandwidth can be examined in any given recording session. It is also worth noting that FbEEG is not based on a trade-off that would favor any frequency band at the expense of another.

Slow Activity in the Preterm Human EEG

In a recent study with FbEEG recordings from preterm neonates, we found that the most salient frequency range that dominated the total spectral power was much below the conventional EEG frequency band (Fig. 25.1; Vanhatalo et al., 2002). This is consistent with the previous well-known observations that an abundance of slow activity is a major feature of EEG activity in the immature brain (Lamblin et al., 1999; Watanabe et al., 1999; see also Chapters 11 and 50). In preterms at an age of 33 gestational weeks, the spectral power peaks at frequencies as low as 0.01 to 0.1 Hz (Fig. 25.1B). It is obvious that when recorded using conventional EEG, this kind of activity must be highly attenuated and distorted by filtering. Hence, only some faint echoes of the slow neonatal EEG activity can be detected at around the lower edge of the conventional recording bandwidth.

Most notably, FbEEG showed that the perinatal human EEG exhibits very slow (up to 5 seconds) spontaneous activity transients (SAT). Furthermore, most of the faster EEG activity is nested within these slow events, and hence practically all of the EEG activity of the immature cortex is associated with the SATs (Fig. 25.1A; Vanhatalo et al., 2002). This is an extremely interesting finding in itself, and in light of animal experiments that have demonstrated that endogenously driven, spontaneous activity is crucial in shaping neuronal connectivity in the developing brain wiring at an early immature stage where sensory input has little or no role at all (Katz and Shatz, 1996).

FbEEG recordings not only unravel a fully novel type of activity in the immature human cortex in the low-frequency bandwidth, but also it is obvious that these data call for a revised nomenclature for the perinatal EEG. Future studies will show whether work of this kind might set the stage for the identification and diagnostics of activity-dependent diseases and malfunctions of the immature brain of the kind proposed by Shatz and collaborators (Penn and Shatz, 1999).

Infraslow EEG Oscillations and Voltage Shifts During Sleep

Using FbEEG, infraslow oscillations (ISOs) that take place at a wide range of frequencies (0.02-0.2 Hz) with an

A

Conventional bandwidth

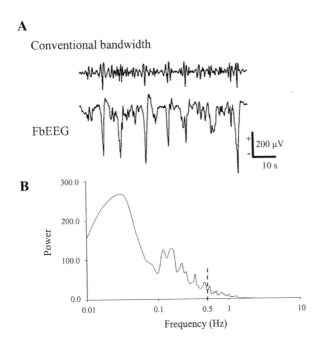

FbEEG

B

Figure 25.1. Slow activity in the perinatal human cortex. Specimen recording of full-band EEG (FbEEG) activity (at O1 vs. Cz) of a premature neonate at 33 weeks of conceptional age shows prominent spontaneous activity transients. FbEEG data (**A,** *lower trace*) was high-pass filtered offline at 0.5 Hz (**A,** *upper trace*) in order to demonstrate the pronounced loss (attenuation, distortion) of slow activity. This is also clearly seen in the power spectrum of FbEEG data from the same experiment (**B**). Note the small fraction of the total EEG power above the conventional cutoff frequency of 0.5 Hz *(dashed line)*. FFT was obtained from three 3-minute segments, using 60-second Hanning window. (Modified from Vanhatalo, S., Rivera, C., Palva, J.M., et al. 2004a. Large-scale spontaneous activity and up-regulation of KCC2 in the developing human cortex. *Submitted.*)

amplitude of up to several tens of microvolts are readily observed during non-rapid-eye-movement (REM) sleep (Vanhatalo et al., 2004b). Interestingly, the phase of ISO shows a robust correlation with higher frequency EEG activities (Fig. 25.2) as well as with phasic brain events, such as the K complex or interictal epileptiform activity. ISOs recorded by FbEEG in humans may thus reflect slow cyclic modulation of cortical excitability under both physiological and patho-

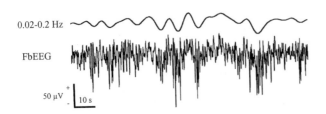

Figure 25.2. Infraslow oscillation during sleep. A 2-minute epoch of FbEEG activity recorded during slow-wave sleep (midfrontal derivation against a calculated linked mastoid reference, adult subject). Data is shown as FbEEG and following band-pass filtering at 0.02 to 0.2 Hz to visualize the prominent infraslow oscillation and its phase locking to activity at higher frequencies. (Modified from Vanhatalo, S., Palva, J.M., Holmes, M.D., et al. 2004b. Infraslow oscillations modulate interictal epileptic activity in the human cortex during sleep. *Submitted.*)

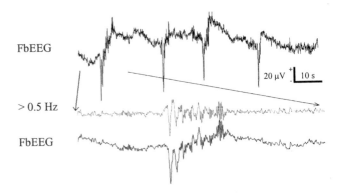

Figure 25.3. Direct current (DC) shifts associated with arousals during sleep. Large positive DC shifts are seen at vertex during transient arousals. One event is shown on an expanded time scale in the *middle* and *lower traces* to illustrate how only the faster activity that is associated with the ascending phase of the positive shift can be seen when using a conventional EEG bandwidth. (Unpublished observations of S. Vanhatalo, J.M. Palva, J. Voipio, and K. Kaila.)

physiological conditions. This idea fits well with results obtained in *in vivo* experiments on rats (Penttonen et al., 1999) and monkeys (Leopold et al., 2003).

Transient arousals during sleep are associated with a vertex-positive DC shift with an amplitude that may exceed hundred microvolts, and a duration of several tens of seconds (Fig. 25.3). A comparable, very slow positive DC shift is also seen during awakening or change in sleep stage to more superficial one, while a vertex negative DC shift takes place when the person falls asleep or shifts to deeper sleep stages (Marshall et al., 1998). Finally, it should be noted that spontaneous infraslow oscillations have been reported in awake subjects (Girton et al., 1973).

Slow EEG Signals Generated by Seizure Activity

Invasive recordings in experimental animals (Caspers et al., 1987; Gumnit and Takahashi, 1965; Mayanagi and Walker, 1975) and humans (Goldring 1963; Wieser et al., 1985) have established that seizures are associated with very slow EEG responses. Early pioneering work in the 1960s (Bates, 1963; Chatrian et al., 1968; Cohn, 1964) demonstrated that ictal DC shifts may be recorded also from the scalp during generalized seizures, but technical difficulties have limited noninvasive, ictal recordings of focal seizures until recently (Ikeda et al., 1999; Vanhatalo et al., 2003a). In addition, some more recent invasive studies using DC-incompatible electrodes (Tallgren et al., 2002) and long time constant alternating current (AC) amplifiers have demonstrated variable low-frequency fluctuations at the seizure focus (Gross et al., 1999; Ikeda et al., 1999).

Our recent study (Vanhatalo et al., 2003a) using FbEEG recordings on epilepsy patients undergoing presurgical evaluation demonstrated that focal seizures are associated with DC shifts that confine to the area with seizure activity (Fig. 25.4). The ictal DC shifts usually begin within seconds after the initiation of electrographic seizure activity, continuing throughout the seizure with slow fluctuation of the ampli-

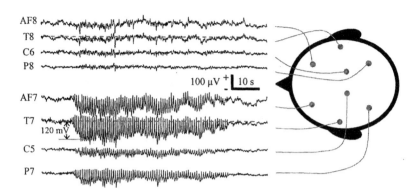

Figure 25.4. Lateralized DC shift during a seizure. FbEEG recording from scalp during a subclinical partial seizure from an adult patient with temporal lobe epilepsy reveals an unilateral negative DC shift with a clear spatiotemporal correlation with spiking activity. All traces are shown against a linked Cz + Oz reference. (Modified from Vanhatalo, S., Holmes, M.D., Tallgren, P., et al. 2003a. Very slow EEG responses lateralize temporal lobe seizures: an evaluation of non-invasive DC-EEG. Neurology 60:1098–1102.)

tude that can reach a level of over hundred microvolts (Fig. 25.4). While the polarity of the ictal DC shifts has been invariably negative when recording directly on the cortical surface above the ictal focus, it may vary when recording seizures from the scalp.

Using simultaneous intracranial and FbEEG recordings, we found that the onset of the scalp-recorded DC shift can often disclose the side (lateralization) of seizure initiation (Fig. 25.4), even in cases where other noninvasive studies (such as video-EEG and neuroimaging) are equivocal. These findings strongly suggest that in noninvasive recordings of ictal EEG activity (see also Lagerlund and Gross, 2003), the bandwidth should be extended to the low frequencies that are readily seen in FbEEG.

Nonneuronal EEG Signals Associated with Changes in Respiration and Hemodynamics

While it is evident that fast EEG activity has a neuronal origin, slow EEG signals may arise from a variety of sources, including both neuronal and nonneuronal generators. Below, we use the term *nonneuronal* when referring to generators of EEG signals that do not arise from the brain tissue parenchyma, i.e., neurons and glial cells (Voipio et al., 2003).

To study the contribution of nonneuronal potential shifts to human FbEEG signals, we have used manipulations known to induce pH shifts at the level of the BBB as well as large hemodynamic changes in healthy subjects (Voipio et al., 2003; Vanhatalo et al., 2003b; Fig. 25.5). Voluntary hyperventilation for a few minutes induced a progressive negative shift with an astonishingly high peak value of up to 2 mV at vertex, whereas hypoventilation caused positive shifts (Voipio et al., 2003). As discussed in detail elsewhere (Voipio et al., 2003), the high amplitude and duration (several minutes) of these scalp-recorded signals cannot be explained on the basis of any neuronal generator mechanism, such as a change in the state of tonic excitation of apical dendrites in cortical pyramidal neurons (Birbaumer et al., 1990; Caspers et al., 1987). Furthermore, bilateral jugular vein compression, head-up and head-down tilt, and Valsalva and Mueller maneuvers all resulted in pronounced DC shifts that were highest at midline derivations and showed a temporal correlation with hemodynamic changes monitored using near-infrared spectroscopy (Vanhatalo et al., 2003b).

The results described above are in agreement with early work (Besson et al., 1970; Sorensen et al., 1978; Woody et al., 1970) which has demonstrated large shifts in the potential of brain tissue that correlate strikingly well with changes in cerebral blood flow and/or CO_2/pH, and are generated across the blood-brain barrier (BBB). Such nonneuronal changes in the potential of brain parenchyma are readily conducted to scalp, which fully accounts for the large DC shifts seen in FbEEG recordings (Voipio et al., 2003).

The fact that slow EEG signals can arise at the level of the BBB has a number of implications. For instance, it is easy to envisage that epileptic activity, known to cause a large change in local blood flow (Duncan, 1997), may produce a DC shift (see above) that is at least to some extent generated by the BBB in the region associated with neuronal hyperactivity. Also, slow signals related to cognitive paradigms may be prone to "contamination" by BBB-generated potentials that arise in response to uncontrolled changes in respiration and end-tidal CO_2 during the cognitive tasks (see also Voipio et al., 2003).

In light of the available data, it is clear that much more work is needed to elucidate the relative contributions and interactions of nonneuronal and neuronal/glial generators to DC shifts seen in both invasive and noninvasive recordings of brain activity.

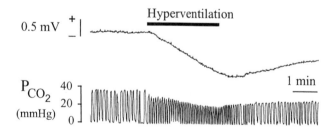

Figure 25.5. Large nonneuronal DC shift caused by hyperventilation. Voluntary hyperventilation gives rise to a progressively increasing negative DC shift that has a millivolt-scale amltitude at vertex (mastoid reference, healthy adult subject). The DC shift is closely paralleled by a fall in end-tidal partial pressure of CO_2 (P_{CO_2}; continuous capnograph signal). (Modified from Voipio, J., Tallgren, P., Heinonen, E., Vanhatalo, S., and Kaila, K. 2003. Ultraslow DC shifts in the human EEG: evidence for a non-neuronal generator. J. Neurophysiol. 89:2208-2214.)

Slow EEG Activity, Cognitive States, and Event-Related Potentials

During the last decades, much if not most of the research on low-frequency EEG has focused on slow potentials that are associated with various kinds of cognitive tasks and states (Birbaumer et al., 1990, 2003; Cui et al., 1999), such as contingent stimulation (contingent negative variation, CNV), motor movements (Bereitschaftspotential), and the orienting paradigm. Subjects may also learn to deliberately induce slow scalp-recorded potentials, which has been used in attempts to construct functional brain-computer interfaces (Hinterberger et al., 2003). All these potentials have a duration of up to several seconds and often an amplitude in the order of only a few microvolts, hence requiring an FbEEG as well as electrodes with an optimal DC performance (Tallgren et al., 2002) for their accurate recording. In addition, the fact that nonneuronal EEG signals are readily elicited by changes in respiration patterns (see section above) calls for caution in the interpretation of slow EEG signals related to cognitive tasks and preparatory states (Vanhatalo et al., 2003c; Voipio et al., 2003).

In addition to slow EEG responses seen in cognitive studies of the kind referred to above, careful analysis of long-latency components (up to ~2,500 msec) of sensory evoked potentials may possess significant potential for clinical monitoring of brain functions. For instance, it has been shown that long latency components of auditory evoked potential correlate nicely with deepening of anesthesia as well as with emergence from anesthesia (Fitzgerald et al., 2001), thus raising the possibility that they could be effectively utilized in anesthesia monitoring. In addition, large slow potential shifts, which may share a number of characteristics with the ISOs described above, have also been reported during anesthesia (Roughan and Laming, 1998).

Conclusions

It is obvious that FbEEG with its capability to record slow activity of the human brain has a wide range of potential applications in both basic science and in the clinic. Above, we have shown that FbEEG is mandatory for faithful, nondistorted, and nonattenuated recording of the most salient aspects of EEG activity seen under a wide variety of circumstances. These include recordings of immature human cortical activity and epileptic seizures, as well as EEG studies of sleep and of various kinds of cognitive tasks and states.

It is likely that the scope of FbEEG measurements will strongly expand in the near future. For instance, animal studies have shown that large waves of spreading depression take place in ischemic brain tissue, giving rise to high-amplitude, infraslow electrical responses (Nedergaard, 1988). It is likely that such events can be readily measured from the human scalp during early phases of ischemia. It will also be of interest to use FbEEG in a reexamination of the hitherto unresolved question of whether slow DC shifts related to cortical spreading depression take place during migraine attacks in humans (Hadjikhani et al., 2001; Lauritzen, 2001).

The technical problems related to FbEEG recording of slow activity can be readily solved (Bauer et al., 1989; Vanhatalo et al., 2003a; Voipio et al., 2003). Hence, it is likely that FbEEG will become a standard technique in various fields of research including neurophysiology, neurology, as well as experimental psychology.

Acknowledgments

Our research is supported by the Academy of Finland, by the Sigrid Jusélius Foundation, and by Arvo and Lea Ylppö Foundation.

References

Bates, J.A.V. 1963. The unidirectional potential changes in petit mal epilepsy. UCLA Forum Sci. 1:237–279.

Bauer, H., Korunka, C., and Leodolter, M. 1989. Technical requirements for high-quality scalp DC recordings. Electroencephalogr. Clin. Neurophysiol. 72:545–547.

Besson, J.M., Woody, C.D., Aleonard, P., et al. 1970. Correlations of brain d-c shifts with changes in cerebral blood flow. Am. J. Physiol. 218:284–291.

Birbaumer, N., Elbert, T., Canavan, A.G., et al. 1990. Slow potentials of the cerebral cortex and behavior. Physiol. Rev. 70:1–41.

Caspers, H., Speckmann, E.-J., and Lehmenkuhler, A. 1987. DC potentials of the cerebral cortex: seizure activity and changes in gas pressures. Rev. Physiol. Biochem. Pharmacol. 106:127–178.

Chatrian, G.E., Somasundaram, M., and Tassinari, C.A. 1968. DC changes recorded transcranially during "typical" three per second spike and wave discharges in man. Epilepsia 9:185–209.

Cohn, R. 1964. DC recordings of paroxysmal disorders in man. Electroencephalogr. Clin. Neurophysiol. 17:17–24.

Cui, R.Q., Huter, D., Egkher, A., et al. 2000. High resolution DC-EEG mapping of the Bereitschaftspotential preceding simple or complex bimanual sequential finger movement. Exp. Brain Res. 134:49–57.

Duncan, J.S. 1997. Imaging and epilepsy. Brain 120:339–377.

Fitzgerald, R.D., Lamm, C., Oczenski, W., et al. 2001. Direct current auditory evoked potentials during wakefulness, anesthesia, and emergence from anesthesia. Anesth. Analg. 92:154–160.

Girton, D.G., Benson, K.L., and Kamiya, J. 1973. Observation of very slow potential oscillations in human scalp recordings. Electroencephalogr. Clin. Neurophysiol. 35:561–568.

Goldring, S. 1963. Negative steady potential shifts which lead to seizure discharge. UCLA Forum Sci. 1:215–236.

Gross, D.W., Gotman, J., Quesney, L.F., et al. 1999. Intracranial EEG with very low frequency activity fails to demonstrate an advantage over conventional recordings. Epilepsia 40:891–898.

Gumnit, R.J., and Takahashi, T. 1965. Changes in direct current activity during experimental focal seizures. Electroencephalogr. Clin. Neurophysiol. 19:63–74.

Hadjikhani, N., Sanchez Del Rio, M., Wu, O., et al. 2001. Mechanisms of migraine aura revealed by functional MRI in human visual cortex. Proc. Natl. Acad. Sci. USA 98:4687–4692.

2003. A brain-computer interface (BCI) for the locked-in: comparison of different EEG classifications for the thought translation device. Clin. Neurophysiol. 114:416–425.

Ikeda, A., Taki, W., Kunieda, T., et al. 1999. Focal ictal direct current shifts in human epilepsy as studied by subdural and scalp recording. Brain 122:827–838.

James, M.F., Smith, J.M., Boniface, S.J., et al. 2001. Cortical spreading depression and migraine: new insights from imaging? Trends Neurosci. 24:266–271.

Katz, L.C., and Shatz, C.J. 1996. Synaptic activity and the construction of cortical circuits. Science 274:1133–1138.

Lagerlund, T.D., and Gross, R.A. 2003. DC-EEG recording: a paradigm shift in seizure localization? Neurology 60:1062–1063.

Lamblin, M.D., Andre, M., Challamel, M.J., et al. 1999. Electroencephalography of the premature and term newborn. Developmental features and glossary. Neurophysiol. Clin. 29:123–219.

Lauritzen, M. 2001. Cortical spreading depression in migraine. Cephalalgia 21:757–760.

Leopold, D.A., Murayama, Y., and Logothetis, N.K. 2003. Very slow activity fluctuations in monkey visual cortex: implications for functional brain imaging. Cereb. Cortex 13:422–433.

Marshall, L., Molle, M., Fehm, H.L., et al. 1998. Scalp recorded direct current brain potentials during human sleep. Eur. J. Neurosci. 10:1167-1178.

Mayanagi, Y., and Walker, A.E. 1975. DC potentials of temporal lobe seizures in the monkey. J. Neurol. 209:199–215.

Nedergaard, M. 1988. Mechanisms of brain damage in focal cerebral ischemia (review). Acta Neurol. Scand. 77:81–101.

Penn, A.A., and Shatz, C.J. 1999. Brain waves and brain wiring: the role of endogenous and sensory-driven neural activity in development. Pediatr. Res. 45:447–458.

Penttonen, M., Nurminen, N., Miettinen, R., et al. 1999. Ultra-slow oscillation (0.025 Hz) triggers hippocampal afterdischarges in Wistar rats. Neuroscience 94:735–743.

Picton, T.W., and Hillyard, S.A. 1972. Cephalic skin potentials in electroencephalography. Electroencephalogr. Clin. Neurophysiol. 33:419–424.

Roughan, J.V., and Laming, P.R. 1998. Large slow potential shifts occur during halothane anaesthesia in gerbils. J. Comp. Physiol. 182:839–848.

Tallgren, P., Vanhatalo, S., Kaila, K., et al. 2002. Evaluation of commercially available EEG electrodes for AC- and DC-EEG measurements. The Nordic Baltic Conference on Biomedical Engineering and Medical Physics, Reykjavik (abst).

Sorensen, E., Olesen, J., Rask-Madsen, J., et al. 1978. The electrical potential difference and impedance between CSF and blood in unanesthetized man. Scand. J. Clin. Lab. Invest. 38:203–207.

Vanhatalo, S., Tallgren, P., Andersson, S., et al. 2002. DC-EEG unmasks very slow activity patterns during quiet sleep in preterm infants. Clin. Neurophysiol. 113:1822–1825.

Vanhatalo, S., Holmes, M.D., Tallgren, P., et al. 2003a. Very slow EEG responses lateralize temporal lobe seizures: An evaluation of non-invasive DC-EEG. Neurology 60:1098–1102.

Vanhatalo, S., Tallgren, P., Becker, C., et al. 2003b. Scalp-recorded slow EEG responses generated in response to hemodynamic changes in the human brain. Clin. Neurophysiol. 114:1744–1754.

Vanhatalo, S., Voipio, J., Dewaraja, A., et al. 2003c. Topography and elimination of slow EEG responses related to tongue movements. NeuroImage 20:1419–1423.

Vanhatalo, S., Rivera, C., Palva, J.M., et al. 2004a. Large-scale spontaneous activity and up-regulation of KCC2 in the developing human cortex. *(Submitted)*

Vanhatalo, S., Palva, J.M., Holmes, M.D., et al. 2004b. Infraslow oscillations modulate interictal epileptic activity in the human cortex during sleep. *(Submitted)*

Voipio, J., Tallgren, P., Heinonen, E., et al. 2003. Ultraslow DC shifts in the human EEG: evidence for a non-neuronal generator. J. Neurophysiol. 89:2208–2214.

Watanabe, K., Hayakawa, F., and Okumura, A. 1999. Neonatal EEG: a powerful tool in the assessment of brain damage in preterm infants. Brain Dev. 21:361–372.

Wieser, H.G., Elger, C.E., and Stodieck, S.R. 1985. The "foramen ovale electrode": a new recording method for the preoperative evaluation of patients suffering from mesio-basal temporal lobe epilepsy. Electroencephalogr. Clin. Neurophysiol. 61:314–322.

Woody, C.D., Marshall, W.H., Besson, J.M., et al. 1970. Brain potential shift with respiratory acidosis in the cat and monkey. Am. J. Physiol. 218:275–283.

26. Ultrafast EEG Activities

Gabriel Curio

Overview

Human electroencephalographic (EEG) and magnetoencephalographic (MEG) somatosensory responses evoked by electrical median nerve stimulation comprise a brief (10-15 msec) burst of high-frequency (approximately 600 Hz) spike-like wavelets ("σ-burst"), overlapping in time with both, the thalamic P15 component and the primary cortical response N20. Converging evidence from recent recordings in animals and humans shows that these macroscopic σ-bursts reflect the timing of highly synchronized and rapidly repeating population spikes generated by cuneothalamic and thalamocortical relay cells, cortical bursting pyramidal cells, and, possibly, fast-spiking inhibitory interneurons. Theoretical analyses suggest that cellular burst coding relays information with high efficiency; moreover, intraburst frequency can index graded sensory stimulus attributes. The human EEG σ-burst comprises multiple components with differential sensitivity to stimulus rate, vigilance, intensity, tactile interference, subject age, drugs, and certain movement disorders. As these ultrafast EEG activities can be assessed using routine somatosensory evoked potential (SEP) equipment, σ-burst recordings open a unique and easy approach for noninvasive studies of human cerebral population spike responses in clinical conditions.

Definition and Significance

"Ultrafast" EEG activity as defined here covers the frequency band from 400 to 1,000 Hz. Below 400 Hz EEG and MEG reflect predominantly synchronized mass excitatory postsynaptic potentials (EPSPs) and, partially, inhibitory postsynaptic potentials (JPSP et al., 1997). These macroscopically summed responses could contain modulations of the membrane potential lingering below the spike threshold, which are not transmitted into the cortical network (Curio, 1999). It is in this context that the 600-Hz component in SEPs or somatically evoked fields (SEFs)—hereafter referred to as σ-bursts, given their spike-like wavelet appearance—provide an opportunity to monitor noninvasively the timing of population spikes in the human cerebral somatosensory system. This chapter provides a condensed guide with key references to σ-burst recordings that can be added easily to the diagnostic repertoire in order to further advance both the physiological and clinical implications of σ-bursts.

Recording and Analysis

Standard SEP procedures can be used to record σ-bursts: the median nerve is stimulated at the wrist above the motor threshold with 0.1-msec square-wave constant-current electrical stimuli. Depending on the signal-to-noise ratio required to clarify the study objective, 1,000 to 8,000 averages are acquired (in 2 to 16 minutes for one trace at a 8.1-Hz stimulus rate). Subjects shall stay awake with eyes open in a brightly lit room; as σ-bursts are sensitive against vigilance fluctuations (see below), a continuously high degree of wakefulness is of critical importance.

EEG channels are recorded using a wide bandpass (5-1,500 Hz; sampling rate 5 kHz; impedances <5 kΩ). A digital high-pass filter (at approximately 400 Hz) can be applied off-line to isolate the σ-burst. If such postprocessing is not available, one channel could be recorded with the acquisition high-pass filter set to 300 to 400 Hz. Analog filters could shift the burst peak latencies, but gross burst amplitude changes can still be assessed. If multichannel EEG is available, it permits multidipolar source reconstructions (Gobbele et al., 1998); yet, even one single channel, e.g., F3-C3′ contralateral to right median nerve stimuli, can identify responses from Brodmann area 3b, because in this montage contributions of the radially oriented area 1 source are negligible (Klostermann et al., 2001a).

Various burst analysis procedures are published, designed for the specific question under study. Determining the number of peaks above noise level and wavelet peak picking for latency/amplitude readings are straightforward with most analysis programs. Alternatively, the mean burst power can be computed as root-mean-square value (Klostermann, et al., 1998).

Early EEG Studies

Short-latency wavelets at 13 to 20 msec after electrical median nerve stimulation have been interpreted as volume-conducted far-field potentials generated sequentially in brainstem and diencephalic structures (Cracco and Cracco, 1976), such as dorsal column nuclei or medial lemniscus (N14-P15), thalamus (N16), and the thalamocortical radiation (N17, N18, Abbruzzese et al., 1978; Stoehr and Riffel, 1982; Maccabee et al., 1983; Eisen et al., 1984), as confirmed by depth recordings (Katayama and Tsubokawa, 1987). Additionally, scalp SEP mappings in patients receiving thoracic epidural spinal cord stimulation exhibited high-frequency wavelets, probably arising from subcortical structures (Paradiso et al., 1995).

Magnetoencephalogram Studies

First multichannel MEG burst recordings showed a close colocalization of σ-burst and the primary cortical response

N20 (Curio et al., 1993, 1994a,b, 1995, 1996); in particular, a link of the macroscopic σ-burst to burst discharge properties of specific neuron classes was proposed, referring to thalamocortical relay (TCR) neurons, bursting cortical pyramidal cells (e.g., chattering cells), and fast-spiking (FS) cortical inhibitory interneurons. Burst generators were suggested to reside at area 3b because the colocated N20 is generated by EPSPs in apical dendrites of area 3b pyramidal neurons (Wood et al., 1985; Allison et al., 1991; Hari and Forss, 1999). A study using magnetic resonance imaging (MRI)-derived gyral anatomy indeed proved that generators for both σ-burst and N20 were colocated at the postcentral gyrus (Hashimoto et al., 1996).

These seemingly diverging results on burst generator loci (SEF: cortex; SEP scalp and depth recordings: thalamocortical radiation) were reconciled by simultaneous SEP/SEF recordings (Curio et al., 1994a) showing that the magnetic

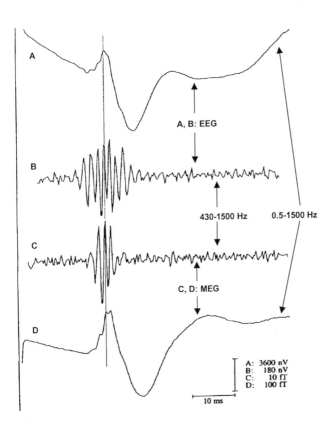

Figure 26.1. Simultaneous magnetoencephalogram (MEG)/EEG recordings of somatosensory responses (8.000 averages) after electrical left median nerve stimulation. Somatosensory evoked potentials (SEPs) (traces **A/B**) were obtained using a C4′–C3′ derivation (negativity at C4′ upward). Magnetic somatically evoked field (SEF) (traces **C/D**) were recorded at the N20 field maximum over the lower part of the right central sulcus (upward deflections: magnetic field lines entering the head). **A/D:** Original records (0.5-1.500 Hz). **B/C:** High-pass-filtered versions (>430 Hz). The *thin line* at 21 msec demonstrates the peak latency preservation before vs. after digital filtering. The *solid line* to the left indicates median nerve electrical stimulation (artifacts clipped). The magnetic σ burst (**C**) is shorter than the simultaneously recorded electrical burst (**B**), which starts earlier and lasts longer. While MEG detects activity mainly from tangential generators (e.g., area 3b), early EEG burst wavelets correspond to radially oriented thalamocortical afferences, and later EEG peaks reflect radially oriented sources in area 1 at the crown of the postcentral gyrus. (Modified from Curio et al., 1994a).)

burst can be substantially shorter than the electrical burst, which starts earlier than its magnetic counterpart and can outlast it (Fig. 26.1); while MEG records mainly activity from tangentially oriented generators (i.e., in fissural neocortex such as area 3b), the EEG picks up also radially oriented sources, such as thalamocortical afferences and sources in area 1 at the crown of the postcentral gyrus.

Human σ-Burst Source Reconstructions

This emerging concept of multiple anatomically distinct EEG σ-burst sources was corroborated using dipole source analysis (Gobbele et al., 1998).

Brainstem

A deep burst source close to the foramen magnum showed an early onset concomitant with the brainstem P14 component; this finding agrees with intraventricular records showing P13/P14 to reflect population spikes in the medial lemniscus (Hashimoto, 1984).

Thalamus

A subsequent subcortical burst source (close to the presumed position of the thalamus) was most active around 16 msec; it might originate from deep axonal segments of thalamocortical fibers (Tsuji et al., 1984; Katayama and Tsubokawa, 1987; Vanderzant et al., 1991). Intrathalamic electrodes implanted for tremor treatment showed a brief (7 msec) polyphasic SEP burst (mean frequency >1,000 Hz) superimposed onto the thalamic P16, which probably reflects a superposition of asynchronous population spikes (Klostermann et al., 1999a); this intrathalamic burst can be functionally dissociated from the surface 600 Hz σ-burst (Klostermann et al., 2000a,b, 2002a,b) and facilitates identifying the thalamic ventral intermediate (VIM) nucleus based on macroscopic SEP criteria (Klostermann et al., 2003).

Cortex

Later burst activity at the primary somatosensory (S-I) hand cortex accompanied the N20 with similar phase reversal across the central sulcus. One high-frequency wavelet at the central region showed no centroparietal phase reversal, suggesting that bursts are superimposed also on the radial P22 source at area 1 (Ozaki et al., 1998), as verified recently by subdural recordings (Maegaki et al., 2000; Kojima et al., 2001). Notably, the orientations of dipoles fitted to burst peaks show a more divergent pattern than the N20 (Ozaki et al., 2001), suggesting that σ-bursts cannot be generated solely by the N20 cell population.

Cortical Somatotopy

Iσ-Bursts can be recorded after stimulation of median and peroneal nerves (Eisen et al., 1984), superficial radial, posterior tibial, and even digital nerves (Curio, 1999; Nakano and Hashimoto, 1999b; Tanosaki et al., 2001; Sakuma and Hashimoto, 1999). Furthermore, median and ulnar nerve evoked σ-bursts exhibit a somatotopic source arrangement at S-I (Curio et al., 1997) resembling the N20 somatotopy (Hari et al., 1993; Hari and Forss, 1999). Thus, σ-bursts are a ubiquitous phenomenon along the somatotopic S-I cortex. As analogous responses occur after clicks in rat auditory cortex (Jones and Barth, 1999), high-frequency bursts represent a general response mode across sensory modalities.

Subcortical Burst Neurons

At all σ-burst locations suggested by these EEG/MEG source analyses, single-cell recordings in animal models have identified neurons discharging high-frequency spike bursts.

Brainstem

Bursts at >500 Hz with low first-spike jitter were observed in dorsal column nuclei (DCNs) of cats, raccoons, and humans (Calvin and Loeser, 1975; Rasmusson and Northgrave, 1997; Canedo et al., 1998) and piglet trigeminal nuclei (Kato et al., 2003). Importantly, natural mechanical receptive field (RF) stimulation evokes DCN burst discharges as well (Pubols et al., 1989). Thus, burst discharges of cuneothalamic relay neurons could generate the deep and early (12–15 ms) σ-burst component (Sonoo et al., 1997; Gobbele et al., 1998).

Somatosensory Thalamus

After electrical digit stimulation, raccoon TCR cells can fire bursts of up to five spikes at 600 Hz with low first-spike latency jitter (Rasmusson, 1996). The human P15 wave (Buchner et al., 1995) has an analog in the form of a large SEP spike from the ventroposterolateral (VPL) nucleus output in cats; subsequent spikes recorded dorsal to VPL correspond to the human P16-P18 complex and could reflect burst discharges of VPL neurons (Allison and Hume, 1981). Accordingly, TCR burst output in the deep thalamocortical radiation could generate σ-burst components at 15 to 18 msec.

Visual Thalamus

Thalamic burst activity is a more general response mode encountered also outside VPL: in awake attentive cats, 77% of lateral geniculate nucleus (LGN) TCR cells discharge bursts during visual stimulation (Guido and Weyand, 1995). Moreover, neighboring LGN neurons with overlapping receptive fields often fire spikes synchronized to within 1 msec (Alonso et al., 1996; Reinagel and Reid, 2000); such precise firing events are reproducible also across cells of the same class (Reinagel and Reid, 2002), favoring the preservation of spike timing for a macroscopic summation.

Cortical Burst Generators

Several cortical sources could contribute to σ-bursts (Curio, 2000), such as presynaptic (thalamocortical) spikes, cortical monosynaptic EPSPs and/or disynaptic IPSPs, bursting cortical neurons (excitatory or inhibitory interneurons, pyramidal cells), rapid sequential intracolumnar spread of activation (Bode-Greuel et al., 1987; Mitzdorf et al., 1979; Mitzdorf, 1985), or reverberatory activity in the local cortical microcircuitry (Langdon and Sur, 1990).

Thalamocortical Inflow at S-I

Notches on early epidural SEPs in S-I of awake monkeys might reflect TCR bursts as they correlate to presynaptic multiunit activity from white matter through most cortical layers (Peterson et al., 1995). TCR terminals make contacts with pyramidal cells dendrites (White, 1979) so that TCR bursts could trigger a sequence of overlapping EPSPs, the sharp-onset transients of which (Stern et al., 1992; Armstrong-James et al., 1993) may be detectable as high-frequency far-fields. Indeed, high-frequency burst responses in piglet S-I (Ikeda et al., 2002) have an initial component insensitive to cortically injected kynurenic acid (Kyna; an antagonist of glutamatergic receptors). This component was localized in cortical layer IV, compatible with spikes produced by thalamocortical axonal terminals. The subsequent Kyna-sensitive (i.e., postsynaptic) component was localized in layer IV initially and spread to superficial and deeper layers.

Cortical Cells

Four neuron classes are known in neocortex (Gray and McCormick, 1996; Nowak et al., 2003): regular-spiking (RS) cells, which are spiny stellate cells in layer 4 and pyramidal cells; fast-spiking (FS) cells, which are sparsely spiny or aspiny nonpyramidal cells, presumably inhibitory interneurons; intrinsic bursting (IB) cells; and chattering (CH) cells, which are layer 2 to 4 pyramidal or spiny stellate neurons that generate repetitive (30–80 Hz) high-frequency (350–700 Hz) spike burst responses.

Bursting Inhibitory Interneurons

Thirty percent of neurons in primate neocortex are inhibitory using γ-aminobutyric acid (GABA) as transmitter (Jones, 1993). In awake rabbits suspected interneurons (SINs) respond almost uniformly with a 500- to 900-Hz burst of three or more short-duration (0.45 msec) spikes (Swadlow, 1989, 1990). SINs in S-I can follow tactile RF stimulation as high as 50 Hz (Swadlow, 1990). In layer 4, SINs are among the first cortical neurons to respond to a peripheral stimulus (Swadlow, 1995). For SIN pairs with monosynaptic thalamic input, spikes can be synchronized sharply, i.e., within ±1 msec (Swadlow et al., 1998). Additionally, intracellular recordings from some FS cells (*n* = 4) in rat barrel cortex revealed bursts responses approximating the periodicity of 400- to 600-Hz surface EEG wavelets (Jones et al., 2000), and putative interneurons in the neocortex of epilepsy-prone rats discharge with repetitive bursts of 300 to 500 Hz (Kandel and Buzsaki, 1997). In principle, these findings could corroborate the proposal that synchronous spikes conducted in vertical axons of inhibitory interneurons contribute to σ-bursts (Hashimoto et al., 1996; Hashimoto, 2000).

Quantitatively, the contribution of such population spikes to the surface σ-burst appears open, as the conduction velocity of inhibitory fibers is only 0.1 m/sec (Salin and Prince, 1996). Accordingly, spike depolarization and repolarization currents would be separated longitudinally in the axon only by 100 μm, implying a substantial field cancellation for such quadripolar source configuration. Furthermore, this kind of interneuronal sharp synchrony survives general anesthesia

(Swadlow et al., 1998), in contrast to human σ-bursts (Klostermann et al., 2000a). While the sharp synchrony of SIN spikes (Swadlow et al., 1998) implies highly synchronous IPSPs in target neurons, GABAergic postsynaptic currents do not underlie fast oscillations because the GABA$_A$ antagonist bicuculline increased the number of burst wavelets without altering amplitude or intraburst frequency (Jones and Barth, 2002).

Bursting Pyramidal Cells

In rat barrel cortex vibrissal displacements evoke early EEG wavelets in two bands (200–400 and 400–600 Hz) phase-locked to stimulus onset (Jones and Barth, 1999; Jones et al., 2000; for separate high-frequency bands in human SEF cf. Haueisen et al., 2001). RS pyramidal cells (*n* = 58) exhibited spikes and/or subthreshold events clustering at latencies separated by successive oscillatory cycles; thus, fast oscillations define preferred latencies for RS spike generation (Jones et al., 2000). Interestingly, the rat somatosensory cortex can initiate and sustain fast oscillations: after

lesions of the somatosensory thalamus epicortical stimuli still generate fast oscillations (Staba et al., 2003).

Neocortical Bursts in Nonhuman Primates

Laminar field potential recordings in monkeys located burst peaks 1 to 4 in area 3b and peaks 3 to 5 in area 1 (Shimazu et al., 2000). Single-cell recordings in awake monkeys (Baker et al., 2003) showed that a subset of S-I units fires both bursts and single spikes phase-locked to surface EEG wavelets in response to electrical median nerve stimuli (Fig. 26.2). Spike width was >0.6 ms in five of six cells, suggesting that "thin-spike" GABAergic interneurons (Swadlow, 1990; Nowak et al., 2003) are at least not the main burst generator. Remaining candidates with long duration spikes are pyramidal neurons and spiny stellate cells (Nowak et al., 2003); the open field structure of elongated pyramidal dendrites favors dipolar far-field visibility. Most interestingly, S-I cells can fire bursts in response to tactile stimuli applied to small skin regions (Fig. 26.2). Hence, burst responses may be important for the processing of natural stimuli, possibly

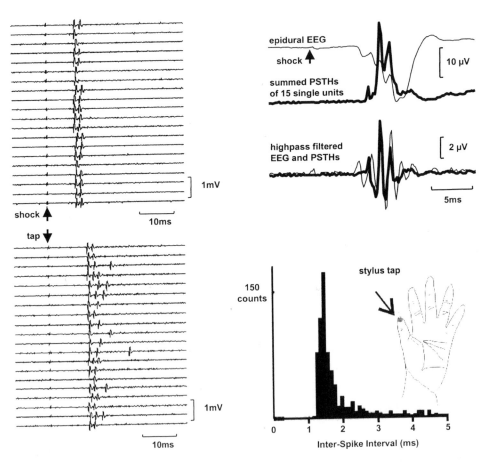

Figure 26.2.   Single-trial single cell burst responses to electrical (**upper left panel**) and natural tactile stimuli (**lower left panel**) recorded in S-I of an awake monkey. Peristimulus time histograms (PSTHs) summed over 15 single units (*thick lines,* **upper right panel**) coincide with the middle part of epidural EEG burst averages (*thin lines*); **middle right panel** depicts the results of high-pass filtering (>428 Hz) the upper panel traces. **Lower right panel** shows the interspike interval histogram of burst responses to natural (tap) stimuli at the cell's receptive field (cf. hand figurine): the unimodal distribution peaks at 1.5 msec corresponding to an intraburst frequency of 660 Hz. (Modified from Baker et al. 2003).)

setting a reference timeframe capable of coding stimulus interactions on a submillisecond time scale (Barth, 2003).

Parameters Influencing σ-Bursts

Stimulus Intensity

The amplitude recruitment of both N20 and σ-burst can be modeled as a sigmoidal function of intensity of electrical median nerve stimuli. Although most subjects showed a parallel recruitment, two of ten subjects required higher stimulation intensities for burst than for N20 recruitment (Klostermann et al., 1998), possibly reflecting slight vigilance decrements in open-eyed "awake" subjects.

Stimulus Rate

The amplitude of the first major burst peak remains remarkably stable when the stimulus rate is increased from 1.5 to 9 Hz; this again points to a presynaptic origin of this early burst peak, reflecting, for example, population spikes conducted in superficial segments of thalamocortical fibers (Gobbele et al., 1999). When the burst refractory behavior was tested over a wider range (Fig. 26.3); (Klostermann et al., 1999b), only a brief high-frequency (700 Hz) early burst component remained discernible above 10 Hz, which gradually decreased with rates up to 25 Hz; burst rate sensitivity was corroborated by recent subdural recordings (Urasaki et al., 2002). At stimulation frequencies <4 Hz, a late burst component became apparent with only 494 Hz intraburst frequency (Klostermann et al., 1999b). Comparably long refractory periods and low intraburst frequencies have been described for bursting cells driven by low-threshold calcium currents (McCormick and Feeser, 1990).

Double Stimulation

After mixed median nerve stimulation the thalamic P14 recovers with very short interstimulus intervals (ISIs), whereas progressively longer ISIs are required for full recovery of later burst peaks (Emori et al., 1991). A recent SEP study (Mackert et al., 2000) revealed a different burst recovery for sensory-only nerves; the rapid burst recovery observed at ISIs as short as 20 msec favors an SEP burst generation by cell populations such as chattering cells and/or inhibitory interneurons, both of which are capable of discharging rapidly repeating (50 Hz) high-frequency (600 Hz) bursts of fast sodium spikes.

Sleep and Macroscopic Bursts

σ-Bursts are diminished in sleep whereas the N20 is not (Emerson et al., 1988). Specifically, EEG σ-bursts decrease from sleep stage II to IV and reappear partially in rapid-eye-movement (REM) sleep (Yamada et al., 1988; Halboni et al., 2000). Also the MEG σ-burst decreased during sleep, whereas the N20 moderately increased; this reciprocal burst/N20 modulation led to the suggestion that SEF bursts are generated mainly by synchronized spikes in vertically arranged axons of area 3b inhibitory interneurons, providing feed-forward inhibition to pyramidal cells (Hashimoto et al., 1996; Hashimoto, 2000). At present, however, the N20-sleep

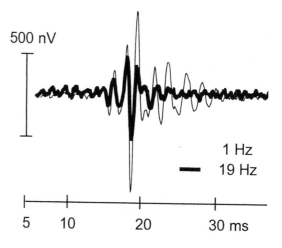

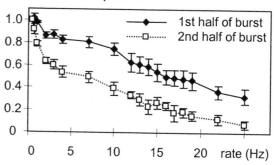

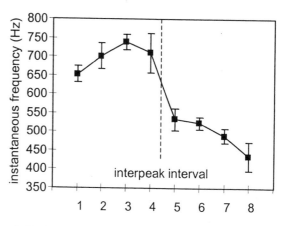

Figure 26.3. **Upper panel:** Superimposed burst responses for 1 Hz and 19 Hz median nerve stimuli show that at 19 Hz the second burst half is attenuated more than the first. **Middle panel:** Recovery functions (six subjects; ± standard error of the mean) for early vs. late burst, normalized at 0.5 Hz. The late burst showed a more pronounced decrement between 0.5 and 2 Hz. **Lower panel:** Grand average of instantaneous intraburst frequencies determined as inverse of successive interpeak intervals at 0.5-Hz stimulus rate. Interpeak intervals 1 to 4 have a higher (mean 700 Hz) instantaneous frequency than intervals 5 to 8 (mean 494 Hz). *Dashed vertical line* defines the separation of early and late burst component. (Modified from Klostermann et al. 1999b).)

relation appears undecided as other studies found the P14–N20 amplitude to decline when subjects fall asleep (Goff et al., 1966; Nakano et al., 1995; Noguchi et al., 1995). Likewise, dipole source analysis yielded no evidence for an N20 increase during sleep; this study revealed also that σ-bursts decreased during sleep at thalamus and cortex but not brainstem (Halboni et al., 2000). State fluctuations are relevant also in awake subjects; σ-bursts are increased for eyes opened vs. closed (Gobbele et al., 2000), and are more variable than the N20. Thus, the more fluctuating σ-burst could index variable factors of processing, such as floating vigilance and/or attention (Klostermann et al., 2001b).

Sleep and Cellular Bursting

These consistent findings of decreased σ-bursts during sleep need not reflect decreased single-cell bursting. Alternatively, it could result from increased burst jitter, leading to partial cancellation during averaging; artificially imposed, slow sinusoidal subthreshold oscillations in neocortical neurons, which resemble sleep delta-waves, increase response jitter (Volgushev et al., 1998). While at the thalamic level bursts can occur during wakefulness, neurons discharge in bursts mostly during sleep; however, because the thalamic relay function is partially shut down during slow-wave sleep (Timofeev et al., 1996), the actual thalamocortical output of evoked cellular bursts may be reduced during sleep, as are macroscopic σ-bursts.

Although σ-bursts are diminished during non-REM sleep, they are partially recovered during REM sleep (Yamada et al., 1988; Halboni et al., 2000). Because adrenergic brainstem afferences are shut down during REM sleep (Hobson et al., 1983), a remaining candidate for σ-burst modulation is acetylcholine (ACh). ACh enhances cell responses in S-I by 200%, and burst responses (400 Hz) are more common during ACh application (Metherate et al., 1988). Stimulation of the nucleus basalis facilitates (via muscarinic receptors) cortical EPSPs and increases the probability and synchrony of evoked spikes (Metherate and Ashe, 1993), in particular also for chattering cells (McCormick and Nowak, 1996). Thus, various ACh effects could converge to strengthen macroscopic σ-bursts (Restuccia et al., 2003).

Sensorimotor Interference

Brushing of palm and fingers decreased the median nerve N20, whereas σ-bursts showed more peaks, possibly reflecting a tonic interneuron facilitation (Hashimoto et al., 1999). During phasic finger movements σ-bursts decreased (Inoue et al., 2002; Tanosaki et al., 2002); specifically, the cortical late burst component was attenuated while the brainstem P14 and the early burst component remained unaffected (Gobbele et al., 2003b). Isometric motor innervation attenuated N20, P25, and P70 waves, while σ-bursts were unaffected; thus, movement-specific gating operates on particular SEP components and might reflect an "efference copy" mechanism (Klostermann et al., 2001a).

Age

In children 6 to 12 years of age, bursts were larger, longer in duration, and had more peaks than in adult subjects; in addition, the interpeak latency was longer in children (Nakano and Hashimoto, 2000). In older subjects, number and amplitudes of burst peaks after the N20 peak were larger than in younger subjects (Nakano and Hashimoto, 1999a). Thus, the physiology of σ-burst maturation and aging calls for further study and must be considered in clinical studies.

Drugs

Bursts are not affected by increased GABAergic inhibition after lorazepam (Restuccia et al., 2002b) or tiagabine (Restuccia et al., 2002a). Dosage, however, appears critical because higher lorazepam levels can delay later burst peaks (Haueisen et al., 2000). The acetylcholinesterase inhibitor rivastigmine increased selectively later burst wavelets between 18 and 28 msec; interestingly, pyramidal chattering cells can be cholinergically activated, whereas ACh does not modify the firing rate of fast-spiking GABAergic interneurons (Restuccia et al., 2003). Apart from these single-dose studies in healthy subjects, one report found in patients with epilepsy that the anticonvulsant drugs valproate and carbamazepine did not alter σ-bursts at blood levels in the lower therapeutic range (Klostermann et al., 2001b).

Burst Pathophysiology

Deafferentation

In patients with pain after spinal cord transection, thalamic cells show high-frequency bursting (Lenz et al., 1994). Generally, thalamic spike bursts may constitute a common denominator for the pathophysiology of positive symptoms in neurogenic pain, tinnitus, movement disorders, epilepsy, and some neuropsychiatric syndromes (Jeanmonod et al., 1996; McCormick, 1999). The probability of encountering burst neurons increases after peripheral deafferentation also in S-I (Martinson et al., 1997; Webster et al., 1997).

Epilepsy

The EEG of Metrazol-treated rats exhibits power up to 800 Hz during spiking but not interictally (Huang and White, 1989), and the EEG spike in epileptic rats is associated with 400- to 600-Hz "ripples" (Kandel and Buzsaki, 1997). In patients with mesial temporal lobe epilepsy, "fast ripples" (FR; 200–500 Hz) may reflect hypersynchronous population spikes of bursting pyramidal cells in the epileptogenic region (Bragin et al., 1999a), and FR generating areas become broader after application of the GABA$_A$ antagonist bicuculline (Bragin et al., 2002). Thus, fast ripples could indicate the epileptic region (Bragin et al., 1999b).

Multiple Sclerosis

σ-Bursts are either absent or showed a prolonged interpeak time in multiple sclerosis (MS) patients even when low-frequency components were normal (Rossini et al., 1985), indexing a subtle deficiency of impulse conduction due to demyelination. Conversely, the N20 was reduced with preserved σ-bursts in 13% of stimulated limbs of 50 MS patients, possibly indicating instances of a mainly axonal lesion type (Gobbele et al., 2003a).

Movement Disorders

Bursts are unaltered in patients with essential tremor or dystonia (Mochizuki et al., 1999b). However, in some patients with Parkinson's disease (PD), σ-bursts were enlarged (Mochizuki et al., 1999a; Mochizuki et al., 1999b), and in patients with PD or multiple system atrophy the duration of illness was positively correlated with burst amplitudes (Inoue et al., 2001). In three patients with myoclonus epilepsy (ME) showing giant P25 waves, enlarged burst wavelets were seen at longer latencies (7–14 msec after N20 onset). The authors suggest that early wavelets near N20 relate to basal ganglia (dys)function and are enlarged in PD patients, and later wavelets are enhanced superimposed on the giant P25–N33 wave in ME patients. However, the stimulus rate was lower for ME patients than for controls (0.53 vs. 2.7 Hz), so that the physiological recovery of late-burst wavelets (Klostermann et al., 1999b) could have contributed to the increase of late-burst peaks in ME patients. Interestingly, two patients with mitochondriopathy without myoclonus showed giant SEP with abolished 600-Hz activity (Liepert et al., 2001). Enlarging the patient database will help to clarify the pathophysiological implications of these findings.

Burst Responses: Mechanisms and Functions

How can a peripheral stimulus trigger a phase-locked high-frequency SEP/SEF response (which requires a timing precision of less than 1 msec to avoid phase cancellation) when conduction delays could disperse the ascending input volley, and cumulative synaptic variability might destroy the coherence in the sequentially activated neuronal populations?

Neurons can discharge spikes with 25 µsec precision if the presynaptic signals arrive coherently; during ontogenetic development unsupervised Hebbian learning selects connections with matching delays from input axons with random delays (Gerstner et al., 1996; Kistler and van Hemmen, 2000); thus, the ratio of postsynaptic to presynaptic spike jitter can become less than one (Marsalek et al., 1997; Burkitt and Clark, 1999).

And why might the brain appreciate precise burst coding? Many central synapses transmit bursts but filter out single spikes (Lisman, 1997). Thalamic bursts potently activate cortical circuits (Swadlow and Gusev, 2001) and can produce long-term synaptic modifications. Thalamic bursts can have a threefold higher encoding efficiency than single spikes (Reinagel et al., 1999). Most importantly, intraburst frequency can code graded sensory information, e.g., on visual contrast (Funke and Kerscher, 2000). Furthermore, bursts of different durations can code different stimulus features (Kepecs and Lisman, 2003); e.g., bursts occur preferentially on the positive slopes of time-varying input signals, and the spike number per burst can signal the slope magnitude (Kepecs et al., 2002). Thus, a highly efficient and information-loaded code for driving a postsynaptic cell may be coincident bursts (Lisman, 1997).

Outlook

Although many variables of stimulation protocol and subject state influence σ-bursts and hence need to be controlled precisely, the approach is fundamentally simple, and significant scientific progress can be expected from routine single-channel SEP recordings under a variety of clinical conditions.

Acknowledgment

This work is supported by Deutsche Forschungsgemeinschart (DFG) grant SFB 618, TP B4.

References

Abbruzzese, M., Favale, E., Leandri, M., et al. 1978. New subcortical components of the cerebral somatosensory evoked potential in man. Acta Neurol. Scand. 58:325–332.

Allison, T., and Hume, A. L. 1981. A comparative analysis of short-latency somatosensory evoked potentials in man, monkey, cat, and rat. Exp. Neurol. 72:592–611.

Allison, T., McCarthy, G., Wood, C.C., et al. 1991. Potentials evoked in human and monkey cerebral cortex by stimulation of the median nerve. A review of scalp and intracranial recordings. Brain 114:2465–2503.

Alonso, J.M., Usrey, W.M., and Reid, R.C. 1996. Precisely correlated firing in cells of the lateral geniculate nucleus. Nature 383:815–819.

Armstrong-James, M., Welker, E., and Callahan, C.A. 1993. The contribution of NMDA and non-NMDA receptors to fast and slow transmission of sensory information in the rat SI barrel cortex. J. Neurosci. 13:2149–2160.

Baker, S.N., Curio, G., and Lemon, R.N. 2003. EEG oscillations at 600 Hz are macroscopic markers for cortical spike bursts. J. Physiol. 550:529–534.

Barth, D.S. 2003. Submillisecond synchronization of fast electrical oscillations in neocortex. J. Neurosci. 23:2502–2510.

Bode-Greuel, K.M., Singer, W., and Aldenhoff, J.B. 1987. A current source density analysis of field potentials evoked in slices of visual cortex. Exp. Brain Res. 69:213–219.

Bragin, A., Engel, J., Jr., Wilson, C.L., et al. 1999a. High-frequency oscillations in human brain. Hippocampus 9:137–142.

Bragin, A., Engel, J., Jr., Wilson, C.L., et al. 1999b. Hippocampal and entorhinal cortex high-frequency oscillations (100-500 Hz) in human epileptic brain and in kainic acid-treated rats with chronic seizures. Epilepsia 40:127–137.

Bragin, A., Mody, I., Wilson, C.L., et al. 2002. Local generation of fast ripples in epileptic brain. J. Neurosci. 22:2012–2021.

Buchner, H., Waberski, T.D., Fuchs, M., et al. 1995. Origin of P16 median nerve SEP component identified by dipole source analysis—subthalamic or within the thalamo-cortical radiation? Exp Brain Res. 104:511–518.

Burkitt, A.N., and Clark, G.M. 1999. Analysis of integrate-and-fire neurons: synchronization of synaptic input and spike output. Neural Comput. 11:871–901.

Calvin, W.H., and Loeser, J.D. 1975. Doublet and burst firing patterns within the dorsal column nuclei of cat and man. Exp. Neurol. 48:406–426.

Canedo, A., Martinez, L., and Marino, J. 1998. Tonic and bursting activity in the cuneate nucleus of the chloralose-anesthetized cat. Neuroscience 84:603–617.

Cracco, R.Q., and Cracco, J.B. 1976. Somatosensory evoked potential in man: far field potentials. Electroencephalogr. Clin. Neurophysiol. 41:460–466.

Curio, G. 1999. High frequency (600 Hz) bursts of spike-like activities generated in the human cerebral somatosensory system. Electroencephalogr. Clin. Neurophysiol. Suppl. 49:56–61.

Curio, G. 2000. Linking 600-Hz "spikelike" EEG/MEG wavelets ("sigmabursts") to cellular substrates: concepts and caveats. J. Clin. Neurophysiol. 17:377–396.

Curio, G., Mackert, B.-M., Burghoff, M., et al. 1993. Neuromagnetic detection of high-frequency (600 Hz) oscillations evoked in the human primary somatosensory cortex. Eur. J. Neurosci. Suppl. 6:228.

Curio, G., Mackert, B.-M., Abraham-Fuchs, K., et al. 1994a. High-frequency activity (600 Hz) evoked in the human primary somatosensory cortex—a review of electric and magnetic recordings. In *Oscillatory Event Related Brain Dynamics*, Ed. C. Pantev, T. Elbert, and B. Luetkenhoener, vol. 271, pp. 205–218. New York: Plenum Press.

Curio, G., Mackert, B.M., Burghoff, M., et al. 1994b. Localization of evoked neuromagnetic 600 Hz activity in the cerebral somatosensory system. Electroencephalogr. Clin. Neurophysiol. 91:483–487.

Curio, G., Mackert, B.-M., Burghoff, M., et al. 1995. Neuromagnetic detection of cerebral high-frequency activity (600 Hz) superimposed on the N20-activity from SI in man. In *Biomagnetism: Fundamental Research and Clinical Applications*, Eds. C. Baumgartner, L. Deecke, G. Stroink, et al., pp. 91–95. Amsterdam: Elsevier Science, IOS Press.

Curio, G., Drung, D., Koch, H., et al. 1996. Magnetometry of evoked fields from human peripheral nerve, brachial plexus and primary somatosensory cortex using a liquid nitrogen cooled superconducting quantum interference device. Neurosci. Lett. 206:204–206.

Curio, G., Mackert, B.M., Burghoff, M., et al. 1997. Somatotopic source arrangement of 600 Hz oscillatory magnetic fields at the human primary somatosensory hand cortex. Neurosci. Lett. 234:131–134.

Eisen, A., Roberts, K., Low, M., et al. 1984. Questions regarding the sequential neural generator theory of the somatosensory evoked potential raised by digital filtering. Electroencephalogr. Clin. Neurophysiol. 59: 388–395.

Emerson, R.G., Sgro, J.A., Pedley, T.A., et al. 1988. State-dependent changes in the N20 component of the median nerve somatosensory evoked potential. Neurology 38:64–68.

Emori, T., Yamada, T., Seki, Y., et al. 1991. Recovery functions of fast frequency potentials in the initial negative wave of median SEP. Electroencephalogr. Clin. Neurophysiol. 78:116–123.

Funke, K., and Kerscher, N. 2000. High-frequency (300–800 Hz) components in cat geniculate (dLGN) early visual responses. J. Physiol. Paris 94:411–425.

Gerstner, W., Kempter, R., van Hemmen, J.L., et al. 1996. A neuronal learning rule for sub-millisecond temporal coding. Nature 383:76–81.

Gobbele, R., Buchner, H., and Curio, G. 1998. High-frequency (600 Hz) SEP activities originating in the subcortical and cortical human somatosensory system. Electroencephalogr. Clin. Neurophysiol. 108:182–189.

Gobbele, R., Buchner, H., Scherg, M., et al. 1999. Stability of high-frequency (600 Hz) components in human somatosensory evoked potentials under variation of stimulus rate—evidence for a thalamic origin. Clin. Neurophysiol. 110:1659–1663.

Gobbele, R., Waberski, T.D., Kuelkens, S., et al. 2000. Thalamic and cortical high-frequency (600 Hz) somatosensory-evoked potential (SEP) components are modulated by slight arousal changes in awake subjects. Exp. Brain Res. 133:506–513.

Gobbele, R., Waberski, T.D., Dieckhofer, A., et al. 2003a. Patterns of disturbed impulse propagation in multiple sclerosis identified by low and high frequency somatosensory evoked potential components. J. Clin. Neurophysiol. 20:283–290.

Gobbele, R., Waberski, T.D., Thyerlei, D., et al. 2003b. Functional dissociation of a subcortical and cortical component of high-frequency oscillations in human somatosensory evoked potentials by motor interference. Neurosci. Lett. 350:97–100.

Goff, W.R., Allison, T., Shapiro, A., et al. 1966. Cerebral somatosensory responses evoked during sleep in man. Electroencephalogr. Clin. Neurophysiol. 21:1–9.

Gray, C.M., and McCormick, D.A. 1996. Chattering cells: superficial pyramidal neurons contributing to the generation of synchronous oscillations in the visual cortex. Science 274:109–113.

Guido, W., and Weyand, T. 1995. Burst responses in thalamic relay cells of the awake behaving cat. J. Neurophysiol. 74:1782–1786.

Halboni, P., Kaminski, R., Gobbele, R., et al. 2000. Sleep stage dependent changes of the high-frequency part of the somatosensory evoked potentials at the thalamus and cortex. Clin. Neurophysiol. 111:2277–2284.

Hari, R., and Forss, N. 1999. Magnetoencephalography in the study of human somatosensory cortical processing. Philos. Trans. R. Soc. Lond. B Biol. Sci. 354:1145–1154.

Hari, R., Karhu, J., Hamalainen, M., et al. 1993. Functional organization of the human first and second somatosensory cortices: a neuromagnetic study. Eur. J. Neurosci. 5:724–734.

Hashimoto, I. 1984. Somatosensory evoked potentials from the human brain-stem: origins of short latency potentials. Electroencephalogr. Clin. Neurophysiol. 57:221–227.

Hashimoto, I. 2000. High-frequency oscillations of somatosensory evoked potentials and fields. J. Clin. Neurophysiol. 17:309–320.

Hashimoto, I., Mashiko, T., and Imada, T. 1996. Somatic evoked high-frequency magnetic oscillations reflect activity of inhibitory interneurons in the human somatosensory cortex. Electroencephalogr. Clin. Neurophysiol. 100:189–203.

Hashimoto, I., Kimura, T., Fukushima, T., et al. 1999. Reciprocal modulation of somatosensory evoked N20m primary response and high-frequency oscillations by interference stimulation. Clin. Neurophysiol. 110:1445–1451.

Haueisen, J., Heuer, T., Nowak, H., et al. 2000. The influence of lorazepam on somatosensory-evoked fast frequency (600 Hz) activity in MEG. Brain Res. 874:10–14.

Haueisen, J., Schack, B., Meier, T., et al. 2001. Multiplicity in the high-frequency signals during the short-latency somatosensory evoked cortical activity in humans. Clin. Neurophysiol. 112:1316–1325.

Hobson, J.A., McCarley, R.W., and Nelson, J.P. 1983. Location and spike-train characteristics of cells in anterodorsal pons having selective decreases in firing rate during desynchronized sleep. J. Neurophysiol. 50:770–783.

Huang, C.M., and White, L.E., Jr. 1989. High-frequency components in epileptiform EEG. J. Neurosci. Methods 30:197–201.

Ikeda, H., Leyba, L., Bartolo, A., et al. 2002. Synchronized spikes of thalamocortical axonal terminals and cortical neurons are detectable outside the pig brain with MEG. J. Neurophysiol. 87:626–630.

Inoue, K., Hashimoto, I., and Nakamura, S. 2001. High-frequency oscillations in human posterior tibial somatosensory evoked potentials are enhanced in patients with Parkinson's disease and multiple system atrophy. Neurosci. Lett. 297:89–92.

Inoue, K., Harada, T., Kaseda, Y., et al. 2002. Effects of movement on somatosensory N20m fields and high-frequency oscillations. Neuroreport 13:1861–1864.

Jeanmonod, D., Magnin, M., and Morel, A. 1996. Low-threshold calcium spike bursts in the human thalamus. Common physiopathology for sensory, motor and limbic positive symptoms. Brain 119:363–375.

Jones, E.G. 1993. GABAergic neurons and their role in cortical plasticity in primates. Cereb. Cortex 3:361–372.

Jones, M.S., and Barth, D.S. 1999. Spatiotemporal organization of fast (>200 Hz) electrical oscillations in rat vibrissa/barrel cortex. J. Neurophysiol. 82:1599–1609.

Jones, M.S., and Barth, D.S. 2002. Effects of bicuculline methiodide on fast (>200 Hz) electrical oscillations in rat somatosensory cortex. J. Neurophysiol. 88:1016–1025.

Jones, M.S., MacDonald, K.D., Choi, B., et al. 2000. Intracellular correlates of fast (>200 Hz) electrical oscillations in rat somatosensory cortex. J. Neurophysiol. 84:1505–1518.

Kandel, A., and Buzsaki, G. 1997. Cellular-synaptic generation of sleep spindles, spike-and-wave discharges, and evoked thalamocortical responses in the neocortex of the rat. J. Neurosci. 17:6783–6797.

Katayama, Y., and Tsubokawa, T. 1987. Somatosensory evoked potentials from the thalamic sensory relay nucleus (VPL) in humans: correlations with short latency somatosensory evoked potentials recorded at the scalp. Electroencephalogr. Clin. Neurophysiol. 68:187–201.

Kato, S., Wang, Y., Papuashvili, N., et al. 2003. Stable synchronized high-frequency signals from the main sensory and spinal nuclei of the pig activated by Abeta fibers of the maxillary nerve innervating the snout. Brain Res. 959:1–10.

Kepecs, A., and Lisman, J. 2003. Information encoding and computation with spikes and bursts. Network 14:103–118.

Kepecs, A., Wang, X.J., and Lisman, J. 2002. Bursting neurons signal input slope. J. Neurosci. 22:9053–9062.

Kistler, W.M., and van Hemmen, J.L. 2000. Modeling synaptic plasticity in conjunction with the timing of pre- and postsynaptic action potentials. Neural Comput. 12:385–405.

Klostermann, F., Nolte, G., Losch, F., et al. 1998. Differential recruitment of high frequency wavelets (600 Hz) and primary cortical response (N20) in human median nerve somatosensory evoked potentials. Neurosci Lett. 256:101–104.

Klostermann, F., Funk, T., Vesper, J., et al. 1999a. Spatiotemporal characteristics of human intrathalamic high-frequency (>400 Hz) SEP components. Neuroreport 10:3627–3631.

Klostermann, F., Nolte, G., and Curio, G. 1999b. Multiple generators of 600 Hz wavelets in human SEP unmasked by varying stimulus rates. Neuroreport 10:1625–1629.

Klostermann, F., Funk, T., Vesper, J., et al. 2000a. Propofol narcosis dissociates human intrathalamic and cortical high-frequency (>400 Hz) SEP components. Neuroreport 11:2607–2610.

Klostermann, F., Funk, T., Vesper, J., et al. 2000b. Double-pulse stimulation dissociates intrathalamic and cortical high-frequency (>400 Hz) SEP components in man. Neuroreport 11:1295–1299.

Klostermann, F., Gobbele, R., Buchner, H., et al. 2001a. Differential gating of slow postsynaptic and high-frequency spike-like components in human somatosensory evoked potentials under isometric motor interference. Brain Res. 922:95–103.

Klostermann, F., Nolte, G., and Curio, G. 2001b. Independent short-term variability of spike-like (600 Hz) and postsynaptic (N20) cerebral SEP components. Neuroreport 12:349–352.

Klostermann, F., Gobbele, R., Buchner, H., et al. 2002a. Dissociation of human thalamic and cortical SEP gating as revealed by intrathalamic recordings under muscle relaxation. Brain Res. 958:146–151.

Klostermann, F., Gobbele, R., Buchner, H., et al. 2002b. Intrathalamic nonpropagating generators of high-frequency (1000 Hz) somatosensory evoked potential (SEP) bursts recorded subcortically in man. Clin. Neurophysiol. 113:1001–1005.

Klostermann, F., Vesper, J., and Curio, G. 2003. Identification of target areas for deep brain stimulation in human basal ganglia substructures based on median nerve sensory evoked potential criteria. J. Neurol. Neurosurg. Psychiatry 74:1031–1035.

Kojima, Y., Uozumi, T., Akamatsu, N., et al. 2001. Somatosensory evoked high frequency oscillations recorded from subdural electrodes. Clin. Neurophysiol. 112:2261–2264.

Langdon, R.B., and Sur, M. 1990. Components of field potentials evoked by white matter stimulation in isolated slices of primary visual cortex: spatial distributions and synaptic order. J. Neurophysiol. 64:1484–1501.

Lenz, F.A., Kwan, H.C., Martin, R., et al. 1994. Characteristics of somatotopic organization and spontaneous neuronal activity in the region of the thalamic principal sensory nucleus in patients with spinal cord transection. J. Neurophysiol. 72:1570–1587.

Liepert, J., Haueisen, J., Hegemann, S., et al. 2001. Disinhibition of somatosensory and motor cortex in mitochondriopathy without myoclonus. Clin. Neurophysiol. 112:917–922.

Lisman, J.E. 1997. Bursts as a unit of neural information: making unreliable synapses reliable. Trends Neurosci. 20:38–43.

Maccabee, P.J., Pinkhasov, E.I., and Cracco, R.Q. 1983. Short latency somatosensory evoked potentials to median nerve stimulation: effect of low frequency filter. Electroencephalogr. Clin. Neurophysiol. 55:34–44.

Mackert, B.M., Weisenbach, S., Nolte, G., et al. 2000. Rapid recovery (20 ms) of human 600 Hz electroencephalographic wavelets after double stimulation of sensory nerves. Neurosci. Lett. 286:83–86.

Maegaki, Y., Najm, I., Terada, K., et al. 2000. Somatosensory evoked high-frequency oscillations recorded directly from the human cerebral cortex. Clin. Neurophysiol. 111:1916–1926.

Marsalek, P., Koch, C., and Maunsell, J. 1997. On the relationship between synaptic input and spike output jitter in individual neurons. Proc. Natl. Acad. Sci. U S A 94:735–740.

Martinson, J., Webster, H.H., Myasnikov, A.A., et al. 1997. Recognition of temporally structured activity in spontaneously discharging neurons in the somatosensory cortex in waking cats. Brain Res. 750:129–140.

McCormick, D.A. 1999. Are thalamocortical rhythms the Rosetta stone of a subset of neurological disorders? Nat. Med. 5:1349–1351.

McCormick, D.A., and Feeser, H.R. 1990. Functional implications of burst firing and single spike activity in lateral geniculate relay neurons. Neuroscience 39:103–113.

McCormick, D.A., and Nowak, L.G. 1996. Possible cellular mechanisms for arousal induced higher frequency oscillations: acetylcholine and ACPD induce repetitive burst firing in visual cortical neurons. Soc. Neurosci. Abstr. 22:644.

Metherate, R., and Ashe, J.H. 1993. Nucleus basalis stimulation facilitates thalamocortical synaptic transmission in the rat auditory cortex. Synapse 14:132–143.

Metherate, R., Tremblay, N., and Dykes, R.W. 1988. Transient and prolonged effects of acetylcholine on responsiveness of cat somatosensory cortical neurons. J. Neurophysiol. 59:1253–1276.

Mitzdorf, U. 1985. Current source-density method and application in cat cerebral cortex: investigation of evoked potentials and EEG phenomena. Physiol. Rev. 65:37–100.

Mitzdorf, U., and Singer, W. 1979. Excitatory synaptic ensemble properties in the visual cortex of the macaque monkey: a current source density analysis of electrically evoked potentials. J. Comp. Neurol. 187:71–83.

Mochizuki, H., Ugawa, Y., Machii, K., et al. 1999a. Somatosensory evoked high-frequency oscillation in Parkinson's disease and myoclonus epilepsy. Clin. Neurophysiol. 110:185–191.

Mochizuki, H., Ugawa, Y., Machii, K., et al. 1999b. Somatosensory evoked high-frequency oscillation in movement disorders. Electroencephalogr. Clin. Neurophysiol. Suppl. 49:90–94.

Nakano, S., and Hashimoto, I. 1999a. The later part of high-frequency oscillations in human somatosensory evoked potentials is enhanced in aged subjects. Neurosci. Lett. 276:83–86.

Nakano, S., and Hashimoto, I. 1999b. Comparison of somatosensory evoked high-frequency oscillations after posterior tibial and median nerve stimulation. Clin. Neurophysiol. 110:1948–1952.

Nakano, S., and Hashimoto, I. 2000. High-frequency oscillations in human somatosensory evoked potentials are enhanced in school children. Neurosci. Lett. 291:113–116.

Nakano, S., Tsuji, S., Matsunaga, K., et al. 1995. Effect of sleep stage on somatosensory evoked potentials by median nerve stimulation. Electroencephalogr. Clin. Neurophysiol. 96:385–389.

Noguchi, Y., Yamada, T., Yeh, M., et al. 1995. Dissociated changes of frontal and parietal somatosensory evoked potentials in sleep. Neurology 45:154–160.

Nowak, L.G., Azouz, R., Sanchez-Vives, M.V., et al. 2003. Electrophysiological classes of cat primary visual cortical neurons in vivo as revealed by quantitative analyses. J. Neurophysiol. 89:1541–1566.

Okada, Y.C., Wu, J., and Kyuhou, S. 1997. Genesis of MEG signals in a mammalian CNS structure. Electroencephalogr. Clin. Neurophysiol. 103:474–485.

Ozaki, I., Suzuki, C., Yaegashi, Y., et al. 1998. High frequency oscillations in early cortical somatosensory evoked potentials. Electroencephalogr. Clin. Neurophysiol. 108:536–542.

Ozaki, I., Yaegashi, Y., Kimura, T., et al. 2001. Dipole orientation differs between high frequency oscillations and N20m current sources in human somatosensory evoked magnetic fields to median nerve stimulation. Neurosci. Lett. 310:41–44.

Paradiso, C., De Vito, L., Rossi, S., et al. 1995. Cervical and scalp recorded short latency somatosensory evoked potentials in response to epidural spinal cord stimulation in patients with peripheral vascular disease. Electroencephalogr. Clin. Neurophysiol. 96:105–113.

Peterson, N.N., Schroeder, C.E., and Arezzo, J.C. 1995. Neural generators of early cortical somatosensory evoked potentials in the awake monkey. Electroencephalogr. Clin. Neurophysiol. 96:248–260.

Pubols, B.H., Jr., Haring, J.H., and Rowinski, M.J. 1989. Patterns of resting discharge in neurons of the raccoon main cuneate nucleus. J. Neurophysiol. 61:1131–1141.

Rasmusson, D.D. 1996. Changes in the response properties of neurons in the ventroposterior lateral thalamic nucleus of the raccoon after peripheral deafferentation. J. Neurophysiol. 75:2441–2450.

Rasmusson, D.D., and Northgrave, S.A. 1997. Reorganization of the raccoon cuneate nucleus after peripheral denervation. J. Neurophysiol. 78:2924–2936.

Reinagel, P., Godwin, D., Sherman, S.M., et al. 1999. Encoding of visual information by LGN bursts. J. Neurophysiol. 81:2558–2569.

Reinagel, P., and Reid, R.C. 2000. Temporal coding of visual information in the thalamus. J. Neurosci. 20:5392–5400.

Reinagel, P., and Reid, R.C. 2002. Precise firing events are conserved across neurons. J. Neurosci. 22:6837–6841.

Restuccia, D., Valeriani, M., Grassi, E., et al. 2002a. Contribution of GABAergic cortical circuitry in shaping somatosensory evoked scalp responses: specific changes after single-dose administration of tiagabine. Clin. Neurophysiol. 113:656–671.

Restuccia, D., Valeriani, M., Grassi, E., et al. 2002b. Dissociated changes of somatosensory evoked low-frequency scalp responses and 600 Hz bursts after single-dose administration of lorazepam. Brain Res. 946:1–11.

Restuccia, D., Della Marca, G., Valeriani, M., et al. 2003. Influence of cholinergic circuitries in generation of high-frequency somatosensory evoked potentials. Clin. Neurophysiol. 114:1538–1548.

Rossini, P.M., Basciani, M., Di Stefano, E., et al. 1985. Short-latency scalp somatosensory evoked potentials and central spine to scalp propagation characteristics during peroneal and median nerve stimulation in multiple sclerosis. Electroencephalogr. Clin. Neurophysiol. 60:197–206.

Sakuma, K., and Hashimoto, I. 1999. High-frequency magnetic oscillations evoked by posterior tibial nerve stimulation. Neuroreport 10:227–230.

Salin, P.A., and Prince, D.A. 1996. Electrophysiological mapping of GABA-A receptor-mediated inhibition in adult rat somatosensory cortex. J. Neurophysiol. 75:1589–1600.

Shimazu, H., Kaji, R., Tsujimoto, T., et al. 2000. High-frequency SEP components generated in the somatosensory cortex of the monkey. Neuroreport 11:2821–2826.

Sonoo, M., Genba-Shimizu, K., Mannen, T., et al. 1997. Detailed analysis of the latencies of median nerve somatosensory evoked potential components, 2: analysis of subcomponents of the P13/14 and N20 potentials. Electroencephalogr. Clin. Neurophysiol. 104:296–311.

Staba, R.J., Brett-Green, B., Paulsen, M., et al. 2003. Effects of ventrobasal lesion and cortical cooling on fast oscillations (>200 Hz) in rat somatosensory cortex. J. Neurophysiol. 89:2380–2388.

Stern, P., Edwards, F.A., and Sakmann, B. 1992. Fast and slow components of unitary EPSCs on stellate cells elicited by focal stimulation in slices of rat visual cortex. J. Physiol. (Lond.) 449:247–278.

Stoehr, M., and Riffel, B. 1982. Short-latency somatosensory evoked potentials to median nerve stimulation: components N13/P13, N14/P14, P15, P16 and P18 with different recording methods. J. Neurol. 228:39–47.

Swadlow, H.A. 1989. Efferent neurons and suspected interneurons in S-1 vibrissa cortex of the awake rabbit: receptive fields and axonal properties. J. Neurophysiol. 62:288–308.

Swadlow, H.A. 1990. Efferent neurons and suspected interneurons in S-1 forelimb representation of the awake rabbit: receptive fields and axonal properties. J. Neurophysiol. 63:1477–1498.

Swadlow, H.A. 1995. Influence of VPM afferents on putative inhibitory interneurons in S1 of the awake rabbit: evidence from cross-correlation, microstimulation, and latencies to peripheral sensory stimulation. J. Neurophysiol. 73:1584–1599.

Swadlow, H.A., and Gusev, A.G. 2001. The impact of "bursting" thalamic impulses at a neocortical synapse. Nat. Neurosci. 4:402–408.

Swadlow, H.A., Beloozerova, I.N., and Sirota, M.G. 1998. Sharp, local synchrony among putative feed-forward inhibitory interneurons of rabbit somatosensory cortex. J. Neurophysiol. 79:567–582.

Tanosaki, M., Hashimoto, I., Iguchi, Y., et al. 2001. Specific somatosensory processing in somatosensory area 3b for human thumb: a neuromagnetic study. Clin. Neurophysiol. 112:1516–1522.

Tanosaki, M., Kimura, T., Takino, R., et al. 2002. Movement interference attenuates somatosensory high-frequency oscillations: contribution of local axon collaterals of 3b pyramidal neurons. Clin. Neurophysiol. 113:993–1000.

Timofeev, I., Contreras, D., and Steriade, M. 1996. Synaptic responsiveness of cortical and thalamic neurones during various phases of slow sleep oscillation in cat. J. Physiol. (Lond.) 494:265–278.

Tsuji, S., Shibasaki, H., Kato, M., et al. 1984. Subcortical, thalamic and cortical somatosensory evoked potentials to median nerve stimulation. Electroencephalogr. Clin. Neurophysiol. 59:465–476.

Urasaki, E., Genmoto, T., Akamatsu, N., et al. 2002. The effects of stimulus rates on high frequency oscillations of median nerve somatosensory-evoked potentials—direct recording study from the human cerebral cortex. Clin. Neurophysiol. 113:1794–1797.

Vanderzant, C.W., Beydoun, A.A., Domer, P.A., et al. 1991. Polarity reversal of N20 and P23 somatosensory evoked potentials between scalp and depth recordings. Electroencephalogr. Clin. Neurophysiol. 78:234–239.

Volgushev, M., Chistiakova, M., and Singer, W. 1998. Modification of discharge patterns of neocortical neurons by induced oscillations of the membrane potential. Neuroscience 83:15–25.

Webster, H.H., Salimi, I., Myasnikov, A.A., et al. 1997. The effects of peripheral deafferentation on spontaneously bursting neurons in the somatosensory cortex of waking cats. Brain Res. 750:109–121.

White, E.L. 1979. Thalamocortical synaptic relations: a review with emphasis on the projections of specific thalamic nuclei to the primary sensory areas of the neocortex. Brain Res. 180:275–311.

Wood, C.C., Cohen, D., Cuffin, B.N., et al. 1985. Electrical sources in human somatosensory cortex: identification by combined magnetic and potential recordings. Science 227:1051–1053.

Yamada, T., Kameyama, S., Fuchigami, Y., et al. 1988. Changes of short latency somatosensory evoked potential in sleep. Electroencephalogr. Clin. Neurophysiol. 70:126–136.

27. Epileptic Seizure Disorders

Ernst Niedermeyer

Basic Considerations

Definition

There is no disease named "epilepsy." Rather, epileptic seizures are abnormal reactions of the brain caused by a large number of diseases. The entire brain or parts of it may be involved; the extent of involvement largely determines the type of seizure. The basic disorder is most commonly localized in the brain, but the failure of important organ systems outside the brain and associated metabolic-toxic changes may lead to secondary encephalopathies and thus to epileptic seizures. Genetic predisposition, which is now being elucidated in these years of clinical genetic progress, also plays a role in epileptic seizures.

The prevalence of epileptic seizures has been estimated to be between 0.5% (core group) and 5% (fringe group with at least one seizure during life). More precise figures of Juul-Jensen and Foldspang (1983) lie between 1.27% and 2.44%. Gumnit (1984) feels that core and fringe group may add up to 9% of the population.

An overview of various epilepsy prevalence studies (Annegers, 1993) shows fairly consistent figures: Bombay, India 3.7; Rochester, Minnesota, 6.66; Denmark, 6.9; Poland, 7.8; Nigeria, 5.3; Mississippi, 6.78; and China, 4.57 (prevalence per 1,000). Similar figures were presented by Greulich and Gerber (1994) and Hauser (1998).

Introduction and Historical Remarks

Electroencephalography (EEG) has revolutionized the entire field of epileptology. No one can deny that ingenious and even great concepts arose in the pre-EEG era; clinical acumen and keen analysis of the observed phenomena resulted in the separation of minor seizures from the tonic-clonic grand mal convulsion. Bravais (1827) has been credited with the description of *focal motor seizures,* while Falret (1860) and Herpin (1867) attempted to individualize *psychomotor seizures* ("aura intellectuel"). Hughlings Jackson deepened insight into such forms of minor attack and their focal origin (Jackson, 1866; Jackson and Beevor, 1889; Jackson and Stewart, 1899). Jackson's work laid the foundation for the linkage of temporal lobe pathology and psychomotor seizures (complex partial seizures); these relationships were further supported by the work of Knapp (1905, 1918) and Stauder (1935).

Petit mal absences were described and categorized prior to the advent of the EEG. Friedmann (1906) gave a detailed account of these absences; he stressed the predominantly benign course of the disorder and felt that these attacks were basically nonepileptic. The term *pyknolepsy* (Sauer, 1916) became quite popular in the German literature; again, em-phasis was placed on the categorical differences between these absences and true epilepsy. The term *pyknolepsy* was used only for children who never developed grand mal. This concept was completely shattered by the EEG observations of Gibbs et al. (1935) and Jung (1939), which demonstrated the same ictal EEG abnormalities in pyknolepsy and epileptic petit mal absences.

The clinical epileptological picture of infantile spasms was described by West (1841); its clinical uniqueness was almost unmistakable, although EEG confirmation by hypsarrhythmic EEG was lacking. On the other hand, the individualization of the *Lennox-Gastaut syndrome* as a clinical epileptological entity depends too heavily on the availability of EEG studies; for the reason, this syndrome has long remained unrecognized (Lennox, 1960; Gastaut et al., 1966, following this EEG observations of Gibbs et al., 1939).

This brief historical review shows very clearly how the progress of clinical epileptology was severely hampered by the unavailability of electrophysiological data. Although the conventional EEG has opened new vistas, modern EEG techniques have made further important epileptological contributions; these include prolonged monitoring of epileptics. These noninvasive techniques have been complemented by recordings from cortex and deep structures of the brain.

Basic Mechanisms of Epileptogenesis

Electrophysiological Methods

Epileptogenesis expresses itself in macro- and microphenomena. Macrophenomena usually alter the EEG, i.e., the macro-EEG, even though they may escape detection by scalp, cortical, or depth electrodes. The discovery of the EEG spike in animal experimentation (Fischer, 1933) catapulted EEG into basic epileptological research aiming at the understanding of the electrical macrophenomena of epileptic activity.

This era of macroevent orientation ended with the introduction of microelectrodes. Tungsten- and glass-pipette electrodes of 5 to 10 μm and eventually around 1 μm in diameter made possible the recording from outside and inside a single neuron. These electrodes have a high ohmic resistance (up to 60 megaohm), which is incompatible with the commercially available EEG amplifiers; the biological potentials would be short-circuited, resulting in noisy recordings. The introduction of the cathode follower (impedance changer) (Toennies, 1938) made possible the recording from single neurons.

Extracellular neuronal recordings were introduced by Li et al. (1952), Jung et al. (1952), and Moruzzi (1952). These microrecordings shed a lot more light on neuronal behavior in the genesis of EEG phenomena and epileptic activity. A by far greater breakthrough was achieved with the introduction of the intraneuronal recording technique: first at the spinal level (Brock et al., 1952; Eccles, 1957, 1958), later at the cortical level (Li, 1962; Philips, 1961). This new technique permitted insights into the behavior of the membrane potential. The biophysical characteristics of the latter were already known from recordings of amphibian giant neurons (Hodgkin and Huxley, 1952; also see Hodgkin, 1964, and Woodbury, 1969).

The Paroxysmal Depolarization Shift

In epileptic conditions, the membrane potential of cortical and deeper seated neurons changes enormously, to an extent that by far exceeds the usual physiological changes occurring with neuronal excitation and associated depolarization. A large paroxysmal depolarization shift (PDS) (Goldensohn and Purpura, 1963; Matsumoto and Ajmone Marsan, 1964) is capable of changing the resting membrane potential of -85 mV to $+30$ mV. This enormous shift is accompanied by massive bursts of rapid neuronal spikes (this is the "spike of the electroneurophysiologist": arising from a single neuron with a duration of about 1 msec, in contrast with the "spike of the electroencephalographer," seen in the conventional EEG; see Chapter 13, "Abnormal EEG Patterns: Epileptic and Paroxysmal"). PDSs originating from a more or less wide cortical region are associated with spike discharges recorded from the surface or scalp EEG (Fig. 27.1).

The nature of the PDS has been hotly debated. Is this paroxysmal phenomenon based on endogenous membrane instability or is it of exogenous and secondary character? What would be the prime mover in the latter case? Is the PDS a specific epileptic entity or is it just an enormous excitatory postsynaptic potential (EPSP): a vastly exaggerated and basically physiological excitatory postsynaptic potential without intrinsic epileptic connotation? A synthesis of these originally opposed views has developed during the last decades.

Neurobiochemical Factors of Epileptogenesis

There is no longer a struggle between the proponents of the "sparks" (primary electrical action) and the "soup" (primary action of the chemical substances). It is now established that neurobiochemical phenomena are primary, giving rise to electrical manifestations. These latter, however, are readily recordable and permit a splendid documentation of the events.

Ions are of great importance. The role of sodium is pivotal in the excitation of the membranes. The sodium pump has been thought to be of special significance in epileptogenesis. It is interesting to note that special interest in the role of sodium in intracellular activities was most active in the 1950s; this era was followed by a period of special interest in potassium and its effect. In the 1970s, special emphasis was placed on calcium and its influx into the neuron as the cause of neuronal depolarization (Lux, 1984; Lux and Heinemann, 1983; Schwartzkroin and Wyler, 1980; Witte, 1987). The role of chloride in penicillin-induced neuronal discharges was also emphasized (Uhlìg et al., 1988; Witte, 1991).

The ionic environment of the neuron is thought to be regulated by glial cells (Futamachi and Pedley, 1976; Prince et al., 1977; Somjen, 1984).

From the technical viewpoint, the use of voltage-clamp, current-clamp, and especially the patch-clamp technique (Neher et al., 1978), has made it possible to demonstrate minute currents in the picoampere range as well as the opening and closing of ionic membrane channels. Voltage-gated ion channels and voltage-gated currents are being regarded as important elements in the understanding of epileptic activity (Heinemann and Eder, 1998).

Neurotransmitters

Excitatory neurotransmitters are naturally involved in epileptogenesis. Glutamate and aspartate [and especially N-methyl-D-aspartate (NMDA)] have been recognized as the most active neuroexcitatory transmitters in the experimental animal as well as in humans (Fisher, 1991a; Sherwin et al., 1988).

γ-Aminobutyric acid (GABA) is considered the most powerful inhibitor of epileptic mechanisms; naturally, its failure may strongly contribute to epileptogenesis. Its depressive effect on neuronal excitability was discovered by Elliott and Jaspers (1959). It has been proposed that GABA is a macromolecular complex with an (a) GABA binding site; (b) a chloride channel, which opens when GABA binds; and (c) a regulatory site (Fariello et al., 1991). A subdivision of GABA receptors refers to the traditional GABA receptors as $GABA_A$ with baclofen as agonist; $GABA_B$ has been linked to potassium and calcium currents. The effect of glutamate and GABA on a single neuron is shown in Figure 27.2; note the massive excitatory depolarization with glutamate and the inhibitory hyperpolarization with GABA.

Figure 27.1. A schematic representation of simultaneously recorded intracellular, extracellular, and field potentials in an epileptiform hippocampal slice. The field potential may be studied as an analogue of the EEG interictal spike. (From Fisher, R.S. 1987. The hippocampal slice. Am. J. EEG Technol. 27:1–14.)

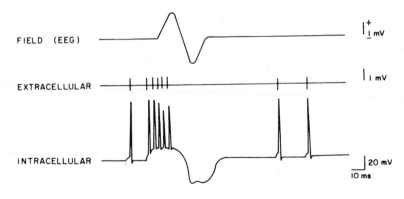

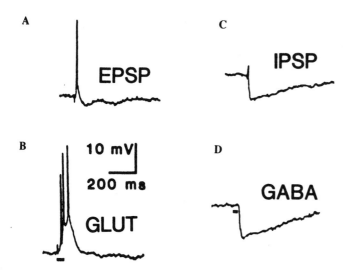

Figure 27.2. Local application of putative neurotransmitters to slice neurons can mimic electrically evoked synaptic transmission. **A:** A shock-evoked excitatory postsynaptic potential (EPSP) in a CA1 pyramidal cell. **B:** A depolarization produced by brief pressure-application of glutamate (GLUT) to the dendritic tree of a CA1 pyramidal neuron. Glutamate was prepared as a 10 mM solution, buffered to pH 7.0, and applied by pressure (10 ps for 5 msec). **C:** A shock-evoked inhibitory postsynaptic potential (IPSP) in a CA1 neuron. **D:** A hyperpolarization, closely resembling the native IPSP, is produced by a brief (10 psi, 20 msec) application of 10 mM γ-aminobutyric acid (GABA) to the cell body region. (From Fisher, R.S. 1987. The hippocampal slice. Am. J. EEG Technol. 27:1–14.)

According to Johnston (1993), neurotransmitters are likely to (a) contribute to epileptogenesis (establishment of epileptic state), (b) contribute to initiation of seizures, (c) modify spread and duration of seizures, and (d) contribute to termination of seizures.

There has been accumulating evidence that focal epileptiform activity is antagonized by GABA and its agonists (Fariello et al., 1991). Generalized epilepsies (without demonstrable focal onset), however, may be enhanced by GABA agonists. The work of Fromm and his co-workers (Faingold and Fromm, 1992; Fromm, 1974, 1986) has provided evidence of an inverse situation in petit mal absence epilepsy with generalized 3/sec spike waves—this form of epilepsy is being conceived as an inhibitory seizure disorder (which indeed requires a special therapeutic approach). While glutamate/aspartate (NMDA) represents the leading excitatory and GABA the eminent inhibitory neurotransmitter, a concept of an imbalance of these two substances as the cause of epileptic seizures would be extremely simplistic. Fisher and Coyle (1991) have emphasized the enormous complexity in the biochemical regulation of paroxysmal activities; the fact remains that "epilepsy involves multiple neurotransmitter systems." Norepinephrine is believed to exert inhibitory effects (Chauvel et al., 1982; Jimenez-Rivera and Waterhouse, 1991). Acetylcholine was thought to have powerful convulsive properties (Tower, 1960) but more recent work has ascribed both excitatory and inhibitory (and seizure-protective) functions to this substance (Segal, 1991).

Protein systems (neuromodulators, second messengers) appear to be involved in epileptiform activity (Delgado—

Escueta et al., 1986; Wasterlain and Mazarati, 1998). The protein calmodulin is presumed to mediate the action of calcium (DeLorenzo, 1986; Kennedy and Greengard, 1981). Peptides related to opiates (endogenous opioid-like peptides) may have both convulsive and anticonvulsive effects (Siggins and Zieglgansberger, 1981; Snead and Simonato, 1991). Postictal electrical depression and refractoriness could result from the release of opioid peptides (Bajorek et al., 1986).

"Second messenger systems" may alter neuronal functioning leading to divergent region-specific effects (Kubo et al., 1986; Vornov and Coyle, 1991). It is presumed that second messenger systems and especially nitric oxide (dual role as endogenous anticonvulsant and neurotoxin?) can modulate neuronal excitability, thus becoming a major factor in the epileptogenesis (Baraban et al., 1991; Vornov, 1991; Wasterlain and Mazarati, 1998).

Neuronal excitability—and hence epileptogenicity—is governed by the interaction of voltage- and ligand-gated ion channels (Traub et al., 1996). In this manner, at least some epileptic syndromes have been thought to be channelopathies (Celesia, 2001, Köhling, 2002; Steinlein and Noebels, 2000).

Seizure Initiation

With increasing influx of afferent signals and massive neuronal depolarization, a negative direct current (DC) shift (this is an ultraslow EEG potential that defies conventional amplification and requires specific direct-coupled "DC recording") starts heralding an epileptic event with or without behavioral ictal signs. The transition from interictal spiking on the cortical surface to ictal spike activity (clinical or subclinical) may be related to a breakdown of local inhibitory mechanisms. Depression of calcium concentration in the extracellular space might contribute to the depression of inhibitory mechanisms (Louvel and Heinemann, 1983). The cerebral localization of the beginning ictal activity may play a role and differs between neocortical epileptogenesis (Connors and Gutnick, 1984) and epileptic activity found in hippocampic slices (Fisher, 1987; Wong et al., 1984).

Precipitation by Influx of Special Afferent Impulses ("Reflex Epilepsy")

The West African baboon *Papio papio,* the epitome of a photosensitivity on a genetic basis, is discussed below (see Primary Generalized Epilepsy). Photosensitive epilepsies are of clinical importance in the human and rare in the kingdom of animals.

Audiogenic (sonogenic) seizures are found in certain strains of mice and rats (Collins, 1972; Faingold and Meldrum, 1990; Krushinsky, 1962; Millan, 1988). The integrity of the inferior colliculus is essential for the development of audiogenic seizures in sound-sensitive animals (Millan, 1988). Human forms of epilepsies caused by unusual triggering factors are discussed later in this chapter.

Spread and Generalization of Epileptic Activity

Intracortical propagation of epileptic activity may occur from dendrite to dendrite (Petsche et al., 1976) or from soma to soma. According to Jasper (1969), the most important mechanism of epileptic spread is synaptic propagation along conducting pathways while spread of potential fields by volume conduction plays a lesser role. Spreading depression (Leão, 1944, 1972) is a very slowly moving process of propagation and may also be involved in epileptic spread (Goldensohn, 1969).

A. Earl Walker and his co-workers have made extensive studies of the spread of epileptic activity induced mainly by penicillin (but also by strychnine and electrical stimulation) in the monkey (Udvarhelyi and Walker, 1965; Walker, 1970; Walker and Udvarhelyi, 1965; Walker et al., 1952). Emphasis was placed on typical "low threshold areas" and "high threshold areas" in the brain. In this manner, the propensities for epileptic responses in various areas of neocortex, limbic system, basal ganglia, thalamus, brainstem, and cerebellum were explored.

Mirror Focus and Secondary Epileptogenesis

Secondary epileptogenic foci may result from the spread of epileptic activity. Morrell (1959) produced foci of homologous areas of the cerebrum with the freezing technique. A secondary focus was found in the region of callosal terminations of the neurons involved in the primary focus ("mirror focus"; Morrell, 1969; Wilder, 1972). The role of secondary epileptogenesis in the human is still an area of controversy (Morrell, 1978, 1985).

The transcallosal "transfer" of cortical spike discharges to the contralateral cortex is doubtful, according to the observations of Ono et al. (2002) in patients undergoing callosotomy.

Cortical Epileptic Activity Propagating into Spinal Cord and Lower Motor Neuron

According to Fromm (1987), the brainstem reticular formation plays a leading role in the propagation of epileptic activity to spinal motor units. This work seems to confirm earlier views of Gastaut and Fischer-Williams (1959).

Special Inhibitory (Anticonvulsive) Mechanisms

Small penicillin-induced foci of cortical epileptic activity are counteracted by a ring of inhibitory action ("surround inhibition"; Prince and Wilder, 1967). The mechanism of "vertical inhibition" (Elger and Speckmann, 1983) plays a major role in the prevention of descending epileptic neuronal activity into the spinal cord.

Seizure-Terminating Inhibitory Mechanisms

The termination of a generalized tonic-clonic convulsion (grand mal seizure) was thought to be due to the depletion of metabolic supplies and increasing hypoxia (Meyer and Portnoy, 1959). It was difficult, however, to reconcile such a view with the abrupt and virtually generalized-synchronous transition from pronounced epileptic EEG activity to sudden flatness—demonstrable in the EEG on the scalp as well as in deep structures.

An active inhibition as the cause of seizure termination was postulated by Efron (1961) and is now widely accepted (Levy and O'Leary, 1965). Cortical norepinephrine strongly increases with the termination of epileptic discharges (Chauvel et al., 1982).

Ablation of the cerebellum enhances epileptic activity in the animal (Dow, 1965). A considerable bulk of literature has dealt with the inhibitory role of the cerebellum in epileptic activity (Babb et al., 1974; Dow et al., 1962; Snider and Cooke, 1953).

The neurobiochemical component of seizure inhibition and termination must not be ignored. Endogenous opioid peptides (which also have seizure-provoking effects) are likely to play a role in seizure termination (Tortella, 1988). This is another example of apparently antagonistic effects caused by the same substance. The species of the experimental animal and the dosage of the substance are important factors. The warning that experimental models may not be relevant to human epilepsy (Johnston, 1993) cannot be overemphasized.

Synchronization of Epileptic Activity

Synchronization of neuronal discharges is of pivotal importance in the generation of substantial and clinical epileptic activity. Synchronization is a still poorly understood epileptogenic mechanism. According to Dichter and Ayala (1987), synchronization may be caused by any of the following mechanisms: (a) recurrent synaptic and nonsynaptic mechanisms (especially via recurrent collaterals and positive feedback mechanisms), (b) antidromic activation of afferent fibers, (c) ephaptic interactions caused by large currents flowing through extracellular space, (d) changes in extracellular ionic concentrations, (e) electrical coupling between neurons, and (f) diffuse release of liberators.

A mathematical model of synchronization was developed by Traub and Wong (1982) and Wong et al. (1986). It was shown that, in the hippocampal slice, as few as four neurons could suffice to sustain paroxysmal burst activity. It is interesting to note, however, that Wyler (1986) was unable to find evidence of enhanced synchronous neuronal firing in epileptogenic foci produced in monkeys.

Confronted with the question "What is Epilepsy?" Schwartzkroin (1993) has singled out hyperexcitability and hypersynchrony as the most important factors in the genesis of epileptic phenomena. These two factors do not have to coincide (with hypersynchrony being of much greater significance in generalized spike-wave discharges).

Experimental Animal Models for Focal Epilepsies

Limitations in the usefulness of animal models in epilepsy research are indubitable; this can be gleaned from the work of Dudek et al. (2002).

Penicillin

Topical application of penicillin on cortex and other cerebral structures has become a classical demonstration of acute epileptogenesis (since the first report of Walker et al., 1946). Prominent negative spikes arise from the affected cerebral region, becoming periodic and stereotyped (Prince and Wilder, 1971; Speckmann and Elger, 1987), firing along with the aforementioned massive paroxysmal depolarization shifts and heralded by slow negative DC shifts (Gumnit and Takahashi, 1965).

Maximal Electroshock

This model for generalized as well as focal epileptic seizures was developed by Spiegel (1937) and proved to be substantial in the discovery of phenytoin and its antiepileptic effects (Merritt and Putnam, 1938). As Fisher (1991b) has pointed out, this method is a model for acute seizures rather than for epileptic seizure disorders. This objection is true for most animal models.

Pentylenetetrazol (Metrazol)

Von Meduna (1935, 1937) used intravenous (i.v.) pentylenetetrazol (PTZ) as convulsive therapy for psychotic patients. Its effects on the central nervous system (CNS) is multifold but there is a very important special effect on the "generalizing system" generating generalized spike waves and myoclonus before a tonic-clonic seizure occurs. This system is most important in the human (in whom focal epileptogenic responses may also be obtained) (Ajmone Marsan and Ralston, 1957). Cortex (forebrain), brainstem, and spinal cord are involved in the epileptic response of the cat (Magistris et al., 1988). By contrast, Miller and Ferrendelli (1988) have stressed a leading role of the medial thalamus and brainstem in PTZ-induced seizures.

Strychnine

Large negative spikes are elicited by topical cortical application of strychnine (Dusser de Barenne and McCulloch, 1939), whereas pronounced rhythmical spiking develops in the reticular formation (cat) with systemic application (Bremer, 1941). Strychnine appears to be antagonistic to the widely (but not consistently) inhibitory effect of glycine.

Ouabain

Ouabain's convulsive effect is probably related to inhibition of sodium and potassium transport and potassium depletion in the brain (Tower, 1969).

Tetrodotoxin

Tetrodotoxin acts on neuronal sodium channels (McIlwain, 1969).

Estrogens

Convulsive action was reported first by Woolley and Timiras (1962).

Kainic Acid

Kainic acid is used mainly for microinjections into limbic structures, producing "limbic status epilepticus" (Menini et al., 1980). The mechanism of action is unclear (an "enigmatic excitotoxin," Olney et al., 1986).

Pilocarpine

Pilocarpine is a muscarinic agent with cholinergic effect, producing seizures in rats (Turski et al., 1983), after hours of convulsions leading to neuronal loss in hippocampus, amygdala, thalamus, neocortex, and substantia nigra (Meldrum, 1988).

Nicotine

Injection of nicotine into the globus pallidus or pars reticularis of the substantia nigra (dogs, monkeys) produces clonic convulsions (Hayashi, 1953; cited by Meldrum, 1988).

Other Convulsive Substances

Other important convulsive substances are picrotoxin (Hahn, 1960), bemegride (Megimide) (Rodin et al., 1958), bicuculline (Meldrum and Horton, 1971), thiosemicarbazide (Wood and Abrahams, 1971), allylglycine (Alberici et al., 1969), methionine sulfoxide (Gershoff and Elvehjem, 1951), and homocysteine (Sprince et al., 1969). Their mode of action has been discussed by Fisher (1991b). The convulsive effect of bicuculline is markedly enhanced by extracellular application of cesium (Hwa and Avoli, 1991).

Kindling

Kindling denotes repeated subthreshold electrical stimulation of various cerebral regions and especially in limbic areas (mostly in the cat). The word *kindling* was introduced by Goddard (1967) following earlier work of Delgado and Sevillano (1961). The amygdaloid region is particularly responsive to kindling (McNamara, 1986; Wada and Sato, 1974).

The kindling technique aims at the gradual escalation of epileptic activity culminating in spontaneous seizures. A reduction of calcium and norepinephrine materializes in the course of kindling (Sato and Ogawa, 1984). There is also a depletion of dopamine in the amygdala. There is evidence that the substantia nigra is capable of regulating the kindling seizure threshold (Gale, 1986; McNamara, 1986). The generalization of epileptic discharges may occur via the midbrain reticular formation (Wada and Sato, 1975, 1975b). GABA agonists have protective effect against kindling.

The kindling effect is less readily demonstrable in higher mammals and may be absent in the human (Le Gal la Salle et al., 1982).

Experimental Models Based on Epileptogenic Lesions Produce Epileptic Responses after a Certain Delay

Alumina Cream

Pure metals tend to produce epileptogenic effects following topical application to the cerebrum. Focal or generalized seizures start 2 to 8 weeks after topical injection. The seizures usually run a self-limited course and respond to antiepileptic medication. Kopeloff et al. (1941) introduced this method, which became widely used (Ward, 1972). The underlying biochemical changes are unclear (Delgado-Escueta et al., 1986).

Cobalt

Seizures induced by topically injected cobalt start 24 to 48 hours after injection (Kopeloff, 1960; Mutani, 1967) and may be of focal or generalized character.

Tungstic Acid

Topical injection produces acute and stormy epileptogenic effects starting 2 to 3 hours after injection (Blum and Liban, 1960).

Freeze or Cold Lesion

Powerful epileptic responses are produced by freezing of cerebral cortex, starting several hours afterward (Goldensohn and Purpura, 1962; Morrell, 1959; Speranski, 1943). Acute edema and chronic gliosis develop at the site of the lesion (Pedley et al., 1976).

Animal models aiming at the elucidation of generalized epilepsies are discussed below (see Primary Generalized Epilepsy).

The Building Blocks of Epileptic EEG Activity: Spikes (Spike Waves, Polyspikes) but Also Ultraslow and Ultrafast Activity

Spikes and spike-related potentials are not the only basic EEG mechanism of epileptic phenomena. There has been growing evidence that ultraslow activity (CD potentials of near-zero frequency; also see Chapter 2 of Speckmann and Elger and Chapter 25 of Vanhatolo et al.) plays a major role by generating a negative baseline shift with superimposed spikes.

Ultrafast activity in the 80- to 1000-Hz range is another building block of epileptic activity (see Chapter 26 of Curio). Figure 27.3 shows paroxysmal activity induced by pentylenetetrazol in a Sprague-Dawley rat (Niedermeyer and Sherman, 2001). Spike activity of fast, slender character (note parameter of time!) are shown in the rat's neocortex, whereas ultrafast activity in the range of 200 to 300/sec is noted in the hippocampus (CA1, CA2). A special relationship between neocortical spiking and hippocampic ultrafast activity could not be demonstrated.

Traub (2003) found such ultrafast "ripples" in the mice rendered epileptic, chiefly in the CA1, faster than 200 Hz but not exceeding 400 Hz. Ultrafast ripples have also been observed in the feline seizures (Grenier et al., 2003). These authors have also studied the intracellular correlates of the ultrafast activity.

Figure 27.4 shows and overview of the "epileptic building blocks," which are not limited to spike discharges and longer. These are exciting times: new light is being thrown on the electrophysiology of epilepsy, and our comprehension of epileptic phenomena is about to deepen considerably.

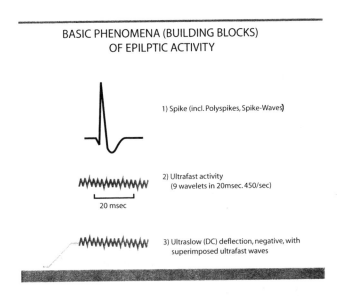

BASIC PHENOMENA (BUILDING BLOCKS) OF EPILPTIC ACTIVITY

1) Spike (incl. Polyspikes, Spike-Waves)

2) Ultrafast activity (9 wavelets in 20msec. 450/sec)

20 msec

3) Ultraslow (DC) deflection, negative, with superimposed ultrafast waves

Figure 27.4.   Basic phenomena (building blocks) of epileptic activity.

Types of Epileptic Seizures

The character of an epileptic seizure is more or less strongly determined by the chief cerebral area involved. Another important factor is the underlying basic epileptic condition, which is the topic of a large section of this chapter. As a matter of fact, the underlying basic condition may be of paramount significance, especially in an infant with infantile spasms-hypsarrhythmia and jackknife seizures, which are not found outside this basic epileptic condition, or in a child with Lennox-Gastaut syndrome and atonic drop attacks, which are germane to this condition and alien to others (also see Wolf, 1985). These basic epileptic conditions are age-determined; for this reason, age is an important factor that is capable of modifying the character of epileptic seizures. Furthermore, the nature and extent of an underlying cerebral lesion may be a negligible factor in the determination of the seizure type in the group of age-determined epileptic conditions.

Figure 27.3. Ongoing paroxysmal activity in rat after pentylenetetrazol. The neocortical tracing at the top shows periodic spikes at a rate of nearly 5/sec. Keep in mind that the entire trace spans a time course of about 0.9 sec. Also keep in mind that these spikes are indeed fast and slender rather than blunted. There is a minimal spread of some neocortical spikes into the anterior thalamic region. Ultrafast ripples reaching frequencies of 200 to 300/sec are quite prominent in the hippocampic lead, while just hints are found in the posterior thalamic tracing. There is no relationship between neocortical spikes and ultrafast ripples in this sample (but noted at other occasions). (Reprinted with permission of the Am. J. End Technol.)

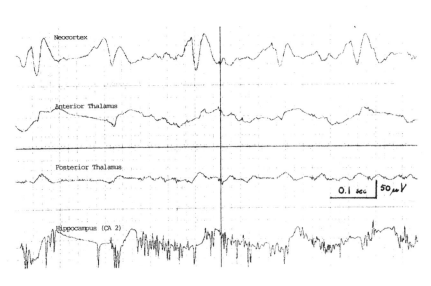

Neocortex

Anterior Thalamus

Posterior Thalamus

0.1 sec 50 μV

Hippocampus (CA 2)

Certain types of seizures, such as focal motor and psychomotor seizures, are highly indicative of special cerebral areas, whereas others are of much less localizing value. The localization depends heavily on such confirming EEG evidence as local spikes and recorded ictal episodes and, in some special cases, on the demonstration of regional changes with depth electrodes. Structural neurodiagnostic tests are needed for the demonstration of significant morphological changes.

Focal seizures may be a prelude to an ensuing grand mal convulsion. The term *aura* has been used for such initiating focal seizures, especially for attacks impinging on afferent systems (visual, acoustic, olfactory, somatosensory, gustatory, and so forth).

Simultaneous EEG recording and functional magnetic resonance imaging (MRI) is beset with problems since the EEG is being obtained in a high-field magnet and during scanning. Baudewig et al. (2001) have reported a method demonstrating simultaneous blood-oxygenation-dependent ("BOLD") MRI sequences and EEG activity with very little artifactual distortion (in epileptic patients).

Classification of Epileptic Seizures

The classification of epileptic seizures is a thankless job. The preferences of "splitters" and "lumpers" must be reconciled in the tedious work of an international committee entrusted with this task by the International League Against Epilepsy, progressing from the older classifications of reputed epileptologists that have sometimes been marred by personal biases. The following classification has been proposed by the Commission on Classification and Terminology (1981). More recent classifications have added relatively little to this straightforward list.

I. Partial (focal, local) seizures
  A. Simple partial seizures (consciousness not impaired)
    1. With motor signs
      a. Focal motor without march
      b. Focal motor with march (jacksonian)
      c. Versive
      d. Postural
      e. Phonatory (vocalization or arrest of speech)
    2. With somatosensory or special sensory symptoms (simple hallucinations, e.g., tingling, light flashes, buzzing)
      a. Somatosensory
      b. Visual
      c. Auditory
      d. Olfactory
      e. Gustatory
      f. Vertiginous
    3. With autonomic symptoms or signs (including epigastric sensation, pallor, sweating, flushing, piloerection, and pupillary dilatation)
    4. With psychic symptoms (disturbance of higher cerebral function), rarely occurring without impairment of consciousness and more commonly experienced as complex partial seizures
      a. Dysphasic
      b. Dysmnesic (e.g., déjà vu)
      c. Cognitive (e.g., dreamy states, distortions of time sense)
      d. Affective (fear, anger)
      e. Illusions (e.g., macropsia)
      f. Structured hallucinations (e.g., music, scenes)
  B. Complex partial seizures (with impairment of consciousness; may sometimes begin with simple symptomatology)
    1. Simple partial onset, followed by impairment of consciousness
      a. With simple partial features (A.1–A.4 above) followed by impaired consciousness
      b. With automatisms
    2. With impairment of consciousness at onset
      a. With impairment of consciousness only
      b. With automatisms
  C. Partial seizures evolving to secondarily generalized seizures (tonic-clonic, tonic, or clonic)
    1. Simple partial seizures evolving to generalized seizures
    2. Complex partial seizures evolving to generalized seizures
    3. Simple partial seizures evolving to complex partial seizures evolving to generalized seizures
II. Generalized seizures (convulsive or nonconvulsive)
  A. Absence seizures
    1. Typical absences, alone or in combination
      a. Impairment of consciousness only
      b. With mild clonic components
      c. With atonic components
      d. With tonic components
      e. With automatisms
      f. With autonomic components
    2. Atypical absence
      a. May have changes in tone that are more pronounced than in A.1
      b. Onset and/or cessation that is not abrupt
  B. Myoclonic seizures (myoclonic jerks, single or multiple)
  C. Clonic seizures
  D. Tonic seizures
  E. Tonic-clonic seizures
  F. Atonic seizures (astatic)
Combinations of the above may occur, e.g., B and F, B and D
III. Unclassified epileptic seizures
IV. Addendum, with respect to occurrence of seizures (cyclic, fortuitous) or precipitation by triggering events

Although widely used and officially recommended (and essentially reiterated by Dreifuss, 1994), this classification has not yet found general acceptance. This might be due to an excess of new terms and the use of cumbersome formulations. Familiar expressions such as "grand mal" and "petit mal" have been all but eliminated in the classification, but numerous neurologists still cling to these terms, even if they are often erroneously used. Unfortunately, the introduction of new terms does not necessarily shed more light on the nature of the seizure types. A breakdown into small ictal-behavioral or ictal-EEG detail may render a classification more nebulous. There are, of course, limitations for every attempt at seizure type classifications. The classification of 1981 cannot accommodate a considerable number of seizures, which then must be listed as unclassifiable because they do not fit the procrustean bed.

We will hence use a double-track system utilizing both old customary and modern terms.

Grand Mal (Tonic-Clonic Seizure)

Clinical Manifestations

The sequence of clinical manifestations has been masterfully described by Gowers (1881, see also republication in 1964) and is given in detail below. Further detailed descriptions were given by Janz (1969), Gastaut and Broughton (1972), and Karbowski (1985). The tonic-clonic seizure lasts about 40 to 70 seconds, or sometimes up to 90 seconds. Initial massive generalized tonic spasm is sometimes initiated with a cry ("a wild, harsh, screaming sound," Gowers, 1881). It is immediately associated with loss of consciousness (profound coma); the arms are usually in semiflexion and the legs in extension. After about 10 to 20 seconds, it is supplanted by the clonic phase in which "the vibratory phenomenon (noted with palpation of the extremely tense muscles) becomes sufficiently prolonged to interrupt completely the tonic contraction" (Gastaut and Broughton, 1972).

This leads to a succession of brief and violent flexor spasms of the entire body. Accompanying apnea leads to a grayish livid complexion, while the rhythmical clonic spasms slow down until a final massive myoclonus marks the end of the seizure. According to Gastaut and Broughton (1972), tongue biting usually materializes during the clonic phase. Mydriasis, arterial hypertension, and tachycardia accompany the attack. Enuresis usually occurs at the termination of the seizure (Gastaut and Broughton, 1972); there may occasionally be loss of feces. The patient is completely flaccid after the last clonic jerk, after which respiration returns. Only a few seconds after the beginning of the flaccid, immediate postictal phase, a tonic muscle spasm returns that is most intense and prolonged in the masseter (Gastaut and Broughton, 1972). This postictal trismus temporarily blocks respiratory effect. The respiration becomes regular in the ensuing recuperative phase, during which the patient returns to consciousness unless he slips directly into a period of postictal sleep. A fall caused by grand mal can be traumatizing; even epidural hematoma has been reported (Tabbador and Balagura, 1981).

Tonic-clonic seizures may occasionally show *unilateral predominance* of the clinical manifestations. Gastaut and Broughton (1972) feel strongly that these attacks (which are more common in children and infants) are in fact generalized seizures with unilateral expression. Do attenuated or mitigated grand mal seizures exist? The answer is affirmative according to Karbowski (1985). These attacks are characterized by shorter duration and rudimentary tonic or clonic phases, possibly due to the effect of anticonvulsive medication.

EEG Manifestations

The grand mal attack is initiated by an abrupt loss of voltage (desynchronization, electrodecremental period) of a few seconds duration; there is evidence of very fast (20–40/sec) activity in all leads. In patients with primary generalized epilepsy, several generalized bursts of polyspike wave complexes with massive bilateral myoclonus may precede the phase of desynchronization.

Muscle activity rapidly obscures the recording; the vertex derivation, however, may remain artifact-free due to the lack of underlying muscles. Informative grand mal recordings can be secured only from patients with muscle relaxation from curarization and artificial respiration. Removal of muscle artifact by means of digital filtering has been achieved by Gotman et al. (1981).

After the phase of desynchronization, which may be as short as 1 to 3 seconds, rhythmical activity at about 10/sec with rapidly increasing amplitude dominates the EEG. Gastaut and Broughton (1972) have laid much stress on this frequency ("epileptic recruiting rhythm," Gastaut and Fischer-Williams, 1959), which is better discernible with the use of automatic frequency analysis.

About 10 seconds after the onset of a seizure, slower frequencies are noted, gradually slowing into the theta and delta range. Once the frequency of 4/sec is reached, "each slow wave interrupts the recruiting rhythm, giving rise to polyspikes and wave complexes, themselves decreasing in frequency" (Gastaut and Broughton, 1972). The clonic activity corresponds with generalized polyspike bursts at each myoclonic jerk (Fig. 27.5).

The last clonic contraction is followed by postictal flatness for several seconds (Zifkin and Dravet, 1998). Very slow irregular delta activity ("postseizure stupor," Gibbs and Gibbs, 1952) then dominates the EEG, with gradual frequency increase into the theta and alpha band; the appearance of an organized posterior alpha rhythm signals the return to the waking state.

In the aforementioned *tonic-clonic seizures with unilateral predominance,* the EEG shows the same type of activity as in regular grand mal seizures except for some degree of lateralization, i.e., more pronounced ictal spiking over the more intensively involved hemisphere (Gastaut and Broughton, 1972).

Atypical Grand Mal

In children, the tonic phase is more pronounced and may last twice as long as the clonic phase (Gastaut and Broughton, 1972). Due to smaller amounts of muscle mass, the convulsive movements are not as impressive as in adolescents and adults. Some asymmetries may be present at the beginning of a seizure.

Grand Mal and Sleep

Grand mal attacks in sleep are common in patients with a primary focus and secondary generalization, but rare in patients with primary generalized epilepsy; in such an event, the seizures occur in non–rapid-eye-movement (REM) sleep only, never in REM sleep (Gastaut and Broughton, 1972).

Prevalence and Age Factor

Grand mal seizures are common at any age, except for the first 5 to 6 months of life, during which they are com-

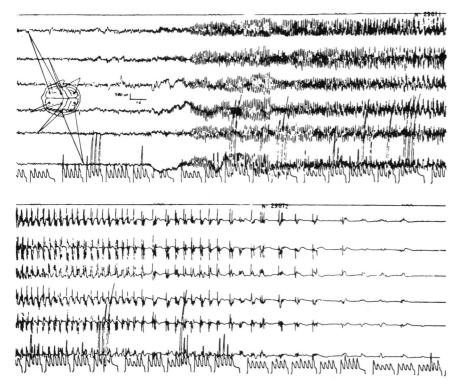

Figure 27.5. The EEG correlate of a grand mal (generalized tonic-clonic) seizure, recorded in a curarized patient and almost free of superimposed muscle activity. The bottom channel of this continuous recording shows the deflections of a frequency analyzer (after W. Grey Walter). The seizure activity is characterized by fast spiking of increasing amplitude during the tonic phase. There are repetitive bursts of spikes mixed with persisting weak muscle potentials during the clonic phase *(lower portion)*. There is unremarkable EEG activity prior to the seizure; the termination of the convulsion is characterized by general voltage depression. (From Gastaut, H., and Broughton, R. 1972. *Epileptic Seizures.* Springfield, IL: Charles C Thomas, with permission.)

pletely absent. Insufficient demyelination of the brain precludes grand mal at this early age. The earliest appearance in infancy is most commonly linked with a sudden rise of temperature (see febrile convulsions). In the research of Gibbs and Gibbs (1952), 5,598 patients of a population of 11,612 epileptics (48.2%) had grand mal only; another 3,290 patients (28.3%) had grand mal in combination with other types of seizures.

Neurophysiological Aspects

One is tempted to regard the grand mal seizure as a standardized maximal and global epileptic response of the brain. Electroconvulsion studies in the cat, however, have shown that the cerebellum and the lower brainstem do not fully participate in the ictal activity (Jung, 1949). The view of a standardized all-out response of the brain requires some correction. Schmidt and Wilder (1968) feel that grand mal convulsions "vary in their severity and in the degree to which they incorporate the various tonic and clonic phases." Variations of the degree of cerebral cortical participation in grand mal seizures have been demonstrated in the cat as well as in the human by Rodin et al. (1966). This view has been supported by the experimental findings of Petsche (1968).

This implies that grand mal seizures are graded rather than maximal cerebral epileptic responses. These variations could explain differences in the response to electroconvulsive therapy in psychiatric illness; following the electrically induced grand mal convulsion, the EEG may show little or marked slowing, probably depending on the degree of neuronal participation in the seizure. It is interesting to note in this context that "there is some evidence that organic

changes manifested in part by an abnormal EEG must occur for success of electroconvulsive therapy" (Solomon, 1967).

Quite different is the view of Gastaut and his co-workers. The emphasis placed on rhythmical 10/sec activity during a large portion of the grand mal attack has been discussed; this "epileptic recruiting rhythm" will follow stimulation only in nonspecific reticular thalamic structures projecting diffusely to both hemispheres over still uncertain connecting pathways. It was felt that the motor, autonomic, and EEG phenomena of the tonic phase could be explained by massive discharge of the thalamic and subthalamic brainstem reticular structures; this would also account for the loss of consciousness. In the clonic phase, the appearance of slow waves has been attributed to cortical inhibitory systems via thalamic and lower brainstem structures or, more specifically, via a thalamocaudate circuit branched from the thalamocorticospinal system. These views have been laid down by Gastaut et al. (1958), Gastaut and Fischer-Williams (1959), and, in condensed form, by Gastaut and Broughton (1972).

Although the tonic phase of a major convulsion can be produced in decorticate animals, there is no cogent reason to accept the concept of a thalamoreticular origin of the tonic phase in which, according to Gastaut and Broughton (1972), the cortex would participate in a "reciprocal feedback fashion."

Absences (Petit Mal)

Terminology

The term *petit mal* arose from the jargon of physicians and attendants in the hospitals of Paris early in the 19th century. According to Temkin (1971), Esquirol (1815) distinguished more or less severe epileptic attacks as "grand mal" and "petit mal," but his definition of these two terms "is obviously vague." Esquirol lumped together all sorts of minor attacks as "vertige épileptique" and "petit mal," used synonymously. The term *absence* was introduced by Calmeil (1824). The modern nomenclature (Gastaut et al., 1970) recommends the term *absence*, but the term *petit mal* is deeply rooted. *Petit mal absence* seems to be an acceptable compromise.

Clinical Manifestations

The petit mal absence occurs mainly in children older than 4 years, with a declining incidence throughout adolescence and early adulthood; persistence beyond middle adult life is very rare.

The attack consists of a sudden lapse of consciousness with impairment of mental functions. Its usual duration ranges from 5 to 20 seconds; longer absences may occur over 1 to 2 minutes, but such an unusual length is a sign of a somewhat complicated epileptic seizure disorder with some degree of automatism-like ictal behavior. The absence is associated with interruption of ongoing activity and, due to moderate impairment of consciousness, the patient is unable to see or hear. There is usually a blank facial expression that contradicts the frequently used term *staring spells*; a true stare is more likely to occur in temporal lobe epileptics with psychomotor seizures. The eyes drift upward ("star gazing," Bamberger and Matthes, 1959; Janz, 1969); rhythmical beating of the eyelids at 3/sec is very common and may be the only apparent motor manifestation of the attack. Marked orofacial movements during the absence are suggestive of a more complex type with poorer response to therapy.

There is good reason to assume that the unique nature of loss of consciousness during the classical absence is based on a temporary suspension of the "working memory" due to the powerful accentuation of spike-wave activity in the frontal cortex (Niedermeyer 1998b, 2003; Pavone and Niedermeyer, 2000). This explains the unmatched immediate restoration of the working memory along with consciousness at the end of the absence (no other form of brief loss of consciousness—syncope, for instance—reverses so quickly). As to the crucial function of working memory (see Fuster, 1995).

The postural control is grossly maintained, but swaying and stumbling movements may be noted in the standing patient (Schmidt and Wilder, 1968). The posture may be altered by sustained or saccadic retroflexion of the head ("retropulsive petit mal," Janz, 1955). Autonomic and especially vasomotor changes are common during the petit mal absence (Jung, 1939; Mirsky and Van Buren, 1965).

Impairment of the level of awareness has been the object of some studies (Cornil et al., 1951; Fischgold, 1957; Lehmann, 1963; Mirsky and Van Buren, 1965; Schwab, 1939; Shimazono et al., 1953). A variety of tests, such as rhythmically pressing a button, have been used to demonstrate the lapse of consciousness (Oller-Daurella and Oller-Ferrer-Vidal, 1977). Mirsky and Tecce (1968) demonstrated the persistence of visual evoked potentials during spike-wave discharges.

EEG Manifestations

The ictal EEG of the petit mal absence is characterized by the generalized synchronous 3/sec spike-wave discharge. The electrographic features of this discharge are more extensively discussed in this chapter on abnormal paroxysmal EEG patterns. No petit mal absence can materialize without this classical pattern but, on the other hand, the 3/sec spike-wave pattern may occur, usually in bursts of less than 5-second duration, without an accompanying petit mal absence. This should serve as a stern warning not to equate generalized 3/sec spike waves with petit mal absences; the latter cannot occur without the former, but the former frequently occur without clinical absences (Clark and Knott, 1955; Lundervold et al., 1959; Silverman, 1954) (Fig. 27.6).

The spike-wave discharge is maximal over the frontal midline and may start at a rate of around 4/sec, quickly slow down to 3 to 3.5/sec, and, during the final phase of the attack, slow to about 2.5/sec. Onset and termination are abrupt; the attacks may be preceded and immediately followed by normal EEG activity, especially when recorded in the waking-resting state rather than during hyperventilation or sleep.

In the rare cases of petit mal absences of middle or old age, the spike-wave complexes are somewhat less impressive, with the spike component being slower and less prominent (Fig. 27.6).

Precipitating Factors

Hyperventilation is an extremely potent activator of the 3/sec spike-wave discharge with or without clinical petit mal absences. This is discussed in greater detail below (see Primary Generalized Epilepsy; also see Chapter 14, "Activation Methods." Further powerful facilitating mechanisms are non-REM sleep and hypoglycemia. In some cases, intermittent photic stimulation is very effective; see Primary Generalized Epilepsy.

Age Factor and Prevalence

Petit mal absences frequently start at the age of 4 years; they are almost never found prior to the age of 3.5 years. Some of these children have a history of febrile convulsion in infancy. There is decline of petit mal epilepsy during the second decade, aside from treatment effects of drastic reduction of attacks. In some cases, the absences start around age 9 to 10 years; German schools (see Janz, 1969) have studied the differences in the course of children with onset earlier (around 4 years) and later (9–15 years). This and the occasional persistence of petit mal into adult life are discussed below (see Primary Generalized Epilepsy) (Rütti, 1982; Rütti and Karbowski, 1983).

Janz et al. (1994) have de-emphasized the significance of the dichotomy of pyknolepsy and juvenile absences. These two forms are conceived as a double leaf arising from the same stem (in analogy to the ginkgo biloba leaf).

A clinical absence with generalized 3/sec spike waves was triggered by tapping the head of a 2½-year-old child. This well-documented case of DeMarco (1990) makes one wonder if such an unusually early manifestation (and precipitation) belongs in the category of primary generalized epilepsy.

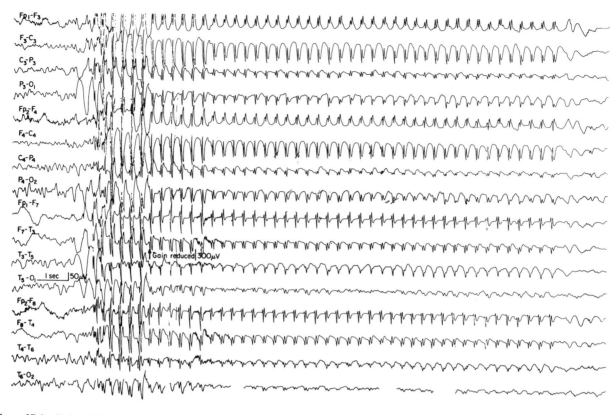

Figure 27.6. Petit mal absence, in an 8-year-old patient. The spike-wave burst is preceded by an aborted run of rhythmical posterior slow 3/sec waves; after two slow waves, the attack begins.

The prevalence can be gleaned from the figures of Gibbs and Gibbs (1952). Among a total of 11,612 epileptics, only 335 (2.9%) had petit mal absences without other types of seizures. There were 896 patients (7.7%) with petit mal in combination with other seizures; 706 of them (6.1%) had a combination of petit mal and grand mal attacks. These figures increase moderately when one deals with a population of children and adolescents.

Neurophysiological Aspects and Clinical Significance

These subjects are discussed in the section on primary generalized epilepsy.

Psychomotor Seizures (Complex Partial Seizures, Temporal Lobe Seizures)

Historical Remarks and Terminology

Falret (1860) has been widely credited with the first description of psychomotor seizures ("aura intellectuel"). From the medicohistorical work of Temkin (1971), however, one cannot derive a clear picture as to whether Falret (1824–1902) successfully individualized the psychomotor seizure with all its complexities. This also is true for B. A. Morel (1809–1879) and Herpin (1799–1865), who made important early contributions on psychomotor seizures. Samt (1876) became familiar with Falret's work; his observations on psychomotor seizures and mental epileptic changes

exude a repulsive image of "the epileptic" as having all sorts of criminal tendencies in combination with sanctimonious behavior. These investigators were medical directors of asylums with particular types of patients who were without modern antiepileptic treatment and perhaps with additional impairment from excessive bromide therapy.

Hughlings Jackson was familiar with the work of Falret. He recognized the role of the temporal lobe and uncinate structures in the pathogenesis of these seizures (Jackson, 1866; Jackson and Beevor, 1889; Jackson and Stewart, 1899). Turner (1907) gave an excellent description of automatisms and "psychical epilepsy," which essentially encompasses the wide range of psychomotor seizures. Foerster (1926) used the term *psychomotor equivalents*. The term *psychomotor seizures* was introduced by Gibbs et al. (1937) on the basis of ictal EEG findings. Anterior temporal random spikes or sharp waves were demonstrated by Gibbs and Gibbs (1947) and Gibbs et al. (1948) as the typical interictal EEG abnormality.

The work of the Montreal School generated special interest in the localization of ictal phenomena; this has prompted the term *temporal lobe epilepsy*, used first by Jasper et al. (1951). The now internationally recommended term *complex partial seizures* (Gastaut, 1970) has been given strong support by Penry (1975); an important monograph on this subject bears this name (Penry and Daly, 1975). This work also reports the reluctance to accept this term in its subdivisions as found in the discussion remarks. Jovanovic (1974) still used the term *psychomotor epilepsy* in his extensive study and Wieser's (1983) brilliant depth EEG study is entitled "Electroclinical Features of Psychomotor Seizure." For these reasons, both the older term (*psychomotor seizures*) and the newer term (*complex partial seizures*) are used in this chapter.

It must be kept in mind that not all psychomotor (complex partial) seizures originate from the temporal lobe. There is some evidence that typical automatisms may arise from frontal and especially fronto-orbital structures (Ludwig et al., 1975; Williamson et al., 1985).

Clinical Ictal Manifestations

The variety of psychomotor seizure manifestations is remarkable. The simplest approach to the multitude of ictal signs and symptoms is to divide them into automatisms with impaired consciousness and experienced seizures. This subdivision is a bit oversimplified. Magnus (1954) proposed the following breakdown of ictal features:

Psychical symptoms
Motor phenomena
Autonomic symptoms
Sensory symptoms

In more recent overviews, the complex manifestations of psychomotor seizures have been presented by Kotagal (1992, 1993), and Bauer (1994). Similar to the earlier work of Wieser (1983), an analysis of the clinical-ictal symptomatology was demonstrated in conjunction with depth EEG findings by Munari et al. (1994).

Description of the clinical seizure manifestations starts with the *psychomotor automatisms* characterized by "automatic" behavior in a state of impaired consciousness. The patient's postural reflexes are preserved; he or she may continue standing, sitting, or even walking and may execute more or less complex motions. Hughlings Jackson (quoted by Daly, 1975) was the first to recognize the automatic character of the patient's ictal actions. Attacks of automatic behavior usually last from 30 seconds to 5 minutes (from 54 to 148 seconds in pentylenetetrazol-induced automatisms of epileptic patients studies by Ajmone Marsan and Ralston, 1957).

According to Gastaut and Broughton (1972), five types of automatism are distinguished: alimentary, mimetic, gestural, ambulatory, and verbal. Penry and Dreifuss (1969) make a distinction between perseverative automatisms, in which the patient continues his action or repeats it in a stereotyped manner, and de novo automatisms, in which a new action is initiated. The patient's clothing seems to invite action during an automatism; buttoning or unbuttoning, fumbling with clothing, undressing, and even exhibitionism occur. Very often, the automatisms are limited to the oral and oropharyngeal sphere; there is swallowing, chewing, smacking, licking, and so forth.

Automatisms can also be classified according to the degree of the level of CNS functioning:

With purposeless and uncoordinated movements
With purposeless and coordinated movements
With purposeful and uncoordinated movements
With purposeful and coordinated movements

This subdivision, however, contributes little to the assessment of the seizure disorder. Automatic behavior in connection with a psychomotor seizure is not necessarily ictal. Quite often it is found to be postictal when the entire sequence of ictal events can be recorded in the EEG laboratory or, even better, documented by EEG telemetry with split screen. Oral movements or other types of automatic behavior may start at a time when the ictal EEG discharge (associated with tonic characteristics, after Rodin, 1975) has already stopped.

Prolonged states of automatic behavior may defy a convincing clinical analysis unless an ictal EEG is available. Trance-like states with socially inconspicuous behavior may last for hours and days, necessitating a very laborious differential diagnosis between hysterical dissociative states, petit mal absence status, global amnesia, and the extremely rare temporal lobe status epilepticus. Running attacks (epilepsia procursiva) are usually limited to mentally deteriorated or institutionalized epileptics.

Experienced seizures (psychosensory seizures) are based on altered perception and consist of illusional misinterpretation or frank hallucinations (perceptions without object). Visual illusions include phenomena such as micropsia and macropsia or strange distortions of the form of objects. In the case of somesthetic illusions, parts of the body or the entire body may be seen as smaller or larger. Similarly, there are auditory illusions, with sounds perceived as from a distance (micro-teleacousia, etc.); vertiginous illusions (among others, the astronautic illusions, which is a feeling like going into space, a product of the last two decades); olfactory illusions, which are not as important as olfactory hallucinations; and gustatory illusions.

Hallucinatory experiences of all sensory modalities have a wide range. Lilliputian hallucinations, in which the world is viewed through the wrong end of binoculars, and autoscopia, seeing one's own image, are examples of visual misperceptions. Distinction of hallucinations from illusions is often difficult. Hearing a symphony enjoyed a long time previously (Gastaut and Broughton, 1972) may be a misperception of time. Most important are olfactory hallucinations, which are almost always unpleasant (burned rubber, rotten eggs, etc.). These hallucinations have some etiological implications, since they occur mainly in tumors impinging on the uncinate region. What has been termed "attacks with cognitive symptomatology" in the international terminology are based on a misperception of time. In the common and widely known "déjà vu" attack, the present merges with the past in the patient's experience. This is an overpowering feeling and quite different from the common, although misleading and inappropriate, experience of having seen this before. Such misinterpretations are normal events, especially in adolescence. Much less common are ictal experience of "jamais vu" (never seen and totally unfamiliar) or "jamais vecu" (never lived, never experienced).

Seizures with "ideational symptomatology" consist of sudden abnormal thought processes, such as forced thinking, with the patient being unable to get rid of a certain thought for the duration of the attack, and, occasionally, metaphysic or transcendental thoughts about death or eternity. The memory function may be subject to ictal changes. There may be inability to recall the past or memories of the past may be recalled in the greatest detail. Such ictal hyperamnesias may extend into panorama-like views of the past.

Seizures with affective symptomatology comprise states of extreme sadness or pleasure (Williams, 1956), but this is a rather uncommon seizure content. *Gelastic epilepsy* (attacks of laughter) are more often reported, but these seizures are not necessarily associated with foci in the temporal lobe or adjacent limbic structures (discussed later) and thus do not convincingly belong in the category of psychomotor seizures (Daly and Mulder, 1957; Gascon and Lombroso, 1971; Jacome et al., 1980; Müller and Müller, 1980; Mutani et al., 1979). This view has not been shared by Chen and Forster (1973). Fear is the most common affective ictal manifestation of psychomotor seizures. According to Gastaut and Broughton (1972), the symptom of fear can be derived from the patient's fearful expression but is rarely mentioned by the patient, who is confused in the ictal state and shows postictal amnesia. Williams (1956) and Daly (1958, 1975), however, have given good examples of experienced ictal fear. Ictal states of bliss and ecstasy have been reported by Gastaut (1978) and Jaffe (1984).

Rage, violence, and aggressiveness as ictal manifestations of psychomotor (temporal lobe) seizures have been reported and discussed by various investigators (Ervin et al., 1955; Mark and Ervin, 1970; Meyer, 1957; Lechner, 1959; Serafetinides, 1965). This work has prompted the term *episodic dyscontrol syndrome* (Bach-y-Rita et al., 1971). Ictal aggression is a very uncommon event (Gibbs and Gibbs, 1964; King and Ajmone Marsan, 1977; Riley and Niedermeyer, 1978; Rodin, 1973). If it materializes, actions are carried out clumsily and ineffectively (Gibbs and Gibbs, 1964). Effective acts of violence and aggression can be executed with lightning-like speed in prolonged postictal confusional states following a series of grand mal attacks, but such postictal states have become quite rare as a consequence of improved therapy.

Visceral (autonomic, vegetative) ictal symptoms are very frequently encountered. Most common is a rising epigastric sensation; however, this also occurs as an aura of other types of seizures. Gastrointestinal hypermotility produces a variety of ictal or postictal sensations (Bauset et al., 1971; Penfield and Faulk, 1955; Van Buren, 1963; Van Buren and Ajmone Marsan, 1960). Pharyngeal dysesthesias were found to arise from the mesiotemporal region (Carmant et al., 1996). A variety of vasomotor, cardiovascular, respiratory, and other autonomic ictal dysfunctions are known. Visceral ictal symptomatology was found in 41% of the patients with psychomotor seizures (King and Ajmone Marsan, 1977), with epigastric sensations occurring in 34%. Cases of "abdominal epilepsy" (Feng, 1980; Moore, 1945) must be carefully differentiated from migraine. "Emetic seizures" with vomiting, preceded by a choking sensation and followed by tonic spasms of trunk and head, have been described by Fiol et al. (1986) and strongly emphasized by Panayiotopoulos (2002) as an important feature of the "Panayiotopoulos syndrome." A right temporal focus was

demonstrated; the seizures disappeared after right temporal lobectomy. On the other hand, Jacome and Suarez (1988) reported an ictus emeticus induced by photic stimulation and accompanied by generalized spikes, spike waves, and polyspikes.

In addition to ictal emesis, "ictal spitting" has also been observed, especially in patients with foci in the right (nondominant) temporal lobe (Kellinghaus et al., 2003).

True syncopal attacks may be triggered by the epileptic activity, and the patient may simply faint and fall to the floor. Other forms of simple falling are caused by sudden tonic rigidity or by atonia (see Lennox-Gastaut Syndrome, below). The "ictal bradycardia syndrome" (Reeves et al., 1996) has been described as potentially life-threatening. In most cases, the epileptic EEG discharges arise from the temporal lobe. *Ictal eroticism* as a psychomotor seizure content is very rare. Following a few reports about ictal orgasic sensations in females (Currier et al., 1971; Freemon and Nevis, 1969; Mulder et al., 1954), Spencer et al. (1981) and Remillard et al. (1983) presented more extensive data on sexual ictal manifestations in women with temporal lobe epilepsy. Remillard et al. (1983) hypothesized that preferential occurrence of ictal eroticism in the female might be due to sexually dimorphic structures located in the limbic portion of the temporal lobe.

Epileptic laughter (gelastic epilepsy) may arise from various areas of the brain. Predominant involvement of the temporal lobe has been reported by Arroyo et al. (1993). *Ictal speech arrest* (ictal aphasia) is not a symptom of psychomotor seizure and belongs to the category of focal seizures (partial elementary seizures). However, ictal speech, in which words or sentences are spoken, is a form of automatism; surprisingly, it is more common in foci within the nondominant temporal lobe or in bilateral temporal foci (Serafetinides and Falconer, 1963). *Tonic manifestations* and *adversive movements* are common manifestations of psychomotor seizures in about 20% of the cases, according to Janz (1969). *Running* (epilepsia procursiva, cursive epilepsy) is a rare manifestation of temporal lobe epilepsy (Chen and Forster, 1973).

Attacks of simple *impairment of consciousness* usually consist of confusional states. In some patients with temporal lobe epilepsy, ictal activity may start with *focal motor manifestations* originating from the adjacent motor cortex. Bossi et al. (1984) have demonstrated such cases with the use of depth EEG; these investigators believe that this type of focal seizure initiation represents a negative prognostic factor because the seizure disorder evidently is not confined to the temporal lobe. This view is congruent with the observations of Bergzon et al. (1968), as well as Delgado-Escueta and Walsh (1985).

Ictal EEG Manifestations

The variability of the EEG correlates of psychomotor seizures is at least "as variable as the clinical features" (Gastaut and Broughton, 1972). This view has developed gradually over the past 40 years.

The work of Gibbs et al. (1937) and Gibbs and Gibbs (1952) stressed the occurrence of 4/sec "flat-topped waves" and trains of spikes in ictal episodes; rhythmical 6/sec activity was also noted. Mazars (1950) and Jasper et al. (1951) emphasized attenuation of amplitudes or desynchronization at the beginning of a psychomotor seizure. The suppression of activity may be noted over most of the involved temporal lobe, while the uncinate region exhibits focal spiking (Jasper et al., 1951). Due to presumed secondary diencephalic involvement, the epileptic discharges become widespread in the course of the attack.

Gastaut and Vigouroux (1958) were impressed by the variability of the ictal EEG discharges. According to Klass et al. (1973) and Klass (1975), no EEG change may be noted at the onset of the attack in about 10% of the cases. Diffuse flattening at the beginning of the ictal discharge was emphasized by Landré et al. (1991). Gastaut and Broughton (1972) have pointed out that complete lack of any recordable EEG discharge during partial complex seizures was found in about 5%. Differences between interictal spiking and ictal rhythmical activity in patients with mesiotemporal lobe epilepsy were pointed out by Kawamura et al. (2002).

Christian (1975) pointed out that spike-wave discharges of generalized synchronous character are not uncommon during psychomotor seizures; similar observations are reported by Fuster et al. (1954), Niedermeyer (1954a), Glaser and Golub (1955), Garsche (1956), and Matthes (1961). These patients also show bilateral synchronous spike-wave patterns in the interictal interval; some of them may have ad-

ditional bilateral temporal foci (Christian, 1975). According to this investigator, most of the patients with spike-wave discharges are children or adolescents. Experience has taught us that most of these patients exhibit the characteristics of the Lennox-Gastaut syndrome, although the spike-wave discharges may not always be of the slow 1 to 2.5/sec type. Psychomotor seizures are not uncommon in the Lennox-Gastaut syndrome; these patients show criteria of temporal lobe epilepsy and signs of generalized epilepsy (secondary generalized epilepsy).

A typical ictal EEG tracing of a psychomotor (complex partial) seizure with automatism is shown in Figure 27.7.

Two basic types of psychomotor (complex partial) seizures have been distinguished by Delgado-Escueta et al. (1983a), Walsh and Delgado-Escueta (1984), and Delgado-Escueta and Walsh (1985). Type I is characterized by initial motionless staring, followed by oral-alimentary automatisms and reactive quasi-purposeful movements in a state of impaired consciousness. Type II features more complex automatisms (postural, adversive head and eye movements, automatic ambulation, focal motor manifestations, bicycling action, or "bringing in a catch of fish"). It was demonstrated that type I is strictly temporal-limbic and benefits from temporal lobectomy, whereas type II is largely extratemporal and hence not suitable for temporal lobectomy. Delgado-Escueta et al. (1983b) also established a type III character-

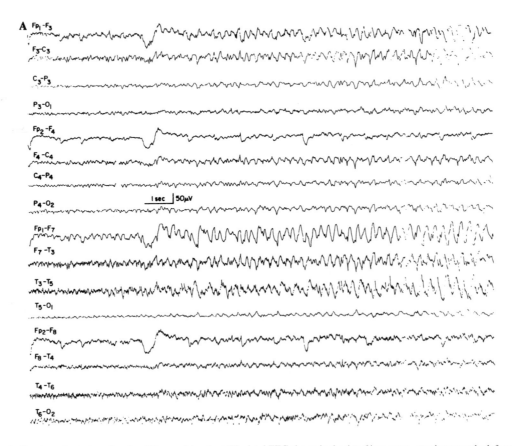

Figure 27.7.   **A:** Psychomotor automatism in a 27-year-old patient. The ictal EEG shows in the 4 to 6/sec range, starting over the left anterior temporal-midtemporal region (F7–T3) with rapid spread into the left frontocentral and right temporal regions.

ized by drop attacks followed by confusion and amnesia. Presumably type III also begins outside the temporal lobe.

A more complex subdivision of psychomotor seizures was proposed by Wieser (1983), who distinguishes five seizure types on the basis of his depth EEG observations: temporal mediobasal limbic type, temporal pole type, temporal neocortical posterior type, opercular-insular type, and frontobasal-cingulate type. Wieser's work is reflected in the proposal made by the Commission on Classification and Terminology of the International League Against Epilepsy (1985). The following subdivision of temporal lobe epilepsies has been suggested: (a) *hippocampic (mediobasal) limbic* or *primary rhinencephalic psychomotor epilepsy,* commonly in combination with amygdalar epilepsy: strange indescribable feelings, experiential hallucinations, or interpretative illusions, followed by motionless stare and oral and alimentary automatisms, lasting about 2 minutes; (b) *amygdalar (anterior polar-amygdalar) seizures:* rising epigastric discomfort, nausea, marked autonomic signs, borborygmi, belching, pallor, or flushing of face, gradually followed by staring, oral-alimentary automatism, and confusion; (c) *lateral posterior temporal seizures:* auditory or visual hallucinations, language dysfunction (if on dominant side), followed by dysphasia, confusion, head movement to one side, and sometimes staring with automatism; (d) *opercular (insular) seizures:* vestibular or auditory hallucina-

tions, borborygmi, belching and autonomic signs, unilateral face twitching, and paresthesiae. Olfactory and gustatory hallucinations may occur. These subdivisions have brought more order into the chaotic abundance of psychomotor seizure manifestations in epilepsies of the temporal lobe or its immediate vicinity.

Age and Prevalence

Psychomotor seizures start most often between the ages of 15 and 30 years. As the most characteristic seizure type of temporal lobe epilepsy, psychomotor seizures are most common in early and middle adulthood. There is also good evidence that psychomotor seizures are not uncommon in adolescence and childhood and may occur even in infancy. Jeras and Tivadar (1973) reported 189 children with psychomotor seizures. In early childhood, the nature of the attack remains poorly defined in most cases because automatisms are not as distinctly developed and subjective manifestations cannot be expressed by the patient. Fear appears to be one of the earliest seizure manifestations (Beaumanoir, 1976); the infant or child may suddenly scream with a fearful facial expression or run to his mother with outward signs of being frightened. Gibbs and Gibbs (1952) show a rather high proportion of psychomotor seizures starting in childhood, with a peak age of onset reached by age 20 to 25. There is certainly a marked decline in the age of onset after

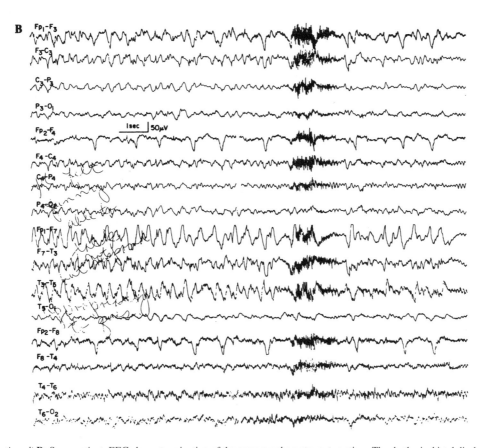

Figure 27.7. *(continued)* **B:** Same patient. EEG shows termination of the same psychomotor automatism. The rhythmical ictal discharges show augmentation in amplitude, slight slowing, and a subtle sharp component.

age 30. This stands in striking contrast to the increase of anterior temporal spike foci with advancing age (Gibbs and Gibbs, 1964). These old-age anterior temporal spike foci, which are mostly due to cerebral arteriosclerosis, are clinically silent in the vast majority of the cases. More recent studies of children with psychomotor seizures showed no major differences from the ictal semeiology of adults (Brockhaus and Elger, 1995; Bye and Foo, 1994).

Many patients with psychomotor seizures also have grand mal attacks; however, these occur much less often. In the research of Gibbs and Gibbs (1952), grand mal attacks as additional seizure types occurred in 70% and focal seizures in 2% of the total number of patients with psychomotor seizures. This is discussed in great detail below (see Temporal Lobe Epilepsy).

The *prevalence* of psychomotor seizure without admixture of other types was found to be 5.8% (678 among a total of 11,612 epileptics) in the research of Gibbs and Gibbs (1952). This figure rose to 23.2% when the number of cases of psychomotor seizures mixed with others (17.4%) was added. The combination of psychomotor and grand mal seizures reached 15.5% in their patient material. A prevalence of 20% was found by Jasper et al. (1951), whereas Magnus (1954) reported a range from 14% to 25% of all epilepsies.

Neuropathological, Etiological, and Neurophysiological Aspects, and Clinical Significance

These aspects are discussed below (see Temporal Lobe Epilepsy).

Epileptic Aura and Pre-Aura

The Aura

An epileptic aura precedes the seizure and may be regarded as the first portion of the seizure. The patient experiences strange sensations of whatever sensory modality is involved. The patient thus is aware of such an event that eludes bystanders. The EEG, however, most commonly reveals the presence of epileptic activity of focal character. An aura may remain an isolated event but, more commonly, it is the prelude to a clinical epileptic seizure. Auras play no role in primary generalized epilepsies. The term *aura* is quite old and has been ascribed to Galen (122–199 AD).

The Pre-Aura

This term was introduced by Niedermeyer (2002) and is used for the designation of earliest "preictal" (better: apparently preictal) manifestations that escape detection by EEG and subjective sensations. A pre-aura may precede the seizure onset by 1 to 20 minutes. Important work on the nature of the pre-aura has been done by Wallstedt et al. (1995), Baumgartner et al. (1998), Le Van Quyen et al. (2001), and Lehnertz et al. (2001).

Table 27.1 provides further information about pre-aura and aura.

Focal Motor and Other Focal Seizures (Partial Seizures with Elementary Symptomatology)

Focal (partial elementary) seizures are also discussed in the section dealing with aspects of cerebral localization and in connection with age-determined epileptic conditions.

It is almost self-evident that every cortical region is capable of producing its own form of focal epileptic seizures; their ictal symptomatology would be the expression of the cortical function. Hughlings Jackson in his *Selected Writings* distinguished discharging cerebral lesions from paralytic lesions: "An epilepsy is a sudden, excessive and rapid discharge of grey matter of some part of the brain; it is a local discharge."

This view could lead to the concept of a cortical mosaic of focal epilepsies in which an almost limitless variety of seizure types could be generated according to the locus of discharge. Experience, however, has taught us that most focal seizures fall into certain standard categories except for some rather whimsical mixtures of focal manifestations. In other words, cortical areas do not share a democratic equality as far as epileptogenic properties are concerned; some areas are simply more epileptogenic than others. This may be due to local neurobiochemical characteristics that may result in low and high thresholds for epileptic manifestations. The motor cortex seems to be a region of comparatively low threshold and is therefore a frequent generator of epileptic activity.

Table 27.1.   Distinctive Features of Pre-Aura, Aura, and Clinical Seizures

	Pre-Aura	Aura	Clinical Seizure
Time Scale	*1–10 (20) min*	*Seconds to about 1 minute*	*Seconds to minutes*
Behavior	Unremarkable	OBJECTIVELY: Unremarkable SUBJECTIVELY: Ictal experience	Ictal behavior according to extent of seizure
SPECT Focal region	Perifocal hyperemia (macrocirculation)	Hyperemia (macrocirculation)	Hyperemia (macrocirculation)
Laser-Doppler immediate vicinity	Perifocal ischemia (microcirculation)	Enhanced ischemia (microcirculation)	Further enhanced ischemia (microcirculation)
Quantified EEG	Suspect/abnormal "neuronal dyssynchrony"	Changing to ictal pattern	Ictal pattern
Conventional EEG	Unremarkable, may be electrodecremental	Changing to ictal pattern	Ictal pattern

(With kind permission of "Clinical Electroencephalography.")

Epileptogenic Focus and Structural Lesions

When cerebral lesions are demonstrated by means of computed tomography (CT) or MRI in cases of focal epilepsy, the epileptogenic focus found in the EEG frequently does not correspond with the CT scan lesion. According to Munari (1985), (a) many epileptogenic lesions cannot be diagnosed by CT scan; (b) topographic relationships between CT scan lesion and the area of seizure onset are not readily demonstrable; and (c) when multiple CT scan lesions coexist in the same patient, the epileptogenic lesion cannot be convincingly determined. Munari assumes that the relationship between location of the epileptogenic zone and the clinical ictal signs and symptoms is more important. The complexity of an epileptogenic zone has been pointed out by Lueders and Awad (1992).

In this vein, the complex relationship between depth EEG foci and ictal behavior in patients with psychomotor (complex partial) seizures has been elucidated by the work of Wieser (1983), Delgado-Escueta et al. (1983a), and Munari and Bancaud (1985). New clinical-topographic subdivisions of these seizures have resulted from this work.

Improved MRI technology ("echo-planar imaging") has added a functional component to the traditionally structural methods of MRI: "functional magnetic resonance imaging" (Cohen, 1992). This has proved to be very helpful in the determination of an epileptogenic focus.

Focal cortical seizure activity has been thought to be coupled with ictal activity in thalamic level on the basis of functional MRI data and cross-correlation analysis (Detre et al., 1996). The association of focal motor seizures and crossed cerebellar diaschisis was demonstrated with MRI (Stübgen, 1995). Studies of the regional cerebral glucose metabolism (with CMR Glu) in focal epilepsy showed marked hypometabolism in both cerebellar hemispheres, especially in children (Seitz et al., 1996).

Focal Motor Seizures (Rolandic Motor Seizures)

Clonic twitching of the contralateral muscles of the body is the typical seizure manifestation of a localized discharge within the precentral gyrus. Bravais (1827) studied focal motor seizures in his thesis. Jackson's work, however, and the classical electrical stimulation studies of Fritsch and Hitzig (1870), Ferrier (1873), and Luciani (1878) have brought the excitability of the human cortex into the right perspective.

In accordance with the somatotopic arrangement within the precentral gyrus, the clonic movements are initially limited to the corresponding area of the body and tend to spread during the attack. Such a spread (for instance, from the facial muscles to the leg) is well known as the *jacksonian march*.

Such a jacksonian march does not materialize in many cases and the attacks remain limited to one body region, usually thumb, fingers, lips, eyelids, or great toe. The cortical representation of these functions, according to Gastaut and Broughton (1972), represents a phylogenetic acquisition of humans, who have been endowed with a particularly large cortical motor zone. Any region may be involved; even trunk muscles may participate. There is no impairment of consciousness during these attacks. Involuntary lingual movements were described as "lingual seizures" occurring in conjunction with contralateral centrofrontal ictal spiking (Neufeld et al., 1988).

A status of constant clonic activity in one muscular region is known as *epilepsia partialis continua* or *Koshevnikov syndrome*. Bilateral focal motor attacks are very rare. Focal motor seizures may be caused by an ipsilateral lesion (Ahuja and Tharakan, 1981), but such cases are exceptional.

The *ictal EEG* is expected to show impressive spiking contralaterally over the involved motor cortex, but such cases with precise focal EEG documentation are seldom observed. Widespread EEG changes with desynchronization, spiking, and more or less rhythmical theta or delta activity may be noted, or there may be a complete lack of ictal EEG activity, also caused in part by movement artifact. The discharge may be subcortical in a three-dimensional involvement of cortical and deep structures (discussed under rolandic epilepsy), or cortical spiking may be too small and desynchronized. In older persons with ischemic cerebrovascular accidents of the watershed type, the EEG picture is even more confusing. The dissociation between spiking over the motor cortex and corresponding motor effects has been investigated by Elger and Speckmann (1980) in the rat; spiking in lamina V after local penicillin gives rise to contralateral twitching without concomitant spiking on the cortical surface. With spike activity in superficial and deep cortical layers, there are accompanying motor effects. These authors also introduced the term *vertical inhibition* for a mechanism responsible for the failure of descending neuronal activity during epicortical epileptiform potentials (Elger and Speckmann, 1983). Quiet epileptogenic foci within the motor cortex can be activated by transcranial magnetic stimulation (Classen et al., 1995).

Adversive Seizures (Versive, Ipsiversive, or Contraversive Seizures)

Adversive seizures may be limited to conjugated eye movements; there is usually extreme lateral gaze to the side contralateral to the lesion. The eye movement may be tonic (oculogyric) or clonic (oculoclonic, also called epileptic nystagmus). These manifestations must be carefully distinguished from nonepileptic nystagmus and oculogyric crises such as brainstem disease and basal ganglia disease.

More commonly, the adversion consists of deviation of head and eyes; even the entire body may rotate to one side (usually contralateral, i.e., opposite side of the focus). Sometimes, the contralateral arm is raised in tonic extension, with the subject apparently looking at his raised hand (Gastaut and Broughton, 1972). This has been impressively demonstrated by the illustrations of Aird and Woodbury (1974) and Matthes (1977).

These attacks may occur with a loss of consciousness (frontopolar region, middle and superior frontal gyrus) or in a conscious state (posterior portion of frontal lobe, vicinity of precentral gyrus) (Penfield and Jasper, 1954; Penfield and Kristiansen, 1951).

The *ictal EEG* usually shows more or less rhythmical slowing with spikes over the affected area and, in most cases, over a large neighboring region. For this reason, a precise focal EEG diagnosis is difficult or impossible.

Adversive seizure phenomena are not limited to the frontal region; oculoclonic seizures may be frontal as well as occipital. The occipital origin of combined oculoclonic and adversive seizures has been clearly shown by Fossas et al. (1985). The initiation of grand mal seizures by a brief adversive movement is quite common and cannot be regarded as a reliable localizing sign. This has been further corroborated by Robillard et al. (1982), as well as by Ochs et al. (1981). Further considerations of this topic are found in the work of Quesney et al. (1992).

Epileptic Spasm/Partial Seizures

A combination of flexor spasms with preceding or subsequent partial clonic seizures has been described by Pachatz et al. (2002), showing in the EEG a juxtaposition of focal and generalized ictal activity. These attacks occur in childhood/adolescence with cryptogenic or residual-acquired etiologies; their prognosis is relatively favorable.

Hypomotor Seizures

This term was introduced by Kallen et al. (2002) and pertains to seizures of infancy and childhood consisting of diminished motor activity along with an undetermined level of consciousness. The EEG shows typical ictal changes of focal or generalized character indicating focal, multifocal, or generalized epileptic disorders.

Somatic Inhibitory Seizures (Ictal Paralysis)

Ictal inhibition of motor activity and resulting ictal paralysis of one limb or one half of the body is a rare and controversial phenomenon. Janz (1969) doubts the existence of such seizures. The observation of "hemiparetic seizures due to excessive inhibitory discharge" (Hanson and Chodos, 1978) has opened new vistas and the observation of Tinuper et al. (1987) demonstrates beyond doubt the existence of ictal paralysis. Under the heading of "negative motor phenomena" (Fahn et al., 1995), this concept has been extended to a striking (and especially excessive) extent.

Postictal paralysis (Todd's paralysis) is common in the wake of unilateral motor seizure activity. Such paretic deficits are found mainly in children and infants; their duration ranges from minutes to hours and seldom exceeds 24 hours. Marked focal slowing over the involved cortical region usually accompanies this transient state (Gustavson et al., 2003).

Aphasic and Phonatory Seizures

Sudden aphasic arrest of ongoing speech, ictal use of unintelligible or inappropriate words, and ictal inability to write or read may occur in patients with epileptogenic lesions of temporal, inferior frontal, or inferior parietal localization of the dominant hemisphere. Sudden anarthric speech arrest may be caused by epileptic activity in the inferior rolandic cortex. Seizures originating in the supplementary motor region may occasionally lead to iterative vocalization or countless repetitions of a certain word (Gastaut and Broughton, 1972).

Verbal automatisms, with utterance of words and whole sentences as seizure content, represent complex partial seizure manifestations and are therefore discussed under the heading of psychomotor seizures.

Sensory (Somatosensory) Focal Seizures

A wide variety of sensations in contralateral body regions to the epileptogenic lesion have been described (Hallen, 1952; Janz, 1969; Russell and Whitty, 1953). Tingling, "pins and needles," numbness, and other paresthesiae have been reported; sensations of pain, burning, or cold may also occur. Strictly sensory focal attacks are uncommon; nonepileptic mechanisms, especially local ischemic disturbances and affections of the peripheral nervous system (Hallen, 1953), must be carefully ruled out. Pain as an ictal sensation may also originate from a temporal lobe focus (Sahota and Stacy, 1993).

Ictal sensations in the genital region may be due to a focus in the superior and interhemispheric fissure portion of the postcentral gyrus but may also occur in the limbic discharges (psychomotor seizures, temporal lobe epilepsy). Ictal EEG changes for somatosensory attacks may be very minor or virtually nonexistent.

Other Afferent Modalities

Elementary visual sensations may be scotomatous or of positive luminous nature, as phosphenes. Spots, balls, stars, and disks in brilliant white or colors may be static or whirling around. These phenomena may occur in the visual field contralateral to the firing occipital cortical lesion or simultaneously in both fields.

Thunderous or hissing noises and other acoustic sensations are reported as *simple auditory phenomena* due to involvement of the auditory projection cortex in the superior temporal cortex. *Olfactory sensations* (parosmias) are mostly disagreeable. The discharges originate from the anterosuperior portion of the uncus. These attacks are also discussed under headings such as psychomotor seizures, temporal lobe epilepsy, and intracranial tumors as the cause of seizures.

Gustatory sensations are very uncommon in seizures. The discharge may arise from the parietal operculum or from the superior peri-insular cortex. *Vertiginous ictal sensations* are short and massive ("tornado-like"). These attacks are very rare (Niedermeyer and Hinchcliffe, 1965). A variety of nonepileptic conditions may cause vertigo and dizziness.

Myoclonic Seizures

Myoclonus is characterized by a rapid involuntary muscle contraction, subtle or massive, usually with locomotor effect, generalized or limited to certain muscular segments, mostly predominant in flexor muscles, and more pronounced in upper extremities. The resulting jerk may be synchronous or moderately asynchronous.

Myoclonus may be epileptic or it may represent a dyskinetic disturbance caused by the breakdown of the motor control systems of the cerebellum. A combination of epileptic and apparently nonepileptic myoclonus may occur. The term *myoclonic* stresses the singular nature (one distinct jerk), whereas *clonic* refers to the repetitive type of muscular twitching.

The complexities of the underlying neurophysiological mechanisms can be gleaned from the work of Watson and Denny-Brown (1955), Halliday (1967a–c, 1975), Shibasaki and Kuroiwa (1975), Chadwick et al. (1977), Hallett et al. (1977), and Kelly et al. (1981). Progress in myoclonus research was sparked by the introduction of myoclonus-triggered back averaging of the concomitant EEG (Shibasaki and Kuroiwa, 1975; also independently developed by Chadwick et al. (1977). Hallett (1985) has summarized the most recent insights into the physiological nature of myoclonus. Three major mechanisms have been pointed out: (a) cortical reflex myoclonus, often occurring in focal motor epilepsy and associated with giant somatosensory evoked potentials (based on hyperexcitability of the sensorimotor cortex; (b) reticular reflex myoclonus, thought to be due to hyperexcitability of the caudal brainstem reticular formation; EEG spikes are not time-locked with myoclonus and are maximal over vertex; (c) primary generalized epileptic myoclonus, as found in primary generalized epilepsy with bilateral predominantly frontocentral EEG event preceding the myoclonus. Hallett's (1985) subdivision of myoclonic phenomena is strictly physiological and not etiologically oriented. This author has made it clear that either cortical reflex myoclonus or reticular reflex myoclonus may occur in clinical disorders associated with myoclonus (Table 27.2).

The clinical-semiological details of the myoclonic movements have been extensively described by Gastaut (1968a) and cinematographically demonstrated by Oller-Daurella and Oller-Ferrer-Vidal (1977, 1981).

Myoclonic phenomena are found in various epileptic conditions such as primary generalized epilepsy, infantile spasms with hypsarrhythmia, and Lennox-Gastaut syndrome, and in degenerative CNS disease, such as Tay-Sachs disease, forms of CNS lipidosis, essential hereditary myoclonus epilepsy (Lafora-Unverricht-Lundborg), encephalitis, acute or chronic renal failure, acute cerebral anoxia, or postanoxic states. More extensive studies on the clinical significance of myoclonus have been presented by Weingarten (1957), Aigner and Mulder (1960), Gastaut (1968a), Bauer (1974), Kinsbourne and Rosenfield (1975), Sulibhavi and Schneck (1975), Farrell and Swanson (1975), Charlton (1975), Niedermeyer et al. (1979a), and Aicardi (1983). It has been pointed out that, in neonates, nonketotic hyperglycinemia represents the most common cause of myoclonus. In infants and young children, progressive myoclonic encephalopathies are usually due to gangliosidoses and ceroid-lipofuscinoses; in older children, Lafora's disease and its variants are in the foreground as the cause of myoclonus (Aicardi, 1983). This investigator has also emphasized that a majority of myoclonic epilepsies do not belong in the group of neurodegenerative disorders; consequently, their prognosis is much better.

This wide clinical range necessitates a discussion of myoclonic phenomena in various sections of this chapter and in Chapter 16, "The EEG in Cerebral Inflammatory Processes," Chapter 19, "Degenerative Disorders of the Central Nervous System," Chapter 22, "Metabolic Central Nervous System Disorders," and Chapter 23, "Cerebral Anoxia: Clinical Aspects." Photomyoclonus will be discussed under the headings Activation Procedures and Primary Generalized Epilepsy (also see Shibasaki et al., 1987).

From the EEG viewpoint, myoclonus is associated with massive spike discharges and especially with bursts of bilateral or generalized synchronous polyspikes in patients with pri-

Table 27.2. Characteristics of Major Neurophysiological Types of Myoclonus[a]

	Cortical Reflex Myoclonus	Reticular Reflex Myoclonus	Primary Generalized Epilepsy Myoclonus
Clinical setting of occurrence	Fragment of focal (partial) epileptic seizures	Fragment of bilateral or generalized epileptic manifestations (aside from primary generalized epilepsy)	Fragment of primary generalized epilepsy
Localization of myoclonus	Involves only a few adjacent muscles	Myoclonus tends to affect the whole body	Small bilateral myoclonic, often fingers only, minimyoclonus (mimicking tremulousness). Also major whole-body myoclonic jerks
Precipitation	Spontaneous or induced (accentuated) by voluntary movement (motor action)	Spontaneous or induced (accentuated) by voluntary movement (motor action)	No extrinsic precipitation except for photosensitivity
Bilateral synchrony of myoclonus	Asynchronous; usually unilateral	Usually synchronous, but synchrony may be quite imperfect	Synchronous (fairly precise bilateral synchrony)
Somatosensory evoked potentials (SSEP)	Enhanced ("giant SSEP")	Unremarkable	Unremarkable
Focal time-locked EEG event	Well demonstrable, with preceding spontaneous and reflex-induced jerks located over appropriate motor cortex region	EEG event (spike) often associated with myoclonus but not time-locked. Spike generalized maximal over vertex	Negative event precedes myoclonus, with bilateral frontocentral maximum, lasting 30–100 msec for major jerks (well time-locked) and 100–250 msec for minimyoclonus (less well time-locked)
CNS origin of neurophysiological event	Focal: motor cortex (local hyperexcitability)	? Caudal brainstem reticular formation	Presumably cortical (frontal, supplementary motor cortex as starting point)
Clinical significance	Focal motor (elementary partial) epileptic seizure, probably also Jakob-Creutzfeldt disease and others	Postanoxic action (intention) myoclonus, renal encephalopathy (uremia), others	Primary generalized epilepsy and related epileptic seizure disorders

[a]Modified from Hallett, M. 1985. Myoclonus: Relation to epilepsy. Epilepsia (New York) 11:567–577.

mary generalized epilepsy and thus with the related photoconvulsive response to intermittent photic stimulation, and also in patients with Lennox-Gastaut syndrome. In infantile spasms with hypsarrhythmia (West syndrome), the EEG correlate of the myoclonus is variable and reaches from sudden flattening or desynchronization to massive spiking and unaltered ictal records. Myoclonus may occur with or without spiking in the EEG in degenerative CNS disease and in Jakob-Creutzfeldt encephalopathy due to slow virus infection; it is associated with very pronounced compounded complexes of mixed slow and sharp activity in subacute sclerosing panencephalitis. Prominent spiking is also the rule in myoclonus caused by hypoglycemia, toxic-metabolic states, and acute cerebral anoxia. More details are presented in the corresponding chapters.

The term *negative myoclonus* was introduced by Tassinari (1981) and denotes brief repetitive lapses of postural

Table 27.3. Clinical and EEG Characteristics of Chronic Conditions with Myoclonus[a]

	Age	Epileptological Symptomatology	Neurological or Mental Deficits	EEG
Primary generalized epilepsy (synonyms: common generalized, centrencephalic, corticoreticular epilepsy)	Mainly 4–16 years; in cases with grand mal, 10–50 years	Petit mal absences Petit mal-grand mal-myoclonus Grand mal-myoclonus Absence (petit mal) status, often with myoclonus	None	Principally generalized or bilateral anterior synchronous spikes, spike-waves (3/sec, 4/sec), polyspikes. Activated by hyperventilation, flicker, sleep (non-REM)
Infantile spasms	Age 4 months to 2.5 years (hypsarrhythmia)	Myoclonic, mainly head nodding Jackknifing with tonic component	Varying from normal findings to forms of cerebral palsy, hydrocephaly, microcephaly, mental retardation	Hypsarrhythmia: high voltage output, irregular slowing with massive spikes, polyspikes, mostly occipital maximum. Asleep: enhanced bursts with stretches of depressed voltage
Lennox-Gastaut syndrome	Onset mostly age 1–10 years, becoming poorly distinct after age 30	Numerous minor motor types of seizures. Tonic, atonic-akinetic, myoclonic, also psychomotor, grand mal petit mal	Varying from normal or more or less severe neurological deficits, types of cerebral palsy, etc. Mental retardation	Slow spike-wave complex ("petit mal variant" after Gibbs and co-workers). 1–2.5/sec. In sleep, runs of rapid spikes, 10–20/sec. Also polyspikes. Frequently general slowing
Cherry red spot-myoclonus syndrome	Childhood to adolescence	Massive myoclonus, also facial; grand mal may occur	Fundi: cherry red spot. Relatively mild neurological deficit, normal intelligence	Positive spikes over vertex, in brief bursts
Essential hereditary myoclonus epilepsy (Lafora-Unverricht-Lundborg)	Onset in childhood or adolescence (the earlier the onset, the more serious the progression)	Myoclonus Grand mal	Cerebellar symptomatology of varying degree: dysmetria, intentional tremor, speech and gait disturbance. Progressive dementia	Severely disorganized, predominantly slow with numerous single spikes, often with needle-like spikes of myogenic character. Few or no polyspikes. Sometimes more rhythmical slow activity with spikes
Benign myoclonus (Hartung) probably related to paramyoclonus multiplex (Friedreich)	Onset in childhood	Myoclonus	None	Mostly normal (a personal observation of an abnormal record is an exception)
Postanoxic myoclonus	Any age	Myoclonus, intention or action type. EEG spikes maximal over vertex	Cerebellar deficit, possibly other posterior anoxic deficits Dementia	Disorganized, with numerous spikes, bilateral synchronous, vertex or frontocentral

tone time-locked to spikes over the contralateral central region (Aguglia et al., 1995; Baumgartner et al., 1996). In some patients, this phenomenon is associated with acute valproate encephalopathy (valproate stupor). According to Rubboli et al. (1995), epileptic negative myoclonus is accompanied by an inhibitory frontal spike component.

Table 27.3 shows the EEG correlates in a variety of clinical conditions with myoclonic seizures. In rare instances,

chronic alcoholism may cause a cerebellar syndrome with ataxia and massive myoclonus without EEG changes (Bartolomei et al., 1996).

Seizures Occurring in Infantile Spasms Only (Jackknifing, Salaam)

These are discussed below [see Infantile Spasms (Hypsarrhythmia)].

EEG Correlates of Myoclonus	Pathological Substratum	Neurophysiological Mechanisms	Cause	Therapy	Prognosis
Myoclonus always associated with spikes, mostly polyspikes, frontal maximum Elicited by flicker: (*a*) photoconvulsion response (with cerebral spikes), (*b*) photomyoclonic response (with myogenic spikes)	None	Controversial, thalamocortical circuitry, ? reticulocortical circuitry; paroxysmal arousal ("dyshormia"); flicker sensitivity	Unknown Probably biochemical deficit. Genetic factor present especially in flicker-sensitive forms	Sodium valproate, ethosuximide (petit mal), phenytoin, phenobarbital, carbamazepine (grand mal component)	Good to fair to good
Mostly desynchronized EEG during myoclonus or jackknifing, occasionally unaltered EEG, or enhanced spike discharges	Varying. Depending on cause, often severe pathology (porencephaly, cortical atrophy), often very minor changes	Unknown	Polyetiological, often with no known cause. See pathological substratum. Genetic predisposition possible.	ACTH, steroids, nitrazepam, clonazepam	Poor or guarded (after age 2.5) and EEG ictal characteristics changing to other epileptic form
Mostly with bursts of polyspikes, never without concomitant spikes	Varying. Depending on cause, often severe forms of pathology, but sometimes no changes; 50% of scans normal	Unknown. Presumed to represent a form of "secondary generalized epilepsy," but precise mechanisms are ill understood	Polyetiological, more than 50% unknown, genetic predisposition possible	Clonazepam, diazepam, sodium valproate	Mostly poor, seizures mostly intractable, mental deterioration
Bursts of vertex spikes associated with myoclonus	Unique inclusions in cortical neurons	Unknown	Probably a mucolipidosis	Anticonvulsant may control grand mal but not myoclonus	Relatively benign although progressive disease
Poorly defined. Myoclonus may occur without any EEG change	Degenerative changes: cerebellum, brainstem, thalamus, cortex, in that order Lafora bodies (?mucopolysaccharides). Dyssynergia cerebellaris myoclonica. R. Hunt: dentate atrophy, cerebellar cortex intact	Controversial and hypothetical. Multilevel dysfunction	Genetic syndrome (autosomal recessive), may be an inborn error of metabolism	No effective therapy known	Poor, progression to death (fast progression in Lafora-Glück form, slowest in Lundborg form)
No EEG correlate	Probably none	Controversial	Genetic syndrome (autosomal dominant), may be an inborn error of metabolism	No effective therapy known, attempts with clonazepam or 5-hydroxytryptophan (5-HTP) might be worthwhile	Excellent: functioning in life not disturbed by persisting myoclonus
Spike bursts may or may not accompany myoclonus	Cerebellar lesions, hippocampic lesion, partial laminary necrosis of cerebral cortex	Controversial	Acute cerebral anoxia, followed by modest recovery (to be differentiated from myoclonus in acute anoxic coma)	L-Dopa, 5-HTP, clonazepam, stereotaxic lesions (nucleus ventr. lat. thal.) (all of unproven effect)	Poor or guarded

*a*From Niedermeyer, E., Fineyre, F., Riley, T., and Bird, B.L. 1979a. Myoclonus and the electroencephalogram. Clin. Electroencephalogr. 10:75–95.

Seizures Occurring in the Lennox-Gastaut Syndrome Only

The discussion of these special types of seizures (tonic, clonic, atonic, akinetic) is found below (see Lennox-Gastaut Syndrome).

Unclassifiable Seizures

Elements of the above seizure types may be mixed, resulting in a protean semiology that defies classification. The EEG plays a crucial role in the determination of the epileptic character and the differentiation of the nonepileptic seizures.

Combining EEG with Functional Magnetic Resonance Imaging

Simultaneous EEG recording and functional MRI is beset with problems since the EEG is being obtained in a high-field magnet and during scanning. Baudewig et al. (2001) have reported a method demonstrating simultaneous blood-oxygenation-dependent ("BOLD") MRI sequences and EEG activity with very little artifactual distortion.

Etiologies of Epileptic Seizures

For centuries, epilepsy has been regarded as an inherited illness. Such a blunt statement is erroneous, despite a grain of truth; yet, it is still widely accepted among laypersons, and even some physicians cling to this view. Hand in hand goes the notion of epilepsy as an incurable disease. To repeat: there is no disease named epilepsy. What is called epilepsy is the chronic recurrence of sudden abnormal reactions of the brain as epileptic seizures. These are caused by large number of brain disorders and facilitated by the presence of a genetic predisposition.

The notion of epilepsy as a disease is difficult to eradicate. Gowers (1881) felt that the entire brain was affected, "that epilepsy is thus a disease of grey matter, and has not any uniform seat. It is a disease of tissue, not of structure." Once again, let us drop the notion of a disease. All epileptics share the fear of an impending attack, but they cannot logically form a society of patients with the same disease. Patients with cerebral palsy and seizures of early onset, war veterans with posttraumatic epilepsy, patients with neurocutaneous degenerative syndromes such as tuberous sclerosis, patients with recent onset of seizures as early brain tumor manifestations—all these patients form a heterogeneous legion of sufferers. Most of them may benefit from anticonvulsants. The medical director of a seizure clinic must look upon these patients with a keen awareness of all the possible epileptogenic manifestations of neurological disease.

The term *epilepsy* should be used with caution in order to avoid the notion of a disease entity. Terms such as *the epilepsies* or *epileptic seizure disorders* are preferable. The relationships between etiologies and age of onset are demonstrated in Table 27.4. Brain damage acquired during the earliest phases of life plays a leading role among the causes of epileptic seizure disorder. It is therefore not surprising that the most common age of onset of epileptic seizure disorders is the first year of life. This has been demonstrated by Oller-Daurella and Oller-Ferrer-Vidal (1981) and Ellenberg et al. (1984).

Table 27.4. The Most Common Causes of Epileptic Seizure According to Age of Onset, Listed in Presumed Order of Importance[a]

First week

Perinatal asphyxia
Perinatal trauma (often with intracranial bleeding)
Very early CNS infection
Cerebral malformations
Hypocalcemia
Hypoglycemia
Other early metabolic changes

Second week

Early CNS infection
Intracranial infection (with electrolyte derangement)
Hypocalcemia (alimentary)
Kernicterus
Cerebral malformation

Third week to 3 months

CNS infection
Subdural collections after CNS infection
Cerebral malformations

4 months to 2 years

Febrile convulsions (triggered by trivial febrile diseases)
CNS infection
Residual epilepsy due to early CNS damage (cerebral palsy)
Cerebrovascular problems: arterial occlusion, venous thrombosis
Inborn errors of metabolism
Neurocutaneous disorders
Note: in predisposed children, seizure disorders may appear as infantile spasms or Lennox-Gastaut syndrome

3 to 10 years

Benign rolandic epilepsy (dysfunction predisposition)
Primary generalized epilepsy (dysfunction predisposition)
Residual epilepsy due to early CNS damage
Trauma
Inborn errors of metabolism
Neurocutaneous disorders
CNS infection
CNS poisoning (lead, etc.)
Note: in predisposed children, seizure disorders may appear as Lennox-Gastaut syndrome

11 to 20 years

Primary generalized epilepsy (dysfunction-predisposition)
Trauma
Residual epilepsy due to early CNS damage (cerebral palsy)
CNS infection
Arteriovenous malformation

21 to 40 years

Trauma
Brain tumor
Chronic alcoholism (in certain areas)
Residual epilepsy due to early CNS damage (cerebral palsy)
Arteriovenous malformations

41 to 60 years

Brain tumor
Chronic alcoholism (in certain areas, leading cause)
Trauma
Cerebrovascular disease (also vasculitis)

Above age 60

Cerebral arteriosclerosis
Brain tumor, primary
Brain tumor, metastatic

[a]Cause frequently remains unknown. In tropical and subtropical countries CNS parasites may be the leading cause.

Chronic Versus Acute Epilepsies

Epileptic seizure disorders may be acutely exacerbated as "status epilepticus," necessitating hospital admission or even intensive care treatment. Acute epileptic manifestations, however, may also occur as a concomitant or complication of acute diseases and catastrophic events involving the brain.

Work on acute convulsions (Bauer and Niedermeyer, 1979) has shown that 83 of 146 patients had grand mal attacks; focal motor attacks occurred in 44 and myoclonic seizures in 11 patients. Cerebrovascular disorder was the most common etiology, followed by metabolic, anoxic, or infectious CNS disease, status-like exacerbations of chronic epileptic seizure disorder, and intracranial trauma. Cerebrovascular accidents were often complicated by metabolic problems and vice versa. Focal motor seizures were most common in acute cerebral anoxia and focal motor (partial elementary) seizures in cerebrovascular accidents. The EEG showed marked lateralization mainly in cerebrovascular accidents and burst-suppression activity mainly in cerebral anoxia.

These patients in acute epileptic states make it even clearer that the notion of epilepsy as a disease must be abandoned. Every human being and every animal is capable of producing epileptic seizures under certain conditions; acute brain disease strongly facilitates the appearance of seizures.

Historical View of Genetic Versus Acquired Epileptic Seizure Disorders

During the period from about 1850 to 1950, leading authors in the field of epileptology were divided into two groups, those who felt epilepsy was inherited and those who felt it was an acquired seizure disorder. There were a few extremes of diametrically opposed views, such as the very strong emphasis on inheritance of Grasset and Rauzier (1920a,b) and Wilson's (1935) virtual denial of a genetic-idiopathic epilepsy, coupled with the expectation that all epilepsies without demonstrable acquired or organic cause (cryptogenetic epilepsies) would eventually show recognizable brain lesions. In general, however, the lines were drawn between idiopathic (genuine, essential) epilepsy with presumed inheritance and acquired forms of epileptic seizures. German schools in the first half of the 20th century (especially Bumke, 1942) stressed the "genuine" forms and laboriously attempted to attribute special personality characteristics to sufferers from "genuine epilepsy." We will return to the question of genetic factors in the discussion of primary generalized epilepsy, which is etiologically characterized by the absence of acquired structural brain lesions.

Not every investigator was satisfied with the dualism of idiopathic versus symptomatic epilepsies. At a remarkably early stage, Delasiauve (1854) divided the epilepsies into the following three categories: (a) essential or idiopathic epilepsy, (b) symptomatic epilepsy due to a cerebral lesion, and (c) "sympathetic" epilepsy due to an extracerebral disturbance secondarily acting on the brain. This was most plausible in metabolic or toxic disturbances, as, for instance, seizures in renal insufficiency.

Foerster (1926) distinguished three principal pathogenetic-pathophysiological components in epileptics: (a) predisposition to seizures; (b) irritative noxa (i.e., an epileptogenic lesion); and (c) a seizure-triggering factor such as flickering light or a special constellation of metabolic factors. Whenever epileptic seizures occur in a neurological disorder, one is inclined to ascribe the seizures to the underlying disease. Such a causal relationship may become quite enigmatic, as for instance in the case of myasthenia gravis, which occasionally may be associated with seizures; there were two patients with seizures among 118 myasthenics, according to Tartara et al. (1982). The possibility of mere coincidence has to be considered; all the pros and cons must be weighed before elimination of a possible true relationship.

The Role of Genetic Factors

A large bulk of literature became obsolete during the end of the 1980s when genetic-epileptological research gathered strong momentum. One of the first impressive results of this work was the genetic linkage of juvenile myoclonic epilepsy (Janz syndrome) to the small arm of chromosome 6 (Delgado-Escueta et al., 1989). Research strategies for the "challenging genetics of epilepsy" (DeLorenzo, 1991) were mapped out by Anderson et al. (1991). Malafosse et al. (1994) emphasized the differences between genetic strategies for diseases with (a) simple and (b) complex modes of inheritance. For the latter (including human epilepsies), "the trait segregation is not sufficient for inferring the way the susceptibility to the disease is inherited." More realistic appears to be the investigation of the role of other potential factors (Malafosse et al., 1994). It is an often forgotten fact that epilepsy is not a disease, as I pointed out at the beginning of this chapter. The nondisease status of epileptic seizure disorder clearly renders genetic epilepsy research more difficult.

The concise and lucid demonstration of the basic concepts of molecular biology for the epileptologist (Lowenstein, 1994) do not appear to be readily applicable to inherited forms of human epilepsy. Progress in mapping human epilepsy genes was reported by Delgado-Escueta et al. (1994) reporting that "seven epilepsy genes have been identified in chromosomes 1q, 6p, 8q, 16p, 20q, 21q and 22q" (a number which has risen to 60 according to Noebels, 2003). This includes the existence of two loci (20q, 8q) for the rare syndrome of benign familial neonatal convulsions. The long arm of chromosome 21 is the locus for both Baltic and Mediterranean form of progressive myoclonus epilepsy (Unverricht-Lundborg disease—not including the Lafora type). It might have come as a surprise to the clinical epileptologist that absence epilepsy is genetically still unclear and thus quite different from juvenile myoclonic epilepsy (its clinically close relative).

On the other hand, Berkovic et al. (1994) have reemphasized the significance of twin research in their genetic-epileptological studies. These authors found a high concordance (65%) for idiopathic generalized epilepsies and (71%) for symptomatic-cryptogenic epilepsies whereas localization related epilepsies showed a low concordance rate of 20%. This latter figure reconfirms the long-upheld view that, even in acquired forms of epileptic seizure disorder, a certain degree of genetic predisposition or susceptibility has to be taken into account.

Very dynamic progress was made in the 1990s and the first years of this millennium in the field of genetics of focal epilepsies. Bygone is the time when focal character was thought to be the exclusive criterion of underlying structural damage. And even if the latter does exist, modern work has shown evidence of additional genetic factors of predisposition.

The work of Berkovic, Genton, Hirsch, and Picard (1999) has been a powerful thought provoker in this respect: for epileptologists but also for electroencephalographers who try to progress in the electroclinical understanding of their patients. When we return to idiopathic/primary generalized epilepsy, the genetic clarification seems to have become even more complex. The work of Sander et al. (2003) has cast doubt on a major locus for primary generalized epilepsy (PGE) forms on non—juvenile-myoclonic-epilepsy character (chromosomal region 8p12).

According to Durner et al. (2001), there is reason to assume that the genetic classification of different forms of primary generalized epilepsy is likely to cut across the clinical classification of its subforms. For example, "a patient with the clinical features of absence epilepsy might have the disease that maps the chromosomes 18 and 5, or the patient might have the disease that is on chromosome 18 and 6." This depends on a familial relationship to juvenile myoclonus epilepsy. Other combinations of loci also result in the absence phenotype.

Epileptic Seizures in Inborn Errors of Metabolism (Degenerative CNS Diseases)

These causes of epileptic seizures are discussed in Chapter 19, "Degenerative Disorders of the Central Nervous System."

Early Infantile Brain Damage

The reader will find pertinent information in the section on neonatal convulsions in this chapter but also in Chapter 19, in Chapter 20, and in discussion of pararhinal and mesiotemporal sclerosis in the section on temporal lobe epilepsy.

Infectious Central Nervous System Disease (Encephalitis)

CNS infection may give rise to epileptic seizures in the acute stage. These attacks belong in the above-mentioned category of acute convulsions and are discussed in the section on EEG and CNS infection.

Inflammatory CNS pathology may turn into a postinfectious residual lesion with epileptogenic properties. Prenatal, perinatal, and infantile postnatal CNS infections may be the cause of epileptic seizure disorders starting years or even decades after the acute infection.

CNS infections and complicating vascular pathology may cause coma, hemiplegia, and acute hemiconvulsive seizure activity (clonic activity in the affected limbs), especially between ages 6 and 24 months. This picture is known as hemiconvulsions, hemiplegia, and epilepsy (HHE) syndrome (Gastaut et al., 1957, 1960) (also called HH syndrome; Beaumanoir, 1976). In this case, the hemiconvulsions constitute the acute infectious and the epilepsy the chronic postinfectious paroxysmal manifestations.

Measles encephalitis used to be a fairly common cause of brain damage in infancy or childhood, frequently accompanied by chronic seizure disorder. This cause is about to disappear with the widespread use of immunization. On the other hand, encephalitis with convulsions or followed by convulsions due to *smallpox vaccination* has disappeared because of the discontinuation of this type of immunization. *Tuberculous meningitis* contracted in infancy or early childhood and with inadequate tuberculostatic treatment, such as a late start of the treatment, may result in brain damage with severe epileptic disorder.

Epileptic seizures are common in *herpes simplex encephalitis* regardless of whether acquired perinatally by passage through the infected birth canal or later in life. In survivors of this CNS infection, epileptic seizures and especially temporal lobe epilepsy may play a major role. Exceptionally, herpes simplex II can cause a chronic smoldering infection resulting in temporal lobe epilepsy (Cornford and McCormick, 1997).

Mosquito-borne encephalitides (St. Louis as well as Eastern, Western, and Venezuela type of equine encephalitis) may become epileptogenic. Japanese encephalitis and Siberian and European *spring-summer encephalitis* are often followed by epileptic manifestations. The Siberian form is the classic cause of Koshevnikov syndrome (epilepsia partialis continua, discussed elsewhere). Epileptic seizures used to occur after incomplete recovery from *Reye's syndrome*.

Seizures may also occur during and after severe *Rickettsia diseases*, such as Rocky Mountain spotted fever and Eurasian typhus. Acute *bacterial purulent meningitis* may lead to massive epileptic seizures; postinfectious epileptic seizures are particularly common in the case of brain abscess formation.

Neurosyphilis used to be a very common source of epileptic seizures (mainly focal but also grand mal), regardless of acquisition in fetal or adult life. *Toxoplasmosis*, a protozoan disease, may cause epileptic seizures in children with transplacentar infection. The role of *malaria* as a cause of chronic epileptic seizure disorders is indubitable, especially in the wake of *Plasmodium falciparum* infection. In primary CNS involvement with *AIDS (HIV infection)*, epileptic seizures may occur along with paroxysmal EEG abnormalities without any complicating opportunistic infections (Parisi et al., 1991). In *Behçet disease*, seizures are rare and a sign of ominous prognosis (Aykutlu et al., 2002).

Cysticercosis (Taenia solium) with cerebral involvement was formerly a widespread disease and still occurs rather frequently in certain Latin American countries (Asenjo and Rocca, 1946; Trelles et al., 1952) and other parts of the world. Rocca (1973) found seizures of focal and generalized character in 40% of the cases. Headaches and psychomotor seizures were reported as initial manifestations (Lore, 1995). Arseni and Marinescu (1974) reported epileptic seizures in 22 of 62 patients (35%) with *cerebral hydatidosis*.

Acute allergic phenomena, especially after insect stings, may be associated with grand mal convulsions in very rare cases when acute edematous changes affect the brain (Kennedy, 1926, 1938; Stevens, 1965a,b).

Multiple sclerosis, pathogenetically a still unclarified demyelinating disease with a presumed relationship to immune reactions, may alter the EEG (Levic, 1978) and infrequently gives rise to epileptic seizures (Bronisch and Rauch, 1970; Drake and Macrae, 1961; Elian and Dean, 1977; Hopf et al., 1970; Trouillas and Courjon, 1972). Bilateral periodic EEG complexes of long duration (500–1,500 msec) were demonstrated in an indubitable case of multiple sclerosis along with seizures responding to carbamazepine (Prier et al., 1992). A special variety of tonic seizures without concomitant EEG changes may occur in this disease (Joynt and Green, 1962; Matthews, 1958, 1962). The prevalence of epileptic seizures in multiple sclerosis ranges from 0.5% (Hopf et al., 1970) to 10.8% (Fuglsand-Frederiksen and Thygesen, 1952).

In most cases of acute encephalitis, the *EEG recovery* or failure to recover provides an excellent prognostic clue. Thus, the persistence of EEG abnormalities after the acute stage may foreshadow the appearance of epileptic seizures.

Craniocerebral Trauma

Again we have to distinguish between convulsions in the acute stage of craniocerebral trauma and those occurring as a sequel to the injury. According to the period of occurrence, trauma-induced seizures are to be divided into the categories described in this subsection. The role of predisposing genetic factors in posttraumatic epilepsy should not be underestimated (Angeleri and Giaquinto, 1981).

In a population of epileptic patients, traumatic etiology varies from 4.3% to 8.5%, but may reach 17% and even 23% (Majkowski, 1991).

Immediate Seizures

Grand mal seizures may begin during the first few seconds after the injury. This type of earliest traumatic seizure has been ascribed to a direct mechanical stimulation of cerebral structures with low epileptogenic threshold (Walker, 1949); other investigators have stressed the role of acetylcholine released from damaged brain cells (Bornstein, 1946; Brenner and Merritt, 1942; Purpura, 1953). Such early attacks may occur in approximately 1% of the victims of craniocerebral trauma (Rowbotham, 1964). According to Jennett (1975), immediate seizures are an uncommon phenomenon, usually following a mild injury in an adult. None of Jennett's patients with an immediate seizure had any further attacks. The latency period allotted for the occurrence of immediate posttraumatic seizures should not be extended beyond 5 minutes (Majkowski, 1991).

Early Epileptic Response to Acute Traumatic Pathology

These attacks mainly develop 12 to 28 hours after injury (Adeloge and Odeku, 1971; Courjon and Scherzer, 1972; Jennett and Lewin, 1960) in severely traumatized patients with cerebral contusion, intracerebral hematoma, or brain laceration. Grand mal attacks signal diffuse cerebral edema, whereas focal attacks are more likely to occur in local edema around a traumatic lesion (Evans, 1963; Jennett,

1975; Rish and Caveness, 1973). No psychomotor seizures occur in this state.

Jennett (1975) maintains the view that these early epileptic responses to traumatic pathology facilitate the occurrence of late posttraumatic epilepsy, against the opinion of Penfield and Jasper (1954). The prevalence of such early traumatic seizures has been reported as 5% (Jennett, 1975) and 9% (Courjon and Scherzer, 1972).

Early Posttraumatic Epilepsy

These seizures develop after the acute traumatic phase, approximately 1 week to 3 months later. Early posttraumatic structural changes are likely to be the cause of these attacks. In Walker's (1958) research, onset of seizures within the first 3 months after the injury occurred in 75% of cases. A much smaller figure (27%) was found by Jennett (1975).

Late Posttraumatic Epilepsy

These attacks start from 3 months to 2 years after the trauma. A prolonged latency period after penetrating head wounds was reported in Vietnam War veterans; in more than 25% of the cases, the seizures started more than 2 years after the injury (Salazar et al., 1985). These seizures are caused by delayed pathological processes such as scarring. Penetrating wounds with cerebral laceration are most apt to lead to brain dura mater cicatrix formation and are most common in high-velocity projectile head wounds in wartime. According to Walker (1949), parietal wounds are more likely to give rise to posttraumatic seizures than frontal, temporal, and occipital injuries.

About 30% to 75% of these patients have focal onset of grand mal attacks or various forms of focal or partial seizures (including psychomotor) (Jennett, 1975). This figure is higher in patients with injuries due to missiles. According to the Vietnam War data of Jabbari et al. (1986), brain volume loss, presence of early hematoma, and retained metal fragments significantly correlated with posttraumatic epilepsy. Preventive anticonvulsive therapy after a severe craniocerebral trauma is of questionable value and, according to Kristiansen et al. (1969) and Salazar et al. (1985), is even worthless. The difficulties of seizure prevention are also demonstrated in the experimental work of Lockard et al. (1976) in alumina gel-induced seizures in the monkey. According to these authors, only high doses of anticonvulsants proved efficacious.

Some forms of posttraumatic epilepsy require special considerations. *Epileptic seizures associated with chronic subdural hematoma* are fairly common; both grand mal and focal seizures may be present. Seizures may develop after the evacuation of subdural as well as acute epidural hematomas. In the latter case, even complete general and neurological recovery may be marred by a subsequent seizure disorder (Jennett, 1975).

A rare form of posttraumatic epileptic seizures is characterized by an unusual degree of severity and a rather poor response to anticonvulsants (Niedermeyer et al., 1970a). These patients usually have a history of a closed craniocerebral trauma sustained in childhood, adolescence, or early adulthood, followed after a relatively long interval of up to several years by seizures, which are mostly of grand mal or psychomotor (automatism) character. These patients show very typical EEG findings with slow spike waves and runs of rapid spikes; they thus resemble the Lennox-Gastaut syndrome.

The *general incidence of posttraumatic epilepsy* based on a 4-year minimum follow-up is around 5% of craniocerebrally injured patients (Jennett, 1975).

The general *course of posttraumatic epilepsy* is fairly benign. Under adequate treatment, the seizure frequency is likely to diminish progressively in 75% of the patients (Courjon, 1969). Jennett's view (1975), however, is more cautious. The aforementioned form of posttraumatic epilepsy with slow spike-wave complexes is of severe and progressive character, but these cases are exceptional. Genetic predisposition might play a role in the pathogenesis of posttraumatic epilepsy.

Now it can be stated that the literature dealing with posttraumatic epilepsy has become scarce. This is fortunately due to the absence of major wars and also to the constant improvement of neurosurgical technique resulting in cleaner and less irritative cranial wounds.

The *EEG* reflects the degree of acute brain damage (see Chapter 21, "Craniocerebral Trauma") but it is often disappointing in the detection of candidates for late posttraumatic epilepsy. Spike activity in an early posttraumatic state of 1 to 3 weeks may be of no prognostic significance whatsoever. On the other hand, the first late posttraumatic attack may appear without preceding ominous changes in the serial EEG. Even after the first late posttraumatic seizure, the EEG changes may be surprisingly mild; spikes are usually scanty, and foci are not readily demonstrable. Jennett (1975) has clearly pointed out the weakness of the EEG in the prediction of posttraumatic epilepsy. In children, head injuries are sometimes followed by seizure disorders with generalized synchronous spike-wave complexes or spike-wave—like bursts (Dumermuth, 1972; Karbowski et al., 1981). This must be distinguished from the aforementioned rare instances of posttraumatic epilepsy with slow spike waves. Epileptic seizures may be the cause of a craniocerebral trauma. In 14 of 811 patients with acute head injury, the trauma was caused by a seizure (Hauser et al., 1984a).

Intracranial Tumors

Epileptic seizures are a well-known manifestation of brain tumors and other space-occupying lesions such as brain abscesses, intracranial hematomas, and parasites. The prevalence of seizures in patients with brain tumors ranges from 20% to 50% (Hess, 1970; Hoefer et al., 1947; Kirstein, 1942; Lund, 1952; Penfield and Jasper, 1954; Sargent, 1921). In chronic epileptics, a brain tumor occasionally emerges as the cause of the seizure disorder. Figures concerning the role of brain tumors as the cause of the epileptic seizures vary considerably due to the composition of the patient material; they range from 0.74% to 15% (Krayenbuehl, 1957; Lund, 1952; Stubbe-Taeglbjerg and Biligaard, 1944). Age is an important factor because brain tumors are listed among the rare causes of seizures in childhood. The incidence of brain tumor is low in a well-screened population of institutionalized epileptics and high in neurosurgical patient material. Special work on seizures due to childhood brain tumors was done by Millichap et al. (1962). A series of re-

cent studies on brain tumor and epileptic seizures can be found (in abstract form) in the proceedings of the Italian EEG Society (1985).

Any type of seizure may be associated with tumors, but focal (partial) attacks are most common (Hess, 1970). It has been demonstrated that "aura"-like episodes of olfactory and gustatory character are most likely to be caused by tumors (Hess, 1970; LeBlanc and Rasmussen, 1974). Type and frequency of the seizures are determined by site, growth rate, and histological type of neoplasm. Slowly growing tumors in the vicinity of the rolandic fissure are most likely to develop seizures (Ketz, 1974; LeBlanc and Rasmussen, 1974).

In adults, the importance of seizures as a sign of brain tumor can hardly be overemphasized. Seizures proved to be the initial symptom in 40% of brain tumors with epileptic attacks (LeBlanc and Rasmussen, 1974). According to Ketz (1974), the average period between first seizure and hospital admission has remained as long as 33 to 38 months, but there is good reason to presume that the use of CT and MRI has already begun to shorten this span. On the other hand, when one investigates a population of patients with adult onset of seizures, there will be a sizable number of cases with seizures caused by a brain tumor (16% in a group of 221 patients with seizures starting past age 25; Dam et al., 1985).

Tumor epilepsies tend to evolve into status epilepticus (Gastaut et al., 1967a,b; Heintel, 1972; Janz, 1960, 1962, 1969), especially in frontal lobe tumors (Janz, 1960, 1969). Brain tumor was found to be the most frequent cause of status epilepticus in the series of Heintel (1972). Focal seizure discharges in the EEG occur mainly in the immediate vicinity of the tumor (Daly, 1975; Hess, 1975). Some investigators (Arfel and Fischgold, 1961; Goldensohn, 1979; Hess, 1975) de-emphasize the localizing value of interictal spike foci in intracranial tumors. According to Kershman et al. (1949), slowly growing tumors such as astrocytomas and oligodendrogliomas are more common causes of epileptic discharges in the EEG than rapidly growing tumors such as glioblastoma multiforme or metastases.

Bilateral synchronous anterior spike activity may occur in frontal and parasagittal tumors (Goldensohn, 1979; Tükel and Jasper, 1952).

After brain surgery, spike discharges in the EEG may be enhanced for some time. Certain surgical procedures are very likely to be followed by postsurgical spike activity. Lifting of the temporal lobe in the Frazier-Spiller operation (retrogasserian rhizotomy) for trigeminal neuralgia used to be a cause of typical anterior temporal sharp waves and spikes; even temporal lobe epilepsy was reported after this procedure (Kubicki, 1963; Kubicki and Münter, 1976; Kubicki and Schulze, 1962). Spikes and intermingled minor spiky activity are naturally enhanced by postsurgical bone defects. After surgical removal of supratentorial meningiomas, paroxysmal EEG activity may occasionally reappear after several years (Zouhar, 1981). *Radiation* (x-ray therapy) may cause *cerebral radiation necrosis,* which, in severe cases, is associated with very pronounced EEG slowing, massive spiking, and clinical seizure disorder.

Dysembryoplastic Neuroepithelial Tumors

This group of tumors (Daumas-Duport, 1993) have been thought to belong to the neuronal migration disorders. Degen et al. (2002) have clearly shown that all of these tumors must be placed into the group of low-grade brain tumors.

Other Space Occupying Lesions

Epileptic seizures are very common in acute and chronic *brain abscesses;* after surgical removal, scar formation quite often leads to chronically recurrent epileptic attacks. EEG evaluations are useful in such cases; spike foci develop in up to 80% of the cases, even in the absence of clinical seizures (Gaches et al., 1965; Legg et al., 1973). According to Christian (1975), one third of the patients with brain abscess develop postsurgical spike foci.

Chronic granulomatous lesions may be the cause of epileptic seizure disorder (tuberculoma or syphilitic gumma) or cystic lesions caused by cysticercosis. Epileptic seizures may occasionally occur in *sarcoidosis* (Besnier-Boeck-Schaumann disease); focal spiking may be present in the EEG (Schwarz and Elsässer, 1961).

Cerebrovascular Disorders

Three forms of epileptic seizure disorder are distinguished in *cerebrovascular accidents* (strokes): (a) seizures preceding the catastrophe, (b) seizures occurring acutely during the stroke, and (c) seizures developing as a sequel of the destructive vascular lesion due to subsequent scar formation (Barolin and Scherzer, 1963; Barolin et al., 1971, 1975; Lesser et al., 1985; Pit'hova et al., 1981). In the acute stage of the stroke, the clinical differentiation between irritative-epileptic phenomena and motor deficits may be difficult (Barolin et al., 1975; Kugler, 1972; Robb and McNaughton 1974).

Premonitory seizures occur weeks or even years before the stroke; their prognostic value has been stressed by Barolin et al. (1971). These premonitory seizures are mostly of focal-motor character and foreshadow the side of the impending motor deficit. These attacks are partially related to compromised blood flow caused by arterial plaques. In the case of an extracranial carotid plaque, prompt surgical intervention can prevent the cerebrovascular accident. This justifies a thorough arteriographic workup. Burri et al. (1989), however, were unable to demonstrate premonitory seizures in patients with strokes.

Seizures accompanying the acute cerebrovascular insult have been well known since the work of Gowers (1881). Strokes are complicated by seizures in 12.5% (Richardson and Dodge, 1954) or 20% (Hudson and Hyland, 1958) of the cases.

The illuminating findings of Burri et al. (1989) are based on 90 stroke patients seen in the acute stage and during subsequent rehabilitation. Seizures occurred in 25 (27.8%) patients; in one patient in the acute stage only (1.1%), in two during acute and late stage (2.2%), and in 22 (24.4%) in the late stage only. Focal-motor seizures dominated in the early phase. Focal EEG signs were helpful in the clarification of late seizures, which occurred after a latency from 10 weeks to 3 years.

Acute epileptic seizures in patients with strokes are by far more common in hemorrhagic rather than ischemic strokes (Vespa et al., 2003). Intrinsic factors as well as unpredictable events are involved in the occurrence of seizures in hemorrhagic strokes (Passero et al., 2002).

Most impressive is seizure activity in *watershed type ischemias.* The pathogenetic mechanisms are indicated in the section on the EEG in cerebrovascular disorder. In such infarctions along the boundary between major arterial territories of the cerebrum, focal motor seizures are very common. These attacks are usually associated with periodic lateralized epileptiform discharges (PLEDs, after Chatrian et al., 1964). Further discussion is also found in Chapter 13, "Abnormal EEG Patterns: Epileptic and Paroxysmal." From the EEG viewpoint, the PLED pattern is the most striking discharge type in acute strokes with epileptic manifestations.

Classical hemiplegic strokes within the middle cerebral artery are typically based on lenticulostriate infarcts. According to Giroud and Dumas (1995), 13 out of 56 patients with lenticulostriate infarcts had seizures. The MRI demonstrated, in patients with seizures, larger infarct size and cortical involvement.

Chronic cerebrovascular disorder and especially *arteriosclerotic changes* are common causes of epileptic seizures with onset in old age (Pit'hova et al., 1981). These patients may not present with a history of typical hemiplegic strokes or transient ischemic attacks in the middle cerebral artery or internal carotid territory, but there is usually good evidence of memory impairment and mental decline. According to Fischer (1959), 4% of patients with cerebral arteriosclerosis of major proportions necessitating hospitalization at some time suffer from epileptic seizures of late onset. Grand mal attacks are predominant and, in spite of the well-known predominance of anterior temporal spike foci in the EEG (Gibbs and Gibbs, 1964; Niedermeyer, 1961; Takahashi et al., 1965), the occurrence of psychomotor seizures (partial complex seizures) is not especially common. Focal motor seizures are more frequently encountered and raise the question of premonitory (prestroke) or poststroke attacks (as described by Barolin et al., 1971, 1975). Poststroke epileptic seizures are most often found in patients with middle cerebral artery infarctions; cardiac emboli play an important role (Agnetti et al., 1985).

Delta foci in cerebrovascular disease are potentially epileptogenic, according to Fischer-Williams (1982), who investigated the transition from an ischemic slow focus into an epileptogenic zone. In a population of 2,291 patients with cerebrovascular accidents, however, only 171 (7.5%) developed epileptic seizures of predominantly focal (partial) character (Iemolo et al., 1985).

In *systemic lupus erythematosus,* seizures, mostly of grand mal character, may be the initial manifestation of the disease (Randow et al., 1965). Kogeorgos and Scott (1982) noted epileptic seizures in 44% of their patients with lupus erythematosus and cerebral involvement. In *morphea* (localized form of *scleroderma*), epileptic seizures were found in 6 of 24 patients (Hwang et al., 1981). In children and adolescents, chronic epileptic seizure disorders may be caused by *sickle cell anemia (SS hemoglobinopathy)* (Baird et al., 1964; Neidengard and Niedermeyer, 1975; Portnoy and Herion, 1972), which is limited to the black race.

In survivors of *subarachnoid hemorrhage caused by intracranial aneurysms,* epileptic seizures were found in 12.5% (Walton, 1953), usually associated with marked EEG changes such as spiking (Kiloh et al., 1972). According to Scott and Cabral (1975), seizures are not uncommon after intracranial aneurysm surgery. De Santis and Rampini (1983) have pointed out that a smaller number of patients operated on for intracranial aneurysms will have subsequent epileptic seizures if the procedure is carried out with microsurgical technique (8% versus 14%).

Arteriovenous malformations of the cerebral hemispheres are very often associated with grand mal or focal seizures; their onset is mainly between the ages of 10 and 35 years. EEG foci are usually present in patients with seizures, but spiking may not be impressive; paroxysmal discharges may even occur on the "wrong" hemisphere (Groethuysen et al., 1955; also see the section on cerebrovascular disorder and EEG). In some cases with unsuccessful surgical treatment, a poorly controllable epileptic seizure disorder may be associated with pronounced focal spiking.

Cortical venous thrombosis may give rise to serious neurological deficits and epileptic seizures after recovery from the acute stage.

Metabolic and Toxic Encephalopathies

Seizures due to acute metabolic and toxic disturbance are discussed in the section on the EEG in metabolic disorders and CNS poisoning. A variety of chronic seizure disorders due to metabolic and/or toxic disorders are presented here.

Chronic renal disease is one of the most common causes in this context. Various types of pathology may be found; chronic glomerulonephritis, nephrosis, polycystic kidney disease, and obstructive nephropathy may be the primary cause. Arterial hypertension may or may not be present. Chronic renal insufficiency may occur at practically any age.

In renal encephalopathies, myoclonus is the most common type of epileptic seizure, with grand mal in second place, whereas focal or partial seizures are uncommon. About one third of the patients with renal insufficiency develop seizures (Locke et al., 1961; Prill et al., 1969), but this figure is based on both chronic and acute cases.

Hepatic encephalopathy causes seizures much less frequently and plays no role as the cause of the chronic seizure disorders.

Eclampsia gravidarum not only causes grand mal attacks acutely but also may lead to posteclamptic seizures as a chronic sequel (Ledermair and Niedermeyer, 1956).

The epileptogenic potentialities of *hypoparathyroidism* and *hyperparathyroidism* are discussed in the section on EEG and metabolic disorders. *Adrenocortical insufficiency (Addison's disease)* may lead to chronic encephalopathy with occasional seizures. Sporadically recurrent convulsion may be caused by bouts of *acute intermittent porphyria* (central form) (Kaplan and Lewis, 1986). *Hyperthyroidism* may give rise to major convulsions and focal seizures (Jabbari and Huott, 1980) and may increase the seizure frequency in a chronic epileptic seizure disorder. A case (age 66) of hypercalcemia with massive biooccipital spiking with grand mal seizures, cortical blindness, hypertension, hallucinosis, and occipital cerebral ischemia has been reported by

Kaplan (1998), who was impressed by certain similarities to eclampsia. The symptoms resolved promptly.

Chronic lead poisoning (lead encephalopathy) is frequently associated with major convulsions. This condition occurs in poor areas with substandard housing; flakes of lead-based paint, now illegal in most countries, are ingested by toddlers. The serum lead level may exceed 1 mg/1,000 mL. An acute encephalopathy with convulsions, lethargy, mental deterioration, ataxia, and moderate to severe EEG abnormalities eventually converts into a chronic encephalopathy with poorly responsive grand mal attacks and usually mild to moderate EEG abnormalities. In children, encephalopathies develop before the emergence of other signs of lead toxicity, such as peripheral neuropathy with wrist drop, anemia with stippling of erythrocytes, hypertension, and colicky abdominal pain. *Coeliac disease* may be associated in some cases with neurological complications and especially with epileptic seizures (Gobbi et al., 1997).

Long-term psychiatric treatment with *phenothiazines,* especially chlorpromazine (Thorazine), leads to generalized paroxysmal bursts in the EEG (Bente and Itil, 1954) and, in some patients, to major convulsions (Itil, 1970; Schlichther et al., 1956; Spatz et al., 1984). In more recent years, the CNS toxicity of *lithium* has been increasingly recognized. In the treatment of manic-depressive illness, lithium often leads to toxic encephalopathy with lethargy, dyskinesias, myoclonus, and major epileptic convulsions. The EEG may respond quite dramatically to lithium; there is massive slowing that is often associated with a sharp component, sometimes resulting in triphasic waves. Frank spike activity may also be present. These changes are usually more prominent over frontal regions. Even at apparent nontoxic serum levels, abnormalities of major proportions may occur. Today, lithium-induced abnormalities probably represent the most important segment of abnormal records found in psychiatric referrals to a general EEG laboratory. More detail is found in the work of Spatz et al. (1978).

In an earlier era of psychiatry, chronically recurrent epileptic attacks were occasionally noted after prolonged and excessive *electroconvulsive treatment (electroshock)* and after *prefrontal lobotomy.* Electroconvulsive treatment has been on the rise during the 1980s and the vast majority of these patients show more or less prominent EEG slowing after a series of treatments. According to Drake and Shy (1989), EEG normality or abnormality does not predict post–electroconvulsive therapy (ECT) confusion. *The occurrence of seizures after convulsive treatment* has been reviewed by Devinsky and Duchowny (1983); there have been 81 documented cases in 19 studies. Epileptic seizures have been reported after *severe and extensive burns* (Hughes et al., 1973). The EEG may show marked abnormalities about 3 to 10 days after the accident (Petersen et al., 1964).

Barbiturate withdrawal and especially the abrupt discontinuation of short- and ultrashort-acting barbiturates in previously seizure-free addicts give rise to grand mal epileptic seizures in more than 50% of these individuals (Kalinowsky, 1942), usually 48 hours after abrupt withdrawal. The EEG shows generalized bursts with spikes at this stage (Faught, 1984; Isbell et al., 1950; Van Sweden and Dumon-Radermecker, 1981; Wikler and Essig, 1970; Wulff, 1957). Nonbarbituric sedatives and hypnotics may give rise to similar withdrawal seizures and EEG changes.

Chronic Alcoholism

Alcohol withdrawal seizures are common events in chronic alcoholics. These are usually full-blown grand mal attacks that occur between 6 and 30 hours after the last drink (Victor and Brausch, 1967). Therefore, withdrawal seizures are noted after a prolonged bout of drinking or after hospitalization due to other illness. Postdrinking proneness to seizures is preceded by heightened flicker sensitivity with photomyoclonic responses with lowered magnesium blood levels; the arterial pH shifts to alkaline values in the range from 7.45 to 7.55. All of these changes may eventually be superseded by the symptomatology of delirium tremens, with a peak onset 72 to 96 hours after the last drink, but this stage may not materialize. These observations are based chiefly on the work of Victor and Brausch (1967) and Victor (1970). An extensive review of the literature has been presented by Chan (1985).

Alcohol withdrawal seizures may occur in all strata of society, but are most common in patients of low socioeconomic status. The role of the type of alcoholic beverages is not quite clear. A subacute encephalopathy with seizures in chronic alcoholics (SESA) has been reported by Niedermeyer et al. (1981). This syndrome is characterized by lethargy, motor deficits, and marked EEG abnormalities such as focal slowing, spikes, and PLED. Focal seizures and grand mal attacks are common. This syndrome is not withdrawal related.

The SESA syndrome was also observed in Europe (Boroojardi et al., 1998; Homma and Niedermeyer, 1993; Mindrich and Schact, 1994; Otto and Kozian, 2001; Rothmeier et al., 2001).

Withdrawal seizures must be distinguished from epileptic seizures due to other causes occurring in chronic epileptics who have become alcoholics. The EEG is very helpful in the differentiation. Deisenhammer et al. (1984) have stressed the role of sleep deprivation in the distinction between true alcohol withdrawal seizures and seizures in epileptics who happen to be chronic alcoholics. Patients with typical alcohol withdrawal seizures are usually sent to the EEG laboratory at a stage when no spontaneous seizure can be recorded. Even the above-mentioned flicker sensitivity may no longer be detectable. According to personal experience, an EEG recording done in the 6- to 30-hour period after the last drink shows massive photomyoclonic responses that may escalate into a typical grand mal, even some minutes after termination of flickering. Most chronic alcoholics with a history of withdrawal seizures show EEG findings best termed within broad normal limits of variability (also see Hauser et al., 1982). There is in most cases a low-voltage tracing with much fast activity.

The lack of interictal paroxysmal burst activity and spike discharges in patients with alcohol withdrawal seizures, even in the critical period, stands in contrast to the wealth of paroxysmal bursts in barbiturate withdrawal.

In alcoholic epileptic patients with seizures unrelated to alcohol withdrawal, abnormal records are the rule, and focal or generalized spiking is the usual finding. The possibility of

seizures due to a chronic subdural hematoma must always be considered in alcoholics, especially in those past the prime of life.

General Remarks on the EEG and the Etiologies of Epileptic Seizures

The diagnostic evaluation of a patient presenting a history of seizures must be based on the following questions: Are the reported attacks epileptic or nonepileptic? If epileptic, is there evidence of a focus? Finally, what is the cause of the seizures? The third question remains unanswered in the majority of the cases. Nevertheless, there are some patterns apt to reveal the nature of the underlying cause.

Most, but not all, generalized synchronous 3 to 4/sec and 4 to 5/sec spike-wave discharges reflect primary generalized epilepsy due to inherited predisposition. PLEDs are most often, but not always, suggestive of a watershed type of infarction. Certain degenerative diseases such as the Bielschowsky-Jansky form of cerebromacular degeneration and Lafora-Unverricht essential hereditary myoclonus epilepsy show very suggestive patterns. In brain tumors, spiking may be completely superseded by polymorphic focal delta activity. In posttraumatic epilepsy of late onset, the spike discharge tends to be fairly inconspicuous. In patients with alcohol withdrawal seizures, the absence of interictal spiking is typical.

Much greater, however, is the EEG contribution to the differentiation of epileptic syndromes, which is discussed below.

Neonatal Seizures

General Considerations

Neonatal seizures are characterized by diverse etiologies and a strikingly different long-term prognosis (Lombroso, 1983a). Epileptic phenomena may be found in healthy infants and in babies with transient metabolic derangement; such phenomena are also found in seriously ill newborns with congenital cerebral malformation, severe perinatal CNS trauma, CNS asphyxia at birth, or massive early CNS infections.

Neonatal convulsions may be divided into essentially severe ("malignant") and essentially benign forms. The EEG has proved very useful in predicting whether the baby will be brain damaged in the future. The work of Dreyfus-Brisac and Monod (1964), Rose and Lombroso (1970), Monod and Dreyfus-Brisac (1972), Lombroso (1983a), Plouin (1985), and Kellaway and Mizrahi (1987) has helped clarify the prognosis of the convulsing newborn. Neonatal convulsions usually are seen in full-term newborns but are not uncommon in premature babies. Epileptic movements during fetal life may be recognized as unusual or suspect by an experienced and observing mother.

Clinical Ictal Characteristics

An overview of the clinical ictal features of neonatal convulsions is shown in Table 27.5 It must be pointed out that physiological movements of newborns are not easily distinguishable from convulsive motions. Some tremulousness

Table 27.5.   Common Neonatal Seizure Patterns[a]

Clonic	Focal (rarely implying focal brain lesions)
	Multifocal (fragmentary, anarchic; must be differentiated from jitteriness)
	Hemiconvulsive (rare in newborns; more frequent in young infants—may be hemiclonic or hemitonic)
Subtle	Abnormal eye movements; mild posturing; oral lingual movements; pedaling and rowing movements; brief tremors, apneas (difficult to diagnose without EEG)
Tonic	Focal or generalized (resemble decerebrate posturing; often with abnormal eye movements, apnea, cyanosis)
Myoclonic	Often fragments of infantile spasms seen later in infancy (must be differentiated from Moro and startles of non-REM sleep)
Ictal apnea	May be combined with cyanosis and hypotonia
Absence-like	Staring with pallor and muscular hypotonia
Oculomotor	Upward eye movement ("eyes rolling up")
Further ictal manifestations	Slight finger contractions; alternating "warding off" arm movements; sudden awakening with crying; eye opening; paroxysmal blinking; nystagmus; vasomotor changes: chewing, limb movements resembling "swimming, rowing, and pedaling"; abrupt changes in respiration, skin color, salivation

[a]Adapted from Lombroso, C.T. 1983a. Prognosis in neonatal seizures. In *Status Epilepticus*, Eds. A.V. Delgado-Escueta, C.G. Wasterlain, D.M. Treiman, and R.G. Porter, pp. 101–113. New York: Raven Press; Kellaway, P., and Mizrahi, E.M. 1987. Neonatal seizures. In *Epilepsy: Electroclinical Syndromes*, Eds., H. Lueders and R.P. Lesser, pp. 13–47. New York: Raven Press.

and jitteriness may or may not be of epileptic character, and the EEG will provide useful information in this respect. Epileptic activity in the newborn is, in general, more prolonged than later in life. The seizures themselves are not so strongly demarcated from the interictal periods, and status epilepticus develops more readily at this age. A full-blown grand mal with a tonic and clonic stage does not materialize during the first 5 months of life because of the underdeveloped cortical function and lack of hemisphere myelination. Kellaway and Mizrahi (1987) limit the grand mal-free period to the first 3 months. There are, of course, no petit mal absences and no proven psychomotor (complex partial) seizures in the neonate. As seen in Table 27.5, an extremely flexible seizure terminology is needed to encompass the epileptic manifestations of this early age.

As is evident from the ictal semiology shown in Table 27.5, there are *obvious and unmistakable neonatal seizures* as well as *subtle, hidden, or debatable ictal phenomena.* When the differentiation of ictal motions from physiological neonatal movements is particularly difficult, there may be ictal autonomic changes such as apnea, change of heart rate, changing complexion, or sudden bouts of arterial hypertension. A very impressive case of ictal hypertension was demonstrated by Kellaway and Mizrahi (1987). Of course, all of these autonomic changes could occur on a nonictal basis. The differential diagnosis is of particular importance in cases of neonatal apnea. This potentially life-threatening condition is more often found to be of a nonepileptic nature.

EEG Correlates of Neonatal Convulsions

The EEG is of great importance in the assessment of neonatal convulsions. Its interpretation requires a special fa-

miliarity of the EEG specialist with problems of cerebral maturation (especially in the case of seizures occurring in prematurely born neonates), physiological neonatal waking and sleep patterns, and the special characteristics of interictal and ictal paroxysmal patterns of the newborn. The combined clinical and EEG assessment is not just of merely academic value; it is very helpful in the prognostication since there are patterns of severe-malignant and benign neonatal seizures.

Rhythmical spiking over a given area of the cerebrum (Fig. 27.8) is a classical EEG pattern of neonatal seizures, especially in focal clonic seizures in which accompanying ictal spiking tends to occur over the contralateral central region (exactly where one would expect it). In the course of such seizures, the spiking may show abrupt changes of location; neither the spikes nor the focal clonic movement follow the rules of a jacksonian march—type migration (Kellaway and Mizrahi, 1987). A fast rate of clonus (3–4/sec) is usually associated with the twitching of a circumscript muscle group; most commonly, a rate of 1 to 3/sec is found. According to Kellaway and Mizrahi (1987), tremor is faster than epileptic clonus and will stop when the limb is restrained (nonepileptic clonus due to a pyramidal system deficit may be arrested with repositioning of the extremity).

Neonatal seizures with rhythmical spiking are often multifocal and the spike activity may shift from one area to an-

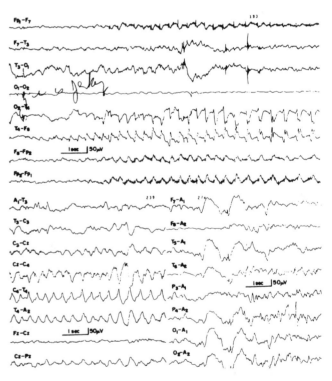

Figure 27.8.   Severe neonatal convulsions (age 11 days, full-term, neonatal herpes simplex encephalitis contracted from mother). Hemiclonic seizures started on the ninth day, mainly on the left side. Upper tracing, onset of left-sided clonic hemiconvulsion with jerking of tongue. Note rhythmical spiking starting over the right temporal region. *Lower tracing (left),* record taken during a left-sided hemiconvulsion; note right central maximum of rhythmical slow activity with a sharp component. *Lower tracing (right),* widespread single spikes in the interictal interval.

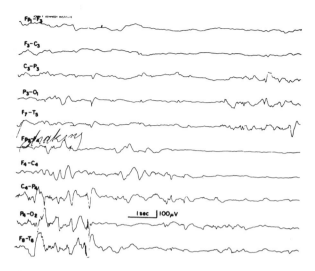

Figure 27.9. EEG of a 10-week-old baby with almost constantly repetitive brief convulsions since birth, with irregularly mixed tonic and clonic elements. Note the stretches of depressed voltage between irregular bursts of slow activity mixed with spikes.

other; central and occipital regions may be most often involved (Dreyfus-Brisac and Monod, 1972), but the temporal lobe is also quite often involved. In some of the newborns, the rhythmical ictal spike discharges occur against a background of ill-defined low-voltage activity. One may also observe an ictal pattern in alpha frequency of chiefly centrotemporal localization (Kellaway and Mizrahi, 1987; "pseudoalpha discharge," after Holmes, 1987). Tonic seizures and a variety of subtle seizures (oral-perioral movements in particular) are often accompanied by shifting rhythmical ictal spiking.

Discontinuous EEG activity punctuated with high voltage bursts of spikes and mixed slow activity (Fig. 27.9) represents the correlate of very severe forms of neonatal seizure disorder. This irregular pattern with repetitive, nearly flat stretches appears to be a foretaste of hypsarrhythmia; this has been confirmed by the work of Hughes (1985). West syndrome with infantile spasms and hypsarrhythmia tends to evolve out of this EEG type.

The limitations of EEG are laid bare by the fact that occasional minor seizures of clinically convincing epileptic character are unassociated with paroxysmal EEG abnormalities. In general, however, the EEG of the neonatal period has proved to be an outstanding tool for further prognostication. This has been well recognized since the work of Rose and Lombroso (1970). Liu et al. (1992) have utilized computerized autocorrelation EEG analysis for the detection of neonatal seizures.

Etiologies of Neonatal Convulsions

Table 27.6 presents an overview of the most common causes of seizures in newborns. This condensed list requires some further details.

The group of *congenital CNS malformations* also comprises conditions such as hydranencephaly, prosencephaly, and dysgenetic cortical anomalies such as agyria, pachygyria, and polymicrogyria. Trisomies should also be added

to this group. The incidence of such malformations as a cause of neonatal seizures is about 5% (Kellaway and Mizrahi, 1987).

A rather large number of *metabolic derangements* are capable of giving rise to seizures in the newborn. *Hypoglycemia* may be due to various causes such as small body size (for gestational age), prematurity as such, hyperinsulinemia due to a diabetic mother, status post—exchange infusion, perinatal asphyxia or trauma, and CNS infection. There may be transient or persistent metabolic disorders; typical for acute metabolic problems are *hyponatremia* and *hypernatremia* due to inappropriate fluid intake and antidiuretic hormone dysfunction. Hypocalcemia presents a rather serious problem when it occurs in the first week of life (usually secondary to perinatal CNS asphyxia or trauma), whereas a mild type of hypocalcemia causes seizures starting around the beginning of the second week of life; the cause of the latter is alimentary (low calcium-phosphate ratio) (Kellaway and Prakash, 1974). *Hypomagnesemia* may be associated with hypocalcemia. It is interesting to note that premature newborns tolerate more serious degrees of hypocalcemia (5.0 mg/100 mL or less) than full-term babies with clonic seizures at calcium levels of less than 7.4 mg/100 mL (Kellaway and Mizrahi, 1987).

Table 27.6. Causes of Neonatal Seizures

Asphyxia at birth	Common, often severe
Immediately before birth, Apgar values improving	
At birth, poor Apgar values	
Perinatal trauma, often with intracranial bleeding	Less common, may be severe
Congenital CNS malformation (porencephaly, hydrocephalus, etc.)	Common, very often severe
Metabolic causes	Rare to common: varying degree of severity, course often benign
Hypoglycemia	
Hypocalcemia	
Hyponatremia	
Urea cycle disturbance with hyperammonemia	
Phenylketonuria	
Kernicterus	
Pyridoxine dependence (deficiency; seizures may occur in utero)	
Nonketotic hyperglycinemia	Often very severe
Infectious CNS disease	Common, often severe
Earliest: *E. coli*, beta-strep	
Somewhat later: *H. influenzae*	
Seizure may be postinfectious if subdural collection is present	
Extracranial infection	Common, quite benign
Otitis	
Gastroenteritis	
Pneumonia	
Vascular CNS disease	
Intraventricular bleeding	Prematurity, very common pathology but not often associated with seizures
Intracerebral bleeding	
Intracerebral infarction	
Subdural bleeding	
Subarachnoid bleeding	Common, often severe

In addition to these transient forms of metabolic disorders, there are also metabolic changes caused by inborn errors of metabolism with very early manifestations. *Phenylketonuria* is the best known of these disorders. *Further aminoacidurias* are maple sugar urine disease, congenital lysinuria, and hyperglycinemia. The nonketotic form of hyperglycinemia is capable of a severe neonatal status epilepticus; its outcome may be fatal. There are various forms of *urea cycle defects* such as carbamyl phosphate synthetase deficiency, ornithine carbamoyltransferase deficiency, argininosuccinic aciduria, and transient hyperammonemia of preterm (associated with perinatal asphyxia). *Organic acidurias* comprise conditions such as propionic acidemia, methylmalonic acidemia, and methylmalonic—coenzyme A (CoA) mutase deficiency. The rare but well-known dysfunctions of *pyridoxine* (vitamin B_6) metabolism encompass pyridoxine deficiency and the autosomal-recessive pyridoxine dependency.

Progress in obstetrical and neonatological management has steadily diminished the incidence of *perinatal asphyxia and trauma*. This condition (also known as hypoxic-ischemic encephalopathy, according to Volpe, 1981) has diminished from about two thirds of cases of neonatal convulsions (Burke, 1954; Craig, 1960; Harris and Tizard, 1960) to about 20% to 30% following the late 1960s (Rose and Lombroso, 1970). A subsequent rise to 50% (Bergman et al., 1983; Watanabe, 1981) simply reflects the better management and prevention of metabolic seizure-inducing conditions (Kellaway and Mizrahi, 1987). At the same time, there was an increase of *intracranial hemorrhages* (another cause of neonatal seizures) due to improvement of survival figures and better detection of such conditions in babies with intracranial bleeding (Dubowitz et al., 1981). Also among these vascular accidents of the CNS are true strokes with arterial infarctions and seizures (Clancy et al., 1985; Mannino and Trauner, 1983). It has been found that stroke-induced seizures in the newborn are of typical clonic character and occur without a detectable neurological (hemiplegic) deficit. Neonatal *subarachnoid hemorrhages* are presently a particular common etiology of seizures (of mostly benign outcome; Aicardi, 1994).

Phacomatoses (neurocutaneous diseases) comprise *tuberous sclerosis, Sturge-Weber disease,* and *neurofibromatosis von Recklinghausen* (in order of diminishing epileptogenicity); seizure onset occurs more commonly after the newborn period. *Incontinentia pigmenti* with typical patterns of cutaneous pigment often affects the CNS in a very severe form, with intractable seizures and with subsequent spasticity and profound mental retardation.

Among *toxic-metabolic causes, kernicterus* (bilirubin encephalopathy) occupies a leading position as the cause of neonatal seizures. Exogenous toxins may exert epileptogenic effects on the newborn (mercury, hexachlorophene, penicillin); *maternal drug dependency* must also be mentioned, especially in the babies of mothers with barbiturate addiction.

The group of *CNS infections* still plays a major role among the causes of seizures in the newborn. The occurrence of seizures automatically indicates that a presumed meningitis has assumed the character of a meningoen-cephalitis. Among *bacterial* infections, β-hemolytic streptococci and *Escherichia coli* are the most epileptogenic agents in the newborn. Of the *viral* etiologies, *herpes simplex, cytomegalovirus,* and *Coxsackie B* are of paramount significance. *Toxoplasmosis* (a protozoan agent), transmitted across the placenta, may also cause seizures in the neonate. The severe bacterial *Haemophilus influenzae* meningoencephalitis with seizures usually begins after the newborn period.

All of the severe neonatal meningoencephalitides may be complicated by a *subdural collection* (hygroma, hematoma), which tends to cause a flare-up of the seizures.

Generally, tonic seizures are most likely to be associated with serious structural etiologies, whereas clonic seizures are most commonly found in more benign and nonstructural neonatal disorders (Lombroso, 1983; Mizrahi and Kellaway, 1998). On the other hand, tonic manifestations of the newborn may also be nonepileptic in nature indicating "forebrain depression" (Kellaway and Hrachovy, 1983)—prognostically just as serious as tonic seizures with ictal EEG patterns.

This overview indicates a mixture of *transient-dysfunctional* mild encephalopathies and those caused by *structural CNS damage*. There is also a factor of variability in the reported composition of neonatal seizure etiologies due to the fluctuations caused by modern progress in management.

Do neonatal seizures as such produce or aggravate brain damage? According to Aicardi (1994), this question is still unanswered.

Benign Versus Severe Neonatal Epileptic Conditions

This section heralds the problems involved in epileptological syndromatology, which is discussed further below. Certain causes of neonatal seizures do produce more severe or more benign types of seizure disorders than others, but this falls into the category of etiologies of seizures, presented in the preceding section. Epileptic syndromes essentially develop more or less independently of the variety of causes, and the etiology may be either unknown or of minor significance.

Plouin (1985) has presented an overview of *benign neonatal convulsions*. They are principally defined by their good prognosis, which implies normal psychomotor development and absence of secondary forms of epilepsy. A typical example of benign neonatal epilepsy is the syndrome of "fifth day seizures." Their incidence varies from 4% to 20% in a population of babies with neonatal convulsions. These seizures are of clonic character and unilateral (focal or multifocal), and there are no EEG abnormalities in the interseizure interval. More information on this syndrome is found in the work of Dehan et al. (1977), Dreyfus-Brisac et al. (1981), Navelet et al. (1981, 1982), and Pryor et al. (1981).

There is also a *familiar type of benign neonatal convulsion* that was first described by Rett and Teubel (1964). The findings of these observers were corroborated by the work of Bjerre and Corelius (1968), Rose and Lombroso (1970), Carton (1978), and Pettit and Fenichel (1980). Plouin (1985) has reviewed this topic. The seizures are mostly of clonic character and, according to Vigevano et al. (1992), mostly unilateral. A dominant autosomal hereditary transmission has been presumed. Several neonatal epileptic syndromes tend to extend into infancy, and these syndromes are discussed in the following section.

Seizures Versus Status Epilepticus in the Neonate

Neonatal seizures are often unusually prolonged or consist of a seemingly endless succession of seizures with a brief interictal interval. For this reason, the term *neonatal status epilepticus* has been used frequently (Dreyfus-Brisac and Monod, 1972; Olmos-Garcia de Alba et al., 1984b).

It simply appears to be the nature of severe neonatal convulsions to show status-like character. The convulsions themselves do not reach the degree of severity found in status epilepticus of a more mature age, especially grand mal status. The severity of the clinical condition lies in the disorder that causes the seizures rather than in the seizure as such.

Prognosis of Neonatal Convulsions

The immediate or short-range mortality from neonatal seizures used to be quite high, reaching 54% in the reports of Burke (1954). This grim overall mortality has fallen to values below the 20% mark in later studies—for instance, 16% in the patient population of Lombroso (1983). An impressive breakdown of mortality, morbidity (neurological deficits, mental retardation), and normal outcome according to the major etiologies has been presented by Kellaway and Mizrahi (1987).

Indicators of a poor prognosis are tonic seizure, presence of congenital CNS malformations, severe CNS infection (meningoencephalitis), nearly flat or pronounced low-voltage character of the EEG, and a discontinuous EEG with bursts of high voltage spikes and slow activity ("prehypsarrhythmic character").

Indicators of a good prognosis are hypocalcemia (alimentary type), other transient metabolic changes, extracranial infections with seizures (otitis, pneumonia, gastroenteritis, etc.), "seizures of the fifth day," benign neonatal convulsion syndrome, familial type of benign neonatal convulsions, clonic character of seizures (not too prolonged and not too often repeating themselves), and a normal EEG in the interseizure interval.

Indicators of an intermediate or guarded prognosis are more serious metabolic CNS disturbances, moderately severe CNS infections, most of the intracranial hemorrhages (or infarctions), persistence of immature patterns in the EEG, frequent clonic seizures, and clonic status epilepticus.

In general, *the more CNS structural pathology is present, the worse the prognosis.* One is also tempted to pose the question of whether neonatal seizures, as such, generate organic cerebral impairment—immediately following or after some delay. Such concern seems to be justified in the light of the experimental work of Wasterlain and Dwyer (1983), who produced seizures in immature rabbits, Wistar rats, and marmoset monkeys (mostly with bicuculline) while studying brain glucose and its transport. A profound depletion of intracellular glucose in the brain was demonstrated in these animals. This experimental work, however, does not necessarily pertain to human neonatal seizures.

Patient populations vary from investigator to investigator, but it is sound to assume that about 50% of all cases of neonatal seizures will have a normal outcome without any form of morbidity. The morbidity rate lies between 30% and 40% and the mortality between 10% and 20%.

Epileptic Syndromes

The syndromatological approach to the epilepsies is of fairly recent origin. It has been recognized over the last few decades that certain forms of epileptic seizure disorders have special clinical and EEG characteristics regardless of their polyetiological background. These forms represent epileptological entities or epileptic syndromes with important differences in course and prognosis. The correct diagnosis of these syndromes is therefore of considerable practical significance. Furthermore, these syndromes are age-dependent and chiefly occur in certain age ranges, especially infancy and childhood but frequently persisting through adolescence into adult life.

The common denominators of these syndromes are certain types of seizures, certain EEG patterns, and a characteristic course and prognosis. Some of these syndromes show both *idiopathic* (no significant underlying structural lesions or CNS diseases) and *symptomatic* forms.

Table 27.7 shows the latest proposal for the classification of epileptic syndromes. This proposal was presented by Wolf (1985). These changes in classification show that the domain of epileptic syndromes is still growing but is also beset with major problems caused by lack of understanding of the physiopathogenesis.

This proposal contains epileptic conditions that I do not consider to be true epileptic syndromes (especially 3.2, 4.2, 4.3, and 4.4). A proposal for Revised Classification of Epilepsies and Epileptic Syndrome by the Commission on Classification and Terminology of the International League Against Epilepsy (Epilepsia 1989;30:389–399) has gone much further in the weakening of a modern epileptological syndromatology. The inclusion of conditions such as temporal or frontal lobe epilepsy creates confusion; these are epileptic seizure disorders determined mainly by regional-localizational factors and strong etiological components (rather than by the inherent dynamics of a true epileptic syndrome with its predominantly benign or severe tendencies).

Early Myoclonic Encephalopathy

This syndrome almost always has its onset in the newborn period. It was first described by Aicardi and Goutières (1978) and is characterized by a *myoclonus of fragmentary or partial erratic character,* massive body myoclonus, partial motor seizures, and tonic spasms. Erratic partial myoclonus (face, limbs, sometimes just a finger or the orbicular area) may appear in the very first hours of life (Aicardi, 1985) and may persist during sleep (Dalla Bernardina et al., 1982a, 1983). The twitches "shift incessantly from one part of the body to another in an anarchic and asynchronous manner" (Aicardi, 1985). Massive myoclonus may not always be present. Tonic spasms usually appear later, mostly

Table 27.7. International Classification of Epilepsies and Epileptic Syndromes

1. Localization-related (focal, local, partial) epilepsies and syndromes
   1.1 Idiopathic with age-related onset
       At present, two syndromes are established, but more may be identified in the future:
       • Benign childhood epilepsy with centrotemporal spike
       • Childhood epilepsy with occipital paroxysms
   1.2 Symptomatic
       This category comprises syndromes of great individual variability, which will mainly be based on anatomical localization, clinical features, seizure types, and etiological factors (if known).
2. Generalized epilepsies and syndromes
   2.1 Idiopathic, with age-related onset, listed in order of age:
       • Benign neonatal familial convulsions
       • Benign neonatal convulsions
       • Benign myoclonic epilepsy in infancy
       • Childhood absence epilepsy (pyknolepsy)
       • Juvenile absence epilepsy
       • Juvenile myoclonic epilepsy (impulsive petit mal)
       • Epilepsy with grand mal seizures (GTCS) on awakening
       Other generalized idiopathic epilepsies, if they do not belong to one of the above syndromes, can still be classified as generalized idiopathic epilepsies.
   2.2 Idiopathic and/or symptomatic, in order of age of appearance:
       • West syndrome (infantile spasms, Blitz-Nick-Salaam Krümpfe)
       • Lennox-Gastaut syndrome
       • Epilepsy with myoclonic-astatic seizures
       • Epilepsy with myoclonic absences
   2.3 Symptomatic
       2.3.1. Nonspecific etiology:
           • Early myoclonic encephalopathy
       2.3.2. Specific syndromes:
           • Epileptic seizures may complicate many disease states.
       Included under this heading are those diseases in which seizures are a presenting or predominant feature.
3. Epilepsies and syndromes undetermined as to whether they are focal or generalized
   3.1 With both generalized and focal seizures:
       • Neonatal seizures
       • Severe myoclonic epilepsy in infancy
       • Epilepsy with continuous spike-waves during slow wave sleep
       • Acquired epileptic aphasia (Landau-Kleffner syndrome)
   3.2 Without unequivocal generalized or focal features
       This heading covers all cases with GTCS where clinical and EEG findings do not permit classification as clearly generalized or localization-related, such as in many cases of sleep grand mal.
4. Special syndromes
   4.1 Situation-related seizures (Gelegenheitsanfälle):
       • Febrile convulsions
       • Seizures related to other identifiable situations such as stress, hormonal changes, drugs, alcohol, or sleep deprivation
   4.2 Isolated, apparently unprovoked epileptic events
   4.3 Epilepsies characterized by specific modes of seizure precipitation
   4.4 Chronic progressive epilepsia partialis continued of childhood

*a*From Commission on Classification and Terminology of the International League Against Epilepsy (headed by F.E. Dreifuss). 1985. Proposal for classification of epilepsies and epileptic syndromes. Epilepsia (New York) 26:267–278.

around the age of 3 months, and are similar to those found in infantile spasms (West syndrome). The occurrence of focal (partial) motor seizures was stressed by Dalla Bernardina et al. (1982a); these attacks may be limited to eye deviation. Autonomic phenomena such as apnea or flushing of the face may be present (Aicardi, 1985).

There are *very typical EEG changes* (Fig. 27.10) with constantly repetitive generalized bursts of high-voltage slow waves with spikes, lasting a few seconds and separated from each other by brief stretches of sudden voltage depression or near flatness. Although the bursts are synchronous, the spikes themselves show no bilateral synchrony. There is also good evidence that the bursts of this burst-suppression are not associated with the motor manifestations.

There is *pronounced impairment* of the neurological and mental status; marked muscular hypotonia is common; pyramidal signs are the rule. Microcephaly may develop. CT scan and MRI findings are mostly unremarkable.

The prevalence of this syndrome is quite low. Familial occurrence has been reported and there is some evidence of an autosomal-recessive inheritance. Aicardi (1985) is inclined to assume a syndrome of diverse causes rather than a single disorder. Thus far, it has been impossible to demonstrate a progressive neurodegenerative CNS disease with a specific biochemistry. The prognosis is very poor; most children die prior to the age of 2 years. Surgical resection of the precentral gyrus at age 1 month was done with seizure control and little motor deficit (Pédespan et al., 1995).

Early Infantile Epileptic Encephalopathy (Ohtahara Syndrome)

This syndrome has been known since the work of Ohtahara et al. (1976) and Ohtahara (1978), who introduced the term *early infantile epileptic encephalopathy* (EIEE). Its main features are *tonic spasms* occurring before the age of 20 days and EEG changes quite similar to those occurring in early myoclonic encephalopathy (Aicardi and Goutières, 1978; Tallada Serra, 1985).

This syndrome could represent a glycine encephalopathy (Aicardi, 1985); the clinical picture and EEG closely resemble those of nonketotic hyperglycinemia. The prognosis is extremely poor, with a mortality of 50% before the age of 1 month. Its prevalence is very low.

Murakami et al. (1993) have emphasized the essentially different nature of early myoclonic encephalopathy and Ohtahara syndrome. Transition into West syndrome and Lennox-Gastaut syndrome is common in the Ohtahara syndrome and rare in early myoclonic encephalopathy (Murakami et al., 1993).

Infantile Spasms (Hypsarrhythmia)

Historical Remarks

The first known case report of sudden massive spasms in infancy was presented in a letter by Dr. D. J. West to *Lancet* on January 26, 1841, and pertained to the doctor's own child. Further reports were quite scanty; according to Gastaut and Poirier (1964), only four reports are known in the period from 1840 to 1920, compared with 18 reports between 1920 and 1950 and 137 reports between 1950 and 1960. The work of Zellweger (1948), Zellweger and Hess (1950), Lennox and Davis (1950), Hess and Neuhaus (1952), Gibbs and Gibbs (1952), Sorel and Dusaucy-Bauloye (1958), Gastaut et al. (1964), Jeavons and Bower (1964, 1974), Charlton (1975), Lacy and Penry (1976), and Lombroso (1983b) gives testimony of an enormous upsurge of clinical interest in this condition.

Infantile spasms consist of sudden tonic and myoclonic phenomena. The term *infantile spasms* is quite satisfactory from the clinical viewpoint and should be preserved. *Hypsar-*

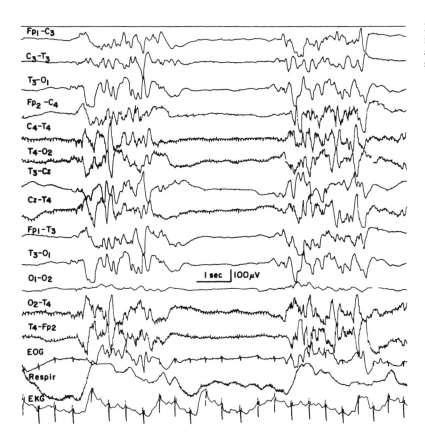

Figure 27.10. Early infantile myoclonic encephalopathy in a 3-month-old patient. Note the burst-suppression-like alternation of mixed slow activity (with some intermingled slow and spiky discharges) and stretches of flattening.

rhythmia (Gibbs and Gibbs, 1952) is an EEG term that denotes the EEG correlate of the condition. It has found surprisingly wide acceptance with clinicians; a clinical term such as *infantile spasms* is certainly preferable as far as the clinical condition, as such, is concerned. Other suggested terms are *minor motor seizures* and *minor motor epilepsy* (Livingston et al., 1958), with the drawback that no separating line is drawn between the attacks occurring in infantile spasms and Lennox-Gastaut syndrome. There are also terms such as *infantile myoclonic encephalopathy of childhood* (proposed by Gastaut) and *propulsive petit mal* (Janz and Matthes, 1955). The term *West syndrome* is now widely used.

The prevalence of infantile spasms or hypsarrhythmia must be gleaned from figures obtained at major epilepsy centers. According to Gastaut et al. (1975), figures of 2.8% among epileptics below age 15 years and 1.3% among all epileptics were found. Boys are more often affected than girls in a 2:1 ratio (Bamberger and Matthes, 1959).

Blacks appear to be less affected than whites (Santiago and Niedermeyer, 1988). A general decrease of the incidence of the infantile spasm-hypsarrhythmia complex was noted by Hughes and Tomasi (1985).

Age

Infantile spasms are found in the age range from 4 to 30 months; earlier and later occurrences of the condition are exceptional. This age range is particularly valid when one looks upon this condition from the combined clinical-electroencephalographic viewpoint. Then it becomes clear that a truly hypsarrhythmic EEG pattern does not develop before age 4 months, although at 3 months a very similar EEG pic-

ture may already be present. From a purely clinical viewpoint, one could define infantile spasms as beginning right after birth; this is exactly what some authors have done (Druckman and Chao, 1955; Weinberg and Harwell, 1965). The hypsarrhythmic pattern tends to develop out of the irregular pattern with bursts and flat stretches in neonatal convulsions as mentioned in the preceding section.

The end of the period of infantile spasms essentially parallels the disappearance of the hypsarrhythmic pattern; this usually occurs in the second half of the third year of life. In exceptional cases, the pattern may linger on for a year or even longer (up to 8 years, according to Jeavons and Bower, 1964, and even up to age 14 years, according to Talwar et al., 1995).

Clinical Ictal Manifestations

Both clonic and tonic phenomena may occur in infantile spasms. The most common type is a *massive flexion myoclonus* of head, trunk, and extremities, known as *jackknifing*. Perhaps the most detailed description of this motion and certain rudimentary variants has been given by Gastaut and Roger (1964). The lightning-like character of this sequence of movements permits an exact analysis only with the use of cinematographic or videotape documentation (see Gastaut and Roger, 1964; Oller-Daurella and Oller-Ferrer-Vidal, 1977). The tonic phenomena are slower and may last 2 to 5 seconds with accompanying autonomic changes such as flushing or lacrimation (Matthes, 1977).

The clonic spasm may show some variation. Instead of abduction of the extremities, adduction may occur to such a degree that the infant appears to be embracing himself (Ladwig et al., 1962), whereas the abduction pattern seems to stimulate the Moro reflex. Extensor spasms are also observed; there is sudden extension of neck and trunk with symmetrical forward extension and extension of lower extremities at the hips and knees ("cheerleader spasm," after Druckman and Chao, 1955). Head nodding may also occur. Brief atonia may also be noted (Hakamada et al., 1981).

The ictal manifestations of infantile spasms are short but tend to repeat themselves in rapid succession. Unilateral spasms have been described by Jeavons and Bower (1964). Up to several hundred or even several thousand spasms per day may occur (Stamps et al., 1959).

Infantile spasms are not void of focal elements. Partial seizures (focal motor) may also occur and may precede the typical spasms (Ohtsuka et al., 1996). This conjunction may indicate a less favorable prognosis. Coupling of focal paroxysmal EEG discharges with infantile spasms is rare (Hrachovy et al., 1994). On the other hand, there has been evidence of areas of focal decrease of cerebral glucose metabolism [positron emission tomography (PET) scanning] without corresponding structural abnormalities (Chugani et al., 1993).

The presence of such focal elements has been the basis for the use of hemispherectomy in these cases (Chugani et al., 1993).

Clinical Signs of Nonictal Character

The general clinical picture of the baby depends on the degree of accompanying brain damage. A sizable number of infants with infantile spasms and hypsarrhythmia (about one third, according to Jeavons and Bower, 1964) are brain damage from birth; many of them have passed through a period of severe neonatal convulsions. Severe cerebral malformations or CNS infections are common causes in such cases. Signs of cerebral palsy in its various forms may be demonstrable.

In many other cases, infantile spasms suddenly start in a previously healthy baby and, at that time, the hypsarrhythmic EEG pattern is already present. When untreated, the psychomotor development of the infant shows signs of retardation starting with the onset of attacks.

EEG Findings

The EEG findings are quite unique and essentially unmistakable, although there is a certain gray zone of questionable or borderline cases. The term *hypsarrhythmia* (Gibbs and Gibbs, 1952) is derived from the Greek word *hypselos,* which means "high," thus indicating the high voltage that generally predominates. No hypsarrhythmic recording can be appropriately obtained with the standard sensitivity of the EEG apparatus; lowering the sensitivity is required. Bursts of very high voltage slow waves occur in irregular fashion with a varying degree of bilateral synchrony, which usually increases in sleep. The stages of early non-REM sleep are particularly conducive to a typical hypsarrhythmic recording. Long stretches of high-voltage slow and intermixed spike activity may suddenly be interrupted by a brief stretch of near flatness in all leads or less commonly near flatness in a few leads or over one hemisphere; these flat stretches are practically limited to sleep tracings (Fig. 27.11).

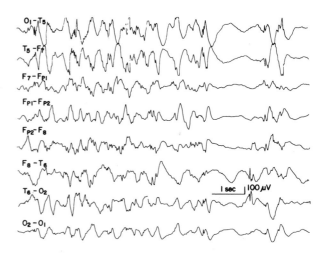

Figure 27.11. Markedly depressed stretches in an 8-month-old patient with infantile spasms–hypsarrhythmia. Record was obtained in sleep.

The spike activity shows single spikes and sharp waves, as well as very brief sequences of polyspikes that are usually of smaller amplitude. The spike activity is almost always of posterior accentuation (Fig. 27.12). The posterior maximum of spike activity is quite helpful in differentiation from the Lennox-Gastaut syndrome, which sometimes starts exceptionally early (i.e., between the ages of 6 and 12 months), when one usually sees the onset and evolution of infantile spasms with hypsarrhythmia. Large slow spike waves of frontal accentuation are found in babies with the Lennox-Gastaut syndrome. This is important since distinction helps clarify the differentiation of these two conditions; Lacy and Penry (1976) have stressed the difficulties in the differential diagnosis.

The ictal EEG, the concomitant of infantile spasms, is quite variable. Fast activity and high-voltage spikes may accompany the attacks (Gibbs and Gibbs, 1952), polyspikes and slow waves may be present (Kellaway, 1959), and no

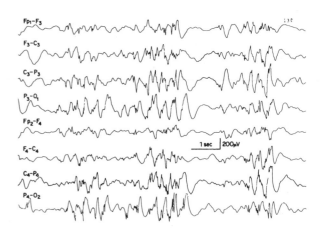

Figure 27.12. Infantile spasms–hypsarrhythmia in an 8-month-old patient. Note high-voltage output (see parameter of sensitivity) and posterior maximum of spikes. Sleep record.

change of the hypsarrhythmic interval EEG may occur, but, most commonly, a sudden suppression of the EEG activity may be seen for several seconds (Jeavons and Bower, 1964; Kellaway, 1959). A sleep recording is a necessity because in some cases the waking record may be unreadable while hypsarrhythmia is confined to the sleep portion (Jeavons and Bower, 1964). The great variability of EEG abnormalities in long-term recordings has been pointed out by Hrachovy et al. (1984).

A fine clinical-electrical analysis of infantile spasms was carried out by Fusco and Vigevano (1993). It was found that, in cryptogenic and symptomatic cases, the EEG pattern that really corresponded to the spasms consists of a slow wave. Asymmetrical spasms and focal signs suggest symptomatic etiology. The persistence of the hypsarrhythmic pattern during a cluster of spasms is found in both symptomatic and idiopathic/cryptogenic groups. Persistence of EEG hypsarrhythmia during a cluster of spasm appears to indicate a favorable prognosis in the idiopathic group (Fusco and Vigevano, 1993). According to Koo and Hwang (1996), occipital lesions are found to be associated with earliest onset of spasms and frontal lesions with late onset.

Hypsarrhythmia is not always a reliable EEG correlate of infantile spasms. There are clinically convincing cases with no hypsarrhythmia, but in these rare exceptions the voltage output is unusually high. Unless there is a rapid response to treatment, the hypsarrhythmic pattern is likely to appear in the further course of such infants.

On the other hand, the clinician could be the one to be blamed when the expected hypsarrhythmia is not found; his presumptive diagnosis may be wrong. The *clinical differential diagnosis* of infantile spasms or hypsarrhythmia has been beautifully demonstrated by Roger et al. (1964) and includes a variety of conditions. In spasmus nutans, the EEG is normal. Jactatio capitis nocturna also has a normal EEG. With salaam tic or "salutatory" spasms (Moro), there are nonspecific EEG abnormalities, sometimes with spikes in combination with epileptic seizures, but no hypsarrhythmia. In myoclonic encephalopathy (Kinsbourne, 1962), the EEG is normal. In recent years, Kinsbourne's syndrome has been supplanted by the syndrome of polymyoclonia-opsoclonus, which (especially with occurrence in early childhood) is associated with a neuroblastoma and represents a distant effect (via third messenger systems). The EEG is of little help in such cases.

Etiological and Neuropathological Considerations

Lacy and Penry (1976) have divided the etiologies into the idiopathic group and the symptomatic group. There is general consensus among investigators that the symptomatic group with known neurological disease or evidence of any kind of brain damage is the larger one. The ratio is approximately one third of cases with idiopathic forms to two thirds with symptomatic forms (Jeavons and Bower, 1964; Kellaway, 1959; Livingston et al., 1958). The introduction of CT can detect structural anomalies in cases that might have been diagnosed as idiopathic in earlier years. With the use of CT scan, it was found that the vast majority of children with infantile spasms show cerebral atrophy or, more seldom, other types of cerebral pathology (Cincinnati et al., 1982).

The number of etiological factors is enormous. Traumatic or asphyxia perinatal brain damage may lead to cerebral palsy associated with hypsarrhythmia; many developmental and congenital CNS anomalies may lead to this condition, with tuberous sclerosis as a more common cause. Inborn errors of metabolism and postinfectious states must also be mentioned. More detailed data are found in the work of Gastaut et al. (1964) and Lacy and Penry (1976). The idiopathic form with no evidence of structural brain damage remains an enigma. This form was conceived as a nosological entity ("infantile myoclonic encephalopathy"), but this concept has not found general approval. (See the discussion of Gastaut et al., 1964.) Familial occurrence is not common, but certainly not negligible; it ranges from 3% to 6%.

Even with an initially normal MRI, PET scan studies and repeated MRIs may show cortical hypometabolism and delayed myelination around age 8 to 10 months (Natsume et al., 1996). Ohtahara et al. (1993) have placed new emphasis on the concept of West syndrome as an age-specific condition (similar to the view of Bamberger and Matthes (1959).

Aicardi Syndrome as a Special Form of Infantile Spasms

Aicardi et al. (1969) described a syndrome in 15 female infants that consisted of infantile spasms (flexor spasms), a genesis of the corpus callosum, and chorioretinal anomalies.

According to Aicardi et al. (1969), the EEG showed hypsarrhythmia in only ten of the 15 infants; four of the remaining five babies showed other types of severe EEG abnormality. Some of the hypsarrhythmia records showed remarkable asymmetries. Even the flexor spasms were often asymmetrical or limited to one half of the body.

The Aicardi syndrome is now considered the expression of a chromosomal aberration (see Chapter 19, "Degenerative Disorders of the Central Nervous System").

Pathogenic Concepts

Infantile spasms with hypsarrhythmia (West syndrome) are now listed as secondary generalized epilepsy, in company with the Lennox-Gastaut syndrome and specific epileptogenic encephalopathies, such as essential, hereditary myoclonus epilepsy or Tay-Sachs disease (Gastaut, 1970). This implies that there must be a primary focus that is eventually superseded by generalization of the EEG phenomena as well as the clinical manifestations, which are void of any specific focal character.

This basic concept of secondary generalization is not proven, although many of these cases show focal structural lesions. One could speculate, however, that a special genetic component predisposes certain infants to this type of epileptic reaction. Thus, a case of cerebral palsy may be accompanied by any type of epileptic seizure or infantile spasms-hypsarrhythmia if a special genetic predisposition is present.

Therapy and Prognosis

Infantile spasms used to be regarded as therapeutically hopeless in view of the poor response to the classical anticonvulsants, such as phenobarbital and diphenylhydantoin. The observation of an excellent response to adrenocorticotropic hormone (ACTH) (Sorel and Dusaucy-Bauloye,

1958) represents one of the most important steps forward in the history of modern anticonvulsive therapy. Unfortunately, the high hopes of the late 1950s have not been completely fulfilled; there has been a backlash of disillusionment. Such pessimism as expressed by Lacy and Penry (1976) ("infantile spasms remain a refractory form of epilepsy") is not justified. Doose (1970) felt that 50% to 70% of the cases could be brought under control with ACTH and corticosteroids, while about 50% could be controlled with nitrazepam. Transient improvement is noted with the ketogenic diet, which is still used in the wake of the work of Livingston (1972).

According to Aicardi (1994), the prognosis remains grave. Mental retardation may persist in 70% to 85%, profound mental retardation in 50%. The assessment of surgical therapy (hemispherectomy) in children with focal characteristics is still premature.

The EEG shows almost immediate improvement under effective therapy. This does not necessarily reflect clinical improvement. Complete normalization may occur, but such responses are mostly temporary; return of spike activity, mostly over posterior regions, is a common event. In many cases with poor therapeutic response and especially in those with preexisting brain damage and a history of neonatal convulsions, transition into the Lennox-Gastaut syndrome is common. This occurs in 58.7% according to Ohtahara et al. (1980) and in 50% to 70% according to Hughes (1985).

Severe Myoclonic Epilepsy in Infants

This syndrome was described first by Dravet (1978) and subsequently confirmed by Dalla Bernardina et al. (1982b). It is a rare, but not extremely rare, condition that starts during the first year of life, especially around the age of 6 months. Predisposing genetic factors are slight to moderate.

The first clinical manifestations are seizures of clonic character, followed by frequently repetitive single myoclonic jerks that may proceed to a full convulsion. In addition, there may be attacks of pallor, cyanosis, atonic phenomena, and automatisms (Dravet et al., 1985). Moderate fever may accompany the first attacks.

EEG findings are initially normal; paroxysmal abnormalities tend to develop during the second year of life with generalized spikes, polyspikes, and spike-wave—like activity. Photosensitivity is common and develops in the first phase of the disorder.

There is a slowdown in the child's psychomotor development with speech decline. Neurologically, ataxia, pyramidal signs, and segmental myoclonus are common. The further evolution is unfavorable and the children are bound to become institutionalized. There is no response to antiepileptic drugs. In the differential diagnosis, the Lennox-Gastaut syndrome (see below) ranks high. Photosensitivity militates for severe myoclonic epilepsy, whereas generalized bursts of slow spike waves and runs of rapid spikes are hallmarks of the Lennox-Gastaut syndrome.

Febrile Convulsions

Age and Definition

This condition is probably the most common epileptic seizure disorder; about 3% to 4% of all children have at least one febrile seizure in infancy or early childhood (2.2–4% according to Knudsen, 1991). The attacks tend to occur between the ages of 6 months and 5 years, especially between 6 months and 3 years. The onset falls into the range of 6 to 24 months. Beaumanoir (1976) feels that it is unwise to call fever-induced convulsions after the age of 4 years "simple febrile convulsions."

Febrile convulsions must be strictly distinguished from epileptic seizures in infants or children with an acute severe febrile disease giving rise to structural lesions. The differences are indicated in Table 27.8. Lumping together both groups would tarnish the predominantly excellent diagnosis of simple febrile convulsions. Even the extensive work of Lennox-Buchthal (1977) and Yamamura et al. (1981) lacks strict separation of these forms. The connection of febrile

Table 27.8.   Differences between Febrile Convulsions and Seizures Due to Febrile Brain Disease

	Febrile Convulsions	Seizures in Febrile Brain Disease
Typical age range	6 months to 3 years (seldom 5 years)	Mainly 0–3 years
Genetic predisposition to seizures	May be strong	Mostly minor or insignificant
Type of seizure	Tonic-clonic (modified or attenuated grand mal)	Tonic-clonic (grand mal-like) or hemiconvulsions
Duration of seizure	Mostly 1–3 min seldom prolonged	Often prolonged, 10 min to hours, status-like or in rapid succession
Clinical setting in which seizures occur	At the onset of a febrile disease, mostly upper respiratory illness, often coinciding with the first sharp rise of temperature	In a variety of CNS infections (encephalitis, meningoencephalitis), intracranial venous thrombosis, cerebrovascular accidents of infancy. Also in exanthema subitum and after smallpox vaccination, but usually less severe.
Type of underlying cerebral pathology	None	Various types of inflammatory and vascular changes, in milder cases limited to edema
Postictal neurological deficit (Todd's paralysis)	Very uncommon	Common and often mixed with pathology-determined neurological defect
EEG	Rapidly normalizes after convulsion normal interval tracings in 80–90%	Abnormal throughout febrile episode, abnormal in interval (except for mild encephalitis)
Anticonvulsive medication	Not necessary (neither for acute convulsions nor for prevention of further seizures)	Acutely needed (preferably benzodiazepines, phenobarbital), long-term treatment required afterward (except for mild encephalitis)
Prognosis	Excellent in the vast majority (especially those with normal interval EEG)	Guarded. Neurological defects and further seizures common

convulsions and hippocampal sclerosis (Fernandez et al. 1998) is categorically unacceptable.

The simple febrile convulsion occurs in an infant during the steep rise of temperature at the beginning of a trivial infection involving mainly the upper respiratory tract. The mother may not even know that the child is running a fever when the convulsion occurs. The academic physician hardly ever has a chance to see these convulsions, which do not necessitate hospitalization but are usually followed by a visit to the doctor's office and subsequent clinical evaluation.

Clinical Manifestations

Simple febrile convulsions represent a tonic-clonic seizure, essentially an infantile version of grand mal attack. Some degree of lateralization may be present, but a strict hemiconvulsion or focal-motor type of seizure would militate against the assumption of a febrile convulsion. Most of these infants and children have two attacks; many have one or more seizures in the course of a few years. Under the heading of "complex febrile seizures" (Berg and Shinnar, 1996; Nelson and Ellenberg, 1976), febrile seizures with focal onset or long duration or rapid repetition are lumped together into a special subgroup.

EEG Findings

Ictal EEG tracings are hard to obtain in a truly simple febrile convulsion; grand mal—like EEG changes are most likely to occur. Tracings obtained in the hospital in the acute febrile state with convulsions show severe lateralized EEG changes (see samples of Lennox-Buchthal, 1977), but these cases are most likely to fall into the category of epileptic seizures in infants with acute structural lesions [also see the HHE syndrome of Gastaut et al. (1957, 1962), discussed earlier].

In the interictal stage, the records are usually normalized and one seldom encounters abnormal tracings. When sedation is used, one is very often surprised to see the very large amount of sedation-induced fast activity, even using chloral hydrate. Gibbs and Gibbs (1964) have pointed out that short spike-wave—like bursts in drowsiness and sleep may occur ("pseudo petit mal discharge"). Des Termes et al. (1978) found 31 children with spike foci among 500 patients with febrile convulsions. The most common site was the occipital lobe and, in 88%, the spike focus disappeared within 3 years. This was often followed by the appearance of a spike-wave focus. Yamatogi et al. (1982) have stressed the excellent prognosis of children with febrile convulsions and perfectly normal EEG tracings. Yamatogi and Ohtahara (1990) have placed emphasis on the clinical value of follow-up EEG studies.

Abnormal interictal tracings are likely to indicate underlying cerebral impairment with paroxysmal properties; these infants might be candidates for a febrile epileptic manifestation (i.e., for a chronic epileptic seizure disorder) in the future. According to Des Termes et al. (1978), the prognosis for these children is mostly favorable.

Etiological and Pathophysiological Considerations

A genetic predisposition to febrile convulsions is indubitable (Frantzen et al., 1970; Giardini, 1983; Lennox, 1953; Lennox-Buchthal, 1971; Metrakos and Metrakos, 1961; Ounsted, 1952; Schuman and Miller, 1966). Details are discussed in the comprehensive work of Lennox-Buchthal (1977).

The *seizure-precipitating action of hyperthermia* is not yet fully understood. The limitation of this action to infancy and early childhood is particularly enigmatic. Brisk changes of the water and electrolyte balance (Millichap et al., 1960) may play an important part. Further theories are discussed extensively by Lennox-Buchthal (1977). The role of vagotonia with enhanced oculocardiac reflex was pointed out by Gastaut and Gastaut (1957).

In addition to trivial upper respiratory tract infections, there are some diseases of infancy of potentially epileptogenic character. The mild and short-lasting roseola infantum (exanthema subitum) is quite often associated with convulsions of infancy and early childhood. The question remains as to whether this represents a true febrile convulsion or a mild or larval encephalitic component. A seizure at the beginning of the first steep rise of fever would support the diagnosis of a simple febrile convulsion, while a seizure at the height of the hyperthermia would militate against it (Table 27.8).

Gérard et al. (2002) have investigated the pedigrees of children with febrile convulsions and nonfebrile generalized epilepsy. These have shown the existence of a new genetic locus for the generalized epilepsy with febrile seizures (GEFS).

Therapy and Prognosis

The vast majority of febrile convulsions have an excellent prognosis. The question of whether or not to treat is not discussed in this context.

Lennox-Gastaut Syndrome

This epileptological entity has been recognized as such over the past two decades, following earlier EEG observations and presumptive electroclinical correlations (Gibbs et al., 1939). These authors noticed the severity and poor prognosis of the seizure disorder in patients with slow spike-wave complexes (called by them "*petit mal variant*," in contrast to the classical 3–4/sec spike-wave complexes in patients with petit mal absences and the prognostically more favorable "primary generalized epilepsy"). A detailed account of the clinical and ictal symptomatology of these epileptics was given by Lennox (1960), and further important work in this field was done by Gastaut et al. (1966). Terms such as *Lennox syndrome* (Beaumanoir et al., 1968) and *épilepsie myokinétique grave* (Sorel, 1964) were proposed and temporarily used. The term *Lennox-Gastaut syndrome* was introduced by Niedermeyer (1968, 1969). The work of Oller-Daurella (1967a, 1973, 1976) deserves special mention in this context. Further aspects are found in a revisitation of this syndrome by Gibbs (1971) and Gastaut (1971), as well as in the studies of Schneider et al. (1970), Chevrie and Aicardi (1972), Blume et al. (1973), Markand (1977), Kurokawa et al. (1980), Beaumanoir (1984), and Niedermeyer (1986).

The diagnosis of this syndrome is based on the occurrence of certain types of seizures, some of them practically syndrome-specific, and typical EEG changes; typically poor treatment response accompanying mental retardation and frequently demonstrable neurological deficits both lend strong support to the diagnosis. A multitude of etiologies may cause this condition, and in many cases the cause remains unknown. According to the research of Gastaut et al. (1975), the prevalence of the Lennox-Gastaut syndrome in a major epilepsy center (5.1% with 10.2% of patients below age 15 and 0.6% of patients above this age) lies above that of infantile spasms. These figures differ from the findings of Kurokawa et al. (1980), who found more cases of infantile spasms-hypsarrhythmia ($n = 757$) than of Lennox-Gastaut syndrome ($n = 320$) in their survey of Japan.

Age

This condition usually starts between the ages of 1 and 10 years; onset in the second decade of life is much less common (16% after Komai, 1977) and adult onset is rare (Bauer et al., 1988). Onset at age 6 to 12 months has been observed and requires solid EEG documentation for differentiation from hypsarrhythmia-infantile spasms. About 10% to 20% of the cases have passed through a period of infantile spasms-hypsarrhythmia before the Lennox-Gastaut syndrome become evident (Niedermeyer, 1969, 1972a, 1974). The transition from infantile spasms to Lennox-Gastaut syndrome has been investigated by Olmos-Garcia de Alba et al. (1984a).

Ictal Manifestations

The types of seizure occurring in the Lennox-Gastaut syndrome are best divided into the following groups (Table 27.9).

Of seizures also occurring in other epileptic conditions, we find grand mal (playing a major role only at the onset of the seizure disorder, often completely absent), psychomotor automatisms (in some cases dominating the picture, quite commonly myoclonus), focal (partial elementary) seizures such as adversive, and rolandic focal motor attacks.

The *occurrence of more than one type of seizure* is almost the rule in the Lennox-Gastaut syndrome; many children have more than two different types of seizures. Seizures also occurring in other epileptic conditions are described in the

Table 27.9. Types of Seizure Occurring in Lennox-Gastaut Syndrome

	Incidence in Lennox-Gastaut Syndrome
Seizures occurring in other seizure disorders	
Grand mal (generalized tonic-clonic)	+
Psychomotor (complex partial)	+
Myoclonus	+ +
Focal motor and other focal (elementary partial)	+
Adversive	±
Seizures occurring almost exclusively in the Lennox-Gastaut syndrome	
Tonic	+ + +
Atonic drop (with tonic and myoclonic elements)	+ + +
Clonic (rapidly repetitive clonic movements)	+
Hemiclonic	+
Atypical absences (with slow spike-waves)	+ +

section on types of epileptic seizures. The more specific seizures, however, need a detailed presentation.

Atonic seizures are divided into a brief and more prolonged type (Gastaut and Broughton, 1972; Oller-Daurella and Oller-Ferrer-Vidal, 1977). This seizure type was first described by Hunt (1922), who used the term *static fit*. Lennox (1945) called it an "astatic absence" as a part of the "petit mal triad"; other terms are *akinetic seizures* (Bridge, 1949), *akinetic petit mal* (Doose, 1964), and *myoclonic-astatic petit mal* (Kruse, 1968). The term *atonic-akinetic seizures* (Niedermeyer, 1969, 1972a, 1974) is imprecise and needs revision, because a special type of akinetic seizure has been individualized. These attacks occur mainly in children; late onset (age 16–35 years) has been reported by Lipinski (1977), Stenzel and Panteli (1981), and Bauer et al. (1983).

The attacks usually occur without provocation. In the brief atonic seizure, there is sudden, more or less intense, muscular hypotonia that may be preceded by a brief myoclonic jerk (Gastaut and Broughton, 1972). Generalized severe hypotonia leads to an abrupt, almost lightning-like, fall; the knees buckle, the torso and head slump forward, and the head may hit the floor or an object in a traumatizing manner. There may be, instead, a fall on the buttocks or a rudimentary seizure with sudden head drop on the chest.

Preceding myoclonus is usually associated with generalized spikes or polyspikes (Gastaut and Broughton, 1972); the atonia (best recorded in a supine patient) is accompanied by spikes, a few spike waves (Oller-Daurella and Oller-Ferrer-Vidal, 1977), and a succession of slow waves (Gastaut and Broughton, 1972). The attack usually lasts only 1 to 2 seconds; the patients probably do not lose consciousness and they pick themselves up immediately afterward. Egli et al. (1985) have provided interesting polygraphic and split-screen video data supporting the view of a predominant tonic component in atonic drop attacks (also see Nolte et al., 1988). According to these authors, axial spasm plays the principal role in the sequence of ictal motions.

In spite of the impressive documentation (or better, because of it), there is good reason to presume that the attacks of axial spasm are different from the sudden traumatizing atonic (or myoclonic) falls of children with Lennox-Gastaut syndrome. The clinical and EEG aspects of axial spasms are more likely to be related to the seizures found in startle epilepsy, discussed later in this chapter.

More prolonged atonic seizures are also called atonic absence or atonic epileptic seizures (according to the dictionary of Gastaut, 1975). Sudden atonia results in a fall, but the patient may remain lying on the floor, flaccid and immobile.

Generalized spikes, sharp waves, slow waves, and activity in the 10/sec range are found in these prolonged atonic seizures, which may last from 30 seconds to a few minutes. The EEG changes and the traumatizing abruptness of fall distinguish this attack from the cataplectic attack, which is strictly nonepileptic (see sleep disorders). These children need to wear protective headgear. In a recent proposal for classification of epilepsies and epileptic syndromes, the commission of the International League against Epilepsy (1985) (headed by F. E. Dreifuss) has suggested separately listing "epilepsy with myoclonic-astatic seizures." This may be a controversial issue because there is some reason to presume that this group of patients truly belongs in the domain of the Lennox-Gastaut syndrome. The EEG shows slow spike-wave complexes, especially in status-like conditions. The proposal stresses a frequently present hereditary predisposition. The outcome is thought to be more favorable than in the Lennox-Gastaut syndrome. The ictal EEG findings are not absolutely conclusive. A very rhythmical slow spike-wave discharge (1–2/sec) may be present in generalized synchrony for the duration of the attack. [See Gastaut and Broughton's (1972) case at the rather unusual age of 25 years.] Oller-Daurella and Oller-Ferrer-Vidal (1977) stress the occurrence of polyspike-wave complexes in these attacks. There has been no general consensus among epileptologists concerning the justification for listing akinetic seizures as a special seizure type.

Tonic seizures show a variety of manifestations; see Gastaut and Broughton (1972) and their subdivision into axial, axorhizomelic, and global tonic seizures. Such purely tonic attacks of bilateral character are limited to children with the Lennox-Gastaut syndrome when properly differentiated from lateralized tonic attacks due to mesiofrontal epileptogenic foci and a variety of nonepileptic attacks (tetanic, decerebration, and so on).

The attacks are short and last from about 5 to 20 seconds. There is extension of the axial musculature with some opisthotonus; moderate flexion of the arms is noted, and this may be followed by extension. Tracheobronchial hypersecretion occurs with repeated attacks, and a fairly dangerous status may evolve (Gastaut et al., 1964).

These attacks or very short rudiments are quite common in non-REM sleep and often are observed in a routine sleep tracing. Bilateral synchronous fast or moderately fast spike activity of about 10 to 25/sec of medium to high voltage and frontal accentuation is the EEG concomitant of these attacks ("runs of rapid spikes"; also see Chapter 13, "Abnormal EEG Patterns") (Fig. 27.13). Simple flattening or desynchronization may also occur. A diffuse slow ictal pattern has been mentioned by Gastaut and Broughton (1972), who consider it extremely rare. De Marco (1980) reported generalized synchronous 3/sec spike waves in a 14-month-old child with frequent axial tonic seizures.

Clonic seizures consist of prolonged myoclonic activity bilaterally. These jerks occur in very rapid succession; asymmetries are not uncommon (Gastaut and Broughton, 1972). The clonic motions are of small amplitude and may involve the entire body or certain (sometimes even distant) parts. There is loss of consciousness. The attacks occur mainly in non-REM sleep and are seen chiefly in childhood. The ictal EEG shows much generalized activity in the 10/sec range, mixed with spike-wave—like discharges, slower and faster frequencies. The duration lies around 1 minute.

Seizures resembling petit mal absences are not uncommon (also see Gastaut and Broughton, 1972; Gastaut et al., 1966). Onset and termination are less abrupt than in classical absences. Episodes of petit mal absence status in the Lennox-Gastaut syndrome will be discussed in the section on status epilepticus.

Clinical Signs of Nonictal Character

About half of the infants, children, or adolescents with Lennox-Gastaut syndrome show no neurological deficit and no evidence of structural brain disease. This is supported by normal findings in CT in approximately 50% of the cases

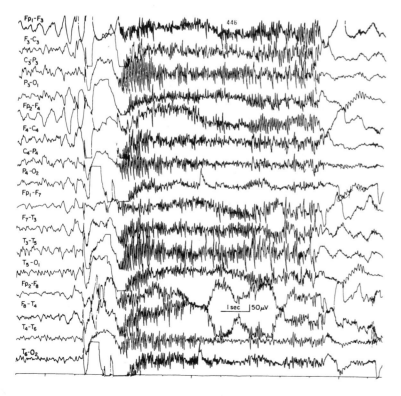

Figure 27.13. A tonic seizure in light sleep in a 20-year-old patient with Lennox-Gastaut syndrome. A generalized run of rapid spikes is preceded by a few large slow waves mixed with spikes.

(Gastaut and Gastaut, 1976; Zimmerman et al., 1977). The others show a wide variety of residual infantile brain lesions, which are often associated with neurological deficits such as forms of cerebral palsy (similar figures are found with the use of MRI).

Mental retardation ranges from the most profound to the slightest degree, essentially depending on the age at onset; the earlier the seizures start, the more serious the intellectual deficit appears to be. In patients with onset after age 10, no mental deficit may be present.

EEG

EEG findings have been crucial in the individualization of the Lennox-Gastaut syndrome as a clinical entity. The outstanding feature is the *slow spike-wave complex* ranging from 1 to 2.5/sec, which is more extensively described in Chapter 13, "Abnormal EEG Patterns." It is more often an interictal rather than an ictal discharge and is most often of generalized synchronous character, although lateralization is also fairly common; local slow spike-wave activity is quite

Figure 27.14. A: Tracing of an 8-year-old boy with Lennox-Gastaut syndrome (mentally retarded, uncontrolled psychomotor automatisms, and occasion grand mal). Note irregular slow (1.5–2.5/sec) spike-wave complexes. **B:** Pronounced slow (about 1.5/sec) spike-wave complexes in generalized synchrony with superior frontal maximum in an 11-year-old patient with Lennox-Gastaut syndrome. The patient was awake at the time of this recording; there were no clinical ictal manifestations.

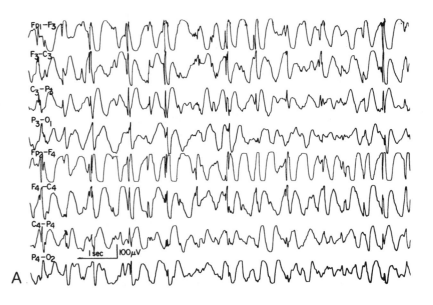

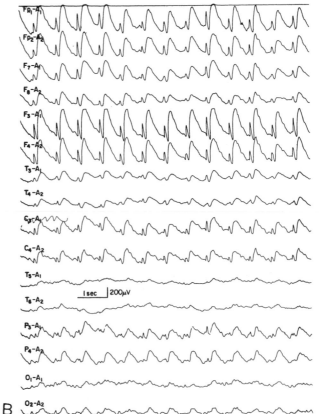

rare. A maximum over the frontal midline is the rule (Fig. 27.14).This discharge is enhanced in non-REM sleep and may become almost continuous. Such an abundance of generalized slow spike-wave activity in non-REM sleep, however, must be carefully distinguished from the condition known as *electrical status epilepticus during sleep in children (ESES) syndrome* (Patry et al., 1971; Tassinari et al., 1984). In the Lennox-Gastaut syndrome, the spike component shows considerable variation; it may be slow ("blunted") or quite fast with true spike character. The slow spike-wave discharge may be present in early infancy between the ages of 6 and 12 months. Classical 3/sec or 3 to 4/sec spike-wave complexes may also be discernible.

Another important pattern is *runs of rapid spikes* (Fig. 27.15, and 27.13), which are seen in non-REM sleep only. This pattern is more common in older children, adolescents, or adults. More information can be found in Chapter 13. The EEG as such ("background EEG") is often disorganized and excessively slow, but a sizable number of patients show a normal frequency spectrum with unremarkable posterior alpha rhythm, the basic rhythm. The degree of general slowing and disorganization usually underscores the severity or advanced stage of the case. These children are often seen in a state of overtreatment with anticonvulsants, resulting in toxic anticonvulsant levels. Interestingly, high and toxic levels of phenobarbital may be completely unassociated with fast EEG activity; this absence of barbiturate-induced fast frequencies is quite characteristic in advanced cases with considerable cerebral impairment (Niedermeyer et al., 1977b).

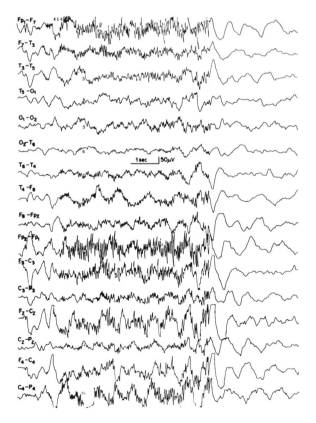

Figure 27.15.   A run of rapid spikes in a 14-year-old patient.

Etiological and Neuropathological Considerations

The aforementioned normal CT scan (or MRI) findings in 50% of the cases further support the view that about half of the cases are idiopathic and hence without structural cerebral changes. The nature of idiopathic forms is completely unclear. Genetic predisposition is certainly more than just a hypothesis; a genetic approach by means of the major histocompatibility complex was made by Smeraldi et al. (1975, 1976).

Acquired pathology of residual character is present in a considerable number of cases; known CNS disease was found in 36 of 125 cases in the material of Niedermeyer (1972a), with CNS infection and birth trauma/asphyxia as the leading problems. One could argue that such pathology alone can hardly account for this severe form of epileptic seizure disorder and that a genetic predisposition is a prerequisite. Even progressive pathology such as intracranial tumors may be associated occasionally with Lennox-Gastaut syndrome (Angelini et al., 1979; Niedermeyer, 1972a). Phenylketonuria, forms of lipidosis (Levy, 1989; Niedermeyer, 1972a), tuberous sclerosis (Cavazutti, 1972; Gastaut et al., 1973), lead encephalopathy (Fejerman et al., 1973), and toxoplasmosis (Cavazutti, 1972) have been specifically mentioned as etiological factors. In essence, this is the same dichotomy of idiopathic and symptomatic forms as in infantile spasms-hypsarrhythmia.

The combination of Lennox-Gastaut syndrome (typical slow spike waves) with *gelastic seizures* in children and adolescents is usually associated with a *hypothalamic hamartoma*. This syndrome used to offer little hope, but advances in neurosurgery have markedly improved the gloomy outlook. According to Berkovic et al. (2003), in the hands of highly experienced neurosurgeons, destruction of the lesion with transcallosal or with transventricular approach and especially with use of gamma knife can render the patients seizure-free along with behavioral improvement.

Pathogenic Concepts

The debatable concept of secondary generalized epilepsy is discussed earlier in the section on infantile spasms. All that was said there also applies to the Lennox-Gastaut syndrome.

Differential Diagnosis

A posttraumatic form of epilepsy with slow spike-wave complexes and runs of rapid spikes in sleep (Niedermeyer et al., 1970a) is discussed in the section on etiologies of epileptic seizures (posttraumatic epilepsy).

There is a possibility that frontal lobe foci may give rise to generalized slow spike-wave complexes; this mechanism of "secondary bilateral synchrony" is discussed below (see Primary Generalized Epilepsy). Gastaut (1984) presented cases of apparent Lennox-Gastaut syndrome but with a presumed primary focus and secondary bilateral synchrony. The reader will find more information in Table 27.10.

Therapy and Prognosis

Most cases of Lennox-Gastaut syndrome are not responsive to therapy. Gastaut et al. (1966) found diazepam (Valium) as a long-term oral anticonvulsant effective in some cases. Preferable are more recently introduced benzo-

Table 27.10.   Steps in the Differential Diagnosis of Spike-Wave Complexes Other Than 6/sec

Step 1. A principal distinction between "classical" and slow spike-wave complexes
  3–4/sec; mostly primary generalized epilepsy
  1–2.5/sec; mostly Lennox-Gastaut syndrome
Step 2. Distinction of two major subgroups of primary generalized epilepsy
  a. 3–3.5/sec or 3–4/sec: most commonly found in children with petit mal absences and adolescents with a history of petit mal absences in childhood. As spike-wave frequency is measured, keep in mind that the first 1 to 3 complexes of a given burst may be "too fast" (about 4–4.5/sec) and the last complexes "too slow" (down to 2.5/sec).
  b. 4–4.5/sec or 4–5/sec: most commonly found in adolescents or young adults with myoclonus and/or tonic-clonic convulsions occurring mainly some time after awakening. There is usually no history of petit mal absences.
Step 3. Differential diagnosis of primary generalized epilepsy
  a. Frontal lobe epilepsy with secondary bilateral synchrony. EEG differentiation may be very difficult or impossible
    Occasional intermixed bursts of rhythmical spiking at about 10/sec support the diagnosis of frontal lobe focus—secondary bilateral synchrony
    Clinically, petit mal absences of rather late onset in life (past age 10 years) and/or unusually long duration (20 sec and longer) support diagnosis of secondary bilateral synchrony with primary frontal focus
      Petit mal absences with immediate transition into major tonic-clonic convulsions (a very rare event) favor the diagnosis of secondary bilateral synchrony with primary frontal focus
  b. Hypothalamic lesions (not thalamic lesions)
    Very rare cases; hypothalamic disorders with endocrine manifestations plus petit mal absences with 3/sec spike-waves
  c. Metabolic disturbances
    Renal encephalopathies with spike-wave bursts
    Barbiturate withdrawal with spike-wave bursts (usually with some degree of photosensitivity).
Step 4. Differential diagnosis of the Lennox-Gastaut syndrome
  a. Post-traumatic epilepsy with slow spike-wave complexes
    Imitates Lennox-Gastaut syndrome electrically but not clinically (seizures types usually grand mal or psychomotor)
  b. Frontal lobe epilepsy with secondary bilateral synchrony EEG and clinical differentiation very difficult or even impossible
  c. ESES syndrome ("electrical status epilepticus of sleep")
    Children with almost continuous generalized slow spike-wave-like (i.e., no typical spike-wave complexes) activity throughout non-REM sleep, not in waking state and REM
    No upper frontal maximum as in Lennox-Gastaut syndrome (instead, posterior or vertex maximum)
    Clinically, seizure disorder much milder than Lennox-Gastaut syndrome
  d. Aphaxia-convulsion syndrome (Landau-Kleffner syndrome)
    In children with aphasia and seizure disorder which is rather mild
    Slow spike-wave activity most impressive in sleep, often generalized and continuous but with maximum over midtemporal area
    In most cases, a self-limited disease
  e. Benign occipital lobe epilepsy
    A benign epileptic condition with some relationship to migraine, often associated with slow spike-waves with occipital or posterior temporal maximum, especially in the waking state
    Clinically, seizures usually initiated with visual symptomatology and often followed by severe headache
  f. Rett syndrome
    A degenerative CNS disease (only in girls)
    Slow spike-wave activity common in earlier stages; the maximum of spike-wave activity varies (mainly temporal or occipital)
  g. Radiation necrosis encephalopathy
    A severe encephalopathy with epileptic seizure disorder (grand mal and various types of focal seizures) may develop following radiation treatment
    These changes occur mainly in deep-seated midline tumors of childhood or adolescence
    Slow spike-wave complexes are particularly slow and may become very pronounced, usually generalized with frontal maximum; asymmetries are common (Niedermeyer, 1988)
  h. Epileptic seizure disorder (along with precocious puberty) caused by hypothalamic hamartoma
  i. Myoclonic astatic epilepsy of childhood
    A controversial clinical entity; must be considered in the differential diagnosis even though the occurrence of slow spike-wave complexes has not been clearly demonstrated

diazepines, chlorazepate dipotassium (Tranxene), and especially clonazepam (Klonopin). Even the removal of operable pathology such as a brain tumor does not guarantee lasting success. Unexpected sudden turns for the better are not uncommon. Long stretches of seizure freedom are occasionally noted but are not attributable to therapy. Because of the bilateral-synchronous character of the seizure discharges, severance of commissural fiber systems has been thought to be beneficial. The *commissurotomy* introduced by Mann et al. (1969) results in a split brain. Splitting of the corpus callosum (*callosotomy*) has been carried out (Gates et al., 1982; Harbaugh and Wilson, 1982); the acute effects on the EEG have been described by Sussmann and Harner (1982). The results of these procedures are debatable.

This is a gloomy picture; the course quite often leads to institutionalization, especially in patients with very early onset. The course of the disease, however, should not be conceived as a linear progression of deterioration. Observation of adult patients shows certain interesting trends.

In adulthood, the EEG may gradually lose the characteristics of the Lennox-Gastaut syndrome. The slow spike-wave complex may disappear after age 20 or 15; instead, runs of rapid spikes in sleep only may become more prominent. This pattern, too, may gradually vanish and spikes or sharp waves of temporal and especially anterotemporal localization may then become predominant. Interestingly, this change may be associated with the appearance of psychomotor (complex partial) seizures as a new phenomenon or enhancement of preexisting seizures of this type. Thus, the patient seems to merge into the mainstream of temporal lobe epilepsy but will remain a deteriorated case with mental deficit or behavioral changes, often fostered by years of institutionalization (Niedermeyer, 1974).

This process has been described as "secondary temporalization" (Niedermeyer, 1966b, 1972a; Nogueira de Melo and Niedermeyer, 1991a). It is doubtful whether all patients take this course. The author has seen a 39-year-old patient who, despite early onset, still had the ictal and EEG characteristics of a typical Lennox-Gastaut syndrome. According to Hughes and Patil (2002) secondary temporalization is a very common development (78% of their patients). Much more impressive is the observation of Benbadis and Dinner (1994): A 64-year-old patient who experienced seizure onset at 14 years. Seizures consisted of staring, sudden falls, and generalized convulsions. There was no mental deficit. The EEG showed widespread and mainly bifrontal 2/sec spike waves, single spikes shifting in frontotemporal leads, and classical runs of rapid spikes.

New Vistas Regarding the Lennox-Gastaut Syndrome

Clinical entities need revisiting from time to time. Refreshing new thoughts have been presented by Ohtahara et al. (1995) who have reemphasized the wide borderland of this syndrome, the role of focal-cortical elements and secondary bilateral synchrony. These authors therefore advocate a more refined subclassification, especially in view of the suitability of neurosurgical treatment (callosotomy).

The highly critical approach of Hirt (1996) attempts to cast doubt on practically all of the electroclinical diagnostic pillars of the diagnosis of Lennox-Gastaut syndrome. Such negativistic analyses could be done in most clinical diagnostic entities; with sufficient destructive nihilism, the "gestalt" of diseases and syndromes could be turned into an empty and worthless construct. Criticism is always welcome but has to be coupled with a constructive attitude.

Atypical Astatic Epilepsy of Childhood

This rather controversial syndrome has been described by Doose (1964) ("akinetic petit mal"). Is this an entity as such or does it represent a benign variant of the Lennox-Gastaut syndrome? Clinical and EEG features may appear to be identical with the Lennox-Gastaut syndrome, but the outcome is milder. Doose (1985) feels that this epileptic condition is taxonomically closer to primary generalized epilepsy rather than to the Lennox-Gastaut syndrome. Deonna et al. (1986) reported a combination of myoclonic-astatic epilepsy and "benign focal epilepsy of childhood."

There are now indications that the Lennox-Gastaut syndrome and the syndrome of myoclonic-astatic epilepsy are indeed two separate entities with different neurophysiological generating the myoclonus. In the Lennox-Gastaut syndrome, myoclonus originates from a stable generator in the frontal cortex. Spreading to contra- and ipsilateral cortical areas, whereas in myoclonic-astatic epilepsy, myoclonus appears to be a primary generalized epileptic phenomenon (Bonanni et al., 2002).

The Panayiotopoulos Syndrome

In an excellent overview of benign childhood partial seizures, Panayiotopoulos (1999) also presented an introduction to a special type of early-onset occipital seizures for which he coined the term *Panayiotopoulos syndrome*. This syndrome was subsequently highlighted in a special study (Panayiotopoulos, 2002) with the following initial characterization of this syndrome: "Panayiotopoulos syndrome is a childhood-related idiopathic benign susceptibility to partial, mainly autonomic, seizures that may be genetically determined. The children have normal physical and neuropsychological development."

The age of onset shows a range from 1 to 14 years with a peak at 4 to 5; 76% start between ages 3 to 6 years. Children of all races are vulnerable. The prevalence is about 13% among children with a seizure onset between age 3 to 6 years and 0.2% to 0.3% of the general population of children may be affected. This figure may be much higher if children with atypical and inconspicuous presentation are included.

The aforementioned "mainly autonomic" seizures consist of feeling sick, looking pale, nausea, retching, and vomiting. There may also be cyanosis, mydriasis (or miosis), cardiorespiratory and thermoregulatory alterations, incontinence of urine and/or feces. Apnea and cardiac asystole may be exceptionally severe. Two thirds of the seizures occur in sleep. Unilateral eye deviation is common. The seizures commonly end with hemiconvulsions or with jacksonian march or generalized convulsions, which, quite rarely, may assume the form of status epilepticus. The duration varies from 1 to 30 minutes (mean 9 minutes) and in some cases much longer, up to 7 hours with an autonomic status. The final portion of the seizure may consist of an ictal syncope with flaccidity. After sufficient sleep, the child is perfectly normal.

The EEG is the most useful test (MRI findings being normal). In 90% of the cases, the EEG shows multifocal spikes and spike waves with posterior accentuation. The ictal EEG "consists mainly of rhythmic delta activity intermixed with usually small spikes." Onset is unilateral, often posterior, but may also be anterior and not strictly localized to one electrode.

The family history is usually negative and there is no relationship to migraine in the family.

In a proposal for a diagnostic scheme of epileptic seizures and syndromes (Engel, 2001), the Panayiotopoulos syndrome has been included as "early-onset benign childhood occipital lobe epilepsy (Panayiotopoulos type)" in contrast with "late-onset childhood epilepsy (Gastaut type)" (see Benign Occipital Lobe Epilepsy, below). This emphasis being laid upon the occipital character has been thought to be excessive, according to Panayiotopoulos (2002).

Having worked in EEG-epileptology (with patients of all ages) for 45 years, and having seen only a handful of children who perhaps could have fitted this syndrome, I have my doubts. Nevertheless, I fully trust the author's scientific veracity and cannot imagine an EEG text that omits discussion of the syndrome.

Primary Generalized Epilepsy ("Idiopathic Generalized Epilepsy")

The entire concept of a primary generalized epilepsy has its foundation in the EEG. Who would have thought that a simple petit mal absence with its rather subtle clinical symptomatology could be the result of massive generalized synchronous epileptic discharges? The first observation of the ictal EEG pattern of petit mal by Gibbs et al. (1935) has been the starting point for numerous attempts to explain the phenomenon of primary generalized seizure discharges. As to history, Brazier (1961) and Gloor (1978) feel that Berger (1933) was truly the first observer of the spike-wave discharge, but the recording with the simultaneous use of a coil galvanometer and an oscilloscope shows only paroxysmal rhythmical high-voltage 3/sec waves without the spike component; the bilateral synchronous character of the burst cannot be derived from the tracing, and the ictal symptomatology in an 18-year-old girl, "rapidly tapping her thigh with her left hand," is not convincing.

Gloor's (1978) historical review clearly shows the subsequent development and the emergence of a subcortical pacemaker theory that eventually was incorporated in Penfield's (1952) concept of the centrencephalic system. This concept had been formulated much earlier in conjunction with the regulation of consciousness (Penfield, 1938); the diencephalic and upper brainstem level were viewed as the "highest level of integration"; this resulted in a blend with the older jacksonian concepts.

Controversy arose over the centrencephalic theory; neuroanatomists and neurophysiologists became involved in the question of whether upper brainstem and thalamic midline structures could serve as the origin of bilateral synchronous cortical seizure discharges. This will be discussed in greater detail.

Terminology

The term *primary generalized epilepsy* has been introduced by the International League Against Epilepsy (1969, 1970, headed by Gastaut; see Gastaut, 1969, 1970). This term deserves general acceptance. It implies that the clinical and EEG phenomena of the seizures occurring in this epileptic condition are generalized from the start. This term has superseded older terms such as *centrencephalic epilepsy* (Penfield, 1952), *cortico-reticular epilepsy* (Gloor, 1968), and *common generalized epilepsy* (Niedermeyer, 1972a). Its weakness lies in the fact that it seems to burn all bridges for a retreat if a truly focal cortical onset with extremely rapid generalization should ever be convincingly demonstrated in the future. Oller-Daurella (1971) has pointed out some weaknesses in the concept of primary generalized epilepsy. The term *primary generalized epilepsy* also implies that there is no structural epileptogenic focus in a disorder based on a dysfunctional state. The view of total lack of structural lesions has been challenged by Meencke and Janz (1984), who found areas of minor dysgenetic changes in autopsy studies of patients with presumed primary generalized epilepsy. This observation has sparked some controversy; Lyon and Gastaut (1985) have minimized the significance of microdysgenesis, which may occur just as well in other conditions or in neurologically normal controls. Meencke and Janz (1985) have further stressed the pathological significance of microdysgenesis. Be this as it may, the widely scattered findings of microdysgenesis cannot explain the distribution type of the abnormal EEG discharges and the

practically immediate appearance of bilateral or generalized synchrony.

Older terms such as *genuine, essential,* or *idiopathic epilepsy* might have been intended as synonyms for the same condition, but are beset by hyperflexibility. These terms stem from the pre-EEG era, when the concept of primary generalized epilepsy in a modern sense was barely thinkable. Therefore, these terms should be discouraged.

Surprisingly, the term *idiopathic* has been strongly resurrected in the International Classification of Epilepsies and Epileptic Syndromes (1985) (Table 27.7).

Age and Prevalence

The age depends on the type of seizure. Classical petit mal absences mostly start at age 4 to 6 years; a special group starts at age 9 to 15 years. (Also see the section on types of seizure.) Myoclonus and grand mal attacks usually start at age 11 to 14 years. Improvement or full seizure control after age 20 to 25 years is very common. There is, however, indubitable evidence of rare cases of petit mal absence seizures in adulthood. A remarkably large population of 42 patients with absences in adult life was analyzed by Rütti (1982); 20 patients were presumed to suffer from primary generalized epilepsy and 22 patients with acquired (symptomatic) forms of seizure disorder. Gastaut et al. (1986) presented the data of 26 patients with primary generalized epilepsy, aged between 35 and 50 years, with follow-up observations of 20 to 37 years. A special manifestation is the petit mal absence status, which may occur in older children, adolescents, adults, and even the elderly over age 80; this will be discussed under the heading of status epilepticus.

Primary generalized epilepsy is sometimes preceded by a period of febrile convulsions in infancy and early childhood. "Benign myoclonic epilepsy of infancy" (Dravet and Bureau, 1982; Lombroso and Fejerman, 1977; Oguni et al., 1985) may also precede primary generalized epilepsy. It is never preceded by severe conditions such as infantile spasms or the Lennox-Gastaut syndrome. A report of petit mal epilepsy during early infancy by De Marco (1980) is misleading. The observed patient was 14 months old, and a very rhythmical generalized-synchronous spike-wave discharge occurred during frequent seizures of tonic character without the typical clinical features of petit mal absences. The episodes were preceded by a short buildup of rapid spiking. Furthermore, the spike-wave discharge is slower than 3/sec (based on the indicated parameter of time).

According to Gastaut et al. (1975), research at a major epilepsy center shows a prevalence of 28.4% for all ages, with 11.3% for grand mal, 9.9% for petit mal absence, 4.1% for myoclonus, and 3.2% for other manifestations.

Table 27.11 lists forms of generalized epilepsies and their relationship to primary generalized epilepsy.

Ictal Manifestations

The *petit mal* absence was discussed in detail in the section dealing with types of seizures. The two different forms are (a) simple petit mal absences, starting at age 4 or shortly thereafter, with a large number of absences per day (sometimes exceeding 100/day); and (b) juvenile petit mal absences with an onset at age 9 to 15 years, more prolonged or

Table 27.11. Epileptic Syndromes and Their Relationship to Primary Generalized Epilepsy (PGE)

Epileptic Syndromes	Relationship to PGE[a]
Benign myoclonic epilepsy of early childhood (Dravet and Bureau, 1981)	+++
Febrile convulsions, simple	+−++
Childhood absence epilepsy (classical petit mal)	++++
Epilepsy with myoclonic absences (myoclonic form of petit mal: Lennox, 1945; "impulsive petit mal": Bamberger and Matthes, 1959)	++
Photosensitive epilepsy, pure	+++
Photosensitive epilepsy with eyelid myoclonus-absence (Jeavons, 1977)	+++
Juvenile absence epilepsy (prepuberty absence: Doose et al., 1965)	++++
Juvenile myoclonic epilepsy (Janz syndrome) (Gastaut, 1968; Janz, 1969)	++++
Epilepsy with grand mal on awakening (Hopkins, 1933; Janz, 1953)	++++
Grand mal-absence epilepsy (Doose et al., 1965)	+++

[a]++++ indicates an integral part of PGE; +++ a very close relationship to PGE; ++ a close or moderately close relationship to PGE.

mixed with more motor activity. The absences of the first type have been called "pycnoleptic" (Janz, 1969; Kuhlo, 1970; Matthes, 1977), using an old term introduced by Sauer (1916), which characterizes the high frequency of the attacks. The absences with onset around age 10 to 15 have been called "spanioleptic" ("spanios," meaning seldom, because of their smaller number of daily seizures) (Doose, 1964). A cyclic change of the frequency has also been noted ("cycloleptic attacks") (Janz, 1969; Matthes, 1977). This distinction (pycnoleptic vs. spanioleptic absences) has been doubted by Loiseau et al. (1995).

Petit mal absences show a wide variety of mild to moderate motor accompaniment; rhythmical eye blinking in synchrony with the spike waves is the most common motor component. Retropulsion of the head is quite common ("retropulsive petit mal"; Janz, 1969); adversive movements and some rhythmically repetitive oral motions may also occur.

Children with petit mal absences often start having *grand mal seizures* in early adolescence. Figures range from 31% (Paal, 1957) to 54% (Livingston et al., 1965); Matthes (1977) goes even further and feels that about two thirds of the children with petit mal absences will have grand mal attacks. In most of these cases, the grand mal seizures do not pose a major problem and are readily brought under control. Janz (1953, 1962) has stressed the role of the stage of awakening as a strongly facilitating factor in these major convulsions. This view has shed much light on the pathophysiological basis of these attacks and deserves full support.

Grand mal attacks in patients with primary generalized epilepsy are very often preceded by sudden bilateral *myoclonus*. These myoclonic jerks may also occur as isolated events, especially in the morning hours after a night of insufficient sleep. Not all seizures at awakening in PGE have to occur in the morning hours; the later afternoon is another critical phase. The crucial factor is the combination of tiredness and repeated escalating arousals with EEG bursts (to be

discussed later). Thus, the dichotomy of awakening grand mal and random grand mal (Greenberg et al., 1995) could be irrelevant. Many patients with the combination of grand mal and myoclonus may never have experienced any petit mal absences earlier in childhood. This petit mal—free form is a special variant of primary generalized epilepsy that also shows slightly different interictal bursts in the EEG. These bursts are relatively short and dominated by 4/sec or 4 to 5/sec spike-wave complexes that are, contrary to the classical 3/sec or 3 to 4/sec spike waves, not readily activated by hyperventilation. Many of these patients are flicker-sensitive (photoconvulsive response), and positive family histories are more often obtained in this group. A special form of "minimyoclonus" with jitter-like twitching (often limited to fingers) has been described by Wilkins et al. (1985). This form may be seen quite frequently in primary generalized epilepsy; the myoclonus is preceded by a small negative spike-like event over upper frontal areas (Table 27.2).

In PGE/Janz syndrome, the origin of myoclonus-associated spike activity is the frontal-premotor and motor cortex (Panzica et al., 2001). These authors also noted similarities between PGE-related myoclonus and myoclonic activity in progressive myoclonus epilepsies.

A remarkably new approach has been taken by Sevim et al. (2002), who subjected epileptic patients and normal controls to motor unit number estimate analysis by means of special electromyography (EMG) investigation. Patients with juvenile myoclonic epilepsy showed significantly lower motor unit counts. These authors pointed out that a genetic tendency to contract juvenile myoclonic epilepsy is associated with a disorganization of lower motor units.

Myoclonus may also be associated with brief petit mal absences. Lennox (1945) conceived of this combination ("myoclonic petit mal") as a part of his "petit mal triad." Janz (1969) has extensively investigated this type of attack and uses the term *impulsive petit mal*; Matthes (1977) prefers the term *Janz syndrome*. An extensive study on myoclonic petit mal in 399 patients with genetic evaluation has been carried out by Tsuboi (1977). Delgado-Escueta and Enrile-Bascal (1984) have stressed the good response to sodium valproate and hence the ultimately good prognosis. This is congruent with the findings of Asconapé and Penry (1984). Further information is found in the work of Schmitz and Sander (2000).

Very prolonged absence-like stages, attacks of petit mal–like stupor, or petit mal automatisms have been termed *petit mal status* (Lennox, 1945), whereas the modern terminology recommends the term *absence status*. These states are discussed in the section on status epilepticus. Whereas all of the ictal manifestations of primary generalized epilepsy tend to occur in children and adolescents, the absence status not only occurs in elderly patients but may even have its onset in old age.

With the exception of simple febrile convulsions, the syndromes listed in Table 27.11 form one large family: PGE, a condition with occasionally fuzzy delineation (Reutens and Berkovic, 1995).

EEG

Most of the relevant EEG findings have been described in detail in Chapter 13, "Abnormal EEG Patterns." It may suffice to reiterate that the 3/sec or 3 to 4/sec spike-wave pattern is the EEG correlate of the classical petit mal absence and also occurs, often abundantly, in the interval, sometimes in drowsiness and sleep. These generalized bursts, with or without clinical absence, are readily triggered by hyperventilation and may materialize after a few deep breaths in untreated patients (Fig. 27.16A).

Intermittent photic stimulation may occasionally trigger petit mal absences with 3/sec spike waves; more often, it is associated with generalized polyspikes of frontal accentuation, with or without clinical myoclonic jerking, most often at frequencies of 14 to 18 flashes/sec. As was pointed out above, photosensitivity is more often noted in patients with 4/sec or 4 to 5/sec spike-wave bursts and a history of grand mal and/or myoclonus.

The phenomenon of myoclonus is almost invariably linked with *polyspike discharges* as far as patients with primary generalized epilepsy are concerned. Polyspikes also contaminate the spike-wave sequences in children with massive myoclonus as a variant of petit mal ("impulsive petit mal," "Janz syndrome," see above), as Matthes (1977) has pointed out (also see Tsuboi, 1977).

A comparison of spike-wave patterns in classic adolescent-onset and adult-onset patients with idiopathic generalized epilepsy showed no differences according to Yenjun et al. (2003). This statement, however, can be questioned when one looks at the authors' EEG illustrations, which show generalized synchrony in the adolescence group and clearly less impressive spike-wave activity of bilateral-anterior synchrony in an aged patient with late onset.

In the majority of patients with primary generalized epilepsy, the EEG frequency spectrum appears to be normal aside from the generalized paroxysmal bursts, the so-called *background activity*. A remarkable exception is the occurrence of prolonged stretches of rhythmical high-voltage 3/sec waves in occipital leads with moderate spread into the vicinity; these bursts occur in a sizable number of children with petit mal absences, sometimes ranging from 2 to 4/sec. This posterior rhythm has been investigated mainly by Subirana and Oller-Daurella (1953), Elston et al. (1956), and Aird and Gastaut (1959). According to Vizioli (1967), this rhythm is found in 55% of the patients with petit mal absences and persists in 60% of the cases after seizure control. Dalby (1969) found occipital delta activity in 38.5% of the patients with petit mal. On the other hand, Oller-Daurella (1967b) observed this pattern in only 20% and Niedermeyer (1972a) in no more than 11.5% of the patients with petit mal absences. Hyperventilation almost invariably activates this rhythm (Lugaresi, 1967). In some cases, a very small spike component is discernible between the large rhythmical delta waves. Lugaresi (1967) also noted that the rhythmical posterior activity may be enhanced under treatment with ethosuximide (Zarontin), although the 3/sec spike-wave complex disappears; these views were also confirmed by Gastaut (1967). Oller-Daurella (1967b) feels that children with petit mal absences and rhythmical occipital delta trains fall into a special epileptological category; this author saw better therapeutic responses to hydantoins, especially mephenytoin (Mesantoin) rather than to the diones. Sorel (1967) considers the occipital rhythmical slow activity to be a very favorable prognostic sign (Fig. 27.16B).

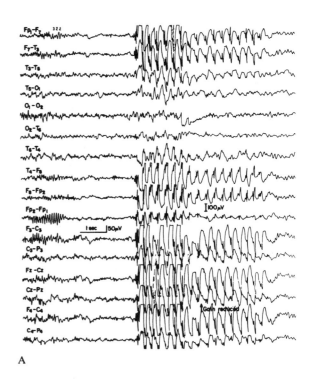

A

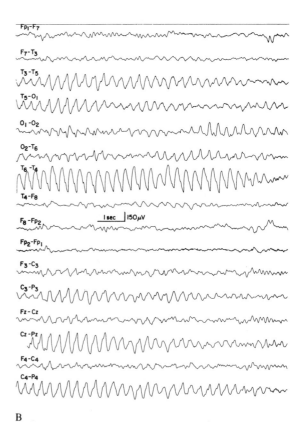

B

Figure 27.16. **A:** A burst of generalized synchronous 3 to 3.5/sec spike-wave complexes with typical frontal maximum, occurring in sleep with subsequent arousal. Note triple spike at the very onset of the burst. Age 17 years, history of petit mal absences and occasional grand mal. **B:** Petit mal absences in a 6-year-old patient. Prolonged runs of rhythmical posterior 2.5 to 3/sec with a spiky component.

The *sleep records* of patients with primary generalized epilepsy show frequent bursts of spikes, polyspikes, and spike waves (Fig. 27.17); this was first pointed out by Gibbs and Gibbs (1952) and subsequently stressed by Niedermeyer (1965, 1966a, 1972a, 1996a), who has placed particular emphasis on the conjunction with the K complex and the frontal midline maximum of the spike discharges. This maximum over the frontal midline is almost invariably present, not only in sleep but also in the waking state. This indicates that arousal plays an important role in the generation of these discharges; this mechanism is discussed in this chapter in the discussion of the basic mechanism. REM sleep is

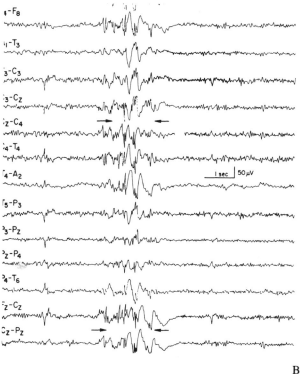

B

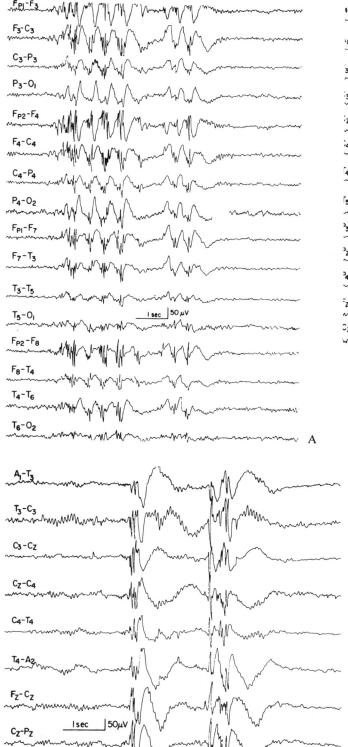

A

C

Figure 27.17. **A:** Spike-wave discharges with frequently intermixed polyspikes in a 30-year-old patient with unusually late onset of petit mal absences at age 18. Stage 2, non-rapid-eye-movement (REM) sleep. Marked frontal maximum. **B:** Same patient, stage 2, non-REM sleep. Transversal montages clearly demonstrate a voltage peak (based on phase reversal) of spike waves and polyspikes over frontal and central midline, but when F_z and C_z are run against each other (channels 15–16), it becomes clear that the frontal midline is the maximally involved area. **C:** Spikes and polyspikes riding on K complexes in stage 2, non-REM sleep in an 18-year-old patient. Well-defined maximum of spiking over frontal midline (F_z). (From Niedermeyer, E. 1979. Generalisierte Epilepsien. EEG Labor 1:119–131.)

associated with an attenuation or total suppression of bilateral synchronous paroxysmal bursts. In exceptional cases, the maximum of the 3/sec spike-wave bursts lies in the vertex region rather than in frontal midline; these children also show rolandic spikes (Niedermeyer, 1981). A stepwise differentiation of spike-wave complexes and their corresponding clinical correlates is presented in Table 27.10.

Etiology and Genetic Predisposition

Primary generalized epilepsy practically means absence of structural pathology. The cause, therefore, must be a dysfunction, which may be conceived of as biochemical and based on a genetic predisposition. Neurological deficits are incompatible with primary generalized epilepsy, but behavior disorder is quite common, especially in adolescents and young adults.

The EEG picture of primary generalized epilepsy with the impressive generalized synchronous 3 to 4/sec spike-wave paroxysms can be mimicked, however, by structural lesions. These lesions must be located in certain strategic areas in order to trigger these discharges. Even under such favorable circumstances, there is some reason to presume that generalized synchronous spike-wave bursts materialize only when a certain genetic predisposition is also present. This sounds very speculative and such a hypothesis is difficult to prove.

It has been noted that generalized synchronous seizure discharges, regardless of their wave morphology and thus comprising single spikes, polyspikes, and spike-wave complexes, may be found in patients with frontoparasagittal, mesiofrontal, and mesiotemporal lesions (Jasper, 1949; Jasper et al., 1951). Tükel and Jasper (1952) introduced the term *secondary bilateral synchrony.* More clinical observations were reported by Ajmone Marsan and Lewis (1960), Stewart and Dreifuss (1967), and Madsen and Bray (1966).

This mechanism is not convincingly demonstrable in the EEG, although Klass (1975) believes that a consistently preceding spike on one side provides evidence of secondary bilateral synchrony. More exceptional are cases with pathology around the third ventricle region involving hypothalamus and rostral mesencephalic portions, but not the thalamus. Tumors and other structural lesions in this area may give rise to 3 to 4/sec spike-wave bursts and clinical petit mal absences; diencephalic-endocrine disturbances are noted in such patients (Boudin et al., 1954; Hann, 1959; Niedermeyer, 1972a; Scherman and Abraham, 1963). According to Y. Mazars et al. (1966) and G. Mazars (1969, 1970), lesions of the cingulate gyrus and particularly within the anterior cingulate region may lead to generalized spike waves, atypical petit mal absences, and grand mal seizures. This concept of "cingulate epilepsy," however, has never been widely accepted.

Primary hypothalamic lesions giving rise to generalized synchronous 3/sec spike-wave complexes and clinical petit mal absences are very rare, but the possibility of a primary frontal lobe focus with secondary bilateral synchrony must be considered more seriously. In such cases, the EEG alone may not offer much help in the differentiation from true primary generalized epilepsy. Occasionally, bursts of spike waves are mixed with rhythmical generalized-synchronous spiking at a rate of about 10/sec; such intermingled brief stretches favor the diagnosis of a primary frontal focus with secondary generalization. More important is the age of onset; petit mal absences starting after age 10 and especially after age 15 are quite suggestive of primary frontal lobe epilepsy with secondary generalization. The same is true for petit mal absences of unusually long duration (more than 20 seconds). Furthermore, an immediate transition from a petit mal absence into a grand mal attack (a very rare event) is suggestive of frontal lobe epilepsy with secondary generalization. The precise mechanisms of secondary bilateral synchrony are poorly understood; one even wonders about an additional genetic predisposition to generalized spike-wave activity. Bilateral synchrony secondary to a frontal lobe focus may also occur in the Lennox-Gastaut syndrome, where it also poses a problem of differential diagnosis. Table 27.10 presents the steps to be taken in the differential diagnosis of spike-wave complexes.

In the presence of *metabolic disturbances,* generalized synchronous seizure discharges may also emerge. Acute withdrawal from barbiturates or similar sedatives may trigger bursts of generalized spikes and spike-wave–like discharges, along with clinical grand mal (Essig and Fraser, 1958; Wikler and Essig, 1970; Wulff, 1957). Renal encephalopathies are associated with marked EEG slowing (Cadilhac and Ribstein, 1961; Gloor et al., 1969; Hughes, 1980; Prill et al., 1969) and may occasionally show generalized synchronous spike-wave activity (Hughes, 1980; Niedermeyer, 1972a). In general, spike-wave formation in patients with metabolic problems lacks the precise rhythmicity found in primary generalized epilepsy with classical petit mal.

A decrease of *N*-acetyl aspartate has been found in the frontal region in patients with juvenile myoclonic epilepsy (Savic et al., 2000). It would be quite important to know if these changes are also found in other forms of primary generalized epilepsy.

Obviously, *genetic* factors are particularly important in the field of primary generalized epilepsy. In this domain, the work of Metrakos and Metrakos (1961) has caused many repercussions. This study includes systematic EEG studies in patients, siblings, and parents, and it was found that generalized synchronous seizure discharges follow an autosomal-dominant pattern of genetic transmission, with variable penetrance regardless of presence or absence of seizures. As Metrakos and Metrakos (1961) have pointed out, there is "the unusual characteristic of a very low penetrance at birth which rises to nearly complete penetrance (close to 50%) for ages 4.5 to 16.5 years" with a gradual decline to almost no penetrance at age 40. These figures are in excellent agreement with the incidence of generalized synchronous seizure discharges of the 3 to 4/sec spike-wave type as well as the clinical seizure manifestations of primary generalized epilepsy.

These results, however, did not find general acceptance. Matthes (1969) felt that his data suggest a recessive rather than a dominant genetic trait. It was also objected that Metrakos and Metrakos (1961) lumped together patients with classical, atypical, and perhaps marginal spike-wave complexes.

Doose et al. (1972) have placed great emphasis on the significance of "abnormal theta rhythm," which is also discussed in Chapter 11, "Maturation of the EEG: Development of Waking and Sleep Patterns," and Chapter 12, "Nonspecific Abnormal EEG Patterns." They presume that this rhythm ("rhythmical monomorphic" 4–7/sec activity of parietal accentuation in children from age 2 to 7) is most often found in the epilepsies of early childhood. Much of this work has been reviewed by Newmark and Penry (1980). In a multifactorial model of inheritance, the heritability of primary generalized epilepsy was found to be 62% with regard to seizures and 73% with regard to EEG abnormalities (E. Andermann, 1980).

All these considerations are quickly becoming obsolete in view of the demonstration of a genetic linkage between juvenile myoclonic epilepsy (Janz syndrome) and the small arm of chromosome 6 (Delgado-Escueta et al., 1989). This linkage could pertain to the entire domain of primary generalized epilepsy (also see under Etiologies in this chapter).

Neuropharmacological Considerations

Generalized spike-wave complexes are readily elicited by the intravenous administration of pentylenetetrazol (Metrazol) in epileptic as well as in nonepileptic individuals. These bursts become increasingly associated with myoclonic jerking; with continuing injection, a grand mal attack materializes (Cure et al., 1948; Kaufmann et al., 1947; Ziskind and Bercel, 1947). The threshold for convulsive phenomena is particularly low in patients with primary generalized epilepsy. Gastaut (1949) used combined pentylenetetrazol injection and presentation of flashes for the determination of the "photometrazolic threshold" for the elicitation of the first myoclonic jerk. The threshold was found to be very low in patients with primary generalized epilepsy and highest, surprisingly, in patients with focal epilepsies, with psychiatric patients and normal controls in second and third place, respectively. This test, however, has gradually fallen into disuse.

Ethyl-methyl-glutarimide (Megimide) was also used as an activating substance for convulsive activity (Delay et al., 1956). Adjmone Marsan and Ralston (1957) have studied the effect of intravenous pentylenetetrazol on a variety of epileptic seizures; they found that this substance quite readily triggered epileptic activity in the supplementary motor region eliciting clinical seizures that were often different from the spontaneous seizure type.

Lombroso and Erba (1970) used intravenous barbiturates as a test in order to distinguish patients with primary and secondary generalized epilepsy; after suppression of the generalized burst, a true epileptogenic focus was found to be demonstrable in the EEG. Waltrégny et al. (1969) used intracarotid sodium in patients with Lennox-Gastaut syndrome and provided evidence of a primary epileptogenic focus.

The internal carotid route was also used for pentylenetetrazol (Bennett, 1953; Gloor, 1968, 1969); injections into the vertebral artery were also carried out (Gloor, 1968, 1969). This work lent support for the theory of a cortical genesis of generalized synchronous seizure discharges. Deactivation with intravenous diazepam (Valium) was used on a larger scale by Niedermeyer (1970a) in patients with generalized synchronous or focal spikes in the EEG. Very small

dosages (2–5 mg) immediately blocked photoconvulsive responses and also generalized synchronous 3 to 4/sec spike-wave bursts for about 20 to 30 minutes; "benign" (rolandic) focal spikes in children showed a good response, but not as dramatic as flicker responses and spike-wave bursts. Inconsistent responses were found in the Lennox-Gastaut syndrome, and poor responses were found in epileptics with a chronic epileptogenic focus, such as temporal or frontal lobe epileptics.

Benzodiazepines might be an endogenous protective substance of the brain. The detection of benzodiazepine receptors (Squires and Braestrup, 1977; Squires et al., 1979) could be of particular importance in the pathogenesis of primary generalized epilepsy.

Special EEG Considerations: True Versus False Bilateral Synchrony and the Role of Ultraslow (DC) Potentials

Bilateral or generalized synchrony in bursts of spikes, spike waves, or polyspikes is more apparent than real. With the oscilloscopic technique, Cohn (1954) and Lueders et al. (1980) found remarkable asynchronies ranging from 5 to 20 msec. There was no consistency of the leading and following hemisphere, and constant shifts from side to side were the rule. With toposcopic technique, spike-wave discharges were found to be traveling waves with certain spatial characteristics (Petsche, 1962; Petsche and Marko, 1959; Petsche and Rappelsberger, 1970; Petsche and Sterc, 1968). Vertex and frontal region were most frequently involved as generators of spike-wave complexes.

Further fine details of generalized synchronous seizures discharges were revealed by the use of the difficult and delicate DC recording technique (Bates, 1963; Chatrian et al., 1968; Cohn 1954, 1964). There was evidence of a negative slow DC shift initiating every burst of generalized synchronous spike-wave complexes.

Experimental Studies and the Search for Animal Models of Primary Generalized Epilepsy

The historical aspects of basic studies of primary generalized epilepsy have been presented by Ajmone Marsan (1969), Niedermeyer (1972a), Myslobodsky (1976), and Gloor (1978, 1984). Penfield's (1938) concept of a centrencephalic system governing the function of consciousness was subsequently supported by the demonstration of thalamocortical connections. Slow electrical stimulation of the intralaminar thalamic nuclei gave rise to the "recruiting response" (Morison and Dempsey, 1942). This provided a certain basis for the followers of a deep pacemaker theory in the genesis of generalized synchronous seizure discharges. Spike-wave–like discharges of bilateral synchronous distribution were produced by slow electrical stimulation of the intralaminar thalamic nuclei in the cat (Jasper and Droogleever-Fortuyn, 1947; subsequently confirmed by Ingvar, 1955; Pollen et al., 1963). Guerrero-Figueroa et al. (1963) produced lesions with aluminum oxide in the brainstem of kittens and observed generalized spike waves without the use of electrical stimulation.

This work gave further support to the concept of a centrencephalic system, placing the emphasis on thalamic structures with diffuse cortical connections. This concept, however, was not generally accepted and other experimental work provided accumulating evidence of the leading role of the cortex (Marcus and Watson, 1968; Okuma et al., 1961; Pradhan and Ajmone Marsan, 1963; Starzl et al., 1953). Participation of deep structures in experimental electroconvulsions showed the rather minor role of the thalamic level (Jung, 1949), and propagation of seizure activity from deep primary foci in *Macaca mulatta* (Walker and Udvarhelyi, 1965) further de-emphasized the role of the thalamus as a pacemaker of epileptic generalization.

During the 1970s, two very important developments took place in this field. One major step was the discovery of photogenic epilepsy in the West African baboon, *Papio papio* (Bert and Naquet, 1970; Killam et al., 1966, 1967). Certain specimens of this species show a form of flicker sensitivity leading to myoclonus and short convulsions, but never to grand mal, which is to some degree comparable to the photosensitivity encountered in a sizable number of patients with primary generalized epilepsy. Bilateral synchronous seizure discharges are triggered mainly with a flash rate around 25/sec over the frontorolandic cortex, whereas spontaneous interictal paroxysmal bursts are common in sleep in particularly photosensitive animals; these discharges also show frontorolandic origin (Fischer-Williams et al., 1968; Menini, 1976; Menini et al., 1983; Naquet, 1973; Naquet et al., 1972). In summary, the work of Naquet and his co-workers has strongly emphasized the role of the frontorolandic cortex and minimized the contribution of the deep-seated pacemaker system. A remarkable feature of this work lies in the fact that the animal's seizure disorder is a naturally occurring disease. This seizure disorder is similar to human primary generalized epilepsy and yet shows marked dissimilarities in that there is no equivalent of petit mal absences, no well-formed spike-wave complexes, and different dynamics of evolution. The papionic seizure disorder does show a strong genetic factor (Naquet, 1975).

The feline model of PGE can be subdivided as follows: (a) thalamic electrical stimulation (Jasper and Droogleever-Fortuyn, 1947; Pollen et al., 1963), causing bisynchronous spike-wave–like activity elicited by stimuli; (b) arrest reaction (Hunter and Jasper, 1949), caused by stimulation of the mesial anterior thalamus (in unanesthetized cats but also in monkeys), which is similar to human petit mal absence but without spike waves; and (c) feline spike waves following intramuscular penicillin (Fisher and Prince, 1977; Prince and Farrell, 1969; subsequently used on a large scale by Gloor and co-workers; Gloor et al., 1977).

The method introduced by Prince and Farrell (1969) consists of intramuscular (i.m.) administration of penicillin in the cat (about 300,000–400,000 IU/kg). Generalized synchronous spike-wave–like bursts are subsequently triggered by the electrical stimulation of thalamic nuclei and parts of the putamen; it was found that the most effective areas were the same as those from which barbiturate spindles and "recruiting responses" (Morison and Dempsey, 1942; see above) could be elicited (Avoli and Gloor, 1981; Avoli et al., 1981; Gloor, 1978, 1984; Gloor et al., 1977; Kostopoulos and Gloor, 1982; Kostopoulos et al., 1982; Quesney et al., 1977; and the comprehensive work of Avoli et al., 1990).

After intramuscular administration of penicillin, cats show signs of flicker sensitivity, blocked or prevented by antidopaminergic agents such as apomorphine or haloperidol (Quesney, 1980). Fisher and Prince (1977a) provided evidence for the leading role of the cortex in the genesis of spike-wave discharges experimentally induced by intramuscular penicillin in the cat. Recordings from cortical neurons showed sequences of EPSP—inhibitory postsynaptic potential (IPSP) in the generation of the spike-wave rhythm (Fisher and Prince, 1977b). These conclusions may appear to be incongruent with the fact that penicillin suppresses inhibition and hence IPSP. This, however, might be true only for GABAergic inhibition, which is suppressed by penicillin, whereas non-GABAergic mechanisms of inhibition may escape the suppressing effect of penicillin.

The feline spike-wave bursts resemble human primary generalized epilepsy more closely than the *Papio papio* model of Naquet and his collaborators, but the fact remains that the model of Gloor's group has the disadvantage of being the mere product of experimentation.

A quite different animal model has been used by Fromm and his collaborators, who have studied the responses of the spinal trigeminal nucleus in the cat to the stimulation of excitatory and inhibitory corticofugal pathways (Faingold and Fromm, 1992; Fromm, 1974, 1986; Fromm and Kohli, 1972; Fromm et al., 1979). This work has resulted in the concept of petit mal absences as a dysfunction of cortical inhibitory pathways.

Rodent models of spike-wave discharges have also entered the scenery. There are two subtypes of models: (a) Wistar rats with spontaneous spike waves (at 6–7/sec), and (b) the "tottering mouse" with neurological signs developing in homozygotes (ataxia, episodes of tonic limb flexion, myoclonus). Spike-wave bursts are in the 6 to 7/sec range.

There has been during the 1990s and into the new millennium a swing toward the concept of generalized spike-wave activity being driven by the frontal lobe. This was shown in Sprague-Dawley rats under intravenous picrotoxin (Medvedev et al., 1996) and also in spontaneous absence seizures of inbred WAG/Rij rats (Meeren, 2002; Meeren et al., 2002). These similarities to the mechanisms proposed in human PGE by the writer of these lines are evidently greater than expected.

The potential fallacies found in all forms of PGE animal models are manifold (see Niedermeyer, 1996a). There is no doubt that human PGE is fundamentally different from all animal models; a more profound understanding can be derived only from the investigation of the human disorder (Niedermeyer, 1996a).

Primary generalized epilepsy is indeed a disorder of *Homo sapiens* with specific dynamics of evolution such as age determination and important relationships to factors such as flickering light, hyperventilation, sleep, and arousing stimuli. Gloor (1984) has cautiously discussed the relevance of experimental studies of the spike-wave discharge in his feline penicillin epilepsy model to primary generalized epilepsy in the human. A possible stumbling block in such inferences on human generalized epilepsy is the dual meaning of the term *spindles*; the spontaneously occurring spindle runs in the human must be carefully distinguished from barbiturate spindles (mostly elicited by thiopental) in the animal experiment (also see Jankel and Niedermeyer, 1985).

Observations in Patients with Implanted Depth Electrodes

Depth EEG studies in patients with petit mal absences have remained somewhat inconclusive. Williams (1953) presumed that the slow component of the spike-wave complex was of thalamic origin, whereas the spike component originates in the cortex. Primary cortical involvement in these discharges was stressed by Hayne et al. (1949), Bickford (1956), Bancaud et al. (1965), and Bancaud (1972). I strongly believe in the primordial role of the frontal cortex. Angeleri et al. (1964) and Rossi et al. (1967) were impressed with the significant role of limbic structures in the genesis of generalized synchronous spike waves. Walker and Marshall (1964) assumed that both cortical and deep foci could give rise to generalized discharges. The leading role of thalamic and mesencephalic structures was emphasized by Wilson and Nashold (1968). Blumenfeld (2002) has reemphasized the role of the thalamus in absence seizures with 3/sec spike waves.

It has been pointed out previously (Niedermeyer, 1972a; Niedermeyer et al., 1969) that the insertion of depth leads into the brain of chronic epileptic patients is unlikely to yield precise information on origin and propagation of the seizure discharges in primary generalized epilepsies. Occasionally, a frontal primary focus with strong secondary bilateral synchrony may be demonstrable, and subsequent partial frontal lobectomy may be quite effective (Niedermeyer, 1972a). In general, however, there are too many pitfalls in the depth EEG technique in the human, such as missing crucial areas by a short distance and recording discharges of rather secondary character; patients with typical primary generalized epilepsy are usually not suitable candidates for depth implants because of the predominantly benign character of their seizure disorder. Interestingly, thalamic atrophy may occur in temporal lobe epilepsy, but not in PGE (on the basis of MRI volumetry evidence) (Natsume et al., 2003).

Role of Sleep and Arousal

It was mentioned before under primary generalized epilepsy and EEG that bilateral synchronous spikes, polyspikes, and spike-wave complexes are usually enhanced in light non-REM sleep (mainly stage 2) and that these bursts are found in conjunction with K complexes. The role of arousal in these patients has been pointed out in detail by Niedermeyer (1966a, 1970b, 1972a, 1982, 1984, 1996a), who introduced the term *dyshormia*, which means faulty or deviant arousal. It has been felt that arousing stimuli generate K complexes contaminated with spikes. These K complexes are maximal over the frontal midline (F_z electrode) and thus differ from the vast majority of K complexes with a vertex (C_z) maximum (Fig. 27.17). A schematic view is shown in Figure 27.18. These data and the resulting concept have been confirmed by the work of Halász and his coworkers (Halász, 1972, 1981, 1984; Halász and Devényi, 1974; Nowack, 1996; Sato et al., 1973). Nocturnal (all night) sleep recordings also demonstrate an increase of generalized paroxysmal discharges in light non-REM sleep (Passouant and Cadilhac, 1970; Tomka, 1983).

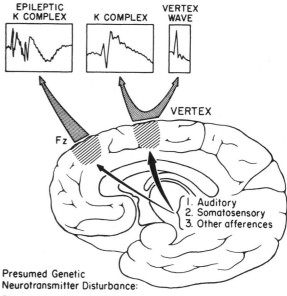

PRESUMED MECHANISMS IN PRIMARY GENERALIZED EPILEPSY

Figure 27.18. Schematic view of the paroxysmal arousal response over frontal midline and the physiological arousal responses in sleep over vertex (K complex, vertex waves). Individual predisposition for paroxysmal responses might be based on a local biochemical defect. (From Niedermeyer, E. 1979. Generalisierte Epilepsien. EEG Labor 1:119–131.)

The frontal midline location indicates involvement of the supplementary motor region in the interhemispheric fissure, where apparently numerous arousing stimuli generate compounded evoked potentials, suppressed in waking state and REM sleep but very prominent in non-REM sleep. Much less potential epileptogenicity is noted in the more common K complexes recorded over the posterior portion of the frontal supplementary motor cortex by means of the vertex electrode. Cirignotta et al. (1982) noted inhibition of muscle tone during generalized bursts of spikes in the sleep records of patients with generalized epilepsy. The EMG was recorded from the mylohyoid muscle. During the loss of tone, the H reflex was also inhibited.

Arousing stimuli may also play a major role in spike-wave bursts occurring in the waking state, although K complexes are naturally undetectable in this stage, with rare exceptions. The aforementioned negative DC shifts (Bates, 1963; Chatrian et al., 1968; Cohn, 1954, 1964; Pagniez et al., 1938) preceding the generalized synchronous spike-wave bursts signal arousal (Caspers and Speckmann, 1970) and suggest an increment of afferent specific and nonspecific inflow from the thalamus to the cortex; this is thought to be associated with increasing neuronal depolarization (Caspers, 1963; Caspers and Speckmann, 1969, 1970; O'Leary and Goldring, 1964).

It has also been shown that a very brief period of arousal precedes petit mal absences in the waking patient; this is naturally not demonstrable in the EEG (no K complexes) but

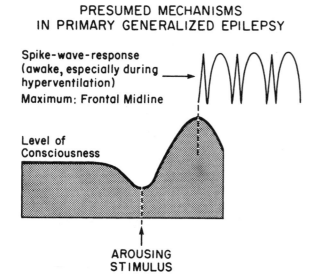

PRESUMED MECHANISMS IN PRIMARY GENERALIZED EPILEPSY

Spike-wave-response
(awake, especially during
hyperventilation)
Maximum: Frontal Midline

Level of
Consciousness

AROUSING
STIMULUS

Figure 27.19. Schematic view of the role of fluctuations of the level of awareness (a short drowsy period with subsequent arousal) as a triggering mechanism in primary generalized epilepsy.

by determination of the audiomotor reaction time, which is shortened immediately before the absence (Lehmann, 1963). This arousal is probably preceded by a brief period of slackened awareness (Fig. 27.19).

During hyperventilation, the delta slowing may be associated with reduced vigilance (Epstein et al., 1994). Lum et al. (2002) have shown distinctive features of hyperventilation-delta drowsiness and spike-wave absence. This sequence of events fits readily into the aforementioned drowsiness-arousal concept, especially when an arousing task is presented to the hyperventilating patient (Niedermeyer and Vaughan-Matthews, 1992).

What causes the paroxysmal type of arousal response that immediately sets off an avalanche of generalized synchronous discharges? One could speculate that genetic predisposition impinges on protective benzodiazepine receptors, possibly resulting in defective receptors (see Squires et al., 1979). Still missing is the demonstration of particularly abundant benzodiazepine receptors in the interhemispheric portion of the frontal lobe in healthy individuals.

Massive arousal leading to immediate awakening usually does not produce epileptic K complexes; more subtle arousing stimuli are more effective. This is comprehensible in the light of experimental data on arousal and DC potentials (Speckmann, personal communication). The investigation of metabolic correlates of the 3/sec spike-wave discharge with the use of PET and ^{18}F-fluorodeoxyglucose did not reveal a specific site of seizure generation (Engel et al., 1982).

The *age factor* ties into these considerations. The sharp component of the K complex is particularly prominent after the age of 4 years and starts to decline during the second decade. Such naturally sharp K complexes apparently facilitate paroxysmal responses. This would parallel the course of primary generalized epilepsy, especially those cases with petit mal absences as the initial seizure manifestation. On the other

hand, course and prognosis of petit mal absences are not quite as benign as one used to assume; this has been pointed out by Lugaresi et al. (1973). In some patients, absences persist into adulthood and even into old age (Gastaut et al., 1986). A careful analysis of lifestyle and habits of such patients shows that their length of nocturnal sleep is well below the required mark (see case reported by Ghigo and Niedermeyer, 2000).

Figure 27.20 schematically demonstrates the plight of an adolescent or young adult with PGE after a night of poor or insufficient sleep. My numerous personal observations have shown the gradual escalation from paroxysmal spike bursts to myoclonus and, in some cases, even to grand mal (Niedermeyer, 1996a).

Spike-Wave Bursts and Sleep Spindles

It has been demonstrated that, in childhood absence epilepsy (and thus in PGE), generalized epileptiform discharges occur when spindles are present (Nobili et al., 2001). Both spindles and K complexes occur in non-REM sleep, mainly in stage 2, but a direct relationship exists between paroxysmal bursts and K complexes (rather than spindles).

Nevertheless, the association of spike bursts and spindles is still being proposed, even in human epileptology (Kellaway et al., 1990). The fact is that arousal in its light forms is the principal generator of spike/spike-wave bursts in PGE, best seen in non-REM sleep or in postsleep drowsiness. Sleep spindles do not have an arousing function and might promote preservation of sleep (Jankel and Niedermeyer, 1985). As it was pointed out earlier, K complexes consist of a sharp, a slow, and a fast component, the latter being identical with superimposed spindles, probably counteracting the arousal effect of the first component. Automatic frequency analysis may pick up the spindle activity in connection with the spike burst—in truth, however, at the tail end of the K complex, i.e., after the spike burst.

Experimental work in animals by Gloor and his co-workers has shown relationships between spindles and spikes (Avoli et al., 1983; Gloor et al., 1990; Kostopoulos et al., 1981; and, above all, the very thoughtful analysis of Kostopoulos, 2000). Human PGE, however, is a unique disorder and EEG investigations with sleep section in these patients will always corroborate the role of arousal with K complexes as the primary force in PGE.

A relationship between generalized-synchronous spike-wave bursts and sleep spindles in patients with generalized epilepsies has been investigated by Kellaway et al. (1990). This may sound to be akin to the aforementioned dyshormia concept, even though sleep spindles are not limited to arousal mechanisms and may also promote preservation of sleep (Jankel and Niedermeyer, 1985). The emphasis on the conjunction of spindles and spike-wave bursts appears to be bolstered by the experimental work of Gloor and his co-workers (Avoli et al., 1983; Gloor et al., 1990; Kostopoulos et al., 1981). With the use of intracellular recording, Steriade (1990) has further endorsed the relationship of spindles and spike-wave discharges (see Chapter 3, "Cellular Substrates of Brain Rhythms").

In human generalized epilepsies with spike-wave bursts, there is little doubt that arousal responses are the prime mover of generalized spikes and spike waves. These

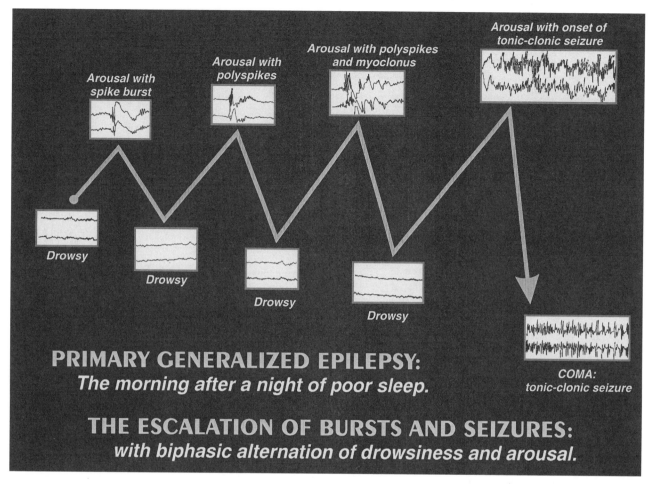

Figure 27.20. The morning after a night of poor sleep in a patient with primary generalized epilepsy (PGE). In reality, the sequence of dozing off and subsequent spike-producing arousal repeats itself more frequently and may go on for 20 to 30 minutes or longer. A full-blown generalized tonic-clonic seizure may never materialize but myoclonus (or absence) are quite common. (Reprinted with permission of Clin. Electroencephalography.)

discharges are certainly by far more likely to be associated with K complexes rather than with spindles. Automatic frequency analysis of such tracings naturally will pick up the spindle frequencies (12–14/sec), which are consistently found in almost every trailing slow wave of a K complex.

Role of Photosensitivity

The dyshormia mechanism of abnormal paroxysmal arousal responses does not pertain to all cases of primary generalized epilepsy. Photosensitivity is another important mechanism and, in some cases, is the predominant or sole demonstrable mechanism of paroxysmal precipitation (Fig. 27.21).

Both mechanisms are often present in the same patient. Patients with photosensitivity only are more likely to suffer from grand mal and myoclonus, with petit mal absences playing a minor role. Spike-wave discharges chiefly show 4 to 5/sec frequencies with a frontal midline maximum. Hyperventilation does not enhance this activity and sleep records may be entirely normal (Fig. 27.22).

These patients show strong photoconvulsive responses to photic stimulation (see Chapter 15, "Brain Tumors and Other Space-Occupying Lesions"), often with concomitant myoclonus. The age factor is not quite as important; grand mal seizures may linger on through adulthood and are not easily suppressed by medication. The genetic factor is potent and, according to Doose et al. (1969), there is, from the genetic viewpoint, good evidence of a special epileptological entity. The genetic factors have been further investigated by Hauser et al. (1983). It was found that siblings of patients with generalized spike-wave patterns were apt to exhibit photoconvulsive responses in a large percentage. Extensive studies and review of the literature on photosensitivity have been carried out by Rabending and Klepel (1978) and Newmark and Penry (1979).

Since that time, a new wave of clinical-electrical research has considerably deepened our understanding of epileptic photosensitivity thus widening the spectrum of its clinical and its EEG accompaniment. Eyelid myoclonia with absences is known since the work of Jeavons (1977), who has further reviewed this topic (Jeavons, 1996); this phenome-

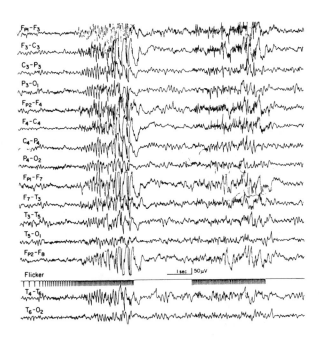

Figure 27.21. A prominent photoconvulsive flicker response in a 16-year-old patient (occasional grand mal since age 14; brother also suffers from grand mal seizures). Bursts of spikes with anterior maximum starts when the flicker frequency rises to about 18/sec. (From Niedermeyer, E. 1979. Generalisierte Epilepsien. EEG Labor 1:119–131.)

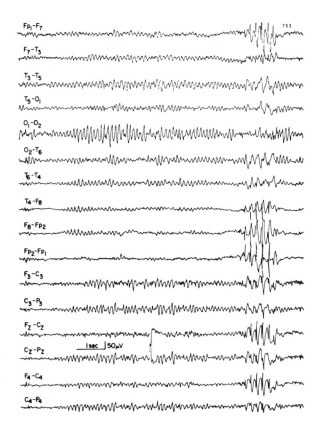

Figure 27.22. A brief burst of bilateral synchronous 4/sec spike-waves (resting awake) in a 57-year-old patient who experienced myoclonic jerking at age 16 to 18 years and a total of six grand mal attacks between ages 31 and 50.

non is often associated with fairly widespread myoclonus. Spikes, polyspikes, and spike-wave–like discharges are generalized with prominent frontal maximum. Eyelid fluttering appears to be a mild form of myoclonia.

The work of Panayiotopoulos and his co-workers is particularly linked with these studies (Panayiotopoulos et al., 1996). These absence-like seizures are most common in childhood and adolescence but may persist into adult life (Giannakodimos and Panayiotopoulos, 1996).

This form with its minor clinical variants is essentially responsive to valproate like most of the manifestations of PGE.

Presence of Focal Spikes in Patients with Primary Generalized Epilepsy

A certain type of focal spikes in childhood ("benign rolandic spikes") may be present occasionally in children who suffer from petit mal absences, especially after suppression of the absences and the spike waves with medication. One cannot construe a case of "secondary bilateral synchrony" in such children. The central spikes may denote nothing but a temporary paroxysmal irritability of the motor cortex extending into the midtemporal region.

This view would shed more light on the demonstration of genetic factors in children with midtemporal spikes (Bray and Wiser, 1965). On the other hand, a strict boundary lies between true focal epilepsies and primary generalized epilepsy in spite of occasional "gray zones" and occasional cases of "crossover" (Nogueira de Melo and Niedermeyer, 1991b). The reader will find more information in the section on benign rolandic epilepsy.

Concluding Remarks

The challenging problem of primary generalized epilepsy remains unsolved. Genetic predisposition and age (chiefly 4–20 years) are significant factors.

Clinical genetics have raised the problem of "splitting versus lumping" the subforms of primary generalized epilepsy (Schmitz et al., 2000). Many genetic data favor the splitter's attitude—clinical (and also EEG) manifestations are conducive to "lumping" and thus preserving the unity of PGE.

It is a specifically human disorder; for this reason, animal models can provide only partial insight into pathogenetic mechanisms. In the human, the generalized synchronous seizure discharge originates from the interhemispheric frontal portion bilaterally. Arousing stimuli play a crucial role in the detonation of these discharges. In some patients, however, the mechanism of photosensitivity is paramount (Fig. 27.23).

Benign Rolandic Epilepsy

In children with spikes over the central region and/or adjacent midtemporal and parietal areas, a benign and readily controllable type of epileptic seizure disorder with focal motor seizures and/or grand mal is the rule. An increasing number of reports over the past 20 years give testimony to growing awareness of this special form of childhood epilepsy. Earlier

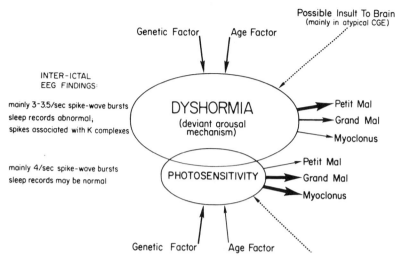

PRESUMED PHYSIOPATHOGENETIC MECHANISMS
IN COMMON GENERALIZED EPILEPSY

Figure 27.23. Presumed physiopathogenetic mechanisms involved in primary generalized epilepsy. The dyshormic and the photosensitive subgroups show considerable overlap. Note the greater significance of the age factor in the dyshormic group; also note differences of spike-wave frequencies and types of seizures. CGE, common generalized epilepsy.

observations of Y. Gastaut (1952), Hess (1958), Nayrac and Beaussart (1958), Isler and Hess (1960), and Gibbs and Gibbs (1964) have set the stage for more recent work in this field (Beaumanoir et al., 1974; Beaussart, 1972; Blom and Brorson, 1966; Blom and Hejbel, 1982; Dalla Bernardina and Beghini, 1976; Hejbel et al., 1975; Lairy and Harrison, 1968; Lombroso, 1967; Loiseau and Beaussart, 1973; Niedermeyer, 1970b, 1972b, 1974). This work has outlined the characteristics of benign rolandic epilepsy, as this condition has been termed over the past few years.

Beaumanoir (1976) has listed this form of childhood epilepsy among the primary generalized epilepsies despite its prominent focal features in the ictal and EEG semiology. Such a classification certainly appears to be provocative. There are indeed certain relationships between benign rolandic epilepsy and primary generalized epilepsies, and conversion from one form to the other may occur (Gastaut, 1982a; Loiseau et al., 1983; Niedermeyer, 1981; Nogueira de Melo and Niedermeyer, 1991b). There is certainly good reason to separate benign rolandic epilepsies from the bulk of focal (partial) epileptic seizure disorders, which will be presented somewhat later. In this section, we also discuss benign seizure disorders in children with spikes outside the rolandic region.

Age and Prevalence

Benign rolandic epilepsy occurs at age 3 to 12 years. The majority of these children are from 6 to 10 years old. Disappearance of the seizures during adolescence or even prior to puberty is the rule. The seizures may occasionally recur much later in life, probably due to seizure-facilitating factors such as severe illness or toxic-metabolic factors.

The sex distribution shows that boys are more often affected. The prevalence is not quite clear and might be somewhere between 5% and 10% in a population of epileptics below age 15. Beaumanoir (1976) goes even further; she

feels that the prevalence of benign rolandic epilepsy exceeds that of petit mal absences and reaches 14% to 15% of all childhood epilepsy cases.

Ictal Manifestations

The seizures, regardless of focal or grand mal character, tend to occur during nocturnal sleep (Loiseau and Beaussart, 1973), mostly during the last hour of sleep or in the first 2 hours. About 80% of the attacks occur in sleep; of the remaining 20%, about 10% take place shortly after awakening. (Note the similarities with primary generalized epilepsy.) Nocturnal seizures may awaken the child afterward.

Preservation of consciousness and hence the ability to describe the experienced seizure was found in 58% (Loiseau and Beaussart, 1973); this indicates the predominance of focal seizures. Grand mal (tonic-clonic) seizures were noted in 26% (Loiseau and Beaussart, 1973).

The seizures are hardly ever seen by the physician, even by the epileptologist who sees sizable numbers of these children (Aicardi et al., 1969; Blom et al., 1972; Loiseau and Beaussart, 1973). One therefore depends heavily on descriptions by the patient or the patient's family; nocturnal videotape or biotelemetry recordings are quite helpful.

Focal seizures often involve the face. The midtemporal spike localization has been thought to be related to paroxysmal activity in the very closely located lower portion of the motor strip (faciolaryngopharyngeal muscles); this has been stressed by Lombroso (1967), who uses the term Sylvian seizures. Hemifacial twitching is definitely more common than clonic motions in the contralateral arm; least common is clonic activity in the leg. In some cases, the entire half of the body participates, but a typical jacksonian march does not seem to occur. Speech arrest is quite common (39% of the seizures; Loiseau and Beaussart, 1973). This is apparently an ictal anarthria with preserved internal speech.

Oropharyngeal involvement is very often reported (53%, Loiseau and Beaussart, 1973), with sounds described as "guttural," "gargling," "throaty," "wheezing," or "as if going to vomit." The feeling of suffocation is reported as coming from the mouth but not from the chest.

These patients also have focal seizures that are not rolandic, with blindness, vertigo, and torsion of the body as ictal signs. This underscores the complexity of the underlying neurophysiological mechanisms.

EEG

Spiking over the central-midtemporal area in children is of limited epileptogenicity. It is reasonable to presume that 50% to 70% of these children have seizures and the remaining 30% to

50% are seizure-free. These latter patients are referred to the EEG laboratory because of a variety of symptoms such as behavior disorder, headaches, and other complaints or deviations.

The spatial distribution of the spike activity requires an appropriate number of electrodes; the International Electrode System is particularly suitable. Otherwise, the rolandic cortex may lie between a frontal and a parietal electrode, and strictly local spiking may escape detection, especially when the midtemporal region is not explored ideally. In my personal experience, a central maximum of spike discharge is slightly more often noted than a midtemporal maximum.

The spikes themselves are large and may be either spikes in the strict sense or sharp waves (see Chapter 13, "Abnormal EEG Patterns: Epileptic and Paroxysmal") (Fig. 27.24).

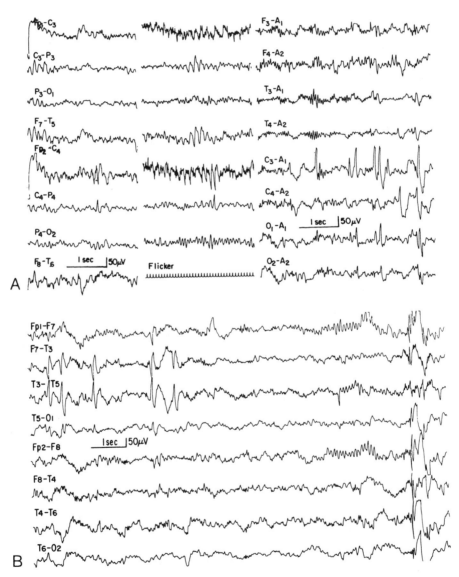

Figure 27.24. A: *Left,* a few suggestions of right central spikes in a 9-year-old boy. *Center,* some activity over right central area during flicker (same patient). *Right,* marked spikes and sharp waves over central regions, especially on the left, during non-REM sleep (same patient). (From Niedermeyer, E., and Koshino, Y. 1975. My-Rhythmus: Vorkommen und klinische Bedeutung. EEG-EMG 6:69–78.) **B:** Sleep tracing in a 7-year-old boy with grand mal attacks since age 3. Postictally, the patient was temporarily aphasic and hemiparetic on the right side. Note left midtemporal spikes and a burst of generalized spikes mixed with slow activity.

Central spiking with dipole formation has been reported by Gregory and Wong (1984, 1992). As a matter of fact, Gregory and Wong (1992) have stressed the clinical relevance of presence or absence of dipole fields in children with epileptic seizure disorder and rolandic spikes. According to their data, the presence of dipole discharges (usually located over frontal or temporal regions) is associated with a benign functional rolandic focus with little or no clinical problems, whereas absence of a dipole discharge is more likely to be found in children with neurological and behavioral abnormalities. In my personal opinion, however, the differential diagnosis of benign rolandic epilepsy should not hinge on central spikes of dipole or nondipole type.

In the course of the 1990s, presence and orientation of dipoles of rolandic spikes have become a widely debated issue. According to Wong (1993), the dipole-dependent topography of rolandic spikes "contains information on the behavior or functional state of brain tissue even distant to the brain region responsible for the spike generation." Van der Meij et al. (1992) feel that sequential mapping can differentiate between epileptic and nonepileptic rolandic spikes. Classically, rolandic spikes considered pathognomonic for benign rolandic epilepsy show dipole configurations with the negative pole over the central (centrotemporal) region and a positive pole over the frontal region (Baumgartner et al., 1996; Lüders et al., 1987). Typical spikes indicating benign rolandic seizure disorder start with a spike of centroparietal negativity and superior frontal negativity, changing within 12 msec to sole central negativity and after further 16 msec to a dipole of central negativity and frontomedian positivity (Van der Meij et al., 1992). Similar findings were observed with visual analysis during ictal manifestations of benign rolandic epilepsy (Gutierrez et al., 1990). According to Legarda and Jayakar (1995), the dipolar distribution of rolandic spikes was not found to be a reliable indicator of potential epileptogenicity.

Yoshinaga et al. (1992) have given strong support to the importance of dipole tracing in benign rolandic and other types of childhood epilepsies. Confusing elements in the assessment of rolandic spikes and their dipoles may arise from the assumption of a single dipole—a concept presently widely supplanted by the concept of multiple sources and extended source geometry (Baumgartner et al., 1996; Gregory and Wong, 1992). It has to be added that every investigator of the cerebral dipole problem has to take into account the stringent limitations of dipole theory (Niedermeyer, 1996b).

Spiking is usually enhanced in light non-REM sleep, during which the discharges may become extremely abundant. Their random character may give way to quasirhythmic or periodic spiking at intervals of less than 1 second; previously unilateral spikes become bilateral synchronous or asynchronous (Beaumanoir, 1976). In many children, rolandic spikes are found in the sleep portion only. According to Beaumanoir (1976), REM sleep restores the unilateral character of the spiking. Beaumanoir (1976) also described the occurrence of bilateral parieto-occipital 4/sec spike-wave-like discharges of moderate voltage seen in the waking patient (Fig. 27.25).

In some patients, interictal rolandic spikes can be blocked with contralateral finger or hand movements (Niedermeyer, 1970), either actively or passively (in sleep) performed. The reactivity of rolandic spikes was studied by Fonseca et al. (1996), who noted a strong spike blocking response tongue movements inside or outside the mouth. On the other hand, Nadkarni et al. (1994) reported a child with centro-midtemporal spikes that could be triggered by blinking.

The rest of the tracing is usually normal in these patients, and the frequency spectrum corresponds to age. Central mu rhythm is sometimes present (Beaumanoir, 1976; Niedermeyer, 1972b), and there is reason to presume that central spikes of childhood may be gradually replaced by mu rhythm, at least in some of the patients (Fig. 27.26). There is indubitable evidence that, in a limited number of patients, the central spike activity can be blocked by contralateral fist

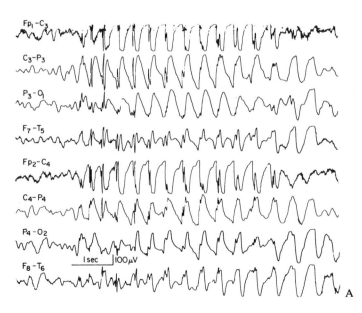

Figure 27.25. **A:** A 5-year-old patient with recent onset of petit mal absences. The recorded generalized spike-wave burst was subclinical. *(Figure continues.)*

Figure 27.25. *(Continued)* **B:** The same patient at age 8 years. There are numerous independent spikes over left central and right centroparietal regions. This case is a typical example of crossover between primary generalized epilepsy and benign rolandic epilepsy.

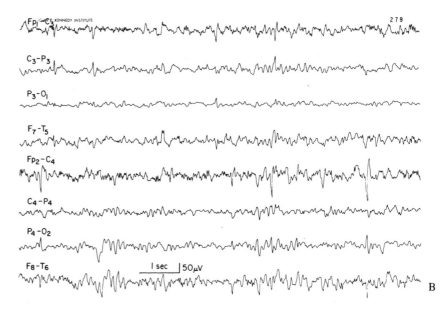

clenching or, even better, by alternate clenching and opening of the fist (Niedermeyer, 1972a,b). This provides further evidence for the functional character of the spikes (Fig. 27.27).

Mitsudome et al. (1997) have pointed out that, in benign rolandic epilepsy, central spikes may be associated with local slowing. Both rolandic spikes and local slowing were found to respond to clonazepam.

In a small number of cases, the spike activity shows a consistent maximum over the vertex (Nelson et al., 1984; Pedley et al., 1980; Pourmand et al., 1984) or over the centroparietal midline region, which may be the sole region of spiking, so that omission of midline leads would result in missing the abnormality (Ehle, 1980). Some of these patients show focal motor or sensory ictal activity of leg predominance; more often, the ictal symptoms do not correspond with the spike localization. Even the parietal midline may be strongly involved in the spike activity (Pourmand et al., 1984).

Clinical Signs of Nonictal Character

One must agree with Beaumanoir (1976) when she points out that neurological deficits are not compatible with benign rolandic epilepsy. This condition is based on dysfunction rather than structural pathology. It is worthwhile, however, to search carefully for a true intracranial lesion. Arteriovenous malformation occasionally may be the cause of discharges and associated seizure.

Central, midtemporal, or parietal spikes or spikes over the midline may also occur in children with evidence of cerebral palsy, in mostly diplegic, quadriplegic, or choreoathetoid forms. In these children, rolandic spikes have a different connotation and do not herald a good prognosis for the seizure disorder. The reader will find more extensive discussion in the section on cerebral palsy.

Behavior disorders are very common in children with true rolandic spikes; they may range from hyperkinetic behavior and signs of minimal cerebral dysfunction to severe

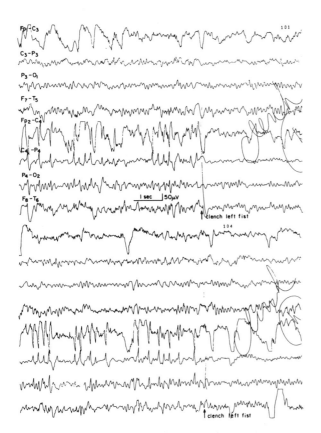

Figure 27.26. A 14-year-old patient with severe personality disorder but no history of epileptic seizures. The *lower portion* was recorded with identical montage, sensitivity, and paper speed. Note abundance of right central spikes and excellent blocking response to contralateral movement (clenching left fist).

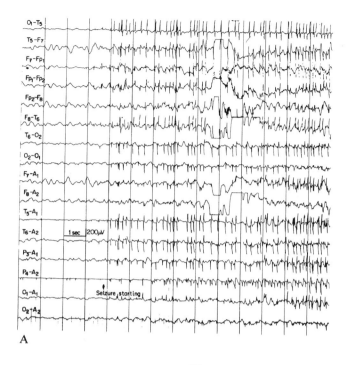

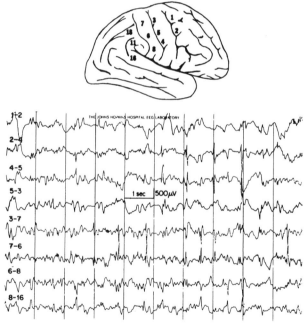

Figure 27.27. **A:** An 8-year-old boy with epilepsia partialis continua or focal motor status (clonic motions, left arm). The EEG shows considerable slowing (note lowered gain). There is evidence of constant muscle activity, but no authentic cerebral spikes are demonstrable. **B:** Same patient. Electrocorticography. In general anesthesia, suppression of focal motor attacks but prominent spiking, especially in leads 4 (precentral gyrus) and 7 (postcentral gyrus).

anxiety neurosis. Various types of headaches may occur; see the symptom profile of Gibbs and Gibbs (1964), who, however, lump together the pure form with cases of cerebral palsy and other organic brain damage. The intelligence is normal in true benign rolandic epilepsy.

Course

The seizures are easily controlled with routine anticonvulsive treatment; hydantoins are preferable over phenobarbital, which often enhances irritability in children. Treatment may even be withheld unless seizures repeat themselves (Beaumanoir, 1976).

Freedom from seizures in adolescence is the rule. The return of a single major convulsion may occasionally occur under the influence of infections, stress, or toxic substances. These cases show no resurgence of the central spike focus, which renders the EEG diagnosis very difficult. The presence of central mu rhythm may serve as a hint that the patient has had central spikes in the past, but such conclusions can be made only with reservations.

Etiological Considerations

This form of epilepsy is due to dysfunction rather than to pathology. A genetic basis is the most logical thought. The work of Bray and Wiser (1965) on familial occurrence of midtemporal spikes has pioneered in this area, and other studies will certainly follow suit. The work of Doose et al. (1977) has further substantiated the significance of genetic factors. A positive family history of epilepsy was reported in 11.3% of 80 children with benign rolandic epilepsy (Gereby, 1985). Gelisse et al. (2003) have pointed out that benign rolandic epilepsy can also affect children with static brain lesions, which, however, have no influences on the benign course. These authors feel that neuroimaging procedures are usually unnecessary in children with benign rolandic epilepsy.

Problems of Differential Diagnosis

Children with benign rolandic epilepsy must be differentiated from the following groups:

1. Children with rolandic spikes and no seizures whatsoever (these children are certainly not epileptics; about 30% to 50% of the children with rolandic spikes have no overt clinical seizures; also see Lerman and Kivity-Ephraim, 1981);
2. Children with rolandic spikes and a history of antecedent brain damage or cerebral palsy (see above);
3. Children who have typical psychomotor seizures and evidence of temporal lobe epilepsy that may gradually progress in severity; these children may have atypical spike localization (central, midtemporal), whereas the classical anterotemporal sharp wave focus does not materialize before adolescence (see below);
4. Children with midtemporal spikes, marked tendency to generalization of spike-wave formation, clinically with aphasia (Landau-Kleffner syndrome, see below);
5. Children with frequent focal motor seizures that become progressively worse: "malignant" rolandic epilepsy of childhood (see below); and

6. Children with centroparietal spikes elicited by tactile stimulation of corresponding cutaneous areas of the body (see under benign parietal epilepsy).

The differentiation of these conditions rests on a careful combined clinical-electroencephalographic assessment of each case.

Spike Foci Outside the Rolandic Region in Children

Occipital spike foci are usually found between the ages of 2 and 5 years. These children show no neurological or ophthalmological deficit; about 40% of them have clinical seizures, mostly grand mal, with good prognosis.

According to Gibbs and Gibbs (1964), frontal spike foci in children are associated with epileptogenicity, with about 80% having overt seizures, and a guarded prognosis. Multiple spike foci (two or more areas of independent spiking) are also highly epileptogenic; the prognosis is guarded and probably fairly good if rolandic spikes predominate.

A theory of spike migration of childhood from occipital to midtemporal and then to conversion into 14 and 6/sec positive spikes, with good prognosis, or anterior temporal spike activity, with poor prognosis, was advanced by Gibbs (1958) but has found little acceptance (see Isler and Hess, 1960). "Focus-migration" must be understood strictly in terms of dysfunction-induced epileptogenesis, which may undergo changes of spatial origin and distribution. A structurally determined epileptogenic focus is unlikely to display any wanderlust. Andermann and Oguni (1991) and Blume (1991) have discussed the pros and cons of the focus migra-

tion theory; both authors have cautioned against the facile use of this term.

Considerations of Basic Mechanisms

True benign rolandic epilepsy is likely to be based on temporary paroxysmal hyperirritability of the motor cortex, which naturally has a lower threshold of epileptic excitability. This is merely a working hypothesis in need of further substantiating evidence.

"Malignant" Rolandic Epilepsy: Rasmussen Encephalitis and Other Causes

Cases of progressively worsening focal motor seizures and prolonged episodes of epilepsia partialis continua (Kozhevnikov syndrome) are quite rare but probably constitute a special epileptological entity (Niedermeyer and Rocca, 1980; Niedermeyer et al., 1977c; Rocca and Niedermeyer, 1982). Motor deficits and mental decline are associated with the seizure disorder (Figs. 27.28 and 27.29).

Their etiology is poorly defined; chronic localized encephalitis may be one of the causes (Andrews et al., 1997; Aguilar and Rasmussen, 1960; Rasmussen et al., 1958). Hemispherectomy seems to be the only effective treatment; limited cortical excisions or lobectomies are ineffective (Fig. 27.29).

The EEG shows endless sequences of ictal spike discharges during focal motor attacks but becomes uninformative in states of epilepsia partialis continua, which probably originate from deep structures or possibly from lamina V of the motor cortex without participation of the superficial lay-

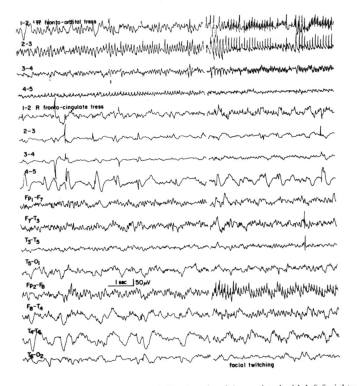
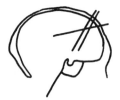

Figure 27.28. Ictal spiking in right frontal leads (depth and scalp) associated with left facial twitching in an 8-year-old boy with chronic encephalitis, not relieved by right frontal lobectomy. Much improved after right hemispherectomy at age 15.

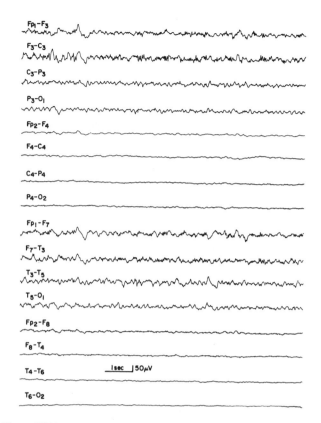

Figure 27.29. Same patient as in Figure 27.28 after right hemispherectomy. Note almost complete loss of activities on the right.

ers, as one is tempted to infer from the experimental work of Elger and Speckman (1979, 1980, 1983). A variant of Rasmussen chronic encephalitis with progressive relentless focal seizures and rather uncommon occipital onset has been reported (Hart et al., 1997). Less convincing is the report of another variant of Rasmussen syndrome with bilateral involvement, cerebral atrophy, and severe psychomotor regression (Silver et al., 1998).

Benign Occipital Lobe Epilepsy

This epileptological entity has been individualized by Gastaut (1982b). It occurs in children and adolescents; there is no persistence into adult life. Seizures are mostly initiated by visual symptoms (amaurosis, phosphenes, or figurative hallucinations), which may be followed by other seizure manifestations (mostly hemiclonic attacks, but also psychomotor seizures and grand mal). Migrainous or pseudomigrainous symptoms with headache, nausea, and vomiting often follow the seizure.

The EEG shows very characteristic changes. In the interval, there are frequently recurrent stretches of rhythmical and well-formed spike-wave discharges of high voltage, at 1.5 to 3/sec, located over occipital regions and the immediate vicinity. Moderate lateralization is common. Ictal EEG discharges consist of continuous spike-wave activity over one occipital region even though the interictal spike-wave pattern is bilateral (Gastaut, 1982b). Figure 27.30 shows an example of the occipital spike-wave discharge.

When one considers the indubitably existing relationship to migraine, the question arises as to whether there is a continuum of more or less epileptogenic conditions between benign occipital lobe epilepsy and forms of basilar artery migraine with paroxysmal posterior EEG changes (Niedermeyer et al., 1988; Panayiotopoulos, 1980; Riggio et al., 1987; also see Chapter 29, "The EEG in Patients with Migraine and Other Forms of Headache"). Lugaresi et al. (1984) reported cases of "scotosensitive seizures" elicited by darkness and eye closure; these authors feel that this seizure type is closely related to benign occipital lobe epilepsy.

Benign occipital lobe epilepsy is unassociated with photosensitivity; there are no paroxysmal responses to flickering light.

Benign Occipital Lobe Epilepsy with Photosensitivity

This appears to be a rare variant of the aforementioned benign occipital lob epilepsy. Such cases (children, adolescents, and young adults) were reported by Ricci and Vigevano (1993) and Guerrini et al. (1995).

Occipital Evoked Spike Epilepsy in Childhood

DeMarco (1983) described four children (of a total of 15,500 children) with pronounced uni- or bilateral occipital spikes elicited by intermittent photic stimulation. In the fur-

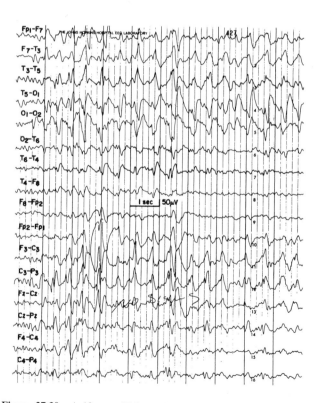

Figure 27.30. A 13-year-old boy with benign occipital lobe epilepsy. There are widespread 1.5 to 2/sec spike-wave complexes with occipital-posterotemporal maximum, occurring in long bursts during wakefulness. The spike waves are lateralized to the left (but the lateralization was not consistent). At other times, the patient had a well-developed posterior alpha rhythm.

ther course, seizures developed; these were mostly visual, such as phosphenes, but there were also occasional automatisms. The seizure disorder gradually vanished within 1 to 2 years; the affected children were neurologically and psychologically normal.

The mechanism of occipital spiking elicited by flashes also occurs in the neurodegenerative disorder Bielschowsky-Jansky disease (see Chapter 19, "Degenerative Disorders of the Central Nervous System").

Benign Parietal Epilepsy

The elucidation of this entity must be credited to Negrin and DeMarco (1977) and DeMarco et al. (1980), who observed the occurrence of spikes over the parietal region (parasagittal zone) after contralateral tactile stimuli. The vast majority of these patients were children between the ages of 4 and 8 years. This phenomenon was found in 96 of 12,500 children (0.8%) in the material of DeMarco et al. (1980). The paroxysmal response to tactile stimuli was found to be enhanced in non-REM sleep. Only 20 of the 96 children had clinical seizures; the remaining children were referred because of behavior problems.

The detection of benign parietal epilepsy depends on a special activation. It is most advisable to use heel tapping as an additional mandatory activation in the EEG laboratory in all children between ages 2 and 10 years.

The findings of DeMarco and his co-workers were impressively confirmed by Fonseca and Tedrus (1994), who studied 186 children with frequent EEG paroxysms evoked by tapping of the feet or hands; there was a history of clinical seizures in 75 (40.3%). Spontaneous epileptiform EEG discharges occurred in 39.6% of the children and mostly in those with seizures (85.3%).

The pattern of parietal (centroparietal) spikes has also been found in a 9-year-old mentally retarded boy with fragile X syndrome (Musumeci et al., 2000).

Benign Psychomotor Epilepsy

Psychomotor (complex partial) seizures due to temporal lobe epilepsy or stemming from the immediate vicinity of the temporal lobe usually indicate a serious or even severe (if not intractable) seizure disorder. There have been, however, reports on a benign type with psychomotor seizures characterized by affective and autonomic ictal symptoms (Dalla Bernardina et al., 1984; Plouin et al., 1980).

In some children with a history of migraine, experienced psychomotor (affective, psychosensory, or cognitive) seizures may occur; these children also exhibit interictal EEG abnormalities consisting mainly of temporal sharp transients (Seshia et al., 1985).

Children with Midtemporal Spikes, Progressive Aphasia, and Seizures (Landau-Kleffner Syndrome)

This syndrome of childhood epilepsy with progressive aphasia has stimulated much interest over the past 20 years and may be regarded as an epileptological entity unless the discovery of a consistently present pathogenic agent such as a virus turns this condition into a specific disease entity. The work of Landau and Kleffner (1957), Alajouanine and Lhermitte (1965), Worster-Drought (1971), Gascon et al. (1973), Deonna et al. (1975), Foerster (1977), and Lou et al. (1977) has been fundamental in the delineation of this syndrome.

This condition is found in children around ages 4 to 6. Speech becomes less intelligible and eventually is limited to a few words. Myoclonic jerking and other forms of brief seizures (akinetic, etc.) are reported. The EEG shows marked spiking, mainly over the left midtemporal region, but there are numerous generalized spike-wave-like bursts, first 3 to 4/sec and later in the 1.5 to 3/sec range, suggestive of a Lennox-Gastaut syndrome (Fig. 27.31) (see Rodriguez and Niedermeyer, 1982).

Cortical biopsy may show inflammatory changes and gliosis with mildly abnormal appearance of the meninges over the left temporal region (Lou et al., 1977). In the course of years, the speech function starts to improve, the seizure frequency diminishes, and the EEG abnormalities gradually vanish. The possibility of a slow viral disease is under consideration.

Riley and Massey (1979) reported three cases of aphasia, headaches, and left temporal spikes in adults. The course was benign, and one wonders if these patients had a milder and shortened form of the childhood syndrome, with spikes but without seizures.

Electrical Status Epilepticus During Sleep (ESES Syndrome)

This syndrome is characterized by continuous slow spike-wave activity during non-REM sleep. The spike-wave complexes are not well formed, and the spike component is usually more pronounced than the slow wave component. The maximum is variable; a maximum over the vertex but also over the occipital region may be present, according to personal observations.

This electroclinical condition has been described by Patry et al. (1971) and Tassinari et al. (1982, 1984). It occurs in children (mostly around age 8 years) with chiefly nocturnal but also diurnal seizures and mild mental retardation. The seizures consist of myoclonus, grand mal, and petit mal-like absences. The unique EEG manifestations during non-REM sleep are coupled with rather bland EEG findings in the waking state and REM sleep; occasional focal or bilaterally synchronous spikes may be present while awake. The dramatic changes in non-REM sleep disappear during adolescence. From the viewpoint of the sleep researcher, it is interesting to note that these children awaken from such a severely disturbed nocturnal sleep pattern in a normally refreshed state.

There has been a recent upsurge of interest in ESES and the aforementioned Landau-Kleffner syndrome. New waves of research in this domain have resulted in a book dealing with both conditions that was edited by Beaumanoir et al. (1995). There have been advocates of a unified syndrome comprising both conditions (Hirsch et al., 1995) and also opponents of this idea. Beaumanoir (1996) as well as Tassinari (1996) have expressed a cautious view aiming at preservation of the status quo.

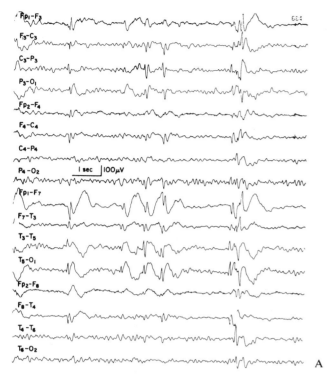

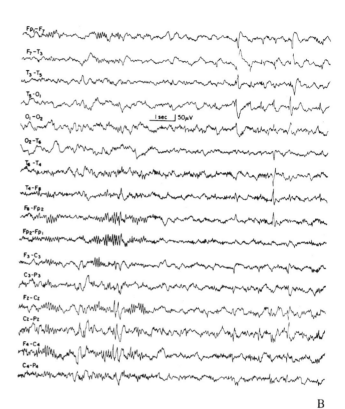

B

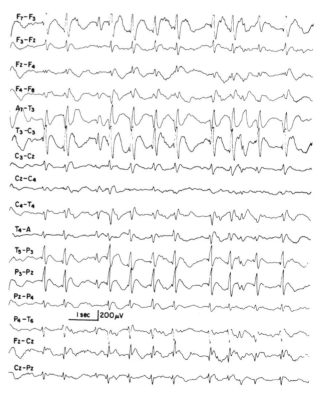

C

Figure 27.31. **A:** Aphasia-convulsion syndrome in an 8-year-old patient. Seizures (grand mal and akinetic), starting at age 7 years, receptive aphasia with onset at age 7.5 years. There is marked spiking, more over left hemisphere with left temporal maximum. **B:** Aphasia-convulsion syndrome in a 6-year-old patient. Onset of grand mal and onset of aphasia at age 5.5 years. Also has atypical absences and akinetic seizures. Sleep record with well-developed spindles and frequent spikes independently over temporal area, more on the left with midtemporal maximum. **C:** Aphasia-convulsion syndrome in an 8-year-old patient. Onset of grand mal seizures and aphasia around age 7.5 years. Sleep record shows generalized slow spike-wave-like activity, lateralized to the left.

Children with Multifocal Spikes

Abundant spike activity of multiple focality and often changing areas of maximal development are sometimes observed in children, mostly between 2 to 10 years. Some of these children have evidently been brain damaged since infancy, and the type of accompanying seizures may vary. Other children with these rather dramatic EEG findings show surprisingly normal neurological and mental findings. In the latter group, the widespread generation of spike activity is likely to be due to temporary paroxysmal hyperexcitability. Genetic predisposition has been suggested by Hauser et al. (1984b).

In some children, multifocal spikes may develop in the wake of West syndrome or in association with Lennox-Gastaut syndrome.

Considerations of Functional Versus Autochthonous Seizure Discharges

The presentation of age-determined epileptic conditions clearly shows benign and vicious forms. Generalized synchronous spikes and spike waves in primary generalized epilepsy and focal spikes in benign rolandic epilepsy can be easily suppressed for a limited period with small doses of intravenous diazepam, whereas many cases of chronic epileptogenic foci are not touched by such small amounts.

This dichotomy of responses of human epileptogenic EEG discharges reminds us of a similar dichotomy that has been widely discussed among neurophysiologists and basic science workers in the field of epileptology. Are we dealing with basically normal neurons that fire excessively due to hypersynchronous synaptic input? Such an epileptogenic focus would consist of a hyperexcitable "neuronal aggregate" (Ayala et al., 1973). On the other hand, one could view the epileptogenic focus as composed of intrinsically abnormal neurons (Atkinson and Ward, 1964; Matsumoto and Ajmone Marsan, 1964). This subject has been masterfully discussed by Schwartzkroin and Wyler (1980). One wonders if the benign therapeutically recalcitrant forms, especially in cases of chronic temporal or frontal lobe epilepsy, are caused by truly abnormal neurons in the area of the focus. Glial dysfunction or scarring could be the cause of epileptic neuronal behavior.

There is accumulating evidence that epileptic seizure disorders based on neuronal hyperexcitability do exist. The key areas of predisposition to epileptic neuronal hyperexcitability may be summarized as follows:

1. Frontal lobe—Supplementary motor area in interhemispheric fissure
   Presumed trigger: arousing stimuli in a state of reduced vigilance
   Generalization: very common and pronounced, exemplified by 3/sec spike-waves, with or without petit mal absence (perhaps via cingulate and thalamocortical connections).
2. Occipital lobe
   Trigger: flickering light and other visual stimuli
   Generalization: common, exemplified by polyspikes with or without myoclonus, occasionally by spike waves with or without petit mal absence, via occip-

itofrontocentral connections and/or geniculate-thalamocortical fiber systems.
3. Rolandic region
   Trigger: unclear; possibly sensorimotor idling
   Generalization: not quite as common; seizures, if occurring, are most often of focal motor character.

Hyperexcitability of all three key areas may occasionally exist in certain patients with primary generalized epilepsy. Such cases epitomize the significance of predisposition (i.e., genetic factors). The hyperexcitability of the sensory-parietal cortex with local spike responses to contralateral tactile stimuli seems to be a related phenomenon.

Epileptic Seizures and Site of Focus

The localization of an epileptogenic focus may strongly determine the character of the seizures. For this reason, epileptology is also a mirror of cerebral-cortical localization. This aspect provides complementary evidence in addition to insights stemming from the observation of cortical deficits due to local pathology or surgical ablation of cerebral regions.

Experimentation of the human brain, unintentional or as a by-product of therapeutic procedures, laid the foundation for investigation of focal epilepsies. According to A. Earl Walker (1957), Fritsch was dressing a cranial wound of a victim of the Prussian-Danish War (1864) when he provoked contralateral muscular contractions in the patient. Hitzig (1871) noticed eye movements to the opposite side when he applied current to electrodes placed over the temples of a subject (O'Leary and Goldring, 1976; Walker, 1957). These observations prompted both investigators to carry out animal experiments demonstrating the motor responses to cortical stimulation. This work was followed by Ferrier's studies of the motor cortex of monkeys and apes (Ferrier and Yeo, 1884). These pioneering studies generated further keen interest in the motor cortex, projection areas, and presumed association areas and eventually culminated in the study of Penfield and Jasper (1954) on epilepsy and the functional anatomy of the human cortex. This combination of special surgery for seizure foci and human neurophysiology in the locally anesthetized patient has remained an unrivaled model of a two-pronged approach aiming at a deeper comprehension of cortical physiology and the processes in and around the epileptogenic focus in humans.

This work also gave new impulse to electroencephalography. The search for patterns, especially with respect to ictal episodes, was complemented by an intensified search for a correct delineation of abnormal function such as an epileptogenic zone. In this chapter we are looking at the epileptic seizure disorder from the viewpoint of cerebral localization.

It is stated in the foregoing section that a spike focus does not necessarily denote a stable epileptogenic focus; benign rolandic epilepsy stands as the epitome of the truth of this statement. Zones of cortical hyperexcitability (hyperirritability) may behave like a focus in the EEG, but these dysfunctions may burn themselves out with advancing age. Not so an epileptogenic focus that is based on cerebral pathology. The types of pathology have never been so lucidly demonstrated as in the work of Penfield and Jasper (1954). Most of this pathology is residual, although the possibility of a space-occupying lesion must always be kept in mind. But are residual epileptogenic lesions quiet residues of a bygone active disease? Electromicroscopic work has shown that "residual" gliosis is a very active process, which provides a better understanding for the epileptic irritation of neurons (Scheibel and Scheibel, 1973).

According to Babb and Brown (1987), ongoing synaptic reorganization leads to epileptogenic connections in further neurons (in the case of hippocampal sclerosis of early life). These authors, however, do not consider hippocampal sclerosis a progressive type of damage.

Temporal Lobe Epilepsy

The temporal lobe is far more often than any other area the seat of an epileptogenic focus. What renders the temporal lobe so prone to harbor epileptogenic foci? The answer probably lies in (a) special anatomicophysiological properties of the limbic (arche- and paleocortical) portion of the temporal lobe, and (b) a certain vulnerability of neocortical and limbic parts of the temporal lobe to some forms of pathology.

Seizures arising from the temporal lobe have captivated the interest of epileptologists, electroencephalographers, neurologists, neurosurgeons, and even psychiatrists during the past two decades. The impressive multitude of temporal lobe functions in the human are reflected by the enormous variety of seizure patterns. Temporal lobe functions are in part higher cortical functions; they are also functions of the limbic system with its crossroads of autonomic nervous system regulations and emotionality.

Terminology

The term temporal lobe epilepsy (introduced by Jasper et al., 1951) is correct as far as seizures arising from the temporal lobe are concerned. It should not be used as a synonym for psychomotor (complex partial) seizures, because (a) not all seizure manifestations of the temporal lobe fall into this category (many patients also have grand mal seizures and a few have grand mal only), and (b) psychomotor (complex partial) seizures may occasionally originate from the vicinity of the temporal lobe, usually as extensions of the limbic system into the fronto-orbital region. The reader will find more information and details on the historical development in the section on types of psychomotor seizures.

Clinical Ictal Manifestations

The wide variety of seizure manifestations is presented in the section on types of psychomotor seizures.

Ictal EEG Manifestations

See also the section on types of psychomotor seizures.

Although psychomotor (complex partial) seizures represent the classical ictal manifestation of temporal lobe epilepsy, the occurrence of grand mal seizures in combination with psychomotor seizures is very common. According to Schmidt et al. (1983), the presence or absence of grand mal does not significantly influence the outcome. An important prognostic factor lies in the frequency of the grand mal at-

tacks; patients with psychomotor and frequent grand mal seizures are not as readily controlled by medication as those with psychomotor and infrequent generalized tonic-clonic convulsions (Schmidt et al., 1983). Even severe cases of temporal lobe epilepsy (candidates for temporal lobectomy) may have experienced psychomotor (complex partial) seizures only. In some of the patients, the history reveals that the only grand mal attacks occurred after abrupt reduction or discontinuation of medications such as phenobarbital or primidone.

Interictal EEG Manifestations

The anterior temporal spike or, more often, sharp-wave discharge, randomly firing, is the classical EEG finding in the interseizure interval. With the use of the International Electrode System, this discharge is recorded from the F7 or F8 electrode, which is essentially frontobasal and slightly in front of the tip of the temporal lobe. This minor shortcoming of the International Electrode System has been pointed out by Silverman (1960), who recommended the use of a special lead slightly behind and below the F7–F8 electrodes. Gibbs and Gibbs (1947), as well as Gibbs et al. (1948), must be credited with the first demonstration of the anterotemporal spike focus; these authors rightly stressed the importance of sleep lest this crucial finding is missed in a tracing obtained solely in the waking state (Fig. 27.32). With the use of additional (total of 75) electrodes (see Fig. 7.2, Chapter 7) this problem shrinks to irrelevance. According to Sammaritano et al. (1991), spike foci in temporal lobe epilepsy are most reliably found in REM sleep rather than in wakefulness and non-REM sleep. In some cases, hyperventilation has been found to be a powerful activating test, resulting in enhancement of the anterotemporal lobe discharges (Lys and Karbowski, 1981; Smith and Scott, 1981) and occasionally in clinical psychomotor seizures.

The spike (sharp wave) discharge is bilateral in about 25% to 35% of the cases (Gastaut, 1953; Gibbs et al., 1948; Jasper et al., 1951). Gibbs and Gibbs (1952) pointed out that patients with bilateral anterior temporal spikes (sharp waves) are more likely to have both psychomotor and grand mal seizures. These authors also stressed the role of sleep in the facilitation of temporal spikes (also see Niedermeyer and Rocca, 1972; and Autret et al., 1983) (Figs. 27.32 and 27.33).

It may be interesting in this context that REM sleep is decreased in patients with complex partial seizures regardless of nocturnal or diurnal occurrence (Bazil et al., 2000).

Bilateral anterior temporal spiking may be bilateral independent or synchronous. Bilateral synchrony has been divided into real synchrony and discharges transmitted from one side to the other. Jasper et al. (1951), using electrocorticographic technique over the operated side, found that the spike discharge occurred over one temporal lobe only in 34%, whereas transmission from side to side was noted in 24%, synchrony in 19%, and bilateral independence in 23%.

The "true" and primary temporal lobe focus presents itself with initial negative DC shifts and requires the recording of ultraslow frequencies (Vanhatalo et al., 2003; also see Chapter 25).

The findings of Jasper et al. (1951) also pertain to the type of underlying pathology. No brain tumor was discov-

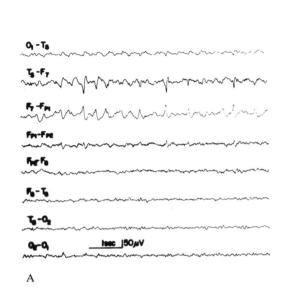

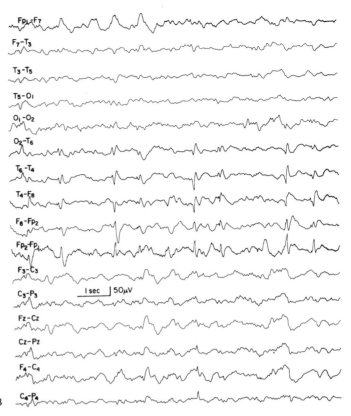

Figure 27.32. **A:** Typical anterior temporal sharp waves in a 29-year-old patient with psychomotor automatisms and grand mal seizures since age 2 years. **B:** Massive sharp-wave activity over right temporal regions, maxi- mal in the anterior temporal lead. Recorded in light sleep in a 32-year-old patient with a history of temporal lobe epilepsy.

ered in patients with bilateral independent temporal spikes. Patients with unilateral spikes often proved to have atrophy; the superior aspects of the temporal lobe showed a maximum of corticographic spike activity. Patients with lesions of the basomesial surface and the tip of the temporal lobe revealed spikes transmitted secondarily to the opposite side or bilateral synchronous spiking. These patients may show less prominent or even equivocal scalp EEG findings.

The paroxysmal EEG abnormalities may exceed the boundaries of the temporal lobe. According to Gabor and Ajmone Marsan (1968), psychomotor or complex partial seizures are more likely to occur when focal EEG abnormalities are limited to the temporal lobe. Sadler et al. (1984) studied the potential fields of anterior temporal spikes with the use of a grid array and subsequent computer analysis. These authors found that anterior temporal spikes most often arose from a point located one-third the distance from the A1 electrode to the Fp1 electrode. Other common origins were near T3 and at a point two thirds the distance from A1 to Fp1. A bipolar anteroposterior montage using the 10–20 electrode system would incompletely record about 40% to 55% of anterior temporal spikes.

In some patients, anterotemporal spikes are scanty, while consistent focal slowing is present over this area. This pattern is usually not good evidence for a space-occupying lesion unless progression of the focal slow (mainly delta) activity is demonstrable (Hill, 1963; Klass, 1975; Klass and

Daly, 1960; Kooi, 1971). The role of temporal interictal rhythmic delta activity (TIRDA) in the EEG diagnosis of temporal lobe epilepsy has been stressed by Reiher and Beaudry (1988). According to Rosati et al. (2003), intractable temporal lobe epilepsies with rare spikes are less severe than those with frequent spikes.

It was pointed out previously that children and young adolescents with temporal lobe epilepsy and unequivocal complex partial seizures often have inconclusive EEG findings. Spikes or sharp waves may be over midtemporal or central regions (thus falsely suggesting benign rolandic epilepsy) or diffuse. Even generalized spike-wave discharges may occur (Kohlheb et al., 1985; Niedermeyer, 1954a), and slow spike-wave complexes may overshadow all other abnormalities in Lennox-Gastaut syndrome, giving rise to psychomotor seizures.

It evidently takes a while until the classical anterotemporal spike (sharp wave) focus is fully developed. The author has seen two cases (ages 4 and 7 years) with exceptional anterotemporal spiking and psychomotor seizures (Fig. 27.33). Very rarely, the opposite happens, with anterotemporal spiking being just a form of benign temporal spiking, even without any seizures and with full EEG normalization at age 11 years (personal observation). With advancing age, the anterotemporal spike focus increasingly becomes the impressive hallmark of temporal epilepsy, until an overabundance of this discharge occurs. Above age 50 to 60 years, the an-

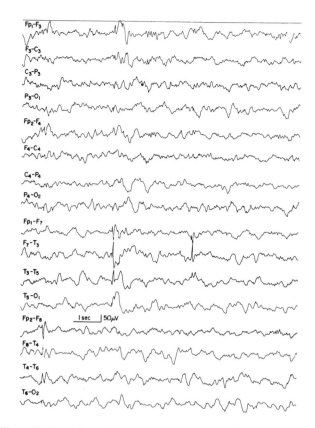

Figure 27.33. A 4-year-old patient has a history of major convulsions and "staring attacks." In sleep, there is evidence of independent left and right anterior temporal spikes.

arise from a wide region, including deep structures, as demonstrated by Westmoreland et al. (1979), and might indicate only some degree of neuronal hyperexcitability.

An unusual EEG pattern in temporal lobe epileptics was described by Ciganek (1961), who noticed frontal midline theta activity with an average frequency of 5.78/sec in 36% of these patients. Hughes and Olson (1981) analyzed eight different paroxysmal temporal lobe discharges and pointed out the varying degrees of epileptogenicity of each discharge type. It was found that the anterior temporal sharp wave or spike discharge was clearly more epileptogenic than other patterns.

Research in the 1990s shed a lot more light on pathological anatomical changes underlying temporal lobe epilepsy; volumetric MRI has been the basis for the evaluation of hippocampal size and mesiotemporal atrophy. In the presence of mesiotemporal atrophy, the EEG quite frequently shows trains of rhythmical delta waves over anterior temporal and midtemporal region, lateralizing with accuracy equal to that of the spikes to the site of atrophy (Gambardella et al., 1995). This was found to be true for unilateral as well as for bilateral temporal lobe foci, which featured bilaterally shifting delta runs (Gambardella et al., 1995). With combined use of MRI and PET, interictal temporal lobe hypometabolism was found to be associated mesiotemporal sclerosis (atrophy) (Semah et al., 1995). In mesiotemporal sclerosis, the characteristic initial EEG seizure pattern is of hypersynchronous character

terotemporal spike or sharp wave is, in most cases, a simple exaggeration of temporal minor sharp activity, which is extremely common in elderly patients with mild or moderate degrees of cerebrovascular disorder and no seizure disorder whatsoever. In epileptics above age 50, temporal lobe spiking is a very common finding, but this does not necessarily mean that one is dealing with a temporal lobe epileptic; on the contrary, grand mal seizures outnumber psychomotor seizures by a wide margin (Niedermeyer, 1958; Takahashi et al., 1965).

The combination of total absence of paroxysmal discharges, marked unilateral temporal polymorphic delta activity, and recent onset of psychomotor seizures is very suggestive of a rapidly growing temporal lobe tumor. Very slowly growing tumors such as certain astrocytomas may show EEG patterns undistinguishable from those of temporal lobe epileptics with residual lesions. Meningiomas of the medial sphenoid wing position and psychomotor seizures may have very little or no EEG abnormality.

Small sharp spikes (see Chapter 13, "Abnormal EEG Patterns: Epileptic and Paroxysmal") may appear over the temporal region and its neighborhood in early sleep as forerunners of typical large anterotemporal sharp waves, giving support to the diagnosis of temporal lobe epilepsy (Fig. 27.34). The occurrence of small sharp spikes alone, however, contributes nothing to this diagnosis. These small discharges

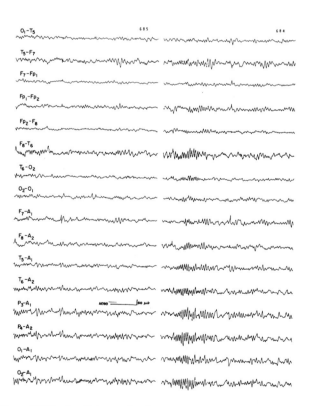

Figure 27.34. Small sharp spikes in the sleep tracing of a 46-year-old patient, maximal over F_7, slightly more prominent in the referential *(bottom)* than in the bipolar montage *(top).* (From Koshino, Y., and Niedermeyer, E. 1975. The clinical significance of small sharp spikes in the electroencephalogram. Clin. Electroencephalogr. 6:131–140.)

with repetitive spiking (Ebner and Hoppe, 1995) (rather than of electrodecremental nature).

With the presently widespread use of combined video-EEG monitoring in potential candidates for temporal lobectomy, the question of uni- versus bilateral involvement and the relevance or irrelevance of spiking over the other side has become an eminent issue. More information is found in the comprehensive works of Engel (1987), Niedermeyer (1990), Lüders (1992), and Wyllie (1993) in order to understand the diversity of epileptological-neurosurgical approaches. In the presence of consistently unilateral ictal epileptiform discharges, the presence of bitemporal spikes has to be assessed with great care (Steinhoff et al., 1995).

The dignity of the routine EEG remains untouched even in these days of increasingly sophisticated and expensive technologies; this becomes clearly evident from the data of Cascino et al. (1996)—such a statement presupposes EEG training of highest quality and the involvement of highly experienced electroencephalographers.

The EEG from scalp, cortex, and depth has been playing a major role in attempts at the differentiation of limbic structures (amygdala, hippocampus), cingulate gyrus and temporal neocortex. The subdivisions of Wieser (1983) into six forms of temporal lobe epilepsy have been mentioned earlier. The detection of lesions in the amygdala might require special structural methods (Van Paesschen et al., 1996). Walczak (1995) has attempted a characterization of a "syndrome of neocortical temporal lobe epilepsy."

With the use of combined depth EEG and proton magnetic resonance spectroscopic imaging, Guye et al. (2002) assumed that metabolic abnormalities are linked to ictal/interictal paroxysmal activities rather than to structural alterations in temporal lobe epileptics.

Is subdivision of temporal lobe epilepsies of highest importance? Are there strong repercussions on treatment—be it noninvasive or surgical? Especially on the basis of surgical electrocorticograms, there is good reason to presume that, in the majority of cases, temporal lobe epilepsy is not limited to a restricted area; it rather affects most structures of the lobe regardless of whether the starting point lies in limbic or neocortical areas (Graf et al., 1983).

Occasionally, the EEG may remain stubbornly normal in patients with clinically unequivocal evidence of temporal lobe epilepsy. Even prolonged EEG recording including video-EEG monitoring may remain noncontributory. Depth EEG implants may miss the true epileptogenic focus and subdural/epidural electrodes may also fail. The use of PET or single photon emission computed tomography (SPECT) scanning is likely to show areas of hypo- and/or hypermetabolism, but this may or may not correspond with the true epileptogenic focus. These, however, are extreme cases that should not detract from the enormous diagnostic effectiveness of EEG in conjunction with nonelectrophysiological methods.

Age and Prevalence

Temporal lobe epilepsy spans a period from early childhood to senility, but classical cases are usually found in older adolescents and in young and middle-aged adults; childhood and senium tend to dilute the clinical and EEG semiology. The prevalence can be derived from the figures given in the discussion of psychomotor seizures. The occurrence of temporal lobe epilepsy in infants has been documented by Karbowski et al. (1988). Special features of temporal lobe seizures occurring in childhood were discussed above (see Psychomotor Seizures).

Neurological Deficits

Neurological deficits are very subtle unless extensive cerebral pathology is present. A rather common neurological sign is facial asymmetry (Remillard et al., 1977) due to a mild upper motor neuron type VIIth nerve weakness, found contralaterally in 73% and ipsilaterally in 13% of a population of temporal lobe epileptics.

Psychological and Psychiatric Features

A review of the copious literature on this subject could fill a monograph; in this context, we must confine ourselves to a few basic statements. According to personal impression, the most common psychological features are irritability and hyposexuality (Niedermeyer et al., 1967); these data were derived from patients considered candidates for temporal lobectomy because of the severity of their seizure disorder. Extensive overviews of the psychiatric dimension of the epilepsies and the special psychiatric aspects of temporal lobe epilepsy are found in the work of Toone (1981), Bear et al. (1984), Blumer (1984), Ferguson and Rayport (1984), Himmelhoch (1984), Trimble (1985), Taylor (1987), Trimble (1991), and Trimble and Schmitz (1998).

A constant state of irritability renders these patients more volatile; some of them exhibit hostility and are prone to aggressive acts, but it must be stated very clearly that these cases are exceptional and not the rule. In recent decades, the conjunction of acts of violence or crime and temporal lobe epilepsy has been widely accepted without sufficient support from clinical data. Single observations of aggressive acts (Mark and Ervin, 1970; Saint-Hilaire et al., 1980; Serafetinides, 1965) must be considered exceptional. Studies of large patient groups have clearly shown the rarity of aggressive acts in patients with temporal lobe epilepsy (Currie et al., 1970; Rodin, 1973; Treiman and Delgado-Escueta, 1983a).

The significance of hyposexuality was pointed out first by Gastaut and Collomb (1954) and Gastaut (1958a); this subject was discussed in greater detail by Blumer and Walker (1967). Blumer (1970) also confirmed occasional earlier reports on hypersexual episodes in these patients. Increased occurrence of homosexuality in male patients with temporal lobe epilepsy and limbic involvement has been reported by Remillard et al. (1984). The erectile dysfunction in men with temporal lobe epilepsy is of neurogenic rather than vasogenic nature (Guldner and Morrell, 1996).

According to J. Stevens (1975), "patients with major psychomotor epilepsy are subject to an increased risk of psychiatric disturbance but . . . except the immediate postictal psychotic state, the risk appears to reflect the site and extent of brain damage and the individual's psychosocial history and opportunities more than a diagnosis of epilepsy." This author also feels that "temporal lobe epilepsy makes a very small contribution to the pool of psychiatric disturbances, including violence."

Relationships to the schizoid personality have been frequently reported and combination with overt schizophrenia is well known, although not common (Dongier, 1959,

1959/60; Ervin et al., 1955; Flor-Henry, 1969; Gibbs and Gibbs, 1952; Hill, 1952; Landolt, 1955, 1960; Rodin et al., 1957; Taylor, 1977). Stevens (1975, 1980) has tried to demonstrate a joint neurobiochemical basis for temporal lobe epilepsy and schizophrenia.

The electroencephalographer will occasionally find that patients with temporal lobe epilepsy and schizophrenia show marked EEG improvement or completely normal tracings when the psychiatric condition is at its worst, while the patient is practically seizure-free, and vice versa (enhanced seizure disorder, massive spiking, and psychiatric improvement). This "seesaw phenomenon" has been observed by Landolt (1955) ("forced normalization") and was confirmed by Dongier (1959/60) and Flor-Henry (1969). This mechanism of "forced normalization," however, is infrequently encountered according to the studies of Libus and Libus (1981) and Ramani and Gumnit (1981).

Postictal forms of psychosis in temporal lobe epileptics have been studied with SPECT, which documented bitemporal and bifrontal hyperperfusion (Leutmezer et al., 2003). This leaves the question as to whether one is dealing with a hidden epileptic phenomenon or a secondary response to enhanced psychological activity.

A comparison of left- and right-sided temporal epilepsies (dominant versus nondominant temporal lobe) has shown some psychological-psychiatric differences (Bingley, 1958). Serafetinides (1970) feels that epileptogenic foci in the temporal lobe in the dominant hemisphere are more likely to be associated with aggressive behavior.

The often-popularized association of temporal lobe epilepsy with aggression and violence is absolutely wrong; the vast majority of patients exhibiting acts of aggression are nonepileptic (Riley and Niedermeyer, 1978; Steinert and Froescher, 1994).

According to Kanemoto et al. (1996), mesial temporal sclerosis may play a role in the genesis of postictal psychosis, which can be associated with aggressive tendency.

Moser et al. (2000) have compared neuropsychological indicators with EEG and MRI concerning the focus lateralization in temporal lobe epileptics. While EEG and MRI were found to be of high lateralizing value, neuropsychological data were of limited use in this regard.

Etiologies and Pathological Substrata

The vast material of the Montreal Neurological Institute (857 cases) was broken down by Mathieson (1975a,b) as follows:

No histopathological abnormality	173
Unspecified minor abnormalities	167
Cortical neuronal loss and gliosis	164
Gliomas and ganglioglioma	105
Cortical neuronal loss, gliosis, and hippocampal sclerosis	73
Hippocampal sclerosis	67
Meningocerebral cicatrix and remote contusion	39
Vascular formation of brain and/or pia	19
Hamartomas	14
Tumors other than gliomas	10
Residuum of brain abscess	10
Postmeningitic cerebral atrophy	4
Tuberous sclerosis and formes frustes	4
Subacute and chronic encephalitides	3
Ulegyria	2
Anomalous cases	2
Residuum of old infarct	1

The large number of tumors warrants special attention when one considers their progressive and eventually life-threatening nature. A sizable portion of these tumors, however, are of very mildly progressive nature and behave almost like a nontumoral lesion. Small tumors as the cause of seizures are found mainly in the mesioinferior areas such as the uncus and amygdaloid region (Cavanagh, 1958). Temporal lobe seizures may also be caused by a pituitary tumor with a large supradiaphragmatic portion and, furthermore, by lipomas of the corpus callosum (Gastaut et al., 1980).

Certain pathogenetic mechanisms have been singled out as highly contributory to some forms of residual epileptogenic lesions. Peiffer (1963) extensively discussed the role of transtentorial herniation (Hill, 1896; Meyer, 1920; Wolback, 1908; also see Finney and Walker, 1962), which may be the result of perinatal brain damage. This mechanism leads to circulatory disturbances and edema involving mesial (hippocampic) portions of the temporal lobe. The term incisural herniation, with incisural alluding to the free edge of the tentorium, was introduced by Earle et al. (1953), but the specific pathogenetic role of this mechanism has been de-emphasized by Veith (1959) and Peiffer (1963).

Hippocampic changes were recognized quite early, and sclerosis of the field (Sommer's sector) was thought to play an important part in the genesis of otherwise unexplained epilepsies. The work of Bouchet and Cazauveilh (1825), Sommer (1880), and Pfleger (1880) must be mentioned in this context. The secondary character of this disturbance was subsequently stressed by Pfleger (1880), Alzheimer (1907), Spielmeyer (1933), Scholz (1951), Peiffer (1963), and Malamud (1966), who indicated the significance of these changes in the pathogenesis of temporal lobe epilepsy. Ammon's horn sclerosis was found in the majority of the cases of temporal lobe epilepsy in the material of Stauder (1935) and Sano and Malamud (1953). The work of Stauder (1935) is remarkable when one considers that this author had a clear concept of temporal lobe epilepsy at a time when the EEG was unknown or at best on the very edge of being discovered. Other investigators reported a lesser incidence of Ammon's horn sclerosis in temporal lobe epileptics (Cavanagh, 1958; Cavanagh and Meyer, 1956; Haberland, 1962; Peiffer, 1963). More comprehensive terms such as pararhinal sclerosis (Gastaut, 1956) and mesiotemporal sclerosis (Falconer, 1968, 1974) are widely used and denote various residual pathologies in mesiotemporal (limbic) regions. There is no evidence of apoptotic cell death in mesial temporal sclerosis (Uysal et al., 2003).

According to Babb and Brown (1987), all proven cases of temporal lobe epilepsy show anatomical evidence of Ammon's horn damage.

The excitatory projection from the dentate gyrus to the hippocampus ("mossy fibers") is thought to be an important component in seizure generation (Henze et al., 2000). This epileptiform alteration of the hippocampus in human temporal lobe epilepsy may result in increased levels of chondroitin and hyaluronic acid ("extracellular matrix components") in hippocampus, neocortex, and cerebrospinal fluid of these patients (Perosa et al., 2002).

Certain etiologies have been stressed by various investigators. Gastaut and Gastaut (1951) felt that bouts of severe otitis media would cause epileptogenic temporal lobe changes. Encephalitis ranks high as a cause of temporal lobe seizures in Malamud's research (1966). Courville (1958), who concentrated on CNS trauma, stressed the infrequent occurrence of pure psychomotor epilepsy in posttraumatic cases. Occult encephaloceles of the middle cranial fossa have been described as the cause of temporal lobe epilepsy (Hyson et al., 1982).

The neuropathological study of Mathieson (1975a,b) is about to be supplanted by data obtained with more modern methodologies. It has demonstrated that the most epileptogenic forms of neuropathological changes are dysembryoplastic neuroepithelial tumors, glioneuronal hamartomas (resembling tuberous sclerosis) and glioneuronal hamartias (Wolf, 1996). Pilocytic astrocytomas, low-grade diffusely infiltrating astrocytomas, oligodendrogliomas, cavernomas scar-like residual states are further frequent causes of chronic epilepsies (Wolf, 1996; Wolf and Wiestler, 1996).

Neurophysiological Mechanisms

Limbic and neocortical portions of the temporal lobe (and, frequently, of the adjacent fronto-orbital region) are actively involved in the ictal and interictal epileptic phenomena of temporal lobe epilepsy. The uncinate region, comprising the amygdaloid complex, uncinate gyrus, and anteroinsular and peri-insular portions of the temporal lobe, appears to be mostly involved in typical psychomotor automatisms, whereas the lateral temporal neocortex appears to be most active in experienced psychomotor seizures (Feindel and Penfield, 1954; Jasper, 1958).

The role of the hippocampus remains enigmatic. Hippocampic electrical stimulation in humans almost never results in afterdischarges or seizures (Jasper, 1958); this structure is most likely to be secondarily involved. Its role, "to consolidate memory traces" (Gloor, 1975), is often jeopardized in ictal activity. It must be added that the left and right hippocampus apparently serve special memory functions, with verbal memory on the dominant and nonverbal visual memory on the nondominant side (Carsi, 1972; Milner, 1975). Amygdalo-hypothalamic connections are likely to account for emotional responses, in normal physiology as well as in a morbid and exaggerated form, during ictal activity. Connections between amygdala and basal ganglia (putamen, globus pallidus, caudate nucleus) might serve the behavioral-motor component of temporal lobe seizures. Autonomic manifestations are probably served by the amygdala through the hypothalamus or originate from the insular cortex (Fig. 27.35). Bilateral temporal lobe involvement is very common; its hypothetical basis was discussed earlier. The secondary character of hippocampic damage due to primary "cryptogenic seizures" has been stressed by Kalviäinen et al., 1998).

Frontal Lobe Epilepsy

Frontal lobe epilepsy is much less common than temporal lobe epilepsy. In the study of Rasmussen (1970), there were 211 nontumoral epileptogenic lesions in the frontal lobe as compared with 551 patients with nontumoral temporal lobe lesions. This is also true for a nonneurosurgical patient population (Fegersten and Roger, 1961). Moreover, frontal lobe epilepsy is less significant as a distinct epileptological en-

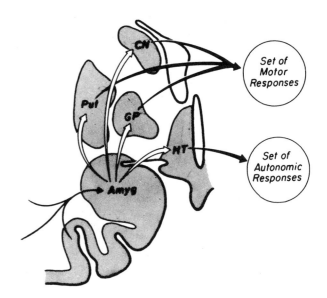

Figure 27.35. The final common pathway of emotional responses. There is widespread neocortical input into the amygdala (Amyg) (topical subdivisions within the amygdala are not indicated). The output encompasses connections with the hypothalamus (HT) as well as putamen (Put), globus pallidus (GP), and caudate nucleus (CN). (Modified from Jasper, H.H. 1958. Functional subdivisions of the temporal region in relation to seizure patterns and subcortical connections. In *Temporal Lobe Epilepsy*, Eds. M. Baldwin and P. Bailey, pp. 40–57. Springfield, IL: Charles C Thomas, with permission of Clin. Electroencephalogr. Chicago; Dr. F.A. Gibbs, chief editor.)

tity. The observation of Penfield and Kristiansen (1951) that frontal lobe seizures often consist of immediate grand mal attacks, thus obscuring any focal initiation, has been widely confirmed.

Clinical Ictal Manifestations

According to Rasmussen (1975b), six different clinical seizure patterns are distinguished:

1. Immediate unconsciousness followed by a grand mal with minimal or no lateralizing signs.
2. Immediate unconsciousness associated with initial turning of the head and eyes (sometimes of the body) to the opposite side, promptly followed by a grand mal, probably originating from the anterior one third or one fourth of the frontal lobe contralateral to the adversive movement.
3. Initial adversion of head and eyes to the opposite side, preserved consciousness, and conscious adversive (contraversive) attack, which after 5 to 20 seconds may or may not be followed by grand mal. The origin usually lies in the convexity of the intermediate frontal region.
4. Posturing movement of the body with tonic elevation of the contralateral arm, downward extension of the ipsilateral arm, and turning of the head away from the side of the lesion as if looking at the raised hand. This type of seizure arises from the medial aspect of the intermediate frontal region in the vicinity of the supplementary motor region. This type of seizure has also been described as "mesiofrontal epilepsy" by Niedermeyer and Walker (1971), who attributed these attacks to the supplemen-

tary motor region within the interhemispheric fissure. (Also see Fusco et al., 1990.)

5. Brief attacks of dizziness, a flush, or a weak feeling. This vague sensation may stop after a few seconds, or it may be followed by brief arrest of activity, confusion, and staring. This attack imitates the petit mal absence clinically and even electroencephalographically. In contrast with true petit mal absences, these attacks may be followed by a grand mal.

6. Sudden alteration of thought process, such as "forced thinking" ("my thoughts suddenly became fixed"). This may be followed by a petit mal-like absence or by a grand mal.

A different subdivision with 14 subgroups has been presented by Geier et al. (1977b) and includes the seizure manifestations that are most likely to arise from distant cortical regions (Table 27.12). Rasmussen (1975b) does not indicate the origin of patterns 5 and 6. These manifestations are rare, and there is reason to presume that the focus is mesiofrontal in the interhemispheric fissure, probably impinging on the cingulate gyrus and triggering "secondary bilateral synchrony" (see Primary Generalized Epilepsy) via mechanisms experimentally studied in cats and monkeys by Lennox and Robinson (1951) and Ralston (1961). In clinical cases, the term cingulate epilepsy (C. Mazars, 1969, 1970; Y. Mazars et al., 1966) has been used. Seizures arising from the fronto-orbital cortex may be indistinguishable from temporal lobe epilepsy (Schneider et al., 1961, 1965). Tharp (1972) has introduced the term fronto-orbital epilepsy as a special entity. Ludwig et al. (1975) have extensively investigated fronto-orbital epileptogenic foci with depth electrodes. A quite different picture of fronto-orbital epilepsy has been presented by Wieser and Hajek (1995) and Harner and Riggio (1995) (screaming, laughing, genital manipulation and pelvic thrusting).

A case with petit mal absence status-like ictal symptomatology due to a left frontal epileptogenic focus was demonstrated by Niedermeyer et al. (1979a,b). Similar cases but with less generalization were reported by Geier et al. (1977a).

In a major study of frontal lobe seizures and their semiology, Bancaud and Talairach (1992) have broken down frontal epileptic manifestations according to their focal origin in the following manner:

1. Seizures originating from areas 4 and 6 (53 patients)
2. Inferior frontal gyrus seizures (18 patients)
3. Medial intermediate frontal seizures (39 patients)
4. Dorsolateral intermediate frontal seizures (25 patients)
5. Anterior cingulate gyrus seizures (area 24) (16 patients)
6. Frontopolar seizures (14 patients)
7. Orbitofrontal seizures (18 patients)
8. Operculo-insular region (27 patients)

Salanova et al. (1995) have divided frontal lobe epilepsy (based on subdural recordings of 150 seizures in 24 patients) into three principal groups: (a) supplementary motor area (tonic uni-, bilateral arm motions, laughing, crying, version of head and eyes), (b) focal motor (unilateral arm and face clonic activity, speech arrest, version of head and eyes), and

Table 27.12. Subdivision of Frontal Lobe Seizures[a,b]

More Frequent	Less Frequent
Deviation of head and eyes	Simple motor automations
Clonic and/or ionic manifestations	Autonomic manifestations
	Subjective sensations
Falls	Disturbances in normal motor behavior
Breaking off of contact	Complex motor automations
Phenatory manifestations	Visual sensations
Immobility	Laughter
Memory disturbances	

[a]More frequently occurring seizure manifestations are listed in the left column; these seizures were observed in more than 75% of the patients of Geier et al. (1977b).

[b]From Geier, S., Bancaud, J., Talairach, J., Bonis, A., Szikis, G., and Enjelvin, J. 1977b. The seizures of frontal lobe epilepsy. A study of clinical manifestations. Neurology (Minneapolis) 27:951–958.

(c) psychomotor (including repetitive movements, bipedal movements, laughing, crying, adversion). These categories might be debatable. Personal observations strongly support the occurrence of clonic convulsions (in fast sequence) arising from the frontal supplementary motor cortex (Ikeda et al., 1999). Repetitive motor activity was found to be a typical ictal manifestation of frontal lobe epilepsy (Riggio et al., 1991; Riggio and Harner, 1995). Chassagnon et al. (2003) have pinpointed a circumscribed pericingulate area and the anterior-ventral portion of the supplementary motor area as the origin of seizures and dyskinetic behavior.

The repetitive character of motions may be due to the eminent role of the frontal lobe (its prefrontal as well as its premotor portion) in the sequential design of movements. Interference with this mechanism could indeed lead to repetitious movements (at present, a conjectural statement).

The relationship between primary (idiopathic) generalized epilepsy and frontal lobe epilepsy has been reinvestigated by Roger and Bureau (1992). It was pointed out earlier (in the discussion of primary generalized epilepsy) that the generalized spike-wave discharges are preponderant over superior frontal regions where the paroxysm appears to originate (cued by arousing stimuli). In cases of secondary bilateral synchrony, a true frontal focus can give rise to the generalized-synchronous spike-wave pattern (corresponding with types 5 and 6 in the list of seizure patterns of frontal lobe epilepsy, according to Rasmussen, 1975b).

The unique form of disturbance of consciousness with immediate return to the normal preictal state in classical petit mal absences might also be related to frontal lobe mechanisms. One has to realize that impairment of consciousness (of whatever cause) requires some time to recover—unlike the petit mal absence. The prefrontal portion of the frontal lobe appears to be the crucial region for the function known as working memory (Baddeley, 1986; Fuster, 1995a,b). The concept of working memory implies that each action initiated by the prefrontal area is checked against existing memory imprints; new action cannot be carried out without such an extremely brief memory check (Niedermeyer, 1998a). The experimental work of Fuster (1995a,b) has made it clear the dorsolateral region of the prefrontal cortex is the area where "past and future meet." Let us suppose that the working memory is totally suspended for the duration of a spike-wave absence. This could readily explain the unique character of "suspended consciousness" during an absence (Niedermeyer, 1998b; Pavone and Niedermeyer, 2000).

Tonic postural seizures in sleep in otherwise healthy children are associated with rhythmical ictal activity (mainly 6–7/sec) of frontal accentuation, which has been described by Vigevano and Fusco (1993). The tonic attacks consist mainly of flexor spasms. Interictally, there may be frontal spikes. These authors have stressed the benign character of this syndrome: a benign frontal lobe epilepsy, akin to benign rolandic epilepsy (also see Epileptic Spasm/Partial Seizures, above). In frontal lobe epilepsy caused by intracranial tumors, the long-term outcome is more favorable than in nontumoral forms of the frontal lobe epilepsy (Zaatreh et al., 2002).

EEG Observations

Frontal lobe spiking may be found in various forms. Spike activity is particularly scarce and the search for an EEG focus often elusive in mesiofrontal (interhemispheric) foci (Niedermeyer and Walker, 1971). If demonstrable at all, spikes are found over the superior frontal or frontal midline region; their size is small.

Large and somewhat blunted sharp waves have been demonstrated by Tharp (1972) in cases of presumed fronto-orbital epilepsy. Generalized synchronous spike-wave bursts are found in patients with bilateral synchrony. In such cases, the Pentothal test of Lombroso and Erba (1970) or the Valium deactivation test (Niedermeyer, 1970a) may demonstrate the primary EEG focus when the bilateral synchronous discharge is selectively silenced. In some of the cases, only depth EEG can demonstrate the primary focus. The ictal patterns of frontal lobe epilepsy are not basically different from other forms of neocortical focal seizure disorders.

The Special Case of Frontotemporal Epilepsies Affecting Speech

If either the frontal or temporal speech area (dominant hemisphere) is inactivated, the patient becomes aphasic (Penfield and Jasper, 1954). Ajmone Marsan and Ralston (1957) also include the parietal lobe. Electrical stimulation of the supplementary motor zone has been found to produce speech arrest for the duration of the attack only, whereas aphasia persists for some minutes after a seizure electrically induced from the inferior frontal and temporal speech areas (Ajmone Marsan and Ralston, 1957).

Ictal speech arrest alone is but seldom associated with typical ictal symptomatologies of psychomotor seizures (Hécaen and Angelergues, 1960). These authors examined 208 epileptics with ictal speech disturbances. A substantial number (28.3%) of the patients with ictal speech arrest had rolandic focal seizures. The interictal EEG in patients with ictal speech arrest due to a focus in the supplementary motor area may be normal (Peled et al., 1984).

Ictal speech automatisms with linguistically correct words, sentences, or fragments of sentences are usually associated with typical psychomotor automatisms and, somewhat surprisingly, arise in the majority of the cases from the nondominant temporal lobe (Serafetinides and Falconer,

1963). Racy et al. (1980) reported two cases of "epileptic aphasia" in old adults and presumed a "monosymptomatic status epilepticus" on the basis of the paroxysmal and slow EEG activity over the left hemisphere. There is, however, no evidence of truly ictal activity in their tracings.

The Special Case of Autosomal-Dominant Nocturnal Frontal Lobe Epilepsy

This form of epileptic seizure disorder is not uncommon and has thwarted painful attempts at diagnostic clarification through decades. Normal EEG findings and lack of structural pathology have plagued the epileptologists for years. For some time, the somewhat atypical motor attacks (falling short of a full grand mal) have raised the specter of a paroxysmal basal ganglia dyskinesia (Lugaresi and Cirignotta, 1981) or that of a sleep disorder.

The work of Ingrid E. Scheffer and her co-workers (1994) has opened new avenues of thought with the description of the autosomal-dominant nocturnal epilepsy. This epochal discovery has also shown that the genetic forms of epilepsy may occur in the disguise of focal seizure disorders. In this vein, there have been further reports on (a) familial temporal lobe epilepsy (Berkovic et al., 1996) and (b) autosomal-dominant rolandic epilepsy with speech dyspraxia (Scheffer et al., 1995)—to name only two of an evolving group of further regional epilepsies of genetic character (Berkovic et al., 1999).

Is Frontal Lobe Epilepsy an Entity or Are There More Than One Clinical-Epileptological Entities?

While temporal lobe epilepsy—despite a multitude of clinical-ictal manifestations—ought to be considered as a whole (with combined limbic and neocortical features), frontal lobe epilepsy should be conceived as consisting of at least three major forms. Frontal lobe regions simply produce special types of epileptic seizures (Niedermeyer, 1998b).

There is a frontal-premotor type of seizure that is chiefly adversive and associated with loss of consciousness if the prefrontal portion is included. There is a mesiofrontal epilepsy that comprises the supplementary motor region, and there is a fronto-orbital epilepsy with chiefly limbic character. Finally, one should add those forms of frontal lobe epilepsy that cause secondary bilateral synchrony (usually associated with a generalized synchronous spike-wave pattern). Is this due to a special localization or to a certain genetic predisposition for generalized spike-waves?

For the time being, this question remains unanswered.

Epileptic Seizures Arising from the Rolandic (Sensorimotor) Cortex

This subsection essentially pertains to rolandic epilepsies of adult life; benign rolandic epilepsy of childhood and rare cases of progressive rolandic epilepsy in children are presented in the section on age-determined epileptic conditions.

Focal motor seizures arising from the precentral motor region have been well known since the observations of Bravais (1827) and Jackson (1870). These seizures beautifully reflect the somatotopic arrangement of the motor cortex. Jackson (1870) made a clear distinction between seizures starting with twitching of facial and glossal muscles and those starting with finger, hand, or foot movements of the opposite side. His work coincided with the experimental findings of Fritsch and Hitzig (1870), Ferrier (1876), and Hitzig (1874). Further animal work on electrical stimulation of the motor cortex was done by Luciani (1878), Grünbaum and Sherrington (1901, 1903), and Horsley (1909); studies on the exposed human motor cortex were carried out by Foerster (1936a,b), Penfield and Rasmussen (1950), Penfield and Kristiansen (1951), Penfield and Jasper (1954) (also see Chapter 39, "Subdural Electrodes").

The somatotopic arrangement of the motor cortex must not be conceived of as a mosaic in which the smallest focus of epileptic irritation will give rise to contralateral twitching of extremely small corresponding muscular segments. In other words, there does not seem to be full equality among the cortical segments. The experimental work of Liddell and Phillipps (1951) has demonstrated that some segments have lower thresholds to electrical stimulation than others. Areas with a large corticorolandic representation also have low thresholds for electrical stimulation (index finger, thumb, then face and foot). This is probably also true for the less commonly focal sensory seizures arising from the postcentral gyrus.

Clinical-Ictal Manifestations

Clonic twitching of contralateral muscle segments with preserved consciousness is the principal manifestation of cortical motor rolandic epilepsy. This clonic activity may (a) remain localized, (b) spread over the rest of the contralateral half of the body, and (c) eventually culminate in grand mal seizure. The precise semiology of the movements was extensively studied by Holmes (1927), long before movie and videotape (see Oller-Daurella and Oller-Ferrer-Vidal, 1977) could be used for the documentation of fine details. The spread of clonic activity from one body region to another is widely known as jacksonian march (see also Gastaut and Broughton, 1972).

Focal rolandic motor seizures usually last from 10 seconds to several minutes. Attacks exceeding a duration of 30 minutes must be regarded as focal motor status or even as epilepsia partialis continua or Koshevnikov syndrome. According to Janz (1969) (analysis of 365 cases), most attacks started in the hand (62 cases), followed by mouth (58 cases), arm (54 cases), fingers (42 cases), foot (35 cases), face (37 cases), and leg (24 cases). Involvement of trunk muscles was uncommon.

As to epileptic manifestations of the sensory rolandic cortex (postcentral gyrus), a variety of paresthesias or dysesthesias have been observed. Janz (1969) listed the sensations experienced by 150 patients with sensory cortical attacks. "Formication," or the sensation of running ants, was the most common symptom (99 patients), followed by numbness (74 patients), pain (47 patients), and sensations of heat or cold (29 patients). Janz (1969) has pointed out that pain as a sensoricortical ictal symptom is more common than one would expect from experimental data concerning pain perception and the postcentral gyrus. This view, however, is not shared by Michelucci et al. (1985), who have pointed out that pain is an uncommon epileptic manifestation.

Focal motor or sensory attacks can stop at any stage. Sensory focal attacks are usually quickly associated with focal motor activity. According to Hallen (1953), uncontaminated sensory cortical seizures are so rare that one should thoroughly rule out possibilities such as ischemic cerebral attacks or peripheral neuritic pain.

Bilateral focal motor seizures are extremely rare. In such cases, the clonic motions spread from one side gradually to the other half of the body. Janz (1969) observed only three cases of this category; they were caused by multiple cerebral metastasis, multiple sclerosis, and head injury, with the third case being a child of 6. Ipsilateral focal motor and sensory seizures have been reported by Ahuja and Tharakan (1981); their underlying mechanisms are controversial.

Focal motor seizures in infants and children may be found, in rare instances in association with a cerebellar mass or lesion. Such an observation was reported by Harvey et al. (1996), who also provided similar observations from the earlier literature. One wonders if the presence of a cerebellar lesion (in childhood) can cause hyperexcitability of the cerebral motor cortex. A true cerebellar origin (as contended by the authors) is unlikely.

Postepileptic paralysis (Todd's paralysis) has been known since the original observations of Todd (1856). Postictal paresis of the ictally involved muscle segments has been thought to be caused by metabolic exhaustion, but in recent years the concept of active inhibition has prevailed. Postictal motor deficits are more common in active pathology such as vascular lesions, arteriovenous malformations, or tumors. In general, these motor deficits are more common in children and last for minutes, hours, or a few days. Strokes initiated by focal motor seizures do not belong in this category. Further information can be derived from the study of Yarnell (1975).

Is Todd's paralysis always postictal or could it be an ictal phenomenon? This question was raised by C. M. Fisher (1978). Hemiparetic seizures have been reported by Hanson and Chodos (1978), Globus et al. (1982), and Smith et al. (1997). Such "negative epileptic phenomena" (akin to the earlier mentioned "negative epileptic myoclonus") appear to be well documented. The EEG may show contralateral delta waves, spikes, or sharp waves. In general, contralateral slowing represents the usual EEG of Todd's paralysis (Gustavson et al., 2003)

EEG Findings

The ictal EEG shows astounding variations. Lack of ictal EEG changes is a well-known weakness of electroencephalography (Gastaut and Tassinari, 1975; Gibbs and Gibbs, 1952), probably due to the smallness of the cortical spiking (Thomas et al., 1977). In the majority of the cases, ictal repetitive spiking is present over the affected motor cortex. Interictal spike activity also shows variations ranging from absence to pronounced focal spiking, which, incidentally, is most common in children with benign rolandic epilepsy. In patients with acute watershed-type infarctions, focal motor seizures are often accompanied by PLED, discussed in Chapter 13, "Abnormal EEG Patterns: Epileptic and Paroxysmal," and Chapter 17, "Cerebrovascular Disorders and EEG."

Neurophysiological Considerations

Focal motor seizures are usually strictly cortical, but the structural lesion causing the seizures may not be precisely located in the rolandic region. Neighboring lesions may cause the precentral cortex to erupt in epileptic discharges due to its low threshold. Participation of the deep structure is likely to complicate focal motor seizures. Such attacks have been described in acute thalamic vascular lesions (Niedermeyer, 1957). This has been more clearly demonstrated in cases with progressive "malignant" rolandic epilepsy of childhood (Rocca and Niedermeyer, 1992); this subject is more extensively discussed in the sections on status epilepticus and epilepsia partialis continua.

In cortical rolandic focal motor seizure activity and also in focal motor status or epilepsia partialis continua, with negative scalp EEG findings, the use of myoclonus-locked averaging can demonstrate regional spike discharges preceding the myoclonus (Shibasaki and Kuroiwa, 1975; Shibasaki et al., 1978).

Etiology

Onset of focal motor or focal sensory seizures in adulthood must always raise the suspicion of a tumor involving or in the vicinity of the rolandic cortex. This is supported by the data of Hess (1970).

Arteriovenous malformations should also be considered one of the more common causes of focal motor seizures. Posttraumatic epilepsy and cerebral arteriosclerosis are also common causes; neurosyphilis and tuberculoma previously ranked high in the list of causes.

Prevalence

Prevalence is probably between 3% and 10% of a population of epileptics, depending on the sampling.

Parietal Lobe Epilepsy

Epileptic phenomena of parietal origin do not form a well-defined epileptological entity. Parietal lobe functions are complex (Critchley, 1979; Denny-Brown and Chambers, 1958); functional differences between the dominant and the nondominant parietal lobe compound the problems of parietal lobe function.

There is, therefore, no typical parietal lobe seizure symptomatology. In most cases, the seizures affect visual functions, and a variety of complex visual disturbances may be found, such as scintillation or oscillopsia. Short attacks of extremely severe vertigo may occur. Geier et al. (1977c) reported automatisms and ictal tonic postural changes of the upper limbs as parietal lobe phenomena.

Rasmussen (1970) reported 84 surgically treated patients (8.5%) with parietal lobe epilepsy of a total of 989 cases with nontumoral epileptogenic lesions. Trauma was the most common cause of these seizures. Posttraumatic epilepsy caused by lacerating wounds from high-velocity projectiles and shell fragments most often affects the centroparietal region. There are no particular signs from the EEG viewpoint. With the use of MEG (with a whole head neuromagnetometer), Hari et al. (1993) could demonstrate a left parietal mirror spike focus in a patient with a right centroparietal epileptogenic focus. This is unusual when one considers that true mirror foci are believed not to exist outside neurophysiological animal experiments.

Occipital Lobe Epilepsy

Seizures arising from the occipital lobe are not common. When the attacks originate from the calcarine fissure, elementary visual sensations such as bright light, sparks, or a ball of fire are experienced. The sensations may move across the visual field or remain stationary for the duration of the seizure. Spread from a temporal lobe focus into the occipital region with elementary visual ictal sensations has been reported by Gastaut (1958b) (Fig. 27.36). On the other hand, paroxysmal discharges originating from an occipital epileptogenic focus may propagate into the temporal lobe; this has been documented in a patient with psychomotor seizures by means of depth EEG including microelectrodes (Babb et al., 1981).

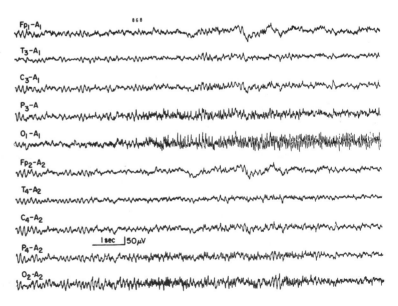

Figure 27.36. Occipital lobe epilepsy; onset of a seizure during which the 39-year-old patient experienced flashing red lights, blurring of vision, and severe headache. Note left occipital onset of fast ictal spiking and subsequent propagation to right occipital and left parietal areas. These attacks occurred during the patient's third pregnancy only. (Patient of the Walter Reed General Hospital, Neurological Service, Washington, D.C; courtesy of Dr. A.D. Huott.) (From Huott, A.D., Madison, D.S., and Niedermeyer, E. 1974. Occipital lobe epilepsy. A clinical and electroencephalographic study. Eur. Neurol. [Basel] 9:325–339.)

Attacks of blindness may be accompanied by generalized spike-wave activity (Strauss, 1963) but this is probably the expression of "benign occipital lobe epilepsy" (see Epileptic Syndromes, above). Bilateral synchronous occipital spike-wave activity has been reported during visual hallucinations (Huott et al., 1974). Epileptic nystagmus, also called oculo-clonic seizures, may occur during occipital lobe seizures (Beun et al., 1984; Chatrian and Spence, 1984; Gastaut, 1960; Giove, 1960; Huott et al., 1974; Penfield and Kristiansen, 1951; White, 1971). The EEG correlates of occipital lobe epilepsy have been extensively studied by Ludwig and Ajmone Marsan (1975), Ikeda et al. (1982), and Marshall (1989).

Occipital lobe epilepsy tends to occur in acute or subacute cerebral disorders (Huott et al., 1974). Occipital lobe epilepsy must be carefully distinguished from migrainous or ischemic disturbances. The differential diagnosis may be quite complex. Hypercalcemia (Barolin and Karbowski, 1973) and nonketotic hyperglycemia (Krendel et al., 1990) have been described as causes of occipital lobe epilepsy with focal spiking.

The occipital lobe is chiefly involved in epilepsies caused (in rare cases) by celiac disease (Gobbi et al., 1997)—an etiology that has been doubted by Cross and Golumbek (2003). In Sturge-Weber disease, epileptic seizures originating from the occipital lobe are the rule; in the vast majority, the occipital lobe foci are unilateral. More information may be found in Chapter 19, "Degenerative Disorders of the Central Nervous System." A progressive form of occipital lobe epilepsy with bilateral symmetrical curvilinear cortical calcifications in the occipital lobe has been described by Sammaritano et al. (1985); there were no cutaneous manifestations in the observed cases, but the possibility of a very atypical form of Sturge-Weber disease cannot be ruled out. Occipital lobe seizures have also been documented in Lafora's form of myoclonus epilepsy (Tinuper et al., 1985). Strictly occipital epileptic discharges are most common before the age of 7 years (Nagendran et al., 1989).

The concept of benign occipital lobe epilepsy (Gastaut, 1982) is presented in another section of this chapter. The differential diagnosis between occipital lobe epilepsy and migraine (especially forms of basilar artery migraine) may be difficult (also see Chapter 29, "The EEG in Patients with Migraine and Other Forms of Headache").

Epilepsies of Deep (Subcortical) Origin

Epileptic seizures of deep subcortical origin are very unusual events. Hypothalamic lesions may occasionally give rise to generalized synchronous seizure discharges with petit mal absences or grand mal. Diencephalic epilepsy with autonomic manifestations (Penfield, 1929) is a rather controversial form of seizure. The epileptogenic character of lipomas of the corpus callosum has been pointed out by Gastaut et al. (1980).

Cerebellar fits is an obsolete term for decerebrate tonic posturing. Trigeminal neuralgia ("tic douloureux") is fundamentally based on epileptic neuronal firing at the pontine level (Fromm, 1992), which explains the good response to some anticonvulsants, but there is no spread whatsoever and no need to list this horrifying disorder among the epilepsies.

In human epileptology, seizures do not arise from the cerebellum. As a matter of fact, it is reasonable to assume that the cerebellum is the origin of seizure-inhibiting impulses (Niedermeyer and Uematsu, 1974). This is congruent with the observation that cerebellar dysfunction increases risk for seizures (Labiner et al., 1987).

Spinal epilepsy is associated with segmental myoclonus and deserves a place in the semiology of spinal cord disease. Shivapour and Teasdall (1980) demonstrated vacuolar degeneration of anterior horn cells as the cause of spinal myoclonus. A special form of spinal epilepsy with tonic attacks, either inhibited or triggered by proprioceptive stimuli, has been described by Egli et al. (1974) in a cervical vascular myelopathy (anterior spinal artery syndrome). Quattrocolo et al. (1987) reported a segmental myoclonus as a sequel of acute anterior poliomyelitis.

For those who are interested in basic epileptic mechanisms at the spinal cord level, the work of Bremer (1958b) and Schwindt and Crill (1984) is recommended.

Considerations of Electrophysiological Characteristics of Temporal Lobe Epilepsy and Other Focus-Determined Epilepsies (Compared with Strictly Dysfunctional Epilepsies)

Characteristics of single spikes may vary according to their degree of complexity; a particularly high degree of complexity was found in spikes over frontal areas and unassociated with cerebral pathology (Rodin et al., 1995). These authors associate spike complexity with a tendency toward generalization (apparently indicating primary generalized epilepsy). In this manner—with the use of the singular value decomposition method—single spikes reveal their relationship to forms of epileptic seizure disorder.

It was mentioned earlier that spikes and/or spike waves may be preceded by negative DC shifts, which are demonstrable even in humans (although with technical difficulties) (Bauer et al., 1989; Chatrian et al., 1964; Cohn, 1954). Such a preceding slow potential could not be found in children with spikes indicating benign rolandic epilepsy (Feucht et al., 1996). The preceding slow DC shift apparently denotes the afferent influx of excitatory messages.

With small dosages of diazepam intravenously given, dysfunction-determined spikes and spike waves are reduced or even blocked for a short period of time unlike structurally determined spikes (as in temporal or frontal lobe epilepsy) which are resistant to the diazepam effect (Niedermeyer, 1970a).

Dysfunctional spikes as a response to arousing stimuli or intermittent photic stimulation (as in primary generalized epilepsy) are the effect of a rapid stimulus-response process. This does differ from spike activity in long-standing structural epileptogenic foci.

With the use of subdural electrodes in epileptic patients, Blume and Kaibara (1993) reported a start-stop-start pattern in the evolution of focal seizure activity: initial spikes first coming to a halt and then resuming their activity with further escalation. The propagation patterns of spikes occurring in temporal lobe epilepsy were studied by Emerson et al. (1995) (with the use of spike averaging—not apparent on visual analysis).

Triggering Mechanisms of Epileptic Seizures

Most epileptic seizures occur without any obvious precipitating mechanisms. Some patients have seizures in a certain set of circumstances, according to circadian cycle or menstrual cycle, in states of tension, or during sudden withdrawal of sedatives or alcohol in addicts and alcoholics. In smaller groups of epileptics, the seizures are triggered by one well-defined precipitating mechanism.

The number of triggering factors is remarkable. Some of them are so rare, perhaps even limited to one person, and so bizarre that only the more important can be discussed. Studies of Gastaut and Tassinari (1966), Bickford and Klass (1969), and especially Forster (1977) have dealt extensively with this subject.

Visually Induced Epilepsies

Convulsive responses to intermittent photic stimulation have been described by W. G. Walter et al. (1946). Subsequent important work was done by Gastaut et al. (1948), Gastaut and Corriol (1948), Gastaut and Gastaut (1949), and Gastaut and Remond (1949). Two major paroxysmal responses were distinguished by Bickford et al. (1952); these are the photomyoclonic and the photoconvulsive responses. These terms are somewhat imprecise because myoclonus and major convulsions may occur in both types, but, in view of the wide acceptance of these designations, no change should be made. This subject has been reviewed by Newmark and Penry (1979).

The photomyoclonic response occurs mainly at flash rates around 14 to 18/sec and consists of marked phase-locked anterior spiking that is most pronounced in the frontopolar leads. The myogenic nature of these driven spikes has been demonstrated by Bickford et al. (1952). Although genuine cerebral spikes are absent on the scalp, depth EEG studies have shown evidence of some deep spiking during the photomyoclonic response (Chatrian and Perez-Borja, 1964). The response does not outlast the flashes, but a gradual buildup of true cerebral spiking may occur afterward.

The photomyoclonic response is, in most instances, a paroxysmal response in a patient who is not suffering from a chronic epileptic seizure disorder. Instead, metabolic changes strongly influence this response, often on a day-to-day basis; even changes from hour to hour may occur. Withdrawal from barbiturates and other sedatives may give rise to a potent photomyoclonic response for a brief period; the same is true for the immediate period after alcohol withdrawal in chronic alcoholics. A photomyoclonic response may be followed by a grand mal seizure in alcohol withdrawal. The myoclonus may show various degrees and tends to be massive rather than subtle. Emotional tension heightens the predisposition to photomyoclonic responses. This response is typically found in adult life. The response may be found in normal volunteers as a transient phenomenon that does not require medication.

The photoconvulsive response is also most readily elicited with flash rates around 14 to 18/sec. The EEG shows prominent generalized bursts of spikes, polyspikes, and irregularly shaped spike-wave discharges with frontal or fron-

tocentral maximum. The response is often accompanied by massive or subtle myoclonus. The paroxysmal discharges tend to outlast the flashes; gradual buildup of prolonged ictal clinical or subclinical activity may occur.

The response is usually found in patients suffering from primary generalized epilepsy and especially in those with a history of grand mal and myoclonic seizures. Children or adolescents with petit mal absences may also show photoconvulsive responses, and, in certain cases, a full-blown petit mal absence with clock-like generalized 3/sec spike waves may be precipitated by the flashes. Major tonic-clonic convulsions (grand mal) may be triggered in certain cases. Poorly classifiable automatism-like seizures may also occur under these conditions, but their EEG correlates are not focal (partial). Sleep, especially non-REM sleep, attenuates all paroxysmal flicker responses. Less epileptogenic are localized occipital or posterior spike responses to stroboscopic photic stimulation (Naquet et al., 1960). Aside from the realm of primary generalized epilepsy, photosensitivity with myoclonus and major convulsions may also occur in children with severe myoclonic epilepsy (Dravet, 1978).

The variety of responses to strobe light and the technique of stimulation are discussed in greater detail in Chapter 14, "Activation Methods." Its author's emphasis on low-luminance visual stimuli has been reasserted at a larger scale (Takahashi, 2002).

Epileptic Responses to Environmental Flickering Light

In these patients, a variety of stimuli triggers the seizures; most often the stimulus is sunlight falling through moving foliage or various artificial flickering lights (Newmark and Penry, 1979). The most common seizures are grand mal convulsions. According to Jeavons and Harding (1975), 84% had grand mal, 6% had petit mal absences, 1.5% had myoclonus, and 2.5% had some form of focal (partial seizures). It is interesting to note that patients with "natural" visual seizure precipitation do not necessarily show massive photoconvulsive responses in the EEG laboratory under strobe light; their flicker responses may be quite mild.

Self-Induction of Visually Evoked Epileptic Phenomena

In rare instances, hand-waving, finger-waving, or rapid blinking while looking at a bright light is used to produce epileptic attacks. These patients appear to be magnetically attracted to this type of manipulation. It is not known if sexual pleasure is derived from these attacks, which are, in most cases, of absence-like character. Petit mal with sexual arousal was habitually produced in a case reported by Ehret and Schneider (1961). Some but not all of these patients are mentally retarded. More about this subject is found in the work of Forster (1977) and Newmark and Penry (1979).

Paroxysmal Responses to Eye Closure

Bursts of generalized spikes and spike-wave-like activity may be precipitated by eye closure in predisposed patients. This is probably a small subgroup of patients with primary generalized epilepsy. Petit mal-like absence is usually produced by this mechanism.

Observations on this subject have been reported by Atzev (1962), Crighel (1963), Gastaut and Tassinari (1966), and Green (1968). Tieber (1972) described this type of precipitation in three siblings. In a patient reported by Vignaendra et al. (1976), this response occurred in the absence of a photoconvulsive response to flicker, which is usually present to a greater or lesser extent. On the other hand, Darby et al. (1980) found induction of bursts and/or seizures by eye closure in seven of 22 flicker-sensitive patients.

This topic attracted renewed interest during the late 1980s and the 1990s. Eyelid closure epilepsy with paroxysmal EEG bursts was mentioned earlier (in its presumed relationship to primary generalized epilepsy). Eyelid closure-induced myoclonias with absences dominate the clinical picture. A special form is characterized by the "fixation-off-sensitive epilepsies" occurring while the eyes are being closed. Panayiotopoulos (1994), the leading proponent in this domain, has placed great emphasis on the differentiation of (a) eyelid-closure photosensitivity (the process of closing the eyes being essential) and (b) eyes-closed-related EEG abnormalities with or without clinical epilepsy (an earlier observation having been reported by Gumnit et al., 1965). The finely detailed differences have to be read in the work of Panayiotopoulos (1994) (together with the important comments of Binnie and T. Takahashi in the same article). This also includes seizures triggered by hand waving.

Television-Induced Seizures

Seizures caused by watching television have been well known since the early observations of Raou and Prichard (1955), Ismay (1958), Klapetek (1959), and Gastaut et al. (1961, 1962). The induced seizures are mainly of the grand mal type. The involved mechanisms are complex; flickering light and certain visual patterns might play a major role. According to Newmark and Penry (1979), these attacks are almost always an indication of general photosensitivity.

Parain et al. (1982) have distinguished two types of television-induced epilepsy. One group has seizures in the vicinity of the screen and is sensitive to the alternating appearance of odd and even lines, but there is usually no hypersensitivity to photic stimulation at 50/sec; the second group is characterized by seizures occurring relatively distant from the screen and there is a definite hypersensitivity to photic stimulation at 50/sec. In this context, it is interesting to note that different frequencies of the AC power source (50/sec in almost all European countries, 60/sec in North America) may influence the occurrence of television-induced epileptic seizures.

Seizures Induced by Visual Exploration

Gastaut and Tassinari (1966) separate these intrinsically triggered attacks from photosensitivity to extrinsic stimuli. A 4-year-old patient of these authors had myoclonic seizures while looking at a colored scarf. A patient of Klass and Daly (1960) had tonic spasms when he was viewing his left hand. Seizures evoked by horizontal gaze have been reported by

Schiff et al. (1982); the partly tonic attacks were initiated by left frontal spiking.

Seizures Induced by Viewing Geometrical Patterns

This rare form of seizure precipitation has been described by Bickford et al. (1953), Bickford and Klass (1969), Ernst (1969), Chatrian et al. (1970a,b), and Dreyer (1972). General photosensitivity and photoconvulsive responses may be present or absent in these patients. Vertical black and white lines are the potent precipitating stimuli. The clinical ictal effect usually consists of myoclonus.

This form can be detected by presentation of tables with patterns or by the combination of flicker stimulation with patterns (see Chapter 14, "Activation Methods"). Half-tone patterns are useful for the activation of occipital lambda waves but fail to induce epileptic activity.

Blinking Causing Rolandic Spikes

Such extremely rare observations were reported by Nadkarni et al. (1994) and Yamagata et al. (1997). These authors ascribed their observations to benign rolandic epilepsy. The report of Vetrugno et al. (1999) showed blinking eliciting central spikes in a 7-year-old boy with psychomotor retardation and dysmorphic features but no clinical seizures. There was evidence of a chromosomopathy.

Reading Epilepsy

The precipitation of epileptic seizures by reading was first reported by Bickford (1954); further cases were subsequently observed by Chavany et al. (1956), H. Stevens (1957), Alajouanine et al. (1959), Critchley (1962), and Atassi (1981). Forster (1977) has added 11 personal observations of reading epilepsy to the thus far known 48 cases. This author lists this type of seizure induction as "epilepsy evoked by higher cognitive function" or "communication-evoked epilepsy (language epilepsy)."

On the other hand, Bickford et al. (1956) have placed the emphasis on peripheral proprioceptive mechanisms. Hypermotility of the jaw and "jaw clinking" or strange laryngeal sensations often precede the first paroxysmal EEG discharges and the seizures. The attacks themselves start with widespread myoclonic or tonic movements and tend to proceed to a grand mal.

The EEG should be accompanied by videotape documentation. The reading material should be selected according to the test procedure designed by Forster (1977). There is focal spiking (left parietal, according to Gastaut and Tassinari, 1966), as well as bilateral synchronous bursts of spikes. This indicates the enigmatic physiopathogenesis of a rare mechanism of seizure precipitation. Some authors noted spike-wave activity during the stage of jaw clicking. A careful study of Epstein and Moore (1982) has shown that the spike-wave activity is not authentically cerebral; these discharges are caused by phasic muscle contraction and correlated head movements.

A new concept of reading epilepsy has emerged: reading epilepsy as an epileptic syndrome with reflex-epilepsy-like mechanisms (Wolf, 1994). According to this investigator, reading epilepsy "has to be warmed up before it fires." Such a rather lengthy warm-up process sets reading epilepsy apart from quick paroxysmal responses.

Eating Epilepsy

Four cases of seizures (myoclonus, absence, psychomotor, or grand mal attacks) triggered by presentation of food, eating, chewing, swallowing, or gastroesophageal distention have been observed by Binnie et al. (1982b). Fiol and Leppik (1984) documented numerous seizures by long-term recording methods in a young adult; the attacks were triggered mostly but not always by the ingestion of food and consisted of head drop followed by confusion and automatism.

Language-Induced Epilepsy

This type of seizure induction was first described by Geschwind and Sherwin (1967) but has been lumped together with reading epilepsy by Forster (1977). Graphogenic seizures induced by writing have been listed among language-induced attacks (Cirignotta et al., 1986; Guterman et al., 1983).

Decision-Making-Induced Epilepsy

This form of seizure induction is closely related to language- and reading-induced epilepsy and probably also to arithmetic-induced epilepsy, described by Ingvar and Nyman (1962). Forster (1977) feels that "the stimulus lies in the higher cognitive functions" under very specific conditions. The EEG of the only observation of these authors shows generalized synchronous spike-wave bursts triggered by chess playing and other forms of decision making. The seizures were of myoclonic character, and there was also a history of a grand mal attack.

Musicogenic Epilepsy

This rare form of seizure precipitation was described by Critchley (1937) following a much earlier report by Merzheevski (1884). The cases described since then (Joynt et al., 1962; Titeca, 1965; Weber, 1956) are somewhat heterogeneous, although listening to music has definitely been the precipitating factor in all of them.

The attacks are mostly psychomotor (complex partial) automatisms, and the induced EEG changes consist of anterotemporal spiking on either side. The spike discharges are usually not present without activation by certain tunes. Music of all styles has been found to be potentially epileptogenic in these cases. The attacks are not consistently reproducible, and an additional emotional factor is very likely.

Wieser et al. (1997) found strong relationships between musicogenic epilepsy and the temporal lobe (especially the right one).

Tapping Epilepsy

A particularly rare form of seizure induction is tapping epilepsy, described by Dawson (1947). Widespread myoclonus was noticed in his patient during examination of the deep tendon reflexes. Contralateral parietal spikes but no seizures were elicited by Negrin and DeMarco (1977) in mostly nonepileptic children by tactile stimulation of the contralateral foot; this is most effective in non-REM sleep. DeMarco (1990) triggered a spike-wave absence with tapping (perhaps a dyshormic arousal response).

Movement-Induced Epilepsy

This seizure-precipitating mechanism has been noted in connection with tonic seizures (Burger et al., 1972) and also with paroxysmal choreoathetosis (Perez-Borja et al., 1967; H. Stevens, 1965), although the latter disorder is not of epileptic nature.

Tooth-Brushing-Induced Epilepsy

Holmes et al. (1982) reported the case of a 12-year-old boy with focal motor seizures induced by oral stimulation and, above all, by tooth brushing. A right frontal low-grade tumor was demonstrated by O'Brien et al. (1996).

Auditory Epilepsy

Pure auditory elicitation of seizures with the use of repetitive stimuli (clicks, etc.) is virtually nonexistent in the human, but is very common in rodents such as the house mouse, deer mouse, rat, or rabbit; the experimental basis has been extensively reviewed by Collins (1972). In the human, a startle mechanism is almost always necessary in order to produce seizures by auditory stimuli.

Startle Epilepsy

After decades of neglect, the precipitation of seizures by startling stimuli has begun to attract considerable interest. Startle mechanisms may be generated by a sudden loud noise or by softly addressing the patient. Somatosensory stimuli may be very effective: simple unexpected touch or stepping into an unexpected hole may trigger an attack.

Most commonly, the attacks are of tonic character with stiffening of the arm or leg contralateral to the epileptogenic focus. These patients tend to have old residual foci due to infantile brain damage with or without porencephalic cysts (Alajouanine and Gastaut, 1958). A myoclonic form of startle epilepsy has been described by Bejar et al. (1985). Bancaud et al. (1967) demonstrated an epileptogenic focus in the frontal supplementary motor region in a patient who benefited from surgical removal of the lesion. A hemiparetic deficit ranging from minimal weakness to hemiplegia is common in patients with startle epilepsy.

In addition to frontal lobe foci, lesions in the vicinity of the parietal interhemispheric fissure may also represent the basis of startle epilepsy. The startle mechanism may occasionally occur in children with Lennox-Gastaut syndrome or Sturge-Weber disease. A study by Aguglia et al. (1984a) deserves special attention (also from the therapeutic viewpoint). Forster (1977) also studied a number of startle epilepsy cases.

It is interesting to note that startle-induced seizures often start with a single spike over the vertex region; this is followed by general desynchronization while toxic spasm develops uni- or bilaterally. A rhythmical spike-wave or spike-wave-like discharge over the vertex may also be noted.

Startle epilepsy must be separated from nonepileptic startle disorder (Alajouanine and Gastaut, 1958) (hyperexplexia). Nonepileptic startle may represent a form of startle-reflex-hyperexcitability on a genetic basis. Such a dysfunction may occur regionally as in the "jumping Frenchmen of Maine." Further research on these jumpers has shown that their startle responses were largely psychologically determined (Saint-Hilaire et al., 1986). Graf et al. (1990) reported startle responses (without paroxysmal EEG accompaniment) in a patient with Lennox-Gastaut syndrome and massive interictal slow spike-wave activity.

Hot Water Immersion–Induced Epilepsy

Epileptic seizures induced by immersion into hot water (about 40°C) may precipitate psychomotor (complex partial) or grand mal seizures (Mofenson et al., 1965; Morimoto et al., 1985).

Vasovagal Syncope Triggering Psychomotor Seizure

This unusual observation was documented by Bergey et al. (1997).

Concluding Remarks

The domain of reflex epilepsy is briefly discussed in the first section of this chapter under basic considerations of epileptic seizure disorders with regard to the animal experiment. In humans, the factors involved in seizure precipitation by external stimuli are particularly complex. Circumscript epileptogenic foci or a general predisposition to seizures may be present.

Ingenious methods have been used to defuse the noxious extrinsic stimuli. The work of Forster and his associates (summarized in Forster, 1977) has been exemplary in this field. These methods include the use of conditioning techniques. This type of custom-tailored therapy is often laborious and expensive; its effectiveness may also wear off over the years, and an epileptic predisposition may find other ways of seizure generation. Therefore, anticonvulsant therapy remains the basic treatment.

Status Epilepticus

The term status epilepticus denotes an "epileptic seizure that is so prolonged or so frequently repeated as to create a fixed and lasting epileptic condition" (see dictionary of Gastaut, 1973, 1975). This author does not specifically mention the duration of these conditions; a length of 30 minutes to 1 hour has generally been regarded as a minimum requirement to justify the use of the term status epilepticus.

There are as many forms of status epilepticus as there are different types of epileptic seizures. Prolongation or a seemingly endless repetition of the attacks, however, is of varying clinical significance according to the type of seizure involved. The term status epilepticus must not be used indiscriminately. Series of major convulsions are often erroneously called status epilepticus; some epileptics tend to have their attacks in clusters, usually of several seizures within a few hours. Neonates show a natural tendency to have prolonged seizures, which may or may not be called "status." All this indicates that there is a certain continuum from clusters of seizures or unusually prolonged seizures to a true status. Extensive studies on status epilepticus have been carried out by Gastaut et al. (1967a-c), Heintel (1972), and Delgado-Escueta et al. (1983c). Froescher's (1979) work is confined to therapeutic approaches.

The electroclinical features of status epilepticus have been reviewed by D. M. Treiman (1995) and new work on its epidemiology has been presented by DeLorenzo et al. (1995). An incidence of 50 patients per 100,000 residents per year was reported. Fountain and Lothman (1995) have reviewed the pathophysiology of status epilepticus; neuronal injury is believed to be the result of a "neurotoxic cascade consisting of multiple parallel process" (this apparently does not pertain to spike-wave absence status according to these authors).

Grand Mal Status (Tonic-Clonic Status)

A full-blown status epilepticus grand mal is a very serious condition that previously had a fairly high mortality rate. Modern advances in the treatment of seizure disorders have reduced the incidence of status epilepticus grand mal.

According to Gastaut et al. (1967a), about 30% of these patients suffer from primary generalized epilepsy and related conditions and 70% suffer from primarily focal epilepsies with secondary generalization. Interestingly, in 56% of the patients of Gastaut et al. (1967a), the grand mal status occurred in patients with no previous history of epilepsy; in other words, status was the first epileptic manifestation. This makes one wonder if such a brain has not "learned" how to stop a single seizure. The most common causes were found to be trauma (posttraumatic epilepsy, status occurring 2–20 months after trauma), brain tumor, and cerebral arteriosclerosis, in that order (Gastaut et al., 1967a). Heintel (1972) found tumor the most frequent cause, followed by trauma and arteriosclerosis. In Celesia's (1976) study, cerebrovascular disorder was the most common etiology. Frontal foci are particularly prone to induce status (Janz, 1960, 1983).

In patients with long-standing destructive brain lesions and epilepsy, status epilepticus as well as the extent of the supratentorial primary lesion play major roles in the development of crossed (contralateral) cerebellar atrophy (Texeira et al., 2002). When one considers the failure of cerebellar structures in generalized-convulsive status epilepticus (Niedermeyer, 1960), one is tempted to stress such a cerebellar-cerebral connection. Still, there remain difficulties understanding the unilaterality of the cerebellar atrophy.

Changes in the gastrointestinal absorption of anticonvulsants caused by trivial infections and incautious withdrawal from anticonvulsants are probably the most common precipitating factors (Hunter, 1959/60; Janz, 1960, 1961, 1983).

In an ongoing status (i.e., after a sizable number of seizures), the patient is in profound coma during and between the attacks. Hyperthermia often develops even above 39°C without apparent cause; the fever is presumably hypothalamic if pneumonia and electrolyte problems can be ruled out. Blood leucocytosis and albuminuria may be present without apparent reason. In such cases, one major convulsion follows another at intervals of a few minutes. The duration of each grand mal, usually 60 to 90 seconds, may be slightly shortened.

The EEG shows slowing and disorganization in the interval until fast low-voltage spiking with focal onset or primary generalizations indicate the onset of a new attack (see previous discussions of types of seizures). Only patients who are curarized permit a good recording of the ictal epi-

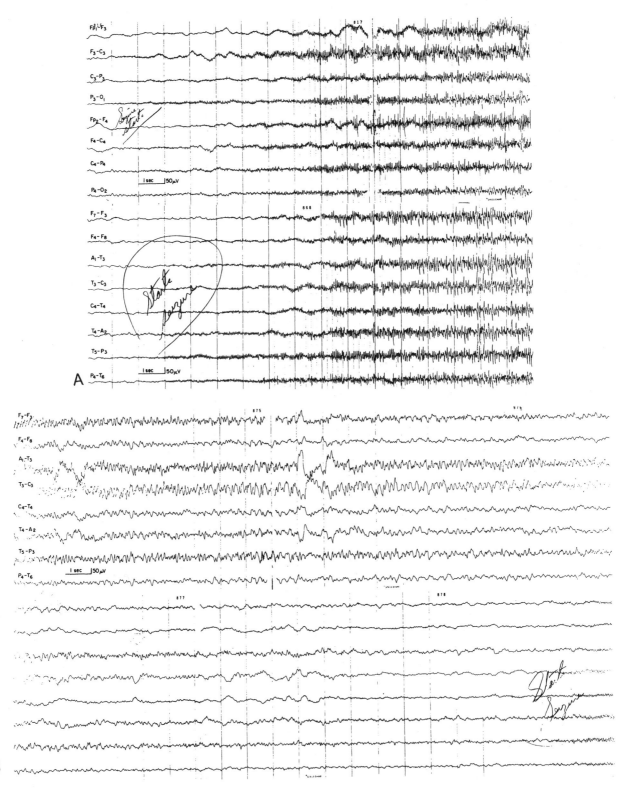

Figure 27.37. **A:** Status epilepticus grand mal in a 20-year-old woman in a state of curarization and artificial respiration. The cause of the status was obscure; the patient was not a known epileptic. Both the upper and the lower eight channels show the onset of two different grand mal attacks during the status. In both instances, the seizure is initiated by left parietal fast spiking with subsequent spread, generalization, and increase of voltage. **B:** Same patient. The bottom part is the continuation of the upper part. It shows the final stage and the termination of a grand mal seizure during the same episode of status as in **A**. Note the general decrescendo of seizure activity and the lack of abrupt termination (compare with Figure 27.5). There is no postictal flatness; instead, there is transitory mixed activity of moderate voltage for a few seconds only until the start of a new seizure. (Patient of the Fitzsimons General Hospital, Neurological Service, Denver, CO; courtesy of Dr. D.S. Madison.)

sodes. Postictally, the record often lacks the postconvulsive flatness or voltage depression that is typical after a single grand mal (Madison and Niedermeyer, 1974; Niedermeyer, 1959, 1960) (Fig. 27.37). These authors have placed much emphasis on the default of postictal flattening and have attributed it to the failure of active inhibition in the postictal stage. One could theorize that this type of inhibition stems from cerebellar structures that, in advanced status, are weakened by hypoxia.

The incidence of grand mal status is not readily determined; the severe form is quite rare. In these advanced cases, intensive care treatment is imperative.

Absence Status (Petit Mal Status)

Following the observation of Lennox (1945), many publications have dealt with petit mal status or absence status. This term implies petit mal lapses in rapid succession and, more often, a prolonged state of impaired consciousness with sluggish mentation or stuporous behavior that must not be regarded as a prolonged petit mal absence. Such twilight states may last for hours or even days.

The first observation of Lennox (1945) was subsequently confirmed by other reports (Bornstein et al., 1956; Dazzi and Lugaresi, 1956; Friedlander and Feinstein, 1956; Goldensohn and Gold, 1960; Jaffe, 1962; Kellaway and Chao, 1955; Landolt, 1956, 1963; Niedermeyer and Khalifeh, 1965; Schwab, 1953; Scott and Masland, 1953; Shev, 1964; Vizioli and Magliocca, 1953; Zappoli, 1955). More extensive reviews of the subject were presented by Lob et al. (1967), Andermann and Robb (1972), Roger et al. (1974), and Karbowski (1985).

Prolonged states of obnubilation are by far more common than series of brief repetitive petit mal absence and present considerable differential diagnostic difficulties. These prolonged twilight states are unique because their ictal-clinical content cannot be related to any type of epileptic seizure. In a strict sense, one is dealing with a special type of epileptic seizure that occurs only as a prolonged episode. Terminological problems can hardly be solved when one considers the petit mal status in all of its three facets: (a) as a status, (b) as a state of altered consciousness, and (c) as a type of seizure that exists only in a prolonged form.

The term petit mal status (Lennox, 1945) was prompted by the observation of almost constant generalized synchronous 3/sec spike-wave activity for the duration of the status. The term spike-wave stupor was suggested by Niedermeyer and Khalifeh (1965) and reemphasized by Kugoh et al. (1987), but the spike-wave discharge is often not present (Lob et al., 1967; Roger et al., 1974).

The clinical symptomatology of a continuous petit mal absence status underlies some inter- and intraindividual variations. The impairment of consciousness has been carefully investigated by Dongier (1967), who distinguishes light obnubilation, with slow mentation, marked obnubilation with confusion, a combination of somnolence-stupor confusion, and a form of "vigil coma" in which the patient is unresponsive to verbal commands, in contrast to the former states, while the response to nociceptive stimuli is preserved. The slow and perturbed mentation also reveals itself

in the domain of speech and design of complex motor actions. In a personal observation, the patient could cook a meal, but the results were disastrous. According to Karbowski (1995), petit mal absence status may occur without any impairment of vigilance.

Rapid eye blinking may be an expression of subtle myoclonus, and there are sometimes more prominent myoclonic body jerks, especially in the myoclonic form described by Terzano et al. (1978). A grand mal attack may occasionally occur at the height of the status. According to Lob et al. (1967), the duration of the episodes in 148 observations ranged from 15 minutes to 31 days; most cases lasted between 2 and 8 hours, but 35 cases exceeded 2 days. Possible triggering factors are onset of the menstrual period, withdrawal or sharp reduction of anticonvulsive treatment, activation with Metrazol or Megimide, hyperventilation, hypoglycemia, intermittent photic stimulation, and electroconvulsive treatment. The termination of the absence status is sudden and abrupt; the patient is then completely his or her old self, and the EEG shows amazing improvement or even normalization. Occasionally a petit mal absence status may occur in the wake of a grand mal convulsion (Bauer et al., 1981); occurrence following childbirth has also been reported (Beaumanoir et al., 1981).

The EEG findings in the ictal episode are more complex than was originally thought. Classical and continuous spike-wave activity is seen in less than half of the cases (41% according to Lob et al., 1967). Fragmented spike waves occurring in repetitive bursts are also quite common (28% according to Lob et al., 1967). Spike-wave activity shows the typical frontal midline maximum, and there is often some polyspike admixture in frontal leads (Fig. 27.38). Irregularly shaped and fragmented spike waves were noted in 10.4%, while in 1.4% (two cases) the record was dominated by repetitive spikes with some degree of intermixed slowing (also see the cases of Rennick et al., 1969). Rhythmical slow activity in the delta or theta range of either frontal or occipital predominance was found in 15.6% (Lob et al., 1967); these records were occasionally punctuated by bursts of rapid spikes at 10 to 20/sec, but, in some cases, rhythmical slow activity appears to be the only striking EEG feature, and spikes are altogether absent.

Unilateral superofrontal onset of spike-wave activity and continuous predominance of spike-wave discharges over this area for the duration of the status are very unusual (Aguglia et al., 1984b; Niedermeyer et al., 1979b) (Fig. 27.39). These observations appear to be incompatible with the concept of petit mal absence status as a primary generalized epileptic event by definition. Another variant of absence status occurs in children with Lennox-Gastaut syndrome. These episodes may be unusually prolonged, exceeding 1 week. The EEG is characterized by generalized slow spike-wave complexes.

As far as age is concerned, Lob et al. (1967) found most observations (31 of 57) in the first two decades of life; the rest were scattered over the span from 21 to 70 years. Even older patients have been reported (Jaffe, 1962; Niedermeyer et al., 1979b).

Figure 27.38. **A:** *Left tracing:* a 47-year-old patient with a history of petit mal absences starting at age 6 years and grand mal since age 15. Patient in petit mal absence status. There are generalized synchronous spikes of frontal accentuation, often forming double and triple spikes, as well as rudimentary spike-wave complexes. *Right tracing:* the same patient during the same recording after diazepam 10 mg i.v. Note total disappearance of spike activity and much drug-induced fast activity. **B:** Same patient. This record was obtained 3 days later; generalized synchronous spike-wave bursts occurred during hyperventilation only. Eyelid fluttering indicates a mild myoclonic component.

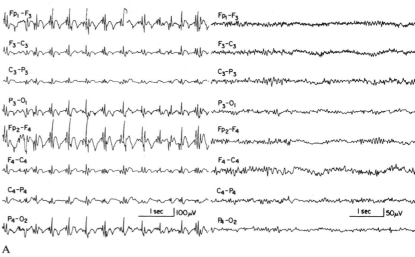

A

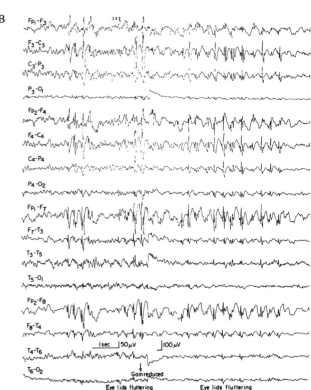

B

Most cases of petit mal absence status (except those of middle or old age) occur in patients with primary generalized epilepsy. These patients have a previous history of simple petit mal absences and/or grand mal and/or myoclonus. Combination with a focal seizure disorder may occur (Berkovic et al., 1985; Niedermeyer et al., 1979b).

In some patients, the absence status occurs without any epileptic antecedents; there are also no underlying structural lesions. The petit mal absence status occurring in children with Lennox-Gastaut syndrome (Brett, 1966) is practically a separate form of status epilepticus. Its response to intravenous benzodiazepines is probably much poorer than in the regular cases, which show an almost immediate cessation of the clinical and EEG changes. Lagerstein and Iffland (1977), however, found an equally good response to intravenous diazepam and clonazepam in both forms of petit mal absence status.

Absence status with generalized polyspike-wave activity may occur in patients with juvenile myoclonic epilepsy (Kimura and Kobayashi, 1996).

Patients with petit mal absence status may be easily misdiagnosed unless EEG tracings are carried out. The differentiation from other prolonged epileptic episodes and from psychiatric conditions is shown in Table 27.13.

The etiology of de novo absence status with onset in middle or old age has been investigated by Thomas et al. (1992). Two factors were stressed by these authors: (a) the emergence of additional epileptogenic factors, and (b) a new and uncommon complication of benzodiazepine withdrawal. Long-term antiepileptic medication may not be required.

Complex Partial (Psychomotor) Status

Lugaresi et al. (1971) pointed out that convincing cases of prolonged temporal lobe automatism could not be found in the literature at that time. On the other hand, status-like series of psychomotor seizures without complete recovery of consciousness in the interval have been reported by Gastaut et al. (1956), Dreyer (1965), and Lugaresi et al. (1971) themselves. This topic was reviewed by Wolf (1970), who discussed several cases including two personal observations.

Within 10 to 20 years, the topic of psychomotor status has become a more widely discussed issue. Karbowski (1980) presented eight personal observations and considered three of them as unequivocal cases of psychomotor status. This author points out that, in most cases, psychomotor status is discontinuous and consists of a series of successive psychomotor automatisms (Fig. 27.40). The existence of a continuous psychomotor status is not ruled out, but Karbowski (1980) felt that a detailed analysis of videotaped data showed that the clinical and EEG picture may camouflage a sequence of single attacks. A primary focus in the hippocampus was demonstrated by Wieser (1980) with depth EEG. In exceptional cases, psychomotor status may be camouflaged as a transient state of aphasia (Dinner et al., 1981).

In a comprehensive review of psychomotor status, Treiman and Delgado-Escueta (1983b) pointed out that

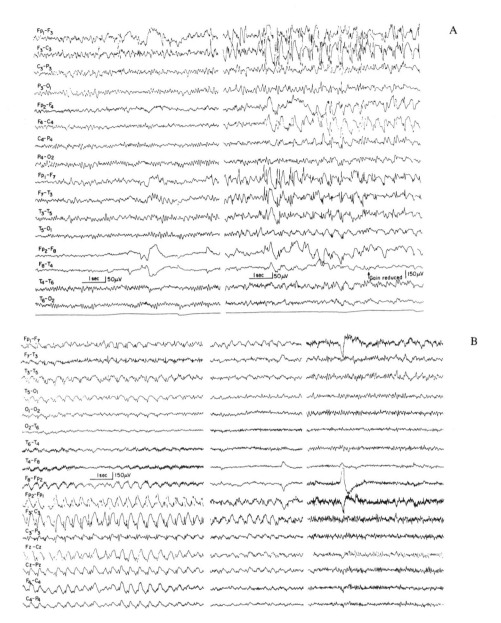

Figure 27.39. **A:** EEG recording from a 23-year-old woman with prolonged episodes of impaired consciousness, associated with frequent smiling, transient aphasic deficits, and right hemiparetic deficits. *Left tracing:* hyperventilation. Appearance of spikes over left superior frontal region (F₃). *Right tracing:* recorded almost immediately afterward. Note onset of rhythmical spike-wave activity (3/sec) with left superior frontal maximum. **B:** *Left tracing:* continuing spike-wave activity with persisting left superior frontal maximum. The last three spike-wave complexes show declining am-

plitude (onset of the effect of i.v. diazepam). *Center tracing:* following diazepam administration, the very last spike waves are noted over the left superior frontal area. *Right tracing:* recorded shortly afterward. Much diazepam-induced fast activity and subtle left frontotemporal slowing. (From Niedermeyer, E., Fineyre, F., Riley, T., et al. 1979b. Absence status (petit mal status) with focal characteristics. Arch. Neurol. (Chicago) 36:417–421.)

about 50 possible cases of this condition had been reported earlier.

Focal Motor Status (Epilepsia Partialis Continua, Koshevnikov Syndrome, Rasmussen Syndrome)

A continuous and circumscript type of focal motor epilepsy has been a classical finding in the wake of Siberian spring-summer encephalitis. This is characterized by constantly repetitive clonic activity of a limited muscular seg-

ment contralateral to the focus. This epileptic activity may be sustained for months and years. Following the first report of Koshevnikov (1895), Russian authors have frequently discussed the role of the cortical and subcortical levels in the physiopathogenesis of this type of focal status (Choroshko, 1908; Omorokov, 1927). Other nonencephalitic types of pathology have also been found as causes of epilepsia partialis continua. For a review of the subject, see the authoritative papers of Juul-Jensen and Denny-Brown (1966) and

Table 27.13.   Petit Mal Absence Status and Its Differential Diagnosis

Epileptic ictal episodes
Petit mal absence status, discontinuous (consisting of repetitive short petit male absences)
Petit mal absence status, continuous (state of obnubilation) (*a*) in a patient with history of primary generalized epilepsy, (*b*) in a patient with no previous history, (*c*) in a patient with a history of focal seizures, (*d*) in a patient with a frontal lobe focus (unilateral), (*e*) in Lennox-Gastaut syndrome
Psychomotor status, discontinuous
Psychomotor status, continuous

Epileptic nonictal episodes
Postconvulsive confusions or delirium after grand mal
Epileptic psychosis, subacute
Chronic psychosis (mostly schizophrenia) in epileptics, mostly with temporal lobe epilepsy

Nonepileptic episodes
Amnestic episodes (global amnesia)
Psychogenic (hysterical) stupor

Thomas et al. (1977). Various tumoral, vascular, and inflammatory lesions have been etiologically linked with focal motor status, but in most of these cases the duration cannot match the length of the Siberian observations (Barolin et al., 1976). Pathological studies may fail to reveal a plausible cause of the focal motor status (Meienberg and Karbowski, 1977). In a sizable number of cases, Singh and Strobos (1980) found nonketotic hyperglycemia as the cause of focal motor status.

The role of Rasmussen encephalitis has been discussed earlier. Various form of local pathology may be the cause of epilepsia partialis continua; among others; neuronal migration anomalies have been reported (Fusco et al., 1992).

Epilepsia partialis continua may be associated with a completely normal EEG, even when the entire rolandic region is carefully explored (Niedermeyer, 1954b). In such cases, the use of myoclonus-locked averaging (Shibasaki and Kuroiwa, 1975) may be helpful in the demonstration of an otherwise hidden focal cortical spike discharge. In other cases, prominent rolandic spiking occurs in conjunction with contralateral twitching (Kugelberg and Widén, 1954). In some cases, even electrocorticographic recording from the precentral gyrus in the waking unanesthetized patient may be spike-free despite ongoing clonic motions (Rocca and Niedermeyer, 1982). On the other hand, Bancaud et al. (1970) and Wieser et al. (1978) have beautifully demonstrated cortical rolandic spikes corresponding with clonic twitching using depth leads. According to Watanabe et al. (1983), a precise time-locked positive spike over the vertex precedes the discharge in the involved flexor hallucis brevis muscle by 32 msec. These data were obtained with jerk-locked computer averaging. An epileptogenic focus in the motor cortex may give rise to transcortical long-loop reflexes, which, according to Watanabe et al. (1984), play an important part in the generation of epilepsia partialis continua.

A remarkable study of 21 adult patients with epilepsia partialis continua and a wide variety of etiologies was carried out by Gurer et al. (2001). There were 16 patients with unilateral lateralized/localized EEG abnormalities during the focal motor seizures. Only one patient had a normal EEG. Lethargy/coma and large infarcts carried a poor prognosis.

Patients with acute cerebrovascular lesions and watershed-type infarctions often exhibit prolonged focal motor attacks that are usually associated with PLEDs (Chatrian et al., 1964). A more extensive discussion of these potentials is found in Chapter 14, "Activation Methods."

Figure 27.40.   Psychomotor (complex partial) status epilepticus in an 18-year-old woman. Patient in light non-REM sleep. There is massive generalized spiking with subtle but indubitable and consistent left posterior temporal accentuation. There are only traces of physiological sleep patterns. Note sudden onset of rhythmical 6/sec activity of spiky character in all leads.

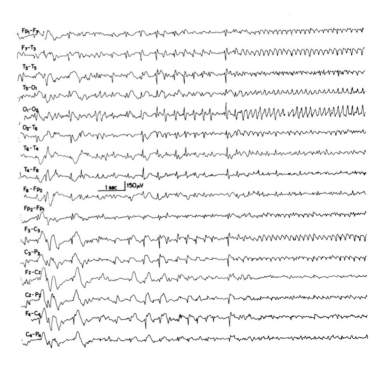

According to Snodgrass et al. (1989), PLEDs represents an intrinsic part of the focal status epilepticus conditions and "could be considered as a form of 'fatigued' clonic phase or as the terminal portion of the latter."

Paradoxical ipsilateral localization of spike (sharp wave) activity in epilepsia partialis continua has been reported by Adelman et al. (1982); these authors explained their surprising findings by the presence of a dipole.

Focal Sensory Status

An exceptional observation of a focal sensory status epilepticus was made by Luengo et al. (1984) in a young adult who had sustained a severe craniocerebral trauma 3 years earlier. The status consisted of recurrent episodes of pain and paresthesiae in the left upper limb. A right-sided occipital lobe status with focal spiking and of 6 days' duration was characterized by left tonic deviation of gaze and prosopagnosia (Garrel et al., 1987).

Various Other Types of Focal (Partial) Status Epilepticus

For more detailed description, see Passouant et al. (1967) and Roger et al. (1974).

1. Hemiconvulsive status: practically a variant of focal motor status, but more severe and potentially fatal, with chiefly clonic activity in one-half of the body. The EEG shows widespread ictal spiking over the affected hemisphere; the onset is chiefly frontal. This type occurs mainly in acute CNS syndrome of infancy and early childhood (also see HHE syndrome).
2. Hemiclonic status: strictly clonic status with widespread repetitive spike activity over the involved hemisphere.
3. Adversive status: often in older adults with cerebrovascular disorder, with adversive attacks in rapid succession, arising from the primarily involved frontal region when the ictal EEG discharge starts before becoming widespread over the entire hemisphere (Takahashi et al., 1990).

With the use of CT scanning and MRI, postepileptic cerebral edema can be documented in cases of focal (partial) status epilepticus (even in the absence of preexisting structural lesion). The area of maximal cerebral edema corresponds with the clinical and electroencephalographic localization of the focal epileptogenic disturbance (Sammaritano et al., 1984).

Tonic Status

Tonic status is uncommon, found mainly in adolescents, and characterized by brief attacks of bilateral tonic spasms associated with runs of rapid spikes or very fast polyspikes on the EEG, in generalized synchrony with frontal maximum (see Gastaut et al., 1967c). These patients usually show the characteristics of the Lennox-Gastaut syndrome. Tonic status epilepticus may last for 1 to 3 weeks.

Myoclonic Status

Massive myoclonus may repeat itself for days or hours. This form of status is very rare in patients with primary generalized epilepsy and usually occurs in children with Lennox-Gastaut syndrome (Gastaut, 1983; Roger et al., 1967; Storm van Leeuwen et al., 1969).

Almost continuously repetitive myoclonic activity is common in forms of progressive myoclonus epilepsy (Lafora-Unverricht-Lundborg disease, dyssynergia cerebellaris myoclonica Ramsay Hunt) (see Chapter 19, "Degenerative Disorders of the Central Nervous System") and in metabolic and toxic encephalopathies. In acute anoxia, myoclonus may be constantly noted while the patient is in profound coma (Gaches, 1971; Krumholz et al., 1984; Madison and Niedermeyer, 1970; Pampiglione and Harden, 1968). Permanent myoclonus may be the outstanding feature in chronic postanoxic myoclonus ("action myoclonus," "intention myoclonus"; Lance and Adams, 1963). The EEG shows a variety of patterns in these conditions.

Nonconvulsive Status Epilepticus

There are only two forms of status epilepticus that fall into the category of nonconvulsive status: (a) absence status (petit mal status), and (b) complex partial status (psychomotor status). The former is rare and the latter is very, if not extremely, rare. Both of these terms are accordingly quite seldom used nowadays while, on the other hand, the term nonconvulsive status became very fashionable during the 1980s and 1990s (Kaplan, 1996). With this changing picture of nonconvulsive status, the prognosis has become very grave and commonly fateful.

As strange as it may sound, much of the blame for this confusion and misnaming has to be put on the EEG! This statement, however, is more apparent than real. It is not the EEG that has to be blamed, but rather the lack of clinical-EEG integration! The clinical findings widely differ from those of the benign transient situation of absence and complex partial status, which respond readily to i.v. benzodiazepine treatment. In some ways, however, there are EEG similarities between the benign true nonconvulsive status and that what is falsely called nonconvulsive status. Figure 27.41 easily explains the difference (Niedermeyer and Ribeiro, 2000).

The false nonconvulsive status does not even represent a real status epilepticus. Practically all of the cases are being caused by cerebral anoxia, associated with coma and an extremely severe acute anoxic encephalopathy, which naturally tends to lead to a fatal outcome. Spike waves, double spike waves, and similar repetitive spike patterns show a superficial similarity to the patterns of true nonconvulsive status. Leaving aside extremely unusually profound forms of true nonconvulsive status, these patients are not comatose. They are confused but ambulatory and not in a protracted profound coma (Niedermeyer and Ribeiro, 2000). Furthermore, those comatose anoxic patients are frequently not even nonconvulsive, since subtle myoclonus is a common accompaniment of the spikes and spike waves (Madison and Niedermeyer, 1974).

Pragmatic Use of the EEG in Diagnosis

Clinical evaluation of a presumed epileptic individual without the use of the EEG is almost unthinkable. As a func-

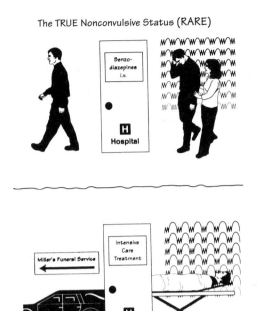

The TRUE Nonconvulsive Status (RARE)

The FALSE Nonconvulsive Status (COMMON)

Figure 27.41. This figure clearly shows the differences between the true and the false nonconvulsive status epilepticus. Striking EEG similarities can be quite misleading in such cases. (Reprinted with permission of *Clinical Electroencephalography.*)

tion-oriented test, the EEG is ideally suited for the demonstration of paroxysmal abnormalities.

Epileptic events are necessarily accompanied by paroxysmal discharges; however, these may be undetectable on the scalp because of small focus in a buried cortical sulcus or in deep limbic or subcortical regions. Limitation of the ictal firing to lamina V may be the cause of lack of spikes on the cortical surface (Elger and Speckmann, 1979; also see Chapter 2, "Introduction to the Neurophysiological Basis of the EEG and DC Potentials"). Without concomitant involvement of larger cortical contingents, deep discharges can be missed. The use of nasopharyngeal and/or sphenoidal leads in presumed inferomesiotemporal discharges is helpful only in a limited number of cases. The use of depth EEG must be restricted to the small number of patients who are candidates for seizure surgery, and even a sizable number of depth leads may miss certain local epileptic events.

On the other hand, paroxysmal discharges may also occur in a substantial number of patients without an epileptic seizure disorder (Lugaresi and Pazzaglia, 1975; Zivin and Ajmone Marsan, 1968). Hence, epileptic discharges may be either too concealed or too readily available, enticing the electroencephalographer to imprudent interpretations. It must be kept in mind, however, that paroxysmal discharges in nonepileptic patients are false-positive findings in a very limited sense only; they are not meaningless. Spikes in nonepileptics clearly indicate a certain degree of proneness or predisposition to epileptic seizure or may even foreshadow a future seizure disorder. The diagnosis of an epileptic seizure disorder must never be made on the sole basis of spikes in the EEG. Useful practical guides

for routine studies in epilepsy have been presented by Engel (1984) and Dinner and Lüders (1985).

In the course of the development of epilepsy monitoring units, the clinical value of interictal spikes has been belittled by most investigators, who, in these special units, are hunting for seizure documentation, i.e., ictal rather than interictal patterns. The interictal spike discharges, however, must not be underrated as an important indicator of paroxysmal activity (Hughes, 1989; Niedermeyer, 1990a).

Use of Activation Methods

Various methods of activation have been used to enhance otherwise undetectable paroxysmal activity. These methods are more extensively discussed in Chapter 14, "Activation Methods." Some of them constitute a part of the standard EEG recording in each major laboratory. Hyperventilation is mandatory in every cooperative presumed-epileptic patient, and the same is true for intermittent photic stimulation. In most major North American EEG laboratories, sleep, either natural or with sedation, is a part of the recording of an epileptic and is regarded as a complementary exploration of states of consciousness other than the waking state. Sleep deprivation further facilitates paroxysmal activities and is a true activation. A whole list of procedures can be put together; all of them aim at the demonstrability of otherwise hidden epileptic discharges (Table 27.14). The timing of the recording may be important. Focal as well as generalized spiking may be activated shortly after an epileptic seizure (Ajmone Marsan and Zivin, 1970; Bauer, 1975; Kaibara and Blume, 1988), but postictal suppression or attenuation of a focus may also occur. A very useful review of the practical value of EEG studies in epileptic patients has been presented by Engel (1984).

Eye opening and closure will demonstrate certain forms of visually induced epilepsies, especially with eye closure. Hyperventilation is the classical activation for petit mal absences and the 3/sec spike-wave discharge; it is much less effective in other forms of epileptic seizure disorder and yet may be capable of inducing practically every type of seizure or the EEG correlate of rudimentary attacks. In some cases of temporal lobe epilepsy, hyperventilation may prove to be remarkably informative. Children below the age of 3.5 years usually do not cooperate with this test; some older children almost enjoy it and may even overdo it a bit. The yield of intermittent photic stimulation is enormous, although limited to a rather small domain of epileptology. However, it may prompt paroxysmal responses in some nonepileptics.

Sleep records made in periods of deep drowsiness, stage 1 and non-REM sleep and stage 2, usually 10 to 30 minutes, are an important part of the EEG evaluation. In generalized as well as in focal (partial) epilepsies, the paroxysmal discharges may be limited to light sleep. The informative value of short sleep tracings with or without sedation has been emphasized by Gastaut et al. (1983, 1984) and Niedermeyer and Höller (1984). Long-term EEG monitoring has demonstrated the increase of spike activity during nocturnal sleep (Martins da Silva et al., 1984).

Sleep deprivation works differently; in this case, the important element in facilitation of paroxysmal discharges is not sleep itself, but fatigue; the patient should be kept from

Table 27.14. EEG Activation Methods for Enhancement of Paroxysmal Discharges

A. *First-line methods*
    Eye opening and closure
    Hyperventilation
    Intermittent photic stimulation (flicker)
    Sleep (short diagnostic non-REM sleep)
    Cautious reduction of anticonvulsive medication (timing depending on
        type of medication and its metabolism)
    Sleep deprivation
    Timing of EEG recording to menstrual cycle (premenstrual hydration)
B. *Second-line methods*
    Convulsants
        Pentylenetetrazol (Metrazol) i.v.
        Bemegride (Megimide) i.v.
    Combined flicker and pentylenetetrazol i.v.
    Methohexital (Brevital) i.v.
    Use of special trigger mechanisms (cutaneous stimuli, viewing
        geometrical structures, visual exploration, startling stimuli)
    Induced hypoglycemia (insulin, fasting)
    Hypoxia (breathing nitrogen)
    Alpha-Chloralose
C. Use of special technology for greater length of recording
    Long-term monitoring

falling asleep in the laboratory. An impressive bulk of literature on sleep deprivation has accumulated during the past 10 years. More information is found in the work of Binnie et al. (1982a), Degen and Degen (1984), and Ellingson et al. (1984), to name just a few of the numerous investigators in this field.

The reduction of long-standing anticonvulsive medication must be handled with great caution, especially when primidone (Mysoline) and phenobarbital are involved. The EEG should be scheduled on the day after reduction of these drugs by 50% for 1 day. More radical reduction for a longer period of time may prompt seizures or even a dangerous status epilepticus grand mal. Interestingly, interictal focal spike activity is not significantly enhanced during the withdrawal phase despite the enormously heightened risk of grand mal seizures (Marciani et al., 1984). No effect on spike localization and seizure symptomatology was noted with acute withdrawal of antiepileptics (Marks et al., 1991).

In candidates for seizure surgery with depth implants, the production of seizures may be necessary in order to study the origin of the attacks. One must not forget that activation by reduced medication gives rise to a certain epileptic rebound and hence does not necessarily reflect the natural state of the patient's seizure disorder.

There are certain mysterious day-to-day changes in the degree of a patient's epileptic activity. It may require a detective's acumen to obtain some insight into certain cycles of epileptogenicity in a given patient. In menstruating women, the premenstruum may be an optimal time for a high-yield EEG recording due to increased hydration with some degree of cerebral edema. In epileptic patients with improvement of seizure frequency after initiation of antiepileptic medication, the interpretation of repeat tracings requires particular caution and restraint because the congruence of clinical improvement and the amount of paroxysmal EEG activity is quite limited (Van Parys, 1981).

Second-line activations are of value only in a few patients; the use of the right trigger mechanism may be very effective. Other methods are of dubious value, especially the use of convulsants, which often activate mechanisms involved in primary generalization before an active cortical focus is put into action. The work of Ajmone Marsan and Ralston (1957) clearly shows the limitations and pitfalls of this method. The combined flicker-pentylenetetrazol method of Gastaut (1949) is interesting for the determination of the individual paroxysmal threshold, but fails as a pragmatic method in the diagnosis of epileptic seizure disorders. Methohexital (Brevital) intravenously tends to activate temporal lobe spikes (Wilder, 1969; also see earlier work of Kajtor, 1956, 1957, and Kajtor et al., 1957, 1958, with recordings from the human hippocampus) and generalized seizures (Celesia and Paulsen, 1972), but it is probably not superior to sleep induced by oral sedatives or unsedated sleep (Table 27.14).

Repetition of EEG recordings in a patient who stubbornly refuses to show the expected paroxysmal discharges will gradually lead to success, but this philosophy is neither elegant nor economical; it may even suggest monetary greed. The EEG obtained in the laboratory is a small window in the patient's daily EEG activity, but this limited recording period can be exploited with the crafty use of numerous channels for better localization and an arsenal of activating methods. This window can be enlarged by prolonged recording in the laboratory over, say, several hours. Instead of the laboratory record, EEG biotelemetry can be done for hours or a full day, permitting much deeper insight into the actual incidence of paroxysmal events in addition to the videotaped behavioral ictal or nonictal changes. In the wake of earlier studies (Köhler and Penin, 1970; Stevens et al., 1971), this method has been used in a number of major institutions (Penry, 1980; Penry and Porter, 1977; Porter, 1980). Personal experience has been a mixture of gratification and disappointment. More remarkable is the cassette approach, for instance with four-channel 24-hour ambulatory cassette recording (Gotman et al., 1980; Ives and Wood, 1980; Sato and Penry, 1980; Woods and Ives, 1977).

These monitoring devices represent considerable progress as far as the documentation of the patient's daily ictal or nonictal epileptic activity is concerned. Their shortcomings are somewhat academic and lie in the limitation of channels and the loss of fine detail in the enormous wealth of data. Some of these shortcomings have been remedied over the past years. Further information is found in the work of Stefan and Burr (1982), Ebersole et al. (1983), Brey and Laxer (1984), Drake (1984), Van der Weide and Kamp (1984), Kamp (1984), and particularly in Chapter 40. EEG monitoring had totally overshadowed all of the earlier mentioned procedures. "Principles of Computerized Epilepsy Monitoring." In many countries, special epilepsy monitoring units have superseded the ambulatory method.

Epileptic Versus Nonepileptic Seizures

With our insight into the morphology and distribution of epileptic EEG discharges, nothing ought to be easier than the differentiation of truly epileptic seizures from nonepileptic attacks such as syncope, hypoglycemia, and hysterical psychogenic and faked attacks.

In the majority of cases, the EEG is indeed extremely helpful in this differential diagnosis, but the difficulties are greater than might be expected. Even with the use of EEG monitoring, there are occasional problem cases. Some of these patients are epileptics who also happen to have psychogenic attacks. In these patients, there may be indubitable interictal spiking, but the attacks themselves are psychogenic. The use of excessive amounts of anticonvulsants leading to a state of drug toxicity may result in an inability to cope with stressful situations, culminating in classical hysterical seizures in somewhat predisposed individuals (Niedermeyer et al., 1970b). Moreover, persons with stigmata of hysteria and individuals with a tendency toward malingering may have misleading minor paroxysmal abnormalities in the resting EEG, perhaps as an indication of their "neuronal excitability" and lack of impulse control. For these reasons, the differential diagnosis may be a bit blurred.

Influence of Anticonvulsive Medication on the EEG of Epileptic Patients

The use of anticonvulsants tends to reduce seizures as well as paroxysmal EEG discharges. These two effects are mostly congruent but discrepancies are sometimes seen. The drug-induced changes are described in detail in Chapter 33, "EEG and Neuropharmacology," and Chapter 34, "EEG, Drug Effects, and Central Nervous System Poisoning."

Anticonvulsant toxicity may reach the degree of severe encephalopathy. In the case of barbiturates, beta activity may disappear when some degree of toxic cerebral impairment is reached (Niedermeyer et al., 1977b). Phenytoin first slows the alpha frequency down to the theta range and, with progressive signs of encephalopathy, such as euphoria, depression, dysarthria, dizziness, vertigo, or ataxia (Roseman, 1961), marked delta activity of anterior accentuation appears. In sleep, one may look in vain for physiological spindles that may be supplanted by widespread rhythmical activity in the 8 to 10/sec range or even slower.

In patients with such a degree of phenytoin toxicity and serum level concentrations above 40 mg/1,000 mL, the EEG is usually spike free and the clinical seizure disorder is well controlled. With increasing toxicity, however, seizures may return and high-voltage spiking may be present (Levy and Fenichel, 1965). Even fatal status epilepticus has been observed at this stage (Utterback, 1958). Ambrosetto et al. (1977) noted phenytoin encephalopathy despite low serum levels (presumably idiosyncratic). While the predominantly cerebellar effects of phenytoin CNS toxicity (acute or subacute) are well known, the nature of a subacute or chronic phenytoin encephalopathy has been widely ignored. In this condition, cerebral impairment may be very pronounced, with mental deterioration, choreoathetoid movements, dystonic movements, opisthotonus, and facial grimacing. More information is found in the work of Lühdorf and Lund (1977) and Niedermeyer (1983, 1990b). Yoshida et al. (1985) have stressed the occurrence of orofacial dyskinesias. The EEG is usually devoid of spike activity and dominated by disorganized diffuse slowing. Unfortunately, the patient's uncontrolled movements are sometimes mistaken for epileptic manifestations, resulting in an increase of phenytoin medication with disastrous results. At apparently nontoxic serum levels, carbamazepine (Tegretol) may occasionally enhance diffuse slow activity (Besser et al., 1995). Furthermore, paroxysmal discharges may be enhanced (especially generalized synchronous patterns), and the seizure disorder may take a turn for the worse (Sachdeo and Chokroverty, 1986; Snead and Hosey, 1985). As to the newest generation of antiepileptic medication, more time is needed for a fair assessment.

It is very important to consider the possibility of such iatrogenic encephalopathies in the evaluation of epileptic patients; the EEG can greatly assist the clinician by providing such clues, even when monitoring of anticonvulsant serum levels is done almost routinely. Let us not forget that therapeutic monitoring shows the drug level in the serum but not in the target organ, the brain.

Magnetoencephalography as an Alternative to EEG in Epileptic Conditions?

There is no doubt that magnetoencephalography (MEG) can provide us with outstanding insights into localization and mechanisms of epileptic activity (see Chapter 57). Barkley and Baumgartner (2003), point out that "the combined use of whole-head MEG systems and multichannel EEG in conjunction with advanced source modeling techniques is an area of active development and will allow a better noninvasive characterization of the irritative zone in presurgical epilepsy evaluation." In spite of its comparative simplicity and its generally affordable price range, the EEG has proved to be an equal partner in this friendly competition.

Concluding Remarks

The pragmatist may ask for a numerically precise answer to the following questions: such as "How useful is the EEG in epileptic seizure disorder? How many false-positive or false-negative EEG findings occur in the EEG evaluation for presumed seizures?" Unfortunately, there are no simple answers. According to Bickford (1963), a normal EEG excludes epilepsy in 70% without activation and in 90% with activation. These are somewhat misleading figures. When we consider a population of epileptic children with a large segment of febrile convulsions, then the usually normal character of the EEG in febrile convulsions will sharply reduce the percentage of abnormal EEG records.

The same is true for a population of patients with alcohol withdrawal seizures and normal interictal tracings, yet the normalcy of the EEG in febrile convulsions and in patients with alcohol withdrawal seizures is an asset and not a shortcoming of the EEG diagnosis of epileptic conditions. Leaving aside febrile convulsions and alcohol withdrawal seizure, the occurrence of a normal EEG in a patient referred because of epileptic seizures must be viewed prudently. Hughes and Gruener (1985) found 300 abnormal (84%) and 58 normal (16%) records in patients considered to have

Table 27.15.   Usefulness of EEG in Various Epileptic Conditions

	Overall Usefulness	False Negatives	False Positives	Comments
Neonatal convulsions	+++	Normal in benign forms	±	Most valuable in differentiation of severe and benign forms
West syndrome (infantile) spasms)	++++	May occur (normal but very high voltage)	±	Hypsarrhythmic pattern practically diagnostic
Febrile convulsions	+	Normal EEG the rule!	Abnormal EEG suggestive of febrile seizures	Value of EEG lies in predominantly normal findings
Lennox-Gastaut syndrome	+++	Almost negligible	+ (difficult differential diagnosis)	A diagnosis grossly based upon EEG. Sleep record helpful
Primary generalized epilepsy (in general)	+++	Almost negligible	+ (seizure-free relatives, other conditions)	Often sleep record needed for EEG evidence, photic stimulation helpful
Pure petit mal absences	++++	No petit mal absence without spike-waves	+	Extremely reliable correlation
Juvenile myoclonic epilepsy	++	?	+	Sleep record, photic simulation helpful
Benign rolandic epilepsy	+++	Almost negligible	++ (seizure-free despite predisposition)	Often sleep record needed for EEG evidence
Benign occipital lobe epilepsy	++	+	+	
Temporal lobe epilepsy	++	+ (repeat records often needed)	+	Sleep record a necessity, EEG diagnosis may require patience
Frontal lobe epilepsy	+	+	+	Difficult EEG diagnosis
Epilepsy of motor cortex	0–++	May be ++	?	A weak spot in the EEG diagnosis
Other focal epilepsies	0–++	+	+	May or may not be reliable
Epilepsies due to unusual triggering factors	++	+	?	Value of EEG depends on imaginative use of activation
Alcohol-withdrawal epilepsy	+	Normal EEG the rule! (mostly of low voltage)	Abnormal record suggests different genesis of epilepsy	Value of EEG lies in predominantly normal findings
Status epilepticus convulsive	+	/	Negligible	May indicate severity of status—helps differential grand mal/tonic/myoclonic
Status epilepticus nonconvulsive	+++	Negligible	±	Excellent in detection of absence status, good in detection of psychomotor status
Psychogenic seizures (pseudoseizures)	+	Normal EEG expected to be the rule but there are many exceptions	Abnormal records not uncommon in patients with psychogenic seizures	EEG useful in spite of its limitations (EEG-video monitoring may be needed)

seizures. Follow-up studies, however, revealed that 28 of the 58 patients with normal records were eventually found to have no seizures, and only nine (2.5%) proved to have indubitable epileptic seizures. These figures stem from a laboratory of highest expertise and underscore the significance of EEG in the diagnosis of seizure disorders. Without the EEG, the differentiation of age-determined epileptic conditions would be almost impossible; this breakdown of epileptological entities is of great practical therapeutic and prognostic significance. Table 27.15 demonstrates the degree of usefulness of EEG findings in various forms of epileptic seizure disorder.

We will therefore avoid simplistic answers to simplistic questions. The value of EEG is determined by intangibles such as the technical quality of the laboratory technicians and the caliber of the electroencephalographer; on his or her experience and effort hinge the thoroughness and trustfulness of the EEG interpretation. For such obvious reasons, the reader will look in vain for easy answers; there are none. There are no shortcuts on the thorny path to expertise in EEG.

References

Adelman, S., Lueders, H., Dinner, D.S., et al. 1982. Paradoxical lateralization of parasagittal sharp waves in a patient with epilepsia partialis continua. Epilepsia (New York) 23:291–295.

Adeloge, E., and Adeku, E.L. 1971. Epilepsy after missile wounds of the head. J. Neurol. Neurosurg. Psychiatry 34:98–103.

Agnetti, V., Mannu, L., and Murrighile, M.R. 1985. Post-stroke epilepsy. Electroencephalogr. Clin. Neurophysiol. 60:71P(abst).

Aguglia, U., Tinuper, P., and Gastaut, H. 1984a. Startle-induced epileptic seizures. Epilepsia (New York) 25:712–720.

Aguglia, U., Tinuper, P., and Farnarier, G. 1984b. Ictal status with frontal onset in acute prolonged confusion in later life. Electroencephalogr. Clin. Neurophysiol. 57:51P–52P(abst).

Aguglia, U., Gambardella, A., Zappia, M., et al. 1995. Negative myoclonus during valproate-related stupor. Neurophysiological evidence of a cortical non-epileptic origin. Electroencephalogr. Clin. Neurophysiol. 94: 103–108.

Aguilar, M.J., and Rasmussen, T. 1960. Role of encephalitis in pathogenesis of epilepsy. Arch. Neurol. (Chicago) 2:663–676.

Ahuja, G.K., and Tharakan, J. 1981. Ipsilateral seizures. Epilepsia (New York) 23:555–561.

Aicardi, J. 1983. Myoclonus as a manifestation of degenerative disorders of the central nervous system in childhood. Electroencephalogr. Clin. Neurophysiol. 56:2P.

Aicardi, J. 1985. Early myoclonic encephalopathy. In *Epileptic Syndromes in Infancy, Childhood, and Adolescence,* Eds. J. Roger, C. Dravet, M. Bureau, et al., pp. 12–21. London: Libbey.

Aicardi, J. 1994. *Epilepsy in Children,* 2nd ed. New York: Raven Press.

Aicardi, J., and Goutières, F. 1978. Encéphalopathie myoclonique néonatale. Rev. EEG Neurophysiol. 8:99–101.

Aicardi, J., Chevrie, J.J., and Rousselie, F. 1969. Le syndrome spasmes en flexion, agénésie calleuse, anomalies chioriorétiniennes. Arch. Franç. Pédiatr. 26:1103–1120.

Aigner, B.R., and Mulder, D.W. 1960. Myoclonus: clinical significance and approach to classifications. Arch. Neurol. (Chicago) 2:600–615.

Aird, R.B., and Gastaut, Y. 1959. Occipital and posterior electroencephalographic rhythms. Electroencephalogr. Clin. Neurophysiol. 11:637–656.

Aird, R.B., and Woodbury, D.M. 1974. *The Management of Epilepsy.* Springfield, IL: Charles C Thomas.

Ajmone Marsan, C. 1969. Pathophysiology of the EEG pattern characteristics of petit mal epilepsy, a critical review of some of the experimental data. In *The Physiopathogenesis of the Epilepsies,* Eds. H. Gastaut, H.H. Jasper, J. Bancaud, et al., pp. 236–248. Springfield, IL: Charles C Thomas.

Ajmone Marsan, C., and Lewis, M.R. 1960. Pathologic findings in patients with centrencephalic seizure patterns. Neurology (Minneapolis) 10:922–930.

Ajmone Marsan, C., and Ralston, B.L. 1957. *The Epileptic Seizure.* Springfield, IL: Charles C Thomas.

Ajmone Marsan, C., and Zivin, L.S. 1970. Factors related to the occurrence of typical paroxysmal abnormalities in the EEG records of epileptic patients. Epilepsia (Amsterdam) 11:361–381.

Alajouanine, T., and Gastaut, H. 1958. La syncinésie-sursaut et l'épilepsie-sursaut à déclenchement sensoriel ou sensitif inopiné. In *Bases Physiologiques et Aspects Cliniques de l'Épilepsie,* Ed. T. Alajouanine, pp. 199–231. Paris: Masson.

Alajouanine, T., and Lhermitte, F. 1965. Acquired aphasia in children. Brain 88:653–662.

Alajouanine, T., Nehlil, J., and Gabersek, V. 1959. À propos d'un cas d'epilepsie déclenchée par la lecture. Rev. Neurol. (Paris) 101: 463–467.

Alberici, M., Rodrigues de Loress Arnaiz, G., and De Robertis, E. 1969. Glutamic acid decarboxylase inhibition and ultrastructural changes by the convulsant allylglycine. Biochem. Pharmacol. 18:137–143.

Alström, C.H. 1950. A study of epilepsy in its clinical, social and genetic aspects. Acta Psychiatr. Scand. (Copenhagen) 63:284.

Alzheimer, A. 1907. Die Gruppierung der Epilepsie. Allg. Z. Psychiatr. 64:418–435.

Ambrosetto, G., Tassinari, C.A., Baruzzi, A., et al. 1977. Phenytoin encephalopathy as probable idiosyncratic reaction. Epilepsia (New York) 18:405–408.

Andermann, E. 1980. Multifactorial inheritance in the epilepsies. In *Advances of Epileptology; XIth Epilepsy International Symposium,* Eds. R. Canger, F. Angeleri, and J.F. Penry, pp. 297–309. New York: Raven Press.

Andermann, E.D., and Metrakos, J.D. 1969. EEG studies of relatives of probands with focal epilepsy who have been treated surgically. Epilepsia (Amsterdam) 10:415–420.

Andermann, F., and Oguni, H. 1991. Do epileptic foci migrate? The pros. Electroencephalogr. Clin. Neurophysiol. 76:96–99.

Andermann, F., and Robb, J.P. 1972. Absence status: appraisal following review of 38 patients. Epilepsia (Amsterdam) 13:177–187.

Anderson, V.E., Hauser, W.A., Leppik, I.E., et al. (Eds.). 1991. *Genetic Strategies in Epilepsy Research.* London: Elsevier.

Andrews, P.I., McNamara, J.O., and Lewis, D.V. 1997. Clinical and electroencephalographic correlates in Rasmussen's encephalitis. Epilepsia 38:189–194.

Angeleri, F., and Giaquinto, S. 1981. Predisposition in traumatic epilepsy: an individual and family study. Electroencephalogr. Clin. Neurophysiol. 51:55P(abst).

Angeleri, F., Ferro-Milone, F., and Parigi, S. 1964. Electrical activity and reactivity of the rhinencephalic, pararhinencephalic and thalamic structures: prolonged implantation of electrodes in man. Electroencephalogr. Clin. Neurophysiol. 16:100–129.

Angelini, L., Broggi, G., Riva, D., et al. 1979. A case of Lennox-Gastaut syndrome successfully treated by removal of a parietotemporal astrocytoma. Epilepsia (New York) 20:665–669.

Annegers, J.F. 1993. The epidemiology of epilepsy. In *The Treatment of Epilepsy,* Ed. E. Wyllie, pp. 157–164. Philadelphia: Lea and Febiger.

Arfel, G., and Fischgold, H. 1961. EEG signs in tumours of the brain. In *Electroencephalography and Cerebral Tumours,* Eds. O. Magnus, W. Storm van Leeuwen, and W.A. Cobb, pp. 36–50. Amsterdam: Elsevier.

Arroyo, S., Lesser, R.P., Gordon, B., et al. 1993. Mirth, laughter and gelastic seizures. Brain 116:757–780.

Arseni, C., and Marinescu, V. 1974. Epilepsy in cerebral hydatiodosis. Epilepsia (New York) 15:45–54.

Asconapé, J., and Penry, J.K. 1984. Some clinical and EEG aspects of benign juvenile myoclonic epilepsy. Epilepsia (New York) 25:108–114.

Asenjo, A., and Rocca, E.D. 1946. Compromiso de los pares creneanos en la cisticercosis cerebral. Rev. Med. Chile 9:605–615.

Atassi, M. 1981. Primäre Lese-Epilepsie. Eine Kasuistik. Z. EEG-EMG 12:128–131.

Atkinson, J.R., and Ward, A.A., Jr. 1964. Intracellular studies of cortical neurons in chronic epileptogenic foci in the monkey. Exp. Neurol. 10:285–295.

Atzev, E.S. 1962. The influence of nonspecific afference on epileptic activity of the brain. Epilepsia (Amsterdam) 3:281–292.

Autret, A., Lafont, F., and Roux, S. 1983. Influence of waking and sleep stages on the inter-ictal paroxysmal activity in partial epilepsy with complex seizures. Electroencephalogr. Clin. Neurophysiol. 55:406–410.

Avoli, M., and Gloor, P. 1981. The effects of transient functional depression of the thalamus on spindles and on bilateral synchronous epileptic discharges of feline generalized penicillin epilepsy. Epilepsia (New York) 22:443–452.

Avoli, M., and Gloor, P. 1982. Thalamic involvement in feline generalized epilepsy: Data from unilaterally and bilaterally decorticated animals. Electroencephalogr. Clin. Neurophysiol. 54:39P(abst).

Avoli, M., Siatitsas, I., Kostopoulos, G., et al. 1981. Effects of post-ictal depression on experimental spike and wave discharges. Electroencephalogr. Clin. Neurophysiol. 52:372–374.

Avoli, M., Gloor, P., Kostopoulos, G., et al. 1983. An analysis of penicillin-induced generalized spike and wave discharges using simultaneous recordings of cortical and thalamic single neurons. J. Neurophysiol. 50: 819–837.

Avoli, M., Gloor, P., Kostopoulos, G., et al. (Eds.). 1990. *Generalized Epilepsy. Neurobiological Approaches.* Boston: Birkhäuser.

Ayala, G.F., Dichter, M., Gumnit, R.J., et al. 1973. Genesis of epileptic interictal spikes. New knowledge of cortical feedback system suggests a neurophysiological explanation of brief paroxysms. Brain Res. 52:1–17.

Aykutlu, E., Baykan, B., Serdaroclu, et al. 2002. Epileptic seizures in Behcet disease. Epilepsia 43:832–835.

Babb, T.L., and Brown, W.J. 1987. Pathological findings in epilepsy. In *Surgical Treatment of the Epilepsies,* Ed. J. Engel., Jr., pp. 511–540. New York: Raven Press.

Babb, T.L., Mitchell, A.G., Jr., and Crandall, P.H. 1974. Fastigiobulbar and dentatothalamic influences on hippocampal cobalt epilepsy in the cat. Electroencephalogr. Clin. Neurophysiol. 36:141–154.

Babb, T.L., Halgren, E., Wilson, C., et al. 1981. Neuronal firing patterns during the spread of an occipital lobe seizure to the temporal lobes in man. Electroencephalogr. Clin. Neurophysiol. 51:104–107.

Bach-y-Rita, G., Lion, J.F., Climent, C.E., et al. 1971. Episodic dyscontrol: a study of 130 violent patients. Am. J. Psychiatry 127:1473–1478.

Baddeley, A.D. 1986. *Working Memory.* Oxford: Oxford University Press.

Baird, R.L., Weiss, D.L., Ferguson, A.D., et al. 1964. Studies in sickle cell anemia. XXI. Clinicopathological aspects of neurological manifestations. Pediatrics 34:92–100.

Bajorek, J.G., Lee, R.J., and Lomax, P. 1986. Neuropeptides. Anti-convulsant and convulsant mechanisms in epileptic model systems and in humans. In *Basic Mechanisms of the Epilepsies,* Eds. A.V. Delgado-Escueta, A.A. Ward, Jr., D.M. Woodbury, et al., pp. 189–500. New York: Raven Press.

Bamberger, P., and Matthes, A. 1959. *Anfälle im Kindesalter.* Basel: S. Karger.

Bancaud, J. 1972. Mechanisms of cortical discharges in "generalized" epilepsies in man. In *Synchronization of EGG Activity in Epilepsies,* Eds. H. Petsche and M.A.B. Brazier, pp. 368–381. Vienna: Springer.

Bancaud, J., and Talairach, J. 1992. Clinical semiology of frontal lobe seizures. In *Frontal Lobe Seizures and Epilepsies,* Eds. P. Chauvel, A.V. Delgado-Escueta, E. Halgren, et al., pp. 3–58. New York: Raven Press.

Bancaud, J., Talairach, J., Bonis, A., et al. 1965. *La stéréo-électroencéphalographie dans l'éilepsie.* Paris: Masson.

Bancaud, J., Talairach, J., and Bonis, A. 1967. Physiopathogénie des épilepsie-sursaut (à propos d'une épilepsie de l'aire motrice supplémentaire). Rev. Neurol. (Paris) 117:441–453.

Bancaud, J., Bonis, A., Talairach, J., et al. 1970. Syndrome de Kojevnikow et accès somatomoteurs (étude clinique, E.E.G. et S.E.E.G.). Encephale 5:391–438.

Baraban, J.M., Cole, A.J., Stratton, K.R., et al. 1991. Neuronal excitability: focus on second messenger systems. In *Neurotransmitters and Epilepsy,* Eds. R.S. Fisher and J.T. Coyle, pp. 33–45. New York: Wiley-Liss.

Barkley, G.L. and Baumgartner, C. 2003. MEG and EEG in epilepsy. J. Clin. Neurophysiol. 20:163–178.

Barolin, G.S., and Karbowski, K. 1973. Okzipitale Krisen im "Grenzland der Epilepsie." Z. EEG-EMG 4:1–8.

Barolin, G.S., and Scherzer, E. 1963. Epileptische Anfälle bei Apoplektikern. Wien. Z. Nervenheilk. 20:35–47.

Barolin, G.S., Scherzer, E., and Schnaberth, G. 1971. Epileptische Manifestationen als Vorboten von Schlaganfällen. Fortschr. Neurol. Psychiatr. 39:199–216.

Barolin, G.S., Scherzer, E., and Schnaberth, G. 1975. *Die zerebrovaskulär bedingten Anfälle.* Bern: Huber.

Barolin, G.S., Scholz, H., Breitfellner, G., et al. 1976. Epilepsia partialis continua Kojevnikow. 7 Fälle. Nervenarzt 47:609–613.

Bartolomei, F., Azulay, J.-P., Barrie, M., et al. 1996. Myoclonic alcohol epilepsy. Epilepsia 37:406–409.

Bates, J.A.V. 1963. Special investigation techniques: indwelling electrodes and electrocorticography. In *Electroencephalography,* Eds. D. Hill and G. Parr, pp. 429–479. New York: Macmillan.

Baudewig, J., Bittermann, H.J., Paulus, W., et al. 2001. Simultaneous EEG and functional MRI of epileptic activity: a case report. Clin. Neurophysiol. 112:1196–1200.

Bauer, G. 1974. Myoklonien: Erscheinungsbild, Pathophysiologie und klinische Bedeutung. Wien. Klin. Wochenschr. 124:577–581.

Bauer, G. 1975. Der Wert von EEG-Kontrollen mglichst bald nach einem epileptischen Anfall. Z. EEG-EMG 6:125–130.

Bauer, G. 1994. Symptomatik der epileptischen Anfallsformen nach dem ILAE Schema. Fokale Anfalle mit komplexer Symptomatik. In *Die Epilepsien,* Ed. W. Froescher, pp. 152–158. De Gruyter: Berlin.

Bauer, G., and Niedermeyer, E. 1979. Acute convulsions. Clin. Electroencephalogr. 10:127–144.

Bauer, G., Hengl, W., and Mayr, U. 1981. Non-convulsive status epilepticus following generalized tonic-clonic seizures. Electronencephalogr. Clin. Neurophysiol. 52:36P(abst).

Bauer, G., Aichner, F., and Saltuari, L. 1983. Epilepsies with diffuse slow spikes and waves of late onset. Eur. Neurol. 22:344–350.

Bauer, G., Benke, T., and Bohr, K. 1988. The Lennox-Gastaut syndrome in adulthood. In *The Lennox-Gastaut Syndrome,* Eds. E. Niedermeyer and R. Degen, pp. 317–327. New York: Alan R. Liss.

Bauer, H., Korunka, C., and Leodolter, M. 1989. Technical requirements for high-quality scalp DC recordings. Electroencephalogr. Clin. Neurophysiol. 72:545–547.

Baumgartner, C., Podreka, I., Olbrich, A., et al. 1996. Epileptic negative myoclonus. An EEG-single-photon-emission CT study indicating involvement of premotor cortex. Neurology 46:753–758.

Baumgartner, C., Graf, M., Doppelbauer, A., et al. 1996. The functional organization of the interictal spike complex in benign rolandic epilepsy. Epilepsia 37:1164–1174.

Baust, W., Bohnke, J., and Rabe, F. 1971. Polygraphische Registrierung vegetativer Begleiterscheinungn bei Isoliertern Epigastrischen Auren. Nervenarzt 42:492.

Bazil, C.W., Castro, L.H.M., and Walczak, T.S., 2000. Reduction of rapid eye movement sleep by diurnal and nocturnal seizures in temporal lobe epilepsy. Arch. Neurol. 57:363–368.

Bear, D., Freeman, R., and Greenberg, M. 1984. Behavioral alterations in patients with temporal lobe epilepsy. In *Psychiatric Aspects of Epilepsy,* Ed. D. Blumer, pp. 197–227. Washington, DC: American Psychiatric Press.

Beaumanoir, A. 1976. *Les épilepsies infantiles. Problèmes de Diagnostic et de Traitement.* Basel: Editiones Roche.

Beaumanoir, A. 1984. Le syndrome de Lennox-Gastaut. In *Les syndromes épileptiques de l'enfant et de l'adolescent,* Eds. J. Roger, C. Dravet, M. Bureau, et al., pp. 89–100. London: John Libbey Eurotext.

Beaumanior, A., Martin, F., Panagopoulos, M., et al. 1968. Le syndrome de Lennox (étude évolutive de trente cas). Schweiz. Arch. Neurol. Neurochir. Psychiatr. 102:31–62.

Beaumanoir, A., Ballis, T., Varfis, G., et al. 1974. Benign epilepsy of childhood with rolandic spike. A clinical electroencephalographic and telencephalographic study. Epilepsia (Amsterdam) 15:301–315.

Beaumanoir, A., Jenny, P., and Jekiel, M. 1981. Study of 4 cases of postpartum petit mal status. Electroencephalogr. Clin. Neurophysiol. 52:55P (abst).

Beaumanoir, A., Bureau, M., and Mira, L. 1995a. Identification of the syndrome. In *Continuous Spikes and Waves During Slow Sleep. Electrical Status Epilepticus During Sleep,* Eds. A. Beaumanoir, M. Bureau, T. Deonna, et al., pp. 243–249. London: Libbey.

Beaumanoir, A., Bureau, M., Deonna, T., et al. (Eds.). 1995b. In *Continuous Spikes and Waves During Slow Sleep. Electrical Status Epilepticus During Sleep.* London: Libbey.

Beaussart, M. 1972. Benign epilepsy of children with rolandic (centro-temporal) paroxysmal foci. A clinical entity. Study of 221 cases. Epilepsia (Amsterdam) 13:795–811.

Bejar, J.M., Lai, C.-W., and Ziegler, D.K. 1985. Sustained myoclonus in a woman with startle epilepsy. Ann. Neurol. 18:101–103.

Benbadis, S.R., and Dinner, D.S. 1994. Lennox-Gastaut syndrome in the elderly? Clin. Electroencephalogr. 25:142–147.

Bengzon, A.R.A., Rasmussen, T., Gloor, P., et al. 1968. Prognostic factor in the surgical treatment of temporal lobe epileptics. Neurology (Minneapolis) 18:717–731.

Bennett, F.E. 1953. Intracarotid and intravertebral Metrazol in petit mal epilepsy. Neurology (Minneapolis) 3:668–673.

Bente, D., and Itil, T. 1954. Zur Wirkung des Phenothiazinkörpers Megaphen auf das menschliche Hirnstrombild. Arzneimitt. Forsch. 4:418–423.

Berg, A.T., and Shinnar, S. 1996. Complex febrile seizures. Epilepsia 37: 126–133.

Berger, H. 1933. Über das Elektroenzephalogramm des Menschen (7th report). Arch. Psychiatr. Nervenkrankh. 100:301–320.

Bergey, G.K., Krumholz, A., and Fleming, C.P. 1997. Complex partial seizure provocation by vasovagal syncope: video-EEG and intracranial electrode documentation. Epilepsia 38:118–121.

Bergman, I., Painter, M.J., Hirsch, R.P., et al. 1983. Outcome in neonates with convulsions treated in an intensive care unit. Ann. Neurol. 14:642–647.

Berkovic, S.F., Andermann, F., Aube, M., et al. 1985. Nonconvulsive confusional frontal status. Epilepsia (New York) 26:529(abst).

Berkovic, S.F., Howell, R.A., Hay, D.A., et al. 1994. Epilepsies in twins. In *Epileptic Seizures and Syndromes,* Ed. P. Wolf, pp. 157–164. London: Libbey.

Berkovic, S.F., McIntosh, A.M., Howell, R.A., et al. 1996. Familial temporal lobe epilepsy: a common disorder in twins. Ann. Neurol. 40:227–232.

Berkovic, S.F., Genton, P., Hirsch, E., et al. 1999. *Genetics of Focal Epilepsies.* London: Libby.

Berkovic, S.F., Arzimanoglu, A., Kuzniecky, R., et al. 2003. Hypothalamic hamartoma and seizures: a treatable epileptic encephalopathy. Epilepsia 44:969–973.

Bert, J., and Naquet, R. 1970. Geographical variations in the photo-sensitivity of the baboon Papio papio. Electroencephalogr. Clin. Neurophysiol. 29:102(abst).

Besser, R., Hornung, K., Theisohn, M., et al. 1992. EEG changes in patients during the introduction of carbamazepine. Electroencephalogr. Clin. Neurophysiol. 83:19–23.

Beun, A.M., Beintema, D.J., Binnie, C.D., et al. 1984. Epileptic nystagmus. Epilepsia (New York) 25:609–614.

Bickford, R.G. 1954. Sensory precipitation of seizures. J. Mich. Med. Soc. 53:1018–1021.

Bickford, R.G. 1956. The application of depth electrography in some varieties of epilepsy. Electroencephalogr. Clin. Neurophysiol. 8: 526–527.

Bickford, R.G. 1963. Electroencephalography. In *Clinical Examinations in Neurology,* Eds. J.A. Bastron et al., pp. 297–310. Philadelphia: W.B. Saunders.

Bickford, R.G., and Klass, D.W. 1969. Sensory precipitation and reflex mechanisms. In *Basic Mechanisms of the Epilepsies,* Eds. H.H. Jasper, A.A. Ward, Jr., and A. Pope, pp. 543–564. Boston: Little, Brown.

Bickford, R.G., Sem-Jacobsen, C.W., White, P.T., et al. 1952. Some observations on the mechanisms of photic and photo-metrazol activations. Electroencephalogr. Clin. Neurophysiol. 4:275–282.

Bickford, R.G., Daly, D., and Keith, H. 1953. Convulsive effects of light stimulation in children. Am. J. Dis. Child. 86:170.

Bickford, R.G., Whelan, J.L., Klass, D.W., et al. 1956. Reading epilepsy: clinical and electroencephalographic study of a new syndrome. Trans. Am. Neurol. Assoc. 81:100–102.

Bingley, T. 1958. *Mental Symptoms in Temporal Lobe Epilepsy and Temporal Lobe Gliomas.* Copenhagen: Munksgaard.

Binnie, C.D., Veldhuizen, R., and Beintema, D.J. 1982a. Evaluation of recording after sleep deprivation in the diagnostic EEG assessment of epilepsy. Electroencephalogr. Clin. Neurophysiol. 54:21P–22P(abst).

Binnie, C.D., Rowan, A.J., and Van Wieringen, A. 1982b. Eating epilepsy: report of 4 cases with review of the literature. Electroencephalogr. Clin. Neurophysiol. 53:47P(abst).

Blom, S., and Brorson, L.O. 1966. Central spikes or sharp waves (rolandic spikes) in children's EEG and their clinical significance. Acta Pediatr. Scand. 55:385–393.

Blom, S., and Heijbel, J. 1982. Benign epilepsy of children with centrotemporal EEG foci: a follow-up study in adulthood of patients initially studied as children. Epilepsia (New York) 23:629–632.

Blom, S., Heijbel, J., and Bergfors, P.G. 1972. Benign epilepsy of children with centrotemporal EEG foci. Prevalence and follow-up study of 40 patients. Epilepsia (Amsterdam) 13:609–613.

Blum, B., and Liban, E. 1960. Experimental baso-temporal epilepsy in the cat. Discrete epileptogenic lesions produced in the hippocampus or amygdaloid by tungstic acid. Electroencephalogr. Clin. Neurophysiol. 10:546–554.

Blume, W.T. 1991. Do epileptic foci migrate? The cons. Electroencephalogr. Clin. Neurophysiol. 76:100–105.

Blume, W.T., and Kaibara, M. 1993. The start-stop-start phenomenon of subdurally recorded seizures. Electroencephalogr. Clin. Neurophysiol. 86:94–99.

Blume, W.T., David, R.B., and Gomez, M.R. 1973. Generalized sharp and slow wave complexes, associated with clinical features and long term follow-up. Brain 96:289–306.

Blumenfeld, H. 2002. The thalamus and seizures. Arch. Neurol. 59:135–137.

Blumer, D. 1970. Hypersexual episodes in temporal lobe epilepsy. Am. J. Psychiatry 126:1099–1106.

Blumer, D. 1984. The psychiatric dimension of epilepsy: historical perspective and current significance. In *Psychiatric Aspects of Epilepsy,* Ed. D. Blumer, pp. 1–65. Washington, DC: American Psychiatric Press.

Blumer, D., and Walker, A.E. 1967. Sexual behavior in temporal lobe epilepsy. Arch. Neurol. (Chicago) 16:37–43.

Bobbi, G., Andermann, F., Naccarato, S., et al. 1997. *Epilepsy and Other Neurological Disorders in Coeliac Disease.* London: Libbey.

Bonanni, P., Parmeggiani, L., and Guerrini, R. 2002. Different neurophysiological patterns of myoclonus characterize Lennox-Gastaut syndrome and myoclonic astatic epilepsy. Epilepsia 43:609–615.

Bornstein, M.B. 1946. Presence and action of acetylcholine in experimental brain trauma. J. Neurophysiol. 9:349–366.

Bornstein, M., Coddors, D., and Song, S. 1956. Prolonged alterations in behavior associated with a continuous electroencephalographic (spike and dome abnormality). Neurology (Minneapolis) 6:444–448.

Boroojerdi, B., Hungs, M., Biniek, R., et al. 1998. Subakute Enzephalopathie mit epileptischen Anfaellen bei einem Patienten mit Chronischem Alkoholismus (SESA Syndrom). Nervenarzt 69:162–165.

Bossi, L., Munari, C. Stoffels, C., et al. 1984. Somatomotor manifestations in temporal lobe seizures. Epilepsia (New York) 25:70–76.

Bouchet and Cazauvielh. 1825. De l'épilepsie considérée dans ces rapports avec l'aliénation mentale. Arch. Gen. Med. 9:510–542.

Boudin, G., Barbizet, J., and Labet, R. 1954. L'association épilepsie-endocrinopathie. Épilepsie d'origine profonde avec tracé épileplique de type petit mal et endocrinopathie d'origine diencéphalique. Rev. Neurol. (Paris) 91:330–346.

Branch, C., Milner, B., and Rasmussen, T. 1964. Intracarotid sodium Amytal for the lateralization of cerebral speech dominance. J. Neurosurg. 21:399–405.

Bravais, L.F. 1827. *Recherches sur les Symptomes et le Traitement de l'Épilepsie Hémiplégique.* Paris: Thèse de Paris No. 118.

Bray, P.F., and Wiser, W.C. 1965. The relation of focal to diffuse epileptiform EEG discharges in genetic epilepsy. Arch. Neurol. (Chicago) 13:223–237.

Brazier, M.A.B. 1961. *A History of the Electrical Activity of the Brain.* New York: Macmillan.

Bremer, F. 1941. Le tetanos strychnique et le méchanisme de la synchronization neuronique. Arch. Int. Physiol. 51:211–260.

Bremer, F. 1958. Les processus d'excitation et d'inhibition dans les phénomènes épileptiques. In *Bases Physiologiques et Aspects Cliniques de l'Épilepsie,* Ed. T. Alajouanine, pp. 1–35. Paris: Masson.

Brenner, C., and Merritt, H.H. 1942. Effect of certain cholin derivates on electrical activity of the cortex. Arch. Neurol. Psychiatry (Chicago) 48:383–395.

Brett, E.M. 1966. Minor epileptic status. J. Neurol. Sci. 3:53–75.

Brey, R.I., and Laxer, K.D. 1984. EEG telemetry and video recording: evaluation of routine use. Electroencephalogr. Clin. Neurophysiol. 58:12P(abst).

Bridge, E.M. 1949. *Epilepsy and Convulsive Disorders in Children.* New York: McGraw-Hill.

Brock, L.G., Coombs, J.S., and Eccles, J.C. 1952. The recordings of potentials from motoneurons with an intracellular electrode. J. Physiol. 117:431–460.

Brockhaus, A., and Elger, C.E. 1995. Complex partial seizures of temporal lobe origin in children of different age groups. Epilepsia 36:1173–1181.

Bronisch, F.W., and Rauch, H.J. 1970. Zur Pathogenese der epileptischen Anfälle bei multipler Sklerose. Deutsch. Z. Nervenheilk. 158:322–344.

Bumke, O. 1942. *Lehrbuch der Geisteskrankheiten,* 5th ed. Munich: Bergmann.

Burger, L.J., Lopez, R.I., and Elliott, F.A. 1972. Tonic seizures induced by movement. Neurology (Minneapolis) 22:656–659.

Burke, J.B. 1954. Prognostic significance of neonatal convulsions. Arch. Dis. Child. 29:342–345.

Burri, H., Schaffler, L., and Karbowski, K. 1989. Epileptische Anfälle bei Patienten mit zerebrovaskulären Insulten. Schweiz. Med. Wochenschr. 119:500–507.

Bye, A.M.E., and Foo, S. 1994. Complex partial seizures in young children. Epilepsia 35:482–488.

Cadilhac, J., and Ribstein, M. 1961. The EEG in metabolic disorders. World Neurol. 2:296–308.

Calmei, L.-F. 1824. *De l'Épilepsie, Étudiée sous la Rapport de son Siège et de son Influence sur la Production de l'Aliénation Mentale.* Paris: Thèse de Paris.

Carmant, L., Carrazana, E., Kramer, U., et al. 1996. Pharyngeal dysesthesia as an aura in temporal lobe epilepsy. Epilepsia 37:911–913.

Cascino, G.D., Trenerry, M.R., So, E.L., et al. 1996. Routine EEG and temporal lobe epilepsy: Relation to long-term EEG monitoring, quantitative MRI and operative outcome. Epilepsia 37:651–656.

Caspers, H. 1963. Über die Beziehungen zwischen Dendritenpotential und Gleichspannung an der Hirnrinde. Pflueger Arch. Gesamte Physiol. Menschen Tiere 269:157–181.

Caspers, H., and Speckmann, E.J. 1969. DC potential shifts in paroxysmal states. In *Basic Mechanisms of the Epilepsies,* Eds. H.H. Jaspers, A.A. Ward, Jr., and A. Pope, pp. 375–388. Boston: Little, Brown.

Caspers, H., and Speckmann, E.J. 1970. Postsynaptische Potentiale einzelner Neurone und ihre Beziehungen zum EEG. Z. EEG-EMG (Stuttgart) 1:55–65.

Cavanagh, J.B. 1958. On certain small tumors encountered in the temporal lobe. Brain 81:389–405.

Cavanagh, J.B., and Meyer, A. 1956. Aetiological aspects of Ammon's horn sclerosis associated with temporal lobe epilepsy. Br. Med. J. 2:1403–1407.

Cavazutti, C.B. 1972. La sindrome di Lennox-Gastaut, encefalopatia epilettica infantile. La Clin. Pediatr. 54:237–245.

Celesia, C.G. 1976. Modern concepts of status epilepticus. JAMA 235:1571–1574.

Celesia, G.C., and Paulsen, R.E. 1972. Electroencephalographic activation with sleep and methohexital. Arch. Neurol. (Chicago) 27:361–363.

Celesia, G.G. 2001. Disorders of membrane channels or channelopathies. Clin. Neurophysiol. 112:2–18.

Chadwick, D., Mallett, M., Harris, R., et al. 1977. Clinical biochemical and physiological features distinguishing myoclonus response to 5-hydroxytryptophan, tryptophan with a monoamino oxidase inhibitor and clonazepam. Brain 100:455–487.

Chan, A.W.K. 1985. Alcoholism and epilepsy. Epilepsia (New York) 26:323–333.

Charlton, M.H. 1975. Infantile spasms. In *Myoclonic Seizures,* Ed. M.H. Charlton, pp. 111–120. Amsterdam: Excerpta Medica.

Chassagnon, S., Minotti, L., Kremer, S., et al. 2003. Restricted frontomesial epileptogenic focus generating dyskinetic behavior and laughter. Epilepsia 44:859–863.

Chatrian, G.E., and Perez-Borja, C. 1964. Depth electrographic observations in two cases of photo-oculoclonic response. Electroencephalogr. Clin. Neurophysiol. 17:71–75.

Chatrian, G.E., and Spence, A.M. 1984. Two cases of epileptic nystagmus associated with occipital EEG seizure activity. Electroencephalogr. Clin. Neurophysiol. 53:63P(abst).

Chatrian, G.E., Shaw, C.M., and Leffman, H. 1964. The significance of periodic lateralized epileptiform discharges in EEG: an electrographic, clinical and pathological study. Electroencephalogr. Clin. Neurophysiol. 17:177–193.

Chatrian, G.E., Somasundaram, M., and Tassinari, C.A. 1968. DC changes recorded transcranially during "typical" three per second spike and wave discharges in man. Epilepsia (Amsterdam) 9:185–209.

Chatrian, G.E., Lettich, E., Miller, L.H., et al. 1970a. Pattern-sensitive epilepsy. Part 1 (An electrographic study of its mechanisms). Epilepsia (Amsterdam) 11:125–150.

Chatrian, G.E., Lettich, E., Miller, L.H., et al. 1970b. Pattern-sensitive epilepsy. Part 2 (Clinical changes, tests of responsiveness and motor output, alterations of evoked potentials and therapeutic measures). Epilepsia (Amsterdam) 11:151–162.

Chauvel, P., Trottier, S., Nassif, S., et al. 1982. Is an alteration of nonadrenergic afferents involved in focal epilepsies? Electroencephalogr. Clin. Neurophysiol. 53:78P(abst).

Chavany, J.A., Fischgold, H., Messimy, R., et al. 1956. Étude clinque et EEG d'un cas d'épilepsie provoquée électivement par la lecture. Rev. Neurol. (Paris) 95:381–386.

Chen, R.-C., and Forster, F.M. 1973. Cursive epilepsy and gelastic epilepsy. Neurology (Minneapolis) 23:1019–1029.

Chevrie, J.J., and Aicardi, J. 1972. Childhood epileptic encephalopathy with slow spike-wave: a statistical study of 80 cases. Epilepsia (Amsterdam) 13:259–271.

Choroschko. 1908. Zur Differentialdiagnose per polyclonia epileptoides continua (Koschewnikowi). Neurol. Centralbl. 27:29.

Christian, W. 1975. *Klinische Elektroenzephalographie, Lehrbuch und Atlas,* 2nd ed. Stuttgart: Thieme.

Chugani, H.T., Shewmon, D.A., Shields, W.D., et al. 1993. Surgery for intractable infantile spasms: neuroimaging perspectives. Epilepsia 34:764–771.

Ciganek, L. 1961. Theta-discharges in the middle-line EEG symptom of temporal lobe epilepsy. Electroencephalogr. Clin. Neurophysiol. 13:669.

Cincinnati, P., Giannotti, A., Gisondi, A., et al. 1982. The contribution of CAT scan in the study of West's syndrome. Electroencephalogr. Clin. Neurophysiol. 54:1P(abst).

Cirignotta, F., Moschen, R., and Sacquegna, T. 1982. Spike related inhibition of tone during sleep. Electroencephalogr. Clin. Neurophysiol. 54:1P(abst).

Cirignotta, F., Zucconi, M., Mondini, S., et al. 1986. Writing epilepsy. Clin. Electroencephalogr. 17:21–23.

Clancy, R., Malin, S., Laraque, D., et al. 1985. Focal motor seizures heralding stroke in full-term neonates. Am. J. Dis. Child. 139:601–606.

Clark, E.C., and Knott, J.R. 1955. Paroxysmal wave and spike activity and diagnostic subclassification. Electroencephalogr. Clin. Neurophysiol. 7:161–164.

Classen, J., Witte, O.W., Schlaug, G., et al. 1995. Epileptic seizures triggered directly by focal transcranial stimulation. Electroencephalogr. Clin. Neurophysiol. 94:19–25.

Cohen, M. 1992. Functional magnetic resonance imaging of the human brain. Epilepsia 33(suppl 3):2(abst).

Cohn, R. 1954. Spike-dome complex in the human electroencephalogram. Arch. Neurol. Psychiatry (Chicago) 71:699–706.

Cohn, R. 1964. DC recordings of paroxysmal disorders in man. Electroencephalogr. Clin. Neurophysiol. 17:17–24.

Collins, R.L. 1972. Audiogenic seizures. In *Experimental Models of Epilepsy,* Eds. D.H. Purpura, J.K. Penry, D. Tower, et al., pp. 347–372. New York: Raven Press.

Commission on Classification and Terminology of the International League Against Epilepsy. 1981. Proposal for revised clinical and electroencephalographic classification of epileptic seizures. Epilepsia (New York) 22:489–501.

Commission on Classification and Terminology of the International League Against Epilepsy (headed by F.E. Dreifuss). 1985. Proposal for classification of epilepsies and epileptic syndromes. Epilepsia (New York) 26:268–278.

Connors, B.W., and Gutnick, M.J. 1984. Cellular mechanisms of neocortical epileptogenesis in an acute experimental model. In *Electrophysiology of Epilepsy,* Eds. P.A. Schwartzkroin and H.V. Wheal, pp. 79–105. London: Academic Press.

Conrad, K. 1940. Die erbliche Fallsucht. Erbbiologischer Teil. In *Handbuch der Erbkrankheiten,* vol. 3, pp. 103–176. Leipzig: Thieme.

Cornford, M.E., and McCormick, G.F. 1997. Adult-onset temporal lobe epilepsy associated with smoldering herpes simplex 2 infection. Neurology 48:425–430.

Cornil, L., Gastaut, H., and Corriol, J. 1951. Appréciation du degré de conscience au cours des paroxysmes épileptiques "Petit Mal." Rev. Neurol. (Paris) 84:149–151.

Corsi, P.M. 1972. *Human Memory and the Medial Temporal Region of the Brain.* Unpublished thesis. Montreal: McGill University. Quoted in Milner, 1975.

Courjon, J. 1969. Posttraumatic epilepsy in electro-clinical practice. In *The Late Effects of Head Injury,* Eds. A.E. Walter, W.F. Caveness, and M. Critchley, pp. 215–229. Springfield, IL: Charles C Thomas.

Courjon, J., and Scherzer, E. 1972. Traumatic disorders. In *Handbook of Electroencephalography and Clinical Neurophysiology,* vol. 14B, Ed.-in-Chief, A. Remond. Amsterdam: Elsevier.

Courville, C.B. 1958. Traumatic lesions of the temporal lobe as the essential cause of psychomotor epilepsy. In *Temporal Lobe Epilepsy,* Eds. M. Baldwin and P. Bailey, pp. 220–239. Springfield, IL: Charles C Thomas.

Craig, W.S. 1960. Convulsive movements occurring in the first 10 days of life. Arch. Dis. Child. 35:336–344.

Crighel, E. 1963. The EEG activating phenomenon on closing the eyes. Electroencephalogr. Clin. Neurophysiol. 15:531.

Critchley, M. 1937. Musicogenic epilepsy. Brain 60:13–27.

Critchley, M. 1962. Reading epilepsy. Epilepsia (Amsterdam) 3:402–405.

Critchley, M. 1979. *The Divine Banquet of the Brain,* pp. 92–105, 115–120. New York: Raven Press.

Cross, A.H. and Golumbek, P.T. 2003. Neurologic manifestations of celiac disease: proven on just a gut feeling. Neurology 60:1566–1568.

Cure, C., Rasmussen, T., and Jasper, H.H. 1948. Activation of seizures and electroencephalographic disturbances in epileptic and control subjects with "Metrazol." Arch. Neurol. Psychiatry (Chicago) 59:691–717.

Currie, S., Heathfield, K.W.G., Henson, R.A., et al. 1970. Clinical course and prognosis of temporal lobe epilepsy. Brain 94:173–190.

Currier, R.D., Little, S.C., Suess, J.F., et al. 1971. Sexual seizures. Arch. Neurol. (Chicago) 25:260–264.

Dalby, M.A. 1969. *Epilepsy and 3 per Second Spike and Wave Rhythms.* Copenhagen: Munksgaard.

Dalla Bernardina, B., and Beghini, G. 1976. Rolandic spikes in children with and without epilepsy (20 subjects photographically studied during sleep). Epilepsia (New York) 17:161–168.

Dalla Bernardina, B., Capovilla, G., Gattoni, M.B., et al. 1982a. Épilepsie myoclonique grave de la prémière année. Rev. EEG Neurophysiol. 12:21–25.

Dalla Bernardina, B., Dulac, O., Bureau, M., et al. 1982b. Encephalopathie myoclonique précoce avec épilepsie. Rev. EEG Neurophysiol. 12:8–14.

Dalla Bernardina, B., Dulac, O., Fejerman, N., et al. 1983. Early myoclonic epileptic encephalopathy (E.M.E.E.). Eur. J. Pediatr. 140:248–252.

Dalla Bernardina, B., Colamaria, V., Capovilla, G., et al. 1984. Sleep and benign partial epilepsies of childhood. In *Epilepsy, Sleep and Sleep Deprivation,* Eds. R. Degen and E. Niedermeyer, pp. 119–133. Amsterdam: Elsevier.

Daly, D.D. 1958. Ictal affect. Am. J. Psychiatry 115:97–108.

Daly, D.D. 1975. Ictal clinical manifestations of complex partial seizures. In *Complex Partial Seizures and Their Treatment,* Eds. J.K. Penry and D.D. Daly, pp. 57–82. New York: Raven Press.

Daly, D., and Mulder, D.W. 1957. Gelastic epilepsy. Neurology (Minneapolis) 7:189–192.

Dam, A.M., Fuglsang-Frederiksen, A., Svarre-Olsen, U., et al. 1985. Late-onset epilepsy: etiologies, types of seizure, and value of clinical investigation, EEG and computerized tomography scan. Epilepsia (New York) 26:227–231.

Darby, C.E., De Korte, R.A., Binnie, C.D., et al. 1980. The self-induction of epileptic seizures by eye closure. Epilepsia (New York) 21:31–42.

Daumas-Duport, C. 1993. Dysembryoplastic neuroepithelial tumors. Brain Pathol. 3:283–295.

Dawson, G.D. 1947. Investigations on a patient subject to myoclonic seizures after sensory stimulation. J. Neurol. Neurosurg. Psychiatry 10: 141–162.

Dazzi, P., and Lugaresi, E. 1956. Sullo "stato di piccolo male" (Revisione criticosintetico con presentazione di due casi). Riv. Neuropsichiatr. 2: 144–179.

Degen, R., and Degen, H.-E. 1984. Sleep and sleep deprivation in epileptology. In *Epilepsy, Sleep and Sleep Deprivation,* Eds. R. Degen and E. Niedermeyer, pp. 273–286. Amsterdam: Elsevier.

Degen, R., Ebner, A., Lahl, R., et al. 2002. Various findings in surgically treated epilepsy patients with dysembryoplastic neuroepithelial tumors in comparison with those of patients with other low-grade brain tumors and other neuronal migration disorders. Epilepsia 43:1379–1384.

Dehan, M., Quilleron, D., Navelet, Y., et al. 1977. Les convulsions de 5e jour de vie: un nouveau syndrome? Arch. Fr. Pédiatr. 34:730–742.

Deisenhammer, E., Klingler, D., and Trügner, H. 1984. Epileptic seizures in alcoholism and diagnostic value of EEG after sleep deprivation. Epilepsia (New York) 25:526–530.

Delasiauve. 1854. *Traité de l'épilepsie.* Paris.

Delay, J., Schuller, E., Drossopoulo, G., et al. 1956. Un nouvel activant des électroencéphalogrammes: l'imide de l'acide éthyl-méthyl glutarique (N.P. 13) ou megimide. Rev. Neurol. (Paris) 94:315–318.

Delgado, J.M.R., and Sevillano, M. 1961. Evolution of repeated hippocampal seizures in the cat. Electroencephalogr. Clin. Neurophysiol. 13:722–733.

Delgado-Escueta, A.V., and Enrile-Bascal, F. 1984. Juvenile myoclonic epilepsy of Janz. Neurology (Cleveland) 34:285–294.

Delgado-Escueta, A.V., and Walsh, G.O. 1985. Type I complex partial seizures of hippocampal origin: excellent results of anterior temporal lobectomy. Neurology (Cleveland) 35:143–154.

Delgado-Escueta, A.V., Treiman, D.M., and Walsh, G.O. 1983a. The treatable epilepsies, parts I and II. N. Engl. J. Med. 308:1576–1584.

Delgado-Escueta, A.V., Bascal, F.E., and Treiman, D.M. 1983b. Complex partial seizures in closed-circuit television and EEG: a study of 691 attacks in 79 patients. Ann. Neurol. 11:292–300.

Delgado-Escueta, A.V., Wasterlain, C.G., Treiman, D.M., et al. (Eds.) 1983c. *Status Epilepticus.* New York: Raven Press.

Delgado-Escueta, A.V., Ward, A.A., Jr., Woodbury, D.M., et al. 1986. New wave of research in the epilepsia. In *Basic Mechanisms of the Epilepsies,* Eds. A.V. Delgado-Escueta, A.A. Ward, Jr., D.M. Woodbury, et al., pp. 3–55. New York: Raven Press.

Delgado-Escueta, A.V., Greenberg, D.A., Treiman, L., et al. 1989. Mapping the gene for juvenile epilepsy. Epilepsia (New York) 30 (Suppl. 4): S8–S18.

Delgado-Escueta, A.V., Serratosa, J.M., Liu, A., et al. 1994. Progress in mapping human epilepsy genes. Epilepsia 35 (Suppl. 1):S29–S40.

DeLorenzo, R.J. 1986. A molecular approach to the calcium signal in brain. Relationship to synaptic modulation and seizure discharges. In *Basic Mechanisms of the Epilepsies,* Eds. A.V. Delgado-Escueta, A.A. Ward, Jr., D.M. Woodbury, et al., pp. 435–464. New York: Raven Press.

DeLorenzo, R.J. 1991. The challenging genetics of epilepsy. In *Genetic Strategies in Epilepsy Research,* Eds. V.E. Anderson, W.A. Hauser, I.E. Leppik, et al., pp. 3–17. Amsterdam: Elsevier.

DeLorenzo, R.J., Pellock, J.M., Towne, A.R., et al. 1995. Epidemiology of status epilepticus. J. Clin. Neurophysiol. 12:316–325.

DeMarco, P. 1980. Petit mal epilepsy during early infancy. Clin. Electroencephalogr. 11:38–40.

DeMarco, P. 1983. Occipital evoked spike epilepsy in childhood. Clin. Electroencephalogr. 14:221–224.

DeMarco, P. 1990. Reflex petit mal absence? Clin. Electroencephalogr. 21: 74–76.

DeMarco, P., Lorenzi, E., and Miotello, P. 1980. Eine besondere Form von Epilepsie in der späten Kindheit. Z. EEG-EMG 11:107–109.

Denny-Brown, D., and Chambers, R.A. 1958. The parietal lobe and behavior. Res. Publ. Assoc. Res. Nerv. Ment. Dis. 26:35–117.

Deonna, T., Beaumanoir, A., Gaillard, F., et al. 1975. Syndrome of acquired aphasia in childhood with seizure disorder and EEG-abnormalities. Proc. Eur. Group of Child Neurologists, 2nd conference, Zurich, Sept. 1975.

Deonna, T., Ziegler, A.L., and Despland, P.A. 1996. Combined myoclonic-astatic and "benign" focal epilepsy of childhood ("atypical benign partial epilepsy of childhood"). A separate syndrome? Neuropediatrics 17:144–151.

De Santis, A., and Rampini, P.M. 1983. Long-term EEG follow-up in 100 patients following surgery for intracranial aneurysm: correlation between patients operated with and without operating microscope. Electroencephalogr. Clin. Neurophysiol. 55:1P–2P(abst).

Des Termes, H., Mises, J., Plouin, P., et al. 1978. The "spike focus" during the evolution of febrile convulsions: an electrophysiological and clinical study of 35 patients. Electroencephalogr. Clin. Neurophysiol. 45:370 (abst).

Detre, J.A., Alsop, D.C., Aguirre, G.K., et al. 1996. Coupling of cortical and thalamic ictal activity in human partial epilepsy: demonstration by functional magnetic resonance imaging. Epilepsia 37:657–661.

Devinsky, O., and Duchowny, M.S. 1983. Seizures after convulsive therapy: a retrospective case survey. Neurology 33:921–925.

Dichter, M.A., and Ayala, G.F. 1987. Cellular mechanisms of epilepsy: a status report. Science 237:157–164.

Dinner, D.S., and Lueders, H. 1985. The electroencephalogram in the routine evaluation of patients with epilepsy. In *The Epilepsies,* Eds. R.J. Porter and P.L. Morselli, pp. 142–173. London: Butterworth.

Dinner, D.S., Lueders, H., Lederman, R.J., et al. 1981. Aphasic status epilepticus: a case report. Electroencephalogr. Clin. Neurophysiol. 52: 86P(abst).

Donaldson, H.H. 1924. Quoted by Collins, R.L. 1972.

Dongier, S. 1959. *Étude Clinique et E.E.G. des Episodes Psychotiques Présentes par les Épileptiques.* Marseille: Thèse, Université de Marseille.

Dongier, S. 1959/60. Statistical study of clinical and electroencephalographic manifestations of 536 episodes occurring in 516 epileptics between seizures. Epilepsia (Amsterdam) 1:117–142.

Dongier, S. 1967. À propos des états de mal généralisés à expression confusionelle. Étude psychologique de la conscience au cours de l'état de petit mal. In *Les États de Mal Épileptiques,* Eds. H. Gastaut, J. Roger, and H. Lob, pp. 110–118. Paris: Masson.

Doose, H. 1964. Das Akinetische Petit mal. Arch. Psychiatr. Nervenkr. 205: 625–654.

Doose, H. 1970. Spezielle Probleme der antikonvulsiven Therapie. In *Epilepsy. Recent Views on Theory, Diagnosis, and Therapy of Epilepsy,* Ed. E. Niedermeyer, pp. 246–260. Basel: S. Karger.

Doose, H. 1985. Myoclonic astatic epilepsy of early childhood. In *Epileptic Syndromes in Infancy, Childhood and Adolescence,* Eds. J. Roger, C. Dravet, M. Bureau, et al., pp. 78–88. London: Libbey.

Doose, H., Gerken, H., Hien-Vlpel, K.F., et al. 1969. Genetics of photosensitive epilepsy. Neuropediatrie 1:56–73.

Doose, H., Gerken, H., and Völzke, E. 1972. On the genetics of EEG anomalies in childhood. I. Abnormal theta rhythms. Neuropediatrie 3:386–401.

Doose, H., Gerken, H., Horstmann, T., et al. 1973. Genetic factors in spike-wave absences. Epilepsia (Amsterdam) 14:57–75.

Doose, H., Gerken, H., Kiefer, R., et al. 1977. Genetic factors in childhood epilepsy with focal sharp waves. II. EEG findings in patients and siblings. Neuropediatrie 8:10–20.

Dow, R.S. 1965. Extrinsic regulatory mechanisms of seizure activity. Epilepsia (Amsterdam) 6:122–140.

Dow, R.S., Fernandez-Guardiola, A., and Manni, E. 1962. The influence of cerebellum on experimental epilepsy. Electroencephalogr. Clin. Neurophysiol. 14:383–398.

Drake, M.E., Jr. 1984. Ambulatory cassette EEG monitoring in initial assessment of suspected seizures. Electroencephalogr. Clin. Neurophysiol. 58:8P(abst).

Drake, M.E., and Shy, K.E. 1989. EEG and electroconvulsive response. Electroencephalogr. Clin. Neurophysiol. 73:66P(abst).

Drake, W.E., and MacRae, D. 1961. Epilepsy in multiple sclerosis. Neurology (Minneapolis) 11:810–816.

Dravet, C. 1978. Les épilepsies graves de l'enfant. Vie Med. 8:543–548.

Dravet, C., and Bureau, M. 1982. The benign myoclonic epilepsy of infancy. Electroencephalogr. Clin. Neurophysiol. 53:81P(abst).

Dravet, C., Bureau, M., and Roger, J. 1985. Severe myoclonic epilepsy in infants. In *Epileptic Syndromes in Infancy, Childhood, and Adolescence,* Eds. J. Roger, C. Dravet, M. Bureau, et al., pp. 58–67. London: Libbey.

Dreifuss, F.E. 1994. The international classification of seizures and epilepsies: Advantages. In *Epileptic Seizures and Syndromes,* Ed. P. Wolf, pp. 9–14. London: Libbey.

Dreyer, R. 1965. Zur Frage des Status epilepticus mit psychomotorischen Alfällen. Nervenarzt 36:221–223.

Dreyer, R. 1972. Mustersehen als Provokationsmittel zur Auslösung epileptischer Phänomene. Arch. Psychiatr. Nervendr. 216:58–69.

Dreyfus-Brisac, C., and Monod, N. 1964. Electroclinical studies of status epilepticus and convulsions in the newborn. In *Neurologic and Electroencephalographic Correlative Studies in Infancy,* Eds. P. Kellaway and I. Petersén, pp. 250–272. New York: Grune & Stratton.

Dreyfus-Brisac, C., and Monod, N. 1972. Neonatal status epilepticus. In *Handbook of Electroencephalography and Clinical Neurophysiology,* vol. 15B. Ed.-in-Chief, A. Remond, pp. 38–52. Amsterdam: Elsevier.

Dreyfus-Brisac, C., Peschanski, N., Radvanyi, M.F., et al. 1981. Convulsions du nouveauné. Aspects cliniques, électroencéphalographiques, étiopathogéniques et pronostiques. Rev. EEG Neurophysiol. 11: 367–378.

Druckman, R., and Chao, D. 1955. Massive spasms in infancy and childhood. Epilepsia (Boston) 4:61–72.

Dubowitz, L.M.S., Levene, M.I., Morante, A., et al. 1981. Neurologic signs in neonatal intraventricular hemorrhage: a correlation with real-time ultrasound. J. Pediatr. 99:127–133.

Dudek, F.E., Staley, K.J., and Sutula, T.P. 2002. The search for animal models of epileptogenesis and pharmacoresistance: are there biologic barriers to simple validation strategies? Epilepsia 43:1275–1277.

Dumermuth, G. 1972. *Elektoenzephalographie im Kindesalter,* 2nd ed. Stuttgart: Thieme.

Durner, M., Keddache, M.A., Tomasini, L., et al. 2001. Genome scan of idiopathic generalized epilepsy: evidence for major susceptibility gene and modifying genes influencing the seizure type. Ann. Neurol. 49:328–335.

Dusser de Barenne, D., and McCulloch, W.S. 1939. Physiological delimitation of neurons in the central nervous system. Am. J. Physiol. 127:620–628.

Earle, K.M.M., Baldwin, M., and Penfield, W. 1953. Incisural sclerosis and temporal lobe seizures produced by hippocampal herniation at birth. Arch. Neurol. (Chicago) 69:27–42.

Ebersole, J.S., Bridgers, S.L., and Silva, C.G. 1983. Differentiation of epileptiform abnormalities from normal transients and artifacts on ambulatory cassette EEG. Am. J. EEG Tech. 23:113–125.

Ebner, A., and Hoppe, M. 1995. Noninvasive electroencephalography and mesial temporal sclerosis. J. Clin. Neurophysiol. 12:23–31.

Eccles, J.C. 1957. *The Physiology of Nerve Cells.* Baltimore: Johns Hopkins Press.

Eccles, J.C. 1958. The behavior of nerve cells. In *Neurological Basis of Behavior,* Eds. G.E.W. Wostenholme and C.M. O'Connor, pp. 28–47. London: Churchill.

Eeg-Olofsson, O., Säfwenberg, J., and Wigertz, A. 1982. HLA and epilepsy: an investigation of different types of epilepsy in children and their families. Epilepsia (New York) 23:27–34.

Efron, R. 1961. Post-epileptic paralysis: theoretical critique and report of a case. Brain 84:381–394.

Egli, M., Bernoulli, C., and Baumgartner, G. 1974. Spinale Epilepsie-Tonische Anfälle nach zervikalem Spinalis-anterior-Syndrom. Z. EEG-EMG 5:87–95.

Egli, M., Mothersill, I., O'Kane, M., et al. 1985. The axial spasm—the predominant type of drop seizure in patients with secondary generalized epilepsy. Epilepsia (New York) 26:401–415.

Ehle, A.L. 1980. Midline spike foci in children. Electroencephalogr. Clin. Neurophysiol. 50:153P(abst).

Ehret, R., and Schneider, E. 1961. Photogene Epilepsie mit suchtartiger Selbstauslösung kleiner Anfälle und wiederhoten Sexualdelikten. Arch. Psychiatr. Nervenkr. 202:75–94.

Elger, C.E., and Speckmann, E.-J. 1979. Interiktale epileptiforme Potentiale im corticalen Oberflächen-EEG und ihre Beziehungen zu spinalen Feldpotentialen bei der Ratte. In *Epilepsie 1978,* Eds. M. Doose and G. Gross-Selbeck, pp. 245–249. Stuttgart: Thieme.

Elger, C.E., and Speckmann, E.-J. 1980. Focal interictal epileptiform discharges (FIED) in the epicortical EEG and their relations to spinal field potentials in the rat. Electroencephalogr. Clin. Neurophysiol. 48: 447–460.

Elger, C.E., and Speckmann, E.-J. 1983. Vertical inhibition in motor cortical epileptic foci and its consequences for descending neuronal activity to the spinal cord. In *Epilepsy and Motor System,* Eds. E.-J. Speckmann and C.E. Elger, pp. 152–160. Munich: Urban & Schwarzenberg.

Elian, M., and Dean, G. 1977. Multiple sclerosis and seizures. In *Epilepsy. The Eighth International Symposium,* Ed. J.K. Penry, pp. 341–344. New York: Raven Press.

Ellenberg, J.H., Hirtz, D.G., and Nelson, K.B. 1984. Age of onset of seizures in young children. Ann. Neurol. 15:127–134.

Ellingson, R.J. 1979. EEGs of premature and full-term newborns. In *Current Practice of Clinical Electroencephalography,* Eds. D.W. Klass and D.D. Daly, pp. 149–177. New York: Raven Press.

Ellingson, R.J., Wilken, K., and Bennett, D.R. 1984. Efficacy of sleep deprivation as an activation and procedure in epilepsy patients. J. Clin. Neurophysiol. 1:83–101.

Elliott, K.A.C., and Jasper, H.H. 1959. Gamma-aminobutyric acid. Physiol. Rev. 39:383–406.

Emerson, R.G., Turner, C.A., Pedley, T.A., et al. 1995. Propagation patterns of temporal spikes. Electroencephalogr. Clin. Neurophysiol. 94:338–348.

Engel, J., Jr. 1984. A practical guide for routine EEG studies in epilepsy. J. Clin. Neurophysiol. 1:109–142.

Engel, J., Jr. 1987. *Surgical Treatment of the Epilepsies.* New York: Raven Press.

Engel, J., Jr. 2001. A proposed diagnostic scheme for people with epileptic seizures and with epilepsy: report of the ILAE task force on classification and terminology. Epilepsia. 42:796–803.

Engel, J., Jr., Kuhl, D.E., Phelps, M.E., et al. 1982. Metabolic correlates of the 3 per sec spike and wave absences. Electroencephalogr. Clin. Neurophysiol. 53:20P(abst).

Epstein, C.M., and Moore, R.J. 1982. Pseudo-spike-and-wave in reading epilepsy. Electroencephalogr. Clin. Neurophysiol. 53:85P(abst).

Epstein, C.M., Duchowny, M., Jaykar, P., et al. 1994. Altered responsiveness during hyperventilation-induced EEG slowing: a non-epileptic phenomenon in normal children. Epilepsia 35:1204–1206

Ernst, J. 1969. Un cas d'épilepsie photosensible avec phénomène d'aimentation visuelle. J. Sci. Med. Lille 87:559–564.

Ervin, F., Epstein, A.W., and King, H.E. 1955. Behavior of epileptic and nonepileptic patients with "temporal spikes." Arch. Neurol. Psychiatry (Chicago) 74:488–497.

Esquirol. 1815. Quoted in Temkin, O. 1971.

Essig, C.F., and Fraser, H.F. 1958. Electroencephalographic changes in man during use and withdrawal of barbiturates in moderate dosage. Electroencephalogr. Clin. Neurophysiol. 10:649–656.

Evans, J.P. 1963. *Acute Head Injury,* 2nd ed. Springfield, IL: Charles C Thomas.

Fahn, S., Hallett, M., Lueders, H.O., et al. (Eds.). 1995. *Negative Motor Phenomena.* Philadelphia: Lippincott-Raven.

Faingold, C.L., and Fromm, G.H. (Eds.). 1992. *Drugs for the Control of Epilepsy: Actions on Neuronal Networks Involved in Seizure Disorders.* Boca Raton, FL: CRC Press.

Faingold, C.L., and Meldrum, B.S. 1990. Excitant amino acids in epilepsy. In *Generalized Epilepsy,* Eds. M. Avoli, P. Gloor, G. Kostopoulos, et al., pp. 102–117. Boston: Birkhäuser.

Falconer, M.A. 1968. The significance of mesial temporal sclerosis (Ammon's horn sclerosis) in epilepsy. Guy's Hosp. Rep. 117:1–12.

Falconer, M.A. 1974. Mesial temporal (Ammon's horn) sclerosis as a common cause of epilepsy. Aetiology, treatment and prevention. Lancet 2: 767–770.

Falret, J. 1860. De l'état mental des épileptiques. Arch. Gen. Med. 16:661–679.

Fariello, R.C., Forchetti, C.M., and Fisher, R.S. 1991. GABAergic function in relation to seizure phenomena. In *Neurotransmitters and Epilepsy,* Eds. R.S. Fisher and J.T. Coyle, pp. 77–93. New York: Wiley-Liss.

Farrell, D.F., and Swanson, P.D. 1975. Infectious diseases associated with myoclonus. In *Myoclonic Seizures,* Ed. M.H. Charlton, pp. 77–110. Amsterdam: Excerpta Medica.

Faught, E. 1984. Photoparoxysmal responses and high-amplitude visual evoked potentials during metaqualone withdrawal. Electroencephalogr. Clin. Neurophysiol. 58:35P–36P(abst).

Fegersten, L., and Roger, A. 1961. Frontal epileptogenic foci. Electroencephalogr. Clin. Neurophysiol. 13:905–913.

Feindel, W., and Penfield, W. 1954. Localization of discharge in temporal lobe automatism. Arch. Neurol. Psychiatry (Chicago) 72:605–630.

Fejerman, N., Gimenez, E.R., Vallejo, N.E., et al. 1973. Lennox-Gastaut and lead intoxication. Pediatrics 52:227.

Feng, Y.K. 1980. Abdominal epilepsy. Chin. Med. J. 93:135–148.

Ferguson, S.M., and Rayport, M. 1984. Psychosis in epilepsy. In *Psychiatric Aspects of Epilepsy,* Ed. D. Blumer, pp. 229–270. Washington, DC: American Psychiatric Press.

Fernandez, G., Effonberger, O., Vinz, B., et al. 1998. Hippocampal malformation as a cause of familial febrile convulsions and hippocampal sclerosis. Neurology 50:909–917.

Ferrier, D. 1873. Experimental researches in cerebral physiology and pathology. West Riding Lunatic Asylum Med. Reports 3:30–96.

Ferrier, D. 1876. *The Functions of the Brain.* London: Smith Elder.

Ferrier, D., and Yeo, C.F.A. 1884. A record of experiments on the effects of lesions of different regions of the cerebral hemispheres. Philos. Trans. R. Soc. Lond. (Biol.) 175:479–564.

Feucht, M., Spoljaric, A.M., Benninger, F., et al. 1996. Gehen epileptische Spitzen langsame Potentialverschiebungen voraus? Negative Ergebnisse bei Kindern mit benigner rolandischer Epilepsie. Z. EEG-EMG 27:62–64.

Finney, L.A., and Walker, A.E. 1962. *Transtentorial Herniation.* Springfield, IL: Charles C Thomas.

Fiol, M.E., and Leppik, I.E. 1984. Eating epilepsy—EEG and clinical study. Electroencephalogr. Clin. Neurophysiol. 57:43P–44P(abst).

Fiol, M.E., Mireles, R., Leppik, I., et al. 1986. Ictus emeticus: clinical and electroencephalographic findings on surface and electrocorticography. Electroencephalogr. Clin. Neurophysiol. 63:42P–43P(abst).

Fischer, M. 1959. Symptomatische Epilepsie bei cerebralen Gefäprozessen. Arch. Psychiatr. Nervenkr. 199:296–310.

Fischer, M.H. 1933. Elektrobiologische Auswirkungen von Krampgiften am Zentralnervensystem. Med. Klin. 25:15–19.

Fischer-Williams, M. 1982. Localized and generalized seizures associated with cerebral ischaemia. Electroencephalogr. Clin. Neurophysiol. 54: 21P(abst).

Fischer-Williams, M., Poncet, M., Riche, D., et al. 1968. Light-induced epilepsy in the baboon, Papio papio: cortical and depth recordings. Electroencephalogr. Clin. Neurophysiol. 25:557–569.

Fischgold, H. 1957. La conscience et ses modifications. Systèmes de références en E.E.G. clinique. *Proc. First Internat. Congr. Neurol. Sci., Brussels 1957. Reports and discussions,* vol. 2, pp. 181–213. Brussels: Les Éditions Acta Med. Belg.

Fisher, C.M. 1978. Transient paralytic attacks of obscure nature: the question of nonconvulsive seizure paralysis. Can. J. Neurol. Sci. 5:267–273.

Fisher, R.S. 1987. The hippocampal slice. Am. J. EEG Technol. 27:1–14.

Fisher, R.S. 1991a. Glutamate and epilepsy. In *Neurotransmitters and Epilepsy,* Eds. R.S. Fisher and J.T. Coyle, pp. 131–145. New York: Wiley-Liss.

Fisher, R.S. 1991b. Animal models of epilepsy. In *Neurotransmitters and Epilepsy,* Eds. R.S. Fisher and J.T. Coyle, pp. 61–76. New York: Wiley-Liss.

Fisher, R.S., and Coyle, J.T. 1991. Summary: neurotransmitters and epilepsy. In *Neurotransmitters and Epilepsy,* Eds. R.S. Fisher and J.T. Coyle, pp. 247–252. New York: Wiley-Liss.

Fisher, R.S., and Prince, D.A. 1977a. Spike-wave rhythms in cat cortex induced by parenteral penicillin. I. Electroencephalographic findings. Electroencephalogr. Clin. Neurophysiol. 42:608–624.

Fisher, R.S., and Prince, D.A. 1977b. Spike-wave rhythms in cat cortex induced by parenteral penicillin. II. Cellular features. Electroencephalogr. Clin. Neurophysiol. 42:625–639.

Flor-Henry, P. 1969. Psychosis and temporal lobe epilepsy. Epilepsia (Amsterdam) 10:363–395.

Foerster, C. 1977. Aphasia and seizure disorders in childhood. In *Epilepsia, The Eighth International Symposium,* Ed. J.K. Penry, pp. 305–306. New York: Raven Press.

Foerster, O. 1926. Die Pathogenese des epileptischen Krampfanfalles. Deutsch. Z. Nervenheilk. 94:15–53.

Foerster, O. 1936a. Motorische Felder und Bahnen. In *Handbuch der Neurologie,* vol. 6, Eds. O. Bumke and O. Foerster, pp. 1–357. Berlin: Springer.

Foerster, O. 1936b. The motor cortex in man in the light of Hughlings Jackson's doctrines. Brain 59:135–159.

Fonseca, L., and Tedrus, G.M.A. 1994. Epileptic syndromes in children with somatosensory evoked spikes. Clin. Electroencephalogr. 25:54–58.

Fonseca, L.C., Tedrus, G.M., Bastos, A., et al. 1996. Reactivity to rolandic spikes. Clin. Electroencephalogr. 27:116–120.

Forster, F.M. 1977. *Reflex Epilepsy, Behavioral Therapy and Conditional Reflexes.* Springfield, IL: Charles C Thomas.

Fossas, P., Sanchez, M.E., and Oller, L. 1985. Occipital origin of partial oculoclonic versive epileptic seizures in a case of post-traumatic epilepsy. Electroencephalogr. Clin. Neurophysiol. 60:58P.

Fountain, N.B., and Lothman, E.W. 1995. Pathophysiology of status epilepticus. J. Clin. Neurophysiol. 12:326–342.

Frantzen, E., Lennox-Buchthal, M., Nygaard, A., et al. 1970. A genetic study of febrile convulsions. Neurology (Minneapolis) 20:909–917.

Freemon, F.R., and Nevis, A.H. 1969. Temporal lobe sexual seizures. Neurology (Minneapolis) 19:87–90.

Friedlander, W.J., and Feinstein, G.H. 1956. Petit mal status. Epilepsia minoris continua. Neurology (Minneapolis) 6:357–362.

Friedmann, M. 1906. Über die gehäuften kleinen nicht epileptischen Absencen oder kurzen narkoleptischen Anfälle. Deutsch. Z. Nervenheilk. 30:462–492.

Fritsch, G., and Hitzig, E. 1870. Über die elekrische Erregbarkeit des Großhirns. Arch. Anat. Physiol. 37:300–332.

Fromm, G.H. 1974. Animal models of generalized convulsive disorders. In *Models of Human Neurological Disease,* Ed. H.L. Klawans, Jr., pp. 149–165. Amsterdam: Excerpta Medica.

Fromm, G.H. 1986. Role of inhibitory mechanisms in staring spells. J. Clin. Neurophysiol. 3:297–311.

Fromm, G.H. 1987. The brain-stem and seizures: Summary and synthesis. In *Epilepsy and the Reticular Formation,* Eds. G.H. Fromm, C.L. Faingold, R.A. Browning, et al., pp. 203–218. New York: Alan R. Liss.

Fromm, G.H. 1992. Trigeminal nuclei, trigeminal neuralgia and epileptic mechanism. Am. J. EEG Technol. 32:186–195.

Fromm, G.H., and Kohli, C.M. 1972. The role of inhibitory pathways in petit mal epilepsy. Neurology (Minneapolis) 22:1012–1020.

Fromm, G.H., Glass, J.D., and Chattha, A.S. 1979. The role of cholinergic mechanisms in the corticofugal inhibition of the spinal trigeminal nucleus. Electroencephalogr. Clin. Neurophysiol. 46:302–309.

Froescher, W. 1979. *Treatment of Status Epilepticus.* Baltimore: University Park Press.

Fuglsang-Frederiksen, V., and Thygesen, P. 1952. Seizures and psychopathology in multiple sclerosis. An electroencephalographic study. Discussion of pathogenesis. Acta Psychiatr. Neurol. Scand. 27:17–41.

Fusco, L., and Vigevano, F. 1993. Ictal clinical electroencephalographic findings of spasms in West syndrome. Epilepsia 34:671–673.

Fusco, L., Iani, C., Faedda, M.T., et al. 1990. Mesial frontal lobe epilepsy: a clinical entity not sufficiently described. J. Epilepsy 3:123–135.

Fusco, L., Bertini, E., and Vigevano, F. 1992. Epilepsia partialis continua and neuronal migration anomalies. Brain Dev. 14:323–328.

Fuster, B.C., Castells, C., and Rodriguez, B. 1954. Psychomotor attacks (primary automatisms) of subcortical origin. Arch. Neurol. Psychiatry (Chicago) 71:466–472.

Fuster, J.M. 1995a. Memory and planning. Two temporal perspectives of frontal lobe function. In *Epilepsy and the Functional Anatomy of the Frontal Lobe,* Eds. H.H. Jasper, S. Riggio, and P.S. Goldman-Rakic, pp. 85–96. New York: Raven Press.

Fuster, J.M. 1995b. *Memory in the Cerebral Cortex.* Cambridge, MA: MIT Press.

Futamachi, K.J., and Pedley, T.A. 1976. Glial cells and extracellular potassium: their relationship in mammalian cortex. Brain Res. 109:311–322.

Gabor, A.J., and Ajmone Marsan, C. 1968. Co-existence of focal bilateral diffuse paroxysmal discharges in epileptics. Epilepsia (Amsterdam) 10: 453–472.

Gaches, J., LeBeau, J., Daum, S., et al. 1965. Étude des sequelles épileptiques dans une série de 20 abscès du corveau suivis depuis plus de 10 ans. Neuro-Chirurgie 11:441–452.

Gale, K. 1986. Role of the substantia nigra in GABA-mediated anticonvulsant actions. In *Basic Mechanisms of the Epilepsies,* Eds. A.V. Delgado-Escueta, A.A. Ward, Jr., D.M. Woodbury, et al., pp. 343–364. New York: Raven Press.

Gambardella, A., Gotman, J., Cendes, F., et al. 1995. Focal intermittent delta activity in patients with mesiotemporal atrophy: a reliable marker of the epileptogenic focus. Epilepsia 36:122–129.

Garrel, S., Pellat, J., and Lavernhe, G. 1987. Occipital status with prosopagnosia. Electroencephalogr. Clin. Neurophysiol. 67:55P(abst).

Garretson, H., Gloor, P., and Rasmussen, T. 1966. Intracarotid amobarbital and Metrazol test for the study of epileptiform discharges in man: a note on its techniques. Electroencephalogr. Clin. Neurophysiol. 21:607–610.

Garsche, R. 1956. Das Elektroenzephalogramm bei den psychomotorischen Anfällen im Kindesalter. Arch. Kinderheilk. 153:27–40.

Gascon, C., Victor, D., Lombroso, C.T., et al. 1973. Language disorders. Convulsive disorder and electroencephalographic abnormalities. Arch. Neurol. (Chicago) 28:156–172.

Gascon, G.C., and Lombroso, C.T. 1971. Epileptic (gelastic) laughter. Epilepsia (Amsterdam) 12:63–76.

Gastaut, H. 1949. Effects des stimulations physiques sur l'E.E.G. de l'homme. Electroencephalogr. Clin. Neurophysiol. Suppl. 2:69–82.

Gastaut, H. 1953. So-called "psychomotor" and "temporal" epilepsy—a critical study. Epilepsia (Boston) 2:59–99.

Gastaut, H. 1956. État actuel des connaissances sur l'anatomie pathologique des épilepsies. Acta Neurol. Psychiatr. Belg. 1:5–20.

Gastaut, H. 1958a. À propos des symptomes cliniques recontrés chez les épileptiques psychomoteurs dans l'intervalle de leurs crises. In *Bases Physiologiques et Aspects Cliniques de l'Épilepsie,* Ed. T.Alajouanine, pp. 139–169. Paris: Masson.

Gastaut, H. 1958b. À propose des décharges neuroniques dévéloppées à distance d'une lésion et des symptomes qui en résultent. In *Bases Physiologiques et Aspects Cliniques de l'Épilepsie,* Ed. T. Alajouanine, pp. 163–184. Paris: Mason.

Gastaut, H. 1960. Un aspect méconnu des décharges neuroniques occipitales: la crise oculo-clonique ou "nystagmus épileptique." In *Les Grandes Activités du Lobe Occipital,* Ed. T. Alajouanine, pp. 169–186. Paris: Masson.

Gastaut, H. 1967. Discussion remark. In *Les Activités Électriques Cérébrales Spontanées et évoquées Chez l'Homme,* Eds. H. Gastaut, A.Waltrégny, R. Poiré, et al., pp. 217–218. Paris: Gauthier-Vallars.

Gastaut, H. 1968a. Séméiologie des myoclonies et nosologie analytique des syndromes myocloniques. Rev. Neurol. (Paris) 119:1–30.

Gastaut, H. 1968b. Clinical and electroencephalographic correlates of generalized spike and wave bursts occurring spontaneously in man. Epilepsia (Amsterdam) 9:179–184.

Gastaut, H. 1969. Classification of the epilepsies. Proposal for international classification. Epilepsia (Amsterdam) (suppl 10):514–521.

Gastaut, H. 1970. Clinical and electroencephalographic classification of epileptic seizures. Epilepsia (Amsterdam) 11:102–113.

Gastaut, H. 1971. Comments on "petit mal variant revisited." Epilepsia (Amsterdam) 12:97–99.

Gastaut, H. 1973. *Dictionary of Epilepsy.* Geneva: World Health Organization.

Gastaut, H. 1975. *Wörterbuch der Epilepsie.* Stuttgart: Hippokrates.

Gastaut, H. 1978. Fyodor Mikhailovitch Dostoevsky's involuntary contribution to the symptomatology and prognosis of epilepsy. Epilepsia (New York) 19:186–201.

Gastaut, H. 1982a. Individualization of so-called benign and functional epilepsy at different times of life. Electroencephalogr. Clin. Neurophysiol. 53:79P(abst).

Gastaut, H. 1982b. A new type of epilepsy: benign partial epilepsy of childhood with occipital spike-waves. .Clin. Electroencephalogr. 13: 13–22.

Gastaut, H. 1983. Classification of status epilepticus. In *Status Epilepticus,* Eds. A.V. Delgado-Escueta, C.G. Wasterlain, D.M. Treiman, et al., pp. 15–35. New York: Raven Press.

Gastaut, H. 1984. L'épilepsie partielle avec synchronie bilatérale secondaire. Proceed. Symposium "Le sindromi epilettiche: aspetti clinici ed evolutivi." Bologna, Sept. 1984.

Gastaut, H., and Broughton, R. 1972. *Epileptic Seizures.* Springfield, IL: Charles C Thomas.

Gastaut, H., and Collomb, H. 1954. Étude du comportement sexuel chez les épileptiques psychomoteurs. Ann. Med. Psychol. 112:657–696.

Gastaut, H., and Corriol, H.H. 1948. Sur la forme des ondes induites sur le cortex cerebral par des stimulations lumineuses rhythmées. C.R. Soc. Biol. (Paris) 142:351–353.

Gastaut, H., and Fischer-Williams, M. 1959. The physiopathology of epileptic seizures. In *Handbook of Physiology,* vol. 1, Eds. J. Field, H.W. Magoun, and V.E. Hall, pp. 329–364. Baltimore: Williams & Wilkins.

Gastaut, H., and Gastaut, H. 1949. Un cas d'épilepsie photogénique pour illustrer l'activation de l'électroencéphalogramme par la stimulation lumineuse intermittente. Sem. Hop. Paris 65:2707–2710.

Gastaut, H., and Gastaut, J.L. 1976. Computerized transverse axial tomography in epilepsy. Epilepsia (New York) 17:325–336.

Gastaut, H., and Gastaut, Y. 1951. Corrélations électroencéphalographiques et cliniques de 100 cas d'épilepsie dite "psychomotrice" avec foyers sur la région temporale du scalp. Rev. Oto-Neuro-Ophthal. 23:257–282.

Gastaut, H., and Gastaut, Y. 1957. Syncopes et convulsions. À propos de la nature syncopale de certaines spasmes du sanglot et des certaines convulsions essentielles hyperthermiques ou à froid. Rev. Neurol. (Paris) 96: 158–163.

Gastaut, H., and Poirier, F. 1964. Historique. In *L'Encéphalopathie Myoclonique Infantile avec Hypsrrhythmie (Syndrome de West),* Eds. H. Gastaut, J. Roger, R. Soulayrol, et al., pp. 2–14. Paris: Masson.

Gastaut, H., and Remond, A. 1949. L'activation de l'électroencéphalogramme dans les affections cérébrales non-epileptogènes (vers une neurophysiologie clinique). Rev. Neurol. (Paris) 81:594–598.

Gastaut, H., and Roger, J. 1964. Séméiologie neurologique. In *L'Encéphalopathie Myoclonique Infantile avec Hypsarrhythmie (Syndrome de West),* Eds. H. Gastaut, J. Roger, R. Soulayrol, et al., pp. 36–52. Paris: Masson.

Gastaut, H., and Tassinari, C.A. 1975. The significance of the EEG and of ictal and interictal discharges with respect to epilepsy. In *Handbook of Electroencephalography and Clinical Neurophysiology,* vol. 13A, Ed.-in-chief, A. Remond, pp. 3–6. Amsterdam: Elsevier.

Gastaut, H., and Tassinari, C.T. 1966. Triggering mechanisms vs. epilepsy. The electroclinical point of view. Epilepsia (Amsterdam) 7:85–138.

Gastaut, H., and Vigouroux, M. 1958. Electro-clinical correlations in 500 cases of psychomotor seizures. In *Temporal Lobe Epilepsy,* Eds. M. Baldwin and P. Bailey, pp. 118–128. Springfield, IL: Charles C Thomas.

Gastaut, H., Roger, J., Corriol, J.H., et al. 1948. Les formes expérimentales de l'épilepsie humaine. L'épilepsie induite par la stimulation lumineuse

intermittente ou épilepsie photogénique. Rev. Neurol. (Paris) 80:161–183.

Gastaut, H., Roger, J., and Roger, A. 1956. Sur la signification de certaines fugues épileptiques. À propos d'une observation électroclinique d' "état de mal temporal." Rev. Neurol. (Paris) 94:298–301.

Gastaut, H., Vigouroux, M., Trevisan, C., et al. 1957. Le syndrome "hémiconvulsion- hémiplegie-épilepsie" (H.H.E. syndrome). Rev. Neurol. (Paris) 97:37–52.

Gastaut, H., Naquet, R., and Fischer-Williams, M. 1958. The pathophysiology of grand mal seizures generalized from the start. J. Nerv. Ment. Dis. 127:21–33.

Gastaut, H., Poirier, F., Payan, H., et al. 1960. H.H.E. syndrome. Hemiconvulsions, hemiplegia, epilepsy. Epilepsia (Amsterdam) 1:418–447.

Gastaut, H., Regis, H., Bostem, J., et al. 1961. À propos des crises surrenante au cours des spectacles télévisés et de leur mécanism. Presse Med. 69:1581–1583.

Gastaut, H., Regis, H., and Bostem, F. 1962. Attacks provoked by television and their mechanism. Epilepsia (Amsterdam) 3:438–445.

Gastaut, H., Roger, J., Soulayrol, R., et al. (Eds.). 1964. *L'Encéphalopathie Myoclonique Infantile avec Hypsarrhythmie (Syndrome de West).* Paris: Masson.

Gastaut, H., Roger, J., Soulayrol, R., et al. 1966. Childhood epileptic encephalopathy with diffuse slow spike-waves (otherwise known as "petit mal variant") or Lennox syndrome. Epilepsia (Amsterdam) 7: 139–179.

Gastaut, H., Poiré, R., Roger, J., et al. 1967a. Les états de mal généralisés tonico-cloniques. In *Les États de Mal Épileptiques,* Eds. H. Gastaut, J. Roger, and H. Lob, pp. 11–43. Paris: Masson.

Gastaut, H., Roger, J., and Lob, H. 1967b. *Les États de Mal Épileptiques.* Paris: Masson.

Gastaut, H., Roger, J., Lob, H., et al. 1967c. Les États de Mal Généralisés Toniques. In *Les États de Mal Épileptiques,* Eds. H. Gastaut, J. Roger, and H. Lob, pp. 44–74. Paris: Masson.

Gastaut, H., Gastaut, J.L., Gonçalves e Silva, E., et al. 1975. Relative frequency of different types of epilepsy: a study employing the classification by the International League against Epilepsy. Epilepsia (New York) 16:457–461.

Gastaut, H., Regis, H., Gastaut, J.L., et al. 1980. Lipomas of the corpus callosum and epilepsy. Neurology (Minneapolis) 30:132–138.

Gastaut, H., Gomez-Almanzar, M., and Taury, M. 1983. Der provozierte Mittagsschlaf: Eine einfache erfolgreiche Methode zur Schlafaktivierung bei Epileptikern. Z. EEG-EMG 14:1–5.

Gastaut, H., Gomex-Almanzar, M., and Taury, M. 1984. The enforced nap: a simple effective method of inducing sleep activation in epileptics. In *Epilepsy, Sleep and Sleep Deprivation,* Eds. R. Degen and E. Niedermeyer, pp. 75–83. Amsterdam: Elsevier.

Gastaut, H., Zifkin, B.G., Mariani, E., et al. 1986. The long-term course of primary generalized epilepsy with persisting absences. Neurology 36: 1021–1028.

Gastaut, Y. 1952. Un élément déroutant de la séméiologie électro-encéphalographique: les pointes rolandiques sans signfication focale. Rev. Neurol. (Paris) 87:448–450.

Gates, J.R., Leppik, I.E., Yap, J., et al. 1982. Effect of total corpus callosectomy on EEG. Epilepsia (New York) 23:441(abst).

Geier, S., Bancaud, J., Bonis, A., et al. 1977a. Enrégistrements télé-E.E.G. de trois crises épileptiques prolongées classées comme des épisodes de petit mal status. Rev. E.E.G. Neurophysiol. 2:201–202.

Geier, S., Bancaud, J., Talairach, J., et al. 1977b. The seizures of frontal lobe epilepsy. A study of clinical manifestations. Neurology (Minneapolis) 27:951–958.

Geier, S., Bancaud, J., Talairach, J., et al. 1977c. Ictal tonic postural changes and automatisms of the upper limb during epileptic parietal lobe discharges. Epilepsia (New York) 18:517–524.

Gelisse, P., Corda, D., Raybaud, C., et al. 2003. Abnormal neuroimaging in patients with benign epilepsy with centrotemporal spikes. Epilepsia 44: 372–378

Gerard, F., Pereira, S., Robaglia-Schlupp, A., et al. 2002 Clinical and genetic analysis of a new multigenerational pedigree with GEFS (generalized epilepsy with febrile seizures plus). Epilepsia 43:581–586

Gereby, G. 1985. Benign centro-temporal epilepsy of childhood. EEG and clinical follow-up of 80 cases. Electroencephalogr. Clin. Neurophysiol. 61:7P(abst).

Gershoff, S.N., and Elvehjem, C.A. 1951. The relative effect of methionine sulfimine on different species. J. Nutr. 45:451–458.

Geschwind, N., and Sherwin, I. 1967. Language induced epilepsy. Arch. Neurol. 16:25.

Ghigo, J., and Niedermeyer, E. 2000. Juvenile myclonic rpilepsy. Am. J. Electroneurodiagn. Technol. 40:372–378.

Giannakodimos, S., and Panayiotopulos, C.P. 1996. Eyelid myoclonia in adults: clinical and EEG features. In *Eyelid Myoclonia with Absences*, Eds. J.S. Duncan and C.P. Panayiotopoulos, pp. 57–68. London: Libbey.

Giardini, M. 1983. High incidence of febrile convulsions in a family. Electroencephalogr. Clin. Neurophysiol. 56:39P(abst).

Gibbs, E.L., and Gibbs, F.A. 1947. Diagnostic and localizing value of electroencephalographic studies in sleep. Publ. Assoc. Res. Nerv. Ment. Dis. 26:366–376.

Gibbs, E.L., Fuster, B., and Gibbs, F.A. 1948. Peculiar low temporal localization of sleep-induced seizure discharges of psychomotor epilepsy. Arch. Neurol. Psychiatry (Chicago) 60:95–97.

Gibbs, F.A. 1958. Differentiation of mid-temporal, anterior temporal and diencephalic epilepsy. In *Temporal Lobe Epilepsy*, Eds. M. Baldwin and P. Bailey, pp. 109–117. Springfield, IL: Charles C Thomas.

Gibbs, F.A. 1971. Petit mal variant revisited. Epilepsia (Amsterdam) 12:89–96.

Gibbs, F.A., and Gibbs, E.L. 1952. *Atlas of Electroencephalography*, 2nd ed., vol. 2. Cambridge, MA: Addison-Wesley.

Gibbs, F.A., and Gibbs, E.L. 1964. *Atlas of Electroencephalography*, 2nd ed., vol. 3. Reading, MA: Addison-Wesley.

Gibbs, F.A., Davis, H., and Lennox, W.G. 1935. The electroencephalogram in epilepsy and in conditions of impaired consciousness. Arch. Neurol. Psychiatry (Chicago) 34:1133–1148.

Gibbs, F.A., Gibbs, E.L., and Lennox, W.G. 1937. Epilepsy, a paroxysmal cerebral dysrhythmia. Brain 60:377–388.

Gibbs, F.A., Gibbs, E.L., and Lennox, W.G. 1939. The influence of the blood sugar level on the wave and spike formation in petit mal epilepsy. Arch. Neurol. Psychiatry (Chicago) 47:1111–1116.

Giove, C. 1960. Contributo alla genesi delle crise oculo-cloniche delle epilettica. Rass. Stud. Psichiatr. 49:940–952.

Giroud, M., and Dumas, R. 1995. Role of associated cortical lesions in motor partial seizures and lenticulostriate infarcts. Epilepsia 36:465–470.

Glaser, G.H., and Golub, L.J. 1955. The electroencephalogram and psychomotor seizures in childhood. Electroencephalogr. Clin. Neurophysiol. 7:329.

Globus, M., Lavi, E., Fich, E., et al. 1982. Ictal hemiparesis. Eur. Neurol. 21:165–168.

Gloor, P. 1968. Generalized cortico-reticular epilepsies. Some considerations on the pathophysiology of generalized bilaterally synchronous spike and wave discharge. Epilepsia (Amsterdam) 9:249–263.

Gloor, P. 1969. Neurophysiological bases of generalized seizures termed centroencephalic. In *The Physiopathogenesis of the Epilepsies*, Eds. H. Gastaut, H.H. Jasper, J. Bancaud, et al., pp. 209–236. Springfield, IL: Charles C Thomas.

Gloor, P. 1975. Contributions of electroencephalography and electrocorticography to the neurosurgical treatment of the epilepsies. In *Neurosurgical Management of the Epilepsies*, Eds. P.O. Purpura, J.K. Penry, and R.D. Walter, pp. 59–105. New York: Raven Press.

Gloor, P. 1978. Evolution of the concept of the mechanisms of generalized epilepsy with spike and wave discharge. In *Modern Perspectives in Epilepsy*, Ed. J.A. Wada, pp. 99–137. St. Albans and Montreal: Eden Press.

Gloor, P. 1984. Electrophysiology of generalized epilepsy. In *Electrophysiology of Epilepsy*, Eds. P.A. Schwartzkroin and H.V. Wheal, pp. 107–136. London: Academic Press.

Gloor, P., Jacob, J.C., Elwan, O.H., et al. 1969. The electroencephalogram in chronic renal failure. In *The Physiopathogenesis of the Epilepsies*, Eds. H. Gastaut, H.H. Jasper, J. Bancaud, et al., pp. 50–59. Springfield, IL: Charles C Thomas.

Gloor, P., Quesney, L.F., and Zumstein, H. 1977. Pathophysiology of generalized penicillin epilepsy in the cat: the role of cortical and subcortical structures. II. Topical application of penicillin to the cerebral cortex and subcortical structures. Electroencephalogr. Clin. Neurophysiol. 43:79–94.

Gloor, P., Avoli, M., and Kostopoulos, G. 1990. Thalamocortical relationships in generalized epilepsy with bilaterally synchronous spike-and-wave discharge. In *Generalized Epilepsy*, Eds. M. Avoli, P. Gloor, G. Kostopoulos, et al., pp. 190–212. Boston: Birkhauser.

Goddard, G.V. 1967. The development of epileptic seizures through brain stimulation at low intensity. Nature 214:1020–1021.

Goldensohn, E.S. 1969. Experimental seizure mechanisms. In *Basic Mechanisms of the Epilepsies*, Eds. H.H. Jasper, A.A. Ward, Jr., and A. Pope, pp. 289–298. Boston: Little, Brown.

Goldensohn, E.S. 1979. Use of the EEG for evaluation of focal intracranial lesions. In *Current Practice of Clinical Electroencephalography*, Eds. D.W. Klass and D.D. Daly, pp. 307–341. New York: Raven Press.

Goldensohn, E.S., and Gold, A.P. 1960. Prolonged behavioral disturbances as ictal phenomena. Neurology (Minneapolis) 10:1–9.

Goldensohn, E.S., and Purpura, D.P. 1963. Intracellular potentials of cortical neurons during focal epileptogenic discharges. Science 193:840–842.

Goldensohn, E.S., and Ward, A.A., Jr. 1975. Pathogenesis of epileptic seizures. In *The Nervous System*, vol. 1, Ed.-in-chief, D.B. Tower, pp. 249–260. New York: Raven Press.

Gotman, J., Ives, J.R., and Gloor, P. 1980. Long-term monitoring of interictal epileptic EEG activity. In *Advances in Epileptology. The Xth Epilepsy International Symposium*, Eds. J. Wada and J.K. Penry, pp. 129–130 (abst). New York: Raven Press.

Gotman, J., Ives, J.R., and Gloor, P. 1981. Frequency content of EEG and EMG at seizure onset: possibility of removal of EMG artifact by digital filtering. Electroencephalogr. Clin. Neurophysiol. 52:626–639.

Gowers, W.R. 1881 (reprinted 1964). *Epilepsy and Other Chronic Convulsive Diseases: Their Causes, Symptoms and Treatment*. New York: Dover (American Academy of Neurology reprint series).

Graf, M., Niedermeyer, E., Schiemann, J., et al. 1983. Electrocorticography. Information derived from intraoperative recordings during seizure surgery. Clin. Electroencephalogr. 15:83–91.

Graf, M., Grisold, W., Jelinek, V., et al. 1990. Startle Response und Epilepsie. Wien. Klin. Wochenschr. 102:233–237.

Grasset, J., and Rauzier, G. 1902a. Étiologie et pathogénie de la névrose comitiale (épilepsie dite idiopathique ou essentielle). Montpellier Med. 15:937–953.

Grasset, J., and Rauzier, G. 1902b. Étiologie et Pathogénie de la névrose comitiale (épilepsie dite idiopathique ou essentielle). Montpellier Med. 15:961–982.

Green, J.B. 1968. Seizures on closing the eyes. Neurology (Minneapolis) 18:391–396.

Greenberg, D.A., Durner, M., Resor, S., et al. 1995. The genetics of idiopathic generalized epilepsies of adolescent onset: differences between juvenile myoclonic epilepsy with random grand mal and with awakening grand mal. Neurology 45:942–946.

Gregory, D.L., and Wong, P.K. 1984. Topographical analysis of the centrotemporal discharges in benign rolandic epilepsy of childhood. Epilepsia (New York) 25:705–711.

Gregory, D.L., and Wong, P.K.H. 1992. Clinical relevance of a dipole field in rolandic spikes. Epilepsia (New York) 33:36–44.

Grenier, F., Timofeev, I., and Steriade, M. 2003. Neocortical very fast oscillations (ripples, 80–200 hz) during seizures. Intra-cellular correlates. J. Neurophysiol. 89:841–852.

Greulich, W., and Gerber, U. 1994. Epidemiologie der Epilepsien. In *Die Epilepsien*, Eds. W. Froescher and F. Vassella, pp. 43–55. Berlin: De Gruyter.

Groethuysen, U.C., Bickford, R.G., and Svien, H.J. 1955. The EEG in arteriovenous anomalies of the brain. Arch. Neurol. Psychiatry (Chicago) 74:506–513.

Grünbaum, A.S.F., and Sherrington, C.S. 1901. Observations on the physiology of the cerebral cortex of some of the higer apes. Proc. Roy Soc. 69:206–209.

Guerrero-Figueroa, R., Barros, A., DeBalbian Verster, H., et al. 1963. Experimental "Petit mal" in kittens. Arch. Neurol. (Chicago) 9:297–306.

Guerrini, R., Dravet, C., Genton, P., et al. 1995. Idiopathic photosensitive occipital lobe epilepsy. Epilepsia 36:883–891.

Guldner, G.T., and Morrell, M.J. 1996. Nocturnal penile tumescence and rigidity evaluation in men with epilepsy. Epilepsia 37:1211–1214.

Gumnit, R.J. 1984. *The Epilepsy Handbook*. New York: Raven Press.

Gumnit, R.J., and Takahashi, T. 1965. Changes in direct current activity during experimental focal seizures. Electroencephalogr. Clin. Neurophysiol. 19:63–74.

Gumnit, R.J., Niedermeyer, E., and Spreen, O. 1965. Seizure activity uniquely inhibited by patterned vision. Arch. Neurol. 13:363–368.

Gurer, G., Saygi, S., and Ciger, A. 2001. Epilepsia partialis continua: clinical and electrophysiological features of adult patients. Clin Electroencephalogr. 32:1–9.

Gustavson, A.R., McIntyre, B.B., and Roberts, H.W. 2003. Electrographic correlates of seizures with Todd's paralysis. A case report. Clin Neurophysiol. 114:393(abst).

Guterman, A., Ramsay, R.E., and Colter, R.M. 1983. Graphogenic epilepsy: report of a "scriptogenic" variant after a stroke. Electroencephalogr. Clin. Neurophysiol. 56:9P(abst).

Gutierrez, A.R., Brick, J.F., and Bodensteiner, J. 1990. Dipole reversal: an ictal feature of benign partial epilepsy with centrotemporal spikes. Epilepsia 31:544–548.

Guye, M., Le Fur, Y., Confort-Gouny, S., et al. 2002. Metabolic and electrophysiological alterations in subtypes of temporal lobe epilepsy: a combined proton magnetic resonance spectroscopic imaging and depth electrodes study. Epilepsia 43:1197–1209.

Haberland, C. 1962. Cerebellar degeneration with clinical manifestations in chronic epileptic patients. Psychiatr. Neurol. (Basel) 143:29–44.

Hahn, F. 1960. Analeptics. Pharmacol. Rev. 12:447–530.

Hakamada, S., Watanabe, K., Hara, K., et al. 1981. Brief atonia associated with electroencephalographic paroxysm in an infant with infantile spasms. Epilepsia (New York) 22:285–288.

Halász, P. 1972. The generalized spike-wave mechanisms and the sleep-wakefulness system. Acta Physiol. Acad. Sci. Hung. 42:293–314.

Halász, P. 1981. Generalized epilepsy with spike-wave paroxysms as an epileptic disorder of the function of sleep promotion. Acta Physiol. Acad. Sci. Hung. 57:51–86.

Halász, P. 1984. Sleep, arousal and electroclinical manifestations of generalized epilepsy with spike wave pattern. In *Epilepsy, Sleep and Sleep Deprivation*, Eds. R. Degen and E. Niedermeyer, pp. 97–107. Amsterdam: Elsevier.

Halász, P., and Devényi, E. 1974. Petit mal absences in night sleep with special reference to transitional sleep and REM periods. Acta Med. Acad. Sci. Hung. 31:31–45.

Hallen, O. 1952. Über Jackson-Anfälle. Dtsch. Z. Nervenheilk. 167:143.

Hallen, O. 1953. Zur Differentialdiagnose der Jackson-Anfälle. Dtsch. Med. Wochenschr. 78:260.

Hallett, M. 1985. Myoclonus: relation to epilepsy. Epilepsia (New York) 26:S67–S77.

Hallett, M., Chadwick, D., and Marsden, C.D. 1977. Ballistic movement overflow myoclonus: a form of essential myoclonus. Brain 100:299–312.

Halliday, A.M. 1967a. The electrophysiological study of myoclonus. Brain 90:241–284.

Halliday, A.M. 1967b. Cerebral evoked potentials in familial progressive myoclonic epilepsy. J. R. Coll. Physicians Lond. 1:123–134.

Halliday, A.M. 1967c. The clinical incidence of myoclonus. In *Modern Trends in Neurology*, Ed. D. Williams, pp. 69–105. London: Butterworth.

Halliday, A.M. 1975. The neurophysiology of myoclonus—a reappraisal. In *Myoclonic Seizures*, Ed. M.H. Charlton, pp. 1–29. Amsterdam: Excerpta Medica.

Hann, J. 1959. Petit mal Anfälle bei hypothalamisch bedingter Pubertas praecox. *Proc. First Internat. Congr. Neurol. Sciences, Brussels 1957*, vol. 3, pp. 701–704. London: Pergamon Press.

Hanson, P.A., and Chodos, R. 1978. Hemiparetic seizures. Neurology (Minneapolis) 28:920–923.

Harbaugh, R.E., and Wilson, D.H. 1982. Telencephalic theory of generalized epilepsy: observations in split-brain patients. Neurosurgery 10:725–732.

Hari, R., Ahonen, A., Forss, N., et al. 1993. Parietal mirror focus detected with a whole-head neuromagnetometer. NeuroReport 5:45–48.

Harris, R., and Tizard, J.P. 1960. The electroencephalogram in neonatal convulsions. J. Pediatr. 57:501–520.

Hart, Y.M., Andermann, F., Fish, D.R., et al. 1997. Chronic encephalitis and epilepsy in adults and adolescents: a variant of Rasmussen's syndrome? Neurology 48:418–424.

Harvald, B. 1954. *Heredity in Epilepsy*. Copenhagen: Munksgaard.

Harvey, A.S., Jayakar, P., Duchowny, M., et al. 1996. Hemifacial seizures and cerebellar ganglioglioma: an epilepsy syndrome of infancy with seizures of cerebellar origin. Ann. Neurol. 40:91–98.

Hauser, W.A. 1998. Incidence and prevalence. In *Epilepsy. A Comprehensive Textbook (3 vol.)*, Eds. J. Engel, Jr. and T. Pedley, vol. 1, pp. 47–57. Philadelphia: Lippincott-Raven.

Hauser, W.A., Rich, S., Nicolosi, A., et al. 1982. Electroencephalographic findings in patients with ethanol withdrawal seizures. Electroencephalogr. Clin. Neurophysiol. 54:64P(abst).

Hauser, W.A., Anderson, V.A., and Rich, S.S. 1983. Effect of photoconvulsive response (PCR) on the occurrence of seizures and of generalized EEG patterns in siblings of generalized spike and wave (GSW) probands. Electroencephalogr. Clin. Neurophysiol. 56:27P(abst).

Hauser, W.A., Tabbador, K., Factor P.R., et al. 1984a. Seizures and head injury in an urban community. Neurology (Cleveland) 34:746–751.

Hauser, W.A., Rich, S., and Anderson, V.E. 1984b. The multifocal spike pattern and sibling risk for epilepsy. Electroencephalogr. Clin. Neurophysiol. 57:44P–45P(abst).

Hayashi, T. 1953. The efferent pathway of epileptic seizures for the face following cortical stimulation differs from that for limbs. Jpn. J. Pharmacol. 4:306–321.

Hayne, R.A., Belinson, L., and Gibbs, F.A. 1949. Electrical activity of subcortical areas in epilepsy. Electroencephalogr. Clin. Neurophysiol. 1: 437–445.

Hécaen, H., and Angelergues, R. 1960. Épilepsie et troubles du language. Encephale 49:138–169.

Heintel, H. 1972. *Der Status Epilepticus*. Stuttgart: Fischer.

Heinemann, U., and Eder C. 1998. Control of neuronal excitability. In *Epilepsy. A Comprehensive Textbook (3 vol.)*, Eds. J. Engel, Jr. and T. Pedley, vol. 1, pp. 237–250. Philadelphia: Lippincott-Raven.

Hejbel, J., Blom, S., and Bergfors, P.G. 1975. Benign epilepsy of children with centrotemporal EEG foci. A study of incidence rate in outpatient care. Epilepsia (New York) 16:657–664.

Henze, D.A., Urban, N.N., and Barrionuevo, G. 2000. The multifarious hippocampal mossy fiber pathway: a review. Neuroscience 98:407–427.

Herpin, T. 1876. *Les Accès Incomplets d'Épilepsie*. Paris: Baillière.

Hess, R. 1958. Verlaufsuntersuchungen über Anfälle und EEG bei kindlichen Epilepsien. Arch. Psychiatr. Nervenkr. 197:568–593.

Hess, R. 1970. Die epileptogenen Hirntumoren. In *Epilepsy, Recent View on Theory, Diagnosis and Therapy of Epilepsy*, Ed. E. Niedermeyer, pp. 200–231. Basel: S. Karger.

Hess, R. 1975. Localization of cerebral tumors. In *Handbook of Electroencephalography and Clinical Neurophysiology*, vol. 14C, Ed.-in-chief, A. Remond, pp. 17–28. Amsterdam: Elsevier.

Hess, R., and Neuhaus, T. 1952. Das Elektroenzephalogramm bei Blitz-Nick Salaamkrämpfen und bei andren Anfallsformen des Kindesalters. Arch. Psychiatr. Nervenkr. 189:37–58.

Hill, D. 1952. EEG in episodic psychotic and psychopathic behavior. Electroencephalogr. Clin. Neurophysiol. 4:419–442.

Hill, D. 1963. The EEG in Psychiatry. In *Electroencephalography, A Symposium on Its Various Aspects*, Eds. D. Hill and G. Parr, pp. 368–428. New York: Macmillan.

Hill, V. 1896. *Physiology and Pathology of the Cerebral Circulation*. London: Churchill. Quoted in Pfeiffer, J., 1963.

Himmelhoch, J.M. 1984. Major mood disorders related to epileptic changes. In *Psychiatric Aspects of Epilepsy*, Ed. D. Blumer, pp. 271–294. Washington, DC: American Psychiatric Press.

Hirsch, E., Maquet, P., Metz-Lutz, M.-N., et al. 1995. The eponym "Landau-Kleffner syndrome" should not be restricted to childhood-acquired aphasia with epilepsy. In *Continuous Spikes and Waves During Slow Sleep. Electrical Status Epilepticus During Slow Sleep*, Eds. A. Beaumanoir, M. Bureaus, T. Deonna, et al., pp. 57–62. London: Libbey.

Hirt, H.R. 1996. Zur Nosologie des Lennox-Gastaut Syndromes. Nervenarzt 67:109–122.

Hitzig, E. 1871. Über beim Galvanisieren des Kopfes entstehende Störungen der Muskelinnervation und der Vorstellungen vom Verhalten im Raume. Arch. Anat. Physiol. Wiss. Med. 716–770.

Hitzig, E. 1874. *Untersuchungen über das Gehirn*. Berlin.

Hodgkin, A.L. 1964. The conduction of the nervous impulse. Liverpool: University Press.

Hodgkin, A.L., and Huxley, A.F. 1952. Currents carried by sodium and potassium ions through the membrane of the giant axon of Loligo. J. Physiol. 116:449–472.

Hoefer, P.F.A., Schlesinger, E.B., Pennes, H.H., et al. 1947. Correlation of clinical and EEG findings in a large series of cases of verified cerebral tumors. Arch. Neurol. Psychiatry (Chicago) 58:118–120.

Holmes, G. 1927. Local epilepsy. Lancet 1:957–973.

Holmes, G.L. 1987. *Diagnosis and Management of Seizures in Children*. Philadelphia: W.B. Saunders.

Holmes, G.L., Blair, S., Eisenberg, E., et al. 1982. Tooth-brushing-induced epilepsy. Epilepsia (New York) 23:657–661.

Homma, G., and Niedermeyer, E. 1993. Subakute Enzephalopathie mit Anfaellen bei Chronischem Alkoholismus. Nervenarzt 64:391–393.

Hooshmand, H. 1972. Apneic seizures treated with atropine. Report of a case. Neurology (Minneapolis) 22:1217–1221.

Hopf, H.C., Stamatovic, A.M., and Wahren, W. 1970. Die Cerebralen Anfälle bei der multiplen Sklerose. J. Neurol. (Berlin) 198:256–279.

Horsley, V. 1909. The function of the so-called motor area of the brain. Br. Med. J. 2:125–132.

Hrachovy, R.A., Frost, J.D., Jr., and Kellaway, P. 1984. Hypsarrhythmia: variations on a theme. Epilepsia (New York) 25:317–325.

Hudson, A.J., and Hyland, H.H. 1958. Hypertensive cerebrovascular disease: a clinical and pathological review of 100 cases. Arch. Intern. Med. 49:1049–1072.

Hughes, J.R. 1980. Correlations between EEG and chemical changes in uremia. Electroencephalogr. Clin. Neurophysiol. 48:583–594.

Hughes, J.R. 1985. Natural history of hypsarrhythmia. Clin. Electroencephalogr. 16:128–130.

Hughes, J.R. 1989. The significance of the interictal spike discharge: a review. J. Clin. Neurophysiol. 6:207–226.

Hughes, J.R., and Gruener, G. 1985. The success of EEG in confirming epilepsy—revisited. Clin. Electroencephalogr. 16:98–103.

Hughes, J.R., and Olson, S.F. 1981. An investigation of eight different types of temporal lobe discharges. Epilepsia (New York) 22:421–435.

Hughes, J.R., and Patil, V.K. 2002. Long-term electro-clinical changes in the Lennox-Gastaut syndrome before, during, and after the flow spike-wave pattern. Clin Electroencephalogr. 33:1–7.

Hughes, J.R., and Tomasi, L.G. 1985. The diminishing incidence of hypsarrhythmia. Clin. Electroencephalogr. 16:178–182.

Hughes, J.R., Cayaffa, J.J., Pruitt, A., Jr., et al. 1973. "Post-ignitic" epilepsy—seizures following burns of the skin. Epilepsia (Amsterdam) 14:97–98(abst).

Hunt, I.R. 1922. On the occurrence of static seizures in epilepsy. J. Nerv. Ment. Dis. 56:351–356.

Hunter, R.A. 1959/60. Status epilepticus. History, incidence and problems. Epilepsia (Amsterdam) 1:162–188.

Huott, A.D., Madison, D.S., and Niedermeyer, E. 1974. Occipital lobe epilepsy. A clinical and electroencephalographic study. Eur. Neurol. (Basel) 9:325–339.

Hwa, G.G.C., and Avoli, M. 1991. Cesium potentiates epileptiform activities induced by bicuculline methiodide in rat neocortex maintained in vitro. Epilepsia (New York) 32:747–754.

Hwang, P., Andermann, F., Mentrakos, K., et al. 1981. The seizures of morphea. Electroencephalogr. Clin. Neurophysiol. 52:47P(abst).

Hyson, M., Andermann, F., Olivier, A., et al. 1982. Occult encephaloceles and temporal lobe epilepsy: developmental and acquired lesions in the middle fossa. Electroencephalogr. Clin. Neurophysiol. 54:42P(abst).

Iemolo, F., Chelazzi, C., d'Onofrio, S., et al. 1985. Epileptic seizures in cerebrovascular accidents. Electroencephalogr. Clin. Neurophysiol. 60:71P(abst).

Ikeda, A., Nagamine, T., Kunieda, T., et al. 1999. Clonic convulsion caused by epileptic discharges from the human supplementary motor area as studied by subdural recording. Epileptic Disord. 1:21–26.

Ikeda, R., Oana, Y., Sakaue, N., et al. 1982. The foci of 40 epileptic patients with visual symptoms. Electroencephalogr. Clin. Neurophysiol. 54:27P(abst).

Ingvar, D.N. 1955. Reproduction of the 3 per second spike and wave EEG pattern by subcortical stimulation in cats. Acta Physiol. Scand. 33:137–150.

Ingvar, D.N., and Nyman, G.E. 1962. Epilepsia arithmetices. A new psychological trigger mechanism in a case of epilepsy. Neurology (Minneapolis) 12:282–287.

Isbell, H., Altschul, S., Kornetsky, C.H., et al. 1950. Chronic barbiturate intoxication. An experimental study. Arch. Neurol. Psychiatry (Chicago) 64:1–28.

Isler, W., and Hess, R. 1960. Verlaufsuntersuchungen über Anfälle und EEG bei fokalen Epilepsien im Kindesalter. Arch. Psychiatr. Nervenkr. 200:257–266.

Ismay, G. 1958. Photogenic epilepsy [letter to the editor]. Lancet 2:376.

Italian EEG Society Proceedings. 1985. Electroencephalogr. Clin. Neurophysiol. 61:92P–95P(abst).

Itil, T.M. 1970. Convulsive and anticonvulsive properties of neuropsychopharmacy. In Epilepsy. Recent Views on Theory, Diagnosis and Therapy of Epilepsy, Ed. E. Niedermeyer, pp. 270–305. Basel: S. Karger.

Ives, J.R., and Woods, J.F. 1980. The results of 6000 hours of continuous EEG recordings in 100 patients suspected of having temporal lobe epilepsy. Electroencephalogr. Clin. Neurophysiol. 50:159P(abst).

Jabbari, B., and Huott, A.D. 1980. Seizures in thyrotoxicosis. Epilepsia (New York) 21:91–96.

Jabbari, B., Vengrow, M.L., Salazar, A.M., et al. 1986. Clinical and radiological correlates of EEG in late phase of head injury: a study of 105 Vietnam veterans. Electroencephalogr. Clin. Neurophysiol. 64:285–293.

Jackson, J.H. 1866. Clinical remarks on the occasional occurrence of subjective sensations of smell in patients who are liable to epileptiform seizures or who have symptoms of mental derangement and in others. Lancet 1:659–660.

Jackson, J.H. 1870. A study of convulsions. Fr. St. Andrew Med. Grad. Assoc. 3:1–45. (Reprinted in Selected Writings of John Hughlings Jackson, Ed. J. Taylor, pp. 8–36. London: Hodder and Stroughton.)

Jackson, J.H., and Beevor, C.E. 1889. Case of tumour of the right temporal-sphenoidal lobe bearing on the localization of the sense of smell and on the interpretation of a particular variety of epilepsy. Brain 12:346–357.

Jackson, J.H., and Stewart, P. 1899. Epileptic attacks with a warning of a crude sensation of smell and with the intellectual aura (dreamy state) in a patient who had symptoms pointing to gross organic disease of right temporo-sphenoidal lobe. Brain 22:534–539.

Jacome, D.E., and Suarez, M. 1988. Ictus emeticus induced by photic stimulation. Electroencephalogr. Clin. Neurophysiol. 69:79P–80P(abst).

Jacome, D.E., McLain, L.W., Jr., and Fitzgerald, R. 1980. Postural reflex gelastic seizures. Arch. Neurol. (Chicago) 37:249–251.

Jaffe, R. 1962. Ictal behaviour disturbance as the only manifestation of seizure disorder: case report. J. Nerv. Ment. Dis. 134:470–476.

Jaffe, R. 1984. "Epileptic ecstasy": evidence from 5 cases. Electroencephalogr. Clin. Neurophysiol. 58:44P(abst).

Jankel, W.R., and Niedermeyer, E. 1985. Sleep spindles. J. Clin. Neurophysiol. 2:1–35.

Janz, D. 1953. Aufwach-Epilepsien. Arch. Psychiatr. Nervenkr. 191:73–98.

Janz, D. 1955. Die klinische Stellung der Pyknolepsie. Dtsch. Med. Wochenschr. 80:1392–1400.

Janz, D. 1960. Status, epilepticus und Stirnhirn. Dtsch. Z. Nervenheil. 180:562–594.

Janz, D. 1961. Conditions and causes of status epilepticus. Epilepsia (Amsterdam) 2:170–177.

Janz, D. 1962. The grand mal epilepsies and the sleeping-waking cycle. Epilepsia (Amsterdam) 3:69–109.

Janz, D. 1969. Die Epilepsien. Stuttgart: Thieme.

Janz, D. 1983. Etiology of convulsive status epilepticus. In Status Epilepticus, Eds. A.V. Delgado-Escueta, C.G. Wasterlain, D.M. Trieman, et al., pp. 47–54. New York: Raven Press.

Janz, D., and Matthes, A. 1955. Die propulsiv-Petit-Mal-Epilepsie. Klinik und Verlauf der sog. Blitz-. Nick- und Salaam Krämpfe. Basel: S. Karger.

Janz, D., Beck-Mannagetta, G., Spröder, B., et al. 1994. Childhood absence epilepsy (pyknolepsy) and juvenile absence epilepsy: One or two syndromes? In Epileptic Seizures and Syndromes, Ed. P. Wolf, pp. 115–126. London: Libbey.

Jasper, H.H. 1949. Étude anatomo-physiologique des épilepsies. Electroencephalogr. Clin. Neurophysiol. Supp. 2:99–111.

Jasper, H.H. 1958. Functional subdivisions of the temporal region in relation to seizure patterns and subcortical connections. In Temporal Lobe Epilepsy, Eds. M. Baldwin and P. Bailey, pp. 40–57. Springfield, IL: Charles C Thomas.

Jasper, H.H. 1969. Mechanisms of propagation. Extracellular studies. In Basic Mechanisms of the Epilepsies, Eds. H.H. Jasper, A.A. Ward, Jr., and A. Pope, pp. 421–438. Boston: Little, Brown.

Jasper, H.H. 1991. Current evaluation of the concepts of centrencephalic and cortico-reticular seizures. Electroencephalogr. Clin. Neurophysiol. 78:2–11.

Jasper, H.H., and Droogleever-Fortuyn, J. 1947. Experimental studies on the functional anatomy of petit mal epilepsy. Publ. Assoc. Res. New Ment. Dis. 26:272–298.

Jasper, H.H., Pertuiset, B., and Flanigin, H. 1951. EEG and cortical electrograms in patients with temporal lobe seizures. Arch. Neurol. Psychiatry (Chicago) 65:272–290.

Jeavons, P.M. 1977. Nosological problems of myoclonic epilepsies in childhood and adolescence. Dev. Med. Child Neurol. 19:38.

Jeavons, P.M. 1996. Eyelid myoclonia and absences: the history of the syndrome. In *Eyelid Myoclonia,* Eds. J.S. Duncan, and C.P. Panayiotopoulos, pp. 13–15. London: Libbey.

Jeavons, P.M., and Bower, B.D. 1964. *Infantile Spasms. A Review of the Literature and a Study of 112 Cases.* London: Heinemann.

Jeavons, P.M., and Bower, B.D. 1974. Infantile spasms. In *Handbook of Clinical Neurology,* Eds. P.J. Vinken and G.W. Bruyn, pp. 219–234. New York: American Elsevier.

Jeavons, P.M., and Harding, G.F.A. 1975. *Photosensitive Epilepsy. A Review of the Literature and a Study of 460 Patients.* London: Heinemann.

Jennett, W.B. 1975. *Epilepsy After Non-Missile Head Injuries.* Chicago: Year Book.

Jennett, W.B., and Lewin, W.S. 1960. Traumatic epilepsy after head injuries. J. Neurol. Neurosurg. Psychiatry 23:295–301.

Jeras, J., and Tivedar, I. 1973. *Epilepsy in Children.* Hanover, NH: University Press of New England.

Jimenez-Rivera, C.A., and Waterhouse, B.D. 1991. The role of non-adrenergic systems in seizure disorders. In *Neurotransmitters and Epilepsy,* Eds. R.S. Fisher and J.T. Coyle, pp. 109–129. New York: Wiley-Liss.

Johnston, M.V. 1993. Neurotransmitters and Epilepsy. In *The Treatment of Epilepsy,* Ed. E. Wyllie, pp. 111–125. Philadelphia: Lea and Febiger.

Jovanovic, U.J. 1974. *Psychomotor Epilepsy.* Springfield, IL: Charles C Thomas.

Joynt, R.J., and Green, D. 1962. Tonic seizures as a manifestation of multiple sclerosis. Arch. Neurol. (Chicago) 2:293–299.

Joynt, R.J., Green, D., and Green, R. 1962. Musicogenic epilepsy. JAMA 179:601–604.

Jung, R. 1939. Über vegetative Reaktionen und Hemmungswirkungen von Sinnesreizen im kleinen epileptischen Anfall. Nervenarzt 12:169–185.

Jung, R. 1949. Hirnelekrische Untersuchungen über den Elektrokrampf. Die Erregungsabläufe in corticalen und subcorticalen Hirnregionen bei Katze und Hund. Arch. Psychiatr. Nervenkr. 183:206–244.

Jung, R., Baumgarten, R.V., and Baumgartner, G. 1952. Mikroableitunger von einzelnen Nervenzellen im optischen Cortex der Katze. Die lichtakiverten B-Neurone. Arch. Psychiatr. Z. Ges. Neurol. 189:521–539.

Juul-Jensen, P., and Denny-Brown, D. 1966. Epilepsia partialis continua. Arch. Neurol. (Chicago) 15:563–578.

Juul-Jensen, P., and Foldspang, A. 1983. Natural history of epileptic seizures. Epilepsy (New York) 24:297–312.

Kaibara, M., and Blume, W.T. 1988. The postictal electroencephalogram. Electroencephalogr. Clin. Neurophysiol. 70:99–104.

Kajtor, F. 1956. Aktivierung und Analyse der steilen Wellen und Krampfspitzen in Evipannarkose bei Temporallappen-Epilepsie. Arch. Psychiatr. Nervenkr. 193:238–262.

Kajtor, F. 1957. Krampfpotentiale des menschlichen Ammonshorns im Wachzustand und im Evipanschlaf. Arch. Psychiatr. Nervenkr. 196:135–153.

Kajtor, F., Mullay, J., Farago, L., et al. 1957. Effect of barbiturate sleep on the electrical activity of the hippocampus of patients with temporal lobe epilepsy (a preliminary report). Electroencephalogr. Clin. Neurophysiol. 9:441–451.

Kajtor, F., Mullay, J., Farago, L., et al. 1958. Electrical activity of the hippocampus of patients with temporal lobe epilepsy. Arch. Neurol. Psychiatry (Chicago) 80:25–38.

Kalinowsky, L.B. 1942. Convulsions in nonepileptic patients on withdrawal of barbiturates, alcohol and other drugs. Arch. Neurol. Psychiatry (Chicago) 48:946–956.

Kallén, C., Wyllie, E., Lüders, H.O., et al. 2002. Hypomotor seizures in infants and children. Epilepsia 43:882–888.

Kalviäinen, R., Slamenperä, T., Partanen, K., et al. 1998. Recurrent seizures may cause hippocampal damage in temporal lobe epilepsy. Neurology 50:1377–1382.

Kamp, A. 1984. Long-term supervised domiciliary EEG monitoring in epileptic patients employing radio telemetry and telephone telemetry. II. Radio telemetry system. Electroencephalogr. Clin. Neurophysiol. 57: 584–586.

Kanemoto, K., Takeuchi, J., Kawasaki, J., et al. 1996. Characteristics of temporal lobe epilepsy with mesial temporal sclerosis, with special reference to psychotic episodes. Neurology 47:1199–1203.

Kaplan, P.W. 1996. Nonconvulsive status epilepticus in the emergency room. Epilepsia 37:643–650.

Kaplan, P.W. 1998. Reversible hypercalcemic cerebral vasoconstriction with seizures and blindness: a paradigm for eclampsia? Clin. Electroencephalogr. 29:120–123.

Kaplan, P.W., and Lewis, D.V. 1986. Juvenile acute intermittent porphyria with hypercholesterolemia and epilepsy. A case report and review of the literature. J. Child Neurol. 1:38–45.

Karbowski, K. 1980. Status psychomotoricus. Klinische und elektroenzephalographische Aspekte. In *Status Psychomotoricus und seine Differentialdiagnose,* Ed. K. Karbowski, pp. 39–71. Bern: Huber.

Karbowski, K. 1985. *Epileptische Anfalle.* Berlin: Springer.

Karbowski, K. 1995. Typische und atypische Petit mal Staten. Z. EEG-EMG 26:249(abst).

Karbowski, K., Pavlincova, E., and Vassella, F. 1981. Zur Frage einer posttraumatischen Absenzenepilepsie. Nervenarzt 52:718–722.

Karbowski, K., Vassella, F., and Pavlincova, E. 1988. Psychomotor seizures in infancy and early childhood. Electroencephalogr. Clin. Neurophysiol. 70:10P(abst).

Kaufman, I.C., Marshall, C., and Walker, A.E. 1947. Metrazol activated electroencephalography. Publ. Assoc. Res. Nerv. Ment. Dis. 21: 476–486.

Kawamura, T., Onishi, H., Hirose, G., et al. 2002. The relationship between interictal spiking and ictal rhythmic activity in the mesial temporal lobe epilepsy. Clin. Neurophysiol. 113:978(abst).

Kellaway, P. 1959. Neurologic status of patients with hypsarrhythmia. In *Molecules and Mental Health,* Ed. F.A. Gibbs, pp. 134–149. Philadelphia: J.B. Lippincott.

Kellaway, P., and Chao, D. 1955. Prolonged status epilepticus in petit mal. Electroencephalogr. Clin. Neurophysiol. 7:145(abst).

Kellaway, P., and Hrachovy, R.A. 1983. Status epilepticus in newborns: a perspective on neonatal seizures. In *Status Epilepticus,* Eds. A.V. Delgado-Escueta, C.G. Wasterlain, D.M. Treiman, et al., pp. 93–99. New York: Raven Press.

Kellaway, P., and Mizrahi, E.M. 1987. Neonatal seizures. In *Epilepsy: Electroclinical Syndromes,* Eds. H. Lueders and R.P. Lesser, pp. 13–47. New York: Raven Press.

Kellaway, P., and Prakash, M. 1974. Hypocalcemia and seizures in the newborn. Electroencephalogr. Clin. Neurophysiol. 37:419–420.

Kellaway, P., Frost, J.D., Jr., and Crawley, J.W. 1990. The relationship between sleep spindles and spike-and-wave bursts in human epilepsy. In *Generalized Epilepsy,* Eds. M. Avoli, P. Gloor, G. Kostopoulos, et al., pp. 36–84. Boston: Birkhauser.

Kellinghaus, C., Loddenkemper, T., and Kotagal, P. 2003. Ictal splitting: clinical and electroencephalographic features. Epilepsia 44:1064–1069.

Kelly, J.J., Jr., Sharbrough, F.W., and Daube, J.R. 1981. A clinical and electrophysiological evaluation of myoclonus. Neurology (New York) 31: 581–589.

Kennedy, F. 1926. Cerebral symptoms induced by angioneurotic edema. Arch. Neurol. Psychiatry (Chicago) 15:28–33.

Kennedy, F. 1938. Allergy and its effect on the central nervous system. Arch. Neurol. Psychiatry (Chicago) 39:1361–1372.

Kennedy, M.B., and Greengard, P. 1981. Two calcium/calmodulin-dependent protein kinases, which are highly concentrated in brain, phosphorylate protein I at distinct sites. Proc. Natl. Acad. Sci. U.S.A. 78:1293–1297.

Kershman, J., Conde, A., and Gibson, W.C. 1949. Electroencephalography in differential diagnosis of supratentorial tumors. Arch. Neurol. Psychiatry (Chicago) 62:255–268.

Ketz, E. 1974. Brain tumors and epilepsy. In *Handbook of Clinical Neurology,* vol. 16I, Eds. P.J. Vinken and G.W. Bruyn, pp. 254–269. Amsterdam: North Holland.

Killam, K.F., Naquet, R., and Bert J. 1966. Paroxysmal responses to intermittent light stimulation in a population of baboons (Papio papio). Epilepsia (Amsterdam) 7:215–219.

Killam, K.F., Killam, E.K., and Naquet, R. 1967. An animal model of light sensitive epilepsy. Electroencephalogr. Clin. Neurophysiol. 22:497–513.

Kiloh, L.G., McComas, A.J., and Osselton, J.W. 1972. *Clinical Electroencephalography,* 3rd ed. London: Butterworth.

Kimura, S., and Kobayashi, T. 1996. Two patients with juvenile myoclonic epilepsy and nonconvulsive status epilepticus. Epilepsia 37:275–279.

King, D.W., and Ajmone Marsan, C. 1977. Clinical features and ictal patterns in epileptic patients with EEG temporal lobe foci. Neurology (Minneapolis) 2:138–147.

Kinsbourne, M. 1962. Myoclonic encephalopathy of infants. J. Neurol. Neurosurg. Psychiatry 25:271–276.

Kinsbourne, M., and Rosenfield, D.B. 1975. Nonprogressive myoclonus. In *Myoclonic Seizures,* Ed. M.H. Charlton, pp. 30–59. Amsterdam: Excerpta Medica.

Kirstein, L. 1942. Epilepsie bei intrakraniellen expansiven Prozessen. Acta Med. Scand. 110:56–68.

Klapetek, J. 1959. Photogenic epileptic seizures provoked by television. Electroencephalogr. Clin. Neurophysiol. 11:809(abst).

Klass, D.W. 1975. Electroencephalographic mechanisms of complex partial seizures. In *Complex Partial Seizures and Their Treatment,* Eds. J.K. Penry and D.D. Daly, pp. 113–140. New York: Raven Press.

Klass, D.W., and Daly, D.D. 1960. Electroencephalography in patients with brain tumor. Med. Clin. North Am. 52:949–957.

Klass, D.W., Espinosa, R.E., and Fischer-Williams, M. 1973. Analysis of concurrent electroencephalographic and clinical events occurring sequentially during partial seizures. Electroencephalogr. Clin. Neurophysiol. 34:728(abst).

Knapp, A. 1905. *Die Geschwülste des rechten und linken Schläfenlappens.* Wiesbaden: Bergmann.

Knapp, A. 1918. Die Tumoren des Schläfenlappens. Arch. Psychiatr. Nervenkr. 42:226–240.

Knudsen, F.U. 1991. Febrile convulsions. In *Comprehensive Epileptology,* Eds. M. Dam and L. Gram, pp. 133–143. New York: Raven Press.

Kogeorgos, J., and Scott, D.F. 1982. Neuropsychiatric and EEG features in 74 cases of systemic lupus erythematosus with cerebral involvement. Electroencephalogr. Clin. Neurophysiol. 53:1P(abst).

Kohlhéb, O., Farkas, V., and Szég, L. 1985. An EEG study of temporal lobe epilepsy in childhood. Electroencephalogr. Clin. Neurophysiol. 61:8P(abst).

Köhler, G.-K., and Penin, H. 1970. Über Grundlagen und Anwendungsbereiche von EEG-Grenzwertwarnung und synchroner Doppelbildaufzeichnung. Z. EEG-EMG 1:102–106.

Köhling, R. 2002. Voltage-gated channels in epilepsy. Epilepsia 43:1278–1295.

Komai, S. 1977. Lennox-Gastaut's syndrome. Prognosis of the secondary generalized epilepsies. Epilepsia (New York) 18:131(abst).

Koo, B., and Hwang, P. 1996. Localization of focal cortical lesions influences age of onset of infantile spasms. Epilepsia 37:1068–1071.

Kooi, K.A. 1971. *Fundamentals of Electroencephalography.* New York: Harper & Row.

Kopeloff, L.M. 1960. Experimental epilepsy in the mouse. Proc. Soc. Exp. Biol. Med. 104:500–504.

Kopeloff, L.M., Barrera, S.E., and Kopeloff, N. 1941. Recurrent convulsive seizures in animals produced by immunological and chemical means. Am. J. Psychiatry 98:891–902.

Koshevnikov. 1895. Eine besondere Form von corticaler Epilepsie. Neurol. Centralb. 14:47–48.

Kostopoulos, G.K. 2000. Spike-and-wave discharges of absence seizures as a transformation of sleep spindles: the continuing development of a hypothesis. Clin. Neurophysiol. 111:S27-S38.

Kostopoulos, G., and Gloor, P. 1982. A mechanism for spike-wave discharge in feline penicillin epilepsy and its relationship to spindle generation. In *Sleep and Epilepsy,* Eds. M.B. Sterman, M.N. Shouse, and P. Passouant, pp. 11–27. New York: Academic Press.

Kostopoulos, G., and Psarropoulou, C. 1990. In vitro electrophysiology of a genetic model of generalized epilepsy. In *Generalized Epilepsy. Neurobiological Approaches,* Eds. M. Avoli, P. Gloor, G. Kostopoulos, et al., pp. 137–157. Boston: Birkhauser.

Kostopoulos, G., Gloor, P., Pellegrini, A., et al. 1981. A study of the transition from spindles to spike and wave discharges in feline generalized penicillin epilepsy: EEG features. Exp. Neurol. 73:43–54.

Kostopoulos, G., Avoli, M., Pellegrini, A., et al. 1982. Laminar analysis of spindles and spikes of the spike and wave discharge of feline generalized penicillin epilepsy. Electroencephalogr. Clin. Neurophysiol. 53:1–13.

Kotagal, P. 1992. Seizure symptomatology of temporal lobe epilepsy. In *Epilepsy Surgery,* Ed. H. Lüders, pp. 143–156. New York: Raven Press.

Kotagal, P. 1993. Psychomotor seizures: clinical and EEG findings. In *The Treatment of Epilepsy,* Ed. E. Wyllie, pp. 378–392. Philadelphia: Lea and Febiger.

Krendel, D.A., Racke, M.K., and Malkoff, M.D. 1990. Complex visual hallucinations due to seizures: clinical-EEG correlations. Electroencephalogr. Clin. Neurophysiol. 75:75S(abst).

Kristiansen, K., Henriksen, S.F., and Ringkjobm, R. 1969. Traumatic epilepsy. Prophylaxis. In *The Late Effect of Head Injury,* Eds. A.E. Walker, W.F. Caveness, and M. Critchley, pp. 261–276. Springfield, IL: Charles C Thomas.

Kruse, R. 1968. *Das Myoklonisch-Astatische Petit Mal.* Berlin: Springer.

Krushinsky, L.V. 1962. Study of pathophysiological mechanism of cerebral haemorrhages provoked by reflex epileptic seizures in rats. Epilepsia (Amsterdam) 3:363–380.

Kubicki, S. 1963. Über seltene Entstehung von Anfallsleiden nach Eingriffen am Ganglion Gasseri. Dtsch. Z. Nervenheilk. 185:502–512.

Kubicki, S., and Münter, M. 1976. EEG-Befunde und epileptische Anfälle nach Operationen am Ganglion Gasseri. Z. EEG-EMG 7:72–80.

Kubicki, S., and Schulze, A. 1962. Über temporale EEG-Herde nach Operationen am Ganglion Gasseri. Neurochirurgia 5:146–161.

Kubo, T., Fukuda, K., Mikami, A., et al. 1986. Cloning, sequencing and expression of complementary DNA encoding the muscarinic acetylcholine receptor. Nature 323:411–416.

Kugelberg, E., and Widén, L. 1954. Epilepsia partialis continua. Electroencephalogr. Clin. Neurophysiol. 6:503–506.

Kugler, J. 1972. Zerebrale ischämische Krisen. Von der aktivierten Krise zur spontanen Synkope. Z. EEG-EMG 3:109–120.

Kugoh, T., Yamamoto, M., and Hosokawa, K. 1987. Spike-wave status syndrome: appearance in non-epileptic patients. Electroencephalogr. Clin. Neurophysiol. 66:87P(abst).

Kuhlo, W. 1970. Petit-mal-Epilepsie. In *Epilepsy, Recent Views on Theory, Diagnosis and Therapy of Epilepsy,* Ed. E. Niedermeyer, pp. 120–138. Basel: S. Karger.

Kurokawa, T., Goya, N., Fukuyama, Y., et al. 1980. West syndrome and Lennox-Gastaut syndrome: a survey of natural history. Pediatrics 65:81–88.

Labiner, D.M., Ng, S.K.C., Hauser, W.A., et al. 1987. Cerebellar dysfunction increases risk for seizures. Epilepsia 28:634(abst).

Lacy, J.R., and Penry, J.-K. 1976. *Infantile Spasms.* New York: Raven Press.

Ladwig, H.A., Vanslager, L., Thomas, J., et al. 1962. Infantile spasms with hypsarrhythmia. Nebr. Symp. Motiv. 47:614–621.

Lagerstein, I., and Iffland, E. 1977. Die intravenöse Behandlung des Petit-Mal-Status mit Diazepam und Clonazepam. Z. EEG-EMG 8:82–88.

Lairy, G.C., and Harrison, A. 1968. Functional aspects of EEG foci in children. In *Clinical Electroencephalography in Children,* Eds. P. Kellaway and I. Petersén, pp. 197–212. New York: Grune & Stratton (Stockholm: Almqvist & Wiksell).

Landau, W.M., and Kleffner, F.R. 1957. Syndrome of acquired aphasia with convulsive disorder in children. Neurology (Minneapolis) 7:523–530.

Landolt, H. 1955. Über Verstimmungen, Dämmerzustände und schizophrene Zustandsbilder bei Epilepsie (Ergebnisse klinischer und elektroenzephalographischer Untersuchungen). Schweiz. Arch. Neurol. Psychiatr. 76:313–321.

Landolt, H. 1956. Über die Symptomatologie der epileptischen Absenz mit Spike-and-wave-Komplexen im EEG. Schweiz. Arch. Neurol. Psychiatr. 78:377.

Landolt, H. 1960. *Die Temporallappenepilepsie und ihre Psychopathologie.* Basel: S. Karger.

Landolt, H. 1963. Die Dämmer- und Verstimmungszustände bei Epilepsie und ihre Elektroenzephalographie. Dtsch. Z. Nervenheilk. 185:411–430.

Landré, E., Munari, C., and Bancaud, J. 1991. Ictal clinical-EEG patterns of partial seizures in temporal lobe epilepsy. Electroencephalogr. Clin. Neurophysiol. 78:11P(abst).

Leão, A.A.P. 1944. Spreading depression of activity in the cerebral cortex. J. Neurophysiol. 7:359–390.

Leão, A. 1972. Spreading depression. In *Experimental Models of Epilepsy,* Eds. D.P. Purpura, J.K. Penry, D.M. Woodbury, et al., pp. 172–196. New York: Raven Press.

LeBlanc, F.E., and Rasmussen, T. 1974. Cerebral seizures and brain tumors. In *Handbook of Clinical Neurology,* Eds. P.J. Vanken and G.W. Bruyn, vol. 15, pp. 295–301. Amsterdam: North Holland.

Lechner, H. 1959. Der lobus limbicus und seine funktionelle Beziehungen zur Affektivität. Wien. Z. Nervenheilk. 16:281–320.

Ledermair, O., and Niedermeyer, E. 1956. Posteklamptische Epilepsie. Geburtsh. Frauenheilk. 16:679–685.

Le Gal la Salle, G., Cavalheiro, E.A., Tanaka, T., et al. 1982. General considerations on the kindling effect. Possible extrapolation to man of data obtained by animal experimentation. Electroencephalogr. Clin. Neurophysiol. 53:78P(abst).

Legarda, S., and Jayakar, P. 1995. Electroclinical significance of rolandic spikes and dipoles in neurodevelopmentally normal children. Electroencephalogr. Clin. Neurophysiol. 95:257–259.

Legg, N.J., Gupta, P.C., and Scott, D.F. 1973. Epilepsy following cerebral abscess. A clinical and EEG study of 70 patients. Brain 96:259–268.

Lehmann, H.J. 1963. Präparoxysmale Weckreaktionen bei pyknoleptischen Absenzen. Arch. Psychiatr. Nervenkr. 204:417–426.

Lehnertz, K., Andrzejak, R.G., Arnhold, J., et al. 2001. Nonlinear EEG analysis in epilepsy. J. Clin. Neurophysiol. 18:209–222.

Lennox, M.A., and Robinson, F. 1951. Cingulate-cerebellar mechanisms in the physiological pathogenesis of epilepsy. Electroencephalogr. Clin. Neurophysiol. 3:197–205.

Lennox, W.G. 1945. The petit mal epilepsies; their treatment with tridione. JAMA 129:1069–1074.

Lennox, W.G. 1951. The heredity of epilepsy, as told by relatives and twins. JAMA 146:529–536.

Lennox, W.G. 1953. Significance of febrile seizures. Pediatrics 11:341–357.

Lennox, W.G. 1960. *Epilepsy and Related Disorders.* Boston: Little, Brown.

Lennox, W.G., and Davis, J.P. 1950. Clinical correlates of the fast and the slow spike wave electroencephalogram. Pediatrics 5:626–644.

Lennox-Buchthal, M.A. 1971. Febrile and nocturnal convulsions in monozygotic twins. Epilepsia (Amsterdam) 12:147–156.

Lennox-Buchthal, M.A. 1973. *Febrile Convulsions. A Reappraisal.* Amsterdam: Elsevier.

Lennox-Buchthal, M.A. 1977. *Fieberkrämpfe.* Stuttgart: Hippokrates.

Lerman, P., and Kivity-Ephraim, S. 1981. Focal epileptic EEG discharges in children not suffering from clinical epilepsy: etiology, clinical significance and management. Epilepsia (New York) 22:551–558.

Lesser, R.P., Lueders, H., Dinner, D.S., et al. 1985. Epileptic seizures due to thrombotic and embolic cerebrovascular disease in older patients. Epilepsia (New York) 26:622–630.

Leutmezer, F., Asenbaum, S., Pietrzyk, U., et al. 2003. Postictal psychosis in temporal lobe epilepsy. Epilepsia 44:582–590.

Le Van Quyen M., Martinerie, M., Navarro, V., et al. 2001. Characterizing neurodynamic changes before seizures. J. Clin. Neurophysiol. 18:191–208.

Levic, Z.M. 1978. Electroencephalographic studies in multiple sclerosis. Specific changes in benign multiple sclerosis. Electroencephalogr. Clin. Neurophysiol. 44:471–478.

Levy, L.L., and Fenichel, G.J. 1965. Diphenylhydantoin activated seizures. Neurology (Minneapolis) 15:716–722.

Levy, L., and O'Leary, J.L. 1965. Arrest of seizure activity. Epilepsia (Amsterdam) 6:116–121.

Levy, S.R. 1989. A case of Lennox-Gastaut syndrome secondary to a temporal lobe tumor. Electroencephalogr. Clin. Neurophysiol. 72:5P(abst).

Li, C.L. 1962. Cortical intracellular synaptic potentials and direct cortical stimulation. J. Comp. Physiol. 60:1–16.

Li, C., McLennan, J., and Jasper, H.H. 1952. Brain waves and unit discharge in cerebral cortex. Science 116:656–657.

Libus, E., and Libus, J. 1981. EEG in epileptic psychical changes. Electroencephalogr. Clin. Neurophysiol. 52:12P(abst).

Liddell, E.G.T., and Phillips, C.G. 1951. Overlapping areas in the motor cortex of the baboon. J. Physiol. (Lond.) 112:392–399.

Lipinski, C.G. 1977. Epilepsies with astatic seizures of late onset. Epilepsia (New York) 18:13–20.

Liu, A., Hahn, J.S., Heldt, G.P., et al. 1992. Detection of neonatal seizures through computerized EEG analysis. Electroencephalogr. Clin. Neurophysiol. 82:30–37.

Livingston, S. 1972. *Comprehensive Management of Epilepsy in Infancy, Childhood, and Adolescence.* Springfield, IL: Charles C Thomas.

Livingston, S., Eisner, V., and Pauli, L. 1958. Minor motor epilepsy: diagnosis, treatment and prognosis. Pediatrics 21:916–928.

Livingston, S., Torres, I., Pauli, L., et al. 1965. Petit mal epilepsy. Results of a prolonged follow-up of 117 patients. JAMA 194:227–232.

Lob, H., Roger, J., Soulayrol, R., et al. 1967. Les états de mal généralisés à expression confusionnelle. In *Les États de Mal Épileptiques,* Eds. H. Gastaut, J. Roger, and H. Lob, pp. 91–109. Paris: Masson.

Locke, J., Merrill, J.P., and Tyler, H.R. 1961. Neurologic complication of acute uremia. Arch. Intern. Med. 108:519–530.

Lockhard, J.S., DuCharme, L.L., Congdon, W.C., et al. 1976. Prophylaxis with diphenylhydantoin and phenobarbital in alumina-gel monkey model. II. Four-month follow-up period: Seizure, EEG, blood, and behavioral data. Epilepsia (New York) 17:49–57.

Loiseau, P., and Beaussart, M. 1973. The seizures of benign childhood epilepsy with Rolandic paroxysmal discharges. Epilepsia (Amsterdam) 14:381–389.

Loiseau, P., Pestre, M., Dartigues, F., et al. 1983. Long-term prognosis in two forms of childhood epilepsy: typical absence seizures and epilepsy with rolandic (centrotemporal) EEG foci. Ann. Neurol. 13:642–648.

Loiseau, P., Duché, B., and Pédespan, J-M. 1995. Absence epilepsies. Epilepsia 36:1182–1186.

Lombroso, C.T. 1967. Sylvian seizures and midtemporal spike foci in children. Arch. Neurol. (Chicago) 17:52–59.

Lombroso, C.T. 1983a. Prognosis in neonatal seizures. In *Status Epilepticus,* Eds. A.V. Delgado-Escueta, C.G., Wasterlain, D.M. Tremain, et al., pp. 101–113. New York: Raven Press.

Lombroso, C.T. 1983b. A prospective study of infantile spasms. Epilepsia (New York) 24:135–158.

Lombroso, C.T., and Erba, G. 1970. Primary and secondary bilateral synchrony. A clinical and electroencephalographic study. Arch. Neurol. (Chicago) 22:321–344.

Lombroso, C.T., and Fejerman, N. 1977. Benign myoclonus of early infancy. Ann. Neurol. 1:138–143.

Lore, T. 1995. A rare presentation in neurocysticercosis: complex partial seizures. Am. J. EEG Technol. 35:270–282.

Lou, H.C., Brandt, S., and Bruhn, P. 1977. Progressive aphasia and epilepsy with a self-limited course. In *Epilepsy. The Eighth International Symposium,* Ed. J.K. Penry, pp. 295–303. New York: Raven Press.

Louvel, J., and Heinemann, U. 1983. Changes in Ca^{2+}, K^+ and neuronal activity during oenanthotoxin-induced epilepsy in cat sensorimotor cortex. Electroencephalogr. Clin. Neurophysiol. 56:457–463.

Lowenstein, D.H. 1994. Basic concepts of molecular biology for the epileptologist. Epilepsia 35 (Suppl. 1):S7–S19.

Luciani, L. 1878. Sulla patogenesi dell'epilessia. Riv. Speriment. di Freniatria e Medicina Legale 4:617–646.

Ludwig, B.I., and Ajmone Marsan, C. 1975. Clinical ictal patterns in epileptic patients with occipital electroencephalographic foci. Neurology (Minneapolis) 25:463–471.

Ludwig, B., Ajmone Marsan, C., and Van Buren, J. 1975. Cerebral seizures of probable orbitofrontal origin. Epilepsia (New York) 16:141–158.

Lüders, H.O., ed. 1992. *Seizure Surgery.* New York: Raven Press.

Lueders, H., and Awad, I. 1992. Conceptual considerations. In *Epilepsy Surgery,* Ed. H. Lueders, pp. 51–62. New York: Raven Press.

Lüders, H., Daube, J., Johnson, R., et al. 1980. Computer analysis of generalized spike-and-wave complexes. Epilepsia (New York) 21:183 (abst).

Lüders, H., Lesser, R.P., Dinner, D.S., et al. 1987. Benign focal epilepsy of childhood. In *Epilepsy. Electroclinical Syndromes,* Eds. H. Lüders and R.P. Lesser, pp. 303–346. Berlin: Springer.

Luengo, A., Picornell, M., Picornell, I., et al. 1984. Partial sensory status. Polygraphic study of wakefulness and spontaneous sleep. Electroencephalogr. Clin. Neurophysiol. 58:4P(abst).

Lugaresi, E. 1967. Discussion remark. In *Les Activités Électriques Cérébrales Spontanées et Évoquées Chez l'Homme,* Eds. H. Gastaut, F. Bostem, A. Waltrégny, et al., pp. 214–217. Paris: Cauthiers-Villars.

Lugaresi, E., and Cirignotta, F. 1981. Hypnogenic paroxysmal dystonia: epileptic seizure or a new syndrome? Sleep 4:129–138.

Lugaresi, E., and Pazzaglia, P. 1975. The EEG in the positive and differential diagnosis of epilepsy. In *Handbook of Electroencephalography and Clinical Neurophysiology,* Ed.-in-chief, A. Remond, vol. 13A, pp. 69–71. Amsterdam: Elsevier.

Lugaresi, E., Pazzaglia, P., and Tassinari, C.A. 1971. Differentiation of "absence status" and "temporal lobe status." Epilepsia (Amsterdam) 12: 77–87.

Lugaresi, E., Pazzaglia, P., Frank, L., et al. 1973. Evolution and prognosis of primary generalized epilepsies of the petit mal absence type. In *Evolution and Prognosis of the Epilepsies,* Eds. H. Gastaut, P. Pazzaglia, and C.A. Tassinari, pp. 3–22. Bologna: Gaggi.

Lugaresi, E., Cirignotta, F., and Montagna, P. 1984. Occipital lobe epilepsy with scotosensitive seizures: the role of central vision. Epilepsia (New York) 25:115–120.

Lühdorf, K., and Lund, M. 1977. Phenytoin-induced hyperkinesia. Epilepsia (New York) 18:409–415.

Lum, L.M., Connolly, M.B., Farrell, K., et al. 2002. Hyperventilation-induced high-amplitude rhythmic slowing with altered awareness: a video-EEG comparison with absence seizures. Epilepsia 43: 1372–1378.

Lund, M. 1952. *Epilepsy in Association with Intracranial Tumor.* Acta Psychiatr. (Copenhagen), Suppl. 81.

Lundervold, A., Henriksen, G.F., and Fegersten, L. 1959. The spike wave complex. A clinical correlation. Electroencephalogr. Clin. Neurophysiol. 11:13–22.

Lux, H.D. 1984. An invertebrate model of paroxysmal depolarization shifts. In *Electrophysiology of Epilepsy,* Eds. P.A. Schwartzkroin and H.V. Wheal, pp. 343–352. London: Academic Press.

Lux, H.D., and Heinemann, U. 1983. Consequences of calcium electrogenesis for the generation of paroxysmal depolarization shift. In *Epilepsy and Motor System,* Eds. E.-J. Speckmann and C.E. Elger, pp. 100–117. Munich: Urban & Schwarzenberg.

Lyon, G., and Gastaut, H. 1985. Considerations on the significance attributed to unusual histological findings recently described in eight patients with primary generalized epilepsy. Epilepsia (New York) 26: 365–367.

Lys, R., and Karbowski, K. 1981. Comments on the problem of the activating effect of hyperventilation on psychomotor seizures. Electroencephalogr. Clin. Neurophysiol. 51:70P(abst).

Madison, D.S., and Niedermeyer, E. 1974. Considerations of "true" status epilepticus (grand mal). Electroencephalogr. Clin. Neurophysiol. 37:431 (abst).

Madsen, J.A., and Bray, P.F. 1966. The coincidence of diffuse electroencephalographic spike wave paroxysms and brain tumors. Neurology (Minneapolis) 16:546–555.

Magistris, M.R., Mouradian, M.S., and Gloor, P. 1988. Generalized convulsions induced by pentylenetetrazol in the cat: participation of forebrain, brainstem and spinal cord. Epilepsia (New York) 29:379–388.

Magnus, O. 1954. Temporal lobe epilepsy. Folia Psychiatr. Neurol. Neurochir. Neerland 57:264–297.

Majkowski, J. 1991. Posttraumatic epilepsy. In *Comprehensive Epileptology,* Eds. M. Dam and L. Gram, pp. 281–288. New York: Raven Press.

Malafosse, A., Mandel, J.-L., Greenberg, D., et al. 1994. Molecular and statistical methods for mapping human genes. In *Idiopathic Generalized Epilepsies,* Eds. A. Malafosse, P. Genton, E. Hirsch, et al., pp. 27–36. London: Libbey.

Malamud, N. 1966. The epileptogenic focus from a pathological standpoint. Arch. Neurol. (Chicago) 14:190–195.

Mann, L.B., Bogen, J.E., and Vogel, P.J. 1969. Cerebral commissurotomy in man: EEG findings. Electroencephalogr. Clin. Neurophysiol. 27:660 (abst).

Marciani, M.-G., J., and Andermann, F. 1984. Changes in interictal and ictal activity during anticonvulsant withdrawal in epileptic patients. Electroencephalogr. Clin. Neurophysiol. 58:32P(abst).

Marcus, E.M. 1972. Experimental models of petit mal epilepsy. In *Experimental Models of Epilepsy,* Eds. D.P. Purpura, J.K. Penry, D. Tower, et al., pp. 113–146. New York: Raven Press.

Marcus, E.M., and Watson, C.W. 1968. Bilateral symmetrical epileptogenic foci in monkey cerebral cortex: mechanisms of interactions and regional variations in capacity for synchronous spike slow wave discharges. Arch. Neurol. (Chicago) 19:99–116.

Marcus, E.M., Watson, C.W., and Simon, S.A. 1968. An experimental model of some varieties of petit mal epilepsy. Epilepsia (Amsterdam) 9: 233–248.

Mark, V.H., and Ervin, F.R. 1970. *Violence and the Brain.* New York: Harper & Row.

Markand, O.N. 1977. Slow spike wave activity in EEG and associated clinical features, often called "Lennox" or "Lennox-Gastaut" syndrome. Neurology (Minneapolis) 27:746–757.

Marks, D.A., Katz, A., Scheyer, R., et al. 1991. Clinical and electrographic effects of acute anticonvulsant withdrawal in epileptic patients. Neurology 41:508–512.

Marshall, D.W. 1989. Occipital epileptiform activity in adults. Electroencephalogr. Clin. Neurophysiol. 72:21P(abst).

Mathieson, G. 1975a. Pathology of temporal lobe foci. In *Complex Partial Seizures and Their Treatment,* Eds. J.K. Penry and D.D. Daly, pp. 163–181. New York: Raven Press.

Mathieson, G. 1975b. Pathological aspects of epilepsy with special reference to the surgical pathology of focal cerebral seizures. In *Neurosurgical Management of the Epilepsies,* Eds. D.P. Purpura, J.K. Penry, and R.D. Walter, pp. 107–138. New York: Raven Press.

Matsumoto, H., and Ajmone Marsan, C. 1964. Cortical cellular phenomena in experimental epilepsy. Ictal manifestations. Exp. Neurol. 9:305–326.

Matthes, A. 1961. Die psychomotorische Epilepsie des Kindesalters. Z. Kinderheilk. 85:455, 472, 668.

Matthes, A. 1969. Genetic studies in epilepsy. In *The Physiopathogenesis of the Epilepsies,* Eds. H. Gastaut, H.H. Jasper, J. Bancaud, et al., pp. 26–30. Springfield, IL: Charles C Thomas.

Matthes, A. 1977. *Epilepsie,* 3rd ed. Stuttgart: Thieme.

Matthews, W.B. 1958. Tonic seizures in disseminated sclerosis. Brain 81: 193–206.

Matthews, W.B. 1962. Epilepsy and disseminated sclerosis. Q. J. Med. 31: 144–155.

Mazars, G. 1969. Cingulate gyrus epileptogenic foci as an origin for generalized seizures. In *Physiopathogenesis of the Epilepsies,* Eds. H. Gastaut, H.H. Jasper, J. Bancaud, et al., pp. 186–189. Springfield, IL: Charles C Thomas.

Mazars, C. 1970. Criteria for identifying cingulate epilepsies. Epilepsia (Amsterdam) 11:41–47.

Mazars, Y. 1950. Interpretation de phénoméne d'extinction dans la phase initiale de crises focales corticales. Rev. Neurol (Paris) 85:520–522.

Mazars, Y., Mazars, G., Gotusso, C., et al. 1966. La place de l'épilepsie cingulaire dans le cadre des épilepsies focales. Rev. Neurol. (Paris) 114: 215–217.

McIlwain, H. 1969. Central energy metabolism and membrane phenomena. In *Basic Mechanisms of the Epilepsies,* Eds. H.H. Jasper, A.A. Ward, Jr., and A. Pope, pp. 83–97. Boston: Little, Brown.

McNamara, J.O. 1986. Kindling model of epilepsy. In *Basic Mechanisms of the Epilepsies,* Eds. A.J. Delgado-Escueta, A.A. Ward, Jr., D.M. Woodbury, et al., pp. 308–318. New York: Raven Press.

Meencke, H.-J., and Janz, D. 1984. Neuropathological findings in primary generalized epilepsy: a study of eight cases. Epilepsia (New York) 25: 8–21.

Meencke, H.J., and Janz, D. 1985. The significance of microdysgenesis in primary generalized epilepsy: an answer to the considerations to Lyon and Gastaut. Epilepsia (New York) 26:368–371.

Meeren, H.K.M. 2002. *Cortico-Thalamic Mechanisms Underlying Generalized Spike-Wave Discharges of Absence Epilepsy.* Thesis, Nijmegen University.

Meeren, H.K.M., Pijn, J.P., Van Luijtelaar, E.L.J.M., et al. 1992. Cortical focus drives widespread corticothalamic networks during spontaneous absence seizures in rats. J. Neurosci. 22:1148–1495.

Meienberg, O., and Karbowski, K. 1977. Die epilepsia partialis continua Kozevnikov. Dtsch. Med. Wochenschr. 102:781–784.

Meldrum, B.S. 1988. *In vivo and in vitro* models of epilepsy and their relevance to man. In *Anatomy of Epileptogenesis,* Eds. B.S. Meldrum, J.A. Ferrendelli, and H.G. Wieser, pp. 27–42. London: Libbey.

Meldrum, B.S., and Horton, R.W. 1971. Convulsive effects of 4-deoxypyridoxine and of bicuculline in photosensitive baboons (*Papio papio*) and in rhesus monkeys (*Macaca mulatta*). Brain Res. 97:407–418.

Menini, C. 1976. Role du cortex frontal dans l'épilepsie photosensible du singe Papio papio. J. Physiol. (Paris) 72:5–44.

Menini, C., Meldrum, B.S., Riche, D., et al. 1980. Sustained limbic seizures induced by intra-amygdaloid kainic acid in the baboon: symptomatology and neuropathological consequences. Ann. Neurol. 8:501–509.

Menini, C., Silva-Comte, C., Velluti, J.C., et al. 1983. Fronto-rolandic cortex and myoclonus in the photosensitive Papio papio. Electroencephalogr. Clin. Neurophysiol. 56:1P(abst).

Merritt, H.H., and Putnam, T.J. 1938. A new series of anticonvulsant drugs tested by experiments on animals. Arch. Neurol. Psychiatry 39:1003–1015.

Merzeevski. 1884. Quoted in Forster, F.M. 1977.

Metrakos, J.D., and Metrakos, K. 1960. Genetics of convulsive disorders. Introduction to problems, methods and baselines. Neurology (Minneapolis) 10:228–240.

Metrakos, J.D., and Metrakos, K. 1970. Genetic factors in epilepsy. In *Epilepsy, Recent Views on Theory, Diagnosis and Therapy of Epilepsy,* Ed. E. Niedermeyer, pp. 71–86. Basel: S. Karger.

Metrakos, K., and Metrakos, J.D. 1961. Genetics of convulsive disorders. II. Genetic and electroencephalographic studies in centrencephalic epilepsy. Neurology (Minneapolis) 11:474–483.

Meyer, A. 1920. Herniation of the brain. Arch. Neurol. Psychiatry (Chicago) 4:387–400.

Meyer, J.E. 1957. Zur forensischen Bedeutung der Temporallappen-Epilepsie. Dtsch. Z. Gerichtl. Med. 46:212–225.

Meyer, J.S., and Protnoy, H.D. 1959. Post-epileptic paralysis. A clinical and experimental study. Brain 82:162–185.

Michelucci, R., Mennonna, P., Roger, J., et al. 1985. Epileptic pain in parietal tumours. Electroencephalogr. Clin. Neurophysiol. 61: 92P(abst).

Millan, M.H. 1988. Sound-induced seizures in rodents. In *Anatomy of Epileptogenesis,* Eds. B.S. Meldrum, J.A. Ferrendelli, and H.G. Wieser, pp. 43–56. London: Libbey.

Miller, J.W., and Ferrendelli, J.A. 1988. Brain stem and diencephalic structures regulating experimental generalized (pentylenetetrazol) seizures in rodents. In *Anatomy of Epileptogenesis,* Eds. B.S. Meldrum, J.A. Ferrendelli, and H.G. Wieser, pp. 57–69. London: Libbey.

Millichap, J.G., Madsen, J.A., and Aledort, L.M. 1960. Studies in febrile seizures. V. Clinical and electroencephalographic study in unselected patients. Neurology (Minneapolis) 10:643–653.

Millichap, J.G., Bickford, R.G., Miller, R.H., et al. 1962. The electroencephalogram in children with intracranial tumors and seizures. Neurology (Minneapolis) 12:329–336.

Milner, B. 1975. Psychological aspects of focal epilepsy and its neurosurgical management. In *Neurosurgical Management of the Epilepsies,* Eds. D.P. Purpura, J.K. Penry, and R.D. Walter, pp. 299–321. New York: Raven Press.

Mindach, M., and Schacht, A. 1994. Bemerkungen zu der Arbeit von G. Homma und E. Niedermeyer. Nervenarzt 65:146–147.

Mirsky, A.F., and Tecce, J.J. 1968. The analysis of visual potentials during spike and wave activity. Epilepsia (Amsterdam) 9:211–220.

Mirsky, A.F., and Van Buren, J.M. 1965. On the nature of the "absence" in centrencephalic epilepsy. A study of some behavioral, electroencephalographic and autonomic factors. Electroencephalogr. Clin. Neurophysiol. 18:334–348.

Mitsudome, A., Ohu, M., Yasumoto, S., et al. 1997. Rhythmic slow activity in benign childhood epilepsy with centrotemporal spikes. Clin. Electroencephalogr. 28:44–48.

Mizrahi, E.M. and Kellaway, P. 1998. *Diagnosis and Management of Neonatal Seizures.* Philadelphia: Lippincott-Raven.

Mofenson, H.C., Weymuller, C.A., and Greensher, J. 1965. Epilepsy due to water immersion. JAMA 191:600–601.

Moore, M.T. 1945. Paroxysmal abdominal pain. A form of symptomatic epilepsy. JAMA 129:1233–1240.

Morimoto, T., Hayakawa, T., Sugie, H., et al. 1985. Epileptic seizures precipitated by constant light, movement in daily life and hot water immersion. Epilepsia (New York) 26:237–242.

Morison, R.S., and Dempsey, E.W. 1942. A study of thalamocortical relations. Am. J. Physiol. 135:281–292.

Morrell, F. 1959. Secondary epileptogenic lesions. Epilepsia (Amsterdam) 1:538–560.

Morrell, F. 1969. Physiology and histochemistry of the mirror focus. In *Basic Mechanisms of the Epilepsies,* Eds. H.H. Jasper, A.A. Ward, Jr., and A. Pope, p. 370. Boston: Little, Brown.

Morrell, F. 1978. Aspects of experimental epilepsy. 1977. In *Modern Perspectives in Epilepsy,* Ed. J.A. Wada, pp. 24–75. Montreal, Quebec/St. Albans, VT: Eden Press.

Morrell, F. 1985. Secondary epileptogenesis in man. Arch. Neurol. (Chicago) 42:318–335.

Moruzzi, G. 1952. L'attività dei neuroni corticali durante il sonno e durante la reazione elettroencefalografica di risveglio. Ric. Sci. 22:1165–1173.

Moser, D.J., Bauer, R.M., Gilmore, R.L., et al. 2000. Electroencephalographic, volumetric, and neuropsychological indicators of seizure focus lateralization in temporal lobe epilepsy. Arch. Neurol. 57: 707–712.

Mulder, D.W., Daly, D., and Bailey, A.A. 1954. Visceral epilepsy. Arch. Intern. Med. 93:481–493.

Müller, D., and Müller, J. 1980. *Lachen als epileptische Manifestation.* VEB G. Fischer: Jena.

Munari, C. 1985. Relationship between the symptomatology of partial seizures and local cerebral lesions. Electroencephalogr. Clin. Neurophysiol. 61:91P(abst).

Munari, C., and Bancaud, J. 1985. Localizing value of clinical symptoms during partial seizures in man. Electroencephalogr. Clin. Neurophysiol. 61:91P–92P(abst).

Munari, C., Tassi, L., Kahane, P., et al. 1994. Analysis of clinical symp-tomatology during stereo-EEG recorded mesiotemporal seizures. In *Epileptic Seizures and Syndromes,* Ed. P. Wolf, pp. 335–357. London: Libbey.

Murakami, N., Ohtsuka, Y., and Ohtahara, S. 1993. Early infantile epileptic syndromes with suppression-bursts. Jpn. J. Psychiatr. Neurol. 47:197–200.

Musumeci, S.A., Scuderi, C., Ferri, R., et al. 200. Does a peculiar EEG pattern exist also for FRAXE mental retardation? Clin. Neurophysiol. 111: 1632–1636.

Mutani, R. 1967. Cobalt experimental hippocampal epilepsy in the cat. Epilepsia (Amsterdam) 8:223–240.

Mutani, R., Agnetti, V., Durelli, L., et al. 1979. Epileptic laughter: electroclinical and cinefilm report of a case. J. Neurol. (Berlin) 220:215–222.

Myslobodsky, M. 1976. *Petit Mal Epilepsy.* New York: Academic Press.

Nadkarni, M.A., Postolache, V., Gold, A., et al. 1994. Central mid-temporal spikes triggered by blinking. Electroencephalogr. Clin. Neurophysiol. 90:36–39.

Naquet, R. 1973. Contribution of experimental epilepsy to understanding some particular forms in man. In *Epilepsy, Its Phenomena in Man,* Ed. M.A. Brazier, pp. 37–65. New York: Academic Press.

Naquet, R. 1975. Genetic study of epilepsy: Contributions of different models, especially the photosensitive Papio papio. In *Growth and Development of the Brain,* Ed. M.A.B. Brazier, pp. 219–230. New York: Raven Press.

Naquet, R., Fegersten, L., and Bert, J. 1960. Seizure discharges localized to the posterior regions in man, provoked by intermittent photic stimulation. Electroencephalogr. Clin. Neurophysiol. 12:305–316.

Naquet, R., Menini, C., and Catier, J. 1972. Photically-induced epilepsy in Papio papio: the initiation of discharges and the role of the frontal cortex and of the corpus callosum. In *Synchronization of EGG Activity in Epilepsies,* Eds. H. Petsche and M.A.B. Brazier, pp. 347–366. Wien: Springer.

Natsume, J., Watanabe, K., Maeda, N., et al. 1996. Cortical hypometabolism and delayed myelination in West syndrome. Epilepsia 37:1180–1184.

Natsume, J., Bernasconi, M., Andermann, F., et al. 2003. MRI volumetry of the thalamus in temporal, extratemporal, and idiopathic generalized epilepsy. Neurology 60:1296–1300.

Navelet, H., D'Allest, A.-M., Dehan, M., et al. 1981. À propos du syndrome des convulsions néonatales du cinquième jour. Rev. EEG Neurophysiol. 11:390–396.

Navelet, Y., D'Allest, A.-M., Dehan, M., et al. 1982. What's new about the fifth day seizures syndrome? Electroencephalogr. Clin. Neurophysiol. 53:80P(abst).

Nayrac, P., and Beaussart, M. 1958. Les pointes-ondes prérolandiques. Expression EEG trés particulière. Étude électroclinique de 21 cas. Rev. Neurol. (Paris) 99:201–206.

Negendran, K., Gordon, A.J., and Prior, P.F. 1989. The clinical significance of occipital epileptiform abnormalities: a retrospective study. Electroencephalogr. Clin. Neurophysiol. 73:59P(abst).

Negrin, P., and De Marco, P. 1977. Parietal focal spikes evoked by tactile somatotopic stimulation in sixty non-epileptic children: the nocturnal sleep and clinical and EEG evolution. Electroencephalogr. Clin. Neurophysiol. 43:312–316.

Neher, E., Sakmann, B., and Steinbach, J.H. 1978. The extracellular patch clamp: a method for resolving current through individual open channels in biological membrane. Pflügers Arch. 375:219–228.

Neidengard, L., and Niedermeyer. E. 1975. The electroencephalogram in neurological complications of sickle cell anemia (SS-hemoglobinopathy). Clin. Electroencephalogr. 6:68–74.

Nelson, K.B., and Ellenberg, J.H. 1976. Predictors of epilepsy of children who have experienced febrile seizures. N. Engl. J. Med. 259:1029–1033.

Nelson, K.R., Brenner, R.P., and De La Paz, D. 1984. Midline spikes—electroencephalographic and clinical features. Electroencephalogr. Clin. Neurophysiol. 57:42P–43P(abst).

Neufeld, M.Y., Blumen, S., and Nisipeanu, P. 1988. Lingual seizures. Electroencephalogr. Clin. Neurophysiol. 69:59P(abst).

Newmark, M.E., and Penry, J.K. 1979. *Photosensitivity and Epilepsy: A Review.* New York: Raven Press.

Newmark, M.E., and Penry, J.K. 1980. *Genetics of Epilepsy: A Review.* New York: Raven Press.

Niedermeyer, E. 1954a. Psychomotor seizure with generalized synchronous spike and wave-discharges. Electroencephalogr. Clin. Neurophysiol. 6:495–496.

Niedermeyer, E. 1954b. Kasuistischer Beitrag zur Epilepsia partialis continua mit EEG-Untersuchung. Dtsch. Z. Nervenheilk. 171:482–489.

Niedermeyer, E. 1957. Motorische Herdepilepsie bei Thalamus-Syndrom (Kasuistische Mitteilung zur Frage der "diencephalen Jackson-Epilepsie"). Wien. Klin. Wochenschr. 69:702–705.

Niedermeyer, E. 1958. Ber epilepsie im Höheren Lebensalter. Arch. Psychiatr. Nervenkr. 197:248–262.

Niedermeyer, E. 1959. Ein Fall von Status epilepticus, durch Tracheotomie und Sauerstoffbeatmung geheilt. Elektroencephalographische und pathophysiologische Erwägungen. Wien. Klin. Wochenschr. 71:530–533.

Niedermeyer, E. 1960. Remarques à propos de la pathophysiologie de l'état de mal. Rev. Neurol. (Paris) 102:681–684.

Niedermeyer, E. 1961. Cerebrovasculäre Altersveränderungen als Epilepsieursache. Acta Neurochir. Suppl. 7:201–206.

Niedermeyer, E. 1965. Sleep electroencephalograms in petit mal. Arch. Neurol. (Chicago) 12:625–630.

Niedermeyer, E. 1966a. Generalized seizure discharges and possible precipitating mechanisms. Epilepsia (Amsterdam) 7:23–29.

Niedermeyer, E. 1966b. Considerations of the centrencephalic (generalized) type of epilepsy. Del. Med. J. 38:341–348.

Niedermeyer, E. 1968. The Lennox-Gastaut syndrome: a severe type of childhood epilepsy. Electroencephalogr. Clin. Neurophysiol. 24:283 (abst).

Niedermeyer, E. 1969. The Lennox-Gastaut syndrome: a severe type of childhood epilepsy. Dtsch. Z. Nervenheilk. 195:263–282.

Niedermeyer, E. 1970a. Intravenous diazepam and its anticonvulsive action. Johns Hopkins Med. J. 127:79–96.

Niedermeyer, E. 1970b. Spitzen über der Zentralregion und mu Rhythmus: Gedanken zum Problem der "funktionellen" Spitzen. Z. EEG-EMG 1:133–141.

Niedermeyer, E. 1972a. *The Generalized Epilepsies.* Springfield, IL: Charles C Thomas.

Niedermeyer, E. 1972b. Focal and generalized seizure discharges in the electroencephalogram and their responses to intravenous diazepam. Int. Med. Digest 7:49–61.

Niedermeyer, E. 1974. *Compendium of the Epilepsies.* Springfield, IL: Charles C Thomas.

Niedermeyer, E. 1981. Complexities of primary generalized epilepsy. Clin. Electroencephalogr. 12:177–191.

Niedermeyer, E., 1982. Petit mal, primary generalized epilepsy and sleep. In *Sleep and Epilepsy,* Eds. M.B. Sterman, M.N. Shouse, and P. Passouant, pp. 191–207. New York: Academic Press.

Niedermeyer, E. 1983. *Epilepsy Guide.* Baltimore: Urban & Schwarzenberg.

Niedermeyer, E. 1984. Awakening epilepsy ("Aufwach-Epilepsie") revisited 30 years later. In *Epilepsy, Sleep and Sleep Deprivation,* Eds. S.R. Degen and E. Niedermeyer, pp. 85–94. Amsterdam: Elsevier.

Niedermeyer, E. 1986. The Lennox-Gastaut syndrome and its frontiers. Clin. Electroencephalogr. 17:117–126.

Niedermeyer, E. 1990a. Clinical relevance of EEG signals in epilepsies. In *Handbook of Electroencephalography and Clinical Neurophysiology,* revised series, vol.4, Eds. J.A. Wada and R.J. Ellingson, pp. 237–261. Amsterdam: Elsevier.

Niedermeyer, E. 1990b. *The Epilepsies.* Baltimore: Urban & Schwarzenberg.

Niedermeyer, E. 1992. Mechanisms of primary generalized (idiopathic) epilepsy. Epilepsia (New York) 33 (suppl. 3):57(abst).

Niedermeyer, E. 1996a. Primary (idiopathic) generalized epilepsy. Clin. Electroencephalogr. 27:1–21.

Niedermeyer, E. 1996b. Dipole theory and electroencephalography. Clin. Electroencephalogr. 27:121–131.

Niedermeyer, E. 1998a. Frontal lobe functions and dysfunctions. Clin. Electroencephalogr. 29:79–90.

Niedermeyer, E. 1998b. Frontal lobe epilepsy: the next frontier. Clin. Electroencephalogr. 29:163–169.

Niedermeyer, E. 2002. The epileptic pre-aura. Clin Electroencephalogr. 33:58–61.

Niedermeyer, E. 2003. Electrophysiology of the frontal lobe. Clin Electroencephalogr. 34:5–12.

Niedermeyer, E., and Höller, L. 1984. Kurzschlaf im EEG-Eine Fundgrube sonst Übersehener EEG-Abnormalitäten. Z. EEG-EMG 15: 57–66.

Niedermeyer, E., and Hinchcliffe, R. 1965. Vertigo and the electroencephalogram. Electroencephalogr. Clin. Neurophysiol. 18:78–81.

Niedermeyer, E., and Khalifeh, R. 1965. Petit mal status ("spike-wave stupor"). An electro-clinical appraisal. Epilepsia (Amsterdam) 6:250–262.

Niedermeyer, E., and Ribeiro, M. 2000. Considerations of nonconvulsive status epilepticus. Clin. Electroencephalogr. 31:192–195.

Niedermeyer, E., and Rocca, U. 1972. The diagnostic significance of sleep electroencephalograms in temporal lobe epilepsy. Eur. Neurol. (Basel) 7:119–129.

Niedermeyer, E., and Rocca, U. 1980. Scalp, cortical and depth EEG contribution to focal motor epilepsy and epilepsia partialis continua. Electroencephalogr. Clin. Neurophysiol. 50:160P(abst).

Niedermeyer, E., and Sherman, D.L. 2001. Ultrafast EEG frequencies—not to be neglected in the future. Am. J. END Technol. 41:192–198.

Niedermeyer, E., and Uematsu, S. 1974. Electroencephalographic recordings from deep cerebellar structures in patients with uncontrolled epileptic seizures. Electroencephalogr. Clin. Neurophysiol. 37:355–365.

Niedermeyer, E., and Vaughan-Matthews, S. 1992. Generalized synchronous paroxysmal bursts and the role of arousal. Electroencephalogr. Clin. Neurophysiol. 82:103P(abst).

Niedermeyer, E., and Walker, A.E. 1971. Mesio-frontal epilepsy. Electroencephalogr. Clin. Neurophysiol. 31:104–105P(abst).

Niedermeyer, E., Walker, A.E., and Blumer, D. 1967. EEG and behavioral findings in temporal lobe epileptics (before and after temporal lobectomy). Electroencephalogr. Clin. Neurophysiol. 23:493(abst).

Niedermeyer, E., Walker, A.E., and Burton, C. 1970a. The slow spike wave complex as a correlate of frontal and fronto-temporal post-traumatic epilepsy. Eur. Neurol. (Basel) 3:330–346.

Niedermeyer, E., Blumer, D., Holscher, E., et al. 1970b. Classical hysterical seizures facilitated by anticonvulsant toxicity. Psychiatr. Clin. (Basel) 3: 71–84.

Niedermeyer, E., Yarworth, S., and Zobniw, A.M. 1977a. Absence of drug-induced beta activity in the electroencephalogram. Eur. Neurol. (Basel) 15:77–84.

Niedermeyer, E., Freeman, J.M., Long, D.M., et al. 1977b. EEG studies in recalcitrant and disabling focal motor seizures. Epilepsia (New York) 18:289(abst).

Niedermeyer, E., Fineyre, F., Riley, T., et al. 1979a. Myoclonus and the electroencephalogram. Clin. Electroencephalogr. 10:75–95.

Niedermeyer, E., Fineyre, F., Riley, T., et al. 1979b. Absence status (petit mal status) with focal characteristics. Arch. Neurol. (Chicago) 36:417–421.

Niedermeyer, E., Freund, G., and Krumholz, A. 1981. Subacute encephalopathy with seizures in alcoholics: a clinical-electroencephalographic study. Clin. Electroencephalogr. 12:113–129.

Niedermeyer, E., Riggio, S., and Santiago, M. 1988. Benign occipital lobe epilepsy. J. Epilepsy 1:3–11.

Nobili, L., Baglietto, M.G., Beelke, M., et al. 2001. Temporal relationship of generalized epileptiform discharges to spindle frequency activity in childhood absence epilepsy. Clin. Neurophysiol. 112:1912–1916.

Noebels, J.L. 2003. Exploring new gene discoveries in idiopathic generalized epilepsy. Epilepsia 44 (suppl 2):16–21.

Noebels, J.L., and Sidman, R.L. 1979. Inherited epilepsy: spike-wave and focal motor seizures in the mutant mouse tottering. Science 204:1334–1336.

Nogueira de Melo, A., and Niedermeyer, E. 1991a. Considerations of secondary temporalization. Clin. Electroencephalogr. 22:161–171.

Nogueira de Melo, A., and Niedermeyer, E. 1991b. Crossover phenomena in epileptic syndromes in childhood epilepsies. Clin. Electroencephalogr. 22:75–82.

Nolte, R., Wolff, M., and Kraegeloh-Mann, I. 1988. The atonic (astatic) drop attacks and their differential diagnosis. In *The Lennox-Gastaut Syndrome,* Eds. E. Niedermeyer and R. Degen, pp. 95–108. New York: Alan R. Liss.

Nowack, W.J. 1996. Dyshormia revisited: generalized seizures and arousal. Clin. Electroencephalogr. 27:22–25.

O'Brien, T.J., Hogan, R.E., Sedal, L., et al. 1996. Tooth-brushing epilepsy: a report of a case with structural imaging and electrophysiology demonstrating a right frontal focus. Epilepsia 37:694–697.

Ochs, R.F., Gloor, P., and Ives, J.R. 1981. The diagnostic value of head turning in the localization of seizures. Electroencephalogr. Clin. Neurophysiol. 51:21P–22P(abst).

Oguni, H., Hara, H., Hayakawa, T., et al. 1985. A clinical and electroencephalographic study of myoclonic epilepsy in infancy. Brain Dev. 7: 75–76.

Ohtahara, S. 1978. Clinico-electrical delineation of epileptic encephalopathies in childhood. Asian Med. J. 21:499–509.

Ohtahara, S., Ishida, T., Oka, E., et al. 1976. On the specific age-dependent epileptic syndrome. The early infantile epileptic encephalopathy with suppression-burst [in Japanese]. *No-to-Hattatsu (Tokyo)* 8:270–280.

Ohtahara, S., Yamatogi, Y., Ohtsuka, Y., et al. 1980. Prognosis of the West syndrome with special reference to Lennox syndrome: a developmental study. In *Advances in Epileptology. Xth Epilepsy International Symposium,* Eds. J.A. Wada and J.K. Penry, pp. 149–154. New York: Raven Press.

Ohtahara, S., Ohtsuka, Y., Yamatogi, Y., et al. 1993. Prenatal etiologies of West syndrome. Epilepsia 34:716–722.

Ohtahara, S., Ohtsuka, Y., and Kobayashi, K. 1995. Lennox-Gastaut syndrome: a new vista. Psychiatry Clin. Neurosci. 49:S179–S183.

Ohtsuka, Y., Murashima, I., Asano, T., et al. 1996. Partial seizures in West syndrome. Epilepsia 37:1060–1067.

Okuma, T., Llinas, R., and Ervin, F.R. 1961. Effect of mesencephalic reticular formation lesion on epileptic seizure threshold. Electroencephalogr. Clin. Neurophysiol. 13:304–305.

O'Leary, J.R., and Goldring, S. 1964. DC potentials of the brain. Physiol. Res. 44:91–125.

O'Leary, J.R., and Goldring, S. 1976. *Science and Epilepsy.* New York: Raven Press.

Oller-Daurella, L. 1967a. *Sindrome de Lennox.* Barcelona: Editorial Espaxs.

Oller-Daurella, L. 1967b. Discussion remark. In *Les activités électriques cérébrales spontanées et évoquees chez l'homme,* Eds. H. Gastaut, R. Poiré, A. Waltrégny, et al., p. 220. Paris: Gauthier-Villars.

Oller-Daurella, L. 1971. Critique du concept de l'épilepsie généralisée primaire, fondée sur la révision d'une série de cas personnels, dont le diagnostic clinique et EEG semble indubitable. Rev. Neurol. (Paris) 124: 487–494.

Oller-Daurella, L. 1973. Evolution et pronostic du syndrome de Lennox-Gastaut. In *Evolution and Prognosis of the Epilepsies,* Ed. E. Lugaresi, pp. 155–164. Bologna: Gaggi.

Oller-Daurella, L. 1976. Las fronteras entre et petit mal y el sindrome de Lennox-Gastaut. Rev. Esp. Oto-Neuro-Oftalmol. Neurocir. 34:27–44.

Oller-Daurella, L., and Oller-Ferrer-Fidal, L. 1977. *Atlas de Crisis Epilepticas.* Basel: Geigy.

Oller-Daurella, L., and Oller-Ferrer-Fidal, L. 1981. *Altas de Crisis Epilepticas,* 2nd ed. Basel: Geigy.

Olmos-Garcia de Alba, G., Valdez, J.M., and Crespo, F.V. 1984a. West syndrome evolving into the Lennox-Gastaut syndrome. Clin. Electroencephalogr. 15:61–68.

Olmos-Garcia de Alba, G., Mora, E.U., Valdez, J.M., et al. 1984b. Neonatal status epilepticus. II. Electroencephalographic aspects. Clin. Electroencephalogr. 15:197–201.

Olney, J.W., Collins, R.C., and Sloviter, R.S. 1986. Excitotoxic mechanisms of epileptic brain damage. In *Basic Mechanisms of the Epilepsies,* Eds. A.V. Delgado-Escueta, A.A. Ward, Jr., D.M. Woodbury, et al., pp. 857–877. New York: Raven Press.

Omorokov, L. 1927. Kojewnikoffsche Epilepsie in Sibirien. Z. Gesamte Neurol. Psychiatr. 107:487.

Ono, T., Matsuo, A., Baba, H., et al. 2002. Is a cortical spike discharge "transferred" to the contralateral cortex via the corpus callosum? an intraoperative observation of electrocorticogram and callosal compound action potentials. Epilepsia 43:1536–1542.

Otto, F.G., and Kozian, R. 201. Subacute encephalopathy with epileptic seizures in alcoholism (SESA): case report. Clin. Electroencephalogr. 32:184–185.

Ounsted, C. 1952. The factor of inheritance in convulsive disorders in childhood. Proc. R. Soc. Med. 45:865–868.

Ounsted, C. 1955. Genetic and social aspects of the epilepsies of childhood. Eugen. Rev. 47:33–49.

Paal, G. 1957. Katamnestische Untersuchungen und EEG bei Pyknolepsie. Arch. Psychiatr. Nervenkr. 196:48–62.

Pachatz, C., Fusco, L., and Vigevano, F. 2003. Epileptic spasms and partial seizures as a single ictal event. Epilepsia 44:693–700.

Pagniez, R., Liberson, W., and Plichet, A. 1938. Contribution a l'etude des electroencephalogrammes des epileptiques. C. R. Soc. Biol. (Paris) 128: 1084–1087.

Panayiotopoulos, C.P. 1980. Basilar migraine, seizures and severe epileptic EEG abnormalities. Neurology (Minneapolis) 30:1122–1125.

Panayiotopoulos, C.P. 1994. Fixation-off-sensitive epilepsies: clinical and EEG characteristics. In *Epileptic Seizures and Syndromes,* Ed. P. Wolf, pp. 55–66. London: Libbey.

Panayiotopoulos, C.P. 1999. *Benign Childhood Partial Seizures and Related Epileptic Syndromes.* London: Libbey.

Panayiotopoulos, C.P. 2002. *The Panyiotopoulos Syndrome.* London: Libbey.

Panayiotopoulos, C.P., Agathonikou, A., Koutroumanidis, M., et al. 1996. Eyelid myoclonus with absences: the symptoms. In *Eyelid Myoclonia with Absences,* Eds. J.S. Duncan and C.P. Panayiotopoulos, pp. 17–26. London: Libbey.

Panzica, F., Rubboli, G., Avanzini, G., et al. 2001. Cortical myoclonus in Janz syndrome. Clin. Neurophysiol. 112:1803–1809.

Parain, D., Zorrilla, F., Samson-Dollfus, D., et al. 1982. EEG findings in 6 cases of television epilepsy. Electroencephalogr. Clin. Neurophysiol. 54:46P(abst).

Parisi, A., Strosselli, M., Pan, A., et al. 1991. HIV-related encephalitis presenting as convulsant disease. Clin. Electroencephalogr. 22:1–4.

Passero, S., Rocchi, R., Rossi, S., et al. 2002. Seizures after spontaneous supratentorial intracerebral hemorrhage. Epilepsia 43:1175–1180.

Passouant, P., and Cadilhac, J. 1970. Décharges épileptiques. In *Epilepsy. Recent Views on Theory, Diagnosis and Therapy of Epilepsy,* Ed. E. Niedermeyer, pp. 87–104. Basel: S. Karger.

Passouant, P., Cadilhac, J., Ribstein, M., et al. 1967. Les états de mal partiels. In *Les États de Mal Épileptiques,* Eds. H. Gastaut, J. Roger, and H. Lob, pp. 152–181. Paris: Masson.

Patry, G., Lyagoubi, S., and Tassinari, C.A. 1971. Subclinical "electrical status epilepticus" induced by sleep in children. Arch. Neurol. (Chicago) 24:242–252.

Pavone, A., and Niedermeyer, E. 2000. Absence seizures and the frontal lobe. Clin. Electroencephalogr. 31:153–156.

Pédespan, J.M., Loiseau, H., Vital, A., et al. 1995. Surgical treatment of an early epileptic encephalopathy with suppression-bursts and focal cortical dysplasia. Epilepsia 36:37–40.

Pedley, T.A., Fisher, R.S., and Prince, D.A. 1976. Focal gliosis and potassium movement in mammalian cortex. Exp. Neurol. 50:346–351.

Pedley, T.A., Tharp, B.R., and Herman, K.R., 1980. Electroencephalographic and clinical correlates of vertex spike foci. Electroencephalogr. Clin. Neurophysiol. 50:153P(abst).

Peiffer, J. 1963. *Morphologische Aspekte der Epilepsien.* Berlin: Springer.

Peled, R., Harnes, B., Borovich, B., et al. 1984. Speech arrest and supplementary motor area seizures. Neurology (Cleveland) 34:110–111.

Penfield, W. 1929. Diencephalic autonomic epilepsy. Arch. Neurol. Psychiatry (Chicago) 22:358–374.

Penfield, W. 1938. The cerebral cortex in man. I. The cerebral cortex and consciousness. Arch. Neurol. Psychiatry (Chicago) 40:417–442.

Penfield, W. 1952. Epileptic automatism and the centrencephalic integrating system. Publ. Assoc. Res. Nerv. Ment. Dis. 30:513–528.

Penfield, W., and Faulk, M.E., Jr. 1955. The insula. Further observations on its function. Brain 78:445–470.

Penfield, W., and Jasper, H.H. 1954. *Epilepsy and the Functional Anatomy of the Human Brain.* Boston: Little, Brown.

Penfield, W., and Kristiansen, K. 1951. *Epileptic Seizure Patterns.* Springfield, IL: Charles C Thomas.

Penfield, W., and Rasmussen, T. 1950. *The Cerebral Cortex of Man.* New York: Macmillan.

Penry, J.K. 1975. Perspectives in complex partial seizures. In *Complex Partial Seizures and Their Treatment,* Eds. J.K. Penry and D.D. Daly, pp. 1–14. New York: Raven Press.

Penry, J.K. 1980. Intensive monitoring of epileptic patients. In *Advances in Epileptology, Xth Epilepsy International Symposium,* Eds. J.A. Wada and J.K. Penry, pp. 29–33. New York: Raven Press.

Penry, J.K., and Daly, D.D. (Eds.). 1975. *Complex Partial Seizures and Their Treatment.* New York: Raven Press.

Penry, J.K., and Dreifuss, F.E. 1969. A study of automatisms associated with the absence of petit mal. Epilepsia (Amsterdam) 10:417–418(abst).

Penry, J.K., and Porter, R.V. 1977. Intensive monitoring of patients with intractable seizures. In *Epilepsy: The VIIIth International Symposium,* Ed. J.K. Penry, pp. 95–101. New York: Raven Press.

Perez-Borja, C., Tassinari, C.A., and Swanson, A.G. 1967. Paroxysmal choreoathetosis and seizures induced by movements. Epilepsia (Amsterdam) 8:260–270.

Perosa, T.S.R., Porcionatto, M.A., Cukier, A., et al. 2002. Extracellular matrix components are altered in the hippocampus, cortex, and cerebrospinal fluid of patients with mesial temporal epilepsy. Epilepsia 43: (suppl 5):159–161.

Petersén, I., Sørbye, R., Gelin, L.E., et al. 1964. EEG and burns. Electroencephalogr. Clin. Neurophysiol. 17:210(abst).

Petsche, H. 1962. Pathophysiologie und Klinik des Petit mal. Toposkopische Untersuchungen zur Phänomenologie des Spike-Wave-Musters. Wien. Z. Nervenheilk. 19:345–442.

Petsche, H. 1968. Epileptischer Anfall und kortikale Neuronenpopulation. Wien. Z. Nervenheilk. 26:45–55.

Petsche, H., and Marko, A. 1959. Zur dreidimensionalen Darstellung des Spike and Wave Feldes. Wien. Z. Nervenheilk. 16:427–435.

Petsche, H., and Rappelsberger, P. 1970. Influence of cortical incisions on synchronization pattern and travelling waves. Electroencephalogr. Clin. Neurophysiol. 28:592–600.

Petsche, H., and Sterc, J. 1968. The significance of the cortex for the travelling phenomenon of brain-waves. Electroencephalogr. Clin. Neurophysiol. 25:11–22.

Petsche, H., Pockberger, H., Rappelsberger, P., et al. 1976. Zur intrakortikalen Elektrogenese: Spontantätigkeit, Schlaf und epileptischer Anfall. Z. EEG-EMG 7:107–121.

Pfleger, L. 1880. Beobachtungen ber Schrumpfung und Sklerose des Ammonshorns bei Epilepsie. Allg. Z. Psychiatr. 36:359–380.

Phillips, CG. 1961. Some properties of pyramidal neurones of the motor cortex. In *The Nature of Sleep.* Eds. G.E.W. Wolstenholme and M. O'Connor, pp. 4–29. Boston: Little, Brown and Co.

Pit'hova, B., Bevilaqua, L., and Wolfova, E. 1981. Epileptic signs in cerebral circulatory disturbances. Electroencephalogr. Clin. Neurophysiol. 52:13P(abst).

Plouin, P., Lérique, A., and Dulac, O. 1980. Étude électroclinique et évolution dans 7 observations des crises partielles complexes dominées par un comportement de terreur chez l'Penfant. In *Progressi in Epilettologia,* Eds. R. Canger, G. Avanzini, and C.A. Tassinari, pp. 29–30, 139–143. Bollettino LICE.

Pollen, D.A., Perot, P., and Reid, K.H. 1963. Experimental bilateral wave and spike from thalamic stimulation in relation to arousal. Epilepsia (Amsterdam) 9:221–232.

Porter, R.J. 1980. Methodology of continuous monitoring with videotape recording and electroencephalography. In *Advances in Epileptology. The Xth Epilepsy International Symposium,* Eds. J.A. Wada and J.K. Penry, pp. 35–42. New York: Raven Press.

Portnoy, B.A., and Herion, J.C. 1972. Neurological manifestations of sickle cell disease. With a review of the literature and emphasis on the prevalence of hemiplegia. Ann. Intern. Med. 76:643–652.

Pourmand, R.A., Markand, O.N., and Thomas, C. 1984. Midline spike discharges: clinical and EEG correlates. Clin Electroencephalogr. 15:232–236.

Pradhan, S.N., and Ajmone Marsan, C. 1963. Chlorambucil toxicity and EEG "centrencephalic" patterns. Epilepsia (Amsterdam) 4:1–14.

Prichard, J.S. 1964. The character and significance of epileptic seizures in infancy. In *Neurological and Electroencephalographic Correlative Studies in Infancy,* Eds. P. Kellaway and I. Petersén, pp. 273–286. New York: Grune & Stratton.

Prier, S., Benoit, C., Dehen, H., et al. 1992. Bilateral periodic stereotyped EEG complexes in multiple sclerosis. Proceed. 6th Eur. Congress Clin. Neurophysiol., Lisbon, Sept. 1992. Clin. Neurophysiol., vol. 22, Suppl. 1–1992, p. 107s. Amsterdam: Elsevier.

Prill, A., Quellhorst, E., and Scheler, F. 1969. Epilepsy: Clinical and electroencephalographic findings in patients with renal insufficiency. In *The Physiopathogenesis of the Epilepsies,* Eds. H. Gastaut, H.H. Jasper, J. Bancaud, et al., pp. 60–68. Springfield, IL: Charles C Thomas.

Primrose, D.C., and Ojeman, G.A. 1992. Outcome of resective surgery for temporal lobe epilepsy. In *Epilepsy Surgery,* Ed. H. Lueders, pp. 601–611. New York: Raven Press.

Prince, D.A., and Farrell, D. 1969. "Centrencephalic" spike wave discharges following parenteral penicillin injection in the cat. Neurology (Minneapolis) 19:309–310.

Prince, D.A., and Wilder, B.J. 1967. Control mechanisms in cortical epileptogenic foci "surround" inhibition. Arch. Neurol. (Chicago) 16:194–202.

Prince, D.A., Pedley, T.A., and Ransom, B.R. 1977. Fluctuations of ion concentrations during excitation and seizures. In *Dynamic Properties of Glial Cells,* Eds. E. Schoffeniels, G. Franck, L. Hertz, et al., pp. 281–303. London: Pergamon Press.

Pryor, D.S., Don, N., and Macourt, D.C. 1981. Fifth day fits: a syndrome of neonatal convulsions. *Arch. Dis. Child.* 56:753–758.

Purpura, D.P. 1953. Activation of epileptogenic foci by topical application of acetylcholine to the exposed cerebral cortex in man. Electroencephalogr. Clin. Neurophysiol. Supp. 3:36(abst).

Quatrocolo, G., Gusmaroli, G., Durelli, L., et al. 1987. Spinal myoclonus: report of a case. Electroencephalogr. Clin. Neurophysiol. 66:53P (abst).

Quesney, L.F. 1980. Photosensitive epilepsy in the cat after systemic and cortical penicillin application. Role of dopaminergic mechanisms in photosensitivity. Epilepsia (New York) 21:185(abst).

Quesney, L.F., Gloor, P., Kratzenberg, E., et al. 1977. Pathophysiology of generalized penicillin epilepsy in the cat. The role of cortical and subcortical structures. I. Systemic application of penicillin. Electroencephalogr. Clin. Neurophysiol. 42:640–655.

Quesney, L.F., Constain, M., and Rasmussen, T. 1992. Seizures from the dorsolateral frontal lobe. In *Frontal Lobe Seizures and Epilepsies,* Eds. P. Chauvel, A.V. Delgado-Escueta, E. Halgren, et al., pp. 233–243. New York: Raven Press.

Rabending, G., and Klepel, H. 1970. Photoconvulsive and photo myoclonic reactions: age dependent variations of genetically determined photosensitivity. Neuropaediatrie 2:164–172.

Rabending, G., and Klepel, H. 1978. *Die Fotostimulation als Aktivierungsmethode in der Elektroenzephalographie.* Jena: Fischer.

Racy, A., Osborn, M.A., Vern, B.A., et al. 1980. Epileptic aphasia. First onset of prolonged monosymptomatic status epilepticus in adults. Arch. Neurol. (Chicago) 37:419–422.

Ralston, B.L. 1961. Cingulate epilepsy and secondary bilateral synchrony. Electroencephalogr. Clin. Neurophysiol. 13:591–598.

Ramani, V., and Gumnit, R.J. 1981. Interictal psychosis during intensive seizure monitoring. Electroencephalogr. Clin. Neurophysiol. 52:86P (abst).

Randow, R., Sonnichsen, N., and Schulz, H. 1965. Epilepsie als Frühsymptom des Lupus erythematodes. Dermatol. Wochenschr. 151:1283–1289.

Raou, K.S., and Prichard, J.S. 1955. Photogenic epilepsy. J. Pediatr. 47: 619–623.

Rasmussen, T. 1970. The neurosurgical treatment of focal epilepsy. In *Epilepsy, Recent Views on Theory, Diagnosis and Therapy of Epilepsy,* Ed. E. Niedermeyer, pp. 306–325. Basel: S. Karger.

Rasmussen, T. 1975. Surgery of frontal lobe epilepsy. In *Neurosurgical Management of the Epilepsies,* Eds. D.P. Purpura, J.K. Penry, and R.D. Walter, pp. 197–205. New York: Raven Press.

Rasmussen, T., Olszewski, J., and Lloyd-Smith, D. 1958. Focal seizures due to chronic localized encephalitis. Neurology (Minneapolis) 8:435– 445.

Reeves, A.L., Nollet, K.E., Klass, D.W., et al. 1996. The ictal bradycardia syndrome. Epilepsia 37:983–987.

Reiher, J., and Beaudry, M. 1988. TIRDA or temporal interictal rhythmic delta activity; specificity and predictive value. Electroencephalogr. Clin. Neurophysiol. 69:96P(abst).

Remillard, G.M., Andermann, F., Rhi-Sausi, A., et al. 1977. Facial asymmetry in patients with temporal lobe epilepsy: a clinical sign useful in the lateralization of temporal epileptogenic lesions. Epilepsia (New York) 18:284(abst).

Remillard, G.M., Andermann, F., Testa, G.F., et al. 1983. Sexual ictal manifestations in women with temporal lobe epilepsy: a finding suggesting sexual dimorphism in the human brain. Neurology (Cleveland) 33:323– 330.

Remillard, G., Andermann, F., Bradwejn, J., et al. 1984. Homosexuality and limbic epilepsy: a study of 12 patients. Electroencephalogr. Clin. Neurophysiol. 57:4P(abst).

Rennick, Ph.M., Perez-Borja, C., and Rodin, E.A. 1969. Transient mental deficits associated with recurrent prolonged epileptic clouded state. Epilepsia (Amsterdam) 10:397–405.

Reutens, D.C., and Berkovic, S.F. 1995. Idiopathic generalized epilepsy of adolescence: are the syndromes clinically distinct? Neurology 45:1469–1476.

Ricci, S., and Vigevano, F. 1993. Occipital seizures provoked by intermittent light stimulation: ictal and interictal findings. J. Clin. Neurophysiol. 10:197–209.

Richardson, E.P., Jr., and Dodge, P.R. 1954. Epilepsy in cerebral vascular disease. Epilepsia (Boston) 3:49–74.

Riggio, S., and Harner, R.S. 1995. Repetitive motor activity in frontal lobe epilepsy. In *Epilepsy and the Functional Anatomy of the Frontal Lobe,* Eds. H.H. Jasper, S. Riggio, and P.S. Goldman-Rakic, pp. 153–164. New York: Raven.

Riggio, S., Santiago, M., and Niedermeyer, E. 1987. Benign occipital lobe epilepsy. Neurology 37 (suppl I):106(abst).

Riggio, S., Harner, R.N., and Cooper, S.A. 1991. Repetitive motor activity and semiology of frontal lobe epilepsy. Epilepsia (New York) 32:64– 65(abst).

Riley, T., and Niedermeyer, E. 1978. Rage attacks and episodic violent behavior: electroencephalographic findings and general considerations. Clin. Electroencephalogr. 9:131–139.

Riley, T.L., and Massey, E.W. 1979. The syndrome of aphasia, headaches and left temporal spikes. Proc. Am. EEG Soc., Atlanta, Georgia.

Rish, B.L., and Caveness, W.F. 1973. Relation of prophylactic medication to the occurrence of early seizures following craniocerebral trauma. J. Neurosurg. 38:155–158.

Robb, P.F., and McNaughton, F. 1974. Vascular diseases. In *Handbook of Clinical Neurology,* Eds. P.J. Vinken and G.W. Bruyn, vol. 15, pp. 302–305. Amsterdam: North Holland.

Robillard, A., Saint-Hilaire, J.-M., Mercier, M., et al. 1982. The lateralizing and localizing value of adversion in seizures. Electroencephalogr. Clin. Neurophysiol. 54:41P(abst).

Rocca, U. 1973. *Tratamiento Quirurgico de la Neurocisticercosis.* Lima (Peru): doctoral thesis.

Rocca, U., and Niedermeyer, E. 1982. Severe forms of focal motor seizure disorders in childhood. Proceed. Congr. Latin. Amer. (Buenos Aires), pp. 277–291.

Rodin, E.A. 1973. Psychomotor epilepsy and aggressive behavior. Arch. Gen. Psychiatry 28:210–213.

Rodin, E.A. 1975. Discussion remark. In *Complex Partial Seizures and Their Treatment*, Eds. J.K. Penry and D.D. Daly, p. 82. New York: Raven Press.

Rodin, E.A., Dejong, R.N., Waggoner, R.W., et al. 1957. Relationship between certain forms of psychomotor epilepsy and schizophrenia. Arch. Neurol. Psychiatry (Chicago) 77:449–463.

Rodin, E.A., Rutledge, L.T., and Calhoun, H.D. 1958. Megimide and metrazol: a comparison of their convulsant properties in man and cat. Electroencephalogr. Clin. Neurophysiol. 10:719–723.

Rodin, E.A., Gonzales, S., Caldwell, D., et al. 1966. Photic evoked responses during induced epileptic seizures. Epilepsia (Amsterdam) 7: 202–214.

Rodin, E., Litzinger, M., and Thompson, J. 1995. Complexity of focal spikes suggests relative epileptogenicity. Epilepsia 36:1078–1083.

Rodriguez, I., and Niedermeyer, E. 1982. The aphasia-convulsion syndrome in children: electroencephalographic aspects. Clin. Electroencephalogr. 13:23–35.

Roger, J., and Bureau, M. 1992. Distinctive characteristics of frontal lobe epilepsy versus idiopathic generalized epilepsy. In *Frontal Lobe Seizures and Epilepsies*, Eds. P. Chauvel, A.V. Delgado-Escueta, E. Halgren, et al., pp. 399–410. New York: Raven Press.

Roger, J., Soulayrol, R., and Pinsard, N. 1964. Diagnostic différential. In *L'Encéphalopathie Myoclonique Infantile avec Hypsarrhythmie (Syndrome de West)*, Eds. H. Gastaut, R. Soulayrol, J. Roger, et al., pp. 143–149. Paris: Masson.

Roger, J., Lob, H., Regis, H., et al. 1967. Les états de mal généralisées myocloniques. In *Les États de Mal Épileptiques*, Eds. H. Gastaut, J. Roger, and H. Lob, pp. 77–84. Paris: Masson.

Roger, J., Lob, H., and Tassinari, C.A. 1974. Status epilepticus. In *Handbook of Clinical Neurology*, vol. 15, Eds. P.J. Vinken and G.W. Bruyn, pp. 145–182. Amsterdam: North Holland.

Rosanoff, A.J., Handy, L.M., and Rasanoff, I.A. 1934. Etiology of epilepsy with special reference to its occurrence in twins. Arch. Neurol. Psychiatry (Chicago) 31:1165–1193.

Rosati, A., Aghakani, Y., Bernasconi, A., et al. 2003. Intractable temporal lobe epilepsy with rare spikes is less severe than with infrequent spikes. Neurology 50:1590–1295.

Rose, A.L., and Lombroso, C.T. 1970. Neonatal seizure state. A study of clinical, pathological and electroencephalographic features in 137 full-term babies with long-term follow-up. Pediatrics 45:404–425.

Roseman, E. 1961. Dilantin toxicity. A clinical and electroencephalographic study. Neurology (Minneapolis) 11:912–921.

Rossi, C.F., Walter, R.D., and Crandall, P.H. 1967. Generalized spike and wave discharge and non-specific thalamic nuclei. Arch. Neurol. (Chicago) 19:174–183.

Rothmeier, J., Friese, M., Willemsen, F., et al. 2001. Subacute encephalopathy with seizures in chronic alcoholism (SESA syndrome). Clin. Electroencephalogr. 32:186–190.

Rovit, R., Gloor, P., and Rasmussen, T. 1961. Intracarotid amobarbital in epilepsy. Arch. Neurol. (Chicago) 5:606–625.

Rowbotham, S.F. 1964. *Acute Injuries of the Head*. Edinburgh: Livingstone.

Rubboli, G., Parmeggiani, L., and Tassinari, C.A. 1995. Frontal inhibitory spike component associated with epileptic negative myoclonus. Electroencephalogr. Clin. Neurophysiol. 95:201–205.

Russell, W.R., and Whitty, C.W.M. 1953. Studies in traumatic epilepsy. Part II. Focal motor and somatic sensory fits: a study of 85 cases. J. Neurol. Neurosurg. Psychiatry 16:73.

Rütti, W. 1982. Absenzen-Epilepsie im Erwachsenenalter. Schwiez. Med. Wochenschr. 112:434–441.

Rütti, W., and Karbowski, K. 1983. Absence epilepsy in adults. Electroencephalogr. Clin. Neurophysiol. 55:18P(abst).

Sachdeo, R., and Chokroverty, S. 1986. Carbamazepine and EEG epileptiform activities. Electroencephalogr. Clin. Neurophysiol. 64:20P(abst).

Sadler, R.M., Lemieux, J.F., and Blume, W.T. 1984. Potential fields of anterior temporal spikes. Electroencephalogr. Clin. Neurophysiol. 58:47P–48P(abst).

Sahota, P.K., and Stacy, M.A. 1993. Pain as a manifestation of seizure disorder. Clin. Electroencephalogr. 24:63–65.

Saint-Hilaire, J.M., Gilbert, M., and Bouvier, G. 1980. Aggression as an epileptic manifestation: two cases with depth electrode study. Epilepsia (New York) 21:184(abst).

Saint-Hilaire, M.-H., Saint-Hilaire, J.M., and Granger, L. 1986. Jumping Frenchmen of Maine. Neurology 36:1269–1271.

Salanova, V., Morris, H.H., Van Ness, P., et al. 1995. Frontal lobe seizures: electroclinical syndromes. Epilepsia 36:16–24.

Salazar, A.M., Jabbari, B., Vance, S.C., et al. 1985. Epilepsy after penetrating head injury. I. Clinical correlates. A report of the Vietnam head injury study. Neurology 35:1406–1414.

Sammaritano, M., Andermann, F., Melanson, D., et al. 1985. The syndrome of epilepsy and bilateral occipital cortical calcifications. Proceed. Annual Meeting Amer. Epilepsy Society, New York.

Sammaritano, M., Gigli, G.L., and Gotman, J. 1991. Interictal spiking during wakefulness and sleep and the localization of foci in temporal lobe epilepsy. Neurology 41:290–297.

Sammaritano, M.R., Andermann, F., Melançon, D., et al. 1984. Partial status epilepticus can cause prolonged focal cerebral oedema. Electroencephalogr. Clin. Neurophysiol. 57:5P(abst).

Samt, P. 1876. Epileptische Irreseinsformen. Arch. Psychiatr. Nervenheilk. 6:110–216.

Sander, T., Windemuth, C., Schulz, H., et al. 2003. Exploration of putative susceptibility locus for idiopathic generalized epilepsy on chromosome 8p12. Epilepsia 44:32–39.

Sano, K., and Malamud, N. 1953. Clinical significance of sclerosis of the Cornu Ammonis. Ictal "psychic" phenomena. Arch. Neurol. Psychiatry (Chicago) 70:40–53.

Santiago, M., and Niedermeyer, E. 1988. Racial factors and epileptic seizure disorders. J. Epilepsy 1:31–33.

Sargent, P. 1921. Some observations on epilepsy. Brain 44:312–328.

Sato, M., and Ogawa, T. 1984. Abnormal behavior in epilepsy and catecholamines. In *Neurotransmitters, Seizures and Epilepsy II*, Eds. R.G. Fariello, P.L. Morselli, K.G. Lloyd, et al., pp. 1–10. New York: Raven Press.

Sato, S., and Penry, J.K. 1980. 24-hour 8-channel EEG digital cassette recording in patients with complex partial seizures. In *Advances in Epileptology. The Xth Epilepsy International Symposium*, Eds. J. Wada and J.K. Penry, p. 129(abst). New York: Raven Press.

Sato, S., Dreifuss, F.E., and Penry, J.K. 1973. The effect of sleep on spike wave discharges in absence seizures. Neurology (Minneapolis) 23:1335–1345.

Sauer, H. 1916 Über gehäufte kleine Anfälle bei Kindern (Pyknolepsie). Mschr. Psychiat. Neurol. 40:267–300.

Savic, I., Lekvall, A., Greitz, D., et al. 2000. MR spectroscopy shows reduced frontal lobe concentrations of N-acetyl aspartate in patients with juvenile myoclonic epilepsy. Epilepsia 41:290–296.

Scheibel, M.E., and Scheibel, A.B. 1973. Hippocampal pathology in temporal lobe epilepsy. A Golgi survey. In *Epilepsy: Its Phenomena in Man*, Ed. M.A.B. Brazier, pp. 311–337. New York: Academic Press.

Scheffer, I.E., Bhatia, K.P., Lopes-Cendes, I.L., et al. 1994. Autosomal dominant frontal epilepsy misdiagnosed as sleep disorder. Lancet 343: 515–517.

Scheffer, I.E., Jones, L., Possebon, M., et al. 1995. Autosomal dominant rolandic epilepsy and speech apraxia: a new syndrome with anticipation. Ann. Neurol. 38:633–642.

Scherman, R., and Abraham, K. 1963. "Centrencephalic" electroencephalographic patterns in precocious puberty. Electroencephalogr. Clin. Neurophysiol. 15:559–567.

Schiff, J., Lechtenberg, R., and Cracco, R. 1982. Gaze-evoked reflex epilepsy. Electroencephalogr. Clin. Neurophysiol. 54:36P(abst).

Schlichther, W., Bristow, M.E., Schultz, S., et al. 1956. Seizures occurring during intensive chlorpromazine therapy. Can. Med. Assoc. J. 74:364–366.

Schmidt, D., Tsai, J.-J., and Janz, D. 1983. Generalized tonic-clonic seizures in patients with complex-partial seizures. Natural history and prognostic relevance. Epilepsia (New York) 24:43–48.

Schmitz, B., and Sander, T. (eds.). 2000. *Juvenile Myoclonic Epilepsy.* Wrightson: Petersfield.

Schmitz, B., Sailer, U., Sander, T., et al. 2000. Clinical genetics in subtypes of idiopathic generalized epilepsies. In *Juvenile Myoclonic Epilepsy*, Eds. B. Schmitz and T. Sander, pp. 129–144. Petersfield: Wrightson.

Schneider, H., Vassella, F., and Karbowski, K. 1970. The Lennox syndrome, a clinical study of 40 children. Eur. Neurol. (Basel) 4:289–300.

Schneider, R.C., Crosby, E.C., Bagchi, B.K., et al. 1961. Temporal or occipital hallucinations triggered from frontal lesions. Neurology (Minneapolis) 11:172–179.

Schneider, R.C., Crosby, E.C., and Farhat, S.M. 1965. Extratemporal lesions triggering the temporal lobe syndrome. J. Neurosurg. 22:246–263.

Scholz, W. 1951. *Die Krampfschädigungen des Gehirns*. Berlin: Springer.

Schuman, S.H., and Miller, L.J. 1966. Febrile convulsions in families. Clin. Pediatr. 5:604–608.

Schwab, R.S. 1939. Methods of measuring consciousness in attacks of petit mal. Arch. Neurol. Psychiatry (Chicago) 41:215–217.

Schwab, R.S. 1953. A case of status epilepticus in petit mal epilepsy. Electroencephalogr. Clin. Neurophysiol. 5:441–442.

Schwartz, H., and Elsässer, K.H. 1961. Klinischer und neuropathologischer Beitrag zur zerebralen Symptomatik beim Melkerson-Rosenthal B Syndrom. Arch. Psychiatr. Neurol. 202:281–304.

Schwartzkroin, P.A. 1993. Basic mechanisms of epileptogenesis. In *The Treatment of Epilepsy*, Ed. E. Wyllie, pp. 83–98. Philadelphia: Lea and Febiger.

Schwartzkroin, P.A., and Wyler, A.R. 1980. Mechanisms underlying epileptiform burst discharges. Ann. Neurol. 7:95–107.

Schwindt, P.C., and Crill, W.E. 1984. The spinal cord model of experimental epilepsy. In *Electrophysiology of Epilepsy*, Eds. P.A. Schwartzkroin and H.V. Wheal, pp. 219–251. London: Academic Press.

Scott, D., and Cabral, R. 1975. Development and prevention of seizures after neurosurgical procedures including ruptured cerebral aneurysms. Proc. Amer. Epilepsy Society, New York.

Scott, J.S., and Masland, R.L. 1953. Occurrence of "continuous symptoms" in epilepsy patients. Neurology (Minneapolis) 3:297–301.

Segal, M. 1991. Serotonin and epilepsy. In *Neurotransmitters and Epilepsy*, Eds. R.S. Fisher and J.T. Coyle, pp. 103–108. New York: Wiley-Liss.

Seitz, R.J., Piel, S., Arnold, S., et al. 1996. Cerebellar hypometabolism in focal epilepsy is related to age of onset and drug intoxication. Epilepsia 37:1194–1199.

Semah, F., Baulac, M., Hasboun, D., et al. 1995. Is interictal temporal hypometabolism related to mesial temporal sclerosis? A positron emission tomography/magnetic resonance imaging confrontation. Epilepsia 36: 447–456.

Serafetinides, E.A. 1965. Aggressiveness in temporal lobe epilepsy and its relation to cerebral dysfunction and environmental factors. Epilepsia (Amsterdam) 6:33–42.

Serafetinides, E.A. 1970. Psychiatric aspects of temporal lobe epilepsy. In *Epilepsy. Recent View on Theory, Diagnosis and Therapy of Epilepsy*, Ed. E. Niedermeyer, pp. 155–169. Basel: S. Karger.

Serafetinides, E.A., and Falconer, M.A. 1963. Speech disturbances in temporal lobe seizures. Brain 86:333–346.

Seshia, S.S., Reggin, J.D., and Stanwick, R.S. 1985. Migraine and complex seizures in children. Epilepsia (New York) 26:232–236.

Sevim, S., Ertas, N.K., and Ertas, M. 2002. Decreased motor unit number estimates in juvenile myoclonic epilepsy. J. Clin. Neurophysiol. 19:178–181

Sherwin, A., Robitaille, Y., Quesney, F., et al. 1988. Excitatory amino acids are elevated in human epileptic cerebral cortex. Neurology 38:920–923.

Shev, E.E. 1964. Syndrome of status petit mal in the adult. Electroencephalogr. Clin. Neurophysiol. 17:466(abst).

Shibasaki, H., and Kuroiwa, Y. 1975. Electroencephalographic correlates of myoclonus. Electroencephalogr. Clin. Neurophysiol. 39:455–463.

Shibasaki, H., Yamashita, Y., and Kuroiwa, Y. 1978. Electroencephalographic studies of myoclonus. Myoclonus-related cortical spikes and high amplitude somatosensory evoked potentials. Brain 101:447–460.

Shibasaki, H., Neshige, R., and Katabuchi, Y. 1987. Electrophysiological study of photosensitive myoclonus. Electroencephalogr. Clin. Neurophysiol. 67:65P(abst).

Shimazono, Y., Hirai, T., Okuma, T., et al. 1953. Disturbance of consciousness in petit mal epilepsy. Epilepsia (Boston) 2:49–55.

Shivapour, E., and Teasdall, R.D. 1980. Spinal myoclonus with vacuolar degeneration of anterior horn cells. Arch. Neurol. (Chicago) 37:451–453.

Siggins, C.R., and Zieglgansberger, W. 1981. Morphine and opioid peptides reduced inhibitory synaptic potentials in hippocampal pyramidal cells in vitro without alteration of membrane potential. Proc. Natl. Acad. Sci. U.S.A. 78:5235–5239.

Silver, K., Andermann, F., Meugher-Villemurek. 1998. Familial alternating epilepsia partialis continua with chronic encephalitis. Another variant of Rasmussen syndrome. Ann. Neurol. 55:733–736.

Silverman, D. 1954. Clinical correlates of the spike-wave complexes. Electroencephalogr. Clin. Neurophysiol. 6:663–669.

Silverman, D. 1960. The anterior temporal electrode and the ten-twenty system. Electroencephalogr. Clin. Neurophysiol. 12:735.

Singh, B.M., and Strobos, R.J. 1980. Epilepsia partialis continua associated with non-ketotic hyperglycemia: clinical and biochemical profile of 21 patients. Ann. Neurol. 8:155–160.

Smeraldi, E., Scorza-Smeraldi, R., Cazzullo, C.L., et al. 1975. Immunogenetics of the Lennox-Gastaut syndrome: frequency of HL-A antigens and haplotypes in patients and first degree relations. Epilepsia (New York) 16:699–703.

Smeraldi, E., Scorza-Smeraldi, R., Cazzullo, C.L., et al. 1976. A genetic approach to the Lennox-Gastaut syndrome by the "major histocompatibility complex" (MHC). In *Epileptology*, Ed. D. Janz, pp. 33–37. Stuttgart: Thieme.

Smith, N.J., and Scott, D.F. 1981. Hyperventilation: its value in temporal lobe epilepsy. Electroencephalogr. Clin. Neurophysiol. 52: 99P(abst).

Smith, R.F., Devinsky, O., and Luciano, D. 1997. Inhibitory motor status: two new cases a new review of inhibitory motor seizures. J. Epilepsy 10: 15–21.

Snead, O.C., III, and Hosey, L.C. 1985. Exacerbation of seizures in children by carbamazepine. N. Engl. J. Med. 313:916–921.

Snead, O.C., III, and Simonato, M. 1991. Opioid peptides and seizures. In *Neurotransmitters and Epilepsy*, Eds. R.S. Fisher and J.T. Coyle, pp. 181–200. New York: Wiley-Liss.

Snider, R.S., and Cooke, P.M. 1953. Cerebellar activity in relation to the electrocorticogram before, during and after seizure states. Electroencephalogr. Clin. Neurophysiol. Suppl. 3:78(abst).

Snodgrass, S.M., Tsuburaya, K., and Ajmone Marsan, C. 1989. Clinical significance of periodic lateralized epileptiform discharges: relationships with status epilepticus. J. Clin. Neurophysiol. 6:159–172.

Solomon, S. 1967. The neurological evaluation. In *Comprehensive Textbook of Psychiatry*, Eds. A.M. Freedman and H.I. Kaplan, pp. 420–443 (see p. 440). Baltimore: Williams & Wilkins.

Somjen, C.G. 1984. Interstitial ion concentration and the role of neuroglia in seizures. In *Electrophysiology of Epilepsy*, Eds. P.A. Schwartzkroin and H.V. Wheal, pp. 303–341. London: Academic Press.

Sommer, W. 1880. Erkrankungen des Ammonshornes als ätiologisches Moment der Epilepsie. Arch. Psychiat. Nervenkrankh. 10:631–675.

Sorel, L. 1964. L'épilepsie myokinétique grave de la prémière enfance avec pointeonde lente (petit mal variant) et son traitement. Rev. Neurol. (Paris) 99:136–138.

Sorel, L. 1967. Discussion remark. In *Les Activités Électriques Cérébrales Spontanées et Évoquées Chez l'Homme*, Eds. H. Gastaut, F. Bostem, R. Poiré, et al., pp. 219–220. Paris: Gauthier-Villars.

Sorel, L., and Dusaucy-Bauloye, A. 1958. À propos de 21 cas d'hypsarrhythmie de Gibbs, son traitement spectaculaire par l'ACTH. Rev. Neurol. (Paris) 99:136–138.

Spatz, R., Kugler, J., Greil, W., et al. 1978. Das Elektroenzephalogramm bei der Lithium-Intoxikation. Nervenarzt 49:539–542.

Spatz, R., Grohmann, R., and Kugler, J. 1984. Paroxysmal EEG activities and epileptic seizures during antidepressant and neuroleptic therapy. Electroencephalogr. Clin. Neurophysiol. 57:32P(abst).

Speckmann, E.J., and Elger, C.E. 1987. Introduction into the neurophysiological basis of the EEG and DC potentials. In *Electroencephalopathy*, 2nd ed., Eds. E. Niedermeyer and F. Lopes deSilva, pp. 1–13. Baltimore: Urban & Schwarzenberg.

Spencer, S.S., Spencer, D.D., Williamson, P.D., et al. 1981. Sexual automatism in partial complex epilepsy. Proceed. Amer. Epilepsy Society.

Speransky, A.D. 1943. *A Basis for the Theory of Medicine*. New York: International Publishers.

Spiegel, E.A. 1937. Quantitative determination of the convulsive reactivity by electrical stimulation of the brain with the skull intact. J. Lab. Clin. Med. 22:1274–1276.

Spielmeyer, W. 1933. Funktionelle Kreislaufstörungen und Epilepsie. Z. Gesamte Neurol. Psychiatr. 148:285–298.

Sprince, H., Parker, C.M., Josephs, J.A., et al. 1969. Convulsant activity of homocysteine and other short chain mercaptoacids: protection therefrom. Ann. N.Y. Acad. Sci. 166:323–325.

Squires, R.F., and Braestrup, C. 1977. Benzodiazepine receptors in rat brain. Nature 266:732–734.

Squires, R.F., Naquet, R., Riche, D., et al. 1979. Increased thermolability of benzodiazepine receptors in cerebral cortex of a baboon with spontaneous seizures: a case report. Epilepsia (New York) 20:215–221.

Stamps, F.W., Gibbs, E.L., Rosenthal, I.M., et al. 1959. Treatment of hypsarrhythmia with ACTH. JAMA 171:408–411.

Starzl, T.E., Niemer, W.T., Dell, M., et al. 1953. Cortical and subcortical electrical activity in experimental seizures induced by Metrazol. J. Neuropathol. Exp. Neurol. 12:262–276.

Stauder, K.H. 1935. Epilepsie und Schläfenlappen. Arch. Psychiatr. Nervenkrankh. 104:181–212.

Stefan, H., and Burr, W. (Eds.). 1982. *Mobile Long-Term EEG Recording*. Stuttgart: Fischer.

Stefanis, C., and Jasper, H.H. 1964. Recurrent collateral inhibition in pyramidal tract neurons. J. Neurophysiol. 27:855–877.

Steinert, T., and Froescher, W. 1994. Aggression bei Epilepsie. Nervenheilkunde 13:199–205.

Steinhoff, B.J., So, N.K., Lim, S., et al. 1995. Ictal scalp EEG in temporal lobe epilepsy with unitemporal versus bitemporal interictal epileptiform discharges. Neurology 45:889–896.

Steinlein, O.K., and Noebels, J.L. 2000. Ion channels and epilepsy in man and mouse. Curr. Opin. Genet. Dev. 10:286–291.

Stenzel, E., and Panteli, C. 1981. Lennox-Gastaut Syndrome des 2. Lebensjahrzehntes. In *Epilepsie 1981,* Eds. H. Remschmidt, L. Rentz, and F. Jungmann, pp. 99–101. Stuttgart: Thieme.

Stériade, M. 1990. Spindling, incremental thalamocortical responses, and spike-wave epilepsy. In *Generalized Epilepsy: Neurobiological Approaches,* Eds. M. Avoli, P. Gloor, G. Kostopoulos, et al., pp. 161–10. Boston: Birkhauser.

Stevens, H. 1957. Reading epilepsy. N. Engl. J. Med. 257:165–170.

Stevens, H. 1965a. Allergy and epilepsy. Epilepsia (Amsterdam) 6:205–216.

Stevens, H. 1965b. Paroxysmal choreoathetosis: a form of reflex epilepsy induced by movements. Trans. Am. Neurol. Assoc. 90:92–93.

Stevens, J.R. 1975. Interictal clinical manifestations of complex partial seizures. In *Complex Partial Seizures and Their Treatment,* Eds. J.K. Penry and D.D. Daly, pp. 85–107. New York: Raven Press.

Stevens, J.R. 1980. Psychoses in epilepsy and epilepsy in psychiatric patients: a re-examination. Epilepsia (New York) 21:184(abst).

Stevens, J.R., Kodama, H., Lonsbury, B., et al. 1971. Ultradian characteristics of spontaneous seizure discharges recorded by radio telemetry in man. Electroencephalogr. Clin. Neurophysiol. 31:313–325.

Stewart, L.F., and Drefuss, F.E. 1967. "Centrencephalic" seizure discharges in focal hemispheric lesions. Arch. Neurol. (Chicago) 17:60–68.

Storm van Leeuwen, W., Jemmekens, F., and Elink Sterk, C. 1969. A case of petit mal status with myoclonus. Epilepsia (Amsterdam) 10:407–414.

Strauss, H. 1963. Paroxysmal blindness. Electroencephalogr. Clin. Neurophysiol. 15:921(abst).

Stubbe-Taeglbjerg, H.P., and Biligaard, K. 1944. Epilepsy as a symptom of intracranial tumors. Arch. Psychiatr. Scand. 19:379–387.

Stübgen, J.-P. 1995. Crossed cerebellar diaschisis related to recurrent focal seizures. Epilepsia 36:316–318.

Subirana, A., and Oller-Daurella, L. 1953. Diagnostico diferencial, clinico y electroencefalografico de la ausencia des "petit mal." Sanciones terapeuticas que comporta. Rev. Espan. Oto-Neuro. Oftal. Neurocir. 12: 278–292.

Sulibhavi, D.C., and Schneck, L. 1975. Myoclonus epilepsy in progressive disease. In *Myoclonic Seizures,* Ed. M.H. Charlton, pp. 60–76. Amsterdam: Excerpta Medica.

Sussmann, N.M., and Harner, R.N. 1982. Acute effects of corpus callostomy on the EEG in a patient with intractable epilepsy. Electroencephalogr. Clin. Neurophysiol. 53:28P(abst).

Tabbador, K., and Balagura, S. 1981. Acute epidural hematoma following epileptic seizures. Arch. Neurol. (Chicago) 38:198–199.

Takahashi, A., Muraski, M., Inami, M., et al. 1990. Adversive seizure status: case reports. Electroencephalogr. Clin. Neurophysiol. 75: S148(abst).

Takahashi, T. 2002. Photosensitive epilepsy. Tokyo: Igaku-Shoin.

Takahashi, T., Niedermeyer, E., and Knott, J.R. 1965. The EEG in older and younger adults with convulsive disorder. Epilepsia (Amsterdam) 6:24–32.

Talada Serra, M. 1985. Early epileptic encephalopathy with a pattern of periodic bursts (Ohtahara syndrome). Electroencephalogr. Clin. Neurophysiol. 60:55P(abst).

Talwar, D., Baldwin, M.A., Hutzler, R., et al. 1995. Epileptic spasms in older children: persistence beyond infancy. Epilepsia 36:151–155.

Tartara, A., Mola, M., Moglia, A., et al. 1982. EEG findings in 118 cases of myasthenia gravis. Electroencephalogr. Clin. Neurophysiol. 54: 5P(abst).

Tassinari, C.A. 1981. New perspectives in epileptology. In *Trends in Modern Epileptology,* Ed. Japanese Epilepsy Association, pp. 42–59. Tokyo: Proceedings of the International Public Seminar of Epileptology.

Tassinari, C.A. 1995. The problems of "continuous spikes and waves during slow sleep" or "electrical status epilepticus during slow sleep" today. In *Continuous Spikes and Waves During Slow Sleep. Electrical Status Epilepticus During Slow Sleep,* Eds. A. Beaumanoir, M. Bureau, T. Deonna, et al., pp. 251–255. London: Libbey.

Tassinari, C.A., Bureau, M., Dravet, C., et al. 1982. Electrical status epilepticus during sleep in children (ESES). In *Sleep and Epilepsy,* Eds. M.B. Sterman, M.N. Shouse, and P. Passouant, pp. 465–479. New York: Academic Press.

Tassinari, C.A., Daniele, O., Dravet, C., et al. 1984. Sleep polygraphic studies in some epileptic encephalopathies from infancy to adolescence. In *Epilepsy, Sleep and Sleep Deprivation,* Eds. R. Degen and E. Niedermeyer, pp. 175–189. Amsterdam: Elsevier.

Taylor, D.C. 1977. Epileptic experience, schizophrenia and the temporal lobe. McLean Hosp. J. (Boston, MA) special issue, June 1977, pp. 22–50.

Taylor, D.C. 1987. Psychiatric and social issues in measuring the input and the outcome of epilepsy surgery. In *Surgical Treatment of the Epilepsies,* Ed. J. Engel, Jr., pp. 485–503. New York: Raven Press.

Temkin, O. 1971. *The Falling Sickness,* 2nd ed. Baltimore: Johns Hopkins Press.

Terzano, M.C., Gemignani, F., and Mancia, D. 1978. Petit mal status with myoclonus: case report. Epilepsia (New York) 19:385–392.

Texeira, R.A., Li, M.L., Santos, S.L.M., et al. 2002. Crossed cerebellar atrophy in patients with precocious destructive brain insults. Arch. Neurol. 59:843–847.

Tharp, B.R. 1972. Orbital frontal seizures. A unique electroencephalographic and clinical syndrome. Epilepsy (Amsterdam) 13:627–642.

Thomas, J.E., Reagan, T.J., and Klass, D.W. 1977. Epilepsia partialis continua. A review of 32 cases. Arch. Neurol. (Chicago) 34:266–275.

Thomas, P., Beaumanoir, A., Genton, P., et al. 1992. "De novo" absence status of late onset. Report of 11 cases. Neurology 42:104–110.

Tieber, E. 1972. Seizure activity on closing of the eyes (report on three cases on one family). Neuropaediatrie 3:305–312.

Tinuper, P., Gobbi, G., Aguglia, U., et al. 1985. Occipital lobe seizures in Lafora disease: a further case documented by EEG. Clin. Electroencephalogr. 16:167–170.

Tinuper, P., Aguglia, U., Laudadio, S., et al. 1987. Prolonged ictal paralysis: electroencephalographic confirmation of its epileptic nature. Clin. Electroencephalogr. 18:12–14.

Titeca, J. 1965. L'épilepsie musicogénique. Revue générale à propos d'un cas personnel suivi pendant quatorze ans. Acta Neurol. Belg. 65:598–648.

Todd, R.B. 1856. *Clinical Lectures on Paralysis. Certain Diseases of the Brain, and Other Affections of the Nervous System,* Ed. 2. London. (Quoted in Penfield, W., and Jasper, H.H., 1954.)

Toennies, J.F. 1938. Differential amplifier. Rev. Sci. Instr. 9:95–97.

Tomka, I. 1983. Die funktionelle Beziehung zwischen Petit mal-Epilepsie und Schlaf. Z. EEG-EMG 14:154–159.

Toone, B. 1981. Psychoses and epilepsy. In *Epilepsy and Psychiatry,* Eds. E.H. Reynolds and M.R. Trimble, pp. 113–137. Edinburgh: Churchill Livingstone.

Tortella, F.C. 1988. Endogenous opioid peptides and epilepsy: Quieting the seizing brain? TIPS 9:366–372.

Tower, O.B. 1960. *Neurochemistry of Epilepsy.* Springfield, IL: Charles C Thomas.

Traub, R.D. 2003. Fast oscillations and epilepsy. Epilepsy Currents 3: 77–79.

Traub, R.D., Borck, C., Colling, S.B., et al. 1996. On the structure of ictal events in vitro. Epilepsia 37:879–891.

Trieman, D.M. 1995. Electroclinical features of status epilepticus. J. Clin. Neurophysiol. 12:343–362.

Treiman, D.M., and Delgado-Escueta, A.V. 1983a. Violence and epilepsy. A critical review. In *Recent Advances in Epilepsy,* vol. 1, Eds. I.A. Pedley and B.S. Meldrum, pp. 179–209. Edinburgh: Churchill Livingstone.

Treiman, D.M., and Delgado-Escueta, A.V. 1983b. Complex partial status epilepticus. In *Status Epilepticus,* Eds. A.V. Delgado-Escueta, C.G. Wasterlain, D.M. Treiman, et al., pp. 69–81. New York: Raven Press.

Trelles, J.O., Rocca, E.D., and Ravens, R. 1952. Estudio sobre neurocisticercosis. Rev. Neuro-Psiquiatr. 15:1–132.

Trimble, M.R. 1985. Psychiatric and psychological aspects of epilepsy. In *The Epilepsies,* Eds. R.J. Porter and P.L. Morselli, pp. 322–355. London: Butterworth.

Trimble, M.R. 1991. *The Psychoses of Epilepsy.* New York: Raven Press.

Trimble, M.R., and Schmitz, B. 1998. The psychoses of epilepsy/schizophrenia. In *Epilepsy. A Comprehensive Textbook (3 vol.),* Eds. J. Engel, Jr. and T. Pedley, vol. 2, pp. 2071–2082. Philadelphia: Lippincott-Raven.

Trouillas, P., and Courjon, J. 1972. Epilepsy with multiple sclerosis. Epilepsia (Amsterdam) 13:325–333.

Tsuboi, T. 1977. *Primary Generalized Epilepsy with Sporadic Myoclonias of Myoclonic Petit Mal Type.* Stuttgart: Thieme.

Tükel, K., and Jasper, H.H. 1952. The electroencephalogram in parasagittal lesions. Electroencephalogr. Clin. Neurophysiol. 4:481–494.

Turner, W.A. 1907. *Epilepsy. A Study of Idiopathic Disease.* London: Macmillan. (Reprinted New York: Raven Press, 1973.)

Turski, W.A., Cavalheiro, E.A., Schwarz, M., et al. 1983. Limbic seizures produced by pilocarpine in rats: behavioral, electroencephalographic and neuropathological study. Behav. Brain Res. 9:315–335.

Udvarhelyi, G.B., and Walker, A.E. 1965. Dissemination of acute focal seizures in the monkey. I. From cortical foci. Arch. Neurol. (Chicago) 12:333–356.

Uhlig, S., Witte, O.W., and Valle, E. 1988. Cl-dependent after-potentials of epileptic discharges in the motor cortex of the rat. In *Proceedings of the Society of Neuroscience,* Toronto, November 1988.

Utterback, R.A. 1958. Parenchymatous cerebellar degeneration complicating diphenylhydantoin (Dilantin) therapy. Arch. Neurol. Psychiatry (Chicago) 80:180–181.

Uysal, H., Cevik, I.S., Soylemezogly, F., et al. 2003. Is the cell death in mesial temporal sclerosis apoptotic? Epilepsia 44:778–784.

Van Buren, J.H. 1963. The abdominal aura. A study of abdominal sensations occurring in epilepsy and produced by depth stimulation. Electroencephalogr. Clin. Neurophysiol. 15:1–19.

Van Buren, J.M., and Ajmone Marsen, C. 1960. A correlation of autonomic and EEG components in temporal lobe epilepsy. Arch. Neurol. (Chicago) 3:683–703.

Van der Meij, W., Van Huffelen, A.C., Wieneke, G.H., et al. 1992. Sequential EEG mapping may differentiate "epileptic" from "nonepileptic" rolandic spikes. Electroencephalogr. Clin. Neurophysiol. 82: 408–414.

Vanhatalo, S., Holmes, M.D., Tallgren, P., et al. 2003. Very slow EEG responses lateralize temporal lobe seizures: an evaluation of non-invasive DC-EEG. Neurology 60:1098–1104.

Van Paesschen, W., Connelly, A., Johnson, C.L., et al. 1996. The amygdala and intractable temporal lobe epilepsy: a quantitative magnetic resonance imaging study. Neurology 47:1021–1031.

Van Parys, J.A.P. 1981. The use of EEG as a method of control in epilepsy. Electroencephalogr. Clin. Neurophysiol. 52:41P(abst).

Van Sweden, B. 1985. Toxic "ictal" confusion in middle age, treatment with benzodiazepines. J. Neurol. Neurosurg. Psychiatry 48:472–476.

Van Sweden, B., and Dumon-Radermecker, M. 1981. Drug-withdrawal syndromes, EEG and clinical aspects. Clin. Electroencephalogr. 12: 50–56.

Van Sweden, B., and Mellerio, F. 1988. Toxic ictal confusion: a symptomatic, situation related subtype of nonconclusive "absence" status epilepticus. J. Epilepsy 1:157–163.

Van Sweden, B., and Mellerio, F. 1989. Toxic ictal delirium. Biol. Psychiatry 154:449–458.

Veith, G. 1959. Die Residualepilepsie vom Standpunkt des Pathologen. Nervenarzt 30:551–554.

Vespa, P.M., O'Phelan, K., Shah, M., et al. 2003. Acute seizures after intracerebral hemorrhage: a factor in progressive midline shift and outcome. Neurology 60(9):1441–1446.

Vetrugno, R., Meletti, S., Plazzi, G., et al. 1999. Bilateral centrotemporal spikes triggered by blinking: an unusual form of sensory input with related cortical EEG activity. Clin. Neurophysiol. 110(11):1995–1999.

Victor, M., and Brausch, J. 1967. The role of abstinence in the genesis of alcohol epilepsy. Epilepsia (Amsterdam) 8:1–20.

Vigevano, F., and Fusco, L. 1993. Hypnic tonic postural seizures in healthy children provide evidence for a partial epileptic syndrome of frontal lobe origin. Epilepsia 34:110–119.

Vigevano, F., Fusco, L., DiCapua, M., et al. 1992. Benign infantile familial convulsions. Eur. J. Pediatr. 151:608–612.

Vignaendra, V., Chee, L.T., Lee, T.C., et al. 1976. Epileptic discharges triggered by blinking and eye closure. Electroencephalogr. Clin. Neurophysiol. 40:491–498.

Vizioli, R. 1967. Discussion remark. In *Les activités électriques cérébrales spontanées et évoquées chez l'homme,* Eds. H. Gastaut, R. Poiré, A. Wlatrégny, et al., p. 214. Paris: Gauthier-Villars.

Vizioli, R., and Magliocco, E.B. 1953. A case of prolonged petit mal seizures. Electroencephalogr. Clin. Neurophysiol. 5:139–140.

Volpe, J.J. 1981. *Neurology of the Newborn.* Philadelphia: Saunders.

Von Meduna, L. 1935. Biologic control of outcome of schizophrenia by producing epileptic attacks with injections of camphor and Metrazol. Z. Neurol. Psychol. 152:235–262.

Von Meduna, L. 1937. *Die Konvulsionstherapie der Schizophrenie.* Halle, 1937.

Vornov, J.J. 1991. Effectors of second messenger system action. In *Neurotransmitters and Epilepsy,* Eds. R.S. Fisher and J.T. Coyle, pp. 47–60. New York: Wiley-Liss.

Vornov, J.J., and Coyle, J.T. 1991. Mechanisms of neurotransmitter receptor action. In *Neurotransmitters and Epilepsy,* Eds. R.S. Fisher and J.T. Coyle, pp. 17–31. New York: Wiley-Liss.

Wada, J. 1949. A new method for the determination of the side of cerebral speech dominance—a preliminary report on the intracarotid injection of sodium Amytal in man. Med. Biol. (Tokyo) (Igaku to Seibutsaki) 14: 221–222.

Wada, J., and Rasmussen, T. 1960. Intracarotid injection of sodium Amytal for lateralization of cerebral speech dominance: Experimental and clinical observation. J. Neurosurg. 17:266–282.

Wada, J., and Sato, M. 1974. Generalized convulsive seizure induced by daily electrical stimulation of the amygdala in cats: correlative electrographic and behavioral feature. Neurology (Minneapolis) 24:565–574.

Wada, J., and Sato, M. 1975a. The generalized convulsive seizure state by daily electrical stimulation of the amygdala in split brain cats. Epilepsia (New York) 16:417–430.

Wada, J., and Sato, M. 1975b. Effects of unilateral lesion in the midbrain reticular formation on kindled amygdaloid convulsion in cats. Epilepsia (New York) 16:693–697.

Walczak, T.S. 1995. Neocortical temporal lobe epilepsy: characterizing the syndrome. Epilepsia 36:633–635.

Walker, A.E. 1949. *Post-Traumatic Epilepsy.* Springfield, IL: Charles C Thomas.

Walker, A.E. 1957. Stimulation and ablation. Their role in the history of cerebral physiology. J. Neurophysiol. 20:435–449.

Walker, A.E. 1958. Posttraumatic epilepsy. Administrative considerations. In *Surgery in World War II: Neurosurgery,* vol. 1, pp. 279–317.

Walker, A.E. 1970. The propagation of epileptic discharge. In *Epilepsy. Recent Views on Theory, Diagnosis and Therapy of Epilepsy,* Ed. E. Niedermeyer, pp. 13–28. Basel: S. Karger.

Walker, A.E., and Marshall, C. 1964. The contribution of depth recording to clinical medicine. Electroencephalogr. Clin. Neurophysiol. 16:88–99.

Walker, A.E., and Udvarhelyi, G.B. 1965. Dissemination of acute focal seizures in monkeys. II. From subcortical foci. Arch. Neurol. (Chicago) 12:357–380.

Walker, A.E., Johnson, H.C., Care, T.J., and Kollros, J.J. 1946. Convulsive effects of antibiotic agents on the cerebral cortex. Science 103:116.

Walker, A.E., Poggio, G.F., and Andy, O.J. 1952. Structural spread of cortically induced epileptic discharges. Neurology (Minneapolis) 2:612–626.

Wallstedt, L., Gazelius, B., Lind, G., et al. 1995. Chronic multifocal recordings of cortical microcirculation and subdural EEG during epileptic seizures in humans. Epilepsia 36(suppl 3):S146–S147(abst).

Walter, W.C., Dovey, V.J., and Shipton, H. 1946. Analysis of electrical responses of the human cortex to photic stimulation. Nature 158:540–541.

Walsh, G.O., and Delgado-Escueta, A.V. 1984. Type II complex partial seizures: poor results of anterior temporal lobectomy. Neurology (Cleveland) 34:1–13.

Walton, J.N. 1953. The electroencephalographic sequelae of spontaneous subarachnoid hemorrhage. Electroencephalogr. Clin. Neurophysiol. 5:41.

Waltrégny, A., Regis, H., Dravet, C., et al. 1969. The contribution of intracarotid sodium Amytal tests in the physiopathogenic study of petit mal variant (Lennox syndrome). In *The Physiopathogenesis of the Epilepsies,* Eds. H. Gastaut, H. Jasper, J. Bancaud, et al., pp. 277–283. Springfield, IL: Charles C Thomas.

Ward, A.A., Jr. 1972. Topical convulsant metals. In *Experimental Models of Epilepsy,* Eds. D.P. Purpura, J.K. Penry, D. Tower, et al., pp. 13–35. New York: Raven Press.

Wasterlain, C.G., and Dwyer, B.E. 1983. Brain metabolism during prolonged seizures in neonates. In *Status Epilepticus,* Eds. A.J. Delgado-Escueta, C.G. Wasterlain, D.M. Treiman, et al., pp. 241–260. New York: Raven Press.

Wasterlain, C.G., and Mazarati, A.M. 1998. Neuromodulation and Second Messengers. In *Epilepsy. A Comprehensive Textbook (3 vol.),* Eds. J. Engel, Jr. and T. Pedley, vol. 1, pp. 277–289. Philadelphia: Lippincott-Raven.

Watanabe, K. 1981. Seizures in the newborn and young infants. *Folia Psychiatr. Neurol.* 35:275–280.

Watanabe, K., Kuroiwa, Y., Shimpo, T., et al. 1983. Epilepsia partialis continua: an electrophysiological study. Electroencephalogr. Clin. Neurophysiol. 56:54P(abst).

Watanabe, K., Kuroiwa, Y., and Toyokura, Y. 1984. Epilepsia partialis continua. Epileptogenic focus in the motor cortex and its participation in transcortical reflexes. Arch. Neurol. (Chicago) 41:1040–1044.

Watson, C.W., and Denny-Brown, D. 1955. Studies of the mechanism of stimulus-sensitive myoclonus in man. Electroencephalogr. Clin. Neurophysiol. 7:341–356.

Weber, R. 1956. Musikogene Epilepsie. Nervenarzt 27:337–340.

Weinberg, W.A., and Harwell, U.L. 1965. Diazepam (Valium) in myoclonic seizures. Am. J. Dis. Child 109:123–127.

Weingarten, K. 1957. *Die Myoklonischen Syndrome.* Vienna: Maudrich.

West, W.J. 1841. On a peculiar form of infantile convulsions. Lancet 1:724.

Westmoreland, B.F., Reiher, J., and Klass, D. 1979. Recording small sharp spikes with depth electroencephalography. Epilepsia (New York) 20: 599–606.

White, J.C. 1971. Epileptic nystagmus. Epilepsia (Amsterdam) 12:157–164.

Wieser, H.G. 1980. Temporal lobe or psychomotor status epilepticus. A case report. Electroencephalogr. Clin. Neurophysiol. 48:558–572.

Wieser, H.G. 1983. *Electroclinical Features of the Psychomotor Seizure.* London: Butterworth.

Wieser, H.G., and Hajek, M. 1995. Frontal lobe epilepsy: compartmentalization, presurgical evaluation and operative results. In *Epilepsy and the Functional Anatomy of the Frontal Lobe.* Eds. H.H. Jasper, S. Riggio, and P.S. Goldman-Rakic, pp. 297–318. New York: Raven.

Wieser, H.G., Graf, H.P., Bernoulli, C., et al. 1978. Quantitative analysis of intracerebral recordings in epilepsia partialis continua. Electroencephalogr. Clin. Neurophysiol. 44:14–22.

Wieser, H.G., Hungerbühler, H., Siegel, A.M., et al. 1997. Musicogenic epilepsy: review of the literature and case report with single photon emission computed tomography. Epilepsia 38:200–207.

Wikler, A., and Essig, C.F. 1970. Withdrawal seizures following chronic intoxication with barbiturates and other sedative drugs. In *Epilepsy. Recent Views on Theory, Diagnosis and Therapy of Epilepsy,* Ed. E. Niedermeyer, pp. 170–184. Basel: S. Karger.

Wilder, B.J. 1969. Activation of epileptic foci in psychomotor epilepsy. Epilepsia (Amsterdam) 10:418(abst).

Wilder, B.J. 1972. Projection phenomena and secondary epileptogenesis—Mirror foci. In *Experimental Models of Epilepsies,* Eds. D.P. Purpura, J.K. Penry, D. Tower, et al., pp. 85–111. New York: Raven Press.

Wilkins, D.E., Hallett, M., and Erba, G. 1985. Primary generalized epileptic myoclonus: a frequent manifestation of minimyoclonus of central origin. J. Neurol. Neurosurg. Psychiatry 48:506–516.

Wilkus, R.J., and Thompson, P.M. 1985. Sphenoidal electrode position and basal EEG during long term monitoring. Epilepsia (New York) 26:137–142.

Williams, D. 1953. A study of thalamic and cortical rhythms in "petit mal." Brain 76:50–69.

Williams, D. 1956. The structure of emotions reflected in epileptic experiences. Brain 79:29–67.

Williamson, P.D., Spencer, D.D., Spencer, S.S., et al. 1985. Complex partial seizures of frontal lobe origin. Ann. Neurol. 18:497–504.

Wilson, S.K. 1935. The epilepsies. In *Handbuch der Neurologie,* vol. 17, Eds. O. Bumke and O. Foerster. Berlin: Springer.

Wilson, W.P., and Nashold, B.S. 1968. Epileptic discharges occurring in the mesencephalon and thalamus. Epilepsia (Amsterdam) 9:265–273.

Witte, O. 1987. Calcium ion involvement in epileptogenesis. Am. J. EEG Technol. 27:223–238.

Witte, O. 1991. *Hemmungsmechanismen cortikaler neurone und ihre Bedeutung fuer die Entsehung interictaler und ictaler epileptischer Entladungsformen.* Düsseldorf (Univers.): Thesis (Venia legendi).

Wolbach, S.B. 1908. Multiple hernias of the cerebrum and cerebellum due to intracranial pressure. J. Med. Res. 19:153. Quoted in Peiffer, J. 1963.

Wolf, H.K. 1996. Hypothese zur Epileptogenese glioneuraler Laesionen. Dtsch. Aerzteblatt 93:A2544–A2547.

Wolf, H., and Wiestler, O.D. 1996. Die Neuropathologie chronischer phamakotherapie-resistenter Epilepsien. Dtsch. Aerztebl. 93:B1997–B1999.

Wolf, P. 1970. Zur Klinik und Psychopathologie des Status psychomotoricus. Nervenarzt 41:603–610.

Wolf, P. 1985. The classification of seizures and the epilepsies. In *The Epilepsies,* Eds. R.J. Porter and P.L. Morselli, pp. 107–124. London: Butterworth.

Wolf, P. 1994. Reading epilepsy. In *Epileptic Seizures and Syndromes,* Ed. P. Wolf, pp. 67–73. London: Libbey.

Wong, P.K. 1993. The importance of source behavior in distinguishing populations of epileptic foci. J. Clin. Neurophysiol. 10:314–322.

Wong, R.K.S., Traub, R.D., and Miles, R. 1984. Epileptogenic mechanisms as revealed by studies of the hippocampal slice. In *Electrophysiology of Epilepsy,* Eds. P.A. Schwartzkroin and H.V. Wheal, pp. 253–275. London: Academic Press.

Wong, R.K.S., Traub, R.D., and Miles, R. 1986. Cellular basis of neuronal synchrony in epilepsy. In *Basic Mechanisms of the Epilepsies,* Eds. A.V. Delgado-Escueta, A.A. Ward, Jr., D.M. Woobury, et al., pp. 583–592. New York: Raven Press.

Wood, J.D., and Abrahams, D.E. 1971. The comparative effects of various hydrazides on gamma-aminobutyric acid and its metabolism. J. Neurochem. 18:1017–1025.

Woodbury, J.W. 1969. Biophysics of nerve membrane. In *Basic Mechanisms of the Epilepsies,* Eds. H.H. Jasper, A.A. Ward, Jr., et al., pp. 41–75. Boston: Little, Brown.

Woods, J.F., and Ives, J.R. 1977. Prolonged monitoring of the EEG in ambulatory patients. In *Epilepsy, The VIIIth International Symposium,* Ed. J.K. Penry, pp. 109–113. New York: Raven Press.

Woolley, D.E., and Timiras, P.S. 1962. Estrous and circadian periodicity electroshock convulsions in rats. Am. J. Physiol. 202:379–382.

Worster-Drought, C. 1971. An unusual form of acquired aphasia in children. Dev. Med. Child. Neurol. 13:563–571.

Wulff, M.H. 1957. The barbiturate withdrawal syndrome. Electroencephalogr. Clin. Neurophysiol. Suppl. 14:173.

Wyler, A.R. 1986. Synchrony between cortical neurons in normal and epileptogenic cortex of monkey. Epilepsia (New York) 27:171–176.

Wyllie, E., (Ed.). 1993. *The Treatment of Epilepsy.* Philadelphia: Lea & Febiger.

Yamagata, T., Momoi, M.Y., Miyao, M., et al. 1997. Blink induced centrotemporal spikes in benign childhood epilepsy with centrotemporal spikes. J. Neurol. Neurosurg. Psychiatry. 63:528–530.

Yamamura, H., Nakanishi, M., Yoshimizu, S., et al. 1981. A follow-up of febrile convulsions in relation to epilepsies—Longitudinal clinico-electroencephalographic observations. Electroencephalogr. Clin. Neurophysiol. 52:71P–72P(abst).

Yamatogi, Y., and Ohtahara, S. 1990. EEG in febrile convulsions. Am. J. EEG Technol. 30:267–280.

Yamatogi, Y., Ishida, S., Terasaki, T., et al. 1982. An electroencephalographic study of febrile convulsions. Electroencephalogr. Clin. Neurophysiol. 54:27P–28P(abst).

Yarnell, P.R. 1975. Todd's paralysis: a cerebrovascular phenomenon? Stroke 6:301–303.

Yenjun, S., Harvey, A.S., Marini, C., et al. 2003 EEG in adult-onset idiopathic generalized epilepsy. Epilepsia 44:252–256.

Yoshida, M., Yamada, S., Ozaki, Y., et al. 1985. Phenytoin-induced ovofacial dyskinesia. A case report. J. Neurol. (Berlin) 231:340–342.

Yoshinaga, H., Amano, R., Oka, E., et al. 1992. Dipole tracing in childhood epilepsy with special reference to rolandic. Brain Topography 4: 193–199.

Zaatreh, M.M., Spencer, D.D., Thompson, J.L., et al. 2002. Frontal lobe tumoral epilepsy: clinical neurophysiologic features and predictors of surgical outcome. Epilepsia 43:727–733.

Zappoli, R. 1955. Two cases of prolonged epileptic twilight state with almost continuous "wave-spikes," an EEG study. Electroencephalogr. Clin. Neurophysiol. 7:421–423.

Zellweger, H. 1948. *Die Krämpfe im Kindesalter.* Basel: Schwabe.

Zellweger, H., and Hess, R. 1950. Familiäre. Blitz-Nick-und Salaam-Krampfe. Helv. Paediatr. Acta 5:85–93.

Zifkin, B., and Dravet, C. 1998. Generalized convulsive seizures. In *Epilepsy. A Comprehensive Textbook (3 vol.),* Eds. J. Engel, Jr. and T. Pedley, vol. 1, pp. 567–577. Philadelphia: Lippincott-Raven.

Zimmerman, A.W., Niedermeyer, E., and Hodges, F.J. 1977. Lennox-Gastaut syndrome and computerized axial tomography. Epilepsia (New York) 18:463–464.

Ziskind, E., and Bercel, N.A. 1947. Preconvulsive paroxysmal electroencephalographic changes after Metrazol injection. Publ. Assoc. Res. Nerv. Ment. Dis. 21:487–501.

Zivin, L., and Ajmone Marsan, C. 1968. Incidence and prognostic significance of "epileptiform" activity in the EEG in non-epileptic subjects. Brain 91:751–777.

Zouhar, A. 1981. The dynamics of EEG changes after surgical operations for meningioma, with a view to tumour localization. Electroencephalogr. Clin. Neurophysiol. 52:88P(abst).

28. Nonepileptic Attacks

Ernst Niedermeyer

Sudden brief loss of consciousness, sudden behavioral changes, or strange subjective sensations are not necessarily epileptic. This should be a truism, but there is a present trend to ascribe too many transient conditions to an epileptic mechanism. Here the differential diagnosis of epileptic seizures is discussed briefly.

In the case of sudden transient loss of consciousness, nonepileptic attacks are essentially due to one of the following disturbances:

1. Circulatory insufficiency giving rise to acute cerebral ischemia;
2. Sudden changes of blood chemistry;
3. Disturbances related to the narcolepsy-cataplexy complex;
4. Psychogenic alterations; or
5. Central motor disorders: dyskinetic and imitating epileptic seizures (often unassociated with loss of consciousness).

These principal disturbances are discussed in this chapter, except for the narcolepsy-cataplexy complex, which is discussed in Chapter 48, "Polysomnography: Principles and Applications in Sleep and Arousal Disorders."

Syncopal Attacks

Principal Clinical Manifestations and Causes

Syncope has been defined as a sudden brief loss of consciousness due to a discrete episode of generalized cerebral ischemia; it is hence a manifestation of acute insufficiency of the cerebral circulation (Naquet and Vigouroux, 1972).

The *vasodepressor* type of syncope has also been termed *vasovagal* because of prominent vagal mechanisms. There are well-known triggering factors, such as venipuncture, the sight of blood, sudden pain caused by (usually minor) injuries, or the receipt of frightening news. The attacks are characterized by muscle weakness, epigastric discomfort, sweating, nausea, restlessness, facial pallor, sighing respiration, and yawning (Engel, 1962). This may proceed to light-headedness, blurring of vision, and sudden loss of consciousness with muscular flaccidity and falling to the ground. In attacks exceeding 15 to 20 seconds, irregular clonic movements are quite common (Engel, 1962). In a special type of *convulsive syncope* (Naquet and Vigouroux, 1972), a tonic spasm is noted, usually 2 to 3 seconds after onset of fainting; this spasm is followed by a few generalized jerks. This type of convulsive syncope tends to occur in attacks caused by transient asystole. According to Naquet and Vigouroux (1972), the convulsive type indicates a longer duration of the circulatory insufficiency.

There is no doubt that syncopal attacks with convulsive movements are not related to the epilepsies; intervening epileptic mechanisms are a strictly secondary response to acute cerebral ischemia (Gastaut, 1958; Gastaut and Gastaut, 1957; Naquet and Bostem, 1964).

The differentiation of syncope and epileptic seizures has been rendered more difficult by the observation of true grand mal (generalized tonic-clonic) seizures triggered by syncopal attacks in children (Battaglia et al., 1989). The electroencephalogram (EEG) showed distinct epileptic phenomena.

A combined form of vasodepressor and orthostatic syncope has been reported in male patients during nocturnal urination. These attacks are known as *micturition syncope* (Donker et al., 1972; Eberhart and Morgan, 1960; Gastaut and Gastaut, 1956; Lukash et al., 1964; Lyle et al., 1961). These patients are otherwise in good health, like most patients with simple vagovasal attacks.

Vasovagal reflex mechanisms result in a "white" or "pallid" syncope. On the other hand, "blue" or "cyanotic" syncope may be caused by a Valsalva maneuver, producing increased intrathoracic pressure and reduced venous return to the heart (Daly, 1990; also see Johnson et al., 1984). EEG slowing but no flattening occurs in the "blue" form (Daly, 1990).

A comprehensive review of syncopal attacks and their mechanisms has been presented by Mumenthaler (1984). Table 28.1 (derived from Mumenthaler's work) presents an overview of the differentiation of syncopal and epileptic seizures. A refreshing review of syncope and vasovagal mechanisms has been presented by Landau and Nelson (1996).

Pathophysiological Mechanisms

Special pathophysiological mechanisms involved in syncopal attacks have been analyzed by Naquet and Vigouroux (1972). These authors distinguish the following mechanisms:

1. Cardiac syncope (mainly in Stokes-Adams syndrome);
2. Bulbopontine syndrome (brainstem tumors, syringobulbia, poliomyelitis, intracranial hypertension during general anesthesia, hypocapnia, cerebral hyper- or hypothermia);
3. Reflex syncope acting on bulbopontine centers: trigeminal, vagal, abdominal, sensory, and especially barosensitive zones (carotid sinus, aortic arch); and
4. Mechanical syncopes, for instance cough (tussive) syncope.

This list of pathogenic mechanisms can be further reduced as follows:

Table 28.1.   Distinct Characteristics in the Differentiation of Major Epileptic Seizures (Grand Mal) and Syncopal Attacks[a]

	Syncope (Fainting)	Grand Mal (Generalized Tonic-Clonic Seizure)
Prodromal symptoms	Dizziness, tinnitus, blackout, abdominal sensation	None or aura (according to focal seizure onset)
Loss of consciousness	Mostly preceded by daze	Very sudden
Duration of loss of consciousness	From seconds to 1 min	Several minutes (seizure 40–90 sec, followed by postictal loss of consciousness)
Complexion	Pale, may become cyanotic Profuse perspiration	Ashen, cyanotic
Muscle tone	Hypotonia, may become hypertonic after 10–20 sec	Immediate hypertonia
Eyes	Eyes rolled upward	Often lateral (horizontal) deviation
Clonic jerks	Rare, in irregular manner	Obligatory in clonic phase
Tongue bite	Exceptional	Very common
Loss of urinary sphincter control	Infrequent	Moderately frequent
Postictal confusion	None or very short	Always, may be prolonged
Postictal aching of musculature	None	Common
Postictal headache	Rare	Common
Rising postictally	After complete mental recovery	Before complete mental recovery
Postictal creatine phosphokinase	Normal	May be increased
Ictal EEG	Diffuse slowing with no or little paroxysmal activity; slowing may be followed by flattening	Pronounced fast spiking in tonic phase, interrupted in clonic phase

[a]Modified from Mumenthaler, M. (ed.) 1984. *Synkopen und Sturzanfälle*. Stuttgart: Thieme.

a. Neurally mediated syncope: occurs in essentially healthy normotensive individuals in whom a certain, often consistently specific, triggering event causes a sudden change in the activity of efferent autonomic neurons (Kaufmann, 1997). Most of these syncopes are vasodepressor attacks ("vasovagal syncope").
b. Autonomic failure: usually based on a disorder of noradrenergic transmission (for further details see Kaufmann, 1997). Among the causes are Shy-Drager syndrome, Riley-Day disease, multiple system atrophy, and high cervical spinal cord lesion.
c. Neurocardiogenic syncope: based on a presumed dysfunction of sensory receptors within the heart such as the Bezold-Jarisch reflex (Bezold and Hirt, 1867; Jarish and Zotterman, 1948; Grimm, 1997). The neurocardiogenic reflex mechanisms are still somewhat controversial.

The bulbopontine centers are divided into a portion with a depressor function (cardioinhibitory fibers via dorsal nucleus of the vagus nerve) and another portion with sympathicotonic effects (multisynaptic reticulospinal tracts projecting into spinal ganglia). Ocular compression produces a strong cardioinhibitory effect, mainly in young individuals, whereas the effect of carotid sinus stimulation in hypersensitive individuals, mostly in older adults, is chiefly vasodepressive. There have been very rare observations of cardioinhibitory (vasovagal) syncope triggered by intermittent photic stimulation (Ossentjuk et al., 1966; Rabending and Klepel, 1978; Rabending et al., 1968). In general, cardiogenic syncope constitutes a more serious medical problem than neurogenic syncope.

Immediately in the wake of a major convulsion, there may be a brief episode of asystolia leading to syncope ("seizure-driven asystolia") (after Schomer, 2003).

EEG in Syncopal Attacks

The EEG in patients with syncopal attacks has been investigated by Hann and Franke (1953), Gastaut and Gastaut (1956, 1957), Broser (1958), Gastaut (1958), Durst and Krump (1961), Gastaut et al. (1961), Naquet and Bostem (1964), Naquet and Vigouroux (1972), and Andriola (1983). Recording during the attack requires a polygraphic approach (Barolin et al., 1970); electrocardiogram (ECG) is absolutely mandatory, and blood pressure measurements are important. In recent years, combined video-EEG-ECG recording has proved to be useful (Dinner et al., 1984). The electroencephalographer should be familiar with the pathophysiology of cerebral anoxia and its EEG correlates in experimental animals and in the human.

The sequence of EEG events in vasodepressor or cardioinhibitory attacks is as follows:

1. Alpha depression,
2. Low-voltage fast activity (possibly due to a transient phase of activation),
3. Theta activity of rising voltage, and
4. High-voltage delta activity, with subsequent EEG recovery.

Alternatively, the following may be found:

1. Delta activity of decreasing voltage (onset of tonic convulsive activity), and
2. Transient electrical silence (tonic motion, followed by clonic twitching), with subsequent EEG recovery.

This is essentially the EEG scenario of simple and more complex convulsive syncopal attacks. In general, a period of 10 seconds elapses before high-voltage delta waves appear.

A special study of *tussive (cough) syncope* was carried out by De Maria et al. (1984). With coughing, cerebrospinal fluid (CSF) pressure rises and impedes cerebral circulation, resulting in cerebral ischemia and syncope.

Brenner (1997) has elucidated the EEG in syncope with fine examples of tracings.

The EEG of a syncope caused by a Stokes-Adams syndrome is shown in Fig. 28.1.

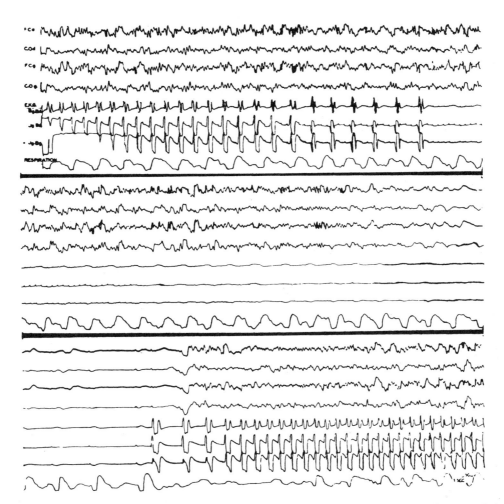

Figure 28.1. Polygraphic recording of a complete cycle. The first four channels record the EEG. The following three, are the electrocardiogram (ECG), in these derivations: left arm-right arm; left leg-right arm; left leg-left arm. The last channel records the respiration. The three parts of the record are recorded continuously. Especially well represented in this record are the isolated P waves on the ECG at the beginning of the asystolia, the mode of appearance of the electric silence, and the apnea during the arousal of the ventricular contractions. (From Regis, H., Toga, M., and Righini, C. 1961. Clinical, electroencephalographic and pathological study of a case of Adams-Stokes syndrome. In *Cerebral Anoxia and the Electroencephalogram,* Eds. J.S. Meyer and H. Gastaut, pp. 295–303. Springfield, IL: Charles C Thomas, with permission.)

Interval EEG of Patients with Syncopal Attacks

Patients with cardiovascular-cerebrovascular disorders are likely to show some abnormalities, as discussed in Chapter 17, "Cerebrovascular Disorders and EEG." Syncope is not uncommon in patients with vertebrobasilar artery insufficiency; these patients often experience some dizziness prior to blacking out. Some of these patients have massive syncopal attacks of extremely abrupt onset triggered by head movements that impinge on the vertebral artery. These patients have mostly normal records; quite often, the tracings are of low voltage. In elderly patients, the differentiation between epileptic seizures and syncope can be made on EEG grounds but, according to Hughes and Zialcita (2000), "Epileptiform activity in elderly patients with syncope is likely to be mildly epileptogenic."

In patients with orthostatic syncope accompanied by dizziness, EEG recordings in erect posture are not helpful in the early stages; subjective dizziness and light-headedness are unassociated with significant EEG changes. The same is true for dizziness induced by active or passive head movements. Marked slowing induced by orthostatic posture in the EEG, however, is noted in patients with *Shy-Drager syndrome.* These patients lack compensatory heart rate changes; the heart pulse rate remains stable, while the blood pressure falls dramatically, giving rise to considerable cerebral ischemia. Marked EEG abnormalities are also found in patients with *Riley-Day syndrome,* who often suffer from syncopal attacks. These patients are usually too frail for an EEG recording under orthostatic stress. The use of the *tilt table* is extremely conducive to syncopal manifestations.

The differentiation of nonepileptic *drop attacks* is aided by the EEG (Wenzel, 1981; also see Mumenthaler, 1984) (Table 28.2).

Breath Holding Attacks of Early Childhood as a Special Form of Syncope

Breath holding attacks are related to syncope and occur rather frequently in older infants and small children. Emo-

Table 28.2.   Differential Diagnosis of Drop Attacks

Type	Mechanism	Age	EEG	Degree of Traumatization
Atonic seizures	Strictly epileptic Lennox-Gastaut syndrome	Mostly children, adolesc.	Markedly abnormal with slow spike-waves	++–++++
Temporal lobe epilepsy with falls	Strictly epileptic, fall rigid or flaccid	Mostly adults	Interictal temporal spikes, ictal repetitive spikes	+++
Vertebrobasilar artery insufficiency	Vascular	Mostly older adults	Mostly low-voltage records	0–+
Basilar art. migraine	Vasomotor	Mostly fem., age 15–30 yrs	Undetermined	0
Cervical spondylosis	Vasomotor (Barré-Liéou syndrome)	Adults (middle, old age)	Mostly low-voltage records	+–++++
Cryptogenic drop attacks of women	Unclear, falls lightning-like	Mostly menopausal women	Undetermined	++
Vestibulo-cerebral syndrome	Vestibular disturbance (very sudden fall)	Mostly adults	Undetermined	+++
Falls in Parkinson syndrome	In early stages very sudden falls	Older adults	Often with excessive slow activity	+++

tional stress and crying trigger these attacks. A division into the "pale type" and "cyanotic type" has been proposed (Gastaut, 1968; Lombroso and Lerman, 1967; Low et al., 1955; Pozo et al., 1981). The underlying pathophysiological mechanisms are complex and not fully understood. The children almost always have normal EEG findings in the interval.

Apneic seizures of infancy are usually distinguishable from epileptic events. According to Hooshmand (1972) and Toyka and Forster (1974), these attacks respond to anticholinergic medication such as atropine. The underlying pathophysiology is poorly understood. Apneic attacks may be induced by crying (Andriola, 1983). These attacks are most common in the neonatal period and in early infancy. A differentiation between these apneic attacks and sleep apnea is necessary; sleep apnea is discussed in Chapter 48, "Polysomnography: Principles and Applications in Sleep and Arousal Disorders."

Sudden Changes of Blood Chemistry

Hypoglycemia

The hypoglycemic attack is characterized by sweating, jitteriness, tremulousness, nervousness, irritability, imperative hunger, mental fatigue, muscular weakness, and, less often, headache, nausea, and vomiting. The clinical symptoms and signs are the same regardless of the underlying cause (Fajans and Thorn, 1966). Table 28.3 shows a classification of the hypoglycemic states according to these authors. Hypoglycemic states may trigger a grand mal attack and often produce paroxysmal EEG activity. The EEG of hypoglycemia is discussed in greater detail in Chapter 22, "Metabolic Central Nervous System Disorders."

Hyperventilation Syndrome

The hyperventilation syndrome lies at the boundary between neurology and psychiatry and has been regarded as a typical psychosomatic disorder. The anxiety-inducing stress of modern life in an industrialized society is particularly conducive to the hyperventilation syndrome.

Earlier work on this condition was done by Finesinger and Mazick (1940) and Engel et al. (1947). Lewis (1953, 1954) placed special emphasis on the chronic hyperventilation syndrome with an undercurrent of depression. Further information is found in the work of Riley (1982) and especially in the study of Fried (1987).

It was demonstrated that anxiety produces a deep sighing respiration; the patients may complain of inability to get enough air. Prolonged hyperventilation leads to hypocapnia. In this state, the patients appear to be extremely tense, frightened, and even panicky; tachycardia, pallor, or blushing is noted.

In daily EEG laboratory work, such attacks are easily provoked by hyperventilation. Interestingly, the EEG of these patients does not show any delta response; it is usually void of any slow activity. This seems to be paradoxical; it is

Table 28.3.   Classification of Hypoglycemic States[a]

Organic hypoglycemia
    Pancreatic islet cell tumor, functioning
    Nonpancreatic tumors associated with hypoglycemia
    Anterior pituitary hypofunction
    Adrenocortical hypofunction
    Acquired extensive liver disease
Hypoglycemia due to specific hepatic enzyme defects
    Glycogen storage disease
    Hereditary fructose intolerance
    Galactosemia
    Familial fructose and galactose intolerance
Functional hypoglycemia
    Reactive functional (postprandial hypoglycemia)
    Reactive secondary to mild diabetes
    Alimentary hypoglycemia (after gastroenterostomy, subtotal gastrectomy)
    "Idiopathic hypoglycemia" of infancy and childhood
    Alcoholism and poor nutrition
Exogenous hypoglycemia (due to insulin or sulfonylurea compounds)
    Iatrogenic
    Factitious

[a]After Fajans, S.S., and Thorn, G.W. 1966. Hyperinsulinism and hypoglycemia. In *Principles of Internal Medicine,* 5th ed. Eds., T.R. Harrison et al., pp. 507–512. New York: McGraw-Hill.

tempting to hypothesize that this might be due to the spillage of epinephrine in the patient's state of anxiety. The epinephrine could presumably counteract the EEG slowing, which has been thought to be mediated through the ascending brainstem reticular formation (Bonvallet and Dell, 1956). Breathing exhaled air from a bag quickly terminates these attacks.

Hyperventilation during physical exercise does not induce alkalosis (and hence no undesirable effects) because it is adapted to the energetic needs (Esquivel et al., 1991). The well-known precipitating effect of absence seizures with 3/sec spike-waves is found in Chapter 27.

Other Humoral Attacks

Tetanic attacks are also produced by hyperventilation; for a discussion of tetany and hypocalcemia, see Chapter 22, "Metabolic Central Nervous System Disorders." Syncopal attacks may be due to tetany (Alajouanine et al., 1958). Attacks that occur in the dumping syndrome, carcinoid syndrome, and hypertensive episodes due to pheochromocytoma are not known to be associated with EEG changes.

Narcolepsy-Cataplexy-Sleep Paralysis Complex

These attacks represent a specific nosological entity that has its place among the sleep disorders. It will be discussed in Chapter 48, "Polysomnography: Principles and Applications in Sleep and Arousal Disorders." Routine laboratory EEG tracings are normal in this condition.

Psychogenic Attacks

Major Hysterical Attacks

The symptomatology of the hysterical attack has been well known since the work of Briquet (1859) and Charcot (1887–1889). Briquet's approach to this problem has proved to be a more solid foundation for modern theories than the work of Charcot, which is beset with iatrogenic artifacts.

Other concepts were essentially based on psychodynamic mechanisms such as dissociation (Janet, 1893/1894) and conversion (Breuer, 1895; Breuer and Freud, 1895, which were critically discussed by Chodoff and Lyons (1958) and Ziegler et al. (1960). The concept of Kretschmer (1923, 1956) with emphasis on "hyponoic" and "hypobulic" mechanisms warrants particular attention.

Hysterical seizures are associated with loss of impulse, usually in stressful situations. These attacks used to be attributed solely (and by definition) to females; this clearly has been proved to be untrue, although female adolescents and young adults are most often involved.

The attacks themselves consist of storms of movements that defy any precise description. Arching the back and pelvic movements may or may not be present; these motions are suggestive of a subconscious sexual content. Rotatory head movements and bicycling and kicking leg movements are also common but not regarded any longer as diagnostic (see below). According to Walczak and Bogolioubov (1996), weeping appears to be a reliable sign of psycho-

genicity. According to a general consensus, falls in a psychogenic attack are never traumatizing and tongue bite as well as urinary incontinence do not occur—a view challenged by Peguero et al. (1995), who found tongue bite, self-injuries, and urinary incontinence in a sizable number of cases. It might be worthwhile to investigate such patient populations for intentional malingering. True malingerers can be very resourceful in producing behavioral changes imitating those found in bona fide epileptic attacks (including a voluntary Babinski sign; Lesser, 1996). The validity of classical hysterical signs has been under scrutiny for many years (Gould et al., 1986; Miller, 1988; Slavney, 1990). The boundaries between subconscious and conscious behavior in psychogenic seizures can be very fuzzy; Slavney's (1990) thoughts are highly elucidating in this challenging domain. Further information is found in the reports of Scott (1982), Karbowski (1984), Rodin (1984), and in the detailed review of Lesser (1996). Psychogenic seizures have been EEG-video documented right after aroused from sleep (Orbach et al., 2003).

Concept of Pseudoseizures

The term *pseudoseizures* denotes a conglomeration of noncerebral or nonepileptic attacks. It was introduced by Liske and Forster (1964), who were aware of the fact that many, but not all, of the patients had psychogenic (hysterical) attacks. Unfortunately, this term is not conducive to a differentiation of the nonepileptic attacks with certain distinctive features.

The term *pseudoseizures* has been more or less equated with psychogenic attacks. This may have been the result of a search for a euphemistic term since older terms such as *hysterical* or *psychogenic attacks* have been thought to have a derogatory connotation. Interestingly, the term *pseudoseizures* has been fading since 1990, while the term *psychogenic seizures* once again is being used more frequently.

Eventually, the term *pseudo-pseudoseizures* emerged (French et al., 1991). These investigators reported patients with typical psychogenic ictal semiology such as side-to-side head shaking and directed hostility; their ictal scalp EEG findings were bland (no ictal pattern). These patients were ultimately found to have exclusively epileptic seizures.

Saygi et al. (1991) have demonstrated major difficulties in the differential diagnosis of psychogenic attacks and frontal lobe seizures. Even pelvic thrusting was found to occur in frontal lobe seizures. "Bizarre automatisms" were reported in frontal lobe epileptics (Riggio et al., 1990). These observations clearly underscore the difficulties in the diagnosis of psychogenic seizures.

Coexistence of epileptic and hysterical seizures in the same patient is not uncommon; in 44 psychogenic seizure patients, 18 (41%) also had true epileptic seizures (Krumholz and Niedermeyer, 1983). In these cases, the hysterical attacks appear to be engrafted on the epileptic seizure disorder, which is obviously the primary problem (Schulte, 1964, 1966). Rabe (1970) has thoroughly investigated the occurrence of epileptic and hysterical seizures in 41 patients who exhibited both types. The true prevalence of this combination remains unclear and may lie between 1% and 2% of the intake of epileptic patients in a major medical institution.

The occurrence of nonepileptic and chiefly psychogenic attacks in patients thought to have posttraumatic epilepsy has been reported by Barry et al. (1991). In these cases, the preceding head injury was mild but the patients remained largely nonfunctional and few went back to work. Males predominated in this group, by a wide margin. In five of 96 cases of seizure surgery (mostly temporal lobectomy), psychogenic seizures emerged after surgery. All of these patients (three males, two females) had an IQ in the range from 66 to 82 (Ney et al., 1998).

In patients with epileptic seizures and perhaps some predisposition to psychogenic attacks, classical hysterical seizure manifestations have been reported by Niedermeyer et al. (1970) (and confirmed by Merskey, 1979) as a consequence of toxic anticonvulsant levels. It seems that these patients are unable to cope with stress in their toxic condition; their response to stress is an escape mechanism that causes the archaic motor pattern of major hysterical attacks. Patients with no epileptic seizures at all but with psychogenic attacks misdiagnosed as epileptic may show aggravated hysterical manifestations with even mildly toxic anticonvulsant levels.

Hysterical Stupor

Hysterical stupor is a dissociative reaction (West, 1967) in which the patient appears to have no rapport with other persons. It is a state of altered consciousness, but definitely not a state of impaired or lowered vigilance. This condition is comparable to hypnosis-induced alterations of consciousness. Its differentiation from absence status and psychomotor status may be difficult (Lesser, 1996; Rabe, 1980). Forceful eye closure in psychogenic stupor is a common finding, emphasized by De Toledo and Ramsay (1996), who investigated the different types of involvement of facial muscles in epileptic and nonepileptic attacks.

Hysterical stupor is closely related to major hysterical attacks but lacks the outbursts of motor activity of the latter. The stuporous states are of longer duration, and there may be signs of blindness or analgesia/anesthesia.

Electroencephalographic Observations

Differential diagnosis between hysterical and epileptic episodes is sometimes more difficult than it seems to be at first glance. The easiest differentiation between these two conditions is in stuporous hysterical patients who are very quiet. These patients usually have a normal tracing with well-developed alpha rhythm that shows normal blocking responses even in cases with psychogenic blindness. One is confronted with the same psychophysiological conditions that prevail in hypnotic states. These patients are fully awake unless they fall into physiological sleep (as hypnotized patients may also fall asleep).

The diagnostic problems are greater in patients with major psychogenic attacks. Such attacks may be triggered by skillful persuasiveness or the intravenous injection of saline (Bazil et al., 1994; Cohen and Suter, 1982; Slater et al., 1995; Suter and Cohen, 1981). This activation procedure, however, has raised ethical questions. Unfortunately, the storm of movements obscures the tracing almost as badly as a grand mal convulsion (Rodin, 1984). One may be able to

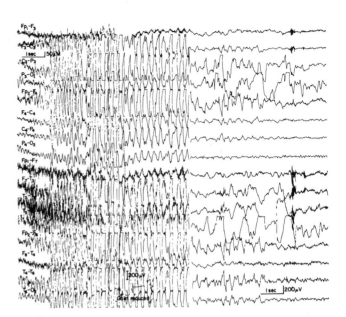

Figure 28.2. A psychogenic attack in a 17-year-old girl. The attack was associated with pronounced bicycle movements of the legs. Note posterior alpha rhythm preceding onset of attack. The rhythmical high-voltage activity in theta and delta range is caused by shaking movements of the entire body. This causes swinging of the electrode wires. A few posterior alpha waves are visible even after onset of the attack. The right tracing shows the immediate postictal period with much artifact. Alpha rhythm is noticeable, although poorly defined because of the lowered gain.

see perfect alpha rhythm right at the onset of the attack and even between violent motor outbursts (Figs. 28.2 and 28.3). Clinical acumen is very helpful. When attempts are made to open the eyes passively, active squeezing is often encountered. Absence of a gag reflex between seizures is a very helpful clinical sign in patients with hysterical states. This is, incidentally, a poorly understood sign that clearly shows that certain deviant neurophysiological mechanisms are put into action.

Prolonged forms of EEG recording such as split-screen video-EEG and intensive monitoring have proved to be very helpful (Holmes et al., 1980; Wilkus et al., 1984). Monitoring has become the diagnostic procedure of choice (Lesser, 1996; Meierkord et al., 1991), provided that this expensive technology is available.

The interval findings of hysterics are not always normal. Minor sharp transients of more localized (mainly temporal) or diffuse character are often found. Intermittent photic stimulation sometimes elicits mildly paroxysmal bursts. Gastaut (1949) found a low "myoclonic threshold" to combined photic and pentylenetetrazol (Metrazol) activation in these individuals. In patients with generalized spike-wave bursts (with or without clinical evidence of primary generalized epilepsy), psychogenic attacks have been reported (Sperling, 1984). Repetitive motor activity has been recognized as an important feature of seizures arising from the anterior portion of the frontal lobe (Riggio and Harner, 1995; Williamson, 1995).

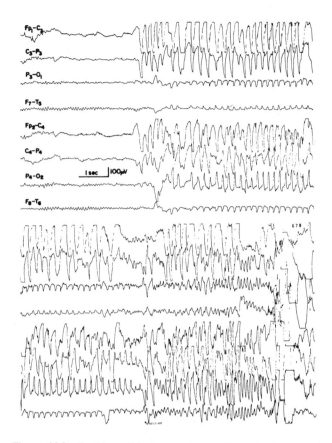

Figure 28.3. Factitious (faked) convulsion with predominant clonic motor activity. The attack was purposefully performed by an EEG technician. Note preictal stretch with posterior alpha rhythm. The dramatic EEG changes are movement artifacts.

Central Motor Disorders: Dyskinetic and Imitating Epileptic Seizures

Basal ganglia dyskinesias are constantly present in the waking state but there are also paroxysmal forms.

Paroxysmal choreoathetosis (described first by Mount and Reback, 1940) usually consists of episodic storms of involuntary movements of mixed character: choreic, athetoid, clonic, and tonic. These attacks are mostly precipitated by certain active or passive movements (kinesiogenic precipitation). Adults, adolescents, and children are affected and there seems to be no sex predominance. There are normal neurological findings in the interval and the EEG is normal, even during the attacks. In a personal observation, in one patient there was persistent posterior alpha rhythm, clearly demonstrable despite massive movement artifact; interestingly, there was also a history of indubitable generalized tonic-clonic seizures.

An unusual form of tonic attacks (extension of one or more extremities) is found in some patients with multiple sclerosis, and it is associated with an unchanged EEG [a type of so-called brainstem attacks (Matthews, 1958; Mumenthaler, 1983)].

Acknowledgment

The assistance of Dr. Fowzia Siddiqui is gratefully acknowledged.

References

Alajouanine, T., Contamin, F., and Cathala, H.P. 1958. *Le Syndrome Tétanie.* Paris: Baillère.

Andriola, M. 1983. Pseudo-seizures secondary to cardiac asystole and apnea. Electroencephalogr. Clin. Neurophysiol. 56:7P(abst).

Barolin, G.S., Lechner, H., and Ott, E. 1970. Polygraphie bei funktionell cerebrovaskulären Syndromen. Wien. Z. Nervenheilkd. 28:271–282.

Barry, E., Bergey, G.K., and Krumholz, A. 1991. Nonepileptic posttraumatic seizures. Epilepsia (New York) 32:54(abst).

Battaglia, A., Guerrini, R., and Gastaut, H. 1989. Syncopal attacks triggering epileptic seizures in childhood: usefulness of EEG investigations. Electroencephalogr. Clin. Neurophysiol. 73:60P(abst).

Bazil, C.W., Kothari, M., Luciano, D., et al. 1994. Provocation of nonepileptic seizures by suggestion in a general population. Epilepsia 35: 768–770.

Bezold, A., and Hirt, L. 1867. Über die physiologischen Wirkungen des essigsauren Veratrins. Untersuch. Physiol. Lab. Würzburg1: 73–156.

Bonvallet, M., and Dell, P. 1956. Reflections on the mechanism of the action of hyperventilation upon the EEG. Electroencephalogr. Clin. Neurophysiol. 8:170(abst).

Brenner, R.P. 1997. Electroencephalography in syncope. J. Clin. Neurophysiol. 14:197–209.

Breuer, J. 1895. *Studien über Hysterie,* 2nd ed. Vienna: Deuticke.

Breuer, J., and Freud, S. 1895. Studies on hysteria. In *Standard Edition of the Complete Psychological Works of Sigmund Freud,* vol. 7. London: Hogarth, 1955.

Briquet, P. 1859. Traité de l'Hystérie. Paris.

Broser, F. 1958. *Die cerebralen vegetativen Anfälle.* Berlin: Springer.

Charcot, J.M. 1887–1889. Leçons du Mardi à la Salpêtrière, Policlinique Paris: Bureaux du Progrès Médical. Paris: Lecroisnier and Babe.

Chodoff, P., and Lyons, H. 1958. Hysteria, the hysterical personality and "hysterical" conversion. Am. J. Psychiatry 114:734.

Cohen, R.J., and Suter, C. 1982. Hysterical seizures: suggestion as a provocative test. Ann. Neurol. 11:391–395.

Daly, D.D. 1990. Epilepsy and syncope. In *Current Practice of Clinical Electroencephalography,* 2nd ed., Eds. D.D. Daly and T.A. Pedley, pp. 269–334.

De Maria, A.A., Westmoreland, B.F., and Sharbrough, F.W. 1984. EEG in cough syncope. Neurology (Cleveland) 34:371–374.

DeToledo, J.C., and Ramsay, R.E. 1996. Patterns of involvement of facial muscles during epileptic and nonepileptic seizures: review of 654 events. Neurology 47:621–625.

Dinner, D.S., Lesser, R.P., Morris, H.H., et al. 1984. Electroclinical study of convulsive syncope: a case report. Electroencephalogr. Clin. Neurophysiol. 57:44P(abst).

Donker, D.N.J., Robles de Medina, E.O., and Kieft, J. 1972. Micturition syncope. Electroencephalogr. Clin. Neurophysiol. 33:328–331.

Durst, W., and Krump, J.E. 1961. Elektroenzephalographische und polygraphische Untersuchungen bei kreislaufbedingten Synkopen und vegetativen Anällen. Nervenarzt 32:401–405.

Eberhart, C., and Morgan, J. 1960. Micturition syncope. JAMA 174:2076–2077.

Engel, G.L. 1962. *Fainting,* 2nd ed. Springfield, IL: Charles C Thomas.

Engel, G.L., Ferris, E.B., and Logan, M. 1947. Hyperventilation. Analysis of clinical symptomatology. Ann. Intern. Med. 27:683–704.

Esquivel, E., Chaussain, M., Plouin, P., et al. 1991. Physical exercise and voluntary hyperventilation in childhood absence epilepsy. Electroencephalogr. Clin. Neurophysiol. 79:127–132.

Fajans, S.S., and Thorn, G.W. 1966. Hyperinsulinism and hypoglycemia. In *Principles of Internal Medicine,* 5th ed., Eds. T.R. Harrison et al., pp. 507–512. New York: McGraw-Hill.

Finesinger, J.E., and Mazick, S.G. 1940. The respiratory response of psychoneurotic patients to ideational and sensory stimuli. Am. J. Psychiatr. 97:27.

French, J.A., Sperling, M.R., and Williamson, P.D. 1991. Pseudo-pseudo-seizures: epileptic seizures masking as psychogenic events. Epilepsia (New York) 32:51(abst).

Fried, R. 1987. *The Hyperventilation Syndrome.* Baltimore: Johns Hopkins University Press.

Gastaut, H. 1949. Effets des stimulations physiques sur l'EEG de l'homme. Electroencephalogr. Clin. Neurophysiol. Suppl. 2:69–82.

Gastaut, H. 1958. Syncope and seizure. Electroencephalogr. Clin. Neurophysiol. 10:571–572.

Gastaut, H. 1968. A physiopathogenetic study of reflex anoxic cerebral seizures in children (syncope, sobbing spasms, breath holding spells). In *Electroencephalography of Children,* Eds. P. Kellaway and I. Petersén, pp. 257–274. New York: Grune & Stratton (Stockholm: Almqvist & Wiksell).

Gastaut, H., and Gastaut, Y. 1956. Étude électroencéphalographique des syncopes. Rev. Neurol. 95:420–421, 547–549.

Gastaut, H., and Gastaut, Y. 1957. Syncopes et convulsions. À propos de la nature syncopale de certaines spasmes du sanglot et des certaines convulsions essentielles hyperthermiques ou à froid. Rev. Neurol. 96:158–163.

Gastaut, H., Vigouroux, R.A., and Dell, M.G. 1961. Polygraphic study of carotid sinus hypersensitivity produced by extra-sinus stimulation (compression of carotid sinus). In *Cerebral Anoxia and the Electroencephalogram,* Eds. H. Gastaut and J.E. Meyer, pp. 185–207. Springfield, IL: Thomas.

Gould, R., Miller, B.L., Goldberg, M.A., et al. 1986. The validity of hysterical signs and symptoms. J. Nerv. Ment. Dis. 174:593–597.

Grimm, D.R. 1997. Neurally mediated syncope: a review of cardiac and arterial receptors. J. Clin. Neurophysiol. 14:170–182.

Hann, J., and Franke, H. 1953. The electroencephalogram in patients with hypersensitive carotid sinus syndrome of cardiac type with prolonged cessation of heartbeat. Electroencephalogr. Clin. Neurophysiol. Suppl. 3:50(abst).

Holmes, G.L., Sackellares, J.C., McKiernan, J., et al. 1980. Evaluation of childhood pseudoseizures using EEG telemetry and video tape monitoring. Pediatrics 97:554–558.

Hooshmand, H. 1972. Apneic seizures treated with atropine. Report of a case. Neurology (Minneapolis) 22:1217–1221.

Hughes, J.R., and Zialcita, M.L. 2000. EEG in the elderly: seizures vs. syncope. Clin. Electroencephalogr. 31:131–137

Janet, P. 1893/1894. *L'état Mental des Hystériques.* Paris.

Jarisch, A., and Zotterman, Y. 1948. Depressor reflexes from the heart. Acta Physiol. Scand. 16:31–51.

Johnson, R.H., Lambie, D.G., and Spaulding, J.M.K. (Eds.). 1984. *Neurocardiology.* London: Saunders.

Karbowski, K. 1984. Diagnostische Probleme bei hysterischen Krampfanfällen. Schweiz. Mech. Wschr. 114:1297–1300.

Kaufmann, H. 1997. Neurally mediated syncope and syncope due to autonomic failure: differences and similarities. J. Clin. Neurophysiol. 14:183–196.

Kretschmer, E. 1923. *Hysterie, Reflex und Instinkt,* 6th ed. Stuttgart: Thieme, 1958.

Kretschmer, E. 1956. *Medizinische Psychologie,* 11th ed. Stuttgart: Thieme.

Krumholz, A., and Niedermeyer, E. 1983. Psychogenic seizures: a clinical study with follow-up data. Neurology (Cleveland) 33:498–502.

Landau, W.M., and Nelson, D.A. 1996. Clinical neuromythology XV. Feinting science: neurocardiogenic syncope and collateral vasovagal confusion. Neurology 46:609–618.

Lesser, R.P. 1996. Psychogenic seizures. Neurology 46:1499–1597.

Lewis, B.I. 1953. The hyperventilation syndrome. Ann. Intern. Med. 38:918–927.

Lewis, B.I. 1954. Chronic hyperventilation syndrome. JAMA 155:1204–1208.

Liske, E., and Forster, F.M. 1964. Pseudoseizures: a problem in the diagnosis and management of epileptic patients. Neurology (Minneapolis) 14:41–49.

Lombroso, C.T., and Lerman, P. 1967. Breathholding spells (cyanotic and pallid infantile syncope). Pediatrics 29:563–581.

Low, N.L., Gibbs, E.L., and Gibbs, A.F. 1955. Electroencephalographic findings in breath holding spells. Pediatrics 15:595–599.

Lukash, W.M., Sawyer, G., and Davis, J. 1964. Micturition syncope produced by orthostasis and bladder distension. N. Engl. J. Med. 270:341–344.

Lyle, C., Monroe, J., Flinn, D., et al. 1961. Micturition syncope N. Engl. J. Med. 265:982–986.

Matthews, W.B. 1958. Tonic seizures in disseminated sclerosis. Brain 81:193–206.

Meierkord, H., Will, B., Fish, D., et al. 1991. The clinical features and prognosis of pseudoseizures diagnosed using video-EEG telemetry. Neurology 41:1643–1646.

Merskey, H. 1979. *The Analysis of Hysteria.* London: Balliere-Tindall.

Miller, E. 1988. Defining hysterical symptoms. Psychol. Med. 18:275–277.

Mount, L.A., and Reback, S. 1940. Familial paroxysmal choreoathetosis. Arch. Neurol. Psychiatr. 44:841–847.

Mumenthaler, M. 1983. *Neurology,* 2nd ed. Stuttgart: Thieme.

Mumenthaler, M. (ed.) 1984. *Synkopen und Sturzanfälle.* Stuttgart: Thieme.

Naquet, R., and Bostem, F. 1964. Étude électroencéphalographique des syncopes. Electroencephalogr. Clin. Neurophysiol. 16:140–152.

Naquet, R., and Vigouroux, R.A. 1972. Acute cerebral anoxia and syncopal attacks. In *Handbook of Electroencephalography and Clinical Neurophysiology,* vol. 14A, Ed. A. Remond, pp. 68–71. Amsterdam: Elsevier.

Ney, G.C., Barr, W.B., Napolitano, C., et al. 1998. New onset psychogenic seizures after surgery for epilepsy. Arch. Neurol. 55:726–730.

Niedermeyer, E., Blumer, D., Holscher, E., et al. 1970. Classical hysterical seizures facilitated by anticonvulsant toxicity. Psychiatr. Clin. (Basel) 3:71–84.

Orbach, D., Ritaccio, A., and Devinsky, D. 2003. Psychogenic nonepileptic seizures associated with video-EEG-verified sleep. Epilepsia 44:64–68.

Ossentjuk, E., Elink Sterk, C.J.O., and Storm van Leeuwen, W. 1966. Flicker-induced cardiac arrest in patient with epilepsy. Electroencephalogr. Clin. Neurophysiol. 20:257–259.

Peguero, E., Abbou-Khalil, B., Fakhoury, T., et al. 1995. Self-injury and incontinence in psychogenic seizures. Epilepsia 36:586–591.

Pozo, D., Pascual, J., and Cantos, M. 1981. Diagnostic value of EEG in reflex (vagal) anoxic cerebral seizures. Electroencephalogr. Clin. Neurophysiol. 52:95P(abst).

Rabe, F. 1970. *Die Kombination hysterischer und epileptischer Anfälle.* Berlin: Springer.

Rabe, F. 1980. Hysterische Dämmerzustände. Differentialdiagnose gegenüber Status psychomotoricus. In *Status Psychomotoricus,* Ed. K. Karbowski, pp. 103–116. Bern: Huber.

Rabending, G., and Klepel, H. 1978. *Die Fotostimulation als Aktivierungsmethode in der Elektroenzephalographie.* Jena: VEB Gustav Fischer.

Rabending, G., Krell, D., and Müller, O. 1968. Durch Fotostimulation ausgelöste Bradykardie mit nachfolgender Asystolie. Psychiatr. Neurol. Med. Psychol. 20:331–335.

Regis, H., Toga, M., and Righini, C. 1961. Clinical, electroencephalographic and pathological study of a case of Adams-Stokes syndrome. In *Cerebral Anoxia and the Electroencephalogram,* Eds. J.S. Meyer and H. Gastaut, pp. 295–303. Springfield, IL: Charles C Thomas.

Riggio, S., and Harner, R.N. 1995. Repetitive motor activity in frontal lobe epilepsy. In *Epilepsy and the Functional Anatomy of the Frontal Lobe,* Ed. H.H. Jasper, S. Riggio, and P.S. Goldman-Rakic, pp. 153–164. Raven Press: New York.

Riggio, S., Harner, R.N., and Privitera, M. 1990. Frontal lobe epilepsy: difficulties with diagnosis and a proposal for classification. Epilepsia (New York) 31:626–627(abst).

Riley, T.L. 1982. Syncope and hyperventilation. In *Pseudoseizures,* Eds. T.L. Riley and A. Roy, pp. 34–61. Baltimore: Williams & Wilkins.

Rodin, E. 1984. Epileptic and pseudoepileptic seizures: Differential diagnostic considerations. In *Psychiatric Aspects of Epilepsy,* Ed. D. Blumer, pp. 179–195. Washington, DC: American Psychiatric Press.

Saygi, S., Katz, A., Marks, D.A., et al. 1991. Frontal lobe complex partial seizures and psychogenic seizures: comparison of the clinical and ictal characteristics. Epilepsia (New York) 32:96–97(abst).

Schomer, D.L. 2003. Hospital and Outpatient-Based Recording Techniques. Proceedings of the American Clinical Neurophysiology Society. San Francisco, CA. September 2003.

Schulte, W. 1964. *Epilepsie und ihre Randgebiete in Klinik und Praxis.* Munich: Lehmann.

Schulte, W. 1966. Psychogene Anfälle beim Epileptiker. Nervenarzt 37: 147.

Scott, D.F. 1982. Recognition and diagnostic aspects of nonepileptic seizures. In *Pseudoseizures,* Eds. T.L. Riley and A. Roy, pp. 21–33. Baltimore: Williams & Wilkins.

Slater, J.D., Brown, M.C., Jacobs, W., et al. 1995. Induction of pseudoseizures with intravenous saline placebo. Epilepsia 36:580–585.

Slavney, P.R. 1990. *Perspectives on Hysteria.* Baltimore: Johns Hopkins University Press.

Sperling, M.R. 1984. Diagnosis of pseudoseizures during EEG recording in a patient with generalized epileptiform discharges in the EEG. Electroencephalogr. Clin. Neurophysiol. 58:37P(abst).

Suter, C., and Cohen, R. 1981. A standardized EEG test for hysterical attacks (pseudoseizures). Electroencephalogr. Clin. Neurophysiol. 51:37P (abst).

Toyka, K.V., and Forster, C. 1974. Apnoeic seizures in the neonatal period: therapy with atropine. Electroencephalogr. Clin. Neurophysiol. 37:442–443(abst).

Walczak, T.S., and Bogolioubov, A. 1996. Weeping during psychogenic nonepileptic seizures. Epilepsia 37:208–210.

Wenzel, U. 1981. Drop attacks in adults. Electroencephalogr. Clin. Neurophysiol. 52:41P(abst).

West, L.J. 1967. Dissociative reaction. In *Comprehensive Textbook of Psychiatry,* Eds. A.M. Freedman and H.I. Kaplan, pp. 885–889. Baltimore: Williams & Wilkins.

Wilkus, R.J., Dodrill, C.B., and Thompson, P.M. 1984. Intensive EEG monitoring and psychological studies of patients with pseudoepileptic seizures. Epilepsia (New York) 25:100–107.

Williamson, P.D. 1995. Frontal lobe epilepsy. Some clinical characteristics. In *Epilepsy and the Functional Anatomy of the Frontal Lobe,* Eds. H.H. Jasper, S. Riggio, and P.S. Goldman-Rakic, pp. 127–150. New York: Raven Press.

Ziegler, F., Imboden, J., and Meyer, E. 1960. Contemporary conversion reactions: a clinical study. Am. J. Psychiatry 116:901.

29. The EEG in Patients with Migraine and Other Forms of Headache

Ernst Niedermeyer

Patients with headaches are usually referred to the electroencephalography (EEG) laboratory in order to rule out underlying cerebral pathology rather than for a clarification of the type of headache. This type of referral has become less frequent with the greater availability of modern neuroimaging.

Headache is one of the most common complaints. As a symptom, it may herald a wide variety of infectious, neoplastic, and vascular intracranial lesions, but it also may be a sign of various dysfunctions impinging on neural, vascular, and muscular structures. It may arise from the vicinity of the cranial cavity or even from distant structures. Metabolic, toxic, and hormonal disturbances are further causes. In other words, headache is a challenge for the diagnostic acumen of neurologists and other specialists. It has been stated that about 20% of the U.S. population complains of headache, and about half of them receive some form of symptomatic medical treatment (Diamond, 1979). Table 29.1 shows a classification of the types of headache. New criteria of classification have been proposed by Silberstein et al. (1996).

Migraine (Classical and Complicated Forms)

General Considerations and Clinical Features

Migraine has been known to humanity for ages; a Sumerian poem written 5,000 years ago gives an account of this disorder. In spite of a remarkable upsurge of research interest in this field, migraine has remained a poorly understood disorder. A plethora of clinical data is found in the work of Sacks (1985).

The clinical symptomatology of the migrainous attack is well known. In the classical form, visual symptoms herald the attack; there are scintillating scotoma with teichoscopy and other forms of visual field cuts. Within a short time (about 5–20 minutes), this stage is supplanted by headache, which is mostly unilateral, with shifting lateralization from attack to attack in most cases. This is accompanied by severe nausea, vomiting, irritability, and photophobia. This stage lasts for hours or a full day. Wolff (1948) has ascribed the initiating visual symptoms to intracerebral local vasoconstriction and the ensuing phase of headache and nausea to an abnormal degree of extracranial vasodilation, which can easily be palpated along the temporal artery on the painful side.

A genetic predisposition is present or even pronounced, but the mode of genetic transmission is not fully understood. The attacks tend to start in adolescence; in childhood, attacks

of abdominal pain may be precursors of migraine. It has been thought that a fall of the plasma serotonin level (Anthony et al., 1967) plays a crucial role in the physiopathogenesis of the migrainous attack, but this concept has not been generally accepted. Allergic (antigen-antibody) reactions, free fatty acids, and prostaglandin E are also believed to be involved in migraine (Anthony, 1970). Activation of 5-hydroxytryptamine receptors has been stressed by Fozard (1980). According to Moskowitz (1984), migraine is caused by a disturbance of the "trigeminovascular system" (connections between trigeminal ganglia and cerebral blood vessels) involving the neurotransmitter peptide, substance P. Experimentally, "neuroinflammation" was produced in animals by electrical stimulation of the trigeminal ganglion causing the release of sensory neuropeptides from nerve terminals (the model of "neurogenic inflammation"; Moskowitz et al., 1993). Biggs and Johnson (1984) have placed special emphasis on the adrenergic system and its role in migraine pathogenesis. A unified neurogenic concept of migraine has been proposed by Diamond and Dalessio (1982).

Not all cases of migraine are due to an inherited dysfunction; neuropathological processes such as arteriovenous malformations of neurosyphilis are known as cases of "symptomatic migraine." This differential diagnosis may occasionally become difficult, because migraine attacks are capable of proceeding to a state of ischemic infarction (Schumacher and Wolff, 1941; Whitty, 1953) and of producing regional computed tomography (CT) scan changes (Skinhøj et al., 1970). In regional cerebral blood flow studies using xenon-133 intraarterially, reduced blood flow was demonstrable during migraine attacks starting posteriorly and very slowly spreading to the rolandic region (Lauritzen et al., 1983). According to Hansen et al., (1984) and Olesen (1991), spreading depression is considered a useful model of migraine aura and presumably also for the subsequent headache. This concept was reemphasized by Olesen (1994), especially on the basis of the positron emission tomography (PET) scan observation (oxygen-15-labeled water) of Woods et al. (1994). There is good evidence of hypoperfusion within the occipital lobe (Woods et al., 1994), which can just as well (if not better) be used as supportive of the vascular concept.

Special involvement of the central visual system is a very common feature of classical migraine with visual initiation. Huang et al. (2003) have shown with the use of functional magnetic resonance imaging (fMRI) the excessive responses to visual stimuli and a particular sensitivity to a pattern of regularly spaced parallel lines of stripes. (See also Lashley, 1941).

Table 29.1. Classification of Headache[a]

Vascular Headache	Muscle Contraction (Psychogenic) Headache	Traction and Inflammatory Headache
Migraine	Cervical osteoarthritis	Mass lesions (tumors, edema, hematomas, cerebral hemorrhage)
1. Classic		
2. Common		
3. Hemiplegic	Complicated migraine	
4. Ophthalmoplegic		
Cluster (histamine)	Chronic myositis	Diseases of the eye, ear, nose, throat, teeth
Toxic vascular	Depressive equivalents and conversion reactions	Infection
Hypertensive		Arteritis, phlebitis; cranial neuralgias; occlusive vascular disease

[a]Modified from Dalessio, D.J. 1979. Classification and mechanism of migraine. Headache 19:114–120.

Whoever reads the original experimental techniques used in the production of spreading depression (Leão, 1944, 1972) will have nagging doubts concerning the appropriateness of the spreading-depression model for a neurogenic migraine concept. The mode of elicitation implies all sorts of mechanical and chemical trauma to the brain tissue; electrocorticographic recording (Leão, 1972) shows flattening of the record followed by several recurrent prominent spikes (against a flat background) and another phase of flattening before the baseline character of the record is restored. It is difficult to imagine that similar electrical processes would occur in migrainous human beings. The primordial nature of vasomotor changes according to H. G. Wolff's (1948) original theory seems to be a lot more plausible.

On the basis of data derived from animal experiments (Wistar rats), Ebersberger et al. (2001) doubt that spreading depression initiates migraine.

Electroencephalographic Findings

The literature in this field is very confusing because almost equal numbers of reports stress the predominance of normal and abnormal tracings. Relatively few records have been obtained during the attacks; these data are discussed later. Daly and Markand (1990) have pointed out that previous studies of migraine and EEG were frequently flawed by sampling problems and heterogeneous populations of migrainous persons.

The contrast between various reports on the EEG in migraine in the interval between attacks is due to (a) composition of material (adults versus children, inclusion or exclusion of hemiplegic cases), (b) different criteria for normality and abnormality in the investigators' EEG interpretation, and (c) difficulties in the delineation of migraine as a nosological entity (inclusion or strict exclusion of cluster headaches or symptomatic forms of migraine with cerebral pathology). Keeping all this in mind, it is still difficult to understand the disparity of the reports.

The predominance of normal-interval EEG records was stressed by Ulett et al. (1952), Jung (1953), Becher (1955), Krischek (1956), Wissfeld and Neu (1960), Bille (1962), and Gibbs and Gibbs (1964). The work of other authors places the emphasis on a variety of abnormalities. Heyck (1956, 1958) found mainly "hypersynchronous bursts" and occasional focal slowing. Weil (1952, 1962) noted pronounced delta responses to hyperventilation. Various types of abnormality were noted by Dow and Whitty (1947) and Selby and Lance (1960). A high incidence of abnormal EEG records was also emphasized by Barolin (1966), Gschwend (1972), and Pithova (1983). Almost equal numbers of normal and abnormal records (with about 45% abnormal tracings) were reported in the extensive work of Smyth and Winter (1964). The reported abnormalities, however, were predominantly mild to moderate, with some bursts, slowing, or sharp transients. With the use of computer frequency analysis, Jonkman and Lelieveld (1981) demonstrated abnormal interval EEG findings in 55% of migrainous patients. According to Drake et al. (1987), the EEG of patients with migraine does not differ significantly from the EEG of normal individuals. This is essentially congruent with my personal views.

Intermittent photic stimulation often shows an occipital driving response extending into the range above 20 flashes/sec ("H response" after Golla and Winter, 1959); according to Smyth and Winter (1964), this is almost specific for migraine. This has been substantiated by Slater (1968). Personal observations essentially support this view. Further substantiation of these findings has been provided by Simon et al. (1982) with the use of spectral analysis during photic stimulation (Fig. 29.1).

EEG findings in the migraine attack range from normal to mildly abnormal (alpha depression) in the initiating ophthalmic phase; even severely abnormal findings have been reported in special cases (Kugler, 1979; Scollo-Lavizzari, 1975; Westmoreland, 1978). Based on his large material, Heyck (1956) found normal tracings in the ophthalmic-vasoconstrictive as well as in the headache-nausea phase. Schoenen et al. (1990) found reduced alpha activity over one occipital region in 19 out of 22 patients recorded during an attack of common migraine. In the light of these observations, the statement that "EEGs have almost always been normal in migraineurs during attacks" (Gorman and Welch, 1993) might be slightly exaggerated, but EEG abnormalities should be viewed as exceptions.

A neuronal dysfunction as the cause of migraine was assumed by Soysal et al. (2001) on the basis of significantly prolonged P100 latencies of visual evoked potentials in the interval between attacks. On the other hand, EEG abnormalities were observed in only four of the 13 patients.

When the migraine attack is complicated by mild hemiparetic or dysphasic deficits (*"migraine accompagnée"*), the EEG may remain normal (Farkas et al., 1985). In cases with pronounced *hemiplegia* and *aphasia,* there is good evidence of delta and theta activity over the affected hemisphere (Bradshaw and Parsons, 1965; Degen et al., 1980; Heron, 1966; Heyck, 1956; Rosenbaum, 1960). The delta activity over the affected hemisphere may be very impressive (see cases of Isler, 1969). The neurological deficit subsides

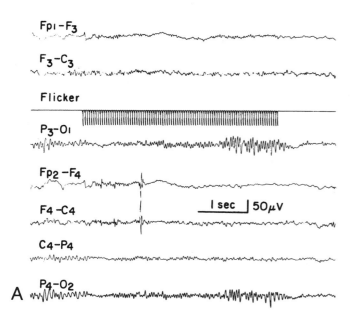

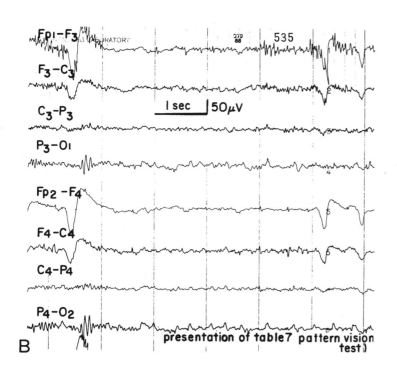

Figure 29.1. **A:** A 31-year-old woman with a history of classical migraine (experiences flashing lights and also some left-sided numbness). EEG obtained in interval. Note good occipital photic driving response to a flash rate of 22/sec ("H response"). The right frontal spiky discharge is artifactual. **B:** Same patient. Very good occipital lambda activation presentation of pattern-vision test tables.

within days (sometimes within weeks), and the focal or lateralized slowing my also linger on for some period of time (Fig. 29.2). Cases of *familial hemiplegic migraine* have been reported by Whitty (1953), Rosenbaum (1960), Bradshaw and Parsons (1965), and Müller and Müller (1977). It has been pointed out that in familial hemiplegia the lateralization of the affected hemisphere remains unchanged in every attack and is the same in all involved family members. This is not congruent with a personal observation. EEG studies in familial hemiplegia show a varying degree of slowing over the brain's affected side.

The contingent negative variation (CNV) has been used for the differential diagnosis of headaches (Maertens de Nord-hout et al., 1986). Ahmed (1999) clearly demonstrated an enhanced CNV in patients with classic and common migraine; their CNV was moderately larger than in patients with tension headaches and much larger than in normal controls. These statements pertain to the pain-free interval between migraine attacks. The CNV changes are believed to reflect catecholamine hyperactivity. According to CNV research, this slow potential measures expectancy, attention, preparation, and motivation. When one considers that, according to

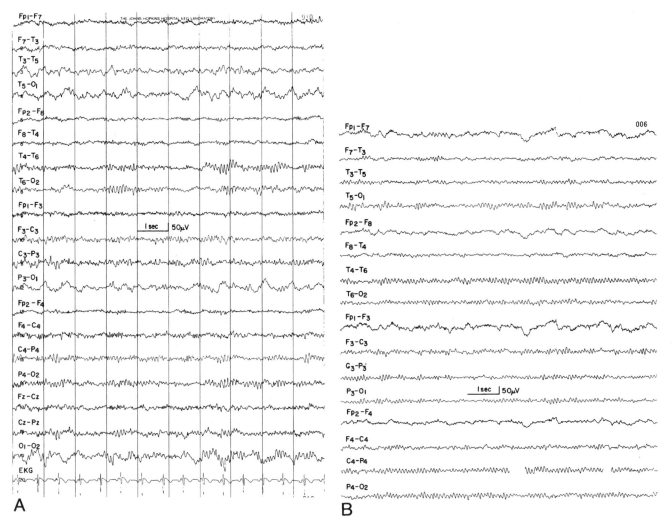

Figure 29.2. **A:** A 13-year-old boy with migraine attacks. EEG recorded during a migraine attack with moderate right hemiparesis and global aphasia. Note marked delta activity over left occipital-posterotemporal region. **B:** EEG taken 5 days later. Clinically normal, EEG normalized.

Ahmed (1999), the enlargement of the CNV would persist after successful antimigraine treatment, then one wonders if enhanced motivation and a powerful desire to perform tasks perfectly are personality traits of migrainous persons.

Atypical Forms of Migraine

Abdominal manifestations of migraine are relatively common in children. Headache is usually absent in these attacks, whereas abdominal pain is in the foreground. Such attacks may last for hours. Temporary agitation and obnubilation during the attack have been noted by Lérique-Koechlin and Mises (1964).

In *childhood migraine,* normal EEG records are the rule (89%), but "benign" focal spikes, mostly rolandic, were found in 9% (Kinast et al., 1982). Kellaway et al. (1960) stressed the high incidence of 14 and 6/sec positive spikes in the sleep records of these children. During the attack of abdominal pain, the EEG is unremarkable (personal observa-

tions). Gibbs and Gibbs (1964) separate abdominal pain attack (with frequent 14 and 6/sec positive spike discharges in the interval) from migraine with normal interval tracings. Lérique-Koechlin and Mises (1964) reported a very high incidence of paroxysmal EEG changes in children with a history of abdominal pain attacks. Moore (1945) introduced the term *abdominal epilepsy* for such cases of acute abdominal pain, but this has not been widely accepted. This term is rather misleading, and its use should be discouraged. In migrainous children, temporal lobe-type seizures have been described (Seshia et al., 1985). These children experienced strange sensations or misperceptions; the EEG in most cases showed sharp activity over the temporal region. "Benign paroxysmal vertigo of childhood" has been found to be a migrainous equivalent (Koehler, 1980).

Basilar migraine represents a syndrome described by Bickerstaff (1961a), consisting of a sudden transient blurring of vision or blindness, vertigo, gait ataxia, dysarthria, acroparesthesias, and pulsatile occipital headache with vomiting. Even syncopal states and loss of consciousness may occur (Bickerstaff, 1961b). Basilar migraine manifestations are more common in older children, adolescents, and young adults; females are more often affected. In adulthood, these attacks may be supplanted by attacks of classical or common migraine. According to Caplan (1991), basilar migraine is not always benign. It affects both sexes and a wider age range; it also may be associated with strokes.

The EEG literature is meager in this domain; a case of Slater (1968) was recorded during a presumed attack and showed diffuse 1.5 to 4/sec activity with subsequent normalization. This patient, however, was 46 years old; this age could cast some doubt on the diagnosis. Lapkin et al. (1977) reported two cases (ages 12 and 10) with diffuse and chiefly posterior slowing in the 1.5 to 2/sec and 3 to 4/sec ranges, respectively, during the attack. This activity vanished with serial recordings. Camfield et al. (1978) observed four adolescents (two girls and two boys) with presumed basilar migraine. These cases were complicated by epileptic seizures (mostly grand mal, but also focal motor). The EEG showed very prominent spike activity and slowing accentuated over the posterior regions. All of these patients had a strongly positive history of classical or common migraine. Similar paroxysmal findings over posterior regions were reported by Panayatopoulos (1980). Another form with predominant beta activity during the attack was delineated by Parain and Samson-Dollfus (1984). Gastaut (1982) has cast much doubt on the observations of Camfield et al. (1978); he feels that these patients were suffering from benign occipital lobe epilepsy (see Chapter 27, "Epileptic Seizure Disorders"). Simple partial status epilepticus in the occipital lobe can be misdiagnosed as migraine (Walker et al., 1995).

According to Ramelli et al. (1998), the EEG of children (11–13 years) with basilar artery migraine showed diffuse subdelta-delta activity during the attack and occipital delta-theta activity hours afterward. The authors warn against concepts of structural lesions (infarction, inflammation) and presume a temporary disfunction.

Cernibori and Bouquet (1984) observed children ages 2 to 14 years with episodes of loss of consciousness ranging from 1 hour to several days; these episodes were attributed to basilar artery migraine of childhood. Diffuse or lateralized slow activity was noted in the EEG, which improved over the ensuing days. Slightly abnormal interval EEG tracings were found in four of 12 children. Episodic comatose states have also been reported by Ganji et al. (1993).

Status Migrainosus

On the basis of personal observations, there is good reason to presume that prolonged or constantly recurrent migraine attacks are the result of severe mental-emotional stress. In this condition, EEG findings are bland and noncontributory.

Whatever neurological-organic basis may be demonstrated in migraine, the involvement of psychogenic factors must not be counted out. Evidence of a link between migraine and neuroticism has been reported by Breslau et al. (1996). Let us assume that, while many migrainous persons are in full control of such subthreshold mechanisms, others

may lose their control temporarily (under stress) or perhaps even permanently. Olesen's (1994) concept of a "clean neurological" migraine—uncontaminated with psychogenic features—cannot be upheld in view of the clinical facts.

Relationships Between Migraine and Epileptic Seizure Disorders

A combination of migraine and epileptic seizure disorder may occur, but it is uncommon (Alvarez, 1959; Barolin, 1966; Giardina and Sideri, 1985). A true link between both disorders is highly debatable (Basser, 1969; Lance and Anthony, 1966; Lees and Watkins, 1963). There is some reason to support the view of Camfield et al. (1978) that, under certain circumstances, migraine can trigger an epileptic attack. This subject has been reviewed by Hess (1977), who presumes that headache may be a secondary symptom in patients with epileptic seizure disorder. There is no cogent need to establish a special form called "dysrhythmic migraine" (Weil, 1952, 1962).

The entire subject of migraine and epilepsy was reinvestigated in extensive work edited by Andermann and Lugaresi (1987) and in the overview of Andermann and Andermann (1992).

An entity named "migraine-triggered epilepsy" has been described by Niedermeyer (1983, 1990, 1993). Typical grand mal seizures occur after a very short visual initiation; migrainous headache and nausea follow the seizure. The EEG is mostly normal in the interval and the response to antiepileptic medication leaves much to be desired. Postepileptic headaches are quite common and there is also a possibility of "epilepsy-triggered migraine" (based on the cases of Jacobs et al., 1996).

On the basis of very extensive data collected (1957 adult probands with epilepsy), Ottman and Lipton (1996) were unable to support the theory of a shared genetic susceptibility for migraine and epileptic disorders. Table 29.2 demonstrates the differentiation of migrainous and certain epileptic conditions.

The EEG in Other Types of Headache

The EEG in nonmigrainous forms of headaches has been thus far a barren field; one is unable to correlate any type of headache with some type of EEG change during the attacks or in the interval. *Cluster headache* is a well-defined entity, but has no special EEG correlate. *Hyperventilation-related headache* associated with EEG slowing has been reported by Sbrascini and Bassi (1983). *Hypnic headache* has been described by Raskin (1988) and related to REM sleep; the EEG is normal (Evers and Goadsby, 2003).

In general, patients with habitual headaches and no organic disease may show EEG patterns that are believed to reveal some degree of "neuronal hyperexcitability"; this is a vague term without any precise scientific foundation, but with some merit in the domain of medical practice. Rolandic mu rhythm is quite often found in patients referred for headaches without demonstrable organic cause. Other patients show mildly paroxysmal flicker responses; still others show

Table 29.2.   Differentiation of Migrainous and Certain Epileptic Conditions

Condition	Occurrence	Sex	Age	Scintillating Scotoma	Visual Hallucination, (Elementary, Figurative)	Headache	Nausea (Vomiting)
Common migraine	Very common	Probably females preponderant	Mostly after age 15 years	0	0	+++	+++
Classic migraine	Common	Mostly males if without headache-nausea	Mostly after age 15 years	+++	?+	0–+++	0–++
Basilar artery migraine	Moderately common	Probably females only	15–35 years	0–+++	0–++	0–++	0–++
Migraine-triggered epilepsy	Very rare	? (? Mainly females)	? 15–40 years	++ (immediately followed by grand mal)	?	+–++ (after grand mal)	0–++ (after grand mal)
Benign occipital lobe epilepsy	Rare	No sex preponderance	5–40 years	0	+–+++	+–++ (after seizure)	+ (after seizure)
Benign rolandic epilepsy–migraine	Very rare	? (? Mainly females)	5–20 years for epileptic past 15 for migrainous manifestations	0 (for epileptic ++ for migrainous attacks)	0	0–++ (after seizure) +++ (in migraine)	0–+ (after seizure) +++ (in migraine)

Syncope	Epileptic Seizures	EEG (Interval)	EEG (During Episodes)	Therapy	Prognosis
0 reduction	0	Mostly normal	Mostly normal	Antimigrainous, stress reduction	Mostly very good (albeit no real cure)
0 (? +)	0	Mostly normal	Mostly normal	Antimigrainous, stress reduction	Mostly very good (albeit no real cure)
0–++	0–+	Normal to slightly abnormal (nonspecific)	Normal to slightly abnormal (with changes due to syncope or convulsion)	Antimigrainous, stress reduction, may require antiepileptics	Mostly very good (? spontaneous cure in middle adulthood)
0	++ (grand mal)	Normal	Typical EEG of a tonic-clonic convulsion	Probably preventive antimigrainous therapy, antiepileptics ineffective	Unclear
0	+++ (mostly visual, also others)	Abnormal with recurrent posterior spike-waves or spikes	Abnormal with bilateral posterior spikes or spike-waves	Antiepileptics	Mostly good
0	+ (focal motor)	Normal or abnormal with rolandic spikes, in adulthood normal	Probably abnormal during focal motor attacks, normal during migraine	Antiepileptics, in later phase antimigrainous, stress reduction	Probably very good (albeit no real cure for migraine)

14 and 6/sec positive spikes or even categorical EEG abnormalities such as psychomotor variant pattern and 6/sec spike waves. The possibility of *vasomotor headaches* as a symptom of larval epilepsy has been discussed by Heyck and Hess (1955). A physiopathogenetic basis of such dysfunctional states with headache is still obscure.

A rather nonspecific type of headache ("fullness of head, pressure, heat, pounding") was found to be an ictal epileptic manifestation in the limbic portion of the right temporal lobe recorded with depth electrodes (Laplante et al., 1982). These patients benefited from surgical resection.

It was found that EEG studies done with spectral analysis in patients with tension headaches did not differ from normal persons (and were also not significantly different from the EEG of migrainous patients) (Drake et al., 1987).

Acknowledgment

The assistance of Dr. Fowzia Siddiqui is gratefully acknowledged.

References

Ahmed, I. 1999. Contingent negative variation in migraine: effect of beta blocker therapy. Clin. Electroencephaologr. 30:21–23.

Alvarez, W.C. 1959. Migraine plus epilepsy. Neurology (Minneapolis) 9:487–491.

Andermann, F., and Andermann, E. 1992. Migraine and epilepsy with special reference to the benign epilepsies of childhood. In *Benign Localized and Generalized Epilepsies of Early Childhood*. Eds. R. Degen and F.E. Dreifuss, pp. 207–214. Amsterdam: Elsevier.

Andermann, F., and Lugaresi, E. (Eds.). 1987. *Migraine and Epilepsy*. Boston: Butterworth.

Anthony, M. 1970. Plasma fatty acids and prostaglandin E in migraine and stress. Headache 16:58.

Anthony, M., Hinterberger, H., and Lance, J.W. 1967. Plasma serotonin in migraine and stress. Arch. Neurol. (Chicago) 16:544–552.

Barolin, G.S. 1966. Migraines and epilepsies—a relationship? Epilepsia (Amsterdam) 7:53–66.

Basser, L.S. 1969. The relation of migraine and epilepsy. Brain 92:285–300.

Becher, F. 1955. Hirnelektrische und elektromyographische Untersuchungen beim Migränesyndrom. Dtsch. Z. Nervenheilk. 172:556.

Bickerstaff, E.R. 1961a. Basilar artery migraine. Lancet 1:15–17.

Bickerstaff, E.R. 1961b. Impairment of consciousness in migraine. Lancet 2:1057–1059.

Biggs, M.J., and Johnson, E.S. 1984. The autonomous nervous system and migraine pathogenesis. In *The Pharmacological Basis of Migraine Therapy*, Eds. W.K. Amery, J.M. Van Nueten, and A. Wauquier, pp. 99–107. London: Pitman.

Bille, B. 1962. Migraine in school children. Acta Paediatr. Suppl. (Uppsala) 51:136.

Bradshaw, P., and Parsons, M. 1965. Hemiplegic migraine: a clinical study. J. Med. 34:65–85.

Breslau, N., Chilcoat, H.D., and Andreski, P. 1996. Further evidence on the link between migraine and neuroticism. Neurology 47:663–667.

Camfield, P.R., Metrakos, K., and Andermann, F. 1978. Basilar migraine, seizures and severe epileptiform EEG abnormalities. Neurology (Minneapolis) 28:584–588.

Caplan, L.R. 1991. Migraine and vertebrobasilar ischemia. Neurology 41:55–61.

Cernibori, A., and Bouquet, F. 1984. Loss of consciousness during basilar artery migraine attack in childhood: EEG and clinical studies. Electroencephalogr. Clin. Neurophysiol. 58:72P(abst).

Dalessio, D.J. 1979. Classification and mechanism of migraine. Headache 19:114–120.

Daly, D.D., and Markand, O.N. 1990. Focal brain lesions. In *Current Practice of Clinical Electroencephalography*, 2nd ed., Eds. D.D. Daly and T.A. Pedley, pp. 35–370. New York: Raven Press.

Degen, R., Degen, H.E., Palm, D., et al. 1980. Die Migraine hémiplégique im Kindesalter. Dtsch. Med. Wochenschr. 105:640–645.

Diamond, S. 1979. Headache: its diagnosis and management (introduction to symposium). Headache 19:113.

Diamond, S., and Dalessio, D.J. 1982. *The Practicing Physician's Approach to Headache.* Baltimore: Williams & Wilkins.

Dow, D.J., and Whitty, C.W. 1947. Electroencephalographic changes in migraine. Review of 51 cases. Lancet 2:52–54.

Drake, M.E., Huber, S.J., Pakalnis, A., et al. 1987. Computerized EEG spectral analysis in migraine and tension headaches. J. Clin. Neurophysiol. 4:301.

Ebersberger, A., Schaible, H.G., Averbeck, B., et al. 2001. Is there a correlation between spreading depression, neurogenic inflammation, and nociception that might cause migraine headache? Ann. Neurol. 49:7–13.

Evers, S., and Goadsby, P.J. 2003. Hypnic headache. Neurology 60:905–909.

Farkas, V., Szeg, L., and Kohlhéb, O. 1985. Hemiplegic migraine in childhood. Differential diagnosis and EEG aspects. Electroencephalogr. Clin. Neurophysiol. 61:4P–5P(abst).

Fozard, J.R. 1980. Proceedings of the International Headache Congress, Florence, 1980. Clin. Psychiatry News 8(9).

Ganji, S., Hellman, S., Stagg, S., et al. 1993. Episodic coma due to acute basilar artery migraine: correlation of EEG and brain stem auditory evoked potentials. Clin. Electroencephalogr. 24:44–48.

Gastaut, H. 1982. A new type of epilepsy: benign partial epilepsy of childhood with occipital spike-waves. Clin. Electroencephalogr. 13:13–22.

Giardina, M., and Sideri, S. 1985. Migraine and epilepsy. Electroencephalogr. Clin. Neurophysiol. 60:71P(abst).

Gibbs, F.A., and Gibbs, E.L. 1964. *Atlas of Electroencephalography*, vol. 3. Reading, MA: Addison-Wesley.

Golla, F.L., and Winter, A.L. 1959. Analysis of cerebral responses to flicker in patients complaining of episodic headache. Electroencephalogr. Clin. Neurophysiol. 11:539–549.

Gorman, M.J., and Welch, K.M.A. 1993. Cerebral blood flow and migraine. In *The Regulation of Cerebral Blood Flow*, Ed. J.W. Phillips, pp. 399–410. Boca Raton: CRC Press.

Gschwend, J. 1972. EEG-Befunde und ihre Interpretation bei einfacher Migräne. J. Neurol. (Berlin) 201:279–292.

Hansen, A.J., Lauritzen, M., and Tfeldt-Hansen, P. 1984. Spreading cortical depression and antimigrainous days. In *The Pharmacological Basis of Migraine Therapy*, Eds. W.K. Amery, J.M. Van Neuten, and A. Wauquier, pp. 161–170. London: Pitman.

Heron, J.R. 1966. Migraine and cerebrovascular disease. Neurology (Minneapolis) 16:1097–1104.

Hess, R. 1977. Epilepsie und Kopfschmerzen. A. EEG-EMG 8:125–136.

Heyck, H. 1956. *Neue Beiträge zur Klinik und Pathogenese der Migräne.* Stuttgart: Thieme.

Heyck, H. 1958. *Der Kopfschmerz.* Stuttgart: Thieme.

Heyck, H., and Hess, R. 1955. Vasomotorische Kopfschmerzen als Symptom larvierter Epilepsien. Schweiz. Med. Wochenschr. 85:573–575.

Huang, J., Cooper, T.G., Santana, B., et al. 2003. Visual distortion provoked by a stimulus in migraine associated with hyperneuronal activity. Headache 43:664–671.

Isler, W. 1969. *Akute Hemiplegien und Hemisyndrome im Kindesalter.* Stuttgart: Thieme.

Jacobs, J., Goadsby, P.J., and Duncan, J.S. 1996. Use of sumatriptan in post-ictal migraine headache. Neurology 47:1104.

Jonkman, E.J., and Lelieveld, M.H.J. 1981. EEG computer analysis in patients with migraine. Electroencephalogr. Clin. Neurophysiol. 52:652–655.

Jung, R. 1953. Neurophysiologische Untersuchungsmethoden. In Handbuch der Inneren Medizin, 4th ed., vol. 5/1, pp. 1206–1314. Berlin: Springer.

Kellaway, P., Crawley, J.W., and Kagawa, N. 1960. Paroxysmal pain and autonomic disturbances of cerebral origin. A specific electroclinical syndrome. Epilepsia (Amsterdam) 1:466–483.

Kinast, M., Lueders, H., Rothner, A.D., et al. 1982. Benign focal epileptiform discharges in childhood migraine (BFEDC). Neurology (NY) 32:1309–1311.

Koehler, B. 1980. Benign paroxysmal vertigo of childhood: a migraine equivalent. Eur. J. Pediatr. 134:149–151.

Krischek, J. 1956. Elektroenzephalographische Befunde bei Migräne. Dtsch. Z. Nervenheilk. 175:43.

Kugler, J. 1979. Elektroenzephalographie und Beziehungen zur Epilepsie. In *Die Migräne*, Ed. D. Soyka, pp. 51–62. Dusseldorf: Labaz.

Lance, J.W., and Anthony, M. 1966. Some clinical aspects of migraine. A prospective survey of 500 patients. Arch. Neurol. (Chicago) 15:356–361.

Lapkin, M.L., French, J.H., Golden, G.S., et al. 1977. The electroencephalogram in childhood basilar artery migraine. Neurology (Minneapolis) 27:580–583.

Laplante, P., Saint-Hilaire, J.M., and Bouvier, G. 1982. Headache as an epileptic manifestation—two cases studied with depth electrodes. Electroencephalogr. Clin. Neurophysiol. 54:36P–37P(abst).

Lashley, K.S. 1941. Patterns of cerebral integration indicated by scotomas of migraine. Arch. Neurol. Psychiatry (Chicago) 46:331–339.

Lauritzen, M., Skyhoj Olsen, T., Lassen, N.A., et al. 1983. Changes in regional cerebral blood flow during the course of classic migraine attacks. Ann. Neurol. 13:633–641.

Leão, A.A.P. 1944. Spreading depression of activity in the cerebral cortex. J. Neurophysiol. 7:359–390.

Leão, A.A.P. 1972. Spreading depression. In *Experimental Models of Epilepsy*, Eds. D.P. Purpura, J.K. Penry, D. Tower, et al., pp. 173–196. New York: Raven Press.

Lees, R., and Watkins, S.M. 1963. Loss of consciousness in migraine. Lancet 2:647–650.

Lérique-Koechlin, A., and Mises, J. 1964. L'EEG dans une manifestation paroxystique non-épileptique de l'enfant: La migraine. Electroencephalogr. Clin. Neurophysiol. 16:203–204.

Martens de Nordhout, A., Timsit-Bertheir, M., Timsit, M., et al. 1986. Contingent negative variation in headache. Ann. Neurol. 19:78–80.

Moore, M.T. 1945. Paroxysmal abdominal pain. A form of symptomatic epilepsy. JAMA 129:1233–1240.

Moskowitz, M.A. 1984. The neurobiology of vascular head pain. *Ann. Neurol.* 16:157–168.

Moskowitz, M.A., Nozaki, K., and Draig, R.P. 1993. Neocortical spreading depression provokes the expression of c-*fos*-protein-like immunoreactivity within trigeminal nucleus caudalis via trigeminovascular mechanisms. J. Neurosci. 13:1167–1177.

Müller, D., and Müller, J. 1977. Die familiäre hemiplegische Migräne. Z. Artzl. Fortibild. 71:763–767.

Niedermeyer, E. 1983. *Epilepsy Guide.* Baltimore: Urban & Schwarzenberg.

Niedermeyer, E. 1990. *The Epilepsies.* Baltimore: Urban & Schwarzenberg.

Niedermeyer, E. 1993. Migraine-triggered epilepsy. Clin. Electroencephalogr. 24:37–43.

Olesen, J. 1991. Conclusions and prospects for the future. In *Migraine and Other Headaches,* Ed. J. Olesen, pp. 347–349. New York: Raven Press.

Olesen, J. 1994. Understanding the biologic basis of migraine. N. Engl. J. Med. 331:1713–1714.

Olesen, J., Tfelt-Hansen, P., and Welch, D.M.A. (Eds.). 1993. *The Headaches.* New York: Raven Press.

Ottman, R., and Lipton, R.B. 1996. Is the comorbidity of epilepsy and migraine due to shared genetic susceptibility? Neurology 47:918–924.

Panayatopoulos, C.P. 1980. Basilar migraine, seizures and severe epileptic EEG abnormalities. Neurology (Minneapolis) 30:1122–1125.

Parain, D., and Samson-Dollfus, D. 1984. Electroencephalograms in basilar artery migraine. Electroencephalogr. Clin. Neurophysiol. 58:392–399.

Pithova, B. 1983. Clinico-EEG correlation in migraine. Electroencephalogr. Clin. Neurophysiol. 55:31P(abst).

Ramelli, G.P., Sturzenegger, M., Donati, F., et al. 1998. EEG findings during basilar migraine attacks in children. Electroencephalogr. Clin. Neurophysiol. 107:374–378.

Raskin, N.H. 1988. The hypnic headache syndrome. Headache 28:534–536.

Rosenbaum, H.E. 1960. Familial hemiplegic migraine. Neurology (Minneapolis) 10:164–170.

Sacks, O. 1985. *Migraine.* Stuttgart: Kohlhammer. (Original English version: *Migraine. The Evolution of a Common Disorder.* London: Faber & Faber.)

Sbrascini, S., and Bassi, P. 1983. Headache and slow hypersynchronization of the EEG during hyperventilation. Electroencephalogr. Clin. Neurophysiol. 55:3P(abst).

Schoenen, J., Jamart, B., De Pasqua, V., et al. 1990. Mapping of EEG and auditory event-potentials in migraine. Electroencephalogr. Clin. Neurophysiol. 75:S134(abst).

Schumacher, G.A., and Wolff, H.G. 1941. Experimental studies on headache. Arch. Neurol. Psychiatry (Chicago) 45:199–214.

Scollo-Lavizzari, G. 1975. Das Elektroenzephalogramm bei der Migräne. Schweiz. Rdsch. Med. (Praxis) 64:234–237.

Selby, G., and Lance, J.W. 1960. Observations on 500 cases of migraine and allied vascular headache. J. Neurol. Neurosurg. Psychiatry 23:23–32.

Seshia, S.S., Reggin, J.D., and Stanwich, R.S. 1985. Migraine and complex seizures in children. Epilepsia (New York) 26:232–236.

Silberstein, S.D., Lipton, R.B., and Sliwinski, M. 1996. Classification of daily and near-daily headaches: field trial of revised IHS criteria. Neurology 47:871–875.

Simon, R.H., Zimmerman, A., Tasman, A., et al. 1982. Spectral analysis of photic stimulation in migraine. Electroencephalogr. Clin. Neurophysiol. 53:270–276.

Skinhoj, E., Hoedt-Rasmussen, K., Paulson, O.B., et al. 1970. Regional cerebral blood flow and its autoregulation in patients with transient focal ischemic attacks. Neurology (Minneapolis) 20:485–493.

Slater, K.H. 1968. Some clinical and EEG findings in migraine. Brain 91: 85–98.

Smyth, V.O.G., and Winter, A.L. 1964. The EEG in migraine. Electroencephalogr. Clin. Neurophysiol. 16:194–202.

Soysal, A., Atay, T., Ozturk, M., et al. 2001. Pattern reversal visual evoked potentials and EEG in migraine with and without visual aura. J. Neurol. Sci. (Turkish) 18:1–8.

Ulett, G.A., Evans, D., and O'Leary, J.L. 1952. Survey of EEG findings in 1,000 patients with chief complaint of headache. Electroencephalogr. Clin. Neurophysiol. 4:463–470.

Walker, M.C., Smith, S.J.M., Sisodiya, S.M., et al. 1995. Case of simple partial status epilepticus in electrophysiological, and magnetic resonance imaging characteristics. Epilepsia 36:1233–1236.

Weil, A.A. 1952. EEG findings in a certain type of psychosomatic headache: dysrhythmic migraine. Electroencephalogr. Clin. Neurophysiol. 4: 181–186.

Weil, A.A. 1962. Observation on dysrhythmic migraine. J. Neurol. Ment. Dis. 134:277–281.

Westmoreland, B. 1978. EEG in the evaluation of headaches. In *Current Practice of Clinical Electroencephalography,* Eds. D.W. Klass and D.D. Daly, pp. 381–394. New York: Raven Press.

Whitty, C.W.M. 1953. Familial hemiplegic migraine. J. Neurol. Neurosurg. Psychiatry 16:172–177.

Wissfeld, E., and Neu, O. 1960. Über die EEG-Verändeungen bei Migräne und die Bedeutung occipitaler Delta-Wellen im EEG. Nervenarzt 31:418.

Wolff, H.G. 1948. *Headache and Other Head Pain.* New York: Oxford University Press.

Woods, R.P., Iacoboni, M., and Mazziota, J.C. 1994. Brief report: bilateral spreading cerebral hypoperfusion during spontaneous migraine headache. N. Engl. J. Med. 331:1689–1692.

30. Psychiatric Disorders and EEG

Joyce G. Small

The place of electroencephalography (EEG) in psychiatry has been consolidated by changes in the official nomenclature beginning with the publication of the third edition of the *Diagnostic and Statistical Manual of Mental Disorders* (DSM-III) (American Psychiatric Association, 1980) followed by the revised edition (DSM-III-R) in 1987, and DSM-IV in 1994. Taken together these diagnostic schema represent major changes in American psychiatry, leading the field away from dynamic speculation and toward the medical model. Although DSM-III, DSM-III-R, and DSM-IV claim to be atheoretical about the causality of psychiatric disorders, it is clear that they have a strong biological orientation. DSM-IV modifies that trend to some extent with the introduction of cultural and ethnic influences and spiritual issues. As in previous editions, DSM-IV retains the multiaxial approach with Axis I devoted to clinical syndromes, Axis II to personality constellations, Axis III to physical illnesses, Axis IV to psychosocial stressors, and Axis V to levels of adaptive functioning. Publication of DSM-V is anticipated between 2007 and 2010. A multidimensional taxonomy is under consideration, which may include more etiological data with findings from epidemiology, neuroimaging, genetics, and other areas. Comorbidity and longitudinal course over the life span may also be incorporated (Helzer and Hudziak, 2002).

These changes have been introduced within a relatively short period of time, so the impact upon the practice of psychiatry is still to be realized. Thus far, users of these systems have found their strengths to include provision of a common language for diagnosis and specific criteria leading to improved diagnostic reliability (Jampala et al., 1992). Detractors object to the use of a "cookbook" approach, which detracts from a deeper understanding of patients' problems and the contribution of specific circumstances to emotional disturbances. It is true that the focus has become relatively superficial with loss of the comprehensive approach of psychoanalysis and Meyerian psychiatry, which emphasize psychodynamics and longitudinal development (Wilson, 1993). However, the DSM methodology facilitates the educational process in psychiatry and encourages a more data oriented, systematic process.

These changes in psychiatry have reaffirmed the importance of electroencephalography along with contributions from genetics, neuroimaging, biochemistry, endocrinology, and other disciplines. As Preskorn (1995) has observed, clinical diagnosis can be viewed as composed of four hierarchical stages, namely symptomatic, syndromic, pathophysiological, and pathoetiological. DSM-IV attends to the first two, whereas EEG and other laboratory investigations deal with the third. The fourth is still elusive in psychiatry but may eventually follow from meticulous application of the other three combined with findings from basic and clinical research as proposed for DSM-V. The concept of endophenotype in psychiatry combines diagnostic classification with genomic analysis that may include multidimensional data to clarify pathways between disease presentation and genotype (Gottesman and Gould, 2003).

Paralleling the above developments there has been an increased interest in EEG applied to psychiatry. Several compendia have appeared about EEG screening and indications for referral in psychiatric populations (Boutros, 1992; Boutros and Struve, 2002; Hughes, 1996; Hughes and John, 1999; Warner et al., 1990). An annotated bibliography of significant EEG-psychiatric references was published (Hughes, 1995). In 1999 two professional groups, the American Psychiatric Electrophysiological Association (APEA) and the American Medical EEG Association (AMEEGA) merged to form the EEG and Clinical Neuroscience Society (Boutros, 2000; Khoshbin, 2000). This combined neurological and psychiatric group is concerned with establishing standards for practice and training in diagnostic and therapeutic electrophysiological procedures and with advancing basic and applied research.

Disorders Usually First Diagnosed in Infancy, Childhood, or Adolescence

The first section of the DSM-IV discusses disorders that usually originate in infancy, childhood, or adolescence.

Mental Retardation

Mental retardation is subdivided into levels of severity up to a maximum I.Q. of 70. Borderline intellectual functioning (I.Q. in the 71 to 84 range) is not listed as a specific diagnosis but is included in a supplementary V-code to be used whenever intellectual limitations at this level contribute to deficits in adaptive behavior.

Clinical investigations of mental retardation involve formal psychological assessments of intellectual level and judgments of adaptive capacities in multiple areas. EEG findings are of importance in many syndromes associated with mental retardation, with an increasing incidence of EEG abnormalities and seizure disorders proportional to the degree of intellectual impairment. EEG is necessary to classify seizures and to identify electroclinical syndromes associated with developmental delay that may or may not exhibit seizures (Sheth, 1998). Video-EEG monitoring has been found useful in defining paroxysmal episodes of uncertain etiology especially in mentally retarded children (Bye et al., 2000; Paolicchi, 2002; Thirumalai et al., 2001). Moreover, the EEG is helpful in monitoring conditions in which deterioration or changes over time may be expected, particularly if individuals display such distinctive manifestations as hypsarrhythmia, petit mal variant discharges, or periodic EEG complexes. In other situations there may be some common EEG features, as for example a relative lack of positive spiking in Down's syndrome (Gibbs and Gibbs, 1964). Alzheimer fibrillary changes and mental deterioration may occur in the latter disorder, often accompanied by EEG abnormalities. In some cases, the development of paroxysmal EEG abnormalities may forecast the onset of seizure disorders (Pueschel et al., 1991). Katada et al. (2000) demonstrated progressive slowing of occipital alpha frequencies at an earlier age in Down's syndrome than in other kinds of mental retardation. Fragile X syndrome is associated with epileptiform EEGs and increased seizure incidence, but centrotemporal spikes resembling benign rolandic epilepsy are the most common EEG manifestations (Berry-Kravis, 2002). In this regard, technically adequate EEG studies of retarded and other severely impaired groups, particularly in disturbed children, are difficult to obtain. Generally, repeated studies with long sampling times must be used to acquire technically adequate recordings during waking, activation procedures, drowsiness, and light sleep.

Learning Disorders
(Formerly Academic Skills Disorders)

The learning disorders section of the DSM-IV includes reading disorder, mathematics disorder, disorder of written expression, and learning disorder not otherwise specified (NOS). EEGs and other assessments of central nervous system (CNS) integrity are appropriate investigations in children with these disabilities. A comprehensive description of the causes, diagnostic investigations, and therapeutic interventions in cases of learning disabilities was contributed by Gillberg and Soderstrom (2003).

Developmental reading disorder or dyslexia has received the most neurophysiological attention. Hughes (1971) studied a large number of children with reading disabilities and found an excess (37%) of usually mild, nonspecific abnormal EEG features that were correlated with lower scholastic achievement. Hemispheric specialization in children with dyslexia has also been investigated. Some experimental evidence suggests that in boys there may be left hemispheric dysfunction, lack of functional specialization of the right hemisphere, or possibly both, whereas left hemispheric dysfunction is sufficient for dyslexia in girls (Witelson, 1977).

Sections that follow in the DSM-IV discuss developmental coordination disorder and receptive and expressive language disabilities including phonological disorder, stuttering, and nonspecific communication disorders. Epileptiform EEG abnormalities occur in the Landau-Kleffner syndrome (acquired epileptic aphasia), which is classified as a mixed receptive-expressive language disorder (Gordon, 2000; Nass et al., 1998). Epileptiform and nonspecific EEG abnormalities were also more common in stutterers than in normal controls (Okasha et al., 1974), suggesting underlying cerebral dysfunction. Studies of slow potentials preceding stuttered speech revealed fewer lateralized asymmetries than with normal speech (Zimmermann and Knott, 1974).

Pervasive Developmental Disorders

The next section of the DSM-IV deals with developmental disorders. This category replaces previous ambiguous

and misleading terms such as *symbiotic psychosis* and *childhood schizophrenia*. The section has been expanded since the last edition of the manual to include Rett's disorder, childhood disintegrative disorder, and Asperger's disorder. The purpose of these changes was to improve differential diagnosis and to avoid overuse of NOS. Autistic disorder is the first listed diagnosis; it is characterized by onset prior to 3 years of age with typical features of markedly abnormal development of social interaction and communication and restricted interests and activities. There are associated diagnoses of mental retardation and seizure disorders in 25% to 40% of cases followed to adolescence (Giovanardi et al. 2000). Predisposing factors include neurological disorders such as maternal rubella, untreated phenylketonuria, tuberous sclerosis, anoxic birth, encephalitis, meningitis, infantile spasms, and fragile X syndrome. EEG characteristics are not mentioned specifically, but this is a disorder in which there have been extensive studies of EEG characteristics. The incidence of EEG abnormalities among autistic subjects ranges from 10% to 83%, with an average of 50% (Small, 1975; Small et al., 1977).

There is disagreement in the literature about the kinds of EEG abnormalities and their clinical correlations, which may be explained in part by technical difficulties in obtaining adequate studies during waking, activation procedures, and sleep in uncooperative subjects. Findings from the major studies with assessment of technical adequacy are shown in Table 30.1 (derived from Netley et al., 1975; Small et al., 1977; Tsai and Tsai, 1985; Waldo et al., 1978). Pooling of the data revealed that EEG abnormalities were most prominent in the autistic subjects, followed by children with other psychiatric disorders and normal controls ($p < .005$). Hashimoto et al. (2001) found epileptiform activity during sleep EEG recordings in 43% of autistics, mostly localized frontal spikes. Data from these kinds of studies and quantitative investigations of neurophysiological data have added significantly to the evidence that autistic disorder is characterized by severe CNS impairment (James and Barry, 1980). Abnormal EEG features were significantly associated with poorer outcome as measured by quantitative assessments of intelligence, speech and educational achievement, and follow-up functioning in one of the largest series, compiled by DeMyer et al. (1973, 1981).

Rett's disorder is characterized by the development of multiple deficits following a period of normal postnatal functioning, unlike autistic disorder in which delays are present earlier. Severe mental retardation, EEG abnormalities, and seizures are more frequent than in autistic disorder, although the two syndromes have not been systematically compared. Rett's disorder is much less common than autistic disorder and has been reported almost entirely in females (Glaze, 2002). A report of EEG findings in ten girls with Rett's syndrome showed persistent rhythmic theta activity during both waking and sleep (Neidermeyer et al., 1997). Childhood disintegrative disorder consists of marked deterioration in multiple areas of functioning following a period of at least 2 years of normal development. Other terms for this condition are Heller's syndrome, dementia infantilis, and disintegrative psychosis. It is a rare disorder occurring mostly in males, associated with severe

Table 30.1. EEG Studies of Autism and Childhood

Study	Autistic Children		Other Psychiatric Diagnoses		Normal Children		Technique of EEG Examination			
	n	% Abnormal EEG	n	% Abnormal EEG	n	% Abnormal EEG	Photic	Sleep	Repeated Tracings	Blind Interpretation
White et al., 1964	102	53	47	47	13	0	—	Most	Done	Done
Fish and Shapiro, 1965	29	30	—	—	—	—	—	—	—	Done
Hutt et al., 1965	10	10	—	—	60	0	—	70%	Done	—
Small, 1968	33	79	67	72	25	0	Done	100%	Done	Done
Creak and Pampiglione, 1969	35	83	—	—	—	—	Most	Few	—	—
Stevens and Milstein, 1970	100	39	97	47	87	10	Done	50%	—	—
Ritvo et al., 1970	86	34	98	37	—	—	—	Attempted in all	Done	Done
Gubbay et al., 1970	22	77	—	—	23	13	—	When possible	—	Done
Treffert, 1970	29	14	211	36	—	—	—	—	—	—
Kolvin, 1971	44	32	28	32	—	—	—	—	—	—
Small, 1975	147	65	87	46	34	6	Done	Done	Done	Done
Netley et al., 1975	15	67	—	—	—	—	—	—	—	—
Waldo et al., 1978	48	50	55	43	—	—	Done	—	Done	—
Tsai et al., 1985	100	47	—	—	—	—	Done	Done	—	—
Subjects of all studies combined[a]	800	50	690	44	242	6				

[a]Comparisons of autistics vs other diagnoses, vs normals, $p < .005$. Comparisons of autistics vs diagnoses, $p < .025$.

mental retardation and increased incidence of EEG abnormalities and seizures.

Asperger's disorder also features severe and sustained impairments in social interaction and restricted repetitive patterns of behavior, interests, and activities with significant deficits in multiple areas of functioning. It is usually recognized at an older age than autistic disorder since there are no clinically significant delays in language or cognitive development. Deficits in social spheres are continuous throughout life but patients are capable of better functioning than in other categories. Sleep EEG studies showed sleep disruptions and periodic leg movements in sleep in a series of eight Asperger patients compared to matched normal controls (Godbout et al., 2000).

Attention-Deficit and Disruptive Behavior Disorders

The next section of DSM-IV is devoted to attention-deficit/hyperactivity disorder (ADHD), conduct disorder, oppositional defiant disorder, and disruptive behavior disorder NOS. The first mentioned replaces a number of popular labels that misleadingly implied an etiological basis for these problems without good scientific foundation. Some of the terms attached to this kind of behavior include hyperkinetic reaction of childhood, hyperkinetic syndrome, hyperactive child syndrome, minimal brain damage, minimal brain dysfunction (MBD), minimal cerebral dysfunction, and minor cerebral dysfunction. These disorders are characterized essentially by developmentally inappropriate inattention, impulsivity, and hyperactivity. In DSM-IV the definition of this disorder has become more circumscribed, with more explicit requirements that there must be clinically significant impairments, onset before age 7, and symptoms that occur in two or more different settings. There is now a single diagnostic category with three subtypes: predominantly inattentive type,

hyperactive-impulsive type, and combined type. These conditions may follow at least three typical courses: all symptoms can persist into adolescence or adult life; the disorder may be self-limiting, with all symptoms disappearing at puberty; or hyperactivity may disappear, but attentional difficulties and impulsivity persist. Moreover, this syndrome may evolve into other kinds of adult psychopathology. The relative frequency of these outcomes is still unknown, although a substantial number of affected individuals become delinquent in adolescence. Recent longitudinal data confirm that ADHD children are at a high risk of developing multiple impairments in cognition, interpersonal, school, and family functioning. Associated psychiatric comorbidity can be present during childhood (Biederman et al., 1996).

Although EEG is not mentioned in DSM-IV, EEG abnormalities are frequent associated features. Such children were the subjects of controlled EEG studies well before publication of DSM-III. With remarkable uniformity, the majority reported an excess of abnormal EEGs in the affected children. The most commonly encountered abnormality was diffuse generalized and/or intermittent slowing outside of normal limits for chronological age in 30% to 60% of cases (Small et al., 1978a). There have been conflicting reports of deviant photic excitability (Milstein and Small, 1974; Shetty, 1971). EEG abnormalities tend to disappear with advancing age (Hechtman et al., 1978; Small et al., 1978a; Weiss and Hechtman, 1979). Several authors ascribed prognostic significance to the EEG findings, particularly in predicting response to stimulant drug therapy, but findings were contradictory with reports of good, poor, or no relationship between abnormal EEGs and therapeutic response (Small et al., 1978a).

Satterfield and Schell (1984) published a pivotal long-term follow-up study in which 110 boys with attention deficits and hyperactivity and 75 normal children were studied with clinical EEGs, auditory event-related potentials (AERPs), and EEG power spectral data. Diagnostic criteria applied were similar to DSM-IV. The children were studied between the ages of 6 and 12 years and followed at ages 14 to 20, by which time 31 (28%) had become seriously delinquent, with multiple arrests for felony offenses. Baseline EEG and other data were compared for the children who became delinquent, nondelinquent hyperactives, and normals. The patients who became delinquent in their teens were characterized in childhood by normal EEGs and power spectral and AERP measures similar to normals. The nondelinquent group had more clinical EEG abnormalities and abnormal EEG power spectral values, as well as significantly lower amplitudes of the second negative potential of the AERP. The authors speculated that the nondelinquent children may have had underlying brain dysfunctions, whereas the children with normal EEG and AERP findings may have had problems secondary to environmental and social factors and/or familial and genetic influences. Observations that abnormal EEG and other neurophysiological indications of brain dysfunctions are predictive of better outcome than normal findings in psychiatric patients are not unique to children with attention deficits, as will be elucidated later in this chapter.

Barry et al., (2003) contributed an extensive description of the electrophysiological features of ADHD. They began with the earliest study of EEG abnormalities by Jasper et al. (1938) and reviewed the older literature progressing to recent quantitative EEG (qEEG) and evolved potentials (EP). The most consistent EEG finding was increased slowing with increased relative theta power in ADHD groups relative to normal children. Two models of ADHD were proposed based on the EEG studies, namely maturational lag and developmental deviation. Cortical underarousal was been proposed to account for the maturational lag subgroup, whereas other clinical groups may have a different pathophysiology. Clarke et al. (2002a) also proposed two major subtypes consisting of a cortically hypoaroused group and a group with delayed CNS maturation. These conclusions were based on EEG clusters in a study of 100 boys with ADHD of the inattentive type. Clarke et al. (2002b) also studied 100 girls with ADHD and matched controls, finding that the neurophysiological characteristics of girls were more homogeneous than in boys with cortical hypoarousal as the main underlying pathophysiology. They assumed that girls with maturational lags in CNS development are not as frequently referred for therapeutic intervention because their behavior is less disruptive. Niedermeyer and Naidu, (1997) offered a neurological concept of ADHD etiology proposing dysfunctional connections between frontal and motor cortical pathways. A functionally "lazy" frontal lobe accounts for disinhibited motor activity and impaired attention. Stimulant therapy may energize or "whip" the frontal cortex thereby enhancing inhibition.

Conduct Disorders

The essential features of conduct disorder are repetitive and persistent patterns of behavior wherein the basic rights of others or age-appropriate societal norms or rules are violated. The diagnostic criteria involve deviant behavior in several categories, namely aggressive conduct, threatening people or animals, behavior leading to property loss or damage, deceitfulness or theft, and serious rule violations. DSM-

IV adds two subtypes depending on age of onset. Identification prior to age 10 is predictive of increased likelihood of aggressive behavior, familial loading of conduct disorders, and later development of antisocial personality disorder. Adolescent onset is generally more benign. EEG studies of these subtypes have not yet been accomplished. DSM-IV mentions lower levels of physiological arousal in children with conduct disorder compared to normals, but does not mention EEG. However, the older literature suggested that delinquent subgroups have EEG characteristics typical of individuals of younger chronological age. Temporal and posterior temporal abnormalities and paroxysmal features have been described. However, some authors have concluded that EEG studies in these situations are of limited value in the absence of positive neurological findings (Phillips et al., 1993).

For several years it was argued that 14 and 6/sec positive spikes were associated with antisocial conduct, impulsive and aggressive behavior, and even homicidal violence, but controlled investigations failed to support these relationships (Klass and Westmoreland, 1985). Nevertheless, the controversy continues with the DeLong et al. 1987 study showing that prominent 14 & 6 complexes in children are associated with temper outbursts and mood, learning, and sleep abnormalities. Krynicki (1978) observed that aggressive behavior in hospitalized adolescents, whether associated with CNS disorders or not, was associated with paroxysmal EEG activity in the frontal areas, whereas nonassaultive behavior disorder patients did not display these EEG patterns. The remainder of this section is taken up with oppositional defiant disorder, a less severe pattern of disruptive behavior that does not violate the basic rights of others. Unlike in adults, DSM-IV does not stress underlying medical conditions in children with behavior problems. However Austin et al. (2002) reported a controlled study of 224 children with recent onset of seizures compared to 159 sibling controls. Patients experiencing seizures had more conduct problems than controls implicating underlying neurological disorders for both seizures and aberrant behavior.

Feeding and Eating Disorder of Infancy or Early Childhood

This DSM-IV section begins with pica, defined as the persistent eating of nonnutritive substances for an extended period of time. EEG studies of this condition have not been conducted per se, although some associated conditions such as mental retardation, lead poisoning, and malnutrition may be associated with EEG abnormalities. Likewise rumination disorder characterized by regurgitation and rechewing of food in an infant or child is not known to be associated with EEG abnormalities. Another listed category is feeding disorder of infancy or early childhood, which is essentially a failure to thrive.

Tic Disorders

This DSM-IV section includes Tourette's disorder, chronic motor or vocal tic disorder, transient tic disorder, and tic disorder NOS. Historically, many of these conditions have been considered as purely psychological, but now there is considerable evidence that at least some of them involve underlying neurological disorders. Tourette's disorder is a case in point; the evidence for neurological dysfunction includes (a) findings of subtle neurological abnormalities in 50% of cases; (b) one third of such patients are left-handed or ambidextrous; (c) EEG abnormalities occur in 25% to 75% of cases; and (d) such patients are often hyperactive during infancy and childhood with perceptual abnormalities (Gilroy and Meyer, 1975). EEG findings typically consist of bilateral or unilateral paroxysmal sharp activity and generalized or focal slowing. However, effects of medications and associated conditions may account for some or all observed EEG abnormalities (Drake et al., 1991). One study showed no differences between Tourette's patients and normal controls (Neufeld et al., 1990). However, a cross-cultural investigation found a uniformly increased incidence of nonspecific EEG abnormalities (Staley et al., 1997). Further, investigations of 12 sets of monozygotic twins with Tourette's syndrome revealed more abnormal EEGs in the twin with the more severe tic disorder (Hyde et al., 1994). Abnormalities consisted mostly of generalized and regional theta slowing emphasized in the frontocentral areas associated with more serious impairments and poorer neuropsychological test performance. This suggested dysfunctions extending beyond the basal ganglia to the thalamus and/or cortex. Medication effects did not appear to contribute significantly. Semerci (2000) studied 40 children and adolescents with Tourette's disorder, finding nonspecific EEG abnormalities and neurological soft signs in 58%, which were significantly associated with low performance IQ scores. Drake et al. (1992) used cassette EEGs to record sleep EEGs in 20 Tourette's disorder outpatients, finding multiple sleep disturbances that varied with different Tourette's disorder symptomatology.

Elimination Disorders

This DSM-IV section concludes with entities of encopresis and enuresis. Functional enuresis has been demonstrated to occur during non-rapid-eye-movement (REM) or beginning REM stages of sleep. The diagnostic workup must rule out possible seizure disorders. On the other hand, functional encopresis is more frequently under voluntary control.

There have been a number of recent polysomnographic studies of enuretic children. Bader et al. (2002) studied 21 children with primary nocturnal enuresis and age-matched controls. Micturition occurred during the first half of the night and was not linked to any specific sleep stage. Tachycardia and brief EEG arousal sometimes preceded voiding. The authors concluded that the sleep of enuretic children is normal but autonomic arousal occurs prior to micturition. Clinical and qEEGs were examined in children with primary nocturnal enuresis by Hallioglu et al. (2001), who concluded that the EEG evidence suggested delayed cerebral maturation. Imada et al. (1998) identified subtypes of enuresis classified by overnight EEG monitoring and cystometry. Best therapeutic results were achieved in patients with normal cystometrograms and EEG arousal responses without awakening before enuresis. Poorest outcome was associated with abnormal cystometry and no EEG arousal (Kawauchi et al., 1998).

Other Disorders of Infancy, Childhood, or Adolescence

The DSM-IV section on childhood disorders concludes with a miscellaneous category that includes separation anxiety disorder, selective mutism, reactive attachment disorder of infancy or early childhood, stereotypic movement disorder, and an NOS category. There have been few EEG studies of these kinds of children. As a matter of fact they tend to be included more often in control groups, as for example, in studies in which autistic children were the experimental subjects.

Stereotypic movement disorder can be associated with medical conditions such as fragile X syndrome, de Lange syndrome, and Lesch-Nyhan syndrome, which may have EEG concomitants. Similar movements also occur in association with mental retardation, pervasive developmental disorders, and obsessive-compulsive disorder, from which they must be differentiated. Other diagnostic considerations include simple and complex motor tics, specific repetitive behavior such as trichotillomania, and involuntary movements associated with neurological conditions such as Huntington's disease. Factitious disorder and self-mutilation in association with other psychiatric illnesses must also be ruled out before this diagnosis is assigned.

Delirium, Dementia, and Amnestic and Other Cognitive Disorders

Major changes have taken place in DSM-IV in these categories. The term *organic mental disorder* has been eliminated because of the misleading implication that other psychiatric disorders do not have an organic basis, recognizing that most if not all have biological as well as psychological and social components. Several conditions listed in DSM-III and DSM-III-R have been shifted to other parts of the manual wherein conditions with similar phenomenological features are grouped together (tabulated in Frances et al., 1995). These changes have shortened this section, which is now limited to the syndromes listed in the title.

It is in these areas that the EEG has perhaps the most to contribute to clinical psychiatry. Simple reliance on descriptive criteria of each syndrome will lead to considerable misdiagnosis. Unsuspected organic conditions may be missed in the case of conditions resembling functional psychiatric illnesses, whereas situations that resemble delirium or dementia may turn out to be functional psychoses or pseudodementias. EEG provides an important inexpensive, noninvasive test to increase the accuracy of diagnostic assessment (Itil, 1982; Koshino, 1989; Lipowski, 1980; Pro and Wells, 1977). Many researchers advise that all hospitalized psychiatric patients should receive such studies, reasoning that it is not possible to discriminate clinically among a wide variety of physical illnesses that present with psychiatric disturbances and functional disorders. Moreover, it has been shown that simply referring suspect cases for EEG examinations does not identify even half of the patients who demonstrate presumptive evidence of some degree of organic involvement on the basis of EEG (Boutros, 1992; Boutros and Struve, 2002; Gibbs and Novick, 1977; Hughes and John, 1999; Small et al., 1966; Struve, 1976, 1977).

However, Warner et al. (1990) found that routine EEG screening of adult psychiatric patients led to a change in diagnosis or treatment in only 2% of cases and questioned its utility. Letters in rebuttal challenged this viewpoint (Schwitzer et al., 1992; Serafetinides, 1993).

Woods and Short (1985) proposed that major psychiatric illnesses are associated with a high incidence of neurological abnormalities that cannot be attributed to psychoses per se, medications, or neurological disease, but have important implications for understanding causation and for guiding prognosis and choice of treatment. This neurological dimension of psychiatry is even more important in the elderly, where the EEG and other studies are valuable in distinguishing pseudodementia, a clinical picture indistinguishable from organic dementia but usually produced by primary affective illness or other functional disorder. To illustrate, Weiner et al. (1991) found that 6% of patients attending a dementia clinic had no cognitive impairment, and that 42% suffered from depression. Such a distinction is enormously important, given the potential for effective treatment of the latter. The converse, however, is also true. Organic mental states, particularly in the elderly, may present as typical mood disorders, which turn out on careful investigation to have an underlying organic basis, often with negative implications for treatment (Holschneider and Leuchter, 1999; Katz et al., 2001; Rosen, 1997; Shulman and Post, 1980). Depression can also be a risk factor or prodrome of vascular dementia and Alzheimer's disease (Kennedy and Scalmati, 2001) especially onset of depression after age 60 (Muller et al., 1997).

Delirium is a syndrome in which the EEG most often corresponds with the clinical picture of clouding of consciousness; changes in psychomotor activity, alterations in sleep, speech, and perception; and disorientation and memory impairment. DSM-IV divides delirium into five categories: general medical conditions, substance intoxication, substance withdrawal, multiple etiologies, and NOS. Deliria from almost all causes are accompanied by generalized theta and/or delta EEG slowing, background disorganization, and loss of reactivity to eye opening and closing proportional to the degree of severity (Jacobson and Jerrier, 2000). Patients may also exhibit reversed or irregular sleep-wake patterns frequently accompanied by wandering and other disruptive behavior (Sato et al., 1996). These manifestations are usually short-lived, resolving at a rate corresponding to clearing of clinical symptoms. However, there are exceptions. An example is delirium tremens, which frequently is not associated with much EEG slowing despite profound mental disturbance (Allahyari et al., 1976). Findings of normal or low-voltage fast EEGs are usual, although dominant background frequencies may be 1 or 2 Hz slower than in the unintoxicated baseline state. Thus an excessively fast or normal EEG in the presence of acute delirium can be clinically useful in raising the question of a state of alcohol withdrawal. Conversely, a grossly slow EEG in a patient suspected of delirium tremens should arouse suspicion of more complicated etiology, such as hepatic encephalopathy or Wernicke's syndrome (Hughes, 1996; Kelley and Reilly, 1983). Another atypical situation is delirium produced by anticholinergic drugs, which is associated with paradoxical EEG findings with reduction of slow-wave ac-

tivity and desynchronization (Fink, 1979). Delirium may be superimposed upon a chronic demented state. In this instance EEG findings are similar to delirium without dementia (Trzepacz et al., 1998). Liptzin et al. (1991) and Liptzin and Levkoff (1992) recommended that better operational criteria for delirium are needed since different nosological systems do not identify the same patients.

Unlike previous editions, DSM-IV specifically mentions the neuroleptic malignant syndrome (NMS), a condition with prominent delirious features. Differential diagnosis includes encephalitis, heat stroke, malignant hyperthermia with anesthetics, abrupt discontinuation of antiparkinsonian medications, and lethal catatonia. The diagnosis depends on both clinical and laboratory evidence, the latter mainly consisting of leukocytosis and evidence of muscle injury with elevated creatine phosphokinase (CPK). The literature indicates that EEGs are either normal or reveal mild nonspecific abnormalities (Addonizio et al., 1987; Fleischhacker et al., 1990; Kurlan et al., 1984; Rosebush and Stewart, 1989). However, nonconvulsive status epilepticus in patients without histories of epilepsy have been reported as complications of NMS (Yoshino et al., 1998, 2000). Nevertheless, the EEG may provide the only indication of CNS involvement aside from changes in levels of consciousness. DSM-IV estimates the mortality as 10% to 20%, acknowledging that fatality rates have decreased with improved recognition and treatment.

While NMS would be classified in DSM-IV as a substance-induced delirium, it is less clear where the phenomenon of water intoxication should be placed except under the NOS heading. Water intoxication is a life-threatening phenomenon resulting from compulsive water drinking associated with hyponatremia and increased vasopressin secretion, which is not uncommonly encountered in psychotic patients. It may be accompanied by worsening of psychosis (Goldman et al., 1997) as well as neuropsychological impairments and delirious features, which can progress to grand mal seizures, coma, and death (Shutty et al., 1993). EEGs may be normal or exhibit mild to profound abnormalities that do not correspond closely to electrolyte changes but may reflect the severity of cerebral edema. Yoshino (1989) summarized the EEG and clinical literature on this subject, pointing out that water intoxication belongs in the differential diagnosis of seizures in psychiatric patients.

Dementia

This section in DSM-IV is organized under headings of dementia of the Alzheimer's type, vascular dementia, dementia due to HIV, head trauma, and various disease entities such as Parkinson's, Huntington's, Pick's, Creutzfeldt-Jakob, as well as general medical conditions, and substance-induced persisting dementia. In addition there are categories of dementia due to multiple etiologies and NOS. The EEG is not mentioned as a specific diagnostic procedure except for the typical periodic discharges in Creutzfeldt-Jakob disease. However, triphasic waves may also appear in elderly psychiatric patients with other severe forms of dementia (Blatt and Brenner, 1996). Diagnosis of delirium, dementia, and seizure disorders is the major role of EEG in clinical and geriatric psychiatry as expounded in Holschneider and

Leuchter (1999). Moreover, treatable dementias associated with late-onset epilepsy and sleep apnea can be identified with EEG investigations.

Differentiation of dementia of the Alzheimer's type and vascular dementia is difficult during life. Reviews by Liston and LaRue (1983a,b) conclude that critical examination of representative pathological studies published over the last 40 years does not support the position that primary degenerative and multi-infarct dementias can be differentiated on the basis of clinical or laboratory criteria. Separating these conditions is important, both for clinical management and for research purposes, but until specific biological markers are used clinically for distinguishing primary degenerative dementia, this diagnosis will probably continue to be made by exclusion. Focal or lateralized EEG abnormalities may be more typical of multi-infarct dementia, but they occur frequently enough in degenerative dementia to lack diagnostic specificity. Moreover, in one study more than 60% of patients with angiographic evidence of ischemic lesions and reduced cerebral blood flow did not show focal EEG changes. Diffuse EEG abnormalities were equally common in groups with and without angiographic and other evidence of vascular disease (Loeb, 1980).

Clinical criteria such as abrupt onset, history of stroke, and focal symptoms are also unreliable, occurring in only about half of cases that ultimately receive a confirmed diagnosis of multi-infarct dementia. A study of 75 autopsy confirmed cases with Alzheimer's disease and 56 matched normal controls revealed that waking EEG abnormalities had a diagnostic sensitivity of 0.87 and specificity of 0.83, which exceeds the yield of other more expensive and invasive imaging procedures. This implies that a diagnosis of Alzheimer's should not be conferred on apparently demented patients with normal EEGs without considerable investigation. Moderate or severe abnormalities are much more likely to be present in Alzheimer's dementia (Robinson et al., 1994; Soininen et al., 1992). Dementia with Lewy bodies is sometimes associated with bilateral frontal intermittent rhythmic delta activity (FIRDA) (Calzetti et al., 2002).

In recent years qEEG studies of dementia predominate. Lindau et al. (2003) found that qEEG and neuropsychological test evidence discriminated between frontotemporal dementia (Pick's disease) and Alzheimer's. However, clinical EEG has advantages of practicality, patient acceptance, availability, and low cost, and is recommended if there is a question of seizures, loss of consciousness, episodic confusion, or rapid deterioration (Kawas, 2003). Rae-Grant et al. (1987) studied 139 patients with Alzheimer's dementia and age-matched controls over a period of 1 to 4 years. EEGs were significantly more abnormal in probands than controls, and severity of EEG disturbance was significantly correlated with impaired psychometric test performance. Diagnosis was confirmed by autopsy in 29 patients in whom EEG abnormalities were shown to be correlated with neuron density but not neurofibrillary tangles. Helkala et al. (1991) followed 24 Alzheimer patients with EEGs, half of whom displayed index EEG abnormalities. Cognitive decline was more prominent in the latter, although clinical severity of dementia increased in both groups. They concluded that an abnormal EEG at an early stage of Alzheimer's may predict a more severe course of cognitive deterioration. Robinson et al. (1994) reported waking EEG findings in 75 patients with Alzheimer's and 13 with mixed Alzheimer and multi-infarct dementia (autopsy confirmed), showing that waking EEG abnormalities are highly predictive of Alzheimer's dementia. Claus et al. (1999) showed that EEG slowing and reactivity discriminated between Alzheimer patients and controls. Kowalski et al. (2001) also studied cases of mild marked and severe dementia. Significant correlations were identified between cognitive impairment and the degree of EEG abnormalities in background, theta and delta waves, focal and lateralized changes, synchronization, and presence of sharp waves and spikes. Matousek et al. (2001) found that EEG slowing was more strongly associated with parietal lobe syndromes than with other neurological deficits and types of cognitive impairment.

Amnestic Disorders

This section deals with disturbances in memory secondary to general medical conditions or persisting effects of toxic substances divided into sections of amnestic disorder due to a general medical condition, substance-induced persisting amnestic disorder, and a NOS category. DSM-IV divides these states into transient—memory impairments lasting for a month or less—and chronic—lasting for longer periods of time. A special instance of transient amnestic states in psychiatry develops after electroconvulsive therapy (ECT). These are prone to occur with closely spaced, frequent seizures induced with high-energy, bilateral, sine wave electrical stimulation (Small et al., 1978b). Generalized and paroxysmal EEG slowing appears after a series of five or fewer treatments; it is more prominent 24 hours after seizures than 1 or 2 hours postictal. Interictal slowing is less pronounced with unilateral ECT and brief pulse electrical stimuli. Post-ECT cognitive impairments are associated with increased EEG delta and theta power, which varies with electrode placement and stimulus intensity (Sackeim et al., 2000). Rare cases of nonconvulsive status epilepticus (NCSE) after ECT have been reported (Povlsen et al., 2003). Similar situations with postictal amnesic phenomena and NCSE occur in epileptic patients, which can be misdiagnosed as transient global amnesia without appropriate EEG studies (Kapur, 1993; Lancman, 1999). Cognitive side effects and EEG changes may also accompany repetitive transcranial magnetic stimulation. EEG monitoring is recommended for therapeutic and safety reasons (Boutros et al., 2000a; Krystal et al., 2000).

Mental Disorders Due to a General Medical Condition

These conditions were formerly listed under the organic disorders, a term eliminated in DSM-IV. Clinical pictures may vary widely including delirium, dementia, and amnestic disorder as previously described as well as psychotic disorder, mood disorder, anxiety disorder, sexual dysfunction, and sleep disorder. The major consideration is that there be evidence from the history, physical examination, or laboratory findings that the observed disturbances are direct physiological consequences of a general medical condition, and not better accounted for by another mental disorder and not occurring exclusively during the course of a delirium. Each syndrome is discussed in detail in the appropriate DSM-IV sections except for catatonic disorder and personality change, which are elucidated in this part of the manual.

The DSM-IV recognizes that catatonic disorder does not occur exclusively in schizophrenia but is a form of delirium encountered in affective disorders and in medical and neurological conditions such as neoplasms, head trauma, cerebral vascular disease, encephalitis, and numerous toxic and metabolic disturbances. Although not mentioned specifically, EEG studies are indicated for diagnosis. Moreover, the older literature contains repeated mention of a high incidence of paroxysmal EEG abnormalities and lower seizure threshold in catatonia that can be associated with altered nitrogen balance and thyroid dysfunctions. NMS, discussed previously, may be a malignant variant of catatonia since the two conditions have many features in common (White and Robins, 1991), including abnormal EEGs (Carroll and Boutros, 1995). Moreover, benzodiazepines can temporarily reverse catatonic symptoms from whatever cause, including those secondary to neuroleptics and epilepsy (Fricchione, 1989). ECT is often an effective therapeutic intervention (Bush et al., 1996; Fink, 1995). Fink and Taylor (2003) provide explicit diagnostic criteria for catatonia, which as so defined may occur in 10% of acute psychiatric hospitalized patients.

The next section discusses personality changes due to general medical conditions. For this diagnosis to be assigned there must be a distinct change from the individual's previous personality pattern or, in the case of children, a marked deviation from normal development. Further, this must be attributed directly to the consequences of a general medical condition and not accounted for by another mental disorder or occur exclusively within a delirium or dementia. Subtypes include labile, disinhibited, aggressive, apathetic, paranoid, other, combined, and NOS. A case in point is HIV infection, which has received much multidisciplinary attention; EEG studies have demonstrated late-stage abnormalities accompanying neurological manifestations (Harrison et al., 1998; Mirsattari et al., 1999).

EEG studies contribute to the identification of underlying medical or neurological problems particularly in patients with seizure disorders. Bear and Fedio (1977) described personality changes with heightened emotionality and hyposexuality with irritability, viscosity, circumstantiality, hypergraphia, religiosity, and propensity for dissociative reactions in patients with temporal lobe epilepsy. They also proposed that the clinical characteristics in temporal lobe epilepsy are governed to some extent by the side of the epileptic focus, with mood disturbances associated with right-sided foci and disturbed thinking with left temporal and bilateral abnormalities.

Some investigators (Rodin and Schmaltz, 1984; Stevens and Hermann, 1981) do not agree with these conclusions. Moreover, the issue of whether epilepsy predisposes to psychiatric problems is controversial. It is well known that chronic medical illness is associated with an increased incidence of psychiatric disorders, but it is not agreed whether patients with epilepsy have any greater predisposition to such problems than persons with other disabling medical conditions. Whitman et al. (1984) pooled the results of numerous investigations and suggested a possible resolution of the conflict. They examined the results of the Minnesota Multiphasic Personality Inventory (MMPI) in 2,796 patients with generalized and temporal lobe epilepsy, other neurological disorders, and chronic physical illnesses. Overall rates of psychopathology were not any higher in epilepsy. However, when psychopathology was present, incidence and severity of psychosis was greatest in the patients with epilepsy. This topic was expanded by Lancman (1999), who delineated multiple types of psychoses associated with epileptic phenomena including ictal, interictal, and postictal states, nonconvulsive status epilepticus, postictal delirium, and peri-ictal aggression. Nevertheless, the most common emotional problem in patients with epilepsy is depression, which is more frequent in persons with epilepsy than other chronic diseases (Robertson et al., 1994).

Substance-Related Disorders

These disorders encompass mental conditions produced by drugs of abuse, side effects of prescribed and over-the-counter medications, and a wide range of chemical toxins. The drugs of abuse are grouped into 11 classes including alcohol, caffeine, and nicotine, helpfully tabulated in DSM-IV under headings of dependence, abuse, intoxication, and withdrawal syndromes. The same clinical pictures are itemized in the section on disorders due to general medical conditions. The need for laboratory confirmation of diagnosis is reiterated frequently, although the major diagnostic criteria involve history and clinical observations. Although seizures are often mentioned as complications of these disorders, the EEG is not recommended specifically, but its role in both diagnosis and treatment monitoring is well established. The two situations in which the EEG is mentioned in DSM-IV are much less clinically relevant. For example, acute use of cannabis is said to produce diffuse EEG background slowing and REM suppression along with hormonal and immunological changes. Extensive qEEG investigations of chronic marihuana use have been reported by Struve et al. (1998), showing increased power and coherence of EEG frontocentral alpha and theta activity and reduced suppression of auditory gating (Patrick and Struve, 2000).

The only other DSM-IV comment about EEG is in a discussion of discontinuation of chronic use of cocaine, in which EEG changes are said to accompany alterations in secretion of prolactin and downward regulation of dopamine receptors. As in the case of marihuana, qEEG and EP studies have been described in cocaine users identifying subtypes with differing likelihood of relapse (Prichep et al., 2002). Gender differences were noted by King et al. (2000), who found increased beta and reduced alpha in male but not female cocaine abusers. Boutros et al. (2000b) reported auditory evoked potential (AEP) changes. Numerous electrophysiological investigations of abused substances are available in the literature, mainly involving qEEG and EPs.

Schizophrenia and Other Psychotic Disorders

This section of DSM-IV is minimally changed from DSM-III-R, except for minor alterations to achieve compatibility with the International Classification of Diseases (ICD-10)

(World Health Organization, 1992). This chapter includes schizophrenia and schizophreniform, schizoaffective, delusional, brief psychotic, shared psychotic, and substance-induced disorders as well as psychosis NOS. Diagnostic criteria require at least two of the following: delusions, hallucinations, disorganized speech and behavior, and negative symptoms as well as socio-occupational dysfunction lasting at least 6 months. Onset is usually in adolescence and early adult life, but rarely appears in childhood and can be delayed until age 50 or later. Earlier onset is associated with poorer outcome, more evidence of structural brain abnormalities and cognitive impairment. Conversely, late onset has less evidence of CNS impairment and better outcome. Late-onset schizophrenia occurs more in females with predominantly paranoid and affective manifestations (Howard et al., 2000).

Psychotic disorders due to medical and neurological impairments are considered separately, which is not to overlook the fact that various forms of schizophrenia are associated with structural brain abnormalities with neurophysiological and other impairments. For example, ventricular enlargement, decreased neuropsychological test performance, and other indications of organicity are commonly encountered in schizophrenic populations (Williams et al., 1985). Interestingly, EEGs in patients with enlarged ventricles were more apt to be normal than in patients with normal computed tomography (CT) findings (Weinberger et al., 1982). Investigations of monozygotic twins discordant for schizophrenia indicated that the schizophrenic twin almost always had the larger ventricles (Suddath et al., 1990). Other studies have shown that schizophrenic patients with premorbid asocial status are prone to have neurological soft signs and I.Q. and other test scores suggestive of brain damage, as well as poorer or delayed response to neuroleptics and more negative symptoms (Merriam et al., 1990; Merlo et al., 1998; Quitkin et al., 1976; Sponheim et al., 2000). Such patients may have less genetic loading for schizophrenia than patients without evidence of CNS disorder (Quitkin et al., 1980), although some workers disagree (Roy and Crowe, 1994). It has been proposed that familial cases of schizophrenia tend to have normal EEGs, whereas sporadic cases more often show EEG abnormalities and other indications of CNS dysfunction (Kendler and Hays, 1982), but this too is controversial (Woods et al., 1991).

Others report that patients with schizophrenia with EEG abnormalities appearing either before or during neuroleptic treatment have more evidence of brain dysfunction than do patients without such EEG findings (Neil et al., 1978). Comorbid hypertension and older age increase the likelihood of EEG abnormalities (Centorrino et al., 2002). However, paroxysmal features developing during treatment with clozapine, an atypical neuroleptic, may predict favorable therapeutic response (Denney and Stevens, 1995). Freudenreich et al. (1997) found that 13% of patients on clozapine developed spikes and more than half displayed EEG slowing, more with higher serum levels. Spontaneous epileptic seizures occurred in about 1% of patients taking neuroleptics, especially clozapine and other low-potency sedating phenothiazines (Itil and Soldatos, 1980). Spike-wave complexes, diffuse delta activity, and FIRDA can develop with high dosages of antipsychotic drugs (Koshino et al., 1993; Matsuura et al., 1994).

Studies of EEG spectral displays in chronic schizophrenics have also shown regional differences that are not evident in the clinical EEG. qEEG has shown more midfrontal theta activity in schizophrenics compared to normals (Westphal et al., 1990). Further details about these kinds of investigations are provided elsewhere in this volume. However, before the advent of qEEG analysis, it was reported that chronic schizophrenics had lower mean alpha frequencies than comparison groups (Javitt, 1997; Shagass, 1977) but not to the degree seen in dementia. In one study slower alpha frequencies were associated with larger lateral ventricles (Karson et al., 1988).

Considerable attention has been devoted to the hypothesis that schizophrenia is primarily associated with dominant hemispheric dysfunction. Abrams and Taylor (1979), using a system of classification similar to DSM-IV, showed that schizophrenic patients had twice as many EEG abnormalities, mostly in left temporal regions, than patients with affective disorders. This study suffered from a number of methodological limitations, including visual analysis of EEG data and brief sampling times. Several qEEG studies have now been published generally supporting bilateral and dominant involvement in schizophrenia (Koles et al., 1994). Further discussion of qEEG findings is beyond the scope of this chapter.

There have been numerous EEG studies of populations of patients diagnosed as schizophrenic according to criteria less stringent than DSM-III-R, comparing them with other patient groups and with controls. Generally, an increase of nonspecific abnormalities has been reported (Small, 1983). However, most of these studies did not employ specific diagnostic criteria. In the past, several researchers reported that EEG abnormalities and paroxysmal dysrhythmias may have a favorable impact on prognosis in schizophrenia. Small et al. (1984) reclassified a population of 759 patients who had received a final DSM-I or DSM-II clinical diagnosis of schizophrenia using Feighner et al. (1972) criteria with long-term follow-up of selected subgroups. Abnormal EEGs occurred mostly in the patients who were reassigned to diagnoses other than schizophrenia. In patients remaining in the Feighner-defined schizophrenia category, EEG abnormality was associated with better outcome than normal EEG findings. Conversely, EEG abnormalities in other diagnostic groups predicted poorer prognosis.

Another study using criteria more like DSM-IV was reported by Struve and Becka (1968), in which B-mitten patterns occurred more frequently in patients with schizophreniform psychoses, which often have more affective characteristics than chronic schizophrenia. Inui et al. (1998) also found more epileptiform EEG variants in patients with atypical psychosis. Later, Struve et al. (1977) found that tardive dyskinesia was associated with B-mitten patterns, which they regarded as a physiological indication of central autonomic dysregulation that was found more with affective disorders than with schizophrenia (Wegner et al., 1979). In this regard definitive EEG abnormalities have not been established in patients with tardive dyskinesia (Kaartinen et al., 1984; Wolf et al., 1984). Likewise, EEG findings are not predictive of whether or not the condition is reversible (Jeste et al., 1979).

Stevens et al. (1979) showed by 24-hour telemetry that temporal EEG abnormalities occur in as many as 30% of schizophrenic patients but demonstrated no correspondence between clinical phenomena and the occurrence of EEG spiking or between either of these manifestations and spontaneous saccadic ocular movements. This study also highlights the important point that EEG observations in disturbed individuals are prone to artifact contamination and difficulties with interpretation that can often be resolved only by repeated efforts to obtain reliable data under conditions of wakefulness, activation procedures, drowsiness, and sleep. The same cautions apply to qEEG and EP investigations.

The DSM-IV section on psychotic disorders due to general medical conditions specifically mentions temporal lobe epilepsy. Patients with psychomotor seizures may develop a psychotic state resembling schizophrenia, which develops years after the onset of seizures, usually at a time when seizure frequency is low. Despite manifestations of thought disorder and impaired reality testing with delusions and hallucinations, such patients have preserved affect and frequently good interpersonal rapport, i.e., relatively few negative symptoms (Stevens, 1988). An interesting EEG association has been observed historically by Landolt (1958), who described "forced normalization" of the EEG, in which normal EEGs were observed during psychotic exacerbations, whereas EEG abnormalities and seizures were associated with improved mental status. Kanemoto et al. (2001) confirmed these observations, especially in temporal lobe epilepsy patients with medial temporal foci. Trimble (1977) suggested that these relationships may develop via mechanisms resembling kindling. When spike occurrence is reduced to a critical interval, permanent alterations in the brain may occur. EEG monitoring in the treatment of psychosis in association with epilepsy can be helpful; if reciprocal relationships are observed between paroxysmal EEG abnormalities and improvement in mental status, therapeutic maneuvers can be used to alter that balance with adjustment of neuroleptic and anticholinergic medications, reduction of anticonvulsant agents, electroconvulsive therapy, or other interventions.

Dominant or bilateral temporal EEG foci in patients with psychomotor epilepsy may predispose to psychosis and severe psychiatric difficulties (Umbricht et al., 1995), whereas mood disorders may be more common with right-sided lesions. Perez et al. (1985) found that left-sided foci were associated with nuclear schizophrenia but did not observe a relationship between right-sided abnormalities and depression. Roberts et al. (1990) stated that schizophrenia-like psychoses in patients with temporal lobe epilepsy were associated with developmental lesions in the medial temporal lobes and larger ventricles. Bruton et al. (1994) found larger ventricles, increased periventricular gliosis, and focal cerebral damage in epileptic patients with schizophrenic-like psychosis. Postictal psychotic states may occur characterized by pleomorphic psychotic phenomena, spontaneous resolution, and a tendency to recur (Logsdail and Toone, 1988). These disorders are relatively rare (chronic interictal psychoses occur 12 times more frequently). As stated previously the most common psychiatric problem in epileptic patients is depression (Kanner and Balabanov, 2000).

The DSM-IV mentions a variety of other medical and neurological conditions that may cause psychotic symptoms, many of which have EEG concomitants, e.g., neoplasms, cerebrovascular disease, Huntington's disease, migraine, infections, and endocrine, metabolic, and electrolyte disturbances. EEG has a significant role in diagnosis and monitoring of treatment in these situations and in substance-induced psychotic disorders in which states of intoxication and withdrawal may complicate the clinical picture.

Mood Disorders

The DSM-IV includes more affective categories than previous DSMs with added descriptions about circumstances of onset and longitudinal course. This section encompasses major depressive disorder, dysthymic disorder, bipolar I and II disorders, cyclothymic disorders, mood disorders due to general medical conditions or substance induced, and NOS categories.

EEG provides important information about depression, more so than in most other psychiatric illnesses. Sleep EEG abnormalities occur in more than half of depressed patients. They include polysomnographic features of sleep continuity disturbances, reduced non-REM (NREM) stages 3 and 4 sleep, decreased REM latency, increased phasic REM activity, and increased duration of REM sleep early in the night. Sleep EEG abnormalities may be more "trait than state" variables since they often persist into phases of remission.

As in the case of schizophrenia, EEG studies suggest that there may be groups within the affective disorders that may have underlying CNS abnormalities. Dalen (1965) studied 35 young patients hospitalized with recurrent manic conditions that likely met DSM-IV criteria for diagnosis of bipolar I disorder. Some patients had normal EEGs and familial loading for affective disorders, suggesting a specific genetic propensity, whereas others had EEG abnormalities and a history of perinatal complications without evidence of hereditary predisposition. Significant correlations among perinatal hazard, abnormal or borderline EEGs, and negative family history of affective disease were demonstrated. This study had a number of limitations, including its restriction to young hospitalized patients not representative of bipolar illnesses as a whole, lack of a control group, and failure to consider EEG effects of psychotropic medications. Hays (1976) and Small et al. (1997) also found positive associations between EEG abnormalities and absent family histories of affective illnesses. However, Waters et al. (1982) reported no significant relationships between perinatal complications and vulnerability to affective illness.

Results from other studies suggest there are individuals with EEG abnormalities within the affective disorder group in whom the etiology of the disorder and symptomatology may differ. This is not to say that individuals with paroxysmal and other EEG abnormalities are more prone to the development of mental illnesses or symptoms, for studies of other populations have not revealed such trends. Rather, it seems that within a psychiatric population, subgroups who have different familial characteristics, clinical features, and prognosis can be identified by EEG methods. Struve et al. (1977) reported associations between EEG paroxysmal characteristics, including variants such as small sharp spikes and 6/sec spike waves, and suicidal ideation and behavior.

Struve (1985) also observed that patients with EEG dysrhythmias who were taking oral contraceptives had a significantly higher incidence of suicidal behavior than did women with normal EEGs. Inui et al. (1998) described more epileptiform variants in patients with atypical psychoses with mixed features of mood disorders and schizophrenia.

Suggestive evidence of EEG associations with bipolar illness was provided by Small et al. (1975), in which both probands and family members showed a nearly 50% incidence of small sharp spike EEG variants. The occurrence of these features was much lower in later studies (17%), possibly related to the increased use of anticonvulsant drugs in bipolar disorder (Small et al., 1997). An interesting observation in two manic patients was made by Van Sweden (1986), who described the rapid development of EEG sleep spindles during behavioral wakefulness. Small et al. (1997) reported that 19% of EEGs in a series of hospitalized manic patients exhibited this phenomenon of "microsleep." Himmelhoch et al. (1980) described a late stage of bipolar illness associated with chronic mania, EEG abnormalities, and treatment resistance. These and other observations suggest that structural brain changes may take place after repeated episodes (Altshuler, 1993; El-Badri et al., 2001). In a large series of acutely manic patients, Small et al. (1997) reported EEG abnormalities in 94 of 202 cases significantly correlated with older age and female gender. Lateralized abnormalities were present in 17 patients, 14 on the left side. From this and qEEG evidence it was concluded that dominant temporal lobe dysfunctions may underlie manifestations of mania (Koles et al., 1994; Small et al., 1997; Small et al., 1998a).

Several investigations suggest that depression may be a disorder of right hemispheric function or of interactions between the hemispheres with relative right-sided or nondominant impairment. Abrams and Taylor (1979) found more right-sided EEG abnormalities among patients diagnosed with affective disorders. Flor-Henry (1972, 1985) postulated right-sided abnormalities in depressive disorders based on observations that patients with temporal lobe epilepsy with right-sided foci were more apt to be depressed. It has also been shown that nondominant unilateral ECT is more therapeutically effective than dominant ECT in depressed patients (Halliday, 1968) in some but not all studies (Abrams, 1989). Nevertheless, bilateral ECT is more effective than unilateral nondominant induction in the treatment of mania (Milstein et al., 1987).

Other evidence comes from studies of patients with temporal lobe epilepsy and other neurological disorders. Wada's group (Hurwitz et al., 1985), using unilateral carotid barbiturate injections, concluded that the dominant hemisphere subserves positive feelings and the nondominant hemisphere negative affects (Lee et al., 1993). Hermann et al. (1991) showed that left frontal lobe dysfunction was associated with depression in patients with temporal lobe epilepsy, whereas a positron emission tomography (PET) study by Bromfield et al. (1992) concluded that depressed patients with complex partial seizures had bilaterally reduced inferior frontal cortex glucose metabolism, noting similar findings in Parkinson's disease and in uncomplicated depression. Strauss et al. (1992) found that men but not women with left focal temporal lobe epilepsy were more vulnerable

to depression. Altshuler et al. (1990) discussed interactions among gender, handedness, seizure focus, and the likelihood of depression. Further discourse on this subject is available in a report by Victoroff et al. (1994), who demonstrated that laterality of ictal onset and the degree of interictal temporal lobe hypometabolism on PET scanning both contribute to the risk of depression.

Poststroke depression has been the subject of numerous clinical and neuroimaging studies. The prevalence of depression following stroke is about double the rate of depression in the general population (Robinson, 2003). EEG studies of the early and late course of depression after stroke as well as poststroke fatigue may provide more insights into ultimate levels of functional recovery (Bogousslavsky, 2002). Conclusive evidence of the pathophysiological substrates of poststroke depression have yet to be elucidated. However, lesions near the frontal pole and basal ganglia on the left side appear to predispose to severe depressive symptoms. Large right hemispheric lesions may also be associated with depression (Lyketsos et al., 1998; MacHale et al., 1998).

Mood disorders due to general medical conditions include a number of entities in which EEG findings are helpful for clarifying diagnosis. An example is the differentiation between depressive pseudodementia and dementia with secondary depression, which was the subject of a study by Brenner et al. (1989). Patients with depression or depressive pseudodementia had normal or mildly abnormal EEGs, whereas most patients with dementia with or without secondary depression had EEG abnormalities, one third of which were moderate or severe. Cornelius et al. (1993) compared clinical symptoms and EEG and CT findings in depressed patients with and without organic syndromes. Focal EEG abnormalities in the temporal and frontal areas were observed in the organic cases without lateralized differences.

EEG changes associated with ECT warrant consideration in this section because the affective disorders are the clinical states most favorably influenced by this treatment. EEG recordings before ECT, during the ictal phase, postictal, and interictal all have clinical relevance. Preexisting EEG abnormalities may predict less favorable response to ECT (Drake and Shy, 1989). Therapeutic adequacy can be evaluated during the ictal phase by means of EEG measures of seizure duration, postictal electrical silence and quantitative assessments of EEG spectral energy (Kellner and Fink, 1996; Kolbeinsson and Petursson, 1988; Suppes et al., 1996). Short-term increases in delta and theta activity after ECT generally accompany improvement in depression (Sackeim et al., 1996). However, post-ECT EEG spikes may indicate the possibility of kindling phenomena (Kubota et al., 2003), as does the rare development of NCSE (Povlsen et al., 2003). Vagus nerve stimulation (VNS) and transcranial magnetic stimulation (TMS) are becoming accepted treatment modalities for depression. EEG studies of these procedures are in progress.

Other treatments of affective disorders are also associated with EEG changes. Lithium induces EEG slowing and paroxysmal activity in patients and normal volunteers. High-voltage delta activity emphasized anteriorly, generalized background slowing, and spike-wave paroxysms are associated with both therapeutic and toxic levels of lithium (Gansaeuer and Alsaadi, 2003; Small, 1986). EEG abnormalities with lithium treatment are also associated with increased levels of trace elements, particularly bromine (Harvey et al., 1992). Tricyclic antidepressant drugs produce EEG disruptions that are correlated with high plasma concentrations and side effects (Preskorn et al., 1984). Seizures with antidepressant drugs can occur depending on predisposing factors, the particular antidepressant drug in question, and the bioavailability of that drug (Rosenstein et al., 1993).

In summary, the importance of the EEG in the study of affective disorders is primarily to rule out organic mental disorders. After this is accomplished, a subgroup of patients with EEG abnormalities may differ from other patients with the same diagnosis in terms of familial constellation, possible etiology, and response to treatment. ECT, lithium, and antidepressant drugs are also associated with EEG changes.

Anxiety Disorders

This DSM-IV section contains the following categories: panic disorder with and without agoraphobia, agoraphobia without panic, specific phobia, social phobia, obsessive-compulsive disorder, posttraumatic stress disorder, acute stress disorder, generalized anxiety disorder, and anxiety disorders with general medical conditions, substance induced or NOS.

Panic disorders have been the subject of several EEG and brain imaging studies. Lepola et al. (1990) reported that most patients with panic disorder have normal EEG and CT findings. However, some authors proposed associations between panic attacks and partial complex seizures because of their clinical similarities (Toni et al., 1996). The differential diagnosis of panic attacks and partial seizures can sometimes be difficult, requiring telemetered EEG monitoring during attacks (Weilburg et al., 1993) since routine EEGs may be uninformative. Polysomnographic studies may also be helpful since nocturnal panic with awaking occurs in 18% to 45% of patients with panic disorder (Craske et al., 2002). However, focal paroxysmal EEG changes were detected in one third of patients during actual panic attacks (Weilburg et al., 1995). Dantendorfer et al. (1996) reported an increased incidence of EEG abnormalities in panic disorder patients as well as MRI abnormalities in septo-hippocampal regions. Goddard and Charney (1997) provided a synopsis of neuroimaging findings in panic disorder. Patients with social anxiety exhibited marked right anterior qEEG activation in the alpha-1 power band and autonomic responses during anticipation of public speaking compared with controls (Davidson et al., 2000). EEG studies have also been conducted in obsessive-compulsive disorder with findings of increased nonspecific abnormalities (Jenike and Brotman, 1984). Neuroimaging (PET) studies suggest dysfunction in the frontal lobes, basal ganglia, and prefrontal regions (Hymas et al., 1991; Sawle et al., 1991).

In cases of posttraumatic stress disorder (PTSD) associated with actual physical and sexual abuse, EEG abnormalities may be present primarily in the frontotemporal regions as well as abnormalities on neurological exams, neuropsychological tests, and imaging studies (Ito et al., 1993). Neurological soft signs were present in men and women who had experienced trauma in childhood and adult life (Gurvits et al., 2000). qEEG studies of combat-related PTSD showed increased theta activity in the central regions compared with controls (Begic et al., 2001). Neuroanatomical substrates of stress-related disorders and neural circuitry in hippocampus, amygdala, cingulate, and medial frontal cortex were described in detail by Bremner (2003).

The major role of EEG in the anxiety disorders is to rule out associated medical conditions that may be considered etiological or contributing to the clinical picture. Medical illnesses causing anxiety symptoms are wide ranging, including endocrinological, cardiovascular, respiratory, metabolic, and neurological conditions. The same is true of substance-induced anxiety disorders in which EEG can provide a sensitive monitor, e.g., in caffeine-induced panic reactions (Christensen et al., 1993). qEEG investigations of asymmetries in anxiety disorders implicate right hemispheric dysfunctions (Bruder et al., 1997; Cutting, 1992; Davidson, 1998).

Somatoform Disorders

This section of the DSM-IV is little changed from the last edition of the manual. It contains somatization disorder, undifferentiated somatoform disorder, conversion disorder, pain disorder, hypochondriasis, body dysmorphic disorder, and somatoform disorder NOS. The essential feature of each of these conditions is the presence of physical symptoms that suggest medical illness but are not etiologic. Clearly, exclusion of such illnesses is essential for diagnosis, particularly since these disorders are usually encountered in nonpsychiatric settings. Although the symptoms of these disorders are physical, the specific pathophysiological processes involved are unknown, but it is assumed that the symptoms are linked to psychological factors or conflicts. Symptom production is not thought to be under voluntary control.

The major area in which EEG is relied on for diagnosis is in the category of conversion disorder, in which symptoms or deficits suggest neurological disease, such as blindness, paralysis, or seizures. In the case of the latter, there may be an antecedent physical disorder that provides a prototype, or genuine and nonepileptic attacks may coexist. The diagnostic separation of pseudoseizures, psychogenic nonepileptic seizures (NES), or hysterical attacks from true seizures can be difficult if not impossible from observation of the episodes. It is important to obtain recordings during attacks, sometimes with split-screen videotaped EEG and patient observations. Repeated recordings during multiple attacks may be necessary to exhibit the presence or absence of stereotyped clinical and EEG features. Attempts to provoke typical attacks with Metrazol or bemegride have not met with widespread acceptance nor do they have established clinical usefulness. Plasma prolactin levels are known to rise within a half-hour after generalized seizures, which may offer further accuracy in hospitalized patients (Trimble, 1978). Serum creatine kinase is also elevated following seizures

(Libman et al., 1991). Ictal single photon emission computed tomography (SPECT) has been shown to differentiate between true and nonepileptic seizures (DeLeon et al., 1997).

Leis et al. (1992) reviewed serial video-EEGs in 47 patients ultimately diagnosed with psychogenic seizures. Lack of responsiveness without motor manifestations was the most common ictal manifestation in this group. Groppel et al. (2000) identified three symptom clusters in prolonged videotapes of NES consisting of motor movements of head, pelvis, and extremities, trembling and falling. Eisendrath and Valan (1994) compared psychiatric observations in patients with genuine and pseudoseizures established by video-EEG telemetry. The patients with pseudoepileptic episodes without genuine seizures met diagnostic criteria for either somatization disorder or personality disorder and frequently had a history of significant childhood loss or physical or psychological trauma. Perhaps as a consequence of brain injury, an increased incidence (8–37%) of nonspecific EEG abnormalities has been observed in patients with pseudoseizures (Bowman, 1993). Harden et al. (2003) found different viewpoints about psychogenic pseudoseizures among neurologists and psychiatrists; the latter having less regard for the accuracy of video-EEGs.

All of the somatoform disorders are conditions with recurrent and multiple somatic complaints generally of many years' duration for which medical attention has been repeatedly sought without confirmation of physical etiologies. For this reason baseline physical and laboratory findings are of particular value not only in ruling out abnormalities on initial workup but also in confirming the absence of significant changes thereafter. Further investigations of the psychobiological disease processes in these conditions are of particular importance, given the suffering and disabilities involved and their contribution to health care costs (Bell, 1994).

Dissociative Disorders

After a brief section on factitious disorder (the deliberate feigning of physical or psychological signs and/or symptoms), DSM-IV continues with the dissociative disorders, mostly unchanged from DSM-III-R except for terminology. This section includes dissociative amnesia, fugue, identity disorder, and depersonalization disorder as well as an NOS category. Diagnosis may be strengthened by structured interviews and rating scales, e.g., the Multidimensional Inventory of Dissociation (Dell, 2002), the Dissociative Experiences Scale (DES) (Alper et al., 1997), and the Structured Clinical Interview for DSM-IV Dissociative Disorders (SCID-D) (Steinberg, 1994). This is another area in which EEG is important for diagnosis and treatment monitoring. In these conditions, there are sudden temporary alterations in consciousness, identity, and/or motor behavior. In dissociative amnesia, there is a loss of memory beginning suddenly, usually following psychosocial stress. It is the latter that usually differentiates this condition from an organic mental disorder. However, epileptiform EEG activity may be precipitated or accentuated by emotional stress, particularly with seizures of focal onset and in patients with schizophrenia or schizoid personality disorders (Small et al., 1964).

Repeated EEG studies at rest, during activation procedures, during sleep, and under circumstances tailored to be evocative for the particular individual can yield diagnostic information.

Bowman and Coons (2000) and Brown and Trimble (2000) provide detailed guidelines for the differential diagnosis of epilepsy, pseudoseizures, dissociative identity disorder, and dissociative disorder NOS with careful observance of DSM criteria, video-EEG, and assessment of symptoms with the SCID-D and DES. Similar workup is called for in dissociative fugue, which is characterized by sudden unanticipated travel with assumption of a new identity and inability to recall the past. Such elaboration is unusual in temporal lobe epilepsy, but it must be ruled out (Kuyk et al., 1999). Coons (1999) described five cases of dissociative fugue in which EEGs and brain scans were normal. Comorbid psychiatric diagnoses included affective disorders and alcohol and drug abuse with criminal activity as well. Coons and Milstein (1992) studied 25 psychogenic (dissociative) amnesia patients, observing many similarities to multiple personality disorder (dissociative identity disorder) including stressful psychological precipitants. None of their patients had seizure histories and only three had abnormal EEG findings.

Dissociative identity disorder is the term now applied to individuals with two or more distinct personalities. Rosenstein (1994) reviewed clinical and neurophysiological findings in this condition, which has fascinated medical and literary writers for a long time. Perhaps the best known is the case described by Thigpen and Cleckley (1957) in *The Three Faces of Eve*, who found no gross EEG differences among the three personalities. Since that time, there have been quantitative assessments of EEG data during emergence of various personalities. Such studies have not yielded convincing evidence of significant electrophysiological concomitants of personality change. Coons et al. (1982) showed that EEG spectral densities differed between simulated personalities in a normal subject; these were probably related to intensity of concentration, contrived moods, and other factors. Discriminations between personalities in patients were less impressive. There is a high incidence of comorbid seizure disorders and various confusional and delirious conditions associated with these states, some of which may be secondary to physical abuse. This diagnosis has been noted to wax and wane over the years, seemingly in keeping with contemporary fashions. It is well known that psychiatrists who show a particular interest in these phenomena are the ones most likely to encounter them. EEG studies are not likely to cast more light upon this situation, except to identify coexisting organic disorders such as epilepsy or posttraumatic lesions, which may be contributing factors. A kindling-like model of dissociation linked to freeze/immobility phenomena and maintained by increased vagal tone and endorphin secretion was proposed by Scaer (2001).

Depersonalization disorders are included among the dissociative disorders. The diagnosis is made when the symptom of depersonalization is not secondary to any other disorder. Mild depersonalization without functional impairment occurs at some time in as many as 70% of young adults and does not warrant a psychiatric diagnosis. EEG studies may be of value in discriminating organic conditions or may lead to suspicion of substance intoxication or withdrawal.

Sexual and Gender Identity Disorders

The DSM-IV includes sexual dysfunctions corresponding to various phases of the sexual response cycle, the paraphilias, gender identity disorders, and sexual disorders NOS. It might be expected that EEG studies would have little bearing on this area of psychiatry. However, organic mental disorders are frequently accompanied by psychosexual dysfunctions. Interictal hyposexuality is often present in temporal lobe epilepsy (Blumer and Walker, 1975). Heath (1972) recorded spikes from depth electrodes during orgasm, an example of EEG spiking that is not of ictal significance. Cohen et al. (1976) showed that there are right-hemispheric qEEG changes during orgasm. These kinds of studies have not received widespread attention, nor have they been applied clinically.

The DSM-IV defines the paraphilias as recurrent intense sexually arousing fantasies, urges, or behavior that may involve nonhuman objects, suffering or humiliation of partners, children, or nonconsenting participants. The most common categories are pedophilia, exhibitionism, voyeurism, sexual masochism and/or sadism, transvestic fetishism, and frotteurism. Nonparaphilic compulsive sexual behavior involves normative conventional sexual behavior taken to compulsive extremes. The estimated incidence of these problems is 5% of the population (Coleman, 2000). The etiology is probably multidimensional and heterogeneous involving elements of obsessive-compulsive disorder, impulse control disorder, and addictive disorders. The neurobiological mechanisms may involve brain neurotransmitter dysregulation and sometimes neurological abnormalities such as in Alzheimer's disease, Huntington chorea, and epilepsy. Disturbances in serotonin, epinephrine and monoamine oxidase may underlie some types of aberrant sexual behavior (Kafka, 2003). Electrophysiological neuroimaging studies may contribute further understanding of these diverse and socially distressing behaviors.

Langevin (1992) summarized the literature on biological factors contributing to paraphilic behavior including physical, neurological, neuropsychological and EEG studies. He referred to case reports of unusual sexual behavior with temporal lobe epilepsy. Studies of qEEG differences between exhibitionists and controls were also described. It appeared that pedophilia is associated with more structural brain abnormalities and neuropsychological test impairments than any of the other paraphilic subtypes (Hendricks et al., 1988). Maes (2001) suggested underlying catecholamine abnormalities and increased sympathoadrenal activity based on studies of pedophiles compared to normal men.

Polysomnography has been utilized in the diagnosis of impotence with the commonly held belief that patients with penile erections during REM sleep are not likely to have an organically based disorder. Spark et al. (1980) raised doubts about these opinions as well as other popular beliefs that impotence is primarily psychogenic. Thirty-seven cases of 105 consecutive patients (35%) with complaints of impotence were found to have significant abnormalities of the hypo-thalamic-pituitary-gonadal axis. Moreover, 14 patients had structural CNS lesions, primarily pituitary tumors. Some of these patients did experience occasional early morning erections and had sporadically successful sexual intercourse. The authors stressed that workup for psychosexual dysfunction should include hormonal assays, and that such cases should not be dismissed as psychogenic even though there are prominent associations between psychosocial stressors and the development of the condition, as this does not necessarily imply cause-effect relationships. By the same token, the high incidence of pituitary tumors warrants further investigation of the integrity of the nervous system, including neuroimaging studies.

Eating Disorders

The DSM-IV has a separate section on this subject; formerly it was included under disorders of childhood and adolescence. This category includes anorexia nervosa, with restricting and binge-eating/purging types, and bulimia nervosa, with purging and nonpurging types. EEGs are not mentioned in discussions of laboratory findings or differential diagnosis, although such patients have been the subjects of EEG studies including an early controlled investigation by Crisp et al. (1968). Fifty-nine percent of their cases had abnormal EEG background activity, 31% had unstable responses to hyperventilation, and 12% had paroxysmal abnormalities, considered attributable to reversible secondary manifestations of starvation, such as electrolyte imbalance, metabolic alkalosis, and relative hypoglycemia. However, other findings suggest there may be a subgroup of anorectics in which underlying organic and neurological difficulties may have etiological importance. Halmi et al. (1977) identified the triad of perinatal complications, childhood attentional deficits, and relative failure to thrive. EEG data were not included, but this group may have sustained some early CNS insult. Treatment with the antihistamine cyproheptadine was more effective than behavior modification for these patients. Other studies have shown that intractable binge eating is associated with neurological soft signs and EEG abnormalities (Rau and Green, 1978).

There is evidence that anticonvulsant drugs may inhibit excessive appetite, perhaps more so in patients with paroxysmal EEG abnormalities or positive spikes (Johnson et al., 1985; Rau et al., 1979). CNS dysfunction in anorexia is also suggested by polysomnographic studies showing abnormalities in slow-wave sleep and phasic REM parameters, with resolution of the former but not the latter with improved nutritional status (Neil et al., 1980). Comparisons with normal EEG anorectics did not suggest that starvation was responsible for the dysrhythmias, even though patients with EEG abnormalities demonstrated more bulimia and laxative and diuretic abuse. Tongoe et al. (1999) studied contingent negative variation (CNV) responses in eight anorexic children and normal controls, showing reduced early and late amplitudes between warning and imperative stimuli in the former but no differences in postimperative amplitudes. They hypothesized that reduced levels of dopaminergic and noradrenergic transmission might underlie the electrophysiological findings and lead to impaired cognitive and appetitive behavior. Asymmetrically increased right prefrontal EEG activity in chronic dieters relative to normal eaters has also been reported (Silva et al., 2002).

Another line of evidence has emerged from neuroimaging studies in which reversible ventricular dilation was described in anorectics, suggesting possible intracranial fluid retention (Enzmann and Lane, 1977; Heinz et al., 1977; Kerem and Katzman, 2003). Other studies indicate that some patients with eating disorders respond to antidepressant medications and that there may be some overlap between eating and affective disorders. However, polysomnographic studies have shown conflicting results (Delvenne et al., 1992; Lauer et al., 1990).

Sleep Disorders

In addition to those conditions listed in the previous edition, DSM-IV lists narcolepsy and breathing-related sleep disorder because of their importance in differential diagnosis. Another important diagnostic consideration is epilepsy, particularly in children, in which there may be difficulty differentiating between abnormal sleep behavior and seizures (Stores, 1991). EEG and other studies are essential for diagnosis of these conditions, as discussed in Chapter 48 on polysomnography.

Impulse-Control Disorders Not Elsewhere Classified

This section of the DSM-IV includes intermittent explosive disorder, kleptomania, pyromania, pathological gambling, trichotillomania, and an NOS category. The EEG is specifically mentioned in connection with intermittent explosive disorder, previously designated by Monroe and others as the episodic dyscontrol syndrome (Monroe et al., 1977; Tucker et al., 1986). The incidence of seizures may be increased in these individuals. The evidence about whether or not EEG abnormalities predict a favorable response with anticonvulsant medications is contradictory (Corrigan et al., 1993; Reeves et al., 2003). EEG studies of the other impulse control disorders have not been encountered except for a pilot qEEG study of pathological gambling reported by Goldstein et al. (1985), which suggested deficits in task-appropriate hemispheric differentiation.

This part of the DSM-IV concludes with a section on adjustment disorders defined as emotional or behavioral responses to psychosocial stressors. The distinction is made between psychological factors affecting a medical condition and adjustment disorder in which the reverse applies; that is, psychological symptoms develop in response to the stress of having a physical illness. Some individuals may present with both. In this instance EEG monitoring may be useful to assess the relative severity of the physical components.

Personality Disorders

The DSM-IV concludes its formal description of diagnostic categories with consideration of the adult personality disorders. Unlike many of the previously described conditions, these categories encompass enduring maladaptive personality traits generally of lifelong duration, although diagnoses are not applied definitively until an individual is at least 18 years of age. Many childhood disorders merge into these conditions, but they are not so designated until maturity because the adult outcome is not inevitable. There are 11 personality constellations described, including an NOS category, with three major clusters of interpersonal behavior and personality characteristics or traits that are common to these conditions. Persons characterized as having paranoid, schizoid, or schizotypal disorders often seem eccentric or odd, whereas those with histrionic, narcissistic, antisocial, and borderline personalities appear dramatic, emotional, or erratic. Anxiety and fearfulness characterize the avoidant, dependent, and obsessive compulsive.

There are relatively few EEG studies of these specifically defined personality disorders. Numerous EEG reports are published about prisoners and individuals exhibiting criminal behavior, but definitive psychiatric diagnostic criteria have generally not been employed. However, studies by Guze (1976) have shown that antisocial personality disorders can be diagnosed in about 50% of prisoners. DSM-IV estimates the prevalence of this disorder as 3% in males and 1% in females. Flagrant antisocial behavior may diminish after age 30. EEG studies of criminal populations have described a variety of nonspecific abnormal EEG features, particularly electrical characteristics that would be regarded as within normal limits in persons of younger chronological age. Whether these findings parallel the onset, course, and decline of antisocial behavior is not known. EEG abnormalities may also reflect frequently coexisting substance abuse, head trauma, and toxic and metabolic disorders. Pillmann et al. (1999) studied relationships between EEG abnormalities and violent criminal behavior in 222 defendants. Left hemispheric focal abnormalities were significantly associated with violent offenses. Comorbid diagnoses included mental retardation, epilepsy, and brain damage.

Raine et al. (1990) showed that adolescents with low levels of physiological reactivity engaged in more adult antisocial behavior than other young people. A combination of physiological measures tested at age 15 of heart rate, skin resistance, and EEG power spectral densities identified 65% of future criminals and 77% of nonoffenders. Adult criminal behavior was associated with lower heart rates, more EEG slowing, and higher galvanic skin resistance. These physiological measures were not correlated with environmental predictors of criminality such as social class, neighborhood, or level of schooling. The authors speculated that abnormal brain arousal mechanisms may underlie antisocial activity in young men. Snyder and Pitts (1984) studied patients with borderline personality disorder, finding more EEG slowing than in depressed controls. However, later studies failed to confirm an excess of EEG abnormalities in borderline personality (Archer et al., 1988; Cornelius et al., 1986). Diffuse slowing was found in 40% of borderlines by De la Fuente et al. (1998), which was unchanged by carbamazepine. Conflicting findings may be related to overly inclusive definitions of this diagnostic category (Hudziak et al., 1996). Russ et al. (1999) investigated pain sensitivity in self-mutilating borderline women, finding more EEG theta power spectral density during a pain procedure in those who self-injured than in controls. A recent review of 24 published electrophysiological studies of borderlines (Boutros et al., 2003) revealed numerous abnormal and atypical EEG and other physiological attributes, but most were inadequately controlled or failed to account for comorbidity.

The area of personality disorders is important for future investigations with EEG and other methods for examining brain function in view of the current lack of effective therapeutic interventions and the poor prognosis. DSM-IV operational definitions of these conditions can provide a framework for future studies. In this way the present nosological system promotes the acquisition of new knowledge that will appear in future DSM editions.

References

Abrams, R. 1989. Lateralized hemispheric mechanisms and the antidepressant effects of right and left unilateral ECT. Convulsive Ther. 5: 244–249.

Abrams, R., and Taylor, M.A. 1979. Differential EEG patterns in affective disorder and schizophrenia. Arch. Gen. Psychiatry 36:1355–1358.

Addonizio, G., Susman, V.L., and Roth, S.D. 1987. Neuroleptic malignant syndrome: Review and analysis of 115 cases. Biol. Psychiatry 22:1004–1020.

Allahyari, H., Deisenhammer, E., and Weiser, G. 1976. EEG examination during delirium tremens. Psychiatr. Clin. (Basel) 9:21–31.

Alper, K., Devinsky, O., Perrine, K., et al. 1997. Dissociation in epilepsy and conversion nonepileptic seizures. Epilepsia 38:991–997.

Altshuler, L.L. 1993. Bipolar disorder: are repeated episodes associated with neuroanatomic and cognitive changes? Biol. Psychiatry 33:563–565.

Altshuler, L.L., Devinsky, O., Post, R.M., et al. 1990. Depression, anxiety, and temporal lobe epilepsy. Arch. Neurol. 47:284–288.

American Psychiatric Association. 1980. Diagnostic and Statistical Manual of Mental Disorders, 3rd ed. Washington, DC: American Psychiatric Association.

American Psychiatric Association. 1987. Diagnostic and Statistical Manual of Mental Disorders, 3rd rev. ed. Washington, DC: American Psychiatric Association.

American Psychiatric Association. 1994. Diagnostic and Statistical Manual of Mental Disorders, 4th ed. Washington, DC: American Psychiatric Association.

Archer, R.P., Struve, F.A., Ball, J.D., et al. 1988. EEG in borderline personality disorder. Biol. Psychiatry 24:731–732.

Austin, J.K., Dunn, D.W., Caffrey, H.M., et al. 2002. Recurrent seizures and behavior problems in children with first recognized seizures: a prospective study. Epilepsia 43:1564–1573.

Bader, G., Neveus, T., Kruse, S., et al. 2002. Sleep of primary enuretic children and controls. Sleep 25:579–583.

Barry, R., Clarke, A.R., and Johnstone, S.J. 2003. A review of electrophysiology in attention-deficit/hyperactivity disorder: I. Qualitative and quantitative electroencephalography. Clin. Neurophysiol. 114:171–183.

Bear, D.M., and Fedio, P. 1977. Quantitative analysis of interictal behavior in temporal epilepsy. Arch. Neurol. 34:454–467.

Begic, D., Hotujac, L., and Jokic-Begic, N. 2001. Electroencephalographic comparison of veterans with combat-related post-traumatic stress disorder and healthy subjects. Int. J. Psychophysiol. 40:167–172.

Bell, I. 1994. Somatization disorder: health care costs in the decade of the brain. Biol. Psychiatry 35:81–83.

Berry-Kravis, E. 2002. Epilepsy in fragile X syndrome. Dev. Med. Child Neurol. 44:724–728.

Biederman, J., Faraone, S., Milberger, S., et al. 1996. A prospective 4-year study of attention-deficit hyperactivity and related disorders. Arch. Gen. Psychiatry 53:437–446.

Blatt, I., and Brenner, R.P. 1996. Triphasic waves in a psychiatric population: a retrospective study. J. Clin. Neurophysiol. 13:324–329.

Blumer, D., and Walker, A.E. 1975. The neural basis of sexual behavior. In Psychiatric Aspects of Neurologic Disease, Ed. M. Greenblatt, pp. 199–217. New York: Grune and Stratton.

Bogousslavsky, J. 2003. Emotions, mood, and behavior after stroke. Stroke 34:1046–1050.

Boutros, N.N. 1992. A review of indications for routine EEG in clinical psychiatry. Hosp. Community Psychiatry 43:716–719.

Boutros, N.N. 2000. Part II: the American Psychiatric Electrophysiology Association (APEA): history and mission. Clin. Electroencephalogr. 31: 67–70.

Boutros, N.N., and Struve, F. 2002. Electrophysiological assessment of neuropsychiatric disorders. Semin. Clin. Neuropsychiatry 7:30–41.

Boutros, N.N., Berman, R.M., Hoffman, R., et al. 2000a. Electroencephalogram and repetitive transcranial magnetic stimulation. Depression Anxiety 12:166–169.

Boutros, N., Campbell, D., Petrakis, I., et al. 2000b. Cocaine use and the mid-latency auditory evoked responses. Psychiatry Res. 96:117–126.

Boutros, N.N., Torello, M., and McGlashan, T.H. 2003. Electrophysiological aberrations in borderline personality disorder: state of the evidence. J. Neuropsychiatry Clin. Neurosci. 15:145–154.

Bowman, E.S. 1993. Etiology and clinical course of pseudoseizures. Relationship to trauma, depression, and dissociation. Psychosomatics 34: 333–342.

Bowman, E.S., and Coons, P.M. 2000. The differential diagnosis of epilepsy, pseudoseizures, dissociative identity disorder, and dissociative disorder not otherwise specified. Bull. Menninger Clin. 64:164–180.

Bremner, J.D. 2003. Functional neuroanatomical correlates of traumatic stress revisited 7 years later, this time with data. Psychopharmacol. Bull. 37:6–25.

Brenner, R.P., Reynolds, C.F., and Ulrich, R.F. 1989. EEG findings in depressive pseudodementia and dementia with secondary depression. Electroencephalogr. Clin. Neurophysiol. 72:298–304.

Bromfield, E.B., Altshuler, L., Leiderman, D.B., et al. 1992. Cerebral metabolism and depression in patients with complex partial seizures. Arch. Neurol. 49:617–623.

Brown, R.J., and Trimble, M.R. 2000. Dissociative psychopathology, nonepileptic seizures, and neurology. J. Neurol. Neurosurg. Psychiatry 69: 285–288.

Bruder, G.E., Fong, R., Tenke, C.E., et al. 1997. Regional brain asymmetries in major depression with or without an anxiety disorder: a quantitative electroencephalographic study. Biol. Psychiatry 41:939–948.

Bruton, C.J., Stevens, J.R., and Frith, C.D. 1994. Epilepsy, psychosis, and schizophrenia: clinical and neuropathologic correlations. Neurology 44: 34–42.

Bush, G., Fink, M., Petrides, G., et al. 1996. Catatonia. II. Treatment with lorazepam and electroconvulsive therapy. Acta Psychiatr. Scand. 93:137–143.

Bye, A.M., Kok, D.J., Ferenschild, F.T., et al. 2000. Paroxysmal nonepileptic events in children; a retrospective study over a period of 10 years. J. Pediatr. Child Health 36:244–248.

Calzetti, S., Bortone, E., Negrotti A., et al. 2002. Frontal intermittent rhythmic delta activity (FIRDA) in patients with dementia with Lewy bodies: a diagnostic tool? Neurol. Sci. 23(suppl 2):S65–66.

Carroll, B.T., and Boutros, N.N. 1995. Clinical electroencephalograms in patients with catatonic disorders. Clin. Electroencephalogr. 26:60–64.

Centorrino, F., Price, B.H., Tuttle, M., et al. 2002. EEG abnormalities during treatment with typical and atypical antipsychotics. Am. J. Psychiatry 159:109–115.

Christensen, L., Bourgeois, A., and Cockroft, R. 1993. Electroencephalographic concomitants of a caffeine-induced panic reaction. J. Nerv. Ment. Dis. 181:327–330.

Clarke, A.R., Barry, R.J., McCarthy, R., et al. 2002a. EEG activity in girls with attention-deficit/hyperactivity disorder. Clin. Neurophysiol. 114:319–328.

Clarke, A.R., Barry, R.J., McCarthy, R., et al. 2002b. EEG evidence for a new conceptualisation of attention deficit hyperactivity disorder. Clin. Neurophysiol. 113:1036–1044.

Claus, J.J., Strijers, R.L.M., Jonkman, E.J., et al. 1999. The diagnostic value of electroencephalography in mild senile Alzheimer's disease. Clin. Neurophysiol. 110:825–832.

Cohen, H.D., Rosen, R.C., and Goldstein, L. 1976. Human EEG laterality changes during sexual orgasm. Arch. Sex. Behav. 5:189–199.

Coleman, E. 2000. Psychiatry and human sexuality. Curr. Opin. Psychiatry 13:277–278.

Coons, P.M. 1999. Psychogenic or dissociative fugue: a clinical investigation of five cases. Psychol. Rep. 84:881–886.

Coons, P.M., and Milstein, V. 1992. Psychogenic amnesia: a clinical investigation of 25 cases. Dissociation 5:73–79.

Coons, P.M., Milstein, V., and Marley, C. 1982. EEG studies of two multiple personalities and a control. Arch. Gen. Psychiatry 39:823–825.

Cornelius, J.R., Brenner, R.P., Soloff, P.H., et al. 1986. EEG abnormalities in borderline personality disorder: specific or nonspecific. Biol. Psychiatry 21:977–980.

Cornelius, J.R., Fabrega, H., Jr., Mezzich, J., et al. 1993. Characterizing organic mood syndrome, depressed type. Compr. Psychiatry 34:432–440.

Corrigan, P.W., Yudofsky, S.C., and Silver, J.M. 1993. Pharmacological and behavioral treatments for aggressive psychiatric inpatients. Hosp. Community Psychiatry 44:125–133.

Craske, M.G., Lang, A.J., Jayson, L., et al. 2002. Does nocturnal panic represent a more severe form of panic disorder? J. Nerv. Ment. Dis. 190:611–618.

Crisp, A.H., Fenton, G.W., and Scotton, L.A. 1968. A controlled study of the EEG in anorexia nervosa. Br. J. Psychiatry 114:1149–1169.

Cutting, J. 1992. The role of right hemisphere dysfunction in psychiatric disorders. Br. J. Psychiatry 160:583–588.

Dalen, P. 1965. Family history, the electroencephalogram and perinatal factors in manic conditions. Acta Psychiatr. Scand. 41:527–563.

Dantendorfer, K., Prayer, D., Kramer, J., et al. 1996. High frequency of EEG and MRI brain abnormalities in panic disorder. Psychiatry Res. Neuroimag. Sect. 68:41–53.

Davidson, R.J. 1998. Anterior electrophysiological asymmetries, emotion, and depression: conceptual and methodological conundrums. Psychophysiology 35:607–614.

Davidson, R.J., Marshall, J.R., Tomarken, A.J., et al. 2000. While a phobic waits: regional brain electrical and autonomic activity in social phobics during anticipation of public speaking. Biol. Psychiatry 47:85–89.

De la Fuente, J.M., Tugendhaft, P., and Mavroudakis, N. 1998. Electroencephalographic abnormalities in borderline personality disorder. Psychiatry Res. 77:131–138.

DeLeon, O.A., Blend, M.J., Jobe, T.H., et al. 1997. Application of ictal brain SPECT for differentiating epileptic from nonepileptic seizures. J. Neuropsychiatry Clin. Neurosci. 9:99–101.

Dell, P.F. 2002. Dissociative phenomenology of dissociative identity disorder. J. Nerv. Ment. Dis. 190:10–15.

DeLong, G.R., Rosenberger, P.B., Hildreth, S. and Silver, I. 1987. The 14 & 6 associated clinical complex: a rejected hypothesis revisited. J. of Child. Neurol. 2:117–127.

Delvenne, V., Kerkhofs, M., Appelboom-Fondu, J., et al. 1992. Sleep polygraphic variables in anorexia nervosa and depression: a comparative study in adolescents. J. Affect. Disord. 25:167–172.

DeMyer, M.K., Barton, S., DeMyer, W.E., et al. 1973. Prognosis in autism: a followup study. J. Autism Child Schizophr. 3:199–246.

DeMyer, M.K., Hingtgen, J.N., and Jackson, R.K. 1981. Infantile autism reviewed: a decade of research. Schizophr. Bull. 7:388–451.

Denney, D., and Stevens, J.R. 1995. Clozapine and seizures. Biol. Psychiatry 37:427–433.

Drake, M.E., and Shy, K.E. 1989. Predictive value of electroencephalography for electroconvulsive therapy. Clin. Electroencephalogr. 20:55–57.

Drake, M.E., Hietter, S.A., Padamadan, H., et al. 1991. Computerized EEG frequency analysis in Gilles de la Tourette syndrome. Clin. Electroencephalogr. 22:250–253.

Drake, M.E., Hietter, S.A., Bogner, J.E., et al. 1992. Cassette EEG sleep recordings in Gilles de la Tourette syndrome. Clin. Electroencephalogr. 23:142–146.

Eisendrath, S.J., and Valan, M.N. 1994. Psychiatric predictors of pseudoepileptic-seizures in patients with refractory seizures. J. Neuropsychiatry Clin. Neurosci. 6:257–260.

El-Badri, S.M., Ashton, C.H., Moore, P.B., et al. 2001 Electrophysiological and cognitive function in young euthymic patients with bipolar affective disorder. Bipolar Disord. 3:79–87.

Enzmann, D.R., and Lane, B. 1977. Cranial computed tomography findings in anorexia nervosa. J. Comput. Assist. Tomogr. 1:410–414.

Feighner, J.P., Robins, E., Guze, S.B., et al. 1972. Diagnostic criteria for use in psychiatric research. Arch. Gen. Psychiatry 26:57–63.

Fink, M. 1979. *Convulsive Therapy: Theory and Practice.* New York: Raven Press.

Fink, M. 1995. Recognizing NMS as a type of catatonia. Neuropsychiatry Neuropsychol. Behav. Neurol. 8:75–76.

Fink, M., and Taylor, M.A. 2003. *Catatonia: A Clinician's Guide to Diagnosis and Treatment.* Cambridge, UK: Cambridge University Press.

Fleischhacker, W.W., Unterweger, B., Kane, J.M., et al. 1990. The neuroleptic malignant syndrome and its differentiation from lethal catatonia. Acta Psychiatr. Scand. 81:3–5.

Flor-Henry, P. 1972. Ictal and interictal psychiatric manifestations in epilepsy: specific or non-specific? Epilepsia 13:773–783.

Flor-Henry, P. 1985. Psychiatric aspects of cerebral lateralization. Psychiatr. Ann. 15:429–434.

Frances, A., First, M.B., and Ross, R. 1995. Getting up to speed on DSM-IV. J. Pract. Psychiatry Behav. Health 1:2–9.

Freudenreich, O., Weiner, R.D., and McEvoy, J.P. 1997. Clozapine-induced electroencephalogram changes as a function of clozapine serum levels. Biol. Psychiatry. 42:132–137.

Fricchione, G. 1989. Catatonia: a new indication for benzodiazepines? Biol. Psychiatry 26:761–765.

Gansaeuer, M., and Alsaadi, T.M. 2003. Lithium intoxication mimicking clinical and electrographic features of status epilepticus: a case report and review of the literature. Clin. Electroencephalogr. 34:28–31.

Gibbs, F.A., and Gibbs, E.L. (Eds.). 1964. *Atlas of Electroencephalography vol. 3., Neurological and Psychiatric Disorders.* Reading, MA: Addison-Wesley.

Gibbs, F.A., and Novick, R.G. 1977. Electroencephalographic findings among adult patients in a private psychiatric hospital. Clin. Electroencephalogr. 8:79–88.

Gillberg, C., and Soderstrom, H. 2003. Learning disability. Lancet 362:811–821.

Gilroy, J., and Meyer, J.S. 1975. *Medical Neurology.* New York: Macmillan.

Giovanardi, R.P., Posar, A., Parmeggiana, A. 2000. Epilepsy in adolescents and young adults with autistic disorder. Brain Dev. 22:102–106.

Glaze, D.G. 2002. Neurophysiology of Rett syndrome. Ment. Retard. Dev. Disabil. Res. Rev. 8:66–71.

Godbout, R., Bergeron, C., Limoges E., et al. 2000. A laboratory study of sleep in Asperger's syndrome. Neuroreport 11:127–130.

Goddard, A.W., and Charney, D.S. 1997. Toward an integrated neurobiology of panic disorder. J. Clin. Psychiatry 58:4–11.

Goldman, M.B., Robertson, G.L., Luchins, D.J., et al. 1997. Psychotic exacerbations and enhanced vasopressin secretion in schizophrenic patients with hyponatremia and polydipsia. Arch. Gen. Psychiatry 54:443–449.

Goldstein, L., Manowitz, P., Nora, R., et al. 1985. Differential EEG activation and pathological gambling. Biol. Psychiatry 20:1232–1234.

Gordon, N. 2000. Cognitive functions and epileptic activity. Seizure (3): 184–188.

Gottesman, I.I., and Gould, T.D. 2003. The endophenotype concept in psychiatry: etymology and strategic intentions. Am. J. Psychiatry 160:636–645.

Groppel, G., Kapitany, T., and Baumgartner, C. 2000. Cluster analysis of clinical seizure semiology of psychogenic nonepileptic seizures. Epilepsia 41:610–614.

Gurvits, T.V., Gilbertson, M.W., Lasko, N.B., et al. 2000. Neurologic soft signs in chronic posttraumatic stress disorder. Arch. Gen. Psychiatry 57:181–186.

Guze, S.B. 1976. *Criminality and Psychiatric Disorders.* New York: Oxford University Press.

Halliday, A.M. 1968. A comparison of the effects on depression and memory of bilateral ECT and unilateral ECT to the dominant and non-dominant hemispheres. Br. J. Psychiatry 114:997–1012.

Hallioglu, O., Ozge, A., Comelekoglu, U., et al. 2001. Evaluation of cerebral maturation by visual and quantitative analysis of resting electroencephalography in children with primary nocturnal enuresis. J. Child Neurol. 16:714–718.

Halmi, K.A., Goldberg, S.C., Eckert, E., et al. 1977. Pretreatment evaluation in anorexia nervosa. In *Anorexia Nervosa,* Ed. R.A. Vigersky, pp. 43–54. New York: Raven Press.

Harden, C.L., Burgut, F.T., and Kanner, A.M. 2003. The diagnostic significance of video-EEG monitoring findings on pseudoseizure patients differs between neurologists and psychiatrists. Epilepsia 44:453–456.

Harrison, M.J.G., Newman, S.P., Hall-Craggs, M.A., et al. 1998. Evidence of CNS impairment in HIV infection: clinical, neuropsychological, EEG, and MRI/MRS study. J. Neurol. Neurosurg. Psychiatry 65:301–307.

Harvey, N.S., Jarratt, J., and Ward, N.I. 1992. Trace elements and the electroencephalogram during long-term lithium treatment. Br. J. Psychiatry 160:654–658.

Hashimoto, T., Sasaki, M., Sugai, K., et al. 2001. Paroxysmal discharges on EEG in young autistic patients are frequent in frontal regions. J. Med. Invest. 48:175–180.

Hays, P. 1976. Etiological factors in manic-depressive psychoses. Arch. Gen. Psychiatry 33:1187–1188.

Heath, R.G. 1972. Pleasure and brain activity in man: deep and surface electroencephalograms during orgasm. J. Nerv. Ment. Dis. 154:3–18.

Hechtman, L., Weiss, G., and Metrakos, K. 1978. Hyperactive individuals as young adults: current and longitudinal electroencephalographic evaluation and its relation to outcome. Can. Med. Assoc. J. 118:919–923.

Heinz, E.R., Martinez, J., and Maenggeli, A. 1977. Reversibility of cerebral atrophy in anorexia nervosa and Cushing's syndrome. J. Comput. Assist. Tomogr. 1:415–418.

Helkala, E-L., Laulumaa, V., Soininen, H., et al. 1991. Different patterns of cognitive decline related to normal or deteriorating EEG in a 3-year follow-up study of patients with Alzheimer's disease. Neurology 41:528–532.

Helzer, J.E., and Hudziak, J.J. 2002. *Defining Psychopathology in the 21st Century.* Washington, DC: American Psychiatric Association Publishing.

Hendricks, S.E., Fitzpatrick, D.F., Hartmann, K., et al. 1988. Brain structure and function in sexual molesters of children and adolescents. J. Clin. Psychiatry 49:108–112.

Hermann, B.P., Seidenberg, M., Haltiner, A., et al. 1991. Mood state in unilateral temporal lobe epilepsy. Biol. Psychiatry 30:1205–1218.

Himmelhoch, J.M., Neil, J.F., May, S.J., et al. 1980. Age, dementia, dyskinesia, and lithium response. Am. J. Psychiatry 137:941–945.

Holschneider, D.P., and Leuchter, A.F. 1999. Clinical neurophysiology using electroencephalography in geriatric psychiatry: neurobiologic implications and clinical utility. J. Geriatr. Psychiatry Neurol. 12:150–164.

Howard, R., Rabins, P.V., Seeman, M.V., et al., and the International Late-Onset Schizophrenia Group. 2000. Late-onset schizophrenia and very-late-onset schizophrenia-like psychosis: an international consensus. Am. J. Psychiatry 157:172–178.

Hudziak, J.J., Boffeli, T.J., Kriesman, J.J., et al. 1996. Clinical study of the relation of borderline personality disorder to Briquet's syndrome (hysteria), somatization disorder, antisocial personality disorder, and substance abuse disorders. Am. J. Psychiatry 153:1598–1606.

Hughes, J.R. 1971. Electroencephalography and learning disabilities. In *Progress in Learning Disabilities,* vol. 2, Ed. H.R. Myklebust, pp. 18–55. New York: Grune and Stratton.

Hughes, J.R. 1995. The EEG in psychiatry: an outline with summarized points and references. Clin. Electroencephalogr. 26:92–101.

Hughes, J.R. 1996. A review of the usefulness of the standard EEG in psychiatry. Clin. Electroencephalogr. 27:35–39.

Hughes, J.R., and John, E.R. 1999. Conventional and quantitative electroencephalography in psychiatry. J. Neuropsychiatry Clin. Neurosci. 11:190–208.

Hurwitz, T.A., Wada, J.A., Kosaka, B.D., et al. 1985. Cerebral organization of affect suggested by temporal lobe seizures. Neurology 35:1335–1337.

Hyde, T.M., Emsellem, H.A., Randolph, C., et al. 1994. Electroencephalographic abnormalities in monozygotic twins with Tourette's syndrome. Br. J. Psychiatry 164:811–817.

Hymas, N., Lees, A., Bolton, D., et al. 1991. The neurology of obsessional slowness. Brain 114:2203–2233.

Imada, N., Kawauchi, A., Kitamori, T., et al. 1996. Long-term results of systematic treatment for nocturnal enuresis based on overnight simultaneous monitoring of electroencephalography and cystometry. Jpn. J. Urol. 87:1114–1119.

Imada, N., Kawauchi, A., Tanaka, Y., et al. 1998. Classification based on overnight simultaneous monitoring by electroencephalography and cystometry. Eur. Urol. 33(suppl 3):45–48.

Inui, K., Motomura, E., Okushima, R., et al. 1998. Electroencephalographic findings in patients with DSM-IV mood disorder, schizophrenia, and other psychotic disorders. Biol. Psychiatry 43:69–75.

Itil, T.M. 1982. The use of electroencephalography in the practice of psychiatry. Psychosomatics 23:799–813.

Itil, T.M., and Soldatos, C. 1980. Epileptogenic side effects of psychotropic drugs: practical recommendations. JAMA 244:1460–1463.

Ito, Y., Teicher, M.H., Glod, C.A., et al. 1993. Increased prevalence of electrophysiological abnormalities in children with psychological, physical, and sexual abuse. J. Neuropsychiatry Clin. Neurosci. 5:401–408.

Jacobson, S., and Jerrier, H. 2000. EEG in delirium. Semin. Clin. Neuropsychiatry 5:86–92.

James, A.L., and Barry, R.J. 1980. A review of psychophysiology in early-onset psychosis. Schizophr. Bull. 6:506–525.

Jampala, V.C., Zimmerman, M., Sierles, F.S., et al. 1992. Consumers' attitudes toward DSM-III and DSM-III-R: a 1989 survey of psychiatric educators, researchers, practitioners, and senior residents. Compr. Psychiatry 33:180–185.

Jasper, H.H., Solomon, P., and Bradley, C. 1938. Electroencephalographic analyses of behavior problem children. Amer. J. Psychiat. 95:641–658.

Javitt, D.C. 1997. Psychophysiology of schizophrenia. Curr. Opin. Psychiatry 10:11–15.

Jenike, M., and Brotman, A., 1984. The EEG in obsessive-compulsive disorder. J. Clin. Psychiatry 45:122–124.

Jeste, D.V., Potkin, S.G., Sinha, S., et al. 1979. Tardive dyskinesia—reversible and persistent. Arch. Gen. Psychiatry 36:585–590.

Johnson, C., Stuckey, M., and Mitchell, J.E. 1985. Psychopharmacology of anorexia and bulimia. In *Anorexia Nervosa and Bulimia. Diagnosis and Treatment,* Ed. J.E. Mitchell, pp. 134–151. Minneapolis, MN: University of Minnesota Press.

Kaartinen, P., Valsanen, E., Reunanen, M., et al. 1984. Tardive dyskinesia and EEG. Clin. Electroencephalogr. 15:226–231.

Kafka, M.P. 2003. The monoamine hypothesis for the pathophysiology of paraphilic disorders: an update. Ann. N.Y. Acad. Sci. Sexually Coercive Behavior: Understanding and Management 989:86–94.

Kanemoto, K., Tsuji, T., and Kawasaki, J. 2001. Reexamination of interictal psychoses based on DSM IV psychosis classification and international epilepsy classification. Epilepsia 42:98–103.

Kanner, A., and Balabanov, A. 2002. Depression and epilepsy: How closely related are they? Neurology 58(suppl):S27–S39.

Kapur, N. 1993. Transient epileptic amnesia—a clinical update and a reformulation. J. Neurol. Neurosurg. Psychiatry 56:1184–1190.

Karson, C.N., Coppola, R., and Daniel, D.G. 1988. Alpha frequency in schizophrenia: an association with enlarged cerebral ventricles. Am. J. Psychiatry 145:861–864.

Katada, A., Hasegawa, S., Ohira, D., et al. 2000. On chronological changes in the basic EEG rhythm in persons with Down syndrome—with special reference to slowing of alpha waves. Brain Dev. 22:224–229.

Katz, I.R., Curyto, K.J., TenHave, T., et al. 2001. Validating the diagnosis of delirium and evaluating its association with deterioration over a one-year period. Am. J. Geriatr. Psychiatry 9:148–159.

Kawas, C.H. 2003. Early Alzheimer's disease. N. Engl. J. Med. 349:1056–1063.

Kawauchi, A., Imada, N., Tanaka, Y., et al. 1998. Effects of systematic treatment based on overnight simultaneous monitoring of electroencephalography and cystometry. Eur. Urol. 33(suppl 3):58–61.

Kelley, J.T., and Reilly, E.L. 1983. EEG, alcohol, and alcoholism. In *EEG and Evoked Potentials in Psychiatry and Behavioral Neurology,* Eds. J.R. Hughes and W.P. Wilson, pp. 55–77. Boston: Butterworths.

Kellner, C., and Fink, M. 1996. Seizure adequacy: Does EEG hold the key? Convulsive Ther. 12:203–206.

Kendler, K.S., and Hays, P. 1982. Familial and sporadic schizophrenia: a symptomatic, prognostic, and EEG comparison. Am. J. Psychiatry 139:1557–1562.

Kennedy, G.L., and Scalmati, A., 2001. The interface of depression and dementia. Curr. Opin. Psychiatry 14:367–369.

Kerem, N.C., and Katzman, D.K. 2003. Brain structure and function in adolescents with anorexia nervosa. Adolesc. Med. State of the Art Rev. 14:109–118.

Khoshbin, S. 2000. The history of the Electroencephalography and Clinical Neuroscience Society (ECNS). Part I: A brief history of the American Medical Electroencephalographic Association (AMEEGA). Clin. Electroencephalogr. 31:63–66.

King, D.E., Herning, R.I., Gorelick, D.A., et al. 2000. Gender differences in the EEG of abstinent cocaine abusers. Neuropsychobiology 42:93–98.

Klass, D.W., and Westmoreland, B.F. 1985. Nonepileptogenic epileptiform electroencephalographic activity. Ann. Neurol. 18:627–635.

Kolbeinsson, H., and Petursson, H. 1988. Electroencephalographic correlates of electroconvulsive therapy. Acta Psychiatr. Scand. 78:162–168.

Koles, Z.J., Lind, J.C., and Flor-Henry, P. 1994. Spatial patterns in the background EEG underlying mental disease in man. Electroencephalogr. Clin. Neurophysiol. 91:319–328.

Koshino, Y. 1989. EEG in psychiatry. Am. J. EEG Technol. 29:219–234.

Koshino, Y., Murata, I., Murata, T., et al. 1993. Frontal intermittent delta activity in schizophrenic patients receiving antipsychotic drugs. Clin. Electroencephalogr. 24:13–18.

Kowalski, J.W., Gawel, M., Pfeffer, A., et al. 2001. The diagnostic value of EEG in Alzheimer disease: correlation with the severity of mental impairment. J. Clin. Neurophysiol. 18:570–575.

Krynicki, V.E. 1978. Cerebral dysfunction in repetitively assaultive adolescents. J. Nerv. Ment. Dis. 166:59–67.

Krystal, A.D., West, M., Prado, R., et al. 2000 EEG effects of ECT: implications for rTMS. Depression Anxiety 12:157–165.

Kubota, F., Shibata, N., Akata, T., et al. 2003. Spikes immediately after electroconvulsive therapy in psychotic patients. Clin. Electroencephalogr. 34:23–27.

Kurlan, R., Hamill, R., and Shoulson, I. 1984. Neuroleptic malignant syndrome. Clin. Neuropharmacol. 7:109–120.

Kuyk, J., Spinhoven, P., van Emde Boas, W., et al. 1999. Dissociation in temporal lobe epilepsy and pseudo-epileptic seizure patients. J. Nerv. Ment. Dis. 187:713–720.

Lancman, M. 1999. Psychosis and peri-ictal confusional states. Neurology 53(suppl 2):S33–S38.

Landolt, H. 1958. Serial electroencephalographic investigations during psychotic episodes in epileptic patients and during schizophrenic attacks. In *Lectures on Epilepsy Suppl. 4, Psychiat. Neurol. Neurochir. Suppl. 4,* Ed. A.M. Lorentz De Hass, pp. 91–133, Amsterdam: Elsevier.

Langevin, R. 1992. Biological factors contributing to paraphilic behavior. Psychiatr. Ann. 22:307–314.

Lauer, C.J., Krieg, J.C., Riemann, D., et al. 1990. A polysomnographic study in young psychiatric inpatients: major depression, anorexia nervosa, bulimia nervosa. J. Affect. Disord. 18:235–245.

Lee, G.P., Loring, D.W., Dahl, J.L., et al. 1993. Hemispheric specialization for emotional expression. Neuropsychiatry Neuropsychol. Behav. Neurol. 6:143–148.

Leis, A.A., Ross, M.A., and Summers, A.K. 1992. Psychogenic seizures: ictal characteristics and diagnostic pitfalls. Neurology 42:95–99.

Lepola, U., Nousiainen, U., Puranen, M., et al. 1990. EEG and CT findings in patients with panic disorder. Biol. Psychiatry 28:721–727.

Libman, M.D., Potvin, L., Coupal, L., et al. 1991. Seizure vs. syncope: measuring serum creatine kinase in the emergency department. J. Gen. Intern. Med. 6:408–412.

Lindau, M., Jelic, V., Johansson, S.E., et al. 2003. Quantitative EEG abnormalities and cognitive dysfunctions in frontotemporal dementia and Alzheimer's disease. Dement. Geriatr. Cogn. Disord. 15:106–114.

Lipowski, Z.J. 1980. Delirium updated. Compr. Psychiatry 21:190–196.

Liptzin, B., and Levkoff, S.E. 1992. An empirical study of delirium subtypes. Br. J. Psychiatry 161:843–845.

Liptzin, B., Levkoff, S.E., Cleary, P.D., et al. 1991. An empirical study of diagnostic criteria for delirium. Am. J. Psychiatry 148:454–457.

Liston, E.H., and LaRue, A. 1983a. Clinical differentiation of primary degenerative and multi-infarct dementia: a critical review of the evidence. Part I: Clinical studies. Biol. Psychiatry 18:1451–1465.

Liston, E.H., and LaRue, A. 1983b. Clinical differentiation of primary degenerative and multi-infarct dementia: a critical review of the evidence. Part II: pathological studies. Biol. Psychiatry 18:1467–1484.

Loeb, C. 1980. Clinical diagnosis of multi-infarct dementia. In *Aging of the Brain and Dementia,* Eds. L. Amaducci, A.N. Davison, and P. Autuono, pp. 251–260. New York: Raven Press.

Logsdail, S.J., and Toone, B.K. 1988. Post-ictal psychoses. A clinical and phenomenological description. Br. J. Psychiatry 152:246–252.

Lyketsos, C.G., Treisman, G.J., Lipsey, J.R., et al. 1998. Does stroke cause depression? J. Neuropsychiatry 10:103–107.

MacHale, S.M., O'Rourke, S.J., Wardlaw, J.M., et al. 1998. Depression and its relation to lesion location after stroke. J. Neurol. Neurosurg. Psychiatry 64:371–374.

Maes, M. 2001. Pedophilia: a biological disorder? Curr. Opin. Psychiatry 14:571–573.

Matousek, M., Brunovsky, M., Edman, A., et al. 2001. EEG abnormalities in dementia reflect the parietal lobe syndrome. Clin. Neurophysiol. 112:1001–1005.

Matsuura, M., Yoshino, M., Ohta, K., et al. 1994. Clinical significance of diffuse delta EEG activity in chronic schizophrenia. Clin. Electroencephalogr. 25:115–121.

Merlo, M.C., Kleinlogel, H., and Koukkou, M. 1998. Differences in the EEG profiles of early and late responders to antipsychotic treatment in first-episode, drug-naive psychotic patients. Schizophr. Res. 30:221–228.

Merriam, A.E., Kay, S.R., Opler, L.A., et al. 1990. Neurological signs and the positive-negative dimension in schizophrenia. Biol. Psychiatry 28:181–192.

Milstein, V., and Small, J.G. 1974. Photic responses in "minimal brain dysfunction." Dis. Nerv. Syst. 35:355–357.

Milstein, V., Small, J.G., Klapper, M.H., et al. 1987. Uni-versus bilateral ECT in the treatment of mania. Conv. Ther. 3:1–9.

Mirsattari, S.M., Berry, M.E., Holden, J.K., et al. 1999. Paroxysmal dyskinesias in patients with HIV infection. Neurology 52:109–114.

Monroe, R.R., Hulfish, B., Balis, G., et al. 1977. Neurologic findings in recidivist aggressors. In *Psychopathology and Brain Dysfunction,* Eds. C. Shagass, S. Gershon, and A.J. Friedhoff, pp. 241–253. New York: Raven Press.

Muller, H.F., Engelsmann, F., Nair, N.P., et al. 1997. Psychogeriatric clinical, electro-encephalographic and autopsy findings. Neuropsychobiology 35:95–101.

Nass, R., Gross, A., and Devinsky, O. 1998. Autism and autistic epileptiform regression with occipital spikes. Dev. Med. Child Neurol. 40:453–458.

Neil, J.F., Merlkangas, J.R., Davies, R.K., et al. 1978. Validity and clinical utility of neuroleptic-facilitated electroencephalography in psychotic patients. Clin. Electroencephalogr. 9:38–48.

Neil, J.F., Merlkangas, J.R., Foster, F.G., et al. 1980. Waking and all-night sleep EEG's in anorexia nervosa. Clin. Electroencephalogr. 11:9–15.

Netley, C., Lockyer, L., and Greenbaum, G.H.C. 1975. Parental characteristics in relation to diagnosis and neurological status in childhood psychosis. Br. J. Psychiatry 127:440–444.

Neufeld, M.Y., Berger, Y., Chapman, J., et al. 1990. Routine and quantitative EEG analysis in Gilles de la Tourette's syndrome. Neurology 40:1837–1839.

Niedermeyer, E., and Naidu, S.B. 1997. Attention-deficit hyperactivity disorder (ADHD) and frontal-motor cortex disconnection. Clin. Electroencephalogr. 28:130–136.

Niedermeyer, E., Naidu, S.B., and Plate, C. 1997. Unusual EEG theta rhythms over central region in Rett syndrome: considerations of the underlying dysfunction. Clin. Electroencephalogr. 2836–2843.

Okasha, A., Moneim, A.S., Bishry, Z., et al. 1974. Electroencephalographic study of stammering. Br. J. Psychiatry 124:534–535.

Paolicchi, J.M. 2002. The spectrum of nonepileptic events in children. Epilepsia 43:60–64.

Patrick, G., and Struve, F.A. 2000. Reduction of auditory P50 gating response in marihuana users: further supporting data. Clin. Electroencephalogr. 31:88–93.

Perez, M.M., Trimble, M.R., Murray, N.M.F., et al. 1985. Epileptic psychosis: an evaluation of PSE profiles. Br. J. Psychiatry 146:155–163.

Phillips, B.B., Drake, M.E., Jr., Hietter, S.A., et al. 1993. Electroencephalography in childhood conduct and behavior disorders. Clin. Electroencephalogr. 24:25–30.

Pillmann, F., Rohde, A., Ullrich, S., et al. 1999. Violence, criminal behavior, and the EEG; significance of left hemispheric focal abnormalities. J. Neuropsychiatry Clin. Neurosci. 11:454–457.

Povlsen, U.J., Wildschiodtz, G., Hogenhaven, H., et al. 2003. Nonconvulsive status epilepticus after electroconvulsive therapy. J. ECT 19:164–169.

Preskorn, S.H. 1995. Beyond DSM-IV: What is the cart and what is the horse? Psychiatr. Ann. 25:53–62.

Preskorn, S.H., Othmer, S.C., Lai, C., et al. 1984. Tricyclic-induced electroencephalogram abnormalities and plasma drug concentrations. J. Clin. Psychopharmacol. 4:262–264.

Prichep, L.S., Alper, K.R., Sverdlov, L., et al. 2002, Outcome related electrophysiological subtypes of cocaine dependence. Clin. Electroencephalogr. 33:8–20.

Pro, J.D., and Wells, C.E. 1977. The use of the electroencephalogram in the diagnosis of delirium. Dis. Nerv. Syst. 38:804–808.

Pueschel, S.M., Louis, S., and McKnight, P. 1991. Seizure disorders in Down's syndrome. Arch. Neurol. 48:318–320.

Quitkin, F., Rifkin, A., and Klein, D.F. 1976. Neurologic soft signs in schizophrenia and character disorders. Arch. Gen. Psychiatry 33:845–853.

Quitkin, F.M., Rifkin, A., Tsuang, M.T., et al. 1980. Can schizophrenia with premorbid asociality be genetically distinguished from the other forms of schizophrenia? Psychiatr. Res. 2:99–105.

Rae-Grant, A., Blume, W., Lau, C., et al. 1987. The electroencephalogram in Alzheimer-type dementia. Arch. Neurol. 44:50–54.

Raine, A., Venables, P.H., and Williams, M. 1990. Relationships between central and autonomic measures of arousal at age 15 and criminality at age 24 years. Arch. Gen. Psychiatry 47:1003–1007.

Rau, J.H., and Green, R.S. 1978. Soft neurological correlates of compulsive eaters. J. Nerv. Ment. Dis. 166:435–437.

Rau, J.H., Struve, F.A., and Green, R.S. 1979. Electroencephalographic correlates of compulsive eating. Clin. Electroencephalogr. 10:180–189.

Reeves, R.R., Struve, F.A., and Patrick, G. 2003. EEG does not predict response to valproate treatment of aggression in patients with borderline and antisocial personality disorders. Clin. Electroencephalogr. 34:84–86.

Roberts, G.W., Done, D.J., Burton, C., et al. 1990. A "mock-up" of schizophrenia: temporal lobe epilepsy and schizophrenia-like psychosis. Biol. Psychiatry 28:127–143.

Robertson, M.M., Channon, S., Baker, J. 1994. Depressive symptomatology in a general hospital sample of outpatients with temporal lobe epilepsy: a controlled study. Epilepsia 35:771–777.

Robinson, D.J., Merskey, H., Blume, W.T., et al. 1994. Electroencephalography as an aid in the exclusion of Alzheimer's disease. Arch. Neurol. 51:280–284.

Robinson, R.G. 2003. Poststroke depression: prevalence, diagnosis, treatment, and disease progression. Biol. Psychiatry 54:376–387.

Rodin, E., and Schmaltz, S. 1984. The Bear-Fedio personality inventory and temporal lobe epilepsy. Neurology 34:591–596.

Rosebush, P., and Stewart, T. 1989. A prospective analysis of 24 episodes of neuroleptic malignant syndrome. Am. J. Psychiatry 146:717–725.

Rosen, I. 1997. Electroencephalography as a diagnostic tool in dementia. Dement. Geriatr. Cogn. Disord. 8:110–116.

Rosenstein, L.D. 1994. Potential neuropsychologic and neurophysiologic correlates of multiple personality disorder. Neuropsychiatry Neuropsychol. Behav. Neurol. 7:215–229.

Rosenstein, D.L., Nelson, J.C., and Jacobs, S.C. 1993. Seizures associated with antidepressants: a review. J. Clin. Psychiatry 54:289–299.

Roy, M.A., and Crowe, R.R. 1994. Validity of the familial and sporadic subtypes of schizophrenia. Am. J. Psychiatry 151:805–814.

Russ, M.J., Campbell, S.S., Kakuma, T., et al. 1999. EEG theta activity and pain insensitivity in self-injurious borderline patients. Psychiatry Res. 89:201–214.

Sackeim, H.A., Luber, B., Katzman, G.P., et al. 1996. The effects of electroconvulsive therapy on quantitative electroencephalograms. Arch. Gen. Psychiatry 53:814–824.

Sackeim, H.A., Luber, B., Moeller, J.R., et al. 2000. Electrophysiological correlates of the adverse cognitive effects of electroconvulsive therapy. J. ECT 16:110–120.

Sato, K., Kamiya, S., Okawa, M., et al. 1996. On the EEG component waves of multi-infarct dementia seniles. Int. J. Neurosci. 86:95–109.

Satterfield, J.H., and Schell, A.M. 1984. Childhood brain function differences in delinquent and non-delinquent hyperactive boys. Electroencephalogr. Clin. Neurophysiol. 57:199–207.

Sawle, G.V., Hymas, N.F., Lees, A.J., et al. 1991. Obsessional slowness. Functional studies with positron emission tomography. Brain 114:2191–2202.

Scaer, R.C. 2001. The neurophysiology of dissociation and chronic disease. Appl. Psychophysiol. Biofeedback 26:73–91.

Schwitzer, J., Neudorfer, C., Schett, P., et al. 1992. Usefulness of screening EEGs in psychiatric inpatients. J. Clin. Psychiatry 53:327–328.

Semerci, Z.B. 2000. Neurological soft signs and EEG findings in children and adolescents with Gilles de la Tourette syndrome. Turkish J. Pediatr. 42:53–55.

Serafetinides, E.A. 1993. EEG in psychiatry. J. Clin. Psychiatry 54:397.

Shagass, C. 1977. Twisted thoughts, twisted brain waves? In Psychopathology and Brain Dysfunction, Eds. C. Shagass, S. Gershon, and A.J. Friedhoff, pp. 353–378. New York: Raven Press.

Sheth, R.D. 1998. Electroencephalogram in developmental delay: specific electroclinical syndromes. Semin. Pediatr. Neurol. 5:45–51.

Shetty, T. 1971. Photic responses in hyperkinesis of childhood. Science 174:1356–1357.

Shulman, K., and Post, F. 1980. Bipolar affective disorder in old age. Br. J. Psychiatry 136:26–32.

Shutty, M.S., Jr., Briscoe, L., Sautter, S., et al. 1993. Neuropsychological manifestations of hyponatremia in chronic schizophrenic patients with the syndrome of psychosis, intermittent hyponatremia and polydipsia (PIP). Schizophr. Res. 10:125–130.

Silva, J.R., Pizzagalli, D.A., Larson, C.L., et al. 2002. Frontal brain asymmetry in restrained eaters. J. Abnorm. Psychol. 111:676–681.

Small, I.F., Small, J.G., Fjeld, S.P., et al. 1966. Organic cognates of acute psychiatric illness. Am. J. Psychiatry 122:790–797.

Small, J.G. 1975. EEG and neurophysiological studies of early infantile autism. Biol. Psychiatry 10:385–397.

Small, J.G. 1983. EEG in schizophrenia. In EEG and Evoked Potentials in Psychiatry and Behavioral Neurology, Eds. J.R. Hughes and W.P. Wilson, pp. 25–40. Woburn, MA: Butterworths.

Small, J.G. 1986. EEG and lithium CNS toxicity. Am. J. EEG Technol. 26: 225–239.

Small, J.G., Stevens, J.R., and Milstein, V. 1964. Electro-clinical correlates of emotional activation of the EEG. J. Nerv. Ment. Dis. 138:146–155.

Small, J.G., Small, I.F., Milstein, V., et al. 1975. Familial associations with EEG variants in manic depressive disease. Arch. Gen. Psychiatry 32:43–48.

Small, J.G., Milstein, V., DeMyer, M.K., et al. 1977. Electroencephalographic (EEG) and clinical studies of early infantile autism. Clin. Electroencephalogr. 8:27–35.

Small, J.G., Milstein, V., and Jay, S. 1978a. Clinical EEG studies of short and long term stimulant drug therapy of hyperkinetic children. Clin. Electroencephalogr. 9:186–194.

Small, J.G., Small, I.F., and Milstein, V. 1978b. Electrophysiology of EST. In Psychopharmacology: A Generation of Progress, Eds. M.A. Lipton, A. DeMascio, and K.F. Killam, pp. 759–769. New York: Raven Press.

Small, J.G., Milstein, V., Sharpley, P.H., et al. 1984. Electroencephalographic findings in relation to diagnostic constructs in psychiatry. Biol. Psychiatry 19:471–487.

Small, J.G., Milstein, V., and Medlock, C.E. 1997. Clinical EEG findings in mania. Clin Electroencephalogr. 28:229–235.

Small, J.G., Milstein, V., Klapper, M.H., et al. 1998. Topographic EEG studies of mania. Clin. Electroencephalogr. 29:1–9.

Snyder, S., and Pitts, W.M., Jr. 1984. Electroencephalography of DSM-III borderline personality disorder. Acta Psychiatr. Scand. 69:129–134.

Soininen, H., and Riekkinen, P.J. 1992. EEG in diagnostics and follow-up of Alzheimer's disease. Acta Neurol. Scand. Suppl. 139:36–39.

Spark, R.F., White, R.A., and Connolly, P.B. 1980. Impotence is not always psychogenic. JAMA 243:750–755.

Sponheim, S.R., Clementz, B.A., Iacono, W.G., et al. 2000. Clinical and biological concomitants of resting state EEG power abnormalities in schizophrenia. Biol. Psychiatry 48:1088–1097.

Staley, D., Wand, R., and Shady, G. 1997. Tourette disorder: a cross-cultural review. Compr. Psychiatry 38:6–16.

Steinberg, M. 1994. Structured Clinical Interview of DSM-IV Dissociative Disorders-Revised (SCID-D-R). Washington, DC: American Psychiatric Association Press.

Stevens, J. 1988. Epilepsy, psychosis and schizophrenia. Schizophr. Res. 1:79–89.

Stevens, J.R., and Hermann, B.P. 1981. Temporal lobe epilepsy, psychopathology, and violence: The state of the evidence. Neurology 31:1127–1132.

Stevens, J.R., Bigelow, L., Denney, D., et al. 1979. Telemetered EEG-EOG during psychotic behaviors of schizophrenia. Arch. Gen. Psychiatry 36: 251–262.

Stores, G. 1991. Confusions concerning sleep disorders and the epilepsies in children and adolescents. Br. J. Psychiatry 158:1–7.

Strauss, E., Wada, J., and Moll, A. 1992. Depression in male and female subjects with complex partial seizures. Arch. Neurol. 49:391–392.

Struve, F.A. 1976. The necessity and value of securing routine electroencephalograms in psychiatric patients: a preliminary report on the issue of referrals. Clin. Electroencephalogr. 7:115–130.

Struve, F.A. 1977. EEG findings detected in routine screening of psychiatric patients—relationship to prior expectation of positive results. Clin. Electroencephalogr. 8:47–50.

Struve, F.A. 1985. Possible potentiation of suicide risk in patients with EEG dysrhythmias taking oral contraceptives: a speculative empirical note. Clin. Electroencephalogr. 16:88–90.

Struve, F.A., and Becka, D.R. 1968. The relative incidence of the B-mitten EEG pattern in process and reactive schizophrenia. Electroencephalogr. Clin. Neurophysiol. 24:80–82.

Struve, F.A., Saraf, K.R., Arko, R.S., et al. 1977. Relationship between paroxysmal electroencephalographic dysrhythmia and suicide ideation and attempts in psychiatric patients. In Psychopathology and Brain Dysfunction, Eds. C. Shagass, S. Gershon, and A.J. Friedhoff, pp. 199–221. New York: Raven Press.

Struve, F.A., Patrick, G., Straumanis, J.J., et al. 1998. Possible EEG sequelae of very long duration marihuana use: pilot findings from topographic quantitative EEG analyses of subjects with 15 to 24 years of cumulative daily exposure to THC. Clin. Electroencephalogr. 29:31–36.

Suddath, R.L., Christison, G.W., Torrey, E.F., et al. 1990. Anatomical abnormalities in the brains of monozygotic twins discordant for schizophrenia. N. Engl. J. Med. 322:789–794.

Suppes, T., Webb, A., Carmody, T., et al. 1996. Is postictal electrical silence a predictor of response to electroconvulsive therapy? J. Affect. Disord. 41:55–58.

Thigpen, C.H., and Cleckley, H.M. 1957. *The Three Faces of Eve.* New York: McGraw-Hill.

Thirumalai, S., Abou-Khalil, B., Fakhoury, T., et al. 2001. Video-EEG in the diagnosis of paroxysmal events in children with mental retardation and in children with normal intelligence. Dev. Med. Child Neurol. 43: 731–734.

Tongoe, K., Numata, O., Sato, T., et al. 1999. Contingent negative variation in children with anorexia nervosa. Pediatr. Int. 41:285–291.

Toni, C., Cassano, G.B., Perugi, G., et al. 1996. Psychosensorial and related phenomena in panic disorders and in temporal lobe epilepsy. Compr. Psychiatry 37: 125–133.

Treffert, D. 1970. Epidemiology of infantile autism. Arch. Gen. Psychiat. 22:431–438.

Trimble, M. 1977. The relationship between epilepsy and schizophrenia: a biochemical hypothesis. Biol. Psychiatry 12:229–304.

Trimble, M.R. 1978. Serum prolactin in epilepsy and hysteria. Br. Med. J. 2:1682.

Trzepacz, P.T., Mulsant, B.H., Dew, M.A., et al. 1998. Is delirium different when it occurs in dementia? J. Neuropsychiatry Clin. Neurosci. 10:199–204.

Tsai, L.Y., and Tsai, M.C. 1985. Implication of EEG diagnoses in the subclassification of infantile autism. J. Autism Dev. Dis. 15:339–344.

Tucker, G.J., Price, T.R.P., Johnson, V.B., et al. 1986. Phenomenology of temporal lobe dysfunction: a link to atypical psychosis—a series of cases. J. Nerv. Ment. Dis. 174:348–356.

Umbricht, D., Degreef, G., Barr, W.B., et al. 1995. Postictal and chronic psychoses in patients with temporal lobe epilepsy. Am. J. Psychiatry 152: 224–231.

Van Sweden, B. 1986. Disturbed vigilance in mania. Biol. Psychiatry 21: 311–313.

Victoroff, J.I., Benson, D.F., Grafton, S.T., et al. 1994. Depression in complex partial seizures. Arch. Neurol. 51:155–163.

Waldo, M.C., Cohen, D.J., Caparulo, B.K., et al. 1978. EEG profiles of neuropsychiatrically disturbed children. J. Am. Acad. Child Psychiatry 17: 656–670.

Warner, M.D., Boutros, N.N., Peabody, C.A. 1990. Usefulness of screening EEGs in a psychiatric inpatient population. J. Clin. Psychiatry 51:363–364.

Waters, B.G.H., Marcenko-Bouer, I., and Smiley, D. 1982. Perinatal complications are not associated with affective disorders in the offspring of bipolar manic-depressives. Neuropsychobiology 8:1–9.

Wegner, J.T., Struve, F.A., Kantor, J.S., et al. 1979. Relationship between the B-mitten EEG pattern and tardive dyskinesia. Arch. Gen. Psychiatry 36:599–603.

Weilburg, J.B., Schachter, S., Sachs, G.S., et al. 1993. Focal paroxysmal EEG changes during atypical panic attacks. J. Neuropsychiatry Clin. Neurosci. 5:50–55.

Weilburg, J.B., Schachter, S., Worth, J., et al. 1995. EEG abnormalities in patients with atypical panic attacks. J. Clin. Psychiatry 56:358–362.

Weinberger, D.R., Wayner, R.L., Stevens, J.R., et al. 1982. Neurological abnormalities in schizophrenia. Society of Biological Psychiatry, 37th Annual Meeting, Toronto, Canada.

Weiner, M.F., Bruhn, M., Svetlik, D., et al. 1991. Experiences with depression in a dementia clinic. J. Clin. Psychiatry 52:234–238.

Weiss, G., and Hechtman, L. 1979. The hyperactive child syndrome. Science 205:1348–1354.

Westphal, K.P., Grozinger, B., Diekmann, V., et al. 1990. Slower theta activity over the midfrontal cortex in schizophrenic patients. Acta Psychiatr. Scand. 81:132–138.

White, D.A.C., and Robins, A.H. 1991. Catatonia and neuroleptic malignant syndrome. Br. J. Psychiatry 158:858–859.

Whitman, S., Hermann, B.P., and Gordon, A.C. 1984. Psychopathology in epilepsy: How great is the risk? Biol. Psychiatry 19:213–236.

Williams, A.O., Reveley, M.A., Kolakowska, T., et al. 1985. Schizophrenia with good and poor outcome II: cerebral ventricular size and its clinical significance. Br. J. Psychiatry 146:239–246.

Wilson, M. 1993. DSM-III and the transformation of American psychiatry: a history. Am. J. Psychiatry 150:399–410.

Witelson, S.F. 1977. Neural and cognitive correlates of developmental dyslexia: age and sex differences. In *Psychopathology and Brain Dysfunction,* Eds. C. Shagass, S. Gershon, and A.J. Friedhoff, pp. 15–49. New York: Raven Press.

Wolf, M.E., Koller, W.C., and Mosnaim, A.D. 1984. Electroencephalogram in tardive dyskinesia. Clin. Electroencephalogr. 15:222–225.

Woods, B.T., and Short, M.P. 1985. Neurological dimensions of psychiatry. Biol. Psychiatry 20:192–198.

Woods, B.T., Kinney, D.K., and Yurgelun-Todd, D.A. 1991. Neurological "hard" signs and family history of psychosis in schizophrenia. Biol. Psychiatry 30:806–816.

World Health Organization. 1992. *The ICD-10 Classification of Mental and Behavioural Disorders: Clinical Descriptions and Diagnostic Guidelines.* Geneva: WHO.

Yoshino, Y. 1989. EEG in psychiatry. Amer. J. EEG. Technology 29:219–234.

Yoshino, A., and Yoshimasu, H. 2000. Nonconvulsive status epilepticus complicating neuroleptic malignant syndrome improved by intravenous diazepam. J. Clin. Psychopharmacol 20:389–390.

Yoshino, A., Yoshimasu, H., Tatsuzawa, Y., et al. 1998. Nonconvulsive status epilepticus in two patients with neuroleptic malignant syndrome. J. Clin. Psychopharmacol. 18:347–349.

Zimmermann, G.N., and Knott, J.R. 1974. Slow potentials of the brain related to speech processing in normal speakers and stutterers. Electroencephalogr. Clin. Neurophysiol. 37:599–607.

31. Neurocognitive Functions and the EEG

Eckart O. Altenmüller, Thomas F. Münte, and Christian Gerloff

According to the results of our investigations of the human EEG, we are confronted with material processes of smallest dimensions linked to psychological processes, yet these being the most wonderful and the most powerful phenomena on this planet. [Hans Berger 1938, p. 306]

The significance of the electroencephalogram (EEG) for investigating neurocognitive functions was already recognized by its discoverer, Hans Berger himself. In his first communication on the human EEG he introduced the topic of this chapter as a question: "Will it be possible to demonstrate intellectual processes by means of the EEG?" (1929, p. 569). And he gave a positive answer in the very same publication when he described the alpha-blockade during cognitive processing as a first objective correlate of mental states. Thus, the "Berger-effect" was the starting point of neurocognitive EEG-research.

In this discipline, the parallelism of methodological improvements and scientific progress can clearly be demonstrated: following Berger's work, research first focused on the relation between EEG frequencies and behavior. The development of averaging-techniques and the ensuing improvement of the signal-to-noise ratio was the prerequisite for the discovery of the small endogenous event-related potential shifts (ERPs), ranging within a few microvolts in amplitude, and reflecting neurocognitive processes. Improvements in direct current (DC) recording techniques during the mid-1980s encouraged several groups to investigate sustained DC-potential shifts in relation to complex cognitive processes. The rapid improvement of other brain-imaging methods such as positron emission tomography (PET) and functional magnetic resonance imaging (fMRI) in the late 1980s forced EEG researchers to compete with or utilize these techniques (Wikswo et al., 1993). This development resulted in an increasing number of cooperating research teams, using co-registration of EEG and magnetoencephalography (MEG), PET, fMRI, and transcranial magnetic stimulation to solve their scientific questions. We are convinced that the future of our discipline lies in a synergistic use of methods providing the excellent temporal resolution of EEG and MEG, and the excellent spatial resolution of MRI and PET.

This chapter provides a systematic review of the field of EEG correlates of neurocognitive processes. It cannot be exhaustive, but nevertheless tries to distill the important general information on neurocognitive EEG research and the most significant recent contributions to this area from a huge body of literature. Some aspects have been reviewed in detail recently. We refer to a concise review article in the new *Handbook of Neuropsychology* by Münte et al. (2000) and to a recently published book, *The Cognitive Electrophysiology of Mind and Brain*, edited by Alberto Zani and Alice Mado Proverbio (2002).

According to the methodological criteria mentioned above, the different approaches of EEG research and the new developments of combined applications of methods in psychophysiology will be presented in separate sections:

(a) the analysis of EEG-frequencies, (b) the endogenous event-related potentials (ERPs), (c) the sustained cortical DC-potential shifts prior to or during mental performance, and (d) the combination of EEG and other brain imaging methods in psychophysiology

EEG Frequencies and Neurocognitive Processes

Neurocognitive research by analysis of the EEG frequencies started with Hans Berger's observation of the alpha-blockade during the performance of mental arithmetic. The electrophysiological basis of wave generation is not completely clarified, but there is general agreement that synchronous discharges of cortical cell assemblies driven by afferent thalamocortical inputs play an important role (see Chapter 2 by Speckmann and Elger). The thalamic pacemakers in turn are controlled by the inhibitory inputs from the substantia reticularis in the midbrain. Activation of the substantia reticularis leads to disinhibition of the thalamic pacemakers and causes desynchronization of the EEG (Singer and Dräger, 1972).

It has been demonstrated that alpha-blocking or event-related desynchronization (ERD) (Pfurtscheller and Aranibar, 1977) is related to arousal mechanisms mediated by the reticular activating system (Lindsley et al., 1949; Moruzzi and Magoun, 1949). The close relationship of ERD with the orienting response is reflected by the fact that ERD is habituating over trials, but recovers when the stimulus changes in quality (Simons et al., 1987). In searching for electrophysiological correlates of focal cortical activation, the topographical distribution of ERD in relation to different mental tasks involving the two hemispheres specifically soon attracted interest. The introduction of the fast Fourier transform algorithm in 1965 facilitated the data analysis and contributed to a wider utilization of frequency analysis in psychophysiological research. Overall, the results were disappointing, exhibiting only small effects that often could not be reproduced by different investigators (Donchin et al., 1977; Gevins et al., 1979). In consequence, many researchers switched over to the developing field of endogenous ERP.

In the past decade, promoted by a rapidly increasing number of manufacturers offering commercial mapping systems that include multichannel frequency analysis and algorithms calculating the interelectrode coherence, mapping has experienced a renaissance. Furthermore, the concept that periodic neural activity in the high-frequency range (>20 Hz) may indicate specific cognitive processes has given new impulses to frequency analysis of the ongoing EEG and MEG (Singer and Gray, 1995). Presently, there is evidence (Engel and Singer, 2001) that neuronal oscillations and synchronization in the gamma frequency range (30–70 Hz) distributed over multiple cortical regions provide a general platform for functional cooperation or large-scale integration, which is an essential requirement for the successful accomplishment of any complex cognitive task (Varela et al., 2001).

However, the results produced by spectral mapping and coherence analysis of the surface EEG have to be interpreted cautiously, since a virtually indefinite number of parameters within variable frequency bands can be generated. Due to methodological and theoretical reasons, a direct comparison of results obtained with scalp electrodes in humans to data from intracortical multielectrode recordings in animals remains questionable.

Local Changes in Frequency and Coherence: Correlation to Mental Performance

Hemispheric differences in alpha power in relation to tasks requiring predominant processing in one hemisphere were observed by many investigators. Diminution of alpha power over the left hemisphere was found during mental arithmetic (Butler and Glass, 1987; Morgan et al., 1974), word search tasks (McKee et al., 1973), verbal fluency tasks (Beaumont et al., 1978), and listening to a tape recording of speech (Duffy et al., 1981). Reading elicited bilateral occipital and parietal alpha diminution (Pfurtscheller and Klimesch, 1987). Diminution of the alpha power over the right hemisphere could be observed during spatial imagery (Rebert and Low, 1978) and music processing (Duffy et al., 1981; McKee et al., 1973). At a closer look, these apparently clear results were far from consistent. The sources of divergent results are manifold: the cognitive demands were confounded with motor task demands (Gevins et al., 1979); the number of electrodes was too small or bipolar recordings were used (Petsche et al., 1986); only narrow bands of the whole alpha activity were preselected (Jürgens et al., 1995); different methods of data analysis, especially the transformation of data into left/right ratios, obscured the results (Donchin et al., 1977); finally, varying definitions of "resting states" representing the baseline were used. Unfortunately, due to the lack of generally accepted standardized methods of data acquisition and data analysis, this Babylonian confusion has further increased and the comparison of results from different laboratories has become more and more difficult.

A recent development in neurocognitive EEG research is the increasing interest in the high-frequency gamma band (>20 Hz). Berger's (1929) hypothesis that high-frequency oscillations may indicate mental processes was nurtured by findings that coherent periodic neural activity in the 40-Hz range accompanies information processing in the visual cortex of vertebrates (Eckhorn et al., 1988). In animal experiments, neuronal oscillations in this frequency range could be related to feature linking and gestalt perception (Singer and Gray, 1995). EEG measurements in humans revealed local enhancement of cortical gamma band activity during preparation and execution of movements (Kristeva-Feige, 1993) during language processing (Pulvermüller et al., 1996), during visual tasks (Tallon et al., 1995), and during music perception, especially in professional musicians (Bhattacharya et al., 2001).

In elegant EEG and MEG experiments, Pulvermüller et al. (1996) could demonstrate that spectral responses in the 30-Hz range were specifically elicited by linguistic processing of meaningful words, but not of meaningless nonwords. Spectral responses to meaningful gestalt-like figures, such as Kanisza's triangle, produced a similar increase in 30-Hz power, but not the responses to matched figures that did not constitute a coherent gestalt (Tallon et al., 1995). In contrast, processing of simple stimuli affects the spectral power in the higher frequency range of the gamma band. Tones or moving bars, as well as preparation and performance of simple repetitive movements, are usually accompanied by enhanced spectral activity in the 40-Hz range or above (Pantev, 1995). It therefore seems that task-related high-frequency oscillations can be subdivided into two functionally separated entities, a 30-Hz and a 40-Hz component. As an explanation, Pulvermüller (1995) proposes that in complex cognitive tasks, e.g., during language processing, Hebbian neuronal cell assemblies are activated—"ignited"—and form a loop from Broca's region to Wernicke's region and back. The round-trip time in such a loop will be 20 to 40 msec or less, equaling a circulation frequency of 25 to 30 Hz. In contrast, if cell assemblies are less widely dispersed, as it can be assumed in primary sensory processing, round-trip times may be substantially shorter so that high-frequency oscillatory cortical activity in the 40- to 60-Hz range will be generated. There are still many questions unresolved with respect to the functional significance of increased gamma activity. Recent studies suggest that an increase in gamma power phase synchronization of induced gamma activity may represent a general mechanism enabling transient associations of neural assemblies. New findings indicate, furthermore, that synchronized gamma activity is specifically involved in selective attention. While feature binding appears to depend primarily on induced gamma synchronization, attentional processes seem to involve both induced and evoked gamma oscillations (Fell et al., 2003). The growing importance of even faster ("ultrafast," 80–1,000 Hz) frequencies has become evident during the first years of the 21st century (see Chapter 26 by Curio).

Endogenous Event-Related Potentials (ERPs) and Neurocognitive Functions

While the early portions of the evoked potential waveform are mainly dependent on physical stimulus characteristics such as loudness or brightness and are therefore often called exogenous potentials, the later portions of the evoked potential have been shown to vary with a variety of psychological variables. Therefore, these later parts (from 100 msec onward) are often called (late, endogenous) ERPs. This is due to the fact that they depend largely on psychological variables, while physical stimulus properties play little or no role in their generation. In relation to the ongoing background EEG, the ERPs exhibit very small amplitudes ranging between 2 and 20 μV in magnitude. Analysis of ERPs, therefore, requires an improvement of the signal-to-noise ratio, which is usually achieved by simple signal averaging (Münte et al., 2000). This procedure leads to time-voltage diagrams, which are characterized by positive and negative deflections, each of which with a specific scalp topography. Several systems of labeling the peaks and troughs of the ERP waveform coexist. Most often, the polarity of a component is denoted by the letters "N" (i.e., negative) or "P" (i.e., positive). The different negative and positive deflections are then labeled in the order of their appearance (e.g., P1, N1, P2, N2, etc.), by their characteristic peak latencies (e.g., N100 or P300), or by their actual peak latencies in a specific experiment (e.g., N148, P125; see Fig. 31.1 for a systematic overview). One has to keep in mind, however, that the label "P1" signifies completely different neurophysiological phenomena in somatosensory, visual, or auditory modalities. Also, sometimes peaks labeled according to their characteristic latencies might occur considerably earlier or later. For example, in difficult visual classification experiments, the P300 effect is often seen as late as 800 msec. In everyday use, the ERP peaks are often identified as components. This is somewhat misleading, since originally the term *component* had been reserved for ERP phenomena that show a unique behavior as a function of experimental manipulations. Therefore, a component might span several ERP peaks ("N2/P3" component) or, because of the dipolar nature of the underlying electromagnetic sources, may manifest itself as a negative peak at one recording site and as a positive peak in others. For example, the mismatch "negativity" component has actually a positive polarity at subsylvian recording sites when a nose-tip reference is employed.

While a lot of ERP research in the past has been devoted to the delineation of the cognitive correlates of certain components, more recent work has circumvented the difficulties of the definition of components by operationally defining ERP effects as markers for task-dependent differences in cognitive processes without making too much reference to the classic components. A case in point is the so-called *Dm* effect [for difference based on later memory performance (Paller et al., 1987); see memory section below]. We have therefore decided to organize this chapter according to the cognitive processes under study and not according to the ERP components. These will be mentioned at the appropriate places.

Neural Generators

While ERPs afford exquisite time resolution on the order of 1 msec, a major drawback has been the lack of knowledge regarding the anatomical generators responsible for the different effects. With the advent of multichannel recordings, the topographical definition of ERP effects has been greatly improved. Nevertheless, it has been known since von Helmholtz (1853) that the problem of recovering the current sources from superficial electromagnetic measurements is

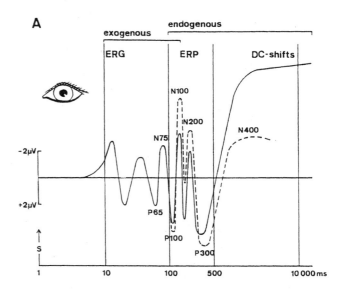

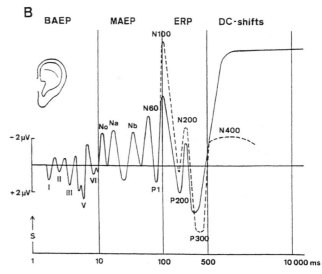

Figure 31.1. Averaged event-related responses to visual **(A)** and acoustic **(B)** stimuli. Schematic potential traces on a logarithmic time-scale. **A:** Exogenous components comprise the electroretinogram (ERG) and the P 65 and N 75. Components with latencies longer than 100-msec latency are considered as endogenous components. The P 100 and N 100 component can be modified by orienting and selective attention *(dashed lines)*, the N 200 by stimulus evaluation and the P 300 by context updating. The N 400 is related to semantic expectancy. Large direct current (DC) shifts occur when complex cognitive tasks have to be solved. **B:** In the acoustic modality exogenous components comprise the acoustic brainstem auditory evoked potentials (BAEPs) and the midlatency auditory evoked potentials (MAEPs). Endogenous components can be modified analogous to the visual modality but have a tendency toward shorter latencies. Whereas exogenous event-related potentials (ERPs) exhibit modality-specific potential traces, endogenous components are very similar in both modalities.

intrinsically based with great difficulties. It is impossible to uniquely determine the spatial configuration of neural activity based on EEG recordings alone (Nunez, 1981). This is also known as the inverse problem.

In spite of this dictum, significant progress has been made in source localization by making certain a priori assumptions about the solution. For example, a common ap-

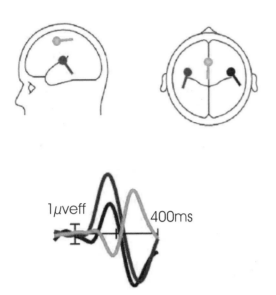

Figure 31.2. Example of the estimation of neural generators of ERPs using multiple equivalent current dipoles as implemented by the brain electric source analysis program package (e.g., Scherg et al., 1999). Data are from a study in which a combined mismatch negativity and P3a response was found for deviant stimuli (Nager et al., 2003). **Upper panel:** Three dipoles were found in an iterative procedure. Two symmetrical dipoles in the auditory cortex explained the activity related to the mismatch negativity. A third frontal source was associated with the P3a. **Lower panel:** Activity of these point dipoles over time.

proach is to assume that an ERP is generated by a small number of focal sources, which can be modeled by equivalent current point dipoles (ECD) (Scherg and Ebersole, 1994; Scherg et al., 1999). The location, orientation, and activity over time of each ECD is iteratively determined by minimizing the difference between the predicted and the actual ERP. This approach, implemented in the popular BESA software, has been successful when comparatively early ERP effects with a circumscribed scalp topography were targeted (Fig. 31.2). For late and widely distributed ERP effects, for which many spatially and temporally overlapping sources can be assumed, this approach becomes increasingly problematic for computational and plausibility reasons.

Another approach, therefore, is to consider a priori all possible fixed source locations. In such continuous current source models the strength of each dipole is estimated according to some mathematical constraint. A unique solution is obtained by minimizing the deviation from these constraints. A number of approaches have been proposed including (among others) weighted minimum L2 norm, i.e., a least squares approach (Brooks et al., 1999; Hämäläinen and Ilmoniemi, 1994; Sarvas, 1987), and maximum smoothness. The latter is implemented in the *low-resolution electromagnetic tomography* (LORETA) software package (Pascual-Marqui, 1999; Pascual-Marqui et al., 1994; see Chapter 59 by Lopes da Silva).

Neuroanatomical considerations suggest that sources of brain electromagnetic activity should be located in gray matter and, because of the orientation of the cortical columns,

oriented orthogonally to the cortical sheet. Moreover, they should be locally coherent, leading to "smooth" activity along the cortical sheet. These considerations can be used to further constrain the solution space (Phillips et al., 2002) by using realistic head models derived from actual brain anatomy. For example, the current version of LORETA computes the current distribution across 2,394 voxels distributed only in gray matter as determined from a standard average brain template provided by the Montreal Neurological Institute.

Stimulus Selection: Attentive and Preattentive Mechanisms

One of the core tasks of our nervous system is to select important information and to discard stimuli that are not deemed important. This filtering out of information has been termed selective attention. At the same time it is also necessary to scan the environment for novel or deviant events in order to redirect attention towards these possibly important stimuli.

Visual Attention

In a typical visual selective attention task, stimuli are represented rapidly in at least two "channels" defined by, for example, their spatial location. Paying attention to stimuli from one channel in order to perform a target detection task ("look and see!" in colloquial English; editorial comment, E. Niedermeyer) gives rise to enhanced amplitudes of several ERP peaks, compared with ERPs to the same stimuli when the other location is detected. The earliest component to be affected by visuospatial attention is an occipitotemporal positivity component that has a latency of about 120 msec (P1) (Fig. 31.3). This component has been shown to be

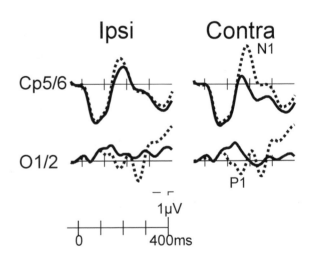

Figure 31.3. Visual ERPs in a selective spatial attention task requiring the subjects to fixate the center of a video screen and to attend either to stimuli appearing to the right or to the left of the fixation cross in order to identify rare target stimuli. ERPs from left and right visual fields are averaged together yielding ERPs for electrodes ipsi- and contralateral to the stimuli. The first attention-modulated ERP component is the occipital P1 component, which is more pronounced for attended stimuli. This is followed by a centroparietal N1 component that is similarly enhanced (unpublished data by Nager and Münte).

generated in secondary visual cortex (Gomez-Gonzalez et al., 1994) and is followed by a similarly enhanced negativity at about 170 msec (N1). While visuospatial attention modulates the amplitude of obligatory components of the ERP, the attention to other stimulus features such as motion, color, or stimulus orientation results in the elicitation of so-called selection negativities (Hillyard and Münte, 1984). These differ in their specific scalp topography, and source modeling suggests that these effects are generated by secondary visual areas dedicated to the processing of the corresponding stimulus features. When multidimensional stimuli are used, e.g., stimuli that are characterized by their location and color, a hierarchical dependency of color selection on location selection has been shown using ERPs.

In addition to maintaining an attentional focus at a specific location or on another specific stimulus feature, a subject often also has to direct the attentional spotlight either as a function of an alerting stimulus or voluntarily. This directive aspect of attention has been studied in cuing tasks, in which a target stimulus is preceded by an attention-directing cue. In such tasks some target stimuli are preceded by valid cues, i.e., the target appears at the designated location, while in a minority of trials the cue is invalid, i.e., the target appears on the other side. Under such circumstances again an attention-dependent modulation of the P1 and N1 components is found (Mangun and Hillyard, 1987).

While attention in the visual domain has been discussed mostly in relation to attention to specific features, more recently it has been stressed that whole objects in the environment may be attended selectively and thus perceived as unified ensembles of their constituent features. In a combined ERP/fMRI study that required subjects to attend to one of two superimposed transparent surfaces formed by arrays of dots moving in opposite directions, neural activity was found for an irrelevant feature (color) of an attended object. This activity could be localized to the color area of the fusiform gyrus. Thus, these ERP data suggest that attention links relevant and irrelevant features to form a unified perceptual object (Schoenfeld et al., 2003).

Auditory Attention

In the auditory modality, selective attention tasks have been conducted using ERPs that are quite similar in design to the visual tasks mentioned above. For example, subjects are instructed to attend to one of two concurrent auditory streams of information defined by their location or pitch in order to detect slightly deviant target tones. In such a scenario, which is similar to the dichotic listening task that has been extensively used in cognitive psychology, the ERPs to stimuli in the attended stimulus "channel" are associated with a more negative waveform starting approximately 100 msec after the onset of the stimulus (Hansen and Hillyard, 1980, 1983; Hillyard et al., 1973). This processing negativity often extends for several hundred milliseconds and can be subdivided into subcomponents. While spatial location has a special status in the visual modality, this is not the case in the auditory modality, as the processing negativity is very similar for the selection according to different auditory features (e.g., pitch, timbre, loudness, duration; Fig. 31.4). It has been used to investigate the processing of multidimen-

sional auditory stimuli, i.e., situations in which stimulus channels are characterized by the factorial combination of different stimulus attributes (e.g., location and pitch; Hansen and Hillyard, 1983). Moreover, a number of studies have addressed the spatial gradient of auditory attention in central and peripheral auditory space (e.g., Teder-Sälejärvi and Hillyard, 1998). Interestingly, the gradient of auditory spatial attention in peripheral auditory space has been found to be much steeper in congenitally blind subjects (Röder et al., 1999) as well as in professional music conductors (Münte et al., 2001; Nager et al., 2003).

Preattentive Auditory Processing

It is of exquisite importance to humans as well as other species to screen the auditory environment for potentially important events. This global surveillance function is conducted without the use of attentional resources and this processing mode therefore has been labeled "preattentive." Two important ERP effects have been investigated in relation to preattentive auditory processing: the mismatch negativity (MMN) and the P3a response.

The MMN is found exclusively in the auditory domain. It is elicited by rare deviant stimuli that deviate physically from a monotonous context, e.g., in duration, pitch, timbre, or loudness. Importantly, the MMN is also found, if the subjects attend elsewhere. Experimentally, this is achieved by having subjects watching a movie or reading a book (reviewed in Näätänen and Winkler, 1999; Picton et al., 2001). The onset latency of the MMN varies but is typically around 130 msec with regard to the stimulus onset. Its duration is between 100 and 200 msec. The MMN shows a frontocen-

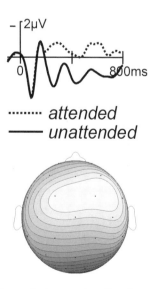

Figure 31.4. Auditory selective attention effect. Data are from a study requiring subjects to attend to one of two interspersed streams of stimuli defined by their pitch in order to identify target stimuli within the attended stream. Attended stimuli give rise to a long-standing negativity (**upper panel**, processing negativity), which has been interpreted as indicating prolonged processing of the attended stimuli. **Lower panel:** A spline-interpolated isovoltage map of the processing negativity is displayed with darker colors indicating positive and lighter colors negative voltage.

tral maximum and, if recorded against a nose-tip reference, a polarity inversion around the sylvian fissure suggesting a generator in the auditory cortex, which has been confirmed by dipole modeling and brain imaging studies (Opitz et al., 2002). In the classical experiments the deviant stimuli were presented against uniform standard stimuli. It therefore has been proposed that the invariant features of the standard stimuli form some kind of memory trace against which the incoming stimuli are compared. If a mismatch between the features of the actual stimulus and the memory trace is detected, an MMN is triggered. More recently, it has been shown that the MMN can also be elicited if repetitive sequences (e.g., tonal scales) are used to create the standard background stimuli (Tervaniemi et al., 1994). Thus, memory formation at the level of the auditory cortex includes the ability to extract complex sequential information (Picton et al., 2001).

A different mode of preattentive auditory processing is marked by the P3a component (Fig. 31.5). This is typically observed for so-called novel stimuli (e.g., the honking of a car, a dog's bark) occurring out of context in a series of stimuli. The P3a is a positivity with a peak latency of about 200 to 250 msec and thus considerably earlier than that of the classical P3b (P300) component. It has a frontocentral distribution. Combined fMRI/ERP recordings have suggested that the main neural generators of the P3a are in the superior temporal gyrus bilaterally and in the right frontal cortex

(Opitz et al., 1999). The P3a response has been interpreted as an electrophysiological correlate of the orienting response (Squires et al., 1975, 1977), which helps the subject to direct attention toward potentially important sources of information (Schröger, 1997).

Somatosensory Attention

If series of electric shocks are presented in a random sequence to different fingers of both hands with one of the fingers being relevant for the task, shocks in the attended "channel" produce an enhanced N140 component of the somatosensory evoked potential (SEP) (Desmedt and Tomberg, 1989). The topographical distribution reveals a maximal amplitude over the prefrontal cortex. In addition to this effect on the N140, earlier ERP signs of selective attention have been demonstrated in the somatosensory modality. At a latency of 30 msec an attention-related positive wave of small amplitude can be recorded over the contralateral parietal lobe (Desmedt and Tomberg, 1989). More recent investigations, combining multichannel recordings with spatiotemporal source modeling have shown attention-dependent modulations of the SEP waveform between 30 and 260 msec. Dipole modeling revealed six brain regions related to selective attention, among them the contralateral postcentral gyrus, the contralateral mesial frontal gyrus, the right posterior parietal cortex and the anterior cingulate gyrus. This suggests that attentional gain setting mechanisms act on different levels of the somatosensory pathway.

Memory

Psychological models distinguish between different memory systems that are presumably subserved by different neural systems and show differential involvement in neurological diseases. Memory systems can be classified according to whether or not their content can be verbalized (the declarative vs. procedural distinction) or whether or not the subject voluntarily accesses the memory content (explicit vs. implicit distinction). Further distinctions refer to the span that an item is kept in memory (working vs. short-term vs. long-term memory) and to the different processes involved in the administration of a memory trace (encoding vs. maintenance vs. retrieval). All of these different levels have been studied using ERPs over the past two decades (for reviews see Friedman and Johnson, 2000; Rugg and Allan, 2000; Rugg and Coles, 1995). Here we can highlight only a number of selected findings.

Event-Related Potential Effects During Retrieval

An important paradigm for memory research calls for the serial presentation of words, faces, or objects in a list with some of the items being repeated during the list. The task of the subject is to explicitly decide by button-press whether a given item is old (repeated) or new (first presentation). Across studies, three ERP effects distinguishing old and new items have been consistently observed: first, a decrease of the amplitude of the N400 component (between 300 and 500 msec, see language section of this chapter); second, an increase of a parietal positive slow wave (between 500 and 800 msec) that has been given different labels such as *late positive component, P300, late positivity,* or *parietal*

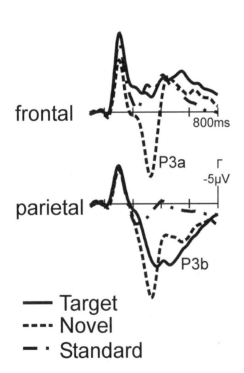

Figure 31.5. ERPs from a modified auditory oddball study: within a series of frequent "standard" stimuli (1,000 Hz, 80% probability) subjects had to identify by button press rare target stimuli (1,500 Hz, 10% probability). These target stimuli give rise to a typical P3b component, which is maximal at parietal recording sites. In addition, 10% of the stimuli comprised so-called novel stimuli; these were environmental noises that were not repeated during the experiment. These novel stimuli are associated with an earlier positivity (P3a) that is maximal at frontal and central recording sites.

old/new effect. Finally, in a number of studies a right frontal positivity has been found in paradigms that extend beyond simple recognition judgments and involve the retrieval of source information (i.e., under what circumstances was the item learned), or require postretrieval decision-making processes. A large body of research (summarized in Münte et al., 2000) has been directed at determining the relation of these three components to different qualities of recognition such as recollection and familiarity. Moreover, it has been asked which of these components is related to repetition in the absence of conscious recognition and which is related to repetition in the presence of conscious recognition. To answer these questions, variants of the old/new task have been used. For example, Düzel et al. (1997) required subjects to perform an old/new recognition judgment in some blocks of their study (explicit task), while in other blocks subjects had to make a living/nonliving judgment. In these latter runs the occasional repetition of items was not task-relevant (implicit task). In the explicit task both the N400 and late positive component were modulated by repetition, while in the implicit task only the N400 effect was seen. This suggests that the N400 modulation indexes repetition independent of recognition.

In so-called source monitoring tasks subjects are required not only to decide whether they have encountered an item before or not, but also to decide about specific aspects of the encoding episode of that item (e.g., the visual background or the speaker's voice). Wilding and Rugg (1996) found a right frontal positivity for those items that were classified as new and attributed to the right source. Consequently, this ERP effect has been discussed as reflecting retrieval of specific perceptual information regarding the memory source.

Effects During Encoding

Instead of presenting words or other stimuli in a continuous series, it is also possible to devise experiments with separate *study* and *test (retrieval)* phases. The registration of EEG during the study phase affords the possibility of averaging the single-trial activity according to whether or not the specific item was subsequently remembered during the retrieval phase. Using this method, Paller et al. (1987) found an increased late positivity (between approximately 300 and 800 msec) for those items that were later remembered, which was termed the Dm effect (see above). When words during the study phase had to be processed at a deep, semantic level (requiring a living, nonliving distinction), the Dm effect was larger and the memory performance better compared to a condition that used a shallow, nonsemantic task (first and last letter of word in alphabetical order). The Dm during encoding, therefore, appears to reflect the retrieval of information about the item from long-term memory.

Working Memory

It can be said that working memory holds, tags, and/or activates sensory information of the information retrieved from long-term memory for current processing. Working memory also actively maintains information, and this information can be changed or updated. An influential view posits that the P300 ERP component reflects this information processing function (Donchin and Coles, 1988), although not everybody agrees with this view (Verleger, 1988).

Typically the P300 is elicited by low probability deviant stimuli in a series of standard, higher probability stimuli when the deviants have to be attended and actively answered. This is called an oddball paradigm. The P300 is widely distributed but is most pronounced over parietal scalp regions. The amplitude of the P300 to the target events in an oddball sequence is inversely related to the global probability of its occurrence. The P300 amplitude is also modulated by the temporal interval between targets and by the local structure of the series (local probability). In an oddball task, in which more than two different stimuli are involved, the P300 amplitude is determined by the probability of the relevant stimulus category (target or standard) and not by the probability of the individual stimulus.

The relation to working memory becomes clearer if one assumes that whenever a target stimulus is encountered in an oddball task, the current target count maintained in working memory must be incremented, leading to an update of the model of the environment. Fine-grained inspection of the P300 "complex" often reveals different portions, which have been labeled P3a, P3b, and slow wave. Intracranial recordings have revealed multiple sites showing P300-like activity (Smith et al., 1990). The latency of the P3b component has been shown to vary systematically with task difficulty in stimulus categorization tasks. Thus, in a very difficult task, the P3b peak latency may well extend beyond 600 msec (Kutas et al., 1977). While manipulations of the difficulty of stimulus classification have profound effects on P3b latency, manipulation of the response selection difficulty has virtually no effect (McCarthy and Donchin, 1981). The P3b latency, therefore, can be used as an index of the timing of information processing as well as to assign task manipulations either to the stimulus evaluation or response selection stages.

Besides the updating of working memory, presumably indexed by the P300 response, information also needs to be actively maintained in working memory. Following Baddeley (1986), the working memory system comprises three major components: the central executive, the visuospatial sketchpad, and the phonological loop. The latter two systems are thought to maintain information over several seconds. In a series of studies Ruchkin and colleagues (1997) found that the scalp topography of the slow ERPs recorded during the retention interval depended on the type of material to be maintained. For example, retention of phonological material leads to a slow wave topography with a left frontal maximum, while retention of visuospatial material leads to a maximum over the right parietal scalp, suggesting that these effects index the activity of the visuospatial sketchpad and the phonological loop.

Language Comprehension and Production

Among all cognitive processes language is unique, as this function is available only to humans. Neurophysiological studies of language, therefore, are confined to humans and have to take advantage of noninvasive measures such as brain potential recordings. Linguists and psycholinguists have dissected the language faculty into several subdomains. While different theories make varying assumptions regarding the exact functional architecture of the language comprehension and production systems, there is a consensus that different types of information are needed that require specialized processing routines. These types of information have been identified as semantic, syntactic, pragmatic, phonological, and prosodic.

Semantic and Pragmatic Effects

A hallmark finding in the development of a neurophysiology of language has been the discovery of the N400 component by Kutas and Hillyard (1980). This is a widely distributed centroparietal negativity with a maximum at 400 msec (Fig. 31.6), which was first found in a sentence reading study. Terminal words that did not match the preceding context (e.g., "I drink my coffee with cream and <u>mud</u>") were associated with an N400, while congruous terminal words ("... with cream and <u>sugar</u>") were not. While this component was originally thought of as a marker of semantic incongruency, further research has shown that the N400 amplitude varies as a function of a number of factors (reviewed in Kutas et al., 2000). For example, the semantic incongruency effect is modulated by the relatedness of the expected word to the actual incongruent word such that a smaller N400 effect is obtained for the sentence "The pizza is too hot to drink" than for the sentence "The pizza is too hot too sing." Another factor is word frequency: words that are more common give rise to a smaller N400. Also, within a sentence the N400 amplitude decreases as a function of the serial position of the eliciting word within the sentence.

The N400 is reduced by the repetition of a word even if a number of other words are presented in between. Recently, it has been shown that N400 is sensitive to processes that require integration of information across several sentences (van Berkum et al., 1999). It has also been found that the N400 varies with pragmatic factors, i.e., with the difficulty of integrating a piece of discourse with general world knowledge (St. George et al., 1994). Taken together, the N400 amplitude appears to be negatively correlated with the ease with which an incoming stimulus can be integrated in the preceding context.

Syntax and Morphology

To establish links between words and ultimately to determine "who did what to whom" in a sentence, syntax is required. Many ERP studies in the syntactic domain have used the violation paradigm, i.e., the induction of grammatical errors. In relation to such errors a late positivity with an onset of approximately 500 msec with a maximum at 600 msec after onset of the critical word at centroparietal sites has been reported (P600 or syntactic positive shift). Syntactic errors that induce a P600 effect can be simple, such as in number agreement violations ("The cat chase_ the dog," Hagoort et al., 1993). The P600 is also observed in situations, in which a highly likely initial reading of a sentence has to be revised ("The woman persuaded to answer the door ...," Osterhout and Holcomb, 1992). The initial reading of the word *persuaded* is that it is very likely the verb of the main clause. This becomes untenable at the word *to*. Now, the syntactic interpretation of the sentence needs to be revised, with *persuaded* being the first word of a truncated relative clause. Precisely upon the presentation of the word *to*, a P600 is obtained in the ERP.

Concerning the functional significance of this P600 effect, it therefore has been proposed as a marker for syntactic reanalysis (Friederici, 1995), or syntactic integration difficulty (Kaan et al., 2000). Although no consensus has been reached yet on the exact functional significance of the P600, common to these views is that the P600 is primarily associated with syntactic processing. Evidence that is challenging this view has been presented, however (Kolk et al., 2003; Münte et al., 1998). A second component that is sometimes observed in grammatical errors is a left anterior negativity, which occurs with an earlier latency but seems to be less stable (King and Kutas, 1995; Kluender and Kutas, 1993; Münte et al., 1993).

Phonology and Prosody

Spoken language allows the speaker to code both syntactic information (e.g., whether a sentence is a question or a

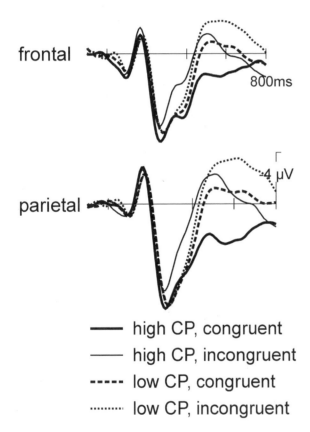

Figure 31.6. ERPs from a sentence processing study. All words except for the terminal word of a sentence were presented visually on a computer monitor. The last word of the sentence was presented via loudspeakers. Sentences were either highly coherent, leading to a high predictability of the terminal word (e.g., "The programmer was unhappy with his new computer": high CP sentence), or were less predictable (e.g., "He went to the store because he needed new socks": low CP sentence). Terminal words of low CP sentences are associated with an increased negativity (N400), which is maximal at parietal sites. In addition, terminal words were manipulated for semantic congruency. Incongruent words (e.g., "The programmer was unhappy with his new cockroach"; "He went to the store because he needed new love") lead to additional negativity in the N400 range.

frontal

800ms

4 µV

parietal

—— high CP, congruent

—— high CP, incongruent

----- low CP, congruent

········ low CP, incongruent

simple declarative sentence) and emotional information (e.g., whether he/she is sad or happy) by modulating the pitch of his/her voice. This is called prosody. An ERP effect, termed the closure positive shift, has been found that indexes an intonational phrase boundary (Steinhauer et al., 1999). These boundaries can be used to guide the initial syntactic analysis of spoken language.

Executive Functions

The term *executive function* denotes a heterogeneous group of higher order, "meta-cognitive" functions that are needed to orchestrate and supervise the behavior of humans (Smith and Jonides, 1999). These functions include planning, supervising, self-monitoring, the ability to inhibit a prepotent response, and the ability to shift a mental set, among others. Two processes, inhibition and self-monitoring, are briefly discussed here.

Inhibition

A popular paradigm to investigate inhibition is the so-called go/no-go task, in which one class of trials requires a response (go trial), while a motor response has to be withheld for another, similar class. No-go trials are characterized by a frontal negativity of about 1 to 4 µV in amplitude. The onset and peak latency of this no-go N200 effect depend on the time at which the information determining the go/no-go decision becomes available (Gemba and Sasaki, 1989; Kok, 1986; Simson et al., 1977). Several lines of evidence link this frontal "N200" to inhibitory processes. For example, invasive studies in behaving monkeys have revealed activity related to response inhibition in the prefrontal cortex in a go/no-go paradigm that gives rise to an N200 in humans (Sasaki et al., 1989). Also, destruction of prefrontal cortex in animals has been found to lead to a profound disturbance of performance in delayed response tasks (Fuster, 1989), and to an enhancement of disinhibition and impulsive behavior (Luria, 1973). Finally, brain imaging (fMRI) has pinpointed the frontal lobe as being important for inhibition in go/no-go trials (Garavan et al., 1999; Konishi et al., 1999).

Self-Monitoring

Recent ERP investigations of executive processes have focused on error detection and action monitoring. By averaging time-locked to the motor response in a cognitive task rather than to the stimulus onset, a negative component has been isolated appearing immediately after committing errors that therefore has been labeled error-related negativity (ERN) (Falkenstein et al., 2000; Gehring et al., 1993). One model associates the ERN to an error-detection mechanism (Falkenstein et al., 2000; Gehring et al., 1993), which compares an internal goal (a computed "best response") with the predicted consequences of the actual response. An internal "error signal" is generated if a mismatch is detected by the system. An alternative interpretation holds that the ERN merely reflects the degree of response conflict experienced by subjects (Botvinick et al., 2001). It has been shown that the process indexed by the ERN is also important for error correction (Rodriguez-Fornells et al., 2002a). Importantly, source modeling techniques have suggested that the ERN

emanates from the anterior cingulate gyrus (ACG). This coincides with findings from fMRI investigations, which also have found activations of the ACG in error trials and conditions that induced a high degree of response conflict (Carter et al., 1998).

Clinical Applications of Event-Related Brain Potentials

Clinical studies with ERPs have not fulfilled initial hopes and, as a general rule of thumb, ERPs have no utility in the diagnostic process of an individual patient. Nevertheless, a great number of ERP studies in clinical populations have been published, which have revealed important information about the information processing deficits of certain neuropsychiatric conditions.

P300 studies with normal elderly subjects have shown that the latency of the P300 becomes longer with increasing age and that this latency increase correlates with the general neuropsychological status of a subject (Polich and Kok, 1995). In patients with dementia, this latency increase is even more pronounced and a number of studies have provided evidence for a correlation between the cognitive decline and P300 latency. It is has been debated whether the latency increase might provide a useful clinical indicator (Polich, 1998).

Some studies have suggested that P300 amplitude and latency are valuable to distinguish between subcortical (e.g., Parkinson's disease, Huntington's disease) and cortical dementias such as Alzheimer's disease (Goodin and Aminoff, 1986). Another replicated finding is that the P300 can reliably distinguish between patients with dementia and those with a pseudo-dementia in the course of depression (Patterson et al., 1988). Other studies have used the P300 to investigate information processing in a variety of neuropsychiatric disorders, such as alcoholism, schizophrenia, depression, and multiple sclerosis. In general, a prolonged latency and/or amplitude decrement was seen for the patient groups. Thus, the P300 appears to be a very general measure to characterize information processing deficits in neuropsychiatric diseases. It lacks diagnostic specificity, however, which limits its use for differential diagnosis.

Mismatch Negativity (MMN)

In recent years, the MMN has been the most widely used ERP component in clinical studies. This is due to its good reproducibility and to the fact that the subject does not have to fulfill a task. It has been demonstrated in newborns (Kraus and Cheour, 2000) and therefore is of potential use for the investigation of developmental problems in the auditory system (Leppänen and Lyytinen, 1997). Another potential application is in the investigation of comatose patients (Kane et al., 1993) and it has been proposed that the MMN might be a superior predictor of outcome compared to other measures.

The MMN has been shown in group studies to reflect developmental problems in the perception of phonemes, which are related to a disturbed language development (Leppänen and Lyytinen, 1997) and developmental dyslexia (Kujala and Näätänen, 2001). In one study, Schulte-Körne and colleagues (1998) compared the MMN elicited by the syllables

/da/ and /ba/ with the MMN elicited by sine-wave tones of different frequencies. Dyslexic subjects showed a smaller MMN than controls for the syllables but a normal MMN for the sine waves. A strong genetic component has been revealed for dyslexia. In this regard the findings of Näätänen (2003) that babies of dyslexic parents already show abnormalities in the MMN to syllables is of great importance.

Only occasional reports concern the use of other ERP components in clinical context. An interesting study shows the potential utility of the N400 component for the characterization of aphasic disorders (Swaab et al., 1998). In this study Broca aphasics and normal control subjects were exposed to sentences ending with a potentially ambiguous word (e.g., "I put my money in the bank"). This sentence was followed by a test word that either was related to the meaning of the word primed by the sentence (e.g., *robber*) or to the alternative meaning (e.g., *river*). The word related to the alternative meaning gave rise to an N400 in normal subjects, suggesting that this meaning had been blocked by the sentence. In aphasics there was no N400 when the test word was presented immediately after the sentence, but the N400 was present when the word was presented with a considerable delay, indicating a temporal delay in sentence processing in the aphasics.

Slow Cortical DC Potentials in Neurocognitive Research

During the past two decades the investigation of cortical DC-potential shifts related to neuropsychological phenomena has increasingly attracted interest. The history of DC recordings supposedly dates back to 1875, when Caton was able to record epicortical DC potentials related to sensory stimulation in animals (a highly arguable claim). After Berger's discovery, EEG research in humans focused on the phasic phenomena and was soon restricted to AC-coupled recordings (i.e., a time constant in the range of 0.3 to 1.5 seconds was used), but physiologists continued the tradition of DC recordings. In 1959, Caspers and Schulze demonstrated in long-term DC recordings the increase in negative cortical DC potential during the transition from sleep to awakeness and to motor activity in the freely moving rat. Astonishingly, although DC recordings during sensory stimulation and cortical processing of stimuli were pursued by physiologists (e.g., David et al., 1969), this method was not adopted by psychologists and neurophysiologists in testing more complex cortical functions and fell into oblivion for more than 10 years. The renaissance of DC recordings during cognitive, sensory, and motor processing in the late 1980s and in the 1990s was in part due to improved amplifier and electrode technology, which facilitated the recording and the management of artifacts (Bauer et al., 1989; Hennighausen et al., 1993; Tucker, 1993). However, in recent years fMRI has replaced EEG in most experiments investigating integrated neurocognitive functions on a longer time scale.

Therefore, we only briefly discuss the negative shifts in cortical DC potential during cognitive processing, and thereafter in anticipation of psychological or behavioral events.

Slow Waves and DC Potential Shifts During the Performance Interval as Correlates of Complex Cognitive Processing

When cognitive processing requires 1 second or longer, a large increase in the surface-negative cortical DC potential occurs. The topographical distribution of these DC potential shifts or "slow potentials" reveals task-specific patterns related to the cortical structures predominantly involved in processing of the required task. Thus, local changes in DC potential can be used for the functional brain imaging. Compared to short-latency event-related potentials up to 500 msec, the slow DC shifts reflect more global task-related processes. In Fig. 31.7 examples of task-specific activation

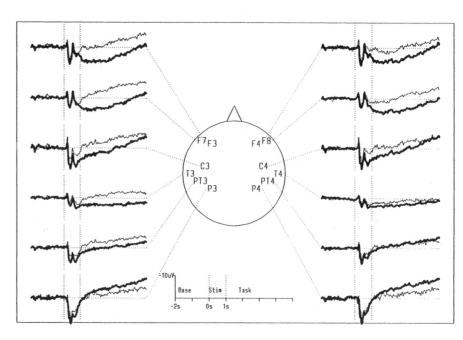

Figure 31.7. Grand-averages of DC-potential shifts during search for synonyms *(thin lines)* and during mental rotation of cubes *(thick lines)* in 16 male right-handed subjects. After recording of a 2-second baseline, stimuli are presented on a computer screen during 1 second. Subsequently, subjects perform the tasks during 4 seconds. Linguistic processing produces a marked increase in surface negativity over inferior left frontolateral brain regions, whereas visuospatial processing produces bilateral parietal activation.

patterns recorded with DC-EEG are displayed topographically. A linguistic task (thin lines) requiring mental search of synonyms to visually presented nouns and a visuospatial task (thick lines) requiring mental rotation of visually presented cubes are compared. The linguistic task causes an increase in DC negativity over the left inferior prefrontal cortex (electrode-position F7). In contrast, the mental rotation task produces maximal activation over the left and the right posterior parietal lobe (electrode positions P3 to P4).

The neurophysiological basis of slow negative DC shifts are long-lasting excitatory postsynaptic potentials at the apical cortical dendrites associated with a surface-negative, depth-positive electric dipole. The depolarization of apical dendrites, in turn, is dependent on sustained afferent input to layer I and/or simultaneous depolarization of large pools of pyramidal neurons (Caspers et al., 1984). The folding of about two thirds of the human cortex renders this simple relationship more complicated: negative-going DC shifts can only be recorded from scalp electrodes, when the sum vector of electric dipoles is perpendicular to the skull. This is the case when large cortical areas are activated during complex and sustained cognitive processes. In contrast, an activation of the planum temporale during decoding of verbal material produces an electric dipole tangentially to the surface of the temporal skull, which may be missed in surface electrode recordings from temporal or parietal locations. These restrictions, however, are common to all electrophysiological investigations of brain activity by means of scalp electrodes. Combination of EEG and MEG measurements, improvement of spatial resolution by multichannel recordings, and application of source localization algorithms with neurophysiologically guided modeling of sources (e.g., Scherg and Ebersole, 1993) have contributed to solve this problem in many respects (see Time and Space: Co-Registration of Synergistic Brain Imaging Results, below).

DC Potentials Related to Language Processing

DC potentials related to language processing were investigated with paradigms ensuring a sustained cognitive activity for several seconds (Altenmüller, 1989; Jung et al., 1984). As demonstrated above, mental search for synonyms produced a predominant activation over the left inferior prefrontal cortex, whereas the semantic category influenced activation patterns (Altenmüller et al., 1993a). Compared to abstract stimuli, search of synonyms to concrete semantic categories generated larger amplitudes over the parietal areas, due to an additional activation of visual association areas when processing highly imaginable words. The predominant activation of the left inferior frontal region is caused by inner speech, i.e., the subjects are silently formulating the synonyms. Correspondingly, in cerebral blood flow studies silent word processing produced an activation of the same cortical areas (Price et al., 1996). Investigation of right- and left-handed patients with known hemispheric dominance revealed that the frontal lateralization of sustained negative DC potential corresponds to hemispheric dominance for language (Altenmüller et al., 1993b); 93% of right-handed subjects ($n = 60$) but only 67% of left-handed subjects ($n = 45$) revealed left-hemispheric lateralization. Developmental changes of cortical activation patterns were found in experiments performed in 6- to 12-year-old children. In contrast to adults, only 60% of right-handed children exhibited left-hemispheric lateralization during the search for synonyms (Altenmüller et al., 1993c). This result supports Lenneberg's (1967) equipotentiality hypothesis, assuming a bilateral language representation in early infancy and a gradually increasing lateralization toward the left hemisphere during intellectual maturation.

Another aspect of language processing was investigated in a study on cortical activation patterns during processing of affective speech prosody (Pihan et al., 2000). Subjects had to identify the emotional category of sentences presented with happy, sad, or neutral intonation. While listening to these sentences, a right hemispheric frontotemporal activation occurred, suggesting that the right hemisphere has a dominant role for the evaluation of the emotional content of language.

Follow-up studies in patients with language disorders can give new insights into cerebral plasticity. In patients with anomic aphasia following left temporoparietal ischemia, DC potentials during the search for synonyms revealed an additional right frontocentral activation in the acute phase of the stroke. Along with complete clinical recovery, a marked decrease of right frontocentral negativity was found (Thomas et al., 1997). The transient activation of the right hemisphere in acute anomic aphasia might be due to an initial disinhibition of contralateral homologous areas and subsequent collateral sprouting and synaptic modulation. Alternatively, an activation of subordinate brain structures related to language processing may occur.

DC Potentials Related to Other Cognitive Functions

EEG correlates of music processing were investigated in a series of experiments. During melody processing, brain activation depends on musical expertise; nonmusicians tended to activate predominantly the right frontotemporal cortex, whereas professional musicians revealed an additional activation of left-hemispheric auditory areas (Altenmüller, 1986). These variations in auditory activation patterns were ascribed to different cognitive strategies and mental representations of music in trained or untrained listeners. Untrained subjects analyzed melodies in a contour-based global manner, a cognitive strategy that relies mainly on right-hemispheric neuronal networks (Heinze et al., 1994). Professionally trained listeners are able to use verbal strategies and inner speech. Furthermore, trained musicians tend to analyze melodies in a sequential interval-based manner, a strategy depending predominantly on left-hemispheric neuronal networks (Altenmüller, 2003). Besides musical expertise, emotional valence during music listening may influence lateralization patterns. When music is eliciting positive feelings, a left-sided frontotemporal lateralization can be observed, and negative feelings are accompanied by a right hemispheric preponderance (Altenmüller et al., 2002). These EEG-findings support the valence hypothesis of affective processing, saying that positive emotions are primarily processed in the left hemisphere and negative in the right hemisphere (Davidson, 1999).

In longitudinal studies during acquisition of musical skills, it could be demonstrated not only that brain plasticity during learning can be monitored with EEG, but also that the method is sensitive enough to record differences in declarative and procedural processing strategies (Altenmüller et al., 2000). The impact of specific musical skills on brain activation patterns is impressively documented in longitudinal studies during piano training. Piano playing requires high-speed control of complex movement patterns under continuous auditory feedback. As a prerequisite, audiomotor integration at cortical and probably subcortical levels has to be established. This audiomotor coupling, which is comparable to the oral-aural loop in language processing, is established after as little as 20 minutes of training, demonstrated by topographic analysis of DC-EEG potentials (Bangert and Altenmüller, 2003). After the first training session, there was additional activity over motor areas while subjects listened to simple piano tunes. Likewise, finger movements on a mute keyboard were associated with an increase of activity over auditory areas. The effect could be enhanced and stabilized during 5 weeks of training. Similar coactivation has also been demonstrated in professional pianists, who displayed magnetoencephalographic activity in sensorimotor cortical regions while listening to piano music (Haueisen and Knösche, 2001). These neural networks thus appear to behave similarly to the so-called mirror neurons in monkey frontal cortex (area F5) that are active during the execution of complex movements as well as the visual observation of the same movements (Umilta et al., 2001).

DC potentials during different learning paradigms were investigated by the Vienna group. M. Lang et al. (1987) demonstrated a task-specific left frontal negativation when subjects had to learn to transform letters into Morse code. Similarly, a left frontal negativation occurred when subjects had to learn word pairs and nonword pairs. Compared to nonwords, the left frontal negativation was considerably larger when meaningful word pairs had to be learned (W. Lang et al., 1988). In a subsequent study, Uhl et al. (1990) were able to demonstrate that frontal activation during paired associate learning is sensitive to interference; when the word pairs to be learned interfered with previously learned word pairs, the left frontal negativation was significantly more pronounced during learning compared to the no-interference condition. The role of the left frontal lobe in the learning studies cited above remains speculative. As discussed in this paper and in accordance with experiments assessing DC shifts during search for synonyms (Altenmüller, 1989), it is probable that silent speech during internal reverberation contributes to the left frontal activation.

Long-term memory function is another field investigated with DC-EEG recordings. Rösler and co-workers (1993, 1997) found during long-term memory retrieval a task-specific topography of surface negative slow potentials. A plateau-like negativity was found over frontal areas with semantic material, over parietal areas with spatial material, and over occipital areas with color material. The amplitude of the negative DC potential was found to be systematically related to the difficulty of the retrieval process. From the results it can be concluded that cortical neuronal networks involved during explicit memory retrieval are also those necessary for perception.

In conclusion, the measurement of sustained cortical DC potentials provides an excellent tool for the noninvasive assessment of cortical activation patterns during various types of cognitive processing. Furthermore, monitoring of the dynamic changes in cortical activation patterns provides information on neural mechanisms underlying learning and cerebral plasticity.

Slow Potentials in Anticipation of Events: The Contingent Negative Variation and the Bereitschaftspotential

As mentioned above, changes in cortical DC potential during sensory processing were known from physiological experiments but were ignored by neurologists and psychologists for a long time. In the middle and late 1960s, their research focused on slow potential shifts in anticipation of motor or cognitive performance. In 1964, Grey Walter and co-workers recorded a negative-going DC shift when a first stimulus or warning stimulus (S1) was followed by a second stimulus or imperative stimulus (S2) that required a motor response. The negativity started to rise 200 to 500 msec after S1 and terminated after S2. This slow potential shift was termed by Walter et al. (1964) the "contingent negative variation" (CNV) and was believed to be related to conditioning, preparation, and expectancy (therefore labeled sometimes "expectancy wave"). Around the same time, Kornhuber and Deecke (1965) described a negative-going slow potential shift starting about 800 to 1,000 msec prior to self-initiated movements. This potential was named "Bereitschaftspotential" (readiness potential) and was related to the "internal event" of a decision to act. We will give only a brief summary concerning their psychophysiological aspects. CNV studies in the field of psychiatric and neurological disorders will not be reviewed here.

The CNV: Expectancy and the Allocation of Cortical Resources

The experimental paradigm that most reliably elicits a CNV consists of a warning stimulus (S1) followed by an imperative stimulus (S2) one or several seconds later to which the subject is required to respond. This response does not need to be motor, and can be any type of cognitive performance, e.g., mental arithmetic. In general, the amplitude of the CNV increases with increasing probability of the occurrence of S2 and with increasing difficulty to discriminate S2. An aversive S2 causes higher amplitudes when compared to a neutral one (Knott and Tecce, 1978). Equally, a highly incentive value of the response produces an increase in amplitude, whereas no task or response following the S2 causes a decrease of CNV negativity. When the S1–S2 interval is extended to 3 or more seconds, a biphasic CNV with an initial negative peak, an intermittent positive slope, and a terminal negative slope emerge. The topography of these two negative components can be distinguished. Whereas the initial negative wave, also termed iCNV, exhibits an almost modality-independent distribution with the largest amplitudes over the frontal lobes, the terminal negative slope (tCNV) reveals a widespread surface distribution with maximal amplitudes over the brain regions involved in the anticipated tasks (Rohrbaugh et al., 1976, reviewed in Rockstroh et al., 1989, pp. 99–125). A motor response with the right hand, for example, elicits a maximal tCNV over the contralateral precentral region. The cerebral generator structures of the CNV cannot be localized with certainty. Animal experiments show that a CNV linked to a motor response is generated in the prestriate and prefrontal cortices contralateral to the moving hand. This activation, however, depends on an intact cerebrocerebellar loop and is abolished when cerebellar hemispherectomies are performed (Sasaki and Gemba, 1984). In humans, it is thought to be controlled by the basal ganglia-thalamocortical loop involving a complex interaction among incoming sensory inputs, motor initiation, output, and personal expectations (Ikeda et al., 1994).

Different and in many conditions certainly overlapping psychophysiological mechanisms seem to underlie the CNV. Walter and colleagues interpreted the CNV as a sign of expectancy. Evidence was provided by the increasing amplitude of the CNV with increasing stimulus probability. Tecce and co-workers related the early negative wave of the CNV to arousal, and the late negative slope to attentional processes. Finally, considering that an aversive S2 or a highly incentive S2, e.g., in the context of monetary reward, yields larger amplitudes of the CNV, the CNV was supposed to reflect motivational states (Rebert et al., 1967). An interesting feature of the late negative slope of the CNV is its area-specific cortical distribution, which apparently reflects task-specific preparation and allocation of resources (Birbaumer et al., 1981, 1988; Lutzenberger et al., 1985). The term *resources* has to be understood as the amount of processing facilities available in a defined time interval to optimize cortical function. The implications of this anticipatory activation is discussed below in the context of the threshold regulation model (Birbaumer et al., 1994).

The Bereitschaftspotential (BP) and the Decision to Act

The Bereitschaftspotential (BP) is a ramp-like negative-going DC shift that precedes a self-paced voluntary motor activity. According to the time course and the scalp topography, Deecke et al. (1969) distinguished four components of the BP: (a) a bilaterally symmetrical negative going ramp-like potential with maximal amplitude over the vertex starting 500 to 1,000 msec prior to electromyogram (EMG) onset (BP in the strict sense); (b) a contralateral preponderance of negativity over the precentral and parietal areas, starting about 200 to 500 msec prior to EMG onset; (c) a small positive deflection beginning around 90 msec prior to the EMG onset with a maximal amplitude over the postcentral areas (premotion positivity, PMP); and (d) a smaller negative potential starting about 50 msec prior to EMG and predominating over the primary motor cortex (motor potential, MP). It must be stressed that these four components are not present in all subjects and that superimposition may complicate the scalp configuration of the compound potential. There is still some debate on the generator structures of these components. The first bilateral negative shift seems to be generated in the supplementary motor area within the mesial cortical surface of both hemispheres (Deecke and Kornhuber, 1978; Kristeva et al., 1991). The second lateralizing component is probably generated in the primary motor

and the postrolandic sensory areas (Neshige et al., 1988). The generator structures of the PMP are not clear. This component is supposed to reflect the deactivation of precentral areas (Deecke et al., 1984), but animal experiments and MEG studies could not prove this hypothesis so far. The motor potential finally seems to be closely related to the pyramidal tract volley, initiating the movement.

According to the generating structures, the amplitude and topography of the BP depend on the type of movement and on the muscle group to be activated, but complicating the situation to a large extent are psychological variables. In most studies, the BP amplitude is positively correlated with the force of different voluntary isometric contractions (Becker and Kristeva, 1980; Wilke and Lansing, 1973). However, as discussed by Rockstroh et al. (1989, pp. 95–98), it is not easy to decide whether the physical parameters themselves or psychological variables, e.g., motivation or attention, cause these effects. McAdam and Seales (1969) showed that BP amplitudes were larger when the motor response was associated with a financial reward. The outcome result of the movement considerably influences the amplitudes of the BP. When the voluntary response was followed by a painful shock, the BP amplitude was four times higher as compared to the responses followed by a neutral tone (Elbert et al., 1984). Task complexity, skillfulness of the movement, and learning influence the amplitude of the BP as well. Rockstroh et al. (1989, p. 98) pointed out that "the BP should rather be considered in terms of action-preparatory processes in which motor preparation may be but one component."

Traditionally, the BP was related to the intentional decision processes of willed action. In intriguing experiments Benjamin Libet et al. (1983) demonstrated that the BP starts about 350 msec prior to conscious awareness of the intention to act. When the subjects "vetoed" their decision to act, the BP, which had normally developed prior to this veto, collapsed and no motion occurred. Libet (1985) concluded that voluntary acts can be initiated by unconscious cerebral processes before conscious intention appears, but that conscious control over the actual motor performance of the acts remain possible. This experimental design has had a long and often controversial history; after all, it has remained unclear whether the urge to act and the action itself represent actual differences in brain states (for a concise review see Eagleman, 2004).

Slow Potentials and the Cortical Threshold Regulation Model

In all the studies presented so far, changes in brain potentials were considered as a dependent variable associated with varying behavior. A different approach was chosen by Bauer (1975) when he developed the "brain-trigger design." He presented a learning task in which the subjects had to learn nonsense syllables. The task presentation was triggered by either the absence or presence of alpha activity. Bauer was able to demonstrate that the ability to learn is increased in the absence of alpha but reduced in the presence of alpha. In a further-developed approach, the level of cortical DC potential was used as a trigger. During high-level cortical negativation, paired associate learning of syllables and numbers was considerably facilitated as compared to learning during positive shifts (Bauer and Nirnberger, 1980). Similar results were obtained in experiments manipulating the local distribution of negative DC potentials with biofeedback (Elbert et al., 1980). Subjects were required to watch a television display on which a small rocket moved from left to right over a period of 6 seconds. The task was to direct the rocket into one of two goals; which goal to take was indicated by a simultaneously presented high- or low-pitched tone. Without the subject's knowledge, the trajectory of the rocket was governed by the DC shift produced during watching the rocket. Within 60 to 160 feedback trials on the average, subjects had learned to control their DC level and were able to direct the rocket into the goal required.

Further experiments demonstrated that subjects could acquire hemisphere-specific control of DC potentials mainly over the central region. The level of surface-negative potential influenced behavior and speed of cognitive processing. Left precentral negativity improved tactile performance and response speed of the right hand and vice versa (Rockstroh et al., 1990). Birbaumer and colleagues (1994) interpret these results in the context of a threshold regulation model; whether a given neuronal network or cell assembly will be activated—"ignited"—by a stimulus or not depends on the threshold of the neuronal assembly. Cortical DC potentials are the objective measure of such thresholds: negativity represents lowering and positivity represents augmenting of thresholds. The local threshold of a certain neuronal assembly is determined by priming: stimuli indicating that a certain cognitive operation will be required in the future initiate a local lowering of thresholds reflected in an increase in negative DC potential. Threshold regulation can be trained via biofeedback. Using operant conditioning, Birbaumer and colleagues developed a thought translation device that trains locked-in patients to self-regulate slow cortical potentials of their electroencephalogram. After training, patients otherwise unable to communicate can select letters, words, or pictograms in a computerized language support program (Kübler et al., 2001).

Time and Space: Co-Registration of Synergistic Brain Imaging Results

As Albert Einstein pointed out, the timing of events, particularly their simultaneity, has no meaning except in relation to a given coordinate system. With respect to the study of complex brain functions, we may translate this into the necessity of considering both the time course and the topographical distribution of neuronal activation. Especially for the understanding of higher cognitive functions, technologies are required that are capable of measuring moment-by-moment changes in the distributed networks that are adaptively configured in response to environmental demands and in the context of purposeful behavior.

During the past 20 years, rapid advances have been made in functional neuroimaging techniques such as PET and fMRI. Their spatial resolution reaches several millimeters, but their effective temporal resolution has remained in the range of seconds or minutes. Only EEG and MEG provide a temporal resolution in the millisecond range, and thus can be used to analyze the rapidly changing neuronal activity that generates complex behavior. The amount of spatial information that can be recovered from the scalp-recorded EEG or MEG has often been underestimated. In the last decade, this situation has prompted a number of research laboratories to aim at an improved spatial resolution of these techniques. Without questioning the fundamental limitations of inferences about electrical sources that may be obtained from scalp-recorded brain electrical or magnetic activity, we have learned that cortical generators of EEG or MEG signals can be determined with centimeter or even subcentimeter accuracy (Cohen et al., 1990; Gevins et al., 1994; Gerloff et al., 1997c).

There are at least three general approaches that have been utilized to increase the reliability of spatial information obtained from scalp recordings: (a) improving the spatial accuracy of the electrical or magnetic data themselves; (b) comparative electrophysiological and imaging studies (Cohen et al., 1997; Manganotti et al., 1998; Rodriguez-Fornells et al., 2002b); and (c) direct co-registration techniques to combine results from different neuroimaging techniques, e.g., EEG and fMRI (Gerloff et al., 1996; Ullsperger and von Cramon, 2001; Opitz et al., 1999, 2002), or MEG and PET (Walter et al., 1992).

Improving the Spatial Accuracy of EEG and MEG

The traditional 10–20 system of electrode placement with only 19 channels results in interelectrode distances of typically 6 to 7 cm, and limits the spatial resolution of the EEG substantially. The major advances in computer technology within the past 20 years now allow recordings of more than a hundred channels simultaneously (currently up to 256 for EEG, up to 306 for MEG), so that with both EEG and MEG whole-head recordings at interelectrode distances of 3 cm and less can be practically accomplished. This is within the 3-dB point on the cortex to point on the scalp spread function, that is, within the size of the scalp representation of a small, discrete neuronal source at the level of the cortex (Gevins, 1990). The appropriate number of channels, however, is not an absolute number. It relates to the spatial distribution of the EEG or MEG component under study. The optimal interelectrode spacing for any given component can be mathematically determined by means of the spatial Nyquist value (Spitzer et al., 1989; Gerloff et al., 1997b). Figure 31.8 illustrates the gain of topographic resolution for a movement-related cortical potential (MRCP), when the channel number is increased from 28 to 122. Only with high-resolution EEG, it is possible to differentiate between discrete bilateral activation foci over the sensorimotor regions.

In addition to the appropriate number of recording channels, the surface-recorded electrical or magnetic signals can be spatially deblurred. This is particularly important for EEG data, since the inhomogeneous volume conduction properties of the different compartments of the human head distort the electrical field on its way from the brain to the outside of the head. There are a number of methods for re-

EEG premovement potentials

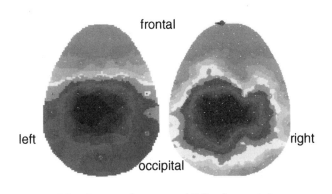

frontal

left

right

occipital

28 channels   122 channels

Figure 31.8. Topographic maps of the premovement component [60 msec before electromyogram (EMG) onset] of movement-related cortical potentials associated with finger extensions of the right hand at a movement rate of 2 Hz (Gerloff et al., 1997). Data from one subject. Only the 122-channel recording discriminates clearly two separate activation maxima (negative peaks, blue) over the sensorimotor region of the left and right hemisphere. With 28 channels, the potential map could as well be generated by a single activity focus in the left hemisphere close to the midline. (See Color Figure 31.8.)

ducing this distortion, from the computationally simple to the very complex. The spatial *Laplacian operator* lies at the simpler end. As the second derivative of the potential field in space, it is proportional to the current entering and exiting the scalp at each electrode site, and makes the recorded field independent of the location of the reference electrode. A simplified version of computing the Laplacian derivation assumes an equidistant and rectangular electrode montage (Hjorth, 1975), but computations based on the true interelectrode relations have become available and are more accurate (Le et al., 1994). Computationally more demanding are methods such as finite element deblurring (FED) (Gevins et al., 1994), a mathematical spatial enhancement procedure that uses an anatomically realistic model of the passive conducting properties of each subject's head and the finite element method to estimate potentials at the cortical surface from scalp potentials. The more sophisticated spatial localization methods have in common that they take into account the individual anatomy of each subject studied (Yvert et al., 1995; Bara-Jimenez et al., 1998; Mirkovic et al., 2003), so that they inherently require co-registration of electrophysiological and anatomical (MRI) data. Figure 31.9 shows a three-dimensional (3D) reconstructed cortical surface together with the corresponding realistic head model, which was computed on the basis of the MRI (Curry software, by Philips, Germany).

Comparative Electrophysiological and Imaging Studies

In many instances, fMRI or PET studies have identified brain regions that are activated during a particular task, but left questions open with regard to the time course of activation, the functional coupling ("crosstalk") between activated areas, and the functional relevance of each regional activation for successful behavioral output. Evidently, all of the latter aspects are essential in order to reveal the cortical processes underlying complex cognitive behavior. The missing information can often be obtained from comparative electrophysiological studies. While it is desirable but not always mandatory to study the same group of subjects with the different methods, the paradigms must be designed as similarly as possible to allow for correlative interpretation of the results.

A good example of how comparative electrophysiological and imaging studies can complement each other is a set of PET, EEG, and transcranial magnetic stimulation experiments that were aimed at the understanding of neuronal plasticity across different sensory modalities in blindness (Sadato et al., 1996; Cohen et al., 1997, 1999; Koyama et al., 1997). Blind subjects who lost their vision early in life have an extraordinary capability for tactile discrimination. The most impressive evidence for that is the speed at which they read Braille. The neural basis for this particularly developed skill has not been known until recently. The first finding in this series of experiments was that the primary visual cortex showed increased regional cerebral blood flow (rCBF) during Braille reading in group of blind subjects, but not in a sighted control cohort (Sadato et al., 1996). This was rather unexpected and exciting since the visual cortex in these blind subjects had never received any meaningful visual input and was thought to be mute. It was therefore suggested that, as a consequence of plastic reorganization of the

3D-reconstructed cortical surface and realistically shaped volume conductor model

vertex

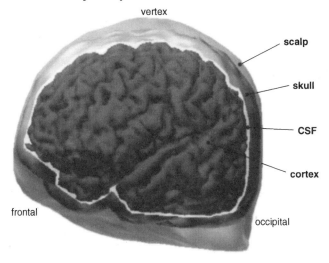

scalp

skull

CSF

cortex

frontal

occipital

Figure 31.9. Three-dimensional reconstruction of the cortical surface, embedded in a realistic head model. Both were computed on the basis of magnetic resonance imaging (MRI) data that were acquired in a conventional 1.5-Tesla scanner. Note the variable thickness of each single layer [cerebrospinal fluid (CSF); skull; scalp] of the head model. This approximation of the true anatomical head shape and individual anatomical details enhances the spatial accuracy of inverse problem solutions substantially.

"blind brain," the visual cortex might have acquired somatosensory functions. From the PET data alone, it could not be determined if the visual cortex is in fact part of the functionally coupled network that mediates Braille reading. A subsequent EEG study demonstrated coherent oscillatory activity between occipital and central regions during Braille reading in the blind (Koyama et al., 1997), supporting the hypothesis that the activation of the visual cortex is functionally coupled with the activation of the sensorimotor cortex and therefore most likely behaviorally meaningful.

The remaining question, namely, how crucial is this regional activation and network-like integration of the visual cortex for the behavioral output, could be addressed using repetitive transcranial magnetic stimulation (rTMS) over the visual cortex (Cohen et al., 1997). Stimulation of cortical areas with rTMS can transiently disrupt specific cognitive functions, such as naming objects (Pascual-Leone et al., 1991), performing complex finger movement sequences on a piano (Gerloff et al., 1997a, 1998), or sensory functions, e.g., auditory perception (Plewnia et al., 2003). Cohen et al. (1997) showed that temporary disruption of the function of the visual cortex induced errors during Braille reading in blind subjects, but did not interfere with any form of tactile discrimination in the sighted control group.

The integration of PET, EEG, and rTMS provided, therefore, for the first time, evidence that brain plasticity across sensory modalities is involved in functional compensation. Figure 31.10 gives a schematic drawing of combined PET, EEG, and TMS results in a blind subject.

Co-Registration

Other than with comparative group studies, formal co-registration must be based on the acquisition of data with different techniques in the same individuals. Since task-related neuronal activation patterns and, to a certain extent, even anatomical features in an individual brain are subject to dynamic changes, the data to merge should be acquired within a narrow time window.

A first and fundamental step of co-registration is to combine functional and anatomical images. For example, Gevins et al. (1990) have mapped the spatial distribution of scalp-recorded EEG data onto the cortical surface, and Reite et al. (1988) have mapped MEG dipole sources onto MR images. Commercial software is now available to accomplish this type of co-registration, which most likely will become a standard procedure in whole-head MEG and high-resolution EEG in the near future. Figure 31.11 gives an example of MEG-MRI co-registration in a motor paradigm (Gerloff et al., 1997c). Less well established is the technique of co-registering several types of functional data together with anatomical images (Walter et al., 1992; Toro et al., 1994; Beisteiner et al., 1995; Gerloff et al., 1996; Wassermann et al., 1996). The latter, however, provides the most comprehensive view into complex brain function, since it allows for a coherent description of subsecond changes in neuronal activity with subcentimeter spatial accuracy (Nunez and Silberstein, 2000; Thees et al., 2003).

Any given 3D measurement (e.g., EEG potentials distributed over the scalp, rCBF changes in the brain as demonstrated by PET) has its own reference coordinate system. Two or more 3D measurements can be brought together by

Schematic of correlative evaluation of cross-modal plasticity of the occipital cortex in a blind person

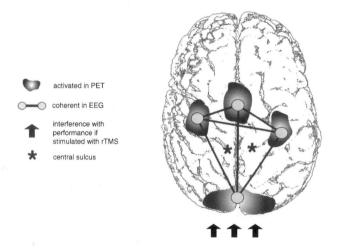

activated in PET

coherent in EEG

interference with performance if stimulated with rTMS

* central sulcus

Figure 31.10. Plastic reorganization of the visuomotor system. Schematic of correlative positron emission tomography (PET), EEG, and repetitive transcranial magnetic stimulation (rTMS) results in a blind subject. The multimodal approach allows for a detailed analysis of the phenomenon of cross-modal plasticity. The occipital ("visual") cortex in people who lost their vision early in life appears to be integrated into the cortical network that mediates tactile discrimination skills (e.g., Braille reading). This type of plasticity is most likely relevant for functional compensation (Sadato et al., 1996; Cohen et al., 1997; Koyama et al., 1997).

Coregistration of MEG dipole sources and anatomical MRI

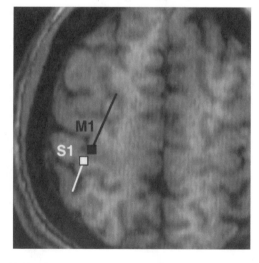

Figure 31.11. Co-registration of the equivalent current dipoles (ECDs) in the primary motor (M1) and primary sensory (S1) cortex. The ECDs were computed from movement-related magnetic fields associated with repetitive movements of the right thumb and co-registered with the high-resolution anatomical MRI of the individual subject. Note how M1 and S1 ECDs are located just anterior and posterior to the central sulcus of the left hemisphere.

matching a minimum of three common points, usually referred to as *fiducial markers*. Typical fiducial markers are the nasion, the left and right preauricular points, and the inion. For EEG and MEG measurements, these points can be registered together with electrode or sensor positions by means of a commercial magnetic digitizer, with an accuracy of about 3 mm (Gevins et al., 1994). Since the position of a 3D volume in space is unambiguously defined by three points, this approach is theoretically accurate and simple to implement. In practice, its disadvantage is that for co-registration the landmarks need to be localized in the anatomical MRI by hand (with a cursor). This can be ambiguous and cause inaccuracies in the centimeter range, particularly with respect to the anterior-to-posterior position of the preauricular points and to the lateral position of the nasion or inion. It is therefore recommended to mark the reference points with a paramagnetic (MR signal-intense) substance (e.g., vitamin E capsules; commercially available adhesive "fiducial markers"), before the subject is studied in the MR scanner.

Alternatively, it is possible to digitize a large number (e.g., 1,000) of randomly located points on the scalp surface. The head surface reconstructed from these points can be mathematically matched with the head surface of the same individual as extracted from the high-resolution MRI. This method of determining a "best fit" between digitized and MRI-derived head surfaces is computationally intensive but less subjective, and the spatial co-registration errors are as small as 2 to 3 mm (Wang et al., 1994). Once the digitized coordinate system of the ("real world") head has been matched with the anatomical MR images, the electrophysiological data can be mapped onto the scalp surface, and can be related to the underlying brain tissue or the underlying activation foci in PET or fMRI. Despite the known coupling of neuronal activity and rCBF, it is rather unclear if we should really expect that electrical sources and rCBF maxima are exactly in the same location in the brain. For example, in a variety of studies cortical generators of movement-related electrical or magnetic fields were no closer to the centers of rCBF maxima than 4.0 to 20.0 mm (EEG vs. PET) (Toro et al., 1994), 18.6 ± 7.6 mm (EEG vs. fMRI) (Gerloff et al., 1996), 17.3 ± 6.3 mm (MEG vs. PET) (Walter et al., 1992), and 16.7 ± 6.8 mm (MEG vs. fMRI) (Beisteiner et al., 1995). Similarly, the localization of the primary motor cortex with transcranial magnetic stimulation differed by 5.0 to 22.0 mm from the corresponding PET activation maxima (Wassermann et al., 1996). It is likely that these discrepancies are mostly related to co-registration problems and the use of simple spheric rather than realistically shaped head models for dipole calculations. Other sources of co-registration inaccuracies include head motion during data acquisition in MRI and PET (Lee et al., 1996; Picard and Thompson, 1997), distortion of the real anatomy in MR images (Maurer et al., 1996; West et al., 1997), and changes of the brain position inside the skull depending on the head position (e.g., upright for EEG vs. supine in the MR scanner). Finally and perhaps most importantly, there might be a systematic difference between rCBF maxima and electrical generator locations, which needs to be further determined.

Recently, the correlations between electrical neuronal activity and rCBF (more specifically, the BOLD signal of fMRI) have been studied by simultaneous recordings from depth electrodes and metabolic changes inside a high-field 4.7-T MRI scanner in monkeys (Logothetis et al., 2001). These findings suggested that the fMRI signal reflects the input and intracortical processing of a given area rather than its spiking output. This is encouraging for EEG-fMRI co-registration because the EEG signal also reflects the processing of afferent information in apical dendrites [excitatory postsynaptic potential (EPSPs)] of pyramidal cells rather than spiking output. Thus, taking fMRI or PET data as a (tentative) reference for adequacy of locating regional activation noninvasively in the human brain with EEG, MEG, or magnetic stimulation is a valuable approach and should be aimed at in future experiments.

Despite the enormous progress in this field, co-registration of different functional imaging results still remains an experimental procedure. It needs further improvement, not only with respect to technical aspects, but even more so regarding our understanding of the different parameters measured, such as equivalent dipole sources of electrical and magnetic fields, the neural substrates of magnetic stimulation effects, and the relation of neuronal activity to rCBF and blood oxygenation level changes in different brain regions. It is important to be aware of some intrinsic limits for each single method that may, for theoretical reasons, be impossible to overcome. For example, increasing the EEG channel number further or improving the deblurring algorithms cannot master the mathematical problem of the ambiguity of inverse problem solutions. Or, with relevance to PET and fMRI, task-related rCBF changes occur relatively slowly and with some delay, which blurs the intrinsic hemodynamic response (Kim et al., 1997; Logothetis et al.; 2001, 2004) so that rapid changes of neuronal activity within a few milliseconds will probably always go undetected in PET or fMRI. At present, co-registration techniques and comparative study designs, based on high-resolution electrophysiological and imaging methods, offer promising ways to bypass these limitations and thereby "relate time and space" in psychophysiological research.

Acknowledgments

The authors are grateful to Leonardo G. Cohen, M.D., and William Bara-Jimenez, M.D., for support regarding the illustrations, and to Mark Hallett, M.D., for constructive comments on the manuscript. E. Altenmüller and C. Gerloff were supported by the DFG (German Research Foundation) grant (AI 269/5, SFB 550/C5).

References

Altenmüller, E. 1986. Hirnelektrische Korrelate der cerebralen Musikverarbeitung beim Menschen. Eur. Arch. Psychiatr. Sci. 235:342–354.
Altenmüller, E. 1989. Cortical DC-potentials as electrophysiological correlates of hemispheric dominance of higher cognitive function. Int. J. Neurosci. 47:1–14.

Altenmüller, E. 2003. How many music centers are in the brain. In *The Biological Foundations of Music,* Eds. R. Zatorre and I. Peretz, pp. 267–279. Oxford: Oxford University Press.

Altenmüller, E., Pfäfflin, H., and Uhl, H. 1993a. Cortical DC-potentials during mental search for synonyms reveal sex differences. In *New Developments in Event Related Potentials,* Eds. H.J. Heinze and T.F. Münte, pp. 9–16. Boston: Birkhauser.

Altenmüller, E., Kriechbaum, W., Helber, U., et al. 1993b. Cortical DC-potentials in identification of the language-dominant hemisphere. Linguistical and clinical aspects. Acta Neurochir. 56:20–33.

Altenmüller, E., Marckmann, G., Uhl, H., et al. 1993c. DC-Potentiale zeigen Entwicklungsabhängige Änderungen kortikaler Aktivierungsmuster während Sprachverarbeitung. Z. EEG-EMG 24:41–48.

Altenmüller, E., Bangert, M., Liebert, G., et al. 2000. Mozart in us: how the brain processes music. Med. Prob. Performing Artists 15:99–106.

Altenmüller, E., Schürmann, K., Lim, V., et al. 2002. Hits to the left—flops to the right. Different emotions during music listening are reflected in cortical lateralisation patterns. Neuropsychologia 40:2242–2256.

Baddeley, A. 1986. *Working Memory.* Oxford: Oxford University Press.

Bangert, M., and Altenmüller, E. 2003. Mapping perception to action in piano practice: a longitudinal DC-EEG study. BMC Neurosci. 4:26–36.

Bara-Jimenez, W., Catalan, M.J., Hallett, M., et al. 1998. Abnormal somatosensory homunculus in dystonia of the hand. Ann. Neurol. 44:826–821.

Bauer, H. 1975. Lernen unter Berücksichtigung hirnphysiologischer Zustände. Paper presented at the Austrian Society for Electroencephalography and Clinical Neurophysiology, Salzburg.

Bauer, H., and Nirnberger, G. 1980. Paired associate learning with feedback of DC potential shifts of the cerebral cortex. Arch. Psychol. 132:237–239.

Bauer, H., Korunka, C., and Leodolter, M. 1989. Technical requirements for high-quality scalp DC-recordings. Electroencephalogr. Clin. Neurophysiol. 72:545–547.

Beaumont, J.G., Mayes, A.R., and Rugg, M.D. 1978. Asymmetry in EEG alpha-coherence and power: effects of task and sex. Electroencephalogr. Clin. Neurophysiol. 45:393–401.

Becker, W., and Kristeva, R. 1980. Cerebral potentials prior to various force deployments. In *Motivation, Motor and Sensory Processing of the Brain: Electrical Potentials, Behaviour and Clinical Use*, Eds. H.H. Kornhuber and L. Deecke, pp. 189–195. Prog. Brain. Res. Vol. 54. Amsterdam: Elsevier.

Beisteiner, R., Gomiscek, G., Erdler, M., et al. 1995. Comparing localization of conventional functional magnetic resonance imaging and magnetoencephalography. Eur. J. Neurosci. 7:1121–1124.

Berger, H. 1929. Über das Elektrenkephalogramm des Menschen. Arch. Psychiatry 87:527–570.

Berger, H. 1938. Das Elektrenkephalogramm des Menschen. Nova Acta Leopoldina 6:173–309.

Berkum Van, J.J., Hagoort, P., and Brown, C.M. 1999. Semantic integration in sentences and discourse: evidence from the N400. J. Cogn. Neurosci. 11:657–671.

Bhattacharya, J., Petsche, H., and Pereda, E. 2001. Long-range synchrony in the gamma band: role in music perception. J. Neurosci. 21:6329–6337.

Birbaumer, N., Lang, P., Cook, E., et al. 1988. Slow brain potentials, imagery and hemispherical differences. Int. J. Neurosci. 39:212–219.

Birbaumer, N., Lutzenberger, W., Elbert, T., et al. 1981. EEG and slow cortical potentials in anticipation of mental tasks with different hemispheric involvement. Biol. Psychol. 13:251–260.

Birbaumer, N., Lutzenberger, W., Elbert, T., et al. 1994. Threshold variations in cortical cell assemblies and behaviour. In *Cognitive Electrophysiology,* Eds. H.J. Heinze, T.F. Münte, and G.R. Mangun, pp. 248–264. Boston: Birkhauser.

Botvinick, M.M., Braver, T.S., Barch, D.M., et al. 2001. Conflict monitoring and cognitive control. Psychol. Rev. 108:624–652.

Brooks, D.H., Ahmad, G.F., Macleod, R.S., et al. 1999. Inverse electrocardiography by simultaneous imposition of multiple constraints. IEEE Trans. Biomed. Eng. 46:3–17.

Butler, S., and Glass, A. 1987. Individual differences in the asymmetry of alpha activation. In *Individual Differences in Hemispheric Specialization,* Ed. A. Glass, pp. 103–120. New York: Plenum.

Carter, C.S., Braver, T.S., Barch, D.M., et al. 1998. Anterior cingulate cortex, error detection, and the on-line monitoring of performance. Science 280:747–749.

Caspers, H., and Schulze, H. 1959. Die Veränderungen der corticalen Gleichspannung während der natürlichen Schaf-Wach-Perioden beim freibeweglichen Tier. Pflugers Arch. 270:103–120.

Caspers, H., Speckmann, E.J., and Lehmenkühler, A. 1984. Electrogenesis of slow potentials of the brain. In *Self-Regulation of the Brain and Behaviour,* Eds. T. Elbert, B. Rockstroh, W. Lutzenberger, et al., pp. 3–16. Heidelberg: Springer.

Caton, R. 1875. The electric currents of the brain. Br. Med. J. 2:278.

Cohen, D., Cuffin, B.N., Yunokuchi, K., et al. 1990. MEG versus EEG localization test using implanted sources in the human brain. Ann. Neuol. 28:811–817.

Cohen, L.G., Celnik, P., Pascual-Leone, A., et al. 1997. Functional relevance of cross-modal plasticity in blind humans. Nature 389:180–183.

Cohen, L.G., Weeks, R.A., Sadato, N., et al. 1999. Period of susceptibility for cross-modal plasticity in the blind. Ann. Neurol. 45:451–460.

David, E., Finkenzeller, P., Kallert, S., et al. 1969. Akustischen Reizen zugeordnete Gleichspannungsänderungen am intakten Schädel des Menschen. Pflugers Arch. 309:362–367.

Davidson, R.J. 1999. The functional neuroanatomy of emotion and affective style. Trends Cogn. Sci. 3:11–21.

Deecke, L., and Kornhuber, H.H. 1978. An electrical sign of participation of the mesial "supplementary" motor cortex in human voluntary finger movements. Brain Res. 159:473–476.

Deecke, L., Scheid, R.P., and Kornhuber, H.H. 1969. Distribution of readiness potential, pre-motion positivity and motor potential of the human cerebral cortex preceding voluntary finger movements. Exp. Brain Res. 7:158–168.

Deecke, L., Heise, B., Kornhuber, H.H., et al. 1984. Brain potentials associated with voluntary manual tracking: Bereitschaftspotential, conditioned pre-motion positivity, directed attention potential and relaxation potential. In *Brain and Information: Event-Related Potentials,* Eds. R. Karrer, J. Cohen, and P. Tueting, pp. 450–464. New York: New York Academy of Science.

Desmedt, J.E., and Tomberg, C. 1989. Mapping early somatosensory evoked potentials in selective attention: critical evaluation of control conditions used for titrating by difference the cognitive P30, P40, P100 and N140. Electroencephalogr. Clin. Neurophysiol. 74:321–346.

Donchin, E. 1981. Surprise!.... Surprise? Psychophysiology 18:493–513.

Donchin, I., and Coles, M.G. 1988. Is the P300 component a manifestation of context updating? Behav. Brain Sci. 11:357–374.

Donchin, E., McCarthy, G., and Kutas, M. 1977. Electroencephalographic investigations of hemispheric specialization. In *Language and Hemispheric Specialization in Man: Cerebral Event-Related Potentials,* Ed. J.E. Desmedt, pp. 212–243. Basel: S. Karger.

Duffy, F.H., Bartels, P.H., and Burchfiel, J.L. 1981. Significance probability mapping: an aid in the topographic analysis of brain electrical activity. Electroencephalogr. Clin. Neurophysiol. 51:455–462.

Düzel, E., Yonelinas, A.P., Mangun, G.R., et al. 1997. Event-related brain potential correlates of two states of conscious awareness in memory. Proc. Natl. Acad. Sci. USA 94:5973–5978.

Eagleman, D.M. 2004. The where and when of intention. Science 303:1144–1146.

Eckhorn, R., Bauer, R., Jordan, W., et al. 1988. Coherent oscillations: a mechanism for feature linking in the visual cortex?. Biol. Cybern. 60:121–130.

Einstein A. 1916. The foundation of the general theory of relativity. In *The Principle of Relativity*, pp. 109–164. Dover: Dover Press.

Elbert, T., Rockstroh, B., Lutzenberger, W., et al. 1980. Biofeedback of slow cortical potentials I. Electroencephalogr. Clin. Neurophysiol. 48:293–341.

Elbert, T., Rockstroh, B., Lutzenberger, W., et al. 1984. Slow brain potentials invoked by voluntary movements and evoked by external stimulation. In *Evoked Potentials II,* Eds. R. Nodar and C. Barber pp. 435–440. London: Butterworth.

Engel, A.K., and Singer, W. 2001. Temporal binding and the neural correlates of sensory awareness. Trends Cogn. Sci. 5:16–25.

Falkenstein, M., Hoormann, J., Christ, S., et al. 2000. ERP components on reaction errors and their functional significance: a tutorial. Biol. Psychol. 52:87–107.

Fell, J., Fernandez, G., Klaver, G., et al. 2003. Is synchronized neuronal gamma activity relevant for selective attention? Brain Res. Rev. 42:265–272.

Friederici, A.D. 1995. The time course of syntactic activation during language processing: a model based on neuropsychological and neurophysiological data. Brain Lang. 50:259–281.

Friedman, D., and Johnson, R. 2000. Event-related potential (ERP) studies of memory encoding and retrieval: a selective review. Microsc. Res. Tech. 51:6–28.

Fuster, J.M. 1989. *The Prefrontal Cortex. Anatomy, Physiology and Neuropsychology of the Frontal Lobe.* New York: Raven Press.

Garavan, H., Ross, T.J., and Stein, E.A. 1999 Right hemispheric dominance of inhibitory control: an event-related functional MRI study. Proc. Natl. Acad. Sci. USA 96:8301–8306.

Gehring, W.J., Gross, B., Coles, M.G.H., et al. 1993. A neural system for error detection and compensation. Psychol. Sci. 4:385–390.

Gemba, H., and Sasaki, K. 1989. Potential related to no-go reaction of go/no–go hand movement task with color discrimination in human. Neurosci. Lett. 101:262–268.

Gerloff, C., Grodd, W., Altenmüller, E., et al. 1996. Coregistration of EEG and fMRI in a simple motor task. Hum. Brain Mapping 4:199–209.

Gerloff, C., Corwell, B., Hallett, M., et al. 1997a. Stimulation over the human supplementary motor area interferes with the organization of future elements in complex motor sequences. Brain 120:1587–1602.

Gerloff, C., Toro, C., Uenishi, N., et al. 1997b. Steady-state movement-related cortical potentials: a new approach to access cortical processing of fast repetitive finger movements. Electroencephalogr. Clin. Neurophysiol. 102:106–113.

Gerloff, C., Uenishi, N., Nagamine, T., et al. 1997c. Bilateral premovement activation in the human motor system: Premotor cortex (PMC) or primary motor cortex (M1)? Soc. Neurosci. Abstr. 23.

Gerloff, C., Corwell, B., Chen, R., et al. 1998. The role of the human motor cortex in the control of complex and simple finger movement sequences. Brain 121:1695–1709.

Gevins, A., Brickett, P., Costales, B., et al. 1990. Beyond topographic mapping: towards functional-anatomical imaging with 124-channel EEGs and 3-D MRIs. Brain Topogr. 3:53–64.

Gevins, A., Cutillo, B., Durousseau, D., et al. 1994. High-resolution evoked potential technology for imaging neural networks of cognition. In *Functional Neuroimaging: Technical Foundations,* Eds. R.W. Thatcher, M. Hallett, T. Zeffiro, et al., pp. 223–231. San Diego: Academic Press.

Gevins, A.S., Zeitlin, G.M., Doyle, J.C., et al. 1979. EEG patterns during "cognitive" tasks. II. Analysis of controlled tasks. Electroencephalogr. Clin. Neurophysiol. 47:704–710.

Gomez-Gonzalez, C.M., Clark, V.P., Fan, S., et al. 1994. Sources of attention-sensitive visual event-related potentials. Brain Topogr. 7:41–51.

Goodin, D.S., and Aminoff, M.J. 1986. Electrophysiological differences between subtypes of dementia. Brain 109:1103–1113.

Hagoort, P., Brown, C.M., and Groothusen, J. 1993. The syntactic positive shift (SPS) as an ERP measure of syntactic processing. Lang. Cog. Proc. 8:439–483.

Hämäläinen, M.S., and Ilmoniemi, R.J. 1994. Interpreting magnetic fields of the brain: minimum norm estimates. Med. Biol. Eng. Comput. 32:35–42.

Hansen, J.C., and Hillyard, S.A. 1980. Endogenous brain potentials associated with selective auditory attention. Electroencephalogr. Clin. Neurophysiol. 49:277–290.

Hansen, J.C., and Hillyard, S.A. 1983. Selective attention to multidimensional auditory stimuli. J. Exp. Psychol. Hum. Percept. Perform. 9:1–19.

Haueisen, J., and Knösche, T.R. 2001. Involuntary motor activity in pianists evoked by music perception. J. Cogn. Neurosci. 13:786–792.

Heinze, H.J., Mangun, G.R., Burchert, W., et al. 1994. Combined spatial and temporal imaging of brain activity during visual selective attention in humans. Nature 372:543–546.

Hennighausen, E., Heil, M., and Rösler, F. 1993. A correction method for DC drift artifacts. Electroencephalogr. Clin. Neurophysiol. 86:199–204.

Hillyard, S.A., and Münte, T.F. 1984. Selective attention to color and location: an analysis with event-related brain potentials. Percept. Psychophys. 36:185–198.

Hillyard, S.A., Hink, R.F., Schwent, V.L., et al. 1973. Electrophysiological signs of selective attention in the human brain. Science 182:177–180.

Hjorth B. 1975. An on-line transformation of EEG scalp potentials into orthogonal source derivations. Electroencephalogr. Clin. Neurophysiol. 39:526–530.

Ikeda, A., Shibasaki, H., Nagamine, T., et al. 1994. Dissociation between contingent negative variation and Bereitschaftspotential in a patient with

cerebellar efferent lesion. Electroencephalogr. Clin. Neurophysiol. 90:359–364.

Jung, R., Altenmüller, E., and Natsch, B. 1984. Zur Hemisphärendominanz für Sprache und Rechnen: elektrophysiologische Korrelate einer Linksdominanz bei Linkshändern. Neuropsychologia 22:755–775.

Jürgens, E., Rösler, F., Hennighausen, E., et al. 1995. Stimulus-induced gamma oscillations: harmonics of alpha activity? NeuroReport 6:813–816.

Kaan, E., Harris, A., Gibson, E., et al. 2000. The P600 as an index of syntactic integration difficulty. Lang. Cogn. Proc. 15:159–201.

Kane, M.N., Curry, S.H., Butler, S.R., et al. 1993. Electrophysiological indicator of awakening from coma. Lancet 341:688.

Kim, S.G., Richter, W., and Ugurbil, K. 1997. Limitations of temporal resolution in functional MRI. Magn. Reson. Med. 37:631–636.

King, J.W., and Kutas, M. 1995. Who did what and when? Using word and clause level ERPs to monitor working memory usage in reading. J. Cogn. Neurosci. 7:376–395.

Kluender, R., and Kutas, M. 1993. Bridging the gap: evidence from ERPs on the processing of unbounded dependencies. J. Cogn. Neurosci. 5:196–214.

Knott, J.R., and Tecce, J.J. 1978. Event-related potentials and psychopathology: a summary of issues and discussion. In *Multidisciplinary Perspectives in Event-Related Brain Potential Research,* Ed. D.A. Otto, pp. 347–354. Washington, DC: Enviromental Protection Agency.

Kok, A. 1986. Effects of degradation of visual stimuli on components of the event-related potential (ERP) in Go/noGo reaction tasks. Biol. Psychol. 23:21–38.

Kolk, H.H.J., Chwilla, D.J., Van Herten, M., et al. 2003 Structure and limited capacity in verbal working memory: a study with event-related potentials. Brain Lang. 8:1–36.

Konishi, S., Nakajima, K., Uchida, Y., et al. 1999. Common inhibitory mechanism in human inferior prefrontal cortex revealed by event-related functional MRI. Brain 122:981–991.

Kornhuber, H.H., and Deecke, L. 1965. Hirnpotentialänderungen bei Willkürbewegungen und passiven Bewegungen des Menschen. Pflugers Arch. 284:1–17.

Koyama, K., Gerloff, C., Celnik, P., et al. 1997. Functional cooperativity of visual, motor and premotor areas during braille reading in patients suffering from peripheral blindness early in life. Neurology 48:A305.

Kraus, N., and Cheour, M. 2000. Speech-sound representation in the brain: studies using mismatch negativity. Audiol. Neuro-Otol. 5:140–150.

Kristeva, R., Cheyne, D., and Deecke, L. 1991. Neuromagnetic fields accompanying unilateral and bilateral voluntary movements: topography and analysis. Electroencephalogr. Clin. Neurophysiol. 81:284–298.

Kristeva-Feige, R., Feige, B., Makeig, S., et al. 1993. Oscillatory brain activity during a motor task. Neuroreport 4:1291–1294.

Kübler, A., Kotchoubey, B., Kaiser, J., et al. 2001. Brain-computer communication: unlocking the locked in. Psychol. Bull. 127:358–375.

Kujala, T., and Näätänen, R. 2001. The mismatch negativity in evaluating central auditory dysfunction in dyslexia. Neurosci. Biobehav. Rev. 25:535–543.

Kutas, M. 1987. Event-related brain potentials elicited during rapid serial visual presentation of congruous and incongruous sentences. In *Current Trends in Event-Related Potential Research,* Eds. R. Johnson, J.W. Rohrbaugh, and R. Parasuraman, pp. 406–411. Amsterdam: Elsevier.

Kutas, M., and Hillyard, S.A. 1980. Reading between the lines: event-related brain potentials during natural sentence processing. Brain Lang. 11:354–373.

Kutas, M., McCarthy, G., and Donchin, E., 1977. Augmenting mental chronometry: the P300 as a measure of stimulus evaluation time. Science 191:792–795.

Kutas, M., Federmeier, K.D., Coulson, S., et al. 2000. Language. In *Handbook of Psychophysiology,* Eds. J.T. Cacioppo, G. Tassinary, and G.G. Berntson, 2nd ed., pp. 576–601. Cambridge: Cambridge University Press.

Lang, M., Lang, W., Uhl, F., et al. 1987. Slow negative potential shifts indicating verbal cognitive learning in a concept formation task. Hum. Neurobiol. 6:183–190.

Lang, W., Lang, M., Kornhuber, A., et al. 1988. Left frontal lobe in verbal associative learning: a slow potential study. Exp. Brain Res. 70:99–108.

Le, J., Menon, V., and Gevins, A. 1994. Local estimate of surface Laplacian derivation on a realistically shaped scalp surface and its performance on noisy data. Electroencephalogr. Clin. Neurophysiol. 92:433–441.

Lee, C.C., Jack, C.R., Jr., and Riederer, S.J. 1996. Use of functional magnetic resonance imaging. Neurosurg. Clin. North Am. 7:665–683.

Lenneberg, E. 1967. *Biological Foundations of Language.* New York: Wiley.

Leppänen, P.H., and Lyytinen, H. 1997. Auditory event-related potentials in the study of developmental language-related disorders. Audiol. Neuro-Otol. 2:308–340.

Libet, B. 1985. Unconscious cerebral initiative and the role of conscious will in voluntary action. Behav. Brain Sci. 8:529–566.

Libet, B., Gleason, C.A., Wright, E.W., et al. 1983. Time of conscious intention to act in relation to onset of cerebral activity (readiness-potential). Brain 106:623–642.

Lindsley, D.B., Bowden, J.W., and Magoun, H.W. 1949. Effect upon the EEG of acute injury to the brain stem activating system. Electroencephalogr. Clin. Neurophysiol. 1:475–486.

Logothetis, N.K., and Wandell, B.A. 2004. Interpreting the BOLD Signal. Annu. Rev. Physiol. 66:735–769.

Logothetis, N.K., Pauls, J., Augath, M., et al. 2001. Neurophysiological investigation of the basis of the fMRI signal. Nature 412:150–157.

Luria, A.R. 1973. *The Working Brain.* London: Penguin Press.

Lutzenberger, W., Elbert, T., Rockstroh, B., et al. 1985. Asymmetry of brain potentials related to sensorimotor tasks. Int. J. Psychophysiol. 2:281–291.

Manganotti, P., Gerloff, C., Toro, C., et al. 1998. Task-related coherence and task-related spectral power during sequential finger movements. Electroencephalogr. Clin. Neurophysiol. 109:50–62.

Mangun, G.R., and Hillyard, S.A. 1987. The spatial allocation of visual attention as indexed by event-related brain potentials. Hum. Factors 29:195–211.

Maurer, C., Aboutanos, G.B., Dawant, B.M., et al. 1996. Effect of geometrical distortion correction in MR on image registration accuracy. J. Comput. Assist. Tomogr. 20:666–679.

McAdam, D.W., and Seales, D.M. 1969. Bereitschaftspotential enhancement with increased level of motivation. Electroencephalogr. Clin. Neurophysiol. 27:73–75.

McCarthy, G., and Donchin, E. 1981. A metric for thought: a comparison of P300 latency and reaction time. Science 211:77–80.

McKee, G., Humphrey, B., and McAdam, D.W. 1973. Scaled lateralization of alpha activity during linguistic and musical tasks. Psychophysiology 10:441–443.

Mirkovic, N., Adjouadi, M., Yaylali, I., et al. 2003. 3-D source localization of epileptic foci integrating EEG and MRI data. Brain Topogr. 16:111–119.

Morgan, A., Macdonald, H., and Hilgaad, E. 1974. EEG alpha-lateral asymmetry related to task and hypnotizability. Psychophysiology 11:275–282.

Moruzzi, G., and Magoun, H.W. 1949. Brainstem reticular formation and activation of the EEG. Electroencephalogr. Clin. Neurophysiol. 1:455–473.

Münte, T.F., Heinze, H.J., and G.R. Mangun, 1993. Dissociation of brain activity related to syntactic and semantic aspects of language. J. Cogn. Neurosc. 5:335–344.

Münte, T.F., Heinze, H.J., Matzke, M., et al. 1998. Brain potentials and syntactic violations revisited: no evidence for specificity of the syntactic positive shift. Neuropsychologia 36:217–226.

Münte, T.F., Urbach, T.P., Düzel., E., et al. 2000. Event-related brain potentials in the study of human cognition and neuropsychology. In *Handbook of Neuropsychology*, Eds. F. Boller, J. Grafmann, and G. Rizolatti, pp. 139–235. Amsterdam: Elsevier Science.

Münte, T.F., Kohlmetz, C., Nager, W., et al. 2001. Neuroperception. Superior auditory spatial tuning in conductors. Nature 409:580.

Näätänen, R. 2003. Mismatch negativity: clinical research and possible applications. Int. J. Psychophysiol. 48:179–188.

Näätänen, R., and Winkler, I. 1999. The concept of auditory stimulus representation in cognitive neuroscience. Psychol. Bull. 125:826–859.

Nager, W., Kohlmetz, C., Altenmüller, E., et al. 2003. The fate of sounds in conductors' brains: an ERP study. Cogn. Brain Res. 17:83–93.

Neshige, R., Lüders, H., Friedman, L., et al. 1988. Recordings of movement-related potentials from the human cortex. Ann. Neurol. 24:439–445.

Nunez, P.L. 1981. *Electric Fields of the Brain: The Neurophysics of EEG.* New York: Oxford University Press.

Nunez, P.L., and Silberstein, R.B. 2000. On the relationship of synaptic activity to macroscopic measurements: does co-registration of EEG with fMRI make sense? Brain Topogr. 13:79–96.

Opitz, B., Mecklinger, A., Friederici, A.D., et al. 1999. The functional neuroanatomy of novelty processing: Integrating ERP and fMRI results. Cereb. Cortex 9:379–391.

Opitz, B., Rinne, T., Mecklinger, A., et al. 2002. Differential contribution of frontal and temporal cortices to auditory change detection: fMRI and ERP results. Neuroimage 15:167–174.

Osterhout, L., and Holcomb, P.J. 1992. Event-related brain potentials elicited by syntactic anomaly. J. Mem. Lang. 34:785–806.

Paller, K.A., Kutas, M., and Mayes, A.R. 1987. Neural correlates of encoding in an incidental learning paradigm. Electroencephalogr. Clin. Neurophysiol. 67:360–371.

Pantev, Ch. 1995. Evoked and induced gamma-band activity of the human cortex. Brain Topogr. 4:321–330.

Pascual-Leone, A., Gates, J.R., and Dhuna, A. 1991. Induction of speech arrest and counting errors with rapid-rate transcranial magnetic stimulation. Neurology 41:697–702.

Pascual-Marqui, R.D. 1999. Review of methods for solving the EEG inverse problem. Int. J. Bioelectromagn. 1:75–86.

Pascual-Marqui, R.D., Michel, C.M., and Lehmann, D. 1994. Low resolution electromagnetic tomography: a new method for localizing electrical activity in the brain. Int. J. Psychophysiol. 18:49–65.

Patterson, J.V., Michalewski, H.J., and Starr, A. 1988. Latency variability of the components of auditory event-related potentials to infrequent stimuli in aging, Alzheimer-type dementia, and depression. Electroencephalogr. Clin. Neurophysiol. 71:450–460.

Petsche, H., Pockberger, H., and Rappelsberger, P. 1986. EEG topography and mental performance. In *Topographic Mapping of Brain Electrical Activity,* Ed. F.H. Duffy, pp. 63–98. London: Butterworths.

Pfurtscheller, G., and Aranibar, A. 1977. Event-related desynchronization detected by power measurements of the scalp EEG. Electroencephalogr. Clin. Neurophysiol. 42:817–826.

Pfurtscheller, G., and Klimesch, W. 1987. Untersuchungen kognitiver Hirnleistungen mit einem dynamischen EEG-mapping-System. In *Zugang zum Verständnis höherer Hirnfunktionen durch das EEG,* Ed. H.M. Weinmann, pp. 75–80. München: Zuckschwerdt.

Phillips, C., Rugg, M.D., and Friston, K.J. 2002. Anatomically informed basis functions for EEG source localization: combining functional and anatomical constraints. Neuroimage 16:678–695.

Picard, Y., and Thompson C.J., 1997. Motion correction of PET images using multiple acquisition frames. IEEE Trans. Med. Imaging 16:137–144.

Picton, T.W., Alain, C., Otten, L., et al. 2001. Mismatch negativity: different water in the same river. Audiol. Neurootol. 5:111–139.

Pihan, H., Altenmüller, E., Hertrich, I., et al. 2000. Cortical activation patterns of affective speech processing depend on concurrent demands on the subvocal rehearsal system: a DC-potential-study. Brain 123:2338–2349.

Plewnia, C., Bartels, M., and Gerloff, C. 2003. Transient suppression of tinnitus by transcranial magnetic stimulation. Ann. Neurol. 53:263–266.

Polich, J. 1998. P300 clinical utility and control of variability. J. Clin. Neurophysiol. 15:14–33.

Polich, J., and Kok, A. 1995. Cognitive and biological determinants of P300: an integrative review. Biol. Psychol. 41:103–146.

Price, C.J., Wise, R.J., Warburton, E.A., et al. 1996. Hearing and saying: the functional neuroanatomy of auditory word processing. Brain 119:919–931.

Pulvermüller, F. 1995. Hebb's concept of cell assemblies and the psychophysiology of word processing. Psychophysiology 33:317–333.

Pulvermüller, F., Eulitz, C., Pantev, Ch., et al. 1996. High-frequency cortical responses reflect lexical processing: an MEG study. Electroencephalogr. Clin. Neurophysiol. 98:76–85.

Rebert, C.S., and Low, D.W. 1978. Differential hemispheric activation during complex visuomotor performance. Electroencephalogr. Clin. Neurophysiol. 44:724–734.

Rebert, C.S., McAdam, D., Knott, J.R., et al. 1967. Slow potential changes in human brain related to level of motivation. J. Comp. Physiol. Psychol. 63:20–23.

Reite, M., Teale, P., Zimmerman, J., et al. 1988. Source location of a 50 msec latency auditory evoked field component. Electroencephalogr. Clin. Neurophysiol. 70:490–498.

Rockstroh, B., Elbert, T., Canavan, A., et al. 1989. *Slow Cortical Potentials and Behaviour.* Baltimore: Urban and Schwarzenberg.

Rockstroh, B., Elbert, T., Birbaumer, N., et al. 1990. Biofeedback-produced hemispheric asymmetry of slow cortical potentials and its behavioural effects. Int. J. Psychophysiol. 9:151–165.

Röder, B., Teder-Sälejärvi, W.A., Sterr, A., et al. 1999. Improved auditory spatial tuning in blind humans. Nature 400:162–166.

Rodriguez-Fornells, A., Kurzbuch, A.R., and Münte, T.F. 2002a. Time course of error detection and correction in humans: neurophysiological evidence. J Neurosci. 22:9990–9996.

Rodriguez-Fornells, A., Rotte, M., Heinze, H.J., et al. 2002b. Brain potential and functional MRI evidence for how to handle two languages with one brain. Nature 415:1026–1029.

Rohrbaugh, J.W., Syndulko, K., and Lindsley, D.B. 1976. Brain wave components of the contingent negative variation in humans. Science 191: 1055–1057.

Rösler, F., Heil, M., and Glowalla, U. 1993. Memory retrieval from long-term memory by slow event-related potentials. Psychophysiology 30: 170–182.

Rösler, F., Heil, M., and Röder, B. 1997. Slow negative potentials as reflections of specific modular resources of cognition. Biol. Psychol. 45:109–141.

Ruchkin, D.S., Berndt, R.S., Johnson, R., et al. 1997. Modality-specific processing streams in verbal working memory: evidence from spatio-temporal patterns of brain activity. Cogn. Brain Res. 6:95–113.

Rugg, M.D., and Allan, K. 2000. Event-related potential studies of long-term memory. In *The Oxford Handbook of Memory,* Eds. E. Tulving and F.I.M. Craik. Oxford: Oxford University Press.

Rugg, M.D., and Coles, M.G. 1995. *Electrophysiology of Mind.* Oxford: Oxford University Press.

Sadato, N., Pascual, L.A., Grafman, J., et al. 1996. Activation of the primary visual cortex by Braille reading in blind subjects. Nature 380:526–528.

Sarvas, J. 1987. Basic mathematical and electromagnetic concepts of the biomagnetic inverse problem. Phys. Med. Biol. 32:11–22.

Sasaki, K., and Gemba, H. 1984. Compensatory motor function of the somatosensory cortex for dysfunction of the motor cortex following cerebellar hemispherectomy in the monkey. Exp. Brain Res. 56:532–538.

Sasaki, K., Gemba, H., and Tsujimoto, T. 1989. Suppression of visually initiated hand movement by stimulation of the prefrontal cortex in the monkey. Brain Res. 495:100–107.

Scherg, M., and Ebersole, J.S. 1993. Models of brain sources. Brain Topogr. 5:419–423.

Scherg, M., and Ebersole, J.S. 1994. Brain source imaging of focal and multifocal epileptiform EEG activity. Clin. Neurophysiol. 24:51–60.

Scherg, M., Bast, T., and Berg, P. 1999. Multiple source analysis of interictal spikes: goals, requirements, and clinical value. J. Clin. Neurophysiol. 16:214–224.

Schoenfeld, M.A., Tempelmann, C., Martinez, A., et al. 2003. Dynamics of feature binding during object-selective attention. Proc. Natl. Acad. Sci. USA 100:11806–11811.

Schröger, E. 1997. On the detection of auditory deviations: a pre-attentive activation model. Psychophysiology 34:245–257.

Schulte-Körne, G., Deimel, W., Bartling, J., et al. 1998. Auditory processing and dyslexia: evidence for a specific speech processing deficit. Neuroreport 9:337–340.

Simons, R.F., Rockstroh, B., Elbert, T., et al. 1987. Evocation and habituation of autonomic and event-related potential responses in a nonsignal environment. J. Psychophysiol. 1:45–60.

Simson, R., Vaughan, H.G., and Ritter, W. 1977. The scalp topography of potentials in auditory and visual go/nogo tasks. Electroencephalogr. Clin. Neurophysiol. 43:864–875.

Singer, W., and Dräger, U. 1972. Postsynaptic potentials in relay neurons of cat lateral geniculate nucleus after stimulation of the mesencephalic reticular formation. Brain Res. 41:214–220.

Singer, W., and Gray, C.M. 1995. Visual feature integration and the temoral correlation hypothesis. Annu. Rev. Neurosci. 18:555–586.

Smith, E.E., and Jonides, J. 1999. Storage and executive processes in the frontal lobes. Science 283:1657–1660.

Smith, M.E., Halgren, E., Sokolik, M., et al. 1990. The intracranial topography of the P3 event-related potential elicited during auditory oddball. Electroencephalogr. Clin. Neurophysiol. 76:235–248.

Sokolov, E.N. 1960. Neuronal model of the orienting reflex. In *The Central Nervous System and Behaviour,* Ed. M. Brazier, pp. 187–276. New York: J. Macy Jr. Foundation.

Spitzer, A., Cohen, L.G., Fabrikant, J., et al. 1989. A method for determining optimal interelectrode spacing for cerebral topographic mapping. Electroencephalogr. Clin. Neurophysiol. 72:355–361.

Squires, N.K., Squires, K.C., and Hillyard, S.A. 1975. Two varieties of long-latency positive wave evoked by unpredictable stimuli in man. Electroencephalogr. Clin. Neurophysiol. 38:387–401.

Squires, N.K., Donchin, E., Herning, R.I., et al. 1977. On the influence of task-relevance and stimulus-probability on event-related-potential components. Electroencephalogr. Clin. Neurophysiol. 42:1–14.

St. George, M., Mannes, S., and Hoffman, J.E. 1994. Global semantic expectancy and language comprehension. J. Cogn. Neurosci. 6:70–83.

Steinhauer, K., Alter, K.A., and Friederici, A.S. 1999. Brain potentials indicate immediate use of prosodic cues in natural speech processing. Nat. Neurosci. 2:191–196.

Swaab, T.Y., Brown, C., and Hagoort, P. 1998. Understanding ambiguous words in sentence contexts: electrophysiological evidence for delayed contextual selection in Broca's aphasia. Neuropsychologia 36:737–761.

Tallon, C., Bertrand, O., Bouchet, P., et al. 1995. Gamma-range activity evoked by coherent visual stimuli in humans. Eur. J. Neurosci. 7:1285–1291.

Teder-Sälejärvi, W.A., and Hillyard, S.A. 1998. The gradient of spatial auditory attention in free field: an event-related potential study. Percept. Psychophysiol. 60:1228–1242.

Tervaniemi, M., Maury, S., and Näätänen, R. 1994. Neural representations of abstract stimulus features in the human brain as reflected by the mismatch-negativity. Neuroreport 5:844–846.

Thees, S., Blankenburg, F., Taskin, B., et al. 2003. Dipole source localization and fMRI of simultaneously recorded data applied to somatosensory categorization. Neuroimage 18:707–719.

Thomas, C., Altenmüller, E., Marckmann, G., et al. 1997. Language processing in aphasia: syndrome-specific lateralization patterns during recovery reflect cerebral plasticity in adults. Electroencephalogr. Clin. Neurophysiol. 102:86–97.

Toro, C., Wang, B., Zeffiro, T., et al. 1994. Movement-related cortical potentials: source analysis and PET/MRI correlation. In *Functional Neuroimaging: Technical Foundations,* Eds. R.W. Thatcher, M. Hallett, T. Zeffiro, et al., pp. 259–267. San Diego: Academic Press.

Tucker, D.M. 1993. Spatial sampling of head electrical fields: the geodesic sensor net. Electroencephalogr. Clin. Neurophysiol. 87:154–163.

Uhl, F., Franzen, P., Serles, W., et al. 1990. Anterior frontal cortex and the effect of proactive interference in paired associate learning: a DC Potential study. J. Cognit. Neurosci. 2:373–382.

Ullsperger, M., and Von Cramon, D.Y. 2001. Subprocesses of performance monitoring: a dissociation of error processing and response competition revealed by event-related fMRI and ERPs. Neuroimage 14:1387–1401.

Umilta, M.A., Kohler, E., Gallese, V., et al. 2001. I know what you are doing. A neurophysiological study. Neuron 31:155–165.

Varela, F., Lachnaux, J.P., Rodriguez, E., et al. 2001. The brainweb: phase synchronization and large-scale integration. Nat. Rev. Neurosci. 2:229–239.

Verleger, R. 1988. Event-related potentials and cognition: A critique of the context updating hypothesis and an alternative interpretation of P3. Behav. Brain Sci. 11:343–427.

Von Helmholtz, H.L.F. 1853. Ueber einige Gesetze der Vertheilung elektrischer Ströme in körperlichen Leitern mit Anwendung auf die thierisch-elektrischen Versuche. Ann. Phys. Chem. 89:211–233.

Waberski, T.D., Gobbele, R., Darvas, F., et al. 2002. Spatiotemporal imaging of electrical activity related to attention to somatosensory stimulation. Neuroimage 17:1347–1357.

Walter, H., Kristeva, R., Knorr, U., et al. 1992. Individual somatotopy of primary sensorimotor cortex revealed by intermodal of MEG, PET and MRI. Brain Topogr. 5:183–187.

Walter, W.G., Cooper, R., Aldridge, V., et al. 1964. Contingent negative variation: an electrical sign of sensorimotor association and expectancy in the human brain. Nature 203:380–384.

Wang, B., Toro, C., Wassermann, E.M., et al. 1994. Multimodal integration of electrophysiological data and brain images: EEG, MEG, TMS, MRI and PET. In *Functional Neuroimaging: Technical Foundations,* Eds.

R.W. Thatcher, M. Hallett, T. Zeffiro, et al., pp. 251–257. San Diego: Academic Press.

Wassermann, E.M., Wang, B.S., Zeffiro, T.A., et al. 1996. Locating the motor cortex on the MRI with transcranial magnetic stimulation and PET. Neuroimage 3:1–9.

West, J., Fitzpatrick, J.M., Wang, M.Y., et al. 1997. Comparison and evaluation of retrospective intermodality brain image registration techniques. J. Comput. Assist. Tomogr. 21:554–566.

Wikswo, J.P., Jr., Gevins, A., and Williamson, S.J. 1993. The future of the EEG and MEG. Electroencephalogr. Clin. Neurophysiol. 87:1–9.

Wilding, E.L., and Rugg, M.D. 1996. An event-related potential study of recognition memory with and without retrieval of source. Brain 119:889–905.

Wilke, J.T., and Lansing, R.W. 1973. Variations in the motor potential with force exerted during voluntary arm movements in man. Electroencephalogr. Clin. Neurophysiol. 35:225–260.

Yvert, B., Bertrand, O., Echallier, J.F., et al. 1995. Improved forward EEG calculations using local mesh refinement of realistic head geometries. Electroencephalogr. Clin. Neurophysiol. 95:381–392.

Zani, A., and Proverbio, A.M. 2002. *The Cognitive Electrophysiology of Mind and Brain.* New York: Academic Press.

32. EEG in Aviation, Space Exploration, and Diving

James D. Frost Jr.

Overview

Human history has been characterized by a continuous expansion of the working environment. Current frontiers encompass air, space, and sea, and each of these domains presents unique problems that limit its effective utilization. The primary role of electroencephalography (EEG) in the exploration and exploitation of these areas has been to serve as a monitoring tool for evaluating adverse effects of the environment upon individuals living within its confines and as a screening device in the selection of crew members for specific tasks. The EEG has not been used extensively in these situations in the past; there were numerous technical problems associated with data acquisition, especially in extralaboratory missions, which sometimes interfered with other objectives of the particular project. Similarly, problems arose in interpreting the data, particularly with respect to the significance of observed changes in the electrographic pattern. However, in spite of these limitations, the EEG has provided valuable information in a number of situations; careful evaluation of the data has facilitated the safe exploration of new areas in aviation, spaceflight, and prolonged undersea missions.

Aviation

Because the pioneering studies in aviation, including both lighter-than-air and early heavier-than-air craft, were conducted before the advent of clinical EEG, this technique did not play a role in evaluating adaptation to the environment above ground level. More recent studies have revealed no EEG changes unique to conventional flying, although, as would be predicted, EEG changes characteristic of acute hypoxia are observed during high-altitude flights when supplemental oxygen is not supplied at appropriate levels (Seege and Wirth, 1977).

The high acceleration values associated with air acrobatics are known to produce slowing in the EEG and even transient flattening (Sem-Jacobsen, 1959; Sem-Jacobson and Sem-Jacobsen, 1963) due to hemodynamic factors. Accelerations of $2g$ to $9g$ in certain orientations can produce rapid loss of consciousness (Whinnery et al., 1987) that may persist for 15 seconds or longer beyond termination of the aerobatic maneuver. Current military fighter aircraft can produce and sustain such high g levels, resulting in a significant risk of crew incapacitation and subsequent accident (Whinnery, 1986). EEG has been utilized in this area primarily to provide an early indication of g-induced cerebral impairment during centrifuge-based flight simulation studies designed to analyze this phenomenon and to evaluate protective measures that can be used during actual flights (Forster and Whinnery, 1988; Guo et al., 1988; Zhang et al., 1991).

The use of the EEG in aviation has focused primarily on its potential value as a screening device for selecting flight-crew candidates and for periodic reevaluation of those already employed (see discussions by Blanc, 1976; Clark and Riley, 2001; Everett and Akhavi, 1982; Everett and Jenkins, 1982; Hendriksen and Elderson, 2001; Rudnyi and Bodrov, 1987; Weber, 2002). A major concern is the detection of abnormalities suggestive of epilepsy or other significant neurological disease and the subsequent rejection or restriction of the flight status of such individuals. Although few would argue against the wisdom of grounding personnel with known neurological disease, there is disagreement concerning the use of the EEG in this setting. Some countries and some private aviation organizations require its use, while others do not. In addition, there is currently no commonly accepted standard of application. Important areas of disagreement exist regarding the correlation of various nonspecific EEG abnormalities with pilot accident rates, and there is even controversy regarding the significance of true epileptiform patterns when they occur occasionally in asymptomatic individuals. Conversely, it is recognized that a routine EEG is subject to significant sampling errors, and thus a "normal" EEG does not exclude the possibility that the individual has a seizure disorder.

In a recent comprehensive review of the use of EEG as a screening device in aircrew selection, Hendriksen and Elderson (2001) pooled data from nine previously published studies, as well as other epidemiological information, to estimate the probability that an asymptomatic candidate pilot with an epileptiform EEG at the time of initial medical evaluation would develop seizures over a subsequent flying career spanning 35 years. They concluded that the risk of developing epilepsy was 25% for such an individual, as compared to 2% in subjects with normal initial EEGs and no prior history of seizures. Based on their findings, which suggest a 12-fold increase of the risk for seizures, these investigators favor rejection of all candidates with epileptiform EEGs, taking the point of view that while such a policy will result in the rejection of a few candidates who will never develop seizures, public safety concerns must take precedence. This viewpoint has been contested by Clark and Riley (2001), who feel that this approach would needlessly exclude many qualified individuals who would never have a seizure, and they favor a selective use of EEG, within the context of a thorough medical evaluation.

Viewed objectively, it seems that the role of the EEG in aviation personnel screening should be no different from its application in general medicine, where it always serves as an adjunct to diagnosis. It is clear that the EEG, when accurately interpreted, can provide objective evidence that is essential to a proper medical evaluation, but it should be utilized only within the framework of a comprehensive medical and neurological examination; the final diagnosis should be based on all available evidence. Thus, the decision to ground a pilot or other crew member should never be based solely on the EEG, nor should a normal EEG ever be considered proof of the absence of disease. Perhaps the most convincing argument for the routine use of the EEG in aviation screening is that it provides a baseline recording with which future tracings may be compared. Such information greatly facilitates the interpretation of minimal findings that may be seen following a subsequent injury or illness and can also serve as the basis for more definitive studies of the prognostic value of the EEG.

In recent years, in-flight EEG recordings have been used to assess the sleep/wake status of pilots during prolonged commercial flights (Gundel et al., 1995; Landstrom and Lofstedt, 1987; Samel et al., 1996, 1997a,b; Wright and Mc-Gown, 2001). These studies have provided information suggesting that aircrew work/rest schedules are not optimal during some long-duration flights, and that a relatively high percentage of pilots may occasionally show objective signs of drowsiness or sleep while on duty. EEG has also been used, both in actual flight and in simulator studies, to provide objective evidence for the efficacy of stimulant medications (e.g., dextroamphetamine and modafinil) in military aviation operations, which sometimes must be conducted by the crew in spite of significant sleep deprivation (Caldwell and Caldwell, 1997; Caldwell et al., 1995, 2000a,b).

Several investigators have explored the potential value of computer-derived quantitative EEG measures as indicators of performance and cognitive workload. Sterman and his colleagues (see review by Sterman and Mann, 1995) have conducted a number of studies under both simulated and actual flight conditions, and have reported specific alterations of EEG activity, including localized suppression of 8- to 13-Hz activity, the magnitudes of which correlate with task difficulty and workload. In similar experimental conditions increases of theta band EEG components have been reported to correlate with increasing cognitive task difficulty in in-flight studies of general aviation pilots (Hankins and Wilson, 1998), and in air military air traffic controllers (Brookings et al., 1996). While these studies are preliminary, the long-term goal is the development of improved methods for the objective evaluation of pilot performance under differing task and environmental conditions.

Space Exploration

EEG recordings have been conducted during a number of United States and Russian space missions. It was apparent from the early studies that clinically significant changes were rare or absent (see review by Maulsby et al., 1976). No abnormalities were observed on visual analysis of approximately 55 hours of continuous EEG recording, including

two sleep periods, during the Gemini 7 flight in 1965 (Maulsby, 1966). However, one of four Russian crew members was reported to have shown an increased amount of theta activity during days 2 and 3 of the flight (Voskrensenskiy et al., 1965), and subsequent computer analysis of the Gemini 7 data revealed some increase in activity in this band (Adey et al., 1967).

An extensive series of EEG recordings was conducted during the three Skylab missions beginning in 1973 (Frost et al., 1974). Because the crews of earlier flights had often complained of insomnia and fatigue, these EEG studies were designed primarily to evaluate sleep characteristics under weightless conditions. In addition to pre- and postflight baseline recordings, multiple all-night recordings were conducted on one astronaut during each of the three flights, for a total of 50 nights, or approximately 400 hours of recording. These data were processed in-flight automatically by an onboard sleep-analysis device (Frost et al., 1975) and postflight by conventional methods after playback of the magnetic tapes. While all three astronauts experienced mild reductions of total sleep time during the flights, it was thought that all subjects obtained adequate sleep (in-flight total sleep times averaged 6.0, 6.3, and 6.7 hours for the three subjects, compared to preflight averages of 6.9, 6.4, and 7.3 hours, respectively), and no significant long-term problems were encountered. Stage 3 sleep tended to be increased above the baseline level during flight, and both stages 3 and 4 were somewhat depressed in the postflight period. Rapid eye movement (REM) sleep, although not consistently altered in flight, increased significantly in the postflight period, along with a decrease in REM latency.

Postflight visual analysis of the recorded EEG data revealed no abnormalities throughout the in-flight or postflight periods. However, it was noted that two astronauts showed a noticeable increase of alpha-rhythm frequency during the early in-flight period as compared to the preflight baseline records. Subsequent quantitative analysis using computer techniques confirmed this observation in two subjects and also revealed small, but significant, increases in beta (13–40 Hz) and delta (0.5–3.5 Hz) amounts in all three individuals (Frost, 1977). For example, the subject of the 84-day Skylab flight had a preflight alpha frequency of 9.2 Hz (average of three baseline values; range, 8.9–9.7 Hz). The first value obtained in flight (day 3) was 10.3 Hz, which was an increase of 1.1 Hz, and values throughout the flight, although tending to decline, were all above the preflight mean. The physiological significance of these findings is unknown, and, without additional data, precise evaluation is not possible because of the many potentially influential factors present in this environment. Such factors included altered metabolic states (Leach and Rambaut, 1974), drugs used for other in-flight problems (Hordinsky, 1974), and fluid shifts secondary to loss of hydrostatic pressure (Thornton et al., 1974).

More recent polysomnographic studies of cosmonauts onboard the Russian MIR space station during flights lasting up to 438 days (Gundel et al., 1993, 1997, 1999, 2002; Stoilova et al., 2000) have reported more frequent sleep disturbances as well as some alteration of the sleep pattern in-flight as compared to the preflight baseline studies. However, the overall average total sleep time of 6.11 hours observed in-flight in four subjects was only slightly below the preflight average of 6.37 hours. The possibility that the observed sleep disturbances onboard MIR might have been a result of elevated CO_2 levels was evaluated in a ground-based chamber study by Gundel et al. (1998). However, they found no significant differences in total sleep time or sleep stage distribution in four subjects who lived for 23 days with an ambient CO_2 level of 1.2% (comparable to the maximum values observed on MIR), in comparison to values observed in the same subjects at a CO_2 level of 0.7%.

EEG, together with other polysomnographic parameters, has been recorded on several astronauts during the current series of NASA space shuttle flights. Four subjects studied during the 17-day STS-78 flight in 1996 (Monk, 1999; Monk et al., 1998, 1999) showed some decrease of sleep time in-flight (average: 6.1 hours, compared to a baseline value of 6.5 hours), although the sleep efficiency (sleep time expressed as a percentage of total time in bed) was high (89.5%), and circadian rhythms were said to have been appropriate for the work/rest schedule. However, all four subjects did exhibit a significant decrease of stages 3 and 4 while in flight. Five additional subjects were studied polysomnographically on several occasions during the 16-day STS-90 and 9-day STS-95 flights in 1998 (Dijk et al., 2001). The average sleep parameters on the four in-flight nights were very similar to the preflight baseline values (total sleep time was 6.5 hours in flight, compared to 6.7 hours preflight, and sleep efficiencies were the same in flight and preflight). However, the authors noted that information obtained from subjective sleep reports and wrist actigraphy on the other in-flight nights (when polysomnography was not obtained) suggested that overall sleep quality was diminished in flight, perhaps a result of less stringent adherence to scheduled bedtimes on nights when recording was not performed. As reported for the Skylab missions (see above), a marked increase of stage REM, together with a decreased REM latency, was seen during the postflight period, along with a decrease of stages 3 and 4.

This series of recordings was also the first to provide a quantitative assessment of sleep-related upper airway resistance changes associated with the microgravity environment (Elliot et al., 2001). All five subjects exhibited some degree of sleep-disordered breathing preflight, with an overall apnea/hypopnea index of 8.3/h (three subjects had values below 5/h, the other two had rates of 6.1/h and 22.7/h, respectively), snoring occurred during 16.5% of the total sleep time, and respiratory-related arousals occurred at a rate of 5.5/h of sleep. The in-flight period was associated with a 55% reduction of the apnea/hypopnea index (average rate 3.4/h in flight), an almost complete absence of snoring (0.7% of sleep time), and fewer respiratory-related arousals (1.8/h in flight). These findings, indicating a significant improvement in sleep-related respiratory function during the flight, appear to demonstrate that gravity plays a crucial causative role in the generation of apnea/hypopnea and snoring.

Considering all of the available data regarding sleep characteristics during spaceflight, it seems reasonable to conclude that this weightless (microgravity) environment is not inherently associated with major disruptions of sleep-wake physiology. While many crew members do complain of occasional sleep problems, polysomnographic studies have documented that average sleep characteristics tend to be only minimally or mildly degraded during the in-flight periods. Factors that probably do contribute to intermittent in-flight sleep problems include altered or changing sleep-wake schedules (Dijk et al., 2001; Gundel et al., 1997; Monk et al., 1998; Prisk, 1998), differing social and light cues (Samel and Gander, 1995), and in-flight medication use (Putcha et al., 1999).

Auditory and visual evoked potentials were studied during an early space shuttle flight in an investigation of the space motion sickness syndrome (Thornton et al., 1985, 1987). The normal test results obtained were cited as evidence suggesting that increased intracranial pressure and/or vestibular hydrops were not likely etiological factors underlying this condition.

Diving

Exploration of the undersea environment has presented more problems with respect to human physiology than either aviation or space exploration. In the latter two situations, the atmosphere can be controlled to closely simulate the normal distribution of gas components (i.e., the partial pressures of nitrogen, oxygen, and carbon dioxide are maintained at values reasonably close to those present at sea level). Although this is also possible in diving, through the use of rigid submersible vehicles such as submarines or diving bells, most recent advances in undersea exploration have aimed at increasing the freedom of movement within the environment through use of self-contained breathing devices (scuba) and pressurized undersea habitats. These latter approaches require delivery of breathing gases at greatly increased pressures, and problems arise due to altered toxicity of the gases, as well as the dangers inherent in the decompression process. The EEG has been used in studies of this environment for approximately 50 years (see review by Maulsby et al., 1976).

When compressed air at a pressure greater than 6 to 7 atm is used as the breathing mixture, symptoms of narcosis such as euphoria, confusion, or incoordination are often observed and are associated with EEG changes. For example, in dives to 250 feet, simulated in a pressure chamber, the onset of symptoms is reported to be accompanied by reduced amplitude and increased frequency of EEG activity and by changes in evoked-potential configuration (Roger et al., 1954, 1955). The key factor, at least for short-term dives (less than 24 hours) with pressure up to approximately 10 atm at a depth of about 290 feet, is the partial pressure of nitrogen. Cabarrou (1966) showed that the EEG alterations (increased alpha frequency, decreased alpha amplitude, and increased theta activity) seen with compressed air were eliminated when a helium-oxygen mixture was used to maintain a normal nitrogen partial pressure, even when the oxygen partial pressure was elevated. However, oxygen toxicity becomes a significant factor with longer exposure, and it, too, must be maintained at a normal partial pressure (Bond, 1964) through the use of an inert gas, e.g., helium. Several studies have shown that, when these factors are properly controlled, it is possible for humans to function normally and conduct useful work during prolonged periods (up to 2 months) at pressures of 2 to 10 atm with no significant EEG abnormalities or major changes in sleep characteristics (Frost et al., 1970; Hock et al., 1966; Johnson and Long, 1966; Naitoh et al., 1970; Serbanescou et al., 1968). At greater depths, even the helium-oxygen mixtures pose problems due to their apparent toxic effects. Brauer et al. (1969) termed the resultant symptoms the "high-pressure nervous syndrome." EEG alterations, primarily an increase of theta-frequency activity, and alterations of sleep patterns (both excessive daytime sleepiness and fragmented nocturnal sleep) occur (Bennett et al., 1986; Matsuoka et al., 1986; Ozawa and Tatsuno, 1989; Rostain and Charpy, 1976; Rostain et al., 1983, 1988a, 1991; Vaernes et al., 1982, 1983, 1985). Alterations of visual and cognitive evoked potentials have also been reported (Vaernes and Hammerborg, 1989). However, these problems can be minimized, even in dives with pressures up to approximately 70 atm (2,251 feet), by using slow compression times of up to 3 days (Bennett et al., 1982; Corriol et al., 1973; Vaernes et al., 1988). Addition of hydrogen (54–56%) to the high-pressure helium-oxygen breathing mixtures was shown to suppress the neurological symptoms of the high-pressure nervous syndrome, although EEG alterations (primarily increased theta activity) persisted (Rostain et al., 1988b). Similarly, incorporation of nitrogen (4.8%) into the helium-oxygen mixture reportedly reduces some symptoms of the high-pressure syndrome, but does not prevent the EEG changes (Pastena et al., 1999; Rostain et al., 1997) or sleep disruption (Rostain et al., 1997). Specific relationships between pressure-induced theta range EEG activity and cognitive performance have been described (Lorenz et al., 1992). Peak EEG power in the theta band correlated positively with increased cognitive demand during a memory search task.

Problems associated with decompression (e.g., "bends" and air embolism) have not been well studied with EEG techniques, but several case reports indicate that the EEG can provide valuable diagnostic information shortly after the suspected event (Bjornstad et al., 2002; Ingvar et al., 1973). Most EEG changes apparently result from localized cerebral ischemia that gives rise to regional or focal slowing, although generalized alterations (e.g., alpha coma pattern) have been reported after presumed involvement of brainstem structures (Synek and Glasgow, 1985). It has been suggested that somatosensory evoked potentials may provide more specific information regarding neurological complications (Yiannikas and Beran, 1988). Long-term residual EEG abnormalities have been reported following decompression illness in some cases (Bjornstad et al., 2002; Sipenen et al., 1999), although in one study EEG abnormalities were no more common in a group of divers with histories of decompression illness than they were in a control group of nondivers (Murrison et al., 1995).

The potential value of the EEG as a screening test for divers has been recognized (Borromei, 1977; Corriol et al., 1976; Malhotra and Kumar, 1975; Todnem et al., 1989, 1990, 1991), but in general the comments made above with respect to its use in aviation apply to this situation as well.

References

Adey, W.R., Kado, T.R., and Walter, D.O. 1967. Computer analysis of EEG data from Gemini flight GT-7. Aerospace Med. 38:345–359.

Bennett, P.B., Coggin, R., and McLeod, M. 1982. Effect of compression rate on use trimix to ameliorate HPNS in man to 686 M (2250 ft.). Undersea Biomed. Res. 9:335–351.

Bennett, P.B., Janke, N., Kolb, M., et al. 1986. Use of EEG digital filtering and display for HPNS diagnosis. Undersea Biomed. Res. 13:99–110.

Bjornstad, J., Nyland, H., Skeidsvoll, H., et al. 2002. [Neurologic decompression sickness in sports divers]. Tidsskr. Nor. Laegeforen 122:1649–1651.

Blanc, D.J. 1976. The EEG in aviation medicine. In *The EEG of the Waking Adult/Handbook of Electroencephalography and Clinical Neurophysiology*, vol. 6, part A, Eds. G.E. Chatrian and G.C. Lairy, pp. 269–274. Amsterdam: Elsevier.

Bond, G.F. 1964. New developments in high pressure living. Arch. Environ. Health 9:310–314.

Borromei, A. 1977. Screening EEG per candidati ad attività subacquee. Minerva Med. 68:1323–1356.

Brauer, R.W., Dimov, S., Fructus, X., et al. 1969. Syndrome neurologique et électrographique des hautes pressions. Rev. Neurol. (Paris) 121:264–265.

Brookings, J.B., Wilson, G.F., and Swain, C.R. 1996. Psychophysiological responses to changes in workload during simulated air traffic control. Biol. Psychol. 42:361–377.

Cabarrou, P. 1966. Étude électro-encephalographique de l'iversse des grandes profondeurs. Maroc. Med. 45:529–536.

Caldwell, J.A., and Caldwell, J.L. 1997. An in-flight investigation of the efficacy of dextroamphetamine for sustaining helicopter pilot performance. Aviat. Space Environ. Med. 68:1073–1080.

Caldwell, J.A., Caldwell, J.L., Crowley, J.S., et al. 1995. Sustaining helicopter pilot performance with Dexedrine during periods of sleep deprivation. Aviat. Space Environ. Med. 66:930–937.

Caldwell, J.A., Caldwell, J.L., Smythe, N.K., et al. 2000a. A double-blind, placebo-controlled investigation of the efficacy of modafinil for sustaining the alertness of aviators: a helicopter simulator study. Psychopharmacology 150:272–282.

Caldwell, J.A., Smythe, N.K., Leduc, P.A., et al. 2000b. Efficacy of Dexedrine for maintaining aviator performance during 64 hours of sustained wakefulness: a simulator study. Aviat. Space Environ. Med. 71:7–18.

Clark, J.B., and Riley, T.L. 2001. Screening EEG in aircrew selection: clinical aerospace neurology perspective. Aviat. Space Environ. Med. 72:1034–1036.

Corriol, J., Chouteau, J., and Catier, J. 1973. Human simulated diving experiments at saturation under oxygen-helium exposures up to 500 meters. Electroencephalographic data. Aerospace Med. 44:1270–1276.

Corriol, J., Papy, J.J., Jacquin, M., et al. 1976. What EEG criteria for diving fitness? Aviat. Space Environ. Med. 47:868–872.

Dijk, D.J., Neri, D.F., Wyatt, J.K., et al. 2001. Sleep, performance, circadian rhythms, and light-dark cycles during two space shuttle flights. Am. J. Physiol. Regul. Integr. Comp. Physiol. 281:R1647–1664.

Elliott, A.R., Shea, S.A., Dijk, D.J., et al. 2001. Microgravity reduces sleep-disordered breathing in humans. Am. J. Respir. Crit. Care Med. 164:478–485.

Everett, W.D., and Akhavi, M.S. 1982. Follow-up of 14 abnormal electroencephalograms in asymptomatic U.S. Air Force Academy cadets. Aviat. Space Environ. Med. 53:277–280.

Everett, W.D., and Jenkins, S.W. 1982. The aerospace screening electroencephalogram: an analysis of the benefits and costs in the U.S. Air Force. Aviat. Space Environ. Med. 53:495–501.

Forster, E.M., and Whinnery, J.F. 1988. Recovery from G_z-induced loss of consciousness: psychophysiologic considerations. Aviat. Space Environ. Med. 59:517–522.

Frost, J.D., Jr. 1977. *Final Report*. Contract NAS 9–13870. Washington, DC: National Aeronautics and Space Administration.

Frost, J.D., Jr., Kellaway, P., and DeLucchi, M.R. 1970. Automatic EEG acquisition and data-analysis system. In *Project Tektite 1*, ONR Report DR 153, Eds. D.C. Pauli and H.A. Cole, pp. A54–A69. Washington, DC: Office of Naval Research.

Frost, J.D., Jr., Shumate, W.H., Salamy, J.G., et al. 1974. Skylab sleep monitoring experiment (M-133). In *The Proceedings of Skylab Life Sciences Symposium*/NASA TM X-58145, vol. 1, pp. 239–285. Washington, DC: National Aeronautics and Space Administration.

Frost, J.D., Jr., Shumate, W.H., Booher, C.R., et al. 1975. The Skylab sleep monitoring experiment. Methodology and initial results. Acta Astronaut. 2:319–336.

Gundel, A., Nalishiti, V., Reucher, E., et al. 1993. Sleep and circadian rhythm during a short space mission. Clin. Invest. 71:718–724.

Gundel, A., Drescher, J., Maas, H., et al. 1995. Sleepiness of civil airline pilots during two consecutive night flights of extended duration. Biol. Psychol. 40:131–141.

Gundel, A., Polyakov, V.V., and Zulley, J. 1997. The alteration of human sleep and circadian rhythms during spaceflight. J. Sleep Res. 6:1–8.

Gundel, A., Parisi, R.A., Strobel, R., et al. 1998. Characterization of sleep under ambient CO_2-levels of 0.7% and 1.2%. Aviat. Space Environ. Med. 69:491–495.

Gundel, A., Drescher, J., Spatenko, Y.A., et al. 1999. Heart period and heart period variability during sleep on the MIR space station. J. Sleep Res. 8:37–43.

Gundel, A., Drescher, J., Spatenko, Y.A., et al. 2002. Changes in basal heart rate in spaceflights up to 438 days. Aviat. Space Environ. Med. 73: 17–21.

Guo, H.Z., Zhang, S.X., Jing, B.S., et al. 1988. A preliminary report on a new anti-G maneuver. Aviat. Space Environ. Med. 59:968–972.

Hankins, T.C., and Wilson, G.F. 1998. A comparison of heart rate, eye activity, EEG and subjective measures of pilot mental workload during flight. Aviat. Space Environ. Med. 69:360–367.

Hendriksen, J.M., and Elderson, A. 2001. The use of EEG in aircrew selection. Aviat. Space Environ. Med. 72:1025–1033.

Hock, R.J., Bond, G.F., and Mazzone, W.F. 1966. Physiological evaluation of Sealab II. Effects of two weeks' exposure to an undersea 7-atmosphere helium-oxygen environment. In *Deep Submergence Systems Project*, pp. 16–18, 41–44. Hawthorne, CA: United States Navy, Northrop Space Labs.

Hordinsky, J.R. 1974. Skylab crew health. Crew surgeons' reports. In *The Proceedings of the Skylab Life Sciences Symposium*/NASA TM X-58154, vol. 1, pp. 61–73. Washington, DC: National Aeronautics and Space Administration.

Ingvar, D.H., Adolphson, J., and Lindemark, C. 1973. Cerebral air embolism during training of submarine personnel in free escape. An electroencephalographic study. Aerospace Med. 44:628–635.

Johnson, L.C., and Long, M.P. 1966. Neurological, EEG, and Psychophysiological Findings Before and After Sealab II. Report 66–19. Washington, DC: Bureau of Medicine and Surgery, Navy Department.

Landstrom, U., and Lofstedt, P. 1987. Noise, vibration and changes in wakefulness during helicopter flight. Aviat. Space Environ. Med. 52: 109–118.

Leach, C.S., and Rambaut, P.C. 1974. Biochemical responses of the Skylab crewmen. In *The Proceedings of the Skylab Life Sciences Symposium*/ NASA TM X-58154, vol. 2, pp. 427–454. Washington, DC: National Aeronautics and Space Administration.

Lorenz, J., Lorenz, B., and Heineke, M. 1992. Effect of mental task load on fronto-central theta activity in a deep saturation dive to 450 msw. Undersea Biomed. Res. 19:243–262.

Malhotra, M.S., and Kumar, C.M. 1975. Electroencephalography in naval divers. Aviat. Space Environ. Med. 46:1000–1001.

Matsuoka, S., Inoue, K., Okuda, S., et al. 1986. EEG polygraphic sleep study in divers under a 31 ATA He O_2 environment with special reference to the automated analysis of sleep stages. Sangyo Ika Daigaku Zasshi 8:293–305.

Maulsby, R.L. 1966. Electroencephalogram during orbital flight. Aerospace Med. 37:1022–1026.

Maulsby, R.L., Frost, J.D., Jr., and Blanc, C.J. 1976. Special environments and selection problems. In *The EEG of the Waking Adult/Handbook of Electroencephalography and Clinical Neurophysiology*, vol. 6, part A, Eds. G.E. Chatrian and G.C. Lairy, pp. 257–274. Amsterdam: Elsevier.

Monk, T.H. 1999. Aging and space flight: findings from the University of Pittsburgh. J. Gravit. Phsiol. 6:137–140.

Monk, T.H, Buysse, D.J., Billy, B.D., et al. 1998. Sleep and circadian rhythms in four orbiting astronauts. J. Biol. Rhythms 13:188–201.

Monk, T.H., Buysse, D.J., and Rose, L.R. 1999. Wrist actigraphic measures of sleep in space. Sleep 22:948–954.

Murrison, A.W., Glasspool, E., Pethybridge, R.J., et al. 1995. Electroencephalographic study of divers with histories of neurological decompression illness. Occup. Environ. Med. 52:451–453.

Naitoh, P., Johnson, L., and Austin, M. 1970. Sleep patterns. In *Project Tektite I*, ONR Report DR 153, Eds. D.C. Pauli and H.A. Cole, pp. A47–A54. Washington, DC: Office of Naval Research.

Ozawa, K., and Tatsuno, J. 1989. Continuous changes in electroencephalographic topograms and auditory reaction time during simulated 21 ATA (atmospheric absolute) heliox saturation dives. Ann. Physiol. Anthropol. 8:247–266.

Pastena, L., Mainardi, G., Faralli, F., et al. 1999. Analysis of cerebral bioelectrical activity during the compression phase of a saturation dive. Aviat. Space Environ. Med. 70:270–276.

Prisk, G.K. 1998. Sleep and respiration in microgravity. Neurosci. News 5:39–45.

Putcha, L., Berens, K.L., Marshburn, T.H., et al. 1999. Pharmaceutical use by U.S. astronauts on space shuttle missions. Aviat. Space Environ. Med. 70:705–708.

Roger, A., Cabarrou, P., and Gastaut, H. 1955. Variations de l'électroencéphalogramme chez l'homme en fonction de la pression. Rev. Neurol. (Paris) 91:475.

Roger, A., Cabarrou, P., and Gastaut, H. 1954. EEG changes in humans due to changes of the surrounding atmosphere pressure. Electroencephalogr. Clin. Neurophysiol. 7:152.

Rostain, J.C., and Charpy, J.P. 1976. Effects upon the EEG of psychometric performance during deep dives in helium-oxygen atmosphere. Electroencephalogr. Clin. Neurophysiol. 40:571–584.

Rostain, J.C., Lemaire, C., Gardette-Chauffour, M.C., et al. 1983. Estimation of human susceptibility to high-pressure nervous syndrome. J. Appl. Physiol. 54:1063–1070.

Rostain, J.C., Gardette-Chauffour, M.C., Gourret, J.P., et al. 1988a. Sleep disturbances in man during different compression profiles up to 62 bars in helium-oxygen mixture. Electroencephalogr. Clin. Neurophysiol. 69: 127–135.

Rostain, J.C., Gardette-Chauffour, M.C., Lemaire, C., et al. 1988b. Effects of a H_2-He-O_2 mixture on the HPNS up to 450 msw. Undersea Biomed. Res. 15:257–270.

Rostain, J.C., Regesta, G., Gardette-Chauffour, M.C., et al. 1991. Sleep organization in man during long stays at 30 and 40 bar in a helium-oxygen mixture. Undersea Biomed. Res. 18:21–36.

Rostain, J.C., Gardette-Chauffour, M.C., and Naquet, R. 1997. EEG and sleep disturbances during dives at 450 msw in helium-nitrogen-oxygen mixture. J. Appl. Physiol. 83:575–582.

Rudnyi, N.M., and Bodrov, V.A. 1987. Current problems in aviation physiology. Kosm. Biol. Aviakosm. Med. 21:4–11.

Samel, A., Gander, P. 1995. Bright light as a chronobiological countermeasure for shiftwork in space. Acta Astronaut. 36:669–683.

Samel, A., Wegmann, H.H., Vejvoda, M., et al. 1996. [Stress and fatigue in long distance 2-man cockpit crew]. Wien. Med. Wochenschr. 146:272–276.

Samel, A., Wegmann, H.-M., Vejvoda, M., et al. 1997a. Two-crew operations: stress and fatigue during long-haul night flights. Aviat. Space Environ. Med. 68:679–687.

Samel, A., Wegmann, H.-M., and Vejvoda, M. 1997b. Aircrew fatigue in long-haul operations. Accid. Anal. Prev. 29:439–452.

Seege, D., and Wirth, D. 1977. Prognostic significance of myoclonias in aerospace altitude studies and others with acute hypoxia-accompanied status. Psychiatr. Neurol. Med. Psychol. Beih. 22–23:43–47.

Sem-Jacobsen, C.W. 1959. Electroencephalographic study of a pilot's stresses in flight. Aerospace Med. 30:797–801.

Sem-Jacobsen, C.W., and Sem-Jacobsen, I.E. 1963. Selection and evaluation of pilots for high performance aircraft and spacecraft by in-flight EEG study of stress tolerance. Aerospace Med. 34:605–609.

Serbanescou, T., Fructus, P., and Naquet, R. 1968. Étude électroencéphalographique du sommeil sous hyperbarie prolongée (opération Ludion II). Rev. Neurol. (Paris) 119:305–306.

Sipinen, S.A., Ahovuo, J., and Halonen, J.-P. 1999. Electroencephalography and magnetic resonance imaging after diving and decompression incidents: a controlled study. Undersea Hyperb. Med. 26:61–65.

Sterman, M.B., and Mann, C.A. 1995. Concepts and applications of EEG analysis in aviation performance evaluation. Biol. Psychol. 40:115–140.

Stoilova, I., Zdravev, T., and Yanev, T. 2000. Evaluation of sleep in space flight. Dokl. Acad. Nauk. 53:59–62.

Synek, V.M., and Glasgow, G.L. 1985. Recovery from alpha coma after decompression sickness complicated by spinal cord lesions at cervical and midthoracic levels. Electroencephalogr. Clin. Neurophysiol. 60:417–419.

Thornton, W.E., Hoffler, G.W., and Rummel, J.A. 1974. Anthropometric changes and fluid shifts. In *The Proceedings of the Skylab Life Sciences Symposium*/NASA TM X-58145, vol. 2, pp. 637–658. Washington, DC: National Aeronautics and Space Administration.

Thornton, W.E., Biggers, W.P., Thomas, W.G., et al. 1985. Electronystagmography and audio potentials in space flight. Laryngoscope 96:924–932.

Thornton, W.E., Moore, T.P., Pool, S.L., et al. 1987. Clinical characterization and etiology of space motion sickness. Aviat. Space Environ. Med. 58:A1–A8.

Todnem, K., Nyland, H., Dick, A.P., et al. 1989. Immediate neurological effects of diving to a depth of 360 metres. Acta Neurol. Scand. 80:333–340.

Todnem, K., Nyland, H., Riise, T., et al. 1990. Analysis of neurologic symptoms in deep diving: implications for selection of divers. Undersea Biomed. Res. 17:95–107.

Todnem, K., Nyland, H., Skeidsvoll, H., et al. 1991. Neurological long term consequences of deep diving. Br. J. Ind. Med. 48:258–266.

Vaernes, R.J., and Hammerborg, D. 1989. Evoked potential and other CNS reactions during a heliox dive to 360 msw. Aviat. Space Environ. Med. 60:550–557.

Vaernes, R., Bennett, P.B., Hammerborg, D., et al. 1982. Central nervous system reactions during heliox and trimix dives to 31ATA. Undersea Biomed. Res. 9:1–14.

Vaernes, R., Hammerborg, D., Ellersten, B., et al. 1983. Central nervous system reactions during heliox and trimix dives to 51 ATA, DEEP EX 81. Undersea Biomed. Res. 10:169–192.

Vaernes, R.J., Hammerborg, D., Ellertsen, B., et al. 1985. CNS reactions at 51 ATA on trimix and heliox and during decompression. Undersea Biomed. Res. 12:25–39.

Vaernes, R.J., Bergan, T., and Warncke, M. 1988. HPNS effects among 18 divers during compression to 360 msw on heliox. Undersea Biomed. Res. 15:241–255.

Voskrensenskiy, A.D., Gazenko, O.G., Izosimov, G.V., et al. 1965. Some physiological data for evaluating the condition and work capacity of cosmonauts in orbital flight. In *Problems of Space Biology*/NASA TT F-368, vol. 4, Ed., N.M. Sisakian, pp. 222–230. Washington, DC: National Aeronautics and Space Administration.

Weber, F. 2002. Routine electroencephalograms of pilots later killed in crashes: a case-control study. Aviat. Space Environ. Med. 73:1114–1116.

Whinnery, J.E. 1986. $+G_z$-induced loss of consciousness in under-graduate pilot training. Aviat. Space Environ. Med. 57:997–999.

Whinnery, J.E., Burton, R.R., Boll, P.A., et al. 1987. Characterization of the resulting incapacitation following unexpected $+G_z$-induced loss of consciousness. Aviat. Space Environ. Med. 58:631–636.

Wright, N., and McGown, A. 2001. Vigilance on the civil flight deck: incidence of sleepiness and sleep during long-haul flights and associated changes in physiological parameters. Ergonomics 44:82–106.

Yiannikas, C., and Beran, R. 1988. Somatosensory evoked potentials, electroencephalography and CT scans in the assessment of the neurological sequelae of decompression sickness. Clin. Exp. Neurol. 25:91–96.

Zhang, S.X., Guo, H.Z., Jing, B.S., et al. 1991. Experimental verification of effectiveness and harmlessness of the Qigong maneuver. Aviat. Space Environ. Med. 62:46–52.

33. EEG and Neuropharmacology

Albert Wauquier

General Considerations

Previous contributions on the electroencephalography (EEG) and neuropharmacology in general (e.g., Longo, 1977; Stumpf and Gogolak, 1987) have reviewed the effects of different drugs on the EEG, often reflecting the historical development in the field of neuropharmacology and focusing on experimental research. This chapter does not deal with detailed historical data, but rather with the variety of methodologies used in the study of drug effects on the EEG and the potential relationship with the purported clinical effects (see also Wauquier and Binnie, 1992).

The study of the effects of drugs on the EEG is termed pharmaco-EEG (PEEG). Berger, in 1931, applied PEEG when he investigated the effects of a subcutaneous administration of cocaine on the alpha activity in the human EEG. Much later, researchers developed quantified techniques to assess drug effects on the EEG. This became known as quantified pharmaco-EEG (QPEEG). QPEEG investigations have concentrated on time-related drug-induced changes in the frequency and amplitude of EEG signals and in developing statistical approaches to the analysis. Attention has also been directed toward functional brain mapping as a technique to depict topographic aspects of drug-induced changes. This chapter gives various examples of these methodologies, from both human studies as well as experimental studies.

The EEG can be used as a measure of central nervous system (CNS) action; both therapeutic and toxic drug levels can be assessed as well as the duration of drug action. Sometimes drugs have a specific effect on the EEG morphology or waves, such as the induction of slow waves (as with serotonin-2 receptor antagonists) or spindles (as seen with γ-hydroxybutyrate). These EEG changes can be used as models to investigate mechanisms of drug action or to study pathologies. In these cases the changes in the EEG are of greater importance than the particular drug causing these changes.

Although the main emphasis here is on the spontaneous and activated EEG, references are also made to the effects of drugs on the changes in vigilance and sleep-wake patterns. The study of drug effects on sleep-wake patterns is not only of direct interest, as demonstrated in the field of hypnotics. Sleep studies may reveal desirable or undesirable drug effects of which the target organ of the drug was not necessarily the brain, as is the case with antihistamines or antihypertensive medication.

The EEG is an excellent method to evaluate central drug action. However, sometimes too much is expected of the EEG. For example, one cannot expect the EEG to be a valuable method to reveal the site of drug action. Another example of the usefulness of the EEG is in the field of neuromonitoring. The EEG is a valuable inexpensive method that can be used to continuously monitor brain function during surgery (open heart, arteries, and brain). It facilitates detecting unwanted effects on the brain, such as ischemia or hypoxia, that otherwise would go unnoticed and may lead to brain damage and neurological consequences.

The limitations of the EEG sometimes lead one to believe it to be unreliable when expectations are not met. It was hoped that the EEG could be used as a simple method to evaluate the depth of anesthesia. However, depth of anesthesia is a complex phenomenon that with difficulty can be assessed using one single parameter. Major advances have been made in that field. An outline of the possibilities and limitations of the use of EEG, therefore, is a topic incorporated throughout this chapter.

There are a number of issues related to the use of the EEG in neuropharmacology that are of more general interest. These issues require (a) a discussion of possible "dissociation" between EEG and behavior, (b) the EEG changes in relationship to plasma levels of a drug, and (c) the EEG changes and underlying biochemical changes. These all can be viewed as subhypotheses related to the field of PEEG, which were derived from the main hypothesis that EEG changes, in a more or less direct way, reflect biochemical, electrophysiological, and behavior processes (Kúnkel, 1982).

In conclusion, the main value of the PEEG is that it allows objective identification of neuropharmacological effects and that these effects can be quantified. It also permits correlation of EEG effects with behavioral variables in order to assess possible psychoactive properties of drugs. Many different techniques are available as research tools. However, QPEEG, as a clinical application, still requires further validation.

Methodological Issues
Detection and Quantification of Pharmacological Actions

The EEG is very sensitive to central actions of pharmacological substances. These include not only psychotropic drugs, hypnotics, anesthetics, and anticonvulsants, but also drugs targeted to organs other than the CNS such as antihypertensives and antihistamines, which have cerebral actions that may be regarded as unwanted side effects. In general, an empirical approach has been adopted for selecting methods of assessment. For instance, the demonstration of a persisting amplitude change in a single-channel EEG, 24 hours after administration of a short-acting drug intended for outpatient anesthesia, provided a timely warning that its effects were more sustained than had been supposed.

In a typical experiment, normal subjects receive several treatments including a placebo and an active substance, given in random order according to a Latin square design. At each session, the EEG is recorded before dosing (administration of substance) and at intervals after dosing. One of the well-publicized statistical methods is to convert changes from baseline to *t* values, which are then plotted against frequency. Typical *t* profiles of power versus frequency are described for different groups of drugs (Saletu et al., 1987). In animal experiments, profiles of different drug classes have been proposed (Krijzer et al., 1983). However, some caution in data analysis interpretation is warranted, for a display of statistical *t* values may overemphasize relatively unimportant changes of data.

There are different schools of thought with respect to the effects of drugs on the "spontaneous" EEG. Spontaneous is defined as an EEG recording in a condition where there are no obvious or known interfering factors. One view is that drug-induced changes are so unspecific, both with respect to a particular drug and drug class, that nothing more can be done than restricting the analysis to a pure descriptive form (e.g., Stumpf and Gogolak, 1987). This does not necessarily imply that drug effects cannot be classified according to a certain principle. Killam (1977), for example, systematized drug effects depending on whether they were producing a stabilization effect of the EEG as compared to a predrug state. In a historical paper, Schallek and Smith (1952) classified drugs according to whether they produced "excitation, depression or convulsive bursts." In sleep-wake analysis of drug effects on stages, which are defined on the basis of typical EEG changes, there are typical drug class related changes (e.g., Wauquier, 1995).

The specificity of drug effects on the EEG has rarely been established, but some changes have led to clinical interpretation. An agent suppressing rapid-eye-movement (REM) sleep or causing EEG arousals is likely to cause reports of disturbed sleep patterns and subjective feelings of poor sleep, either upon drug administration or upon withdrawal. The induction of epileptiform activity or photosensitivity is prima facie evidence of an epileptogenic effect, whereas the suppression of spontaneous or induced epileptiform discharges occurs after acute (but not necessarily chronic) administration of representatives of all the main groups of established antiepileptic drugs.

Another view is that drug effects on the EEG can be differentiated. The EEG is sensitive to subtle differences, provided that objective procedures are applied and that there is a sufficient parameter extraction. Such an approach requires quantified and statistical methods (e.g., Fink, 1980; Herrmann, 1982; Itil, 1982; Saletu, 1976). By using a classification system based on quantified analysis there is a potential for allowing predictions toward therapeutic applications. This carries the danger of leading to erroneous conclusions if not used critically. In addition, one still must regard each drug as a unique entity, such as its characteristic pharmacokinetic profile, which is one of many factors that determines a specific action on the EEG (Herrmann, 1982).

It has thus been claimed that various pharmacological classes of psychotropic drugs can be distinguished by characteristic quantitative changes in the EEG after the acute or chronic administration to normal subjects or, after chronic administration to patients with psychiatric disorders (Herr-

mann, 1982; Itil, 1981; Saletu, 1976). In both acute and chronic administration, baseline EEG characteristics need to be defined, taking into account spontaneous and possible circadian rhythm variations. There are obvious pharmacodynamic differences between the effects of single and multiple doses and it would be surprising if these were not reflected in the EEG. It is, therefore, unlikely that changes in QPEEG after single doses in normal subjects will be identical to the EEG changes in patients after chronic dosing, even where the clinical disorder itself produces no EEG changes. Certainly, the presence of a central drug effect, an effective dose or plasma level, and the minimum duration of action can be established by QPEEG studies. However, the intriguing proposition that single dose effects in healthy persons are predictive of therapeutic action in patients has yet to be reliably verified, despite the intensive research in this area over several decades. Furthermore, the clinical correlate of an EEG change is often more conjecture than based on validation studies. For example, it is still uncertain whether the marked increase of beta activity following intake of benzodiazepines, either by anxious patients or relaxed volunteers, is related to the anxiety-reducing properties of benzodiazepines and whether this is a universal feature of all anxiolytics. The prospective use of QPEEG analysis requires validation with independent measures of psychiatric state and cognitive function. Similar considerations apply to sleep studies: tricyclic antidepressants suppress REM sleep, but REM suppression is a not a valid single criterion for screening potential antidepressants.

Although computer-assisted quantification of drug effects has greatly facilitated PEEG studies, visual analysis remains of importance, particularly when detecting those subtle or transient phenomena most amenable to intuitive clinical interpretation. Different quantification methods, both automatic and visual, have been introduced for parameterization (selecting parameters) and feature extraction (data reduction). Quantitative parameters with predictive value have been developed and are subject of intensive research.

Quantification of PEEG changes uses time series analysis by such methods as power spectra, zero crossing, or normalized sleep descriptors. In most cases the absolute power in different frequency bands is measured, but in some situations quotients between frequency bands or indices of relative power are of greater value. This provides a different type of information concerning changes in the EEG frequency composition independent of overall fluctuations in amplitude. The relative merits of these methods are controversial if used independently of the question asked. For example, changes in absolute power during open heart surgery may be good indicators of changes in body temperature and fluctuations in plasma levels of drug effects, whereas the relative steady state of the relative power might be indicative for stability of the anesthetic condition (Wauquier et al., 1984a).

In 1982, Itil, using a database of QPEEG studies that utilized period analysis and power spectrum data, proposed that a matrix could be created that differentiates the four major categories of psychotropic drugs (antidepressants, anxiolytics, neuroleptics, and psychostimulants). A two-dimensional presentation was used with the coordinates of the grid based on the EEG profiles. The profile of these new drugs was assessed by using the database. Drugs were then positioned within the grid to determine their therapeutic class. It is assumed that such an approach provides an objective method to classify drugs.

QPEEG studies often present major problems for statistical analysis. If EEGs are recorded and analyzed from several channels, in eyes-open and -closed conditions, at several time intervals after dosing and with three or more different treatments, then a dozen features can be extracted and many thousands of numerical values are produced. The problem of distinguishing biologically meaningful results arises from those that attain apparent statistical significance merely because so many statistical tests have been performed ("capitalization on chance"). A strictly mathematical approach, such as the classical Bonferroni correction (see Simes, 1986, for an improved version), may not be helpful because it dictates the setting of significance levels so stringent that significance is unattainable without vast numbers of subjects. In exploratory studies, a pragmatic solution to accept may be those effects that are consistently present at different intervals after dosing, between channels, or that show a relationship to the dose or blood levels of the drugs. The results then need to be confirmed in further studies. Thus, an adaptive statistical approach may be used to focus on a small number of features likely to be biologically relevant and to avoid the pitfall of capitalizing on chance. An international expert committee published recommended standards for conduct and analysis of QPEEG investigations in humans (Stille and Herrmann, 1982).

Spatial Distribution

Technical development lead to color-coded topographical mapping. As a reference for drug effects, the frequency content of the EEG taken in an alert eyes-closed situation is often used (Nuwer, 1990). The commercial availability of brain electrical activity mapping systems has encouraged the use of topographic displays to show drug-induced EEG changes. Often it seems this is done because the equipment provides a convenient way of performing EEG spectra, instead of using the equipment to test any specific hypothesis about the topography of drug effects. Since the frequency composition of both the basal EEG and the drug-induced changes are not uniform over the scalp, regional differences in drug effects are to be expected. To assess these topographic features, or to detect any changes that may be restricted to particular region of the scalp, it is necessary to record from several channels. For exploratory studies, an anterior and posterior bipolar derivation over each hemisphere appears to be a minimum requirement. This does not imply an anatomical localization of drug action. There is little evidence that the objectives of QPEEG are served by analyzing the activity from much greater numbers of channels, or by using mapping to present the overwhelming amount of data that will result. A display of changes at a large number of electrode sites with "significant" values highlighted in color may encourage capitalization on chance variations, an error less likely to occur with more objective statistical analysis of numerical data. Nevertheless, there are pragmatic reasons for analyzing multiple channels. Many drugs produce an increase of beta activity, which might be most conspicuous over the frontal regions, or drugs alter the frequency of the dominant rhythm, which is more clearly seen posterior. It is, therefore, suggested that in spite of numerous factors that may affect brain, drugs produce characteristic and consistent changes.

In accordance with a method produced by Duffy et al. (1981), Saletu et al. (1987) computed statistical probability maps based on *t* values where the significance of a drug effect versus placebo could be evaluated. This statistical approach to topographical distribution remains to be investigated. It appears, however, that in most QPEEG studies topographic mapping is the most widely used way of presenting data. Itil and associates (e.g., Itil, 1982), in particular, have been promoting the idea that drug classification can be done using a brain mapping database. Along similar lines, statistical analysis of standardized quantitative electrophysiological features relative to normative data is proposed to aid in the differential diagnosis of brain dysfunctions (John et al., 1988).

Vigilance

Many definitions of vigilance have been formulated, most of which concern the reactivity of external, chiefly visual, stimuli. In the view of Koella (1982), any definition of vigilance should involve input from many sensory systems and imply a measurable behavioral assessment. He defines vigilance as "the readiness of an organism to respond to a given situation with appropriate behavior, defined in its quantitative and qualitative aspects." During the transition from wakefulness to sleep there are evident fluctuations in the level of vigilance. Vigilance as a functional condition of the brain can be measured by the EEG. Changes are revealed on both a short (minutes) and a very short (seconds) time scale.

In sleep studies the main emphasis is on changes in vigilance and transitions from one stage to another, whereas in PEEG such changes may be regarded as intervening variables. If not experimentally controlled, an adequate description of the level of vigilance is important for interpretation of possible drug effects. However, it can also be considered that the level of vigilance may co-determine a possible drug action. Thus, at low levels of vigilance, possible stimulating actions can be demonstrated more easily, and at high levels, sedative effects are more easily shown.

Classical sleep staging involves a distinction between wakefulness and various levels of sleep, but a more refined differentiation within the waking state is required. More than half a century ago, Loomis was the first to use the EEG to describe vigilance. He distinguished four consecutive stages of lowered awareness progressing to sleep. A more differentiated "vigil sonogram" was developed by Kugler (1981) and applied in the assessment of anesthetics. Changes in vigilance based on the EEG were further developed by several others. Matejcek et al. (1982) used an alpha–slow-wave index by comparing power values in alpha frequency bands to others. In general, assessment has been made using alpha activity and the development of slow waves as indicators.

In a study by Wright et al. (1995), EEG power analysis using absolute and relative power in addition to coherence analysis between homologous brain sites revealed topographical and temporal patterns during the transition from wakefulness to sleep. Brain sites closest to the midline clearly showed an increase in theta and a decrease in alpha power, but few changes were evident lateral of the midline. Decrease in coherence for alpha activity was seen for homologous sites. Decrease of alpha power occurred later in the posterior regions. This study illustrated the value of multiple channel analysis and of quantitative EEG analysis.

Herrmann (1982) has described a vigilance index based on automatic data classification, taking into account the amount and amplitude of alpha, theta, and frontal beta activity. Matousek and Petersén (1979) developed a computerized method for assessing levels of vigilance. They defined 22 variables based on EEG spectral analysis, and subsequently studied the correlation between spectral values and lowered vigilance (over sleep stages 0 and 1). This method appeared well suited for describing organic brain syndromes and for demonstrating changes in vigilance following drug treatment. Other authors used not only the EEG but also other polygraphic parameters to describe different states of vigilance. For example, Simon et al. (1977) classified waking stages on the basis of polygraphic recordings of the EEG, muscle tone, and eye movements.

Recording facial muscle electromyogram (EMG) responses to nociceptive stimuli may be useful for assessing patient's reactivity, both in sleep and anesthesia. Even in the presence of an apparently efficient neuromuscular blockade, there may be increases in sensory evoked facial muscle EMG (SEMP) indicative of inadequate anesthesia. For this purpose it is not common to employ averaging of evoked responses, but instead to monitor integrated EMG activity during the occurrence of natural (or surgical) stimuli (Edmonds and Wauquier, 1988).

There are difficulties in distinguishing between spontaneous and drug-induced changes of vigilance. It is assumed, however, that under baseline conditions during the first 5 minutes of the recording there is a relatively stable level of vigilance. Any changes occurring within the first 5 minutes of the recording after drug administration are probably pharmacologically induced. Because of the great interindividual variability, some authors object to selecting a particular EEG activity, such as the alpha rhythm, for describing vigilance. Assumptions concerning the normal frequency content of the EEG can be avoided by the use of chronospectrogram analysis (e.g., Matejcek, 1982). This uses spectral analysis to plot changes with time from an initially well-controlled stable state of vigilance. Drug effects are then measured in terms of their vigilance enhancing or diminishing effect by respectively prolonging or shortening the initial state of vigilance. As described before, the study of Wright et al. (1995) clearly showed that multichannel and temporal analysis is required to adequately identify the subtle changes in fluctuation of the wakefulness state.

Many CNS active drugs affect the level of vigilance. It is, therefore, of great importance to standardize test situations such as simplicity of the test and avoidance of tolerance according to various rules. Currently, however, there are no well-validated absolute measures of vigilance.

Analysis of Sleep-Wake Patterns

Two states of sleep can be recognized on the basis of polysomnography by using EEG variables (minimally a central and occipital derivation) and non-EEG variables (eye movements, chin muscle tension). These states are REM sleep and non-REM sleep. In humans non-REM sleep is further divided into four stages. Stage 1 is considered to be the transition to sleep or drowsiness. Stage 2 is light sleep and is also characterized by the presence of transient events, such as K complexes and spindles. Stages 3 and 4 are stages of deep sleep. The latter stages are also known as slow-wave sleep because of the presence of high amplitude waves in the delta frequency domain.

Visual or automatic analysis of sleeping and waking is of great value in detecting both wanted and unwanted central actions and side effects of drugs. Specifically, hypnotics are developed with the purpose of affecting sleep patterns; however, all psychotropic drugs have such actions. There is an ordinate amount of literature published on the effects of psychotropic drugs on sleep patterns (for reviews see Gaillard, 1989; Inoue and Krueger, 1990; Kales, 1995; Nicholson et al., 1989; and Wauquier et al., 1985a,b, 1989a, 1995).

Even where the CNS is not the intended target organ, central sedative side effects may be produced. For instance, traditional antihistamines lead to an increase in slow-wave sleep, a decrease in REM sleep, and eventually a decrease in vigilance during waking (Wauquier et al., 1981b, 1984b). In assessing drugs with known CNS actions, it is important to distinguish therapeutic (e.g., antipsychotic) from nonspecific effects. The study of sleep patterns may not qualify to make such distinctions, but brain mapping or QPEEG studies may make this possible (covered later in this chapter). On the other hand, it is important to understand whether the disturbance of the sleep-wakefulness patterns are caused by a therapeutic effect of the drug or a nontherapeutic pharmacological action, such as is the case with antihypertensives (Monti, 1987).

A change in a sleep pattern does not necessarily reflect a drug action at sites involved in sleep regulation. Some drugs may affect the generators of EEG waves and thereby indirectly increase the amount of slow waves, without affecting the structures involved in slow-wave sleep regulation. Slow-wave sleep enhancing effect is seen with serotonin-2 receptor antagonists (Idzikowski et al., 1986). It was discussed whether this increase in slow-wave sleep is directly related to a mechanism involved in sleep regulation or an unspecific effect on the EEG slow-wave generators (e.g., Borbely et al., 1988). Many experiments using specific serotonin receptor agonists and antagonists demonstrated that the slow-wave sleep maintenance was directly related to an antagonism of the 5-HT2 receptor (Wauquier and Dugovic, 1990). In addition, the effect appeared to be a light/dark modulatory effect of the 5-HT2 receptor antagonist ritanserin, suggesting a role of these receptors in sleep-wakefulness synchronization with the photoperiod (Dugovic et al., 1989).

Whether drugs are affecting the EEG aspects of the sleep-wakefulness stages or whether they are acting on the substrate and mechanism of these stages and therefore also modulate the EEG aspects on which stage definition is partly based, is a continuing issue. There is evidence suggesting that certain transmitter action affects the EEG and behavior by acting on different brain structures. This is the case with the role of noradrenergic neurons in wakefulness. Dopamine agonists and antagonists have a more direct effect on systems involved in the regulation of sleep and wakefulness (Wauquier, 1995).

Several drugs affect phasic events during sleep. For example, benzodiazepines enhance both the amount of K complexes and spindles (Johnson et al., 1976). Because such phasic events are essential determinants of a sleep stage, a change in their occurrence, therefore, may affect the scoring of that particular stage. However, additional features codetermine the scoring of a particular stage. Other drugs may affect non-EEG variables, such as REM or muscle atonia, and therefore interfere with the occurrence of a particular stage. One may take advantage of these observations by analyzing the drug effect on those phasic events or other non-EEG variables independent of sleep staging.

It is equally important to differentiate between EEG aspects and behavior. If a drug stimulates motor activity or causes behavioral excitement (e.g., psychostimulants), it may prevent sleep. However, some drugs may cause persistent wakefulness apparently independent of behavioral excitation. This occurs, for example, with high doses of L-dopa (e.g., Wauquier et al., 1985b). If a drug (e.g., the antihistamine diphenhydramine) causes behavioral quiescence or drowsiness, it may promote sleep without possessing hypnotic properties. But often it is unclear what the primary or secondary effects are, in particular, when there are no overt behavioral changes or when these changes are subtle. In this case it is important to find out whether a drug affects typical features of seep. Some drugs cause "dissociation" among the characteristics that define a sleep stage. Dissociation refers to the simultaneous occurrence of apparent incompatible features. A typical example is seen with anticholinergic drugs such as scopolamine. These drugs may produce slow waves on the EEG of perfectly awake animals. Other typical examples can be found in the field of anesthesia where behavioral sleep may be associated with an activated EEG pattern.

There is a particular problem related to the assessment of sleep-wake patterns. The description of the effects of drugs on sleep often deals with quantitative aspects, in particular, the amount of time spent in different stages. Expressed in percentage of control condition, changes may vary between 0% and 100%. However, the possibilities of observable changes are limited due to the constraints of the measures themselves. For example, when a drug enhances the amount of slow-wave sleep, it invariable does so at the expense of wakefulness or other stages of sleep. The question often is: What are the primary and secondary effects? If a drug enhances slow-wave sleep or decreases wakefulness, is it because the drug enhances slow-wave sleep, facilitates the induction of slow waves, or decreases arousability? These possibilities all suggest that EEG and non-EEG variables, as well as the behavior, need to be measured in order to adequately assess a drug effect on sleep-wake patterns.

Other factors such as age have to be taken into account. In this case scoring criteria may influence the assessment of the amount of slow-wave sleep. It is well known that the delta frequency in non-REM sleep shows an age-related shift toward 2 to 4 Hz versus 1 to 2 Hz in younger people. The amplitude of the delta waves also decreases in an age-related way. Yet, when a scoring criterion of 75 µV is used it will substantially underestimate the time spent in slow-wave sleep. Similarly, the characteristics of spindles, a hallmark of stage 2 non-REM (or light sleep), show an age-related change, thus affecting scoring of that stage (Wauquier, 1993).

An alternative but seldom used approach is to study drug effects on patterns of EEG activity independent of sleep stages. An example of such an approach is based on the observation that there is an organization of phasic events and arousals within the different stages of sleep. Terzano et al. (1985) described the occurrence, within each stage of sleep as a "cyclic alternating pattern" (CAP). There is an alternation between the background EEG activity, typically for a single sleep stage; another phase consisting of clusters of synchronized activity (series of K complexes, slow waves); desynchronized patterns of arousals; and phasic events. An analysis in terms of CAPs represents a structured way of looking at fluctuations of EEG patterns during sleep.

Depoortere et al. (1991) were the first to study drugs using the concept of CAPs independent of sleep stages in rats. He essentially applied Hjorth's analysis, which uses normalized slope descriptors. In particular, he used unstable and alternating amplitude segments as an indicator of a CAP sequence. Both CAPs and these unstable amplitude segments are sensitive indicators of sleep quality. Analysis of CAPs is one of the new avenues in the analysis of drug effects on the features of sleep and wakefulness, which are independent of the traditional sleep scoring criteria (Parrino and Terzano, 1996).

Monitoring

One of the most widely used techniques in documenting the effects of anesthetics has been to monitor and quantify the EEG (reviews by Edmonds and Wauquier, 1986; Edmonds et al., 1996). The simplest analyzers provide a single measure of the amplitude or frequency content of one channel of the EEG. The mean frequency may be determined by measuring the period between zero-crossings and amplitude by the integrated voltage or by the squared value (power). Period amplitude analysis is used by some researchers, whereas others derive frequency and amplitude information from the power spectrum. In many monitoring applications, important information is provided by short-term fluctuations in the EEG, which are on a time scale less than a second. As a consequence, period-amplitude analysis, which resolves individual waves, may have advantages over spectral methods using a fixed epoch length generally greater than 1 second.

Various special-purpose instruments, using spectral edge (the upper frequency boundary containing 90% of the power), have been developed to display supposed univariate measures in a form suitable for reading by a clinician unsophisticated in EEG. Such techniques may serve the patients' safety, giving a warning of imminent brain damage during surgery by detecting abnormal patterns of cerebral electrical activity. However, their use as measures of depth of anesthesia has been controversial (Wauquier, 1986). Over the past decade many studies using spectral edge and other related parameters, such as bispectral index (BIS), in relationship to depth of anesthesia, sedation, hypnotic effect, etc. evaluated the validity of the relationship. The BIS is a measure of the degree to which frequency components in the EEG are phase-locked. It is a single number that represents an integrated measure designed to correlate with end points of anesthesia (e.g., Bruhn et al., 2003).

The utility and validity of a particular technique is linked to the questions posed. There are measures for assessing inadequacy of anesthesia or for detecting the occurrence of cerebral ischemic events (Edmonds and Wauquier, 1986; Edmonds et al., 1996; Wauquier, 1986). QPEEG studies are essential in order to develop the criteria for monitoring graded levels of anesthesia, to assess the adequacy of anesthesia, and to detect cerebral ischemia. Neuromonitoring during surgery adequately assists the surgeon and anesthesiologist in safeguarding the patient from neurological and cognitive deficit (Edmonds et al., 1996).

Effects of Drugs Targeted for the Central Nervous System on the EEG

Many, if not all, CNS active drugs affect the EEG. In fact, such an effect could even be used to define a CNS action of a drug. A summarizing view on the EEG effects of a number of important drug classes is given and includes psychotropic drugs, nootropics, antiepileptics, anesthetics and analgesics, and hypnotics (benzodiazepines and barbiturates). More extensive reviews on different drug classes can be found in the literature (Herrmann, 1982; Krueger et al., 1989; Mendelson, 1989; Stumpf and Gogolak, 1987; Wauquier et al., 1985a).

Psychotropics

It is well documented that psychoactive compounds exhibit an effect on the EEG. The most typical effects of several classes of psychotropic agents obtained in humans are summarized in Table 33.1. They represent an overall consensus based on several papers cited here, but they do not necessarily represent the activity of an individual drug. Since most of the results were obtained after a single dose administration to normal volunteers, little can be said about the relationship between the EEG effects and pharmacodynamics of a drug (Saletu et al., 1987). It can also be concluded that these results do not necessarily reflect therapeutic CNS effects in patients.

On the basis of data similar to these shown in Table 33.1, various researchers have developed classification systems using discriminant analysis. The analysis used by Herrmann and Schaerer (1986) is based on relative power values obtained from occipital EEG recordings in healthy volunteers resting with eyes closed. QPEEG performed in this way is not necessarily a direct indicator of psychotropic properties of a drug. However, a particular drug effect might be used as a model for potential therapeutic efficacy. Herrmann and Schaerer (1986) describe different examples including the

suggestion that beta activity could be a relevant model for predicting therapeutic efficacy of neuroleptic drugs. More complex patterns are revealed by using topographical mapping (Kúnkel, 1982). Some researchers (e.g., Fink and Erwin, 1982) even suggest that QPEEG is a better predictor of antidepressant activity than any other pharmacological tests.

Using the results obtained following the administration of single doses of different drug classes, topographical pharmaco-EEG maps were constructed by Saletu et al. (1987). The mapping revealed a differential effect between low-potency and high-potency neuroleptics. Low-potency neuroleptics (chlorprothixene) increased absolute and relative delta and theta power. It also decreased alpha power, and less consistently, increased beta activity. The delta augmentation was maximum over the posterior regions, whereas the theta power increase was maximum over the temporal region. High-potency neuroleptics such as haloperidol, in contrast, increased alpha power.

Saletu et al. (1987) compared the maps on neuroleptic activity to those obtained after antidepressants, tranquilizers, psychostimulants, and nootropics. The information gathered from maps may provide valuable information with respect to the therapeutic efficacy of a drug in individual cases. The significance of specific topographical changes requires further exploration, particularly with respect to a possible correlation with clinical data.

Gogolak (1980) reviewed the experimental literature on neuroleptics and antidepressant drugs. Very few studies applied QPEEG techniques to these drug classes since this historical review. Krijzer and Van Der Molen (1986) and Krijzer et al. (1983) displayed t values resulting from an analysis of variance (ANOVA) using relative power values over a frequency range of 0.2 to 100 Hz, which were derived from different intracranial electrodes in order to describe an antidepressant drug profile. Typically, they did not use fixed frequency bands, but applied a moving window over power spectra. A t value analysis occasionally poses the problem of capitalizing on small effects. However, their technique appears to be able to differentiate various groups of psychotropic drugs. The advantage of their methodology is that a more precise description of the frequency changes is provided.

Many researchers have described the effects of psychoactive drugs on sleep-wake patterns in animals (Kales, 1995;

Table 33.1. Effects of Psychotropic Agents on the EEG[a]

Drug Class	Synchr.	Delta/ Theta	Alpha 8–13 Hz	Beta 1 13–20 Hz	Beta 2 >20 Hz
Neuroleptics					
Sedative	+	+ +	− −	−	+
Nonsedative	0	0	−	+ +	+
Antidepressants	−	+	−	0	+
Psychostimulants					
LSD type	−	−	+	+	+
Amphetamine	−	−	−	+	+
Anxiolytics	−	0	−	+ +	+ +
Hypnotics	+	+ +	− −	+ +	+ +
Nootropics	0	−	+	+	+

[a]Key: 0, no effect or not typical; +, increase; −, decrease; + +, strong increase; − −, strong decrease.

Polc et al., 1979; Wauquier et al., 1985a). Few developed a methodology for large-scale drug assessment using computerized methods of sleep-wake analysis (Ruigt et al., 1989). Furthermore, a pharmacological model using sleep patterns or sleep stages was seldom used. Kleinlogel (1982) differentiated psychotropic drugs on the basis of their catecholaminergic effect by using a quantified analysis of EEG during REM sleep in rats. They used this stage of sleep because of its sensitivity to drug effects. A normalized slope descriptor computed the Hjorth parameters of activity, mobility, and complexity of epochs selected during REM sleep. Postdrug values taken at several time intervals were compared to predrug values. This methodology allowed for a dissociation between neuroleptics and antidepressants. Within these classes, differences appeared to be related to activation or inhibition of catecholaminergic systems.

Nootropics

In general, a slowing of the EEG frequency and localized delta activity might be related to the oxygen supply to the brain and mental function. Drugs affecting these changes, and thereby enhancing vigilance, might be able to improve mental function. Nootropics are proposed to be such drugs. Some of these drugs, such as Hydergine, were shown to reduce slow-wave activity and increase the dominant alpha frequency (Saletu and Grünberger, 1980). In experimental research, nootropics were also found to increase cortical alpha activity.

Using topographical brain mapping, Saletu et al. (1987) investigated the effects of a single dose of pyritinol (600 mg p.o.). Slow alpha power increased over the whole brain, predominantly in the parietal, vertex, and central regions. Relative delta power appeared to decrease in the same regions. Similarly, Herrmann et al. (1988) demonstrated that the chronic treatment of pyritinol decreased the absolute delta power and increased the alpha slow-wave index. They further showed that this effect was related to both performance and clinical symptoms.

Although the EEG changes by nootropics have not yet been shown to bear any functional significance to the aged person, the vigilance-improving effects in the elderly might be related to the improvement of mental function. However, the EEG changes in humans did not always correlate with clinical improvement. Although it is not an overall finding, there appears to be dissociation between EEG and behavior.

Antiepileptics

Antiepileptic drugs (AEDs) belong to several different chemical and pharmacological classes and show some specificity of action on different types of seizures, epileptic syndromes, and epileptiform EEG discharges. Therefore, it may be unrealistic to expect a QPEEG profile characteristic of antiepileptic action. Thus far, none has been found for AEDs in general or for their various pharmacological subgroups. QPEEG changes, however, have been reported for several AEDs in clinically relevant concentrations, but these should probably be regarded as evidence of sedative rather than anticonvulsive action. Interestingly, QPEEG may serve as an objective means for studying the time course of AED effects (Van Wieringen et al., 1987).

Chronic administration of AEDs has little consistent effect on spontaneous interictal discharges, provided that the actions of 3/sec spike-wave activity of drugs that are effective in absence are excluded on the grounds that the discharges in question are not strictly interictal. In contrast, acute quantitative studies of spike counts and photosensitivity have proven to be useful in providing preliminary evidence of efficacy in many people (Binnie et al., 1986a,b) and in determining the speed of action after alternative routes of administration were used (Milligan et al., 1982, 1983). Such techniques also provide a useful guide to the duration of action, which may be of particular importance in the decision on whether to proceed with the development of an AED with a short half-life.

Because sleep-wake patterns are often disturbed in epileptic patients, it is of interest to assess whether antiepileptic drugs are normalizing disturbed sleep-wake patterns as well as affecting ictal activity. In a study of epileptic beagles, it appeared that the changes in sleep-wake patterns reflected a psychotropic drug action independent of the antiepileptic action (Wauquier et al., 1986).

Many researchers have described changes in sleep patterns in humans following chronic antiepileptic treatment (Baldy-Moulinier, 1982; Declerck and Wauquier, 1991; Johnson 1982; Wolf et al., 1984). Most antiepileptics give rise to a normalization and stabilization of sleep patterns (Johnson, 1982). This normalization may consist of an improved sleep architecture, a restoration of sleep cycle sequence, and a reduced frequency of awakenings. The hypotheses is then that stabilization is a consequence of an increase in arousal threshold. Since spindles and K complexes may be considered signs of inhibition and activation, respectively, an analysis of these phasic events in epileptic patients may shed further light on the arousal hypothesis. Some antiepileptics, however, may disrupt sleep patterns rather than improve them. Ethosuximide, due to its activating properties on the reticular formation, may enhance light sleep and increase the number of awakenings (Wolf et al., 1984). Carbamazepine, in contrast to a study in cats (Gigli et al., 1988), hardly affects sleep patterns in humans (Declerck and Wauquier, 1991).

Anesthetics and Analgesics

There are two approaches to QPEEG studies in anesthesia. The first is an attempt to find EEG changes characteristic of anesthesia (Edmonds and Wauquier, 1986). Unfortunately, a unitary explanation for the varied pharmacological actions of anesthetics has not yet been found. In contrast to the graded depression of behavior, in which parallel EEG slowing was seen with some anesthetics, others produce behavioral unresponsiveness with activated or even epileptiform EEG patterns. Furthermore, in clinical practice many anesthetic agents are used in combination with each other.

The second approach is to use QPEEG as a guide to the safe and effective administration of anesthetics. The basic concept is that for each of the pharmacological classes there exist EEG features that change in univariate manner with graded levels of anesthesia (Scott et al., 1985).

Inhalational anesthetics are often used as adjuvants to supplement other agents. There are some limited similarities among the effects obtained with various inhalation agents (Pichlmayer et al., 1983; Rampil and Smith, 1985). There are characteristic changes from the relaxed wake pattern; for example, the first EEG change induced by nitrous oxide is the disappearance of the alpha rhythm. This is followed by a decrease in the EEG amplitude and an increase in the dominant frequency most noted anterior. Thereafter, slow waves in the theta and delta ranges gradually develop while the amplitude increases. Often, faster activities are superimposed on slower components. The sequence of events may differ between various anesthetics. In the instance of halothane, for example, before continuous delta activity appears, a mixture of delta and monorhythmic alpha frequency is seen to produce a striking "mitten pattern." Some agents produce very different characteristic patterns. Isoflurane, for instance, at 1.5 to 2.0 minimal alveolar concentration (MAC), often causes a sudden depression of the EEG. On the other hand, enflurane at the same concentration may result in activation with an increasing frequency and paroxysmal bursts. In contrast, halothane and short-acting barbiturates cause gradual development of burst suppression at high doses.

There have been several QPEEG studies on narcotics. The most striking finding is an increase in amplitude of low-frequency components (<3.5 Hz). In experimental studies the indication of slow-wave activity was seen with different types of narcotics including morphine and fentanyl-type agents (Wauquier et al., 1981a). The induction of theta rather than delta activity and the occurrence of spindles are associated with a diminished anesthetic effect. Therefore, total power and power in the low-frequency bands (or ratios between delta and theta power) may be useful in comparing graded levels of anesthesia. The value of such measures for generally assessing depth of anesthesia has not been established (Wauquier, 1986). In contrast, relative power in discrete frequency bands seems better suited to assess the stability of anesthetic effects (and incidentally for detecting hazardous situations as cerebral ischemia) (Bovill et al., 1982; Wauquier et al., 1984a). It has been suggested that univariate measures, such as spectral edge frequency, might be suitable for monitoring depth of anesthesia over the full range of narcotic effects.

An important preliminary step in developing the methods for EEG monitoring of anesthesia is to define the anesthetic effect in objective clinical terms (e.g., lack of movement or absence of an increase in heart rate in response to a stimulation, etc.). Suitable EEG measures must then be identified in order to detect significant changes in the anesthetic state. For instance, onset and duration of an anesthetic or hypnotic action can be calculated by documenting the beginning of slow activity and studying its evolution, respectively. Thus, a continuous display of power (absolute or relative) in the delta or theta band may be illustrative of both the onset and duration of the action. However, in assessing recovery from anesthesia, return of alpha or beta activity may be of greater value. It has been suggested that transient phenomena, such as K complexes, may be useful in detecting recovery (Bovill et al., 1982).

Ideally, a QPEEG measure that shows a univariate relationship to anesthetic effect and plasma level is required. Unfortunately, simple descriptors extracted from EEG spec-

tra often show a multimodal relationship to the depth of anesthesia. Therefore, a change seen at low concentrations does not progressively increase, but rather is reversed at higher blood levels (Levy, 1984). Several studies show hysteresis effects, which are QPEEG changes lagging behind those of plasma levels. Acute tolerance also occurs, which may diminish EEG changes, although constant plasma levels are maintained. Thus, different concentrations may coincide with the same absolute QPEEG values. Also different QPEEG measures taken from identical concentrations of anesthesia can be obtained from the same individual at different points in time. There are ceiling effects, which occur when an EEG measure (for instance, delta power) attains a maximum and then shows no further change with increasing dosages of the drug. Maximal change may occur before maximal anesthesia has been reached (Wauquier et al., 1988). Consequently, since the point at which these changes occur depends on both the total amount of the agent and the rate at which it is administered, plasma levels associated with a maximal EEG change may not result in a level of anesthesia that is adequate for major surgical interventions.

The application of QPEEG techniques to anesthesia has advanced by using a variety of EEG measures. Some parameters, including relative power and bispectral edge, are suggested to be valuable in assessing adequacy of anesthesia. The predictive value of such measures needs further validation.

Benzodiazepines and Barbiturates

Benzodiazepines were shown to increase the cortical EEG frequency in the beta range of different animal species. However, the actual frequency varied considerably within the studies, and the maximum effect is seen in different regions. One of the most prominent effects of benzodiazepines is the appearance of spindle activity consistently seen in the frontal leads as was reported decades ago (Joy et al., 1971).

Barbiturates, such as pentobarbital, given at high doses produce an overall increase in power that is dominant in delta and alpha bands (Schallek and Johnson, 1976). Short-acting barbiturates like thiopental induce burst-suppressions, which appear to be associated with prominent metabolic depression. The progressive slowing of the EEG, which ends eventually in isoelectricity, is in line with the unidirectional CNS depression.

QPEEG effects from barbiturates and benzodiazepines include a generalized increase in beta activity. Those produced by long-acting barbiturates have a frequency of 18 to 30/sec, an amplitude of 20 to 50 μV and are maximal in the frontal regions. Benzodiazepine-induced beta activity, in contrast, is slower (14–25 cycles/sec) and more diffuse, albeit usually with a frontal emphasis. The frequency and amplitude of benzodiazepine-induced beta activity is influenced by various factors such as age, type of medication, and environmental conditions.

Janssen et al. (1989) developed a methodology controlling for environmental factors that possibly affect the induction by benzodiazepines. Conditions of eyes open, eyes closed, and a task performance were alternated prior to and following drug intake. The recordings were kept at 90 seconds in order to maintain a constant condition. Power spectral analysis revealed the range of beta induction during these conditions.

An important issue is whether the induction of beta activity in benzodiazepines is related more to their anxiolytic properties than to their sedative properties. However, vigilance is determined not only by drug concentrations but also by chronobiological factors. This may introduce ambiguity in the relationship between EEG changes and apparent clinical effects. In some studies of benzodiazepines, peak power of the beta activity appeared to be correlated with an anticonvulsant action that increased as epileptiform activity was reduced.

Hypnotics are also used, intravenously, as induction agents in anesthesia. Doenicke et al. (1973), for example, studied the EEG effects of the short-acting nonbarbiturate hypnotic etomidate in human volunteers. They used a visual analysis of the EEG, classifying the changes according to a vigilance scale. They demonstrated a rapid evolution toward deep sleep (delta waves) with a progressive return to baseline within 20 minutes. Thus, they applied a quantification of a visual analysis. Doenicke et al. (1973) hypothesized that etomidate caused an inhibition in the neocortical areas.

Wauquier et al. (1978) performed a QPEEG study in dogs, comparing etomidate with the short-acting barbiturate methohexital. Both drugs produced sustained theta activity with underlying beta activity. Power spectral analysis showed that in the frontal cortex, basolateral amygdala, caudate nucleus, and dorsal hippocampus, both drugs produced a significant decrease in relative delta power with an increase in relative power in theta- and alpha-frequency bands. It could not be stated where the effect was generalized, although it was probably because of the use of the average common reference.

It is important to distinguish between drugs such as barbiturates and benzodiazepines, which are used to treat sleep disorders, and those drugs used in the induction of anesthesia (see above). In general, hypnotics are prescribed for people who have delayed sleep onset, interrupted sleep, or lack of deep sleep. The quality of hypnotic drug effects may be evaluated by a subjective assessment through questionnaires or analog scales. However, polysomnography has been shown to make a useful contribution to the objective characteristics of disturbed sleep patterns and to the effects of hypnotics upon them. An ideal hypnotic should not disturb normal sleep at all while restoring disturbed sleep to normal. It should also induce sleep that has normal physiological characteristics.

In general, chronic treatment of benzodiazepines for insomnia shortens sleep latency, diminishes the number of awakenings, and decreases nocturnal restlessness (Oswald et al., 1982). Benzodiazepines often prolong total sleep and may prolong REM latency. Some benzodiazepines may shorten the duration of REM sleep and decrease the amount of slow-wave sleep (stages non-REM 3 and 4). They are also known to increase the number of sleep spindles and K complexes in stage 2 (Johnson et al., 1976). Hence, their effect is not restoring the normality. Similar considerations apply to barbiturates; however, these drugs substantially reduce REM sleep.

Few studies have considered the distribution of stages 3 and 4 of non-REM sleep following the administration of benzodiazepines. Gaillard and Blois (1989) found that flunitrazepam promotes deep sleep at the beginning of the night and increases light sleep during the second and third parts of the night. Similar findings were reported by Declerck et al. (1992).

Although standardized controlled procedures for the evaluation of drug effects on normal volunteers is desirable, it is of equal importance to assess the effects of benzodiazepines used routinely. Few studies have addressed this question. Wauquier and Declerck (1991) studied sleep patterns in patients who were prescribed a variety of benzodiazepines by general practitioners. An objective assessment of sleep patterns revealed that 1 week after drug intake, sleep onset was shorter while stage 2 increased as did sleep efficiency. In spite of the disappearance of the subjective complaint, the changes could no longer be objectively measured 6 weeks later. It is of interest to note that the prescription of a short-acting benzodiazepine was done irrespective of the type, severity, duration, and probable cause of insomnia.

Several recently developed hypnotics bind to the benzodiazepine receptor, but at different subsites. They produce a more nocturnal sleep profile than the traditional benzodiazepines. These third-generation hypnotics such as zolpidem and zopiclone shorten sleep onset, increase total sleep time and sleep efficiency, and do not affect the physiological sleep architecture (Declerck et al., 1992; Kryger et al., 1991). Kryger et al. (1991) compared the subjective with the objective evaluation of the hypnotic efficacy of zolpidem in 16 patients with chronic insomnia. The long-standing effects were shortening of the sleep latency and increased total sleep time. The objective parameters correlated with the subjective variables. But, when asked, the patients overestimated the sleep latency and time spent awake while underestimating total sleep time. There was also a high coefficient of variation between the subjective and objective measures. However, because the maintenance of sleep variables and sleep architecture cannot reliably be measured subjectively, polysomnographic recordings remain essential to determine the efficacy of hypnotics.

Along similar lines, Declerck et al. (1992) used polygraphic recordings in women who subjectively complained of insomnia, in a study of their sleep patterns after administration of a single dose of zolpidem. The recordings did not substantiate the complaint, and, although sleep latency was shortened, there was no change in sleep architecture. In contrast, flunitrazepam increased stage 2, prolonged the latency of REM sleep, reduced the total amount of REM sleep, and increased stages 3 and 4 during the first 2 hours of sleep. This study further reinforces the utility of polysomnographic recordings. Much research evaluated endogenous sleep modulating substances, like adenosine, which by definition act in a more physiological way (Inoué, 1989; Wauquier et al., 1989b).

With respect to EEG morphology, the most striking effect of benzodiazepines is the decrease in delta amplitude, and the reduction of the number of delta waves (Johnson et al., 1976). According to Feinberg et al. (1977) the decrease in delta activity in stage non-REM 4 is compensated by an increase in stage non-REM 2. Furthermore, they claim that there is a decrease in amplitude of delta waves without a reduction in their number. Whether these alterations in delta activity reflect any change in sleep quality is not clear (Feinberg, 1989).

The pharmacokinetic properties of hypnotics are important because it is desirable to limit the duration of action to the night, without having a hangover or a residual sedation the following day. Short-acting (2–3 hours) benzodiazepines, on the other hand, may lead to an initial suppression, which is followed by a compensatory rebound increase of, for example, REM sleep at the end of the night. This is suggested not to be the case with the new generation of hypnotics. To investigate hangover effects, it may be helpful to use continuous ambulatory EEG monitoring or a multiple sleep latency test to assess fluctuation of diurnal vigilance following the night of administered hypnotic therapy. Neither barbiturates nor benzodiazepines show a close relationship between blood levels and EEG changes. Typically they show hysteresis, as EEG slowing lags behind the increasing blood levels.

Conclusions

Pharmacoelectroencephalography is a discipline developed from a pragmatic and empirical point of view. It has generated a wealth of descriptive information. Yet, as Kúnkel (1982) formulated, few hypotheses justify the use of these particular methodologies in the assessment of psychoactive drugs. A description of a drug effect on the EEG, even when quantified or when topographic patterns are analyzed, does not lead to a better understanding of the mechanism or site of action for a drug. However, the changes in the EEG do reflect a functional change in brain.

Basically, the earlier assumption was that there is a relationship, albeit not necessarily direct, between an EEG change and behavior, which by itself is a consequence of a biochemical effect in brain. A direct relationship between an EEG effect and the therapeutic effect of a drug is not always evident. This should not lead to the conclusion that PEEG profiles are typical descriptors of a drug effect on brain that could not be generated.

QPEEG effects might be related to pharmacokinetics, dynamics, and bioavailability. When critically used, QPEEG analysis in conjunction with clinical observations, may serve as a predictor of therapeutic drug effects. It is suggested that psychoactive drugs have different types of profiles of activity. Topographic patterns of drug effects require standardized testing conditions. Statistical methods of analysis need to be developed further to ascertain that typical drug EEG patterns can be differentiated. It remains to be seen if this methodology will improve therapeutic predictability.

References

Baldy-Moulinier, M. 1982. Temporal lobe epilepsy and sleep organization. In *Sleep and Epilepsy,* Eds. M.B. Sterman, M.N. Shouse, and P. Passouant, pp. 347–359. New York: Academic Press.

Binnie, C.D., Kasteleijn-Nolst Trenite, D.G.A., and De Korte, R. 1986a. Photosensitivity as a model for acute anti-epileptic drug studies. Electroencephalogr. Clin. Neurophysiol. 63:35–41.

Binnie, C.D., Van Emde Boas, W., Kasteleijn-Nolst Trenite, D.G.A., et al. 1986b. Acute effects of Lamotrigine (BW430C) in persons with epilepsy. Epilepsia 27:248–254.

Bovill, J.G., Sebel, P.S., Wauquier, A., et al. 1982. Electroencephalographic effects of sufentanil anaesthesia in man. Br. J. Anaesth. 54:45–52.

Bruhn, J., Bouillon, T.W., Radulescu, L., et al. 2003. Correlation of approximate entropy, bispectral index, and spectral edge frequency 95 (SEF95) with clinical signs of "anesthetic depth" during coadministration of propofol and remifentanil. Anesthesiology 98:621–627.

Declerck, A.C., and Wauquier, A. 1991. Antiepileptics and sleep. In *Epilepsy, Sleep and Sleep Deprivation,* Eds. R. Degen and Rodin, E.A. (Epilepsy Res. Suppl. 2), pp. 153–163. Amsterdam: Elsevier.

Declerck, A.C., Ruwe, F., O'Hanlon, J.F., et al. 1992. Effects of Zolpidem and flunitrazepam on nocturnal sleep of women subjectively complaining of insomnia. Psychopharmacology, 106:497–501.

Depoortere, H., Granger, P., Leonardon, J., et al. 1991. Evolution of the cyclic alternating pattern in rats by automatic analysis of sleep amplitude variation: effects of Zolpidem. In *Phasic Events and Dynamic Organization of Sleep,* Eds. M.G. Terzano, P.L. Halasz, and A.C. Declerck, pp. 17–33. New York: Raven Press.

Doenicke, A., Kugler, J., Penzel, G., et al. 1973. Hirnfunktion und Toleranzbreite nach Etomidate, einem neuen barbiturartreien i.v. applizierbaren Hypnoticum. Anaesthesist 22:357–368.

Duffy, F.H., Bartels, P.H., and Burchfiel, J.L. 1981. Significance probability mapping: an aid in the topographic analysis of brain electrical activity. Electroencephalogr. Clin. Neurophysiol. 51:455–462.

Dugovic, C., Leysen, J.E., Janssen, P.F.M., et al. 1989. The light-dark cycle modulates effect of ritanserin on sleep-wakefulness patterns in the rat. Pharm. Bioch. Behavior 34:533–537.

Edmonds, H.L., Jr., and Wauquier, A. 1986. Computerized EEG monitoring. Applications in anesthesia and intensive care, p. 116. Helsinki Instrumentarium Science Foundation.

Edmonds, H.L., Jr., Rodriguez, R.A., and Audenaert, S.M. 1996. The role of neuromonitoring in cardiovascular surgery. [review]. J. Cardiothorac. Vasc. Anesth. 10:15–23.

Feinberg, I. 1989. Effects of maturation and aging on slow wave sleep in man: Implications for neurobiology. In *Slow Wave Sleep: Physiological, Pathophysiological and Functional Aspects,* Eds. A. Wauquier, C. Dugorvic, and M. Radulovacki, pp. 31–48. New York: Raven Press.

Feinberg, I., Fein, G., Walker, J.M., et al. 1977. Flunazepam effects on slow wave sleep: stage 4 suppressed, but number of delta waves constant. Science 198:847–848.

Fink, M. 1980. The significance of quantitative pharmacoelectroencephalography in establishing dose-time relations and its impact on clinical pharmacology: critical review and perspectives. Psychopharmacol. Bull. 17:94.

Fink, M., and Erwin, P. 1982. Pharmaco-EEG study of 6-azamianserin (Org 3770): dissociation of EEG and pharmacologic predictors of antidepressant activity. Psychopharmacology 78:44–48.

Gaillard, J.M. 1989. Benzodiazepines and GABA-ergic transmissions. In *Principles and Practice of Sleep Medicine,* Eds. M.G. Kryger, T. Roth, and W.C. Dement, pp. 213–218. Philadelphia: W.B. Saunders.

Gaillard, J.M., and Blois, R. 1989. Differential effects of flunitrazepam on human sleep in combination with flumazenil. Sleep 12:120–132.

Gigli, G.L., Gotman, J., and Thomas, S.T. 1988. Sleep alterations after acute administration of carbamazepine in cats. Epilepsia 29:748–752.

Gogolak, G. 1980. . Neurophysiological properties (in animals). In *Psychotropic Agents: I. Antipsychotics and Antidepressants,* Eds. F. Hoffmeister and G. Stille, pp. 415–428. Berlin: Springer-Verlag.

Herrmann, W.M. 1982. *Electroencephalographyin Drug Research.* Stuttgart: Fischer.

Herrmann, W.M., and Schaerer, E. 1986. Pharmaco-EEG computer EEG analyses to describe the projection of drug effects on a functional cerebral level in humans. *In Clinical Applications of Computer Analysis of EEG and Other Neurophysiological Signals. Handbook of Electroencephalography and Clinical Neurophysiology,* vol. 2, Eds. F.H. Lopes da Silva, W. Storm van Leeuwen, and A. Remond, pp. 385–445. Amsterdam: Elsevier.

Herrmann, W.M., Kern, V., and Rohmel, J. 1988. The effects of pyritinol on the functional deficits of patients with organic mental disorders. Pharmacopsychiatry 19:378–385.

Idzikowski, C., Mills, E.D., and Glennard, R. 1986. 5-Hydroxytryptamine-2 antagonist increases human slow wave sleep. Brain Res. 378:164–168.

Inoué, S. 1989. *Biology of Sleep Substances.* Boca Raton: CRC Press.

Inoué, S., and Krueger, J.M. 1990. *Endogenous Sleep Factors.* The Hague: SPB Academic Publishing.

Itil, T.M. 1981. The use of computerized bio-electrical potentials (CEEG) in the discovery of psychotropics. Drug Dev. Res. 4:373–407.

Itil, T.M. 1982. The significance of quantitative pharmaco-EEG in the discovery and classification of psychotropic drugs. In *Electroencephalography in Drug Research,* Ed. W.M. Herrmann, pp. 131–158. Stuttgart: Fischer.

Janssen, F.H., Beeker, L., Griep, P.A.M., et al. 1989. Short term effects of temazepam in the EEG of healthy volunteers. Neuropsychobiology 22: 72–76.

John, E.R., Prichep, L.S., Fridman, J., et al. 1988. Neurometrics: computer-assisted differential diagnosis of brain dysfunctions. Science 239:162–169.

Johnson, L.C. 1982. Effects of anticonvulsant medication in sleep patterns: In *Sleep and Epilepsy,* Eds. M.B. Sterman, M.N. Shouse, and P. Passouant, pp. 381–394. New York: Academic Press.

Johnson, L.C., Hanson, J., and Bickford, R.G. 1976. Effects of flurazepam on sleep spindles and K-complexes. Electroencephalogr. Clin. Neurophysiol. 40:67–77.

Joy, R.M., Hance, A.J., and Killam, K.F. 1971. A quantitative electroencephalographic comparison of some benzodiazepines in the primate. Neuropharmacology 10:483–497.

Kales, A. 1995. *The Pharmacology of Sleep.* New York: Springer-Verlag.

Killam, K.F. 1977. Introduction. In *Handbook of Electroencephalography and Clinical Neurophysiology,* vol. 7c, ed., V.G. Longo, pp. 3–6. Amsterdam: Elsevier.

Kleinlogel, H. 1982. The rat paradoxical sleep as a pharmacological test model. In *EEG in Drug Research,* Ed. W.M. Herrmann, pp. 75–88. Stuttgart: Fischer.

Koella, W.P. 1982. A modern concept of vigilance. Experientia 38:1426–1437.

Krijzer, F., and Van Der Molen, R. 1986. Classification of psychotropic drugs by EEG analysis: learning sex development. Neuropsychobiology 16:205–214.

Krijzer, F., Van Der Molen, R. Van Oorschot, R., et al. 1987. Effects of antidepressants on the EEG of the rat. Neuropsychobiology 9:167–173.

Krueger, J.M., Obol, F., Jr., Johanssen, L., et al. 1989. Endogenous slow wave sleep substances: a review. In *Slow Wave Sleep. Physiological, Pathophysiological and Functional Aspects,* Eds. A. Wauquier, C. Dugovic, and M. Radulovacki, pp. 75–90. New York: Raven Press.

Kryger, M.H., Steljes, D., Pouliot, Z., et al. 1991. Subjective versus objective evaluation of hypnotic efficacy: experience with Zolpidem. Sleep 14:399–407.

Kugler, J., 1981. *Electroenzephalographie in Klinik und Praxis.* Stuttgart: Thieme.

Kúnkel, H. 1982. On some hypotheses underlying pharmaco-electroencephalography. In *Electroencephalography in Drug Research,* Ed. W.M. Herrmann, pp. 1–16. Stuttgart: Fischer.

Levy, W.J. 1984. Intraoperative EEG patterns: implications for EEG monitoring. Anesthesiology 60:430–434.

Longo, V.G. (Ed.) 1977. Effect of drugs on the EEG. In *Handbook of Electroencephalography and Clinical Neurophysiology.* Vol. 7C, Ed.-in-chief, A. Remond, Amsterdam: Elsevier.

Matejcek, M. 1982. Vigilance and EEG. In *Electroencephalography in Drug Research,* Ed. W.M. Herrmann, pp. 405–508. Stuttgart: Fischer.

Matousek, M., and Petersén, I. 1979. Automatic measurement of the vigilance level and its possible application in psychopharmacology. Psychopharmacology 12:148–154.

Mendelson, W.B. 1989. Pharmacology of slow wave sleep in illness and health. In *Slow Wave Sleep. Physiological, Pathophysiological and Functional Aspects,* Eds. A. Wauquier, C. Dugovic, and M. Radulovacki, pp. 155–166. New York: Raven Press.

Milligan N., Dhillon, S., Oxley, J., et al. 1982. Absorption of diazepam from the rectum and its effect on interictal spikes in the EEG. Epilepsia 23:323–331.

Milligan, N., Oxley, J., and Richens, A. 1983. Acute effects of intravenous phenytoin on the frequency of inter-ictal spikes in man. Br. J. Pharmacol. 16:285–289.

Monti, J.M. 1987. Disturbance of sleep and wakefulness associated with the use of antihypertensive agents. Life Sci. 41:1979–1988.

Nicholson, A.N., Bradley, C.M., and Pascoe, P.A. 1989. Medications: effect on sleep and wakefulness. In *Principles and Practice of Sleep Medicine,*

Eds. M.H. Kryger, T. Roth, W.C. Dement, pp. 223–236. Philadelphia: W.B. Saunders.

Nuwer, M.R. 1990. The development of EEG brain mapping. J. Clin. Neurophysiol. 7:459–471.

Oswald, I., French, C., Adam K., et al. 1982. Benzodiazepine hypnotics remain effective 24 weeks. Br. Med. J. 284:860–861.

Parrino, L., and Terzano, M. 1996. Polysomnographic effects of hypnotic drugs: a review. Psychopharmacology 126:1–16.

Pichlmayer, I., Lip, V., and Kúnkel, H. 1983. *Das Electroenzephalogram in der Anesthesie.* Berlin: Springer.

Polc, P., Schneeberger, J., and Haefely, W. 1979. Effects of several centrally active drugs on the sleep-wakefulness cycle of rats. Neuropharmacology 18:259–267.

Rampil, I.J., and Smith, N.T. 1985. Comparison of EEG indices during halothane anesthesia. J. Clin. Monit. 1:89.

Ringt, G.S.F., Van Proosdiji, J.N., and Von Wesenbeek, L.A.C.M. 1989. A large scale, high resolution, automated system for rat sleep staging. Part II: validation and application. Electroencephalogr. Clin. Neurophysiol. 73:64–71.

Saletu, B. 1976. *Psychopharmaka, Hirntatigkeit und Schlaf.* Basel: S. Karger.

Saletu, B., and Grünberger, J. 1980. Antiypoxidotic and nootropic changes: proof of this encephalotropic and pharmacodynamic properties by quantitative EEG investigations. Prog. Neuro-Psycho-pharmacol. 4:469–489.

Saletu, B., Anderer, P., Kinsperger, K., et al. 1987. Topographic brain mapping of EEG in neuropsychopharmacology—part II. Cerebral applications (Pharmaco EEG mapping). Mech. Find. Clin. Pharmacol. 9:385–408.

Schallek, W., and Johnson, T.C. 1976. Spectral density analysis of the effects on barbiturates and benzodiazepines on the electroencephalogram of the squirrel monkey. Arch. Int. Pharmacodyn. 223:301–310.

Schallek, W., and Smith, T.H.F. 1952. Electroencephalographic analysis of side effects of spasmolytic drugs. J. Pharmacol. Exp. Ther. 106:291–298.

Scott, J.C., Ponganis, K.V., and Stanski, D.R. 1985. EEG quantification of narcotic effect: the comparative pharmacodynamics of fentanyl and alfentanil. Anesthesiology 62:234–241.

Simes, R.J. 1986. An improved Bonferroni procedure for multiple tests of significance. Biometrica 73:751–754.

Simon, O., Schulz, H., and Rassmanm, W. 1977. The definition of waking stages on the basis of continuous recordings in normal subjects. Electroencephalogr. Clin. Neurophysiol. 42:48–56.

Stille, G., and Herrmann, W.M. 1982. Guidelines for pharmaco-EEG studies in man. Pharmaco-psychiatry 15:107–108.

Stumpf, C., and Gogolak, G. 1987. EEG and neuropharmacology. In *Electroencephalography,* Eds. E. Niedermeyer and F. Lopes da Silva, 2nd ed., pp. 553–565. Baltimore: Urban & Schwarzenberg.

Terzano, M.G., Mancia, D., Salati, M.R., et al. 1985. The cyclic alternative pattern as a physiological component of normal NREM sleep. Sleep 8: 137–145.

Van Wieringen, A., Binnie, C.D., De Boer, P.T.E., et al. 1987. Electroencephalographic findings in six antiepileptic drug trials. Epilepsy Res. 1: 3–15.

Wauquier, A. 1986. Monitoring depth of anesthesia with the EEG. *In Anesthesiology 1986. Drugs, Devices, Concepts and Problems,* Eds. T.H. Stanley and W.I. Petty, pp. 242–254. Dordrecht: Martinus Nijhoff.

Wauquier, A. 1993. Aging and phasic events during sleep. Physiol. Behav. 54:803–806.

Wauquier, A. 1995. Pharmacology of the catecholaminergic system. In *The Pharmacology of Sleep,* Ed. A. Kales, pp. 65–90. New York: Springer-Verlag.

Wauquier, A., and Binnie, C. 1992. Neurophysiological evaluation of drugs. In *Clinical Neurophysiology, Pediatric Neurophysiology, Special Techniques and Applications,* Eds. J. Osselton, C. Binnie, R. Cooper, et al. London: Butterworth-Heinemann Medical.

Wauquier, A., and Declerck, A.C. 1991. Objective assessment of sleep patterns resulting from benzodiazepines prescribed by the general practitioners. Neuropsychobiology 24:57–60.

Wauquier, A. and Dugovic, C. 1990. Serotonin and sleep-wakefulness. In *The Neuropharmacology of serotonin.* Ann NY Acad Sci 600:447–459.

Wauquier, A., Van den Broeck, W.A.E., Verheyen, J.L., et al. 1978. Electroencephalographic study of the short-acting hypnotics etomidate and methohexital in dogs. Eur. J. Pharmacol. 47:367–377.

Wauquier, A., Niemegeers, C.J.E., and Janssen, P.A.J. 1981a. Neuropharmacological comparison between domperidone and metoclopramide. Jpn. J. Pharmacol. 31:201–210.

Wauquier, A., Van den Broeck, W.A.E., Niemegeers, C.J.E., et al. 1981b. A comparison between astemizole and other antihistamines on sleep-wakefulness cycles in dogs. Neuropharmacology 20:853–859.

Wauquier, A., Van den Broeck, W.A.E., Niemegeers, C.J.E., et al. 1981c. Effects of morphine, fentanyl, sufentanil and the short-acting morphine-like, analgesic alfentanil on the EEG in dogs. Drug Dev. Res. 1:167–179.

Wauquier, A., Bovill, J.G., and Sebel, P.J. 1984a. Electroencephalographic effects of fentanyl, sufentanil and alfentanil anaesthesia in man. Neuropsychobiology 11:203–206.

Wauquier, A., Van den Broeck, W.A.E., Awouters, F., et al. 1984b. Further studies on the distinctive sleep-wakefulness profiles of antihistamines (astemizole, ketotifen, terfenadine) in dogs. Drug. Dev. Res. 4:617–625.

Wauquier, A., Gaillard, J.M., Monti, J.M., et al. 1985a. *Sleep: Neurotransmitters and Neuromodulators,* p. 334. New York: Raven Press.

Wauquier, A., Clincke, G.H., Van den Broeck, W.A.E., et al. 1985b. An active and permissive role of dopamine in sleep wakefulness regulation. In *Sleep: Neurotransmitters and Neuromodulators,* Eds. A. Wauquier, J.M. Gaillard, J.M. Monti, et al., pp. 107–120. New York: Raven Press.

Wauquier, A., Van den Broeck, W.A.E., and Edmonds, H.L. 1986. Sleep in epileptic beagles and antiepileptics. Funct. Neurol. 1:53–61.

Wauquier, A., De Ryck, M., Van den Broeck, W.A.E., et al. 1988. Relationships between quantitative EEG measures and pharmacodynamics of alfentanil in dogs. Electroencephalogr. Clin. Neurophysiol. 69:550–560.

Wauquier, A., Dugovic, C., and Radulovacki, M. 1989a. *Slow Wave Sleep: Physiological, Pathophysiological and Functional Aspects,* p. 331. New York: Raven Press.

Wauquier, A., Dugovic, C., Van den Broeck, W.A.E., et al. 1989b. Effects of adenosine transport inhibition on sleep. In *Slow Wave Sleep: Physiological, Pathophysiological and Functional Aspects,* Eds. A. Wauquier, C. Dugovic, and M. Radulovacki, pp. 287–299. New York: Raven Press.

Wolf, P., Roder-Wanner, U.V., and Brede, M. 1984. Influence of therapeutic phenobarbital and phenytoin medication on the polygraphic sleep of patients with epilepsy. Epilepsia 25:407–475.

Wright K.P., Badia, P., and Wauquier, A. 1995. Topographical and temporal patterns of brain activity during the transition from wakefulness to sleep. Sleep 18: 880–889.

34. EEG, Drug Effects, and Central Nervous System Poisoning

Gerhard Bauer and Richard Bauer

A large number of the patients examined in an electroencephalography (EEG) laboratory are under treatment with drugs that alter EEG activity. Therefore, it is important to know the effects of the particular drug(s) used, possible changes due to chronic overdosage, and the patterns of overt intoxication. This chapter discusses the EEG findings that are most important clinically and the classes of drugs most frequently used in modern medicine, and provides an overview of toxic encephalopathies of clinical importance.

Drugs Acting on the Central Nervous System

General Anesthetics

Molecular and cellular mechanisms of general anesthesia have been reviewed by Franks and Lieb (1994) and Campagna et al. (2003). Anesthetics exert their effects on the spinal cord and the brain primarily at the neuronal ion channels via neurotransmitter receptors and by binding directly to the protein site. Initially, anesthetics induce amnesia, euphoria, analgesia, hypnosis, excitation, and hyperreflexia. Surgical anesthesia consists of deep sedation, muscle relaxation, and diminished or abolished motor and autonomous responses to noxious stimuli. Specific effects of different substances (nitrous oxide, halothane, enflurane, isoflurane, sevoflurane, desflurane, propofol) are due to specific binding sites and genetic peculiarities of the patient.

Numerous investigations deal with the correlation of EEG signs and the stages of anesthesia (Clark and Rosner, 1973; Clark et al., 1971; Faulconer and Bickford, 1960; Gibbs et al., 1937; Glaze, 1997; Marshall et al., 1965; Sadove et al., 1967). The initial phase is dominated by the appearance of frontal fast activity, gradually becoming more generalized and associated with dissolution of the alpha rhythm. During excitation, paroxysmal activities become discernible with experimental animals (Schütz and Caspers, 1957), and in nonepileptic and epileptic patients with enflurane (Burchiel et al., 1977; Ito et al., 1988), sevoflurane (Jääskeläinen et al., 2003) and propofol (Walder et al., 2002). As anesthesia deepens, activity becomes slower and the voltage increases. Eventually, a burst–suppression pattern can be observed (Brazier, 1955; Derbyshire et al., 1936; Ellington, 1968; Fischer–Williams, 1963; Swank, 1949). At the deepest level, EEG activity ceases. The burst–suppression pattern exhibits no differences from those seen with deep comatose states under pathological circumstances (see Chapters 21 and 24) or intoxication with sedative drugs (see below). Chapter 56 discusses neuroanesthesia problems.

Hypnotics and Sedatives

Barbiturates

In most countries, barbiturates remained on the market only as antiepileptic drugs and anesthetics. As hypnotics, barbiturates have been replaced by benzodiazepines. Combinations with barbiturates also have disappeared from the pharmacopoeia.

Barbiturates apparently act at all levels of the neuraxis. They exert their effects by binding to a specific site on the γ-aminobutyric acid $GABA_A$ receptor, different from the binding site of benzodiazepines (Macdonald and Kelly, 1994; McKernan and Whiting, 1996). Low blood concentrations produce inhibition of higher cortical functions and disinhibition of more primitive behavior. With increasing blood levels, clinical signs are determined by generalized inhibition.

EEG Changes with Therapeutic Doses

When administered in small doses, the barbiturates produce an increase in fast activities in the range of 25 to 35 cycles per second (cps), soon shifting to 15 to 25 cps. This activity is predominant over the frontal cortex and spreads to parietal and occipital areas (Adams and Hubach, 1960; Fink, 1968). Increasing doses are accompanied by intermixed slow activities and dissolution of the alpha rhythm, indicating drowsiness and sleep. In children, in the elderly, and in patients with organic brain lesions, barbiturates even in low doses may induce irritability, hyperactivity, or delirium (Ban and Amin, 1979; Livingston, 1966). Lack of barbiturate–induced fast activity indicates a diffuse organic brain lesion; asymmetries are suggestive of a focal lesion (Pampiglione, 1952).

Chronic Overdosage

Signs of chronic barbiturate intoxication in epileptic patients mostly are the result of overdosage, and might be misinterpreted as personality changes incorrectly attributed to the epileptic disorder. Signs include general sluggishness, lethargy, difficulty in thinking, poor memory, learning disabilities, and cerebellar deficits (Ban and Amin, 1979; Bruni and Wilder, 1979; Myers and Stockard, 1975). Chronic neurotoxicity may result in insidiously developing disturbances of higher cognitive functions without concomitant abnormalities (Novelly et al., 1986; Reynolds, 1983; Trimble, 1991). Compared with other antiepileptic drugs, cognitive adverse effects are pronounced with phenobarbital (for review see Cramer and Mattson, 1995). EEG changes are similar to those seen in the first stage of acute intoxication. In epileptic patients, an increase in slow activity in serial recordings without increase or even with reduction in seizure frequency is indicative of overdosage and should prompt an evaluation of the serum level.

EEG Changes After Withdrawal

After long–term ingestion of barbiturates, abrupt withdrawal leads to paroxysmal abnormalities. Myoclonic jerks, even as myoclonic status, generalized tonic–clonic seizures, and delirium are major complications (Wikler et al., 1955). The EEG frequently shows generalized paroxysmal activities and spikes, especially with photic stimulation (Braesco and Lairy, 1959; Kurtz, 1976a; Wikler and Essig, 1970; Wulff, 1960). These changes are usually transient in nature and most often occur within the first few days after withdrawal, but they may occasionally persist for 3 to 4 weeks. They also occur without clinical seizures and even with medically controlled gradual withdrawal (Fig. 34.1).

Acute Intoxication

Sedatives such as barbiturates, anxiolytic drugs, phenothiazines, and tricyclic antidepressants can all produce coma. They directly depress cellular oxidative metabolism and do not permanently damage neuronal functions. The mere functional character of central nervous system (CNS) depression

after an acute overdose indicates a less grave prognosis even in the presence of very serious clinical and EEG signs.

According to the multilevel action of barbiturates, the clinical syndrome encompasses cortical, reticular, vestibular, and other brainstem dysfunctions. Coma due to overdose with sedatives is fairly characteristic if one considers the depth of unresponsiveness in combination with flaccid muscle tone, absent plantar responses, and preserved pupillary reactions (Plum and Posner, 1972). With fast-acting barbiturates cerebral functions can be depressed in a rostrocaudal fashion and motor signs may initially evolve (Plum and Posner, 1972) (Fig. 34.2). In severe cases, circulatory effects lead to a typical shock syndrome (Harvey, 1975). Subsequent cerebral hypoxia may turn the functional disturbance into structural damage with serious prognostic implications.

EEG signs in different stages of acute intoxication closely resemble those observed with other CNS depressant substances. Initial dissolution of the alpha rhythm and appearance of interspersed theta frequencies are followed by predominant slow activities superimposed by 10 to 16 cps rhythmical activity maximal over the anterior regions. Such an EEG is suggestive of intoxication with depressant drugs of any type (Fig. 34.2). However, the so–called spindle coma after head injury and the alpha coma pattern with cerebral hypoxia may look similar. Superimposed fast activities after intoxications have also been termed "drug–induced alpha

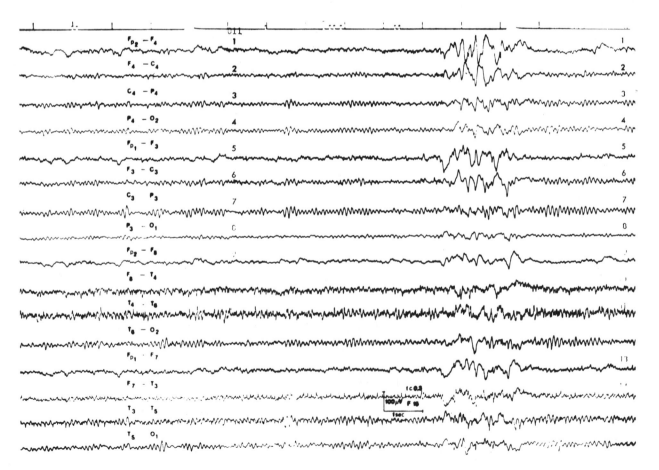

Figure 34.1. W.M., a 33-year-old woman and chronic abuser of alcohol and barbiturates (Optalidon). EEG at the sixth day after admission for withdrawal. No seizures. Paroxysmal 2 to 3 cps waves with intermingled small spikes.

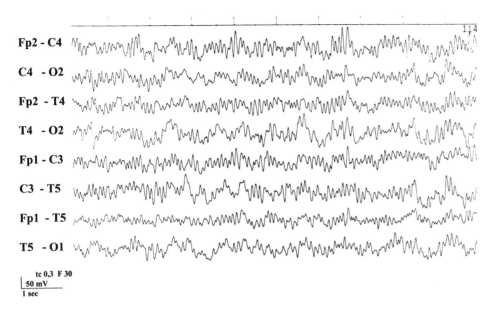

Figure 34.2. E.A., a 24-year-old woman who made a suicide attempt by ingesting a combination of cyclobarbital, hexobarbital, meprobamate, and carbromal (Somnupan, banned in Austria for several years). Coma with decerebrate posturing (with fast-acting barbiturates cerebral functions can be depressed in a rostrocaudal fashion and motor signs may initially evolve; Plum and Posner, 1972). EEG with diffuse slow activity superimposed by high-voltage 10 to 13 cps activities. Patient recovered completely.

coma" (Kuroiwa et al., 1981). The separation from alpha coma pattern with hypoxic states has prognostic significance with a much more favorable outlook of superimposed fast rhythms with intoxications (Austin et al., 1988; Kuroiwa et al., 1981; Lersch and Kaplan, 1984). With deepening coma, fast frequencies disappear and diffuse delta activity becomes prominent. With impending breakdown of vegetative func-

tions, periods of flattening, and, eventually, a burst–suppression pattern appear (Denny–Brown et al., 1947; Ellington, 1968; Krump, 1954; Mantz et al., 1965; Mellerio, 1964). Preceding or following the development of a burst–suppression pattern, the record may be characterized by bi– or triphasic sharp transients (Kubicki, 1967) (Fig. 34.3). Electrocerebral silence signifies the most advanced cases. The prognostic

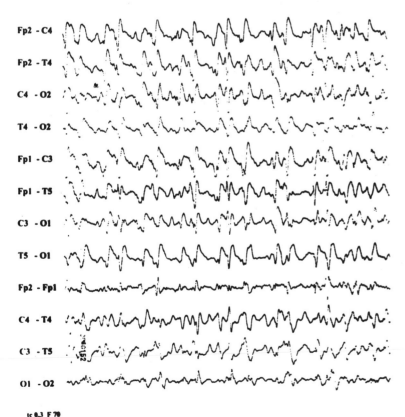

Figure 34.3. B.H., a 33-year-old woman who is in a coma after a suicide attempt by ingesting barbiturates. Diffuse slow activity with triphasic waves.

meaning of this otherwise ominous sign is less grave with intoxication. Several patients survived without permanent neurological sequelae (Bennett et al., 1976; Bird and Plum, 1968; Ellington, 1968; Haider et al., 1971; Mantz et al., 1965; Mellerio, 1970; Sament and Huott, 1969).

Attempts have been made to correlate the EEG with clinical signs and blood levels (Haider et al., 1971; Kubicki and Rieger, 1968; Kubicki et al., 1970; Kurtz, 1976a; Sament and Huott, 1969). In the earliest phases, clinical signs are superior to the EEG in the assessment of the severity of the functional disturbance, whereas the EEG alone permits grading of stages during the later phases.

Miscellaneous Hypnotic Drugs

Melatonin

Melatonin has been extensively discussed in the popular media. Melatonin is the hormone of darkness (Utiger, 1992). The substance may act as a phase–setter for sleep–wake cycles in subjects with a delayed sleep phase syndrome (Dahlitz et al., 1991). A carefully timed dose of melatonin can improve the symptoms of jet lag (Arendt et al., 1995). However, controlled studies with the substance are the exception (Waldhauser et al., 1990). Formulations of the substance lack the standards of the pharmaceutical industry, and safety remains uncertain (Arendt, 1996), although the hypnotic effect of melatonin in humans seems to be established (Brzezinski, 1997). Effects on the conventional EEG have not been reported.

Bromides

Bromide was the drug of choice as anticonvulsant and sedative during the second half of the 19th century. It is still used in the treatment of therapy–resistant tonic–clonic seizures (Boenick et al., 1985; Dreifuss and Bertram, 1986). With acute bromide intoxication, the EEG shows mixed slow and fast activity. Very pronounced EEG slowing is found in chronic bromide encephalopathies. Drug level determinations have improved the handling of the drug, so the typical bromism of the old days has disappeared.

Antipsychotic Drugs

Antipsychotic drugs are used for the treatment of schizophrenia. They are listed as typical, classic, or first-generation antipsychotic agents (chlorpromazine, perphenazine, trifluoperazine, thiothixene, haloperidol) and as atypical or second-generation drugs (clozapine, risperidone, olanzapine, quetiapine, ziprasidone, aripiprazole, amisulpride). Major progress has been made in elucidating their mechanism of action (for review see Freedman, 2003). Typical antipsychotic drugs act by blocking the dopamine D2 receptor and are connected with parkinsonian side effects. The newer antipsychotic compounds bind to many different receptors including members of the dopamine receptor family and 5-HT2A receptors.

Typical Antipsychotic Drugs

EEG changes due to neuroleptics are not particularly different for the numerous substances under this pharmacological heading and therefore are discussed jointly.

EEG Changes with Therapeutic Doses

A great number of visual as well as automatic analyses of EEG changes due to therapeutic doses of neuroleptics can be summarized as follows. Neuroleptics increase the alpha activity with a slight shift to the lower range and increase the amount of slow activity and the general voltage output, but decrease the percent time of beta activity, variability of frequencies, and the average frequency (Bente, 1975; Fink, 1968, 1969; Itil, 1971; Saletu, 1976; Terzian, 1952).

Epileptogenic Potency

Paroxysmal slow waves and sharp waves have been observed (Bente, 1975; Itil, 1970). Although the risk of seizures under treatment with typical antipsychotic drugs does not differ substantially from the general population (Alldredge, 1999), with high doses seizures may occur (Chang and Davis, 1979; Itil and Soldatos, 1980; Kugler et al., 1979; Kurtz, 1976a; Logothetis, 1967; Oliver et al., 1982; Toone and Fenton, 1977; Van Sweden, 1984; Van Sweden and Dumon–Radermecker, 1982). EEG and seizure frequency can deteriorate in chronic epileptic patients. Several cases of nonconvulsive status epilepticus have been reported under neuroleptic treatment (Laan and DeWeerd, 1990; Van Sweden 1984, 1985).

Acute Intoxication

Overdosage with neuroleptics usually leads to sedation and coma. In milder cases, patients can be agitated, delirious, or confused (Angst and Hicklin, 1967; Helmchen, 1961; Lang and Moore, 1961). Involuntary extrapyramidal movements, parkinsonism, and generalized tonic–clonic seizures can be prominent. Fatalities are rare if the neuroleptics alone are taken; death is attributable to cardiac effects. The EEG is dominated by slow waves, frequently occurring as generalized paroxysmal activities. Fast frequencies as in barbiturate poisoning are not recorded (Kurtz, 1976a; Mellerio, 1964).

Atypical Antipsychotic Drugs

A long list of newer antipsychotic drugs are on the market (clozapine, amisulpride, olanzapine, quetiapine, risperidone, sertindol, ziprasidone, zotepine). In a systematic meta-analysis only clozapine exhibited fewer parkinsonian symptoms and a higher antipsychotic effect than conventional drugs (Leucht et al., 2003). Compared wit the classic antipsychotics, the newer drugs are less extensively studied with quantitative EEG methods. Some EEG data exist on clozapine and risperidone.

Clozapine

Clozapine has affinity for serotonin (5–HT2a, 5–HT6, 5–HT7, 5–HT2c, 5–HT3), α–adrenergic, and dopamine D4 receptors, but weak affinity for the D2 receptor (Schmidt et al., 1995). Clozapine causes no extrapyramidal symptoms and tardive dyskinesia (Leucht et al., 2003). The major adverse effect of clozapine relates to its potential for damaging the granulocyte cell line. A cumulative risk figure for agranulocytosis of 0.8% at 1 year and 0.9% at 18 months was calculated (Alvir et al., 1993).

EEG power spectra show an increase in delta, theta, and above 21 cps beta activity. In chronically treated patients, the EEG became abnormal in up to 57% of the patients, which is greater than with other antipsychotics (Isermann and Haupt, 1976; Koukkou et al., 1979; Naber and Hippius, 1990; Schmauss et al., 1989; Spatz et al., 1978b). Increased theta- and delta activities were prominent over the frontal, central, and parietal areas (Joutsiniemi et al., 2001). These abnormalities included paroxysmal slowing and spikes. Clozapine can provoke seizures (Devinsky et al., 1991; Günther et al., 1993; Haller and Binder, 1990; Lindstrom, 1988; Liukkonen et al., 1992; Markowitz and Brown, 1987; Pacia and Devinsky, 1994). Seizure frequency amounts up to 4% (Baldessarini and Frankenburg, 1991), increases with doses over 600 mg per day and seems to be greater than with other antipsychotic drugs. In addition to generalized tonic–clonic seizures, myoclonic jerks have been observed (Berman et al., 1992).

Risperidone

Risperidone is a benzisoxazole derivative with combined dopamine D2 receptor and serotonin 5–HT2 receptor blocking properties (Mortimer, 1994). The substance has an established efficacy in acute psychotic states. Risperidone does not induce EEG changes in the waking state and no seizures occurred during treatment (Cunningham Owens, 1996). Some changes in sleep profile have been reported.

Antidepressant Drugs

Since the introduction of the first–generation tricyclic antidepressants, several new drugs have been marketed. New antidepressants might be classified according to their central mode of action into selective serotonin reuptake inhibitors (fluoxetine, fluvoxamine, paroxetine, citalopram, sertraline), dual serotoninergic antidepressants (reuptake inhibitors plus receptor antagonism; nefazodone), selective serotonin and noradrenaline reuptake inhibitors (venlafaxine), noradrenergic and specific serotonergic antidepressants (mirtazapine), selective noradrenaline reuptake inhibitors (reboxetine), and reversible specific monoamine oxidase inhibitors (moclobemide) (for review see Frazer, 1997; Schmitz, 2002). Antidepressants, especially amitriptyline, and several antiepileptic drugs (see below) are also important in the treatment of neuropathic pain (McQuay and Moore, 1997; Sindrup and Jensen, 2000).

Tricyclic Antidepressants

EEG Changes with Therapeutic Doses

Tricyclic antidepressants such as imipramine, amitriptyline, doxepin, desipramine, nortriptyline, and protriptyline increase the amount of slow and fast activity along with instability of frequencies and voltage. Furthermore, they slow down the frequency of the alpha rhythm (Bente, 1975; Fink, 1968, 1969; Itil, 1970; Kiloh et al., 1961; Saletu, 1976).

Epileptogenic Potency

Paroxysmal slow waves, spikes, and polyspikes occur with therapeutic doses (Bente, 1975; Davison, 1965; Harrer, 1960; Itil, 1970; Kiloh et al., 1961; Kugler, 1960;

Kurtz, 1976a; VanMeter et al., 1959). The seizure frequency may increase in chronic epileptic patients. Furthermore, single or multiple seizures occur in nonepileptic patients, especially with high doses (Chang and Davis, 1979; Edwards et al., 1986; Jabbari et al., 1985; Kiloh et al., 1961; Skowron and Stimmel, 1992). Status epilepticus was reported with amitriptyline (Scharfetter, 1965) and with imipramine (Michon et al., 1959). Several cases of absence status have been thought to be due to treatment with tricyclic agents (Bourrat et al., 1986; Rumpl and Hinterhuber, 1981; Thomas et al., 1992).

Acute Intoxication

Unlike the phenothiazines, tricyclic antidepressants have much narrower therapeutic ranges and quickly reach toxic levels. Overdosage may result in serious life–threatening conditions. This is of great concern, because depression is notorious for suicidal attempts. The clinical picture is characterized by hyperpyrexia, hypertension, seizures, and coma (Byk, 1975; Chang and Davis, 1979; Davies and Allaye, 1963). The prognosis depends largely on the effects on the cardiovascular system. Even with therapeutic doses, there is an increased tendency toward cardiac arrhythmias, and there have been several reports of unexpected death. Greater than tenfold differences in the number of deaths per million prescriptions have been shown between the different tricyclic antidepressants and between the newer antidepressants (Buckley and McManus, 2002). The EEG during acute intoxication shows widespread, poorly reactive, irregular 8 to 10 cps activity and paroxysmal abnormalities including spikes as well as unspecific coma patterns (Kurtz, 1976a; Mellerio, 1964) (Fig. 34.4).

New Antidepressants

Second–generation antidepressants might be differentiated from the first–generation antidepressants by means of quantitative EEG parameters (Herrmann et al., 1979; Kerhofs et al., 1990). With the newest drugs, emphasis has shifted away from quantitative EEG investigations.

Similar to the first–generation antidepressants, a number of the newer drugs can induce epileptic seizures. There are differences in seizure propensity within the substances, particularly pronounced with maprotiline and bupropion and low with trazodone, nefazodone, mirtazapine, and the selective serotonin reuptake inhibitors (for review see Frazer, 1997; Montgomery, 1995; Schmitz, 2002; Skowron and Stimmel, 1992). Vollmer–Haase and Folkerts (1997) reported focal seizures evolving to generalized seizures under the treatment of paroxetine, a 5–HT reuptake inhibiting substance. The EEG exhibited corresponding focal sharp waves.

In general, the new antidepressant drugs have a higher therapeutic index than the tricyclic compounds. Overdosage with several of the new drugs have been reported, and deaths have been reported (for review see Frazer, 1997). Fatal toxicity index for venlafaxine is higher than those for other serotoninergic antidepressants (Buckley and McManus, 2002). EEG signs during the intoxicated state are rarely demonstrated and show no particular features.

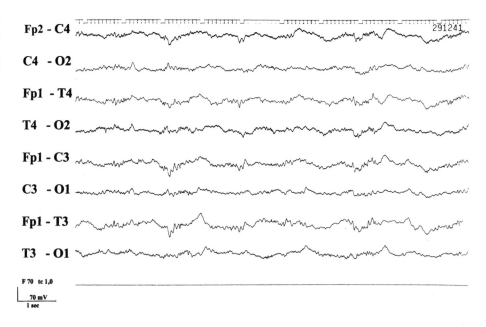

Figure 34.4. P.M., a 22-year-old man who is comatose due to intoxication with an unidentified amount of tricyclic antidepressants. Unresponsive slowing with superimposed fast activities. The patient survived and was transferred to the psychiatric ward the next day.

Lithium

Lithium is commonly used in the prophylactic treatment of bipolar mood disorders. EEG changes during the treatment are frequent and marked (Corcoran et al., 1949; Fetzer et al., 1981; Helmchen and Kanowski, 1971; Henninger, 1969; Johnson et al., 1970; Mayfield and Brown, 1966; Shopsin et al., 1970; Ulrich et al., 1982). In general, they parallel the blood serum levels, but there are also remarkable discrepancies.

Acute intoxication with lithium salts can be a life–threatening condition. Early symptoms include fatigue, muscular weakness, and tremor. When plasma concentrations rise above 2 mEq/L, more serious toxic effects occur. Disturbances in renal elimination or fever with liberation of tissue–bound lithium are the most frequent causes of intoxication. Obtundation, stupor, or delirium is always present. Neurological signs show a bewildering variety of cortical and subcortical dysfunctions (Bejar, 1985; Poewe and Bauer, 1982; Sansone and Ziegler, 1985), optomotor disturbances (Coppeto et al., 1983; Lee and Lessel, 2003; Sandyk, 1984; Williams et al., 1988), and peripheral neuropathies (Chang et al., 1988, 1990; Sansone and Ziegler, 1985). Movement disorders are especially dramatic. Choreiform hyperkinesis (Walevski and Radwan, 1986), myoclonic jerks (stimulus–sensitive and occurring in prolonged bursts) (Caviness and Evidente, 2003), convulsions, bizarre and complex extrapyramidal movements, and several other signs may be observed. Such conditions have been called lithium–induced Creutzfeldt–Jakob syndrome (Casanova et al., 1996; Smith and Kocen, 1988) or nonconvulsive status epilepticus (Lee, 1985). Permanent neurological sequelae due to lithium toxicity have also been reported (Donaldson and Cunningham, 1983; Gille et al., 1997; Habib et al., 1986; Kores and Lader, 1997; Nagaraja et al., 1987; Peiffer, 1981).

The EEG is always markedly abnormal with lithium intoxication (Koufen and Consbruch, 1972; Spatz et al., 1978a) and shows diffuse slowing and paroxysmal abnormalities including spikes and triphasic waves. Focal slowing also occurs and does not have to be taken as a sign of focal brain lesion (Helmchen and Kanowski, 1971; Koufen and Consbruch, 1972; Low, 1979). Improvement of electrical activity parallels clinical improvement, but the EEG abnormalities regularly outlast the abnormal serum levels (Fig. 34.5).

Anxiolytic Drugs
Benzodiazepines

The main actions of benzodiazepines can be described as hypnotic, anxiolytic, anticonvulsant, myorelaxant, and amnesic. They exert their actions by binding at specific sites at the $GABA_A$ receptor chloride ionophore (Gardner et al., 1993; Haefely, 1989). The distribution of $GABA_A$ receptors within brain regions and changing compositions of receptor subunits might contribute to differences in the efficacy of the numerous benzodiazepines (Doble and Martin, 1992; Gale, 1989; McKernan and Whiting, 1996). Furthermore, pharmacokinetic properties like rapidity of absorption, half-life time, binding to fat deposits, and activities of metabolites (Maczaj, 1993) are important. In general, all benzodiazepines exert actions mentioned above and share the same side effects, although with different relations. Therefore, those on the huge list of benzodiazepines (clobazam, clonazepam, diazepam, estazolam, flunitrazepam, flurazepam, lorazepam, nitrazepam, quazepam, temazepam, triazolam among others) are considered together.

EEG Changes with Therapeutic Doses

The benzodiazepine derivatives are potent activators of beta activity, which persist in the EEG as long as 2 weeks after the last ingestion. As with barbiturates, benzodiazepine–induced fast activities are reduced over the site of a

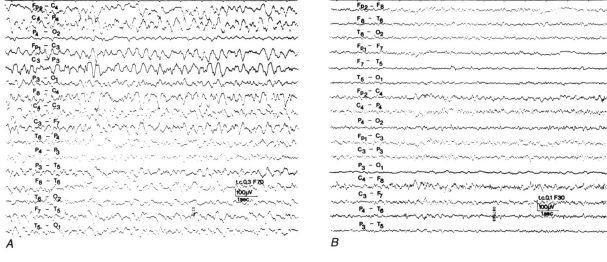

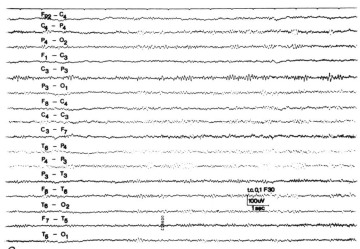

Figure 34.5. E.R., a 43-year-old woman with intoxication from lithium carbonate. **A:** Delirious, multiple hyperkinesia, general rigidity. Blood serum level of Li 2.95 mval/L. Diffuse slowing with rhythmical 1 to 3 cps activity maximal over anterior regions. Some triphasic–like waves. **B:** Four days after **A**. Clinically improved, but still slow mentation and scattered myoclonic jerks. Blood serum level of Li 0.5 mval/L. Some diffuse 2.5 to 7 cps activity. **C:** Nine days after **A**. No abnormal results at neurological examination. No more Li could be found in the blood. The EEG was also normal.

cerebral lesion (Gotman et al., 1982). Furthermore, benzodiazepines produce a decrease in alpha activity and general voltage, and a slight increase of 4 to 7 cps activity (Fink, 1968; Itil, 1970; Saletu, 1976). After long–term treatment, paroxysmal rhythmical slow waves have been reported (Hollister and Barthel, 1959; Jörgensen and Wulff, 1958).

Effect on Seizures

Benzodiazepines have a favorable influence on seizures, but have no effect on interictal focal spikes (Niedermeyer, 1970). Despite the antiepileptic action, they may provoke tonic status epilepticus if intravenously administered to children with absence status in Lennox–Gastaut syndrome (Prior et al., 1972; Tassinari et al., 1971, 1972). Lorazepam has been reported to be superior in the treatment of status epilepticus because it is less extensively bound to fat (Treiman et al., 1998). Withdrawal of benzodiazepines has been considered an etiological factor of de novo absence status of late onset (Thomas et al., 1992, 1993). Absence status should not be confused with delirious withdrawal syndromes without spikes (Hauser et al., 1989).

Side Effects of Benzodiazepines

All benzodiazepines share a long list of side effects consisting of tiredness during the day following ingestion (hangover), rebound anxiety, anterograde amnesia, rebound insomnia, low-dose dependency, and withdrawal syndromes. The profile of side effects depends on the specific binding site, the dose, the half-life time, and other pharmacokinetic variables. With short-acting substances, the amnesic effects are comparatively marked (Bixler et al., 1991; Gillin, 1991; Greenblatt et al., 1991; Häcki, 1986; Oswald, 1989; Scharf et al., 1988; Van der Kroef et al., 1979). In general, benzodiazepines have significantly fewer side effects than barbiturates, and it is appropriate to prefer them as hypnotics.

Acute Intoxication

The clinical picture resembles those seen with other CNS depressant drugs and is not truly specific for benzodiazepines (Bruni and Wilder, 1979; Plum and Posner, 1972). The prognosis is generally good, although in patients with decreased respiratory reserve and, in the very young, even therapeutic doses may dangerously depress cardiorespiratory function (Mattson, 1972). The EEG shows prominent fast activity with no response to stimuli. With larger doses, coma patterns, as in other intoxications, are recorded (Kurtz, 1976a; Mellerio, 1964).

Zolpidem

Zolpidem belongs to the class of imidazopyridines (Langtry and Benfield, 1990). It binds to the alpha-1 unit of the $GABA_A$ receptor complex (McKernan and Whiting, 1996). Similar side effects to those with benzodiazepines have been reported. Sleep architecture is claimed to resemble normal patterns more closely. Nothing is known about the influence on the EEG in the waking state or during intoxication.

Zopiclone

Zopiclone belongs to a new class of hypnotics, the cyclopyrrolones. The final pathway constitutes an opening of the chloride ionophore. The most frequent adverse effects include bitter taste, dry mouth, and complaints comparable to those with the benzodiazepines (Allain et al., 1991). EEG changes are not reported. Microstructural analysis of sleep architecture and decrease of EEG arousals allow distinguishing benzodiazepines, zolpidem, and zopiclone (Parrino et al., 1997).

Baclofen

Baclofen is a selective $GABA_B$ receptor agonist and is used for treatment of spasticity (Misgeld et al., 1995). With oral therapeutic doses, no increase of seizure frequency has been reported in chronic epileptic patients (Terrence et al., 1983). Baclofen is also given intrathecally via a drug delivery system. Seizures have been observed with intrathecal baclofen application (Kofler et al., 1994). Structural brain damage seems prerequisite for baclofen to exert epileptogenic activity. The same is true for overdose due to a failure

of the drug delivery system (Fig. 34.6). Under these circumstances the EEG can exhibit periodic lateralized epileptiform discharges without overt seizures (Fakhoury et al., 1998).

Psychotogenic Drugs

Lysergic Acid Diethylamide (LSD) and Mescaline

These agents cause decreased amplitude and depression of slow waves as well as acceleration of the dominant frequencies during the drug–induced psychotic state (Borenstein and Cujo, 1969; Brown, 1968; Denber et al., 1953; Itil, 1970; Ketz, 1974).

Marijuana

Cannabis exerts its central effects through the CB1 cannabinoid receptor (for review see Iversen, 2003). These effects include disruption of psychomotor behavior, short-term memory impairment, stimulation of appetite, and antinociceptive and antiemetic actions. There is little evidence of irreversible mental deficits and any causal link with an increased risk of psychiatric illness. Cannabis is effective in the treatment of neuropathic pain and spasticity (Karst et al., 2003).

Administration by smoking produces no visible effects on the conventional EEG (Fink, 1974; Low, 1979; Rodin et al., 1970; Volavka et al., 1972). EEG slowing reported by Deliyannakis et al. (1970) was mild and inconclusive; most of these subjects showed no EEG changes.

Central Nervous System Stimulants

Central stimulants potentiate central dopamine activity. Different modes of dopaminergic potentiation have been shown in such drugs as the amphetamines, methylphenidate, and cocaine (Nausieda, 1979).

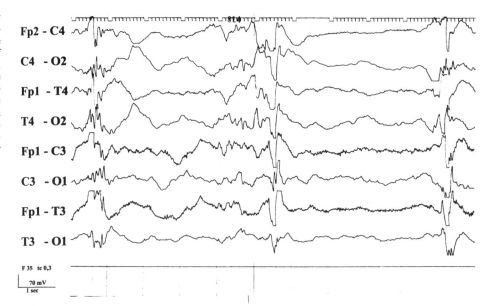

Figure 34.6. M.C., a 17-year-old boy who had a severe brain trauma 1 year earlier. Marked spasticity. Now comatose due to an overdose of baclofen (failure of the intrathecal drug delivery system). Had left–sided focal motor seizures the first day after intoxication. The EEG taken the second day exhibits periodic paroxysmal slow and spiky waves on a severely abnormal slow background activity. Recovered up to the habitual condition after the brain trauma. No further seizures.

Low-Dose Effects on EEG

CNS stimulants increase the amounts of beta and alpha activity, reduce the general voltage and the amount of slow waves, and tend to suppress seizure discharges in pertinent cases, especially the 3-cps spike and wave complexes (Chauncy and Leake, 1958; Fink, 1968; Longo and Silvestrini, 1957; Saletu, 1976). Abnormal slow waves during stupor and coma are diminished by the administration of methylphenidate. So–called recreational drugs illegally offered as Ecstasy contain CNS stimulants, especially methamphetamines. Therefore, most CNS stimulants have been banned from the market because of their addictive potential. Modafinil, a pharmacologically unique wake-promoting agent has replaced the traditional amphetamines for the treatment of narcolepsy (U.S. Modafinil in Narcolepsy Multicenter Study Group, 2000) and attention-deficit disorder.

Acute Intoxication

Intoxications with CNS stimulants have increased due to their use as Ecstasy. In a 1996 survey nearly 5 millions Americans have reported using methamphetamine at some time in their lives (Office of Applied Studies, 1996). Symptoms of mild intoxications are those of sympathetic activity. In more severe poisoning, hypertension, confusion, cardiac anomalies, and finally hyperthermia, convulsions, circulatory failure, and coma occur. Death due to amphetamines is related either to direct pharmacologic effects (Kalant and Kalant, 1975) or to secondary complications in drug addicts (Schifano et al., 2003). The EEG with overdose of stimulant drugs shows the usual coma pattern without any particular features (Ketz, 1974). Methamphetamines can damage dopaminergic and serotoninergic neurons (Ernst et al., 2000) and produce corresponding permanent neurological abnormalities.

Cocaine

Cocaine has become a major substance in the field of drug addiction. Cocaine binds strongly to the dopamine–reuptake transporter and blocks such reuptake after normal neuronal activity. High dopamine concentrations at the synapse produce the characteristic cocaine "high" (Leshner, 1996). Common neural substrates seems to exist for the addictive properties of nicotine and cocaine (Pich et al., 1997). Variants of the *DRD2* gene have been associated with cocaine, nicotine, and opioid dependency (for review see Noble, 2003).

Berger's historic experiments on the EEG effects of cocaine intake have been confirmed. Cocaine increases beta power correlated with the area under the cocaine plasma versus time curve (Herning et al., 1985). Several neurological complications are associated with chronic cocaine intake. It induces strokes (Caplan et al., 1982; Daras et al., 1994b; Globe and Merkin, 1986; Konzen et al., 1995; Mody et al., 1988; Qureshi et al., 1997), orbital infarction (Van Stavern and Gorman, 2002), subarachnoid and intracerebral hemorrhages (Aggarwal et al., 1996; Daras et al., 1994b; Nolte et al., 1996; Schwartz and Cohen, 1984), vasospasm after aneurysmal subarachnoid hemorrhage (Conway and Tamargo, 2001), cerebral vasculitis (Krendel et al., 1990), choreoathetoid movements (Daras et al., 1994a), persistent dyskinesias (Weiner et al., 2001), oculomotor nerve palsies (Migita et al., 1997), spinal and medullary vascular syndromes (Di Lazzaro et al., 1997; Mody et al., 1988), and can provoke seizures or exacerbate a preexisting seizure disorder (Eidelberg et al., 1961; Koppel et al., 1996; Lesse and Collins, 1979; Myers and Earnest, 1984; Nausieda, 1979; Stevens et al., 1996). Seizure activity can present as complex partial status epilepticus (Ogunyemi et al., 1989).

Antiepileptic Drugs

Drug therapy of epilepsies represents the long–term therapy par excellence. Dose– or interaction–related CNS toxic effects are common. Delayed toxic effects and drug–induced diseases are not dose related, are occasionally life threatening, and are not always reversible. Antiepileptic drugs act directly on voltage–gated ion channels and by influencing GABA–mediated effects. Effects upon the GABA system are manyfold. Antiepileptic drugs can bind at the GABA$_A$ receptor at different binding sites, can inactivate GABA–metabolizing enzymes and inhibit uptake of GABA into nerve cells and glia cells. Other antiepileptic drugs influence the glutaminergic system via *N*-methyl-D-aspartate (NMDA) or α-amino-3-hydroxy-5-methyl-4-isoxazole proprionate (AMPA) receptors. For detailed and comprehensive information, the reader is referred to Levy et al. (1995).

Several antiepileptic drugs are used in the treatment of neuropathic pain syndromes (Tremont-Lukats et al., 2000) and migraine, and as so-called mood stabilizers.

Actions of antiepileptic drugs on the EEG have to be divided into effects of therapeutic doses on background activity and on frequency and morphology of preexisting spikes as well as into the effects of overdoses, overt intoxication, and withdrawal. In general, the standard antiepileptic drugs slow down the frequency of the occipital basic rhythm even with nontoxic serum levels and increase the percentage of power in the theta and delta bands with visual (Herkes et al., 1993; Salinsky et al., 1994) and with quantitative analysis (Salinsky et al., 2003). These changes correlate with cognitive effects and subjective complaints. The effect on interictal spikes varies considerably with a positive correlation between seizure frequency and the number of spikes in some patients (Duncan, 1987).

Hydantoins

Signs of cerebellovestibular dysfunction signal initial hydantoin overdosage. Occasionally, this condition may be confused with a cerebellar tumor (Hess, 1974). Cerebellar atrophy occurs with chronic hydantoin use but also with acute intoxication (Kuruvilla and Bharucha, 1997; Luef et al., 1996). An overt hydantoin intoxication is further characterized by altered higher cognitive function, pyramidal signs, and several extrapyramidal movement disorders (Murphy et al., 1991). Epileptic seizures may be exacerbated (Bauer, 1996; Osorio et al., 1989; Stilman and Masdeu, 1985; Zwarts and Sie, 1985). Cardiovascular toxicity is rare unless the substance has been given parenterally (Wyle and Berk, 1991).

In contrast to barbiturates and benzodiazepines, the EEG shows no increase in fast activities (Roseman, 1961). With spectral analyses, however, an increased power in the fast frequencies was found at serum levels in excess of 32 mmol/L (Fink et al., 1979). Phenytoin increases the power in the theta and delta bands with blood levels in the usual range and without clinical signs of overt intoxication (Herkes et al., 1993; Salinsky et al., 1994). There are conflicting reports on the influence of phenytoin on interictal epileptiform discharges. No changes (Wilkus et al., 1978), an increase (Bente, 1975; Carrie, 1976), and a decrease of spikes (Buchthal et al., 1960; Wilkus and Green, 1974) have been found.

No changes in background activity occurred with phenytoin reduction (Duncan et al., 1989). Withdrawal of antiepileptic drugs routinely is used as a seizure provoking method in intensive epilepsy monitoring. No misleading information was gained with this procedure localizing single epileptogenic foci (Spencer et al., 1981). The same was true withdrawing carbamazepine and valproate.

At toxic levels, phenytoin can cause marked diffuse delta activity and paroxysmal slow-wave abnormalities (Bente, 1975; Müller and Müller, 1972; Roseman, 1961). This is also true in cases of chronic encephalopathy with near-normal serum levels (Ambrosetto et al., 1977).

Carbamazepine

Carbamazepine is related to the tricyclic antidepressants and shares their EEG effects (Bente, 1975). Carbamazepine may cause diffuse slowing (Bente, 1975; Besser and Krämer, 1987; Pryse–Phillips and Jeavons, 1970; Rodin et al., 1974; Salinsky et al., 1994; Wilkus et al., 1978). Besser et al. (1992) found no correlation between serum levels of carbamazepine or the epoxide and the increase of powers in the theta and delta bands. Furthermore, EEG slowing was not associated with increase in seizure frequency (Bente, 1975; Cereghino et al., 1974; Duncan, 1987; Saunders and Westmoreland, 1979). Generalized paroxysmal activities including spikes can be increased during successful treatment with carbamazepine (Wilkus et al., 1978). Most studies have found that carbamazepine either increases the amount of

preexisting interictal focal spikes or has no effect (Jongmans, 1964; Sachdeo and Chokroverty, 1985; Wilkus et al., 1978).

Carbamazepine was claimed to have fewer adverse neuropsychological effects than phenobarbital (Meador et al., 1991). However, carbamazepine has cognitive side effects (O'Dougherty et al., 1987), and these effects might be due to depression of cerebral glucose metabolism (Theodore et al., 1989). Differences to phenytoin are not clinically significant (Dikmen et al., 1991; Dodrill and Troupin, 1991; Meador et al., 1990). Clinical signs of acute poisoning include ataxia, nystagmus, diplopia, drowsiness, and diffuse slowing in EEG (Fig. 34.7). Cardiovascular complications are common (Leslie et al., 1983). Carbamazepine intoxication may exacerbate seizures (Bauer, 1996).

Succinimides

The use of succinimides directed against absence seizures has declined in recent years due to antiepileptic drugs with a broader efficacy spectrum (valproate, lamotrigine). The succinimides sometimes cause somnolence, lethargy, and emotional instability accompanied by signs of altered vigilance in EEG. Acute intoxication has been reported rarely.

Valproic Acid

Valproate in the usual doses did not significantly change background activity (Bruni et al., 1980; Herkes et al., 1993; Villarreal et al., 1978). Others reported diffuse slowing (Miribel and Marinier, 1968; Sackellares et al., 1980; Sannita et al., 1989). The most important change of the EEG of epileptic patients with valproate consists of reduction or even disappearance of generalized spikes along with seizure reduction (Adams et al., 1978; Braathen et al., 1988; Bruni et al., 1980; Erenberg et al., 1982; Sato et al., 1982; Stefan et al., 1983; Villarreal et al., 1978). Photosensitive spikes like-

Figure 34.7. K.B., a 17-year-old girl with temporal lobe epilepsy with rare seizures. Self–poisoning with a huge amount of a slow-release preparation of carbamazepine (CBZ). CBZ level the next day 16 µg/mL. Soporous. Diffuse slowing and 5 to 6 cps rhythmical activities over the posterior regions. Recovered promptly.

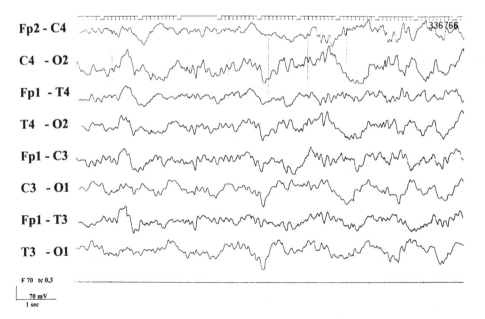

wise disappear with valproate treatment (Harding et al., 1978).

Intoxication with valproate was occasionally accompanied by marked diffuse slowing (Adams et al., 1978), considered to be partly caused by drug interactions (Simon and Penry, 1975). Drowsiness, stupor, and coma occur in rare cases with normal doses of valproic acid, with or without evident metabolic changes such as hyperammonemia and low carnitine (for review see Dreifuss, 1995). In the diagnosis of valproate-associated encephalopathy the EEG plays an important role. It is characterized by bilaterally synchronous high–voltage, slow-wave activity. The 2-EN-valproate metabolite may play a role in neurotoxicity. Fatal liver failure with valproate therapy has been reported (Dreifuss et al., 1987; Scheffner et al., 1988). There are no indications that repeated EEG records can herald this insidious complication. Enormous interindividual differences have been observed with acute valproate poisoning. The effects may range from severe coma to simple tiredness (Garnier et al., 1982).

Clonazepam

Clonazepam is a benzodiazepine and produces similar EEG changes (Pindar et al., 1976). It has little influence on focal epileptic activity (Gogolak et al., 1973; Petsche, 1972). Given intravenously, the substance is a powerful blocker of status epilepticus, but the effect remains temporary in absence status occurring in patients suffering from Lennox–Gastaut syndrome. Furthermore, like diazepam (Prior et al., 1972) clonazepam can produce tonic seizures given intravenously in this setting (Martin and Hirt, 1973).

Vigabatrin

Vigabatrin binds irreversibly to GABA transaminase and inhibits the catabolism of the neurotransmitter. GABA is increased in the brain after vigabatrin exposure (for review see Grant and Heel, 1991).

In animals, vigabatrin slows down the background activity (Halonen et al., 1992) and induces generalized spikes (Myslobodsky et al., 1979). In humans, one study reports diffuse slowing with vigabatrin (Marciani et al., 1997), whereas several other studies found no influence on background EEG activity (Hammond and Wilder, 1985; Kälviäinen et al., 1993; Mervaala et al., 1989). No consistent influence on interictal spikes was reported by Ben–Menachem and Treiman (1989) and Marciani et al. (1997). On the other hand, the development of generalized spikes was seen, occasionally accompanied by myoclonic jerks or absence seizures, even in patients with focal epilepsies (Luna et al., 1989; Marciani et al., 1995; Michelucci and Tassinari, 1989; Sälke–Kellermann et al., 1993). Excess GABA content in the brain was held responsible for the induction of generalized spikes (see also tiagabine).

Acute encephalopathies characterized by electroencephalographic abnormalities occurred after starting vigabatrin (Sälke–Kellermann et al., 1993; Sharief et al., 1993). The few reported cases do not allow a decision whether these encephalopathies are related to co–medication or to a preexisting cerebral anomaly. Overdose with vigabatrin or intoxications has not come to our attention.

Observations of concentric and irreversible visual field deficits (Malmgren et al., 2001) limited the use of the substance to the West syndrome and to otherwise untreatable focal epilepsies.

Lamotrigine

Lamotrigine blocks voltage–gated sodium channels (for review see Fitton and Goa, 1995). Rash is the most common cause of withdrawal of lamotrigine treatment. Co-medication with valproic acid and rapid titration are risk factors.

Widespread EEG attenuation was reported in nonepileptic individuals with lamotrigine intake. No slowing in background activity was seen in volunteers (Mervaala et al., 1995) and in epileptic patients (Foletti and Volanschi, 1994). Lamotrigine has a marked decreasing effect on the occurrence and frequency of spontaneous and photosensitive generalized spikes and waves (Besag, 1991; Binnie et al., 1986) as well as on interictal epileptiform activity in young patients with drug-resistant epilepsy (Erikson et al., 2001).

Lamotrigine can lead to exacerbation of myoclonic epilepsies (Biraben et al., 2000; Guerrini et al., 1998; Jansky et al., 2000) and produce nonconvulsive status epilepticus (Trinka et al., 2002). One report deals with self–poisoning with lamotrigine (Buckley et al., 1993). No serious toxicity was observed. There was a prolongation of QRS in the electrocardiogram (ECG), but no EEG examination was reported.

Gabapentin

Gabapentin is a chemical derivative of GABA, which penetrates the blood-brain barrier. The substance has proven antiepileptic properties. There are several lines of evidence for its mechanisms of action. Gabapentin has been shown to elevate GABA levels in various brain regions (Petroff et al., 1996), it binds to a unique and novel site in rat brain (Suman–Chauhan et al., 1993), and the binding protein has been identified as a subunit of a voltage-dependent calcium channel (Gee et al., 1996).

Gabapentin toxicity is low (for review see Ramsey, 1995). The most common adverse events are somnolence, dizziness, and ataxia. Overdoses showed no serious toxicity (Fischer et al., 1994). Prolonged therapy with gabapentin induced EEG slowing that correlates with cognitive complaints (Salinsky et al., 2002). Gabapentin-treated subjects had an increase in slow-wave sleep compared with baseline (Foldvary-Schaefer et al., 2002). Saletu et al. (1986) investigated the EEG under gabapentin with computer–assisted spectral analysis and found an attenuation of total power, augmentation of delta and theta activity, and a decrease of alpha activity.

Felbamate

Felbamate is the first drug with proven efficacy against seizures occurring in Lennox–Gastaut syndrome (Felbamate Study Group in the Lennox–Gastaut Syndrome, 1993). Observations of aplastic anemia and liver failure including fatalities have been reported after the drug was marketed in the U.S. (Kaufman et al., 1997). The use of felbamate now is limited to patients with otherwise intractable epilepsies (French et al., 1999). Some overdoses have been reported with low toxicities. EEG investigations have been published only in animal experiments.

Tiagabine

Tiagabine has an established mode of anticonvulsant action via inhibition of GABA uptake (for review see Suzdak and Jansen, 1995). The substance has a proven antiepileptic potency in focal seizures and a low toxicity (Leppik, 1995). Overdose has been reported (Laech et al., 1995).

The effects of tiagabine on electroencephalogram and spike–wave discharges have been studied in animals (Coenen et al., 1995; Walton et al., 1994). In a rat model of absence epilepsy, spike waves and other forms of paroxysmal activity were facilitated by tiagabine. As with vigabatrin, an increase of GABA content in the brain can result in generalized EEG abnormalities and seizures in epilepsy patients. Several cases of nonconvulsive status epilepticus have been reported during therapy with tiagabine (Kellinghaus et al., 2002; Zhu and Vaughn, 2002). In partial epilepsies, however, no rhythmic slow waves or other new EEG abnormalities have been found (Kälviäinen et al., 1996).

Topiramate

Topiramate is a broad-spectrum antiepileptic drug with multiple modes of action. Cognitive and behavioral effects are slightly worse than with valproic acid (Meador et al., 2003). Word-finding difficulties are a specific side effect in several patients treated with topiramate (Mula et al., 2003). So far, no comprehensive reports have been published with regard to EEG.

Levetiracetam

Levetiracetam is chemically related to piracetam and was screened for second-generation nootropic substances. It is devoid of anticonvulsant activities in traditional seizure screening models but exhibits a broad antiepileptic spectrum and so-called antiepileptogenic properties in experimental and clinical investigations (for review see Dooley and Plosker, 2000). Levetiracetam has become a major antiepileptic drug for partial and probably also for generalized seizures. Antimyoclonic efficacy has been reported anecdotally (Frucht et al., 2001; Kinrions et al., 2003).

In animal models levetiracetam did not change the baseline EEG, whereas it markedly suppressed spikes and waves (Gower et al., 1995). It also can inhibit spikes in human neocortical tissue (Gorji et al., 2002), and reduce the corticospinal response to magnetic stimulation (Sohn et al., 2001) and the amount of interictal spikes in epilepsy patients (Stodieck et al., 2001).

Other Drugs

A great number of drugs produce EEG changes and CNS intoxications (for review see Kurtz, 1976a,b). This section selects details of several drugs with particular interest for neurologists.

Morphine and the Opiates

Morphine and the opiates produce only mild to moderate effects on the EEG; the frequency of the alpha rhythm may be slowed down, and paroxysmal changes may occasionally appear. Rapid-eye-movement (REM) sleep depression has been observed. In neonates, morphine produces profound reversible EEG alterations, which have to be taken into consideration in the interpretation of abnormalities in these age groups (Young and Da Silva, 2000). Morphine and heroin addicts usually show unremarkable EEG tracings unless they present in a comatose state after overdose, which produces diffuse slowing. EEG abnormalities observed in an alert addict should prompt the suspicion of a HIV–related brain disease.

Aminophylline

Aminophylline is a bronchodilator commonly used for the treatment of chronic destructive pulmonary disease. Agitation, tremor, delirium, and even coma occur with therapeutic doses (Gleason et al., 1969). Acute convulsions may complicate the comatose state (Jakobs and Senior, 1974; McKee and Hagerty, 1957; White and Daeschner, 1956). In some cases, repetitive focal seizures were reported (Schwartz and Scott, 1974; Yarnell and Nai–Shin–Chu, 1975) (Fig. 34.8). These partial motor seizures were uniformly resistant to anticonvulsants and accompanied by periodic lateralized epileptiform discharges in the EEG. An underlying structural brain disease could be demonstrated in most cases.

Isoniazid (INH)

INH, a highly effective tuberculostatic drug, is known to interact with several antiepileptic drugs. This interaction may lead to intoxication from previously well-tolerated doses of anticonvulsants. Overdose of INH can produce coma complicated by acute convulsions, metabolic acidosis, hyperglycemia, and acetonuria (Katz and Carver, 1956; Kurtz et al., 1967; Livingston et al., 1956). The interictal EEG is characterized by diffuse slowing and generalized paroxysmal slow waves with intermingled bilateral sharp waves (Mellerio, 1964). With a large overdose of INH, status epilepticus has been observed (Grimminger, 1953; Kubicki et al., 1964; Scheibe, 1953; Schneider et al., 1971; Terman and Teitelbaum, 1970).

Penicillin

The parenteral administration of very large doses of penicillin G (40–80 million units/day) may produce jerks, generalized seizures, or even status epilepticus (Gastaut et al., 1967; Niedermeyer, 1974; Weinstein, 1975). Intrathecal or intraventricular application is even more likely to produce status epilepticus (Haguenau and Bouygues, 1947; Schwob et al., 1948; Vallery–Radot et al., 1951). In the treatment of status epilepticus of other etiologies, penicillin should not be administered as an antibiotic drug.

Antineoplastic Agents

A rapidly growing number of antineoplastic substances increase the armamentarium fighting cancer. Many if not all

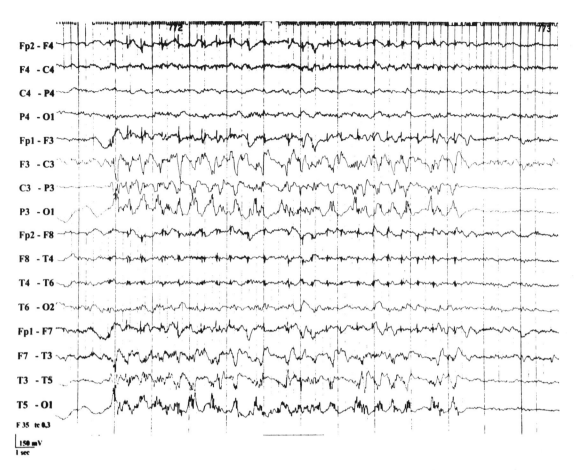

Figure 34.8. K.H., a 58-year-old man who is a chronic asthmatic and alcoholic. Relapsing episodes of focal motor status with epilepsia partialis continua–like features with twitchings of left facial and upper extremity muscles. Euphyllin overdose due to self-medication. No abnormalities with computed tomography and magnetic resonance imaging scan. The EEG exhibited constantly repeated episodes of left parietotemporal slow and superimposed fast activities accompanied by periodic twitches (see muscle artifacts).

of these drugs cause encephalopathies with personality changes, confusions, hallucinations, and coma (see also Chapter 15, "Brain Tumors and Other Space-Occupying Lesions"). Detailed reports exist for ifosfamide. It causes nonconvulsive status epilepticus (Wengs et al., 1993) and encephalopathy characterized by periodic generalized triphasic waves and negative myoclonus (Meyer et al., 2002).

Salicylate

Salicylate overdose occurs with suicidal attempts or accidentally. Most persons lack prominent neurological symptoms, but severe illness with coma and seizures can occur (Plum and Posner, 1972). Two reports mention EEG changes (Brown and Wilson, 1971; Münthe and Knehans, 1997). The records showed diffuse slowing accentuated over the anterior regions and occasionally in rhythmical trains.

Metrizamide

Metrizamide (Amipaque) is a nonionic water–soluble radiological contrast agent. Metrizamide is used for myelography. Nausea, vomiting, myoclonus, and seizures are symptoms of metrizamide–induced encephalopathy acutely occurring after its use. Several cases of nonconvulsive status epilepticus have also been reported (Elian and Fenwick, 1985; Obeid et al., 1988; Vollmer et al., 1985) (Fig. 34.9).

Toxic Encephalopathies

Several forms of CNS poisoning due to toxic agents are dealt with above and in other chapters. A selection of the remaining toxic encephalopathies relevant for neurologists is given in the following paragraph. For a comprehensive review the reader is referred to textbooks of toxicology and to the handbook articles of Mellerio and Kubicki (1977) and Kurtz (1976b).

Toxic encephalopathies present themselves as acute, subacute, or chronic disorders. Neurological and EEG abnormalities indicate alterations of neuronal structures, receptor composition, and sensitivity or neuronal death. In general, clinical signs may be classified as coma, organic mental impairment, seizures, movement disorders, involvement of cranial and spinal peripheral nerves, and neuromuscular

Figure 34.9. E.A., a 56-year-old woman who is comatose after myelography with metrizamide. Continuous repetitive triphasic waves. These conditions have also been called symptomatic nonconvulsive status (see text).

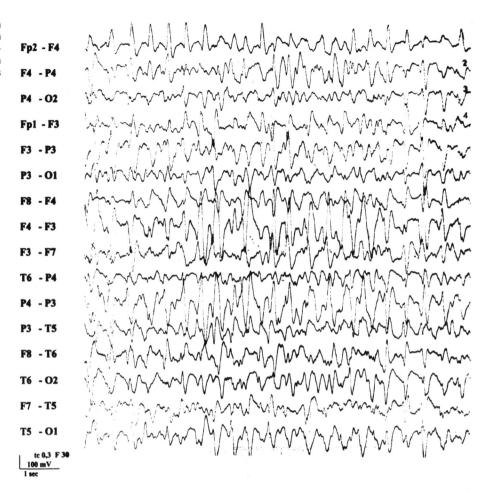

dysfunction (Johnson, 1981; Lane and Routledge, 1983; Morrow and Routledge, 1983; Paulseth and Klawans, 1985; Tanner, 1986). EEG changes are confined to coma, acute encephalopathies and severe chronic deficit syndromes.

Lead

The neurotoxic actions of lead include apoptosis, excitotoxicity, influences on neurotransmitter storage and release processes, mitochondria, second messengers, cerebrovascular endothelial cells, astroglia and oligoglia (for review see Lidsky and Schneider, 2003). Chronic exposure to lead is associated with intellectual impairment. Declines in IQ have been correlated to blood lead concentrations, even those below 10 μg per deciliter (Canfield et al., 2003).

Lead acts on voltage-sensitive ion channels (Audesirk, 1993). In acute intoxications, the EEG shows the usual signs of diffuse encephalopathies. Fejerman et al. (1973) reported lead encephalopathy as a cause of a Lennox-Gastaut syndrome with slow spikes and waves. In chronic forms, the EEG is inconclusive (Benignus et al., 1981; Burchfiel et al., 1980).

Mercury

Exposure to high doses of methylmercury causes devastating damage to the nervous system, resulting in abnormalities in motor function and impairment in the visual, auditory,

and somatosensory systems (for review see Mahaffey, 1999). Chronic toxicity is related to industrial exposure and mainly affects the kidney. Exposure to mercury from dental amalgams and fish consumption has been a concern for decades. Recent data do not support the hypothesis of prenatal mercury as a neurodevelopmental risk factor (Myers et al., 2003).

The EEG abnormalities consist of unspecific diffuse slowing and reflect the clinical state (Brenner and Snijder, 1980). Quantified EEG may document early effects of exposure to mercury vapor (Pirkivi and Tolonen, 1989).

Manganese

The most characteristic manifestations of manganese poisoning is parkinsonism. After prolonged exposure spasticity, epileptic seizures, and dementia may be associated (Lee, 2000). Myoclonus along with high-intensity signals in the globus pallidus on T1-weighted magnetic resonance imaging (MRI) have been reported (Ono et al., 2002). EEG slowing and fast activity (Mellerio and Kubicki, 1977) as well as normal EEG findings (Fuenzalida and Mena, 1967) were observed.

Aluminium

Toxic effects of aluminium have been recognized particularly with chronic renal failure on treatment with hemodialysis. The dialysis encephalopathy syndrome (Alfrey et al., 1976) shows EEG changes with diffuse slowing and spikes. However, the disease virtually has disappeared with improvement of dialysis technique. Aluminium and other metal ions promote the aggregation of β-amyloid protein *in vitro* (Manthy et al., 1993) and accumulate in the neurofibrillary tangles of patients with Alzheimer's disease (Good et al., 1992). Aluminium was considered an etiological factor in Alzheimer's disease and in the amyotrophic lateral sclerosis and Parkinson-dementia complex (Guam's disease). So far, this hypothesis did not stand the test of time.

Thallium

Thallium has been widely used as a raticide. Ingestion of thallium occurs with suicidal or murderous intention. The clinical picture and the EEG signs are essentially of nonspecific character (Prick, 1979).

Carbon Monoxide

Carbon monoxide intoxication was a frequent incident during the times of traditional heating. It is also encountered in wine cellars. The CNS effects are related to its extremely strong affinity to hemoglobin leading to hypoxic states. If the acute intoxication with different comatose stages is survived, vegetative states, diffuse encephalopathies, focal abnormalities, and extrapyramidal syndromes may persist (Bokonjic, 1963). The cortex and/or the white matter may show intensive ischemic necrosis. Pallidum necrosis is particularly frequent (Meyer, 1966). Diffusion MRI findings revealed disappearance of initially seen white matter lesions (Sener, 2003). Clinical symptoms and MRI findings demonstrated a delayed encephalopathy after a symptom free period (Kim et al., 2003; Zagami et al., 1993).

EEG abnormalities in acute and protracted encephalopathies are well known (Bokonjic, 1963; Lennox and Petersen, 1958). Diffuse or focal epileptiform abnormalities may be interspersed in the usual coma patterns (Bokonjic, 1963). Leweke et al. (1999) found a good correlation of the clinical and electroencephalographic course.

Methyl Alcohol (Methanol)

Methyl alcohol is metabolized to formaldehyde and formic acid. Formaldehyde is particularly toxic for retinal cells, and formic acid causes acidosis, generally considered the main cause of CNS involvement (Schneck, 1979). Intoxications mostly occur with low social status and may acquire an epidemic character. The symptoms are characterized mainly by visual disturbances and consecutive permanent blindness. Epileptic seizures, stupor, and coma are signs of severe acute intoxication. Necrosis of the putamen and cerebellar cortex (Orthner, 1950) and corresponding parkinsonian syndromes (Ley and Gali, 1983) have been reported.

The EEG shows marked slowing that correlates mainly with acidosis rather than with blood and cerebrospinal fluid methanol level (Jameson and Kane, 1969).

Ethylene Glycol

Ethylene glycol is used as antifreeze. Intoxications occur in developing countries, if the substance is used for elixir preparations of drugs (Hanif et al., 1995; O'Brien et al., 1998), with suicidal attempts, and if the substance is criminally added to wine (Van der Linden-Cremers and Sangster, 1985). Glycol causes renal failure and death (Hanif et al., 1995; O'Brien et al., 1998) and peripheral nerve palsies mimicking polyradiculitis (Lewis et al., 1997; Rollins et al., 2002; Spillane et al., 1991; Zhou et al., 2002). Little is known about the EEG changes with acute intoxication. With comatose states, the usual patterns without any specific signs can be observed.

Ethyl Alcohol (Ethanol)

Hallucinosis, delirium tremens, and epileptic seizures are usually understood as withdrawal signs following dependence and habituation. EEG activity is desynchronized, voltages are low, and spikes may be encountered, if recording occurs within the first 48 hours after withdrawal (Chan, 1985; Krauss and Niedermeyer, 1991; Van Sweden 1983a,b). Photomyogenic responses have been thought to occur frequently with alcohol withdrawal. However, this correlation could not be corroborated (Fisch et al., 1989). A constantly abnormal EEG in an alcoholic with seizures suggests epilepsy or symptomatic seizures unrelated to alcohol (Sand et al., 2002). Chronic alcohol use was no risk factor for a first symptomatic epileptic seizure (Leone et al., 2002).

Wernicke encephalopathy, Korsakov syndrome, sensorimotor polyneuropathy, retrobulbar neuritis, and cerebral pellagra are clearly related to nutritional deficiencies, mainly aneurine deficiency, which serves as a cofactor in many enzyme systems. In the Wernicke–Korsakov encephalopathy the EEG is variable, showing mainly diffuse slowing. The polyneuropathy shows mixed myelin and axonal degeneration. The pathophysiology of dementia, cerebellar degeneration, pontine myelinolysis, and Marchiafava–Bignami disease remains uncertain. A severe dysfunction is reflected in EEG slowing.

Alcohol encephalopathy represents most likely a continuum showing a spectrum of clinical presentations depending on the degree of involvement of multiple affected systems (Lishman, 1986; Van Sweden, 1983a,b). A subacute encephalopathy may occur showing focal seizures, transient focal cortical deficits, and periodic lateralized epileptiform discharges (PLEDs) in the EEG (Niedermeyer et al., 1981). Moreover, alcohol withdrawal has been shown to activate PLEDs in chronic focal cerebral lesions (Mani et al., 2003). Although still controversial, in some instances the relation of alcohol abuse and epilepsy may be causal (Chan, 1985; Hauser et al., 1988; Ng et al., 1988).

Organic Solvents

Trichloroethylene and methylbenzene (toluene) are used as industrial solvents. Workers are at an occupational hazard for intoxication. A major source of intoxication is the solvent abuse by children and young adults in developing countries (Ashton, 1990). Neurotoxicity leads to cranial and peripheral neuropathies; cerebellar, pyramidal, and extrapyramidal signs; as well as cognitive decline. MRI revealed white matter lesions, brain atrophy, and thalamic hypointensity (Aydin et al., 2002). Persistent EEG alterations have been reported (Stracciari et al., 1985).

Organophosphate Pesticides

Organophosphates exhibit anticholinesterase activity. Originally introduced as pesticides, they now are produced as chemical warfare agents. Sarin was used in terrorist attacks in Japan and found and destroyed in the Gulf War. Three different syndromes can be recognized (Lockwood, 2002). Acute poisoning includes muscle weakness, respiratory failure, massive bronchorrhea, epileptic seizures, coma, and death. An intermediate syndrome is characterized by pre- and postsynaptic neuromuscular junction failure. Late syndromes show delayed polyneuropathy and parkinsonism.

EEG changes in organophosphorous poisoning show nonspecific enhancement of slow activity as well as paroxysmal discharges (Bartels and Friedel, 1979; Cossa and Camuzard, 1957; Kurtz, 1976b; Mellerio, 1964; Puskas and Rusnak, 1969; Roussel, 1959). According to Okonek and Rieger (1975), there is a characteristic sequence of EEG patterns in alkylphosphate poisonings. Unlike other acute intoxications, the first stage of deep coma shows relatively fast rhythmical activity. Paroxysmal EEG activity was found to be exceptional although massive myoclonic jerks and other convulsive manifestations were noted (Okonek and Rieger, 1975).

Further details about environmental toxins may be gleaned from Lockwood (1997).

References

Adams, A.E., and Hubach, H. 1960. Hirnelektrische Korrelate der Wirkungen zentral dämpfender Substanzen im normalen EEG des Erwachsenen. Dtsch. Z. Nervenheilk. 181:71–92.

Adams, D.J., Lüders, H., and Pippenger, Ch. 1978. Sodium valproate in the treatment of intractable seizure disorders: a clinical and electroencephalographic study. Neurology (Minneapolis) 28:152–157.

Aggarwal, S.K., Williams, V., Levine, St.R., et al. 1996. Cocaine–associated intracranial hemorrhage: absence of vasculitis in 14 cases. Neurology 46:1741–1743.

Alfrey, A.C., Le Gendre, G.R., and Kachny, W.D. 1976. The dialysis encephalopathy syndrome. Possible aluminum intoxication. N. Engl. J. Med. 294:184–188.

Allain, H., Delahaye, C.H., LeCoz, F., et al. 1991. Postmarketing surveillance of zopiclone in insomnia: analysis of 20513 cases. Sleep 14:408–413.

Alldredge, B.K. 1999. Seizure risk associated with psychotropic drugs: clinical and pharmacokinetic considerations. Neurology 53(suppl 2): S68–S75.

Alvir, J., Liebermann, J., Saffermann, A.Z., et al. 1993. Clozapine–induced agranulocytosis: incidence and risk factors in the United States. N. Engl. J. Med. 329:162–167.

Ambrosetto, C., Tassinari, C.A., Baruzzi, A., et al. 1977. Phenytoin encephalopathy as probable idiosyncratic reaction: case report. Epilepsia 18:405–408.

Angst, J., and Hicklin, A. 1967. Deliriöse Psychosen unter Neuroleptika und Antidepressiva. Schweiz. Med. Wschr. 97:546–549.

Arendt, J. 1996. Melatonin. Claims made in the popular media are mostly nonsense (editorial). Br. Med. J. 312:1242–1243.

Arendt, J., Deacon, S., English, J., et al. 1995. Melatonin and adjustment to phase shift. Work hours, sleepiness and accidents. Proceedings of the International workshop, Karolinska Institute, Stockholm, September 1994. J. Sleep Res. 4(suppl 2):74–79.

Ashton, C.H. 1990. Solvent abuse. Br. Med. J. 20:135–136.

Audesirk, G. 1993. Electrophysiology of lead intoxication: effects on voltage sensitive ion channels. Neurotoxicology 14:137–147.

Austin, E.J., Wilkus, R.J., and Longstreth, W.T. 1988. Etiology and prognosis of alpha coma. Neurology 38:773–777.

Aydin, K., Sencer, S., Demir, T., et al. 2002. Cranial MR findings in chronic toluene abuse by inhalation. AJNR. 23:1173–1179.

Baldessarini, R.J., and Frankenburg, F.R. 1991. Clozapine: a novel antipsychotic agent. N. Engl. J. Med. 324:746–754.

Ban, T.A., and Amin, M. 1979. Hypnotics, minor tranquilizers and sedatives. In Handbook of Clinical Neurology, vol. 37, Eds. P.J. Vinken and G.W. Bruyn, pp. 347–364. Amsterdam: North Holland.

Bartels, M., and Friedel, B. 1979. Langauernde EEG-Veränderungen bei einer E605/Vergifung. Z. EEG-EMG 10:22–25.

Bauer, J. 1996. Seizure–inducing effects of antiepileptic drugs. Acta Neurol. Scand. 94:367–377.

Bejar, J.M. 1985. Cerebellar degeneration due to acute lithium toxicity. Clin. Neuropharmacol. 8:379–381.

Ben–Menachem, E., and Treiman, D.M. 1989. Effect of gamma–vinyl GABA on interictal spikes and sharp waves in patients with intractable complex partial seizures. Epilepsia 30:79–83.

Benignus, V.A., Otto, D.A., Müller, K.E., et al. 1981. Effects of age and body lead burden on CNS functions is young children. II. EEG spectra. Electroencephalogr. Clin. Neurophysiol. 52:240–248.

Bennett, D.R., Hughes, J.R., Korein, J., et al. 1976. Atlas of Electrocephalography in Coma and Cerebral Death. New York: Raven Press.

Bente, D. 1975. Antikonvulsiva und Elektroencephalogramm. In Antiepileptische Langzeitmedikation, Ed. H. Helmchen, pp. 182–189. Basel: S. Karger.

Berman, I., Zalma, A., DuRuland, C.J., et al. 1992. Clozapine–induced myoclonic jerks and drop attacks (letter). J. Clin. Psychiatry 53:329–330.

Besag, F.M. 1991. Use of the "Monolog" spike wave monitor to evaluate lamotrigine for absence seizures. Epilepsia 32(suppl 1):S89–S90(abst).

Besser, R., and Krämer, G. 1987. Carbamazepin und EEG. In Carbamazepin in der Neurologie, Eds. G. Krämer and H.Ch. Hopf, pp. 142–146. Stuttgart, New York: Thieme.

Besser, R., Hornung, K., Theison, M., et al. 1992. EEG changes in patients during the introduction of carbamazepine. Electroencephalogr. Clin. Neurophysiol. 83:19–23.

Binnie, C.D., van–Emde–Boas, W., and Kasteleijn–Nolste–Trenite, D.G. 1986. Acute effects of lamotrigine (BW 430C) in persons with epilepsy. Epilepsia 27:248–254.

Biraben, A., Allain, H., Scarabin, J.M., et al. 2000. Exacerbation of juvenile myoclonic epilepsy with lamotrigine. Neurology 55:1758.

Bird, T.D., and Plum, F. 1968. Recovery from barbiturate overdose with prolonged isoelectric electroencephalogram. Neurology (Minneapolis) 18:456–460.

Bixler, E.O., Kales, A., Manfredi, R.L., et al. 1991. Next–day memory impairment with triazolam use. Lancet 337:827–831.

Boenick, H.E., Lorenz, H.J., and Jürgens, U. 1985. Bromide–heute als antiepileptische Substanzen noch nützlich? Nervenarzt 10:579–582.

Bokonjic, N. 1963. Stagnant Anoxia and Carbon Monoxide Poisoning. Amsterdam: Elsevier.

Borenstein, P., and Cujo, P. 1969. Électroencéphalographie clinique et substances psychotropes. Sem. Hôp. Paris 45:1315–1330.

Bourrat, Ch., Garde, P., Boucher, M., et al. 1986. États d'absence prolongée chez des patients agés sans passé épileptique. Rev. Neurol. 142:696–702.

Braathen, G., Theorell, K., Persson, A., et al. 1988. Valproate in the treatment of absence epilepsy in children: a study of dose–response relationship. Epilepsia 29:548–552.

Braesco, M., and Lairy, G.C. 1959. Aspects electroencephalogarphiques lors due sevrage barbiturique chez les malades nonepileptiques. Rev. Neurol. (Paris) 100:335–336(abst).

Brazier, M.A.B. 1955. Studies of electrical activity of the brain in relation to anesthesia. In Conference on Neuropharmacology, Ed. H.A. Abramson, pp. 107–144. New York: Josiah Macy Jr. Foundation.

Brenner, R.P., and Snijder, R.D. 1980. Late EEG-findings and clinical status after organic mercury poisoning. Arch. Neurol. 37:282–284.

Brown, B.B. 1968. Subjective and EEG responses to LSD in visualizer and nonvisualizer subjects. Electroencephalogr. Clin. Neurophysiol. 25:372–379.

Brown, G.L., and Wilson, W.P. 1971. Salicylate intoxication and the CNS with special reference to EEG findings. Dis. Nerv. System. 32:135–140.

Bruni, J., and Wilder, B.J. 1979. The toxicology of antiepileptic drugs. In Handbook of Clinical Neurology, vol. 37, Eds. P.J. Vinken and G.W. Bruyn, pp. 199–222. Amsterdam: North Holland.

Bruni, J., Wilder, B.J., Baumann, A.W., et al. 1980. Clinical efficacy and long–term effects of valproic acid therapy on spike–and–wave discharges. Neurology 30:42–46.

Brzezinski, A. 1997. Melatonin in humans. N. Engl. J. Med. 336:186–195.

Buchthal, F., Svensmark, O., and Schiller, P.J. 1960. Clinical and electro-encephalographic correlations with serum levels of diphenylhydantoin. Arch. Neurol. 2:624–630.

Buckley, N.A., and McManus, P.R. 2002. Fatal toxicity of serotoninergic and other antidepressant drugs: analysis of United Kingdom mortality data. Br. Med. J. 325:1332–1333.

Buckley, N.A., Whyte, I.M., and Dwason, A.H. 1993. Self–poisoning with lamotrigine (letter). Lancet 342:1552–1553.

Burchfiel, J.L., Duffy, F.H., Bartels, P.H., et al. 1980. The combined descrita rating power of quantitative EEG and neuropsychologic measures in evaluating CNS effects of lead in low levels. In *Low Level Lead Exposure*, Ed. H.C. Needleman. New York: Raven Press.

Burchiel, F., Stockard, J.J., Calverley, R.K., et al. 1977. Relationship of pre– and postanesthetic EEG abnormalities of enflurane–induced seizure activity. Anesth. Analg. 56:509–514.

Byk, R. 1975. Drugs and the treatment of psychiatric disorders. In *The Pharmacological Basis of Therapeutics,* Eds. L.S. Goodman and A. Gilman, pp. 152–200. New York: Macmillan.

Campagna, J.A., Miller, K.W., and Forman, St.A. 2003. Mechanisms of action of inhaled anesthetics. N. Engl. J. Med. 348:2110–2124.

Canfield, R.L., Henderson, C.R., Cory-Slechta, D.A., et al. 2003. Intellectual impairment in children with blood lead concentrations below 10 ug per deciliter. N. Engl. J. Med. 348:1517–1526.

Carrie, J.R.G. 1976. Computer–assisted EEG sharp transient detection and quantification during overnight recordings in an epileptic patient. In *Quantitative Analytic Studies in Epilepsy,* Eds. P. Kellaway and I. Petersen, pp. 225–235. New York: Raven Press.

Caplan, L.R., Heir, D.B., and Banks, G. 1982. Stroke and drug abuse. Stroke 13:869–872.

Casanova, B., de Entrambasaguas, M., Perla, C., et al. 1996. Lithium–induced Creutzfeldt–Jakob syndrome. Clin. Neuropharmacol. 19:356–359.

Caviness, J.N., and Evidente, J.N. 2003. Cortical myoclonus during lithium exposure. Arch. Neurol. 60:401–404.

Cereghino, J.J., Bock, J.T., Van Meter, J.C., et al. 1974. Carbamazepine for epilepsy. Neurology (Minneapolis) 24:401–410.

Chan, A.W.K. 1985. Alcoholism and epilepsy. Epilepsia 26:323–333.

Chang, S.S., and Davis, J.M. 1979. Toxicity of psychotherapeutic agents (antipsychotics, tricyclic antidepressants, MAO inhibitors and disulfiram). In *Handbook of Clinical Neurology,* vol. 37, Eds. P.J. Vinken, and G.W. Bruyn, pp. 299–327. Amsterdam: North Holland.

Chang, Y.–Ch., Yip, P.–K., Chiu, Y.–N., et al. 1988. Severe generalized polyneuropathy in lithium intoxication. Eur. Neurol. 28:39–41.

Chang, Y.–Ch., Lin, H.–N., and Deng, H.–C. 1990. Subclinical lithium neurotoxicity: correlation of neural conduction abnormalities and serum lithium levels in manic–depressive patients with lithium treatment. Acta Neurol. Scand. 82:82–86.

Chauncy, D., and Leake, P.D. 1958. *The Amphetamines.* Springfield, IL: Charles C Thomas.

Chu, N.S., Squires, K., and Starr, A. 1978. Auditory brain stem potentials in chronic alcohol intoxication and alcohol withdrawal. Arch. Neurol. 35:596–602.

Clark, D.L., and Rosner, B.S. 1973. Neurophysiologic effects of generalized anesthetics. I. The electroencephalogram and sensory evoked responses in man. Anesthesiology 38:564–582.

Clark, D.L., Hosick, E.C., and Rosner, B.S. 1971. Neurophysiological effects of different anesthetics in unconscious man. J. Appl. Physiol. 31:884–891.

Coenen, A.M.L., Blezer, E.H.M., and van Luijtelaar, E.L.J.M. 1995. Effects of the GABA–uptake inhibitor tiagabine on the electroencephalogram, spike–wave discharges and behavior of rats. Epilepsy Res. 21:89–94.

Conway, J.E., and Tamargo, R.J. 2001. Cocaine use is an independent risk factor for cerebral vasospasm after aneurysmal subarachnois hemorrhage. Stroke 32:2338–2343.

Coppeto, J.R., Monteiro, M.L.R., Lessell, S., et al. 1983. Downbeat nystagmus during long–term therapy with moderate–dose lithium carbonate. Arch. Neurol. 40:754–755.

Corcoran, A.C., Taylor, R.D., and Page, I.H. 1949. Lithium poisoning from the use of salt substitutes. JAMA. 139:685–688.

Cossa, P., and Camuzard, M. 1957. Formes neurologiques subaigues des intoxications par les esters phosphoriques. Rev. Neurol. 96:163–167.

Cramer, J.A., and Mattson, R.H. 1955. Phenobarbital toxicity. In *Antiepileptic Drugs,* 4th ed., Eds. R.H. Levy, R.H. Mattson, and B.S. Meldrum, pp. 409–420. New York: Raven Press.

Cunningham Owens, D.G. 1996. Adverse effects of antipsychotic agents. Drugs 51:895–930.

Dahlitz, M., Alvarez, B., Vignau, J., et al. 1991. Delayed sleep phase syndrome response to melatonin. Lancet 337:1121–1124.

Daras, M., Koppel, B.S., and Atos–Radzion, E. 1994a. Cocaine–induced choreoathetoid movements ("crack dancing"). Neurology 44:751–752.

Daras, M., Tuchman, A.J., Koppel, B.S., et al. 1994b. Neurovascular complications of cocaine. Acta Neurol. Scand. 90:124–129.

Davies, D.M., and Allaye, R. 1963. Amitriptyline poisoning. Lancet 2:543.

Davison, K. 1965. EEG activation after intravenous amitriptyline. Electroencephalogr. Clin. Neurophysiol. 19:298–300.

Deliyannakis, E., Panagopoulos, C., and Huott, A.D. 1970. The influence of hashish on the human EEG. Clin. Electroencephalogr. 1:128–140.

Denber, H.C.B., Merlis, S., and Hunter, W. 1953. The action of mescaline and brain wave patterns of schizophrenic patients before and after electroconvulsive treatment. Electroencephalogr. Clin. Neurophysiol. Suppl. 3:30.

Denny–Brown, D.E., Swan, R.L., and Foley, J.M. 1947. Respiratory and electrical signs in barbiturate intoxications. Trans. Am. Neurol. Assoc. 77:77.

Derbyshire, A.J., Rempel, B., Forbes, A., et al. 1936. The effects of anesthetics on action potentials in the cerebral cortex of the cat. Am. J. Physiol. 116:577–596.

Devinsky, O., Honigfeld, G., and Patin, J. 1991. Clozapine–related seizures. Neurology 41:369–371.

Dikmen, S.S., Temkin, N.R., Miller, B., et al. 1991. Neurobehavioral effects of phenytoin prophylaxis of posttraumatic seizures. JAMA. 265:1271–1277.

Di Lazzaro, V., Restuccia, D., Oliviero, A., et al. 1997. Ischaemic myelopathy associated with cocaine: clinical, neurophysiological, and neuroradiological features. J. Neurol. Neurosurg. Psychiatry 63:531–533.

Doble, A., and Martin, I.L. 1992. Multiple benzodiazepine receptors: no reason for anxiety. TiPS 13:76–81.

Dodrill, C.B., and Troupin, A.S. 1991. Neuropsychological effects of carbamazepine and phenytoin: A reanalysis. Neurology 41:141–143.

Donaldson, I.M., and Cunningham, J. 1983. Persisting neurologic sequelae of lithium carbonate therapy. Arch. Neurol. 40:747–751.

Dooley, M., and Plosker, G.L. 2000. Levetiracetam. A review of its adjunctive use in the management of partial seizures. Drugs 60:871–893.

Dreifuss, F.E. 1995. Valproic acid. Toxicity. In *Antiepileptic Drugs,* 4th ed., Eds. R.H. Levy, R.H. Mattson, and B.S. Meldrum, pp. 641–648. Philadelphia: Lippincott-Raven.

Dreifuss, F.E., and Bertram, E.H. 1986. Bromide therapy for intractable seizures. Epilepsia 27:593.

Dreifuss, F.E., Santili, N., Langer, D.H., et al. 1987. Valproic acid fatalities: a retrospective review. Neurology 37:379–385.

Duncan, J.S. 1987. Antiepileptic drugs and the electroencephalogram. Epilepsia 28:259–266.

Duncan, J.S., Smith, S.J., Forster, A., et al. 1989. Effects of removal of phenytoin, carbamazepine, and valproate on the electroencephalogram. Epilepsia 30:590–596.

Edwards, J.G., Long, S.K., Sedgwick, E.M., et al. 1986. Antidepressants and convulsive seizures: clinical, electroencephalographic, and pharmacological aspects. Clin. Neuropharmacol. 9:329–360.

Eidelberg, E., Lesse, H., and Gault, F.P. 1961. Convulsant effects of cocaine. Fed. Proc. 20:322.

Elian, M., and Fenwick, P. 1985. Metrizamide and the EEG: three case reports and a review. J. Neurol. 232:341–345.

Ellington, A.L. 1968. Electroencephalographic pattern of burst suppression in a case of barbiturate coma. Electroencephalogr. Clin. Neurophysiol. 25:491–493.

Erenberg, G., Rothner, A.D., Henry, C.E., et al. 1982. Valproic acid in the treatment of intractable absence seizures in children. Am. J. Dis. Child. 136:526–529.

Erikson, A.S., Knutson, E., and Nergardth, A. 2001. The effect of lamotrigine on epileptiform discharges in young patients with drug-resistant epilepsy. Epilepsia 42:230–236.

Ernst, Th., Chang,L., Leonido-Yee,M., et al. 2000. Evidence for long-term neurotoxicity associated with methamphetamine abuse. Neurology 54: 1344–1349.

Fakhoury, T., Abou-Khalil, B., and Blumenkopf, B. 1998. EEG changes in intrathecal baclofen overdose: a case report and review of the literature. EEG Clin. Neurophysiol. 107:339–342.

Faulconer, A. Jr., and Bickford, R.G. 1960. *Electroencephalography in Anesthesiology.* Springfield, IL: Charles C Thomas.

Fejerman, N., Gimenez, E.R., Vallejo, N.E., et al. 1973. Lennox-Gastaut syndrome and lead intoxication. Pediatrics 52:227–234.

Felbamate Study Group in the Lennox–Gastaut Syndrome. 1993. Efficacy of felbamate in childhood epileptic encephalopathy (Lennox–Gastaut syndrome). N. Engl. J. Med. 328:29–33.

Fetzer, J., Kader, G., and Danahy, S. 1981. Lithium encephalopathy: a clinical, psychiatric and EEG evaluation. Am. J. Psychiatry 138:1622–1623.

Fink, M. 1968. EEG classification of psychoactive compounds in man: a review and theory of behavioral associations. In *Psychopharmacology: A Review of Progress 1957–1967*, Ed. D.H. Effron, pp. 497–507. U.S. Public Health Service publication No. 1836. Washington, DC: U.S. Government Printing Office.

Fink, M. 1969. EEG and human psychopharmacology. Ann. Rev. Pharmacol. 9:241–258.

Fink, M. 1974. EEG profiles and bioavailability measures of psychoactive drugs. Mod. Probl. Psychopharmacopsychiatry 8:76–98.

Fink, M., Irwin, P., Sannita, W., et al. 1979. Phenytoin: EEG effects and plasma levels in volunteers. Ther. Drug Monit. 1:93–103.

Fisch, B.J., Hauser, W.A., Brust, J.C.M., et al. 1989. The EEG response to diffuse and patterned photic stimulation during acute untreated alcohol withdrawal. Neurology 39:434–436.

Fischer, J.H., Barr, A.N., Rogers, S.L., et al. 1994. Lack of serious toxicity following gabapentin overdose. Neurology 44:982–983.

Fischer–Williams, M. 1963. Burst–suppression activity as an indication of undercut cortex. Electroencephalogr. Clin. Neurophysiol. 15:723–724.

Fitton, A., and Goa, K.L. 1995. Lamotrigine. An update of its pharmacology and therapeutic use in epilepsy. Drugs 50:691–713.

Foldvary-Schaefer, N., De Leon Sanchez, I., Karafa, M., et al. 2002. Gabapentin increases slow-wave sleep in normal adults. Epilepsia 43:1493–1497.

Foletti, G., and Volanschi, D. 1994. Influence of lamotrigine addition on computerized background EEG parameters in severe epileptogenic encephalopathies. Eur. Neurol. (suppl. 1):S87–S89.

Franks, N.P., and Lieb, W.R. 1994. Molecular and cellular mechanisms of general anesthesia. Nature 367:607–613.

Frazer, A. 1997. Pharmacology of antidepressants. J. Clin. Pharmacol. 17(suppl 1):S1–S18.

Freedman, R. 2003. Schizophrenia. N. Engl. J. Med. 349:1738–1749.

French, J., Smith, M., Faught, E., et al. 1999. Practice advisory: The use of felbamate in the treatment of patients with intractable epilepsy. Neurology 52:1540–1545.

Frucht, St.J., Louis, E.D., Chuang, C., et al. 2001. A plot tolerability and efficacy study of levetiracetam in patients with chronic myoclonus. Neurology 57:1112–1114.

Fuenzalida, S., and Mena, I. 1967. Intoxication cronica por manganeso y sus relaciones con las enfermedades del sistema extrapiramidal. Rev. Med. Chile 95:667.

Gale, K. 1989. GABA in epilepsy: the pharmacological basis. Epilepsia 30(suppl 3):S1–S11.

Gardner, C.R., Tully R.W., and Hedgecock, J.R. 1993. The rapidly expanding range of neuronal benzodiazepine receptor ligands. Prog. Neurobiol. 40:1–61.

Garnier, R., Boudignat, O., and Fornier, P.E. 1982. Valproate poisoning. Lancet 320:97.

Gastaut, H., Roger, J., and Lob, H. 1967. *Les États de Mal Épileptiques*. Paris: Masson.

Gee, N.S., Brown, J.B., Dissanayake, V.U.K., et al. 1996. The novel anticonvulsant drug, gabapentin (Neurontin), binds to the alpha 2 delta subunit of a calcium channel. J. Biol. Chem. 271:5768–5776.

Gibbs, F.A., Gibbs, E.L., and Lennox, W.G. 1937. Effects on the electroencephalogram of certain drugs which influence nervous activity. Arch. Intern. Med. 60:154–166.

Gille, M., Ghariani, S., Piéret, F., et al. 1997. Encéphalomyopathie aigue et syndrome cérébelleux persistant après intoxication par sel de lithium et haloperidol. Rev. Neurol. (Paris) 153:268–270.

Gillin, J.Ch. 1991. The long and the short of sleeping pills. N. Engl. J. Med. 324:1735–1737.

Glaze, D.G. 1997. Drug effects. In *Current Practice of Clinical Electroencephalography,* 2nd ed., Eds. D.D. Daly and T.A. Pedley, pp. 489–512. Philadelphia: Lippincott–Raven.

Gleason, M.M., Gosselin, R.E., and Hodge, H.C. 1969. *Clinical Toxicology of Commercial Products*. Baltimore: Williams & Wilkins.

Globe, L.I., and Merkin, M. 1986. Cerebral infarction in a user of free–base cocaine ("crack"). Neurology 36:1602–1604.

Gogolak, G., Stumpf, C., and Tschakaloff, C. 1973. Antikonvulsive Wirkung von Clonazepam und Ro 8–4192 gegen Penicillin– und Lidocaine–Krämpfe. Arneimittel–Forsch. (Drug Res.) 23:545.

Good, P.F., Perl, D.P., Bierer, L.M., et al. 1992. Selective accumulation of aluminium and iron in the neurofibrillary tangles of Alzheimer´s disease: a laser microprobe (LAMMA) study. Ann. Neurol. 31:286–292.

Gorji, A., Höhling, J.-M., Madeja, M., et al. 2002. Effect of levetiracetam on epileptiform discharges in human neocortical slices. Epilepsia 43:1480–1487.

Gotman, J., Gloor, P., Quesney, L.F., et al. 1982. Correlations between EEG changes induced by diazepam and the localization of epileptic spikes and seizures. Electroencephalogr. Clin. Neurophysiol. 54:614–621.

Grant, S.M., and Heel, R.C. 1991. Vigabatrin. A review of its pharmacodynamic and pharmacokinetic properties, and therapeutic potential in epilepsy and disorders of motor control. Drugs 41:889–926.

Greenblatt, D.J., Harmatz, J.S., Shapiro, L., et al. 1991. Sensitivity to triazolam in the elderly. N. Engl. J. Med. 324:1961–1698.

Gower, A.J., Hirsch, E., Boehrer, A., et al. 1995. Effects of levetiracetam, a novel antiepileptic drug, on convulsant activity in two genetic rat models of epilepsy. Epi. Res. 22:207–213.

Grimminger, A. 1953. Toxische Wirkungen des Isonicotinsäurehydrazids (Suicid mit Neoteben). Beitr. Klin. Tuberk. 110:387–393.

Guerrini, R., Dravet, C., Genton, P., et al. 1998. Lamotrigine and seizure aggravation in severe myoclonic epilepsy. Epilepsia 39:508–512.

Habib, M., Khalil, R., LePensec Bertrand, D., et al. 1986. Syndrome neurologique persistant après traitement par les sels de lithium. Rev. Neurol. (Paris) 142:61–64.

Häcki, M. 1986. Amnestische Episoden nach Einnahme des Hypnotikums Midazolam. Wirkung oder Nebenwirkung? Schweiz. Med. Wochenschr. 116:42–44.

Haefely, W.E. 1989. Pharmacology of the benzodiazepine receptor. Eur. Arch. Psychiatr. Neurol. Sci. 238:294–301.

Haguenau, J., and Bouygues, P. 1947. Méningite à entérocoques guérie par la penicilline. Bull. Soc. Méd. Hôp. Paris 4 Ser. 63:186–189.

Haider, J., Matthew, H., and Oswald, J. 1971. Electroencephalographic changes in acute drug poisoning. Electroencephalogr. Clin. Neurophysiol. 30:23–31.

Haller, E., and Binder, R.L. 1990. Clozapine and seizures. Am. J. Psychiatry 147:1069–1071.

Halonen, T., Pitkänen, A., Koivisto, E., et al. 1992. Effect of vigabatrin on the electroencephalogram in rats. Epilepsia 33:122–127.

Hammond, E.J., and Wilder, B.J. 1985. Effects of gamma–vinyl–GABA on the human electroencephalogram. Neuropharmacology 24:975–984.

Hanif, M., Mobarak, M.R., Ronan, A., et al. 1995. Fatal renal failure caused by diethylene glycol in paracetamol elixir: the Bangladesh epidemic. Br. Med. J. 311:88–91.

Harding, G.F.A., Herrick, C.E., and Jeavons, P.M. 1978. A controlled study of the effect of sodium valproate on photosensitive epilepsy and its prognosis. Epilepsia 19:555–565.

Harrer, G. 1960. Zur Chemotherapie der Depressionen. Wien. Med. Wschr. 110:255–259.

Harvey, S.C. 1975. Hypnotics and sedatives. The barbiturates. In *The Pharmacological Basis of Therapeutics,* Eds. L. S. Goodman and A. Gilman, pp. 102–123. New York: Macmillan.

Hauser, P., Devinsky, O., DeBellis, M., et al. 1989. Benzodiazepine withdrawal delirium with catatonic features. Occurrence in patients with partial seizure disorders. Arch. Neurol. 46:696–699.

Hauser, W.A., Ng, S., Ki. C., et al. 1988. Alcohol, seizures and epilepsy. Epilepsia 29:S66–S78.

Helmchen, H. 1961. Delirante Abläufe unter psychiatrischer Pharmakotherapie. Arch. Psychiatr. Z. Nervenheilk. 202:395–411.

Helmchen, H., and Kanowski, S. 1971. EEG–Veränderungen unter Lithium–Therapie. Nervenarzt 43:145–152.

Henninger, G.R. 1969. Lithium effects on cerebral cortical function in manic depressive patients. Electroencephalogr. Clin. Neurophysiol. 27:670(abst).

Herkes, G.K., Lagerlund, T.D., Sharbrough, F.W., et al. 1993. Effects of antiepileptic drug treatment on the background frequency of EEGs in epileptic patients. J. Clin. Neurophysiol. 10:210–216.

Herning, R.I., Jones, R.T., Hooker, W.D., et al. 1985. Cocaine increases EEG beta: a replication and extension of Hans Berger's historic experiments. Electroencephalogr. Clin. Neurophysiol. 60:470–477.

Herrmann, W.M., Fichte, K., Itil, T.M., et al. 1979. Development of a classification rule for four clinical therapeutic psychotropic drug classes with

EEG power–spectrum variables of human volunteers. Pharmacopsychiatry 12:20–34.

Hess, R. 1974. Electroencephalography. In *Handbook of Clinical Neurology*, Eds. P.J. Vinken and G.W. Bruyn, pp. 498–532. Amsterdam: North Holland.

Hollister, L.E., and Barthel, C.A. 1959. Changes in the electroencephalogram during chronic administration of tranquilizing drugs. Electroencephalogr. Clin. Neurophysiol. 11:792–795.

Isermann, H., and Haupt, R. 1976. Auffällige EEG–Veränderungen unter Clozapin–Behandlung bei paranoid–halluzinatorischen Psychosen. Nervenarzt 47:268.

Itil, T.M. 1970. Convulsive and anticonvulsive properties of neuro–psycho–pharmaca. In *Epilepsy. Modern Problems in Pharmacopsychiatry*, vol. 4, Ed. E. Niedermeyer, pp. 270–305. Basel: Karger.

Itil, T.M. 1971. Quantitative pharmaco–electroencephalography in assessing new anti–anxiety agents. In *Advances in Neuro–Psychopharmacology*, Eds. O. Vinar, Z. Votova, and P.B. Bradley, pp. 199–209. Amsterdam: North Holland.

Itil, T.M., and Soldatos, 1980. Epileptogenic side effects of psychotropic drugs. JAMA. 244:1460–1463.

Ito, B.M., Sato, S., Kufta, L.V., et al. 1988. Effect of isoflurane and enflurane on the electroencephalogram of epileptic patients. Neurology 38:924–928.

Iversen,L. 2003. Cannabis and the brain. Brain 126:1252–1270.

Jääskeläinen, S.K., Kaistoi, K., Suni, L., et al. 2003. Sevoflurane is epileptogenic in healthy subjects at surgical levels of anesthesia. Neurology 61:1073–1078.

Jabbari, B., Byran, G.E., Marsh, E.E., et al. 1985. Incidence of seizures with tricyclic and tetracyclic antidepressants. Arch. Neurol. 42:480–481.

Jakobs, M.H., and Senior, R.M. 1974. Theophylline toxicity due to impaired theophylline degradation. Am. Rev. Respir. Dis. 110:342–345.

Jameson, H.D., and Kane, R. 1969. EEG records during an epidemic of methanol intoxication. Electroencephalogr. Clin. Neurophysiol. 26:112 (abst).

Jansky, J., Rásonyi, G., Halàsz, P., et al. 2000. Disabling erratic myoclonus during lamotrigine therapy with high serum level—report of two cases. Clin. Neuropharmacol. 23:86–89.

Johnson, D.A.W. 1981. Drug-induced psychiatric disorders. Drugs 22:57–69.

Johnson, G., Maccario, M., Gershon, S., and Korein, J. 1970. The effect of lithium on the electroencephalogram, behavior and serum electrolytes. J. Nerv. Ment. Dis. 151:273–289.

Jongmans, J.W.M. 1964. Report of the antiepileptic action of Tegretol. Epilepsia 5:74–82.

Jörgensen, R.S., and Wulff, M.H. 1958. The effect of orally administered chlorpromazine on the electroencephalogram of man. Electroencephalogr. Clin. Neurophysiol. 10:325–329.

Joutsiniemi, S.-L., Gross, A., and Appelberg, B. 2001. Marked clozapine-induced slowing of EEG background over frontal, central, and parietal scalp areas in schizophrenic patients. J. Clin. Neurophysiol. 18:9–13.

Kalant, H., and Kalant, O.H. 1975. Death in amphetamine users: Causes and rates. Can. Med. Assoc. J. 112:299–304.

Kälviäinen, R., Keränen, T., and Riekkinen, P.J. 1993. Place of newer antiepileptic drugs in the treatment of epilepsy. Drugs 46:1009–1024.

Kälviäinen, R., Äikiä, M., Mervaala, E., et al. 1996. Long–term cognitive and EEG effects of tiagabine in drug–resistant partial epilepsy. Epilepsy Res. 25:291–297.

Karst, M., Salim, K., Burstein, S., et al. 2003. Analgesic effect of the synthetic cannabinoid CT-3 on chronic neuropathic pain. JAMA. 290:1757–1762.

Katz, B.E., and Carver, M.W. 1956. Acute poisoning with isoniazid treated with exchange transfusions. Pediatrics 18:77.

Kaufman, D., Kelly, J.P., Levy, M., et al. 1997. Evaluation of case reports of aplastic anemia among patients treated with felbamate. Epilepsia 38: 1265–1269.

Kellinghaus, C., Dziewas, R., and Lüdemann, P. 2002. Tiagabin-related non-convulsive status epilepticus in partial epilepsy: three case reports and a review of the literature. Seizure 11:243–249.

Kerkhofs, M., Rilaert, Ch., DeMaertelaer, V., et al. 1990. Fluoxetine in major depression: efficacy, safety and effects on sleep polygraphic variables. Int. Clin. Psychopharmacol. 5:253–260.

Ketz, E. 1974. Wirkung von Antikonvulsiva und psychotropen Drogen auf das EEG. Z. EEG–EMG 5:99–106.

Kiloh, L.G., Davison, K., and Osselton, J.W. 1961. An electroencephalographic study of the analeptic effects of imipramine. Electroencephalograph. Clin. Neurophysiol. 13:216–223.

Kim, J., Chang, K., Song, I.Ch., et al. 2003. Delayed encephalopathy of acute carbon monoxide intoxication: diffusivity of cerebral white matter lesions. AJNR. 24:1592–1597.

Kinrions, P., Ibrahim, N., Murphy, K., et al. 2003. Efficacy of levetiracetam in a patient with Unverricht-Lundborg progressive myoclonic epilepsy. Neurology 60:1394–1395.

Kofler, M., Kronenberg, M.F., Rifici, C., et al. 1994. Epileptic seizures associated with intrathecal baclofen application. Neurology 44:25–27.

Konzen, J.P., Levine, St.R., and Garcia, J.H. 1995. Vasospasm and thrombus formation as possible mechanisms of stroke related to alkaloid cocaine. Stroke 26:1114–1118.

Koppel, B.S., Samkoff, L., and Daras, M. 1996. Relation of cocaine use to seizures and epilepsy. Epilepsia 37:875–878.

Kores, B., and Lader, M.H. 1997. Irreversible lithium neurotoxicity: an overview. Clin. Neuropharmacol. 20:283–299.

Koufen, H., and Consbruch, U. 1972. Die Lithium–Intoxikation. Beobachtungen an 6 Fällen. Nervenarzt 43:145–152.

Koukkou, M., Angst, J., and Zimmer, D. 1979. Paroxysmal EEG activity and psychopathology during treatment with clozapine. Pharmacopsychiatry 12:173–183.

Krauss, G.L., and Niedermeyer, E. 1991. Electroencephalogram and seizures in chronic alcoholism. Electroencephalogr. Clin. Neurophysiol. 78:97–104.

Krendel, D.A., Ditter, S.M., Frankel, M.R., et al. 1990. Biopsy–proven cerebral vasculitis associated with cocaine abuse. Neurology 40:1092–1094.

Krump, J.E. 1954. Das Hirnstrombild im Verlauf der Schlafmittelvergiftung und seine differentialdiagnostische Bedeutung. Verh. Dtsch. Ges. Inn. Med. 2:323.

Kubicki, S. 1967. Triphasic potentials following a state of deep coma (coma depasse) in patients with intoxications by hypnotics. Electroencephalogr. Clin. Neurophysiol. 23:382(abst).

Kubicki, S., and Rieger, H. 1968. The EEG during acute intoxication with hypnotics. Electroencephalogr. Clin. Neurophysiol. 25:94(abst).

Kubicki, S., Ibe, K., and Götze, W. 1964. EEG–Veränderungen bei einer INH–bedingten Psychose und nach einem Suizidversuch mit Neoteben. Arch. Toxicol. 20:197–209.

Kubicki, S., Rieger, H., Busse, G., et al. 1970. Elektroencephalographische Befunde bei schweren Schlafmittelvergiftungen. Z. EEG–EMG 1: 80–93.

Kugler, J. 1960. Chemotherapie der Depression und EEG. Wien. Klin. Wochenschr. 72:465–468.

Kugler, J., Lorenzi, E., Spatz, R., et al. 1979. Drug–induced paroxysmal EEG activities. Pharmacopsychiatry 12:165–172.

Kuroiwa, Y., Furukawa, T., and Inaki, K. 1981. Recovery from drug–induced alpha coma. Neurology 31:1359–1361.

Kurtz, D. 1976a. The EEG in acute and chronic drug intoxications. In *Metabolic, Endocrine and Toxic Diseases/Handbook of Electroencephalography and Clinical Neurophysiology*, vol. 15, Ed. G.H. Glaser, pp. 88–104. Amsterdam: Elsevier.

Kurtz, D. 1976b. The EEG in intoxication by pesticides and raticides. In *Metabolic, Endocrine and Toxic Diseases/Handbook of Electroencephalography and Clinical Neurophysiology*, vol. 15, Ed. G.H. Glaser, pp. 105–107. Amsterdam: Elsevier.

Kurtz, D., Feuerstein, J., Weber, M., et al. 1967. Interêt de la surveillance électroencéphalographique dans la cadre de la réanimation des comas par intoxication médicamenteuse aigue. Rev. Neurol. (Paris)117:531–532.

Kuruvilla, Th., and Bharucha, N.E. 1997. Cerebellar atrophy after acute phenytoin intoxication. Epilepsia 38:500–502.

Laan, L.A.E.M., and DeWeerd, A.W. 1990. Medikamentös induzierter Absenzenstatus: Die Bedeutung des EEGs für Diagnose und Behandlung. Z. EEG–EMG 21:131–133.

Laech, J.P., Stolarek, I., and Brodie, M.J. 1995. Deliberated overdose with the novel anticonvulsant tiagabine. Seizure 4:155–157.

Lane, R.J.M., and Routledge, P.A. 1983. Drug induced neurological disorders. Drugs 26:124–147.

Lang, A.W., and Moore, R.A. 1961. Acute toxic psychoses concurrent with phenothiazine therapy. Am. J. Psychiatry 117:939–940.

Langtry, H.D., and Benfield, P. 1990. Zolpidem: a review of its pharmacodynamic and pharmacokinetic properties and therapeutic potential. Drugs 40:291–313.

Lee, J.W. 2000. Manganese intoxication. Arch. Neurol. 57:597–599.

Lee, M.S., and Lessel, S. 2003. Lithium-induced periodic alternating nystagmus. Neurology 60:344.

Lee, S.I. 1985. Nonconvulsive status epilepticus. Ictal confusion in later life. Arch. Neurol. 42:778–781.

Lennox, M.A., and Petersen, P.B. 1958. Electroencephalographic findings in acute carbon monoxide poisoning. Electroencephalogr. Clin. Neurophysiol. 10:63–68.

Leone, M., Tonini, C., Bogliun, G., Monaco, F., et al., for the ARES (Alcohol Related Seizures) Study Group. 2002. Chronic alcohol use and first symptomatic epileptic seizure. J. Neurol. Neurosurg. Psychiatry 73:495–499.

Leppik, I.E. 1995. Tiagabine: the safety landscape. Epilepsia 36(suppl 6): S10–S13.

Lersch, D.R., and Kaplan, A.M. 1984. Alpha–pattern coma in childhood and adolescence. Arch. Neurol. 41:68–70.

Leshner, A.I. 1996. Molecular mechanisms of cocaine addiction. N. Engl. J. Med. 335:128–129.

Leslie, P.H., Heyworth, R., and Prescott, L.F. 1983. Cardiac complications of carbamazepine intoxication: treatment by hemoperfusion. Br. J. Med. 286:1018.

Lesse, H., and Collins, J.P. 1979. Effects of cocaine on propagation of limbic seizure activity. Pharmacol. Biochem. Behav. 11:689–694.

Leucht, St., Wahlbeck, K., Hamann, J., et al. 2003. New generation antipsychotics versus low-potency conventional antipsychotics: a systematic review and meta-analysis. Lancet 361:1581–1589.

Levy, R.H., Mattson, R.H., and Meldrum, B.S. (Eds.). 1995. *Antiepileptic Drugs*, 4th ed. New York: Raven Press.

Leweke, F., Damian, M.S., Kern, A., et al. 1999. Zweizeitige Kohlenmonoxid-intoxikation: Akinetisches Syndrom und Leukenzephalopathie. Akt. Neurol. 26:86–90.

Lewis, L.D., Smith, B.W., and Mamourian, A.C. 1997. Delayed sequelae after acute overdoses or poisonings: cranial neuropathy related to ethylene glycol ingestion. Clin. Pharmacol. Ther. 61:692–699.

Ley, C.O., and Gali, F.G. 1983. Parkinsonin syndrome after methanol intoxication. Eur. Neurol. 22:405–409.

Lidsky, T.I., and Schneider, J.S. 2003. Lead neurotoxicity in children: basic mechanisms and clinical correlates. Brain 126:5–19.

Lindstrom, L.H. 1988. The effect of long–term treatment with clozapine in schizophrenia: a retrospective study in 96 patients treated with clozapine for up to 13 years. Acta Psychiat. Scand. 77:542–529.

Lishman, W.A. 1986. Alcoholic dementia: a hypothesis. Lancet 1:1184–1186.

Liukkonnen, J., Koponen, H.J., and Nousiainen, U. 1992. Clinical picture and long–term course of epileptic seizures that occur during clozapine treatment. Psychiatry Res. 44:107–112.

Livingston, S. 1966. *Drug Therapy for Epilepsy*. Springfield, IL: Charles C Thomas.

Livingston, S., Petersen, D., and Peck, J.L. 1956. Convulsive prevention in two year old child following ingestion of isoniazid. Pediatrics 18: 77–79.

Lockwood, A.L. 1997. Exposure to environmental toxins. Curr. Opin. Neurol. 10:507–511.

Lockwood, A.L. 2002. Editorial comment: organophosphate pesticides and public policy. Curr. Opin. Neurol. 15:725–726.

Logothetis, J. 1967. Spontaneous epileptic seizures and electroencephalographic changes in the course of phenothiazine therapy. Neurology (Minneapolis) 17:869–877.

Longo, V.G., and Silvestrini, B. 1957. The action of eserine and amphetamine on the electrical activity of the rabbit brain. J. Pharmacol. Exp. Ther. 120:160–170.

Low, M.D. 1979. Evaluation of psychiatric disorders and the effects of psychotherapeutic and psychomimetic agents. In *Current Practice of Clinical Electroencephalography*, Eds. D.W. Klass and D.D. Daly, pp. 395–410. New York: Raven Press.

Luef, G., Burtscher, J., Kremser, Ch., et al. 1996. Magnetic resonance volumetry of the cerebellum in epileptic patients after phenytoin overdosage. Eur. Neurol. 36:273–277.

Luna, D., Dulac, O., Pajot, N., et al. 1989. Vigabatrin in the treatment of childhood epilepsies: a single–blind placebo–controlled study. Epilepsia 30:430–437.

Macdonald, R.L., and Kelly, K.M. 1994. Mechanisms of action of currently prescribed and newly developed antiepileptic drugs. Epilepsia 35(suppl 4):S41–S50.

Maczaj, M. 1993. Pharmacological treatment of insomnia. Drugs 45:44–55.

Mahaffey, K. 1999. Methylmercury: a new look at the risk. Public Health Rep. 114:397–413.

Malmgren, K., Ben-Menachem, E., and Frisén, L. 2001. Vigabatrin and visual toxicity: evolution and dose dependence. Epilepsia 42:609–615.

Mani, J., Sitajayalakshmi, S., Borgohain, R., et al. 2003. Subacute encephalopathy with seizures in alcoholism. Seizure 12:126–129.

Manthy, P.W., Ghilardi, J.R., and Rogers, S. 1993. Aluminium, iron, and zinc ions promote aggregation of physiological concentrations of β-amyloid peptide. J. Neurochem. 61:1171–1174.

Mantz, J.M., Kurtz, D., Otteni, J.C., et al. 1965. EEG aspects of six cases of barbiturate coma. Electroencephalogr. Clin. Neurophysiol. 18:426(abst).

Marciani, M.G., Maschio, M., Spanedda, F., et al. 1995. Development of myoclonus in patients with partial epilepsy during treatment with vigabatrin: an electroencephalographic study. Acta Neurol. Scand. 91:1–5.

Marciani, M.G., Stantione, P., Maschio, M., et al. 1997. EEG changes induced by vigabatrin monotherapy in focal epilepsy. Acta Neurol. Scand. 95:115–120.

Markowitz, J.C., and Brown, R.P. 1987. Seizures with neuroleptics and antidepressants. Gen. Hosp. Psychiatry 9:135–141.

Marshall, M., Longley, B.P., and Stanton, W.H. 1965. Electroencephalography in anesthetic practice. Br. J. Anaesth. 37:845–857.

Martin, D., and Hirt, H.R. 1973. Clinical experience with clonazepam (Rivotril) in the treatment of epilepsies in infancy and childhood. Neuropediatrie 4:245–266.

Mattson, R.H. 1972. Other antiepileptic drugs. Benzodiazepines. In *Antiepileptic Drugs*, Eds. D.M. Woodbury, J.K. Penry, and R.P. Schmidt, pp. 497–518. New York: Raven Press.

Mayfield, D., and Brown, R.G. 1966. The clinical, laboratory and electroencephalographic effects of lithium. J. Psychiatr. Res. 4:207–219.

McKee, M., and Hagerty, R.J. 1957. Aminophylline poisoning. N. Engl. J. Med. 256:956–957.

McKernan, R.M., and Whiting, P.J. 1996. Which GABA–A receptor subtypes really occur in the brain? Trends Neurosci. 19:139–143.

McQuay, H.J. and Moore, R.A.1997. Antidepressants and chronic pain. Br. Med. J. 314:763–764

Meador, K.J., Loring, D.W., Huh, K., et al. 1990. Comparative cognitive effects of anticonvulsants. Neurology (Minneapolis) 40:391–394.

Meador, K.J., Loring, D.W., Allen, M.E., et al. 1991. Comparative cognitive effects of carbamazepine and phenytoin in healthy adults. Neurology (Minneapolis) 41:1537–1540.

Meador, K.J., Loring, D.W., Hulihan, J.F., et al. 2003. Differential cognitive and behavioral effects of topiramate and valproate. Neurology 60:1483–1488.

Mellerio, F. 1964. L'électroencéphalographie dans les intoxications aigues. Paris: Masson.

Mellerio, F. 1970. Étude électroclinique d'une intoxication aigue avec silence cérébral électrique, survie de guérison. Rev. Neurol. 122:533–535.

Mellerio, F., and Kubicki, S. 1977. Encephalopathy due to poisoning. In *Handbook of Electroencephalography and Clinical Neurophysiology*, vol. 15A, Ed.-in-chief, A. Remond, pp. 108–135. Amsterdam: Elsevier.

Mervaala, E., Partanen, J., Nousiainen, U., et al. 1989. Electrophysiologic effects of gamma–vinyl GABA and carbamazepine. Epilepsia 30:189–193.

Mervaala, E., Koivisto, K., and Hänninen, T. 1995. Electrophysiological and neuropsychological profiles of lamotrigine in young and age–associated memory impairment (AAMI) subjects. Neurology 46(suppl 4): S259.

Meyer, A. 1966. Intoxication. In *Greenfield's Neuropathology*. Eds., W. Blackwood, W.H. McMenemy, R.M. Norman, and D.S. Russell. pp. 235–287. Baltimore: Williams & Wilkins.

Meyer, Th., Ludolph, A.C., and Münch, C. 2002. Ifosfamide encephalopathy presenting with asterixis. J. Neurol.Sci. 1999:85–88.

Michelucci, R., and Tassinari, C.A. 1989. Response to vigabatrin in relation to seizure type. Br. J. Clin. Pharmacol. 27:119–124.

Michon, P., Larcan, A., Huriet, C., et al. 1959. Intoxication volontaire mortelle par imipramine. Bull. Soc. Méd. Hôp. Paris. 4 Ser. 75:989–992.

Migita, D.S., Devereaux, M.W., and Tomsak, R.L. 1997. Cocaine and pupillary-sparing oculomotor nerve palsies. Neurology 49:1466–1467.

Miribel, J., and Marinier, R. 1968. Modifications electroencephalographiques chez des enfants epileptiques traites par le depakine. Rev. Neurol. (Paris) 119:313–320.

Misgeld, U., Bijak, M., and Jarolimek, W. 1995. A physiological role for GABA–B receptors and the effects of baclofen in the mammalian central nervous system. Prog. Neurobiol. 46:423–462.

Mody, C.K., Miller, B.L., McIntyre, H.B., et al. 1988. Neurologic complications of cocaine abuse. Neurology 38:1189–1193.

Montgomery, S.A. 1995. Safety of mirtazapine: a review. Int. Clin. Psychopharmacol. 10(suppl 4):S37–S45.

Morrow, Y.I., and Routledge, P.A. 1988. Drug-induced neurological disorders. Adverse Drug React. Acute Poisoning Rev. 3:105–133.

Mortimer, A.M. 1994. Newer and older antipsychotics. A comparative review of appropriate use. CNS Drugs 2:381–396.

Mula, M., Trimble, M.R., Thompson, P., et al. 2003. Topiramate and word-finding difficulties in patients with epilepsy. Neurology 60:1104–1107.

Müller, J., and Müller, D. 1972. Hirnelektrische Korrelate bei Überdosierung von antikonvulsiven Medikamenten. Nervenarzt 43:270–272.

Münthe, Th.F., and Knehans, A. 1997. EEG–Befunde bei rezidivierender Salizylat–Intoxication. Z. EEG–EMG 28:52–54.

Murphy, J.M., Motiwala, R., and Devinsky, O. 1991. Phenytoin intoxication. South Med. J. 84:1199–1204.

Myers, F.B., and Stockard, J.J. 1975. Neurologic and electroencephalographic correlates in glutethimide intoxication. Clin. Pharmacol. Ther. 17:212–220.

Myers, G.J., Davidson, P.W., Cox, Ch., et al. 2003. Prenatal methylmercury exposure from ocean fish consumption in the Seychelles child development study. Lancet 361:1686–1692.

Myers, J.A., and Earnest, M.P. 1984. Generalized seizures and cocaine abuse. Neurology (Minneapolis) 34:675–676.

Myslobodsky, M.S., Ackermann, R.F., and Engel, J. Jr. 1979. Effects of gamma–acetylenic GABA and gamma–vinyl GABA on Metrazol–activated, and kindled seizures. Pharmacol. Biochem. Behav. 11:265–271.

Naber, D., and Hippius, H. 1990. The European experience with the use of clozapine. Hosp. Community Psychiatry 24:265–267.

Nagaraja, D., Taly, A.B., Sahu, R.N., et al. 1987. Permanent neurological sequelae due to lithium toxicity. Clin. Neurol. Neurosurg. 98:31.

Nausieda, P.A. 1979. Central stimulant toxicity. In Handbook of Clinical Neurology, vol. 37, Eds. P.J. Vinken and G.W. Bruyn, pp. 223–297. Amsterdam: North Holland.

Ng, S.K.C., Hauser, W.A., Brust, Y.C.M., et al. 1988. Alcohol consumption and withdrawal in new-onset seizures. N. Engl. J. Med. 319:637–666.

Niedermeyer, E. 1970. Electroencephalographic studies on the anticonvulsive action of diazepam. Eur. Neurol. 3:88–96.

Niedermeyer, E. 1974. Compendium of the Epilepsies. Springfield, IL: Charles C Thomas.

Niedermeyer, E., Freund, G., and Krumholz, A. 1981. Subacute encephalopathy with seizures in alcoholics: a clinical electroencephalographic study. Clin. Electroencephalogr. 12:113–129.

Noble, E.P. 2003. D2 dopamine receptor gene in psychiatric and neurologic disorders and its phenotypes. Am. J. Med. Genet. 116B:103–125.

Nolte, K.B., Brass, L.M., and Fletterick, C.F. 1996. Intracranial hemorrhage associated with cocaine abuse: a prospective autopsy study. Neurology 46:1291–1296.

Novelly, R.A., Schwartz, M.M., Mattson, R.H., et al. 1986. Behavioral toxicity with antiepileptic drugs: concepts and methods of assessment. Epilepsia 27:331–340.

Obeid, T., Yaqub, B., Panayiotopoulos, Ch., et al. 1988. Absence status epilepticus with computed tomographic brain changes following metrizamide myelography. Ann. Neurol. 24:582–584.

O´Brien, K.L., Selanikio, J.D., Hecdivert, Ch., et al., for the Acute Renal Failure Investigation Team. 1998. Epidemic of pediatric deaths from acute renal failure caused by diethylene glycol poisoning. JAMA. 279:1175–1180.

O'Dougherty, M., Wright, F.S., Cox, S., et al. 1987. Carbamazepine plasma concentration. Relationship to cognitive impairment. Arch. Neurol. 44:863–867.

Office of Applied Studies. 1996. Preliminary results from the 1996 National Household Survey on Drug Abuse. Substance Abuse and Mental Health Administration.

Ogunyemi, A.O., Locke, G.E., Kramer, L.D., et al. 1989. Complex partial status epilepticus provoked by "crack" cocaine. Ann. Neurol. 26:785–786.

Okonek, S., and Rieger, H. 1975. EEG Veränderungen bei Alkylphosphatvergiftungen. Z. EEG-EMG 6:19–27.

Oliver, A.P., Luchius, D.J., and Wyatt, R.J. 1982. Neuroleptic–induced seizures. Arch. Gen. Psychiatry 39:206–209.

Ono, K., Komai, K., and Yamada, M. 2002. Myoclonic involuntary movement associated with chronic manganese poisoning. J. Neurol. Sci. 199:93–96.

Orthner, H. 1950. Die Methylalkoholvergiftung. Berlin: Springer.

Osorio, I., Burnstine, Th.H., Remler, B., et al. 1989. Phenytoin–induced seizures. A paradoxical effect at toxic concentrations in epileptic patients. Epilepsia 30:230–234.

Oswald, I. 1989. Triazolam syndrome 10 years on. Lancet 2:451–452.

Pacia, S.V. and Devinsky, O. 1994. Clozapine-related seizures: experience with 5629 patients. Neurology 44:2247–2249.

Pampiglione, G. 1952. Induced fast activity in the EEG as an aid in the location of cerebral lesions. Electroencephalogr. Clin. Neurophysiol. 3:79–82.

Parrino, L., Boselli, M., Spaggiari, M.C., et al. 1997. Multidrug comparison (lorazepam, triazolam, zolpidem, and zopiclone) in situational insomnia: polysomnographic analysis by means of the cyclic alternating pattern. Clin. Neuropharmacol. 20:253–263.

Paulseth, J.E., and Klawans, H.L. 1985. Drug-induced behavioral disorders. In Handbook of Clinical Neurology, vol. 2 (46), Ed. J.A.M. Frederiks, pp. 591–608. Amsterdam: Elsevier.

Peiffer, J. 1981. Clinical and neuropathological aspects of long–term damage to the central nervous system after lithium medication. Arch. Psychiatr. Nervenkr. 231:41–60.

Petroff, O.A.C., Rothman, D.L., Behar, K.L., et al. 1996. The effect of gabapentin on brain gamma–aminobutyric acid in patients with epilepsy. Ann. Neurol. 39:95–99.

Petsche, H. 1972. Zum Nachweis des kortikalen Angriffspunktes des antikonvulsiven Benzodiazepinderivats Clonazepam (Ro 5–4023). Z. EEG–EMG 3:145.

Pich, E.M., Pagliusi, S.R., Tessari, M., et al. 1997. Common neural substrates for the addictive properties of nicotine and cocaine. Science 275:83–86.

Pindar, R.M., Brogden, R.N., Speight, T.M., et al. 1976. Clonazepam: a review of its pharmacological properties and therapeutic efficacy in epilepsy. Drugs 12:321–361.

Pirkivi, L., and Tolonen, U. 1989. EEG findings in chlor-alkali workers subjected to low long term exposure to mercury vapour. Br. J. Ind. Med. 46:370–375.

Plum, F., and Posner, J.P. 1972. Diagnosis of Stupor and Coma, 2nd ed. Philadelphia: F.A. Davis.

Poewe, W., and Bauer, G. 1982. Neurologische Befunde bei akuter Lithium–Intoxikation. Neuropsychiatr. Clin. 1:53–57.

Prick, J.J.G. 1979. Thallium poisoning. In Handbook of Neurology, vol. 36, Eds. P.J. Vinken and G.W. Bruyn, pp. 239–278. Amsterdam: North Holland.

Prior, P.F., Maclaine, G.N., Scott, D.F., et al. 1972. Tonic status epilepticus precipitated by intravenous diazepam in a child with petit mal status. Epilepsia 13:467–472.

Pryse–Phillips, W.E.M., and Jeavons, P.M. 1970. Effect of carbamazepine (Tegretol) on the electroencephalograph and ward behavior of patients with chronic epilepsy. Epilepsia 11:263–273.

Puskas, G., and Rusnak, C. 1969. Certain electroencephalographic aspects in accidental poisoning with Ecatox in children. Electroencephalogr. Clin. Neurophysiol. 27:630(abst).

Qureshi, A.I., Akbar, M.S., Czander, E., et al. 1997. Crack cocaine use and stroke in young patients. Neurology 48:341–345.

Ramsey, R.E. 1995. Gabapentin. Toxicity. In Antiepileptic Drugs, 4th ed., Eds. R.H. Levy, R.H. Mattson, and B.S. Meldrum, pp. 857–860. New York: Raven Press.

Reynolds, E.H. 1983. Mental effects of antiepileptic medication: a review. Epilepsia 24(suppl 2):S85–S95.

Rodin, E.A., Domino, E.F., and Porzak, J.P. 1970. The marihuana–induced "social high." Neurological and electroencephalographic concomitants. JAMA. 213:1800.

Rodin, E.A., Rim, C.S., and Rennick, P.M. 1974. The effects of carbamazepine on patients with psychomotor epilepsy. Neurology (Minneapolis) 11:547–561.

Rollins, Y.D., Filley, C.M., McNutt, J.T., et al. 2002. Fulminant ascending paralysis as a delayed sequela of diethylene glycol (Sterno) ingestion. Neurology 59:1460–1463.

Roseman, E. 1961. Dilantin toxicity: a clinical and electroencephalographic study. Neurology (Minneapolis) 11:912–921.

Roussel, J. 1959. Tentatives de suicides par insecticides. Acta Neurol. Psychiatr. Belg. 59:1067–1077.

Rumpl, E., and Hinterhuber, H. 1981. Unusual "spike–wave stupor" in a patient with manic–depressive psychosis treated with amitriptyline. J. Neurol. 226:131–135.

Sachdeo, R., and Chokroverty, S. 1985. Increasing epileptiform activities in EEG in presence of decreasing clinical seizures after carbamazepine. Epilepsia 26:522(abst).

Sackellares, J.C., Sato, S., Dreifuss, F.E., et al. 1980. The effect of valproic acid on the EEG background. In *Advances in Epileptology: Xth Epilepsy International Symposium*, Eds. J.A. Wada and J.K. Penry, p. 132. New York: Raven Press.

Sadove, M.S., Becka, D., and Gibbs, F.A. 1967. *Electroencephalography for Anesthesiologists and Surgeons*. London–Philadelphia: Pitman–Lippincott.

Saletu, B. 1976. *Psychopharmaka, Gehirntätigkeit und Schlaf. Bibliotheka Psychiatrica*, No. 155. Basel: S. Karger.

Saletu, B., Grünberger, J., and Linzmayer, L. 1986. Evaluation of encephalatrophic and psychotropic properties of gabapentin in man by pharmaco–EEG and psychometry. Int. J. Clin. Pharmacol. Toxicol. 24:362–373.

Salinsky, M.C., Oken, B.S., and Morehead, L. 1994. Intraindividual analysis of antiepileptic drug effects on EEG background rhythms. Electroencephalogr. Clin. Neurophysiol. 90:186–193.

Salinsky, M.C., Binder, L.M., Oken, B.S., et al. 2002. Effects of gabapentin and carbamazepine on the EEG and cognition in healthy volunteers. Epilepsia 43:482–490.

Salinsky, M.C., Oken, B.S., Storzbach, D., et al. 2003. Assessment of CNS effects of antiepileptic drugs by using quantitative EEG measures. Epilepsia 44:1042–1050.

Sälke–Kellermann, A., Baier, H., Rambeck, B., et al. 1993. Acute encephalopathy with vigabatrin (letter). Lancet 342:185.

Sament, S., and Huott, A.D. 1969. The EEG in acute barbiturate intoxication with particular reference to isoelectric EEGs. Electroencephalogr. Clin. Neurophysiol. 27:695(abst).

Sand, T., Brathen, G., Michler, R., et al. 2002. Clinical utility of EEG in alcohol-related seizures. Acta Neurol. Scand. 105:18–24.

Sandyk, R. 1984. Oculogyric crisis induced by lithium carbonate. Eur. Neurol. 23:92–94.

Sannita, W.G., Gervasio, L., and Zagnoni, P. 1989. Quantitative EEG effects and concentration of sodium valproate: acute and long–term administration to epileptic patients. Neuropsychobiology 22:231–235.

Sansone, M.E.G., and Ziegler, D.K. 1985. Lithium toxicity: a review of neurologic complications. Clin. Neuropharmacol. 8:242–248.

Sato, S., White, B.G., Penry, J.K., et al. 1982. Valproic acid versus ethosuximide in the treatment of absence seizures. Neurology 32:157–163.

Saunders, M.G., and Westmoreland, B.F. 1979. The EEG in the evaluation of disorders affecting the brain diffusely. In *Current Practice of Clinical Electroencephalography*, Eds. D.W. Klass and D.D. Daly, pp. 343–379. New York: Raven Press.

Scharf, M.B., Fletcher, K., and Graham, J.P. 1988. Comparative amnesic effects of benzodiazepine hypnotic agents. J. Clin. Psychiatry 49:134–137.

Scharfetter, C. 1965. Vergiftung mit einem Antidepressivum:Status epilepticus bei suicidaler Amitriptylinintoxication. Bemerkungen zur Neurologie schwerer Vergiftungen. Arch. Psychiatr. Nervenkr. 207:79–98.

Scheffner, D., König, S., Rauterberg–Ruland, I., et al. 1988. Fatal liver failure in 16 children with valproate therapy. Epilepsia 29:530–542.

Scheibe, F. 1953. Tod nach 15 g Isonicotinsäurehydrazid. Z. Gesamte Inn. Med. 8:283.

Schifano, F., Oyefeso, A., Webb,L., et al. 2003. Review of deaths related to taking ecstasy, England and Wales, 1997-2000. Br. Med. J. 326:80–81.

Schmauss, M., Wolff, R., Erfurth, A., et al. 1989. Tolerability of long term clozapine treatment. Psychopharmacology 99:105–108.

Schmidt, Ch.J., Sorensen, St.M., Kehne, J.H., et al. 1995. The role of 5–HT 2a receptors in antipsychotic activity. Life Sci. 56:2209–2222.

Schmitz, B. 2002. Antidepressant drugs: indications and guidelines for use in epilepsy. Epilepsia 43(suppl 2):14–18.

Schneck, S.A. 1979. Methyl alcohol. In *Handbook of Neurology*, vol. 36, Eds. P.J. Vinken and G.W. Bruyn, pp. 351–360. Amsterdam: North Holland.

Schneider, E., Jungbluth, H., and Oppermann, F. 1971. Die akute Isoniazid–Intoxikation. Eine neurologische, elektroencephalographische und toxikologische Verlaufsuntersuchung. Klin. Wochenschr. 49:904–910.

Schütz, E., and Caspers, H. 1957. Tierexperimentelle Untersuchungen über die Provokation und Aktivierung pathologischer EEG–Phänomene, insbesondere von Krampfströmen durch Narkose und im medikamentösen Schlaf. Klin. Wochenschr. 30:811.

Schwartz, K.A., and Cohen, J.A. 1984. Subarachnoid hemorrhage precipitated by cocaine snorting. Arch. Neurol. 41:705.

Schwartz, K.A., and Scott, D.F. 1974. Aminophylline–induced seizures. Epilepsia 15:501–505.

Schwob, R.A., Bonduelle, M., and Vernant, P. 1948. État de mal épileptiques à evolution fatale après injection intraarachidienne de penicilline. Bull. Soc. Méd. Hôp. Paris 4 Ser. 64:687–691.

Sener, R.N. 2003. Acute carbon monoxide poisoning: diffusion MR imaging findings. AJNR. 24:1475–1477.

Sharief, M.K., Sander, J.W.A., and Shorvon, S.D. 1993. Acute encephalopathy with vigabatrin (letter). Lancet 342:619.

Shopsin, B., Johnson, G., and Gershon, S. 1970. Neurotoxicity with lithium: differential drug responsiveness. Int. Pharmacopsychiatry 5:170–182.

Simon, D., and Penry, J.K. 1975. Sodium–di–N–propylacetate (DPA) in the treatment of epilepsy. A review. Epilepsia 16:549–573.

Sindrup, S.H., and Jensen, T.S. 2000. Pharmacologic treatment of pain in polyneuropathy. Neurology 55:915–920.

Skowron, D.M., and Stimmel, G.L. 1992. Antidepressants and the risk of seizures. Pharmacotherapy 12:18–22.

Smith, S.J.M., and Kocen, R.S. 1988. A Creutzfeldt–Jakob like syndrome due to lithium toxicity. J. Neurol. Neurosurg. Psychiatry 51:120–123.

Sohn, Y.H., Kaelin-Lang, A., Jung, H.Y., et al. 2001. Effect of levetiracetam on human corticospinal excitability. Neurology 57:858–863.

Spatz, R., Kugler, J., Greil, W., et al. 1978a. Das Elektroencephalogram bei der Lithium–Intoxikation. Nervenarzt 49:539–542.

Spatz, R., Lorenzi, E., Kugler, J., et al. 1978b. Häufigkeit und Form von EEG–Anomalien bei Clozapintherapie. Arzneim. Forsch. (Drug Res.) 28:1499–1500.

Spencer, S.S., Spencer, D.D., Williamson, P.D., et al. 1981. Ictal effects of anticonvulsant medication withdrawal in epileptic patients. Epilepsia 22:297–307.

Spillane, L., Roberts, J.R., and Meyer, A.E. 1991. Multiple cranial nerve deficits after ethylene glycol poisoning. Ann. Emerg. Med. 20:208–210.

Stefan, H., Hoffmann, F., Fichsel, H., et al. 1983. Therapie generalisierter Epilepsien mit Langzeit–EEG–gesteuerter Einmalgabe von Natrium–Valproat. Nervenarzt 54:430–434.

Stevens, J.R., Denney, D., and Szot, P. 1996. Kindling with clozapine: behavioral and molecular consequences. Epilepsy Res. 26:295–304.

Stilman, N., and Masdeu, J.C. 1985. Incidence of seizures with phenytoin toxicity. Neurology (Minneapolis) 35:1769–1772.

Stodieck, S., Steinhoff, B.J., Kolmsee, S., et al. 2001. Effect of levetiracetam in patients with epilepsy and interictal epileptiform discharges. Seizure 10:583–587.

Stracciari, A., Gallassi, R., Ciardulli, C., et al. 1985. Neuropsychological and EEG evaluation in exposure to trichloroethylene. J. Neurol. 232:120–122.

Suman–Chauhan, N., Webdale, L., Hill, D.R., et al. 1993. Characterization of (3H)gabapentin to a novel site in rat brain: homogenate binding studies. Eur. J. Pharmacol. 244:293–301.

Suzdak, P.D., and Jansen, J.A. 1995. A review of the preclinical pharmacology of tiagabine: a potent and selective anticonvulsant GABA uptake inhibitor. Epilepsia 36:612–626.

Swank, R.L. 1949. Synchronization of spontaneous electrical activity of cerebrum by barbiturate narcosis. J. Physiol. (Lond.) 12:161.

Tanner, C.M. 1986. Drug induced movement disorders. In *Handbook of Clinical Neurology*, vol. 5(49), Eds. P.J. Vinken, G.W. Bruyn, and H.L. Klawans, pp. 185–204. Amsterdam: Elsevier.

Tassinari, C.A., Gastaut, H., Dravet, C., et al. 1971. A paradoxical effect: status epilepticus induced by benzodiazepines (Valium and Mogadon). Electroencephalogr. Clin. Neurophysiol. 31:182.

Tassinari, C.A., Dravet, C., Roger, J.A., et al. 1972. Tonic status epilepticus by intravenous benzodiazepine in five patients with Lennox–Gastaut syndrome. Epilepsia 13:421–435.

Terman, D., and Teitelbaum, D.T. 1970. Isoniazid self–poisoning. Neurology (Minneapolis) 20:299–304.

Terzian, H. 1952. Studio eletroencefalografico dell'azione del Largactil (4560 RP). Rass. Neurol. Veg. 9:211–215.

Terrence, Ch.F., Fromm, G.H., and Roussan, M.S. 1983. Baclofen. Its effect on seizure frequency. Arch. Neurol. 40:28–29.

Theodore, W.H., Bromfield, E., and Onorati, L. 1989. The effect of carbamazepine on cerebral glucose metabolism. Ann. Neurol. 25:516–520.

Thomas, P., Beaumanoir, A., Genton, P., et al. 1992. "De novo" absence status of late onset: report of 11 cases. Neurology 42:104–110.

Thomas, P., Lebrun, C., and Chatel, M. 1993. De novo absence status epilepticus as a benzodiazepine withdrawal syndrome. Epilepsia 34:355–358.

Toone, B.K., and Fenton, G.W. 1977. Epileptic seizures induced by psychotropic drugs. Psychol. Med. 7:271–273.

Treiman, D.M., Meyers, P.D., Walton, N.Y., et al., for the Veterans Affairs Status Epilepticus Cooperative Study Group 1998. A comparison of four treatments for generalized convulsive status epilepticus. N. Engl. J. Med. 339:792–798.

Tremont-Lukats, I.W., Megeff, C., and Backonja, M.-M. 2000. Anticonvulsants for neuropathic pain syndromes. Drugs 60:1029–1052.

Trimble, M.R. 1991. Neurobehavioral effects of anticonvulsants. JAMA. 13:1307–1308.

Trinka, E., Dilitz, E., Unterberger, I., et al. 2002. Nonconvulsive status epilepticus after replacement of valproate with lamotrigine. J. Neurol. 249:1417–1422.

Ulrich, G., Scheuler, W., and Müller–Oerlinghausen, B. 1982. Zur visuell–morphologischen Analyse des hirnelektrischen Verhaltens bei Patienten mit manisch–depressiven und schizoaffektiven Psychosen unter Lithiumprophylaxe. Fortschr. Neurol. Psychiatr. 50:24–36.

U.S. Modafinil in Narcolepsy Multicenter Study Group. 2000. Randomized trial of modafinil as a treatment for the excessive daytime somnolence of narcolepsy. Neurology 54:1166–1175.

Utiger, R.D. 1992. Melatonin—the hormone of darkness (editorial). N. Engl. J. Med. 327:1377–1379.

Vallery–Radot, Pasteur, L., Milliez, P., et al. 1951. État de mal épileptique fatal après une injection arachidienne de penicilline concentrée au cours d'une ménengite cérébrospinale à méningocoques. Bull. Soc. Méd. Hôp. Paris 4 Ser. 67:769–771.

Van der Kroef, C. 1979. Reactions to triazolam. Lancet 2:526.

Van der Linden-Cremers, P.M.A., and Sangster, B. 1985. Medical sequelae of the contamination of wine with diethylene glycol. Ned. Tijdschr. Geneeskd. 129:1890–1891.

VanMeter, W.G., Owens, H.F., and Himwich, H.E. 1959. Effects of Tofranil, an antidepressant drug, on electrical potentials of rabbit brain. Can. Psychiatr. Assoc. J. Suppl. 4:113–119.

Van Stavern, G.P., and Gorman, M. 2002. Orbital infarction after cocaine use. Neurology 59:642–643.

Van Sweden, B. 1983a. The EEG in chronic alcoholism. 1. The EEG in alcohol addicts presenting with psychosis. Clin. Neurol. Neurosurg. 85:3–11.

Van Sweden, B. 1983b. The EEG in chronic alcoholism. 1. The EEG in alcohol addicts presenting with psychosis. Clin. Neurol. Neurosurg. 85:12–20.

Van Sweden, B. 1984. Neuroleptic neurotoxicity, electro–clinical aspects. Acta Neurol. Scand. 69:137–146.

Van Sweden, B. 1985. Toxic "ictal" confusion in middle age: treatment with benzodiazepines. J. Neurol. Neurosurg. Psychiatry 48:472–476.

Van Sweden, B., and Dumon–Radermecker, M. 1982. The EEG in chronic psychotropic drug intoxication. Clin. Electroencephalogr. 13:206–215.

Villarreal, H.J., Wilder, B.J., Willmore, L.J., et al. 1978. Effects of valproic acid on spike and wave discharges in patients with absence seizures. Neurology 28:886–891.

Volavka, J., Dornbusch, R., Feldstein, S., et al. 1972. Effects of delta–9 tetrahydrocannabinol on EEG, heart rate, and mood. Electroencephalogr. Clin. Neurophysiol. 33:453.

Vollmer, M.E., Weiss, H., Beanland, C., et al. 1985. Prolonged confusion due to absence status following metrizamide myelography. Arch. Neurol. 42:1005–1008.

Vollmer–Haase, J., and Folkerts, H. 1997. Primär fokale, sekundär generalisierte epileptische Anfälle unter Paroxetin. Akt. Neurol. 24:167–169.

Walder, B., Tramer, M.R., and Seeck, M. 2002. Seizure-like phenomena and propofol. Neurology 58:1327–1332.

Waldhauser, F., Saletu, B., and Trinchard–Lugan, I. 1990. Sleep laboratory investigations on hypnotic properties of melatonin. Psychopharmacology 100:222–226.

Walevski, A., and Radwan, M. 1986. Choreoathetosis as toxic effect of lithium treatment. Eur. Neurol. 25:412–415.

Walton, N.Y., Gunawan, S., and Treiman, D.M. 1994. Treatment of experimental status epilepticus with the GABA uptake inhibitor, tiagabine. Epilepsy Res. 19:237–244.

Weiner, W.J., Rabinstein, A., Levin, B., et al. 2001. Cocaine-induced persistent dyskinesias. Neurology 56:964–965.

Weinstein, L. 1975. Penicillins and cephalosporins. In *The Pharmacological Basis of Therapeutics,* Eds. L.S. Goodman and A. Gilman, pp. 1130–1166. New York: Macmillan.

Wengs, W.J., Talwar, D., and Bernard, J. 1993. Ifosfamide-induced nonconvulsive status epilepticus. Arch. Neurol. 50:1104–1105.

White, P.H., and Daeschner, C.W. 1956. Aminophylline (theophylline ethylenediamine) poisoning in children. J. Pediatr. 49:262–271.

Wikler, A., and Essig, C.F. 1970. Withdrawal seizures following chronic intoxication with barbiturates and other sedative drugs. In *Epilepsy, Modern Problems in Pharmacopsychiatry,* vol. 4, Ed. E. Niedermeyer, pp. 185–199. Basel: Karger.

Wikler, A., Fraser, H.F., Isbell, H., et al. 1955. Electroencephalograms during cycles of addiction to barbiturates in man. Electroencephalogr. Clin. Neurophysiol. 7:1–13.

Wilkus, R.J., and Green, J.R. 1974. Electroencephalographic investigations of the antiepileptic agent Sulthiame. Epilepsia 15:13–25.

Wilkus, R.J., Dodrill, C.B., and Troupin, A.S. 1978. Carbamazepine and the electroencephalogram of epileptics: a double–blind study in comparison to phenytoin. Epilepsis 25:467–475.

Williams, D.P., Troost, B.T., and Rogers, J. 1988. Lithium–induced down–beat nystagmus. Arch. Neurol. 45:1022–1023.

Wulff, M.H. 1960. The barbiturate withdrawal syndrome: a clinical and electroencephalographic study. Electroencephalogr. Clin. Neurophysiol. Suppl. 14:57.

Wyie, C.D., and Berk, W.A. 1991. Severe oral phenytoin overdose does not cause cardiovascular morbidity. Ann. Emerg. Med. 20:508–512.

Yarnell, P.R., and Nai–Shin-Chu. 1975. Focal seizures and aminophylline. Neurology (Minneapolis) 25:819–822.

Young, G.B., and Da Silva, O.P. 2000. Effects of morphine on the electroencephalograms of neonates: a prospective, observational study. Clin. Neurophysiol. 111:1955–1960.

Zagami, A.S., Lethlan, A.K., and Mellick, R. 1993. Delayed neurological deterioration following carbon monoxide poisoning: MRI findings. J. Neurol. 240:113–116.

Zhou, L., Zabad, R., and Lewis, R.A. 2002. Ethylene glycol intoxication: electrophysiological studies suggest a polyradiculopathy. Neurology 59:1809–1810.

Zhu, Y., and Vaughn, B.V. 2002. Non-convulsive status epilepticus induced by tiagabine in a patient with pseudoseizure. Seizure 11:57–59.

Zwarts, M.J., and Sie, O. 1985. A case report of phenytoin encephalopathy. Correlation between serum levels, seizure increase and EEG spike and wave activity. Clin. Neurol. Neurosurg. 87:205–208.

35. Nasopharyngeal, Sphenoidal, and Other Electrodes

Edward L. Reilly

The traditional application of electrodes to the scalp provides a good representation of the electrical activity from the lateral surface of the cerebral hemispheres. Once the surface cortex origin of the electroencephalogram (EEG) was recognized, it was understood that many areas of the cortex are not well recorded from scalp electrodes as usually placed. It has been a common practice for a number of years to add additional electrodes to those traditionally applied either in the International 10-20 system (American EEG Society, 1986; Jasper, 1958) or in the various anatomical placements of EEG electrodes (APEEGE) (Gibbs and Gibbs, 1984).

When a specific area of involvement is suspected because of the patient's symptomatology, some of these less typical electrodes should be placed.

Current research in the use of computer-assisted topographical maps has also led to interest in increased electrode number, but this is an area of continued research. The American EEG Society Guidelines for Standard Electrode Position Nomenclature were developed with a standard terminology for the identification of 75 electrodes including the two earlobe electrodes as noted in Chapter 7 (American EEG Society, 1990).

Unusual Focal Activity

In some instances, the placement of additional electrodes is indicated by suggestions in the ongoing record of an unusual pattern or, more commonly, by detection of some activity that is isolated in a single electrode. The latter is rare enough to make its presence suspicious, and it is desirable to rule out the possibility that the observation is simply some sort of electrode artifact. The easiest solution to either one of these difficulties is the immediate application of a "prime" electrode. The technologist places another electrode as close as possible to the electrode source of the questionable activity. The technologist must use caution to be sure the original electrode and the added electrode remain isolated from each other; otherwise, the two electrodes will be shorted out, and the exercise will serve no purpose. Once this prime electrode is attached, the technologist again records from the channels that demonstrated the suspicious activity. For example, the activity may have shown up in the P_3 electrode in a T_5 to P_3 and P_3 to P_z montage. The prime electrode is placed adjacent to the P_3 electrode, and the montage is now modified to run T_5 to P_3 and P_3 to P_z again, but in other channels one runs T_5 to P_3 (prime) and P_3 (prime) to P_z. The persistence of the unusual feature in both the channels with the P_3 electrode and (simultaneously) in the channels with the

prime electrode can reassure both technologist and reader that the activity is genuine and not an electrode artifact.

Applications of Specific Additional Scalp Electrodes

In a discussion of the International 10-20 System earlier in this book, it was observed that the system was designed to allow for and perhaps even encourage use of additional scalp electrodes under specific circumstances.

The prime electrode mentioned above is not a specific electrode, except to confirm something seen in a particular electrode rather than to explore areas not covered by the routinely used electrodes. One common instance in which additional electrodes are used is in a patient thought to have a lesion in the longitudinal fissure, perhaps provoking focal motor or sensory symptomatology involving the foot or lower leg. Such lesions may sometimes provoke abnormalities in the midline vertex (C_z) electrode or a disturbance in the left (C_3) or right (C_4) central electrodes. The latter tend to lie over the central sulcus or fissure of Rolando. In some instances, however, no abnormality is seen in any of these electrodes. In patients with such a history or observed focal jerking of the foot in the laboratory, it may be prudent to add electrodes. Generally, additions are made at a point between the vertex and traditional central electrodes. The additional electrodes would be C_1 and C_2 electrodes. It is also advisable when adding these extra electrodes to place electrodes equidistant between the F_z and C_z and C_z and P_z electrodes, which would be the FC_z and CP_z, respectively. The additional closely spaced electrodes may sometimes show correlation with the clinical history or observed clinical seizure that would not be evident from routine 10-20 placements.

Temporal Lobe Interest

Documentation of epileptiform abnormality from the temporal lobe is frequently difficult to obtain. A classic study showed that when repeated EEGs were done over a period in excess of 1 year, temporal lobe epileptiform discharge could be found in 98% of the people who appeared to have seizures of temporal origin (Ajmone Marsan and Zivin, 1970). Attempts to prove or improve the observation have not been demonstrated in large studies.

The methodologies to locate this sometimes difficult-to-define activity include normal recording, special insertion of electrodes through the nostril but not invasively, and invasive electrodes of various types including through tissue and by vascular passage (Nakase et al., 1995).

In the psychiatric population in which the confounding possibility of psychomotor seizures is a concern, there is generally not a great desire to use invasive procedures. Special electrode positions and nasopharyngeal electrodes are probably the maximum extent to which such a patient would be investigated.

On the other hand, in an individual for whom the possibility of surgery for a seizure disorder might prove worthwhile, additional recordings, including sphenoidal electrodes of various types that do require penetration of the skin or dura and carry some risks if misplaced, become an option and perhaps a necessity.

T1 and T2 Electrodes

The clear clinical importance of the temporal lobe and particularly the anterior temporal area to those interested in seizure disorders, and to some extent those interested in sudden behavior change and behavioral disorders, has led to a preoccupation with recording from the temporal pole. Nonepileptiform abnormalities in patients over 40 are enhanced by these electrodes as well (Nowack et al., 1988).

It has been argued that the International 10-20 System neglects the anterior temporal pole because the F_7 and F_8 electrodes lie anterior to the anatomical temporal pole. Many electroencephalographers feel that it is relatively rare for anterior temporal abnormality not to involve the F_7 and F_8 electrode as much as, and perhaps more than, it involves the midtemporal T_3 and T_4 leads. It is, however, certainly worthwhile in cases of suspected temporal activity unconfirmed by traditional electrodes to attempt a closer examination of the temporal area in the same manner that one would view the central area, as described earlier.

Traditionally, placement of electrodes close to the temporal pole has led to those electrodes being called T_1 and T_2. It is important in every laboratory placing such electrodes that there be documentation as to the placement method used because the method varies. In the International 10-20 System, it would be expected that T_1 would be one-half the distance from F_7 to T_3 and that the electrode would lie on the 10% circumferential line created during electrode application in that system (Jasper, 1958), but in the updated terminology there is no T_1 or T_2 and that position is called FT_7 and FT_8 (American EEG Society, 1991).

In the United States, a common placement of the T_1 and T_2 electrode is that described by Silverman (1965). This placement of the T_1 and T_2 electrode is based on the distance from the lateral canthus of the eye to the external auditory canal. An electrode is placed one third of this total distance anterior to the auditory canal and 1 cm up from a line connecting those two landmarks.

As is the case for some of the special basal temporal electrode placements to be discussed subsequently, there is debate about the value of the T_1 and T_2 electrodes. It is uncertain how often an abnormality seen with these placements is not seen at all in traditional configurations. It is clear that these electrodes sometimes give a very spectacular and clearer demonstration of temporal epileptiform activity,

but some studies have found significantly greater detection from the T_1 and T_2 than from the standard 10-20 system temporal electrodes (Homan et al., 1988; Sadler and Goodwin, 1989). Whether the demonstrated activity is isolated to these electrodes or only more nicely demonstrated, it is useful for technologists and readers to be familiar with the methodology and have experience in the interpretation of the activity from these additional electrode placements.

Anterior Zygomatic Electrodes

Twenty-one patients with temporal lobe epilepsy were studied with sphenoidal electrode and surface electrodes placed over the anterior part of the zygomatic arch bilaterally. Both methods identified abnormality in 18 of the 21; the abnormality was epileptiform in all 18 observations with sphenoidal leads but epileptiform in only 16 of the 18 recorded in the anterior zygomatic electrode and nonepileptiform in the other two (Manzano et al., 1986).

Mandibular Notch Electrodes

Recordings from the mandibular notch achieved results not statistically different from sphenoidal and T_1 and T_2 electrodes (Sadler and Goodwin, 1989). Surface electrodes were placed over the mandibular notch surface 2½ cm anterior to the tragus of the ear and just below the zygoma [mandibular notch surface (MNS)], and platinum alloy subdermal needle electrodes [mandibular notch subdermal (MNSD)] were similarly placed with virtually identical results.

Basilar Temporal Lobe Electrodes

Some electroencephalographers are convinced that not all abnormal discharges are reflected on the lateral surface of the scalp regardless of the scalp electrodes used. One solution to this problem is the use of depth electrodes, as discussed in other chapters in this text. On the other hand, attempts have been made to apply electrodes in such a way that activity from less surface aspects of the cortex can be recorded without penetrating the dura mater, preferably without entering the cranial cavity. It is possible to do this without breaking tissue at all; in some instances the attempt is made through insertion of a needle that does not enter the cranial cavity.

The two most commonly used systems for closer and sometimes longer term investigation of temporal lobe activity are the nasopharyngeal and sphenoidal electrodes. The nasopharyngeal electrode, as presently used, has the advantage of being noninvasive. The tip of this electrode lies in the nasopharyngeal space, and the electrode is a blunt-tipped one that does not penetrate the mucosa. The sphenoidal electrode requires penetration of skin and muscle but does not enter the cranial cavity.

Nasopharyngeal Electrodes

In one of the earlier attempts to improve understanding of deep structures and their function, Grinker (1938) inserted a probe in animals to a point in the posterior part of the hard palate. This probe made a circular opening of several millimeters in the mucosa. The probe was used both for stimulation and for subsequent recording of activity that was felt to be a much closer representation of hypothalamic activity than could be obtained from scalp electrodes.

For humans, the technique was varied; a slightly curved cylinder with a sharp pointed silver-plated tip was passed through the nostril and pressed through the mucous tissue in the back of the vault of the pharynx at the junction of the roof and posterior wall (Grinker, 1938). It was noted that this early electrode did not prevent the patient from being able to walk around and swallow while it was in place. Subsequent to Grinker's work, there has been continuing debate as to whether the nasopharyngeal (NP) electrode is a true hypothalamic electrode, a hippocampal electrode, or predominately an electrode measuring activity from the mesial inferior temporal lobe. Currently used NP electrodes are designed to rotate laterally from the midline. Certainly, for many of the patients who have temporal lobe symptomatology and evidence that the epileptiform discharge seen is also reflected in lateral electrodes on the scalp surface over the temporal region, the temporal region is clearly the source.

It is not necessary to penetrate the mucosa; most NP electrodes currently in use have a silver ball at the tip of the otherwise insulated electrode that is the actual recording source (Bach-Y-Rita et al., 1969; MacLean, 1949). NP electrodes are readily available from a number of commercial sources. Some of the models with weights on the external end were designed with the well-intentioned view that it would help hold the electrode against the nasopharynx. They are probably more cumbersome to use and more uncomfortable for the patient than the simple bent electrode in each nostril. It is relatively common in recording from NP electrodes to use bipolar montages that connect the NP electrodes to the other traditional temporal electrodes. It is important to record conventional temporal chains simultaneously because the nasopharyngeal

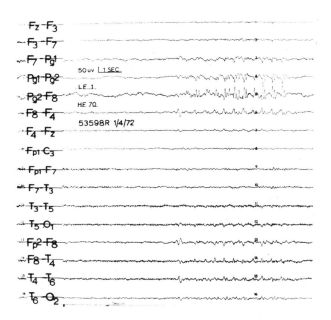

Figure 35.2. Multiple spikes in channels 4 and 5 associated with surface negative sharp wave activity. The scalp activity is far less striking than that seen with NP electrodes.

electrode will often reassure the clinician that what may be perhaps minimal in the scalp electrode deflections represent significant epileptiform discharge (Figs. 35.1 to 35.3).

The comparison of some of the standard scalp activity with that derived from the NP electrode is important, but it

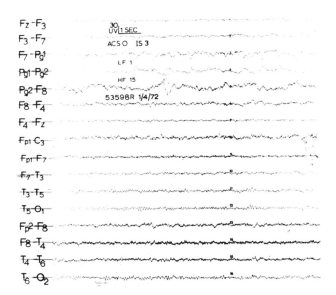

Figure 35.1. A short burst of multiple spikes in the Pg$_2$ [right nasopharyngeal (NP)] electrode. There is no reflection in the right temporal scalp electrodes.

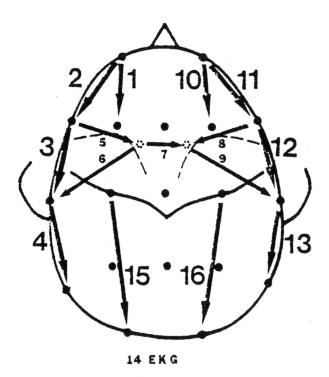

Figure 35.3. This montage includes anterior to posterior trains of conventional scalp temporal activity and simultaneous recording from the NP electrodes.

also is important to use both bipolar and reference recording techniques. In attempting to develop reference recording, there is the initial problem that in the instance of scalp, as well as NP electrode abnormality, the standard ipsilateral earlobe reference, may be equally involved. There may be some advantage to using contralateral ears, vertex, nasion, or midline occipital electrodes as the reference.

The S or Z shape of the electrode can intimidate the technologist or electroencephalographer inserting it for the first time. This change in direction by the bend of the electrode makes it far more comfortable within the nostril than an electrode that over time has become straightened or that has been somewhat straightened by a well-meaning "humanitarian." It is useful to draw a template of the initial bends so that they can be restored after straightening through repeated use and handling in the washing and sterilization process.

The distinct Z shape should be maintained; and the electrode should lie perfectly flat on a surface. In initial work, it was thought necessary to x-ray the placement to be sure that the tip was placed laterally, but this is unnecessary. With the Z-shaped electrode, the lateral rotation of the electrode tip is clearly demonstrated by the fact that the external portions of the electrodes cross the midline and each other if the rotation has been properly carried out. If the outer end of an electrode does not cross the midline but is rotated outward, the electrode tip has rotated medially. Similarly, if the end of the electrode is pointing up, then the electrode has failed to rotate properly.

Actual description of the insertion of the electrodes has been published (Mavor and Hellen, 1964; MacLean, 1949). The most common and most useful insertion for recording from the temporal lobes involves placement of the tip of the electrode on the inferior aspect of the nostril. Insertion is greatly facilitated by putting a pillow or folded blanket under the patient's shoulders so that the neck is hyperextended. The patient needs to be reassured that this position will be held for only a few minutes and the patient can return to a comfortable position with the pillow under the head rather than the shoulders as soon as the insertion is complete. The patient needs to be forewarned that there will be a sensation as if something is crawling through the nostril, which in many people provokes tearing or sneezing. This is of no consequence as long as the patient expects it and is not frightened that something is wrong.

The patient should be carefully instructed to immediately report any pain to the technologist inserting the electrode. Insertion should be stopped and the electrode promptly withdrawn for another attempt if it actually hurts. The partially inserted electrode is far more uncomfortable than having the electrode withdrawn and passed the entire distance in the proper location on the second or third attempt. Passage of the electrode requires steady pressure both in keeping the tip of the electrode down and passing it through the nasal passage. Because the tearing and sneezing persists only while the electrode is moving, there is an advantage to moving it as swiftly as possible; as soon as the patient indicates pain or there is a clear obstruction, however, the pressure should cease. The technologist advancing the electrode is required to keep very firm control of the downward and forward pressure while at the same time being alert to let the

electrode rotate at will to the right or left as it negotiates the nasal pathway. Although it is possible to insert the electrode from the written directions, it is clearly an advantage if the technologist can watch someone else insert an electrode before inserting the second one. As long as the technologist is willing to stop as soon as the patient experiences pain, he or she is not apt to penetrate the mucosa, much less to have any effect on the bone. It has been suggested that insertion should be done by a physician, but this does not appear to be necessary. It is far safer to allow a technologist to insert nasopharyngeal electrodes than it is to allow technologists to determine the amount of sedation that a patient might receive for sleep.

There is argument as to the frequency with which epileptiform activity is demonstrated with nasopharyngeal electrodes in instances in which there is absolutely no evidence for such irritative discharge from scalp electrodes. That long-running debate appears to be no closer to a resolution than at the onset of the argument.

Several reports of fairly large series have appeared. One of the largest involved the routine use of NP electrodes in patients who were over 15 and who accepted the procedure (de Jesus and Masland, 1970). In this instance, the electrodes were used in 934 records of the 1,245 run in the index population. According to the laboratory, 57% of the records involving NP use were abnormal in some way or another. Of the abnormal records, eight showed spikes in the nasopharyngeal electrodes and nothing from the scalp electrodes, and 22 showed clear NP electrode abnormality but no scalp abnormality that was clear without the added evidence from the NP electrodes. Thus, in this unselected series of patients, 5.6% of the abnormal records showed crucial temporal abnormality only on the basis of the nasopharyngeal electrodes.

Additional studies have been carried out on patients with known (Kashing and Celesia, 1976) or suspected (Schraeder and Humphries, 1977) partial complex seizures. In the series of known partial complex seizure patients, the NP electrodes in sleep showed specific discharge in 31 patients (25%) who had normal awake and sleep discharge. Of these 31 patients 16 had exclusive nasopharyngeal electrode abnormality and another 15 had low-voltage spike discharges on the scalp that had been missed without the evidence of the NP electrodes. Schraeder and Humphries (1977) studied patients suspected of partial complex seizures and 12 of the 72 patients (16.7%) suspected of partial complex seizures showed paroxysmal discharges. Of those 12, eight (11% of the total number of patients) demonstrated abnormality in the NP electrode, and for five of them the abnormality was in the NP electrode only. Three demonstrated the abnormality both in scalp and NP electrodes. Thus in this series 6.9% demonstrated the abnormality only in NP leads. Another 4.2% demonstrated it in scalp plus NP leads, and the remaining 5.6% demonstrated the abnormality solely in scalp electrodes.

Escueta et al. (1977) reviewed 76 epileptic attacks in 14 epileptics with two electroclinical types of psychomotor attacks. The more common type consisted of an initial motionless stare, stereotyped movements, and reactive automatisms, and in this type focal temporal or lateralizing features were common. The less common type started with stereotyped and reactive automatisms and there were only diffuse changes in the EEG. The nasopharyngeal electrodes had a high yield for focal-lateralizing/EEG features.

Gupta et al. (1989) examined 648 psychiatric patients and they found that the nasopharyngeal lead revealed a greater percentage of epileptiform abnormalities than were seen in the routine wake scalp EEG.

Goodin et al. (1990) found that anterior temporal and nasopharyngeal electrodes in combination with routine scalp electrodes detected 97% of the interictal spikes, whereas the standard electrode placements detected only 58%.

Sperling and Engel (1985, 1986) felt that the recordings with ear and temporal electrodes were sufficient and that the nasopharyngeal electrode as a routine procedure was unnecessary. Similarly, Sadler and Goodwin (1989) suggested that NP electrodes did not show a significant difference between better tolerated scalp derivations. This latter study included other nonstandard scalp derivations with good yields approaching sphenoidal electrode rates and better than those found in standard 10-20 placements.

The NP electrode has been used to investigate evoked potential responses (Perrault and Picton, 1984; Peters and Reilly, 1973; Smith et al., 1971; Starr and Squires, 1982). In some instances, polarity of the particular waves between the scalp electrodes and the nasopharyngeal electrodes have been compared in order to gain better insight into those waves that appear to come from a single underlying process, in contrast to others that may represent more than one cerebral process (Perrault and Picton, 1984; Smith et al., 1971). This technique has been used as part of a process attempting to determine those evoked potential components that have lateralized generator sources or sources that move through the brainstem (Starr and Squires, 1982).

It has been suggested that the appearance of far-field median nerve somatosensory evoked potentials show better identification of P_{13} in NP electrode recordings, and this appears useful in assessing focal lesions in the higher cervical cord or the cervicomedullary junction (Restucci et al., 1995).

Nasopharyngeal electrodes have been used in recording of a somatosensory evoked potentials. Wagner (1988) felt the electrodes proved useful due to their position medioventrally to the lower brainstem and provide further information about generator dipole location. Porkkola et al. (1997) felt that the P14 could be reliably recorded with NP electrodes during isoflurane anesthesia even during EEG burst-suppression when the N20 wave was attenuated.

Tympanic and Ear Canal Electrodes

Another method of attempting to get closer to portions of the brain not easily examined from the traditional scalp electrodes involves the development of a tympanic lead (Arellano, 1949). As originally described, an S-shaped, 6-cm-long insulated tube with a soft felt ball 7 mm in diameter at the tip was used. The tip is soaked in normal saline and the electrode, as originally described, is inserted until the patient "feels a slight momentary pain." It is probably unwise to make such extreme attempts to make sure that the electrode is directly against the tympanic membrane. Good judgment in this regard must be exercised. This electrode is

very close to the middle and posterior cranial fossa. This lead has perhaps been more favorably received for use in measurements of brainstem auditory evoked potentials (BAEPs) than for traditional EEG recordings. In some individuals, use of this electrode provides better identification of peak 1.

Other varieties of electrodes in the ear canal appear to provide accurate latency measurements and some amplitude enhancement of wave I and V in BAEP measurement (Bauch and Olsen, 1990; Beattie and Lipp, 1990). It is possible with ear canal electrodes to both record and provide stimulus delivery from the electrode (Bauch and Olsen, 1990).

Nasoethmoidal Electrodes

Lethinen and Bergstrom (1970) described a technique for recording from the inferior frontal lobe. As with some of the other special electrode derivations, the electrodes demonstrated activity not seen at all from scalp electrodes or, in more instances, provided additional information and confirmation.

These electrodes have a terminal curve; after the use of nasoconstrictive drops and local anesthetic, the electrodes are passed between the septum nasi and the conchae. They are passed upward until they are inserted against the lamina cribrosa of the ethmoidal bone. Because they tend to be firmly held between the conchae and the septum nasi, no further fastening is necessary. There has been some conjunctival irritation associated with their use, but otherwise, like the nasopharyngeal electrodes, these are not uncomfortable when in place.

Sphenoidal Electrodes

The sphenoidal electrode is referred to at times as an "ala magna" electrode. It was introduced by Jones (1951). Investigators were trying various ways of gaining closer access to the temporal lobe or access to portions of the temporal lobe not readily examined with scalp electrodes (Fig. 35.4). The preceding electrodes took advantage of natural body orifices for insertion of the electrode, but Jones introduced recording from fine-gauge needles insulated except at the tip. They are inserted between the zygoma and the sigmoid notch in the mandible until they are in contact with the base of the skull lateral to the foramen ovale. Modifications of this technique have involved insertion of an electrode directed mesially to the base of the skull just anterior and lateral to the pterygopalatine fossa, as well as inserting electrodes aimed for the posterior rim of the foramen ovale (Rovit et al., 1961). When these two different sphenoidal electrodes are inserted, the one anterior to the pterygopalatine fossa is referred to as an anterior sphenoidal electrode, whereas the latter, posterior to the foramen ovale, is referred to as a posterior sphenoidal electrode. Technique and modifications are described in a number of studies (King et al., 1986; Kristensen and Sindrup, 1978; Rovit and Gloor, 1960; Rovit et al., 1960, 1961; Sperling and Engel, 1986; Sperling et al., 1986).

In the initial technique described by Jones (1951), and in some subsequent recording techniques where actual needles

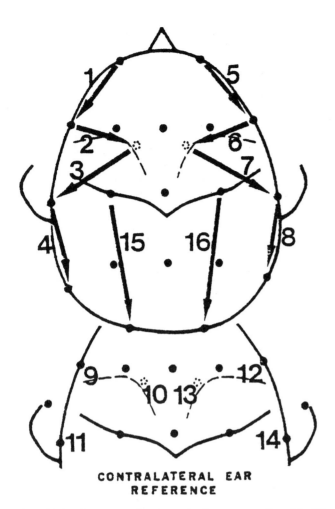

Figure 35.4. This montage involves a simultaneous recording of the NP electrodes in a bipolar configuration and in a reference configuration to the opposite ear in an effort to increase the chances of having an uninvolved reference electrode.

were used as electrodes, it was common to use a local anesthetic that was injected through the needle itself as it was advanced. Subsequently, many of the electrodes used are not hollow needles, but are solid electrode material, requiring the laboratory to decide whether anesthesia will be carried out as a separate procedure or dispensed with. It has been suggested that avoidance of local anesthesia or its use only subcutaneously allows pain as a desirable warning if the trigeminal nerve is being approached by the electrode (Christodoulou, 1967; Iriarte et al., 1996; King et al., 1986).

In many instances, it is desirable to record from a patient over a series of days. As an attempt to develop a method of doing this with electrodes more conducive to long-term use, the introduction of electrodes made from platinum and stainless steel wires was suggested (Ives and Gloor, 1977, 1978). As is sometimes done with depth electrodes, these very small wires are inserted by a needle that is withdrawn after the long-term electrode is in place. Another study raised some serious questions about the long-term location of such small electrodes. In a study of 33 patients with the electrode in place for an average of more than 5 days, it was found that

while the original electrode had been, on the average, within 7 mm of the foramen ovale, the electrodes were, on the average, 15.8 mm from that point at the time they were due to be removed (Wilkus and Thompson, 1985). It could not be demonstrated in the latter study that the EEG recordings were adversely affected by this migration of the electrode tip. Acupuncture needles have been used as the sphenoidal electrode and were felt to be well tolerated and to provide an additional incidence of abnormality (Feng et al., 1981, 1983).

Some studies of sphenoidal electrodes show an increase in abnormality in as many as 40.5% of the seizure patients who had no other specific changes in waking or sleep EEGs. It was noted, however, that although a high rate of abnormality was seen in patients who have seizures with automatisms and amnesias, the rate of abnormality was 80% less in patients whose seizures consisted of psychic seizures with hallucinations and illusions rather than automatisms (Kristensen and Sindrup, 1978).

Clearly the value of use of sphenoidal electrodes is more reasonable in patients being considered for surgery, but even in those patients the increased yield over scalp electrodes remains open for debate. Binnie et al. (1989) found only two instances in 111 patients where less than 90% of the sphenoidal discharges were visible from surface electrodes. In contrast, in a study of 20 patients, Sadler and Goodwin (1989) found that the sphenoidal electrodes detected significantly more spikes than nasopharyngeal, ear lobe, or F_2 and F_8 electrodes, but showed no advantage over T_1 and T_2, MNS, or MNSD electrodes. Another study reported that the "start-stop-start" phenomenon seen in some patients in the sphenoidal electrode first might improve seizure onset localization (Atalla et al., 1996).

Another study comparing surface and chronic sphenoidal electrodes in 74 seizures from 42 patients found 19% of the seizures were not apparent from the surface (Ives et al., 1996). The authors compared the records of 74 EEG recordings of temporal lobe seizures from 42 patients. The coronal sphenoidal montage allowed recognition of temporal lobe seizures not seen in the surface temporal electrodes in 19% of the seizures and led to earlier identification of the seizure onset in 70%. Sirven et al. (1997) recorded EEGs with the 10-20 system and sphenoidal electrodes recording 734 seizures for 166 patients. Seizure onset location was reproducible in 68% of the cases and variable patterns of seizure onset were seen in 32% of the patients. Patients with unilateral interictal spikes were more likely to have consistent ictal onset patterns than those with bilateral interictal spikes. Sixty-eight percent of the patients had unilateral interictal and 27% had bilateral interictal spikes.

Kanner et al. (1995) demonstrated that sphenoidal electrodes placed under fluoroscopic guidance, so that the recording tip was immediately below the foramen ovale, yield a significant advantage over blind placement later.

Kanner and Jones (1997) found this placement was most useful when the interictal foci had a significantly narrower field contour.

Kanner et al. (2002) compared ictal recordings of 156 seizures with sphenoidal electrodes placed under fluoroscopic guidance and anterior temporal electrodes, and found that interrater agreement among the four raters was significantly greater with sphenoidal electrodes than with the anterior temporal electrode. The number of seizures correctly localized was 144 with the sphenoidal electrodes and 99 with the anterior temporal electrodes. In this series sphenoidal electrodes added ictal data not identified by anterior temporal electrodes in about one fourth of the patients.

Fenton et al. (1997) felt that fluoroscopically guided placement of sphenoidal electrodes offered distinct advantages over standard techniques, such as more precision in placement, reduced likelihood of facial pain, and fewer complications from vessel perforation or nerve injury. Pacia et al. (1998) found that seizure rhythms confined to sphenoidal electrode ictal onset without involvement of scalp electrodes occurred only in patients with mesial temporal lobe epilepsy. They also noted that a small subset of the patients had seizure onset localized exclusively to one sphenoidal electrode before involvement of the T1/2 and temporal scalp electrodes. Fernandez Torre et al. (1999), in their series evaluating 2,280 epileptiform discharges from 20 patients, found that only on 29 occasions (4.15%) were the discharges recorded at the foramen ovale and not at the anterior temporal electrode. They also noted that a large proportion of the discharges seen at the deepest foramen ovale contacts are not seen either on the scalp or at the superficial foramen ovale contact. Kissani et al. (2001) looked at 314 seizures obtained from 110 patients. They found that electrodes located next to the foramen ovale as the electrode site yield improvement over surface electrodes only in the 5.4% to 7% of seizures. It was felt the improvement derives from the fact that the low-amplitude signals often seen at seizure onset may show higher amplitude on sphenoidal rather than scalp recordings.

Yoshinaga et al. (2001), in an attempt to subclassify four cases with temporal spikes on the scalp EEG, also used sphenoidal electrodes and dipole localization, and they concluded that sphenoidal electrodes are useful for differentiating between mesial and lateral temporal lobe foci but ought to be used in combination with dipole localization to identify frontal lobe foci.

Mintzer et al. (2002) looked at 101 ictal tracings in 31 patients with possible temporal lobe epilepsy, and they concluded that the sphenoidal electrodes were unnecessary to detect seizures that met a strict mesial temporal onset criteria and did not yield useful information for surgical evaluation beyond that provided by temporal electrodes.

The use of sphenoidal electrode recording in combination with other function tests such as positron emission tomography shows promise for avoiding false localization of ictal onset as recorded from sphenoidal EEG recordings alone and may decrease the need for depth electrode confirmation before surgery for epilepsy (Engel et al., 1990).

Some researchers scoff at the idea that special electrodes and, in particular, NP electrodes can show abnormalities in a record totally free of scalp abnormality and with unequivocal changes limited to the nonscalp electrodes. It appears that such a result is not common, but that such records occur in a number of patients. Many investigators report that the use of such electrodes clarifies and confirms equivocal scalp abnormalities in a number of instances, so that at least some percentage of isolated abnormalities that could have otherwise been missed are identified. It then becomes a question of what patient population is being studied and whether or not the findings of the small extra percentage will have a treatment and outcome impact in a particular setting.

Although all these electrodes appear to show some additional abnormalities, there is one frequent design error that must be watched for by consumers of the data. The most blatant and consistent error is to use the additional technique only on those individuals whose initial studies were normal. This type of sequence can never have any result but to show a greater rate of abnormality with the index procedure. It is well known that serial recordings enhance the likelihood of finding abnormalities, particularly epileptiform abnormalities, in records (Ajmone Marsan and Zivin, 1970). Only when the patients and controls are repeatedly tested with both the standard and the test procedure can one truly identify the value of the new procedure in finding abnormalities. Such a study in regard to use of sleep deprivation demonstrated that drug-induced sleep is as provocative as the difficult but long-supported habit of sleep-deprivation provocation (Degen and Degen, 1983). It is to be hoped that this type of comparison study will be done more often for other recording techniques including NP and sphenoidal recording.

References

Ajmone Marsan, C., and Zivin, L.S. 1970. Factors related to the occurrence of typical paroxysmal abnormalities in the EEG records of epileptic patients. Epilepsia 11:361–381.

American EEG Society Electrode Nomenclature Committee. 1990. American Electroencephalographic Society Guidelines for Standard Electrode Position Nomenclature. J. Clin. Neurophysiol. 8:200–202.

American EEG Society Guidelines Committee. 1986. American Electroencephalographic Society Guidelines in EEG and evoked potentials. J. Clin. Neurophysiol. 3:1–147.

Arellano, A.P. 1949. A tympanic lead. Electroencephalogr. Clin. Neurophysiol. 1:112–113.

Atalla, N., Abou-Khalil, B., and Fakhoury, T. 1996. The start-stop-start phenomenon in scalp-sphenoidal ictal recordings. Electroencephalogr. Clin. Neurophysiol. 98(1):9–13.

Bach-Y-Rita, G., Lion, J., Reynolds, J., et al. 1969. An improved nasopharyngeal lead. Electroencephalogr. Clin. Neurophysiol. 26:220–221.

Bauch, C.D., and Olsen, W.O. 1990. Comparison of ABR amplitudes with TIPtrode and mastoid electrodes. Ear Hear. 11:463–467.

Beattie, R.C., and Lipp, L.A. 1990. Effects of electrode placement on the auditory brainstem response using ear canal electrodes. Am. J. Otol. 11:314–319.

Binnie, C.D., Marston, D., Polkey, C.E., et al. 1989. Distribution of temporal spikes in relation to the sphenoidal electrode. Electroencephalogr. Neurophysiol. 73:403–409.

Christodoulou, G. 1967. Sphenoidal electrodes. Acta Neurol. Scand. 43:587–593.

Degen, R., and Degen, H.E. 1983. The diagnostic value of the sleep EEG with and without sleep deprivation in patients with atypical absences. Epilepsia 24:557–565.

de Jesus, P.V., and Masland, W.S. 1970. The role of nasopharyngeal electrodes in clinical electroencephalography. Neurology 20:869–878.

Engel, J., Jr., Henry, T.R., Risinger, M.W., et al. 1990. Presurgical evaluation for partial epilepsy: relative contributions of chronic depth-electrode recordings versus FDG-PET and scalp-sphenoidal ictal EEG. Neurology 40:1670–1677.

Escueta, A.V., Kunza, U, Waddell, G., et al. 1977. Lapse of consciousness and automatisms in temporal lobe epilepsy: a videotape analysis. Neurology 27(2):144–155.

Feng, Y.K., Hsu, C.C., and Kuo, T.H. 1981. Innovation in electroencephalography. The use of acupuncture needles as sphenoidal electrodes. A report of observations on 648 cases. Clin. Exp. Neurol. 17:39–45.

Feng, Y.K., Xu, J.Q., and Guo, D.H. 1983. The use of acupuncture needles as sphenoidal electrodes in electroencephalography. Observation of 2,000 cases. Chin. Med. J. (Engl.) 96:211–218.

Fenton, D.S., Geremia, G.K., Dowd, A.M., et al. 1997. Precise placement of sphenoidal electrodes via fluoroscopic guidance. AJNR 18(4):776–778.

Fernandez Torre, J.L., Alarcon, G., Binnie, C.D., et al. 1999. Comparison of sphenoidal, foramen ovale and anterior temporal placements for detecting interictal epileptiform discharges in presurgical assessment for temporal lobe epilepsy. Clin. Neurophysiol. 110(5):895–904.

Gibbs, E.L., and Gibbs, T.J. 1984. Universal APEEGE (anatomical placement of EEG electrodes) system. Clin. Electroencephalogr. 15:1–20.

Goodin, D.S., Aminoff, M.J., and Laxer, K.D. 1990. Detection of epileptiform activity by different noninvasive EEG methods in complex partial epilepsy. Ann. Neurol. 27(3):330–334.

Grinker, R.R. 1938. Scientific apparatus and laboratory methods. Science 87:73–74.

Gupta, B.K., Yerevaian, B., and Charlton, M. 1989. Nasopharyngeal EEG recording in psychiatric patients. J. Clin. Psychiatry 50(7):262–264.

Homan, R.W., Jones, M.C., and Rawat, S. 1988. Anterior temporal electrodes in complex partial seizures. Electroencephalogr. Clin. Neurophysiol. 70:105–109.

Iriarte, J., Parra, J., and Kanner, A.M. 1996. Transient facial palsy in sphenoidal electrode placement. Epilepsia 37(12):1239–1241.

Ives, J.R., and Gloor, P. 1977. New sphenoidal electrode assembly to permit long-time monitoring of the patient's ictal or interictal EEG. Electroencephalogr. Clin. Neurophysiol. 42:575–580.

Ives, J.R., and Gloor, P. 1978. Update: chronic sphenoidal electrodes. Electroencephalogr. Clin. Neurophysiol. 44:789–790.

Ives, J.R., Drislane, F.W., Schachter, S.C., et al. 1996. Comparison of coronal sphenoidal versus standard anteroposterior temporal montage in the EEG recording of temporal lobe seizures. Electroencephalogr. Clin. Neurophysiol. 98(5):417–421.

Jasper, H.H. 1958. The ten-twenty electrode system of the International Federation. Electroencephalogr. Clin. Neurophysiol. 10:371–375.

Jones, D.P. 1951. Recording of the basal electroencephalogram with sphenoidal needle electrodes. Electroencephalogr. Clin. Neurophysiol. 3:100.

Kanner, A.M., and Jones, J.C. 1997. When do sphenoidal electrodes yield additional data to that obtained with antero-temporal electrodes? Electroencephalogr. Clin. Neurophysiol. 102(1):12–19.

Kanner, A.M., Ramirez, L., and Jones, J.C. 1995. The utility of placing sphenoidal electrodes under the foramen ovale with fluoroscopic guidance. J. Clin. Neurophysiol. 12(1):72–81.

Kanner, A.M., Parra, J., Gil-Nagel, A., et al. 2002. The localizing yield of sphenoidal and anterior temporal electrodes in ictal recordings: a comparison study. Epilepsia 43(10):1189–1196.

Kashing, D.M., and Celesia, G.G. 1976. Nasopharyngeal electrodes in the diagnosis of partial seizures with complex symptoms. Arch. Neurol. 35:519–520.

King, D.W., So, E.L., Marcus, R., et al. 1986. Techniques and applications of sphenoidal recording. J. Clin. Neurophysiol. 3:51–65.

Kissani, N., Alarcon, G., Dad, M., et al. 2001. Sensitivity of recording at sphenoidal electrode site for detecting seizure onset: evidence from scalp, superficial and deep foramen ovale recordings. Clin. Neurophysiology. 112(2):232–240.

Kristensen, O., and Sindrup, E.H. 1978. Psychomotor epilepsy and psychosis. II. Electroencephalographic findings (sphenoidal electrode recordings). Acta Scand. 57:370–379.

Lethinen, O.J., and Bergstrom, L. 1970. Clinical and laboratory notes. Naso-ethmoidal electrode for recording the electrical activity of the inferior surface of the frontal lobe. Electroencephalogr. Clin. Neurophysiol. 29:303–305.

MacLean, P.D. 1949. A new nasopharyngeal lead. Electroencephalogr. Clin. Neurophysiol. 1:110–112.

Manzano, G.M., Ragazzo, P.C., Tavares, S.M., et al. 1986. Anterior zygomatic electrodes: a special electrode for the study of temporal lobe epilepsy. Appl. Neurophysiol. 49:213–217.

Mavor, H., and Hellen, M.K. 1964. Nasopharyngeal electrode recording. Am. J. EEG Technol. 4:43–50.

Mintzer, S., Nicholl, J.S., Stern, J.M., et al. 2002. Relative utility of sphenoidal and temporal surface electrodes for localization of ictal onset in temporal lobe epilepsy. Clin. Neurophysiol. 113(6):911–916.

Nakase, H., Ohnishi, H., Touho, H., et al. 1995. An intra-arterial electrode for intracranial electro-encephalogram recordings. Acta Neurochir. 136 (1–2):103–105.

Nowack, W.J., Janati, A., Metzer, W.S., et al. 1988. The anterior temporal electrode in the EEG of the adult. Clin. Electroencephalogr. 19:199–204.

Pacia, S.V., Jung, W.J., and Devinsky, O. 1998. Localization of mesial temporal lobe seizures with sphenoidal electrodes. J. Clin. Neurophysiol. 15(3):256–261.

Perrault, N., and Picton, T.W. 1984. Event-related potentials recorded from the scalp and nasopharynx. Electroencephalogr. Clin. Neurophysiol. 59: 261–278.

Peters, J., and Reilly, E.L. 1973. Nasopharyngeal electrodes in auditory evoked response research. Laryngoscope 12:1923–1928.

Porkkola, T., Kaukinen, S., Hakkinen, V., et al. 1997. Median nerve somatosensory evoked potentials during isoflurane anaesthesia. Can. J. Anaesth. 44(9):963–968.

Restucci, D., Di Lazzaro, V., Valeriani, M., et al. 1995. Origin and distribution of P13 and P14 far-field potentials after median nerve stimulation. Scalp, nasopharyngeal and neck recording in healthy subjects and in patients with cervical and cervico-medullary lesions. Electroencephalogr. Clin. Neurophysiol. 96(5):371–384.

Rovit, R.L., and Gloor, P. 1960. Temporal lobe epilepsy. A study using multiple basal electrodes. II. Clinical findings. Neurochirurgia 3:19–34.

Rovit, R.L., Gloor, P., and Henderson, L.R., Jr. 1960. Temporal lobe epilepsy. A study using multiple basal electrodes. I. Description of method. Neurochirurgia 3:6–19.

Rovit, R.L., Gloor, P., and Rasmussen, T. 1961. Sphenoidal electrodes in the electrographic study of patients with temporal lobe epilepsy. J. Neurosurg. 18:1512–1518.

Sadler, R.M., and Goodwin, J. 1989. Multiple electrodes for detecting spikes in partial complex seizures. Can. J. Neurol. Sci. 16:326–329.

Schraeder, P.L., and Humphries, M. 1977. Nasopharyngeal sleep EEGs in a community hospital setting. Arch. Neurol. 34:788.

Silverman, D. 1965. The anterior temporal electrode and the ten-twenty system. Am. J. EEG Technol. 5:11–514.

Sirven, J.I., Liporace, J.D., French, J.A., et al. 1997. Seizures in temporal lobe epilepsy: I. Reliability of scalp/sphenoidal ictal recording. Neurology 48(4):1041–1046.

Smith, D.B., Allison, T., and Goff, W.R. 1971. Nasopharyngeal recording of odorant-evoked responses in normal subjects and in patients with olfactory or trigeminal deficit. Electroencephalogr. Clin. Neurophysiol. 31: 415–416.

Sperling, M.R., and Engel, J. Jr. 1985. Electroencephalographic recording from the temporal lobes: a comparison of ear, anterior temporal, and nasopharyngeal electrodes. Ann. Neurol. 17(5):510–513.

Sperling, M.R., and Engel, J. 1986. Sphenoidal electrodes. J. Clin. Neurophysiol. 3:67–73.

Sperling, M.R., Mendius, J.R., and Engel, J. 1986. Mesial temporal spikes: a simultaneous comparison of sphenoidal, nasopharyngeal, and ear electrodes. Epilepsia 27:81–86.

Starr, A., and Squires, K. 1982. Distribution of auditory brainstem potentials over the scalp and nasopharynx in humans. Ann. N.Y. Acad. Sci. 42: 388–427.

Wagner, W. 1988. Recording of subcortical somatosensory evoked potentials using nasopharyngeal electrodes—a study in sedated patients. EEG-EMG Z. EEG EMG Verwandte Gebiete 19(3):141–147.

Wilkus, R.J., and Thompson, P.M. 1985. Sphenoidal electrode positions and basal EEG during long term monitoring. Epilepsia 26:137–142.

Yoshinaga, H., Hattori, J., Nakahori, T., et al. 2001. Combined use of sphenoidal electrodes and the dipole localization method for the identification of the mesial temporal focus. Eur. J. Neurol. 8(2):149–156.

36. Depth Electroencephalography

Ernst Niedermeyer

Electroencephalographers have always been painfully aware of the limitations of scalp recordings. It is generally felt that electroencephalogram (EEG) activity recorded from the scalp represents only a fraction of the activity within the brain. For this reason, clinical electroencephalographers have often jealously and admiringly looked at the work of their colleagues in experimental neurophysiology, who document EEG potentials from every thinkable cerebral region with such apparent ease. The suspicion that scalp EEG potentials are not truly authentic and perhaps are altered on their journey from the locus of origin to the scalp has often filled electroencephalographers with feelings of inferiority. On the other hand, true cerebral activity recorded directly from the cortex or depth has been viewed as a prestigious form of EEG recording.

A brief historical review shows the stages of development and the changing goals of this special branch of EEG. This chapter discusses the important ethical restrictions in this field, the laborious technical prerequisites, and the present state of affairs, along with the fields in which depth EEG is considered valuable and ethically justifiable. In the 1970s, interest in depth EEG was on the decline, but this trend turned around in the 1980s, with more widespread use of seizure surgery.

There has been an astounding surge of interest and activities in the field of depth EEG along with the emergence of new methods of prolonged EEG recording and combined video documentation. This development started around 1980 and has breathed new life into epilepsy surgery. An impressive International Conference on the Surgical Treatment of Epilepsy was held in February 1986 in Palm Desert, California, to celebrate the centennial of epilepsy-oriented brain surgery, which was originated by Horsley (1886). This conference ushered in a new era of presurgical EEG evaluation, with renewed emphasis being placed on depth electroencephalography. It also resulted in a comprehensive work on the state of affairs of depth electroencephalography edited by Engel (1987a).

Similar conferences followed. The Second International Cleveland Clinic Epilepsy Symposium in June 1990 was the basis for another enormous comprehensive work edited by Lüders (1992). These two overviews give testimony to the highly dynamic development of a hitherto but modestly active subspecialty.

Historical Aspects

EEG exploration of the depth of the human brain was initiated by experimental neurophysiologists using various animals. Soon after Berger's first reports, experimental workers applied the new tool with a variety of technical modifications (Bishop, 1935; Gerard et al., 1936; Jung and Kornmüller, 1938; Kornmüller, 1939; Spiegel, 1937). This work meant the dawning of a new era in electrophysiological neurophysiology.

Attempts at depth recording in the human started in the 1940s. Earlier recordings consisted of short tracings obtained during neurosurgical explorations, such as the widely known recording from the exposed cerebellum by Foerster and Altenburger (1935), which in reality is of little use (Niedermeyer 2004).

Short recordings from the depths of the human brain were obtained by Meyers and Hayne (1948), Hayne et al. (1949a,b), Knott et al. (1950), and Jung et al. (1950). This early work placed particular emphasis on the basal ganglia. This soon led to exploration of thalamic structures by Okuma et al. (1954), Williams (1953), Ishikawa (1957), and Matsui (1957). These studies were acute, short, depth recordings, essentially limited to one recording session after the insertion. These attempts were aimed at clarifying physiological mechanisms involved in motor activity and the role of thalamic structures in the epilepsies.

The insertion of chronic indwelling electrodes into the human brain was prompted by a wave of interest in such psychosurgical procedures as prefrontal leukotomy. These patients were, in most cases, sufferers from chronic psychotic states, and it was hoped that depth recordings would shed some light on these conditions. The most important work in this field was done by Delgado et al. (1952), Dodge et al. (1953), Heath et al. (1953), Sem-Jacobsen et al. (1955, 1956), Heath (1963, 1972), Walter and Crow (1964), and Sem-Jacobsen (1968).

Since the mid-1950s, however, the use of depth EEG recording has focused on the epilepsies. This development parallels an epoch in seizure surgery initiated by the introduction of the temporal lobectomy (Ajmone Marsan and Van Buren, 1958; Bailey, 1953; Bailey and Gibbs, 1951; Penfield and Baldwin, 1952; Rasmussen and Jasper, 1958; Walker, 1967; Walker and Marshall, 1964). Growing awareness of both the complications caused by depth implants and of ethical considerations made it imperative that a depth implant serve a therapeutic purpose, such as the accurate localization of an epileptogenic focus for seizure surgery (an indirect therapeutic goal) or use in combination with stereotaxic coagulation (a direct therapeutic goal).

This brief review must not end without due appreciation of the comprehensive atlas of intracranial electroencephalography by Sperling (1993). This work is based on epileptological patient records. In these days (at the time of the writing of this edition), depth EEG data almost exclu-

Table 36.1.   Purpose and Clinical Domain of Depth Implant

1. Epileptic conditions
   Main purpose: diagnostic
2. Basal ganglia disease
   Main purpose: therapeutic subthalamic nucleus
3. Intractable pain
   Main purpose: therapeutic
4. Psychosis and deviant behavior
   Main purpose: scientific-academic
Always consider principles of medical ethics

Table 36.2.   Purpose of Implant

1. For recording only
2. For recording and electrical stimulation (to activate epileptogenic foci)
3. In association with prolonged therapeutic electrical stimulation (inhibition of pain from thalamus, inhibition of seizure activity from cerebellum)
4. In association with therapeutic lesions (thermocoagulation)

Table 36.3.   Single Use Electrodes Versus Reusable Depth Probes

Single Use Electrodes	Reusable Depth Probes
Mostly bundles (tresses) of thin wires	Stable (electrically)
Flexible	Solid and bulky (locations easily determined)
Sometimes electrically unstable	Expensive
Inexpensive	More traumatic to brain tissue
Easily bent or broken	More conducive to infection and transmission of slow virus (Jakob-Creutzfeldt) and therefore virtually out of use today
Site determination not always easy	
Small risk of infection	

sively originate from presurgical diagnostic work performed in epilepsy monitoring units.

Tables 36.1 and 36.2 summarize the purpose of and rationale for depth implants.

Technical Considerations

Choice of Material for Electrodes

Noble metals such as copper, silver, gold, and platinum are excellent conductors for use in depth EEG. Dodge et al. (1953) used 38-gauge enameled copper wire inserted as four-strand cables or tresses. The use of copper, however, is not recommended because of possible oxidation and secondary cellular tissue reactions. Despite satisfactory tracings and the avoidance of adverse effects on the patients, Dodge et al. (1954) later preferred the use of stainless steel electrodes with diameters of 50 and 37 μm. This group of investigators at the Mayo Clinic then turned to somewhat larger stainless steel strands (40 gauge, 0.003 inch, 74 μm) insulated with enamel varnish. The use of stainless steel was prompted by concern about possible toxic effects on brain parenchyma from copper, silver, gold, and possibly also platinum. While alloys are generally avoided, an admixture of chromium (18%) and nickel (8%) to stainless steel has proved to be valuable (Bates, 1963). The avoidance of toxic material is particularly important in the case of chronic implants.

Tresses and Probes

There was formerly some controversy about the advantages and disadvantages of tresses and probes. Table 36.3 shows a comparison of these two forms of implant. This debate came to an abrupt end when it became clear that reusable solid probes could transmit slow virus infections, as has been observed in the case of Jakob-Creutzfeldt disease (Bernoulli et al., 1977). This grave risk, however, can be prevented by intensive autoclaving (Murray et al., 1986).

There is no doubt, however, that probes were once extremely useful in depth EEG. These semiflexible or rigid shafts had several recording surfaces, usually spaced some millimeters apart. A plastic shaft with eight silver rings was used by Hayne et al. (1949a,b). A multicontact probe made of platinum, introduced by Ray et al. (1965), is capable of yielding excellent records. This probe has a diameter of 0.75 mm and a hollow core. Most such probes are made with 18 electrode contacts, each 1 mm long and 0.075 mm wide. The electrode surface is "platinized" and gradually becomes covered with microscopic particles of platinum black, a process that enlarges the conducting surface. In general, these probes appear more suitable for acute recording sessions rather than prolonged implantation.

However, as mentioned before, strands of thin wires forming tresses have completely supplanted the expensive reusable probes. For this reason, all further discussion concerns tresses.

Electrode Construction

Earlier editions of this book featured a description of depth electrode construction. The described technique has been superseded by more modern and also commercially available depth electrodes. For this reason, a detailed presentation is omitted in this chapter (Zobniw et al., 1975).

Choice of Electrode Sites

The electrode sites are determined by the purpose of the implant. Other determining factors are avoidance of exceedingly delicate and vulnerable cerebral structures where even a little insertion trauma could lead to serious problems such as certain brainstem areas subserving vital functions or the precentral motor cortex and the vicinities of major arteries.

The use of depth EEG in chronic epileptic patients, in whom the target areas are rather large (even permitting free-hand insertion), is the main topic of discussion in this section. The most commonly explored regions are the temporal and frontal lobes. In *temporal lobe epilepsy* the temporal cortex, limbic structures (amygdala, hippocampus), and fronto-orbital cortex (probably an extension of the limbic system) may be jointly or separately involved in the generation of spikes. For this reason, a combination of tresses is advisable, with one tress on each side aiming at the amygdaloid complex, and with the tip reaching the inferior temporal cortex, and one tress on each side aiming at the fronto-orbital cortex. These tresses can be inserted through the same superior frontal bur hole.

Occasionally, the amygdaloid tress is inserted through a lateral temporal bur hole. In rare cases with the use of the long RIM (Ray-IBM-Mayo) (Ray et al., 1965) platinum probe, the limbic region has been explored by a posterior implant reaching the hippocampic gyrus, hippocampus, and amygdala. In exceptional cases, special epidural electrodes have been introduced through a bur hole to pick up cortical activity, especially over the motor cortex, in addition to depth implants at other places. Thalamic tresses are sometimes used to determine the participation of the thalamic level in special forms of epileptic seizure disorder. Velasco et al. (1990) reported interesting findings concerning frontothalamic paroxysmal discharges with the use of depth electrode recordings from the centromedian nuclei in children with Lennox-Gastaut syndrome.

In *frontal lobe epilepsy,* a fronto-orbital tress can be used, provided that the electrodes are spaced in the aforementioned manner, with a hiatus between leads 3 and 4 (leads at 4, 11, 18, 40, 50, and 60 mm from the tip). This permits exploration of the superiorfrontal region and especially of the supplementary motor area.

The mesial portion of the frontal supplementary motor area is better investigated with the use of a special mesiofrontal tress. This tress can be inserted through a superofrontal bur hole in a posterior direction and with almost horizontal orientation. With this localization, special attention must be paid to the vicinity of the anterior cerebral (pericallosal) artery. The mesiofrontal region can also be explored through a parietal bur hole and with a downward-anterior direction of the tress. Exploration of the occipital lobe is rarely performed (Perez-Borja et al., 1962).

Other authors have focused their interest on special small structures such as the fornix in combination with a fornicotomy in patients with temporal lobe epilepsy, described by Umbach and Riechert (1964) and Umbach (1966).

Chapter 37 discusses the technique of *stereoelectroencephalography* developed by Bancaud et al. (1962, 1965, 1969, 1973), Bancaud and Talairach (1973, 1975), Wieser (1983), and Munari and Bancaud (1985).

Good communication between the neurosurgeon and the epileptologist-electroencephalographer is paramount in the planning stage. Their basic philosophies concerning the use of depth EEG should be similar, because good teamwork is one of the most important prerequisites for depth implants and seizure surgery with electrocorticographic control.

Selection of Patients

Tables 36.1 and 36.2 review the reasons for and purposes of depth implants. Here the discussion is limited to the *epileptological indications* for depth implants. Principally, depth implants are reserved for potential candidates for seizure surgery. This requires a few words on indications for seizure surgery (see also Andermann, 1987; Gumnit, 1987; McNaughton and Rasmussen, 1975; Walter, 1973). There is agreement in the field that *the primary therapy for a patient suffering from recurrent epileptic seizure is medical and consists of anticonvulsants.* This kind of therapy must be linked to a more comprehensive approach that includes psychological guidance and counseling and occupational rehabilitation. The choice of anticonvulsant must be optimal for every given case; the amount of medication must avoid toxic levels, and the therapy must be monitored by repeated drug level determination.

If anticonvulsants are not effective and reduction of seizure frequency is nil to moderate, the option of seizure surgery may be considered. At this point, the morphological basis of the seizure disorder should be well understood; patients with nonfocal forms are eliminated from further considerations for surgery. This includes patients with Lennox-Gastaut syndrome and other severe forms of nonfocal epilepsy. Patients with serious intellectual deficits may have to be rejected, and this may also be true for psychotic epileptics. Thus, a relatively small number of patients will remain as candidates for seizure surgery; these are mostly temporal lobe epileptics, some frontal lobe epileptics, and a few patients with other forms of focal epilepsies.

The *time factor* is also important; some time must pass before a patient can be considered suitable for surgery. Not only must all possibility of a reasonable medical approach be explored, but there is also the possibility that an initially progressive type of seizure disorder may become milder over the ensuing years. This is particularly true for childhood epilepsies; the question of early versus delayed seizure surgery in children with severe focal epilepsies is not easily answered.

Walker (1972) compared the situation with a barrel of apples containing a single rotten fruit. "Unless the bad apple is removed, shortly all the apples will become affected with the rot." This basic philosophy may be correct in some and erroneous in other cases of childhood epilepsy. The possibility of spontaneous mitigation of the seizure disorder must be considered, especially in certain forms of childhood epilepsies with focal spikes, as discussed in Chapter 27, "Epileptic Seizure Disorders."

Furthermore, the factor of *motivation* ranks very high. Candidates for seizure surgery should be highly motivated. Such patients or their relatives may sometimes urge the neurosurgeon too strongly and try to manipulate medical decisions; caution and prudence are needed. Unfortunately, very passive and unmotivated patients are likely to have poor or below-average surgical results.

All these considerations are also valid for the implantation of depth electrodes. In general, motivated patients tolerate implants particularly well. Undesirable side effects and complications, possibly necessitating early removal of the electrodes may occur in 5% to 10% of the patients. This underscores the need for the patient's informed consent; such consent must be based not simply on a brochure or a few words said in passing, but on a long, friendly conversation. The patient should be informed that depth EEG can outline the epileptogenic zone better than scalp EEG and can detect deep spikes on "the other side" as an unexpected finding after a series of scalp tracings with consistently unilateral spiking.

There should be a natural awareness of the *ethical implications* of depth EEG. In the field of epileptology, the public will understand the need for well-indicated depth implants.

Truly humane physicians act according to their own conscience and never impose any invasive procedure on any patient because of academic or scientific curiosity.

The implantations of depth leads in candidates for temporal or frontal lobectomy is not generally considered an absolute necessity. There are straightforward cases of left or right temporal lobe epilepsy diagnosed on the basis of consistent scalp EEG findings, sometimes supported by positive neuroimaging findings. Even in such cases, however, depth EEG sometimes demonstrates considerable contralateral spiking, even to the degree that the planned lobectomy may have to be dropped. In other words, depth implants further limit the number of candidates for seizure surgery, and the selection of truly suitable cases further improves the results of seizure surgery.

On the basis of their broad investigations, Bouvier et al. (1981) concluded that depth electrode exploration should always be done before seizure surgery. According to these authors, 29 of a total of 97 patients were classified as "clear-cut cases" prior to depth exploration, "but 83% of them were false clear-cut." These figures represent an eloquent warning against temporal lobectomy without preceding depth implant. In view of the potential risks of the depth implant, a real dilemma may arise, particularly with patients older than 50. As a compromise solution, the innocuous insertion of *epidural cup electrodes* (i.e., regular scalp EEG electrodes) through a bur hole with placement over strategic areas may provide information that is quite superior to scalp EEG findings as far as correct lateralization and left-to-right spiking ratio is concerned (Niedermeyer and Uematsu, 1989a,b).

Subdural electrodes are presently in extensive use and are discussed in Chapter 39.

According to Engel et al. (1990), temporal lobectomy is justifiable even without preceding intracranial recording provided that focal scalp-sphenoidal EEG findings show consistent ictal onset and that localized hypometabolism [positron emission tomography (PET) scan] predominantly involves the same temporal lobe, and no other conflicting findings are present (focal functional deficit, structural imaging, and seizure semiology). As to lateralization, more precise answers have come from the use of DC potentials (Vanhatab et al., see Chapter 25).

Insertion of Depth Electrodes

There used to be three main insertion techniques: freehand, freehand with guides, and stereotaxic. Ojeman and Engel (1987) have pointed out that "chronic depth electrodes are usually inserted according to stereotaxic coordinates and the practice of freehand insertion is to be discouraged." Details of stereotaxic insertion techniques cannot be given in this context (see McCarthy et al., 1992).

In the 1990s, the advent of computerized "navigational systems" further improved the precision of depth implants.

EEG Recording Technique

Twenty channels or more are needed for depth recordings when more than one tress is used. A few channels always should be reserved for simultaneous scalp EEG recordings, although the number of scalp electrodes is limited by the bandages. With the superior frontal insertion technique, the frontopolar, temporal, and occipital regions are usually bandage-free. This leaves, in general, 10 or 12 channels for depth recording. Occasionally, one channel must be sacrificed for monitoring [electrocardiogram (ECG), electrooculogram, electromyogram (EMG), etc.].

The author recommends bipolar montages running adjacent electrodes against each other, with, for instance, 1–2, 2–3, 3–4, 4–5, and 5–6 in each tress. In the bottom channels, use scalp linkages such as Fp_1–F_7, F_7–T_3, T_3–O_1, or Fp_1–F_7, F_7–O_1, with corresponding linkages on the right. The role of the scalp leads is discussed below; the scalp leads yield information concerning the posterior alpha rhythm, which, after insertion, may slow down into the theta range as a temporary cerebral response to insertion. Activations such as hyperventilation and intermittent photic stimulation usually reveal very little in these patients.

Provocation of a seizure with intravenous pentylenetetrazol (Metrazol or Cardiazol) or ethyl-methyl-glutarimid (Megimide) may produce misleading results concerning the seizure focus. Major convulsion or tonic attacks (Ajmone-Marsan and Ralston, 1957) are readily produced with these drugs. The motor activity may lead to a strong pull on the electrodes and even to extraction; for this reason, such methods must be reserved for the last recording day. With the modern emphasis of ictal episodes rather than interictal spiking as a guideline for the focal origin (Crandall, 1973), spontaneous seizures are facilitated by gradual reduction of the anticonvulsant dosage. *Cautious reduction of anticonvulsive medication* may be effectively used to provoke seizures.

For the distinction between presumed primary and secondary seizure discharges, the deactivation test with intravenous diazepam may be helpful (Niedermeyer, 1970). Long-standing focal spiking in an epileptogenic zone is more resistant to small dosages of diazepam (2–5 mg i.v.) than presumably secondary spikes, which may be suppressed or attenuated for several minutes (Niedermeyer, 1970). According to Gotman et al. (1982), the area of seizure onset shows the poorest beta response to i.v. diazepam, as shown by frequency analysis. Sperling et al. (1986) have used intravenous injections of thiopental; with larger dosages, the region of the epileptogenic focus develops a local burst-suppression pattern.

The *intracarotid sodium Amytal tests* (Wada, 1949) *for determination of cerebral dominance* are done prior to surgery, but the author schedules this test after termination of the depth recording period and monitors the scalp EEG only. This test may also yield important information concerning whether spikes on "the other side" are independent or bilateral-synchronous (Rovit et al., 1961). A staff of neuropsychologists should be present during the sodium Amytal test (see Jones-Gotman, 1987).

Fiol et al. (1983) also studied the effect of intracarotid sodium Amytal on presumed primary and secondary epileptogenic foci.

Hufnagel et al. (1990) used subdural recordings during the Wada test. The sodium Amytal test has been even further refined by the use of selective arterial injection (balloon technique, selective catheterization technique). This has led to selective sodium Amytal tests for the anterior cerebral artery (Wieser, 1992) and posterior cerebral artery (Petersen and Sharbrough, 1992). The incidence of complications increases in these selective arterial injections.

Duration of Depth Implant

Depth EEG evaluation of a chronic epileptic can be done in one prolonged recording period shortly after insertion ("acute study") or in daily repeated recording sessions over a period of weeks ("chronic study"). Acute studies have the advantage of utilizing a greater number of electrodes. Bancaud and Talairach (1975) have been proponents of acute studies with the use of eight to 12 tresses or probes, each with ten to 15 leads. Thus, up to 180 depth electrode contacts can be used in one patient. The number of explored targets is truly awe inspiring. It is easy to understand that such a large number of tresses may produce considerable discomfort for the patient and facilitate infection over a long period of time. According to Bancaud and Talairach (1975), in the case of unsatisfactory information, "an acute study can be repeated without difficulty at intervals of several days or months and made to incorporate any necessary changes in electrode placement. Since the stereotaxic landmarks remain constant, the same entry point of the electrodes with respect to the double grid can be used repeatedly." Munari and Bancaud (1985) have advocated the use of acute as well as chronic implants. A thorough discussion of acute and chronic intracranial recording techniques is found in the work of Ojeman and Engel (1987).

Extremely long depth EEG studies, several months or even up to 2 years in duration (Becker et al., 1957; Heath, 1972), have been used, mainly in chronic psychotics. Quite often, chemical changes at the electrode recording surface develop in chronic recording, and the declining quality for the recording sets a limit. For the sake of the patient's well being, the length of the implant should not exceed the period needed for observation; 1 to 3 weeks is usually sufficient in a chronic epileptic and, in an epilepsy monitoring unit, 1 week is seldom exceeded.

Complications of Insertion

The complication rate in depth EEG may reach 5% to 10%. Bleeding from punctured vessels and infection are the most common causes. Fatal outcome is extremely rare. Chronic morbidity is also uncommon, because intracerebral hematomas are mostly small and evolving infection is usually quickly controlled by removal of electrodes and appropriate antibiotic treatment.

The small diameter of the inserting needles has been considered an advantage, but this view has been refuted by Sem-Jacobsen (1968); according to him, "introducers smaller than 0.5 mm more easily penetrate vessels and cause bleeding; needles larger than 1 mm may also cause more damage."

Infection with slow virus material (Jakob-Creutzfeldt disease) caused by reusable depth probes has been mentioned before. All this reemphasizes that implantation of depth electrodes should not be undertaken lightly.

In 135 depth implants, Flanigin (1989) reported the following incidence of complications:

Deaths	0
Hemorrhage	4
Mild memory deficit	1
Recovery without residual	2
Surgical evacuation with slight residual	1
Infarction with residual paresis	1
Abscess	2
Resolved without residual	1
Excised without residual	1

Electrical Stimulation

Penfield and Jasper (1954) described extensively the search for the cortical epileptogenic zone with the use of cortical electrical stimulation during surgery in the locally anesthetized patient. Stress was laid upon the elicitation of the same type of seizure that the patient used to experience under ordinary conditions. Results of stimulation are more impressive after temporary reduction of the patient's anticonvulsive medication.

Electrical stimulation of depth leads aims at determining low threshold areas and eliciting a seizure that is identical with the patient's regular seizure pattern. Unfortunately, the information obtained from electrical stimulation is somewhat limited and may be confusing. Strong spike afterdischarge may be noted in an area where no interictal spikes or no ictal EEG activity is found. Work by Wieser et al. (1979) clearly shows the superiority of spontaneous over electrically induced ictal discharges with regard to their localizing value.

The author uses a stimulation frequency of 40 pulses/sec. A pulse duration of 1 msec is advisable. The duration of each series of pulses is 5 seconds. Stimulation is bipolar, stimulating two adjacent contacts of a given tress. Bates (1963) recommends the use of constant voltage for bipolar and constant current for unipolar stimulation; modern stimulators have controls for this choice.

An initial voltage of 1 or 2 V and a current of 0.5 mA may be used with gradual increase of these values. The terminals of the stimulator are connected into specific plug-in holes for each channel of the EEG machine, which should be designed for this type of use. In this manner, the stimuli are conducted to the depth electrodes. The EEG amplifiers are turned off for the 5 seconds of stimulation and immediately afterward turned on again, unless stimulation artifact can be minimized by special installations.

Electrically stimulated areas briefly remain refractory for another stimulation; it is therefore advisable to stimulate, for instance, leads 1 to 2 of tress 1, then 1 to 2 of tress 2 (instead of 2 to 3 of tress 1), and to proceed in this manner. The threshold for epileptic afterdischarges is lowered by reduced intake of anticonvulsants. The author never uses currents exceeding 2 mA or voltages exceeding 15 V. Higher voltages could act as a stimulus used for electroconvulsions. One must keep in mind that the goal is the detection of low threshold areas.

Isolated electrical stimuli have been delivered by human depth leads to study anatomicophysiological relationships such as amygdala-hippocampus connections (Buser and Bancaud, 1983).

The use of electrical stimulation has reached new heights with the thorough exploration of large cortical regions by means of subdural grids. This technique (see Lüders et al., 1987) is most useful for the delineation of motor cortex and the speech regions. Chapter 39 is dedicated to the subdural recording technique.

Determination of the Electrode Sites

With the use of stereotaxic technique, localization can be accomplished with the direct and the indirect method (Bancaud and Talairach, 1975). The direct method is more precise but requires intracranial angiography and pneumoencephalography under stereotaxic conditions (head in stereotaxic frame); this is sometimes supplemented by lipiodol ventriculography in order to obtain a more precise outline of structures. Indirect stereotaxic localization is based on the demonstration of the line connecting the anterior and posterior commissures (bicommissural line; Talairach et al., 1952, 1967). This line is the basis for a grid system that also takes into account individual variations of cranial configuration.

For the determination of the site of depth leads introduced with freehand methods, the radiological evaluation is combined with the use of human atlases; however, these may not do justice to interindividual variations. The atlas of Schaltenbrand and Bailey (1959) is most useful because such differences are taken into account.

All this has been dramatically overshadowed by three-dimensional magnetic resonance imaging (MRI) techniques capable of demonstrating lesions as well as introduced material in cortex and depth.

Basic Differences Between Depth and Scalp EEG Data

At first glance, depth EEG tracings do not look much different from the scalp EEG. A more careful look reveals a wider frequency spectrum; the mixture of slow, medium, and fast frequencies is usually more striking in depth leads. The voltage may or may not be higher in the depth; this depends greatly on the tress location, which may be either close to or some distance from gray masses that include buried neocortical gyri.

Essentially, special characteristics of the depth EEG are determined by (a) the size and material of the depth electrode, influencing impedance and time constant of the electrode (with attenuation of slow activity, due to time constant characteristics); (b) the special type of surrounding cerebral parenchyma (gray versus white matter, special forms of EEG activity determined by certain deep structures, although there is no true EEG specificity of deep structures); and (c) the role of attenuation factors, such as vicinity or distance of EEG generator areas and attenuating effects of tissue.

The *attenuation factors* require special discussion. An abundance of deep spikes often stands in stark contrast to scarcity of spikes on the scalp (see Niedermeyer and

Rocca, 1972) due to the fact that many deep spikes never reach the scalp. Very often, such local spikes do not propagate far. According to Abraham and Ajmone-Marsan (1958) and Cooper et al. (1965), the size of a deep or cortical generator is of prime importance. Amplitude and degree of neuronal synchrony are also important factors facilitating spread. Propagation is opposed by such attenuation factors as tissues or fluids. The propagation of signals in the depth does not support dipole theories (Cooper et al., 1965; Niedermeyer, 1996, 1997). Further work in this field has been done by Gloor (1975), Pfurtscheller and Cooper (1975), and Smith et al. (1983). Specificity of depth EEG patterns in different brain structures is "rather poor" (Ciganek et al., 1981).

Physiological Characteristics of Depth EEG Activity

Posterior alpha rhythm is demonstrable in posterior implants and can be found throughout the occipital lobe. Albe-Fessard (1975) found some "true" alpha rhythm in medial portions of the pulvinar. Otherwise, electrothalamograms fail to show organized alpha rhythm (Gücer et al., 1978; Wieser and Siegfried, 1979a,b). The hippocampus is not reached by the posterior alpha rhythm. Wagner (1984) has given an eloquent account of the data collected on the human hippocampic EEG patterns. Fast activity (18–25/sec or faster) is particularly common in the depth of the frontal lobes (Cooper et al., 1965). Lambda waves (Chatrian et al., 1960; Fourment et al., 1976; Perez-Borja et al., 1962) are quite impressive in occipital lobe depth recording. In drowsiness and sleep, massive large sharp activity is quite widespread, evidently corresponding with positive occipital sharp transients of sleep (POSTS) on the scalp. Rolandic mu rhythm usually shows a fast (about 20/sec) equivalent over the cortex; this may be picked up from parietal depth implants close to the rolandic cortex; the customary frequency in the alpha range may also be found.

In sleep, spindles and K complexes are noted mainly over the frontal lobes. Deep frontal spindles are recorded at a time when the scalp EEG shows deepening drowsiness without the characteristics of stage 2 sleep. Even in the waking state (with demonstrable posterior alpha rhythm in simultaneous scalp recording), unequivocal sleep spindle activity may be recorded from superior frontal regions (supplementary motor cortex) with depth leads (Caderas et al., 1982; Jankel and Niedermeyer, 1985; Niedermeyer and Jankel, 1984; Niedermeyer et al., 1986). Deep frontal spindles and spindles on the scalp do not necessarily occur in synchrony, and there is reason to presume a number of spindle generators. This becomes particularly evident with thalamic recordings (Gücer et al., 1978) demonstrating spindle trains in the ventrobasal complex and its vicinity without corresponding spindles on the scalp. Wieser and Siegfried (1979a) demonstrated vertex waves and K complexes in periaqueductal gray structures.

Independent alpha-like rhythmical activity in the waking state and some spindle-like activity in sleep have been recorded from deep cerebellar structures (Niedermeyer and

Uematsu, 1974). These findings were surprising in view of the widely known experimental findings of cerebellar activity in animals showing predominant very fast activity beyond the EEG range around 200 to 300/sec (Adrian, 1934; Bremer, 1958; Dow, 1938; Niedermeyer, 2004; Snider, 1950).

Abnormal Patterns and Paroxysmal Discharges in Depth Leads

In chronic epileptics, deep spike discharges usually outnumber spikes on the scalp by a wide margin, at a ratio of 20:1 or even more (Niedermeyer and Rocca, 1972). A variety of spikes can be recorded, ranging from needle-like fast spikes to much slower discharges that fall into the sharp-

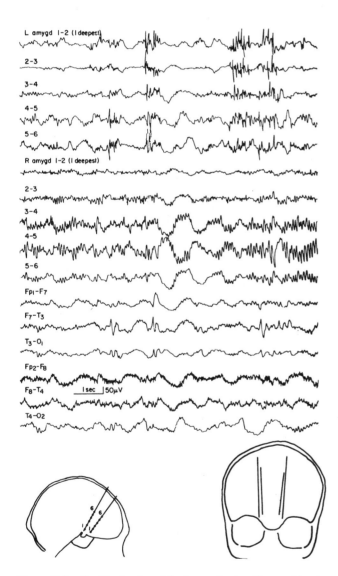

Figure 36.1. Combined scalp and depth recording in a 38-year-old patient with temporal lobe epilepsy since age 3 (rare grand mal but numerous and therapeutically unresponsive psychomotor automatisms). Three sharp waves are shown in scalp leads over the left anterior temporal area (F_7); numerous polyspikes occur in all leads of the left amygdaloid tress. The implant was performed by Dr. A. Earl Walker.

wave category. From the viewpoint of wave morphology, deep spikes may be indistinguishable from spikes recorded on the scalp (Fig. 36.1).

The question of synchrony versus asynchrony of deep spike activity has been of great importance. With the use of computer analysis, Brazier (1972) investigated the coherence function of deep spike activity in the limbic system. These attempts aim to determine which structure is driven by which other structure, in order to shed some light on the primary, secondary, or tertiary character of certain spike discharges. These questions are not easy to answer. The use of a ruler to determine which spike comes first usually achieves nothing. Depth electroencephalographers tend to forget that, even with a maximum allowable number of inserted electrodes, a quite insufficient number of targets are reached; the true origin of interictal or ictal spiking often remains elusive.

A simple focus of seizure discharges such as an anterior temporal sharp-wave focus on the scalp in a case of temporal lobe epilepsy tends to become more complex with several subfoci in the depth (Fig. 36.2). Even in "elementary" focal motor epilepsy, the spatial distribution of depth EEG discharges is more complex than one would expect from the clinical and scalp EEG data (Wieser, 1981). On the other hand, an amazing degree of synchrony between individual depth leads and between depth and scalp leads may be noted in some cases of generalized epilepsy.

Deep temporal spiking is often enhanced in sleep, but maximum spike activity may be located contralateral to the real focus; rapid-eye-movement (REM) sleep has been presumed to be a more trustworthy indicator of the side of the focus (Lieb et al., 1980; Rossi et al., 1984a,b). Wieser (1984) observed a relationship between deep temporal spikes and arousal responses in sleep.

King and Spencer (1995) investigated the discharge patterns during ictal activity in medial temporal structures where spike discharge rates of 13 to 25/sec where common. It was found that temporal neocortical seizures have significantly faster discharge frequencies than those with hippocampal onset.

On the scalp, the main phase of single spikes or sharp waves is almost always negative. Not so in the depth, where a prominent positive phase is not uncommon. The 14 and 6/sec positive spike discharge may be found in a variety of deep structures (Niedermeyer et al., 1967); these discharges sometimes show negative polarity in the depth.

Occasionally, one is struck by very pronounced slow activity in the depth. This could be due to a local lesion giving rise to delta activity. It must be kept in mind, however, that such findings could be by-products of the implants. Furthermore, the physical characteristics of the thin wires affect the time constant and limit the ability to faithfully record slow activity.

In their assessment of a practical value of depth EEG in the workup of patients with intractable seizures, Spencer et al. (1982) conclude that "of the presently available localizing criteria, depth EEG appears to be the most accurate." There are limitations, however, and Gloor (1983) has pointed out that "depth EEG is no panacea for difficult localization problems."

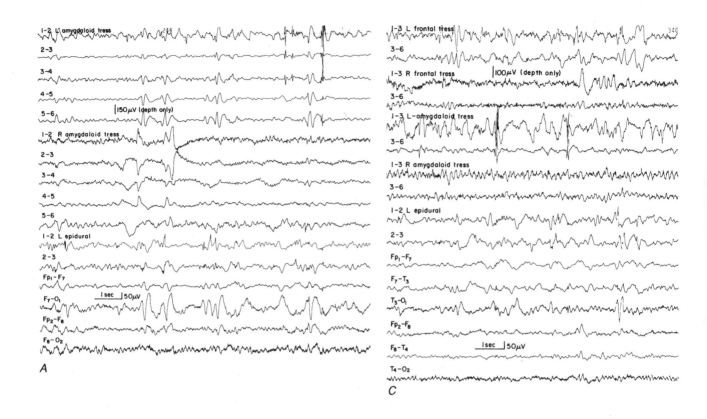

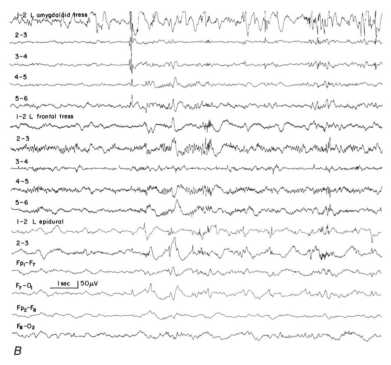

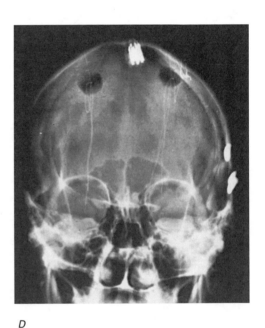

Figure 36.2. Implant performed by Dr. S. Uematsu in a 38-year-old patient with temporal lobe epilepsy, unresponsive to appropriate anticonvulsive medication. Attacks about two to three times per day, beginning with loss of memory, followed by a bad taste in the mouth, staring expression, and automatic behavior, occasionally culminating in a grand mal convulsion. **A:** (For electrode localization, see **D–F.**) The scalp lead shows four paroxysmal events in F_7 (left anterior temporal); Fp_1 appears to be almost equally involved. Their EEG expression is a sharp wave, except for the discharge on the right, which is a spike. Note that these sharp waves on the scalp are associated with similarly shaped sharp waves in the left amygdaloid tress. Also note a few independent spikes in left epidural lead 1 and in the deeper contacts of the left amygdaloid tress. **B:** Note independent spiking in left amygdaloid tress and left epidural leads. **C:** Considerable independent spikes and/or sharp waves occurring in left frontal tress, left amygdaloid tress, left epidural leads, and scalp leads. **D–F:** Electrode location.

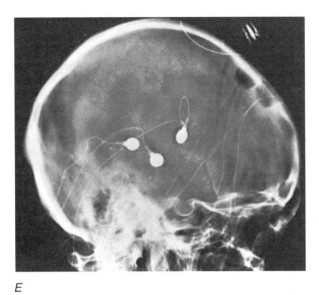

E

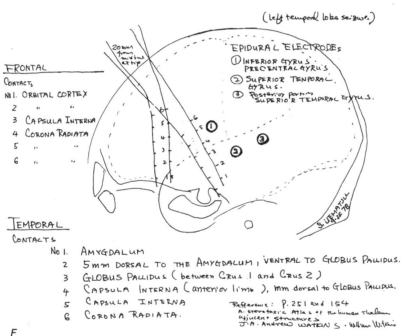

F

Figure 36.2. *(continued)* **E** and **F**.

Epileptic Activity in Deep Structures Such as Basal Ganglia, Diencephalon, Brainstem, and Cerebellum

The role of the *thalamus* in cases of presumed primary generalized epilepsy has been discussed at length during the past 30 years; it is reviewed in great detail by Gloor (1978, 1984). Much of the controversy has arisen from experimental data, but depth EEG in human epileptics has also made some contributions to this field. This is of special importance when one considers that primary generalized epilepsy is a typically human disorder and animal models are beset with limitations.

Hayne et al. (1949a,b) explored with one tress of electrodes cortical and deep structures of patients with petit mal absences and other generalized seizures; these authors found the cortex predominantly involved in the generation of spike-wave complexes. Williams (1953) presumed that, in patients with petit mal, the slow component of the spike-wave complex was of thalamic origin and the spike component was of cortical origin. Bickford (1956) stressed the role of the frontal lobe as the most likely origin of the spike-wave discharge. According to Walker and Marshall (1964), both cortical and deep foci could give rise to generalized synchronous seizure discharges. Angeleri et al. (1964) emphasized the role of limbic structures in such patients. Rossi et al. (1967) observed independent deep temporal spike activity in patients with generalized-synchronous seizure patterns. Bancaud et al. (1965) and Bancaud (1972) placed very strong emphasis on the frontal lobes with the role of thalamic and mesencephalic structures in the genesis of generalized spike-wave discharges. Wilson and Nashold (1968) investigated epileptic discharges in thalamic and midbrain level. Dinner et al. (2002) demonstrated ictal and interictal epileptic activity in the subthalamic nucleus with electrodes implanted for therapeutic subthalamic stimulation.

The elucidation of generalized epilepsies by depth EEG can be seriously impeded by the heterogeneity of the patient material. An attempt must be made to divide the patients into true cases of primary generalized epilepsy, spurious cases mimicked by secondary bilateral synchrony—see

Chapter 27—and cases of Lennox-Gastaut syndrome (Niedermeyer, 1972; Niedermeyer et al., 1969). It must be kept in mind that primary generalized epilepsies with classical petit mal absences are fairly benign seizure disorders in the vast majority of cases. It is unlikely that these patients will become candidates for depth implants and seizure surgery except under very unusual clinical circumstances, such as poor response to medication or a search for a hidden deep focus because of the poor response. In severe cases of Lennox-Gastaut syndrome, the cerebellum participates in cortical and deep epileptic ictal and interictal activity (Niedermeyer and Uematsu, 1974) (Fig. 36.3). In such patients, depth EEG evaluations have been done in more recent years in view of surgical treatment with callosotomy (Fischer and Niedermeyer, 1986, 1987). Drlickova et al. (1983) electri-

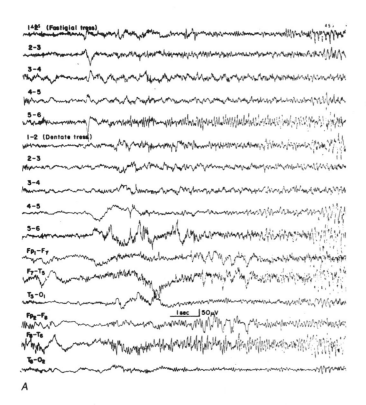

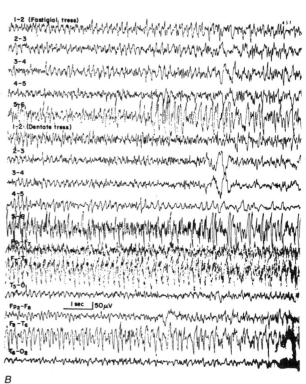

A

B

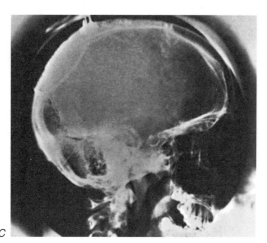

C

Figure 36.3. Combined cerebellar depth leads and scalp leads in a 16-year-old patient with intractable seizure disorder. The implant was carried out by Dr. S. Uematsu; the cerebellar electrodes were subsequently used for local stimulation for therapeutic purposes. **A:** Onset of a spontaneous seizure occurring while patient was in light sleep. He opened his eyes and showed a blank stare; there were rhythmical twitching movements of his right shoulder. Ictal EEG activity at around 27/sec was first noted in right anterior temporal scalp lead (F_8), spreading within 0.5 seconds to left anterior temporal and then presumably to the shallowest lead (6) of the fastigial tress inserted paramedian, about 5 mm to the left of midline. There is marked buildup of ictal spiking in this area (cerebellar cortex, close to tuber). **B:** There is rhythmical ictal spiking in all scalp and depth leads. **C:** Electrode sites. Fastigial tress: 1, rostral portion of central lobulus; 2, caudal (lower) portion of central lobulus; 3, culmen, 5.5 mm dorsal to fastigial nucleus; 4, medullary substance between declive and tuber; 5 and 6, tuber, cerebellar cortex. Dentate tress: 1, culmen; 2, declive; 3, dentate nucleus; 4, paramedian portion of biventer. Sites 5 and 6, extracerebellar.

cally stimulated the dentate nucleus of the cerebellum in six epileptics and investigated the stimulation effects on the hippocampic EEG and the scalp tracing.

Interictal Versus Ictal Discharges

The observation and recording of a typical clinical seizure (indistinguishable from seizures occurring outside the hospital) have been regarded by Penfield and Jasper (1954) as extremely important goals in electrocortico-graphic exploration. As to the depth EEG, the same emphasis on recorded and observed seizures is still expressed in the work of Crandall (1973), Walter (1973), Bancaud and Talairach (1975), Lieb et al. (1981), and Wieser (1983).

On the other hand, the complex nature of a seizure, even an apparently simple partial seizure, precludes full assessment of the underlying morphology, since so many potentially involved structures may not be reached by the exploring electrodes. Important epileptic activity may be found only a few millimeters distant from a quiet region. Thus, the true physiopathogenesis and true spatial distribution of the seizure activity often remain unfathomable. In some patients, ictal events start from several areas independently (Rossi, 1973). The occurrence of ictal events is facilitated by reduction of anticonvulsants, but in this state, lateralization of seizure onset is not necessarily correct (Ajmone-Marsan, 1984; Engel and Crandall, 1983). Bilaterally independent onset of seizures does not necessarily foreshadow a poor result of seizure surgery (Engel et al., 1981a).

It has been shown that focal interictal spiking in the depth EEG of temporal lobe epileptics declines significantly several minutes prior to a seizure, whereas the rate of bilateral loosely coupled spike activity increases in the preictal period (Lange et al., 1983). Toczek et al. (1997) have shown that, with use of ictal intracranial recordings, a precise localization of ictal onset within the mesiofrontal region can be obtained.

Reliance on interictal spikes can be quite unrealistic, but the localizing value of consistent focal spiking should not be ignored. According to Lieb et al. (1981) "lateralization information in interictal surface and depth records is more closely related to the side of seizure generation than to the degree of seizure relief obtained following lobectomy." Rossi (1973) has given an eloquent account of the localizing value and misleading properties of interictal spikes. Reliance on low threshold or prolonged afterdischarges following electrical stimulation is not advisable (Fig. 36.4).

Ictal discharges recorded from typical temporal-limbic depth implants and those picked up by subdural electrodes have been compared by Eisenschenk et al. (2001). It was found that subdural strip electrodes recordings alone may result in inaccurate focus identification "with potential for possible suboptimal treatment of temporal lobe epilepsy." Thus, the depth implant technique appears to be preferable. If, however, subdural electrode placement includes the parahippocampal region, then the results are not inferior any longer to those of depth implants (Eisenschenk et al., 2001).

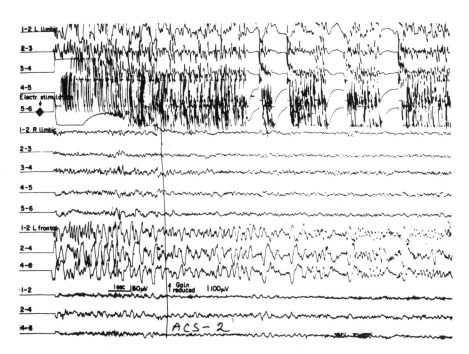

Figure 36.4. Depth recording from a 27-year-old patient; the implant was performed by Dr. A. Earl Walker. Note the pronounced afterdischarge following electrical stimulation of contacts 5 and 6 to the left limbic tress. Electrode sites. Left frontal tress: 1 and 2 in gyrus rectus, 3 in caudate nucleus, 4 in internal capsule, 5 in head of the caudate nucleus, 6 in white matter. Right frontal tress: 1 in suprachiasmatic cistern, 2 in gyrus rectus, 3 in stria terminalis (transition from putamen to caudate nucleus), and 4–6 in caudate nucleus. Left limbic tress: 1 and 3 in inferior temporal cortex, 32 in inferior amygdala, 4 and 5 in inferior hippocampus, 6 in posterior Ammon's formation. Right limbic tress: 1 in inferior temporal cortex, 2 in white matter, 3 in anterior border of amygdala, 4 in inferior posterior amygdala, 5 in inferior hippocampus, and 6 in posterior hippocampus.

Technological Adjuncts of Depth EEG

Use of *oscilloscopic techniques* to study the pathways of seizure discharges in temporal lobe epileptics (involving a four-channel static memory oscilloscope) has been demonstrated by Buser and Bancaud (1967) and Buser et al. (1973).

Exploration of electrophysiological responses to odorants was carried out in association with depth EEG studies in patients with temporal lobe epilepsy by Hughes and Andy (1979). Lieb et al. (1984) determined the *interhemispheric propagation time* from epileptogenic foci in the hippocampic area to the homologous contralateral hippocampus during depth-recorded ictal events. A propagation of 5 seconds or less apparently heralds a good response to temporal lobectomy. Slow propagation (greater than 20 seconds) is usually associated with loss of neurons in the contralateral hippocampus and suggests poor surgical results.

Microelectrodes were used in chronic epileptics by Rayport and Waller (1961, 1967), Ward and Schmidt (1961), Marg and Adams (1967), and Ward (1969). Rayport (1975) leaves no doubt about the laborious nature of this type of cortical and deep exploration in the human.

Computerized data analysis of depth EEG data has been used on various occasions. Coherence studies (Brazier, 1972) have been helpful in the elucidation of deep temporal lobe spike activity in human epileptic. Lopes da Silva et al. (1977) used automatic spike detection techniques in combined depth and scalp recording. Lieb et al. (1978) studied deep temporal spikes with automatic spike detection. Power spectral analysis and coherence studies were used for the analysis of brainstem data (Wieser, 1983; Wieser and Siegfried, 1979a). Prolonged EEG monitoring from depth electrodes with or without videotapes (using biotelemetry or cable connection) has been used frequently, especially by Ives et al. (1981) and by Engel et al. (1981b). For further advances in the field, see Engel (1987b), Lüders (1992), and, in particular, the condensed analysis of Gotman (1993).

Depth EEG Work Outside the Field of Epileptology

It has been pointed out that the implantation of depth electrodes in the human brain involves very important ethical considerations that automatically restrict the use of the technique unless a therapeutic effect, such as stereotaxy of lesions or stimulation of deep structures for therapeutic purposes, can be combined with the recording.

Recordings from the *basal ganglia* and the *thalamus* in combination with stereotaxic surgery for the Parkinson syndrome were carried out by Umbach (1966), following earlier work by Ishikawa (1957) and Jinnai (1966), with demonstration of spontaneous EEG activity in the pallidum, caudate nucleus, and thalamic regions.

Albe-Fessard (1975) has given an impressive account of her work on stereotaxic recording from thalamic regions. Her studies (Albe-Fessard et al., 1962, 1966) have made an important contribution to the electrophysiological distinction between various thalamic nuclei. Narabayashi and Kubota (1967) picked up somatosensory evoked potentials from the postventralis lateralis region of the thalamus in parkinso-

nians. Andy and Jurko (1982) studied thalamic EEG discharges in painful dyskinesias. A conjunction of "minor motor movements" and thalamic discharges was reported by Andy (1984).

Thalamic recordings (ventrobasal complex) in patients with cerebrovascular disease and Dejerine-Roussy syndrome may show considerable slowing in thalamic structures (Gücer et al., 1978); these studies were done in combination with electrical stimulation therapy for thalamic pain. Tassinari et al. (1971) studied the EEG of brainstem structures in patients with dyssynergia myoclonica and action myoclonus.

The bulk of depth EEG work done in the field of psychiatry can be mentioned only in passing. Much of this work was done in the early period of human intracerebral recording. Hope of an electrophysiological clarification of the major psychoses has remained unfulfilled, although the work of Heath (1958, 1966) and Heath and Guerrero-Figueroa (1965) showed paroxysmal changes in certain limbic structures and especially in the septal region. Walter and Crow (1964) used indwelling electrodes in psychotic patients in combination with polarization treatment and multiple small coagulations.

Some of these studies aimed at the investigation of human behavior in conjunction with self-stimulation techniques (mapping of pleasure and displeasure areas) (Bishop et al., 1963; Heath, 1963; Sem-Jacobsen, 1968). Self-stimulation leading to sexual arousal and orgasm has been reported by Heath (1972), who found paroxysmal responses mainly in the septum, but also in the amygdaloid nucleus. These studies naturally raise ethical questions. Avramov (1966) and Bechtereva (1974) recorded direct current (DC) shifts from various deep areas (including pons and thalamus) of the human brain with particular emphasis on the waking state and on non-REM and REM sleep. Hippocampic DC shift studies in epileptic patients were carried out by Machek et al. (1983).

Summary

Depth studies have opened a new dimension in clinical electroencephalography, but this technique can be used only in association with a therapeutic procedure or, in epileptology, as a final screening test for the suitability of candidates for seizure surgery. In addition to ethical restrictions, there are also considerable electrophysiological limitations, because the number of explored targets will always remain insufficient.

An interesting comparison of data derived from epileptic patients with conventional and with intracranial EEG was carried out by Rektor et al. (1997). The scalp EEG did fairly well in the localization of epileptogenic lesions; there were confirming findings with stereoencephalography in most cases but even the invasive recordings showed limitation (in a population of 87 patients).

An intracerebral electrode may miss a nearby epileptic event if the spike generator is not large enough. Such a deep spike may be propagated along pathways to a far-distant brain region; in other words, a signal of clinical significance may escape detection by a nearby depth lead. On the other hand, the probing electrode may pick up spikes of little relevance in the process of epileptogenesis.

Whoever uses EEG recordings from the depth of the brain to demonstrate the "true" or "real" epileptogenic focus is bound to be disappointed. The presumed circumscript primary focus and origin of the seizure disorder may turn out to be an illusion. In most cases of a severe focal (partial) epileptic seizure disorder, there may be a wide zone of paroxysmal dysfunction with various "subfoci" sometimes apt to appear and disappear in a "will-o'-the-wisp"-like manner. Such concepts have been expressed by Graf et al. (1984), Engel (1987b), Lüders and Awad (1992), and Ebersole (1997), who have advocated a much broader and more three-dimensional idea of focus.

Missing the truly epileptogenic zone just by a few millimeter is a source of deep concern and anxiety for the depth electroencephalographer. Those who use PET should interpret cortical areas with hypometabolism as regions not involved in epileptiform activity, although such epileptic activity commonly occurs in the surrounding cortex. The cortical tissue adjacent to the hypometabolic regions can be highly epileptogenic-based on a profound and very important study of Juhasz et al. (2000).

Authenticity is the great asset of depth EEG. The recorded potentials are truly cerebral, without distortion on their way to the scalp. On the other hand, ignorance of the relevance or lack of relevance of an intracerebrally recorded spike discharge is the nemesis of the interpreter of depth recordings. From this point of view, the value of regular scalp EEG recordings is by no means diminished by comparison to depth EEG data; the lack of absolute authenticity and the loss of enormous amounts of deep cerebral EEG information is compensated for by the demonstration of the most relevant type of electrical brain activity: the potentials produced by the most powerful generators and capable of reaching the cranial surface. Depth and scalp EEG are therefore complementary methods in the exploration of brain pathology.

References

Abraham, K., and Ajmone-Marsan, C. 1958. Patterns of cortical discharges and their relation to routine scalp electroencephalography. Electroencephalogr. Clin. Neurophysiol. 10:447–461.

Adrian, E.D. 1934. Discharge frequency in cerebral and cerebellar cortex. Physiol. (London) 83:32(abst).

Ajmone-Marsan, C. 1984. Electroencephalographic studies in seizure disorders: additional considerations. J. Clin. Neurophysiol. 1:143–157.

Ajmone-Marsan, C., and Ralston, B.L. 1957. *The Epileptic Seizure.* Springfield, IL: Charles C Thomas.

Ajmone-Marsan, C., and Van Buren, J.M. 1958. Epileptiform activity in cortical and subcortical structures in the temporal lobe of man. In *Temporal Lobe Epilepsy,* Eds. M. Baldwin and P. Bailey, pp. 78–108. Springfield, IL: Charles C Thomas.

Albe-Fessard, D. 1975. Electrophysiological techniques used to differentiate thalamic nuclei. In *Handbook of Electroencephalography and Clinical Neurophysiology,* vol. 10B, Ed. A. Remond, pp. 46–58. Amsterdam: Elsevier.

Albe-Fessard, D., Arfel, G., Guidot, G., et al. 1962. Dérivations d'activités spontanées et évoquées dans les structures cérébrales de l'homme. Rev. Neurol. (Paris) 106:89–105.

Albe-Fessard, D., Guiot, G., Lamarre, Y., et al. 1966. Activation of thalamocortical projections related to tremorogenic processes. In *The Thalamus,* Eds. D.P. Purpura and M.D. Yahr, pp. 237–253. New York: Columbia University Press.

Andermann, F. 1987. Identification of candidates for surgical treatment of epilepsy. In *Surgical Treatment of the Epilepsies,* Ed. J. Engel, Jr., pp. 51–70. New York: Raven Press.

Andy, O.J. 1984. Diencephalic discharges and minor motor movements. Electroencephalogr. Clin. Neurophysiol. 58:34P(abst).

Andy, O.J., and Jurko, M. 1982. Thalamic EEG changes in painful dyskinesias (case report). Electroencephalogr. Clin. Neurophysiol. 53:95P(abst).

Angeleri, F., Ferro-Milone, F., and Parigi, S. 1964. Electrical activity and reactivity of the rhinencephalic, pararhinencephalic and thalamic structures: prolonged implantation of electrodes in man. Electroencephalogr. Clin. Neurophysiol. 16:100–129.

Avramov, S.R. 1966. Steady potential dynamics in the human deep brain structures during wakefulness, at rest and in response to stimulation. Abtoreferat dissertatsii, Leningrad, 24 pp. (in Russian, quoted after N.P. Bechtereva).

Bailey, P. 1953. Treatment of psychomotor states by anterior temporal lobectomy. Res. Publ. Assoc. Neuro. Ment. Dis. 31:341–346.

Bailey, P., and Gibbs, F.A. 1951. The surgical treatment of psychomotor epilepsy. JAMA 145:365–370.

Bancaud, J. 1972. Mechanisms of cortical discharges in "generalized" epilepsies in man. In *Synchronization of EEG Activity in Epilepsies,* Eds. H. Petsche and M.A.B. Brazier, pp. 368–381. Vienna: Springer.

Bancaud, J., and Talairach, J. 1973. L'électroencéphalographie de profondeur (S.E.E.G.) dans l'épilepsie. In *Modern Problems of Pharmacopsychiatry-Epilepsy.* vol. 4, pp. 29–41. Basel: S. Karger.

Bancaud, J., and Talairach, J. 1975. Macro-stereoelectroencephalography in epilepsy. In *Handbook of Electroencephalography and Clinical Neurophysiology,* Ed. A. Remond, vol. 10B, pp. 3–33. Amsterdam: Elsevier.

Bancaud, J., Talairach, J., Schaub, C., et al. 1962. Stereotaxic functional exploration of the epilepsies of the supplementary areas of the mesial surface of the hemisphere. Electroencephalogr. Clin. Neurophysiol. 14: 788.

Bancaud, J., Talairach, J., Bonis, A., et al. 1965. *La Stéréoélectroencéphalographie dans l'Épilepsie.* Paris: Masson.

Bancaud, J., Talairach, J., Bonis, A., et al. 1969. Constitution chez l'homme des foyers épileptogènes secondaires. Rev. Neurol. (Paris) 121:297–306.

Bancaud, J., Talairach, J., Geier, S., et al. 1973. *E.E.G. et S.E.E.G. dans les Tumeurs Cérébrales et L'Épilepsie.* Paris: Edifor.

Bates, J.A.V. 1963. Special investigation techniques: indwelling electrodes and electrocorticography. In *Electroencephalography. A Symposium on Its Various Aspects,* Eds. D. Hill and G. Parr, pp. 429–471. New York: Macmillan.

Bechtereva, N.P. 1974. DC changes associated with the sleep wakefulness cycle. In *Handbook of Electroencephalography and Clinical Neurophysiology,* Ed. A. Remond, vol. 10A, pp. 25–32. Amsterdam: Elsevier.

Becker, H.C., Founds, W.L., Peacock, S.M., et al. 1957. A roentgenographic stereotaxic technique for implanting and maintaining electrodes in the brain of man. Electroencephalogr. Clin. Neurophysiol. 9:533–543.

Bernoulli, C., Siegfried, G., Baumgartner, G., et al. 1977. Danger of accidental person-to-person transmission of Creutzfeldt-Jakob disease by surgery. Lancet 1:478–479.

Bickford, R.G. 1956. The application of depth electrography in some varieties of epilepsy. Electroencephalogr. Clin. Neurophysiol. 8:526–527.

Bishop, G.H. 1935. Electrical responses accompanying activity of the optic pathway. Arch. Ophthalmol. 14:992–1019.

Bishop, M.P., Elter, S.T., and Heath, R.G. 1963. Intracranial self-stimulation in man. Science 140:394–396.

Bouvier, G., Saint-Hilaire, J.-M., Maltais, R., et al. 1981. Depth electrode exploration before surgery for epilepsy: always, sometimes or never. Electroencephalogr. Clin. Neurophysiol. 52:45P(abst).

Brazier, M.A.B. 1972. Interactions of deep structures during seizures in man. In *Synchronization of EEG Activity in Epilepsies,* Eds. H. Petsche and M.A.B. Brazier, pp. 409–424. Vienna: Springer.

Bremer, F. 1958. Cerebral and cerebellar potentials. Physiol. Rev. 38: 357–388.

Buser, P., and Bancaud, J. 1967. Bases techniques et méthodologiques de l'exploration stéréotaxique du télencéphale (données électrophysiologiques et électro-cliniques). In *Atlas d'anatomie Stéréotaxique du Télencéphale,* Eds. J. Talairach, G. Szikla, P. Tournoux, et al., pp. 251–323. Paris: Masson.

Buser, P., and Bancaud, J. 1983. Unilateral connections between amygdala and hippocampus in man. A study of epileptic patients with depth electrodes. Electroencephalogr. Clin. Neurophysiol. 55:1–12.

Buser, P., Bancaud, J., and Talairach, J., 1973. Depth recordings in man in temporal lobe epilepsy. In *Epilepsy: Its Phenomena in Man,* Ed. M.A.B. Brazier, pp. 67–97. New York: Academic Press.

Caderas, M., Niedermeyer, E., Uematsu, S., et al. 1982. Sleep spindles recorded from deep cerebral structures in man. Clin. Electroencephalogr. 13:216–225.

Chatrian, G.E., Bickford, R.G., and Uihlein, A. 1960. Depth electrographic study of a fast rhythm evoked from the human calcarine region by steady illumination. Electroencephalogr. Clin. Neurophysiol. 12:167–176.

Ciganek, L., Sramka, M., and Nadvornik, P. 1981. Stereoelectroencephalography (SEEG)—a method in clinical electrophysiology of the human brain. Electroencephalogr. Clin. Neurophysiol. 52:4P(abst).

Cooper, R., Winter, A.L., Crow, H.J., et al. 1965. Comparison of subcortical, cortical and scalp activity using chronic indwelling electrodes in man. Electroencephalogr. Clin. Neurophysiol. 18:217–228.

Crandall, P.H. 1973. Developments in direct recordings from epileptogenic regions in the surgical treatment of partial epilepsies. In *Epilepsy: Its Phenomena in Man,* Ed. M.A.B. Brazier, pp. 287–310. New York: Academic Press.

Delgado, J.M.R., Hamlin, H., and Chapman, W.P. 1952. Technique of intracranial electrode emplacement for recording and stimulation and its possible therapeutic values in psychotic patients. Confin. Neurol. 12:315–319.

Dinner, D.S., Neme, S., Nair, D., et al. 2002. EEG and evoked potential recording from the subthalamic nucleus for deep brain stimulation of intractable epilepsy. Clin Neurophysiol. 113:1391–1402.

Dodge, H.W., Bailey, A.A., Bickford, R.G., et al. 1953. Neurosurgical and neurological application of depth electrography. Proc. Staff Med. Mayo Clin. 28:88–91.

Dodge, H.W., Bickford, R.G., Bailey, A.A., et al. 1954. Techniques and potentialities of intracranial electrography. Postgrad. Med. 15:291–300.

Dow, R.S. 1938. The electrical activity of the cerebellum and its functional significance. J. Physiol. (London) 94:67–86.

Drlickova, V., Sramka, M., and Nadvornik, P. 1983. Dynamics of EEG and SEEG changes in dentate nucleus stimulation for the treatment of epilepsy. Electroencephalogr. Clin. Neurophysiol. 55:30P(abst).

Ebersole, J.S. 1997. Diffuse epileptogenic foci: past, present, future. J. Clin. Neurophysiol. 14:470–483.

Eisenschenk, S., Gilmore, R.L., Cibula, J.F., et al. 2001. Lateralization of temporal lobe foci: depth versus subdural electrodes. Clin. Neurophysiol. 112:836–844.

Engel, J. (ed.) 1987a. *Surgical Treatment of the Epilepsies.* New York: Raven Press.

Engel, J., Jr. 1987b. New concepts of the epileptogenic focus. In *The Epileptic Focus,* Eds. H.G. Wieser, E.-J. Speckmann, and J. Engel, Jr., pp. 83–94. London: Libbey.

Engel, J., Jr., and Crandall, P.H. 1983. Falsely localizing ictal onsets with depth EEG telemetry during anticonvulsant withdrawal. Epilepsia (New York) 24:344–355.

Engel, J., Jr., Crandall, P.H., and Brown, W.J. 1981a. Significance of focal, regional and bilaterally independent ictal EEG onsets recorded from mesial temporal depth electrodes (SEEG). Electroencephalogr. Clin. Neurophysiol. 51:21P(abst).

Engel, J., Jr., Rausch, R., Lieb, J.P., et al. 1981b. Correlation of criteria used for localizing epileptic foci in patients considered for surgical therapy of epilepsy. Ann. Neurol. 9:215–224.

Engel, J., Jr., Henry, T.R., Risinger, M.W., et al. 1990. Presurgical evaluation for partial epilepsy: relative contributions of chronic depth-electrode recordings vs. FDG-PET and scalp-sphenoidal ictal EEG. Neurology 40:1670–1677.

Fiol, M.E., Gates, J.R., and Torres, F. 1983. Intracarotid amobarbital effect on epileptiform discharges. Electroencephalogr. Clin. Neurophysiol. 56: 26P–27P(abst).

Fisher, R.S., and Niedermeyer, E. 1986. Depth EEG studies in the Lennox-Gastaut syndrome. Epilepsia (New York) 27:637–638(abst).

Fisher, R.S., and Niedermeyer, E. 1987. Depth EEG studies in the Lennox-Gastaut syndrome. Clin. Electroencephalogr. 18:191–200.

Flanigin, H.F. 1989. Depth electrode studies in pre-surgical evaluations. Electroencephalogr. Clin. Neurophysiol. 73:67P(abst).

Foerster, O., and Altenburger, H. 1935. Elektrobiologische Vorgänge an der menschilchen Hirnrinde. Dtsch. Z. Nervenheilk. 135:277–288.

Fourment, A., Calvet, J., and Bancaud, J. 1976. Electrocorticography of waves associated with eye movements in man during wakefulness. Electroencephalogr. Clin. Neurophysiol. 40:457–469.

Gerard, R.W., Marshall, W.H., and Saul, L.J. 1936. Electrical activity of the cat's brain. Arch. Neurol. Psychiatry (Chicago) 36:675–738.

Gloor, P. 1975. Contribution of electroencephalography to the neurosurgical treatment of the epilepsies. In *Neurosurgical Management of the Epilepsies,* Eds. D.P. Purpura, J.K. Penry, and R.D. Walter, pp. 59–105. New York: Raven Press.

Gloor, P. 1978. Evolution of the concept of the mechanism of generalized epilepsy with bilateral spike and wave discharge. In *Modern Perspectives in Epilepsy,* Ed. J.A. Wada, pp. 99–137. Montreal: Eden Press.

Gloor, P. 1983. Electroencephalography and the role of depth recordings. Abstracts, 15th Epilepsy International Symposium, Washington, DC, 1983, p. 76.

Gloor, P. 1984. Electrophysiology of generalized epilepsy. In *Electrophysiology of Epilepsy,* Eds. P.A. Schwartzkroin and H.V. Wheal, pp. 107–136. London: Academic Press.

Gotman, J. 1993. Computer-assisted EEG analysis. In *The Treatment of Epilepsy,* Ed. E. Wyllie, pp. 268–277. Philadelphia: Lea and Febiger.

Gotman, J., Gloor, P., Quesney, L.F., et al. 1982. Correlations between EEG changes induced by diazepam and the localization of spikes and seizures. Electroencephalogr. Clin. Neurophysiol. 54:614–621.

Graf, M., Niedermeyer, E., Schiemann, J., et al. 1984. Electrocorticography: information derived from intraoperative recordings during seizure surgery. Clin. Electroencephalogr. 15:83–91.

Gücer, G., Niedermeyer, E., and Long, D.M. 1978. Thalamic recordings in patients with chronic pain. J. Neurol. (Berlin) 219:47–61.

Gumnit, J. 1987. Postscript: Who should be referred for surgery? In *Surgical Treatment of the Epilepsies,* Ed. J. Engel, Jr., pp. 71–74. New York: Raven Press.

Hayne, R., Belinson, L., and Gibbs, F.A. 1949a. Electrical activity of subcortical areas in epilepsy. Electroencephalogr. Clin. Neurophysiol. 1: 437–445.

Hayne, R., Meyers, R., and Knott, J.R. 1949b. Characteristics of electrical activity of human corpus striatum and neighboring structures. J. Neurophysiol. 12:185–195.

Heath, R.G. 1958. Correlation of electrical recordings from cortical and subcortical regions of the brain with abnormal behavior in human subjects. Confin. Neurol. 18:305–315.

Heath, R.G. 1963. Electrical self-stimulation of the brain in man. Am. J. Psychiatry 120:571–577.

Heath, R.G. 1966. Schizophrenia: biochemical and physiologic aberrations. Int. J. Neuropsychiatry 2:597–610.

Heath, R.G. 1972. Pleasure and brain activity in man. Deep and surface electroencephalogram during orgasm. J. Nerv. Ment. Dis. 154:3–18.

Heath, R.G., and Guerrero-Figueroa, R. 1965. Psychotic behavior with evoked septal dysrhythmia: Effects of intracerebral acetylcholine and gamma aminobutyric acid. Am. J. Psychiatry 121:1080–1086.

Heath, R.G., Peacock, S.M., and Miller, W. 1953. Induced paroxysmal electrical activity in man recorded simultaneously through subcortical and scalp electrodes. Trans. Am. Neurol. Assoc. 78:247.

Horsley, V. 1886. Brain-surgery. Br. Med. J. 2:670–675.

Hufnagel, A., Helmstadter, C., Elger, C.E., et al. 1990. Electrocorticographic registration of the epileptic focus during intracarotid amobarbital test: its correlation to localized memory and learning deficits. Electroencephalogr. Clin. Neurophysiol. 75:S62(abst).

Hughes, J.R., and Andy, O.J. 1979. The human amygdala. I. Electrophysiological responses to odorants. Electroencephalogr. Clin. Neurophysiol. 46:428–443.

Ishikawa, O. 1957. Electroencephalographical study of human thalamus. Folia Psychiatr. Neurol. Jpn. 11:128–149.

Ives, J., Gloor, P., Quesney, F., et al. 1981. The contribution and importance of an automatic cable-telemetry seizure monitoring system on a group of epileptic patients with stereotaxic depth electrodes. Electroencephalogr. Clin. Neurophysiol. 51:23P–24P(abst).

Jankel, W.R., and Niedermeyer, E. 1985. Sleep spindles. J. Clin. Neurophysiol. 2:1–35.

Jinnai, D. 1966. Clinical results of Forel-H-tomy in the treatment of epilepsy. Confin. Neurol. 27:129–136.

Jones-Gotman, M. 1987. Commentary: Psychological evaluation, testing hippocampal function. In *Surgical Treatment of the Epilepsies.* Ed. J. Engel, Jr., pp. 203–211. New York: Raven Press.

Juhasz, C., Chugani, D.C., Muzik, O., et al. 2000. Is epileptogenic tissue truly hypometabolic on interictal positron emission tomography? Ann. Neurol. 48:88–96.

Jung, R., and Kornmüller, A. E. 1938. Eine Methodik der Ableitung lokalisierter Potentialschwankungen aus subcorticalen Hirngebieten. Arch. Psychiatr. Nervenkrankh. 109:1–30.

Jung, R., Riechert, T., and Meyer-Mickeleit, R.W. 1950. Über intracerebrale Hirnpotentialableitungen bei hirnchirurgischen Eingriffen. Dtsch. Z. Nervenheilk. 162:52–60.

King, D., and Spencer, S. 1995. Invasive electroencephalography in mesial temporal lobe epilepsy. J. Clin. Neurophysiol. 12:32–45.

Knott, J.R., Hayne, R.A., and Meyers, H.R. 1950. Physiology of sleep-wave characteristics and temporal relations of human electroencephalograms recorded from the thalamus, the corpus striatum and the surface of the scalp. Arch. Neurol. Psychiatry (Chicago) 63:526–527.

Kornmüller, A.E. 1939. Bioelektrische Untersuchungen ber den Pathomechanismus des Zentralnervensystems. Dtsch. Z. Nervenheilk. 139:81–89.

Lange, H.H., Lieb, J.P., Engel, J., Jr., et al. 1983. Temporo-spatial patterns of pre-ictal spike activity in human temporal lobe epilepsy. Electroencephalogr. Clin. Neurophysiol. 56:543–555.

Lieb, J.P., Woods, S.C., Siccardi, A., et al. 1978. Quantitative analysis of depth spiking in relation to seizure foci in patients with temporal lobe epilepsy. Electroencephalogr. Clin. Neurophysiol. 44:641–663.

Lieb, J.P., Joseph, J.P., Engel, J., Jr., et al. 1980. Sleep state and seizure foci related to depth spike activity in patients with temporal lobe spikes. Electroencephalogr. Clin. Neurophysiol. 49:539–557.

Lieb, J.P., Engel, J., Jr., and Crandall, P.H. 1981. Rates of false localization in surface and depth interictal EEG records in temporal lobe epilepsy. Electroencephalogr. Clin. Neurophysiol. 51:21P(abst).

Lieb, J.P., Babb, T.L., Engel, J., Jr., et al. 1984. Interhemispheric propagation time of hippocampal seizures: cell density and surgical outcome correlates. Electroencephalogr. Clin. Neurophysiol. 58:38P(abst).

Lopes da Silva, F.H., Van Hulten, K., Lommen, J.G., et al. 1977. Automatic detection and localization of epileptic foci. Electroencephalogr. Clin. Neurophysiol. 43:1–13.

Lüders, H. (Ed.) 1992. *Epilepsy Surgery*. New York: Raven Press.

Lüders, H.O., and Awad, I. 1992. Conceptual considerations. In *Epilepsy Surgery*, Ed. H.O. Lüders, pp. 51–62. New York: Raven Press.

Lüders, H., Lesser, R.P., Dinner, D.S., et al. 1987. Commentary: chronic intracranial recording and stimulation with subdural electrodes. In *Surgical Treatment of the Epilepsies*, Ed. J. Engel, Jr., pp. 297–321. New York: Raven Press.

Machek, J., Vladyka, V., Ojec, E., et al. 1983. Negative slow potential changes (NSPC) in the hippocampus-amygdala complex (HAC) of epileptic patients treated with HAC thermocoagulation. Electroencephalogr. Clin. Neurophysiol. 55:30P(abst).

Marg, E., and Adams, J.E. 1967. Indwelling multiple micro-electrodes in the brain. Electroencephalogr. Clin. Neurophysiol. 23:277–280.

Matsui, I., Yoshioka, H., Ishikawa, O., et al. 1957. Clinical and EEG reactions developed by electrical stimulation of human caudatum and thalamus. Folia Psychiatr. Neurol. Jpn. 11:150–156.

McCarthy, G., Spencer, D.D., and Riker, R.J. 1992. The stereotaxic placement of depth electrodes. In *Epilepsy Surgery*, Ed. H.O. Lüders, pp. 385–393. New York: Raven Press.

McNaughton, F.L., and Rasmussen, T. 1975. Criteria for selection of patients for neurosurgical treatment. In *Neurosurgical Management of the Epilepsies*, Eds. D.P. Purpura, J.K. Penry, and R.D. Walter, pp. 37–48. New York: Raven Press.

Meyers, H.R., and Hayne, R. 1948. Electrical potentials of the corpus striatum and cortex in Parkinsonism and hemiballism. Trans. Am. Neurol. Assoc. 73:10–14.

Munari, C., and Bancaud, J. 1985. The role of stereo-electroencephalography (SEEG) in the evaluation of partial epileptic seizures. In *The Epilepsies*, Eds. R.J. Porter and P.L. Morselli, pp. 267–306. London: Butterworth.

Murray, N.M.F., Kris, A., and Evans, B. 1986. AIDS, Hepatitis B and Creutzfeldt-Jakob disease: guidelines for dealing with patients and electrodes in the clinical neurophysiology laboratory. J. Electrophysiol. Technol. 12:53–59.

Narabayashi, H., and Kubota, K. 1967. Thalamic projections of lowest threshold muscle afferents seen by averaging technique. Confin. Neurol. 29:159(abst).

Niedermeyer, E. 1970. Intravenous diazepam and its anticonvulsive action. Johns Hopkins Med. J. 127:79–96.

Niedermeyer, E. 1972. *The Generalized Epilepsies*. Springfield, IL: Charles C Thomas.

Niedermeyer, E. 1996. Dipole theory and electroencephalography. Clin. Electroencephalogr. 27:121–131.

Niedermeyer, E. 1997. The EEG from scalp, cortex and depth: Comparisons and considerations. Clin. Electroencephalogr. 28:60–61.

Niedermeyer, E. 2004. The electrocerebellogram. Clin. EEG Neurosci. 35:112–915.

Niedermeyer, E., and Jankel, W.R. 1984. Falling asleep: depth EEG and thermographic observations. Electroencephalogr. Clin. Neurophysiol. 58:8P(abst).

Niedermeyer, E., and Rocca, U. 1972. The diagnostic significance of sleep electroencephalogram in temporal lobe epilepsy. Eur. Neurol. (Basal) 7:119–129.

Niedermeyer, E., and Uematsu, S. 1974. Electroencephalographic recordings from deep cerebellar structures in patients with uncontrolled epileptic seizures. Electroencephalogr. Clin. Neurophysiol. 37:355–365.

Niedermeyer, E., and Uematsu, S. 1989a. Epidural recordings in candidates for temporal lobectomy. Electroencephalogr. Clin. Neurophysiol. 72:9P(abst).

Niedermeyer, E., and Uematsu, S. 1989b. Bilateral epidural EEG recordings: a reliable and safe assessment of candidates for temporal lobectomy. Epilepsia (New York) 30:694(abst).

Niedermeyer, E., Ray, C.D., and Walker, A.E. 1967. Depth studies in a patient with fourteen and six per second positive spikes. Electroencephalogr. Clin. Neurophysiol. 22:86–89.

Niedermeyer, E., Laws, E.R., Jr., and Walker, A.E. 1969. Depth EEG findings in epileptics with generalized spike-wave complexes. Arch. Neurol (Chicago) 21:51–58.

Niedermeyer, E., Jankel, W.R., and Uematsu, S. 1986. Falling asleep: observations and thoughts. Am. J. EEG Technol. 26:165–175.

Ojeman, G.A., and Engel, J., Jr. 1987. Acute and chronic intracranial recording and stimulation. In *Surgical Treatment of the Epilepsies*, Ed. J. Engel, Jr., pp. 263–288. New York: Raven Press.

Okuma, T., Shimazono, Y., Fukuda, T., et al. 1954. Cortical and subcortical recordings in non-anesthesized and anesthetized periods in man. Electroencephalogr. Clin. Neurophysiol. 6:269–286.

Penfield, W., and Baldwin, M. 1952. Temporal lobe seizures and the technic of subtotal temporal lobectomy. Ann. Surg. 136:625–634.

Penfield, W., and Jasper, H.H. 1954. *Epilepsy and the Functional Anatomy of the Human Brain*. Boston: Little, Brown.

Perez-Borja, C., Chartrian, G.E., Tyce, F.A., et al. 1962. Electrographic patterns of the occipital lobe in man. A topographic study based on the use of implanted electrodes. Electroencephalogr. Clin. Neurophysiol. 14:171.

Petersen, R.C., and Sharbrough, F.W. 1992. Posterior cerebral artery amobarbital test. In *Epilepsy Surgery*, Ed. H.O. Lüders, pp. 525–529. New York: Raven Press.

Pfurtscheller, G., and Cooper, R. 1975. Frequency dependence of the transmission of the EEG from cortex to the scalp. Electroencephalogr. Clin. Neurophysiol. 38:93–96.

Rasmussen, T., and Jasper, H.H. 1958. Temporal lobe epilepsy: Indication for operation and surgical technique. In *Temporal Lobe Epilepsy*, Eds. P. Bailey and M. Baldwin, pp. 440–460. Springfield, IL: Charles C Thomas.

Ray, C.D., Bickford, R.G., Clark, L.C., Jr., et al. 1965. A new multicontact multi-purpose brain depth probe. Mayo Clin. Proc. 40:781–790.

Rayport, M. 1975. Stereotaxic microelectrode recording in human focal epilepsy. In *Handbook of Electroencephalography and Clinical Neurophysiology*, Ed. A. Remond, vol. 10B, pp. 34–35. Amsterdam: Elsevier.

Rayport, M., and Waller, H.J. 1961. Microelectrode analysis of the human epileptiform spike. Excerpta Med., Int. Congress Ser. 37:14.

Rayport, M., and Waller, H.J. 1967. Technique and results of microelectrode recording in human epileptogenic foci. Electroencephalogr. Clin. Neurophysiol. Suppl. 25:143–151.

Rektor, I., Svejdova, M., Kanovsky P., et al. 1997. Can epileptologists without access to intracranial EEG use reliably the International League Against Epilepsy Classification of the localization-related epileptic syndromes? J. Clin. Neurophysiol. 14:250–254.

Rossi, G.F. 1973. Problems of analysis and interpretation of electrocerebral signals in human epilepsy. A neurosurgeon's view. In *Epilepsy: Its Phenomena in Man*, Ed. M.A.B. Brazier, pp. 259–285. New York: Academic Press.

Rossi, G.F., Walter, R.D., and Crandall, P.H. 1967. Generalized spike and wave discharges and non- specific thalamic nuclei. Arch. Neurol. (Chicago) 19:174–183.

Rossi, G.F., Colicchio, G., Pola, P. 1984a. Interictal epilepsy activity during sleep: a stereo-EEG study in patients with partial epilepsy. Electroencephalogr. Clin. Neurophysiol. 58:97–106.

Rossi, G.F., Colicchio, G., Pola, P., et al. 1984b. Sleep and epileptic activity. In *Epilepsy, Sleep and Sleep Deprivation*, Eds. R. Degen and E. Niedermeyer, pp. 35–46. Amsterdam: Elsevier.

Rovit, R., Gloor, P., and Rasmussen, T. 1961. Intracarotid amobarbital in epilepsy. Arch. Neurol. (Chicago) 5:606–626.

Schaltenbrand, G., and Bailey, P. (Eds.). 1959. *Introduction to Stereotaxis with an Atlas of the Human Brain*. Stuttgart: Thieme.

Sem-Jacobsen, C.W. 1968. *Depth-electrographic Stimulation of the Human Brain and Behavior*. Springfield, IL: Charles C Thomas.

Sem-Jacobsen, C.W., Petersen, H., Lazarte, J.A., et al. 1955. Electroencephalographic rhythms from the depths of the frontal lobe in 60 psychotic patients. Electroencephalogr. Clin. Neurophysiol. 7:193–210.

Sem-Jacobsen, C.W., Petersen, M.C., Dodge, H.W., et al. 1956. Electroencephalographic rhythms from the depths of the parietal, occipital and temporal lobes of man. Electroencephalogr. Clin. Neurophysiol. 8:263–278.

Smith, D.B., Sidman, R.D., Henke, J.S., et al. 1983. Scalp and depth recordings of induced cerebral potentials. Electroencephalogr. Clin. Neurophysiol. 55:145–150.

Snider, R.S. 1950. Recent contributions to the anatomy and physiology of the cerebellum. Arch. Neurol. Psychiatry (Chicago) 64:196–219.

Spencer, S.S., Spencer, D.D., Williamson, P.D., et al. 1982. The localizing value of depth electroencephalography in 32 patients with refractory epilepsy. Ann. Neurol. 12:248–253.

Sperling, M.R. 1993. *Intracranial Electroencephalography*. Amsterdam: Elsevier.

Sperling, M.R., Brown, W.J., and Crandall, P.H. 1986. Focal burst-suppression induced by thiopental. Electroencephalogr. Clin. Neurophysiol. 63:203–208.

Spiegel, E.A. 1937. Comparative study of the thalamic, cerebral and cerebellar potentials. Am. J. Physiol. 118:569–579.

Talairach, J., De Ajuriaguerra, J., and David, M. 1952. Études stéréotaxiques et structures encéphaliques profondes chez l'homme. Presse Méd. 28:605–609.

Talairach, J., Szikla, G., Tournoux, P., et al. 1967. *Atlas d'Anatomie Stéréotaxique du Télencéphale*. Paris: Masson.

Tassinari, C.A., Roger, J., Regis, H., et al. 1971. Die myoklonische zerebelläre Dyssynergie nach Ramsay Hunt und die Aktionsmyoklonie beim Lance-Adams-Syndrom. Z. EEG-EMG 2:86–91.

Toczek, M.T., Morrell, M.J., Risinger, M.W., et al. 1997. Intracranial ictal recordings in mesial frontal lobe epilepsy. J. Clin. Neurophysiol. 14:499–506.

Umbach, W. 1966. *Electrophysiologische und vegetative Phänomeme bei stereotaktischen Hirnoperationen*. Berlin: Springer.

Umbach, W., and Riechert, T. 1964. Elektrophysiologische und klinische Ergebnisse stereotaktischer Eingriffe im limbischen System bei temporaler Epilepsie. Nervenarzt 35:482–488.

Velasco, M., Velasco, F., Alcala, H., et al. 1990. Epileptiform EEG activity of the centromedian thalamic nuclei in children with Lennox-Gastaut syndrome. Electroencephalogr. Clin. Neurophysiol. 75:S158(abst).

Wada, J. 1949. A new method for the determination of the side of cerebral speech dominance—a preliminary report on the intracarotid injection of sodium Amytal in man. Med. Biol. (Tokyo) 14:221–222 (in Japanese).

Wagner, W. 1984. Das EEG des menschlichen Hippokampus—eine Zusammenfassung und Diskussion bisher veröffentlichter Ergebnisse bei Patienten mit neurologischen Grunderkrankungen. Z. EEG-EMG 15:8–14.

Walker, A.E. 1967. Temporal lobectomy. J. Neurosurg. 6:641–649.

Walker, A.E. 1972. Surgical treatment of epilepsy. In *Comprehensive Management of Epilepsy in Infancy, Childhood and Adolescence*, Eds. S. Livingston and I.M. Pruce, pp. 406–436. Springfield, IL: Charles C Thomas.

Walker, A.E., and Marshall, C. 1964. The contribution of depth recording to clinical medicine. Electroencephalogr. Clin. Neurophysiol. 16:88–99.

Walter, R.D. 1973. Tactical considerations leading to surgical treatment of limbic epilepsy. In *Epilepsy: Its Phenomena in Man*, Ed. M.A.B. Brazier, pp. 99–119. New York: Academic Press.

Walter, W.G., and Crow, H.J. 1964. Depth recording from the human brain. Electroencephalogr. Clin. Neurophysiol. 16:68–72.

Ward, A.A., Jr. 1969. The epileptic neuron: chronic foci in animal and man. In *Basic Mechanisms of the Epilepsies*, Eds. H.H. Jasper, A.A. Ward, Jr., and A. Pope, pp. 263–288. Boston: Little, Brown.

Ward, A.A., Jr., and Schmidt, R.P. 1961. Some properties of single epileptic neurons. Arch. Neurol. (Chicago) 5:308–313.

Wieser, H.G. 1981. Stereo-electroencephalographic correlates of motor seizures. Electroencephalogr. Clin. Neurophysiol. 52:98P(abst).

Wieser, H.G. 1983. *Electroclinical Features of the Psychomotor Seizure*. Stuttgart: Fisher (London: Butterworth).

Wieser, H.G. 1984. Temporal lobe epilepsy, sleep and arousal: Stereo-EEG findings. In *Epilepsy, Sleep and Sleep Deprivation*, Eds. R. Degen and E. Niedermeyer, pp. 137–167. Amsterdam: Elsevier.

Wieser, G. 1992. Anterior cerebral artery amobarbital test. In *Epilepsy Surgery*, Ed. H.O. Lüders, pp. 515–523. New York: Raven Press.

Wieser, H.G., and Siegfried, J. 1979a. Hirnstamm-Ableitungen (Makroelektroden) beim Menschen. 1. Elektrische Befunde im Wachzustand und Ganznachtschlaf. Z. EEG-EMG 10:8–19.

Wieser, H.G., and Siegfried, J. 1979b. Hirnstamm-Ableitungen (Makroelektroden) beim Menschen. 2. Klinische und elektrische Effekte bei Stimulation im periaquduktalen Grau (PGM); augenbewegungsabhängige Aktivität; visuelle und somatosensorische Reizantworten im PGM. Z. EEG-EMG 10:62–69.

Wieser, H,G., Bancaud, J., Talairach, J., et al. 1979. Comparative value of spontaneous and chemically and electrically induced seizures in establishing the lateralization of temporal lobe seizures. Epilepsia (New York) 20:47–59.

Williams, D. 1953. A study of thalamic and cortical rhythms in "petit mal." Brain 76:50–67.

Wilson, W.P., and Nashold, B.S. 1968. Epileptic discharges occurring in the mesencephalon and thalamus. Epilepsia (Amsterdam) 9:265–273.

Zobniw, A.M., Yarworth, S., and Niedermeyer, E. 1975. Depth electroencephalography. J. Electrophysiol. Technol. 1:215–240.

37. Stereoelectroencephalography and Foramen Ovale Electrode Recording

Heinz Gregor Wieser

The electroencephalogram (EEG) is the most informative laboratory test for the diagnosis of epilepsy because it can help answer the following important questions (Engel, 1989): Does the patient suffer from epilepsy? What kind of epilepsy? How good is therapy? Where is (are) the epileptogenic lesion(s)?

If surgical treatment is envisaged, precise localization, i.e., accurate identification of an interictal EEG spike focus and, in particular, of the seizure onset, becomes the most important issue.

With reference to *exact localization* there are, however, several well-known drawbacks of the standard 10–20 scalp EEG. For example, it does not adequately cover the temporal lobes and the interhemispheric cortex. To compensate for this, several *additional electrodes* and *EEG recording techniques* are in common use. These can be divided into *noninvasive, semiinvasive,* and *invasive* techniques. With the term *noninvasive* we denote all *extracranial techniques*, i.e., additional basal electrodes and special *extracranial electrodes*.

Basal electrodes are placed on the ear lobes (A_1 and A_2), on the mastoid (M_1 and M_2), over the zygoma, or at T_1 and T_2 (true temporals). The most commonly employed *special extracranial electrodes* in the investigation of patients with suspected temporal or frontal epilepsy are *nasopharyngeal* (Pg1-Pg2), *sphenoidal* (Sp1-Sp2), *nasoethmoidal* (NE1-NE2), and *supraorbital* (SO1-SO2) electrodes (Quesney and Gloor, 1987). In addition, the so-called *peg electrodes* have been advocated for presurgical evaluation (Wieser and Morris, 1997). Although they are extracranial, some people prefer to label them intermediately invasive. They seem to have some advantages over the epidural screw electrodes, which are no longer in common use. Furthermore, Ribaric and Sekulovic (1989) have described the use of *orbital electrodes*.

Nasopharyngeal electrodes are inserted through the nose to record from the roof of the nasopharynx. Usually the electrodes are somewhat flexible and can be placed by an EEG technologist (Mavor and Hellen, 1964). The utility of nasopharyngeal electrodes is limited by the fact that these electrodes are uncomfortable, reduce the likelihood that natural sleep recording can be obtained, and cannot be left in place for long periods of time. In addition, pharyngeal muscle contraction and movement produce artifacts that confound interpretation.

Sphenoidal electrodes (Fig. 37.1) are more potent. Sphenoidal electrodes, however, are not recommended for use in the routine EEG laboratory, but are preferred for long-term monitoring. Their main advantage is that they provide more reliable recordings, although they have only a minimally higher yield for detecting mesial temporal spikes, when compared to other basal electrodes (Rovit et al., 1961; Sperling et al., 1986). See King et al. (1986) and Chapter 35, "Nasopharyngeal, Sphenoidal, and Other Electrodes," for details concerning the construction of the electrode, insertion technique and removal, as well as advantages, disadvantages, and potential complications of this procedure.

Epidural screw electrodes have been used at the Montreal Neurological Institute for similar purposes (Quesney, 1987), but protrude from the skull and may produce patient discomfort. *Epidural strip electrodes* (Wyler et al., 1984) require either a craniotomy or a larger bur hole. *Epidural peg electrodes* were developed in order to allow sampling of the EEG of the cortical convexity in some potential candidates for epilepsy surgery, and in particular to help guide placement of subdural grid arrays in patients with neocortical epilepsy. The electroencephalographer decides on the locations for the epidural peg electrodes using all available information including the history and semiology (especially the aura) of the seizures; the neurological examination; the results of neuroimaging; and the results of the prolonged EEG/video recordings with closely spaced scalp and sphenoidal electrodes. The electrode locations are marked on the patient's scalp by the EEG technologist.

Epidural peg electrodes (Fig. 37.2) are mushroom-shaped composites of Silastic plastic with a stainless steel (or platinum) disk that serves as the electrical contact. They are surgically implanted using a 4.5-mm bur hole. These electrodes have been in use at the epilepsy center of the Cleveland Clinic Foundation since 1988 and have been used for sampling ongoing EEG from wide areas of the cerebral hemispheres. The preliminary results from 30 of these cases have been reported in the literature (Awad et al., 1991; Barnett et al., 1990; Wieser and Morris, 1997).

Dissection of the epidural space is not needed for the epidural peg electrodes, and therefore the theoretical risk of epidural hematoma is avoided. The electrodes may be inserted using general or local anesthesia. While individual electrodes may be inserted through a 1- to 2-cm scalp incision, if several are to be used in one region (e.g., the frontal convexity), the surgeon may elect to turn a scalp flap; if electrodes are to be placed below the hair line, a scalp flap is customary.

A 4.5-mm bur hole using a twist drill with a "stop" is made by the surgeon at the predetermined electrode sites and a peg electrode of appropriate length is inserted into the hole. The diameter of the electrode is 4.7 mm at the base and 4.5 mm at the tip; it is made in lengths of 3 to 19 mm in 2-mm increments. The wire is 38 gauge, 15 strand, 50 AWG

Figure 37.1. Placement of sphenoidal electrodes. The needle is inserted approximately 1 inch (2.5 cm) anterior to the tragus immediately under the zygomatic arch (*black dot* in the lateral view, *left*). The tip of the electrode lies close to the foramen ovale (*right*). The *inset* shows the tip of the insertion needle with the multistranded Teflon-coated wire, which is free at the tip and is bent backward.

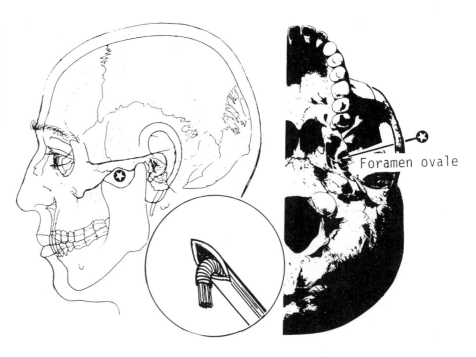

Figure 37.2. Epidural peg electrode. **A:** The electrode consists of a stainless steel or platinum disc embedded into a mushroom-shaped Silastic housing. The stalk has a gradual taper from a maximum diameter (d2) of 4.7 mm to a tip diameter (d1) of 4.5 mm. Stalk heights (h) range from 3 to 19 mm in 2-mm increments to match skull thickness. The cap (d3) has a diameter of 12.7 mm, a radius of curvature of 9.5 mm, and a height of 2.5 mm (MDX4–4210, Dow Corning Corp., Midland, MI). The peg is implanted via 1.5-cm scalp incision (shown in **B**) or under a subgaleal flap. **C:** Im-

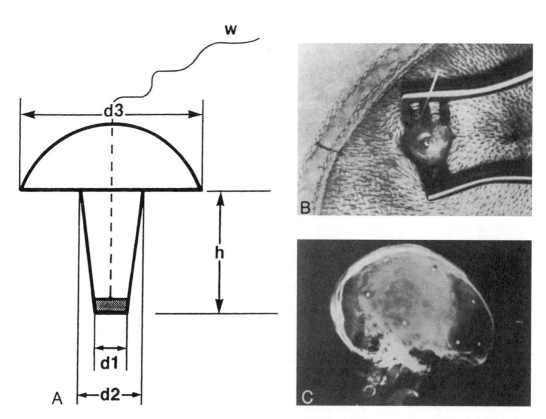

planted epidural pegs are shown in the lateral skull x-ray. (**A** from Barnett, G.H., Burgess, R.C., Awad, I.A., et al. 1990. Epidural peg electrodes for the presurgical evaluation of intractable epilepsy. Neurosurgery 27:113–115. **B** and **C** from Awad, I.A., Assirati, J.A., Burgess, R., et al. 1991. A new class of electrodes of intermediate invasiveness: preliminary experience with epidural pegs and foramen ovale electrodes in the mapping of seizure foci. Neurol. Res. 13:177–183.)

(American wire gauge) Teflon-coated steel and exits from the dome of the electrode. It is threaded through a surgical needle and exits the scalp approximately 2 cm from the electrode itself (Awad et al., 1991; Barnett et al., 1990; Wieser and Morris, 1997). The wound is closed and the patient is sent to the laboratories for recordings.

Most commonly, the epidural peg electrodes are used *in combination with foramen ovale electrodes* and provide complementary and additional information to them. The foramen ovale electrodes are inserted by the surgeon during the same procedure.

The Cleveland Clinic Foundation group has had no serious complications from the epidural peg electrodes used in isolation; with over 500 pegs inserted, there has not been a single instance of a purulent wound infection. In all patients, the peg electrodes are cultured at the time of their removal; approximately one third of patients will have a positive culture, usually *Staphylococcus aureus*. If patients; cultures are positive, patients are treated prophylactically with the appropriate antibiotic for 2 weeks (Awad, personal communication).

The *intracranial recording techniques* can be divided into *extracerebral* and *intracerebral* techniques. The former include *subdural strips* (Wyler et al., 1984) and *grids* (Lüders et al., 1987) and the *foramen ovale electrodes*. The *intracerebral* techniques comprise "*depth electroencephalography,*" in which no stereotactic technique is employed and "*stereoelectroencephalography,*" in its strict sense.

Foramen Ovale Electrode Recording

The foramen ovale (FO) electrode recording technique can be labeled as an *intermediately invasive* or *semiinvasive approach* (Wieser, 1992). Because of the possibility of complications, its use is restricted and we recommend it only for presurgical evaluation of candidates for temporal lobe epilepsy (TLE) surgery.

Rationale for and History of Development of Foramen Ovale Electrode Recording

Based on our stereoelectroencephalographic (SEEG) findings that the majority of complex partial seizures originate in the mesiobasal limbic temporal lobe (Wieser, 1983), we proposed and developed the so-called transsylvian selective amygdalohippocampectomy (AHE) as a surgical treatment for mesiobasal TLE (Wieser, 1986; Wieser and Yasargil, 1982; Yasargil and Wieser, 1987). The first microsurgical operation of this type was performed in 1975 by Yasargil and, by the end of October 2003, 477 patients had been operated on by AHE with good results (Wieser et al., 2003). Before 1984, most of the candidates for AHE had to be evaluated by SEEG. This implied that only a relatively small proportion of the patients with surgically treatable mesiobasal TLE could be operated on. Since then the use of magnetic resonance imaging (MRI), single photon emission computed tomography (SPECT), positron emission tomography (PET), magnetic resonance spectroscopy (MRS), and sophisticated EEG analysis techniques has improved the presurgical evaluation. Despite this progress, it is still mandatory that the relevant epileptogenicity of a structural abnormality and/or functional

deficit zone must be proven. We therefore tried to simplify the neurophysiological part of the presurgical evaluation procedure of possible candidates for AHE by developing the FO recording technique.

In April 1984, we recorded for the first time in humans from a unipolar electrode, which was placed with its tip epicortically in the uncal region and which had been inserted through the right FO according to the technique of Kirschner (1932). Previous experiments in dogs had suggested this approach to be useful for detecting mesiobasal limbic foci. In 1985, we published this technique (Wieser et al., 1985), announcing the FO electrode as a new recording method for the preoperative evaluation of patients suffering from mesiobasal TLE. At that time, on the basis of our experience with ten patients, we attributed to this recording technique several great advantages: FO electrode placement is a relatively simple freehand manipulation, and, in comparison to the stereotactic depth recording (SEEG), it is nontraumatic to the brain. The FO electrodes were well tolerated and no relevant side effects were noted in the first ten patients. The FO electrodes showed extremely stable recording over prolonged periods, thus making them suitable for recording habitual seizures. In addition, satisfactory direct current (DC) recording was possible using Ag/AgCl electrodes and a special reference electrode. In comparison with conventional sphenoidal electrodes, FO electrodes had a much better signal-to-noise ratio and provided more precise localizing information, which is of importance for possible selective AHE (Wieser and Yasargil, 1982). Because of these encouraging early results, we then developed an improved multipolar FO electrode with better mechanical characteristics (Wieser and Moser, 1988; Wieser and Schwarz, 2001).

Thus far, 247 patients have undergone FO electrode implantation and we have made a detailed electroclinical analysis of 320 full-blown seizures and 93 auras recorded by FO electrodes in 77 patients by the end of 1989 (Wieser and Siegel, 1991). From the data forms submitted to the 1992 Palm Desert Conference, 160 of 4,627 anterior temporal lobectomies have been studied with FO electrodes, 121 of 547 AHEs, 50 of 1,011 extratemporal resections, 2 of 217 hemispherectomies, 5 of 795 corpus callosum sections, and 4 of 424 lesionectomies (Engel, personal communication).

FO Electrodes: Their Characteristics, Insertion, and Removal

The previously used FO electrodes (Fig. 37.3) were produced in our technical laboratory. In essence, this FO electrode consisted of four or ten Teflon-insulated, helically wound silver wires (diameter, 0.1143 mm = 0.0045 inch) ending in four or ten poles and mounted on a special stainless steel wire 0.1 mm in diameter. The electrode had adequate mechanical properties (tested in several cadaver experiments), was flexible enough, and had a special end to avoid penetration of the arachnoidal-pial layer. In the standard four-polar electrode, each pole consisted of 90 parallel windings and was 4 mm long. The distance between two contacts was 5 mm. The external diameter of the electrode was such that it passes through a special cleavable 18-gauge cannula of adequately small size (external diameter of the

Figure 37.3. Four-contact foramen ovale electrode with special cleavable cannula (18 gauge with background bevel) used for insertion of the multipolar foramen ovale electrode.

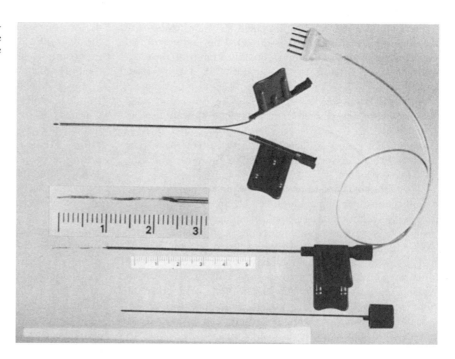

cannula, 1.23 mm; internal diameter, 0.93 mm). The cleavable cannula (produced and marketed by Medialimed SA; CH-1604 Puidoux, Switzerland) permitted the four- or ten-pin connector to be mounted, soldered, and the stabilizing insulator poured in well before implantation, and therefore ensures the best electrode reliability. The electrode impedance ranged from less than 200 ohms to a maximum of 700 ohms, respectively, whereas the DC offset potential was less than 2 mV. Several types of FO electrodes are commercially available.

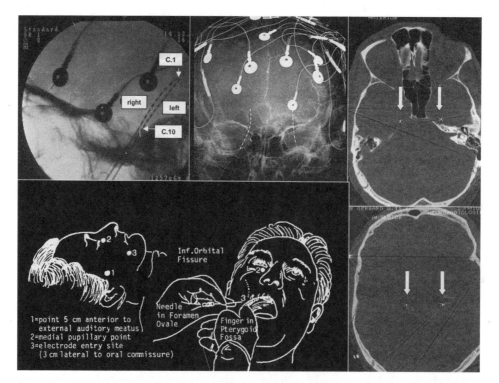

Figure 37.4. Foramen ovale electrodes. Schematic drawing of Härtel's cutaneous landmarks (Härtel, 1914) and mode of insertion to the foramen ovale according to Kirschner (1932). X-ray films and computed tomography (CT) scans showing the inserted ten-contact foramen ovale electrodes *(arrows)*. C.1 and C.10 are contacts 1 and 10, respectively. (From Wieser, H.G., Elger, C.E., and Stodieck, S.R.G., 1985. The "foramen ovale electrode": a new recording method for the preoperative evaluation of patients suffering from mesio-basal TLE. Electroencephalogr. Clin. Neurophysiol. 61:314–322, with permission.)

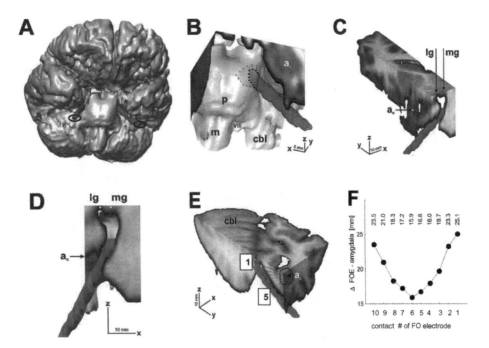

Figure 37.5. Three-dimensional (3D) anatomical location of foramen ovale (FO) electrode. **A:** Intracranial course of both FO electrodes. **B:** Location of the tip of left FO electrode *(large dots)* in the ambient cistern *(small dots)*. **C:** Relation of left FO electrode to the center of amygdala (ac) in CT space, center of lateral geniculate body (lg), center of the medial geniculate body (mg). **D:** Posterior view of left FO electrode within ambient cistern and its relation to ac, lg, and mg. **E:** Linear distance of each individual FO contact (length 2 mm, intercontact spacing 2 mm) to ac. **F:** Mean distance of each FO electrode contact to ac. Other abbreviations/symbols: the ellipse demarcates the foramen ovale; the FO electrode is in red; m, mesencephalon; p, pons; VII, rootlets of left vestibular nerve; 1 and 5, number of FO electrode contact; *, uncus hippocampi. (Modified from Wieser HG, Schwarz U. Topography of *foramen ovale* electrodes by 3D image reconstruction. *Clinical Neurophysiology* 2001;112:2053-2056, with permission.) (See Color Figure 37.5.)

Insertion of the FO electrode can be done under local anesthesia. Currently, however, we prefer the procedure to be done under general anesthesia. With the stylet inside the special cannula, the needle is inserted 3 cm lateral to the oral commissure and directed along the intersection of two orthogonal planes: (a) the plane defined by the insertion point, a point on the lower eyelid corresponding to the medial border of the pupil, and the tip of the electrode; and (b) a plane defined by the insertion point, a point 5 cm anterior to the external meatus acusticus and the tip of the electrode (Fig. 37.4).

The patient usually responds to the passage of the needle through the foramen ovale with a wince and a brief contraction of the masseter muscle. After withdrawal of the stylet, cerebrospinal fluid usually drops and the electrode can then be carefully inserted under radioscopic control. In most instances, the tip of the electrode slips without any resistance into the caudal end of the ambient cistern (Fig. 37.5). The cleavable cannula is then withdrawn and broken and the freed electrode is fixed by the use of a special clamp to the skin. Gauze and adhesive tape cover the electrode where it penetrates the skin. Antibiotic protection is given throughout the recording period and is continued for 3 days after the explantation. For the removal of the FO electrode, anesthesia is not necessary. During the withdrawal of the electrode a short-lasting painful sensation in the ipsilateral teeth is relatively common. Therefore, the patients should be informed about this possibility before the explantation.

Montage, Recording, and Analysis

More sophisticated recording (in particular DC recording) is done hard-wired with 32 or more channels in the laboratory. During radiotelemetric EEG monitoring on the ward (in AC mode), we prefer an uninterrupted bipolar montage connecting the 20 contacts of both FO electrodes, as shown in Fig. 37.6. The other channels are used for simultaneous scalp EEG and polygraphy, if indicated. Three Telefactor Videometry Systems (1094 New Dehaven Ave., W. Conshohocken, PA, 19428; phone: 610–825–4555; Fax: 610–941–0348; sales: 800–425–3334; e-mail: *sales@telefactor.com*; Web site: *http://www.telefactor.com*; Telefactor/Europe: Buitenkant 7, 8011 VH Zwolle, The Netherlands; phone: 31–38–4-231724; Fax: 31–38–4-231152; e-mail: *100667.1567@ compuserve.com*), which have up to 128 channels, have been adopted for our special needs and allow continuous monitoring without additional personnel (Wieser and Moser, 1988). Figure 37.7 gives an example of an ictal EEG recording obtained with this system.

Patient Data

FO electrodes were implanted in 247 patients in Zurich; 245 patients had medically refractory complex partial seizures with or without secondary generalization, one had aggressive outbursts thought to reflect limbic seizures, and one had no epileptic seizures. In most of the patients, prior to FO electrode implantation, there was rather strong suspicion of mesiobasal

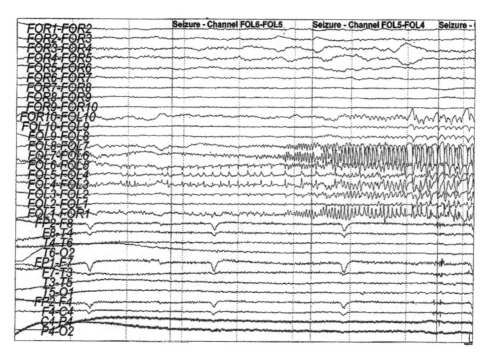

Figure 37.6. Ten-contact foramen ovale electrode recorded left mesial temporal seizure onset. Phase reversal of the initial spike train is at contact 5 of the left foramen ovale electrode (FOL5). Note that the deepest contact is numbered 1, and the contact closest to the foramen ovale is numbered 10. (See also Figs. 37.4 and 37.5.)

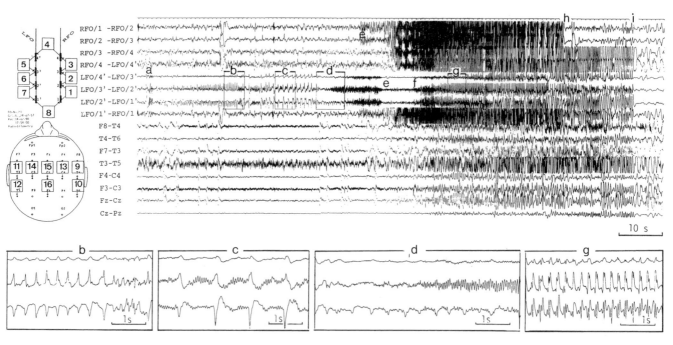

Figure 37.7. Example of a foramen ovale electrode recording showing a complex partial seizure with an onset at the left posterior parahippocampal gyrus. Note the multistaged seizure discharge. *a,* short-lived primary hypersynchronous pattern. *b,* electropositive ictal recruiting. *c,* so-called afterdischarge pattern. *d,* critical decrement and crescendo-like buildup of the high-frequency low-amplitude ("tonic") discharge pattern. *e,* propagation to the contralateral mesiobasal temporal lobe with ipsilateral decrement. *f,* reprise of the discharge left mesiotemporal. *g,* bilateral limbic systemic discharge. *h,* preterm isolated seizure cessation at the right posterior parahippocampal gyrus. *i,* general cessation of seizure discharge. The montage is shown on the left. Channels 1 to 8 are bipolar recordings from the FO electrodes in a closed chain (right contacts 1–4; left contacts 1′–4′). Channels 9–16 are bipolar scalp derivations (10–20 system; collodion-fixed Ag/AgCl cup electrodes). (From Wieser and Siegel, A.M. 1992. Indikationen zur chirurgischen Epilepsiebehandlung. Schweiz. Rundsch. Med. Prax. 81(19): 632–639.)

limbic seizure foci, as evidenced from the seizure symptomatology, interictal and ictal scalp EEG, neuropsychological examinations, and structural [computed tomography (CT), MRI] and functional (SPECT and PET) imaging. These patients were evaluated with the aim of demonstrating a unilateral mesiobasal limbic seizure focus with that degree of confidence necessary for surgical intervention. Twenty-nine patients had less clear evidence for mesiobasal temporal lobe (TL) seizure onset with some contradictory findings pointing to lateral TL or extratemporal seizure onset. The majority of these patients were evaluated simultaneously with FO and stereotactic depth electrodes. Only in 11 patients was mesiobasal limbic seizure onset rather unlikely. These patients underwent long-term monitoring with FO electrodes in order to definitively rule out mesiobasal limbic seizure onset (in which case they would have been no longer candidates for surgical treatment) or to prove a possible secondary pacemaker role of one mesiobasal TL (in which case a so-called palliative AHE would be considered as a treatment option).

Twenty-one percent of this series were considered inoperable and 79% underwent surgery, mostly selective AHE. Patients evaluated by FO electrodes prior to AHE did not differ significantly in their postoperative seizure outcome when compared to the overall AHE series evaluated mainly by SEEG (Wieser et al., 2003) (Table 37.1).

Complications

In the Zurich FO series, we had one serious complication consisting of a subarachnoid hemorrhage, which led to a transient upper pontine syndrome. A transient hypo- or dysesthesia, localized in one corner of the mouth, was reported in 19% of the cases. No other side effects or complications, and, in particular, no persisting trigeminal impairments, occurred. At the Palm Desert Epilepsy Surgery Conference, it was reported that a few other severe complications had occurred at other centers (Schüler et al., 1991).

Do Foramen Ovale Electrodes Yield Better Localizing Data Than Sphenoidal Electrodes?

We examined whether equally useful information might be obtained through sphenoidal electrodes when compared to FO electrodes. We designed a special FO electrode with eight contacts: four intracranial contacts, corresponding to our usual FO electrode, and four extracranial contacts, corresponding to a well-placed sphenoidal electrode (intercontact spacing, 5 mm). We implanted this FO electrode bilaterally in six patients undergoing presurgical evaluation. The recordings were reviewed by three independent raters, who selected for further analysis the most characteristic interictal epileptiform potentials and electroencephalographic seizures, as well as some physiological hippocampal graphoelements, such as spindles and hippocampal mu waves. We plotted the field distribution along the intracranial and extracranial contacts for each class of graphoelements.

Results

A considerable number of the epileptiform events detected in the intracranial contacts remained undetected in the

Table 37.1. Comparison of the Seizure Outcome of Four Patient Groups Operated on by Selective Amygdalohippocampectomy

	N	Type of Presurgical Evaluation (seizure monitoring)			Seizure Outcome (Engel Classes) after 1 year			
					I	II	III	IV
Group I	254				69%	9%	13%	9%
1975–1992		SEEG	32	17%				
(les:non-les = 60%:40%)		SEEG + FO	10					
		FO	87	34%				
		Non-invasive	125	49%				
Group II	165				79%	10%	9%	1%
1993–Aug. 2001		SEEG	0	1%				
(les:non-les = 41%:59%)		SEEG + FO	2					
		FO	77	47%				
		Strips & grids			66%			
		& FO	31	19%				
		Non-invasive	55	33%				
Group III	189				76%	8%	12%	5%
(les = gross lesion)								
Group IV	180				66%	11%	15%	9%
(non-les = no gross lesion other than HS)								

Groups I and II had AHE in different time periods (I: 1975 to 1992; II: 1993 to August 2001). "Non-lesional" patients of Group I have been evaluated mainly by SEEG, those of Group II mainly by FO electrodes. Since the seizure outcome differs depending on the underlying histopathology, "lesional" AHE (Group III) and so-called "non-lesional" AHE, i.e., mesial temporal lobe epilepsy (MTLE) with hippocampal sclerosis (HS) are also shown with their seizure outcome. Note that seizure outcome is better in the period 1993–2001; despite less invasive presurgical evaluation and despite that the proportion of the "non-lesional" AHE is larger, compared to the period 1975–1992. ("Lesional AHE" do better than "non-lesional AHE"). Seizure outcome classes: I, free of disabling seizures; II, rare seizures; III, worthwhile improvement, i.e., more than 75% seizure reduction and a clear-cut improvement of quality of life; IV, no worthwhile improvement.

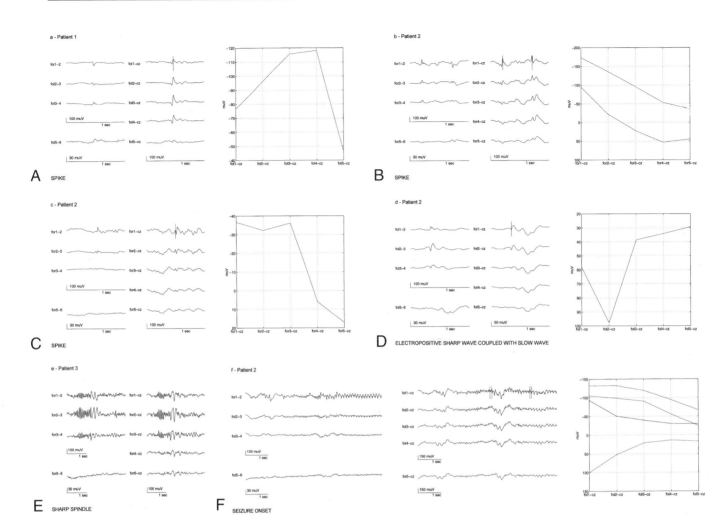

Figure 37.8. Six prototypic examples (**A–F**) showing, from left to right: bipolar tracings, referential tracings (ref = Cz, scalp), and the distribution of peak amplitude in contacts FO1 to FO5. Note that FO1 is the deepest in-tracranial contact, and the FO4 the intracranial contact closest to the fora-men ovale, whereas FO5 and FO6 are extracranial contacts corresponding to well-placed "sphenoidal" electrode contacts (see also Fig. 37.9).

extracranial (sphenoidal) contacts (Figs. 37.8 and 37.9). The likelihood of detection in the extracranial contacts depends on (1) location in the mesiobasal temporal lobe (anterior *versus* posterior), (2) the type of the graphoelement (spike, sharp wave, sharp slow wave, rhythmic spindle-like patterns, etc.), and (3) amplitude. Many electrophysiological events with localizing value are detected in the intracranial contacts, but remain undetected in the extracranial (sphenoidal) contacts. FO electrodes accordingly yield better localizing data than sphenoidal electrodes.

FO electrode recorded spikes show a typical localization in the frontotemporal basal cortices when analyzed by low-resolution electromagnetic tomography (LORETA) in the ascending slope (Fig. 37.10), but a more widespread ipsilateral, a cingulate and a contralateral activity in the descending slope.

Likewise, the dipole analysis of averaged scalp EEG triggered by a FO electrode recorded spike correctly localizes the dipole into the mesial temporal lobe (Fig. 37.11), suggesting that more information can be obtained with sophisticated scalp EEG analysis techniques.

Conclusions

We conclude from our own experience based on strict indications that the semiinvasive technique of FO electrode recording is suitable for the evaluation of potential candidates for AHE. Since this type of resective surgery has dramatically reduced the need for larger TL resections at our institution, we believe that a reasonable proportion of patients considered for surgical treatment of TL epilepsy are candidates for bilateral FO electrode evaluation. The aim of the FO electrode implantation is to record and study the patient's spontaneously occurring habitual seizures. It should be stressed, however, that the nature of the FO electrode recording technique implies that only restricted questions can be answered by this technique, namely (a) do the seizures originate at the mesiobasal TL structures? If yes, (b) are they constantly lateralized? In addition, (c) information is ob-

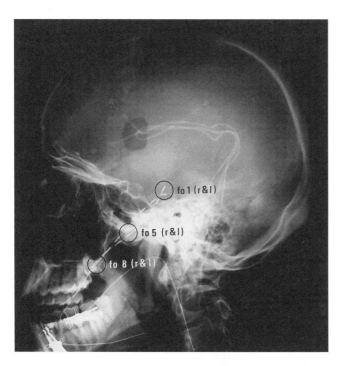

Figure 37.9. The special FO electrode *in situ*: FO1 to FO4 are intracranially, and FO5 to FO8 extracranially contacts with FO5 corresponding to a well placed sphenoidal electrode.

tained as to whether the seizure origin is more anterior or posterior. If the seizures do not originate at one mesiobasal TL, the patient is no longer a suitable candidate for curative selective AHE, and it must then be decided whether further evaluation is indicated with a view toward more extensive TL or even extratemporal surgery.

There is evidently a risk of falsely localizing an apparent seizure origin in the mesiobasal TL and missing the true origin outside these structures when the FO electrode technique is used. The best way to minimize this risk is to carefully study the clinical features accompanying the seizures by recording the occurrence of the subjective auras and/or the objective signal symptoms and to correlate these with the simultaneously recorded EEG. In addition, as already mentioned, FO electrodes can be combined with other recording techniques, such as peg electrodes or subdural strips. As with stereotactic depth recordings, the most reliable seizure onset pattern recorded with the FO electrodes is the high-frequency low-amplitude discharge pattern and the so-called hypersynchronous seizure-onset pattern (Wieser et al., 1993). In the absence of these patterns, the localization of the seizure focus should be questioned. A very local decrement at the FO electrodes is the most frequently observed initial seizure pattern in our FO electrode series. If followed within 3 to 5 seconds by a high-frequency discharge at the same localization, it is also a reliable pattern. From our analysis of simultaneous recordings from depth electrodes inserted directly into limbic structures, such as the amygdala, anterior and posterior hip-

pocampus, and parahippocampal as well as fronto-orbital and cingulate gyrus, and from FO electrodes (Fig. 37.12), it became evident that a very local initial flattening of the EEG record from the FO electrode was nearly always associated with a high-frequency low-amplitude discharge observed in the stereotactic depth recordings from the hippocampal formation and/or amygdala.

Only in the very rare cases of prolonged discharges totally confined to the amygdala and not affecting the hippocampal formation may the FO electrode miss completely the amygdala discharge. This is because the amygdala behaves like a closed electrical field. In our SEEG series, however, these amygdala seizures account for only about 3% of all psychomotor seizures. In summary, we believe that the FO electrode has withstood its practical test and has substantially facilitated the presurgical evaluation of the majority of candidates for TL surgery by decreasing the risks of invasive neurophysiological evaluation without excessive loss of information. Although patients who underwent AHE after SEEG and patients who underwent AHE after FO electrode recording, did not differ significantly with respect to their epileptological outcome, such a comparison does not mean too much because there is the bias according to which more complicated cases are submitted to invasive recordings—at present and in the future. In addition, we should not forget that high-resolution MRI and PET were not available in the early SEEG series, but were nearly always used in the late FO electrode series (Table 37.1).

Stereoelectroencephalography

The term *stereoelectroencephalography* (stereo-EEG, SEEG) was coined by the Paris school (Bancaud, 1959; Talairach et al., 1952). It emphasizes that this method relies on stereotactic principles, but also that the method aims to measure the electrical activity of the brain in a three-dimensional way.

The history of recordings from the human brain, using insulated needles, starts with Berger (1931) and Foerster and Altenburger (1935) and is extensively dealt with in Chapter 36, "Depth Electroencephalography." Most of the early recordings of the pioneers of human depth recording, however, suffered from severe shortcomings. Recording was limited to short intraoperative periods, could only be performed from certain "superficial" targets, could barely cover more than a very limited brain site, and localization of the recorded structure was imprecise or not possible at all.

It was only after the fabrication and application of human stereotactic instruments (Hayne and Meyers, 1959; Hayne et al., 1949; Leksell, 1949; Riechert and Mundinger, 1955; Spiegel and Wycis, 1952; Talairach et al., 1958) that accurate electrode placements were possible. In epilepsy, stereotactic methods were first applied by Spiegel and Wycis (1950, 1951) for the functional investigation of the thalamus and hypothalamus in petit mal epilepsy. Within the same framework, i.e., directed to the treatment of seizures within the concept of "centrencephalic" seizure origin, similar techniques were employed during this time by Williams and Parsons Smith (1949), Jung et al. (1951), and Kirikae and

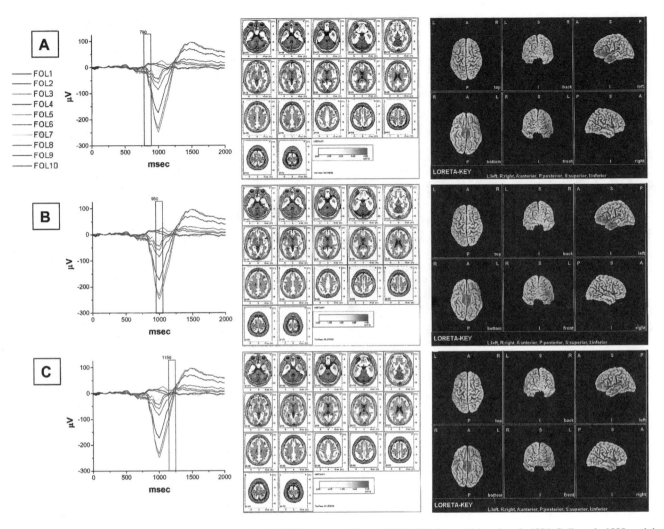

Figure 37.10. Low-resolution electromagnetic tomography (LORETA) localization at beginning of an averaged left FO-recorded spike (790–890 msec) **(A)**, at the peak (950–1,050 msec) **(B)**, and at the end (1,150–1,250 msec). **(C)**, Note that at the end activity propagates backward and to the contralateral temporal tip. [Courtesy of Friedman A., M.D., Ph.D.; see refs. Pascual-Marqui, 1999, 2002; Pascual-Marqui et al., 1994; Strik et al., 1998; and the Web site of low-resolution brain electromagnetic tomography (LORETA), R.D. Pascual-Marqui, the KEY Institute for Brain-Mind Research, University Hospital of Psychiatry, Zurich, Switzerland: *http://www.unizh.ch/keyinst/ NewLORETA/LORETA01.htm.*] (See Color Figure 37.10.)

Wada (1951). Determination of focal cortical epilepsies, however, remained the domain of electrocorticography, as systematized by Jasper et al. (1951).

Multitarget depth electrode studies in humans date back to 1953 (Ribstein, 1960). At that time, however, placement of several flexible electrodes, for instance, in the "rhinencephalic" (mediobasal temporal) structures, was rather imprecise and did not depend on stereotactic principles. The use of simultaneous functional stereotactic exploration of many cortical and subcortical structures had to await the publication of atlases providing their spatial coordinates (Talairach and Tournoux, 1988; Talairach et al., 1967). The simultaneous recording from many stereotactically inserted electrodes together with scalp EEG was pioneered in St. Anne/Paris and became known as stereoelectroencephalography (SEEG).

Despite their invasive nature, SEEG studies of intracerebral electrical activity have been widely applied in the epileptic patient and have contributed enormously to our understanding of the origin and spread of seizure discharges (Ajmone-Marsan, 1980; Angeleri et al., 1964; Babb and Crandall, 1976; Bancaud et al., 1965; Bickford, 1956; Bickford et al., 1953; Brazier, 1956, 1973; Brazier et al., 1954; Buser et al., 1973; Chkhenkeli and Sramka, 1990; Crandall, 1973; Crandall et al., 1963; Delgado, 1956; Delgado-Escueta and Walsh, 1983; Engel and Crandall, 1983; Gloor, 1975; Lieb et al., 1976; Ludwig et al., 1975; Quesney and Gloor, 1985; Rossi, 1973; Sem-Jacobsen, 1968; Spiegel and Wycis, 1952, 1961; Talairach et al., 1958, 1974; Van Buren et al., 1975; Walker, 1962; Wieser, 1983; Williamson et al., 1980).

Rationale

It is important to emphasize that stereo-EEG is not equivalent to depth recording *only*, but, in the understanding of the Paris school, is the *simultaneous* recording of surface

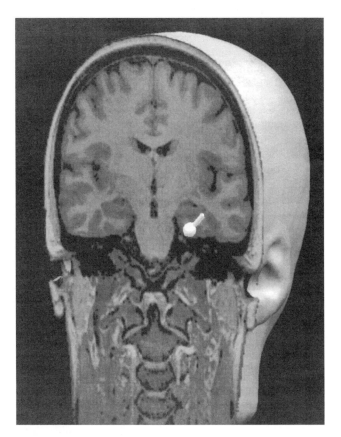

Figure 37.11. Dipole analysis of an averaged epileptic spike recorded by simultaneous scalp and FO electrodes and triggered by a left FO spike with maximum of amplitude at contact 6 (Brain Voyager and BESA Software, see ref. Scherg, 2001, and *http://www.besa.de*. (Courtesy of M. Sitzler.)

Table 37.2. Zurich Epilepsy Surgery Series (Nov. 2003)

Type of Surgery	N		%	
Temporal lobe				
Selective amygdalohippocampectomy	477 ⎱		50.3 ⎱	
Anterior temporal lobectomy	94	197		71.1
Temporal lateral and inferior resections	42		20.8 ⎰	
Others	61 ⎰			
Frontal lobe resections (partial)	114 ⎱		12.0 ⎱	
Rolandic (pre- and postcentral) resections	65	227	6.9	23.9
Parietal resections (partial)	28		3.0	
Occipital resections (partial) and	20 ⎰		2.1 ⎰	
temporo-occipital cortectomies				
Subtotal hemispherectomies and	19 ⎱		2.0 ⎱	
multilobar resections		21		2.2
Hemispherectomies	2 ⎰		0.2 ⎰	
Anterior callosal sections (incl. ACS and	9 ⎱		0.9 ⎱	
limited frontal resections)				
Hypothalamic hamartoma, parasellar tumors	2	26	0.2	2.7
Stereotactic procedures (lesioning)	7		0.7	
Stimulation procedures (DBS 4,	8 ⎰		0.8 ⎰	
Cerebellar Stimulation 1, VNS 3)				
Total	**948**		**100**	

and depth EEG. Since only a limited number of electrodes may justifiably be implanted, recording is possible only from a limited number of a priori designated locations of the brain. Therefore, coherent a priori hypotheses with regard to possible seizure onset in a given patient are mandatory (Wieser, 1987a). Combining the stereotactic depth with the scalp EEG, the *sampling problem* inherent in depth EEG is thus minimized, so that the shortcomings of each are compensated by the other, i.e., the extremely sharp but relatively "tunneled vision" of depth recording (Quesney and Gloor,

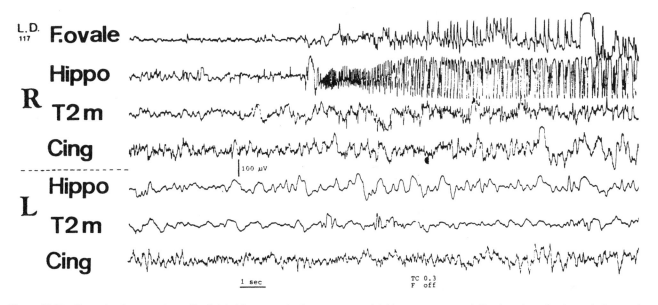

Figure 37.12. Example of a narrowly confined right hippocampal seizure onset simultaneously recorded by stereotactic depth electrodes and FO electrodes. Eight-channel ambulatory Oxford Medilog cassette recording. Channel 8 (ECG) not shown. (Modified from Wieser, H.G. 1986. Selective amygdalohippocampectomy: indications, investigative technique and results. In *Advances and Technical Standards in Neurosurgery*, vol. 13, Eds. L. Symon, L. Brihaye, B. Guidetti, et al., pp. 39–133. Vienna/New York: Springer.)

1985) is balanced by the distorted and "blurred vision" of the scalp EEG.

Insertion and Removal of Electrodes

Although most stereotactic techniques allow the electrodes to be implanted from any angle, most centers prefer to use the orthogonal approach in their routine work. The Yale group has advocated depth probes that are inserted through occipital guide pins and course through the long axes of both hippocampi (McCarthy et al., 1992). Targets most often explored are the medial temporal lobe structures, such as the amygdala, hippocampal pes, and parahippocampal gyrus, usually with anterior, middle, and posterior placements. Additional electrodes may also be placed to record from orbital and mesial frontal cortex if ictal behavior suggests early frontal symptoms. Recording from the cingulate gyrus has been done in a large number of patients in Paris (Mazars, 1969) and in Zurich (Wieser, 1983). In principle, most of the extratemporal structures can be explored stereotactically, but today there is a tendency to use *subdural strips and grids* for extratemporal epilepsies instead of stereotactic depth electrodes or to combine these methods (Lüders, 1992).

According to the Paris school, prior to implantation, the brain and its *vessels* must be known in the stereotactic reference system. To achieve this, the so-called répérage (Fig. 37.13A) has been performed as the first step. This *neuroradiological examination* under stereotactic conditions was a necessary precondition not only for the calculation of the

targets but also for minimizing the risks. It consisted of mounting the stereotactic frame, and then performing pneumencephalography and, if necessary, ventriculography with positive contrast medium. Finally, the vessels were visualized by means of angiography of both the carotid, and if necessary, also of the vertebral arteries (Fig. 37.14).

Some targets could be visualized directly (e.g., pes hippocampus), whereas others could be inferred indirectly by studying the vessels (e.g., rolandic fissure and other sulci) or by applying the atlas information using the proportional grid system based on the anterior and posterior commissure (ap-cp line and its verticals; see Fig. 37.20). This approach has now been replaced by MRI (or at least CT) and digital subtraction angiography (DSA) stereotactic techniques (McCarthy et al., 1992; Olivier and DeLotbinière, 1987) (Fig. 37.15).

Stereo-EEG Electrodes

There is a large variety of commercially available electrodes. Cobalt, copper, nickel, and vanadium should be avoided because of toxic tissue reactions. Stainless steel (316L) and cobalt alloys exhibit a capsule type of response. Gold is also used. Our own electrode has been produced in collaboration with the Straumann Company (Comte et al., 1983). It is a so-called hollow-core electrode, which permits the introduction of the electrode with the guiding stylet inside, thus minimizing the traumatization of the brain (Fig. 37.14). In addition, with minimal adaptation, these electrodes can be used to host in the inner lumen other recording devices, such

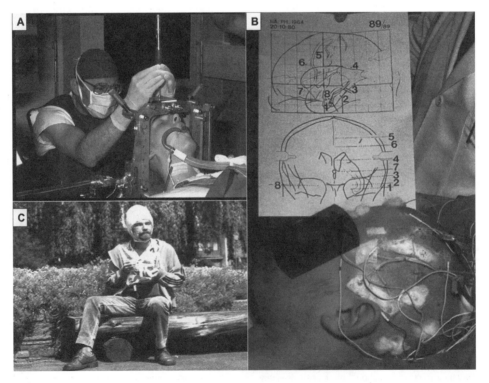

Figure 37.13. **A:** Illustration of the so-called répérage, i.e., neuroradiological examination in the Talairach frame and individual stereotactic reference system. **B:** After implantation of eight 10-contact depth electrodes (see schematic drawing) for stereoelectroencephalograph (SEEG) recording. **C:** Ambulatory cassette recording from depth- and surface electrodes. (See Color Figure 37.13.)

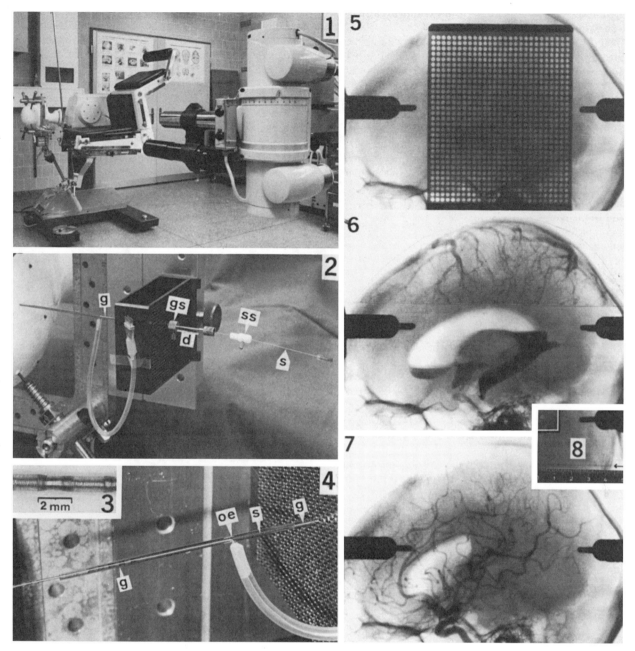

Figure 37.14. Illustration of the so-called répèrage, i.e., the neuroradiological examination under stereotactic conditions, and the implantation of hollow-core depth electrodes using Talairach's principles and system. **1:** Table of Alexander with Talairach's stereotactic frame and the x-ray tube at a distance of 4.75 m, permitting teleradiography with approximately parallel x-rays allowing for a 1:1 picturing without distortion. **2:** Part of the stereotactic frame with the double grid and the guiding device for introduction of the electrode. The guiding cannula (g) enters the bony orificium. Then the distance between the guide stopper (gs) and the end of the guide for the stylet is measured (d) and added to the calculated position of the stylet stopper (ss). To allow placement of the hollow-core electrode with mounted connector on the rigid stylet (s), the double grid had to be moved back by 6 cm. **3:** Visualization of details of the slightly recessed electrode contacts. **4:** Visualization of how the guiding stylet is introduced into the lumen of an electrode (oe). **5–7:** Teleradiographic examination under stereotactic conditions as done prior to the magnetic resonance imaging (MRI)- and CT-guided era. Examples are given showing the holes of the double grid (**5,** see also **2**) and direct delineation of the most important brain structures (lower half of **6**) and the vessels (upper half of **6:** venous phase of the angiography; **7:** early arterial phase). Note that the x-ray films can be directly superposed. **8:** X-ray (in the anteroposterior view) assuring the correct position of the multicontact depth electrode *(arrow)*. The *inset* shows the size of the trepanation made by a special drill introduced through the double grid. After insertion of the electrode to the target, the stylet is withdrawn and the lumen of the electrode is usually closed by a special Silastic wire. The lumen, however, can be used for other devices, for example, a push-pull device can be introduced to examine extracellular fluid.

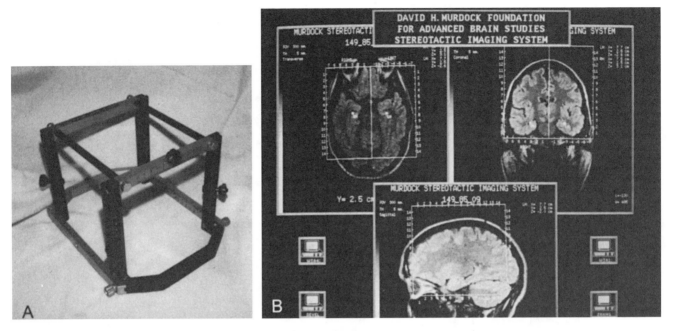

Figure 37.15.   A, B: MRI-guided stereotactic targeting. (Courtesy of David H. Murdock Foundation.)

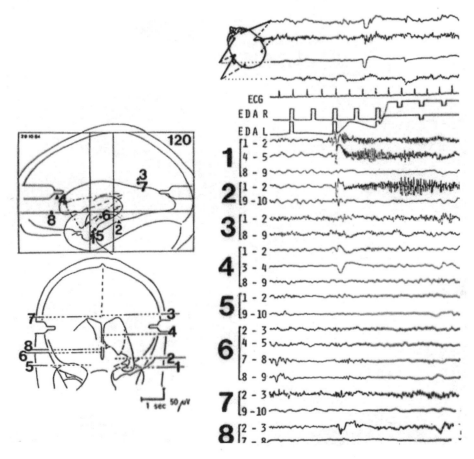

Figure 37.16.   Simultaneous seizure origin in left amygdala (1/1–2) and (1/4–5) and hippocampus (2/1–2). Displayed are four scalp EEG channels; electrocardiogram (ECG); electrodermal activity (EDA) of right (R) and left (L) hand, and depth-EEG channels. Note that the electrodermal re-sponse of the left hand (EDA L) corresponds with the seizure onset. Large numerals correspond to the electrodes, small numerals indicate the contacts, with 1 indicating the most medial and 10 the most lateral contact.

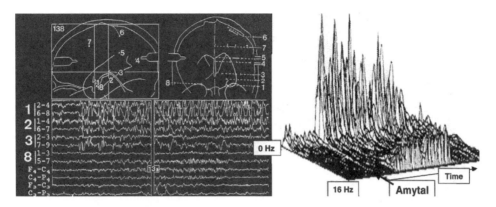

Figure 37.17. SEEG-recorded, Amytal-induced delta activity in the left anterior mesial depth electrodes (1/2–4), 1/6–8, and 2/2–4; *left*) and compressed spectral array of the channel 1/2–4 (amygdala) to visualize the time course of the delta increase (*right*). ↑, injection of 87.5 mg Amytal into the anterior choroidal artery (Wieser et al., 1997).

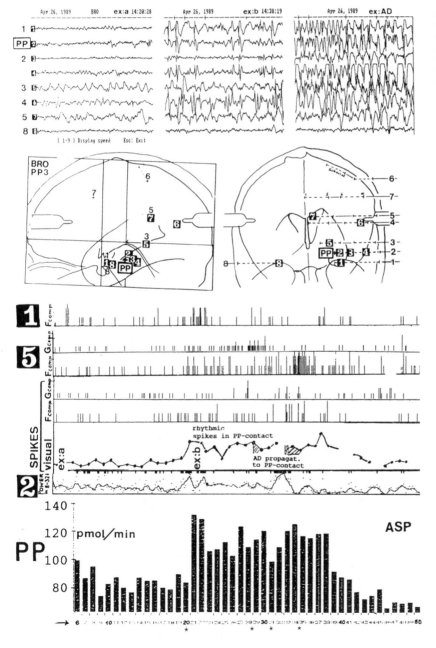

Figure 37.18. Example of a combined EEG and extracellular fluid analysis, showing three depth-recorded EEG sections (during the indicated time ex:a, ex:b, and ex:AD) and the drawing with the position of the depth electrodes. PP indicates the place closest to the push-pull electrode (= 2/1–2). The extracellular fluid was collected at 1-minute fractions at a flow rate of 20 μL/min over a period of 1 hour and analyzed by *o*-phthalaldehyde precolumn derivatization high-pressure liquid chromatography (HPLC), thus allowing detection of known and putative transmitters [aspartate, glutamate, homocysteate, glycine, γ-aminobutyric acid (GABA), β-alanine, and taurine] at the femto-mole level (Do et al., 1991). The *bottom trace* shows the modulation of the aspartate level, which nicely follows the spike rate at the electrode closest to the PP. The spikes are counted visually and by two different automatic spike detection algorithms (Fcomp, Gcomp). *Asterisks (bottom)* indicate the appearance of afterdischarges induced by electrical stimulation of mesiobasal limbic structures.

as push-pull cannula devices, in order to study the extracellular fluid for known and putative transmitters in relation to EEG changes, and in particular to epileptiform events (Cuénod et al., 1990; Wieser et al., 1989) (see Fig. 37.18).

Montage, Recording, and Analysis

There are several methods for recording from stereotactically implanted depth electrodes. Bipolar recording has some advantages and is most often used in routine monitoring, followed by recording against a common average. We use the bipolar mode or a common average electrode, which is fed by inactive contacts situated in the white matter. An important aspect is the fact that the montages can be changed with the aim of *narrowing down* the area of interest, which is most often the area of the onset of the habitual seizures. Today, all available contacts are adequately recorded and stored digitally, so that, according to the question at hand, the most appropriate montages can later be selected and displayed. In reality, however, almost always an a priori selection must be made. Despite all technical progress in daily clinical routine, it is still not practical, if technically possible, to accomplish monitoring with 200 or more simultaneously recorded channels. (This amount of information is usually available if, for example, 15 depth electrodes are implanted and simultaneous scalp-EEG and polygraphic recording is done.) To make the most adequate preselection possible, we had interposed in our hard-wired laboratory a selection board that allowed us to choose every conceivable recording montage (i.e., referential versus bipolar, short distance versus long distance, closed long chains versus isolated local bipolar recordings), and to change the montage with a minimal effort according to new insights or questions. Nowadays, of course, computerized digital technology is used instead. Figures 37.16 to 37.19 give examples of the type of information that can be gained by proper SEEG evaluation.

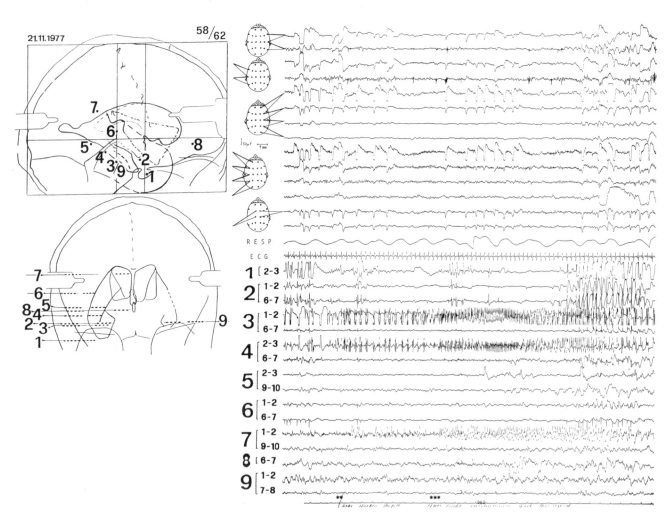

Figure 37.19. Example of a stereoelectroencephalographically recorded ictal event of a 16-year-old girl evaluated for surgical treatment of her medically refractory complex partial seizures. At ** the patient warns that the aura of detachment has changed its character to a "strong fit." At *** she spontaneously explains that she suffers from blurred vision and an epigastric/cardiac pressure. Note that the initial aura of detachment (not shown) was accompanied by a more anterior temporal polar discharge with a maximum in electrodes 1 + 2, and medial contacts of 3, whereas the amplification of subjective sensations (**) coincides with spread of the discharge to the posterior cingulate cortex (7/1–2). (Follow-up: seizure-free since right temporal lobectomy) (06–02–1978).

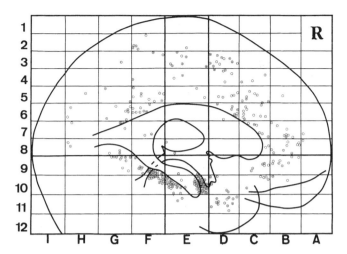
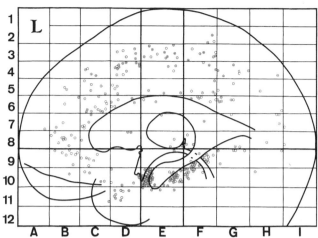

Figure 37.20. Superposition of the targets for the SEEG electrodes in a total of 60 patients shown in the normalized Talairach system based on the anterior (ac) and posterior (pc) commissures and their verticals (vca, vcp). The preferred targets are situated in the mesiobasal temporal lobe and consist of the amygdala, anterior hippocampus (pes), and anterior, middle, and posterior parahippocampal gyrus. The cingulate gyrus (Brodmann's area 32 and 24), the supplementary motor area (SMA; within the field D/3–4), and fronto-orbital regions have been explored relatively frequently. (Modified from Siegfried, J., and Wieser, H.G., 1988. The actual role of stereotactic operations on deep brain structures in the treatment of medically refractory epilepsies. In *The Rational Basis of the Surgical Treatment of Epilepsies*, Ed. G. Broggi, pp. 113–119. London: Libbey.)

Patient Data

My personal experience with SEEG in Zurich is based on 141 SEEG-explored patients. The position of the stereotactically implanted depth electrodes in a total of 61 consecutive patients using the normalized ac-pc line Talairach system is shown in Fig. 37.20. Of 141 SEEG-evaluated patients, 106 patients (75%) were operated on and 35 patients were judged inoperable. From the patients who underwent therapeutic operations, 49 patients had selective amygdalohippocampectomy, and 57 patients had other temporal or extratemporal resections. Table 37.2 lists the epilepsy operations and the number of patients operated on in Zurich to November 2003 and followed by the author.

Complications

We had two more serious complications directly related to SEEG. In one patient, a small intracerebral hematoma and in the other an oculomotor palsy occurred. Furthermore, in our hospital there were two deaths from Creutzfeldt-Jakob disease (CJD) in patients who had undergone SEEG evaluation and subsequent therapeutic TL operations that completely controlled the seizures. The circumstances of this extraordinary complication have been reported (Bernoulli et al., 1977). In short, an electrode used to record from a known CJD-infected person during palliative stereotactic thalamic surgery to ameliorate continuous violent myoclonia was reused after formalin gas sterilization in epilepsy patients, who were then inoculated with this transmissible agent. Two of our patients subsequently died as a consequence of having acquired CJD.

Data Analysis

The analysis of interictal and ictal data is accomplished both by visual analysis of the EEG record and of the split-screen videotape and by computer-aided methods. In our laboratories, the latter consists of continuous compressed spectral array (CSA) "vigilance" programs (spectral power density with parameter extraction using spectral edge frequencies and ratios of certain EEG frequency bands) as well as amplitude and spectral mapping (TWIN EEG Review and Analysis Software—Windows 95/NT) phase- and coherence analysis (PLUS Analysis Software-Telefactor) automatic spike detection (Meles and Wieser, 1982; Wieser, 1987b, 1992), and more recently sophisticated source generator and dipole analyses (Figs. 37.10 and 37.11).

Recognition of auras and seizures is accomplished by automatic seizure detection and inspection of CSA for characteristic changes, button press of the patient and/or observer, and inspection of the split-screen videotape. If indicated, ictal EEGs are further analyzed using phase and coherence analysis to obtain estimates of time delays between the signals of the various EEG channels.

References

Ajmone-Marsan, C. 1980. Depth electrography and electrocorticography. In *Electrodiagnosis in Clinical Neurology*, Ed. M.J. Aminoff, pp. 167–196. Edinburgh: Churchill Livingstone.

Angeleri, F., Ferro-Milone, F., and Parigi, S. 1964. Electrical activity and reactivity of the rhinencephalic, pararhinencephalic, and thalamic structures: prolonged implantation of electrodes in man. Electroencephalogr. Clin. Neurophysiol. 16:100–129.

Awad, I.A., Assirati, J.A., Burgess, R., et al. 1991. A new class of electrodes of intermediate invasiveness: preliminary experience with epidural pegs and foramen ovale electrodes in the mapping of seizure foci. Neurol. Res. 13:177–183.

Babb, T.L., and Crandall, P.H. 1976. Epileptogenesis of human limbic neurons in psychomotor epileptics. Electroencephalogr. Clin. Neurophysiol. 40:225–243.

Bancaud, J. 1959. Apport de l'exploration fonctionelle par voie stéréotaxique à la chirurgie de l'épilepsie. Neurochirurgie 5:55–112.

Bancaud, J., Talairach, J., Bonis, A., et al. 1965. La Stéréo-électro-encéphalographie dans l'Épilepsie, p. 321. Paris: Masson.

Barnett, G.H., Burgess, R.C., Awad, I.A., et al. 1990. Epidural peg electrodes for the presurgical evaluation of intractable epilepsy. Neurosurgery 27:113–115.

Berger, H. 1931. Über das Elektrenkephalogramm des Menschen III. Arch. Psychiatr. Nervenheilk. 94:16–60.

Bernoulli, C., Siegfried, J., Baumgartner, G., et al. 1977. Danger of accidental person-to-person transmission of Creutzfeldt-Jakob disease by surgery. Lancet 1:478–479.

Bickford, R.G. 1956. The application of depth electrography in some varieties of epilepsy. Electroencephalogr. Clin. Neurophysiol. 8:525–527.

Bickford, R.G., Dodge, H.W., Jr., Peterson, M.C., et al. 1953. A new method of recording from subcortical regions of the human brain. Electroencephalogr. Clin. Neurophysiol. 5:464.

Brazier, M.A.B. 1956. Depth recording from the amygdaloid region in patients with temporal lobe seizures. Electroencephalogr. Clin. Neurophysiol. 8:532–533.

Brazier, M.A.B. 1973. Electrical seizure discharges within the human brain: the problem of spread. In Epilepsy, Its Phenomena in Man, Ed. M.A.B. Brazier, pp. 153–170. New York: Academic Press.

Brazier, M.A.B., Schroeder, H., Chapman, W.P., et al. 1954. Electroencephalographic recordings from depth electrodes implanted in the amygdaloid regions in man. Electroencephalogr. Clin. Neurophysiol. 6:702.

Buser, P., Bancaud, J., and Talairach, J. 1973. Depth recordings in man in TLE. In Epilepsy, Its Phenomena in Man, Ed. M.A.B. Brazier, pp. 7–97. New York: Academic Press.

Chkhenkeli, S.A., and Sramka, M. 1990. Epilepsy and Its Surgical Treatment (in Russian; English summary), Slovenskey Akademie.

Comte, P., Siegfried, J., and Wieser, H.G. 1983. Multipolar hollow-core electrode for brain recordings. Appl. Neurophysiol. 46:41–46.

Crandall, P.H. 1973. Developments in direct recordings from the epileptogenic regions in the surgical treatment of partial epilepsies. In Epilepsy, Its Phenomena in Man, Ed. M.A.B. Brazier, pp. 288–310. New York: Academic Press.

Crandall, P.H., Walter, R.D., and Rand, R.W. 1963. Clinical applications of studies on stereotactically implanted electrodes in TLE. J. Neurosurg. 20:827–840.

Cuénod, M., Audinat, E., Do, K.Q., et al. 1990. Homocysteic acid as transmitter candidate in the mammalian brain and excitatory amino acids in epilepsy. In Excitatory Amino Acids and Neuronal Plasticity, Ed. Y. Ben-Ari, pp. 57–63. New York: Plenum Press.

Delgado, J.M.R. 1956. Use of intracerebral electrodes in human patients. Electroencephalogr. Clin. Neurophysiol. 8:528–530.

Delgado-Escueta, A.V., and Walsh, G.D. 1983. The selection process for surgery of intractable complex partial seizures: surface EEG and depth electrography. Assoc. Res. Nerv. Ment. Dis. 61:295–326.

Do, K.Q., Klancnik, J.M., Gähwiler, B., et al. 1991. Release of excitatory amino acids: animal studies and epileptic foci studies in human. In Excitatory Amino Acids, Eds. B.S. Meldrum, F. Moroni, R.P. Simon, et al., pp. 677–685. New York: Raven Press.

Engel, J., Jr. 1989. Seizure and Epilepsy. Philadelphia: F.A. Davis.

Engel, J., Jr., and Crandall, P.H. 1983. Falsely localizing onsets with depth EEG telemetry during anticonvulsant withdrawal. Epilepsia 24:344–355.

Foerster, O., and Altenburger, H. 1935. Elektrobiologische Vorgänge an der menschlichen Hirnrinde. Dtsch. Z. Nervenkeilk.

Gloor, P. 1975. Contributions of electroencephalography and electrocorticography to the neurosurgical treatment of the epilepsies. In Advances in Neurology, vol. 8, Eds. D.P. Purpura, J.K. Penry, and R.D. Walter, pp. 59–105. New York: Raven Press.

Hayne, R., and Meyers, R. 1959. An improved model of a human stereotaxic instrument. J. Neurosurg. 7:463–475.

Hayne, R.A., Belinson, L., and Gibbs, F.A. 1949. Electrical activity of subcortical areas in epilepsy. Electroencephalogr. Clin. Neurophysiol. 1:437–445.

Härtel, F. 1914. Über die intracranielle Injektionsbehandlung der Trigeminusneuralgie. Med. Klin. 10:582–584.

Jasper, H., Pertuiset, B., and Flanigin, H. 1951. EEG and cortical electrograms in patients with temporal lobe seizures. Arch. Neurol. Psychiatr. (Chicago) 65:272–290.

Jung, R., Riechert, T., and Heines, K.D. 1951. Zur Technik und Bedeutung der operativen Elektrocorticographie und subcorticalen Hirnpotentialableitung. Nervenarzt 22:433–436.

King, D.W., So, E.L., Marius, R., et al. 1986. Techniques and applications of sphenoidal recording. J. Clin. Neurophysiol. 3:51–65.

Kirikae, T., and Wada, J. 1951. Electrothalamogram of petit mal seizures. Med. Biol. 20:253.

Kirschner, M. 1932. Electrocoagulation des Ganglion Gasseri. Zbl. Chir. 47:2841–2843.

Leksell, L. 1949. A stereotaxic apparatus for intracranial neurosurgery. Acta Chir. Scand. 99:229–253.

Lieb, J.P., Walsh, G.O., Babb, T.L., et al. 1976. A comparison of EEG seizure patterns recorded with surface and depth electrodes in patients with TLE. Epilepsia 17:137–160.

Lüders, H.O. (Ed.). 1992. Epilepsy Surgery. New York: Raven Press.

Lüders, H., Lesser, R.P., Dinner, D.S., et al. 1987. Commentary: chronic intracranial recording and stimulation with subdural electrodes. In Surgical Treatment of the Epilepsies, Ed. J. Engel, Jr., pp. 297–321. New York: Raven Press.

Ludwig, B.I., Ajmone-Marsan, C., and Van Buren, J.M. 1975. Depth and direct cortical recording in seizure disorders of extratemporal origin. Neurology 26:1085–1099.

Mavor, H., and Hellen, M.K. 1964. Nasopharyngeal electrode recording. Am. J. EEG Technol. 4:43–50.

Mazars, G. 1969. Cingulate gyrus epileptogenic foci as an origin for generalized seizures. In The Physiopathogenesis of the Epilepsies, Eds. H. Gastaut, H. Jasper, J. Bancaud, et al., pp. 186–189. Springfield, IL: Charles C Thomas.

McCarthy, G., Spencer, D.D., and Riker, R.J. 1992. The stereotaxic placements of depth electrodes in epilepsy. In Epilepsy Surgery, Ed. H.O. Lüders, pp. 385–393. New York: Raven Press.

Meles, H.P., and Wieser, H.G. 1982. Computer-generated dynamic presentation of functional versus anatomical distances in the human brain. Appl. Neurophysiol. 45:404–405.

Olivier, A., and DeLotbinière, A. 1987. Stereotactic techniques in epilepsy. Neurosurg. State of the Art Rev. 2(1).

Pascual-Marqui, R.D. 1999. Review of methods for solving the EEG inverse problem. Int. J. Bioelectromagn. 1:75–86.

Pascual-Marqui, R.D. 2002. Standardized low-resolution brain electromagnetic tomography (sLORETA): technical details. Method Find Exp. Clin. 24(suppl D):5–12.

Pascual-Marqui, R.D. 2003. The KEY Institute for Brain-Mind Research. Available at http://www.unizh.ch/heyinst/NewLORETA/LORETA01.htm.

Pascual-Marqui, R.D., Michel, C.M., and Lehmann, D. 1994. Low resolution electromagnetic tomography: a new method for localizing electrical activity in the brain. Int. J. Psychophsiol. 18:49–65.

Quesney, L. 1987. Extracranial EEG evaluation. In Surgical Treatment of the Epilepsies, Ed. J. Engel, Jr., pp. 129–166. New York: Raven Press.

Quesney, L.F., and Gloor P. 1985. Localization of epileptic foci. In Long-Term Monitoring in Epilepsy, Eds. J. Gotman, J.R. Ives, and P. Gloor (EEG suppl 37), pp. 132–156. Amsterdam: Elsevier.

Quesney, L.F., and Gloor, P. 1987. Special extracranial electrodes. In Presurgical Evaluation of Epileptics, Eds. H.G. Wieser and C.E. Elger, pp. 162–176. Berlin/Heidelberg: Springer-Verlag.

Ribaric, I., and Sekulovic, N. 1989. Experience with orbital electrodes in the patients operated on for epilepsy—results of temporofrontal resections. Acta Neurochir. Suppl. 46:21–24.

Ribstein, M. 1960. Exploration du cerveau humain par électrodes profondes. Electroencephalogr. Clin. Neurophysiol. Suppl. 16.

Riechert, T., and Mundinger, F. 1955. Beschreibung und Anwendung eines Zielgerätes für stereotaktische Hirnoperationen: II Modell. Acta Neurochir. Suppl. 3:308–337.

Rossi, G.F. 1973. Problems of analysis and interpretation of electrocerebral signals in human epilepsy: A neurosurgeon's view. In Epilepsy: Its Phenomena in Man, Ed. M.A.B. Brazier, pp. 259–285. New York: Raven Press.

Rovit, R.L., Gloor, P., and Rasmussen, T. 1961. Sphenoidal electrodes in the electrographic study of patients with TLE. An evaluation. J. Neurosurg. 18:151–158.

Scherg, M. 2001. EEG FOCUS, EEG source imaging and review. Version 2.2. User Manual written by P. Berg, N. Ille, M. Scherg; MEGIS Software GmbH, Munich. (BESA is a registered trademark of Dr.rer.nat. Michael Scherg) http://www.besa.de.

Schüler, P., Stefan, H., Neubauer, U., et al. 1991. Vergleich von Foramen-Ovale und subduralen Streifenelektroden zur präoperativen Epilepsiediagnostik. Abstract-Book 36th Annual Meeting German EEG-Society, p. 152, October 10–13, Celle.

Sem-Jacobsen, C.W. 1968. *Depth Electrographic Stimulation of the Human Brain and Behavior.* Springfield, IL: Charles C Thomas.

Siegfried, J., and Wieser, H.G. 1988. The actual role of stereotactic operations on deep brain structures in the treatment of medically refractory epilepsies. In *The Rational Basis of the Surgical Treatment of Epilepsies,* Ed. G. Broggi, pp. 113–119. London: Libbey.

Sperling, M.R., Mendius, J.R., and Engel, J., Jr. 1986. Mesial temporal spikes: a simultaneous comparison of sphenoidal, nasopharyngeal and ear electrodes. Epilepsia 27:81–86.

Spiegel, E.A., and Wycis, H.T. 1950. Thalamic recordings in man, with special reference to seizure discharges. Electroencephalogr. Clin. Neurophysiol. 2:23–29.

Spiegel, E.A., and Wycis, H.T. 1951. Diencephalic mechanisms in petit mal epilepsy. Electroencephalogr. Clin. Neurophysiol. 3:473–475.

Spiegel, E.A., and Wycis, H.T. 1952. *Stereoencephalotomy,* part I. New York: Grune & Stratton.

Spiegel, E.A., and Wycis, H.T. 1961. Chronic implantation of intracerebral electrodes. In *Electrical Stimulation of the Brain,* Ed. D.E. Sheer, pp. 37–44. Austin: University of Texas Press.

Strik, W.K., Fallgatter, A.J., Brandeis, D., et al. 1998. Three-dimensional tomography of event-related potentials during response inhibition: evidence for phasic frontal lobe activation. Evoked Potentials EEG Clin. Neurophysiol. 108:406–413.

Talairach, J., and Tournoux, P. 1988. *Co-Planar Stereotaxic Atlas of the Human Brain.* Stuttgart, New York: Georg Thieme.

Talairach, J., De Ajuriaguerra, J., and David, M. 1952. Études stéréotaxique et structures encéphaliques profondes chez l'homme. Presse Méd. 28: 605–609.

Talairach, J., David, M., and Tournoux, P. 1958. *L'Exploration Chirurgicale Stéréotaxique du Lobe Temporal dans l'Epilepsie Temporale: Rêperage Anatomique Stéréotaxique et Technique Chirurgicale.* Paris: Masson.

Talairach, J., Szikla, G., Tournoux, P., et al. 1967. *Atlas d'Anatomie Stéréotaxique du Télencéphale.* Paris: Masson & Cie.

Talairach, J., Bancaud, J., Szikla, G., et al. 1974. Approche nouvelle de la neurochirurgie de l'épilepsie. Méthodologie stéréotaxique et résultats thérapeutiques. Neurochirurgie 20 (suppl 1): 1–240.

Van Buren, J.M., Ajmone-Marsan, C., Mutsaga, N., et al. 1975. Temporal lobe seizures with additional foci treated by resection. J. Neurosurg. 43:596–607.

Walker, A.E. 1962. Stereotaxic methods for the study of subcortical activity in epilepsy. Confin. Neurol. 22:217–222.

Wieser, H.G. 1983. *Electroclinical Features of the Psychomotor Seizure.* Stuttgart/London: Gustav Fischer/Butterworth.

Wieser, H.G. 1986. Selective amygdalohippocampectomy: indications, investigative technique and results. In *Advances and Technical Standards in Neurosurgery,* vol. 13, Eds. L. Symon, L. Brihaye, B. Guidetti, et al., pp. 39–133. Vienna/New York: Springer.

Wieser, H.G. 1987a. Stereo-electroencephalography. In *Presurgical Evaluation of Epileptics,* Eds. H.G. Wieser and C.E. Elger, pp. 192–204. Berlin/Heidelberg/New York: Springer.

Wieser, H.G. 1987b. Data analysis. In *Surgical Treatment of the Epilepsies,* Ed. J. Engel, Jr., pp. 335–360. New York: Raven Press.

Wieser, H.G. 1992. Computer evaluation and display of seizure activity recorded from chronically implanted depth electrodes. In *Computers in Stereotactic Neurosurgery,* Ed. P. Kelly, pp. 177–190. Oxford: Blackwell.

Wieser, H.G., and Morris, H., III. 1997. Foramen ovale and peg electrodes. In *Epilepsy, A Comprehensive Textbook,* Eds. J. Engel, Jr., and T.A. Pedley, pp. 1707–1717. New York: Raven Press.

Wieser, H.G., and Moser, S. 1988. Improved multipolar foramen ovale electrode monitoring. J. Epilepsy 1:13–22.

Wieser, H.G., and Schwarz, U. 2001. Topography of foramen ovale electrodes by 3D image reconstruction. Clin. Neurophysiol. 112:2053–2056.

Wieser, H.G., and Siegel, A.M. 1991. Analysis of foramen ovale electrode recorded seizures and correlation with outcome following amygdalohippocampectomy. Epilepsia 32:838–850.

Wieser, H.G., and Siegel, A.M. 1992. Indikationen zur chirurgischen Epilepsiebehandlung. Schweiz. Rundsch. Med. Prax. 81(19):632–639.

Wieser, H.G., and Yasargil, M.G. 1982. Selective amygdalohippocampectomy as a surgical treatment of mesiol-basal limbic epilepsy. Surg. Neurol. 17:445–457.

Wieser, H.G., Elger, C.E., and Stodieck, S.R.G. 1985. The "foramen ovale electrode": a new recording method for the preoperative evaluation of patients suffering from mesio-basal TLE. Electroencephalogr. Clin. Neurophysiol. 61:314–322.

Wieser, H.G., Do, K.Q., Perschak, H., et al. 1989. Modulation of extracellular aspartate level during epileptiform events in primary epileptogenic area of patients (abstract). Satellite Symp. on Physiology, Pharmacology and Development of Epileptogenic Phenomena (XXXI Internat. Congr. of Physiological Sciences, Helsinki (1989), Frankfurt, July 4–8, 1989.

Wieser, H.G., Engel, J., Jr., Williamson, P.D., et al. 1993. Surgically remediable temporal lobe syndromes. In *Surgical Treatment of the Epilepsies,* 2nd ed., Ed. J. Engel, Jr., pp. 49–63. New York: Raven Press.

Wieser, H.G., Müller, S., Schiess, R., et al. 1997. The anterior and posterior selective temporal lobe amobarbital tests: angiographical, clinical, electroencephalographical PET and SPECT findings, and memory performance. Brain Cogn. 33:71–97.

Wieser, H.G., Ortega, M., Friedman, A., et al. 2003. Long-term seizure outcome following amygdalohippocampectomy. J. Neurosurg. 98:751–763.

Williams, D., and Parsons Smith, G. 1949. The spontaneous electrical activity of the human thalamus. Brain 72:450–482.

Williamson, P.D., Spencer, D.D., Spencer, S.S., et al. 1980. Presurgical intensive monitoring using depth electroencephalography in TLE. In *Advances in Epileptology: 10th Epilepsy International Symposium,* Eds. J.A. Wada and J.K. Penry, pp. 73–81. New York: Raven Press.

Wyler, A.R., Ojemann, G.A., Lettich, E., et al. 1984. Subdural strip electrodes for localizing epileptogenic foci. J. Neurosurg. 60:1195–1200.

Yasargil, M.G., and Wieser, H.G. 1987. Selective microsurgical resections. In *Presurgical Evaluation of Epileptics,* Eds. H.G. Wieser and C.E. Elger, pp. 352–360. Berlin/Heidelberg: Springer.

38. Electrocorticography

Luis Felipe Quesney and Ernst Niedermeyer

Intraoperative cortical electroencephalogram (EEG) recordings, or electrocorticography (ECoG), was introduced in the 1940s to map the location and extent of the epileptogenic brain tissue prior to surgical removal during the neurosurgical treatment of partial epilepsies (Ajmone Marsan, 1980; Ajmone Marsan and Baldwin, 1958; Ajmone Marsan and O'Connor, 1973; Bates, 1963; Bechtevera, 1962; Gloor, 1975; Graf et al., 1984; Jasper, 1949; Magnus et al., 1962; Marshall and Walker, 1949; Meyers et al., 1950; Niedermeyer, 1982; Penfield and Jasper, 1954; Walker et al., 1947).

Historically, this technique was pioneered in humans by Hans Berger (1929), who performed intraoperative EEG recordings with electrodes placed over the dural surface in patients with skull defects. In recent years, due to increased sophistication of the extracranial and intracranial preoperative EEG investigation, coupled with the progressive development of structural and functional neuroimaging, the role of ECoG in the localization of the epileptogenic zone has been reduced.

In centers performing epilepsy surgery, intraoperative ECoG is used to identify the location and limits of the epileptogenic zone as well as to guide the extent of resection and to assess the completeness of the surgical removal.

Equipment and Recording Techniques

ECoG is usually recorded on paper using a 16- or 21-channel electroencephalograph, ideally located in a gallery adjacent to, but separate from, the operating room (Jasper, 1949). An intercom system provides verbal communication between the clinical neurophysiologist and the neurosurgeon.

A frequency bandpass of 0.5 to 70 Hz ensures adequate recording of epileptiform discharges and background activity. A sensitivity of 30 to 50 μV/mm is commonly used for ECoG recordings since the electrocerebral activity recorded directly from the cortical surface is significantly larger than on scalp recordings.

The recording electrodes must make light contact with the exposed cortex. Flexible electrodes are preferable to rigid ones. The electrodes themselves are made of silver, platinum, or stainless steel; the contact between electrode and brain tissue is achieved with a ball-shaped tip. Carbon tip electrodes are used in some centers.

A set of 16 to 21 cortical electrodes is recommended. In addition, the use of multicontact depth electrodes is very helpful for an acute exploration of deep limbic and neocortical structures during temporal lobectomy (Gloor, 1975; Wennberg et al., 1997a).

After surgery, the ECoG electrodes are cleaned and submitted to autoclaving (Ajmone Marsan and O'Connor, 1973). According to these authors, 24 hours should elapse between gas sterilization and reutilization.

Electrical Stimulation

The rationale behind electrical stimulation of the brain in patients with intractable partial seizures resides in the assumption that human epileptogenic brain tissue might display increased excitability to electrical stimulation, thus generating an afterdischarge, ideally associated with the patient's habitual early ictal manifestations. Several studies have demonstrated that afterdischarge thresholds and durations vary according to anatomical sites (Jasper, 1954; Walker, 1949) and in regard to time (Ajmone Marsan, 1972; Walker, 1949). Electrical stimulation thresholds are elevated in areas that are structurally damaged (Bernier et al., 1990; Cherlow et al., 1977). Afterdischarges may arise from areas with no significant spontaneous interictal epileptic activity (Gloor, 1975) and therefore their role as indicators of the ictal generator is equivocal (Bernier et al., 1990).

Intraoperative electrical stimulation of the brain may also be used for cortical functional mapping. The pioneer work of Penfield and his co-workers (Penfield and Jasper, 1954; Penfield and Kristiansen, 1951), using electrical stimulation during ECoG recordings in patients operated on under local anesthesia, resulted in the intraoperative mapping of speech areas, and in the identification of the somatomotor and somatosensory cortex. Localization of these anatomical regions was important in order to exclude them from the surgical removal. Other studies have shown that cortical tongue mapping is very useful in determining the point of junction of the central and sylvian sulci, a crucial landmark for surgical cortical resections along the temporal lobe convexity (Picard and Olivier, 1983). Ojeman and Dodrill (1985) have used intraoperative electrical stimulation to determine cortical sites involved in memory and speech mechanisms. Recently, presurgical functional mapping of cortical areas that cannot be surgically removed is performed preoperatively using functional magnetic resonance imaging (fMRI), positron emission tomography (PET), or magnetoencephalography (MEG) (Toga and Mazziota, 2002).

Afterdischarges triggered by electrical stimulation are characterized by rhythmically repetitive high-voltage spikes, or polyspike-wave-like complexes with abrupt termination. Such prolonged afterdischarges are usually subclinical or associated with subtle clinical behavioral manifestations (Stefan et al., 1991).

Electrical stimulation is usually performed using biphasic square pulses with a 0.5- to 2-msec duration at a frequency of 40 to 60 Hz. An initial voltage of 2 V, or an initial current of 0.5 mA (with gradual increase to about 10 V and 2 mA) is commonly used. Either constant current or constant voltage stimulation may be used. The length of the stimulation should not exceed 5 to 8 seconds.

General Anesthesia and Cortical EEG Activity

General anesthesia induces abundant fast activity in the 15 to 30/sec range and it reduces or eliminates interictal epileptic discharges. The use of methohexital (Brevital), a short-acting barbiturate, has been recommended by Ajmone Marsan and O'Connor (1973) because of its spike-activating properties (Musella et al., 1971; Wennberg et al., 1997b).

The morphology of interictal epileptiform discharges such as spikes, sharp waves, and spike and slow-wave complexes is very similar in cortical and scalp recorded EEG, aside from the large difference in amplitude that must be compensated for by sensitivity changes. Much cortical EEG activity exceeds 500 µV and it may even reach several millivolts. Over a severely impaired cortex, a virtually flat electrocorticogram may be encountered.

If recordings obtained during the waking state are done under local anesthesia, a posteriorly recorded alpha rhythm may show considerable extension into the temporal lobe. Rolandic mu rhythm may be present over the motor cortex, mostly in a harmonic frequency of about 20/sec and often with spiky discharges. The blocking effect of this rhythm by contralateral movement is dramatic as well as useful.

Localization of the Epileptogenic Brain Tissue
Preexcision Recording

Since recording of spontaneous electrographic seizures during ECoG is rare, intraoperative localization of the epileptogenic brain tissue is largely dependent on recording interictal epileptic activity. The effectiveness of ECoG as a preoperative tool depends on whether the interictal epileptic abnormality provides reliable localizing information regarding the site and extent of the epileptogenic brain tissue to be removed. It has been known since the work of Penfield and Jasper (1954) that the most active spiking area may not coincide with the location of the lesion. Commonly, the interictal epileptic disturbance recorded at ECoG in patients with temporal lobe epilepsy involves mesial temporal and neocortical temporal lobe structures simultaneously or independently (Fig. 38.1) with variable participation of adjacent lobes (Cendes et al., 1993; Devinsky et al., 1992; Engel et al., 1975; Gastaut et al., 1953; Graf et al., 1984; Kajtor et al., 1958; Niedermeyer, 1982, 1987; Quesney and Niedermeyer, 1993; Rasmussen, 1983; Stefan et al., 1991; Tuunainen et al., 1994;

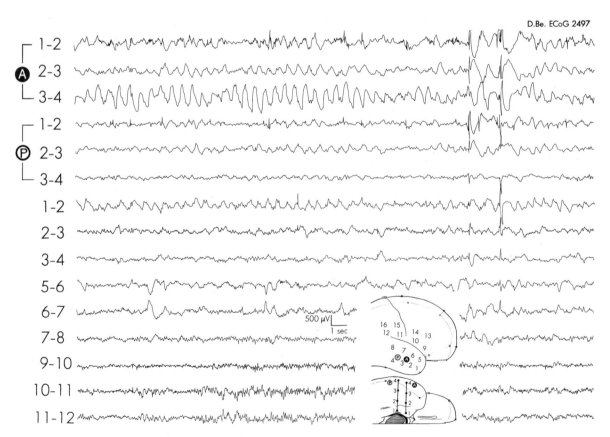

Figure 38.1. Electrocorticograph (ECoG) recording showing spontaneous multifocal interictal spiking involving the second temporal gyrus anteriorly (1–2), electrode 6 in the first temporal gyrus, and the mesial temporal lobe structures synchronously (A1–2, P1–2). In addition, widespread interictal epileptiform bursts involving the mesial temporal lobe structures as well as the temporal neocortex were recorded. (From Stefan, H., Quesney, L.F., Abou-Khalil, B., and Olivier, A. 1991. Electrocorticography in temporal lobe epilepsy surgery. Acta Neurol. Scand. 83:65–72, with permission.)

Walker, 1967, 1974). A similar mesial-neocortical distribution of the interictal epileptic abnormality can be observed in patients investigated with chronically implanted depth electrode prior to surgery performed with ECoG guidance (Wennberg et al., 1997a). In our experience, the cortical distribution of interictal epileptic abnormality in patients with long-standing medically intractable temporal lobe seizures varies from a focal or restricted expression to a more widespread spiking involving the entire temporal lobe with multifocal independent accentuation in different gyri (Quesney et al., 1988; Stefan et al., 1991). We believe that the cortical distribution of interictal epileptic abnormality in temporal lobe epilepsy reflects a topographic continuum of interictal epileptogenicity reminiscent of that observed in frontal lobe epilepsy (Chatrian and Quesney, 1997; Quesney et al., 1988, 1992a).

In the past, several reports have indicated that the interictal epileptic disturbance recorded intraoperatively provides relevant information regarding the extent of the epileptogenic brain tissue that must be surgically removed (Ajmone Marsan, 1980; Bengzon et al., 1968; Fiol et al., 1991; Graf

et al., 1984; Jennum et al., 1993; Ojeman, 1980; Primrose and Ojeman, 1992; Stefan et al., 1991). Other investigators have emphasized that standardized temporal lobectomy could be performed without ECoG control (Engel, 1987a; Spencer and Inserni, 1992).

The success of selective amygdalohippocampectomy in patients with temporal lobe epilepsy secondary to mesial temporal sclerosis (McBride et al., 1991) has led to questions about the need to remove the entire preresection spiking area recorded at ECoG.

It is currently believed that the preresection interictal spiking in temporal lobe epilepsy does not provide reliable clues regarding the extent of epileptogenic brain tissue to be removed and does not predict surgical outcome.

During the ECoG exploration of frontal, central motor, and parietal regions, the distribution of the interictal epileptic disturbance is often widespread (Quesney et al., 1990, 1992b; Salanova et al., 1992, 1995a,b; Wennberg et al., 1997c) even in the presence of circumscribed lesions. In extratemporal epilepsy, preexcision mapping of the interictal epileptogenic

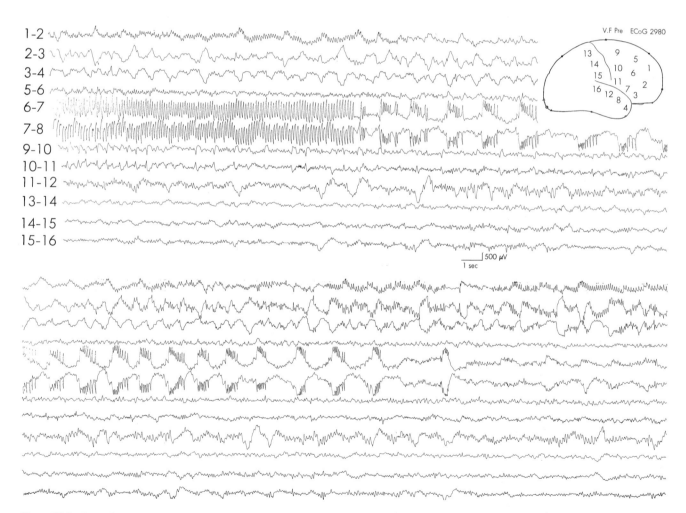

Figure 38.2. Preexcision ECoG in a patient with a right frontocentral cortical dysplastic lesion on magnetic resonance imaging (MRI). The tracing shows electrographic seizure activity recorded multifocally. A 1½–2 Hz rhythmic activity was seen at electrode 3; rhythmic polyspike activity at 10 Hz recorded maximally at electrodes 1 and 7; rhythmic 2–3 Hz spike-and-wave activity recorded at electrode 10. (From Palmini, A., Gambardella, A., Andermann, F., et al. 1995. Intrinsic epileptogenicity of human dysplastic cortex as suggested by corticography and surgical results. Ann. Neurol. 37:476–487, with permission.)

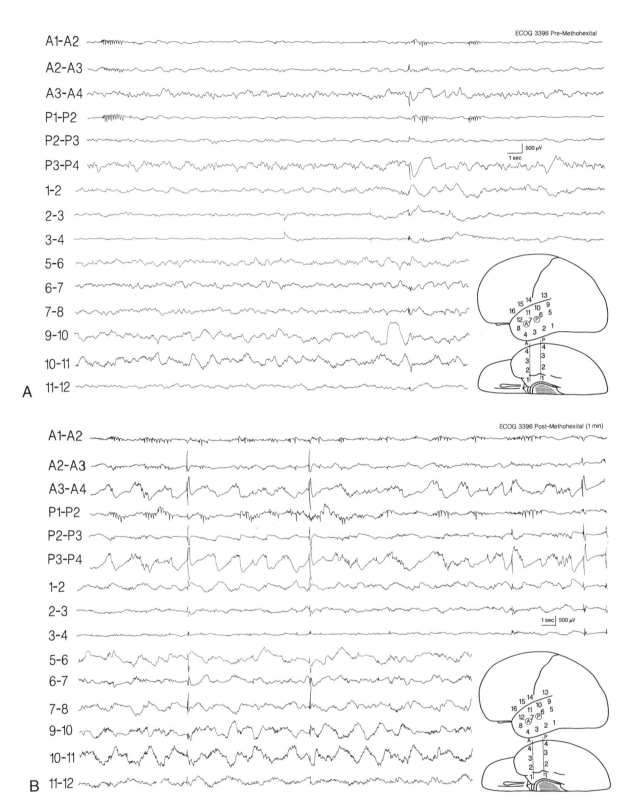

Figure 38.3.   **A:** Baseline preexcision ECoG prior to methohexital injection showing active limbic epileptiform activity and a single independent temporal neocortical spike. **B:** Preexcision ECoG 1 minute after injection of 40 mg methohexital showing activation of epileptiform activity recorded independently from limbic and temporal neocortical structures. A slight burst-suppression pattern developing over neocortex. **C:** Postexcision ECoG showing activation of temporal neocortical epileptiform activity and burst-suppression pattern. (From Wennberg, R., Quesney, F., Olivier, A., and Dubeau, F. 1997b. Induction of burst-suppression and activation of epileptiform activity after methohexital and selective amygdalo-hippocampectomy. Electroencephalogr. Clin. Neurophysiol. 102:443–451, with permission.)

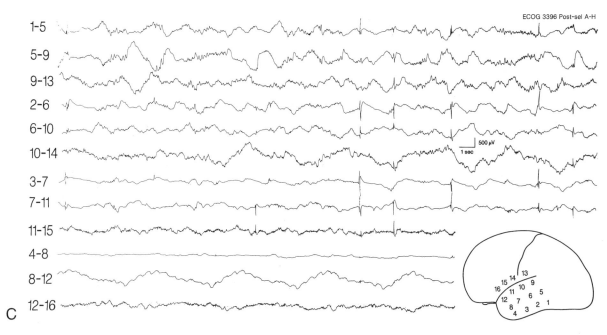

Figure 38.3. *(continued)*

area is useful, particularly if a tailored surgical resection is planned (Quesney et al., 1998). A study comprising 60 patients with frontal lobe epilepsy operated on under ECoG guidance showed that the distribution and abundance of interictal spiking recorded at ECoG was the most powerful prognostic indicator of postsurgical outcome with respect to seizure control (Wennberg et al., 1997c). Preexcision epileptic abnormality recorded from less than two gyri and absence of postexcision epileptic activity distant to the resection border both strongly predicted a favorable (class I or II) outcome, according to Engel's (1987b) classification. Residual spiking limited to the resection border did not significantly correlate with outcome. The presence of a circumscribed frontal lobe lesion was also significantly correlated with favorable outcome (Wennberg et al., 1998).

Electrocorticography is a very useful tool in the anatomical localization of cortical dysplastic lesions. The electrographic correlate of this lesion consists of rhythmic electrographic seizure discharge (Fig. 38.2), which coincides with the anatomical extent and location of the MRI cortical dysplastic lesion. A good surgical outcome in these patients is proportional to the completeness of the lesion's surgical removal, and ECoG is a reliable tool to indicate the presence of underlying dysplastic cortex (Palmini et al., 1995).

The introduction of three-dimensional (3D) image guidance intraoperatively has permitted a better correlation of the ECoG findings with the lesion to be surgically removed and its boundaries. This technique is particularly helpful in the surgical treatment of focal cortical dysplasia and when a tailored cortical resection is planned.

Postexcision Recording

The significance of ECoG recording after a temporal lobe resection is controversial. Some authors believe that the per-

sistence of spike activity after surgical excision is of little or no prognostic value (Ajmone Marsan and Baldwin, 1958; Chatrian and Quesney, 1997; Gibbs et al., 1958; Walker et al., 1960). Other investigators advocate that persistent spike activity after surgical removal predicts an unsatisfactory outcome (Bengzon et al., 1968; Gloor, 1975; Jasper et al., 1961; McBride et al., 1991). Postexcision spike activity involving the insula is known to have no prognostic value (Gloor, 1975; Silfvenius et al., 1964). Activation of interictal spiking in the temporal neocortex following selective amygdalohippocampectomy occurs frequently and it has no prognostic significance (Cendes et al., 1993; Wennberg et al., 1997b).

Recent evidence confirms that in frontal lobe epilepsy, postexcision residual spiking indicates a poor outcome in terms of seizure control (Wennberg et al., 1998).

A burst-suppression EEG pattern (Fig. 38.3) has been reported to be a characteristic finding in patients submitted to functional hemispherectomy (Wennberg et al., 1998).

Concluding Remarks

The anatomical distribution of cortical epileptic abnormality recorded intraoperatively may range from a focal or restricted anatomical site to a widespread epileptogenic area despite the presence of a circumscribed lesion. This very likely represents the ECoG expression of an epileptogenic network, which may have a different anatomical location than the lesion. The opinions in the literature are divided as to whether cortically recorded interictal spiking represents a reliable marker of the brain region to be surgically removed. Most experts, however, agree that in patients with cortical dysplasia presenting as continuous rhythmic epileptic discharges, EcoG is very useful in the planning of the surgical removal. More recently, we have reported similar rhythmic epileptiform discharges in patients with extensive brain gliosis (Guerreiro et al., 2003).

ECoG is not essentially required if en-bloc temporal lobe resections or if a selective amygdalohippocampectomy is planned. ECoG, however, is very helpful in patients with temporal neocortical epilepsy requiring surgery. ECoG provides reliable information regarding the extent of epileptogenic brain tissue to be removed in extratemporal epilepsy and in patients with cortical dysplasia. Small (less than two gyri) cortical epileptogenic areas are associated with a favorable surgical outcome. Cortical subpial transection is usually performed under ECoG guidance.

Wennberg et al. (1998) demonstrated that both pre- and postexcision ECoG data are good predictors of outcome in frontal lobe epilepsy.

References

Ajmone Marsan, C. 1972. Focal electrical stimulation. In *Experimental Models of Epilepsy: A Manual for the Laboratory Worker,* Eds. D.P. Purpura, J.K. Penry, D.B. Tower, D.B., et al., pp. 147–172. New York: Raven Press.

Ajmone Marsan, C. 1980. Depth electrography and electrocorticography. In *Electrodiagnosis in Clinical Neurology,* Ed. M.J. Aminoff, pp. 167–196. New York: Churchill Livingstone.

Ajmone Marsan, C., and Baldwin, M. 1958. Electrocorticography. In *Temporal Lobe Epilepsy,* Eds. M. Baldwin and P. Bailey, pp. 368–395. Springfield, IL: Charles C Thomas.

Ajmone Marsan, C., and O'Connor, M. 1973. Electrocorticography. In *Handbook of Electroencephalography and Clinical Neurophysiology,* Ed. A. Remond, vol. 10C, pp. 3–49. Amsterdam: Elsevier.

Bates, J.A.V. 1963. Special investigation techniques—indwelling electrodes and electrocorticography. In *Electroencephalography: A Symposium on Its Various Aspects,* Eds. H. Hill and G. Parr, pp. 429–479. New York: Macmillan.

Bechtevera, N.P. 1962. *Biopotentials of Cerebral Hemispheres in Brain Tumors.* New York: Constants Bureau.

Bengzon, A.R.A., Rasmussen, T., Gloor, P., et al. 1968. Prognostic factors in surgical treatment of temporal lobe epilepsy. Neurology (Minneapolis) 18:717–731.

Berger, H. 1929. Über das Elektrenkephalogramm des Menschen. Arch. Psychiatr. Nervenkr. 87:527–570 (translated by Gloor, P. 1969. Electroencephalogr. Clin. Neurophysiol. Suppl. 28:37–73).

Bernier, G.P., Richer, F., and Giard, N. 1990. Electrical stimulation of the human brain in epilepsy. Epilepsia 31:513–520.

Cendes, F., Dubeau, F., Olivier, A., et al. 1993. Increased neocortical spiking and surgical outcome after selective amygdalo-hippocampectomy. Epilepsy Res. 16:195–206.

Chatrian, G.-E., and Quesney, L.F. 1997. Intraoperative electrocorticography. In *Epilepsy: A Comprehensive Textbook,* Eds. J. Engel, Jr., and T.A. Pedley. New York: Raven Press.

Cherlow, D.G., Dymond, A.M., Crandall, P.H., et al. 1977. Evoked response and after-discharge thresholds to electrical stimulation in temporal lobe epileptics. Arch. Neurol. 34:527–531.

Devinsky, O., Canevini, M.P., Sato, S., et al. 1992. Quantitative electrocorticography in patients undergoing temporal lobectomy. J. Epilepsy 5: 178–185.

Engel, J. Jr. 1987a. Approaches to the localization of the epileptogenic lesion. In *Surgical Treatment of the Epilepsies,* Ed. Engel, J. Jr., pp. 75–100. New York: Raven Press.

Engel, J. Jr. 1987b. Outcome with respect to epileptic seizures. In *Surgical Treatment of the Epilepsies,* Ed. Engel, J. Jr., pp. 553–571. New York: Raven Press.

Engel, J. Jr., Driver, M.V., and Falconer, M.A. 1975. Electrophysiological correlates of pathology and surgical results in temporal lobe epilepsy. Brain 98:129–156.

Fiol, M.E., Torres, F., Gates, J.R., et al. 1991. The prognostic value of residual spikes in the postexcision electrocorticogram after temporal lobectomy. Neurology 41:512–516.

Gastaut, H., Naquet, R., Vigouroux, R., et al. 1953. Étude électrographique chez l'homme et chez l'animal des décharges épileptiques dites "psychomotrices." Rev. Neurol. 88:310–354.

Gibbs, F.A., Amador, L., and Rich, C. 1958. Electroencephalographic findings and therapeutic results in surgical treatment of psychomotor epilepsy. In *Temporal Lobe Epilepsy,* Eds. M. Baldwin and P. Bailey, pp. 358–367. Springfield, IL: Charles C Thomas.

Gloor, P. 1975. Contributions of electroencephalography and electrocorticography to the neurosurgical treatment of the epilepsies. In *Neurosurgical Management of Epilepsies,* Eds. D.P. Purpura, J.K. Penry, and R.D. Walker, pp. 59–105. New York: Raven Press.

Graf, M., Niedermeyer, E., Schiemann, J., et al. 1984. Electrocorticography: information derived from intraoperative recordings during seizure surgery. Clin. Electroencephalogr. 15:83–91.

Guerreiro, M.M., Quesney, L.F., Salanova, V., et al. 2003. Continuous electrocorticogram epileptiform discharges due to brain gliosis. J. Clin. Neurophysiol.

Jasper, H.H. 1949. Electrocorticogram in man. Electroencephalogr. Clin. Neurophysiol. Suppl. 2:16–29.

Jasper, H.H. 1954. Electrocorticography. In *Epilepsy and the Functional Anatomy of the Human Brain,* Eds. Penfield, W., and Jasper, H.H., pp. 692–738. Boston: Little, Brown.

Jasper, H.H., Arfel-Capdevielle, G., and Rasmussen, T. 1961. Evaluation of EEG and cortical electrographic studies for prognosis of seizures following surgical excision of epileptogenic lesions. Epilepsia 2:130–137.

Jennum, P., Dhuna, A., Davies, K., et al. 1993. Outcome of resective surgery for intractable partial epilepsy guided by subdural electrode arrays. Acta Neurol. Scand. 87:434–437.

Kajtor, F., Hullay, J., Farago, L., et al. 1958. Electrical activity of the hippocampus of patients with temporal lobe epilepsy. AMA Arch. Neurol. Psychiatry 80:25–38.

Magnus, P., De Vet, A.C., Van der Marel, A., et al. 1962. Electrocorticography during operations for partial epilepsy. Dev. Child. Neurol. 4:35–48.

Marshall, C., and Walker, A.E. 1949. Electrocorticography. Bull. John Hopkins Hosp. 85:344–359.

McBride, M.C., Binnie, C.D., Janota, I., et al. 1991. Predictive value of intraoperative electrocorticograms. Electroencephalogr. Clin. Neurol. 30: 526–532.

Meyers, H.R., Knott, J.R., Hayne, R.A., et al. 1950. The surgery of epilepsy. Limitations of the concept of the corticoelectrographic "spike" as an index of the epileptogenic focus. J. Neurosurg. 7:337–346.

Musella, L., Wilder, B.J., and Schmidt, R.P. 1971. Electroencephalographic activation with intravenous methohexital in psycho-motor epilepsy. Neurology (Minneapolis) 21:594–602.

Niedermeyer, E. 1982. Electrocorticography. In *Electroencephalography,* Eds. E. Niedermeyer and F. Lopes da Silva, pp. 537–541. Munich: Urban & Schwarzenberg.

Niedermeyer, E. 1987. Electrocorticography. In *Electroencephalography, Basic Principles, Clinical Applications and Related Fields,* 2nd ed., Eds. E. Niedermeyer, F. Lopes da Silva, pp. 613–617. Baltimore: Urban and Schwarzenberg.

Ojeman, G.A. 1980. Basic mechanisms implicated in surgical treatments of epilepsy. In *Window to Brain Mechanisms,* Eds. J.S. Lockard and A.A. Ward, Jr., pp. 261–277. New York: Raven Press.

Ojeman, G.A., and Dodrill, C.B. 1985. Verbal memory deficits after left temporal lobectomy. Mechanism and intraoperative prediction. J. Neurosurg. 62:101–107.

Palmini, A., Gambardella, A., Andermann, F., et al. 1995. Intrinsic epileptogenicity of human dysplastic cortex as suggested by corticography and surgical results. Ann. Neurol. 37:476–487.

Penfield, W., and Jasper, H.H. 1954. *Epilepsy and the Functional Anatomy of the Human Brain.* Boston: Little, Brown.

Penfield, W., and Kristiansen, K. 1951. *Epileptic Seizure Patterns.* Springfield, IL: Charles C Thomas.

Picard, C., and Olivier A. 1983. Sensory cortical tongue representation in man. J. Neurosurg. 59:781–789.

Primrose, D.C., and Ojeman, G.A. 1992. Outcome of resective surgery for temporal lobe epilepsy. In *Epilepsy Surgery,* Ed. H. Lüders, pp. 601–611. New York: Raven Press.

Quesney, L.F., and Niedermeyer, E. 1993. Electrocorticography. In *Electroencephalography: Basic Principles, Clinical Applications, and Related Fields,* 3rd ed., Eds. E. Niedermeyer and F. Lopes da Silva, pp. 695–699. Baltimore: Williams & Wilkins.

Quesney, L.F., Abou-Khalil, B., Cole, A., et al. 1988. Pre-operative and intracerebral EEG investigation in patients with temporal lobe epilepsy: trends, results and review of pathophysiologic mechanisms. Acta. Neurol. Scand. 78(suppl 117):52–61.

Quesney, L.F., Constain, M., Fish, D.R., et al. 1990. Frontal lobe epilepsy—field of recent emphasis. Am. J. EEG Technol. 30:177–193.

Quesney, L.F., Constain, M., Rasmussen, T., et al. 1992a. Presurgical EEG investigation in frontal lobe epilepsy. In *Surgical Treatment of Epilepsy* (Epilepsy Res. Suppl. 5), Eds. Theodore, W.H., pp. 55–69. Amsterdam: Elsevier Science Publishers.

Quesney, L.F., Constain, M., Rasmussen, T., et al. 1992b. How large are frontal lobe epileptogenic zones? EEG, ECoG and SEEG evidence. In *Advances in Neurology,* vol. 57, Eds. P. Chauvel, A.V. Delgado-Escueta, E. Halgren, et al. New York: Raven Press.

Quesney, L.F., Wennberg, R., Olivier, A., et al. 1998. EcoG findings in extratemporal epilepsy: the MNI experience. In *Electrocorticography: Current Trends and Future Perspectives* (EEG Suppl. 48), Eds. L.F. Quesney, C.D. Binnie, and G.E. Chatrian. Amsterdam: Elsevier Science B.V.

Rasmussen, T. 1983. Surgical treatment of complex partial seizures: results, lessons and problems. Epilepsia 24:S65–S75.

Salanova, V., Andermann, F., Olivier, A., et al. 1992. Occipital lobe epilepsy: electroclinical manifestations, electrocorticography, cortical stimulation and outcome in 42 patients treated between 1930 and 1991. Brain 115:1655–1680.

Salanova, V., Andermann, F., Rasmussen, T., et al. 1995a. Parietal lobe epilepsy. Clinical manifestations and outcome in 82 patients treated surgically between 1929 and 1988. Brain 118:607–627.

Salanova, V., Andermann, F., Rasmussen, T., et al. 1995b. Tumoural parietal lobe epilepsy. Clinical manifestations and outcome in 34 patients treated between 1934 and 1988. Brain 118:1289–1304.

Silfvenius, H., Gloor, P., and Rasmussen, T. 1964. Evaluation of insular ablation in surgical treatment of temporal lobe epilepsy. Epilepsia 5:307–320.

Spencer, D.D., and Inserni, J. 1992. Temporal lobectomy. In *Epilepsy Surgery,* Ed. H.O. Lüders, pp. 533–545. New York: Raven Press.

Stefan, H., Quesney, L.F., Abou-Khalil, B., et al. 1991. Electrocorticography in temporal lobe epilepsy surgery. Acta Neurol. Scand. 83:65–72.

Toga, A.W., and Mazziota, J.C. 2002. *Brain Mapping: The Methods,* 2nd ed. New York: Academic Press.

Tuunainen, A., Nousiainen, U., Mervaala, E., et al. 1994. Postoperative EEG and electrocorticography: relation to clinical outcome in patients with temporal lobe surgery. Epilepsia 35:1165–1173.

Walker, A.E. 1949. Electrocorticography in epilepsy. A surgeon's appraisal. In *Électroencéphalographie et Électrocorticographie de l'Épilepsie,* Ed. H. Fischgold, Electroencephalogr. Clin. Neurophysiol. Suppl. 2:30–37. Langres: l'Expansion Scientifique Française.

Walker, A.E. 1967. Temporal lobectomy. J. Neurosurg. 26:642–649.

Walker, A.E. 1974. Surgery for epilepsy. In *The Epilepsies (Handbook of Clinical Neurology),* vol. 15, Eds. Magnus, O., and Lorentz de Haas, A.M., pp. 739–757. Amsterdam: North Holland.

Walker, A.E., Marshall, C., and Beresford, E.M. 1947. Electrocorticographic characteristics of the cerebrum posttraumatic epilepsy. Assoc. Res. Nerv. Men. Dis. 26:502–515.

Walker, A.E., Lichtenstein, S., and Marshall, C. 1960. A critical analysis of electrocorticography in temporal lobe epilepsy. Arch. Neurol. 2:172–182.

Wennberg, R., Quesney, F., Olivier, A., et al. 1997a. Mesial temporal versus lateral temporal interictal epileptiform activity: comparison of chronic and acute intracranial recordings. Electroencephalogr. Clin. Neurophysiol. 102:486–494.

Wennberg, R., Quesney, F., Olivier, A., et al. 1997b. Induction of burst-suppression and activation of epileptiform activity after methohexital and selective amygdalo-hippocampectomy. Electroencephalogr. Clin. Neurophysiol. 102:443–451.

Wennberg, R., Quesney, L.F., and Villemure, J.-G. 1997c. Epileptiform and non-epileptiform paroxysmal activity from isolated cortex after functional hemispherectomy. Electroencephalogr. Clin. Neurophysiol. 102:437–442.

Wennberg, R., Quesney, L.F., Olivier, A., et al. 1998. Electrocorticography and outcome in frontal lobe epilepsy. Electroencephalogr. Clin. Neurophysiol. 106:357–368.

39. Subdural Electrodes

Ronald P. Lesser and Santiago Arroyo

Localization of the epileptogenic area (EA) is the aim for presurgical evaluation of patients with uncontrolled seizures. To attain accurate localization a variety of noninvasive studies are performed including scalp video-electroencephalogram (EEG) recording and neuroimaging techniques [magnetic resonance imaging (MRI), single photon emission computed tomography (SPECT), and positron emission tomography (PET)]. Concurrent localization with some or all of these techniques to a certain area makes surgery and relief of seizures feasible (Engel et al., 1982), at least in those cases in which the EA is far from sensorimotor or language areas.

Advancement in noninvasive techniques have permitted good EA localization and surgery in many patients with refractory epilepsy (Engel, 1993). However, in some patients seizure origin remains veiled and implanted electrodes are necessary for localization. On the other hand, for those patients with EA near eloquent brain areas, subdural electrodes allow mapping of brain functions through techniques of electrical stimulation, helping to delineate the safety margins of the projected resection. This chapter reviews the types of electrodes, implant techniques, and risks, and analyzes the situations in which we believe subdural electrodes should be implanted in patients with uncontrolled epilepsy.

Electrode Characteristics

Subdural electrodes are made of stainless steel or platinum-iridium. Theoretically, platinum-iridium may have some advantages because of its relative inertness, higher stability for stimulation procedures, and lack of magnetic properties (Mortimer et al., 1970). However, both have been used successfully. Electrode contacts are of different diameters varying from 2 to 5 mm, with center-to-center distances of 0.5 to 2 cm between electrodes. Electrodes are inlaid in a fixed, usually rectangular, array in a thin transparent Silastic plate. This Silastic plate keeps the electrodes in a set place and allows visual inspection of the cortical surface under the electrodes, thus permitting visualization of the actual relations of the electrodes with the brain convolutions and vessels (Fig. 39.1). In addition, Silastic gives flexibility to the plate, making possible its adaptation to the overall brain surface. There are a variety of arrays in which the electrodes are laid out. The most usual designs are 8 × 8, 6 × 8, 2 × 8, here called grids, and 1 × 8 and 1 × 4, called strips.

Technique for Implantation of Subdural/Epidural Electrodes

Subdural electrodes are placed under general anesthesia. Placement of grids is done through a craniotomy. Scalp and bone flaps are tailored depending on the area of interest,

then the dura is opened and the electrodes are placed under direct visual inspection. Special attention is directed to avoid positioning the electrodes over cortical vessels because EEG recordings in this situation may be less informative and functional localization via stimulation is more difficult. In addition, painful sensations can occur when stimulation currents affect the nerves accompanying the cortical vessels (although this effect is not restricted to large vessels) (Lesser et al., 1985). The grid is fixed in place by suturing the corners to the dura and by stitching the dura to the cable. The dura is closed with continuous suture. The craniotomy is sealed with Silastic adhesive, and the scalp incision is closed in two layers. The cables from the grid exit through the craniotomy, each cable with its own exit route. Then, they are tunneled under the scalp and exit at a certain distance from the craniotomy opening (Fig. 39.1). Strict antiseptic procedures are used in caring for the external surgical incisions.

Subdural strips are inserted through a bur hole and slipped into the subarachnoid space under the temporal lobe or over the convexity of the hemisphere. Frequently, bilateral strips are used (Dodrill and Troupin, 1991; Spencer et al., 1990, 1991; Wyler et al., 1984, 1988a,b, 1989a,b) for lateralization between the two hemispheres.

Some laboratories use a standard placement in each case (e.g., bilateral symmetric strips to lateralize side of seizure onset). Although we use fairly standard placements in many cases, in others, we, and many other laboratories, often use placements tailored to reflect the expected region of the patient's seizures and vary the number of electrodes for each case. Depending on the expected location of the patient's seizure focus, the arrangement of the electrodes differs so that placement of the grids or strips is tailored in each case. Unilateral or bilateral placement on the convexity, basal temporal area, or into the interhemispheric fissure can be performed with a wide variety of electrode grid arrangements.

In some centers strips or grids of electrodes are placed in the epidural space (Goldring, Gregorie, and Tempelhoff, 1989; Goldring, 1978, 1987; Goldring and Gregorie, 1984). These epidural electrodes are inserted through a bur hole or craniotomy. The dura may be opened to allow electrical stimulation testing to map movement, sensory, language, or other areas. Somatosensory evoked potentials could be performed with the dura either open or closed. Once these are done, the dura is closed and the electrodes are placed and sewn onto the dura. Grids and strips are of dimensions similar to the ones used in the subdural space and are particularly used over the convexity. Whether to use subdural or epidural electrodes depends on the experience that each center has with these techniques. Subdural electrodes may allow more

Figure 39.1. Intrasurgical photographs of a subdural grid. The electrodes are embedded in a transparent Silastic material that allows visualization of the underlying brain.

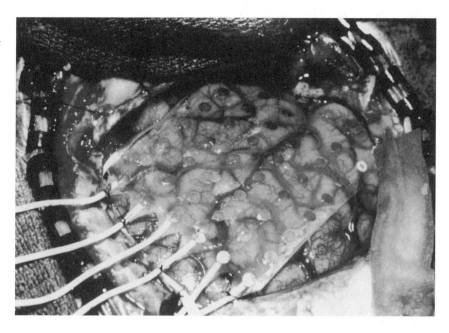

precise functional localization because the relationships of each electrode to the underlying brain can be directly visualized. Besides, they can cover the basal and paramesial regions of the temporal lobe. Epidural electrodes, on the other hand, can be used for stimulation if the dura beneath the grid is completely deafferented. Also, if the dura is not opened, there is theoretical reduction of the risk of infection.

Another approach to subdural recording is by flexible subdural bundles and reeds of electrodes that have been used with depth electrodes. These bundles are introduced at the same time and through the same bicoronal bur hole as the depth electrodes (Van Veelen et al., 1990). Finally, one can use subdural strips and depth electrodes simultaneously (Spencer and Spencer, 1994).

Mushroom-shaped epidural peg electrodes (Awad et al., 1991a; Barnett et al., 1990) are of similar electrode materials and diameter as subdural electrodes. They are placed either under local or general anesthesia and are reported to have minimal risk of infection or hemorrhage. Epidural pegs allow samplings of cortical activity from several different areas of the cortex, although with fewer recording electrodes in any one region, compared to subdural and epidural arrays.

Complications

Surgical implantation of subdural electrodes had been thought to have a low risk of complications, with an overall 1% morbidity, and with a 4% morbidity for grids, similar to that of depth electrodes (Van Buren, 1987). Complications of subdural strips (Wyler et al., 1991) and epidural electrodes (Goldring, 1991) appeared to be lower than that for grids, with a morbidity of 0.85% for strips and 2% for epidural electrodes.

However, studies have shown a higher occurrence of side effects. This has been particularly the case for subdural grids, rather than for strips. In a prospective study that included 58 subdural/epidural electrodes implants, it was shown that the most common complications were fever (42%), cerebrospinal fluid leakage (19%), headache (15%), and nausea (4%) (Swartz et al., 1996). No permanent sequelae were reported. Although in this study there were no infections, this complication has been reported by others (Wyler et al., 1991). Technical details, such as tunneling the cable under the scalp to exit away from the craniotomy incision (Wyllie et al., 1987a,b), reduce the incidence of infection. To prevent infection, it is useful to limit the recording period to less than 2 weeks. In any case, there is usually a good response to antibiotic treatment and removal of the electrodes. Hamer et al. (2002) retrospectively reviewed their experience with 198 subdural grid electrode placements in 187 patients over a 17-year period. They found that the complication rate had decreased; however, in the last 5 years of the study, 19/99 patients (19%) had complications, including two patients (2%) with permanent sequelae. In the last 3 years, the complication rate was 13.5% (5/37) without permanent deficits. Over the entire study, complications occurred in 52 of 198 monitoring sessions (26.3%): infection ($n = 24$; 12.1%), transient neurologic deficit ($n = 22$; 11.1%), epidural hematoma ($n = 5$; 2.5%), increased intracranial pressure ($n = 5$; 2.5%), and infarction ($n = 3$; 1.5%). One patient (0.5%) died during grid insertion. The authors found that complications increased when a greater number of grids/electrodes were used ($p = .021/p = .052$; especially >60 electrodes), when the duration of monitoring was longer ($p = .004$; especially >10 days), when the patient was older ($p = .005$), when grids were placed on the left ($p = .01$), and when there were bur holes in addition to the craniotomy ($p = .022$). No association with complications was found for number of seizures, IQ, anticonvulsants, or grid localization.

Although the need for prophylactic antibiotics is controversial (Fullagar and Wyler, 1993; Wyler et al., 1991), some groups use prophylactic wide-spectrum antibiotics (usually a third-generation cephalosporin) during the whole period while the electrodes are implanted.

Headaches during the period of electrode implantation are probably related to increased intracranial pressure due to the mass effect of the electrodes. Treatment of this condition requires analgesics and fluid restriction. In addition, one can "tent" the dura over the grid by using a dural patch. Mannitol and corticosteroids are occasionally administered to reduce acute brain edema; however, we do not use them routinely. Occasionally, focal symptoms and signs and decreased mental status occur and removal of the electrodes is necessary. Sometimes the reasons for the adverse clinical signs are clear, but this is not always the case, and is an area for further investigation.

Epidural or subdural hematomas and aseptic necrosis of the bone flap are less common (Kramer et al., 1994). Very rarely, a subdural hematoma can produce focal seizures not representative of the patient's habitual seizures (Malow et al., 1995).

Monitoring the Patient with Subdural Electrodes

After electrode implantation the patient stays in the intensive care unit for 24 hours. After postoperative recovery we admit the patient to the video/EEG monitoring, generally for about 1 to 2 weeks. Antiepileptic medication is maintained for the first 24 to 48 hours and, if no seizures occur, it is gradually tapered and withdrawn. Doses of anticonvulsants vary in accordance with individual patient seizure frequency. In principle, one might prefer to stimulate the brain while high anticonvulsant levels are present in order to avoid stimulation-induced seizures. Conversely, it would be preferable to do seizure monitoring at times when levels are low, and thus facilitate seizure occurrence. In practice, the two are done simultaneously in order to complete the assessment in as short a time as possible. There are practical ways to optimize the scheduling. For example, if stimulation will occur during the week, medication levels can be lower over the weekend.

Once EEG recording and stimulation are satisfactorily accomplished, we usually perform any indicated cortical resection at the time that the grid is removed. We observe the position of the electrodes relative to the anatomical landmarks in the operating room. We resect the epileptogenic tissue, taking into account the location of the ictally and interictally active electrodes and the results of the electrical stimulation.

Technical Specifications and Montage Selection

In most laboratories EEG is recorded by cable telemetry, although radiotelemetry is still sometimes used. Since the patient is videotaped during the EEG recordings, movement is in any case somewhat restricted, and radiotelemetry, therefore, conveys no special advantages. In most monitoring units EEG signals are recorded in referential montage and led via shielded cables to standard EEG amplifier box(es) where the signal is amplified and filtered (for example, 0.3 time

constant, and 100–300 Hz low pass filter). The information usually has been digitized at between 200 and 256 Hz. More recent information indicates that higher sampling rates can be useful. For instance, with implanted electrodes, one can record high-frequency activity (at frequencies from 80 to 500 Hz) at the start of some seizures (Arroyo et al., 1994; Bragin et al., 1999, 2002; Fisher et al., 1992).

The large number of contacts available with subdural electrodes can make montage design difficult, and it usually is necessary to have 64 to 128 channels to facilitate montage selection. Montages may be used in referential or bipolar chains or combinations of both. Recording in referential montage implies prior knowledge of which electrode in the array is suitable as a reference. At least initially, that is not always possible. A reference on the scalp or an outside of the head also can be used, but artifacts are more likely to occur.

Interictal and Ictal Recording with Subdural Electrodes

Subdural electrodes allow prolonged monitoring and the recording of interictal and ictal EEG activity. We will briefly review these issues.

Interictal Activity

Only a small percentage of all interictal spikes recorded with subdural electrodes are observed at the scalp when subdural and scalp electrodes are used simultaneously (Devinsky et al., 1989; Lüders et al., 1987). This is due to the attenuation of the cortical activity by the overlaying skull and scalp. The amplitude of discharges recorded at the scalp depends on several variables such as voltage, area of the cortex involved, depth of the source, and the degree of synchronicity of the cortical area affected (Alarcon et al., 1994; Cooper et al., 1965). Subdural electrodes have similar detection rates as depth electrodes for interictal spikes of mesial temporal origin (Privitera et al., 1990).

Interictal epileptiform activity recorded with subdural electrodes gives indispensable complementary information regarding the potential extent of the epileptogenic region (Kanner et al., 1993; Lüders et al., 1987; Wyllie et al., 1987,a,b) (Fig. 39.2). In fact, resection of the areas with prominent interictal discharges has been associated with good surgical outcome (Armon et al., 1996; Lüders et al., 1987). However, the use of interictal spikes for seizure surgery has some limitations: First, some physiological sharp transients may be difficult to differentiate from epileptogenic spikes (Lüders et al., 1987). Second, occasional divergences in localization of the ictal versus interictal activity have been observed, so that the presence of interictal spikes may not necessarily indicate the site of the seizure focus (Kazee et al., 1991; Lüders et al., 1989; Wyllie et al., 1987,a,b). Third, the parameters that define the degree of epileptogenicity of the spikes are not known, although spike frequency is at least a very good index of epileptogenicity (Bustamante et al., 1981). Fourth, in patients with lesions, some workers have found removal of regions with interictal or ictal EEG activity to be less important than removal of the lesion for seizure relief after surgery (Britton et al., 1994;

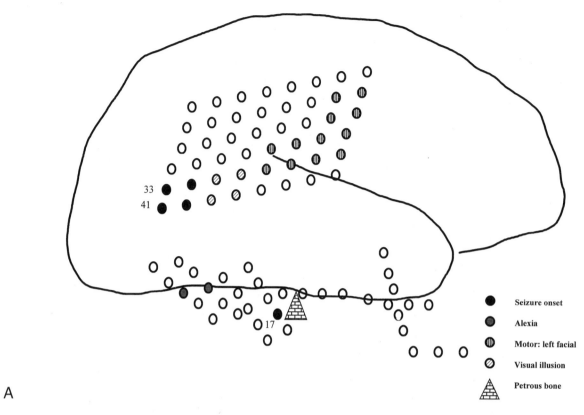

A

B

Figure 39.2. Recordings from a patient with right posterior temporal lobe epilepsy. **A:** The location of subdural electrodes over the lateral cortex and some of the pertinent findings. Observe the locations of the motor face and arm areas and the location of the ictal EEG epileptogenic area. **B:** A basal view of the subdural electrode placement.

Cascino, 1990) (although not all of these patients become seizure free).

Ictal Activity

Interpretation of tracings from subdural electrodes requires familiarity with a variety of normal and abnormal patterns and artifacts (Figs. 39.3 and 39.4). Furthermore, there are a number of observations regarding recorded patterns that sometimes answer but at other times raise questions about how to interpret these recordings.

Site of Seizure Onset

The site where ictal activity is first seen in chronic intracranial recording helps localize the region of maximal epileptogenicity, and, consequently, helps to identify the area that must be resected. However, intracranial electrodes only record from a portion of the brain. Therefore, clinical experience is essential in interpreting recordings. Also, it

has been demonstrated that time lags from the place of onset indicate the pattern of activity spread (Gotman, 1987; Lieb et al., 1987).

Type of EEG Pattern

EEG seizure onset can be focal (involving only one or two electrodes), regional (involving three or more contacts), or generalized. A recent study on ictal patterns recorded with subdural electrodes has shown that most patients show early electrodecremental events, generalized or focal, involving frequencies below 40 Hz (Alarcon et al., 1995). Resection of areas with localized activity between 20 and 80 Hz has been associated with good outcome (Fisher et al., 1992; Alarcon et al., 1995). Generalized electrodecremental events at onset are more frequent in extratemporal (mainly frontal lobe) seizures (Arroyo et al., 1992b; Baumgartner et al., 1996). However, generalized electrodecremental onset might not imply poor outcome in temporal lobe seizures (Alarcon et al., 1995).

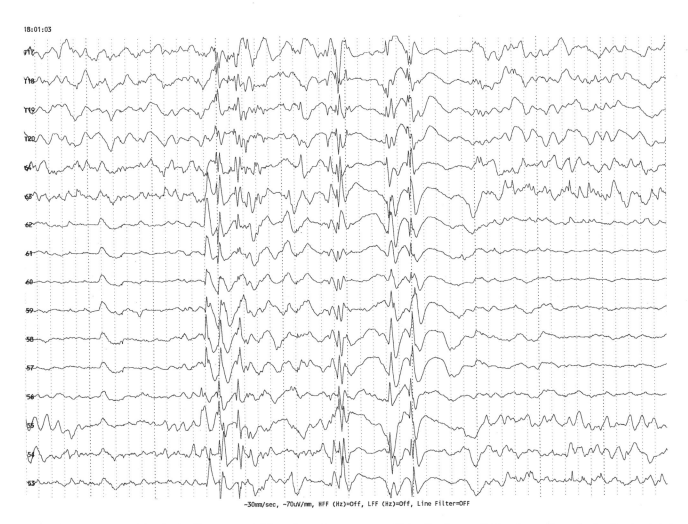

18:01:03

~30mm/sec, ~70uV/mm, HFF (Hz)=Off, LFF (Hz)=Off, Line Filter=OFF

Figure 39.3. A sample of interictal spikes as recorded from these electrodes. The recordings display a subset (16) of all of the recorded channels. The electrodes are over the basal (channels 1–4) and lateral (channels 5–16) temporal lobe. Note bursts of high-voltage spikes and polyspikes located at many different electrodes with no single maximum. Electrode 17 is the first channel.

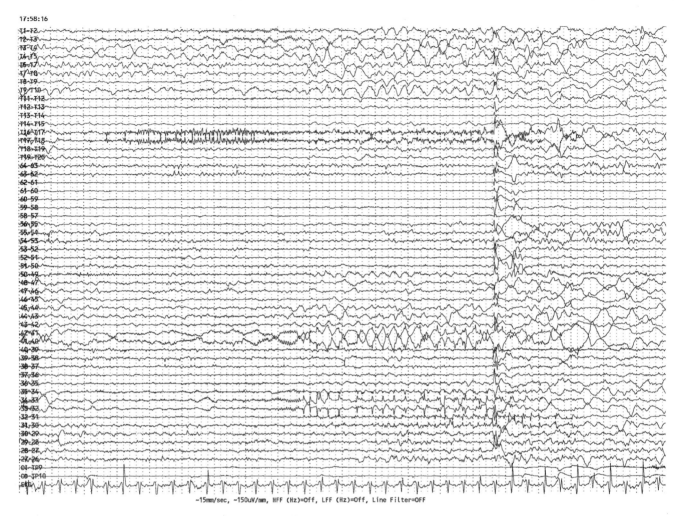

Figure 39.4. An ictal onset, consisting of low-voltage high-frequency activity over T17 (channels 13–14), quickly spreading to electrodes 33 (channels 45–46), 34 (channels 44–45), 41 (channel 37–38), and 42 (channels 36–37). Spikes then occur at electrodes 33, 34, 41, 42, and T10 (channel 8) while high-frequency activity persists at T17.

Type of EEG Recording

Direct current (DC) recording can occasionally be useful for delineating the epileptogenic area in patients with neocortical (mostly extratemporal) seizures in whom a diffuse electrodecremental pattern is frequently observed (Ikeda et al., 1996). A slow-rising negative potential during DC recording has been observed in a more restricted area and occurs seconds before the initial ictal EEG pattern (Ikeda et al., 1996).

Seizure Localization

Ictal patterns may differ between seizures of mesial temporal origin and seizures of extratemporal origin (Spencer et al., 1992). Seizures of patients with mesial temporal origin are more likely to have high-frequency onset and have periodic spikes previous to the definite ictal pattern. Ictal epileptogenic areas in patients with frontal or extratemporal lobe seizures are large, and frequently multifocal widely distributed spikes are observed (Salanova et al., 1993, 1995,a,b).

Extratemporal seizure onset associated with abnormal pathological substrate may be more likely to be associated with lower frequency EEG activity and no periodic spikes before seizure onset when compared to extratemporal seizure onset recorded from areas without pathological findings (Spencer et al., 1992).

Variability of EEG Ictal Onset

When the EA is constant for a patient, there is a better prognosis for seizure control after surgery. However, variability of ictal onset in the same patient is sometimes observed (Quesney and Gloor, 1985; Spencer et al., 1987, 1992). This variability could be related to an increase in the number of seizures taking place in a short period, but could be related to other, unknown, factors. Some have found variability EEG frequency at seizure onset to be more frequent in temporal versus extratemporal seizures (Spencer et al., 1992). An increased number of locations of seizure onset may be associated with a decreased surgical success rate.

Afterdischarge Threshold to Electrical Stimulation and Electrically Induced Seizures

Some consider an increased threshold for afterdischarges to occur at the seizure focus (Engel et al., 1981), but not all agree (Bernier et al., 1987, 1990; Gloor, 1975; Wieser, 1987). One study using subdural electrodes found that thresholds for afterdischarges vary from point to point and from day to day in the same area (Lesser et al., 1984). In contrast, a study using intraoperative single-unit recording found that the epileptogenic cortex was more likely to produce afterdischarges to repetitive stimuli compared with the more normal cortex (Wyler and Ward, 1981). Overall, it is likely that, unless the circumstances for testing are very carefully restricted, stimulation for seizure focus localization has a limited utility.

The reliability of seizures elicited by electrical stimulation for delineating the seizure focus is limited (Gloor, 1975; Halgren, 1982; Jumao-as and Dasheiff, 1988; Lüders et al., 1987; Wieser et al., 1979), and, when it is performed, it is usually for confirmation of the already identified epileptic focus (Bernier et al., 1987, 1990). Low-threshold areas have been associated with regions where there were more active interictal discharges (Wyler and Ward, 1981). However, these variations are frequently difficult to interpret because of the above-mentioned threshold variations (Gloor, 1975; Lesser, 1984). Furthermore, in reports of depth electrode stimulation, it is not clear if there is a consistent relation between stimulation-produced reproduction of clinical manifestations of the patients' seizures, for example an aura, and the localization of the epileptic focus (Halgren, 1982). Overall, many workers believe that seizures caused by electrical stimulation are of little or no use for delineating the seizure focus (Lüders et al., 1987).

Indications for Subdural Electrodes for Localization of the Epileptogenic Area

Scalp video-EEG recording is still the most valuable source of information regarding the site of seizure onset. It gives data about the presence or absence of epileptic seizures (sometimes the patient evaluated for surgery does not have epilepsy!) (Arroyo et al., 1994; Fisher et al., 1992), the type of seizures by analysis of their ictal semiology [for example, temporal versus extratemporal lobe origin (Gil-Nagel and Risinger, 1997)], and the ictal EEG localization. Scalp EEG localization, however, is not possible in some of these patients (Lieb et al., 1976; Spencer et al., 1985). This is especially true in patients with extratemporal lobe seizures in whom EA localization with scalp EEG recording frequently gives diffuse EEG patterns (Arroyo et al., 1994; Salanova et al., 1993, 1995a,b; Sveinbjornsdottir and Duncan, 1993; Williamson et al., 1992). Nowadays, neuroimaging has a significant impact on decision making about the need of invasive monitoring (Spencer, 1994). High-quality MRI, especially using volumetric measurement of the hippocampus (Cascino et al., 1992a; Trenerry et al., 1993) or three-dimensional (3D) reconstructions (Bastos et al., 1995), has shown focal abnormalities related to pathologic findings associated with seizures (Barkovich et al., 1995;

Bastos et al., 1995; Bergin et al., 1995; Berkovic and McIntosh, 1995; Ostertun et al., 1996). Identification of a lesion with MRI changes the presurgical evaluation scheme and the surgical approach and has, for example, reduced the need for invasive procedures such as subdural electrodes (Spencer, 1995). Patients with lesional epilepsy are often good candidates for surgery provided that the EA is neighboring the lesion. If this is the case, complete lesion resection is the main, but not the only, factor that leads to good prognosis after epilepsy surgery (Britton et al., 1994; Cascino et al., 1992b, 1993). It is likely to be the case that failures occur when removal of the lesion did not, in passing, remove a sufficient portion of the EA as well. Other imaging tests for functional deficits (interictal or ictal SPECT or PET) can provide additional confirmatory data.

Figure 39.5 summarizes the indications for subdural electrode implantation in patients with an epileptogenic lesion demonstrated by MRI. These indications should be interpreted in a broad context. In different patients, different options might be possible. In patients with nonlocalized ictal EEG records but in whom the ictal EEG activity is lateralized, we use subdural grids in three situations:

1. in those patients in whom the EA is near eloquent brain areas (or other cortical areas controlling critical functions that need to be mapped for a safe resection);
2. in those patients with lesions that are frequently associated with large EA like migration disorders, porencephalic cysts, or lesions subsequent to trauma or encephalitis (Cendes et al., 1995; Dubeau et al., 1995; Free et al., 1996; Hirabayashi et al., 1993; Marks et al., 1992; Mathern et al., 1994; Mattia et al., 1995; Palmini et al., 1995);
3. in those patients in whom the extent or precise location of resection cannot be determined noninvasively.

A lesion per se is not necessarily reason for a grid. For example, in cases of patients with lesions (tumor, cavernous angioma, for example) located far from sensorimotor or language areas we and others (Britton et al., 1994; Cascino et al., 1992b, 1993) believe that it often is best to proceed directly to surgery without the aid of invasive procedures. It has been shown that temporal or extratemporal lobe seizures can be falsely lateralized using scalp ictal EEG (Adelman et al., 1982; Boon et al., 1991; King and Spencer, 1995; Sammaritano et al., 1987; Spencer et al., 1984; Wyler et al., 1984). For this reason, in patients with EEG ictal onset contralateral to a lesion or with bilateral seizure onsets we often place bilateral subdural strips or bilateral depth electrodes to lateralize seizure onset or assure bilaterality. These cases have occurred in patients with space-occupying lesions, with seizure foci located in the interhemispheric fissure, as well as in patients with temporal lobe foci. If seizures are bilaterally independent, we do not pursue surgery, although other centers remove the lesion without the resection of the contralateral epileptic focus with moderately good results (Boon et al., 1991; Hirsch et al., 1991).

Figure 39.6 presents the indications for subdural electrode implantation in patients with normal MRI, including those with atrophy and high signal intensity of the hippocampus, suggesting hippocampal sclerosis. It is usually

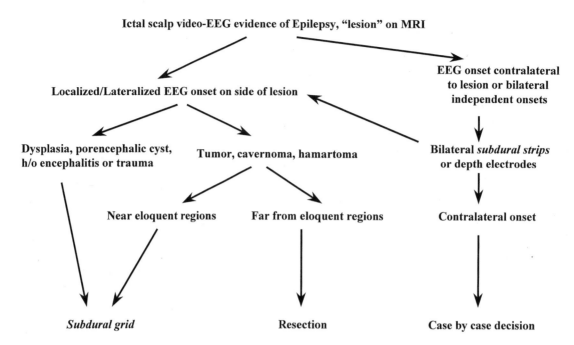

Figure 39.5. Schematic of a presurgical decision-making protocol in patients refractory complex partial seizures with a magnetic resonance imaging (MRI) lesion (other than mesial temporal sclerosis).

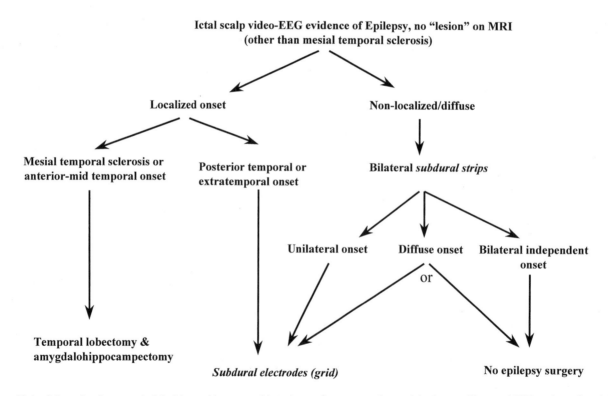

Figure 39.6. Schematic of a presurgical decision-making protocol in patients refractory complex partial seizures with normal MRI or signs of mesial temporal sclerosis.

unnecessary to use intracranial EEG monitoring in patients with an anterior temporal focus on the scalp (Engel et al., 1981, 1990) with or without hippocampal sclerosis. Grids are more useful in patients with evidence for a possible posterior temporal contribution to the region of epileptogenesis (Prasad et al., 2003; Wieser and Siegel, 1991), especially if seizures arise from the dominant hemisphere. In these patients the extent of the EA needs to be defined and in many cases language areas need to be delineated before surgery (Blume et al., 1991; Duchowny et al., 1994). Many patients with normal MRI and nonlocalized seizure onset have extratemporal lobe seizures. In these patients surgical treatment often is less successful (Armon et al., 1996; Zentner et al., 1996). In certain cases, however, surgery can be pursued in view of the poor quality of life of the patient and the intractability of the seizures (Laskowitz et al., 1995). If this is the case, we initially use subdural electrode strips, or a large continuous electrode array over the region or regions where the EA is expected to be. If a unilateral onset is demonstrated a grid can be implanted to define the EA further. If no localized EA is demonstrated, we may not pursue further workup.

Indications for Subdural Electrodes Versus Depth Electrodes

Whether to use subdural electrodes, depth electrodes or combinations of both is not clearly defined and depends on the experience that each center has with these techniques (Barry et al., 1989; Blume et al., 1985; Foerster, 1936; Lüders et al., 1987, 1989; Resnick et al., 1989; Rosenbaum and Laxer, 1989; Schomer et al., 1984; Spencer, 1989; Spencer et al., 1990; Sperling and O'Connor, 1989; Van Veelen et al., 1990; Wyler et al., 1988a,b, 1989b). Simultaneous implantation of intracerebral depth electrodes and subdural grid or strip electrodes is feasible and useful for epileptogenic area localization in selected patients (Barry et al., 1992; Shimizu et al., 1990; Spencer et al., 1990; Van Veelen et al., 1990).

Depth electrodes record directly from within the deep (for example, mesial temporal) structures, and only a portion of these areas (e.g., parahippocampal gyri) can be covered with subdural electrodes. On the other hand, subdural electrodes allow coverage of considerable portions of the lateral and basal temporal or other lobes. Such coverage is minimal with depth electrodes. This broad coverage is especially significant in patients with neocortical, especially extratemporal lobe, seizures (Baumgartner et al., 1996; Uematsu et al., 1990).

Depth electrodes often are directed to the mesial temporal structures because these areas are thought to contribute importantly to the great majority of complex partial seizures of temporal lobe origin (Spencer, 1989, 1991; Spencer et al., 1990). Subdural strips or grids cannot reach the most mesial temporal structures. However, experience with recordings suggests that in a number of patients the epileptogenic region is not limited to the mesial structures (Arroyo et al., 1992; Barry et al., 1992). Depth electrodes may underrepresent neocortical contributions due to their restricted coverage of the neocortex. In addition, even if the epileptogenic

focus is confined to a small area of the brain (e.g., the hippocampus), ictal activity originates or first spreads in most cases to the ipsilateral temporal lobe neocortex (Spencer, 1998; Spencer et al., 1990), so that neocortical recording may be sufficient for localization or lateralization purposes.

Depth electrodes are most useful when trying to lateralize mesial temporal epileptogenic areas (Angeleri et al., 1964; Talairach and Bancaud, 1974). In some centers a large number of depth electrodes are placed over extratemporal regions (Chauvel et al., 1992) but, due to the inherent "nearsightedness" of all intracerebral electrodes and the usually large epileptogenic areas associated with extratemporal lobe seizures (Arroyo et al., 1994; Baumgartner et al., 1996), we do not favor this approach. In fact, depth electrodes have been disappointing in the investigation of extratemporal lobe seizures due to the necessarily incomplete electrode coverage (Hajek and Wieser, 1988; Ludwig et al., 1976). The use of subdural grids in frontal lobe seizures might in theory allow a better seizure focus definition and thus better seizure control postsurgery (Sutherling et al., 1990; Wyllie et al., 1987b), and, in any case, should help to disclose the functionally important areas and subsequently reduce the risk of functional damage (Gates et al., 1988; Lüders et al., 1987; Pfurtscheller, 1977; Rosenbaum and Laxer, 1989; Spencer et al., 1987, 1990), but this remains to be clearly proven. Finally, in patients in whom previous seizure surgery has failed, subdural electrode recording is associated with better seizure control, compared with patients studied with scalp recording (Awad et al., 1991b; Wyler et al., 1989a).

Electrical Stimulation and Functional Localization with Subdural Electrodes

Electrical stimulation of the cortex, although nonphysiological, provides a simple way to disclose some of the functions of the cortex. It has been known since the 19th century that cortical function can be altered by focal application of electrical currents (Fritsch and Hitzig, 1870). Electrical stimulation of the human cortex was not performed until later (Barthlow, 1974; Uematsu et al., 1992b). Foerster and Penfield and collaborators (Foerster, 1936; Foerster and Penfield, 1930; Penfield and Jasper, 1954; Penfield and Roberts, 1959) developed and extended its use for clinical purposes when cortical resection in patients with epilepsy was contemplated. One can use cortical stimulation to identify regions modulating sensory, motor, language, and other cortical functions, thus allowing these areas to be spared, while resecting the maximal amount of epileptogenic brain tissues (Foerster, 1936; Penfield and Boldrey, 1937; Penfield and Jasper, 1954). In the last two decades, due to the expansion of surgery for epilepsy, electrical stimulation has been widely performed and has been confirmed as a reliable technique for functional localization (Ajmone-Marsan, 1980; Allison et al., 1996; Baumgartner et al., 1993; Goldring, 1978; Goldring and Gregorie, 1984; Jack et al., 1994; Jefferson, 1935; Laxer et al., 1984; Lesser et al., 1981, 1987; Lim et al., 1994; Lüders et al., 1982; Malow et al., 1996; Nii et al., 1996; Ojeman, 1983a,b; Ojemann and Mateer, 1979; Penfield and Perot, 1963; Perrine et al., 1994;

Rapport et al., 1983; Rasmussen and Milner, 1975; Rogawski and Porter, 1990; Schäffler et al., 1994; Schomer et al., 1984; Serafetinides, 1966; Urasaki et al., 1994; Van Buren et al., 1975, 1978; Wyler et al., 1984).

Electrical stimulation can be performed while the patient is in the operating room under local anesthesia or by means of chronically implanted subdural electrodes. Intraoperative electrocorticography and stimulation procedures (Berger et al., 1989; Burchiel et al., 1989; Ojeman, 1979, 1983a,b, 1987; Ojemann and Whitaker, 1978; Rogawski and Porter, 1990) have been used successfully for many years, but are subject to the constraints of the operating room. Only about half an hour to 2 hours is allowed for testing, and relatively few sites or modalities can be explored. Also, it requires a high degree of patient cooperation, which is not possible in some cases, for example with children or some mentally retarded patients. By comparison, stimulation with chronic subdural electrodes allows an extensive period for testing (several hours a day over several days), making it possible to use a more extensive testing protocol, which can be customized in response to findings. In individual patients it also is possible to retest areas of interest, and to check for afterdischarges in neighboring electrodes. All of this is accomplished while patients are in a relaxed atmosphere, and permitted to rest whenever tired (Bernier et al., 1987, 1990; Burnstine et al., 1990; Fedio et al., 1990; Kluin et al., 1988; Lim et al., 1991; Lüders et al., 1991; Ojemann and Whitaker, 1978; Uematsu et al., 1992a; Wyler et al., 1991).

Although electrical stimulation is an unnatural way of activating the brain, clinical experience has shown that there is a correspondence between the functional results and the underlying neural activity (Arroyo et al., 1992a; Nathan et al., 1993). Knowledge of the location of a functional area can help the surgeon to weigh risks and benefits of a resection within those regions minimizing the possible sequels of a resection. Techniques based on signal analysis (Crone et al., 1993, 1994) may supplement or replace electrical stimulation in the future since the entire array can be tested simultaneously.

There have been some concerns about the safety of subdural electrode stimulation. Parameters for safe stimulation are known (Agnew and McCreery, 1987; Gordon et al., 1990), and no specific pathological features have been correlated with the presence of the electrodes actually employed, or with the amount of electrical stimulation given (Gordon et al., 1990). Finally, even though it is reasonable to be concerned about the possibility of a kindling effect from electrical stimulation, there are no reports that this in fact occurs in clinical situations. Moreover, the parameters used are not those that are likely to produce this effect (Lesser et al., 1987).

In the last few years there has been a dramatic development of functional MRI (fMRI) for localization of eloquent functions. Functional MRI is useful for localization of the sensorimotor strip, especially the functional representation area for the hand (Rao et al., 1995; Sanes et al., 1995; Yetkin et al., 1995). Functional MRI using a task activation of the sensory motor cortex appears to have similar results to those obtained with subdural electrode electrical stimulation (Jack et al., 1994), although experience is still limited. In some centers fMRI is substituting for cortical electrical stimulation for functional localization, especially in those patients with a lesion. However, its widespread use for language localization, although feasible, has been hampered by technical difficulties and can require a high degree of patient cooperation (Binder et al., 1995, 1996a,b; Desmond et al., 1995).

Summary

EEG recordings with subdural electrodes have been used for seizure focus localization when scalp electrodes do not provide enough localizing or lateralizing data. Subdural electrodes are especially well suited for covering extensive areas of the brain, and thus are particularly useful in patients with neocortical epilepsy. In addition they allow localization of the sensory, motor, and language areas of the brain and permit maximal seizure focus resection with minimal functional damage.

Acknowledgments

This chapter has been supported in part by the National Institutes of Health grant 1-RO1-NS26553 from the National Institute of Neurological Disorders and Stroke, the Whittier Foundation, the Seaver Foundation, and the McDonnel-Pew Program in Cognitive Neuroscience.

Authors' Note

A portion of the material in this chapter represents a compilation of material published previously.

References

Adelman S, Lüders HO, Dinner DS, et al. 1982. Paradoxical lateralization of parasagittal sharp waves in a patient with epilepsia partialis continua. *Epilepsia* 23:291–295.

Agnew WF, and McCreery DB. 1987. Considerations for safety in the use of extracranial stimulation for motor evoked potentials. *Neurosurgery* 20:143–147.

Ajmone-Marsan C. 1980. Depth electrography and electrocorticography, in Aminoff MJ (ed): *Electrodiagnosis in Clinical Neurology.* New York: Churchill Livingstone.

Alarcon G, Guy CN, Binnie CD, et al. 1994. Intracerebral propagation of interictal activity in partial epilepsy: implications for source localisation. *J Neurol Neurosurg Psychiatry* 57:345–449.

Alarcon G, Binnie CD, Elwes RD, et al. 1995. Power spectrum and intracranial EEG patterns at seizure onset in partial epilepsy. *Electroencephalogr Clin Neurophysiol* 94:326–337.

Allison T, McCarthy G, Luby M, et al. 1996. Localization of functional regions of human mesial cortex by somatosensory evoked potential recording and by cortical stimulation. *Electroencephalogr Clin Neurophysiol* 100:126–140.

Angeleri F, Ferro-Milone F, and Parigi S. 1964. Electrical activity and reactivity of the rhinencephalic, pararhinencephalic and thalamic structures: prolonged implantation of electrodes in man. *Electroencephalogr Clin Neurophysiol* 16:100–129.

Armon C, Radtke RA, Friedman AH, et al. 1996. Predictors of outcome of epilepsy surgery: multivariate analysis with validation. *Epilepsia* 37: 814–821.

Arroyo S, Krauss GL, Fisher RS, et al. 1992a. Seizure localization: mapping with scalp vs. arrays of subdural electrodes. *Epilepsia* 33(suppl 3): 90(abst).

Arroyo S, Krauss GL, Lesser RP, et al. 1992b. Simple partial seizures: clinicofunctional correlation—a case report. *Neurology* 42:642–646.

Arroyo S, Lesser RP, Fisher RS, et al. 1994. Clinical and electroencephalographic evidence for sites of origin of seizures with diffuse electrodecremental pattern. *Epilepsia* 35:974–987.

Awad IA, Assirati JA, Burgess R, et al. 1991a. A new class of electrodes of "intermediate invasiveness": preliminary experience with epidural pegs and foramen ovale electrodes in the mapping of seizure foci. *Neurol Res* 13:177–183.

Awad IA, Nayel MH, and Lüders HO. 1991b. Second operation after failure of previous resection for epilepsy. *Neurosurgery* 28:510–518.

Barkovich AJ, Rowley HA, and Andermann F. 1995. MR in partial epilepsy: value of high-resolution volumetric techniques. *AJNR* 16:339–343.

Barnett GH, Burgess RC, Awad IA, et al. 1990. Epidural peg electrodes for the presurgical evaluation of intractable epilepsy. *Neurosurgery* 27:113–115.

Barry E, Bergey GK, and Wolf AL. 1989. Simultaneous subdural grid and depth electrode recordings of patients with refractory complex partial seizures. *Epilepsia* 30:695.

Barry E, Wolf AL, Huhn SL, et al. 1992. Simultaneous subdural grid and depth electrodes in patients with refractory complex partial seizures. *J Epilepsy* 5:111–118.

Barthlow R. 1874. Experimental investigations into functions of the human brain. *Am J Med Sci* 67:305.

Bastos AC, Korah IP, Cendes F, et al. 1995. Curvilinear reconstruction of 3D magnetic resonance imaging in patients with partial epilepsy: a pilot study. *Magn Reson Imaging* 13:1107–1112.

Baumgartner C, Doppelbauer A, Sutherling WW, et al. 1993. Somatotopy of human hand somatosensory cortex as studied in scalp EEG. *Electroencephalogr Clin Neurophysiol* 88:271–279.

Baumgartner C, Flint R, Tuxhorn I, et al. 1996. Supplementary motor area seizures: propagation pathways as studied with invasive recordings. *Neurology* 46:508–514.

Berger MS, Kincaid J, Ojemann GA, et al. 1989. Brain mapping techniques to maximize resection, safety, and seizure control in children with brain tumors. *Neurosurgery* 25:786–792.

Bergin PS, Fish DR, Shorvon SD, et al. 1995. Magnetic resonance imaging in partial epilepsy: additional abnormalities shown with the fluid attenuated inversion recovery (FLAIR) pulse sequence. *J Neurol Neurosurg Psychiatry* 58:439–443.

Berkovic SF, and McIntosh AM. 1995. Preoperative MRI predicts outcome of temporal lobectomy: an actuarial analysis. *Neurology* 45:1358–1363.

Bernier GP, Saint-Hilarie JM, Girard N, et al. 1987. Commentary: intracranial electrical stimulation, in Engel J (ed): *Surgical Treatment of the Epilepsies*, pp. 323–334. New York: Raven Press.

Bernier GP, Richer F, Giard N, et al. 1990. Electrical stimulation of the human brain in epilepsy. *Epilepsia* 31:513–520.

Binder JR, Rao SM, Hammeke TA, et al. 1995. Lateralized human brain language systems demonstrated by task substraction functional magnetic resonance imaging. *Arch Neurol* 52:593–601.

Binder JR, Frost JA, Hammeke TA, et al. 1996a. Function of the left planum temporale in auditory and linguistic processing. *Brain* 119:1239–1247.

Binder JR, Swanson SJ, Hammeke TA, et al. 1996b. Determination of language dominance using functional MRI: a comparison with the Wada test. *Neurology* 46:978–984.

Blume WT, Girvin JP, McLachlan RS, et al. 1985. Use of subdural electroencephalography in candidates for surgical relief of uncontrolled partial epileptic seizures. *Electroencephalogr Clin Neurophysiol* 61:38P.

Blume WT, Whiting SE, and Girvin JP. 1991. Epilepsy surgery in the posterior cortex. *Ann Neurol* 29:638–645.

Boon PA, Williamson PD, Fried I, et al. 1991. Intracranial, intra–axial, space-occupying lesions in patients with intractable partial seizures: an anatomoclinical, neurophysiological, and surgical correlation. *Epilepsia* 32:467–476.

Bragin A, Engel J Jr., Wilson CL, et al. 1999. High-frequency oscillations in human brain. *Hippocampus* 9:137–142.

Bragin A, Mody I, Wilson CL, et al. 2002. Local generation of fast ripples in epileptic brain. *J Neurosci* 22:2012–2021.

Britton JW, Cascino GD, Sharbrough FW, et al. 1994. Low-grade glial neoplasms and intractable partial epilepsy: efficacy of surgical treatment. *Epilepsia* 35:1130–1135.

Burchiel KJ, Clarke H, Ojemann GA, et al. 1989. Use of stimulation mapping and corticography in the excision of arteriovenous malformations in sensorimotor and language-related neocortex. *Neurosurgery* 24:322–327.

Burnstine TH, Lesser RP, Hart J, et al. 1990. Characterization of the basal temporal language area in patients with left temporal lobe epilepsy. *Neurology* 40:966–970.

Bustamante L, Lueders H, Pippenger C, et al. 1981. Quantitative evaluation of anticonvulsant effects on penicillin-induced spike foci in cats. *Neurology* 31:1163–1166.

Cascino GD. 1990. Epilepsy and brain tumors: implications for treatment. *Epilepsia* 31(suppl 3):S37–S44.

Cascino GD, Jack CR Jr, Hirschorn KA, et al. 1992a. Identification of the epileptic focus: magnetic resonance imaging. *Epilepsy Res Suppl* 5:95–100.

Cascino GD, Kelly PJ, Sharbrough FW, et al. 1992b. Long-term follow-up of stereotactic lesionectomy in partial epilepsy: predictive factors and electroencephalographic results. *Epilepsia* 33:639–644.

Cascino GD, Hulihan JF, Sharbrough FW, et al. 1993. Parietal lobe lesional epilepsy: electroclinical correlation and operative outcome. *Epilepsia* 34:522–527.

Cendes F, Cook MJ, Watson C, et al. 1995. Frequency and characteristics of dual pathology in patients with lesional epilepsy. *Neurology* 45:2058–2064.

Chauvel P, Trottier S, Vignal JP, et al. 1992. Somatomotor seizures of frontal lobe origin, in Chauvel P, Delgado-Escueta AV, Halgren E, and Bancaud J (eds): *Frontal Lobe Seizures and Epilepsies*, pp. 185–232. New York: Raven Press.

Cooper R, Winter AL, Crow HJ, et al. 1965. Comparison of subcortical, cortical and scalp activity using chronically indwelling electrodes in man. *Electroencephalogr Clin Neurophysiol* 18:217–228.

Crone NE, Lesser RP, Krauss GL, et al. 1993. Topographic mapping of human sensorimotor cortex with electrocortical spectra. *Epilepsia* 34 (suppl 6):122–123.

Crone NE, Hart J, Lesser RP, et al. 1994. Spectral changes associated with regional cerebral processing results of direct cortical recording in humans. *Epilepsia* 35(suppl 8):103(abst).

Desmond JE, Sum JM, Wagner AD, et al. 1995. Functional MRI measurement of language lateralization in Wada-tested patients. *Brain* 118:1411–1419.

Devinsky O, Sato S, Kufta CV, et al. 1989. Electroencephalographic studies of simple partial seizures with subdural electrode recordings. *Neurology* 39:527–533.

Dodrill CB, and Troupin AS. 1991. Cognitive effects of anticonvulsants. *Neurology* 41:1326

Dubeau F, Tampieri D, Lee N, et al. 1995. Periventricular and subcortical nodular heterotopia. A study of 33 patients. *Brain* 118:1273–1287.

Duchowny M, Jayakar P, Resnick T, et al. 1994. Posterior temporal epilepsy: electroclinical features. *Ann Neurol* 35:427–431.

Duchowny M, Jayakar P, Harvey AS, et al. 1996. Language cortex representation: effects of developmental versus pathology. Ann. Neurol. 1996;40:31–38.

Engel J Jr. 1993. Update on surgical treatment of the epilepsies. Summary of The Second International Palm Desert Conference on the Surgical Treatment of the Epilepsies (1992). *Neurology* 43:1612–1617.

Engel J Jr, Rausch R, Lieb JP, et al. 1981. Correlation of criteria used for localizing epileptic foci in patients considered for surgical therapy of epilepsy. *Ann Neurol* 9:215–224.

Engel J Jr, Kuhl DE, Phelps ME, et al. 1982. Comparative localization of epileptic foci in partial epilepsy by PET and EEG. *Ann Neurol* 12:529–539.

Engel J Jr, Henry TR, Risinger MW, et al. 1990. Presurgical evaluation for partial epilepsy: relative contributions of chronic depth electrode recordings versus FDG-PET and scalp-sphenoidal ictal EEG. *Neurology* 40:1670–1677.

Fedio P, Balish M, Sato S, et al. 1990. Basal temporal stimulation and the effects on memory and language. *Epilepsia* 31:678.

Fisher RS, Webber WRS, Lesser RP, et al. 1992. High-frequency EEG activity at the start of seizures. *J Clin Neurophysiol* 9:441–448.

Foerster O. 1936. The cerebral cortex in the light of Hughling Jackson's doctrines. *Brain* 59:135–159.

Foerster O, and Penfield W. 1930. The structural basis of traumatic epilepsy and results of radical operation. *Brain* 53:99–119.

Free SL, Li LM, Fish DR, et al. 1996. Bilateral hippocampal volume loss in patients with a history of encephalitis or meningitis. *Epilepsia* 37:400–405.

Fritsch G, and Hitzig E. 1870. Uber die elektrische erregbarkeit des Grosshirns. *Arch Anat Physiol Wissenschaftliche Med* 37:300–332.

Fullagar T, and Wyler AR. 1993. Subdural strip electrodes for seizure monitoring. *J Epilepsy* 6:95–97.

Gates JR, Maxwell RE, Fiol ME, et al. 1988. Usefulness of subdural grid electrodes in resecting epileptic lesions adjacent to eloquent cortex. *Epilepsia* 29:660.

Gil-Nagel A, and Risinger MW. 1997. Ictal semiology in hippocampal versus extra–hippocampal temporal lobe epilepsy. *Brain* 120:183–192.

Gloor P. 1975. Contributions of electroencephalography and electrocorticography to the neurosurgical treatment of the epilepsies, in Purpura DP, Penry JK, Walter RD (eds): *Advances in Neurology*, pp. 59–105. New York, Raven Press.

Goldring S. 1978. A method for surgical management of focal epilepsy, especially as it relates to children. *J Neurosurgery* 49:344–356.

Goldring S. 1987. Pediatric epilepsy surgery. *Epilepsia* 28(suppl 1):S82–S102.

Goldring S. 1991. Surgical treatment of epilepsy in the pediatric patient, in Apuzzo MLJ (ed): *Neurological Aspects of Epilepsy*, pp. 199–216. American Association of Neurological Surgeons.

Goldring S, and Gregorie EM. 1984. Surgical management of epilepsy using epidural recordings to localize the seizure focus. Review of 100 cases. *J Neurosurgery* 40:447–466.

Goldring S, Gregorie EM, and Tempelhoff R. 1989. Surgery of epilepsy, in Dudley H, Carter D, Russell RCG (eds): *Operative Surgery*, pp. 427–442. London: Butterworth.

Gordon B, Lesser RP, Rance NE, et al. 1990. Parameters for direct cortical electrical stimulation in the human: histopathologic confirmation. *Electroencephalogr Clin Neurophysiol* 75:371–377.

Gotman J. 1987. Interhemispheric interactions in seizures of focal onset: data from human intracranial recordings. *Electroencephalogr Clin Neurophysiol* 67:120–133.

Hajek M, and Wieser HG. 1988. Extratemporal, mainly frontal, epilepsies: surgical results. *J Epilepsy* 1:103–109.

Halgren E. 1982. Mental phenomena induced by stimulation in the limbic system. *Hum Neurobiol* 1:251–260.

Hamer HM, Morris HH, Mascha EJ, et al. 2002. Complications of invasive video-EEG monitoring with subdural grid electrodes. *Neurology* 58:97–103.

Hirsch LJ, Spencer SS, Spencer DD, et al. 1991. Temporal lobectomy in patients with bitemporal epilepsy as defined by depth electroencephalography. *Ann Neurol* 30:347–356.

Ikeda A, Terada K, Mikuni N, et al. 1996. Subdural recording of ictal DC shifts in neocortical seizures in humans. *Epilepsia* 37:662–674.

Jack CR Jr, Thompson RM, Butts RK, et al. 1994. Sensory motor cortex: correlation of presurgical mapping with functional MR imaging and invasive cortical mapping. *Radiology* 190:85–92.

Jefferson G. 1935. Jacksonian epilepsy: a background and postscript. *Postgrad Med J* 11:150–162.

Jumao-as A, and Dasheiff R. 1988. The utility of depth electrode stimulated seizures contralateral to the proposed site of epilepsy surgery. *Epilepsia* 29:660.

Kanner AM, Morris HH, Lüders HO, et al. 1993. Usefulness of interictal sharp waves of temporal lobe origin in prolonged video-EEG monitoring studies. *Epilepsia* 34:884–889.

Kazee AM, Lapham LW, Torres CF, et al. 1991. Generalized cortical dysplasia. Clinical and pathologic aspects. *Arch Neurol* 48:850–853.

King D, and Spencer S. 1995. Invasive electroencephalography in mesial temporal lobe epilepsy. *J Clin Neurophysiol* 12:32–45.

Kluin K, Abou-Khalil B, and Hood T. 1988. Inferior speech area in patients with temporal lobe epilepsy. *Neurology* 38(suppl 1):277.

Kramer U, Riviello JJ, Carmant L, et al. 1994. Morbidity of depth and subdural electrodes: children and adolescents versus young adults. *J Epilepsy* 7:7–10.

Laskowitz DT, Sperling MR, French JA, et al. 1995. The syndrome of frontal lobe epilepsy: characteristics and surgical management. *Neurology* 45:780–787.

Laxer KD, Needleman R, and Rosenbaum TJ. 1984. Subdural electrodes for seizure focus localization. *Epilepsia* 25:651.

Lesser RP, Hahn JF, Lüders HO, et al. 1981. The use of chronic subdural electrodes for cortical mapping of speech. *Epilepsia* 22:240.

Lesser RP, Lüders HO, Klem G, et al. 1984. Cortical afterdischarge and functional response thresholds: results of extraoperative testing. *Epilepsia* 25:615–621.

Lesser RP, Lüders HO, Klem G, et al. 1985. Ipsilateral trigeminal sensory responses to cortical stimulation by subdural electrodes. *Neurology* 35:1760–1763.

Lesser RP, Lüders HO, Klem G, et al. 1987. Extraoperative cortical functional localization in patients with epilepsy. *J Clin Neurophysiol* 4:27–53.

Lieb JP, Walsh GO, Babb TL, et al. 1976. A comparison of EEG seizure patterns recorded with surface and depth electrodes in patients with temporal lobe epilepsy. *Epilepsia* 17:137–160.

Lieb JP, Hoque K, Skomer CE, et al. 1987. Inter-hemispheric propagation of human mesial temporal lobe seizures: a coherence-phase analysis. *Electroencephalogr Clin Neurophysiol* 67:101–119.

Lim SH, Dinner DS, Lüders HO, et al. 1991. Anatomical location and somatotopic representation of the human supplementary motor area. *Neurology* 41(suppl 1):402.

Lim SH, Dinner DS, Pillay PK, et al. 1994. Functional anatomy of the human supplementary sensorimotor area: results of extraoperative electrical stimulation. *Electroencephalogr Clin Neurophysiol* 91:179–193.

Lüders HO, Hahn JF, Lesser RP, et al. 1982. Localization of epileptogenic spike foci: comparative study of closely spaced scalp electrodes, nasopharyngeal, sphenoidal, subdural, and depth electrodes, in Akimoto H, Kazamatsuri H, Seino M, and Ward A (eds): *Advances in Epileptology: XII Epilepsy International Symposium*. New York: Raven Press.

Lüders HO, Lesser RP, Dinner DS, et al. 1987. Commentary: Chronic intracranial recording and stimulation with subdural electrodes, in Engel J (ed): *Surgical Treatment of the Epilepsies*, pp. 297–321. New York: Raven Press.

Lüders HO, Hahn JF, Lesser RP, et al. 1989. Basal temporal subdural electrodes in the evaluation of patients with intractable epilepsy. *Epilepsia* 30:131–142.

Lüders HO, Lesser RP, Hahn JF, et al. 1991. Basal temporal language area. *Brain* 114:743–754.

Ludwig BI, Ajmone-Marsan C, and Van Buren JM. 1976. Depth and direct cortical recording in seizure disorders of extratemporal origin. *Neurology* 26:1085–1099.

Malow BA, Sato S, Kufta CV, et al. 1995. Hematoma-related seizures detected during subdural electrode monitoring. *Epilepsia* 36:733–735.

Malow BA, Blaxton TA, Sato S, et al. 1996. Cortical stimulation elicits regional distinctions in auditory and visual naming. *Epilepsia* 37:245–252.

Marks DA, Kim J, Spencer DD, et al. 1992. Characteristics of intractable seizures following meningitis and encephalitis. *Neurology* 42:1513–1518.

Mathern GW, Babb TL, Vickrey BG, et al. 1994. Traumatic compared to non-traumatic clinical-pathologic associations in temporal lobe epilepsy. *Epilepsy Res* 19:129–139.

Mattia D, Oliver A, and Avoli M. 1995. Seizure-like discharges recorded in human dysplastic neocortex maintained in vitro. *Neurology* 45:1391–1395.

Mortimer JT, Shealy CN, and Wheeler C. 1970. Experimental nondestructive electrical stimulation of the brain and spinal cord. *J Neurosurg* 32:553–559.

Nathan SS, Sinha SR, Gordon B, et al. 1993. Determination of current density distributions generated by electrical stimulation of the human cerebral cortex. *Electroencephalogr Clin Neurophysiol* 86:183–192.

Nii Y, Uematsu S, Lesser RP, et al. 1996. Does the central sulcus divide motor and sensory functions? *Neurology* 46:360–367.

Ojemann GA. 1979. Individual variability in cortical localization of language. *J Neurosurg* 50:164–169.

Ojemann GA. 1983a. Brain organization for language from the perspective of electrical stimulation mapping. *Behav Brain Sci* 2:189–230.

Ojemann GA. 1983b. Electrical stimulation and the neurobiology of language. *Behav Brain Sci* 6:221–226.

Ojemann GA. 1987. Acute and chronic intracranial stimulation, in Engel J (ed). *Surgical Treatment of the Epilepsies*, pp. 263–288. New York: Raven Press.

Ojemann GA, and Whitaker H. 1978. Language localization and variability. *Brain Language* 6:239–260.

Ostertun B, Wolf HK, Campos MG, et al. 1996. Dysembrioplastic neuroepithelial tumors: MR and CT evaluation. *AJNR* 17:419–430.

Palmini A, Gambardella A, Andermann F, et al. 1995. Intrinsic epileptogenicity of human dysplastic cortex as suggested by corticography and surgical results. *Ann Neurol* 37:476–487.

Penfield W, and Boldrey E. 1937. Somatic motor and sensory representation in the cerebral cortex of man as studied by electrical stimulation. *Brain* 60:389–443.

Penfield W, and Jasper H. 1954. *Epilepsy and the Functional Anatomy of the Human Brain.* Boston: Little, Brown.

Penfield W, and Perot P. 1963. The brain's record of auditory and visual experience—A final summary and discussion. *Brain* 86:595–696.

Penfield W, and Roberts L. 1959. *Speech and Brain Mechanisms.* Princeton, NJ: Princeton University Press.

Perrine K, Devinsky O, Uysal S, et al. 1994. Left temporal neocortex mediation of verbal memory: evidence from functional mapping with cortical stimulation. *Neurology* 44:1845–1850.

Pfurtscheller G. 1977. Graphical display and statistical evaluation of even-related desynchronization. *Electroencephalogr Clin Neurophysiol* 43:759–760.

Prasad A, Pacia SV, Vazquez B, et al. 2003. Extent of ictal origin in mesial temporal sclerosis patients monitored with subdural intracranial electrodes predicts outcome. *J Clin Neurophysiol* 20:243–248.

Privitera MD, Quinlan JG, Yeh H, et al. 1990. Interictal spike detection comparing subdural and depth electrodes during electrocorticography. *Electroencephalogr Clin Neurophysiol* 76:379–387.

Quesney LF, and Gloor P. 1985. Localization of epileptic foci, in Gotman J, Ives JR, Gloor P (eds): *Long-term monitoring in epilepsy (EEG suppl. Q37),* pp. 165–200. Amsterdam: Elsevier Science Publishers, B.V.

Rao SM, Binder JR, Hammeke TA, et al. 1995. Somatotopic mapping of the human primary motor cortex with functional magnetic resonance imaging. *Neurology* 45:919–924.

Rapport RL, Tan CT, and Whitaker HA. 1983. Language function and dysfunction among Chinese- and English-speaking polyglots: Cortical stimulation, Wada testing, and clinical studies. *Brain Language* 18:342–366.

Rasmussen T, and Milner B. 1975. Clinical and surgical studies of the cerebral speech areas in man, in Zulch KJ, Creutzfeldt O, Galbraith GC (eds): *Otfried Foerster Symposium on Cerebral Localization.* New York: Springer-Verlag.

Resnick TJ, Duchowny MS, Alvarez LA, et al. 1989. Comparison of depth and subdural electrodes in recording interictal activity in children being evaluated for surgery. *Epilepsia* 30:659.

Rogawski MA, and Porter RJ. 1990. Antiepileptic drugs: pharmacological mechanisms and clinical efficacy with consideration of promising developmental stage compounds. *Pharmacol Rev* 42:223–286.

Rosenbaum TJ, and Laxer KD. 1989. Subdural electrode recordings for seizure focus localization. *J Epilepsy* 2:129–135.

Salanova V, Morris HH, Van Ness PC, et al. 1993. Comparison of scalp electroencephalogram with subdural electrocorticogram recordings and functional mapping in frontal lobe epilepsy. *Arch Neurol* 50:294–299.

Salanova V, Andermann F, Rasmussen T, et al. 1995a. Parietal lobe epilepsy. Clinical manifestations and outcome in 82 patients treated surgically between 1929 and 1988. *Brain* 118:607–627.

Salanova V, Morris HH, Van Ness P, et al. 1995b. Frontal lobe seizures: electroclinical syndromes. *Epilepsia* 36:16–24.

Sammaritano M, Lotbinière A, Andermann F, et al. 1987. False lateralization by surface EEG of seizure onset in patients with temporal lobe epilepsy and gross focal cerebral lesions. *Ann Neurol* 21:361–369.

Sanes JN, Donoghue JP, Thangaraj V, et al. 1995. Shared neural substrates controlling hand movements in human motor cortex. *Science* 268:1775–1777.

Schäffler L, Lüders HO, Morris HH, et al. 1994. Anatomic distribution of cortical language sites in the basal temporal language area in patients with left temporal lobe epilepsy. *Epilepsia* 35:525–528.

Schomer DL, Erba G, Blume H, et al. 1984. The utility of subdural strip recordings for the localization of epileptic activity. A case report. *Electroencephalogr Clin Neurophysiol* 58:125P.

Serafetinides EA. 1966. Speech findings in epilepsy and electro-cortical stimulation: an overview. *Cortex* 2:463–473.

Shimizu H, Suzuki I, Ishijima B, et al. 1990. Modifications of temporal lobectomy according to the extent of epileptic foci and speech-related areas. *Surg Neurol* 34:229–234.

Spencer DD, Spencer SS, Mattson RH, et al. 1984. Intracerebral masses in patients with intractable partial epilepsy. *Neurology* 34:432–436.

Spencer SS. 1989. Depth versus subdural electrode studies for unlocalized epilepsy. *J Epilepsy* 2:123–127.

Spencer SS, Spencer DD, Williamson PD, Mattson R. 1990. Combined depth and subdural electrode investigation in uncontrolled epilepsy. *Neurology* 40:74–79.

Spencer SS. 1991. Intracranial recording, in Spencer SS, Spencer DD (eds): *Surgery for Epilepsy,* pp. 54–65. Cambridge, MA: Blackwell Scientific Publications.

Spencer SS. 1994. The relative contributions of MRI, SPECT, and PET imaging in epilepsy. *Epilepsia* 35(suppl 6):S72–89.

Spencer SS. 1995. MRI and epilepsy surgery. *Neurology* 45:1248–1250.

Spencer SS, and Spencer DD. 1994. Entorhinal-hippocampal interactions I medial temporal lobe epilepsy. *Epilepsia* 35:721–727.

Spencer SS, Williamson PD, Bridgers SL, et al. 1985. Reliability and accuracy of localization by scalp ictal EEG. *Neurology* 35:1567–1675.

Spencer SS, Williamson PD, Spencer DD, et al. 1987. Human hippocampal seizure spread studied by depth and subdural recording: the hippocampal commissure. *Epilepsia* 28:479–489.

Spencer SS, Spencer DD, Williamson PD, et al. 1990. Combined depth and subdural electrode investigation in uncontrolled epilepsy. *Neurology* 40:74–79.

Spencer SS, Guimaraes P, Katz A, et al. 1992. Morphological patterns of seizures recorded intracranially. *Epilepsia* 33:537–545.

Sperling MR, and O'Connor MJ. 1989. Comparison of depth and subdural electrodes in recording temporal lobe seizures. *Neurology* 39:1497–1504.

Sutherling WW, Risinger MW, Crandall PH, et al. 1990. Focal functional anatomy of dorsolateral fronto-central seizures. *Neurology* 40:87–98.

Sveinbjornsdottir S, and Duncan JS. 1993. Parietal and occipital lobe epilepsy: a review. *Epilepsia* 1993;34:493–521.

Swartz BE, Rich JR, Dwan PS, et al. 1996. The safety and efficacy of chronically implanted subdural electrodes: a prospective study. *Surg Neurol* 46:87–93.

Talairach J, and Bancaud J. 1974. Stereotaxic exploration and therapy in epilepsy, in Magnus O, Lorentz de Haas AM, Vinken PJ, Bruyn GW (eds): *The Epilepsies (Handbook of Clinical Neurology),* pp. 758–782. Amsterdam: North-Holland Publishing Company.

Trenerry MR, Jack CR Jr, Ivnik RJ, et al. 1993. MRI hippocampal volumes and memory function before and after temporal lobectomy. *Neurology* 43:1800–1805.

Uematsu S, Lesser RP, Fisher RS, et al. 1990. Resection of the epileptogenic area in critical cortex with the aid of a subdural electrode grid. *Stereotact Funct Neurosurg* 54/55:34–45.

Uematsu S, Lesser RP, Fisher RS, et al. 1992a. Motor and sensory cortex in humans: topography studied with chronic subdural stimulation. *Neurosurgery* 31:59–72.

Uematsu S, Lesser RP, and Gordon B. 1992b. Localization of sensorimotor cortex: the influence of Sherrington and Cushing on the modern concept. *Neurosurgery* 30:904–913.

Urasaki E, Uematsu S, Gordon B, et al. 1994. Cortical tongue area studied by chronically implanted subdural electrodes—with special reference to parietal motor and frontal sensory responses. *Brain* 117:117–132.

Van Buren JM. 1987. Complications of surgical procedures in the diagnosis and treatment of epilepsy, in Engel J (ed): *Surgical Treatment of the Epilepsies,* pp. 465–475. New York: Raven Press.

Van Buren JM, Ajmone-Marsan C, and Mutsuga N. 1975. Temporal lobe seizures with additional foci treated by resection. *J Neurosurg* 43:596–607.

Van Buren JM, Fedio P, and Frederick GC. 1978. Mechanism and localization of speech in the parietotemporal cortex. *J Neurosurg* 2:233–238.

Van Veelen CWM, Debets RM, Van Huffelen AC, et al. 1990. Combined use of subdural and intracerebral electrodes in preoperative evaluation of epilepsy. *Neurosurgery* 26:93–101.

Wieser HG. 1987. Data analysis, in Engel J (ed). *Surgical treatment of the Epilepsies,* pp. 335–360. New York: Raven Press.

Wieser HG, Siegel AM. 1991. Analysis of foramen ovale electrode-recorded seizures and correlation with outcome following amygdalohippocampectomy. *Epilepsia* 32:838–850.

Wieser HG, Bancaud J, Talairach J, et al. 1979. Comparative value of spontaneous and chemically induced seizures in establishing the lateralization of temporal lobe seizures. *Epilepsia* 20:47–59.

Williamson PD, Boon PA, Thadani VM, et al. 1992. Parietal lobe epilepsy: Diagnostic considerations and results of surgery. *Ann Neurol* 1992;31:193–201.

Wyler AR, and Ward AA. 1981. Neurons in human epileptic cortex. Response to direct cortical stimulation. *J Neurosurg* 55:904–908.

Wyler AR, Ojemann GA, Lettich E, et al. 1984. Subdural strip electrodes for localizing epileptogenic foci. *J Neurosurg* 60:1195–1200.

Wyler AR, Richey ET, Atkinson RA, et al. 1988a. Strip electrodes in acute electrocorticography. *J Epilepsy* 1:95–97.

Wyler AR, Walker G, Richey ET, et al. 1988b. Chronic subdural strip recordings for difficult epileptic problems. *J Epilepsy* 1:71–78.

Wyler AR, Hermann BP, and Richey ET. 1989a. Results of reoperation for failed epilepsy surgery. *J Neurosurg* 71:815–819.

Wyler AR, Richey ET, and Hermann BP. 1989b. Comparison of scalp to subdural recordings for localizing epileptogenic foci. *J Epilepsy* 2:91–96.

Wyler AR, Walker G, and Somes G. 1991. The morbidity of long-term seizure monitoring using subdural strip electrodes. *J Neurosurg* 74:734–737.

Wyllie E, Lüders HO, Dinner DS, et al. 1987a. Cortical electrical stimulation of frontal and temporal speech areas in the evaluation of epilepsy surgery in children. *Epilepsia* 28:622

Wyllie E, Lüders HO, Morris HH, et al. 1987b. Clinical outcome after complete or partial cortical resection for intractable epilepsy. *Neurology* 37:1634–1641.

Yetkin FZ, Mueller WM, Hammeke TA, et al. 1995. Functional magnetic resonance imaging mapping of the sensorimotor cortex with tactile stimulation. *Neurosurgery* 36:921–925.

Zentner J, Hufnagel A, Ostertun B, et al. 1996. Surgical treatment of extratemporal epilepsy: clinical, radiologic, and histopathologic findings in 60 patients. *Epilepsia* 37:1072–1080.

40. Principles of Computerized Epilepsy Monitoring

Ronald P. Lesser and W. Robert S. Webber

The revolution in microprocessor technologies now provides an unprecedented opportunity to clinical neurophysiologists. Some applications of this technology, for example evoked potential recordings, have been employed for years, and the fundamental principles of microprocessor-based recognition of both epileptiform and nonepileptiform electroencephalogram (EEG) signals have been discussed elsewhere (Barlow, 1986; Binnie, 1986; Gevins and Remond, 1987; Gotman et al., 1985; Kaplan and Lesser, 1990; Lopes da Silva, 1987; Panych and Wada, 1990). Current hardware now makes it possible to use computer-based techniques for essentially all clinical and investigational neurophysiological recordings. Over the previous decade microprocessor techniques have largely replaced paper-based recordings in many laboratories, as old equipment aged, and added capability was required, and pricing made digital electrophysiology the preferred choice. Hardware and software continue to change rapidly; however, certain interrelated design principles for electrophysiologic monitoring will remain constant (Table 40.1):

1. The system should be *expandable* with respect to the number of channels of data for each patient, number of patients, the number of review stations, and in terms of the nature of the analysis performed. It should be capable of acquiring, managing, and storing the large amounts of data generated in this setting.
2. The system should be *modular*, with relatively standard parts throughout. Each patient should have an independent processor system, so that breakdown in one system would not result in loss of data from all patients throughout the entire unit. Adding more patients or review stations should merely require connecting the appropriate modules to the system, just as one now can buy additional EEG machines.
3. There should be *redundancy* in the system so that (a) in the case of breakdown of a part, another could be substituted, at least on a temporary basis; (b) if data capture did not occur through one means, it could be accomplished through another; and (c) no single point failure could cause the whole system to become inoperable. To give an analogy, if a paper-based EEG machine malfunctions, another can be brought into its place. Microprocessor-based systems should offer similar functionality.
4. There should be *separation* of the data capture, analysis, and storage functions, so that enhancements in one function do not require modifications to other parts of the system. This in turn leads to better software productivity. In addition, such a separation imitates what we do now: the technologist obtains the EEG on one machine in one place. The electroencephalographer often reads the EEG in an entirely different place, without needing the original "data acquisition machine" to do so.
5. There should be *human data validation*. For example, EEG data of interest (such as seizures, spikes, and normal variant patterns) detected by the patient computer should automatically be made available to the electroencephalographer for confirmation and analysis.
6. There should be *computer-aided analysis* of the captured data, to free the electroencephalographer from the repetitive aspects of EEG evaluation. The results of the computer analysis should be reviewable and revisable by the electroencephalographer. The speed of data presentation should be comparable to paper: that is, the electroencephalographer should be able to page through the computerized data as quickly as through a paper record. Random access with jumping ahead, behind, or to specified places in the record should be possible. The computer should, additionally, offer calculation, measurement, and analysis benefits not possible with paper records. The digital record should also be more flexible, allowing gain, filter, time scale, and montage changes at the time of review.
7. There should be *data reduction*, including both summarization of the captured information and storage via electronic media. Storage should occur automatically under microprocessor control.
8. The system operations should be *usable* by personnel *with a minimum of computer experience* and training. As many as possible of the system operations should be automatic and hidden from the user.
9. Video and EEG are both essential parts of prolonged inpatient seizure monitoring. Although *computer-aided synchronization of video and EEG is helpful*, simultaneous display is *not essential*. More important is the quality of the EEG data, the quality of the video data, and the ease of comparing events recorded at the same time using the differing media. Although digital storage is becoming less expensive, digital video consumes about four times more hard disk space than EEG (MPEG1 compared to 128 channels of 200 sample/second). Digital video technology is relatively mature and available for most of the major EEG system vendors. The quality of digital video is now approaching that of standard videotape and continues to evolve and improve.

Table 40.1.   Criteria for Digitally Based Monitoring

Large data handling capacity
Modular—expandable
Relatively hardware-independent
Redundant parts, resilient against failure
Separate data collection, review, and storage functions
Computer detections reviewable by users
Opportunity for both computer and human event detection and marking
Screen review as clear and as fast as paper review
Automatic management and archiving of data files
Reasonably easy to use
Video and EEG recordings should complement one another
Reliable service and support

Oken, B.S., and Chiappa, K.H. 1986. Statistical issues concerning computerized analysis of brainwave topography. Ann. Neurol. 19:493–497.
Lesser, R.P., Webber, W.R.S., and Fisher, R.S. 1992. Design principles for computerized monitoring. Electroencephalogr. Clin. Neurophysiol. 82: 239–247.

10. The vendor should have a reputation for making *reliable equipment* and for giving *good service*. Information about this can only be obtained by speaking with your colleagues. You also should consider what the capabilities are within your institution. If you are buying equipment for a seizure-monitoring unit, keep in mind that such units generally are open 24 hours per day, 7 days per week. Think about how you would go about repairing a machine that stopped functioning at the start of a holiday weekend.

The System

System design ideally proceeds from task to software to hardware. Specific requirements include acquisition of up to 128 channels (typically 32–64) of EEG data per patient, with capacity for on-line (real-time) and off-line display of data.

Data Acquisition

A major hardware issue relates to the speed and capacity of the data bus to transfer acquired data to memory or long-term storage. Use of 64 channels at 200 samples per second requires 12,800 data points per second. Scalp EEG voltages can be represented adequately with a dynamic range of 70 dB, which then requires 12 bits of resolution for analog-to-digital conversion (ADC). Subdural recordings can be as high as 2,000 to 4,000 µV. Since the noise in good commercial EEG amplifiers is 0.1 µV or less, the full dynamic range is 92 dB. To use this full range requires 16 bits of resolution (96 dB dynamic range). Our own experience and that of others with subdural recordings indicate that higher sample rates up to 1,000 sample/second are needed to capture low-voltage fast activity (Bragin et al., 1999; Fisher et al., 1992; Medvedev, 2002). High-resolution recordings, that is 1,000 samples/second and 16-bit ADC, once considered exotic, should now be taken as the norm for intracranial recordings.

EEG/Seizure Analysis Software

No "perfect" computer-based analyzer of spikes, seizures, EEG background, sleep, or other physiological parameters is yet available, and improvements in analysis software still are needed. A second practical limitation in using computers in the EEG laboratory has been the computing power of the microprocessor. This remains a possible limitation but microprocessors are becoming more powerful and less expensive at a rapid pace. Furthermore, multiprocessor systems make it possible to increase the amount of processing of patient data by buying an extra plug-in board rather than an extra computer.

Seizure detection software usually is designed to detect both interictal and ictal epileptiform activity. A "circular buffer" often is implemented in memory so that data from before the time of detection of an event also can be reviewed (Gotman, 1982; Gotman et al., 1979; Ives et al., 1976). Data storage can be initiated by the computer, the patient, or a family or staff member. If no events of interest occur, the memory is overwritten with more recent data as the memory becomes full. Provisions for human initiation of data-saves are important because microprocessor detection remains imperfect, and because the EEG during nonepileptic clinical events that imitate epilepsy also must be captured and analyzed. For example, a circular buffer might save approximately 2 to 5 minutes of data before the save trigger, and 1 to 3 minutes after. In the case of a single epileptiform potential, a 2-second segment might be saved, with the event in the center. Save times should be programmable by menu choice, but are also dependent on number of EEG channels, digital sampling rate, and amount of computer memory. Random saves of data also should occur, with the timing and duration of these saves under control of program menus.

EEG Files and Their Management

Patients may have multiple seizures per day. Interictal spikes also must be detected, stored, and analyzed. Samples of routine "baseline" EEG also should be saved. This volume of information mandates a carefully planned file system (Lesser et al., 1990; Webber et al., 1989). The following is a description of one such system, as developed at our institution.

We developed a number of filing conventions. First, each patient has a "housekeeping" file. This is an ASCII file (American Standard Characters for Information Interchange) that contains patient information such as the patient name and hospital unit number, patient montage information, computer and amplifier settings, and a list of all the EEG files saved on that patient. All changes to computer and amplifier settings are recorded in this file together with the time and date when the changes were made. The housekeeping file is the single complete record of the equipment settings for the patient's admission. It is used as a table of contents and reference source by computer programs.

Second, we also developed an annotation file, which logs the times and locations of EEG items that have been identified by the computer or clinician, together with text descriptions added by the clinician who reviews the EEG data. The annotation file becomes the basis for the final report for the monitoring. There is only one annotation file for each patient, growing with each computer or human addition.

Third, there are patient EEG files comprising baseline EEG segments, interictal spikes detected by computer, or ictal segments detected by computer or human observers. These formats have been designed to serve several functions, including fast routine viewing of the EEG, to provide rapid access to one or more channels of EEG data, to support future research needs, to be reasonably compact, and to store continuous and noncontinuous segments of EEG.

Fourth, a method of naming the patient data files in a unique way is necessary. This requirement might seem obvious, but not all EEG equipment vendors provide systems that guarantee this when multiple machines are used. Suppose that an institution has two EEG machines and John Doe is recorded on one while Jane Doe is recorded on the other. In this case, a file naming system that uses only the last name and first initial will have problems if both data sets are to be archived on one medium at the same time. This is quite possible when EEG machines are networked to a shared file server and the EEG files are archived only by one device attached to the network. Using a single DVD or CD-ROM burner, or similar storage device for each EEG machine, might be a partial solution, but still would require a data management system that would give the full name of each patient, and the machine on which they were recorded. To avoid this kind of problem, we devised what we have found to be a robust approach, user friendly for those who have to work with EEG files directly and amenable to automated file management. It is also in use by at least one EEG vendor.

The file name is made up of five parts. The first part is derived from the patient's last name. (This is helpful for those that manage files directly.) Then a unique identifier for each EEG machine is added. This is followed by a name counter to make all names unique for a given EEG machine, i.e., consecutive John Smiths will get different files names on a given EEG machine. The name counter is only incremented for each new first letter of the last name. For instance, the name counter starts at 01 for John Smith, then goes to 02 for Jane Smyth. However, the system keeps 26 separate name counters, one for each letter of the alphabet. In the above example, the third patient, John Doe, would have a name counter of 01. This method allows the name counter to last much longer than if it were incremented for each new patient. The fourth part of the file name identifies the file type if more than one type of record is produced on the machine, i.e., EEGs and evoked potentials. The fifth and last part of the name is a file counter to distinguish between consecutive files of the same type on a given machine. For example, in long-term monitoring some systems create a new EEG file every few minutes. A further refinement to this system uses radix 36 for the name and file counters. That is, the count goes from 00 to 09 in ten steps then 0A to 0Z in 26 steps, then on to 10 through to 19 in ten more steps, and 1A to 1Z in 26 more steps, and so on. This makes the counters last much longer than a more conventional radix 10 count. Using these principles, our original four-bed epilepsy monitoring unit operated for 8 years with all file names generated automatically and no identical name collisions occurring. The name system would have lasted another 70 years before any of the counters rolled over.

In some long-term monitoring centers many intracranial patients are evaluated with a custom montage. After a few years of use, the system will have accumulated several tens

of montages, and the list of montages grows unwieldy. An ideal system would store patient-specific montages with the patient's EEG data while general-purpose montages would be stored with the system. When the patient's data are removed to an archive, their montages would move with EEG data. This design means that only the current patients' and system montages appear in the selection list, while all other montages are archived.

We utilized the above-described locally developed system when we opened our monitoring unit. Commercial systems differ in their implementation of the preceding principles. From the practical point of view, when considering a system, the electroencephalographer should evaluate how a given system has approached the issues described above, with a view toward ease of use and of retrieval.

Digital Video

First-generation long-term video/EEG monitoring systems used VCR tape recorders. Digital video has advanced sufficiently to a point where all the major EEG system vendors now include it and have abandoned VCR tapes. There are several video formats in use, some of them proprietary. The most popular standard format is MPEG (Moving Picture Experts Group) that is not controlled by any one vendor and thus is available to all vendors. The MPEG format uses compression to save disk space and achieves compression factors of between 8:1 and 30:1. Marketing literature often quotes compression factors of 100:1 or more, but these claims overlook the data reductions that take place when the studio-quality video is converted to consumer-grade video. The compression factors in all MPEG formats are dependent on the image complexity and motion in the image. The more features or more motion in the image, the less compression is achievable. The amount of compression can vary by about a factor of two or more (Fogg, 1996).

The first standard, MPEG1, appeared in 1992 and covered video data stored simply as sequence of frames and was intended for use with video disks and CD-ROMs. This standard allows for very high resolution images up to $4,096 \times 4,096$ pixels per frame, but the most common subset of the standard, called "constrained parameters bit streams," which gained popular support uses 352×240 pixels per frame, 30 frames/second, and has a compressed data rate of about 1.5 megabits/second (MPEG1, 1993). The second standard, MPEG2, released in 1995, was aimed at digital TV, and extended MPEG1 to cover interlaced images used in television (MPEG2, 2002). The MPEG2 format being derived from MPEG1 also supports different frame sizes. The most popular one used with MPEG2 is 720×480 pixels per frame, 30 frames/second. MPEG2 is perceived as a higher quality format mostly because it is used with a larger frame size rather than because of any improvement in the compression methods used. Due to the larger frame size the compressed data rate of MPEG2 is in the range 3.4 to 4.5 megabits/second.

There are others MPEG standards namely MPEG4, MPEG7, and MPEG21. These cover interactive uses of video information and are beyond the scope of this chapter. However, it is possible that MPEG4 with its ability to represent much more than just the video information (Koenen, 1999) could contain the complete patient EEG data set including reports, computed tomography (CT) scans, magnetic resonance imaging (MRI) scans, and three-dimensional (3D) image analysis.

Data Transfer and Storage

A single bed in a monitoring unit, operating for 24 hours per day and sampling 64 channels of data at 200 samples/second/channel, would generate about 1.5 megabytes of data per minute. The final file size would depend on a number of factors, including the precise storage format used by a system, the presence of built-in data compression, and the like. Therefore, actual size of files would vary. Nonetheless, the amount of data acquired for 64 channels of data would be the equivalent of about 12,000,000 pages of 16-channel EEG paper per year. [For 16 channels: 6 pages/min × (24 × 60) minutes/day × 365 days/year; double for 32 channels and double again for 64.] The digital volume of data is also considerable. For example, a seizure record consists of 5 to 8 minutes of EEG. If 32 to 64 channels of data are acquired, 5 to 8 minutes can occupy from 3.8 to 12.3 megabytes of disk space and some patients have dozens of seizures per day. By way of comparison, 10 megabytes of data would store 5,000 pages of text. One CD-ROM could hold about 600 megabytes of data, the equivalent of about 8,000 pages of 16-channel EEG paper. Each disk could thus hold about 60 routine outpatient EEGs. Because of the size of the data load, careful consideration must be given to data management and storage. Although a DVD holds 4.7 gigabytes of data and thus eases the storage burden, digital video and high-resolution EEG recording, i.e., 128 channels at 1,000 samples/second, restore the burden again. As shown in Table 40.2, the complete video and high-resolution EEG record for one day would require 15 DVDs if it were to be saved in its entirety.

As with traditional EEG recording, data review and interpretation generally occur separately from the data acquisition process. This allows additional records to be obtained while the previous records are being interpreted by the electroencephalographer, and in general allows a more efficient segmentation of functions. In modern systems, the transfer of data from one machine to another (for example, from the data acquisition to the data review machine) is managed automatically by computer software. The program could move data either from the acquisition to the review machine, or from the acquisition machine to a file server. In this latter case, the review machine would read from the file server. There should be automated programs to deal with permanent file storage, for example to CD-ROM or DVD. Software should locate files for transfer automatically, thus freeing the user from the tedious details of file tracking, transfer, and storage. As patient files are reviewed, the user should be prompted for a decision, or have the opportunity to decide, whether to save or delete a given file.

Analysis by the Electroencephalographer

A number of different display modes are possible in most systems, depending on the clinical need. Data may be viewed sequentially forward or in reverse, or clicking the mouse on a time line can permit jumping to a particular point. Using a mouse, it should be possible to tag events of interest (such as spikes), to annotate as to significance, and to analyze. For example, one may wish to analyze location of maximum amplitude of a discharge, determine lead-lag interchannel relationships of ictal or interictal discharges, measure interchannel correlations and coherence (Gevins, 1987; Gotman, 1981, 1983), generate fast Fourier transforms, or perform other analytic tasks. Because there is no paper and no ink, there is, therefore, neither paper pull nor curvilinear pen artifact. Thus, using a screen cursor, events on separate channels can be compared precisely and, if the data acquisition rates are suitable, latency differences in the millisecond range can be accurately determined.

The digital basis of the data allows relatively straightforward manipulation by the reviewer (Lesser et al., 1990; Nuwer, 1990). For example, all data could be obtained using a "reference" montage, and later re-montaged off-line into whatever arrangement appeared appropriate. Data can be displayed at higher or lower gains or display speeds or with different filter characteristics. The same microprocessor techniques that allow precise analysis of the data can facilitate graphical displays of important data and of the relationships of data points to one another. A number of ways of producing such displays have been suggested and discussed (Duffy, 1989; Duffy et al., 1979, 1986; Frost, 1987; Gotman et al., 1978; Guedes de Oliveira and Lopes da Silva, 1980; Lopes da Silva et al., 1977; Nuwer, 1989; Nuwer et al., 1987; Oken and Chiappa, 1986). Finally, output may be produced at low or high resolution on a standard laser printer. Laser printer hardcopy can be forwarded to

Table 40.2.   Digital Video and EEG Sizes (Sorted by Size)

Channels	Sample Rate	K Bytes/Sec	Giga Bytes/Day	DVD Disks (4.7 GB)
20	200	8.0	0.69	0.15
64	200	25.6	2.21	0.47
128	200	51.2	4.42	0.94
MPEG1 1.5 M bits/sec		187	16	3.4
128	1,000	256	22.1	4.7
MPEG2 standard 3.4 M bits/sec		425	36	7.8
MPEG2 high 4.5 M bits/sec		562	48	10.3
MPEG2 with 128 channels	1,000	818	70	15.0

hospital records and to referring physicians, but as digital networks and storage improve, paper will become increasingly unnecessary except as a medium for temporary exchange. Paper storage and consumption is therefore vastly reduced compared to traditional EEG.

Discussion

Digitally based seizure monitoring has numerous benefits, but also several disadvantages. Benefits include the ability to acquire and store prodigious quantities of EEG data efficiently, to alter the appearance of the data at the time of review, to apply computer-based seizure or spike-detection and analysis programs, and to share data among various local and remote stations. Disadvantages include cost, unfamiliarity to many electroencephalographers (EEG interpretation is a visual process and a screen does look different from paper), requirement for at least a minimum of technical sophistication on the part of the user, and the need for support staff. The need for on-site support staff, in the form of sophisticated programmers and training personnel, will be an ongoing necessity until digital EEG systems become more mature and established. In our experience, however, the advantages of digital-based seizure monitoring have far exceeded the disadvantages.

It has become clear to us that a completely digital approach has considerable advantages for data acquisition, data transfer, data analysis, and data storage. An outpatient building was opened some years ago in our institution and this building is several blocks from the offices in which EEGs are interpreted. The EEGs in this outpatient building are digitally acquired and transmitted to the hospital EEG offices for interpretation using digital fiber. However, data transmission does not require a local area network to be useful. EEGs or evoked potentials can be placed on floppy or optic disks, tapes, portable drives, or on other storage media and transferred in this fashion. All of these are relatively portable and all are smaller and lighter than a paper EEG. In all of these cases the data could be acquired in a relatively general format and then subsequently redisplayed and reanalyzed in a quite different format.

As microprocessors allow us to apply increasingly sophisticated algorithms to neurophysiological data in a convenient fashion, we will ourselves have to become still more sophisticated in our ability to assess the significance of the results we obtain. For example, it is important to emphasize that display and mapping techniques summarize data, by extrapolating from the original data. These represent visual aids to the electroencephalographer. They do not necessarily represent new data in themselves and are only as good as the analysis on which the graphics are based. The actual data are only those provided by the number of electrodes attached to the patient. This is usually a smaller number than the number of dots produced by the graphic output; these gradations represent extrapolations from the data and may or may not be accurate reflections of how the data changed in the actual patient or patients represented. Nonetheless, graphical aids can provide a useful way of summarizing information.

These and other similar considerations should serve to underscore the fact that microprocessors have no intrinsic intelligence. Their value is conferred by virtue of speed, consistency in applying repetitive operations, and tirelessness. A processor will not know by itself the most appropriate means of evaluating data, nor whether the data analyzed are appropriate for the analysis, nor whether the obtained results are meaningful. For these reasons, digitized EEG analysis will be a supplement to, rather than a replacement for, human judgment. Nonetheless, experience over recent years suggests that computerized EEG monitoring, properly applied and interpreted, can be a very useful extension to the skills of the clinician.

Acknowledgments

We thank Wanda Novak for secretarial assistance. A portion of the material in this chapter represents a compilation of material published previously (especially Lesser et al., 1990). Drs. Lesser and Webber receive research funding from and are entitled to sales royalty from Bio-logic Systems, Inc., which is developing products related to the research described in this paper. Dr. Webber is also a consultant to the company. The terms of this arrangement have been reviewed and approved by the Johns Hopkins University in accordance with its conflict of interest policy.

References

Barlow, J.S. 1986. Artifact processing (rejection and minimization) in EEG data processing. In *Clinical Applications of Computer Analysis of EEG and Other Neurophysiological Signals. Handbook of Electroencephalography and Clinical Neurophysiology,* revised series, vol. 2, Eds. F.H. Lopes da Silva, W. Storm van Leeuwen, and A. Remond, pp. 15–62. Amsterdam: Elsevier,.

Binnie, C.D. 1986. Computer applications in monitoring. In *Clinical Applications of Computer Analysis of EEG and other Neurophysiological Signals. Handbook of Electroencephalography and Clinical Neurophysiology,* revised series, vol. 2, Eds. F.H. Lopes da Silva, W. Storm van Leeuwen, and A. Remond, pp. 67–91. Amsterdam: Elsevier.

Bragin, A., Engel, J., Jr., Wilson, C.L., et al. 1999. High-frequency oscillations in human brain. Hippocampus 9:137–142.

Duffy, F.H. 1989. Clinical value of topographic mapping and quantified neurophysiology. Arch. Neurol. 46:1133–1134.

Duffy, F.H., Burchfiel, J.L., and Lombroso, C.T. 1979. Brain electrical activity mapping (BEAM): a method for extending the clinical utility of EEG and evoked potential data. Ann. Neurol. 5:309–321.

Duffy, F.H., Bartels, P.H., and Neff, R. 1986. A response to Oken and Chiappa. Ann. Neurol. 19:494–496.

Fisher, R.S., Webber, W.R.S., Lesser, R.P., et al. 1992 High-frequency EEG activity at the start of seizures. J. Clin. Neurophysiol. 9:441–448.

Fogg, C., LeGall, D.J., Mitchell, J.L., et al. 1996. *MPEG Video Compression Standard.* New York: Kluwer Academic Publishers.

Frost, J.D., Jr. 1987. Mimetic techniques. In *Methods of Analysis of Brain Electrical and Magnetic Signals. Handbook of Electroencephalography and Clinical Neurophysiology,* revised series, vol. 1, Eds. A.S. Gevins and A. Remond, pp. 195–209. Amsterdam: Elsevier.

Gevins, A.S. 1987. Correlation analysis. In *Methods of Analysis of Brain Electrical and Magnetic Signals. Handbook of Electroencephalography and Clinical Neurophysiology,* revised series, vol. 1, Eds. A.S. Gevins and A. Remond, pp. 171–193. Amsterdam: Elsevier.

Gevins, A.S., and Remond, A. (Eds.) 1987. *Methods of Analysis of Brain Electrical and Magnetic Signals. Handbook of Electroencephalography and Clinical Neurophysiology,* revised series, vol. 1. Amsterdam: Elsevier.

Gotman, J. 1981. Interhemispheric relations during bilateral spike-and-wave activity. Epilepsia 22:453–466.

Gotman, J. 1982. Automatic recognition of epileptic seizures in the EEG. Electroencephalogr. Clin. Neurophysiol. 54:530–540.

Gotman, J. 1983. Measurement of small time difference between EEG channels: method and application to epileptic seizure propagation. Electroencephalogr. Clin. Neurophysiol. 56:501–514.

Gotman, J., Gloor, P., and Schaul, N. 1978. Comparison of traditional reading of the EEG and automatic recognition of interictal epileptic activity. Electroencephalogr. Clin. Neurophysiol. 44:48–60.

Gotman, J., Ives, J.R., and Gloor, P. 1979. Automatic recognition of interictal epileptic activity in prolonged EEG recordings. Electroencephalogr. Clin. Neurophysiol. 46:510–520.

Gotman, J., Ives, J.R., Gloor, P., et al. 1985. Monitoring at the Montreal Neurological Institute. In *Long-Term Monitoring in Epilepsy* (EEG suppl No. 37), Eds. J. Gotman, J.R. Ives, and P. Gloor, pp. 327–340. Amsterdam: Elsevier.

Guedes de Oliveira, P.H.H., and Lopes da Silva, F.H. 1980. A topographic display of epileptiform transients based on a statistical approach. Electroencephalogr. Clin. Neurophysiol. 48:710–714.

Ives, J.R., Thompson, C.J., and Gloor, P. 1976. Seizure monitoring: a new tool in electroencephalography. Electroencephalogr. Clin. Neurophysiol. 41:422–427.

Kaplan, P.W., and Lesser, R.P. 1990. Prolonged extracranial and intracranial in–patient monitoring. In *Clinical Neurophysiology of Epilepsy. Handbook of Electroencephalography and Clinical Neurophysiology,* revised series, vol. 4, Eds. J.A. Wada and R.J. Ellingson, pp. 121–154. Amsterdam: Elsevier.

Koenen, R. 1999 MPEG-4—multimedia for our time. IEEE Spectrum 36: 26–33.

Lesser, R.P., Webber, W.R.S., Wilson, K., et al. 1990. A microprocessor-based epilepsy monitoring unit. Neurology 40(suppl 1):255.

Lopes da Silva, F. 1987. Computer-assisted EEG diagnosis: pattern recognition in EEG analysis, feature extraction and classification. In *Electroencephalography. Basic Principles, Clinical Applications and Related Fields,* Eds. E. Niedermeyer and F. Lopes da Silva, pp. 899–919. Baltimore: Urban & Schwarzenberg.

Lopes da Silva, F.H., Van Hulten, K., Lommen, J.G., et al. 1977. Automatic detection and localization of epileptic foci. Electroencephalogr. Clin. Neurophysiol. 43:1–13.

Medvedev, A.V. 2002. Epileptiform spikes desynchronize and diminish fast (gamma) activity of the brain. An "anti-binding" mechanism? Brain Res. Bull. 58:115–128.

MPEG1. 1993. Information technology—coding of moving pictures and associated audio for digital storage media at up to about 1.5 Mbit/s. ISO/IEC 11172-1. Web Site: *http://www.iso.org/iso/en/CatalogueDetail Page.CatalogueDetail?CSNUMBER=19180.*

MPEG2. 2000. Information technology—generic coding of moving pictures and associated audio information: Video. ISO/IEC 13818-2. Web Site: *http://www.iso.org/iso/en/CatalogueDetailPage.Catalogue Detail?CSNUMBER=31539.*

Nuwer, M.R. 1989. Uses and abuses of brain mapping. Arch. Neurol. 46: 1134–1136.

Nuwer, M.R. 1990. Paperless electroencephalography. Semin. Neurol. 10: 178–184.

Nuwer, M.R., Jordan, S.E., and Ahn, S.S. 1987. Evaluation of stroke using EEG frequency analysis and topographic mapping. Neurology 37:1153–1159.

Oken, B.S., and Chiappa, K.H. 1986. Statistical issues concerning computerized analysis of brainwave topography. Ann. Neurol. 19:493–497.

Panych, L.P., and Wada, J.A. 1990. Computer applications in data analysis. In *Clinical Neurophysiology of Epilepsy. Handbook of Electroencephalography and Clinical Neurophysiology,* revised series, vol. 4, Eds. J.A. Wada, and R.A. Ellingson, pp. 361–385. Amsterdam: Elsevier.

Webber, W.R.S., Wilson, K., and Lesser, R.P. 1989. A file system for computer-based EEG. Epilepsia 30:739.

41. Digital EEG

Gregory L. Krauss and W. Robert S. Webber

This chapter describes digital electroencephalogram (EEG) and its uses, including (a) EEG and computer hardware components; (b) digital recording principles; (c) how to use digital applications, including filters and review techniques; (d) limitations in current digital recording systems; and (e) directions for future development.

Introduction and History

Digital EEG is the conversion of the electroencephalogram into binary data bits for computer review. The major scientific advantages of digital EEG over paper-based analog EEG are that the digitally acquired signals can be flexibly formatted and measured precisely (Nuwer, 1997). Most EEG laboratories convert from paper-based analog systems to digital systems, however, for practical rather than scientific reasons: to save on costs in storing bulky paper EEG and to avoid messy ink pen recordings with analog EEG recorders. Because of the advantages of digital EEG, it was recognized over 20 years ago that EEG presented on computer would eventually replace paper-based analog EEG (Remond, 1977). This became feasible only in the 1990s, however, as inexpensive and powerful microprocessors with high-capacity storage medium became available. Digital EEG development was also diverted by an early leap into automatic EEG interpretation, particularly by nonvalidated applications of quantitative EEG (QEEG) (Duffy, 1989; Duffy et al., 1994; John, 1989; Nuwer, 1990a; Thatcher, 2003).

First-generation commercial digital EEG systems introduced in the early 1990s were little more than analog EEG systems with poor-resolution screen displays and magnetic data storage (Nuwer, 1990b). Current second-generation commercial EEG systems offer acceptable screen resolution, report-writing programs, and analysis programs that supplement visual EEG review, e.g., automatic spike and seizure detection (Qu and Gotman, 1995; Webber et al., 1996), Laplacian analysis (Babiloni et al., 1996), and spectral topographic maps (Lopes da Silva, 1990; Scherg, 2002). Many of these functions have been available for many years on expensive inpatient epilepsy monitoring systems. Grass Instruments is an example of a pioneer manufacturer of analog EEG recorders that developed a digital EEG system only in 1997 (as a subsidiary of the futuristically named Astro-Med Corporation), integrating an analysis package first developed by Jean Gotman for inpatient video-EEG seizure recording. Computerized EEG has been used for seizure recording and EEG research recording for a much longer period (Gotman, 1987; Künkel, 1977; Lagerlund et al., 1996).

The practical advantages of digital EEG over traditional paper-based systems are not trivial. An EEG laboratory performing 1,000 EEG paper recordings per year produces a volume of paper over 10 m³. These data can be reduced with digital EEG to several computer tapes or CD-ROMs and DVDs (American Electroencephalographic Society, 1994). Digital EEG permits recording and review stations to be at separate sites, with EEG transferred on computer networks and EEG files stored via networks and indexed on a searchable database. The scientific advantages of precise EEG quantification, however, have yet to be realized: precise measurements of EEG frequencies, amplitudes, and locations permit comparisons between patients and reference groups and allow serial comparisons of patient's EEGs (Nuwer et al., 1994). Serial measurements of background slowing in patient groups with Alzheimer's dementia (Salinsky et al., 1992; Soininen et al., 1989) may serve as independent measures of drug treatment response. Future EEG systems with integrated analysis tools and database filing may support this type of data collection.

EEG and Computer Components and Engineering Principles

Digital EEG systems consist of an analog amplifier system with EEG electrodes and jackbox; an analog-to-digital converter (ADC), which samples and measures continuous analog EEG; a computer, which displays the digital signals on a monitor; and computer storage devices (Fig. 41.1). Digital systems record analog signals with moderate amplification and broad bandpass analog filters. Digitized traces are then scaled, filtered and formatted into various montages for optimal review (Fig. 41.2).

Electrodes and Jackbox

Digital EEG recording is performed using standard EEG electrodes and jackbox inputs. Some digital systems have electronically switched jackboxes that allow amplifier input channels to be switched among an array of different electrodes without interrupting the recording. This is useful for special applications such as intraoperative recording in which it is difficult to replace reference or other electrodes.

Analog Amplifiers and Filters

Since digitally converted EEG can be scaled and filtered after its acquisition, analog amplifiers are set to record EEG over a large dynamic range with minimal signal filtering and scaling. Most digital EEG systems amplify analog signals in a 2,000 to 4,000 µV dynamic range, sufficient to capture physiological EEG (<1,000 µV peak to peak). Broad bandpass analog filters settings are used for acquisition. Low filters (high pass) stabilize direct current (DC) drift and

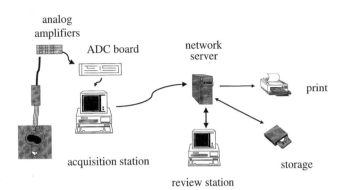

Figure 41.1. A sample digital EEG laboratory using a network server to transfer and store EEG files.

maintain a normal baseline for alternating current (AC) recording. Low filter settings for digital systems range from 0.01 to 5 Hz, and low filters up to 100 Hz are available on advanced systems for special applications. High-frequency filters (low pass) are used to remove noise occurring above physiologic frequencies and to prevent aliasing during signal digitization. High-frequency filters on current systems are 50 to 100 Hz, with filter settings on advanced system up to 3 kHz. Analog notch filters of 50 Hz (Europe) or 60 Hz (North America) are available. There is little EEG energy above 70 Hz on extracranial recording, and so higher filter settings are unnecessary for routine recording. Higher filter settings may be needed to record and detect high-frequency activity on intracranial recordings or to record rapid events, such as short-latency evoked potentials. Amplification gain is 2,000 to 20,000 (2 K to 20 K) for most systems and 50 to 200,00 in advanced systems.

Analog amplifiers are usually electronic circuit boards attached to a control panel with manual switches to control gain and analog filters. Amplifiers may measure impedance and have individual power switches. Newer systems use software to control analog amplifier settings. Some systems use miniature amplifier modules, with 16 to 32 amplifiers fitting in palm-sized or jackbox-sized cases. These systems frequently have relatively fixed amplifier settings and rely on digital scaling and signal filtering to present EEG. For example, EEG is acquired with broad-pass analog filter set-

tings (0.1–100 Hz) and high-frequency activity is subsequently digitally filtered. These systems are adequate for routine EEG recordings, but may be limited for special applications requiring amplifier settings outside the standard range. Ambulatory digital EEG (Iguchi et al., 1994) and some research systems (Dunseath and Kelly, 1995) also use miniature amplifiers, and usually locate preamplifiers next to the head in order to minimize movement artifact and electrical interference.

Analog-to-Digital Converters (ADCs)

Digital converters are usually solid-state circuits placed on a computer board. Digital converters measure the continuous analog EEG signal at discrete time intervals, i.e., sampling the signal at a fixed rate. Sample rates must be high enough to accurately represent complex waveforms without overloading the computer unnecessarily. As shown in Fig. 41.3, five to ten samples are usually required to accurately represent EEG waveforms, depending on waveform complexity. Since skull attenuates high-frequency activity above 40 Hz, sample rates of 200 to 400 are usually sufficient for extracranial recording. For commercial EEG systems, popular sample rates are 256 and a few have additional rates up to 1,000 Hz. Higher sample rates are needed to record higher frequency intracranial activity (Fisher et al., 1992).

ADCs usually employ one analog-to-digital chip working at a rapid, fixed rate. Multiple channels are then scanned in sequence by this single ADC chip. This causes a time delay when a large number of channels are sampled serially. In a 32-channel EEG system, an event that occurred simultaneously at channels 1 and 32 would be displayed offset in time by one sample interval at channel 32 due to its later sampling. Most digital systems overcome the time-delay inherent in serial ADC with a "sample and hold" function for each channel. Samples are obtained simultaneously and held for all analog channels, and then are serially measured. Some converters use intersample interpolation to estimate the sample value at a common instant in time. Another approach is to use high sampling and converter rates, while saving only a fraction of the data.

Aliasing and Undersampling

Signal distortion, called aliasing, occurs when too low sample rates are used to digitize analog signals, which is a critical principle. The highest frequency that can be represented in a digitized signal is half the sample rate, and is called the Nyquist frequency or limit (Bendat and Piersol, 1980; Brigham, 1988). If signals with frequencies higher than the Nyquist frequency for a given sampling system are digitized, they end up with a lower aliased frequency below the Nyquist limit.

Figure 41.4 shows the effects of reducing sample rate and hence Nyquist frequency on an 18-Hz sine wave. At 200 samples/sec the wave is clearly represented. At 50 samples/sec (Nyquist = 25 Hz) the wave is recognizable, but some distortion is present. At 20 samples/sec (Nyquist = 10 Hz) aliasing has set in and the digitized frequency of the wave is now 2 Hz. Figure 41.5 shows how the frequency of signals above the Nyquist limit are folded into the Nyquist

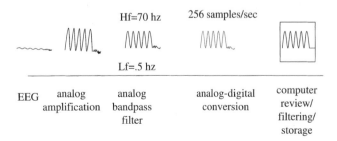

Figure 41.2. The recording design for digital systems: EEG signals are amplified and filtered with broad-pass analog filters. Following digitization, the signal is scaled, filtered, and then reviewed on a computer monitor.

Epileptiform Spike FP2-F8

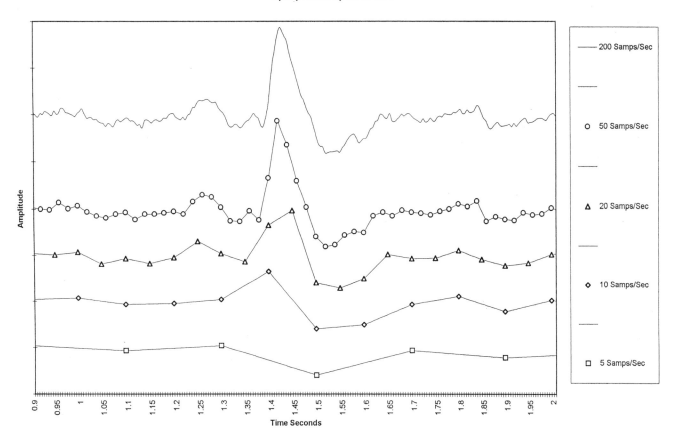

Figure 41.3. The effect of different sample rates on digital representation of a sharp wave. The *top trace* is sampled at 200 samples/sec. The next four traces show where the sample points are for 50, 20, 10, and 5 samples/sec. Each sample point is shown as an *open symbol* and interpolation lines are shown joining up these *open symbols*. As the sample rate is reduced, detail of high-frequency waveforms is lost and low-frequency waves are distorted.

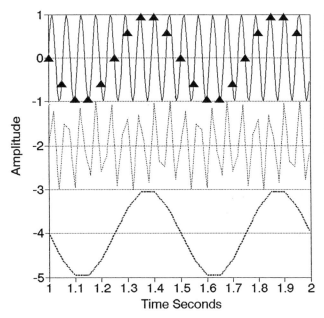

Figure 41.4. The aliasing of an 18-Hz sine wave to 2 Hz is shown when sampled at 20 samples/sec. The *top trace* shows the original 18-Hz sine wave sampled at 200 samples/sec. The next trace shows the same wave sampled at 50 samples/sec. There is some distortion, but the original wave is still visible. The lowest trace shows 20 samples/sec. The wave has been aliased to 2 Hz. The sample points are shown on the original wave *(top trace)* as *small vertical bars*. The Nyquist limit has been violated due to sampling performed at less than two times the signal frequency.

Figure 41.5. Insufficient digital sampling produces aliased signals at frequencies (y axis) proportionate to the signal frequency (x axis) and the sampling frequency (200 samples/sec in this example). The Nyquist limit for 200 samples/sec sampling is 100 Hz; hence, the signal is accurately represented between 0 and 100 Hz. Aliased signal are folded back at the frequencies shown for frequencies >100 Hz. A 101-Hz signal, for example, produces a 99-Hz aliased signal, and a 199-Hz signal produces a 1-Hz aliased signal.

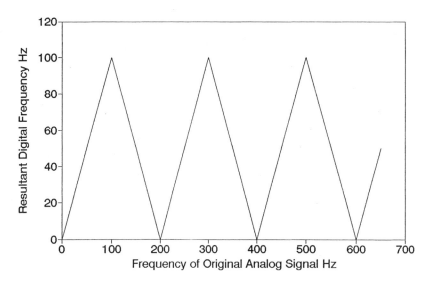

range. Aliasing cannot be removed from the digital signal once present. Aliased signals "fold back" into lower frequencies, so that although this occurs with undersampled high-frequency signals, lower frequency signals are distorted. There are two ways to avoid aliasing: sampling more than 2 times the maximum signal frequency (e.g., >100 samples/second for scalp EEG), and using analog filters to remove high-frequency signals above the Nyquist limit. Most digital systems combine 70- or 100-Hz high filters and sample rates of 200 to 400 Hz to avoid aliasing. One trap is that 70- and 100-Hz analog filters in many commercial systems have gradual roll-offs, permitting high-frequency energy to be aliased into the lower spectrum of an EEG recorded. This may become significant with intracranial recordings that contain signals up to 120 Hz (Fisher et al., 1992) or in recordings marred with high-frequency noise, unless sample rates are increased or sharper cutoff analog filters are used.

In addition to aliasing, undersampled signals do not accurately represent analog waveforms. An extreme example of this is a 100-Hz sine wave that is sampled at 100 samples/sec. The ADC will read the same constant sample value for each sample it takes because it will catch the waveform at the same point with each sample. The digitized frequency of this 100-Hz sine wave will appear to be zero. The effect of an inadequate sample rate of EEG patterns can be seen in Fig. 41.3. As sample rates decrease progressively from 200 samples/sec to 5 samples/sec, more and more detail is lost and distortion appears in the low-frequency range due to aliasing. The Nyquist limit of two times the highest is a lower limit beyond which information is completely lost. Where wave shape is important in the analysis of signals such as EEG it is traditional to sample at least 8 to 10 times the highest frequency component of interest.

Dynamic Range (Amplitude Resolution)

The dynamic range is the full-scale voltage divided by the smallest change in volts. For the vertical scale, i.e., voltage amplitude, dynamic range is sometimes expressed in bits on a binary logarithmic scale. A 6-bit converter mea-

sures voltage in 2^6 (= 64) increments. Each additional bit doubles the dynamic range. Most second-generation digital EEG machines record signals at 8- to 12-bit (256 to 4,096) increments. The dynamic range for commercial systems include physiologically important ranges, which for scalp EEG is approximately 2,000 μV full scale. Advanced EEG systems offer precise vertical recording (e.g., 12–16 bit recording) and a large full-scale range (e.g., 4,000 μV). The lower limit of the dynamic range is set by amplifier noise, and in commercial systems this is around 0.1 μV. Thus the dynamic range of EEG signals, particularly where intracranial signals are concerned, is of order 40,000, which requires 16-bit ADC for faithful recordings.

Digital systems have a much larger dynamic range than paper. This means that the amplifier gain can be kept fixed, and the vertical scale on the display can be adjusted over a wide range to reveal low-voltage signals on the one hand, and reduce high-voltage waves on the other. With traditional analog systems using pen writers, there is a risk that signals will be clipped and data lost if the amplifier gain is too high.

Digital Display Limits

Current color computer monitors display only a fraction of sampled data and at a resolution well below human visual resolution (Table 41.1). Computer monitors used for EEG typically have display screens that are 1,280 to 1,600 pixels wide and 1,024 to 1,200 pixels high. This provides a vertical pixel resolution of about 1 in 64 (about 6 bits, assuming a screen with 16 channels of EEG and 1,024 pixels vertical screen size), whereas a 12-bit converter typically used in computer-based EEG systems has an amplitude resolution of 1 in 4,096 (i.e., resolution 64 times greater than computer monitors). A contemporary 600 dots per inch (dpi) laser printer that is used to print digital EEG has a vertical resolution of about 1 in 600 (about 9 bits) for a channel separation of 1 inch. Laser printing resolution is equivalent to dynamic range, that is, the smallest vertical change compared to vertical span of the EEG signal, also known as full-scale deflection (FSD). A conventional paper EEG machine has an

Table 41.1. Horizontal (Time) Resolution for Displaying EEG (Pixel Equivalent) and Maximum Frequencies Which Can Be Represented

Display System	Pixel/mm	Equivalent Nyquist Frequency Hz (Half Sample Rate)	Visual Frequency Resolution (Assume 10 Samples/Wave; Risk, 1993)
Computer screen 20″ 375 mm, 1,600 pixels wide (10 sec page, 37.5 mm/sec)	4.3	80	16
Ink and paper EEG machine 0.2 mm pen, 30 mm/sec	5.0*	N/A	75
Human eye resolution 1 arc sec at 18″ for 30 mm/sec	7.5	112	22.4
Laser jet printer 600 dpi for 30 mm/sec	23	345	69

* Number of lines/mm.

amplitude resolution of 1 in 115 (about 7 bits, assuming 23 mm channel spacing, 0.2 mm trace), which is about one bit above that of a computer display.

Current display monitors are also limited in horizontal (time) resolution, particularly compared to laser printer output. A monitor with a 1,280-pixel horizontal display displays 10 seconds of EEG at 128 points per second. This is 50% of the typical 256 samples/sec sample rate. A 70-msec duration spike is represented on a 1,280-pixel display screen by 9 points (at 30 mm/sec compression), resulting in irregular steps in the steep portion of the waveform (Fig. 41.6). Laser jet printers at 600 dpi have a maximum resolution of 23.6 dots/mm, giving a maximum frequency of 354 Hz, a

factor of 5.5 times higher than the finest available computer monitors used for EEG (1,600 × 1,200 21-inch monitors). This is higher than typical ADC sampling rates, resulting in accurate representation of spikes and other brief events. Monochrome monitors such as those used in radiology have resolution several times that of color monitors; however, graphic systems with color cathode ray tube (CRT) monitors dominate the commercial EEG market.

Psychometric Limits in Visual EEG Recognition

EEG should be displayed at resolutions near the limits of human visual resolution. Unfortunately, current computer displays do not match human psychometric limits for view-

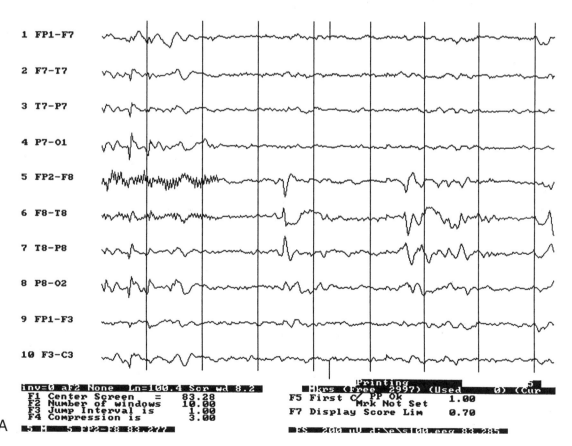

Figure 41.6. Display resolution varies markedly for older and newer computer monitors and for laser jet printing. **A:** A first-generation system with a 1,024 × 768 pixel monitor display produces irregular, distorted sharp waves. *(continued)*

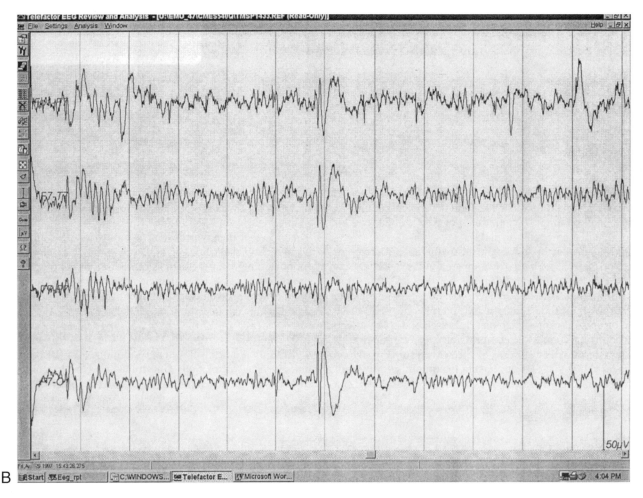

Figure 41.6. *(continued)* **B:** A second-generation system with a 1,600 × 1,200 pixel monitor more accurately displays sharp waves, with some staircasing of vertical lines and distortion of peaks.

ing EEG (Risk, 1993). Normal vision can resolve approximately 7.5 pixels/mm (191 pixels/inch) at 18 inches on a 14-inch display. This is equivalent to 225 pixels/sec for 30 mm/sec compression and a visual resolution of 22.5 cycles/second (c/sec) at 18-inch or 30 c/sec at 13.5-inch viewing distance. This assumes ten samples are needed to accurately represent a wave. Waves at higher frequencies can be detected (e.g., 50-Hz line noise appears distinct from 60-Hz line noise), but their waveforms cannot be visually resolved. Psychometric limits can be compared with paper and computer display, again assuming visual resolution is approximately one-tenth that of the spatial pixel rate (Risk, 1993). The maximum resolution of an analog paper record is 75 Hz running at a paper speed of 30 mm/sec. This is based on a pen line width of 0.2 mm giving 150 lines/mm; then applying the Nyquist limit (max frequency is half sample rate, i.e., lines/mm) gives a max frequency of 75 Hz. For currently available high-resolution computer monitors (1,600 pixels spread over 375 mm, i.e., 4.3 pixels/mm) the maximum resolution is 64 Hz. Though visually detectable, this frequency is higher than can be visually resolved in this case, distin-

guished from other frequencies. Lowering time compression increases visual frequency resolution proportionately, e.g., reducing time compression from 30 mm/sec to 60 mm/sec doubles recognized frequencies to 45 Hz at an 18-inch viewing distance (for a 14-inch screen). Electroencephalographers are trained, however, to recognize patterns presented at 30 mm/sec, and reduced compression increases review time.

EEG Storage

Mass storage tape media have been available for several decades, but digital storage has only recently become affordable and rapidly retrievable (Table 41.2). CD-ROMs, DVD, and tape storage systems all store several hundred routine EEGs. CD-ROM writers are well-established and inexpensive devices and currently store 680 MB for under a dollar. Recently, DVD writers have become available that are not much more expensive than CD-ROMs. These DVD writers store from 4.7 to 9.4 gigabyte per disk, depending on media type; DVD storage capacity can be expected to double in the next few years. Unfortunately, there are several competing DVD record-

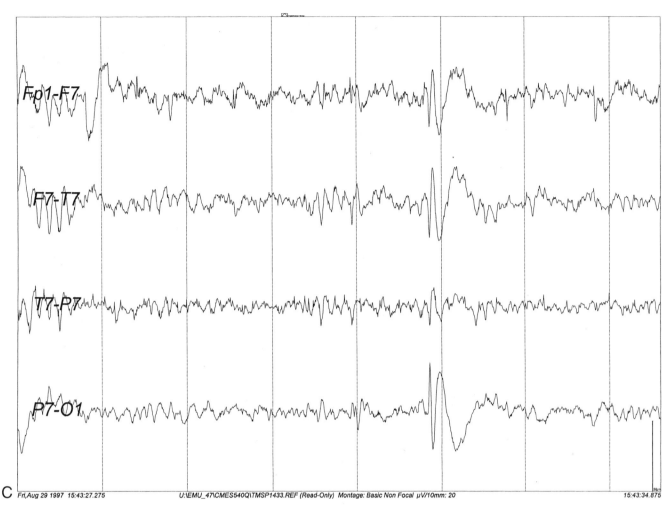

Fp1-F7

F7-T7

T7-P7

P7-O1

C Fri,Aug 29 1997 15:43:27.275   U:\EMU_47\CMES540Q\TMSP1433.REF (Read-Only) Montage: Basic Non Focal µV/10mm: 20   15:43:34.875

Figure 41.6.   *(continued)* **C:** A laser jet printer at 600 dots-per-inch (dpi) produces relatively smooth lines and sharp peaks. All displays are printed using a 600-dpi laser jet.

Table 41.2.   Storage Capacities, Data Rates, and Relative Costs for Various Digital Media for EEG

| Media | Capacity MB | Supports Direct Reading of EEG from Media | Cost Relative to Lowest for 1 MB of EEG | Short-Term Scalp, 20 Channels, One 20-Min Record (8 kb/sec) | | Long-Term Grid/Depth, 64 Channels, 24-Hour Data Set (25.6 kb/sec) | |
				Units Needed for 20-Min Record	Physical Storage Volume (cm³)	Units Needed for 1 Day (24 hours)	Physical Storage Volume (cm³)
(Paper)		Yes	260	1.0	1,200	230*	276,480
Floppy Diskette	1.44	Yes	3,174	6.7	165.5	1,536	38,140
CompactFlash 512 MB	512	Yes	1,714	0.0187	0.089	4.32	20.62
Zip 250 Drive	250	Yes	658	0.0384	4.35	8.85	1,002
JAZ Drive 2 GB	2,000	Yes	274	0.0048	0.989	1.10	227
DVD-RAM	9,400	Yes	7.4	0.0010	0.146	0.235	33.6
CD-Rom	680	Yes	3.6	0.014	1.26	3.25	290
DVD-R, DVD+RW	4,700	Yes	3.4	0.0020	0.182	0.47	42.0
Super DLT Tape	320,000	No	1.0	0.00003	0.011	0.0069	2.55

* Relative to one 20-min, 20-channel record.

ing and storage standards. Two competing organizations, DVDForum *(http://www.dvdforum.org/forum.shtml)* and DVD+RW Alliance *(http://www.dvdrw.com)* promote at least six formats for DVDs with varying degrees of compatibility between these formats and the DVD drives able to read and write them. Of these various formats, DVD-RAM is intended for data and has more error checking than the other formats and is thus a more reliable format for long-term archival storage. DVD-RAM storage can be either single sided (4.7 gigabyte) or double sided (9.4 gigabyte). The single-sided disk is the same size as CD-ROM and commercial multimedia DVD disks. The double-sided DVD disk is contained in a protective cartridge that takes up more physical space than the single-sided disk.

Small portable tape drive storage devices appear optimal for storing EEG, particularly for one or two EEG machines, since they are inexpensive and provide similar high storage capacity at low cost. CD-ROMs and DVD, however, provide more rapid retrieval of EEG than tapes, and tapes may deteriorate after 10 years and must be remastered for secure long storage. Although the Super DLT tape is the least costly and most compact storage medium, EEG cannot be read directly from tape. The files must be transferred to the computer hard disk before they can be read. For all other media, the EEG data can be read directly.

Using Digital EEG Machines

Although flexibly displayed EEG offers a number of advantages over paper-based EEG, electroencephalographers are trained to recognize patterns on the EEG using a limited range of display settings, and readers must be organized when adjusting display settings to avoiding misinterpreting EEG.

Digital Review

EEG can be viewed on computer monitors as serial pages EEG (usually 10 second/page) or with continuous scrolling. EEG can be presented very rapidly as serial pages (up to 3 pages/sec in current systems), but only slowly in a scroll mode due to throughput limits of video-graphic and monitor systems. Full-channel EEG can be read at a maximum rate of approximately 2 page/sec at 30 mm/sec compression. Faster rates invite superficial reading of EEG, but are useful for screening gross EEG events such as seizures or sleep states. Some readers prefer viewing EEG as pages. It is visually easier to scan EEG in a "scroll" mode than "page" mode, however, since the eyes remain forward instead of continuously scanning horizontally. Scroll mode allows readers to visually screen EEG on the right side of the monitor, and then scan to the left to scrutinize possible significant patterns without interrupting the display. A rapid scroll mode also emulates the dynamic, continuous EEG, and does not split EEG patterns across adjacent pages. Significant patterns may be missed and the reading frame must be adjusted when patterns run across page breaks. Partial pagination is an effective compromise: scrolling is emulated by rapidly presenting pages of EEG, with the EEG advanced only several seconds on successive pages.

Constructing Reading Montages

A major advantage of digital EEG is that patterns recorded using a common reference can be displayed optimally using multiple bipolar and reference display montages. EEG during sleep, for example, is often best viewed using a transverse bipolar montage to identify central vertex waves. Temporal lobe sharp waves may be missed with a mastoid reference (A1/A2) due to close spacing between active and reference electrodes, but may be prominent on a Pz-reference montage, since this reference coupling maximizes recording distances between the "active" temporal leads and permits comparisons between left and right hemisphere activity.

Since EEG voltages measure potential differences between two sites, recordings that contain common recording electrodes can be reformatted with simple algebra to display the potential difference between linked electrodes. EEG recorded between desired leads and a common reference electrode (R), for example, is subtracted, canceling the common reference, leaving a new bipolar derivation. To construct a display montage with a F7-T3 tracing, for example, electrode pairs containing a common Pz reference can be subtracted: (F7-Pz) − (T3-Pz) = (F7-T3) + (Pz-Pz) = F7-T3. New reference montages can be constructed similarly. In the above example, a new T6 reference can be constructed by repeatedly subtracting T6-Pz channel from the recording channels: (F7-Pz) − (T6-Pz) = (F7-T6) − (Pz-Pz) = F7-T6. New derivatives can be formed only if they are recorded against a common reference or if they are linked by a continuous chain of bipolar leads. For example, if data are acquired as unlinked chains Fp1-F7, F7-T3, and Fp2-F8, F8-T4, a new T3-T4 derivation, cannot be formed. T3-T4 can be constructed algebraically, however, if the recording included Fp1-Fp2: (Fp1-Fp2) − (F7-T3) − (Fp1-F7) + (Fp2-F8) + (F8-T4) = T3-T4. This method is in use in the Johns Hopkins epilepsy monitoring unit and in the Digitrace ambulatory EEG system.

Using Reading Montages

Most laboratories construct standard longitudinal, transverse, and reference montages incorporating 10–20 system electrodes in their digital systems and do not take advantage of the flexibility of digital montages. Additional montages incorporating closely spaced 10% system electrodes and sphenoidal electrodes improve recording sensitivity by recording placing electrodes directly over areas of interest and by defining field boundaries. Anterior temporal leads such as FT9/FT10 and Ch1/Ch2 improve detection of seizure patterns in basomesial temporal regions (Krauss et al., 1992). Epileptogenic activity associated with sensory/motor seizures is frequently missed by standard electrodes, but may be detected on added central and parietal leads (e.g., C1/2, and CP3/CP4). We routinely use reading montages with both reference and bipolar displays, since the techniques are complementary (Fig. 41.7).

The technician must view and maintain all the recording electrodes used during EEG acquisition, in order for them to be available in various reading montages. A practical way to fit many channels of EEG on a single review screen is to compact standard 10–20 electrodes in standard longitudinal

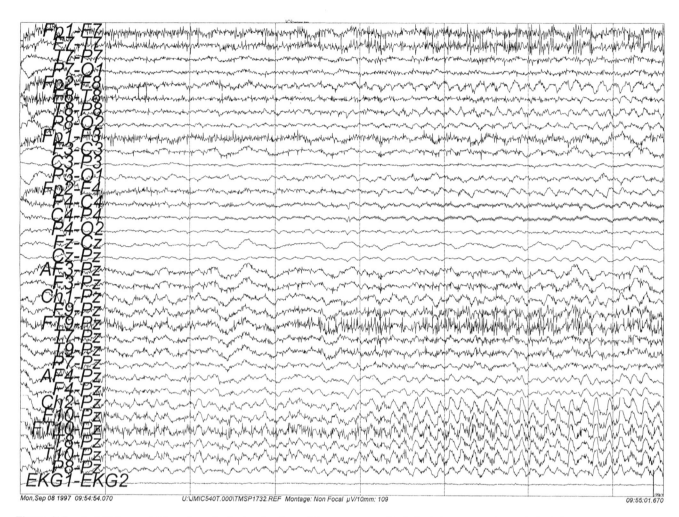

Mon, Sep 08 1997 09:54:54.070   U:\JMIC540T.000\TMSP1732.REF Montage: Non Focal μV/10mm: 109   09:55:01.670

Figure 41.7. A right temporal lobe seizure is displayed using a Johns Hopkins reading montage with bipolar channels and 10–20 system electrodes in the upper half of the EEG page and reference channels with closely spaced 10% electrodes in the lower half of the EEG page. A right temporal lobe ictal theta pattern is seen in both the upper bipolar display and in the lower reference display. Slow-wave phase reversals in bipolar leads and amplitude variations in reference leads provide complementary information in localizing ictal activity to the anterior-midtemporal region.

or transverse displays in the upper screen and to display added leads as reference derivations in the lower screen. A maximum of only 16 to 32 channels can be reviewed on standard monitors at a time (depending on screen size). Additional channels can be monitored using a scroll or zoom function. Although it is helpful to detect and localize abnormalities by recording them at several electrodes in one region, the benefits of using additional electrodes have to be balanced with the difficulties of placing extra electrodes and reviewing additional channels. Technicians must carefully maintain reference electrodes during the recording. Any high-amplitude signal that causes clipping on channels using the reference electrode will corrupt the review montage.

Special Reading Montages

Many special reading montages can be constructed with digitally acquired data, including montages using a common average reference, linked ear references, noncephalic neck references, Laplacian derivatives, and arrays customized to map specific brain regions. The common average reference is very useful for minimizing noise present in a single reference electrode and to display abnormalities around superior head regions where distant, symmetrically placed reference sites are difficult to find. Newer digital systems permit rapid selection and de-selection of leads to include in the common average, making it easy to exclude leads that dominate the average reference. These usually include FP1/FP2 when eye movements or blinks are present, O1/O2 when movement contaminates posterior leads, and extremely active leads (e.g., a T3 site with continuous spiking). It is important to maintain a spatially balanced array of electrodes in the common average. The Laplacian montage acts as a spatial filter, highlighting edges of local fields. Electrodes must be maintained very carefully in Laplacian montages, however, since fields for nonsignificant noise will be highlighted as well as focal abnormalities. Laplacian estimates improve localization with standard 10–20 electrodes only slightly, mostly over superior head regions, due to limited spatial sampling. Laplacian montages constructed using closely spaced 10%

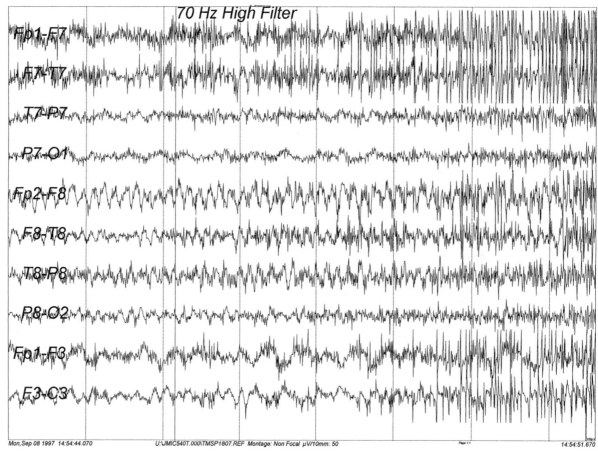

A   Mon,Sep 08 1997 14:54:44.070   U:\JMIC540T.000\TMSP1807.REF   Montage: Non Focal   µV/10mm: 50   Page 1:1   14:54:51.670

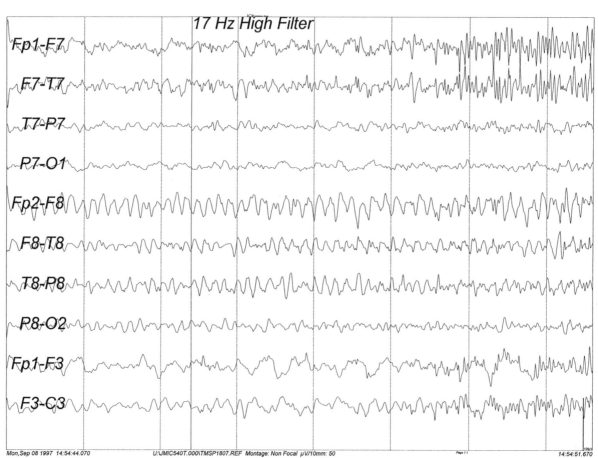

B   Mon,Sep 08 1997 14:54:44.070   U:\JMIC540T.000\TMSP1807.REF   Montage: Non Focal   µV/10mm: 50   Page 1:1   14:54:51.670

electrodes along with spline field estimates improve EEG localization (Gevins et al., 1994).

Digital Filters

EEG is acquired with broad-band analog filters, usually 0.1 to 70 Hz, with subsequent digital filtering. Unlike analog filters, carefully designed finite impulse response (FIR) digital filters do not cause any delay in the signal they pass. Digital filters provide tremendous flexibility, since the EEG can be viewed both with and without filters applied. EEG removed by analog filters during acquisition cannot be recovered, and digital filters remove the need for a technician to anticipate the need for filters. A patient may move during the onset of a seizure and obscure the EEG, for example, something a technician cannot anticipate. Digital high filters are especially useful in screening for important rhythmical patterns in otherwise artifact-marred recordings. Ictal theta patterns or generalized slowing may be evident only with 15- to 25-Hz digital high filters in agitated, moving, or seizing patients (Fig. 41.8). It is important to recognize that high filters <25 Hz can also attenuate spikes and remove significant beta frequency patterns. A more limited range of digital low filters, usually 0.1 to 1.5 Hz, is needed to stabilize movement and slow-wave currents due to sweat or DC phenomena. Occasionally it is useful to remove low-frequency blink or eye-movement signals using low filters in order to screen for epileptiform patterns. It is important to recognize that FIR filters cannot isolate waveforms such as spikes if they are in the frequency range of physiological noise. Myoclonic seizures, for example, are often associated with small polyspike bursts in the same frequency range as electromyogram (EMG). Digital filters also do not obviate the need to have cleanly recorded EEG in which movement and non-EEG physiological artifact is minimized. Advanced filter systems that model and remove eye movement artifact and other unwanted signals may eventually be introduced into clinical (Ille et al., 2002).

A typical filter sequence for routine EEG review is the following: (1) use broad-pass analog filter settings for acquisition (scalp: 0.1–70 Hz, intracranial 0.1–100 Hz); (2) review EEG initially using broad-pass digital filters, 0.3 Hz and 70 Hz; (3) apply notch filter (60 Hz) if there is persistent line artifact; (4) briefly apply high-frequency filters as needed during clinical events, e.g., a 25-Hz high filter during a movement-obscured clinical event; (5) apply a continuous low and high filter only for extremely agitated or uncooperative patients with otherwise unusable recordings. For example, in a continuously moving, unsedated child, stabilize the baseline with a 1.5-Hz low filter and apply a 15-Hz high filter to remove muscle artifact (Fig. 41.9), recognizing that low-frequency slow patterns and high-frequency epileptiform and other phenomena are attenuated. Digital filters should always be returned to a broad bandpass once a usable baseline is restored, e.g., after the agitated or uncooperative patient falls asleep.

Digital EEG File Formats, Compatibility Between Systems

Digital EEG systems all use different file formats for storing the EEG waveform data. Each system can for the most part only read the EEG data created by it. Even within one commercial EEG company it is possible to find several file formats in use. Each file format results form different design compromises between processor and disk speed, and storage cost considerations. Each vendor develops its own EEG file format in isolation for commercial reasons (Itil, 1993).

In large hospitals it is possible to find several different types of digital EEG machines, from several vendors, in use. Each vendor tends to have specific strengths in one area of EEG. For instance, at the Johns Hopkins Hospital, four commercial systems, each from different vendors, are used for ambulatory, outpatient, intraoperative, and long-term monitoring. In addition, there is a fifth system developed in-house for critical care EEG monitoring. Each of these digital systems was brought into use at a different time and fulfilled a different set of requirements.

Within one institution the use of multiple file formats presents some problems. Some EEG systems have more advanced analysis features, but these cannot be used on the EEG data from other systems because the advanced analysis system cannot read those files. In addition staff have to learn many different interfaces as the operation of each EEG machine is also different. Yet other problems exist between institutions. If a pair of hospitals use different EEG equipment, then EEG records from one cannot be read by the other, hence patient data are not transferable between hospitals.

Archiving of EEG data also presents some unique issues. Unlike a paper EEG, you always need an EEG system to read the digital record. As time goes by, and one generation of equipment is replaced by the next, the older EEG records will not be readable by the new equipment. Experience at Johns Hopkins Hospital indicates that the life of digital EEG systems is no more than 8 years, and may be much less. This is because the microcomputer industry changes at such at rate, doubling performance in 18 to 24 months (a trend referred to as Moore's law, and that has been sustained for over 20 years). However pediatric records need to be available for up to 18 years.

As new equipment is brought in to replace older systems, one is faced with either maintaining the older system to preserve access to the old data or having conversion programs that convert the old data to the new system's format. Maintaining old systems is not always possible because parts break and cannot be replaced as they are no longer made. The microcomputer industry continually moves onto faster and larger storage devices and changes operating systems every few years with no interest in producing or supporting older, slower system components.

Figure 41.8.   A: A probable right temporal ictal pattern is partially obscured by muscle artifact when recorded with a 70-Hz high filter. **B:** A right temporal 7 to 8 cycles per second (cps) ictal pattern is more evident after high-frequency noise is removed with a 17-Hz high filter.

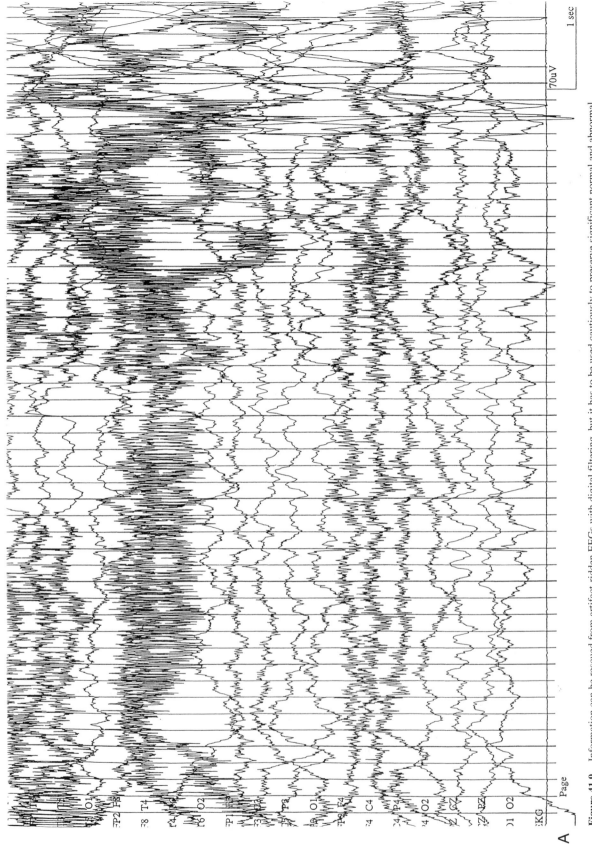

Figure 41.9. Information can be rescued from artifact-ridden EEGs with digital filtering, but it has to be used cautiously to preserve significant normal and abnormal patterns. **A:** An unreadable EEG from an uncooperative, agitated child using a standard 0.5- to 70-Hz filter bandpass.

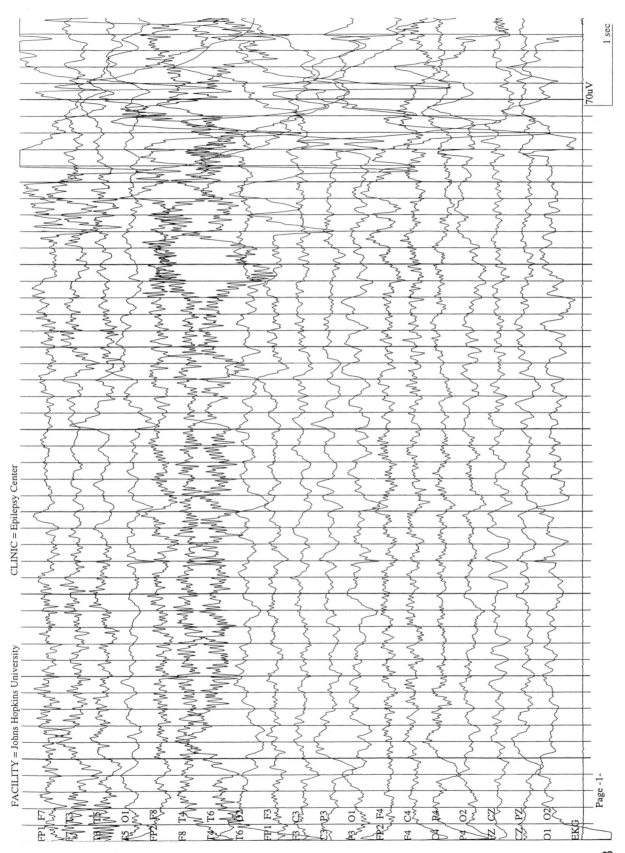

Figure 41.9. *(continued)* **B:** Bilateral 2–3 cps slowing becomes evident when 1.5-Hz low filters and 15-Hz high filters are applied. *(continued)*

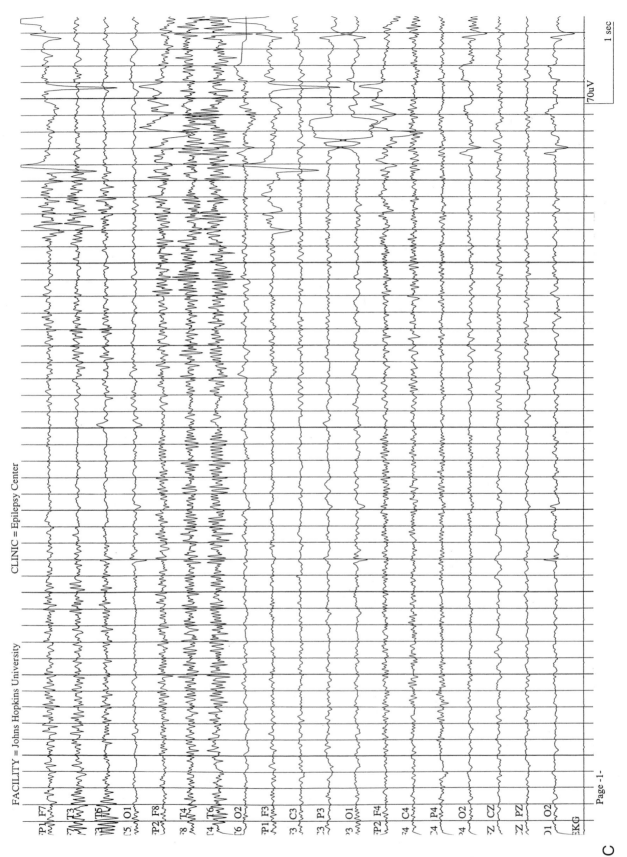

Figure 41.9. *(continued)* **C:** The same recording appears normal when slow activity is removed inappropriately with a 15-Hz low (high pass) filter.

Converting old EEG files to a new system format requires the vendor to write a conversion program if the old and new system vendors are different. It also assumes that the old and new system vendors will exchange the necessary technical information to allow a file conversion program to be written. Then there is the cost of the labor and storage media to hold the newly converted data. These issues make it an expensive, nontrivial task to move an archive of digital EEG data from one vendor's system to another.

These issues have been appreciated by Jacobs (1993) and a solution in the form of a standard file format for EEG has been developed, American Society for Testing and Material (ASTM) E1467-92 (ASTM, 1992). The ASTM standard is ambitious and forward looking in its scope. All the data are stored as ASCII code (American Standard Characters for Information Interchange), as that is the most portable between computer systems both for archive storage and transmission between systems. The standard is comprehensive in that it supports annotations, results, and requests for test and billing along the line of HL7, all for integration into hospital information systems.

The ASTM standard is capable of meeting all archive and transfer functions independent of equipment, but unfortunately, very few vendors and EEG centers have adopted this standard (Lagerlund, 2003). It is likely that the standard will be taken over by the American Clinical Neurophysiology Society (ACNS) and be made available as an ACNS guideline (Lagerlund, 2003).

There is the freely available Extensible Biosignal (EBS) format (Hellmann et al., 1996) that covers much of the same ground as ASTM 1467 with the additional advantage of using the international character set ISO 10646 and supporting the more efficient binary format in a machine-independent way.

Electroencephalographers frequently need to review EEGs from other centers. Some vendors have addressed this need by pairing "mini" EEG reader programs with the EEG on a CD-ROM. These CD-ROM EEG readers have most of the functions of the vendors' standard EEG reader but are usually restricted to the EEG on the CD-ROM. The neurologist has the added burden of having to work with several EEG reader programs, each with its own sets of program menus and quirks.

Several vendors are now supporting the European Data Format (EDF) as a standard EEG data file format (Kemp et al., 1992). Unlike ASTM, this is a simple binary format and can be used as a primary working format. EEG review programs can potentially read EDF files directly, without a slow data conversion required for ASCII formats. Recently, EDF has been extended to EDF+. This format overcomes two limitations of the original EDF specification—the requirement that data be continuous in time and the lack of support for text annotations to the EEG. With EDF+ the EEG data can contain gaps in time, i.e. be interrupted, and annotations can be linked to the EEG. The extensions to the EDF standard, incorporated in EDF+, have been made to preserve as much backward compatibility with EDF as possible. Older EDF reader programs can display EDF+ EEG data, but being unaware of the time gaps, they just show it as one continuous record. If annotations are present, they appear odd-looking waveforms (Kemp and Olivan, 2003).

The need for a standard EEG file format is not yet fully appreciated as many centers are still using their first or only digital system and there are not many requests to transfer digital EEG records between centers. As efficient management of information becomes more critical in health care, the inefficiencies of multiple vendor formats and maintaining access to older archived EEG data will force users of digital EEG to streamline their EEG services and focus on a standard file format, such as EDF/EDF+ or ASTM E1467-92.

Remote EEG Access

The advances in computer and Internet technology, together with increasing availability of faster broadband connections such as DSL, and networking over cable and satellite TV, have made remote access to EEG machines a practical reality. It is now possible with high-speed Internet connections and remote access programs to view the EEG waveforms collected on an EEG machine in another country with a delay of only a few seconds (Elger and Burr, 2000). High-quality digital video still requires more network bandwidth than is available over broadband network connections. However, judging from the history of computer development, transferable digital video will be a reality by time the next edition of this book is published.

EEG system vendors are increasingly using databases to track and manage EEG archives. This helps ensure that records are not lost or deleted before they are archived. However, the database can make the system inflexible when trying to read EEGs from remote locations or sending digital EEG studies to other centers for a second opinion. Problems arise when a digital EEG arrives on the EEG reading system from a remote site or when the EEG reader wants to review a study on a remote computer over the network. In both cases the local database has no entry for this remote EEG and hence cannot see it, even though EEG data are available on the EEG reviewing computer. In our experience at Johns Hopkins Hospital, some vendors provide import mechanisms but these are often complicated and may require the EEG reader to call upon a computer technician alter the EEG program configuration.

The Future

The advances in computer hardware and software technology have resulted in easy-to-use, flexible digital EEG systems. Digital EEG, however, has not significantly expanded the clinical role of EEG, with the possible exceptions of new ambulatory EEG and OR/ICU EEG monitoring systems (Claassen and Mayer, 2002). An expanded clinical role for digital EEG may depend partially on validating advanced analysis techniques, e.g., serially quantifying EEG in patients with dementia or modeling seizure sources (Nunez et al., 1994; Roth et al., 1997; Scherg and Ebersole, 1994; Scherg et al. 2002).

Features in a future ideal EEG system can be envisioned, however, by combining recording and software technologies developed at a number of different research centers (Dunseath

Table 41.3. A Comparison of Early, Current, and "Future" Computer EEG Systems

First-Generation Systems	Second-Generation Systems	Future "Ideal" Systems
Emulate analog EEG	Standard electrodes, high-capacity computer, windows OS	High-impedance recording systems requiring no manual scalp preparation or electrode measurements
Limited sampling, 8 bits	200–400 samples/sec, 12 bits	≥400 samples/sec, ≥12 bits 1,000 samples/sec (has been achieved by a few systems)
Limited filters	Flexible FIR filters	Advanced adaptive and spatial filters
Slow review, poor display resolution	Fast paging, slow scroll review, acceptable display resolution	Rapid page and scroll review display resolution > visual resolution
Not networked	Networked	High-capacity networks
Expensive storage media	Inexpensive, medium capacity storage media	Inexpensive, high capacity storage media, rapid indexing
Proprietary file formats	Proprietary file formats	"Translatable" or generic data formats
No report writers	Limited report writers and database filing	Report writers and integrated database filing, analyzed data in database for serial and population comparisons
Limited analysis tools	Integrated voltage/spectral analysis and mapping, automatic spike detection	Advanced analysis tools: high-resolution EEG and source localization on custom head models and 3D images
		On-line EEG atlas/dictionary with AI waveform matching and screening

and Kelly, 1995; Gevins et al., 1996; Lesser et al., 1992; Qu and Gotman, 1993; Taheri et al., 1994; Towle et al., 1995; Yoo, 1997) (Table 41.3). Ideal systems could include high digital sampling rates, accurate and rapid display modes, and high-capacity networks and clinical databases. Systems could include advanced artificial intelligence with waveform matching tools that call up reference waveforms and definitions from a dictionary similar to word processor spell checking systems. The user could select the correct match, with the patient's specific results compared to a clinical reference database. This software aide could eventually screen EEG for significant normal and abnormal patterns (Nakamura et al., 1996). A major advance would be high-resolution recording systems that do not require skin preparation or manual measurements to place scalp electrodes. A feasible system would use a 32- to 64-channel electrode helmet with high-impedance amplifiers mounted on electrode cylinders as described by Dunseath and Kelly (1995). Electrodes could slide against the scalp, and positions relative to the spherical helmet would be digitally measured. This would provide an accurate 3D head model and multichannel recordings. These could be used alone for routine high-resolution recording and source modeling or integrated with MRI.

References

American Electroencephalographic Society. 1994. Guidelines for recording clinical EEG on digital media. J. Clin. Neurophysiol. 11:114–115.

ASTM Standard Designation. 1992. E1467–92 specification for transferring digital neurophysiological data between independent computer systems. Available from: ASTM, 1916 Race Street, Philadelphia, PA 19103.

Babiloni, F., Babiloni, C., Carducci, F., et al. 1996. Spline Laplacian estimate of EEG potentials over a realistic magnetic resonance–constructed scalp surface model. Electroencephalogr. Clin. Neurophysiol. 98:363–374.

Bendat, J.S., and Piersol, A.G. 1980. *Engineering Applications of Correlation and Spectral Analysis.* New York: John Wiley.

Brigham, E.O. 1988. *The Fast Fourier Transform and Its Applications,* Ed. A.V. Oppenheim. Englewood Cliffs, NJ: Prentice Hall.

Claassen, J., and Mayer, S.A. 2002. Continuous electroencephalographic monitoring in neurocritical care. Curr. Neurol. Neurosci. Rep. 2(6):534–540.

Duffy, F.H. 1989. Clinical value of topographic mapping and quantified neurophysiology. Arch. Neurol. 46:1133–1134.

Duffy, F.H., Hughes, J.R., Miranda, F., et al. 1994. Status of quantitative EEG (QEEG) in clinical practice. Clin. Electroencephalogr. 25:vi–xxii.

Dunseath, W.J., and Kelly, E.F. 1995. Multichannel PC–Based data–acquisition system for high–resolution EEG. IEEE Trans. Biomed. Eng. 42:1212–1217.

Elger, C.E., and Burr, W. 2000. Advances in telecommunications concerning epilepsy. Epilepsia 41(suppl 5):S9–12.

Fisher, R.S., Webber, W.R.S., Lesser, R.P., et al. 1992. High-frequency EEG activity at the start of seizures. J. Clin. Neurophysiol. 9:441–448.

Gevins, A., Le, J., Martin, N.K., et al. 1994. High resolution EEG: 124–channel recording, spatial deblurring and MRI integration methods. Electroencephalogr. Clin. Neurophysiol. 90(5):337–358.

Gevins, A., Smith, M.E., Le, J., et al. 1996. High resolution evoked potential imaging of the cortical dynamics of human working memory. Electroencephalogr. Clin. Neurophysiol. 98(4):327–348.

Gotman, J. 1987. Computer analysis during intensive monitoring of epileptic patients. Adv. Neurol. 46:249–269.

Hellmann, G., Kuhn, M., Prosch, M., et al. 1996. Extensible biosignal (EBS) file format: simple method for EEG data exchange. Electroencephalogr. Clin. Neurophysiol. 99:416–426.

Iguchi, H., Watanabe, K., Kozato, A., et al. 1994. Wearable electroencephalograph system with preamplified electrodes. Med. Biol. Eng. Comput. 32:459–461.

Ille, N., Berg, P., and Scherg, M. 2002. Artifact correction of the ongoing EEG using spatial filters based on artifact and brain signal topographies. J. Clin. Neurophysiol. 19(2):113–124.

Itil, K.Z. 1993. Responses to the views and commentary on "Standard Specification for Transferring Digital Neurophysiological Data Between Independent Computer Systems." J. Clin. Neurophysiol. 10:535–536.

Jacobs, E.C. 1993. Responses to the views and commentary on "Standard Specification for Transferring Digital Neurophysiological Data Between Independent Computer Systems." J. Clin. Neurophysiol. 10:538–539.

John, E.R. 1989. The role of quantitative EEG topographic mapping of "neurometrics" in the diagnosis of psychiatric and neurological disorders: the pros. Electroencephalogr. Clin Neurophysiol. 73:2–4.

Kemp, B., and Olivan, J. 2003. European data format "plus" (EDF+), an EDF alike standard format for the exchange of physiological data. Clin. Neurophysiol. 114:1755–1761. Web site: *http://www.hsr.nl/edf/edfplus.htm.*

Kemp, B., Varri, A., Rosa, A.C., et al. 1992. A simple format for exchange of digitized polygraphic recordings. Electroencephalogr. Clin. Neurophysiol. 82(5):391–393. Web site: *http://www.hsr.nl/edf.*

Krauss, G.L., Lesser, R.P., Fisher, R.S., et al. 1992. Anterior "cheek" electrodes are comparable to sphenoidal electrodes for the identification of ictal activity. Electroencephalogr. Clin. Neurophysiol. 83:333–338.

Künkel, H. 1977. Historical review of principal methods. In *EEG Informatics: A Didactic Review of Methods and Applications of EEG Data Processing,* Ed. A. Remond. New York: Elsevier Scientific.

Lagerlund, T.D. 2003. ACNS Medical Instrumentation Committee Meeting. Minutes of September 17.

Lagerlund, T.D., Cascino, G.D., Cicora, K.M., et al. 1996. Long-term electroencephalographic monitoring for diagnosis and management of seizures. Mayo Clin. Proc. 71:1000–1006.

Lesser, R.P., Webber, W.R.S., and Fisher, R.S. 1992. Design principles for computerized monitoring. Electroencephalogr. Clin. Neurophysiol. 82: 239–247.

Lopes da Silva, F.H. 1990. A critical review of clinical applications of topographic mapping of brain potentials. J. Clin. Neurophysiol. 7:535–551.

Nakamura, M., Sugi, T., Ikeda, A., et al. 1996. Clinical application of automatic integrative interpretation of awake background EEG: quantitative interpretation, report making, and detection of artifacts and reduced vigilance level. Electroencephalogr. Clin. Neurophysiol. 98(2):103–113.

Nunez, P.L., Silberstein, R.B., Cadusch, P.J., et al. 1994. A theoretical and experimental study of high resolution EEG based on surface Laplacians and cortical imaging. Electroencephalogr. Clin. Neurophysiol. 90:40–57.

Nuwer, M.R. 1990a. The development of EEG brain mapping. J. Clin. Neurophysiol. 7:459–471.

Nuwer, M.R. 1990b. Paperless electroencephalography. Semin. Neurol. 10: 178–184.

Nuwer, M.R. 1997. Assessment of digital EEG, quantitative EEG, and EEG brain mapping: report of the American Academy of Neurology and the American Clinical Neurophysiological Society. Neurology 49: 277–292.

Nuwer, M.R., Lehmann, D., Lopes de Silva, F., et al. 1994. IFCN guidelines for topographic and frequency analysis of EEGs and EPs: report of an IFCN Committee. Electroencephalogr. Clin. Neurophysiol. 91:1–5.

Qu, H., and Gotman, J. 1993. Improvement in seizure detection performance by automatic adaptation to the EEG of each patient. Electroencephalogr. Clin. Neurophysiol. 86(2):79–87.

Qu, H., and Gotman, J. 1995. A seizure warning system for long–term epilepsy monitoring. Neurology 45(12):2250–2254.

Remond, A. 1977. *Why Analyze, Quantify, or Process Routine Clinical EEG? EEG Informatics: A Didactic Review of Methods and Applications of EEG Data Processing.* New York: Elsevier Scientific.

Risk, W.S. 1993. Viewing speed and frequency resolution in digital EEG. Electroencephalogr. Clin. Neurophysiol. 87:347–353.

Roth, B.J., Ko, D., von Albertini–Carletti, I.R., et al. 1997. Dipole localization in patients with epilepsy using the realistically shaped head model. Electroencephalogr. Clin. Neurophysiol. 102(3):159–166.

Salinsky, M.C., Oken, B.S., Kramer, R.E., et al. 1992. A comparison of quantitative EEG frequency analysis and conventional EEG in patients with focal brain lesions. Electroencephalogr. Clin. Neurophysiol. 83:358–366.

Scherg, M., and Ebersole, J.S. 1994. Brain source imaging of focal and multifocal epileptiform EEG activity. Neurophysiol. Clin. 24:51–60.

Scherg, M., Ille, N., Bornfleth, H., et al. 2002. Advanced tools for digital EEG review: virtual source montages, whole-head mapping, correlation, and phase analysis. J. Clin. Neurophysiol. 19(2):91–112.

Soininen, H., Partanen, J., Laulumaa, V., et al. 1989. Longitudinal EEG spectral analysis in early stage of Alzheimer's disease: 3–year follow–up and clinical outcome. Electroencephalogr. Clin. Neurophysiol. 72:290–297.

Taheri, B.A., Knight, R.T., and Smith, R.L. 1994. A dry electrode for EEG recording. Electroencephalogr. Clin. Neurophysiol. 90(5):376–383.

Thatcher, R.W., Biver, C.J., and North, D.M. 2003. Quantitative EEG and the Frye and Daubert standards of admissibility. Clin. Electroencephalogr. 34(2):39–53.

Towle, V.L., Cohen, S., Alperin, N., et al. 1995. Displaying electrocorticographic findings on gyral anatomy. Electroencephalogr. Clin. Neurophysiol. 94(4):221–228.

Webber, W.R., Lesser, R.P., Richardson, R.T., et al. 1996. An approach to seizure detection using an artificial neural network. Electroencephalogr. Clin. Neurophysiol. 98:250–273.

Yoo, S., Guttman, C.R., Ives, J.R., et al. 1997. 3D localization of surface 10–20 EEG electrodes on high resolution anatomical MR images. Electroencephalogr. Clin. Neurophysiol. 102(4):335–339.

42. EEG Monitoring During Carotid Endarterectomy and Open Heart Surgery

Warren T. Blume and Frank W. Sharbrough

Carotid Endarterectomy

Purpose

Carotid endarterectomy is a surgical procedure designed to prevent ischemic stroke distal to carotid artery stenosis. The North American Symptomatic Carotid Endarterectomy Trial (1991) found it effective in preventing stroke among patients with recent (<4 months) hemispheric transient ischemic attacks (TIAs) or nondisabling strokes, which have a high-grade stenosis (70–94%) of the internal carotid artery. Such patients who underwent carotid endarterectomy had 17% lower incidence of ipsilateral stroke and 15% lower incidence of any stroke over 2 years' follow-up compared to similar patients treated medically. Of importance is the limitation of this study to centers previously demonstrating a low carotid endarterectomy (CE) complication rate. Barnett et al. (2003) have reaffirmed the effectiveness of CE: "All patients with symptoms related to *severe carotid stenosis* fare better with CE than with medical care alone. In the absence of life-threatening disease they should receive CE." CE risk slightly exceeds that of medical management for moderate (50–69%) stenosis, although CE gave some benefit. Below 50% stenosis no benefit was found. Adequate proof of effectiveness of CE for asymptomatic stenosis has yet to be achieved (Mayberg, 2003).

Controversy surrounds whether a shunt should be used. The electroencephalographer may be involved in this question, which is discussed below.

Procedure

Anesthesia

General anesthesia has been preferred (Ferguson, 1982a; Ferguson and Gamache, 1984), using nitrous oxide and oxygen with isoflurane. This combination may be supplemented equally well by fentanyl or remifentanil (Doyle et al., 2001). An alternative anesthetic regimen consists of nitrous oxide in oxygen and propofol after induction with etomidate and fentanyl (Laman et al., 2001). Propofol may produce less clamp-related delta activity than other anesthetic agents (Laman et al., 2001). As with other anesthetic agents, the sequential diffuse changes as anesthesia deepens are an increase in beta activity, then delta, then burst suppression (Borgeat et al., 1991; Ebrahim et al., 1994; Newman et al., 1995; Reddy et al., 1992). General anesthesia is considered to provide cerebral protection by reducing the patient's metabolism and permitting precise control of systemic blood pressure and arterial gas concentrations throughout the procedure. Depth of anesthesia can be guided by electroencephalography (EEG).

A renewed interest in local anesthesia (LA) via a regional cervical block has emerged (Calligaro et al., 2001; Harbaugh and Pikus, 2001; Krenn et al., 2002; McCarthy et al., 2002; Stoneburner et al., 2002; Wellman et al. 1998). Prospectively comparing local with general anesthesia, McCarthy et al. (2002) found increased tolerance to carotid clamping as indicated by greater postclamp middle cerebral artery velocity with LA, yet major complications occurred equally often but rarely in each group.

Operation

After adequate exposure of the distal common carotid artery, the carotid bifurcation, and the internal carotid artery (well beyond the upper end of the plaque), the common, external, and internal carotid arteries are clamped so that the arteriotomy and endarterectomy can be performed.

Whether or not a shunt should be placed between the distal common carotid and internal carotid arteries during the 30 to 45 minutes that the vessels are clamped is an unresolved controversy. Shunts are placed in the belief that carotid vessel clamping can reduce cerebral blood flow below the threshold of ischemic tolerance. Some surgical teams use shunts routinely (Giannotta et al., 1980; Thompson et al., 1970); others never do (Allen and Preziosi, 1981; Baker et al., 1977; Bland and Lazar, 1981; Ott et al., 1980; Whitney et al., 1980). Still others place shunts if indicated by one or more monitoring techniques (Ojemann et al., 1975; Sundt et al., 1981).

In these three groups of studies, the reported incidence of perioperative stroke was highest among those using shunts routinely and lowest among those never using shunts. These data suggest that intraoperative or postoperative strokes are more likely caused by embolism than diminished cerebral blood flow and thus question the value of shunting and monitoring (Brown et al., unpublished; Ferguson, 1982b) (see Significance of Clamp-Associated EEG Changes, below, for further discussion). Accurate comparison of these methods can be made only by a prospective single surgical team study, as the major factors determining risk of endarterectomy are likely surgical and anesthetic techniques (Ferguson, 1982a; Ferguson and Gamache, 1984).

Supporting this view, the Cochrane Stroke Group trials register (Counsell et al., 2000) found no difference between routine shunting and no shunting for all stroke, ipsilateral stroke, or death within 30 postoperative days. They also indicate that large-scale randomized trials using no shunting as the control group would be required to settle this issue.

Stroke in the postoperative period may occur from thrombus at the operative site. This threat is guarded against by monitoring the neurological examination, retinal artery pressures, and the EEG. Thus, there are at least two times in the procedure when EEG monitoring may prove helpful: during clamping and in the immediate postoperative period.

Intraoperative Monitoring of Cerebral Hemodynamics

For those employing shunts electively, monitoring cerebral blood flow and electrical activity has become an important tool in this decision.

So that the correlative value of EEG findings during carotid endarterectomy can be appreciated, three other monitoring methods for operations under general anesthesia will be described.

Carotid Stump Pressure (CSP)

Measurement of residual pressure in the internal carotid system following temporary occlusion of the common and external carotid arteries has been thought to reflect arterial pressure in the circle of Willis and thus to indicate the collateral blood supply to the hemisphere of the occluded vessel (Wilkinson et al., 1965). Although earlier reports doubted its usefulness (Beebe et al., 1978; Sundt et al., 1977), later studies obtained close correlation of CSP with EEG changes and patency of the contralateral carotid artery. For example, Cherry et al. (1991) and Harada et al. (1995) reported EEG changes in 73% and 58% of patients whose CSP was <25 mm Hg, 32% of those at 25 to 50 mm Hg, and only 2% and 4% when CSP exceeded 50 mm Hg. Similarly, Brown et al. (unpublished), in a study of 487 carotid endarterectomies, found a low incidence of EEG change when mean CSP exceeded 40 mm Hg, and an increasing incidence below that level. Their study found EEG and CSP equally capable of detecting intraoperative hemodynamic stroke.

Transcranial Doppler (TCD)

TCD monitoring of middle cerebral artery flow velocity (MCAV) may also assess dependence of the ipsilateral hemisphere on MCA blood supply (Arnold et al., 1997; Fiori et al., 1997, McCarthy et al., 2002). Stenosis or occlusion of the contralateral carotid artery was associated with larger MCAV decreases upon clamping (Arnold et al., 1997). TCD may also detect signals representing embolic flow after clamp release (Fiori et al., 1997). Near-infrared spectroscopy assesses the hemodynamic effect of carotid clamping as well as does TCD (Hirofumi et al., 2003; Vernieri et al., 2003).

Cerebral Blood Flow (CBF) by Xenon-133

CBF is measured by extracranial detection of xenon-133 injected into either the internal carotid artery above the atheromatous plaque or the common carotid artery below the plaque with the external carotid artery occluded. Mean hemisphere flow is calculated immediately from a 2-minute initial slope technique. Measurements are made before, during, and after clamping (Ferguson and Gamache, 1984; Sharbrough et al., 1973; Sundt et al., 1981). The Mayo group has always placed a shunt for values less than 18 mL $\cdot$ 100 g^{-1} $\cdot$ min^{-1} and commonly for flows less than 30 mL $\cdot$ 100 g^{-1} $\cdot$ min^{-1}

(Sundt et al., 1977) even if the EEG remained unchanged (Sundt et al., 1981). This method is less commonly used now in favor of the above-mentioned procedures.

The relative costs of intraoperative monitoring methods should be considered. In Canada, EEG monitoring costs about one hundred times that of CSP measurement. Thus, Ferguson's group in London measures CSP routinely and adds EEG monitoring only for cases considered preoperatively to be at higher risk for poor collateral blood flow (Brown et al., unpublished).

EEG Monitoring

Intraoperative EEG monitors cerebral cortical function at a time when clinical evaluation is not possible in a patient under general anesthesia. A monitoring system should provide rapid and reliable demonstration of electroencephalographic activity in the operating room while interfering minimally with the course of the endarterectomy. Reliability of such monitoring requires a well-defined set of baseline values for the individual patient and a set of criteria to distinguish mild to moderate from severe alterations. Variations of EEG activity due to nonsurgical factors such as changes in anesthetic level, blood pressure, or other physiological aspects should be known by the monitoring team.

Technique

Because EEG changes during carotid endarterectomy can be diffuse or regional and because the specter of uncorrectable artifact from electrodes under surgical drapes is ever-present, 16 channels of EEG data are preferable. We apply 16 to 19 scalp electrodes according to the 10–20 system, omitting ear placements. Some centers use only frontopolar, central, parietal, occipital and midtemporal placements while adding electrocardiogram (ECG) and a movement transducer (Jenkins et al., 1983). Use of at least 16 recording channels is necessary to adequately depict activity from these regions.

Electrodes are applied with collodion to ensure stable performance throughout the procedure. A bipolar anterior-posterior montage is less prone to artifact and electrical interference and gives easily appreciated interhemispheric comparative data. Agreement about the optimum linear frequency span has yet to be achieved among the several centers. Thus, at University Hospital, London, the low linear frequency is set at 0.3 Hz and the high linear frequency at 70 Hz, whereas the Mayo Clinic span is 1 to 15 or 30 Hz. Sixty-cycle filtering is needed in the operating room electrical environment.

Because reduction of relatively low-amplitude beta activity is the most common initial EEG change with carotid artery clamping, a sensitivity setting of 5 μV/mm or even 3 μV/mm is required.

Because a large amount of EEG data is generated at carotid endarterectomy and because attention is directed to changes in ongoing EEG activity more than morphology of individual waveforms, a paper speed of 5 or 15 mm/sec is preferred to the standard 30 mm/sec for the intraoperative recording (Sharbrough, 1983). If unusual EEG changes develop that are difficult to recognize at 5 mm/sec, simply increase the speed to 15 or 30 mm/sec to identify the pattern

(Guidelines on Intraoperative Electroencephalography by the American Clinical Neurophysiology Society, unpublished).

A preoperative, awake, resting EEG using at least the intraoperative montage can be recorded on the same day as the procedure. Focal or hemispheric abnormalities contralateral to the planned carotid endarterectomy increase the chance of a clamp-associated EEG change (Blume et al., 1986).

An at least 10-minute baseline preclamp recording while the patient is anesthetized is essential to appreciate any clamp-associated changes. The recording is continued for at least 10 minutes after clamp release to assure that any intraoperative changes have resolved. Some centers (Chiappa et al., 1979) record continuously from wakefulness through anesthesia to wakefulness, but the value of the initial transition is uncertain. Ideally, EEG monitoring in the recovery room would help to detect any postoperative carotid occlusion, but other methods are available (see above).

Symmetrical EEG Patterns During Anesthesia

Although much has been written about the different effects of various agents on the EEG during anesthesia, we are struck more by the similarity of the EEG patterns produced by different agents when used at concentrations below their minimal alveolar concentration (MAC) level (the level necessary to prevent movement to painful stimulus in about 50% of subjects). Therefore, the following subsections describe the several types of symmetrical EEG patterns seen when using concentrations of common agents (thiopental, halothane, desflurane, enflurane, isoflurane, sevoflurane, nitrous oxide), which produce a similar subanesthetic or anesthetic effect.

Patterns at Subanesthetic or Minimal Anesthetic Concentrations

Thiopental, halothane, enflurane, isoflurane, as well as 50% nitrous oxide, when administered at subanesthetic concentrations, all produce a similar pattern of drug-induced beta activity that is maximum anteriorly (Stockard and Bickford, 1975). In contrast, short-acting opiates (alfentanil, fentanyl, sufentanil) reportedly decrease beta and slow alpha (VanCott and Brenner, 2003).

EEG Changes with Induction

Most of the usual surgical inductions are carried out relatively rapidly with etomidate, propofol, or thiopental, which results in the following characteristic sequence of changes. Beta activity appears or augments and alpha vanishes. The beta activity, described under the subanesthetic pattern, rapidly becomes more widespread, increases in amplitude, and slows in frequency toward the alpha range. During this phase, the faster rhythm may be intermixed with a burst of high-amplitude, intermittent, rhythmic delta activity, usually frontally maximum [the frontal intermittent rhythmic delta activity (FIRDA) pattern] before a steady-state anesthetic pattern of the type to be described below is established.

Patterns at Sub-MAC Anesthetic Concentrations

At this lighter level of steady-state anesthesia, a characteristic widespread anteriorly maximum rhythmic (WAR) pattern, usually in the lower beta or alpha frequency range, is seen with all agents that we have studied including halothane, enflurane, isoflurane, and even thiopental (Figs.

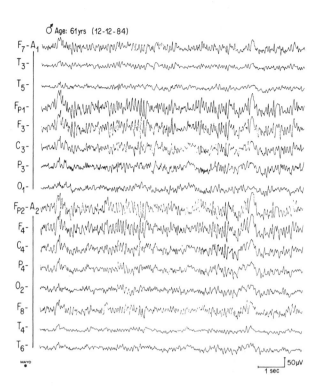

Figure 42.1. Some of the characteristic EEG patterns under anesthesia are well demonstrated in this referential montage and include (1) widespread anteriorly maximum rhythmic (WAR) alpha activity seen maximally in the Fp1,2 and F3,4 derivations; (2) occasional anterior intermittent slow waves (AIS) with a triangular waveform seen in the first second and the last 2 seconds, with highest amplitude in the Fp1,2 regions; (3) the more widespread, persistent slow wave (WPS) of longer wavelength and more irregular form best seen posteriorly.

42.1 and 42.2). The frequency of this pattern tends to slow with increasing concentrations of the agent. This anesthetic WAR pattern is strikingly similar to the postanoxic WAR alpha-coma pattern.

The origin of the postanoxic WAR pattern remains uncertain. However, the anesthetic WAR pattern, usually in the alpha frequency range, may be simply a drug-induced variant of beta activity (Sharbrough, 1982), which with anesthesia has become more widespread, higher in amplitude, and has slowed in frequency from the upper beta range to the lower beta range and finally into the alpha or even theta range. In humans, this anesthetic WAR pattern tends to be much more continuous than normal sleep spindles. In cats, the pattern tends to be more intermittent and bears a closer resemblance to sleep spindles. Even in cats, however, the WAR pattern may not represent the same mechanism as normal sleep spindles and is more closely related to the drug-induced beta activity seen with subanesthetic concentrations of these agents (Stockard and Bickford, 1975).

In addition to the WAR anesthetic pattern, there are often anteriorly maximum intermittent slow (AIS) waves that are commonly diphasic, with a sharply contoured, initially negative phase being followed by a more rounded positive phase (Fig. 42.1). These AIS waves characteristically have a duration of less than 1 second and may occur either singly or

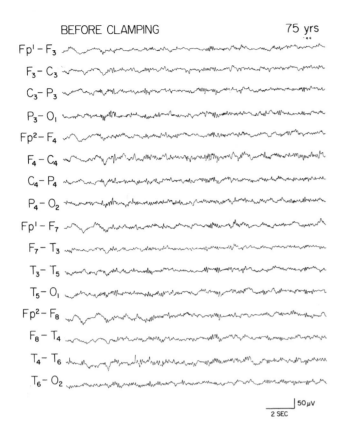

BEFORE CLAMPING   75 yrs

Fp' – F₃

F₃ – C₃

C₃ – P₃

P₃ – O₁

Fp² – F₄

F₄ – C₄

C₄ – P₄

P₄ – O₂

Fp' – F₇

F₇ – T₃

T₃ – T₅

T₅ – O₁

Fp² – F₈

F₈ – T₄

T₄ – T₆

T₆ – O₂

50 μV
2 SEC

Figure 42.2.   Right carotid endarterectomy. WAR, AIS, and WPS patterns on bipolar montage. Note the slower paper speed than used in Figure 42.1.

in brief trains. When preceded by a waxing WAR pattern, they may resemble a mitten pattern.

In addition to the AIS waves described above, more widespread persistent slow (WPS) waves, often of lower amplitude, may become prominent (Figs. 42.1 and 42.2). The duration of these individual polymorphic slow waves usually exceeds 1 second. This activity may be maximally expressed posteriorly and in the temporal regions. This pattern is least obvious with halothane and enflurane and is most prominent with isoflurane. Although nitrous oxide alone is not potent enough to be an anesthetic agent at atmospheric pressure, it potentiates the effects of other inhalation agents. During "balanced anesthesia" 50% nitrous oxide is commonly used in combination with other agents. In this situation, the WPS pattern tends to be more prominent than when only a single agent is used. With deepening levels of anesthesia there is an increase in the amplitude and wavelength of the WPS pattern and a decrease in WAR pattern frequency. Rhythmic delta bursts may occur if anesthesia is suddenly increased.

Patterns with Supra-MAC Concentrations

Anesthetic agents begin to demonstrate their most unique and idiosyncratic effects when concentration levels are pushed above MAC. For instance, enflurane may elicit spike-and-wave activity around 1.5 MAC. Between 2 and 3 MAC, bursts of high-voltage spikes are often separated by periods

of relative inactivity. At this level seizures may be elicited, especially when activated by hyperventilation (Stockard and Bickford, 1975). In contrast, isoflurane tends to exert a prominent antiepileptic effect with intermittent inactivity at 1.5 MAC and frequently loss of all EEG activity between 2 and 2.5 MAC. Halothane also has an antiepileptic effect, but may not produce EEG inactivity even with concentrations as high as 4 MAC. The ability of an agent such as desflurane and isoflurane to more rapidly produce EEG suppression or burst suppression at supra-MAC levels correlates with its tendency to produce more WPS at sub-MAC levels.

Although nitrous oxide itself is not an anesthetic agent, its combination with other agents may produce inactivity at a lower concentration of the primary anesthetic agent.

EEG Patterns with Emergence from Anesthesia and with Other Changes in Anesthetic Level

Discontinuing anesthesia from a sub-MAC level is followed by characteristic changes. The WAR pattern decreases in amplitude and increases in frequency and almost always moves into the beta range before the patient can be aroused. The WPS pattern gradually decreases before the patient is arousable. During the transition from the anesthetic to the arousable state, bursts of intermittent rhythmic delta may occur, which resemble the FIRDA pattern seen with induction. These bursts are less prominent with emergence than with induction, possibly due to the slower rate of emergence than induction.

Other Factors Affecting Symmetrical EEG Patterns

Factors besides the quantity of anesthetics used can alter the EEG diffusely. Thus, decreasing the $Paco_2$ level below 40 mm Hg as well as decreasing the amount of stimulation that would be painful if awake could produce a pattern suggestive of a deeper level of anesthesia. The converse also applies. Such principles apply primarily during lighter sub-MAC levels of anesthesia. Such factors may explain sudden diffuse EEG changes in the absence of any action by the anesthetist. Progressive hypothermia slows the EEG frequency spectrum with gradual reduction in amplitude leading to inactivity at about 25°C. Hypothermia also augments the EEG effects of anesthetic agents.

Preclamp Focal Abnormalities During Anesthesia

The majority of patients undergoing endarterectomy show a symmetrical baseline pattern of the type described above. However, depending on case selection, 30% to 40% may show a focal abnormality of varying degrees of severity (Sundt et al., 1981). The focal abnormality consists of unilateral reduction of the amplitude of the WAR anesthetic pattern by greater than 30% to 40% (Fig. 42.3). This is usually associated with increase in the wavelength and amplitude of persistent polymorphic delta on the side of the reduced amplitude. The delta pattern can generally be distinguished from the usual WPS pattern during anesthesia by its longer wavelength, irregular form, and higher amplitude on the abnormal side. In a majority of cases, a focal baseline EEG abnormality correlates with preoperative clinical deficits. However, a smaller percentage of patients with such baseline abnormalities have only experienced TIAs, presumably on a hemodynamic basis.

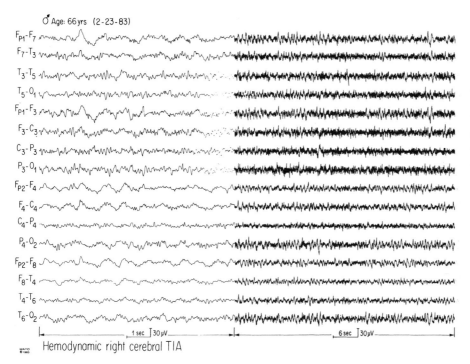

♂ Age: 66 yrs (2-23-83)

Fp1-F7

F7-T3

T3-T5

T5-O1

Fp1-F3

F3-C3

C3-P3

P3-O1

Fp2-F4

F4-C4

C4-P4

P4-O2

Fp2-F8

F8-T4

T4-T6

T6-O2

|— 1 sec ⌐30 µV —| |— 6 sec ⌐30 µV —|

Hemodynamic right cerebral TIA

Figure 42.3. EEG under isoflurane anesthesia. This patient had 98% right carotid stenosis, low right retinal artery pressure, and posturally related right cerebral transient ischemic attacks (TIAs) presumably on a hemodynamic basis. Although there was no preoperative residual clinical deficit, the EEG showed right-sided reduction of faster anesthetic components with increase in amount, duration, and persistence of irregular slowing in the right hemisphere. These abnormalities can be appreciated at the usual paper speed of 30 mm/sec (*left segment*) as well as the slower paper speed of 6 mm/sec (*right segment*).

A preoperative focal anesthetic EEG abnormality usually correlates with a preoperative waking EEG abnormality. However, anesthesia may activate an abnormality that was either inapparent or less apparent during the waking trace. On the other hand, anesthesia may obscure an abnormality apparent on the awake EEG. Anesthesia is likely to activate an abnormality that is minimal or inapparent during the waking state in the case of an anterior hemispheric insult that has left the alpha pattern normal and symmetrical. Despite such a normal awake symmetrical alpha pattern, the anesthetic record may show a major reduction in the WAR pattern and an increase in the irregular slowing in the anterior distribution. In these cases any drug-induced beta activity seen during the preanesthetic state almost always is reduced on the side of a reduced anesthetic WAR pattern, giving further evidence that the anesthetic alpha frequency WAR pattern is more directly related to drug-induced beta rhythm than it is to the normal waking alpha rhythm.

Anesthesia may convert intermittent rhythmic delta in the temporal region on the side of ischemia to a more obvious and more persistent focal slowing, along with reduction in the WAR pattern. On the other hand, a more posterior lesion, producing significant abnormality in the alpha pattern, may leave the anesthetic WAR pattern symmetrical without obvious focal slowing. In such a case, the preanesthetic beta pattern is usually also symmetrical.

Finally, the nonlocalizing FIRDA, or more persistent generalized slowing, which is easily recognized as abnormal during the waking state, cannot be identified as abnormal during anesthesia because these patterns commonly occur in most patients at some stage of anesthesia regardless of whether or not they have had previous central nervous system (CNS) disease.

Intraoperative EEG Changes

When the preclamp EEG shows only the symmetrical anesthetic patterns without overriding focal features, appreciation of clamp-related alterations is usually straightforward. However, when ipsilateral regional abnormalities precede clamping, a 20- to 30-second sample should be visible to the electroencephalographer as such abnormalities commonly fluctuate enough to render comparisons difficult.

Two types of clamp-related alterations may occur: (a) a decreased amplitude of all activity including delta and faster components, and (b) an increase in amplitude and wave duration of delta. These modifications may occur ipsilaterally or bilaterally (Chiappa et al., 1979; Sharbrough et al., 1973). Both modifications often occur together. An increased delta activity is almost always associated with a decrease in amplitude of higher frequency activity (Figs. 42.4 and 42.5). The quantity of delta activity that accompanies reductions in higher frequency activity may depend partly on the high band-pass filter used. Figure 42.6 illustrates a marked reduction of all frequencies including delta using a high band-pass filter of 1.0 Hz, whereas Figure 42.7, with the filter at 0.3 Hz, shows augmentation of very slow delta with reduction of other frequencies. Augmentation of delta reflects a less severe reduction of blood flow than does attenuation of all EEG activity (compare Figs. 42.4 and 42.6).

In the absence of a contralateral carotid occlusion or severe stenosis, EEG changes with clamping are usually only ipsilateral (Figs. 42.5 to 42.8). Bilateral clamp-related changes usually occur with a severe compromise in contralateral blood flow (Fig. 42.4). The incidence of unilateral change is more than twice that of bilateral change (Blume et al., 1986). Some type of visibly apparent clamp-related

Figure 42.4. Right carotid endarterectomy. This EEG (paper speed 15 mm/sec) during right carotid clamping shows the type of EEG change seen with a less severe reduction in cerebral blood flow. There is increased amplitude of slow-wave activity, with a frequency greater than 1 Hz, associated with simultaneous reduction in faster frequency components. The prominent bilateral change in this, as in most such cases, is related to a preexisting carotid occlusion contralateral to clamping. The major change is on the *right*, the side of the clamping, and the less severe change is contralateral where there is relatively preserved background posteriorly.

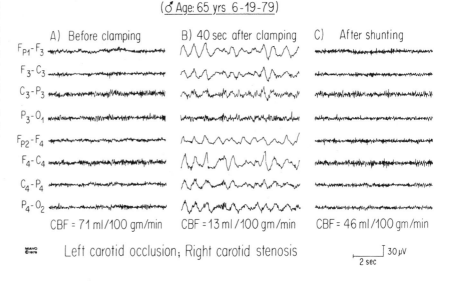

change occurred in 31% of the University Hospital, London, series and in 28% of the Mayo Clinic experience (Blume et al., 1986; Sundt et al., 1981).

Although gradations occur, it is remarkably easy to distinguish major or severe changes from moderate alterations. A major change consists of attenuation of all activity by at least 75% and/or a twofold or more increase of <1 Hz delta activity. Attenuation occurs far more commonly as a major change (Figs. 42.6 to 42.8) and may be accompanied by augmentation of <1 Hz activity. Attenuation of delta activity may occur with especially marked major changes. Major changes appeared in 12.5% of the University Hospital, London, experience but only 3% to 4% of the Mayo series. Many factors could account for this slight difference in incidence of major change: the subjective element in assessing nonprocessed EEG, different high band-pass filter frequencies, varying anesthetic techniques, and different patient populations.

A moderate change is attenuation of nondelta activity to about 50% of its preclamp amount and/or an obvious and persistent increase of delta activity at greater than 1 Hz. Moderate changes occurred in 19% of the London series (Blume et al., 1986) (Fig. 42.5).

Clamp-related changes appear within the first minute of clamping in over 80% of patients and within the first 20 seconds in 69%. As would be expected, major changes begin earlier, over 80% within the first 20 seconds (Blume et al., 1986) (Figs. 42.6 to 42.8).

Transient, focal or regional changes, occurring at times other than with carotid artery clamping, can be seen in a small percentage of cases. The majority of these may be due to asymmetrical effects of changing levels of anesthesia on a preexisting focal abnormality and therefore is of no consequence (Sundt et al., 1981). However, approximately 1% of patients develop a persistent focal EEG change during the endarterectomy itself, which is unassociated with carotid

Figure 42.5. Left carotid endarterectomy. A second example of a moderate change in the left hemisphere after clamping the left internal carotid artery showing a moderate reduction of the WAR pattern in the left hemisphere. A slight diminution in WAR frequency amplitude in the right hemisphere is also evident. The moderate increase in diffuse delta may be due to factors other than clamping (see text). The slightly greater increase in left hemisphere delta may result from clamping.

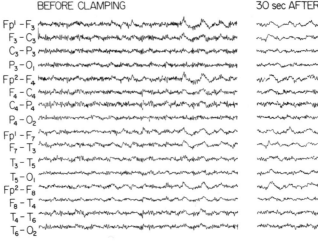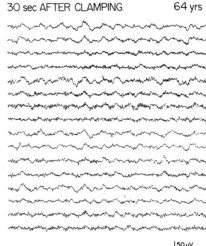

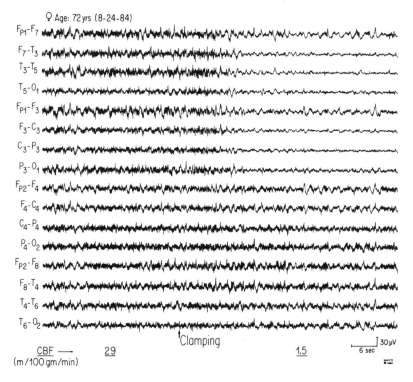

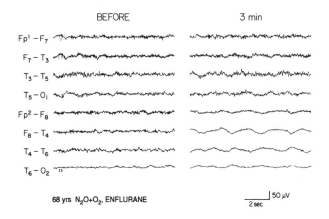

Figure 42.6. Left carotid endarterectomy. This EEG (paper speed 6 mm/sec) during left carotid clamping shows the major change commonly seen with severe reduction of cerebral blood flow (in this case, to 1.5 mL $\cdot$ 100 $g^{-1} \cdot min^{-1}$). The left central head regions show attenuation of all EEG activity (both fast- and slow-wave activity) by greater than 50%. The least affected region on the left is the frontopolar area, and the next least affected is the occipital region. These areas may receive collateral blood supply from the anterior and posterior communicating arteries and the basilar system.

clamping and which is ultimately associated with a neurological deficit in the immediate postoperative period. This change likely represents embolization, probably from the operative site (Brown et al., unpublished).

Cerebral blood flow measurement techniques, when combined with EEG phenomena, may distinguish hemodynamic-related EEG changes from embolism. Ischemic-related EEG changes caused by decreased perfusion pressure beyond the clamped carotid artery are always associated with a low blood flow as measured by the xenon technique or TCD. However, if an EEG change persists and is associated with a measured normal blood flow, this is virtually pathognomonic of embolization. This result occurs because embolic occlusion of a high percentage of vessels may still give normal or increased flow as the xenon technique and TCD study the remaining patent arteries; the occluded vessels do not contribute to the overall measurement of flow.

Figure 42.7. Major change. This EEG (paper speed 15 mm/sec) during right carotid clamping is recorded with a high band-pass filter of 0.3 Hz (EEGs in Figs. 42.4 and 42.6 were recorded with a high band-pass filter of 1 Hz). With clamping, there is reduction in amplitude of faster frequency components, but an increase in amplitude of the long wavelength delta with a frequency of less than 0.5 Hz. Had this EEG been recorded with a high band-pass filter setting of 1 Hz, it is possible that the slow-wave activity would have been instrumentally reduced to a very low voltage level. Effects of different high band-pass filters are discussed in the text.

Predictability of EEG Change

Clamp-related EEG modifications occur more commonly in patients with contralateral abnormalities on the preoperative awake EEG than in patients with only ipsilateral or diffuse abnormalities (Blume et al., 1986). Similarly, when the contralateral carotid artery is more than 90% stenosed, there is greater incidence of a clamp-associated EEG change than when that artery is less than 50% stenosed (Arnold et al., 1997). Cherry et al. (1991) reported a 48% incidence of clamp-related EEG changes with contralateral carotid occlusion compared to 18% to 21% when the artery was only stenotic or normal. Thirty-nine percent of patients with contralateral carotid occlusions had major clamp-related EEG changes compared to 16% with patent carotid arteries in the Schneider et al. (2002) study. Other studies (Brown et al., unpublished; Cherry et al., 1991; Harada et al., 1995) also found that the proportion of patients with severe EEG change and mean CSP <25 mm Hg increased with worsening severity of contralateral carotid artery stenosis. These relationships likely reflect the quantity of vascular disease in the

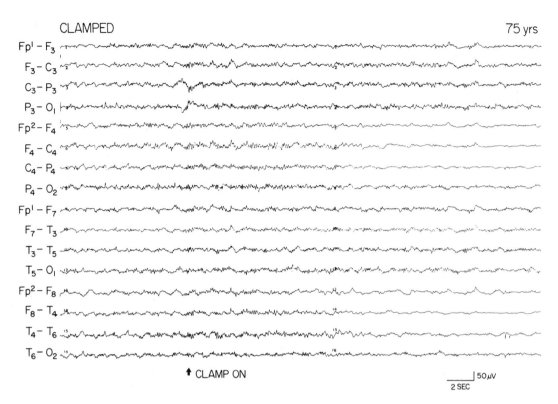

Figure 42.8. Right carotid endarterectomy. A continuously recorded example of a major change in the right hemisphere associated with clamping the right internal carotid artery: >75% reduction of higher frequency activity with some increase in right hemisphere delta activity. The left hemisphere exhibits no definite changes at this time. High band-pass filter = 0.3 Hz.

contralateral carotid system and therefore the capacity for collateral flow. In contrast, Brown et al. (unpublished) obtained no correlation of EEG change with ipsilateral patency.

Pathophysiology

Regional or diffuse clamp-related EEG changes can be due to one or more of the following: (a) decreased regional cerebral blood flow, (b) embolism, and (c) anesthetic level changes.

Two types of data indicate that sudden reduction in regional CBF accounts for the majority of clamp-associated EEG modifications: (a) in the Mayo experience where such changes prompted placement of a shunt, the EEG was almost always restored to its preclamp patterns; and (b) in the University Hospital, London, series without shunts, only 2 of 55 patients with clamp-associated EEG changes awoke with a neurological deficit, both among the 22 with major changes (see below). Therefore, the clinical significance of clamp-associated EEG changes hinges on the tolerance of the cerebral cortex to ischemia and the neuronal alterations that the changes represent.

There is a good correlation between regional cerebral blood flow and clamp-associated EEG changes. In the study of Sundt et al. (1981), all patients with blood flows of less than 10 mL $\cdot$ 100 g^{-1} $\cdot$ min^{-1} had clamp-associated EEG changes, but no patient whose regional cerebral blood flow exceeded 25 mL $\cdot$ 100 g^{-1} $\cdot$ min^{-1} had an EEG change. Shar-

brough et al. (1973) had found major EEG changes at blood flows below 18 mL $\cdot$ 100 g^{-1} $\cdot$ min^{-1}, minor changes from 18 to 23 mL $\cdot$ 100 g^{-1} $\cdot$ min^{-1}, and no change above 23 mL $\cdot$ 100 g^{-1} $\cdot$ min^{-1}. However, there is some range of cerebral blood flows for each EEG finding. Thus, Trojaborg and Boysen (1973) found EEG attenuation at regional cerebral blood flow values of 11 to 19 mL $\cdot$ 100 g^{-1} $\cdot$ min^{-1} and increased delta activity at 16 to 23 mL $\cdot$ 100 g^{-1} $\cdot$ min^{-1}. Such ranges suggest that other factors such as PaO$_2$ and PaCO$_2$ are likely involved. Subsequently, Messick et al. (1987) found EEG changes in six of eight patients with regional CBFs below 10 mL $\cdot$ 100 g^{-1} $\cdot$ min^{-1} but no EEG alterations in 23 patients above that level. This study was carried out during normocapnia and isoflurane-50% nitrous oxide and oxygen anesthesia.

The threshold for EEG changes varies somewhat with anesthetic agent. Michenfelder et al. (1987) defined the "critical cerebral blood flow" as that level below which the majority of patients developed EEG ischemic changes within 3 minutes of carotid occlusion. The critical CBF was approximately 10 mL $\cdot$ 100 g^{-1} $\cdot$ min^{-1} for isoflurane anesthesia, 15 mL $\cdot$ 100 g^{-1} $\cdot$ min^{-1} for enflurane, and 20 mL $\cdot$ 100 g^{-1} $\cdot$ min^{-1} for halothane. At very low flows (0-4 mL) most of the patients developed EEG changes and there were no differences among the anesthetics. However, at flows of 5 to 9, 10 to 14, and 15 to 19 mL $\cdot$ 100 g^{-1} $\cdot$ min^{-1}, the incidence of EEG changes with isoflurane was significantly less than with the other two anesthetics. At flows of 10 to 14 and 15 to 19 mL · 100 g^{-1} · min^{-1}, EEG ischemic changes occurred less commonly with enflurane than with halothane. Similarly, in their experience, isoflurane was associated with a significantly lower incidence of EEG ischemic changes (18%) than with either enflurane or halothane (26% and 25%, respectively). Isoflurane has been found to be a more potent cerebral metabolic depressant than halothane at concentrations up to 1.5 MAC in cats (Todd and Drummond, 1984).

An abrupt decrease in focal CBF restricts delivery of oxygen and glucose, substrates of oxidative phosphorylation upon which the brain almost exclusively depends for energy production (Dirnagl et al., 1999). With energy depletion, neurons and glia depolarize. Consequently, presynaptic and somatodendritic voltage-dependent calcium channels are activated and excitatory amino acids (EAAs) are released into the extracellular space. Energy-dependent EAA reuptake is decreased, adding to the amount of extracellular glutamate. Sodium, chloride, and water enter the neurons, causing cellular edema. Calcium ingress occurs, which (a) activates proteolytic enzymes that degrade cytoskeletal proteins; and (b) activates free radicals, which damage membranes, elicit inflammation, cause apoptosis, and impair mitochondrial function. All these events (and more) occur within minutes of blood flow restriction (Dirnagl et al., 2003).

If such changes reflect acute alteration of cerebral function, why are they reversible? First, there seem to be differences between the threshold of CBF producing EEG change, that leading to ion changes described above, and that producing neuronal damage. Studies in the baboon (Astrup et al., 1977) showed that extracellular potassium concentration in the cortex remained normal or slightly elevated at a point in ischemia when EEG activity ceased. Thus, there exists a range of perfusion values associated with loss of electrical activity, which is sufficient to maintain a close to normal tissue concentration of adenosine triphosphate (ATP). Unfortunately, the range between these levels is only moderate; the threshold for major EEG changes in humans is about 10 to 20 mL · 100 g^{-1} · min^{-1} (see above, and Sharbrough et al., 1973), whereas that for massive ionic changes in the baboon is about 10 mL · 100 g^{-1} · min^{-1} (Astrup et al., 1981).

However, as regional CBF values of a small percentage of patients would fall below both the threshold of producing severe EEG change and that producing energy failure, such margins cannot provide an entire answer to the question of reversibility. Several experimental studies have demonstrated such reversibility. Salford et al. (1973a,b) have shown that even a moderate hypoxia-induced energy imbalance does not lead to neuronal damage. Several authors (Crowell et al., 1970; Hossmann et al., 1977; Jones et al., 1981; Sundt and Michenfelder, 1972; Sundt et al., 1969) have documented full clinical recovery in about half of animals whose cortices were subjected to ischemia for periods ranging from 15 minutes to 3 hours. Heiss and Rosner (1983), using microelectrode recordings of single cell activity, found that postischemic viability was determined not only by residual blood flow but also by duration of ischemia. Their data suggest that for an occlusion time of 30 minutes, the threshold blood flow for functional and histological damage would be about 5 mL · 100 g^{-1} · min^{-1}.

Fortunately, factors exist that protect the brain somewhat from effects of clamp-induced carotid occlusion. First, the collateral blood supply is the most clinically assessable feature. Second, a previous subthreshold ischemic insult may have activated mechanisms constituting "ischemic preconditioning" or "ischemic tolerance," which is associated with some preservation of energy metabolism and mitochondrial function (Dirnagl et al., 2003). Third, 3 hours of exposure to isoflurane limits ischemia-induced damage in mice (Kapinya et al. 2002). Whether a shorter period would protect the human brain remains unknown. General anesthesia may be an additional factor in reversibility of ischemia-produced neuronal dysfunction in the clinical situation. The lowered cerebral metabolic rate by inhalation anesthetics such as halothane, enflurane, and isoflurane, and possibly nitrous oxide, and by the narcotics (Shapiro, 1981) alters carbohydrate metabolism such that brain glucose and glycogen levels rise and lactic acid concentrations fall. As it is possible that cellular lactic acidosis is one of the critical factors causing cell death (Sundt and Michenfelder, 1972), such alterations would reduce the damaging effects of ischemia.

Significance of Clamp-Associated EEG Changes

Despite such potential reversibility, there will likely be a residuum of patients with major clamp-associated EEG changes reflecting very low regional CBF values. As indicated above, the length of time that neural tissue can tolerate ischemia without infarction is inversely related to the severity of the reduction of blood flow during the time of ischemia. For example, at zero flow, as with cardiac arrest, it is approximately 4 minutes. At higher levels of flow (about 15 mL · 100 g^{-1} · min^{-1}), tolerance may be as long as 1 hour or more.

It has been the Mayo Clinic policy to place a shunt whenever a visible EEG change occurs or whenever the CBF with clamping descended below 18 to 20 mL · 100 g^{-1} · min^{-1} (Sundt et al., 1981). Thus, shunts were placed in 511 of 1,145 consecutive carotid endarterectomies (45%). At University Hospital, London, 176 consecutive carotid endarterectomies were performed by a single neurosurgeon with EEG monitoring without placement of a shunt. No postoperative complications occurred among patients without EEG changes or among the 33 patients with moderate clamp-associated EEG changes. However, two of 22 patients (9%) of this series with major clamp-associated EEG changes awoke with a related neurological deficit. Although they may still have been embolic, one must consider at present that these deficits were consequent to severe clamp-associated cerebral ischemia. A more recent study by the London group (Brown et al., unpublished) found only a 0.4% incidence of irreversible clamp-associated ischemia.

Thus, one can conclude that moderate clamp-associated changes can be managed in the same manner as no EEG change. However, major changes may indicate the need for a shunt. These latter changes consist of a marked attenuation of activity at all frequencies except <1 Hz activity, which may increase twofold. Although shunt placement itself may risk embolism, this was known to occur in only two of 511 instances of shunt placement in the Mayo Clinic series (Sundt et al., 1981).

EEG Changes Not Associated With Clamping

In about 1% of endarterectomies, a focal EEG change appears unassociated with carotid clamping and persists throughout the remainder of the procedure. There is a high incidence of new neurological deficits postoperatively in such instances, probably caused by embolization (Sundt et al., 1981). Brown et al's. (unpublished) study of 487 endarterectomies encountered six strokes; neuroimaging determined that four of these were embolic and two ischemic. This finding is in accordance with earlier writings (Archie, 1991; Krul et al., 1989; Steed et al., 1982), which indicate that most perioperative strokes are embolic, not ischemic. A sudden major focal EEG change first appearing after 1 minute of clamping suggests embolism. Late embolism may also account for perioperative deficits that were "undetected" by EEG, i.e., occurring in the recovery room after monitoring has ended.

Small cortical (<3 cm) and subcortical infarcts of either cause may elude EEG detection (Macdonell et al., 1988).

Display Techniques

Compressed spectral arrays using limited channels and computer topographic brain mapping have been used to display EEG changes during carotid endartectomy. These have not gained widespread acceptance among centers with considerable experience in such monitoring, as they inject their own technical complexities and limitations into the process and do not enhance the appreciation of significant EEG alterations. Thus, mild and moderate EEG changes were not reliably detected by observers when displayed as a computer-derived density spectral array (Kearse et al., 1993). Only severe changes were readily revealed by this method. In a Minicucci et al. (2000) study, on-line visual analysis disclosed more clamp-related changes (28%) than computer analysis (20%), the latter including variability and asymmetry indices, spectral edge frequency, and main dominant frequency.

To determine which EEG derivations best distinguish patients with major clamp-related EEG changes from those without such, Laman et al. (2001) studied changes in power of four frequency bands in all possible EEG derivations and considered those producing the greatest area under receiver operating characteristics (ROCs) curves as the best indicators. Anterior, longitudinal, and ipsilateral derivations with large interelectrode distances ranked highest—results generally congruent with visually based intuition.

As automated analysis schemes have not effectively distinguished true changes from artifacts, it is understandable that the American Clinical Neurophysiology Society (1994) in guideline nine indicates that the clinical application of quantitative EEG techniques should be "limited and adjunctive."

Somatosensory Evoked Potentials

Guerit et al. (1997) have denoted the following factors that may create abnormalities to the somatosensory evoked potential (SEP) from median nerve stimuli during a carotid endarterectomy: (a) cross clamping, (b) a systemic blood pressure drop with or without cross clamping, (c) cerebral embolism, (d) head positioning, and (e) modification of the anesthetic regimen.

Branston et al. (1974) found that the cortical SEP reduced progressively when regional CBF fell below 16 mL · 100 g^{-1} · min^{-1}. Clamp-related SEP abnormalities signify a regional cerebral oxygen saturation (rSo$_2$) of <50% to 56% and an rSo$_2$ drop of 10% to 15% as shown by two studies (Beese et al., 1998; Cho et al., 1998). However, the larger Beese study disclosed moderate interpatient variability in rSo$_2$ when SEPs altered and moderate rSo$_2$ overlap between preserved and altered SEPs. An overlap in CSPs and SEP preservation or alteration was found by Dinkel et al. (1992); although CSP descended below 50 mm Hg in all 12 patients with SEP loss, 61 (84%) of 73 patients with <50 mm Hg CSP had normal SEPs. Horsch et al. (1990) studied the value of SEPs in 734 patients. An abnormal SEP occurred in 89 patients (12%), of which six (0.8%) were irreversible; all six patients suffered a postoperative neurological deficit without improvement. Four additional patients without SEP changes also had postoperative deficits; in only one of these four did the deficit persist. Unfortunately, technical factors precluded use of SEP in 59 cases (8%). This group (Haupt and Horsch, 1992) obtained very similar results in a second study. In a study of 32 patients routinely shunted or not, Wober et al. (1998) found no intergroup difference in the proportion with abnormal SEPs. Their meta-analysis disclosed a poor to mediocre positive predictive value of SEP for development of new neurological deficits after CE.

While SEP alterations may reflect cerebral ischemia, evoked potentials do not appear to have any monitoring advantages over the routine EEG. Although placement of only four electrodes is required for SEP and drugs have no effect, ischemia in an unrecorded area would not be detected and the SEP data are updated only every 2 to 5 minutes.

EEG Monitoring During Open Heart Surgery

During cardiopulmonary bypass (CPB), CBF may vary significantly and clinically unsuspected cerebral ischemia may occur.

Stockard et al. (1974) recorded the EEG in 75 patients undergoing CPB for various cardiac procedures. Visual analysis of the bipolar-recorded EEG was supplemented by power spectral analysis, peak power frequency computation, and average EEG amplitude integration. Fifteen of these patients were exposed to significant hypotension during CPB. All had associated bilateral EEG changes consisting of a slowing or decrease in EEG activity. All eight of these patients who developed postoperative neurological deficits had EEG disturbances, which began at the time of the hypotensive episodes during CPB. These persisted postoperatively and correlated with the nature and evolution of the deficits. Diffuse slowing and/or attenuation was associated with impairment of consciousness postoperatively, and regional abnormalities could be correlated with unilateral seizures or hemiparesis. The seven patients whose EEG changes were transient had no postoperative deficits.

Salerno et al. (1978) carried out a prospective EEG study of 118 patients undergoing CPB. Twenty-two (19%) demonstrated some EEG abnormality during the procedure. Five of the six incidences of severe EEG change were traced to obstruction of pump lines or to low perfusion flow and pressure. Ten of the 16 moderate changes occurred only during the establishment of CPB and did not persist, while four continued throughout the procedure. In two, the abnormalities began during the second half of the procedure. The cause of these moderate alterations was not indicated. Again, the EEG abnormalities consisted of sudden-appearing decrease in voltage and/or excessive delta activity occurring regionally or diffusely.

Hypothermia used with CPB contributes considerably to the EEG modifications. Hypothermia alone produces no EEG change until the body temperature falls below 30°C (Kiloh et al., 1972), at which point high-amplitude delta appears. As the temperature falls further, amplitude and frequency of all components diminish to a burst-suppression pattern at about 20°C. Although Levy (1984) also noted EEG modifications at onset of CPB and with hypotension, his study focused on hypothermia-related alterations. During hypothermic bypass, burst suppression occurred in eight of his 33 subjects; duration of suppression periods progressively shortened during rewarming. Total power (sum of power in individual frequencies from 1 to 32 Hz) correlated well with temperature, reflecting the fall in EEG amplitude with hypothermia. Levy also found linear changes with temperature in the peak power frequency of the higher frequencies (8–10 Hz) in 76% of patients, reflecting slowing of such frequencies with hypothermia. Actually, spectral analysis revealed two frequency bands, about 5 Hz and 8 to 10 Hz, both of which decrease in frequency and amplitude with hypothermia. Unfortunately, his automated system used a high band-pass filter with a cutoff at 4 Hz, resulting in a considerable loss of low-frequency activity. Predictably, the effects of fentanyl-midazolam anesthesia on EEG are enhanced by hypothermia (Stephan et al., 1989). Toner et al. (1997) found with anesthesia and hypothermia that intraoperative and end-of-perfusion changes on quantitative EEG did not relate to postoperative cerebral function. Similarly, Miller et al. (1994), studying infants, found that intraoperative EEG changes bore no relationship to postoperative neurological outcome.

Although bispectral analysis (BIS) is useful when the distribution of signal amplitudes deviates from gaussian (normality) as occurs in EEG signals during anesthesia, Barr et al. (1999, 2000a,b) found that BIS failed to distinguish among anesthetic levels or between the anesthetic state and wakefulness. Freye (1999) found that EEG power spectra helped indicate insufficient antinociception with opiates, but an experienced anesthetist would rarely require this distinction in practice.

However, EEG spectral edge EEG analysis proved useful in establishing the necessary sufentanil dose for coronary artery bypass grafting (Chi et al., 1991; Sareen et al., 1997).

The foregoing discussion illustrates that EEG changes during CPB are multifactorial in origin. Hypotension, hemodilution, changes in anesthetic concentrations and in blood gases, hypothermia, air and clot embolism, mechani-cal dysfunction of pump lines, and previous CNS disease may all contribute. Of these, the deep hypothermia is likely the major factor that limits use of EEG in cardiac surgery. Salerno et al. (1978) were apparently able to distinguish the more gradual and progressive EEG changes due to hypothermia from the more abrupt and occasionally regional effects of inadequate cerebral perfusion. However, in the practical situation, communication with the anesthetist and other personnel may well be required to unravel the pathogenesis of the EEG alterations.

The complexity of CPB-related EEG modifications, the possibly different significances of alterations of separate frequency bands, and the importance of regional changes all preclude the use of any excessively simplistic device such as a single-channel cerebral function monitor at this early stage of our knowledge of this subject.

Acknowledgments

We thank Drs. G.G. Ferguson and N. Brown and Mr. D. Kent McNeill for helpful comments. Maria Raffa carefully prepared the manuscript.

References

Allen, G.S., and Preziosi, T.J. 1981. Carotid endarterectomy: a prospective study of its efficacy and safety. Medicine 60:298–309.

American Clinical Neurophysiologion Society. (Unpublished). Guidelines on intraoperative electroencephalography.

American Clinical Neurophysiologion Society 1994. Guideline nine: guidelines on evoked potentials. J. Clin. Neurophysiol. 11:40–73.

Archie, J.P. 1991. Technique and clinical results of carotid stump back-pressure to determine selective shunting during carotid endarterectomy. J. Vasc. Surg. 13:319–327.

Arnold, M., Sturzenegger, M., Schaffler, L., et al. 1997. Continuous intraoperative monitoring of middle cerebral artery blood flow velocities and electroencephalography during carotid endarterectomy. A comparison of the two methods to detect cerebral ischemia. Stroke 28(7):1345–1350.

Astrup, J., Symon, L. Branston, N.M., et al. 1977. Cortical evoked potential and extracellular K+ and H+ at critical levels of brain ischemia. Stroke 8:51–57.

Astrup, J., Siesjo, B.K., and Symon, L. 1981. Thresholds in cerebral ischemia—the ischemic penumbra. Stroke 12:723–725.

Baker, W.H., Dorner, D.B., and Barnes, R.W. 1977. Carotid endarterectomy: is an indwelling shunt necessary? Surgery 82:321–326.

Barnett, H.J.M., Meldrum, H., Eliasziw, M., et al. 2003. Treatment of symptomatic arteriosclerotic carotid artery disease. In *Advances in Neurology. Ischemic Stroke, v*ol. 92, Eds. H.J.M. Barnett, J. Bogousslavsky, and H. Meldrum, pp. 307–317. Philadelphia: Lippincott Williams & Wilkins.

Barr, G., Jakobsson, J.G., Owall, A., et al. 1999. Nitrous oxide does not alter bispectral index: study with nitrous oxide as sole agent and as an adjunct to i.v. anaesthesia. Br. J. Anaesth. 82:827–830.

Barr, G., Anderson, R.E., Owall, A., et al. 2000a. Effects on the bispectral index during medium-high dose fentanyl induction with or without propofol supplement. Acta Anaesthesiol. Scand. 44:807–811.

Barr, G., Anderson, R.E., Samuelsson, S, et al. 2000b. Fentanyl and midazolam anaesthesia for coronary bypass surgery: a clinical study of bispectral electroencephalogram analysis, drug concentrations and recall. Br. J. Anaesth. 84:749–752.

Beebe, H.G., Pearson, J.M., and Coatsworth, J.J. 1978. Comparison of carotid artery stump pressure and EEG monitoring in carotid endarterectomy. Am. Surg. 44:655–660.

Beese, U., Langer, H., Lang, W., et al. 1998. Comparison of near-infrared spectroscopy and somatosensory evoked potentials for the detection of cerebral ischemia during carotid endarterectomy. Stroke 29(10):2032–2037.

Bland, J.E., and Lazar, M.L. 1981. Carotid endarterectomy with shunt. Neurosurgery 8:153–157.

Blume, W.T., Ferguson, G.G., and McNeill, D.K. 1986. Significance of EEG changes at carotid endarterectomy. Stroke 17:891–897.

Borgeat, A., Dessibourg, C., Popovic, V., et al. 1991. Propofol and spontaneous movements: an EEG study. Anesthesiology 74(1):24–27.

Branston, N.M., Symon, L., Crockard, H.A., et al. 1974. Relationship between the cortical evoked potential and local cortical blood flow following acute middle cerebral artery occlusion in the baboon. Exp. Neurol. 45:195–208.

Brown, N., Ferguson, G.G., Blume, W.T. (Unpublished). The efficacy of intra-operative EEG and carotid stump pressure monitoring for carotid endarterectomy.

Calligaro, K.D., Dougherty, M.J., Lombardi, J., et al. 2001. Converting from general anesthesia to cervical block anesthesia for carotid endarterectomy. Vasc. Surg. 35(2):103–106.

Cherry, K.J., Roland, C.F., Hallett, J.W., Jr., et al. 1991. Stump pressure, the contralateral carotid artery, and electroencephalographic changes. Am. J. Surg. 162(2):185–188.

Chi, O.Z., Sommer, W., and Jasaitis, D. 1991: Power spectral analysis of EEG during sufentanil infusion in humans. Can. J. Anaesth. 38:275–280.

Chiappa, K.H., Burke, S.R., and Young, R.R. 1979. Results of electroencephalographic monitoring during 367 carotid endarterectomies. Stroke 10:381–388.

Cho, H., Nemoto, E.M., Yonas, H., et al. 1998. Cerebral monitoring by means of oximetry and somatosensory evoked potentials during carotid endarterectomy. J. Neurosurg. 89(4):533–538.

Counsell, C., Salinas, R., Naylor, R., et al. 2000. Routine or selective carotid artery shunting for carotid endarterectomy (and different methods of monitoring in selective shunting). Cochrane Database Syst Rev. (2): CD000190.

Crowell, R.M., Olsson, Y., Klatzo, I., et al. 1970. Temporary occlusion of the middle cerebral artery in the monkey: clinical and pathological observations. Stroke 1:439–448.

Dinkel, M., Schweiger, H., and Goerlitz, P. 1992. Monitoring during carotid surgery: somatosensory evoked potentials vs. carotid stump pressure. J. Neurosurg. Anesthesiol. 4(3):167–175.

Dirnagl, U., Iadecola, C., and Moskowitz, M.A. 1999. Pathobiology of ischaemic stroke: an integrated view. TINS 22:391–396.

Dirnagl, U., Simon, R.P., and Hallenbeck, J.M. 2003. Ischemic tolerance and endogenous neuroprotection. Trends Neurosci. 26:248–254.

Doyle, P.W., Coles, J.P., Leary, T.M., et al. 2001. A comparison of remifentanil and fentanyl in patients undergoing carotid endarterectomy. Eur. J. Anaesthiol. 18(1):13–19.

Ebrahim, Z.Y., Schubert, A., Van Ness, P., et al. 1994. The effect of propofol on the electroencephalogram of patients with epilepsy. Anesth. Analg. 78(2):275–279.

Ferguson, G.G. 1982a. Extracranial carotid artery surgery. Clin. Neurosurg. 29:543–574.

Ferguson, G.G. 1982b. Intra-operative monitoring and internal shunts: are they necessary in carotid endarterectomy? Stroke 13:287–289.

Ferguson, G.G., and Gamache, F.W., Jr. 1984. Cerebral protection during carotid endarterectomy: intraoperative monitoring, anesthetic techniques, and temporary shunts. In Stroke and the Extracranial Vessels, Ed. R.R. Smith, pp. 187–201. New York: Raven Press.

Fiori, L., Parenti, G., and Marconi, F. 1997. Combined transcranial Doppler and electrophysiologic monitoring for carotid endarterectomy. J. Neurosurg. Anesthesiol. 9(1):11–16.

Freye, E., Dehnen-Seipel, H., Latasch, L., et al. 1999. Slow EEG-power spectra correlate with haemodynamic changes during laryngoscopy and intubation following induction with fentanyl or sufentanil. Acta Anaesthesiol. Belg. 50:71–76.

Giannotta, S.L., Dicks, R.E., and Kindt, G.W. 1980. Carotid endarterectomy: technical improvements. Neurosurgery 7:309–312.

Guerit, J.M., Witdoeckt, D., de Tourtchaninoff, M., et al. 1997. Somatosensory evoked potential monitoring in carotid surgery. I. Relationships between qualitative SEP alterations and intraoperative events. Electroencephalogr. Clin. Neurophysiol. 104(6):459–469.

Harada, R.N., Comerota, A.J., Good, G.M., et al. 1995. Stump pressure, electroencephalographic changes, and the contralateral carotid artery: another look at selective shunting. Am. J. Surg. 170(2):148–153.

Harbaugh, R.E., and Pikus, H.J. 2001. Carotid endarterectomy with regional anesthesia. Neurosurgery 49(3):642–645.

Haupt, W.F., and Horsch, S. 1992. Evoked potential monitoring in carotid surgery: a review of 994 cases. Neurology 42(4):835–838.

Heiss, W.D., and Rosner, G. 1983. Functional recovery of cortical neurons as related to degree and duration of ischemia. Ann. Neurol. 14: 294–301.

Hirofumi, O., Otone, E., Hiroshi, I., et al. 2003. The effectiveness of regional cerebral oxygen saturation monitoring using near-infrared spectroscopy in carotid endarterectomy. J. Clin. Neurosci. 10(1):79–83.

Horsch, S., De Vleeschauwer, P., and Ktenidis, K. 1990. Intraoperative assessment of cerebral ischemia during carotid surgery. J. Cardiovasc. Surg. 31:599–602.

Hossmann, K.A., Sakaki, S., and Zimmermann, V. 1977. Cation activities in reversible ischemia of the cat brain. Stroke 8:77–81.

Jenkins, G.M., Chiappa, K.H., and Young, R.R. 1983. Practical aspects of EEG monitoring during carotid endarterectomies. Am. J. EEG Technol. 23:191–203.

Jones, T.H., Morawetz, R.B., Crowell, R.M., et al. 1981. Thresholds of focal cerebral ischemia in awake monkeys. J. Neurosurg. 54:773–782.

Kapinya, K.J., Prass, K., and Dirnagl, U. 2002. Isoflurane induced prolonged protection against cerebral ischemia in mice: a redox sensitive mechanism? Neuroreport 13(11):1431–1435.

Kearse, L.A., Jr., Martin, D., McPeck, K., et al. 1993. Computer-derived density spectral array in detection of mild analog electroencephalographic ischemic pattern changes during carotid endarterectomy. J. Neurosurg. 78(6):884–890.

Kiloh, L.G., McComas, A.J., and Osselton, J.W. 1972. Clinical Electroencephalography, 3rd ed., p. 155, London: Butterworths.

Krenn, H., Deusch, E., Jellinek, H., et al. 2002. Remifentanil or propofol for sedation during carotid endarterectomy under cervical plexus block. Br. J. Anaesth. 89(4):637–640.

Krul, J.M.J., van Gijn, J., Ackerstaff, R.G.A., et al. 1989. Site and pathogenesis of infarcts associated with carotid endarterectomy. Stroke 20: 324–328.

Laman, D.M., van der Reijden, C.S., Wieneke, G.H., et al. 2001. EEG evidence for shunt requirement during carotid endarterectomy: optimal EEG derivations with respect to frequency bands and anesthetic regimen. J. Clin. Neurophysiol. 18(4):353–363.

Levy, W.J. 1984. Quantitative analysis of EEG changes during hypothermia. Anesthesiology 60:291–297.

Macdonell, R.A.L., Donnan, G.A., Bladin, P.F., et al. 1988. The electroencephalogram and acute ischemic stroke. Distinguishing cortical from lacunar infarction. Arch. Neurol. 45:520–524.

Mayberg, M.R. 2003. Journal watch. Neurology 5(12):89.

McCarthy, R.J., Nasr, M.K., McAteer, P., et al. 2002. Physiological advantages of cerebral blood flow during carotid endarterectomy under local anaesthesia. A randomised clinical trial. Eur. J. Vasc. Endovasc. Surg. 24(3):215–221.

Messick, J.M., Casement, B., Sharbrough, F.W., et al. 1987. Correlation of regional cerebral blood flow (rCBF) with EEG changes during isoflurane anesthesia for carotid endarterectomy: critical rCBF. Anesthesiology 66: 344–349.

Michenfelder, J.D., Sundt, T.M., Fode, N., et al. 1987. Isoflurane when compared to enflurane and halothane decreases the frequency of cerebral ischemia during carotid endarterectomy. Anesthesiology 67:336–340.

Miller, G., Rodichok, L.D., Baylen, B.G., et al. 1994. EEG changes during open heart surgery on infants aged 6 months or less: relationship to early neurologic morbidity. Pediatr. Neurol. 10(2):124–130.

Minicucci, F., Cursi, M., Fornara, C., et al. 2000. Computer-assisted EEG monitoring during carotid endarterectomy. J. Clin. Neurophysiol. 17(1): 101–107.

Newman, M.F., Murkin, J.M., Roach, G., et al. 1995. Cerebral physiologic effects of burst suppression doses of propofol during nonpulsatile cardiopulmonary bypass. CNS subgroup of McSPI. Anesth. Analg. 81(3): 452–457.

North American Symptomatic Carotid Endarterectomy Trial Collaborators. 1991. Beneficial effect of carotid endarterectomy in symptomatic patients with high-grade carotid stenosis. N. Engl. J. Med 325:445–453.

Ojemann, R.G., Crowell, R.M., Roberson, G.H., et al. 1975. Surgical treatment of extracranial carotid occlusive disease. Clin. Neurosurg. 22: 214–263.

Ott, D.A., Cooley, D.A., Chapa, L., et al. 1980. Carotid endarterectomy without temporary intraluminal shunt: study of 309 consecutive operations. Ann. Surg. 191:708–714.

Reddy, R.V., Moorthy, S.S., Mattice, T., et al. 1992. An electroencephalographic comparison of effects of propofol and methohexital. Electroencephalogr. Clin. Neurophysiol. 83(2):162–168.

Salerno, T.A., Lince, D.P., White, D.N., et al. 1978. Monitoring of electroencephalogram during open heart surgery. A prospective analysis of 118 cases. J. Thorac. Cardiovasc. Surg. 76:97–100.

Salford, L.G., Plum, F., and Siesjo, B.K. 1973a. Graded hypoxia oligemia in rat brain. I. Biochemical alterations and their implications. Arch. Neurol. 29:227–233.

Salford, L.G., Plum, F., and Brierley, J.B. 1973b. Graded hypoxia-oligemia in rat brain. II. Neuropathological alterations and their implications. Arch. Neurol. 29:234–238.

Sareen, J., Hudson, R.J., Rosenbloom, M., et al. 1997. Dose-response to anaesthetic induction with sufentanil: haemodynamic and electroencephalographic effects. Can. J. Anaesth. 44:19–25.

Schneider, J.R., Droste, J.S., Schindler, N., et al. 2002. Carotid endarterectomy with routine electroencephalography and selective shunting: influence of contralateral internal carotid artery occlusions and utility in prevention of perioperative strokes. J. Vasc. Surg. 35(6):1114–1122.

Shapiro, H.M. 1981. Anesthesia effects upon cerebral blood flow, cerebral metabolism, and the electroencephalogram. In *Anesthesia*, Ed. R.D. Miller, pp. 795–824. New York: Churchill Livingstone.

Sharbrough, F.W. 1982. Nonspecific abnormal EEG patterns. In *Electroencephalography: Basic Principles Clinical Applications And Related Fields,* Eds. E. Niedermeyer, and F. Lopes da Silva, pp. 135–154. Baltimore and Munich: Urban and Schwarzenberg.

Sharbrough, F.W. 1983. EEG monitoring: II. Intraoperative recordings. American EEG Society Course, American EEG Society, New Orleans, LA.

Sharbrough, F.W., Messick, J.M., and Sundt, T.M. 1973. Correlation of continuous electroencephalograms with cerebral blood flow measurements during carotid endarterectomy. Stroke 4:674–683.

Steed, D.L., Peitzman, A.B., Grundy, B.L., et al. 1982. Causes of stroke in carotid endarterectomy. Surgery 92:634–641.

Stephan, H., Sonntag, H., Lange, H., et al. 1989. Cerebral effects of anaesthesia and hypothermia. Anaesthesia 44:310–316.

Stockard, J.J., and Bickford, R.G. 1975. The neurophysiology of anaesthesia. In *A Basis and Practice of Neuroanaesthesia*, Ed. E. Gordon, pp. 3–46. Amsterdam: Excerpta Medica.

Stockard, J.J., Bickford, R.G., Myers, R.R., et al. 1974. Hypotension-induced changes in cerebral function during cardiac surgery. Stroke 5:730–746.

Stoneburner, J.M., Nichanian, G.P., Cukingnan, R.A., et al. 2002. Carotid endarterectomy using regional anesthesia: a benchmark for stenting. Am. Surg. 68(12):1120–1123.

Sundt, T.M., Grant, W.C., and Garcia, J.H. 1969. Restoration of middle cerebral artery flow in experimental infarction. J. Neurosurg. 31:311–322.

Sundt, T.M., and Michenfelder, J.D. 1972. Focal transient cerebral ischemia in the squirrel monkey. Circ. Res. 30:703–712.

Sundt, T.M., Houser, O.W., Sharbrough, F.W., et al. 1977. Carotid endarterectomy: results, complications and monitoring techniques. In *Advances in Neurology,* Eds. R.A. Thompson, and J.R. Green, pp. 97–119. New York: Raven Press.

Sundt, T.M., Sharbrough, F.W., Piepgras, D.G., et al. 1981. Correlation of cerebral blood flow and electroencephalographic changes during carotid endarterectomy. Mayo Clin. Proc. 56:533–543.

Thompson, J.E., Austin, D.J., and Patman, R.D. 1970. Carotid endarterectomy for cerebrovascular insufficiency: long-term results in 592 patients followed up to thirteen years. Ann. Surg. 172:663–679.

Todd, M.M., and Drummond, J.C. 1984. A comparison of the cerebrovascular and metabolic effects of halothane and isoflurane in the cat. Anesthesiology 60:276–282.

Toner, I., Taylor, K.M., Lockwood, G., et al. 1997. EEG changes during cardiopulmonary bypass surgery and postoperative neuropsychological deficit: the effect of bubble and membrane oxygenators. Eur. J. Cardiothorac. Surg. 11(2):312–319.

Trojaborg, B.W., and Boysen, G. 1973. Relation between EEG, regional cerebral blood flow and internal carotid artery pressure during carotid endarterectomy. Electroencephalogr. Clin. Neurophysiol. 34:61–69.

VanCott, A.C., and Brenner, R.P. 2003. Drug effects and toxic encephalopathies. In *Current Practice of Clinical Electroencephalography,* 3rd ed., Eds. J.S. Ebersole, and T.A. Pedley, pp. 474–477. Philadelphia: Lippincott Williams & Wilkins.

Vernieri, F., Tibuzzi, F., Pasqualetti, P., et al. 2003. Transcranial Doppler and near-infrared spectroscopy can evaluate the hemodynamic effect of carotid artery occlusion. Stroke 35(1):64–70.

Wellman B.J., Loftus, C.M., Kresowik, T.F., et al. 1998. The differences in electroencephalographic changes in patients undergoing carotid endarterectomies while under local versus general anesthesia. Neurosurgery 43(4):769–773.

Whitney, D.G., Kahn, E.M., Estes, J.W., et al. 1980. Carotid artery surgery without temporary indwelling shunt: 1917 consecutive procedures. Arch. Surg. 115:1393–1399.

Wilkinson, H.A., Wright, R.L., and Sweet, W.H. 1965. Correlation of reduction in pressure and angiographic cross-filling with tolerance of carotid occlusion. J. Neurosurg. 22:241–245.

Wober, C., Zeitlhofer, J., Asenbaum, S., et al. 1998. Monitoring of median nerve somatosensory evoked potentials in carotid surgery. J. Clin. Neurophysiol. 15(5):429–438.

43. EEG Source Localization (Model-Dependent and Model-Independent Methods)

Terrence D. Lagerlund and Gregory A. Worrell

One of the goals of electroencephalography (EEG) and evoked potential studies is to obtain information on the localization of abnormal rhythms or transient waveforms or features. In conventional EEG interpretation, this usually involves determining in which of the many recorded channels the rhythm or feature of interest has the greatest amplitude. For bipolar montages, the same information is obtained by locating waveforms of opposite polarity in two channels sharing a common electrode (phase reversals). Localization by conventional EEG requires no special equipment and no models or assumptions about the underlying physiological sources or the properties of the intervening volume-conducting medium. However, the accuracy of localization is limited by several factors. These include the large interelectrode spacing used in conventional EEG (6 to 7 cm for the International 10–20 System electrode placements) and the smearing of potentials by the volume-conducting medium, especially the poorly conducting skull (Nunez et al., 1994). Another factor for deep sources located in sulci or the interhemispheric fissure is that the electrical activity generated by these sources may have maximal amplitude at scalp electrodes placed some distance from the location immediately above the source (so-called tangential dipole generators, for instance). Although recording from arrays of closely spaced intracranial electrodes has been used to circumvent these limitations of scalp EEG in subjects undergoing evaluation for possible epilepsy surgery, this is an invasive technique that poses some risks. Localization by conventional EEG interpretation is also limited by the difficulty in visualizing spatial distributions of waveforms or features using conventional time-series displays, and, in the case of referential recordings, confusion may result from activity recorded by the reference electrode.

Digital computers may aid in extracting information from EEG and evoked potential waveforms that is not readily obtainable with visual analysis alone. The ability to better localize waveforms or features of interest and, ultimately, locate their intracranial sources by processing the digitized signals can be useful for both clinical and research purposes. Analysis of the scalp EEG to improve the ability to localize the sources of waveforms of interest requires special equipment (a digital EEG system) and software, and the analytic techniques may depend on models or assumptions about the sources of the EEG and the volume-conducting medium. Furthermore, instrumental, external interference, and physiological artifacts may be more difficult to recognize after processing the EEG. This is particularly true when display formats other than time-series waveforms, such as topographic maps, are used. There-

fore, the processed EEG or evoked potentials should be interpreted in conjunction with the unprocessed data (displayed as time-series waveforms). This may best be accomplished in actual implementations of analysis techniques by displaying the processed data on the same screen as the unprocessed data from which they were derived.

Model-Dependent Methods

One approach to localization of EEG or evoked potential features of interest is to attempt to solve the *inverse problem*, that is, to attempt to find the intracranial sources generating a known distribution of scalp potentials. Of course, scalp recordings provide potentials only at certain discrete locations on the head surface (the electrode positions), and even at these locations there is significant uncertainty about the actual potential value because of artifacts or noise that may contaminate the recorded signals. Furthermore, even if the distribution of potentials over the entire head surface were known exactly, this would not precisely determine the sources creating the potential distribution. Stated another way, an infinite number of sets of intracranial sources may produce exactly the same potential distribution on the head surface. Thus, the general inverse problem has no unique solution. To obtain a solution, one must place constraints on the number, type, or location of sources; that is, a *source model* must be used.

Dipole Localization Methods

A common approach to the inverse problem is to assume a priori that a feature in the EEG or evoked potential is generated by one or more intracranial dipole sources (a dipole source model). This assumption seems most reasonable for relatively small sources, for example, the generators of certain evoked potential peaks that are located in a deep structure, such as the brainstem or thalamus. Conversely, this assumption seems unreasonable when potentials generated by cerebral cortical neurons are analyzed, because neuronal activity in widespread cortical areas may contribute to the scalp potential. However, dipole localization may be applied to even fairly widespread cortical sources, provided that the source dipoles are viewed as *equivalent* dipoles. Equivalent dipoles may be defined as dipolar sources whose scalp potential distribution corresponds closely to the measured potentials; they may be considered to be the vector sum of all the dipoles representing current flow in individual cortical neurons in which there are synchronous postsynaptic potentials that contribute to a measurable scalp potential.

Nonlinear Dipole Localization Methods

The simplest dipole source localization algorithm attempts to find the location, orientation, and strength of a *single* dipole whose potential field at the scalp surface best accounts for the recorded EEG potentials at a specified instant (for example, the peak of an evoked potential or an epileptic spike discharge). A single dipole source can be completely characterized by six parameters, specifically, the three coordinates of the dipole in a three-dimensional rectangular coordinate system (x, y, and z) and the components of the dipole moment vector (m_x, m_y, and m_z) along each of the three axes in this coordinate system. If these parameters are known and there is an appropriate model of the volume-conducting medium between the dipole source and the scalp surface, the potential at each point on the scalp surface due to the dipole source can be calculated. The algorithm usually computes the potentials at each of the electrode positions and then calculates an error parameter, which is the sum of the squares of the differences between the computed potentials and the measured potentials at the electrode positions at the specified time. Because the computed scalp potentials depend in a nonlinear fashion on the six dipole parameters, a nonlinear least-squares minimization algorithm is used to search the six-dimensional parameter space for optimal values of x, y, z, m_x, m_y, and m_z (those that minimize the error parameter). The final value of the error parameter provides a measure of the "goodness of fit" of the single dipole potential to the measured potentials, which is indicative of how well a single equivalent dipole (Fig. 43.1) represents the recorded potentials (Scherg, 1990; Kavanagh et al., 1978; Scherg and Von Cramon, 1986; Schneider, 1972; Sidman et al., 1978, 1990, 1991).

This approach is relatively computationally demanding, is quite sensitive to noise or artifacts in the measured poten-

tials and to inaccuracies in the head (volume-conductor) model used (Radich and Buckley, 1995; Scherg and Berg, 1991; Zhang and Jewett, 1993), and is also very sensitive to the initial estimates of dipole location, because the least-squares minimization algorithm may find only a local minimum of the error parameter instead of the desired global minimum. The initial estimates are usually supplied by the electroencephalographer on the basis of a guess about the likely source location. A refinement of this approach that saves computational time involves a hybrid linear and nonlinear search: a three-parameter linear least-squares search on the parameters m_x, m_y, and m_z is carried out during the course of a three-parameter nonlinear least-squares search on the parameters x, y, and z (Salu et al., 1990).

The "fixed dipole model" is a variation of this method that uses the measured EEG potentials during a brief epoch rather than potentials at one instant (spatiotemporal dipole analysis). It is assumed that the dipole source responsible for the measured EEG potentials during this epoch remains at a constant location, that its dipole moment vector maintains a constant orientation throughout the epoch, and that only its magnitude (the "dipole strength") varies. This assumption may be valid if sufficiently brief epochs are chosen. This method is less sensitive to noise or artifacts in the EEG recordings than the method of fitting potentials at a single point in time (Scherg and Berg, 1991) but still can have relatively large errors in the fit dipole parameters (Zhang et al., 1994). Another variation is the "rotating dipole" method, in which it is assumed that the dipole source responsible for the measured EEG potentials during the chosen epoch remains at a constant location but that both its magnitude and its direction vary (Scherg and Von Cramon, 1985). Fixed and rotating dipole models also have been applied to data in the frequency domain (Raz et al., 1992; Valdés et al., 1992) as an alternative to time-domain analyses.

When it is not possible to adequately fit the measured EEG potentials by use of a single dipole (as indicated by an excessive value of the summed squared differences between measured and computed potentials), an additional dipole source may be introduced into the model. This may be done, for example, by subtracting the potentials computed from the first best-fit dipole from the measured EEG potentials and fitting the resulting residual potentials to a second dipole. After this, the 12 dipole parameters (six per dipole) may be fine-tuned to achieve the optimal fit with measured potentials. Usually, some artificial constraints on the parameter search algorithm must be applied to prevent the two dipoles from approaching each other so closely in location or orientation, or both, that the algorithm cannot reliably determine the individual dipole parameters. Additional dipoles may be added to the model, up to a theoretical maximum that depends on the number of electrodes (*M*) available. For the fixed dipole model in which one parameter per dipole must be estimated, the maximal number of dipoles is $M - 1$; for the rotating dipole model, in which three parameters per dipole must be estimated, it is $(M - 1)/3$; and for the unconstrained model, in which all six dipole parameters must be estimated, it is $(M - 1)/6$. However, unless the actual number of sources is known a priori, a unique solution to the inverse problem cannot be obtained, and attempting to solve

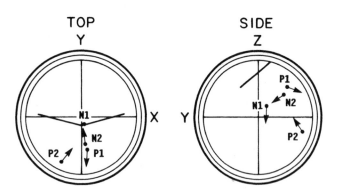

Figure 43.1. Results of dipole source localization applied to averaged visual evoked potential recordings for 20 older healthy volunteers (10 male, 10 female; mean age, 68.1 years). The *arrows* show the locations and orientations of single equivalent dipole sources in top and side views for N1, P1, N2, and P2 peaks in the full field checkerboard pattern reversal visual evoked potential (average of 64 trials). The head is modeled by a concentric sphere, with layers representing brain, skull, and scalp. The *heavy solid lines* represent the approximate location of the central fissure. (From Sidman, R.D., Major, D.J., Ford, M.R., et al. 1991. Age-related features of the resting pattern-reversal visual evoked response using the dipole localization method and cortical imaging technique. J. Neurosci. Methods 37:27–36, with permission of Elsevier Science Publishers BV.)

for more dipole sources than actually exist can lead to non-physiological results (Cabrera Fernández et al., 1995). In addition, the nonlinear least-squares minimization algorithm becomes cumbersome and prone to relatively large errors in the fit dipole parameters when more than a few dipoles are used, particularly when the effect of noise in the recorded EEG is considered (Cabrera Fernández et al., 1995; Zhang and Jewett, 1994a,b). Various methods have been proposed to obtain better initial parameter guesses and to escape from local minima during the nonlinear least-squares minimization procedure (Achim et al., 1991; Mosher et al., 1992).

Equivalent dipole modeling of epileptic spike potentials is one clinical application of this technique (Baumgartner, 1994; Wong, 1991). Information about the location of the epileptogenic region (or regions) of cortex can be more confidently and accurately obtained from equivalent dipole modeling than by visual review alone. In addition, spatiotemporal dipole analysis with fixed or rotating dipole models can be used to determine propagation patterns of epileptic spikes (Fig. 43.2). This technique has been used successfully to differentiate mesial-basal temporal lobe foci (predominantly type 1 spikes with both tangential and radial dipoles) from lateral neocortical temporal or extratemporal foci (predominantly type 2 spikes, which are well modeled by a single radial dipole). This has been shown to be clinically useful in the evaluation of patients with intractable epilepsy for possible epilepsy surgery (Ebersole, 1991, 1994). Ictal discharges may sometimes be analyzed in a fashion similar to that used for interictal spikes.

Dipole sources obtained by these analyses are not mathematically unique solutions. They cannot be interpreted as indicating the actual source (or sources) of any given spike discharge but are only equivalent sources in the sense defined earlier. Furthermore, when the model of the volume-conducting medium between the dipole sources and the scalp surface is simplified sufficiently to make the calculations practical (for example, a spherical shell head model), the equivalent dipoles are frequently displaced by more than 1 cm superiorly from the location of the actual sources in the temporal lobe, so that when they are superimposed on an anatomical image, such as a magnetic resonance imaging (MRI) scan, they appear to be located in the frontal lobe instead. With the advent of relatively inexpensive but powerful computers, increasing emphasis has been placed on developing better volume-conductor models that can improve the accuracy of source localization.

Linear Dipole Analysis Methods

In contrast to the nonlinear methods of dipole source localization, linear methods assume a significantly larger number of dipoles and may be used to model sources distributed more widely within the cortex. In the linear methods, the dipoles representing the solution of the inverse problem are assumed to have known locations and orientations (that is, these parameters are fixed in the model and are not part of the solution set to be found); only the *strength* of each dipole source need be determined to best match the actual recorded scalp EEG. With this assumption, the potential at any scalp electrode position is a linear combination of the individual dipole source strengths, and linear algebraic techniques may be used to solve for the dipole source strengths. The advantages over nonlinear methods are a significantly faster computation of the solution and the ability to determine a solution without the necessity of specifying any initial estimates.

From a mathematical standpoint, three types of linear dipole analysis methods may be defined, depending on the relation between N (the number of source dipoles) and M (the number of recording electrodes):

1. $N < M$ (fewer sources than recording electrodes). In this case, no solution to the inverse problem matches the recorded scalp potentials exactly. Therefore, as in the nonlinear dipole methods, the solution is found that minimizes the sum of the squares of the differences between the computed potentials and the measured potentials at each electrode position. An example of this approach is the algorithm named FOCUS (Scherg, 1994), which typically assumes that there are about 16 dipole sources, with one or two sources located in each brain lobe and hemisphere (for example, a left occipital source, a right

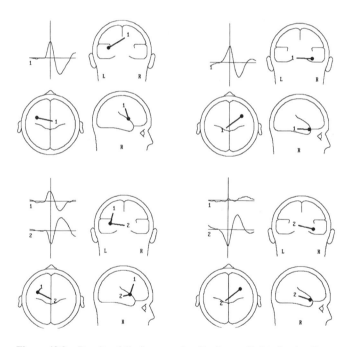

Figure 43.2. Results of dipole source localization applied to focal epileptic spikes from patients with complex partial epilepsy. Spikes are classified as type 1 (with sharply defined negative fields, steep voltage gradients, inferolateral location, and association with distinct, contralateral positive fields that show sagittal maxima) or type 2 (with broad negative fields extending to or beyond the midline, gradual voltage gradients, and no clear positive maxima contralaterally). Type 1 dipole localizations and corresponding source potentials are on the left and type 2 are on the right. *Top*, single dipole models; *bottom*, two-dipole fully constrained tangential-radial models. The oblique, single-dipole solution for the type 1 spike has both tangential and radial components, with activity in the tangential dipole beginning before that of the radial dipole (as seen from the source potentials). Type 2 spikes are well modeled by a radial dipole, with little activity ascribed to a tangential source. (From Ebersole, J.S. 1991. EEG dipole modeling in complex partial epilepsy. Brain Topogr. 4:113–123, with permission of Human Sciences Press.)

occipital source, a left parietal source, and so on). Most sources are assumed to be radially oriented (perpendicular to the cortical surface), but some tangential sources (for example, in the mesial temporal region) are also included. The results of this model are the strengths of all dipole sources as a function of time. These source strengths may be displayed in conventional time-series format as a "dipole source" montage; this format is well suited to visualizing time and frequency characteristics of the putative sources. Alternatively, a topographic "map" may be created that represents in graphical form the source strengths at a given instant (such as at the peak of an epileptic spike).

2. $N = M$ (as many sources as there are recording electrodes). In this case, for appropriately chosen sources, one unique solution to the inverse problem matches the recorded scalp potentials exactly. An example of this approach is the "spatial deconvolution" algorithm, which assumes that there is one radially oriented dipole source located directly beneath each scalp electrode on a spherical surface of fixed radius chosen to approximate that of cerebral cortex (Junghöfer et al., 1997; Nunez, 1986, 1987). The results of this model are the strengths of all dipole sources as a function of time. As for the FOCUS algorithm, these source strengths may be displayed in conventional time-series format as a dipole source montage, or a topographic map may be created that represents in graphical form the source strengths at a given instant (such as at the peak of an epileptic spike).

3. $N > M$ (more sources than recording electrodes). In this case, an infinite number of solutions to the inverse problem match the recorded scalp potentials exactly. The one "minimum norm" solution (which minimizes the sum of the squares of the source dipole strengths) is therefore found. An example of this approach is the cortical imaging technique (CIT) (Sidman, 1991; Sidman et al., 1989), which typically assumes about 160 dipole sources, all radially oriented, uniformly spaced, and located on a hemispherical surface at a given radius (for example, 0.45 × head radius). The results of this model are the strengths of all dipole sources as a function of time. Because the number of sources is large and the minimum norm solution found by the algorithm is only one of an infinite number of possible solutions, a time-series display or topographic map of the source strengths is not very useful. Instead, the source strengths are used to calculate the potentials on a spherical "imaging" surface located somewhere between the source surface and the head surface; the radius of the imaging surface is chosen to approximate that of the cerebral cortex (for example, 0.57 × head radius). These "cortical" potentials may be displayed in conventional time-series format as a "cortical" montage, or a topographic map may be created that represents in graphical form the "cortical" potentials at a given instant, such as at the peak of an evoked potential (Ford et al., 1993; Kearfott et al., 1991; Sidman et al., 1990, 1991, 1992).

Another model using more sources than electrodes is based on iterative refinement of the minimum norm solution of the inverse problem (Srebro, 1994, 1996a,b). In this method, a realistic model of the cortex consisting of N nodes ($N = 1,271$ was used by Srebro) based on sections of a cadaver head is constructed by digitizing the contours, and cortical current sources are modeled as a single dipole at each node, with an orientation vector chosen to be perpendicular to the cortical surface at that node. A minimum norm solution to the inverse problem is found as for CIT, but then the coordinates of the centroid of the distribution of "active" nodes and the second moment of this distribution are calculated and used to define an ellipsoidal volume element that contains within it the most active sources. The minimum norm solution to the inverse problem is then recalculated using *only* those nodes contained within the ellipsoid, which serves to "concentrate" the cortical activity in a smaller region. This approach is repeated many times until the smallest possible ellipsoidal cluster of active nodes has been found that provides an adequate model of the measured scalp potentials. The locations and strengths of active nodes can then be displayed as a representation of the most probable location of the cortical generators. This method has been applied with some success to localizing the generators of certain visual evoked potentials (Srebro and Oguz, 1997).

Low-resolution electromagnetic tomography (LORETA) is another generalized minimum-norm estimate for the source distribution that uses more sources than electrodes. LORETA uses a uniformly distributed, discretized three-dimensional grid of dipole sources within the volume of the brain, with considerably more dipole sources than recording electrodes. A unique solution is chosen by minimizing the Laplacian of the current distribution with a depth weighting by the dipole signal strength (Pascual-Marqui et al., 1994).

Because of the reduced computational complexity of linear source methods, it is possible to combine these with realistic, patient-specific, finite element volume-conductor models based on MRI (Ebersole, 1999; Phillips et al., 2002). With these source localization methods it is possible to combine the temporal resolution of EEG with the spatial resolution of other imaging methods, such as MRI and single-photon emission computed tomography (SPECT). The integration of these imaging methods has shown promise as a clinical tool for localization of epileptogenic brain (Worrell et al., 2000) (Fig. 43.3).

Model-Independent Methods

An alternative approach to the dipole localization methods described previously for localization of EEG or evoked potential sources consists of various methods that do not require any assumptions about the number, type, or configuration of sources in the brain. These may be called model-independent methods, although some of these methods do require a model of the volume-conducting medium between the sources and the recording electrodes.

Topographic Display Methods

Topographic display methods that show the distribution of scalp potentials at one instant during an EEG or evoked potential recording have been used for many years as an adjunct to conventional time-series waveform displays. Such

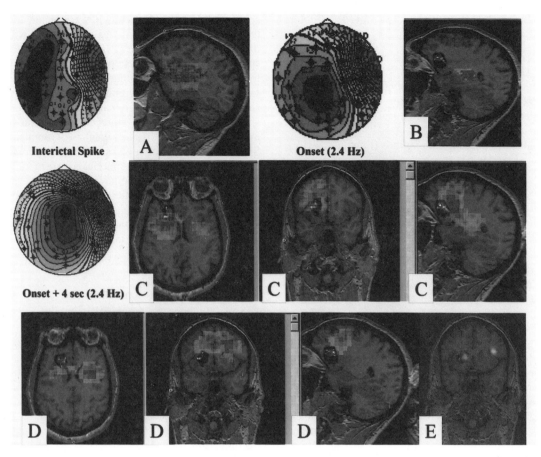

Figure 43.3. **A:** Scalp potential map of an interictal spike and the corresponding low-resolution electromagnetic tomography (LORETA)-derived generator co-registered to the patient's magnetic resonance imaging (MRI) scan. For the scalp map, the right hemisphere is on the reader's right. The co-registered figures use the standard MRI convention; that is, the left hemisphere is on the right. **B:** Phase-encoded frequency analysis scalp potential map and corresponding ictal generator for the lowest frequency (2.4 Hz) spectral peak at onset of the patient's seizure. The LORETA-derived ictal generators are co-registered to the patient's MRI scan. The *dark gray area* indicates maximal neuronal activity. At the onset of the ictal discharge, the generator localizes to the right lateral temporal lobe and not to the right frontal lesion on MRI. **C:** Phase-encoded frequency spectral analysis scalp potential map at seizure onset + 4 seconds, when the spectral power is at a maximum, and the corresponding LORETA-derived ictal generator *(light gray area)* in the horizontal, coronal, and parasagittal planes for the lowest frequency (2.4 Hz) spectral peak. The ictal generator localizes to the lesion on MRI. **D:** The LORETA generator in the horizontal, coronal, and parasagittal planes for the lowest frequency (2.0 Hz) spectral peak at seizure onset + 30 seconds. **E:** The ictal–single-photon emission computed tomography (SPECT) study from this seizure co-registered to the MRI scan. The time of radioisotope injection was at seizure onset + 28 seconds. The SPECT image has a region of ictal hyperperfusion in the contralateral as well as ipsilateral frontal lobes, consistent with the bifrontal generators determined by LORETA. (From Worrell, G.A., Lagerlund, T.D., Sharbrough, F.W., et al. 2000. Localization of the epileptic focus by low-resolution electromagnetic tomography in patients with a lesion demonstrated on MRI. Brain Topogr. 12:273–282, with permission of Human Sciences Press.)

"brain maps" are well suited to visualizing the spatial distribution of an EEG feature or waveform or an evoked potential peak, but a single map cannot convey the time variation or frequency characteristics of EEG activities or waveforms. In itself, topographic mapping is not so much an analysis technique as a display method. However, the results of various analyses may be displayed in topographic map format. For example, frequency spectral analysis may be performed on an epoch or multiple epochs of EEG, and the spectral power (or amplitude) within a particular band of frequencies (such as 8 to 13 Hz) may be calculated for all recorded channels and the results displayed as a topographic map. Methods that display maps of scalp potentials do not require any volume-conductor model.

For the generation of a topographic display, the value of the potential (or other quantity being mapped) must be known at all points on the mapping surface (for example, the scalp surface for conventional scalp potential maps or the cortical surface for maps of cortical potentials estimated by the CIT algorithm described previously). However, scalp recordings provide potentials only at certain discrete locations on the head surface (the electrode positions), and even at these locations there is significant uncertainty about the actual potential value because of artifacts or noise that may contaminate the recorded signals. A topographic mapping technique, therefore, must begin with an algorithm that can interpolate potentials to intermediate points between the scalp electrode positions.

Some of the methods used for interpolating EEG potentials are the following:

- Nearest neighbor inverse distance-weighted (Babiloni et al., 1995; Duffy et al., 1979)
- All-electrode inverse distance-weighted (Lemos and Fisch, 1991)
- Rectangular surface (two-dimensional) splines (Nunez, 1989; Perrin et al., 1987b)
- Rectangular three-dimensional splines (Law et al., 1993; Srinivasan et al., 1996)
- Spherical surface splines (Babiloni et al., 1995; Nunez, 1989; Perrin et al., 1989)
- Spherical harmonic expansion (SHE) (Lagerlund et al., 1995; Pascual-Marqui et al., 1988; Shaw, 1989)
- Single dipole or multidipole source model (Junghöfer et al., 1997)

The nearest neighbor method with four neighbors (Duffy et al., 1979) is most commonly used for interpolation because of the ease of computation (Fig. 43.4). Its disadvantages are that map discontinuities and extrema are always located at electrode sites, and artifacts or noise within the recorded signal from one electrode may significantly affect the map in the vicinity of that electrode. The various spline and SHE methods require more computation time but provide a continuous interpolated potential surface within the region of the map, allow better estimation of the locations of the extrema, and may be less sensitive to artifacts or noise at a single electrode. A surface spline is defined as the surface obtained by minimizing the bending energy of an infinite plate constrained to pass through known points. Rectangular splines are based on a rectangular Cartesian coordinate system (x and y for two-dimensional splines; x, y, and z for three-dimensional splines). Two-dimensional rectangular splines assume that electrodes and intermediate points are located on a flat, rectangular mapping region. Three-dimensional splines assume a mapping volume in three-dimensional space and therefore make no assumptions about head shape, but they require more computational time and are more difficult to display than two-dimensional splines. Spherical splines are based on a spherical coordinate system and therefore assume a spherical surface on which electrodes and intermediate points are located. The SHE method is equivalent to the spherical spline method of order 2 (Lagerlund et al., 1995) and has been demonstrated to produce identical results. Table 43.1 shows the formulas used to represent scalp potentials in each of these methods.

Laplacian Methods

The Laplacian of a function $V(x,y)$ is a new function $\mathcal{L}(x,y)$, which is the curvature of V in the x direction added to the curvature of V in the y direction:

$$\mathcal{L}(x,y) = (\partial^2 V/\partial x^2) + (\partial^2 V/\partial y^2)$$

The Laplacian of the scalp potential is proportional to the current density in the radial direction (in amperes/cm^2) entering or leaving the skull and is thus an indicator of intracranial current sources. Whereas the scalp potential decreases relatively slowly with distance away from an intracranial generator (such as a dipole), the Laplacian of the potential decreases much faster, so that topographic maps of

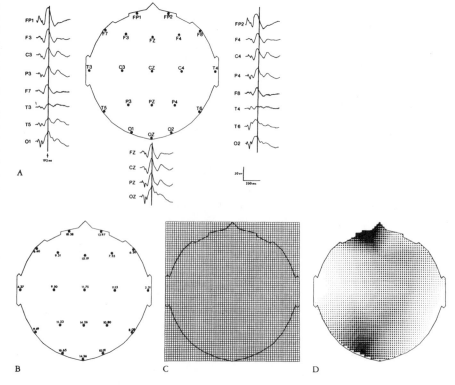

Figure 43.4. Example of the construction of a topographic map for flash visual evoked potential data. **A:** Individual visual evoked potentials for the electrodes indicated on the head diagram. **B:** Mean voltages at these locations for the 4-msec epoch beginning 192 msec after the flash stimulus. **C:** How the head is treated as a 64-by-64 grid, with voltage values calculated at each intersection of the grid lines by linear interpolation from the three nearest known electrodes. **D:** Resulting gray-scale intensity topographic map. (From Duffy, F.H., Burchfiel, J.L., and Lombroso, C.T. 1979. Brain electrical activity mapping (BEAM): A method for extending the clinical utility of EEG and evoked potential data. Ann. Neurol. 5:309–321, with permission of the American Neurological Association.)

Table 43.1. Formulas for Interpolating EEG Potentials

- Nearest neighbor and all-electrode inverse distance-weighted averaging

$$V(x,y) = \sum_{n=1}^{J} A_n[(x - x_n)^2 + (y - y_n)^2]^{-L/2}$$

- Rectangular surface splines

$$V(x,y) = \sum_{i=0}^{L-1} \sum_{j=0}^{i} A_{ij} x^{i-j} y^j$$
$$+ \sum_{n=1}^{N} B_n[(x - x_n)^2 + (y - y_n)^2]^{L-1}$$
$$\log[(x - x_n)^2 + (y - y_n)^2 + r^2]$$

- Rectangular three-dimensional splines

$$V(x,y) = \sum_{i=0}^{L-1} \sum_{j=0}^{i} \sum_{k=0}^{j} A_{ijk} x^{i-j} y^{j-k} z^k$$
$$+ \sum_{n=1}^{N} B_n[(x - x_n)^2 + (y - y_n)^2 + (z - z_n)^2]^{L-1}$$
$$\log[(x - x_n)^2 + (y - y_n)^2 + (z - z_n)^2 + r^2]$$

- Spherical surface splines

$$V(\theta, \varphi) = A_0 + (1/4\pi) \sum_{n=1}^{N} \sum_{l=1}^{\infty} (2l + 1)[l(l + 1)]^{-L} P_l$$
$$[\cos\theta \cos\theta_n - \sin\theta \sin\theta_n \cos(\varphi - \varphi_n)]$$

- Spherical harmonic expansion

$$V(\theta, \varphi) = \sum_{l=0}^{L} \sum_{m=-l}^{l} A_{lm} Y_{lm}(\theta, \varphi)$$

the scalp Laplacian localize underlying generators better than potential maps.

Methods to calculate the scalp Laplacian are similar to those used to interpolate scalp potentials. These include the following:

- Nearest neighbor inverse distance-weighted (Babiloni et al., 1995; Lagerlund et al., 1995)
- All-electrode inverse distance-weighted (Lemos and Fisch, 1991)
- Rectangular surface (two-dimensional) splines (Nunez, 1989; Perrin et al., 1987a)
- Rectangular three-dimensional splines projected onto spherical surface (Law et al., 1993; Srinivasan et al., 1996)
- Rectangular three-dimensional splines projected onto ellipsoidal surface (Law et al., 1993)
- Realistic scalp surface two-dimensional thin plate splines (Babiloni et al., 1996)
- Spherical surface splines (Babiloni et al., 1995; Nunez, 1989; Perrin et al., 1989)
- SHE (Lagerlund et al., 1995; Pascual-Marqui et al., 1988; Shaw, 1989)
- Single dipole or multidipole source model (Junghöfer et al., 1997)

The nearest neighbor method with four neighbors is most commonly used for calculation of the scalp Laplacian because of the ease of computation (Hjorth, 1975; Lagerlund,

1991; Wallin and Stålberg, 1980). For the special case of four equidistant neighbor electrodes located anteriorly, posteriorly, to the left, and to the right, the Laplacian is calculated as $\mathscr{L} = V_1 + V_2 + V_3 + V_4 - 4V_0$, in which V_0 is the potential at the center electrode and V_1 through V_4 are the potentials at the four neighbor electrodes. (It is often convenient to calculate $-\mathscr{L}/4$ rather than $\mathscr{L}$ itself; this is calculated as the center electrode potential minus the average potential at the four neighbors.) A disadvantage of this method is that artifacts or noise within the recorded signal from one electrode may significantly affect the Laplacian calculated at multiple neighboring sites. Also, it is more difficult to calculate Laplacians at electrodes on the edge of the electrode array (where four neighbors cannot be identified). One practical method of determining the Laplacian at an "edge" electrode is to subtract the average potential at *three* neighbors (rather than four) from the potential at the center electrode (Fig. 43.5). The other methods (spline and SHE) involve calculating the Laplacian from an analytical formula for the scalp potential that has been fitted to the measured potentials at the electrode positions. These methods require more computational time but may overcome some of the limitations of the nearest neighbor method.

Topographic maps of the scalp Laplacian provide greater spatial resolution for intracranial generators than do scalp potential maps (Fig. 43.6). However, obtaining significantly greater spatial resolution also requires the use of denser electrode arrays with 64 or 128 electrodes (Junghöfer et al., 1997; Nunez and Westdorp, 1994; Nunez et al., 1991, 1994). Because of the technical difficulties inherent in applying large numbers of electrodes to the head by conventional methods, special sensor (electrode) arrays are typically used (Tucker, 1993) when high spatial resolution EEG or evoked potential studies are performed (Fig. 43.7).

Multivariate Statistical Methods

The potential measured at scalp electrodes represents the linear superposition of cortical potentials, and therefore the signals at various electrodes are usually highly correlated. It is often useful to transform the measured data in an effort to decrease the data redundancy, capture the essential structure of the data, and extract physiologically useful information about the actual sources of the scalp potentials. This represents an example of a fundamental problem in statistical signal processing, in which the goal is often to find a "good" representation of multivariate data by a suitable transformation. Specific methods are usually defined by the criteria used to obtain the optimal transformation.

Principal component analysis (PCA) and, more recently, independent component analysis (ICA) are two examples of multivariate analysis that have been used in EEG and evoked potential studies. ICA and PCA are examples of linear transformation methods that require the following assumptions: (1) Components have fixed spatial projections during the epoch of interest. (2) Signal conduction times are negligible and the potentials from different components combine linearly at the scalp without time delays. (3) The number of components that can be determined is equal to the number of scalp electrodes. (4) Components are temporally independent of each other across the epoch of evaluation. The defi-

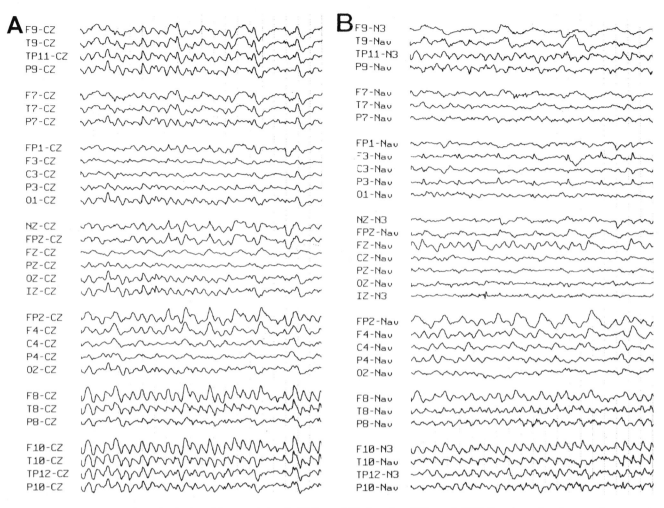

Figure 43.5. A: Four-second epoch of referentially recorded scalp EEG during a right temporal lobe seizure. **B:** The Laplacian of these scalp potentials calculated by the modified nearest neighbor method. Nav, four-neighbor average; N3, three-neighbor average. (From Lagerlund, T.D., Sharbrough, F.W., Busacker, N.E., et al. 1995. Interelectrode coherences from nearest-neighbor and spherical harmonic expansion computation of Laplacian of scalp potential. Electroencephalogr. Clin. Neurophysiol. 95:178–188, with permission of Elsevier Science Ireland.)

The definition of temporal independence distinguishes ICA from PCA. Both PCA and ICA are considered to be methods to remove the correlations introduced into the measured scalp data by mixing of the component signals. In PCA the reduction is accomplished using only second-order statistics (the covariance matrix), which decorrelates the signals. ICA seeks the more ambitious goal of making the outputs statistically independent by including higher order statistics. If the probability functions describing the signals are gaussian, statistical independence is equivalent to being uncorrelated (in the sense used in PCA), because the gaussian distribution is completely described by the signal mean and its covariance. This is clarified below.

An epoch of scalp EEG (with m channels and n time points) is represented by the $m \times n$ matrix $\mathbf{E}$ and is linearly related to the $m \times n$ component matrix $\mathbf{s}$ by an $m \times m$ mixing matrix $\mathbf{W}$, that is, $\mathbf{E} = \mathbf{Ws}$. (This is true under the assumptions described above.) To find an "unmixing matrix" that can be applied to $\mathbf{E}$ to recover information about the components, PCA and ICA make additional requirements on the

statistical properties of $\mathbf{s}$. The statistical properties of $\mathbf{s}$ are completely defined by the function $F(\mathbf{s}^1, \mathbf{s}^2, \ldots, \mathbf{s}^m)$ that gives the joint probability of $(\mathbf{s}^1, \mathbf{s}^2, \ldots, \mathbf{s}^m)$. The variables $(\mathbf{s}^1, \mathbf{s}^2, \ldots, \mathbf{s}^m)$ representing the m columns of the $\mathbf{s}$ matrix are (mutually) independent if the joint probability density function can be factored as follows: $F(\mathbf{s}^1, \mathbf{s}^2, \ldots, \mathbf{s}^m) = F_1(\mathbf{s}^1) F_2(\mathbf{s}^2) F_3(\mathbf{s}^3) \ldots F_m(\mathbf{s}^m)$, where $F_i(\mathbf{s}^i)$ is the marginal probability density, which is independent of the other probability distributions. This simply states that the signal $\mathbf{s}^1$ is mutually independent of all the other signals. This is a stronger statement than uncorrelated, which only means that $< \mathbf{s}^i \mathbf{s}^j > - < \mathbf{s}^i > < \mathbf{s}^j > = 0$ $(i \neq j)$, where $< >$ denotes the average. Statistical independence is a stronger requirement, specifically, that $< g_1(\mathbf{s}^i) g_2(\mathbf{s}^j) > - < g_1(\mathbf{s}^i) > < g_2(\mathbf{s}^j) > = 0$ $(i \neq j)$, for any functions g_1 and g_2 (Papoulis, 1991). If the joint probability distribution functions are gaussian, the statements are equivalent, and in that case ICA is identical to PCA.

PCA is frequently performed using the singular value decomposition (SVD) algorithm (Golub and Van Loan, 1989), which states that it is always possible to find three matrices,

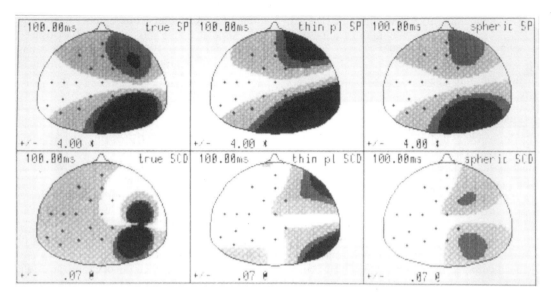

Figure 43.6. Maps of scalp potential (SP) (*top*) and corresponding scalp Laplacians or source current density (SCD) (*bottom*) for simulated data representing a tangential current dipole located in the right part of a sphere, with the 16 electrodes on the left part, in a three-layer concentric shell head model. From left to right: the "true" maps, computed from the model at each point; the rectangular surface or thin plate (thin pl) two-dimensional spline interpolated maps; and the spherical surface spline interpolated maps. (From Perrin, F., Pernier, J., Bertrand, O., and Echallier, J.F. 1989. Spherical splines for scalp potential and current density mapping. Electroencephalogr. Clin. Neurophysiol. 72:184–187, with permission of Elsevier Science Ireland.)

M, A, and **P**, such that $\mathbf{E} = \mathbf{M}\,\mathbf{A}\,\mathbf{P}^T$, in which **M** is an $m \times m$ matrix, such that $\mathbf{M}^T\mathbf{M} = \mathbf{M}\,\mathbf{M}^T = 1$; **A** is an $m \times m$ diagonal matrix; and $\mathbf{P}^T$ is an $m \times n$ matrix with $\mathbf{P}^T\,\mathbf{P} = 1$. Here **P** contains the m normalized orthogonal principal component waveforms, **A** contains m amplitudes that apply to the m principal components, and **M** represents the topographic factors that map the components to m EEG channels; $\mathbf{M}_{ij}$ is the contribution of the jth component to the ith channel. Note that **M** is an orthogonal matrix, $\mathbf{M}^T = \mathbf{M}^{-1}$, unlike the matrix **W** introduced in the ICA transform below. The connection between SVD and the transformation that identifies the component directions of maximal variance can be shown from the covariance matrix $\mathbf{C} = \mathbf{E}^T\mathbf{E}$, where $\mathbf{E}^T$ is the transpose of the measured EEG matrix. From the SVD relation above, $\mathbf{C} = (\mathbf{PAM}^T)\,(\mathbf{MAP}^T) = \mathbf{PA}^2\mathbf{P}^T$, and the principal components defined by SVD are the eigenvectors of the covariance matrix, where the first principal component is chosen to be the component associated with the maximal eigenvalue (the component with maximal variance).

Whereas PCA decorrelates the component outputs (using an orthogonal transformation matrix **M**), ICA attempts to find a transform that makes the component outputs statistically independent; that is, the joint probability function can be factored as $F(\mathbf{s}^1, \mathbf{s}^2, \ldots, \mathbf{s}^m) = F_1(\mathbf{s}^1)\,F_2(\mathbf{s}^2)\,F_3(\mathbf{s}^3)\,\ldots\,F_m(\mathbf{s}^m)$. ICA finds an unmixing matrix, $\mathbf{W}^{-1}$, that when applied to the measured EEG decomposes the multichannel scalp data into a sum of temporally independent and spatially fixed components, $\mathbf{u} = \mathbf{W}^{-1}\mathbf{E}$. Here **u** is identical to **s** introduced above, except for an unknown scaling factor. Unlike PCA, the transformation matrix in ICA is not orthogonal ($\mathbf{W}^T \neq \mathbf{W}^{-1}$), because of consideration of higher order statistics. A commonly used algorithm for ICA is a gradient-descent method called INFOMAX and is based on maximization of the entropy (Bell and Sejnowski, 1995). The algorithms used in ICA have been discussed and compared in reviews (Hyvärinen, 1999; Lee et al., 2000).

PCA using the SVD algorithm and ICA have been applied to EEG and evoked potential data as a means of decomposing an epoch of multichannel EEG or evoked potential data into a linear combination of features defined in terms of their

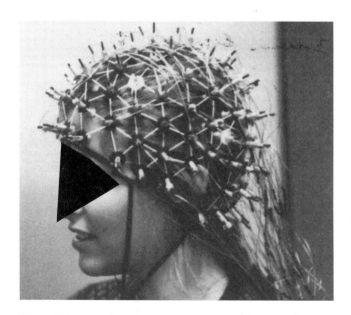

Figure 43.7. An example of a special sensor array used for high-resolution EEG studies: the 128-channel geodesic sensor net. The net is applied with the lower band placed across the brow ridge and along the canthomeatal line. (From Tucker, D.M. 1993. Spatial sampling of head electrical fields: the geodesic sensor net. Electroencephalogr. Clin. Neurophysiol. 87:154–163, with permission of Elsevier Science Ireland.)

spatial distribution, temporal profile, and amplitude (Harner, 1988, 1990; Harner and Riggio, 1989; Jung et al., 2001; Makeig et al., 2002; Mckeown et al., 1999).

PCA and ICA may be used to analyze an epoch of multichannel EEG into multiple linearly independent (spatially and temporally uncorrelated in PCA and statistically independent in ICA) components or features. The original EEG may be reconstructed as a linear combination of all components. The results of PCA and ICA are the components, which may be displayed as time-series waveforms, and topographic factors that determine how much each component contributes to each EEG channel. These factors may be displayed as a topographic map after suitable interpolation to points other than the electrode positions.

Because each component is independent of every other component, the topographic factors for the various components may be used as a starting point for dipole analysis or other source localization techniques (Achim et al., 1988; Baumgartner et al., 1989; Soong and Koles, 1995; Wong, 1991; Zhukov et al., 2000). PCA has also been used to deter-

mine empirically the actual number of sources (dipoles) before dipole analysis is performed (Mosher et al., 1992; Scherg and Picton, 1991). In addition, PCA has been used as a means for separation of "abnormal" from "normal" components of an EEG (Koles, 1991). However, a one-to-one correspondence does not necessarily exist between components and individual anatomical sources. A single source (for example, the eyes as generators of ocular movement artifacts) may produce waveforms that separate into several components (for example, one for horizontal eye movements and another for vertical eye movements). Conversely, multiple sources may contribute to one of the components. Thus, ascribing any physiological significance directly to the individual components determined by PCA is inappropriate (Lamothe and Stroink, 1991), and, although it remains to be clarified, similar arguments can most likely be made about ICA components.

One practical application of PCA (Lagerlund et al., 1997) and ICA (Jung et al., 1998) is to remove unwanted artifacts, such as ocular movement or electrocardiographic signals,

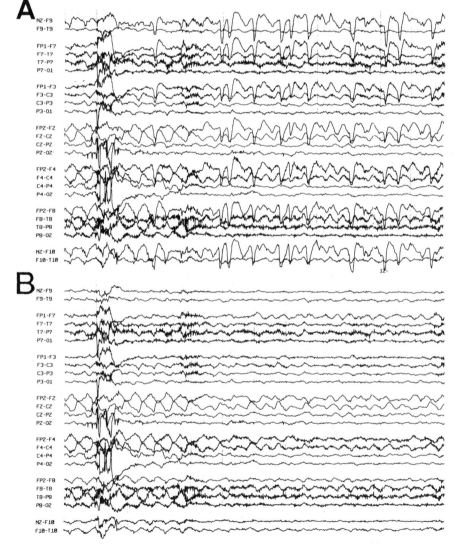

Figure 43.8. Spatial filtering of ocular movement artifacts by principal component analysis. For this analysis, the singular value decomposition method was applied to a 5-second epoch of EEG with a 24-channel bipolar montage; the resulting 24 components were inspected to determine that components 1 through 3 represented ocular movement artifacts, and a spatial filter was created by omitting the first three components from the EEG. **A:** This spatial filter was then applied to a 12-second epoch of EEG recorded from the same subject at the end of a partial seizure, which shows rhythmic and polymorphic delta activity obscured by ocular movement artifacts. **B:** In the resulting spatially filtered EEG, ocular movement artifacts have been largely removed, allowing the underlying slow waves to be seen. Some slow components in the frontal channels are attenuated but not removed; they are probably not ocular movement artifacts. (From Lagerlund, T.D., Sharbrough, F.W., and Busacker, N.E. 1997. Spatial filtering of multichannel electroencephalographic recordings through principal component analysis by singular value decomposition. J. Clin. Neurophysiol. 14:73–82, with permission of the American Clinical Neurophysiology Society.)

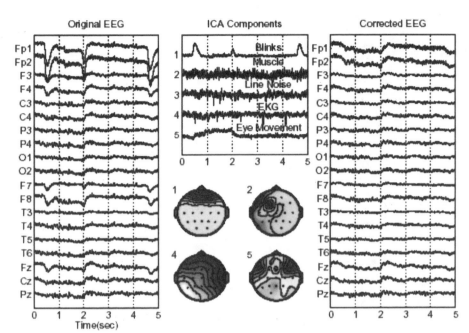

Figure 43.9. *Left:* Five-second epoch of an EEG time series. *Center:* Independent component analysis (ICA) components accounting for eye movements, cardiac signals, and line noise sources. EKG, electrocardiogram. *Right:* The same EEG signals "corrected" for artifacts by removing the five selected components. (From Jung, T.-P., Humphries, C., Lee, T.-W., et al. 1998. Extended ICA removes artifacts from electroencephalographic recordings. In *Advances in Neural Information Processing Systems 10:* Proceedings of the 1997 conference, Eds., M.I. Jordan, M.J. Kearns, and S.A. Solla, pp. 894–900. Cambridge, Massachusetts: MIT Press, with permission of MIT Press.)

from the EEG on the basis of their *spatial* characteristics (that is, their distribution across channels). This is done by omitting the components representing these artifacts from the linear combination when reconstructing the EEG from the component waveforms. This technique has been used for artifact recognition and removal, and with PCA has been found to be superior to other methods, such as dipole modeling and propagation factors (Lagerlund et al., 1997; Lins et al., 1993), and does not depend on assuming a one-to-one relationship between principal components and sources (Figs. 43.8 and 43.9).

Cortical Projection Methods

Although the inverse problem, as stated previously, does not have a unique solution, the *inward continuation* problem can be solved uniquely under appropriate conditions. That is, one can uniquely calculate the potential at all points on a surface inside the head (for example, the cortical surface) from the potentials on the outer head (scalp) surface if no intervening generators exist and if the geometry and electrical properties of all intervening tissues are known. In principle, this does not require knowledge of the location or number of generators (other than the assumption that all generators are located *inside* the cortical surface). In addition to calculating the potential on the cortical surface, one may calculate the Laplacian of this potential.

In practice, several methods have been proposed to estimate cortical potentials from measured scalp potentials. The *spatial deconvolution* algorithm, mentioned earlier (Junghöfer et al., 1997; Nunez, 1986, 1987), is a model-dependent method to do this; it assumes a single radial dipole under each electrode and estimates the cortical potentials from the calculated dipole strengths. The CIT, mentioned previously, assumes a hemispheric array of radial dipoles to estimate cortical potentials (Fig. 43.10) (Ford et al., 1993; Kearfott et

al., 1991; Sidman, 1991; Sidman et al., 1990). In addition to their uses for interpolation and calculation of the Laplacian of the scalp potentials, the SHE and spherical spline algorithms can be coupled with a three-sphere or similar volume-conductor model to estimate cortical potentials (Pascual-Marqui et al., 1988; Lagerlund et al., 1995); however, this method is not very sensitive to deep sources. The *iterative refinement of the minimum norm solution*, mentioned previously, assumes a large number of dipoles in a realistic cortical model (Srebro, 1994, 1996a,b; Srebro and Oguz, 1997) and could be used to estimate cortical potentials as well. Finally, the *deblurring* algorithm (Gevins et al., 1991; Le and Gevins, 1993) uses a finite element model of the scalp, skull, and cortical surface to estimate potentials at the cortical surface (Fig. 43.11). Many of these methods have been applied to somatosensory, visual, and long-latency auditory evoked potentials to localize cortical sources of various evoked potential peaks.

Volume Conductor Models

The only electrical property of the volume conductor that is usually modeled is the electrical conductivity. The assumption is made that, at the frequencies of interest for EEG, capacitive effects within the head tissues are negligible. Models of the head as a volume conductor may be classified as *homogeneous* or *inhomogeneous*. Homogeneous models assume uniform electrical conductivity throughout and ignore the markedly different conductivity of various tissues, such as the poorly conducting skull. Inhomogeneous models assume that the head may be divided into regions that are homogeneous in themselves, but each region may have different electrical conductivities.

Models also differ in the geometry assumed for the head. The most common models are based on spherical surfaces.

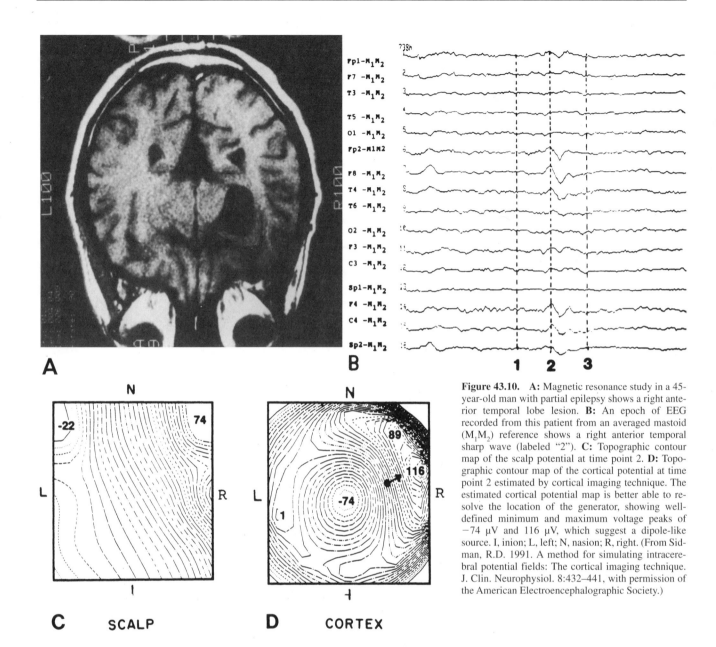

Figure 43.10. **A:** Magnetic resonance study in a 45-year-old man with partial epilepsy shows a right anterior temporal lobe lesion. **B:** An epoch of EEG recorded from this patient from an averaged mastoid (M_1M_2) reference shows a right anterior temporal sharp wave (labeled "2"). **C:** Topographic contour map of the scalp potential at time point 2. **D:** Topographic contour map of the cortical potential at time point 2 estimated by cortical imaging technique. The estimated cortical potential map is better able to resolve the location of the generator, showing well-defined minimum and maximum voltage peaks of −74 μV and 116 μV, which suggest a dipole-like source. I, inion; L, left; N, nasion; R, right. (From Sidman, R.D. 1991. A method for simulating intracerebral potential fields: The cortical imaging technique. J. Clin. Neurophysiol. 8:432–441, with permission of the American Electroencephalographic Society.)

The simplest is the homogeneous sphere model, which assumes that the head is a perfect sphere with uniform electrical conductivity throughout. This model has the computational advantage that the potential on the scalp surface due to a single dipole of arbitrary location and orientation may be expressed in analytical (closed) form rather than as an infinite series expansion (Wilson and Bayley, 1950). More complex models assume concentric spherical shells. For example, in a three-sphere model (Fig. 43.12), the inner sphere represents the brain, the middle spherical shell the skull, and the outermost spherical shell the scalp (Kavanagh et al., 1978; Rush and Driscoll, 1969). In a four-sphere model, an additional inner spherical shell representing cerebrospinal fluid is included between brain and skull (Cuffin and Cohen, 1979). Most models assume that each spherical shell is isotropic in its electrical properties, although some multisphere models allow anisotropic conductivity values (Zhou and van Oosterom, 1992). The homogeneous sphere model is used by CIT and some dipole localization algorithms, whereas the three-sphere (or four-sphere) model is used by the spatial deconvolution, SHE, iterative refinement of the minimum norm solution, and many dipole localization algorithms. Although neglecting the skull clearly leads to mislocalization of intracranial dipole generators, a simple relationship has been found between the location and strength of the best-fit dipole in a homogeneous sphere and that in a three-sphere volume conductor, which allows dipoles obtained from the homogeneous sphere model to be easily converted to a more realistic model (Ary et al., 1981).

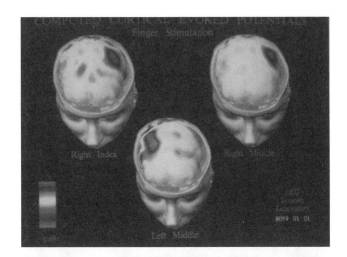

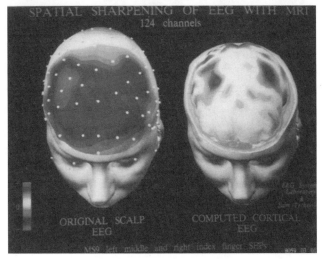

Figure 43.11. **Top:** Estimated cortical steady-state somatosensory evoked potentials (SEPs) elicited by 14.92-Hz stimulation (with occasional missing stimuli) of the left middle, right middle, and right index fingers of a normal subject with use of the deblurring method; all three show the expected contralateral maximum in activity. **Bottom:** Scalp (*left*) and estimated cortical (*right*) SEPs of this subject in response to 14.92-Hz stimulation of the left middle and right index fingers; the *white dots* on the left represent the 124 scalp EEG recording electrode positions. The increase in spatial detail produced by the deblurring method is apparent. (From Le, J., and Gevins, A. 1993. Method to reduce blur distortion from EEG's using a realistic head model. IEEE Trans. Biomed. Eng. 40:517–528, with permission of IEEE.)

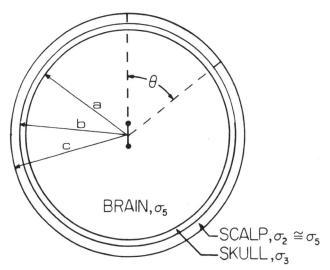

Figure 43.12. Three concentric spheres head model. The sphere radii are *a*, brain; *b*, skull; and *c*, scalp. The scalp and brain conductivities (σ_2 and σ_5) are approximately equal but are about 80 times the skull conductivity (σ_3) in this model. (From Nunez, P. 1981. *Electric Fields of the Brain: The Neurophysics of EEG*, pp. 140–175. New York: Oxford University Press, with permission of the publisher.)

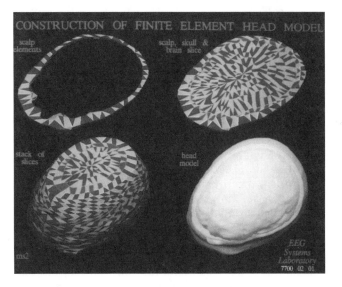

Figure 43.13. Method of automated construction of finite elements in brain, skull, and scalp volumes using magnetic resonance images. *Upper left:* A single ring of scalp. *Upper right:* The addition of skull and brain elements within one slice bounded by two consecutive horizontal magnetic resonance images. *Lower left:* All slices except the topmost horizontal slice. *Lower right:* A shaded depiction of all three surfaces superimposed. (From Le, J., and Gevins, A. 1993. Method to reduce blur distortion from EEG's using a realistic head model. IEEE Trans. Biomed. Eng. 40:517–528, with permission of IEEE.)

The finite element (boundary element) method assumes that important head regions (typically scalp, skull, and brain) may be decomposed into multiple small adjacent elements, typically in the form of small tetrahedrons of approximately 1 to 2 cm in length and thickness, each of which is homogeneous. The actual geometry of the scalp, skull, and brain surfaces as obtained from MRI of the head may be modeled in this fashion with reasonable accuracy when sufficient elements are used, producing a volume-conductor model tailored to an individual subject (Fig. 43.13). The electrical conductivities of the various elements are assigned one of three values, depending on whether they are located within scalp, skull, or brain (Gevins et al., 1991; Le and Gevins, 1993; Srebro and Oguz, 1997). Finite element models used in dipole localization, LORETA, and deblurring algorithms may lead to significantly more accurate localization of sources than the simpler spherical models, but they are considerably more computationally demanding.

Magnetoencephalographic Source Localization

Magnetoencephalography (MEG) is the recording of the small magnetic fields produced by the electrical activity of neurons in the brain. These magnetic fields are generated by current flowing in neurons (for the EEG, primarily due to postsynaptic potentials generated in cortical pyramidal cells, with little or no contribution from action potentials, because postsynaptic potentials occur synchronously in thousands or tens of thousands of neurons when action potentials reach the cerebral cortex in afferent axons). There is a small contribution to the MEG from extracellular current flow in the volume-conducting medium around the brain, but this is generally less than the contribution of intracellular currents. These magnetic fields are extremely small, typically in the femtotesla or picotesla range (10^{-15} to 10^{-12} T), and must be detected by a magnetic gradiometer connected to a special type of extremely sensitive amplifier called a superconducting quantum interference device (SQUID), which must be cooled by liquid helium. To eliminate "noise" signals due to the much larger magnetic fields associated with electrical equipment, power lines, and Earth's magnetic field, a special magnetically shielded room is also required. This, plus the expensive SQUID devices and the liquid helium cryostat required, makes MEG a very expensive tool. Another disadvantage of MEG is that it cannot readily be used for the long-term recordings needed to capture and localize an epileptic seizure because the subject's head must be kept immobilized near the magnetic gradiometer array during the entire recording. Also, until recently the number of channels available in commercial MEG instruments was relatively small, although now there are systems available with more than 100 channels, and the spatial resolution of such devices is quite good. Finally, because magnetic fields created by a current source are always oriented along a tangent to a circle around the line of current flow, the MEG is insensitive to radially oriented currents in the cerebral cortex and is sensitive only to tangential currents, in contrast to EEG, which is sensitive to both (although more sensitive to radial currents). For this reason, MEG recordings are often combined with simultaneous, conventional EEG recordings.

The most important advantage of MEG is source localization. Unlike the situation for EEG, the accuracy of localization of intracranial sources is not limited by the smearing effects of the volume-conducting medium (especially the poorly conducting skull) on electrical potentials because all the tissues between the sources and the magnetic field detectors are transparent to magnetic fields (Cohen and Cuffin, 1991; Cuffin and Cohen, 1979; Hari, 1994; Lopes da Silva et al., 1991; Stefan et al., 1994). This means that when a dipole localization algorithm is used with MEG data, a simple homogeneous sphere model of the volume conductor is usu-

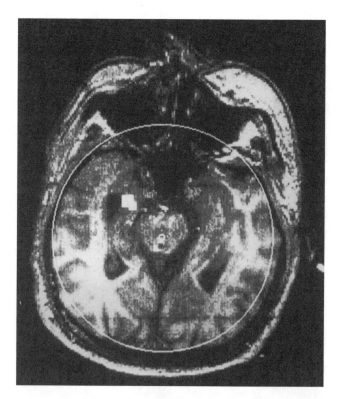

Figure 43.14. Results of magnetoencephalographic source dipole localization after fusion with magnetic resonance image in patient with intractable partial epilepsy and right mesial temporal atrophy (confirmed by tissue pathologic examination after amygdalohippocampectomy). The interictal epileptic activity on magnetoencephalographic recordings (rectangular markers) was localized to the right mesial temporal region. (From Stefan, H., Schuler, P., Abraham-Fuchs, K., et al. 1994. Magnetic source localization and morphological changes in temporal lobe epilepsy: Comparison of MEG/EEG, ECoG and volumetric MRI in presurgical evaluation of operated patients. Acta Neurol. Scand. Suppl. 152:83–88, with permission of Munksgaard.)

ally sufficient to obtain accurate source dipole localization. This result has been demonstrated in subjects with known intracranial lesions (such as tumors) by superimposing the dipole locations determined by the model on the subject's MRI and comparing the dipole locations with the location of the lesion (Fig. 43.14). In addition to recording the spontaneous MEG, one can record evoked magnetic fields in response to visual, auditory, and somatosensory stimuli, and these may also be subjected to dipole localization algorithms to determine the location of visual, auditory, and somatosensory cortical areas (Harding et al., 1991). This technique may be used as part of the surgical planning for patients with tumors or vascular malformations; in these patients, the sensory cortical areas may be significantly displaced from their usual or expected location by the foreign body lesion.

References

Achim, A., Richer, F., and Saint-Hilaire, J.M. 1988. Methods for separating temporally overlapping sources of neuroelectric data. Brain Topogr. 1: 22–28.

Achim, A., Richer, F., and Saint-Hilaire, J.M. 1991. Methodological considerations for the evaluation of spatio-temporal source models. Electroencephalogr. Clin. Neurophysiol. 79:227–240.

Ary, J.P., Klein, S.A., and Fender, D.H. 1981. Location of sources of evoked scalp potentials: corrections for skull and scalp thicknesses. IEEE Trans. Biomed. Eng. 28:447–452.

Babiloni, F., Babiloni, C., Fattorini, L., et al. 1995. Performances of surface Laplacian estimators: a study of simulated and real scalp potential distributions. Brain Topogr. 8:35–45.

Babiloni, F., Babiloni C., Carducci, F., et al. 1996. Spline Laplacian estimate of EEG potentials over a realistic magnetic resonance-constructed scalp surface model. Electroencephalogr. Clin. Neurophysiol. 98:363–373.

Baumgartner, C. 1994. EEG dipole localization: discussion. Acta Neurol. Scand. Suppl. 152:31–32.

Baumgartner, C., Sutherling, W.W., Di, S., et al. 1989. Investigation of multiple simultaneously active brain sources in the electroencephalogram. J. Neurosci. Methods 30:175–184.

Bell, A.J., and Sejnowski, T.J. 1995. An information-maximization approach to blind separation and blind deconvolution. Neural Comput. 7: 1129–1159.

Cabrera Fernández, D., Grave de Peralta Menendez, R., and Gonzalez Andino, S.L. 1995. Some limitations of spatio temporal source models. Brain Topogr. 7:233–243.

Cohen, D., and Cuffin, B.N. 1991. EEG versus MEG localization accuracy: theory and experiment. Brain Topogr. 4:95–103.

Cuffin, B.N., and Cohen, D. 1979. Comparison of the magnetoencephalogram and electroencephalogram. Electroencephalogr. Clin. Neurophysiol. 47:132–146.

Duffy, F.H., Burchfiel, J.L., and Lombroso, C.T. 1979. Brain electrical activity mapping (BEAM): a method for extending the clinical utility of EEG and evoked potential data. Ann. Neurol. 5:309–321.

Ebersole, J.S. 1991. EEG dipole modeling in complex partial epilepsy. Brain Topogr. 4:113–123.

Ebersole, J.S. 1994. Non-invasive localization of the epileptogenic focus by EEG dipole modeling. Acta Neurol. Scand. Suppl. 152:20–28.

Ebersole, J.S. 1999. EEG source modeling: the first word. J. Clin. Neurophysiol. 16:201–203.

Ford, M.R., Sidman, R.D., and Ramsey, G. 1993. Spatio-temporal progression of the AEP P300 component using the cortical imaging technique. Brain Topogr. 6:43–50.

Gevins, A., Le, J., Brickett, P., et al. 1991. Seeing through the skull: Advanced EEGs use MRIs to accurately measure cortical activity from the scalp. Brain Topogr. 4:125–131.

Golub, G.H., and Van Loan, C.F. 1989. *Matrix Computation*, 2nd ed. Baltimore: Johns Hopkins University Press.

Harding, G.F., Janday, B., and Armstrong, R.A. 1991. Topographic mapping and source localization of the pattern reversal visual evoked magnetic response. Brain Topogr. 4:47–55.

Hari, R. 1994. Comment: MEG in the study of epilepsy. Acta Neurol. Scand. Suppl. 152:89–90.

Harner, R.N. 1988. Brain mapping or spatial analysis? Brain Topogr. 1: 73–75.

Harner, R.N. 1990. Singular value decomposition—a general linear model for analysis of multivariate structure in the electroencephalogram. Brain Topogr. 3:43–47.

Harner, R.N., and Riggio, S. 1989. Application of singular value decomposition to topographic analysis of flash-evoked potentials. Brain Topogr. 2:91–98.

Hjorth, B. 1975. An on-line transformation of EEG scalp potentials into orthogonal source derivations. Electroencephalogr. Clin. Neurophysiol. 39: 526–530.

Hyvärinen, A. 1999. Survey on independent component analysis. Neural. Comput. Surv. 2:94–128.

Jung, T.-P., Humphries, C., Lee, T.-W., et al. 1998. Extended ICA removes artifacts from electroencephalographic recordings. In *Advances in Neural Information Processing Systems 10*: Proceedings of the 1997 conference, Eds. M.I. Jordan, M.J. Kearns, and S.A. Solla, pp. 894–900. Cambridge, MA: MIT Press.

Jung, T.-P., Makeig, S., Mckeown, M.J., et al. 2001. Imaging brain dynamics using independent component analysis. Proc. IEEE 89:1107–1122.

Junghöfer, M., Elbert, T., Leiderer, P., et al. 1997. Mapping EEG-potentials on the surface of the brain: a strategy for uncovering cortical sources. Brain Topogr. 9:203–217.

Kavanagh, R.N., Darcey, T.M., Lehmann, D., et al. 1978. Evaluation of methods for three-dimensional localization of electrical sources in the human brain. IEEE Trans. Biomed. Eng. 25:421–429.

Kearfott, R.B., Sidman, R.D., Major, D.J., et al. 1991. Numerical tests of a method for simulating electrical potentials on the cortical surface. IEEE Trans. Biomed. Eng. 38:294–299.

Koles, Z.J. 1991. The quantitative extraction and topographic mapping of the abnormal components in the clinical EEG. Electroencephalogr. Clin. Neurophysiol. 79:440–447.

Lagerlund, T.D. 1991. Montage reformatting and digital filtering. In *Epilepsy Surgery*, Ed. H. Lüders, pp. 317–322. New York: Raven Press.

Lagerlund, T.D., Sharbrough, F.W., Busacker, N.E., et al. 1995. Interelectrode coherences from nearest-neighbor and spherical harmonic expansion computation of Laplacian of scalp potential. Electroencephalogr. Clin. Neurophysiol. 95:178–188.

Lagerlund, T.D., Sharbrough, F.W., and Busacker, N.E. 1997. Spatial filtering of multichannel electroencephalographic recordings through principal component analysis by singular value decomposition. J. Clin. Neurophysiol. 14:73–82.

Lamothe, R., and Stroink, G. 1991. Orthogonal expansions: their applicability to signal extraction in electrophysiological mapping data. Med. Biol. Eng. Comput. 29:522–528.

Law, S.K., Nunez, P.L., and Wijesinghe, R.S. 1993. High-resolution EEG using spline generated surface Laplacians on spherical and ellipsoidal surfaces. IEEE Trans. Biomed. Eng. 40:145–153.

Le, J., and Gevins, A. 1993. Method to reduce blur distortion from EEG's using a realistic head model. IEEE Trans. Biomed. Eng. 40:517–528.

Lee, T., Girolami, M., Bell, A., et al. 2000. A unifying information-theoretic framework for independent component analysis. Comput. Math. Applicat. 39:1–21.

Lemos, M.S., and Fisch, B.J. 1991. The weighted average reference montage. Electroencephalogr. Clin. Neurophysiol. 79:361–370.

Lins, O.G., Picton, T.W., Berg, P., et al. 1993. Ocular artifacts in recording EEGs and event-related potentials. I: Scalp topography. II: source dipoles and source components. Brain Topogr. 6:a, 51–63; b, 65–78.

Lopes da Silva, F.H., Wieringa, H.J., and Peters, M.J. 1991. Source localization of EEG versus MEG: empirical comparison using visually evoked responses and theoretical considerations. Brain Topogr. 4:133–142.

Makeig, S., Westerfield, M., Jung, T.P., et al. 2002. Dynamic brain sources of visual evoked responses. Science 295:690–694.

Mckeown, M.J., Humphries, C., Iragui, V., et al. 1999. Spatially fixed patterns account for the spike and wave features in absence seizures. Brain Topogr. 12:107–116.

Mosher, J.C., Lewis, P.S., and Leahy, R.M. 1992. Multiple dipole modeling and localization from spatio-temporal MEG data. IEEE Trans. Biomed. Eng. 39:541–557.

Nunez, P. 1986. Removal of reference electrode and volume conduction effects from evoked potentials. I. Derivation of method and computer simulation. Technical Note LTN 71–85–13. San Diego: Navy Personnel Research and Development Center.

Nunez, P. 1987. Removal of reference electrode and volume conduction effects by spatial deconvolution of evoked potentials using a three-concentric sphere model of the head. Electroencephalogr. Clin. Neurophysiol. Suppl. 39:143–148.

Nunez, P.L. 1989. Estimation of large scale neocortical source activity with EEG surface Laplacians. Brain Topogr. 2:141–154.

Nunez, P.L., and Westdorp, A.F. 1994. The surface Laplacian, high resolution EEG and controversies. Brain Topogr. 6:221–226.

Nunez, P.L., Pilgreen, K.L., Westdorp, A.F., et al. 1991. A visual study of surface potentials and Laplacians due to distributed neocortical sources: computer simulations and evoked potentials. Brain Topogr. 4:151–168.

Nunez, P.L., Silberstein, R.B., Cadusch, P.J., et al. 1994. A theoretical and experimental study of high resolution EEG based on surface Laplacians and cortical imaging. Electroencephalogr. Clin. Neurophysiol. 90:40–57.

Papoulis, A. 1991. *Probability, Random Variables, and Stochastic Processes*, 3rd ed. New York: McGraw-Hill.

Pascual-Marqui, R.D., Gonzalez-Andino, S.L., Valdes-Sosa, P.A., et al. 1988. Current source density estimation and interpolation based on the spherical harmonic Fourier expansion. Int. J. Neurosci. 43:237–249.

Pascual-Marqui, R.D., Michel, C.M., and Lehmann, D. 1994. Low resolution electromagnetic tomography: a new method for localizing electrical activity in the brain. Int. J. Psychophysiol. 18:49–65.

Perrin, F., Bertrand, O., and Pernier, J. 1987a. Scalp current density mapping: value and estimation from potential data. IEEE Trans. Biomed. Eng. 34:283–288.

Perrin, F., Pernier, J., Bertrand, O., et al. 1987b. Mapping of scalp potentials by surface spline interpolation. Electroencephalogr. Clin. Neurophysiol. 66:75–81.

Perrin, F., Pernier, J., Bertrand, O., et al. 1989. Spherical splines for scalp potential and current density mapping. Electroencephalogr. Clin. Neurophysiol. 72:184–187.

Phillips, C., Rugg, M.D., and Friston, K.J. 2002. Anatomically informed basis functions for EEG source localization: combining functional and anatomical constraints. Neuroimage 16:678–695.

Radich, B.M., and Buckley, K.M. 1995. EEG dipole localization bounds and MAP algorithms for head models with parameter uncertainties. IEEE Trans. Biomed. Eng. 42:233–241.

Raz, J., Turetsky, B., and Fein, G. 1992. Frequency domain estimation of the parameters of human brain electrical dipoles. J. Am. Stat. Assoc. 87:69–77.

Rush, S., and Driscoll, D.A. 1969. EEG electrode sensitivity—an application of reciprocity. IEEE Trans. Biomed. Eng. 16:15–22.

Salu, Y., Cohen, L.G., Rose, D., et al. 1990. An improved method for localizing electric brain dipoles. IEEE Trans. Biomed. Eng. 37:699–705.

Scherg, M. 1990. Fundamentals of dipole source potential analysis. In *Auditory Evoked Magnetic Fields and Electric Potentials. Advances in Audiology*, Eds. F. Grandori, M. Hoke, and G.L. Romani, vol. 6, pp. 40–69. Basel: Karger.

Scherg, M. 1994. From EEG source localization to source imaging. Acta Neurol. Scand. Suppl. 152:29–30.

Scherg, M., and Berg, P. 1991. Use of prior knowledge in brain electromagnetic source analysis. Brain Topogr. 4:143–150.

Scherg, M., and Picton, T.W. 1991. Separation and identification of event-related potential components by brain electric source analysis. Electroencephalogr. Clin. Neurophysiol. Suppl. 42:24–37.

Scherg, M., and von Cramon, D. 1985. A new interpretation of the generators of BAEP waves I-V: results of a spatio-temporal dipole model. Electroencephalogr. Clin. Neurophysiol. 62:290–299.

Scherg, M., and Von Cramon, D. 1986. Evoked dipole source potentials of the human auditory cortex. Electroencephalogr. Clin. Neurophysiol. 65:344–360.

Schneider, M.R. 1972. A multistage process for computing virtual dipolar sources of EEG discharges from surface information. IEEE Trans. Biomed. Eng. 19:1–12.

Shaw, G. 1989. Spherical harmonic analysis of the electroencephalogram. Ph.D. thesis, University of Alberta, Edmonton.

Sidman, R.D. 1991. A method for simulating intracerebral potential fields: the cortical imaging technique. J. Clin. Neurophysiol. 8:432–441.

Sidman, R.D., Giambalvo, V., Allison, T., et al. 1978. A method for localization of sources of human cerebral potentials evoked by sensory stimuli. Sens. Processes 2:116–129.

Sidman, R.D., Kearfott, R.B., Major, D.J., et al. 1989. Development and application of mathematical techniques for the non-invasive localization of the sources of scalp-recorded electric potentials. In *Biomedical Modelling and Simulation*, Eds. J. Eisenfeld, and D.S. Levine, pp. 133–157. Basel: J.C. Baltzer.

Sidman, R.D., Ford, M.R., Ramsey, G., et al. 1990. Age-related features of the resting and P300 auditory evoked responses using the dipole localization method and cortical imaging technique. J. Neurosci. Methods 33:23–32.

Sidman, R.D., Major, D.J., Ford, M.R., et al. 1991. Age-related features of the resting pattern-reversal visual evoked response using the dipole localization method and cortical imaging technique. J. Neurosci. Methods 37:27–36.

Sidman, R.D., Vincent, D.J., Smith, D.B., et al. 1992. Experimental tests of the cortical imaging technique—applications to the response to median nerve stimulation and the localization of epileptiform discharges. IEEE Trans. Biomed. Eng. 39:437–444.

Soong, A.C., and Koles, Z.J. 1995. Principal-component localization of the sources of the background EEG. IEEE Trans. Biomed. Eng. 42:59–67.

Srebro, R. 1994. Continuous current source inversion of evoked potential fields in a spherical model head. IEEE Trans. Biomed. Eng. 41:997–1003.

Srebro, R. 1996a. An iterative approach to the solution of the inverse problem. Electroencephalogr. Clin. Neurophysiol. 98:349–362.

Srebro, R. 1996b. Iterative refinement of the minimum norm solution of the bioelectric inverse problem. IEEE Trans. Biomed. Eng. 43:547–552.

Srebro, R., and Oguz, R.M. 1997. Estimating cortical activity from VEPS with the shrinking ellipsoid inverse. Electroencephalogr. Clin. Neurophysiol. 102:343–355.

Srinivasan, R., Nunez, P.L., Tucker, D.M., et al. 1996. Spatial sampling and filtering of EEG with spline Laplacians to estimate cortical potentials. Brain Topogr. 8:355–366.

Stefan, H., Schuler, P., Abraham-Fuchs, K., et al. 1994. Magnetic source localization and morphological changes in temporal lobe epilepsy: comparison of MEG/EEG, ECoG and volumetric MRI in presurgical evaluation of operated patients. Acta Neurol. Scand. Suppl. 152:83–88.

Tucker, D.M. 1993. Spatial sampling of head electrical fields: the geodesic sensor net. Electroencephalogr. Clin. Neurophysiol. 87:154–163.

Valdés, P., Bosch, J., Grave, R., et al. 1992. Frequency domain models of the EEG. Brain Topogr. 4:309–319.

Wallin, G., and Stålberg, E. 1980. Source derivation in clinical routine EEG. Electroencephalogr. Clin. Neurophysiol. 50:282–292.

Wilson, F.N., and Bayley, R.H. 1950. The electric field of an eccentric dipole in a homogeneous conducting medium. Circulation 1:84–92.

Wong, P.K. 1991. Source modelling of the rolandic focus. Brain Topogr. 4:105–112.

Worrell, G.A., Lagerlund, T.D., Sharbrough, F.W., et al. 2000. Localization of the epileptic focus by low-resolution electromagnetic tomography in patients with a lesion demonstrated on MRI. Brain Topogr. 12:273–282.

Zhang, Z., and Jewett, D.L. 1993. Insidious errors in dipole localization parameters at a single time-point due to model misspecification of number of shells. Electroencephalogr. Clin. Neurophysiol. 88:1–11.

Zhang, Z., and Jewett, D.L. 1994a. DSL and MUSIC under model misspecification and noise-conditions. Brain Topogr. 7:151–161.

Zhang, Z., and Jewett, D.L. 1994b. Model misspecification detection by means of multiple generator errors, using the observed potential map. Brain Topogr. 7:29–39.

Zhang, Z., Jewett, D.L., and Goodwill, G. 1994. Insidious errors in dipole parameters due to shell model misspecification using multiple time-points. Brain Topogr. 6:283–298.

Zhou, H., and van Oosterom, A. 1992. Computation of the potential distribution in a four-layer anisotropic concentric spherical volume conductor. IEEE Trans. Biomed. Eng. 39:154–158.

Zhukov, L., Weinstein, D., and Johnson, C. 2000. Independent component analysis for EEG source localization. IEEE Eng. Med. Biol. Mag. 19:87–96.

44. Spinal Cord Monitoring

Marc R. Nuwer and James W. Packwood

Continuous monitoring of the spinal cord provides a surgeon with warnings about potential damage to the spinal cord. Such warnings can trigger corrective actions before the impairment becomes permanent (American Academy of Neurology, 1990; Jones et al., 1994; Møller, 1995; Nuwer, 1986; Russell and Rodichok, 1995). Several different methods of spinal cord monitoring are now available (American EEG Society, 1994; Nuwer et al., 1993). The most commonly used method is stimulation of the posterior tibial nerve while recording from the scalp and neck. A more recent development is transcranial cortical stimulation with recording from leg muscles or large nerves. Some monitorists use the alternate technique of recording or stimulating at the spinal cord itself.

Intraoperative neurophysiological monitoring is valuable and cost-effective when the nervous system is at risk during an operation. Spinal cord monitoring is useful during procedures around the spinal cord. It potentially can reduce the risk of ischemia from compression of feeding blood vessels, compression or stretch injury, or other damage to the spinal cord. In general the risk of serious damage to a nervous system pathway should be at least 1% to justify monitoring that pathway. In addition it must be possible for the surgeon or anesthesiologist to alter the operating plan if the evoked potential (EP) monitoring shows a possible impairment.

Monitoring Techniques

Somatosensory Evoked Potential Techniques

Electrical stimulation is delivered to the posterior tibial nerve at the ankles. Unilateral stimulation is preferred to test each half of the spinal cord. Bilateral simultaneous stimulation paradigms may fail to detect a significant change from baseline if one half of the cord is impaired while the other half of the cord is still functioning well. Bilateral stimulation produces higher amplitude scalp responses that can be helpful when the response to independent unilateral stimulation is poorly defined.

Stimulation is delivered usually alternately to each leg. The separation of stimulation to the other leg is half the stimulus interval for each leg separately. In this way, monitoring can be accomplished for each leg quickly. One disadvantage to this technique is that the two EPs tend to overlap one another. This is so especially if open filters are used (e.g., a low filter set at 1 Hz). The overlap is less prominent when the low filter is restricted (e.g., a low filter set at 30 Hz with a left-right stimulus delay greater than 30 msec).

Cortical somatosensory evoked potential (SEP) amplitudes increase as the stimulus intensity increases but only up to a certain point; beyond that there is little or no gain in EP amplitude. However, that point differs among patients and even among various nerves within the same patient. That point is approximately twice the motor threshold in typical outpatients. For outpatients the stimulus intensity is kept below that point to allow the patient to relax. The unconscious patient can well tolerate stimulation at twice the motor threshold. Neuromuscular junction blocking agents reduce the muscle artifact but interfere with checking the motor threshold and application site. Technologists may assess the placement of the stimulating electrodes prior to the use of neuromuscular blocking agents, e.g., prior to surgery. In the absence of noticeable motor movement, optimal intensity can be gauged by gradually increasing the intensity until the EP amplitude no longer increases.

There is an inherent trade-off in increasing the stimulation rate. At fast rates, the EP amplitude is attenuated. The EP is harder to find at fast rates; slower is better. Yet, operating room (OR) monitoring is usually undertaken to identify complications as quickly as possible. The faster the stimulation, the more quickly a new EP can be averaged and the more quickly a clinical problem can be identified; faster is better. The correct stimulus rate is a compromise between those two competing goals. The trade-off point for stimulus rate is 5/sec for typical patients (Nuwer and Dawson, 1984a). The actual optimal stimulus rate varies among patients. The older and the more symptomatic the patient, the slower and stronger the stimulation will have to be to elicit acceptable responses. If a patient has a particularly low amplitude EP, a lower stimulation rate is useful to increase the EP amplitude. Likewise, if a patient has a very large easily defined EP, faster rates of stimulation can be employed.

For posterior tibial nerve stimulation, the maximum amplitude of the early cortical peak is often slightly contralateral to the hemisphere generating it, a phenomenon called "paradoxical localization." Arriving somatosensory impulses generate a dipole pointing in varying directions, sometimes in a more anterior-posterior direction and other times in a lateral direction. This variability presumably depends on the subtleties of where the primary sensory cortex lies among the sulci or gyri in an individual patient. The highest amplitude recording sites are often at CPz, CP1, and CP2. (CPz is halfway between CZ and PZ. CP1 is halfway between CZ and P3. CP2 is halfway between CZ and P4.) Some users prefer instead to use the sites most often used in outpatients. In this way, the midline recording site is at the point 2 cm behind Cz, referred to as Cz'. For the off-midline recording sites, many users prefer C3' and C4', located 2 cm posterior to C3 and C4, respectively. A reference electrode is often located on the forehead (Fz, Fpz), or at the ear, neck, or shoulder.

Recordings from the neck or other noncephalic sites may pick up far-field cortical or subcortical signals. These potentials have the distinct advantage of being less affected by anesthesia than the near-field cortical potentials. Unfortunately, in some patients these noncephalic channels are too noisy for reliable monitoring. A monitorist will usually try several recording channels early in the procedure, and follow those that are most suitable.

Filtering removes unwanted noise while keeping most of the desired signal. Noise can be caused by muscle, movement, electrocardiogram (ECG), and other nonphysiological and physiological sources. In the intraoperative monitoring setting, noise can also be from true nervous system signals that vary from time to time in a clinically meaningless manner. This is particularly true of the components of EPs, which are rather slow and late (e.g., 60 msec or more after a lower extremity stimulus). One study has investigated the ordinary reproducibility or variability of EP recordings during portions of operations in which there was no reason to believe that the nervous system pathways were at any risk of injury (Nuwer and Dawson, 1984a). When wide-open filters were used (e.g., 1-Hz low filters), considerable variability of the scalp-recorded EPs was seen. By using restricted filters (e.g., 30-Hz low filters), much of the slower, later, taller components of the EP were eliminated, and the reproducibility of the remaining faster, earlier components were substantially improved. Figure 44.1 demonstrates this effect and suggests that the optimum trade-off of low filtering occurs at about 30 Hz. At low-filter settings of 75 Hz (or higher) the EP often became too attenuated.

There is an advantage to placing additional recording electrodes over the lower half of the body. Commonly sites are popliteal fossa or lumbosacral spine. This helps when interpreting changes in cervical and cortical EPs. These caudal recordings show that stimulation remains technically adequate. During some operations the temperature of the ex-

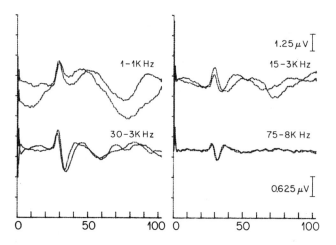

Figure 44.1. Effects of four different filter settings run simultaneously in one patient during spinal cord SEP monitoring. Recordings are from a cortical bipolar montage (CZ-PZ). Amplitude scale is doubled for the lower two sets of tracings. The figure demonstrates the general principal that a 30 Hz low filter is often the best at eliminating variability while preserving amplitude. (From Nuwer and Dawson, 1984b with permission.)

tremities gradually drops several degrees. This can cause a decrease in the peripheral conduction velocity, as is well known to electromyographers. Documentation of this gradual slowing of the peripheral conduction velocity is useful in interpreting gradual delays seen in cervical or cortical EPs.

Transcranial Motor Techniques

Monitoring motor pathways is often accomplished by stimulation of the motor cortex and recording at the lower extremity muscles. These techniques have become more popular in recent years. Motor cortex is activated through the intact skull using high-voltage electrical stimulation. Another way to do this is with direct motor cortex stimulation with muscle recording. Again, this limits the monitoring to just the pyramidal pathway, the one pathway for which there is the greatest clinical concern.

The motor cortex can be stimulated electrically in the OR through the intact skull, using a stimulus intensity severalfold higher than that used for peripheral nerve stimulation. In the particular technique popularized by Burke and colleagues (1992), the stimulating cathode is placed above the motor cortex to be stimulated. This is accomplished without discomfort in the anesthetized patient in the OR, whereas an awake patient would find this a painfully large stimulus intensity.

Stimulation is delivered through the intact skull through small corkscrew-shaped electrodes at C3 and C4. Special high-voltage stimulators are often used to achieve 600- to 1,000-V pulses. Brief trains of three or four 50-μsec electrical pulses are delivered with an interstimulus interval or 2 to 4 msec. The intensity is set to produce a maximal compound muscle action potential (CMAP) as would be typical of routine nerve conduction study (NCS) clinical tests. Recordings are made over upper or lower extremity muscles in a manner typical for NCS. Often the same type of NCS recording equipment is used synchronized to the special transcranial stimulator. To record from muscles in surgery, neuromuscular blockade needs to be carefully controlled. Typically, the anesthesiologists' train-of-four device is used to keep blockade at 1.5 twitches or less for median nerve stimulation.

Recording can also be made from nerves instead of muscles. This avoids the dual problem of body movement during surgery from the stimulation, and the lack of recordable signals when neuromuscular blockade is used.

These techniques are not used as continuously as SEP throughout the cases. Rather, they are often used intermittently and in conjunction with concomitant SEP monitoring.

Some investigations have also tried to use transcranial magnetic stimulation. The magnetic technique is not painful for the awake subject. Unfortunately, general anesthetics abolish the motor responses in this technique. The only successful cases reported in the OR have been done with extremely light general anesthesia. A quadripulse (four successive pulses) transcranial magnetic stimulation has been more successful than single pulses. Overall, the magnetic techniques have not been as successful as the transcranial electrical techniques.

Spinal Stimulation Techniques

Stimulation and recording electrodes for spinal cord monitoring also can be placed around the spinal cord. These

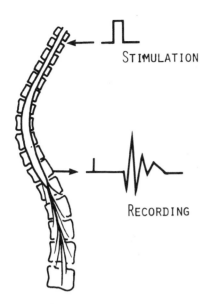

Figure 44.2. Schematic drawing of the basic concept for direct spinal cord monitoring of descending pathways. Stimulation of the spinal cord is carried out from the extradural space, while recording is made from the subdural space. (From Tamaki et al., 1981 with permission.)

invasive procedures involve placement of needles, wires, or other electrode apparatus into the epidural space, subarachnoid space, or elsewhere within the surgical field. Stimulation and recording at the spinal cord and cauda equina are relatively safe.

The evoked spinal potential, generated from within the spinal cord itself, is a complex polyphasic waveform. The several different components of the complex are probably generated from different pathways within the spinal cord. The fastest ascending EP peak may be from the dorsal spinocerebellar tract. Some invasive techniques directly monitor the pyramidal tract.

Japanese investigators pioneered and developed techniques for recording from the caudal spinal cord after stimulating the rostral spinal cord (Fig. 44.2). This paradigm directly monitors orthodromic pyramidal tract activity along with antidromic conductions along the posterior columns and other pathways. Tamaki et al. (1981) summarized the methods and surgical experience with such a technique. An 18-gauge polyethylene tubing was modified to create the electrodes used for this technique. Two coils of fine platinum wire were placed on the tubing, one coil at the end of the catheter and the other 15 mm from the end. The stimulating electrode was placed in the extradural space at an upper thoracic level, often using a Tuohy needle inserted percutaneously. Another recording electrode was put into the epidural space, at a low lumbar level and then advanced rostrally to the level of the conus medullaris. Stimulation was delivered in square wave pulses 0.3 msec wide at a rate of 30 to 50 pulses/sec with an intensity of 30 to 120 V. The caudal record demonstrated polyphasic EPs 100 to 150 μv in amplitude. Such large amplitude was due to the very effective direct spinal cord stimulation, resulting in conduction along multiple simultaneous spinal cord pathways. Also the recording electrodes were placed in the subarachnoid space at the conus medullaris, thereby removing the amplitude attenuation effect of any intervening tissue. Because the potentials were so large, only 50 to 100 stimuli were needed for each averaged EP trace. With a stimulus rate of 30 to 50 pulses/sec, a new averaged EP trace could be recorded every few seconds.

Recording can also be made peripherally from nerve or muscle. Muscle recording can be done with electromyography (EMG) techniques, and have the advantage that they are a way to monitor motor pathways per se without influence from other pathways. Machida et al. (1985) compared EPs to recordings from muscle and reported that the former was the superior monitoring method, from a practical view.

Spinal cord can also be stimulated from ligamentum flavum or interspinous ligaments (Nagle et al., 1996; Owen et al., 1991, 1995; Péréon et al., 2002). Stimulation effectively reaches the nearby spinal cord and triggers ascending and descending volleys. Recording can be obtained at caudal spinal cord, cauda equina, or peripherally. Lower extremity muscle recording increases the reassurance that the pyramidal tract is monitored, although reflex contributions from other tracks cannot be excluded. Because of the proximity to paraspinous muscles, these stimulating techniques require effective neuromuscular blockade. If recording is to be accomplished from lower extremity muscles, this blockade must be incomplete, and thereby leaving some residual twitches of paraspinous muscle during stimulation.

Epidural Recording with Peripheral Stimulation

EPs from the spinal cord can be measured using stimulation of posterior tibial nerves (Bradshaw et al., 1984; Jones, 1982; Jones et al., 1982, 1983). Recording electrodes were fine wires introduced through a 16-gauge catheter into the epidural space at a lower cervical or upper thoracic level. The recording electrodes were easy to insert at the rostral end of the surgical field, the leads were unobtrusive to the surgeon, and technically adequate recordings could be obtained in 95% of cases. A reference needle was inserted into muscle at the same level. The posterior tibial nerve was stimulated as quickly as 20/sec without degradation of the recordings. Filters used were 200 Hz and 2,000 Hz. The epidural recordings in most cases had three well-defined peaks, averaging 2.4 μv in amplitude. An acute EP attenuation greater than 50% was a distinctly unusual event, and any such amplitude reduction was considered an indication of potential neurological complications.

Whittle et al. (1984a,b, 1986) used subdural electrodes in place of the epidural recording electrodes. This technique is suitable for neurosurgical procedures when the dura is open. In other respects the technique resembled those with epidural recordings.

Macon et al. (1980, 1982) took a different approach in neurosurgical cases. After a laminectomy was performed exposing the spinal epidural space, 1-mm-diameter platinum wire electrode pairs were placed both rostral and caudal to the surgical site. Recordings were made to the time of the onset of the EP complex at both the rostral and caudal sites, and those latency values were used to calculate conduction velocity across the surgical site. Those authors believe that such latency or velocity measures are more stable than amplitude measures used in other techniques. They also advocated use of a bipolar electrode in the epidural space rather than a single epidural electrode referenced to a subcutaneous needle.

Comparisons Among Invasive Techniques

The invasive spinal cord monitoring techniques differ from each other in the amplitude of recorded EPs and in the technical difficulties encountered. Highest amplitudes are seen with direct spinal cord stimulation with epidural recording. Tall, well-defined potentials are clearly seen after only 100 trials. At 20 stimuli/sec, a new EP might take only 3 to 4 seconds to collect. Epidural recording with peripheral stimulation yields smaller EPs, but they can be obtained after just 10 to 20 seconds.

Epidural electrodes carry a theoretical risk of bleeding, infection, or trauma associated with placement, or from electrical tissue damage (burns) from direct cord stimulation. But there are no reported cases of actual damage. The epidural and ligament electrodes can become dislodged. The surgeon needs to secure them firmly in place.

The direct cord stimulation may activate antidromic and orthodromic, ascending and descending tracts often bilaterally. This contrasts with peripheral techniques in which each leg can be stimulated one at a time, providing separate left-right information about pathway integrity. Minahan et al. (2001) warned that many "motor" techniques monitor non-motor pathways too, and the user should be aware of that possibility. They reported a case of paraplegia without monitoring warnings in a spinal stimulation case.

Overall, epidural recordings are quick and reliable. They are used especially during neurosurgical procedures when the epidural space is already exposed. They provide large EPs quickly but are yet to be widely accepted in litigation-prone regions.

Patient-Related Factors

Age

Intraoperative spinal cord monitoring can be performed reasonably well in patients ranging from as young as 1 month old to elderly ages. In infants, there is a tendency to have significantly larger stimulus artifacts and a greater effect of inhalation anesthetics in reducing cortical SEPs. In the elderly cortical EPs may be small and more difficult to find.

Drugs

Some drugs and anesthetic agents used in the operating room can impair monitoring of cortical SEPs. This occurs especially for the inhalation agents enflurane, isoflurane, and halothane. Newer agents desflurane and sevoflurane seem to act similarly to isoflurane in EPs. It is important to understand the effects of these and other drugs commonly used during monitoring.

Barbiturates and benzodiazepines at low doses cause little or no change in the latency or amplitude of the early SEP peaks. Moderate to high barbiturate doses, or an acute intra-venous bolus, can have noticeable effects. At doses sufficient to cause EEG burst suppression, pentobarbital does not alter the N_2O EPs but may cause a mild attenuation of the middle and long latency SEPs. At very high doses barbiturate effects are more pronounced. Even the spinal epidural EPs can be attenuated by acute intravenous boluses of barbiturates.

Narcotics administered by bolus or by continuous infusions increased primary cortical peak latencies but produced unpredictable amplitude changes.

SEPs are clearly attenuated by nitrous oxide. Even during the 30 minutes after discontinuation of nitrous oxide, EP amplitudes remained 30% less than baseline values (Herwig et al., 1984; Sloan and Koht, 1985). When a 30-Hz low filter was used, the nitrous oxide caused a 70% average amplitude attenuation. The higher the filter setting, the greater the amplitude attenuation (Nuwer and Dawson, 1984a). Spinal EP peaks are relatively well preserved despite nitrous oxide administration (Johnson et al., 1983).

Nitrous oxide (50%) caused a greater degree of amplitude loss than did enflurane or isoflurane given at the minimum dose to achieve hemodynamic stability (0.5 to 1.0%). The nitrous oxide caused a 40% amplitude attenuation, whereas the other two inhalation anesthetics caused only a 20% amplitude loss in a study by McPherson et al. (1985).

For lower extremity SEPs, the EP may disappear when the isoflurane is raised to 0.75% (Nuwer and Dawson, 1984a). Isoflurane affects lower extremity EP testing more than upper extremity testing. This may be due to the anatomical location of the lower extremity generators, buried deep in the interhemispheric fissure. Enflurane at doses up to 4% causes a moderate loss of amplitude for the early peaks but a complete loss of middle and long latency peaks at the cortex, whereas the spinal epidural response was decreased much less (Fujioka et al., 1994). Similar results were seen with halothane (Baines et al., 1985; Salzman et al., 1986; Wang et al., 1985). Contaminant use of the nitrous oxide plus other inhalation anesthetics is particularly problematic for cortical recordings.

Neuromuscular junction blocking agents are especially helpful to EP recording. They have no direct effect on the EP itself. They can, however, very substantially reduce the amount of muscle artifact present as well as movement due to the electrical stimulation.

Boluses of medication are to be avoided in general, especially of agents that clearly change central nervous system (CNS) function. This includes barbiturates, lidocaine, and narcotic agents. Obviously in some situations these medications must be given in bolus form. The interpretation of the EP record during the 5 to 10 minutes after bolus administration of such medications is difficult. It is recommended that such medications be given as a constant infusion.

Temperature

Patients in surgery often experience a drop in their core temperature 1°C or more over the course of an operation. Limb temperature may drop several degrees. This can decrease conduction velocity and increase the latency to peaks. This gradual temperature-dependent increase in latency is usually accompanied by no significant amplitude change. Slowing peripherally can be monitored with peripheral recording channels, e.g., electrodes over the lumbar spine or on the leg. SEP central delays in conduction due to temperature are usually of a smaller degree. Motor EPs can also still be recorded at moderate hypothermia (Meylaerts et al., 1999a). Below 30°C, it is difficult or impossible to record cortical EPs.

Interpretation of Changes

Causes of Change

For most techniques, an acute 50% amplitude drop or 5% to 10% latency increase is considered clinically important. Smaller degrees of background variability in latency and amplitude are common but not generally of clinical interest.

Changes during monitoring can be from new clinical impairment, anesthetic or systemic medical changes, or technical problems.

Equipment or techniques can fail for a variety of reasons. A stimulating or recording electrode can fall off of the leg or the cable leading to the electrode can be accidentally cut or unplugged. With a constant voltage stimulus, increasing stimulating electrode impedance can reduce nerve stimulation and decrease EP amplitude. Attenuation or loss of the stimulus artifact is an important hint that the stimulator is not properly functioning. Lowering of the temperature and blood pressure, systemic hypoxia, or other severe metabolic derangements can change EPs. Acute administration of drugs, especially as a bolus of barbiturates or benzodiazepines, can lead to acute EP changes. A common cause for change is deepening the anesthetic or adding a new agent.

Once technical, anesthetic, and systemic reasons for change have been reasonably excluded, EP changes should be considered to be from spinal cord impairment. Surgical causes of change include direct trauma to the cord with a scalpel, electrocautery device, retraction, blunt trauma, compression, stretching of the cord from spinal distraction, or vascular insufficiency from compression, embolus, or thrombosis. If EPs return to baseline latency and amplitude within 15 minutes of an acute change, then the patient is unlikely to have postoperative impairment, even if the EPs had disappeared briefly. If EPs very gradually return to baseline by the end of the surgical procedure, new neurological postoperative deficits occasionally follow. If EPs disappear and remain absent indefinitely, then the patient is at a substantial risk for postoperative impairment, perhaps greater than a 50% risk of significant impairment. If the EPs become attenuated by more than 50% but are still present to some small degree, then the patient is still at some risk for new postoperative neurological impairment, with approximately 25% risk of an amplitude decrease less than 50%. An amplitude drop of 30% to 50% would be reason to monitor the patient's neurological status very closely during the immediate postoperative period.

In the OR, the monitorist tracks the latencies and amplitudes continuously. Many techniques allow for new EPs every 2 minutes—some faster than that. Tracings are printed for later review and used to evaluate gradual changes. A written flow sheet of latency and amplitude values can help the monitorist identify gradual changes. Tracking anesthetic changes, blood pressures, and temperature also help understand significant changes when they occur.

False-Negative Cases

False-negative cases (Ben-David et al., 1987; Ginsburg et al., 1985; More et al., 1988; Nuwer, 1986) are those in which postoperative neurological deficits occur despite stable EPs. In the most serious false-negative cases, postoperative paraparesis or paraplegia occurs despite the spinal cord EP monitoring persistently having been normal and unchanged. In theory this could occur because the EPs usually travel the posterior column or other ascending pathway, rather than directly in the pyramidal tract. One spinal cord tract may be impaired without impairing all tracts.

In minor false-negative cases, mild, transient postoperative neurological sequelae occur despite stable EPs (Harper

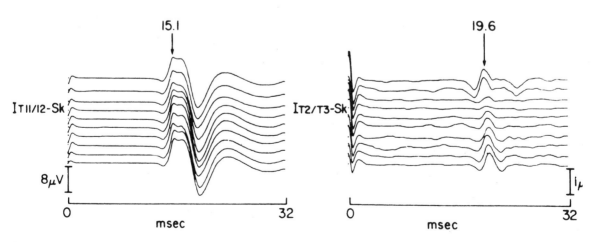

Figure 44.3. Consecutive tracings obtained immediately before, during and after compression of the spinal cord. Pressure was applied after trace 2 (reading down) and released after trace 4. Recordings were made from interspinous ligaments T2–3 and T11–12 using a skin reference. The T2–3 channel shows the effects of cord impairment due to the pressure. The T11–12 channel shows no impairment caudal to the compression. (From Lueders et al., 1982 with permission.)

et al., 1988; Tamaki et al., 1984; Wilber et al., 1984). Many such patients had patches of dysesthesia for days or weeks postoperatively, possibly due to segmental spinal wiring.

One review presented six cases from four institutions occurring in more than 600 cases (Lesser et al., 1986). In three of the six cases, impairment probably developed postoperatively, with motor function preserved initially and deteriorating over ensuing hours. In two cases the EPs had changed intraoperatively, with 30% to 50% transient amplitude losses that were not considered at the time to be a predictor of postoperative neurological problems.

Another reported false-negative case occurred during bilateral simultaneous posterior tibial nerve monitoring. The patient suffered a hemicord syndrome. The EPs at the scalp did not substantially change. This serves to warn that the two legs should be stimulated separately, not simultaneously (Molaie, 1986).

Two cases of temporary quadriparesis were reported after cervical discectomy and grafting (Jones et al., 2003). These two cases were among more than 2,000 procedures performed, so that the apparent risk of such false-negative SEP monitoring was less than 0.1%.

EPs rarely remain stable when postoperative neurological sequelae nevertheless occur. Often such cases are of transient sensory changes only. Occasionally more serious sequelae occur. Physicians who deal with monitoring should be aware of this possibility. Neurological impairment also can occur during the hours after monitoring has stopped.

Clinical Settings

Neurological postoperative deficits are substantially reduced when intraoperative somatosensory monitoring is used in patients undergoing surgery that puts the spinal cord at risk. For scoliosis surgery, SEP monitoring reduced paraplegia by 60% (Nuwer et al., 1995). Monitoring also is efficacious for neurosurgical spinal procedures and for thoracic procedures endangering spinal cord blood flow. Monitoring is not fail-safe, as shown by true positive cases in which neurological deficits did occur despite early warnings from monitoring. Rare false-negative cases also occur, in which monitoring fails to warn of new complications.

Scoliosis

Permanent paraplegia is the most feared postoperative complication after orthopedic spinal deformity surgery. Risk factors for paraplegia are kyphosis, congenital scoliosis, preexisting neurological impairment, and preoperative traction. The impairment may be from direct stretching of the spinal cord, compression of the cord, trauma during fitting of the orthopedic instrumentation, or interference with blood flow. EPs can monitor spinal cord function to prevent some complications. Figure 44.4 shows an example of normal, stable cortical SEP peaks during 2 hours of a monitored scoliosis procedure. The main alternative to EP monitoring is the wake-up test, discussed in more detail below.

Various series reports on scalp EP monitoring have been supportive of its usefulness (Brown and Nash, 1979; Brown et al., 1984; Engler et al., 1978; Mostegl and Bauer, 1984;

Nash et al., 1977a,b; Spielholz et al., 1979; Wilber et al., 1984).

The largest part of the literature on scoliosis and other evoked potential spinal monitoring is composed of case series reported by individual surgeons and institutions. Earlier reports were mainly about SEPs, epidural recordings, and spinal stimulation techniques (Abel et al., 1990; Albanese et al., 1991; Apel et al., 1991; Bieber et al., 1986; Bradshaw et al., 1984; Cheliout-Heraut, et al., 1989; Dawson et al., 1991; Dinner et al., 1986; Engler et al., 1978; Forbes et al., 1991; Fujioka et al., 1994; Gonzalez et al., 1984; Halonen et al., 1990; Hicks et al., 1991; Johnston et al., 1986; Jones et al., 1982, 1983; Keith et al., 1990; LaMont et al., 1983; Loder et al., 1991; Lubicky et al., 1989; Lueders et al., 1982; Machida et al., 1988; Mostegl et al., 1987; Nuwer et al., 1995; Phillips et al., 1995; Roy et al., 1987; Ryan and Britt, 1986; Tamaki, 1989; Tamaki et al., 1981, 1984; Whittle et al., 1986; Wilber et al., 1984).

More recent reports have compared SEPs to transcranial motor evoked potentials (Burke and Hicks, 1998; Lang et al., 1996; Langeloo et al., 2001; Pelosi et al., 2001, 2002; Péréon et al., 2002). Generally the motor and somatosensory techniques changed acutely in parallel. Recovery of motor EPs by the end of the procedure was a better predictor of no deficits. On the basis of the long-term successful use of these techniques, Padberg et al. (1998) have recommended that the wake-up test is no longer needed in routine cases when reliable monitoring data are stable. Noonan et al. (2002) recommended wake-up tests when SEPs changed, even when the SEPs had returned to normal by the end of the procedure.

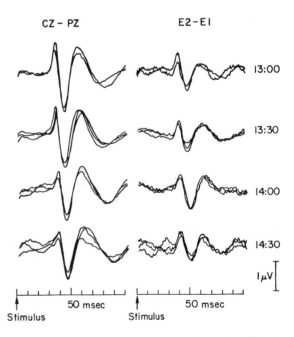

Figure 44.4. Stable cortical SEP potentials are shown here. These were recorded during a routine Harrington rod procedure. Sets of 2–3 repetitions are shown for a bipolar AP (CZ-PZ) and a bipolar transverse (CP1-CP2) channel over 90 minutes. (E1-E2 is an old nomenclature for CP1-CP2.) (From Nuwer, 1986 with permission.)

Such reports include patients in whom spinal cord monitoring showed changes that prompted the surgeon's intervention. Some intervention was not completely successful, so some patients did have postoperative neurological sequelae. Recognizing the limitations in such single-center surveys, a large multicenter survey was carried out to study spinal cord monitoring clinical outcomes.

The Multicenter Study of Spinal Cord Monitoring in Scoliosis Surgery surveyed members of the Scoliosis Research Society (SRS), which represents surgeons with a special interest in scoliosis surgery. Annual reporting of surgical complications is required for society membership. Previous SRS surveys of neurological complications are also available. The multicenter study has published results in two ways: (a) results for U.S. institutions only (Nuwer et al., 1995), and (b) aggregate results for the U.S. and 23 other nations (Dawson et al., 1991).

Among 173 surveyed U.S. surgeons, 153 (88%) used SEP spinal cord monitoring. They had 1 to 18 years of experience using SEP monitoring (median 7 years). During this time they conducted 97,586 spinal surgery cases, in which SEP spinal monitoring was used in 51,263 (53%). The median number of monitored cases was 250 cases per surgeon. Most patients had scoliosis, but others had kyphosis, spinal fractures, or other similar spinal problems. Table 44.1 presents the neurological outcomes from the spinal monitoring. In delayed-onset cases neurological complications were not

Table 44.1. Neurological Outcome Prediction Rates for SEP Monitoring in Spinal Surgery

Total Procedures	51,263	(100%)
False-Negative Rate (FN): Neurological Postoperative Deficits Despite Stable SEPs		
Definite	34	(0.066%)
Equivocal	13	(0.025%)
Delayed onset	18	(0.035%)
Total:	65	(0.127%)
False-Positive Rate: No Neurological Deficits Despite SEP Changes		
Definite	504	(0.983%)
Equivocal	270	(0.527%)
Total:	774	(1.510%)
True-Positive (TP) Rate: Neurological Deficits Predicted by SEP Changes		
Definite	150	(0.293%)
Equivocal	67	(0.131%)
Total:	217	(0.423%)
Neurological Deficits (FN plus TP)		
Definite	184	(0.359%)
Equivocal	80	(0.156%)
Delayed onset	18	(0.035%)
Total:	282	(0.550%)
True-Negative Rate: No Neurological Deficit and Stable SEPs		
Total:	50,207	(97.94%)

These data are from the multicenter outcome study of SEP spinal cord monitoring in scoliosis organized through the Scoliosis Research Society (33). They were obtained from 153 U.S. surgeon respondents. Note the very low rate of definite false negative cases (0.063%).

Table 44.2. SEP Monitoring in Scoliosis

Sensitivity: 417/451	92.5%
Specificity: 50,207/50,781	98.9%
Positive Predictive Value 417/991	42.1%
Negative Predictive Value 50,207/50,241	99.93%

These outcome measures are from the multicenter outcome survey of 153 U.S. surgeons organized through the Scoliosis Research Society (33). Table 44.1 shows a further breakout of validity measures from that survey. The very high negative predictive value here indicates the high reliability of the monitoring when the SEP remains normal and stable. The outcome survey report (33) discusses in detail these data and related assumptions.

present immediately after surgery but developed in subsequent days. In false-negative cases, patients suffered neurological complications even though there was no warning from EP monitoring. In false-positive cases, the patient had no new neurological problems despite EP changes. Some false-positive cases were instances in which the surgeon was alerted and intervened successfully to avert neurological deficits. Ideally these would not be called false-positive cases. Other false-positive cases were EP changes due to anesthetic changes or technical problems. In true-positive cases, the EP changed, warning the surgeon, but the patient nevertheless suffered postoperative complications. In some of the latter cases, the EP monitoring may have reduced the severity of the neurological complications, but this issue is not clarified by this survey. Table 44.2 presents validity measures reported in that study.

In this survey, the overall rate of new postoperative neurological deficits was about 50% lower among the patients operated on by experienced SEP monitoring teams, as compared either to historical controls or to contemporaneous control teams that had made little use of SEP monitoring. The major neurological deficits, i.e., paraplegia and paraparesis, were reduced more than 60% among the surgical groups regularly employing SEP monitoring. Serious neurological deficits appear to be prevented entirely by monitoring for about one patient out of every 200 undergoing surgery for scoliosis.

Outcomes for the different SEP monitoring techniques have been compared to each other (Aminoff, 1989). Techniques commonly used in the United Kingdom or Japan are more invasive than those used in the U.S. In the Multicenter Survey, U.S. and overseas physicians each had similar rates of neurological deficits (Nuwer and Carlson, 1992). The study concluded that the various spinal cord monitoring techniques are comparable in their ability to conduct monitoring.

Among these epidural techniques, one series (Forbes et al., 1991) reported 1,168 scoliosis cases over 16 years. SEP changes occurred in 119 cases, in which 32 had new postoperative neurological deficits. No false-negative cases occurred, i.e., each neurological deficit was predicted by the SEPs. Several epidural series report successful use of spinal cord electrical stimulation techniques (Baba et al., 1994a,b; Fujioka et al., 1994; Koyanagi et al., 1993; Matsuda and Shimazu, 1989; Murakami et al., 1994; Tamaki, 1989; Tamaki et al., 1981, 1984). These techniques have been in use for over 20 years, many using spinal cord stimulation through electrodes in the spinal canal. Others used spinal stimulation with electrodes at the interspinous ligaments, ligamentum flavum, or spinous processes (Nagle et al., 1996; Owen et al., 1991, 1995; Phillips et al., 1995), or even transcranial electrical stimulation of motor cortex (Burke et al., 1992). These techniques all have been reported to be effective monitoring techniques.

Neurosurgical Procedures

Spinal cord damage can also occur during spinal neurosurgical procedures such as for tumors, trauma, syrinx, and malformations. Early reports on monitoring for such cases used SEP, spinal stimulation, and epidural recording techniques (Baba et al., 1994a,b; Bennett and Benson, 1989; Chabot et al., 1986; Daube, 1991; Desmedt, 1989; Ducker et al., 1986; Epstein et al., 1993; Erwin and Erwin, 1993; Harper and Daube, 1989; Koyanagi et al., 1993; Kurthen and Schramm, 1994; Macon and Poletti, 1982; Matsuda and Shimazu, 1989; McDonnell et al., 1986; Meyer et al., 1988; Møller, 1995; Murakami et al., 1994; Nuwer, 1989; Prestor and Golob, 1999; Raudzens, 1982; Russell and Rodichok, 1995; Schramm and Møller, 1991; Spetzler et al., 1979; Witzmann and Reisecker, 1989; Young and Mollin, 1989; Zentner, 1989). Endovascular procedures can also benefit from monitoring the nervous system during times of risk (Sala et al., 2001; Zentner et al., 1988). The postoperative rate of new neurological impairment in these procedures is considerably higher than that for scoliosis surgery. There is no multicenter survey or meta-analysis available for these reports. A good historical control series was provided by Epstein and colleagues (Macon and Poletti, 1982) for cervical spinal procedures. Before SEP monitoring 8/218 (3.7%) patients became quadriplegic postoperatively. For the first 100 consecutive cases with SEP monitoring, no patient became quadriplegic, which was both medically and statistically a significant improvement. Spinal cord monitoring did successfully identify complications early enough to allow prompt intervention and subsequent lack of neurological deficits in these patients.

Several studies specifically evaluated motor EPs in spinal neurosurgery. Zentner (1989) reported good success clinically and technically with transcranial motor cortex stimulation in 87% of his cases. In the others, the anesthesia abolished the desired muscle signals. A 50% or greater amplitude drop accompanied each case of postoperative deficits. Calancie et al. (1998, 2001) found that somatosensory and motor EP techniques were complementary. Somatosensory monitoring failed to detect some motor deficits, whereas motor EP monitoring failed to detect some sensory deficits.

Wiedemayer et al. (2002) evaluated the impact of monitoring on the decisions surgeons made in 423 cases. The largest group of their patients had spinal surgery. About 10% had EP changes that prompted surgical interventions, and some had postoperative deficits. Another 12% had EP changes, no intervention was possible, and most of those patients had postoperative deficits. About 4% of these neurosurgical cases had no EP changes but did have some postoperative deficits. The interventions initiated by monitoring changes included changing the dissection, increasing perfusion pressure, deciding to limit the surgery, adjusting clips and retractors, treating vasospasm, and in one case stopping the procedure. They estimated that 5.2% of their surgical population was spared postoperative neurological deficits because of monitoring.

Overall, the literature for neurosurgical procedures is smaller than for scoliosis but the method, goal, and outcomes appear to be similar, and the studies identify complications early enough to allow prompt intervention and subsequent lack of neurological deficits in these patients.

Thoracic Procedures

The spinal cord is placed at risk during some vascular procedures involving the thoracic aorta, e.g., repairs of aneurysms and congenital anomalies such as coarctations. Spinal cord monitoring has been evaluated systematically for these procedures (Coles et al., 1982; Cunningham et al., 1982, 1987; Dasmahapatra et al., 1987; de Mol et al., 1989; Dolman et al., 1986; Drenger et al., 1992; Galla et al., 1994; Kaplan et al., 1986; Kopf et al., 1985; Krieger and Spencer, 1985; Laschinger et al., 1983a,b, 1984, 1987; Livesay et al., 1985; Maeda et al., 1989; Matsui et al., 1994; Mizoi and Yoshimoto, 1993; North et al., 1991; Okamoto et al., 1992; Schepens et al., 1994; Shiiya et al., 1995; Stühmeier et al., 1993; Wilson et al., 1988; Yamamoto et al., 1994). Monitoring has substantial benefit, warning surgeons when insufficient collateral circulation occurs. Interventions include shunting, raising blood pressure, adjusting retractors, or reimplantation of critical intercostal vessels. The speed and duration of SEP loss is predictive of neurological deficits in such cases. Figure 44.5 shows tracings from a patient while the aorta is cross-clamped.

There are problems with lower extremity ischemia abolishing SEP or motor evoked potential (MEP) monitoring without significant spinal cord ischemia. SEP monitoring with popliteal fossa channels can help to assess when that is occurring.

In three series with somatosensory monitoring in 232 patients (Faberowski et al., 1999; Guerit et al., 1999; Wada et al., 2001), 25% of the patients in each series had adverse SEP changes. Most had a resolution of the SEP changes with raising the perfusion pressure, moving clamps, or reimplanting critical vessels. None of those patients suffered a postoperative deficit. Two patients had a complete and permanent SEP loss, and another lost SEPs for 200 minutes. Those three had postoperative paraplegia. In these three series, three patients also had delayed paraplegia with onset during the immediate postoperative period. The SEP did not predict those delayed deficits.

In five reports with transcranial electrical MEP monitoring in 196 patients (de Haan et al., 1997; MacDonald and

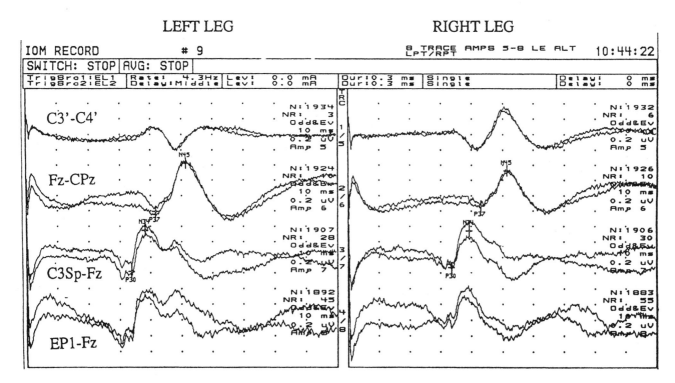

Figure 44.5. SEP spinal cord monitoring from a 20-year-old man while his thoracic aorta is cross clamped during repair of a coarctation. The technique here shows the bilaterally recording of peaks from each leg, using a delay between left and right posterior tibial nerve stimulation. Four chan-

nels are recorded for each leg. Principal peaks are marked. These peaks did not change in latency or amplitude during the procedure, correctly predicting no new neurologic deficit postoperatively.

Janusz, 2002; Meylaerts et al., 1999b; Sueda et al., 2000; van Dongen et al., 2001), about 40% of cross-clamping was associated with MEP changes. About 5% of patients suffered paraplegia, all of which were predicted by monitoring. Some of these studies assessed both SEP and MEP, and found similar monitoring outcomes.

Overview

There are many ways to conduct spinal cord monitoring. Some are adaptations of outpatient SEP testing. Others involve direct spinal cord stimulation, epidural spinal recording, or similar invasive techniques.

Outcome using monitoring is favorable. Neurological postoperative deficits are cut in half for surgeons using monitoring. The rate of paraplegia is cut by 60%. Rare false-negative cases have been reported, however. When compared, the various techniques of monitoring seem to have similar efficacy in preventing deficits. Applications are for scoliosis correction, neurosurgical procedures around the spinal cord, and cardiothoracic or vascular procedures in which the spinal cord's blood supply is threatened.

References

Abel, M.F., Mubarak, S.J., Wenger, D.R., et al. 1990. Brainstem evoked potentials for scoliosis surgery: a reliable method allowing use of halogenated anesthetic agents. J. Pediatr. Orthop. 10:208–213.

Albanese, S.A., Spadaro, J.A., Lubicky, J.P., et al. 1991. Somatosensory cortical evoked potential changes after deformity correction. Spine 16: S371–S374.

American Academy of Neurology. 1990. Intraoperative neurophysiology. Neurology 40:1644–1646.

American Electroencephalographic Society. 1994. Guidelines for intraoperative monitoring of sensory evoked potentials. J. Clin. Neurophysiol. 11(1):77–87.

Aminoff, M.J. 1989. Intraoperative monitoring by evoked potentials for spinal cord surgery. Electroencephalogr. Clin. Neurophysiol. 73:378–380.

Apel, D.A., Marrero, G., King, J., et al. 1991. Avoiding paraplegia during anterior spinal surgery. The role of somatosensory evoked potential monitoring with temporary occlusion of segmental spinal arteries. Spine 16:S365–S370.

Baba, H., Kawahara, N., Nagata, S., et al. 1994a. Spinal cord evoked potentials in cervical and thoracic myelopathy. In *Handbook of Spinal Cord Monitoring,* Eds. S.J. Jones, S. Boyd, M. Hetreed, et al., pp. 99–103. London: Kluwer.

Baba, H., Kawahara, K., Tomita, K., et al. 1994b. Spinal cord evoked potentials in spinal cord intermittent claudication. In *Handbook of Spinal Cord Monitoring,* Eds. S.J. Jones, S. Boyd, M. Hetreed, et al., pp. 104–109. London: Kluwer.

Baines, D.B., Whittle, I.R., Chaseling, R.W., et al. 1985. Effect of halothane on spinal somatosensory evoked potentials in sheep. Br. J. Anaesth. 57:896–899.

Ben-David, B., Haller, G., and Taylor, P. 1987. Anterior spinal fusion complicated by paraplegia. A case report of a false–negative somatosensory evoked potential. Spine 12:536–539.

Bennett, H.L., and Benson, D.R. 1989. Somatosensory evoked potentials for orthopaedic spine trauma. J. Orthop. Trauma. 3:11–18.

Bieber, E., Tolo, V., and Uematsu, S. 1986. Spinal cord monitoring during posterior spinal instrumentation and fusion. Clin. Orthop. Rel. Res. 229: 121–124.

Bradshaw, K., Webb, J.K., and Fraser, A.M. 1984. Clinical evaluation of spinal cord monitoring in scoliosis surgery. Spine 9:636–643.

Brown, R.N., and Nash, C.L., Jr. 1979. Current status of spinal cord monitoring. Spine 4:466–470.

Brown, R.H., Nash, C.L., Jr., Berrilla, J.A., et al. 1984. Cortical evoked potential monitoring: a system for intraoperative monitoring of spinal cord function. Spine 9:256–261.

Burke, D., and Hicks, R.G. 1998. Surgical monitoring of motor pathways. J. Clin. Neurophysiol. 15:194–205.

Burke, D., Hicks, R., Stephen, J., et al. 1992. Assessment of corticospinal and somatosensory conduction simultaneously during scoliosis surgery. Electroencephalogr. Clin. Neurophysiol. 85:388–396.

Calancie, B., Harris, W., Broton, J.G., et al. 1998. "Threshold-level" multipulse transcranial electrical stimulation of motor cortex for intraoperative monitoring of spinal motor tracts: description of method and comparison to somatosensory evoked potential monitoring. J. Neurosurg. 88:457–470.

Calancie, B., Harris, W., Brindle, G.F., et al. 2001. Threshold-level repetitive transcranial electrical stimulation for intraoperative monitoring of central motor conduction. J. Neurosurg. (Spine 1) 95:161–168.

Chabot, R.J., John, E.R., and Prichep, L.S. 1986. Real-time intraoperative monitoring during neurosurgical and neuroradiological procedures. In *Neurophysiology and Standards of Spinal Cord Monitoring.* Eds. T.B. Ducker and R.H. Brown, pp. 207–215. New York: Springer-Verlag.

Cheliout-Heraut, F., Vital, J.M., Pouliquen, J.C., et al. 1989. Surveillance per-operatoire des scolioses chez l'adulte jeune par les potentiels evoques somesthesiques: a propos de 33 cas. Neurophysiol. Clin. 19:297–310.

Coles, J.G., Wilson, G.J., Sima, A.F., et al. 1982. Intraoperative detection of spinal cord ischemia using somatosensory cortical evoked potentials during thoracic aortic occlusion. Ann. Thorac. Surg. 34:299–306.

Cunningham, J.N., Jr., Laschinger, J.C., Merkin, H.A., et al. 1982. Measurement of spinal cord ischemia during operations upon the thoracic aorta. Ann. Surg. 196:285–296.

Cunningham, J.N., Jr., Laschinger, J.C., and Spencer, F.C. 1987. Monitoring of somatosensory evoked potentials during surgical procedures on the thoracoabdominal aorta. J. Thorac. Cardiovasc. Surg. 94:275–285.

Dasmahapatra, H.K., Coles, J.G., Taylor, M.J., et al. 1987. Identification of risk factors for spinal cord ischemia by the use of monitoring of somatosensory evoked potentials during coarctation repair. Circulation 76: SIII-14–18.

Daube, J.R. 1991. Monitoring of spine surgery with evoked potentials. In *Intraoperative Neurophysiologic Monitoring in Neurosurgery;* Eds. J. Schramm, AR Møller, p. 127–137. New York: Springer-Verlag.

Dawson, E.G., Sherman, J.E., Kanim, L.E.A., et al. 1991. Spinal cord monitoring results of the Scoliosis Research Society and the European Spinal Deformity Society survey. Spine 16:S361–S364.

De Haan, P., Kalkman, Cor J., de Mol, B.A., et al. 1997. Efficacy of transcranial motor-evoked myogenic potentials to detect spinal cord ischemia during operations for thoracoabdominal aneurysms. J. Thorac. Cardiovasc. Surg. 133:87–101.

de Mol, B.A.J.M., Boezeman, E.H.J.F., Hamerlijnck, R.P.H.M., et al. 1989. Experimental and clinical use of somatosensory evoked potentials in surgery of aneurysms of the descending thoracic aorta. Thorac. Cardiovasc. Surg. 38:146–150.

Desmedt, J.E. (Ed.). 1989. *Neuromonitoring in Surgery.* Amsterdam: Elsevier.

Dinner, D.S., Lüders, H., Lesser, R.P., et al. 1986. Intraoperative spinal somatosensory evoked potential monitoring. J. Neurosurg. 65:807–814.

Dolman, J., Silvay, G., Zappulla, R., et al. 1986. The effect of temperature, mean arterial pressure, and cardiopulmonary bypass flows on somatosensory evoked potential latency in man. Thorac. Cardiovasc. Surg. 34: 217–222.

Drenger, B., Parker, S.D., McPherson, R.W., et al. 1992. Spinal cord stimulation evoked potentials during thoracoabdominal aortic aneurysm surgery. Anesthesiology 76:689–695.

Ducker, T.B., and Brown, R.H. (Ed.). 1986. *Neurophysiology and Standards of Spinal Cord Monitoring.* New York: Springer-Verlag.

Engler, G.L., Spielholz, N.I., Bernhard, W.N., et al. 1978. Somatosensory evoked potentials during Harrington instrumentation for scoliosis. J. Bone Joint Surg. [Am.]. 60A:528–532.

Epstein, N.E., Danto, J., and Nardi, D. 1993. Evaluation of intraoperative somatosensory-evoked potential monitoring during 100 cervical operations. Spine 18:737–747.

Erwin C.W., and Erwin, A.C. 1993. Up and down the spinal cord: intraoperative monitoring of sensory and motor spinal cord pathways. J. Clin. Neurophysiol. 10:425–436.

Faberowski, L.W., Black, S., Trankina, M.F., et al. 1999. Somatosensory-evoked potentials during aortic coarctation repair. J. Cardiothor. Vasc. Anesthes. 13:538–543.

Forbes, H.J., Allen, P.W., Waller, S.C., et al. 1991. Spinal cord monitoring in scoliosis surgery. J. Bone Joint Surg. [Br]. 73B:487–491.

Fujioka, H., Shimoji, K., Tomita, S., et al. 1994. Spinal cord potential recordings from the extradural space during scoliosis surgery. Br. J. Anesthesia. 73:350–356.

Galla, J.D., Ergin, A., Sadeghi, A.M., et al. 1994. A new technique using somatosensory evoked potential guidance during descending and thoracoabdominal aortic repairs. J. Cardiac Surg. 9:662–672.

Ginsburg, H.H., Shetter, A.G., and Raudzens, P.A. 1985. Postoperative paraplegia with preserved intraoperative somatosensory evoked potentials. J. Neurosurg. 6:296–300.

Gonzalez, E.G., Hajdu, M., Keim, H., et al. 1984. Quantification of intraoperative somatosensory evoked potential. Arch. Phys. Rehabil. 65: 721–725.

Guerit, J.M., Witdoeckt, C., Verhelst, R., et al. 1999. Sensitivity, specificity, and surgical impact of somatosensory evoked potentials in descending aorta surgery. Ann. Thorac. Surg.67:1943–1946.

Halonen, J.P., Jones, S.J., Edgar, M.A., et al. 1990. Multi-level epidural recordings of spinal SEPs during scoliosis surgery. New Trends Adv. Tech. Clin. Neurophysiol. 41:342–347.

Harper, C.M., and Daube, J.R. 1989. Surgical monitoring with evoked potentials: the Mayo Clinic experience. In *Neuromonitoring in Surgery*, Ed. J.E. Desmedt, pp. 275–301. Amsterdam: Elsevier.

Harper, C.M., Daube, J.R., Lichy, W.J., et al. 1988. Lumbar radiculopathy after spinal fusion for scoliosis. Muscle Nerve 11:386–391.

Herwig, L.D., Milam, S.B., and Jones, D.L. 1984. Time course of recovery following nitrous oxide administration. Anesth. Prog. 133–135.

Hicks, R.G., Burke, D.J., and Stephen, P.H. 1991. Monitoring spinal cord function during scoliosis surgery with Cotrel-Dubousset instrumentation. Med. J. Aust. 154:82–86.

Johnson, R.M., McPherson, R.W., and Szymanski, J. 1983. The effects of stimulus intensity on somatosensory evoked potentials during intraoperative monitoring. Anesthesiology 59:A365.

Johnston, C.E. II, Happel, L.T., Jr., Norris, R., et al. 1986. Delayed paraplegia complicating sublaminar segmental spinal instrumentation. J. Bone Joint Surg. [Am.]. 68:556–563.

Jones, S.J. 1982. Clinical applications of short-latency somatosensory evoked potentials. Ann. N.Y. Acad. Sci. 388:369–387.

Jones, S.J., Edgar, M.A., and Ransford, A.O. 1982. Sensory nerve conduction in the human spinal cord: epidural recordings made during scoliosis surgery. J. Neurol. Neurosurg. Psychiatry 45:446–451.

Jones, S.J., Edgar, M.A., Ransford, A.O., et al. 1983. A system for the electrophysiological monitoring of the spinal cord during operations for scoliosis. J. Bone Joint Surg. B65:134–139.

Jones, S.J., Boyd, S., Hetreed, M., et al. (Eds.). 1994. *Handbook of Spinal Cord Monitoring.* London: Kluwer.

Jones, S.J., Buonamassa, S., Crockard, H.A. 2003. Two cases of quadriparesis following anterior cervical discectomy, with normal perioperative somatosensory evoked potentials. J. Neurol. Neurosurg. Psychiatry 74:273–276.

Kaplan, B.J., Friedman, W.A., Alexander, J.A., et al. 1986. Somatosensory evoked potential monitoring of spinal cord ischemia during aortic operations. Neurosurgery 19:82–90.

Keith, R.W., Stambough, J.L., and Awender, S.H. 1990. Somatosensory cortical evoked potentials: a review of 100 cases of intraoperative spinal surgery monitoring. J. Spinal Dis. 3:220–226.

Kopf, G.S., Hume, A.L., Durkin, M.A., et al. 1985. Measurement of central somatosensory conduction time in patients undergoing cardiopulmonary bypass: an index of neurologic function. Am. J. Surg. 149:445–448.

Koyanagi, I., Iwasaki, Y., Isu, T., et al. 1993. Spinal cord evoked potential monitoring after spinal cord stimulation during surgery of spinal cord tumors. Neurosurgery 33:451–460.

Krieger, K.H., and Spencer, F.C. 1985. Is paraplegia after repair of coarctation of the aorta due principally to distal hypotension during aortic cross-clamping? Surgery 97:2–7.

Kurthen, M., and Schramm, J. 1994. Application of intraoperative spinal cord monitoring to neurosurgery. In *Handbook of Spinal Cord Monitor-*

ing, Eds. S.J. Jones, S. Boyd, M. Hetreed, et al., pp. 59–70. London: Kluwer.

LaMont, R.L., Wasson, S.L., and Green, M.A. 1983. Spinal cord monitoring during spinal surgery using somatosensory spinal evoked potentials. J. Pediatr. Orthop. 3:31–36.

Lang, E.W., Beutler, A.S., Chesnut, R.M., et al. 1996. Myogenic motor-evoked potential monitoring using partial neuromuscular blockade in surgery of the spine. Spine 21:1676–1686.

Langeloo, D.D., Journee, H.L., Polak, B., et al. 2001. A new application of TCE-MEP: spinal cord monitoring in patients with severe neuromuscular weakness undergoing corrective spine surgery. J. Spinal Dis. 14:445–448.

Laschinger, J.C., Cunningham, J.N., Jr., Isom, O.W., et al. 1983a. Definition of the safe lower limits of aortic resection during surgical procedures on the thoracoabdominal aorta: use of somatosensory evoked potentials. J. Am. Coll. Cardiol. 2:959–965.

Laschinger, J.C., Cunningham, J.N., Jr., Nathan, I.M., et al. 1983b. Experimental and clinical assessment of the adequacy of partial bypass in maintenance of spinal cord blood flow during operations on the thoracic aorta. Ann. Thorac. Surg. 36:417–426.

Laschinger, J.C., Cunningham, J.N., Jr., Nathan, I.M., et al. 1984. Intraoperative identification of vessels critical to spinal cord blood supply—use of somatosensory evoked potentials. Curr. Surg. 41:107–109.

Laschinger, J.C., Izumoto, H., and Kouchoukos, T. 1987. Evolving concepts in prevention of spinal cord injury during operations on the descending thoracic and thoracoabdominal aorta. Ann. Thorac. Surg. 44:667–674.

Lesser, R.P., Raudzens, P., Lueders, H., et al. 1986. Postoperative neurological deficits may occur despite unchanged intraoperative somatosensory evoked potentials. Ann. Neurol. 19:22–25

Livesay, J.J., Cooley, D.A., Ventemiglia, R.A., et al. 1985. Surgical experience in descending thoracic aneurysmectomy with and without adjuncts to avoid ischemia. Ann. Thorac. Surg. 39:37–46.

Loder, R.T., Thomson, G.J., and LaMont, R.L. 1991. Spinal cord monitoring in patients with nonidiopathic spinal deformities using somatosensory evoked potentials. Spine 16:1359–1364.

Lubicky, J.P., Spadaro, J.A., Yuan, H.A., et al. 1989. Variability of somatosensory cortical evoked potential monitoring during spinal surgery. Spine 14:790–798.

Lueders, H., Gurd, A., Hahn J., et al. 1982. A new technique for intraoperative monitoring of spinal cord function. Spine 7:2;110–115.

MacDonald, D.B., and Janusz, M. 2002. An approach to intraoperative neurophysiologic monitoring of thoracoabdominal aneurysm surgery. J. Clin. Neurophysiol. 19:43–54.

Machida, M., Weinstein, S.L., Yamada, T., et al. 1985. Spinal cord monitoring. Spine 10:407–413.

Machida, M., Weinstein, S.L., Yamada, T., et al. 1988. Monitoring of motor action potentials after stimulation of the spinal cord. J. Bone Joint Surg. 70A:911–918.

Macon, J.B., and Poletti, C.E. 1982. Conducted somatosensory evoked potentials during spinal surgery. Part 1: control conduction velocity measurements. J. Neurosurg. 57:349–353.

Macon, J.B., Poletti, C.E., Sweet, W.H., et al. 1980. Spinal conduction velocity measurement during laminectomy. Surg. Forum. 31:453–455.

Maeda, S., Miyamoto, T., Murata, H., et al. 1989. Prevention of spinal cord ischemia by monitoring spinal cord perfusion pressure and somatosensory evoked potentials. J. Cardiovasc. Surg. 30:565–571.

Matsuda, H., and Shimazu, A. 1989. Intraoperative spinal cord monitoring using electric responses to stimulation of caudal spinal cord or motor cortex. In *Neuromonitoring in Surgery*, Ed. J.E. Desmedt, pp. 175–190. Amsterdam: Elsevier.

Matsui, Y., Goh, K., Shiiya, N., et al. 1994. Clinical application of evoked spinal cord potentials elicited by direct stimulation of the cord during temporary occlusion of the thoracic aorta. J. Thorac. Cardiovasc. Surg. 107:1519–1527.

McDonnell, D.E., Flanigin, H.F., and Sullivan, H.G. 1986. Somatosensory evoked potentials (SEP) intraoperative monitoring during cranial vertebral compression and instability. In *Neurophysiology and Standards of Spinal Cord Monitoring*, Eds. T.B. Ducker and R.H. Brown, pp. 251–260. New York: Springer-Verlag.

McPherson, R.W., Mahla, M., Johnson, R., et al. 1985. Effects of enflurane, isoflurane and nitrous oxide on somatosensory evoked potentials during fentanyl anesthesia. Anesthesiology 62:626–633.

Meyer, P.R. Jr., Colter, H.B., and Gireesan, G.T. 1988. Operative neurological complications resulting from thoracic and lumbar spine internal fixation. Clin. Orthop. Rel. Res. 237:125–131.

Meylaerts, S.A., De Haan, P., Kalkman, C.J., et al. 1999a. The influence of regional spinal cord hypothermia on transcranial myogenic motor-evoked potential monitoring and the efficacy of spinal cord ischemia detection. J. Thorac. Cardiovasc. Surg. 118:1038–1045.

Meylaerts, S.A., Jacobs, M.J., Iterson, V.V., et al. 1999b. Comparison of transcranial motor evoked potentials and somatosensory evoked potentials during thoracoabdominal aortic aneurysm repair. Ann. Surg. 6:742–749.

Minahan, R.E., Sepkuty, J.P., Lesser, R.P., et al. 2001. Anterior spinal cord injury with preserved neurogenic motor evoked potentials. Clin. Neurophysiol. 112:1442–1450.

Mizoi, K., and Yoshimoto, T. 1993. Permissible temporary occlusion time in aneurysm surgery as evaluated by evoked potential monitoring. Neurosurgery 33:434–440.

Molaie, M. 1986. False negative intraoperative somatosensory evoked potentials with simultaneous bilateral stimulation. Clin. Electroencephalogr. 17:6–19.

Møller, A.R. (Ed.). 1995. *Intraoperative Neurophysiologic Monitoring*. Luxemburg: Harwood.

More, R.C., Nuwer, M.R., and Dawson, E.G. 1988. Cortical evoked potential monitoring during spinal surgery: sensitivity, specificity, reliability, and criteria for alarm. J. Spinal Disorders 1:75–80.

Mostegl, A., and Bauer, R. 1984. The application of somatosensory-evoked potentials in orthopedic spine surgery. Arch. Orthop. Trauma Surg. 103–179–184.

Mostegl, A., Bauer, R., and Eichenauer, M. 1987. Intraoperative somatosensory potential monitoring. A clinical analysis of 127 surgical procedures. Spine 13:396–400.

Murakami, M., Mochizuki, M., Okamoto, Y., et al. 1994. Spinal cord monitoring during surgery for intramedullary spinal cord tumours. In *Handbook of Spinal Cord Monitoring*, Eds. S.J. Jones, S. Boyd, M. Hetreed, et al., pp. 197–204. London: Kluwer.

Nagle, K.J., Emerson, R.G., Adams, D.C., et al. 1996. Intraoperative monitoring of motor evoked potentials: a review of 116 cases. Neurology 47:999–1004.

Nash, C.L., Jr., Lorig, R.A., Schatzinger, L.A., et al. 1977a. Spinal cord monitoring during operative treatment of the spine. Clin. Orthop. 126:100–105.

Nash, C.L., Jr., Schatzinger, L.H., Brown, R.H., et al. 1977b. The unstable thoracic compression fracture: its problems and the use of spinal cord monitoring in the evaluation of treatment. Spine 2:261–265.

Noonan, K.J., Walker, T., Feinberg, J.R., et al. 2002. Factors related to false-versus true-positive neuromonitoring changes in adolescent idiopathic scoliosis surgery. Spine 8:825–830.

North, R.B., Drenger, B., Beattie, C., et al. 1991. Monitoring of spinal cord stimulation evoked potentials during thoracoabdominal aneurysm surgery. Neurosurgery 28:325–330.

Nuwer, M.R. (Ed.). 1986. *Evoked Potential Monitoring in the Operating Room*. New York: Raven Press.

Nuwer, M.R. 1989. Monitoring spinal cord surgery with cortical somatosensory evoked potentials. In *Neuromonitoring in Surgery*, Ed. J.E. Desmedt, pp. 151–164. Amsterdam: Elsevier.

Nuwer, M.R., and Carlson, L.G. 1992. A multicentre survey of spinal cord monitoring outcome. In *Handbook of Spinal Cord Monitoring*, Eds. S.J. Jones, S. Boyd, M. Hetreed, et al., pp. 78–87. London: Kluwer.

Nuwer, M.R., and Dawson, E. 1984a. Intraoperative evoked potential monitoring of the spinal cord: enhanced stability of cortical recordings. Electroencephalogr. Clin. Neurophysiol. 59:318–327.

Nuwer, M.R., and Dawson, E. 1984b. Intraoperative evoked potential monitoring of the spinal cord: a restricted filer, scalp method during Harrington instrumentation for scoliosis. Clin. Orthop. 183:42–50.

Nuwer, M.R., Daube, J., Fischer, C., et al. 1993. Neuromonitoring during surgery. Electroencephalogr. Clin. Neurophysiol. 87:263–276.

Nuwer, M.R., Dawson, E.G., Carlson, L.G., et al. 1995. Somatosensory evoked potential spinal cord monitoring reduces neurologic deficits after scoliosis surgery: results of a large multicenter survey. Electroencephalogr. Clin. Neurophysiol. 96:6–11.

Okamoto, Y., Murakami, M., Nakagawa, T., et al. 1992. Intraoperative spinal cord monitoring during surgery for aortic aneurysm: application of spinal cord evoked potential. Electroencephalogr. Clin. Neurophysiol. 84:315–320.

Owen, J.H., Bridewell, K.H., Grubb, R., et al. 1991. The clinical application of neurogenic motor evoked potentials to monitor spinal cord function during surgery. Spine 16:S285–S390.

Owen, J.H., Sponseller, M.D., Szymanski, J., et al. 1995. Efficacy of multimodality spinal cord monitoring during surgery for neuromuscular scoliosis. Spine 20(13):1480–1488.

Padberg, A., Holden-Wilson, T., Lenke, L., et al. 1998. Somatosensory- and motor-evoked potential monitoring without a wake-up test during idiopathic scoliosis surgery. Spine 23:1392–1400.

Pelosi, L., Stevenson, M., Hobbs, G.J., et al. 2001. Intraoperative motor evoked potentials to transcranial electrical stimulation during two anesthetic regimens. Clin. Neurophysiol. 112:1076–1087.

Pelosi, L., Lamb, J., Grevitt, M., et al. 2002. Combined monitoring of motor and somatosensory evoked potentials in orthopaedic spinal surgery. Clin. Neurophysiol. 113:1082–1091.

Péréon, Y., Nguyen The Tich, S., Delecrin, J., et al. 2002. Combined spinal cord monitoring using neurogenic mixed evoked potentials and collision techniques. Spine 27:1571–1576.

Phillips, L.H. III, Blanco, J.S., and Sussman, M.D. 1995. Direct spinal stimulation for intraoperative monitoring during scoliosis surgery. Muscle Nerve 18:319–325.

Prestor, B., and Golob, P. 1999. Intra-operative spinal cord neuromonitoring in patients operated on for intramedullary tumors and syringomyelia. Neurol. Res. 21:125–129.

Raudzens, P.A. 1982. Intraoperative monitoring of evoked potentials. Ann. N.Y. Acad. Sci. 338:308–326.

Roy, E.P. III, Gutmann, L., Riggs, J.E., et al. 1987. Intraoperative somatosensory evoked potential monitoring in scoliosis. Clin. Orthop. Rel. Res. 229:94–98.

Russell, G.B., and Rodichok, L.D. 1995. *Intraoperative Neurophysiologic Monitoring*. Boston: Butterworth-Heinemann.

Ryan, T.P., and Britt, R.H. 1986. Spinal and cortical somatosensory evoked potential monitoring during corrective spinal surgery with 108 patients. Spine 11:352–361.

Sala, F., Niimi, Y., Berenstein, A., et al. 2001. Neuroprotective role of neurophysiological monitoring during endovascular procedures in the spinal cord. Ann. N.Y. Acad. Sci. 939:126–136.

Salzman, S.K., Beckman, A.L., Marks, H.G., et al. 1986. Effects of halothane on intraoperative scalp-recorded somatosensory evoked potentials to posterior tibial nerve stimulation in man. Electroencephalogr. Clin. Neurophysiol. 65:36–45.

Schepens, M., Boezeman, E., Hamerlijnck, R., et al. 1994. Somatosensory evoked potentials during exclusion and reperfusion of critical aortic segments in thoracoabdominal aortic aneurysm surgery. J. Cardiac Surg. 9:692–702.

Schramm, J., and Møller, A.R. (Eds.). 1991. *Intraoperative Neurophysiologic Monitoring in Neurosurgery*. New York: Springer-Verlag.

Shiiya, N., Yasuda, K., Matsui, Y., et al. 1995. Spinal cord protection during thoracoabdominal aortic aneurysm repair: results of selective reconstruction of the critical segmental arteries guided by evoked spinal cord potential monitoring. J. Vasc. Surg. 21:970–975.

Sloan, T.B., and Koht, A. 1985. Depression of cortical somatosensory evoked potentials by nitrous oxide. Br. J. Anaesth. 57:849–852.

Spetzler R.F., Selman, W.R., Nash, C.L. Jr., et al. 1979. Transoral microsurgical odontoid resection and spinal cord monitoring. Spine 4:506–510.

Spielholz, N.I., Benjamin, M.V., Engler, G.L., et al. 1979. Somatosensory evoked potentials during decompression and stabilization of the spine. Spine 4:500–505.

Stühmeier, K.D., Grabitz, K., Mainzer, B., et al. 1993. Use of the electrospinogram for predicting harmful spinal cord ischemia during repair of thoracic or thoracoabdominal aortic aneurysms. Anesthesiol. 79:1170–1176.

Sueda, T., Okada, K., Watari, M., et al. 2000. Evaluation of motor- and sensory-evoked potentials for spinal cord monitoring during thoracoabdominal aortic aneurysm surgery. Japan. J. Thorac. Cardiovasc. Surg. 48:60–65.

Tamaki, T. 1989. Spinal cord monitoring with spinal potentials evoked by direct stimulation of the spinal cord. In *Neuromonitoring in Surgery*, Ed. J.E. Desmedt, pp. 139–149. Amsterdam: Elsevier.

Tamaki, T., Tsuji, H., Inoue, S., et al. 1981. The prevention of iatrogenic spinal cord injury utilizing the evoked spinal cord potential. Int. Orthop. 4:313–317.

Tamaki, T., Noguchi, T., Takano, H., et al. 1984. Spinal cord monitoring as a clinical utilization of the spinal evoked potentials. Clin. Orthop. 184:58–64.

Van Dongen, E.P., Schepens, M.A., Morshuis, W.J., et al. 2001. Thoracic and thoracoabdominal aortic aneurysm repair: use of evoked potential monitoring in 118 patients. J. Vasc. Surg. 34:1035–1040.

Wada, T., Yao, H., Miyamoto, T., et al. 2001. Prevention and detection of spinal cord injury during thoracic and thoracoabdominal aortic repairs. Ann. Thorac. Surg. 72:80–85.

Wang, A.D., Costa e Silva, I., Symon, L., et al. 1985. The effects of halothane on somatosensory and flash visual evoked potentials during operations. Neurol. Res. 7:58–62.

Whittle, I.R., Johnston, I.H., Besser, M., et al. 1984a. Intraoperative spinal cord monitoring during surgery for scoliosis using somatosensory evoked potentials. Aust. N.Z. J. Surg. 54:553–557.

Whittle, I.R., Johnston, I.H., and Besser, M. 1984b. Spinal cord monitoring during surgery by direct recording of somatosensory evoked potentials. J. Neurosurg. 60:440–443.

Whittle, I.R., Johnston, I.H., and Besser, M. 1986. Recording of spinal somatosensory evoked potentials for intraoperative spinal cord monitoring. J. Neurosurg. 64:601–612.

Wiedemayer, H., Fauser, B., Sandalcioglu, I.E., et al. 2002. The impact of neurophysiological intraoperative monitoring on surgical decisions: a critical analysis of 423 cases. J. Neurosurg. 96:255–262.

Wilber, R.G., Thompson, G.H., Shaffer, J.W., et al. 1984. Postoperative neurological deficits in segmental spinal instrumentation. J. Bone Joint Surg. [Am.]. 66A:1178–1187.

Wilson, G.J., Rebeyka, I.M., Coles, J.G., et al. 1988. Loss of the somatosensory evoked response as an indicator of reversible cerebral ischemia during hypothermic, low-flow cardiopulmonary bypass. Ann. Thorac. Surg. 45:206–209.

Witzmann, A., and Reisecker F. 1989. Somatosensory and auditory evoked potentials monitoring in tumor removal and brainstem surgery. In *Neuromonitoring in Surgery*, Ed. J.E. Desmedt, pp. 219–241. Amsterdam: Elsevier.

Yamamoto, N., Takano, H., Kitagawa, H., et al. 1994. Monitoring or spinal cord ischemia by use of the evoked spinal cord potentials during aortic aneurysm surgery. J. Vasc. Surg. 20:826–833.

Young, W., and Mollin, D. 1989. Intraoperative somatosensory evoked potentials monitoring of spinal surgery. In *Neuromonitoring in Surgery*, Ed. J.E. Desmedt, pp. 165–173. Amsterdam: Elsevier.

Zentner, J. 1989. Scalp recorded somatosensory evoked potentials in response to cauda equina stimulation in neurosurgical operations on the spinal cord. Br. J. Neurosurg. 3:39–43.

Zentner, J., Schumacher, M., and Bien, S. 1988. Motor evoked potentials during interventional neuroradiology. Neuroradiology 30:252–255.

45. Transcranial Electrical and Magnetic Stimulation

Aleksandar Beric and Manoj Raghavan

The physiological responses of the nervous system to controlled stimuli yield valuable insights into its functional organization. Delivery of stimuli to the peripheral nervous system or exposed nervous tissue is relatively easy. However, noninvasive stimulation of the central nervous system (CNS) poses several challenges. So, while direct electrical stimulation of surgically exposed cerebral cortex has been used by neurosurgeons as early as the latter half of the 19th century (Bartholow, 1874; Horsley, 1886), it took another century of technological advances before focal transcranial stimulation (TCS) became a reality. Instances of noninvasive brain stimulation prior to the 1980s were at best crude, if not accidental. The earliest instances of TCS are probably reports of phosphenes, or even syncope, in subjects whose heads were placed at the center of powerful induction coils (d'Arsonval, 1896). Although focal cortical stimulation was not the objective, the introduction of electroconvulsive therapy (ECT) in the 1930s (Cerletti, 1940) is another step in the evolution of transcranial brain stimulation. ECT and its benefits in psychiatric conditions demonstrated that brain stimulation may not only be interesting as a technique for studying brain physiology, but may indeed have therapeutic potential in neuropsychiatric disorders. It was several more decades before controlled and focal excitation of the brain by TCS was first accomplished in the 1980s. This chapter discusses clinically relevant issues in TCS methodologies and reviews a spectrum of results that have potential clinical applications.

Principles of Transcranial Stimulation: Electrical Versus Magnetic Stimulation

There are two choices in TCS techniques: electrical and magnetic. As demonstrated by ECT, strong electrical currents delivered via scalp electrodes can depolarize neurons in the brain. This is the basis of transcranial electrical stimulation (TES). Merton and Morton (1980) successfully demonstrated focal nonconvulsive TES of the primary motor cortex. For any voltage applied at the scalp, the electrical impedance of the path taken by the current determines its magnitude. With TES this path includes scalp, skull, dura, and cerebrospinal fluid (Saypol et al., 1991). TES typically requires high voltages at the scalp to produce depolarization of cortical neurons, and tends to excite a broad area of cortex (Nathan et al., 1993). Stimulation of pain receptors, and consequent discomfort to the patient or subject is inevitable. While electrode size appears to have little impact on this, briefer pulses may reduce the discomfort (Suihko, 2002; Zentner and Neumuller, 1989). However, in anesthetized pa-

tients undergoing spinal cord surgery, TES has been extensively used for the intraoperative monitoring of corticospinal tract (CST) integrity.

Unlike electrical currents, magnetic fields are neither deflected nor attenuated by intervening tissue. A time-varying magnetic field is always accompanied by an orthogonally oriented time-varying electromotive force in accordance with Faraday's law. When this secondary electric field is generated in a conducting medium, an electrical current is induced in the direction of the field in accordance with Lenz's law. In transcranial magnetic stimulation (TMS), neuronal depolarization is caused by currents generated in this manner within the nervous system, in response to an externally applied time-varying magnetic field. Excitation of the motor cortex using magnetic stimulation was first reported in 1985 (Barker and Jalinous, 1985). To generate the magnetic field, a brief high-intensity current, typically lasting a few hundred microseconds, is passed through a conducting coil. Traditionally, these have been air-core coils and the maximal magnetic field intensities generated are of the order of 2 tesla (comparable to the static field-strengths used for magnetic resonance imaging).

In its early applications, TCS provided a physiological technique for assessing CST function in humans without surgical exposure. A motor evoked potential (MEP) is a compound muscle action potential (CMAP) recorded from limb or trunk muscles elicited by TCS of the motor cortex. The same basic technique can also be used for spinal cord and proximal-root stimulation, adding to the repertoire of nerve conduction studies for assessment of peripheral nervous system dysfunctions (Cros and Chiappa, 1993). TCS when combined with proximal-root stimulation can help to assess the central segment of the descending motor system (Abbruzzese et al., 1991; Hess et al., 1987a; Mayr et al., 1991; Schadi et al., 1991), giving clinicians and neuroscientists unprecedented insight into motor control. Currently, TCS is used in a wide variety of physiological and clinical studies. In addition to the corticospinal system, visual, somatosensory, language, memory, and learning systems are being explored using TCS. Repetitive TCS (rTCS) provides additional diagnostic techniques and more importantly, potential new therapeutic approaches that are discussed later in the chapter.

In addition to the fundamental differences between TES and TMS described earlier, there are differences in how they excite corticospinal neurons (Rothwell, 1991; for a review see Di Lazzaro et al., 2003). Electrical stimulation depolarizes corticospinal neurons directly (vertical fiber depolarization), whereas magnetic stimulation indirectly depolarizes corticospinal neuron afferents (horizontal fiber depolarization) (Day et al., 1987, 1989a; Rothwell et al., 1991; Thompson et al., 1991). This notion is supported by a difference in the latencies of the muscle responses recorded after TES and TMS. The latency of MEP is shorter after TES than TMS, regardless of whether it is performed during complete muscle relaxation or voluntary contraction facilitation (Fig. 45.1). However, it is also possible that the difference is due to a CST axon being more distally depolarized with electrical stimulation and very proximally depolarized with magnetic stimulation (Edgely et al., 1990). Early evidence of the presence of D direct waves recorded from the descending CST only after electrical stimulation and absence of the D wave after magnetic stimulation was later disputed by Amassian et al. (1990). Their findings suggested that with different orientation of the magnetic coil, it is possible to obtain direct stimulation of CST axons with consequently

shorter MEP latencies comparable to electrical MEPs. The controversy regarding the exact site of neuronal depolarization still exists considering the many different approaches to either electrical or magnetic stimulation (Epstein et al., 1990; Rothwell et al., 1994; Rudiak and Marg, 1994; Wilson et al., 1996). The intensity of the magnetic pulse, the shape of the magnetic field produced by the coil, and coil-orientation relative to the brain determine the brain region excited by TMS. Similarly, the current intensity and location of anode and cathode on the scalp determines the brain region stimulated in TES. The differences in facilitatory responses to magnetic TCS and electrical TCS have been used to ascertain the role of afferents in modulating cortical excitability (Brasil-Neto et al., 1993a; Cohen et al., 1993).

Some of the early data pertaining to the multiple descending volleys generated by TCS of the human motor areas was obtained in the context of intraoperative monitoring (IOM) (Fig. 45.2) of patients under general anesthesia (Berardelli et al., 1990; Burke et al., 1990). In anesthetized patients, recordings may be obtained from CST axons at different sites along the descending pathway. The orientation of the TMS coil is responsible for either predominantly direct CST stimulation with generation of D waves (comparable to electrical stimulation) or predominantly indirect stimulation with generation of I waves and longer latency MEPs (Di Lazzaro et al., 2003; Nakamura et al., 1996). TES in anesthetized patients introduces the possibility that the stimulus may be supramaximal. Considering that it produces vertical-fiber depolarization, there have been speculations about extremely distal sites of depolarization, such as the brainstem or pyramidal decussation (Rothwell et al., 1994). Distally generated volleys that arrive early may have excitatory or inhibitory effects in the spinal cord that modify response to the descending volley (D wave), comparable to the effects of a conditioning stimuli. These theoretical considerations do not appear relevant when comparing electrical and magnetic stimulation in awake subjects with threshold, or just suprathreshold stimulus intensities.

The level of discomfort caused by the stimulation is a major difference between electrical and magnetic TCS. TES requires high-voltage short-duration pulses in order to produce a current that is strong enough to produce depolarization of the CST. Because of the spread of the current and the resulting depolarization of muscles and sensory nerve terminals in the scalp, moderate-to-severe discomfort or even frank pain can occur. It appears that the pain originates from receptors in the scalp underlying the stimulating electrodes (Hakkinen et al., 1995). In contrast, magnetic stimulation causes minimal discomfort during TCS, except at higher frequencies. This has led to widespread adoption of TMS as the preferred technique for TCS except in anesthetized patients.

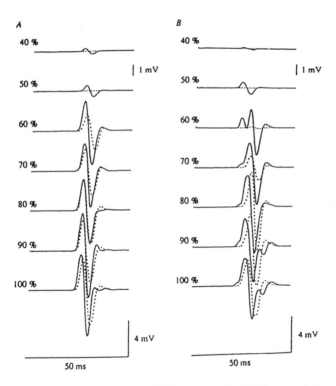

Figure 45.1. Electromyogram (EMG) responses in right first dorsal interosseus (FDI) to counterclockwise magnetic (**A**) and anodal (**B**) stimulation at different stimulus intensities when contracting *(continuous lines)* and when relaxing *(dashed lines)*. Each trace is an average of five trials. The response threshold is lower in contracting muscle for both forms of stimulation, and the response waveform is more complex with anodal stimulation in the contracting muscle at a stimulus intensity of 100%. The response latency is some 1 to 8 msec shorter for anodal (20 msec) than magnetic (21.8 msec) stimulation. The latencies when relaxed were 23 msec for anodal and 22.6 msec for magnetic stimulation. As the intensity of the magnetic stimulus was increased the response latency shortened from 23 msec in the contracting muscle to 21.8 msec, and from 25 to 22.6 msec in relaxed muscle. As the intensity of electrical stimulation was increased, the response latency in the relaxed muscle shortened from 25.6 to 23 msec. The latency remained constant in the contracting muscle at all intensities of stimulation. (From Rothwell, J.C., Thompson, P.D., Day, B.L., Boyd, S., and Marsden, C.D. 1991. Stimulation of the human motor cortex through the scalp. Exp. Physiol. 76:159–200, with permission.)

Stimulator Designs and Related Instrumentation
Electrical Stimulators

Electrical stimulators for TES may be either constant current or constant voltage devices. Constant current devices adjust the voltage to ensure a predetermined current flow

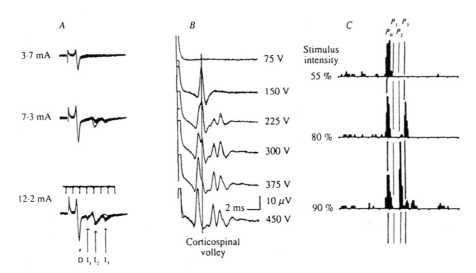

Figure 45.2. Comparison of direct recording of the descending volleys set up in monkey (**A**) and human (**B**), with the changes in firing probability of a human single motor unit in the FDI (**C**) after electrical transcranial stimulation (TCS) of the motor cortex. **A:** Bipolar recordings from the dorsolateral funiculus at the C4-C5 level after surface anodal stimulation of the exposed motor cortex of the baboon at three different intensities (mA). Negativity downward; time scale, milliseconds. At the lowest intensities, a single D wave is seen, at high intensities the later I_2 and I_3 waves are recruited and finally I_1 waves. (From Kernell, D., and Wu, C.-P., 1967. Responses of the pyramidal tract to stimulation of the baboon's motor cortex. J. Physiol. 191:653–672.). **B:** Bipolar recordings from the high thoracic epidural space in a patient undergoing corrective surgery for scoliosis. High-voltage electrical stimulation was given over the scalp at the intensities shown. Note the early recruited D wave followed by I waves at the higher intensities. Also note the shortening of D-wave latency by about 0.8 msec at the highest intensities. (From Burke, D., Hicks, R.G., and Stephen, J.P.H. 1990. Corticospinal volleys evoked by anodal and cathodal stimulation of the human motor cortex. J. Physiol. (Lond.) 425:283–299.) **C:** Poststimulus time histograms of single motor unit firing behavior in the FDI muscle following electrical stimulation of the scalp at different intensities (percentage output of stimulator). All traces start 10 msec after the stimulus was given, and the horizontal calibration markers are at 2.5-msec intervals. With low intensities of stimulation, an early single peak in firing probability is seen (P_0). At higher intensities, later peaks become clear (P_2 and P_3). (From Rothwell, J.C., Thompson, P.D., Day, B.L., Boyd, S., and Marsden, C.D. 1991. Stimulation of the human motor cortex through the scalp. Exp. Physiol. 76:159–200, with permission.)

through the scalp electrodes regardless of the impedance of the circuit. The current generated by a constant voltage device, on the other hand, depends on the impedance of the circuit, which includes the scalp and skull. The pulsed currents may be monophasic or biphasic. Typical pulse widths are of the order of few tens of microseconds with voltages up to 1,000 V, and peak currents of the order of an ampere. Both square wave pulses and exponentially decaying pulses have been used. Small pulse widths ensure that the total dissipated energy is within safe limits despite the high currents. Available stimulators often allow protocols that use pulse trains. Data from intraoperative monitoring support the greater efficacy of pulse pairs and pulse trains in eliciting MEPs (Haghighi and Gaines, 2003). The electrical pulses are delivered via cutaneous electrodes. The location of the stimulating anode and cathode determine the current path and the resulting area of cortical stimulation. Several different geometries of scalp electrodes have been used for stimulus delivery, including disc-shaped electrodes, screw-type electrodes that penetrate the scalp, and monofocal anodal electrodes with circumferential or headband cathodes (Rossini et al., 1985). Self-adhesive electrodes are very commonly used. Electrode geometry, however, does not appear to significantly modify the level of discomfort associated with TES as much as shorter pulse durations (Suihko, 2002; Zentner and Neumuller, 1989).

Magnetic Stimulators

The essential components of a magnetic stimulator are the magnetic coil itself, circuitry that allows one to control the intensity and parameters of the current pulses sent through the coil, and the capacitors that accumulate the charge required to produce the high currents. Additional features often available are coil positioning mounts, or arms that help stabilize the coil with respect to the head, temperature sensors within coils that prevent overheating during extended pulse train delivery, cooling measures to prevent heating, hardware interfaces to computers with software control of stimulation parameters, and navigational tools to accurately target specific locations in the brain.

One difference between commercially available magnetic stimulators is whether the current flow is biphasic, dampened, or monophasic (Claus et al., 1990). Pulse configuration and the direction of resulting magnetic fields significantly affects the responses elicited (Antal et al., 2002; Di Lazzaro et al., 2003; Maccabee et al., 1991). Stimulator designs also differ in the maximal rate of stimulation that is achievable. Single and bi-pulse stimulators are relatively inexpensive. Stimulators capable of extended rapid rate pulse trains are currently available, but cost significantly more.

A major design feature is the stimulating coil itself. Coil design variables include coil size, shape, and the use of multicoils (Cadwell, 1991; Jalinous, 1991; Rosler et al., 1989a), all of which are relevant to the focality of the stimulation. The size of the coil is also correlated to its capacity to handle high currents, and the maximal field intensities that it can thus generate. MEPs from the lower extremities require higher intensity stimuli because of the anatomical representation of the foot deep in the interhemispheric fissure. Once the feasibility of TMS had been demonstrated, the focality of stimulation became a central issue. Technical improvements have evolved to stimulate different areas of hand and arm representation for basic physiology as well as for precise clinical localization (Wassermann et al., 1992). The direction of the magnetic field, and the orientation of the coil determine the direction of current flow inside the brain and can have major effects on MEP responses (Meyer et al., 1991). The magnetic field intensity produced by circular coils is typically maximal at the inner rim of the coil. Butterfly or figure-of-eight coils produce peak magnetic field intensities at a point between the two halves if the magnetic field produced by the two halves is in the same direction. These and other modifications (Jalinous, 1991; Meyer et al., 1990) have resulted in the ability to deliver more focal stimulation.

Roth et al. (2002) recently suggested an innovative coil design that allows stimulation of deeper brain targets. The use of extended pulse trains in research employing rTMS has placed new demands on coil design. Several distinct factors determine the rate and duration of a stimulus pulse train that can be delivered by a magnetic stimulator. The high current required to drive the stimulating coil is generated by discharging capacitors that accumulate charge constantly. The larger these capacitors, the more stimuli they can deliver in any given interval of time. Heating of the coil limits the number of stimuli in a pulse train. As a result, the use of magnetic stimulation has, until recently, seen limited use in the operating room where at times a large number of stimuli may be required for response averaging. Higher frequency stimulation causes more rapid heat buildup. Coils that use circulated air or liquid to cool the coils are now commercially available. To compensate for the very low efficiency and high power requirements of the air-core coils typically used with today's stimulators, there are new designs developed with a coil built around a highly saturable (>0.5 T) core material (Epstein and Davey, 2002). This allows the coil to produce a strong magnetic field with a fraction of the input power while reducing losses to heat when compared to air-core coils. This technology also reduces the size and weight of the stimulator drive circuitry, and facilitates extended stimulation protocols as thermal buildup in the coil is minimized. The need for realistic "placebo" or sham stimulation in clinical trials of rTMS has prompted other innovations in coil design. Ruohonen et al. (2000) have suggested a figure-of-eight coil design where the current direction in the two halves can be switched, allowing the same coil to double for both "treatment" and "placebo" stimulation.

Regardless of the variations in coil design and shape of the magnetic field produced, it is important to be able to reproduce the same stimulus intensity on different trials. In some early designs, consecutive stimuli of the same dialed intensity did not yield the same magnetic field intensities. The first stimulus after changing the intensity, however, often produced a variable, usually stronger than the dialed, magnetic field (Reutens et al., 1993). This, however, is no longer a major consideration for currently available designs.

Magnetic Resonance Imaging-Guided Stereotactic TMS

As discussed earlier, coil dimension, shape, stimulus intensity, as well as coil position and orientation relative to the head, determine the volume of brain tissue that can be electrically excited by transcranially delivered magnetic pulses. In principle, the reproducibility of phenomena resulting from brain stimulation, both within and between subjects, depends on being able to excite the same brain regions, at the same intensity, at different times. Accurate targeting of specific brain locations demands that there be a known system of correspondence between the location and orientation of the coil at the scalp, stimulus intensity, and the brain volume that is effectively stimulated. This is especially of concern when very focal stimulation is desired using small coils.

A simple way to specify the stimulated region is based on scalp anatomical landmarks. The standardized 10–20 EEG electrode placement system has been widely used in reporting coil position. There are some known correspondences between these locations and underlying cerebral structures (Homan et al., 1987). However, these correspondences are highly variable. Furthermore, individual variability in brain anatomy, and functional reorganization that often accompanies brain pathologies, add to the imprecision of navigational systems based on scalp landmarks.

Magnetic resonance imaging (MRI) based stereotactic navigational techniques have been developed by several laboratories in recent years. The level of precision afforded by these navigational techniques makes it feasible to evaluate TMS as a tool for the presurgical mapping of eloquent cortical areas (Ettinger et al., 1998; Krings et al., 1997, 1998, 2001a,b; Miranda et al., 1997; Potts et al., 1998). The navigational techniques essentially determine the transformation required between a coordinate system based on skull or scalp landmarks and one defined in terms of brain anatomy. This is typically based on MRI. Once this transformation is known, one can calculate and display the volume of brain tissue that would receive stimulation given the position and orientation of the coil relative to the head. This minimizes the uncertainty arising from the inconsistent relationship between scalp structures and underlying brain anatomy. A comparison between guided and unguided stimulation based on measurement of MEPs demonstrated the marked superiority of guided stimulation in being able to revisit specific motor areas accurately (Gugino et al., 2001). Commercial products have recently become available for MRI-guided TMS.

TMS Compatible EEG

The ability to record EEG data during magnetic or electrical stimulation offers additional insights into the immediate effects of TMS on cortical physiology. Magnetic pulse artifacts, induction of high currents in recording wires and their effects, and possible heating of scalp electrodes during pulse trains are of concern when applying TMS during EEG recordings. The technique of using high-resolution EEG in combination with stereotactically guided TMS has been studied by Ilmoniemi et al. (1997). Surprisingly, source localization of the EEG response over time shows a delayed response in the contralateral sensorimotor areas after a single pulse delivered to homologous areas on one side (Ilmoniemi et al., 1997; Komssi et al., 2002).

Overview of Stimulation Protocols and Their Effects

Over the course the last couple of decades several distinct stimulation protocols have evolved in the various applications of TCS. The effects of these stimulation protocols in different cortical areas will be discussed with reference to specific applications during the course of this chapter. A summary outline of the different protocols is provided here.

Single-Pulse TMS

The earliest applications of TCS mainly studied MEP responses to single-pulse stimulation (Barker and Jalinous, 1985; Barker et al., 1986). The primary effect of single-pulse stimulation of the motor cortex is the excitation of the CST. The motor threshold using single-pulse TMS and the amplitude and latency of MEP responses have been studied extensively in this way. The effects of single-pulse stimulation have been studied in other cortical areas as well. In visual areas the positive phenomena elicited are phosphenes (Kammer, 1999). Unlike MEPs, which can be measured physiologically, phosphenes are perceptual events that can be quantified only on the basis of subjective reports. The interference produced by single pulses can be inferred from their effects on specific tasks that recruit that particular area. For instance, visual detection thresholds are elevated when the visual stimulus presentation is paired with single magnetic pulses delivered to the occipital cortex (Kammer and Nusseck, 1998; Kastner et al., 1998). Given the very short duration of single pulses and their immediate effects, this typically requires synchronization of magnetic pulse delivery and delivery of task-related stimuli. With stimulation of frontal eye fields, saccadic eye movements can be either delayed or evoked (Li et al., 1997; Priori et al., 1993; Ro et al., 2003). TMS during more complex memory-guided saccades can show site-specific increase in errors, suggesting involvement of different cortical regions in learning, memorization, and execution of sequences (Muri et al., 1995, 1996). Single-pulse stimulation has been used in a wide array of experimental settings including the study of verbal working memory (Mottaghy et al., 2003), visuospatial perception (Fierro et al., 2001a,b), and BOLD functional MRI (fMRI) responses to TMS (Bohning et al., 2000; Brandt et al., 1996).

Paired-Pulse TMS

The paired-pulse (or bi-pulse) paradigm evolved as a means of studying cortical responses to a single pulse. These responses include intracortical facilitation and inhibition (Nakamura et al., 1997; Wassermann et al., 1996c). The technique looks at the MEP response to a TMS pulse applied with varying delays after a conditioning pulse. MEP responses using this technique has been studied extensively as a means of characterizing local cortical excitation and inhibition in normal subjects, as well as in several neurological disorders. Typically the second pulse is delivered by the same coil and at the same location. However, a second coil may be used to deliver a conditioning pulse at a different location in order to study corticocortical connectivity, inhibition, or facilitation. Neither single nor paired-pulse stimulation has been shown to produce changes in brain physiology beyond the immediate effects of the stimulation itself.

Repetitive TMS (rTMS)

When a longer duration of interference with local cortical processing is desired, a repetitive train of magnetic pulses may be used. The development of stimulators that allow the magnetic coil to be discharged at rates exceeding 30 Hz has facilitated several new areas of exploration. Rapid-rate rTMS has been used especially in studying language and higher cognitive functions including learning and memory, where it has been used to differentiate stages of cognitive processing (Grafman et al., 1994; Pascual-Leone and Hallett, 1994; Pascual-Leone et al., 1994a, 1996d). Rapid-rate rTMS has a much stronger, longer, and more widespread effect on the cortex (Fig. 45.3) (Jennum et al., 1995; Pascual-Leone et al., 1994d). The experience from several initial studies suggested no significant adverse effects of rTMS in relation to cognitive performance, seizure risk, hormonal levels, and cardiac rhythms (Pascual-Leone et al., 1993b; Wassermann et al., 1996b). However, there have been reports of seizure provocation in healthy subjects who had no known seizure risk (Pascual-Leone et al., 1993b; Wassermann et al., 1996a). As we shall discuss in later sections, there is a growing body of evidence indicating that the effects of the long pulse trains extend beyond the immediate effects on cortical function or the increased seizure risk associated with stimulation. These prolonged effects appear to be strongly frequency and intensity dependent. An emerging principle appears to be that high-frequency rTMS causes a temporary focal increase in cortical excitability, while low-frequency rTMS (1 Hz or less) typically leads to a decrease in cortical excitability (for a review see Chen, 2000). These effects were initially described in the motor cortex (Chen et al., 1997), but have since reproduced in other areas including somatosensory (Satow et al., 2003), visual (Antal et al., 2002; Fumal et al., 2003), and language areas (Knecht et al., 2002; Sparing et al., 2001). The precise duration of these effects has yet to be established. The sustained effects of rTMS represent novel brain mechanisms whose underlying physiology remains as yet undetermined (Wassermann and Lisanby, 2001). Though there are several parallels between these effects and phenomena of activity-dependent synaptic plasticity such as long-term potentiation (LTP) and long-term depression (LTD) of synapses (for reviews see Kirkwood et al., 1993; Tsumoto, 1992), no direct link has yet been established. The release of neuromodulatory substances and the expression of specific gene products are other hypothetical mechanisms. While the mechanisms underlying these effects of rTMS are by themselves of great interest, they also provide noninvasive ways to create "virtual le-

Figure 45.3. Time course of the increase in excitability after a 10-pulse repetitive transcranial magnetic stimulation (rTMS) train at 150% intensity and 20 Hz. The increase in excitability was demonstrated by measuring the amplitude of the motor evoked potentials (MEPs) produced by single-pulse TMS stimuli at 90% intensity and 0.2 Hz. **A:** Representative example in one subject. **B:** Plot of the MEP amplitudes in the three subjects tested. Note the normalization of the excitability ~3 to 4 minutes after the rTMS train. (From Pascual-Leone, A., Valls-Sole, J., Wassermann, E.M., et al. 1994d. Responses to rapid-rate transcranial stimulation of the motor cortex. Brain 117:847–858, with permission.)

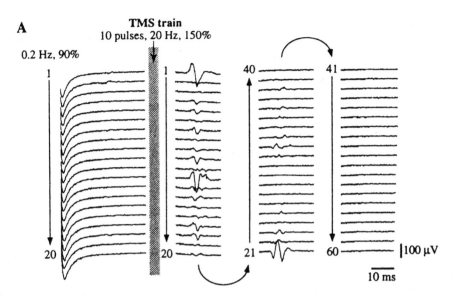

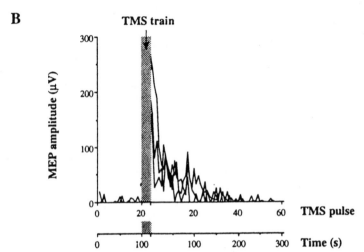

sions" that aren't permanent. They also provide a means to modulate focal cortical excitability for therapeutic benefit in various neuropsychiatric conditions. The last decade has seen an explosion of research activity utilizing repetitive magnetic TCS as an investigational tool in both clinical and basic neuroscience. However, our discussion in the following sections primarily focuses on clinical applications.

Safety Issues and Guidelines

Brain stimulation by any means always raises several concerns about its safety for patients and normal human subjects. Foremost among these is the risk of provoking seizures. Other concerns relate to possible changes in brain tissue that may cause either temporary or long-lasting brain dysfunction. These could arise at many conceivable levels. Possible effects to be considered include direct electrical tissue damage, expression of specific gene products including mediators of inflammation, epileptogenesis, alteration of the normal physiological properties of neural circuits, modula-

tion of neuroendocrine function, and secondary effects on autonomic function including heart rate and blood pressure regulation. There are also concerns pertaining to effects on structures outside the brain, including effects on the inner ear related to the sharp clicks produced during magnetic stimulation, or scalp injury and discomfort that may result from both TMS and TES. In patients with metallic foreign bodies or implanted devices such as deep brain stimulators, cardiac pacemakers, or vagus nerve stimulators, TMS also poses risks related to secondary currents induced in them by pulsed magnetic fields, and the possibility of displacing ferromagnetic objects.

Safety issues in TES methodologies have been outlined by Jajakar (1993), and were recently reviewed by MacDonald (2002) based on clinical experience from more than 15,000 cases of intraoperative MEP monitoring. Seizures and cardiac arrhythmias are rare, and tongue and lip lacerations, which have been reported, can be prevented by soft bite-blocks. No recognized neuropsychological or endocrine effects have been reported. Relative contraindications include a history of epilepsy, cardiac arrhythmia, proconvulsant medications, intracranial electrodes, raised intracranial pressure, and implanted biomedical devices such as pacemakers. There has been much speculation about the long-term effects of electrical stimulation of peripheral nerves and deleterious effects on the CNS (Agnew and McCreery, 1987; Agnew et al., 1989). As good pathological studies of stimulated nervous system tissues are lacking, brain stimulation protocols should always record data meticulously, so that adverse events can be reviewed in the context of the stimulation parameters and specifics of the patient or subject.

The risks associated with TMS depend to a great degree on the stimulation protocol used. With single pulse, or low-frequency repetitive stimulation (<1 Hz), no significant effects on short-term memory or cognitive functions have been found (Bridgers, 1991; Ferbert et al., 1991). No permanent hearing loss has been found with TMS despite prolonged exposure to the loud clicks in some volunteers (Pascual-Leone et al., 1992a). Patients with ferromagnetic intracranial metal implants should not be stimulated. It does not appear that patients with epilepsy are at higher risk for seizure (Hufnagel and Elger, 1991); however, a few reports suggest the possibility of inducing seizures in patients with recent large hemispheric infarcts (Homberg and Netz, 1989), which should be considered a relative contraindication. Patients with implanted stimulators and pacemakers should be avoided. In recording MEPs, fewer repetitions and low frequency of stimulation is recommended. Lower stimulus intensities may be used if some facilitatory maneuvers are simultaneously employed. However, long-term deleterious effects appear very unlikely with single pulse TMS or paired-pulse stimulation.

Repetitive TMS represents a different situation for several reasons: (1) there are short-term changes in excitatory responses (Jennum et al., 1995; Pascual-Leone et al., 1994d); (2) interruption of higher cognitive functions can accompany rapid rate stimulation, (3) generalized seizures have been reported in subjects with no known seizure risk (Pascual-Leone et al., 1993b; Wassermann et al., 1996a), and (4) there is growing evidence that the effects of long pulse trains on the cortical excitability may long outlast the stimulus itself. Rightfully, this type of stimulation requires closer scrutiny. Detailed guidelines to ensure patient safety during rTMS were published by Wassermann (1998), based on the deliberations of an international workshop on the safety of rTMS, held in June 1996. In a subsequent study of rTMS safety in normal subjects, Jahanshahi et al. (1997) found that after 50 consecutive trains of 20 Hz, quadrupulse TMS, at intensities between 5% and 10% above motor threshold, neurological, cognitive, motor function, and electrocardiogram remained unchanged despite an increase in MEP amplitudes. Heart rate and blood pressure changes during rapid-rate rTMS appear to be correlated more to the subject's level of discomfort during stimulus rather than to central autonomic stimulation (Foerster et al., 1997). Serum hormone levels have been studied during 10- and 20-Hz left dorsolateral prefrontal rTMS (Evers et al., 2001). Significant decreases were noted only in the levels of cortisol and thyroid-stimulating hormone (TSH). In a unique study of 21 patients undergoing intracranial EEG studies for medically refractory partial epilepsy,

single and quadrupulse TMS was applied over the epileptic focus and ipsilateral motor cortex, at stimulus intensities as high as 100% of stimulator output (Schulze-Bonhage et al., 1999). The stimulation failed to trigger complex-partial or generalized seizures. Only one patient with mesial-temporal sclerosis experienced an aura accompanied by a brief electrographic event in the hippocampus. A recent study in patients undergoing rTMS trials for depression tracked several neurocognitive variables using a comprehensive battery that included tests of attention, working memory, executive function, objective memory, and motor speed (Martis et al., 2003). No significant changes in these variables were found during the course of the treatment. Nevertheless, surprising adverse outcomes of rTMS in therapeutic trials should always be monitored for, as illustrated by a report of worsened complex movements in parkinsonian patients that persisted for a week after 10 Hz rTMS to the supplementary motor areas (Boylan et al., 2001).

In the United States, as with other clinical devices, the use of TMS technologies is regulated by the Food and Drug Administration (FDA). The single-pulse magnetic stimulators are currently considered low-risk devices. The use of single pulse, paired-pulse, or low-frequency (<1.0 Hz) repetitive stimulation requires only an institutionally approved protocol. On the other hand, the use of rapid-rate stimulators in human applications of rTMS at frequencies above 1.0 Hz, requires investigational device exemption status as well as institutionally approved protocols. Further studies that characterize the long-term effects of TMS, and careful monitoring of adverse events from human studies are clearly indicated.

Motor Evoked Potentials (MEPs)

Measurement Technique

MEPs represent recordings of compound muscle action potentials (CMAPs) and therefore are measured and analyzed accordingly. The onset latency is a reliable measure and is usually taken as the mean of at least three consecutive responses. Peak-to-peak amplitude of the response is measured, but because of the complex and dispersed nature of the waveform, especially for lower extremity MEPs, the area under the curve is probably a better measure. To obtain accurate estimates of maximal MEP response when faced with near maximal but submaximal responses, Eisen et al. (1991) proposed measuring 20 consecutive MEPs and taking the largest as a measure of the maximal MEP. Frequently, MEP amplitude is expressed as a percentage of the maximal peripherally induced CMAP (Britton et al., 1991), which takes into account the amount of available motor units in the particular muscle for a particular subject.

A more precise approach usually used in basic research uses single-unit recordings and presentation of data through peri- or poststimulus histograms (Awiszus and Feistner, 1994; Brouwer and Ashby, 1991; Day et al., 1989b; Garland and Miles, 1997; Mills et al., 1991). This approach allowed recognition of clusters of time-dependent discharges (Fig. 45.2) thought to reflect the arrival of subsequent repetitive depolarizations from cortex to the spinal motoneuron (D and

I waves). This approach can be combined with single muscle-fiber recording where the jitter of the consecutive discharges could be measured (Brower and Ashby, 1990; Zarola et al., 1989; Zidar et al., 1987) and the number of synapses preceding an MEP inferred. Still another technique uses measurement of muscle twitch tension and results in an interesting observation that the tension after TCS was higher than after a single peripheral stimulus of approximately the same CMAP amplitude. An explanation lies in the repetitive nature of not only the corticospinal volley (Berardelli et al., 1991) but also the transmission of repetitive discharge to the spinal motoneuron and muscle cell now summating twitch tension of more than one depolarization. This leads to a partial lack of correlation between the twitch amplitude and the MEP amplitude (Kiers et al., 1995).

Central conduction time can be calculated as a difference in latency of onset of MEP elicited by TCS and spinal cord or proximal root stimulation. F-wave latency can also be used as a measure of peripheral conduction time. Therefore, central conduction time can be easily calculated for both upper and lower extremity MEPs (Booth et al., 1991; Robinson et al., 1988).

Motor evoked potentials can also be recorded epidurally as traveling descending volleys before they reach the spinal motoneuron (Berardelli et al., 1990; Burke et al., 1990; Deletis, 1993; Rothwell et al., 1994). In that situation, we measure onset and peak latencies of each wave in the series, peak-to-peak amplitude of the entire complex, and each component separately. In recording of epidural as well as muscle MEPs, it is important to verify whether the responses are supramaximal or submaximal up to the maximal output of the stimulator. In awake subjects, it is crucial to quantify whether the MEP responses were obtained during full target-muscle relaxation or, if not, what the intensity of the contraction as the percentage of the maximal voluntary contraction was.

For conditioning studies, the timing interval has to be precisely defined as it changes not only amplitudes but also the latencies of the responses. Because different results can be obtained depending on the intensity of the conditioning stimulus, all the characteristics of that stimulus should be defined (Reutens et al., 1993) and a reasonable number of different intensities explored. This applies to both peripheral nerve conditioning and double-pulse TCS studies (Claus and Brunholzl, 1994; Inghilleri et al., 1990).

A problem with MEP measurement and testing paradigms is the inherent variability of MEP amplitude. This has an impact on latency measurements as well. This is a complex problem because there is a large variability in amplitude of descending volleys in patients under general anesthesia (Burke et al., 1995). Because epidural recording is limited to only descending tracts, it does not take into account any additional variability of the alpha motoneuron excitability that certainly adds to the total variability of recorded MEPs. It is well recognized that MEPs are more variable in the relaxed state, while any attempt to increase the probability of motoneuron discharge will result in decreased variability (Kiers et al., 1993), regardless of whether it is by muscle contraction or afferent conditioning.

Age-Dependent MEP Changes

Motor evoked potentials mature during the first decade of life, reaching full maturity between the ages of 8 and 11 years (Khater-Boidin and Duron, 1991; Koh and Eyre, 1988). Before the age of 1 year, MEPs can be absent (Müller et al., 1991). They mature long after myelinization of the descending pathways, with delays similar to, although even longer than, cortical somatosensory evoked potentials (SEPs) (Cindro et al., 1985). There are two aspects of MEP maturation: (1) the latency of the response, which is chiefly dependent on the peripheral and central conduction velocity; and (2) the appearance of the response, which depends on the excitability of the circuitry. It appears that both are immature until the age of 8 years (Koh and Eyre, 1988). That is the time that some children attain the adult range of conduction velocity and also the time when it is possible to obtain MEP without additional facilitation. As central myelinization is complete at the age of 3, it would indicate slow maturation of motor circuitry and some age-dependent changes of nervous system excitability, most likely at the cortical level, as peripheral conduction and spinal circuitry have been already well established. This explanation is supported by results from macaque monkeys in which there is comparatively similar slow maturation of CST conduction in a rostrocaudal direction demonstrated both morphologically and physiologically (Armand et al., 1994; Olivier et al., 1997).

On the other side of the spectrum, there are slow changes seen at age 60 onward, dominated by slow, progressive loss of fibers and decrease in MEP amplitudes. This finding significantly impacts the interpretation of data in patients with amyotrophic lateral sclerosis (ALS) and Parkinson's disease (PD) (Eisen et al., 1991).

Stimulation at Rest Versus Voluntary Facilitation

Early studies of TCS demonstrated that slight voluntary background contraction of the target muscle increases the MEP amplitude and decreases the latency by 2 to 4 msec (Fig. 45.1). Therefore, defining the recording paradigm is crucial, for example, as the shortest latencies of MEPs are obtained with electrical TCS during voluntary contraction (Caramia et al., 1989). The paradigm affects both normative values and left-right intrasubject comparisons. Frequently, electrical TCS is submaximal due to the increase in pain coinciding with the increase in intensity of stimulation limiting subject tolerance to obtain the maximal MEP. In addition, the maximal output of stimulators usually does not produce maximal MEP in relaxed subjects. This is true for both electrical and magnetic stimulators. Boosting output of electrical stimulator, however, further increases discomfort that occurs with higher output. Therefore, today electrical stimulation is almost exclusively used during IOM in general anesthesia. Magnetic stimulators are notorious for being submaximal for lower extremity stimulation, and contrary to expectations, further development of the focal stimulators reduced the availability of larger coils potentially being able to deliver enough output to obtain maximal leg MEPs. The inherited variability of submaximal responses alters the recorded amplitudes and therefore the reproducibility of the MEPs, both short term and long term.

One way to approach maximal MEPs is to facilitate the response; this may allow less output to reach the maximal MEP up to the maximal stimulator output or up to subjects' maximal tolerance in case of electrical stimulation. Because it is believed that voluntary contraction facilitates MEPs at both the cortical and spinal levels, the downside is that the results of MEPs at rest do not reflect the same physiological processes as those during contraction. During voluntary contraction, there may be both an increase in the size of the descending volley and decrease in the spinal motoneuron threshold. Therefore, the lesser size of the descending volley will result in an MEP. It is speculated that as the descending volley consists of a number of successive waves (Fig. 45.2), e.g., D and I 1, I 2, I 3 (Burke et al., 1990; Day et al., 1989a; Inghilleri et al., 1989; Rothwell et al., 1991; Thompson et al., 1991) during facilitation, the depolarization occurs at the arrival of the D or I 1 wave and does not require summation with later waves. This will result in the shorter onset latency of the MEP and variable latency of the submaximal MEPs with respect to the stimulus intensity and the amount of facilitation. Maximal facilitation can be reached with no more than 10% of the maximal voluntary contraction (Helmers et al., 1989; Ravnborg et al., 1991), making it easier to control the variability during voluntary contraction, as it does not make any difference if the patient exerts, for example, 15% or 40% of the maximal contraction. On the other hand, MEPs at rest require very rigorous control of the background EMG activity, as minor changes can result in both amplitude and latency differences. Usually the surface EMG is checked for the presence of any activity at 50 µV per division of the display. This is clearly arbitrary, however, and some changes in excitability can still be attributed to unrecognized voluntary activation (Chiappa et al., 1991).

Some controversy remains regarding facilitation of the MEP by activation of nontarget muscles that may be either proximal, contralateral homologous, or nonhomologous. It seems that there are no significant excitatory effects with any of these activations (Chiappa et al., 1991). Yet, there appears to be contralateral inhibition, most likely transcallosally mediated, that is shown both physiologically by changes in the silent period (Chiappa et al., 1995) and in blood flow (Dettmers et al., 1996). There is a lack of either postexercise facilitation or depression, however, after contralateral homologous muscle activation (Samii et al., 1997). Interestingly, the cortical topography of MEPs at rest and during facilitation may not be exactly the same (Wilson et al., 1995).

A special case of facilitation involves the soleus muscle, because it is considered mainly a postural, antigravity muscle with mainly vestibulospinal input. However, a short-latency MEP was obtained that behaved similarly to other extremity muscles, i.e., latency shortened with activation (Lavoie et al., 1995; Valls-Solé et al., 1994). In addition, facilitation was linear over the wider range of muscle activity efforts. The short-latency responses were also obtainable during postural tasks, suggesting that the motor cortex might be able to exert rapid adjustment of soleus activity whether it is either voluntary or postural (Lavoie et al., 1995). Soleus MEP usually consists of two components, the ubiquitous early MEP and the late component MEP. The late component generation in healthy subjects is debatable because it is believed to be a stretch reflex due to preferential activation of the tibialis anterior muscle during TCS (Sammut et al., 1995). This may not be an explanation, however, for the presence of late component MEPs in other leg muscles (Dimitrijevic et al., 1992).

Other Forms of Reinforcement/Conditioning

In paralyzed patients, forms of reinforcement other than voluntary contraction are the only alternative for facilitation. Vibration of the muscle or tendon can facilitate an MEP (Caramia et al., 1991; Claus et al., 1988). It is not as powerful as voluntary contraction but may bring the response that otherwise would be considered absent. Withdrawal reflex and other nonspecific facilitations can also be used as they increase the spinal excitability, letting the small descending volley reach the threshold and result in measurable MEP (Hufnagel et al., 1990; Kasai et al., 1992). The underlying mechanism of this form of facilitation is different from voluntary activation, and the results should be interpreted accordingly. A special form of facilitation is conditioning with an electrical stimulus (Fig. 45.4); it could be timed in such a way as to coincide with the arrival of the TCS descending volley at the spinal level or to reach the cortex at the time of TCS delivery (Deletis et al., 1987, 1992; Deuschl et al., 1991; Komori et al., 1992; Rossini et al., 1991). In both instances, a significant reproducible facilitation was observed, providing an avenue for facilitation in myelopathic and uncooperative patients. It also allows for objective assessment of sensorimotor integration, which has enormous basic importance and possible clinical implications (Gracies et al., 1994; Mazevet et al., 1996; Mazzocchio et al., 1994; Mercuri et al., 1997).

Conditioning paradigm results raise a few questions. It appears that at late cortical facilitatory intervals, there is no shortening of MEP latency. During early spinal facilitation, however, there is a significant decrease in the MEP latency (Deletis et al., 1992). This approach may allow exploration of the effect of an increased descending volley independently from increased spinal excitability and may lead to better understanding of peripheral-versus-cortical silent periods. A special form of conditioning is the effect of speech on MEPs. Reading aloud consistently increased the size of MEPs only in the dominant hand, providing additional avenues for studies of cerebral dominance (Tokimura et al., 1996). Intracortical excitatory and inhibitory phenomena can be studied with double-pulse magnetic and/or electrical TCS, describing the precise timing of inhibition and facilitation (Claus and Brunholzl, 1994; Valzania et al., 1997; Wassermann et al., 1996c; Ziemann et al., 1996a,b).

Excitatory and Inhibitory Effects

Suprathreshold single pulse TCS of motor areas is usually followed by positive phenomena such as a movement. Similarly, under special conditions sensory experience can be evoked during TCS (Amassian et al., 1989a, 1991; Gandevia et al., 1993). Shortening of the reaction time (RT) with subthreshold motor cortex TCS has been also observed (Pascual-Leone et al., 1992b). These are all considered to be

Figure 45.4. Representative electromyographic responses from right abductor pollicis brevis *(left)* after focal magnetic stimulation of the scalp positions located 1 cm apart on the contralateral hemisphere. Scalp positions are described by their location on the x and y axes (0, 0 represents the C_z position). The map on the *right* shows the amplitude of MEPs evoked after stimulation of different scalp positions on the left hemisphere. Note that the largest MEP was obtained after stimulation of position −5, 2. The label on the head's cartoon shows the scalp area stimulated. (From Cohen, L., Brasil-Neto, J., Pascual-Leone, A., et al. 1993. Plasticity of cortical motor output organization following deafferentation, cerebral lesions, and skill acquisition. In *Electrical and Magnetic Stimulation of the Brain and Spinal Cord (Adv. Neurol. Vol. 63)*. Eds., O. Devinsky, A. Beric, and M. Dogali, pp. 187–200. New York: Raven, with permission.)

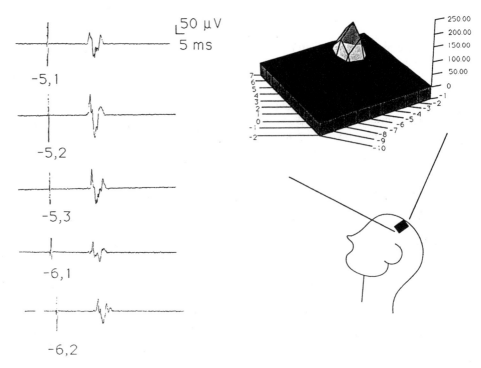

excitatory effects of TCS, which are similar or identical to those elicited by direct stimulation of the exposed cortex. However, inhibitory effects can also be elicited by TCS (Mills, 1988), such as a delay or interruption of muscle contraction during the reaction-time paradigm (Day et al., 1989b). TCS suppression of spatial localization of a cutaneous stimulus (Seyal et al., 1997) is another inhibitory effect of TCS. A more subtle phenomenon of inhibition elicited by TCS is that of the long-latency response to stretch through hypothesized transcallosal inhibition (Taylor et al., 1995).

The silent period seen during continuous muscle contraction and concomitant TCS has been explored extensively (Fig. 45.5) (Brasil-Neto et al., 1995; Fritz et al., 1997; Fuhr et al., 1991; Garland and Miles, 1997; Inghilleri et al., 1993, 1997; Priori et al., 1995; Roick et al., 1993; Triggs et al., 1993a,b; Wassermann et al., 1991; Wilson et al., 1993a,b). Changes in the silent period have been examined in different neurologic conditions including stroke, multiple sclerosis, ALS, and sensory neuropathy (Braune and Fritz, 1995; Haug and Kukowski, 1994; Triggs et al., 1992).

Effects of Sleep and Pharmacological Agents on MEPs and Relevance to Intraoperative Monitoring

The amplitude of MEPs varies between trials. The threshold for the appearance of an MEP is also variable, especially during relaxation. Often-recognized subtle variation in state of consciousness can affect the recording. We have observed larger variability of the responses and more unpredictable conditioning paradigm responses in first-time subjects of TCS recordings, especially with electrical stimulation. Not

unexpectedly, there are changes in excitability during sleep as documented by increased excitability and larger MEPs in the rapid eye movement (REM) phase compared to the slow-wave phase of sleep (Hess et al., 1987b).

Benzodiazepines suppress cortical SEPs after an initial increase in size that probably reflects both better relaxation and some disinhibition. Short-acting midazolam decreased MEPs without latency change, suggesting cortical effect (Schonle et al., 1989). In addition, diazepam shortened the silent period after TCS (Fig. 45.5), an effect reversible with flumazenil, but without effect on paired TCS paradigm (Inghilleri et al., 1996). Thiopental slightly decreased the amplitude of MEPs. Interestingly, hyperventilation reduced the duration of the silent period after TCS (Priori et al., 1995). Antiepileptics were also studied in healthy subjects (Mavroudakis et al., 1997; Zieman et al., 1996a). Carbamazepine, diphenylhydantoin, lamotrigine, and losigamone all increased the TCS thresholds, while vigabatrin and baclofen reduced intracortical excitability measured by effect of paired TCS.

The better-studied agents are anesthetics, considering their profound influence on any neurophysiological function. They result in a decrease or absence of MEPs, an effect similar to their demonstrated suppression of SEPs and interference with IOM. In an everlasting effort to find the ultimate IOM procedure, muscle MEPs were tried, with modified and improved techniques, but their reliability is still debated. The problem is that MEPs are influenced by all currently used anesthetic agents (Kalkman et al., 1992; Taniguchi et al., 1993) primarily because they depend on cortical excitability, spinal excitability, and secure neuromuscular transmission. All three levels are affected by anesthetic agents, and the low amplitude or absence of

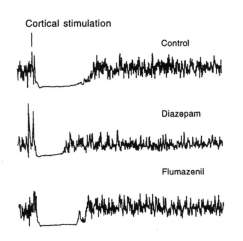

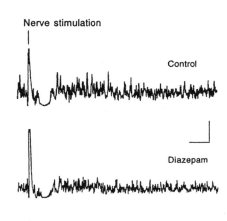

Figure 45.5. Silent period after cortical *(left)* and peripheral *(right)* stimulation in a normal subject before and after diazepam and flumazenil injection. Note the shortening of the cortical silent period after diazepam administration and its normalization after flumazenil injection. Traces are the average of ten single rectified EMG trials from the first dorsal interosseus muscle. Horizontal calibration is 100 msec, vertical calibration is 400 μV. (From Inghilleri, M., Berardelli, A., Marchetti, P., et al. 1996. Effects of diazepam, baclofen and thiopental on the silent period evoked by transcranial magnetic stimulation in humans. Exp. Brain Res. 109:467–472, with permission.)

response is most likely a cumulative effect at all levels. Nitrous oxide and low-concentration or halogenated agents decrease the amplitude of MEPs even without affecting a neuromuscular junction (Calancie et al., 1991; Zentner et al., 1989). Higher concentrations of halogenated agents abolish MEPs, making them no more attractive than SEPs, which are also abolished at these levels of anesthetics. If neuromuscular blockade is used, MEPs are absent, a frequent practice in major back surgeries. A promising approach is the use of TCS with epidural recording (Deletis, 1993; Kitagawa et al., 1989; Loughnan et al., 1989). However, in scoliosis surgery, which is probably the riskiest orthopedic surgery for spinal cord dysfunction, it is difficult to obtain reliable recordings from the lower end of the field. Although the risk of paraplegia may not lie in the lower end of the field, epiconus, and conus, its exclusion from monitoring allows the possibility of false-negative responses, a drawback also associated with SEPs. There are some reasonable modifications to the standard awake MEP technique, such as use of paired and repetitive electrical TCS that may be due to the temporal summation, and that facilitate the muscle MEPs even under usual anesthesia conditions (Jones et al., 1996; Kalkman et al., 1995). On the other hand, if neuromuscular blockade is used, it might be titrated to the desired amplitude of the twitches in routine train-of-four testing (Lang et al., 1996). Overall, IOM is the only field in which electrical MEPs are extensively used today; practically all TCS in awake patients or healthy subjects is performed with magnetic stimulators.

Intraoperative Monitoring of MEPs

Measurement of MEPs during spine surgery offers a physiological technique for monitoring the integrity of the CST (Jellinek et al., 1991; Zentner, 1991). Since the patient is under anesthesia, stimulus-related discomfort that restricts the use of TES in awake patients is not a concern. However, anesthetic agents variably attenuate the amplitudes of MEPs recorded. Given the lower cost of instrumentation, and especially a possibility of use of in-built electrical stimulators, TES has been extensively used for intraoperative monitoring.

Until recently TES stimulators also had the advantage of being able to sustain extended stimulus trains. Earlier TMS coil designs suffered from overheating during repeated pulse delivery. With the introduction of rapid rate stimulators, and provisions for cooling the coil, this is no longer a major concern. Over recent years, TMS has increasingly been used in operating rooms. In a study of combined SEPs and threshold-level MEP measurements during spine surgery, Calancie et al. (2001) found that MEPs were recordable in all but 9 of 194 patients while SEPs were recordable in only 42 of the patients, suggesting that TES may be a more reliable measure for monitoring spinal cord health. The combined use of SEPs and MEPs increases the odds of successfully recording responses that allow spinal cord monitoring (Pelosi et al., 2002).

In a series of 34 cases of spine surgery that were monitored intraoperatively using SEPs and MEPs, Calancie et al. (1998) found that TES was recordable in 32 of these patients and accurately predicted all instances of postoperative motor deficits, but missed four instances of sensory deficits. In this series baseline SEPs were recordable in only 25 of the 34 patients, and failed to predict five instances of motor deficits, again supporting the complementary nature of these measurements.

The immaturity of the corticospinal tract may limit the utility of TES in very young children. In 19 children under the age of 36 months, attempts to record D waves using TES during resection of intramedullary spinal cord tumors were successful in seven children (aged 21–36 months), but unsuccessful in the other 12 (aged 8–31 months) (Szelenyi et al., 2003). MEPs elicited by TES have also been recorded during brain tumor surgery. Zhou and Kelly (2001) found that persistent reduction of MEP amplitude greater than 50% of baseline during brain tumor resections was predictive of postoperative motor deficits.

MEP monitoring during TES has been found to be an effective technique for detecting spinal cord ischemia during surgery for thoracoabdominal aneurysms (de Haan et al., 1997; van Dongen et al., 2001). One of the considerations in monitoring for spinal cord ischemia is that motor neurons in the anterior horn are more likely to signal the onset of ischemic injury, and therefore MEPs that depend on their integrity are likely to be more sensitive for this particular application compared to SEPs (de Haan and Kalkman, 2001). Myogenic MEPs, as opposed to MEPs recorded from the spinal cord or cauda equina, are more likely to be sensitive to spinal ischemia (Dong et al., 2002).

TMS has been increasingly adopted for intraoperative MEP monitoring in recent years. In a comparison of SEPs and TMS-based MEP monitoring in 27 patients, Aglio et al. (2002) concluded that as with TES, the two techniques are complementary, and postoperative motor outcome is accurately predicted by MEP measurements, but not SEPs. Qayumi et al. (1997) showed that TMS-based MEPs can rapidly detect spinal ischemia in a porcine model of spinal cord ischemia. MEPs produced by TMS have also been studied during spinal angiography, and support the notion that anterior spinal cord function is better monitored using MEP measurements rather than SEPs.

Central Fatigue

MEP technique intuitively appears to be *the* technique to measure and understand central fatigue. However, in light of the constraints of almost every technique it is not surprising that it has not met expectations. There is a whole series of experiments and subsequent reports pertaining to changes in the amplitude of MEPs during and after muscle fatiguing (Brasil-Neto et al., 1993a, 1994; Samii et al., 1996). Very plausible explanations have been presented regarding postexercise facilitation and depression. Although there is some similarity between decremental response to TCS and neuromuscular transmission decrement in myasthenia gravis, it appears to be only a superficial resemblance and oversimplification.

Another approach consists of fatiguing during maximal voluntary contraction combined with twitch interpolation technique after peripheral stimulation and TCS (Gandevia et al., 1996; Taylor et al., 1996). These experiments as well as a report on central fatigue in multiple sclerosis patients (Sheean et al., 1997) suggest that there is an impairment of cortical drive upstream from the motor cortex that is responsible for observed abnormalities.

Cortical Plasticity

Topographic mapping of MEPs is an ideal method for short- and long-term assessment of motor cortex plasticity under very different circumstances (Fig. 45.6). Enlargement or shrinkage of muscle maps can be followed in chronic or acute deafferentations. Changes in maps after spinal cord lesions were obtained with enlargements of muscle maps of regions just proximal to the lesion level as well as larger amplitudes of MEPs (Topka et al., 1991). Similar changes were found with amputation together with some sensory experiences (Cohen et al., 1993). The dynamics of cortical changes can also be followed in an acute experiment, such as with limb anesthesia (Brasil-Neto et al., 1993b) or following traumatic amputation (Pascual-Leone et al., 1996b). Apart from deafferentation, it is possible to follow cortical reorganization in subjects with highly specialized, overlearned skills, such as in blind persons proficient in braille reading (Pascual-Leone et al., 1993a; Pascual-Leone and Torres, 1993).

Special MEPs

Usually MEPs are recorded in limb muscles after stimulation of the appropriate scalp or cortical areas. The largest number of studies of both healthy subjects and patients were obtained from the hand, especially the thenar muscles. However, there are a number of important contributions obtained by specialized recordings from nonlimb muscles, such as diaphragm or abdominal muscles demonstrating essentially the same MEP behavior as for limb muscles (Plassman and Gandevia, 1989). Facial and trigeminal innervated muscles were investigated for evidence of unilateral or bilateral innervation (Benecke et al., 1988; Cruccu et al., 1989, 1990; Meyer et al., 1994; Rossler et al., 1989b, 1991; Urban et al., 1997). A similar approach was also used to investigate the tongue muscle (Meyer et al., 1997; Muellbacher et al., 1994). Even esophageal MEPs were studied during swallowing and vagal stimulation (Aziz et al., 1995).

Also investigated were pelvic floor muscles (Mathers et al., 1990), both the urogenital diaphragm muscles without tonic activity and the sphincter muscles with ongoing tonic activity. Different results were obtained depending on bladder fullness (Thiry and Deltenre, 1989). Relatively slow conduction velocities (CVs) with long latencies were obtained from pelvic floor muscles (Herdmann et al., 1991) reminiscent of the long latencies of SEPs after pudendal nerve stimulation. As there is no major slowing at the peripheral level for sensory and motor fibers, it is most likely that the delay is central and characteristic of sacral segmental organization.

Effects of Repetitive TMS on Motor Cortical Excitability

Repetitive TMS of sensorimotor areas produces sustained effects on regional excitability that far outlast the stimulus train. Chen et al. (1997) showed that sustained low-frequency near-motor-threshold rTMS at 0.9 Hz can reduce MEP amplitudes by as much as 20% lasting for at least 15 minutes, while stimulation at 0.1 Hz had no apparent effect. These sustained effects of low-frequency rTMS have since been confirmed by several other studies (Di Lazzaro et al., 2002; Fitzgerald et al., 2002; Gerschlager et al., 2001). Increased excitability has been demonstrated after high-frequency suprathreshold pulse trains (Berardelli et al., 1998; Chen, 2000; Jahanshahi et al., 1997; Jennum et al., 1995). The effects are not only frequency dependent, but also stimulus intensity dependent (Fitzgerald et al., 2002).

There are also accompanying changes in the cortical silent period after both high- and low-frequency rTMS. Low-frequency rTMS near motor threshold appears to shorten cortical silent period, while high-frequency stimulating produced alternating fluctuations of the silent period (Fierro et al., 2001a,b). At a much lower frequency of 0.3 Hz, Cincotta et al. (2003) found that a 30-minute-long suprathreshold pulse train (115% motor threshold) produced lengthened cortical silent periods both immediately

A.   Conditioned Magnetic Trans-cranial Stimulation

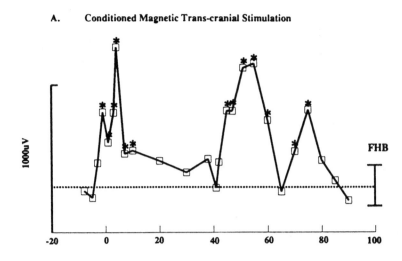

B.   Conditioned Electrical Trans-cranial Stimulation

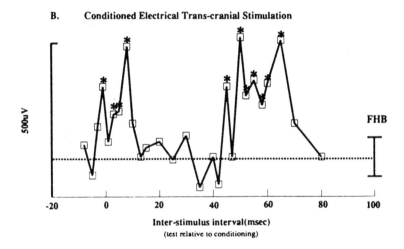

Inter-stimulus interval(msec)
(test relative to conditioning)

Figure 45.6. Comparison of averaged (*n* = 3) MEP amplitudes recorded from flexor hallucis brevis (FHB) muscle of an individual subject, magnetic (**A**) and electrical (**B**) TCS as a function of condition-test interstimulus interval. The conditioning stimulus was electrical stimulation of the ipsilateral tibial nerve at the ankle. *Asterisks* identify those intervals that exhibited MEP amplitudes significantly different (*p* < .0015) from control values. (From Deletis, V., Schild, J.H., Beric, A., et al. 1992. Facilitation of motor evoked potentials by somatosensory afferent stimulation. Electroencephalogr. Clin. Neurophysiol. 85:302–310, with permission.)

after stimulation as well as 90 minutes later, indicating a long-lasting enhancement of the inhibitory mechanisms responsible for the silent period. Using a paired-pulse paradigm and MEP measurements, Wu et al. (2000) found that 5- and 15-Hz rTMS for motor areas both decreased intracortical inhibition, while the 15-Hz train increased intracortical facilitation with a different time course. The effects are again clearly frequency dependent. This was explored further by looking at the effects of a range of frequencies from 1 to 15 Hz (Romeo et al., 2000). Pulse trains at frequencies above 2 Hz prolonged the silent period, while only 1-Hz stimulation produced a shortening of silent period. The same study also examined the effect of stimulus intensity and found a trade-off between frequency and intensity in bringing about inhibition or facilitation; facilitation could be produced at lower frequencies by increasing stimulus intensity. Subthreshold 1-Hz pulse trains appear to decrease cortical excitability mainly by decreasing facilitation (Romero et al., 2002). A trade-off has also

been reported between pulse intensity and the duration of the pulse train, with inhibition being seen with shorter trains (Modugno et al., 2001). Low-frequency near-threshold rTMS of motor areas also appears to produce suppressive effects on adjoining sensory areas as measured using tactile thresholds (Satow et al., 2003) and SEPs (Enomoto et al., 2001; Tsuji and Rothwell, 2002).

Effects of rTMS over one motor cortex appears to have simultaneous effects in the homologous cortical areas. Suprathreshold 1-Hz rTMS of the motor cortex on one side not only decreased MEP amplitudes ipsilaterally, but also increased MEP amplitudes on the opposite side (Plewnia et al., 2003). Using subthreshold 0.5- and 5-Hz rTMS, Gorsler et al. (2003) found high-frequency stimulation increased contralateral excitability, while low-frequency stimulation decreased it. These effects, which outlast the stimuli by at least several minutes, appear also to depend on whether the stimuli are subthreshold or suprathreshold. These interhemispheric effects parallel the delayed EEG response on homologous cortex that has been seen within 30 msec of stimulating one side (Ilmoniemi et al., 1997).

A recent result of enormous interest to therapeutic applications of rTMS showed that repeated trains of 1-Hz rTMS can have cumulative suppressive effects on motor cortex excitability if repeated within 24 hours to 7 days (Baumer et al., 2003). This finding suggests a physiological basis for repeating "treatment sessions" of rTMS in various experimental therapeutic trials such as those in the treatment of epilepsy, dystonia, or other neuropsychiatric disorders where the goal of stimulation is to decrease regional cortical excitability.

TMS for Surgical Planning
Noninvasive Mapping of the Motor Cortex

MEP measurement can be used for noninvasive topographic mapping of the motor cortex. Maps of both proximal and distal arm muscles have been obtained that are in concordance with known topography of the motor cortex (Brasil-Neto et al., 1992; Wassermann et al., 1992). Usually the number of excitable scalp positions, amplitude of MEPs, scalp position for evoking the largest MEP, and the threshold for evoking MEPs are reported and plotted on a two- or three-dimensional model (Fig. 45.6). It can be used to distinguish excitatory and inhibitory maxima for a single muscle (MEP vs. silent period) (Wassermann et al., 1993) or to distinguish small differences in topography of neighboring muscles (Wilson et al., 1993a,b). This approach has far-reaching implications in assessment of cortical reorganization after trauma and amputation and investigation of cortical plasticity in general (Cohen et al., 1993).

Using scalp landmark-based navigation, Macdonell et al. (1999) compared fMRI localization of motor areas with TMS localization in a patient with a dysplastic right hemisphere and concluded that the methods are complementary: fMRI identified the cortical areas activated by the motor task, while TMS identified primarily the areas that give rise to the corticospinal tract. A similar conclusion about the complementary nature of fMRI- and TMS-derived representational maps was arrived at by Lotze et at. (2003). The development of MRI-based stereotactic guidance tools for TMS in recent years has dramatically altered the scope of functional motor mapping using this technique (Ettinger et al., 1998; Krings et al., 1998, 2001a,b). Comparison of rTMS-based motor maps with those acquired from direct cortical stimulation suggest that navigated TMS can provide comparable results, and may thus have a role in noninvasive presurgical planning (Krings et al., 1997). A comparison of navigated rTMS- with fMRI-based motor mapping suggests that the technique may be a useful adjunct, or even an alternative to fMRI in preoperative assessments (Krings et al., 2001a). The technique of rTMS has also been applied intraoperatively prior to exposure of the cortical surface, and found to be highly sensitive for the localization of the primary motor cortex (Rohde et al., 2003).

Language Lateralization and Localization Using TMS

Noninvasive lateralization of language can be of great value to neurosurgical planning in cortical areas close to lan-

guage representations. Currently, the gold standard for making this assessment is the intracarotid amobarbital procedure (IAP) (for reviews see Trenerry and Loring, 1995; van Emde Boas, 1999), which is invasive, associated with the risks of angiography, and time consuming. Functional MRI techniques for locating language areas, while still experimental, appears extremely promising (Binder, 1997; Sabsevitz et al., 2003; Sabbah et al., 2003). Repetitive TMS (rTMS) has been explored as an alternative noninvasive technique for mapping language and speech areas (Epstein et al., 1996; Jennum et al., 1994; Pascual-Leone et al., 1991). The initial studies employed rapid-rate rTMS to produce interference with language tasks such as picture naming or expressive speech. Pascual-Leone (1991) screened six adult epileptic patients for induction of speech arrest and counting errors after stimulation. He found that lateralization of expressive speech by rTMS correlated very well with the IAP, suggesting that rTMS may be helpful for noninvasive determination of hemispheric language dominance. Michelucci et al. (1994) found that rTMS with rapid-rate stimulation was effective in producing speech arrest concordant with side of manual preference in only seven of 14 patients. Epstein et al. (2000) compared inferior frontal speech arrest from rTMS with bilateral IAP in 17 epilepsy surgical candidates. They found that while rTMS lateralized frontal language areas in a manner consistent with IAP in most of the subjects, rTMS also tended to favor the right hemisphere at a rate significantly greater than the IAP test. They concluded that available methods for inducing speech arrest with rTMS do not replicate the result of IAP tests.

As in other cortical areas, the effects of rTMS on language cortex is frequency dependent. Sparing et al. (2001) compared the effects of 1- and 20-Hz extended pulse trains delivered to language and visual areas, and tested picture naming immediately after the stimulus trains. They found that 20-Hz stimulation of Wernike's area facilitated picture naming in a significant way. Clearly, speech arrest by itself is an insufficient paradigm for mapping language function. In patients with epilepsy or developmental abnormalities, bilateral representations, or even dissociations between receptive and expressive language functions may often be encountered (Rutten et al., 2002; Springer et al., 1999). Further limitations of rapid-rate rTMS in this application are the discomfort from temporalis muscle contraction that may be associated with frontotemporal stimulation, and the possibility of triggering seizures in a patient group that is already prone to seizures. Remote effects on the contralateral homologous cortex may be an additional confounding factor. Suppression of local cortical excitability, or "virtual lesions," produced by extended low-frequency rTMS (<1 Hz) offers one way around these issues. This offers the possibility of performing cortical mapping by inactivation as opposed to stimulation. The results of Knecht et al. (2002) suggest that focal suppression of language areas using this paradigm may be used to identify language lateralization in ways that are consistent with fMRI. Refinement of stimulation parameters to maximize focal suppression and the use of sensitive automated tests of language after low-frequency rTMS could potentially make this technique more robust in its ability to localize language areas.

Visual Cortex Mapping

Phosphenes elicited by TMS of the occipital cortex are some of the earliest reported responses elicited by magnetic stimulation. Over the years, TMS has found several applications in the study of visual cortical function (for reviews see Cowey and Walsh, 2001; Merabet et al., 2003). Single-pulse TMS can elicit several effects in the visual system, from suppression and delay of visual perception (Amassian et al., 1989b, 1993, 1994) to unmasking as described by Maccabee et al. (1991) and Cracco et al. (1993). Improvements in coil design allowing more focal excitation in combination with stereotactic navigation now offer the potential for mapping visual areas noninvasively using TMS. Elicitation of scotoma that can be directly visualized by the subject in the presence of a patterned stimulus displayed briefly approximately 100 msec after a pulse of occipital TMS was demonstrated by Kamitini and Shimojo (1999). The scotoma were found to shift with coil position according to known topography of the visual cortex. Phosphene mapping using image-guided delivery of TMS has been shown to yield topographic maps of hemifield representations (Fernandez et al., 2002; Potts et al., 1998). However, in this application, fMRI techniques in development may prove to be much faster (DeYoe et al., 1996; Kollias et al., 1998; Roux et al., 2001).

Other Potential Clinical Applications

Neurological Disorders

In epilepsy, initial studies of TMS as a tool for localizing partial epilepsies indicated limited value (see Jennum and Winkel, 1994). However, motor thresholds, MEP amplitudes, and intracortical inhibition or facilitation quantitated using TMS can potentially be of value in understanding the cortical mechanisms underlying different epilepsy syndromes. Paired TCS of the motor cortex has been used to demonstrate decreased intracortical inhibition in juvenile myoclonic epilepsy (Caramia et al., 1996), progressive myoclonic epilepsies (Manganotti et al., 2001), as well as idiopathic generalized epilepsies (Macdonell et al., 2001). Some studies suggest cryptogenic localization related epilepsy to be associated with both a decrease in cortical inhibition as well as increased facilitation (Cantello et al., 2000; Cincotta et al., 1998). The same methods may also provide insights into mechanisms by with specific anticonvulsants act (Reis et al., 2002; Rizzo et al., 2001), and possibly allow exploration of synergies between different agents.

Trials of rTMS as a therapeutic intervention in medically refractory partial epilepsy is motivated by the observation that cortical excitability can be decreased focally by low-frequency (<1 Hz) stimulation. In animal experiments, chronic treatment with low-frequency rTMS has an inhibitory effect on seizure induction by both electroconvulsive shock and pentylene-tetrazole in rats (Akamatsu et al., 2001; Fleishmann et al., 1999). However, chronic high-frequency rTMS facilitates the time of onset of pentylene-tetrazole-induced seizures in rats (Ebert and Ziemann, 1999). Tergau et al. (1999) studied the effects of 5 consecutive days of rTMS on nine patients with medically refractory partial epilepsy using 0.33-Hz submotor threshold pulses delivered at the vertex. They found a mean reduction in seizure frequency of 36.6% in the 4-week period following stimulation compared to a similar period prior to the stimulation. Within 6 to 8 weeks, they also noted a return of the seizure frequency to baseline. Menkes and Gruenthal (2000) examined the effect of TMS in a patient with focal cortical dysplasia using 0.5-Hz pulses at a stimulus intensity 5% below the motor threshold using a 9-cm coil positioned over the region of the dysplasia. Stimuli were applied biweekly for a period of 4 weeks. They found a 70% reduction in seizure frequency over the 4-week period of stimulation. Seizure frequency returned toward the baseline frequency during the month following stimulation. However, a placebo-controlled study using 15 minutes of 1-Hz rTMS, at 120% of motor threshold and delivered twice daily for a week, failed to show any statistically significant differences in seizure frequency between treatment and placebo groups (Theodore et al., 2002). The authors did note, however, a transient trend toward improvement in the treatment group that was greater in patients with lateral as opposed to mesial seizure foci. Both the stimulus intensity and frequency of the pulses were substantially higher in this study compared to the two previous studies. Further investigations are warranted to explore stimulus parameters that yield therapeutic effects in epilepsy, if any.

Movement disorders are a fertile ground for diagnostic use of TCS (for reviews see Berardelli, 1999; Cantello, 2002). Parkinson's disease patients show a number of abnormalities, from silent period shortening to RT abnormalities that can be improved with either subthreshold single TCS or rTCS (Pascual-Leone et al., 1994b,c). Interesting observations have been made in movement disorders, with shortening of the silent period in PD (Cantello et al., 1991; Nakashima et al., 1995) and a tendency for normalization after treatment with L-dopa (Priori et al., 1994a). On the contrary, the silent period in Huntington's disease was prolonged (Priori et al., 1994b). Abnormal MEPs were found in focal dystonia with both excitatory and inhibitory disturbances (Ikoma et al., 1996; Mavroudakis et al., 1995; Odergren et al., 1997). Changes in intracortical cortical inhibition have also been reported in hand dystonia and blepharospasm (Sommer et al., 2002) as well as cervical dystonia (Cakmur et al., 2004).

There have been several studies looking for therapeutic effects of rTMS in movement disorders, especially Parkinson's disease (for a review see Berardelli, 1999; Cantello, 2002). Bilateral frontal stimulation with low-frequency rTMS showed improvement of motor performance in patients with PD (Dragasevic et al., 2002; Ikeguchi et al., 2003). Short-term improvements in motor function have been reported after 5-Hz stimulation of primary motor areas (Pascual-Leone et al., 1994c; Siebner et al., 1999a, 2000). However, Boylan et al. (2001) found that 10-Hz rTMS over the supplementary motor areas worsened parkinsonian symptoms for up to a week, raising concerns of safety. In a small series of patients with essential tremor, 1-Hz rTMS of the cerebellum was shown to significantly reduce symptoms acutely (Gironell et al., 2002). In dystonias, there is a growing body of evidence suggesting decreased intracortical inhibition. Given the ability of rTMS to modulate cortical excitability, potential therapeutic applications of low-frequency rTMS have been sought with some evidence of improvements (Filipovic et al., 2004; Siebner et al., 1999b).

TMS studies in migraine with visual auras suggest that the disorder is associated with increased excitability of the occipital cortex, as indicated by lower phosphene threshold (Aurora et al., 1998, 2003). Using extended 1-Hz rTMS of the occipital cortex, Brighina et al. (2002) found that while phosphene thresholds are elevated in normal subjects by the stimulation, the thresholds were lowered by the procedure in migraineurs. They also document that while phosphenes were reported during stimulation by 47% of normal subjects, all patients with migraine reported phosphenes, again indicating hyperexcitability of the occipital cortex in this patient group. This result also suggests that 1-Hz rTMS is unlikely to have therapeutic effects in migraine with aura, given that it further increases occipital cortex excitability. However, as has been observed in the motor cortex, modulation of occipital cortex excitability may depend on stimulus intensity and frequency in ways that have not been explicitly explored

Three-month outcome of stroke was assessed in motor thresholds to single-pulse TMS during rest and voluntary facilitation (Catano et al., 1995, 1996). The single most important predictive parameter was the presence or absence of MEPs with or without facilitation (Catano et al., 1995). In addition, a follow-up of MEP threshold had some prognostic significance (Catano et al., 1996).

Amyotrophic lateral sclerosis shows a variety of MEP abnormalities that correspond to the severity of the disease. Interestingly, the duration of the silent period has been shown to be markedly shortened, beyond what is seen in PD and therefore may be a more reliable marker of ALS (Desiato and Caramia, 1997). The shortening of the silent period has also been seen in patients with hepatic cirrhosis even before manifestation of hepatic encephalopathy at which point all MEP parameters were abnormal (Nolano et al., 1997).

After head injury, a number of patients developed apallic syndrome with major motor deficits. Surprisingly, almost half of the small studied group showed well-preserved MEPs (Inghilleri et al., 1994). Disappointingly, TCS does not have a prognostic or diagnostic value in spinal cord injury patients as has been also shown in a study by Macdonell and Donnan (1995).

Chronic pain is another area of potential therapeutic application of rTMS. A few recent published reports have documented relief of chronic pain following high-frequency stimulation of the motor and parietal cortices (Lefaucheur 2001; Rollnik et al., 2002; Topper et al., 2003).

Psychiatric Disorders

Therapeutic effects of rTMS have been sought in the treatment of depression, obsessive-compulsive disorders, psychosis, and medically refractory hallucinations. In depression, two factors motivate studies of rTMS as a possible therapeutic measure. The benefits of ECT in refractory depression raise the possibility that nonconvulsive focal stimulation of specific brain areas may accomplish the same effect. A guiding rationale in designing stimulation paradigms has been the notion that high-frequency stimulation produces increased cortical excitability and that low-frequency stimulation produces a local decease in excitability. Regional cerebral blood flow (rCBF) studies in depression suggest hypometabilism in the left dorsolateral frontal lobe (Bench et al., 1992, 1995). Repetitive TMS has been shown to modify rCBF in ways that parallel changes in cortical excitability. These effects on rCBF also appear to be strongly frequency dependent (Loo et al., 2003). Stimulation of the left prefrontal cortex at 20 Hz at 100% motor threshold produced persistent increases in rCBF in bilateral frontal, limbic, and paralimbic regions, while 1-Hz rTMS produced more circumscribed decreases in rCBF (Speer et al., 2000).

Both rapid-rate stimulation on the left and low-frequency stimulation on the right have been studied in treating depression. Early studies with prefrontal cortex stimulation suggested promising therapeutic effects (Alonso et al., 2001; Conca et al., 1996; George et al., 1995; Greenberg et al., 1997; Klein et al., 1999; Menkes et al., 1999; Pascual-Leone et al., 1996a,c; Sachdev et al., 2001). However, further evaluations of the effects of rTMS in several studies have shown marked variability of efficacy in depression, from none to significant, as well as conflicting dependencies on stimulation parameters. For example, on one extreme, Nahas et al. (2003) recently found no statistically significant effects on depression in a placebo-controlled study of patients with bipolar affective disorder using left dorsolateral prefrontal rTMS at 5 Hz at 110% of motor threshold. However, other trials where patients with major depression were randomized to ECT and rTMS, reported a clear and comparable response to both ECT and rTMS, which was above 55% (Dannon et al., 2002; Grunhaus et al., 2003; Janicak et al., 2002).

Another "placebo" or sham-stimulation controlled study demonstrated a significant benefit of rTMS, but did not see any difference between 20-Hz and 5-Hz stimulation (George et al., 2000). On the other extreme, patients with depression treated with rTMS have been reported to show not only improvement in the depression but also simultaneous appearance of manic symptoms (Ella et al., 2002; Sakkas et al., 2003). A meta-analysis based on a review of 16 studies (Martin et al., 2002) concluded that there was no strong evidence of the benefit of rTMS, but that given the small sample size of the studies, a therapeutic effect could not be excluded. A more recent meta-analysis concluded that the available data seem to support an antidepressant effect of high-frequency rTMS of the left dorsolateral prefrontal cortex (Gershon et al., 2003). High-frequency (20 Hz at 80% motor threshold) stimulation for 20 minutes daily for 2 weeks, in schizophrenic patients with psychotic symptoms, showed a statistically significant decrease in psychotic symptoms, but no significant effects on depression or anxiety (Rollnik et al., 2000). In the treatment of obsessive-compulsive disorder, a recent appraisal of the evidence based on a meta-analysis concluded that there are insufficient data from controlled trials to draw any definitive conclusions about the therapeutic benefit of rTMS (Martin et al., 2003). Efficacy of rTMS has also been explored with variable results in the treatment of medication-resistant hallucinations (Franck et al., 2003; Hoffman et al., 2003; Schreiber et al., 2002).

A study in patients with Tourette syndrome failed to demonstrate any clinical benefit of 20 minutes of rTMS of frontal areas at 1 Hz, 20% below motor threshold (Munchau et al., 2002).

It is conceivable that clinical response in any of these conditions is sensitive to stimulus parameters in ways that have yet to be systematically explored. Patient variables that are different in the various trials also have to be considered. Further data that help identify these variables are clearly required before any definitive conclusions can be drawn about the therapeutic value of rTMS in the treatment of any neurological or psychiatric disorder.

References

Abbruzzese, G., Morena, M., DallAgata, D., et al. 1991. Motor evoked potentials (MEPs) in lacunar syndromes. Electroencephalogr. Clin. Neurophysiol. 81:202–208.

Aglio, L.S., Romero, R., Desai, S., et al. 2002. The use of transcranial magnetic stimulation for monitoring descending spinal cord motor function. Clin. Electroencephalogr. 33:30–41.

Agnew, W.F., and McCreery, D.B. 1989. Considerations for safety in the use of extracranial stimulation for motor evoked potentials. Neurosurgery 20:143–147.

Agnew, W.F., McCreery, D.B., Yuen, T.G.H., et al. 1989. Histological and physiologic evaluation of electrically stimulated peripheral nerve: considerations for the selection of parameters. Ann. Biomed. Eng. 17:39–60.

Akamatsu, N., Fueta, Y., Endo, Y., et al. 2001. Decreased susceptibility to pentylenetetrazol-induced seizures after low-frequency transcranial magnetic stimulation in rats. Neurosci. Lett. 310:153–156.

Alonso, P., Pujol, J., Cardoner, N., et al. 2001. Right prefrontal repetitive transcranial magnetic stimulation in obsessive-compulsive disorder: a double-blind, placebo-controlled study. Am. J. Psychiatry 158:1143–1145.

Amassian, V.E., Cracco, R.Q., and Maccabee, P.J. 1989a. A sense of movement elicited in paralyzed distal arm by focal magnetic coil stimulation of human motor cortex. Brain Res. 479:355–360.

Amassian, V.E., Cracco, R.Q., and Maccabee, P.J. 1989b. Suppression of visual perception by magnetic coil stimulation of human occipital cortex. Electroencephalogr. Clin. Neurophysiol. 74:458–462.

Amassian, V.E., Quirk, G.J., and Stewart, M. 1990. A comparison of corticospinal activation by magnetic coil and electrical stimulation of monkey motor cortex. Electroencephalogr. Clin. Neurophysiol. 77:390–401.

Amassian, V.E., Somasundaram, M., Rothwell, J.C. 1991. Paraesthesias are elicited by single pulse, magnetic coil stimulation of motor cortex in susceptible humans. Brain 114:2505–2520.

Amassian, V.E., Maccabee, P.J., Cracco, R.Q. 1993. Measurement of information processing delays in human visual cortex with repetitive magnetic coil stimulation. Brain Res. 605:317–321.

Amassian, V.E., Maccabee, P.J., Cracco, R.Q. 1994. The polarity of the induced electric field influences magnetic coil inhibition of human visual cortex: implications for the site of excitation. Electroencephalogr. Clin. Neurophysiol. 93:21–26.

Antal, A., Kincses, T.Z., Nitsche, M.A., et al. 2002. Pulse configuration-dependent effects of repetitive transcranial magnetic stimulation on visual perception. Neuroreport 13:2229–2233.

Armand, J., Edgley, S.A., Lemon, R.N., et al. 1994. Protracted postnatal development of the corticospinal projections from the primary motor cortex to hand motoneurones in the macaque monkey. Exp. Brain Res. 101:178–182.

Aurora, S.K., Ahmad, B.K., Welch, K.M., et al. 1998. Transcranial magnetic stimulation confirms hyperexcitability of occipital cortex in migraine. Neurology 50:1111–1114.

Aurora, S.K., Welch, K.M., Al-Sayed, F. 2003. The threshold for phosphenes is lower in migraine. Cephalalgia 23:258–263.

Awiszus, F., and Feistner, H. 1994. Quantification of D- and I-wave effects evoked by transcranial magnetic brain stimulation on the tibialis anterior motoneuron pool in man. Exp. Brain Res. 101:153–158.

Aziz, Q., Rithwell, J.C., Barlow, J., et al. 1995. Modulation of esophageal responses to magnetic stimulation of the human brain by swallowing and by vagal stimulation. Gastroenterology 109:1437–1445.

Barker, A.T., and Jalinous, R. 1985. Noninvasive magnetic stimulation of human motor cortex. Lancet 1:1106–1107.

Barker, A.T., Freeston, I.L., Jalinous, R., et al. 1986. Clinical evaluation of conduction time measurements in central motor pathways using magnetic stimulation of human brain. Lancet 1:1325–1326.

Bartholow, R. 1874. Experimental investigations into the functions of the human brain. Am. J. Med. Sci. 67:305–313.

Baumer, T., Lange, R., Liepert, J., et al. 2003. Repeated premotor rTMS leads to cumulative plastic changes of motor cortex excitability in humans. Neuroimage 20:550–560.

Bench, C.J., Friston, K.J., Brown, R.G., et al. 1992. The anatomy of melancholia—focal abnormalities of cerebral blood flow in major depression. Psychol. Med. 22:607–615.

Bench, C.J., Frackowiak, R.S., Dolan, R.J. 1995. Changes in regional cerebral blood flow on recovery from depression. Psychol. Med. 25:247–261.

Benecke, R., Meyer, B-U., Schonle, P., et al. 1988. Transcranial magnetic stimulation of the human brain: responses in muscles supplied by cranial nerves. Exp. Brain Res. 71:623–632.

Berardelli, A. 1999. Transcranial magnetic stimulation in movement disorders. Electroencephalogr. Clin. Neurophysiol. Suppl. 51:276–280.

Berardelli, A., Inghilleri, M., Cruccu, G., et al. 1990. Descending volley after electrical and magnetic transcranial stimulation in man. Neurosci. Lett. 112:54–58.

Berardelli, A., Inghilleri, M., Rothwell, J.C., et al. 1991. Multiple firing of motoneurones is produced by cortical stimulation but not by direct activation of descending motor tracts. Electroencephalogr. Clin. Neurophysiol. 81:240–242.

Berardelli, A., Inghilleri, M., Rothwell, J.C., et al. 1998. Facilitation of muscle evoked responses after repetitive cortical stimulation in man. Exp. Brain Res. 122:79–84.

Binder, J. 1997. Functional magnetic resonance imaging. Language mapping. Neurosurg. Clin. North Am. 8:383–392.

Bohning, D.E., Shastri, A., Wassermann, E.M., et al. 2000. BOLD-f MRI response to single-pulse transcranial magnetic stimulation (TMS). J. Magn. Reson. Imaging 11:569–574.

Booth, K.R., Streletz, L.J., Raab, V.E. 1991. Motor evoked potentials and central motor conduction: studies of transcranial magnetic stimulation with recording from the leg. Electroencephalogr. Clin. Neurophysiol. 81:57–62.

Boylan, L.S., Pullman, S.L., Lisanby, S.H., et al. 2001. Repetitive transcranial magnetic stimulation to SMA worsens complex movements in Parkinson's disease. Clin. Neurophysiol. 112:259–264.

Brandt, S.A., Davis, T.L., Obrig, H. 1996. Functional magnetic resonance imaging shows localized brain activation during serial transcranial stimulation in man. NeuroReport 7:734–736.

Brasil-Neto, J.P., McShane, L.M., Fuhr, P., et al. 1992. Topographic mapping of the human motor cortex with magnetic stimulation: factors affecting accuracy and reproducibility. Electroencephalogr. Clin. Neurophysiol. 85:9–15.

Brasil-Neto, J.P., Pascual-Leone, A., Valls-Sole, J. 1993a. Post-exercise depression of motor evoked potentials: a measure of central nervous system fatigue. Exp. Brain Res. 93:181–184.

Brasil-Neto, J.P., Valls-Sole, J., Pascual-Leone, A. 1993b. Rapid modulation of human cortical motor outputs following ischaemic nerve block. Brain 116:511–525.

Brasil-Neto, J.P., Cohen, L.G., and Hallett, M. 1994. Central fatigue as revealed by post-exercise decrement of motor evoked potentials. Muscle Nerve 17:713–719.

Brasil-Neto, J.P., Cammarota, J., Valls-Sole, J. 1995. Role of intracortical mechanisms in the late part of the silent period to transcranial stimulation of the human motor cortex. Acta Neurol. Scand. 92:383–386.

Braune, H.J., and Fritz, C. 1995. Transcranial magnetic stimulation-evoked inhibition of voluntary muscle activity (silent period) is impaired in patients with ischemic hemispheric lesion. Stroke 26:550–553.

Bridgers, S.L. 1991. The safety of transcranial magnetic stimulation reconsidered: evidence regarding cognitive and other cerebral effects. In *Magnetic Motor Stimulation: Basic Principles and Clinical Experience (EEG Suppl 43)*, Eds. W.J. Levy, R.Q. Cracco, A.T. Barker, et al., pp. 170–179. New York: Elsevier.

Brighina, F., Piazza, A., Daniele, O., et al. 2002. Modulation of visual cortical excitability in migraine with aura: effects of 1 Hz repetitive transcranial magnetic stimulation. Exp. Brain Res. 145:177–181.

Britton, T.C., Meyer, B.-U., and Benecke, R. 1991. Variability of cortical evoked motor responses in multiple sclerosis. Electroencephalogr. Clin. Neurophysiol. 81:186–194.

Brouwer, B., and Ashby, P. 1990. Corticospinal projections to upper and lower limb spinal motoneurons in man. Electroencephalogr. Clin. Neurophysiol. 76:509–519.

Brouwer, B., and Ashby, P. 1991. Altered corticospinal projections to lower limb motor neurons in subjects with cerebral palsy. Brain 114:1395–1407.

Burke, D., Hicks, R.G., and Stephen, J.P.H. 1990. Corticospinal volleys evoked by anodal and cathodal stimulation of the human motor cortex. J. Physiol. (Lond.) 425:283–299.

Burke, D., Hicks, R., Stephen, J., et al. 1995. Trial-to-trial variability of corticospinal volleys in human subjects. Electoencephalogr. Clin. Neurophysiol. 97:231–237.

Cadwell, J. 1991. Optimizing magnetic stimulator design. In *Magnetic Motor Stimulation: Basic Principles and Clinical Experience (EEG Suppl 43),* Eds. W.J. Levy, R.Q. Cracco, A.T. Barker, et al., pp. 238–248. New York: Elsevier.

Cakmur, R., Donmez, B., Uzunel, F., et al. 2004. Evidence of widespread impairment of motor cortical inhibition in focal dystonia: a transcranial magnetic stimulation study in patients with blepharospasm and cervical dystonia. Adv. Neurol. 94:37–44.

Calancie, B., Klose, K.J., Baier, S., et al. 1991. Isoflurane-induced attenuation of motor evoked potentials caused by electrical motor cortex stimulation. J. Neurosurg. 74:897–904.

Calancie, B., Harris, W., Broton, J.G., et al. 1998. "Threshold-level" multipulse transcranial electrical stimulation of motor cortex for intraoperative monitoring of spinal motor tracts: description of method and comparison to somatosensory evoked potential monitoring. J. Neurosurg. 88:457–470.

Calancie, B., Harris, W., Brindle, G.F., et al. 2001. Threshold-level repetitive transcranial electrical stimulation for intraoperative monitoring of central motor conduction. J. Neurosurg. 95:161–168.

Cantello, R. 2002. Applications of transcranial magnetic stimulation in movement disorders. J. Clin. Neurophysiol. 19:272–293.

Cantello, R., Gianelli, M., Bettucci, D. 1991. Parkinson's disease rigidity: magnetic motor evoked potentials in a small hand muscle. Neurology 41:1449–1456.

Cantello, R., Civardi, C., Cavalli, A., et al. 2000. Cortical excitability in cryptogenic localization-related epilepsy: interictal transcranial magnetic stimulation studies. Epilepsia 41:694–704.

Caramia, M.D., Pardal, A.M., Zarola, F., et al. 1989. Electric vs magnetic transcranial stimulation of the brain in healthy humans: a comparative study of central motor tracts "conductivity" and "excitability." Brain Res. 479:98–104.

Caramia, M.D., Cicinelli, P., Paradiso, C. 1991. "Excitability," changes of muscular response to magnetic brain stimulation in patients with central motor disorders. Electroencephalogr. Clin. Neurophysiol. 81:243–250.

Caramia, M.D., Gigli, G., Iani, C. 1996. Distinguishing forms of generalized epilepsy using magnetic brain stimulation. Electroencephalogr. Clin. Neurophysiol. 98:14–19.

Catano, A., Houa, M., Caroyer, J.M., et al. 1995. Magnetic transcranial stimulation in non-haemorrhagic sylvian strokes: interest of facilitation for early functional prognosis. Electroencephalogr. Clin. Neurophysiol. 97:349–354.

Catano, A., Houa, M., Caroyer, J.M., et al. 1996. Magnetic transcranial stimulation in acute stroke: early excitation threshold and functional prognosis. Electroencephalogr. Clin. Neurophysiol. 101:233–239.

Cerletti, U. 1940. L'Elettroshock. Riv. Speriment. Frenatria 1:209–310.

Chen, R. 2000. Studies of human motor physiology with transcranial magnetic stimulation. Muscle Nerve Suppl. 9:S26–32.

Chen, R., Classen, J., Gerloff, C., et al. 1997. Depression of motor cortex excitability by low-frequency transcranial magnetic stimulation. Neurology 48:398–403.

Chiappa, K.H., Cros, D., Day, B. 1991. Magnetic stimulation of the human motor cortex: ipsilateral and contralateral facilitation effects. In *Magnetic Motor Stimulation: Basic Principles and Clinical Experience (EEG Suppl 43),* Eds. W.J. Levy, R.Q. Cracco, A.T. Barker, et al., pp. 186–201. New York: Elsevier.

Chiappa, K.H., Cros, D., Kiers, L. 1995. Crossed inhibition in the human motor system. J. Clin. Neurophysiol. 12:82–96.

Cincotta, M., Borgheresi, A., Lori, S., et al. 1998. Interictal inhibitory mechanisms in patients with cryptogenic motor cortex epilepsy: a study of the silent period following transcranial magnetic stimulation. Electroencephalogr. Clin. Neurophysiol. 107:1–7.

Cincotta, M., Borgheresi, A., Gambetti, C., et al. 2003. Suprathreshold 0.3 Hz repetitive TMS prolongs the cortical silent period: potential implications for therapeutic trials in epilepsy. Clin. Neurophysiol. 114:1827–1833.

Cindro, L., Prevec, T.S., and Beric, A. 1985. Maturation of cortical potentials evoked by tibial nerve stimulation in newborns, infants and children aged four and eight years. Dev. Med. Child Neurol. 27:740–745.

Claus, D., and Brunholzl, C. 1994. Facilitation and disfacilitation of muscle responses after repetitive transcranial cortical stimulation and electrical peripheral nerve stimulation. Electroencephalogr. Clin. Neurophysiol. 93:417–420.

Claus, D., Mills, K.R., and Murray, N.M.F. 1988. Facilitation of muscle responses to magnetic brain stimulation by mechanical stimuli in man. Exp. Brain Res. 71:273–278.

Claus, D., Murray, N.M.F., Spitzer, A., et al. 1990. The influence of stimulus type on the magnetic excitation of nerve structures. Electroencephalogr. Clin. Neurophysiol. 75:342–349.

Cohen, L., Brasil-Neto J., Pascual-Leone, A., et al. 1993. Plasticity of cortical motor output organization following deafferentation, cerebral lesions, and skill acquisition. In *Electrical and Magnetic Stimulation of the Brain and Spinal Cord (Adv. Neurol. Vol. 63),* Eds. O. Devinsky, A. Beric, and M. Dogali, pp. 187–200. New York: Raven.

Conca, A., Koppi, S., Konig, P., et al. 1996. Transcranial magnetic stimulation: a novel antidepressive strategy? Neuropsychobiology 34:204–207.

Cowey, A., Walsh, V. 2001. Tickling the brain: studying visual sensation, perception and cognition by transcranial magnetic stimulation. Prog. Brain Res. 134:411–425.

Cracco, R.Q., Amassian, V., Maccabee, P.J. 1993. Insights into cerebral function revealed by magnetic coil stimulation. In *Electrical and Magnetic Stimulation of the Brain and Spinal Cord (Adv. Neurol. Vol. 63).* Eds. O. Devinsky, A. Beric, and M. Dogali, pp. 43–50. New York: Raven.

Cros, D., and Chiappa, K.H. 1993. Clinical applications of motor evoked potentials. In *Electrical and Magnetic Stimulation of the Brain and Spinal Cord (Adv. Neurol. Vol. 63).* Eds. O. Devinsky, A. Beric, and M. Dogali, pp. 179–185. New York: Raven.

Cruccu, G., Berardelli, A., Inghilleri, M., et al. 1989. Functional organization of the trigeminal motor system in man. Brain 112:1333–1350.

Cruccu, G., Inghilleri, M., Berardelli, A., et al. 1990. Cortico-facial and cortico-trigeminal projections. A comparison by magnetic brain stimulation in man. In *New Trends and Advanced Techniques in Clinical Neurophysiology (EEG Suppl 41),* Eds. P.M. Rossini and F. Mauguiere, pp. 140–144. New York: Elsevier.

Dannon, P.N., Dolberg, O.T., Schreiber, S., et al. 2002. Three and six-month outcome following courses of either ECT or rTMS in a population of severely depressed individuals—preliminary report. Biol. Psychiatry 51:687–690.

d'Arsonval, A. 1896. Dispositifs pour la mesure des courants alternatifs de toutes fréquences. C. R. Soc. Biol. (Paris) 3:450–457.

Day, B.L., Thompson, P.D., Dick, J.P., et al. 1987. Different site of activation of electrical and magnetic stimulation of the human brain. Neurosci. Lett. 75:101–106.

Day, B.L., Dressier, D., Maertens de Noordhout, A. 1989a. Electric and magnetic stimulation of human motor cortex: surface EMG and single motor unit responses. J. Physiol. (Lond.) 412:449–473.

Day, B.L., Rothwell, J.C., Thompson, P.D. 1989b. Delay in the execution of voluntary movement by electrical or magnetic brain stimulation in intact man. Brain 112:649–663.

de Haan, P., Kalkman, C.J. 2001. Spinal cord monitoring: somatosensory- and motor-evoked potentials. Anesthesiol. Clin. North Am. 19:923–945.

de Haan, P., Kalkman, C.J., de Mol, B.A., et al. 1997. Efficacy of transcranial motor-evoked myogenic potentials to detect spinal cord ischemia during operations for thoracoabdominal aneurysms. J. Thorac. Cardiovasc. Surg. 113:87–100.

Deletis, V. 1993. Intraoperative monitoring of the functional integrity of the motor pathways. In *Electrical and Magnetic Stimulation of the Brain and Spinal Cord (Adv. Neurol. Vol. 63),* Eds. O. Devinsky, A. Beric, and M. Dogali, pp. 201–214. New York: Raven.

Deletis, V., Dimitrijevic, M.R., and Sherwood, A.M. 1987. Effects of electrically induced afferent input from limb nerves on the excitability of the human motor cortex. Neurosurgery 20:195–197.

Deletis, V., Schild, J.H., Beric, A., et al. 1992. Facilitation of motor evoked potentials by somatosensory afferent stimulation. Electroencephalogr. Clin. Neurophysiol. 85:302–310.

Desiato, M.T., and Caramia, M.D., 1997. Towards a neurophysiological marker of amyotrophic lateral sclerosis as revealed by changes in cortical excitability. Electroencephalogr. Clin. Neurophysiol. 105:1–7.

Dettmers, C., Ridding, M.C., Stephan, K.M. 1996. Comparison of regional cerebral blood flow with transcranial magnetic stimulation at different forces. J. Appl. Physiol. 81:596–603.

Deuschl, G., Michels, R., Berardelli, A. 1991. Effects of electric and magnetic transcranial stimulation on long latency reflexes. Exp. Brain Res. 83:403–410.

DeYoe, E.A., Carman, G.J., Bandettini, P., et al. 1996. Mapping striate and extrastriate visual areas in human cerebral cortex. Proc. Natl. Acad. Sci. U.S.A. 93:2382–2386.

Di Lazzaro, V., Oliviero, A., Berardelli, A., et al. 2002. Direct demonstration of the effects of repetitive transcranial magnetic stimulation on the excitability of the human motor cortex. Exp. Brain Res. 44:549–553.

Di Lazzaro, V., Oliviero, A., Pilato, F., et al. 2003. Corticospinal volleys evoked by transcranial stimulation of the brain in conscious humans. Neurol. Res. 25:143–150.

Dimitrijevic, M.R., Kofler, M., McKay, W.B. 1992. Early and late lower limb motor evoked potentials elicited by transcranial magnetic motor cortex stimulation. Electroencephalogr. Clin. Neurophysiol. 85:365–373.

Dong, C.C., MacDonald, D.B., Janusz, M.T. 2002. Intraoperative spinal cord monitoring during descending thoracic and thoracoabdominal aneurysm surgery. Ann. Thorac. Surg. 74:S1873–1876.

Dragasevic, N., Potrebic, A., Damjanovic, A., et al. 2002. Therapeutic efficacy of bilateral prefrontal slow repetitive transcranial magnetic stimulation in depressed patients with Parkinson's disease: an open study. Mov. Disord. 17:528–532.

Ebert, U., Ziemann, U. 1999. Altered seizure susceptibility after high-frequency repetitive transcranial magnetic stimulation in rats. Neurosci. Lett. 273: 155–158.

Edgely, S.A., Eyre, J.A., Lemon, R.N., et al. 1990. Excitation of the corticospinal tract by electromagnetic and electrical stimulation of the scalp in the macaque monkey. J. Physiol. (Lond.) 425:301–320.

Eisen, A., Siejka, S., Schulzer, M., et al. 1991. Age-dependent decline in motor evoked potential (MEP) amplitude: with a comment on changes in Parkinson's disease. Electroencephalogr. Clin. Neurophysiol. 81:209–215.

Ella, R., Zwanzger, P., Stampfer, R., et al. 2002. Switch to mania after slow rTMS of the right prefrontal cortex. J. Clin. Psychiatry 63:249.

Enomoto, H., Ugawa, Y., Hanajima, R., et al. 2001. Decreased sensory cortical excitability after 1 Hz rTMS over the ipsilateral primary motor cortex. Clin. Neurophysiol. 112:2154–2158.

Epstein, C.M., Davey, K.R. 2002. Iron-core coils for transcranial magnetic stimulation. J. Clin. Neurophysiol. 19:376–381.

Epstein, C.M., Schwartzenberg, D.G., Davey, K.R., et al. 1990. Localizing the site of magnetic brain stimulation in humans. Neurology 40:666–670.

Epstein, C.M., Lah, J.J., Meador, K. 1996. Optimum stimulus parameters for lateralized suppression of speech with magnetic brain stimulation. Neurology 47:1590–1593.

Epstein, C., Woodard, J., Stringer, A., et al. 2000. Repetitive transcranial magnetic stimulation does not replicate the Wada test. Neurology 55: 1025–1027.

Ettinger, G.J., Leventon, M.E., Grimson, W.E., et al. 1998. Experimentation with a transcranial magnetic stimulation system for functional brain mapping. Med. Image Anal. 2:133–142.

Evers, S., Hengst, K., Pecuch, P.W. 2001. The impact of repetitive transcranial magnetic stimulation on pituitary hormone levels and cortisol in healthy subjects. J. Affect. Disord. 66:83–88.

Ferbert, A., Mussmann, N., Menne, A., et al. 1991. Short-term memory performance with magnetic stimulation of the motor cortex. Eur. Arch. Psychiatry Clin. Neurosci. 241:135–138.

Fernandez, E., Alfaro, A., Tormos, J.M., et al. 2002. Mapping of the human visual cortex using image-guided transcranial magnetic stimulation. Brain Res. Protoc. 10:115–124.

Fierro, B., Brighina, F., Piazza, A., et al. 2001a. Timing of right parietal and frontal cortex activity in visuo-spatial perception: a TMS study in normal individuals. Neuroreport 12:2605–2607.

Fierro, B., Piazza, A., Brighina, F., et al. 2001b. Modulation of intracortical inhibition induced by low- and high-frequency repetitive transcranial magnetic stimulation. Exp. Brain Res. 138:452–457.

Filipovic, S.R., Siebner, H.R., Rowe, J.B., et al. 2004. Modulation of cortical activity by repetitive transcranial magnetic stimulation (rTMS): a review of functional imaging studies and the potential use in dystonia. Adv. Neurol. 94:45–52.

Fitzgerald, P.B., Brown, T.L., Daskalakis, Z.J., et al. 2002. Intensity-dependent effects of 1 Hz rTMS on human corticospinal excitability. Clin. Neurophysiol. 113:1136–1141.

Fleischmann, A., Hirschmann, S., Dolberg, O.T., et al. 1999. Chronic treatment with repetitive transcranial magnetic stimulation inhibits seizure induction by electroconvulsive shock in rats. Biol. Psychiatry 45:759–763.

Foerster, A., Schmitz, J.M., Nouri, S., et al. 1997. Safety of rapid-rate transcranial magnetic stimulation: heart rate and blood pressure changes. Electroencephalogr. Clin. Neurophysiol. 104:207–212.

Franck, N., Poulet, E., Terra, J.L., et al. 2003. Left temporoparietal transcranial magnetic stimulation in treatment-resistant schizophrenia with verbal hallucinations. Psychiatry Res. 120:107–109.

Fritz, C., Braune, H.J., Pylatiuk, C., et al. 1997. Silent period following transcranial magnetic stimulation: a study of intra- and inter-examiner reliability. Electroencephalogr. Clin. Neurophysiol. 105:235–240.

Fuhr, P., Agostino, R., and Hallett, M. 1991. Spinal motor neuron excitability during the silent period after cortical stimulation. Electroencephalogr. Clin. Neurophysiol. 81:257–262.

Fumal, A., Bohotin, V., Vandenheede, M., et al. 2003. Effects of repetitive transcranial magnetic stimulation on visual evoked potentials: new insights in healthy subjects. Exp. Brain Res. 150:332–340.

Gandevia, S.C., Killian, K., McKenzie, D.K. 1993. Respiratory sensations, cardiovascular control, kinaesthesia and transcranial stimulation during paralysis in humans. J. Physiol. (Lond.) 470:85–107.

Gandevia, S.C., Allen, G.A., Butler, A.E., et al. 1996. Supraspinal factors in human muscle fatigue: evidence for suboptimal output from the motor cortex. J. Physiol. (Lond.) 490:529–536.

Garland, S.J., and Miles, T.S. 1997. Responses of human single motor units to transcranial magnetic stimulation. Electroencephalogr. Clin. Neurophysiol. 105:94–101.

George, M.S., Wasserman, E.M., Williams, W.A. 1995. Daily repetitive transcranial magnetic stimulation (rTMS) improves mood in depression. NeuroReport 6:1853–1856.

George, M.S., Nahas, Z., Molloy, M., et al. 2000. A controlled trial of daily left prefrontal cortex TMS for treating depression. Biol. Psychiatry 48:962–970.

Gerschlager, W., Siebner, H.R., Rothwell, J.C. 2001. Decreased corticospinal excitability after subthreshold 1 Hz rTMS over lateral premotor cortex. Neurology 57:449–455.

Gershon, A.A., Dannon, P.N., Grunhaus, L. 2003. Transcranial magnetic stimulation in the treatment of depression. Am. J. Psychiatry 160:835–845.

Gironell, A., Kulisevsky, J., Lorenzo, J., et al. 2002. Transcranial magnetic stimulation of the cerebellum in essential tremor: a controlled study. Arch. Neurol. 59:413–417.

Gorsler, A., Baumer, T., Weiller, C., et al. 2003. Interhemispheric effects of high and low frequency rTMS in healthy humans. Clin. Neurophysiol. 114:1800–1807.

Gracies, J.K., Meunier, S., and Pierrot-Deseilligny, E. 1994. Evidence for corticospinal excitation of presumed propriospinal neurones in man. J. Physiol. (Lond.) 475:509–518.

Grafman, J., Pascual-Leone, A., Alway, D. 1994. Induction of a recall deficit by rapid-rate transcranial magnetic stimulation. NeuroReport 5: 1157–1160.

Greenberg, B.D., George, M.S., Martin, J.D. 1997. Effect of prefrontal repetitive transcranial magnetic stimulation in obsessive-compulsive disorder: a preliminary study. Am. J. Psychiatry 154:867–869.

Grunhaus, L., Schreiber, S., Dolberg, O.T., et al. 2003. A randomized controlled comparison of electroconvulsive therapy and repetitive transcranial magnetic stimulation in severe and resistant nonpsychotic major depression. Biol. Psychiatry 53:324–331.

Gugino, L.D., Romero, J.R., Aglio, L., et al. 2001. Transcranial magnetic stimulation coregistered with MRI: a comparison of a guided versus blind stimulation technique and its effect on evoked compound muscle action potentials. Clin. Neurophysiol. 112:1781–1792.

Haghighi, S.S., Gaines, R.W. 2003. Repetitive vs. single transcranial electrical stimulation for intraoperative monitoring of motor conduction in spine surgery. Mo. Med. 100:262–265.

Hakkinen, V., Eskola, H., Yli-Hankala, A., et al. 1995. Which structures are sensitive to painful transcranial electric stimulation? Electromyogr. Clin. Neurophysiol. 35:377–383.

Haug, B.A., and Kukowski, B. 1994. Latency and duration of the muscle silent period following transcranial magnetic stimulation in multiple sclerosis, cerebral ischemia, and other upper motoneuron lesions. Neurology 44:936–940.

Helmers, S.L., Chiappa, K.H., Cros, D., et al. 1989. Magnetic stimulation of the human motor cortex: facilitation and its relationship to a visual motor task. J. Clin. Neurophysiol. 6:321–332.

Herdmann, J., Bielefeldt, K., and Enck, P. 1991. Quantification of motor pathways to the pelvic floor in humans. Am. J. Physiol. 260:720–723.

Hess, C.W., Mills, K.R., Murray, N.M., et al. 1987a. Magnetic brain stimulation: central motor conduction studies in multiple sclerosis. Ann. Neurol. 22:744–752.

Hess, C.W., Mills, K.R., Murray, N.M.F., et al. 1987b. Excitability of the human motor cortex is enhanced during REM sleep. Neurosci. Lett. 82: 47–52.

Hoffman, R.E., Hawkins, K.A., Gueorguieva, R., et al. 2003. Transcranial magnetic stimulation of left temporoparietal cortex and medication-resistant auditory hallucinations. Arch. Gen. Psychiatry 60:49–56.

Homan, R.W., Herman, J., Purdy, P. 1987. Cerebral location of international 10–20 system electrode placement. Electroencephalogr. Clin. Neurophysiol. 66:376–382.

Homberg, V., and Netz, J. 1989. Generalized seizures induced by transcranial magnetic stimulation of motor cortex. Lancet 11:1223.

Horsley, V. 1886. Brain surgery. Br. Med. J. 2:670–675.

Hufnagel, A., and Elger, C.E. 1991. Responses of the epileptic focus to transcranial magnetic stimulation. In *Magnetic Motor Stimulation: Basic Principles and Clinical Experience (EEG Suppl 43)*, Eds. W.J. Levy, R.Q. Cracco, A.T. Barker, et al. pp. 86–99. New York: Elsevier.

Hufnagel, A., Jaeger, M., and Elger, C.E. 1990. Trans-cranial magnetic stimulation: specific and non-specific facilitation of magnetic motor evoked potentials. J. Neurol. 237:416–419.

Ikeguchi, M., Touge, T., Nishiyama, Y., et al. 2003. Effects of successive repetitive transcranial magnetic stimulation on motor performances and brain perfusion in idiopathic Parkinson's disease. J. Neurol. Sci. 209: 41–46.

Ikoma, K., Samii, A., Mercuri, B., et al. 1996. Abnormal cortical motor excitability in dystonia. Neurology 46:1371–1376.

Ilmoniemi, R.J., Virtanen, J., Ruohonen, J., et al. 1997. Neuronal responses to magnetic stimulation reveal cortical reactivity and connectivity. Neuroreport 8:3537–3540.

Inghilleri, M., Berardelli, A., Cruccu, G., et al. 1989. Corticospinal potentials after transcranial stimulation in humans. J. Neurol. Neurosurg. Psychiatry 52:970–974.

Inghilleri, M., Berardelli, A., Cruccu, G., et al. 1990. Motor potentials evoked by paired cortical stimuli. Electroencephalogr. Clin. Neurophysiol. 77:382–389.

Inghilleri, M., Berardelli, A., Cruccu, G., et al. 1993. Silent period evoked by transcranial stimulation of the human cortex and cervicomedullary junction. J. Physiol. (Lond.) 466:521–534.

Inghilleri, M., Formisano, M., Berardelli, A. 1994. Transcranial electrical stimulation in patients with apallic syndrome. Acta Neurol. Scand. 89: 15–17.

Inghilleri, M., Berardelli, A., Marchetti, P., et al. 1996. Effects of diazepam, baclofen and thiopental on the silent period evoked by transcranial magnetic stimulation in humans. Exp. Brain Res. 109:467–472.

Inghilleri, M., Cruccu, G., Argenta, M., et al. 1997. Silent period in upper limb muscles after noxious cutaneous stimulation in man. Electroencephalogr. Clin. Neurophysiol. 105:109–115.

Jahanshahi, M., Ridding, M.C., Limousin, P., et al. 1997. Rapid rate transcranial magnetic stimulation—a safety study. Electroencephalogr. Clin. Neurophysiol. 105:422–429.

Jajakar, P. 1993. Physiologic principles of electrical stimulation. In *Electrical and Magnetic Stimulation of the Brain and Spinal Cord (Adv. Neurol. Vol. 63)*, Eds. O. Devinsky, A. Beric, and M. Dogali, pp. 17–27. New York: Raven.

Jalinous, R. 1991. Technical and practical aspects of magnetic nerve stimulation. J. Clin. Neurophysiol. 8:10–25.

Janicak, P.G., Dowd, S.M., Martis, B., et al. 2002. Repetitive transcranial magnetic stimulation versus electroconvulsive therapy for major depression: preliminary results of a randomized trial. Biol. Psychiatry 51:659–667.

Jellinek, D., Jewkes, D., Symon, L. 1991. Noninvasive intraoperative monitoring of motor evoked potentials under propofol anesthesia: effects of spinal surgery on the amplitude and latency of motor evoked potentials. Neurosurgery 29:551–557.

Jennum, P., Winkel, H. 1994. Transcranial magnetic stimulation. Its role in the evaluation of patients with partial epilepsy. Acta. Neurol. Scand. Suppl. 152:93–96.

Jennum, P., Friberg, L., Fuglsang-Fredriksen, A., et al. 1994. Speech localization using repetitive transcranial magnetic stimulation. Neurology 44:269–273.

Jennum, P., Winkel, H., and Fuglsang-Fredriksen, A. 1995. Repetitive magnetic stimulation and motor evoked potentials. Electroencephalogr. Clin. Neurophysiol. 97:96–101.

Jones, S.J., Harrison, R., Koh, K.F., et al. 1996. Motor evoked potential monitoring during spinal surgery: responses of distal limb muscles to transcranial cortical stimulation with pulse trains. Electroencephalogr. Clin. Neurophysiol. 100:375–383.

Kalkman, C.J., Drummond, J.C., Ribberink, A.A. 1992. Effects of propofol, etomidate, midazolam, and fentanyl on motor evoked responses to transcranial electrical or magnetic stimulation in humans. Anesthesiology 76:502–509.

Kalkman, C.J., Ubags, L.H., Been, H.D., et al. 1995. Improved amplitude of myogenic motor evoked responses after paired transcranial electrical stimulation during sufentanil/nitrous oxide anesthesia. Anesthesiology 83:270–276.

Kamitani, Y., Shimojo, S. 1999. Manifestation of scotomas created by transcranial magnetic stimulation of human visual cortex. Nat. Neurosci. 2: 767–771.

Kammer, T. 1999. Phosphenes and transient scotomas induced by magnetic stimulation of the occipital lobe: their topographic relationship. Neuropsychologia 37:191–198.

Kammer, T., Nusseck, H.G. 1998. Are recognition deficits following occipital lobe TMS explained by raised detection thresholds? Neuropsychologia 36:1161–1166.

Kasai, T., Hayes, K.C., Wolfe, D.L., et al. 1992. Afferent conditioning of evoked motor potentials following transcranial magnetic stimulation of motor cortex in normal subjects. Electroencephalogr. Clin. Neurophysiol. 85:95–101.

Kastner, S., Demmer, I., Ziemann, U. 1998. Transient visual field defects induced by transcranial magnetic stimulation over human occipital pole. Exp. Brain Res. 118:19–26.

Kernell, D., and Wu, C.-P. 1967. Responses of the pyramidal tract to stimulation of the baboon's motor cortex. J. Physiol. 191:653–672.

Khater-Boidin, J., and Duron, B. 1991. Postnatal development of descending motor pathways studied in man by percutaneous stimulation of the motor cortex and the spinal cord. Int. J. Dev. Neurosci. 9:15–24.

Kiers, L., Cros, D., Chiappa, K.H., et al. 1993. Variability of motor potentials evoked by transcranial magnetic stimulation. Electroencephalogr. Clin. Neurophysiol. 89:415–423.

Kiers, L., Clouston, P., Chiappa, K.H., et al. 1995. Assessment of cortical motor output: compound muscle action potential versus twitch force recording. Electroencephalogr. Clin. Neurophysiol. 97:131–139.

Kirkwood, A., Dudek, S.M., Gold, J.T., et al. 1993. Common forms of synaptic plasticity in the hippocampus and neocortex in vitro. Science 260:1518–1521.

Kitagawa, H., Itoh, T., Takano, H. 1989. Motor evoked potential monitoring during upper cervical spine surgery. Spine 14:1078–1083.

Klein, E., Kreinin, I., Chistyakov, A., et al. 1999. Therapeutic efficacy of right prefrontal slow repetitive transcranial magnetic stimulation in major depression: a double-blind controlled study. Arch. Gen. Psychiatry 56:315–320.

Knecht, S., Floel, A., Drager, B., et al. 2002. Degree of language lateralization determines susceptibility to unilateral brain lesions. Nat. Neurosci. 5:695–699.

Koh, T.H.H.G., and Eyre, J.A. 1988. Maturation of corticospinal tract assessed by electromagnetic stimulation of the motor cortex. Arch. Dis. Child. 63:1347–1352.

Kollias, S.S., Landau, K., Khan, N., et al. 1998. Functional evaluation using magnetic resonance imaging of the visual cortex in patients with retrochiasmatic lesions. J. Neurosurg. 89:780–790.

Komori, T., Watson, B.V., and Brown, W.F. 1992. Influence of peripheral afferent on cortical and spinal motoneuron excitability. Muscle Nerve 15: 48–51.

Komssi, S., Aronen, H.J., Huttunen, J., et al. 2002. Ipsi- and contralateral EEG reactions to transcranial magnetic stimulation. Clin. Neurophysiol. 113(2):175–184.

Krings, T., Buchbinder, B.R., Butler, W.E., et al. 1997. Stereotactic transcranial magnetic stimulation: correlation with direct electrical cortical stimulation. Neurosurgery 41:1319–1325.

Krings, T., Naujokat, C., von Keyserlingk, D.G. 1998. Representation of cortical motor function as revealed by stereotactic transcranial magnetic stimulation. Electroencephalogr. Clin. Neurophysiol. 109:85–93.

Krings, T., Foltys, H., Reinges, M.H., et al. 2001a. Navigated transcranial magnetic stimulation for presurgical planning—correlation with functional MRI. Minim. Invasive Neurosurg. 44:234–239.

Krings, T., Chiappa, K.H., Foltys, H., et al. 2001b. Introducing navigated transcranial magnetic stimulation as a refined brain mapping methodology. Neurosurg. Rev. 24:171–179.

Lang, E.W., Beutler, A.S., Chesnut, R.M. 1996. Myogenic motor-evoked potential monitoring using partial neuromuscular blockade in surgery of the spine. Spine 21:1676–1686.

Lavoie, B.A., Cody, F.W.J., and Capaday, C. 1995. Cortical control of human soleus muscle during volitional and postural activities studied using focal magnetic stimulation. Exp. Brain Res. 103:97–107.

Lefaucheur, J.P., Drouot, X., Keravel, Y., et al. 2001. Pain relief induced by repetitive transcranial magnetic stimulation of precentral cortex. Neuroreport 12:2963–2965.

Li, J., Olson, J., Anand, S., et al. 1997. Rapid-rate transcranial magnetic stimulation of human frontal cortex can evoked saccades under facilitating conditions. Electroencephalogr. Clin. Neurophysiol. 105:246–254.

Loo, C.K., Sachdev, P.S., Haindl, W., et al. 2003. High (15 Hz) and low (1 Hz) frequency transcranial magnetic stimulation have different acute effects on regional cerebral blood flow in depressed patients. Psychol. Med. 33:997–1006.

Lotze, M., Kaethner, R.J., Erb, M., et al. 2003. Comparison of representational maps using functional magnetic resonance imaging and transcranial magnetic stimulation. Clin. Neurophysiol. 114:306–312.

Loughnan, B.A., Anderson, S.K., Hetreed, M.A. 1989. Effects of halothane on motor evoked potential recorded in the extradural space. Br. J. Anaesth. 63:561–564.

Maccabee, P.J., Amassian, V.E., Cracco, R.Q. 1991. Stimulation of the human nervous system using the magnetic coil. J. Clin. Neurophysiol. 8:38–55.

MacDonald, D.B. 2002. Safety of intraoperative transcranial electrical stimulation motor evoked potential monitoring. J Clin. Neurophysiol. 19:416–429.

Macdonell, R.A.L., and Donnan, G.A. 1995. Magnetic cortical stimulation in acute spinal cord injury. Neurology 45:303–306.

Macdonell, R.A., Jackson, G.D., Curatolo, J.M., et al. 1999. Motor cortex localization using functional MRI and transcranial magnetic stimulation. Neurology 53:1462–1467.

Macdonell, R.A., King, M.A., Newton, M.R., et al. 2001. Prolonged cortical silent period after transcranial magnetic stimulation in generalized epilepsy. Neurology 57:706–708.

Manganotti, P., Tamburin, S., Zanette, G., et al. 2001. Hyperexcitable cortical responses in progressive myoclonic epilepsy: a TMS study. Neurology 57:1793–1799.

Martin, J.L., Barbanoj, M.J., Schlaepfer, T.E., et al. 2002. Transcranial magnetic stimulation for treating depression. Cochrane Database Syst. Rev. (2):CD003493.

Martin, J.L., Barbanoj, M.J., Perez, V., et al. 2003. Transcranial magnetic stimulation for the treatment of obsessive-compulsive disorder. Cochrane Database Syst. Rev. (3):CD003387.

Martis, B., Alam, D., Dowd, S.M., et al. 2003. Neurocognitive effects of repetitive transcranial magnetic stimulation in severe major depression. Clin Neurophysiol. 114:1125–1132.

Mathers, S.E., Ingram, D.A., and Swash, M. 1990. Electrophysiology of motor pathways for sphincter control in multiple sclerosis. J. Neurol. Neurosurg. Psychiatry 53:955–960.

Mavroudakis, N., Caroyer, J.M., Brunko, E., et al. 1995. Abnormal motor evoked responses to transcranial magnetic stimulation in focal dystonia. Neurology 45:1671–1677.

Mavroudakis, N., Caroyer, J.M., Brunko, E., et al. 1997. Effects of vigabatrin on motor potentials evoked with magnetic stimulation. Electroencephalogr. Clin. Neurophysiol. 105:124–127.

Mayr, N., Baumgartner, C., Zeitlhofer, J., et al. 1991. The sensitivity of transcranial cortical magnetic stimulation in detecting pyramidal tract lesions in clinically definite multiple sclerosis. Neurology 41:566–569.

Mazevet, D., Pierrot-Deseilligny, E., and Rothwell J.C. 1996. A propriospinal-like contribution to electromyographic responses evoked in wrist extensor muscles by transcranial stimulation of the motor cortex in man. Exp. Brain Res. 109:495–499.

Mazzocchio, R., Rossi, A., and Rothwell, J.C. 1994. Depression of Renshaw recurrent inhibition by activation of corticospinal fibres in human upper and lower limb. J. Physiol. (Lond.) 481:487–498.

Menkes, D.L., Gruenthal, M. 2000. Slow-frequency repetitive transcranial magnetic stimulation in a patient with focal cortical dysplasia. Epilepsia 41:240–242.

Menkes, D.L., Bodnar, P., Ballesteros, R.A., et al. 1999. Right frontal lobe slow frequency repetitive transcranial magnetic stimulation (SF r-TMS) is an effective treatment for depression: a case-control pilot study of safety and efficacy. J. Neurol. Neurosurg. Psychiatry 67:113–115.

Merabet, L.B., Theoret, H., Pascual-Leone, A. 2003. Transcranial magnetic stimulation as an investigative tool in the study of visual function. Optom. Vis. Sci. 80:356–368.

Mercuri, B., Wassermann, E.M., Ikoma, K., et al. 1997. Effects of transcranial electrical and magnetic stimulation on reciprocal inhibition in the human arm. Electroencephalogr. Clin. Neurophysiol. 105:87–93.

Merton, P.A., and Morton, H.B. 1980. Stimulation of cerebral cortex in intact human subject. Nature 285:227–228.

Meyer, B.-U., Kloten, H., Britton, T.C., et al. 1990. Technical approaches to hemisphere-selective transcranial magnetic brain stimulation. Electromyogr. Clin. Neurophysiol. 30:311–318.

Meyer, B.-U., Britton, T.C., Kloten, H., et al. 1991. Coil placement in magnetic brain stimulation related to skull and brain anatomy. Electroencephalogr. Clin. Neurophysiol. 81:38–46.

Meyer, B.-U., Werhahn, K., Rothwell, J.C., et al. 1994. Functional organisation of corticonuclear pathways to motoneurones of lower facial muscles in man. Exp. Brain Res. 101:465–472.

Meyer, B.-U., Liebsch, R., and Roricht, S. 1997. Tongue motor responses following transcranial magnetic stimulation of the motor cortex and proximal hypoglossal nerve in man. Electroencephalogr. Clin. Neurophysiol. 105:15–23.

Michelucci, R., Valzania, F., Passarelli, D., et al. 1994. Rapid-rate transcranial magnetic stimulation and hemispheric language dominance: usefulness and safety in epilepsy. Neurology 44:1697–1700.

Mills, K.R. 1988. Excitatory and inhibitory effects on human spinal motoneurones from magnetic brain stimulation. Neurosci. Lett. 94:297–302.

Mills, K.R., Boniface, S.J., and Schubert, M. 1991. The firing probability of single motor units following transcranial magnetic stimulation in healthy subjects and patients with neurological disease. In *Magnetic Motor Stimulation: Basic Principles and Clinical Experience (EEG Suppl 43)*, Eds. W.J. Levy, R.Q. Cracco, A.T. Barker, et al., pp. 100–110. New York: Elsevier.

Miranda, P.C., de Carvalho, M., Conceicao, I., et al. 1997. A new method for reproducible coil positioning in transcranial magnetic stimulation mapping. Electroencephalogr. Clin. Neurophysiol. 105:116–123.

Modugno, N., Nakamura, Y., MacKinnon, C.D., et al. 2001. Motor cortex excitability following short trains of repetitive magnetic stimuli. Exp. Brain Res. 140:453–459.

Mottaghy, F.M., Gangitano, M., Krause, B.J., et al. 2003. Chronometry of parietal and prefrontal activations in verbal working memory revealed by transcranial magnetic stimulation. Neuroimage 18:565–575.

Muellbacher, W., Mathis, J., and Hess, C.W. 1994. Electrophysiological assessment of central and peripheral motor routes to the lingual muscles. J. Neurol. Neurosurg. Psychiatry 57:309–315.

Müller, K., Homberg, V., and Lenard, H-G. 1991. Magnetic stimulation of motor cortex and nerve roots in children. Maturation of cortico-motoneuronal projections. Electroencephalogr. Clin. Neurophysiol. 81:63–70.

Munchau, A., Bloem, B.R., Thilo, K.V., et al. 2002. Repetitive transcranial magnetic stimulation for Tourette syndrome. Neurology 59:1789–1791.

Muri, R.M., Rivaud, S., Vermesch, A.I., et al. 1995. Effects of transcranial magnetic stimulation over the region of the supplementary motor area during sequences of memory-guided saccades. Exp. Brain Res. 104:163–166.

Muri, R.M., Vermesch, A.I., Rivaud, S., et al. 1996. Effects of single-pulse transcranial magnetic stimulation over the prefrontal and posterior parietal cortices during memory-guided saccades in humans. J. Neurophysiol. 76:2101–2106.

Nahas, Z., Kozel, F.A., Li, X., et al. 2003. Left prefrontal transcranial magnetic stimulation (TMS) treatment of depression in bipolar affective disorder: a pilot study of acute safety and efficacy. Bipolar Disord. 5:40–47.

Nakamura, H., Kitegawa, H., Hawaguchi, Y., et al. 1996. Direct and indirect activation of human corticospinal neurons by transcranial magnetic and electrical stimulation. Neurosci. Lett. 210:45–48.

Nakamura, H., Kitagawa, H., Kawaguchi, Y., et al. 1997. Intracortical facilitation and inhibition after transcranial magnetic stimulation in conscious humans. J. Physiol. 498:817–823.

Nakashima, K., Wang, Y., Shimoda, M., et al. 1995. Shortened silent period produced by magnetic cortical stimulation in patients with Parkinson's disease. J. Neurol. Sci. 130:209–214.

Nathan, S.S., Sinha, S.R., Gordon, B., et al. 1993. Determination of current density distributions generated by electrical stimulation of the human cerebral cortex. Electroencephalogr. Clin. Neurophysiol. 86:183–192.

Nolano, M., Guardascione, M.A., Amitrano L., 1997. Cortico-spinal pathways and inhibitory mechanisms in hepatic encephalopathy. Electroencephalogr. Clin. Neurophysiol. 105:72–78.

Odergren, T., Rimpilainene, I., and Borg, J. 1997. Sternocleidomastoid muscle responses to transcranial magnetic stimulation in patients with cervical dystonia. Electroencephalogr. Clin. Neurophysiol. 105:44–52.

Olivier, E., Edgley, S.A., Armand, J., et al. 1997. An electrophysiological study of the postnatal development of the corticospinal system in the macaque monkey. J. Neurosci. 17:267–276.

Pascual-Leone, A. 1991. Induction of speech arrest and counting arrest with rapid rate transcranial magnetic stimulation. Neurology 41:607–702.

Pascual-Leone, A., and Hallett, M. 1994. Induction of errors in a delayed response task by repetitive transcranial magnetic stimulation of the dorsolateral prefrontal cortex. NeuroReport 5:2517–2520.

Pascual-Leone, A., and Torres, F. 1993. Plasticity of the sensory–motor cortex representation of the reading finger in Braille readers. Brain 116:39–52.

Pascual-Leone, A., Gates, J.R., and Dhuna, A. 1991. Induction of speech arrest and counting errors with rapid-rate transcranial magnetic stimulation. Neurology 41:697–702.

Pascual-Leone, A., Cohen, L.G., Shotland, L.I. 1992a. No evidence of hearing loss in humans due to transcranial magnetic stimulation. Neurology 42:647–651.

Pascual-Leone, A., Brasil-Neto, J.P., Wassermann, E.M., et al. 1992b. Effects of focal transcranial magnetic stimulation on simple reaction time to visual, acoustic, and somatosensory stimuli. Brain 115:1045–1059.

Pascual-Leone, A., Cammarota, A., Wassermann, E.M. 1993a. Modulation of motor cortical outputs to the reading hand in braille readers. Ann. Neurol. 34:33–37.

Pascual-Leone, A., Houser, C.M., Reeves, K. 1993b. Safety of rapid-rate transcranial magnetic stimulation in normal volunteers. Electroencephalogr. Clin. Neurophysiol. 89:120–130.

Pascual-Leone, A., Gomez-Tortosa, E., Grafman, J. 1994a. Induction of visual extinction by rapid-rate transcranial magnetic stimulation of parietal lobe. Neurology 44:494–498.

Pascual-Leone, A., Valls-Sole, J., Brasil-Neto, J.P. 1994b. Akinesia in Parkinson's disease. I. Shortening of simple reaction time with focal, single-pulse transcranial magnetic stimulation. Neurology 44:884–891.

Pascual-Leone, A., Valls-Sole, J., Brasil-Neto, J.P. 1994c. Akinesia in Parkinson's disease. II. Effects of subthreshold repetitive transcranial motor cortex stimulation. Neurology 44:892–898.

Pascual-Leone, A., Valls-Sole, J., Wassermann, E.M., et al. 1994d. Responses to rapid-rate transcranial stimulation of the motor cortex. Brain 117:847–858.

Pascual-Leone, A., Catala, M.D., and Pascual, A.P. 1996a. Lateralized effect of rapid-rate transcranial magnetic stimulation of the prefrontal cortex on mood. Neurology 46:499–502.

Pascual-Leone, A., Peris, M., Tormos, J.M., et al. 1996b. Reorganization of human cortical motor output maps following traumatic forearm amputation. NeuroReport 7:2068–2070.

Pascual-Leone, A., Rubio, B., Pallardo, F., et al. 1996c. Beneficial effect of rapid-rate transcranial magnetic stimulation of the left dorsolateral prefrontal cortex in drug-resistant depression. Lancet 348:233–238.

Pascual-Leone, A., Wassermann, E.M., Grafman, J., et al. 1996d. The role of the dorsolateral prefrontal cortex in implicit procedural learning. Exp. Brain Res. 107:479–485.

Pelosi, L., Lamb, J., Grevitt, M., et al. 2002. Combined monitoring of motor and somatosensory evoked potentials in orthopaedic spinal surgery. Clin. Neurophysiol. 113:1082–1091.

Plassman, B.L., and Gandevia, S.C. 1989. Comparison of human motor cortical projections to abdominal muscles and intrinsic muscles of the hand. Exp. Brain Res. 78:301–308.

Plewnia, C., Lotze, M., Gerloff, C. 2003. Disinhibition of the contralateral motor cortex by low-frequency rTMS. Neuroreport 14:609–612.

Potts, G.F., Gugino, L.D., Leventon, M.E., et al. 1998. Visual hemifield mapping using transcranial magnetic stimulation coregistered with cortical surfaces derived from magnetic resonance images. J. Clin. Neurophysiol. 15:344–450.

Priori, A., Bertolasi, L., Rothwell, J.C., et al. 1993. Some saccadic eye movements can be delayed by transcranial magnetic stimulation of the cerebral cortex in man. Brain 116:355–367.

Priori, A., Berardelli, A., Inghilleri, M., et al. 1994a. Motor cortical inhibition and the dopaminergic system. Brain 117:317–323.

Priori, A., Berardelli, A., Inghilleri, M., et al. 1994b. Electromyographic silent period after transcranial brain stimulation in Huntington's disease. Mov. Disord. 9:178–182.

Priori, A., Berardelli, A., Mercuri, B., et al. 1995. The effect of hyperventilation on motor cortical inhibition in humans: a study of the electromyographic silent period evoked by transcranial brain stimulation. Electroencephalogr. Clin. Neurophysiol. 97:69–72.

Qayumi, K.A., Janusz, M.T., Jamieson, E.W., et al. 1997. Transcranial magnetic stimulation: use of motor evoked potentials in the evaluation of surgically induced spinal cord ischemia. J. Spinal Cord Med. 20:395–401.

Ravnborg, M., Blinkenberg, M., and Dahl, K. 1991. Standardization of facilitation of compound muscle action potentials evoked by magnetic stimulation of the cortex. Results in healthy volunteers and in patients with multiple sclerosis. Electroencephalogr. Clin. Neurophysiol. 81:195–201.

Reis, J., Tergau, F., Hamer, H.M., et al. 2002. Topiramate selectively decreases intracortical excitability in human motor cortex. Epilepsia 43:1149–1156.

Reutens, D.C., Macdonell, R.A.L., and Berkovic, S.F. 1993. The influence of changes in the intensity of magnetic stimulation on coil output. Muscle Nerve 16:1338–1341.

Rizzo, V., Quartarone, A., Bagnato, S., et al. 2001. Modification of cortical excitability induced by gabapentin: a study by transcranial magnetic stimulation. Neurol. Sci. 22:229–232.

Ro, T., Farne, A., Chang, E. 2003. Inhibition of return and the human frontal eye fields. Exp. Brain Res. 150:290–296.

Robinson, L.R., Jantra, P., and MacLean, I.C. 1988. Central motor conduction times using transcranial stimulation and F wave latencies. Muscle Nerve 11:174–180.

Rohde, V., Mayfrank, L., Weinzierl, M., et al. 2003. Focused high frequency repetitive transcranial magnetic stimulation for localisation of the unexposed primary motor cortex during brain tumour surgery. J. Neurol. Neurosurg. Psychiatry 74:1283–1287.

Roick, H., von Giesen, H.J., and Benecke R. 1993. On the origin of the postexcitatory inhibition seen after transcranial magnetic brain stimulation in awake human subjects. Exp. Brain Res. 94:489–498.

Rollnik, J.D., Huber, T.J., Mogk, H., et al. 2000. High frequency repetitive transcranial magnetic stimulation (rTMS) of the dorsolateral prefrontal cortex in schizophrenic patients. Neuroreport 11:4013–4015.

Rollnik, J.D., Wustefeld, S., Dauper, J., et al. 2002. Repetitive transcranial magnetic stimulation for the treatment of chronic pain—a pilot study. Eur. Neurol. 48:6–10.

Romeo, S., Gilio, F., Pedace, F., et al. 2000. Changes in the cortical silent period after repetitive magnetic stimulation of cortical motor areas. Exp. Brain Res. 135:504–510.

Romero, J.R., Anschel, D., Sparing, R., et al. 2002. Subthreshold low frequency repetitive transcranial magnetic stimulation selectively decreases facilitation in the motor cortex. Clin. Neurophysiol. 113:101–107.

Rosler, K.M., Hess, C.W., Heckmkann, R., et al. 1989a. Significance of shape and size of the stimulating coil in magnetic stimulation of the human motor cortex. Neurosci. Lett. 100:347–352.

Rosler, K.M., Hess, C.W., and Schmid, U.D. 1989b. Investigation of facial motor pathways by electrical and magnetic stimulation: sites and mechanisms of excitation. J. Neurol. Neurosurg. Psychiatry 52:1149–1156.

Rosler, K.M., Schmid, U.D., and Hess, C.W. 1991. Transcranial magnetic stimulation of the facial nerve: where is the actual excitation site? In *Magnetic Motor Stimulation: Basic Principles and Clinical Experience (EEG Suppl 43)*, Eds. W.J. Levy, R.Q. Cracco, A.T. Barker, et al., pp. 362–368. New York: Elsevier.

Rossini, P.M., Marciani, M.G., Caramia, M., et al. 1985. Nervous propagation along "central" motor pathways in intact man: characteristics of motor responses to bifocal and "unifocal" spine and scalp non-invasive stimulation. Electroencephalogr. Clin. Neurophysiol. 61:272–286.

Rossini, P.M., Paradiso, C., Zarola, F. 1991. Brain excitability and long latency muscular arm responses: non-invasive evaluation in healthy and parkinsonian subjects. Electroencephalogr. Clin. Neurophysiol. 81:454–465.

Roth, Y., Zangen, A., Hallett, M. 2002. A coil design for transcranial magnetic stimulation of deep brain regions. J. Clin. Neurophysiol. 19:361–370.

Rothwell, J.C. 1991. Physiological studies of electrical and magnetic stimulation of the human brain. In *Magnetic Motor Stimulation: Basic Principles and Clinical Experience (EEG Suppl 43)*, Eds. W.J. Levy, R.Q. Cracco, A.T. Barker, et al., pp. 29–35. New York: Elsevier.

Rothwell, J.C., Thompson, P.D., Day, B.L., et al. 1991. Stimulation of the human motor cortex through the scalp. Exp. Physiol. 76:159–200.

Rothwell, J., Burke, D., Hicks, R. 1994. Transcranial electrical stimulation of the motor cortex in man: further evidence for the site of activation. J. Physiol. (Lond.) 481:243–250.

Roux, F.E., Ibarrola, D., Lotterie, J.A., et al. 2001. Perimetric visual field and functional MRI correlation: implications for image-guided surgery in occipital brain tumours. J. Neurol. Neurosurg. Psychiatry 71:505–514.

Rudiak, D., and Marg, E. 1994. Finding the depth of magnetic brain stimulation: a re-evaluation. Electroencephalogr. Clin. Neurophysiol. 93:358–371.

Ruohonen, J., Ollikainen, M., Nikouline, V., et al. 2000. Coil design for real and sham transcranial magnetic stimulation. IEEE Trans. Biomed. Eng. 47:145–148.

Rutten, G.J., Ramsey, N.F., van Rijen, P.C., et al. 2002. FMRI-determined language lateralization in patients with unilateral and mixed language dominance according to the Wada test. Neuroimage 17:447–460.

Sabbah, P., Chassoux F., Leveque C., et al. 2003. Functional MR imaging in assessment of language dominance in epileptic patients. Neuroimage 18:460–467.

Sabsevitz, D.S., Swanson, S.J., Hammeke, T.A., et al. 2003. Use of preoperative functional neuroimaging to predict language deficits from epilepsy surgery. Neurology 60:1788–1792.

Sachdev, P.S., McBride, R., Loo, C.K., et al. 2001. Right versus left prefrontal transcranial magnetic stimulation for obsessive-compulsive disorder: a preliminary investigation. J. Clin. Psychiatry 62:981–984.

Sakkas, P., Mihalopoulou, P., Mourtzouhou, P., et al. 2003. Induction of mania by rTMS: report of two cases. Eur. Psychiatry 18:196–198.

Samii, A., Wassermann, E.M., Ikoma, K., et al. 1996. Characterization of post-exercise facilitation and depression of motor evoked potentials to transcranial magnetic stimulation. Neurology 46:1376–1382.

Samii, A., Canos, M., Ikoma, K., et al. 1997. Absence of facilitation or depression of motor evoked potentials after contralateral homologous muscle activation. Electroencephalogr. Clin. Neurophysiol. 105:241–245.

Sammut, R., Thickbroom, G.W., Wilson, S.A., et al. 1995. The origin of the soleus late response evoked by magnetic stimulation of human motor cortex. Electroencephalogr. Clin. Neurophysiol. 97:164–168.

Satow, T., Mima, T., Yamamoto, J., et al. 2003. Short-lasting impairment of tactile perception by 0.9 Hz-rTMS of the sensorimotor cortex. Neurology 60:1045–1047.

Saypol, J.M., Roth, B.J., Cohen, L.G., et al. 1991. A theoretical comparison of electric and magnetic stimulation of the brain. Ann. Biomed. Eng. 19:317–328.

Schadi, W., Dick, J.P., Sheard, A., et al. 1991. Central motor conduction studies in hereditary spastic paraplegia. J. Neurol. Neurosurg. Psychiatry 54:775–779.

Schonle, P.W., Isenberg, C., Crozier, T.A. 1989. Changes of transcranially evoked motor responses in man by midazolam, a short acting benzodiazepine. Neurosci. Lett. 101:321–324.

Schreiber, S., Dannon, P.N., Goshen, E., et al. 2002. Right prefrontal rTMS treatment for refractory auditory command hallucinations—a neuro-SPECT assisted case study. Psychiatry Res. 116:113–117.

Schulze-Bonhage, A., Scheufler, K., Zentner, J., et al. 1999. Safety of single and repetitive focal transcranial magnetic stimuli as assessed by intracranial EEG recordings in patients with partial epilepsy. J. Neurol. 246:914–919.

Seyal, M., Siddiqui, I., and Hundal N.S. 1997. Suppression of spatial localization of a cutaneous stimulus following transcranial magnetic pulse stimulation of the sensorimotor cortex. Electroencephalogr. Clin. Neurophysiol. 105:24–28.

Sheean, G.L., Murray, N.M., Rothwell, J.C., et al. 1997. An electrophysiological study of the mechanism of fatigue in multiple sclerosis. Brain 120:299–315.

Siebner, H.R., Mentschel, C., Auer, C., et al. 1999a. Repetitive transcranial magnetic stimulation has a beneficial effect on bradykinesia in Parkinson's disease. Neuroreport 10:589–594.

Siebner, H.R., Tormos, J.M., Ceballos-Baumann, A.O., et al. 1999b. Low-frequency repetitive transcranial magnetic stimulation of the motor cortex in writer's cramp. Neurology 52:529–537.

Siebner, H.R., Rossmeier, C., Mentschel, C., et al. 2000. Short-term motor improvement after sub-threshold 5-Hz repetitive transcranial magnetic stimulation of the primary motor hand area in Parkinson's disease. J. Neurol. Sci. 178:91–94.

Sommer, M., Ruge, D., Tergau, F., et al. 2002. Intracortical excitability in the hand motor representation in hand dystonia and blepharospasm. Mov. Disord. 17:1017–1025.

Sparing, R., Mottaghy, F.M., Hungs, M., et al. 2001. Repetitive transcranial magnetic stimulation effects on language function depend on the stimulation parameters. J. Clin. Neurophysiol. 18:326–330.

Speer, A.M., Kimbrell, T.A., Wassermann, E.M., et al. 2000. Opposite effects of high and low frequency rTMS on regional brain activity in depressed patients. Biol. Psychiatry 48:1133–1141.

Springer, J.A., Binder, J.R., Hammeke, T.A., et al. 1999. Language dominance in neurologically normal and epilepsy subjects: a functional MRI study. Brain 122:2033–2046.

Suihko, V. 2002. Modelling the response of scalp sensory receptors to transcranial electrical stimulation. Med. Biol. Eng. Comput. 40:395–401.

Szelenyi, A., Bueno de Camargo, A., Deletis, V. 2003. Neurophysiological evaluation of the corticospinal tract by D-wave recordings in young children. Childs Nerv. Syst. 19:30–34.

Taniguchi, M., Nadstawek, J., Langenbach, U., et al. 1993. Effects of four intravenous anesthetic agents on motor evoked potentials elicited by magnetic transcranial stimulation. Neurosurgery 33:407–415.

Taylor, J.L., Fogel, W., Day, B.L., et al. 1995. Ipsilateral cortical stimulation inhibited the long-latency response to stretch in the long finger flexors in humans. J. Physiol. (Lond.) 483:821–831.

Taylor, J.L., Butler, J.E., Allen, G.M., et al. 1996. Changes in motor cortical excitability during human muscle fatigue. J. Physiol. (Lond.) 490:519–528.

Tergau, F., Naumann, U., Paulus, W., et al. 1999. Low-frequency repetitive transcranial magnetic stimulation improves intractable epilepsy. Lancet 353:2209.

Theodore, W.H., Hunter, K., Chen, R., et al. 2002. Transcranial magnetic stimulation for the treatment of seizures: a controlled study. Neurology 59:560–562.

Thiry, A.J., and Deltenre, P.F. 1989. Neurophysiological assessment of the central motor pathway to the external urethral sphincter in man. Br. J. Urology 63:515–519.

Thompson, P.D., Day, B.L., Crockard, H.A. 1991. Intra-operative recording of motor tract potentials at the cervical medullary junctions following scalp electric and magnetic stimulation of the motor cortex. J. Neurol. Neurosurg. Psychiatry 54:618–623.

Tokimura, H., Tokimura, Y., Oliviero, A., et al. 1996. Speech-induced changes in corticospinal excitability. Ann. Neurol. 40:628–634.

Topka, H., Cohen, L.G., Cole, R.A., et al. 1991. Reorganization of corticospinal pathways following spinal cord injury. Neurology 41:1276–1283.

Topper, R., Foltys, H., Meister, I.G., et al. 2003. Repetitive transcranial magnetic stimulation of the parietal cortex transiently ameliorates phantom limb pain-like syndrome. Clin. Neurophysiol. 114:1521–1530.

Trenerry, M.R., Loring, D.W. 1995. Intracarotid amobarbital procedure. The Wada test. Neuroimag. Clin. North. Am 5:721–728.

Triggs, W.J., Macdonell, R.A.L., Cros, D. 1992. Motor inhibition and excitation are independent effects of magnetic cortical stimulation. Ann. Neurol. 32:345–351.

Triggs, W.J., Kiers, L., Cros, D., et al. 1993a. Facilitation of magnetic motor evoked potentials during the cortical stimulation silent period. Neurology 43:2615–2620.

Triggs, W.J., Cros, D., Macdonell, R.A.L. 1993b. Cortical and spinal motor excitability during the transcranial magnetic stimulation silent period in humans. Brain Res. 628:39–48.

Tsuji, T., Rothwell, J.C. 2002. Long lasting effects of rTMS and associated peripheral sensory input on MEPs, SEPs and transcortical reflex excitability in humans. J. Physiol. 540:367–376.

Tsumoto, T. 1992. Long-term potentiation and long-term depression in the neocortex. Prog. Neurobiol. 1992;39:209–228.

Urban, P.P., Beer, S., and Hopf, H.C. 1997. Cortico-bulbar fibers to orofacial muscles: recordings with enoral surface electrodes. Electroencephalogr. Clin. Neurophysiol. 105:8–14.

Valls-Sole, J., Alvarez, R., and Tolosa, E.S. 1994. Responses of the soleus muscle to transcranial magnetic stimulation. Electroencephalogr. Clin. Neurophysiol. 93:421–427.

Valzania, F., Strafella, A.P., Quatrale, R. 1997. Motor evoked responses to paired cortical magnetic stimulation in Parkinson's disease. Electroencephalogr. Clin. Neurophysiol. 105:37–43.

van Dongen, E.P., Schepens, M.A., Morshuis, W.J., et al. 2001. Thoracic and thoracoabdominal aortic aneurysm repair: use of evoked potential monitoring in 118 patients. J. Vasc. Surg. 34:1035–1040.

van Emde Boas, W. 1999. John A. Wada and the sodium Amytal test in the first (and last?) 50 years. J. Hist. Neurosci. 8:286–292.

Wassermann, E.M. 1998. Risk and safety of repetitive transcranial magnetic stimulation: report and suggested guidelines from the International Workshop on the Safety of Repetitive Transcranial Magnetic Stimulation, June 5–7, 1996. Electroencephalogr. Clin. Neurophysiol. 108:1–16.

Wassermann, E.M., Lisanby, S.H. 2001. Therapeutic application of repetitive transcranial magnetic stimulation: a review. Clin Neurophysiol. 112:1367–1377.

Wassermann, E.M., Fuhr, P., Cohen, L.G., et al. 1991. Effects of transcranial magnetic stimulation on ipsilateral muscles. Neurology 41:1795–1799.

Wassermann, E.M., McShane, L.M., Hallett, M., et al. 1992. Noninvasive mapping of muscle representations in human motor cortex. Electroencephalogr. Clin. Neurophysiol. 85:1–8.

Wassermann, E.M., Pascual-Leone, A., Valls-Sole, J. 1993. Topography of the inhibitory and excitatory responses to transcranial magnetic stimulation in a hand muscle. Electroencephalogr. Clin. Neurophysiol. 89:424–433.

Wassermann, E.M., Cohen, L.G., Flitman, S.S., et al. 1996a. Seizures in healthy people with repeated "safe" trains of transcranial magnetic stimulation. Lancet 347:825–826.

Wassermann, E.M., Grafman, J., Berry, C. 1996b. Use and safety of a new repetitive transcranial magnetic stimulator. Electroencephalogr. Clin. Neurophysiol. 101:412–417.

Wassermann, E.M., Samii, A., Mercuri, B. 1996c. Responses to paired transcranial magnetic stimuli in resting, active and recently activated muscles. Exp. Brain Res. 109:158–163.

Wilson, S.A., Lockwood, R.J., Thickbroom, G.W., et al. 1993a. The muscle silent period following transcranial magnetic cortical stimulation. J. Neurol. Sci. 114:216–222.

Wilson, S.A., Thickbroom, G.W., and Mastaglia, F.L. 1993b. Transcranial magnetic stimulation mapping of the motor cortex in normal subjects. The representation of two intrinsic hand muscles. J. Neurol. Sci. 118:134–144.

Wilson, S.A., Thickbroom, G.W., and Mastaglia, F.L. 1995. Comparison of the magnetically mapped corticomotor representation of a muscle at rest and during low-level voluntary contraction. Electroencephalogr. Clin. Neurophysiol. 97:246–250.

Wilson, S.A., Day, B.L., Thickbroom, G.W., et al. 1996. Spatial differences in the sites of direct and indirect activation of corticospinal neurones by magnetic stimulation. Electroencephalogr. Clin. Neurophysiol. 101:255–261.

Wu, T., Sommer, M., Tergau, F., et al. 2000. Lasting influence of repetitive transcranial magnetic stimulation on intracortical excitability in human subjects. Neurosci. Lett. 287:37–40.

Zarola, F., Caramia, M.D., Paradiso, C. 1989. Single fibre motor evoked potentials to brain, spinal roots and nerve stimulation. Comparisons of the "central" and "peripheral" response jitter to magnetic and electric stimuli. Brain Res. 495:217–224.

Zentner, J. 1991. Motor evoked potential monitoring during neurosurgical operations on the spinal cord. Neurosurg. Rev. 14:29–36.

Zentner, J., Neumuller, H. 1989. Modified impulse diminishes discomfort of transcranial electrical stimulation of the motor cortex. Electromyogr. Clin. Neurophysiol. 29:93–97.

Zentner, J., Kiss, I., and Ebner, A. 1989. Influence of anesthetics—nitrous oxide in particular—on electromyographic response evoked by transcranial electrical stimulation of the cortex. Neurosurgery 24:253–256.

Zhou, H.H., Kelly, P.J. 2001. Transcranial electrical motor evoked potential monitoring for brain tumor resection. Neurosurgery 49:1488–1489.

Zidar, J., Trontelj, J.V., and Mihelin, M. 1987. Percutaneous stimulation of human corticospinal tract: a single-fibre EMG study of individual motor unit response. Brain Res. 422:196–199.

Ziemann, U., Lonnecker, S., Steinhoff, B.J., et al. 1996a. Effects of antiepileptic drugs on motor cortex excitability in humans: a transcranial magnetic stimulation study. Ann. Neurol. 40:367–378.

Ziemann, U., Rothwell, J.C., and Ridding, M.C. 1996b. Interaction between intracortical inhibition and facilitation in human motor cortex. J. Physiol. (Lond.) 496:873–881.

46. Corticomuscular and Intermuscular Frequency Analysis: Physiological Principles and Applications in Disorders of the Motor System

Pascal Grosse and Peter Brown

General Considerations

A decade or so ago, it was first demonstrated in humans (Farmer et al., 1993; McLachlan and Leung, 1991) and other primates (Murthy and Fetz, 1992; Sanes and Donoghue, 1993) that the central nervous system synchronizes motor units. Nevertheless, the fact that muscle discharge tends to be rhythmic had already been demonstrated some 200 years earlier. In 1810, William Wollaston, using a precursor of the stethoscope, determined a rhythm in the β-band by comparing the pitch of the sound picked up over his muscles with that from a horse drawn carriage driven over the cobbled streets of London at different speeds (Wollaston, 1810). About a century later, the German neurophysiologist Hans Piper (Fig. 46.1) delineated a further modulation of motor unit discharges in the low γ-band at around 40 Hz (Piper, 1907).

Oscillatory drives from the central nervous system to muscle are best defined by frequency analysis techniques, and the application of these has led to new pathophysiological insights in the arena of movement disorders and may eventually contribute to routine clinical neurophysiological practice. Frequency analysis looks at synchrony within the different elements of the nervous system and is based on the cross-correlation between two signals such as electroencephalography (EEG) and EEG, EEG and electromyography (EMG), or EMG and EMG in the time and frequency domain. The principal measure of correlation between two signals in the frequency domain is coherence. It is mathematically bounded between 0 and 1, where 1 indicates a perfect linear relationship and 0 indicates that the two signals are not at all linearly related at a given frequency. Thus, oscillatory coupling between motor elements of the central nervous system and EMG discharge is most clearly measured as coherence. Additionally, frequency analysis provides an estimate of the phase difference and therefore temporal relation between the two signals.

Most studies on frequency analysis of the motor system have used one signal of cerebral origin [e.g., scalp EEG, MEG, electrocorticography (EcoG), or basal ganglia local field potential (LFPs)] and EMG as the second signal. However, in the routine neurophysiological setting, in which only scalp EEG is available, the signal can easily be marred by muscle artifact. Thus, it is fortunate that the same drive that leads to coherence between cortex and muscle also leads to coherence between the EMG signals of agonist muscles coactivated in the same task (Kilner et al., 1999). The principle that intermuscular coherence may give comparable information about descending cortical drives as cor-

ticomuscular coupling has been validated in disease (Grosse et al., 2003a). Nevertheless, it should be remembered that oscillatory presynaptic drives to spinal motoneurons other than those of cortical origin will also be reflected in the synchronization of motor unit discharge. Thus EMG-EMG coherence may give an additional insight into subcortical motor drives (Grosse and Brown, 2003; Sharott et al., 2003; Spauschus et al., 1999).

Physiological Drives to Muscle

The human central nervous system drives muscle discharges at a number of different frequencies, although the physiological function of these oscillations is far from clear (Brown et al., 2000; Farmer, 1998). One of the interests from the clinical point of view is that these different activities may be characteristic of functional activities in distinct circuits within the motor system. The different physiological oscillatory drives between the central nervous system and muscle are summarized in Table 46.1. The first is a low frequency drive at 2 to 3 Hz that has been, in retrospect, rather confusingly termed "common drive" (De Luca and Erim, 1994). This rhythm can be picked up during isometric contraction or slow movements. The site of its generation is unclear, but as it is preserved in patients with cortical or capsular strokes (Farmer et al., 1993), it is not likely to be related to the corticospinal system.

Oscillations in the 6- to 12-Hz range have been related to the pulsatile organization of slow movements at ~10 Hz (Vallbo and Wessberg, 1993)—identical to physiological action tremor—and to the central component of physiological postural tremor (Conway et al., 1995a). The olivary-cerebellar system has been suggested as a possible generator for the 6- to 12-Hz oscillations (Llinás and Pare, 1995). Consistent with this, some studies have failed to show a cortical correlate at ~10 Hz (Kilner et al., 1999; Mima et al., 2000). Nevertheless, the exclusivity of the subcortical generation of this drive has been challenged since other studies have detected significant corticomuscular coherence at this frequency (Raethjen et al., 2000; Salenius et al., 1997) indicative of some sensorimotor cortex involvement.

In contrast, there is general agreement that motor unit synchronization in the β (15-30 Hz) and low γ (30-60 Hz) bands is predominantly driven from the primary motor cortex, with less influential contributions possibly from supplementary motor and premotor cortices (Feige et al., 2000; Marsden et al., 2000). Coupling between primary motor cortex and muscle has been demonstrated by both magnetoen-

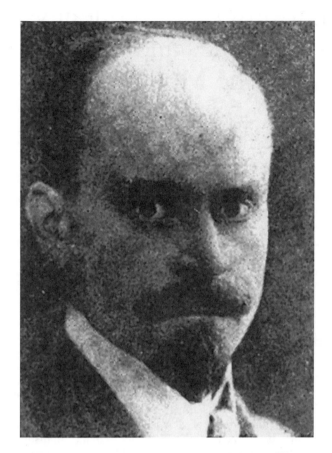

Figure 46.1. Hans Edmund Piper, German physiologist (1877–1915). Read biology, then research assistant at the Institute for Physiology, Berlin. In 1908 he became head of the Department of Physics at this institution. Initially he focused his research on embryology, his later work encompassed mostly physiological topics, in particular optics, the physiology of muscles and nerves, and a theory on electrical currents in the retina where he developed Piper's law. (From Abeßer, Elke/Schubert, Ernst. 1977. Das Berliner Physiologische Institut der Humboldt-Universität. 100 Jahre nach seiner Gründung. Wissenschaftliche Schriftenreihe der Humboldt-Universität zu Berlin, p. 29. Berlin.)

cephalography (MEG) (Brown et al., 1998b; Conway et al., 1995b; Salenius et al., 1997) and surface EEG (Halliday et al., 1998; Mima et al., 1998), although coherence in the γ-band is best seen with the former technique due to the low-pass filtering characteristics of the skull and scalp. Corticomuscular coherence seems ubiquitous and is even demonstrated by those muscles with small representation in the motor cortex such as the paraspinal and abdominal wall muscles (Murayama et al., 2001). The coherence in the β-band appears during weak tonic contraction and is abolished by movement, whereas that in the γ-band is more obvious in strong contractions and may persist during slow movements (Baker et al., 1997; Brown et al., 1998b; Kilner et al., 1999). EMG-EMG frequency analysis in the striated ocular muscles (Brown and Day, 1997; Spauschus et al., 1999) and respiratory muscles (Carr et al., 1994) have demonstrated high-frequency drives (>60 Hz) of brainstem origin. However, the brainstem may also be responsible for some low-frequency drives between 12 and 18 Hz, demonstrable during postural instability (Sharott et al., 2003) or the acoustic startle response (Grosse and Brown, 2003).

Methodology

Parameters of Frequency Analysis

Spectra are usually determined using the fast Fourier transform (FFT). Representative spectral examples are illustrated in Fig. 46.2. Data are divided into serial, usually nonoverlapping windows, transformed, and then averaged. The basic trade-off to be considered in the FFT approach is between frequency resolution and spectral variance. As the size of the windows decrease, the variance decreases, but the spectral resolution becomes poorer. Spectra derived from an FFT approach are defined pointwise, and the frequency difference between two adjacent points is given by the sampling rate divided by the FFT window size.

Alternatively, spectra can be determined using multivariate autoregressive (MAR) models. The latter have the desirable property of representing the characteristics of a signal

Table 46.1. Physiological oscillatory drives synchronizing motor units in humans

Frequency range [Hz]	Origin	Task in which manifest	Method	References
~2 ("common drive")	Unknown	Isometric contraction, slow movements	EMG-EMG	De Luca et al., 1982
6–12	Unknown	Isometric contraction, slow movements	MEG-EMG, EMG-EMG	Vallbo and Wessberg, 1993; Conway et al., 1995b; Marsden et al., 2001a
12–18	Brainstem	Postural instability, acoustic startle response	EMG-EMG	Sharott et al., 2003; Grosse and Brown, 2003
15–30	Motor cortex	Submaximal voluntary contraction	MEG-EMG EEG-EMG	Conway et al., 1995b; Halliday et al., 1998
30–60 ("Piper rhythm")	Motor cortex	Strong voluntary contraction, slow movements	MEG-EMG	Brown et al., 1998b
60–90	Brainstem	Eye movements	EMG-EMG	Brown and Day, 1997; Spauschus et al., 1999
60–100	Brainstem	Respiration	EMG-EMG	Carr et al., 1994

EMG, electromyogram; MEG, magnetoencephalogram.

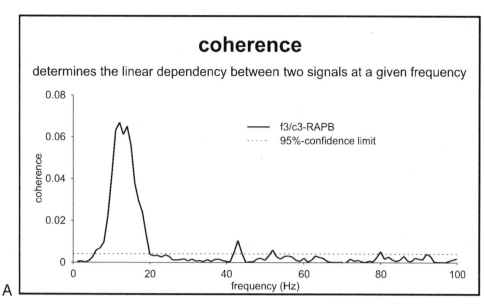

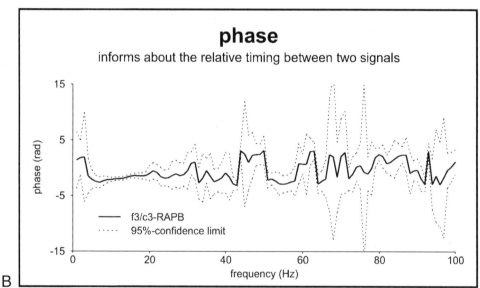

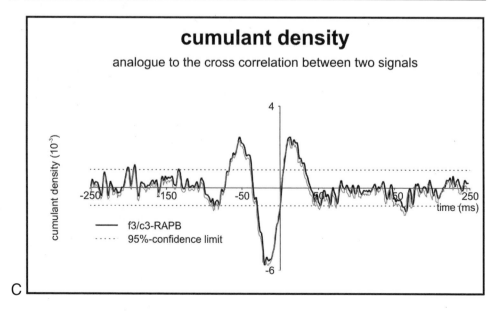

Figure 46.2. Examples of measures derived from autospectra and the cross-spectrum in a patient with cortical myoclonus. In this case the coherence (**A**) between the two signals (EEG at f3/c3 and electromyogram (EMG) from the right abductor pollicis brevis, RAPB) is above the 95%-confidence limit between 6 and 20 Hz with a peak at 12 Hz. The relevant phase relation (**B**) between 6 and 20 Hz shows very narrow 95% confidence limits where EEG (f3/c3) leads EMG by 15.7 ± 2.8 seconds (95% confidence limit). **C:** Cumulative density function *(black line)* shows a negative EEG deflection with a peak at ~15 msec before EMG. *Gray line* is the back-averaged EEG with EMG as the trigger, which is almost identical to the cumulative density function. The *dotted lines* are the 95% confidence limit of the cumulative density function. Record length is 275 seconds.

with just a few coefficients, which can then be used to calculate the relevant spectra. Because of this property, MAR models are often useful for modeling short data sets. In addition, MAR spectra are continuous functions of frequency, and thus avoid the spectral resolution problems encountered with the FFT approach. In practice, however, the calculation of true confidence limits is problematic, and the approximate limits that can be calculated are generally wider than their FFT counterparts (Cassidy and Brown, 2002). Also, the computation time for FFT methods is much faster than for MAR modeling. The MAR representation can be embedded into more complex nonstationary models, which are often necessary in the analysis of signals whose statistical properties change substantially over time.

Finally, coherence estimation can also be achieved using wavelet analysis. The major advantage of this technique is that, as opposed to FFT-based analysis, the data do not have to be stationary and that short, significant episodes of coherence can be detected. For a detailed introduction to this technique see Lachaux et al. (2001). Whichever technique is used, autospectra and cross-spectra may be derived, and from these, coherence and phase (Fig. 46.2).

The *coherence* between signals a and b at frequency l is an extension of Pearson's correlation coefficient and is defined as the absolute square of the cross-spectrum normalized by the autospectra:

$$|R_{ab}(\lambda)|^2 = \frac{|f_{ab}(\lambda)|^2}{f_{aa}(\lambda)\,f_{bb}(\lambda)}$$

In this equation, f_{aa}, f_{bb}, and f_{ab} give the values of the auto and cross-spectra as a function of frequency l.

Phase, $f_{ab}(l)$, is expressed mathematically as the argument of the $\phi_{ab}(\lambda) = \arg\{f_{ab}(\lambda)\}$ cross-spectrum.

The phase comprises two factors—the constant time lag given by the slope of the phase spectrum, when linear, and a constant phase shift, which is reflected in the intercept and is due to differences in the shapes of the signals (Mima and Hallett, 1999). A negative gradient indicates that the input/reference signal leads. To calculate the *temporal delay* between the two signals the following equation is used (where the phase is in radians):

$$\frac{\Delta\phi}{\Delta frequency x 2\pi}$$

The *cumulative density estimate*, equivalent to the cross-correlation between signals, is calculated from the inverse Fourier transform of the cross-spectrum. When the input/reference signal is EMG this cumulative density estimate resembles a back-averaged EEG record. For a general introduction to coherence readers are referred to Challis and Kitney (1991), and for a more detailed discussion of the measures derived from frequency analysis to Rosenberg et al. (1989) and Halliday et al. (1995) for FFT approaches and Cassidy and Brown (2002) for MAR approaches.

Problems of Recording and Interpretation

Some common problems of recording and interpretation specific to frequency analysis of the motor system merit closer consideration.

Signal Collection

The first problem is the signal itself and the question of how closely it matches the activity to be modeled. For example, the skull and scalp act as a low-pass filter so that scalp EEG may not reflect cortical activities at higher frequencies that are otherwise evident in EcoG or MEG recordings. Another factor is the focality of the cortical area sampled by scalp EEG. This can be increased by Laplacian derivations such as the current source density and Hjorth transformation. The latter also tend to give higher EEG-EMG coherence estimates, whereas common average references and balanced noncephalic references may give misleading results because of possible EMG contamination (Mima and Hallett, 1999). Surface EMG is best rectified prior to analysis to emphasize synchronizing influences (Myers et al., 2003). In addition, it is necessary to sample the signal at a rate that is greater than twice the low-pass filter setting so as to avoid aliasing and the identification of spurious spectral elements.

Coherence

Any artifact common between signals leads to high coherence values over the relevant frequency band. This is most commonly evident in the case of mains artifact, but any volume conduction of signals between electrodes or crosstalk within leads or amplifiers also leads to falsely inflated coherences. Such artifacts occur with zero phase delay, and are obvious in paradigms in which biologically related signals would be expected to demonstrate phase differences, such as when investigating the coupling between EEG and EMG.

EMG-EMG frequency analysis, in particular, may be limited by volume conduction between muscles. This can be ruled out if there is a constant phase lag between the two EMG signals in the range of significant coherence. Thus it is generally best to choose muscle pairs that are separated (e.g., forearm extensors and intrinsic hand muscles), where one would expect physiological coupling to involve a phase difference. Alternatively, volume conduction can be limited by appropriate leveling of both signals and analyzing the coherence between the resulting point processes (Fig. 46.3).

In addition, because coherence ranges between 0 and 1, its variance must be stabilized by transformation before statistical comparison. In practice, this makes relatively small difference to small coherences, but is important with coherences >0.6. The usual transform used is the arc hyperbolic tangent transformation (Rosenberg et al., 1989), which can then lead to transformed coherences greater than 1.

Phase

Two factors must be remembered when the temporal delay between two signals is calculated from the phase. First, low-pass filters, such as the skull and scalp, may introduce phase shifts that may underestimate real conduction delays (Lopes da Silva, 1989). Second, more than one coherent activity may overlap in the same frequency band, in which case the phase estimate is a mixture of the different phases. This may help explain why the temporal differences

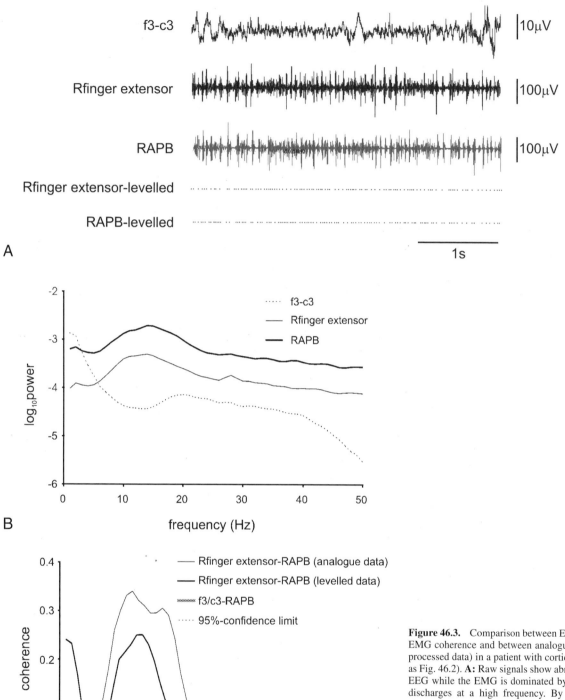

Figure 46.3. Comparison between EEG-EMG and EMG-EMG coherence and between analogue and leveled (point processed data) in a patient with cortical myoclonus (same as Fig. 46.2). **A:** Raw signals show abnormally slow waves EEG while the EMG is dominated by rhythmic burst-like discharges at a high frequency. By leveling these, discharges are transformed into a point process *(dots)*, which represents only those EMG bursts above a certain threshold, thus avoiding volume conduction. **B:** Autospectra of EEG and analogue EMG. **C:** EMG-EMG and EEG-EMG coherences exhibit the same peak at ~12 Hz, but EMG-EMG coherence is far higher and covers a broader range. With leveling EMG-EMG coherence drops slightly compared to the analogue signal but the pathological peak at ~12 Hz is preserved.

calculated between EEG or MEG and EMG are often shorter than those predicted from transcranial stimulation of the motor cortex (Brown et al., 1998b), as both efferent and afferent corticomuscular coupling may occur in overlapping frequency bands. Coexisting bidirectional oscillatory flows between neural networks can be separated through application of the directed transfer function (Kaminski and Blinowska, 1991; Mima et al., 2001a).

Frequency Analysis in Disorders of the Motor System

Pathological oscillatory drives manifest themselves either as a shift in frequency of the physiological coherence or as elevated coherence at a given frequency. In some disorders of the motor system frequency analysis has already identified some abnormal features of the oscillatory drive from the central nervous system to muscle (Table 46.2 and Fig. 46.4).

Cortical Myoclonus (Fig. 46.4A)

Frequency analysis shows the greatest potential as a diagnostic tool in cortical myoclonus. To date, the diagnosis of cortical myoclonus has relied on the detection of giant cortical sensory evoked potentials and/or of a cortical correlate upon back-averaging (Shibasaki and Kuroiwa, 1975). Frequency analysis, however, may have several advantages over the time domain technique of back-averaging as high-frequency myoclonic discharges do not preclude analysis and no arbitrary trigger level has to be chosen so that jitter is less. Thus, a cortical correlate related to myoclonic jerking was demonstrated in cumulative density estimates in eight patients in whom classical back-averaging failed to show a cortical correlate in five (Brown et al., 1999). Six of the patients in this study also showed exaggerated coherence. This report described patients with large amplitude jerks of low frequency typical of postanoxic myoclonus and progressive myoclonic epilepsy and ataxia. Recently, significant coherence between EEG and EMG has also been reported in the rhythmic high-frequency low-amplitude myoclonus typical of cortical tremor (Guerrini et al., 2001). Patients with cortical myoclonus also have exaggerated coherence between ipsilat-

eral muscles coactivated by myoclonic jerks (Brown et al., 1999). Thus, EMG-EMG coherence analysis has been shown to be a very useful surrogate marker of coherence between motor cortex and EMG (Grosse et al., 2003a) with, under some circumstances, a greater sensitivity and specificity than back-averaging and EEG-EMG frequency analysis.

Tremor (Fig. 46.4B)

Corticomuscular coherence in tremor with maximal coherence at the frequency of the tremor was first demonstrated in parkinsonian rest tremor using MEG (Volkmann et al., 1996). This finding has since been confirmed in studies of MEG-/EEG-EMG coherence (Hellwig et al., 2000; Salenius et al., 2002), but the time delays between cortex and muscle are very variable, suggestive of mixed efferent and afferent corticomuscular drives (Hellwig et al., 2000). Findings in essential and exaggerated physiological tremor have been more contradictory. A single channel MEG-EMG study failed to demonstrate corticomuscular coherence at tremor frequency in essential tremor (Halliday et al., 2000). In contrast, a recent EEG-EMG study with extensive head coverage showed coherence between the contralateral sensorimotor cortex and the tremulous arm (Hellwig et al., 2001). The same authors could not, however, demonstrate EEG-EMG coherence at tremor frequency in enhanced physiological postural tremor, although this is at odds with studies on physiological tremor using EMG-EMG coherence analysis in patients with mirror movement (Köster et al., 1998; Mayston et al., 2001) and with MEG-EMG coherence studies in physiological postural tremor (Marsden et al., 2001a).

Parkinson's Disease

Parkinson's disease is characterized by a reduction in the normal cortical oscillatory drive to muscles in the beta and gamma band. Instead, in untreated Parkinson's disease MEG-EMG coherence tends to be at ≤ 10 Hz. Such synchronization of muscle discharge at rest and action tremor frequencies leads to a suboptimal unfused pattern of muscle activation, thereby slowing the onset of voluntary actions and decreasing contraction strengths (Brown et al., 1998a). Treatment with L-dopa or therapeutic stimulation of the subthalamic nucleus re-

Table 46.2. Pathological oscillatory drives in humans

Disease	Frequency range (Hz)	Method	Comment	Reference
Dystonia	4–7	EMG-EMG	Manifest in cervical dystonia and some limb dystonia	Tijssen et al., 2000; Tijssen et al., 2002; Grosse et al., in press
Parkinson's disease	~3–6	MEG-EMG EEG-EMG EMG-EMG	When tremor is present	Volkmann et al., 1996; Hellwig et al., 2000; Raethjen et al., 2000
Essential tremor	8–12	EEG-EMG EMG-EMG		Hellwig et al., 2001; Raethjen et al., 2000
Orthostatic tremor	16	EMG-EMG		McAuley et al., 2000
Cortical myoclonus	10–175	EEG-EMG EMG-EMG		Brown et al., 1999; Grosse et al., 2003a
Myoclonus of corticobasal degeneration	0–60	EMG-EMG	Inflated EMG-EMG coherence in the absence of significant EEG-EMG coherence	Grosse et al., 2003b

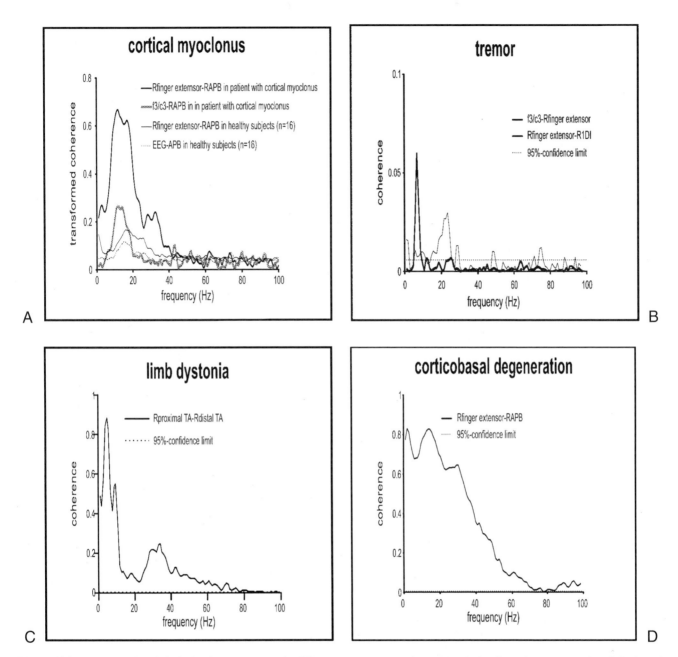

Figure 46.4. Examples of pathological coherence spectra in different movement disorders. **A:** In cortical myoclonus coherence is exaggerated compared to a sample of healthy subjects, note the shift of the physiological peak in the β-band to a lower frequency for both EEG-EMG and EMG-EMG-coherence spectra. **B:** Patient with generalized tremor with arms outstretched; note a discrete peak at the tremor frequency at ~7 Hz in EMG-EMG coherence, whereas in EEG-EMG there is no such peak; instead a peak appears in the β-band mirroring voluntary contraction. **C:** In dystonia EMG-EMG coherence in the lower leg characteristically discloses inflated coherence at ~5 Hz with other physiological peaks in the ~8–10 Hz β- and low γ-bands. **D:** In corticobasal degeneration with myoclonus there is an excessively inflated EMG-EMG coherence in the affected limb over a wide frequency range in the absence of any significant EEG-EMG coherence.

stores the normal cortical drive and enables cortical motor elements to oscillate at higher frequencies (Salenius et al., 2002). Muscles can then be activated at higher frequencies, improving bradykinesia. Motor cortical elements are also freer to form dynamic patterns of synchronized activity at frequencies above 20 Hz that might be important in higher-order aspects of motor control (Brown and Marsden, 1998).

Dystonia (Fig. 46.4C)

Patients with upper limb dystonia show abnormal coherence between extensor carpi radialis and flexor carpi radialis over 1 to 12 Hz and 14 to 32 Hz, leading to the suggestion that cortical drives may be responsible for the cocontraction of antagonistic muscles in this condition (Farmer et al.,

1998). In contrast, in writer's cramp the only abnormality was a discrete peak in EMG-EMG coherence at 11 to 12 Hz when tremor was present.

EMG-EMG frequency analysis has been used to distinguish idiopathic dystonic torticollis from voluntary torticollis in agonistic muscles. Patients with dystonic torticollis exhibit an abnormal synchronized drive in agonistic sternocleidomastoid and splenius capitis muscles between 4 and 7 Hz (Tijssen et al., 2000). The same common 4- to 7-Hz drive can also be found in complex cervical dystonia (Tijssen et al., 2002) and some forms of limb dystonia (Grosse et al., 2004).

Corticobasal Degeneration (Fig. 46.4D)

Patients with corticobasal degeneration with myoclonus can exhibit dramatically inflated EMG-EMG coherence in the absence of any evidence of a pathological corticospinal drive as determined by EEG-EMG coherence. This constellation raises the possibility of prominent involvement of the subcortical motor system in the generation of the myoclonus in corticobasal degeneration (Grosse et al., 2003b).

Stroke

Transcranial magnetic stimulation and imaging studies have suggested that the ipsilateral motor cortex may show compensatory activity in stroke patients after recovery. This hypothesis was explicitly tested in patients with long-standing subcortical lacunar, pure motor strokes, but no coherence between muscle and ipsilateral motor cortex could be found (Mima et al., 2001b). Coherence between EMG and contralateral EEG was smaller for distal but not proximal muscles on the affected side, in line with the view that pyramidal pathways are differently organized to proximal and distal muscles.

Functional Neurosurgery

In the future a specific clinical application of frequency analysis in patients with movement disorders treated with deep brain stimulation might be to identify the optimal electrode contact for stimulation. It has recently been shown that the degree of coherence between the local potential picked up by contacts on subthalamic nucleus macroelectrodes and EEG recorded over the midline scalp is correlated with the degree of clinical improvement derived from stimulation at that contact (Marsden et al., 2001b). A comparable finding for coherence between GPi and EEG in dystonia would be particularly useful as stimulation effects may be delayed for many months in this condition.

References

Baker, S.N., Olivier, E., and Lemon, R.N. 1997. Coherent oscillations in monkey motor cortex and hand muscle EMG show task-dependent modulation. J. Physiol. 501:225–241.

Brown, P. 2000. The Piper rhythm and related activities in man. Prog. Neurobiol. 60:97–108.

Brown, P., and Day, B.L. 1997. Eye acceleration during large horizontal saccades in man. Exp. Brain Res. 113:153–157.

Brown, P., and Marsden, C.D. 1998. What do the basal ganglia do? Lancet 351:1801–1804.

Brown, P., Corcos, D., and Rothwell, J.C. 1998a. Does parkinsonian action tremor contribute to muscle weakness in Parkinson's disease? Brain 120:401–408.

Brown, P., Salenius, S., Rothwell, J.C., et al. 1998b. Cortical correlate of the Piper rhythm in humans. J. Neurophysiol. 80:2911–2917.

Brown, P., Farmer, S.F., Halliday, D.M., et al. 1999. Coherent cortical and muscle discharge in cortical myoclonus. Brain 122:461–472.

Carr, L.J., Harrison, L.M., and Stephans, J.A. 1994. Evidence for bilateral innervation of certain homologous motoneurone pools in man. J. Physiol. 475:217–227.

Cassidy, M.J., and Brown, P. 2002. Hidden Markov based autoregressive analysis of stationary and non-stationary signals for coupling studies. J. Neurosci. Methods 116:35–53.

Challis, R.E., and Kitney, R.I. 1990. Biomedical signal processing (in four parts). Part 1: time-domain methods. Med. Biol. Eng. Comput. 28:509–524.

Challis, R.E., and Kitney, R.I. 1991. Biomedical signal processing (in four parts). Part 3: The power spectrum and coherence function. Med. Biol. Eng. Comput. 29:225–241.

Conway, B.A., Farmer, S.F., Halliday, D.M., et al. 1995a. On the relation between motor-unit discharge and physiological tremor. In *Alpha and Gamma Motor Systems*, Eds. A. Taylor, M.H. Gladden, R. Durbaba, pp. 596–598. New York: Plenum Press.

Conway, B.A., Halliday, D.M., Farmer, S.F., et al. 1995b. Synchronization between motor cortex and spinal motoneuronal pool during the performance of a maintained motor task in man. J. Physiol. 489:917–924.

De Luca, C.J., Erim, Z. 1994. Common drive of motor units in regulation of muscle force. Trends Neurosci. 17:299–305.

De Luca, C.J., LeFever, R.S., McCue, M.P., et al. 1982. Control scheme governing concurrently active human motor units during voluntary contractions. J. Physiol. 329:129–142.

Farmer, S.F. 1998. Rhythmicity, synchronization and binding in human and primate motor systems. J. Physiol. 509:3–14.

Farmer, S.F., Bremner, F.D., Halliday, D.M., et al. 1993. The frequency content of common synaptic inputs to motoneurons studies during isometric voluntary contraction in man. J. Physiol. 470:127–155.

Farmer, S.F., Sheean, G.L., Mayston, M.J., et al. 1998. Abnormal motor unit synchronization of antagonist muscles underlies pathological co-contraction in upper limb dystonia. Brain 121:801–814.

Feige, B., Aertsen, A., and Kristeva-Feige, R. 2000. Dynamic synchronisation between multiple cortical motor areas and muscle activity in phasic voluntary movements. J. Neurophysiol. 84:2622–2629.

Grosse, P., and Brown, P. 2003. The acoustic startle evokes bilaterally synchronous oscillatory EMG activity in the healthy human. J. Neurophysiol. 90:1654–1661.

Grosse, P., Guerrini, R., Parmiggiani, L., et al. 2003a. Abnormal corticomuscular and intermuscular coupling in high frequency rhythmic myoclonus. Brain 126:326–342.

Grosse, P., Kühn, A., Cordivari, C., et al. 2003b. Synchronising influences in the myoclonus of corticobasal degeneration. Mov. Disord. 18:1345–1350.

Grosse, P., Edwards, M., Tijssen, M.A.J., et al. In press. Patterns of EMG-EMG-coherence in dystonia. Mov. Disord. 19:758–769.

Guerrini, R., Bonanni, P., Patrignani, A., et al. 2001. Autosomal dominant cortical myoclonus and epilepsy (ADCME) with complex partial and generalized seizures: a newly recognized epilepsy syndrome with linkage to chromosome 2p11.1-q12.2. Brain 124:2459–2475.

Halliday, D.M., Rosenberg, J.R., Amjad, A.M., et al. 1995. A framework for the analysis of mixed time series/point process data—theory and application to the study of physiological tremor, single motor unit discharges and electromyograms. Prog. Biophys. Mol. Biol. 64:237–278.

Halliday, D.M., Conway, B.A., Farmer, S.F., et al. 1998. Using electroencephalography to study functional coupling between cortical activity and electromyograms during voluntary contractions in humans. Neurosci. Lett. 241:5–8.

Halliday, D.M., Conway, B.A., Farmer, S.F., et al. 2000. Coherence between low-frequency activation of the motor cortex and tremor in patients with essential tremor. Lancet 355:1149–1153.

Hellwig, B., Häußler, S., Lauk, M., et al. 2000. Tremor-correlated cortical activity detected by electroencephalography. Clin. Neurophysiol. 111:806–809.

Hellwig, B., Häußler, S., Schelter, B., et al. 2001. Tremor-correlated cortical activity in essential tremor. Lancet 357:519–523.

Kaminski, M., and Blinowska, K.J. 1991. A new method of the description of the information flow in the structures. Biol. Cybern. 65:203–210.

Kilner, J.M., Baker, S.N., Salenius, S., et al. 1999. Task-dependent modulation of 15–30 Hz coherence between rectified EMGs from human hand and forearm muscles. J. Physiol. 516:559–570.

Köster, B., Lauk, M., Timmer, J., et al. 1998. Central mechanisms in human enhanced physiological tremor. Neurosci. Lett. 241:135–138.

Lachaux, J., Lutz, A., Rudauf, D., et al. 2001. Estimating the time-course of coherence between single trial brain signals: an introduction to wavelet coherence. Neurophysiol. Clin. 32:157–174.

Llinàs, R., and Pare, D. 1995. Role of intrinsic neuronal oscillations and network ensembles in the genesis of normal and pathological tremor. In *Handbook of Tremor Disorders*, Eds. L.J. Findley and W.C. Koller, pp. 7–36. New York: Marcel Dekker.

Lopes da Silva, F., Pijn, J.P., and Boeijinga, P. 1989. Interdependence of EEG signals: linear vs nonlinear associations and the significance of time delays and phase shifts. Brain Topogr. 2:9–18.

Marsden, J.F., Werhahn, K.J., Ashby, P., et al. 2000 Organisation of cortical activities related to movement in humans. J. Neurosci. 20:2307–2314.

Marsden, J.F., Brown, P., and Salenius, S. 2001a. Involvement of the sensorimotor cortex in physiological force and action tremor. Neuroreport 12:1937–1941.

Marsden, J.F., Limousin-Dowsey, P., Ashby, P., et al. 2001b. Subthalamic nucleus, sensorimotor cortex and muscle interrelationships in Parkinson's disease. Brain 124:378–388.

Mayston, M.J., Harrison, L.M., Stephens, J.A., et al. 2001. Physiological tremor in human subjects with X-linked Kallmann's syndrome and mirror movements. J. Physiol. 530:551–563.

McAuley, J.H., Britton, T.C., Rothwell, J.C., et al. 2000. The timing of primary orthostatic tremor bursts has a task-specific plasticity. Brain 123:254–266.

McLachlan, R.S., and Leung, L. 1991. A movement-associated fast rolandic rhythm. J. Can. Sci. Neurol. 18:333–336.

Mima, T., and Hallett, M. 1999. Electroencephalographic analysis of cortico-muscular coherence: reference effect, volume conduction and generator mechanism. Clin. Neurophysiol. 110:1892–1899.

Mima, T., Gerloff, C., Steger, J., et al. 1998. Frequency-coding of motor control system-coherence and phase estimation between cortical rhythm and motoneuronal firing in humans. Soc. Neurosci. Abstr. 24:1768(abst).

Mima, T., Goldstein, S., Toma, K., et al. 2000. The lack of cortico-muscular coherence coupling of 8–12 Hz central component of physiological tremor. Mov. Disord. 15(suppl 3):78.

Mima, T., Matsuoka, T., and Hallett, M. 2001a. Information flow from the sensorimotor cortex to muscle in humans. Clin. Neurophysiol. 112:122–126.

Mima, T., Keiichiro, T., and Koshy, B. 2001b. Coherence between cortical and muscular activities after subcortical stroke. Stroke 32:2597–2601.

Murayama, N., Lin, Y.Y., Salenius, S., et al. 2001. Oscillatory interaction between human motor cortex and trunk muscles during isometric contraction. Neuroimage 14:1206–1213.

Murthy, V.N., and Fetz, E.E. 1992. Coherent 25- to 35-Hz oscillations in the sensorimotor cortex of awake behaving monkeys. Proc. Natl. Acad. Sci. USA 89:5670–5674.

Myers, L.J., Lowery, M., O'Malley, M., et al. 2003. Rectification and nonlinear pre-processing of EMG signals for cortico-muscular analysis. J. Neurosci. Methods 124:157–165.

Piper, H.E. 1907. Über den willkürlichen Muskeltetanus. Pflugers Gesamte Physiol. Menschen Tiere 119:301–338.

Raethjen, J., Lindemann, M., Dumplemann, M., et al. 2000. Cortical correlates of physiological tremor. Mov. Disord. 15(suppl 3):90.

Rosenberg, J.R., Amjad, A.M., Breeze, P., et al. 1989. The Fourier approach to the identification of functional coupling between neuronal spike trains. Prog. Biophys. Mol. Biol. 53:1–31.

Salenius, S., Portin, K., Kajola, M., et al. 1997. Cortical control of human motoneuron firing during isometric contraction. J. Neurophysiol. 77:3401–3405.

Salenius, S., Avikainen, S., Kaakkola, S., et al. 2002. Defective cortical drive to muscle in Parkinson's disease and its improvement with levodopa. Brain 125:491–500.

Sanes, J.N., and Donoghue, J.P. 1993. Oscillations in local field potentials of the primate motor cortex. Proc. Natl. Acad. Sci. USA 90:4470–4474.

Sharott, A., Marsden, J., and Brown, P. 2003. Primary orthostatic tremor is an exaggeration of a physiological response to instability. Mov. Disord. 18:195–199.

Shibasaki, H., and Kuroiwa, Y. 1975. Electroencephalographic correlates of myoclonus. Electroencephalogr. Clin. Neurophysiol. 39:455–463.

Spauschus, A., Marsden, J.F., Halliday, D.M., et al. 1999. The origin of ocular microtremor in man. Exp. Brain Res. 126:556–562.

Tijssen, M.A.J., Marsden, J.F., and Brown, P. 2000. Frequency analysis of EMG activity in patients with idiopathic torticollis. Brain 123:677–686.

Tijssen, M.A.J., Münchau, A., Marsden, J.F., et al. 2002. Descending control of muscles in patients with cervical dystonia. Mov. Disord. 17:493–500.

Vallbo, A.B., and Wessberg, J. 1993. Organisation of motor output in slow finger movements in man. J. Physiol. 469:673–691.

Volkmann, J., Joliot, M., Mogilner, A., et al. 1996. Central motor loop oscillations in parkinsonian resting tremor revealed by magnetoencephalography. Neurology 46:1359–1370.

Wollaston, W.H. 1810. On the duration of muscle action. Philos. Trans. R. Soc. Lond. 1–5.

47. Polygraphy

Anton Kamp, Gert Pfurtscheller, Günter Edlinger, and Fernando Lopes da Silva

Polygraphy denotes the simultaneous recording of several physiological and/or behavioral variables. The main reasons for the simultaneous recording of several variables are to obtain information on behavioral aspects and to differentiate artifacts in the electroencephalographic (EEG) data. These objectives usually do not require precise representation; in many instances, the relevant information concerns only the occurrence of a certain phenomenon or is easily obtained from clearly discernible characteristics of a variable. Therefore, most polygraphic data of interest in EEG studies can be obtained using simple recording methods that allow appreciable distortion of the original data. If, however, the polygraphic variables are of primary concern, then sophisticated and precise recording methods are necessary. In view of the techniques used and the interpretation of the recorded data, these methods go far beyond the simple polygraphic methodology commonly applied to EEG studies. This chapter discusses these simple methods and presents a number of examples of variables that are of interest in certain EEG studies. A classic survey of variables of interest in polygraphic studies and of corresponding recording methods can be found in *Manual of Psychophysiological Methods,* edited by Venables and Martin (1967a).

In practice, polygraphic recordings are made with an EEG apparatus; this may be of primary interest for determining the temporal relations between the EEG and the other signals, which reflect different physiological functions and/or behavioral states. Unfortunately, the frequency characteristics and the magnitude ranges of many signals of interest for polygraphic studies fall outside those provided by a conventional EEG recording system; moreover, they might not be recordable due to the electrical characteristics of the input circuit of the EEG recorder. Such signals, therefore, require special provisions, such as the use of specialized preamplifiers or input couplers to obtain an adaptation or a conversion; in this way, the recording of such signals can be carried out with the EEG apparatus. Many variables of interest in polygraphic studies, such as blood pressure, respiratory parameters, temperature, and electrodermal signals, vary slowly as a function of time; therefore, their recording requires highly sensitive universal DC amplifiers that are equipped with means of sensitivity control and adjustable high- and low-pass filters for selection of the appropriate frequency response. Modern EEG recorders have low sensitivity auxiliary input terminals that also permit direct current (DC) recording; these inputs can be used to record other signals of sufficiently large amplitude (for example, in Fig. 47.8, the traces indicated by EDG, STIM, BUTTON PRESS, and TIME CODE). When the EEG is used to record different physiological and/or behavioral variables simultaneously, employing separate recording systems, the time relations between the various types of signals must be preserved by using a form of time indexing or time marking on both recording media.

Cardiovascular Variables

Electrocardiogram and Heart Rate

There are several reasons for recording the electrocardiogram (ECG) simultaneously with the EEG. It may be desirable in specific cardio- or cerebrovascular studies. In most cases, however, the ECG recording is not intended to carry out a vascular study but only serves as an indicator of ECG artifacts in EEG records or as a general parameter of vegetative functions; in these latter circumstances, one is mainly interested in the heart rate. An ECG can be recorded perfectly using an EEG system because the electrical characteristics of its input circuit and the provisions commonly available for adjustment of frequency response and gain are adequate. The bandwidth required for appropriate ECG recording goes from 0.8 to 60 Hz; the recording sensitivity required is approximately 1 mV/cm using conventional ECG electrode placements. When the ECG electrodes are placed on the chest wall, a higher sensitivity may be necessary. The subject's behavioral activities might lead to artifacts in the ECG record, owing to muscular activity or electrode motion. The latter can be reduced significantly by using an appropriate type of electrode, such as cup electrodes with a jelly bridge between skin and electrode surface. Interference caused by electromyographic potentials can be minimized by choosing electrode positions carefully and lowering the high-frequency response of the recording system (20 Hz; -3 dB) in order to attenuate the high-frequency electromyogram (EMG) potentials. High-frequency filtering can be obtained by means of the EEG apparatus's adjustable high-frequency filters.

Heart rate recording is best carried out by using a series of pulses generated at the top of clearly distinguishable R waves of the ECG. If, however, owing to less favorable electrode positions, the R wave cannot be easily distinguished, extra signal processing must be applied. This processing may consist of high-pass filtering and/or the introduction of a refractory period, during which the instrument is insensitive. Commercially available heart frequency meters or heart rate counters usually have such provisions. Heart rate measurements may be given in terms of the number of beats over a certain period of time (heart rate, HR) or in terms of heart period (HP), the average interval between a number of successive heartbeats $\left(\overline{T} = \dfrac{1}{N} \sum_{n=1}^{n} T_{int}(n) \right)$. Because HR and

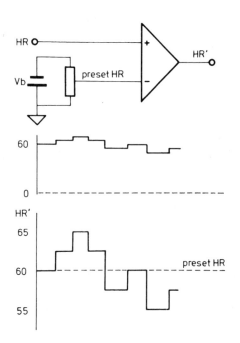

Figure 47.1. Method for recording instantaneous heart rate (HR); the momentary heart period (HP) value, transformed into HR, is plotted in relation to an adjustable preset mean HR value.

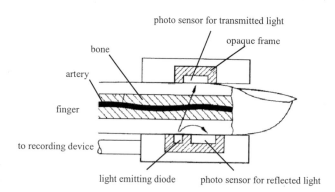

Figure 47.2. Principle of finger photoplethysmography for transmission and reflexion of light.

HP are reciprocal, the instrument, although calibrated in terms of heart rate, may have a meter deflection or another output signal proportional to T_{int} the interval between successive heartbeats. In the available instruments, heart rate is more commonly presented than heart period. In some applications of polygraphy, the main interest is not in the nominal HR, but rather in heart rate changes and the relation to other physiological, psychological, or behavioral variables. So that relatively small HR changes can be distinguished, the recording is best carried out with a preadjusted preset HR value. The model given in Fig. 47.1 demonstrates a simple method for subtracting a preset value from the HR meter's electrical output.

Plethysmography

Plethysmography is the measurement of the variations in organ or limb volume due to changes in the quantity of blood it contains. Because such volume changes are related to increased or decreased blood flow, plethysmographic methods can be used to obtain estimates of the mean blood flow rate and of pulsatile and transient flow changes. Plethysmography may be of interest in psychophysiological studies because mental processes and behavioral responses are often accompanied by changes in such cardiovascular parameters as blood flow, accompanied by measurable changes in limb volume. Continuous measurement of the latter is known as pulse volume plethysmography; under certain restricted conditions, an index of the blood flow rate can also be obtained in this way (Melrose et al., 1954). In most psychophysiological studies, however, the variable of interest relates to changes in blood volume and in blood volume pulses. The most common methods for measuring limb vol-

ume changes are pneumatic and photoelectric. Pneumatic methods are the more complicated and are not suited to psychophysiological studies. Therefore, although providing more precise information, they are much less frequently used in polygraphy. Figure 47.2 shows the principle of finger photoplethysmography. Two photo sensors measure the transmission and reflection of the light emitted from a light emitting diode. The fraction of transmitted light through the tissue and the fraction of reflected light from the tissue depend on the amount of blood in the tissue. Extensive discussions of the measuring principles, amplifier recorder requirements, and recorded waveforms have been provided by Lader (1967) (pneumatic plethysmography) and Weiman (1967) (photoplethysmography).

Impedance plethysmography of the thorax for impedance cardiography is the basis for noninvasive beat-to-beat monitoring of the stroke volume (Gratze et al., 1998). An electric current is introduced into the thorax and the corresponding voltage is measured. The ratio of voltage to current yields the impedance (Z) that varies (in a very simplified model) with the amount and distribution of blood in the thorax. Based on the ECG, the phonocardiogram (PCG) and impedance cardiogram (ICG), the stroke volume can be determined noninvasively (Fig. 47.3).

Blood Pressure

The catheter-manometer system is, at present, the fundamental method for continuous accurate measurement of the full arterial pressure waveform. It is, however, an invasive procedure and should be avoided unless the introduction of a catheter into an artery is absolutely necessary. The Riva-Rocci-Korotkoff method (using an upper arm cuff and a stethoscope) is noninvasive and commonly used, but it does not provide continuous blood pressure information. However, most automatic methods developed for determining blood pressure have been based primarily on the Riva-Rocci-Korotkoff method. For instance, Roy and Weiss (1962) described a technique for providing intermittent determinations of the systolic and diastolic blood pressure obtained over several heartbeats. Such systems have also become commercially available. The method indicated above, however, is sensitive to motion artifacts and not continuous.

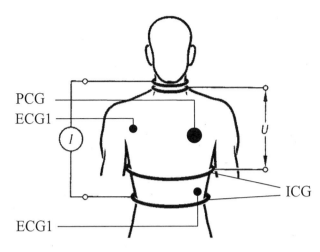

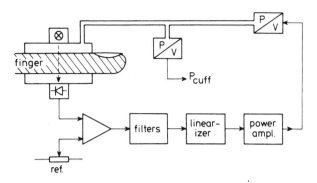

Figure 47.3. Principle of impedance cardiography. (Adapted from Gratze, G., Fortin, J., Holler, A., et al. 1998. A software package for non-invasive, real-time beat-to-beat monitoring of stroke volume, blood pressure, total peripheral resistance and for assessment of autonomic function. Comp. Biol. Med. 28:121–142.)

Figure 47.4. Block diagram of a system for noninvasive continuous recording of blood pressure based on the Penaz principle. (From Wesseling, K.H., van Bemmel, R.A., van Dieren, A., et al. 1978. Two methods for the assessment of hemodynamic parameters for epidemiology. Acta Cardiol. 33:84–87).

Penaz (1973) developed an important improvement in the noninvasive determination of blood pressure, using continuous measurement of the blood pressure in the finger. This method uses a finger cuff. By means of a servosystem the cuff pressure is maintained equal to the arterial pressure. This is achieved by minimizing arterial diameter changes using a photoelectric plethysmographic feedback method. The working principle is shown in the block diagram of Fig. 47.4. The further development and evaluation of methods based on this approach (Reeben and Epler, 1975; Wesseling et al., 1978) are of great interest to those interested in the continuous measurement and recording of beat-to-beat diastolic, systolic, and mean arterial pressure. This is indicated in Fig. 47.5 by the similarity between continuous blood pressure and curves recorded simultaneously by way of noninvasive and invasive methods.

The noninvasive blood pressure measurement was first applied during anesthesia (Wesseling et al., 1986) and was also used for long-term sleep monitoring in patients with systemic hypertension and sleep-related breathing disorders (Penzel et al., 1991a). The new system gives valuable results if the position of the finger cuff is carefully controlled. An example of blood pressure recordings combined with respiratory measurements is displayed in Fig. 47.6. A review of noninvasive continuous blood pressure measurements is found in Ruddel and Curio (1991) and more recently in Parati et al. (2003).

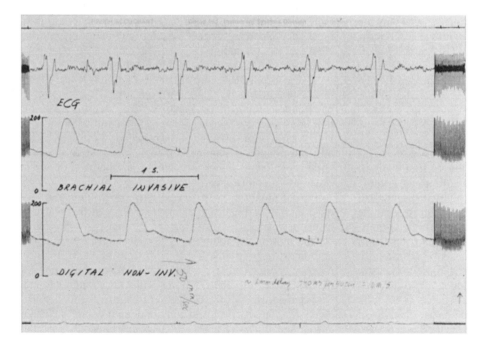

Figure 47.5. Example of a comparison of continuous recordings of blood pressure, simultaneously obtained by an invasive (intraarterial) and a noninvasive method. The latter was performed according to the method introduced by Penaz.

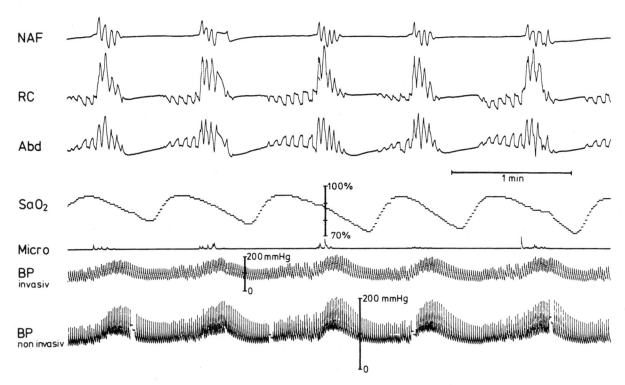

Figure 47.6. Recording of a patient with obstructive apneas and systemic hypertension. The trace of nasal airflow (NAF) shows complete cessation of respiratory flow, whereas rib cage (RC) and abdominal (Abd) movement show obstructive efforts. Noninvasive (FINA-PRES) and invasive BP were recorded in parallel. Sao₂, oxygen saturation; Micro, snoring noise. (From Penzel, T., Ducke, E., Peter, J.J., et al. 1991a. Non-invasive monitoring of blood pressure in a sleep laboratory. In *Non-invasive Continuous Blood Pressure Measurement,* Eds. H. Ruddel and I. Curio. Frankfurt am Maim: Peter Lang.)

The capacity for measuring acute and immediate changes in autonomic, EEG, and hemodynamic physiological variables during different sleep stages on a continuous basis has played an important role in enabling us to understand the interplay between changes in EEG and changes in circulatory variables and in autonomic neural functions. In this way the possibility of recording simultaneously with the EEG, heart rate (HR) variability, and blood pressure (BP), among other cardiovascular physiological variables, has advanced our understanding of mechanisms linking sleep and cardiovascular physiology (Murali et al., 2003).

Respiration

The polygraphic recording of respiration patterns is usually carried out to obtain information on frequency or changes in inhalation depth. Changes in thoracic volume due to respiratory movements are usually estimated in terms of changes in the perimeter of the chest; this can be measured easily using transducers working on the principle of a strain gauge. This type of respiration transducer, which is commercially available, consists of a tube with an inner diameter of a few millimeters; the tube is elastic and is filled with an electrically conductive liquid substance with measurable electrical resistance. The tube forms part of a belt strapped around the chest; changes in resistance resulting from changes in chest perimeter are

measured by means of the Wheatstone bridge circuit. The rather smooth slow respiration rhythm can be recorded with most EEGs without further measures; in case of insufficient frequency response of the apparatus, an alternating current (AC) voltage can be applied to the measuring bridge instead of a DC voltage. If respiration must be recorded from moving subjects, chest size changes not related to respiration can easily occur; in these cases other methods should be chosen.

A simple and easily implemented solution is to use a thermistor or equivalent temperature-sensitive device placed in the mouth and/or nostrils. Such a device works as a respiration transducer by signaling the characteristic differences in temperature of the inspired and expired air. With such methods, information is obtained on frequency and on depth of chest movements. Other methods should be used to obtain exact information concerning respiratory volume.

For information concerning respiratory volume and thoracic and abdominal diameter, variations can be measured by using elastic strips provided with strain gauges that encircle the thorax and abdomen at the level of the nipple and umbilicus, respectively. Using both measurements, the respiratory volume can be calculated. This method of spirometry determines the contributions of the chest and abdomen separately, then adds them together to mimic the total spirometric volume. As the chest and abdominal volumes change during breathing, changes in electrical impedance of the bands are related to changes in the spirometric volume contributions using a calibration and gain adjustment procedure. A combination of techniques is commonly used, namely the measurement of oral and nasal airflow and, in parallel, of abdominal and thoracic movements (Fig. 47.4). The best method to analyze the respiratory effort is the use of an esophageal pressure probe (Roberts and Davies, 1989).

Pulse oximetry is a noninvasive method to measure the arterial hemoglobin oxygen saturation (SaO_2). Continuous pulse and oxygen saturation measurements are obtained by ear, finger, or soft probes (Fig. 47.4 contains an example). The widely used pulse oximeter quantifies the SaO_2 as a percentage based on spectrophometric and photoelectric plethysmography (West et al., 1987). The SaO_2 measurement yields information about the effectiveness of respiration and is recommended for all types of sleep monitoring (Penzel et al., 1991b).

Electrodermal Activities

The variations of skin electrical properties in relation to psychological variables, commonly known as the galvanic skin response (GSR) or psychogalvanic response (PGR), consist of changes of the electrical conductivity of the skin or of the electrical skin potential, which can be measured by means of electrodes placed on the palms or the soles in reference to an electrode placed elsewhere, such as on the back of the hand.

For such measurements, the skin should be intact; when placing the electrodes, the skin must not be abraded. The skin potential can be recorded easily, but it is unstable and of little use; therefore, skin electrical conductance is much

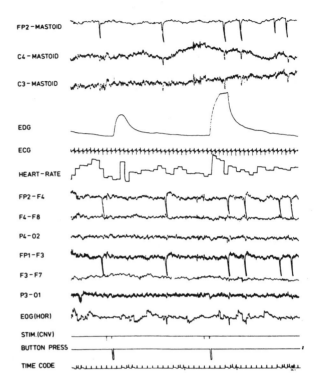

Figure 47.8.   Polygraphic recording obtained during a contingent negative variation (CNV) investigation carried out in a normal subject. EEG activities were recorded from three direct coupled CNV derivations (FP_2, C_4, and C_3 against linked mastoids) and six anteroposterior symmetrical derivations. Other variables recorded were electrodermogram (EDG), electrocardiogram (ECG), instantaneous heart rate, electro-oculogram horizontal eye movements [EOG(HOR)], CNV stimulus presentation [STIM.(CNV)], the button press, and a time code (1-second intervals).

more useful in this respect. It can be estimated by applying a constant voltage across two electrodes and by measuring the resulting electrical current. This is, of course, equivalent to estimating the skin electrical resistance by applying a constant current through the electrodes and measuring the voltage across the electrodes. Skin resistance can vary considerably among subjects, assuming values from kilo- to megaohms. Transient skin resistance responses related to sudden changes in psychological state are on the order of 100 ohms. In practice, it is preferable to measure skin electrical conductance by applying a constant voltage, instead of measuring resistance by applying a constant electrical current. The circuit of Fig. 47.7A illustrates a constant voltage measuring procedure. An example of electrodermal responses recorded during the performance of a contingent negative variation (CNV) paradigm from a normal subject is shown in Fig. 47.8. Classic extensive basic and practical information about electrodermal response recording can be found in the publications by Venables and Martin (1967b) and Montagu (1964) on skin resistance potential. Interesting applications of the GSR in psychophysiological studies have been published by Deschaumes-Molinaro et al. (1992) and Vernet-Maury et al. (1999).

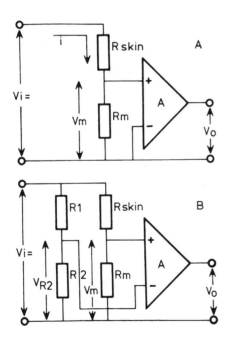

Figure 47.7.   A: Schematic diagram of a basic electronic circuit for the recording of electrodermal conductance using a constant voltage source. **B:** Bridge circuit for the recording of relatively small changes in electrodermal conductance.

Eye Movements

In various behavioral studies, particularly in sleep research for the recognition of sleep stages, eye movement recording (i.e., by means of the electro-oculogram, EOG) is necessary. Eye movement recording is also useful in EEG recording, for identifying eye movement artifacts and studying lambda waves. An example of the former is the recording of eye movement in relation to that of the CNV; in this case, it is possible either to reject the EEG epochs, where the amount of eye movement exceeds a certain predetermined threshold in order to carry out selective averaging (Papakostopoulos et al., 1973), or to average the EOG along with the CNV to obtain an indication of the reliability of the latter (see also Chapter 48, "Polysomnography"). Preferably, the method chosen for identifying eye movement artifacts will make use of the electrical field generated by the eyes. The EOG is, in general, easy to measure. The usual principle of EOG measurement is demonstrated by the model in Fig. 47.9. As a result of the corneoretinal standing potential (the cornea is positive relative to the fundus), a DC potential difference can be measured either between the pair of electrodes (EH) placed in a horizontal plane near the canthi of the eyes or between the two electrodes (EV) placed in a vertical plane, depending on the position of the eyeballs. Any change in eyeball position results in a corresponding change of these two potential differences. DC recording is necessary to measure exact eye positions, whereas AC recording suffices for determining changes in eye position.

To carry out a DC recording of the EOG, nonpolarizable electrodes must be used, and the drift of the electrodes' offset potential should be taken into account. To obtain sufficiently high recording sensitivity, the electrodes must be placed as close to the eye as possible. To record horizontal movements, the electrodes should be placed near the external canthus of each eye; for vertical movements, the electrodes should be placed closely above and below one or both eyes. The EOG measured in this way has an amplitude of about 20 µV per degree of eyeball rotation. A frequency response up to about 30 Hz is adequate to record the most rapid eye movements, and thus an EEG recording channel can be used without further provision [see, for example, trace EOG (HOR) in Fig. 47.8]. Other principles for monitoring eye movement in clinical EEG are the measurement of changes in impedance related to eye movements (Sullivan and Weltman, 1963) and use of a pressure transducer system (Winter and Kellenyi, 1971). In the latter system, a thin membrane covering one end of a tube held in a spectacle frame is adjusted to touch the closed eyelid lightly. A pressure transducer connected at the other end of the tube detects pressure changes from eye movements. Robinson (1963) describes eye movement recording systems that also provide information on exact eye position; eye position is determined from the voltage generated by an alternating magnetic field in a coil embedded in a scleral contact lens worn by the subject. A similar photoelectric device (Gauthier and Voile, 1975) consists of four small infrared detecting cells mounted on a light spectacle frame together with a miniature infrared (9,000 Å) emitting diode. This system, which preserves maximum vision field size, has a resolution less than 1 min of arc, a band width of 1,000 Hz, and 5% linearity of the maximum range. Currently, systems are available for recording and analysis of a wide range of eye movements, both saccadic and smooth pursuit movements, where these are measured using a scleral reflection technique (IRIS instrument) (Muir et al., 2003). Saccades are rapid eye movements that move the line of sight between successive points of fixation; they are among the best understood of movements, possessing dynamic properties that are easily measured (Leigh and Kennard, 2003). Saccades have become a popular means to study motor control and cognitive functions, particularly in conjunction with other techniques such as EEG, evoked potentials, functional imaging, and transcranial magnetic stimulation.

Muscle Activity and Body Movements

EMG Activity

Part of the electrical activity of muscles (EMG) can be recorded easily, by means of either surface electrodes placed on the surrounding skin or needle electrodes inserted into muscle. The frequency range of EMG potentials, particularly those recorded by means of intramuscular needles, goes far beyond the frequency response of most EEG recording systems. Even an EEG apparatus having an ink-jet writing system with a frequency response up to 1,000 Hz does not provide a faithful representation of EMG potentials. However, using a filter giving the highest possible EEG frequency response (usually 70–100 Hz), the recording of EMG activity in most instances adequately indicates the presence of muscular activity and may even provide a rough quantitative measure of the amount of such activity. In certain applications, the latter can be better obtained by passing the EMG potentials through a two-way rectifier, the output of which is integrated with a specified time window. In this way, a rectified smoothed EMG record is obtained. It is important to recognize that the recording of EMG along with EEG signals may be necessary for the interpretation of some specific features of the latter, particularly in those applications such as EEG-based brain-computer interfaces that rely on automated measurements of EEG features (Goncharova et al., 2003).

In behavioral studies, EMG activity is often used to monitor the onset of certain motor activities such as limb move-

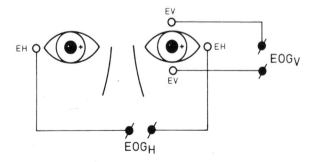

Figure 47.9. Positions of EOG electrodes for recording horizontal and vertical eye movements.

ments. Another way of determining limb movements and tremor (Oppel and Umbach, 1977) makes use of displacement transducers or accelerometers. A special form of tremor is the microtremor (microvibration), which is a phenomenon of the sensorimotor system that is modulated by central mechanisms (Burne et al., 1984). This microtremor is in the frequency range of 8 to 12 Hz (amplitudes of 1–10 μm) and can be recorded by an accelerometer fixed, e.g., at the wrist. The measurement range of such an accelerometer should be between ±5 g, such that the microtremor in the range of 10 mV/g can be recorded. Using accelerometry and EMG recordings of the forearm, the characteristics of physiological tremor have been studied (Elble, 2003). In addition to the microtremor, also ballistic movements can be measured with this technique.

Body Movements

The detection of limb or whole-body movements can be of interest in sleep studies. With a simple wrist actigraph, a discrimination between sleep and wakefulness is possible (Sadeh et al., 1989). Actigraphy has been found to be reliable for evaluating sleep patterns in patients with insomnia, for studying the effect of treatments designed to improve sleep, in the diagnosis of circadian rhythm disorders, including shift work (Ancoli-Israel et al., 2003). Such a wrist actigraph can be used, not only in the sleep laboratory, but also with outpatients to obtain a picture of the degree of sleep disturbances within, e.g., a 24-hour period (Penzel et al., 1991b). The recording of movements along with the EEG can also be important in differentiating authentic EEG activity from movement artifacts (Buchtal et al., 1973), which, on the basis of their waveforms and amplitude, cannot easily be identified as noncerebral. When monitoring movements of epileptic patients to determine the occurrence of seizures during the night, transducers indicating global body movements may be used. With this objective, conventional pressure or displacement transducers or other special methods developed for the detection of whole-body (van Nimwegen et al., 1975) or limb movements (Kripke et al., 1978) have been used.

Another method used for recording body movements is the static charge-sensitive bed, which consists of a mattress with two electrically active layers (Alihanka et al., 1981) with the use of filters, the ballistocardiogram, respiratory signals, and movement signals can be differentiated.

For movement quantification in epileptic seizures advanced video analysis methods can be applied (Li et al., 2002). Markers at landmark points are attached to the patient. Then EEG is acquired and the movement of the body parts is monitored using special cameras. Quantified motion trajectories of body parts can be extracted based on the fiducial markers. The trajectories reflect the motion pattern of patients during seizures yielding additional movement information that cannot be obtained from standard video EEG analysis.

Temperature

Temperature can be measured with sensors placed on the skin or with a rectal probe. Temperature measure-

ments are especially important in sleep studies. Detailed studies of rectal temperature recordings over 24 hours are reported by Stephan and Dorow (1985). Experiments with long-term isolation of subjects have revealed a relationship between the body temperature and the duration and stage of sleep (Zulley et al., 1981). To assess core temperature, for instance during monitoring under anesthesia, the recording of tympanic temperature may be carried out.

References

Alihanka, J., Vaahtoranta, K., and Saarikivi, J. 1981. A new method of long-term monitoring of the ballistocardiogram, heart rate, and respiration. Am. J. Physiol. 240:348–392.

Ancoli-Israel, S., Cole, R., Alessi, C., et al. 2003. The role of actigraphy in the study of sleep and circadian rhythms. Sleep 26(3):342–392.

Buchthal, F., Dahl, E., and Projaborg, W. 1973. Simultaneous recording of acceleration and brain waves. Electroencephalogr. Clin. Neurophysiol. 34:550–552.

Burne, J.A., Lippold, O.C., and Pryor, M. 1984. Proprioceptors and normal tremor. J. Physiol. 348:559–572.

Deschaumes-Molinaro, C., Dittmar, A., and Vernet-Maury, E. 1992. Autonomic nervous system response patterns correlate with mental imagery. Physiol. Behav. 51(5):1021–1027.

Elble, R.J. 2003. Characteristics of physiologic tremor in young and elderly adults. Clin. Neurophysiol. 114(4):624–635.

Gauthier, G.M., and Volle, M. 1975. Two-dimensional eye movement monitor for clinical and laboratory recordings. Electroencephalogr. Clin. Neurophysiol. 39:285–291.

Goncharova, I.I., McFarland, D.J., Vaughan, T.M., et al. 2003. EMG contamination of EEG: spectral and topographical characteristics. Clin. Neurophysiol. 114(9):1580–1593.

Gratze, G., Fortin, J., Holler, A., et al. 1998. A software package for non-invasive, real-time beat-to-beat monitoring of stroke volume, blood pressure, total peripheral resistance and for assessment of autonomic function. Comp. Biol. Med. 28:121–142.

Kripke, D.R., Mullaney, D.J., Messin, S., et al. 1978. Wrist actigraphic measures of sleep and rhythms. Electroencephalogr. Clin. Neurophysiol. 44:674–676.

Lader, M.H. 1967. Pneumatic plethysmography. In *A Manual of Psychophysiological Methods,* Eds. P.H. Venables and I. Martin, pp. 159–183. Amsterdam: North Holland.

Leigh, R.J., and Kennard, C. 2003. Using saccades as a research tool in the clinical neurosciences. Brain 127(3):460–477.

Li, Z., da Silva A.M., and Cunha, J.P.S. 2002. Movement quantification in epileptic seizures: a new approach to video-EEG analysis. IEEE Trans. Biomed. Eng. 49:565–573.

Melrose, D.G., Lynn, R.B., Rainbow, R.L.G., et al. 1954. A sensitive digital plethysmograph. Lancet 1:810–812.

Montagu, J.D. 1964. The psycho-galvanic reflex: a comparison of d.c. and a.c. methods of measurement. J. Psychosom. Res. 8:49–65.

Muir, S.R., MacAskill, M.R., Herron, D., et al. 2003. EMMA—an eye movement measurement and analysis system. Australas Phys. Eng. Sci. Med. 26(1):18–24.

Murali, N.S., Svatikova, A., and Somers, V.K. 2003. Cardiovascular physiology and sleep. Front Biosci. 8:s636–652.

Oppel, F., and Umbach, W.W. 1977. A quantitative measurement of tremor. Electroencephalogr. Clin. Neurophysiol. 43:885–888.

Papakostopoulos, D., Winter, A., and Newton, P. 1973. New techniques for the control of eye potential artifacts in multichannel CNV recordings. Electroencephalogr. Clin. Neurophysiol. 34:651–653.

Parati, G., Ongaro, G., Bilo, G., et al. 2003. Non-invasive beat-to-beat blood pressure monitoring: new developments. Blood Pressure Monitoring 8(1):31–36.

Penaz, J. 1973. Photoelectric measurement of blood pressure volume and flow in the finger. In Digest of the 10th International Conference on Medicine and Biological Engineering, Eds. R. Alben, W. Vogt, and W. Helbig, p. 104. Dresden.

Penzel, T., Ducke, E., Peter, J.J., et al. 1991a. Non-invasive monitoring of blood pressure in a sleep laboratory In *Non-invasive Continuous Blood Pressure Measurement,* Eds. H. Ruddel and I. Curio. Frankfurt am Main: Peter Lang.

Penzel, T., Stephan, K., Kubicki, S., et al. 1991b. Integrated sleep analysis, with emphasis on automatic methods. In *Epilepsy, Sleep and Sleep Deprivation,* 2nd ed. (Epilepsy Res. Suppl. 2), Eds. R. Degen and E.A. Roding, pp. 177–204. Amsterdam: Elsevier.

Reeben, V., and Epler, M. 1975. Detection and many-side use of signals from controlled counter pressure finger cuffs. Proc. Biocapt. Paris 1: 265–270.

Roberts, S., and Davies, W.L. 1989. Comparison of simple (slope based) and more complex (simple syntactic) algorithms for central apnoea detection. In *Sleep Research,* Eds. M.H. Chase, R. Lydic, and C. O'Connor, p. 398. Los Angeles: Brain Information Service/Brain Research Inst.

Robinson, D.A. 1963. A method of measuring eye movement using a scleral search coil in a magnetic field. IEEE Trans. Biomed. Eng. BME 10:137–145.

Roy, R., and Weiss, M. 1962. Automatic blood pressure indicator. IRE Trans. Biomed. Electron. 9:244–246.

Ruddel, H., and Curio, I. 1991. *Non-invasive Continuous Blood Pressure Measurement.* Frankfurt am Main: Peter Lang.

Sadeh, A.J., Alster, J., Urbach, D., et al. 1989. Actigraphically based automatic bedtime sleep-wake scoring: Validity and clinical applications. Ambulatory Monitoring 2:209–216.

Stephan, K., and Dorow, R. 1985. Circadian variations of core body temperature, performance and subjective ratings of fatigue in "morning" and "evening" types. In *Circadian Rhythms in the Central Nervous System,* Eds. P.A. Redfern et al., pp. 233–236. Weinheim: VCH.

Sullivan, G.H., and Weltman, G. 1963. Impedance oculograph—a new technique. J. Appl. Physiol. 18:215.

van Nimwegen, C.. Boter, J., and van Eijnsbergen, B. 1975. A method of detecting epileptic seizures. Epilepsia 16:689–692.

Venables, P.H., and Martin, I. (Eds.). 1967a. *A Manual of Psychophysiological Methods.* Amsterdam: North Holland.

Venables, P.H., and Martin, I. 1967b. Skin resistance and skin potential. In *A Manual of Psychophysiological Methods,* Eds. P.H. Venables and I. Manin, pp. 53–102. Amsterdam: North Holland.

Vernet-Maury, E., Alaoui-Ismaili, O., Dittmar, A., et al. 1999. Basic emotions induced by odorants: a new approach based on autonomic pattern results. J. Auton. Nerv. Syst. 15; 75(2–3):176–183.

Weiman, J. 1967. Photoplethysmography. In *A Manual of Psychophysiological Methods,* Eds. P.H. Venables and I. Martin, pp. 185–217. Amsterdam: North Holland.

Wesseling, K.H., van Bemmel, R.A., van Dieren, A., et al. 1978. Two methods for the assessment of hemodynamic parameters for epidemiology. Acta Cardiol. 33:84–87.

Wesseling, K.H., Settels, J.J., and de Wit, B. 1986. The measurement of continuous finger arterial pressure noninvasively in stationary subjects. In *Biological and Psychological Factors in Cardiovascular Disease,* Eds. T.H. Schmidt, T.M. Dembroski, and G. Blumchen, pp. 355–375. Berlin: Springer-Verlag.

West, P., George, C.F., and Kryger, M.H. 1987. Dynamic in vivo response characteristics of three oximeters: Hewlett-Packard 47201A, Biox III, and Nellcor N-100. Sleep 10:263–271.

Winter, A.L., and Kellenyi, L. 1971. Eye movement monitoring. Proc. Electrophysiol. Technol. Assoc. 18:121.

Zulley, J., Wever, R.A., and Aschoff, J. 1981. The dependence of onset and duration of sleep on the circadian rhythm of rectum temperature. Pflugers Arch. 391:314–318.

48. Polysomnography: Principles and Applications in Sleep and Arousal Disorders

Roger J. Broughton and Janet M. Mullington

This chapter discusses polygraphic (i.e., multiple event) recordings of the sleep-wake cycle and the various patterns encountered in normal subjects and in patients with sleep disorders. When polygraphic techniques are used to document sleep patterns, the studies have come to be referred to as polysomnographic recordings (Dement, 1976). Polysomnograms are most frequently performed overnight, but are sometimes obtained during daytime naps or continuous 24-hour monitoring. This chapter considers the personnel, space and equipment needs, recording techniques for the different polysomnographic variables, normal sleep staging and means of data presentation, age-related changes, dissociated or otherwise atypical sleep patterns, excessive daytime sleepiness, and sleep-waking patterns in clinical sleep disorders. Other descriptions of the fundamentals of polygraphic recording techniques can be found in Gastaut and Broughton (1972), McGregor et al. (1978), Guilleminault (1982), Howard (1985), and Broughton et al. (1985), as well as in polysomnographic atlases (Butkov, 1996; Shepard, 1991). The American Sleep Disorders Association (ASDA), subsequently renamed the American Academy of Sleep Medicine (AASM), has published several position papers in the journal *Sleep*, including practice parameters for the indications for polysomnography (ASDA, 1997). The AASM has a Web site *(http://www.aasmnet.org)* with links to helpful guidelines and resources for sleep medicine clinicians, scientists, technical personnel, and laboratory managers.

Technical Personnel

The selection of mature, motivated, and competent technologists is crucial. They must be both continuously present and vigilant through 8- to 10-hour overnight recording sessions, usually working alone and often with patients who are quite ill. The technologist is responsible for observing and describing in detail the nature and timing of such behavioral events as sleep terrors and nocturnal seizures and must be able to recognize and handle emergencies and perform cardiopulmonary resuscitation if necessary. The work is mentally and physically demanding. The technologist requires particularly strong support in this arduous task and should be treated as a professional in a demanding field of work.

Technologists chosen for performing diagnostic sleep recordings should preferably have full electroencephalography (EEG) technician training and registration and may also come from a respiratory therapy background. They should receive additional well-supervised training in the numerous specialized polygraphic studies, in visual sleep staging, and in techniques used in overnight patient care. In North America, a professional body, the Association of Polysomnographic Technologists, has developed standards of training and practice and devised examinations for registration.

For each recording session, the technologist should receive information and, when available, reading material about the patient's presenting symptoms, plus an explanation of any unusual variables to be recorded and of the reasons for these choices. The technologist should ensure that all equipment is functioning and should have backup equipment in case of technical problems in the middle of the night; indeed, he or she should be responsible for equipment maintenance in general. Technologists must be sensitive in interpersonal relations with patients, who sometimes feel quite uneasy with such studies. For all these reasons (ensuring quality of recordings, documenting behavior during sleep, assisting in medical emergencies), unattended polysomnography is considered unethical and unacceptable.

Equipment and Recording Room

Polysomnography is increasingly performed using commercial digital equipment developed specifically for this purpose. It is still often done using traditional ink-pen EEG equipment or, when variables such as body temperature or pressure data, which require direct current (DC) recording and large excursion pens, must be documented, using either a physiological polygraphic recorder or a hybrid apparatus having both types of preamplifiers and oscillographs. Both the apparatus and technologist should be housed in a room separate from that of the sleeping subject. It is very important that the subject's room be as homelike and uninstitutional as possible. A regular home bed, closet, and night stand should be present. The room should be soundproofed to avoid noise disturbance, include an intercommunication system for contact with the patient, and have rheostatically controlled lighting. Toilet facilities and preferably a shower should be nearby.

For overnight recordings, the subject comes to the preparation room about 1 hour prior to the usual hour of retiring, is shown around the recording suite to become familiar with the environment, has the electrodes attached, and then is put to bed; the lights are then turned off. It is important to note the time of "lights out" for later measurement of latency to sleep onset and other variables.

Polygraphic Variables

To visually stage sleep adequately, one must monitor at least one central and ipsilateral occipital referential (usually to an earlobe or mastoid) EEG linkages, an oculogram for rapid eye movements, and a submental electromyogram (EMG) for axial muscle tone, all of which are essential for sleep staging. These channels are supplemented by others required for diagnosis of specific sleep disorders and are several in type: monitoring further superficial EMGs for movement disorders in sleep (e.g., anterior tibialis, gastrocnemius, and wrist entensor muscles) or for respiratory effort (intercostal muscle EMGs); detection of respiratory problems by documenting upper airway air exchange (thermistors or thermocouples), monitors of chest or abdominal, respiratory movement (inductive plethysmography or strain gauges), and transcutaneous arterial oxygen level (oxygen saturation or oxygen tension); screening for cardiac arrhythmias or other abnormalities by electrocardiogram (ECG); and assessment of male impotence (nocturnal penile tumescence measures by strain gauges). Whatever the phenomena monitored, all electrode wires should be sufficiently long to allow free movement in bed and should be gathered together at the back of the head into a "pony tail" arrangement going to the connector box in order to avoid entanglement.

EEG Monitoring

The widely followed scoring manual of Rechtschaffen, Kales, and collaborators (1968) uses a single central EEG lead. However, because subjects may show a waking alpha rhythm localized to the occipital area that does not diffuse anteriorly to the central electrode, such a single central lead is often insufficient to separate wakefulness from stage 1 (drowsiness). The international 10–20 system (Jasper, 1958) should be used to position electrodes. Standard gold or nonpolarizable Ag/AgCl electrodes (Broughton et al., 1976) are attached with collodion-soaked gauze using compressed air to ensure good contact. For recordings exceeding 10 hours, it is helpful to use electrodes (such as the Montreal Neurological Institute type) with holes in the back through which further electrolyte paste may be added during the session. Particularly careful application of all electrodes is essential in polysomnography, because the recordings are very long and electrode reapplication during the night will lead to prolonged awakening and consequent disturbance of habitual sleep patterns. Electrode resistance should be kept below 5,000 ohms. Some patients, for instance those with possible nocturnal epileptic seizures, require a much larger than average number of scalp electrodes. Even when staging alone is required, it is good practice to put on bilateral central and occipital electrodes so that if electrode artifacts are a problem during sleep, the homologous contralateral electrode can be selected manually, without awakening the subject. It is self-evident that needle type electrodes must never be employed.

Electro-Oculogram Monitoring

Electro-oculogram (EOG) recordings can serve either to document the simple presence or absence of eye movements in sleep staging or to allow detailed analysis of separate horizontal and vertical eye movements. For routine recordings, the Rechtschaffen–Kales manual recommends referential recordings from each outer canthus to the ipsilateral ear. These derivations have the advantage of showing horizontal eye movements as out-of-phase potentials in the two channels, but have the disadvantage of containing much artifact in the

leads, especially in slow-wave sleep when the EEG reaches maximum amplitude. These circumstances also apply to the referential supraorbital and infraorbital derivations recommended for vertical eye movements. If, as in routine sleep recordings, only presence or absence of eye movements needs to be recorded, a bipolar linkage may be done from an electrode 1 cm lateral and 1 cm superior to one outer canthus to a second electrode 1 cm lateral and 1 cm inferior to the other outer canthus. Because all normal eye movements in sleep are conjugate, such a derivation doubles the EOG potential (the electrode toward which the eyes move becoming relatively positive, the other relatively negative) compared to referential recording. Any EEG pickup, originating largely in the frontal lobes, tends to be equipotential between these two periocular electrodes and to cancel out. A substantial signal-to-noise gain, therefore, is obtained at the relatively trivial trade-off of not recording the small proportion of oblique eye movements in the axis of the electrodes. A recent further improvement on this approach has been made (Häkkinen et al., 1993).

EOG electrodes should not be attached with collodion-soaked gauze, because collodion may damage the cornea. Moreover, collodion attachment is inflexible, causing discomfort and possible lifting off during facial movements in sleep. Use of sticky tape avoids these problems. Tape should be at least double the width of the electrode diameter and be cut so that it extends 4 to 5 mm around the electrode and usually 5 to 8 cm along the wire. A length of tape added at right angles over the end of the first tape helps anchor the latter. Best results have been obtained with micropore surgical tape that has maintained good contact for more than 48 hours of continuous recording. Normally, a high-frequency filter of 35 Hz is used to reduce EMG contamination, and a 0.3- to 0.5-second low-frequency filter (time constant) permits recording of both the slow rolling eye movements of drowsiness and the rapid ocular motion of REM sleep.

In special situations during which one wishes to document eye position, such as in the investigation of nocturnal eye movement disturbances in neurological patients, nonpolarizable electrodes and DC recordings must be used. Eye movements may also be recorded using strain gauges or infrared light-sensitive devices with an external source. Although the latter techniques are less sensitive to EEG, EMG, or ECG artifacts, the equipment is more cumbersome and is seldom used.

EMG Monitoring

Submental EMG is recorded using regular EEG electrodes placed submentally on the skin overlying the mylohyoid muscle. EMG electrodes can be secured with flexible sticky tape running along the electrode plus an anchoring tape. Three electrodes may be attached, one just behind the tip of the jaw and the other two more posteriorly and laterally. This arrangement allows the technologist to select the bipolar electrode combination giving the best tonic EMG. Some laboratories place pairs of electrodes on the tip of the jaw or on the side of the face over the masseter muscles to record axial muscle tone (Bliwise et al., 1974; Mouret et al., 1965).

The tonic EMG level in axial muscles usually decreases from wakefulness through stages 1, 2, 3, and 4 of non-rapid-eye-movement (REM) sleep, and is normally absent in REM sleep (Berger, 1961; Jacobson et al., 1964). There is, however, wide interindividual variability in resting chin EMG levels, which depends on the amount of subcutaneous adipose tissue, muscle tone, age, and other factors. In some subjects, tonic EMG activity is absent in all stages other than wakefulness and stage 1 drowsiness except, of course, during body movements. EMG recordings use a short time constant to reduce respiratory and other movement artifacts; minimal filtering permits passage of the higher frequency EMG activity. The amplification should be adjusted for good background levels in presleep drowsiness; 20 μV/cm is a typical setting.

Extra long leads are required to record limb EMGs, which are needed, for instance, to diagnose so-called periodic limb movements in sleep (nocturnal myoclonus) or the restless leg syndrome, to investigate movement disorders, to document the hand and arm gestures of REM sleep behavior disorder, and to record convulsive movements during nocturnal epileptic seizures.

Respiratory Monitoring

Measurements of upper airway exchange and of respiratory effort are routine in diagnostic polysomnography. They are essential to document spontaneous respiratory changes in sleep and to detect and assess various forms of sleep apnea and hypopnea, upper airway resistance syndrome, breathing problems in chronic obstructive pulmonary disease (COPD), and to investigate near-miss cases of sudden infant death syndrome (SIDS). For adults, syndrome definitions and measurement techniques are described for sleep disordered breathing in an AASM task force report (AASM, 1999).

It is important to distinguish among central, mixed, and obstructive sleep apnea. In central apnea, recurrent absence of central respiratory drive causes all mechanical respiratory efforts to cease, and no air exchange occurs at the mouth or nose. In obstructive apnea, respiratory efforts continue but no air exchange occurs due to collapse of the upper airway. Mixed apnea is defined as a central apnea evolving into an obstructive apnea. Differentiating the forms of apnea, therefore, requires monitoring both upper airway airflow and thoracoabdominal movement. Endoesophageal (intrathoracic) pressure recording may also be necessary to detect the partial obstructions of upper airway resistance syndrome that can exist in the absence of actual apneas or hypopneas.

By definition, an apneic episode is characterized by lack of upper airway exchange of 10 seconds or more. The frequency of apneic episodes is usually expressed as an apnea index consisting of the number of apneas per hour of sleep. An apnea-plus-hypopnea index or respiratory disturbance index (RDI), should also be calculated. Hypopneas are defined as reductions of respiratory movement by at least 50% of baseline in the absence of respiratory acceleration and in association with a detectable drop (3-4% or more) in transcutaneous oxygen level (usually measured as O_2 saturation) or with signs of transient EEG arousal. Partial obstructions are defined as a detectable reduction in upper airway airflow associated with detectable decreased O_2 saturation or with an increase in intrathoracic negative pressure monitored by esophageal probe. Episodes of significantly low arterial

oxygen levels occurring in the absence of apnea and hypopnea may be seen in sleep of patients with chronic obstructive pulmonary disease.

Respiratory monitoring, therefore, most frequently combines recordings of upper airway air exchange, thoracic and abdominal movement, and transcutaneous O_2 saturation measures. Differentiation of obstructive and mixed versus central apnea is facilitated by using an endoesophageal balloon to measure intrathoracic pressure changes and/or intercostal EMG recordings to measure respiratory effort. Highly specialized centers and fully trained personnel can determine hemodynamic changes by recording pressure in the radial artery, pulmonary artery, or other vessels. All measures of upper airway airflow and of chest and abdominal movement use a bandpass of DC to 0.5 Hz. Recordings of oxygen saturation, oxygen tension, $TcCO_2$, and systemic pulmonary artery or other pressure measurements all require DC recording.

Upper Airway Air Flow
Thermistor

Thermistor resistance fluctuations are induced by temperature changes of air passing in and out through the mouth and nostrils. They are useful only for monitoring respiratory rate. Thermistors are attached with sticky tape in front of one, or preferably both, nostrils, and also in front of the mouth to ensure pickup in both nasal and mouth breathers. A small plastic mask funneling upper airway air movement to a single sensor can be substituted, but may be less comfortable for the patient. A DC voltage source and Wheatstone bridge complete the circuit.

Thermocouple

Thermocouples are thermoelectric generators constructed of dissimilar metals (e.g., constantin and copper) that generate a potential in response to temperature change. Usually, two thermocouples are attached at the nostrils by nontraumatic clips and a third is held by sticky tape in front of the mouth. They can be connected directly to the plug-in box and used with AC voltage, provided the amplifier has a filter for frequencies <0.16 Hz, with a time constant of <1 second. Like thermistors, these detectors measure only respiratory rate.

Capnography

Capnography, using a CO_2 analyzer, is only rarely used to determine respiratory rate. It is employed, however, to document CO_2 retention in various sleep-related respiratory disorders, especially COPD and hypoventilation syndromes.

Pneumotachography

Pneumotachography is the only technique allowing direct quantification of ventilation during sleep. It can measure flow rate, tidal volume, and other respiratory variables. However, the technique involves a very uncomfortable airtight mask and a flow-to-pressure transducer system that offers considerable resistance to respiration. The technique is seldom used except with continuous positive airway pressure (CPAP) treatment of sleep apnea, since a mask is already employed. Many CPAP machines now have a flow transducer for this purpose, the flow pattern of which can be helpful to indicate airway resistance.

Nasal Flow

Nasal flow can be monitored using a simple cannula, as is used to deliver oxygen, attached to a pressure transducer. The method does not provide a quantifiable signal, but is considered to be more informative and reliable than thermistors and thermocouples by many clinicians. The primary concern in using this technology is that the signal may drop due to mouth breathing. However, a simple oral thermister/thermocouple can be used in addition, to resolve this problem.

Thoracoabdominal Movement

Inductive Plethysmography

Inductive plethysmography is currently a common means of monitoring respiratory movement. It is, in fact, an improved method of spirometry, which separates chest and abdominal movement and then adds them together, mimicking total spirometric volume. The sensors are two wire coils, one placed around the chest and the other around the abdomen. They are sometimes housed together in a fabric vest. A change in mean cross-sectional coil area produces a proportional variation in coil inductance, which is converted into a voltage change by a variable frequency oscillator. Careful presleep calibration is essential. There are three output channels: rib cage movement, abdominal movement, and total volume. Obstructive apnea is recorded as continued respiratory movement of both chest and abdomen with no significant change in the total volume signal (because the movements are paradoxical). In central apnea, all three signals are suppressed. Mixed apneas show a succession of the two patterns. Hypopneas can also be quantified using this apparatus.

Strain Gauge

Strain gauges are also widely used to monitor chest and abdominal movement. Most consist of a silicone rubber tube filled with a conductor, for instance mercury or packed graphite, the resistance of which varies with the core diameter. The tube is incorporated into belt-like structures, one of which is placed around the chest and another around the abdomen. Sticky tape should be applied at right angles to the belts so that the detectors will remain stable during nocturnal movement. As each inspiration stretches the tube, its core diameter decreases and resistance increases, and vice versa. A similar belt, incorporating a piezoelectric crystal of quartz or sapphire, and creating a current when distorted by inspiration or expiration, may also be used. These are more sensitive to movement artifact whether from general body movements or cardiac contractions (ballistocardiac effect).

Impedance Plethysmography

Impedance plethysmography is a seldom-used technique that involves measure of transthoracic and transabdominal impedance changes with respiration.

Magnetometry

Magnetometry involves measuring the magnetic field generated between two sides of a body by chest and abdominal movement. The technique uses ferrite wire coils held in rubber sleeves and attached to aluminum plates. The apparatus is quite cumbersome and the technique is rarely used.

Intrathoracic Pressure Monitoring

Monitoring using an endoesophageal pressure probe permits the currently most sensitive detection of heightened respiratory effort (measured as increases in intrathoracic negative pressure) to overcome increased upper airway resistance, whether or not the level reaches that of obstructive hypopnea or even full apnea. An endoesophageal tube is led through the nose with local anesthesia and then, when reaching the posterior pharynx, is swallowed with the probe lying about 5 cm above the esophageal-gastric junction. Sticky tape at the nose fixates the probe.

Snoring Monitors

Excessive inspiratory-expiratory snoring suggests reduced upper airway diameter, as well as hypotonia of the muscles of the soft palate and posterior and lateral pharyngeal walls. Bursts of loud guttural inspiratory snoring following quiescent periods are characteristic of obstructive sleep apnea. Such sounds may be detected by a room microphone and recorded directly on the polysomnogram tracing, as described by Lugaresi et al. (1978) and Weitzman et al. (1980). Krumpe and Cumminskey (1980) introduced an approach using a stethoscope head pickup taped to the lateral surface of the neck and connected to a microphone. Other systems use a vibration sensor, which involves a small rubber disk containing a piezocrystal and is taped to the patient's throat area, which vibrates during prerecording simulated snoring. In all approaches, the signal is appropriately filtered, rectified, and integrated before display.

Indirect Arterial Blood Gas Monitoring

To fully assess the severity of the various forms of sleep-related breathing impairment, arterial oxygen levels should be measured. Techniques are available to continuously detect both O_2 saturation (%) and O_2 tension (mm Hg, torr) with the results superimposed directly on the polysomnogram. Transcutaneous $TcCO_2$ can also be monitored and is useful for a number of pulmonary or muscular diseases (e.g., COPD, myotonic dystrophy).

Oxygen Saturation

A finger or ear probe is worn, which computes and displays oxygen saturation (O_2 sat) using an optical device involving computation of absorption of certain wavelengths of light. One part of the probe usually consists of two fiberoptic bundles enclosed in Teflon or, in other commercial equipment, contains light-emitting diodes. The other portion houses the light-sensing apparatus, the output of which is led to the oximeter. The system is standardized across a band of wavelengths and continuously compares the new intensity information with the stored standardized results and computes, displays, and graphs, using a DC channel, the oxygen saturation. The skin should be carefully cleaned with 70% isopropyl alcohol and may be arterialized by brisk rubbing before the monitoring device is placed on the finger or pinna. Continuous oxygen saturation monitoring has become essentially a routine procedure.

Oxygen Tension

Transcutaneous oxygen tension can also be measured. Oxygen diffuses across tissues to the skin surface, so that it is possible to detect arterial oxygen tension in millimeters of mercury or torr by means of an oxygen-sensitive electrode applied to the external skin surface. The chest wall is most often used. The electrode contains a thermistor-regulated heating resistor to ensure necessary skin arterialization, in combination with a Clarke-type oxygen electrode. The system must be calibrated before each use; sometimes the electrode site must be altered during the night to avoid heat blistering. With the proper precautions, this technique may quite accurately assess clinically significant hypoxemia in sleep disorder patients (Kapoor et al., 1984). Because of its cumbersome and at times uncomfortable nature, the technique is much less often used than O_2 saturation monitoring.

CO_2 Monitoring

Transcutaneous CO_2 measures may also be monitored indirectly by a number of commercial systems. In some systems pO_2 and CO_2 detections are performed by two parts of the same probe. Others combine a transcutaneous CO_2 electrode and another for O_2 saturation in the same physical probe. Using transcutaneous monitors, and especially for $Tcco_2$, it is good practice to obtain arterial blood gas measures when starting the study to calibrate the unit's values. In general, Tco_2 saturation devices are very reliable other than for very low levels (below about 50–60%), whereas O_2 and CO_2 tension devices are rather less accurate in predicting actual blood gas levels.

Systemic and Pulmonary Arterial Pressure

These highly specialized techniques should be used in carefully selected patients only when highly qualified and experienced technicians are available. These techniques are described by Lugaresi et al. (1978).

Electrocardiogram

It may be important to monitor the ECG for a number of clinical situations. Sleep apnea patients often have marked sinus arrhythmia or extra systoles. They may also show more serious abnormalities, such as prolonged asystolic episodes or atrial or ventricular fibrillation. Patients with nocturnal angina may show ST segment deviation. Those with sleep terrors, idiopathic central nervous system (CNS) hypersomnia, or psychophysiological (stress-related) insomnia may exhibit distinctive heart rate patterns across the night. In polysomnography, the usual ECG derivation uses two electrodes, one on each shoulder or side of the chest referenced right to left (modified lead I), or from right shoulder or chest to a lower electrode below the heart area or to a left leg site (modified lead II). Such an ECG is sufficient to monitor heart rate, extra systoles, and other arrhythmias. Because of differences in display speed and amplifier frequency response characteristics, this ECG is not directly comparable to a routine ECG. If PQRST complex abnormalities must be interpreted, the latter should be monitored independently.

Esophageal pH

Patients may have insomnia due to nocturnal reflux of acidic stomach contents into the lower esophagus, usually in relation to a hiatus hernia. If this phenomenon is suggested clinically, a pH probe is introduced nasally and swallowed to about 5 cm above the esophageal sphincter. Recording using the technique described by Orr et al. (1982) can con-

firm the diagnosis and facilitate decisions regarding appropriate therapy.

Penile Tumescence

Nocturnal penile tumescence (NPT) may be measured in males to help differentiate psychogenic from organic causes of impotence. Normal REM sleep-related erections persist in psychogenic cases, whereas patients with organic impotence experience no such erections. Karacan (1982) has described in detail the strain gauge technique used for calibrating, recording, and scoring NPT. Some laboratories supplement this with monitoring of the bulbocavernosus EMG activity. Penile tumescence monitoring requires particular care and sensitive handling by both physician and technologist.

Core Body Temperature

The 24-hour pattern of rectally measured body temperature, which approximates core body temperature, can help define several disorders of the circadian sleep-wake cycle and may be abnormal in various neurological lesions, such as loss of the circadian pattern resulting from damage to the suprachiasmatic nuclei. A number of commercially available recording devices exist, usually as part of an ambulant monitoring system.

Montages

It is important that montages be developed for diagnostic purposes; the montages are selectable according to the patient's presenting symptoms. A typical screening montage regularly used to detect and quantify both respiratory variables in sleep and leg motor abnormalities is provided in Table 48.1. The preamplifier time constants, filter positions, and usual gain settings are also provided. Such a basic mon-

Table 48.1. Ottawa General Hospital Screening Montage

Channel	Derivation	Time Constant (Hz)	Filter (Hz)	Gain (μV/mm)
1	Fp_2-A_1	0.3	70	7
2	C_4-A_1	0.3	70	7
3	O_2-A_1	0.3	70	7
4	Fp_1-A_2	0.3	70	7
5	C_3-A_2	0.3	70	7
6	O_1-A_2	0.1	70	7
7	Right eye A_2	0.1	70	10
8	Left eye A_1	0.1	70	10
9	Submental EMG	5.0	70	3
10	Precordial ECG	0.3	70	50–70
11	Right nostril[a]	0.1	15	~5
12	Left nostril[a]	0.1	15	~5
13	Mouth[a]	0.1	15	~5
14	Chest movement[b]	0.1	70	~5
15	Abd. movement[b]	0.1	15	~5
16	Right ant. tib. EMG	5.0	70	5
17	Left ant. tib. EMG	5.0	70	5
18	Transcutaneous O_2 sat or PO_2 (through DC amplifier direct to paper)			

[a]By thermocouple.
[b]By inductive plethysmography or strain gauge. Respiratory variables 11–15 adjusted by gain control for a 2–3 cm baseline excursion.
ECG, electrocardiogram; EMG, electromyogram.

tage is very useful and is easily modified to other purposes. In epileptic patients, the respiratory and peripheral EMG channels can be reduced and more ample EEG coverage is made, taking into account the location of abnormalities in waking EEGs. Patients with mainly motor abnormalities may have eight to ten EMGs recorded bilaterally over agonists and antagonists. In the investigation of patients with impotence, three or more DC channels can be dedicated to measure penile tumescence.

Sleep Staging

Basic Sleep Stages

Most laboratories use the guidelines set down in the manual for the visual scoring of sleep edited by Rechtschaffen and Kales (1968). Recording is generally done at a speed of 10 or sometimes 15 mm/sec providing scoring epochs of 30 or 20 seconds, respectively. The details of the EEG features during the different sleep stages are included in Chapter 10. This discussion reviews the main criteria of the different sleep stages and the other most often measured sleep variables. The EEG criteria mentioned must be met at referential central lead other than presence or absence of an alpha rhythm, which is best determined at an occipital lead.

An overnight recording usually includes periods of wakefulness and fluctuating drowsiness before definitive sleep onset (defined below). Polygraphic recordings of wakefulness normally contain an alpha rhythm (however, this may be blocked if the individual is looking about, and some persons lack this rhythm), the presence or absence of scanning eye movements, a sustained tonic submental EMG pattern, and the absence of EEG features of sleep. Similar patterns are seen in awakenings during the night. Only that portion after sleep onset is scored as nocturnal wakefulness; it is usually referred to as wakefulness after sleep onset (WASO) or stage 0.

Sleep onset is defined somewhat differently by various centers, depending mainly on whether or not their members agree with Johnson (1973) and others that behavioral sleep begins only once sigma waves (sleep spindles) appear, i.e., in stage 2. Others define nocturnal sleep onset as the moment at which the first continuous 90 seconds of stage 1 or 30 seconds of any other sleep stage are present. Sleep latency is defined as the time in minutes from lights out to one of these end points or to direct entry into REM sleep (sleep-onset REM period, SOREMP), when this abnormal pattern occurs.

The total sleep period (TSP) is the number of minutes from sleep onset to the final morning awakening. It includes wakefulness after sleep onset, stages 1, 2, 3, and 4 of non-REM sleep, REM sleep, and movement time, all of which are generally expressed both in minutes and as a TSP percentage. Various abnormal dissociated patterns may also occur and are discussed later.

WASO (Stage 0)

The polygraphic patterns seen in nocturnal wakefulness are similar to those of presleep wakefulness.

Stage 1

This stage may be usefully divided into substages 1A and 1B (Gastaut and Broughton, 1965; Valley and Broughton,

1983). In substage 1A, the alpha rhythm diffuses to anterior head regions, often slows (compared to presleep wakefulness) by 0.5 to 1.5 cycles/sec, and then fragments before disappearing. In a significant portion of subjects another pattern of alpha activity appears that is maximum frontally, symmetrical across the scalp, and 1 to 2 Hz slower than the posterior waking alpha rhythm (Broughton and Hasan, 1995; Hasan and Broughton, 1994). It has been referred to as "anterior slow alpha of drowsiness." When less than 50% of an epoch contains any rhythmic alpha activity and the EEG consists of medium amplitude mixed frequency (mainly theta) activity, sometimes with (negative) vertex sharp waves, it is scored as substage 1B. This substage is equivalent to stage 1 of the Rechtschaffen–Kales manual. Roth (1961) divides substage 1B into three further substages depending on EEG content and reactivity. During substages 1A and 1B, there may be slow rolling eye movements.

Stage 2

Stage 2 is characterized by one or more sleep spindles, K complexes, and less than 20% of the epoch containing delta waves to criterion (see below). Sleep spindles are 11.5 to 15.0 cycles/sec central bursts, which must last longer than 0.5 seconds to be scored. Although the Rechtschaffen–Kales scoring manual does not give an amplitude criterion for spindles, most visual scorers and automatic systems use 15 μV. K complexes consist of all or any two of three main components, i.e., a negative vertex sharp-wave maximum at the midline central electrode, a following negative slow-wave maximal frontally, and a sleep spindle maximal in the central regions. They must be of at least 0.5-second duration to be scored.

Stage 3

Stage 3 is scored when 20% to 50% of the epoch contains delta waves of 0.5 to 2.5 cycles/sec frequency and of 75 μV or greater peak-to-peak amplitude.

Stage 4

Stage 4 is scored when more than 50% of the epoch contains delta waves to these criteria.

REM Sleep

REM sleep contains medium amplitude mixed frequency, mainly theta and low-voltage delta EEG patterns associated with rapid eye movements either in bursts or in isolation, plus general absence of sustained axial muscle tone in the submental EMG. Bursts of so-called saw-toothed waves may occur, generally just before REM bursts (Berger and Oswald, 1962). The initial REM period (REMP) at times contains some low-voltage spindles. In REM sleep, and indeed in sleep in general, a distinction is often made between ongoing "tonic" events, such as the relatively desynchronized EEG and atonia of REM sleep, and brief "phasic" events, such as REM bursts, muscular twitching, and transitory cardiorespiratory irregularity. Phasic periods of low-amplitude rapid respiration are often seen normally accompanying REM bursts and may be incorrectly scored as abnormal respiratory events. The topic of phasic events in sleep is elaborated in Terzano et al. (1991).

Movement Time

Movement time (MT) is scored for each epoch in which more than 50% of the EEG is obscured by artifacts that make staging impossible. Such movement artifacts must be preceded and followed by epochs of definite EEG sleep. Movement time, therefore, is to be distinguished both from movement arousals with awakening and from movements during wakefulness. The artifacts impeding EEG analysis usually consist of high-amplitude patterns of tonic EMG over 45 to 50 µV or of preamplifier blocking.

The main stages of the sleep-wake cycles are illustrated in Fig. 48.1. The illustration shows typical wakefulness, stage 2, stage 4, and REM sleep. Falling asleep is normally progressive, from alert wakefulness with searching eye movements and a more or less blocked alpha rhythm (Fig. 48.2) through quiet wakefulness with sustained alpha rhythm (Fig. 48.3), increased amplitude, anterior diffusion,

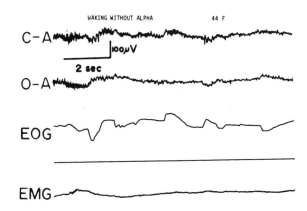

Figure 48.2. Wakefulness without alpha. This illustration and subsequent figures (Figs. 48.3 and 48.6) in the same narcoleptic subject show a non-REM sleep onset. In aroused wakefulness, as in this segment, there is little alpha, which is largely blocked, plus eye movements related to visual exploration of the environment and sustained submental muscle tone.

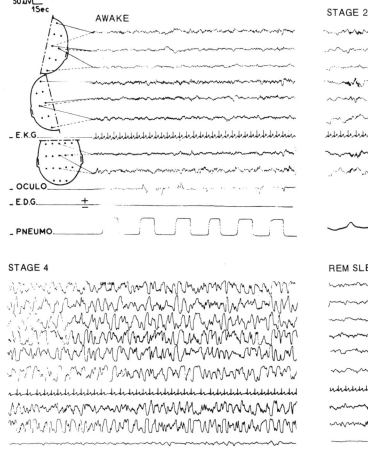

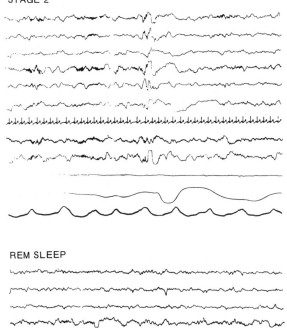

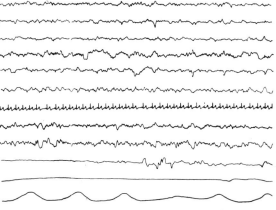

Figure 48.1. Sleep stages in humans. **Upper left:** The fragment shows an EEG of wakefulness, searching eye movements, tachycardia, tachypnea, and absence of electrodermographic (EDG) activity. **Upper right:** Stage 2 is illustrated, showing sleep spindles and a K complex associated with an EDG response. **Lower left:** Stage 4 shows continuous delta waves, car-

dioréspiratory slowing, and much EDG activity. **Lower right:** In rapid-eye-movement (REM) sleep there is mixed-frequency, medium-voltage EEG activity, a REM burst, cardiorespiratory irregularity, and reduction of EDG activity.

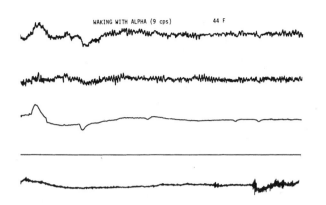

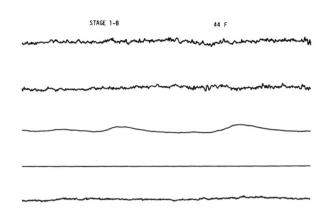

Figure 48.3. Wakefulness with alpha. With relaxed wakefulness and eye closure occurring before falling asleep, as in this segment, subjects show sustained alpha of waking frequency (9.0 cycles/sec in this subject).

Figure 48.5. In substage 1B, the alpha has fragmented and more or less disappeared and, as in this polygraphic strip, consists of mixed-frequency, medium-voltage EEG, and may include negative vertex sharp waves.

and at times slowing of the alpha rhythm in substage 1A (Fig. 48.4), loss of alpha rhythm and its replacement by mixed-frequency activity and slow rolling eye movements in substage 1B (Fig. 48.5), and the appearance of K complexes and spindles with entry into stage 2 sleep (Fig. 48.6). Epochs are initially scored individually by the above criteria and then are to some extent further restaged by contextual rules detailed in Rechtschaffen and Kales (1968). Such rules indicate, for instance, that if a single epoch of stage 1 is preceded and followed by epochs of stage 2, then this epoch lacking spindles or K complexes is nevertheless counted as stage 2 sleep. Similarly a stage 1 epoch lacking eye movements and axial muscle tone preceded and followed by REM sleep would be scored as REM sleep.

Other Sleep Parameters

Apart from conventional sleep stages, other variables are often measured that characterize sleep structure or "architecture" (cf. Williams et al., 1974). These include:

1. Delta latency: latency (minutes) from sleep onset to initial stage 3 patterns.

2. REM latency: latency (minutes) from sleep onset to initial epoch of REM sleep.
3. Number of stage shifts (a measure of sleep stability): often measured as number of shifts within or out of non-REM (NREM) sleep/100 min non-REM sleep, and similarly for REM sleep.
4. Number of awakenings: number of episodes after sleep onset of sustained waking patterns lasting 1 minute or longer.
5. Time in bed (TIB): time from recording onset (lights out) to termination of recording.
6. Total sleep time (TST): total minutes of stages 1, 2, 3, 4, REM, and MT, plus any abnormal or dissociated sleep states (some authors do not include stage 1 in TST).
7. Sleep efficiency: best expressed as the percentage of TSP spent asleep, i.e., TST/TSP. Some centers use TST/TIB, which makes no sense in many clinical conditions.
8. Number of REM periods: the number of REM periods (that is, REM sleep patterns separated by at least 15 minutes from any preceding and subsequent REM sleep). In cases of substantial sleep fragmentation, a

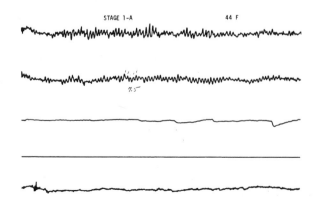

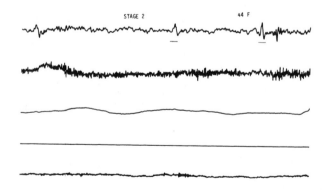

Figure 48.4. Substage 1A. In this stage, the alpha often increases in amplitude and becomes more diffuse over anterior head regions; its frequency may slow relative to wakefulness (here to 7.5 cycles/sec).

Figure 48.6. Stage 2. This stage contains sleep spindles, K complexes, and less than 20% delta activity. The recordings show K complexes and spindling. Note the more or less progressive decrease in muscle tone from Figs. 48.2 to 48.6.

REM period may include numerous epochs other than REM sleep (usually stage 1 or waking patterns).

9. REM sleep efficiency: because REM periods may be particularly fragmented, as in narcolepsy-cataplexy (Broughton and Mamelak, 1980; Montplaisir et al., 1978; Passouant et al., 1967), a REMP efficiency index is sometimes measured. It can be defined (Broughton and Mamelak, 1980) as the percentage of true REM epochs in an overall REM period; this measure reflects the percentage of brief transitions into wakefulness, stage 1, stage 2, or other patterns that are not REM sleep.

10. REM period duration: measured from the first to last epoch in each REMP.

11. REM cycle duration: the mean interval from the onset of consecutive REMPs across the night.

12. REM density: The percentage during REM sleep periods of "mini-epochs" (usually of 2 seconds' duration) containing one or more rapid eye movements.

13. Cyclic alternating pattern (CAP): throughout NREM sleep periods of an approximately 30- to 180-seconds cyclic alternation of quiescent sleep and arousals may occur, which shows a number of properties including alternation of a number of significant polysomnographic variables. The CAP rate can be measured as follows: (Total CAP time/Total NREM sleep time) × 100 (Terzano et al., 1985).

14. Microarousals: these consist of brief arousals typically lasting 5 to 10 seconds that do not lead to change of sleep stage. The clinical importance of such microarousals is clear as, even where there is no significant decrease in total sleep time or other traditional sleep measures, they may lead to daytime sleepiness (Bonnet, 1985, 1987). Scoring guidelines are available (ASDA, 1992).

In young and middle aged normal adults the main nocturnal sleep measures typically show that sleep latency is less than 20 minutes, total sleep time is 360 to 550 minutes, WASO is 5% to 8% of the TSP, stage 1 is 5% to 10%, stage 2 40% to 55%, stage 3 5% to 10%, stage 4 5% to 10%, and REM sleep 18% to 25%. There are, however, important age related changes.

Histograms

Histograms were initially done manually (Fig. 48.7) from scoring sheets but now have become a routine part of commercially available computer systems, which also permit the creation of a useful database. The histogram, patient data, and comparative normative data are appended to the polysomnographer's clinical report sent to the referring physician. Histograms permit rapid visual analysis of a night of sleep and stress the main organizational features of duration, continuity, cyclicity, and depth. Visual analysis of a typical normal young adult histogram (Fig. 48.7, center) demonstrates that slow-wave sleep is typically clustered in the first third of the night; that a sustained period of non-REM sleep occurs before the first REMP; that REMPs usually lengthen from the first to the second and the second to the third, but thereafter remain more or less constant in length; and that the last third of the night is passed mainly in REM and stage 2 sleep.

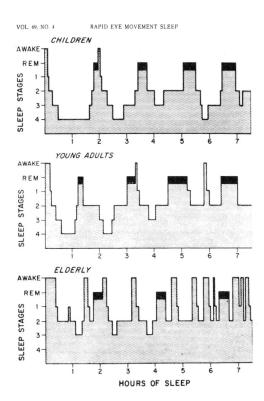

Figure 48.7. Histograms of normal sleep cycles. REM sleep *(darkened area)* occurs cyclically through the night at all stages. Slow-wave sleep is concentrated in the first third of the night and is greatest in childhood. With aging, stage shifts and awakenings increase, reflecting sleep fragmentation and a reduction of stages 3 and 4. (From Kales, A., and Kales, J. 1974. Recent findings in the diagnosis and treatment of disturbed sleep. N. Engl. J. Med. 209:487–499.)

Ontogeny of Normal Sleep

Marked changes occurring in normal sleep as a function of age require a summary description. Further details may be found in Roffwarg et al. (1966), Feinberg (1969a), Anders et al. (1971), Williams et al. (1974), Prinz et al. (1982), and in other sources referred to in those publications. There are age-dependent changes in total sleep amount and timing, as well as in distribution of the individual sleep stages. The normal overall temporal evolution of sleep is illustrated in Figure 48.8, from Kleitman (1963). It shows clearly that newborns sleep a great deal (mean about 17.5 hours per 24 hours) at intervals distributed more or less equally around the circadian day. In very early childhood, there is coalescence into a nocturnal sleep period plus several daytime naps. With early growth and development, the number of daytime naps decreases and the length of night sleep increases. The last nap given up (usually before the child must attend school throughout the day) is almost inevitably the early to midafternoon nap; sleep then becomes monophasic. Most adults maintain a monophasic pattern unless they belong to a siesta culture, have the opportunity to nap, do shift work, or have some other evident cause of polyphasic sleep. In older age (after retirement), napping again becomes common. The topic of napping and polyphasic sleep is comprehensively reviewed in Dinges and Broughton (1989) and in

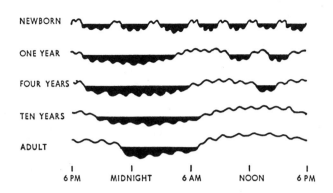

Figure 48.8. A schematic representation of the ontogenetic evolution from the polyphasic sleep pattern of the newborn infant to the monophasic sleep pattern of the late childhood and adulthood. The last nap given up is almost always in the afternoon. The secondary undulations represent the basic rest-activity periodicity of some 45 to 60 minutes in the newborn, which gradually lengthens to 85 to 110 minutes in the adult. *Black areas* represent sleep. (From Kleitman, N. 1963. *Sleep and Wakefulness.* Chicago: University of Chicago Press.)

Stampi (1992). This typical ontogenetic evolution of sleep as a whole also involves impressive changes in sleep architecture. Reviews of the changes in infancy and young childhood are found in Dittrichova (1969), Dreyfus-Brisac and Curzi-Dascalova (1975), Ellingson (1975), Dreyfus-Brisac (1979), and Hakamada et al. (1980).

In premature infants, complete sleep staging by adult criteria is impossible. The EEG shows periods of electrical silence replaced by high-amplitude mixed-frequency activity, a pattern called "tracé alternant." Using polygraphic variables of limb twitching, eye movement, cardiorespiratory irregularity, and other measures, one can separate "active sleep" (infantile REM sleep) from "quiet sleep" (equivalent to later non-REM sleep). The lack of EEG definition does not permit further substaging of quiet sleep. Based on such criteria, the REM percentage of total sleep is very high (40–50%) and the REM cycle period is very short (40–45 minutes). SOREMPs may occur.

Term neonates also show tracé alternant; as well, they lack sleep spindles and an alpha rhythm, making detailed staging impossible. Active sleep represents some 35% to 45% of total sleep time, with the remainder being quiet sleep. The REM cycle is 45 to 50 minutes in length. The tracé alternant pattern usually disappears by 2 to 3 months of age. Definite sleep spindles are regularly present from about 3 to 4 months (Metcalf, 1970; Ellingson, 1975) and spontaneous K complexes from 6 months onward (Metcalf et al., 1971). SOREMPs continue to occur up to the age of 3 to 4 months, especially at the time of nursing.

By 1 year of age, the infant's alpha rhythm and sleep spindles are fully developed (Lenard, 1970; Metcalf, 1970). The terms *REM sleep* and *NREM sleep*, rather than *active* and *quiet sleep*, are then used. It becomes possible to reliably divide non-REM sleep into stages 1 to 4 and to do complete sleep staging as in an adult record. Night sleep shows very high amounts of both slow-wave (stages 3 and 4) and of REM sleep, accounting for 30% to 40% and 30% to 45% of total sleep, respectively (Fig. 48.7, top). As well as high

amounts of REM sleep, the REM cycle remains rapid, with a period of 50 to 60 minutes. Nocturnal wakefulness is low. The first REM period may not occur for some 3 hours after sleep onset, apparently being suppressed by the high amounts of slow-wave sleep.

Through childhood to adolescence, the amounts of slow-wave and of REM sleep decrease progressively, so that correspondingly greater portions of the night sleep period consist of lighter NREM stages 2 and 1. Brief awakenings become more common with this lightening of sleep. The REM cycle period also decelerates progressively; it averages 60 to 75 minutes around age 6 and lengthens to the adult periodicity of 85 to 110 minutes by adolescence and young adulthood (Fig. 48.7). It does not significantly alter thereafter.

As exemplified by Figs. 48.9 and 48.10, diminution of deep slow-wave sleep and increase in wakefulness continues through the entire life span after 1 year of age. These changes also can be seen by comparing the typical sleep histograms of children, young adults, and the elderly, as shown in Fig. 48.7. In the elderly, slow-wave sleep is markedly suppressed. This has been shown to be due exclusively to a reduced slow-wave amplitude, rather than to a decrease in slow-wave abundance (Feinberg et al., 1968; Kahn and Fisher, 1969; Webb, 1982). The number of awakenings exceeding 1 minute's duration increases dramatically. Although the amount of REM sleep drops only slightly after age 85, normal REM latency shortens, indicating a "phase advance" of the ultradian REM cycle. This is probably secondary to weakened slow-wave sleep (SWS) in the first third of the night. Sleep also lightens behaviorally, as reflected in a lowered threshold for awakening stimuli. Finally, central and obstructive apneas, periodic leg movements, and restless leg activity all increase, any of which can further disrupt sleep. Many normal elderly persons perceive this normal sleep fragmentation and lightening as insomnia. If there is no ex-

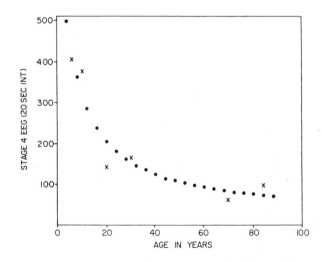

Figure 48.9. Stage 4 sleep as a function of age (total number of 20-second epochs). Stages 3 and 4 both decrease markedly with age. However, the decreases in the elderly have been shown to be related to reduced delta wave amplitude, rather than number. (From Feinberg, I., and Carlson V.R. 1968. Sleep variables as a function of age in man. Arch. Gen. Psychiatry 187:239–250.)

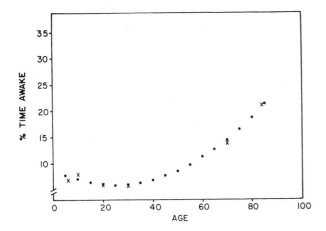

Figure 48.10. Wakefulness after sleep onset expressed as a percentage of time in bed as a function of age. Wakefulness increases progressively after about 40 years of age. (From Feinberg, I., and Carlson, V.R. 1968. Sleep variables as a function of age in man. Arch. Gen. Psychiatry 18:239–250.)

cessive daytime sleepiness, they can usually be reassured that their nighttime sleep is normal. The daytime naps taken by many elderly persons also show relatively low amounts of SWS and are more fragmented than those of younger subjects. All of these changes are markedly accentuated in presenile dementia of the Alzheimer's type (Prinz et al., 1982).

Further details on age- and sex-related sleep changes are available in the references provided above and in the Williams et al. (1974) volume on normative patterns, which has comprehensive sleep stage and other measures.

Dissociated or Otherwise Atypical Sleep Patterns

In a variety of situations (e.g., sleep deprivation, altered sleep habits, drug and drug withdrawal effects) and in certain sleep pathologies, a number of dissociated, abnormal, or atypical polygraphic sleep patterns may be observed. Some of these represent unusual combinations of otherwise apparently normal individual phenomena, such as a marked intrusion of the alpha rhythm upon the slow waves of stages 3 and 4 (so-called alpha–delta or alpha–non-REM sleep), or the appearance of marked sleep spindles in otherwise normal REM sleep after the first sleep cycle (REM–spindle sleep). Other phenomena consist of one of the components of a sleep state occurring in isolation, as when the REM sleep atonia appears subclinically in polygraphic recordings in the fully developed symptoms of cataplexy or sleep paralysis. Sleep stage timing may also become abnormal, as when a REM period occurs at the start of night sleep (SOREMP) in adulthood. The normal ultradian NREM/REM cyclicity may be altered or lost. Sleep may appear inappropriately in the daytime, either as sleep attacks, need for naps, brief "microsleep" episodes, partial sleep states, or unstable alertness with waxing and waning between various levels of alertness/sleepiness. These are only a few of the many possible documented sleep patterns.

Alpha-Delta Sleep

This pattern is characterized by the coexistence of alpha activity and delta waves in what otherwise would be normal stage 3 or 4 sleep. Although initially described in association with depression (Hauri and Hawkins, 1973), it has now been found in a number of conditions, all of which are associated subjectively with nonrestorative sleep. It appears to be particularly characteristic of the so-called fibrositis syndrome or fibromyalgia (Moldofsky et al., 1975). These authors have shown that the alpha-delta pattern can be induced in normal individuals, without awakening them, using auditory stimuli (Fig. 48.11). Such subjects will then complain of daytime aches and pains, feelings of being "washed out" in the morning, reduced pain threshold, and other features of the fibrositis syndrome.

REM-Spindle Sleep

In a number of conditions, the barriers between the features of NREM and REM sleep appear to break down, and various stages referred to as intermediate sleep or transitional sleep appear. A large number of subvarieties have been documented, particularly by Lairy, de Barros-Ferreira, and their colleagues in Paris. The most usual phenomenon is the appearance of substantial spindling in REM sleep throughout the night. When care is taken to identify this state in normal patients, it in fact ranges from 1% to 8% of total sleep time, as reported by Snyder (1966) (1–7%), Goldsteinas et al. (1969) (1.7%), de Barros-Ferreira and Mattos (1969) (7.7%), and Petre-Quadrans (1969) (7.3%). Although this sleep stage is often ignored, it nevertheless forms an important component of even normal sleep and is often as abundant as nocturnal wakefulness. It increases markedly in a number of sleep pathologies, including the daytime sleep of hypersomniacs (Schwartz, 1968) and in the night sleep patterns of schizophrenia (Ey et al., 1975; Koresko et al., 1963) and narcolepsy (de Barros-Ferreira and Lairy, 1976). The abundance of intermediate sleep seen in some narcoleptics is illustrated in Fig. 48.12.

REM Sleep Without REMs

In a number of conditions, long periods of EEG patterns identical to those of REM sleep, generally occurring when REM sleep would be expected, but lacking REM bursts, are recorded. These patterns often alternate with periods of stage 2 or 3 sleep. Their occurrence in various mental diseases has been described in detail by the Paris group (Ey et al., 1975; Lairy et al., 1968). Snyder (1968) has reported on "ambiguous" REM sleep in depression; Petre-Quadrans and Jouvet (1966) have noted similar patterns in mental retardation. The cause of the more or less selective loss of REM burst activity is unknown. Other causes include various forms of ophthalmoplegia.

REM Sleep Without Atonia

In some conditions, normal axial muscle atonia in REM sleep is not present. This appears to be particularly common in recordings of patients treated with tricyclic antidepressants (Guilleminault et al., 1976c), monoamine oxidase (MAO) inhibitors (Akindele et al., 1970), and phenothiazines. An example is given in Fig. 48.13. The situation

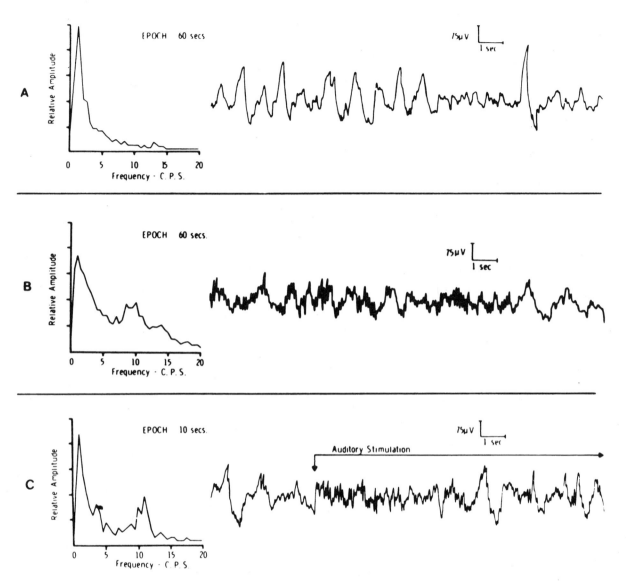

Figure 48.11. Alpha-delta sleep. **A:** Frequency spectra and raw EEG from a healthy 25-year-old subject. **B:** A 42-year-old fibrositis patient. **C:** A 21-year-old control during stage 4 sleep suppression by auditory stimulation. All three exhibit delta peaks at 1 cycle/sec. The fibrositis patient shows alpha-delta patterns in raw EEG and a 10 cycle/sec spectral peak.

The stage 4 suppressed control shows similar alpha-delta patterns with auditory stimulation. (From Moldofsky, H., Scarisbrick, R., England, R., et al. 1975. Musculoskeletal symptoms and non-REM sleep disturbances in patients with "fibrositis syndrome" and healthy subjects. Psychosom. Med. 37:341–351.)

implies selective pharmacological suppression of the mechanisms of REM atonia. Another condition characterized by absence of REM atonia is REM sleep behavior disorder.

REM Bursts During Non-REM Sleep

Normal and depressed persons taking clomipramine (Passouant et al., 1972) and narcoleptics being treated with that medication to suppress REM-based symptoms (Guilleminault et al., l976c) have at times been found to exhibit REM activity more or less throughout sleep (Fig. 48.14).

Isolated REM Atonia

The evidence is conclusive that cataplexy represents the selective triggering, during wakefulness and by emotional stimuli, of REM sleep atonia (Guilleminault, 1976) and that

sleep paralysis is the isolated appearance of REM atonia associated with full wakefulness either before entry into REM sleep or during awakenings from REM sleep (Hishikawa et al., 1968). In narcoleptic-cataplectic patients, who have a propensity for this dissociation, brief, isolated atonia may occur as a subclinical event, as illustrated in Fig. 48.15 from Montplaisir (1976).

Sleep-Onset REM Periods

In normal adults following regular night sleep patterns, REM sleep does not appear until after at least 60 minutes, and often only after 90 to 100 minutes, of NREM sleep. Thereafter, REMPs occur cyclically during the night. However, in conditions with increased pressure for REM sleep or reduced pressure for deep slow-wave sleep, early or even

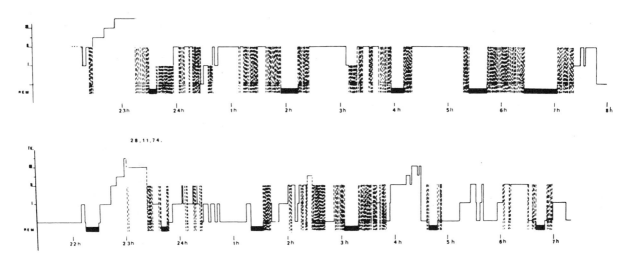

Figure 48.12. Intermediate sleep (REM-spindle sleep). The histograms show two consecutive nights in a 26-year-old narcoleptic. The sleep stages are plotted inverted from the usual, and intermediate sleep is shown as *vertical dotted lines.* The second night showed a sleep-onset REM period. Both nights contained large amounts of intermediate sleep. (From De Barros-Ferreira, M., and Lairy, G.C. 1976. Ambiguous sleep in narcolepsy. In *Narcolepsy,* Eds. C. Guilleminault, W.C. Dement, and P. Passouant, pp. 57–75. New York: Spectrum.)

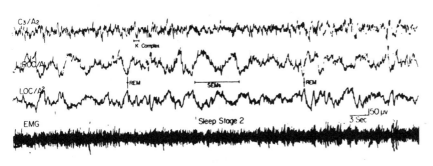

Figure 48.13. REM sleep without atonia. The recording shows typical EEG and electro-oculogram (EOG) patterns of REM sleep; however, these were associated with sustained submental EMG potentials rather than with the atonia normally accompanying that state. The recording was taken from a patient with narcolepsy-cataplexy on treatment with clomipramine. (From Guilleminault, C., Reynal, D., Takahashi, S., et al. 1976c. Evaluation of short-term and long-term treatment of the narcolepsy syndrome with clomipramine hydrochloride. Acta Neurol. Scand. 54:71–87.)

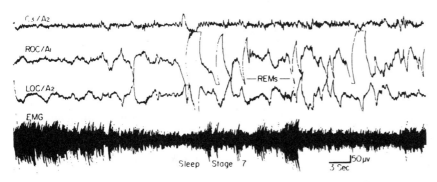

Figure 48.14. REM activity during non-REM sleep. Both REMs and slow eye movements are recorded in association with stage 2 EEG patterns of K complexes, spindles, and several isolated delta waves. The recording was in a patient with narcolepsy-cataplexy on treatment with clomipramine. (From Guilleminault, C., Reynal, D., Takahashi, S., et al. 1976c. Evaluation of short-term and long-term treatment of the narcolepsy syndrome with clomipramine hydrochloride. Acta Neurol. Scand. 54:71–87.)

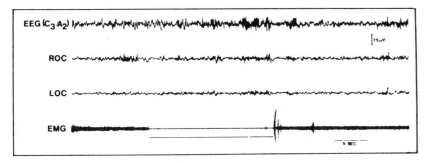

Figure 48.15. Isolated atonia in a case of narcolepsy-cataplexy. During stage 2 sleep with sleep spindles and absence of eye movements from either outer canthus, there is a 20-second period of isolated atonia recorded on the submental electromyogram (EMG) and terminated by a high amplitude myoclonic potential and return of sustained EMG. (From Montplaisir, J. 1976. Disturbed nocturnal sleep. In *Narcolepsy,* Eds. C. Guilleminault, W.C. Dement, and P. Passouant, pp. 42–56. New York: Spectrum.)

direct entry from wakefulness into REM sleep may occur. A SOREMP is usually defined as REM sleep within 10 minutes after sleep onset. If previous REM deprivation, alcoholism, drug withdrawal, very irregular sleep-waking habits, or severe depression can be ruled out, the appearance of SOREMPs is highly supportive of a diagnosis of narcolepsy-cataplexy; it characterizes about 50% of onsets of night sleep in these patients (Rechtschaffen et al., 1963). The diurnal sleep attacks of this condition also often begin in REM sleep, as do many voluntary naps recorded in the Multiple Sleep Latency Test (described below).

Altered Ultradian REM Cyclicity

The normal cyclic reappearance of REM sleep may be disturbed under certain conditions. Poor REM cyclicity is particularly characteristic of the night sleep of patients with narcolepsy-cataplexy (Hishikawa et al., 1976; Meier-Ewert et al., 1975; Montplaisir, 1976). Medications, such as MAO inhibitors, that completely suppress REM sleep (Akindele et al., 1970) obviously abolish the cyclicity. It has been said that loss of REM cyclicity after head injury implies a very bad prognosis (Bergamasco et al., 1968). Nocturnal cyclic REM sleep may also be affected by the repeated (REM) awakenings seen in so-called REM interruption insomnia (Greenberg, 1967) and in other medical conditions occurring typically in that sleep state. These include cluster headache (Dexter and Weitzman, 1970), angina pectoris (Nowlin et al., 1965), and painful nocturnal penile erections (Karacan, 1971).

Other Special Recording and Data Analysis Techniques

Several techniques other than traditional polysomnography exist for studying sleep and its disorders.

Long Cables

Long and relatively lightweight cables, carefully shielded and grounded to reduce movement artifact, can be used in sleep studies of paroxysmal behavioral events; they have, for example, been successfully applied to studies of sleepwalking (Jacobson et al., 1965). Such a cable system has the advantage of very low cost. Movement, however, is obviously restricted to the length of the cable.

Ambulatory In-Home Unattended Monitoring (Portable Recorders)

In a number of situations (e.g., in some patients with narcolepsy or various clinical forms of hypersomnia), documentation of sleep distribution over 24 hours may be desired. In other instances, the presence of infrequent paroxysmal behavioral events of unknown, possibly epileptic, origin might make long-duration recordings desirable. Portable recorders, usually worn on a belt, harness or shoulder slung, may be the answer in such cases. These devices have the advantages of recording subjects in their normal environment at their usual activity levels and of low recording cost, especially concerning technologists' time.

The main limitations of portable recording systems are (a) they are sometimes restricted to eight channels of information; (b) behavioral episodes cannot be noted by an observer (although the use of written logs and an event marker superimposed upon one channel may help locate these); and (c) technical problems may develop while the subject is away from the laboratory and not be picked up until the recording is downloaded. Nevertheless, entirely acceptable recordings for sleep staging may be obtained using portable equipment even with four channels (two EEG, one EOG, and one EMG) (Broughton, 1989). Ambulant assessment of sleep apnea, periodic movements in sleep, and a number of other sleep pathologies may also be performed. The EMG and electrode artifacts present during movements in active wakefulness disappear when the subject becomes quiet and relaxed or falls asleep, thereby permitting high-quality sleep recordings.

Ambulatory digital polysomnographic monitoring technology has made considerable advancements over the last decade. Several systems are now able to store large amounts of data, sampled at frequencies ≥ 100 Hz on several channels. Some of these systems have, in addition, software that permits computer-assisted scoring, and database construction toolkits. Some also have the ability to perform spectral analysis and other customized functions that are useful for researchers. In 1990 the ASDA published a position statement in the journal *Sleep* (Roffwarg, 1990), announcing its view that automatic scoring was insufficiently validated with respect to clinical sleep scoring, and therefore not acceptable. There have been no position papers published in the interim that have reversed that statement. Computerized scoring is not yet at a level accepted by the field, and needs to be carefully proofed on a page-by-page basis by a trained sleep technician or polysomnographer.

While the unattended home recording is not considered acceptable for diagnostic testing of sleep disordered breathing (AASM, 2003), it is useful for other indications. Further development of home monitoring devices gives promise of reducing hospital costs while permitting the study of sleep disorders in the patient's normal home environment. The laboratory environment is known to influence sleep patterns, including the "first-night" effect of longer sleep latency, more fragmented sleep, increased REM latency (Rechtschaffen and Verdone, 1964; Agnew et al., 1966), and inhibition of such episodic behavioral disturbances as sleepwalking and sleep terrors (Broughton, 1968; Gastaut and Broughton, 1965; Jacobson et al., 1965).

Telemetry (and Video-Telemetry)

The advantages of telemetry include free patient movement, a greater number of channels than most portable recorders, and, above all, the ability to combine split-screen video and polygraphic recording for behavioral-polygraphic correlations. The major disadvantages are those having to do with laboratory, rather than home, recording and the need for the subject to remain within range of the receiver station. These can, to some extent, be circumvented by using home telemetry combined with telephone transmission (Roy, 1976). There are a large number of commercial telemetric systems available.

Home Apnea Detectors

A final stream of development is the quite recent appearance of dedicated systems for home monitoring of sleep apnea and often O_2 saturation level without sleep staging capabilities. Such instrumentation has mainly been assessed for screening purposes prior to in-laboratory assessment or for follow-up studies for treatment effects after the diagnosis has been established by a laboratory polysomnogram. Until recently, uncertainty about the use and limitations of such approaches is reflected in the lack of unanimity of guidelines (Ferber et al., 1994; Pack et al., 1995; Stradling, 1992). The AASM, in a new position paper on the use of portable monitoring devices in the assessment of obstructive sleep apnea, found that devices with sufficient recording capability and quality may be useful when used for attended, but not for unattended, recordings (AASM, 2003).

Excessive Daytime Sleepiness and Its Investigation

Excessive daytime sleepiness (EDS) in sleep-wake disorders is the most common symptom of referral for diagnosis to sleep clinics and requires separate discussion. An understanding of EDS requires some knowledge of normal alertness/sleepiness patterns across the waking period.

Alertness normally fluctuates across the day, reflecting both endogenous biological rhythms and the timing of the major sleep period. The marked daily pressure for sleep late in the evening, and the appearance of sleep itself express, the influence of an endogenous once-a-day circadian ("circa," around; "dias," day) rhythm (Aschoff, 1976). It is now recognized that humans also have a two per day (circasemidian) pattern of sleep propensity, with a second period of increased pressure for sleep in the midafternoon (Broughton, 1975). This is detectable even in persons who remain awake in the midafternoon; at this time, there is a transitory drop in performance, the "post-lunch dip" (Blake, 1967). It is also the moment of the last nap given up in growth and development (Kleitman, 1963), napping in college students (Evans et al., 1977), return of napping in the elderly (Webb, 1983), and of the siesta in cultures that limit their mean quota of nighttime sleep (Broughton, 1983). After morning awakening and both before and after this afternoon lull, normal subjects usually remain alert, with the highest levels shown in the morning by so-called "larks" ("morning types") and in the evening by "owls" ("evening types"). The mechanism of this afternoon period of sleep facilitation is uncertain but appears to represent the reversal of the effects of increasing duration of wakefulness across the day by a circadian arousal process (Broughton, 1994; Broughton and Krupa, 2003). There is also strong evidence for a more rapid endogenous ultradian ("ultra," more than; "dias," day) rhythm of oscillations in daytime alertness with a periodicity of 90 to 140 minutes, i.e., about that of the nocturnal non-REM/REM cycle. This phenomenon is well documented for EEG signs of drowsiness (Kripke, 1972; Manseau and Broughton, 1984; Okawa et al., 1984), pupillary changes of alertness (Lavie, 1979), and rapidity of sleep onset (Lavie and Scherson, 1981).

Many sleep disorders are associated with markedly increased subjective and objective daytime sleepiness and/or with actual daytime sleep. Although most typical of the large variety of hypersomnias, increased sleepiness can also be encountered in disorders of inadequate nighttime sleep (insomnias), disturbances of circadian sleep-waking patterns (as in shift work), some parasomnias leading to considerable sleep fragmentation, and in disorders of the wakefulness maintaining system, such as the subwakefulness syndrome (Roth, 1961), also called subvigilance syndrome (Mouret et al., 1972). Moreover, EDS is a major cause of human misery. It has extreme psychosocial impact in such areas as occupation (efficiency, fear of job loss, actual job loss, and disability insurance), education (poor marks and problems with teachers), recreation, driving, accidents, and so on. These are well documented in controlled studies of narcolepsy-cataplexy (Broughton et al., 1981a, 1983) and idiopathic hypersomnia (Broughton et al., 1980), two conditions characterized by extreme EDS. Indeed, EDS psychosocial disability in narcolepsy has been shown to exceed even that of comparable epilepsies (Broughton et al., 1984).

The evident importance of EDS has led over the years to the development of a number of techniques to investigate and quantify the phenomenon:

1. *Subjective assessment.* A widely used method of subjective assessment is the seven-point Stanford Sleepiness Scale (Hoddes et al., 1972). Although this scale accurately assesses acute sleepiness induced in normal individuals by one night of total sleep deprivation (Glenville and Broughton, 1979; Hoddes et al., 1973), it becomes rather unreliable in normals after only five nights of partial sleep deprivation (Herscovitch and Broughton, 1981) and is not at all reliable for studying chronic sleepiness in narcoleptics (Valley and Broughton, 1981; VanDongen et al., 2003) or sleep apneics (Roth et al., 1980). It therefore appears that, in prolonged sleepiness, subjects lose their ability to accurately assess their own level of impairment. Similar findings pertain for the 10-cm visual-analog scale of subjective sleepiness of Monk et al. (1983).

2. *Self-assessed behavioral sleepiness.* The Epworth Sleepiness Scale assesses the probability of falling asleep during situations ranging in activity level from inactive to very active; it is considered reliable and correlates with the MSLT (Johns 1991, 1992). The Functional Outcomes Sleep Questionnaire assesses the impact of sleepiness on everyday activities, is reliable, and is considered useful in the assessment of treatment efficacy (Weaver et al., 1997).

3. *Performance deficits.* Performance measures can be used to quantify objective deficits from EDS (Billiard, 1976; Guilleminault et al., 1975a; Valley and Broughton, 1981, 1983; Wilkinson, 1965). In direct comparison of sleepy untreated narcoleptics to controls, it was found that narcoleptics have problems with relatively long, boring, and repetitive tasks (e.g., the Wilkinson auditory vigilance test), but perform short challenging ones at normal levels (Valley and Broughton, 1981). Such a pattern resembles

that of sleep-deprived normals. Moreover, it has been found (Valley and Broughton, 1983) that performance of untreated narcoleptics on vigilance tasks reaches normal levels during periods of sustained wakefulness, decreases with increasing levels of somnolence or light sleep, and exhibits transient carryover impairment after arousal from even light somnolence into full wakefulness. The latter phenomenon of drowsiness-inertia is analogous to the more intense sleep inertia effects of nocturnal arousals.

4. *Pupillometry.* This technique to determine level of sleepiness has long been used to assess narcoleptics in uncontrolled studies (Schmidt, 1982; Yoss et al., 1969). In a carefully controlled study the only significant change in untreated narcoleptics compared to controls was an increase in spontaneous oscillations, i.e., hippus (Newman and Broughton, 1991). Measures of pupillary size and reactivity had no statistical validity to separate groups.

5. *EEG.* Routine EEG has been used for many years to help document EDS. The increase in drowsy patterns is well documented in the narcolepsy EEG literature (Daly and Yoss, 1957; Gastaut and Roth, 1957; Roth, 1964) and in studies of a large number of other patient groups. Tests, however, have generally been unstructured and unquantified.

6. *Multiple Sleep Latency Test (MSLT).* The MSLT was developed by Carskadon and Dement (1977) and first formally tested in an EDS patient group by Richardson et al. (1978). The subject's polysomnogram (EEG, EOG, and submental EMG) is recorded several times a day at regular 2-hour intervals (generally 10 a.m., 12 noon, 2 p.m., 4 p.m., and 6 p.m.). The lights are turned out and the subject is asked to go to sleep as quickly as possible. Recording in early reports was stopped after 10 minutes of sleep or 20 minutes of recording time, whichever occurred first. Dependent measures are latency to stage 1 (sleep latency) and presence or absence of SOREMPs. If no sleep occurs, sleep latency is scored as 20 minutes. The original protocol has been refined by a consensus guidelines committee (Carskadon et al., 1986), and ASDA has published a report on clinical indications for the test (Thorpy, 1992). Patients with EDS show much shorter mean sleep latencies across the nap periods (Fig. 48.16) with a mean sleep latency of 6 minutes or less generally considered reflecting "pathological sleepiness." Patients with narcolepsy-cataplexy or other causes of excessive pressure for REM sleep may show SOREMPs with two or more in a five-nap MSLT characterizing narcolepsy (Mitler et al., 1979). The MSLT is currently the most widely used objective measure of sleepiness.

7. *Tests of ability to remain awake.* Two variants of the MSLT follow a similar recording paradigm, but the patients are asked to remain awake. Patients with true EDS are unable to fight off sleep and, as in the MSLT, show much shorter sleep latencies than normals. These two tests, the Maintenance of Wakefulness Test (MWT) introduced by Mitler et al. (1982) and the Repeated Test of Sustained Wakefulness (RTSW) introduced by

Hartse et al. (1982), try to mimic more closely the efforts to suppress sleep pressure experienced in everyday circumstances by EDS patients. To date, they lack the large body of age- and sex-related normative data available for the MSLT and so are less widely used.

8. *Afternoon nap test.* A period of increased pressure for sleep in the afternoon is normal. Roth et al. (1986) introduced a simple midafternoon 2-hour nap recording to measure EDS. The sleepiness index of this technique uses not only sleep latency, but also a factorial weighing of both the latencies and amounts of all sleep stages recorded. The index obtained clearly separates various patient groups (i.e., narcoleptics, idiopathic hypersomniacs, and sleep apneics) from normal individuals. Because it requires only 2, rather than 8, hours in the laboratory, the technique has definite advantages, although it appears to be little used.

9. *Evoked potential studies.* Broughton et al. (1981b, 1982) first used cerebral evoked potentials as a more rapid quantitative approach to assess EDS in sleep disorder patients. Simple auditory evoked potentials (AEPs) to tone stimuli showed significant differences between controls and narcoleptics—even to stimuli presented during sustained EEG wakefulness, when no performance differences were present according to the most sensitive tests available. High variability, however, made the simple AEP technique insufficiently sensitive for EDS diagnosis. Complex evoked potentials of both the P300 and CNV type have also been assessed (Aguirre and Broughton, 1984; Broughton and Aguirre, 1987). EDS was shown to cause a significant amplitude reduction in component P3, which clearly distinguished

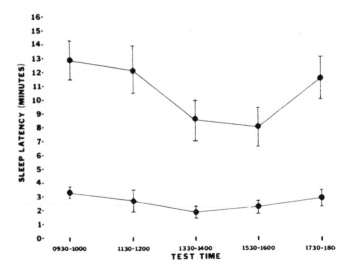

Figure 48.16. Multiple sleep latency test comparing mean [± standard error of the mean (SEM)] sleep latencies for control *(upper curve)* and narcoleptic *(lower curve)* subjects. For each opportunity to sleep, patients with narcolepsy fell asleep significantly more quickly than normal control subjects. (From Richardson, G., Carskadon, M., Flagg, W., et al. 1978. Excessive daytime sleepiness in man: multiple sleep latency measurement in narcoleptic and control subjects. Electroencephalogr. Clin. Neurophysiol. 45:621–627.)

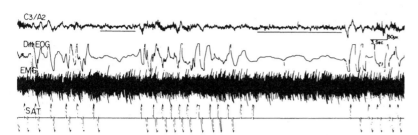

Figure 48.17. Microsleep episodes. The narcoleptic patient was performing a serial alternation task (SAT). The recording shows two microsleep episodes *(underlined)* lasting about 9 and 18 seconds, respectively. Each is associated with EEG slowing and loss of waking artifacts, slow eye movements, and loss of serial alternation. (From Guilleminault, C., Billiard, M., Montplaisir, J., et al. 1975a. Altered states of consciousness in disorders of daytime sleepiness. J. Neurol. Sci. 26:337–393.)

awake narcoleptics from controls. P3 amplitude reduction from a single 7-minute P300 paradigm was subsequently shown by discriminant analysis to be almost as powerful as mean MSLT sleep latency (across 8 hours) in distinguishing groups (Broughton et al., 1988a).

10. *Power spectral EEG analysis.* In drowsiness, quantitative spectral EEG analysis has documented that theta and low-voltage delta activities increase as alpha rhythm slows and disappears (Matousek and Petersen, 1983; Ogilvie et al., 1991; Torsvall and Ackerstedt, 1987). The alpha attenuation test (AAT), which quantifies spectral power in the alpha band during wakefulness as an eyes closed/opened ratio, has been shown to closely parallel MSLT results (Alloway et al., 1997; Stampi et al., 1995), but, like a number of other tests of sleepiness, it is not yet in widespread clinical practice.

Nature of EDS and Episodes of Abnormal Sleep

Pathological sleepiness and sleep show numerous important features. Very brief microsleeps, lasting but a few seconds and associated with mental lapses, may occur. These were first described by Ganado (1958) and have been studied particularly by Guilleminault and Dement (1977), who consider them characteristic of narcolepsy. Microsleeps are best documented by combining EEG with a continuous performance task (Fig. 48.17). Studies of seated performing narcoleptics attempting to stay awake, however, have mainly shown slow waxing and waning patterns of alertness (Fig. 48.18) lasting dozens of seconds or minutes (Valley and Broughton, 1983). Under such circumstances, microsleeps are essentially absent and the performance deficit is not explicable by the microsleep-lapse hypothesis alone. Even more prolonged episodes of drowsiness may occur and be expressed as amnesic automatisms, for instance driving a car to some unusual place and not knowing how one got there. Such episodes in sleepy patients have been referred to as "fugue-like states" by Ganado (1958), "fugue states" by Levin (1959), and "altered states of consciousness" by Guilleminault et al. (1975a). It has been postulated that a prolonged series of microsleeps may cause such episodes.

More or less involuntary longer sleep attacks may occur, especially in narcolepsy. It has been shown that in patients with narcolepsy-cataplexy (and therefore with abnormal REM pressure), daytime sleep attacks may begin with either non–REM or REM sleep. Especially in narcoleptics who are able to sleep when they want to, sleep attacks may recur with an ultradian 90- to 140-minute periodicity throughout the day (Baldy-Moulinier et al., 1976; Passouant et al., 1969; Volk et al., 1984) as an apparent intensification of the normal ultradian oscillation in alertness mentioned above.

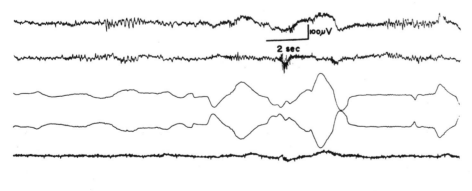

Figure 48.18. Waxing and waning patterns. The recording was taken in a patient with narcolepsy-cataplexy during Wilkenson's auditory vigilance task (artifact of stimuli at bottom). The top five channels are C3-A1, O1-A1, left outer canthus-A1, right outer canthus-A2, and submental EMG. In the first 6 seconds, the EEG contains stage 1B patterns with some theta activity and slow eye movements. Thereafter, there are 6 seconds of diffuse but mainly occipital alpha and then further EEG desynchronization associated with REMs. The last 4 seconds contain return to stage 1B patterns. EMG is unaltered throughout.

Figure 48.19. Cyclic sleep attacks in mono-symptomatic narcolepsy. The 24-hour clock shows the nocturnal period with sleep onset into non-REM sleep. In the daytime, four sleep attacks occurred at about 2-hour intervals, all consisting of non-REM sleep. (From Baldy-Moulinier, M., Arguner, A., and Besset, A. 1976. Ultradian and circadian rhythms in sleep and wakefulness. In *Narcolepsy,* Eds. C. Guilleminault, W.C. Dement, and P. Passouant, pp. 485–497. New York: Spectrum.)

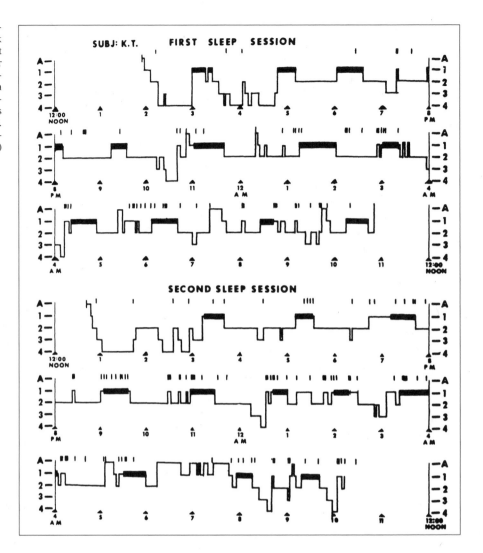

Ultradian sleep episodes beginning in non-REM or REM sleep are illustrated respectively in Figs. 48.19 and 48.20. All excessively sleepy patients, including narcoleptics, display a propensity for particularly long midafternoon sleep episodes involving mainly non-REM sleep (Broughton et al., 1986). It is evident, therefore, that the underlying circasemidian and ultradian rhythms continue to be manifested, and indeed are intensified, in these conditions.

Until recently, it has been assumed that sleepiness was a unitary phenomenon varying only in intensity. There is reason to believe, however, that there are qualitatively different forms of sleepiness, primarily expressing pressure for non-REM sleep, pressure for REM sleep, and de–arousal by impaired reticulocortical activation (Broughton, 1982a). The evidence for such diverse states of sleepiness is increasing. Differences in sleepiness prior to REM sleep (i.e., in REM sleepiness) versus prior to non-REM sleep (non-REM sleepiness) have been shown for simple evoked potentials to click stimuli (Pressman et al., 1982) and for P300 and CNV measures (Aguirre and Broughton, 1984). The latter include increased component P2 amplitude, decreased P3 amplitude, and essential suppression of CNV in REM sleepiness compared to non-REM sleepiness (Broughton and Aguirre, 1987). REM sleepiness has also been found to be greater both subjectively (higher ratings) and objectively (shorter MSLT sleep latencies), although that study also found that once sleep occurs, REM sleep is relatively more refreshing (Broughton and Aguirre, 1987). This may explain the more imperative nature of sleep attacks in narcoleptic-cataplectic patients in whom pressure for REM sleep is present, whereas in monosymptomatic non-REM narcolepsy, idiopathic hypersomnia, and sleep apnea the sleep episodes are less pressing and more or less exclusively involve non-REM sleep. Further evidence for qualitatively different states of sleepiness has been reviewed (Broughton, 1992). The presence in narcolepsy of both REM and non-REM sleepiness and also the possibility of coexistent subwakefulness (Broughton, 1976; Broughton et al., 1995) may help explain why its associated EDS is particularly refractory to treatment.

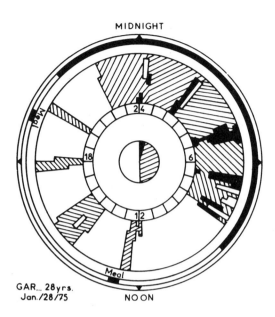

Figure 48.20. Cyclic sleep attacks in narcolepsy-cataplexy. The nocturnal period shows a sleep-onset REM period (in *black*) at 22 hours and much nocturnal wakefulness. In the daytime, there are six sleep episodes, all beginning in REM sleep and recurring at about 2-hour intervals. (From Passouant, P., Cadilhac, J., and Baldy-Moulinier, M. 1967. Physiopathologic des hypersomnies. Rev. Neurol. (Paris) 6:585–629.)

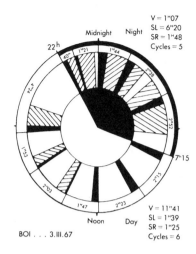

Figure 48.21. Idiopathic hypersomnia. In this 25-year-old woman, two recordings at 2-week intervals showed extreme hypersomnia lasting some 21 hours. The *vertical lines* over the sleep stages mark major body movements. The normal cyclicity of sleep is maintained, and little fragmentation occurs. (From Roth, B., Nevsimalova, S., and Rechtschaffen, A. 1972. Hypersomnia with "sleep drunkenness." Arch. Gen. Psychiatry 26:456–462.)

Polysomnography of Specific Sleep and Arousal Disorders

Early explicit attempts to classify sleep disorders include those by Broughton (1972a), Williams et al. (1974), and Cadilhac (1976). In 1979 the Association of Sleep Disorders Centers and the Association for the Psychophysiological Study of Sleep (now the Sleep Research Society) published a detailed classification (Roffwarg et al., 1979) that separates the conditions into (a) disorders of initiating and maintaining sleep (insomnias); (b) disorders of excessive somnolence (hypersomnias); (c) disorders of the sleep-wake schedule (circadian rhythm disorders); and (d) dysfunctions associated with sleep, sleep stages, or partial arousals from sleep (parasomnias).

One of the difficulties in classifying sleep disorders symptomatically is that a single medical condition may present under more than one such category. For example, periodic movements in sleep (nocturnal myoclonus) or sleep apnea may lead to a primary complaint of either insomnia (group a) or excessive daytime somnolence (group b). Similarly, such conditions as sleep terrors or dream anxiety attacks, which primarily characterize the parasomnias (group d), may cause such severe sleep disruption that they present as a form of insomnia (group a). A subsequent classification initiated by the American Sleep Disorders Association and later involving significant international input has been published (ICSD, 1990) and an updated version is in press. Textbooks of sleep medicine with detailed polysomnographic features of individual sleep disorders are available

(Billiard, 1994; Chokroverty, 1994; Kryger et al., 1994; Thorpy, 1990). The following presentation uses a breakdown rather similar to the Roffwarg et al. (1979) approach.

The Hypersomnias (Increased Duration and/or Depth of Nocturnal Sleep)

Idiopathic Hypersomnia

Most thoroughly documented by B. Roth and collaborators (Roth, 1962, 1976, 1980; Roth et al., 1969), so-called idiopathic CNS hypersomnia no doubt represents the purest form of hypersomnia. Sleep is markedly lengthened, often to 12 to 16 hours or exceptionally, as in Fig. 48.21, to more than 20 hours per day. Such patients are typically very deep sleepers awakened only with great difficulty. About 50% exhibit sleep drunkenness on morning awakening (Roth et al., 1972). Patients experience EDS and may take long unrefreshing naps. True irresistible sleep attacks, however, are generally absent, as always are narcolepsy's dissociative symptoms of cataplexy or sleep paralysis. Many cases are familial; others are sporadic. Overnight sleep recordings (Fig. 48.21) show marked sleep extension with normal cyclicity, very few awakenings, and lack of an early REM period; relative tachycardia might also be noted.

Narcolepsy

Narcolepsy is characterized by inappropriate and more or less irresistible daytime sleep attacks superimposed upon chronic EDS. When these attacks occur alone, the condition is variously referred to as monosymptomatic narcolepsy, isolated narcolepsy, or non-REM narcolepsy. Night sleep tends to be normal or extended, and daytime sleep attacks to consist of sustained NREM sleep (Fig. 48.19). The latter are generally less overwhelming than are the REM onset attacks common in narcolepsy-cataplexy. Some consider mono-symptomatic narcolepsy to be a form of idiopathic hypersomnia, although it can evolve to narcolepsy-cataplexy; in the latter condition, approximately 50% of sleep attacks also consist of NREM sleep with the other half containing REM sleep.

In polysymptomatic, compound, or REM narcolepsy, sleep attacks and EDS are joined by one or several further symptoms, in particular cataplexy, sleep paralysis, and vivid hypnagogic hallucinations. Nocturnal sleep is typically disturbed and unrestorative with frequent awakenings and terrifying dreams. Night sleep studies in compound narcolepsy typically show decreased REM latency or SOREMPs (Figs. 48.20 and Fig. 48.22); even distribution of stages 3 and 4 throughout the night; frequent stage shifts; fragmentation, especially of REM sleep; and poor REM cyclicity (Broughton and Mamelak, 1980; Hishikawa et al., 1976; Meier-Ewert et al., 1975; Montplaisir et al., 1978; Passouant

et al., 1967; Rechtschaffen et al., 1963). Daytime recordings (as in the Multiple Sleep Latency Test) in polysymptomatic cases show that sleep attacks or naps frequently also contain SOREMPs or very short REM latencies (Fig. 48.20); 20% to 100% (depending on the study) of the sleep attacks themselves begin with REM sleep. Daytime recordings also show recurrent drowsiness with waxing and waning vigilance (Fig. 48.18) and may contain microsleeps (Fig. 48.17). The peak distribution of day sleep occurs earlier than that of naps in normals (Mullington et al., 1990).

The details of the polygraphic recordings and many other aspects of the condition may be found in Guilleminault et al. (1976a) and Roth (1980). Narcolepsy-cataplexy is not a rare condition; recent prevalence studies give a figure of just under 0.1%, making it somewhat more common than multiple sclerosis. Familial cases may occur. Genetic influences in general are strong. The condition has an almost 100% association with presence of the human leukocyte antigen (HLA)-DR2 (DWI5) (Honda et al., 1984) and, more particularly the DQw*0602 allele DQB1*0602 HLA marker (Mignot et al., 1994). Because total sleep per 24 hours is not necessarily increased, but rather is fragmented at night and distributed through the 24-hour day, some consider narcolepsy-cataplexy to be a dyssomnia rather than a true hypersomnia.

Sleep Apnea

Sleep apnea can be obstructive, central, or mixed (central then obstructive). An apneic episode is defined as a cessation of breathing of longer than 10 seconds' duration. Although the condition combining excessive daytime sleepiness with (usually obstructive) apnea is at times termed "hypersomnia with sleep apnea" (Lugaresi et al., 1978), such patients may awaken dozens to hundreds of times per night with such apneic episodes, and the condition may present equally as a sleep maintenance form of insomnia. Careful respiratory monitoring of oronasal airflow by thermistors or thermocouples (Fig. 48.23) and of chest and movement by strain gauge, inductive plethysmography, or other techniques is necessary to define the precise nature of an apnea.

In obstructive apnea, airflow at the nose and mouth ceases due to upper airway collapse. Respiratory drive is initially unchanged and thoracoabdominal movements continue but are ineffectual, being out of phase (paradoxical breathing). In central apnea, the medullary respiratory centers temporarily cease to function, abolishing thoracoabdominal movement and, consequently, oronasal airflow. In the mixed form, central apnea evolves into obstructive apnea.

Especially during obstructive and mixed apneas, blood oxygen levels may fall rapidly (Fig. 48.24). It is the resultant hypoxia and hypercapnia that cause intensification of breathing efforts by activating the reticular formation and medullary respiratory centers with consequent awakening, return of upper airway airflow, and return to waking respiratory reflexes, which are altered in sleep. The resultant sudden relief of obstruction causes a characteristic intense guttural inspiratory snort usually easily detectable by the history or by portable tape recording. The obstruction is

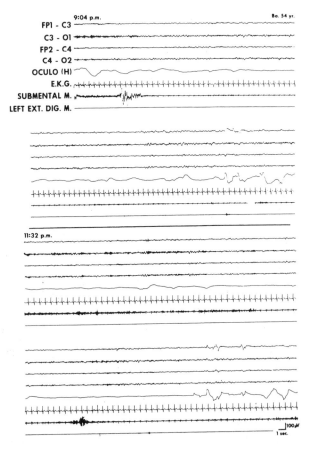

Figure 48.22. Sleep-onset REM periods (SOREMPs) in a 54-year-old patient with narcolepsy-cataplexy. At 9:04 p.m., there is direct passage from a waking alpha rhythm through about 20 seconds of stage 1 patterns with slow eye movements to full-blown REM sleep. After this SOREMP, the patient has some 80 minutes of non-REM sleep (mainly stages 3 and 4) followed by a long period of nocturnal wakefulness. Then at 11:32 p.m., he again passed from wakefulness directly into REM sleep.

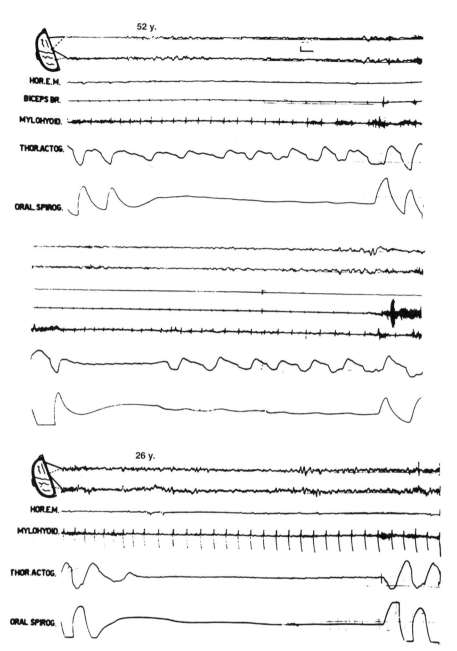

Figure 48.23. The three types of sleep apnea. The *upper tracing* shows typical obstructive sleep apnea with loss of upper airway airflow (oral spirogram) associated with continuing thoracic movement. The *middle tracing* shows mixed apnea, in which an initially central apnea (no chest movement or oral airflow) evolves into obstructive apnea (return of thoracic movements). The *lower tracing* shows central apnea with loss of thoracic movement and oral airflow. (From Coccagna, G.G., Petrella, A., Berti-Ceroni, G., et al. 1968. Polygraphic contributions to hypersomnia and respiratory troubles in the Pickwickian syndrome. In *The Abnormalities of Sleep in Man,* Eds. H. Gastaut, E. Lugaresi, G. Berti-Ceroni, et al., pp. 215–221. Bologna: Aulo Gaggi.)

often due to backward movement of the base of the tongue or collapse of the posterior pharynx in sleep superimposed upon a predisposing decreased diameter of the upper airways from such mechanical factors as obesity, e.g., as part of the so-called Pickwickian syndrome of Burwell et al. (1956), enlarged adenoids and tonsils, micrognathia, laryngeal stenosis, or other. If left untreated, the condition may evolve to pulmonary, then systemic, hypertension, to cardiac arrhythmias, and to death in sleep. These patients have normal waking ventilatory responses and lack discernible cerebral or spinal cord lesions.

Upper airway resistance syndrome is a sleep apnea variant first described by Guilleminault et al. (1982) and consists of a number of features similar to obstructive sleep apnea including similar causes of upper airway obstruction; negative intrathoracic pressure changes during respiratory efforts in sleep; similar symptoms such as snoring, restlessness, and night sweats; poor school performance and behavioral problems in children; the frequent association of night sleep fragmentation and daytime sleepiness; and a similar response to the same therapeutic measures (Downey et al., 1993). However, the apnea and apnea plus hypopnea indices remain normal and O_2 desaturations are much less common or absent despite the other evidence of difficulty in breathing (episodes of negative intrathoracic pressure and, at times, a marked increase in heart rate variability).

Alveolar hypoventilation may also cause apparent hypersomnia and EDS. Patients display reduced chemical control

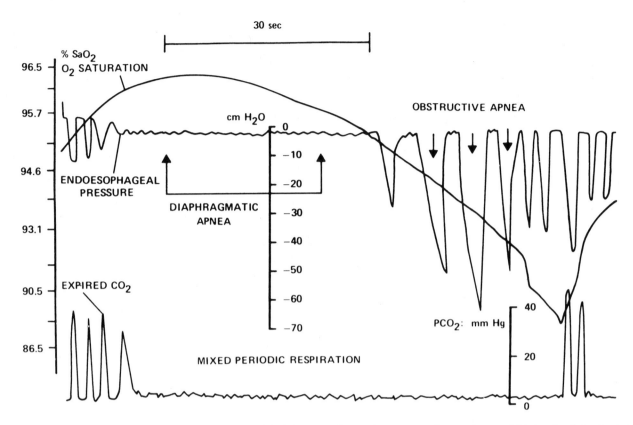

Figure 48.24. Hypoxia during mixed sleep apnea. The polygraph includes blood O_2 saturation, expired CO_2, and endoesophageal pressure. The apnea lasted about 140 seconds, as seen by absence of expired CO_2 with a shorter early central component lasting about 20 seconds, i.e., the duration of di-aphragmatic apnea, as written on the record. During the obstructive apnea, component O_2 saturation decreased. (From Guilleminault, C., Eldridge, F.L., Simmon, F.B., et al. 1975b. Sleep apnea syndrome: Can it induce hemodynamic changes? West J. Med. 123:7–16.)

(hypocapnic drive) in both wakefulness and sleep. Spirometric and other tests in wakefulness are normal. In sleep, however, hypoventilation, hypercapnia, and hypoxemia appear, at times associated with central apneas. REM sleep in particular aggravates the hypoxemia and hypercapnia. Patients may lack known CNS or pulmonary lesions and present with true primary hypoventilation, the so-called Ondine's curse (Severinghaus and Mitchell, 1962). Others have neurological lesions in the brainstem or upper spinal cord, including those from cordotomy, or may have mechanical respiratory problems involving rib cage movement (as in scoliosis), muscular efficiency (as in muscular dystrophy or obesity), or similar problems.

A general discussion of sleep apnea and hypoventilation syndromes with emphasis on polygraphic changes may be found in volumes by Lugaresi et al. (1978), Guilleminault and Dement (1978), and Saunders and Sullivan (1994).

Motor Abnormalities

Periodic Movements in Sleep

Periodic movements in sleep (PMS) consist of periods of repetitive, stereotyped, mainly leg movements present more or less exclusively during sleep. They may lead to marked EDS, especially when associated with repeated microarousals. One or (usually) both legs may be involved. The movement resembles a withdrawal response with toe exten-sion and ankle, knee, and hip flexion. The movements are relatively slow, lasting 0.5 to 2.0 seconds, and tonic rather than myoclonic. Use of the term *nocturnal myoclonus* is therefore inappropriate, particularly considering that nocturnal forms of true pathological myoclonus exist. The movements are usually pseudorhythmic, recurring every 20 to 80 seconds over extended periods of sleep (Lugaresi et al., l966). Anterior tibialis EMGs document their presence and temporal distribution (Fig. 48.25). At times each leg movement is associated with a brief EEG microarousal; at other times, no EEG change is seen. Patients are typically unaware of such movements, and they may first be suggested in a history from the sleeping partner. PMS has been found to be common in EDS patients referred to sleep disorder clinics (Coleman et al., 1980). It appears in fact that PMS may both be a cause of EDS (especially when repeated microarousals are present) and may also be a nonspecific result of any cause of chronic sleep fragmentation.

Fragmentary Non-REM Myoclonus

Brief (less than 200 msec) twitch-like myoclonus in non-REM sleep, involving various muscle groups in asynchronous and asymmetrical fashion, may be associated with marked EDS (Broughton and Tolentino, 1984). The twitchings generally do not cause EEG arousal and are seldom noted by the sleeper, although the sleeping partner may

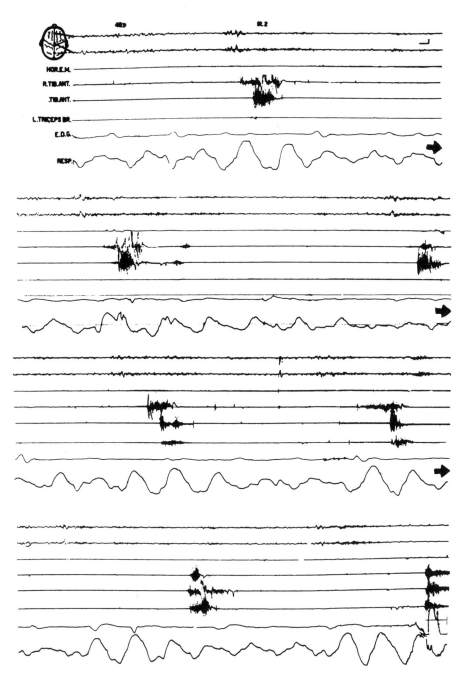

Figure 48.25. Periodic movements in sleep (Symond's nocturnal myoclonus) in a case of restless leg syndrome. The patient shows recurrent leg muscle contractions repeated every 20 to 25 seconds involving both sides, mainly the right. Each tonic leg spasm lasts 2 to 3 seconds and is preceded by increased respiratory excursion and K complexes. (From Cocagna, G., Ceroni, G.R., and Ambrosetto, C. 1968. Restless legs syndrome and nocturnal myoclonus. In *The Abnormalities in Sleep in Man,* Eds. H. Gastaut, E. Lugaresi, G. Berti-Ceroni, et al., pp. 285–294. Bologna: Aulo Gaggi.)

complain. They may be associated with benign fasciculations. The jerks do not occur in bursts as does physiological REM myoclonus. Like PMS, with which they may be associated, they can be encountered in a large variety of other causes of EDS (Broughton et al., 1985) or may occur alone. Typical patterns are illustrated in Fig. 48.26.

Recurrent Hypersomnias

Menstrual Hypersomnia

Recurrent menstrual hypersomnia, detailed by Billiard et al. (1975), is a rare form of hypersomnia involving increases in both sleep states and that recurs in the premenstrual or menstrual periods. It appears to be related to cyclic increases in serum progesterone.

Kleine-Levin Syndrome

This is a rare form of recurrent hypersomnia that appears as bouts of several days or weeks in duration. During these periods, sleep is greatly extended and is associated with compulsive and increased eating (megaphagia), hypersexuality, loss of sexual inhibitions, and often irritability and/or apathy. It is seen almost exclusively in adolescent males. Patients are normal between attacks. The condition appears to reflect intermittent dysfunction of the hypothalamus

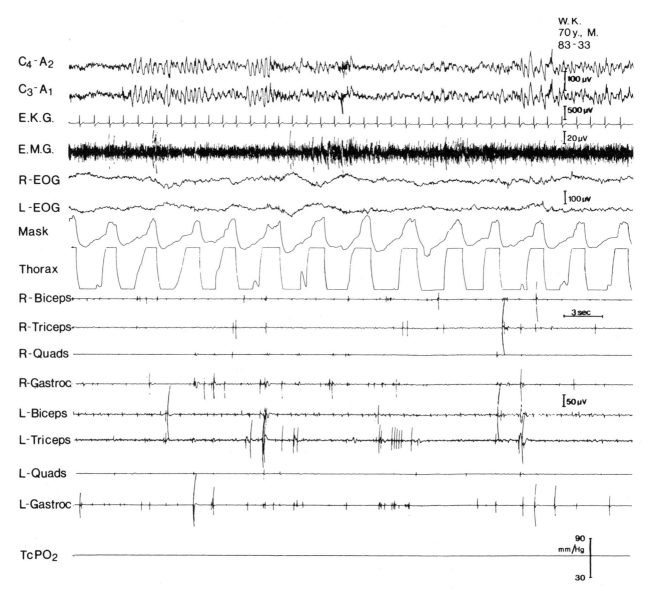

Figure 48.26. Fragmentary non-REM myoclonus. The polysomnogram includes multiple superficial EMG leads. There are multiple asynchronous brief potentials recorded over various body muscles. The largest amplitude of these were associated with visible myoclonus. (From Broughton, R., To-lentino, M.A., and Krelina, M. 1985. Excessive fragmentary myoclonus in NREM sleep: a report on 38 cases. Electroencephalogr. Clin. Neurophysiol. 61:123–133.)

(Critchley, 1962; Kleine, 1925; Levin, 1936). Polysomnography shows increased total 24-hour sleep time usually with fragmentation of night sleep and increased day sleep and daytime drowsiness.

Hypersomnia in the Bipolar Affective Disorder

Episodes of hypersomnia involving both non-REM and REM sleep are also encountered during depressive phases of bipolar affective disorder (major depression, manic-depressive illness). Patients then show increased sleep length with conservation of its continuity, a short REM latency, and some reduction of slow-wave sleep (Kupfer et al., 1972). If

manic periods are not prominent, a condition of more or less exclusively cyclic hypersomnia may be present.

Miscellaneous Non-REM Hypersomnias

Hypersomnias involving (mainly or exclusively) increased non-REM, especially stages 3 and 4, sleep can be caused by lesions and/or dysfunctions (e.g., posttraumatic, metabolic, or toxic) of the mesencephalic reticular formation, posterior hypothalamus, and other brainstem structures involved in arousal (Roth, 1980; Vein, 1966). This represents by far the largest group of hypersomnias and includes many classical forms, such as Von Economo's encephalitis lethargica, trypanosomiasis, and drug-related states (excessive effects of hypnotics, sedatives, or tranquilizers; tolerance to CNS stimulants). Some consider monosymptomatic narcolepsy, in which the attacks occur exclusively in NREM sleep, as a form of non-REM hypersomnia.

Pseudohypersomnia

So-called pseudohypersomnia may occur in neurotic individuals who remain in bed for long periods and show normal overnight sleep followed by prolonged morning drowsiness. It also occurs in normal individuals who are natural long sleepers and show simple sleep extension without features of idiopathic hypersomnia such as long afternoon naps, excessive daytime sleepiness, and morning sleep drunkenness (Hartmann et al., 1972; Webb and Friel, 1971). The latter situation appears to represent one extreme end of the normal distribution curve for sleep need, which sometimes appears to be genetically determined. Such normal individuals regularly require 10 to 12 hours or more of sleep and may seek medical attention because of concern over their unusual sleep need. As in the case of natural short sleepers (Stuss and Broughton, 1978), proof that the sleep habit represents the person's optimal amount can be shown by deterioration on daytime performance tests after both sleep extension or partial sleep deprivation from the habitual amount—in this case down to the normal range of 6.5 to 8 hours.

The Insomnias (Fragmented or Reduced Night Sleep; A Complaint of Poor Sleep)

In many sleep disorders, polygraphic sleep patterns are characterized by greatly delayed sleep onset, sleep fragmentation, and/or reduced total sleep; patients usually complain of poor-quality, nonrestorative, and often restless sleep. Persistent poor-quality sleep may lead to marked daytime sleepiness, making the presenting complaint one of apparent excessive daytime sleepiness. Insomnia may be classified by temporal features into sleep onset, sleep maintenance (i.e., frequent within sleep arousals), and early morning awakening forms. Disruption of sleep continuity by multiple brief arousals without significant sleep loss can produce performance decrements similar to those of marked sleep deprivation (Bonnet, 1985, 1987). The results of polygraphic recordings vary substantially with the etiology and the clinical form of insomnia.

Acute Situational Insomnia

Situational insomnia (transient psychophysiological insomnia) is very common and is associated with emotional arousal related to some apparent or real threat or conflict. This may be due to loss of a loved one, divorce, student examinations, threatened job loss, or other obvious factors. The "first-night effect" of stress in the new laboratory situation (Agnew et al., 1966; Rechtschaffen and Verdone, 1964) represents a specific example. Night sleep usually shows increased sleep latency, decreased stages 3 and 4, increased REM latency with decreased REM percentage, and more

frequent stage shifts and awakenings. No serious mood disorder is present, and the psychophysiological arousal and insomnia disappear in a few days or weeks.

Chronic Psychophysiological Insomnia

In some individuals, especially those with apparent constitutionally weak sleep abilities, acute situational insomnia evolves into chronic insomnia. As in the first group, medical, toxic, drug-related, and other similar types of insomnia are absent. Most such patients appear to develop a conditioned response to the initial stress-related insomnia. They might try too hard to sleep, thereby perpetuating excessive nocturnal arousal; or the sleeping environment itself can become a conditioning stimulus associated with poor sleep (Hauri, 1985). The polygraphic changes are similar to those of transient insomnia.

Depression

Depression is regularly associated with poor sleep. In neurotic (reactive) depression, there is increased sleep latency, reduced stages 3 and 4 and varying amounts of REM sleep, frequent awakenings and stage shifts, and, often, early morning awakening (Gresham et al., 1965; Mendels and Hawkins, 1967; Zung et al., 1964). The major affective disorders of psychotic depression and bipolar affective disease cause great sleep disturbance. The hypomanic pole of bipolar affective disorder is generally associated with extreme and sometimes total insomnia (Hawkins et al., 1967; Mendels and Hawkins, 1971; Snyder, 1968), which may precede the manic swing by several days (Snyder, 1968). As mentioned above, hypersomnia characterizes the depressive pole. In endogenous and acute psychotic depression, sleep is very fragmented, stages 3 and 4 are reduced, and REM latency is typically very short. Indeed, short REM latency may be considered as a hallmark or biological marker of endogenous depression (Kupfer and Foster, 1978).

Drug-Related Insomnia

Insomnia induced by drug intake is common. CNS stimulants taken chronically or too late in the day may lead to severe insomnia. This may occur with prescription stimulants such as methylphenidate and amphetamines or with chronic abuse of either caffeine or nicotine. Repeated use of stimulants may lead to tolerance, so that increasing doses are required to maintain the same level of daytime alertness. Insomnia may give way to "crashes" or sudden excessive urges to sleep in the daytime; toxic or psychotic reactions may also appear. Indeed, the first case of amphetamine psychosis was reported in a narcoleptic patient taking excessive amounts of the prescribed stimulant (Young and Scoville, 1938). Night sleep is generally very fragmented with reduced REM sleep and SWS (Oswald, 1969). Sustained use of or withdrawal from numerous other drugs can also lead to insomnia. These substances include thyroid preparations, oncotherapeutic drugs, MAO inhibitors, adrenocorticotropic hormone (ACTH), alpha-methyl-DOPA, oral contraceptives, propranolol, alcohol, and many others.

Motor Abnormalities

Restless Leg Syndrome

The restless leg syndrome (RLS) of Ekbom (1960), described earlier by Allison (1943) as "leg jitters," consists of deep dysesthesias in the lower limbs during immobility. These are accentuated by recumbency and by somnolence, resulting in a virtually irresistible urge to move the legs. This usually leads to severe sleep onset insomnia (Fig. 48.27) (Coccagna and Lugaresi, 1968; Frankel et al., 1974). Restless legs are often associated with periodic movements in sleep (PMS) (Montplaisir et al., 1994), which may lead to awakening and return of the restless leg activity. Some RLS patients have peripheral vascular or neuropathic disease. The condition is more common in pregnancy and typically improves during febrile illnesses.

Periodic Movements in Sleep (PMS)

In a small proportion of cases, PMS (described above) causes marked sleep fragmentation. Insomnia may then be the primary complaint.

Hypnagogic Generalized Myoclonus

A rare motor cause of insomnia involves the normal brief generalized myoclonus at sleep onset ("nocturnal starts," "hypnic jerks"), appearing more or less exclusively in stage 1 drowsiness (Gastaut and Broughton, 1965; Oswald, 1959), which intensify and increase in frequency. Excessive intensification and repetition of the physiological sleep-onset jerks can cause sleep-onset insomnia, as first described clinically by Mitchell (1890) and demonstrated polygraphically by Broughton (1988).

Sleep Apnea

Insomnia may be a complaint of obstructive sleep apnea due to the frequent repeated awakenings associated with inspiratory snoring. Central sleep apnea, however, is the most common form of respiratory-related insomnia. It may be induced repeatedly in drowsiness, leading to arousal and repetition of the cycle. Alternatively, it may occur in deeper sleep stages and lead to a sleep maintenance, rather than sleep onset, form of insomnia (Guilleminault et al., 1973).

CNS Lesions

Rarely, neurological lesions occur in brain structures necessary for sleep induction or maintenance and cause true organic insomnias. These structures include the basal forebrain (preoptic) areas and bulbar (probably tractus solitarius) synchronizing areas in the first group and, in the second group, the midline raphe nuclei. Some of Von Economo's encephalitis lethargica patients were in fact insomniac; most of those had basal forebrain lesions. Bricolo (1967) has described insomnia lasting 96 hours in a parkinsonian patient after thalamotomy. Feldman (1971), Wilkus et al. (1971), and Schott et al. (1972) found marked sleep reduction in traumatic or vascular lesions of the ventral pons, with sleep consisting mainly of stage 1 or 2 and with reduced or absent REM sleep. Adey et al. (1968) noted that high spinal cord lesions ostensibly affecting the bulbar synchronizing areas lead to severe insomnia. Morvan's fibrillary chorea is characterized by severe or total insomnia, often attributed to raphe lesions. A carefully studied case with temporary return of sleep with 5-hydroxytryptophan was published by Fischer-Perroudon et al. (1974). Finally, Lugaresi et al. (1986) have described a fatal form of familial insomnia with lesions restricted to the anterior and dorsomedial thalamic nuclei, areas shown by Hess (1944) to be sleep inducing.

Medical, Toxic, and Related Diseases

A wide variety of disease conditions may lead to insomnia; in many, the polygraphic changes have not yet been fully documented. Sleep improves with resolution of the underlying processes. These disorders can range from peripheral nerve and muscular problems (neuritis, carpal tunnel syndrome, compression neuropathy, night cramps/growing pains, or myotonic dystrophy), low back or other pain, endocrine and metabolic diseases (hyperthyroidism, Cushing's syndrome, or Addison's disease), early stages of renal and hepatic failure (often showing marked PMS), gastrointestinal diseases of various types, pulmonary conditions with paroxysmal nocturnal dyspnea, and others. The conditions tend to disturb sleep by causing pain, dysthymia, or movement disorders, or by directly affecting sleep-wake regulation mechanisms.

A further group of medical disorders that can produce insomnia from repeated awakening, and that were included among the parasomnias in the classification of Roffwarg et al. (1979), include the sleep-related abnormal swallowing syndrome (Guilleminault et al., 1976b), gastroesophageal reflux in sleep (Orr et al., 1979), sleep-related asthma (Kales et al., 1968, 1970), and such REM-related phenomena as cluster headache, nocturnal angina, and painful erections.

Childhood-Onset Insomnia

A small proportion of patients suffer from insomnia since childhood and appear to have a permanent and endogenously regulated high level of wakefulness. There may also

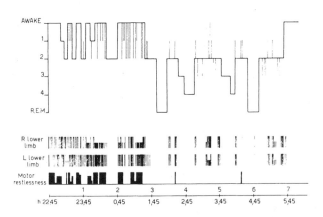

Figure 48.27. Insomnia in restless legs associated with periodic movements in sleep. Myoclonus of the lower limbs and overall restlessness are noted below the sleep histogram. Until 0150 hours, the patients shows mainly wakefulness, stage 1, and some stage 2 sleep. REM sleep was associated with little myoclonus. Slow-wave sleep occurs only some 4 hours after retiring. The picture is one of marked sleep onset insomnia. (From Coccagna, G., and Lugaresi, E. 1968. Insomnia in the restless leg syndrome. In *The Abnormalities of Sleep in Man,* Eds. H Gastaut, E. Lugaresi, G. Berti-Ceroni, et al., pp. 285–294. Bologna: Aulo Gaggi.)

be soft neurological signs (Hauri and Olmstead, 1980). Such subjects are exquisitely sensitive to caffeine in tea, coffee, soft drinks, and chocolate, and display sleep patterns similar to those of chronic psychophysiological insomnia.

Insomnia Complaints Without Objective Findings

At times, statements of having slept little or not at all are contradicted by observers' descriptions of the person having slept or even snored all night long, or by essentially normal polysomnographic sleep patterns despite sleep denial (Borkovec, 1979; Carskadon et al., 1976). The personality profile is not that of hypochondriasis. This well-documented, still little-understood condition appears to represent a dissociative phenomenon of relative mental wakefulness associated with behavioral and physiological sleep.

Natural Short Sleepers

A number of apparently normal subjects appear to require only a very small amount of sleep relative to the general norm. Such subjects do not complain of EDS, sleep problems, or difficulties with mood or performance. Like naturally long sleepers, they appear to represent one end of the normal distribution of sleep need. Sleep studies (Fig. 48.28) show very efficient sleep consisting of short latency, rapid descent into stages 3 and 4, few or no awakenings, and varying amounts of REM sleep (Jones and Oswald, 1968; Meddis et al., 1973; Stuss and Broughton, 1978; Webb and Friel, 1971). It has been shown in at least one extreme natural short sleeper that performance was unimpaired by either sleep reduction or sleep extension, even from a habitual amount of 2 to 3.5 hours (Stuss and Broughton, 1978), thereby proving that the subject was obtaining his optimal sleep amount, in this case only about 2.5 hours. Such subjects have a form of pseudoinsomnia, as, apparently, do patients with a subjective insomniac complaint but normal sleep recordings (Carskadon et al., 1976).

Disorders of the Circadian Sleep-Wake Cycle

Jet Lag

Jet lag from flying across time zones causes temporary sleep problems during adaptation to the new timing of sleep-wake activities (McFarland, 1975). The clinical picture is one of desynchronization between previous sleep-wake cycles and local demands, so that patients initially tend to be awake during the local sleeping time and be sleepy during the local waking period. The disturbance is generally greater after eastward than westward flights. This is apparently because travel is then in opposition to the direction of the sun, causing environmental light/darkness cues to be more out of phase for a given time zone difference, and also because the endogenous circadian rhythm is slightly longer than 24 hours, making sleep delay easier than sleep advance. Polysomnograms typically show long sleep latencies, a degree of sleep fragmentation, and (locally) inappropriate wakening hours.

Shift Work and Irregular Sleep

Some individuals maintain very irregular sleep-wake patterns, leading to severe sleep problems. In shift work, rotat-

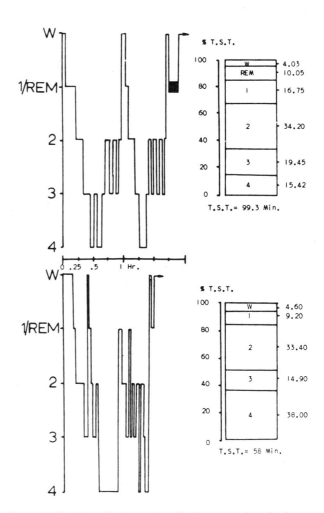

Figure 48.28. Naturally shorter sleep. The histograms show the sleep patterns of a healthy 57-year-old man who adopted a 1.5- to 2.0-hour sleep pattern during World War II. He shows normal total amounts of stages 3 and 4 sleep for his age and reached only REM sleep the first night. (From Stuss, D., and Broughton, R. 1978. Extreme short sleep: personality profiles and a case of sleep requirement. Waking Sleeping 2:101–105.)

ing schedules cause marked deterioration of circadian sleep-wake patterns and may also lead to severe insomnia. A main difference from jet lag is that the local sleep-wake cycles are regularly out of synchrony with what the shift worker wishes to maintain. Subjects often revert to the social norm on weekends, making it difficult to keep biorhythms entrained to the work schedule. Daytime sleep is lighter and more fragmented (Weitzman et al., 1970), due to a combination of higher core body temperature and environmental light and noise. Both irregular sleep patterns and shift work may be associated in normal persons with sleep-onset REM periods. Dissociated REM sleep may also occur. Sleep paralysis may be induced in normals by irregular or fragmented sleep patterns (Takeuchi et al., 1992). It also appears that irregular sleep habits may help trigger development of narcolepsy-cataplexy in genetically predisposed subjects (Broughton et al., 1981a).

Delayed and Advanced Sleep Phase Syndromes

Some individuals present with debilitating functional disorders in which their fixed hours of sleeping and awakening are either much later or earlier than desired. Attempts to voluntarily reset their circadian sleep timing to the norm generally prove unsuccessful. In the delayed sleep phase syndrome (Thorpy et al., 1988; Weitzman et al., 1981), patients cannot get to sleep until the early morning hours and so complain of sleep-onset insomnia. Thereafter, they sleep soundly and, if unawakened, have 7 to 8 hours of normal sleep. If they must awaken early in order to work yet cannot fall asleep until 2 to 3 a.m., they obviously undergo a great deal of sleep deprivation. Attempts to go to sleep at the normal hour are unsuccessful, and patients may resort to sleeping pills. In some cases, the sleep cycle can be rephased by moving the hour of retirement progressively later (Czeisler et al., 1981) until the desired temporal placement of sleep is established ("chronotherapy"). Morning bright light therapy, which advances the phase of the circadian system, may also help normalize sleep patterns to the desired clock time. In the advanced sleep phase syndrome (Moldofky et al., 1986), subjects experience more or less imperative pressure to sleep in the early evening and rise excessively early; this condition is seen most often in the elderly. Again sleep structure is normal, but the temporal placement of sleep is not. Chronotherapy or evening bright light therapy may help to delay the nocturnal sleep period.

Non–24-Hour Sleep-Wake Syndrome

The endogenous circadian periodicity of sleep in humans, as shown in environments free of all time cues, is 24.1 to 24.3 hours. The 24-hour periodicity characterizing normal social sleep patterns is entrained by forced awakening at consistent morning hours either by natural stimuli (especially light) or by an alarm. In some individuals (Kokkoris et al., 1978), the endogenous greater than 24-hour periodicity is maintained (Fig. 48.29), apparently due to lack of CNS response to time cues. Such subjects sleep later by 0.1 to 0.5 hours every day and so will progressively move into a daytime sleep pattern and then back into night sleep. Like the delayed sleep phase syndrome, this so-called hypernychthemeral syndrome makes maintenance of a conventional work-rest schedule impossible. The phenomenon may reflect impairment of the suprachiasmatic nucleus that controls circadian periodicity. The condition has also been reported in blindness (Miles et al., 1977).

Episodic Behavioral Disorders in Sleep ("Parasomnias")

Three types of attacks occur preferentially with arousals from stages 3 and 4 of SWS: confusional arousals (nocturnal sleep drunkenness), sleep terrors, and sleepwalking. All involve some degree of confusion, disorientation, and retrograde amnesia. Recurrent attacks can often be provoked in

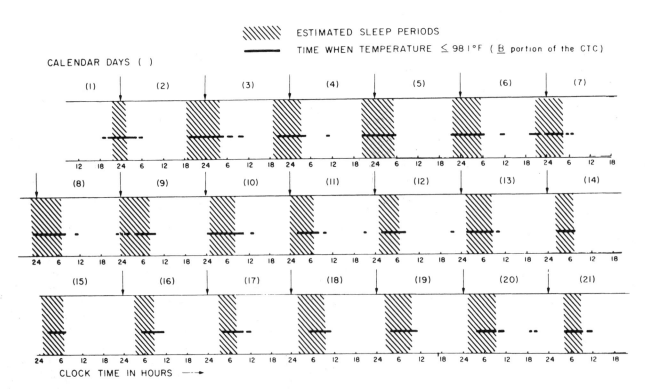

Figure 48.29. Non–24-hour sleep/wake syndrome. The figure gives the sleep period (from sleep logs) and the periods of circadian hypothermia (less than 98.1°F) as recorded by a rectal indwelling continuous temperature monitor (core temperature curve [CTC]). Note on calendar days 8 through 21 that the sleep period comes later and later during the 24 hours. (From Kokkoris, C.P., Weitzman, E.D., Pollak, C.P., et al. 1978. Long-term ambulatory temperature monitoring in a subject with a hypernychthemeral sleep-wake cycle disturbance. Sleep 1:177–180.)

subjects suffering from these parasomnias by simple forced awakening during SWS, thereby providing strong evidence against a necessary psychogenic origin in sleep (one would have to postulate that the forced arousals were timed when unknown mental activity was about to generate an episode), and for an abnormality of the SWS arousal process itself (Broughton, 1968; Gastaut and Broughton, 1965). Because of these features, the conditions have been considered pathophysiologically as "disorders of arousal" (Broughton, 1968). Even when occurring in epileptic individuals, these parasomnias represent coexistent nonepileptic phenomena (Gastaut and Broughton, 1965). They must therefore be distinguished respectively from nocturnal episodes of confusion, complex automatisms, or fear (very rare) related to nocturnal epileptic seizures.

Confusional Awakenings (Nocturnal Sleep Drunkenness)

Individuals awakened from deep sleep may experience prolonged confusion, disorientation, poor coordination, automatic behavior, and varying degrees of amnesia. Nocturnal confusional awakenings typically occur with arousals in the first part of the night, during sleep stages 3 and 4 (Gastaut and Broughton, 1965), and are particularly common in children. After such awakenings, even normal individuals show substantially impaired performance (Feltin and Broughton, 1968; Scott and Snyder, 1968) as well as visual evoked potentials intermediate between sleep and wakefulness (Broughton, 1968; Saier et al., 1968). During these behavioral states, the EEG may show either so-called stage 1B patterns or an alpha rhythm that is nonreactive to bright illumination, a pattern that has been called stage IA3 (Gastaut and Broughton, 1965). Such nocturnal episodes of sleep drunkenness should be distinguished from morning sleep drunkenness, which occurs in about 50% of patients with idiopathic hypersomnia (Roth et al., 1972).

A different type of confusional awakening is occasionally seen during arousal from REM sleep. These are particularly frequent in the elderly (Feinberg, 1969b) and in REM-rebound hypersomnias (e.g., in withdrawal states from REM-suppressant drugs) characterized by hallucinatory experiences during states intermediate between REM sleep and wakefulness. The latter is particularly well documented for alcoholic hallucinosis (Gross et al., 1966).

Sleep Terrors (Pavor Nocturnus, Incubus Attack)

The sleep terror is characterized by abrupt arousals with a piercing scream or cry followed by behavior indicative of acute anxiety. Attacks occur during sleep, generally in the first third of the night. The individual has a frightened expression, marked tachycardia and tachypnea, often profuse sweating, and dilated pupils. Full consciousness is usually not attained for 5 to 10 minutes after the start of an attack. During this time, the person is inconsolable; the attack must simply run its course. Little imagery is recalled. Often it consists of a single scene (Fisher et al., 1970; Gastaut and Broughton, 1965) resembling a photograph rather than an organized sequence, as is experienced in a dream. There may be feelings of choking, being crushed or other respiratory difficulty, palpitations, paralysis, or acute dread. The at-

tacks (Figs. 48.30 and 48.31) arise during stages 3 and 4 sleep and are associated with rapid desynchronization to low-voltage fast waking patterns combined with marked increase in heart rate, tachypnea, increased muscle tone, and other polygraphic patterns of acute arousal (Gastaut and Broughton, 1965; Fisher et al., 1970). The intensity of a sleep terror, as measured by the degree of increase in heart rate, is proportional to the duration of preceding SWS (Fisher et al., 1970). Patients generally do not remember attacks the next day. If multiple attacks occur during a single night, they may also arise in stage 2.

Sleepwalking

Sleepwalking consists of complex behavior, including leaving the bed and walking about, usually during the first third of the night. The subject may perform various, often stereotypic, activities such as clearing off a table, dressing, or eating. Attempts to attract the subject's attention are unsuccessful. If awakened, the subject is amnesic for the attack and does not recall anything beyond fragmented imagery. Violence may occur (Broughton and Shimizu, 1995) and even homicide has been reported (Broughton et al., 1994). Attacks begin during stages 3 and 4 sleep (Broughton, 1968; Gastaut and Broughton, 1965; Jacobson et al., 1965; Kales et al., 1966). During the episodes, the EEG (Fig. 48.32) becomes relatively desynchronized and shows stage 1 patterns with mixed, mainly theta, frequencies or a continuous nonreactive alpha rhythm (substage IA3) (Gastaut and Broughton, 1965). As in Fig. 48.30, the episodes may be precipitated in predisposed individuals by artificial forced awakening from slow-wave sleep (Gastaut and Broughton, 1965).

Terrifying Dreams (Dream Anxiety Attacks)

Organized frightening dreams, sometimes having content threatening to the sleeper's life, may disturb sleep and lead to awakening. Such dreams may be accompanied by moaning or other vocalizations, but are not associated with the piercing cry or behavioral intensity characterizing the sleep terror. The autonomic activation is not nearly as intense, although some degree of tachycardia and tachypnea during preceding sleep or upon awakening is common. The attacks, moreover, are not accompanied by the confusion and disorientation of sleep terrors; the sensorium rapidly or immediately clears after awakening. Attacks characteristically take place in the second half of the night (Fig. 48.33) and are associated with REM sleep (Fisher et al., 1970). They may occur in predisposed persons during periods of insecurity or daytime conflicts (Hartmann, 1984) and are particularly common during situations of increased REM sleep, as in REM rebound from previous REM suppression due to stress, or from drugs (sleeping pills, stimulants, or alcohol). Terrifying dreams are also more common in patients receiving beta-blockers (e.g., propranolol) for hypertension.

REM Sleep Behavioral Disorder

Another category of parasomnia first described by Hishikawa et al. (1981) and more fully detailed by Schenck et al. (1986) consists of unusual aggressive behavioral episodes arising in the REM sleep. They are most common in older patients lacking daytime aggression or

Figure 48.30.   Sleep terror (initial part). The attack was one of a number that night in a 25-year-old subject; it arose in stage 3. It was associated with sitting up and screaming. The order of phenomena in the polygraph is noted with letters. There was a series of K complexes (followed rapidly by desynchronization of waking patterns), eye movement, tachycardia, drop in skin resistance, bed movement on the actogram, marked increase in muscle tone, and tachypnea, all occurring in 5 to 6 seconds. This reflects the extreme intensity and rapidity of the arousal. The cardiac and respiratory rates essentially doubled. The attack is continued in Fig. 48.31. (From Gastaut, H., and Broughton, R. 1965. A clinical and polygraphic study of episodic phenomena during sleep: academic address. Recent Adv. Biol. Psychiatry 7:197–221.)

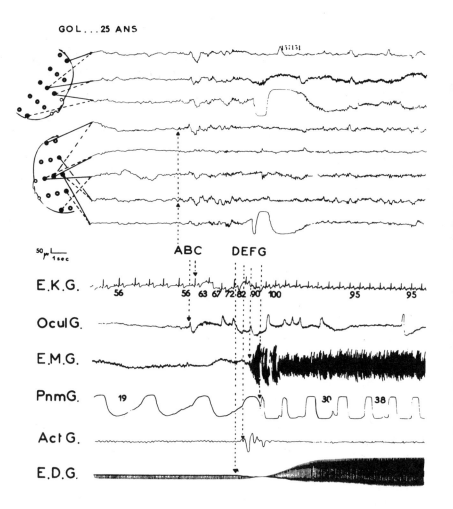

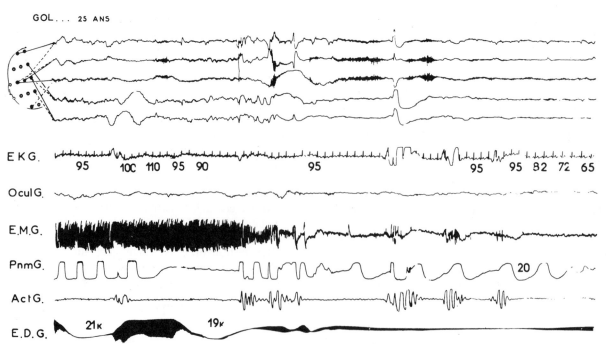

Figure 48.31.   Sleep terror (continued). The continuation of the polygraphic recording in Fig. 48.30 is shown. During the attack, there is persistent tachycardia (reaching 110 beats/min) and tachypnea with one period of apnea; sustained, markedly increased muscle tone; and falling skin resistance. The entire attack lasted some 25 seconds. (From Gastaut, H., and Broughton, R. 1965. A clinical and polygraphic study of episodic phenomena during sleep: academic address. Recent Adv. Biol. Psychiatry 7: 197–221.)

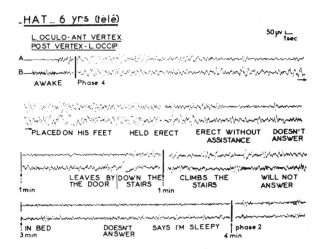

Figure 48.32. Experimentally induced confusional arousal with sleep-walking. The recording was done by telemetry with two channels: left outer canthus to midline frontal (anterior vertex) and midline parietal (posterior vertex) to left occipital. The initial fragment shows eye movements and an occipital alpha rhythm. About 1 hour later, when this 6-year-old sleep-walker was in stage 4, the experimenter entered the bedroom, giving rise to some desynchronization of the EEG *(upper right)*, placed the subject on his feet, and initially held him erect. After several seconds, the subject was able to stand without assistance and did not answer questions; 1 minute later, he walked out of the bedroom and down the stairs. After 1 minute of wandering around, mainly with stage 1B patterns, he climbed back up the stairs, showing patterns of unreactive alphas (stage 1A/e3) to bright lights for filming. After 3 minutes, he was in bed; he would not answer until finally offered simply an almost inaudible, "I'm sleepy." After 4 minutes, he was in stage 2. There was no recall the following morning. (From Gastaut, H., and Broughton, R. 1965. A clinical and polygraphic study of episodic phenomena during sleep: academic address. Recent Adv. Biol. Psychiatry 7: 197–221.)

psychiatric problems and in chronic alcoholics. The attacks generally occur in the second half of the night and consist of incomplete awakenings with violent kicking, punching, diving out of bed, rapid ambulatory collisions, and similar wild behaviors. They have also been seen in conjunction with a variety of neurological pathologies, including dementia, subarachnoid hemorrhage, olivopontocerebellar degeneration, and Guillain-Barré syndrome; and a significant proportion of patients go on to develop Parkinson's disease. Polysomnograms show marked phasic REM bursts and myoclonic potentials on peripheral EMGs plus

movement artifacts associated with EEG patterns of continuing REM sleep or of wakefulness after REM sleep (Mahowald and Schenck, 1994). The attacks resemble those induced in cats by suppressing REM sleep atonia and paralysis by pontine tegmental lesions first reported by Jouvet and Delorme (1965).

Sleep-Related Enuresis (Enuresis Nocturna)

The condition consists of involuntary micturition at night after the age—usually more than 3 years—at which bladder control should have been attained. The loss of urine occurs diffusely in all sleep stages (Kales et al., 1977; Mikkelson et al., 1980). The person may or may not show full electrographic awakening during the enuretic episode (Fig. 48.34). Clinically, the enuretic is initially very difficult to arouse and, when awake, often shows confusion and disorientation and lack of organized dream recall. There is evidence that enuretics' bladders are more reactive than those of normal subjects to a number of stimuli (Gastaut and Broughton, 1965), that their bladders are smaller (Muellner, 1960) and so fill more rapidly in sleep, and that their sensation of bladder stimuli is impaired (Bradley, 1977; Di Perri and Meduri, 1975). The main physiopathogenic issue is why, unlike normals, enuretics with full bladders do not awaken either rapidly or completely enough to either suppress the micturition reflex or get out of bed and void (Broughton, 1982b).

Sleep-Related Head-Banging (Jactatio Capitis Nocturna)

This term denotes to-and-fro rocking of the head or, less commonly, of the entire body. It may occur either just at sleep onset in stages 1A and 1B drowsiness (predormitional form) or throughout all sleep stages (dormitional form), as described by Gastaut and Broughton (1965) and Baldy-Moulinier et al. (1970). It interferes little or not at all with ongoing sleep. The condition is seen at times in normal children, especially in situations of stress or family disharmony, and more frequently in mental retardation. Retarded individuals are particularly prone to the dormitional form (Thorpy and Glovinsky, 1989).

Hypnogenic Paroxysmal Dystonia

Lugaresi and Cirignotta (1981) described a previously unrecognized form of parasomnia in which subjects present

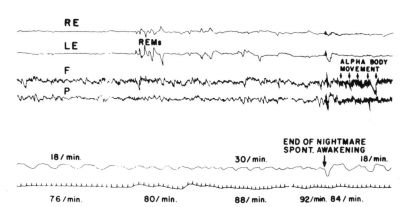

Figure 48.33. Dream anxiety attack. The polygraph recording was taken during a dream anxiety attack (REM nightmare). Normal frontal and parietal EEGs of REM sleep and REM bursts are recorded initially with increasing respiratory and cardiac rates. The dream is terminated with spontaneous awakening. Note that the autonomic arousal is not nearly as intense as for the sleep terror. (From Fisher, C.F., Byrne, J., Edwards, T., et al. 1970. A psychophysiological study of nightmares. J. Psychoanal. Assoc. 18:747–782.)

Figure 48.34. Enuresis nocturna. This 7-year-old enuretic child had an enuretic episode in slow-wave sleep. After some 12 seconds of stage 4 sleep, there is a series of higher amplitude delta waves of K complex type associated with onset of tachycardia. The micturition begins at the point where the "miction" indicator loses the mainline artifact and becomes a flat line showing only movement artifact. Passage into stage 2 occurs at the time of arousal. Although some EEG movement artifact and eye movements are associated with the global body movement, neither EEG nor behavioral wakening occurred. (From Gastaut, H., and Broughton, R. 1965. A clinical and polygraphic study of episodic phenomena during sleep: academic address. Recent Adv. Biol. Psychiatry 7:197–221.)

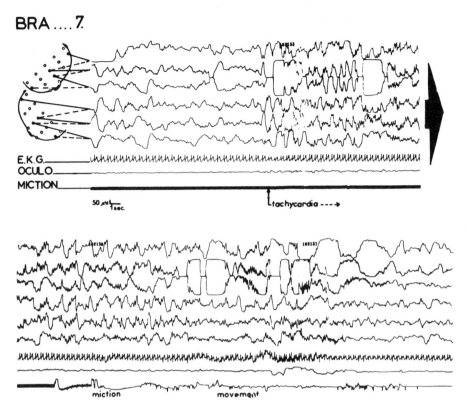

with sleep-related dystonic movements, for instance slow rotation of the head or trunk with frequent abductor limb movements in extension or flexion, usually lasting 15 to 45 seconds. These arise during tranquil sleep. Subjects may sit up in bed and then fall back. Their eyes may be open, but they remain unresponsive. Attacks typically occur during stage 2 or 3 sleep (Fig. 48.35) and have not been encountered in REM sleep. Concomitant sleepwalking or sleep terrors have not been reported. In a short form the EEG generally lacks any discharges, although most subjects re-

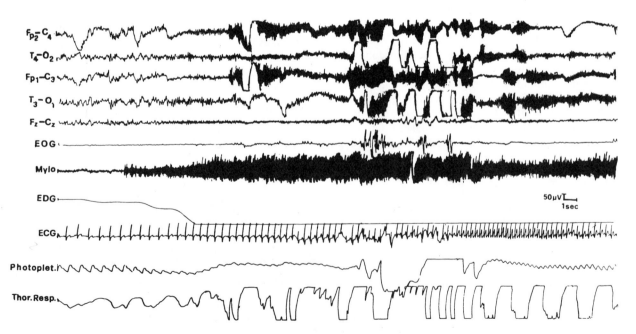

Figure 48.35. Paroxysmal nocturnal dystonia. This brief attack begins in stages 3 and 4 non–REM sleep and consists polygraphically of a drop in skin resistance on the electrodermogram (EDG), decreased pulsation on the finger plethysmogram (photoplet), and an increase in chin muscle tone (mylo). This is associated with EEG arousal, tachypnea, and tachycardia. (E. Lugaresi and F. Cirignotta, unpublished observation.)

spond to carbamazepine and some patients have been shown to have a frontal epileptic focus at times difficult or impossible to detect with routine scalp EEG (Tinuper et al., 1990). A longer form has also been described (Lugaresi and Cirignotta, 1982), which does not respond to the same medication, has never been associated with an EEG discharge and is believed to reflect an underlying neurochemical disorder.

Sleep-Related Epileptic Seizures

About 20% to 25% of epileptics have seizures exclusively or mainly at night (sleep epilepsies), and a further 30% to 40% have seizures distributed around the clock in both sleep and wakefulness (diffuse epilepsies). The remaining 35% to 50% of epileptics have seizures exclusively or mainly during wakefulness (waking epilepsies). Therefore, nocturnal seizures are not infrequent (Gibberd and Bateson, 1974; Janz, 1962). The relationships between epileptic seizures and sleep, arousal from sleep, biological rhythms, and sleep deprivation have been reviewed extensively elsewhere (Broughton, 1972b, 1984). In brief, there is evidence that tonic-clonic (grand mal), tonic, and myoclonic generalized epileptic seizures are activated in NREM sleep, whereas typical absences (petit mal discharges) may be seen in REM sleep. The partial seizures tend to have more complex relationships with sleep states, which depends on their location of onset. Seizures, particularly generalized tonic-clonic seizures and generalized myoclonic attacks, may occur regularly in association with morning awakening; in other seizure patients, sleep deprivation is a recurrent precipitating factor.

Rarely, sleep-related epileptic seizures can give rise to behavioral patterns that mimic nonepileptic attacks, for instance, urinary incontinence leading to diagnostic confusion with enuresis nocturna, psychomotor automatisms of complex partial seizures with sleepwalking, or ictal fear from partial complex seizures with sleep terrors or dream anxiety attacks. Examples are cases of nocturnal wanderings of epileptic origin (Plazzi et al., 1995) and a form of autosomal-dominant frontal epilepsy presenting as an apparent nonepileptic sleep disorder (Scheffer et al., 1994). One of the more common reasons for patient referral to an EEG laboratory for a sleep recording is, in fact, to determine whether nocturnal attacks of unknown etiology are epileptic or nonepileptic.

References

AASM. 1999. Sleep-related breathing disorders in adults: recommendations for syndrome definition and measurement techniques in clinical research. Sleep 22:667–689.

AASM. 2003. Practice parameters for the use of portable monitoring devices in the investigation of suspected obstructive sleep apnea in adults. A joint project sponsored by the American Academy of Sleep Medicine, the American Thoracic Society, and the American College of Chest Physicians. Sleep 26:907–913.

Adey, W.R., Bors, E., and Porter, R.W. 1968. EEG patterns after high spinal cord lesions in man. Arch. Neurol. 19:377–383.

Agnew, H.W., Webb, W.B., and Williams, R.L. 1966. The first night effect: an EEG study of sleep. Psychophysiology 2:263–266.

Aguirre, M., and Broughton, R.J. 1984. Objective and subjective measures of (REM and NREM) sleepiness in narcolepsy-cataplexy. Sleep Res. 13:128.

Akindele, M.O., Evans, J.J., and Oswald, I. 1970. Monoamine oxidase inhibition, sleep and mood. Electroencephalogr. Clin. Neurophysiol. 29:47–56.

Allison, F.G. 1943. Obscure pains in chest, back or limbs. Can. Med. Assoc. J. 48:36–54.

Alloway, C.E.D., Ogilvie, R.D., and Shapiro, C.M. 1997. The alpha attenuation test: assessing excessive daytime sleepiness in narcolepsy-cataplexy. Sleep 20:258–266.

Anders, T., Emde, R., and Parmalee, A. (Eds.). 1971. A *Manual of Standardized Terminology, Techniques and Criteria for Scoring States of Sleep and Wakefulness in Newborn Infants.* Los Angeles: UCLA Brain Information Service, NINDS Neurological Information Network.

Aschoff, J. 1976. Circadian systems in man and their implications. Hosp. Pract. 11:51–58.

ASDA. 1992. EEG arousals: scoring rules and examples: a preliminary report from the Sleep Disorders Atlas Task Force of the American Sleep Disorders Association. Sleep 15:173–184.

ASDA. 1997. ASDA Standards of Practice Committee. Practice parameters for the indications for polysomnography and related procedures. Sleep 20:406–422.

Baldy-Moulinier, M., Levy, M., and Passouant, P. 1970. A study of jactacio capito during night sleep. Electroencephalogr. Clin. Neurophysiol. 28:87(abst).

Baldy-Moulinier, M., Arguner, A., and Bisset, A. 1976. Ultradian and circadian rhythms in sleep and wakefulness. In *Narcolepsy,* Eds. C. Guilleminault, W.C. Dement, and P. Passouant, pp. 485–497. New York: Spectrum.

Bergamasco, B., Bergamini, L., Doriguzzi, T., et al. 1968. EEG sleep patterns as a prognostic criterion in post-traumatic coma. Electroencephalogr. Clin. Neurophysiol. 24:374–377.

Berger, R.J. 1961. Tonus of extrinsic laryngeal muscles during sleep and dreaming. Science 134:840.

Berger, R.J., and Oswald, I. 1962. Eye movements during active and passive dreams. Science 137:601.

Billiard, M. 1976. Competition between the two types of sleep and the recuperative function of REM versus NREM sleep in narcoleptics. In *Narcolepsy,* Eds. C. Guilleminault, W.C. Dement, and P. Passouant, pp. 77–96. New York: Spectrum.

Billiard, M. (Ed.). 1994. *Le Sommeil et Ses Troubles.* Paris: Masson.

Billiard, M., Guilleminault, C., and Dement, W.C. 1975. A menstruation-linked periodic hypersomnia. Neurology (Minneapolis) 25:436–443.

Blake, M.J.F. 1967. Time of day effects on performance in a range of tasks. Psychon. Sci. Sect. Hum. Exp. Psychol. 9:349–350.

Bliwise, D., Coleman, R., Bergmann, B., et al. 1974. Facial muscle tonus during REM and NREM sleep. Psychophysiology 11:497–508.

Bonnet, M.H. 1985. The effect of sleep disruption on sleep, performance and mood. Sleep 8:11–19.

Bonnet, M.H. 1987. Sleep restoration as a function of periodic awakening, movement or electroencephalographic change. Sleep 10:364–373.

Borkovec, T.D. 1979. Pseudo (experiential) insomnia and idiopathic (objective) insomnia: theoretical and therapeutic issues. Adv. Behav. Res. Ther. 2:27–55.

Bradley, W.E. 1977. Electroencephalography and bladder innervation. J. Urol. 118:412–414.

Bricolo, A. 1967. Insomnia after bilateral stereotactic thalamotomy in man. J. Neurol. Neurosurg. Psychiatry 10:154–158.

Broughton, R. 1968. Sleep disorders: disorders of arousal? Science 159:326–338.

Broughton, R. 1972a. A proposed classification of sleep disorders. Sleep Res. 1:146(abst).

Broughton, R. 1972b. Sleep and neurological states. In *The Sleeping Brain,* Ed. M. Chase, pp. 363–376. Los Angeles: Brain Information Service/Brain Research Institute, UCLA.

Broughton, R.J. 1975. Biorhythmic variations in consciousness and psychological functions. Can. Psychol. Rev. 16:217–230.

Broughton, R.J. 1976. Discussion. In *Narcolepsy,* Eds. C. Guilleminault, W.C. Dement, and P. Passouant, pp. 667. New York: Spectrum.

Broughton, R. 1982a. Performance and evoked potential measures of various states of daytime sleepiness. Sleep 5(suppl 2):135–146.

Broughton, R. 1982b. Pathophysiology of enuresis nocturna, sleep terrors and sleepwalking: Current status and the Marseille contribution. In *Henri Gastaut and the Marseille School's Contribution to the Neurosciences,* Ed. R.J. Broughton, pp. 401–410. Amsterdam: Elsevier.

Broughton, R. 1983. The siesta: social or biological phenomenon? Sleep Res. 12:28(abst).

Broughton, R. 1984. Epilepsy and sleep: a synthesis and prospectus. In *Epilepsy—Sleep—Sleep Deprivation,* Eds. R. Degen and E. Niedermeyer, pp. 317–356. Amsterdam: Elsevier.

Broughton, R. 1988. Pathological fragmentary myoclonus, intensified "hypnic jerks" and hypnogenic foot tremor. Three unusual sleep–related movement disorders. In *Sleep 86,* Ed. W.R. Koella, pp. 41–43. Stuttgart: Fischer Verlag.

Broughton, R.J. 1989. Ambulatory sleep-wake monitoring in the home environment. In *Ambulatory Home Monitoring,* Ed. J.S. Ebersole, pp. 277–298. New York: Raven.

Broughton, R. 1992. Qualitatively different states of sleepiness. In *Sleep, Arousal and Performance: A Tribute to Bob Wilkinson,* Eds. R. Broughton and R. Ogilivie, pp. 45–59. Boston: Birkhauser.

Broughton, R.J. 1994. Some important underemphasized aspects of sleep onset. In *Sleep Onset Mechanisms,* Eds. R. Ogilvie and J. Harsh, pp. 19–36. Arlington, VA: American Psychological Association.

Broughton, R., and Aguirre, M. 1987. Differences between REM and NREM sleepiness measured by event-related potentials (P300 CNV), MSLT and subjective estimate in narcolepsy-cataplexy. Electroencephalogr. Clin. Neurophysiol. 67:317–326.

Broughton, R., and Hasan, J. 1995. Quantitative topographical electroencephalographic mapping during drowsiness and sleep onset. J. Clin. Neurophysiol. 12:372–386.

Broughton, R., and Krupa, S. 2003. The apparent mechanism of the afternoon "nap zone." Sleep 26(suppl):A96.

Broughton, R., and Mamelak, M. 1980. Effects of nocturnal gamma-hydroxybutyrate on sleep/waking patterns in narcolepsy-cataplexy. Can. J. Neurol. Sci. 7:23–31.

Broughton, R., and Shimizu, T. 1995. Sleep-related violence: a medical and forensic challenge. Sleep 18:727–730.

Broughton, R., and Tolentino, M.A. 1984. Fragmentary pathological myoclonus in NREM sleep. Electroencephalogr. Clin. Neurophysiol. 57: 303–309.

Broughton, R., Hanley, J., Quanbury, O., et al. 1976. Electrodes. In *Handbook of Electroencephalography and Clinical Neurophysiology,* vol. 3A, Ed. R. Broughton, pp. 5–27. Amsterdam: Elsevier.

Broughton, R., Nevsimalova, S., and Roth, B. 1980. The socio-economic effects of idiopathic hypersomnia: comparisons with controls and with compound narcoleptics. In *Sleep 1978,* Eds. L. Popoviciu, B. Asgian, and G. Badiu, pp. 229–233. Basel: S. Karger.

Broughton, R., Ghanem, Q., Hishikawa, Y., et al. 1981a. Life effects of narcolepsy in 180 patients from North America, Asia and Europe compared to controls. Can. J. Neurol. Sci. 8:299–304.

Broughton, R., Low, R., Valley, V., et al. 1981b. Sensitivity of the AEP compared to performance during Wilkinson's auditory vigilance task in narcoleptics and normals. Electroencephalogr. Ciin. Neurophysiol. 51:17R.

Broughton, R., Low, R., Valley, V., et al. 1982. Auditory evoked potentials compared to performance measures and EEG in assessing excessive daytime sleepiness in narcolepsy-cataplexy. Electroencephalogr. Clin. Neurophysiol. 54:572–582.

Broughton, R., Ghanem, Q., Hishikawa, Y., et al. 1983. Life-effects of narcolepsy: relationships to geographic origin (North America, Asia or European) and to other patient and illness variables. Can. J. Neurol. Sci. 10:100–104.

Broughton, R., Guberman, A., and Roberts, J. 1984. Comparison of psychosocial effects of epilepsy and narcolepsy-cataplexy: a controlled study. Epilepsia 25:423–433.

Broughton, R., Tolentino, M.A., and Krelina, M. 1985. Excessive fragmentary myoclonus in NREM sleep: a report on 38 cases. Electroencephalogr. Clin. Neurophysiol. 61:123–133.

Broughton, R., Valley, V., Aguirre, M., et al. 1986. On the excessive daytime sleepiness and the pathophysiology of narcolepsy: a laboratory perspective. Sleep 9:205–215.

Broughton, R., Aguirre, M., and Dunham, W. 1988a. A comparison of multiple and single sleep latency and cerebral evoked potential (P300) measures in the assessment of excessive daytime sleepiness in narcolepsy-cataplexy. Sleep 11:537–545.

Broughton, R., Dunham, W., Lutley, K., et al. 1988b. Ambulatory 24-hour sleep/wake recordings in narcolepsy-cataplexy. Electroencephalogr. Clin. Neurophysiol. 70:473–81.

Broughton, R., Billiard, M., Frost, J., et al. 1989. Monitoring sleep and sleep related disorders. In *Recommendations in the Practice of Clinical Neurophysiology,* 2nd ed., Ed. R. Ellingson, pp. 696–701. Amsterdam: Elsevier.

Broughton, R., Billings, R., and Cartwright, R. 1994. Homicidal somnambulism: a case report. Sleep 17:235–264.

Broughton, R.J., Dunham, W., Krupa, S., et al. 1995. Impairment of waking arousal in narcolepsy. Sleep Res. 24:206(abst).

Burwell, C.S., Robin, E.D., Whaley, R.D., et al. 1956. Extreme obesity associated with alveolar hypoventilation: a Pickwickian syndrome. Am. J. Med. 21:811–818.

Butkov N. 1996. *The Atlas of Clinical Polysomnography.* Ashland, OR: Synapse Media (2 vols).

Cadhilac, J. 1976. Classification des troubles du sommeil. Therapie 31: 7–25.

Carskadon, M.A., and Dement, W.C. 1977. Sleep tendency: an objective measure of sleep loss. Sleep Res. 6:200(abst).

Carskadon, M., Dement, W., Mitler, M., et al. 1976. Self-report versus sleep laboratory findings in 122 drug free subjects with the complaint of chronic insomnia. Arch. J. Psychiatry 133:1382–1388.

Carskadon, M., Dement, W.C., Mitler, M., et al. 1986. Guidelines for the Multiple Sleep Latency Test (MSLT): a standard measure of sleepiness. Sleep 9:519–524.

Chokroverty, S. (Ed.). 1994. *Sleep Disorders Medicine.* Stoneham, MA: Butterworth, Heinemann.

Coccagna, G., and Lugaresi, E. 1968. Insomnia in the restless leg syndrome. In *The Abnormalities of Sleep in Man,* Eds. H. Gastaut, E. Lugaresi, G. Berti-Ceroni, et al., pp. 139–147. Bologna: Aulo Gaggi.

Coccagna, G., Petrella, A., Berti-Ceroni, G., et al. 1968. Polygraphic contributions to hypersomnia and respiratory troubles in the Pickwickian syndrome. In *The Abnormalities of Sleep in Man,* Eds. H. Gastaut, E. Lugaresi, G. Berti Ceroni, et al., pp. 215–221. Bologna: Aulo Gaggi.

Coleman, R.M., Pollak, C., and Weitzman, E.D. 1980. Periodic movements in sleep (nocturnal myoclonus): relation to sleep-wake disorders. Ann. Neurol. 8:416–421.

Critchley, M. 1962. Periodic hypersomnia and megaphagia in adolescent males. Brain 85:627–656.

Czeisler, C.A., Richardson, G.S., Colman, R.M. 1981. Chronotherapy: resetting the circadian clock of patients with delayed sleep phase syndrome. Sleep 4:1–21.

Daly, D.D., and Yoss, R.E. 1957. The electroencephalogram in narcolepsy. Electroencephalogr. Clin. Neurophysiol. 9:109–120.

De Barros-Ferreira, M., and Lairy, G.C. 1976. Ambiguous sleep in narcolepsy. In *Narcolepsy,* Eds. C. Guilleminault, W.C. Dement, and P. Passouant, pp. 57–75. New York: Spectrum.

De Barros-Ferreira, M., and Mattos, E. 1969. Etude évolutive du sommeil de nuit au cours d'épisodes maniaques ou depressif aigues. Rev. Neurol. (Paris) 121:348–357.

Dement, W.C. 1976. Daytime sleepiness and sleep attacks. In *Narcolepsy,* Eds. C. Guilleminault, W.C. Dement, and P. Passouant, pp. 17–42. New York: Spectrum.

Dexter, J.D., and Weitzman, E.D. 1970. The relationship of nocturnal headache to sleep stage patterns. Neurology (Minneapolis) 20:513–518.

Dinges, D., and Broughton, R. (Eds.). 1989. *Sleep and Alertness: Chronobiological, Behavioral and Medical Aspects of Napping.* New York: Raven Press.

Di Perri, R., and Meduri, M. 1975. A polygraphic approach to the study of nocturnal enuresis. In *Sleep 1974,* Eds. P. Levin and W.P. Koella, pp. 413–416. Basel: S. Karger.

Dittrichova, J. 1969. Development of sleep in infancy. In *Brain and Early Behavior,* Ed. R.J. Robinson, pp. 193–201. London: Academic Press.

Downey, R., Perkin, R.M., and MacQuarrie, J. 1993. Upper airway resistance syndrome: sick, symptomatic but under–recognized. Sleep 16: 620–623.

Dreyfus-Brisac, C. 1979. Ontogenesis of brain bioelectrical activity and sleep organization in neonates and infants. In *Human Growth,* vol. 3, Eds. F. Falkner and J.M. Tanner, pp. 157–182. New York: Plenum Press.

Dreyfus-Brisac, C., and Curzi-Dascalova, L. 1975. The EEG during the first year of life. In *Handbook of Electroencephalography and Clinical Neurophysiology,* Ed. A. Remond, vol. 6B: *The Evolution of the EEG from Birth to Adulthood,* Ed. G. Lairy, pp. 24–30. Amsterdam: Elsevier.

Ekbom, K.A. 1960. Restless leg syndrome. Neurology (Minneapolis) 10: 868–873.

Ellingson, R. 1975. Ontogenesis of sleep in the human. In *Experimental Study of Human Sleep: Methodological Problems,* Eds. G. Lairy and P. Salzarulo, pp. 129–146. Amsterdam: Elsevier.

Evans, F., Cook, M., Cohen, H., et al. 1977. Appetitive and replacement naps: EEG and behavior. Science 197:687–689.

Ey, H., Lairy, G., de Barros-Ferreira, M., et al. 1975. *Psychophysiologie du Sommeil et Psychiatrie.* Paris: Masson.

Feinberg, I. 1969a. Effects of age on human sleep patterns. In *Sleep: Physiology and Pathology,* Ed. A. Kales, pp. 39–52. Philadelphia: J.B. Lippincott.

Feinberg, I. 1969b. Sleep in organic brain conditions. In *Sleep: Physiology and Pathology,* Ed. A. Kales, pp. 131–147. Philadelphia: J.B. Lippincott.

Feinberg, I., Koresko, R., and Heller, N. 1968. EEG sleep patterns as a function of normal and pathological aging in man. Arch. Gen. Psychiatry 18:239–250.

Feldman, M.H. 1971. Physiological observations in a chronic case of "locked-in" syndrome. Neurology (Minneapolis) 21:459–478.

Feltin, M., and Broughton, R. 1968. Differential effects of arousal from slow wave versus REM sleep. Psychophysiology 5:231(abst).

Ferber, R., Millman, R., Coppola, M., et al. 1994. Portable recording in the assessment of obstructive sleep apnea. An American Sleep Disorders Association review. Sleep 17:378–392.

Fischer-Perroudon, C., Mouret, J., and Jouvet, M. 1974. Sur un cas d'agrypnie au cors d'une maladie de Morvan. Effet favorable du 5-hydroxytryptophane. Electroencephalogr. Clin. Neurophysiol. 36:1–18.

Fisher, C.F., Byrne, J., Edwards, T., et al. 1970. A psychophysiological study of nightmares. J. Psychoanal. Assoc. 18:747–782.

Frankel, B.L., Patton, B.N., and Gillin, J.C. 1974. Restless leg syndrome: sleep electroencephalographic and neurologic findings. JAMA 230: 1302–1303.

Ganado, W. 1958. The narcolepsy syndrome. Neurology (Minneapolis) 8: 487–492.

Gastaut, H., and Broughton, R. 1965. A clinical and polygraphic study of episodic phenomena during sleep: academic address. Recent Adv. Biol. Psychiatry 7:197–221.

Gastaut, H., and Broughton, R. 1972. *Epileptic Seizures,* pp. 11–18. Springfield, IL: Charles C Thomas.

Gastaut, H., and Roth, B. 1957. A propos des manifestations électroencéphalographiques de 150 cas de narcolepsie avec ou sans cataplexie. Rev. Neurol. (Paris) 97:388–393.

Gibberd, F.B., and Bateson, M.C. 1974. Sleep epilepsy: its pattern and prognosis. Br. Med. J. 2:402–405.

Glenville, M., and Broughton, R.J. 1979. Reliability of the Stanford Sleepiness Scale compared to short duration performance tests and the Wilkinson auditory vigilance task. In *Pharmacology of the States of Alertness,* Eds. P. Passouant and I. Oswald, pp. 235–247. Oxford: Pergamon Press.

Goldsteinas, L., Boissenot, Y., and Chabert, F. 1969. Privation expérimentale de certaines stades de sommeil chez le sujet normal. Rev. Neurol. (Paris) 121:219–226.

Greenberg, R. 1967. Dream interruption insomnia. J. Nerv. Ment. Dis. 144: 18–21.

Gresham, S.C., Agnew, H.W., and Williams, R.L. 1965. The sleep of depressed patients. Arch. Gen. Psychiatry 13:503–507.

Gross, M.M., Goodenough, D., Tobin, M., et al. 1966. Sleep disturbances and hallucinations in the acute alcoholic psychoses. J. Nerv. Ment. Dis. 142:493–514.

Guilleminault, C. 1976. Cataplexy. In *Narcolepsy,* Eds. C. Guilleminault, W.C. Dement, and R. Passouant, pp. 125–147. New York: Spectrum.

Guilleminault, C. (Ed.). 1982. *Sleeping and Waking Disorders: Indications and Techniques.* Menlo Park: Addison-Wesley.

Guilleminault, C., and Dement, W.C. 1977. Amnesia and disorders of excessive daytime sleepiness. In *Neurobiology of Sleep and Memory,* Eds. R.R. Drucker-Colin and J.L. McGaugh, pp. 441–456. New York: Academic Press.

Guilleminault, C., and Dement, W.C. (Eds.). 1978. *Sleep Apnea Syndromes.* New York: Alan R. Liss.

Guilleminault, C., Eldridge, F.L., and Dement, W.C. 1973. Insomnia with sleep apnea: a new syndrome. Science 181:856–858.

Guilleminault, C., Billiard, M., Montplaisir, J., et al. 1975a. Altered states of consciousness in disorders of daytime sleepiness. J. Neurol. Sci. 26:377–393.

Guilleminault, C., Eldridge, F.L., Simmon, F.B., et al. 1975b. Sleep apnea syndrome: can it induce hemodynamic changes? West J. Med. 123:7–16.

Guilleminault, C., Dement, W.C., and Passouant, R (Eds.). 1976a. *Narcolepsy.* New York: Spectrum.

Guilleminault, C., Eldridge, F.L., Phillips, J.R., et al. 1976b. Two occult cases of insomnia and their therapeutic problems. Arch. Gen. Psychiatry 33:1241–1245.

Guilleminault, C., Reynal, D., Takahashi, S., et al. 1976c. Evaluation of short-term and long-term treatment of the narcolepsy syndrome with clomipramine hydrochloride. Acta Neurol. Scand. 54:71–87.

Guilleminault, C., Winkle R., Korobkin R., et al. 1982. Children and nocturnal snoring—evaluation of the effects of sleep related respiratory resistive load and daytime functioning. Eur. J. Pediatr. 139:165–171.

Hakamada, S., Watanabe, K., Hara, K., et al. 1980. The evolution of some EEG features in normal and abnormal infants. Brain Behav. 2:373–377.

Häkkinen, V., Hirvonen, K., Hasan, J., et al. 1993. Effects of small differences in electrode positions on EOG signals: application to vigilance studies. Electroencephalogr. Clin. Neurophysiol. 86:294–300.

Hartmann, E. 1984. *The Nightmare.* New York: Basic Books.

Hartmann, E., Baekeland, F., and Zwilling, G.K. 1972. Psychological differences between long and short sleepers. Arch. Gen. Psychiatry 26: 463–468.

Hartse, K.M., Roth, T., and Zorick, F.J. 1982. Daytime sleepiness and daytime wakefulness: the effect of instruction. Sleep 5(suppl 2):107–118.

Hasan, J., and Broughton, R. 1994. Quantitative topographical mapping during drowsiness and sleep onset. In *Sleep Onset Mechanisms,* Eds. R. Ogilvie and J. Harsh, pp. 219–236. Arlington, VA: American Psychological Association.

Hauri, P. 1985. Primary sleep disorders and insomnia. In *Clinical Aspects of Sleep and Sleep Disturbance,* Ed. T.L. Riley, pp. 81–112. Boston: Butterworth.

Hauri, P., and Hawkins, D.R. 1973. Alpha-delta sleep. Electroencephalogr. Clin. Neurophysiol. 34:233–238.

Hauri, P., and Olmstead, E. 1980. Childhood-onset insomnia. Sleep 3: 59–65.

Hawkins, D.F., Mendels, J., Scott, J., et al. 1967. The psychophysiology of sleep in psychotic depression: a longitudinal study. Psychosom. Med. 29:329–347.

Herscovitch, J., and Broughton, R. 1981. Sensitivity of the Stanford Sleepiness Scale to the effects of cumulative partial sleep deprivation and recovery oversleeping. Sleep 4:83–92.

Hess, W.R. 1944. Das Schlafsyndrom als Folge dienzephaler Reizung. Helv. Physiol. Acta 2:305–347.

Hishikawa, Y., Nan'no, H., Tachibana, M., et al. 1968. The nature of the sleep attack and other symptoms of narcolepsy. Electroencephalogr. Clin. Neurophysiol. 24:1–10.

Hishikawa, Y., Wakamatsu, H., Furuya, H., et al. 1976. Sleep satiation in narcoleptic patients. Electroencephalogr. Clin. Neurophysiol. 41:1–18.

Hishikawa, Y., Sugita, Y., Teshima, Y., et al. 1981. Sleep disorders in alcoholic patients with delirium tremens. In *Psychophysiological Aspects of Sleep,* Ed. I. Karacan, pp. 109–122. Park Ridge, NJ: Noyes Medical.

Hoddes, E., Dement, W.C., and Zarcone, V. 1972. The history and use of the Stanford Sleepiness Scale. Psychophysiology 9:150(abst).

Hoddes, E., Zarcone, V., Smyth, H.R., et al. 1973. Quantification of sleepiness—a new approach. Psychophysiology 10:431–436.

Honda, Y., Doi, Y., Guji, T., et al. 1984. Narcolepsy and HLA: positive DR2 as a prerequisite for the development of narcolepsy. Folia Psychiatr. Neurol. Jpn. 38:360.

Howard, G.F. 1985. Laboratory assessment of sleep and related functions. In *Clinical Aspects of Sleep and Sleep Disturbance,* Ed. T.L. Riley, pp. 197–228. Boston: Butterworth.

ICSD—International Classification of Sleep Disorders: Diagnostic and Coding Manual. 1990. Diagnostic classification steering committee, Thorpy, M.J., chairman. Rochester, MN: American Sleep Disorders Association.

Itil, T.M., Shapiro, D.M., Fink, M., et al. 1969. Digital computer classification of EEG sleep stages. Electroencephalogr. Clin. Neurophysiol. 27:76–83.

Jacobson, A., Kales, A., Lehmann, D., et al. 1964. Muscle tonus in human subjects during sleep and dreaming. Exp. Neurol. 10:371–375.

Jacobson, A., Kales, A., Lehmann, D., et al. 1965. Somnambulism: all night electroencephalographic studies. Science 148:975–977.

Janz, D. 1962. Grand mal epilepsies and the sleeping-waking cycle. Epilepsia 3:69–109.

Jasper, H.H. 1958. The ten-twenty electrode system of the International Federation. Electroencephalogr. Clin. Neurophysiol. 10:371–375.

Johns, M.W. 1991. A new method for measuring daytime sleepiness: the Epworth sleepiness scale. Sleep 14:540–545.

Johns, M.W. 1992. Reliability and factor analysis of the Epworth sleepiness scale. Sleep 15:376–381.

Johnson, L. 1973. Are stages of sleep related to waking behavior? Am. Sci. 61:326–338.

Jones, H., and Oswald, J. 1968. Two cases of healthy insomnia. Electroencephalogr. Clin. Neurophysiol. 24:378–380.

Jouvet, M., and Delorme, F. 1965. Locus coeruleus et sommeil paradoxal. C.R. Soc. Biol. (Paris) 159:885–899.

Kahn, E., and Fisher, C. 1969. The sleep characteristics of the normal aged male. J. Nerv. Ment. Dis. 148:477–499.

Kales, A., Jacobson, A., Paulson, M.J., et al. 1966. Somnambulism: psychophysiological correlates. Arch. Gen. Psychiatry 14:586–594.

Kales, A., Beall, G.N., Bajor, G.F., et al. 1968. Sleep studies in asthmatic adults: relationships of attacks to sleep stage and time of night. J. Allergy 41:164–173.

Kales, A., Kales, J.D., and Sly, R.M. 1970. Sleep patterns of asthmatic children: all-night studies. J. Allergy 40:300–308.

Kales, A., Kales, J.D., Jacobson, A., et al. 1977. Effects of imipramine on enuretic frequency and sleep stages. Pediatrics 60:431–436.

Kapoor, A., Barker, D., and Broughton, R. 1984. Reliability of thoracic transcutaneous oxygen tension monitoring during overnight recordings. Electroencephalogr. Clin. Neurophysiol. 57:5P(abst).

Karacan, I. 1971. Painful nocturnal penile erections. JAMA 215:1831.

Karacan, I. 1982. Evaluation of nocturnal penile tumescence and impotence. In Sleep and Waking Disorders: Indications and Techniques, Ed. C. Guilleminault, pp. 343–372. Menlo Park: Addison Wesley.

Kleine, W. 1925. Periodische Schlafsucht. Monatsschr. Psychiatr. Neurol. 57:285–320.

Kleitman, N. 1963. Sleep and Wakefulness. Chicago: University of Chicago Press.

Kokkoris, C.R., Weitzman, E.D., Pollak, C.P., et al. 1978. Long-term ambulatory temperature monitoring in a subject with a hypernychthemeral sleep-wake cycle disturbance. Sleep 1:177–180.

Koresko, R.L., Snyder, F., and Feinberg, I. 1963. Dream time in hallucinating and non-hallucinating schizophrenic patients. Nature 199:1118–1119.

Kripke, D.F. 1972. An ultradian biological rhythm associated with perceptual deprivation and REM sleep. Psychosom. Med. 3:221–234.

Krumpe, P., and Cumminskey, J. 1980. Use of laryngeal sound recordings to monitor sleep apnea. Am. Rev. Respir. Dis. 122:797–801.

Kryger, M.H., Roth, T., and Dement, W.C. (Eds.). 1994. Principles and Practice of Sleep Medicine, 2nd ed. Philadelphia: W.B. Saunders.

Kupfer, D.J., and Foster, F.G. 1978. EEG sleep and depression. In Sleep Disorders: Diagnosis and Treatment, Eds. R.L. Williams and I. Karacan, pp. 163–204. New York: John Wiley & Sons.

Kupfer, D.I., Himmelhoch, J.M., Swanzburg, M., et al. 1972. Hypersomnia in manic-depressive disease. Dis. Nerv. Syst. 33:720–724.

Lairy, G.C., de Barros-Ferreira, M., and Goldsteinas, L. 1968. Les phases intermédiaires du sommeil. In The Abnormalities of Sleep in Man, Eds. H. Gastaut, E. Lugaresi, G. Berti-Ceroni, et al., pp. 275–284. Bologna: Aulo Gaggi.

Lavie, P. 1979. Ultradian rhythms in alertness—a pupillometric study. Biol. Psychol. 9:49–56.

Lavie, R., and Scherson, A. 1981. Ultrashort sleep-waking schedule. I. Evidence of ultradian rhythmicity in "sleepability." Electroencephalogr. Clin. Neurophysiol. 52:163–174.

Lenard, H.G. 1970. The development of sleep spindles in the EEG during the first two years of life. Neuropediatrie 1:264–276.

Levin, M. 1936. Periodic somnolence and morbid hunger: a new syndrome. Brain 59:494–515.

Levin, M. 1959. Aggression, guilt and cataplexy. Am. J. Psychiatry 116:133–136.

Lugaresi, E., and Cirignotta, F. 1981. Hypnogenic paroxysmal dystonia. Sleep 4:129–136.

Lugaresi, E., and Cirignotta, F. 1982. Two variants of nocturnal paroxysmal dystonia with attacks of short and long duration. In Epilepsy, Sleep and Sleep Deprivation, Eds. R. Degen and E. Niedermeyer, pp. 169–173. Amsterdam: Elsevier.

Lugaresi, E., Coccagna, G., Gambi, D., et al. 1966. A propos de quelques manifestations nocturnes myocloniques (nocturnal myoclonus de Symonds). Rev. Neurol. (Paris) 115:547–555.

Lugaresi, E., Coccagna, G., Berti Ceroni, G., et al. 1968. Restless legs syndrome and nocturnal myoclonus. In The Abnormalities of Sleep in Man, Eds. H. Gastaut, E. Lugaresi, G. Berti Ceroni, et al., pp. 285–294. Bologna: Aulo Gaggi.

Lugaresi, E., Coccagna, G., and Mantovani, M. 1978. Hypersomnias with Periodic Apneas. New York: SP Medical and Scientific Press.

Lugaresi, E., Medori, R., Montagna, P., et al. 1986. Fatal familial insomnia and dysautonomia with selective degeneration of thalamic nuclei. N. Engl. J. Med. 315:997–1003.

Mahowald, M.W., and Schenck, C.H. 1994. REM sleep behavior disorder. In Principles and Practice of Sleep Medicine, 2nd ed., Eds. M.H. Kryger, T. Roth, and W.C. Dement, pp. 574–588. Philadelphia: W.B. Saunders.

Manseau, C., and Broughton, R. 1984. Bilaterally synchronous ultradian EEG rhythms in awake adult humans. Psychophysiology 21:265–273.

Matousek, M., and Petersen, I. 1983. A method for assessing alertness fluctuations from EEG spectra. Electroencephalogr. Clin. Neurophysiol. 55:108–113.

McFarland, R.A. 1975. Air travel across time zones. Am. Sci. 63:23–30.

McGregor, P.A., Weitzman, E.D., and Pollak, C.R. 1978. Polysomnographic recording techniques used for diagnosis of sleep disorders in a sleep disorders center. Am. J. EEG Technol. 18:107.

Meddis, R., Pearson, A., and Langford, G. 1973. An extreme case of healthy insomnia. Electroencephalogr. Clin. Neurophysiol. 36:213–214.

Meier-Ewert, K., Schopfer, B., and Ruther, R. 1975. Drei narkoleptische Syndrome. Nervenarzt 46:624–635.

Mendels, T., and Hawkins, D.R. 1967. Sleep and depression: a followup study. Arch. Gen. Psychiatry 16:536–542.

Mendels, J., and Hawkins, D.R. 1971. Longitudinal study in hypomania. Arch. Gen. Psychiatry 19:445–452.

Metcalf, D.R. 1970. EEG sleep spindle ontogenesis. Neuropediatrie 1:428–433.

Metcalf, D., Mondale, J., and Butler, F.K. 1971. Ontogenesis of spontaneous K-complexes. Psychophysiology 8:340–347.

Mignot, E., Lin, X., Arrigoni, J., et al. 1994. DQB1*0602 and DQA1*0102 (DQ1) are better markers than DR2 for narcolepsy in Caucasian and black Americans. Sleep 17:S60-S67.

Mikkelson, E.J., Rapoport, J.L., Nu, L., et al. 1980. Childhood enuresis: sleep patterns and psychopathology. Arch. Gen. Psychiatry 37:1139–1147.

Miles, L.M., Raynal, D.M., and Wilson, M.A. 1977. Blind man living in normal society has circadian rhythm of 24.9 hours. Science 198:421–423.

Mitchell, S.W. 1890. Some disorders of sleep. Am. J. Med. Sci. 100:109–127.

Mitler, M.M., van der Hoed, J., Carskadon, M.A., et al. 1979. REM sleep episodes during the multiple sleep latency test in narcoleptic patients. Electroencephalogr. Clin. Neurophysiol. 46:479–481.

Mitler, M.M., Gujarty, K.S., Sampson, M.G., et al. 1982. Multiple daytime nap approaches to evaluating the sleepy subject. Sleep 5(suppl 2):119–127.

Moldofsky, H., Scarisbrick, P., England, R., et al. 1975. Musculoskeletal symptoms and non-REM sleep disturbance in patients with "fibrositis syndrome" and healthy subjects. Psychosom. Med. 37:341–351.

Moldofsky, H., Musisi, S., and Philipson, E.A. 1986. Treatment of advanced sleep phase syndrome by phase advance chronotherapy. Sleep 9:61–65.

Monk, M.M., Leng, V.C., Folkard, S., et al. 1983. Circadian rhythms in alertness and core body temperature. Chronobiologia 4:45–55.

Montplaisir, J. 1976. Disturbed nocturnal sleep. In Narcolepsy, Eds. C. Guilleminault, W.C. Dement, and P. Passouant, pp. 42–56. New York: Spectrum.

Montplaisir, J.Y., Billiard, M., Takahashi, S., et al. 1978. Twenty-four hour recording in REM narcoleptics with special reference to nocturnal sleep disruption. Biol. Psychiatry 13:73–89.

Montplaisir, J., Godbout, R., Pelletier, G., et al. 1994. Restless leg syndrome and periodic movements in sleep. In Principles and Practice of Sleep Medicine, 2nd ed., Eds. M. Kryger, T. Roth, and W. Dement, pp. 589–597. Philadelphia: W.B. Saunders.

Mouret, J., Delorme, F., and Jouvet, M. 1965. Activité des muscles de la face au cours du sommeil paradoxal chez l'homme. Compt. Rend. Soc. Biol. (Paris) 159:391–394.

Mouret, J.R., Renard, B., Quenin, P., et al. 1972. Monoamines et regulation de la vigilance I. Apport et interprétation biochimique des données polygraphiques. Rev. Neurol. (Paris) 172:139–155.

Muellner, S.R. 1960. Development of urinary control in children: a new concept in cause, prevention and treatment of primary enuresis. J. Urol. 84:714–716.

Mullington, J., Dunham, W., and Broughton, R.J. 1990. Phase timing and duration of naps in narcolepsy-cataplexy: preliminary findings. In *Sleep 90*, Ed. J.A. Home, pp. 158–160. Stuttgart: Fischer–Verlag.

Newman, J., and Broughton, R. 1991. Pupillometric assessment of excessive day time sleepiness in narcolepsy-cataplexy. Sleep 14:121–129.

Nowlin, J.B., Troyer, W.G., Collins, W.S., et al. 1965. The association of nocturnal angina pectoris with dreaming. Ann. Intern. Med. 63:1040–1046.

Ogilvie, R.D., Simons, I.A., Kuderian, R.H., et al. 1991. Behavioral, event-related potential and EEG/FFT changes at sleep onset. Psychophysiology 28:54–64.

Okawa, M., Matousek, M., and Petersen, I. 1984. Spontaneous vigilance fluctuations in the daytime. Psychophysiology 21:207–211.

Orr, W.C., Robinson, M.G., and Johnson, L.F. 1979. Acid clearing with esophagitis and controls. Gastroenterology 96:12–13.

Orr, W.C., Bollinger, C., and Stahl, M. 1982. In *Sleeping and Waking Disorders. Indications and Techniques,* Ed. C. Guilleminault, pp. 331–343. Menlo Park: Addison-Wesley.

Oswald, I. 1959. Sudden bodily jerks on falling asleep. Brain 82:92–103.

Oswald, I. 1969. Drugs and dependence on amphetamine and other drugs. In *Sleep: Physiology and Pathology,* Ed. A. Kales, pp. 317–330. Philadelphia: J.B. Lippincott.

Pack, A.I., Remmers, J.E., Roth, T., et al. 1995. Guidelines for in-home testing: a need for reassessment. Sleep 18:136–137.

Passouant, P., Cadhilac, J., and Baldy-Mouliner, M. 1967. Physiopathologie des hypersomnies. Rev. Neurol. (Paris) 6:585–629.

Passouant, P., Halberg, F., Genicot, R., et al. 1969. La periodicité des accès narcoleptiques et le rhythme ultradien du sommeil rapide. Rev. Neurol. (Paris) 121:155–164.

Passouant, R., Cadhilac, J., and Ribstein, M. 1972. Les privations de sommeil avec mouvements oculaires par les antidepresseurs. Rev. Neurol. (Paris) 121:173–192.

Petre-Quadrans, O. 1969. Contribution à l'étude de la phase dite paradoxale du sommeil. Thesis, Brussels.

Petre-Quadrans, O., and Jouvet, M. 1966. Paradoxical sleep and dreaming in the mentally retarded. J. Neurol. Sci. 3:608–612.

Plazzi, G., Tinuper, P., Montagna, P., et al. 1995. Epileptic nocturnal wanderings. Sleep 18:749–756.

Pressman, M.R., Spielman, A.I., Pollak, C., et al. 1982. Long-latency evoked response during sleep deprivation and in narcolepsy. Sleep 5 (suppl. 2):147–156.

Prinz, P., Peskind, E.R., Vitaliano, R.R., et al. 1982. Changes in sleep and waking EEGs of non-demented and demented elderly subjects. J. Am. Geriatr. Soc. 30:86–92.

Rechtschaffen, A., and Kales, A. (Eds.). 1968. A *Manual of Standardized Terminology, Techniques and Scoring System for Sleep Stages in Human Subjects.* U.S. Department of Health, Education and Welfare, Public Health Service. Washington, DC: U.S. Government Printing Office.

Rechtschaffen, A., and Verdone, R. 1964. Amount of dreaming: effect of incentive, adaptation to laboratory and individual differences. Percept. Motor Skills 19:947–958.

Rechtschaffen, A., Wolpert, E.A., Dement, W.C., et al. 1963. Nocturnal sleep of narcoleptics. Electroencephalogr. Clin. Neurophysiol. 15:599–609.

Reding, G., Zepelin, H., Robinson, J.E., et al. 1968. Nocturnal teeth-grinding: all night psychophysiological studies. J. Dent. Res. 47:786–797.

Richardson, G., Carskadon, M.A., Flagg, W., et al. 1978. Excessive daytime sleepiness in man: multiple sleep latency measurement in narcoleptic and control subjects. Electroencephalogr. Clin. Neurophysiol. 45:621–627.

Roessler, R., Collins, F., and Ostman, R. 1970. A period analysis classification of sleep stages. Electroencephalogr. Clin. Neurophysiol. 29:358–362.

Roffwarg, H.P. 1990. ASDA position statement: automatic scoring. Sleep 13:284–285.

Roffwarg, H.P., Muzio, J.N., and Dement, W.C. 1966. Ontogenetic development of the human sleep-dream cycle. Science 152:604–619.

Roffwarg, H.P., Clark, R.W., Guilleminault, C., et al. 1979. Diagnostic classification of sleep and arousal disorders. Sleep 2:5–127.

Roth, B. 1961. The clinical and theoretical importance of EEG rhythms corresponding to states of lowered vigilance. Electroencephalogr. Clin. Neurophysiol. 13:395–399.

Roth, B. 1962. *Narkolepsie und Hypersomnie vomStandpunkt der Physiologie des Schlafes.* Berlin: VEB Verlag Volk und Gesundheit.

Roth, B. 1964. L'EEG dans la narcolepsie-cataplexie. Electroencephalogr. Clin. Neurophysiol. 16:170–190.

Roth, B. 1976. Functional hypersomnia. In *Narcolepsy,* Eds. C. Guilleminault, W.C. Dement, and P. Passouant, pp. 333–349. New York: Spectrum.

Roth, B. 1980. (Trans. R. Broughton) *Narcolepsy and Hypersomnia.* Basel: S. Karger.

Roth, B., Bruhova, S., and Lehovsky, M. 1969. REM sleep and NREM sleep in narcolepsy and hypersomnia. Electroencephalogr. Clin. Neurophysiol. 26:176–182.

Roth, B., Nevsimalova, S., and Rechtschaffen, A. 1972. Hypersomnia with "sleep drunkenness." Arch. Gen. Psychiatry. 26:456–462.

Roth, B., Nevsimalova, S., Sonka, K., et al. 1986. Polygraphic indexing of sleepiness and polygraphic score of sleepiness in narcolepsy and hypersomnia. Sleep 9:243–245.

Roth, T., Harstse, K.M., Zorick, F., et al. 1980. Multiple naps and the evaluation of daytime sleepiness in patients with upper airway sleep apnea. Sleep 3:425–439.

Roy, O. 1976. Biotelemetry and telephone transmission. In *Handbook of Electroencephalography and Clinical Neurophysiology,* vol. 3A, Ed. R. Broughton, pp. 46–66. Amsterdam: Elsevier.

Saier, J., Regis, H., Mano, I., et al. 1968. Potentiels évoqués visuels pendant les differentes phases du sommeil chez l'homme: etude de la réponse visuelle évoquée après le reveil. In *The Abnormalities of Sleep in Man,* Eds. H. Gastaut, E. Lugaresi, G. Berti Ceroni, et al., pp. 55–66. Bologna: Aulo Gaggi.

Saunders, N.A., and Sullivan, C. Eds. 1994. *Sleep and Breathing.* New York: Marcel Dekker.

Scheffer I.E., Kailash, P.B., and Lopes-Cendes, I. 1994. Autosomal dominant frontal epilepsy misdiagnosed as sleep disorder. Lancet 343:515–517.

Schenck, C.H., Bundlie, S.R., and Ettinger, M.C. 1986. Chronic behavioral disorders of human REM sleep: a new category of parasomnia. Sleep 9:293–308.

Schmidt, H.S. 1982. Pupillometric assessment of disorders of arousal. Sleep 5(suppl 2):157–164.

Schott, B., Michel, D., Mouret, J., et al. 1972. Monoamines et regulation de la vigilance. I. Syndromes lésionnels du système nerveux central. Rev. Neurol. (Paris) 127:157–171.

Schwartz, B.A. 1968. Afternoon sleep in certain hypersomnolent states: "intermediate sleep." Electroencephalogr. Clin. Neurophysiol. 24:569–581.

Scott, J., and Snyder, F. 1968. "Critical reactivity" (Piéron) after abrupt awakenings in relation to EEG stage 4 sleep. Psychophysiology 4:370(abst).

Severinghaus, J.W., and Mitchell, R.A. 1962. Ondine's curse: Failure of respiratory center automaticity while awake. Clin. Res. 10:122.

Shepard, J.W. 1991. *Atlas of Sleep Medicine.* Mount Kisco, NY: Futura Publishing.

Snyder, F. 1966. Toward an evolutionary theory of dreaming. Am. J. Psychiatry 123:121–136.

Snyder F. 1968. Electrographic studies of sleep in depression. In *Computers and Other Electronic Devices in Psychiatry,* Eds. E.S. Kleine and R. Lasky, pp. 272–304. New York: Grune & Stratton.

Stampi, C. (Ed.) 1992. *Why We Nap.* Boston: Birkhauser.

Stampi, C., Stone, P., and Michimori, 1995. A new quantitative method for assessing sleepiness: the alpha attenuation test. Work Stress 9:368–376.

Stradling, J.R. 1992. Sleep studies for sleep-related breathing disorders. J. Sleep Res. 1:265–273.

Stuss, D., and Broughton, R. 1978. Extreme short sleep: personality profiles and a case study of sleep requirement. Waking Sleeping 2:101–105.

Takeuchi, T., Miyasita, A., Sasaki, Y., et al. 1992. Isolated sleep paralysis elicited by sleep interruption. Sleep 15:217–225.

Terzano, M.G., Mancia, D., Salati, M.R., et al. 1985. The cyclic alternating pattern as a physiologic component of normal NREM sleep. Sleep 8:137–145.

Terzano, M.G., Halasz, P., and DeClerck, A.C. (Eds.). 1991. *Phasic and Dynamic Aspects of Sleep.* New York: Raven Press.

Thorpy, M.J. (Ed.). 1990. *Handbook of Sleep Disorders.* New York Basel: Marcel Dekker.

Thorpy, M.J. 1992. The clinical use of the Multiple Sleep Latency Test. The Standards of Practice Committee of the American Sleep Disorders Association. Sleep 15:268–276.

Thorpy, M.J., and Glovinsky, R.B. 1989. Headbanging (jactacio capitus nocturna). In *Principles and Practice of Sleep Medicine,* Eds. M.H. Kryger, T. Roth, and W.C. Dement, pp. 648–654. Philadelphia: W.B. Saunders.

Thorpy, M., Korman, E., Spielman, A.J., et al. 1988. Delayed sleep phase syndrome in adolescents. J. Adolesc. Med. 9:22–27.

Tinuper, P., Cerullo, A., and Cirignotta, F. 1990. Nocturnal paroxysmal dystonia with short-lasting attacks: three cases with evidence for an epileptic frontal lobe origin of seizure. Epilepsia 31:549–556.

Torsvall, L., and Ackerstedt, T. 1987. Sleepiness on the job: Continuously measured EEG changes in train drivers. Electroencephalogr. Clin. Neurophysiol. 66:502–511.

Valley, V., and Broughton, R. 1981. Daytime performance deficits and physiological vigilance in untreated patients with narcolepsy-cataplexy compared to controls. Rev. EEG Neurophysiol. (Paris) 11:133–139.

Valley, V., and Broughton, R. 1983. The physiological (EEG) nature of drowsiness and its relation to performance deficits in narcoleptics. Electroencephalogr. Clin. Neurophysiol. 55:243–251.

Van Dongen, H.P., Maislin, G., Mullington, J.M., et al., 2003. The cumulative cost of additional wakefulness: dose-response effects on neurobehavioral functions and sleep physiology from chronic sleep restriction and total sleep deprivation. Sleep 26:117–126.

Vein, A.M. 1966. *Syndrome of Hypersomnia, Narcolepsy and Other Forms of Pathological Sleepiness.* Moscow: Izdatelstvo Meditsina (in Russian).

Volk, S., Simon, O., Schulz, H., et al. 1984. The structure of wakefulness and its relationship to daytime sleep in narcoleptic patients. Electroencephalogr. Clin. Neurophysiol. 57:119–128.

Weaver, T.E., Laizner, A.M., Evans, L.K., et al., 1997. An instrument to measure functional status outcomes for disorders of excessive sleepiness. Sleep 20:835–843.

Webb, W.B. 1982. Sleep in older persons: sleep structure of 50- to 60-year-old men and women. J. Gerontol. 37:581–586.

Webb, W. 1983. Discussion. The siesta: social or biological phenomenon? Sleep Res. 12:28(abst).

Webb, W.B., and Friel, J. 1971. Sleep stage and personality changes of natural long and short sleepers. Science 171:587–588.

Weitzman, E., Kripke, D., Goldmacher, D., et al. 1970. Acute reversal of the sleep-waking cycles in man. Arch. Neurol. 22:483–489.

Weitzman, E.D., Pollak, C.R., and McGregor, R. 1980. The polysomnographic evaluation of sleep disorders in man. In *Electrodiagnosis in Clinical Neurology,* Ed. M.J. Aminoff, pp. 496–524. New York: Churchill Livingstone.

Weitzman, E.D., Czeisler, C.A., and Colman, R.M. 1981. Delayed sleep phase syndrome, a chronobiological disorder with sleep-onset insomnia. Arch. Gen. Psychiatry 38:737–746.

Wilkinson, R.T. 1965. Sleep deprivation. In *The Physiology of Human Survival,* Eds. O.G. Eldholm and A.L. Bacharach, pp. 339–530. London: Academic Press.

Wilkus, R.J., Harvey, F., Ojemann, L.M., et al. 1971. Electroencephalogram and sensory evoked potentials. Findings in an unresponsive patient with pontine infarct. Arch. Neurol. 24:538–547.

Williams, R.L., Karacan, I., and Hursch, C.J. 1974. *EEG of Human Sleep.* New York: John Wiley.

Yoss, R.E., Moyer, N.J., and Ogle, K.N. 1969. The pupillogram and narcolepsy. Neurology (Minneapolis) 19:921–928.

Young, D., and Scoville, W.B. 1938. Paranoid psychosis in narcolepsy and the possible danger of benzedrine treatment. Med. Clin. North Am. 22:637–646.

Zung, W.W.K., Wilson, W.R., and Dodson, W.E. 1964. Effect of depressive disorders on the sleep EEG responses. Arch. Gen. Psychiatry 10:439–445.

49. Electroencephalography of the Newborn: Normal and Abnormal Features

Mark S. Scher

Electroencephalography/Polysomnography (EEG Sleep) of the Newborn

Advances in neonatal intensive care have led to improved survival for high-risk infants. Concomitant with these medical improvements has been an increasing awareness of two groups of neonates at risk for neurodevelopmental problems. One group is comprised of acutely ill neonates who have survived neonatal disease because of sophisticated intensive care management. These children remain subsequently at risk for sequelae (Scher et al., 1988d). Long-term follow-up studies of these infants have indicated that 10% to 50% of such children manifest variable degrees of long-term neurodevelopmental sequelae (Coolman et al., 1985; Drillien et al., 1980; Eilers et al., 1986; Ford et al., 1985; Hack, 1997; Hack et al., 1997, 1999, 1983; Lefebvre et al., 1988; Marlow et al., 1988; Michelsson et al., 1984; Nickel et al., 1982; Rantakallio and von Wendt, 1985; Watanabe and Iwase, 1972). Problems range from hearing loss in 3% and visual loss in 5%, to delay in psychomotor development or neurological damage in as many as 50% of survivors (Coolman et al., 1985; Lefebvre et al., 1988). Once these survivors reach school age, there are estimates that one fifth to one third require special education assistance despite normal intelligence with no clearly defined neurological handicap (Lefebvre et al., 1988; Hack et al., 1999). To what degree antepartum maldevelopment or injury contributes to the morbidity of this group remains a confounding variable (Freeman, 1985).

More frustrating to health care providers is a larger group of children who comprise the "silent majority" with neurodevelopmental problems despite no obvious antepartum, intrapartum, or neonatal difficulties (Freeman, 1985). These children usually present during early childhood with developmental delay, mental retardation, cerebral palsy, or recurrent seizures. Despite appearing clinically asymptomatic during the neonatal and infancy periods, congenital or acquired lesions, which were contracted during the antepartum period, only become clinically apparent at older ages (Freeman, 1985).

Therefore, while some infants can be identified as high risk by epidemiological or clinical factors, many appear neurologically intact based on the neonate's limited clinical repertoire (Nelson and Ellenberg, 1987). There remains a need for more sensitive diagnostic evaluations of the central nervous system (CNS) that can supplement clinical observations (Scher and Barmada, 1987).

Structural and Functional Assessment of Neonatal Brain

Brain imaging techniques developed over two and a half decades have revolutionized the diagnosis of major structural disorders of the neonatal brain. Cranial ultrasonography (Edwards et al., 1980; Hill et al., 1983; Rumack et al., 1985), cranial computed tomography (CT) (Pape et al., 1983), magnetic resonance imaging (MRI) (Gooding et al., 1984; Hope et al., 1984; Johnson et al., 1983), and positron emission tomography (PET) (Doyle et al., 1983; Watt and Strongman, 1985) extend the clinician's ability to detect either acquired or congenital lesions in specific brain regions. More recently, techniques utilizing spectroscopy and volumetric MRI analyses add additional biochemical or anatomical information regarding regional brain function (Huppi et al., 1998; Novotny et al., 1998).

Newborn brain abnormalities, however, may also be expressed in functional terms, with or without demonstrable structural correlates. Specifically, neurophysiological studies can provide continuous documentation of CNS function and complement structural studies. Recent advances in the neurophysiological assessment of newborn brain function offer unique opportunities for the coordinated evaluation of the dysfunctional CNS (Scher and Barmada, 1987). Innovative methods of assessing brain structure and function, nonetheless, should always be based on sound clinical judgment. When neuroimaging and EEG are used together, interpretation of results can be more accurate (Baumgart and Graziani, 2001; Biagioni et al., 2001). Reliable and rapid identification of infants by these methods will then allow the clinician to develop strategies of cerebral resuscitation that can be provided at a time when injury may be potentially reversible (Johnston et al., 1995). Protocols for neonatal neurointensive care, however, have yet to be tested and implemented.

Normal Neonatal EEG-Sleep Features

Neonatal EEG studies have been reported for more than half a century (Okamato and Kirikae, 1951). Seminal work by researchers throughout the world offer a wealth of information concerning the developmental neurophysiology of the immature brain (Anders et al., 1971; Dreyfus-Brisac, 1955, 1956, 1957, 1962, 1964, 1968, 1970, 1972, 1979; Ellingson, 1958, 1960, 1964; Ellingson et al., 1974; Ellingson and Peters, 1980; Kellaway and Crawley, 1964; Kellaway and Petersen, 1964; Parmelee, 1967; Parmelee et al.,

Table 49.1. Guidelines for the Interpretation of Normal Neonatal EEG

1. EEG features reflect gestational or conceptional age, not birthweight.
2. Estimates of electrical maturity should be within 2 weeks for preterm neonate's stated EGA, and 1 week for full-term neonate's EGA.
3. Knowledge of neonatal behavioral state during the recording is essential.
4. Serial EEG studies more accurately document ontogeny of rhythms than single studies.
5. Attention to both temporal and spatial characteristics of the EEG record should be explicitly stated in the electrographic interpretation (e.g., occipital theta, delta brushes, synchrony, sleep cycle, etc.)
6. Concordance between specific electrographic and polygraphic components of EEG-sleep begins as early as 30 weeks (EGA), but is not complete after 36 weeks (EGA).

EGA, estimated gestational age.

1968, 1969; Parmelee and Stern, 1972; Prechtl, 1974, 1984; Prechtl and Lenard, 1967; Prechtl and Nijhuis, 1983; Prechtl et al., 1969, 1979; Watanabe and Iwase, 1972; Watt and Strongman, 1985; Werner et al., 1977). Earlier studies, however, predated the creation of the modern neonatal intensive care unit (NICU) (Dreyfus-Brisac et al., 1955, 1956, 1957, 1962, 1964, 1968, 1970, 1972, 1979; Ellingson, 1958, 1960, 1964; Ellingson et al., 1974; Ellingson and Peters, 1980; Kellaway and Crawley, 1964; Kellaway and Petersen, 1964). As a consequence, the neonatal electroencephalographer has assumed a more limited consultative role in the neurological care of the sick neonate.

With the evolution to our present-day tertiary level NICU, technical improvements in the recording apparatus and standardization of recording procedures now assist the neurological consultant with sophisticated continuous neurophysiological assessments. Proper instrumentation and technique performed by electrodiagnostic technologists provide reliable neonatal EEG-sleep studies, which can be used to evaluate CNS functioning.

Several basic tenets can assist in one's understanding of the principal applications of neonatal EEG interpretation (Table 49.1). Maturational changes in scalp-generated EEG patterns should be anticipated at different ages of maturity. For the trained electroencephalographer, the electrical maturity of the neonatal brain should be estimated within 2 weeks of the gestational age for preterm (PT) infants and 1 week for full-term (FT) infants (Hrachovy et al., 1990; Lombroso, 1985). Electrographic patterns reflect the postconceptional age (PCA) of the infant, rather than the somatic growth. Concordance between electrographic and polygraphic physiological measures require a sufficient degree of CNS maturation beyond 36 weeks' conceptional age (CA). Finally, serial studies can more accurately document either normal ontogeny or the evolution of encephalopathic patterns than by single recordings.

A strategy for visual analysis of neonatal EEG records has been discussed (Hrachovy et al., 1990; Lombroso, 1985). One should develop a consistent style of physiological pattern recognition and clinical correlation by repetitive exposures to a wide variety of EEG-sleep records. Before beginning an electrographic assessment, it is of paramount importance to have the knowledge of the PCA and state of arousal of the neonatal patient. The time of the infant's delivery, last feeding, medication administration, and medical procedures may all alter the EEG background. Close communication between the electroneurodiagnostic technologist and the neonatal nurse/physician team add an important level of interaction that will improve the interpretation of the study.

Instrumentation and Recording Techniques

At least ten electrodes are required as the minimum number for adequate EEG recordings (Anders et al., 1971). More surface area over which additional electrodes can monitor cerebral activities is potentially desirable, but this strategy must be balanced with the more limited ability to visualize electrographic activity, because of the smaller head size of the neonate, which results in less potential differences between adjacent electrodes. A 10–20 system electrode placement remains the standard method of application of scalp electrodes, but specific electrodes (i.e., parietal, anterior, or posterior temporal) may need to be eliminated to increase interelectrode distance. Specific locations such as the occipital, temporal, midline, and frontal regions should always be included for monitoring because of the abundant activity occurring in these brain regions. Other technical aspects are stressed in Table 49.2.

Silver-silver chloride electrodes are most commonly used, and their application to the scalp can be achieved with either paste or collodion. Needle electrodes are no longer recommended. The electrode arrays or montages can be either bipolar or referential, although the former montage choice is preferable given the importance of regional localization. Multiple montages may be utilized depending on the specific interpretative needs; however, a single bipolar or combined bipolar-tangential montage allows the technologist and the electroencephalographer to more readily observe changes in EEG-sleep state without interruptions when an alternative montage is chosen.

Alternative instrumental control settings are preferred on neonatal recordings than for the older child and adult. Adjustments in sensitivity, paper speed, and filter settings may help facilitate the electrographic interpretation (Lombroso, 1989; Scher, 1985a). Sensitivity settings should begin with the standard 7 μV/mm, but may need to be periodically adjusted throughout the record, because of state changes or scalp edema. Both high- and low-frequency filters should be appropriately chosen to allow accurate representation of an appropriate range of frequencies of cerebral origin. Overzealous use of filter settings may eliminate brain-generated activities while attempting to minimize undesirable noncerebral artifactual signals. For the newborn patient, lower frequency filter settings, commonly referred to as time constants, should preferably remain at 0.25 to 0.5 rather than 0.1 to avoid the elimination of commonly occurring slow-frequency waveforms. Fifteen rather than the conventional 30 mm/second paper speed may be advantageous, since slower paper speeds permit easier visualization of slowly reoccurring normal features, such as the discontinuity during quiet sleep or abnormal features, such as seizures or periodic discharges.

Important noncerebral information can be derived from recording motility, cardiorespiratory, and eye movements.

Table 49.2. Technical Aspects of Neonatal EEG Recordings

A. The recording environment
  1. a. Maintain positive working relationship with medical staff.
     b. Coordinate EEG studies with other testing procedures.
     c. Position monitoring equipment in a way that least affects working conditions.
  2. Recognize potential sources of artifact.
  3. Recordings in an open bed warmer vs. an isolette require different concerns with respect to artifacts.
  4. Technologist should recognize situations when additional help is needed to place equipment or reposition the patient.
  5. Anticipate a 1.5- to 2-hour time commitment.
B. Recording equipment
  1. Devices should be properly shielded to minimize artifact from other monitoring devices.
  2. Technologist should be proficient in operating evoked potential and synchronized EEG-monitoring equipment.
  3. a. Careful attention to patient and electrical safety guidelines.
     b. Communication with clinical engineering of the hospital to maintain hospital guidelines for equipment safety (JCOHA: Joint Commission on Hospital Accreditation).
     c. Maintain infection control standards.
     d. Close attention to hand washing and electrode cleaning.
C. Instrumentation-electrode application
  1. Use of collodion or paste—either technique is acceptable but collodion is less desirable in isolette recordings due to inadequate ventilation.
  2. Neonatal electrode sizes strongly suggested.
  3. Use hypoallergenic skin tape to minimize skin irritation.
  4. Minimum of ten scalp electrodes.
  5. Fp1 and Fp2 often replaced by Fp3 and Fp4 due to smaller frontal brain regions.
  6. Select one or two montages for best assessment of sleep state changes.
  7. Use 15 mm/sec paper speed to depict state changes, synchrony and periodic discharges.
  8. Use long time constant (0.3) to assess slow activity.
  9. Attention to cardiorespiratory, electromyogram, and electro-oculogram monitoring during the recordings.
D. Technologist notations
  1. Occipital-frontal circumference should be accurate. Note skull deformities that might affect this measurement.
  2. Review chart for documentation of gestational maturity.
  3. Assist electroencephalographer by identifying which medical personnel (nurse *and* physician) has most information with respect to questionable seizure activity or clinical status.
  4. Document areas of scalp edema, cephalhematomas, extraventricular drains, etc.
  5. Record blood studies obtained during or around recording session, including blood gases, antiepileptic drug (AED) levels, and other metabolic values.
  6. Include ventilatory status including ventilator rate changes.
  7. Frequent notations during recording are of paramount importance, especially head position, respiratory excursions, suspicious clinical activity, and personnel around recording equipment.
  8. Note start and finish times of recordings, medication administrations, clinical changes (i.e., bradycardia, apnea, etc.).
  9. Actively attempt to identify and correct artifact-providing situations.

Such monitors assist in the identification of specific segments of the EEG sleep cycle. Noncerebral physiological observations may have relevance to the clinical problem that prompted the request for the EEG study. Important sources of artifact can more readily be identified or eliminated by using noncerebral monitors. As with adults, physiological and nonphysiological artifacts must be properly identified on neonatal recordings because they may interfere with the interpretation of cerebral activity. Three basic forms of artifacts—instrumental, external, and physiological—may occur in the neonate. Accurate descriptions by the technologist assist the neurologist in the diagnosis of a neurological disorder in the neonate (Scher, 1985a). The technologist should try not only to identify the source of an artifact, but also to eliminate such phenomena during the recording.

Both skill and speed are required by the electroneurodiagnostic technologist to obtain a quality recording in a busy NICU. Ample time should be allowed for proper electrode application because of the special challenges with recordings of medically ill preterm neonates confined to an isolette. Information from the medical record should include the neonate's gestational and postconceptional ages as well as the state of arousal. The physician who ordered the study should be identified so that a clearly written request for the EEG study states the clinical concerns. Many patients may have been administered medications. Each of these drugs should be listed by the technologist. Skull defects, vital signs, and pertinent laboratory studies should all be described since they may affect the electrographic and clinical interpretations of the recording.

Frequent and accurate annotations by the technologist throughout the study must corroborate changes in state of the neonatal patient. Eye opening and closure as well as repositioning of the patient's head are some examples of annotations that are essential for proper interpretation. Consensual validation of suspicious cerebral activity between the electroencephalographer and technologist is always a high priority at the time of the review of the record (Scher, 1985a).

Assessment of Central Nervous System Maturation

Several fundamental principles should be followed for an accurate interpretation of neonatal EEG-sleep studies. The following discussion is an introduction to its potential application in abnormal clinical situations, which will be discussed subsequently.

The pediatrician defines the child's PCA as the infant's estimated gestational age at birth plus the number of days or weeks of postnatal life (i.e., estimated gestational at birth plus postnatal age equals PCA). Changes in electrographic and polysomnographic patterns reflect increasing CAs of the neonate independent of somatic growth; preterm neonates at postconceptional term ages are expected to express similar EEG-sleep patterns as appropriate for gestational age term newborns. Subtle physiological differences, however, also exist, which will be later discussed.

Pioneering investigations by several independent researchers offer a wealth of information regarding developmental neurophysiology of the immature brain (Anders et al., 1971; Dreyfus-Brisac, 1955, 1956, 1957, 1962, 1964, 1968, 1970, 1972, 1979; Ellingson, 1958, 1960, 1964; Ellingson et al., 1974; Ellingson and Peters, 1980; Kellaway and Crawley, 1964; Kellaway and Petersen, 1964; Krieger et al., 1987; Lombroso, 1979, 1985, 1989; Lombroso and Matsumiya, 1985; Parmelee, 1967; Parmelee et al., 1968, 1969; Parmelee and Stern, 1972; Prechtl 1974, 1984; Prechtl and Lenard, 1967; Prechtl and Nijhuis, 1983; Prechtl et al., 1969, 1979; Werner et al., 1977). Specific features of the

EEG in the asymptomatic neonate relate to the gestational age of the neonate. It is generally accepted that a combination of intrahemispheric and interhemispheric electrographic features correlate with CNS maturation within 2 weeks of the clinically derived gestational age.

Current methods for assessing CNS maturation include the gestational age calculation from the mother's last menstrual period, fetal ultrasonographic changes in head and body size, and a variety of obstetrical signs that correlate with overall fetal maturation. Clinical examination of the neonate at birth also offers an estimation of CNS maturation assessed by convolutional measurements. A variety of clinical scoring techniques emphasize neurological parameters of tone and postural reflexes (Ballard et al., 1979; Dubowitz et al., 1970; Saint-Anne Dargassies, 1974). However, these standard methods are inaccurate for the early premature infant as well as misleading in specific clinical situations. In these circumstances, electrographic/polysomnographic estimates of CNS maturation can be especially useful to verify clinical estimates of gestational age. Before considering if a neonate is encephalopathic, one must initially determine if an EEG-sleep pattern is age-appropriate, reflecting the healthy medical status for a given CA. Two EEG-sleep studies demonstrate how electrographic polysomnographic estimates of gestational maturity were obtained for both healthy and ill preterm neonates (Scher and Barmadaet, 1987; Scher et al., 1995a,b). EEG-polysomnographic patterns were compared with fetal and obstetrical data. Without knowledge of clinical examination criteria for both healthy and ill preterm infants, EEG estimates of maturity were as accurate as clinical and/or anatomical estimates. This interpretative information, therefore, can be extremely helpful for the clinician in the following ways: First, many high-risk pregnancies do not include accurate information with respect to gestational maturity. Second, the symptomatic infant may be too medically ill or too premature to permit accurate clinical assessment of maturity by examination criteria alone. Third, electrographic, rather than polygraphic assessment of brain maturity is more reliable for the infant of <36 weeks' CA.

Ontogeny of EEG Features

Evolving EEG sleep patterns in the asymptomatic, presumably healthy, preterm infant has been the subject of many excellent reviews (Hrachovy et al., 1990; Lombroso, 1985; Volpe et al., 1983; Watanabe and Iwase, 1972; Werner et al., 1977). Improvements in neonatal intensive care, however, require periodic revisions that include more premature neonates (Anderson et al., 1985; Marret et al., 1997; Vecchierini et al., 2003). This is particularly relevant for the premature infant of less than 32 weeks' gestation in whom tremendous improvements in survival have occurred over the last decade. It is important, however, to verify which EEG-sleep patterns are normal only *after* systematic neurodevelopmental assessment of such children. Studies of healthy infants with normal developmental status are still required.

We now describe regional and hemispheric EEG patterns for preterm and full-term neonates, arbitrarily assigned within specific gestational age ranges. Temporal, spatial, and state organization of the EEG recordings are high-

lighted, with appropriate illustrations that comprise the cerebral activities noted during each age range.

Gestational Age of <28 Weeks

Neonates with a gestational age of <25 weeks fall below the limits of viability. Therefore, few infants survive on whom even one EEG recording can be obtained. However, useful information is now available to characterize the neurophysiological profile of these very premature neonates (Marret et al., 1997). An undifferentiated EEG sleep profile is observed with no distinctive features noted between waking or sleep state segments. The record remains largely discontinuous, with short periods of continuous EEG activity that may last for as long as 1 minute. Patterns of motility consist of segmental myoclonic movements of the face or body, as well as generalized myoclonic and tonic posturing either in an axial or appendicular distribution.

A pattern of alternating active and inactive EEG periods in preterm infants is termed electrographic discontinuity or tracé discontinu (Dreyfus-Brisac, 1968; Ellingson, 1964). Anderson et al. (1985) found that 60% of EEG recordings consist of discontinuity; the average interburst interval during this age range was between 8 and 16 seconds, with the longest interburst intervals being between 15 and 88 seconds. Similar ranges for the duration of interburst intervals have been found by other authors (Anderson et al., 1985; Benda et al., 1989; Connell et al., 1987; Eyre et al., 1988; Hughes et al., 1983a,b, 1987; Vecchierini et al., 2003), as listed in Table 49.3, which is in sharp contrast to earlier descriptions of interburst intervals as long as 2 minutes in duration (Lombroso, 1989). Such a difference may be, in part, based on the medical condition of the neonate at the time of the recording and/or the lack of information concerning long-term follow-up.

Activity predominates in the vertex, central, and occipital regions. Bitemporal attenuation is common (Scher and Barmada, 1987). While the traditional explanation for this feature is that it reflects intrahemispheric asynchrony, underdevelopment of the inferior frontal and superior temporal gyri (Scher and Barmada, 1987) may also help explain the

Table 49.3. Guidelines for the Use of EEG to Assess for an Encephalopathy in the Sick Neonate

1. Information concerning gestational age, state of arousal, and medical conditions, including medications, needs to be considered before offering an electrographic interpretation.
2. Serial recordings are far more advantageous than single recordings to document the progression or resolution of an encephalopathic process.
3. The EEG abnormality may reflect an encephalopathy due to antepartum, intrapartum, and/or neonatal difficulties.
4. Abnormal EEG patterns are rarely pathognomonic for specific diagnoses and complement clinical and imaging evaluations.
5. Partial or complete normalization of EEG disturbances commonly occurs over time.
6. Both diffuse and focal disturbances can coincidentally affect background EEG activity.
7. Significant EEG abnormalities may be seen in the absence of clinical expression of neurological disturbances in the neonate.
8. Mild to moderately severe EEG abnormalities are not always reliable for prognostic purposes and should be closely matched with the evolving clinical condition.

relative quiescence of activity in this brain region (Figs. 49.1 and 49.2).

EEG activity consists of mixed frequencies, predominated by delta activities in the parasagittal and occipital regions. Occipital delta is either isolated to one or two waveforms and is rarely longer than 5 to 6 seconds in duration or rhythmic in nature. Faster frequencies in the theta, alpha, and beta ranges are also intermixed in multiple head regions. Diffuse theta bursts are commonly seen during either continuous or discontinuous periods. Beta/delta complexes are transient patterns that identify premature neonates of varying postconceptional ages. This pattern is the principal landmark regional electrographic feature of the preterm infant. Random or briefly rhythmic 0.3 to 1.5 Hz delta activity of 50 to 250 µV (Hrachovy et al., 1990) have superimposed bursts of low- to moderate-amplitude faster frequencies with a frequency range of 10 to 20 Hz. The amplitude of such activity on bipolar recordings rarely exceed 60 to 75 µV. Historically, various terms have been applied to such complexes, such as *spindle delta bursts, brushes, spindle-like fast waves,* and *ripples of prematurity.* These complexes can be readily seen as early as 24 to 26 weeks, largely in the central and midline regions as well as the occipital regions.

Runs of monorhythmic alpha and/or theta activities are seen independent of delta brushes principally in the occipital regions in the neonate <28 weeks' gestation (Fig. 49.2). This transient pattern has been described in more detail and given the acronym STOP (i.e., sharp theta activity of the premature neonate) (Hughes et al., 1990); it can last for up to 6 to 10 seconds in either an asynchronous or asymmetric manner. Such activity should be distinguished from the more diffuse bursts of moderate- to high-amplitude theta, which are also commonly noted at this early age of prematurity.

Intra- and interhemispheric synchrony have been variably described by different authors. Lombroso (1979, 1985) described synchronous bursts as morphologically similar bursts of activity appearing within 1.5 seconds; synchronous periods noted from 50% at 31 to 32 weeks' CA to 100% at 40 to 43 weeks' CA with a midpoint of 70% to 85% at 35 to 36 weeks' CA. This is in sharp contrast to another description that interhemispheric synchrony has a mean of 93% for 1-minute epochs at 27 weeks' CA with a mean of 94% at 29 to 32 weeks' CA (Anderson et al., 1985). The hypersynchronous pattern in the infant <30 weeks' CA may be related to brainstem activity, while the greater instances of asynchrony between 30 and 36 weeks' CA reflect cortical synaptogenesis and myelination.

The methodology for defining synchrony varies between authors, but one must consider that a high degree of intrahemispheric synchrony does exist in the premature infant of even 30 weeks' gestation. However, it should be accepted that greater asynchrony may occur as the distance from the midline increases with rapid brain growth beyond 30 weeks' CA. Rapid growth of temporal and parietal structures may contribute to more frequent episodes of physiological asynchrony (Hrachovy et al., 1990). Measures of asynchrony

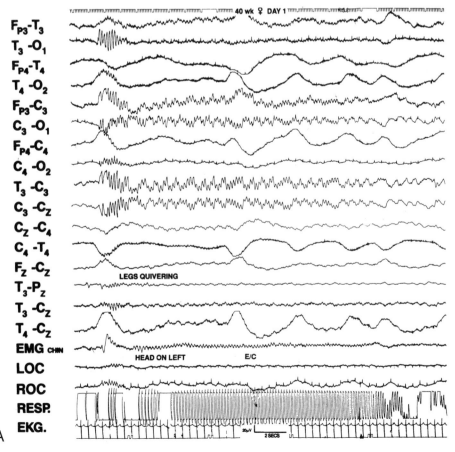

Figure 49.1. A: Physiological artifact secondary to clonus of the legs in a 40-week, 1-day-old female infant after a severe hypoxic ischemic episode at delivery. Electrodes in contact with the mattress generate a rhythmic signal secondary to movement of the head during tremulous episodes. (*continued*)

Figure 49.1. (*continued*) **B:** Physiological artifact consisting of myogenic potentials seen on multiple channels of a recording of a 27-week, 12-day-old infant with herpes encephalitis. Although the background is markedly abnormal because of severe suppression of background activity, the muscle-generated artifacts are not of cerebral origin, despite a spike-like morphology. (From Scher MS. 1985. Physiologic artifacts in neonatal electroencephalography. Am J EEG Technol 25:257–277, with permission.)

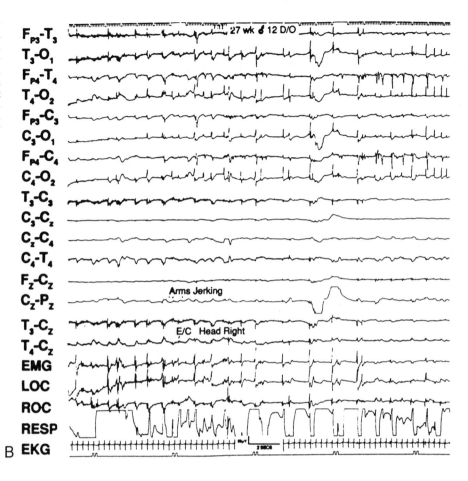

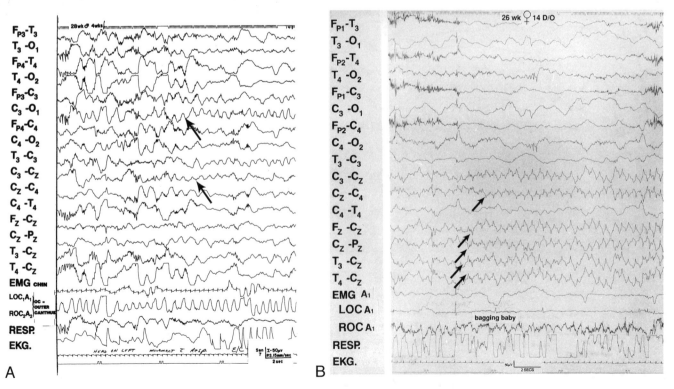

Figure 49.2. **A:** Ventilatory artifact noted in the left central region on an EEG recording of a 28-week, 28-day-old male infant synchronized to the respiratory excursions (*arrows*). **B:** Physiological artifacts created during ventilatory assistance using an Ambu bag by a neonatal nurse. Unusual waveforms are noted at the midline and in the parasagittal regions.

must include not only information about CA but also EEG state changes. Definitions of asynchrony should involve all background rhythms rather than only bursts during discontinuous epochs (Anderson et al., 1985; Lombroso, 1985).

Gestational Age of 28 to 31 Weeks

While the cyclic organization of state remains largely undifferentiated (Lombroso 1985, 1989), periods of body and eye movements coincide more consistently with irregular respirations during continuous periods of EEG. Computer classification of state by spectral and polysomnographic analyses recently demonstrated a high correlation among rapid eye movements (REMs) and EEG continuity in preterm infants, even at these earlier CAs (Scher, 1997a; Scher et al., 2003a,b).

Discontinuous epochs still predominate but decrease in duration as compared to the very premature neonate of <28 weeks' CA. Interbursts become progressively briefer with a dramatic increase in low- to moderate-amplitude faster rhythms primarily in the theta range (Figs. 49.3 and 49.4).

By 32 weeks, the degree of discontinuity has decreased to 45% of the record (Anderson et al., 1985). Dreyfus-Brisac (1970) found an alternating pattern in 24% of records at 32 to 34 weeks' gestation. The average interburst intervals at 29 to 31 weeks' CA ranged between 5 and 14 and 4 and 11 seconds, respectively, with means of 9 and 7 seconds, while the longest interburst periods for these two CA groups were found to be between 16 to 57 and 6 to 41 seconds with means of 36 and 20 seconds, respectively (Table 49.3).

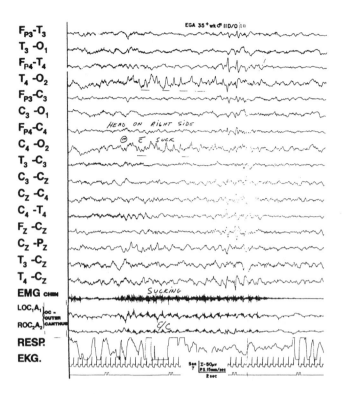

Figure 49.4. Buccolingual artifact from sucking in a 35-week, 11-day-old infant resulting in sharp-wave discharges in the right occipital area. (From Scher MS. 1985. Physiologic artifacts in neonatal electroencephalography. Am J EEG Technol 25:257–277, with permission.)

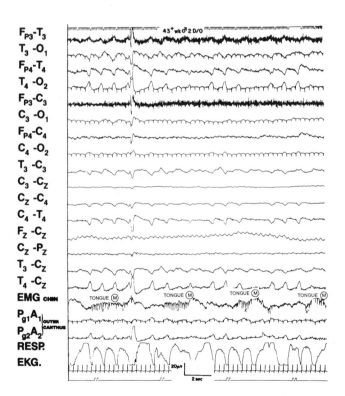

Figure 49.3. Hiccoughing artifact in a 43-week, 2-day-old infant creating diffuse repetitive sharp wave discharges. (Note: the "x" marks under the EMG line indicate the occurrence of each hiccough.)

Monorhythmic occipital delta is now quite abundant at 28 to 31 weeks with durations that are greater than 30 seconds. Delta brush patterns continue to be abundant involving not only the vertex and central regions, but also the occipital and temporal regions (Werner et al., 1977). It may, at times, be difficult to differentiate superimposed delta brushes in the temporal region particularly because of the abundance of temporal theta bursts (Scher, 1991).

Another useful developmental marker is the appearance of rhythmic 4.5- to 6-Hz activity occurring independently as well as synchronously in each midtemporal region. Although this activity is noted at <28 weeks' CA, it is expressed maximally between 28 weeks' and 32 weeks' CA. Historically, this feature has been described as "temporal sawtooth waves" (Yakovlev and Lacour, 1967). Amplitudes range from roughly 20 to 200 µV, and with maturation, these bursts may reach the alpha frequency. In a study of 436 infants (Hughes et al., 1987), a parabolic polynomial function has described the age incidence of temporal theta activity, strongly reflecting the pattern as a maturational landmark. Temporal theta can obtain a maximum incidence of 36% (Anderson et al., 1985) at 29 to 30 weeks after which it diminishes rapidly. At 32 weeks, only 12% of the record persists in this pattern (Anderson et al., 1985). This rhythmic theta activity should be distinguished from repetitive sharp activity in the theta range seen at near term and term ages in the midline and rolandic regions, particularly during the quiet sleep segment.

The clinical significance of sharp-wave transients in healthy preterm infants has been poorly understood at these early preterm ages. Regional patterns associated with maturation as discussed above must be considered before assigning sharp-wave criteria to a transient waveform. Sharply contoured delta brushes or temporal or occipital theta bursts may appear epileptiform without clearly satisfying morphological criteria for a spike or sharp wave (Scher, 1991).

Sporadic multifocal spikes and sharp waves can be seen at any gestational age (Ellingson, 1964; Harris and Tizard, 1960; Monod et al., 1960; Parmelee et al., 1968; Petre-Quadens and de Lee, 1970; Prechtl 1974, 1984; Prechtl and Lenard, 1967; Prechtl and Nijhuis, 1983; Prechtl et al., 1969, 1979; Rantakallio and von Wendt, 1985; Richards et al., 1986; Robertson, 1982, 1987; Rumack et al., 1985; Saint-Anne Dargassies, 1974; Samson-Dollfus, 1955; Volpe et al., 1983; Yakovlev and Lacour, 1967), but few studies include preterm infants less than 32 weeks' estimated gestational age (EGA). Anderson et al. (1985) studied the incidence and location of spikes and sharp waves in 33 preterm infants, 27 to 32 weeks' EGA. Both features were infrequent, with spikes less common that sharp waves. Both morphologies were most abundant in frontal and temporal regions, with frontal and temporal sharp waves increasing in incidence from 27 to 32 weeks. Central sharp waves decreased in number over time, while occipital and vertex discharges had the lowest incidence. Unfortunately, only 55% of infants were verified as normal on follow-up at 6 to 8 months of age. Scher et al. (1993) tabulated sharp-wave transients from 94 three-hour studies on 52 healthy neonates from 29 to 43 weeks' PCA. Sharp waves in four anatomical regions accounted for 94%, 83%, and 84% in full-term, preterm, and preterm at postconceptional term ages (i.e., F_{P1}, F_P, T_4, and C_3). For neonates <32 weeks, sharp-wave transients in the right occipital and temporal regions accounted for more than half of transients noted at that age range. Brain maturation alters the location and morphology of sharp-wave transients in healthy neonates, who were neurodevelopmentally normal at 18 months of age. Corroboration with other studies involving large preterm populations with neurodevelopmental follow-up are needed before assigning clinical significance to sharp waves in asymptomatic preterm infants.

Gestational Age 32 to 34 Weeks

Body and eye movements take on a more phasic rather than tonic pattern with better differentiation between continuous EEG activity as active sleep and discontinuous EEG activity as quiet or non-REM sleep segments, the latter segment with fewer movements, except for buccolingual movements and occasional myoclonic jerks (Curzi-Dascalova et al., 1988). Scher et al. (1997a–d) described fewer REMs and more facial movements as the degree of electrographic discontinuity increases. Variable respirations persist, but short periods of regular respirations are now present during discontinuous portions of the recording.

EEG background is more continuous, with cyclic periods of tracé discontinu (Figs. 49.5 and 49.6). Synchronous delta frequencies of varying amplitude still predominate, interrupted by random inactive periods. Faster frequencies of variable amplitudes are also present, represented by the faster component of a delta brush pattern. Regional patterns (i.e., brushes, theta bursts) predominate in the rolandic and occipital regions as well as the temporal and midline regions.

The most characteristic feature at this age range is the increase in multifocal sharp waves (see section below) as well as the appearance of reactivity to stimulation, characterized by transient periods of attenuation independent of discontinuity.

Sharply contoured activity predominates in the temporal and central regions, with positive temporal sharp waves frequently seen in synchronous or independently occurring runs (Fig. 49.7). The sharp activity in the central regions is more likely negative in polarity and should be carefully distinguished from physiological artifacts that can occur due to fontanel pulsation or ventilatory excursions. Positive temporal sharp waves in healthy neonates need to be differentiated from pathological rolandic and vertex positive sharp waves that are seen in the sick neonate with either intraventricular hemorrhage or periventricular leukomalacia. Scher et al. (1994) described the maturational trends of positive temporal sharp waves on serial recordings for 52 healthy neonates who were normal by at least 18 months of age.

Reactivity to stimulation appears during this gestational age range. Nonspecific EEG changes are induced by tactile or painful stimulation, usually with an abrupt attenuation or desynchronization of background. This can be difficult to distinguish from low-amplitude quiescent periods, but becomes more obvious with maturation, allowing a better distinction between active and quiet sleep. Uncommonly, bursts of higher amplitude delta activity may also characterize this reactivity. It is unknown whether these are the precursors of more discrete arousal patterns such as K complexes and hypersynchronous delta that are seen at older ages.

Reactivity to photic stimulation has been studied more systematically (Anderson et al., 1985). Responses to photic stimulation are clearly seen in the EEG of the early premature infant (Ellingson, 1958). Responses to isolated flashes have a prominent negative wave component. Ellingson (1960) described the later positive component occurring with maturation, with decreasing latency in proportion to increasing CA. In contrast to isolated flashes, repetitive flashes or photic driving have also been investigated by several authors, but such responses are difficult to detect in the EEG of the neonate (Ellingson, 1960, 1964). Only between 4% and 5% of premature and full-term infants exhibit photic driving with a wide range of flicker frequencies. Anderson et al. (1985) found that even early premature infants between 27 to 32 weeks exhibit driving in 65% of 34 neonates when the frequencies are limited to two to ten flashes per second. Some authors have claimed that these driving responses are more readily seen in the premature infant because of the more continuous higher amplitude mixture of background frequencies (Monod et al., 1960).

Responses to other forms of sensory stimulation such as auditory or painful stimulation have been the object of less attention in both the premature or full-term neonate. Monod and Garma (1971) investigated behavioral and physiological responses to auditory clicks in the premature neonate. They found vertex spikes in response to auditory clicks readily noted in neonates at 32 to 34 weeks' CA. This is in contrast to a less distinctive response with more mature ages. Sudden, loud auditory stimuli more effectively produce EEG changes than visual (Ellingson, 1960) or tactile (Dreyfus-Brisac et al., 1957) stimuli. Such periods of desynchronization have been postulated to be associated with the psychophysiological property of habituation and may represent electrographic representation of perceptual memory and discriminatory functions of the neonate (Anderson et al., 1985).

Gestational Age 34 to 37 Weeks' CA

Cyclic alterations between wakefulness and sleep as well as longer periods of continuous periods of EEG predominate during this age range. More concordant segments between cerebral and noncerebral signals now begin to resemble active and quiet sleep segments of the term infant. For

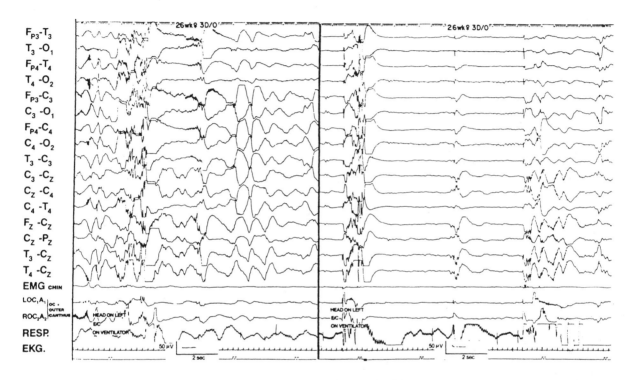

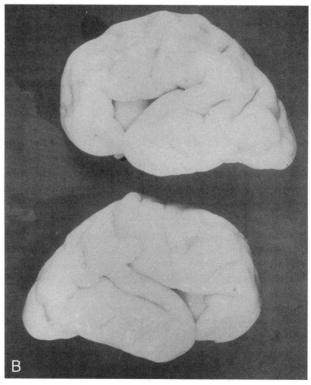

Figure 49.5. **A:** Two EEG tracings for a 26-week, 3-day-old female. The first frame demonstrates generalized theta and delta slowing with prominent vertex central slow activity. Note the bitemporal attenuation. In the second frame, synchronous interburst intervals of <30 seconds in duration are noted. Note prominent delta brush patterns in the vertex region. **B:** Lateral view of the brain for the same patient in **A**. Underdeveloped frontal and temporal lobes with a clearly visible insula. Immature sulcation pattern, especially involving the rolandic, calcarine, and superior temporal sulci. (From Scher MS, and Barmada A. 1987. Estimation of gestational age by electrographic, clinical, and anatomical criteria. Pediatr Neurol 3:256–262, with permission.)

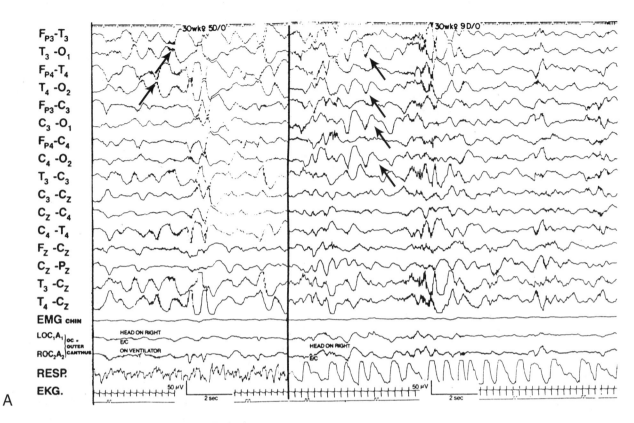

A

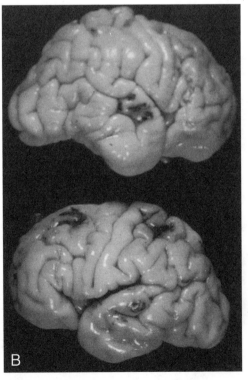

B

Figure 49.6. **A:** Two EEG tracings for a 30-week, 5-day-old female. In the first frame, continuous EEG activity with prominent temporal delta brush and delta patterns are noted *(arrows)*. In the second frame, occipital delta and theta brush patterns are recorded *(arrows)*. **B:** Lateral view of the brain for the patient in **A**. Greater degree of sulcation evident than Figure 49.5B. Note the more complete elaboration of the rolandic, superior temporal, and calcarine sulci. There is shortening of the anterior to posterior brain length and a persistently visible insula, both of which reflect dysmaturity of the brain. (From Scher MS, and Barmada A. 1987. Estimation of gestational age by electrographic, clinical, and anatomical criteria. Pediatr Neurol 3:256–262, with permission.)

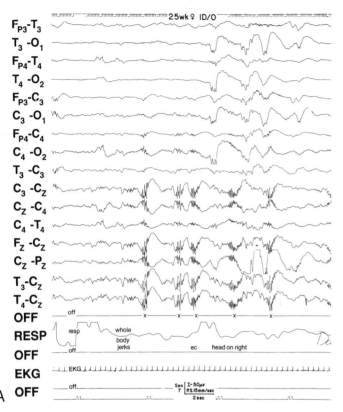

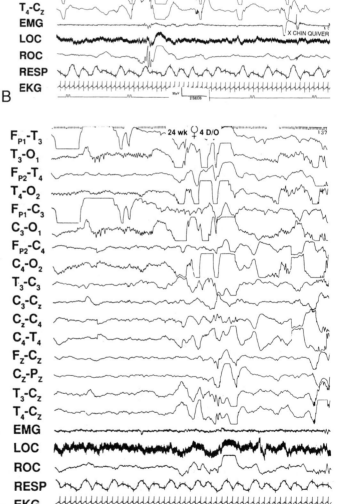

Figure 49.7. **A:** EEG tracing of a 25-week, 1-day-old female depicting prominent vertex delta brushes, as well as occipital theta and delta brushes. Briefly rhythmic occipital delta are noted, as well as myoclonic movements (x marks), which appear coincident with the delta brush patterns. **B:** EEG tracing of a 24-week, 4-day-old female demonstrating features characteristic of this gestational age (i.e., <28 weeks estimated gestational age). Isolated occipital delta with theta/alpha bursts are noted. Bitemporal attenuation and parasagittal delta brushes are also recorded. **C:** An EEG tracing of a 24-week, 4-day-old infant with a more prolonged occipital theta/alpha that is asymmetric in amplitude. Shifting asymmetries of such features are common.

instance, motility patterns take on a distinctive phasic quality with movements that predominate during active sleep. An absence of motility except for generalized myoclonic and facial movements are seen during quiet sleep. Myogenic activity measured at the chin characteristically remains low during the periods of active sleep, while higher and more phasic activity occurs during quiet sleep. The cyclic nature of the active and quiet sleep periods still lacks the well-defined 30- to 70-minute cycle seen in the term infant.

Electrographic components of the EEG sleep cycle in this gestational age range show a predominance of continuous EEG activity composed of mixed delta and theta waves activity usually lower in amplitude (20-100 µV) than at younger gestational ages. Low-amplitude faster rhythms of alpha and beta activities are also present, with fewer delta brushes persisting primarily over the temporal and occipital regions. Brushes also more commonly appear during quiet sleep than during active sleep.

Frontal sharp transients of 50 to 150 µV are predominantly noted at 34 to 35 weeks' gestation (250 µV), but may be seen at earlier gestational ages. Historically, these waveforms were termed "encoches frontales" (Monod et al., 1960) and popularly identified as "frontal sharp transients" (Kellaway and Crawley, 1964; Kellaway and Petersen, 1964) as well as "pointes lents diphasiques frontales" (Arfel et al., 1977; Monod and Tharp, 1977). These sharp waves usually have an initial surface positive component followed by a negative component, but are also associated with rhyth-

mic sharply contoured frontal delta activity (Goldie et al., 1971) and can occasionally be high amplitude (250 µV). Scher et al. (1994c) described the predominance of these frontal sharp transients, particularly in term neonates.

In contrast, fewer multifocal sharp transients occur, and, as with more preterm neonates, are sometimes difficult to distinguish from the intermixed background theta or beta background frequencies.

The discontinuous quality of the EEG sleep tracing during this CA range indicates the appearance of a tracé alternant rather than a tracé discontinu pattern noted in younger premature infants. The quiescent periods now consist of more activity that may exceed 15 µV/mm, with a greater mixture of low-amplitude faster rhythms noted. Also, during this age range, quiet sleep segments may alternate as a tracé discontinu pattern, rather than a tracé alternant pattern.

Gestational Age 38 to 42 Weeks' CA

Electrographic/polygraphic patterns are fully elaborated during this age range. Alternating periods of wakefulness and sleep as well as cyclic changes between four segments of sleep state and indeterminate sleep can be identified. Two active sleep and quiet EEG segments compose most of this cycle, with a total length varying from 30 to 70 minutes, associated with the presence or absence of rapid eye movements, body movements, autonomic signs, and arousal episodes.

While conventional wisdom dictates that only the term and near-term infant express such an organized EEG sleep

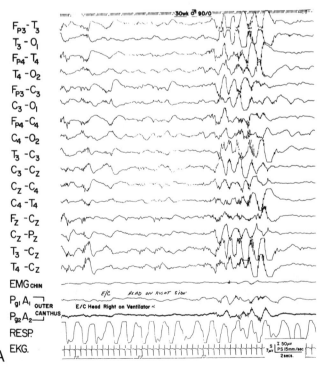

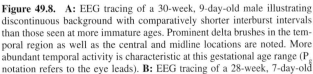

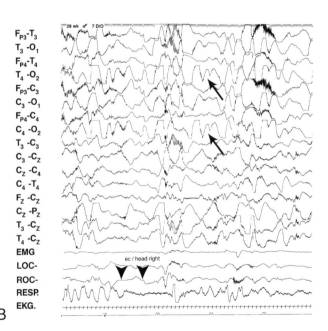

Figure 49.8. **A:** EEG tracing of a 30-week, 9-day-old male illustrating discontinuous background with comparatively shorter interburst intervals than those seen at more immature ages. Prominent delta brushes in the temporal region as well as the central and midline locations are noted. More abundant temporal activity is characteristic at this gestational age range (P$_g$ notation refers to the eye leads). **B:** EEG tracing of a 28-week, 7-day-old male showing continuous activity composed of prominent rhythmic occipital delta lasting >20 seconds *(arrows)*. Rapid eye movements (REM) *(arrowhead)* commonly occur during continuous EEG tracing of the premature neonate.

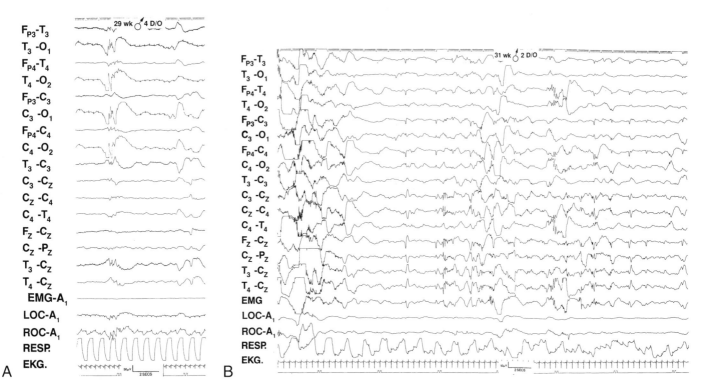

Figure 49.9. **A:** EEG tracing for a 29-week, 4-day-old male with sharply contoured occipital theta giving the appearance of pathological sharp activity. Superimposed waveforms may appear sharp in morphology and must be clearly distinguished from abnormal epileptiform discharges in this young age group. **B:** EEG tracing of a 31-week, 2-day-old male demon-strating prominent frontal and central sharp activity intermixed with delta brush and other intermixed frequencies characteristic for the age. Note the prominent frontal parasagittal and midline sharp waves in this healthy asymptomatic premature infant.

cycle, concordance among specific EEG and polygraphic parameters has been described in the preterm infant as early as 25 to 30 weeks' gestation (Curzi-Dascalova et al., 1988; Johnson et al., 2003; Scher et al., 1997a–d). This concordance reflects the temporal coordination of specific neural systems that subserve these physiological behaviors. A more rudimentary sleep cycle may be better detected in the premature neonate by using more quantitative techniques (Johnson et al., 2003; Scher et al., 1990, 1997a–d).

The EEG sleep organization of the full-term neonate has traditionally been well described, and sleep architecture is similar for the premature infant who has matured to a full-term age. Two active sleep segments occupy 50% of the sleep time of the full-term infant, composed of mixed frequency pattern (M) and a low-voltage regular (LVI) pattern that begin and end the sleep cycle. Quiet sleep segments, consisting of high-voltage slow (HVS) and tracé alternant (TA) segments, occupy 35% to 40% of the cycle. Transitional or indeterminate segments (i.e., discordance between EEG and polygraphic criteria of sleep state) compose 10% to 15% of the cycle. While the mixed-frequency active sleep pattern is composed of moderate-amplitude delta and lower amplitude theta, alpha, and beta range activities, this EEG background is also associated with wakefulness (Fig. 49.8).

The LVI pattern is characterized by a continuous low-amplitude admixture of frequencies (15 to 30 mV) mostly in the theta and beta ranges (Fig. 49.9). Considerable amounts of alpha activity are intermixed both posteriorly and anteri-orly. This pattern can be seen either during wakefulness or active sleep.

Two quiet sleep segments, high-voltage slow and tracé alternant (Fig. 49.10), occupy the second and third positions in this idealized EEG sleep cycle. The high-voltage slow pattern (HVS) is composed of diffuse continuous high-amplitude 50 to 150 μV delta activity, intermixed with theta and beta range activity of lower amplitude. The HVS segment is quite brief (4–6% of the cycle) and is rapidly re-placed by the TA pattern. During the TA segment, delta and theta range activities alternate with lower amplitude faster frequencies seen synchronously over both hemispheres.

Frontal sharp waves may be abundant especially during quiet sleep. These waveforms are bilateral and synchronous, but also can be asymmetric. Frontal sharp waves are seen less often during active and indeterminate sleep segments and are least likely to be noted during LVI active sleep (Arfel et al., 1977; Stratton, 1982). During sleep, frontal sharp transients are noted until the beginning of the second month of life (Erkinjuntti and Kero, 1985; Yakovlev and Lacour, 1967).

As with preterm infants, the clinical significance of spikes and sharp waves in asymptomatic full-term neonatal populations remains controversial. Most groups do not have adequate follow-up data or were selected based on clinical problems. Clancy et al. (1985) identified 69 healthy infants who had an acute life-threatening event [i.e., near-miss sudden infant death syndrome (SIDS) event]. Analyses of 10 minutes of active sleep documented more frequent sharp

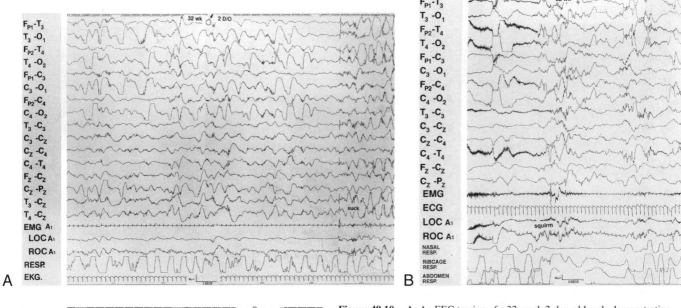

A

B

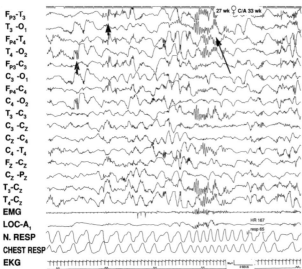

C

Figure 49.10. **A:** An EEG tracing of a 32-week 2-day-old male demonstrating a continuous background of fast and slow frequencies. **B:** Discontinuous EEG segment of a 32-week-old female demonstrating reactivity. **C:** An EEG tracing for a 33-week corrected-age female demonstrating an abundance of regional patterns characteristic at this gestational age including temporal theta and brushes. Frontal sharp activity and frontal brushes, occipital theta, and occipital brushes are also noted in the context of a continuous EEG background.

waves in near-term than term infants. Temporal sharp waves were more abundant than centrally located discharges, persisting until 50 weeks' CA.

Karbowski and Nencka (1980) studied 1-hour sleep recordings in 82 full-term healthy newborns without subsequent follow-up. Eighty-one percent had predominantly right centrotemporal sharp waves with an average interval of 3 minutes and 47 seconds (Figs. 49.11 through 49.15). Only 12% had predominantly left central waves with an average interval of 15 minutes. All discharges were noted primarily in indeterminate sleep.

Statz et al. (1982) followed 24 full-term healthy infants to 9 to 12 months of age after obtaining a neonatal sleep recording. They noted sporadic multifocal nonrepetitive discharges during quiet sleep in all infants, while only 25% of infants had discharges during active sleep. The parietal region had the most abundant discharges with intervals between 25 seconds and 38 minutes.

Scher et al. (1994c) described the incidence of sharp waves in a healthy neonatal population, with mean numbers per hour for full-term, preterm, and preterm at postconceptional term ages as 11.7 ± 12, 10.0 ± 7, and 13 ± 10. Clearly, some healthy neonates may have higher numbers of sharp-wave transients despite the absence of encephalopathic patterns with normal neurodevelopment.

Clearly, the clinical significance of spikes and sharp waves for both preterm and full-term infants needs more investigation. As Karbowski and Nencka (1980) emphasized, sporadic sharp waves may be either normal or abnormal, depending on the clinical context, the EEG background activity, location, morphology, and CA. Unless discharges are repetitive, periodic, or positive in polarity, pathological significance should be cautiously assigned (see section on abnormal neonatal EEG patterns, below).

Central sharp-wave transients and rhythmic sharply contoured theta in the parasagittal and vertex regions are also

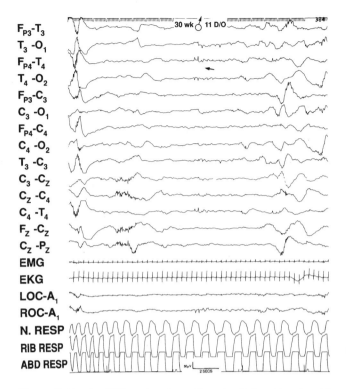

Figure 49.11. An EEG tracing for a 30-week, 11-day-old male with briefly repetitive positive temporal sharp waves in this healthy asymptomatic neonate *(arrows)*. Normal neurodevelopment has been documented at one year of age.

seen. This midline pattern is rhythmic and has a spindle-like appearance (Hayakawa et al., 1987). It is unknown whether these rhythmic activities are rudimentary sleep spindles seen between 2 and 4 months of age. Sleep spindles commonly noted at 2 to 4 months of age may be seen as early as 4 to 6 weeks of age, and frontal sharp waves are normally noted 3 to 4 weeks following birth.

Delta brush patterns are occasionally noted during the quiet sleep segment, but are rare and isolated primarily to the temporal and occipital regions.

As described above, synchrony should be 100% during sleep of the full-term neonate. Transient asymmetries, mainly in the temporal regions, can be observed, particularly during the initial minutes of quiet sleep (Challamel et al., 1984; O'Brien et al., 1987).

Ontogeny of EEG-sleep organization through the termination of the neonatal period (i.e., 28 days following a full-term birth) has been systematically investigated by only a few researchers (Beckwith and Parmelee, 1986; Ellingson and Peters, 1980; Lombroso and Matsumiya, 1985). Gradual disappearance of tracé alternant by 3 to 6 weeks following a full-term birth as well as a change from active to quiet sleep onset have been described.

Brain Adaptation to Conditions of Prematurity

Several longitudinal sleep studies without polygraphy report no differences in sleep organization between preterm and full-term infants (Anders and Keener, 1985; Ungerer et

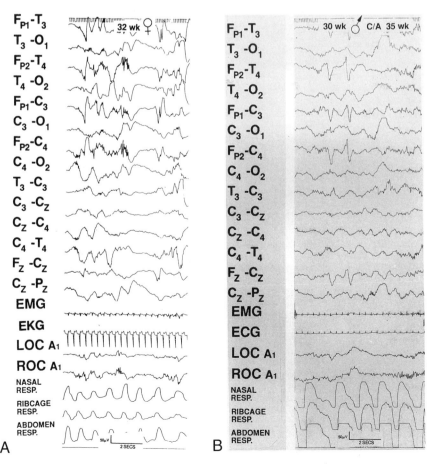

Figure 49.12. **A:** An EEG tracing of a 32-week infant with frontal sharp waves. **B:** EEG tracing of a 35-week corrected age infant with frontal sharp waves.

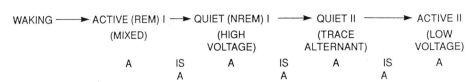

ULTRADIAN SLEEP CYCLE
(FULL TERM)

WAKING ⟶ ACTIVE (REM) I ⟶ QUIET (NREM) I ⟶ QUIET II ⟶ ACTIVE II
          (MIXED)   (HIGH   (TRACE   (LOW
                             VOLTAGE)   ALTERNANT)   VOLTAGE)

          A   IS   A   IS   A   IS   A
                   A   A   A

Figure 49.13. Ultradian sleep cycle of a fullterm neonate indicating the four segment sleep cycle beginning and ending with an active sleep period with two intervening quiet sleep periods. Arousals (A) occur as periods of reactivity either within or between sleep segments that can be on either a spontaneous or an evoked basis. Transitional or indeterminate sleep periods punctuate changes in sleep state segments. (From Scher MS. 1988. Neonatal EEG sleep cycling—a developmental marker of central nervous system maturation [part II]. Pediatr Neurol 4:329–336, with permission.)

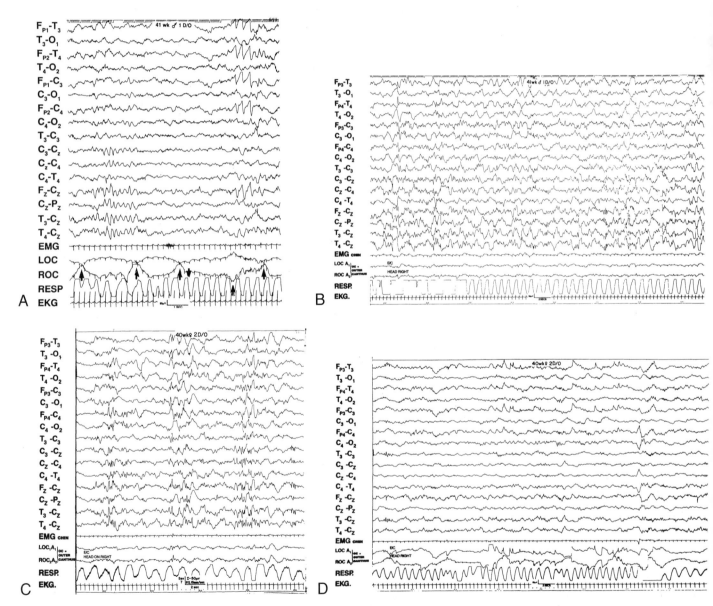

Figure 49.14. A: Example of a mixed-frequency active sleep state in a 41-week, 1-day-old male. Note the rhythmic theta activity in the midline and the frontal sharp waves during a transition to indeterminate sleep. (*Arrows* indicate the horizontal eye movements characteristic of rapid eye movements of sleep.) **B:** High-voltage EEG tracing in a healthy full-term infant, 41-week, 1-day-old male characteristic of a quiet sleep segment with absence of movements and regular respiratory and cardiac rhythms. **C:** EEG tracing of a 40-week, 2-day-old female depicting a tracé alternant quiet sleep segment. Note the occasional delta brush patterns as well as sharp transients that can be seen in various head regions in the sleep segment, particularly in the right hemisphere. **D:** EEG tracing of a 40-week, 2-day-old female depicting the low-voltage irregular activity sleep segment. Rapid eye movements are prominent during this portion of the sleep cycle with frontopolar sharp waves reflecting eye movement-induced artifact.

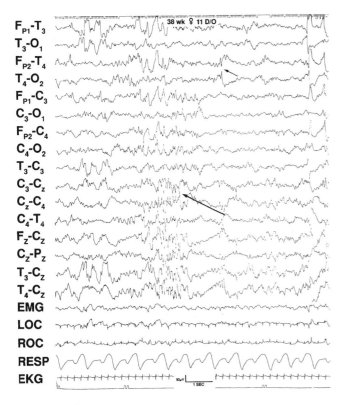

Figure 49.15. EEG tracing for a 38-week, 11-day-old infant with sharply contoured midline and parasagittal sharply contoured theta *(long arrow)*. Also note the isolated sharp waves seen in the right temporal region *(short arrow)*. Both patterns can be seen in healthy patients and have no prognostic significance.

al., 1983). Using polygraphic recordings, however, differences between the preterm and full-term cohorts at matched postconceptional term ages have been described, with respect to sleep architecture, continuity, phasic, spectral, cardiorespiratory, and temperature measures (Curzi-Dasclova et al., 1993; Scher et al., 1992, 1994e–i). Longer bursts during tracé alternant, early sleep spindle appearance, more immature patterns for the conceptional age, better phase stability, and specific frequency bands have been described (Joseph et al., 1976). Behavioral criteria of sleep are also different between the groups (Willekens et al., 1984). The sleep cycle in the preterm and postconceptional term age infant has been noted to be one third longer than the full-term infant, with a greater percentage of quiet sleep (Scher et al., 1992). Preterm neonates have fewer movements, fewer and shorter arousals, higher mean rectal temperatures, less cardiorespiratory regularity during quiet sleep (Scher et al., 1994e–g), and lower spectral EEG energies (Scher, 1994) during specific sleep state segments than full-term infants. While these differences are subtle, each reflects a condition of prematurity on brain maturation for a specific neuronal system. Adaptation of brain function of the preterm infant as expressed on EEG-sleep studies may reflect physiological dysmaturity to biological/environmental stresses that may occur because of intrauterine and/or extrauterine factors (Amiel-Tison and Pettigrew, 1991). Dysmature EEG-sleep

measures may also predict neurodevelopmental performance, as suggested by EEG-sleep studies on healthy preterm infants (Scher, 1996), as well as recovering newborns for various clinical risk factors, such as prenatal substance exposure (Scher et al., 1988a,b, 2000), chronic lung disease (Hahn and Tharp, 1990), SIDS (Scher et al., 1997c,d), or general medical complications (Beckwith and Parmelee, 1986). A dysmaturity index has been proposed that combines polygraphic and spectral data analyses to distinguish preterm infants who have altered brain maturation (Scher et al., 2003b).

Neonatal EEG Sleep as an Ultradian Rhythm

During the last several decades, extensive information has been published with respect to the existence and functional significance of ultradian (less than 24 hours) rhythms in humans (Sterman et al., 1977). Durations of ultradian rhythms are between 30 minutes and 24 hours and may represent an important portion of the entire spectrum of human biological rhythms (Hildebrandt, 1986). The human sleep cycle fits into a longer ultradian period lasting over an hour, while individual EEG frequencies that compose continuous EEG activity represent markedly shorter periods of duration lasting only seconds.

Two biorhythmic processes define the temporal organization of sleep in the neonate: a weak circadian sleep-wake rhythm and a stronger ultradian REM-non-REM (NREM) rhythm (Glotzbach et al., 1995). Both biorhythms evolve over increasing ages. Internal biological clocks become better organized around environmental cues, such as the light-dark cycle, temperature, noise, and social interaction (Anders et al., 1995). In normal full-term newborns, sleep alternates with waking states over a 3- to 4-hour cycle, both at night and during the day. Within the first month or two of life after birth for the full-term infant, sleep-wake state organization begins to adapt to the light and dark cycles, as well as regularly recurring social cues. Circadian rhythmicity of body temperature and heart rate is noted in approximately 50% of preterm infants at 29 to 35 weeks' CA (Mirimiran and Kok, 1991). However, stronger ultradian rhythms of 3 to 4 hours' duration correspond to feeding and social interventions (Glotzbach et al., 1995). Increases in body movement activity, as well as heart rate, and decreases in rectal skin temperature are noted during interventions, reflecting changes in the infant's microenvironment and the infant-caregiver interactions. Even the ultradian EEG-sleep cycle length of the preterm infant as defined by changes in EEG discontinuity show a positive correlation of cycle length and increasing CA (Scher et al., 1994f,h,i). By postconceptional term age, the ultradian EEG-sleep cycle is longer for the preterm than the full-term infant (Scher et al., 1992). Regardless of the cycle length, sleep architecture remains the same between preterm and full-term groups, composed of active sleep segments interrupted by transitional or indeterminate sleep segments. Reactivity or arousal periods punctuate within and between sleep segments. Both indeterminate sleep and arousal phenomena represent important expressions of sleep continuity.

Mathematical relationships among sleep components better define the development of this ultradian neonatal sleep cycle in the infant (Harper et al., 1981). Sleep parameters including EEG-sleep state, motility, rapid eye movements, and arousal can be expressed more quantitatively. For a particular gestational age range, specific period, phase, and amplitude relationships may better define ontogeny of the EEG sleep cycle. With maturation of the CNS, relationships solidify among these parameters. Specific temporal relationships exist at early gestational ages (i.e., <30 weeks) (Johnson and Scher, 2003).

Comparisons of sleep cycles in preterm neonates at corrected term ages with those of full-term infants can assess the degree to which premature neonates adapt to this extrauterine environment. What is more, such studies can also be compared with fetal state patterns (Prechtl, 1984). Differences between groups reflect differences in CNS maturation that are, in part, due to maternal circadian influences on fetal development that have been altered in children prematurely born.

Maturation of Specific Physiological Behaviors in Preterm Infants

An earlier review of ultradian physiological rhythms in term neonates and young infants emphasized the concordance among groups of physiological behaviors (Stratton, 1982). Relationships may exist among specific combinations of physiological behaviors in the preterm infants, even though state transitions in newborns of <36 weeks are not easily defined. While circadian influence may not be established until sometime after birth (Hellbrugge, 1960, 1968), selected aspects of sleep organization are already expressed by the preterm infant. The following summary of several physiological behaviors highlights how state differentiation evolves in the preterm infant.

Rapid eye movements represent one of the main identifying features of active sleep. Active sleep constitutes the majority of the neonatal sleep cycle. Rapid eye movements appear to be time locked to continuous EEG activity as early as 31 to 32 weeks' gestation (Curzi-Dascalova et al., 1988; Johnson and Scher, 2003; Scher, 1997a–c). REM activity is not a random rhythm (Prechtl et al., 1967) and may have predictable intervals of occurrence (Dittrichova et al., 1972), even at early gestational ages (Johnson and Scher, 2003). Different classes of REM at different times of the sleep cycle may exist, and the numbers and types of REM increase with maturation (Ersyukova, 1980; Lynch and Aserinsky, 1986). This feature also can be measured during fetal life, as well as being associated with continuous EEG activity in preterm neonates as early as 30 weeks' EGA (Prechtl, 1984). Closer identification of REM occurrence during each EEG pattern is needed to better understand the importance of this developing ultradian rhythm. Positive correlations with maturation were noted with REM/minute during transitional indeterminate segments of EEG sleep; conversely, negative correlations for REM/minute were noted with increasing conceptional age during discontinuous EEG sleep (Scher et al., 1994f).

Motility patterns are also an integral part of the neonatal sleep cycle (Anders et al., 1971). Different motility patterns appear at successively older neonatal ages up until term. These developing patterns are seen in both extrauterine-reared neonates as well as fetuses (Robertson 1982, 1987). Myoclonic and whole-body movements predominate in the preterm infant (Fukumoto et al., 1981; Hayakawa et al., 1987; Prechtl et al., 1979), while smaller, slower body movements are seen in the full-term neonate. Attention to specific segments of the EEG sleep cycle of the neonate is important since motility patterns may differ during different segments of the cycle (Hayakawa et al., 1987). Similar motility patterns have been documented *in utero* by fetal ultrasonography (Prechtl, 1974; Robertson, 1982, 1987), reflecting continuity of brain function from fetal to neonatal life (Precht, 1984).

Maturational trends in cardiorespiratory behavior have also been studied in preterm infants using spectral analyses; decreased variability of cardiorespiratory behavior is seen with increasing postconceptional age (Scher et al., 1994g). Spectral EEG measures are stronger indicators of functional brain maturity compared with noncerebral measures, such as cardiorespiratory behavior. Periodic breathing and respiratory pauses are physiological events that commonly occur in preterm infants (Glotzbach et al., 1989; Martin et al., 1986). Also, cardiorespiratory measures, as well as motility and temperature changes, do not correlate with changes in EEG continuity, REMs, or spectral EEG energies of the preterm infant, or at any specific postconceptional age (Scher et al., 1997).

Computer Strategies for EEG Sleep Analyses of the Neonate

Comparatively less attention has been directed to automated analyses of neonatal EEG-sleep studies, compared with those of older persons (Agarwal and Gotman, 2002). Since an earlier review of this topic (Scher et al., 1990), further advancements in both computerized devices and mathematical programming have been developed. To succeed in the development of an automated state detector for neonates, technical innovations must recognize the unique neurophysiological expressions of state transitions of the newborn that do not exist for the older patient. A short list of these unique electrographic/polysomnographic behaviors includes a shorter sleep cycle, prominent EEG delta rhythms in different regional locations, intra- and interhemispheric electrographic asynchrony, discrete neonatal waveform patterns (i.e., delta brush and theta burst patterns), a high percentage of periodic breathing, a greater number and heterogeneity of rapid eye movements, and unique motor patterns that reflect fetal postural reflexes that precede the expression of more sophisticated movement patterns.

Previous neonatal sleep studies initially applied automated techniques to assess functional brain maturation using analyses that were based on assumptions of stationarity, without consideration of time-dependent changes (Bes et al., 1988; Connell et al., 1987; Eyre et al., 1988; Giaquinto et al., 1977; Havlicek et al., 1975; Kuks et al., 1988; Lombroso, 1979; Sterman et al., 1977; Willekens et al., 1984). The preferred methodological approach has been fast Fourier transform analyses, studied initially with full-term neonates (Eiselt et al., 2001; Field et al., 2002; Ktonas et al., 1995; Lehtonen et al., 1998; Witte et al., 1997), followed by reports in preterm infants (Eiselt et al., 1997; Holthausen et

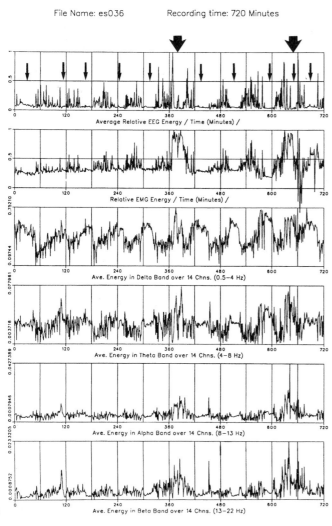

Figure 49.16. **A:** Total EEG energy distributions of 14 channels of EEG averaged over a 12-hour neonatal EEG sleep study. Note that the average EEG energy has periodic segments of relatively lower energy *(arrows)*. These correspond to the quiet sleep segments of each EEG sleep cycle through the night. The average energy in the delta band, however, appears to rise to a maximum at these times of low total energy. *(Arrowheads* indicate feeding periods.) **B:** A quiet sleep (i.e., tracé alternant) segment occurring during one of these low EEG energy periods described in **A.** (Channels 1 through 14 are EEG channels, while channels 15 through 25 are noncerebral signals.)

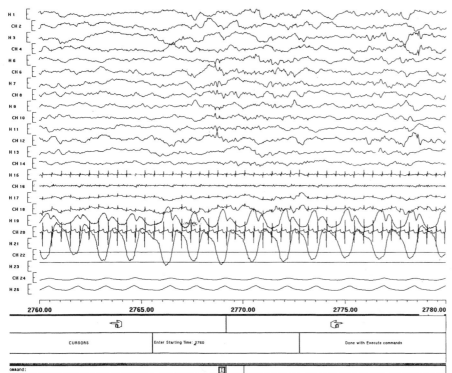

al., 2000; Kuhle et al., 2001; Myers et al., 1997; Sawaguchi et al., 1996; Schramm et al., 2000; Vanhatalo et al., 2002). Similar calculations, based primarily on assumptions of stationarity, were also described for specific neonatal and infant risk groups for SIDS (Schechtman et al., 1995), apnea (Schramm et al., 2000), hyperbilirubinemia (Gurses et al., 2002), white matter necrosis (Inder et al., 2003), and asphyxia (Hellström-Westas, 1992) applying power analyses to one particular physiological behavior, with little attention to the multiple neuronal networks that contemporaneously express state transitions. Single-channel monitoring devices have demonstrated that important maturational trends can be documented using standard spectral values (Burdjalov et al., 2003) without regional or hemispheric specificity.

Few reports have combined cerebral and noncerebral measures to more comprehensively study newborn sleep states (Pan and Ogawa, 1999; Regalado et al., 2001). One research group has applied automated analysis methods of neonatal sleep to both cerebral and noncerebral measures, combining computations to detect and quantify both stationary and nonstationary signal behaviors. Simultaneous assessment of multiple cerebral and noncerebral measures is emphasized to define neonatal state (Scher et al., 1992). Spectral analyses of EEG (Scher et al., 1994h,i, 1995b, 1996, 2003b), cardiorespiratory behavior (Scher et al., 1994g), temperature (Scher et al., 1994e, 2003a), arousal behavior (Scher et al., 1992, 1995b, 2003d), and REMs (Scher, 1992, 2003b; Scher et al., 1996), establish that there are important physiological differences during sleep between healthy preterm and full-term cohorts. Nonlinear computations for feature extraction of EEG signals (Turnbull et al., 2001), arousals (Scher et al., 2003d), and state/outcome prediction (Turnbull et al., 2001) have also been suggested as a part of the overall strategy to develop an automated neonatal state detector.

Differences in the functional brain organization between neonatal cohorts have been incorporated into a statistical model that offers a mathematical paradigm to define physiological brain dysmaturity of preterm neonates at corrected full-term ages. This dysmaturity index is based on seven selected physiological measures (Scher 1997a-c; Scher et al., 2003b-d) that best represent differences in functional brain organization and maturation between healthy preterm and full-term cohorts. This statistical model characterizes any particular physiological behavior of the preterm infant as either delayed or accelerated in relation to full-term controls. Automated methodologies that can capture these selected behaviors over time offer an opportunity to characterize the process of developmental neuroplasticity within the immature brain of a neonate who has been stressed by environmental or disease conditions.

Advances in developmental neuroscience over the last 15 years have expanded our knowledge base regarding the sequential steps in brain maturation. The later developmental stages of this complicated process of maturation encompass remodeling or resculpting of the brain, sometimes termed plasticity or activity-dependent development, which include signaling processes within neuronal cells and networks. Use or disuse of specific neuronal populations or networks will lead to pruning and remodeling of the brain's neuronal circuitry. Apoptosis or programmed cell death also contributes to modifying brain structure or function, during both prenatal and postnatal periods (Bredesen, 1995; Hughes et al., 1999). During the last trimester of pregnancy and into the first year of life, dendritic arborization, synaptogenesis, myelinization, and neurotransmitter development rapidly evolve in the immature brain (Goldman-Rakic, 1987), during which adverse conditions of prematurity (i.e., both prenatal and postnatal time periods), medical illnesses, and environmental stresses collectively alter the process of activity-dependent development and apoptosis on specific neuronal circuitry. Given that remodeling of neuronal connectivity is ultimately required for the expression of complex neurobehaviors including cognitive abilities at older ages (Caviness, 1989), aberrant remodeling will alternatively be expressed as neurocognitive and neurobehavioral deficits.

Automated neurophysiological methodologies can assess brain organization and maturation in the newborn, offering a surrogate marker for activity-dependent development of the fetal and neonatal brain. Computational algorithms applied to selected physiological measures of neonatal sleep can provide insights into the process by which neuronal networks change and adapt over longer periods of time during extrauterine life under adverse medical and socioeconomic conditions, and in the context of genetic endowment. Applications and methods of nonlinear dynamics to experiments in neurobiology will help better characterize the biological process of neuroplasticity (Abarbanel and Rabinovich, 2001). Computational analyses of complex stimuli that reflect changes in neuronal circuitry can enhance our understanding of the encoding and transmission of information by neuronal networks that subserve complex functions that range from sleep to cognitive performance. The application of these processing techniques to the neonatal intensive care setting will permit better assessment of EEG-sleep state organization and maturation, and transform neonatal intensive care units into neurointensive care facilities.

Summary of Normal Neonatal EEG Sleep

Neonatal electroencephalography can accurately document the ontogeny of both regional and hemispheric electrographic patterns by visual analyses of paper records, as well as ultradian EEG-sleep rhythms by automated analyses of digitized records. Such patterns can serve as templates for normal extrauterine brain development. Furthermore, comparisons with physiological profiles of fetal state behavior obtained by abdominal sonographic studies can follow intrauterine brain maturation. Such strategies will ultimately improve our diagnostic skills for the successful care of the high-risk fetus as well as the neonate.

Electroencephalography remains the *only* bedside neurodiagnostic procedure that provides a continuous record of cerebral function over long periods of time. While other advanced methods of anatomical or functional inquiry provide detailed, but brief, snapshots of cerebral physiology, EEG provides the important aspect of its evolution and structure in time (Gloor, 1985). Knowledge of the temporal dimensions of developmental changes or pathological processes is essential to acquire an understanding of both the significance of normal ontogeny as well as deviations from

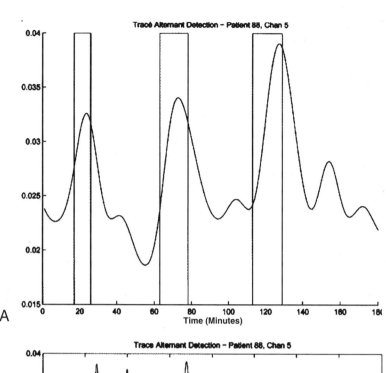

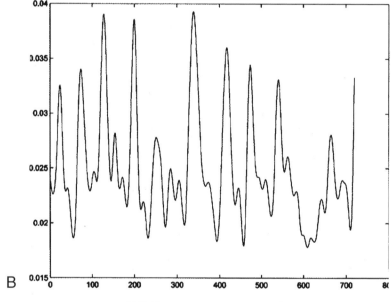

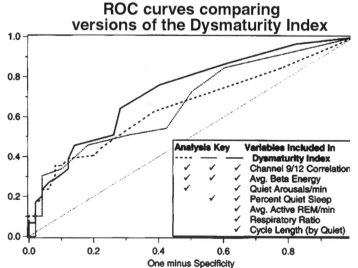

Figure 49.17. **A:** Discrete wavelet-transform calculation after smoothing showing periods of tracé alternant represented by boxed areas. **B:** Multiple-hour sleep study indicating the presence of tracé alternant quiet sleep with intervals that approximate the ultradian sleep cycle of the full-term newborn. **C:** Sleep study: receiver-operator characteristic curves for the dysmaturity index (DI) demonstrating a greater area under the curve when seven vs. three sleep behaviors were compared between neonatal cohorts. Note the y axis represents the preterm cohort while the x axis represents fullterm infants. (From Turnbull JP, Loparo KA, Johnson MW, and Scher MS. 2001. Automated detection of tracé alternant during sleep in healthy full term neonates using discrete wavelet transform. Clin Neurophysiol 112:1893–1900, with permission.)

these biologically programmed processes in pathological conditions. Correlations with sophisticated MRI volumetric analyses (Huppi et al., 1998) will compare functional and anatomical ontogenies.

Abnormal Neonatal Electroencephalography/Polysomnography

Abnormal Neonatal EEG-Sleep Features

The neurophysiologist's interpretive abilities concerning abnormal neonatal EEG/polysomnographic patterns can assist in the neurological care of the sick neonate. As discussed in the section on normal neonatal EEG sleep, several guidelines help frame the overall advantages and limitations of such a laboratory tool for diagnostic and prognostic purposes (Table 49.3).

Single EEG recordings obtained randomly during the acute or convalescent neonatal periods may be helpful, but are less advantageous than serial recordings (Hrachovy et al., 1990; Lombroso, 1985; Scher and Barmada, 1987; Tharp, 1981; Westmoreland et al., 1986). Multiple recordings at appropriate intervals during the neonatal period offer a wealth of information concerning neurophysiological maturation and integrity. The resolution or persistence of abnormal patterns have important prognostic implications.

Even with this ability to follow the progression of an encephalopathy with serial recordings, newborns may have had the onset of an encephalopathic process prior to birth (Scher, 1994, 2001). EEG abnormalities, seen shortly after birth, reflect antepartum and/or intrapartum insults to the CNS. Current methods of fetal surveillance (i.e., abnormal fetal heart rate tracings, placental abnormalities, antepartum fetal ultrasound findings, etc.) may suggest intrapartum and/or antepartum difficulties that must be integrated into the clinical correlation of EEG findings.

Abnormal EEG-sleep patterns in the neonate are rarely pathognomonic, and a specific diagnosis is infrequently associated with particular pattern. Diverse etiologies can contribute to the encephalopathic state. Every attempt should be made to incorporate pertinent clinical correlations into the interpretive section of the EEG report, uniting all known clinical and laboratory facts together with the electrographic interpretation. However, it is not necessarily the goal of the clinical neurophysiologist to offer specific diagnoses based on only electrographic interpretations. Rather, EEG studies complement clinical and imaging evaluations to broaden one's diagnostic and prognostic profile of the high-risk infant.

It has been widely observed that even severe EEG pattern abnormalities rapidly disappear over time. This normalization of EEG disturbances occurs even in infants who suffer severe neurological sequelae (Lombroso, 1985; Tharp, 1981). It is advisable, therefore, to obtain serial studies beginning early during the acute phase of an illness and systematically repeat studies daily or weekly depending on clinical priorities with respect to the management of the infant (Pezzani et al., 1986; Pressler et al., 2001). EEG studies initially obtained late in the convalescent period prior to discharge are less effective; severe abnormalities may have completely or partially resolved.

Assessment of Neonatal Encephalopathies: Diagnostic and Prognostic Goals

Determination of the sick neonate's level of consciousness is an enormously difficult task. The clinical repertoire of the neonate is largely limited to the infant's level of arousal, muscle tone, and postural reflexes. There are also the practical limitations to performing the neonatal examination because of the NICU setting. The neonate, particularly the preterm infant, may be confined to an isolette environment. The newborn infant may be intubated with multiple catheters and require paralytic agents for ventilatory control.

All of these factors can seriously disrupt the efficient assessment of the neonate's level and content of arousal. Consequently, the dearth of clinical findings and the hostile NICU environment limit the clinician's ability to assess the level and stability of neurological state in the sick neonate. Such restrictions, therefore, emphasize the important role of neurophysiological studies for the assessment of an encephalopathic process.

Many varied medical situations contribute to the encephalopathic state of the sick neonate on a hemispheric, regional, diffuse, or multifocal basis. It is not uncommon to have multiple events contribute to the expression of an encephalopathic state. For example, metabolic derangements give more diffuse EEG disturbances, while cerebrovascular accidents express more focal abnormalities. These conditions can, in fact, be present concurrently. Comparisons of serial recordings, therefore, may emphasize a variety of different abnormalities depending on both the time of the recording and the predominant encephalopathic process that is electrographically expressed.

Electroencephalographic disturbances are generally graded as mild, moderate, or marked. Unfortunately, interpretations may vary from laboratory to laboratory, particularly with respect to the grading of mild or moderate abnormalities based on visual analyses (Tharp, 1989). Quantitative measurements of regional and hemispheric activities by computer techniques will improve one's ability to assign a more reliable threshold for degrees of abnormality concerning specific physiological measures. Nonetheless, general categories of abnormalities are listed below that can assist in the assessment of preterm and full-term neonates. Table 49.4 lists the major EEG abnormalities that are used as reference points for the neurophysiologist with respect to the severity of an encephalopathy.

Classification of Background EEG Abnormalities in Term Infants

Discussions have highlighted the variety of background disturbances that can be seen in term infants (Holmes, 1989; Hrachovy et al., 1990; Lombroso, 1985). Attempts at grading these abnormalities are also included. Although preterm infants may have similar abnormalities, they will be discussed separately. A discussion of neonatal seizures concludes this chapter.

Table 49.4. Major EEG Abnormalities

	Near term and full term[a] (36–41+ weeks)	Preterm (30–36 weeks)
Inactive[c]	X	X
Burst suppression	X	X
Slow[b]	X	X
Low voltage[e]	X	
Monorhythmic	X	
No spatial/temporal organization	X	
Asymmetry	X	X (>50%)
Interhemispheric asynchrony	X	X
Abnormal superimposed patterns	X	X
Focal spikes	X	X
Seizures	X	X

[a] Monod N, Pajor N, and Guidasci S. 1972. The neonatal EEG: statistical studies and prognostic value in full-term and preterm babies. Electroencephalogr Clin Neurophysiol 32:529.

[b] Tharp BR, Cukier F, and Monod N. 1981. The prognostic value of the electroencephalogram in premature infants. Electroencephalogr Clin Neurophysiol 51:219.

[c] Below 5 µV or isoelectric.

[d] 0.5–1 Hz.

[e] Maximal 25 µV.

From Scher MS, Painter MJ, and Guthrie RD. 1988. Cerebral neurophysiological assessment of the high-risk neonate. In *Recent Advances in Neonatal Care,* ed. RD Guthrie, in the series, *Clinics in Critical Care Medicine.* New York: Churchill Livingstone, with permission.

Markedly Abnormalities in Term Infants

Electrocerebral Inactivity (Isoelectric Recording)

Cerebral activity below 5 µV despite high sensitivity settings and long interelectrode distances may be noted on neonatal recordings. The lack of reactivity to sensory stimulation usually accompanies this severe degree of abnormality. Minimal amplitude criteria (i.e., <5 µV) have been used by several authors (Holmes et al., 1982; Lombroso, 1985; Monod et al., 1972; Rose and Lombroso, 1970), while others have required the total absence of all cerebral electrical activity (Aso et al., 1989). Once the possibilities of a postictal situation, hypothermia, or a reversible metabolic-toxic disorder can be eliminated, this abnormal pattern carries grave prognostic implications (Lombroso, 1985). Most infants either die or have severe neurological sequelae (Aso et al., 1989; Barabas et al., 1993; Holmes et al., 1982; Monod et al., 1972;

O'Brien et al., 1987; Rose and Lombroso, 1970). These studies indicate that an isoelectric record noted during the early neonatal course is associated with high mortality in a high percentage of patients. In one study, 17 of 19 patients (89%) died (Pezzani et al., 1986), with only one survivor being developmentally normal at 6 years of age, while two others had seizures and developmental delay. Another study involving both preterm and full-term infants with isoelectric records showed a survival rate of 15% (2/20) with only one normal survivor at 5 years of age (Barabas et al., 1993).

A neuropathological study from the same laboratory (Aso et al., 1989) found that infants with isoelectric records who died had widespread encephalomalacia and ischemic neuronal necrosis. In this study, ten different anatomical sites were systematically studied in six neonates who had an isoelectric EEG (Table 49.5). The cerebral cortex, corpus callosum, thalamus, midbrain, and pons were moderate to markedly affected in all of these cases. Other locations such as the white matter, cerebellum, hypothalamus, and medulla were also damaged. These sites, however, were spared in a least one infant who initially had an isoelectric record with qualitative improvement on a subsequent recording.

A variety of clinical situations ranging from massive intracranial hemorrhage and asphyxia to fulminant meningitis may all be expressed as an inactive or isoelectric EEG. Even major CNS malformations such as hydranencephaly, as well as severe inborn errors of metabolism disorders such as nonketotic hyperglycinemia, may result in such an abnormal recording. These conditions resemble the experimentally induced asphyxial insults that result in isoelectric EEG tracings. This is followed by the reemergence of seizures and other abnormal background activities (Volpe, 2001).

Barabas et al. (1993) reported that 15 of 20 infants had at least one isoelectric record during the first several days of life, with clinical evidence of partially preserved brain function (Figs. 49.18 to 49.21). These infants, therefore, could not satisfy the criteria of brain death. Most infants in this group had demonstrable brain insults that occurred at times prior to labor and delivery. Seven of 20 had evidence of only antepartum brain injury; timing of the insult was based on obstetrical (i.e., loss of fetal movements), placental/cord pathology (meconium-laden macrophages, small placental weight), and/or clinical findings [i.e., intrauterine growth retardation (IUGR), joint contractures]. All but three infants died in the immediate neonatal period, with only one of the

Table 49.5. Neuropathological Findings in Patients with Isoelectric Tracings

Case #	GA (weeks)	CE	HERN	Auto	INN	PVL	PSN	CI	PVH-IV H	NDS
S1	24	+	−	−	+	−	+	−	III	5
S4	26	+	−	−	+	−	−	−	IV	9
S6	31	−	−	−	+	+	+	−	IV	10
S8	38	+	+	−	+	+	+	+	−	9
S10	39	+	+	+	+	−	−	+	−	9
S11	40	+	−	−	+	+	−	−	−	9

CE, cerebral edema; HERN, herniation; Auto = autolysis; INN, ischemic neuronal necrosis; PVL, periventricular leukomalacia; PSN, pontosubicular necrosis; CI, cerebral infarction; PVH-IVH, periventricular-intraventricular hemorrhage; NDS, numbers of damages structure; +, damage present; − damage absent.

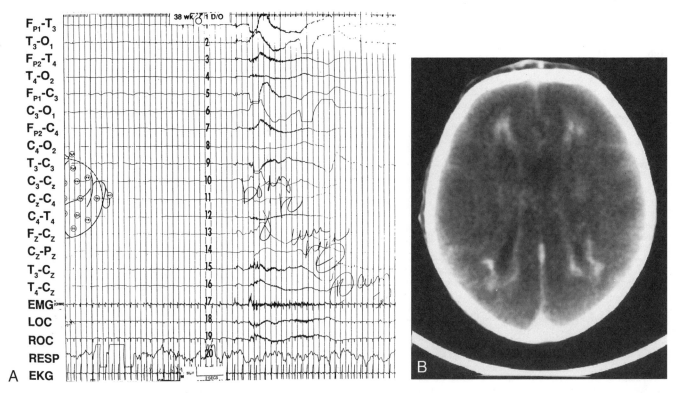

Figure 49.18. **A:** An EEG recording of a 38-week, 1-day-old male infant with nonimmune hydrops fetalis. The patient demonstrated an isoelectric EEG tracing in the context of a partially preserved neurological examination. C_3 artifact from respiratory movements is noted. Prominent whole-body jerks with head turning and arm stiffening were also noted, suggestive of seizures. Partially intact neurological function was documented by clini-cal examination. However, no electrographic seizure correlate was noted on coincident EEG recordings, as depicted in this example. **B:** Computed tomography (CT) scan for patient in **A** documenting significant cortical hypodensities and prominent periventricular enhancement. Postmortem examination revealed widespread cavitation and calcification.

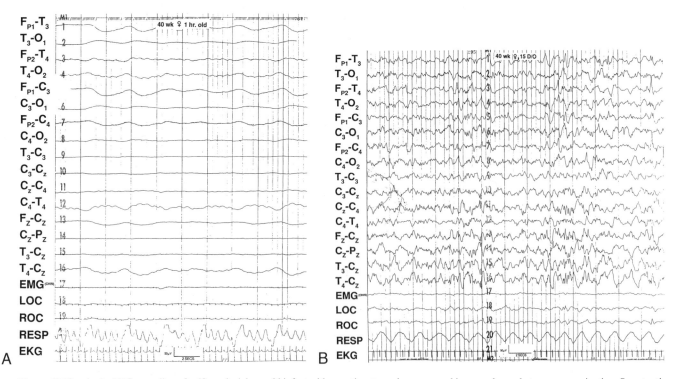

Figure 49.19. **A:** An EEG recording of a 40-week, 1-hour-old infant with a history of a severe abruptio placenta and velamentous insertion of the umbilical cord. Sudden exsanguination and cardiac arrest after delivery necessitated cardiopulmonary resuscitation. An EEG was obtained within 30 minutes of life, indicating an isoelectric background in the context of agita-tion, tremulousness, and increased muscle tone on examination. Sweat artifact is noted on multiple channels. **B:** Follow-up record for the same patient at 15 days of age showing a well-developed quiet sleep segment. Subsequently, the patient developed spasticity of the lower extremities, which resolved by 2 years of age. She is functionally normal at 6 years of age.

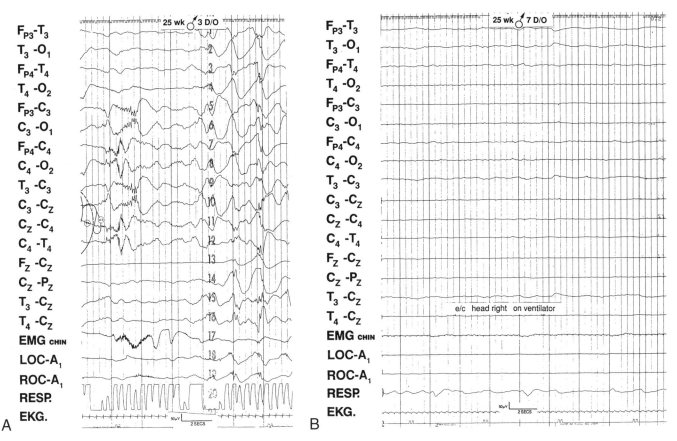

Figure 49.20. **A:** A portion of an EEG tracing for a 25-week, 3-day-old male infant demonstrating an age-appropriate tracé discontinu background activity. **B:** Following a severe hypotensive episode secondary to disseminated intravascular coagulation, a repeat record demonstrated an isoelectric background. Same calibration as **A**. Note respiratory excursions producing artifact. The patient later expired. Permission for postmortem examination was denied.

survivors being developmentally normal. Clearly, antepartum insults may result in an isoelectric EEG pattern rather than an emergent insult during labor and delivery. The presence of brain function on examination puts into question the legitimacy of using an isoelectric EEG to help define brain death in the immediate neonatal period for both preterm and full-term infants.

Paroxysmal or Suppression-Burst Pattern

The original descriptive term *paroxysmal background disturbance* was used by French neonatal neurophysiologists (Monod et al., 1972), while the same pattern is now more commonly identified as *burst suppression* (Werner et al., 1977). The gestational age of the infant must be known before describing this abnormality, since the preterm infant commonly expresses discontinuous electrographic tracing (Figs. 49.22 and 49.23). Earlier descriptions of the suppression burst pattern consisted of a nonreactive discontinuous tracing, with long periods of quiescence >20 seconds in duration (Monod et al., 1972; Werner et al., 1977) interrupted by synchronous or asynchronous bursts of poorly organized background activity. Modified forms of this pattern have also been more recently described that are composed of more organized bursts of background activity with shorter

quiescent periods; such modified forms of suppression burst patterns may in part be due to more aggressively managed clinical situations, such as metabolic-toxic encephalopathies that are potentially reversible (i.e., drug intoxication). These abnormal patterns should be distinguished from the discontinuous quiet sleep segment (i.e., tracé alternant) during which reactivity to stimuli and rich mixtures of frequencies appear.

The paroxysmal or suppression burst pattern has been traditionally associated with poor prognosis (Aso et al., 1989; Holmes et al., 1982; Monod et al., 1972; Pezzani et al., 1986; Rose and Lombroso, 1970). Pezzani et al. (1986) found that four of six full-term infants with this pattern died while the survivors had severe neurological sequelae. Aso et al. (1989) found that of seven infants with suppression burst patterns, five had neuronal necrosis, four had periventricular hemorrhage-intraventricular hemorrhage (PVH-IVH), three had periventricular leukomalacia (PVL), three had cerebral infarction, and two had pontosubicular necrosis. This neuropathological study emphasizes the diverse types of severe deficits that can be seen with suppression burst activity.

Modified forms of the suppression burst pattern have been described (Holmes, 1989; Holmes et al., 1982). These patients tend to have a pattern that changes with stimulation.

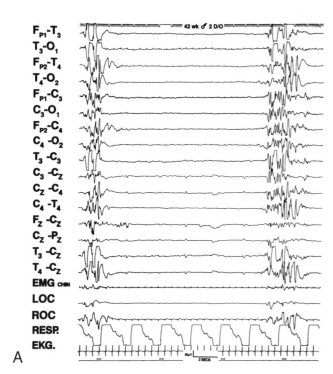

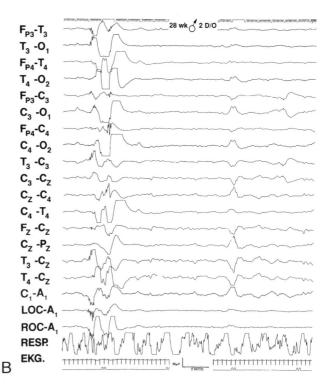

Figure 49.21.   A: A 42-week, 2-day-old male infant with a suppression-burst pattern on an EEG recording that did not react to sensory stimulation. Note the low-amplitude sharp-wave morphology from respiratory excursion at the midline electrode. (From Scher MS. 1994. Pediatric electroencephalography and evoked potentials. In *Pediatric Neurology, Principles* *and Practice,* vol. 1, ed. KF Swaiman. St. Louis: Mosby Year-Book, with permission.) **B:** An age-appropriate tracé discontinu pattern for a 28-week, 2-day-old male as compared with the invariant suppression-burst pattern noted in **A.**

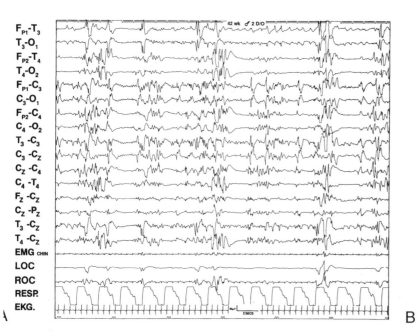

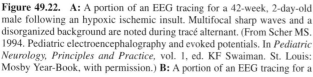

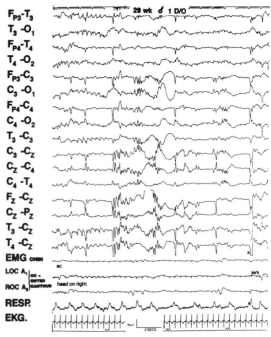

Figure 49.22.   A: A portion of an EEG tracing for a 42-week, 2-day-old male following an hypoxic ischemic insult. Multifocal sharp waves and a disorganized background are noted during tracé alternant. (From Scher MS. 1994. Pediatric electroencephalography and evoked potentials. In *Pediatric Neurology, Principles and Practice,* vol. 1, ed. KF Swaiman. St. Louis: Mosby Year-Book, with permission.) **B:** A portion of an EEG tracing for a 29-week, 1-day-old male twin following twin-to-twin transfusion. The patient was clinically hypotonic and less responsive. Prominent vertex and frontal sharp waves were noted. The patient had a CT scan showing white matter hypodensities. Follow-up examination was within normal limits at 3 years of age.

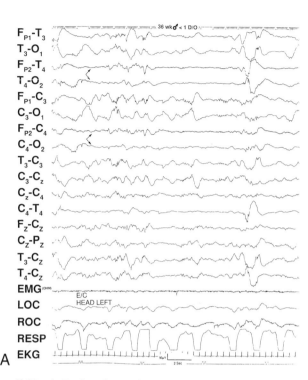

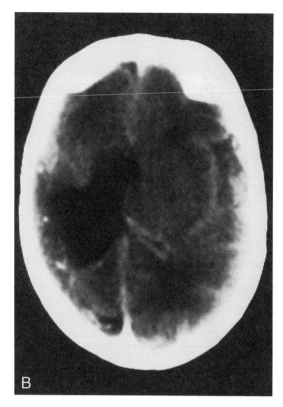

Figure 49.23. **A:** Portion of an EEG recording of a 36-week, 1-day-old male with congenital porencephaly. Note the attenuation in the right hemisphere both above and below the sylvian fissure *(twin arrow marks).* **B:** CT scan obtained on the patient in **A** showing a porencephaly in the right hemisphere following the distribution of the right middle cerebral artery.

Five infants had discontinuous tracings consistent with suppression burst that became a continuous pattern with tactile stimulation. Although none of the infants were normal at follow-up, only one had severe deficits.

Hypsarrhythmia

The hypsarrhythmic pattern associated with infantile spasms usually appears after at least 3 to 4 months of age (Watanabe et al., 1982). Although rarely noted during the neonatal period, it can be observed in children of <44 weeks' CA. Asynchronous bursts of high-amplitude slow activity mixed with multifocal spikes and sharp waves have been described. Periods of suppression that vary in duration may be generalized or lateralized. Generalized myoclonic movements may appear during periods of attenuation. One report differentiated neonatal hypsarrhythmia from burst suppression by the appearance of high-amplitude activity exceeding 1,000 μV (Ohtahara, 1978), and suggested a syndrome of infantile spasms and suppression burst activity in the EEG of the neonate, which differs from those in older patients termed "early infantile epileptic encephalopathy." Other authors described a similar syndrome called "neonatal myoclonic encephalopathy" beginning during the first weeks of life. Such patients have fragmentary myoclonus associated with a variety of seizures other than infantile spasms with a burst-suppression pattern on the EEG. This pattern is expressed with infants with either brain malformations or inborn errors of metabolism.

Spikes and Sharp Waves

In most situations, the electroencephalographer will have difficulty assigning clinical significance to sporadic epileptiform features on recordings of the preterm or full-term neonate. Such features have already been discussed in the section on normal neonatal EEG and can be seen in asymptomatic, apparently healthy infants. However, as outlined in Table 49.6, several features can help distinguish normal from abnormal spike and sharp-wave discharges. Epileptiform discharges that are frequent and multifocal, or persistently occur in every state, may have pathological significance. Several authors (Rowe et al., 1985; Werner et al., 1977) have suggested that more than five spike or sharp-wave discharges per hour may suggest an abnormality (Fig. 49.22A). Other features such as positive sharp waves, periodic discharges, and midline discharges commonly reflect CNS insults. These will be discussed below under preterm EEG abnormalities.

Spike and sharp-wave discharges have been described in specific neonatal populations that were identified based on serious medical disorders, principally seizures. Hughes et al. (1983a,b) described spike and sharp-wave discharges in 236 neonates whose CA ranged from 24 to 48 weeks. Fifty-five percent had recordings because of the clinical suspicion of neonatal seizures. Sporadic sharp waves, more frequent in the right hemisphere, were principally in the centrotemporal region in 85% of the total population (Fig. 49.22B). An ad-

Table 49.6. Physiological versus Pathological Significance of Neonatal Sharp Transients

Physiological
Regional patterns of maturation
    Delta brushes
    Occipital theta bursts
    Temporal theta bursts
    Positive temporal bursts
    Frontal sharp transients
Spike and sharp waves
    Sporadic, multifocal, nonrepetitive
    Frequency < 5 hours*
Most frequent during quiet sleep (QS)
    Multifocal during bursts of tracé alternant (TA)
    Least frequent during low-voltage regular (LVI) pattern

Pathological
Altered patterns of maturation
    Increased incidence
    Asymmetric presentation
        Altered morphology
        Spikes and sharp waves
        Frequent multifocal in any state (>5 hours)*
    Positive sharp waves
        Parasagittal
        Rolandic
        Periodic discharges

* Data from Rowe et al., 1985.

ditional 15% had either positive sharp waves or repetitive discharges. Unfortunately, coincident EEG seizures were not documented; no control group in which epileptiform discharges were tabulated was included, nor was follow-up reported for this population.

Rowe et al. (1985) documented sharp wave discharges in 51% of 74 neonates (30–40 weeks' CA) with clinical seizures. Follow-up data was available to 33 months of age. Sharp waves were predictive of neurodevelopmental outcome when considered independently. However, the authors stressed that EEG background abnormalities were more predictive of neurodevelopmental outcome than were epileptiform features.

Spike discharges rarely occur in neonates at any gestational age, while sharp-wave discharges are frequently noted in frontopolar, right temporal, and left central regions. Sharp waves in occipital or midline locations are rarely seen in otherwise healthy neonates and may have greater clinical significance (Scher et al., 1994c).

Low-Amplitude Recording

This electrographic pattern is characterized by background frequencies that are of 5 to 15 µV in amplitude during the wakeful state and 10 to 25 µV during the sleep states (Lombroso, 1985; Monod et al., 1972). Although differences in amplitude between sleep states may be seen, most records have a low-amplitude background with no state differentiation. One must distinguish pattern from the cyclic ultradian neonatal EEG-sleep rhythm during which the low-voltage irregular active sleep background is seen for approximately 10% to 15% of the cycle.

This background abnormality has grave prognostic significance (Holmes et al., 1982; Monod et al., 1972; Rose and

Lombroso, 1970), particularly if it persists beyond the first week of life (Lombroso, 1985). At times, this low-amplitude recording may have intermixed monotonous nonreactive theta activity (Monod et al., 1972; Tharp et al., 1981).

One should be alert to a variety of situations that can result in low-amplitude records. Postictal records following seizures, barbiturate administration, and hypothermia are examples of situations that can also result in an inactive record. Ample recording times should help distinguish clinically significant records from nonpathological situations.

Excessive Discontinuity

Although excessive discontinuity implies that such a pattern is neither isoelectric, inactive, nor suppression burst, this background abnormality may still represent a significant encephalopathy. Permanently discontinuous activity has been described (Biagioni et al., 1999; Pezzani et al., 1986; Selton and André, 1997), consisting of short bursts. This is contrasted by Aso et al. (1989), who defined an interburst interval to be 60 seconds or greater. Pezzani et al. (1986) found no children with this background pattern survived without sequelae, and five of eight of these children expired. These authors went on to describe additional abnormalities superimposed on the permanent discontinuous background, such as sharp waves in the frontal and central regions, as well as frontally predominant slow activity. Selton and André (1997) and Biagioni et al. (1999) reported similar results. These authors claimed that the longer the interburst interval, the more compromised the neurological outcome. No child escaped major sequelae when interburst intervals were longer than 40 seconds. Fourteen of 15 children (93%) with permanently discontinuous background and absent normal physiological patterns either expired or had severe sequelae.

Diffusely Slow Background

A diffusely slow pattern composed of delta activity during either wakefulness or sleep, with little activity in the theta range, has been described by several authors (Holmes et al., 1982; Lombroso, 1985; Monod et al., 1972; Rose and Lombroso, 1970). Invariant and diffusely distributed delta rhythms are noted acutely during the first week of life, but can be seen during the convalescent period several weeks after birth. These patterns were initially described in studies that predated the establishment of the modern NICU (Monod and Garma, 1971); other authors (Holmes, 1989; Lombroso, 1985) have claimed that this pattern is uncommon.

Hemispheric Amplitude Asymmetry

Hemispheric amplitude asymmetry, defined as >50% difference in amplitude and/or frequencies in each hemisphere, has been described with neuropathological correlates (Aso et al., 1989, 1990; Scher and Tharp, 1982). This pattern can be seen with lateralized pathology. Four infants had cerebral lesions that were either hemorrhagic or ischemic in nature, with attenuated amplitude over the more pathologically involved hemisphere (Fig. 49.23). Congenital lesions such as porencephaly may also contribute to hemispheric attenuation of background amplitudes. As previously emphasized in

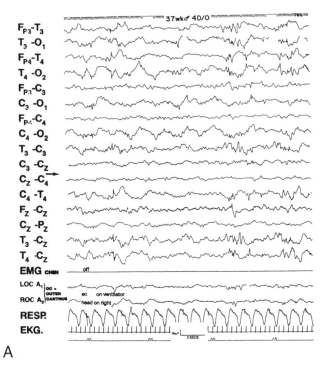

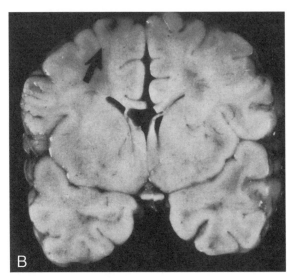

A

B

Figure 49.24. **A:** Portion of an EEG tracing for a 37-week, 4-day-old male with vertex attenuation *(arrow)*. Multifocal sharp waves are also noted at T_4 and 0. The patient had persistent pulmonary hypertension of the newborn and subsequently expired. **B:** A brain section of the patient de-scribed in **A** showing multifocal infarctions. The *arrow* indicates one such infarction in the parasagittal region of the right hemisphere, corresponding with the attenuation noted on the EEG described in **A**.

the chapter on normal neonatal EEG features, notation of cephalhematomas, scalp edema, or technical conditions such as head positioning, electrode paste smearing, sweat, or asymmetric electrode placement must be documented. With any technical questions concerning these EEG asymmetries, follow-up records are strongly recommended.

It should also be stressed that asymmetries may accompany seizure phenomena with transient suppression of activity in areas where an ictal pattern was recently documented. While an asymmetry usually implies that the pathology exists on the more attenuated regions, conversion of focal background attenuation to slowing has also been described (Scher and Tharp, 1982). Finally, transient asymmetries have been described in asymptomatic previously healthy neonates (Challamel et al., 1984; O'Brien et al., 1987) and may be noted during the first several minutes of quiet sleep in the absence of structural lesions.

Focal Attenuation

There are records that are persistently attenuated over only one scalp region without involvement of the entire hemisphere (Fig. 49.24). Such focal attenuation is commonly associated with focal or lateralized neuropathological lesions. Aso et al. (1989) found that five infants with at least one EEG with a focal attenuation were noted to have neuropathological lesions. Three of these patients had extensive lesions that were unilateral to the attenuation, and one infant showed more severe white matter infarction in the opposite hemisphere. An additional infant showed no pathological

changes that could be correlated with the attenuation of the EEG. Conversely, these authors described unilateral lesions on postmortem examination involving either necrosis or hemorrhage in the cortex or white matter with the absence of a demonstrable EEG attenuation. The accuracy of detecting a morphological lesion was estimated to be 74% with a specificity of 85%.

Interhemispheric Asynchrony

Asynchrony has been arbitrarily described as morphologically similar bursts that are temporally separated by more than 1.5 seconds. Some authors claim the infant's postconceptional age helps predict the degree of asynchrony; this has been recently challenged. Asynchrony in the term infant is considered abnormal (Fig. 49.25); the neuropathological findings associated with patients with marked asynchrony include a study in which nine patients with excessive asynchrony were described (Aso et al., 1989); two patients with lesions within the corpus callosum expressed asynchrony. In general, white matter lesions and PVH-IVH were noted in infants with asynchrony compared to infants who did not manifest this abnormality. Normative values for interhemispheric asynchrony need to be more firmly established by multiple authors at successive gestational age ranges before assigning pathological significance.

Absent or Disrupted EEG State Cycling

Although it has been emphasized that a rudimentary sleep cycle in the preterm neonate is difficult to ascertain,

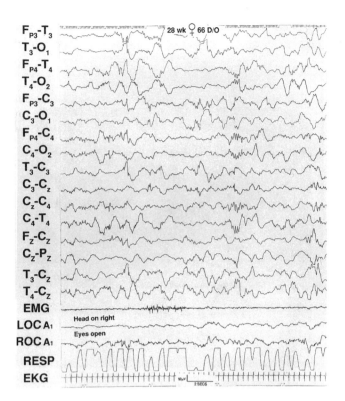

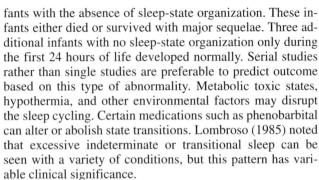

Figure 49.25. A 28-week, 66-day-old female who suffered a grade IV intraventricular hemorrhage. The patient had a normal neurological examination. This EEG tracing indicates a significant asynchrony with alternating attenuation in homologous temporal and central regions. The patient demonstrates a significant hemiparesis at 3 years of age.

fants with the absence of sleep-state organization. These infants either died or survived with major sequelae. Three additional infants with no sleep-state organization only during the first 24 hours of life developed normally. Serial studies rather than single studies are preferable to predict outcome based on this type of abnormality. Metabolic toxic states, hypothermia, and other environmental factors may disrupt the sleep cycling. Certain medications such as phenobarbital can alter or abolish state transitions. Lombroso (1985) noted that excessive indeterminate or transitional sleep can be seen with a variety of conditions, but this pattern has variable clinical significance.

Excessively labile EEG sleep states have also been described, with rapid transitions over seconds to minutes. This usually reflects transient forms of encephalopathy, but may also be associated with infants with more chronic problems such as with hypoplastic left heart syndrome (Olson et al., 1989), maternal substance use (Scher et al., 1988a), or maternal preeclampsia (Schulte et al., 1971). Normative values for sleep-state architecture include estimates of active sleep at 50% and quiet sleep at 30% to 35%. However, antepartum, intrapartum, or neonatal conditions may influence both sleep architecture and continuity measures.

Abnormalities of Maturational Development

As described previously, an experienced electroencephalographer should be able to determine postconceptional age within 2 weeks in the premature infant and within 1 week for the term infant. Disorders of electrographic maturation suggest cerebral insults during intrauterine life or the immediate neonatal period. Dysmaturity of more than 2 weeks of the stated postconceptional age of the infant defines an abnormality (Fig. 49.27). Dysmature patterns may be transient in infants who suffer severe but reversible hyaline membrane disease and have little prognostic significance (Holmes et al., 1979). However, persistently dysmature patterns based on either electrographic or sleep-state criteria are worrisome with respect to neurodevelopmental sequelae. For instance, dysmature patterns on the EEG have been noted in neonates with

state differentiation can be seen as early as 31 to 32 weeks' gestation. By postconceptional term ages, cyclicity between active and quiet sleep segments is expected. The absence or disruption of this cyclicity can be diagnostic of an encephalopathy with prognostic implications (Fig. 49.26).

Pezzani et al. (1986) found that EEGs obtained during the first 24 hours of life in 80 full-term infants included 24 in-

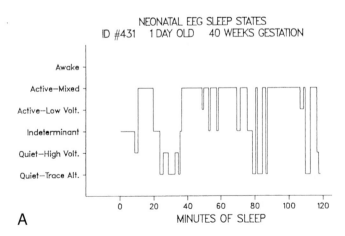

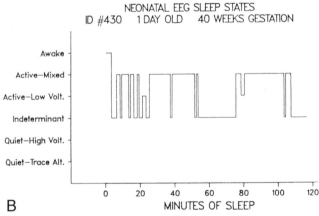

Figure 49.26. A: A histogram of a normal neonatal sleep cycle indicating the alteration between active and quiet sleep segments with intermixed transitional or indeterminate sleep periods. **B:** A histogram of an abnormal EEG cycle indicating no quiet sleep segments and excessively long transitional sleep periods. (From Scher MS. 1988. Neonatal EEG sleep cycling—a developmental marker of central nervous system maturation (part II). Pediatr Neurol 4:329–336, with permission.)

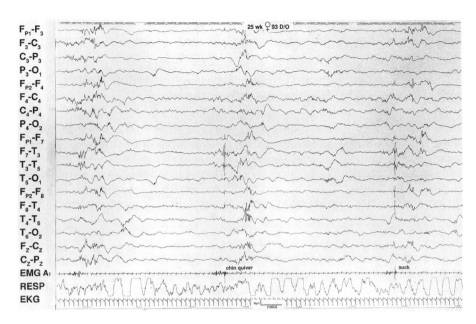

Figure 49.27. A portion of an EEG tracing of a 25-week, 93-day-old female with a dysmature EEG tracing during quiet sleep consisting of a lack of background, excessive delta brush patterns, and asynchrony for a corrected term age. The patient was abnormal at 3 years of age with delayed cognitive and motor development.

chronic lung disease who had compromised neurodevelopmental sequelae at 3 years of age (Tharp, 1989). One report suggested that a postnatal undernutritional condition was associated with electrographic dysmaturity (Hayakawa et al., 2003). Dysmature sleep-state organization has also been noted in neonates with chronic lung disease (Scher and Barmada, 1987) and asymptomatic preterm infants at postconceptional term ages (Scher et al., 1997c,d, 2003b).

Strict guidelines for assessing EEG maturation need to be developed. While normative values for certain patterns such as delta brush have been described, systematic investigations by multiple authors of other EEG waveforms such as occipital (Hughes et al., 1987) and temporal theta bursts (Scher et al., 1994d) are still needed. Computer analyses that can better quantitate regional and hemispheric power spectra at specific EEG frequencies may help establish more strict maturation criteria for frequency and amplitude. Normative data derived from both analog and digital analyses can then more easily assess for electrographic and polysomnographic dysmaturity (Scher et al., 1996).

Background Abnormalities in Preterm Infants

As illustrated in Table 49.2, electrographic abnormalities of the preterm infant have not been as widely studied as in term infants; certain abnormalities overlap with those of term infants. Most features, however, require that the neurophysiologist have knowledge of the expected electrographic and polygraphic features for a particular gestational age.

The most comprehensive study (Tharp et al., 1981) reviewed 181 serial EEGs performed during the neonatal period on 81 infants with an estimated gestational age of <36 weeks. Infants with normal serial EEGs during the neonatal period were usually normal or had minor sequelae. Children with at least one markedly abnormal record either expired or had significant neurodevelopmental dysfunction. Moderately abnormal records in this study were not as predictive. The authors classified severely abnormal records as having at least one of the following patterns: isoelectric backgrounds, positive rolandic sharp waves, electroencephalographic seizures, paroxysmal discharges on isoelectric background, excessive intrahemispheric asynchrony (i.e., >50% of the record), persistent hemispheric voltage amplitude asymmetries, and excessively slow background of variable amplitudes that was unreactive to stimulation. Moderately abnormal records were classified: generalized low-amplitude activity with normal background, low-amplitude background with permanent asymmetry that is <50% of the record, excessive asynchrony for the age, dysmaturity, and low-amplitude records with preservation of patterns appropriate for the infant's PCA.

Isoelectric Pattern

Based on criteria described in the section on term infants, few preterm infants with isoelectric records have been described. Tharp et al. (1981) described two infants, both of whom expressed this pattern. Barabas et al. (1993) described seven preterm infants with isoelectric records, all of whom expired or had major neurological sequelae (Fig. 49.20).

Suppression Burst or Paroxysmal Pattern

As previously described for term infants, bursts of high-amplitude chaotic delta activity with intermixed spike or faster rhythms on an isoelectric background with interburst intervals >20 seconds are described. Such a pattern may be difficult to classify in the preterm infant because of tracé discontinu, which commonly occurs at more immature gestational ages. If such activity is invariant, unresponsive to stimulation, and contained prolonged interburst intervals, such a pattern may be equivalent to the suppression burst patterns seen at older ages. Such a pattern was described by Tharp et al. (1981) in six infants and resulted in death or severe neurological sequelae in all patients.

Low-Amplitude Recording

Electrographic studies with background activity <20 μV, with occasional bursts of rhythmic activity or sharp-wave features have been classified as low amplitude. Such a pattern was considered severely or moderately abnormal, depending on the persistence of patterns compared with particular post-conceptional age. Tharp et al. (1981) found five infants with unreactive low-amplitude records consisting of delta activity. One child survived with only minor sequelae.

Slow Frequency Background

Background activity consisting of diffuse delta between 20 and 100 µV in amplitude with superimposed theta activity unreactive to sensory stimuli would fit this classification.

Age-appropriate discrete patterns such as delta brush and theta burst patterns would be diminished or absent during such recordings. As with term infants, this pattern is unusual in the preterm infant. Tharp et al. (1981) described two infants with this pattern, both of whom survived with major neurological sequelae.

Asymmetric Records

EEG studies were considered markedly abnormal with interhemispheric amplitude asymmetries exceeding 50% throughout the entire recording in all demonstrable EEG-sleep states. More regional or focal asymmetries were considered only moderately abnormal, with <50% difference in amplitude. Asymmetric patterns have been associated with a compromised neurological outcome. Tharp found that all nine infants with at least one record with a significant amplitude asymmetry either expired or had severe sequelae. Aso

et al. (1989) also found that hemispheric asymmetry was associated with significant brain pathology in all four preterm patients with this EEG abnormality.

Positive Sharp Waves in the Midline Central Regions and Other Regions

Waveforms between 50 and 150 µV that are surface positive lasting 100 to 250 msec are important abnormal features to identify on the preterm neonatal EEG record. Such discharges occur unilaterally or bilaterally in either the central or midline regions (Fig. 49.28). Waveform morphologies can be complex with surface negative components following the positive phase. Such patterns are seen singly or in brief runs. Historically, authors initially associated central sharp waves with IVH (Blume and Dreyfus-Brisac, 1982; Clancy and Tharp, 1984; Clancy et al., 1984; Cukier et al., 1972; Marret et al., 1986). However, this finding has also been associated with white matter necrosis in neonates with meningitis, hydrocephalus, aminoacidopathies, and asphyxia (Marret et al., 1997; Novotny, et al., 1987; Scher, 1988a-c).

Cukier et al. (1972) first suggested positive rolandic sharp waves (PRS) and the association with IVH. Blume and Dreyfus-Brisac (1982) described two types of PRS; the first type occurred singly, clearly differentiated from the background, while the second type was admixed with fast and slow background activity. Clancy and Tharp (1984) and Clancy et al. (1984) found central positive sharp waves in 13 of 22 infants with IVH on 30 EEG studies. Only one other

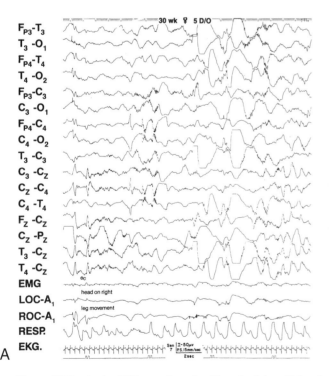

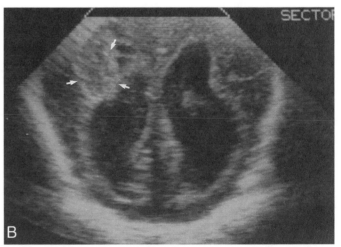

Figure 49.28. A: An EEG recording of a 30-week, 5-day-old female showing midline and rolandic positive sharp waves in the context of relatively preserved background rhythms during active sleep. **B:** A coronal view on cranial ultrasound demonstrating a grade IV intraventricular hemorrhage of the patient described in **A** *(arrowheads)*. (From Scher MS, Painter MJ, and Guthrie RD. 1988. Cerebral neurophysiological assessment of the high-risk neonate. In *Recent Advances in Neonatal Care,* ed. RD Guthrie, in the series *Clinics in Critical Care Medicine.* New York: Churchill Livingstone, with permission.)

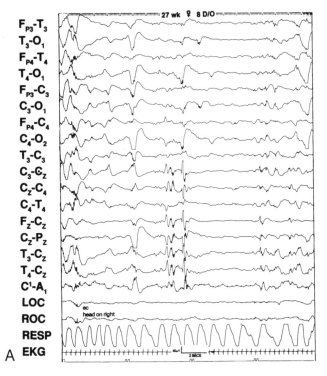

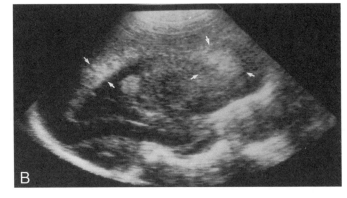

Figure 49.29. A: Portion of an EEG tracing of a 27-week, 8-day-old female with a prominent parasagittal positive sharp wave that is also recorded using an adjacent electrode close to the midline. **B:** A sagittal view on cranial ultrasound of the patient described in **A** documenting extensive periventricular echo densities in both the anterior and posterior regions. The patient had significant spastic quadriplegia on follow-up examination at 4 years of age. (From Scher MS, Painter MJ, and Guthrie RD. 1988. Cerebral neurophysiological assessment of the high-risk neonate. In *Recent Advances in Neonatal Care*, ed. RD Guthrie, in the series *Clinics in Critical Care Medicine*. New York: Churchill Livingstone, with permission.)

infant had positive rolandic sharp waves without IVH. The authors suggested, therefore, that PRS has a high specificity but low sensitivity. They later described 30 premature infants with multifocal white matter necrosis with and without IVH on ultrasound or autopsy with central positive sharp waves (Novotny et al., 1987). Infants with grade III to IV IVH had a higher prevalence (69.2%) for central positive sharp waves than the entire group of patients (31.8%), with the greatest prevalence occurring between the fifth and eighth postnatal day.

Scher (1988a–c) reported that positive sharp waves with a midline field of distribution were associated with a variety of pathological lesions including white matter necrosis (Fig. 49.29). Fourteen of 16 patients (88%; 25 records) with a mean gestational age had cerebral lesions, IVH in eight infants, PVL in five infants, and cerebral infarction in one infant. The amplitude of these discharges ranged from 20 to 180 μV with an anterior-posterior electrical field maximal at CZ extending from FZ to PZ. Myoclonic movements were sometimes associated with these discharges. Predominantly biphasic, but also triphasic and polyphasic, waveforms were noted. In patients with IVH, PRSs had a mean repetitive rate of 1.3/minute, with vertex positive sharp waves displaying a mean repetitive rate of 1.9/minute in patients. However, those patients with PVL displayed midline discharges with a mean repetitive rate of 2.5/minute. Seventy-six percent of records with positive vertex sharp waves were obtained on

infants who were older than 1 week. This feature was one of several midline electrographic abnormalities that frequently occurred in association with parasagittal cerebral lesions in the newborn. Midline electrographic abnormalities also have been noted in older patients (de la Paz and Brenner, 1981; Eble et al., 1981; Kennedy, 1959; Tukel and Jasper, 1952). In addition, midline discharges of positive or negative polarity can also occur coincident with myoclonus, suggesting the phenomenon of neonatal cortical myoclonus (Scher, 1985a–c). This may carry the same clinical significance as myoclonic phenomena noted in older patients (Halliday, 1967; Monod et al., 1960; Shibasaki et al., 1985).

More recent reports of neonates with PVL who were studied with EEG claimed good outcome predictions. These groups reported accurate prognostic information based on either the location of positive sharp waves in the frontal or occipital regions (Okumura et al., 2003) or the frequency of positive waves (Vermeulen et al., 2003).

Prolonged Quiescent Periods During Discontinuous Sleep in the Preterm Infant

This abnormality, sometimes seen with monorhythmic theta activity in the preterm infant, was described by Benda et al. (1989). Three subdivisions of interburst intervals of increasing duration in activity suggest a more unfavorable outcome. EEGs of 46 infants (25–35 weeks' CA) were reviewed and the interburst intervals were divided into groups of <20 seconds, 20 to 29 seconds, and those ≥30 seconds. Favorable outcome was seen with intervals that were <20 seconds, with a more unfavorable outcome in intervals ≥30 seconds. These findings support other reports that also describe interburst intervals for preterm infants. All investigators describe an expected interburst interval of <20 seconds in duration for the healthy asymptomatic neonate (see section on normal neonatal EEG, Table 49.3).

Periodic Discharges in Preterm and Fullterm Infants

Periodic EEG patterns are regularly recurrent generalized or focal/lateralized transient complexes, associated with various neurological disorders (Au et al., 1980; Bickford and Butt, 1968; Celesia, 1973; Chatrian et al., 1964; Cobb, 1979; de la Paz and Brenner, 1981; Kennedy, 1959; Kuroiwa and Celesia, 1980; Lesse et al., 1958; Markand and Daly, 1971; PeBenito and Cracco, 1979; Schwartz et al., 1973; Westmoreland et al., 1986). Generalized periodic EEG patterns have clinical significance primarily for degenerative disorders in older patients (Au et al., 1980; Celesia, 1973; Cobb, 1979). Generalized periodic patterns can also be seen with a variety of metabolic encephalopathies (Bickford and Butt, 1968; Radermecker, 1955; Schwartz et al., 1973).

Periodic lateralized epileptiform discharges (PLEDS) are usually associated with acute vascular, infectious, or traumatic lesions of the brain (Chatrian et al., 1964; Kennedy, 1959; Radermecker, 1955; Schwartz et al., 1973). While usually associated with acute structural brain lesions, PLEDS can also occur following seizures with or without structural lesions, as well as in patients with chronic encephalopathies (PeBenito and Cracco, 1979; Westmoreland et al., 1986).

Children with focal or lateralized periodic patterns have been reported, but descriptions are limited to chronic diffuse lesions of the brain in older children (PeBenito and Cracco, 1979), term neonates with hypoxic ischemic encephalopathy (McCutcheon et al., 1984), or preterm and term neonates with herpes encephalitis (Estivill et al., 1977; Mizrahi and Tharp, 1982; Sainio et al., 1983).

These discharges are stereotypic paroxysmal complexes separated by nearly identical intervals between individual recurrent complexes. Lateralized periodic discharges of at least 10 minutes in duration or 20% of the recording time are defined as PLEDS (Celesia, 1973; Chatrian et al., 1964). Scher et al. (1989) reviewed 1,114 recordings of 592 neonates and found focal periodic discharges in 57 (5%) of the recordings for 34 neonates, 26 preterm neonates, and eight term infants. PLEDS were noted in only four of these infants. Sixteen patients (47%) with focal periodic discharges also had electrographic seizures on the same or subsequent record. Stroke was the most common brain lesion (53%) in this neonatal population (Fig. 49.30). Preterm neonates had discharges that were <60 seconds in duration and located in the parasagittal regions, while discharges in term neonates were longer than a minute and located in the temporal re-

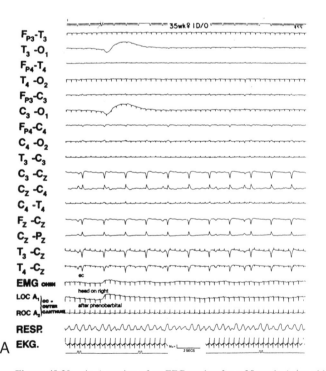

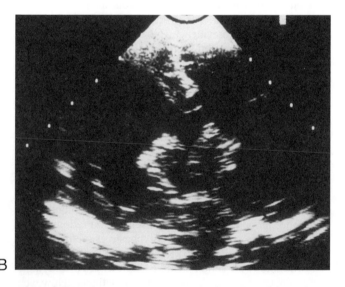

Figure 49.30. **A:** A portion of an EEG tracing for a 35-week, 1-day-old female with trisomy 13/15 demonstrating a periodic discharge in the midline. **B:** A coronal view of the cranial ultrasound for the patient described in **A** showing lobar holoprosencephaly. The patient expired with verification of this malformation on postmortem examination. (From Scher MS, and Beggarly M. 1989. Clinical significance of focal periodic patterns in the newborn. J Child Neurol 4:175–185, with permission.)

gions. Of the 34 neonates, 15 (44%) died and 58% (11/19) of these infants were abnormal with respect to neurological development. The authors suggest that focal periodic discharges in the neonate have the same clinical significance as PLEDS recorded on older children and adults. PLEDS are less common in the neonatal population with an incidence rate of 0.3%, which is below the reported range of 0.6% to 8.5% in older patients (Chatrian et al., 1964). While these discharges usually indicate a lesion in the neonatal brain, the neurological examination findings may or may not be helpful depending on the gestational maturity of the infant. While term infants with periodic discharges appear to have decreased levels of arousal or hypotonia in all cases, only 50% of preterm neonates demonstrated a neurological abnormality at the time the discharges were noted.

Other differences include the high percentage of seizures in term (80%) as compared with preterm infants (35%). Shewmon (1990) argued that periodic discharges may represent electrographic seizures with a markedly slower evolution that are not easily discernible on standard EEG recordings.

Acute hypoxic ischemic encephalopathy was the predominant etiology associated with periodic discharges in term infants. More varied etiologies were present in the preterm infants. While some authors (Estivill et al., 1977; McCutcheon et al., 1984; Mizrahi and Tharp, 1982; Sainio et al., 1983) have described periodic discharges in neonates with either neonatal herpes simplex encephalitis or asphyxia, these authors also argue that periodic discharges are not pathognomonic of any specific condition.

Bilateral periodic high-amplitude slow and sharp and slow, as well as spike and slow-wave complexes, can also be seen in neonates with severe metabolic encephalopathies due to inborn errors of metabolism (Scher et al., 1986a,b). Such complexes are maximally expressed in the frontal regions with intervals between 5 and 20 seconds. Some authors have described these generalized periodic discharges as "suppression burst variant of hypsarrhythmia" (Aicardi, 1985; Ohtahara, 1978).

Generalized Monorhythmic Background Frequencies

Generalized or focal monorhythmic activities in the theta or alpha ranges are unusual patterns that are associated with severe neonatal brain disease. These rhythms occur synchronously as well as independently in each hemisphere, sometimes prominently in the central and temporal regions. Although alpha range activity has been seen with chromosomal abnormalities and multiple congenital abnormalities (Hrachovy et al., 1990), more diffuse theta activities can be seen in preterm infants following significant hypoxic ischemic encephalopathies (Fig. 49.31).

Assessment of Prognosis in Preterm and Full-Term Infants

As emphasized several times during this discussion, serial EEGs offer more information than an isolated recording. Some reports, nonetheless, emphasize the prognostic significance of even single recordings that demonstrate severely abnormal features (Harris and Tizard, 1960; Schulte et al.,

1971; Watanabe et al., 1980). Other reports, however, suggest that serial studies provide the clinician with a more sensitive prognostic indication of neurodevelopmental outcome (Monod et al., 1972; Tharp, 1981). One report even suggested that serial recordings can assist in estimating the timing of brain injury in preterm infants (Hayakawa et al., 1999). As previously summarized in Table 49.2, the major abnormalities in these two significant studies indicate that a normal neonatal EEG is highly correlated with favorable outcome. Major abnormalities were prognostic for poor outcomes in both term and preterm infants. Other authors have relied on specific patterns recorded as part of interictal EEG patterns to predict developmental outcome. Rose and Lombroso (1970) stated that the neonates with seizures and a normal EEG had an 86% chance of normal development at 4 years of age regardless of the clinical history at the time of their illness. Rowe et al. (1985) evaluated the prognostic value of EEG in both term and preterm infants with clinically observed seizures and also found that in 74 infants between 30 and 43 weeks of age, the background activity was highly correlated with outcome. Ortibus et al. (1996) similarly reported that EEG background was a strong predictor of outcome for neonates with EEG-confirmed seizures, particularly when combined with specific neuroimaging and clinical findings. Watanabe et al. (1980) reviewed EEGs of 422 full-term infants with neonatal asphyxia, also claiming that background EEG was an excellent predictor of outcome. Biagioni et al. (1994, 1996) and Marret et al. (1997)

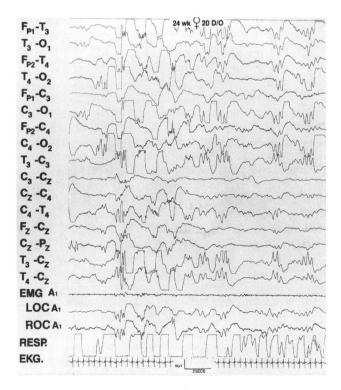

Figure 49.31. A 24-week, 20-day-old female with a diffuse monotonous theta background lacking in other rhythms. High-amplitude delta produced blocking of the pens. Patient had suffered septic shock and disseminated intravascular coagulation, and later expired. No autopsy was available.

suggested that selected maturational features, including negative and positive sharp transients, correlate with outcome.

Certain authors have stressed the superiority of the EEG over neurological examination to assess outcome. Holmes et al. (1982) found that in 38 full-term infants with neonatal asphyxia who had EEGs during the first 2 weeks, the EEG was a more sensitive predictor of sequelae than the neurological examination. Tharp et al. (1989) also emphasized the superiority of EEG over the neurological examination findings in preterm infants. Scher et al. (1989) found that although all preterm infants with periodic discharges either expired or had major sequelae, only 50% of preterm infants were clinically symptomatic at the time of these discharges. While earlier studies stress the clinical criteria to help predict outcome in term infants with asphyxia (Brown, 1973; Brown et al., 1972, 1974), such examinations may be difficult to elicit or standardize in a busy NICU. Constant manipulation of the infant, aggressive use of medications that affect muscle tone or strength, and multiple indwelling catheters severely hamper one's ability to examine an ill neonate, masking or altering neurological findings. EEG studies, therefore, can assist when such examinations are difficult to impossible to perform.

Medication Effects on EEG-Sleep Patterns

Electroencephalographers must consider that certain CNS-active medications, particularly in the toxic range, may alter background activity (Lombroso, 1985; Tharp, 1981). Holmes (1989) discussed how medications can significantly alter neonatal EEG activities.

Few drugs, however, used in neonatal care have been studied. Prolonged inactivity usually occurs following a loading dose of phenobarbital, which may last longer than 1 hour following administration. Staudt et al. (1981) argued that infants with phenobarbital plasma levels above 6 mg/dL show significant background suppression. Other authors also reported the appearance of an isoelectric record or invariant discontinuous record with high doses of antiepileptic medications (Pezzani et al., 1986). Benda et al. (1989) on the other hand, in studying 46 preterm infants, found that a mean therapeutic phenobarbital level did not prolong interburst intervals during tracé discontinu in preterm infants.

No studies have systematically investigated the effects of other nonepileptic medications that may also affect the EEG tracing. In a case report, nafcillin-induced seizures were reported after intraventricular administration (Brozanski et al., 1988). Other commonly used drugs in the neonatal patient, such as morphine, fentanyl, and theophylline, have not been systematically studied. Quantitative analyses using computer techniques will be better able to monitor EEG changes relative to loading and maintenance doses, as well as establish dose-response effects on EEG frequencies and amplitudes.

In summary, neurophysiological assessments using EEG/polysomnographic studies permit the clinician to recognize expected patterns of brain maturation in the healthy neonate. By comparison, one can detect encephalopathic behaviors of newborns who are medically at risk. Severe physiological expressions of encephalopathy are associated with neuropathological lesions on postmortem examinations,

brain lesions documented on neuroimaging studies, and major neurodevelopmental sequelae of survivors. When interpreted in the context of history, clinical findings, and other laboratory information, neurophysiological studies augment our understanding of both the severity and perhaps the timing of the encephalopathic process (Scher, 1994).

Neonatal Seizures: Controversies/Opportunities for the Neurophysiologist

A newborn with seizures is one of the few neurological emergencies in this age group (Scher, 2001, 2002). There is an urgency to establish rapid diagnostic and therapeutic plans, emphasizing the crucial role played by the clinical neurophysiologist. The clinician's strategy for the recognition and management of neonatal seizures demands heightened diagnostic acumen. The neurophysiologist can be aided by two current technological advances. Synchronized video/EEG/polygraphic monitoring and computer analyses will occupy a central role in neonatal neurological intensive care over the next decade. As discussed below, controversial aspects concerning neonatal seizures must be resolved (Camfield and Camfield, 1987; Scher et al., 1989) to achieve a consensus with respect to a universal diagnostic approach to neonates with suspected seizures.

Despite the need to establish the diagnosis of neonatal seizures, several unique aspects of this condition impede proper recognition. Multiple etiologies may lead to the expression of seizures. Efficacy of antiepileptic drugs and the prediction of outcome are also controversial. Experimental research in developing and mature animals suggests both subcortical (Browning, 1985) as well as deep cortical gray matter (Caveness et al., 1980; Hosokawa et al., 1980) input into the propagation of seizures. All of these problems impede the establishment of accepted diagnostic and treatment criteria of this neonatal medical emergency.

Previous studies have fallen short of resolving these issues because of limited preterm populations, technological resources, patients pretreated with antiepileptic medications, or limited follow-up capabilities. Certain pioneering investigations predated the development of portable EEG or synchronized video polygraphic monitoring (Brown, 1973; Dennis, 1978; Eriksson and Zetterström, 1979; Keene and Lee, 1973; Rose and Lombroso, 1970; Seay and Bray, 1977) or did not use such devices available at the time of the studies (Bergman et al., 1983; Goldberg et al., 1982; Holden et al., 1982). Traditionally, many centers chose only clinical criteria to diagnose neonatal seizures and, therefore, could not address problems of overestimation and underestimation of seizure incidence based on coincident paper EEG or synchronized video EEG polygraphic recordings (Mizrahi, 1984; Mizrahi and Kellaway, 1987; Radvanyi-Bouvet et al., 1985; Scher and Barmada, 1987; Scher et al., 1986a,b). Few studies recruited preterm infants (Helström-Westas et al., 1985; Radvanyi-Bouvet et al., 1985; Scher et al., 1989), particularly infants who were <30 weeks' gestation. No center has attempted to study efficacy of treatment by controlling the type of antiepileptic medications used to treat seizures. In fact, most studies included patients who were already treated with such medications prior to neurophysiological assessments (Clancy and Legido, 1987; Mizrahi and Kellaway, 1987). No published reports have investigated the use of computer analysis of neonatal seizures, although a variety of quantitative techniques have been studied in epileptic populations at older ages (Gottman, 1983) and in healthy neonates (Eyre et al., 1988; Havlicek et al., 1975; Kuks et al., 1988; Willekens et al., 1984). Finally, most studies have not conducted statistical analyses of antepartum, intrapartum, and neonatal conditions that would help better predict efficacy of response to medications, survival, or neurological morbidity of patients with seizures. All of the above-mentioned concerns must be considered by the clinical neurophysiologist when comparing clinical and electrographic aspects of neonatal seizure detection.

Clinical Versus EEG Criteria

The international classification of epileptic seizures does not apply to newborn seizures (Commission on Classification, 1981). Neonates are unable to sustain organized generalized discharges as in older patients and, therefore, do not manifest tonic-clonic seizures. As a result, clinical seizure phenomena are difficult to detect. Until recently, neonatal seizure criteria have been commonly grouped into five clinical types based on behavioral observations (Scher, 2001). More recently, studies utilizing EEG and behavioral monitoring by synchronized video-EEG polygraphic technique monitoring have improved these classifications, but more comprehensive diagnostic criteria utilizing both clinical and electrical categories are needed that represent a more balanced approach to neonatal seizure diagnosis.

Subtle or Fragmentary Seizures

Subtle seizures are considered the most frequently observed clinical category. Seizures of this clinical type are commonly characterized by repetitive facial activity, unusual bicycling or pedaling movements, momentary fixation of gaze, or apnea (Scher, 2001) (Fig. 49.32). A specific behavior such as apnea, a common respiratory finding, rarely occurs as the only clinical expression of a seizure (Fenichel et al., 1979). Convulsive apnea is usually associated with other clinical seizure categories.

In general, subtle seizures are quite unimpressive in their clinical appearance and may be overlooked, but may reflect significant brain injury. The inconsistent relationship of subtle behaviors with scalp-recorded electrographic seizures (Mizrahi and Kellaway, 1987) emphasizes the need to study more closely the temporal and spatial characteristics of both criteria using video/EEG/polygraphic recordings.

Clonic Seizures

Clonic seizures consist of rhythmic movements of muscles that are either focal or multifocal in distribution, involving one or multiple extremities (Fig. 49.33). A rapid followed by a slow phasic movement distinguishes clonic activities from the symmetric to-and-fro motion of nonepileptic tremulousness or jitteriness. Gentle flexion of the body part suppresses tremors but not clonic activity. Tonic components are usually quite subtle and may be absent. Generalized clonic movements may be seen in the absence of any tonic activity. While multifocal clonic activity has been described to have no predictable anatomical pattern, focal clonic activity may suggest a specific regional or hemispheric brain lesion.

Tonic Seizures

Tonic seizures involve sustained extension or flexion of axial or appendicular muscles. EEG confirmation is required, since tonic activity may occur in the absence of cortical seizures in a high percentage of patients; one study by Kellaway and Hrachovy (1983) noted only a 30% correlation between tonic seizures and coincident electrographic correlates (Fig. 49.18). Tonic seizures respond poorly to antiepileptic drug (AEDs), and if associated with electrographic seizures, signify poor prognosis.

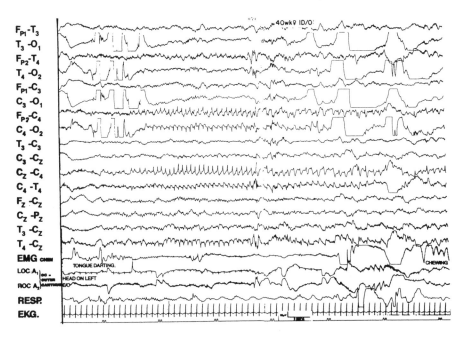

Figure 49.32. An EEG tracing of a 40-week, 1-day-old female described in Figure 49.19A, documenting lingual and lateral eye movements (note eye channels) coincidental with an electrographic seizure in the right central region. (From Scher MS, and Painter MJ. 1990. Electrographic diagnosis of neonatal seizures. Issues of diagnostic accuracy, clinical correlation and survival. In *Neonatal Seizures*, ed. CG Wasterlain, and P Vert. New York: Raven Press, with permission.)

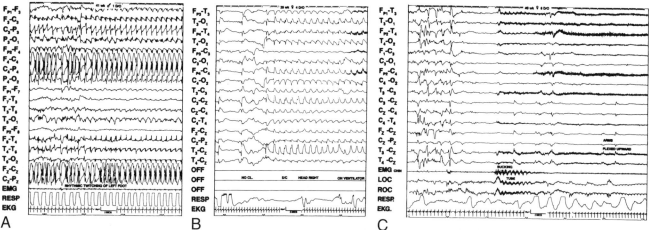

Figure 49.33. **A:** EEG tracing of a 41-week, 1-day-old male with clonic movements of the left foot seen coincidentally with bihemispheric electrographic seizures, with higher amplitude in the right central region. **B:** EEG tracing of a 25-week, 4-day-old female with an electrographic seizure noted without coincident clinical seizure activity. **C:** An EEG tracing of a 40-week, 6-day-old female with repetitive arm flexion and buccolingual movements in the absence of any coincident electrographic seizures. (From Scher MS. 1994. Pediatric electroencephalography and evoked potentials. In *Pediatric Neurology, Principles and Practice,* vol. 1, ed. KF Swaiman. St. Louis: Mosby Year-Book, with permission.)

Myoclonic Seizures

These movements are rapid, isolated jerks, most frequently noted in preterm infants, but also seen in severely ill term infants (Fig. 49.34). Consequently, myoclonic seizures are associated with major CNS insults. Simultaneous EEG recordings are necessary since nonepileptic pathological myoclonus of the newborn may also exist in the sick infant (Scher, 1985a–c). What is more, both healthy preterm as well as term infants may manifest either age-appropriate myoclonus of prematurity or clinically benign sleep myoclonus (Coulter and Allen, 1982; Holmes, 1987).

Synchronized EEG-Video Monitoring: Distinguishing Seizures from Other Nonepileptic Neonatal Behavior

Synchronized EEG-video monitoring is used in pediatric populations at risk for different neurological diseases (Mizrahi, 1984). Mizrahi and Kellaway (1987) proposed a classification of seizure and nonseizure activity based on the temporal relationships between clinical and electrical criteria documented by synchronized video EEG correlations. Their investigations using a bedside EEG/polygraphic/video monitoring technique provide insights into the interpretation of abnormal clinical findings in relation to electrographic activity. In one study, 415 clinical seizures in 71 infants were monitored, showing that clonic seizure activity had the best correlation with coincident electrographic seizures, while subtle seizures had an inconsistent relationship with coincident EEG seizure activity. Whether such clinical phenomena should then be interpreted as nonepileptic brainstem release behavior or represent subcortical seizure onset with inconsistent propagation to the surface has yet to be resolved (Figs. 49.35 and 49.36).

Nonepileptic behaviors and conditions of neonates may be difficult to diagnose without the use of coincident EEG monitoring. Determining whether the behavior is normal for neonates or is part of an encephalopathic process rests on the exercise of clinical judgment.

Benign Neonatal Sleep Myoclonus

Myoclonic activity may involve a single or multiple body part of portions of those parts. During early infancy, such movements generally occur during sleep that can be bilateral and asynchronous, as well as asymmetric, sometimes migrating from one muscle group to another. Rhythmic movements may not be prolonged, but may cluster during active versus quiet sleep. Myoclonic movements are more common in preterm infants (Hakamada et al., 1981), but can be observed in the full-term neonate, as well; the EEG shows no coincident epileptiform activity. When aroused, the infant's movements cease, and are rarely noted during the wakeful alert state. Benign myoclonus of the neonate typically disappears over several months (Resnick et al., 1986).

Tremulousness or Jitteriness

Rapid generalized tremulousness may be often mistaken for clonic seizure activity, but such movements do not have a fast and slow phase, as with clonic activity. Also, flexion extension of the limb or body part involved in the tremulous movement will diminish or eliminate the movement. Tremulousness may be spontaneous or provoked by stimulation and should be suspected in infants who are small for gestational age or following asphyxial stress, metabolic encephalopathy, drug intoxication or withdrawal, or intracranial hemorrhage. In one study of 38 full-term infants (Shuper et al., 1991) with excessive tremulousness after 6 weeks of age, movements resolved by a mean age of 7.2 months, with 92% of children demonstrating normal neurodevelopment at 3 years of age.

Neonatal Dyskinesias: Dystonia or Choreoathetosis

Dystonia and choreoathetosis are commonly occurring movement disorders that can be misdiagnosed as seizures. These nonepileptic movement disorders can be associated with either acute or chronic disease states involving basal

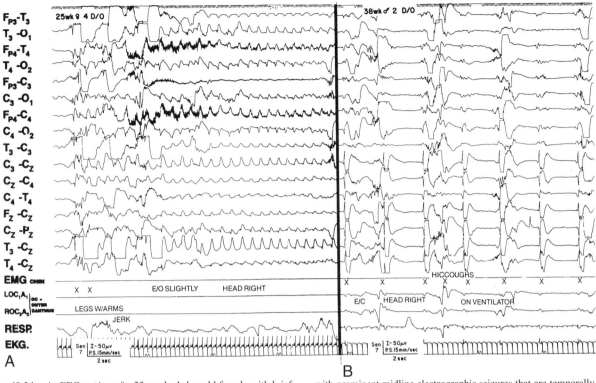

Figure 49.34. **A:** EEG tracing of a 25-week, 4-day-old female with brief myoclonic movements prior to an electrographic seizure seen diffusely over both hemispheres. **B:** An EEG tracing of a 38-week, 2-day-old male with prominent midline electrographic seizures that are temporally related to myoclonic movements of the diaphragm (x marks).

ganglia structures, or the extrapyramidal pathways that innervate these regions. Either antepartum or intrapartum adverse events such as severe asphyxia can damage the basal ganglia (i.e., status marmoratus) (Volpe, 2001); rarely, specific inherited metabolic diseases (e.g., glutaric aciduria) also can injure these structures. Sustained posturing or dys-

tonia also may reflect lack of functional inhibition of subcortical motor pathways due to disease or malformation of the neocortex. Documentation of these movements without electrographic seizures using video-EEG-polygraphic recordings will help avoid misdiagnosis and inappropriate treatment (Fig. 49.35).

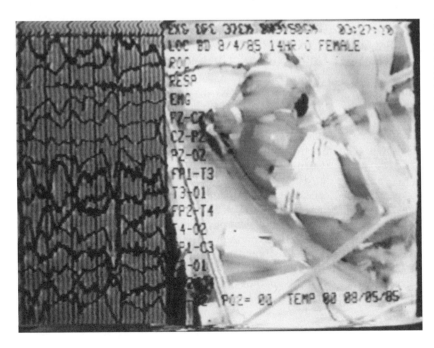

Figure 49.35. Sample of a video EEG of a full-term 14-hour-old female who has demonstrated posturing of the back and left arm in the absence of a coincident electrographic seizure. (From Scher MS, and Painter MJ. 1989. Controversies concerning neonatal seizures. In *Seizure Disorders. The Pediatric Clinics of North America*, vol. 36(2), ed. JM Pellock, pp. 281–310. Philadelphia: WB Saunders, with permission.)

Figure 49.36. A sample of a synchronized video EEG recording documenting an electrographic seizure prominently noted in the P_ZO_2 region in the absence of any coincident clinical activity.

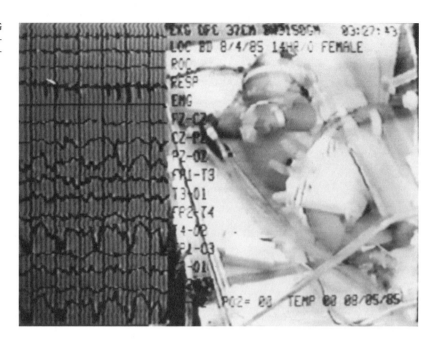

Incidence of Neonatal Seizures

Problems with the recognition of neonatal seizures result from both overestimation and underestimation of the incidence of this disorder. Previous investigations have reported a wide range of incidence from 0.5% in term infants to 20.2% in preterm infants (Bergman et al., 1983; Hill and Volpe, 1981). Such wide discrepancies may in part be due to the varying postconceptional ages of newborns included in such studies as well as criteria for selection. Furthermore, hospital-based studies that specialize in evaluating the high-risk infant may report a higher rate than population studies that are based on newborns admitted to general nurseries and who are less medically ill. Most importantly, previous incidence figures have been based on clinical criteria that may not adequately distinguish seizures from normal or pathological nonepileptic neonatal behavior. A report of the inborn incidence of neonatal seizures in a hospital-based population of high-risk newborns (Scher et al., 1989) estimates that 2% of the neonatal population admitted to an NICU had electrographic seizures. This is 0.2% of all liveborns at this obstetrical center. Future studies must compare the incidence of seizures for both inborn and outborn populations, utilizing both electrographic and clinical criteria.

Studies of Overestimation of Seizures

Studies emphasize the difficulty in identifying suspicious movements without coincident EEG monitoring. Careful evaluation of suspicious behaviors, such as tremors myoclonus or dystonia, may be abnormal, but nonepileptic. Only 30% of infants with tonic behavior have coincident EEG seizure activity (Kellaway et al., 1983) (Figs. 49.33C and 49.35), prompting these investigators to emphasize the experimental animal evidence for brainstem release phenomena as an explanation for these neonatal behaviors.

In another study from the same center, only 17% with subtle movements had a consistent relationship with EEG seizures in 71 term and near-term infants (Mizrahi and Kellaway, 1987), emphasizing again a nonepileptic pathophysiological mechanism. Another study also stressed the limitations of scalp recorded EEGs by reporting that only 10% of the EEGs obtained on 80 neonates with suspicious movements had coincident electrographic seizures (Scher et al., 1989). All these studies emphasize the risk of overestimating seizures if suspicious movements are identified without coincident EEG monitoring. In fact, it has been suggested that synchronized video polygraphic monitoring should be required to fully characterize the electrographic and clinical phenomena associated with questionable seizure activity (Mizrahi and Kellaway, 1987).

Underestimation of Seizures

Newborns may have electrographic seizures that would go undetected unless the EEG is used (Coen et al., 1982; Scher et al., 1989; Seay and Bray, 1977). Although some of these patients may be pharmacologically paralyzed for ventilatory support (Goldberg, 1983; Staudt et al., 1981), other electrographic seizures have no observable clinical activity (Coen et al., 1982; Helström-Westas et al., 1985; Scher et al., 1989; Shewmon, 1990) (Fig. 49.33B). One report indicates that 50% of neonates with electrographic seizures are unaccompanied by clinical phenomena (Scher et al., 1989). Clinical and electrographic criteria were noted in 20 of 62 (32%) of preterm and 16 of 30 (53%) of full-term infants. This population was defined over a 4-year period in which 92 neonates with seizures using EEG criteria were identified in the NICU with a total population of 4,020. Seventeen infants in this group had seizures documented while paralyzed.

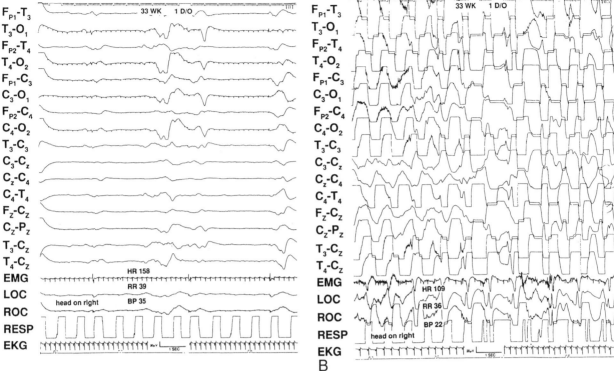

A

Figure 49.37. **A:** An EEG tracing of a 33-week, 1-day-old female indicating a lack of background. Note the vital sign values for blood pressure, heart, and respiratory rates. **B:** Same patient as described in **A** showing a precipitous drop in heart rate and blood pressure coincident with a generalized electrographic seizure. An evolution in this generalized seizure was noted over 3 minutes. (From Scher MS, and Painter MJ. 1989. Controversies concerning neonatal seizures. In *Seizure Disorders. The Pediatric Clinics of North America,* vol. 36(2), ed. JM Pellock, pp. 281–310. Philadelphia: WB Saunders, with permission.)

In part, underestimation of seizures may result because of inadequate monitoring of autonomic changes coincident with electrographic seizures. Autonomic changes may consist of alterations in respiration, blood pressure, or heart rate, as well as changes in pupillary size or salivation (Fig. 49.37). Paroxysmal autonomic events that are periodic or recurring should always be treated as possible seizure phenomena when a seizure recording is obtained (Perlman and Volpe, 1983).

Electroclinical Disassociation of Neonatal Seizures

Experimental evidence suggests that the brain is dependent on deep gray matter and brainstem structures for seizure propagation (Browning, 1985), as well as surface cortical tissue (Caveness et al., 1980; Hayakawa et al., 1987), but clinical investigations into the possibility of subcortical epileptic foci have been limited to anecdotal reports (Danner et al., 1985). Although depth recordings in adults and adolescents have documented subcortical seizures, direct or indirect evidence in the neonate has not yet been available. The phenomenon of electroclinical disassociation (ECD) (Weiner et al., 1991), attempts to address this controversial topic. One hundred and ten infants with electrographically confirmed seizures were investigated with respect to ECD. A seizure was defined as an electrographic event characterized by the sudden appearance of repetitive waveforms that had a demonstrable evolution in frequency, morphology, amplitude, and field, with a minimum duration of 10 seconds. ECD was defined as a clinical seizure that occurred at times with and other times without electrographic signature. Since the study focused on the relationship of clinical movements to their electrographic expression, 34 infants with only electrical seizures and 25 pharmacologically paralyzed infants were excluded.

Of the remaining 51 infants, 33 satisfied the criteria for electroclinical (EC) seizures, having movements consistently coupled to an electrographic discharge. This group was compared to 18 infants who had ECD. The ECD group comprised 16% of infants with electrographically confirmed seizures and 19% of 243 electrographic seizures. Extremity movements occurred at a significantly higher rate with EC seizures, while clinical features that preceded electrical seizures were associated with the ECD group to a statistically significant degree.

Uncoupling of clinical and electrographic expressions of neonatal seizures after antiepileptic medication administration also contributes to the underestimation of the true seizure occurrence. One study estimated that 25% of neonates had persistent electrographic seizures despite resolutions of their clinical seizure behaviors after receiving one or more antiepileptic medications (Scher et al., 2002a,b); this phenomenon is termed electroclinical uncoupling.

The phenomena of ECD and uncoupling may contribute to a more balanced seizure taxonomy that includes both EEG and clinical seizure criteria. Rather than specific clinical behaviors being interpreted as nonepileptic because of the inconsistent association of these movements with coincident EEG seizure activity, one might alternately suggest that certain clinical activity lacks a consistent EEG correlate because of ECD, with epileptic foci that are not detected by scalp EEG. The inconsistent electrographic capture on scalp recordings may represent seizures emanating from foci deep within the brain, only inconsistently discharging through final anatomical effector pathways (Weiner et al., 1991). State-of-the-art monitoring equipment utilizing video, audio, and electrographic data may provide the necessary temporal resolution necessary to characterize such behavioral and electrographic events.

Seizure Duration and Topography

Little attention has been directed toward quantifying the ictal and interictal periods on an EEG recording. One study measured the exact duration of these periods in primarily term and near-term infants (Clancy et al., 1984); the majority of the population (87%) received one or more antiepileptic medications prior to obtaining the EEG tracings. Seizures were recurrent but relatively brief, lasting 137 seconds, separated by interictal recovery periods of variable duration, but 8 minutes on the average. The minimum duration of seizures was defined as 10 seconds.

In another study seizure durations were reviewed in 68 neonates consisting of 34 full-term neonates and 34 preterm neonates (15 patients were ≤31 weeks' gestation) (Scher et al., 1993). This study considered the effect of gestational age, serial seizures, and antiepileptic medication on seizure durations. Serial series were defined as either continuous seizure activity for at least 30 minutes or recurrent seizures for 50% or more of the recording time. Thirty-six percent, 12 of 33 full-term infants, had serial seizures with a mean duration of 29.6 minutes prior to antiepileptic drug use. Only 9% (3/33) preterm had status epilepticus with a mean duration of 5.2 minutes. Excluding patients with serial seizures, mean seizure durations were similar at different gestation ages (2.8 and 3.9 minutes for preterm and full-term infants, respectively). Phenobarbital was used as the antiepileptic drug in 90% of the population. Ictal duration was shorted by 77% to 0.6 minutes in preterm infants and by 41% to 1.1 minutes in full-term infants. Surprisingly, interictal durations were paradoxically shortened in preterm infants after drug use (i.e., 16.5 minutes versus 12.9). However, the mean durations were longer in full-term infants after drug administration (i.e., 11.3–18 minutes).

A third report emphasized the location, duration, and response of seizures to antiepileptic medications (Bye and Flanagan, 1995). Seizures were frequent and limited electrographic spread; although seizure variables remained stable over time, drug therapy shortened seizure duration, increased interictal periods, decreased the spread of discharges, and reduced coincident clinical features. Uncoupling of the clinical and electrographic expression of seizures may be anticipated following antiepileptic medication administration (Scher et al., 2002a,b).

More recent reports offer greater descriptive details of differences of seizure onset, duration, and topography between preterm and full-term neonates (Patrizi et al., 2003).

Additional studies of ictal and interictal durations are needed to facilitate the development of automated seizure detection programs. Computer techniques may more accurately measure ictal and interictal durations, but must first be based on visually analyzed records (Altenburg et al., 2003; Liu et al., 1993). Such computer strategies will then better assess the efficacy of AEDs as measured by their effects on seizure duration, electrographic field, as well as clinical expression (Scher et al., 1995a,b).

Ictal Patterns

Ictal patterns in the newborn are rhythmic discharges consisting of waveforms of similar morphology that change an evolution with respect to frequency, amplitude, and electrical field (Fig. 49.28). Four basic categories of ictal patterns have been traditionally described (Scher, 2001): focal ictal patterns with normal background, focal ictal patterns with abnormal backgrounds, focal monorhythmic patterns of various frequencies, and multifocal ictal patterns.

Shewmon (1990) framed several problems concerning the definition of an electrographic seizure, even among experienced clinical neurophysiologists. The author emphasizes the ictal/interictal dichotomy by suggesting that brief but intermittent rhythmic discharges <10 seconds, as well as prolonged periodic discharges with longer slow evolutions, may also represent neonatal seizures. Although such concerns will remain, most electroencephalographers traditionally identify ictal patterns as having at least 10 seconds in duration with an evolution in the above-mentioned electrographic features (Fig. 49.38).

Focal Ictal Patterns

Discharges originating in one region may spread to homologous regions in both preterm and term infants. In general, discharges seen with normal EEG background and the absence of a structural lesion have a more favorable prognosis (Rose and Lombroso, 1970). Conversely, focal ictal patterns with low amplitude and disorganized backgrounds are associated with structural lesions and a higher risk for sequelae (Fig. 49.39).

Focal Monorhythmic Charges of Varying Frequencies

Such discharges may be expressed in any frequency range, without specific association with gestational age. On rare occasions, specific frequencies have been associated with particular clinical phenomena (i.e., alpha frequency seizures associated with apnea). In general, during an EEG-documented seizure, the frequency and morphology of waveforms gradually change, as do the electrical field and amplitude of the discharges. Focal ictal patterns also may vary only slightly with respect to these electrographic descriptions. Lombroso (1985), for example, emphasizes that specific ictal patterns of repetitive discharges that are slow delta range frequency are usually superimposed on low-amplitude disorganized background; such patterns are described in children with compromised neurological outcome.

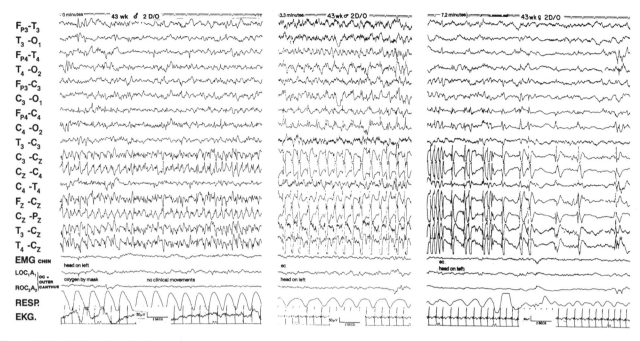

Figure 49.38. EEG tracing of a 43-week, 2-day-old male demonstrating the evolution of electrographic discharge with an onset in the midline spreading to the central and temporal regions. Note the evolution in morphology frequency and field. (From Scher MS, Painter MJ, Bergman I, et al. 1989. EEG diagnoses of neonatal seizures: clinical correlations and outcome. Pediatr Neurol 5:17–24, with permission.)

Multifocal Ictal Discharges

Electrical seizure activity may originate from anatomically unrelated brain regions. Such a pattern is usually associated with a high instance of neurological sequelae (Hrachovy et al., 1990; Scher et al., 1989).

Etiologies of Neonatal Seizures

Issues exist with respect to the causes of neonatal seizures. As with background EEG abnormalities, seizures are also not disease specific. A neonate who is ill may have a variety of medical difficulties that predisposes to seizures

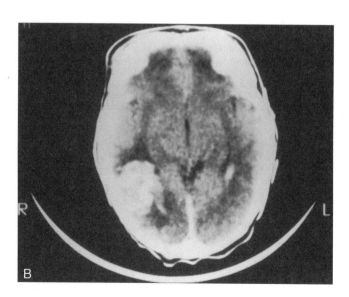

Figure 49.39. **A:** EEG tracing of a 43-week, 1-day-old male with an onset of two seizures at the midline and the right posterior quadrant. This patient had severe pulmonary hypertension of the newborn. **B:** A CT scan of the patient in **A** showing a hemorrhagic infarction in the right posterior quadrant. This patient has severe spastic quadriparesis at 7 years of age.

(Volpe, 2001). Despite the large number of possibilities that can be associated with neonatal seizures, a small subset of etiologies most commonly is noted. Medical conditions that occur with hypoxic ischemic insults (i.e., asphyxia) contribute significantly to the seizure diathesis. The presence of hypoglycemia, hypocalcemia, intracranial hemorrhage, or cerebral infarction commonly occurs in patients with asphyxia (Brown et al., 1972, 1974; Cockburn et al., 1973). Rarely, a genetic form of autosomal-dominant neonatal seizures can occur (Bjerre and Corelius, 1968; Pettit and Fenichel, 1980). Most asphyxia occurs before or during labor and delivery, with only 10% of neonates suffering asphyxia during the neonatal period (Volpe, 1989). Therefore, intrauterine factors that lead to asphyxia may contribute to

seizures, including placental or maternal disease. With the advent of more sophisticated fetal ultrasonography, antenatal intracranial brain lesions associated with infants with seizures have been detected.

Cerebral infarction has an important association with neonates with seizures (Clancy et al., 1985; Larroche, 1968; Levy et al., 1985; Ment et al., 1984; Scher et al., 1986a) (Fig. 49.40). Ischemic brain lesions in one particular study were noted in 77% of full-term and 39% of preterm infants (Scher et al., 1986a). Grade III to IV subependymal hemorrhage was also seen in 45% of preterm infants with neonatal seizures. Documentation of these structural lesions is important, together with other clinical and demographic data in relation to immediate and long-term outcome.

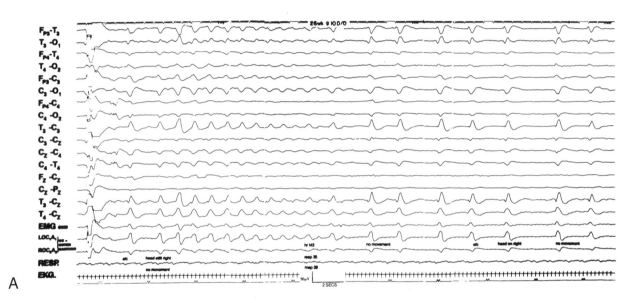

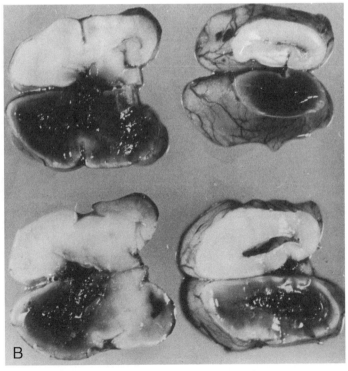

Figure 49.40.   **A:** An EEG tracing for a 26-week, 10-day-old female with necrotizing enterocolitis and disseminated intravascular coagulation. An electrographic seizure was seen predominantly in the left hemisphere both above and below the sylvian fissure with spread to involve the homologous right hemispheric regions. The patient subsequently expired, but no autopsy was obtained. (From Scher MS, Painter MJ, Bergman I, et al. 1989. EEG diagnoses of neonatal seizures: clinical correlations and outcome. Pediatr Neurol 5:17–24, with permission.) **B:** A coronal section of the brain of the patient described in **A** indicating a significant hemorrhagic infarction of the left hemisphere. (From Scher MS, and Painter MJ. 1989. Controversies concerning neonatal seizures. In *Seizure Disorders. The Pediatric Clinics of North America,* vol. 36(2), ed. JM Pellock, pp. 281–310. Philadelphia: WB Saunders, with permission.)

Table 49.7. Causes of Neonatal Seizures

Trauma
Subdural hematoma
Intracortical hemorrhage
Cortical vein thrombosis
Hypoxic–ischemic encephalopathy, subependymal hemorrhage
Congenital abnormalities (cerebral dysgenesis)
Hypertension
Metabolic
Hypocalcemia
Hypomagnesemia
High phosphate load
Infant of a diabetic mother
Hypoparathyroidism
Maternal hyperparathyroidism
Idiopathic
Hypoglycemia
Galactosemia
Intrauterine growth retardation
Infant of a diabetic mother
Glycogen storage disease
Idiopathic
Electrolyte imbalance
Hypernatremia
Hyponatremia
Infections
Bacterial meningitis
Cerebral abscess
Herpes encephalitis
Coxsackie meningoencephalitis
Cytomegalovirus
Toxoplasmosis
Syphilis
Drug withdrawal
Methadone
Heroin
Barbiturate
Propoxyphene
Pyridoxine dependency
Amino acid disturbances
Maple syrup urine disease
Urea cycle abnormalities
Nonketotic hyperglycinemia
Ketotic hyperglycinemia
Toxins
Local anesthetics
Isoniazid
Bilirubin
Maternal cocaine
Familial seizures
Neurocutaneous syndromes
Tuberous sclerosis
Incontinentia pigmenti
Genetic syndromes
Zellweger syndrome
Smith–Lemli–Opitz syndrome
Neonatal adrenoleukodystrophy
Benign familial epilepsy (fifth day convulsions)

From Painter MJ, and Gaus L. 1991. J Child Neurol 1991;6:104, with permission.

Neonatal seizures are not disease specific and may be caused by a combination of medical conditions. Table 49.7 lists the major etiologies associated with seizures in the newborn, some of which have already been discussed, and may be reviewed in greater detail elsewhere (Scher, 2001; Scher et al., 1996). Some examples include CNS infections acquired *in utero* or postnatally, CNS malformations, inborn errors of metabolism, drug withdrawal and intoxication,

early myoclonic encephalopathy, and familial neonatal seizures. The last two entities are quite unusual, but should be included in the differential diagnosis of neonatal seizures, representing progressive epileptic syndromes associated with severe myoclonic seizures (Ohtahara, 1978), or autosomal-dominant neonatal seizures, which are a rare form of epilepsy in neonates (Tibbles, 1980).

Prognosis of Neonates with Seizures

While it has recently been suggested that the mortality rate for clinical seizures has dropped from 40% to 15% (Volpe, 2001), this trend is not based on the electrographic diagnoses of seizures. In fact, in one report, the EEG criteria for seizures found 50% mortality in preterm and 40% in full-term infants (Scher et al., 1989). Furthermore, the incidence of adverse neurological sequelae was noted in 65% of survivors.

A change in the etiologies of seizures over the last several decades must be considered before assessing the prognosis of infants with seizures. While there are substantial reductions in seizures caused by late-onset hypocalcemia or birth trauma, proportionally higher numbers of neonates with hemorrhagic or ischemic cerebrovascular lesions are now associated with neonatal seizures (Clancy and Spitzer, 1985; Larroche, 1968; Levy et al., 1985; Ment et al., 1984; Scher et al., 1986).

Specific clinical criteria of neonatal seizures have prognostic implications. Tonic, myoclonic, and subtle seizures imply a more diffuse or multifocal brain insult suggesting a poorer prognosis (Hrachovy et al., 1990; Lombroso, 1985; Scher et al., 1989). Such seizure types have also been noted in association with inborn errors of metabolism, malformations, and severe asphyxia.

Interictal EEG findings are particularly useful in predicting neurological outcome in neonates with seizures. Background EEG activity is an excellent indicator of outcome, as emphasized in earlier sections in this chapter. Certain major disturbances such as suppression burst are highly predictive of poor outcome. Neither ictal patterns alone nor interictal spikes and sharp waves fully predict the risk for sequelae. In a study of 137 full-term infants with neonatal seizures, Rose and Lombroso (1970) found that neonates with seizures who had a normal EEG had an 86% chance of normal development at age 4. Conversely, neonates with low-amplitude, periodic, or multifocal spikes in the interictal EEG background had only a 7% chance for normal development. Rowe et al. (1985) supported these findings in their discussion of prognosis in 74 term and preterm neonates with seizures. They emphasized that EEG background actually was more predictive of outcome than interictal sharp waves.

As previously mentioned, Monod et al. (1972) and Tharp et al. (1981) emphasized for full-term and preterm infants, respectively, the importance of serial records in assessing neurological outcome. These authors found that normal neonatal EEGs were highly correlated with favorable outcomes, while markedly abnormal records are associated with poorer outcomes for both term and preterm infants.

The clinician treating patients with neonatal seizures is appropriately concerned about the risk of epilepsy. Few studies have attempted to predict subsequent epilepsy in neonates with seizures as confirmed by electrographic studies. Using clinical criteria only, some reports estimate that as many as

20% to 30% of neonates with seizures will develop epilepsy (Camfield and Camfield, 1987; Holden et al., 1982; Holmes, 1987). Excluding seizures with fever, the incidence of epilepsy at 4 years of age appears to range from 15% to 20% of neonates with electrographically confirmed seizures (Scher et al., 1990) to >50% of neonates (Clancy et al., 1996).

Brain imaging techniques have revolutionized the diagnosis of major structural diseases of the brain, thereby improving the accuracy of outcome prediction. Techniques that apply both structural and functional studies, such as MRI (Huppi et al., 1998; Young et al., 1987; Younkin et al., 1986) and PET (Volpe, 1989; Wasterlain, 1976), extend our abilities to detect structural and metabolic disturbances of the brain due to seizures. Comparisons of these techniques will augment our ability to describe the metabolic and neurophysiological consequences of structural lesions of the brains of neonates with seizures.

Efficacy of Treatment

A number of issues still remain with respect to the treatment of neonatal seizures (Camfield and Camfield, 1987; Scher, 2001; Scher et al., 1989). While some argue that neonates should be treated only if seizures are clinically expressed and prolonged in duration, others suggest that all seizures should be treated because of the possibility of their detrimental effects on the immature brain (Collins, 1986; Johnston and Silverstein, 1985). It is equally controversial as to how long to treat a neonate with seizures. Rapid dis-

continuation after 1 week following the seizure occurrence has been suggested (Scher et al., 1996).

Different medications are available to treat neonatal seizures. Phenobarbital and phenytoin remain the most widely used, but the benzodiazepines have certain theoretic advantages in treating neonatal seizures. Published studies in which the efficacy of phenobarbital was reported are conflicting. Based on clinical seizure criteria, only 36% of neonates at one institution responded to phenobarbital alone (Painter et al., 1999). Similarly, Lockman et al. (1979) found cessation of seizures with phenobarbital in 32%. By contrast, Gal et al. (1982) reported that seizure control was achieved with phenobarbital monotherapy in 85% of patients with loading doses that were as much as twice that reported in infants.

Free drug fractions that determine efficacy and toxicity have been studied in pediatric populations (Scher et al., 1989). Binding of drugs in neonates with seizures has been reported. Binding can be significantly altered in a sick neonatal patient. Such alterations may cause toxic side effects by affecting cardiovascular or respiratory functions. Efficacy of treatment must not only utilize appropriate total, free, and bound fractions to verify the cortical representation of seizures, but also guard against toxicity if free fractions are dangerously high. Serial drug level determinations combined with analog and digital EEG analyses will better assess efficacy and toxicity of AEDs in future studies, as suggested by Painter et al. (1999) (Fig. 49.41).

Figure 49.41. A histogram of 41-week male indicating both seizure duration and frequency before and following diazepam infusion. Note the resolution of the periodic drops in pulse oximetry values but only a slight reduction in seizure frequency. The seizure duration remained unchanged. (From Scher MS, and Painter MJ. 1990. Electrographic diagnosis of neonatal seizures. Issues of diagnostic accuracy, clinical correlation and survival. In *Neonatal Seizures,* ed. CG Wasterlain, and P Vert. New York: Raven Press, with permission.)

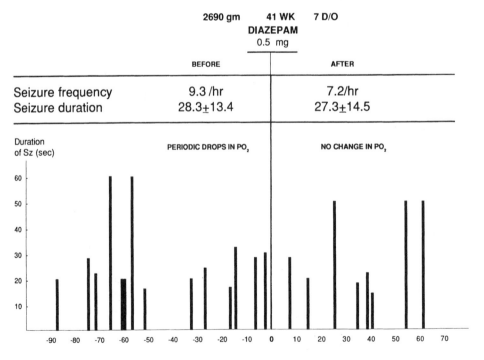

Summary

Electrophysiological monitoring is the only technique that can assess cerebral function continuously over time. This advantage must also be stressed in the context of the neurophysiological assessment of the sick neonate. To objectively identify pathophysiological concomitants of episodic or periodic disease phenomena such as seizures, noninvasive methods of electrophysiological recordings adapt most readily to the complicated environment of the neonatal intensive care unit.

Pathophysiological events may occur intermittently at unpredictable times (i.e., neonatal seizures) (Gloor, 1985). Furthermore, maladaptive physiological interrelationships among cortical and subcortical neuronal tract systems may subtly herald disturbances of biological rhythm (i.e., neonatal EEG sleep), which can be detected only by quantitative EEG recordings over extended periods, while the clinical examination remains age–appropriate. Other methods of measuring both brain structure and function (i.e., PET and spectral nuclear magnetic resonance) provide detailed, but brief snapshots of information that may be better interpreted in the context of continuous electrophysiological recordings. As with other physiological monitoring techniques in cardiology, neuroanesthesia, and epilepsy, which rely on long-term monitoring in the intensive care unit and epilepsy suites, long-term neurophysiological monitoring deserves an important place in the neonatal intensive care unit.

Acknowledgment

Preparation of this chapter, was aided, in part, by research grants NS01110, NS26793, MO1RR00084, NS34508, NR01894, and HL07193 funded by the National Institutes of Health.

References

Abarbanel ADI, and Rabinovich MI. 2001. Neurodynamics: nonlinear dynamics and neurobiology. Curr Opin Neurobiol 11:423–430.

Agarwal R, and Gotman J. 2002. Digital tools and polysomnography. J Clin Neurophysiol 19:136–143.

Aicardi J. 1985. Early myoclonic encephalopathy. In *Epileptic Syndromes in Infancy, Childhood and Adolescence,* Eds. Roger J, Dravet C, Bureau M, et al., pp. 12–22. London: John Libbey.

Altenburg J, Vermeulen RJ, Strijers RLM, et al. 2003. Seizure detection in the neonatal EEG with synchronization likelihood. Clin Neurophysiol 114:50–55.

American Electroencephalographic Society Guidelines in EEG and Evoked Potentials. 1986. Ajmone Marsan C, ed. J Clin Neurophysiol 3 (Suppl 1):1–152.

Amiel-Tison C, and Pettigrew AG. 1991. Adaptive changes in the developing brain during intrauterine stress. Brain Dev 13:67–76.

Anders T, Ende R, and Parmelee A. 1971. A Manual of Standardized Terminology, Technique, and Criteria for Scoring of States of Sleep and Wakefulness in Newborn Infants. UCLA Brain Information Service. Los Angeles: NINDS, Neurological Information Network.

Anders TF, and Keener M. 1985. Developmental course of nighttime sleep-wake patterns in full-term and premature infants during the first year of life. I. Sleep 8:173–192.

Anders TF, Sadeh A, and Appareddy V. 1995. Normal sleep in neonates and children. In: Ferber R, Kryger M (eds). Principles and Practice of Sleep Medicine in the Child. Philadelphia: Saunders.

Anderson CM, Torres F, and Faoro A. 1985. The EEG of the early premature. Electroencephalogr Clin Neurophysiol 60:95–105.

Arfel G, Leondardon N, and Mousali E. 1977. Densité et dynamique des encoches pointues frontales dans le sommeil du nouveau-né et du nourisson. Rev EEG Neurophysiol 7:351–360.

Aso K, Scher MS, and Barmada M. 1989. Neonatal electroencephalography and neuropathology. J Clin Neurophysiol 6:103–123.

Aso K, Scher MS, and Barmada M. 1990. Cerebral infarcts and seizures in the neonate. J Child Neurol 5:224–228.

Au WJ, Gabor AJ, Vijayan N, et al. 1980. Periodic lateralized epileptiform discharges (PLEDs) in Creutzfeldt-Jakob disease. Neurology 30:611–617.

Ballard JL, Novak KK, and Driver M. 1979. A simplified score for assessment of fetal maturation of newly born infants. J Pediatr 95:769–774.

Barabas RE, Barmada MA, and Scher MS. 1993. Timing of brain insults in severe neonatal encephalopathies with an isoelectric EEG. Pediatr Neurol 9:39–44.

Barlow JS. 1985. Methods of analysis of nonstationary EEGs with emphasis on segmentation techniques: a comparative review. J Clin Neurophysiol 2:267–304.

Baumgart S, and Graziani LJ. 2001. Predicting the future for term infants experiencing an acute neonatal encephalopathy: electroencephalogram, magnetic resonance imaging, or crystal ball? Pediatrics 107:588–590.

Beckwith L, and Parmelee AH Jr. 1986. EEG patterns of preterm infants, home environment, and later IQ. Child Dev 57:777–789.

Benda GI, Engel RCH, and Zhang Y. 1989. Prolonged inactive phases during the discontinuous pattern of prematurity in the electroencephalogram of very-low-birthweight infants. Electroencephalogr Clin Neurophysiol 72:189–197.

Bennett FC, and TeKolste K. 1988. Preschool motor skills of children born prematurely and not diagnosed as having cerebral palsy. Dev Behav Pediatr 9(4):189–193.

Bergman I, Painter MJ, Hirsch RP, et al. 1983. Outcome in neonates with convulsions treated in an intensive care unit. Ann Neurol 14:642–647.

Bes F, Baroncini P, Dugovic C, et al. 1988. Time course of night sleep EEG in the first year of life: a description based on automatic analysis. Electroencephalogr Clin Neurophysiol 69(6):501–507.

Biagioni E, Bartalena L, Boldrini A, et al. 1994. Background EEG activity in preterm infants: correlation of outcome with selected maturational features. Electroencephalogr Clin Neurophysiol 91:154–162.

Biagioni E, Boldrini A, Bottone U, et al. 1996. Prognostic value of abnormal EEG transients in preterm and full-term neonates. Electroencephalogr Clin Neurophysiol 99:1–9.

Biagioni E, Bartalena L, Boldrini A, et al. 1999. Constantly discontinuous EEG patterns in full-term neonates with hypoxic-ischaemic encephalopathy. Clin Neurophysiol 110:1510–1515.

Biagioni E, Mercuri E, Rutherford M, et al. 2001. Combined use of electroencephalogram and magnetic resonance imaging in full-term neonates with acute encephalopathy. Pediatrics 107(3):461–468.

Bickford RG, and Butt HR. 1968. Hepatic coma: the electroencephalographic pattern. J Clin Invest 1955;34:790–799.

Bjerre I, and Corelius E. 1968. Benign familial neonatal convulsions. Acta Paediatr Scand 57:557–561.

Blume WT, and Dreyfus-Brisac C. 1982. Positive rolandic sharp waves in neonatal EEG: types and significance. Electroencephalogr Clin Neurophysiol 53:277–282.

Bredesen DE. 1995. Neural apoptosis. Ann Neurol 38:839–851.

Brown JK. 1973. Convulsions in the newborn period. Dev Med Child Neurol 15:823–846.

Brown JK, Cockburn F, and Forfar JO. 1972. Clinical and chemical correlates in convulsions of the newborn. Lancet 1:135–139.

Brown JK, Purvis RJ, Forfar JO, et al. 1974. Neurological aspects of perinatal asphyxia. Dev Med Child Neurol 16:567–580.

Browning RA. 1985. Role of the brainstem reticular formation in tonic-clonic seizures: lesion and pharmacological studies. Fed Proc 44:2425–2431.

Brozanski B, Scher MS, and Albright L. 1988. Intraventricular Nafcilin-induced seizures in a neonate. Pediatr Neurol 4(3):188–190.

Burdjalov VF, Baumgart S, Spitzer AR. 2003. Cerebral function monitoring: a new scoring system for the evaluation of brain maturation in neonates. Pediatrics 112(4):855–861.

Bye AME, and Flanagan D. 1995. Spatial and temporal characteristics of neonatal seizures. Epilepsia 36(10):1009–1016.

Camfield PR, and Camfield CS. 1987. Neonatal seizures: a commentary on selected aspects. J Child Neurol 2:244–251.

Caveness WF, Kato M, Malamut BL, et al. 1980. Propagation of focal motor seizures in the pubescent monkey. Ann Neurol 7:213–221.

Caviness VS Jr. 1989. Normal development of cerebral neocortex. In: Developmental Neurobiology, Eds. Evrard P, Minkowski A, pp. 1–10. New York: Raven Press.

Celesia CG. 1973. Pathophysiology of periodic EEG complexes in subacute sclerosing panencephalitis (SSPE). Electroencephalogr Clin Neurophysiol 35:293–300.

Challamel MJ, Isnard H, Brunon AM, et al. 1984. Asymétrie EEG transitoire a l' entrée dans le sommeil calme chez le nouveau-né: étude sur 75 observations. Rev Electroencephalogr Neurophysiol Clin 14:17–23.

Chatrian GE, Shaw CM, and Leffman H. 1964. The significance of periodic lateralized epileptiform discharges in EEG: an electrographic, clinical and pathological study. Electroencephalogr Clin Neurophysiol 17:177–193.

Chi JG, Dooling EC, and Gilles GH. 1977. Gyral development of the human brain. Ann Neurol 1:86–93.

Clancy RR. 1996. The contribution of EEG to the understanding of neonatal seizures. Epilepsia 37:S52–S59.

Clancy RR, and Fischer RA. 1984. Midline sagittal epileptogenic foci in children. Epilepsia 25:652.

Clancy R, and Legido A. 1987. The exact ictal and interictal duration of electroencephalographic neonatal seizures. Epilepsia 18:537–541.

Clancy RR, and Spitzer AR. 1985. Cerebral cortical function in infants at risk for sudden infant death syndrome. Ann Neurol 18:41–47.

Clancy RR, and Tharp BR. 1984. Positive rolandic sharp waves in the electroencephalograms of premature neonates with intraventricular hemorrhage. Electroencephalogr Clin Neurophysiol 57:395–404.

Clancy RR, Tharp BR, and Enzman D. 1984. EEG in premature infants with intraventricular hemorrhage. Neurology 34:583–590.

Clancy R, Malin S, Laraque D, et al. 1985. Focal motor seizures heralding stroke in full-term neonates. Am J Dis Child 139:601–606.

Cobb WA. 1979. Evidence on the periodic mechanism in herpes simplex encephalitis. Electroencephalogr Clin Neurophysiol 46:345–350.

Cockburn F, Brown JK, Belton NR, et al. 1973. Neonatal convulsions associated with primary disturbance of calcium phosphorus and magnesium metabolism. Arch Dis Child 48:99–118.

Coen RW, McCutchen CB, Wermer D, et al. 1982. Continuous monitoring of electroencephalogram following perinatal asphyxia. J Pediatr 100:628–630.

Collins RC. 1986. Selective vulnerability of the brain: new insights from the excitatory synapse. Metab Brain Dis 1:231–240.

Commission on Classification and Terminology of the International League Against Epilepsy. 1981. Proposal for Revised Clinical and Electroencephalographic Classification of Epileptic Seizures. Epilepsia 22:489–501.

Connell JA, Oozeer R, and Dubowitz V. 1987. Continuous 4-channel EEG monitoring: a guide to interpretation with normal values in preterm infants. Neuropediatrics 18:138–145.

Coolman RB, Bennett FC, Sells CJ, et al. 1985. Neuromotor development of graduates of the neonatal intensive care unit: patterns encountered in the first two years of life. Dev Behav Pediat 6:327–333.

Coulter DL, and Allen RJ. 1982. Benign neonatal sleep myoclonus. Arch Neurol 39:191–192.

Cukier F, Andre M, Monod N, et al. 1972. Apport de l'EEG au diagnostic des hemorragies intra-ventriculaires du prématuré. Rev Electroencephalogr Neurophysiol 2:318–322.

Curzi-Dascalova L, Peirano P, and Morel-Kahn Inserm F. 1988. Development of sleep states in normal premature and full-term newborns. Develop Psychobiol 21:431–444.

Curzi-Dascalova L, Figueroa JM, Eiselt M, et al. 1993. Sleep state organization in premature infants of less than 35 weeks' gestational age. Pediatr Res 34:624–628.

Danner R, Shewmon DA, and Sherman MP. 1985. Seizures in an atelencephalic infant: Is the cortex essential for neonatal seizures? Arch Neurol 42:1014–1016.

De la Paz D, and Brenner RP. 1981. Bilateral independent periodic lateralized epileptiform discharges: clinical significance. Arch Neurol 38:713–715.

Dennis J. 1978. Neonatal convulsions: aetiology, late neonatal status and long-term outcome. Dev Med Child Neurol 21:153–158.

De Weerd AW. 2000. EEG in neonates. What does the neonatal EEG tell about prognosis? In: Clinical Neurophysiology at the Beginning of the 21st Century (Supplements to Clinical Neurophysiology Vol. 53), pp. 243–249.

Dittrichova J, Paul K, and Pavlikova E. 1972. Rapid eye movements in paradoxical sleep in infants. Neuropaediatrie 3:248–257.

Dooling EC, Chi JG, and Gilles FH. 1983. Telencephalic development: changing gyral patterns. In: Gilles FH, Leviton A, Dooling EC (eds.) The Developing Brain, p. 94. Boston: Wright.

Dorovini-Zis K, and Dolman CL. 1977. Gestational development of brain. Arch Pathol Lab Med 101:192–195.

Doyle LW, Nahmias C, Firnau G, et al. 1983. Regional cerebral glucose metabolism of newborn infants measured by positron emission tomography. Dev Med Child Neurol 25:143–151.

Dreyfus-Brisac C. 1964. The electroencephalogram of the premature infant and full-term newborn: normal and abnormal development of waking and sleeping patterns. In: Kellaway P, Petersén I (eds.). Neurological and Electroencephalographic Correlative Studies in Infancy, pp 186–206. New York: Grune & Stratton.

Dreyfus-Brisac C. 1968. Sleep ontogenesis in early human prematurity from 24 to 27 weeks of conceptional age. Dev Psychobiol 1:162–169.

Dreyfus-Brisac C. 1970. Ontogenesis of sleep in human prematures after 32 weeks of conceptional age. Dev Psychobiol 3:91–121.

Dreyfus-Brisac C. 1979. Neonatal electroencephalography. In: Scarpelli EM, Cosmie EV (eds). Reviews in Perinatal Medicine, Vol 3, pp. 397–430. New York: Raven Press.

Dreyfus-Brisac C, and Blanc C. 1956. Électroencéphalogramme et maturation cerebrale. Encephale 45:205–241.

Dreyfus-Brisac C, and Larroche JC. 1972. Discontinuous EEGs in premature and full-term neonates. Electro-anatomo-clinical correlations. Electroencephalogr Clin Neurophysiol 32:575.

Dreyfus-Brisac C, and Monod N. 1970. Sleeping behavior in abnormal newborn infants. Neuropadiatrie 1:354–366.

Dreyfus-Brisac C, Samson-Dreyfus D, and Fischgold H. 1955. Activite electrique cerebrale du premature et du nouveau-ne. Ann Pediatr 31:1–7.

Dreyfus-Brisac C, Fischgold H, Samson-Dollfus D, et al. 1957. Veille, sommeil, réactivité sensorielle chez le prématuré, le nouveaune le nourrisson. Electroencephalogr Clin Neurophysiol [Suppl.] 6:417–440.

Dreyfus-Brisac C, Flescher J, and Plassart E. 1962. L'électroencéphalogramme Crité d'âge conceptionnel du nouveau-né à terme et du prématuré. Biol Neonat 4:154–173.

Drillien CM, Thompson AJM, and Burgoyne K. 1980. Low-birthweight children at early school age: a longitudinal study. Dev Med Child Neurol 22:26–47.

Dubowitz LMS, Dubowitz V, and Goldberg C. 1970. Clinical assessment of gestational age in the newborn infant. Pediatrics 77:1–10.

Dwyer BE, and Wasterlain CG. 1982. Electroconvulsive seizures in the immature rat adversely affect myelin accumulation. Exp Neurol 78:616–628.

Eble A, Co S, and Jones MG. 1981. Clinical correlates of midline spikes. An analysis of 21 patients. Arch Neurol 38:355–357.

Edwards MK, Brown DL, Muller J, et al. 1980. Cribside neurosonography: realtime sonography for intracranial investigation of the neonate. AJNR 1:501.

Eilers BL, Desai NS, Wilson MA, et al. 1986. Classroom performance and social factors of children with birthweights of 1,250 grams or less: follow-up at 5 to 8 years of age. Pediatrics 77:203–208.

Eiselt M, Schendel M, Witte H, et al. 1997. Quantitative analysis of discontinuous EEG in premature and full-term newborns during quiet sleep. Electroencephalogr Clin Neurophysiol 103(5):528–534.

Eiselt M, Schindler J, Arnold M, et al. 2001. Functional interactions within the newborn brain investigated by adaptive coherence analysis of EEG. Neurophysiol Clin 31(2):104–113.

Ellingson RJ. 1958. Electroencephalograms of normal full-term newborns immediately after birth with observations on arousal and visual evoked responses. Electroencephalogr Clin Neurophysiol 10:31–50.

Ellingson RJ. 1960. Cortical electrical responses to visual stimulation in the human infant. Electroencephalogr Clin Neurophysiol 12:663–677.

Ellingson RJ. 1964. Studies of the electrical activity of the developing human brain. In: Himwich WA and EH (eds.) The Developing Brain-Progress in Brain Research, pp. 26–53. Amsterdam: Elsevier.

Ellingson RJ, and Peters JF. 1980. Development of EEG and daytime sleep patterns in low risk premature infants during the first year of life: Longitudinal observations. Electroencephalogr Clin Neurophysiol 50:165.

Ellingson RJ, Dutch SJ, and McIntire MS. 1974. EEGs of prematures: 3–8 year follow-up study. Develop Psychobiol 7:529–538.

Erkinjuntti M, and Kero P. 1985. Heart rate response related to body movements in healthy and neurologically damaged infants during sleep. Early Hum Dev 12:31–37.

Eriksson M, and Zetterström R. 1979. Neonatal convulsions. Incidence and causes in the Stockholm area. Acta Paediatr Scand 68:807–811.

Ersyukova II. 1980. Oculomotor activity and autonomic indices of newborn infants during paradoxical sleep. Hum Physiol 6:57–64.

Estivill E, Monod N, and Amiel-Tison C. 1977. Etude électro-encéphalographique d'un cas d'encéphalite herpétique néo-natale. Rev EEG Neurophysiol 7:380–385.

Eyre JA, Oozen RC, and Wilkinson AR. 1983. Continuous electroencephalographic recording to detect seizures in paralyzed newborns. Br Med J 286:1017–1018.

Eyre JA, Nanei S, and Wilkinson AR. 1988. Quantification of changes in normal neonatal EEGs with gestation from continuous five-day recordings. Dev Med Child Neurol 30:599–607.

Fenichel GM, Olson BJ, and Fitzpatrick JE. 1979. Heart rate changes in convulsive and nonconvulsive apnea. Ann Neurol 7:577–582.

Field T, Diego M, Hernandez-Reif M, et al. 2002. Relative right versus left frontal EEG in neonates. Dev Psychobiol 41(2):147–155.

Ford GW, Rickards AL, Kitchen WH, et al. 1985. Handicaps and health problems in 2 year old children of birthweight 500 to 1500 g. Aust Paediatr J 21:15–22.

Freeman M, ed. 1985. *Prenatal and Perinatal Factors Associated with Brain Disorders.* Bethesda, MD: NIH Publications, No. 85–1149.

Fukumoto M, Mochizuki N, Takeishi M, et al. 1981. Studies of body movements during night sleep in infancy. Brain Dev 3:37–43.

Gal P, Toback J, Boer HR, et al. 1982. Efficacy of phenobarbital monotherapy in treatment of neonatal seizures. Relationship to blood levels. Neurology 32:1401–1404.

Giaquinto S, Marciano F, Monod N, et al. 1977. Applications of statistical equivalence to newborn EEG recordings. Electroencephalogr Clin Neurophysiol 42:406–413.

Gloor P. 1985. General introduction. In: Gotman J, Ives JR, Gloor P (eds). *Long-Term Monitoring in Epilepsy.* Elsevier, Amsterdam, New York. Electroencephalogr Clin Neurophysiol, suppl 37:xiii–xx.

Glotzbach SF, Tansey PA, Baldwin RB, et al. 1989. Periodic breathing cycle duration in preterm infants. Pediatr Res 25:258–261.

Glotzbach SF, Edgar DM, and Ariagno RL. 1995. Biological rhythmicity in preterm infants prior to discharge from neonatal intensive care. Pediatrics 95:231–237.

Goldberg HJ. 1983. Convulsions: a ten year review. J Arch Dis Child 58:976–978.

Goldberg RN, Goldman SL, Ramsay RE, et al. 1982. Detection of seizure activity in the paralyzed neonate using continuous monitoring. Pediatrics 69:583–586.

Goldie L, Svedsen-Rhodes U, Easton J, et al. 1971. The development of innate sleep rhythms in short gestation infants. Dev Med Child Neurol 13:40–50.

Goldman-Rakic PS. 1987. Development of cortical circuitry and cognitive function. Child Dev 58:601–622.

Gooding CA, Brasch RC, Lallemand DP, et al. 1984. Nuclear magnetic resonance imaging of the brain in children. J Pediatr 104:509–515.

Gottman J. 1983. Measurement of small time differences between EEG channels: method and application to epileptic seizure propagation. Electroencephalogr Clin Neurophysiol 56:501–514.

Gurses D, Kilic I, Sahiner T. 2002. Effects of hyperbilirubinemia on cerebrocortical electrical activity in newborns. Pediatr Res 52(1):125–130.

Hack M. 1997. Effects of intrauterine growth retardation on mental performance and behavior, outcomes during adolescence and adulthood. Eur J Clin Nutr 52:S1, 65–71.

Hack M, Fanaroff AA. 1999. Outcomes of children of extremely low birth weight and gestational age in the 1990's. Early Hum Dev 53:193–218.

Hack M, Caron B, Rivers A, et al. 1983. The very low birthweight infant: the broader spectrum of morbidity during infancy and early childhood. Dev Behav Pediat 4:243–249.

Hack M, Friedman H, and Fanaroff AA. 1996. Outcomes of extremely low birth weight infants. Pediatrics 98:931–937.

Hahn JS, and Tharp BR. 1990. The dysmature EEG pattern in infants with bronchopulmonary dysplasia and its prognostic implications. Electroencephalogr Clin Neurophysiol 76:106–113.

Hahn JS, Monyer H, and Tharp BR. 1989. Interburst interval measurements in the EEGs of premature infants with normal neurological outcome. Electroencephalogr Clin Neurophysiol 73:410–418.

Hakamada S, Watanabe K, Hara K, et al. 1981. Development of the motor behavior during sleep in newborn infants. Brain Dev 3:345–350.

Halliday AM. 1967. The electrophysiological study of myoclonus in man. Brain 90:241–284.

Harper RM, Leake B, Miyahara L, et al. 1981. Development of ultradian periodicity and coalescence at 1 cycle per hour in electroencephalographic activity. Exp Neurol 73:127–143.

Harris R, Tizard JP. 1960. The electroencephalogram in neonatal convulsions. J Pediatr 50:501–520.

Havlicek V, Chiliaeva R, and Chernick V. 1975. EEG frequency spectrum characteristics of sleep states in full-term and pre-term infants. Neuropaediatrie 6:24–40.

Hayakawa F, Watanabe K, Hakamada S, et al. 1987. FZ theta/alpha bursts: A transient EEG pattern in healthy newborns. Electroencephalogr Clin Neurophysiol 67:27–31.

Hayakawa F, Okumura A, Kato T, et al. 1999. Determination of timing of brain injury in preterm infants with periventricular leukomalacia with serial neonatal electroencephalography. Pediatrics 104:1077–1081.

Hayakawa M, Okumura A, Hayakawa F, et al. 2003. Nutritional state and growth and functional maturation of the brain in extremely low birth weight infants. Pediatrics 111:991–995.

Hellbrugge T. 1960. The development of circadian rhythms in infants. Cold Spring Harbor Symp Quant Biol 25:311–323.

Hellbrugge T. 1968. Ontogenese des rhythmes circadaires chez l'enfant. In: Ajuriaguerra J de (ed.). *Cycle Biologiques et Psychiatrie,* pp. 159–183. Geneva and Paris: Masson.

Hellström-Westas L. 1992. Comparison between tape recorded amplitude integrated EEG monitoring and sick newborn infants. Acta Pediatr 81:812–819.

Helström-Westas L, Rosen I, and Sweningen NW. 1985. Silent seizures in sick infants in early life. Acta Paediatr Scand 74:741–748.

Hildebrandt G. 1986. Functional significance of ultradian rhythms and reactive periodicity. J Interdisc Cycle Res 17:307–319.

Hill A, and Volpe JJ. 1981. Seizures, hypoxic-ischemic brain injury and intraventricular hemorrhage in the newborn. Ann Neurol 10:109–121.

Hill LM, Breckle R, and Gehrking WC. 1983. The prenatal detection of congenital malformations by ultrasonography. Mayo Clin Proc 58:805.

Holden KR, Mellits ED, and Freeman JM. 1982. Neonatal seizures. I. Correlation of prenatal and perinatal events with outcomes. Pediatrics 70:165–176.

Holmes G. 1987. Diagnosis and management of seizures in childhood. In: Markowitz M (ed.). *Major Problems in Clinical Pediatrics,* vol. 30. Philadelphia: WB Saunders.

Holmes G. 1989. Electrodiagnosis in neurologic prognosis: Prognostic value of EEG and EPs in newborns and young infants. Reproduced in part from "EEG Abnormalities in Neonates." American EEG Society course text.

Holmes G, Logan WJ, Kirkpatrick BV, et al. 1979. Central nervous system maturation in the stressed premature. Ann Neurol 6:518–522.

Holmes G, Rowe J, Hafford J, et al. 1982. Prognostic value of electroencephalogram in neonatal asphyxia. Electroencephalogr Clin Neurophysiol 53:60–72.

Holthausen K, Breidbach O, Scheidt B, et al. 2000. Brain dysmaturity index for automatic detection of high-risk infants. Pediatr Neurol 22(3):187–91.

Hope PL, Costello AM, Cady EB, et al. 1984. Cerebral energy metabolism studied with phosphorus NMR spectroscopy in normal and birth-asphyxiated infants. Lancet 2:366–370.

Hosokawa S, Iguchi T, Caveness WF, et al. 1980. Effects of manipulation of sensorimotor system on focal motor seizures in the monkey. Ann Neurol 7:222–229.

Hrachovy RA, Mizrahi EM, and Kellaway P. 1990. Electroencephalography of the Newborn. In: Daly DD, Pedley TA (eds). *Current Practice of Clinical Electroencephalography,* 2nd ed., pp. 201–242. New York: Raven Press.

Hughes JR, Fino J, and Gagnon L. 1983a. The use of the electroencephalogram in the confirmation of seizures in premature and neonatal infants. Neuropediatrics 14:213–219.

Hughes JR, Fino J, and Gagnon L. 1983b. Periods of activity and quiescence in the premature EEG. Neuropediatrics 14:66–72.

Hughes JR, Fino JJ, and Hart LA. 1987. Premature temporal theta. Electroencephalogr Clin Neurophysiol 67:7–15.

Hughes JR, Miller JK, Fino JJ, et al. 1990. The sharp theta rhythm on the occipital areas of prematures (STOP): a newly described waveform. Clin Electroencephalogr 21:77–87.

Hughes PE, Alexi T, Walton M, et al. 1999. Activity and injury-dependent expression of inducible transcription factors, growth factors and apoptosis-related genes within the central nervous system. Prog Neurobiol 57: 421–450.

Huppi PS, Warfield S, Kikinis R, et al. 1998. Quantitative magnetic resonance imaging of brain development in premature and mature newborns. Ann Neurol 43:224–235.

Inder TE, Buckland L, Williams CE, et al. 2003. Lowered electroencephalographic spectral edge frequency predicts the presence of cerebral white matter injury in premature infants. Pediatrics 111(1):27–33.

Johnson MA, Pennock JM, Bydder GM, et al. 1983. Clinical NMR imaging of the brain in children: Normal and neurological disease. AJR 141: 1005–1018.

Johnson MW, Scher MS. 2003. Cyclicity of neonatal sleep behaviors at 25 to 30 weeks corrected gestational age. Sleep 26(suppl):A144–145.

Johnston MV, and Silverstein FS. 1985. New insights into mechanisms of neuronal damage in the developing brain. Pediatr Neurosci 12:87–89.

Johnston MV, Trescher WH, and Taylor GA. 1995. Hypoxic and ischemic central nervous system disorders in infants and children. Acta Pediatr 42:1–45.

Joseph JP, Lesevre N, and Dreyfus-Brisac C. 1976. Spatio-temporal organization of EEG in premature infants and full-term newborns. Electroencephalogr Clin Neurophysiol 40:153–168.

Karbowski K, and Nencka A. 1980. Right mid-temporal sharp EEG transients in healthy newborns. Electroencephalogr Clin Neurol 48:461–469.

Keene JH, and Lee D. 1973. The sequelae of neurological convulsions. The study of 112 infants. Arch Dis Child 48:541–542.

Kellaway P, and Crawley JW. 1964. *A Primer of Electroencephalography of Infants, Sections I & II: Methodology and Criteria of Normality.* Houston: Baylor University College of Medicine.

Kellaway P, and Petersen I. 1964. *Neurological and Electroencephalographic Correlative Studies in Infancy.* New York: Grune & Stratton.

Kellaway P, Hrachovy RA. 1983. Status epilepticus in newborns: a perspective on neonatal seizures. In Delgado-Escueta AV, Wasterlain CG, Treiman DM, Porter RJ (Eds). Status Epilepticus: Mechanisms of Brain Damage and Treatment. New York: Raven Press, 34:93–99.

Kennedy WA. 1959. Clinical and electroencephalographic aspects of epileptogenic lesions of the medial surface and superior border of the cerebral hemisphere. Brain 82:147–161.

Krieger DN, Lofink RM, Doyle EL, et al. 1987. Neuronet: implementation of an integrated clinical neurophysiology system. Med Instrum 217:296–303.

Ktonas PY, Fagioli I, Salzarulo P. 1995. Delta (0.5–1.5 Hz) and sigma (11.5–15.5 Hz) EEG power dynamics throughout quiet sleep in infants. Electroencephalogr Clin Neurophysiol 95(2):90–96.

Kuhle S, Klebermass K, Olischar M, et al. 2001. Sleep-wake cycles in preterm infants below 30 weeks of gestational age. Preliminary results of a prospective amplitude-integrated EEG study. Wien Klin Wochenschr 113 (7–8):219–223.

Kuks JBM, Vos JE, and O'Brien MJ. 1988. EEG coherence functions for normal newborns in relation to their sleep state. Electroencephalogr Clin Neurophysiol 69:295–302.

Kuroiwa Y, and Celesia CG. 1980. Clinical significance of periodic EEG patterns. Arch Neurol 37:15–20.

Larroche JC. 1967. Maturation cerebrale et hypodeveloppement ponderal du nouveaune. J Neurol Sci 5:39–59.

Larroche JC. 1968. Nécrose cérébrale massive chez le nouveau-né. Biol Neonat 13:340.

Lefebvre F, Bard H, Veilleux A, et al. 1988. Outcome at school age of children with birthweights of 1000 grams or less. Dev Med Child Neurol 30:170–180.

Lehtonen J, Kononen M, Purhonen M, et al. 1998. The effect of nursing on the brain activity of the newborn. J Pediatr 132(4):646–651.

Lehtonen L, Johnson MW, Martin RJ, et al. 2002. Sleep state disruptions impair oxygenation in ventilated ELBW infants as detected by behavioral/EEG analyses. J Pediatrics141(3):363–368.

Lesse S, Hoefer PFA, and Austin JH. 1958. The electroencephalogram in diffuse encephalopathies. AMA Arch Neurol Psychiatr 79:359–375.

Levy SR, Abroms IF, Marshall PC, et al. 1985. Seizures and cerebral infarction in the full-term newborn. Ann Neurol 17:366–370.

Liu A, Hahn JS, Heldt GP, et al. 1993. Detection of neonatal seizures through computerized EEG analysis. Electroencephalogr Clin Neurophysiol 24:19–24.

Lockman LA, Kriel R, Zaske D, et al. 1979. Phenobarbital dosage for control of neonatal seizures. Neurology 29:1445–1449.

Lombroso CT. 1979. Quantified electrographic scales on 10 pre-term healthy newborns followed up to 40–43 weeks of conceptional age by serial polygraphic recordings. Electroencephalogr Clin Neurophysiol 46: 460–474.

Lombroso CT. 1985. Neonatal polygraphy in full-term and preterm infants: A review of normal and abnormal findings. J Clin Neurophysiol 2: 105–155.

Lombroso CT. 1989. Neonatal electroencephalography. In: Niedermeyer E, Lopez-Desilva F (eds.). *Electroencephalography, Basic Principles, Clinical Applications in Related Fields,* pp. 599–637. Baltimore and Munich: Urban and Schwarzenberg.

Lombroso CT, and Matsumiya Y. 1985. Stability in waking-sleep states in neonates as a predictor of long-term neurologic outcome. Pediatrics 76:52–63.

Lynch JA, and Aserinsky E. 1986. Developmental changes of oculomotor characteristics in infants when awake and in the active state of sleep. Behav Brain Res 20:175–183.

Markand ON, and Daly DD. 1971. Pseudoperiodic lateralized paroxysmal discharges in electroencephalogram. Neurology 21:975–981.

Marlow N, Hunt LP, and Chiswick ML. 1988. Clinical factors associated with adverse outcome for babies weighing 2000 g or less at birth. Arch Dis Child 63:1131–1136.

Marret S, Parain D, Samson-Dollfus D, et al. 1986. Positive rolandic sharp waves and periventricular leukomalacia in the newborn. Neuropediatrics 17:199–202.

Marret S, Parain D, Ménard J-F, et al. 1997. Diagnostic value of neonatal electroencephalography in premature newborns less than 33 weeks of gestational age. Electroencephalogr Clin Neurophysiol 102:178–185.

Martin RJ, Miller MJ, and Carlo WA. 1986. Pathogenesis of apnea in preterm infants. J Pediatr 109:733–741.

McCutcheon CB, Coen R, and Iragui VJ. 1984. Periodic lateralized epileptiform discharges in asphyxiated neonates. Electroencephalogr Clin Neurophysiol 61:201–217.

McLachlan RS, Rose KJ, Derry PA, et al. 1997. Health-related quality of life and seizure control in temporal lobe epilepsy. Ann Neurol 41:482–489.

Ment LR, Duncan CC, and Ehrenkranz RA. 1984. Perinatal cerebral infarction. Ann Neurol 16:559–568.

Michelsson K, Lindahl E, Parre M, et al. 1984. Nine-year follow-up of infants weighing 1500 g or less at birth. Acta Paediatr Scand 73:835–841.

Mirimiran M, and Kok JH. 1991. Circadian rhythm in early human development. Early Hum Dev 262:121–128.

Mizrahi EM. 1984. Electroencephalographic/polygraphic/video monitoring in childhood epilepsy. J Pediatr 105:1–12.

Mizrahi EM, and Kellaway P. 1987. Characterization and classification of neonatal seizures. Neurology 37:1837–1844.

Mizrahi EM, and Tharp BR. 1982. Characteristic EEG pattern in neonatal herpes simplex encephalitis. Neurology 32:1215–1220.

Monod N, and Garma L. 1971. Auditory responsivity in the human premature. Biol Neonate 292–316.

Monod N, and Tharp B. 1977. Activité électroencéphalographique normale du nouveau-né et du prématuré au cours des états de veille et de sommeil. Rev EEG Neurophysiol 7:302–315.

Monod D, Dreyfus-Brisac C, Ducas P, et al. 1960. L'EEG du nouveauné à terme. Étude comparative chez le nouveau-né en présentation céphalique et en présentation de siége. Rev Neurol 102:375–379.

Monod N, Pajot N, and Guidasci S. 1972. The neonatal EEG: statistical studies and prognostic value in full-term and preterm babies. Electroencephalogr Clin Neurophysiol 32:529–544.

Myers MM, Fifer WP, Grose-Fifer J, et al. 1997. A novel quantitative measure of trace-alternant EEG activity and its association with sleep states of preterm infants. Dev Psychobiol 31(3):167–174.

Neidermeyer E, Bauer G, Burnite R, et al. 1977. Selective stimulus-sensitive myoclonus in acute cerebral anoxia. Arch Neurol 34:365–368.

Nelson KB, and Ellenberg JH. 1987. The asymptomatic newborn and risk of cerebral palsy. AJDC 141:1333–1335.

Nelson KR, Brenner RP, and de la Paz D. 1983. Midline spikes. EEG and clinical features. Arch Neurol 40:473–476.

Nickel RE, Bennett FC, and Lamson FN. 1982. School performance of children with birthweights of 1,000 g or less. Am J Dis Child 136:105.

Novotny E, Ashwal S, and Shevell M. 1998. Proton magnetic resonance spectroscopy: an emerging technology in pediatric neurology research. Pediatr Res 44:1–10.

Novotny EJ Jr, Tharp BR, Coen RW, et al. 1987. Positive rolandic sharp waves in the EEG of the premature infant. Neurology 37:1481–1486.

Nowack WJ, Abdorasool J, and Angtuaco T. 1989. Positive temporal sharp waves in neonatal EEG. Clin Electroencephalogr 20(3):196–201.

Nunes ML, Da Costa JC, and Moura-Ribeiro MVL. 1997. Polysomnographic quantification of bioelectrical maturation in preterm and full-term newborns at matched conceptional ages. Electroencephalogr Clin Neurophysiol 102:186–191.

O'Brien MJ, Lems YL, and Prechtl HFR. 1987. Transient flattenings in the EEG of newborns—a benign variation. Electroencephalogr Clin Neurophysiol 67:16–26.

Ohtahara S. 1978. Clinico-electrical delineation of epileptic encephalopathies in childhood. Asian Med J 21:7–17.

Okamato Y, and Kirikae T. 1951. Electroencephalographic studies on brain of foetus, of children of premature birth and newborn, together with a note on reactions of foetus brain upon drugs. Folia Psychiatr Neurol Jpn 5:135–146.

Okumura A, Hayakawa F, Kato T, et al. 2003. Abnormal sharp transients on electroencephalograms in preterm infants with periventricular leukomalacia. J Pediatr 143:26–30.

Olson DM, and Shewmon DA. 1989. Electroencephalographic abnormalities in infants with hypoplastic left heart syndrome. Pediatr Neurol 5(2):93–98.

Ortibus EL, Sum JM, and Hahn JJ. 1996. Predictive value of EEG for outcome and epilepsy following neonatal seizures. Electroencephalogr Clin Neurophysiol 98:175–185.

Painter MJ, Scher MS, Alvin J, et al. 1999. A comparison of the efficacy of phenobarbital and phenytoin in the treatment of neonatal seizures. N Engl J Med 341(7):485–489.

Pan XL, Ogawa T. 1999. Microstructure of longitudinal 24 hour electroencephalograms in healthy preterm infants. Pediatr Int 41(1):18–27.

Pape KE, Bennett-Britton S, Szymonowicz W, et al. 1983. Diagnostic accuracy of neonatal brain imaging: a postmortem correlation of computed tomography and ultrasound scans. J Pediatr 102:275–280.

Parmelee AH Jr. 1967. Changes in sleep patterns in premature infants as a function of brain maturation. In Minkowski A (ed.): *Regional Development of the Brain in Early Life*, p. 459. Oxford: F.A. Davis.

Parmelee AH, and Stern R. 1972. Development of states in infants. In: Clemente DC, Purpurer DP, Mayer EE (eds.). *Sleep and the Maturing Nervous System*, pp. 199–228. New York: Academic Press.

Parmelee AH, Schulte FJ, Akiyama Y, et al. 1968. Maturation of EEG activity during sleep in premature infants. Electroencephalogr Clin Neurophysiol 24:319–329.

Parmelee AH, Akiyama Y, Stern E, et al. 1969. A periodic cerebral rhythm in newborn infants. Exp Neurol 25:575–584.

Patrizi S, Holmes GL, Orzalesi M, et al. 2003. Neonatal seizures: characteristics of EEG ictal activity in preterm and full-term infants. Brain Dev 25:427–437.

Paul K, Krajca V, Roth Z, et al. 2003. Comparison of quantitative EEG characteristics of quiet and active sleep in newborns. Sleep Med 4:543–552.

PeBenito R, and Cracco JB. 1979. Periodic lateralized epileptiform discharges in infants and children. Ann Neurol 6:47–50.

Pedley TA, Tharp BR, and Herman K. 1981. Clinical and electroencephalographic characteristics of midline parasagittal foci. Ann Neurol 9:142–149.

Perlman JM, and Volpe JJ. 1983. Seizures in the preterm infant: effects on cerebral blood flow velocity, intracranial pressure, and arterial blood pressure. J Pediatr 102:288–293.

Petre-Quadens O, and de Lee C. 1970. Eye movements during sleep: a common criterion of learning capacities and endocrine activity. Dev Med Child Neurol 12:730–740.

Pettit RE, and Fenichel GM. 1980. Benign familial neonatal seizures. Arch Neurol 37:47–48.

Pezzani C, Radvanyi E, Bouvet MF, et al. 1986. Neonatal electroencephalography during the first twenty-four hours of life in full-term newborn infants. Neuropediatrics 17:11–18.

Prechtl HFR. 1974. The behavioral states of the newborn infant. Brain Res 76:185–212.

Prechtl HFR. 1984. Continuity of neural functions from prenatal to postnatal life. In: *Spastics International Medical Publications*, pp. 1–255.

Oxford: Blackwell Scientific Publications Ltd., Philadelphia: J.B. Lippincott.

Prechtl HFR, and Lenard HG. 1967. A study of eye movements in sleeping newborn infants. Brain Res 5:477–493.

Prechtl HFR, and Nijhuis JG. 1983. Eye movements in the human fetus and newborn. Behav Brain Res 10:119–124.

Prechtl HFR, Weinmann H, and Akiyama Y. 1969. Organization of physiological parameters in normal and neurologically abnormal infants. Neuropaediatrie 1:101–109.

Prechtl HFR, Fargel JW, Weinmann HM, et al. 1979. Postures, motility and respiration of low risk preterm infants. Dev Med Child Neurol 21:3–27.

Pressler RM, Boylan GB, Morton M, et al. 2001. Early serial EEG in hypoxic ischaemic encephalopathy. Clin Neurophysiol 112:31–37.

Radermecker J. 1955. The EEG in the encephalitides and related cerebral conditions. Electroencephalogr Clin Neurophysiol 7:488.

Radvanyi-Bouvet MF, Vallecalle MH, Morel-Kahn F, et al. 1985. Seizures and electrical discharges in preterm infants. Neuropediatrics 16:143–148.

Rantakallio P, and von Wendt L. 1985. Prognosis for low-birthweight infants up to the age of 14: a population study. Dev Med Child Neurol 27:655–663.

Regalado MG, Schechtman VL, Khoo MC, et al. 2001. Spectral analysis of heart rate variability and respiration during sleep in cocaine-exposed neonates. Clin Physiol 21(4):428–436.

Resnick TJ, Moshe SL, Perotta L, et al. 1986. Benign neonatal sleep myoclonus: relationship to sleep states. Arch Neurol 43:266–268.

Richards JE, Parmelee AH Jr, and Beckwith L. 1986. Spectral analysis of infant EEG and behavioral outcome at age five. Electroencephalogr Clin Neurophysiol 64:1–11.

Robertson SS. 1982. Intrinsic temporal patterning in the spontaneous movement of awake neonates. Child Dev 53:1016–1021.

Robertson SS. 1987. Human cyclic motility: fetal-newborn continuities and newborn state differences. Dev Psychobiol 20:425–442.

Rose AL, and Lombroso CT. 1970. Neonatal seizure states. A study of clinical, pathological, and electroencephalographic features in 137 full-term babies with a long-term follow up. Pediatrics 45:404–425.

Rowe JC, Holmes GL, Hafford J, et al. 1985. Prognostic value of electroencephalogram in term and preterm infants following neonatal seizures. Electroencephalogr Clin Neurophysiol 60:183–196.

Rumack CM, Manco-Johnson ML, Manco-Johnson MJ, et al. 1985. Timing and course of neonatal intracranial hemorrhage using realtime ultrasound. Radiology 154:101–105.

Sainio K, Granstrom E, Pettay O, et al. 1983. EGG in neonatal herpes simplex encephalitis. Electroencephalogr Clin Neurophysiol 56:556–561.

Saint-Anne Dargassies S. 1974. *Le developpement neurologique du nouveaune a term et premature*. Paris: Masson et Cie.

Samson-Dollfus D. 1955. L'électroencéphalogramme du prématuré jusqu'à l'âge de trois mois et du nouveau-né à terme. Thesis Med. Paris: Foulon.

Sawaguchi H, Ogawa T, Takano T, et al. 1996. Developmental changes in electroencephalogram for term and preterm infants using an autoregressive model. Acta Paediatr Jpn 38(6):580–589.

Schechtman VL, Harper RK, Harper RM. 1995. Aberrant temporal patterning of slow-wave sleep in siblings of SIDS victims. Electroencephalogr Clin Neurophysiol 94(2):95–102.

Scher MS. 1985a. Physiologic artifacts in neonatal electroencephalography. AM J EEG Technol 25:257–277.

Scher MS. 1985b. The value of midline electrodes in neonatal electroencephalography. Am J EEG Technol 25:241–255.

Scher MS. 1985c. Pathological myoclonus of the newborn: electrographic and clinical correlations. Pediatr Neurol 1:342–348.

Scher MS. 1988a. A developmental marker of central nervous system maturation: Part I. Pediatr Neurol 4:265–273.

Scher MS. 1988b. A developmental marker of central nervous system maturation: Part II. Pediatr Neurol 4:329–336.

Scher MS. 1988c. Midline electrographic abnormalities and cerebral lesions in the newborn brain. J Child Neurol 3:135–146.

Scher MS. 1991. Spikes and sharp waves in the neonatal EEG: physiologic and clinical significance. Am J EEG Technol 31:145–172.

Scher MS. 1994. Neonatal encephalopathies as classified by EEG-sleep criteria. Severity and timing based on clinical/pathologic correlations. Pediatr Neurol 11:189–200.

Scher MS. 1996. Normal electrographic-polysomnographic patterns in preterm and full-term infants. Semin Pediatr Neurol 3(1):12.

Scher MS. 1997a. Seizures in the newborn infant. Diagnosis, treatment, and outcome. Clin Perinatol 24:735–772.

Scher MS. 1997b. Neurophysiological assessment of brain function and maturation. I. A measure of brain adaptation in high risk infants. Pediatr Neurol 16:191–198.

Scher MS. 1997c. Neurophysiological assessment of brain function and maturation. II. A measure of brain dysmaturity in healthy preterm neonates. Pediatr Neurol 16:287–295.

Scher MS. 2001. Perinatal asphyxia: timing and mechanisms of injury in neonatal encephalopathy. Curr Neurol Neurosci Rep 1:175–184.

Scher MS. 2002. Controversies regarding neonatal seizure recognition. Epileptic Disord 4:138–158.

Scher MS, and Barmada M. 1987. Estimation of gestational age by electrographic, clinical, and anatomical criteria. Pediatr Neurol 3:256–262.

Scher MS, and Beggarly M. 1989. Clinical significance of focal periodic patterns in the newborn. J Child Neurol 4:175–185.

Scher MS, and Painter MJ. 1989. Controversies concerning neonatal seizures. In: Pellock JM (ed.). Seizure Disorders. The Pediatric Clinics of North America, 36(2):281–310. Philadelphia: WB Saunders.

Scher MS, and Painter MJ. 1990. Electrographic diagnosis of neonatal seizures. Issues of diagnostic accuracy, clinical correlation and survival. In: Wasterlain CG, Vert P (eds.). Neonatal Seizures. New York: Raven Press.

Scher MS, and Tharp B. 1982. Significance of focal abnormalities in neonatal EEG-radiologic correlation and outcome. Ann Neurol 12:217.

Scher MS, Barmada M, Fria T, et al. 1986a. Neonatal nonketotic hyperglycinemia: correlation of neurophysiological and neuropathological findings. Neuropediatrics 17:137–144.

Scher MS, Klesh KW, Murphy TF, et al. 1986b. Seizures and infarction in neonates with persistent pulmonary hypertension. Pediatr Neurol 2:332–339.

Scher MS, Painter MJ, and Guthrie RD. 1988a. Cerebral neurophysiological assessment of the high-risk neonate. In Guthrie RD (ed). Recent Advances in Neonatal Care. In the series, Clinics in Critical Care Medicine. New York: Churchill Livingstone.

Scher MS, Richardson GA, Coble PA, et al. 1988b. The effects of prenatal alcohol and marijuana exposure: Disturbances in neonatal sleep cycling and arousal. Pediatr Res 24:101–105.

Scher MS, Painter MJ, Bergman I, et al. 1989. EEG diagnoses of neonatal seizures: Clinical correlations and outcome. Pediatr Neurol 5:17–24.

Scher MS, Sun M, Hatzilabrou GM, et al. 1990. Computer analyses of EEG sleep in the neonate: Methodological considerations. J Clin Neurophysiol 7(3):417–441.

Scher MS, Steppe DA, Dahl RE, et al. 1992. Comparison of EEG-sleep measures in healthy full-term and preterm infants at matched conceptional ages. Sleep 15(5):442–448.

Scher MS, Hamid MY, Steppe DA, et al. 1993. Ictal and interictal durations in preterm and term neonates. Epilepsia 34(2):284–288.

Scher MS, Alvin J, Gaus L, et al. 1994b. Uncoupling of electrical and clinical expression of neonatal seizures after antiepileptic drug administration. Pediatr Neurol 11(2):83.

Scher MS, Bova JM, Dokianakis SG, et al. 1994c. Physiological significance of sharp wave transients on EEG recordings of healthy preterm and full-term neonates. Electroencephalogr Clin Neurophys 90:179–185.

Scher MS, Bova JM, Dokianakis SG, et al. 1994d. Positive temporal sharp waves on EEG recordings of healthy neonates: a benign pattern of dysmaturity in preterm infants at postconceptional term ages. Electroencephalogr Clin Neurophys 90:173–178.

Scher MS, Dokianakis SG, Sun M, et al. 1994e. Rectal temperature changes during sleep state transitions in full-term and preterm neonates at postconceptional term ages. Pediatr Neurol 10:191–194.

Scher MS, Steppe DA, Dokianakis SG, et al. 1994f. Maturation of phasic and continuity measures during sleep in preterm neonates. Pediatr Res 36:732–737.

Scher MS, Steppe DA, Dokianakis SG, et al. 1994g. Cardiorespiratory behavior during sleep in full-term and preterm neonates at comparable postconceptional term ages. Pediatr Res 36:738–744.

Scher MS, Sun M, Steppe DA, et al. 1994h. Comparisons of EEG state-specific spectral values between healthy full-term and preterm infants at comparable postconceptional ages. Sleep 17(1):47–51.

Scher MS, Sun M, Steppe DA, et al. 1994i. Comparisons of EEG spectral and correlation measures between healthy term and preterm infants. Pediatr Neurol 10:104–108.

Scher MS, Sinha S, Martin J, et al. 1995a. Estimation of gestational maturity of preterm infants by five fetal sonographic measurements compared with neonatal EEG and the last menstrual period. Electroencephalogr Clin Neurophysiol 95:408–413.

Scher MS, Steppe DA, Banks DL, et al. 1995b. Maturational trends of EEG-sleep measures in the healthy preterm neonate. Pediatr Neurol 12(4):314–322.

Scher MS, Dokianakis SG, Sun M, et al. 1996. Computer classification of sleep in preterm and full-term neonates at similar postconceptional term ages. Sleep 19(1):18–25.

Scher MS, Dokianakis SG, Steppe DA, et al. 1997a. Computer classification of state in healthy preterm neonates. Sleep 20(2):132–141.

Scher MS, Steppe DA, Sclabassi RJ, et al. 1997b. Regional differences in spectral EEG measures betweenhealthy full-term and preterm infants. Pediatr Neurol 17:218–223.

Scher MS, Steppe DA, Banks DL. 1997c. Brain dysmaturity as expressed by EEG-sleep differences between healthy preterm and full-term neonatal cohorts. J SIDS Infant Mortal 2:141–149.

Scher MS, Steppe DA, Sun M, et al. 1997d. Changes in spectral EEG energy during sleep over the first two months of life in healthy neonatal cohorts. J SIDS Infant Mortal 2:133–139.

Scher MS, Trucco J, Beggarly ME, et al. 1998. Neonates with electrically-confirmed seizures and possible placental associations. Pediatr Neurol 19:37–41.

Scher MS, Richardson GA, Day NL. 2000. Effects of prenatal cocaine/crack and other drug exposure on electroencephalographic sleep studies at birth and one year. Pediatrics 105:39–48.

Scher MS, Wiznitzer M, Bangert BA. 2002a. Cerebral infarctions in the fetus and neonate: Maternal-placental-fetal considerations. Clin Perinatol 29:1–32.

Scher MS, Steppe DA, Beggarly ME, et al. 2002b. Neonatal EEG-sleep disruption mimicking hypoxic-ischemic encephalopathy after intrapartum asphyxia. Sleep Med 3:411–415.

Scher MS, Steppe DA, Salerno DG, et al. 2003a. Temperature differences during sleep between full-term and preterm neonates at matched conceptional ages. Clin Neurophysiol 114:17–22.

Scher MS, Jones BL, Steppe DA, et al. 2003b. Functional brain maturation in neonates as measured by EEG-sleep analyses. Clin Neurophysiol 114:875–882.

Scher MS, Alvin J, Painter MJ. 2003c. Uncoupling of clinical and EEG seizures after antiepileptic drug use in neonates. Pediatric Neurology 28:277–280.

Scher MS, Kelso RS, Turnbull JP, et al. 2003d. Automated arousal detection in neonates. Sleep 26(suppl):A143.

Scholten CA, Vos JE, and Prechtl HFR. 1985. Compiled profile of respiration, heart beat and motility in newborn infants: a methodological approach. Med Biol Eng Comput 23:15–22.

Schramm D, Scheidt B, Hubler A, et al. 2000. Spectral analysis of electroencephalogram during sleep-related apneas in pre-term and term born infants in the first weeks of life. Clin Neurophysiol 111:1788–1791.

Schulte FJ, Heinze G, and Schrempf G. 1971. Maternal toxemia, fetal malnutrition, and bioelectric brain activity of the newborn. Neuropaediatrie 2:439–460.

Schulz H, and Labie P. 1985. Ultradian Rhythms in Physiology and Behavior. Berlin: Springer-Verlag.

Schwartz MS, Prior PF, and Scott DF. 1973. The occurrence and evolution in the EEG of a lateralized periodic phenomenon. Brain 96:613–622.

Seay AR, and Bray PF. 1977. Significance of seizures in infants weighing less than 2500 grams. Arch Neurol 34:381–382.

Selton D, André M. 1997. Prognosis of hypoxic-ischaemic encephalopathy in full-term newborns—value of neonatal electroencephalography. Neuropediatrics 28:276–280.

Shewmon DA. 1990. What is a neonatal seizure? Problems in definition and quantification for investigative and clinical purposes. J Clin Neurophysiol 7(3):315–368.

Shibasaki H, Neshige R, and Hashiba Y. 1985. Cortical excitability after myoclonus: jerk-locked somatosensory evoked potentials. Neurology 35:36–41.

Shuper A, Zalzberg J, Weitz R, et al. 1991. Jitteriness beyond the neonatal period: a benign pattern of movement in infancy. J Child Neurol 6:243–245.

Statz A, Dumermuth G, Mieth D, et al. 1982. Transient EEG patterns during sleep in healthy newborns. Neuropediat 13:115–122.

Staudt F, Roth G, and Engle RC. 1981. The usefulness of electroencephalography in curarized newborns. Electroencephalogr Clin Neurophysiol 51:205–208.

Sterman MB, Harper RM, Haven SB, et al. 1977. Quantitative analysis of infant EEG development during quiet sleep. Electroencephalogr Clin Neurophysiol 43:371–385.

Stratton P. 1982. Rhythmic functions in the human newborn. In: Stratton P (ed.): *Psychobiology of the Human Newborn*. New York: John Wiley.

Sun M, Li CC, Sekhar LN, et al. 1989. A Wigner spectral analyzer for nonstationary signals. IEEE Transactions on Instrumentation and Measurement 38:961–966.

Tharp BR. 1981. Neonatal Electroencephalography. In: Korobkin R, Guillinaut C (eds.). *Progress In Perinatal Neurology*, pp. 31–64. Baltimore: Williams & Wilkins.

Tharp BR. 1989. Electroencephalography in the assessment of the premature and full-term infant. In: Stevenson D, Sunshine P (eds.). *Fetal and Neonatal Brain Injury*, pp. 175–184. Toronto/Philadelphia: B.C. Decker.

Tharp BR, and Laboyrie PM. 1983. The incidence of EEG abnormalities and the outcome of infants paralyzed with neuromuscular blocking agents. Crit Care Med 11:926–929.

Tharp BR, Cukier F, and Monod N. 1981. The prognostic value of the electroencephalogram in premature infants. Electroencephalogr Clin Neurophysiol 51:219–236.

Tharp BR, Scher MS, and Clancy RR. 1989. Serial EEGs in normal and abnormal infants with birth weights less than 1200 grams—a prospective study with long term follow-up. Neuropediatrics 20:64–72.

Tibbles JAR. 1980. Dominant benign neonatal seizures. Dev Med Child Neurol 22:664–667.

Torres F, and Anderson C. 1985. The normal EEG of the human newborn. J Clin Neurol Physiol 2:89–103.

Tukel K, and Jasper H. 1952. The electroencephalogram in parasagittal lesions. Electroencephalogr Clin Neurophysiol 4:481–494.

Turnbull JP, Loparo KA, Johnson MW, et al. 2001. Automated detection of tracé alternant during sleep in healthy full term neonates using discrete wavelet transform. Clin Neurophysiol 112:1893–1900.

Ungerer JA, Sigman M, Beckwith L, et al. 1983. Sleep behavior of preterm children at three years of age. Dev Med Child Neurol 25:297–304.

Vanhatalo S, Tallgren P, Andersson S, et al. 2002. DC-EEG discloses prominent, very slow activity patterns during sleep in preterm infants. Clin Neurophysiol 113:1822–1825.

Vecchierini MF, Curzi-Dascalova L, Trang-Pham H, et al. 2001. Patterns of EEG frequency, movement, heart rate, and oxygenation after isolated short apneas in infants. Pediatr Res 49(2):220–226.

Vecchierini MF, D'Allest AM, Verpillat P. 2003. EEG patterns in 10 extreme premature neonates with normal neurological outcome: qualitative and quantitative data. Brain Dev 25:330–337.

Vermeulen RJ, Sie LTL, Jonkman EJ, et al. 2003. Predictive value of EEG in neonates with periventricular leukomalacia. Dev Med Child Neurol 45:586–590.

Vohr BR, and Garcia Coll CT. 1985. Neurodevelopmental and school performance of very low-birthweight infants: a seven-year longitudinal study. Pediatrics 76:345–350.

Volpe JJ. 1989. Neonatal seizures: current concepts and revised classification. Pediatrics 84:422–428.

Volpe JJ. 2001. *Neurology of the Newborn*. Philadelphia: WB Saunders.

Volpe JJ, Herscovitch P, Perlman JM, et al. 1983. Positron emission tomography in the newborn: Extensive impairment of regional cerebral blood flow with intraventricular hemorrhage and hemorrhagic intracerebral involvement. Pediatrics 72:589–601.

Wasterlain CG. 1976. Effects of neonatal status epilepticus on rat brain. Dev Neurol 26:975–986.

Wasterlain CG. 1978. Neonatal seizures in brain growth. Neuropediatrics 9:213–228.

Wasterlain CG, and Plum F. 1973. The vulnerability of developing rat brain to electroconvulsive seizures. Arch Neurol 19:38–45.

Watanabe K, and Iwase K. 1972. Spindle-like fast rhythms in the EEGs of low birth weight infants. Dev Med Child Neurol 14:373–381.

Watanabe K, Hara K, Miyazaki S, et al. 1977. Electroclinical studies of seizures in the newborn. Folia Psychiatr Neurol Jpn 31:383–392.

Watanabe K, Miyazaki S, Hara K, et al. 1980. Behavioral state cycles, background EEGs, and prognosis of newborns with perinatal hypoxia. Electroencephalogr Clin Neurophysiol 49:618–625.

Watanabe K, Kuroyanagi M, Hara K, et al. 1982. Neonatal seizures and subsequent epilepsy. Brain Dev 4:341–346.

Watanabe K, Inokuma K, Takeuchi T, et al. 1985. Neurophysiology of neonates and sequelae of early brain damage. In: Arima M, Suzuki Y, Yabuuchi H (eds.). *The Developing Brain and Its Disorders*. Basel: S. Karger.

Watt J, and Strongman K. 1985. The organization and stability of sleep states in full-term, preterm and small-for-gestational-age infants: a comparative study. Dev Psychobiol 18:151–162.

Weiner SP, Painter MJ, and Scher MS. 1991. Neonatal seizures: electroclinical disassociation. Pediatr Neurol 7:363–368.

Werner SS, Stockard JE, and Bickford RG. 1977. *Atlas of Neonatal Electroencephalography*. New York: Raven Press.

Westmoreland BF, Klass DW, and Sharbrough FW. 1986. Chronic periodic lateralized epileptiform discharges. Arch Neurol 43:494–496.

Willekens H, Oumermuth G, Duc G, et al. 1984. EEG spectral powers and coherence analysis in healthy full-term neonates. Neuropediatrics 15:180–190.

Willis J, and Gold JP. 1980. Periodic alpha seizures with apnea in the newborn. Dev Med Child Neurol 22:214–222.

Witte H, Putsche P, Eiselt M, et al. 1997. Analysis of the interrelations between a low-frequency and a high-frequency signal component in human neonatal EEG during quiet sleep. Neurosci Lett 236:175–179.

Yakovlev PI, and Lacour AR. 1967. The myelogenetic cycles of regional maturation of the brain. In: Minkowski A (ed.). *Regional Development of the Brain in Early Life*, pp. 3–70. Symposium. Philadelphia: FA Davis.

Young RS, Cowan BE, Petroff OA, et al. 1987. In vivo 31P and in vitro 1H, nuclear magnetic resonance study of hypoglycemia during neonatal seizure. Ann Neurol 22:622–628.

Younkin DP, Delivoria-Papadopoulos M, Maris J, et al. 1986. Cerebral metabolic effects of neonatal seizures measured with in vivo 31P NMR spectroscopy. Ann Neurol 20:513–519.

Zubrick SR, Macartney H, and Stanley FJ. 1988. Hidden handicap in school-age children who received neonatal intensive care. Dev Med Child Neurol 30:145–152.

50. Event-Related Potentials: Methodology and Quantification

Fernando Lopes da Silva

Electroencephalography as a general method for the investigation of human brain function includes ways of determining the reaction of the brain to a variety of stimuli. Few such stimuli may be associated with clearcut changes in the EEG; some, however, provoke changes that are difficult to visualize. The research field dedicated to the detection, quantification, and physiological analysis of those slight EEG changes that are related to particular events has been of growing interest in recent years. These EEG changes may be treated globally under the common term *event-related potentials* (ERPs); a subset of the ERPs is sensory (visual, auditory, somatosensory) evoked potentials (EPs). This chapter considers some general aspects of the analysis of EPs. Regan (1977) prepared an authoritative specialized textbook on this topic; other general sources include Storm van Leeuwen et al. (1975), John and Thatcher (1977), Callaway et al. (1978), and Barber (1980). Reviews of the applications of computer methods to ERP detection and analysis are those of Barrett (1986), Gevins and Cutillo (1986), and Regan (1989).

Evoked Potential Analysis: General Aspects

EPs are usually defined in the time domain as the brain electrical activity that is triggered by the occurrence of particular events or stimuli. The basic problem of analysis is detecting ERP activity within the often much larger ongoing or background activity (i.e., the activity not related to the stimulus). Dawson (1951) attempted to solve this problem by the photographic superposition of a number of time-locked responses. This method has the advantage of enhancing response in contrast to the ongoing activity and, at the same time, providing an indication of response variability. It is, however, difficult to quantify the results in this way. Since the introduction of the summation method (Dawson, 1954) and the development of digital computer techniques (Barlow, 1957; Brazier, 1960; Clark, 1958), EPs are obtained in special-purpose digital computers and expressed as time-varying functions. In general terms, there is no fundamental argument to justify the preference for either time or frequency EP analysis. Both reflect the same reality. The choice of analytic domain, therefore, is determined by practical considerations. Nevertheless, implicit in the choice of EP analysis method is a certain general model of the generation of these potentials.

According to the most widely accepted model, EPs are signals generated by neural populations that become active time-locked to the stimulus; this signal is summed to the ongoing EEG activity. In another view, however, EPs are assumed to result from reorganizing part of the ongoing activity. The latter model has received particular attention since the investigation of Sayers et al. (1974), which showed that, when Fourier analysis was applied to the EEG segments recorded immediately after high- and low-intensity auditory stimuli, the distribution of phase spectral values differed markedly according to stimulus intensity; the distribution of amplitude values did not. They concluded that effective auditory stimuli generate an EP mainly by reorganizing the phase spectra of the existing (spontaneous) EEG activity. According to this concept, EPs result from a process incorporating phase control. In this manner, the notion of signal-to-noise ratio in terms of power, or amplitude, does not provide much information. Following this concept, a method of detecting EPs based on phase spectra evaluation in single-trial realizations may be more fruitful than simple time averaging. Nevertheless, the wide use of time averaging in practical EP work is so overwhelming that this form of analysis is treated extensively in the following section. Vijn et al. (1991) showed that visual stimuli reduce the ongoing EEG amplitude and thus confirm the notion that an EP added simply to the background EEG does not hold. This matter was further investigated and Makeig and collaborators (2002), who demonstrated that ERPs could be generated by stimulus-induced phase resetting of ongoing EEG components. This reinforces the concept that ERPs are produced, at least partially, by resetting of the phase of neuronal oscillations reflected in EEG signals as originally hypothesized by Sayers et al. (1974) and Basar et al. (1980).

Time Averaging of EP

EP analysis begins with two basic assumptions: (a) the electrical response evoked from the brain is invariably delayed relative to the stimulus; and (b) the ongoing activity is a stationary noise, the samples of which may or may not be correlated. In this way, EP can be considered a signal ($s(k)$) corrupted by additive noise ($\underline{n}(k)$), the ongoing activity. (Assume that the signals are sampled, with k as the discrete time variable.) EP detection becomes, in this way, a question of improving signal-to-noise ratio. Usually one assumes a *simple additive model* (stochastic variables are indicated by underlined symbols). The recorded stochastic signal $\underline{x}(k)$ is given as a sum of two terms:

$$\underline{x}(k) = s(k) + \underline{n}(k) \qquad (50.1)$$

The expected value of $\underline{n}(k)$ is zero. The average of $\underline{x}(k)$ over N realizations is then defined as:

$$\underline{x}(k) = \frac{1}{N} \sum_{i=1}^{N} \underline{x}_i(k) \qquad (50.2)$$

The expected value of the average is given as:

$$E[\overline{\underline{x}}(k)] = E\left[\frac{1}{N} \sum_{i=1}^{N} \overline{\underline{x}_i}(k)\right] = s(k) \qquad (50.3)$$

[since $E(\underline{n}(k)) = 0$. The variance of $\overline{\underline{x}}(k)$ is as follows:

$$var[\overline{\underline{x}}(k)] = E\left[\left(\frac{1}{N} \sum_{i=1}^{N} \underline{n}_i(k)\right)^2\right] = \frac{1}{N} var\,[\underline{n}(k)] \quad (50.4)$$

since $s(k)$ is assumed to be invariant. Therefore, the signal-to-noise ratio in terms of amplitude improves proportionally to $\sqrt{N}$. In more general terms, however, it should be assumed that the signal $s(k)$ is a stochastic signal, so that expression 50.1 should be reformulated as follows:

$$\underline{x}(k) = \underline{s}(k) + \underline{n}(k) \qquad (50.5)$$

The importance of this apparently small difference lies in the fact that the model given by expression 50.5 implies that the EP is not fully described by the mean value of $\underline{x}(k)$, but also by the higher statistical moments, as for instance the variance. In most practical cases, the latter model (expression 50.5) gives a better account of reality. As pointed out by John et al. (1978), the former model (expression 50.1) is valid only for anesthetized preparations and possibly for the short latency components of EP that mainly reflect sensory processes; this is, however, not the case for long-latency components.

For a comprehensive study of EP, *multivariate analysis methods* may be used (Donchin, 1966; John et al., 1964; Ruchkin et al., 1964; Streeter and Raviv, 1965). In this case, one considers an EP to be a multidimensional stochastic variable, i.e., a vector $\overline{x}$ where the elements are the values in subsequent time points:

$$\vec{\underline{x}} = (\underline{x}(1) \ldots \underline{x}(NS))^T \qquad (50.6)$$

Thus the expression 50.5 can be rewritten as a vectorial sum:

$$\vec{\underline{x}} = \vec{\underline{s}} + \vec{\underline{n}} \qquad (50.7)$$

assuming that $E(\vec{\underline{n}}) = 0$ as before. Therefore

$$E(\vec{\underline{x}}) = E(\vec{\underline{s}}) \qquad (50.8)$$

The second-order moment of $\vec{\underline{x}}$ is given by the covariance matrix C; considering any two samples represented by k and l, one may write:

$$Cov_{k1} = E[(\underline{x}(k)) - E(\underline{x}(k))\,(\underline{x}(1) - E(\underline{x}(1)))] \quad (50.9)$$

There are multivariate statistical methods that enable the structure of such signals as EPs to be represented as functions of a small number of factors. A technique to achieve this form of representation is the *principal components method*. The essence of the principal components method is to account for the EP as a linear combination of a small number of basis functions. It can be proved (e.g., Morrison, 1967) that, if one chooses as basic functions the eigenfunctions $\vec{\psi}_i$, of the covariance matrix, the following expression gives the best P-dimensional approximation (in a least-squares sense) to the EP ($p < NS$):

$$\vec{\underline{x}} = E(\vec{\underline{x}}) + \sum_{i=1}^{p} \lambda_1 \, \vec{\psi}_i \qquad (50.10)$$

In the expression, the coefficients λ are uncorrelated and the eigenfunctions $\vec{\psi}_1$ are orthogonal. It should be noted, however, that this form of description is only a statistical way of describing EP; one cannot assume that the eigenfunctions necessarily correspond to independent physiological generators (van Rotterdam, 1970). Nevertheless, the method can be very useful for data reduction in EP research where one wants to go further than the mean value of the EP.

In principal components analysis, the first component is the one accounting for the greatest variance; as many components as one wishes can be determined in order to account for a certain percentage of the total variance. In EP analysis, it is usually not necessary to go further than $i = 4$ or 5. In this way, a parsimonious description of EP can be achieved. Principal components analysis, however, is no more than a transformation of the original data. In this form of analysis, no provision can be made for variance components attributable only to the unreliability of the observations (Morrison, 1967). This and other shortcomings of principal components analysis can be solved by way of the mathematical model of *factor analysis*.

In factor analysis, each observation x_i is represented in terms of a linear function of common factor variables and of a signal latent specific variable that can be represented as follows (provided that the means of the observations are zero):

$$\begin{array}{c} x_1 = \lambda_{ij}y_j + \ldots + \lambda_{im}y_m + e_j \\ \hline x_n = \lambda_{nj}y_j + \ldots + \lambda_{nm}y_m + e_n \end{array} \qquad (50.11)$$

where y_j is the jth common factor variable, λ_{ij} is called the loading of the ith observation on the jth common factor, and e_i, is the ith specific factor variable. The covariances of the observations x_i are reflected only on the specific factors. Factor analysis is based on a specific statistical model in which the number of common factors is specified beforehand; an example of factor analysis in EP research is shown in Fig. 50.1. These methods of analysis can be of great usefulness in order to provide a small set of features that can be employed for the classification and clustering of EP as discussed below (Donchin, 1966, 1969; Donchin and Herning, 1975; John et al., 1973; Rebert, 1978). As an illustration of the usefulness of principal components and discriminant analysis, the study of Donchin and Cohen (1967) found that the discriminant between EP recorded to task-relevant and task-irrelevant stimuli was based essentially on time points at 300 msec.

Another form of data reduction of average EP involves describing EP as a sum of a set of analytical functions, such as, for example, damped sinusoids as thoroughly investigated by Freeman (1964, 1975). Later, this chapter discusses the possibility of describing EP as a sum of harmonically related sine waves (i.e., Fourier components).

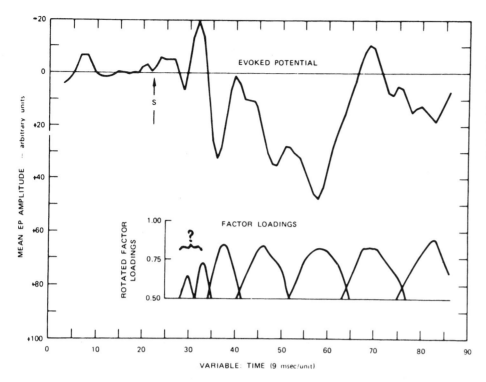

Figure 50.1. Average evoked potential (EP) of one subject (parietal leads; $N = 512$ epochs; epoch length, 765 msec) and the corresponding seven factor loading plots. The reality of the first two factors in the waveform of this example is questionable, because the factors also showed loadings in the prestimulus period. (Adapted from Robert, C.S. 1978. Neuroelectric measures of lateral specialization in relation to performance. Electroencephalogr. Clin. Neurophysiol. 34:231–238.)

Analysis in the Frequency Domain

The introductory remarks discussed the benefit of an analysis in the frequency domain of EP, as shown by Sayers et al. (1974). This section considers, in particular, (a) those EPs that are difficult to detect in the time domain because they occur without a fixed phase or time relation to the trigger, and (b) EPs caused by continuous stimuli that are preferably analyzed in the frequency domain.

EPs consisting of *changes in spectral intensity* in the alpha frequency band in relation to voluntary hand movements (Pfurtscheller, 1977; Pfurtscheller and Aranibar, 1977) exemplify the first category. This type of EP can best be shown by decomposing the EEG in frequency bands and averaging the power (or amplitude) within different bands in relation to the trigger. It is thus necessary to use statistical methods of EP evaluation to test whether or not the changes occurred by chance. This problem has been solved by Kamp and Vliegenthart (1977), who performed a spectral analysis of the EEG occurring before and after the stimulus, averaged the spectral intensities, and tested with a nonparametric method (Mann-Whitney test) whether the spectral intensities measured after the stimulus differed from baseline values.

A novel approach consists in applying independent component analysis (ICA) by means of which spatial filters can be identified that separate the EEG activity into the sum of distinct temporally maximally independent component processes (Bell and Sejnowski, 1995; Makeig et al., 1996; Vigário et al., 2000) (see also Chapter 58).

Steady-state EPs are elicited by such continuous stimuli as sine wave-modulated light or amplitude-modulated tone. These EPs may be described by measuring their amplitudes and phases as functions of the frequency of the stimulus (Lopes da Silva et al., 1970; Regan, 1966, 1977; Spekreijse et al., 1976; Van der Tweel and Verduyn Lunel, 1965). If the physiological systems underlying the generation of the EP were linear, the information from a study of the system by way of transient or continuous stimuli would be the same. However, considering that most of these systems have nonlinear properties, both types of stimuli can provide different information. When investigating steady-state EPs, mainly of the visual system, one can take great advantage of Fourier analysis of responses; an analog Fourier analyzer that is both economical and flexible was used for this purpose (Regan, 1966, 1977, 1989). To construct an amplitude and phase plot of a steady-state visual EP, for example, it is necessary to stimulate successively with different frequencies. An alternative is to stimulate with light, the intensity of which is modulated by gaussian noise. In this way, the stimulus contains all frequencies at the same time. The EP is thus obtained by calculating the cross-correlation function (Equation 58.10 in Chapter 58) or the cross-power spectrum (Equation 58.11) between the stimulus and the corresponding EEG (Lopes da Silva, 1970; Lopes da Silva et al., 1970; Reits, 1975); it can be shown that the result of the cross-correlation in such a case is equivalent to the impulse response of the linear components of the system (Fig. 50.2). The system, however, may contain nonlinear elements; in such a case, its characteristics may be analyzed using noise-modulated light by computing higher order cross-spectra or cross-correlation functions that can be defined similarly to the bispectrum (see Equation 58.16). This question, however, is too specialized to be considered in detail here (see review by Spekreijse et al., 1976, and Regan, 1989).

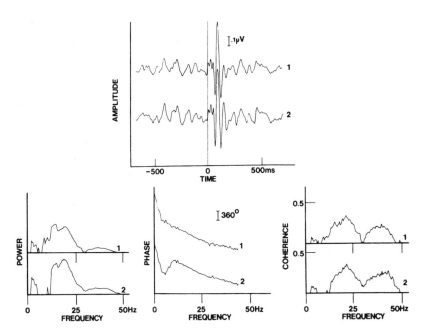

Figure 50.2. A cross-correlation function between the noise-modulated light stimulus field and the EEG. Note that in the cross-correlation responses several components can be distinguished; the values of the cross-correlation responses at negative times give a measure for the variance of the response owing to the finite time length (4 minutes) of the EEG record used for analysis. The responses were derived from two electrodes placed on the midline (occipital region) in relation to a reference placed on the earlobe. Below the Fourier transformation are the cross-correlation responses (i.e., the cross-power and phase spectra are shown along with the normalized cross-power spectrum or coherence function). From the slopes of the phase spectra, estimates of the time delays of the responses can be obtained.

It can be seen that up to about 20 Hz the phase lag increases more rapidly with frequency (i.e., the time delays are longer) than for frequencies above 20 Hz. In the coherence spectra there are two maxima; one is in the range 14 to 20 Hz and the other is in the range of 30 to 45 Hz. The former corresponds to the response components in the medium frequency range that have latencies of 100 to 120 msec; the latter corresponds to the early components of higher frequency content with latency of about 30 msec. (Adapted from Spekreijse, H., Estevez, O., and Reits, D. 1976. Visual evoked potentials and the physiological analysis of visual processes in man. In *Visual Evoked Potentials in Man,* Ed. J.E. Desmedt, pp. 3–15. Oxford: Clarendon Press.)

Special Problems of EP Analysis

Five problems that commonly arise in EP investigation are (a) the question of the relation between EPs and background activity; (b) the problem of detecting and classifying single-trial EPs, particularly in order to improve the averaging procedure; (c) a posteriori filtering (Wiener filtering) to improve the estimation of the average EP; (d) ways of controlling the averaging procedures, and alternative techniques; and (e) the topology of EPs in relation to the corresponding anatomical sources.

In detecting EPs, the main concern, of course, is to increase the signal-to-noise ratio so that the EEG background activity will not contaminate the EP. Equation 50.4 illustrates that the ratio between the variance of the averaged signal and the variance of the noise is 1/N. This holds for the case where the noise samples are uncorrelated. Often, however, this is not the case, as for instance in the presence of a strong rhythmic background such as an alpha rhythm. In such a case, subsequent samples of $n(k)$ are not independent. The degree of independence of the samples of $n(k)$ is given by the autocorrelation function of the background activity (see for a definition Chapter 58, "EEG Analysis: Theory and Practice," and Equation 58.7), which has in this case the following form:

$$R_{xx}(\tau) = \sigma^2 \exp(-\beta|\tau|) \cos(2\pi v_0 \tau) \quad (50.12)$$

where σ^2 is the var$[\underline{n}(k)]$, τv_0 is the mean frequency of the alpha rhythm, β/π is the corresponding bandwidth, and π is the delay parameter. In this way the EP variance [var$(\bar{x}(k))$] has to be given in another form than Equation 50.4 (Spekreijse et al., 1976):

$$\text{var}[\underline{x}(k)] =$$

$$\frac{\sigma^2}{N}\left[\frac{1 - \exp(-2\beta T)}{1 - 2\exp(-\beta T)\cos(2\pi v_0 T) + \exp(-2\beta T)}\right]$$

$$(50.13)$$

where 1/T is the frequency at which stimuli are presented. It is therefore important to emphasize that rhythmicity of the background will influence the signal-to-noise ratio. It can be seen from Equation 50.13 that this variance ratio tends to σ^2/N when βT becomes large. A related problem is whether the stimulation should be periodic or aperiodic; aperiodic stimulation can lead to reduced EP variance as shown theoretically by Ten Hoopen (1975) and experimentally by Arnal and Gerin (1969). More specifically, Ruchkin (1965) has demonstrated that the variance of the averaging estimate is closer to zero when the interstimuli intervals are exponentially distributed.

The detection of single-trial EP is important for two reasons: to remove the effect of latency variations between single-trial EP, which leads to a deterioration of the ensemble average, and to classify single-trial EP.

Variations in Latency

The methods used to remove variations in latency result, of course, in improved performance of the averaging procedure. The first attempt to solve this problem was made by Woody (1967), who used an adaptive filter to preprocess the single-trial EP before averaging. This procedure involves computing the cross-correlation (see Equation 58.10) between a template (e.g., an initial estimate of the average EP) and the EEG segment corresponding to each single trial; the cross-correlation will have a maximum at a certain time sample k_m that will not be the same for different trials. This maximum is found at the time sample at which the template and any data sample are most similar. The single-trial EPs are then readjusted along the time axis so that all k_m samples are aligned (i.e., synchronized); thereafter, the single trials realigned in this way are averaged. This provides a better estimate of the average EP. This new average EP can be used as a new template and the process repeated.

This iterative procedure can lead to a better estimate of the optimal average EP where the latency is the only variable. Woody showed that it was also possible to use the procedure mentioned above to classify single-trial EP by using the magnitude of the cross-correlation function; in this way, different EP subclasses could be separated. Other techniques have been proposed with the aim of further refining Woody's proposed method. McGillem and Aunon (1977), Steeger (1979), and Steeger and Reinhardt (1977) described methods that can provide better estimates of average EP because they take into account the statistical properties of the ongoing EEG activity. According to McGillem and Aunon (1977), the aim is to find a filter that, when applied on a single-trial EP, will lead to an estimate of average EP with a minimum square error. After filtering, individual components (peaks and troughs) are located.

By aligning the corresponding individual components and averaging over the ensemble, a latency-corrected average EP can be obtained. Steeger (1979) introduced a related approach using the maximum likelihood detector proposed by Helstrom (1968). According to this method, a matched filter is created that is adapted optimally to the template (the average EP) as well as to actual ongoing activity, which is estimated by its autocorrelation function. (Woody's adaptive filter was only adapted optimally to the template and to white noise.) Each single-trial EEG segment is then passed through the matched filter and the maximum output signal is found; in this way it is possible to estimate the latency corresponding to that maximum. Thereafter, an optimal average EP can be obtained after correction for latency deviations. Results obtained using this procedure are compared in Fig. 50.3 to those obtained by simple triggered average; it can be seen that the former present about twice the magnitude of the latter.

The problem of measuring the signal-to-noise (S/N) ratio of single-trial EPs has been extensively investigated by Coppola et al. (1978). In this study, equations have been proposed to estimate empirically S/N that may be useful in EP clinical or psychophysiological studies (for details see Coppola et al., 1978). A method related to those described above but also involving classification process was proposed by Pfurtscheller and Cooper (1975) under the term *selective averaging*; according to this technique, single-trial EPs are cross-correlated with different templates. The maxima of the cross-correlation functions are used to estimate the amplitude and latency of particular components. Thereafter, those trials that fall within certain amplitude and/or latency limits are averaged. In this way, different types of selected averages can be obtained that may correspond to different subsystems and/or physiological conditions. In cases where all trials are averaged together, there is a considerable information loss.

EP Classification

The analysis of single-trial EP is also important in determining whether a certain single-trial EP belongs to a specific EP class. This problem of classification can be solved using multivariate statistical methods (Donchin, 1969). In general terms, the question involves: (a) describing EP by a set of features (in the simplest case, the values of the sample points) and establishing a feature profile; and (b) making a learning set where EP corresponding to a priori defined classes are pooled and finding a discriminant function (i.e., a decision rule) that must partition the space occupied by all objects (the EP) so that unique patterns corresponding to different classes can be identified. (c) Finally, the class to which any new object (i.e., a single-trial EP) belongs must be determined; this is accomplished by computing a discriminant score for each object. Thus, each single-trial EP is classified in the subspace within which the discriminant score falls. The EP features used in the procedure described can be simply the corresponding sample values or a reduced amount of data such as can be obtained using factor or principal component analysis.

It has been suggested that a posteriori or Wiener filtering, introduced by Walter (1968), can improve averaging efficiency. The following description uses the concepts of power spectrum and related functions as explained in more detail in Chapter 58. Assume that the additive model of Equation 50.5, in which the EP, $x(k)$, is considered the sum of a signal $s(k)$ and a noise term $n(k)$ is valid, that $s(k)$ and $n(k)$ are uncorrelated, and that both have means of zero. The power spectrum of the average signal $\bar{x}(k)$ obtained by averaging N realizations is given by the following expression:

$$P_{\overline{xx}}(f_i) = P_{ss}(f_i) + \frac{1}{N} P_{nn}(f_i) \qquad (50.14)$$

Therefore, the averaging reduces the power spectrum of the noise term in the unaveraged signal $P_{nn}(f_i)$ by a factor $1/N$. Moreover, assume that the spectrum of each realization has been made and that an average of all these spectra has been computed: $\overline{P_{xx}(f_i)}$; thus, it can be written:

$$\overline{P_{xx}(f_i)} = P_{ss}(f_i) + P_{nn}(f_i) \qquad (50.15)$$

Figure 50.3. Average EPs recorded between vertex and mastoid, stimulus is a sinusoidal tone of 1000 Hz, 40 dB above 2×10^{-4} μ bar, 600 msec. **a:** The results of simple averaging are shown for a number of averaging steps. **b:** The results obtained using an adaptive filter (based on a maximum likelihood detector adapted to broadband colored noise) followed by synchronization and averaging are shown. Note the improvement in EP discrimination. The plots are in relative vertical scale; t_{ST} is the stimulus onset. (Courtesy of G.H. Steeger.)

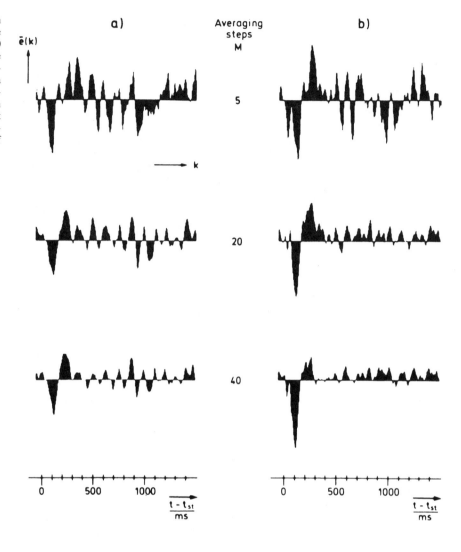

Combining Equations 50.14 and 50.15 one can derive:

$$P_{ss}(f_i) = \frac{N}{N-1} P_{\overline{xx}}(f_i) - \frac{1}{N-1} \overline{P_{xx}(f_i)} \quad (50.16)$$

Wiener (1949) has shown that for a signal $\underline{x}(k) = \underline{s}(k) + \underline{n}(k)$ with power spectra $P_{xx}(f_i)$, $P_{ss}(f_i)$, $P_{nn}(f_i)$, a linear filter can be constructed that provides an optimal estimator of the signal $\underline{s}(k)$; this linear filter has a transfer function h(k), or in the frequency domain $H(f_i)$, which is given by the following expression (Walter, 1968):

$$H(f_i) = \frac{P_{ss}(f_i)}{P_{ss}(f_i) + P_{nn}(f_i)} \quad (50.17)$$

Doyle (1975) has shown, however, that one should use an expression other than 50.17 for defining the filter $H(f_i)$ for use on the *average* EP, based on N realizations:

$$H(f_i) = \frac{P_{ss}(f_i)}{P_{ss}(f_i) + \dfrac{1}{N} P_{nn}(f_i)} \quad (50.18)$$

In this case, notice is taken of the situation after averaging, because the averaging procedure reduces the power of the noise term by a factor 1/N as shown in Equation 50.14. Expression 50.18 has been critically reviewed by Albrecht et al. (1977), who pointed out that in the denominator the term $1/N\ P_{nn}(f_i)$ should be replaced by a more general term $|h_N(f_i)|^2 P_{nn}(f_i)$, where the function $|h_N(f_i)|^2$ reflects the attenuation of the noise due to averaging; this function depends not only on N but also on the length of the realization and on the time interval between the end of one realization and the following stimulus (for details see Albrecht et al., 1977). Using Equation 50.18, the optimal filter according to Doyle becomes:

$$H'(f_i) = \frac{\dfrac{N}{N-1} P_{\overline{xx}}(f_i) - \dfrac{1}{N-1} \overline{P_{xx}(f_i)}}{P_{\overline{xx}}(f_i)} \quad (50.19)$$

The application of filter $H(f_i)$ to the averaged signal $\overline{x}(k)$ can be written formally as follows:

$$\overline{x}(k)*F^{-1}[H'(f_i)] \quad (50.20)$$

where H′(f$_i$) is the impulse response of the Wiener filter according to Doyle, the asterisk represents the convolution operation, and the symbol F^{-1} indicates the inverse Fourier transformation. However, in a theoretical study in which Wiener filtering was compared to EP averaging, Albrecht et al. (1977) demonstrated that the former yields a better estimate of s(k) than the latter, although the difference between both decreases with an increased number of realizations. (It can be seen from Equation 50.18 that as N becomes large, H(f$_i$) tends to unity.) Moreover, they also pointed out, in both cases, the importance of using interstimuli intervals leading to the smallest error of the average (i.e., the intervals should be exponentially distributed), as also shown by Ruchkin (1965). Therefore, it appears that Wiener filtering would be of practical interest in EP analysis only in those cases where a small number of realizations is available. In fact, Strackee and Cerri (1977) have shown in a theoretical study that a posteriori (Wiener) filtering does not improve EP averages, although this technique does improve the signal-to-noise ratio for individual realizations. Albrecht et al. (1977) have performed a number of simulations to study the influence of interstimuli intervals and other factors on average or Wiener-filtered EP; when averaging only five realizations, the mean square error of the estimate was, for the Wiener filter, about 76% that of the straightforward average EP obtained using random interstimuli intervals. If 20 realizations were averaged using randomly distributed stimuli, the error for the Wiener filter was about 86% of that of the average EP. If the interstimuli intervals were constant and 20 realizations were averaged, there was almost no difference between the errors obtained using the two methods. The effectiveness of a posteriori (Wiener) filtering in cases using few (five) stimuli, but not larger sets (20), has also been demonstrated by Hartwell and Erwin (1976) (Fig. 50.4). De-Weerd and co-workers (1979, 1981) have described an adaptive time-varying filter capable of optimizing the estimation of both low-frequency components of relatively long duration and higher frequency components of short duration. Investigation along these lines may help improve substantially the estimation of evoked potentials.

Some critical remarks on time-averaging EP, on ways of controlling averaging procedures, and on alternative techniques must be presented here. The averaging procedure is not as simple as it may appear to the casual observer. Indeed, a simple additive model by means of which an EP is accounted for as the sum of a deterministic signal and an uncorrelated background noise holds only in ideal cases. There may very well be interference between the neural activity evoked by the stimulus and the ongoing activity leading to a reorganization of the latter, as demonstrated by Sayers et al. (1974).

This fact notwithstanding, one may still accept as an extremely simplified EP model one based on linear addition. More research is needed in order to understand the processes of interference between EP and ongoing activity. Nevertheless, investigators who use EP should be aware of the violation of the assumption that the term *noise* consists of an uncorrelated signal. Therefore, it is necessary to take into account the statistical characteristics of the ongoing activity (see Equation 50.13) and the presentation rate of the stimuli.

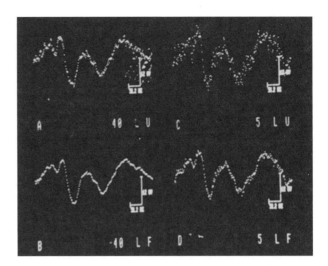

Figure 50.4. Comparison of average visual evoked potentials (VEP) obtained using different techniques. **A:** Unfiltered average of 40 responses to photic stimuli. **B:** Result of applying Wiener filtering to the same 40 responses averaged. **C:** Simple average of five responses of the 40 seen in **A**. **D:** Result of applying Wiener filtering (filter calculated from five responses) to the five responses averaged in **C**. The montage was between C3 and yoked mastoid electrodes that provided the reference. Upward deflection indicates relative negativity at C3. (Adapted from Hartwell, J.W., and Erwin, C.W. 1976. Evoked potential analysis: online signal optimization using a minicomputer. Electroencephalogr. Clin. Neurophysiol. 41:416–421.)

It has been emphasized that the intervals between stimuli should be unrelated to the main frequency components of the ongoing activity (Albrecht et al., 1977; Ruchkin, 1965). Even assuming the simplified additive model of EP, it should be realized that the signal should not be considered deterministic; rather, it is stochastic in nature. In practice, of course, it is not necessary to apply principal components or factor analysis to all EP, but, in general, it is important to measure EP variance along with the average. Previous sections have discussed the possibility of improving averaging by considering EP variability as regards latency (McGillem and Aunon, 1977; Steeger, 1979; Woody, 1967) or by resorting to the method of selective averaging (Pfurtscheller and Cooper, 1975). These methods are recommended for a thorough analysis of time-averaged EP.

Those who apply EP might not have access to the computer facilities necessary to implement the methods indicated above. However, it is highly recommended that the averaging procedure include some form of estimate of EP variability and the ongoing activity. A very simple solution is to compute partial averages of EP (e.g., five sets of N realizations each) and compare numerically the corresponding means and standard deviations or, at least, to compare graphically the different realizations, as in Dawson's old superposition method. This solution has the disadvantage of requiring long stimulation sessions. Another useful procedure, which may be combined with the former, is similar computation of partial averages of EEG segments, but without the application of the stimulus; in this way one can estimate the mean and standard deviation of the ongoing activity in the absence of the stimulus. In any case, it is always best to include in the signal to be averaged a period of time prior to the delivery of the stimulus in order to get an estimate of the mean and variability of the ongoing activity. An interesting method that can be combined with the normal averaging procedure in order to estimate the magnitude and structure of ongoing activity is the plus-minus (±) average proposed by Schimmel (1967). The (±) average is computed by alternate addition and subtraction of each realization and division by N (even number); the deviation of each EP about the average value and the (±) average have the same statistical structure. The latter can be implemented more easily by either manually or automatically setting the averaging computer to "add" or "subtract" mode or by alternating input polarity.

In many instances, the main limitation encountered in practice is the great difficulty of recording a sufficiently large number of EPs under equivalent conditions. Therefore, the methods of improving signal-to-noise ratio using a small number of trials (or even single ones) are of great importance.

Another alternative to simple EP averaging is computing the median, as proposed by Borda and Frost (1968). The median is the middle value in any group of observations. Although for a normal population the average or mean has a smaller variance than the median, it may be useful to compute a median EP because that value is less sensitive to a few unusually large or small realizations than the mean. This

technique can substantially reduce the error in computing average EP that may result from movement, muscle, or technical artifacts. A practical problem, however, is that computing the median requires storage of all realizations. To resolve this difficulty, Walter (1971) proposed a simpler procedure calculating the appropriate median.

EP Topology

A separate section discusses special EP types. This section presents only some of the general aspects to the topological analysis of EP. Different forms of EP involve activity within more or less well-circumscribed areas of the cortical surface and even subcortical areas, as in the case of the far-field EP. Therefore, at scalp level, the ensuing electrical activity can be recorded over a large region due to the presence of volume conduction. In this sense, EP recording using two electrodes may give a very limited image of the real underlying neural activity. It is in some way an equivalent of an EP in the time domain based on the amplitude value at two times samples only. Nevertheless, valuable EP research can be carried out using only one bipolar deviation. To estimate the localization of the neural systems responsible for EP generation, however, it is essential to sample the scalp surface appropriately. As discussed in Chapter 58, sampling of the EEG in space must take into consideration spatial fre-

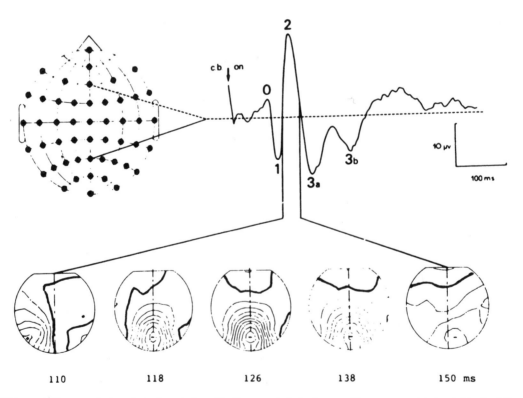

Figure 50.5. VEP recorded between the two electrodes as indicated by the electrode positions; *top,* potential versus time representation of the VEP; *bottom,* potential field distribution of the VEP at the time samples given (100 . . . 150 msec). Time of stimulus onset [a checkerboard (cb) of 20-degree extent and 20-degree checks is lit up] is indicated; the negative and positive signs are also indicated within the spatial chart. The isopotential lines were plotted at 2 μV intervals. The *heavy black line* means zero potential. On the first chart (110 msec after the cb lights up), it can be seen that a

relatively large positive component is located in the left occipital region; this component declines and is followed by a negative posterior median component. This component reaches the peak (2 in VEP plot) at about 126 msec after stimulus onset. (Adapted from Remond, A. 1977. Introduction to a new technique of topography. In *Spatial Contrast,* Eds. H. Spekreijse and L.H. van der Tweel, pp. 66–68. Amsterdam: North Holland; and Ragot, R.A., and Remond, A. 1978. EEG field mapping. Electroencephalogr. Clin. Neurophysiol. 45:417–421.)

quencies present in the EP. To determine these frequencies, it is necessary to have a priori knowledge of the spatial characteristics of the EP in question. This can be achieved by multichannel recordings with small interelectrode distances. In this way, Vaughan (1969), Vaughan et al. (1968), and Vaughan and Ritter (1970) mapped the scalp for several EP types. In these studies, derivations against a common reference were used; the presence of significant activity in the reference (chin or nose) and artifacts (muscular and eye movements) was carefully assessed. It should be noted that, in this type of study, the pitfalls of simple averaging must be taken into consideration. In other words, the fact that the EEG background activity may differ substantially with scalp location should be considered when processing EPs recorded at different sites; as a rule, the number of realizations for an identical S/N improvement should not be the same at all recording sites. Vaughan (1969) was able to make isopotential maps for different time samples of several forms of EP and to relate the spatial distributions with results of a computer model.

The studies of Remond and collaborators (Ragot and Remond, 1978) and of Lehmann (1971, 1972) also provide the spatial gradients characteristic of some EP types (Fig. 50.5). The general problem of spatial properties of EEG signals is discussed in Chapter 58; these theoretical concepts also apply in EP research. In the past two decades, some progress has been made in developing and evaluating methods for localizing within the human brain electrical sources of EPs, mainly visual EP. Kavanagh et al. (1978) demonstrated that, using appropriate algorithms and simultaneous recording of 38 derivations, it is possible to estimate the location of equivalent dipoles in the human visual cortex responsible for generating visual EP. One of the main limitations of such a general approach, however, is that different cortical areas may be involved in the generation of the type of EP studied, so that such a localization cannot be more than a crude approximation of reality. A combination of this type of estimation with a meaningful manipulation of the conditions of stimulation, e.g., pattern simulation of specific areas of the visual fields as Jeffreys and Axford (1972a,b) and Lesèvre (1973) have done, or investigation of specific system abnormalities (Kooi et al., 1973; Lehmann et al., 1969), may provide the best insight into the anatomical sources of the different EP components. Indeed, multiple dynamic sources distributed on the cortex underlie the evoked activity after sensory stimulation in all modalities. Therefore, it is important to test various physiological hypotheses on real data while making multiple source models (Scherg and Berg, 1991). Currently a number of methods are being used in EP topology for the localization of the sources of event-related electric potentials and/or magnetic fields. Some of these methods require specific models of the sources, i.e., discrete equivalent dipoles, such as spatiotemporal dipole best fits and multiple signal classification scans (MUSIC) preferentially using realistic models of the volume conductor (Buchner et al., 1995). Another method can be applied without any model of the sources, the surface Laplacian (Klein and Carney, 1995). Still another assumes the existence of distributed sources on the cortical surface, the minimum norm least square approach (MNLS). An interesting discussion of mod-

els of sources and pitfalls of the methodology was presented by van Dijk et al. (1993). For a more detailed description of these methods the reader is referred to Chapter 58.

In Chapter 5, "Biophysical Aspects of EEG and Magnetoencephalogram Generation," the section on magnetoencephalography (MEG) referred to some new advances in localizing equivalent current dipoles within the brain using magnetic measurements. A review of research on sensory evoked responses can be found in Okada (1983). Of particular interest are those studies in which the localization of equivalent dipoles takes into account both MEG and EEG measurements as performed for the somatosensory (Wood et al., 1985) and for the visual (Stok, 1986) modalities. Using MEG, it has been possible to obtain good insight into the functional somatotopic organization of the human somatosensory cortex (Okada et al., 1987), the organization of the human visual cortex where it appears that the responses to onset and offset of a (checkerboard) patterned stimulus are generated in different areas (Kouijzer et al., 1985; Lopes da Silva and Spekreijse, 1991; Stok et al., 1990), and the tonotopic organization of the auditory cortex (Elberling et al., 1982; Scherg et al., 1989). More recently a number of studies are being carried out in which electric and/or magnetic recordings of event-related phenomena are combined with realistic magnetic resonance imaging (MRI)-based models of the volume conductor. An interesting discussion of these comparative studies, suggesting reasonable but imperfect correlation between electrophysiological and hemodynamic responses, studied with functional MRI (fMRI), is provided by George et al. (1995). Particularly important is the possibility of integrating multiple sources of distributed event-related neural activity under a variety of paradigms and conditions (Tesche et al., 1995). Using these methodologies, new perspectives in studies of human cognitive brain functions are being created (Näätänen et al., 1994). In this way differences between information obtained by means of EEG and MEG can be evaluated in studies of higher order cognitive processing, for example, using P300/N400 complexes (Eulitz et al., 1997). In addition to the early studies mentioned above, the new methodological approaches are contributing to a much finer analysis of processes of sensory information in different modalities, namely in auditory processing (Pantev et al., 1995; Siedenberg et al., 1996; Verkindt et al., 1995), in the analysis of the visual parallel pathways that lead to the striate (V1) and prestriate cortex in the human brain (Ffytche et al., 1995), and of the somatosensory system (Elbert et al., 1995) including pain-related fields (Kitamura et al., 1995). Methodological advances in MEG and EEG analysis of event-related events are reviewed by Kakigi et al. (2000) and by Michel et al. (2001).

References

Albrecht, V., Lansky, P., Indra, M., et al. 1977. Wiener filtration versus averaging of evoked responses. Biol. Cybern. 27:147–154.

Arnal, D., and Gerin, P. 1969. Étude du bruit résiduel des potentiels évoqués moyens. Electroencephalogr. Clin. Neurophysiol. 27:315–321.

Barber, C. (Ed.). 1980. *Evoked Potentials.* Lancaster: MTP Press.

Barlow, J.S. 1957. An electronic method for detecting evoked responses of the brain and for reproducing their average waveforms. Electroencephalogr. Clin. Neurophysiol. 9:340–343.

Barrett, G. 1986. Analytic techniques in the estimation of evoked potentials. In *Clinical Applications of Computer Analysis of EEG and Other Neurophysiological Signals. Handbook of Electroencephalography and Clinical Neurophysiology* (New Series, vol. 2), Eds. F.H. Lopes da Silva, W. Storm van Leeuwen, and A. Remond, pp. 311–334. Amsterdam: Elsevier.

Basar, E, 1980. EEG-Brain dynamics: relation between EEG and brain evoked potentials. Elsevier, Amsterdam.

Borda, R.P., and Frost, J.D. 1968. Error reduction in small sample averaging through the use of the median rather than the mean. Electroencephalogr. Clin. Neurophysiol. 25:391–392.

Brazier, M.A.B. 1960. Some uses of computers in experimental neurology. Exp. Neurol. 2:123–143.

Buchner, H., Waberski, T.D., Fuchs, M., et al. 1995. Comparison of realistically shaped boundary element and spherical head models in source localization of early somatosensory evoked potentials. Brain Topogr. 8:137–143.

Callaway, E., Tueting, P., and Koslow, S.H. (Eds.). 1978. *Event-Related Brain Potentials in Man.* New York: Academic Press.

Clark, W.A. 1958. Average response computer (ARC1). Prog. Rep. Res. Lab. Electron. M.I.T. 114–117.

Coppola, R., Tabor, R., and Buchsbaum, M.S. 1978. Signal to noise ratio and response variability measurements in single trial evoked potentials. Electroencephalogr. Clin. Neurophysiol. 44:214–222.

Dawson, G.D. 1951. A summation technique for detecting small signals in a large irregular background. J. Physiol 115:2–3.

Dawson, G.D. 1954. A summation technique for the detection of small evoked potentials. Electroencephalogr. Clin. Neurophysiol. 6:153–154.

de Weerd, J.P.C. 1981. *Estimation of Evoked Potentials: A Study of a Posteriori "Wiener" Filtering and Its Time-Varying Generalization,* Thesis. University of Nijnegen.

de Weerd, J.P.C., Nuyen, G.J.H., Johannesma, P.J.M., et al. 1979. Estimation of signal and noise spectra by special averaging techniques with application to a posteriori "Wiener" altering. Biol. Cybern. 32:153–164.

Donchin, E. 1966. A multivariate approach to the analysis of average evoked potentials. IEEE Trans. Biomed. Eng. 13:131–139.

Donchin, E. 1969. Discriminant analysis in average evoked response studies: the study of single trial data. Electroencephalogr. Clin. Neurophysiol. 27:311–314.

Donchin, E., and Cohen, L. 1967. Average evoked potentials and intramodality selective attention. Electroencephalogr. Clin. Neurophysiol. 22:537–546.

Donchin, E., and Herning, R.I. 1975. A simulation study of the efficacy of stepwise discriminant analysis in the detection and comparison of event related potentials. Electroencephalogr. Clin. Neurophysiol. 38:51–68.

Doyle, D.J. 1975. Some comments on the use of Wiener-filtering for the estimation of evoked potentials. Electroencephalogr. Clin. Neurophysiol. 38:533–534.

Elbert, T., Junghöfer, M., Scholz, B., et al. 1995. The separation of overlapping neuromagnetic sources in first and second somatosensory cortices. Brain Topogr. 7:275–282.

Eulitz, C., Eulitz, H., and Elbert, T. 1997. Differential outcomes from magneto and electroencephalography for the analysis of human cognition. Neurosci. Lett. 227:185–188.

Elberling, C., Bak, C., Kofoed, B., et al. 1982. Auditory magnetic fields. Source location and "tonotopical organization" in the right hemisphere of the human brain. Scand. Audio. 11:59–63.

Ffytche, D.H., Guy, C.N., and Zeki, S. 1995. The parallel visual motion inputs into areas V1 and V5 of human cerebral cortex. Brain 118:1375–1394.

Freeman, W.J. 1964. Use of digital adaptive filters for measuring pre-pyriform evoked potentials from cats. Exp. Neurol. 10:475–492.

Freeman, W.J. 1975. *Mass Action in the Nervous System.* New York: Academic Press.

George, J.S., Aine, C.J., Mosher, J.C., et al. 1995. Mapping function in the human brain with magnetoencephalography, anatomical magnetic resonance imaging, and functional magnetic resonance imaging. J. Clin. Neurophysiol. 12:406–431.

Gevins, A.S., and Cutillo, B.A. 1986. Signals of cognition. In *Clinical Applications of Computer Analysis of EEG and Other Neurophysiological Signals. Handbook of Electroencephalography and Clinical Neurophysiology* (New Series, vol. 2), Eds. F.H. Lopes da Silva, W. Storm van Leeuwen, and A. Remond, pp. 335–384. Amsterdam: Elsevier.

Hartwell, J.W., and Erwin, C.W. 1976. Evoked potential analysis. Online signal optimization using a minicomputer Electroencephalogr. Clin. Neurophysiol. 41:416–421.

Helstrom, C.W. 1968. *Statistical Theory of Signal Detection,* 2nd ed. Oxford: Pergamon Press.

Jeffreys, D.A., and Axford, J.G. 1972a. Source locations of pattern-specific components of human visual evoked potentials. I. Component of striate cortical origin. Exp. Brain Res. 16:1–21.

Jeffreys, D.A., and Axford, J.G. 1972b. Source locations of pattern-specific components of human visual evoked potentials. II. Component of extrastriate cortical origin. Exp. Brain Res. 16:22–40.

John, E.R., and Thatcher, R.W. 1977. *Functional Neuroscience/Neurometrics,* vol. II. Hillsdale, NJ: Lawrence Erlbaum.

John, E.R., Ruchkin, D.S., and Villegas, J. 1964. Signal analysis and behavioral correlates of evoked potentials configurations in cats. Ann. N.Y. Acad. Sci. 112:362–420.

John, E.R., Walker, P., Cawood, D., et al. 1973. Factor analysis of evoked potentials. Electroencephalogr. Clin. Neurophysiol. 33:33–34.

John, E.R., Ruchkin, D.S., and Vidal, J.J. 1978. Measurement of event-related potentials. In *Event-related Brain Potentials in Man,* Eds. E. Callaway, P. Tueting, and S.H. Koslow, pp. 93–138. New York: Academic Press.

Kakigi, R., Hoshiyama, M., Shimojo, M., et al. 2000. The somatosensory evoked magnetic fields. Prog. Neurobiol. 61(5):495–523.

Kamp, A., and Vliegenthart, W. 1977. Sequential frequency analysis: a method to quantify event related EEG changes. Electroencephalogr. Clin. Neurophysiol. 42:843–846.

Kavanagh, R.N., Darcey, T.M., Lehmann, D., et al. 1978. Evaluation of methods for three-dimensional localization of electrical sources in the human brain. IEEE Trans. Biomed. Eng. 25:421–429.

Kitamura, Y., Kakigi, R., Hoshiyama, M., et al. 1995. Pain-related somatosensory evoked magnetic fields. Electroencephalogr. Clin Neurophysiol. 95:463–474.

Klein, S.A., and Carney, T. 1995. The usefulness of the Laplacian in principal component analysis and dipole source localization. Brain Topogr. 8:91–108.

Kooi, K.A., Yamada, T., and Marshall, R.E. 1973. Field studies of monocularly evoked cerebral potentials in bitemporal hemianopsia. Neurology (Minnesota) 23:1217–1225.

Kouijzer, W.J.J., Stok, C.J., Reits, D., et al. 1985. Neuromagnetic fields evoked by a patterned on-off set stimulus. IEEE Trans. Biomed. Eng. 32:455–458.

Lehmann, D. 1971. Multichannel topography of human alpha EEG fields. Electroencephalogr. Clin. Neurophysiol. 31:439–449.

Lehmann, D. 1972. Human scalp EEG fields: Evoked, alpha, sleep and spike-wave patterns. In *Synchronization of EEG Activity in Epilepsies,* Eds. H. Petsche and M.A.B. Brazier, pp. 307–326. New York: Springer.

Lehmann, D., Kavanagh, R.N., and Fender, D.H. 1969. Field studies of averaged visually evoked potentials in a patient with a split-chiasm. Electroencephalogr. Clin. Neurophysiol. 26:193–199.

Lesèvre, N. 1973. Potentiels évoqués par des patterns chez l'homme: influence de variables caractérisant le stimulus et sa position dans le champ visuel. In *Activités Évoquées et leur Conditionnement,* Eds. A. Fessard and G. Lelord, pp. 1–22. Paris: INSERM.

Lopes da Silva, F.H. 1970. *Dynamic Characteristics of Visual Evoked Potentials.* Thesis. University of Utrecht.

Lopes da Silva, F.H., and Spekreijse, H. 1991. Localization of brain sources of visually evoked responses using single and multiple dipoles. An overview of different approaches. In *Event-Related Brain Research,* Eds. C.H.M. Brunia, G. Mulder, and M.N. Verbaten. Electroencephalogr. Clin. Neurophysiol. Suppl. 42:38–46. Amsterdam: Elsevier.

Lopes da Silva, F.H., van Rotterdam, A., Storm van Leeuwen, W., et al. 1970. Dynamic characteristics of visual EPs in the dog. I. Cortical and subcortical potentials evoked by sine wave modulated light. Electroencephalogr. Clin. Neurophysiol. 29:246–259.

Makeig, S., Bell, A.J., Jung, T.P., et al. 1996. Independent component analysis of electroencephalographic data. In *Advances in Neural Information Processing Systems,* Eds. D. Touretzki, M. Mozer, and M. Hasselmo, pp. 145–151. Cambridge, MA: MIT Press.

McGillem, C.D., and Aunon, J.I. 1977. Measurement of signal components in single visually evoked brain potentials. IEEE Trans. Biomed. Eng. 24(3):232–241.

Michel, C.M., Thut, G., Morand, S., et al. 2001. Electric source imaging of human brain functions. Brain Res. Rev. 36(2–3):108–118.

Morrison, D.F. 1967. *Multivariate Statistical Methods.* New York: McGraw-Hill.

Näätänen, R., Ilmoniemi, R.J., and Alho, K. 1994. Magnetoencephalography in studies of human cognitive function. Trends Neurosci. 17:389–395.

Okada, Y.C. 1983. Influence concerning anatomy and physiology of the human brain based on its magnetic field. II. Nuovo Cimento 2D:379–409.

Okada, Y.C., Lauritzen, M., and Nicholson, C. 1987. MEG source models and physiology. Phys. Med. Biol. 32:43–51.

Pantev, C., Bertrand, O., Eulitz, C., et al. 1995. Specific tonotopic organizations of different areas of the human auditory cortex revealed by simultaneous magnetic and electric recordings. Electroencephalogr. Clin. Neurophysiol. 94:26–40.

Pfurtscheller, G. 1977. Graphical display and statistical evaluation of event-related desynchronization (ERD). Electroencephalogr. Clin. Neurophysiol. 43:486–487.

Pfurtscheller, G., and Aranibar, A. 1977. Event-related conical desynchronization by power measurements of scalp EEG. Electroencephalogr. Clin. Neurophysiol. 42:817–826.

Pfurtscheller, G., and Cooper, R. 1975. Selective averaging of the intracerebral click evoked responses in man: an improved method of measuring latencies and amplitudes. Electroencephalogr. Clin. Neurophysiol. 38:187–190.

Ragot, R.A., and Remond, A. 1978. EEG field mapping. Electroencephalogr. Clin. Neurophysiol. 45:417–421.

Rebert, C.S. 1978. Neuroelectric measures of lateral specialization in relation to performance. Electroencephalogr. Clin Neurophysiol. Suppl. 34: 231–238.

Regan, D. 1966. Some characteristics of average steady-state and transient responses evoked by modulated light. Electroencephalogr. Clin. Neurophysiol. 20:238–240.

Regan, D. 1977. *Evoked Potentials in Psychology, Sensory Physiology and Clinical Medicine.* London: Chapman and Hall.

Regan, D. 1989. *Human Brain Electrophysiology: Evoked Potentials and Evoked Magnetic Fields in Science and Medicine.* New York: Elsevier.

Reits, D. 1975. *Cortical Potentials in Man Evoked by Noise Modulated Light.* Thesis. University of Utrecht.

Remond, A. 1977. Introduction to a new technique of topography. In *Spatial Contrast,* Eds. H. Spekreijse and L.H. van der Tweel, pp. 66–68. Amsterdam: North Holland.

Ruchkin, D.S. 1965. An analysis of average response computations based upon aperiodic stimuli. IEEE Trans. Biomed Eng. 12:87–94.

Ruchkin, D.S., Villegas, J., and John, E.R. 1964. An analysis of average evoked potentials making use of least mean square techniques. Ann. N.Y. Acad. Sci. 15:799–826.

Sayers, P., Beagley, H.A., and Hanshall, W.R. 1974. The mechanisms of auditory evoked EEG responses. Nature 247:481–483.

Schimmel, H. 1967. The (±) reference: accuracy of estimated mean components in average evoked response studies. Science 157:92–94.

Scherg, M., and Berg, P. 1991. Use of prior knowledge in brain electromagnetic source analysis. Brain Topogr. 4:143–150.

Scherg, M., Vajsar, J., and Picton, T.W. 1989. A source analysis of the human auditory evoked potentials. J. Cogn. Neurosci. 1:336–355.

Siedenberg, R., Goodin, D.S., Aminoff, M.J., et al. 1996. Comparison of late components in simultaneously recorded event-related electrical potentials and event-related magnetic fields. Electroencephalogr. Clin. Neurophysiol. 99:1917.

Spekreijse, H., Estevez, O., and Reits, D. 1976. Visual evoked potentials and the physiological analysis of visual processes in man. In *Visual Evoked Potentials in Man,* Ed. J.E. Desmedt, pp. 3–15. Oxford: Clarendon Press.

Steeger, G.H. 1979. *Ein Bettrag zur Verbesserung der Messung akustisch evozierter Potentiate variabler Latenz im Elektroenzephalogramm des Menschen.* Thesis. Universitat ErlangenNrnberg.

Steeger, G.H., and Reinhardt, J. 1977. Ein Mittelwertrechner für reizausgelöste neuroclektrische Signale varibler Latenz. Biomed. Tech. 22:68–74.

Stok, C.J. 1986. *The Inverse Problem in EEG and MEG with Application to Visual Evoked Responses.* Thesis. University of Twente, Enschede, The Netherlands.

Stok, C.J., Spekreijse, H., Peters, M.J., et al. 1990. A comparative EEG/MEG equivalent dipole study of the pattern onset visual response. In *New Trends and Advanced Techniques in Clinical Neurophysiology,* Eds. P.M. Rossini and F. Mauguière. Electroencephalogr. Clin. Neurophysiol Suppl. 41:34–50. Amsterdam: Elsevier.

Storm van Leeuwen, W., Lopes da Silva, F.H, and Kamp, A. 1975. Evoked responses. Part A, vol. 8, Ed. P. Buser. In *Handbook of Electroencephalography and Clinical Neurophysiology,* Ed.-in-chief, A. Remond. Amsterdam: Elsevier.

Strackee, J., and Cerri, S.A. 1977. Some statistical aspects of digital Wiener filtering and detection of prescribed frequency components in time averaging of biological signals. Biol. Cybern. 28:55–61.

Streeter, D.N., and Raviv, J. 1965. *Research on Advanced Computer Methods for Biological Data Processing.* Rept ASTIA, Doc. AD 637452. Springfield, VA: Defense Documentation Center, Defense Supply Agency, Clearing house for Federal Scientific and Technical Information.

Ten Hoopen, M. 1975. Variance in average response computation: Regular versus irregular stimulation. In *Handbook of Electroencephalography and Clinical Neurophysiology,* Part A, vol. 8, Ed. A. Remond, pp. 151–158. Amsterdam: Elsevier.

Tesche, C.D., Uusitalo, M.A., Ilmoniemi, R.J., et al. 1995. Signal space projections of MEG data characterize both distributed and well localized neuronal sources. Electroencephalogr. Clin. Neurophysiol. 95:189–200.

Van Dijk, B.W., Spekreijse, H., and Yamazaki, T. 1993. Equivalent dipole source localization of EEG and evoked potentials: sources of errors or sources with confidence? Brain Topogr. 5:355–359.

van der Tweel, L.H., and Verduyn Lunel, H.F.E. 1965. Human visual responses to sinusoidally modulated light. Electroencephalogr. Clin. Neurophysiol. 18:587–598.

van Rotterdam, A. 1970. Limitations and difficulties in signal processing by means of principal component analysis. IEEE Trans. Biomed. Eng. 17:268–269.

Vaughan, H.G. 1969. The relationship of brain activity to scalp recordings of event-related potentials. In *Averaged Evoked Potentials,* Eds. E. Donchin and D.B. Lindsley, pp. 45–94. NASASP 191.

Vaughan, H.G., and Ritter, W. 1970. The sources of auditory evoked responses recorded from the human scalp. Electroencephalogr. Clin. Neurophysiol. 28:360–367.

Vaughan, H.G., Jr., Costa, D., and Ritter, W. 1968. Topography of the human motor potential. Electroencephalogr. Clin. Neurophysiol. 25:1–10.

Verkindt, C., Bertrand, O., Perrin, F., et al. 1995. Tonotopic organization of the human auditory cortex: N100 topography and multiple dipole model analysis. Electroencephalogr. Clin. Neurophysiol. 96:143–156.

Vigário, R., Sarela, J., Jousmaki, V., et al. 2000. Independent component approach to the analysis of EEG and MEG recordings. IEEE Trans. Biomed. Eng. 47(5):589–593.

Vijn, P.C.M., Van Dijk, B.W., and Spekreije, H. 1991. Visual stimulation reduces EEG activity in man Brain Res. 550:49–53.

Walter, D.O. 1968. A posteriori "Wiener filtering" of averaged evoked responses. Electroencephalogr. Clin. Neurophysiol. Suppl. 27:61–70.

Walter, D.O. 1971. Two approximations of the median evoked response. Electroencephalogr. Clin. Neurophysiol. 30:246–247.

Wiener, N. 1949. *Extrapolation, Interpolation and Smoothing of Stationary Time Series.* New York: John Wiley & Sons.

Wood, C.C., Cohen, D., Cuffin, B.N., et al. 1985. Electrical sources in human somatosensory cortex: identification by combined magnetic and potential recordings. Science 227:1051–1053.

Woody, C.D. 1967. Characterization of an adaptive filter for the analysis of variable latency neuroelectric signals. Med. Biol. Eng. 5:539–553.

51. EEG Event-Related Desynchronization (ERD) and Event-Related Synchronization (ERS)

Gert Pfurtscheller and Fernando Lopes da Silva

EEG desynchronization or blocking of alpha band rhythms due to sensory processing or motor behavior was first reported by Berger (1930), Jasper and Andrew (1938), and Jasper and Penfield (1949). This desynchronization reflects a decrease of oscillatory activity related to an internally or externally paced event and is known as event–related desynchronization (ERD; Pfurtscheller and Aranibar, 1979) The opposite, namely the increase of rhythmic activity, is termed event-related synchronization (ERS, Pfurtscheller and Lopes da Silva, 1999). ERD and ERS are characterized by their fairly localized topography, phasic behavior, and frequency specificity. Both phenomena can be studied as functions of time and space (ERD maps). There is general agreement that EEG alpha desynchronization is a reliable correlate of the increased cellular excitability in thalamocortical systems during cortical information processing (Steriade and Llinas, 1988).

Event-Related Potentials Versus EEG Reactivity

Two types of changes in the electrical activity of the cortex may occur upon sensory stimulation: one change is time-locked and phase-locked (evoked) and can be extracted from the ongoing activity by simple linear methods such as averaging; the other is time-locked but not phase-locked (induced) and can only be extracted through some nonlinear methods such as envelope detection or power spectral analysis. Which mechanisms underlie these types of responses? The time- and phase-locked response can easily be understood in terms of the response of a quasistationary system to an external stimulus that can be accounted for, in a first approximation, by a process of addition of the evoked response to the ongoing activity of the neural networks, albeit the latter may undergo some degree of reorganization as well. The induced changes can be understood as a manifest change of the ongoing activity, resulting from changes in the dynamical state of the neural networks. These changes can be due to a variety of factors; in particular they may depend on modulating influences arising from neurochemical brain systems, on changes in the strength of synaptic interactions, or on changes affecting the intrinsic membrane properties of the local neurons.

A typical example of the occurrence of both phase-locked (evoked) and non-phase-locked (induced) EEG activities is found with visual stimulation; induced EEG oscillations around 40 Hz are found in parallel with the phase-locked visual evoked potentials (VEPs; Gray et al., 1989). Averaging over a number of EEG trials improves the signal-to-noise ratio of the VEP, but not of the oscillatory response.

Quantification of EEG Reactivity

The ERD/ERS can be quantified in time and space. For the quantification, a number of event-triggered EEG trials are necessary, including some seconds before and some seconds after the event (Fig. 51.1). The event can be externally paced (e.g., acoustical, visual, or somatosensory stimulation) or internally paced (e.g., voluntary finger movement). The procedure of processing, once the frequency band has been selected, includes the following steps: (a) bandpass filtering of each event-related trial, (b) squaring of each amplitude sample to obtain power samples, (c) averaging over all trials, and (d) averaging over a small number of consecutive power samples to reduce the variance. An alternative method is based on the calculation of the intertrial variance (Kalcher and Pfurtscheller, 1995; Kaufman et al., 1989). Absolute band power is converted into percentage power by defining the power within a reference interval as 100%. By convention, a power decrease corresponds to an ERD and a power increase to an ERS (Pfurtscheller and Lopes da Silva, 1999).

ERD/ERS time courses can also be calculated by using the Hilbert transform and determining the envelope of a bandpass filtered signal (Clochon et al., 1996). Hilbert-based ERD calculation yields very similar results as the method of bandpass filtering (Knosche and Bastiaansen, 2002).

Selection of EEG Frequency Bands

One way of defining the EEG frequency bands of interest is to search for the most reactive frequency components. This search involves the comparison of two 1-second power spectra to identify frequency bands showing statistically significant differences. The first 1-second power spectrum is calculated during the reference interval (i.e., during rest), while the second is calculated during the period of interest, for example before movement-onset to investigate premovement ERD or after movement to investigate postmovement beta ERS (Fig. 51.2). A frequency band with a significant power decrease is selected for ERD calculation (e.g., 8–12 Hz in Fig. 51.2), while a band with a significant power increase (e.g., 12–19 Hz in Fig. 51.2) is defined for ERS calculation (Neuper and Pfurtscheller, 2001b; Pfurtscheller et al., 1996a, 1997b). Theoretically, the frequency band can be defined for each derivation. In practice, a few derivations overlying the areas of interest—depending on the specific study being performed—are used to determine the frequency bands for all electrodes; for example, temporal and parietal electrodes are selected in a memory task and central electrodes in a movement study.

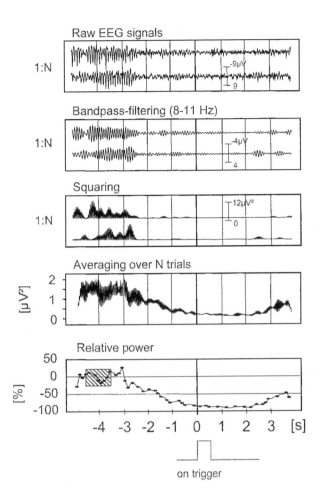

Figure 51.1. Schema for event-related desynchronization (ERD) processing showing an example with movement-related mu desynchronization. The raw EEG signals (0.5–50 Hz) are first band pass filtered (8–12 Hz), then all samples are squared and averaged over all *N* trials. After averaging over consecutive power samples (compression) and specification of a reference interval (e.g., −3.5 to −4.5), the relative band power values are displayed. A power decrease corresponds to ERD.

Another method of frequency band selection can be applied specifically to subdivide the alpha band into subbands, as used by Klimesch et al. (1994). The dominant alpha peak in the power spectrum calculated for the whole trial is first detected. The upper alpha band is then defined as consisting of the frequencies between this alpha peak frequency and the upper edge of the classically defined alpha band, while the lower alpha band is defined as those frequencies between the alpha peak frequency and the lower edge of the alpha band.

To obtain a dynamic representation of changing activity within a broad frequency range, the calculation of time-frequency maps using bandpass filtering (Graimann et al., 2002) (Fig. 51.3) and wavelet transformation (Alegre et al., 2003; Pfurtscheller and Lopes da Silva, 1999) is recommended. A method with high time-frequency resolution is the matching pursuit with stochastic Gabor dictionaries as estimator for the signal's energy density (Durka et al., 2001).

Event-Related Desynchronization (ERD) and Event-Related Synchronization (ERS)

The alpha band rhythm displays a relatively widespread desynchronization (ERD) in perceptual, judgment, and memory tasks (Pfurtscheller and Klimesch, 1992; Van Winsum et al., 1984). An increase of task complexity or of attention demand results in an increased magnitude of ERD (Boiten et al., 1992; Dujardin et al., 1993). Moreover, it has been shown that there is a relationship between the P300 event-related potential and ERD of alpha band activity (Sergeant et al., 1987; Yordanova et al., 2001). It has to be kept in mind, however, that the ERD is measured as a percentage of power relative to the reference interval, and therefore it depends on the amount of rhythmic activity in this interval. To make a reliable estimate of the power at the resting level (reference epoch), the intervals between consecutive events (e.g., cues, self-paced movements, etc.) should be randomized and not shorter than about 8 seconds.

It is important to note that alpha desynchronization is not a unitary phenomenon. If different frequency bands within the range of the extended alpha band are distinguished, two distinct patterns of desynchronization can be observed. Lower alpha desynchronization (in the range of about 6–10 Hz) is obtained in response to almost any type of task. It is topographically widespread over the entire scalp and probably reflects general task demands and attentional processes. Upper alpha desynchronization (in the range of about 10–12 Hz), in contrast, is topographically restricted and is rather related to task-specific aspects (Klimesch, 1999; Klimesch et al., 1992).

It is of interest to note that blocking of alpha band rhythms occurs not only in response to specific stimulation, but also during anticipation of the stimulus. Modality-specific ERD patterns, for instance, have been demonstrated, during anticipatory attention to a feedback stimulus presented in different modalities. Examples are the occipitally maximal ERD preceding visual stimuli and temporally maximal ERD (in MEG data) prior to an auditory feedback stimulus (Bastiaansen et al., 2001).

In a Sternberg-type auditory memory task, where first a memory set consisting of four vowels and 3 seconds later a probe (one vowel) were presented, the subject had to judge whether the probe was present in the memory set (Krause et al., 1996). The presentation of the memory set (auditory encoding) elicited a significant ERS in both alpha-frequency bands. In contrast, the presentation of the probe (auditory retrieval) elicited a bilateral ERD over centroparietal areas, also in both alpha-frequency bands. This ERD can be related to memory scanning processes. The absence of an ERD during the memory set presentation can be explained by the anatomical localization of the auditory cortex below the surface. Desynchronization due to direct auditory processing alone, therefore, is hard to detect in scalp-recorded EEG. The finding that encoding elicits ERS whereas retrieval elicits ERD in the broad alpha-frequency band has been reproduced in subsequent studies (Fingelkurts et al., 2002; Krause et al., 1999, 2001). In recent studies, ERD/ERS was

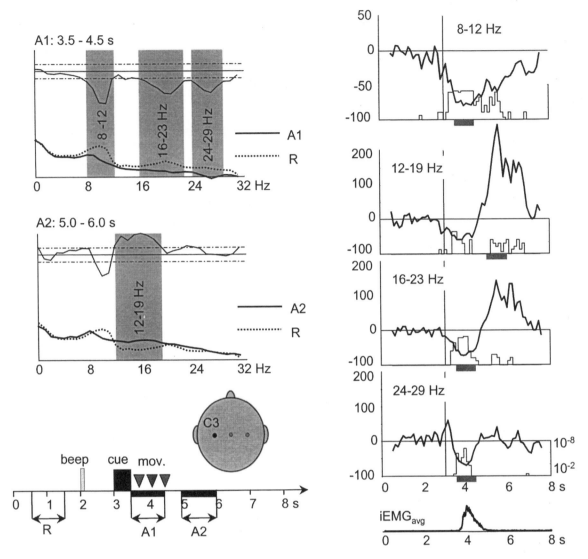

Figure 51.2. **Left side:** Superimposed logarithmic 1-second power spectra calculated in the reference period (R) and in the activity periods A1 and A2 in a cue-paced right finger movement experiment. A1 and A2 correspond to two 1-second time intervals; one is selected during the cue-triggered finger movement (A1) and the other after termination of the movement (A2). In addition, the differences between the two superimposed spectra are displayed with 95% confidence intervals indicated by the *dotted lines.* The frequency ranges displaying significant power decrease or increase are marked. **Right side:** Band power time course calculated for the frequency bands indicated in the spectra on the left. Data are triggered according to cue-onset *(vertical line).* The integrated and averaged electromyogram (EMG) shows the beginning and end of the movements. The step function indicates the significance level (sign test *p* from 10^{-2} to 10^{-8}) for the respective power changes. The *horizontal line* marks the band power in the reference period. Downward deflection indicates power decrease or ERD, upward deflection indicates power increase or event-related synchronization (ERS). (Modified from Neuper and Pfurtscheller, 2001a.)

further investigated in relation to cognitive processes involved in the perceptual and semantic analysis of verbal and nonverbal auditory stimuli (Lebrun et al., 2001) and in relation to emotional stimulus material (Aftanas et al., 2001, 2002).

In addition to sensory and cognitive processing, voluntary movement also results in a circumscribed desynchronization in the upper alpha and lower beta bands, localized over sensorimotor areas (Alegre et al., 2002; Cassim et al., 2001; Derambure et al., 1993; Neuper and Pfurtscheller, 2001a; Pfurtscheller and Aranibar, 1979; Pfurtscheller and Berghold, 1989; Stancak and Pfurtscheller, 1996c; Toro et

al., 1994). The desynchronization starts over the contralateral rolandic region and becomes bilaterally symmetrical with execution of movement. It is of interest that the time course of the contralateral mu desynchronization is almost identical in case of brisk and slow finger movements, and it starts more than 2 seconds prior to movement onset (Stancak and Pfurtscheller, 1996a). Finger movement of the dominant hand is accompanied by a pronounced ERD in the contralateral hemisphere and by a very low ERD in the ipsilateral side, whereas movement of the nondominant finger is preceded by a less lateralized ERD (Stancak and Pfurtscheller, 1996b). Different reactivity patterns have been observed

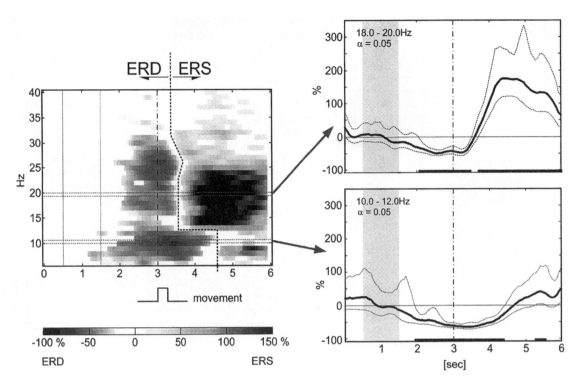

Figure 51.3. Left side: Example of an ERD/ERS time-frequency map based on an ERD/ERS analysis of partially overlapping frequency bands covering the entire frequency range of interest (e.g., 5–40 Hz). This ERD/ERS map is a matrix, the rows of which correspond to ERD/ERS calculations for specific frequency bands. In this example, the ERD/ERS map was constructed from ERD/ERS curves with a bandwidth of 2 Hz and an overlap of 1 Hz. The trigger time point is marked by a *dashed-dotted vertical line*. The reference interval is indicated by two *dotted vertical lines*. **Right side:** Examples of corresponding ERD/ERS time curves for two selected frequency bands (10–12 Hz, 18–20 Hz).

Figure 51.4. ERD/ERS time-frequency maps **(left side)** and topographical maps of mu ERD **(right side)** of a representative subject during execution **(upper panel)** versus imagination of a right-hand movement **(lower panel)**. Time-frequency maps are recorded from electrode position C3; time point 0 indicates movement-onset and the onset of cue presentation in the execution and imagination task, respectively.

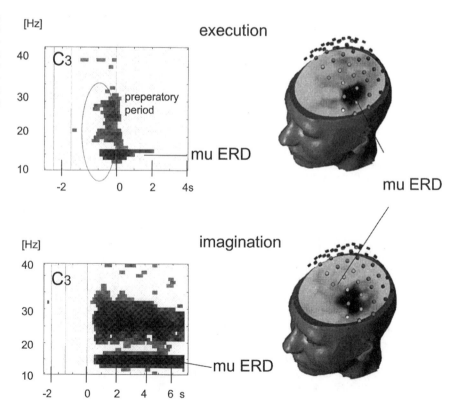

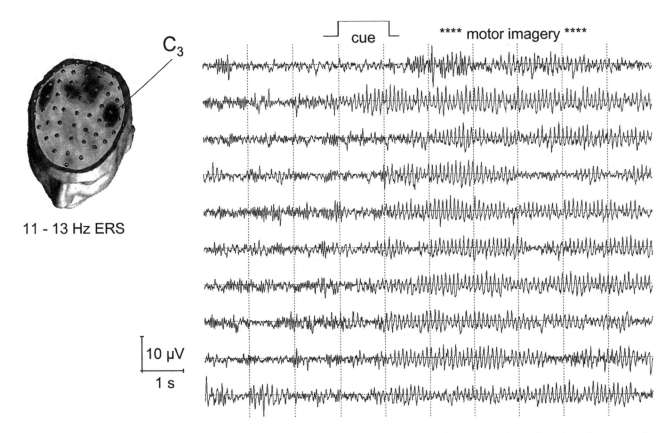

Figure 51.5. Left side: Topographic map indicating the localized 10-Hz ERS on electrode positions C3 and C4 during foot motor imagery. **Right side:** Examples of single EEG trials, recorded from electrode position C3, in a cue-based motor imagery experiment. Note the enhancement of mu rhythm during the imagination of foot movements.

with mu rhythms in the lower and upper alpha frequency band (Pfurtscheller et al., 2000b).

In addition to motor preparation, also mental imagery can produce replicable EEG patterns over primary sensory and motor areas (e.g., Beisteiner et al., 1995; Leocani et al., 1999; Pfurtscheller and Neuper, 1997). This is in accordance with the concept that motor imagery is realized via the same brain structures, which are involved in programming and preparing of movements (Decety, 1996; Jeannerod, 1995). For example, imagination of right and left hand movements result in desynchronization of mu and beta rhythms over the contralateral hand area, very similar in topography to planning and execution of real movements (Neuper and Pfurtscheller, 1999) (Fig. 51.4).

During repeated training sessions with the motor imagery task, the pattern of contralateral desynchronization of alpha band components becomes even more pronounced, and a concomitant power increase (ERS) over the ipsilateral side can develop. These findings strongly indicate the existence of activity of primary motor cortex during mental simulation of movement. Hence, we can assume that the premovement ERD and the ERD during motor imagery reflect a similar type of readiness, or presetting of neural networks, in sensorimotor areas. An involvement of the primary sensorimotor cortex in motor imagery was further supported by functional brain imaging (e.g., Porro et al., 1996; Roth et al., 1996) and

by transcranial magnetic stimulation (TMS) studies that showed an increase of motor responses during mental imagination of movements (Rossi et al., 1998).

The observation that, in parallel with the contralateral ERD, movement imagination also triggers a significant ipsilateral ERS supports the concept of antagonistic behavior of neural networks ("focal ERD/surrounding ERS"; Suffczynski et al., 1999) described in the next subsection. A comparable effect, induced alpha oscillations in the hand area during foot movement, is demonstrated in Fig. 51.5. It is of interest to note that the antagonistic behavior of alpha components (ERD/ERS) is a dominant feature of the upper alpha band and is not seen with lower frequency components.

Interpretation of Desynchronization and Synchronization in the Alpha Band

Increased cellular excitability in thalamocortical systems results in a low-amplitude desynchronized EEG (Steriade and Llinas, 1988). Therefore, ERD can be interpreted as an electrophysiological correlate of activated cortical areas involved in processing of sensory or cognitive information or production of motor behavior (Pfurtscheller, 1992). An increased and/or more widespread ERD could be the result of the involvement of a larger neural network or of more cell assemblies in information processing. Factors contributing to such an enhancement of the ERD are increased task complexity, more efficient task performance (Boiten et al., 1992; Dujardin et al., 1993; Klimesch et al., 1996a; Sterman et al., 1996), and more effort and attention that may be needed in the case of some patients, elderly, or low IQ subjects (Defebvre et al., 1996; Derambure et al., 1993; Labyt et al., 2004; Neubauer et al., 1995).

Explicit learning of a movement sequence, e.g., key pressing with different fingers, is accompanied by an enhancement of ERD over the contralateral central regions. Once the movement sequence has been learned and the movement is performed more automatically, the ERD is reduced. These ERD findings strongly suggest that the activity in primary sensorimotor areas increases in association with learning a new motor task and decreases after the task has

been learned (Zhuang et al., 1997). The involvement of the primary motor area in learning motor sequences was also suggested by Pascual-Leone et al. (1995) who studied motor output maps by TMS.

The opposite phenomenon to desynchronization is synchronization; in this case the amplitude enhancement is likely mediated by the cooperative or synchronized behavior of a large number of neurons. When the summed synaptic events become sufficiently large, the field potentials can be recorded with macroelectrodes not only within the cortex but also over the scalp. To be recorded at the scalp it is necessary that cortical activity is coherent over an appreciable surface of cortical tissue (Cooper et al., 1965; Lopes da Silva, 1991). When patches of neurons display coherent activity in the alpha band, a depressed state of active process-

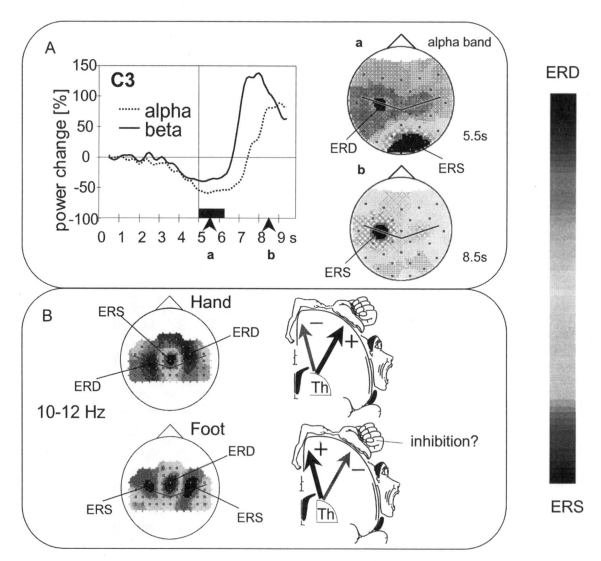

Figure 51.6. A: Grand average (*N* = 9) ERD/ERS curves calculated in the alpha and beta bands during a right-hand movement task *(left side).* Grand average maps calculated for a 125-msec interval during movement (a) and after movement-offset in the recovery period (b) *(right side).* **B:** Maps displaying ERD and ERS for an interval of 125 msec during voluntary movement of the hand *(left,* **upper panel**) and movement of the foot *(left,* **lower panel**). The motor "homunculus" with a possible mechanism of cortical activation/deactivation gated by thalamic structures is shown on the right. (Modified from Pfurtscheller, G., Lopes da Silva, F.H., 1999. Event-related EEG/MEG synchronization and desynchronization: basic principles. Clin. Neurophysiol. 110, 1842–1857.)

ing of information in the underlying cortical neuronal populations can be assumed to exist.

It is of interest to note that about 85% of cortical neurons are excitatory, with the other 15% being inhibitory (Braitenberg and Schuz, 1991). Inhibition in neural networks, however, is very important, not only to optimize energy demands but also to limit and control excitatory processes. Klimesch (1996) suggested that synchronized alpha band rhythms may introduce powerful inhibitory effects, which could act to block a memory search from entering irrelevant parts of neural networks.

Adrian and Matthews (1934) described a system that is neither receiving nor processing sensory information as an "idling system." Localized synchronization of 12- to 14-Hz components in awake cats was interpreted by Case and Harper (1971) as a result of "idling cortical areas." Cortical idling can thus denote the dynamical state of a cortical area, of at least some cm², which is not involved in processing sensory input or preparing motor output. In this sense, occipital alpha rhythms can be considered as idling rhythms of the visual areas, and mu rhythms as idling rhythms of sensorimotor areas (Kuhlmann, 1978). Also sleep spindles during the early sleep stages can also correspond to a blockage of synaptic transmission through the thalamus (Steriade and Llinas, 1988).

Localized desynchronization of the alpha band activity related to a specific sensorimotor event does not occur in isolation, but can be accompanied by an increase of synchronization in neighboring cortical areas that correspond to the same or to another modality of information processing, as indicated above.

To describe this observation the term *focal ERD/surround ERS* was introduced by Suffczynski et al. (1999). An example of this kind of intermodal interaction, in the form of a central desynchronization and a parieto-occipital synchronization of EEG mu activity that occurs in a voluntary finger movement task, is illustrated in (Fig. 51.6A). A similar antagonistic behavior with desynchronization of central mu rhythm and synchronization of parieto-occipital alpha rhythms during repetitive brief finger movement was reported by Gerloff et al. (1998). The opposite phenomenon, the enhancement of central mu rhythm and blocking of occipital alpha rhythm during visual stimulation, was reported by Koshino and Niedermeyer (1975) and Kreitmann and Shaw (1965). Further examples demonstrating intramodal interaction, in terms of a hand area ERD and foot area ERS during hand movement and a hand area ERS and foot area ERD during foot movement, can be seen in Fig. 51.6B (see also Pfurtscheller and Neuper, 1994; Pfurtscheller et al., 1997a).

The focal mu desynchronization in the 10- to 12-Hz band may reflect a mechanism responsible for selective attention focused to a motor subsystem. This effect of focal attention may be accentuated when other cortical areas, not directly involved in the specific motor task, are "inhibited." In this process, the interplay between thalamocortical modules and the corresponding reticular nucleus neurons that form a chain of inhibitory neurons that project not only to the thalamocortical relay neurons but also to neighboring inhibitory neurons may play an important role (Suffczynski et al., 1999).

The Functional Meaning of Theta ERS and Upper Alpha ERD for Memory

Studies of the human scalp EEG regarding event-related synchronization in the theta band (about 4–6 Hz) and desynchronization in the alpha range (about 7–12 Hz) show, in general, that in response to task demands theta band power increases (synchronizes) whereas alpha band power decreases (desynchronizes). This dissociation between EEG frequency ranges (theta versus alpha range) and type of event-related response (ERS versus ERD) is of functional significance. Several studies indicate that different frequency bands in the theta and alpha range are associated with different types of cognitive processes. Whereas event-related changes in the theta band appear to be related to encoding and retrieval processes of general working memory systems (WMS), the upper alpha frequency range (of about 10–12 Hz) reacts selectively to sensory-semantic memory processes of a long-term memory system (LTMS), and the lower alpha band to attentional processes (cf. Klimesch, 1999 for a review). It is important to emphasize that the functional specificity of these frequency bands can better be put in evidence if frequency boundaries are adjusted to the peak of individual alpha frequency (IAF) of a given subject, and if rather narrow bands are used (for a description of the respective methods cf. Doppelmayr et al., 1998; Klimesch et al., 1996b).

The functional specificity of the theta and alpha band with respect to a language processing task was demonstrated by Röhm et al. (2001). These authors found that increased language processing demands, implying an increase in WMS's load, are reflected in a selective increase of theta activity, while an increase in semantic processing is reflected in a selective decrease of upper alpha activity.

ERD and Neural Efficiency

In the so-called neural efficiency concept of human intelligence, it is assumed that brighter individuals as compared to less intelligent ones show a more efficient brain function while solving cognitive tasks. This hypothesis was based on studies employing various brain imaging techniques in exploring potential bases of cognitive abilities. In particular, studies by Haier and co-workers (e.g., Haier et al., 1988) initiated great interest in neural efficiency research. Using positron emission tomography (PET), they found that a person's intelligence level is strongly associated with the amount of brain activation (glucose metabolism rate) while performing a nonverbal intelligence test: the higher the person's intelligence level, the less strongly their brains had to be activated to achieve a good performance. To date, there is a large body of evidence that confirms this negative relationship between cognitive abilities and the extent of brain activation.

Aside from studies applying brain imaging methods, it was found that also the amplitude and spatial distribution of alpha band ERD in cognitively demanding situations reflects interindividual differences in human intelligence (Neubauer et al., 1995). Whereas subjects with relatively lower IQ displayed a rather widespread and unspecific ERD in a visual letter-matching task, subjects with higher IQ produced less pronounced ERD, restricted to parieto-occipital areas (Neubauer et al., 1999). Thus, neural efficiency may be related to a more focused use of specific task-relevant areas in high intelligent as compared to lower intelligent individuals. The negative association between intelligence level and amount of alpha band ERD turned out to be a rather robust finding, being observable in subsequent studies with, for example, different task materials (verbal, numeric, figural) (Jausovec and Jausovec, 2000; Neubauer and Fink, 2003; Neubauer et al., 2002), in different types of cognitive tasks with different degrees of complexity (e.g., from elementary cognitive tasks to complex reasoning tasks). Additionally, it was found that even fine-grained differences in cognitive load are reflected in upper alpha band ERD. As an example, a linearly increasing desynchronization with ascending cognitive load was demonstrated recently in different working memory tasks (Stipacek et al., 2003).

Induced Beta Oscillations

Two different types of induced beta oscillations can be observed: one is short-lasting in the form of bursts, which is found mainly after termination of movement, somatosensory stimulation, or motor imagery; and the other is long-lasting and occurs simultaneously with motor actions. A characteristic feature of the postmovement beta synchronization is its strict somatotopical organization reported in magnetoencephalogram (MEG) (Salmelin et al., 1995) and EEG recordings (Neuper and Pfurtscheller, 1996; Pfurtscheller and Lopes da Silva, 1999). Another feature is its frequency specificity, with a slightly lower frequency over the lateralized sensorimotor areas as compared to the midcentral area (Neuper and Pfurtscheller, 2001b). Frequency bands in the range of 16 to 20 Hz were reported for the hand representation area and of 20 to 24 Hz for the midcentral area close to the vertex. The observation that a self-paced finger movement can activate neuronal networks in hand and foot representation areas with different frequency in both areas (Fig. 51.7; see also Pfurtscheller et al., 2000a), provides further support for the notion that the frequency of these oscillations may be characteristic for the underlying neural circuitry.

The postmovement beta synchronization is found after both active and passive movements (Alegre et al., 2002; Cassim et al., 2001). This indicates that proprioceptive afferences play an important role in the desynchronization of the central beta rhythm and the subsequent beta rebound. However, electrical nerve stimulation (Neuper and Pfurtscheller, 2001b), mechanical finger stimulation (Pfurtscheller et al., 2001), and even motor imagery (Neuper and Pfurtscheller, 1999) also can induce a beta ERD followed by

Figure 51.7. A: Grand average time courses of the relative beta band power calculated for subject-specific frequency bands. Average hand area specific frequency was 16.6 Hz *(full line curves)* and foot area specific frequency was 22.8 Hz *(stripped line curves).* Data are triggered at movement-offset (indicated by the *vertical line).* Note the large band power increase (beta ERS, indicated by upward deflection) over the hand area, with the lower frequency component, and the larger power increase over the foot area with the high-frequency components. The horizontal line marks the average band power in the 1-second reference interval that started 4 seconds before the trigger. **B:** ERS distributions of one representative subject calculated in the bands 14 to 19 Hz and 20 to 24 Hz shown over the cortical surface *(left side).* A light disk marks the location of the maximal beta ERS. Each map corresponds to a time interval of 125 msec. ERS results over the cortical surface were computed based on the linear estimation method. A realistically shaped head model (brain-skull-scalp compartments) was constructed from 200 transversal T1-weighted magnetic resonance (MR) images. For the indicated positions of maximal beta ERS, the corresponding ERD/ERS time courses are shown *(right side).* The *horizontal line* indicates the band power in the reference interval, the *vertical line* the time of movement offset. (Modified from Pfurtscheller, G., Neuper, C., Pichler-Zalaudek, K., et al. 2000a. Do brain oscillations of different frequencies indicate interaction between cortical areas in humans? Neurosci. Lett. 286, 66–68.)

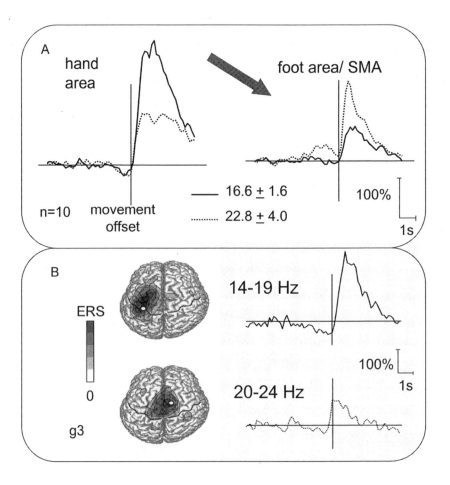

a short-lasting beta ERS or beta rebound. A general explanation for the induced beta bursts in the motor cortex *after* movement, somatosensory stimulation, and motor imagery could be that the beta-generating network shifts from a highly activated state during movement to a deactivated or an inhibited state immediately after movement cessation.

By applying TMS during self-paced movement or median nerve stimulation, it was shown that the excitability of motor cortex neurons was significantly reduced in the first second after termination of movement or of stimulation, respectively (Chen et al., 1998, 1999). This gives support to the interpretation that the beta rebound might represent a deactivated or inhibited cortical state. This is also in line with the finding of the suppression of the beta rebound during continuous sensory motor cortex activation in MEG (Schnitzler et al., 1997) and EEG (Pfurtscheller et al. 2002) (Fig. 51.8).

Such a continuous activation, as for example during cube manipulation with one hand, is accompanied not only by an intense outflow from the motor cortex to the hand muscles but also by an afferent flow from mechano- and proprioreceptors to the somatosensory cortex. This strong activation of the sensorimotor cortex could be responsible for the suppression of the beta rebound. At movement arrest the networks of the motor area may be reset, what would be reflected in the beta rebound or beta bursts in the sensorimotor area. The latter could be interpreted as representing a "resetting of functions" in contrast to a "binding function" that may be related to some types of gamma oscillations.

In contrast to the short-lasting beta rebound interpreted as a correlate of a transient inhibitory state of motor cortex circuitry, also long-lasting trains of beta oscillations associated

with activation of motor areas may be observed. One example is beta oscillations close to the vertex induced by foot motor imagery (Pfurtscheller et al., 2000a). A possible source of these beta oscillations associated with an active brain state could be the supplementary motor area (SMA). It is well documented that the SMA is activated during active movement and motor imagery as demonstrated, for example, by PET measurements (Deiber et al., 1991).

Summarizing, there are two types of central beta reactivity patterns: short lasting beta bursts (beta rebound after performance of different sensorimotor tasks) associated with a deactivated (inhibited) cortical state, and long-lasting beta oscillations induced simultaneously with a motor task during activation of motor cortex networks. It has to be kept in mind, however, that activation of sensorimotor areas results generally in a desynchronized pattern (beta ERD) but can also, under certain circumstances, be accompanied by a synchronized pattern.

Gamma Band Oscillations

In addition to the oscillations in the alpha and lower beta band, induced oscillations are also present in the frequency band around 40 Hz, i.e., in the gamma band. Such oscillations were reported during sensory, cognitive, and motor processing (for a detailed review see Tallon-Baudry and Bertrand, 1999). These gamma oscillations may be related to binding of sensory information and to sensorimotor integration. Indeed, oscillations in the gamma band appear appropriate to mediate rapid coupling or to synchronize spatially separated cell assemblies (Singer, 1993).

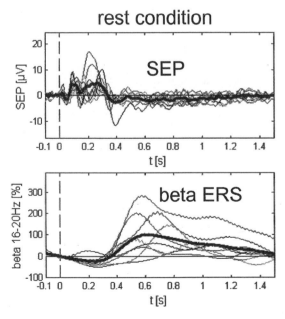
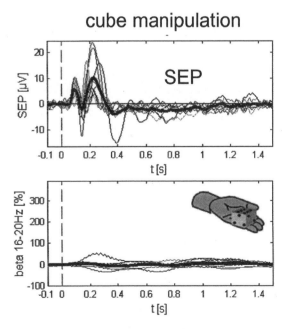

Figure 51.8. Superimposed individual somatosensory evoked potentials (SEPs) (**upper panels,** referential recording, Cpz) and the individual beta ERS curves (**middle** and **lower panels,** bipolar, channel C3, frequency range 16-20 Hz and 20-24 Hz) for six subjects. *Left part* of the figure represents condition A (resting), the *right part* indicates condition B (cube manipulation). The mean curve of each panel is displayed with a *thick line.* (Modified from Pfurtscheller, G., Woertz, M., Müller, G., et al. 2002. Contrasting behavior of beta event-related synchronization and somatosensory evoked potential after median nerve stimulation during finger manipulation in man. Neurosci. Lett. 323:113–116.)

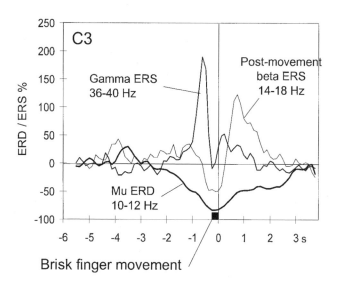

Figure 51.9. Superposition of different band power versus time courses triggered for brisk finger movement offset. The duration of the index finger extension and flexion was 0.2 second. Note the relatively long-lasting mu rhythm (10–12 Hz) desynchronization starting about 2 seconds prior to movement onset, the postmovement beta (14–18 Hz) ERS following a beta ERD, and the short-lasting increase of power around 40 Hz prior to movement onset.

The existence of at least three different types of oscillations at the same electrode location over the sensorimotor hand area during brisk finger lifting is documented in Fig. 51.9. Beside a mu desynchronization (10–12 Hz) and a postmovement beta synchronization (14–18 Hz), also induced gamma oscillations (36–40 Hz) are present. These 36- to 40-Hz oscillations reach a maximum shortly before movement onset, whereas the beta ERS has its maximum after movement offset. Further details on movement-related gamma oscillations in humans can be found in Pfurtscheller et al. (1993) and Salenius et al. (1996).

Gamma oscillations in the frequency range from 60 to 90 Hz associated with movement were observed in subdural recordings (electrocorticography [ECoG]) by Crone et al. (1998b) and Pfurtscheller et al. (2003). In contrast to the alpha band rhythms, the gamma oscillations reflect a stage of active information processing. A prerequisite for the development of gamma bursts may be the desynchronization of alpha band rhythms. The examples in Fig. 51.10 show that induced gamma and beta oscillations are embedded in desynchronized alpha band activity.

Another interesting finding is that separate foci of synchronized gamma activities occurring in cortical regions that are widely separated—often even in different lobes—can display high correlation or coherence during the performance of cognitive or motor tasks. In this context the observations of Rodriguez et al. (1999), who studied EEG gamma activity in subjects viewing visual stimuli that were perceived either as faces or as meaningless shapes, are particularly relevant. These authors found that only face perception induced a long-distance pattern of gamma synchronization, corresponding to the moment of perception itself and to the ensuing motor response. A period of strong gamma desynchronization marked the transition between

the moment of perception and the motor response. They suggested that this desynchronization reflects a process of active uncoupling of the underlying neural ensembles that is necessary to proceed from one cognitive state to another. These results are also in line with the animal studies of Bressler et al. (1993), who reported task-related increases of coherence in high-frequency activities in the monkey neocortex during the performance of a pattern-discrimination task; gamma band activities in the striate and motor cortex were briefly correlated when a motor response occurred and were uncorrelated when no response occurred. Andrew and Pfurtscheller (1996) reported a phasic increase in 40-Hz event-related coherence (ERCoh) between the contralateral sensorimotor and the supplementary motor areas during the performance of unilateral finger movements. In contrast, the 40-Hz coherence between the left and right sensorimotor areas showed no changes in coherence during the movement and remained low throughout. These findings suggest that increases in gamma band coherence are functionally related to the task being performed. Possibly, the coherence between the gamma oscillations in these remote regions is facilitated by specific corticocortical connections between the two separated neural masses sustaining the gamma oscillations.

ERD/ERS Patterns in Intracranial and Subdural Recordings in Humans

Different types of movement-related ERD patterns have been observed in subdural (Crone et al., 1998a; Ohara et al., 2000; Pfurtscheller et al., 2003; Toro et al., 1994) and intracerebral recordings (Sochurkova and Rektor, 2003; Szurhaj et al., 2003). Stereoelectroencephalograph (SEEG) studies with intracerebral depth electrodes in pre- and postcentral gyri and the frontal medial cortex in epileptic patients during self-paced hand movement revealed a relative widespread mu and beta ERD followed by a more focused beta ERS in primary sensorimotor areas and SMA proper (Szurhaj et al., 2003). In a similar SEEG study on one epileptic surgery candidate, Sochurkova and Rektor (2003) reported for the first time a mu and beta ERD recorded by means of depth electrodes located in the basal ganglia (putamen) in a "self-paced" motor task. The postmovement beta ERS was in this case most prominent in the 28- to 32-Hz band.

Intracranial EEG recordings have also shown increased theta band frequencies when patients were navigating through a virtual maze using memory in comparison with the condition where they guided through the maze by specific cues (Caplan et al., 2001; Kahana et al., 1999).

Induced gamma activity (>30 Hz) can be considered an index of cortical activation for auditory perception. Auditory stimuli induced a broad banded gamma activity (40 Hz, as well as 80 to 100 Hz) in ECoG of greater amplitude during presentation of phonemes as compared to tones. The topography of gamma ERS was more focused than that of alpha ERD (Crone et al., 2001). Gamma oscillations, recorded from limbic cortex, appear to be modulated in recordings obtained when patients successfully memorized words, and transient couplings between different functional areas, within the gamma frequency band, have been put in evidence during associative learning (Fell et al., 2001; Miltner et al., 1999).

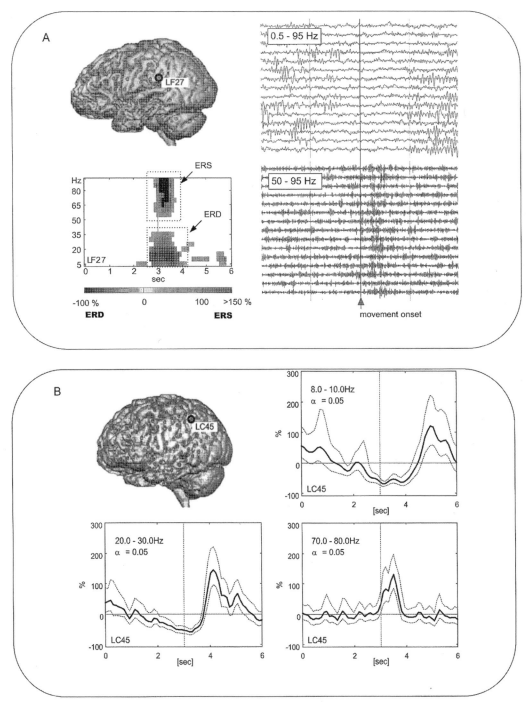

Figure 51.10. Electrocorticography (ECoG) data recorded from electrodes placed over the temporal and frontal lobe neocortex for monitoring purposes in an epileptic patient, and sampled at 200 Hz. The subject performed self-paced movement tasks such as index finger movement and palmar pinch with a minimum of 4 seconds between repetitions. ERD/ERS was quantified from about 40 trials at movement onset and with a statistical significance of *p* = .05. **A:** Raw ECoG trials of different frequency bands (0.5–95 Hz and 50–95 Hz) for channel LF27 of one subject C16 performing palmar pinch *(right side)*. The corresponding ERD/ERS time-frequency map spanning a frequency range of 5 to 90 Hz with a frequency resolution of 5 Hz and frequency bands of 10 Hz *(left side)*. **B:** ERD/ERS curves with 95% confidence intervals for channel LC45 of subject C17 performing index finger movement. In both cases (**A** and **B**) gamma activity (gamma ERS) of around 70 to 80 Hz, which is embedded in alpha and beta ERD, is clearly visible.

EEG Reactivity and Neurological Disorders

The quantification of movement-related desynchronization can improve the diagnosis of functional deficits in patients with cerebrovascular disorders and Parkinson's disease (PD). It was shown that a high correlation exists between morphological (computed tomography [CT]) and functional findings in cerebrovascular disorders. The ERD is reduced or abolished over the affected hemisphere. Based on ERD measurements during voluntary hand movement, it was, for example, possible to differentiate between a superficial and deep vascular lesion (Pfurtscheller et al., 1981). The use of alpha and beta ERD for prediction of motor recovery in stroke patients was reported by Platz et al. (2002). Defebvre et al. (1994, 1996) and Magnani et al. (1998) showed that the premovement ERD in PD is less lateralized over the contralateral sensorimotor area and it is delayed as compared to control subjects. In Parkinson's patients with unilateral predominant clinical signals, Labyt et al. (2003) made an interesting comparison of the ERD/ERS in mu and beta frequency bands elicited by movements (finger extension or visuo-guided targeted movement) of the less akinetic and the more akinetic hand. They found that the simple finger extension made with the less akinetic limb elicited a premovement mu ERD focused over the contralateral central region, while the visuo-guided movement induced additional mu ERD over the contralateral parietal region as well as an earlier ipsilateral mu ERD. When the same movements, however, were performed with the more affected hand, the contralateral ERD was delayed, and the ERD induced by the visuo-guided movement occurred earlier while the contralateral parietal ERD was absent. Furthermore, there was a clear postmovement beta ERS focused on the contralateral central area for the less affected hand, but this was remarkably attenuated for the more akinetic hand. These findings indicate that ERD/ERS studies can give interesting information regarding the pathophysiology of the dynamics of sensorimotor integration in patients with PD. Treatment with L-dopa in patients with idiopathic PD can significantly reduce the delayed ERD onset (Magnani et al. 2002). Recently, it was reported that stimulation of the internal globus pallidus in patients with PD can enhance the mu ERD, before and during self-paced wrist movement (Devos et al., 2002).

Abnormal reactivity of mu and beta rhythms during the planning of voluntary movement has also been shown in epileptic patients (Derambure et al., 1999). Patients who have frequent focal motor seizures show a delayed and more widespread mu rhythm ERD and a delay of recovery of mu and beta rhythms than normal control subjects. These findings may be related to a change in excitability of sensorimotor neural networks that are activated during the spread of the epileptic discharge.

References

Adrian, E.D., and Matthews, B.H. 1934. The Berger rhythm: potential changes from the occipital lobes in man. Brain 57:355–385.

Aftanas, L.I., Varlamov, A.A., Pavlov, S.V., et al. 2001. Affective picture processing: event-related synchronization within individually defined human theta band is modulated by valence dimension. Neurosci. Lett. 303(2):115–118.

Aftanas, L.I., Varlamov, A.A., Pavlov, S.V., et al. 2002. Time-dependent cortical asymmetries induced by emotional arousal: EEG analysis of event-related synchronization and desynchronization in individually defined frequency bands. Int. J. Psychophysiol. 44(1):67–82.

Alegre, M., Labarga, A., Gurtubay, I.G., et al. 2002. Beta electroencephalograph changes during passive movements: sensory afferences contribute to beta event-related desynchronization in humans. Neurosci. Lett. 331(1):29–32.

Alegre, M., Gurtubay, I.G., Labarga, A., et al. 2003. Alpha and beta oscillatory changes during stimulus-induced movement paradigms: effect of stimulus predictability. Neuroreport 14(3):381–385.

Andrew, C., and Pfurtscheller, G. 1996. Event–related coherence as a tool for studying dynamic interaction of brain regions. Electroencephalogr. Clin. Neurophysiol. 98:144–148.

Bastiaansen, M.C.M., Böcker, K.B.E., Brunia, C.H.M., et al. 2001. Event-related desynchronization during anticipatory attention for an upcoming stimulus: a comparative EEG/EMG study. Clin. Neurophysiol. 112:393–403.

Beisteiner, R., Höllinger, P., Lindinger, G., et al. 1995. Mental representations of movements. Brain potentials associated with imagination of hand movements. Electroencephalogr. Clin. Neurophysiol. 96:83–193.

Berger, H. 1930. Uber das Elektrenkephalogramm des Menschen II. J. Psychol. Neurol. 40:160–179.

Boiten, F., Sergeant, J., and Geuze, R. 1992. Event–related desynchronization: the effects of energetic and computational demands. Electroencephalogr. Clin. Neurophysiol. 82:302–309.

Braitenberg, V., and Schuz, A. 1991. Anatomy of the Cortex. New York: Springer.

Bressler, S.L., Coppola, R., and Nakamura, R. 1993. Episodic multi–regional cortical coherence at multiple frequencies during visual task performance. Nature 366:153–156.

Caplan, J.B., Madsen, J.R., Raghavachari, S., et al. 2001. Distinct patterns of brain oscillations underlie two basic parameters of human maze learning. J. Neurophysiol. 86(1):368–380.

Case, M.H., and Harper, R.M. 1971. Somatomotor and visceromotor correlates of operantly conditioned 12–14 c/s sensorimotor cortical activity. Electroencephalogr. Clin. Neurophysiol. 31:85–92.

Cassim, F., Monaca, C., Szurhaj, W., et al. 2001. Does post-movement beta synchronization reflect an idling motor cortex? Neuroreport 12(17):3859–3863.

Chen, R., Yassen, Z., Cohen, L.G., et al. 1998. The time course of corticospinal excitability in reaction time and self-paced movements. Ann. Neurol. 44:317–325.

Chen, R., Corwell, B., and Hallett M. 1999. Modulation of motor cortex excitability by median nerve and digit stimulation. Exp. Brain Res. 129:77–86.

Clochon, P., Fontbonne, J.M., Lebrun, N., et al. 1996. A new method for quantifying EEG event-related desynchronization: amplitude envelope analysis. Electroencephalogr. Clin. Neurophysiol. 98(2):126–129.

Cooper, R., Winter, A.L., Crow, H.J., et al. 1965. Comparison of subcortical, cortical and scalp activity using chronically indwelling electrodes in man. Electroencephalogr. Clin. Neurophysiol. 18:217–228.

Crone, N.E., Miglioretti, D.L., Gordon, B., et al. 1998a. Functional mapping of human sensorimotor cortex with electrocorticographic spectral analysis. I. Alpha and beta event-related desynchronization. Brain 121:2271–2299.

Crone, N.E., Miglioretti, D.L., Gordon, B., et al. 1998b. Functional mapping of human sensorimotor cortex with electrocorticographic spectral analysis. II. Event-related synchronization in the gamma band. Brain 121:2301–2315.

Crone, N.E., Boatman, D., Gordon, B., et al. 2001. Induced electrocorticographic gamma activity during auditory perception. Clin. Neurophysiol. 112:565–582.

Decety, J. 1996. The neurophysiological basis of motor imagery. Behav. Brain Res. 77:45–52.

Defebvre, L., Bourriez, J.L., Dujardin, K., et al. 1994. Spatiotemporal study of Bereitschaftspotential and event-related desynchronization during voluntary movement in Parkinson's disease. Brain Topogr. 6:237–244.

Defebvre, L., Bourriez, J.L., Destee, A., et al. 1996. Movement-related desynchronization pattern preceding voluntary movement in untreated Parkinson's disease. J. Neurol. Neurosurg. Psychiatry 60:307–312.

Deiber, M.P., Passingham, R.E., Colebatch, J.G., et al. 1991. Cortical areas and the selection of movement: a study with positron emission tomography. Exp. Brain Res. 84:393–402.

Derambure, P., Defebvre, L., Dujardin, K., et al. 1993. Effect of aging on the spatio-temporal pattern of event-related desynchronization during a voluntary movement. Electroencephalogr. Clin. Neurophysiol. 89:197–203.

Derambure, P., Bourriez, J.L., Defebvre, L., et al. 1999. Reactivity of central cortical rhythms in epileptic patients with focal seizures. In *Event-Related Desynchronization. Handbook of Electroencephalography and Clinical Neurophysiology*, Eds. G. Pfurtscheller, and F.H. Lopes da Silva, revised ed., vol. 6, pp. 395–400. Amsterdam: Elsevier.

Devos, D., Derambure, P., Bourriez, J.L., et al. 2002. Influence of internal globus pallidus stimulation on motor cortex activation pattern in Parkinson's disease. Clin. Neurophysiol. 113:1110–1120.

Doppelmayr, M., Klimesch, W., Pachinger, T., et al. 1998. Individual differences in brain dynamics: important implications for the calculation of event-related band power measures. Biol. Cybernet. 79:49–57.

Dujardin, K., Derambure, P., Defebvre, L., et al. 1993. Evaluation of event-related desynchronization (ERD) during a recognition task: effect of attention. Electroencephalogr. Clin. Neurophysiol. 86:353–356.

Durka, P.J., Ircha, D., Neuper, C., et al. 2001. Time-frequency microstructure of electroencephalogram desynchronization and synchronization. Med. Biol. Eng. Comput. 39(3):315–321.

Fell, J., Klaver, P., Lehnertz, K., et al. 2001. Human memory formation is accompanied by rhinal-hippocampal coupling and decoupling. Nat. Neurosci. 4(12):1259–1264.

Fingelkurts, A.A., Krause, C.M., and Sams, M. 2002. Probability interrelations between pre-/post-stimulus intervals and ERD/ERS during a memory task. Clin. Neurophysiol. 113(6):826–843.

Gerloff, C., Hadley, J., Richard, J., et al. 1998. Functional coupling and regional activation of human cortical motor areas during simple, internally paced and externally paced finger movements. Brain 121:1513–1531.

Graimann, B., Huggins, J.E., Levine S.P., et al. 2002. Visualization of significant ERD/ERS patterns in multichannel EEG and ECoG data. Clin. Neurophysiol. 113(1):43–47.

Gray, C.M., Konig, P., Engel, A., et al. 1989. Oscillatory responses in cat visual cortex exhibit inter-columnar synchronization which reflects global stimulus properties. Nature 338:334–337.

Haier, R.J., Siegel, B.V., Nuechterlein, K.H., et al. 1988. Cortical glucose metabolic rate correlates of abstract reasoning and attention studied with positron emission tomography. Intelligence 12:199–217.

Jasper, H.H., and Andrew, H.L. 1938. Electro-encephalography III. Normal differentiation of occipital and precentral regions in man. Arch. Neurol. Psychiat. 39:96–115.

Jasper, H.H., and Penfield, W. 1949. Electrocorticograms in man: effect of the voluntary movement upon the electrical activity of the precentral gyrus. Arch. Psychiat. Z. Neurol. 183:163–174.

Jausovec, N., and Jausovec, K. 2000. Differences in event-related and induced brain oscillations in the theta and alpha frequency bands related to human intelligence. Neurosci. Lett. 293:191–194.

Jeannerod, M. 1995. Mental imagery in the motor context. Neuropsychologia 33(11):1419–1432.

Kahana, M.J., Sekuler, R., Caplan, J.B., et al. 1999. Human theta oscillations exhibit task dependence during virtual maze navigation. Nature 399 (6738):781–784.

Kalcher, J., and Pfurtscheller, G. 1995. Discrimination between phase-locked and non-phase-locked event-related EEG activity. Electroencephalogr. Clin. Neurophysiol. 94:381–483.

Kaufman, L., Schwartz, B., Salustri, C., et al. 1989. Modulation of spontaneous brain activity during mental imagery. J. Cogn. Neurosci. 2:124–132.

Klimesch, W. 1996. Memory processes, brain oscillations and EEG synchronization. J. Psychophysiol. 24:61–100.

Klimesch, W. 1999. EEG alpha and theta oscillations reflect cognitive and memory performance: A review and analysis. Brain Res. Rev. 29:169–195.

Klimesch, W., Pfurtscheller, G., and Schimke, H. 1992. Pre- and poststimulus processes in category judgment tasks as measured by event-related desynchronization (ERD). J. Psychophysiol. 6:186–203.

Klimesch, W., Schimke, H., and Schwaiger, J. 1994. Episodic and semantic memory: an analysis in the EEG theta and alpha band. Electroencephalogr. Clin. Neurophysiol. 91:428–441.

Klimesch, W., Doppelmayr, M., Russegger, H., et al. 1996a. Theta band power in the human scalp EEG and the encoding of new information. NeuroReport 7:1235–1240.

Klimesch, W., Schimke, H., Doppelmayr, M., et al. 1996b. Event–related desynchronization (ERD) and the Dm-effect: Does alpha desynchronization during encoding predict later recall performance? Int. J. Psychophysiol. 24:47–60.

Knosche, T.R., and Bastiaansen, M.C. 2002. On the time resolution of event-related desynchronization: a simulation study. Clin. Neurophysiol. 113(5):754–763.

Koshino, Y., and Niedermeyer, E. 1975. Enhancement of rolandic mu-rhythm by pattern vision. Electroencephalogr. Clin. Neurophysiol. 38:535–538.

Krause, M.C., Lang, A.H., Laine, M., et al. 1996. Event–related EEG desynchronization and synchronization during an auditory memory task. Electroencephalogr. Clin. Neurophysiol. 98:319–326.

Krause, C.M., Lang, A.H., Laine, M., et al. 1999. Cortical activation related to auditory semantic matching of concrete versus abstract words. Clin. Neurophysiol. 110:1371–1377.

Krause, C.M., Sillanmäi, L., Häggqvist A., et al. 2001. Test-retest consistency of the event-related desynchronisation/event-related synchronization of the 4–6, 6–8, 8–10 and 10–12 Hz frequency bands during a memory task. Clin. Neurophysiol. 112:750–757.

Kreitmann, N., and Shaw, J.C. 1965. Experimental enhancement of alpha activity. Electroencephalogr. Clin. Neurophysiol. 18:147–155.

Kuhlman, W.N. 1978. Functional topography of the human mu rhythm. Electroencephalogr. Clin. Neurophysiol. 44:83–93.

Labyt, E., Devos, D., Bourriez, J.-L., et al. 2003. Motor preparation is more impaired in Parkinson's disease when sensorimotor integration is involved. Clin. Neurophysiol. 114(12):2423–2433.

Labyt, E., Szurhaj, W., Bourriez, J.-L., et al. 2004. Influence of aging on cortical activity associated with a visuo-motor task. Neurobiol. Aging 25(6):817–827.

Lebrun, N., Clochon, P., Etévenon, P., et al. 2001. An ERD mapping study of the neurocognitive processes involved in the perceptual and semantic analysis of environmental sounds and words. Cogn. Brain Res. 11(2):235–248.

Leocani, L., Magnani, G., and Comi, G. 1999. Event-related desynchronization during execution, imagination and withholding of movement. In *Event-Related Desynchronization. Handbook of Electroencephalography and Clinical Neurophysiology*, Eds. G. Pfurtscheller, and F.H. Lopes da Silva, revised ed., vol. 6, pp. 291–301. Amsterdam: Elsevier.

Lopes da Silva, F. 1991. Neural mechanisms underlying brain waves: from neural membranes to networks. Electroencephalogr. Clin. Neurophysiol. 79:81–93.

Magnani, G., Cursi, M., Leocani, L., et al. 1998. Event–related desynchronization during self-paced movement and CNV-paradigm in Parkinson's disease. Mov. Disord. 13:653–660.

Magnani, G., Cursi, M., Leocani, L., et al. 2002. Acute effects of L-dopa on event-related desynchronization in Parkinson's disease. Neurol. Sci. 23(3):91–97.

Miltner, W.H., Braun, C., Arnold, M., et al. 1999. Coherence of gamma-band EEG activity as a basis for associative learning. Nature 397(6718):434–436.

Neubauer, A.C., and Fink, A. 2003. Fluid intelligence and neural efficiency: effects of task complexity and sex. Personality Individual Diff. 35:811–827.

Neubauer, A., Freudenthaler, H.H., and Pfurtscheller, G. 1995. Intelligence and spatio–temporal patterns of event-related desynchronization (ERD). Intelligence 20:249–266.

Neubauer, A.C., Sange, G., and Pfurtscheller, G. 1999. Psychometric intelligence and event-related desynchronization during performance of a letter matching task. In *Event-Related Desynchronization. Handbook of Electroencephalography and Clinical Neurophysiology*, Eds. G. Pfurtscheller, and F.H. Lopes da Silva, revised ed., vol. 6, pp. 219–231. Amsterdam: Elsevier.

Neubauer, A.C., Fink, A., and Schrausser, D.G. 2002. Intelligence and neural efficiency: the influence of task content and sex on brain-IQ relationship. Intelligence 30:515–536.

Neuper, C., and Pfurtscheller, G. 1996. Post-movement synchronization of beta rhythms in the EEG over the cortical foot area in man. Neurosci. Lett. 216:17–20.

Neuper C., and Pfurtscheller G. 1999. Motor imagery and ERD. In *Event-Related Desynchronization. Handbook of Electroencephalography and*

Clinical Neurophysiology, Eds. G. Pfurtscheller, and F.H. Lopes da Silva, revised ed., vol. 6, pp. 303–325. Amsterdam: Elsevier.

Neuper, C., and Pfurtscheller, G. 2001a. Event-related dynamics of cortical rhythms: frequency-specific features and functional correlates. Int. J. Psychophysiol. 43:41–58.

Neuper, C., and Pfurtscheller, G. 2001b. Evidence for distinct beta resonance frequencies related to specific sensorimotor cortical areas. Clin. Neurophysiol. 112(11):2084–2097.

Ohara, S., Ikeda, A., Kunieda, T., et al. 2000. Movement-related change of electrocorticographic activity in human supplementary motor area proper. Brain 123:1203–1215.

Pascual-Leone, A., Dang, N., Cohen, L.G., et al. 1995. Modulation of muscle responses evoked by transcranial magnetic stimulation during the acquisition of new fine motor skills. J. Neurophysiol. 74:1037–1045.

Pfurtscheller, G. 1992. Event–related synchronization (ERS): an electrophysiological correlate of cortical areas at rest. Electroencephalogr. Clin. Neurophysiol. 83:62–69.

Pfurtscheller, G., and Aranibar, A. 1979. Evaluation of event-related desynchronization (ERD) preceding and following voluntary self-paced movements. Electroencephalogr. Clin. Neurophysiol. 46: 138–146.

Pfurtscheller, G., and Berghold, A. 1989. Patterns of cortical activation during planning of voluntary movement. Electroencephalogr. Clin. Neurophysiol. 72:250–258.

Pfurtscheller, G., and Klimesch, W. 1992. Functional topography during a visuo verbal judgement task studied with event-related desynchronization mapping. J. Clin. Neurophysiol. 9:120–131.

Pfurtscheller, G., and Lopes da Silva, F.H. 1999. Event-related EEG/MEG synchronization and desynchronization: basic principles. Clin. Neurophysiol. 110:1842–1857.

Pfurtscheller, G., and Neuper, C. 1994. Event–related synchronization of mu rhythm in the EEG over the cortical hand area in man. Neurosci. Lett. 174:93–96.

Pfurtscheller, G., and Neuper C. 1997. Motor imagery activates primary sensorimotor area in humans. Neurosci. Lett. 239:65–68.

Pfurtscheller, G., Sager, G., and Wege, W. 1981. Correlations between CT scan and sensorimotor EEG rhythms in patients with cerebrovascular disorders. Electroencephalogr. Clin. Neurophysiol. 52: 473–485.

Pfurtscheller, G., Neuper, C. and Kalcher, J. 1993. 40-Hz oscillations during motor behavior in man. Neurosci. Lett. 162(1–2):179–182.

Pfurtscheller, G., Stancak A. Jr., and Neuper, C. 1996a. Post-movement beta synchronization. A correlate of an idling motor area? Electroencephalogr. Clin. Neurophysiol. 98:281–293.

Pfurtscheller, G., Stancak A. Jr., and Neuper, C. 1996b. Event–related synchronization (ERS) in the alpha band—an electrophysiological correlate of cortical idling: a review. Int. J. Psychophysiol. 24:39–46.

Pfurtscheller, G., Neuper, C., Andrew, C., et al. 1997a. Foot and hand area mu rhythms. J. Psychophysiol. 26:121–135.

Pfurtscheller, G., Stancak A. Jr., and Edlinger, G. 1997b. On the existence of different types of central beta rhythms below 30 Hz. Electroencephalogr. Clin. Neurophysiol. 102:316–325.

Pfurtscheller, G., Neuper, C., Pichler-Zalaudek, K., et al. 2000a. Do brain oscillations of different frequencies indicate interaction between cortical areas in humans? Neurosci. Lett. 286:66–68.

Pfurtscheller, G., Neuper, C., and Krausz, G. 2000b. Functional dissociation of lower and upper frequency mu rhythms in relation to voluntary limb movement. Clin. Neurophysiol. 111:1873–1879.

Pfurtscheller, G., Krausz, G., and Neuper, C. 2001. Mechanical stimulation of the fingertip can induce bursts of beta oscillations in sensorimotor areas. J. Clin. Neurophysiol. 18(6):559–564.

Pfurtscheller, G., Woertz, M., Müller, G., et al. 2002. Contrasting behavior of beta event-related synchronization and somatosensory evoked potential after median nerve stimulation during finger manipulation in man. Neurosci. Lett. 323:113–116.

Pfurtscheller, G., Graimann, B., Huggins, J.E., et al. 2003. Spatiotemporal patterns of beta desynchronization and gamma synchronization in corticographic data during self-paced movement. Clin. Neurophysiol. 114:1226–1236.

Platz, T., Kim, I.H., Engel, U., et al. 2002. Brain activation pattern as assessed with multi-modal EEG analysis predict motor recovery among stroke patients with mild arm paresis who receive the Arm Ability Training. Restor. Neurol. Neurosci. 20(1–2):21–35.

Porro, C.A., Francescato, M.P., Cettolo, V., et al. 1996. Primary motor and sensory cortex activation during motor performance and motor imagery: a functional magnetic resonance imaging study. J. Neurosci. 16:7688–7698.

Rodriguez, E., George, N., Lachaux, J.P., et al. 1999. Perception's shadow: long-distance synchronization of human brain activity. Nature 397 (6718):391–395.

Röhm, D., Klimesch, W., Haider, H., et al. 2001. The role of theta and alpha oscillations for language comprehension in the human electroencephalogram. Neurosci. Lett. 310:137–140.

Rossi, S., Pasqualetti, P., Tecchio, F., et al. 1998. Corticospinal excitability modulation during mental simulation of wrist movements in human subjects. Neurosci. Lett. 243:147–151.

Roth, M., Decety, J., Raybaudi, M., et al. 1996. Possible involvement of primary motor cortex in mentally simulated movement: a functional magnetic resonance imaging study. Neuroreport. 7:1280–1284.

Salenius, S., Salmelin, R., Neuper, C., et al. 1996. Human cortical 40 Hz rhythm is closely related to EMG rhythmicity. Neurosci. Lett. 213: 75–78.

Salmelin, R., Hamalainen, M., Kajola, M., et al. 1995. Functional segregation of movement-related rhythmic activity in the human brain. Neuroimage 2:237–243.

Schnitzler, A., Salenius, S., Salmelin, R., et al. 1997. Involvement of primary motor cortex in motor imagery: a neuromagnetic study. Neuro Image 6(3):201–208.

Sergeant, J., Geuze, R., and Van Winsum, W. 1987. Event–related desynchronization and P300. Psychophysiology 24:272–277.

Singer, W. 1993. Synchronization of cortical activity and its putative role in information processing and learning. Annu Rev. Physiol. 55:349–374.

Sochurkova, D., and Rektor, I. 2003. Event-related desynchronization/synchronization in the putamen. An SEEG case study. Exp. Brain Res. 149(3):401–404.

Stancak A. Jr., and Pfurtscheller, G. 1996a. Mu-rhythm changes in brisk and slow self-paced finger movements. Neuroreport 7:1161–1164.

Stancak A. Jr., and Pfurtscheller, G. 1996b. The effects of handedness and type of movement on the contralateral preponderance of mu-rhythm desynchronization. Electroencephalogr. Clin. Neurophysiol. 99:174–182.

Stancak A. Jr., and Pfurtscheller, G. 1996c. Event–related desynchronization of central beta rhythms in brisk and slow self-paced finger movements of dominant and nondominant hand. Cogn. Brain Res. 4:171–184.

Steriade, M., and Llinas, R. 1988. The functional states of the thalamus and the associated neuronal interplay. Phys. Rev. 68:649–742.

Sterman, M.B., Kaiser, D.A., and Veigel, B. 1996. Spectral analysis of event-related EEG responses during short-term memory performance. Brain Topogr. 9(1):21–30.

Stipacek, A., Grabner, R.H., Neuper, C., et al. 2003. Sensitivity of human EEG alpha band desynchronization to different working memory components and increasing levels of memory load. Neurosci. Lett. 353(3):193–196.

Suffczynski, P., Pijn, P.J.M., Pfurtscheller, G., et al. 1999. Event-related dynamics of alpha band rhythms: a neuronal network model of focal ERD/surround ERS. In *Event-Related Desynchronization. Handbook of Electroencephalography and Clinical Neurophysiology,* Eds. G. Pfurtscheller, and F.H. Lopes da Silva, revised ed., vol. 6, pp. 67–85. Amsterdam: Elsevier.

Szurhaj, W., Derambure, P., Labyt, E., et al. 2003. Basic mechanisms of central rhythms reactivity to preparation and execution of voluntary movement: a stereoencephalographic study. Clin. Neurophysiol. 114(1):107–119.

Tallon-Baudry, C., and Bertrand, O. 1999. Oscillatory gamma activity in humans and its role in object representations. Trends Cognit. Sci. 3(4):151–162.

Toro, C., Deuschl, G., Thatcher, R., et al. 1994. Event–related desynchronization and movement-related cortical potentials on the ECoG and EEG. Electroencephalogr. Clin. Neurophysiol. 93:380–389.

Van Winsum, W., Sergeant, J. and Gueze, R. 1984. The functional significance of event-related desynchronization of alpha rhythms in attentional and activating tasks. Electroencephalogr. Clin. Neurophysiol. 58:519–524.

Yordanova, J., Kolev, V., and Polich, J. 2001. P300 and alpha event-related desynchronization (ERD). Psychophysiology 38(1):143–152.

Zhuang, P., Toro, C., Grafman, J., et al. 1997. Event–related desynchronization (ERD) in the alpha frequency during development of implicit and explicit learning. Electroencephalogr. Clin. Neurophysiol. 102:374–381.

52. Visual Evoked Potentials and Electroretinograms

Gastone G. Celesia and Neal S. Peachey

The visual system can be studied noninvasively by recording field potentials from the surface of the cornea or the scalp overlying the visual cortex. Retinal potentials recorded at the cornea constitute the electroretinogram (ERG) and reflect the initial processes of phototransduction and retinal transmission. Cortical potentials constitute the visual evoked potential (VEP) and reflect the output features of the entire visual pathway.

ERGs were first recorded directly from the eye by Holmgren in 1865. However, the routine use of ERGs in clinical practice did not occur until the development of reliable differential amplifiers and safe contact lenses in the 1950s (Armington, 1974). ERGs evoked by bright flashes are large potentials having an amplitude of several microvolts (μV) and are generated by the photoreceptors and by the retinal glial cells (Granit, 1955; Armington, 1974). Utilization of monochromatic stimuli and scotopic and photopic conditions permits the study of the physiology and pathophysiology of the photoreceptors and the separation of rod and cone contributions to the flash ERG (Armington, 1974; Chatrian et al., 1980a,b; Dowling, 1979; Fishman et al., 2001).

VEPs were first recorded in animals directly from the striate cortex; they could not be recorded from the scalp due to their small amplitude. VEP recording became feasible with the introduction of summation and computer averaging techniques (Ciganek, 1958; Dawson, 1954). The functional integrity of the visual pathways can be evaluated by VEPs (Celesia, 1982; Halliday, 1978; Halliday et al., 1972). Furthermore, manipulation of visual stimuli permits the preferential evaluation of the various segments of the visual pathways (Celesia, 1984).

The clinician applying these technologies to the study of the visual system must be aware that, as Floyd Ratliff (1982) stated, "There is no 'best method' of stimulus control or of data analysis in the study of visual evoked potentials." Recordings and stimulation must be tailored to the clinical problem to be studied. Evaluation of peripheral retinal function, for example, can be achieved best by flash electroretinography, whereas optic nerve function may be assessed by pattern-reversal VEPs. Evaluation of retinal function, anterior visual pathways, and retrochiasmal pathway function are discussed separately.

Retinal Function
Response Characteristics of the Retina

The eye is both an optical and a neuronal device. The light entering the eye must pass through transparent media (the cornea, the aqueous humor, the lens, and the vitreous humor) to reach the retina. A prerequisite for normal retinal function is an intact optic system. Thus, for example, a cataract may prevent a pattern stimulus from reaching the retina and being transformed into electrical signals to be transmitted to the visual cortex and perceived by the subject. In the study of visual function, one must always be aware of the optical status of the eye.

The retina is a neuronal membrane lining the back of the eye chamber (Polyak, 1941; Rodieck, 1973b). The amount of light entering the lens and reaching the photoreceptors is determined by the diameter of the pupil, which is controlled by the iris, a diaphragm that can be contracted or dilated by the ciliary muscles (Graham et al., 1965).

The retina is organized into three cellular layers (Fig. 52.1): the outer nuclear layer (ONL), the inner nuclear layer (INL), and the ganglion cell layer (GCL). Neuronal connections are made primarily in two synaptic layers: the outer plexiform layer (OPL) and the inner plexiform layer (IPL). The ONL contains the cell bodies of the rod and cone photoreceptors. The OPL contains the synapses among photoreceptors, horizontal cells, and bipolar cells. The INL contains the cell bodies of horizontal, bipolar, and amacrine neurons and the cell bodies of the radial class of retinal glial cell, the Müller cell. The IPL contains the synaptic interconnections among bipolar, amacrine, and ganglion cells. The GCL contains the cell bodies of the ganglion cells, as well as of displaced amacrine cells. Detailed reviews of retinal anatomy have been published (Dacey, 2000; Djamgoz, 1995; Dowling, 1987; Rodieck, 1973b). The outer surface of the retina is delimited by the retinal pigment epithelium (RPE). The RPE is critically involved in many activities required for normal retinal function including the flow of nutrients and waste products between the photoreceptors and the choroidal circulation, the visual cycle by which light sensitivity is maintained, and the phagocytosis of shed outer segment disks (reviewed in Marmor and Wolfensberger, 1998).

In the vertebrate retina there are two classes of photoreceptors: cones and rods. The human retina is rod-dominated, containing only about 5% cones (Curcio et al., 1990). Photoreceptors have three main functional sections. The outer segment contains the light-sensitive photopigments along with the phototransduction machinery, which are organized into a series of bi-lipid membrane disks. The inner segment houses the nucleus and cellular organelles. The photoreceptor terminal contains synapses where glutamate is used to communicate with second-order neurons. All rods contain the same type of visual pigment, rhodopsin. The three types of cones (red, green, or blue) are differentiated by the pho-

Figure 52.1. Origin of flash electroretinogram (ERG) waves. **Left:** Diagram of the cellular components of the retina. G, ganglion cells; M, glial Müller cells; A, amacrine cells; B, bipolar cells; H, horizontal cells; E, pigmented epithelium. **Right:** Schematic component analysis of the predominantly rod *(upper)* and cone *(lower)* ERG, as modified from Brown (1980). The ERG represents the algebraic summation of the photoreceptor potential, the b wave, and the direct current (DC) component. Note that the c wave from the pigmented epithelium has been omitted.

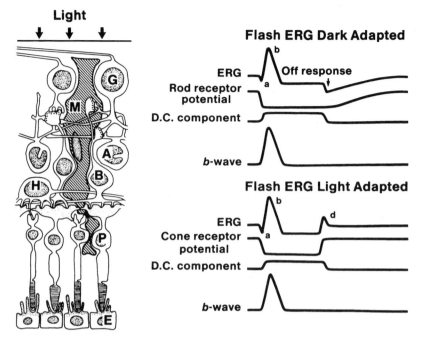

topigment contained in the outer segment, which are differentially sensitive to light of different wavelength (Kraft et al., 1990).

Visual pigments are activated by the absorption of light and initiate the phototransduction cascade. This cascade culminates in the closure of ion channels along the outer segment membrane, membrane hyperpolarization, and a consequent reduction in the rate of neurotransmitter release at the synaptic terminal (Stryer, 1986). In the human eye, the amplification gained from the phototransduction cascade is such that a visual sensation can result from one quantal absorption occurring in only three rod photoreceptors (Hecht et al., 1942).

The response of the photoreceptors is transmitted centrally in a different fashion for rods and cones. Information from rods is carried by one primary pathway, which is from rods to rod depolarizing bipolar cells (DBCs), to rod amacrine cells, and then to on- and off-center ganglion cells via an excitatory synapse to cone DBCs and an inhibitory signal to cone hyperpolarizing bipolar cells (HBCs; Boycott and Dowling, 1969; Dacheux and Raviola, 1986; Wassle et al., 1991). Other pathways have been identified (Deans et al., 2002; Field and Rieke, 2002; Raviola and Gilula, 1973; Soucy et al., 1998). In comparison, cone activity is carried to depolarizing and hyperpolarizing bipolar cells and then, respectively, to the on- and off-center ganglion cells. Lateral inhibitory connections, mediated by horizontal and amacrine cells, form the basis for the development of antagonistic receptive fields, which are instrumental in the coding of spatial patterns and contrast (Shapley and Enroth-Cugell, 1983). Chromatic information is derived from circuits comparing the responses of the different types of cone photoreceptors. The net result is that the output of the photoreceptors is extensively processed by the time that corresponding signals are transmitted from the

ganglion cells via the optic nerve to the lateral geniculate and the visual cortex.

Different regions of the retina are specialized for different functions. These are mirrored by changes in the organization of the retinal architecture. For example, the best acuity is achieved by the central fovea, the foveola (Fig. 52.2). This region contains only cones in a highly ordered packing. Moreover, each foveal cone makes contact with only a single bipolar and ganglion cell of each class (Missotten, 1974; Sterling, 1983). As a result, the response of each foveal cone is transmitted with high fidelity through the retina. Across the retina, Frisen and Frisen (1976) have shown that the decrease in visual acuity that occurs at more peripheral locations is highly correlated with the decrease in ganglion cell density. In comparison, the retinal region with the best sensitivity to light is located some 20 to 30 degrees away. This sensitivity increase reflects the increased concentration of rods in the periphery (Fig. 52.2) and the increased degree of synaptic convergence that is achieved at more peripheral locations.

Ganglion cells transmit information to the lateral geniculate body via action potentials. Each ganglion cell responds to light stimulation only in a certain retinal area called the receptive field. If stimulation of the center of the receptive field induces on-discharges, stimulation of the periphery produces off-discharges (Kuffler, 1953). This center-surround opponent arrangement represents the initial coding step of the central visual system. There are three major classes of cells: the midget cells representing 80% of the ganglion cells and constituting the P or parvocellular pathway, the parasol cells representing 5% to 8% of the ganglion cells and constituting the M or magnocellular pathway, and the bistratified ganglion cells representing 5% of cells and constituting the K or koniocellular pathways (Perry et al., 1984). The P cells have a small receptive field, are slow con-

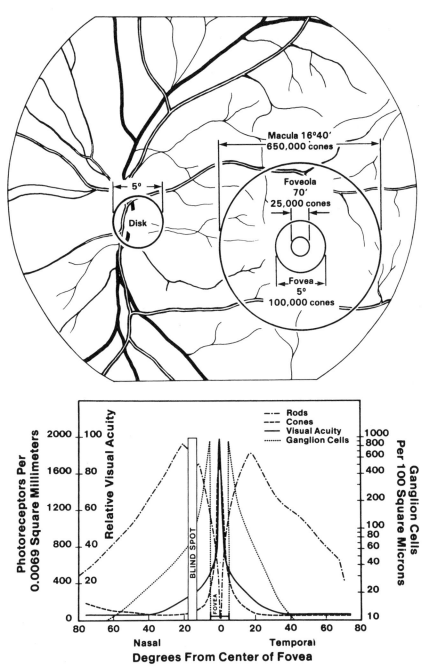

Figure 52.2. **Top:** Ocular fundus. The size of the disk, macula, fovea, and foveola are expressed in degrees of visual angle. **Bottom:** Diagram of the distribution of photoreceptors (rods and cones) and ganglion cells and their relationship to visual acuity. The data on visual acuity are obtained from Jones and Higgins (1952). The distribution of rods and cones is from Osterberg (1935). The distribution of ganglion cells is from Van Buren (1963) and Oppel (1967). Note the logarithmic scale for the ganglion cell distribution.

ducting, have a color opponency mechanism (i.e., red center, green surround spectral opponency) and have a fine spectral discrimination. The M cells have high conduction velocity and a center-surround opponent mechanism and provide analysis of movement. The K cells have no center-surround mechanisms. The function of the K pathway is less clear. Morand et al. (2000) studied the K pathway in humans with electrophysiological techniques and suggested that the K system process moving stimuli via very fast activation of cortical areas. From this study it appears that processing of moving stimuli are mediated by both K and M pathways. The K pathway processes blue-on information from the S-

cone retinal input (Dobkins, 2000); thus, it is also involved in color processing.

This complex retinal physiology can be partially studied by electroretinography. Manipulation of visual stimuli permits evaluation of the functional integrity of photoreceptors and retina neuronal circuitry. Two types of ERGs have been used extensively in clinical practice: flash ERGs and pattern ERGs. They are reviewed below. This chapter focuses on the clinical application of ERGs. The reader is referred to the literature for a more extensive review of the electrophysiology of the retina (Dowling, 1987; Djamgoz et al., 1995).

Flash Electroretinography

In response to the short duration (<1 msec) stimuli typically used in clinical settings, the ERG is composed of two major components, the "a wave" and "b wave," as well as a series of higher frequency oscillatory potentials (Armington, 1974; Fishman et al., 2001). The source of these underlying components has been investigated by intracellular and intraretinal recordings (Brown, 1980; Dowling, 1987; Karwoski et al., 1996) as well as by using pharmacological agents that selectively interfere with different aspects of retinal function (Knapp and Schiller, 1984; Robson et al., 2003; Sieving et al., 1994; Stockton and Slaughter, 1989).

The cornea-negative a wave reflects in large measure the massed response of the rod or cone photoreceptors (Breton et al., 1994; Hood and Birch, 1993, 1994), although postreceptoral contributions are clearly present (Bush and Sieving, 1994; Robson et al., 2003). In comparison, the cells that contribute to the cornea-positive b wave change depending on whether stimulus conditions elicit rod- or cone-mediated potentials. Under dark-adapted conditions, which isolate rod-mediated responses, the b wave reflects the activity of the rod depolarizing bipolar cells (Hood and Birch, 1996; Kofuji et al., 2000; Robson and Frishman, 1995). Under stimulus conditions that isolate cone-mediated activity, the b wave reflects the combined activity of both depolarizing and hyperpolarizing bipolar cells (Bush and Sieving, 1996; Sieving et al., 1994).

A standard ERG testing protocol has been developed for clinical purposes (Marmor and Zrenner, 1998–99). The standard incorporates a series of stimulus conditions designed to isolate rod-mediated responses by presenting stimuli to the dark-adapted eye and cone-mediated responses by rapid flicker and light adaptation. In addition, the standard addresses other important issues such as electrodes, amplifier settings, stimulus calibration, and the establishment of normative data.

In the clinic, the flash ERG is used primarily to evaluate outer retinal function (Fig. 52.3). Flash ERG is particularly useful in the diagnosis of retinal pigmentary degeneration (Fig. 52.4). The ERG is depressed or absent in retinitis pigmentosa (Armington et al., 1961; Berson et al., 1968, 1969, 1979). Retinitis pigmentosa (RP) is a retinal dystrophy affecting predominantly the rods; cones are affected only at advanced stages. RP patients, in the early stages, have in-

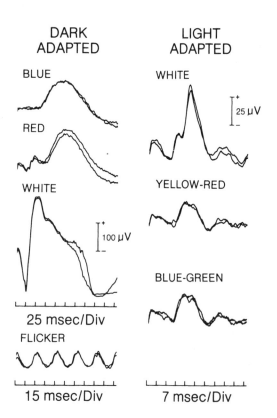

Figure 52.3. Flash ERG in a normal 32-year-old man. Each response represents the average of five ERGs; two averages are superimposed to demonstrate reproducibility. *Left:* ERG to dim suprathreshold and scotopically matched blue and red flashes, to white flashes and to 32-Hz flicker in the absence of background light. *Right:* ERG to white and photopically matched yellow-red and blue-green flashes in the presence of background light. Note the different amplitude and time calibration for the two columns.

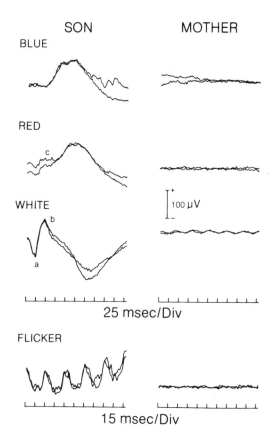

Figure 52.4. Full-field flash ERG in two members of a family. The mother *(right)* suffers from retinitis pigmentosa; her central vision is spared, although her peripheral vision is severely affected. She has nyctalopia. Note the absence of any recognizable ERG. The son *(left),* age 15, has normal fundus and normal visual acuity. The dark-adapted ERGs show small amplitude b wave, particularly to red and white light, suggesting early rod dysfunction. The flicker ERG is normal, indicating normal cone function. a, a wave; b, b wave; c, cone response. (From Celesia, G.G. 1984. Evoked potential techniques in the evaluation of visual function. J. Clin. Neurophysiol. 1:55–76.)

volvement limited to the dark-adapted rod ERG response, accompanied by impaired night vision (nyctalopia). As the disease progresses, they show evidence of impaired cone vision, including reduced amplitude of light-adapted ERG responses. A reduced dark-adapted b wave amplitude with normal b wave latency (often referred to as implicit time) in RP patients indicates a focal disease that leaves segments of the retina normal and able to respond to light with normal latency (Marmor, 1979). A general rule of flash ERG states that preserved latency in the presence of decreased amplitude indicates a focal or patchy retinal disorder, whereas prolonged latency indicates diffuse retinal disease. In the latter case, most of the retinal cells respond abnormally to the stimulus. Early reduction in amplitude and prolongation of latency of dark-adapted rod responses have been found, even before classic funduscopic changes appear, in subjects whose families have dominantly inherited RP. Reduced amplitude and prolonged latencies in the dark-adapted rod responses were also found in female carriers of X-linked retinitis pigmentosa (Berson et al., 1979; Peachey et al., 1988). Therefore, ERG can be used in genetic counseling to detect carriers and early-affected subjects (Fig. 52.4) in families with a history of retinal pigmentary degeneration.

Other inherited retinal diseases demonstrate a more selective involvement of either rod or cone systems. Congenital nyctalopia, a nonprogressive autosomal-dominant disorder of rod function, is characterized by impaired night vision, normal daylight vision, and normal fundi. The ERG shows normal cone function but abnormal rod function with absent or severe reduction of the b wave in dark-adapted testing (Figs. 52.5 and 52.6). Oguchi's disease, another form of night blindness, is characterized by diffuse graying of the fundus and specific ERG changes (Gouras, 1970). The ERG in dark-adapted tests shows low amplitude or absent b waves similar to the ERG of congenital nyctalopes. However, if the eye is allowed to adapt to darkness for an extended period (more than 12 hours), a large amplitude b wave can be obtained in response to dim blue flash.

Congenital achromatopsia (rod monochromatism) affects the cone system selectively. It is characterized by absent color vision and impaired visual acuity. The ERG (Figs. 52.5 and 52.6) shows normal b waves in the dark-adapted state, but no cone oscillations to red flashes and no light-adapted responses, both responses generated via the cone system.

The ERG is also useful in evaluating paraneoplastic retinopathies. Cancer-associated retinopathy (CAR) involves photoreceptor degeneration, with an attendant decline in overall ERG amplitude (Rios et al., 1997; Sawyer et al., 1976; Thirkill et al., 1987). Melanoma-associated retinopathy (MAR) impairs transmission from photoreceptors to depolarizing bipolar cells, and induces a selective reduction in the ERG b wave (Alexander et al., 1992; Milam et al., 1993).

Central retinal occlusion (CRO) produces interesting ERG changes (Armington, 1974; Krill, 1970). In CRO, only

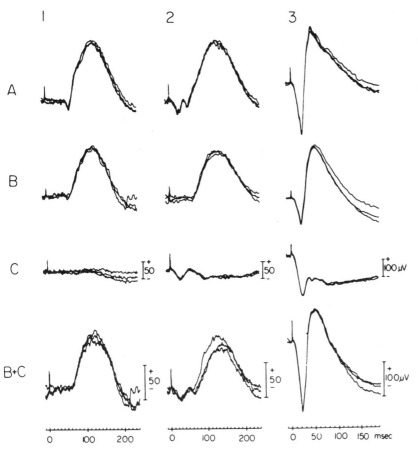

Figure 52.5. Three superimposed single-trace ERGs elicited in dark-adapted conditions by standard, dim, full-field, scotopically matched, blue (1), red (2), and white (3) flashes in a normal subject (**A**), a rod monochromat (**B**), and a congenital nyctalope (**C**). Waveforms in **B** and **C** were obtained by algebraic summation of individual traces from rod monochromat (**B**) and congenital nyctalope (**C**), respectively. (From Chatrian, G.E., Nelson, P.L., Lettich, E., et al. 1980b. Computer assisted electroretinography. II. Separation of rod and cone components of the electroretinogram in congenital achromatopsia and congenital nyctalopia. Am. J. EEG Technol. 20:79–88.)

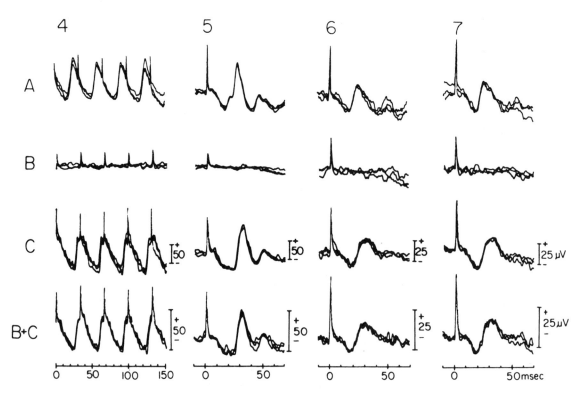

Figure 52.6. Continuation of Figure 52.5. ERGs evoked by standard 30-Hz white flicker stimulus in the absence of background light (4) and by standard single white (5) and photopically matched yellow-red (6) and blue-green (7) flashes in the presence of white background light. (From Chatrian, G.E., Nelson, P.L., Lettich, E., et al. 1980b. Computer assisted electroretinography. II. Separation of rod and cone components of the electroretinogram in congenital achromatopsia and congenital nyctalopia. Am. J. EEG Technol. 20:79–88.)

the retinal circulation supplying the inner retina is impaired; the choroidal circulation remains intact. Sparing of the choroidal circulation results in intact photoreceptors but impaired Müller cells. The ERG, therefore, is characterized by a prominent a wave but depressed or absent b wave. This dramatic effect of retinal anoxia confirms that the a wave represents the leading edge of the large receptor potential (Brown, 1980; Granit, 1955).

ERGs can also help assess degrees of retinal ischemia (Johnson et al., 1988; Sabates et al., 1983). Sabates et al. (1983) have shown in central retinal venous occlusion (CRVO) that the b wave amplitude varies with the amount of retinal ischemia, the presence of which often precedes the development of neurovascular glaucoma. Johnson and Hood (1996) show that ERG changes arise at the photoreceptor level. The possibility that the ERG can be used to select CRVO patients requiring photocoagulation to prevent neurovascular glaucoma is currently being investigated.

Other potentially damaging conditions, particularly those that affect the retina diffusely, may be associated with reduced ERG amplitude (Figs. 52.7 and 52.8A). Damage of the retinal periphery will affect ERG rod components more severely than it will cone components.

Flash ERG testing, therefore, can be utilized in assessing retinal damage and has been shown to be abnormal in many disorders including diabetic and sickle cells retinopathies (Bresnick, 1991; Peachey et al., 1990; Ramsay et al., 1977), retinoschisis (Peachey et al., 1987b), cone and rod degenera-

tions (Fishman et al., 2001; Heckenlively et al., 1991), as well as other disorders. Gouras and Niemeyer (2004) suggest, "Responses less than 10 μV are usually pathological. Responses that are in the range of a μV indicate severe retinal pathology. Those of 0.1 μV or less, often called 'extinguished,' are invariably associated with a severe visual handicap."

Superimposed on the ascending slope of the flash ERG are a series of four to six wavelets, the *oscillatory potentials* (OPs). The OPs are high-frequency responses in the region of 100 to 160 Hz and can be easily isolated from slower ERG components by selective filtering using an amplifier bandpass of 100 to 500 or 1,000 Hz (Celesia, 1988; Karwoski and Kawasaki, 1991; Peachey et al., 1987a). The origin of these signals is not completely clarified, but they appear to be generated in the IPL and most likely are related to depolarizing amacrine and interplexiform neuronal cells (Sakai and Naka, 1988; Wachmeister, 2001). OPs can be utilized as selective probes of the functional integrity of the neuronal circuitry of the proximal retina. Clinically they have been shown to be abnormal in diabetic and ischemic retinopathies (Fig. 52.8B) independently and often before abnormalities of the b wave have been detected (Bresnick, 1991; Bresnick and Palta, 1987; Bresnick et al., 1984; van der Torren and van Lith, 1989).

While the flash ERG provides a useful index of overall retinal function, many retinal disorders impair only the macular region (Fishman et al., 2001). Macular disorders are

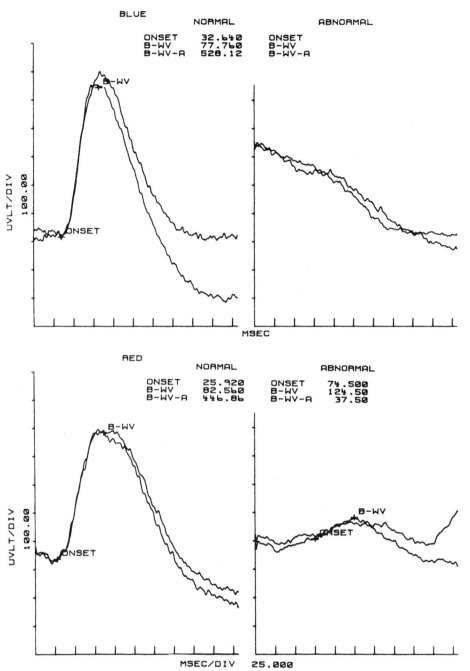

Figure 52.7. ERGs in the dark-adapted state to dim blue and red flashes in a normal subject *(left column)* and in a 54-year-old man with diabetic retinopathy *(right column)*. The diabetic patient complained of impaired night vision and dimmed vision. Visual acuity was 20/25. Note that the b wave is almost absent to blue flashes and very small to red flashes, indicating severe impairment of the rod system. B-WV, latency of b wave; B-WV-A, amplitude of b wave. (From Celesia, G.G. 1985a. Visual evoked responses. In *Evoked Potential Testing. Clinical Applications,* Eds. J.H. Owen and H. Davis, pp. 1–54. Orlando, FL: Grune & Stratton.)

particularly disabling because they affect the high acuity fovea. Flash ERGs in such patients are typically normal. Two related approaches have been developed to address this issue. The focal ERG technique involves presenting a small (~1 degree) high-frequency stimulus to the fovea using a stimulator-ophthalmoscope (Sandberg and Ariel, 1977). An annular surround of steady light reduces the effectiveness of light scattered from the test region. This technique has been useful in evaluating patients with macular disease (Birch et al., 1988; Sandberg et al., 1979). The multifocal ERG (mfERG) technique extends the focal analysis of retinal function by isolating responses to a large number of retinal areas simultaneously, providing a map of retinal function that defines outer retinal involvement in cases of visual loss (Bearse and Sutter, 1996; Keating et al., 2000; Marmor et al., 2003). mfERG is effective for early detection and assessment of a wide range of conditions that involve the retina in focal areas such as such as macular disease, vascular disease, inflammatory disorders, etc.

Pattern Electroretinography

Pattern ERGs (P-ERGs) were first obtained by pattern-reversal stimuli, in which patterns alternate but mean luminance is kept constant (Armington, 1968; Riggs et al.,

Figure 52.8. **A:** Continuation of Figure 52.7. The upper ERGs were obtained in the dark-adapted state with white flashes. The lower ERGs were obtained with 32-Hz white flicker. Both a and b waves to a white flash have a small amplitude. The latency of the b wave to flicker is delayed at 43.2 msec (boundary of normality, 36.0). These findings indicate the presence of a diffuse retinopathy. (From Celesia, G.G. 1985a. Visual evoked responses. In *Evoked Potential Testing. Clinical Applications,* Eds. J.H. Owen and H. Davis, pp. 1–54. Orlando, FL: Grune & Stratton.)

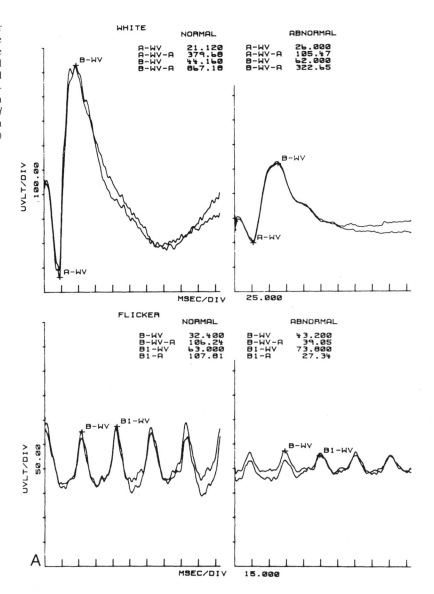

1964; reviewed by Zrenner, 1990). The spatial frequency-amplitude function of the P-ERG shows a band-passing tuning behavior (Celesia and Tobimatsu, 1990; Fiorentini et al., 1981; Hess and Baker, 1984; Tobimatsu et al., 1989) with attenuation at low spatial frequencies. Attenuation at low spatial frequencies indicates that the P-ERG originates in cells with lateral inhibition and center-surround receptive field organization. Bipolar and ganglion cells both have center-surround receptive field organization. Transection of the optic nerve in cats and monkeys results in retrograde degeneration of the ganglion cells and abolition of steady-state and transient P-ERGs (Celesia and Tobimatsu, 1990; Dawson et al., 1986; Hollander et al., 1984; Maffei and Fiorentini, 1981; Tobimatsu et al., 1989). The current source density analysis of P-ERG in monkeys has shown a dipole localized in the proximal 30% of the retina at the GCL/IPL/INL level (Baker et al., 1988; Sieving and Steinberg, 1987). Zrenner and Nelson (1988) recorded the mem-

brane depolarizing potentials of amacrine cells and showed their remarkable similarity to the transient P-ERG. They suggested that P-ERG may be a mixture of ganglion and amacrine cell responses. Holder (2001) suggests that the N95 component of P-ERG arises in the spiking activity of the retinal ganglion cells, whereas some of the b wave (or P50) arises in more upstream retinal structures (Holder, 2001; Viswanathan et al., 2000).

It is now generally agreed that the P-ERG is predominantly a foveal response that originates in the proximal retina. The size of the spatial features of stimuli used to evoke the P-ERG is an important variable that may influence the source of the response (Baker et al., 1988; Celesia, 1988; Celesia and Tobimatsu, 1990; Celesia et al., 1987). P-ERGs to high and medium spatial frequency stimuli (i.e., with small stimulus elements) are dependent on the integrity of ganglion cells with a contribution from amacrine cells (Baker and Hess, 1984; Baker et al., 1988; Celesia and

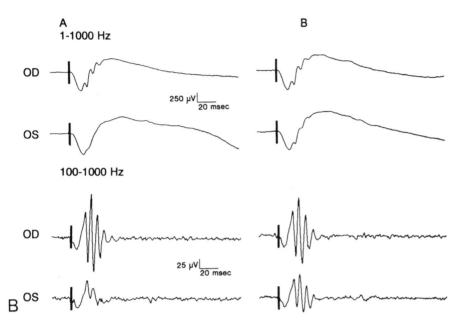

CENTRAL RETINAL VEIN OCCLUSION

Figure 52.8 (continued). **B:** A 32-year-old woman with central retinal vein occlusion in the left eye (OS). Visual acuity in the left eye was 20/200. *A,* ERGs recorded at the onset of the disorder; *B,* ERGs recorded 6 months later when the patient's vision had recovered to 20/30. The *upper half* of the illustration shows the oscillatory potential (OP) riding on the ascending slope of the b wave. The *lower half* of the figure shows the simultaneously recorded OP with the low bandpass at 100 Hz to eliminate the a and b waves. The OPs are then easily recognizable. Note normal responses from the right eye (OD) and the small OPs from the left eye. The a and b waves were normal from both eyes. (From N.S. Peachey, 1991, unpublished.)

Kaufman, 1985; Celesia and Tobimatsu, 1990; Hess and Baker, 1984; Holder, 2001; Viswanathan et al., 2000; Zrenner and Nelson, 1988). However, the pattern reversal to low spatial frequencies stimuli is a mixed response containing a second harmonic response to luminance (Baker et al., 1988; Celesia et al., 1991; Tomoda et al., 1991a,b).

P-ERGs to transient stimuli consist of a negative a wave followed by a positive b wave (Fig. 52.9). Often the b wave of P-ERG is called P50 and is followed by another negative wave called N95. The amplitude and latency of P-ERG waves are tabulated in Table 52.1.

If the P-ERG reflects postreceptor retinal activity and possibly ganglion cell activity, it can be used as a marker to determine retinocortical transient time, provided visual evoked scalp potentials are recorded simultaneously. Retinocortical transient time (RCT) will then reflect activity outside the retina in the visual pathways (Celesia and Kaufman, 1985; Celesia and Tobimatsu, 1990; Celesia et al., 1987; Kaufman and Celesia, 1985). RCT is defined as the difference in milliseconds between VEP and ERG wave latencies. Two retinocortical times have been calculated: RCT(b-N70) equals the latency of N70 minus b wave (or P50) latency, and RCT(b-P100) equals the latency of P100 minus the b wave (or P50) latency.

P-ERGs to steady-state stimulation consist of quasi-sinusoidal deflections as shown in Fig. 52.9. The mean amplitude of a steady-state P-ERG to 15′ checks is 2.5 μV; to 31′ check, it is 3.2 μV. In retinal lesions affecting the macula preferentially, Celesia and Kaufman (1985) described abnormal transient P-ERGs in 89% of cases with checks of 15′ and in 67% of patients with checks of 31′. Small or absent P-ERG has also been noted in senile macular degeneration

(Fig. 52.10). In cases of early macular degeneration, P-ERG was present but delayed (Celesia and Kaufman, 1985; Kaufman and Celesia, 1985). Similar absent or greatly depressed P-ERGs in macular diseases were described by Sherman (1982) and Holder (2001).

P-ERG abnormalities are not limited to maculopathies. They are also present in any optic nerve lesions with associated retrograde ganglion cell degeneration (Bobak et al., 1983; Celesia and Kaufman, 1985; Dawson et al., 1982; Fiorentini et al., 1981; Kaufman et al., 1988; Maffei, 1982). The implications of P-ERG abnormalities in optic nerve dysfunction are discussed in more detail in the section on anterior visual pathway function.

A delayed P-ERG occurs only in macular diseases; absent or markedly depressed P-ERGs are present in either maculopathies or severe optic nerve diseases associated with axonal involvement and retrograde ganglion cell degeneration. It should be emphasized that in macular lesions flash ERGs are normal (Fig. 52.10). Thus P-ERGs are useful in the assessment of macular function and retinal ganglion cell function (Celesia and Brigell, 1999; Holder, 2001). Holder (2001) suggests that the P-ERG P50 (or b wave) can be used as an index of macular function. Reduction in P-ERG N95 with preservation of P50 may indicate dysfunction at the level of the retinal ganglion cells (Holder, 2001).

These data support the principle of selective activation: different structures of the retina can be preferentially, if not exclusively, activated by varying the type of stimulation (Celesia, 1984). Flashes selectively activate retinal luminance and color detectors, whereas small pattern stimuli preferentially activate contrast and edge detectors.

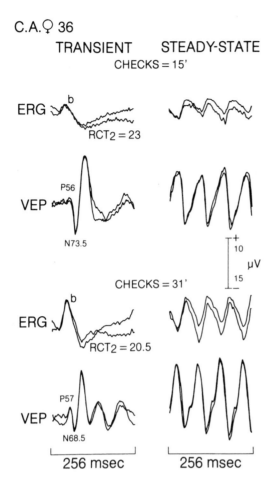

C.A.♀ 36

TRANSIENT   STEADY-STATE

CHECKS = 15'

ERG   b   RCT₂ = 23

VEP   P56   N73.5

+ 10 μV 15 −

CHECKS = 31'

ERG   b   RCT₂ = 20.5

VEP   P57   N68.5

256 msec   256 msec

Figure 52.9. Normal pattern ERG (P-ERG) and visual evoked potential (VEP) to transient and steady-state pattern stimulation in a 36-year-old woman. Positive is upward for both P-ERG and VEP. In the calibration, 5 refers to P-ERG amplitude and 10 to VEP amplitude. Two responses are superimposed to verify reproducibility of the data. The upper half of the figure shows the responses to 15′ checks; the lower half shows response to 31′ checks. RCT₂, retinocortical transmission time in milliseconds from the ERG b wave to the N70 deflection.

Function of Anterior Visual Pathways

Anatomy and Physiology

The optic nerve and chiasma are arbitrarily included in the definition of anterior visual pathways for the purpose of this review. The optic nerve from the eye to the chiasm is about 50 mm long and comprises nerve fibers originating in the ganglion cells. Nerve fibers from ganglion cells in the macula constitute the papillomacular bundle that occupies the entire temporal side of the optic disk. This bundle of fibers then moves toward the center of the optic disk as it approaches the chiasma. Fibers from peripheral ganglion cells occupy less central positions in the optic disk and optic nerve (Hoyt and Luis, 1962; Minckler, 1980). The optic nerve fibers are small myelinated fibers; 92% of the axons are 2 μm or less in diameter, 6% have a diameter around 4 μm, and only 2% have a large axon (>4 μm) (Oppel, 1963). Calculated conduction velocities range from 1.3 to 20 msec (Ogden and Miller, 1966; Ogden, 1984).

The human retina projects to both ipsi- and contralateral sides of the cortex. Fibers from the nasal retina cross in the chiasma; crossed and uncrossed fibers begin to separate at the termination of the optic nerve. Macular fibers also are subdivided into crossed and uncrossed fibers; the macular fibers from the nasal portion of the macula cross in the chiasma into the contralateral optic tract, whereas the macular temporal fibers travel into the ipsilateral optic tract.

The functional integrity of the visual pathways, once they enter the optic nerve, can be assessed using VEPs recorded from the occipital scalp region. It is presumed that these potentials are near-field potentials from the visual cortices (Arroyo et al., 1997; Celesia et al., 1982). It is therefore important to review briefly the physiology of the central visual system. Visual neurons respond selectively to progressively more complex visual patterns, at ascending levels in the cortical hierarchy (Barlow, 1953; Hubel and Wiesel, 1959, 1968, 1974). Individual neurons can be selectively sensitive to movement orientation and direction and the width, length, velocity, and contrast of stimuli. Each neuron must be con-

Table 52.1. Pattern ERGs and VEPS: Normative Data

Parameter	15′ Checks		31′ Checks	
	Range	Mean ± SD	Range	Mean ± SD
ERG				
a wave latency[a]	20.5–37.0	28.3 ± 3.0	20.0–36.0	27.1 ± 2.6
b wave latency	38.0–55.5	47.3 ± 2.7	39.0–54.0	46.1 ± 2.5
b wave amplitude	0.4–5.1	1.8 ± 0.8	0.5–7.1	2.3 ± 1.1
VEP				
P60 latency	50.0–75.0	60.9 ± 4.2	44.5–67.0	56.1 ± 3.5
N70 latency	63.5–87.5	75.5 ± 4.1	60.0–87.5	70.8 ± 3.7
N70 amplitude	1.0–18.2	5.1 ± 3.1	0.7–14.5	3.9 ± 2.2
P100 latency	83.5–107.5	98.1 ± 4.4	81.5–107.0	94.7 ± 5.0
P100 amplitude	1.1–38.1	9.9 ± 5.9	1.9–29.9	8.7 ± 4.7
Retinocortical time				
RCT (b-N70)	17.0–40.5	28.3 ± 3.9	13.5–38.5	24.8 ± 3.3
RCT (b-P100)	39.0–63.0	50.8 ± 4.0	36.5–60.5	48.7 ± 4.4

[a]Latencies are expressed in milliseconds; amplitudes are expressed in microvolts.

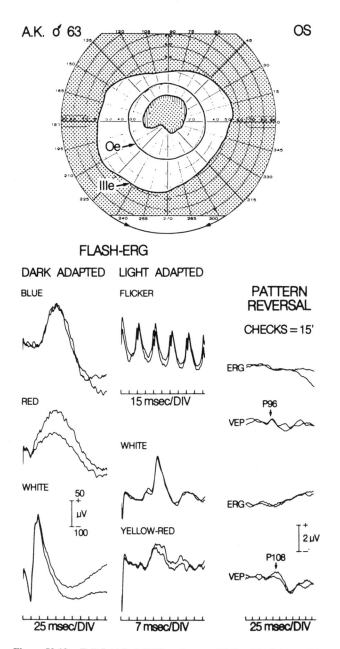

Figure 52.10. Full-field flash ERGs and pattern ERGs of the left eye (OS) in a 63-year-old man with senile macular degeneration. Note the presence of a large central scotoma in the visual field. Flash ERGs are shown in the first and second column and are normal. Normal flash ERGs indicate normal functioning photoreceptors and absence of a diffuse retinal disorder. The third column shows P-ERGs and VEPs. The upper two tracings are the response to 15′ checks, the lower tracings responses to 31′ checks. Note the absence of P-ERG and the very small but still present VEPs. (From Celesia, G.G. 1985a. Visual evoked responses. In *Evoked Potential Testing. Clinical Applications,* Eds. J.H. Owen and H. Davis, pp. 1–54. Orlando, FL: Grune & Stratton.)

striate cortex (Hendrickson, 1985; Livingstone and Hubel, 1982, 1984, 1988; Tootell et al., 1981). The techniques of [¹⁴C]deoxyglucose autoradiography and cytochrome oxidase staining have demonstrated the existence of dots, stripes, and columns representing complex units of cortical organization in the visual system (Hendrickson, 1985; Livingstone and Hubel, 1982, 1984, 1988).

Although there is still debate about whether cortical cells are feature detectors or spatial frequency filters (Albrecht et al., 1980; Campbell and Robson, 1968; Hubel and Wiesel, 1959, 1968; Tootell et al., 1981), it is generally agreed that the visual system is a multichannel device that processes information via parallel channels (Arden, 1978; Regan, 1989; Shapley, 1982) and that each channel constitutes a set of sequential processes (Celesia, 1984).

Empirically, it has been shown that full-field stimulation with patterned stimuli is best suited to evaluating anterior pathway function (Celesia, 1978, 1982; Celesia and Daly, 1977b; Halliday, 1978; Halliday et al., 1972, 1977). VEPs to patterned stimuli are discussed in the next two sections.

Transient VEPs

Transient visual evoked potentials (T-VEPs) result from *transient* changes in brain activity after intermittent stimulation. Pharmacological studies indicate that the recorded waveform reflects the algebraic summation of more fundamental underlying components (Arakawa et al., 1993; Zemon et al., 1980). T-VEPs are critically dependent on many parameters: stimulus brightness or luminance, contrast level, type of photic stimulus (patterned or unpatterned), type and size of patterned stimuli, total field size, and method and presentation rate (Arden et al., 1977; Celesia et al., 1993). We recommend that the guidelines set by the International Society for Clinical Electrophysiology of Vision (Odom et al., 2004) and the International Federation of Clinical Neurophysiology (Celesia and Brigell, 1999) be followed. Although T-VEPs can be elicited by a variety of visual stimuli, including flashes, light emitting diodes (LEDs), and gratings (Bodis-Wollner and Onofrj, 1982; Bodis-Wollner et al., 1979; Camisa et al., 1981; Lesser et al., 1985), the most frequently used stimulus is checkerboard pattern reversal. Checkerboard-patterned stimuli consist of series of black and white checks reversing at a set reversal rate. Checkerboard pattern reversal has become the preferred stimulus because it evokes reproducible and relatively large potentials (Celesia and Brigell, 1999; Odom et al., 2004). Check sizes and contrast are important variables in the use of patterned stimuli. Checks or gratings of less than 30′ of arc stimulate predominantly contrast and spatial frequency detectors, whereas patterns at low spatial frequency (checks larger than 40′) inevitably stimulate luminance channels (Maffei, 1982). Checks equal to or smaller than 15′ of arc not only stimulate contrast and spatial frequency channels but also preferentially stimulate the fovea (Harter and White, 1970; Meredith and Celesia, 1982; Regan and Richards, 1971).

Field and check sizes may have to be changed relative to the region of the visual pathways to be studied. To detect small demyelinating lesions affecting optic nerve fibers originating in ganglion cells subserving the fovea (the papil-

sidered a multichannel coding device responding to specific information presented in the stimulus (Celesia, 1984; Hendrickson, 1985). There is anatomical and electrophysiological evidence that the primate visual cortex is subdivided into distinct anatomical regions that process different types of visual information, and has a separate connection to the pre-

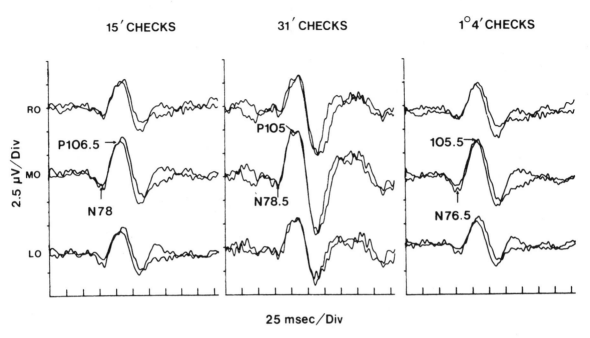

JB ♂ AGE 71 OD

Figure 52.11. Normal P-VEPs to three different size checks in a 71-year-old man. The two major waves N70 and P100 have been labeled. Positive waves have an upward deflection. RO, right occipital; MO, midoccipital; LO, left occipital; OD, right eye. (From Celesia, G.G. and Cone, S. 1985. Visual evoked potentials: a practical approach within the guidelines for clinical evoked potential studies. Am. J. EEG. Technol. 25:93–113.)

lomacular bundle), checks equal to or smaller than 30′ with a small total field should be used. On the other hand, to stimulate areas outside the fovea to detect chiasmal or retrochiasmal lesions, large fields with check sizes greater than 1′ may be preferable (Celesia, 1984).

Normative Data

T-VEPs consist of positive-negative deflections designated by capital letters followed by a number indicating the average latency. The two most frequent waves (Fig. 52.11) are designated N70 (negative wave occurring at about 70 msec) and P100 (positive wave occurring at around 100 msec). Often, a positive wave around 50 msec, named P50, precedes N70.

Normative data values for responses to 15′ and 31′ checks are shown in Table 52.1. Normative data were obtained with bandpass filters of 5 to 250 Hz. Analog filters may drastically modify the wave morphology affecting both response amplitude and latency (Fig. 52.12). If the recording is noisy, an alternative to analog filtering is the use of digital filtering and/or waveform smoothing (De Weerd, 1984; Wastell, 1979). These two methods eliminate some of the noise in the tracing without introducing any latency shift.

N70 and P100 latencies change with age (Allison et al., 1983; Celesia and Daly, 1977a,b; Shaw and Cant, 1980; Shearer and Dustman, 1980; Sokol et al., 1981; Tomoda et al., 1991a,b). Increased latency is most evident after age 45 and is caused by a combination of age-related phenomena: decreased conduction velocity in the optic nerve

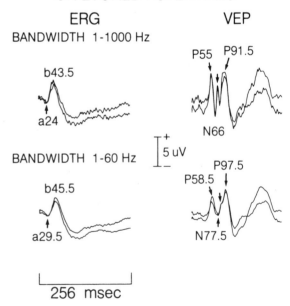

EFFECTS OF HIGH FREQUENCY FILTERS ON EVOKED POTENTIALS

Figure 52.12. Effects of high-frequency analog filters on the amplitude and latency of pattern-evoked ERGs and VEPs in a subject with suspected multiple sclerosis (MS). The responses were recorded simultaneously but with different bandwidths. A sharp positive wave seen between waves P55 and P91.5 with wide bandpass filters is reduced to a notch with high filters of 60 Hz. The filter of 60 Hz also produces a phase shift in the latencies of all waves.

and optic pathways due to defective myelin regeneration (Wisniewski and Terry, 1976) or axonal dystrophy (Dolman et al., 1980; Sung, 1964), corpora amylacea in the optic nerve and chiasm (Andrew, 1971), degeneration of retinal ganglion cells (Gartner and Henkind, 1981; Varbec, 1965), changes in neurotransmitter function and increased synaptic delay (Samorajski, 1977; Wayner and Emmers, 1958), or neuronal loss in the lateral geniculate and striate cortex (Ordy and Brizzee, 1979).

Gender also affects response latency, with females displaying slightly shorter latencies (Allison et al., 1983; Celesia, 1985a). It is suggested that the small differences in latencies between sexes can be accounted for by differences in brain size and the related smaller and shorter pathways in females (Allison et al., 1983).

Clinical Applications

In 1972, Halliday et al. demonstrated the usefulness of T-VEPs to checkerboard pattern reversal in the diagnosis of optic neuritis. Since that time, delayed or absent T–VEPs to pattern-reversal stimulation have been employed effectively to detect optic nerve pathology.

Abnormal pattern T-VEPs have been reported in many disorders affecting the optic nerve, including retrobulbar neuritis, papillitis, ischemic optic neuropathy, toxic and metabolic optic neuropathy, optic nerve compression, and optic atrophy (Bobak et al., 1988; Bodis-Wollner et al.,

1979; Celesia, 1978, 1982; Celesia and Daly, 1977b; Celesia et al., 1987; Franco et al., 1987; Halliday, 1978; Halliday et al., 1976, 1977; Kirkham and Coupland, 1983; Vernant et al., 1997).

T-VEPs are quite useful in helping to establish the diagnosis of multiple sclerosis (MS). The presence of delayed (Fig. 52.13) or absent T-VEPs in the absence of retinal pathology suggests the presence of an optic nerve lesion. The demonstration of an optic nerve lesion in a subject with evidence of central nervous system disorder may establish the presence of multiple lesions, the hallmark of MS diagnosis. In the author's laboratory, T-VEPs were delayed or absent in 72% of patients suffering from MS (Fig. 52.14). More important is the great sensitivity of VEPs to subclinical optic nerve lesions. Indeed, VEPs can reveal silent pathologies in the absence of other clinical signs of visual impairment; 54% to 70% of MS patients without visual dysfunction and with normal neuro-ophthalmological examination had delayed VEPs (Andersson and Siden, 1995; Asselman et al., 1975; Becker and Richards, 1984; Bodis-Wollner et al., 1979; Bottcher and Trojaborg, 1982; Celesia, 1978; Celesia et al., 1986, 1987; Guerit and Argiles, 1988; Halliday et al., 1972, 1977).

By using more than one stimulus parameter in optic nerve function assessment, one can test more than one "parallel information processing channel" and more accurately detect abnormalities (Celesia, 1984). Pathological processes

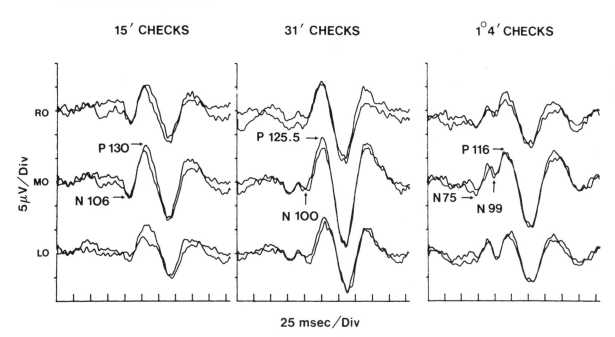

Figure 52.13. T-VEPs in a patient with the diagnosis of definite MS but no evidence of visual dysfunction. Upward deflection indicates positivity. RO, right occipital; MO, midoccipital; LO, left occipital; OD, right eye. Pattern reversal with checks of three different sizes were used. Note that the latency prolongation of wave N70 and P100 is more severe for smaller checks than for larger ones. The major positive wave of the VEPs to 1-degree, 4' stimuli is dispersed into two waves. (From Celesia, G.G., and Cone, S. 1985. Visual evoked potentials: a practical approach within the guidelines for clinical evoked potential studies. Am. G. EEG Technol. 25:93–113.)

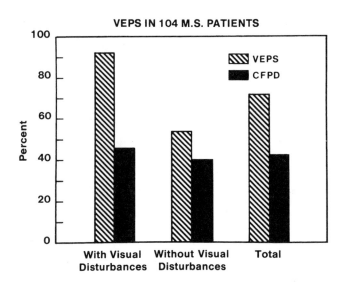

VEPS IN 104 M.S. PATIENTS

Figure 52.14. Results of T-VEPs to pattern reversal with checks of 31′ and to critical frequency of photic driving (CFPD) in 104 patients with suspected MS.

can affect these channels differentially. For instance, patients with suspected MS have been found to have delayed VEPs only when the stimulus pattern was presented in a specific orientation or with a specific spatial frequency (Camisa et al., 1981; Coupland and Kirkham, 1982). A pattern presented in a different orientation or specific frequency often evoked normal potentials.

T-VEPs can also detect chiasmic compression (Gott et al., 1979; Halliday et al., 1976). Patients with computed tomographic (CT) evidence of suprasellar extension and normal visual fields had abnormal VEPs (Gott et al., 1979). Absent or prolonged T-VEPs to full-field pattern stimulation indicate direct optic nerve compression or compromise by vascular impairment. Detection of chiasmatic lesions in the absence of optic nerve involvement requires the use of hemifield stimulation. Absence or prominent amplitude depression of responses to stimulation of both temporal or both nasal hemifields is unequivocal evidence of chiasmatic impairment.

T-VEPs must be interpreted with caution. Refractive errors and retinal diseases may affect both latency and amplitude. Delayed latency and decreased amplitude have been reported with as little as two diopters of refractive error, especially with the use of small checks and low contrast level stimulation (Collins et al., 1979; Van Lith, 1980). Pupil size is another variable that influences the amplitude and latency of T-VEP. Tobimatsu et al. (1988) showed that the increased P100 latency with decreased pupillary diameter is caused by decreased retinal illuminance. They estimated that P100 latency will increase by 10 to 15 msec/log unit of decreased retinal illuminance. *It is of paramount importance to avoid misinterpretation of VEPs abnormalities due to refractory errors, pupillary changes, or lens opacities as related to pathology in the visual pathways.*

We recommend (Celesia, 1999) the following precautions:

1. Measurement of visual acuity and pupil diameter of each eye.

2. Use of corrective lenses to compensate for refractory errors.
3. In cases of refractive errors greater than 20/100, determine whether the acuity can be corrected with a "pinhole."
4. Pupils should not be dilated with midriatics.
5. Use monocular stimulation.

Delayed or absent P100 has been reported in retinal diseases, particularly in maculopathies (Celesia and Kaufman, 1985; Chatrian et al., 1982). Most often, retinal pathology can be excluded by examining the fundus. However, in early maculopathies, the fundus may appear normal. In such cases, the simultaneous use of pattern ERG and VEPs allows differentiation between demyelinating optic nerve diseases and maculopathies. In the former, the pattern ERG is normal; in the latter, the ERG is either delayed or severely depressed.

Simultaneous P-ERG and VEP recordings in patients with MS (Fig. 52.15) reveals three types of abnormalities: (a) normal P-ERG, delayed VEPs, and prolonged RCT; (b) normal P-ERGs and absent VEPs; and (c) absent P-ERGs and VEPs (Celesia and Kaufman, 1985; Celesia et al., 1986; Kaufman and Celesia, 1985). Normal P-ERGs, accompanied by prolonged VEPs and RCT, indicate demyelination of the optic nerve, whereas normal P-ERGs in the absence of VEPs indicate total block of the optic nerve fibers stimulated by the specific pattern. Impaired P-ERGs with absent or delayed VEPs suggest severe axonal involvement with retrograde degeneration of ganglion cells. Kaufman et al. (1985, 1988) have suggested that in cases of recent optic neuritis an abnormal P-ERG (absent or greatly reduced P-ERG) indicates poor prognosis for visual recovery, whereas the preservation of P-ERGs is usually associated with visual function recovery. These authors further demonstrated that progressive loss of P-ERG amplitude correlated with the development of optic nerve atrophy.

In a prospective 12-month study of optic neuritis (Celesia and Tobimatsu, 1990), we simultaneously evaluated visual field, visual acuity, contrast sensitivity, color vision, and VEP to 15′ and 30′ checks. Visual fields, color vision, and VEPs to 15′ checks were initially abnormal in all patients. Contrast sensitivity was abnormal in 95% and visual acuity and VEPs to 30′ in 90% of patients. Recovery of vision occurred in 80% of patients. It was rapid and complete in the majority of cases within the first 2 months. VEPs latency, however, remained prolonged in 19 (95%) patients, even when their vision had returned to normal. VEPs are a reliable indicator of resolved optic neuritis and can be useful to verify a past episode of optic neuritis (Celesia and Tobimatsu, 1990; Hood et al., 2000; Neima and Regan, 1984).

With the advent of magnetic resonance imaging (MRI) and related neuroimaging techniques, the issue has become the usefulness of VEPs in the neurologist armamentarium. Although there are few studies comparing the two modalities, there are data confirming the importance of VEPs in selective cases (Miller et al., 1988). VEPs are diagnostically important in cases of acute transverse myelitis. The American Academy Transverse Myelitis Consortium Group (2002) states: "Brain MRI with gadolinium and visual

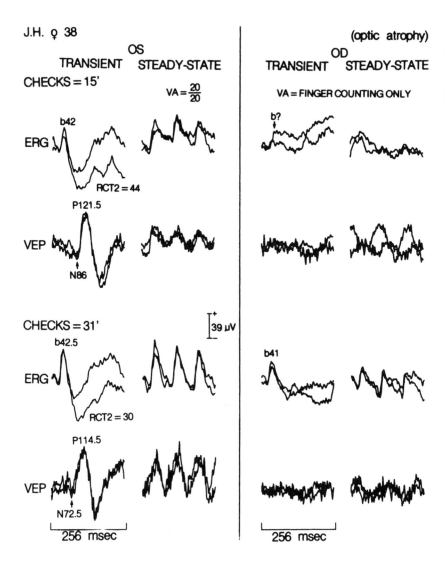

Figure 52.15. Optic atrophy in a 38-year-old woman with retrobulbar neuritis due to MS. Note the probable absence of transient P-ERG at 15' checks stimulation, but its presence at 31' checks in the affected eye (OD). Steady-state P-ERG to 15' checks is also absent. Larger checks of 31' produce a small P-ERG, probably related to stimulation of the perimacular area. There is a total block of nerve conduction through the optic nerve manifested by absence of VEPs to both 15' and 31' checks. Stimulation of the normal left eye (OS) shows normal P-ERGs but prolonged P100 and retinocortical transient time (RCT) to stimulation with 15' checks.

evoked potentials will determine if there is demyelination elsewhere in the neuraxis, therefore, defining the process as multifocal." VEPs have been retained as the only useful sensory evoked potentials in the revised multiple sclerosis diagnostic criteria (McDonald et al., 2001). McDonald et al. (2001) point out that VEPs are not necessary in the diagnosis if the patient has had two or more attacks and has MRI evidence of multiple lesions.

In conclusion, VEPs are very sensitive in detecting dysfunction in the optic nerve, and can objectively demonstrate the presence of a lesion outside the brain and confirm the multiplicity of lesions for the diagnosis of multiple sclerosis.

Steady-State VEPs

Steady-state potentials are electrical events evoked by rapid repetitive sensory stimulation. Continuous rapid stimulation evokes responses of constant amplitude and frequency. Each potential overlaps another so that no individual response can be related to any particular stimulus cycle (Celesia, 1982; Regan, 1989). It is presumed that the brain has achieved a steady state of excitability. Steady-state potentials can be studied by conventional averaging methods or by Fourier analysis.

Steady-state VEPs (S-VEPs) to pattern reversal checks or gratings consist of sinusoidal deflections, usually at double the frequency of the reversal cycle. Thus, an 8-Hz pattern reversal evokes responses having 16 deflections/sec (Fig. 52.9). The rapid stimulation rates possible in steady-state studies permit considerable time savings and therefore a more complete analysis of visual system physiology and pathophysiology (Atkinson et al., 1979; Bodis-Wollner et al., 1972; Kupersmith et al., 1984; Odom et al., 1982; Pirchio et al., 1978; Regan, 1989; Spekreijse et al., 1973). VEPs specific to changes in contrast, and their relation to psychophysical contrast modulation threshold, were demonstrated with steady-state responses (Bodis-Wollner et al., 1972; Spekreijse et al., 1973). Spatial and temporal frequency tuning in the human retina and cortex were also demonstrated using this technique (Odom et al., 1982; Peachey and Seiple, 1987).

Clinically, steady-state responses to grating have been successfully used to establish the contrast sensitivity of in-

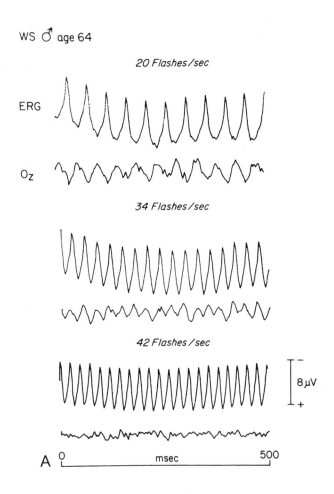

WS ♂ age 64

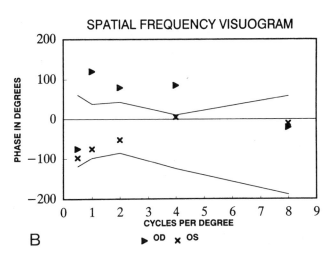

SPATIAL FREQUENCY VISUOGRAM

B

▶ OD ✕ OS

Figure 52.16. **A:** CFPD from stimulation of the right eye in a 64-year-old paraplegic with a 10-year history of progressive chronic myelopathy. Note normal ERG responses (retinal CFPD) while cortical responses were absent after the flash frequency was increased above 34 flashes/second. This dissociation between retinal and cortical CFPD suggests dysfunction of the right optic nerve. (From Celesia, G.G. 1982. Steady state and transient visual evoked potentials in clinical practice. Ann. N.Y. Acad. Sci. 388: 290–305.) **B:** Spatial frequency visuogram in a 52-year-old man with known multiple sclerosis and normal visual acuity in both eyes. Five spatial frequency stimuli were tested. The two lines, one above and one below the zero line, represent the boundary of normality. Note normal responses with stimulation of the left eye (OS), but abnormal phase lag for responses obtained at the middle spatial frequencies with stimulation of the right eye (OD).

fants (Atkinson et al., 1979; Pirchio et al., 1978) and demonstrate contrast sensitivity loss in MS⁻ (Kupersmith et al., 1984).

S-VEPs to flashes are used to determine the critical frequency of photic driving (CFPD). CFPD is defined as the highest frequency at which photic driving is detectable and is measured in flashes per second (Celesia, 1978; Celesia and Daly, 1977a,b; Cohen et al., 1980). CFPD represents the objective counterpart of critical flicker fusion. Simultaneous recording of ERGs and midoccipital VEPs allows assessment of retinal as well as cortical CFPD (Fig. 52.16), the values of which should be the same in normal individuals.

CFPD was abnormal in 42% of a group of 104 MS patients (Fig. 52.14); although it was less sensitive than pattern VEPs, it was the sole abnormality in two patients. Patients with optic opacities cannot be tested with pattern VEPs, but CFPD measurement permits evaluation of the function of the retinal cone system as well as the functional integrity of the visual pathways that process luminance. In optic nerve lesions, retinal CFPD is normal, but cortical CFPD is at least 10 flashes/sec lower than retinal CFPD (Fig. 52.16A).

Fourier analysis has been used to study S-VEPs to harmonically simple light (Regan, 1989); both phase and amplitude can be studied with this method. Responses were found to be phase delayed and of low amplitude in retrobulbar neuritis (Heron et al., 1974; Regan, 1975). The visual deficits of patients are often limited to a discrete subset of

visual function not routinely tested. Orientation-dependent deficits (Camisa et al., 1981) and abnormalities limited to a narrow range of spatial frequencies have been described in multiple sclerosis (Neima and Regan, 1984). The utilization of fast Fourier analysis with interfaced computer-generated visual stimulation permits the rapid evaluation of spatial frequency functions with power spectrum analysis that cannot be done with conventional averaging. Steady-state responses to sinusoidal gratings alternating at 4 Hz with spatial frequencies varying from 0.5 to 8 cycles/degree were studied by Celesia et al. (1992) in 21 normals and 21 patients with multiple sclerosis. Amplitude and phase of the second harmonic responses were plotted as a function of spatial frequency and referred to as amplitude and phase visuograms. Two types of abnormalities were observed in the phase visuograms of multiple sclerosis patients: (a) abnormal responses at all spatial frequencies tested (37%), and (b) abnormal responses only at selective spatial frequencies (52%). Some patients (Fig. 52.16B) had phase lag limited to low, or middle, or high spatial frequencies. These data confirm that multiple sclerosis selectively affects specific neuronal channels within the spatial pathways.

VEPs in Infants

VEPs can be recorded from newborns and infants and utilized to assess their visual function (Banks, 1980; Ellingson et al., 1973; Sokol and Dobson, 1976; Sokol et al., 1981).

VEPs have been used to determine the onset of visual cortical function (Atkinson et al., 2002), the maturation of visual pathways (Crognale, 2002), the development of luminance, color, and contrast sensitivity (Morrone et al., 1996; Suttle et al., 2002), and even to determine visual acuity (Riddell et al., 1997; Skoczenski and Norcia, 1999).

Moskowitz and Sokol (1983) showed that P100 is consistently present at all ages, with longer latency at birth and gradually reduction to adult-like values. P100 latency decreases rapidly during the first year of life for both large and small checks, but the time course varies as a function of the check size. P100 to checks greater than 45′ shows adult latency values by 1 year of age, whereas P100 to checks smaller than 20′ does not reach adult latency levels by age 5.

Pattern VEPs are difficult to obtain in children younger than 5, particularly in infants, due to their inability to fully cooperate. Often VEPs to flashes are used to test infant visual function. Flash VEPs on a term infant are characterized by two major peaks (Engel, 1975), a negative wave labeled N1 (latency 156 ± 26 msec) and a positive wave labeled P1 (latency 180 to 200 msec). CFPDs have also been recorded in premature and term infants, even when they are asleep and their eyes are closed. Interpretation of infant flash VEPs should always be cautious, because VEP preservation does not guarantee normal visual perception; conversely, very abnormal VEPs have been recorded in infants who later developed normal vision.

Function of Retrochiasmal Pathways

Anatomy and Physiology

Definitions of retrochiasmal pathways include the following structures: optic tracts, lateral geniculate bodies, optic radiations, and visual cortex. Information from the contralateral hemifield travels in the optic tract and, after synaptic transfer to lateral geniculate body neurons, continues into the striate area 17 via the geniculocalcarine tract. In humans, information travels to the two other visual areas (areas 18 and 19) via area 17. There is no direct geniculocortical projection to the parastriate (area 18) or peristriate (area 19) cortex.

In the primate brain, 35 visual cortical areas have been identified (Felleman and Van Essen, 1991). Many of these areas have a full retinotopic representation of the visual field. Kaas (1989) proposes that multiple cortical representation is the most efficient way to increase information processing in the phylogenetic scale as mammals require more sophisticated and selective information of the visual environment. *Modular parallel processing* provides a means to increase speed and power of information processing. It therefore has been proposed that new modules (i.e., cortical areas) are added during evolution as primates were able to extract and use information regarding specific features of the environment (Kaas, 1989).

Recent developments in neuroimaging and specifically positron emission tomography (PET), and functional MRI in conjunction with new technologies in histology have improved our understanding of human visual system (Celesia et al., 1996; DeYoe et al., 1994; Fox et al., 1987; Kaas, 1989;

Tootell and Hadjikhani, 2001; Tootell et al., 1996; Zeki et al., 1991). The present knowledge confirms that the complexity of visual cortical representation demonstrated in monkeys is also valid for humans. As shown in Fig. 52.17 visual stimulation in humans not only activates areas 17, 18, and part of 19, but also a lateral temporal region that probably represent area V5 or MT. Approximately one third of the human brain is involved in visual processing. Although it is not yet possible to subdivide the visual cortex with the same details as it has been achieved in monkeys, at least ten cortical areas have been identified in humans by a combination of anatomical, functional, and behavioral studies (Tootell et al., 1995, 1996). V1 is similar to the monkeys (Fox et al., 1987) and correspond to the cytoarchitectonic area 17. V2 occupies part of cytoarchitectonic area 18 (Kaas, 1989). The old anatomical area 19 is a large cortical region that contains different functional areas, including area V3, V3a, and VP. Areas V3 and V3a (also named DM) are located dorsally or superiorly to the calcarine fissure above area V2. These six areas (V1, V2, V3, V3a, VP, V4v) have a detailed retinotopic representation and are very similar to the macaque homologous visual areas (Fig. 52.18) The dimension of the human retinotopic areas are almost double that of primates (DeYoe et al., 1996; Haxby et al., 2001; Sereno et al., 1995; Tootell et al., 1996, 1997; Van Essen and Drury, 1997). Within area 19, and including part of area 37, lies area V4-V8. There are considerable variations between individuals and there is some difficulty in determining the boundaries between area VP (ventroposterior) and V4-V8 (De Yoe et al., 1996; Downing et al., 2001; Van Essen and Drury, 1997).

The M and P pathways, although partially segregated, co-exist in area V1, and V2, but as they exit these regions they take different routes. The M (where) system goes to area V3 and then to the medial temporal region V5, and terminates in the posterior parietal area 7a. This system processes where the stimuli are located and determines if they are moving. The P (what) system goes to area VP-V4-V8 (part of Broadman area 19) and then proceeds to the inferior temporal area 37 via the two streams P-B and P-I and processes the form and color of the visual stimulus.

As we stated in the section on retinal physiology, the function of the K pathway is not clear, but in primates K cells can be subdivided into several classes with different functional properties. Some of these cells contribute to spatial and temporal processing (Xu et al., 2001).

This functional specialization in separate anatomical areas is confirmed by the effect of selected lesions producing deficits limited to color or spatial perception (Kraut et al., 1997; Stein and Walsh, 1997; Zihl et al., 1991). On the other hand, we also must acknowledge that anatomical segregation is far from absolute, and some lesions limited to specific areas produce only temporary effect, and than the patient appears to recover. Anatomical studies in primates have demonstrated 305 interconnecting pathways among the various visual areas (Van Essen et al., 1992).

It is then reasonable to assume that the distribution of surface-recorded potentials to flashes or pattern reflects the complex interaction of electrical field potentials within at least four or five cortical areas, rather than the sole volume transmission of striate dipoles.

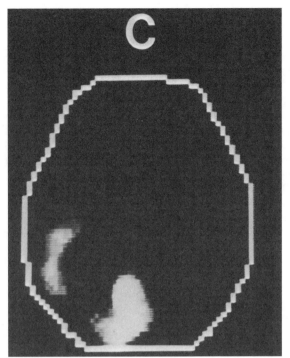
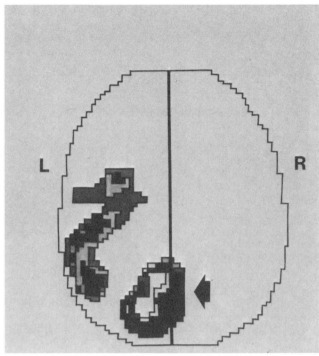

Figure 52.17. Positron emission tomography in a patient with left homonymous hemianopsia with macular splitting. **Left:** The image (C) is the result of computer subtraction of the scan obtained during pattern stimulation from the scan obtained during resting state. Reliable differences between the stimulated and the resting state are shown in the scan as *white areas.* **Right:** The diagram of the scan. The *black arrow* indicates the region of activation on the mesial surface of the occipital lobe. Note that two cortical areas were activated by the pattern stimulation: the occipital lobe (areas 17, 18, and 19) and the lateral temporal region (middle temporal visual area?). (From Celesia, G.G. 1985b. Neuronal generators of human visual evoked potentials: correlation between visual evoked potentials and visualization of regions of cortical activation by positron emission tomography. In *Evoked Potentials. Neurophysiological and Clinical Aspects,* Eds. C. Morocutti and P.A. Rizzo, pp. 245–254, Amsterdam: Elsevier.)

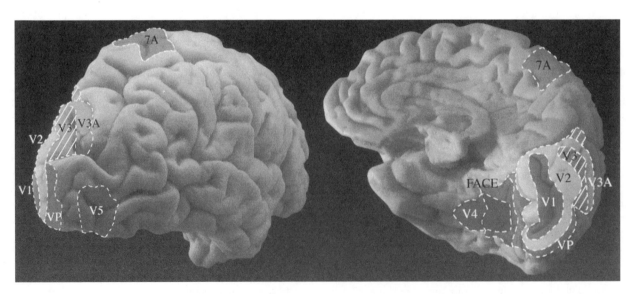

Figure 52.18. Representation of visual cortices in human. The topographical mapping is based on data obtained from positron emission tomography, high-resolution functional MRI, and histochemistry of the human brain (Celesia and Brigell, 1998; De Yoe et al., 1994, 1996; Tootel et al., 1997; Van Essen and Drury, 1997; Zeki et al., 1991). Note that area V3A, VP, and 7A are involved in motion analysis. See text for details.

VEPs to Hemifield Pattern Stimulation

The value of VEPs in retrochiasmatic lesion diagnosis remains highly controversial. Part of the difficulty relates to the complex topographical distribution of VEPs and their variations in normal subjects (Abe and Kuroiwa, 1990; Celesia et al., 1983). Amplitude asymmetry to full-field pattern reversal has proven unreliable as a diagnostic indicator (Kuroiwa and Celesia, 1981, 1987).

Full-field stimulation produces symmetrical amplitude distribution of VEPs over both occipital regions in about 63%, and mild asymmetrical responses in the remaining 37% of subjects (Abe and Kuroiwa, 1990; Celesia and Cone, 1985; Kuroiwa and Celesia, 1981). Hemifield stimulation evokes asymmetrical amplitude responses in 64% of cases (Fig. 52.19), with usually higher amplitude potentials ipsilateral to the hemifield stimulated. Symmetrical responses to hemifield pattern stimulation over both lateral occipital regions are recorded in about 30% of normal individuals (Barrett et al., 1976; Blumhardt et al., 1977, 1982; Celesia et al., 1983; Halliday, 1978). The greater amplitude of P100 over the scalp ipsilateral to the stimulated hemifield (paradoxical lateralization of P100) has been explained by the mesial location of the generators in the hemisphere contralateral to the stimulated hemifield (Barrett et al., 1976).

VEPs to hemifield pattern-reversal stimulation detects 75% to 85% of patients with known visual pathway lesions and homonymous field defects (Bell and Biersdorf, 1989;

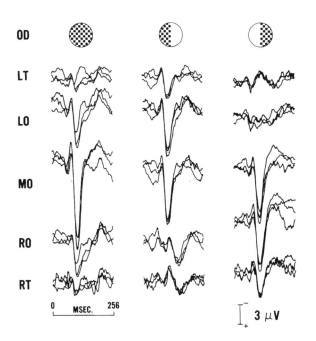

Figure 52.19. T-VEPs amplitude distribution during full- and half-field stimulation in a normal subject. The superimposition of VEPs from three trials demonstrates the reliability of the responses. Note the ipsilateral higher amplitude of the responses to hemifield stimulation. Downward deflection indicates positivity. LT, left temporal; LO, left occipital; MO, mid-occipital; RO, right occipital; RT, right temporal.

Blumhardt et al., 1982; Celesia et al., 1983; Haimovic and Pedley, 1982; Maitland et al., 1982; Streletz, 1981). VEPs to hemifield stimulation are considered abnormal when there is no response to stimulation of the appropriate hemifield (Fig. 52.20A). Topographic mapping of VEPs to hemifield pattern stimulation has been tried, but the complexity and variation of the responses has been an obstacle to clinical application. As shown in Fig. 52.20A, VEPs topographic mapping to hemifield pattern stimulation, in normals, may reveal either an ipsilateral or contralateral occipital lateralization. Dipole source localization can be applied to these potentials to derive the equivalent dipoles underlying surface evoked potentials (Fender, 1987; Scherg, 1989). In a study of 20 normals, we found that the dipole correctly localized the source of P100 to the contralateral occipital lobe, whereas the topographic mapping varied in relation to the dipole vector (Fig. 52.20B).

It is generally acknowledged that the value of VEP in diagnosing retrochiasmatic lesions is poor. The 15% to 25% failure rate of hemifield VEPs probably relates to the topographic variability of the human striate cortex and to the large cortical representation of the macular region in multiple cortical areas (Celesia, 1984, 1985b; Reivich et al., 1981). The striate cortex does not always reach the occipital pole, and often the lateral exposed part of the striate cortex is asymmetrical, being larger in the left hemisphere (Brindley, 1973; Smith, 1907; Stensaas et al., 1974). An even more important factor is the large representation of the macula in the striate cortex (Brindley, 1973; Celesia et al., 1982; Reivich et al., 1981; Stensaas et al., 1974). Pattern-reversal hemifield stimulation activates the hemimacula, and its magnified cortical representation results in normal topographic distribution of VEPs. Improved diagnostic yield in retrochiasmatic lesions requires the development of methodology to preferentially stimulate the periphery of the visual field.

Multifocal VEPs may prove to be useful for detecting visual field defects (Betsuin et al., 2001; Hood et al., 2000). This technique, however, has not been fully evaluated in a large clinical study.

Patients with retrochiasmatic lesions often have additional neurological deficits that interfere with their ability to cooperate during perimetric visual testing or pattern-reversal hemifield stimulation. In such cases, steady-state flash-evoked responses have been evaluated by Fourier analysis; compressed spectrum array has also been employed (Celesia et al., 1978). Visual stimulation consists of 4-second trains of increasingly frequent flashes (Fig. 52.21). At each stimulation frequency, the peak energy is computed as the spectral energy in a window around the frequency of stimulation. Findings are quantified by calculating spectral energy ratios from homologous regions of the right and left hemispheres at each frequency (Celesia et al., 1978, 1982). Abnormal visual evoked spectrum array (VESA) is characterized by small or absent spectral responses, with ratios above 2.5, over the occipital region contralateral to the affected field (Fig. 52.21). VESAs were studied in 39 patients with verified homonymous hemianopsia and found to be abnormal in 26 cases (67%).

Figure 52.20. A: T-VEPs amplitude abnormalities in a 65-year-old man with left homonymous hemianopsia. Monocular stimulation of the affected hemifield failed to produce a reliable response. Abbreviations as in Figure 52.19. **B:** VEPs to right hemifield pattern stimulation (1-degree checks) in two normal subjects. Recording was carried out simultaneously from 20 electrodes placed on the scalp in accordance with the 10–20 international system. In column *A* are selected VEPs (positivity is shown as an upward deflection), in column *B,* the amplitude topographic mapping of P100, and in column *C,* the dipole source localization for P100. The subject in the upper half of the illustration shows the highest P100 amplitude at 02 with a corresponding topographic map showing a positive peak in the right occipital region. The dipole source localization correctly puts the dipole in the left occipital region with the vector oriented toward the right. The subject in the lower half of the illustration shows the highest P100 amplitude at 01 with a corresponding topographic map showing the peak of positivity in the left occipital region. The dipole is correctly localized in the left occipital region with the vector in this subject oriented toward the left. (From Brigell, M., Rubboli, G., and Celesia, G.G. 1991. Application of a single equivalent dipole model to the hemifield pattern VEP. Invest. Ophthalmol. Vis. Sci. 32(suppl):910.)

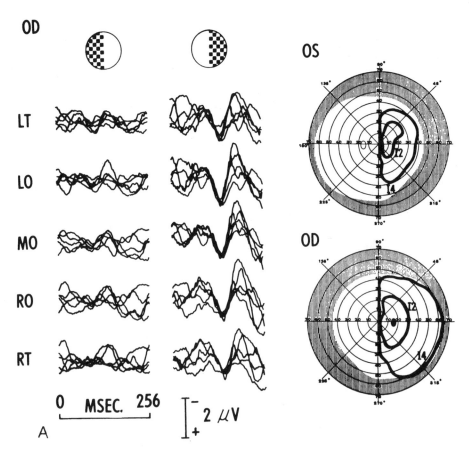

RIGHT HEMIFIELD MONOCULAR STIMULATION

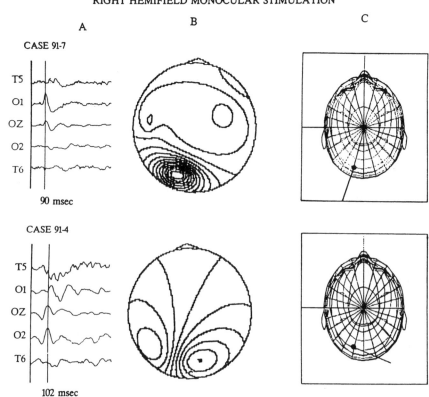

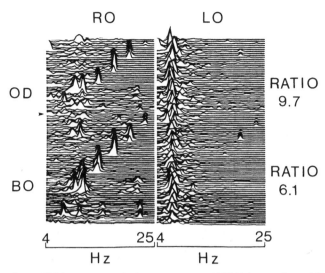

Figure 52.21. Visual evoked spectrum array (VESA) in a patient with right homonymous hemianopsia. Note the almost total absence of response to photic stimulation and the predominant background activity at about 5 to 6 Hz in the left occipital (LO) region. BO, binocular stimulation; the *arrow* on the ordinate indicates the onset of monocular stimulation of the right eye (OD).

VEPs in Cortical Blindness

Bilateral lesions of the occipital lobes, if sufficiently extensive, result in cortical blindness. Surprisingly, VEPs have been found to be present in most of the cases studied (Abraham et al., 1975; Bodis-Wollner et al., 1977; Celesia et al., 1980, 1982; Kooi and Sharbrough, 1966; Spehlmann et al., 1977). Flash responses are often prolonged and simplified. Responses to patterns evoked by small gratings or checks are affected, although responses to larger size patterns remain constant.

There are two possible explanations for VEP preservation in cortical blindness: EPs either originate in extrastriate areas (areas V_2 and V_3) via retinotectal cortical pathways (Celesia et al., 1980; Spehlmann et al., 1977) or are generated by small islands of striate cortex that have survived the pathological process causing the occipital lobe destruction (Celesia, 1984, 1987; Celesia et al., 1982, 1991). The latter hypothesis is supported by the presence of functioning islands of striate cortex demonstrated by PET in a cortically blind patient. In this case, glucose metabolism and regional cerebral blood flow showed a functioning area of cortex in the anterior aspect of the left striate area (Celesia et al., 1982, 1991). These areas most likely represent peripheral retinal fields and are insufficient for conscious visual perception or are capable of only rudimentary visual perception.

Special Applications of VEPs

VEP abnormalities have been reported in disorders affecting neurotransmitters and specifically the dopaminergic and cholinergic systems (Bodis-Wollner et al., 1983, 1986). Parkinson's disease is the prototype of a disorder caused by neurotransmitter dysfunction and specifically related to dopamine depletion. VEPs have been reported to be abnormal in Parkinson's disease and other forms of parkinsonism (Bodis-Wollner et al., 1983, 1986; Calzetti et al., 1990; Nightingale et al., 1986). Abnormalities of visual processing and abnormal pattern electroretinograms and VEPs have also been described in Alzheimer's disease (Gilles et al., 1989; Katz et al., 1989; Philpot et al., 1990; Trick et al., 1989) and attributed to impairment of the cholinergic system. VEPs have been used to study congenital abnormalities of the retinogeniculostriate projections. Albinism is characterized by hypomelanosis and by aberrant retinal projections. Albinos have crossing fibers arising from the temporal retina near the vertical meridian, while the more peripheral temporal retina produces nondecussating projections (Guillery et al., 1975). This disorganization alters the orderly representation within the lateral geniculate body and the striate cortex. Abnormal topographic distribution of VEPs reflecting anomalous visual projections have been demonstrated (Carroll et al., 1980; Coleman et al., 1979; Creel et al., 1978, 1981) in human albinos.

VEPs have also been used to study amblyopia-exanopsia. Abnormal latencies of pattern VEPs have been noted in about half of the patients studied (Sokol, 1978; Spekreijse et al., 1972). P100 amplitude and latencies are particularly affected when the stimuli used are small checks. It is unclear in humans if the amblyopia is due to retinal, geniculate ganglion, or cortical factors. Arden et al. (1982) found abnormal amplitude of pattern ERGs in the amblyopic eye and noted that persistent abnormal pattern ERG was associated with orthoptic treatment failure and poor visual acuity. They argue that these findings may indicate functional retinal deterioration. Further studies are necessary to determine whether or not these techniques can be applied successfully to early detection of amblyopia in infants and young children.

VEPs to flashes and LEDs have been used to monitor visual function during pituitary tumor surgery (Raudenz, 1982). The aim of intraoperative monitoring is to prevent excessive manipulation of the optic nerve and chiasma and to prevent visual loss. Unfortunately, complete absence of VEPs to flashes or LEDs does not preclude the possibility of severe postsurgical visual impairment. The visual stimuli used in the operating room are too crude to permit satisfactory monitoring of visual function. Better technology is needed to improve the sensitivity and reliability of operative VEP monitoring.

Acknowledgment

This work was supported in part by the Veterans Administration.

References

Abe, Y., and Kuroiwa, Y. 1990. Amplitude asymmetry of hemifield patterns reversal VEPs in healthy subjects. Electroencephalogr. Clin. Neurophysiol. 77:81–85.

Abraham, F.A., Melamed, E., and Levy, S. 1975. Prognostic value of visual evoked potentials in occipital blindness following basilar artery occlusion. Appl. Neurophysiol. 32:126–135.

Albrecht, D.G., De Valois, R.L., and Thorell, L.G. 1980. Visual cortical neurons: Are bars or gratings the optimal stimuli? Science 207:88–90.

Alexander, K.R., Fishman, G.A., Peachey, N.S., et al. 1992. 'On' response defect in paraneoplastic night blindness with cutaneous malignant melanoma. Invest. Ophthalmol. Vis. Sci. 33:477–483.

Allison, T., Wood, C.C., and Goff, W.R. 1983. Brainstem auditory, pattern-reversal, and short latency somatosensory evoked potentials: latency in relation to age, sex and brain and body size. Electroencephalogr. Clin. Neurophysiol. 55:919–636.

American Academy Transverse Myelitis Consortium Group. 2002. Proposed diagnostic criteria and nosology of acute transverse myelitis. Neurology 59:499–505.

Andersson, T., and Siden, A. 1995. An analysis of VEP components in optic neuritis. Electroencephalogr. Clin. Neurophysiol. 35:77–85.

Andrew, W. 1971. *The Anatomy of Aging in Man and Animal,* pp. 1–159. New York: Grune & Stratton.

Arakawa, K., Peachey, N.S., Celesia, G.G., et al. 1993. Component-specific effects of physostigmine on the cat visual evoked potential. Exp. Brain Res. 95:271–276.

Arden, G.B. 1978. The importance of measuring contrast sensitivity in cases of visual disturbance. Br. J. Ophthalmol. 62:198–209.

Arden, G.B., Bodis-Wollner, I., Halliday, A.M., et al. 1977. Methodology of patterned visual stimulation. In *Visual Evoked Potentials in Man: New Developments,* Ed. J.E. Desmedt, pp. 3–15. New York: Oxford University Press.

Arden, G.B., Vaegan, A., and Hogg, C.R. 1982. Clinical and experimental evidence that the pattern electroretinogram (PERG) is generated in more proximal retinal layers than the focal electroretinogram (FERG). Ann. N.Y. Acad. Sci. 388:580–601.

Armington, J.C. 1968. The electroretinogram, the visual evoked potential, and the area-luminance relation. Vision Res. 8:263–276.

Armington, J.C. 1974. *The Electroretinogram.* New York: Academic Press.

Armington, J.C., and Biersdorf, W.R. 1958. Long-term adaptation of the human electroretinogram. J. Comp. Physiol. Psychol. 51:1–5.

Armington, J.C., Gouras, P., Tepas, D.I., et al. 1961. Detection of the electroretinogram in retinitis pigmentosa. Exp. Eye Res. 1:74–80.

Arroyo, S., Lesser, R.P., Poon, W.T., et al. 1997. Neuronal generators of visual evoked potentials in humans: visual processing in the human cortex. Epilepsia 38:600–610.

Asselman, P., Chadwick, D.W., and Marsden, C.D. 1975. Visual evoked responses in the diagnosis and management of patients suspected of multiple sclerosis. Brain 98:261–282.

Atkinson, J., Braddick, O., and French, J. 1979. Contrast sensitivity of the human neonate measured by the visual evoked potential. Invest. Ophthalmol. Vis. Sci. 18:210–213.

Atkinson, J., Anker, S., Rae, S., et al. 2002. Cortical visual evoked potentials in very low birth weight premature infants. Arch. Dis. Child Fetal Neonatal Ed. 86:28–31.

Baker, C.L., and Hess, R.F. 1984. Linear and nonlinear components of human electroretinogram. J. Neurophysiol. 51:952–967.

Baker, C.L., Jr., Hess, R.R., Olsen, B.T., et al. 1988. Current source density analysis of linear and non-linear components of the primate electroretinogram. J. Physiol. 407:155–176.

Banks, M.S. 1980. Infant refraction and accommodation. In *Electrophysiology and Psychophysics: Their Use in Ophthalmic Diagnosis,* Ed. S. Sokol, pp. 205–232. Boston: Little, Brown.

Barlow, H.B. 1953. Summation and inhibition in the frog's retina. J. Physiol. 119:60–88.

Barrett, G., Blumhardt, L.D., Halliday, A.M., et al. 1976. A paradox in the lateralization of the visual evoked response. Nature 261:253–255.

Bearse, M.A. Jr., and Sutter, E.E. 1996. Imaging localized retinal dysfunction with the multifocal electroretinogram. J. Opt. Soc. Am. A13:634–640.

Becker, W.J., and Richards, I.M. 1984. Serial pattern shift visual evoked potentials in multiple sclerosis. Can J. Neurol. Sci. 11:53–59.

Bell, R.A., and Biersdorf, W.R. 1989. Homonymous hemianopia and pattern onset hemifield visual evoked potentials. Arch. Ophthalmol. 107:1429–1430.

Berson, E.L., Gouras, P., and Gunkel, R.D. 1968. Rod responses in retinitis pigmentosa, dominantly inherited. Arch. Ophthalmol. 80:58–67.

Berson, E.L., Gouras, P., and Hoff, M. 1969. Temporal aspects of the electroretinogram. Arch. Ophthalmol. 81:207–214.

Berson, E.L., Rosen, J.B., and Simonoff, E.A. 1979. Electroretinographic testing as an aid in detection of carriers of X-chromosome-linked retinitis pigmentosa. Am. J. Ophthalmol. 87:460–468.

Betsuin, Y., Mashima, Y., Ohde, H., et al. 2001. Clinical application of the multifocal VEPs. Curr. Eve. Res. 22:54–63.

Birch, D.G., Jost, B.F., and Fish, G.E. 1988. The focal electroretinogram in fellow eyes of patients with idiopathic macular holes. Arch. Ophthalmol. 106:1558–1563.

Blumhardt, L.D., Barrett, G., and Halliday, A.M. 1977. The asymmetrical visual evoked potential to pattern reversal in one half-field and its significance for the analysis of visual field defects. Br. J. Ophthalmol. 61:456–461.

Blumhardt, L.D., Barrett, G., Kriss, A., et al. 1982. The pattern evoked potential in lesions of the posterior visual pathways. Ann. N.Y. Acad. Sci. 388:264–289.

Bobak, P., Bodis-Wollner, I., Harnois, C., et al. 1983. Pattern electroretinograms and visual evoked potentials in glaucoma and multiple sclerosis. Am. J. Ophthalmol. 96:72–83.

Bobak, P., Friedman, R., Brigell, M., et al. 1988. Visual evoked potentials to multiple temporal frequencies: use in differential diagnosis of optic neuropathy. Arch. Ophthalmol. 106:936–940.

Bodis-Wollner, I., and Onofrj, M. 1982. System diseases and visual evoked potential diagnosis in neurology: changes due to synaptic malfunction. Ann. N.Y. Acad. Sci. 388:327–348.

Bodis-Wollner, I., Hendley, C.D., and Kulikowski, J.J. 1972. Electrophysiological and psychophysical responses to modulation of contrasts of a grating pattern. Perception 1:341–349.

Bodis-Wolner, I., Atkin, A., Raab, E., et al. 1977. Visual association cortex and vision in man: patterned evoked potentials in a blind boy. Science 198:629–631.

Bodis-Wollner, I., Hendley, C.D., Mylin, L.H., et al. 1979. Visual evoked potentials and the visuogram in multiple sclerosis. Ann. Neurol. 5:40–52.

Bodis-Wolner, I., Harnois, C., Bobak, P., et al. 1983. On the possible role of temporal delays of afferent processing in Parkinson's disease. J. Neurol. Transmission. Suppl. 19:243–252.

Bodis-Wolner, I., Ghilardi, M.F., and Mylin, L.H. 1986. The importance of stimulus selection in VEP practice: The clinical relevance of visual physiology. In *Evoked Potentials,* Eds. R.Q. Cracco and I. Bodis-Wolner, pp. 15–27. New York: Alan R. Liss.

Bottcher, J., and Trojaborg, W. 1982. Follow up of patients with suspected multiple sclerosis: a clinical and electrophysiological study. J. Neurol. Neurosurg. Psychiatry 45:809–814.

Boycott, B.D., and Dowling, J.E. 1969. Organization of the primate retina: light microscopy. Philos. Trans. R. Soc. Lond. [B] Biol. Sci. 225:109–184.

Bresnick, G.H. 1991. Diabetic retinopathy. In *Principles and Practice of Clinical Electrophysiology of Vision,* Eds. J.R. Heckenlively and G.B. Arden, pp. 619–635. St. Louis: C.V. Mosby.

Bresnick G.H., and Palta, M. 1987. Oscillatory potential amplitudes. Arch. Ophthalmol. 105:929–933.

Bresnick, G.H., Korth, K., Groo, A., et al. 1984. Electroretinographic oscillatory potentials predict progression of diabetic retinopathy. Preliminary report. Arch. Ophthalmol. 102:1307–1311.

Breton, M.E., Schueller, A.W., Lamb, T.D., et al. 1994. Analysis of ERG a-wave amplification and kinetics in terms of the G-protein cascade of phototransduction. Invest. Ophthalmol. Vis. Sci. 35:295–309.

Brigell, M., Rubboh, G., and Celesia, G.G. 1991. Application of a single equivalent dipole model to the hemifield pattern VEP. Invest. Ophthalmol. Vis. Sci. 32(suppl.):910.

Brindley, G.S. 1973. Sensory effects of electrical stimulation of the visual and paravisual cortex in man. In *Handbook of Sensory Physiology,* Ed. R. Jung, pp. 583–594. Berlin: Springer-Verlag.

Brown, K.T. 1980. Physiology of the retina. In *Medical Physiology,* Ed. V.B. Mountcastle, pp. 504–543. St. Louis: C.V. Mosby.

Bush, R.A., and Sieving, P.A. 1994. A proximal retinal component in the primate photopic ERG a-wave. Invest. Ophthalmol. Vis. Sci. 35:635–645.

Bush, R.A., and Sieving, P.A. 1996. Inner retinal contributions to the primate photopic fast flicker electroretinogram. J. Opt. Soc. Am. A13:557–565.

Calzetti, S., Franchi, A., Taratufolo, G., et al. 1990. Simultaneous VEP and P-ERG investigations in early Parkinson's disease. J. Neurol. Neurosurg. Psychiatry 53:114–117.

Camisa, J., Mylin, L.H., and Bodis-Wollner, I. 1981. The effect of stimulus orientation on the visual evoked potential in multiple sclerosis. Ann. Neurol. 10:532–539.

Campbell, F.W., and Robson, J.C. 1968. Application of Fourier analysis to the visibility of gratings. J. Physiol. 197:551–556.

Carroll, W.M., Jay, B.S., McDonald, W.I., et al. 1980. Pattern evoked potentials in human albinism. Evidence of two topographical asymmetries reflecting abnormal retino-cortical projections. J. Neurol. Sci. 48:265–287.

Celesia, G.G. 1978. Visual evoked potentials in neurological disorders. Am. J. EEG Technol. 18:47–59.

Celesia, G.G. 1982. Steady state and transient visual evoked potentials in clinical practice. Ann. N.Y. Acad. Sci. 388:290–305.

Celesia, G.G. 1984. Evoked potential techniques in the evaluation of visual function. J. Clin. Neurophysiol. 1:55–76.

Celesia, G.G. 1985a. Visual evoked responses. In *Evoked Potential Testing. Clinical Applications,* Eds. J.H. Owen and H. Davis, pp. 1–54. Orlando, FL: Grune & Stratton.

Celesia, G.G. 1985b. Neuronal generators of human visual evoked potentials: correlation between visual evoked potentials and visualization of regions of cortical activation by positron emission tomography. In *Evoked Potentials. Neurophysiological and Clinical Aspects,* Eds. C. Morocutti and P.A. Rizzo, pp. 245–254. Amsterdam: Elsevier.

Celesia, G.G. 1987. Correlation between visual evoked potentials and PET neuro-imaging in subjects with retrochiasmatic lesions. Electroencephalogr. Clin. Neurophysiol. Suppl. 39:276–280.

Celesia, G.G. 1988. Anatomy and physiology of visual evoked potentials and electroretinograms. Neurol. Clin. 6:657–670.

Celesia, G.G. 1999. Visual evoked potentials in clinical neurology. In *Electrodiagnosis in Clinical Neurology,* Ed. M. Aminoff, pp. 421–438. New York: Churchill Livingstone.

Celesia, G.G., and Brigell, M.G. 1998. Cortical visual processing. Proceeding of the 14th International Congress of EEG and Clinical Neurophysiology. Amsterdam: Elsevier.

Celesia, G.G., and Brigell, M.G. 1999. Cortical visual processing. Electroencephalogr. Clin. Neurophysiol. Suppl. 50:202–209.

Celesia, G.G., and Cone, S. 1985. Visual evoked potentials: a practical approach within the guidelines for clinical evoked potential studies. Am. J. EEG Technol. 25:93–113.

Celesia, G.G., and Daly, R.F. 1977a. Effects of aging on visual evoked responses. Arch. Neurol. 34:403–407.

Celesia, G.G., and Daly, R.F. 1977b. VECA: a new electrophysiological test for the diagnosis of optic nerve lesions. Neurology 27:637–641.

Celesia, G.G., and Kaufmann, D. 1985. Pattern ERGs and visual evoked potentials in maculopathies and optic nerve diseases. Invest. Ophthalmol. Vis. Sci. 26:726–735.

Celesia, G.G., and Tobimatsu, S. 1990. Electroretinograms to flash and to patterned visual stimuli in retinal and optic nerve disorders. In *Visual Evoked Potentials,* Ed. J.E. Desmedt, pp. 45–55. Amsterdam: Elsevier.

Celesia, G.G., Bodis-Wollner, I., Chatrian, G.E., et al. 1993. Recommended standards for electroretinograms and visual evoked potentials. Report of an IFCN committee. Electroencephalogr. Clin. Neurophysiol. 87:421–436.

Celesia, G.G., Som, V.K., and Rhode, W.S. 1978. Visual evoked spectrum array (VESA) and interhemispheric variations. Arch. Neurol. 35:678–682.

Celesia, G.G., Archer, C.R., Kuroiwa, Y., et al. 1980. Visual function of the extrageniculocalcarine system in man. Arch. Neurol. 37:704–706.

Celesia, G.G., Polcyn, R.E., Holden, J.E., et al. 1982. Visual evoked potentials and positron emission tomographic mapping of regional cerebral blood flow and cerebral metabolism: Can the neuronal potential generators be visualized? Electroencephalogr. Clin. Neurophysiol. 54:243–256.

Celesia, G.G., Meredith. J.T., and Pluff, K. 1983. Perimetry, visual evoked potentials and visual spectrum array in homonymous hemianopsia. Electroencephalogr. Clin. Neurophysiol. 56:16–30.

Celesia, G.G., Kaufman, D., and Cone, S. 1986. Simultaneous recording of pattern electroretinography and visual evoked potentials in multiple sclerosis. A method to separate demyelination from axonal damage to the optic nerve. Arch. Neurol. 43:1247–1252.

Celesia, G.G., Kaufman, D., and Cone, S.B. 1987. Simultaneous recording of pattern electroretinograms and visual evoked potentials in patients with multiple sclerosis. In *Evoked Potential III,* Eds. C. Barber, and T. Blum, pp. 225–230. Boston: Butterworth.

Celesia, G.G., Bushnell, D., Cone Toleikis, S., et al. 1991. Cortical blindness and residual vision: Is the "second" visual system in humans capable of more than rudimentary visual perception? Neurology 41:862–869.

Celesia, G.G., Brigell, M., Gunnink, R., and Dang, H. 1992. Spatial frequency evoked visuograms in multiple sclerosis. Neurology 42:1067–1070.

Celesia, G.G., Peachey, N.S., Brigell, M., et al. 1996. Visual evoked potentials: recent advances. In *Functional Neuroscience* (EEG Suppl. 46), Eds. C. Barber, G.G. Celesia, G.C. Comi, et al., pp. 3–14. Amsterdam: Elsevier.

Chatrian, G.E., Lettich, E., Nelson, P.L., et al. 1980a. Computer assisted quantitative electroretinography. I. A standardized method. Am. J. EEG Technol. 20:57–77.

Chatrian, G.E., Nelson, P.L., Lettich, E., et al. 1980b. Computer assisted electroretinography. II. Separation of rod and cone components of the electroretinogram in congenital achromatopsia and congenital nyctalopia. Am. J. EEG Technol. 20:79–88.

Chatrian, G.E., Turella, G.S., Nelson, P.L., et al. 1982. Effects of retinal dysfunction on visual evoked potentials. The Cleveland Clinic Foundation. The Second International Evoked Potentials Symposium 2:21.

Ciganek, L. 1958. Potentiels corticaux chez l'homme, évoqués par les stimuli photiques. Rev. Neurol. 99:194–196.

Cohen, J., and Cohen, P. 1983. *Applied Multiple Regression/Correlation Analysis for Behavioral Sciences.* Hillsdale, NJ: Lawrence Erlbaum Associates.

Cohen, S.N., Syndulko, K., Tourtelotte, W.W., et al. 1980. Critical frequency of photic driving in the diagnosis of multiple sclerosis. A comparison to pattern evoked responses. Arch. Neurol. 37:80–83.

Coleman, J., Sydnor, C.F., Wolbarsht, M.L., et al. 1979. Abnormal visual pathways in human albinos studied with visually evoked potentials. Exp. Neurol. 65:667–679.

Collins, D.W., Carroll, W.M., Black, J.L., et al. 1979. Effect of refractory error on the visual evoked response. Br. Med. J. 1:231–232.

Coupland, S.G., and Kirkham, T.H. 1982. The orientation-specific visual evoked potential deficits in multiple sclerosis. J. Neurol. Sci. 9:331–337.

Creel, D., O'Donnell, F.E., Jr., and Witkop, C.J., Jr. 1978 Visual system anomalies in human ocular albinos. Science 201:931–933.

Creel, D., Spekreijese, H., and Reits, D. 1981. Evoked potentials in albinos: efficacy of pattern stimuli in detecting misrouted optic fibers. Electroencephalogr. Clin. Neurophysiol. 52:595–603.

Creutzfeldt, O.D. 1988. Extrageniculo-striate visual mechanisms: compartmentalization of visual functions. In *Vision Within Extrageniculo-striate Systems,* Eds. T.P. Hicks, and G. Benedeck, pp. 307–320. Amsterdam: Elsevier.

Crognale, M.A. 2002. Development, maturation, and aging of chromatic visual pathways: VEP results. J. Vis. 2:438–450.

Cunningham, V.J., Deiber, M.P., Frackowiak, R.S.J., et al. 1990. The motion area (area V5) of human visual cortex. J. Physiol. 423:101–102.

Curcio, C.A., Sloan, K.R., Kalina, R.E., et al. 1990. Human photoreceptor topography. J. Comp. Neurol. 292:497–523.

Dacey, D.M. 2000. Parallel pathways for spectral coding in primate. Annu. Rev. Neurosci. 23:743–775.

Dacheux, R.F., and Raviola, E. 1986. The rod pathway in the rabbit retina: a depolarizing bipolar and amacrine cell. J. Neurosci. 6:331–345.

Dawson, G.D. 1954. A summation technique for the detection of small evoked potentials. Electroencephalogr. Clin. Neurophysiol. 1:65–84.

Dawson, W.W., Maida, T.M., and Rubin, M.L. 1982. Human pattern-evoked retinal responses are altered by optic atrophy. Invest. Ophthalmol. Vis. Sci. 22:796–803.

Dawson, W.W., Startton, R.D., Hope, R.D., et al. 1986. Tissue responses of the monkey retina. Tuning and dependence on inner layer integrity. Invest Ophthalmol. Vis. Sci. 27:734–745.

Deans, M.R., Volgyi, B., Goodenough, D.A., et al. 2002. Connexin36 is essential for transmission of rod-mediated visual signals in the mammalian retina. Neuron 36:703–712.

De Weerd, J.P.C. 1984. Somatosensory evoked potentials: review of techniques. In *International Symposium on Somatosensory Evoked Potentials,* pp. 11–20. Rochester: Custom Printing.

DeYoe, E.A., Neitz, J., Miller, D., et al. 1994. Mapping multiple visual areas in human cerebral cortex. Invest. Ophthalmol. Vis. Sci. 35(suppl): 1813.

DeYoe, E.A., Carman, G.J., Bandettini P., et al. 1996. Mapping striate and extrastriate visual areas in human cerebral cortex. Proc. Natl. Acad. Sci. U.S.A. 93:2382–2386.

Djamgoz, M.B.A., Archer, S.N., and Vallerga, S. 1995. *Neurobiology and Clinical Aspects of the Outer Retina.* Dordrecht: Kluwer Academic Publishers.

Dobkins, K.R. 2000. Moving colors in lime light. Neuron 25:15–18.

Dolman, C.L., McCormick, A.O., and Drance, S.M. 1980. Aging of the optic nerve. Arch. Ophthalmol. 98:2053–2058.

Dowling, J.E. 1979. Information processing by local circuits. The vertebrate retina as a model system. In *The Neurosciences. Fourth Study Program,* Eds. F.O. Schmitt and F.G. Worden, pp. 163–181. Cambridge, MA: MIT Press.

Dowling, J.E. 1987. *The Retina. An Approachable Part of the Brain.* Cambridge, MA: Belknap Press.

Downing, P.E., Jiang, Y., Kanwisher, N., et al. 2001. A cortical area selective for visual processing of the human body. Science 293:2470–2473.

Ederer, F. 1973. Shall we count numbers of eyes or numbers of subjects? Arch. Ophthalmol. 89:1–2.

Ellingson, E.R., Lathrop, G.H., Dahany, T., et al. 1973. Variability of visual evoked potentials in human infants and adults. Electroencephalogr. Clin. Neurophysiol. 34:113–124.

Engel, R.C.H. 1975. *Abnormal Electroencephalograms in the Neonatal Period,* pp. 106–118. Springfield, IL: Charles C Thomas.

Felleman, D.J., and Van Essen, D.C. 1991. Distributed hierarchical in the primate cerebral cortex. Cerebral Cortex, 1:1–47.

Fender, D.H. 1987. Source localization of brain electrical activity. In *Methods of Analysis of Brain Electrical and Magnetic Signals,* Eds. A.S. Gevins, and A. Remond, pp. 355–403. Amsterdam: Elsevier.

Field, G.D., and Rieke, F. 2002. Nonlinear signal transfer from mouse rods to bipolar cells and implications for visual sensitivity. Neuron 34:773–785.

Fiorentini, A., Maffei, L., Pirchio, M., et al. 1981. The ERG in response to alternating gratings in patients with diseases of the peripheral visual pathways. Invest. Ophthalmol. Vis. Sci. 21:490–493.

Fishman, G.A., Birch, D.G., Holder, G.E., et al. 2001. *Electrophysiologic Testing in Disorders of the Retina, Optic Nerve, and Visual Pathway,* 2nd ed. San Francisco: American Academy of Ophthalmology.

Fox, P.T., Miezin, F.M., Allman, J.M., et al. 1987. Retinotopic organization of human visual cortex mapped with positron-emission tomography. J. Neurosci. 7:913–922.

Franco, F., dePalma, P., Mapelli, G., et al. 1987. Evoked potentials in idiopathic optic neuritis. Possibilities of early diagnosis of demyelinating disease. Riv. Neurol. 57:290–297.

Frisen, L., and Frisen, M. 1976. A simple relationship between the probability distribution of acuity and the density of retinal output channels. Acta Ophthalmol. 54:437–444.

Gartner, S., and Henkind, P. 1981. Aging and degeneration of the human macula. I. Outer nuclear layer and photoreceptors. Br. J. Ophthalmol. 65:23–28.

Gilles, C., DeBuyl, O., Genevrois, C., et al. 1989. Specificity of visual evoked potentials alterations in Alzheimer's disease: comparison with normal aging, depression and scopolamine administration in young healthy volunteers. Acta Neurol. Belg. 89:226–227.

Gott, P.S., Weiss, M.H., Apuzzo, M., et al. 1979. Checkerboard visual evoked response in evaluation and management of pituitary tumors. Neurosurgery 5:553–558.

Gouras, P. 1966. Rod and cone independence in the electroretinogram of the dark adapted monkey's perifovea. J. Physiol. 187:455–464.

Gouras, P. 1970. Electroretinography. Some basic principles. Invest. Ophthalmol. Vis. Sci. 9:557–569.

Gouras, P., and Evers, H.U. 1985. The neurocircuitry of primate retina. In *Neurocircuitry of the Retina. A Cajal Memorial,* Eds. A. Gallego and P. Gouras, pp. 233–244. New York: Elsevier.

Gouras, P., and Niemeyer, G. 2004. Electroretinography. In *Disorders of Visual Processing,* Ed. G.G. Celesia. Amsterdam: Elsevier.

Graham, C.H., Bartlett, N.R., Brown, J.L., et al. 1965. *Vision and Visual Perception.* New York: John Wiley.

Granit, R. 1955. *Receptors and Sensory Perception.* New Haven, CT: Yale University Press.

Guerit, J.M., and Argiles, A.M. 1988. The sensitivity of multimodal evoked potentials in multiple sclerosis. A comparison with magnetic resonance imaging and cerebrospinal fluid analysis. Electroencephalogr. Clin. Neurophysiol. 70:230–238.

Guillery, R.W., Okoro, A.N., and Witkop, C.J., Jr. 1975. Abnormal visual pathways in the brain of a human albino. Brain Res. 96:373–377.

Haimovic, I.C., and Pedley, T.A. 1982. Hemifield pattern reversal visual evoked potentials. II. Lesions of the chiasm and posterior pathways. Electroencephalogr. Clin. Neurophysiol. 54:121–131.

Halliday, A.M. 1978. Clinical applications of evoked potentials. In *Recent Advances in Clinical Neurology,* Eds. W.B. Matthews and G.H. Glaser, pp. 47–73. Edinburgh: Churchill Livingstone.

Halliday, A.M., McDonald, W.I., and Mushin, J. 1972. Delayed pattern-evoked responses in optic neuritis in relation to visual acuity. Lancet 1:982–985.

Halliday, A.M., Halliday, E., Kriss, A., et al. 1976. The pattern-evoked potential in compression of the anterior visual pathways. Brain 99:357–374.

Halliday, A.M., McDonald, W.I., and Mushin, J. 1977. Visual evoked potentials in patients with demyelinating disease. In *Visual Evoked Potentials in Man: New Developments,* Ed. J.E. Desmedt, pp. 438–449. Oxford: Clarendon Press.

Harter, M.R., and White, C.T. 1970. Evoked cortical responses to checkerboard patterns: effects of check size as a function of visual acuity. Electroencephalogr. Clin. Neurophysiol. 28:48–54.

Haxby, J.V., Gobbini, M.I., Furey, M.L., et al. 2001. Distributed and overlapping representation of faces and objects in ventrotemporal cortex. Science 293:2425–2430.

Hecht, S., Schlaer, S., and Pirenne, M.H. 1942. Energy, quanta and vision. J. Gen. Physiol. 25:818–840.

Heckenlively, J.R., Feldman, K., and Wheeler, N.C. 1991. Retinitis pigmentosa: cone-rod degenerations: a comparison of clinical findings to electrophysiological parameters. In *Principles and Practice of Clinical Electrophysiology of Vision,* Eds. J.R. Heckenlively and G.B. Arden, pp. 510–527. St. Louis: C.V. Mosby.

Hendrickson, A.E. 1985. Dots, stripes and columns in monkey visual cortex. Trends Neurosci. 8:406–410.

Heron, J.R., Regan, D., and Milner, B.A. 1974. Delay in visual perception in unilateral optic atrophy after retrobulbar neuritis. Brain 97:69–78.

Hess, R.F., and Baker, C.L. 1984. Human pattern-evoked electroretinogram. J. Neurophysiol. 51:939–951.

Holder, G.E. 2001. Pattern ERG and an integrated approach to visual pathway diagnosis. Progr. Retin. Eye Res. 20:531–561.

Hollander, H., Bisti, S., Maffei, S., et al. 1984. ERG and retrograde changes in retinal morphology after intracranial optic nerve section. Exp. Brain Res. 55:483–493.

Holmgren, F. 1865–1866. En method att objektivera effectenaf Ijusintryck pa retina. Upsala Lakareforenings Forhandlingar 1:177–191.

Hood, D.C., and Birch, D.G. 1993. Human cone receptor activity: the leading edge of the a-wave and models of receptor activity. Vis. Neurosci. 10:857–871.

Hood, D.C., and Birch, D.G. 1994. Rod phototransduction in retinitis pigmentosa: estimation and interpretation of parameters derived from the rod a-wave. Invest. Ophthalmol. Vis. Sci. 35:2948–2961.

Hood, D.C., and Birch, D.G. 1996. Beta wave of the scotopic (rod) electroretinogram as a measure of the activity of human on-bipolar cells. J. Opt. Soc. Am. A13:623–633.

Hood, D.C., Odel, J.G., and Zhang, X. 2000. Tracking the recovery of local optic nerve function after optic neuritis: a multifocal VEP study. Invest. Ophthalmol. Vis. Sci. 41:4032–4038.

Hoyt, W.F., and Luis, O. 1962. Visual fiber anatomy in the infrageniculate pathway of the primate: uncrossed and crossed retinal quadrant fibers projections studied with Nauta silver stain. Arch. Ophthalmol. 68:94–106.

Hubbell, W.L., and Bownds, M.D. 1979. Visual transduction in vertebrate photoreceptors. Annu. Rev. Neurosci. 2:17–34.

Hubel, D.M., and Wiesel, T.N. 1959. Receptive fields of single neurons in the cat's striate cortex. J. Physiol. 148:574–591.

Hubel, D.M., and Wiesel, T.N. 1968. Receptive fields and functional architecture of monkey striate cortex. J. Physiol. 195:215–243.

Hubel, D.L., and Wiesel, T.N. 1974. Uniformity of monkey striate cortex: a parallel relationship between field size, scatter and magnification factor. J. Comp. Neurol. 158:295–306.

IFCN Committee Report. 1993. Recommended standards for electroretinograms and visual evoked potentials. Electroencephalogr. Clin. Neurophysiol. 87:421–436.

International Standardization Committee, International Society for Clinical Electrophysiology of Vision. 1989. Standard for clinical electroretinography. Arch. Ophthalmol. 107:816–819.

Johnson, M.A., and Hood, D.C. 1996. Rod photoreceptor transduction is affected in central retinal vein occlusion associated with iris neovascularization. J. Opt. Soc. Am. A13:572–576.

Johnson, M.A., Marcus, S., Elman, M.J., et al. 1988. Neovascularization in central retinal vein occlusions: Electroretinographic findings. Arch. Ophthalmol. 106:348–352.

Jones, L.A., and Higgins, G.C. 1952. Photographic granularity and graininess. III. Some characteristics of the visual system of importance in the evaluation of graininess and granularity. J. Opt. Soc. Am. 37:217–263.

Kaas, J.H. 1989. Why does the brain have so many visual areas? J. Cognitive Neurosci. 1:121–135.

Kaplan, E., Lee, B.B., and Shapley, R.M. 1990 New view of primate retinal function. In *Progress in Retinal Research,* vol. 9, Eds. N. Osborne, and G. Chader, pp. 273–336. Oxford: Pergamon Press.

Karwoski, C., and Karwoski, K. 1991. Oscillatory potentials. In Principles and Practice of Clinical Electrophysiology of Vision, Eds. J.R. Heckenlively and G.B. Arden, pp. 125–131. St. Louis: Mosby.

Karwoski, C.J., Xu, X., and Yu, H. 1996. Current-source density analysis of the electroretinogram of the frog: methodological issues and origins of components. J. Opt. Soc. Am. A13:549–556.

Katz, B., Rimmer, S., Iragui, V., et al. 1989. Abnormal pattern electroretinogram in Alzheimer's disease: evidence for retinal ganglion cell degeneration. Ann. Neurol. 26:221–225.

Kaufman, D., and Celesia, G.G. 1985. Simultaneous recording of pattern electroretinogram and visual evoked responses in neuro-ophthalmologic disorders. Neurology 35:644–651.

Kaufman, D., Lorance, R., and Wray, S.H. 1985. Pattern electroretinogram: a prognostic indicator of optic nerve lesions. Neurology 35(suppl 1):130.

Kaufman, D., Lorance, R., Woods, M., et al. 1988. Pattern electroretinogram: a prognostic indicator of optic nerve lesions. Neurology 38:1764–1774.

Keating, D., Parks, S., and Evans A. 2000. Technical aspects of multifocal ERG recording. Doc. Ophthalmol. 100:77–98.

Kirk, R.E. 1982. *Experimental Design: Procedures for the Behavioral Sciences.* New York: Brooks/Cole.

Kirkham, T.H., and Coupland, S.G. 1983. The pattern electroretinogram in optic nerve demyelination. Can. J. Neurol. Sci. 10:256–260.

Knapp, A.C., and Schiller, P.H. 1984. The contribution of on-bipolar cells to the electroretinogram of rabbits and monkeys. A study using 2-amino-4-phosphobutyrate (APBB). Vision Res. 24:1841–1846.

Kofuji, P., Ceelen, P., Zahs, K.R., et al. 2000. Genetic inactivation of an inwardly rectifying potassium channel (Kir4.1) in mice: phenotypic impact in retina. J. Neurosci. 20:5733–5740.

Kooi, K.A., and Sharbrough, F.W. 1966. Electrophysiological findings in cortical blindness. Report of a case. Electroencephalogr. Clin. Neurophysiol. 20:260–263.

Kraft, T.W., Makino, C.L., Mathies, R.A., et al. 1990. Cone excitations and color vision. Cold Spring Harb. Symp. Quant. Biol. 55:635–641.

Kraut, M., Hart, J. Jr., Soher, B.J., et al. 1997. Object shape processing in the visual system evaluated using functional MRI. Neurol. 48:1416–1420.

Krill, A.E. 1970. The electroretinogram and electrooculogram: Clinical applications. Invest. Ophthalmol. 9:600–617.

Kuffler, S.W. 1953. Discharge patterns and functional organization of mammalian retina. J. Neurophysiol. 16:37–68.

Kupersmith, M.J., Seiple, W.H., Nelson, J.I., et al. 1984. Contrast sensitivity loss in multiple sclerosis. Selectivity by eye, orientation, and spatial frequency measured with the evoked potential. Invest. Ophthalmol. Vis. Sci. 25:632–639.

Kuroiwa, Y., and Celesia, G.G. 1981. Visual evoked potentials after hemifield pattern stimulation in the diagnosis of retrochiasmatic lesions. Arch. Neurol. 38:86–90.

Kuroiwa, Y., and Celesia, G.G. 1987. Amplitude difference between pattern evoked potentials after left and right hemifield stimulation. Neurology 37:795–799.

Lesser, R.P., Lüders, H., Klem, G., et al. 1985. Visual potentials evoked by light-emitting diodes mounted in goggles. Cleve. Clin. Q. 52:223–228.

Livingstone, M.S., and Hubel, D.H. 1982. Thalamic input to cytochrome oxidase-rich regions in monkey visual cortex. Proc. Natl. Acad. Sci. U.S.A. 79:6098–6101.

Livingstone, M.S., and Hubel, D.H. 1984. Anatomy and physiology of a color system in the primate visual cortex. J. Neurosci. 4:309–356.

Livingstone, M.S., and Hubel, D.H. 1988. Segregation of form, color, movement, and depth: anatomy, physiology, and perception. Science 240:740–749.

Maffei, L. 1982. Electroretinographic and visual cortical potentials in response to alternating gratings. Ann. N.Y. Acad. Sci. 388:1–10.

Maffei, L., and Fiorentini, A. 1981. Electroretinographic responses to alternating gratings before and after section of the optic nerve. Science 211:953–955.

Maitland, M.J., Aminoff, C., Kennard, C., et al. 1982. Evoked potentials in the evaluation of visual field defects due to chiasmal or retrochiasmal lesions. Neurology 32:968–991.

Mansfield, R.J.W. 1985. Primate photopigments and cone mechanisms. In *The Visual System,* Eds. A. Fein and J.S. Levine, pp. 89–106. New York: Alan R. Liss.

Marmor, M.F. 1979. The electroretinogram in retinitis pigmentosa. Arch. Ophthalmol. 97:1300–1304.

Marmor, M.F., and Wolfensberger, T.J. 1998. *The Retinal Pigment Epithelium.* Oxford: New York.

Marmor, M.F., and Zrenner, E. 1998–99. Standard for clinical electroretinography International Society for Clinical Electrophysiology of Vision (1999 update). Doc. Ophthalmol. 97:143–156.

Marmor, M.F., Hood, D.C., Keating, D., et al. 2003. Guidelines for basic multifocal electroretinography (mfERG). Doc. Ophthalmol. 106:105–115.

Maunsell, J.H.R., and Van Essen, D.C. 1983. Functional properties of neurons in middle temporal visual area of the macaque monkey II. Binocular interactions and sensitivity to binocular disparity. J. Neurophysiol. 49:1148–1167.

McDonald, W.I., Compston, A., Edan, G., et al. 2001. Recommended diagnostic criteria for multiple sclerosis: guidelines from the International Panel on the diagnosis of multiple sclerosis. Ann. Neurol. 50:121–127.

Meredith, J.T., and Celesia, G.G. 1982. Pattern-reversal visual evoked potentials and retinal eccentricity. Electroencephalogr. Clin. Neurophysiol. 3:243–253.

Milam, A.H., Saari, J.C., Jacobson, S.G., et al. 1993. Autoantibodies against retinal bipolar cells in cutaneous melanoma-associated retinopathy. Invest. Ophthalmol. Vis. Sci. 34:91–101.

Miller, D.H., Newton, M.R., van der Poel, J.C., et al. 1988. Magnetic resonance imaging of the optic nerve in optic neuritis. Neurology 38:175–179.

Minckler, D.S. 1980. The organization of nerve fiber bundles in the primate optic nerve head. Arch. Ophthalmol. 98:1630–1636.

Missotten, L. 1974. Estimation of the ratio of cones to neurons in the fovea of the human retina. Invest. Ophthalmol. Vis. Sci. 13:1045–1049.

Morand, S., Thut, G., Meredith, J.T. 2000. *http://isi1.webofscience.com.* Cereb. Cortex 10:817–825.

Morrone, M.C., Fiorentini, A., Burr, D.C. 1996. Development of the temporal properties of visual evoked potentials to luminance and color contrast in infants. Vision Red. 36:3141–3155.

Moskowitz, A., and Sokol, S. 1983. Developmental changes in the human visual system as reflected by the latency of the pattern reversal VEP. Electroencephalogr. Clin. Neurophysiol. 56:1–15.

Neima, D., and Regan, D. 1984. Pattern visual evoked potentials and spatial vision in retrobulbar neuritis and multiple sclerosis. Arch. Neurol. 41:198–201.

Nightingale, S., Mitchell, K.W., and Howe, J.W. 1986. Visual evoked cortical potentials and pattern electroretinograms in Parkinson's disease and control subjects. J. Neurol. Neurosurg. Psychiatry 49:1280–1287.

Odom, J.V., Maida, T.M., and Dawson, W.W. 1982. Pattern evoked retinal responses (PERR) in human: effect of spatial frequency, temporal frequency, luminance and defocus. Curr. Eye Res. 2:99–108.

Odom, V.J., Bach, M., Barber, C., et al. 2004. Visual evoked potentials Standard. *International Society for Clinical Electrophysiology of Vision.* Doc. Ophthalmol. (in press).

Ogden, T.E. 1984. Nerve fiber layer of the primate retina: morphometric analysis. Invest. Ophthalmol. Vis. Sci. 25:19–29.

Ogden, T.E., and Miller, R.F. 1966. Studies of the optic nerve of the rhesus monkey: nerve fiber spectrum and physiological properties. Vision Res. 6:485–506.

Oppel, O. 1963. Mikroskopische Untersuchungen über die Anzahl und Kaliber der markhaltigen Nervenfasern im fasciculus opticus des Menschen. Graefes Arch. Ophthalmol. 166:19–27.

Oppel, O. 1967. Untersuchungen über die Verteilung und Zahl der retinalen Ganglienzellen beim Menschen, Albrecht v. Graefes Arch. Klin. Exp. Ophthalmol. 172:1–22.

Ordy, J.M., and Brizzee, K.R. 1979. Functional and structural age differences in the visual system of man and nonhuman primate models. In *Sensory Systems and Communication in the Elderly.* Eds. J.M. Ordy and K.R. Brizzee, pp. 13–50. New York: Raven Press.

Osterberg, G. 1935. Topography of the layer of rods and cones in the human retina. Acta Ophthalmol. 13(suppl 6):1–102.

Peachey, N.S., and Seiple, W.H. 1987. Contrast sensitivity of the human pattern electroretinogram. Invest. Ophthalmol. Vis. Sci. 28:151–157.

Peachey, N.S., Alexander, K.R., and Fishman, G.A. 1987a. Rod and cone contributions to oscillatory potentials: an explanation for the conditioning flash effect. Vision Res. 27:859–866.

Peachey, N.S., Fishman, G.A., Derlacki, D., et al. 1987b. Psychophysical and electrophysiological findings in X-linked juvenile retinoschisis. Arch. Ophthalmol. 105:513–516.

Peachey, N.S., Fishman, G.A., Derlacki, D.J., et al. 1988. Rod and cone dysfunction in carriers of X-linked retinitis pigmentosa. Ophthalmology 95:677–685.

Peachey, N.S., Gagliano, D.A., Jacobson, M.S., et al. 1990. Correlation of electroretinographic findings and peripheral retinal nonperfusion in patients with sickle cell retinopathy. Arch. Ophthalmol. 108:1106–1109.

Perry, V.H., Oehler, R., and Cowey, A. 1984. Retinal ganglion cells that project to the dorsal lateral geniculate nucleus in the macaque monkey. Neuroscience 12:1101–1123.

Philpot, M.P., Amin, D., and Levy, R. 1990. Visual evoked potentials in Alzheimer's disease: correlations with age and severity. Electroencephalogr. Clin. Neurophysiol. 77:323–329.

Pirchio, M., Spinelli, D., Fiorentini, A., et al. 1978. Infant contrast sensitivity evaluated by evoked potentials. Brain Res. 141:179–184.

Polyak, S. 1941. *The Retina.* Chicago: University of Chicago Press.

Ramsay, W.J., Ramsay, R.C., Purple, R.L., et al. 1977. Involutional diabetic retinopathy. Am. J. Ophthalmol. 84:851–854.

Ratliff, F. 1982. Radial spatial patterns and multifrequency temporal patterns: possible clinical applications. Ann. N.Y. Acad. Sci. 388:651–656.

Raudenz, P.A. 1982. Intraoperative monitoring of evoked potentials. Ann. N.Y. Acad. Sci. 388:308–326.

Raviola, E., and Gilula, N.B. 1973. Gap junctions between photoreceptor cells in the vertebrate retina. Proc. Natl. Acad. Sci. U.S.A. 70:1677–1681.

Regan, D. 1972. *Evoked Potentials in Psychology, Sensory Physiology and Clinical Medicine.* London: Chapman & Hall.

Regan, D. 1975. Recent advances in electrical recording from the human brain. Nature 253:401–407.

Regan, D. 1989. *Human Electrophysiology. Evoked Potentials and Evoked Magnetic Fields in Science and Medicine.* Amsterdam: Elsevier.

Regan, D., and Richards, W. 1971. Independence of evoked potentials and apparent size. Vision Res. 11:679–684.

Reivich, M., Cobb, W., Rosenquist, A., et al. 1981. Abnormalities in local cerebral glucose metabolism in patients with visual field defects. J. Cereb. Blood Flow Metab. 1(suppl 1):S471–472.

Riddell, P.M., Ladenheim, B., Mast, J., et al. 1997. Comparison of measures of visual acuity in infants: teller acuity cards and sweep visual evoked potentials. Optom. Vis. Sci. 74:702–707.

Riggs, L.A., Johnson, E.P., and Schick, A.M.L. 1964. Electrical responses of the human eye to moving stimulus pattern. Science 144:567.

Rios, J.J., Odel, J.G., Hirano, M., et al. 1997. Rod-sparing paraneoplastic retinopathy, opsoclonus, and peripheral neuropathy due to small cell lung carcinoma. Neuro-ophthalmology 17:101–105.

Robson, J.G., and Frishman, L.J. 1995. Response linearity and dynamics of the cat retina: the bipolar cell component of the dark-adapted ERG. Vis. Neurosci. 12:837–850.

Robson, J.G., Saszik, S.M., Ahmed, J., et al. 2003. Rod and cone contributions to the a-wave of the electroretinogram of the macaque. J. Physiol. 547:509–530.

Rodieck, R.W. 1973a. *The First Steps in Seeing.* Sunderland, MA: Sinauer Associates.

Rodieck, R.W. 1973b. The vertebrate retina: principles of structure and function. San Francisco: W.H. Freeman and Company.

Rosner, B. 1982. Statistical methods in ophthalmology: an adjustment for the intraclass correlation between eyes. Biometrics 38:105–114.

Sabates, R., Hirose, T., and McMeel, W. 1983. Electroretinography in the prognosis and classification of central retinal vein occlusion. Arch. Ophthalmol. 101:232–235.

Sakai, H., Naka, K.I. 1988. Neuron network in codfish retina. Prog. Ret. Res. 7:149–208.

Samorajski, T. 1977. Central neurotransmitter substances and aging: a review. J. Am. Geriatr. Soc. 25:337–352.

Sandberg, M.A., and Ariel, M. 1977. A hand-held, two-channel stimulator ophthalmoscope. Arch. Ophthalmol. 95:1881–1882.

Sandberg, M.A., Jacobson, S.G., and Berson, E.L. 1979. Foveal cone electroretinograms in retinitis pigmentosa and juvenile macular degeneration. Am. J. Ophthalmol. 88:702–707.

Sawyer, R.A., Selhorst, J.B., Zimmerman, L.E., et al. 1976. Blindness caused by photoreceptor degeneration as a remote effect of cancer. Am. J. Ophthalmol. 81:606–613.

Scherg, M. 1989. Fundamental of dipole source potential analysis. In *Auditory Evoked Magnetic Fields and Potentials. Advance Audiology,* Eds. M. Hoke, F. Grandori, and G.L. Romani, pp. 2–30. Basel: S. Karger.

Sereno, M.I., Dale, A.M., Reppas, J.B., et al. 1995. Borders of multiple visual areas in humans revealed by functional magnetic resonance imaging. Science 268:889–893.

Shapley, R. 1982. Parallel pathways in the mammalian visual system. Ann. N.Y. Acad. Sci. 388:11–20.

Shapley, R., and Enroth-Cugell, C. 1983. Visual adaptation and retinal gain controls. Progr. Ret. Res. 3:263–346.

Shaw, N.A., and Cant, B.R. 1980. Age-dependent changes in the latency of pattern visual evoked potential. Electroencephalogr. Clin. Neurophysiol. 48:237–241.

Shearer, D.E., and Dustman, R.E. 1980. The pattern reversal evoked potential: the need for laboratory norm. Am. J. EEG Technol. 20:185–200.

Sherman, J. 1982. Simultaneous pattern-reversal electroretinograms and visual evoked potentials in diseases of the macula and optic nerve. Ann. N.Y. Acad. Sci. 388:214–226.

Sieving, P.A., and Steinberg, R.G. 1987. Proximal retinal contribution to the intraretinal 8 Hz pattern ERG of cat. J. Neurophysiol. 57:104–120.

Sieving, P.A., Murayama, K., and Naarendorp, F. 1994. Push-pull model of the primate photopic electroretinogram: a role for hyperpolarizing neurons in shaping the b-wave. Vis. Neurosci. 11:519–532.

Skoczenski, A.M., and Norcia, A.M. 1999. Development of VEP Vernier acuity and grating acuity in human infants. Invest. Ophthalmol. Vis. Sci. 40:2411–2417.

Slaughter, M.M., and Miller, R.F. 1985. The role of glutamate receptors in information processing in the distal retina. In *Neurocircuitry of the Retina. A Cajal Memorial,* Eds. A. Gallego and P. Gouras, pp. 51–65. New York: Elsevier.

Smith, G.E. 1907. New studies on the folding of the visual cortex and the significance of the occipital sulci in the human brain. J. Anat. 41:198–207.

Sokol, S. 1972. An electrodiagnostic index of macular degeneration. Use of a checkerboard pattern stimulus. Arch. Ophthalmol. 88:619–624.

Sokol, S. 1978. Patterned elicited ERGs and VECPs in amblyopia and infant vision. In *Visual Psychophysics and Physiology,* Eds. J.C. Armington, J. Krauskopf, and B.R. Wooten, pp. 453–462. New York: Academic Press.

Sokol, S., and Dobson, V. 1976. Pattern reversal visual evoked potentials in infants. Invest. Ophthalmol. 15:58–62.

Sokol, S., Moskowitz, A., and Towle, V.L. 1981. Age related changes in the latency of visual evoked potentials: influence of check size. Electroencephalogr. Clin. Neurophysiol. 51:559–562.

Soucy, E., Wang, Y., Nirenberg, S., et al. 1998. A novel signaling pathway from rod photoreceptors to ganglion cells in mammalian retina. Neuron 21:481–493.

Spehlmann, R., Gross, R.A., Ho, S.U., et al. 1977. Visual evoked potentials and postmortem findings in a case of cortical blindness. Ann. Neurol. 2:531–534.

Spekreijse, H., Khoe, L.H., and Van der Tweel, H.L. 1972. A case of amblyopia: electrophysiology and psychophysics of contrast. Adv. Exp. Med. Biol. 24:141–156.

Spekreijse, H., Van der Tweel, H.L., and Zuidema, T. 1973. Contrast evoked responses in man. Vision Res. 13:1577–1601.

Stein, J., and Walsh, V. 1997. To see but not to read; the magnocellular theory of dyslexia. TINS 20:147–152.

Stensaas, S.S., Eddington, D.K., and Dobelle, W.H. 1974. The topography and variability of the primary visual cortex in man. J. Neurosurg. 40:747–755.

Sterling, P. 1983. Microcircuitry of the cat retina. Annu. Rev. Neurosci. 6:149–185.

Stockton, R.A., and Slaughter, M.M. 1989. B-wave of the electroretinogram. A reflection of ON bipolar cell activity. J. Gen. Physiol. 93:101–122.

Streletz, L.J., Bae, S.H., Roeshman, R.M., et al. 1981. Visual evoked potentials in occipital lesions. Arch. Neurol. 38:80–85.

Stryer, L. 1986. Cyclic GMP cascade of vision. Annu. Rev. Neurosci. 9:87–119.

Sung, J.H. 1964. Neuroaxonal dystrophy in mucoviscidosis. J. Neuropathol. Exp. Neurol. 23:567–583.

Suttle, C.M., Banks, M.S., Graf, E.W. 2002. FPL and sweep VEP to tritan stimuli in young human infants. Vision Res. 36:3141–3155.

Thirkill, C.E., Roth, A.M., and Keltner, J.L. 1987. Cancer-associated retinopathy. Arch. Ophthalmol. 105:372–375.

Tobimatsu, S., Celesia, G.G., and Cone, S.B. 1988. Effects of pupil diameter and luminance changes on pattern electroretinograms and visual evoked potentials. Clin. Vis. Sci. 2:293–302.

Tobimatsu, S., Celesia, G.G., Cone, S.B., et al. 1989. Electroretinographs to checkerboard pattern reversal in cats: Physiological characteristics and effect of retrograde degeneration of ganglion cells. Electroencephalogr. Clin. Neurophysiol. 73:341–352.

Tomoda, H., Celesia, G.G., and Cone-Toleikis, S. 1991a. Effects of spatial frequency on simultaneous recorded steady state pattern electroretinograms and visual evoked potentials. Electroencephalogr. Clin. Neurophysiol. 80:81–88.

Tomoda, H., Celesia, G.G., Brigell, M.G., et al. 1991b. The effects of age on the steady-state pattern electroretinograms and visual evoked potentials. Doc. Ophthalmol. 77:201–211.

Tootell, R.B.H., and Hadjikhani, N. 2001. Where is dorsal V4 in human visual cortex? Retinotopic, topographic and functional evidence. Cereb. Cortex 11:298–311.

Tootell, R.B.H., Silverman, M.S., and De Valois, R.L. 1981. Spatial frequency columns in primary visual cortex. Science 214:813–815.

Tootell, R.B.H., Reppas, J.B., Kwong, K.K., et al. 1995. Functional analysis of human MT and related visual cortical areas using magnetic resonance imaging. J. Neurosci. 15:3215–3230.

Tootell, R.B.H., Dale, A.M., Sereno, M.I., et al. 1996. New images from human visual cortex. TINS 19:481–489.

Tootell, R.B.H., Mendola, J.D., Hadjikhani, N.K., et al. 1997. Functional analysis of V3A and related areas in human visual cortex. J. Neurosci. 18:7060–7078.

Trau, R., Van Looy, H., Meckaert, I., et al. 1982. Une nouvelle methode d'exploration clinique: l'ERG et VER simultanes au pattern. Bull. Soc. Belge Ophthalmol. 198:111–121.

Trick, G.L., Barris, M.C., and Bickler-Bluth, M. 1989. Abnormal pattern electroretinograms in patients with senile dementia of the Alzheimer type. Ann. Neurol. 26:226–231.

Van Buren, J.M. 1963. *The Retinal Ganglion Cell Layer.* Springfield, IL: Charles C Thomas.

van der Torren, K., and van Lith, G. 1989. Oscillatory potentials in early diabetic retinopathy. Doc. Ophthalmol. 71:375–379.

Van Essen, D.C., and Drury, H.A. 1997. Structural and functional analyses of human cerebral cortex using a surface based atlas. J. Neurosci. 18:7079–7102.

Van Essen, D.C., Anderson, D.C., and Felleman, D.J. 1992. Information processing in the primate visual system: an integrated systems perspective. Science 255:419–423.

Van Lith, G.H.M. 1980. The application of visually evoked cerebral potentials in ophthalmological diagnosis. Clin. Neurol. Neurosurg. 2:82–85.

Varbec, F. 1965. Senile changes in the ganglion cells of the human retina. Br. J. Ophthalmol. 49:561–572.

Vernant, J.C., Cabre, P., Smadja, D., et al. 1997. Recurrent optic neuromyelitis with endocrinopathies: a new syndrome. Neurology 48:58–64.

Viswanathan, S., Frishman, L.J., and Robson, J.G. 2000. The uniform field and pattern ERG in macaques with experimental glaucoma: removal of spiking activity. Invest. Ophthalmol. Vis. Sci. 41:2797–2810.

Wachtmeister, L. 2001. Some aspects of the oscillatory response of the retina. Prog. Brain Res. 131:465–474.

Wassle, H., Yamashita, M., Greferath, U., et al. 1991. The rod bipolar cell of the mammalian retina. Vis. Neurosci. 7:99–112.

Wastell, D.G. 1979. The application of low-pass linear filters to evoked potential data: filtering without phase distortion. Electroencephalogr. Clin. Neurophysiol. 46:355–356.

Wayner, M.J., and Emmers, R. 1958. Spinal synaptic delay in young and aged rats. Am. J. Physiol. 194:403–405.

Wiesel, T.N., and Gilbert, C.D. 1986. Visual cortex. Trends Neurosci. 9:509–512.

Wisniewski, H.M., and Terry, R.D. 1976. Neuropathology of the aging brain. In *Neurobiology of Aging,* Eds. R.D. Terry and S. Gershon, pp. 265–280. New York: Raven Press.

Xu, X.M., Ichida, J.M., Allison, J.B., et al. 2001. A comparison of koniocellular, magnocellular and parvocellular receptive field properties in the lateral geniculate nucleus of the owl monkey (*Aotus trivirgatus*). J. Physiol. 531:203–218.

Zeki, S. 1990. Colour vision and functional specialization in the visual cortex. J. Neurosci. 6:11–64.

Zeki, S., Watson, J.D.G., Lucek, C.J., et al. 1991. A direct demonstration of functional specialization in human visual cortex. J. Neurosci. 11:641–649.

Zemon, V., Kaplan, E., and Ratliff, F. 1980. Bicuculline enhances a negative component and diminishes a positive component of the visual evoked potential in the cat. Proc. Natl. Acad. Sci. U.S.A. 77:7476–7478.

Zihl, J., von Cramon, D., Mai, N., and Schmid, C. 1991. Disturbance of movement after bilateral posterior brain damage. Brain 114:2235–2252.

Zrenner, E. 1990. The physiological basis of the pattern electroretinogram. Prog. Ret. Res. 9:427–464.

Zrenner, E., and Nelson, R. 1988. Spatial characteristics of scotopic responses in the corneally recorded electroretinogram elicited by multispot patterns. Clin. Visual Sci. 3:29–44.

53. Auditory Evoked Potentials

Gastone G. Celesia and Mitchell G. Brigell

Evoked potentials (EPs) after an auditory stimulus have been recorded directly from the human cortex (Celesia, 1976; Celesia and Puletti, 1969; Howard et al., 2000), the brainstem (Möller and Janetta, 1982, 1983), the eighth nerve (Möller and Jho, 1991; Möller et al., 1981; Spire et al., 1982), the cochlea (Coats, 1974; Ruben et al., 1976), and the scalp. The need to study objectively and noninvasively the function of the auditory system, specifically the cochlea-auditory nerve-brainstem pathways, resulted in an extensive development of scalp recording of both near- and far-field potentials. It is customary to subdivide the auditory evoked responses into different classes in relation to their latencies (Davis, 1976; Picton and Fitzgerald, 1983; Regan, 1989). Early-latency EPs occur in the first 10 to 12 msec after an auditory stimulus, whereas evoked responses occurring between 12 and 50 msec are referred to as middle-latency EPs, and responses occurring 50 msec or more after the stimulus are referred to as slow or late EPs (Table 53.1).

The clinical usefulness of the early potentials has stood the test of time (Chiappa, 1990; Davis and Owen, 1985; Regan, 1989) and receives particular emphasis in this chapter.

Early Auditory Evoked Potentials

Early auditory evoked potentials (early AEPs) have also been referred to as short-latency AEPs and correspond to the responses recorded within the first 12 msec after an auditory stimulus. Responses recorded from the external auditory meatus or the tympanic membrane and occurring within the first 2.5 msec after a stimulus are referred to as the electro-cochleogram (ECochG) because they reflect receptor potentials generated in the cochlea and auditory nerve. The responses recorded from the vertex to the mastoid or earlobe and occurring from 1 to 12 msec are referred to as brainstem auditory evoked potentials (BAEPs) or auditory brain response (ABRs). Although it is possible to record the two types of responses simultaneously, for the sake of clarity they are described separately.

Electrocochleogram

Sound waves travel via the external auditory canal to the tympanic membrane, where they produce changes in air pressure and displacement of the tympanic membrane. Displacements of the tympanic membrane are transmitted via the ossicular chain (malleus, incus, and stapes) to the oval window of the cochlea. The tympanic membrane and ossicular chain are not just passive transmitters of movements; together, they function as an acoustic transformer, permitting efficient conversion of motion from the middle ear to the cochlear liquid (Gelfand, 1981; Morest, 1983).

The cochlea contains an epithelial tube, the cochlear duct, filled with endolymph. The endolymph is suspended within another fluid-filled space, the perilymphatic space, which is a spiral tube closed at one end by the footplate of the stapes in the oval window and at the other end by the round window. It is continuous with the vestibular labyrinth and the cerebrospinal fluid and contains perilymph. Vibration or displacement of the stapedial footplate at the oval window changes the pressure in the perilymphatic space. The cochlea is subdivided into two connected compartments by the cochlear duct. The space above the duct is called the scala vestibuli, and the space below the duct the scala tympani. Within the cochlear duct are the basilar membrane and the organ of Corti. Vibrations transmitted by the stapedial footplate are transformed into a traveling wave at the basilar membrane. The envelope of the vibrations reaches maximum displacement at a particular point along the cochlear duct; high frequencies produce maximum displacement at the base of the cochlea, whereas low frequencies produce maximum displacement toward the apex (von Bekesy, 1960). The organ of Corti contains sensory cells: inner and outer hair cells that carry cilia of graded length. The longest cilia in each cell are embedded in the tectorial membrane. When the basilar membrane vibrates, hair cell cilia bend against the tectorial membrane or are perturbed by the endolymph displacement. Somehow this perturbation, although not completely understood, produces electrical depolarization of the hair cells (receptor potential).

The inner hair cells are in contact with afferent nerve fibers originating in the spiral ganglion cells. The fibers originating in the spiral ganglion form the cochlear nerve. A separate set of spiral ganglion fibers innervates the outer hair cells. It has been shown that the more intense the stimulation, the larger the number of hair cells excited and the more cochlear nerve fibers firing. Information about stimulus frequency and amplitude is transmitted to the central nervous system (CNS) via cochlear nerve discharge patterns.

The first-order afferents of the auditory system are spiral ganglion cells, the central processes of which form the auditory portion of the eighth nerve. The auditory nerve compound action potential represents the close synchronization of nerve impulses within the auditory nerve fibers.

The ECochG is recorded with a needle electrode positioned near the round window (transtympanic ECochG) or a ball electrode placed in the external auditory meatus (extratympanic ECochG) and referred to a second more distant electrode (Chatrian et al., 1982, 1985; Coats, 1974; Deans et al., 1996; Eggermont and Odenthal, 1974; Ruth and Lambert, 1989; Schwaber and Hall, 1990) positioned either at the vertex or the midline frontal area. Noninvasive silver

Table 53.1.   Classification of Auditory Evoked Potentials According to Latency

Type	Latency (msec)	Terminology	Presumed Source
Early	<12		
ECochG	1–4	Cochlear microphonic	AC component receptor potential—cochlear hair cells
		Summating potential	DC component receptor potential—cochlear hair cells
		N_1 or AP	Auditory nerve compound action potential
BAEPs or ABR	1–12		I-auditory nerve action potential
		Waves I to V	II-V-brainstem[a]
Middle	12–50		
Transient		Na (N20), Pa (P30)	Myogenic vs. neurogenic source
Steady-state		40-Hz AEP	
Slow or late	>50		
Late	50–250	N100, P150, N200	Cortical
Long	>250	P300, CNV	Cortical

[a]See text for details.
ABR, auditory brain response; BAEP, brainstem auditory evoked potential; ECochG, electrocochleogram.

ball electrodes placed 2 to 4 mm from the tympanic membrane are preferred for recording ECochG at the present time (Chatrian et al., 1982; Coats, 1974).

Broadband clicks or tone bursts of specific frequencies can be used to elicit an ECochG. As shown in Fig. 53.1, the ECochG consists of three components: the cochlear microphonic (CM) potential, the summating potential (SP), and the auditory nerve compound action potential (AP or N_1). Procedures for separating and enhancing the various components have been described (Chatrian et al., 1982). The CM consists of bursts of high-frequency electrical oscillations of alternating polarity, usually lasting 2 msec or longer. The SP is a negative potential arising from the baseline and followed abruptly by a larger negative wave, the AP or N_1 po-

tential. CM and SP are both graded potentials originating in the hair cells of the organ of Corti. The CM is the alternating current (AC) component of the hair cell receptor potential (Sellick and Russell, 1978); SP represents the direct current (DC) potentials (Dallos, 1973; Davis, 1958). The AP represents the action potential of the auditory nerve and therefore is the same potential as wave I of the BAEPs.

Objective audiometry with frequency-specific tone bursts has been performed with ECochG. The marker has been the AP response, and threshold to tone bursts of 500, 1,000, 2,000, 4,000, and 8,000 Hz corresponding to the subjective audiometry have been obtained (Eggermont, 1976; Naunton and Zerlin, 1976; Yoshie, 1973). The correlation between subjective and ECochG audiogram is excellent, with mean

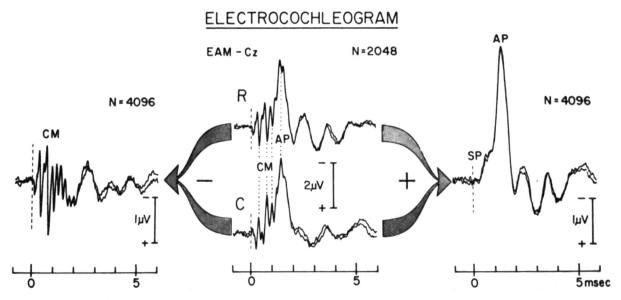

Figure 53.1.   Electrocochleogram (ECochG) elicited by exclusively rarefaction (R) or condensation (C) clicks *(middle section)* are composites of the cochlear microphonic (CM) potential, summating potential (SP), and the auditory nerve compound action potential (AP). *Dotted line* emphasizes reversal of CM polarity and lack of AP polarity reversal when stimulus phase is inverted. SP polarity behaves similarly to that of AP. Algebraically subtracting C from R ECochGs results in summation of CM and cancellation of most of the SP and AP *(left),* whereas adding C to R ECochGs results in summation of SP and AP and cancellation of most CM (right). (From Chatrian, G.E., Wirch, A.L., Lettich, E., et al. 1982. Click-evoked human electrocochleogram. Non-invasive recording method, origin and physiologic significance. Am. J. EEG Technol. 22:151–174.)

differences of about 0 to 5 dB between the two methods. On the other hand, ECochG thresholds determined with broadband clicks do not permit reliable estimation of the audiogram (Eggermont, 1982). The best correspondence between click threshold and audiometry is for 2 and 4 kHz. The use of clicks both for ECochG and BAEPs allows the estimation of hearing loss levels equal to or greater than 2 kHz. Small localized regions of hearing loss or low-frequency hearing loss will be missed (Eggermont, 1982).

Although the study of AP (N_1) does not offer any advantage in comparison to the study of wave I of the BAEPs, the usefulness of ECochG is based on the study of the CM and the SP. These two potentials reflect the function of the receptor potentials and therefore cochlear function. In practice, only the SP has proved useful in differentiating cochlear versus retrocochlear hearing deficits. In Meniere's disease, SPs are often abnormal (Coats, 1981a,b; Ghosh et al., 2002; Eggermont, 1979; Yen et al., 1995) with either greatly increased amplitude (<0.7 mV) or with reversed polarity; that is, they become positive. An absent or reversed SP in Meniere's disease or sudden deafness suggests a poor prognosis for recovery of the lost hearing (Coats, 1981a; Ghosh et al., 2002; Nishida et al., 1976). Camilleri and Howarth (2001) studied 70 patients with severe Meniere's disease to determine if electrocochleography (ECoG) could predict the patients who would be free of vertigo, 2 and 5 years after surgery. At 5 years, 5/8 (63%) patients with normal ECoG were relieved of dizziness compared to 30/30 (100%) with abnormal ECoG (*p* < .001). They concluded that patients with a normal ECoG are less likely to benefit from saccus surgery.

O'Malley et al. (1985) reported greatly enhanced SP in hearing loss associated with X-linked hypophosphatemic osteomalacia, suggesting the presence of endolymphatic hydrops. Changes in the cochlear microphonic and N_1 potential in cases of gentamicin ototoxicity were reported by Keene and Graham (1984).

Eggermont (1983) tried to answer an important and longstanding question in electrocochleography: What particular information can be gained from ECochG that is not available from BAEPs? He concludes that audiogram estimation is as accurate with BAEPs as with ECochGs. ECochG, however, provides SP-based information important in evaluating inner ear disorders, particularly Meniere's disease; the technique is also useful in establishing prognosis in sudden deafness. BAEPs are clearly superior in studying brainstem disorders. Simultaneous ECochG and BAEP recording provides more detailed information about the function of both the cochlea and the auditory pathways (Schlake et al., 2001). Portmann et al. (1985) effectively used simultaneous ECochG and BAEP recording in 61 cases of sudden deafness. They were able to determine that most of the deafness was due to cochlear pathology; however, in 19 cases the data revealed retrocochlear involvement, including four unsuspected acoustic neuromas.

Brainstem Auditory Evoked Potentials (BAEPs) or Auditory Brainstem Responses (ABRs)

BAEPs are a set of seven positive waves recorded from the scalp during the first 12 msec following a click (Jewett and Williston, 1971; Jewett et al., 1970). They represent far-

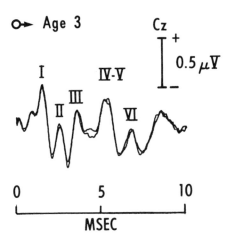

Figure 53.2. Brainstem auditory evoked potential (AEP) in a normal child aged 3. Two tracings are superimposed to show reproducibility of the responses. Recording was between Cz and the ipsilateral ear. Click intensity was 110 dB/sound pressure level (SPL). Note that waves IV and V are fused together in a single complex.

field potentials originating in the brainstem and are labeled I to VII (Fig. 53.2). BEAPs are the tools most frequently used to study the functional integrity of the central auditory pathways.

Origin of BAEPs

There is still considerable debate about the source of BAEP waves (Allen and Starr, 1978; Buchwald, 1983; Davis-Gunter et al., 2001; Hashimoto, 1982a,b; Jewett, 1970; Jewett and Williston, 1971; Legatt et al., 1988; Möller and Janetta, 1982, 1983; Möller and Jho, 1991; Möller et al., 1994; Pratt et al., 1990; Scherg and Von Cramon, 1985a,b; Starr and Achor, 1975). It is now acknowledged that far-field potentials are derived from three possible sources (Table 53.2): afferent volleys (all-or-none action potentials), graded postsynaptic potentials, and changes in the current flow within the surrounding volume conductor. The initial hypothesis, based on the correspondence between human and animal BAEPs and on the time relationship between

Table 53.2. Origin of BAEP Waves

Wave	Generator
I	Compound action potential recorded from the distal end of the acoustic nerve or graded potential of dendritic terminals of acoustic nerve
II	Changes in current flow at the porus acusticus internus, or compound action potential of the auditory nerve at the entrance into the brainstem, or graded potentials from cochlear nucleus
III	Cochlear nucleus and trapezoid body or superior olivary complex and trapezoid body
IV	Lateral lemniscus, ventral lemniscus cells, or superior olivary complex or ascending auditory fibers in the pons
V	Ventrolateral inferior colliculus and ventral lateral lemniscus
VI, VII	Higher brainstem structures (medical geniculate body?)

waves I and V and responses recorded directly from different nuclear regions, suggested that BAEPs arose from multiple generators activated sequentially within the brainstem auditory pathways. The demonstration that intracranial recordings around the inferior colliculus have responses with longer latencies than wave V (Hashimoto, 1982a,b; Möller and Janetta, 1982) and that auditory nerve responses have longer propagation times than previously suspected (Möller and Janetta, 1983; Möller et al., 1981, 1994), together with a study of BAEPs scalp distribution and analysis using a spatiotemporal dipole model, have suggested that BAEPs may have multiple generators with nonsequential interaction among second-order axons and third-order ipsilateral and contralateral axons and neuronal cells (Scherg and Von Cramon, 1985a,b).

Wave I is a negative wave (seen as a positive wave at the vertex) recorded at the ear being stimulated and reflecting eighth nerve activity. Recording in humans (Moller and Jho, 1991; Möller et al., 1981; Spire et al., 1982) and studies of dipole sources (Scherg and Von Cramon, 1985a,b) suggest that wave I reflects the action potential of the distal portion of the acoustic nerve near the cochlea. Buchwald (1983), on the other hand, asserts that wave I represents graded potentials in dendritic terminals of the acoustic nerve in the mammalian cochlea. Whether or not wave I is an action potential or a graded dendritic potential, it nevertheless reflects activity at the distal end of the eighth nerve.

The origins of wave II has been related to postsynaptic potentials in the cochlear nucleus in the brainstem (Achor and Starr, 1980; Buchwald, 1983; Jewett, 1970). However, recordings from the auditory nerve in humans during surgery showed that the action potential of the intracranial portion of the eighth nerve close to the brainstem corresponded to wave II (Möller et al., 1981; Hashimoto et al., 1981; Spire et al., 1982), suggesting that wave II is generated in the proximal portion of the auditory nerve. Scherg and Von Cramon (1985a,b) suggest that wave II may actually represent changes in current flow due to the auditory nerve transition from within the skull into the posterior fossa. Wave II may represent the summation of more than one generator (Ananthanarayan and Durrant, 1991).

Wave III is thought to represent potentials evoked within the superior olivary complex and trapezoid body (Achor and Starr, 1980; Buchwald, 1983; Jewett, 1970). Patients with hereditary motor-sensory neuropathy have shown delayed waves I and II but normal waves III to V (Garg et al., 1982); conversely, patients with pontine hemorrhages sparing the superior olivary nucleus have normal waves I, II, and III (Chiappa, 1982). Data on the dipole sources (Scherg and Von Cramon, 1985a,b) suggest that wave III represents the interaction of two dipoles, one originating in the ventral cochlear nucleus and the other in the ipsi- and contralateral trapezoid body and superior olivary complex. These data suggest that the origin of wave III is within the brainstem (Legatt et al., 1988).

The origins of waves IV and V are still under some debate. Animal data show that wave IV is not affected by destruction of either the inferior colliculi or the superior olivary complex, whereas lesions of the lateral lemniscus (LL) profoundly affect wave IV (Buchwald, 1983; Zaaroor

and Starr, 1991). It is unclear, however, whether wave IV represents postsynaptic potentials in the LL, action potentials from lemniscal fibers, or a combination of the two. Wave V was initially believed to originate in the inferior collicular region (Buchwald, 1983; Jewett, 1970), but direct recording from the human inferior colliculus has showed potentials with latencies longer than wave V (Möller and Janetta, 1982; Möller et al., 1994). These authors therefore suggest that wave V is generated in the lateral lemniscus. Studies of dipole models suggest a close interaction between waves IV and V, with wave V receiving contributions from the ipsi- and contralateral superior olivary complexes and lateral lemnisci.

The sources of waves VI and VII are even less clear. There is speculation that they may originate in the medial geniculate body above the colliculi.

Although it is not possible at this time to absolutely locate the source of each BAEP wave, the knowledge that the first wave is generated in the eighth nerve and that waves III to V are generated in the brainstem is sufficient for clinical applications, as will be demonstrated in the next few pages.

The diagnostic power of BAEPs relies on I to V interpeak latency, which represents brainstem transmission time and therefore brainstem auditory processing.

Normative Data

The widespread application of BAEP recording in clinical practice has led to concern not only about misuse and overuse of the test, but also about its quality and standardization (Chiappa and Young, 1985; Eisen and Cracco, 1983; Jacobson and Northern, 1991). These issues were addressed in the American Electroencephalographic Society's guidelines for clinical evoked potential studies (Pratt et al., 1999). These guidelines mandate clinicians to adhere to rigorous quality control standards when using BAEPs to assist in the diagnosis of otological or neurological disorders.

BAEPs vary considerably in relation to changing auditory stimulus parameters (Chiappa, 1980, 1982; Coats, 1978; Davis and Owen, 1985; Moore, 1983). Each acoustic stimulus can be broken down into three primary components: frequency, intensity, and time (Durrant, 1983; Moore, 1983; Weber et al., 1981). Frequency refers to the spectrum of sound in hertz (Hz) and relates to the location of physical stimulation along the basilar membrane of the cochlea and along the tonotopic representation of the central auditory pathways. Intensity refers to the loudness of the stimulus and is expressed in decibels (dB) relative to a reference. Time includes duration, rise-fall time, repetition rate, and phase of onset of the stimulus. Clicks represent very short acoustic waves, with the first wave usually more prominent than the others. They are usually generated by a square wave electrical pulse and consist of mixed spectral frequencies. Each tone has a specific frequency (e.g., a 1,000- or 2,000-Hz tone burst) with a rising time (the time before the stimulus reaches a plateau), a stable plateau, and a decay or fall time to the baseline. The duration of the stimulus is measured in either microseconds (μsec) or milliseconds (msec). The phase of onset refers to the initial direction of the mechanical displacement of the basilar membrane of the cochlea. A click's phase of onset is referred to as polarity and defined according to the pressure that the first acoustic wave applies to the tympanic membrane. Positive pressure is referred to as condensation, and negative pressure as rarefaction.

The intensity of an acoustic stimulus is measured in three ways: hearing level (HL), sensation level (SL), and sound pressure level (SPL). HL is defined as the average threshold in decibels of a group of normal adults tested in the same laboratory under the identical conditions used to record BAEPs. SL indicates the subject's individual threshold and is measured just before BAEP recording begins. The American EEG Society (1994) recommends that acoustic stimuli be calibrated in decibels peak equivalent sound pressure level (dB/SPL). SPL measurements use as a reference level a physical standard of 20 micropascals. Although this is the most reliable method currently available, it depends on the click's acoustic waveform with possible measurement errors of 3 to 9 dB (Picton et al., 1984). In spite of this pitfall, measurements of click intensity in dB/SPL provide better inter-laboratory comparability than dB HL or dB SL.

Standardized recording techniques are also important in obtaining reproducible BAEPs. Recording electrodes should be placed over the vertex, the right and left earlobes (A1 and A2), or the right and left mastoid processes (M1 and M2). The vertex electrode is referred to the ipsilateral earlobe (or mastoid), as well as the contralateral ear (or mastoid). Simultaneous recordings to ipsi- and contralateral derivations are recommended to improve wave detection. Wave I (Fig. 53.3) is selectively attenuated in contralateral derivation, whereas waves IV and V are separated better in contralateral than in ipsilateral recordings (Stockard et al., 1978). Amplification is variable but on the order of $10^5\times$, with frequency

cutoffs of 100 and 3,000 Hz. A total of 2,000 sweeps of 10-msec duration are averaged at least twice to ensure reproducibility. The stimulus used in BAEP recording is usually a broadband click generated by a 100-μsec rectangular pulse, delivered monaurally. Contralateral masking with 60 dB/SPL white noise is recommended to avoid crossover responses (that is, responses originating from bone-conducted stimulation of the contralateral ear).

BAEPs are relatively independent of consciousness and resistant to drugs, especially sedatives (Cohen and Britt, 1982; Goff et al., 1977; Janssen et al., 1991; Stockard et al., 1979). However, age, sex, intensity, and rate may affect the latency and amplitude of these potentials (Chiappa, 1982; Chiappa et al., 1979; Davis and Owen, 1985; Freeman et al., 1991; Moore, 1983; Sturzebecher and Werbs, 1987).

The acoustic phase of the click affects BAEP latency. Rarefaction clicks evoke shorter latency waves I and V (Coats and Martin, 1977; Maurer et al., 1980; Ornitz et al., 1980), although these changes vary considerably among subjects (Emerson et al., 1982). Phase effect is further increased in patients with high-frequency hearing loss, in whom condensation and rarefaction may produce out-of-phase responses that can cancel each other when algebraically combined (Coats and Martin, 1977; Schwartz et al., 1990). In view of these effects, rarefaction clicks are now generally recommended.

Click presentation rate is another variable that must be considered. Allen and Starr (1978) have shown increased wave V latency associated with increases from 10 to 30 to 50 clicks per second.

BAEP latencies decrease in quasi-linear manner with increasing stimulus intensities (Coats, 1978; Galambos and Hecox, 1978; Moore, 1983). Both wave I and wave V latencies increase as intensity decreases, whereas the I–V interpeak interval remains essentially unchanged (Fig. 53.4). Normative values, therefore, vary relative to stimulus intensity; the relationship between the two is referred to as the latency-intensity function and is summarized in a graph (Fig. 53.5).

The utilization of latency-intensity functions rather than the study of BAEPs to a single-intensity click increases the power of the test (Coats, 1978; Coats and Martin, 1977). Comparing the subject's latency-intensity functions with normal standards permits detection of conductive, cochlear, and retrocochlear dysfunctions (Coats, 1978; Coats and Martin, 1977; Galambos and Hecox, 1978).

Age is another important variable affecting BAEPs. In prematures and newborns, waves II, IV, and VI are less well defined than waves I and V, and the I–V interpeak interval is longer than in adults (Hecox and Galambos, 1974; Mochizuki et al., 1982; Stockard and Stockard, 1983). There is an approximate 0.2 msec/week decrease in wave V latency at 26 to 40 weeks gestational age. After the neonatal period, latencies decrease more slowly, reaching adult values by 1 year of age (Hecox and Galambos, 1974; Mochizuki et al., 1982; Salamy et al., 1978; Sturzebecher and Werbs, 1987; Yamasaki et al., 1991). BAEP values also change, although less dramatically, with advancing age; latency increases gradually as the individual grows older (Kjaer, 1980a; Rowe, 1978). Allison et al. (1984) reported a

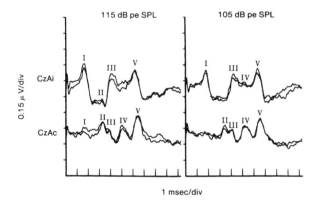

MC ♂ 3 Weeks

Ipsilateral		Contralateral		Ipsilateral		Contralateral	
I	1.64	I	1.66	I	1.72	I	-
III	4.12	III	3.78	III	4.20	III	4.34
V	6.20	V	6.40	V	6.32	V	6.94
I-V	4.56	I-V	4.74	I-V	4.60	I-V	-

Figure 53.3. Brainstem AEPs in a 3-week-old boy. Note the greater amplitude of wave I from ipsilateral recording but the better definition of wave IV in contralateral recording. CZ, vertex; Ai, ipsilateral earlobe; Ac, contralateral earlobe; pe, peak equivalent; SPL, sound pressure level. *Left:* Responses were to clicks of 115 dB/SPL; *right,* responses were to clicks of 105 dB/SPL.

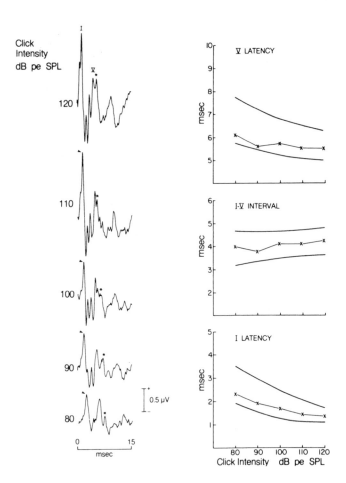

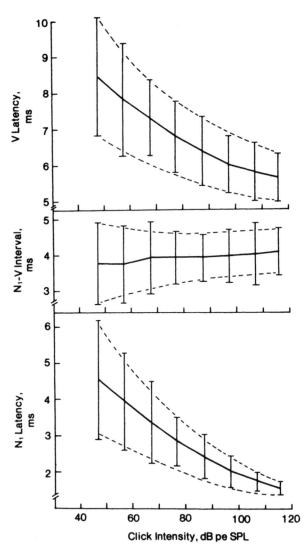

Figure 53.4. Brainstem auditory evoked potentials (BAEPs) in a normal 32-year-old woman. Results to monaural stimulation of the left ear. Recordings were obtained with a plastic-leaf silver electrode placed in the external auditory meatus and referred to the vertex. BAEPs to clicks of decreasing intensity are illustrated *(left)*. Waves I and V are labeled and tagged with an *arrow* and an *asterisk*. Note the SP response preceding wave I. The latency intensity functions of waves I, V, and I–V interval are shown *(right)*. The *thick lines* represent the boundary of normal. Note that the value of the subject marked by an X% is well within the normal range. pe, peak equivalent; SPL, sound pressure level.

Figure 53.5. Latency-intensity curves from 23 normal-hearing ears showing means *(solid lines)* and ±2 standard deviation limits *(crossbar)*. *Dashed lines* show estimated normal ranges. pe, peak equivalent; SPL, sound pressure level.(From Coats, A.C. 1978. Human auditory nerve action potentials and brain stem evoked responses. Arch. Otolaryngol. 104:709–717.)

change in wave V of 0.0072 msec/year for males and a change of 0.0040 msec/year for females. Similarly, Rosenthall et al. (1985) found increased latency with increasing age in waves I, III, and V, but noted that the I–V interval was equal in all age groups. Chu (1985), on the other hand, reported a small increase of the I–V interval with age. It is therefore unclear whether or not central auditory conduction time increases significantly with age. It is agreed that most of the changes that do occur are related to an increase in wave I, which may be related to age-related mechanical and neuronal changes in the cochlea (Schuknecht, 1964).

Gender also influences the various BAEP waves; there are consistently shorter latencies in females (Chu, 1985; Michalewski et al., 1980; Stockard et al., 1979; Sturzebecher and Werbs, 1987). Male-female differences are attributed to different body and brain sizes.

Clinical Applications

BAEPs are effective in evaluating the integrity of the peripheral and central auditory pathways. There is general agreement that BAEPs are useful for (a) hearing assessment in infants; (b) determining hearing loss in uncooperative adult patients; (c) evaluating hearing in functional deafness; (d) evaluating brainstem function in suspected multiple sclerosis; (e) evaluating neuro-otological disorders (acoustic neuromas, cerebellopontine angle tumors, and brainstem lesions); and (f) monitoring the function of the auditory pathway during surgical procedures that may be complicated by damage of the cochlea or auditory nerve and cause deafness.

BAEP interpretation requires identification and measurement of waves I, III, and V and the measurement of I–V and I–III interpeak intervals. These values should then be com-

TYPES OF ABNORMAL
LATENCY-INTENSITY FUNCTIONS

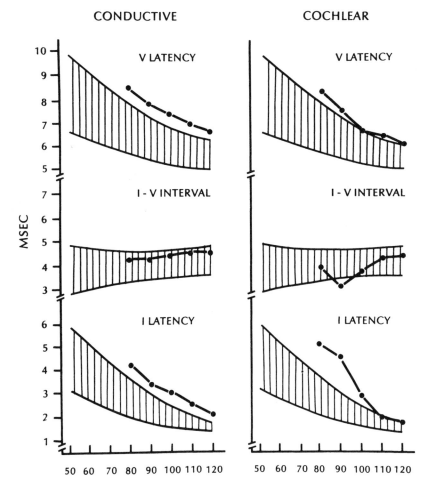

Figure 53.6. Latency-intensity functions in conductive and cochlear hearing loss. The *hatched area* represents the boundary of normality. The *line* connecting the *dots* represents the latency-intensity function for the two types of abnormalities. pe, peak equivalent; SPL, sound pressure level. (See text for details.)

pared with the normal values for the patient's age and sex. Interpretation should be cautious; some practical rules should be followed. First, absence of wave I with normal wave V probably reflects technical problems in recording. The use of an external auditory meatus electrode referred to the vertex in such cases usually reveals a normal wave I. Second, absence of wave III is significant only when wave V is also missing or delayed. Third, BAEPs cannot be interpreted without considering the patient's hearing status; conductive hearing loss and cochlear pathology may profoundly affect BAEP wave latency and amplitude (Coats, 1978; Coats and Martin, 1977; Chatrian et al., 1985; Galambos and Hecox, 1978; Jacobson and Northern, 1991).

The utilization of latency-intensity functions permits differentiation of four types of pathologies:

1. Latency-intensity functions indicating conductive hearing loss (Fig. 53.6). The functions are characterized by prolonged wave I and wave V with latency-intensity

curves parallel to the normal curve. The I–V and I–III intervals are normal.

2. Latency-intensity functions indicating cochlear hearing loss (Fig. 53.6). This type of abnormality accompanies high-frequency hearing loss of cochlear origin. It is characterized by a recruiting curve for wave I; that is, normal or mildly prolonged wave I latencies with loud clicks and greater delays with decreased intensity, resulting in a steep curve. Wave V is not drastically affected, and its curve is less steep, resulting in a shortened I–V interval.

3. Latency-intensity functions indicating retrocochlear deficit type I (Fig. 53.7). Wave I is prolonged with a steep latency-intensity function; wave V is prolonged; therefore, the I–V interval is prolonged. This type of abnormality has been reported in lesions affecting the eighth nerve.

4. Latency-intensity functions indicating retrocochlear deficit type II (Fig. 53.7). The wave I latency-intensity curve is normal. Wave V and the I–V interpeak interval are prolonged. The latency-intensity function of wave V

Figure 53.7. Two types of latency-intensity functions in retrocochlear dysfunction. (See text for details.)

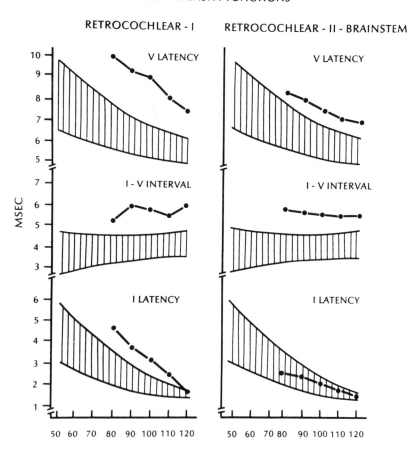

TYPES OF ABNORMAL
LATENCY-INTENSITY FUNCTIONS

RETROCOCHLEAR - I   RETROCOCHLEAR - II - BRAINSTEM

CLICK INTENSITY (dB pe SPL)

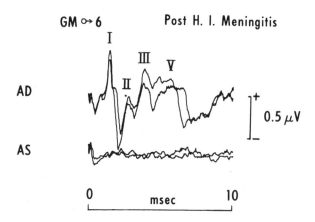

GM ○→ 6   Post H. I. Meningitis

AD

AS

0   msec   10

Figure 53.8. BAEPs in a boy, aged 6, 10 days after recovery from *Haemophilus influenzae* meningitis. Note the total absence of any response to left ear stimulation (AS), suggesting profound damage to the left cochlea or VIII nerve. Stimulation consisted of rarefaction clicks at 75 dB HL. Stimulation of the right ear AD shows a prolonged I–V interval and a dispersed wave V amplitude, suggesting right brainstem damage.

and the I–V interval is variable. A delayed wave V with normal wave I latency signifies that the delay has occurred somewhere after wave I (that is, central to the auditory nerve). A variation of this type of abnormal BAEP is characterized by normal wave I and absence of succeeding waves. Selective elimination of specific waves may help localize the pathology. Absence of all waves suggests a deficit involving the cochlea or the eighth nerve (Fig. 53.8). Preservation of wave I with elimination of all later peaks indicates total functional destruction of the brainstem (Starr, 1976; Starr and Hamilton, 1976) and has been observed in cerebral death (Fig. 53.9).

In more limited brainstem lesions, waves I, II, and III may be preserved while waves IV and V are either absent or prolonged. The most sensitive indicator of brainstem pathology is prolongation of the I–V interpeak interval. Further localization in these cases may be achieved by analyzing the I–III and III–V intervals (Fig. 53.10). Prolongation of the III–V interval alone indicates a deficit at or after the superior olivary complex, in either the high pons or the low midbrain (Chiappa, 1990; Starr and Achor, 1975; Starr and Hamilton, 1976). This detailed interpretation is based on two assump-

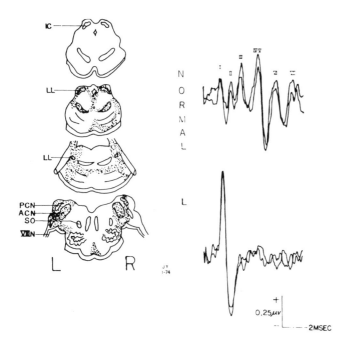

Figure 53.9. The distribution of neuropathology and BAEPs in a patient with anoxic brain damage. The BAEPs were recorded when the neurological examination and EEG were compatible with brain death. Note that the response to a 65-dB hearing level (HL) click consisted of only prolonged latency wave I, compared to the normal record. (From Starr, A., and Hamilton, A.E. 1976. Correlation between confirmed sites of neurologic lesions and abnormalities of far-field auditory brainstem responses. Electroencephalogr. Clin. Neurophysiol. 41:595–608.)

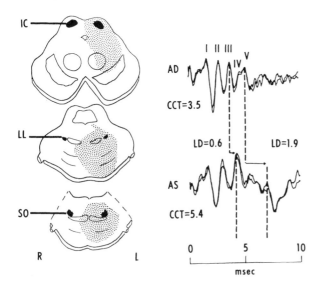

Figure 53.10. BAEPs in a man, aged 31, with a pontine glioma. The diagrams on the *left* show the patient's lesion as seen by computed tomography the same day as the BAEP recordings. Note the progressively increased latencies of waves III and V with stimulation of the left ear (AS), resulting in a prolonged I–V interval central conduction time % (CCT) of 5.4 msec. Wave V is also markedly depressed. The diagnosis was confirmed postmortem. IC, inferior colliculus; LL, lateral lemniscus; SO, superior olive; AD, right ear; LD, latency difference.

tions—that each BAEP wave is generated in a known neuronal location and that detailed identification of a lesion within brainstem structures is important in diagnosis and management of neurological disorders—neither of which is correct. There is no consensus on the origin of BAEPs. Furthermore, the clinician is interested only in whether the lesion is intraaxial (within the brainstem) or extraaxial (in the VIII nerve). BAEPs cannot specify the nature of the lesion but only the type and location of dysfunction.

In adults, BAEPs have been most useful in diagnosing cerebellopontine angle tumors and diseases affecting the brainstem. Cerebellopontine angle tumors include a variety of expanding lesions: acoustic neuromas, meningiomas, cholesteatomas, neurofibromas, and meningiomas. BAEPs have been recorded extensively in cerebellopontine angle tumors (Clemis and McGee, 1979; Eggermont and Don, 1986; Feblot and Uziel, 1982b; Grabel et al., 1991; Harner and Laws, 1983; Sohmer et al., 1974; Starr and Hamilton, 1976; Stockard and Rossiter, 1977), with conflicting results.

Many abnormal findings in acoustic neuromas have been described, with frequent claims of typical BAEP patterns. There are no patterns specific for cerebellopontine angle tumors, only findings that, interpreted with caution, may be compatible with a lesion localized either in the eighth nerve or in the brainstem. A normal wave I with prolonged wave V and I–V interpeak interval (Fig. 53.11), complete absence of any wave following wave I, or even absence of any BAEPs have been noted in cerebellopontine angle tumors. BAEPs were abnormal in 44 of 46 cases (96%) of surgically confirmed acoustic neurinomas (Harner and Laws, 1983). Similarly, a diagnostic yield of 80% was reported in 45 cases of acoustic neuroma by Feblot and Uziel (1982b).

The false-positive result rate has been reported to be as high as 12% to 36% (Clemis and Mitchell, 1977; Selter and Brackmann, 1977), often due to the presence of hearing loss. Selter and Brakmann (1977) suggest that 0.1 msec should he subtracted from wave V latency for every 10 dB of loss over 50 dB for the 4-kHz pure tone threshold. Hyde and Blair (1981) suggested a correction of 0.1 msec for every 5 dB of loss over 55 dB. Using these corrective measures in the presence of hearing loss drastically reduces false-positive rates. The important message here is that BAEPs cannot be interpreted without a proper history and knowledge of the patient's audiogram (Coats, 1978; Coats and Martin, 1977; Eggermont, 1983). Conversely, in a patient suspected of having a cerebellopontine angle tumor, abnormal BAEPs, especially latency-intensity curves suggesting retrocochlear abnormality, should be considered highly compatible with the diagnosis of cerebellopontine angle tumor. The aim of the testing is to identify small acoustic neuromas before they compress the cerebellum and brainstem.

The diagnostic importance of BAEPs in cerebellopontine angle tumor has decreased considerably with the use of magnetic resonance imaging (MRI), which can now easily diagnose intracanicular small eighth nerve tumors. However, BAEPs can be used to prognosticate the expected auditory function following surgery. Matthies and Samii (1997) used BAEPs for evaluation and prediction of auditory function in acoustic neuromas. They studied 420 patients. Patients with good clinical and audiometric hearing and a severe abnormality of BAEPs had severe nerve compression

Figure 53.11.   BAEPs in a man, aged 24, with a left surgically verified acoustic neurofibroma. The patient is affected with von Recklinghausen's neurofibromatosis. BAEPs from monaural stimulation of the left ear are shown on the *left*. The latency-intensity functions are shown on the *right*. Note normal wave I and prolonged wave V and I–V interpeak interval.

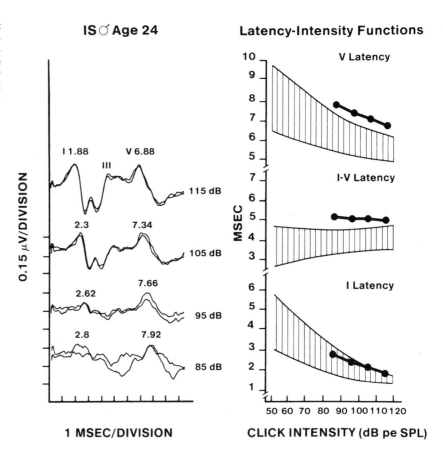

or adhesion by the tumor. Great decrease in amplitude or absence of wave III was a poor prognostic factor. They concluded that BAEPs can be used as a preoperative classification of auditory nerve compromise and a predictor of the chances of hearing preservation following surgery. The same conclusion was reached by Glassock et al. (1993) in 161 cases of acoustic neuromas. Patients with normal BAEPs had a higher probability of hearing preservation in comparison to those with abnormal pre-operative BAEPs.

Starr et al. (1996) have described hearing impairment due to a neuropathy of the auditory nerve. They reported ten children and young adults suffering from hearing impairment due to a disorder of the auditory portion of the VIII nerve. The disorder progressed to a generalized peripheral neuropathy in eight patients (hereditary neuropathy in three and sporadic causes in five). They demonstrated normal cochlear outer heir cell function, and absent or distorted BAEPs.

BAEPs have been used frequently as a diagnostic tool in multiple sclerosis (MS) (Chiappa, 1980; Kjaer, 1980b; Robinson and Rudge, 1977; Stockard and Rossiter, 1977; Stockard et al., 1977). The primary MS abnormality is a prolonged I–V interpeak interval, indicating brainstem dysfunction (Figs. 53.12 and 53.13). Abnormalities are common in patients with the diagnosis of definite MS (Table 53.3), but BAEP testing is most valuable in patients suspected of having a history of MS and who show no evidence of brainstem lesions. The demonstration of a brainstem lesion in these cases increases the diagnostic certainty and often obviates the need for additional testing. BAEPs not only reveal un-

suspected lesions but also are useful in documenting an abnormality when either the history or the clinical findings are equivocal (Chiappa, 1990; Regan, 1989).

BAEP abnormalities indicating a brainstem lesion have also been reported in brainstem infarcts, brainstem hemorrhages, tumors (Fig. 53.10) compressing or invading the brainstem (pinealomas, gliomas, and metastatic lesions), and other degenerative CNS diseases (Chiappa, 1990; De-Pablos et al., 1991; Gadoth et al., 1991; Maurer et al., 1980; Starr and Achor, 1975; Starr and Hamilton, 1976; Stockard and Rossiter, 1977).

Metabolic and toxic encephalopathies can also alter BAEPs (Kohelet et al., 1990; Newman, 1991). Walser et al. (1984) studied the effect of uremia on the BAEPs and demonstrated wave I attenuation consistent with an effect on the cochlea or auditory nerve, as well as slowing of wave V and the I–V interval consistent with brainstem involvement. Peak latencies of wave V and interpeak latencies were shorter after dialysis in a group of 38 chronic renal failure patients (Pratt et al., 1986).

BAEPs have been used in the early prediction of outcome in posttraumatic coma (Facco et al., 1985; Goiten et al., 1983; Karnaze et al., 1982; Yagi and Baba, 1983). Facco et al. (1985) showed that 95% of the survivors among 40 severely head-injured patients had a I–V interpeak interval 4.50 or less at a stimulation intensity of 110 dB/SPL. All the patients with a I–V interpeak interval greater than 4.48 msec died or remained in a vegetative state. However, Yagi and Baba (1983) reported that only 26 of 54 comatose patients with normal I–V intervals

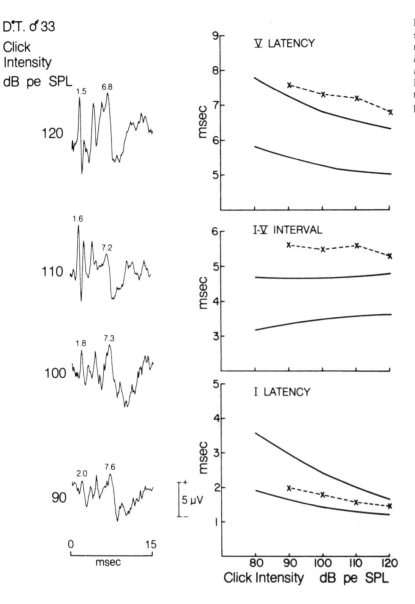

D.T. ♂ 33
Click
Intensity
dB pe SPL

120

110

100

90

$$\begin{matrix}\text{+}\\ 5\ \mu V\\ \text{−}\end{matrix}$$

0   15
msec

Figure 53.12. BAEPs in a man, aged 33, with a diagnosis of possible multiple sclerosis (MS). BAEPs from monaural stimulation of the right ear are shown on the *left.* The latency-intensity functions are illustrated on the *right.* Note normal wave I and prolonged wave V and I–V interpeak interval. The pattern of abnormalities in this case was almost identical to the case in Fig. 53.11. pe, peak equivalent; SPL, sound pressure level.

recovered. Profoundly altered BAEPs may be related to hemotympanum and temporal bone fracture rather than to brainstem dysfunction. In view of these discrepancies, it is unwise to prognosticate outcome solely on the basis of BAEP findings.

In brain death, three types of BAEP abnormalities have been described: total absence of any BAEPs, preservation of wave I and absence of any other wave (Fig. 53.9), and preservation of both waves I and II with absence of any other BAEP component (Chiappa, 1990; Goldie et al., 1981; Starr, 1976). Preservation of wave II in cases with postmortem confirmation of brainstem destruction argues in favor of wave II representing an action potential from the acoustic nerve as it enters the brainstem.

BAEPs in Infants and Children

BAEPs have two important pediatric applications: hearing assessment in neonatal populations and determining brainstem function in newborns and children (Cox, 1984; Galambos and Hecox, 1978; Galambos et al., 1984; Schul-man-Galambos and Galambos, 1975, 1979; Shannon et al., 1984) (also see Chapter 55).

The American Academy of Pediatrics Task Force on Newborn and Infant Hearing (1999), concerned about the harmful effects of hearing loss on normal child development and on subsequent abilities to learn and communicate, endorses the goal of universal detection of hearing loss in infants before 3 months of age, with appropriate intervention no later than 6 months of age. The incidence of hearing impairment in the general neonatal population has been reported at 0.26% (Simmons, 1978); however, this rate is considerably higher in neonatal intensive care units and especially in newborns weighing less than 1,500 g (Galambos et al., 1984; Ment et al., 1982; Roberts et al., 1982; Shannon et al., 1984). The incidence of hearing loss in high-risk neonates has been reported to be as low as 2.3% and as high as 9%. The Centers for Disease Control and Prevention (CDC) reports that in 1999 to 2001 a total of 660,639 newborn were screened in United States and an average of 4% were re-

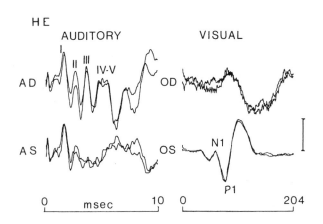

Figure 53.13. BAEPs and visual evoked potentials (VEP) to 31-minute checks in a 44-year-old woman with MS. Note the abnormal BAEPs to stimulation of the left ear (AS). Wave V latency was 8.24 msec, and the I–V interpeak interval was 6.58 msec. (The values for the right ear, AD, were 5.6 and 3.95, respectively.) Stimulation of the right eye showed abnormal VER. These data suggest the presence of two lesions, one in the left auditory pathways of the brainstem and the other in the right optic nerve. OD, right eye; OS, left eye. Upward deflection indicates positive polarity for the BAEPs and negative polarity for VEPs. The calibration bar is 0.25 µV for BAEPs and 3 µV for VEPs.

ferred for audiological evaluation (Centers for Disease Control and Prevention, 2003). Although the true incidence has not been clearly established, the need for early identification of infants with hearing loss is self-evident. Rehabilitative measures must be initiated as early in life as possible to assure normal learning and verbal development. Language acquisition of the infant is permanently affected if the intervention is not done in the first 6 months after birth (Baroch, 2003; Gracey, 2003; Harney, 2000; Helfer et al., 2003).

White (2003) reviewed the current status of the activities of early hearing detection and intervention (EHDI) programs that were developed since the late 1980s. He assessed the implementation by the United States federal government in the last 15 years to promote more effective EHDI programs, and the legislation passed by states related to universal newborn hearing screening. He reported that as of 2002 there were still serious gaps in the implementation of universal screening. He stated, "The most serious obstacles are the shortage of qualified pediatric audiologists, inadequate reimbursement for screening and diagnosis, and lack of knowledge among primary health care providers about EHDI issues." Another

issue remains the methodology of testing the newborn. Helfer et al. (2003) put it clearly in the title of their article: "Wanted: A National Standard for Early Hearing Detection and Intervention Outcomes Data." There are presently two competing methods of screening infants: BAEPs and transient-evoked otoacoustic emissions. The American Academy of Pediatrics Task Force on Newborn and Infant Hearing (1999) states that acceptable methodologies for physiologic screening include "evoked otoacoustic emissions (EOAEs) and auditory brainstem response (BAEPs), either alone or in combination." EOAEs are measured by presenting brief clicks to the ear through a probe inserted in the external ear canal. The probe contains a speaker and a microphone. The speaker generates sounds and the microphone records the EOAEs generated by the cochlea. Hayes (2003) and Clarke et al. (2003) compared BAEPs and EOAEs and found no significant differences between the two systems.

BAEPs have been used effectively to identify high-risk infants (Downs, 1982; Galambos and Hecox, 1978; Galambos et al., 1984; Kramer et al., 1989; Lary et al., 1989; Stueve and O'Rourke, 2003; Schulman-Galambos and Galambos, 1975, 1979). Questions, however, have been raised about the validity and reliability of neonatal BAEP testing, specifically about the technique's low predictive value. Indeed, only 5.26% of infants with initially abnormal BAEPs were later demonstrated to have abnormal hearing (Shannon et al., 1984). In the same study, the predictive value of a negative test was 100%; that is, all of the 115 infants with initially normal BAEPs were later found to have normal hearing.

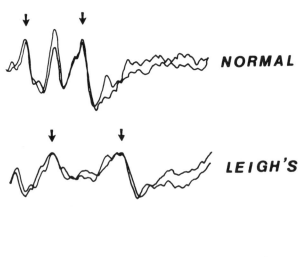

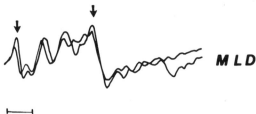

Figure 53.14. BAEPs from two patients with disorders known to affect myelin integrity: Leigh's disease and metachromatic leukodystrophy (MLD). Note the abnormal interwave interval with normal amplitude I/V ratios in both cases. The time scale is 2 msec. (From Hecox, K.E., Cone, B., and Blaw, M.E. 1981. Brainstem auditory evoked responses in the diagnosis of pediatric neurologic diseases. Neurology 31:832–840, with permission.)

Table 53.3. BAEPs Abnormalities in Multiple Sclerosis

| | | Multiple Sclerosis | | | | | |
| | | Definite | | Probable | | Possible | |
Authors		Patients	%	Patients	%	Patients	%
Stockard et al.	1977	30	93	30	77	40	35
Chiappa	1980	81	47	67	21	54	22
Fisher et al.	1981	33	67	54	41	68	19
Lowitzsch and Maurer	1982	10	90	46	63	66	41
Kjaer	1985	95	81	31	68	80	45

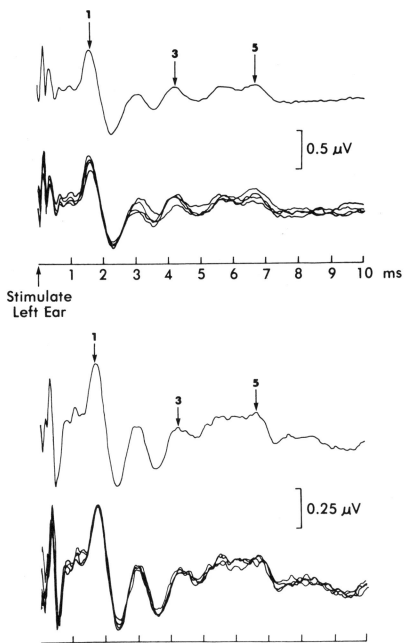

Figure 53.15. BAEPs in a 10-year-old boy with Alexander's disease diagnosed by brain biopsy. Waves I, II, and III are normal (I–III interpeak latency: right, 2.5 msec; left, 2.6 msec). Wave V amplitude is below normal range bilaterally, and I–V interpeak latency was prolonged (5.1 msec bilaterally). Each trial is an average of 2048 responses to 65 dB HL clicks at 11 Hz recorded between vertex and ipsilateral mastoid. *Upper trace,* summation of four trials; *lower traces,* four trials superimposed. (From Davis, S.L., Aminoff, M.J., and Berg, B.O. 1985. Brain-stem or cerebellar dysfunction. Arch Neurol. 42:156–160.)

A cautious approach to newborn testing is advocated, and the following suggestions have been made: all should be tested at, at least, three intensity levels (25, 45, and 65 dB HL), either before discharge or within the first month after discharge. Testing should be "pass-fail"; if the BAEPs are normal, no additional testing is warranted. However, newborns with absent or clearly abnormal BAEPs must be referred for retesting within 3 to 4 months. Retesting must then include not only BAEPs but also full audiologic evaluation (i.e., referred to a pediatric audiologist). No infant should be considered hearing impaired until the problem is confirmed by retesting.

Once an infant is hearing impaired, treatment needs to be instituted as soon as possible. Recently, besides audiological rehabilitation programs, cochlear implants have been applied successfully to both infants and adults (Clark, 2003; Spitzer et al., 2003).

BAEPs have been used effectively to diagnose and evaluate neurological disorders in children (Davis et al., 1985; Garg et al., 1982; Hecox et al., 1981; Warren, 1989). Hecox et al. (1981) suggest that BAEPs can be used to differentiate between neurodegenerative diseases primarily affecting the white matter and gray matter diseases. BAEPs are abnormal in

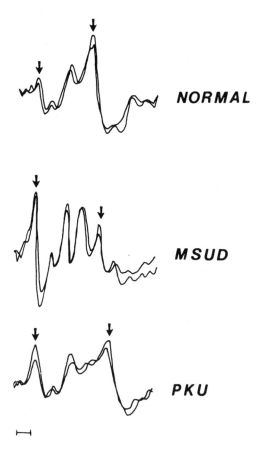

Figure 53.16. BAEPs in dysmyelinating disorders. The *top tracing* was obtained from an age-matched control subject, whereas the two lower tracings were obtained from an 18-month-old and a 14-month-old with maple syrup urine disease (MSUD) and phenylketonuria (PKU), respectively. Note that wave I is larger than wave V and that there is an abnormal interwave I–V interval in the MSUD tracing. The *bottom tracings* were obtained from an untreated PKU patient. Note the prolonged interwave interval in the *lowest tracings*. The time scale is 1.7 msec. (From Hecox, K.E., Cone, B., and Blaw, M.E. 1981. Brainstem auditory evoked response in the diagnosis of pediatric neurologic diseases. Neurology 31:832–840.)

diseases affecting primarily white matter, such as Leigh's disease (Fig. 53.14), the various leukoencephalopathies (Fig. 53.15), maple syrup disease, and phenylketonuria (Fig. 53.16). BAEPs are usually normal in diseases primarily involving brainstem gray matter, such as Wernicke's encephalopathy and neuronal ceroid lipofuscinosis (Davis et al., 1985). BAEP abnormalities in infants and children are nonspecific for individual diseases (Davis et al., 1985; Warren, 1989); abnormal BAEPs have been reported in infective (Fig. 53.17), neoplastic, demyelinating, and degenerative diseases (Fig. 53.18) involving primarily the white matter or the white and gray matter of the brainstem. However, the demonstration of brainstem dysfunction in conjunction with the results of other ancillary tests may aid in the diagnosis of a specific disease. Wellman et al. (2003) have shown that 14% of 79 children with confirmed bacterial meningitis experienced "permanent sensorineuronal hearing loss." To identify these children they used BAEPs and either cortical EP audiometry or standard audiometry. They concluded that early identification of these children is important for rehabilitation aimed at a "better aca-

demic and language outcome." They advocate "routine inpatient audiological screening of postmeningitic children."

Intraoperative Monitoring of BAEPs

Intraoperative BAEP recording has been used to help monitor auditory nerve and brainstem function during surgical procedures within the posterior and middle fossa. Such procedures are occasionally complicated by postoperative neurological deficits of the eighth nerve and brainstem. Such intraoperative monitoring may allow the surgeon to detect dysfunction early enough to prevent permanent damage (Friedman et al., 1985; Grabel et al., 1991; Grundy, 1982; Polo et al., 2004; Spire et al., 1982). BAEPs are recorded continuously during surgery, and the monitoring team alerts the surgeon when changes occur. Reversible complete disappearance of BAEPs is still compatible with complete

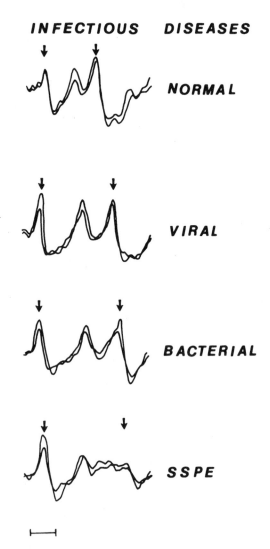

Figure 53.17. BAEPs in infective diseases. Responses from patients with viral meningitis, bacterial meningitis, and subacute sclerosing panencephalitis (SSPE) are shown. Note that all three produce abnormalities of interwave interval. In SSEP, there is also an amplitude ratio abnormality with a low-voltage wave V. (From Hecox, K.E., Cone, B., and Blaw, M.E. 1981. Brainstem auditory evoked response in the diagnosis of pediatric neurologic diseases. Neurology 31:832–840.)

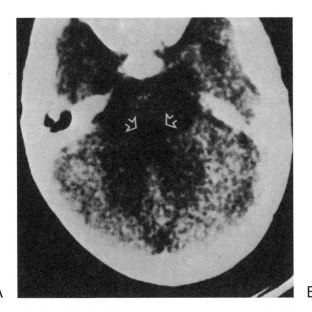

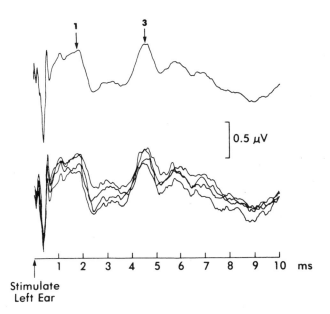

Figure 53.18. Right: BAEPs to left ear stimulation in 6-month-old boy with Leigh's disease when his computed tomographic scan was normal. Waves I and III are normal (I–III interpeak latency, 2.7 msec), but later components are absent. Each trial is the average of 2048 responses to 83 dB HL clicks at 11 Hz recorded between vertex and ipsilateral mastoid. *Upper trace,* summation of four trials; *lower trace,* four trials superimposed. **Left:** same patient, now aged 9 months. Note symmetrical areas of decreased attenuation in brainstem tegmentum adjacent to floor of fourth ventricle (arrowheads). (From Davis, S.L., Aminoff, M.J., and Berg, B.O. 1985. Brain-stem auditory evoked potentials in children with brain-stem or cerebellar dysfunction. Arch. Neurol. 42:156–160.)

neurological recovery, whereas persistent BAEP loss is usually associated with long-term hearing loss and possibly lasting neurological deficit (Polo et al., 2004).

The main benefit of intraoperative BAEPs monitoring is the reduction of the incidence of permanent postoperative neurological deficit (Fisher et al., 1995; Möller, 1996). Polo et al. (2004) suggested that during surgery a delay in latency of peak V of 0.6 msec represents a "warning" signal and that a delay of 1 msec represents a "critical" warning "before irreversibility" and thus permanent hearing loss. They concluded: "These warnings should help the surgeon to avoid or correct maneuvers that are dangerous for hearing function."

Middle-Latency Auditory Evoked Potentials

Middle-latency auditory evoked potentials (MLPs) are potentials occurring between 12 and 50 msec after acoustic stimulation. They can be recorded from transient or from high-frequency stimuli; transient stimuli evoke transient MLPs (usually abbreviated as MLPs) and high-frequency stimuli evoke middle latency auditory steady-state responses (ASSRs).

MLPs to transient stimuli are characterized by multiple negative positive waves termed No, Po, Na, Pa, and Nb. The most often studied deflections are Na, occurring at a latency of 15 to 20 msec and Pa occurring at 25 to 30 msec. These potentials are recorded optimally if a filter bandpass of at least 10 to 300 Hz is selected and stimulus frequency is under 10 per second.

ASSRs can be recorded using 40-Hz acoustic stimuli (Galambos et al., 1981; Picton et al., 2003; Spydell et al., 1985; Stapells et al., 1984). ASSRs have been called the 40-Hz response because they consist of a quasi–sinusoidal response at about 40 Hz. The potentials are of relatively high voltage, often with an amplitude twice that of transient MLP. There is evidence that this increase in amplitude is due to the superimposition of similar phase components of the transient response at this frequency (Galambos et al., 1981). ASSRs can be quickly recorded and have been used to monitor general anesthesia (Picton et al., 2003) and to evaluate hearing loss in medicolegal cases (Dejonckere and Coryn, 2000).

There has been considerable controversy regarding the sources of the transient MLP. Early literature showed that myogenic activity contributes to the response (Bickford et al., 1963, 1964; Celesia and Puletti, 1969; Celesia et al., 1968; Cody and Bickford, 1969; Davis, 1968). However, neurogenic components have been demonstrated in patients who have been administered muscle relaxants or during sleep (Harker et al., 1977; Kraus et al., 1985; Picton et al., 1974). The Na component probably originates from mesencephalic structures including the inferior colliculus (Hashimoto et al., 1981; Kileny et al., 1987; McGee et al., 1991). The origin of the Pa peak appears to be more complex. Although this peak clearly is generated in part by auditory cortex (Celesia et al., 1968; Chatrian et al., 1960; Jacobson et al., 1990; Lee et al., 1984; Scherg and von Cramon, 1985a,b), there is good evidence of subcortical contribution to the response (Parving et al., 1980; Woods et al., 1987). Evidence from work with a guinea pig model has suggested that the Pa peak is composed of a lateral component generated in the temporal lobe and a midline component of subcortical origin through a nonprimary auditory pathway (Kraus and McGee, 1995; Kraus et al., 1988). The Pb component (sometimes referred to as P50) is optimally recorded midline central and frontal head regions to low-frequency stimulation (<1/s). Its generator appears to be in thalamic cholinergic neurons of the ascending reticular activating system (Buchwald et al., 1989; Erwin and Buchwald, 1986).

The MLR has been clinically applied in the assessment of hearing threshold in infants and children, the identification of dysfunction in central auditory pathways, and the evaluation of the central auditory pathways in candidates for cochlear implants. The MLR is more variable that the BAEP in the normal population (Kraus et al., 1985) and has greater test-retest variability (Kavanaugh et al., 1988). This limits its use for hearing thresholds. However, the test has the advantage of producing large responses to pure tone stimuli and to stimuli near threshold. Thus, if repeatable responses are obtained, it can be stated with reasonable certainty that hearing is no worse than the corresponding intensity level (Fifer and Sierra-Irizarry, 1988). Furthermore, the test provides a method to assess thresholds to low frequencies that are crucial for speech perception. Although the response may be reduced in amplitude ipsilateral to the side of a temporal lobe lesion, the response has been reported to be normal in approximately 50% of patients with unilateral temporal lobe lesions (Kraus et al., 1982). The response may also be present in patients with bilateral temporal lobe lesions and cortical deafness (Parving et al., 1980; Woods et al., 1987). Lesions of the thalamus or midbrain are more likely to affect the MLR (Spydell et al., 1985) (Fig. 53.19). The MLR to electrical stimulation has been successfully applied to the assessment of the central auditory pathways in candidates for cochlear implants (Kileny and Kemink, 1987; Lambert et al., 1990; Miller, 1991; Groenen et al., 1997). The response is preferred to the BAER because it is not affected by the large stimulus artifact. A normal electrical MLR is a good prognostic sign for success of the cochlear implant (Firszt et al., 2002).

Failure of adaptation of the Pb component has been suggested to show abnormal sensory gating in schizophrenia (Adler et al., 1985; Cardenas et al., 1993).

Late Auditory Evoked Potentials

Evoked potentials occurring 50 msec or more after acoustic stimulation are called slow or late auditory EPs (Table 53.1) (Davis, 1976; Picton and Fitzgerald, 1983; Picton et al., 1974, 1984). These potentials can be subdivided into exogenous components N1, P1, and P2, which are primarily dependent on characteristics of the external stimulus, and endogenous components, such as P300, N400, CNV, and the mismatch negativity, which are more dependent on internal cognitive processes.

Exogenous late auditory evoked potentials (LAEPs) are best elicited by tone bursts and have the highest amplitude over the vertex, although they are widely distributed over the frontal and central scalp (Polich and Starr, 1983). The N1 is the most prominent of the late potentials. It is generated by multiple sources including the superior temporal plane, the superior temporal gyrus, and perhaps even frontal motor cortex (Goff et al., 1978; Knight et al., 1980; Näätänen and Picton, 1987; Woods, 1995; Yamamoto et al., 1988). The later waves may arise from the auditory association cortex and/or the frontal association cortex (Picton et al., 1974, 1984).

Abnormal LAEPs have been reported in various types of psychopathology; however, dramatic inter- and intrasubject variability has limited the clinical utility of these potentials (Cracco, 1979; Karrer et al., 1984; Roth et al., 1979; Shagass et al., 1978).

Studies of endogenous LAEPs have provided new insights into human cognitive neurophysiology. Although extensive review of this topic is beyond the scope of this chapter (see Jacobson et al., 1997, for a review), some of the more interesting paradigms are briefly described here. The P300 is a potential that is evoked by an infrequently occurring stimulus of interest. The typical paradigm used to obtain a P300 is termed the oddball paradigm. The subject is instructed to count the number of occurrences of a given tone that is presented on 15% to 20% of the trials and to ignore a frequent tone presented on the other trials. The P300 is seen in the response obtained to the infrequent tones only. P300 latency increases by 1 to 2 msec per year in the adult

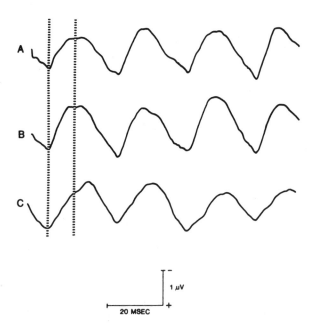

Figure 53.19. Steady-state AEPs of 40 Hz to rarefaction clicks. *A*, response from a normal subject; *B*, response from a patient with a temporal lobe lesion; *C*, response from a patient with a midbrain lesion. The waveforms are aligned so that the positive wave V deflections coincide. Note that the negative peaks of the 40-Hz components are shifted to the right for the midbrain lesion subject in comparison with those for the normal subject and the cortical lesion subject. This shift of the sinusoid-like 40-Hz component, relative to wave V deflection, is what produces the lower phase values found in the midbrain lesion. (From Spydell, J., Pattee, G., and Goldie, W. 1985. The 40 Hertz auditory event related potential: normal values and effects of lesions. Electroencephalogr. Clin. Neurophysiol. 62:193–202.)

population (Goodin et al., 1978) and has been reported to be abnormally delayed in patients with dementia (Goodin et al., 1978) and in children with attention deficit disorder (Loiselle et al., 1980). Other studies have reported successful application of the P300 in monitoring cognitive status of patients following traumatic brain injury (Levin, 1985) and in assessing poststroke (Squires and Hecox, 1983). It should be noted that many of the differences reported in the abovementioned papers are statistical differences between groups rather than significant differences between individual patients and a normal group. Thus, although the P300 may provide some insight to the pathophysiology of cognition, it is not of clinical use at the present time. The N400 is a potential obtained to linguistic stimuli when there is semantic incongruity (Kutas and Hillyard, 1980). Further study of this potential may aid in the understanding of language processing. The mismatch negativity (MMN) is an exogenous potential that occurs when a repetitive auditory stimulus is briefly altered (Näätänen, 1991). Liebenthal et al. (2003) have recorded simultaneous mismatch negative N400 and functional MRI (fMRI) and noted foci of increased BOLD signal in the right superior temporal gyrus and right and left superior temporal plane. These data suggest that the response is due to multiple generators in the temporal lobes. MMN has the potential application for learning about the development of auditory discrimination (Alho et al., 1990).

References

Achor, L.J., and Starr, A. 1980. Auditory brain stem responses in the cat. I. Intracranial and extracranial recordings. Electroencephalogr. Clin. Neurophysiol. 48:154–173.

Adler, L.E., Waldo, M.C., and Freedman R. 1985. Neurophysiologic studies of sensory gating in schizophrenia: comparison of auditory and visual responses. Biol. Psychiatry 20:1284–1296.

Alho, K., Sainio, K., Sajaniemi, N., et al. 1990. Event-related brain potential of human newborns to pitch change of an acoustic stimulus. Electroencephalogr. Clin. Neurophysiol. 77:151–155.

Allen, A.R., and Starr, A. 1978. Auditory brain stem potentials in monkey (*M. mulatta*) and man. Electroencephalogr. Clin. Neurophysiol. 45:53–63.

Allison, T., Hume, A.L., Wood, C.C., et al. 1984. Developmental and aging changes in somatosensory, auditory, and visual evoked potentials. Electroencephalogr. Clin. Neurophysiol. 58:14–24.

American Academy of Pediatrics, Task Force on Newborn and Infant Hear. 1999. Newborn and infant hearing loss: detection and intervention (RE9846). Pediatrics 103:527–530.

American Electroencephalographic Society. 1994. Guideline 9: guidelines on evoked potentials. J. Clin. Neurophysiol. 11:40–73.

Ananthanarayan, A.K., and Durrant, J.D. 1991. On the origin of wave II of the auditory brainstem evoked response. Ear Hear. 12(3):174–179.

Baroch, K.A. 2003. Universal newborn hearing screening: fine-tuning the process. Curr Opin Otolaryngol Head Neck Surg. 11:424–427.

Bickford, R.G., Jacobson, J.L., and Galbraith, R.F. 1963. A new audio motor system in man. Electroencephalogr. Clin. Neurophysiol. 15:921–925.

Bickford, R.G., Jacobson, J.L., and Cody, D.T. 1964. Nature of average evoked potentials to sound and other stimuli in man. Ann. N.Y. Acad. Sci. 112:204–223.

Buchwald, J.S. 1983. Generators. In *Bases of Auditory Brain-Stem Evoked Responses,* Ed. E.J. Moore, pp. 157–195. New York: Grune & Stratton.

Buchwald, J.S., Erwin R.J., Read, S., et al. 1989. Mid–latency auditory evoked responses: differential abnormality of PI in Alzheimer's disease. Electroencephalogr. Clin. Neurophysiol. 74:378–384.

Camilleri, A.E., and Howarth, K.L. 2001. Prognostic value of electrocochleography in patients with unilateral Meniere's disease undergoing saccus surgery. Clin. Otolaryngol. 26:257–260.

Cardenas, V.A., Gerson, J., and Fein, G. 1993. The reliability of P50 suppression as measured by the conditioning/testing ratio is vastly improved by dipole modeling. Biol. Psychiatry 33:335–344.

Celesia, G.G. 1976. Organization of auditory cortical areas in man. Brain 99:403–414.

Celesia, G.G., and Puletti, F. 1969. Auditory cortical areas of man. Neurology 19:211–220.

Celesia, G.G., Broughton, R.J., Rasmussen, T., et al. 1968. Auditory evoked responses from the exposed human cortex. Electroencephalogr. Clin. Neurophysiol. 24:458–466.

Centers for Disease Control and Prevention (CDC). 2003. Infants tested for hearing loss—United States, 1999–2001. MMWR 52:981–984.

Chatrian, G.E., Petersen, M.C., and Lazarte, J.A. 1960. Responses to clicks from the human brain: some depth electrographic observations. Electroencephalogr. Clin. Neurophysiol. 12:479–489.

Chatrian, G.E., Wirch, A.L., Lettich, E., et al. 1982. Click-evoked human electrocochleogram. Non-invasive recording method, origin and physiologic significance. Am. J. EEG Technol. 22:151–174.

Chatrian, G.E., Wirch, A.L., Edwards, K.H., et al. 1985. Cochlear summating potential to broadband clicks detected from the human external auditory meatus. A study of subjects with normal hearing for age. Ear Hear. 6:130–138.

Chiappa, K.H. 1980. Pattern shift visual, brainstem auditory and short-latency somatosensory evoked potentials in multiple sclerosis. Neurology 30:110–123.

Chiappa, K.H. 1982. Physiologic localization using evoked responses: pattern shift visual, brainstem auditory and short latency somatosensory. In *New Perspectives in Cerebral Localization,* Eds. R.A. Thompson and J.R. Green, pp. 63–113. New York: Raven Press.

Chiappa, K.H. 1990. *Evoked Potentials in Clinical Medicine.* New York: Raven Press.

Chiappa, K.H., and Young, R.R. 1985. Evoked responses overused, underused, or misused? Arch. Neurol. 42:76–77.

Chiappa, K.H., Gladstone, K.H., and Young, R.R. 1979. Brain-stem auditory evoked responses: studies of waveform variations in 50 normal human subjects. Arch. Neurol. 36:81–87.

Chu, N.S. 1985. Age-related latency changes in the brain-stem auditory evoked potentials. Electroencephalogr. Clin. Neurophysiol. 62:431–436.

Clark, G. 2003. Cochlear implants in children: safety as well as speech and language. Int. J. Pediatr. Otorhinolaryngol. 67(suppl 1):S7–S20.

Clarke, P., Iqbal, M., and Mitchell, S. 2003. A comparison of transient-evoked otoacoustic emissions and automated auditory brainstem responses for pre-discharge neonatal hearing screening. Int. J. Audiol. 42:443–447.

Clemis, J.D., and McGee, T. 1979. Brainstem electric responses. Audiometry in the differential diagnosis of acoustic tumors. Laryngoscope 89:31–42.

Clemis, J.D., and Mitchell, C. 1977. Electrocochleography and brain stem responses used in the diagnosis of acoustic tumors. J. Otolaryngol. 6:447–459.

Coats, A.C. 1974. On electrocochleographic electrode design. J. Acoust. Soc. Am. 56:708–711.

Coats, A.C. 1978. Human auditory nerve action potentials and brain stem evoked responses. Arch. Otolaryngol. 104:709–717.

Coats, A.C. 1981a. The summating potential and Meniere's disease. I. Summating potential amplitude in Meniere and non-Meniere ears. Arch. Otolaryngol. 107:199–208.

Coats, A.C. 1981b. Meniere's disease and the summating potential. II. Vestibular test results. Arch. Otolaryngol. 107:263–270.

Coats, A.C., and Martin, J.L. 1977. Human auditory nerve action potentials and brain stem evoked responses: effects of audiogram shape and lesion location. Arch. Otolaryngol. 103:605–622.

Cody, D.T., and Bickford, R.G. 1969. Averaged evoked myogenic responses in normal man. Laryngoscope 79:400–416.

Cohen, M.S., and Britt, R.H. 1982. Effects of sodium pentobarbital, ketamine, halothane, and chloralose on brainstem auditory evoked responses. Anesth. Analg. 61:338–343.

Cox, L.C. 1984. The current status of auditory brainstem response testing in neonatal populations. Pediatr. Res. 18:780–783.

Cracco, R.Q. 1979. Evoked potentials in patients with neurological disorders. In *Evoked Brain Potentials and Behavior,* Ed. H. Begleiter. New York: Plenum Press.

Dallos, P. 1973. *The Auditory Periphery. Biophysics and Physiology.* New York: Academic Press.

Davis, H. 1958. Transmission and transduction in the cochlea. Laryngoscope 68:359–382.

Davis, H. 1968. Averaged-evoked-response EEG and audiometry. Acta Otolaryngol. (Stockh.) 65:79–85.

Davis, H. 1976. Principles of electric response audiometry. Ann. Otol Rhinol. Laryngol. 85:1–96.

Davis, H., and Owen, J. 1985. Auditory evoked potentials. In *Evoked Potential Testing. Clinical Applications,* Eds. J.H. Owen and H. Davis, pp. 55–108. New York: Grune & Stratton.

Davis, S.L., Aminoff, M.J., and Berg, B.O. 1985. Brain-stem auditory evoked potentials in children with brain-stem or cerebellar dysfunction. Arch. Neurol. 42:156–160.

Davis-Gunter, M.J., Lowenheim, H., Gopal, K.V., et al. 2001. The I' potential of the human auditory brainstem response to paired click stimuli. Scand Audiol. 30:50–60.

Deans, J.A., Hill, J., Birchall, J.P., et al. 1996. The effect of electrode position in electrocochleography. Clin. Otolaryngol. 21(4):317–323.

Dejonckere, P.H., and Coryn, C.P. 2000. A comparison between middle latency responses and late auditory evoked potentials for approximating frequency-specific hearing levels in medicolegal patients with occupational hearing loss. Int. Tinnitus 6:174–181.

DePablos, C., Berciano, J., and Calleja, J. 1991. Brainstem auditory evoked potentials and blink reflex in Friedreich's ataxia. J. Neurol. 1:238/4: 212–216.

Downs, D.W. 1982. Auditory brainstem response testing in the neonatal intensive care unit: a cautious approach. ASHA 24:1009–1015.

Durrant, D.J. 1983. Fundamentals of sound generation. In *Basis of Auditory Brain-Stem Evoked Responses,* Ed. E.J. Moore, pp. 15–49. New York: Grune & Stratton.

Eggermont, J.J. 1976. Analysis of compound action potential responses to tone bursts in the human and guinea pig cochlea. J. Acoust. Soc. Am. 60:1132–1139.

Eggermont, J.J. 1979. Summating potentials in Meniere's disease. Arch. Otolaryngol. 222:63–75.

Eggermont, J.J. 1982. The inadequacy of click-evoked auditory brainstem responses in audiological applications. Ann. N.Y. Acad. Sci. 388:707–709.

Eggermont, J.J. 1983. Audiologic disorders. In *Basis of Auditory Brain-Stem Evoked Responses,* Ed. E.J. Moore, pp. 287–315. New York: Grune & Stratton.

Eggermont, J.J., and Don, M. 1986. Mechanism of central conduction time prolongation in brainstem auditory evoked potentials. Arch. Neurol. 43:116–120.

Eggermont, J.J., and Odenthal, D.W 1974. Methods in electrocochleography. Acta Otolaryngol. Suppl. 316:16–26.

Eisen, A., and Cracco, R.Q. 1983. Overuse of evoked potentials: caution. Neurology 33:618–621.

Emerson, R.G., Brooks, E.B., Parker, S.W., et al. 1982. Effects of click polarity on brainstem auditory evoked potentials in normal subjects and patients: unexpected sensitivity of wave V. Ann. N.Y. Acad. Sci. 388:710–721.

Erwin, R., and Buchwald, J.S. 1986. Midlatency auditory evoked responses: differential effects of sleep in the human. Electroencephalogr. Clin. Neurophysiol. 65:383–392.

Facco, E., Martini, A., Zuccarello, M., et al. 1985. Is the auditory brainstem response (ABR) effective in the assessment of post-traumatic coma? Electroencephalogr. Clin. Neurophysiol. 62:332–337.

Feblot, P., Uziel, A. 1982b. Detection of acoustic neuromas with brainstem auditory evoked potentials: comparison between cochlear and retrocochlear abnormalities. Adv. Neurol. 32:169–176.

Feblot, P., and Uziel, A. 1982. Detection of acoustic neuromas with brainstem auditory evoked potentials: comparison between cochlear and retrocochlear abnormalities. In *Clinical Applications of Evoked Potentials in Neurology,* Eds. J. Courjon, F. Mauguiere, and M. Revol, pp. 169–176. New York: Raven Press.

Fifer, R.C., and Sierra-Irizarry, B. 1988. Clinical applications of the auditory middle latency response. Am. J. Otol. 9(suppl):47–56.

Firszt, J.B., Chambers, A.R.D., and Kraus, N. 2002. Neurophysiology of cochlear implant users II: comparison among speech perception, dynamic range, and physiological measures. Ear Hear. 23:516–531.

Fisher, C., Blanc, A., Mauguiere, F., et al. 1981. Apport des potentiels evoqués auditifs precoces au diagnostic neurologique. Rev. Neurol. (Paris) 26:229–240.

Fisher, R.S., Raudenz, P., and Nunemacher, M. 1995. Efficacy of intraoperative neurophysiological monitoring. J. Clin. Neurophysiol. 12:97–109.

Freeman, S., Sohmer, H., and Silver, S. 1991. The effect of stimulus repetition rate on the diagnostic efficacy of the auditory nerve brainstem evoked response. Electroencephalogr. Clin. Neurophysiol. 78(4):284–290.

Friedman, W.A., Kaplan, B.J., Gravenstein, D., et al. 1985. Intraoperative brain-stem auditory evoked potentials during posterior fossa microvascular decompression. J. Neurosurg. 62:552–557.

Gadoth, N., Gordon, C.R., Bleich, N., et al. 1991. Three modality evoked potentials in Charcot-Mane-Tooth disease (HMSN-J). Brain Dev. 13: 91–94.

Galambos, R., and Hecox, K.E. 1978. Clinical applications of the auditory brainstem response. Otolaryngol. Clin. North Am. 11:722.

Galambos, R., Makeig, S., and Talmachoff, P. 1981. A 40-Hertz auditory potential recorded from the human scalp. Proc. Natl. Acad. Sci. U.S.A. 78:2643–2647.

Galambos, R., Hicks, G.E., and Wilson, M.S. 1984. The auditory brainstem response reliably predicts hearing loss in graduates of a tertiary intensive care nursery. Ear Hear. 5:254–260.

Garg, B.P., Markand, O.N., and Bustion, P.F. 1982. Brainstem auditory evoked responses in hereditary motor-sensory neuropathy: site of origin of wave II. Neurology 32:1017–1019.

Geisler, C.D., Frishkopf, L.S., and Rosenblith, W.A. 1958. Extracranial responses to acoustic clicks in man. Science 128:1210–1211.

Gelfand, S. 1981. *Hearing.* New York: Marcel Dekker.

Glassock, M.E., Hays J.W., Minor, L.B., et al. 1993. Preservation of hearing in surgery for acoustic neuromas. J Neurosurg. 78:864–870.

Goff, W.R., Allison, T., Lyons, W., et al. 1977. Origins of short latency auditory evoked potentials in man. Prog. Clin. Neurophysiol. 2:30–44.

Goff, W.R., Allison, T., and Vaughan, H.G. 1978. The functional neuroanatomy of event related potentials. In *Event-related Brain Potentials in Man,* Eds. E. Callaway, P. Tueting, and S.H. Koslow, pp. 1–79. New York Academic Press.

Goiten, K.J., Amit, Y., Fainmesser, P., et al. 1983. Diagnostic and prognostic value of auditory nerve brainstem evoked responses in comatose children. Crit. Care Med. 11:91–94.

Goldie, W.D., Chiappa, K.H., Young, R.R., et al. 1981. Brainstem auditory and short latency somatosensory evoked responses in brain death. Neurology 31:248–256.

Goodin, D., Squires, K., and Starr, A. 1978. Long latency event-related components of the auditory evoked potential. Brain 101:635–648.

Ghosh, S., Gupta, A.K., and Mann, S.S. 2002. Can electrocochleography in Meniere's disease be noninvasive? J. Otolaryngol. 31:371–375.

Grabel, J.C., Zappulla, R.A., Ryder, J., et al. 1991. Brainstem auditory evoked responses in 56 patients with acoustic neurinoma. J. Neurosurg. 74(5):749–753.

Gracey, K. 2003. Current concepts in universal newborn hearing screening and early hearing detection and intervention programs. Adv. Neonatal. Care 3:308–317.

Greiman, M.C., and Lusk, R.P. 1991. Pressure-induced modifications of the acoustic nerve. Part II. Auditory brainstem responses. Am. J. Otolaryngol. 12(1):12–19.

Groenen, P., Snik, A., and van den Broek, P. 1997. Electrically evoked auditory middle latency responses versus perception abilities in cochlear implant users. Audiology 36:83–97.

Grundy, B. 1982. Monitoring of sensory evoked potentials during neurosurgery operations: methods and applications. Neurosurgery 11:556–575.

Harker, L., Hosik, E., Voots, R., et al. 1977. Influence of succinylcholine on middle component auditory evoked potentials. Arch. Otolaryngol. 103: 133–137.

Harner, S.G., and Laws, E.R. 1983. Clinical findings in patients with acoustic neurinoma. Mayo Clin. Proc. 58:721–728.

Harney, C.L. 2000. Infant hearing loss: the necessity for early identification. Bol. Assoc. Med. P. R. 92:130–132.

Hashimoto, I. 1982a. Auditory evoked potentials recorded directly from the human VIIIth nerve and brain stem: Origins of their fast and slow components. In *Kyoto Symposia* (EEG Suppl. 36), Eds. P.A. Buser, W.A. Cobb, and T. Okuma, pp. 305–314. Amsterdam: Elsevier.

Hashimoto, I. 1982b. Auditory evoked potentials from the human midbrain: slow brain stem responses. Electroencephalogr. Clin. Neurophysiol. 53: 652–657.

Hashimoto, I., Ishiyama, Y., Yoshimoto, T., et al. 1981. Brain-stem auditory evoked potentials recorded directly from human brain-stem and thalamus. Brain 104:841–859.

Hayes, D. 2003. Screening methods: current status. Ment. Retard. Dev. Disabil. Res. Rev. 9:65–72.

Hecox, K.E., and Galambos, R. 1974. Brain stem auditory evoked responses in human infants and adults. Arch. Otolaryngol. 99:30–33.

Hecox, K.E., Cone, B., and Blaw, M.E. 1981. Brainstem auditory evoked response in the diagnosis of pediatric neurologic diseases. Neurology 31:832–840.

Helfer, T.M., Lee, R.B., Maris, D.C., et al. 2003. Wanted: a national standard for early hearing detection and intervention outcomes data. Am. J. Audiol. 12:23–30.

Howard, M.A., Volkov, I.O., Mirsky R., et al. 2000. Auditory cortex on the human posterior superior temporal gyrus. J. Comp. Neurol. 416:79–92.

Hyde, M.L., and Blair, R.L. 1981. The auditory brainstem response in neuro-otology: perspectives and problems. J. Otolaryngol. 10:117–125.

Jacobson, G.P., Privitera, M., Neils, J.M., et al. 1990. The effects of anterior temporal lobectomy on the middle latency auditory evoked potential. Electroencephalogr. Clin. Neurophysiol. 75:230–241.

Jacobson, G.P., Kraus, N., and McGee T.J. 1997. Hearing as reflected by middle and long latency event-related potentials. In *Electrophysiologic Evaluation in Otolaryngology*, Eds. B.R. Alford, J. Jerger, and H.A. Jenkins. Basel: Karger, Adv. Otorhinolaryngol. 53:46–84.

Jacobson, J.T., and Northern, J.L. 1991. *Diagnostic Audiology*. Austin: Pro-ed.

Janssen, R., Hetzler, B.E., Creason, J.P., et al. 1991. Differential impact of hypothermia and pentobarbital on brainstem auditory evoked response. Electroencephalogr. Clin. Neurophysiol. 80(5):412–421.

Jewett, D.L. 1970. Volume-conducted potentials in response to auditory stimuli as detected by averaging in the cat. Electroencephalogr. Clin. Neurophysiol. 28:609–618.

Jewett, D.L., and Williston, J.S. 1971. Auditory-evoked far fields averaged from the scalp of humans. Brain 94:681–696.

Jewett, D.L., Romano, M.N., and Williston, J.S. 1970. Human auditory evoked potentials: possible brainstem components detected on the scalp. Science 167:1517–1518.

Karnaze, D.S., Marshall, L.F., McCarthy, C.S., et al. 1982. Localizing and prognostic value of auditory evoked responses in coma after closed head injury. Neurology 32:299–302.

Karrer, R., Cohen, J., and Tucting, P. 1984. Brain and information: event-related potentials. Ann. N.Y. Acad. Sci. 425:1–768.

Kavanaugh, K.T., Domico, W.D., Crews, P.L., et al. 1988. Comparison of the intrasubject repeatability of auditory brainstem and middle latency responses elicited in young children. Ann. Otol. Rhinol Laryngol. 97:264–271.

Keene, M., and Graham, J.M. 1984. Clinical monitoring of the effects of gentamicin by electrocochleography J. Laryngol. Otol. 1:11–21.

Kileny, P.R., and Kemink, J.L. 1987. Electrically evoked middle-latency auditory evoked potentials in cochlear implant candidates. Otolaryngol. Head Neck Surg. 113:1072–1077.

Kileny, P., Paccioretti, D., and Wilson A.F. 1987. Effects of cortical lesions on middle-latency auditory evoked responses. Electroencephalogr. Clin. Neurophysiol. 66:108–120.

Kjaer, M. 1980a. Recognizability of brain stem auditory evoked potential components. Acta Neurol. Scand. 62:20–33.

Kjaer, M. 1980b. Variations of brain stem auditory evoked potentials correlated to duration and severity of multiple sclerosis. Acta Neurol. Scand. 61:157–166.

Kjaer, M. 1985. Brainstem auditory evoked potentials in demyelinating diseases of the central nervous system. In *Evoked Potentials Neurophysiological and Clinical Aspects*, Eds. C. Morocutti and P.A. Rizzo, pp. 175–184. Amsterdam: Elsevier.

Knight, R.T., Hillyard, S.A., Woods, D.L., et al. 1980. The effects of frontal and temporal-parietal lesions in the auditory evoked potential in man. Electroencephalogr. Clin. Neurophysiol. 50:112–124.

Kohelet, D., Usher, M., Arbel, E., et al. 1990. Effect of gentamicin on the auditory brainstem evoked response in term infants: a preliminary report. Pediatr. Res. 28(3):232–234.

Kramer, S.J., Vertes, D.R., Condon, M. 1989. Auditory brainstem responses and clinical follow-up of high-risk infants. Pediatrics. 83:385–392.

Kraus, N., and McGee, T. 1995. The middle latency response generating system. In *Perspectives of Event-Related Potential Research*, Eds. G. Karmos, M. Molnar, V. Csepe, et al., EEG Suppl, Elsevier Sciences, 44:93–101.

Kraus, N., Ozdamar, O., Hier, D., et al. 1982. Auditory middle latency responses (MLRs) in patients with cortical lesions. Electroencephalogr. Clin. Neurophysiol. 54:275–287.

Kraus, N., Smith, D., Reed, N., et al. 1985. Auditory middle latency responses in children: effect of age and diagnostic criteria. Electroencephalogr. Clin. Neurophysiol. 62:343–351.

Kraus, N., Smith, D.I., and McGee T. 1988. Midline and temporal lobe MLRs in the guinea pig originate from different generator systems: a conceptual framework for new and existing data. Electroencephalogr. Clin. Neurophysiol. 70:541–558.

Kutas, M., and Hillyard, S.A. 1980. Reading senseless sentences: Brain potentials reflect semantic incongruity. Science 207:203–205.

Lambert, P.R., Ruth, R.A., and Halpin, C.F. 1990. Promontory electrical stimulation in labyrinthectomized ears. Arch. Otolaryngol. Head Neck Surg. 116(2):197–201.

Lary, S., DeVries, L.S., Kaiser, A., et al. 1989. Auditory brainstem responses in infants with posthaemorrhagic ventricular dilatation. Arch. Dis. Child. 64(1):17–23.

Lee, Y.S., Lueders, H., Dinner D.S., et al. 1984. Recording of auditory evoked potentials in man using chronic subdural electrodes. Brain. 107:115–131.

Legatt, A.D., Avezzo, J.C., Vaughn, H.G. Jr. 1988. The anatomic and physiologic bases of brain stem auditory evoked potentials. Neur. Clin. 6:681–704.

Levin, H. 1985. Neurobehavioral recovery. In *Central Nervous System Trauma Status Report*, Eds. D. Becker and J. Povlishock, pp. 281–300. Bethesda: National Institutes of Health.

Liebenthal, E., Ellingson, M.L., Spanaki, M.V., et al. 2003. Simultaneous ERP and fMRI of the auditory cortex in a passive oddball paradigm. Neuroimage 19:1395–1404.

Loiselle, D., Stamm, J., Maitinsky, S., et al. 1980. Evoked potential and behavioral signs of dysfunctions in hyperactive boys. Psychophysiology 17:193–201.

Lowitzsch, K., and Maurer, K. 1982. Pattern-reversal visual evoked potentials in reclassification of 472 MS patients. In *Clinical Applications of Evoked Potentials in Neurology*, Eds. J. Courjon and F. Mauguière, pp. 487–491. New York: Raven Press.

Matthies, C., and Samii, M. 1997. Management of vestibular schwannomas (acoustic neuromas): the value of neurophysiology for evaluation and prediction of auditory function in 420 cases. Neurosurgery 40:919–930.

Maurer, K., Scafer, E., and Leitaner, H. 1980. The effect of varying stimulus polarity (rarefaction vs. condensation) on early auditory evoked potentials. Electroencephalogr Clin. Neurophysiol. 50:330–344.

McGee, T., Kraus, N., Comperatore, C., et al. 1991. Subcortical and cortical components of the MLR generating system. Brain Res. 54:211–220.

Ment, L.R., Scott, D.T., Ehrenkranz, R.A., et al. 1982. Neonates of <1,250 grams birth-weight: prospective neurodevelopmental evaluation during the first year postterm. Pediatrics 70:292.

Michalewski, H.J., Thompson, L.W., Patterson, J.V., et al. 1980. Sex differences in the amplitudes and latencies of the human auditory brain stem potential. Electroencephalogr. Clin. Neurophysiol. 48:351–356.

Miller, J.M. 1991. Physiologic measures of electrically evoked auditory system responsiveness: effects of pathology and electrical stimulation. Am. J. Otol. 12(suppl):28–36.

Mochizuki, Y., Go, T., Ohkubo, H., et al. 1982. Developmental changes of brainstem auditory evoked potentials (BAEPs) in normal human subjects from infants to young adults. Brain Dev. 4:127–136.

Möller, A.R. 1996. Monitoring auditory function during operations to remove acoustic tumors. Am. J. Otol. 17:452–460.

Möller, A.R., and Janetta, P.J. 1982. Evoked potentials from the inferior colliculus in man. Electroencephalogr. Clin. Neurophysiol. 53:612–620.

Möller, A.R., and Janetta, P.J. 1983. Auditory evoked potentials recorded from the cochlear nucleus and its vicinity in man. J. Neurosurg. 59:1013–1018.

Möller, A.R., and Jho, H.D. 1991. Compound action potentials recorded from the intracranial portion of the auditory nerve in man: effects of stimulus intensity and polarity. Audiology 30(3):142–163.

Möller, A.R., Janetta, P.J., Bennett, M., et al. 1981. Intracranially recorded responses from the human auditory nerve: new insights into the origin of brain stem evoked potentials (BSEPs). Electroencephalogr. Clin. Neurophysiol. 52:18–27.

Möller A.R., Jannetta P.J., and Jho H.D. 1994. Click-evoked responses from the cochlear nucleus: a study in human. Electroencephalogr. Clin. Neurophysiol. 92(3):215–224.

Moore, E.J. 1983. Effects of stimulus parameters. In *Basis of Auditory Brain-Stem Evoked Responses,* Ed. E.J. Moore, pp. 221–251. New York: Grune & Stratton.

Morest, D.K. 1983. Functional anatomy of the auditory system. In *Basis of Auditory Brain-Stem Evoked Responses,* Ed. E.J. Moore, pp. 51–66. New York: Grune & Stratton.

Näätänen, R. 1991. Mismatch negativity outside strong attentional focus: a commentary on Woldorff et al. Psychophysiology 28:478–484.

Näätänen, R., and Picton, T. 1987. The NI wave of the human electric and magnetic response to sound. Psychophysiology 24:375–425.

Naunton, R.F., and Zerlin, S. 1976. Basis and some diagnostic implications of electrocochleography. Laryngoscope 86:475–482.

Newman, T.B. 1991. Neonatal jaundice and brainstem auditory responses. J. Pediatr. 118(4):653.

Nishida, H., Kumagami, H., and Katsunori, D. 1976. Prognostic criteria of sudden deafness as deduced by electrocochleography. Arch. Otolarygol. 102:601–607.

O'Malley, S., Ramsden, R.T., Latif, A., et al. 1985. Electrocochleographic changes in the hearing loss associated with X-linked hypophosphataemic osteomalacia. Acta Otolaryngol. (Stockh.) 100:13–18.

Ornitz, E.M., Mo, A., Olson, S.T., et al. 1980. Influence of click sound pressure direction on brain stem responses in children. Audiology 19:254–254.

Parving, A., Solomon, G., Eberling, C., et al. 1980. Middle components of the auditory evoked response in bilateral temporal lesions: report on a patient with auditory agnosia. Scand. Audiol. 9:161–167.

Picton, T., and Fitzgerald, P.G. 1983. A general description of the human auditory evoked potentials. In *Basis of Auditory Brain-Stem Evoked Responses,* Ed. E.J. Moore, pp. 141–156. New York: Grune & Stratton.

Picton, T., Hillyard, S., Krausz, H., et al. 1974. Human auditory evoked potentials. I. Evaluation of components. Electroencephalogr. Clin. Neurophysiol. 36:179–190.

Picton, T.W., Stapells, D.R., Perrault, N., et al. 1984. Human event-related potentials: current perspectives. In *Evoked Potentials.* II, Eds. R.H. Nodar and C. Barber, pp. 3–24. Boston: Butterworth.

Picton, T.W., John, M.S., Purcell, D.W., et al. 2003. Human auditory steady-state responses: the effects of recording technique and state arousal. Anesth. Analg 97:1396–1402.

Polich, J.M., and Starr, A. 1983. Middle, late, and long-latency auditory evoked potentials. In *Basis of Auditory Brainstem Evoked Responses,* Ed. E.J. Moore, pp. 345–361. New York: Grune & Stratton.

Polo, G., Fischer, C., Sindou, M.P., et al. 2004. Brainstem auditory evoked potential monitoring during microvascular decompression for hemifacial spasm: intraoperative brainstem auditory evoked potential changes and warning values to prevent hearing loss-prospective study in a consecutive series of 84 patients. Neurosurgery 54:97–104.

Portmann, M., Dauman, R., and Aran, J.M. 1985. Audiometric and electrophysiological correlations in sudden deafness. Acta Otolaryngol. (Stockh.) 99:363–368.

Pratt, H., Aminoff, M., Nuwer, M.R., Starr, A. 1999. Short-latency auditory evoked potentials. The International Federal of Clinical Neurophysiology. Electroencephalogr. Clin. Neurophysiol. Suppl. 52:69–77.

Pratt, H., Brodsky, G., Goldsher, M., et al. 1986. Auditory brain-stem evoked potentials in patients undergoing dialysis. Electroencephalogr. Clin. Neurophysiol. 63:18–24.

Pratt, H., Bleich, N., and Feingold, K. 1990. Three-channel Lissajous' trajectories of auditory brainstem evoked potentials: Contribution of fast and slow components to planar segment formation. Hear Res. 43(2–3):159–171.

Regan, D. 1989. *Human Brain Electrophysiology. Evoked Potentials and Evoked Magnetic Fields in Science and Medicine.* Amsterdam: Elsevier.

Roberts, J.L., Davis, H., Phon, G.L., et al. 1982. Auditory brainstem responses in preterm neonates: maturation and follow-up. 1982. J. Pediatr. 101:257–263.

Robinson, K., and Rudge, P. 1977. Abnormalities of the auditory evoked potentials in patients with multiple sclerosis. Brain 100:19–40.

Rosenhall, U., Bjorkman, G., Pedersen, K., et al. 1985. Brainstem auditory evoked potentials in different age groups. Electroencephalogr. Clin. Neurophysiol. 62:426–430.

Roth, W.T., Ford, J.M., Pfefferbaum, A., et al. 1979. Event related potential research in psychiatry. In *Human Evoked Potentials: Applications and Problems,* Eds. D. Lehman and E. Callaway, pp. 331–345. New York: Plenum Press.

Rowe, M.J. III. 1978. Normal variability of the brain-stem auditory evoked response in young and old adult subjects. Electroencephalogr. Clin. Neurophysiol. 44:459–470.

Ruben, R.J., Elberling, C., and Salomon, G. 1976. *Electrocochleography.* Baltimore: University Park Press.

Ruth, R.A., and Lambert, P.R. 1989 Comparison of tympanic membrane to promontory electrode recordings of electrographic responses in patients with Meniere's disease. Otolaryngol. Head Neck Surg. 100:546–542.

Salamy, A., McKean, C.M., Pettett, G., et al. 1978. Auditory brainstem recovery processes from birth to adulthood. Psychophysiology 15:214–220.

Scherg, M., and Von Cramon, D. 1985a. A new interpretation of the generators of BAEP waves I–V. Results of spatio-temporal dipole model. Electroencephalogr. Clin. Neurophysiol. 62:290–299.

Scherg, M., and Von Cramon, D. 1985b. Two bilateral sources of the late AEP identified by a spatio-temporal dipole model. Electroencephalogr. Clin. Neurophysiol. 62:290–299.

Schlake, H.P., Milewski, C., Goldbrunner, R.H., et al. 2001. Combined intra-operative monitoring of hearing by means of auditory brainstem responses (ABR) and transtympanic electrocochleography (ECochG) during surgery of intra- and extrameatal acoustic neurinomas. Acta Neurochir. (Wien.) 143:985–995.

Schuknecht, W. 1964. Further observations on the pathology of presbycusis. Arch. Otolaryngol. 80:369–382.

Schulman-Galambos, C., and Galambos, R. 1975. Brain stem auditory responses in premature infants. J. Speech Hear. Res. 18:456–465.

Schulman-Galambos, C., and Galambos, R. 1979. Brain stem evoked response audiometry in newborn hearing screening. Arch. Otolaryngol. 105:86–90.

Schwaber, M.K., and Hall, J.W. 1990. A simplified technique for transtympanic electrocochleography. Am. J. Otol. 11:260–265.

Schwartz, D.M., Morris, M.D., Spydell, J.D., et al. 1990. Influence of click polarity on the brainstem auditory evoked response (BAER) revisited. Electroencephalogr. Clin. Neurophysiol. 77(6):445–457.

Sellick, P.M., and Russell, I.J. 1978. Intracellular studies of cochlear hair cells; filling the gap between basilar membrane mechanics and neuronal excitation. In *Evoked Electrical Activity in the Auditory Nervous System,* Eds. R.F. Nauton and C. Fernandez, pp. 113–139. New York: Academic Press.

Selter, W.A., and Brackmann, D.E. 1977. Acoustic tumor detection with brain stem electric response audiometry. Arch. Otolaryngol. 103:181–187.

Shagass, C., Ornitz, E.M., Sutton, S., et al. 1978. *Event-related Potentials in Man,* Eds. E. Calloway, P. Tueting, and S.H. Koslow, pp. 443–496. New York: Academic Press.

Shannon, D.A., Felix, J.K., Krumholz, A., et al. 1984. Hearing screening of high-risk newborns with brainstem auditory evoked potentials: A follow-up study. Pediatrics 73:22–26.

Simmons, P.B. 1978. Identification of hearing loss in infants and young children. Otolaryngol. Clin. North Am. 11:19–28.

Sohmer, H., Feinmesser, M., and Szabo, G. 1974. Sources of electrocochleographic responses as studied in patients with brain damage. Electroencephalogr. Clin. Neurophysiol. 37:663–669.

Spire, J.P., Dohrmann, G.J., and Prieto, P.S. 1982. Correlation of brainstem evoked response with direct acoustic nerve potential. In *Clinical Applications of Evoked Potentials in Neurology,* Eds. J. Courjon, F. Mauguiere, and M. Revol, pp. 159–167. New York: Raven Press.

Spitzer, J.B., Fayad, J.N., and Wazen, J.J. 2003. The expanding domain of implantable hearing devices: an update on current status in the United States. Rev. Laryngol. Otol. Rhinol. (Bord.) 124:39–44.

Spydell, J., Pattee, G., and Goldie, W. 1985. The 40 Hertz auditory event related potential: normal values and effects of lesions. Electroencephalogr. Clin. Neurophysiol. 62:193–202.

Squires, K., and Hecox, K. 1983. Electrophysiological evaluation of higher level auditory processing. Semin. Hear. 4:415–432.

Stapells, D., Linden, D., Suffield, J., et al. 1984. Human auditory steady state potentials. Ear Hear. 5:105–115.

Starr, A. 1976. Auditory brain-stem responses in brain death. Brain 99:543–554.

Starr, A., and Achor, J. 1975. Auditory brain stem responses in neurological diseases. Arch. Neurol. 32:761–768.

Starr, A., and Hamilton, A.E. 1976. Correlation between confirmed sites of neurologic lesions and abnormalities of far-field auditory brainstem responses. Electroencephalogr. Clin. Neurophysiol. 41:595–608.

Starr, A., Picton, T.W., Sininger, Y., et al. 1996. Auditory neuropathy. Brain. 119:741–753.

Stockard, J.E., and Stockard, J.J. 1983. Recording and analyzing. In *Basis of Auditory Brain-Stem Evoked Responses,* Ed. E.J. Moore, pp. 255–286. New York: Grune & Stratton.

Stockard, J.E., Stockard, J.J., Westmoreland, B.F., et al. 1979. Brainstem auditory evoked responses. Normal variation as a function of stimulus and subject characteristics. Arch. Neurol. 36:823–831.

Stockard, J.J., and Rossiter, V.S. 1977. Clinical and pathologic correlates of brain stem auditory response abnormalities. Neurology 27:316–325.

Stockard, J.J., Stockard, J.E., and Sharbrough, F.W. 1977. Detection and localization of occult lesions with brainstem auditory responses. Mayo Clin. Proc. 52:761–769.

Stockard, J.J., Stockard, J.E., and Sharbrough, F.W. 1978. Nonpathologic factors influencing brainstem auditory evoked potentials. Am. J. EEG Technol. 18:177–209.

Stueve, M.P., O'Rourke, C. 2003. Estimation of hearing loss in children: comparison of auditory steady-state response, auditory brainstem response, and behavioral test methods. Am. J. Audiol. 12:125–136.

Sturzebecher, E., and Werbs, M. 1987. Effects of age and sex on auditory brainstem response. A new aspect. Scand. Audiol. 16(3):153–157.

Von Bekesy, G. 1960. *Experiments in Hearing.* New York: McGraw-Hill.

Walser, H., Kriss, A., Cunningham, K., et al. 1984. A multimodal evoked potential assessment of uremia. In *Evoked Potentials, II,* Eds. R.H. Nodar and C. Barber, pp. 643–649. Boston: Butterworth.

Warren, M.P. 1989. The auditory brainstem response in pediatrics. Otolaryngol. Clin. North Am. 22(3):473–500.

Weber, B.A., Seitz, R.M., and McCutcheon, M.J. 1981. Quantifying click stimuli in auditory brainstem response audiometry. Ear Hear. 2:15–19.

Wellman, M.B., Sommer, D.D., and McKenna, J. 2003. Sensorineural hearing loss in postmeningitic children. Otol. Neurotol. 24:907–912.

White, K.R. 2003. The current status of EHDI programs in the United States. Ment. Retard. Dev. Disabil. Res. Rev. 9:79–88.

Woods, D.L. 1995. The component structure of the N1 wave of the human auditory evoked potential. In *Perspectives of Event-Related Potential Research,* Eds. G. Karmos, M. Molnar, V. Csepe, et al. EEG Suppl. Elsevier Sciences, 44:102–109.

Woods, D.L., Clayworth, C.C., Knight, R.T., et al. 1987. Generators of middle– and long–latency auditory evoked potentials: implications from studies of patients with bitemporal lesions. Electroencephalogr. Clin. Neurophysiol. 68:132–148.

Yagi, T., and Baba, S. 1983. Evaluation of brain-stem function by the auditory brain-stem response and the caloric vestibular reaction in comatose patients. Arch. Otolaryngol. 238:33–43.

Yamamoto, T., Williamson, S.J., Kaufman, L., et al. 1988. Magnetic localization of neuronal activity in the human brain. Proc. Natl. Acad. Sci. USA 85:8732–8736.

Yamasaki, M., Shono, H., Oga, M., et al. 1991. Changes in auditory brainstem response of normal neonates immediately after birth. Biol. Neonate 60(2):92–101.

Yen, P.T., Lin, C.C., and Huang, T.S. 1995. A preliminary report on the correlation of vestibular Meniere's disease with electrocochleography and glycerol test. Acta Otolaryngol. Suppl. 520(pt 2):241–246.

Yoshie, N. 1973. Diagnostic significance of the electrocochleogram in clinical audiometry. Audiology 12:504–539.

Zaaroor, M., and Starr, A. 1991. Auditory brainstem evoked potentials in cat after kainic acid induced neuronal loss. I. Superior olivary complex. Electroencephalogr. Clin. Neurophysiol. 80(5):422–435.

54. Somatosensory Evoked Potentials: Normal Responses, Abnormal Waveforms, and Clinical Applications in Neurological Diseases

François Mauguière

The modern history of clinical somatosensory evoked potential (SEP) testing began over 50 years ago with George Dawson's (1947) recordings, in patients with myoclonus, of what is known today as a giant somatosensory cortical responses. Because of their relatively large amplitude and low frequency compatible with a slow sampling rate of analog-digital conversion, the cortical SEPs were the first studied in normals and patients. In the 1970s and early 1980s the spinal potentials and subcortical far-field potentials were identified. Although the origins and mechanisms of far-field SEPs are still debated in the literature, correlations among abnormal waveforms, lesion site, and clinical findings now can be considered well established. The most recent advances in our knowledge of cortical responses to somatosensory stimulation are issued from development of multichannel recordings of evoked potentials (EPs) and evoked magnetic fields coupled with source modeling and source localization in the three-dimensional (3D) images of brain volume, as provided by magnetic resonance imaging (MRI). This approach, based of the resolution of the inverse problem, which consists in modeling sources from the field distribution, results in models of brain activation that may substantially differ from those issued from clinical correlations between the abnormal waveform and the lesion site. In brief, the approach based on electroclinical correlations tended toward the identification of a single generator for each SEP component, which is acceptable for responses reflecting the sequential activation of fibers and synaptic relays of the somatosensory pathways. Conversely, source modeling often suggests that the evoked field distribution at a given moment may result from activities of multiple distributed sources that overlap in time. This model fits better with the parallel activation and the feedback controls that characterize the processing of somatosensory inputs at the cortical level.

This chapter does not aim at exhaustivity, but focuses on recent findings that might be helpful for the recording and interpretation of SEPs in clinical practice.

Stimulation and Recording Procedures

Only the essential technical requirements for SEPs recording in clinical practice are given here. More technical details concerning electrodes, amplifiers, stimulators, and safety can be found elsewhere in this book as well as in other books (Chiappa, 1990; Halliday, 1993; Mauguière, 1995; Spehlmann, 1985), and in guidelines published by the American Electroencephalographic Society (1984) and the International Federation of Clinical Neurophysiology (Nuwer et al., 1994; Mauguière et al., 1999).

Stimulus Types

Electrical Stimuli

Brevity and strict control in time of stimulus onset and cut-off, and thus of averaging trigger, are the major advantages of electrical stimulation over any other types of stimulus.

SEPs are usually evoked by bipolar transcutaneous electrical stimulation applied on the skin over the trajectory of peripheral nerves. Dermatomal electrical stimulation can also be used to explore root lesions (see below). Monophasic electrical pulses of 100 to 300 μsec can be delivered through rectangular, disk, or needle electrodes connected to the negative (cathode) or positive (anode) pole of the stimulator. Electrical stimuli depolarize nerve fibers directly by generating a potential difference in the medium adjacent to the nerve trunk and thus across the nerve fiber membrane, causing a depolarization close to the site of the cathode. Electrical stimuli thus bypass the peripheral encoding of natural stimuli (pressure, vibrations, joint movements) by the receptors. The different categories of fibers that subserve the different types of sensations can be individualized on the basis of their diameter and thickness of their myelin sheaths. There is an inverse relation between the fiber diameter on the one hand and its threshold to electrical stimulation and conduction velocity on the other hand. In most clinical applications of SEPs electrical stimuli are delivered at intensities equivalent to three to four times the sensory threshold, which produce a twitch in the muscles innervated by the stimulated nerve when it contains a contingent of motor fibers. At this stimulus intensity the rapidly conducting large myelinated fibers, including fibers subserving touch and joint sensation but also muscle afferents, are activated because of their higher resistance.

The contribution of muscle afferents to cortical SEPs after stimulation of upper limb mixed nerves remains a matter of controversy. It is considered negligible by Halonen et al. (1988) and Kunesch et al. (1995). However, selective intrafascicular stimulation of hand muscle afferents at the wrist and motor-point stimulation were shown to produce short-latency cortical SEPs with the same waveforms (Gandevia and Burke, 1988; Gandevia et al., 1984) and modeled dipolar sources (Restuccia et al., 2002a) as those obtained by stimulating the trunk of a mixed nerve. These cortical responses were obtained also after motor-point stimulation of proximal upper limb muscles (Gandevia and Burke, 1988) and muscles of the trunk (Gandevia and Macefield, 1989). They are relatively small as compared with potentials evoked from the whole mixed nerve or digital nerves because only relatively few afferents are activated. Their first cortical component peaks later than for median nerve stimulation at the wrist and at approximately the same latency as for stimulation of the digital nerves (Gandevia and Burke, 1990). Therefore, the possibility remains that, when stimulating a mixed nerve of the upper limb such as the median nerve, the cortical response to muscle afferents inputs could be gated by the response to cutaneous and joint inputs. To conclude, the contribution of muscle afferents median nerve cortical SEPs can be considered as weak, compared to that of cutaneous afferents.

The situation is quite different after electric stimulation of lower limb sensorimotor nerves such as the posterior tibial nerve for which muscle afferents have been shown to have a major contribution to cortical SEPs (Burke et al., 1981, 1982; Gandevia et al., 1984; Macefield et al., 1989). The latency of the earliest cortical response is shorter after stimulation of abductor hallucis muscular fascicle than after stimulation of the posterior tibial nerve, and its amplitude is approximately half that of the tibial nerve response (Burke et al., 1981). It has been shown that, after stimulation of the tibial nerve, inputs conveyed by muscle afferents, which have the fastest conduction velocity, are able to occlude the response to cutaneous inputs (Burke et al., 1982). Because of this gating, the cutaneous afferent volley may make little or no contribution to the cerebral potential evoked by electric stimulation of lower limb mixed nerves. Electric simulation of pure sensory nerves, such as digital nerves for the upper limb and sural nerve for the lower limb, activates exclusively skin and joint peripheral and dorsal column fibers. It is advisable to use this type of stimulus in any attempt to correlate the quality of perception with SEP data in normal subjects as well as in patients with impaired sensation (Mauguière et al., 1983a). At the upper limb, stimulation of the finger tip (Desmedt and Osaki, 1991) or distal phalanx of fingers (Restuccia et al., 1999) activates selectively skin fibers, while stimulation of digital nerves at the level of the first or second phalanx concern both joint and skin afferents.

Paired electrical stimuli delivered to the same nerve at various interstimulus intervals can be used to characterize distinct components of a given response according to their refractoriness after the response to the first stimulus of the pair (conditioning stimulus), and also to combine SEP testing with psychophysical evaluation of time discrimination performances in detecting the second stimulus of the pair (El Kharroussi et al., 1996). The voltage of the response to the second stimulus of the pair is evaluated by subtracting the response to the test stimulus delivered alone in a separate session.

The effect on SEPs of spatial interference between two electrical stimuli delivered simultaneously but at two distinct sites has been first described by Burke et al. (1982) and Gandevia et al. (1983). These authors showed that after simultaneous stimulation of both index and middle fingers of the same hand the size of the early component of the cerebral potential is less than predicted by simple addition of the

potentials produced by stimulation of the fingers individually. A procedure based on this observation has been recently applied to the study of somatosensory processing in patients with dystonia (Tinazzi et al., 2000).

The interfering influences of sensory and motor events on electrically evoked SEPs have been widely used in the context of gating paradigms (see Cheron et al., 2000, for a review). In particular, models of centrifugal and centripetal SEP gating during movement programming or execution are based on the results from these studies (see below).

Natural Stimuli

Physiological stimuli have a higher selectivity than that of electrical stimulation of sensory nerves. SEPs and somatosensory evoked magnetic fields (SEFs) can be obtained in response to a brief mechanical impact on the fingertip (Debecker and Desmedt, 1964; Halliday and Mason, 1964; Kakigi and Shibasaki, 1984; Nakanishi et al., 1973; Pratt and Starr, 1981) or air puffs (Forss et al., 1994b; Hashimoto, 1987; Schieppati and Ducati, 1984). For skin stimulation, there is some difficulty in getting a consistent, quick, and well-defined movement of the striker using an electro-mechanical device, which is why stimulators producing fast rise-time (1 msec) and short-duration (4–5 msec) air puffs have been developed. However, due to the small population of excited fibers, these mechanical stimuli produce low-voltage responses and are not used routinely in the clinical setting, in spite of their potential advantage over conventional electrical stimuli.

Selective stimulation of joint afferent fibers using passive movements of fingers is difficult to achieve mostly because of possible interference between activations of joint, tendinous, and muscle stretch receptors. Dedicated devices have been developed to activate selectively finger joint afferents (Desmedt and Osaki, 1991) or muscle afferents (Mima et al., 1996). These stimulators produce a small and brisk passive flexion movement of finger II, or fingers II and III, proximal interphalangeal joint, with an amplitude of 2 degrees (Desmedt and Osaki, 1991) or 4 degrees (Mima et al., 1996) in 25 msec. In spite of close similarities between stimulation paradigms and evoked responses in these two studies, authors are diverging about the nature of afferent peripheral fibers involved in cortical response genesis, although they discard the hypothesis of a significant participation of cutaneous fibers. Desmedt and Osaki (1991) considered that the small 2-degree flexions they applied to the finger with the wrist in slight extension were unlikely to activate the spindle afferents of finger extensor muscles. Mima et al. (1996) opposed the argument that joint afferents discharge only in extreme flexion or extension positions while a 4-degree flexion of the finger produces a muscle stretch in the extensor muscle far larger than that needed to record evoked cortical response in monkeys (Phillips et al., 1971). Moreover, they observed that responses to finger flexion were preserved after anoxic ischemia blocking the conduction of joint and cutaneous fibers from the moved finger, and concluded that muscle afferents from finger extensor muscles were responsible for cortical evoked responses. Lastly, this latter observation is in partial contradiction to that of an abolition of cortical evoked responses to larger finger displacements (up to 45 degrees) after anoxia of the hand reported earlier by Papakostopoulos et al. (1974).

Pain Stimulation

As performed routinely in clinical neurophysiology laboratories SEPs to electrical stimulation of peripheral nerves do not explore the small myelinated A delta or unmyelinated C afferents to spinothalamic tracts, which subserve temperature and pain sensation. The early report by Halliday and Wakefield (1963) showed that SEPs to electrical stimulation of a peripheral nerve at motor threshold are normal in patients with lesions of the spinothalamic tract and a loss of pain and temperature sensation. The possibility to investigate human pain is attracting increasing attention. There are various methods for evoking pain, including tooth pulp stimulation, cutaneous electrical stimulation, mechanical and electrical stimulation, and cutaneous thermal laser stimulation (Carmon et al., 1976). Bromm and Treede (1983, 1987) have shown that a selective activation of A delta or C fibers can be achieved depending on the energy of brief heat pulses delivered by a CO_2 laser beam applied to the skin surface.

Stimulus Intensity

In most clinical studies the intensity of electrical stimuli is set at motor threshold, or at motor plus sensory threshold (Lesser et al., 1979), for stimulation of mixed sensorimotor nerves, and at three or four times the sensory threshold for stimulation of sensory nerves. At such stimulus intensities all SEP components peaking before 50 msec poststimulus reach their maximal amplitude. The drawbacks of this method are that the physiological threshold can be drastically modified by the disease process and that some patients are unable to cooperate in the evaluation of sensory threshold.

Stimulus Rate

Stimulus rates of 1 to 10/sec are commonly used in clinical neurophysiology laboratories with no significant changes in the amplitudes or latencies of subcortical or primary sensory cortex (SI) responses. These rates are considered as acceptable for clinical studies in most textbooks (Chiappa, 1990; Halliday, 1993). However, lower rates are recommended to study the amplitudes of cortical potentials peaking more than 25 msec after stimulation of the upper limb.

At rates over 3/sec even early cortical potentials peaking after the initial SI response can be depressed, in particular the frontal N30 potential that is one of the SEPs most often reported as affected in movement disorders. The amplitudes of middle- and long-latency responses, in particular those generated in the SII area, reach their saturation level at stimulus rates far below 1/sec (Hari et al., 1984). The effect of stimulus rates on the amplitude of cortical SEPs can be used as a means to distinguish the components one with another. This approach has been applied to identify short-latency SEPs to median nerve (Garcia-Larrea et al., 1992) and tibial nerve (Tinazzi et al., 1996a) stimulation.

Analysis Time and Sampling Rate

Most of the SEP components have proved their clinical utility peak before 50 and 100 msec for upper and lower limb stimulation, respectively. Consequently, there is no necessity to record routinely SEPs over analysis times longer than 100 msec except for the recording of middle-latency responses generated in SII (Hari et al., 1983, 1984), posterior parietal (Forss et al., 1994a), and mesial cortical areas (Forss et al., 1996). Most commercially available devices can calculate 512 sampling points over analysis times in the 10- to 100-msec range. This gives bin widths of 97 and 195 μsec for analysis times of 50 and 100 msec, which are appropriate to obtain far-field and short-latency cortical SEPs without aliasing, respectively (see Spehlman, 1985).

Filters

A broad band-pass, with a high-pass filter set at less than 3 Hz and a low-pass filter set over 2,000 Hz, is optimal to record without distortion all SEP components including fast far-field potentials. Analog filter roll-offs should not exceed 12 and 24 dB/octave for low- and high-frequency filters, respectively. Digital filtering of responses acquired with a broad band-pass filter offers the possibility of selecting offline frequencies of clinical interest.

Gain and Number of Sweeps

Gains between 100.000 and 200.000 are adequate. The number of sweeps to be averaged is variable according to the signal-to-noise ratio of the different SEP components. In practice 500 sweeps are enough, in most instances, to obtain the responses at Erb's point, as well as to extract the main early cortical components. For the recording of spinal and scalp far-field EPs often up to 1,000 to 2,000 sweeps must be averaged.

Electrode Placement

Recording Electrodes

Standard disk electrodes, well attached on the skin and scalp surface, are suitable for most recordings; needle electrodes can also be used. When recording SEP one usually aims to study during the same run peripheral, spinal, brainstem, and early cortical SEPs. Peripheral nerve volleys of action potentials as well as conducted and segmental spinal SEPs can be recorded by placing cutaneous electrodes along the route of the fiber tracts or close to the fixed generators of segmental spinal responses (near-field recording). Electrodes placed on the scalp pick up both SEPs generated in the cortex and thalamocortical fibers, which are picked up as near-field responses located in restricted areas and far-field positivities reflecting the evoked activity generated in peripheral, spinal, and brainstem somatosensory fibers.

The SEP literature is full of discussions about the most appropriate site for the reference electrode to record each of the components of the response; in fact the knowledge of the field distributions and of supposed source locations and orientations is enough for a correct choice of the recording derivation. Considering the field distribution the optimal recording condition is in theory that in which the reference is not influenced by the activity under study. Most of the far-field potentials that have proved to be clinically useful are widely distributed over the scalp. Consequently, they reach their maximal amplitude in referential recordings in which the reference electrode is placed in a noncephalic position and they are canceled, or drastically reduced, when both recording electrodes are placed on the scalp. Furthermore, a noncephalic reference common to all channels is also adequate for all near-field recordings, and there is no theoretical argument against the recommendation of using this type of montage in all situations. However, the electrical and physiological (electrocardiogram, electromyogram, etc.) noise level may be increased by the long distance between the active and reference electrode in noncephalic reference montages. Conversely, differential amplification between the two maxima of a dipolar potential field on the scalp produced by an identified single generator increases the signal voltage and reduces the noise level. Therefore, montages proposed for routine recordings often stem from a compromise between (a) the theoretical optimum represented by a common noncephalic reference and (b) practical considerations in terms of pertinent components to be studied in a given clinical condition and electrical environment.

The routine four-channels montages proposed in the International Federation of Clinical Neurophysiology (IFCN) guidelines (Mauguière et al., 1999) explore the afferent peripheral volley (in the supraclavicular and popliteal fossa for upper and lower limb, respectively), the segmental spinal responses at the neck and lumbar spine levels, as well as the subcortical far-field and early cortical SEPs using scalp electrodes placed in the parietal and frontal regions for upper limb SEPs and at the vertex for lower limb SEPs. Since knowledge of the field distributions and source locations is a prerequisite for a correct choice of derivations, recording montages will be proposed after the description of normal SEP components.

Multiple channel recordings (24, 32, 64, or more) permit assessing the scalp topographic distribution of SEPs; they can be obtained using a cap with electrodes placed according to the modified 10–20 electrode system for SEPs, or whole-head magnetoencephalography (MEG) devices for SEFs. These multiple-channel recordings, eventually assisted by mapping based on computerized voltage or current fields interpolation, have brought invaluable information on the spatial distribution of each component of the response; moreover, they are indispensable for calculating the evoked fields sources coordinates in a spherical or MRI-based realistic model of the head.

Ground Electrode

The position of the ground electrode is more crucial for SEPs than for the recording of any other type of EPs, due to the electrical artifact produced by the stimulation. To minimize the electrical artifact produced by the stimulation, the ground electrode should be placed on the stimulated limb between the stimulation site and the recording electrodes. Flexible metal strips covered with saline-soaked cloth wrapped around the limb close to the stimulus site are recommended. Electrically isolated stimulators allow the use of a ground electrode on the head, which is adequate for eliminating artifact related to the electrical main and radiofrequency interference.

Normal Responses

Short Latency SEPs to Upper Limb Stimulation (Electrical Stimulation of Median, Ulnar, Radial, or Finger Nerves)

The main early SEP components will be described as they appear on recordings using a noncephalic reference

electrode placed at the shoulder on the nonstimulated side after stimulation of the median nerve at the wrist (Fig. 54.1). When necessary we will discuss the modifications of waveform and latency related to the use of other reference electrode sites.

Peripheral N9 Component

Stimulation of a mixed nerve such as the median nerve elicits a compound action potential (CAP) reflecting the pe-

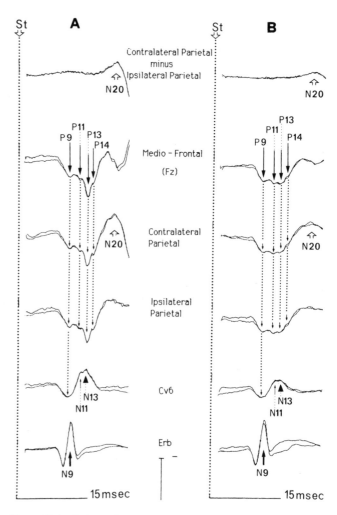

Figure 54.1. Early median nerve somatosensory evoked potential (SEPs) (noncephalic reference recording). This figure illustrates the Erb's point N9, spinal N11, N13, far-field P9, P11, P13, P14, and cortical N20 components (**A**) and the effect of vibrations applied to the stimulated hand (**B**). The far-field potentials are picked up at all cephalic recording sites. Only the potentials reflecting the moving action potentials in peripheral (N9, P9) and central segments (N11, P11) of the first-order neuron are unaffected by the interfering vibrations. Conversely, all potentials reflecting activities generated after the first synapse in the cord dorsal horn (N13), brainstem (P13, P14), and SI cortex (N20) are reduced by the interfering stimulus. In this normal subject the N11 spinal potential, reflecting the ascending volley in dorsal column fibers, is discernible in the ascending slope of the postsynaptic dorsal horn N13 potential. Note that the P9 far-field potentials are recorded at all recording sites above Erb's point. Calibration: 10 µV for Erb's point trace and 5 µV for all other traces. (From Ibañez V., Deiber M.P., and Mauguière F. 1989. Interference of vibrations with input transmission in dorsal horn and cuneate nucleus in man: A study of somatosensory evoked potentials (SEPs) to electrical stimulation of median nerve and fingers. Exp. Brain Res. 75:599–610, with permission.)

ripheral ascending volley that can be recorded at different levels of forearm and arm. In most routine SEP recordings carried out in patients with lesions of the central nervous system (CNS), the peripheral ascending volley is recorded only at Erb's point in the supraclavicular fossa. The CAP appears as a triphasic positive-negative-positive waveform with a negative peak culminating at about 9 msec in normal subjects (N9). If necessary, a CAP with a shape similar to that of the N9 potential peaking at an earlier latency can also be recorded more distally over the trajectory of the nerve. Median nerve CAPs are a mixture of motor antidromic and sensory orthodromic responses, and thus are qualitatively different from SEPs generated in the somatosensory pathways. Because of their large amplitude (5–10 V at Erb's

point) they are usually obtained using runs of 500 stimuli. The amplitude of peripheral CAPs are unaffected by interfering stimuli applied on the stimulated hand (Fig. 54.1) or when the stimulus rate is increased up to 50 Hz (Ibañez et al., 1989).

Spinal Segmental N13 Component

Electrical stimulation of large diameter myelinated fibers of peripheral nerves produces a dorsal horn (DH) potential with a posterior-negative and anterior positive dipolar field perpendicular to the cord axis. This field distribution of DH potentials has been demonstrated by direct spinal recordings at all segmental levels of the cord (Fig. 54.2), and a comprehensive atlas of these responses is now available (Dimitrije-

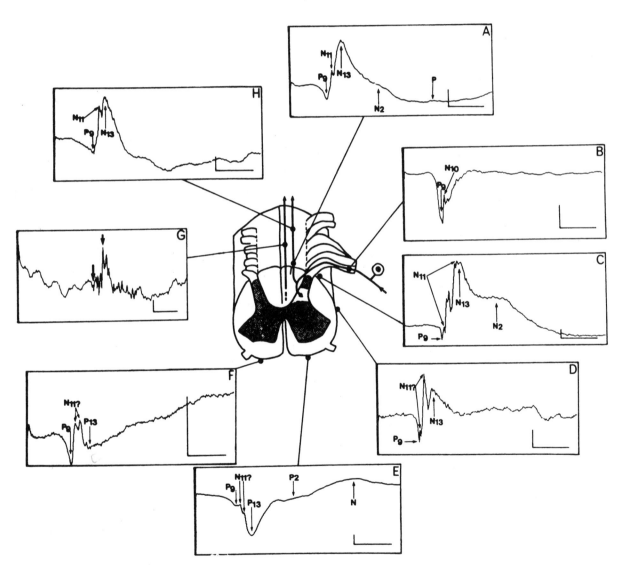

Figure 54.2. Direct recording of spinal potentials on cervical cord surface after stimulation of the median nerve. A cervical cord segment is represented containing one axon from cervical dorsal root ganglion cell on the stimulated side. The dorsal recordings (**A** and **C**) show the P9, N11, N13, and later N2 and P waves. The anterior recordings (**E** and **F**) show the polarity reversal of the dorsal horn N13 response (P13). The recording close to the root spinal entry zone shows the P9 and N10 dorsal root potentials (**B**). The ascending action potentials in dorsal columns corresponding to the surface N11 potential are illustrated in **G**; these fast action potentials are also visible in **A, C,** and **H** on the ascending phase of the N13 potential. The origin of fast N11 activities recorded at lateral and anterior electrode sites (**D–F**) is not firmly assessed (presynaptic afferents in the dorsal horn, spinocerebellar pathways). Calibration: horizontal bars 10 msec, vertical bars 10 μV except in **G**, where it represents 1 μV. (From Jeanmonod D., Sindou M., and Mauguière F. 1991. The human cervical and lumbo-sacral evoked electrospinogram. Data from intra-operative spinal cord surface recordings. Electroencephalogr. Clin. Neurophysiol. 80:477–489, with permission.)

vic and Halter, 1995). The cervical N13 potential is recorded at the posterior neck, with a maximum voltage at the level of C5-C7 spinous processes and decreases in amplitude at more rostral or caudal electrode positions. N13 does not show any latency shift between C6 and C2 recordings in normal subjects (Desmedt and Cheron, 1980a; Desmedt and Nguyen, 1984; Mauguière, 1983). When recorded anterior to the cord by an electrode placed at the anterior aspect of the neck (Desmedt and Cheron, 1980a; Mauguière and Ibañez, 1985), the cervical DH response is recorded as a spinal P13 positivity. This polarity reversal has been demonstrated with esophageal (Desmedt and Cheron, 1981a) and epidural (Cioni and Meglio, 1986) recordings and also by direct recordings from the surface of the cervical cord (Jeanmonod et al., 1989, 1991). Both N13 and P13 spinal components are reduced in amplitude to the same degree when the stimulation rate is increased over 10/sec (Ibañez et al., 1989), both persist in brain death or in cervicomedullary lesions (Buchner et al., 1986; Mauguière and Ibañez, 1985; Mauguière et al., 1983c), and both are selectively reduced or abolished in lesions of the cervical cord gray matter sparing the spinal somatosensory tracts (Restuccia and Mauguière, 1991). Thus the most likely generator of the N13/P13 cervical potentials is the compound segmental postsynaptic potential triggered in the DH gray matter by the afferent volley in fast conducting myelinated fibers. Direct recordings on the cord surface have shown that the characteristics of N13 in humans are very similar to those of the N1 spinal potential described in animal studies, which reflects the postsynaptic neuronal response of DH laminae IV and V neurons to inputs conveyed by group I and II peripheral afferent fibers (Austin and McCouch, 1955; Beall et al., 1977; Gasser and Graham, 1933).

In noncephalic reference recordings the N13 often has a small voltage. A cervical transverse derivation between two electrodes located respectively over the C6 spinal process and above the laryngeal cartilage is the most adapted for recording the spinal N13/P13 segmental response (Fig. 54.3). Substraction of the anterior cervical positivity from the posterior neck negativity increases the signal-to-noise ratio and has the advantage over the more conventional C6-Fz montage of recording a segmental DH response that is not contaminated by SEP components generated above the foramen magnum (see below).

Apart from its field distribution, a second characteristic of the segmental N13 potential is that it shows amplitude reduction, rather than latency prolongation, when the dorsal afferent volley is time dispersed, or when the number of responding DH neurons is reduced. For diagnostic purposes the limitation of N13 amplitude measurements is that distribution of this parameter in a group of normal subjects does not show a gaussian profile. Therefore, the lower limit of normal N13 amplitude values estimated by the mean minus 2 to 3 standard deviations (SDs) is statistically meaningless. The best way to evaluate the N13 amplitude is to calculate the ratio between the N13 amplitude and that of the dorsal root N9/P9 deflection that immediately precedes N13 in transverse cervical montage recordings (Restuccia and Mauguière, 1991). The distribution of the log10 (N13/N9) amplitude ratio has a gaussian profile in normals. The normal lower limit of the normal N13/N9 ratio, defined as the mean

value minus 2.5 SD, is of about 1.2. The N9/P9 deflection shows good test-retest reliability and its amplitude closely reflects the incoming volley in the cervical roots, which is likely to be unaffected in spinal cord diseases. Moreover, the N13/P9 amplitude ratio remains stable when tested at stimulus intensities between motor threshold and twice the motor threshold (Restuccia and Mauguière, 1991). Runs of 1,000 stimuli delivered at 2 per second are appropriate in most cases to obtain well-defined cervical potentials using either a noncephalic or anterior cervical reference site.

Upper Cervical N13 Potential

It has been known for many years that a negative potential peaking at a latency of about 13 msec can be recorded intraoperatively at the dorsal aspect of the cervicomedullary junction (Allison and Hume, 1981; Andersen et al., 1964; Lesser et al., 1981; Moller et al., 1986; Morioka et al., 1991). On the skin surface, however, it is not easy after median nerve stimulation to separate this potential at upper cervical level from the segmental cervical N13, so that the former can be interpreted as a rostral spread of the latter. In particular, there is no evidence of a latency increase of the median nerve N13 negativity from the Cv6 to Cv2 level in noncephalic reference recordings, although in bipolar recordings along the neck the mean N13 peak latency was found to be longer at rostral than at caudal levels (Kaji and Sumner, 1987). An elegant insight to this latency problem was provided by Zanette et al. (1995), who showed that the N13 recorded at upper cervical level peaks 0.8 msec later than the lower cervical N13 after ulnar nerve stimulation, but not after median nerve stimulation, in noncephalic reference recordings. The greater distance from the dorsal root entry zone to the cuneate nucleus for ulnar nerve than for median nerve afferent fibers was proposed to explain this latency shift. Araki et al. (1997) have addressed the question of separate generators for the lower and upper cervical N13 potentials by using a conditioning-test paired stimulus paradigm for stimulation of the median nerve. They confirmed that at interstimulus intervals (ISIs) of 4 to 18 msec the test of the lower cervical segmental N13 to the second stimulus was attenuated by 2% to 34% when compared to the control response, as previously reported by Iragui (1984) and by El-Kharoussi et al. (1996) after stimulation of median nerve and the second and third fingers, respectively. More unexpected was the finding that, while the scalp P13-P14 showed the same attenuation as the lower cervical N13, the N13 recorded at the CV2 level showed an increase of 4% to 25% at these ISI. The upper cervical N13 is supposed to be generated by the presynaptic volley in the dorsal column (DC) fibers close to the cuneate nucleus, but the difficulty of separating it from the DH N13 lessens its clinical reliability in routine clinical recordings (see Mauguière, 2000, for a review).

Conducted Cervical N11 Component

The nuchal N11 potential is recorded all along the posterior aspect of the neck, where it usually appears to encroach upon the ascending slope of N13. In noncephalic reference recordings its onset latency increases from C6 to C1 spinal processes by 0.9 ± 0.15 msec (Desmedt and Cheron, 1980a; Mauguière, 1983). This bottom-up shift of N11 onset la-

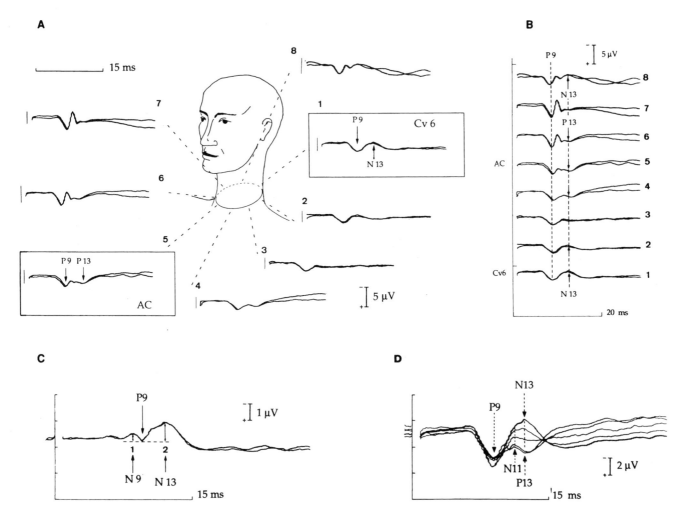

Figure 54.3. Neck recording of the N13/P13 segmental potential. Normal distribution of the N13/P13 recorded using an array of cervical electrodes and a reference at the shoulder contralateral to the stimulated right median nerve **(A)**. The triphasic root activity is picked up at lateral neck electrodes on the stimulated side (6,7) and its initial positivity is synchronous with that of the P9 potentials picked at all other recording sites **(B)**. The N11 potential is not clearly visible in this subject as compared with that illustrated in Fig. 54.1; it appears as a notch on the initial phase of the segmental N13/P13 potential and does not reverse its polarity at anterior neck recording sites **(D)**. The trace obtained using a derivation between the posterior neck electrode at C6 level (1) and the anterior cervical electrode (AC, electrode 5) shows the segmental cord response with a maximal amplitude, which can be quantified by measuring the peak-to-peak P9.N13 /N9.P9 ratio. Note that the surface distribution of the N13/P13 spinal response is very similar to that observed in direct recording on the cord surface illustrated in Fig. 54.2. (From Restuccia D., and Mauguière F. 1991. The contribution of median nerve SEPs in the functional assessment of the cervical spinal cord in syringomyelia. A study of 24 patients. Brain 114:361–379, with permission.)

tency suggests that N11 is generated by the ascending volley of action potentials in the dorsal columns of the cervical spinal cord. As first reported by Cracco (1973), it is often difficult to differentiate the N11 from the following N13 component. This seriously hampers the use of N11 in clinical practice, which is limited to cervical cord lesions that selectively obliterate the N13 potential. In direct recordings on the cervical cord surface during surgery, N11 appears as a fast polyphasic component that overlaps in time with the slower N13 segmental postsynaptic potential.

Far-Field Positive Scalp Positivities (P9, P11, P13, P14)

On scalp noncephalic reference recordings with a high-frequency filter over 1,000 Hz and a fast sampling rate (bin width < 200 μsec) three or four stationary positivities are consistently observed with a wide distribution and a medio-frontal predominance. In normal adults these potentials peak with mean latencies of 9, 11, 13, and 14 msec and are labeled P9, P11, P13, and P14, respectively, according to the polarity-latency nomenclature. There is some interindividual variation in the waveform of the two latest P13 and P14 potentials since either the P13 or P14 peaks can predominate. The amplitude of these far-field positive potentials are not affected when the stimulation rate is increased up to 50 Hz (Ibañez et al., 1989).

The P9 potential is picked up at the neck as well as on the scalp. It reflects the afferent volley in the trunks of the brachial plexus in axilla and supraclavicular fossa (Cracco and Cracco, 1976; Nakanishi et al., 1981). Its peaking latency varies with arm length and its onset latency, but not its peaking latency, is influenced by the respective positions of arm and trunk (Desmedt et al., 1983a).

The P11 potential reflects the ascending volley in the fibers of dorsal columns at the cervical level. Desmedt and Cheron (1980a) first reported that, after median nerve stimulation at the wrist, the P11 potential begins in synchrony with the cervical N11 potential at the C6 level, which is close to the dorsal root entry zone in the cervical cord. The P11 potential is not recorded in about 20% of normal controls and, thus the clinical significance of its absence in patients is questionable. Conversely, its persistence when later scalp components are abnormal is a reliable indicator of preserved dorsal column function in patients with lesions located in the medulla oblongata or at the cervicomedullary junction.

The P13-P14 far-field potentials are consistently recorded in normal subjects (see Restuccia, 2000, for a review). Both may be of similar amplitude, or either of them may be the larger of the two (Fig. 54.1). In some subjects P14 is hardly visible as a notch on the ascending phase of P13; in others P13 and P14 cannot be differentiated. In the same individual the morphology of the P13-P14 complex can display some degree of side-to-side difference, which creates difficulties for interpreting left-right asymmetries in patients. P14, but not P13, always peaks later than the cervical segmental N13 potential (Mauguière, 1987). Since the P13-P14 complex is picked up at the earlobe with a lesser amplitude than in the frontal region of the scalp, it can be recorded with a scalp-earlobe montage (Nakanishi et al., 1978). The P13-P14 complex is the only scalp far-field SEP that is reduced by interfering stimulations, such as vibrations, applied to the hand on the stimulated side (Ibañez et al., 1989). This suggests that it is generated after the synaptic relay in the nucleus cuneatus. Patients with thalamic lesions usually show a normal P14, suggesting that this component originates at subthalamic level (Anziska and Cracco, 1980; Mauguière et al., 1982; Nakanishi et al., 1978). Conversely, in cervicomedullary lesions (Mauguière and Ibañez, 1985; Mauguière et al., 1983c) or in brain-dead patients (Buchner et al., 1986) the P14 potential is absent. These findings suggest that the generator of P14 is situated above the level of the foramen magnum.

Simultaneous scalp and nasopharyngeal SEP recording in deeply comatose and brain dead patients brought some information concerning the origins of the P14 potential (Wagner, 1991). In patients with signs of upper brainstem dysfunction this author observed that the P14 recorded between scalp and nasopharynx is lost while an earlier P13 positivity persists in scalp to shoulder traces. This observation suggests that the P14 recorded between the scalp and the nasopharynx reflects the activity of medial lemniscus pathways at the upper part of the brainstem, whereas the P13 might be generated at the cervicomedullary junction. A normal P13 coexisting with an abnormal P14 has been observed in patients with pontine or mesencephalic lesions (Delestre et al., 1986; Kaji and Sumner, 1987; Mavroudakis et al., 1993; Nakanishi et al., 1983), supporting the hypothesis that P13 and P14 potentials could be generated at different anatomical levels in the cervicomedullary and brainstem somatosensory pathways. This view is reinforced by the

observation, in noncephalic reference recordings, that the P13 positivity recorded at the nasopharynx can be preserved while the scalp P14 is abnormal in lesions of the lower brainstem (Restuccia et al., 1995).

The scalp and nasopharynx P13 potential is different from the segmental P13 positivity recorded at the anterior aspect of the neck. In spite of their similar latencies and polarities, these two components have different distributions and origins and the segmental spinal P13 is preserved in all patients with upper cervical or cervicomedullary lesions.

Thus, according to our present knowledge the most probable mechanism generating the P13-P14 potentials are (1) the ascending volley in upper cervical DC fibers at the cervicomedullary junction or in medial lemniscus fibers in the brainstem; (2) the postsynaptic response of nucleus cuneatus neurons; and (3) junctional stationary potentials related with the moving action potential volley across the border between neck and posterior fossa (Kimura et al., 1983, 1984).

For the sake of clarity, the P13-P14 complex is often labeled as P14, a convention that is adopted here. It can be useful to calculate the P9/P14 amplitude ratio in patients. As with the I/V amplitude ratio of brainstem auditory evoked potential (BAEPs) one compares, by measuring the P9/P14 ratio, the amplitude of a peripheral potential (P9) with that of a brainstem potential (P14). In normals the P9 potential is smaller than the P14 potential when recorded with a broad band-pass of 1.6 to 3,200 Hz, and the distribution of the P9/P14 ratio has a gaussian profile (García-Larrea and Mauguière, 1988).

The N18 Scalp Negativity

This potential identified by Desmedt and Cheron (1981b) is a long-lasting scalp negative shift, which immediately follows P14. In normals N18 can only be identified in the posterior parietal region ipsilateral to the stimulation, where there is no or minimal interference with cortical potentials. The N18 is a long-lasting component (about 20 msec when recorded with a 1- to 3,000-Hz band pass), and when low frequencies are cut off by filtering it can be falsely interpreted as an ipsilateral cortical N20. It is still uncertain whether the N18 negativity contains several subcomponents; several wavelets are superimposed on its plateau at fixed latencies on repeated recordings in the same individual, which favor this interpretation. When all cortical responses are eliminated by deafferentation due to a lesion of the ventroposterolateral (VPL) thalamic nucleus (Mauguière et al., 1983b) or by direct lesion of the centroparietal cortex (Mauguière, 1987), N18 can be recorded on the whole surface of the scalp (Fig. 54.4). After hemispherectomy, which entails retrograde degeneration of the thalamocortical neurons, the N18 potential is most often preserved (Mauguière and Desmedt, 1989); however, N18 can be missing, as well as the P14 potential, long after hemispherectomy including the thalamus (Restuccia et al., 1996) in relation with retrograde degeneration of the cuneate-thalamic projections. These observations rule out the possibility that N18 could reflect a cortical or a thalamic response to lemniscal or extralemniscal inputs.

The earliest hypothesis, concerning the generation of N18, was that of a postsynaptic response of the brainstem

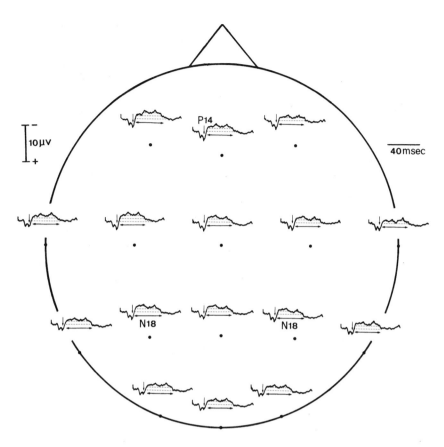

Figure 54.4. Scalp topography of the P14 and N18 potentials. In this patient with a large left centroparietal lobe lesion eliminating all cortical SEPs the N18 is recorded on the whole surface of the scalp, preceded by the P9 and P14 potentials (noncephalic reference recording). Note that the amplitude of the P14 potential is maximal in the frontal region, whereas that of the P9 potential is similar at all recording sites. (From Mauguière F. 1995. Evoked potentials. In *Clinical Neurophysiology: EMG, Nerve Conduction and Evoked Potentials,* Eds. J.W. Osselton, C.D. Binnie, R. Cooper, et al., pp. 325–563. Oxford: Butterworth-Heinemann, with permission.)

nuclei connected with the DC nuclei to ascending inputs conveyed by ancillary fibers of the medial lemniscus. This hypothesis has been supported by intracerebral SEP recordings in humans showing a stationary negativity between the upper pons and the midbrain, peaking at the same latency as the scalp N18 (Urasaki et al., 1990). However, nasopharyngeal recordings (Tomberg et al., 1991a) rather suggested an N18 origin in the medulla oblongata and, more precisely in the nucleus cuneatus (NC). Potentials recorded dorsal and ventral to NC in humans (Morioka et al., 1991) show a biphasic waveform that is very similar to that of NC responses to peripheral nerve stimulation in cats. The first phase of this response in cats represents the postsynaptic potential of NC relay neurons to the DC afferent volley, while the second one reflects the presynaptic inhibition of DC fibers terminals in NC (Andersen et al., 1964). This inhibition consists in a feedback depolarization of DC terminals, triggered by the afferent volley in DC fibers collaterals, and mediated by NC interneurons. To date it is accepted that N18 reflects a similar phenomenon in the human brainstem (see Sonoo, 2000, for a review). Several arguments lend substance to this analogy: (a) The distribution and polarity are similar in cat and human recordings. (b) The presynaptic inhibition of DC terminals in cats, like the human N18, lasts for several tens of milliseconds, probably because it is mediated via a polysynaptic chain of interneurons. (3) The N18 voltage is unaffected by interfering vibrations applied on the hand on the stimulated side (Manzano et al., 1998), contrary to the P14 potential, which is attenuated (Ibañez et al.,

1989); this finding fits with the inference that N18 reflects inhibitory activity upon DC terminals.

In normal subjects noncephalic reference recordings of scalp SEPs show two positivities of cortical origin that are superimposed upon N18 in the central and frontal regions contralateral to stimulation, namely central P22 and frontal P20 (see below). Thus the early portion of N18 appears as a negativity preceding the onsets of P20 and P22 in the midfrontal and central regions, respectively. These frontal and central negativities have been considered as genuine cortical responses and labeled as N15, N16, N17, or N19 components (Iwayama et al., 1988; Yamada et al., 1984). However, superimposition of traces recorded in the posterior parietal region ipsilateral to stimulation, where N18 is not contaminated by contralateral cortical components, clearly shows that there is no actual scalp negativity other than N18 and N20 within the first 22 msec following stimulation. The N18 plateau recorded in the parietal region ipsilateral to stimulus can serve as a baseline to assess the voltage and the shape of cortical components peaking in the 20- to 40-msec latency range. Since most of the N18 is picked at earlobe, the use of the earlobe ipsilateral to stimulation bypasses this baseline problem by eliminating the N18 negative shift in the resulting waveforms.

Early Cortical SEPs

These cortical SEPs are peaking in the 18- to 35-msec latency range and are all obtained with optimal voltage in response to stimuli delivered at a slow rate (less than 2/sec).

They are recorded on the scalp in the parietal region contralateral to stimulation and in a large frontocentral area, mostly contralateral to stimulation. They are superimposed on the widespread N18 in noncephalic reference recordings. Although the scalp distribution of these potentials shows substantial variations between subjects, their profiles and voltages are relatively symmetrical in a given individual, so that side-to-side differences in a group of normal subjects can be used as norms for assessing interhemispheric asymmetries in patients. For latency measurements, calculating the intervals from the peak of the far-field P14 to the peak of each of the cortical components permits eliminating interindividual variability related to arm length and body height differences.

Though studies in normals and patients converge on the conclusion that responses recorded in the parietal region originate in the somatosensory area SI, there is still some controversy as to whether some of the early cortical SEPs recorded in the frontal region might be generated in the prerolandic cortex. Several clinical studies reported that frontal and parietal SEP waveforms can be selectively affected in patients with focal hemispheric lesions (Mauguière and Desmedt, 1991; Mauguière et al., 1983a; Slimp et al., 1986; Tsuji et al., 1988) and suggested prerolandic generators for some of the SEPs recorded in the frontal region. These observations, based on clinical examination, abnormal SEP waveforms analysis, and computed tomography (CT) imaging of lesions were at the origin of the hypothetical sensorimotor model of early SEPs sources. This model had the advantage of fitting with the concept of a short latency control of motor cortex by peripheral somatosensory inputs via transcortical long-loop reflexes. Conversely, direct cortical recordings in humans (see Allison et al., 1991, for a review) supported the view that all sources of early cortical SEPs are located in the parietal cortex, and more precisely in the primary somatosensory area (SI). This controversy, the terms of which are discussed in more detail later in this chapter, should not discourage clinicians from using cortical SEPs as indexes of brain dysfunction in the assessment of patients with sensory or motor disorders for two main reasons. First, correlations between a clinical deficit and a SEP abnormality are clinically pertinent facts, even if they can lead to pathogenetic hypothesis, which are not validated by other approaches. Second, in lesion studies, the extent of the lesion, as well as its functional effects, which were difficult to assess by correlating SEP waveforms with CT images of the early 1980s, are now more accessible by fusing anatomical and functional data from MRI, emission tomography, and source modeling of SEPs.

N20-P20 and P22 Potentials

Two sets of early cortical potentials are consistently recorded in normal subjects on the scalp contralateral to stimulation. The first is made of a parietal N20 and frontal P20 dipolar field; the second is composed of a central P22 positivity (Fig. 54.5). These components are also present after finger stimulation with a latency delay of 2 to 3 msec, as compared with median nerve SEPs, because of finger-to-wrist conduction time.

The parietal N20 and frontal P20 reflect the activity of a dipolar generator in Brodmann's area 3b situated in the posterior bank of the rolandic fissure (Allison et al., 1980; Broughton, 1969; Goff et al., 1977) and represents the earliest cortical potential elicited by median nerve stimulation. This dipolar field distribution is also observed in magnetic recordings. All source modeling studies of electrical and magnetic fields, as well as direct cortical recordings, converge on the conclusion that the N20-P20 field is produced by a dipolar source tangent to the scalp surface reflecting the response of area 3b neurons to cutaneous inputs. This was confirmed by the finding that the N20-P20 response is not evoked by joint inputs produced by passive finger movements (Desmedt and Osaki, 1991). Therefore, the polarity reversal line of the N20-P20 dipolar field recorded on the scalp or directly on the cortex and the equivalent dipolar source modeled from electric or magnetic recordings are now widely used to localize the central fissure in the assessment of patients with a lesion or an epileptogenic area located in the rolandic region.

On scalp (Fig. 54.6) and some direct cortical recordings a P22 recorded in the central region was found to peak 1 to 2 msec later than the N20-P20 potentials (Desmedt and Cheron, 1980b, 1981b; Papakostopoulos and Crow, 1980). This has been taken as an argument to consider P22 as a genuine component generated by a source distinct from that of N20-P20 (Desmedt and Cheron, 1981b), while others denied the existence an independent P22 (Allison, 1982).

Sequential spatial maps of scalp recorded SEPs have shown that the N20-P20 dipolar field is followed in the central region contralateral to stimulation by a positive P22 field peaking 1.0 to 2.5 msec with little or no negative counterpart on the scalp (Deiber et al., 1986). This spatial distribution of this P22 central positivity suggests that its source is radial to the scalp surface. Most studies of SEFs failed to confirm such a source in the central region probably because magnetic recordings are blind to magnetic fields produced by dipolar sources radial to scalp surface (Brenner et al., 1978; Okada et al., 1984; Wood et al., 1985).

The question of whether the radial source of the central P22 is located behind the central sulcus, in the primary somatosensory area, or in front of it, in the primary motor area, is not easy to address by scalp recordings in normals, even when assisted by dipole modeling techniques based on a spherical head-model (Buchner et al., 1995; Franssen et al., 1992). One argument in favor of a precentral origin of the P22 potential is that it may be selectively lost in patients with hemispheric lesions who have normal sensations but signs of upper motor neuron dysfunction, and selectively preserved in patients with hemianesthesia or astereognosis and no motor deficit (Mauguière and Desmedt, 1991; Mauguière et al., 1983a; Slimp et al., 1986; Tsuji et al., 1988). Some direct cortical recordings in monkeys and humans, however, failed to identify a P22 in the precentral cortex (Allison et al., 1989b; McCarthy et al., 1991) but individualized a surface positive potential, labeled as P25, with a source radial to the scalp surface and located at the posterior edge of the rolandic fissure in Brodmann's area 1. In a SEP and positron emission tomography (PET) study Ibañez et al. (1995) reported that at stimulus rates between 4 and 16/sec SI was the only area showing a cerebral blood flow (CBF) increase, while at stimulus rates of 0.2 and 1 Hz no CBF change was induced by electrical stimulation of the median nerve. Lastly, a dipole

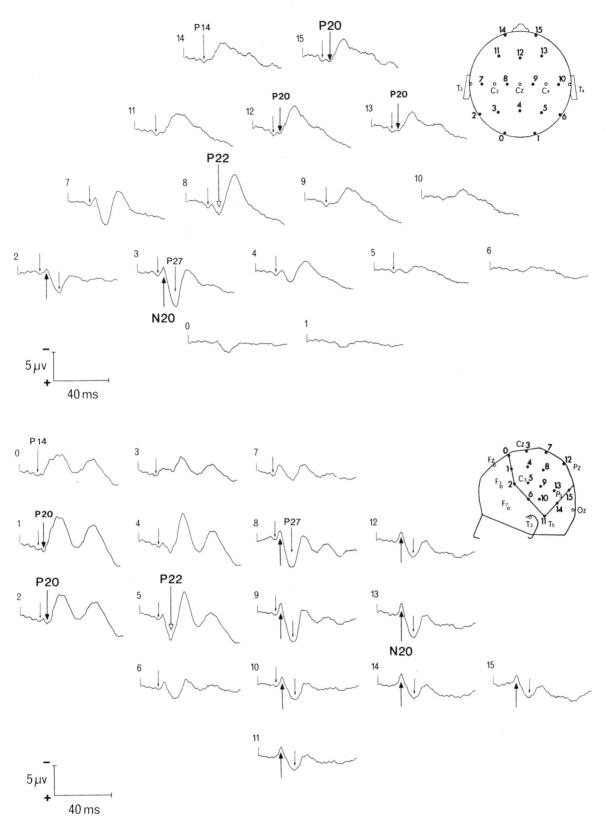

Figure 54.5. Scalp topography of the N20-P20 and P22 potentials (earlobe reference). Responses to stimulation of the third finger of the right hand are illustrated. In the *upper part* of the figure the electrode montage covers the whole scalp surface; in the *lower part* the electrode array is restricted to the left centroparietal area. The P22 positivity peaks in a restricted area at the C3 electrode site (electrodes 8 and 5 in *upper* and *lower parts* of the figure, respectively). The N20-P20 dipolar field has a wider distribution covering the parietal region contralateral to stimulation (N20) and the contralateral central and frontal regions (P20), with a polarity reversal at the level of the scalp projection of the rolandic fissure. (From Deiber M.P., Giard M.H., and Mauguière F. 1986. Separate generators with distinct orientations for N20 and P22 somatosensory evoked potentials to finger stimulation. Electroencephalogr. Clin. Neurophysiol. 65:321–334, with permission.)

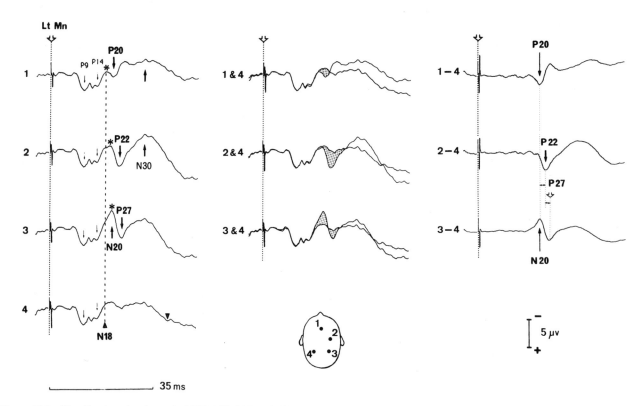

Figure 54.6. Identification of early cortical N20, P22, P27, and N30 potentials (left median nerve stimulation; noncephalic reference recording). Since the subcortical far-field positivities and N18 potentials are recorded uncontaminated by cortical potentials in the parietal region ipsilateral to stimulation *(trace 4, left column)*, responses obtained in this region can be used as a baseline to assess cortical responses, either by superimposition to *(middle column)*, or substraction from *(right column)*, the contralateral responses. This shows that neither the P20 and P22 potentials nor the P27 and N30 potentials peak at the same latencies. Moreover, the negativities *(asterisks)* recorded in the contralateral central (2) and midfrontal region disappears in difference waveforms. They correspond to interruption of the widespread N18 (Fig. 54.4) by the cortical positive responses P27, P22, and P20. Due to the restricted filter band-pass used for this recording, the P14 amplitude is less than that of the P9 potential. (From Mauguière et al. 1997, with permission.)

modeling study of SEPs using realistic head models and constraining the solution in the individual brain MRI volume supported the data from direct cerebral recordings by showing that the P22 source is located at the crown of the postcentral gyrus (Buchner et al., 1996). These data from cortical recordings and modeling of scalp responses are challenged by some experimental data in monkeys: (1) short-latency unit responses to somatosensory inputs can be recorded in the motor cortex (Lemon, 1981; Tanji and Wise, 1981), and (2) early median nerve SEPs are recorded in the motor cortex (Nicholson-Peterson et al., 1995). According to the data of Nicholson-Peterson et al. (1995), the earliest cortical responses to upper limb stimulation are likely to result from the approximately coincident activation of at least three dipolar sources in areas 3b, 4, and 1 with orientations both opposing and orthogonal to each other. Sources in area 3b and 4 have opposite orientations tangent to the scalp surface, while the source located in area 1, at the crown of the postcentral gyrus, is oriented radial to the scalp surface. Thus, even if it would be hazardous to imagine a strict homology between SEP components in monkey and humans, due to the considerable anatomical differences between the two species, these experimental data support the contribution of the motor cortex to the N20-P20 and P22 scalp potentials.

Parietal P24 and P27 Potentials

These potentials are recorded in the parietal region contralateral to stimulation; their peaking latencies show large interindividual variations between 24 and 27 msec. In some subjects two distinct P24 and P27 can be identified while only one of the two peaks is observed in others. This explains why, according to the polarity-latency nomenclature, the first parietal positive potential following N20 has received various labels in literature (P24, P25, or P27). These variations reflect the fact that the activities of several parietal sources overlap in time in this latency range. The P27 potential was found to be abnormal in patients with focal lesions of the parietal cortex, presenting with astereognosis and normal N30 frontal responses (Mauguière et al., 1982, 1983a). A P27 source in the primary somatosensory area (Brodmann's area 1), radial to scalp surface, would accord with these findings. The P24 potential on its own is associated with a frontal N24 potential. The dipolar source of the P24-N24 field is tangent to scalp surface, and thus presumed to be oriented perpendicular to the rolandic fissure. There is no report of a lesion affecting the P24 potential with preserved N20 and P27 potentials.

Frontal N30 Potential (N24-N30 Complex)

The frontal potential, labeled as N30 in most clinical studies, has warranted much attention in the recent SEP literature because it shows some abnormality in patients with various types of motor disorders. It is picked up in the frontal region contralateral to stimulation; however, it often spreads to the midfrontal region and to the frontal region ipsilateral to stimulus. Its waveform show two distinct components of which the earlier one, peaking at about 24 msec (N24), appears as notch on the ascending slope of the later one, which peaks at 30 msec (N30) and has the larger voltage of the two in normal young adults (Fig. 54.7).

There is now some consensus on the conclusions that the frontal negativity with its two N24 and N30 peaks cannot be generated by a single source (Delberghe et al., 1990; Garcia-Larrea et al., 1992; Ozaki et al., 1996a), and that the early part (N24) of the frontal negativity corresponds to the polarity reversal of the parietal P24 potential across the central sulcus. The latter statement is supported by several observations issued from intracranial and scalp recordings:

1. In the latency range of the scalp N30 Allison et al. (1989a), using intracranial recordings during surgery, have identified a dipolar field, frontal negative and parietal positive, and considered it as generated by a source in area 3b, tangent to the scalp surface. Probably because of anesthesia this field reached its maximum at 30 msec and was labeled N30-P30 by these authors.
2. On the scalp the field distribution is clearly dipolar at the peaking latency of the N24 with a parietal positivity and

a midfrontal negativity spreading to the frontocentral region. This dipolar potential field has been labeled N24-P24 (Garcia-Larrea et al., 1992) or N27-P27 (Ozaki et al., 1996a), it corresponds to the N30-P30 of Allison et al. (1989a), and its distribution fits well with a dipolar source perpendicular to the rolandic fissure and tangent to the scalp.
3. The two negative frontal N24 and N30 components react differently to changes in stimulus rate (Delberghe et al., 1990; Garcia-Larrea et al., 1992; Valeriani et al., 1998a). The early N24 remains unaffected if the stimulus frequency is increased up to 10 Hz, while the later N30 decreases at stimulus rates higher than 1 per second and is virtually absent at 10 per second.
4. Source modeling studies of scalp responses converge to the conclusion that the distribution of the scalp N24-P24 can be explained by a single source in the posterior bank of the central sulcus (Buchner et al., 1995; Valeriani et al., 1998b).
5. The administration of tiagabine, which enhances γ-aminobutyric acid (GABA) inhibition, increases selectively the voltage of the N24-P24 dipolar field, suggesting that it could reflect the repolarization of the neuronal population that produces the N20-P20 field in area 3b (Restuccia et al., 2002b).

Conversely the origin of the main N30 negativity of the frontal N24-N30 is still a debated issue. There has been a long controversy as to whether frontal N30 and parietal P27 components could have separate sources. Three early obser-

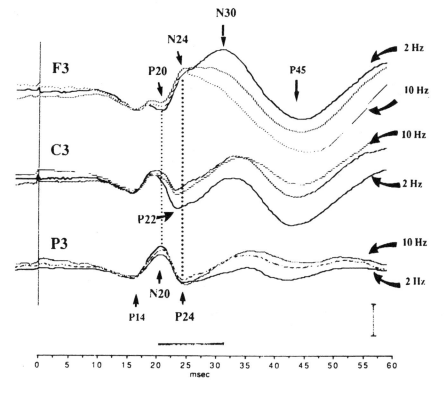

Figure 54.7. Identification of the P24-N24 dipolar field and frontal N30 responses. Responses to right median nerve stimulation have been recorded in the left parietal (P3), central (C3), and frontal (F3) regions at stimulus rates of 2 *(thick traces)*, 5, and 10 Hz. The dipolar P24-N24 response is unaffected, while the frontal N30 is dramatically depressed, by increasing the stimulus rates. Calibration: 2 μV. (From Garcia-Larrea L., Bastuji H., and Mauguière F. 1992. Unmasking of cortical SEP components by changes in stimulus rate a topographic study. Electroencephalogr. Clin. Neurophysiol. 84:71–83 with permission.)

vations have supported the hypothesis that, contrary to the N24/P24 dipolar field, N30 does not represent the frontal counterpart of the parietal P27:

1. N30 amplitude decreases with aging while that of P27 increases (Desmedt and Cheron, 1980b).
2. N30 can be selectively absent, or decreased, with preserved parietal P27, in patients with focal lesions of the frontal lobe (Mauguière et al., 1983a) or of the thalamus or internal capsule (Mauguière and Ibañez, 1990; Mauguière and Desmedt, 1991), presenting with motor symptoms and normal sensation.
3. N30 was found to be selectively reduced in Parkinson's disease with a decrease of the N30/P27 amplitude ratio (see below).

Based on these findings it has been proposed that the N30 and P27 potentials originate in the precentral cortex and in the SI area (Brodmann's area 1), respectively; each of these two dipolar sources being oriented perpendicular to the scalp surface. However, the existence of any N30 potential generated in the precentral cortex has been questioned by Allison et al. (1989a) and McCarthy et al. (1991) on the basis of direct cortical recordings in monkeys and humans. The most convincing evidence that the N30 potential may have a frontal origin stems from several observations (see Cheron et al., 2000, for a review) suggesting that the N30 potential could be related with motor programming and generated in the premotor cortex of area 6, and more precisely in the supplementary motor area (SMA):

1. N30 was reported to be absent in a patient with a falx meningioma compressing the inner aspect of the precentral frontal cortex (Rossini et al., 1989).
2. Voluntary movements of the fingers on the stimulated side was shown to exert a gating effect on frontal SEPs by reducing selectively the amplitude of N30, without effect on parietal potentials (Cheron and Borenstein, 1987; Cohen and Starr, 1985; Rossi et al., 2002; Rossini et al., 1989). This effect, which had been observed and to a certain extent overviewed by Papakostopoulos et al. in 1975, is less for simple than for complex fingers movements. Two mechanisms have been proposed to explain this selective gating of frontal SEPs by active movement. First, cortical motor neurons involved in fingers movements could also account for part of the frontal SEPs and would be unable to respond simultaneously to the afferent volley triggered by the electric stimulation. The second mechanism is that of a corticocortical inhibition by which the motor neurons active during movements would suppress the response of cortical neurons involved in the generation of the N30 potential.
3. A gating of N30, but also of N24, occurs during movement preparation in reaction time paradigms where SEPs are recorded before movement onset (Shimazu et al., 1999).
4. The gating of N30 does not require that the intended movement be executed and also occurs when the subject mentally simulates a complex sequence of finger movements on the stimulated side (Fig. 54.8) (Cheron and Borenstein, 1992; Rossini et al., 1996). When the same mental movement simulation (MMS) concerns the non-

stimulated hand, or when the subject performs a mental task other than motor simulation, this gating effect does not occur. It has long been known that this MMS task increases the cerebral blood flow in the SMA (Roland et al., 1980); this observation has been considered as indirect evidence that the SMA might be the generator of the N30 potential.
5. The N30 potential, as well as the homologue M30 magnetic field, is enhanced when subject observes repetitive grasping movements or complex sequences of fingers movements performed by an examiner during stimulation. This effect is independent of the complexity of the observed movements; it has been interpreted as reflecting storage of subject's somatosensory information connected with the observed movements (Rossi et al., 2002),

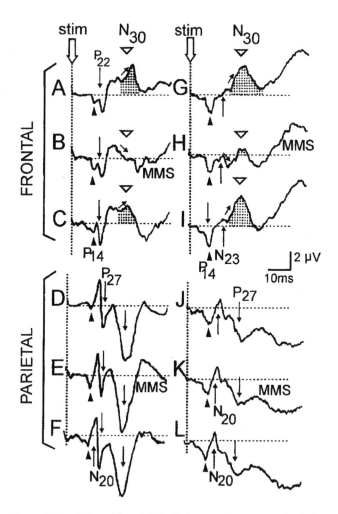

Figure 54.8. Gating of frontal SEPs during mental movement simulation (MMS). These responses were obtained in two distinct normal subjects *(right and left traces)* before **(A,D,G,J)**, during **(B,E,H,K)**, and after **(C,F,I,L)** mental simulation of movement. The *dotted areas* indicate the N30 potential surface above the baseline. Note that the N24 frontal potential, labeled N23 by the authors, and the parietal responses are not affected by mental imagery of movement. (From Cheron, G., and Borenstein, S. 1992. Mental movement stimulation affects the N30 frontal component of the somatosensory evoked potential. Electroencephalogr. Clin. Neurophysiol. 84:288–292, with permission.)

and related to the SMA activation observed in PET studies when subjects observe meaningful actions (Grezes et al., 1998).

However, if there little doubt that the N30 amplitude is linked to motor programming, its origin in the SMA is challenged by data from direct cortical recordings, which favor a N30 dipolar source radial to the scalp surface, located in Brodmann's area 1 of the SI cortex (Allison et al., 1989a, 1991), and do not show a N30 potential in this area (Barba et al., 2001). Moreover, after subtraction of the N24-P24 field, the maximum of the remaining scalp N30 field has the same location as that of the P22 potential in the central region (Ozaki et al., 1996a). This suggests that the N30 potential is generated close to the central sulcus and not in the premotor cortex, a view supported by most of the source modeling studies of early SEPs (Valeriani et al., 2000). Lastly, functional MRI studies have shown that all of cortical areas involved in actual movements, and not only the SMA, are activated during mental simulation of movements (Stephan et al., 1995).

If the origin of N30 in the SMA has not been verified, the possibility that it might be generated in the primary motor area has not been ruled out by direct recordings, or source modeling, of SEPs or SEFs. Conversely, source modeling studies supported this hypothesis (Waberski et al., 1999). The movement-related gating of N30, therefore, could reflect a similar change in motor cortex excitability both during movement and mental motor imagery. Studies using transcranial magnetic stimulation (TMS) converge to the conclusion that the excitability of the motor cortex is increased during actual movement and mental movement simulation (Kasai et al., 1997; Ridding et al., 1995), so that N30 amplitude would reflect the level of motor cortex inhibition. However, the fact that N30 and motor cortex inhibition are decreased during movement and motor imagery does not imply that the underlying mechanisms are the same in the two conditions. A TMS study by Ridding and Rothwell (1999) suggests that, in spite of a similar effect of movement and motor imagery on N30 amplitude, activity in the circuits responsible for GABAergic inhibition of the motor cortex is reduced during voluntary contraction while motor imagery, which activates similar brain regions as overt movement but does not result in afferent input, does not produce significant changes in intracortical inhibition.

Ipsilateral Short Latency Cortical Potentials Evoked by Upper Limb Stimulation in Direct Cortical Recordings

No early cortical potential is observed on the scalp ipsilateral to electrical stimulation of the median nerve in normal subjects as well as in the majority of direct cortical presurgical recordings in epileptic patients (Allison et al., 1989a; Lüders et al., 1986). However, four epileptic patients, of a series of 41 recorded at the Cleveland Clinic Foundation with subdural electrodes placed over the central area showed a clearly identifiable early ipsilateral median nerve potential, the characteristics of which have been reviewed by Noachtar et al. (1997). This response has an amplitude four to 16 times smaller than that of the contralateral

SEP; it begins with a positivity restricted to one or two electrodes of the grid, which peaks 1.2 to 17.8 msec later than the earliest positivity following the N20 potential in the contralateral response. The maxima of ipsi- and contralateral positivities were distributed between 1 and 2 cm apart in the central region and, according to responses to electric stimulation of the cortex, the ipsilateral response was maximal anterior to the rolandic fissure in two of the four patients. The low incidence of ipsilateral responses suggests that they are generated by a small population of cortical neurons and can be missed by subdural recordings when their source is buried in a sulcus. Another possibility is that ipsilateral responses reflect plastic reorganization of the cortex occurring only in a minority of patients with an epileptogenic area in the central region. The functional significance of these ipsilateral responses and the nature of their afferent pathways remain speculative.

Middle- and Long-Latency SEPs to Upper Limb Stimulation

These responses have been identified either by scalp and cortical SEP recordings or through modeling of magnetic SEFs. They have not proved their clinical utility and most of them are modulated by cognitive factors. They are briefly described here to provide the reader with a comprehensive review of the field.

P45 and N60 Potentials

Both P45 and N60 potentials are recorded contralaterally to the stimulation in the central and frontal regions. It is still debated whether they reflect the activation of associative cortical areas, via corticocortical connections, or cortical responses to inputs transmitted directly from the thalamus. Early SEP studies in patients with focal lesions have shown that P45 is preserved in patients with isolated loss of pain and temperature sensations (Giblin, 1964; Halliday and Wakefield, 1963; Noel and Desmedt, 1975). Moreover, it may persist in patients with lesion of the parietal cortex causing pure astereognosis and abnormal N20 or P27 over the damaged hemisphere (Mauguière et al., 1982, 1983a). This latter finding suggests that the P45 potential might be generated by parallel ascending inputs rather than through corticocortical fibers originating from the SI generators of the N20-P27 potentials. Little is known about the N60 potential. The observation that its voltage reaches its plateau only when the intensity of the stimulus is increased up to seven times the sensory threshold has suggested that it might be generated by spinothalamic afferents, but lesion studies have hitherto failed to confirm this hypothesis (Bastuji, Garcia-Larrea, and Mauguière, unpublished data). Recent intracranial recordings coupled with source modeling of scalp responses suggest that three distinct sources contribute to the N60; one is located in the frontocentral cortex contralateral to stimulation, and the two others are located in the suprasylvian cortex (somatosensory area SII) on both sides (Barba et al., 2002a). In scalp recordings two distinct components can be identified on the basis of their latencies and scalp distributions, namely, a frontocentral N60 contralateral to stimulation and a bilateral N70 in the temporal regions. Thus, none of the scalp negative potentials identified as N60 or N70 in the literature has been shown to be generated in the posterior parietal cortex.

Responses of the Second Somatosensory Area (SII)

The most precise available descriptions of the human SII area have long been those by Penfield and Rasmussen (1957) and Woolsey et al. (1979) based, respectively, on electrical stimulation and intracortical recordings of SEPs. They showed a single complete representation of the body located lateral to the end of the rolandic fissure on the dorsolateral surface of the hemisphere and extending to the cortex of the upper bank of the sylvian fissure, contrasting with the multiple body maps identified in the lateral sulcus of monkey's brain (Burton et al., 1995; Krubitzer et al., 1995). The clinical deficit resulting from SII lesions is also more controversial than that observed after SI lesions. Whereas Penfield and Roberts (1959) concluded that removal of SII is followed by "no obvious sensory or motor defect," it has been reported that a lesion of the suprasylvian somatosensory cortex produces a deficit in tactile object recognition by the opposite hand (Caselli, 1993). However, this observation, based on clinical and MRI data, has not been correlated with abnormalities of perisylvian SEPs; moreover, it has not been checked either that the SI responses were normal in these patients.

The existence of short-latency SEPs generated in SII peaking earlier than 40 msec after median nerve stimulus remains a debated issue in the literature. Lüders et al. (1985), using an array of 96 subdural electrodes in a single epileptic patient, recorded responses to contralateral median nerve and finger stimulation in the inferior frontal gyrus, peaking only 2.4 msec later than SI evoked responses that they considered as originating in the SII area. However, these authors failed to record such early responses ipsilateral to stimulation, and the measurement area was clearly anterior to the cortical zone producing longer latency perisylvian responses in human corticograms (Allison et al., 1989b). Of the numerous MEG studies of SII responses to median nerve stimulation, only that of Karhu and Tesche (1999) found neuromagnetic activity in the SII area starting 20 to 30 msec after contralateral stimulus, simultaneously, or even before the first activation in SI area. Lastly, recent stereotactic recordings in the suprasylvian cortex has confirmed early bilateral responses peaking at about 30 msec in area SII (Barba et al., 2002b).

If the existence of early SEPs in SII warrants confirmation, that of SII responses peaking in the 60- to 120-msec latency range has been confirmed by several investigators using various electrophysiological approaches. Because it picks up selectively magnetic fields produced by current sources located in the fissural cortex and tangent to the scalp surface (see Hämäläinen et al., 1993, for a review), MEG was the earlier noninvasive technique that permitted individualizing the somatosensory response from the SII area, which is buried in the sylvian fissure. More than 20 years ago median nerve magnetic SEFs peaking in the 100-msec latency range were recorded with a scalp topography compatible with sources located in the parietal operculum of both hemispheres, more precisely in the superior surface of the sylvian fissure posterior to the crossing point of the

rolandic and sylvian fissures (Hari et al., 1983, 1984). These SEFs originating from parietal opercular sources were shown (a) to be more variable from one subject to another than SI SEFs, (b) to be very sensitive to the ISI, and (c) to have a somatotopic organization (Hari et al., 1990, 1993). Early corticographic recordings on the surface of suprasylvian cortex also showed responses, interpreted as originating in SII, peaking in the 100- to 120-msec latency range, ipsi- and contralateral to the stimulus and sensitive to the ISI and task condition (see Allison et al., 1992, for a review).

These latter potentials identified as SII responses can be recorded in scalp and deep recordings of median nerve SEPs. In scalp recordings P100 and N120 potentials are consistently recorded in the central and temporal regions opposite to finger stimulation, respectively (Garcia-Larrea et al., 1995). The field distribution of the N120 response is compatible with a generator located in the SII area contralateral to stimulus. At a latency of about 140 msec a scalp negativity distributed over both central regions and the vertex is of maximal amplitude when the subject has his attention drawn to the stimulus and is instructed to mentally count the stimuli. This response is modulated by attention and shows the same behavior as the endogenous processing negativity originally described in response to auditory tones (see Näätänen, 1990, for a review). Bilateral activation of SII areas could contribute to the generation of this N140 negativity, but, in the absence of confirmative source modeling or lesions studies, this hypothesis remains conjectural.

Direct intracortical recordings using electrodes stereotactically implanted in the upper bank of the sylvian fissure have shown a N60-P90 response to median nerve stimulation (Fig. 54.9) that represents one of the most robust cortical somatosensory response recorded outside the central parietofrontal cortex in humans (Frot and Mauguière, 1999; Frot et al., 1997). Contrary to that of SI responses, the amplitude of the SII potentials does not saturate at stimulus intensities of three to four times the sensory threshold, but continues to increase up to and above the pain threshold (Frot et al., 2001). Ipsilateral SII responses are consistently recorded by depth electrodes; they peak 10 to 12 msec later than contralateral ones, a delay compatible with a transcallosal interhemispheric transmission. The difference between latencies of surface SII responses recorded by corticography and depth responses obtained by stereotactic recordings is unclear. It is probable that the first N60 potential of depth recording is not picked up on the cortical surface because its amplitude is far less than that of the following P90 response.

Long-Latency Responses of the Posterior Parietal, Mesial, and Frontal Cortex

Using a whole-head 122-superconducting quantum interference device (SQUID) magnetometer, SEF sources has been modeled in the posterior parietal (Forss et al., 1994a) and mesial cortex (Forss et al., 1996) contralateral to stimulation and in both frontal lobes (Mauguière et al., 1997a,b), which are all active in the 70- to 160-msec latency range, in response to stimuli delivered at long ISIs, in particular when mentally counted by the subject. Intracortical recordings lend some substance to these SEF dipole modeling findings (Allison et al., 1992). Scalp recordings of SEPs, however, do

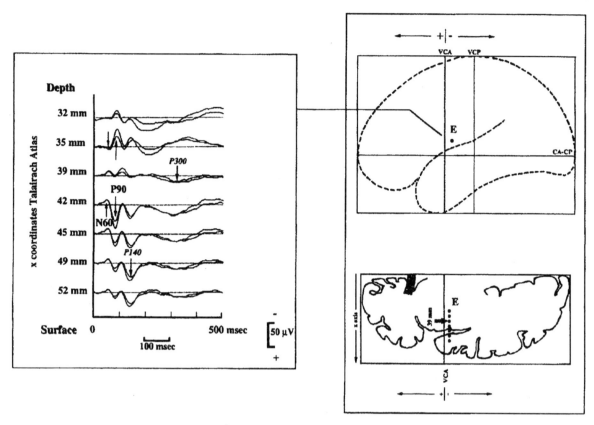

Figure 54.9. N60-P90 intracortical responses recorded in the parietal operculum (SII area) after electric stimulation of the median nerve at the wrist. (From Frot, M., and Mauguière, F. 1999. Timing and spatial distribution of somatosensory responses recorded in the upper bank of the sylvian fissure (SII area) in humans. Cereb. Cortex 9:854–863, with permission.)

not allow one to identify components reflecting specifically the activities of these sources, as identified from SEF modeling, probably because the field distribution reflects simultaneous activation of multiple and largely distributed sources at these latencies. Moreover, there is no available study demonstrating abnormal SEP or SEF profiles associated with focal lesions affecting the cortical regions proposed as generators of these long-latency responses.

Short-Latency SEPs to Lower Limb Stimulation (Fig. 54.10)

Electrical stimulation of the tibial nerve at the ankle is adopted by most authors for the testing of the sensory pathways of the lower limb. However, the electrical stimulation can also be applied to the sural nerve at the ankle, or to the peroneal nerve at the knee without major changes in the general waveform of the spinal or scalp responses. As compared with tibial nerve SEPs, only the peaking latencies are modified; they are delayed by about 3 msec, or shortened by about 5 to 6 msec, respectively, for sural and peroneal nerve stimulation. In what follows, tibial nerve SEPs are taken as the reference for describing the normal waveforms.

Peripheral Nerve Response

A compound action potential corresponding to the activation of tibial nerve fibers is recorded at the posterior aspect

of the knee using a bipolar montage. The negative peak of this near-field potential peaks at a latency of about 7 msec in adults. This N7 potential reflects a mixed response of motor and sensory fibers, which is clinically useful to assess the function of the peripheral segment of the pathway. The afferent volley in cauda equina roots can be recorded using skin electrodes placed at the L5-S1 level and a distant reference site, for instance at the knee opposite to the stimulation.

Spinal Potentials

An electrode situated on the spinal process of T12 or L1 vertebrae and connected to a distal reference electrode records a spinal negative potential peaking at 21 to 24 msec in normal subjects. According to different authors, this segmental response has been labeled N20 (Tsuji et al., 1984), N21 (Small and Matthews, 1984), N22 (Lastimosa et al., 1982; Riffel et al., 1984), N23 (Yamada et al., 1982), or N24 (Desmedt and Cheron, 1983). These differences in nomenclature are mostly due to differences in the mean body height of the subjects sampled for normative studies. In what follows this response is labeled N22. After tibial nerve stimulation the lumbar N22 originates mostly from the spinal segment receiving fibers from the S1 root (Delbeke et al., 1978; Delwaide et al., 1985; Desmedt and Cheron, 1983; Dimitrijevic et al., 1978; Jones and Small, 1978; Lastimosa et al., 1982; Small and Matthews, 1984; Tsuji et al., 1984).

Figure 54.10. Short-latency tibial nerve SEPs. The segmental lumbar P17 response at the spinous process of the L1 vertebra was recorded using a reference electrode at the knee contralateral to stimulation of the tibial nerve at the ankle. For scalp response recording the reference was placed at the right earlobe (A2) (see text for a detailed description). (From Mauguière F. 1995. Evoked potentials. In *Clinical Neurophysiology: EMG, Nerve Conduction and Evoked Potentials,* Eds. J.W. Osselton, C.D. Binnie, R. Cooper, et al., pp. 325–563. Oxford: Butterworth-Heinemann, with permission.)

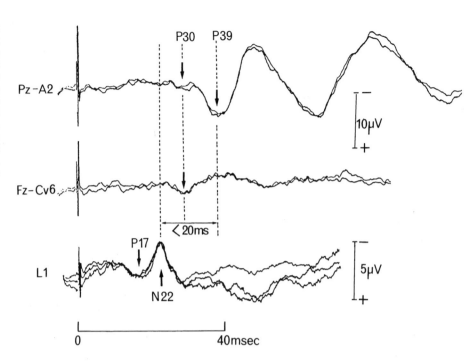

As all segmental DH responses (see Dimitrijevic and Halter, 1995, for a review) the N22 demonstrates a polarity reversal when recorded anterior to the cord, a field distribution consistent with a horizontal dipolar source reflecting the postsynaptic response of DH neurons to incoming inputs. The N22 amplitude is maximal close to the entry zone of the S1 root in cord surface recordings and decreases steeply without any latency shift at more rostral or caudal electrode sites (Jeanmonod et al., 1991). The N22 potential is followed by a slow positivity, known as the P wave, which reverses into a negativity when recorded at the anterior aspect of the cord (Jeanmonod et al., 1989; Shimoji et al., 1977) and may reflect the processes of presynaptic inhibition affecting the primary afferent fibers in the DH. In intraoperative direct recording of the cord, several fast negativities are superimposed on the ascending slope of the N22; they reflect the action potentials ascending in the dorsal columns. In most skin surface recordings these negativities cannot be individualized.

When the reference electrode is not situated on the axis of propagation of the peripheral ascending volley, the N22 potential is preceded by a small positivity peaking around 17 msec. This P17 positivity is a far-field potential originating in lumbosacral plexus trunks, which can also be recorded occasionally on the scalp when the reference electrode is placed at the knee (or iliac crest) on the nonstimulated side (Desmedt and Cheron, 1983; Yamada et al., 1982).

Scalp Far-Field P30 Potential

With appropriate noncephalic reference montages widespread far-field positivities, other than the P17 described above, can be recorded on the scalp that peak before the onset of the earliest cortical potential in the 25- to 32-msec latency range (Desmedt and Cheron, 1983; Kakigi and Shibasaki, 1983; Yamada et al., 1982). Only the latest of

these positivities, identified by Yamada et al. (1982) as the P31 potential, is consistently recorded in normals after tibial nerve stimulation at the ankle. This observation was confirmed by several investigators who labeled this potential as P28 (Chiappa and Ropper, 1982; Kakigi et al., 1982), P30 (Desmedt and Bourguet, 1985; Guérit and Opsomer, 1991; Urasaki et al., 1993; Vera et al., 1983), or P31 (Desmedt and Cheron, 1983; Seyal et al., 1983). The latency of this potential varies according to body height, and is labeled P30 in this chapter, according to the author's normative data.

The utility of the P30 potential has been validated for clinical applications of tibial SEPs in patients with spinal cord and brainstem lesions (Tinazzi and Mauguière, 1995; Tinazzi et al., 1996b). The P30 potential is widely distributed on the scalp with a predominance in the frontal region (Desmedt and Bourguet, 1985; Guérit and Opsomer, 1991) and therefore is drastically reduced in scalp-reference recordings (Seyal et al., 1983). When recorded with electrodes located in the fourth ventricle during surgery, this potential shows the same intracranial spatiotemporal distribution as the P14 component of median nerve SEPs (Urasaki et al., 1993). Therefore, the P30 potential is likely to be generated in the brainstem (Desmedt and Cheron, 1983; Yamada et al., 1982) and can be viewed as the homologue, for the lower limb, of the far-field P14 recorded on the scalp after median nerve stimulation.

Recording of P30 is made easier if the scalp electrode is placed in the midfrontal region at Fz or Fpz, where P30 has its maximal amplitude with minimal contamination by subsequent cortical potentials. If electrodes are too posteriorly situated, P30 may be lost in the descending slope of the cortical P39 potential. The most practical reference site for recording of P30 is the nucha at the spinous process of the sixth cervical vertebra (Seyal et al., 1983; Tinazzi and Mauguière, 1995). Since no segmental response is evoked by lower limb stimulation at the cervical cord level, the neck can be considered as virtually inactive at the peaking latency of P30. The ascending volley in spinal somatosensory pathways reaches the cervical level at a latency of about 27 msec but, due to the time dispersion of afferent impulses, no consistent potential is recorded by a skin cervical electrode at this latency. In some normal subjects a scalp far-field P27 potential distinct from P30 is recordable in the frontal region, which reflects the ascending volley in the cervical cord (Desmedt and Cheron, 1983; Yamada et al., 1982)

N33 Scalp Potential

In noncephalic or earlobe reference recordings a small N33 negativity (Desmedt and Bourguet, 1985; Guérit and Opsomer, 1991) may precede the P39 potential. This negativity is widely distributed over the scalp; part of it is also picked up at the earlobe so that it is reduced in earlobe reference recordings. Because some of the cortical potentials are picked up at the earlobe contralateral to stimulation, it is preferable to use the earlobe ipsilateral to stimulation as the reference site for the recording of cortical tibial nerve SEPs (Tinazzi et al., 1997a). N33 is considered as the homologue of the N18 upper limb SEP and is likely to have a similar origin in the lower brainstem (see above).

Cortical Potentials

The earliest cortical potential elicited by the stimulation of tibial nerve at the ankle is a positive potential usually labeled P37, P39, or P40 for it peaks at a mean latency of 37 to 40 msec in normal subjects (see Yamada, 2000, for a review). In what follows this potential is labeled P39. This potential peaks 6 to 7 msec earlier after stimulation of the tibial nerve at the popliteal fossa, and about 3 msec later after stimulation of the sural nerve at the ankle. In normal subjects P39 is recordable on the vertex and can be reliably obtained midway between Pz and Cz using a scalp to earlobe montage. Frequently the maximum of P39, although close to the midline, is slightly shifted on the side of the scalp ipsilateral to the stimulation (Cruse et al., 1982). The most likely reason for this paradoxical lateralization is that the somatotopic representation of the lower limb in the somatosensory SI, and in particular that of the foot, is situated at the inner aspect of the hemisphere. This paradoxical scalp distribution of P39 is not observed when the proximal leg is stimulated, for instance after stimulation of the femoral nerve or lateral femoral cutaneous nerve (Wang et al., 1989; Yamada et al., 1996). SEP mapping in normals often shows a dipolar field distribution for P39, with a maximum of positivity ipsilateral to the stimulation in the parietal region and a maximum of negativity (N39) in the contralateral frontocentral region (Cruse et al., 1982; Desmedt and Bourget, 1985; Kakigi and Jones, 1986; Seyal et al., 1983; Tinazzi et al., 1996a). Magnetic fields evoked by stimulation of the lower limb also show this distribution (Hari et al., 1984; Huttunen et al., 1987). The negative N39 maximum of this dipole is not consistently obtained, probably because of intersubject differences in the orientation of the leg area in SI with respect to the scalp surface, so that one can envisage all intermediates between a vertical radial dipole with a positive maximum on the vertex, and a

nearly tangential one with a P39 and N39 culminating respectively in the ipsi- and contralateral parietal regions. As for median nerve SEPs, the question is still debated whether all of these potentials reflect the activity of the lower limb area in SI, or whether some could be generated in other cortical areas. Another question is to determine whether the P39-N39 dipolar field has a single source in SI tangent to the scalp (Cruse et al., 1982; Kakigi and Jones, 1986; Kakigi and Shibasaki, 1992; Seyal et al., 1983; Tsumoto et al., 1972), or several (Beric and Prevec, 1981; Desmedt and Bourguet, 1985; Pelosi et al., 1988; Vas et al., 1981). Studies on the effect of the frequency rate on cortical SEP amplitude favor the latter hypothesis by showing the following:

1. N39 and P39 can show some difference in their respective latencies, the former peaking earlier than the latter; this explains why some authors have proposed labeling these potentials N37 and P40, respectively (Yamada, 2000).
2. P39 is selectively reduced with preserved N39 in patients with motor neuron disease (Zanette et al., 1996).
3. P39 is reduced at high stimulation rates (Chiappa, 1990; Chiappa and Ropper, 1982), while the frontal N39 amplitude remains unaffected at stimulus rates up to 7.5 Hz (Tinazzi et al., 1996a).
4. Source modeling studies of scalp responses (Baumgartner et al., 1998) and direct intracerebral recordings (Valeriani et al., 2001) have suggested that two sources located in the central region are quasi-simultaneously involved in the generation of the N39-P39 field on scalp surface. One is indeed tangential to scalp surface and responsible for a dipolar field with a positive maximum in the centroparietal region ipsilateral to stimulus, and a negative maximum in the frontotemporal region contralateral to stimulus. The other is perpendicular to scalp surface and responsible for part of the vertex P39 potential.

Studies of the effects of movement on cortical tibial SEPs have shown that P39, but not N39, is gated during voluntary movement of the stimulated foot (Tinazzi et al., 1997b; Valeriani et al., 1998b, 2001). During tonic contraction this effect is proportional to the level of muscle strength maintained by the subjects. These findings have been interpreted in different ways according to the different source models. Tinazzi et al. (1998) proposed that P39 could be generated in the motor cortex, while N39 could be the equivalent of the median nerve N20 and generated in area 3b in the SI area. Valeriani et al. (1998b, 2001) considered that only the radial central source of the vertex P39, possibly located rostral to the central sulcus, is sensitive to voluntary movements.

P39 is followed by N50 and P60 components, these three waves forming the "W" profile (P39-N50-P60) of the cortical response recorded in the centroparietal region. This waveform has been reported in all studies on tibial nerve SEPs (see Tinazzi et al., 1997a, for a review). Electrical stimulation of the L5 and S1 dermatomes also evokes a consistent, W-shaped response on the scalp with a first positivity at about 50 msec after stimulation (Katifi and Sedgwick, 1986). The N50 and P60 potentials culminate at the vertex (Cz) and do not show the same clear dipolar distribution as the P39-N39 response on the scalp, thus suggesting that the W-shaped P39-N50-P60 waveform could be generated by several sources with distinct orientations (Desmedt and Bourguet, 1985; Guérit and Opsomer, 1991). There is no clinical study demonstrating that the N50 or P60 potential can be selectively affected by a single focal lesion, and these two potentials show the same attenuation as P39 during active movement (Tinazzi et al., 1997b). Conversely it is not exceptional in demyelinating diseases to see a single persisting positivity peaking at the P60 latency while the P39 potential cannot be identified.

Scalp SEPs Evoked by Stimulation of the L5 and S1 Dermatomes

Electrical stimulation of the L5 and S1 dermatomes, applied at the medial side of the first metatarsophalangeal joint and at the lateral side of the fifth metatarsophalangeal joint, respectively, yields consistent W-shaped evoked potentials on the scalp (Katifi and Sedgwick, 1986). These dermatomal potentials are obtainable by using a derivation between electrodes placed at Cz (lead 1) and midway between Fpz and Fz (lead 2), a filter bandpass of 5 to 250 Hz, a stimulus rate of about 3/sec, and a stimulus strength of 2.5 times sensory threshold. This gives about 80% of the maximal response and is tolerated by normal subjects. The first scalp positive potential peaks at mean latencies of about 48.5 and 50 msec, respectively, for stimulation of the L5 and S1 dermatomes. This technique is especially useful for exploring L5 and S1 monoradiculopathies, as stimulation of a single peripheral nerve containing fibers that enter the cord via multiple roots may give normal responses, mediated through the unaffected roots.

Short Latency SEPs to Pudendal Nerve Stimulation

Stimulation of the dorsal nerves of the penis or the clitoris elicits spinal and scalp responses with a waveform very similar to that of SEPs obtained by stimulation of the posterior tibial nerve.

A spinal negative N15 potential equivalent to the tibial nerve N22 potential can be recorded on the skin surface after stimulation of the penis or clitoris (Opsomer et al., 1989, 1990). On direct cord recordings the N15 potential shows a polarity reversal on the anterior aspect of the cord and is preceded by a P10 potential that has the same origin as the tibial nerve P17 potential (Turano et al., 1995).

Electrical stimulation of the dorsal nerve of the penis (or clitoris) yields consistent, W-shaped, evoked potentials on the scalp (Guérit and Opsomer, 1991; Haldeman et al., 1982). The earliest positivity of this response culminates at 40 msec after stimulation. Direct cortical recordings have located the genitalia somatotopic area anterior to the foot area on the mesial aspect of SI (Allison et al., 1996).

SEPs to Trigeminal Nerve Stimulation

A P19 scalp component can be evoked by electrical stimulation of the lips (Stöhr et al., 1981). Other authors using various methods of stimulation described similar cortical

SEP components (Bennett and Jannetta, 1983; Buettner et al., 1982; Dreschler and Neuhauser, 1986). Leandri et al. (1988) pointed out that the scalp response to stimulation of trigeminal afferents recorded by means of surface electrodes could be contaminated by muscular artefacts. To detect, but also to locate, the trigeminal nerve dysfunction, they proposed using the early potentials evoked by stimulation of the infraorbital nerve through needle electrodes inserted into the infraorbital foramen. They described three far-field positive waves reflecting the compound action potential at the entry of the maxillary nerve into the gasserian ganglion (W1), at the entry zone of the trigeminal root into the pons (W2), and in the presynaptic portion of the trigeminal spinal tract (W3).

Measurement of the Central Conduction Time (CCT)

One of the advantages of SEP recording in clinical routine is to permit an evaluation of the transit time of the ascending volley in the central segments of the somatosensory pathways. In most studies this transit time is referred to as the central conduction time (CCT).

Upper Limb SEPs

Various montages and procedures have been proposed for measuring the CCT depending on whether the aim is merely to detect a conduction slowing and to follow-up CCT values during the evolution of a disease in the same individual, or to locate accurately the site where conduction velocity is slowed down. In all types of montages the conduction in the proximal segment of brachial plexus roots can be evaluated by measuring the interval between the peaks of the supraclavicular N9 (or far-field P9) and the spinal N13 potentials. Techniques that provide the investigator with an index of global CCT abnormality are considered to yield enough information in many clinical situations; among these, the measurement of the interpeak interval between the cervical N13 and the parietal N20 components is the most widely used. However, this procedure evaluates the CCT from the peak of the postsynaptic DH potential (N13), which is produced in parallel to the ascending volley in the dorsal columns. In intramedullary cervical cord lesions, for instance, a normal conduction in the dorsal columns may coexist with a clearly abnormal, or even absent, N13 potential (Mauguière and Restuccia, 1991). Moreover, the N13-N20 interval does not allow a separate assessment of conduction times in the intraspinal and intracranial segments of the somatosensory pathways. In spite of these limitations, the N13-N20 interval has progressively become a synonym for CCT since the early studies of Hume and Cant (1978).

In mediofrontal (Fz) reference montages the CCT is usually measured from the peak of the cervical negativity recorded at C6 to the peak of the contralateral parietal N20 (Eisen and Odusote, 1980; Hume and Cant, 1978). The use of a frontal reference may introduce some uncertainty in the identification of the N13 and N20 potentials because the brainstem P14 and cortical P22 potentials recorded by the scalp reference are injected as negative N14 and N22 potentials in the C6-Fz and parietal-Fz traces, respectively; consequently, their peaks can be confused with those of the genuine cervical N13 and parietal N20 potentials. Interindividual variations of waveforms resulting from interferences between potentials picked at the neck and on the scalp may be problematic when sampling normative data, and this difficulty increases when analyzing distorted waveforms in patients. In Fz reference recordings this difficulty can be overcome by measuring the CCT between the onset of the cervical N11-N13 negativity and that of the parietal N20. The onset of N11 corresponds to the spinal entry time of the afferent volley and the onset of N20 to the arrival time of the fastest action potentials at the parietal cortex contralateral to stimulation. The only major inconvenience of this measurement is the presence, in C6-Fz traces, of a N9 potential preceding the N11-N13 potentials that may prevent a reliable measurement of the onset latency of the N11-N13 wave. This N9 potential is a combination of the P9 potentials picked up at the neck and at Fz; the negative polarity of this potential in the C6-Fz trace stems from the fact that the latter is usually larger than the former.

In noncephalic reference recordings three transit times can be calculated to assess central conduction (Fig. 54.11). Conduction from the brachial plexus roots to the brainstem and from the brainstem to the parietal cortex can be explored, respectively, by calculating the P9-P14 and the P14-N20 intervals. Moreover, the global CCT can be evaluated by measuring the intervals either between peaks of N13 and N20 potentials (peak CCT) or between the onsets of N11 and N13 potentials (onset CCT). Although the peak of N13 is easier to identify in this type of montage than in frontal reference recordings (see above), only the interval between the onsets of N11 and of N20 actually assesses the transit time from the spinal entry time to the onset of the cortical response (Desmedt and Cheron, 1980a; Zegers de Beyl, 1988a). In practical terms there may be some difficulty in choosing an onset latency for N11. However, Ozaki et al. (1996b) reported that, of the two procedures, only the onset CCT is able to show that the ulnar nerve CCT is longer than the median nerve CCT, and that the CCT correlates with body height in normal subjects.

Lower Limb SEPs

In most clinical applications of tibial nerve SEPs the CCT from the lumbosacral spinal cord to the cortex is evaluated by the interval between the peak of the lumbar N22 negativity and the peak of the cortical P39 potential (Noel and Desmedt, 1980; Perlik and Fischer, 1987; Small and Matthews, 1984; Veilleux and Daube, 1987; Yiannikas et al., 1986; Yu and Jones, 1985). As for upper limb SEPs, one can argue (1) that the N22 potential reflects a postsynaptic DH response, which can be abnormal in patients with lesions of the lumbosacral spinal cord whose CCT is preserved; and (2) that only the onset of N22 reflects the spinal entry time of the afferent volley. However, because of the presence of the far-field P17 in the lumbar, region this measurement is often problematic and only N22-P39 interpeak CCT has been validated in clinical studies. The peaking latencies of N22 and P39 are correlated with body height in normal subjects (Chiappa, 1990; Tinazzi and Mauguière, 1995; Tsuji et al., 1984), while authors' opin-

ions diverge concerning the correlation between N22-P39 interpeak interval and height.

Several attempts have been made to evaluate separately the intraspinal and intracranial CCT using lower limb SEPs. Measurement of conduction velocity of the propagated volley along the cord by recording tibial SEPs on the skin at different levels of the spine proves to be relatively unsatisfactory. Recordings of a dorsal column CAP, the latency of which increases from caudal to rostral levels of the spine,

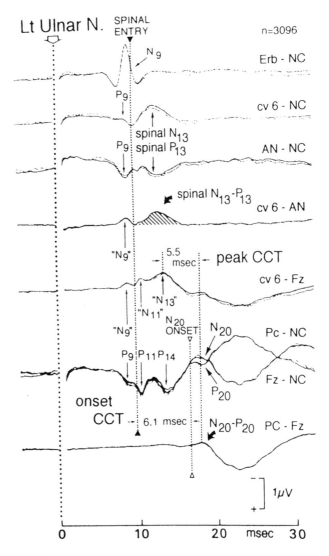

Figure 54.11. Central conduction time (CCT) measurements: ulnar nerve SEPs. The entry time of the afferent volley in the spinal cord corresponds to the onset latency of the N11 potential at C6 or anterior neck (AC) recorded with a noncephalic (NC) or Fz reference, and to the onset of the scalp far-field P11 recorded in the parietal region contralateral to stimulation (Pc) or midfrontal region (Fz) with a NC reference. The N20 onset latency can be measured either after superimposition of contralateral parietal and frontal traces, or by substraction of these two responses (Pc-Fz). In this normal subject the peak CCT between N13 and N20 is 5.5 msec, while the onset CCT measured from the entry time of the afferent volley in the cord and the onset of the cortical N20 is 6.1 msec. (From Ozaki I., Takada H., Shimamura H., et al. 1996b. Central conduction in somatosensory evoked potentials. Comparison of ulnar and median data evaluation of onset versus peak methods. *Neurology* 47:1299–1304, with permission.)

have been reported by several authors (Desmedt and Cheron, 1983; Kakigi et al., 1982; Seyal et al., 1983; Yamada et al., 1982). However, these reports mostly concern young normal volunteers, in whom very small potentials could be recorded up to the cervical level by averaging 2,000 to 6,000 stimulations. The amplitude of the spinal CAP drops dramatically from T12 to T6 (Delbeke et al., 1978; Seyal et al., 1983). Moreover, cervical responses recorded with skin electrodes are small (Desmedt and Cheron, 1983; Sherwood, 1981; Tsuji et al., 1984) or even unrecordable in C6 or C2 shoulder reference recordings (Mauguière and Tinazzi, 1995). This is due to the time-dispersion of the ascending volley at the cervical level, as evidenced by epidural (Macon and Poletti, 1982; Macon et al., 1982; Whittle et al., 1986) or direct recordings of the cord (Turano et al., 1995). By analogy with upper limb SEPs it has been proposed that the transit time from cervical cord to cortex be evaluated by measuring the interval between the negative peak recorded at the neck with a cervicofrontal derivation and the peak of the P39 potential on the vertex (Lüders et al., 1981; Riffel et al., 1984; Small and Matthews, 1984). This cervical negativity does not originate in the cervical cord, it is made of the brainstem P30 potential (see above) picked by the frontal reference electrode and injected as a negativity in the C6-Fz waveform. It has been shown that measuring the N22-P30 and P30-P39 interpeak intervals provides a reliable evaluation of the intraspinal and intracranial CCTs in normals and patients with focal cervical cord, brainstem, and hemispheric lesions (Tinazzi and Mauguière, 1995; Tinazzi et al., 1996b).

Recording Montages

Several recommended montages for short-latency SEP recording have been proposed, including in a previous edition of this book and in guidelines published by the IFCN (Mauguière et al., 1999). In what follows we describe the advantages and limitations of each type of montage according to the SEP components under study. Depending on the clinical question to be solved, the number of channel available and the recording environment users can combine several of these derivations.

Upper Limb SEPs

Peripheral N9 Potential

This potential is picked up at the Erb's point location ipsilateral to the stimulated limb (EPi). The reference electrode can be placed at the contralateral Erb's point (EPc) or at Fz site on the scalp. With the EPc reference only the N9 triphasic wave is recorded; with the Fz reference it is followed by a N14 negativity and a P30 positivity, which correspond to the P14 and N30 potentials recorded at Fz, respectively. When a limited number of channels is available, the EPi-Fz derivation thus permits assessing the far-field P14 and frontal N30 potentials.

Spinal N11 and N13 Potentials

The active electrode is attached to the dorsal neck at the level of C6 (or C5) spinous process. The reference electrode

connected to grid 2 of the amplifier can be positioned at Fz or at various noncephalic sites. The advantage of the Fz position is to yield larger responses, but its main disadvantage is that this higher amplitude is due to injection in the resulting waveform of the far-field P11 and P14 potentials picked up at the Fz site. Therefore, it is preferable to choose a noncephalic reference electrode, which can be positioned either at EPc or at the posterior aspect of the shoulder contralateral to simulation (Shc) or at the anterior aspect of the neck (anterior cervical, AC) in a supraglottal position. The advantage of the AC reference is that the N13 potential is better defined because of its transverse cervical dipolar source. Moreover, normal values of the amplitude ratio between N13 and the preceding N9-P9 have been published for median, ulnar, and radial nerve stimulation (Restuccia and Mauguière, 1991; Restuccia et al., 1992) with this derivation.

Far-Field P9, P11, P14 and N18 Potentials

These potentials are widespread on the scalp; therefore, the reference electrode should be placed in a noncephalic position (EPc or Shc) while the active electrode can be placed in various positions. However, when only a limited number of channels is available, it is recommended to place the active electrode in the parietal region contralateral to stimulation (Pc electrode, see below) in order to record also the cortical N20 and P27 potentials with the same channel. Hitherto available normal values of the P9-P14 amplitude ratio have been obtained with the PC-Shc montage (Garcia-Larrea and Mauguière, 1988). The N18 negativity is better identifiable in traces recorded in the parietal region ipsilateral to stimulation, where there is no interaction with the contralateral N20 cortical potential. With an earlobe reference, either ipsi- or contralateral to stimulation, only the P14 is clearly identifiable.

Cortical Potentials

In the majority of normal subjects the parietal N20-P27 response is obtained with maximal amplitude at a point situated 5 cm behind Cz and 7 cm laterally in the parietal region opposite to stimulation (Pc) and is adequately recorded with a noncephalic or earlobe reference. When recorded with a noncephalic reference electrode (EPc or Shc) the N20-P27 deflection is preceded by the far-field positivities and the N18 is superimposed to the ascending phase of the N20 potential. With an earlobe reference the P9 and P14 potentials are reduced and the N18 potential is almost canceled. Since the cortical SEPs are partly picked up at the earlobe contralateral to stimulation, it is recommended to use the earlobe ipsilateral to stimulation to study the amplitude of the cortical SEPs (Tomberg et al., 1991b). The central P22 potential is picked up with maximal amplitude at a site situated 2 cm in front of Cz and 5 cm laterally, while the maximum of the frontal N30 is obtained on the midline between Cz and Fz. Both P22 and N30 potentials can be recorded using a reference electrode placed either in a noncephalic site or at the earlobe, preferably ipsilateral to stimulation. The widely used Pc-Fz derivation cancels most of the far-field responses and does not allow studying separately the potentials recorded in the frontal region. It has the advantage of increasing the size of the N20 potential because of the dipolar

N20-P20 distribution of this potential on the scalp (see above); this can be useful for monitoring the cortical SI response during surgery. However, the best way of recording this response with no interference with the far-field potentials, including N18, is to use a derivation between the parietal electrodes contra- and ipsilateral to stimulation (Pc-Pi); this methods also permits better identifying the N20 onset. The distribution of middle- and long-latency cortical SEPs shows more interindividual variations than the earlier potentials; thus, mapping studies using an array of electrodes disposed according to the International 10–20 System with an earlobe reference ipsilateral to stimulation is recommended for their recording.

Lower Limb SEPs

Peripheral Potential in the Popliteal Fossa

The near-field action potential evoked by tibial nerve stimulation is recorded by a first electrode on the midline 2 cm above the popliteal crease of the stimulated side and a second one 3 cm more rostral on the midline.

Spinal N22 Potential

The spinal segmental N22 potential is recorded at the spinous process of T12 or L1 vertebra. The reference can be placed at the iliac crest, at the knee contralateral to stimulation, or 1 cm above the umbilicus. In the author's experience this latter derivation is preferable, for it permits obtaining the stationary N22 and the preceding P17 potentials with an optimal amplitude in 85% of normal subjects.

Brainstem P30 Potential

A Fz-C6 (or Fpz-C6) derivation is optimal to obtain the far-field P30 potential. This potential can also be identified on scalp derivation between Cz and the earlobe ipsilateral to stimulation, but with a small amplitude, which impairs its reliability in clinical studies.

Cortical Potentials

In normal subjects the P39 potential is consistently recorded by an electrode on the midline of the scalp located midway between the Cz and Pz locations. A reference electrode at the earlobe ipsilateral to stimulation has been shown to be optimal, since it does not pick up any of the cortical SEPs (Tinazzi et al., 1997a). As for upper limb SEP recording the use of a midfrontal (Fpz) reference increases the size of the P39 response because of the dipolar distribution of the P39-N39 dipolar field on the scalp surface (see above). Due to the possible paradoxical lateralization of P39, a derivation between the centroparietal region ipsilateral to stimulation (2 cm behind Cz and 2 to 4 cm laterally) and the earlobe ipsilateral to stimulation can be useful to better identify this component, in particular when it is reduced in patients.

Potentials Evoked by CO_2 Laser Painful Stimulation

Brief heat pulses delivered by CO_2 laser beam stimulation of the skin offers the possibility of exploring selectively the small myelinated A delta fibers, and eventually non-

myelinated C fibers, responding to painful stimuli at the periphery (Bromm and Treede, 1984; Treede et al., 1988). Cortical responses to CO_2 stimuli are triggered by inputs conveyed in the spinothalamic tracts, which are not explored by conventional electric stimulation of peripheral nerves. Therefore, CO_2 laser SEPs can be viewed as a clinically useful complementary investigation, in particular in patients with dissociated loss of pain and temperature sensation, in whom cortical responses can be selectively affected (Bromm et al., 1991; Kakigi et al., 1991a; Treede et al., 1991). Unfortunately, the number of fibers stimulated by the laser beam is too small to elicit spinal segmental responses of the DH on skin recordings.

As shown in Figure 54.12 the earliest cortical potential evoked by CO_2 laser stimulation of the hand peaks at about 160 msec; it has a dipolar distribution on the scalp with a negative maximum in the temporal region contralateral to stimulation and a positive maximum in the midfrontal region (Kunde and Treede, 1993; Valeriani et al., 1996). It is

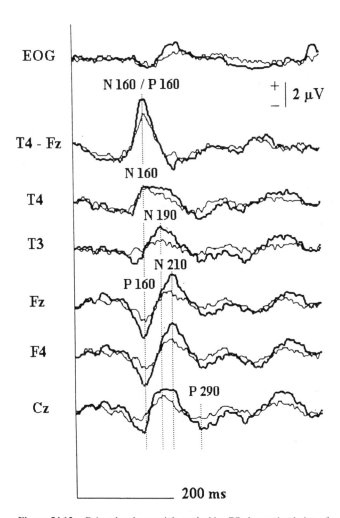

Figure 54.12. Pain-related potentials evoked by CO_2 laser stimulation of the hand. The earliest cortical response is represented by a temporal N160 and frontal P160 dipolar field contralateral to the stimulated side. The vertex N210-P290 response illustrated here corresponds to the N2-P2 potentials (see text for details).

followed by a N2-P2 negative-positive deflexion peaking at about 200 to 250 and 300 to 350 msec. The N2-P2 response is maximal at Fz and Cz electrode sites (see Treede et al., 1995, for a review). The N2-P2 vertex potential represents the largest response and is thus the most reliable one for clinical studies (Kakigi et al., 1991a). The latency of the N160-P160 response is compatible with input transmission via the A delta fibers at the periphery. The N2-P2 deflection, first described by Carmon et al. (1976), could be related with the attentional drive triggered by the painful stimulus and thus considered as a cognitive response. The N160-P160 response was shown to be insensitive to attention fluctuations and to the intensity of pain perception as assessed by a visual analog scale; conversely the N2-P2 vertex response increases when the attention is drawn to the stimulus and its amplitude correlates with pain subjective intensity (Garcia-Larrea et al., 1997). The P2 wave, in spite of its modulation by attention, is different from the later P3 wave peaking at about 500 msec post-CO_2 laser stimulation. This late P3 appears when the subject is detecting actively the stimulus applied on a target hand (Kanda et al., 1996; Towell and Boyd, 1993).

All of the hitherto published source models of CO_2 laser EPs and evoked magnetic fields include dipolar sources in areas SII contra- and ipsilateral to stimulation (Bromm and Chen, 1995; Kitamura et al., 1995; Tarkka and Treede, 1993; Valeriani et al., 1996). The presence of an N140-P170 response to CO_2 laser stimulation of the hand in the cortex of the upper bank of the sylvian fissure has been recently confirmed by direct intracortical recordings (Frot et al., 2001). Very recently a deeper insular source has been identified by intracerebral recordings (Frot and Mauguière, 2003), with a negative-positive response pattern very similar to that of the suprasylvian SII responses, but with later peaking latencies at 180 to 230 msec after the stimulus (N180-P230). Intracerebral recordings have also shown that SII and insular responses ipsilateral to the stimulus peak 10 to 15 msec after the contralateral responses, suggesting a callosal transmission. Other sources of pain EPs have been proposed in SI, cingulate cortex, and mesial temporal lobe on the basis of dipole modeling.

CO_2 laser stimulation can also be applied to explore the function of A delta fibers in the territory of the trigeminal nerve. This stimulation yields consistent negative-positive cortical responses peaking at 160 and 240 msec, respectively (Cruccu et al., 1999, 2001).

Maturation of SEPs

The development of somatosensory pathways from birth to adult life is dominated by two coexisting phenomena, which have opposite effects on SEPs. Myelinogenesis causes a progressive increase in conduction velocities and synchronization of potentials with age, while body growth increases latencies and desynchronization. Differences in recording procedures make difficult the comparison of latency and amplitude values reported in the available studies of SEP maturation. The largest series of SEP normative data in children is that published by Taylor (1993). Previously, only a few SEP maturation studies using a noncephalic reference

montage had been published (Lafrenière et al., 1990; Tomita et al., 1986).

During the first 4 to 5 years of life SEP maturation is marked by a progressive synchronization and a latency reduction of all potentials (Bartel et al., 1987; Cadilhac et al., 1985; Desmedt et al., 1976; Hashimoto et al., 1983; Laureau et al., 1988; Tomita et al., 1986; Zhu et al., 1987). Conduction velocities are known to reach adult values before the age of 3 years in the peripheral nervous system (Desmedt et al., 1973; Thomas and Lambert, 1960), but this acceleration is slower in the central somatosensory pathways (Cracco et al., 1979; Desmedt et al., 1973, 1976). Spinal cord conduction in lower limb fibers reaches adult values at the age of 5 to 6 years (Cracco et al., 1979). Later on, changes in conduction velocity related to fiber maturation interact with those of body growth and the peaking latencies progressively increase, so that adult values are reached at the age of 15 to 17 years (Allison et al., 1983; Tomita et al., 1986).

When divided by arm's length or body height, the latencies of all central SEPs decrease from birth to the age of 10 years and stabilize thereafter (Tomita et al., 1986). The rising time between onsets and peaks of the cortical N20 and P39 evoked respectively by median and tibial nerve stimulations decreases steadily from birth to the age of 16 years (Zhu et al., 1987). In infants aged 7 to 14 years the voltage of the cervical N13 median nerve SEP recorded with an anterior cervical electrode tends to be higher than in adults, while the P14 component tends to be lower with a greater P9/P14 amplitude ratio.

Nonpathologic Factors of SEP Variation

Aging

The effects of age on SEP latencies mainly reflects conduction slowing in the peripheral nerves evidenced by the increase of the N9 component after median nerve stimulation. The central conduction time between the spinal N13 and the parietal N20 was reported as unaffected (Desmedt and Cheron, 1980b; Dorfman and Bosley, 1979), or increased (Hume et al., 1982) during normal aging. Uncertainties as to the measurement of the spinal N13 peaking latency on traces obtained using a cervical to Fz montage may account for these diverging results. The amplitude of the frontal N30 tends to decrease with age, and this component can be virtually absent on both sides in healthy octogenarians whereas the parietal N20 tends to increase (Desmedt and Cherun, 1980b).

Body Height and Gender in Adults

The absolute latencies of SEPs vary according to the distance between the stimulated site and the SEP sources. This effect is naturally more pronounced for lower than for upper limb SEPs. This variability is less for the interpeak intervals used for calculating CCT than for absolute latencies. It is usually not considered when sampling norms of CCT values for upper limb SEPs. Absolute latencies of N22, P30, and P39 potentials evoked by lower limb stimulation are correlated with body height (Chiappa, 1990; Tinazzi and Mauguière, 1995). The upper normal values of the N22-P39 interval vary between 18 and 20 msec for body heights of 1.50 and 1.90 m, respectively (Chiappa, 1990).

Shorter CCTs have been reported in females as compared to males (Green et al., 1982), but this finding was not confirmed by others (Mervaala et al., 1988).

Skin and Core Temperature

Peripheral nerve conduction velocities are known to be affected by changes in limb temperature. Marked decrease in body temperature, as observed during drug-induced hypothermia, increases the absolute and interpeak latencies of both the early cortical N20 and the positive far-field positive potentials. Moreover, the curves of amplitude decrease versus body temperature during hypothermia are not the same for peripheral, spinal, brainstem, and cortical SEPs (Guérit et al., 1990). The N20 potential disappears at temperatures ranging from 17° to 25°C, the P14 at 17° to 20°C. The peripheral N9 and spinal N13 potentials remains identifiable down to body temperature of 17°C. SEP changes related to hypothermia warrant special attention in comatose patients in whom they can combine with those induced by CNS depressant drugs. These effects are described below (see Coma; see Brain Death).

Attention

It has been assumed for years that the cortical SEPs peaking before 50 msec following stimulation of the upper limb are not significantly affected by cognitive processes. However, Desmedt et al. (1983b), in an odd-ball detection task of somatosensory stimuli, have identified a P40 potential in response to target stimuli, suggesting that attention-related processes could affect the early cortical SEPs. This P40 can also be identified in response to nontarget stimuli during "lie" experiments in which the subject is instructed to detect rare deviant target stimuli that are never delivered in a monotonous series of identical stimuli (Desmedt and Tomberg, 1989). Moreover, a positive shift is observed after the peaking latency of N30 in response to nontarget electrical stimuli when the attention of the subject is drawn toward the stimulated area (Garcia-Larrea et al., 1991). However, these attention-related changes of early cortical SEPs are not likely to affect the amplitude of the P27, N30, and P45 potentials as recorded in routine conditions, that is, using runs of 500 stimuli or more with no instruction given to the subject.

Sleep and Vigilance

Some changes in the amplitude, waveform, and latency of the parietal N20 have been reported during natural sleep in normal subjects (Yamada et al., 1988). The main change consisted of a prolongation of N20 latency of about 0.4 msec between the awake state and sleep stage II and in a reduction of N20 latency of about 0.3 msec between stage II and rapid-eye-movement (REM) sleep. The disappearance of sharp inflections superimposed over the rising phase of N20 in non-REM sleep where reported by Emerson et al. (1988), and were further investigated by Yamada et al. (1988) using off-line digital filtering. The physiological significance of these wavelets is not yet elucidated; they may correspond to the negative deflections seen on the plateau of the N18 po-

tential, and thus be of subcortical origin. The latency changes observed during sleep are not likely to affect the interpretation of the SEP waveform in patients. However, a maximal prolongation of 0.9 msec of the N9-N20 interval have been reported between wake and sleep (Emerson et al., 1988), suggesting that the patient state should be monitored using EEG in patients with a fluctuating state of vigilance.

Drugs

Significant group differences in CCT were reported between controls and ambulatory epileptic patients treated with phenobarbital or phenytoin (Green et al., 1982), whereas phenobarbital, primidone, and valproic acid seem to have no demonstrable effect. Similarly, Mavroudakis et al. (1991) have reported latency increase of N13 and N20 potentials after a single intravenous injection of phenytoin with blood levels of the drug between 19 and 25 mg/L. When drug sedation is necessary, low anxiolytic doses of benzodiazepines per os can be used and have not been reported to provoke false SEP abnormalities. A prospective study of median nerve SEPs showed that vigabatrin, as an add-on therapy in patients with refractory partial seizures, did not cause any significant prolongation of CCT over a follow-up period of 2 years (Mauguière et al., 1997c). Only serious overdoses of CNS depressant drugs were reported to be associated to abnormally prolonged N13-N20 CCT in comatose patients (Rumpl et al., 1988a). These effects are clinically relevant for the interpretation of SEPs in coma and brain death (see below).

Abnormal Waveforms and Clinical Applications

By combining SEP recordings at different levels of the somatosensory pathways it is possible to assess the transmission of the afferent volley from the periphery up to the cortex. Consequently, the abnormal SEP waveforms as well as their diagnostic utility will be first described according to the lesion site. The relevance of SEP recording in specific clinical situations or pathologies is discussed at the end of this section.

Peripheral Lesions

SEPs can be useful for the evaluation of peripheral pathology in three circumstances: (1) to measure peripheral conduction velocities when sensory nerve action potentials (SNAPs) cannot be obtained at the periphery because of the neuropathic process; (2) to explore proximal lesions of the peripheral sensory pathways that are not accessible to electromyogram (EMG) studies; (3) to study the whole somatosensory pathway up to the cortex in pathologies combining peripheral and central lesions.

Neuropathies

Early in the history of SEPs it was demonstrated that the N20 potential to stimulation of median, ulnar, or digital nerves could be recorded in neuropathies where SNAPs cannot be obtained from recording the nerve itself (Desmedt et al., 1966; Giblin, 1964). The difference between the latencies of the N20 potentials obtained by stimulation of the same nerve at two different levels permits estimation of the conduction velocity in the segment between the two stimulated points. N20 potential recording can thus be used as a means to assess peripheral conduction velocity in severe hereditary neuropathies, such as Charcot-Marie-Tooth or Dèjerine-Sottas diseases, acquired toxic or metabolic neuropathies (Parry and Aminoff, 1987), and even carpal tunnel syndrome (Desmedt et al., 1966). For this indirect measurement of peripheral conduction velocity the onset latencies of the N20 recorded using a reference electrode positioned at Fz or in the parietal region ipsilateral to stimulation are more accurate than peak latencies. Though it is generally assumed that SEPs to electric stimulation of a mixed nerve mostly reflect the activity of cutaneous and joint afferents, stimulation of muscle afferents was shown to elicit a cortical response after stimulation of the posterior tibial nerve, which peaks a few milliseconds earlier than that evoked by cutaneous inputs (Burke et al., 1981, 1982; Gandevia et al., 1984). Thus the sensory conduction velocities indirectly measured using the latency of the first cortical response to stimulation of a mixed nerve may not be equivalent to those obtained by direct recording of SNAPs after selective stimulation of cutaneous afferents.

In pure sensory neuropathies with conduction abnormalities in the proximal segment of sensory fibers, distal conduction velocities, as assessed by conventional EMG testing, can be normal. SEPs are useful in this condition to assess conduction in the damaged segment of sensory fibers. CO_2 laser cortical EPs can also be useful to explore sensory neuropathies affecting preferentially the A delta myelinated fibers, and reduced responses parallel the impairment of pain and temperature sensation as well as the decreased density of small diameter fibers, as assessed by histological examination of skin biopsy (Kakigi et al., 1991b; Kenton et al., 1980).

Brachial and Lumbosacral Plexus Lesions

Most published reports concern traumatic injuries, but the utility of SEPs has also been demonstrated in metastatic lesions (Synek and Cowan, 1983a).

SEPs are useful to assess the topography of the injury as well as to detect whether some inputs are reaching the CNS. One of the main surgical issues in plexopathies is to know whether the lesion is proximal or distal to dorsal ganglia because only lesions distal to the ganglia are accessible to microneurosurgical intervention. Persistence of a normal Erb's point potential (N9) and far-field P9 at the neck and on the scalp with abolition of all subsequent components indicates a root avulsion proximal to the ganglia with a very poor prognosis for recovery. When N9 and N13 potentials are recordable the N13 attenuation roughly reflects the total proportion of damaged fibers at pre- or postganglionic levels, whereas N9 decrease reflects only distal lesions. The absence of all components including N9 potential indicates a complete lesion distal to the ganglia, but does not rule out the possibility of a more proximal lesion in addition to the distal damage, so that this SEP pattern is not 100% reliable (Jones et al., 1981). Reliability of SEP recording can be increased by stimulating several nerves and/or dermatomes to study selectively different trunks or roots of the brachial

plexus. Stimulation of musculocutaneus, radial, median, and ulnar nerves has been proposed to thoroughly explore the brachial plexus (Eisen, 1986).

In lumbosacral plexopathies the persistence of a reproducible P39 cortical potential, even if delayed or reduced, indicates that ascending inputs are reaching the CNS. Conversely, the lumbar N22 is less reliable since it is not constantly obtained in normal subjects. Only clear side-to-side asymmetries of N22 with reduced or absent N22 on the affected side can be viewed as a sign of spinal deafferentation.

Thoracic Outlet Syndrome

Upper limb SEPs are normal in most patients with thoracic outlet syndrome. The value of SEPs in this syndrome is limited to the patients in whom another pathology is suspected. In the few cases with abnormal SEPs, abnormal responses have been observed only for ulnar nerve stimulation and consist of amplitude reduction or abolition of the N13 potential, associated or not with N9 attenuation (Glover et al., 1981; Siivola et al., 1979; Yiannikas and Walsh, 1983).

Guillain-Barré Syndrome

This pathology predominantly affects roots and proximal nerve segments so that peripheral conduction velocities are often normal at the early stage of the disease. Moreover, F-wave recording assesses motor conduction in proximal nerve segments and ventral roots, but not in dorsal roots. Upper limb SEPs show absent, delayed, or dispersed N9 potential with a reduced or absent N13 and increased N9-N13 interval (when measurable). If lesions are confined to the proximal segments, N9 may be normal. In about half of these patients median nerve SEPs are within normal limits (Brown and Feasby, 1984; Ropper and Chiappa, 1986; Walsh et al., 1984). Tibial SEPs are more frequently abnormal, showing a normal or delayed peripheral response at the popliteal fossa with a reduced or absent lumbar N22 potential (Ropper and Chiappa, 1986). Reports of increased central conduction time in Guillain-Barré syndrome have been published (Ropper and Marmarou, 1984), but no definite evidence exists from large series of patients.

Proximal Lesions of the Lower Limb Nerves and Lumbo-Sacral Plexus

SEPs to femorocutaneous nerve stimulation medial to the anterior iliac crest can be useful in meralgia paresthetica to assess the severity of nerve compression and to decide whether surgery is necessary (Synek, 1985). In retroperitoneal compressive lesions of the femoral nerve scalp, SEPs to saphenous nerve stimulation at the lateral aspect of the knee can be absent or delayed (Synek and Cowan, 1983b).

Radiculopathies

SEPs to stimulation of mixed nerves are seldom useful in radiculopathies since they explore multiple roots, so that a monoradiculopathy may be masked by normal responses mediated through unaffected roots. Selective nerve stimulation using saphenous, superficial peroneal, and sural nerves (Eisen, 1986; Eisen and Elleker, 1980) or dermatomal stimulation (Aminoff et al., 1985; Katifi and Sedgwick, 1986, 1987) are more appropriate for exploring radiculopathies. In spite of dermatomal overlapping between roots and of interindividual variations, these techniques proved to be useful for exploring radiculopathies, especially those that present only with pain or sensory symptoms (Eisen et al., 1983; Katifi and Sedgwick, 1987). The recording of compound nerve action potentials at the periphery and of scalp N20 or P39, respectively, for upper and lower limb stimulations, provides enough information for detecting conduction abnormalities but does not provide information as to the exact site where conduction is impaired. Thus, abnormalities of scalp SEPs must be carefully interpreted when the pathology under investigation may affect conduction in the CNS, in particular at the spinal cord level. If a spinal cord pathology is suspected, it becomes mandatory to control the segmental spinal SEPs and to measure the CCT. For upper limb stimulation, it is possible to obtain reliable N13 and P14 potentials after digit stimulation, but for lower limb studies the reliability of lumbar N22 and far-field P30 to dermatomal stimulation has not been validated in patients.

Combined Involvement of Peripheral and Central Somatosensory Pathways in Hereditary Ataxias

It has been demonstrated in Friedreich's ataxia (FA) that sensory nerve conduction velocity is only moderately decreased, whereas sensory nerve action potentials are reduced or absent. In most patients with a history of more than 10 years of clinical symptoms, no SEPs can be obtained after stimulation of upper or lower limbs. When a parietal N20 persists after median nerve stimulation it peaks with a delayed latency and its amplitude is reduced (Jones et al., 1980; Mastaglia et al., 1978; Noel and Desmedt, 1976; Nuwer et al., 1983; Pedersen and Trojaborg, 1981; Sauer and Schenck, 1977; Taylor et al., 1985; Vanasse et al., 1988). Even when severely reduced the N9 and P9 potentials may have latencies within normal limits. When P14 persists, the N9-P14 (or P9-P14) transit times are usually normal; conversely, the P14-N20 interval is often prolonged. The cervical N13, when recorded with a noncephalic reference, cannot be identified in most cases. Therefore, persistence of a scalp P14 potential is the most likely reason why a cervical negative response can be obtained in some FA patients when SEPs are recorded with a cervical to Fz montage (Jones et al., 1980; Pedersen and Trojaborg, 1981).

SEPs have been studied in hereditary ataxias other than FA (Nuwer et al., 1983; Pedersen and Trojaborg, 1981; Thomas et al., 1988; Vanasse et al., 1988, 1990) and have proved to be of potential value for the classification of subtypes in this group of diseases. In familial spastic paraplegia and hereditary cerebellar ataxia, SEPs differ from those observed in Friedreich's disease in two main respects: (a) the incidence of abnormal responses is smaller (Pedersen and Trojaborg, 1981); and (b) peripheral N9/P9 components are normal in most cases (Dimitrijevic et al., 1982; Pedersen and Trojaborg, 1981). For instance, most of the patients with progressive early-onset hereditary ataxias have a normal N9; P9 and P14 potentials are present but N20 is delayed or absent (Vanasse et al., 1990). SEPs in clinically unaffected members of families with Strümpell's hereditary spastic paraplegia may be used to detect asymptomatic heterozygotes.

Spinal Cord Lesions

Spinal Cord Trauma

In most cases of complete functional transection of the spinal cord scalp, cortical SEPs are absent after stimulation of nerves, the roots of which enter the spinal cord below the lesion while spinal segmental responses recorded caudal to the lesion are unaffected (Sedgwick et al., 1980; York et al., 1983). However, absent segmental lumbosacral spinal responses have been reported in patients with cord trauma at thoracic or cervical level (Beric et al., 1987).

At the early stage the persistence of SEPs on the scalp may suggest some residual spinal cord function when clinical examination would lead to more pessimistic conclusions. In the chronic stage of functionally incomplete lesions SEP abnormalities correlate well with clinical somatosensory signs, in particular discriminative skin and joint sensation (Dimitrijevic et al., 1983; Dorfman et al., 1980). It has been observed in the acute stage that SEPs predict better the sensory recovery than clinical examination (Young, 1982), and that SEP amelioration may antedate clinical improvement (Rowed et al., 1978). However, the prognostic value of SEPs is often considered as limited (McGarry et al., 1984; York et al., 1983) and has not been evaluated prospectively in a large population of patients. SEPs testings can detect a transient deterioration of conduction in spinal somatosensory pathways that occurs between the third and sixth day after injury and is presumed to be related with spinal cord edema (Perot and Vera, 1982).

Tumors of the Spinal Cord

Abnormalities of CCT and of segmental spinal N13 and N22 SEPs can be observed in intramedullary spinal cord tumors (Ibañez et al., 1992). In a series of 63 patients we observed one or several of these abnormalities in more than 75% of cases (Mauguière et al., 1996). In cervical intramedullary tumors median nerve SEPs show uni- or bilateral abnormalities of P14, N13, and N22-P39 CCT, respectively, in 75%, 86%, and 78% of cases. These abnormalities are clinically silent (i.e., not associated with sensory deficit or abnormal reflexes in the explored territory) in more than one third of cases. The highest rate of clinically silent SEP abnormality in cervical intramedullary tumors is that of the N13 potential, which is over 50%. There is no large series of thoracic intramedullary tumors investigated using SEPs in the literature; in our series prolonged N22-P39 interval or absent P39 potential were observed, at least on one side, in 75% of cases, but were clinically silent in only 10%. There is no simple relation between the size of the lesion as assessed by MRI and the severity of SEP abnormalities in intramedullary spinal cord tumors; thus, SEPs are useful to evaluate preoperatively the cord dysfunction (Fig. 54.13). In our experience SEP monitoring during surgery reveals transient or persisting central conduction changes in 71% of patients, and there is a good correlation between these changes and the postoperative clinical and SEP outcome. We did not observe any postoperative deterioration of SEPs or of sublesional cutaneous and joint sensation when no SEP changes had occurred during surgery. Conversely, postoperative clinical or SEP deterioration occurred in 70% and 40%, respectively, after transient intraop-

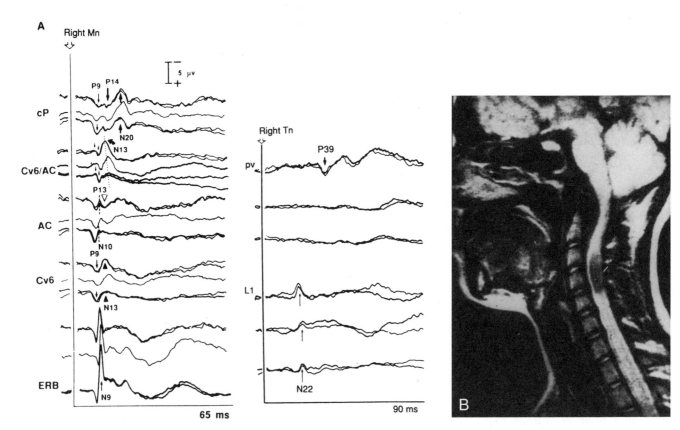

Figure 54.13. Median and tibial nerves SEPs in a case of C3-T5 ependymoma. The spinal magnetic resonance imaging (MRI) shows an enlargement of the cord below a tumoral cyst located at the C3 vertebral level. For each derivation the *lower traces* are those obtained before surgery, the *middle traces* and *upper traces* were obtained 2 weeks and 12 months, respectively, after surgery. The segmental median nerve N13 cervical potential and the cortical P39 potentials were absent before the operation. N13 recovered 2 weeks and P39 12 months after complete surgical removal of the tumor. Erb, Erb's point-Fz derivation; Cv6, posterior neck electrode noncephalic reference at the shoulder contralateral to stimulation (NC); AC, anterior cervical-NC derivation; Cv6-AC, transverse Cv6-AC derivation; cP, contralateral-NC derivation; L1, spinous L1 vertebra process, with knee contralateral to stimulation; pv, posterior vertex (Pz), with earlobe contralateral to stimulation. Note that, in spite of the size of the tumor and of the abolition of the cervical N13 potential, the P9-N20 interval is within normal limits before and after surgery, whereas the cortical tibial nerve P39 was absent before and 2 weeks after surgery. The amplitude of the P14 potential is reduced in all recordings. (From Ibañez V., Fischer G., and Mauguière F. 1992. Dorsal horn and dorsal column dysfunction in intramedullary cervical cord tumours: a SEP study. Brain 115:1209–1234, with permission.)

erative SEP abnormalities; these figures reached 85% when SEP had not returned to baseline values at the end of surgery (Mauguière et al., 1996).

Extrinsic compression of the cord by an extramedullary tumor affects more central conduction than spinal segmental responses (Mauguière et al., 1985; Schramm et al., 1984). Normalization of CCTs after cord decompression (Fig. 54.14) can be observed after surgical decompression and return to normal sensation (Mauguière and Ibañez, 1985). Dermatomal SEPs have been used to determine the upper and lower levels of dorsal column dysfunction in cord compressions (Jorg et al., 1982); this time-consuming technique adds little to more conventional SEP studies and cannot compete with neuroimaging for localizing the lesion.

Syringomyelia

SEPs can be normal when the syrinx does not involve the DH and when the dorsal columns are not constricted by herniation of cerebellar tonsils through the foramen magnum (Arnold-Chiari malformation). However, this eventuality is exceptional, since of a series of 24 patients with cervical syringomyelia that we explored consecutively, only one had normal median nerve SEPs (Restuccia and Mauguière, 1991). The most frequent upper limb SEP abnormality is the amplitude reduction or absence of the segmental N13 potential that we observed in 83% of median nerve SEPs. This abnormality was associated with normal P14 and N20 potential in 75% of cases (Fig. 54.15). This selective abnormality of segmental N13 with preserved dorsal column conduction has been reported by several authors in small series, or in single case reports (Emerson and Pedley, 1986; Kaplan et al., 1988a; Mastaglia et al., 1978; Urasaki et al., 1988). Its frequency has been overlooked in the early study of Veilleux and Stevens (1987) because it becomes obvious only when the cervical response is recorded with a noncephalic reference montage (Mauguière and Restuccia, 1991). N13 abnormalities are correlated with abnormal tendon reflexes and with pain and temperature hypesthesia in

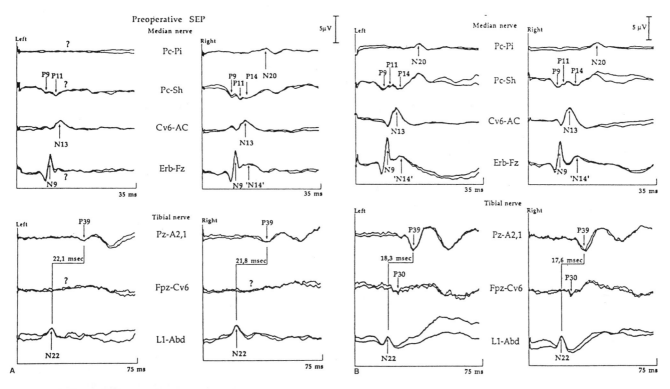

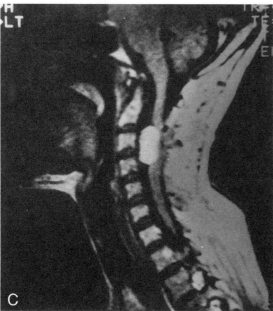

Figure 54.14. Median and tibial nerves SEPs in C2-C3 compression of the cervical cord by a chondrosarcoma. The preoperative SEPs show absent median nerve P14, N20, and tibial nerve P30 potentials with preserved N13 and scalp far-field P11 and delayed P39 on the left side. On the right side the median nerve P14 is reduced, the tibial nerve P30 is absent, and cortical N20 and P39 potentials are delayed. After surgical decompression of the cord all SEP components are obtained, and the only persisting abnormality is an amplitude reduction of the P14 potential on both sides. Pc, contralateral parietal electrode; Sh, shoulder contralateral to stimulation; Pc-Pi, contralateral-ipsilateral parietal derivation. (From Tinazzi, M., Zanette, G., Bonato, C., et al. 1996b. Neural generators of tibial nerve P30 somatosensory evoked potential studied in patients with a focal lesion of the cervico-medullary junction. Muscle Nerve 19:1538–1548, with permission.)

upper limbs. This latter observation is rather unexpected since the N13 potential does not reflect the response of DH spinothalamic cells to A delta and C fibers afferent volley. However, DH neurons are not segregated enough according to the types of their afferents to make possible a selective damage to spinothalamic cells by the syrinx, so that N13 abnormality reflects a global dysfunction of the cord DH in syringomyelia. This interpretation is supported by the observation that cortical responses to CO_2 laser painful stimuli peaking in the 200- to 350- msec latency range are abnormal

in all patients with cervical syringomyelia showing reduced or absent N13 potential (Kakigi et al., 1991a).

Cervical Spondylotic Myelopathy

Cervical spondylotic myelopathy is the most frequent type of myelopathy seen in general hospitals. Several studies have emphasized the diagnostic utility of SEP recording in cervical spondylotic myelopathy (El-Negamy and Sedgwick, 1979; Emerson and Pedley, 1986; Ganes, 1980; Noel and Desmedt, 1980; Perlik and Fischer, 1987; Siivola et al.,

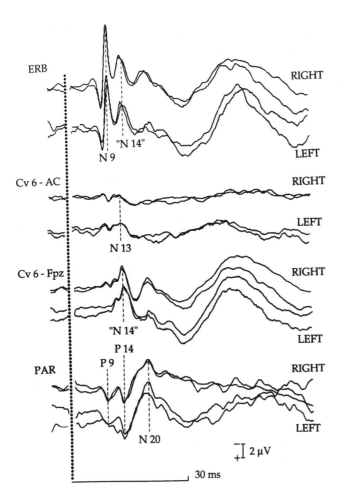

Figure 54.15. Absence of the segmental cervical N13 potential with preserved cervical cord conduction in a case of syringomyelia. This figure illustrates the fact that when the P14 and N20 upper limb SEPs are preserved in intramedullary lesions, the absence of the segmental N13, which is evident in cervical transverse derivation Cv6-AC, is masked in Cv6-Fz recordings due to injection of the scalp P14 potential as an N14 negativity in scalp Fpz reference derivations (Erb and Cv6-Fpz).

1981; Yu and Jones, 1985). Globally these first reports demonstrated abnormalities of median and/or tibial nerve SEPs in about 50% of patients with cervical myelopathy. In spite of differences in recording methods and patients selection, authors converged on the opinion that lower limb stimulation is more effective than upper limb stimulation to disclose abnormalities of central somatosensory conduction in such patients (Perlik and Fischer, 1987; Stöhr et al., 1982; Yu and Jones, 1985). In one study only ulnar nerve SEPs were reported as more sensitive than either median or tibial nerve SEPs in this pathology (Veilleux and Daube, 1987).

The recording of the segmental N13 spinal potential, using an anterior cervical reference electrode, was shown to increase the sensitivity of upper limb SEPs for detecting DH dysfunction in cervical spondylotic myelopathy (Restuccia et al., 1992). Restuccia et al. (1994) reported 84%, 93%, and 65% of N13 abnormality in median, radial, and ulnar nerves SEPs, respectively (Fig. 54.16). In a nonnegligible number

of patients SEP abnormalities are observed in the absence of direct MRI evidence of cord narrowing or of intramedullary hyperintense T2 signal (Berthier et al., 1996). Narrowing of the cervical cord diameter and presence of increased signal intensity on T2-weighted images of the cervical cord are considered as reliable MRI criteria to select candidates to surgical decompression (see Braakman, 1994, for a review). Nevertheless, the relation among MRI abnormalities of the cervical cord, the severity of the myelopathy, and the postoperative outcome remains questionable. Neither narrowing of the cord diameter nor increased intramedullary T2 signal is necessarily associated with median nerve SEP signs of cervical cord dysfunction. However, prolonged CCT after stimulation of the lower limbs is observed in more than two thirds of these patients, so that by combining median and tibial nerve stimulation most of patients with such severe MRI abnormalities have abnormal SEPs. Thus the practical utility of median and tibial nerve SEP recording is definitely more obvious in patients without MRI evidence of a cervical cord lesion due to compression. In more than 60% of these patients, signs of cervical cord dysfunction can be disclosed by SEP recordings (Berthier et al., 1996).

Amyotrophic Lateral Sclerosis (ALS)

SEPs are not indicated as a routine diagnostic procedure in ALS. However, several authors have reported central SEP abnormalities in ALS including abnormal central conduction and/or amplitude reduction of cortical SEPs (Anziska and Cracco, 1983; Bosch et al., 1985; Cosi et al., 1984; Dasheiff et al., 1985; Georgesco et al., 1994; Radtke et al., 1986; Subramian and Yannikas, 1990; Zanette et al., 1990, 1995). These findings were not confirmed by others (Mattheson et al., 1983; Matthews, 1980; Oken and Chiappa, 1986). Abnormal SEPs in a patient with clinical signs of motor neuron disease are expected in various diseases that may mimic ALS, where peripheral or central somatosensory pathways can be affected, such as spondylotic myelopathy, lymphoma, AIDS, paraneoplastic syndromes, and monoclonal paraproteinemia. Abnormal central conduction SEPs are more surprising in the idiopathic form of ALS where the dorsal columns, somatosensory thalamic relays, and SI granular cell layers are known to be spared. Reduced cortical response to tibial nerve stimulation is the most consistent SEP abnormality reported in ALS. Zanette et al. (1996) observed it in 22 of 29 ALS patients, whereas tibial nerve SEPS were unaffected in ten progressive muscular atrophy (PMA) patients. Reduced cortical tibial nerve SEPs could be related to axonal loss in muscle afferent fibers. However, this explanation does not hold for lower limb SEP abnormalities as reported by Georgesco et al. (1997) in response to stimulation of cutaneous nerves such as sural, saphenous internus, and medial plantar nerves. Other proposed explanations for tibial nerve SEPs abnormalities are a neuronal loss in the somatosensory cortex that may selectively affect the generators of the cortical SEPs to lower limb stimulation, or a perturbation of the control exerted by the motor cortex over the subcortical sensory relays and somatosensory cortex.

At the upper limb some authors reported a selective loss or abnormality of the central P22 potential to median nerve stimulation, suggesting, on the assumption that P22 is gen-

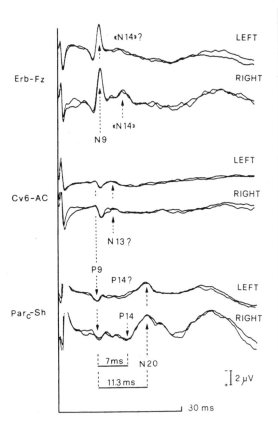

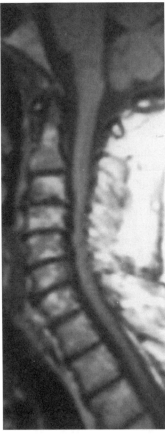

Figure 54.16. Absence of the segmental N13 with impaired cervical cord conduction in a case of spondylotic myelopathy. In this patient the segmental N13 is reduced and the brainstem P14 reduced and delayed, with prolonged CCT on both sides. (From Restuccia, D., Valeriani, M., Di Lazzaro, V., et al. 1994. Somatosensory evoked potentials after multisegmental upper limb stimulation in the diagnosis of cervical spondylotic myelopathy. J. Neurol. Neurosurg. Psychiatry 57:301–308, with permission.)

erated in Brodmann's area 4, that this abnormality might reflect the loss of pyramidal cells in the motor area (Zanette et al., 1990). This view was reinforced by some correlation between SEP abnormalities and the severity or the stage in the evolution of the disease, which is not unanimously accepted.

Lesions of the Cervicomedullary Junction

When the volley of impulses ascending in the cervical dorsal columns is blocked or dispersed at the cervicomedullary junction, the segmental N13 potential to upper limb stimulation is normal, whereas far-field P14 and later components are absent or abnormal (Mauguière et al., 1983c; Yamada et al., 1986). The lower limb P39 SEP is most often abnormal, but can be preserved in association with severe upper limb SEP abnormalities (Mauguière and Ibañez, 1985); this occurs when the lesion compresses only the outer dorsal column fibers. When the P39 potential is abnormal an absent or delayed, P30 is consistently observed (Tinazzi et al., 1996b). This cervicomedullary pattern (Mauguière, 1987) has no etiological specificity.

Brainstem Lesions

Upper limb P14 and N18 potentials and lower limb P30 are generated close to the dorsal columns nuclei in the medulla oblongata. Therefore, these components are clearly reduced, delayed, or absent in lesions of the medulla oblongata affecting somatosensory input transmission at this level. Conversely, they are preserved in most patients with pontine or mesencephalic lesions. When not completely canceled the P14 potential is delayed and the P9/P14 amplitude ratio is abnormally high in such patients. This pattern combining normal spinal N13 potential with absent or clearly abnormal P14 and cortical SEPs is similar to that observed in upper cervical cord lesions (see above). It can be observed in any destructive (Mauguière et al., 1983c) or compressive (Mauguière and Ibañez, 1985) lesion of this region as well as in brain dead patients (Anziska and Cracco, 1980, 1981). Interruption of the spinothalamic tract in medulla oblongata (Wallenberg's syndrome) does not modify P14 and N20 potentials (Halliday and Wakefield, 1963). More than 50% of patients with a lesion located in the pons or in the cerebral peduncles have a reduced or absent N20 after median nerve stimulation, and in most of them the P14 and N18 potentials are normal. Thus, apart from the unequivocal signification of the cervicomedullary pattern, there is no SEP pattern specific of focal upper brainstem lesions. The behavior of the P30 potential evoked by lower limb stimulation is the same as that of the median nerve P14 in brainstem lesions (Tinazzi and Mauguière, 1995; Tinazzi et al., 1996b).

Thalamic, Capsulothalamic, and Cortical Lesions

In our series of 241 patients with a focal hemispheric lesion documented by neuroimaging (Mauguière and Ibañez,

1990) SEPs to median nerve stimulation were abnormal in more than 70% of capsulothalamic and in nearly 90% of posterior thalamic lesions. After stimulation of the affected side, amplitude reduction or loss of both parietal N20-P27 and frontal P22-N30 potentials with preserved scalp far-field positivities including P14 represents the most frequent SEP abnormality in thalamic or capsular lesions interrupting the somatosensory pathways (Graff-Radford et al., 1985; Mauguière and Ibañez, 1990; Mauguière et al., 1982, 1983b; Nakanishi et al., 1978; Stöhr et al., 1983; Yamada et al., 1985). The N18 potential persists in this condition in noncephalic reference recordings (Mauguière et al., 1983b). Reduced or absent parietal N20-P27 SEPs are highly correlated with astereognosis and reduced touch and joint sensation.

Normal early cortical SEPs are consistently recorded in association with normal touch and joint sensation in patients with an anterior thalamic infarction or with a small posterior thalamic lesion sparing the VPL nucleus. Conversely, in the capsulothalamic lesions there are a few patients whose parietal SEPs are normal in spite of impaired joint position or tactile sensations. The reverse situation, i.e., normal sensation with reduced parietal SEP, may also occur in capsulothalamic lesions, suggesting that the cortex is able to compensate for the effects of partial deafferentation due to subcortical lesions. There is no simple relation between thalamic pain and deafferentation of area S1 as evidenced by loss of SEP primary cortical components (Mauguière and Desmedt, 1988). In patients with pure thalamic ischemic stroke there is a fairly good correlation between SEPs and neuroimaging data. Early cortical SEPs, including the N20, P22, P27, N30, and P45 components, are consistently absent or abnormal in posterolateral infarctions of the geniculothalamic artery territory with loss of touch and position sense. Conversely, they are normal in infarctions in other thalamic arterial territories. In capsular infarcts in the territory of anterior choroid artery or in thalamocapsular hematomas there is no such a clear correlation between neuroimaging data and SEP findings. In these patients the degree of hemispheric somatosensory deafferentation cannot be accurately predicted from CT scan or MRI images. Selective loss of frontal or parietal SEPs are infrequently observed in capsulothalamic lesions (Mauguière and Desmedt, 1991).

In large cortical lesions involving the central and parietal areas SEP abnormalities are very similar to those encountered in posterior thalamic lesions deafferenting the hemisphere, showing a loss of all cortical SEPs with preserved P14 and N18 potentials. In lesions situated outside the centroparietal area early cortical SEPs are normal. Most the patients showing dissociated loss of parietal N20-P27 or frontal P22-N30 potentials have cortical lesions (Fig. 54.17). In the 109 patients with cortical lesions of our series (Mauguière and Ibañez, 1990) there was a highly significant correlation between abnormal SEPs and the presence of sensory and/or motor deficits. When elementary touch and joint sensation is preserved astereognosis of the hand opposite to the cortical lesion is consistently associated with abnormal N20 and/or P27 abnormality (Mauguière et al., 1983a). Conversely, precentral lesions eliminating specifically the P22 component are usually associated to central hemiparesis (Mauguière et al., 1983a; Slimp et al., 1986). Abnormal frontal SEPs were

also reported during surgical monitoring of carotid endarterectomy (Gigli et al., 1987) and after a transient ischemic attack (de Weerd and Veldhuizen, 1987).

Less than 10% of patients with focal hemispheric lesions present with dissociated abnormalities of frontal and parietal early cortical SEPs showing either reduced or absent N20-P27 with preserved P22-N30, or the reverse (Mauguière and Ibañez, 1990). This suggests that parietal and frontal SEPs may have distinct generators activated via direct and distinct thalamocortical pathways. When N20 or P27 is lost, patients with cortical lesions usually show no motor deficit but astereognosis, eventually combined with hypesthesia for some elementary sensory modalities. Conversely, sensations are preserved and motoricity impaired in patients with absent or grossly abnormal P22 or N30.

As for cortical lesions, contralateral hypesthesia and astereognosis are commonplace in patients with a thalamocapsular lesion and a selective abnormality of N20-P27 SEPs. However, these patients may also be hemiparetic, or hemiplegic, in spite of persisting frontal P22-N30 SEPs due to interruption of the efferent motor pathways. Patients with a selective loss of frontal P22-N30 SEPs in relation to a subcortical lesion present with various types of motor deficits including hemiplegia, ataxic hemiparesis, and motor neglect, while somatic sensations are usually fairly preserved.

Prognostic Significance of SEPs in Stroke

Some experimental studies have shown that recovery is better when early SEPs remained unaffected during middle cerebral artery occlusion in monkeys (Branston et al., 1976). Several investigators reported a better functional prognosis in stroke patients with persistence or early recovery of cortical SEPs (Crespi et al., 1982; La Joie et al., 1982). However, De Weerd and co-workers (1985) reported that only one patient out of 18 with minor cerebral ischemia achieved complete SEP recovery in spite of good clinical evolution.

Giant SEPs

Since the first description by Dawson in 1947, it has been known that giant SEPs can occur in association with the cortical reflex myoclonus observed in progressive myoclonic epilepsies (PME) and with focal motor seizures in lesions of the perirolandic area (Dawson, 1947; Ikeda et al., 1995; Kakigi and Shibasaki, 1987; Mauguière and Courjon, 1980; Mauguière et al., 1981; Obeso et al., 1985; Rothwell et al., 1984; Seyal, 1995; Shibasaki and Kuroiwa, 1975; Shibasaki et al., 1985a,b; Valeriani et al., 1997a,b).

The giant SEP in PME was first described as a P25-N33 complex by Shibasaki and Kuroiwa (1975), the amplitude of which, when measured from peak to peak, can reach 50 μV or more and is usually of more than 15 μV (Fig. 54.18). Giant SEPs show a large degree of inter- and intraindividual variation; nevertheless, most PME patients with cortical myoclonus show a parietal positive and frontal negative dipolar field peaking at about 25 msec contralateral to median nerve stimulation. Jerk-locked back averaging the EEG prior to the myoclonus shows that spontaneous myoclonus can be associated with an abnormal cortical spike in some patients with cortical myoclonus (Shibasaki and Kuroiwa, 1975).

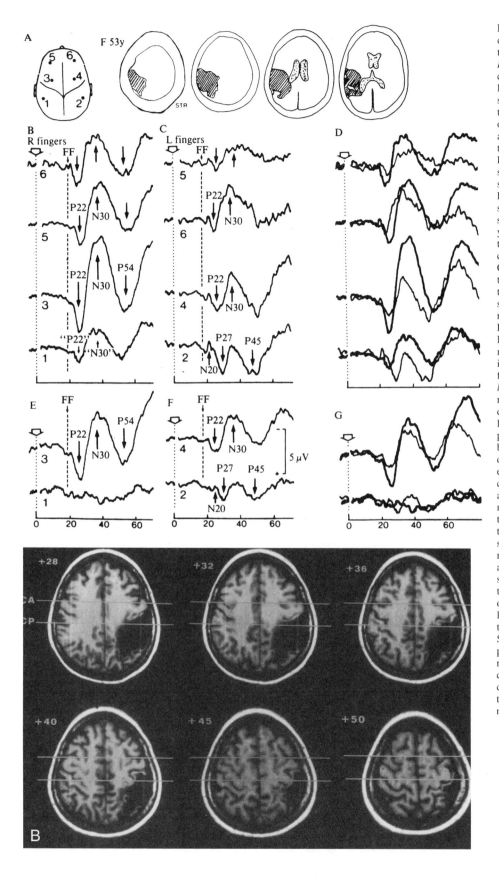

Figure 54.17. The paradigmatic case of dissociated loss of parietal SEPs. These traces are those of case 10 published in *Brain* by Mauguière et al. (1983a) recorded 5 years after a complete ischemic lesion of the left parietal lobe. These responses were obtained after stimulation of the second and third fingers at an intensity of three times the sensory threshold in **B** and **C**, and at the sensory threshold intensity of the normal side in **E** and **F**. Responses of normal and damaged hemispheres, at the two stimulus intensities, are superimposed in **D** and **G**. Parietal N20, P27, and P45 potentials are definitely absent, and frontal P22 and N30 clearly preserved, over the damaged side. Seven years after this recording a brain MRI of this patient was performed in the anterior commissure-posterior commissure (CA-CP) stereotactic planes and showed that the postrolandic cortex, situated between the CA and CP lines in all illustrated slices, is entirely damaged (the left side is represented on the right in MRI slices). Furthermore, the lesion extended far below the lower illustrated MRI slice (+28 mm) in the posterior white matter of the internal capsule and corona radiata. Therefore, there is no doubt that *in this particular patient* the SEPs recorded in the frontal region of the damaged left hemisphere cannot be generated in the left parietal lobe. This case remains unique because the parietal branches of the left middle cerebral artery had been selectively, and accidentally, obstructed during intracarotidian embolization of a malformation of the occipital branch of the left external carotid artery, producing a lesion that is almost never encountered in spontaneous infarctions. In spite of the large ischemic area, this patient was not hemiplegic but presented with a complete anesthesia of her right side. On verbal instruction she was also able to locate approximately tactile stimulations applied on her right anesthetic side; the "blind-touch" phenomenon of this patient has been reported by Paillard et al. (1983) independently of, but in the same year as, our publication of her SEP recordings. The existence of large prerolandic responses in this patient can result from synaptic reorganization of the cortical circuitry long after the stroke and does not necessarily imply that short latency responses are generated in the prerolandic cortex of normal subjects.

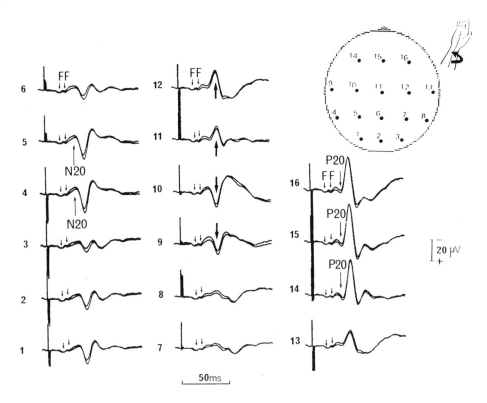

Figure 54.18. Scalp topography of giant SEPs in a case of progressive myoclonic epilepsy. The giant response *(bold arrows)* has a clear dipolar field distribution and shows a phase reversal in the central region contralateral to stimulation with a voltage gradient over 50 μV between the two extrema. This aspect is quite different from that of giant SEPs illustrated in Fig. 54.17. Note that the far-field P9 and P14 and the N20 parietal potentials have normal amplitudes. (From Mauguière F. 1995. Evoked potentials. In *Clinical Neurophysiology: EMG, Nerve Conduction and Evoked Potentials*, Eds. J.W. Osselton, C.D. Binnie, R. Cooper, et al., pp. 325–563. Oxford: Butterworth-Heinemann, with permission.)

The interval between the peak of P25 or the back-averaged cortical spike and the onset of the myoclonus is in the order of 20 msec in the arm, consistent with rapid conduction from motor cortex to muscle down to a direct corticospinal pathway. This observation suggests that giant SEPs and myoclonus-related spikes reflect a cortical hyperexcitability to afferent impulses (pyramidal myoclonus of Halliday, 1967), in these patients.

When identifiable the parietal N20 potential to median nerve stimulation has normal latency and amplitude in most patients with cortical myoclonus (Mauguière et al., 1981; Obeso et al., 1985; Rothwell et al., 1984; Shibasaki et al., 1985a). Similarly, P14 is normal in such patients (Mauguière et al., 1981). The normal size of the N20 component indicates that the sensory input into the cortex as well as the primary cortical response itself are not grossly abnormal. It has been suggested on the basis of waveform decomposition and computerized modeling that the giant SEP results from an abnormal enhancement of certain components of the normal SEPs (Shibasaki et al., 1990). This has been confirmed by dipole modeling showing that the scalp distribution of both normal and giant SEPs can be explained by the same cortical sources and suggesting that giant SEPs mostly reflect an enhanced response of the N24-P24 generator in area 3b (Valeriani et al., 1997a). Enhanced cortical response to proprioceptive inputs can be observed in some of the PME patients with giant median nerve SEPs, in association with exaggerated EMG response to passive movements (Mima et al., 1997). Thus cortical hyperresponses to either cutaneous inputs alone or to both cutaneous (area 3b) and proprioceptive (areas 3a or 2) inputs can occur in PME with cortical re-

flex myoclonus. The various combinations of these two abnormalities, in terms of amplitude, may account for the waveform variations reported in the early literature on this topic.

Intravenously (IV) injected benzodiazepines reduce spontaneous myoclonus and reflex muscle jerking, but their effect on giant SEPs is a matter of controversy. Both reduction (Mauguière and Courjon, 1980; Shibasaki et al., 1985a) and paradoxical enhancement (Rothwell et al., 1984) of SEPs have been reported under the effect of benzodiazepines.

Giant SEPs can be recorded in the absence of myoclonus-related spikes and vice versa. Thus patients who apparently have similar clinical symptoms can show different SEP abnormalities. Complete electrophysiological investigation of patients with myoclonus includes jerk-locked EEG averaging (Shibasaki and Kuroiwa, 1975), conventional SEP recordings to median nerve, and finger stimulation and the recording of the long latency myogenic reflex activity (C reflex) to median nerve stimulation, which reflects the myoclonus itself. Shibasaki et al. (1985a) proposed to classify myoclonus in four subtypes according to electrophysiological data: Type I is the above-described pyramidal myoclonus. In type II giant SEPs are absent and myoclonus-related spike is present, suggesting that myoclonus is not triggered by hyperexcitability of the sensorimotor cortex to afferent inputs. In type III only giant SEPs are present, presumably because the epileptic discharge causing the myoclonic jerk is generated in deep cortical layers and has no recordable scalp correlates. In type IV both giant SEPs and jerk-locked spikes are absent, and the efferent impulses generating myoclonus in response to afferent inputs might be generated in subcortical reticular structures; this type could correspond to the reticular reflex myoclonus of Hallett et al. (1977).

Not all of the patients with myoclonus have giant SEPs. In particular, enhanced SEPs are usually not observed in benign forms of juvenile myoclonic epilepsies and in essential nonprogressive isolated myoclonus. They are inconstant in Creutzfeldt-Jakob disease and posthypoxic myoclonus. In the two latter conditions the existence of giant SEPs probably depends on the evolutive stage of the disease. Conversely, giant SEPs are an almost constant feature in the various forms of PME. At the end of the evolution, the amplitude of SEPs may decrease and even return to normal range in PMEs, and a moderate increase of early scalp SEP components (about 30% more than mean values in controls) can be observed (Mervaala et al., 1984).

Giant SEPs can also be observed over the damaged hemisphere in patients with supratentorial tumors, posttraumatic cortical atrophies, or long after an ischemic or hemorrhagic stroke (Furlong et al., 1993; Laget et al., 1967; Valeriani et al., 1997b). In these patients the enhancement of the cortical response is often less than that observed in PME patients with cortical reflex myoclonus. Loss of inhibitory control and postlesional collateral sprouting of cortical afferents could be responsible for such SEP abnormalities. Various components of the normal cortical SEP waveform can be increased and the resulting aspect often differs from that of the giant P25-N33 observed in cortical myoclonus (Fig. 54.19). A selective increase of a N20-P22 deflection strictly localized in the central region was reported in a patient with a rolandic tumor (Valeriani et al., 1997b). The scalp topography of this abnormal response was compatible with a dipolar source radial to the scalp surface, and interpreted as an abnormal response of Brodmann's area 3a, which is known to receive proprioceptive inputs from muscle afferents. In focal lesions, giant SEPs are often observed in the absence of myoclonus triggered by somatosensory stimuli, but the occurrence of focal motor seizures is frequent in the history of such patients.

In some children aged 3 to 13 years with normal neurological status, vertex and parietal EEG spikes, corresponding to high-voltage SEPs (up to 400 μV), can be evoked by a single tactile stimulation (De Marco and Negrin, 1973). The presence of these "extreme SEPs" might forecast the possible occurrence of partial motor seizures with benign outcome (De Marco and Tassinari, 1981). Median nerve cortical SEPs in these children are usually normal up to a latency of 60 msec and then show a large central negativity, which reaches its maximum only for low stimulation frequencies of 0.2 to 0.5 Hz (Plasmati et al., 1989). "Extreme SEPs" were shown to have the same scalp topography and modeled source as spontaneous rolandic spikes in children with benign rolandic epilepsy (Manganotti et al., 1998a,b).

Multiple Sclerosis (MS) and Central Demyelination

Historically SEPs have been the first evoked responses tested in MS patients (Namerow, 1968). The main effect of central demyelination is to slow down the conduction and thus to increase the time dispersion of impulses in the dorsal columns, medial lemniscus, and thalamocortical fibers. Abnormal SEPs are thus very similar, whatever the causal phenomenon of demyelination, and are frequently observed in the absence of any sensory symptoms. By providing a quan-

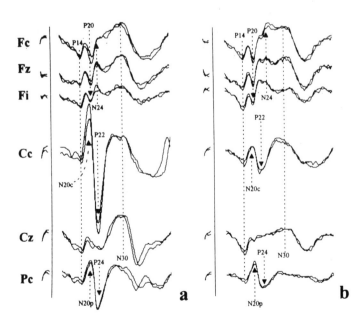

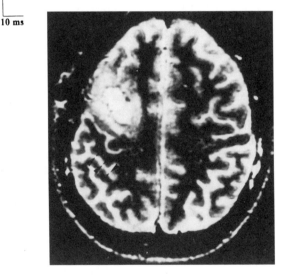

Figure 54.19. Giant SEPs in a case of right frontal astrocytoma without cortical myoclonus. SEPs to right median nerve stimulation *(right column)* have normal amplitudes and topography. After left median nerve stimulation SEPs show normal N20 and P24 potentials in the parietal region contralateral to stimulation (Pc) and normal P20, N24, and N30 potentials in the frontal region (Fi, frontal ipsilateral to stimulation; Fc, frontal contralateral to stimulation). The abnormal giant response has a topography restricted to the central region contralateral to stimulation (Cc). (From Valeriani, M., Restuccia, D., Di Lazzaro V, et al. 1997b. Giant central N20-P22 with normal area 3b N20-P20: an argument in favor of an area 3a generator of early median nerve cortical SEPs? Electroencephalogr. Clin. Neurophysiol. 104:60–67, with permission.)

titative index of central conduction that can be periodically reassessed, SEPs, like all other types of EPs, are useful in all situations where a functional follow-up of the disease is requested, including long-term therapeutic trials of new pharmacological agents.

Types of SEP Abnormalities

The most frequent SEP abnormality in MS is the latency increase or absence of the P39 component evoked by tibial nerve stimulation, which is observed in a majority of SEP-abnormal MS patients (Slimp et al., 1990; Trojaborg and Petersen, 1979), followed by delayed or absent P14 and N20 potentials to median nerve stimulation. Latency abnormalities are associated with prolonged CCT, and peripheral SEPs are normal in central demyelination (see Chiappa, 1990, and Halliday, 1993, for a review). Amplitude reduction of the scalp P14 potential, as evaluated by measuring the P9/P14 amplitude ratio in scalp to shoulder traces, is observed in more than 90% of MS patients with abnormal SEPs (Garcia-Larrea and Mauguière, 1988; Yamada et al., 1986). SEP abnormalities can be uni- or bilateral, and, when unilateral, may concern only one limb. The frequency of abnormal SEPs is maximal when the four limbs are tested and increases by less than 10% by testing the upper limb when tibial SEPs are normal.

Absent or reduced cervical response after median nerve stimulation in neck to front recordings is widely accepted as a frequent finding in MS. This is a priori rather surprising since a N13 reduction would suggest that the postsynaptic DH response is dispersed because of demyelination at the root entry zone in a nonnegligible number of MS patients. In fact, noncephalic reference recording of the cervical responses in MS patients (Garcia-Larrea and Mauguière, 1988) shows that reduction of spinal N13 is infrequent and that in most instances amplitude abnormality of the cervical negativity results from reduction of the P14 potential, which, in a neck to front derivation, is injected as a negativity in the cervical response.

SEP Scores in MS

A first approach to evaluate the diagnostic yield of SEPs in MS consists of calculating the frequency of uni- or bilateral abnormalities according to the different diagnostic classes of MS. Clinical criteria of MS classification vary according to the author, but those first proposed by McAlpine et al. (see Matthews et al., 1985, for a review) are the most widely accepted to evaluate the hit rates of paraclinical tests. SEP scores increase according to the diagnostic classes from possible to definite MS, from 49% to 77% in the review of published series by Chiappa (1990), and from 55% to 70% in the series from our department (Fischer et al., 1986). These figures show that, in spite of laboratory differences in the recording procedures, there is a consensus as to the frequency of SEP abnormalities in MS. Due to the high frequency of progressive paraparetic forms of the disease in the probable MS class and to the high sores of SEPs in this category of patients, the difference between probable and definite MS is less pronounced for SEPs than for other types of EPs.

SEPs may be abnormal in the absence of any clinical somatosensory sign as well as in patients with chronic MS who have never experienced symptoms referable to the sensory system. Conversely, SEPs may be normal in nearly one fourth of patients with sensory complaints or abnormal sensory findings at clinical examination. In that respect, SEPs differ from other EPs that are exceptionally normal in symptomatic patients. This finding reflects the fact that SEPs do not explore all of the somatosensory pathways but preferentially the dorsal column system. It is not uncommon in clinical routine to record normal SEPs during a relapse with somatosensory signs, and this finding must not lead to questioning the organicity of patient's complaints or to discarding the diagnosis of MS.

Several early studies (Bartel et al., 1983; Chiappa, 1990; Fischer et al., 1986; Kjaer, 1987; Purves et al., 1981) converged on the global conclusion that SEPs are less profitable than visual evoked potential (VEPs) when searching for silent demyelination in MS. Score differences among studies mostly reflect differences in patient selection, and the fact that clinically silent lesions, which do not reveal a dissemination of lesions and thus do not contribute in diagnostic clarification, are not considered in some of them.

SEPs Versus MRI

Brain and spinal cord MRI have proved to be, in many clinical situations, more sensitive than EPs for the detection of clinically silent zones of abnormal signal intensity in the CNS of patients with suspected MS. Therefore, the diagnostic utility of EPs at the early stage of the disease has become questionable. The use of MRI is limited by high installation and operative costs as compared with the ease and speed with which EP testing can be carried out. This can be taken as an argument to use EPs as a screening test to select among patients with purely subjective symptoms those in whom MRI should be performed. One can predict, however, that in a near future a high proportion of these patients will be referred for EP testing after that brain MRI has been done. The introduction of MRI has thus dramatically modified the role of EP testing at the early stage of the disease, which is now done more to assess the organicity of subjective symptoms and to follow up the course of the disease than to detect lesion dissemination when MRI is abnormal. SEPs are also useful in screening the many patients consulting the neurologist for paresthesias or sensation of numbness in one limb compatible with CNS dysfunction, in whom the clinical examination is uninformative or unconvincing. Moreover, it must be noted that MRI abnormal signals in the white matter reflect increased water content of the tissue and not demyelination per se and are not specific of MS, but this limitation in specificity also applies to EP abnormalities.

Published series reviewed by Halliday (1993) converge to the conclusion that brain MRI discloses abnormal signals in more than 80% of MS patients. There is little doubt that brain MRI is superior to EPs in detecting silent lesions in patients with clinical evidence of isolated optic neuritis, brainstem, or cord lesions. As a confirmatory test MRI is also more efficient than EPs in detecting the lesion itself except in patients with clinically isolated optic neuritis or thoracolumbar syndrome. In 1987 Miller et al. showed that tibial nerve SEPs detected CCT abnormalities in nearly 70% of patients with signs of thoracolumbar cord dysfunction, while brain and spinal cord MRI failed at that time to detect any lesion in 70% of them. The progress of MRI technique has already increased the impact of MRI in detecting small lesions in the cord and brainstem and has overcome this limitation (Comi et al., 1987).

In spite of these converging arguments in support of MRI as being helpful in diagnosing MS in a larger percentage of doubtful cases than is EP recording, one study concluded that there was no difference in diagnostic rates between brain MRI without contrast injection and brain CT scan with contrast injection plus VEPs, BAEPs, and SEPs (O'Connor et al., 1994). This study also showed that median plus tibial nerve SEPs were more often abnormal (49.5%) than pattern reversal VEPs (38.2%) and BAEPs (22.4%), and that multimodal EPs showed abnormalities suggestive of MS diagnosis in nearly 10% of patients with suspected MS and normal brain MRI.

Predictive Value of EP Abnormalities

The predictive value of EP abnormalities recorded early in the course of the disease has been evaluated in studies where SEPs were part of a multimodality EP evaluation including VEPs and BAEPs. There is some evidence that among patients whose EPs are recorded when the diagnosis of MS can only be suspected, those in whom multimodality EPs disclose a silent lesion have more chances to develop MS than those with normal EPs. The early study by Deltenre et al. (1982) demonstrated that in patients with suspected MS at the beginning of a 4-year follow-up study, multimodal EPs (including VEPs, median and peroneal nerves SEPs, BAEPs, and blink reflexes) disclosed a silent lesion in 82% (36/44) of the patients who were classified as definite MS at the end of the study, but in only 19% (12/64) of those in whom the diagnosis of MS remained pending. This was confirmed in a smaller group by Matthews et al. (1982), using VEPs, BAEPs, and SEPs in patients with possible MS. Deltenre et al. (1984) reported data from multimodal EP recordings in 273 patients with suspected MS, of whom 171 completed the trial after a mean follow-up period of 80 ± 38 months. The diagnostic of MS became definite in 56 patients, of whom 86% had diagnostic EP abnormality (i.e., disclosing a silent lesion) at the beginning of the trial. Diagnostic EP abnormalities were distributed as follows: VEPs, 66%; SEPs, 23%; and BAEPs, 12.5%, thus confirming the superiority of pattern reversal VEPs over SEPs in the diagnosis of the disease. Hume and Waxman (1988) confirmed this finding in a group of 222 patients with suspected MS followed up for an average of 32 months (12–55 months). Nearly 50% of patients who were reclassified as definite MS at the end of the study had diagnostic EP abnormalities at the first test, whereas the diagnosis of definite MS was firmly assessed in only 4% of those who had normal EPs at the first test. In this study diagnostic abnormalities were also observed more frequently for pattern reversal VEPs than for SEPs or BAEPs, and more patients with abnormal VEPs than with abnormal SEPs had deteriorated on follow-up.

Confirmatory and Localizing Value of SEP Abnormalities

Besides their utility as indicators of multifocal clinically silent lesions, EPs are often useful to assess the organicity of poorly reliable or unspecific "soft" symptoms. EPs then represent a confirmatory test aiming at detecting the lesion itself and not lesions elsewhere than in the area suspected of being affected. For this purpose only, abnormal EPs have an absolute diagnostic value.

Whatever the result of brain MRI, SEP abnormalities after stimulation of the symptomatic limb will ascertain that symptoms are related to a conduction abnormality in the central somatosensory pathways. SEPs also help to determine the site of abnormal conduction in MS and to correlate it with clinical symptoms or MRI data. By combining MRI and SEPs it has been confirmed that the most frequent site of dispersed conduction in the somatosensory pathways of the upper limb is the dorsal columns of the cervical cord (Turano et al., 1991).

Adrenoleukodystrophy

Adrenoleukodystrophy (ALD) is a peroxisomal disorder caused by an abnormal gene localized in the Xq28 area, which shows variable clinical features, from severe cerebral symptoms in childhood to progressive peripheral and spinal symptoms in adults (adrenomyeloneuropathy). SEPs have proved their usefulness in detecting subclinical abnormalities of the segmental N13 cervical potential or of CCT in 12 of 19 ALD carriers, which represent the largest series hitherto reported in the literature (Restuccia et al., 1997).

Coma

Interpretation of SEPs in deeply comatose patients must take into account the combined effects of hypothermia and CNS depressant drugs. Hypothermia increases CCT, with a linear relation between the two parameters between 35° and 40°C and an exponential relation below 35°C (Guérit et al., 1990; Hume and Cant, 1981). The use of CNS depressant drugs has considerably increased for the past 20 years in intensive care units (ICUs), in particular that of intravenous barbiturate perfusion, which depresses the EEG activity and brainstem reflexes. Fortunately, short-latency SEPs are rather resistant to barbiturate anesthesia and remains within normal limits in this condition (Drummond et al., 1985; Ganes and Lundar, 1983; Hume and Cant, 1981; Sutton et al., 1982). However, transient SEP latency increases can be observed after injection of barbiturates, which should not be misinterpreted as signs of neurological deterioration when observed in the course of continuous SEP monitoring (Drummond et al., 1985; McPherson et al., 1986; Sutton et al., 1982).

Most SEP studies in coma and brain death have been limited to short latency potentials peaking before 30 msec after stimulation of the median nerve. A review of series published between 1978 and 1988 concerning a total number of 690 patients demonstrated that a single recording of median nerve SEPs in the acute stage of a coma has some prognostic value as to the final outcome (see Mauguière et al., 1995). This review showed that the percentage of deaths or permanent vegetative stages (PVS) is of 90% when the cortical N20 is lost on both sides in head-injured or vascular brain-damaged comatose patients. In these two categories of patients the coma outcome is death, PVS. or severe disability, according to the Glasgow Outcome Scale (Jennett et al.,

1981) in 74% of cases when N20 is absent on one side, 58% when the CCT is increased, 35% when early cortical SEPs are normal on both sides, and in 14% when all cortical SEPs including middle- and late-latency responses are preserved. However, only repeated or serial recordings of SEPs, preferably in combination with recordings of early (BAEPs) and middle-latency auditory potentials, offers the possibility to monitor brainstem and cortical responses and to detect early changes related to deterioration of brainstem or cortical function.

The absence of all early cortical responses to median nerve stimulation on both sides with preserved peripheral N9 and cervical N13 potentials carries a prognosis of death or PVS in 90% of comas due to primary hemispheric lesions identifiable on neuroimaging investigations, and in almost 100% of postanoxic comas (Brunko and Zegers de Beyl, 1987). In this latter condition bilateral loss of the N20 potential heralds PVS more frequently than in posttraumatic or vascular lesions, in particular when associated with preserved BAEPs (Brunko and Zegers de Beyl, 1987; Frank et al., 1985). This SEP pattern has not the same prognostic value when the coma is caused by a primary brainstem lesion, which can interrupt ascending somatosensory pathways or in noncomatose patients presenting with a locked-in syndrome, which, in addition to motor de-efferentation, can include interruption of somatosensory pathways when the lesions involve the tegmentum pontis. In comas due to primary brainstem lesions, moderate disability or good recovery, according to the Glasgow Outcome Scale, have been reported in patients with no recordable early cortical SEPs (Rumpl et al., 1983).

Furthermore, in the interpretation of absent cortical SEPs in a comatose patient whose past medical history is unknown, the possibility should not be overlooked of preexisting pathologies such as multiple sclerosis, heredodegenerative diseases, and Arnold-Chiari malformation, which may themselves lead to absence of N20, and eventually of P14. Logi et al. (2003) have recently reviewed the literature data published since 1984 on the prognostic value of SEPs in 1,818 patients. The positive predictive value of SEP parameters has been evaluated with regard to a bad outcome characterized by the absence of return to consciousness [Glasgow Outcome Scale scores 1 (death) and 2 (persistent vegetative state)], or to a favorable life outcome defined as a return to consciousness with or without disability (Glasgow Outcome Scale scores 3–5). Since neither SEP methodology nor criteria for estimation of clinical outcome are uniform across studies from different authors, the overall results presented are to be taken as a general indication. However, the data are so converging that the prognostic value of SEP recordings can be considered as firmly established. This study confirmed that the value of SEPs for predicting a bad outcome varies according to etiologies and must be analyzed separately in anoxia, which causes mostly diffuse cortical lesions, and in traumatic and vascular lesions that can affect directly the sensory pathways at the brainstem or subcortical levels. In postanoxic coma, all studies converge to a 100% specificity of bilateral N20 absence in predicting poor outcome in postanoxic comatose adult patients (Bassetti et al., 1996; Berek et al., 1995;

Brunko and Zegers de Beyl, 1987; Chen et al., 1996; Logi et al., 2003; Madl et al., 2000; Rothstein et al., 1991; Sherman et al., 2000; Walser et al., 1985). Logi et al. (2003) reported that a peak-to-peak N20-P24 amplitude value below 1.2 μV on both sides had the same prognostic value as bilateral N20 abolition in this group of patients.

In head-injured patients or those with vascular lesions, bilateral absence of N20 also carries a very pejorative prognosis with a predictive value for no return to consciousness in 90% to 100% of patients.

The loss of early cortical SEPs on one side only, with preserved P14 potential, does not provide by itself clear information concerning the vital prognosis in comatose patients with hemispheric traumatic or vascular lesions. Conversely, this pattern indicates a focal lesion of the parietal cortex or thalamic radiations; it is associated with a high incidence of severe sensorimotor lateralized disability in case of survival and usually persists long after the head injury (Jabbari et al., 1987). This SEP feature is quite exceptional in anoxic or metabolic comas (Brunko and Zegers de Beyl, 1987; Frank et al., 1985; Walser et al., 1985).

Increased CCT has been considered as predictive of severe coma outcome in the early SEP studies (Hume and Cant, 1981; Hume et al., 1979; Rumpl et al., 1983). However, 42% of head-injured comatose patients in whom a single SEP recording shows prolonged CCT completely recover or have a moderate disability. The fact that CCT is measurable implies that the N20 response is preserved and some difficulty may occur in identification of the cervical N13 potential, and thus in the measurement of the peak to peak N13-N20 CCT, in cervical to front recordings (see above). Long after recovery of coma in head-injured patients, it is rare to observe a prolonged CCT in the absence of other SEP abnormalities (Jabbari et al., 1987). This low incidence suggests that, contrary to the complete loss of early cortical SEPs, a prolonged CCT is often a reversible phenomenon as shown by repeated measurements in coma (Newlon et al., 1982; Rumpl et al., 1988b). An optimal use of CCT in coma would be to monitor this parameter continuously. Systems permitting a continuous of CCT have been described (Pfurtscheller et al., 1987) but have not yet come into routine use in ICUs.

The recording of normal N20 and early cortical responses in the acute phase of a coma does not provide any certitude of good recovery since only two thirds of these patients will have a good recovery, either complete or with minimal disability. This reflects the fact that contingent events during the course of the coma may worsen the final outcome. The recording of normal middle- and long-latency cortical SEPs increases to about 85% the chances of complete recovery (Greenberg et al., 1982; Pfurtscheller et al., 1985). One drawback is that these components are much more sensitive to CNS depressant drugs than early cortical responses.

Brain Death

Our concepts on the assessment of brain death have considerably evolved from the early clinical description of the "coma dépassé" (coma beyond coma) by Mollaret and Goulon in 1959, where the recording of an isoelectric EEG played a key role by showing the loss of thalamocortical rhythmic activity, toward the idea that the brain is dead when brainstem functions are irreversibly lost (see Pallis et al., 1990, for a review). Neuroimaging techniques now offer the possibility to assess, in comatose patients maintained in life by respiratory assistance, whether a focal brainstem or supratentorial lesion can be considered as responsible for this critical clinical condition. Normal images of the brain, however, can be obtained in the early stage of an irreversible brain damage such as that caused by acute anoxia. In a patient whose comatose state is directly related to an identified brain lesion, the absence of segmental brainstem reflexes tested by two experienced neurologists would be theoretically sufficient to ascertain brainstem death; after that any interference with depressant drug treatment has been definitely eliminated (Pallis, 1990). Such an ideal situation is not met in all instances, and objective proof of brain death has been steadily sought, since the very beginning of the intensive care history, to avoid the unacceptable risk of a false diagnosis of brain death based exclusively on a clinical report. Therefore, the pending question, which is more pragmatic than conceptual, is to identify the neurophysiological tests that are reliable enough to state that no activity persists in the CNS rostral to the foramen magnum, in all conditions where the diagnosis of brain death is at stake. In many ICUs the EEG and multimodal EPs including SEPs are routinely recorded for monitoring cerebral functions in deeply comatose patients, and the eventuality that brain death could be diagnosed without the help of confirmatory electrophysiological techniques is not envisaged.

The responsiveness of brainstem relays and primary somatosensory cortex can be assessed by the scalp recording of P14 and N20 potentials. In this clinical context the loss of cortical and brainstem SEPs is clinically relevant only after peripheral or spinal damage has been eliminated by the recording of normal peripheral N9 and spinal N13 potentials and appropriate neuroimaging investigations.

The disappearance of the P14 and N18 potentials in a comatose patients, whose N20 potentials are absent on both sides, indicates a dysfunction of the lower brainstem. Conversely the segmental spinal N13 can persist long after the P14 potential has disappeared in brainstem death (Fig. 54.20). Therefore, the median nerve SEP pattern of brainstem death consists of the persistence of the spinal N13 at the neck and of far-field P9 and P11 on the scalp, with absent P14, N18, and cortical responses (Anziska and Cracco, 1980). When interpreting SEPs in the context of brain death diagnosis, the possibility of a lesion at the cervicomedullary junction must be eliminated, since it can reproduce the SEP pattern observed in brain death (see above).

Recently, the question has been addressed of whether the later part of the P14 potential could reflect the activity of the medial lemniscal pathways at the upper brainstem level, while only the earlier part of this potential would be generated in the medulla oblongata. The P14 potential recorded several hours before clinical signs of brain death peaks later than the P14 positivity, which may persist after the clinical diagnosis of brain death (Buchner et al., 1988; Wagner, 1991, 1996). This observation suggests that by analyzing the P14 wave only in terms of presence or absence in deeply comatose patients, one overlooks the fact that the P14 deflec-

tion contains at least two distinct components, which overlap in time and produce the P13-P14 waveform when the brainstem somatosensory pathways are functioning normally. The P14 potential recorded between the scalp (Fz) and a nasopharyngeal electrode was shown to disappear in brain death, while it persists in non-brain-dead comatose patients (Wagner, 1991, 1996). It was thus proposed to consider the loss of this rostral P14 as an indicator of brainstem death even in patients whose scalp SEPs recorded with a noncephalic reference show a persisting positivity peaking at 13 to 14 msec. The utility of scalp to nasopharynx recordings of the rostral SEPs in brainstem death diagnosis warrants further validation.

The recording of the EEG, SEPs, and BAEPs is recommended as a confirmatory test of cerebral death in many countries; however, it has been questioned whether electrophysiological explorations are indispensable for the diagnosis of brain death on the following three arguments: (1) that the brain is dead when the brainstem is dead; (2) that "electrocerebral silence" does not demonstrate brainstem death, while clinical examination of brainstem reflexes does; (3) that the recording of SEPs and BAEPs is technically more demanding than the use of the EEG. The reservation that a

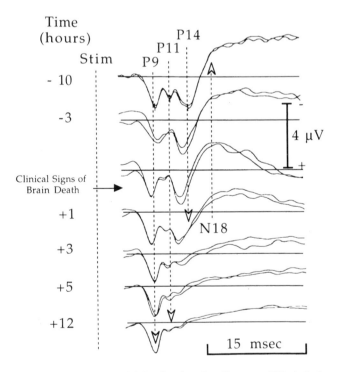

Figure 54.20. Rostrocaudal deterioration of median nerve SEPs in brain death. This figure shows that 1 hour after clinical diagnosis of brain death (time: +1) a P14 potential persists, with a shorter peaking latency than that of the P14 recorded before brain death (time: −10). This potential disappears later on (time: +3). The amplitude of the subcortical N18 potential decreases in parallel with that of the P14 potential. Three hours after clinical diagnosis of brain death, only the P9 (brachial plexus) and P11 (cervical cord) are recordable on the scalp. (Modified from Buchner H., Ferbert A., and Hacke, W. 1988. Serial recording of median nerve stimulated subcortical somatosensory evoked potentials (SEPs) in developing brain death. Electroencephalogr. Clin. Neurophysiol. 69:14–23.)

peripheral, cervical cord or brainstem pathology preexisting to that causing the coma can hamper the use of EPs also applies to the clinical testing of brainstem reflexes, which also have the disadvantage of being less resistant to anesthetic drugs than brainstem and early cortical SEPs. Any neurologist aware of the pitfalls of brainstem reflexes testing is able to interpret correctly SEP and BAEP abnormalities and will be helped in that by modern neuroimaging techniques. Therefore, the question is not whether EPs could replace clinical testing, but rather whether adding SEP and BAEP recording to the list of maneuvers used to assess brainstem function would increase the reliability of brainstem death diagnosis in the hands of an experienced practitioner. Our answer to this question, based on more than 10 years of a routine use of EPs in intensive care patients, is definitely positive.

Parkinson's Disease and Movement Disorders

Parkinson's Disease

Rossini et al. (1989) were the first to report a reduction of the frontal N30 median nerve SEP in patients with Parkinson's disease (PD), in association with parietal SEPs of normal amplitude. These authors hypothesized that the rigidity or akinesia of PD patients could be related to this SEP abnormality, which was confirmed after MPTP (1-methyl-4-phenyl 1,2,3,6-tetrahydropiridine) treatment in monkeys by the recording of the frontal N15, which is the homologue of the human N30 in monkeys (Onofrj et al., 1994). Statistical analysis of SEP topography showed that differences in temporal and power spectrum distributions of SEPs between normal subjects and PD patients are confined to frontal scalp areas (Babiloni et al., 1994). Moreover, the amplitude of the N30 potential was found to be inversely correlated with that of the second component (latency range 50–60 msec) of the long latency reflexes (LLRs) evoked by electrical stimulation of the median nerve (Rossini et al., 1991), which are commonly increased in PD. It has also been shown by Cheron et al. (1994) that, though reduced, the N30 potential in PD shows the same amplitude decrease as in normal subjects during voluntary finger movements, and that this gating effect is not modified by apomorphine, a dopamine receptors agonist.

There are, however, conflicting reports concerning attenuation of the frontal N30 potential in patients with PD. The N30 reduction was confirmed in two successive studies in 69% and 71% of PD patients (Rossini et al., 1993, 1995) emphasizing the utility of evaluating the decrease of the amplitude ratio between the frontal and parietal SEPs, the latter being preserved in such patients. Conversely, a reduced N30 was observed in only 32.5% of PD patients by Onofrj et al. (1995), with no clear relation between N30 amplitude and motor performances, and several authors failed to confirm this N30 reduction, either when comparing PD patients with normal subjects matched for age, or when comparing the SEPs to stimulation of the most affected side with those to stimulation of the less affected side in patients with hemiparkinsonism (Garcia et al., 1995; Huttunen and Teravainen, 1993; Mauguière et al., 1993). SEPs to median nerve stimulation have also been reported as normal in multiple system atrophy (Abbruzzese et al., 1997).

Another open question is whether the amplitude of the N30 potential actually correlates with motor performances in PD and could be used as an objective marker of the evolution state of the disease. Motor fluctuations with "off" periods of severe parkinsonian disability alternating with "on" periods of relative mobility marked by dyskinetic involuntary movements offer the possibility to address directly this question in test-retest studies in individual patients. "On" periods can be obtained by subcutaneous injection of apomorphine, which is an agonist of D1 and D2 dopamine receptors. The effects of subcutaneous apomorphine injection on the amplitude of the frontal N30 have been studied with controversial results. Rossini et al. (1993, 1995), Cheron et al. (1994), and Stanzione et al. (1997) reported a clear-cut and selective amplitude increase of N30 in association with clinical improvement, while other authors did not observe this effect on frontal SEPs, in spite of a clear improvement of motor performances (Mauguière et al., 1993). In line with this latter negative result, acute or chronic administration of L-dopa and bromocriptine did not modify the SEP amplitude in PD patients, in spite of positive clinical effects in the study by Onofrj et al. (1995). Differences in the severity of the disease between patients cohorts included in these studies may account for such divergences. Pierantozzi et al. (1999) provided the most recent evidence in favor of a link between N30 amplitude and motor performances in PD patients treated with deep brain stimulation of the internal globus pallidus or of the nucleus subthalamicus. These authors reported that during stimulation the N30 amplitude increases in correlation with the positive effects on motor abilities; conversely, after interruption of stimulation the N30 enhancement fades nearly in parallel with the clinical effects.

Dystonia

Abnormal central integration of afferent somatosensory inputs is, among others, a possible causative mechanism of dystonia (Hallett, 1995). The first report on SEPs in patients with focal or generalized dystonia is that of Reilly et al. (1992). These authors reported a selective increase of the N30 potential, which could reflect hyperactivity of the striatocortical loops. However, in this study, N30 abnormalities were similar after stimulation of either the affected or unaffected side in patients with unilateral dystonia. This result has been replicated by Kanovsky et al. (1997, 1998) in patients with spasmodic torticollis, but a decreased N30 has also been reported in this condition (Mazzini et al., 1994) and in patients with hand dystonia (Grissom et al., 1995). Tinazzi et al. (1999) reported an increase of tibial nerve P39 and N50 potentials that was unrelated to the severity of the disease and present on both sides in patients with unilateral dystonia. This finding can be interpreted as reflecting an abnormal central processing of somatosensory inputs related to increased excitability of the motor cortex and is quite coherent with the early findings of Reilly et al. (1992). This interpretation makes sense if one assumes that P39 and N50 are generated in the motor cortex, a view that is plausible (see above), and that the decreased activity in the putamen, which is the most commonly affected in secondary dystonia, increases the excitability of the motor cortex.

Responses to paired interfering stimuli have been studied recently by comparing the amplitudes of SEPs to simultaneous stimulation of the median and ulnar nerve on the same side with that of the sum of SEPs amplitudes after stimulation of each nerve individually. In normal subjects the former are smaller than the latter for N13, P14, N20, P27, and N30 potentials, while this does not occur for the peripheral N9 potential. This gating phenomenon, which can be interpreted as reflecting a central surround inhibition of incoming volleys from neighboring territories, was found to be less efficient in dystonic patients than in normal subjects (Tinazzi et al., 2000). This sensory overflow could play a role in the distortion of sensory and motor cortical maps of dystonic patients.

Abnormal movement related gating of SEPs has been carefully investigated in patients with writer's cramp using a reaction time paradigm (Murase et al., 2000). The main finding was that premovement gating of N24 and N30 frontal SEPs, usually observed in normal subjects with this paradigm, is lacking or reduced in patients with writer's cramp. This abnormality was identical in dystonic as well as in simple writer's cramp. Conversely, there was no difference in SEPs gating during voluntary movements between patients and normal subjects. These authors considered that, during movement preparation, changes in SEPs are due mainly to changes in central sensory transmission produced by the intention to move, and unrelated to a centrifugal gating produced by an efferent copy of the motor command, which is preserved in writer's cramp. Thus dystonia could be related to some defect in a premotor subroutine (Kaji et al., 1995), which includes the specification of motor commands for a forthcoming action as well as the specific setting of cortical responsiveness to afferent somatosensory inputs.

Huntington's Disease

Since the first study by Oepen et al. (1981) several authors have reported abnormal early cortical N20-P27 potentials in scalp reference recordings of patients with Huntington's chorea (Bollen et al., 1985; Ehle et al., 1984; Noth et al., 1984). Using an earlobe reference montage Töpper et al. (1980) have shown that the frontal P22 and N30 potentials are selectively depressed in this disease. However, these authors did not find any significant correlation between the severity of the movement disorder and that of the SEP abnormalities. Moreover, abnormal SEPs have also been reported in clinically asymptomatic subjects at risk for the disease, as well as in symptomatic patients during sedation of the choreic movements. Thus there is no proven link between the movement disorder and SEP abnormalities in this pathology.

Trigeminal Neuralgia

Arterial compression of the trigeminal roots in the cerebellopontine angle has been recognized as a frequent etiology of the so-called idiopathic trigeminal neuralgia; pain relief in these cases can be achieved by decompressive microsurgery (Jannetta, 1977). Several attempts have been made to detect conduction slowing reflecting trigeminal compression using trigeminal SEPs. However, the routine

use of trigeminal SEPs remained limited for three main reasons: (1) the clinical presentation of trigeminal neuralgia is in most cases so typical that ancillary techniques are useless to settle the diagnosis; (2) imaging techniques (CT scan or MRI and/or angiography) are usually carried out systematically whenever an extrinsic compressive lesion is suspected and/or a neurosurgical treatment envisaged; and (3) there are still some uncertainties as to the most adequate recording method and identification of normal components of the evoked response (see SEPs to Trigeminal Nerve Stimulation, above). The P19 scalp component evoked by electrical stimulation of the lips was reported as delayed in 40% of patients with trigeminal neuralgia (Stöhr et al., 1981). Later studies confirmed P19 potential abnormalities in trigeminal neuralgia (Bennett and Jannetta, 1983; Buettner et al., 1982; Dreschler and Neuhauser, 1986). Leandri et al. (1988) used the early potentials evoked by stimulation of the infraorbital nerve in these patients. Nine patients out of the 38 of their series with clinically idiopathic trigeminal neuralgia showed abnormal responses on the affected side. The most frequent abnormality was an increase of the interpeak interval between waves W1 and W3, supposed to take origin respectively at the entry of the maxillary nerve into the gasserian ganglion and in the presynaptic portion of the trigeminal spinal tract. The latency of wave W2, thought to take origin at the entry zone of the trigeminal root into the pons, was normal in eight of the nine patients with abnormal responses. These authors reported similar abnormalities in tumors of the cerebellopontine angle, while both waves W2 and W3 were delayed in patients with trigeminal neuralgia or hypesthesia symptomatic of a parasellar tumor.

Pain Syndromes

Two major categories of chronic pain have been recognized on clinical grounds. One is referred to as somatic pain and is thought to be due to prolonged activation of pain receptors or nociceptors; chronic pain in malignant disease, for example, is usually included in this category. The second type of pain, which is often referred to as neurogenic pain, results from direct injury to the nervous system. Gybels and Sweet (1989a,b) have reviewed the arguments supporting this distinction. EPs are useful mainly for investigating the second type of pain syndrome. The most direct approach to neurogenic pain is to record responses evoked by painful stimuli. Laser-evoked potentials (LEPs) have demonstrated their ability to detect lesions in peripheral and central pain pathways, including small-fiber neuropathies (Agostino et al., 2000; Kakigi et al., 1991a; Lankers et al., 1991; Lefaucheur et al., 2002), spinal cord lesions (Kakigi et al., 1991b; Treede et al., 1991), and brainstem infarcts affecting the spinothalamic system (Bromm et al., 1991; Kanda et al., 1996). In healthy subjects the amplitude of cortical LEPs correlates with the subjective sensation of pain, rather than with the physical stimulus intensity (Garcia-Larrea et al., 1997). Hypnotically induced hyperalgesia may also increase the amplitude of LEPs in parallel with the level of pain sensation, in the absence of any real change in the stimulus physical magnitude (Arendt-Nielsen et al., 1990). In patients with spinothalamic lesions, reduction of pain sensation is associated with LEP decrease (Casey et al., 1996; Kakigi et al., 1991b; Treede et al., 1991), whereas enhanced cortical responses to laser have been reported in patients with increased pain sensitivity (Gibson et al., 1994; Lorenz et al., 1996; Treede et al., 1995). All these observations suggest that LEPs magnitude might, in both normal and pathological conditions, be an accurate index of the subjective pain experience, and that, if heat/pain sensitivity is pathologically increased (as in allodynia and hyperalgesia), the amplitude of LEPs may also be increased (Treede et al., 1995). This point of view, however, has been challenged by some reported cases showing a dissociation between decreased cortical LEPs (due to deafferentation) and enhanced pain sensation to laser stimuli in cases of neurogenic pain (Casey et al., 1996; Wu et al., 1999). An alternative view, therefore, has developed suggesting that, while in normal subjects LEPs might accurately reflect the degree of pain sensation, in patients with neuropathic lesions they essentially reveal the degree of spinothalamic deafferentation (Casey et al., 1996; Wu et al., 1999). Recently, Garcia-Larrea et al. (2002) have studied laser-evoked cortical potentials (LEPs) in 54 consecutive patients presenting with either unilateral neurogenic central pain or unilateral pain of nonorganic origin. They compared LEPs obtained by stimulation of painful and non-painful homologous territories in each patient. LEPs were significantly attenuated after stimulation over the painful territory in patients with central pain; in contrast, LEPs were *never* attenuated in patients with nonorganic *(sine materia)* forms of pain, in whom LEPs could even be enhanced to stimulation of the painful territory when hyperalgesia was present. These authors concluded that (1) in patients with organic central pain syndromes, including spontaneous pains and/or hyperalgesia and allodynia, reduced LEPs essentially reflect the dysfunction of the lateral pain system subserved at the periphery by A delta fibers but do not reflect the affective aspects of pain sensation; and (2) normal or enhanced LEPs in patients with nonorganic pain syndromes or pain anesthesia are thus useful to document the psychogenic participation to the syndrome.

Evaluation of Spinal Surgery for Spasticity and Pain

Functional posterior rhizotomy (FPR) consists of sectioning 25% to 75% of the L2-S2 dorsal root fibers in patients with severe spasticity in lower limbs. Microsurgical lesion of the dorsal root entry zone (DREZ-tomy) is a microcoagulation of DH superficial laminae at C5-T1 or L2-S2 levels efficient in the treatment of central pain and spasticity (see Sindou and Jeanmonod, 1989, and Sindou et al., 1976, for a review). Both procedures aims at deafferenting or damaging enough DH cells to obtain relief of pain and spasticity, with sparing of large-diameter fibers subserving joint and touch sensation at and below the operated metameric levels and, at the sacral level, preservation of perineal sensation and bladder tone.

The postoperative amplitude decrease of segmental potentials (upper limb N13, pudendal nerve N15, or lower limb N22) correlates well with the number of operated roots or

metameric segments during FPR and DREZ-tomy. A retrospective survey in 64 consecutive patients followed for 1 year after DREZ-tomy suggests that an amplitude reduction of 60% to 75% of DH potentials gives optimal results on pain and spasticity (Turano et al., 1995). After cervical DREZ-tomy causing a N13 potential reduction of more than 60% sensation and conducted SEPs to sublesional stimulation are fully preserved, however, the P14 and N20 potentials, when recordable before surgery, often deteriorate on the operated side.

Fictitious Hemianesthesia

There is no evidence that short-latency SEPs could be affected in patients suspected of fictitious sensory loss related to hysterical conversion or alleged by the patient in a medicolegal context. Consequently, the finding of normal responses provides a firm basis for the diagnosis of fictitious sensory loss. The question of whether SEP components peaking later than the parietal N20 and P27 could be modified in hysterical hemianesthesia remains open in the absence of quantified indexes of normal interhemispheric variations, based on topographical studies. Usefulness of SEPs for the diagnosis of hysterical sensory loss has been thoroughly and critically discussed by Halliday (1993).

SEPs in Systemic Disorders and Internal Medicine

Multimodal EPs including SEPs have been studied in various diseases and dysmetabolic states of which some may cause or be associated with clinically silent conduction abnormalities in the CNS. Pathologies where SEPs can be useful in follow-up or treatment monitoring will be briefly covered here.

Congenital Hypothyroidism

Increased N13-N20 interval has been reported before substitutive treatment in newborns with congenital hypothyroidism. Amelioration of SEP abnormalities is slower than that of BAEPs under treatment and may remain incomplete after 6 months of hormonal therapy. There is no significant SEPs group differences between controls and children aged 18 months, 3 years, or 5 to 9 years in whom the disease has been detected and treated early (see Laureau et al., 1986, 1987).

Renal Failure

Severe uremia affects both the peripheral and the central nervous system. Multimodal EPs have been studied in untreated, hemodialyzed, and kidney-transplanted patients. Compared to controls, patients with renal failure, when recorded before the first dialysis session, have, as a group, delayed peripheral and central median nerve SEPs with no CCT abnormality (Walser et al., 1982). Patients with successful renal transplant do not differ from controls, whereas patients with long-term hemodialysis show delayed SEPs.

Vitamin Deficiency

Patients with vitamin B_{12} deficiency and megaloblastic anemia may present with clinical signs of subacute combined degeneration. Most of these patients have abnormal scalp SEPs after stimulation of the lower limbs (Krumholz et al., 1984). Abnormal median nerve SEPs are less frequent; abnormalities concern the transit time in the dorsal columns at the cervical level (Zegers de Beyl et al., 1988b). Due to reduced nerve conduction velocities, all SEP latencies can also be delayed.

Vitamin E deficiency is implicated as a pathophysiological agent in neurological deficits encountered in patients with abetalipoproteinemia, biliary atresia, and cystic fibrosis. Prolonged N13-N20 intervals have been reported in these patients (see Kaplan et al., 1988b, for a review). The relation among the degree of neurological deficit, SEP abnormalities, and serum vitamin E level is not firmly established.

Acquired Immune Deficiency Syndrome (AIDS)

SEPs can be useful to detect subclinical lesions of the CNS in asymptomatic HIV-positive subjects and patients with minor general symptoms of the disease (AIDS-related complex) or persistent generalized lymphadenopathy. In asymptomatic HIV-positive patients, tibial nerve SEPs are more sensitive than median nerve SEPs for detecting subclinical lesions (Smith et al., 1988). SEPs may disclose either peripheral or central conduction slowing. Multimodal EP studies combining VEPs, SEPs, and BAEPs detect abnormalities in 20% to 40% of HIV-positive patients, whereas percentages of AIDS patients showing one or several EP abnormalities in multimodal EP testing are of 60% and 85%, respectively, in neurological symptom-free and symptomatic patients (Comi et al., 1987; Farnarier and Somma-Mauvais, 1990; Iragui et al., 1994). In HIV-infected children, SEPs have been reported as normal in most cases, including symptomatic patients (Schmitt et al., 1992). Unlike HIV infection, the HTLV1 associated myelopathy causes CCT abnormalities with no abnormal changes in peripheral conduction (Kakigi et al., 1988).

References

Abbruzzese G., Marchese R., and Trompetto C. 1997. Sensory and motor evoked potentials in multiple system atrophy: a comparative study with Parkinson's disease. Mov. Disord. 12:315–321.

Agostino R., Cruccu G., Iannetti G.D., et al. 2000. Trigeminal small-fibre dysfunction in patients with diabetes mellitus: a study with laser evoked potentials and corneal reflex. Clin Neurophysiol. 111:2264–2267.

Allison T. 1982. Scalp and cortical recordings of initial somatosensory cortex activity to median nerve stimulation in man. Ann. N.Y. Acad. Sci. 338:677–678.

Allison T., and Hume A.L. 1981. A comparative analysis of short latency somatosensory evoked potentials in man, monkey, cat, and rat. Exp. Neurol. 72:592–611.

Allison T., Goff W.R., Williamson P.D., et al. 1980. On the neural origin of early components of the human somatosensory evoked potentials. In *Clinical Uses of Cerebral, Brainstem and Spinal Somatosensory Evoked Potentials, Progr. Clin. Neurophysiol,* vol. 7, Ed. Desmedt J.E. pp 51–68. Basel: Karger.

Allison T., Wood C.C., and Goff W.R. 1983. Brain stem auditory, pattern reversal visual and short latency somatosensory evoked potentials: latencies in relation to age, sex, and brain and body size. Electroencephalogr. Clin. Neurophysiol. 55:619–636.

Allison T., McCarthy G., Wood C.C., et al. 1989a. Human cortical potentials evoked by stimulation of the median nerve. I. Cytoarchitectonic areas generating short-latency potentials. J. Neurophysiol. 62:694–710.

Allison T., McCarthy G., Wood C.C., et al. 1989b. Potentials generated in human somatosensory cortex to stimulation of the median nerve. II. Cytoarchitectonic areas generating long-latency potentials. J. Neurophysiol. 62:711–722.

Allison T., McCarthy G., Wood C.C., et al. 1991. Potentials evoked in human and monkey cerebral cortex by stimulation of the median nerve: a review of scalp and intracranial recordings. Brain 114:2465–2503.

Allison T., McCarthy G., and Wood C.C. 1992. The relationship between human long-latency somatosensory evoked potentials recorded from the cortical surface and from the scalp. Electroencephalogr. Clin. Neurophysiol. 84:301–314.

Allison T., McCarthy G., Luby M., et al. 1996. Localization of functional regions of human mesial cortex by somatosensory evoked potential recording and by cortical stimulation. Electroencephalogr. Clin. Neurophysiol. 100:126–140.

American Electroencephalographic Society. 1984. Guidelines for clinical evoked potentials studies. J. Clin. Neurophysiol. 1:3–53.

Aminoff M.J., Goodin D.S., Barbaro N.M., et al. 1985. Dermatomal somatosensory evoked potentials in unilateral lumbosacral radiculopathy. Ann. Neurol. 17:171–176.

Andersen P., Eccles J.C., Schmidt R.F., et al. 1964. Slow potential waves produced in the cuneate nucleus by cutaneous volley and cortical stimulation. J. Neurophysiol. 27:78–91.

Anziska A., and Cracco R.Q. 1980. Short-latency somatosensory evoked potentials: studies in patients with focal neurological disease. Electroencephalogr. Clin. Neurophysiol. 49:227–239.

Anziska A., and Cracco R.Q. 1981. Short latency SEPs to median nerve stimulation: comparison of recording methods and origin of components. Electroencephalogr. Clin. Neurophysiol. 5:531–539.

Anziska A., and Cracco R.W. 1983. Short-latency somatosensory evoked potentials to median nerve stimulation in patients with diffuse neurologic disease. Neurology 33:989–993.

Araki A., Yamada T., Ito T., et al. 1997. Dissociation between upper and lower neck N13 potentials following paired median nerve stimuli. Electroencephalogr. Clin. Neurophysiol. 104:68–73.

Arendt-Nielsen L., Zachariae R., and Bjerring P. 1990. Quantitative evaluation of hypnotically suggested hyperaesthesia and analgesia by painful laser stimulation. Pain 42:243–251.

Austin G.M., and McCouch G.P. 1955. Presynaptic component of intermediary cord potential. J. Neurophysiol. 18:441–451.

Babiloni F., Babiloni C., Cecchi L., et al. 1994. Statistical analysis of topographic maps of short-latency somatosensory evoked potentials in normal and parkinsonian subjects. IEEE Trans. Biomed. Eng. 41:617–624.

Barba C., Frot M., Guénot M., et al. 2001. Stereotactic recordings of median nerve SEPs in the human supplementary motor area. Eur. J. Neurosci. 13:347–356.

Barba C., Frot M., Valeriani M., et al. 2002a. Distinct fronto-central N60 and suprasylvian N70 middle-latency components of the median nerve SEPs as assessed by scalp topographic analysis, dipolar source modelling and depth recordings. Clin. Neurophysiol. 113:981–992.

Barba C., Frot M., and Mauguière F. 2002b. Early secondary somatosensory area (SII) SEPs. Data from intracerebral recordings in humans. Clin. Neurophysiol. 113:1778–1786.

Bartel D.R., Markand O.N., and Kolar O.J. 1983. The diagnosis and classification of multiple sclerosis: evoked responses and spinal fluid electrophoresis. Neurology 33:611–617.

Bartel P., Conradie J., Robinson E., et al. 1987. The relationship between somatosensory evoked potential latencies and age and growth parameters in young children. Electroencephalogr. Clin. Neurophysiol. 68:180–186.

Bassetti C., Bomio F., Mathis J., et al. 1996. Early prognosis in coma after cardiac arrest: a prospective clinical, electrophysiological, and biochemical study of 60 patients. J. Neurol. Neurosurg. Psychiatry 61:610–615.

Baumgartner V., Vogel H., Ellrich J., et al. 1998. Brain electrical source analysis of primary cortical components of the tibial nerve somatosensory evoked potential using regional sources. Electroencephelogr. Clin. Neurophysiol. 108:588–599.

Beall J.E., Applebaum A.E., Foreman R.D., et al. 1977. Spinal cord potentials evoked by cutaneous afferents in the monkey. J. Neurophysiol. 40:199–211.

Bennett M.H., and Jannetta P.J. 1983. Evoked potentials in trigeminal neuralgia. Neurosurgery 13:242–247.

Berek K., Lechleitner P., Luef G., et al. 1995. Early determination of neurological outcome after prehospital cardiopulmonary resuscitation. Stroke 26:543–549.

Beric A., and Prevec T.S. 1981. The early negative potential evoked by stimulation of the median nerve in man. J. Neurol. Sci. 50:299–306.

Beric A., Dimitrijevic M.R., and Light J.K. 1987. A clinical syndrome of rostral and caudal spinal injury: neurological, neurophysiological and urodynamic evidence for occult sacral lesion. J. Neurol. Neurosurg. Psychiatry 50:600–606.

Berthier E., Turjman F., and Mauguière F. 1996. Diagnostic utility of somatosensory evoked potentials (SEPs) in presurgical assessment of cervical spondylotic myelopathy. Clin. Neurophysiol. 26:300–310.

Bollen E.L., Arts R.J., Roos R.A., et al. 1985. Somatosensory evoked potentials in Huntington's chorea. Electroencephalogr. Clin. Neurophysiol. 62:235–240.

Bosch P.E., Yamada T., and Kimura J. 1985. Somatosensory evoked potentials in motor neuron disease. Muscle Nerve 8:556–562.

Braakman R. 1994. Management of cervical spondylotic myelopathy. J. Neurol. Neurosurg. Psychiatry 57:257–263.

Branston N.M., Symon L., and Crockard H.A. 1976. Recovery of the cortical evoked response following temporary middle cerebral artery occlusion in baboon: relation to local blood flow and PO_2. Stroke 7:2–9.

Brenner D., Lipton J., Kaufman L., et al. 1978. Somatically evoked magnetic fields of the human brain. Science 199:81–83.

Bromm B., and Chen A.C.N. 1995. Brain electrical source analysis of laser evoked potentials in response to painful trigeminal nerve stimulation. Electroencephalogr. Clin. Neurophysiol. 95:14–26.

Bromm B., and Treede R.D. 1983. CO_2-laser radiant heat pulses activate C nociceptors in man. Pflugers Arch. 399:155–156.

Bromm B., and Treede R.D. 1984. Nerve fibre discharge, cerebral potentials and sensations induced by CO_2 laser stimulation. Hum. Neurobiol. 3:33–40.

Bromm B., and Treede R.D. 1987. Human cerebral potentials evoked by CO_2-laser stimuli causing pain. Exp. Brain. Res. 67:153–162.

Bromm B., Frieling A., and Lankers J. 1991. Laser evoked potentials in patients with dissociated loss of pain and temperature sensibility. Electroencephalogr. Clin. Neurophysiol. 100:342–353.

Broughton R.J. 1969. In *Average Evoked Potentials*, Eds. E. Donchin and D.B. Lindsley, pp. 79–84. Washington, DC: U.S. Government Printing Office.

Brown W.F., and Feasby F.E. 1984. Sensory evoked potentials in Guillain-Barré polyneuropathy. J. Neurol. Neurosurg. Psychiatry 47:288–291.

Brunko E., and Zegers de Beyl D. 1987. Prognostic value of early cortical somatosensory evoked potentials after resuscitation from cardiac arrest. Electroencephalogr. Clin. Neurophysiol. 66:15–24.

Buchner H., Ferbert A., Sherg M., et al. 1986. Evoked potential monitoring in brain death. Generators of BAEP and spinal SEP. In *Clinical Problems of Brainstem Disorders*, Eds. K. Kunze, W.H. Zangemeister, and A. Arlt, pp. 130–133. Stuttgart: Georg Thieme Verlag.

Buchner H., Ferbert A., and Hacke, W. 1988. Serial recording of median nerve stimulated subcortical somatosensory evoked potentials (SEPs) in developing brain death. Electroencephalogr. Clin. Neurophysiol. 69:14–23.

Buchner H., Adams L., Müller A., et al. 1995. Somatotopy of human hand somatosensory cortex revealed by dipole source analysis of early somatosensory evoked potentials and 3D-NMR tomography. Electroencephalogr. Clin. Neurophysiol. 96:121–134.

Buchner H., Waberski T.D., Fuchs M., et al. 1996. Postcentral origin of P22: evidence from source reconstruction in a realistically shaped head model and from a patient with a post-central lesion. Electroencephalogr. Clin. Neurophysiol. 100:332–342.

Buettner U.W., Petruch F., Schlegmann K., et al. 1982. Diagnostic significance of cortical somatosensory evoked potentials following trigeminal nerve stimulation. In *Clinical Applications of Evoked Potentials in Neurology. Advances in Neurology*, vol. 32, Eds. J. Courjon, F. Mauguière, and M. Revol, pp. 339–345. New York: Raven Press.

Burke D., Skuse N.F., and Lethlean K. 1981. Cutaneous and muscle afferent components of the cerebral potential evoked by electrical stimulation of human peripheral nerves. Electroencephalogr. Clin. Neurophysiol. 51:579–588.

Burke D., Gandevia S.C., McKeon B., et al. 1982. Interactions between cutaneous and muscle afferent projections to cerebral cortex in man. Electroencephalogr. Clin. Neurophysiol. 53:349–360.

Burton H., Fabri M., and Alloway K. 1995. Cortical areas within the lateral sulcus connected to cutaneous representations in areas 3b and 1: a revised interpretation of the second somatosensory area in macaque monkeys. J. Comp. Neurol. 355:539–562.

Cadilhac J., Zhu Y., Geogesco M., et al. 1985. La maturation des potentiels évoqués somesthésiques cérébraux. Rev. EEG Neurophysiol. 15:1–11.

Carmon A., Mor J., and Goldberg J. 1976. Evoked cerebral response to noxious thermal stimulation in humans. Exp. Brain Res. 25:103–107.

Caselli R.J. 1993. Ventrolateral and dorsomedial somatosensory association cortex damage produces distinct somesthetic syndromes in humans. Neurology 43:762–771.

Casey K.L., Beydoun A., Boivie J., et al. 1996. Laser-evoked cerebral potentials and sensory function in patients with central pain. Pain 64:485–491.

Chen R., Bolton C.F., Young B. 1996. Prediction of outcome in patients with anoxic coma: a clinical and electrophysiologic study. Crit. Care Med. 24:672–678.

Cheron G., and Borenstein S. 1987. Specific gating of the early somatosensory evoked potentials during active movement. Electroencephalogr. Clin. Neurophysiol. 67:537–548.

Cheron G., and Borenstein S. 1992. Mental movement stimulation affects the N30 frontal component of the somatosensory evoked potential. Electroencephalogr. Clin. Neurophysiol. 84:288–292.

Cheron G., Piette T., Thiriaux A., et al. 1994. Somatosensory evoked potentials at rest and during movement in Parkinson's disease: evidence for a specific apomorphine effect on the frontal N30 wave. Electroencephalogr. Clin. Neurophysiol. 92:491–501.

Cheron G., Dan B., and Borenstein S. 2000. Sensory and motor interfering influences on somatosensory evoked potentials. J. Clin. Neurophysiol. 17:280–294.

Chiappa K.H. 1990. *Evoked Potentials in Clinical Medicine*, 2nd ed. New York: Raven Press.

Chiappa K.H., and Ropper A.H. 1982. Evoked potentials in clinical medicine. N. Engl. J. Med. 306:1205–1211.

Cioni B., and Meglio M. 1986. Epidural recordings of electrical events produced in the spinal cord by segmental, ascending and descending volleys. Appl. Neurophysiol. 49:315–326.

Cohen L.G., and Starr A. 1985. Specific gating of the early somatosensory evoked potentials. Neurology 35:691–698.

Comi G., Medaglini S., Locatelli T., et al. 1987. Multimodality evoked potentials in acquired immunodeficiency syndrome. In *Evoked Potentials III*, Eds. C. Barber and T. Blum, pp. 408–412. Boston: Butterworth.

Cosi V., Poloni M., Mazzini L., et al. 1984. Somatosensory evoked potentials in amyotrophic lateral sclerosis. J. Neurol. Neurosurg. Psychiatry 47:857–861.

Cracco R.Q. 1973. Spinal evoked response: peripheral nerve stimulation in man. Electroencephalogr. Clin. Neurophysiol. 35:379–386.

Cracco R.Q., and Cracco J.B. 1976. Somatosensory evoked potential in man: Far-field potentials. Electroencephalogr. Clin. Neurophysiol. 41:460–466.

Cracco J.B., Cracco R.Q., and Stolove R. 1979. Spinal evoked potentials in man: A maturational study. Electroencephalogr. Clin. Neurophysiol. 46:58–64.

Crespi V., Mandelli A., and Minolli G. 1982. Short-latency somatosensory evoked potentials in patients with acute focal vascular lesions of the supratentorial somesthetic pathways. Acta Neurol. Scand. 65:274–279.

Cruccu G., Romaniello A., Amantini A., et al. 1999. Assessment of trigeminal small fiber function: brain and reflex responses evoked by CO_2-laser stimulation. Muscle Nerve 22:508–516.

Cruccu G., Leandri M., Iannetti G.D., et al. 2001. Small fiber dysfunction in trigeminal neuralgia. Carbamazepine effect on laser-evoked potentials. Neurology 56:1722–1726.

Cruse R., Klem G., Lesser R., et al. 1982. Paradoxical lateralization of cortical potentials evoked by stimulation of posterior tibial nerve. Arch. Neurol. 39:222–225.

Dasheiff R.M., Drake M.E., Brendle A., et al. 1985. Abnormal somatosensory evoked potentials in ALS. Electroencephalogr. Clin. Neurophysiol. 60:306–311.

Dawson G.D. 1947. Investigations on a patient subject to myoclonic seizures after sensory stimulation. J. Neurol. Neurosurg. Psychiatry 10:141–162.

Debecker J., and Desmedt J.E. 1964. Les potentials évoqués cérébraus et les potentials de nerf sensible chez l'homme. Acta Neurol. Belg. 64:1212–1248.

Deiber M.P., Giard M.H., and Mauguière F. 1986. Separate generators with distinct orientations for N20 and P22 somatosensory evoked potentials to finger stimulation. Electroencephalogr. Clin. Neurophysiol. 65:321–334.

Delbeke E.J., McComas A.J., and Kopec S.J. 1978. Analysis of lumbosacral evoked potentials in man. J. Neurol. Neurosurg. Psychiatry 41:293–302.

Delberghe X., Mavroudakis N., Zegers de Beyl D., et al. 1990. The effect of stimulus frequency on post- and precentral short latency somatosensory evoked potentials (SEPs). Electroencephalogr. Clin. Neurophysiol. 77: 96–92.

Delestre F., Lonchampt P., and Dubas F. 1986. Neural generator of P14 far-field somatosensory evoked potential studied in a patient with a pontine lesion. Electroencephalogr. Clin. Neurophysiol. 65:227–230.

Deltenre P., Van Nechel C., Vercruysse A., et al. 1982. Results of a prospective study on the value of combined visual, somatosensory, brainstem auditory evoked potentials and blink reflex measurements for disclosing subclinical lesions on suspected multiple sclerosis. In *Clinical Applications of Evoked Potentials in Neurology. Advances in Neurology*, vol. 32, Eds. J. Courjon, F. Mauguière, and M. Revol, pp. 473–479. New York: Raven Press.

Deltenre P., Van Nechel C., Strul S., et al. 1984. A five year prospective study on the value of multimodal evoked potentials and blink reflex, as an aid to the diagnosis of suspected multiple sclerosis. In *Evoked Potentials II: The second International Evoked Potentials Symposium*, Eds. R.H. Nodar and C. Barber, pp. 603–608. Boston: Butterworth.

Delwaide P.J., Schoenen J., and De Pasqua V. 1985. Lumbosacral spinal evoked potentials in patients with MS. Neurology 35:174–179.

De Marco P., and Negrin P. 1973. Parietal focal spike evoked by contralateral tactile somatotopic stimulations in four non-epileptic subjects. Electroencephalogr. Clin. Neurophysiol. 24:308–312.

De Marco P., and Tassinari C.A. 1981. Extreme somatosensory evoked potential (ESEP): an EEG sign forecasting a possible occurrence of seizures in children. Epilepsia 22:569–575.

Desmedt J.E., and Bourguet M. 1985. Color imaging of parietal and frontal somatosensory potential fields evoked by stimulation of median or posterior tibial nerve in man. Electroencephalogr. Clin. Neurophysiol. 62:1–17.

Desmedt J.E., and Cheron G. 1980a. Central somatosensory conduction in man: Neural generators and interpeak latencies of the far-field components recorded from neck and right or left scalp or earlobes. Electroencephalogr. Clin. Neurophysiol. 50:382–403.

Desmedt J.E., and Cheron G. 1980b. Somatosensory evoked potentials to finger stimulation in healthy octogenarians and in young adults: waveforms, scalp topography and transit times of parietal and frontal components. Electroencephalogr. Clin. Neurophysiol. 50:404–425.

Desmedt J.E., and Cheron G. 1981a. Prevertebral (oesophageal) recording of subcortical somatosensory evoked potentials in man: the spinal P13 component and the dual nature of the spinal generators. Electroencephalogr. Clin. Neurophysiol. 52:257–275.

Desmedt J.E., and Cheron G. 1981b. Non-cephalic reference recording of early somatosensory potentials to finger stimulation in adult or aging man: differentiation of widespread N18 and contralateral N20 from the prerolandic P22 and N30 components. Electroencephalogr. Clin. Neurophysiol. 52:553–570.

Desmedt J.E., and Cheron G. 1983. Spinal and far-field components of human somatosensory evoked potentials to posterior tibial nerve stimulation analysed with oesophageal derivations and non-cephalic reference recording. Electroencephalogr. Clin. Neurophysiol. 56:635–651.

Desmedt J.E., and Nguyen T.H. 1984. Bit-mapped colour imaging of the potential fields of propagated and segmental sub-cortical components of somatosensory evoked potentials in man. Electroencephalogr. Clin. Neurophysiol. 58:481–497.

Desmedt J.E., and Osaki I. 1991. SEPs to finger joint input lack the N20-P20 response that is evoked by tactile inputs: contrast between cortical generators in areas 3b and 2 in humans. Electroencephalogr. Clin. Neurophysiol. 80:513–521.

Desmedt J.E., and Tomberg C. 1989. Mapping early somatosensory evoked potentials in selective attention: critical evaluation of control conditions used for titrating by difference the cognitive P30, P40, P100 and N140. Electroencephalogr. Clin. Neurophysiol. 74:321–346.

Desmedt J.E., Manil J., Borenstein S., et al. 1966. Evaluation of sensory nerve conduction from averaged cerebral evoked potentials in neuropathies. Electromyography. 6:263–269.

Desmedt J.E., Noel P., Debecker J., et al. 1973. Maturation of afferent conduction velocity as studied by sensory nerve potentials and by cerebral evoked potentials. In *New Developments in Electromyography and Clinical Neurophysiology*, vol. 2, Ed. J.E. Desmedt, pp. 52–63. Basel: Karger, Basel.

Desmedt J.E., Brunko J., and Debecker J. 1976. Maturation of the somatosensory evoked potential in normal infants and children, with special reference to the early N1 component. Electroencephalogr. Clin. Neurophysiol. 40:43–58.

Desmedt J.E., Tran Huy N., and Carmelier J. 1983a. Unexpected latency shifts of the stationary P9 somatosensory evoked potential far-field with changes in shoulder position. Electroencephalogr. Clin. Neurophysiol. 56:628–634.

Desmedt J.E., Nguyen T.H., and Bourguet M. 1983b. The cognitive P40, N60, P100 components of somatosensory evoked potentials and the earliest signs of sensory processing in man. Electroencephalogr. Clin. Neurophysiol. 56:272–282.

De Weerd A.W., and Veldhuizen R.J. 1987. The frontally recorded somatosensory evoked potential un cerebral ischemia: significance in diagnosis and prognosis. In *Evoked Potentials III*, Eds. C. Barber and T. Blum, pp. 317–322. Boston: Butterworth.

De Weerd A.W., Looyenga A., Veldhuizen R.J., et al. 1985. Somatosensory evoked potentials in minor cerebral ischemia: diagnostic significance and changes in serial records. Electroencephalogr. Clin. Neurophysiol. 62:45–55.

Dimitrijevic M.R., and Halter J.A. (Eds). 1995. *Atlas of Human Cord Evoked Potentials*. Boston: Butterworth-Heinemann.

Dimitrijevic M.R., Larsson L.E., Lehmkuhl D., et al. 1978. Evoked spinal cord and nerve root potentials in humans using a non-invasive recording technique. Electroencephalogr. Clin. Neurophysiol. 45:331–340.

Dimtrijevic M.R., Lenman J.A.R., Prevec T., et al. 1982. A study of posterior column function in familial spastic paraplegia. J. Neurol. Neurosurg. Psychiatry 45:46–49.

Dimitrijevic M.R., Prevec T.S., and Sherwood A.M. 1983. Somatosensory perception and cortical evoked potentials in established paraplegia. J. Neurol. Sci. 60:253–265.

Dorfman L.J., and Bosley T.M. 1979. Age-related changes in peripheral and central nerve conduction in man. Neurology 29:38–44.

Dorfman L.J., Peskask I., Bolsey T.M., et al. 1980. Use of cerebral evoked potentials to evaluate spinal somatosensory function in patients with traumatic and surgical myelopathies. J. Neurosurg. 52:654–660.

Dreschler F., and Neuhauser B. 1986. Somatosensory trigeminal evoked potentials in normal subjects and in patients with trigeminal neuralgia before and after thermocoagulation of the ganglion gasseri. EMG Clin. Neurophysiol. 26:315–326.

Drummond J.C., Todd M.M., and Schubert A. 1985. The effect of high dose sodium thiopental on brainstem auditory and median nerve somatosensory evoked responses in humans. Anesthesiology 63:249–254.

Ehle A.L., Stewart R.M., Lellelid N.A., et al. 1984. Evoked potentials in Huntington's disease: a comparative longitudinal study. Arch. Neurol. 41:379–382.

Eisen A. 1986. SEPs in the evaluation of disorders of the peripheral nervous system. In *Evoked Potentials: Frontiers in Clinical Neuroscience*, vol. 3, Eds. R.Q. Cracco and I. Bodis-Wollner, pp. 409–417. New York: Alan R. Liss.

Eisen A., and Elleker G. 1980. Sensory nerve stimulation and evoked cerebral potentials. Neurology 30:1097–1105.

Eisen A., and Odusote K. 1980. Central and peripheral conduction times in multiple sclerosis. Electroencephalogr. Clin. Neurophysiol. 48:253–265.

Eisen A., Hoirch M., and Moll A. 1983. Evaluation of radiculopathies by segmental stimulation and somatosensory evoked potentials Can. J. Neurol. Sci. 10:178–182.

El Kharoussi M., Ibañez V., Ben Jelloun W., et al. 1996. Potentiels évoqués somesthésiques: Interférences et masquage perceptif des afférences cutanées chez l'Homme. Neurophysiol. Clin. 26:85–101.

El-Negamy E., and Sedgwick E.M. 1979. Delayed cervical somatosensory evoked potentials in cervical spondylosis. J. Neurol. Neurosurg. Psychiatry 42:238–241.

Emerson R.G., and Pedley T.A. 1986. Effect of cervical spinal cord lesions on early components of the median nerve somatosensory evoked potential. Neurology 36:20–26.

Emerson R.G., Sgro J.A., Pedley T.A., et al. 1988. State-dependent changes in the N20 component of the median nerve somatosensory evoked potentials. Neurology 38:64–68.

Farnarier G., and Somma-Mauvais H. 1990. Multimodal evoked potentials in HIV infected patients. In *New Trends and Advanced Techniques in Clinical Neurophysiology*, EEG J. Suppl. 41. Eds. P.M. Rossini and F. Mauguière, pp. 355–369. Amsterdam: Elsevier.

Fischer C., Mauguière F., Ibañez V., et al. 1986. Potentiels évoqués visuels, auditifs précoces et somesthésiques dans la sclérose en plaques (917 cas). Rev. Neurol. 142:517–523.

Forss N., Hari R., Salmelin R., et al. 1994a. Activation of the human posterior parietal cortex by median nerve stimulation. Exp. Brain Res. 99: 309–315.

Forss N., Salmelin R., and Hari R. 1994b. Comparison of somatosensory evoked fields to airpuff and electric stimuli. Electroencepalogr. Clin. Neurophysiol. 92:510–517.

Forss N., Merlet I., Vanni S., et al. 1996. Activation of human mesial cortex during somatosensory attention task. Brain Res. 734:229–235.

Frank L.M., Furgivelle T.L., and Etheridge J.E. 1985. Prediction of chronic vegetative state in children using evoked potentials. Neurology 35:931–934.

Franssen H., Stegeman D.F., Molemen J., et al. 1992. Dipole modelling of median nerve SEPs in normal subjects and patients with small subcortical infarcts. Electroencephalogr. Clin. Neurophysiol. 84:401–417.

Frot M., and Mauguière F. 1999. Timing and spatial distribution of somatosensory responses recorded in the upper bank of the sylvian fissure (SII area) in humans. Cereb. Cortex 9:854–863.

Frot M., and Mauguière F. 2003. Dual representation of pain in the operculo-insular cortex in humans. Brain 126:438–450.

Frot M., Rambaud L., and Mauguière F. 1997. Intracerebral recordings of responses from the parieto-opercular area S2 after electrical and CO_2 laser stimuli in humans. Electroencephalogr. Clin. Neurophysiol. 103: 179.

Frot M., Garcia-Larrea L., Guénot M., et al. 2001. Responses of the supra-sylvian (SII) cortex in humans to painful and innocuous stimuli. A study using intra-cerebral recordings. Pain 94:65–73.

Furlong P.L., Wimalaratna S., and Harding G.F.A. 1993. Augmented P22-N31 SEP component in a patient with unilateral space occupying lesion. Electroencephalogr. Clin. Neurophysiol. 88:72–76.

Gandevia S.C., and Burke, D. 1988. Projection to the cerebral cortex from proximal and distal muscles in the human upper limb. Brain 111:389–403.

Gandevia S.C., and Burke D. 1990. Projection of thenar muscle afferents to frontal and parietal cortex of human subjects. Electroencephalogr. Clin. Neurophysiol. 77:353–361.

Gandevia S.C., and Macefield G. 1989. Projection of low-threshold muscle afferents from intercostal muscles to the cerebral cortex. Resp. Physiol. 77:203–214.

Gandevia S.C., Burke D., and McKeon B.B. 1983. Convergence in the somatosensory pathway between cutaneous afferents from the index and middle fingers in man. Exp. Brain. Res. 50:415–425.

Gandevia S.C., Burke D., and McKeon B.B. 1984. The projection of muscle afferents from hand to cerebral cortex in man. Brain 107:1–13.

Ganes T. 1980. Somatosensory conduction times and peripheral, cervical and cortical evoked potentials in patients with cervical spondylosis. J. Neurol. Neurosurg. Psychiatry 43:683–689.

Ganes T., and Lundar T. 1983. The effect of thiopentone on somatosensory evoked responses and EEGs in comatose patients. J. Neurol. Neurosurg. Psychiatry 46:509–514.

Garcia P.A., Aminoff M.J., and Goodin D.S. 1995. The frontal N30 component of the median-derived SEP in patients with predominantly unilateral Parkinson's disease. Neurology 45:989–992.

Garcia-Larrea L., and Mauguière F. 1988. Latency and amplitude abnormalities of the scalp far-field P14 to median nerve stimulation in multiple sclerosis. Electroencephalogr. Clin. Neurophysiol. 71:180–186.

Garcia-Larrea L., Bastuji H., and Mauguière F. 1991. Mapping study of somatosensory evoked potentials during selective spatial attention. Electroencephalogr. Clin. Neurophysiol. 80:201–214.

Garcia-Larrea L., Bastuji H., and Mauguière F. 1992. Unmasking of cortical SEP components by changes in stimulus rate a topographic study. Electroencephalogr. Clin. Neurophysiol. 84:71–83.

Garcia-Larrea L., Lukaszewicz A.C., and Mauguière F. 1995. Somatosensory responses during selective spatial attention: the N120 to N140 transition. Psychophysiology 32:526–537.

Garcia-Larrea L., Peyron R., Laurent B., et al. 1997. Association between laser-evoked pain potentials and pain perception. Neuroreport 8:3785–3789.

Garcia-Larrea L., Convers P., Magnin M., et al. 2002. Laser-evoked potential abnormalities in central pain patients: the influence of spontaneous and provoked pain. Brain 125: 2776–2781.

Gasser H.S., and Graham H.T. 1933. Potentials produced in the spinal cord by stimulation of the dorsal roots. Am. J. Physiol. 103:303–320.

Georgesco M., Salerno A., Carlander B., 1994. Les potentiels évoqués somesthésiques dans la sclérose latérale amyotrophique et la sclérose latérale primaire. Rev. Neurol. (Paris) 150:292–298.

Georgesco M., Salerno A., and Camu W. 1997. Somatosensory evoked potentials elicited by stimulation of lower-limb nerves in amyotrophic lateral sclerosis. Electroencephalogr. Clin. Neurophysiol. 104:333–342.

Giblin D.R. 1964. Somatosensory evoked potentials in healthy subjects and in patients with lesions of the nervous system. Ann. N.Y. Acad. Sci. 112: 93–142.

Gibson S.J., Littlejohn G.O., Gorman M.M., et al. 1994. Altered heat pain thresholds and cerebral event-related potentials following painful CO_2 laser stimulation in subjects with fibromyalgia syndrome. Pain 58:185–193.

Gigli G.L., Caramia M., Narciani M.G., et al. 1987. Monitoring of subcortical and cortical somatosensory evoked potentials during endarterectomy: comparison with stump pressure levels. Electroencephalogr. Clin. Neurophysiol. 68:424–432.

Glover J.L., Worth R.M., Bendick P.J., et al. 1981. Evoked responses in the diagnosis of thoracic outlet syndrome. Surgery 89:86–93.

Goff G.D., Matsumiya Y., Allison T., et al. 1977. The scalp topography of human somatosensory and auditory evoked potentials. Electroencephalogr. Clin. Neurophysiol. 42:57–76.

Graff-Radford N.R., Damasio H., Yamada T., et al. 1985. Nonhaemorrhagic thalamic infarction: clinical, neuropsychological and electrophysiological findings in four anatomical groups defined by computerized tomography. Brain 108:485–516.

Green J.B., Walcoff M.R., and Lucke J.F. 1982. Comparison of phenytoin and phenobarbital effects on far-field auditory and somatosensory evoked potentials interpeak latencies. Epilepsia 23:417–421.

Greenberg R.P., Newlon P.G., and Becker D.P. 1982. The somatosensory evoked potentials in patients with severe head injury: outcome prediction and monitoring of brain function. Ann. New York Acad. Sci. 388:683–688.

Grezes J., Costes N., and Decety J. 1998. Top-down effect of the strategy on the perception of biological motion: a PET investigation. Cogn. Neuropsychol. 15:553–582.

Grissom, J.R., Toro, C., Tretteau, J., et al. 1995. The N30 and N140-P190 median nerve somatosensory evoked potentials waveforms in dystonia involving the upper extremity (Abstract). Neurology 45(suppl 4):A458.

Guérit J.M., and Opsomer R.J. 1991. Bit-mapped imaging of somatosensory evoked potentials after stimulation of the posterior tibial nerves and dorsal nerve of the penis/clitoris. Electroencephalogr. Clin. Neurophysiol. 80:228–237.

Guérit J.M., Soveges L., Baele P., et al. 1990. Median nerve evoked potentials in profound hypothermia for ascending aorta repair. Electroencephalogr. Clin. Neurophysiol. 77:163–173.

Gybels J.M., and Sweet W.H. 1989a. Neurosurgical treatment of persistent pain. In *Open Anterolateral Cordotomy*, pp. 151–172. Basel: Karger.

Gybels J.M., and Sweet W.H. 1989b. Neurosurgical treatment of persistent pain. In *Thalamotomy*, pp. 221–234. Basel: Karger.

Haldeman S., Bradley W.E., Bhatia N.N., et al. 1982. Pudendal evoked response. Arch. Neurol. 39:280–283.

Hallett M. 1995. Is dystonia a sensory disorder? Ann. Neurol. 38:139–140.

Hallett M., Chadwick D., Adam J., et al. 1977. Reticular reflex myoclonus; a physiological type of human post-hypoxic myoclonus. J. Neurol. Neurosurg. Psychiatry 40:253–264.

Halliday A.M. 1967. The electrophysiological study of myoclonus in man. Brain 90:241–284.

Halliday A.M. 1993. *Evoked Potentials in Clinical Testing*. Edinburgh: Churchill Livingstone.

Halliday A.M., and Mason A.A. 1964. The effect of hypnotic anesthesia on cortical responses. J. Neurol. Neurosurg. Psychiatry 27:300–312.

Halliday A.M., and Wakefield G.S. 1963. Cerebral evoked potentials in patients with dissociated sensory loss. J. Neurol. Neurosurg. Psychiatry 26: 211–219.

Halonen J.P., Jones S., and Shawkat F. 1988. Contribution of cutaneous and muscle afferent fibres to cortical SEPs following medial and radial nerve stimulation in man. Electroencephalogr. Clin. Neurophysiol. 71: 331–335.

Hämäläinen M., Hari R., Ilmoniemi R., et al. 1993. Magnetoencephalography: theory, instrumentation, and applications to non invasive studies of the working humain brain. Rev. Mod. Physics 65:413–497.

Hari R., Hämäläinen M., Kaukoranta E., et al. 1983. Neuromagnetic responses from the second somatosensory cortex in man. Acta Neurol. Scand. 68:207–212.

Hari R., Reinikainen K., Kaukoranta E., et al. 1984. Somatosensory evoked cerebral magnetic fields from SI and SII in man. Electroencephalogr. clin. Neurophysiol. 57:254–263.

Hari R., Hämäläinen H., Tiihonen J., et al. 1990. Separate finger representations at the human second somatosensory cortex. Neuroscience 37:245–249.

Hari R., Karhu J., Hämäläinen M., et al. 1993. Functional organization of the human first and second somatosensory cortices: a neuromagnetic study. Eur. J. Neurosci. 5:724–734.

Hashimoto T., Tayama M., Hiura K., et al. 1983. Short latency somatosensory evoked potential in children. Brain Dev. 5:390–396.

Hashimoto I. 1987. Somatosensory evoked potentials elicited by air-puff stimuli generated by a new high-speed air control system. Electroencephalogr. Clin. Neurophysiol. 67:231–237.

Hume A.L., and Cant B.R. 1978. Conduction time in central somatosensory pathways in man. Electroencephalogr. Clin. Neurophysiol. 45:361–375.

Hume A.L., and Cant B.R. 1981. Central somatosensory conduction after head injury. Ann. Neurol. 10:411–419.

Hume A.L., and Waxman S.G. 1988. Evoked potentials in suspected multiple sclerosis: diagnostic value and prediction of clinical course. J. Neurol. Sci. 83:191–210.

Hume A.L., Cant B.R., and Shaw N.A. 1979. Central somatosensory conduction time in comatose patients. Ann. Neurol. 5:379–384.

Hume A.L., Cant B.R., Shaw N.A., et al. 1982. Central somatosensory conduction time from 10 to 79 years. Electroencephalogr. Clin. Neurophysiol. 54:49–54.

Huttunen J., and Teravainen H. 1993. Pre- and post–central cortical somatosensory evoked potentials in hemiparkinsonism. Mov. Disord. 8:430–436.

Huttunen J., Kaukoranta E., and Hari R. 1987. Cerebral magnetic responses to stimulation of tibial and sural nerves. J. Neurol. Sci. 79:43–54.

Ibañez V., Deiber M.P., and Mauguière F. 1989. Interference of vibrations with input transmission in dorsal horn and cuneate nucleus in man: a study of somatosensory evoked potentials (SEPs) to electrical stimulation of median nerve and fingers. Exp. Brain Res. 75:599–610.

Ibañez V., Fischer G., and Mauguière F. 1992. Dorsal horn and dorsal column dysfunction in intramedullary cervical cord tumours: a SEP study. Brain 115:1209–1234.

Ibañez V., Deiber M.P., Sadato N., et al. 1995. Effects of stimulus rate on regional cerebral blood flow after median nerve stimulation. Brain 118:1339–1351.

Ikeda A., Shibasaki H., Nagamine T., et al. 1995. Peri-rolandic and fronto-parietal components of scalp recorded giant SEPs in cortical myoclonus. Electroencephalogr. Clin. Neurophysiol. 96:300–309.

Iragui V.J. 1984. The cervical somatosensory evoked potential in man, far-field conducted and segmental components. Electroencephalogr Clin. Neurophysiol. 57:228–235.

Iragui V.J., Kalmijn J., Thal L.J., et al. 1994. Neurological dysfunction in asymptomatic HIV-1 infected men: evidence from evoked potentials. HNRC group. Electroencephalogr. Clin. Neurophysiol. 92:1–10.

Iwayama K., Mori K., Iwamoto K., et al. 1988. Origin of frontal N15 component of SEP in man. Electroencephalogr. Clin. Neurophysiol. 71:125–132.

Jabbari B., Vance S.C., Harper M., et al. 1987. Clinical and radiological correlates of somatosensory evoked potentials in the late phase of head injury: a study of 500 Vietnam veterans. Electroencephalogr. Clin. Neurophysiol. 67:289–297.

Jannetta P.J. 1977. Observations on the etiology of trigeminal neuralgia, hemifacial spasm, acoustic nerve dysfunction and glossopharyngeal neuralgia. Definite microsurgical treatment and results in 117 patients. Neurochirurgia 20:145–154.

Jeanmonod D., Sindou M., and Mauguière F. 1989. Three transverse dipolar generators in the human cervical and lumbo-sacral dorsal horn: evidence from direct intraoperative recordings on the spinal cord surface. Electroencephalogr. Clin. Neurophysiol. 74:236–240.

Jeanmonod D., Sindou M., and Mauguière F. 1991. The human cervical and lumbo-sacral evoked electrospinogram. Data from intra-operative spinal cord surface recordings. Electroencephalogr. Clin. Neurophysiol. 80:477–489.

Jennett B., Snoek J., Bond M.R., et al. 1981. Disability after head injury: observations on the use of the Glasgow outcome scale. J. Neurol. Neurosurg. Psychiatry 44:285–293.

Jones S.J., and Small M. 1978. Spinal and subcortical evoked potentials following stimulation of the posterior tibial nerve in man. Electroencephalogr. Clin. Neurophysiol. 44:299–306.

Jones S.J., Baraitser M., and Halliday A.M. 1980. Peripheral and central somatosensory nerve conduction defects in Friedreich's ataxia. J. Neurol. Neurosurg. Psychiatry 43:495–503.

Jones S.J., Wynn Parry C.B., and Landi A. 1981. Diagnosis of brachial plexus traction lesions by sensory nerve action potentials and somatosensory evoked potentials. Injury 12:376–382.

Jorg J., Dullberg W., and Koeppen S. 1982. Diagnostic value of segmental somatosensory evoked potentials in cases with chronic para- or tetraspastic syndromes. *In Clinical Applications of Evoked Potentials in Neurology. Advances in Neurology,* vol. 32, Eds. J. Courjon, F. Mauguière, and M. Revol, pp. 347–358. New York: Raven Press.

Kaji R., Shibasaki H., and Kimura J. 1995. Writer's cramp: a disorder of motor subroutine? Ann. Neurol. 38:837–838.

Kaji R., and Sumner A.J. 1987. Bipolar recording of short-latency somatosensory after median nerve stimulation. Neurology 37:410–418.

Kakigi R., and Jones S.J. 1986. Influence of concurrent tactile stimulation on somatosensory evoked potentials following posterior tibial nerve stimulation in man. Electroencephalogr. Clin. Neurophysiol. 65:118–129.

Kakigi R., and Shibasaki H. 1992. Effects of age, gender and stimulus side on the scalp topography of somatosensory evoked potentials following posterior tibial nerve stimulation. J. Clin. Neurophysiol. 9:431–440.

Kakigi R., and Shibasaki H. 1983. Scalp topography of the short-latency somatosensory evoked potentials following posterior tibial nerve stimulation in man. Electroencephalogr. Clin. Neurophysiol. 56:430–437.

Kakigi R., and Shibasaki H. 1984. Scalp topography of mechanically and electrically evoked somatosensory potentials in man. Electroencephalogr. Clin. Neurophysiol. 59:44–56.

Kakigi R., and Shibasaki H. 1987. Generator mechanisms of giant somatosensory evoked potentials in cortical reflex myoclonus. Brain 110:1359–1373.

Kakigi R., Shibasaki H., and Tanaka K. 1991a. CO_2 laser induced pain-related somatosensory evoked potentials in peripheral neuropathies: correlation between electrophysiological and histopathological findings. Muscle Nerve 14:441–450.

Kakigi R., Shibasaki H., Kuroda Y., et al. 1991b. Pain-related somatosensory evoked potentials in syringomyelia. Brain 114:1871–1889.

Kakigi R., Shibasaki H., Hashizume A., et al. 1982. Short latency somatosensory evoked spinal and scalp-recorded potentials following posterior tibial nerve stimulation in man. Electroencephalogr. Clin. Neurophysiol. 53:602–611.

Kakigi R., Shibasaki H., Kuroda Y., et al. 1988. Multimodality evoked potentials in HTLV1 associated myelopathy. J. Neurol. Neurosurg. Psychiatry 51:1094–1096.

Kakigi R., Shibasaki H., Kuroda Y., et al. 1991a. Pain-related somatosensory evoked potentials in syringomyelia. Brain 114:1871–1889.

Kakigi R., Shibasaki H., and Tanaka K., et al. 1991b. CO2 laser-induced pain-related somatosensory evoked potentials in peripheral neuropathies: correlations between electrophysiological and histopathological findings. Muscle Nerve 14:441–450.

Kanda M., Fujiwara N., Xiaoping X., et al. 1996. Pain-related and cognitive components of somatosensory evoked potentials following CO_2 laser stimulation in man. Electroencephalogr. Clin. Neurophysiol. 100:105–114.

Kanovsky P., Streitova H., Dufek J., et al. 1997. Lateralization of the P22/N30 component of somatosensory evoked potentials of the median nerve in patients with cervical dystonia. Mov. Disord. 12:553–560.

Kanovsky P., Streitova H., Dufek J., et al. 1998. Changes in lateralization of the P22/N30 component of median nerve somatosensory evoked potentials in patients with cervical dystonia after successful treatment with botulinum toxin. Mov. Disord. 13:108–117.

Kaplan P.W., Hosford D.A., Werner M.H., et al. 1988a. Somatosensory evoked potentials in a patient with a cervical glioma and syrinx. Electroencephalogr. Clin. Neurophysiol. 70:563–565.

Kaplan P.W., Rawal K., Erwin C.W., et al. 1988b. Visual and somatosensory evoked potentials in vitamin E deficiency with cystic fibrosis. Electroencephalogr. Clin. Neurophysiol. 71:266–272.

Karhu J., and Tesche C.D. 1999. Simultaneous early processing of sensory input in human primary (SI) and secondary (SII) somatosensory cortices. J. Neurophysiol. 81(5):2017–2025.

Kasai T., Kawai S., Kawanishi M., et al. 1997. Evidence for facilitation of motor evoked potentials (MEPs) induced by motor imagery. Brain Res. 744:147–150.

Katifi H.A., and Sedgwick E.M. 1986. Somatosensory evoked potentials from posterior tibial nerve and lumbosacral dermatomes. Electroencephalogr. Clin. Neurophysiol. 65:249–259.

Katifi H.A., and Sedgwick E.M. 1987. Dermatomal somatosensory evoked potentials in lumbosacral disk disease: diagnosis and results of treatment. In *Evoked Potentials III*, Eds. C. Barber and T. Blum, pp. 285–292. London: Butterworth.

Kenton B., Coger R., Crue B., et al. 1980. Peripheral fibers correlates to noxious thermal stimulation in humans. Neurosci. Lett. 17:301–306.

Kimura J., Mitsudome A., Beck D.O., et al. 1983. Field distribution of antidromically activated digital nerve potentials. Model for far-field recording. Neurology 33:1164–1169.

Kimura J., Mitsudome A., Beck D.O., et al. 1984. Stationary peaks from a moving source in far-field recording. Electroencephalogr. Clin. Neurophysiol. 58:351–361.

Kitamura Y., Kakigi R., Hoshiyama M., et al. 1995. Pain-related somatosensory evoked magnetic fields. Electroencephalogr. Clin. Neurophysiol. 95:463–474.

Kjaer M. 1987. Evoked potentials in the diagnosis of multiple sclerosis. In *The London Symposia*, EEG J. Suppl 39, Eds. R.J. Ellingson, N.M.F. Murray, and A.M. Halliday, pp. 291–196. Amsterdam: Elsevier.

Krubitzer L., Clarey J., Tweedale R., et al. 1995. Redefinition of somatosensory areas in the lateral sulcus of macaque monkeys. J. Neurosci. 15:3821–3839.

Krumholz A., Weiss H.D., Goldstein P.J. et al. 1984. Evoked responses in vitamin B12 deficiency. Ann. Neurol. 9:407–409.

Kunde V., and Treede R.D. 1993. Topography of middle latency somatosensory evoked potentials following painful laser stimuli and nonpainful electrical stimuli. Electroencephalogr. Clin. Neurophysiol. 88:280–289.

Kunesch E., Knecht S., Schnitzler A., et al. 1995. Somatosensory evoked potentials elicited by intraneural microstimulation of afferent nerve fibers. J. Clin. Neurophysiol. 12:476–487.

Lafrenière L., Laureau E., Vanasse M., et al. 1990. Maturation of short-latency somatosensory evoked potentials by median nerve stimulation: a cross-sectional study in a large group of children. In *New Trends and Advanced Techniques in Clinical Neurophysiology*, EEG J. Suppl. 41., Eds. P.M. Rossini, and F. Mauguière, pp. 236–242. Amsterdam: Elsevier.

Laget P., Mamo H., and Houdart R. 1967. De l'intérêt des potentiels évoqués somesthésiques dans l'étude des lésions du lobe pariétal de l'homme. Étude préliminaire. Neurochirurgie 13:841–853.

La Joie W.J., Reddy N.M., and Melvin J.L. 1982. Somatosensory evoked potentials: their predictive value in right hemiplegia. Arch. Phys. Med. Rehab. 63:223–226.

Lankers J., Frieling A., Kunze K., et al. 1991. Ultralate cerebral potentials in a patient with hereditary motor and sensory neuropathy type I indicate preserved C-fibre function. J. Neurol. Neurosurg. Psychiatry 54:650–652.

Lastimosa A.C.B., Bass N.H., Stanback K., et al. 1982. Lumbar spinal cord and early cortical evoked potentials after tibial nerve stimulation: effects of stature on normative data. Electroencephalogr. Clin. Neurophysiol. 54: 499–507.

Laureau E., Vanasse M., Hebert R., et al. 1986. Somatosensory evoked potentials and auditory brainstem responses in congenital hypothyroidism. I: A longitudinal study before and after treatment in six infants detected in the neonatal period. Electroencephalogr. Clin. Neurophysiol. 64:501–510.

Laureau E., Hebert R., Vanasse M., et al. 1987. Somatosensory evoked potentials and auditory brainstem responses in congenital hypothyroidism. II: a cross-sectional study in childhood. Correlations with hormonal levels and developmental quotients. Electroencephalogr. Clin. Neurophysiol. 67:521–530.

Laureau E., Majnermer A., Rosenblatt B., et al. 1988. A longitudinal study of short latency somatosensory evoked responses in healthy newborns and infants. Electroencephalogr. Clin. Neurophysiol. 71:100–108.

Leandri M., Parodi C.I., and Favale E. 1988. Early trigeminal evoked potentials in tumours of the base of the skull and trigeminal neuralgia. Electroencephalogr. Clin. Neurophysiol. 71:114–124.

Lefaucheur J.P., Drouot X., and Jarry A. 2002. Clinical usefulness of Nd:YAG laser-evoked potentials in small-fiber neuropathy. Neurophysiol. Clin. 32:91–98.

Lemon R.N. 1981. Functional properties of monkey motor cortex neurones receiving afferent inputs from the hand and fingers. J. Physiol. 311:313–339.

Lesser R.P., Koehle R., and Lüders H. 1979. Effect of stimulus intensity on short latency somatosensory evoked potentials. Electroencephalogr. Clin. Neurophysiol. 47:377–382.

Lesser R.P., Lueders H., Hahn J., et al. 1981. Early somatosensory evoked potentials by mesian nerve stimulation: intraoperative monitoring. Neurology 31:1519–1523.

Logi F., Fischer C., Murri L., et al. 2003. The prognostic value of evoked responses from primary somatosensory and auditory cortex in comatose patients. Clin. Neurophysiol. 114:1615–1627.

Lorenz J., Grasedyck K., and Bromm B. 1996. Middle and long latency somatosensory evoked potentials after painful laser stimulation in patients with fibromyalgia syndrome. Electroencephalogr. Clin. Neurophysiol. 100:165–168.

Lüders H., Andrish J., Gurd A., et al. 1981. Origin of far-field subcortical potentials evoked by stimulation of tibial nerve. Electroencephalogr. Clin. Neurophysiol. 52:336–344.

Lüders H., Lesser R.P., Dinner D.S., et al. 1985. The second somatosensory area in humans: Evoked potentials and electrical stimulation studies. Ann. Neurol. 17:177–184.

Lüders H., Dinner D.S., Lesser R.P., et al. 1986. Evoked potentials in cortical localization. J. Clin. Neurophysiol. 3:75–84.

Macefield G., Burke D., and Gandevia S.C. 1989. The cortical distribution of muscle and cutaneous afferent projections from the human foot. Electroencephalogr. Clin. Neurophysiol. 72:518–528.

Macon J.B., and Poletti C.E. 1982. Conducted somatosensory evoked potentials during spinal surgery. Part I: Control conduction velocity measurements. J. Neurosurg. 57:349–353.

Macon J.B., Poletti C.E., Sweet W.H., et al. 1982. Conducted somatosensory evoked potentials during spinal surgery: Part II: Clinical applications. J. Neurosurg. 57:354–359.

Madl C., Kramer L., Domanovits H., et al. 2000. Improved outcome prediction in unconscious cardiac arrest survivors with sensory evoked potentials compared with clinical assessment. Crit. Care Med. 28:721–726.

Manganotti P., Zanette G., Beltramello A., et al. 1988a. Spike topography and functional magnetic resonance imaging (fMRI) in benign rolandic epilepsy with spikes evoked by tapping stimulation. Electroencephalogr. Clin. Neurophysiol. 107:88–92.

Manganotti P., Miniussi C., Santorum E., et al. 1988b. Scalp topography and source analysis of interictal spontaneous spikes and evoked spikes by digital stimulation in benign rolandic epilepsy. Electroencephalogr. Clin. Neurophysiol. 107:18–26.

Manzano G.M., Negrão N., and Nòbrega J.A.M. 1998. The N18 component of the median nerve SEP is not reduced by vibrations. Electroencephalogr. Clin. Neurophysiol. 108:259–266.

Mastaglia F.L., Black J.L., Edis R., et al. 1978. The contribution of evoked potentials in the functional assessment of the somatosensory pathways. Clin. Exp. Neurol. 15:279–298.

Matheson J.K., Harrington H., and Hallett M. 1983. Abnormalities of somatosensory evoked potentials visual and brainstem potentials in amyotrophic lateral sclerosis. Muscle Nerve 6:529.

Matthews W.B., Wattam-Bell J.R.B., and Poutney E. 1982. Evoked potentials in the diagnosis of multiple sclerosis: a follow up study. J. Neurol. Neurosurg. Psychiatry 45:303–307.

Matthews W.B., Acheson E.D., Batchelor J.R., et al. 1985. *Mc Alpine's Multiple Sclerosis*. Edinburgh: Churchill Livingstone.

Mauguière F. 1983. Les potentiels évoqués somesthésiques cervicaux chez le sujet normal. Analyse des aspects obtenus selon le siège de l'électrode de référence. Rev. EEG. Neurophysiol. 13:259–272.

Mauguière F. 1987. Short-latency somatosensory evoked potentials to upper limb stimulation in lesions of brainstem, thalamus and cortex. In *The London Symposia*, EEG J. Suppl 39, Eds. R.J. Ellingson, N.M.F. Murray, and A.M. Halliday, pp. 302–309. Amsterdam: Elsevier.

Mauguière F. 1995. Evoked potentials. In *Clinical Neurophysiology: EMG, Nerve Conduction and Evoked Potentials*. Eds. J.W. Osselton, C.D. Binnie, R. Cooper, et al., pp. 325–563. Oxford: Butterworth-Heinemann.

Mauguière F. 2000. Anatomical origin of the cervical N13 potential evoked by upper extremity stimulation. J. Clin. Neurophysiol. 17:236–245.

Mauguière F., and Courjon J. 1980. Effects of intravenously injected clonazepam on the cortical somatosensory evoked response in dyssynergia cerebellaris myoclonica. In *EEG and Clinical Neurophysiology*,

Eds. H. Lechner and A. Aranibar, pp. 433–444. Amsterdam: Excerpta Medica.

Mauguière F., and Desmedt J.E. 1988. Thalamic pain syndrome of Dejérine-Roussy. Differentiation of four subtypes assisted by somatosensory evoked potentials data. Arch. Neurol. 45:1312–1320.

Mauguière F., and Desmedt J.E. 1989. Bilateral somatosensory evoked potentials in four patients with long-standing surgical hemispherectomy. Ann. Neurol. 26:724–731.

Mauguière F., and Desmedt J.E. 1991. Focal capsular vascular lesions can selectively deafferent the prerolandic or the parietal cortex: Somatosensory evoked potentials evidence. Ann. Neurol. 30:71–75.

Mauguière F., and Ibañez V. 1985. The dissociation of early SEP components in lesions of the cervico-medullary junction: a cue for routine interpretation of abnormal cervical responses to median nerve stimulation. Electroencephalogr. Clin. Neurophysiol. 62:406–420.

Mauguière F., and Ibañez V. 1990. Loss of parietal and frontal somatosensory evoked potentials in hemispheric deafferentation. In *New Trends and Advanced Techniques in Clinical Neurophysiology*, EEG J. Suppl. 41. Eds. P.M. Rossini and F. Mauguière, pp. 274–285. Amsterdam: Elsevier.

Mauguière F., and Restuccia D. 1991. Inadequacy of the forehead reference montage for detecting spinal N13 potential abnormalities in patients with cervical cord lesion and preserved dorsal column function. Electroencephalogr. Clin. Neurophysiol. 79:448–456.

Mauguière F., Bard J., and Courjon J. 1981. Les potentiels évoqués somesthésiques dans la dyssynergie cérébelleuse myoclonique progressive. Rev. EEG. Neurophysiol. 11:174–182.

Mauguière F., Brunon A.M., Echallier J.F., et al. 1982. Early somatosensory evoked potentials in thalamocortical lesions of the lemniscal pathways in humans. In *Clinical Applications of Evoked Potentials in Neurology, Advances in Neurology*, vol. 32, Eds. J. Courjon, F. Mauguière, and M. Revol, pp. 321–338. New York: Raven Press.

Mauguière F., Desmedt J.E., and Courjon J. 1983a. Astereognosis and dissociated loss of frontal or parietal components of somatosensory evoked potentials in hemispheric lesions. Brain 106:271–311.

Mauguière F., Desmedt J.E., and Courjon J. 1983b. Neural generators of N18 and P14 far-field somatosensory evoked potentials studied in patients with lesions of thalamus or thalamo-cortical radiations. Electroencephalogr. Clin. Neurophysiol. 56:283–292.

Mauguière F., Schott B., and Courjon J. 1983c. Dissociation of early SEP components in unilateral traumatic section of the lower medulla. Ann. Neurol. 13:309–313.

Mauguière F., Ibañez V., and Fischer C. 1985. Les potentiels évoqués somesthésiques dans les tumeurs intra-rachidiennes. Rev. EEG Clin. Neurophysiol. 15:95–106.

Mauguière F., Ibañez V., Deiber M.P., Garcia-Larrea L. 1987. Noncephalic reference recording and spatial mapping of short-latency SEPs to upper limb stimulation: normal responses and abnormal patterns in patients with nondemyelinating lesions of the CNS. In *Evoked Potentials III: The Third International Evoked Potentials Symposium*. Eds. C. Barber and T. Blum, pp. 40–55. Boston: Butterworth.

Mauguière F., Broussolle E., and Isnard J. 1993. Apomorphine induced relief of the akinetic-rigid syndrome and early median nerve somatosensory evoked potentials in Parkinson's disease. Electroencephalogr. Clin. Neurophysiol. 88:243–254.

Mauguière F., Holder G.E., Garcia-Larrea L., et al. 1995. Evoked potentials diagnostic yield of evoked potentials. In *Clinical Neurophysiology: EMG, Nerve Conduction and Evoked Potentials*, Eds. J.W. Osselton, C.D. Binnie, R. Cooper, et al., pp. 431–563. Oxford: Butterworth-Heinemann.

Mauguière F., Ibañez V., Turano G., et al. 1996. Neurophysiology in intramedullary spinal cord tumours. In *Intramedullary Spinal Cord Tumours*, Eds. G. Fischer and J. Brotchi, pp. 24–33. Stuttgart. Thieme.

Mauguière F., Merlet I., Forss N., et al. 1997a. Activation of a distributed cortical network in the human brain. A dipole modelling study of magnetic fields evoked by median nerve stimulation. Part I: Location and activation timing of SEF sources. Electroencephalogr. Clin. Neurophysiol. 104:281–289.

Mauguière F., Merlet I., Forss N., et al. 1997b. Activation of a distributed cortical network in the human brain. A dipole modelling study of magnetic fields evoked by median nerve stimulation. Part II: Effects of stimulus rate attention and stimulus detection. Electroencephalogr. Clin. Neurophysiol. 104:290–295.

Mauguière F., Chauvel P., Dewailly J., et al. 1997c. No effect of long-term Vigabatrin treatment on central nervous system conduction in patients with refractory epilepsy: results of a multicenter study of somatosensory and visual evoked potentials. Epilepsia. 38:301–308.

Mauguière F., Allison T., Babiloni C., et al. 1999. Somatosensory evoked potentials. In Deuschl G. and Eisen A. (Eds), *Recommendations for the practice of Clinical Neurophysiology*. Electroencephalogr. Clin. Neurophysiol. Suppl. 52:79–90.

Mavroudakis N., Brunko E., Nogueira M.C., et al. 1991. Acute effects of diphenylhydantoin on peripheral and central somatosensory conduction. Electroencephalogr. Clin. Neurophysiol. 78:263–266.

Mavroudakis N., Brunko E., Delberghe X., et al. 1993. Dissociation of P13-P14 far-field potentials: clinical and MRI correlation. Electroencephalogr. Clin. Neurophysiol. 88:240–242.

Mazzini L., Zaccala M., and Balzarini C. 1994. Abnormalities of somatosensory evoked potentials in spasmodic torticollis. Mov. Disord. 9:426–430.

McCarthy G., Wood C.C., and Allison T. 1991. Cortical somatosensory evoked potentials: I. Recordings in the monkey Macaca fascicularis. J. Neurophysiol. 66:53–63.

McGarry J., Friedgood D.L., Woolsey R., et al. 1984. SSEP in spinal cord injuries. Surg. Neurol. 22:341–343.

McPherson R.W., Sell B., and Traystman R.J. 1986. Effects of thiopental, fentanyl and ethomidate on upper extremity somatosensory evoked potentials in humans. Anesthesiology 65:584–589.

Mervaala E., Partanen J.V., Keränen T., et al. 1984. Prolonged cortical somatosensory evoked potential latencies in progressive myoclonus epilepsy. J. Neurol. Sci. 64:131–135.

Mervaala E., Pääkkönen A., and Partanen V. 1988. The influence of height, age and gender on the interpretation of median nerve SEPs. Electronceph. Clin. Neurophysiol. 71:109–113.

Miller D.H., McDonald W.I., Blumhardt L.D., et al. 1987. MRI of brain and spinal cord in isolated non-compressive spinal cord syndromes. Ann. Neurol. 22:714–723.

Mima T., Terada K., Maekawa M., et al. 1996. Somatosensory evoked potentials following proprioceptive stimulation of fingers in man. Exp. Brain Res. 29:440–443.

Mima T., Terada K., Ikeda H., et al. 1997. Afferent myoclonus studied by proprioception-related SEPs. Electroencephalogr. Clin. Neurophysiol. 104:51–59.

Mollaret P., and Goulon M. 1959. Le coma dépassé (mémoire préliminaire). Rev. Neurol. 101:3–10.

Moller A.R., Jannetta P.J., and Burgess J.E. 1986. Neural generator of the somatosensory evoked potentials recording from the cuneate nucleus in man and monkeys. Electroencephalogr. Clin. Neurophysiol. 65:241–248.

Morioka T., Shima F., Kato M., et al. 1991. Direct recordings of the somatosensory evoked potentials in the vicinity of the dorsal column nuclei in man: their mechanisms and contribution to the scalp far-field potentials. Electroencephalogr. Clin. Neurophysiol. 80:221–227.

Murase N., Kaji R., Shimazu H., et al. 2000. Abnormal premovement gating of somatosensory input in writer's cramp. Brain 123:1813–1829.

Näätänen R. 1990. The role of attention in auditory information processing as revealed by event-related potentials and other brain measures of cognitive function. Behav. Brain Sci. 13:201–288.

Nakanishi T., Takita K., and Toyokura Y. 1973. SEPs to tactile tap in man. Electroencephalogr. Clin. Neurophysiol. 34:1–6.

Nakanishi T., Shimada Y., Sakuta M., et al. 1978. The initial positive component of the scalp recorded somatosensory evoked potential in normal subjects and in patients with neurological disorders. Electroencephalogr. Clin. Neurophysiol. 45:26–34.

Nakanishi T., Tamaki M., Arasaki K. et al. 1981. Origins of the scalp-recorded somatosensory far field potentials in man and cat. In *The Kyoto Symposia*, EEG. J. Suppl. 36, Eds. P.A. Buser, W.A. Cobb, and T. Okuma, pp. 336–348. Amsterdam: Elsevier.

Nakanishi T., Tamaki M., Ozaki Y., et al. 1983. Origins of short latency somatosensory evoked potentials to median nerve stimulation. Electroencephalogr. Clin. Neurophysiol. 56:74–85.

Namerow N.S. 1968. Somatosensory evoked responses in multiple sclerosis patients with varying sensory loss. Neurology 18:1197–1204.

Newlon P.G., Greenberg R.P., Hyatt M.S., et al. 1982. The dynamics of neuronal dysfunction and recovery following severe head injury, assessed with serial multimodality evoked potentials. J. Neurosurg. 57:168–177.

Nicholson-Peterson N., Schroeder C.E., and Arezzo J.C. 1995. Neural generators of the early cortical somatosensory evoked potentials in the awake monkey. Electroencephalogr. Clin. Neurophysiol. 96:248–260.

Noachtar S., Lüders H.O., Dinner D.S., et al. 1997. Ipsilateral median somatosensory evoked potentials recorded from human somatosensory cortex. Electroencephalogr. Clin. Neurophysiol. 104:189–198.

Noel P., and Desmedt J.E. 1975. Somatosensory cerebral evoked potentials after vascular lesions of the brainstem and diencephalon. Brain 98:113–128.

Noel P., and Desmedt J.E. 1976. Somatosensory pathway in Friedreich's ataxia. Acta Neurol. Belg. 76:271.

Noel P., and Desmedt J.E. 1980. Cerebral and far-field somatosensory evoked potentials in neurological disorders involving the cervical spinal cord, brainstem, thalamus and cortex. In *Clinical Uses of Cerebral, Brainstem and Spinal Somatosensory Evoked Potentials. Progr. Clin. Neurophysiol.*, vol 7. Ed. Desmedt, pp. 205–230. Basel: Karger.

Noth J., Engel L., Friedemann H.H., et al. 1984. Evoked potentials in patients with Huntington's disease and their offspring. Electroencephalogr. Clin. Neurophysiol. 59:134–141.

Nuwer M.R., Perlman S.L., Packwood J.W., et al. 1983. Evoked potential abnormalities in the various inherited ataxias. Ann. Neurol. 13:20–27.

Nuwer M.R., Aminoff M., Desmedt J., et al. 1994. IFCN recommended standards for short latency somatosensory evoked potentials. Report of an IFCN committee. Electroencephalogr. Clin. Neurophysiol. 91:6–11.

Obeso J.A., Rothwell J.C., and Marsden C.D. 1985. The spectrum of cortical myoclonus: from focal reflex jerks to spontaneous motor epilepsy. Brain 108:193–224.

O'Connor P., Tansey C., Kucharczyk W., et al., and Rochester-Toronto MRI study group. 1994. A randomized trial of test result sequencing in patients with suspected multiple sclerosis. Arch Neurol 51:53–59.

Oepen G., Doerr M., and Thoden U. 1981. Visual (VEP) and somatosensory (SSEP) evoked potentials in Huntington's chorea. Electroencephalogr. Clin. Neurophysiol. 51:666–670.

Okada Y.C., Tanenbaum R., Williamson S.J., et al. 1984. Somatotopic organization of the human somatosensory cortex revealed by neuromagnetic measurements. Exp. Brain. Res. 56:197–205.

Oken B.S., and Chiappa K.H. 1986. Somatosensory evoked potentials in neurological diagnosis. In *Evoked Potentials. Frontiers in Clinical Neuroscience*, vol. 3, Eds. R.Q. Cracco and I. Bodis-Wollner, pp. 379–389. New York: Alan R. Liss.

Onofrj M., Ferracci F., Fulgente T., et al. 1994. Effects of drug manipulation on anterior components of somatosensory evoked potentials in a parkinsonian animal model. Drugs Exp. Clin. Res. 20:29–36.

Onofrj M., Fulgente T., Malatesta G., et al. 1995. The abnormality of N30 somatosensory evoked potential in idiopathic Parkinson's disease is unrelated to disease stage or clinical scores and insensitive to dopamine manipulations. Mov. Disord. 10:71–80.

Opsomer R.J., Caramia M.D., Zarola F., et al. 1989. Neurophysiological evaluation of central-peripheral sensory and motor pudendal fibres. Electroencephalogr. Clin. Neurophysiol. 74:260–270.

Opsomer R.J., Guerit J.M., Van Cangh P.J., et al. 1990. Electrophysiological assessment of somatic nerves controlling the genital and urinary functions. In *New Trends and Advanced Techniques in Clinical Neurophysiology*, EEG Suppl. 41. Eds. P.M. Rossini and F. Mauguière, pp. 298–305. Amsterdam: Elsevier.

Ozaki I., Shimamura H., Baba M., et al. 1996a. N30 in Parkinson's disease. Letter to the editor. Neurology. 47:303–305.

Ozaki I., Takada H., Shimamura H., et al. 1996b. Central conduction in somatosensory evoked potentials. Comparison of ulnar and median data evaluation of onset versus peak methods. Neurology 47:1299–1304.

Paillard J., Michel F., and Stelmach G. 1983. Localization without content. A tactile analogue of "blindsight." Arch. Neurol. 40:548–551.

Pallis C. 1990. Brainstem death. In *Handbook of Clinical Neurology, vol. 13, Head Injury*, Ed. R. Braakman, pp. 441–496. Amsterdam: Elsevier.

Papakostopoulos D., and Crow H.J. 1980. Direct recording of the somatosensory evoked potentials from the cerebral cortex of man and the difference between precentral and postcentral potentials. In *Clinical uses of cerebral, brainstem and spinal somatosensory evoked potentials. Progr. Clin. Neurophysiol*, vol. 7, Ed. J.E. Desmedt, pp. 15–26. Basel: Karger.

Papakostopoulos D., Cooper R., and Crow H.J. 1974. Cortical potentials evoked by finger displacement in man. J. Physiol. 245:70P–72P.

Papakostopoulos D., Cooper R., and Crow H.J. 1975. Inhibition of cortical evoked potentials and sensation by self-initiated movement in man. Nature 258:321–324.

Parry G.J., and Aminoff M.J. 1987. Somatosensory evoked potentials in chronic acquired demyelinating peripheral neuropathy. Neurology 37:313–316.

Pedersen L., and Trojaborg W. 1981. Visual, auditory and somatosensory pathway involvement in hereditary cerebellar ataxia, Friedreich's ataxia and familial spastic paraplegia. Electroencephalogr. Clin. Neurophysiol. 52:283–297.

Pelosi L., Cracco J.B., Cracco R.Q., et al. 1988. Comparison of scalp distribution of short latency somatosensory evoked potentials (SSEPs) to different stimulation of different nerves in the lower extremity. Electroencephalogr. Clin. Neurophysiol. 71:422–428.

Penfield W., and Rasmussen T. 1957. *The Cerebral Cortex of Man: A Clinical Study of Localization*. New York: Macmillan.

Penfield W., and Roberts L. 1959. *Speech and Brain Mechanisms.* Princeton: Princeton University Press.

Perlik S.J., and Fischer M.A. 1987. Somatosensory evoked response evaluation of cervical spondylitic myelopathy. Muscle Nerve 10:481–489.

Perot P.L., and Vera C.L. 1982. Scalp-recorded somatosensory evoked potentials to stimulation of nerves in the lower extremities and evaluation of patients with spinal cord trauma. Ann. N.Y. Acad. Sci. 388:359–368.

Pfurtscheller G., Schwartz G., and Gravenstein N. 1985. Clinical relevance of long latency VEPs and SEPs during coma and emergence from coma. Electroencephalogr. Clin. Neurophysiol. 62:88–98.

Pfurtscheller G., Schwartz G., Schroettner O., et al. 1987. Continuous and simultaneous monitoring of EEG spectra, brainstem auditory and somatosensory evoked potentials in the intensive care unit and the operating room. J. Clin. Neurophysiol. 4:389–396.

Phillips C.G., Powell T.P., and Wiesendanger M. 1971. Projection from low-threshold muscle afferents of hand and forearm to area a of the baboon cortex. J. Physiol. 217:419–446.

Pierantozzi M., Mazzone P., Bassi A., et al. 1999. The effect of deep brain stimulation on the frontal N30 component of somatosensory evoked potentials in advanced Parkinson's disease patients. Electroencephalogr. Clin. Neurophysiol. 110:1700–1707.

Plasmati R., Blanco M., Michelucci R., et al. 1989. SEPs study in idiopathic infantile epilepsies. In *Reflex Seizures and Epilepsies,* Eds. A. Beaumanoir, H. Gastaut H. and R. Naquet, pp. 75–81. Geneva: Editions Médecine et Hygiène.

Pratt H., and Starr A. 1981. Mechanically and electrically evoked somatosensory potentials in humans; scalp and neck distribution of short latency components. Electroencephalogr. Clin. Neurophysiol. 51:138–147.

Purves S.J., Low M.D., Galloway J., et al. 1981. A comparison of visual, brainstem auditory, and somatosensory evoked potentials in multiple sclerosis. Can. J. Neurol. Sci. 8:15–19.

Radtke R.A., Erwin A., and Erwin C.W. 1986. Abnormal somatosensory evoked potentials in amyotrophic lateral sclerosis. Neurology 36:796–801.

Reilly J.A., Hallett M., Cohen L.G., et al. 1992. The N30 component of somatosensory evoked potentials in patients with dystonia. Electroencephalogr. Clin. Neurophysiol. 84:243–247.

Restuccia D. 2000. Anatomic origin of P13 and P14 scalp far-field potentials. J. Clin. Neurophysiol. 17:246–257.

Restuccia D., and Mauguière F. 1991. The contribution of median nerve SEPs in the functional assessment of the cervical spinal cord in syringomyelia. A study of 24 patients. Brain 114:361–379.

Restuccia D., Di Lazzaro V, Valeriani M., et al. 1992. Segmental dysfunction of the cervical cord revealed by abnormalities of the spinal N13 potential in cervical spondylotic myelopathy. Neurology. 42:1054–1063.

Restuccia D., Valeriani M., Di Lazzaro V., et al. 1994. Somatosensory evoked potentials after multisegmental upper limb stimulation in the diagnosis of cervical spondylotic myelopathy. J. Neurol. Neurosurg. Psychiatry 57:301–308.

Restuccia D., Di Lazzaro V, Valeriani M., et al. 1995. Origin and distribution of P13 and P14 far-field potentials after median nerve stimulation. Scalp, nasopharyngeal and neck recordings in healthy subjects and in patients with cervical and cervico-medullary lesions. Electroencephalogr. Clin. Neurophysiol. 96:371–384.

Restuccia D., Di Lazzaro V, Valeriani M., et al. 1996. Brainstem somatosensory dysfunction in a case of long-standing left hemispherectomy with removal of the left thalamus: a nasopharyngeal and scalp SEP study. Electroencephalogr. Clin. Neurophysiol. 100:184–188.

Restuccia D., Di Lazzaro M., Valeriani M., et al. 1997. Neurophysiological abnormalities in adrenoleukodystrophy carriers. Evidence of different degrees of central nervous system involvement. Brain 120:1139–1148.

Restuccia D., Valeriani M., Barba C., et al. 1999. Different contribution of joint and cutaneous inputs to early scalp somatosensory evoked potentials. Muscle Nerve 22:910–919.

Restuccia D., Valeriani M., Insola A., et al. 2002a. Modality-related scalp responses after selective electrical stimulation of cutaneous and muscular upper limb afferents in humans: specific and unspecific components. Muscle & Nerve. 26:44–54.

Restuccia D., Valeriani M., Grassi E., et al. 2002b. Contribution of gabaergic circuitry in shaping scalp somatosensory evokes responses in humans: specific changes after single-dose administration of tiagabine. Clin. Neurophysiol. 113:656–671.

Ridding M.C. and Rothwell J.C. 1999. Afferent input and cortical organization: a study with magnetic stimulation, Exp. Brain Res. 126:536–544.

Ridding M.C., Taylor J.L., and Rothwell J.C. 1995. The effect of voluntary contraction on cortico-cortical inhibition in human motor cortex. J. Physiol. 487:541–548.

Riffel B., Stöhr M., and Körner S. 1984. Spinal and cortical potentials following stimulation of posterior tibial nerve in the diagnosis and localization of spinal cord diseases. Electroencephalogr. Clin. Neurophysiol. 58: 400–407.

Roland P.E., Larsen B., Larsen N.A., et al. 1980. Supplementary motor area and other cortical areas in organization of voluntary movements in man. J. Neurophysiol. 43:118–136.

Ropper A.H., and Marmarou A. 1984. Mechanisms of pseudotumor in Guillain-Barré syndrome. Arch. Neurol. 41:259–261.

Ropper A.H., and Chiappa K.H. 1986. Evoked potentials in Guillain-Barré syndrome. Neurology 36:587–590.

Rossi S., Tecchio F., Pasqualetti P., et al. 2002. Somatosensory processing during movement observation in humans. Clin. Neurophysiol. 113:16–24.

Rossini P.M., Babiloni F., Bernardi G., et al. 1989. Abnormalities of short-latency somatosensory evoked potentials in parkinsonian patients. Electroencephalogr. Clin. Neurophysiol. 74:277–289.

Rossini P.M., Paradiso C., Zarola F., et al. 1991. Brain excitability and long-latency muscular arm responses: non-invasive evaluation in healthy and parkinsonian subjects. Electroencephalogr. Clin. Neurophysiol. 81: 454–465.

Rossini P.M., Traversa R., Boccasena P., et al. 1993. Parkinson's disease and somatosensory evoked potentials: apomorphine-induced transient potentiation of frontal components. Neurology 43:2495–2500.

Rossini P.M., Bassetti M.A., and Pasqualetti P. 1995. Median nerve somatosensory evoked potentials. Apomorphine-induced transient potentiation of frontal components in Parkinson's disease and in parkinsonism. Electroencephalogr. Clin. Neurophysiol. 96:236–247.

Rossini P.M., Caramia D., Bassetti M.A., et al. 1996. Somatosensory evoked potentials during the ideation and execution of individual finger movements. Muscle Nerve 19:191–202.

Rothstein T.L., Thomas E.M., and Sumi S.M. 1991. Predicting outcome in hypoxic-ischemic coma. A prospective clinical and electrophysiologic study. Electroencephalogr. Clin. Neurophysiol. 79:101–107.

Rothwell L.J.C., Obeso J.A., and Marsden C.D. 1984. On the significance of giant somatosensory evoked potentials in cortical myoclonus. J. Neurol. Neurosurg. Psychiatry 47:33–42.

Rowed D.W., McClean J.A.G., and Tator C.H. 1978. Somatosensory evoked potentials in acute spinal cord injury. Prognostic value. Surg. Neurol. 9:203–210.

Rumpl E., Prugger M., Gerstenbrand F., et al. 1983. Central somatosensory conduction time and short-latency somatosensory evoked potentials in post-traumatic coma. Electroencephalogr. Clin. Neurophysiol. 56:583–596.

Rumpl E., Prugger M., Battista H.J., et al. 1988a. Short latency somatosensory evoked potentials and brain stem auditory evoked potentials in coma due to CNS depressant drug poisoning. Preliminary observations. Electroencephalogr. Clin. Neurophysiol. 70:482–489.

Rumpl E., Prugger M., Gerstenbrand F., et al. 1988b. Central somatosensory conduction time and acoustic brainstem transmission time in post-traumatic coma. J. Clin. Neurophysiol. 5:237–260.

Sauer M., and Schenck E. 1977. Electrophysiologic investigations in Friedreich heredoataxia and in hereditary motor and sensory neuropathy. Electroencephalogr. Clin. Neurophysiol. 43:623.

Schieppati M., and Ducati A. 1984. Short latency cortical potentials evoked by tactile air-jet stimulation of body and face in man. Electroencephalogr. Clin. Neurophysiol. 58:418–425.

Schmitt B., Seeger J., and Jacobi G. 1992. EEG and evoked potentials in HIV-infected children. Clin. Encephalogr. 23:11–117.

Schramm J., Assfalg B., and Brock M. 1984. Segmentally evoked preoperative and postoperative somatosensory potentials in spinal tumors. In *Evoked Potentials II*, Eds. R.H. Nodar and C. Barber, pp. 406–412. Boston: Butterworth.

Sedgwick E.M., El-Negamy E., and Frankel H. 1980. Spinal cord potentials in traumatic paraplegia and quadriplegia. J. Neurol. Neurosurg. Psychiatry 43:823–830.

Seyal M. 1995. Cortical reflex myoclonus. A study of the relation between giant somatosensory evoked potentials and motor excitability. J. Clin. Neurophysiol. 55:95–101.

Seyal M., Emerson R.G., and Pedley T.A. 1983. Spinal and early scalp-recorded components of the somatosensory evoked potential following stimulation of the posterior tibial nerve. Electroencephalogr. Clin. Neurophysiol. 55:320–330.

Sherman A.L., Tirschwell D.L., Micklesen P.J., et al. 2000. Somatosensory potentials, CSF creatine kinase BB activity, and awakening after cardiac arrest. Neurology 54:889–894.

Sherwood A.M. 1981. Characteristics of somatosensory evoked potentials recorded over the spinal cord and brain of man. IEEE Trans. 28:481–487.

Shibasaki H., and Kuroiwa Y. 1975. Electroencephalographic correlates of myoclonus. Electroencephalogr. Clin. Neurophysiol. 39:455–463.

Shibasaki H., Yamashita Y., Neshige R., et al. 1985a. Pathogenesis of giant somatosensory evoked potentials in progressive myoclonic epilepsy. Brain 108:225–240.

Shibasaki H., Neshige R., and Hashiba Y. 1985b. Cortical excitability after myoclonus. Jerk-locked somatosensory evoked potentials. Neurology 35:36–41.

Shibasaki H., Nakamura M., Nishida S., et al. 1990. Waveform decomposition of "giant SEP" and its computer model for scalp topography. Electroencephalogr. Clin. Neurophysiol. 77:286–294.

Shimazu H., Kaji R., Murase N., et al. 1999. Pre-movement gating of short-latency somatosensory evoked potentials. Neuroreport 10:2457–2460.

Shimoji K., Matsuki M., and Shimizu H. 1977. Waveform characteristics and spatial distribution of evoked spinal electrogram in man. J. Neurosurg. 46:304–313.

Siivola J., Myllyllä V.V., Sulg I., et al. 1979. Brachial plexus and radicular neurography in relation to cortical evoked responses. J. Neurol. Neurosurg. Psychiatr. 42:1151–1158.

Siivola J., Sulg I., and Heiskari M. 1981. Somatosensory evoked potentials in diagnostics of cervical spondylosis and herniated disk. Electroencephalogr. Clin. Neurophysiol. 52:276–282.

Sindou M., and Jeamonod D. 1989. Microsurgical DREZ–tomy for the treatment of spasticity and pain in the lower limbs. Neurosurgery 24: 655–670.

Sindou M., Fischer G., and Mansuy L. 1976. Posterior spinal rhizotomy and selective posterior rhizidiotomy. Prog. Neurol. Surg. 7:201–250.

Slimp J.C., Tamas L.B., Stolow W.C., et al. 1986. Somatosensory evoked potentials after removal of somatosensory cortex in man. Electroencephalogr. Clin. Neurophysiol. 65:111–117.

Slimp J.C., Janczakowski J., Seed L.J., et al. 1990. Comparison of median and posterior tibial nerve somatosensory evoked potentials in ambulatory patients with definite multiple sclerosis. Am. J. Phys. Med. Rehabil. 69: 293–296.

Small M., and Matthews W.B. 1984. A method of calculating spinal cord transit time from potentials evoked by tibial nerve stimulation in normal subjects and patients with spinal cord disease. Electroencephalogr. Clin. Neurophysiol. 59:156–164.

Smith T., Jakobsen J., Gaub J., et al. 1988. Clinical and electrophysiological studies of human immunodeficiency virus-seropositive men without AIDS. Ann. Neurol. 23:295–297.

Sonoo M. 2000. Anatomic origin and clinical application of the widespread N18 potential in median nerve somatosensory evoked potentials. J. Clin. Neurophysiol. 17:258–268.

Spehlmann R. 1985. *Evoked Potential Primer. Visual, Auditory and Somatosensory Evoked Potentials in Clinical Diagnosis.* Boston: Butterworth.

Stanzione P., Traversa R., Pierantozzi M., et al. 1997. SEPs N30 amplitude in pharmacologically induced rigidity: relationship with the clinical status. Eur. J. Neurol. 4:24–38.

Stephan K.M., Fink G.R., Passingham R.E., et al. 1995. Functional anatomy of the mental representation of upper extremity movements in healthy subjects. J. Neurophysiol. 73:373–386.

Stöhr M., Petruch F., and Scheglman K. 1981. Somatosensory evoked potentials following trigeminal nerve stimulation in trigeminal neuralgia. Ann. Neurol. 9:63–66.

Stöhr M., Buettner U.W., and Riffel B. 1982. Spinal somatosensory evoked potentials in cervical cord lesions. Electroencephalogr Clin Neurophysiol. 54:257–265.

Stöhr M., Dichgans J., Voigt K. et al. 1983. The significance of somatosensory evoked potentials for localization of unilateral lesions within the cerebral hemispheres. J. Neurol. Sci. 61:49–63.

Subramaniam J.C., and Yannikas C. 1990. Multimodality evoked potentials in motor neuron disease. Arch. Neurol. 989–994.

Sutton L.N., Frewen T., Marsh R., et al. 1982. The effects of deep barbiturate coma on multimodality evoked potentials. J. Neurosurg. 57:78–185.

Synek V.M. 1985. Assessing sensory involvement in lower limb nerve lesion using somato-sensory evoked potential techniques. Muscle & Nerve 8:511–515.

Synek V.M., and Cowan J.C. 1983a. Somatosensory evoked potentials in patients with metastatic involvement of the brachial plexus. Electromyogr. Clin. Neurophysiol. 23:545–551.

Synek V.M., and Cowan J.C. 1983b. Saphenous nerve evoked potentials and the assessment of intraabdominal lesions in the femoral nerve. Muscle Nerve 6:453–456.

Tanji J., and Wise S.P. 1981. Submodality distribution in sensorimotor cortex of the unanesthetized monkey. J. Neurophysiol. 45:467–481.

Tarkka I.M., and Treede R.D. 1993. Equivalent electrical source analysis of pain-related somatosensory evoked potentials elicited by a CO_2 laser. J. Clin. Neurophysiol. 10:513–519.

Taylor M.J. 1993. Evoked potentials in paediatrics. In *Evoked Potentials in Clinical Testing,* Ed. A.M. Halliday, pp. 489–521. Edinburgh: Churchill Livingstone.

Taylor M.J., Chan Lui W.Y., and Logan N.J. 1985. Longitudinal evoked potential studies in hereditary ataxias. Can. J. Neurol. Sci. 12:100–105.

Thomas J.E., and Lambert E.H. 1960. Ulnar nerve conduction velocity and H reflex in infants and children. J. Appl. Physiol. 15:1–9.

Thomas P.K., Jefferys J.G.R., Smith I.S., et al. 1981. Spinal somatosensory evoked potentials in hereditary spastic paraplegia. J. Neurol. Neurosurg. Psychiatry 44:243–246.

Tinazzi M., and Mauguière F. 1995. Assessment of intraspinal and intracranial conduction by P30 and P39 tibial nerve somatosensory evoked potentials in cervical cord and hemispheric lesions. J. Clin. Neurophysiol. 12:237–253.

Tinazzi M., Zanette G., Fiaschi A., et al. 1996a. Effects of stimulus rate on the cortical posterior tibial nerve SEPs: a topographic study. Electroencephalogr. Clin. Neurophysiol. 100:210–219.

Tinazzi M., Zanette G., Bonato C., et al. 1996b. Neural generators of tibial nerve P30 somatosensory evoked potential studied in patients with a focal lesion of the cervico-medullary junction. Muscle Nerve 19:1538–1548.

Tinazzi M., Zanette G., Manganotti B., et al. 1997a. Amplitude changes of tibial nerve cortical SEPs when using ipsilateral or contralateral ear as reference. J. Clin. Neurophysiol. 14:217–225.

Tinazzi M., Zanette G., La Porta F., et al. 1997b. Selective gating of lower limb cortical somatosensory evoked potentials (SEPs) during passive and active foot movements. Electroencephalogr. Clin. Neurophysiol. 104:312–321.

Tinazzi M., Fiaschi A., Mauguière F., et al. 1998. Effects of voluntary contraction on tibial nerve somatosensory evoked potentials: gating of specific cortical responses. Neurology 50:1655–1661.

Tinazzi M., Frasson E., Polo A., et al. 1999. Evidence for an abnormal cortical sensory processing in dystonia: selective enhancement of lower limb P37-N50 somatosensory evoked potential. Mov. Disord. 14:473 480.

Tinazzi M., Priori A., Bertolasi L., et al. 2000. Abnormal central integration of a dual somatosensory input in dystonia: evidence for sensory overflow. Brain 123:42–50.

Tomberg C., Desmedt J.E., Ozaki I., et al. 1991a. Nasopharyngeal recordings of somatosensory evoked potentials document the medullary origin of the N18 far-field. Electroencephalogr. Clin. Neurophysiol. 80:496–503.

Tomberg C., Desmedt J.E., and Osaki I. 1991b. Right or left ear reference changes the voltage of frontal and parietal somatosensory evoked potentials. Electroencephalogr. Clin. Neurophysiol. 80:504–512.

Tomita Y., Nishimura S., and Tanaka T. 1986. Short-latency SEPs in infants and children: developmental changes and maturational index of SEPs. Electroencephalogr. Clin. Neurophysiol. 65:335–343.

Töpper R., Schwarz M., Podoll K., et al. 1980. Absence of frontal somatosensory evoked potentials in Huntington's disease. Brain 111:87–101.

Towell A.D., and Boyd SG. 1993. Sensory and cognitive components of the CO_2 laser–evoked cerebral potentials. Electroencephalogr. Clin. Neurophysiol. 88:237–239.

Treede R.D., Kief S., Hölzer T., et al. 1988. Late somatosensory evoked cerebral potentials in response to cutaneous heat stimuli. Electroencephalogr. Clin. Neurophysiol. 70:429–441.

Treede R.D., Lankers J., Frieling A., et al. 1991. Cerebral potentials evoked by painful laser stimuli in patients with syringomyelia. Brain 114:1595–1607.

Treede R.D., Lorenz J., Kunze K., et al. 1995. Assessment of nociceptive pathways with laser-evoked potentials in normal subjects and patients. In *Pain and the Brain. From Nociception to Cognition.* Eds. B. Bromm and J.E. Desmedt, pp. 337–392. New York: Raven Press.

Trojaborg W., and Petersen E. 1979. Visual and somatosensory evoked cortical potentials in multiple sclerosis. J. Neurol. Neurosurg. Psychiatry 42:323–330.

Tsuji S., Lüders H., Lesser R.P., et al. 1984. Subcortical and cortical somatosensory potentials evoked by posterior tibial nerve stimulation: normative values. Electroencephalogr. Clin. Neurophysiol. 59:214–228.

Tsuji S., Muray Y., and Kadoya C. 1988. Topography of somatosensory evoked potentials to median nerve stimulation in patients with cerebral lesions. Electroencephalogr. Clin. Neurophysiol. 71:280–288.

Tsumoto T., Hirose N., Nonaka S., et al. 1972. Analysis of somatosensory evoked potentials to lateral popliteal nerve stimulation in man. Electroencephalogr. Clin. Neurophysiol. 33:379–388.

Turano G., Jones S.J., Miller D.H., et al. 1991. Correlation of SEP abnormalities with brain and cervical cord MRI in multiple sclerosis. Brain 114:663–681.

Turano G., Sindou M., and Mauguière F. 1995. Spinal cord evoked potentials monitoring during spinal surgery for pain and spasticity. In *Atlas of Human Cord Evoked Potentials,* Eds. M.R. Dimitrijevic and J.A. Halter, pp. 107–122. Boston: Butterworth-Heinemann.

Urasaki E., Wada S., Kadoya C., et al. 1988. Absence of spinal N13-P13 and normal scalp far-field P14 in a patient with syringomyelia. Electroencephalogr. Clin. Neurophysiol. 71:400–404.

Urasaki E., Wada S., Kadoya C., et al. 1990. Origin of scalp far-field N18 of SSEPs in response to median nerve stimulation. Electroencephalogr. Clin. Neurophysiol. 77:39–51.

Urasaki E., Tokimura T., Yasukouchi H., et al. 1993. P30 and N33 of posterior tibial nerve SSEPs are analogous to P14 and N18 of median nerve SSEPs. Electroencephalogr. Clin. Neurophysiol. 88:525–529.

Valeriani M., Rambaud L., and Mauguière F. 1996. Scalp topography and dipolar source modelling of potentials evoked by CO_2 Laser stimulation of the hand. Electroencephalogr. Clin. Neurophysiol. 100:343–352.

Valeriani M., Restuccia D., Di Lazzaro V., et al. 1997a. The pathophysiology of giant SEPs in cortical myoclonus: a scalp topography and dipolar source modelling study. Electroencephalogr. Clin. Neurophysiol. 104:122–131.

Valeriani M., Restuccia D., Di Lazzaro V., et al. 1997b. Giant central N20-P22 with normal area 3b N20-P20: an argument in favor of an area 3a generator of early median nerve cortical SEPs? Electroencephalogr. Clin. Neurophysiol. 104:60–67.

Valeriani M., Restuccia D., Di Lazzaro V., et al. 1998a. Dipolar sources of the early scalp SEPs to upper limb stimulation. Effects of increasing stimulus rates. Exp. Brain Res. 120:306–315.

Valeriani M., Restuccia D., Di Lazzaro V., et al. 1998b. Dissociation induced by voluntary movement between two different components of the centro-parietal P40 SEP to tibial nerve stimulation. Electroencephalogr. Clin. Neurophysiol. 108:190–198.

Valeriani M., Restuccia D., Barba C., et al. 2000. Central scalp projection of the N30 SEP source activity after median nerve stimulation. Muscle Nerve 23:353–360.

Valeriani M., Insola A., Restuccia D., et al. 2001. Source generators of the early somatosensory evoked potentials to tibial nerve stimulation: an intracerebral and scalp recording study. Clin. Neurophysiol. 112:1999–2006.

Vanasse M., Garcia-Larrea L., Neuschwander L., et al. 1988. Evoked potentials studies in Friedreich's ataxia and progressive early onset cerebellar ataxia. Can. J. Neurol. Sci. 15:292–298.

Vanasse M., Gabet J.Y., De Léan J., et al. 1990. Utility of short-latency evoked potentials in the classification of progressive, early onset cerebellar ataxias. In *New Trends and Advanced Techniques in Clinical Neurophysiology,* EEG J. Suppl. 41. Eds. P.M. Rossini and F. Mauguière, pp. 223–235. Amsterdam: Elsevier.

Vas G.A., Cracco J.B., and Cracco R.Q. 1981. Scalp recorded short latency cortical and subcortical somatosensory evoked potentials in peroneal nerve stimulation. Electroencephalogr Clin. Neurophysiol. 51:1–8.

Veilleux M., and Daube J.R. 1987. The value of ulnar somatosensory evoked potentials (SEPs) in cervical myelopathy. Electroencephalogr Clin. Neurophysiol. 68:415–423.

Veilleux M., and Stevens J.C. 1987. Syringomyelia: electrophysiologic aspects. Muscle Nerve 10:449–458.

Vera C.L., Perot P.L., and Fountain E.I. 1983. Scalp recorded somatosensory evoked potentials after stimulation of the tibial nerve. Electroencephalogr. Clin. Neurophysiol. 56:159–168.

Wabersky T.D., Buchner H., Perkuhn M., et al. 1999. N30 and the effect of explorative finger movements: a model of the contribution of the motor cortex to early somatosensory potentials. Clin. Neurophysiol. 110:1589–1600.

Wagner W. 1991. SEP testing in deeply comatose and brain dead patients; the role of nasopharyngeal, scalp and earlobe derivations in recording the P14 potential. Electroencephalogr. Clin. Neurophysiol. 80:352–363.

Wagner W. 1996. Scalp, earlobe and nasopharyngeal recordings of the median nerve somatosensory evoked P14 potential in coma and brain death. Brain 119:1507–1521.

Walser H., Kriss A., Cunningham K., et al. 1982. A multimodal evoked potential assessment of uremia. In *Evoked Potentials II,* Eds. R.H. Nodar and C. Barber, pp. 643–649. Boston: Butterworth.

Walser H., Mattle H., Keller H.M., et al. 1985. Early cortical median nerve somatosensory evoked potentials. Prognostic value in anoxic coma. Arch. Neurol. 42:32–38.

Walsh J.C., Yiannikas C., and McLeod J.G. 1984. Abnormalities of proximal conduction in acute idiopathic polyneuritis: Comparison of short-latency evoked potentials and F waves. J. Neurol. Neurosurg. Psychiatry 47:197–200.

Wang J., Cohen L.J., and Hallett M. 1989. Scalp topography of somatosensory evoked potentials following electrical stimulation of femoral nerve. Electroencephalogr. Clin. Neurophysiol. 74:112–123.

Whittle I.R., Johnston I.H., and Besser M. 1986. Recording of spinal somatosensory evoked potentials for intraoperative spinal cord monitoring. J. Neurosurg. 64:601–612.

Wood C.C., Cohen D., Cuffin B.N., et al. 1985. Electrical sources in human somatosensory cortex: identification by combined magnetic and potential recordings. Science 227:1051–1053.

Woolsey C.N., Erickson T.C., and Gilson W.E. 1979. Localization in somatic sensory and motor areas of human cerebral cortex as determined by direct recording of evoked potentials and electrical stimulation. J. Neurosurg. 51:476–506.

Wu Q., Garcia-Larrea L., Mertens P., et al. 1999. Hyperalgesia with reduced laser evoked potentials in neuropathic pain. Pain 80:209–214.

Yamada T. 2000. Neuroanatomic substrates of lower extremity somatosensory evoked potentials. J. Clin. Neurophysiol. 17:269–279.

Yamada T., Machida M., and Kimura J. 1982. Far-field somatosensory evoked potentials after stimulation of the tibial nerve. Neurology 32:1151–1158.

Yamada T., Kayamori R., Kimura J., et al. 1984. Topography of SEPs after stimulation of the median nerve. Electroencephalogr. Clin. Neurophysiol. 59:29–43.

Yamada T., Graff-Radford N.R., Kimura J., et al. 1985. Topographic analysis of somatosensory evoked potentials in patients with well-localized thalamic infarctions. J. Neurol. Sci. 68:31–46.

Yamada T., Ishida T., Kudo Y., et al. 1986. Clinical correlates of abnormal P14 in median SEPs. Neurology. 36:765–771.

Yamada T., Kameyama S., Fuchigami Y., et al. 1988. Changes of short latency somatosensory evoked potentials in sleep. Electroencephalogr. Clin. Neurophysiol. 70:126–136.

Yamada T., Matsubara M., Shiraishi M., et al. 1996. Topographic analysis of somatosensory evoked potentials following stimulation tibial, sural and lateral femoral cutaneous nerve. Electroencephalogr. Clin. Neurophysiol. 100:33–43.

Yiannikas C., and Walsh J.C. 1983. Somatosensory evoked potentials in thoracic outlet syndrome. J. Neurol. Neurosurg. Psychiatry 46:234–240.

Yiannikas C., Shahani B.T., and Young RR. 1986. Short-latency somatosensory-evoked potentials from radial, median, ulnar and peroneal nerve stimulation in the assessment of cervical spondylosis. Comparison conventional electromyography. Arch. Neurol. 43:1264–1271.

York D.H., Watts C., Raffensberg M., et al. 1983. Utilization of SSEP in spinal cord injury. Spine 8:832–837.

Young W. 1982. Correlation of somatosensory evoked potentials and neurological findings in spinal cord injury. In *Early Management of Acute Spinal Cord Injury,* Ed. C.H. Tator, pp. 153–165. New York: Raven Press.

Yu Y.L., and Jones S.J. 1985. Somatosensory evoked potentials in cervical spondylolysis. Correlation of median, ulnar and posterior tibial nerve responses with clinical and radiological findings. Brain 108:273–300.

Zanette G., Polo A., Gasperini M., et al. 1990. Far-field and cortical somatosensory evoked potentials in motor neuron disease. Muscle Nerve 13:47–55.

Zanette G., Tinazzi M., Manganotti P., et al. 1995. Two distinct cervical N13 potentials are evoked by ulnar nerve stimulation. Electroencephalogr. Clin. Neurophysiol. 96:114–120.

Zanette G., Tinazzi M., Polo A., et al. 1996. Motor neuron disease with pyramidal tract dysfunction involves the cortical generators of the early somatosensory evoked potential to tibial nerve stimulation. Neurology 47:932–938.

Zegers de Beyl D., Delberghe X., Herbaut A.G., et al., 1988a. The somatosensory central conduction time: Physiological considerations and normative data. Electroencephalogr. Clin. Neurophysiol. 71:17–26.

Zegers de Beyl D., Delecluse F., Verbanck S., et al. 1988b. Somatosensory conduction in Vitamin B12 deficiency. Electroencephalogr. Clin. Neurophysiol. 69:313–318.

Zhu Y., Geogesco M., and Cadilhac J. 1987. Normal latency values of early cortical somatosensory evoked potentials in children. Electroencephalogr. Clin. Neurophysiol. 68:471–474.

55. Evoked Potentials in Infancy and Childhood

Allan Krumholz

Because neurological function and development are difficult to assess clinically in infants and young children, the use of evoked potentials in pediatric neurology has become an area of great interest and clinical activity. Numerous neurodiagnostic techniques, including imaging and electrophysiological methods, have been investigated in an effort to find objective measures that could help determine or predict cognitive or sensory capabilities in children. However, the acknowledged limitations of even the best modern brain imaging techniques, such as computed tomography (CT), magnetic resonance imaging (MRI), functional magnetic resonance imaging, and positron emission tomography (PET), for assessing specific physiological and neurological functions or more general neurological development have prompted investigation of other methods for neurological evaluation in infants and children. In particular, the demonstrated value of EEG in neonatal neurological assessment (Lombroso, 1987) has stimulated interest in electrophysiological methods, and considerable attention has centered on the field of event-related or evoked potentials.

Evoked potentials are electrophysiological responses to specific sensory stimuli, for instance, sound, light, or tactile stimulation. The evoked potentials that have demonstrated the greatest clinical utility in both adults and children have been brainstem auditory evoked potentials (BAEP), also termed auditory brainstem responses (ABR), visual evoked potentials (VEP), and somatosensory evoked potentials (SEP) (Table 55.1).

History

Evoked potentials were the first forms of electrical signals recorded from the brain. In 1875, Richard Caton described electrical activity from the brain when he recorded evoked potentials to light in animals (Brazier, 1984). Although Caton's early observations lacked the influence and sophistication of Hans Berger's monumental studies of human EEG, they preceded Berger's work by half a century.

Initially, technical difficulties in recording the small, relatively low-voltage electrical potential changes associated with event-related potentials severely limited their utility. Furthermore, early methods of recording these signals involved superimposing tracings, which was tedious and imprecise. However, Dawson, working in the late 1940s, developed a technique that used a mechanical rotator and gave a summated average of repeated stimuli, making evoked potential averaging more reliable and practical (Brazier, 1984). The introduction of digital computing methods and marketing of clinical averaging systems dedicated to evoked potential applications have allowed widespread utilization of evoked potential testing methods in both clinical and experimental neurology.

The first clinical applications for evoked potentials were not in children but in adults. In the early 1970s, Halliday et al. (1973) discovered that subclinical VEP delays occurred in multiple sclerosis and could be used to aid diagnosis. At about the same time, Jewett (1970) reported recordable early electrical potentials to auditory stimulation that did not originate in the cortex and were much more stable and clinically applicable than the previously described later-latency cortical auditory evoked potential (AEP). In addition, early SEP components were demonstrated that originated in subcortical regions of the nervous system and are of considerable clinical utility (Chiappa, 1997). Although these initial clinical applications of evoked potentials were in adult neurology, evoked potential techniques were early recognized to have great promise for pediatric assessments.

Origin of Evoked Potentials

Specific source generators for many recorded and clinically used evoked potentials remain somewhat controversial. Late evoked potential components, for instance the P-100 component of the VEP and the P-300 component widely used in experimental psychology and cognitive neurophysiology, are derived from electrical potential changes from apical dendrites of cortical neurons and have a neurophysiological basis similar to that of conventional EEG. These evoked potentials arise from the cortex and are termed *near-field potentials* because they are best recorded by electrodes nearest the region of cortex from which they originate. In contrast, very early or short-latency components of some evoked potentials, that is, those appearing within the first 20 to 30 msec after stimulation, may derive from axonal potentials generated principally from subcortical fiber tracts of the specific sensory pathways stimulated. Most axonal potentials are traveling impulses and difficult to record from distant electrodes, but sometimes, possibly with changes in direction, geometry, or volume of the conducting medium, fixed or stationary potentials are produced that can be recorded at electrodes quite distant from the site of origin of these potentials, and these types of evoked potentials have been termed *far-field potentials*. Examples of such far-field evoked potentials include the BAEP and the short latency components of the median and posterior tibial nerve SEPs (Kimura et al., 1986).

Although the individual peaks or components of a short-latency evoked potential are often related to a specific part of a subcortical sensory pathway, such as a subcortical relay nucleus, they may actually be more complex and have mul-

Table 55.1. Evoked Potentials Established as Clinically Useful in Infants and Children

Brainstem auditory evoked potentials (BAEP) also called auditory
  brainstem responses (ABR)
Visual evoked potential (VEP)
Somatosensory evoked potential (SEP) (to median or posterior nerve
  stimulation)

tiple source generators, including axonal potentials and synaptic relays. In terms of nomenclature, an individual wave peak is generally designated on the basis of its polarity and approximate mean latency or relative position in the sequence of the characteristic waveform (Figs. 55.1 to 55.3).

General Aspects of Evoked Potential Development

All types of standard evoked potentials, visual, auditory, and somatosensory, have been shown to mature and develop during infancy and childhood (Cracco et al., 1979; Hrbek et al., 1973; Krumholz et al., 1985). In premature infants, evoked potentials may be recorded, but the waveforms are not as well developed as in older subjects and the latencies of individual components tend to be significantly longer. Maturation, particularly as manifested by shortening wave component latencies, is rapid, with most evoked response latencies reaching adult values in the first few years of life (Allison et al., 1984). This dramatic electrophysiological maturation is postulated to relate to several specific developmental changes occurring in the nervous system during this critical growth period. These include myelination, improved synaptic efficiency, and increased axonal diameter. All of these important neurobiological influences may contribute to the electrophysiological changes observed in evoked potential maturation (Eggermont, 1988).

Evoked potentials have many exciting possible applications in pediatric and developmental neurology because they allow correlation of specific electrophysiological measures

with functional abilities. Some of these applications, such as the use of BAEPs in hearing assessment, have already proved useful (Shannon et al., 1984; Vohr et al., 2001), whereas others, such as the use of P-300 for evaluating intellectual ability, are still considered experimental. Because of the rapid growth of evoked potentials as a clinical field and the popular enthusiasm for pediatric applications, it is particularly important to separate those areas in which evoked potentials are already of well-established clinical value from those in which their clinical relevance remains so controversial that they should best be considered experimental or investigational.

The natural development and change of evoked potentials with age and wider variability makes it more difficult to define limits of normality in infants and children than in adults. Because evoked potential stimulation and recording parameters may vary considerably among laboratories, it is generally suggested that the limits of normality for evoked potentials in infants, children, and adults be established by testing large normal populations. The limits of normality may then be defined as 2.5 or 3.0 standard deviations above the mean for a control sample from the normal population (American Electroencephalographic Society, 1994; Chiappa, 1997). However, for infants and young children, these normative values need to be age specific, requiring a large number of subjects at various ages, which poses a major limitation for most laboratories. However, established laboratories have defined age-specific and, in the case of SEPs, height-specific normative evoked potential ranges for infants and children (Gilmore, 1988; Gorga et al., 1989; Krumholz et al., 1985; Thivierge and Côté, 1990). Despite some reservations, such normative values can be used as a guide by other laboratories using the same recording and stimulation methods.

Auditory Evoked Potentials

Description

Auditory evoked potentials have proven useful in determining hearing ability in infants and children, and as determinants of structural brainstem lesion, myelin disorders, and

Figure 55.1. Components of the brainstem auditory evoked potential (BAEP): waves I, III, and V; interpeak intervals I–III, III–V, and I–V; amplitude of waves I and V (IV–V complex).

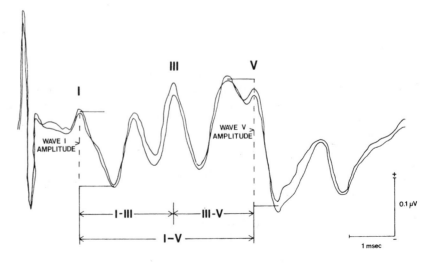

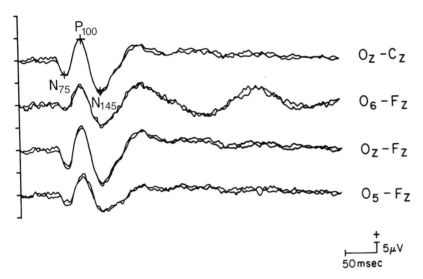

Figure 55.2. The visual evoked potential (VEP) in a multiple channel derivation (O_5 and O_6 are lateral to O_z on the *left* and *right,* respectively).

some specific degenerative or systemic neurological diseases. Their value as predictors of general childhood neurological development (Salamy, 1984) is less well established and remains controversial (Cox et al., 1992; Levy, 1997a; Starr, 1984).

Although both cortical and brainstem auditory evoked potentials have been used effectively in clinical settings, the BAEP has rapidly developed into the favored method of testing. Unlike behavioral audiometry, the BAEP is not limited by lack of language comprehension; its results can be determined more objectively and reviewed more critically than those of behavioral audiometric methods or cortical evoked potentials. In addition, unlike cortical auditory evoked potentials, the BAEP is a very stable response. BAEPs do not vary significantly with state of consciousness or drug administration, so that sedation is possible and often even desirable during the recording procedure (Galambos et al., 1984; Shannon et al., 1984; Vohr et al., 2001). There are now also automated techniques of recording and scoring BAEPs or what are also called auditory brainstem responses (ABRs) that improve the efficiency and cost-effectiveness of this test (Vohr et al., 2001).

The basic BAEP waveform is shown in Figure 55.1. The various components of the BAEP are far-field potentials that have been related to specific source generators or sites in the brainstem auditory pathway: wave I is associated with the auditory nerve action potential; wave II with the cochlear nucleus; wave III with the superior olivary complex; wave IV with ascending auditory pathways in the dorsal and rostral pons or possibly with the nucleus of the lateral lemniscus; and wave V somewhat superior to that area, in the mesencephalon, possibly in the region of the inferior colliculus. Later BAEP components—waves VI and VII, which because of their instability have been of limited clinical use—have been attributed to the regions of the medial lemniscus and primary auditory cortex, respectively. The data supporting the existence of specific sequential generators and their precise location are controversial, and these individual waves and peaks may actually be products of multiple source generators in the auditory pathway. Still, these anatomical generators, although controversial in terms of their precise locations, are generally accepted as approximate BAEP sources (Buchwald and Huang, 1975; Chiappa, 1997; Stern et al., 1982).

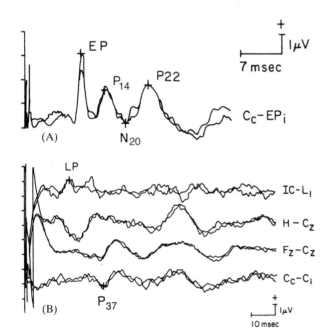

Figure 55.3. Somatosensory evoked potentials to median (**A**) and posterior tibial (**B**) nerve stimulation. In **A**, *EP* is Erb's point, and *Cc* is the central electrode position contralateral to the stimulus. In **B**, *LP* is the lumbar potential, *IC* is the iliac crest, and *H* is the hand.

Technique

The auditory stimulus used with children and neonates is similar to that used with adults, and may be delivered in a standard manner through headphones (American Electroencephalographic Society, 1994). However, because of the infant's and child's small head size, it is important to adapt the earphones to secure a proper fit, and to be particularly careful not to collapse the external auditory canal. In infants particularly, the latter can be a problem; a single, carefully applied earphone may be used to reduce the chance of collapsing the external canal, and some centers use specially made ear inserts.

The standard auditory stimuli are clicks of varying intensity but constant polarity and 100-μsec duration; the standard recording derivation is generally from the vertex (C_z) and the earlobe or mastoid ipsilateral to the ear stimulated, with positivity at the vertex recorded as an upward deflection (Fig. 55.1). This recording is used for routine measurement and tends to demonstrate the auditory nerve potential, wave I, optimally. Simultaneous recordings from the vertex using the opposite ear for a reference help clarify identification of later wave forms, particularly components of the IV–V wave complex.

Standard stimulation parameters and recording methods are generally similar to those for adults (American Electroencephalographic Society, 1994; Krumholz et al., 1985; Levy, 1997a).

In term infants, stimulation rates of approximately 10/sec at standard intensities (60–75 dB, as referenced to normal-hearing controls) produce waves similar to those in adults. In preterm infants, however, individual waves, particularly waves II and IV, may not be as reproducible, and higher stimulation rates might further impair individual wave recognition. Some observers have suggested that condensation clicks may produce better responses in infants, whereas rarefaction clicks are preferable in adults (Stockard, 1981). Either may be used as long as a constant polarity is maintained and polarity is considered when determining standards of normality.

Maturation

The BAEP demonstrates very definite maturational changes in newborns, and particularly in preterm infants. It first appears just before 30 weeks of conceptional (gestational plus chronological) age, but changes most dramatically in infancy, with individual peak latencies reaching near-adult values at about 2 to 3 years of age (Allison et al., 1984; Gorga et al., 1989); the neonatal hearing threshold nears adult values by term (Krumholz et al., 1985). In the preterm stage, before 35 weeks of conceptional age, all BAEP components may not be clearly defined, but by 40 weeks all components are usually discernible (Krumholz et al., 1985). Initially, BAEP latencies were thought to correlate closely with and even predict neonatal conceptional age. However, age has proven not to be the sole determinant of newborn BAEP latency, and it has been postulated that the BAEP may actually be a measure of other critical factors influencing neurophysiological function and development (Goldstein et al., 1979; Salamy, 1984). Numerous specific BAEP components mature in newborn and particularly in preterm infants. These maturing variables include waveform, wave latency, interpeak intervals, and relative wave V/I amplitude (Brivio et al., 1993; Krumholz et al., 1985).

Individual waves between 30 and 40 weeks of conceptional age are better seen using monaural rather than binau-

Table 55.2. Relative Frequency of Appearance of Individual BAEP Waves to a 65 dB nHL Click in Normal Subjects[a]

Conceptional Age	Number	Waves (%)				
		I	II	III	IV	V[b]
30–32 Weeks						
Monaural	11	100	18	100	30	100
Binaural	15	85	20	90	35	80
33–35 Weeks						
Monaural	17	94	41	94	65	100
Binaural	33	100	38	100	53	95
36–38 Weeks						
Monaural	25	96	52	100	72	100
Binaural	29	100	50	100	60	100
Full term						
Monaural	25	100	76	100	84	100
Binaural	25	100	60	100	65	100
Adults						
Monaural	50	100	100	100	93	100
Binaural	50	100	92	100	80	100

[a]From Krumholz, A., Felix, J.K., Goldstein, P.J., and McKenzie, E. 1985. Maturation of the brain-stem auditory evoked potential in premature infants. Electroencephalogr. Clin. Neurophysiol. 62:124–134.
[b]Or IV–V complex.

ral stimulation (Table 55.2). Prior to about 28 to 30 weeks, individual waveforms vary widely and a clearly reproducible response may not be obtainable. This cannot be attributed to hearing loss because infants at that age demonstrate cortical evoked potentials to stimuli of intensity similar to those that fail to produce BAEPs (Starr et al., 1977). In these neonates, the inability to record a BAEP may reflect lack of electrical potential synchronization of subcortical auditory axons. Waveform consistency and reproducibility increases as the infants approach term, with the BAEP waveform approaching its adult form by 38 to 43 weeks of conceptional age. However, even by 30 weeks of conceptional age, nearly 100% of healthy premature infants may be expected to demonstrate reproducible waves I, III, and V; waves II and IV remain somewhat more variable in appearance until term (Table 55.2) (Krumholz et al., 1985).

That latency of individual BAEP waves and their interpeak intervals decrease with patient age can be demonstrated by serial monitoring of individual premature babies (Fig. 55.4). Despite the fact that individual wave latencies demonstrate a clear maturing pattern with advancing gestational age in the preterm infant, the variability of these mean BAEP latencies at various gestational ages continues to be relatively large (Table 55.3). The various interpeak intervals, such as the I–V interval, which have provided such useful clinical measures in adults, also decrease in latency as the preterm infant or newborn ages. Although more stable and consistent than absolute peak latencies, these are still so variable, even among healthy neonates with well-established gestational ages, that their utility for assessing individual infants remains doubtful. It is important to note, however, that this variability decreases substantially as the infant approaches term. Therefore, although the various individual wave components vary considerably, even among healthy preterm infants of similar ages, limiting the clinical

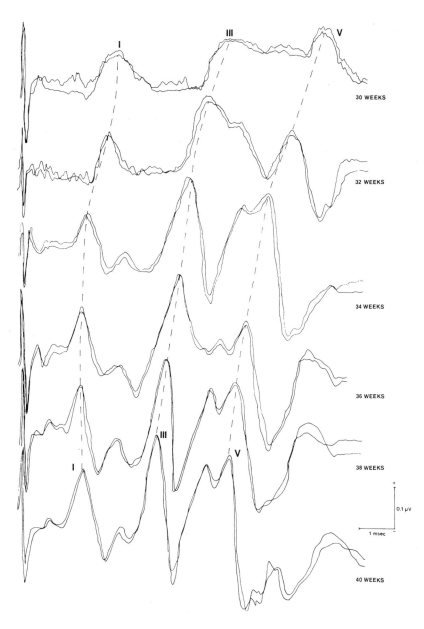

Figure 55.4. Serial BAEP studies in an individual preterm infant between 30 and 40 weeks postconceptional age.

utility of this measure, interpeak intervals are significantly more stable than individual peak latencies. Furthermore, serial change in any individual's interpeak interval may provide a reasonably stable measure (Goldstein et al., 1979; Krumholz et al., 1985).

Although very clear and impressive maturational BAEP changes occur, it has been difficult to consistently correlate infant BAEP observations (except in some specific instances, including hearing loss or severe asphyxia) with clinical state or later outcome. This relates in part to the fact that the BAEP varies so widely among individual preterm infants (much more so than in adults or older children) that the same criteria for abnormality that are of established value in older populations are difficult to apply to newborns. This limits the use of peak or interpeak intervals in the neurological evaluation of preterm infants. However, some investigators report significant clinical correlations with

BAEP conduction delays in newborns, suggesting that latency delays in preterms and newborns can be related to poor neurological outcome (Salamy, 1984; Salamy et al., 1989). This observation, however, has not been universal (Stockard et al., 1983) and remains controversial (Cox et al., 1992; Levy, 1997a; Starr, 1984).

Although definite clinical correlates of latency differences in neonates and children have been difficult to confirm, it has been shown that group differences in BAEP latency may correspond to some central nervous system (CNS) disorders. In one study, apneic preterm infants as a group were shown to have significantly longer latency BAEPs, in terms of both peak and interpeak intervals, than neonates without apnea. This latency difference disappeared as the apneic infants matured and their clinical problems disappeared (Henderson-Smart et al., 1983). Consequently, this study demonstrates that, despite the fact that BAEPs may

Table 55.3. Normal BAEP Interpeak Intervals to a 65 dB nHL Click[a]

Conceptional Age	Number	Interpeak Interval[b]		
		I–III	III–V	I–V
30 Weeks or less				
Monaural	4	3.43 (1.14)	3.60 (0.74)	7.69 (1.23)
Binaural	3	3.03 (0.23)	3.32 (0.81)	6.24 (0.96)
31–32 Weeks				
Monaural	12	3.07 (0.97)	2.97 (0.93)	6.05 (0.92)
Binaural	17	2.87 (0.62)	2.84 (0.62)	5.95 (0.84)
33–34 Weeks				
Monaural	13	2.95 (0.34)	2.61 (0.37)	5.60 (0.35)
Binaural	28	2.90 (0.40)	2.54 (0.35)	5.45 (0.53)
35–36 Weeks				
Monaural	25	2.93 (0.42)	2.50 (0.31)	5.36 (0.48)
Binaural	38	2.76 (0.44)	2.59 (0.37)	5.24 (0.55)
37–38 Weeks				
Monaural	19	2.75 (0.27)	2.28 (0.25)	5.10 (0.42)
Binaural	16	2.51 (0.30)	2.61 (0.31)	5.09 (0.52)
Full term				
Monaural	25	2.76 (0.27)	2.18 (0.27)	4.92 (0.29)
Binaural	25	2.79 (0.31)	2.37 (0.20)	5.13 (0.31)
Adults				
Monaural	50	2.11 (0.13)	1.89 (0.16)	3.99 (0.20)

[a]From Krumholz, A., Felix, J.K., Goldstein, P.J., and McKenzie, E. 1985. Maturation of the brain-stem auditory evoked potential in premature infants. Electroencephalogr. Clin. Neurophysiol. 62:124–134.
[b]Mean (standard deviation); values in msec.

Table 55.4. Criteria for High Risk Hearing Loss

1. Family history of childhood hearing impairment.
2. Congenital perinatal infection.
3. Anatomical malformations involving the head or neck.
4. Birth weight below 1,500 g.
5. Hyperbilirubinemia exceeding indications for exchange transfusion.
6. Bacterial meningitis.
7. Ototoxic medications.
8. Mechanical ventilation lasting 5 days or longer.
9. Apgar scores of 0–4 at 1 minute or 0–6 at 5 minutes.
10. Stigmata or other findings associated with a syndrome known to include hearing loss.

still be of limited value for predicting neurological prognosis for individual infants, it may be possible to use BAEP latencies in preterms and neonates to define group differences in children, yielding insights into factors influencing neurological development. Other studies correlate evoked potentials such as BAEP more closely to outcome from specific disease states, such as hypoxic ischemic coma particularly in combination with SEPs and correlated with imaging, but again there are limitations (Mewasingh et al., 2003).

Audiometric Testing

It is generally accepted that hearing loss is a serious health problem because of both its high incidence and its harmful effects on cognitive and psychological development. Neonatal hearing loss is of particular concern because many of its harmful effects could be corrected by proper early auditory amplification. Although most childhood hearing loss develops as a consequence of otitis media or other local ear problems, a substantial proportion of hearing loss is congenital or occurs neonatally and could be identified by neonatal screening. The prevalence of newborn and infant hearing loss is estimated to range from 1.5 to 6.0 per 1,000 live births (American Academy of Pediatrics Joint Committee on Infant Hearing, 1995). Some infants are known to have a much higher incidence (1–5%) than the general neonatal population; most of these so-called high-risk newborns can be identified using a high-risk registry (American Academy of Pediatrics Joint Committee on Infant Hearing, 1995). High-risk newborns make up approximately 5% of all live births, depending on the population under considera-

tion. The factors that make a newborn high risk for hearing loss are listed in Table 55.4 (American Academy of Pediatrics Joint Committee on Infant Hearing, 1995; American Speech-Language-Hearing Association, 1989; Committee on Hearing, 1987). Similar factors apply to infants and young children.

Numerous techniques have been evaluated in efforts to discover a reliable method of newborn audiometric screening, including behavioral audiometry, impedance audiometry, respiratory response audiometry, cardiac response audiometry, and a crib movement system, the crib-o-gram (Shannon et al., 1984; Swigart, 1986). However, all these methods have serious limitations and are of questionable reliability in young children and particularly infants, so most have been abandoned in neonatal hearing evaluation. The physiological measures that are currently most popular and promising are otoacoustic emissions tests, including both transient evoked otoacoustic emissions and distortion product otoacoustic emissions, and the BAEP (American Academy of Pediatrics Joint Committee on Infant Hearing, 1995; Kennedy et al., 1991, Norton et al., 2000).

The BAEP has been used in many centers in neonatal hearing evaluation and screening, and the results have been impressive. Numerous investigators have confirmed the reliability of the BAEP for diagnosing hearing loss in newborns and other subjects who may be difficult to test with standard behavioral methods (Table 55.4). For example, it has been demonstrated that the BAEP to clicks is reliable to within 5 to 10 dB of the behaviorally determined hearing threshold for frequencies in the mid-to-high frequency range, which includes the important speech frequencies (Sasma, 1990; Swigart, 1986). Furthermore, the BAEP to pure tones of varying frequencies may be useful for more detailed or specific auditory assessment (Yamada et al., 1983). Despite general agreement that the BAEP can detect hearing loss and is useful in the newborn period, some differences persist in interpretation of the results and their significance (Galambos et al., 1984; Gorga et al., 1987; Murray et al., 1985; Norton et al., 2000; Vohr et al., 2001).

Many hearing studies using BAEPs in the newborn period have limited themselves to high-risk newborns and have confirmed a high incidence (2–20%) of hearing loss (Table 55.5). High-risk children are generally identified by a high-risk registry or have graduated from a facility such as a neonatal intensive care unit (Salamy et al., 1989). In those populations, hearing loss screening has been performed

Table 55.5. Results of BAEP Screening for Determining Hearing Loss in High Risk Newborns

Authors	Number Tested	Failing Screening (%)	Abnormal at Follow-up (%)
Schulman-Galambos and Galambos (1979)	75	5.3	5.3
Roberts et al. (1982)	128	39.0	2.3
Galambos et al. (1984)	971	16.7	4.8
Shannon et al. (1984)	168	12.5	1.2
Jacobson and Morehouse (1984)	176	19.9	4.0
Dennis et al. (1984)	200	11.5	5.0

using various protocols. Generally, a BAEP threshold is set, above which an infant is considered to have failed or to have had an abnormal response. Thresholds of anywhere from 25 to 60 dB have been recommended; an abnormality is defined as the absence of response at that intensity in one or both ears. Latency measures may also be considered in identifying an abnormality (Murray et al., 1985; Shannon et al., 1984).

The specific yield and reliability of BAEP hearing screening in newborns remain controversial despite numerous studies (Table 55.5). Although some screening studies identify nearly 20% of high-risk newborns as hearing impaired, the actual incidence of significant hearing loss on follow-up is considerably lower, probably 1% to 5% of all at-risk infants. Significant numbers of these initial screening failures turn out to be false positives (Murray et al., 1985; Norton et al., 2000; Shannon et al., 1984; Vohr et al., 2001). Still, BAEP hearing screening does not seem to produce many false-negative diagnoses or miss children born with significant hearing loss (Galambos et al., 1994; Shannon et al., 1984). Consequently, such screening in infants may be considered highly sensitive, but might not be as specific for subsequent hearing impairment. However, the degree of specificity depends on the criteria used to define abnormality (Kennedy et al., 2000; Shannon et al., 1984).

Some protocols for hearing screening in newborns require testing of all newborns who meet high-risk criteria for hearing loss as recommended by the American Academy of Pediatrics (Table 55.4). Children may be tested in the nursery when stable and nearly ready for discharge. This avoids testing of newborns who may respond abnormally due to immaturity or metabolic or structural disorders that may later resolve. Infants can be tested without sedation. Stimulation parameters vary. The infant is considered to have passed the test if reliable responses are judged to be present. This author tends not to rely on response latency, but unusually long latency responses (more than 2 standard deviations above age-dependent normative values listed in Table 55.6) are viewed with suspicion. If an abnormal or questionable response is obtained at the time of screening, the child is retested with BAEPs for a hearing threshold determination in both ears prior to discharge. A threshold exceeding 30 dB in either ear may be considered a failure or abnormality; the pediatrician and family are informed and the child scheduled

for retesting 3 months after the initial threshold test. If 30 dB or greater hearing loss in either ear is confirmed by retesting, the child is referred for further audiological and speech and language evaluation, follow-up, and habilitation as deemed necessary. Also, in distinguishing conductive from sensorineural hearing impairment, BAEP wave V latency-intensity function measurements may be useful when they can be plotted over a range of at least 30 dB. The slope of the wave V latency-intensity curve can identify recruitment, with slopes exceeding 60 µsec/dB in infants over 37 weeks of gestational age suggestive of sensorineural impairment (Stockard and Stockard, 1986; Van der Drift et al., 1988).

Using such methods, although approximately 15% of high-risk infants fail initial screening, only 7% to 10% demonstrate abnormal thresholds at discharge, and only 3% to 5% are abnormal at the 3-month follow-up test. Of that latter group, some studies find that no more than half will subsequently prove to have significant hearing loss. Thirty decibels might be too conservative a limit of normality for neonatal hearing; the author has found that most false-positive diagnoses have been made in infants with unilateral or mild hearing loss in the 30- to 50-dB range. In fact, infants who consistently demonstrate bilateral hearing losses greater than 60 dB normalized hearing level (nHL) are most likely to subsequently prove to have significant hearing loss (Shannon et al., 1984).

The high incidence of false positives, however, does not necessarily mean that BAEPs are unreliable for neonatal hearing evaluation; it may instead relate to the extreme sensitivity of the technique. It is known that infants, particularly high-risk infants, are prone to accumulating fluid in their middle ears (infantile serous otitis media), which often disappears without permanent hearing loss. This type of transient ear disorder may account for the high incidence of minor, apparently transient, hearing loss observed in high-risk neonates (Shannon et al., 1984; Stockard, 1981).

Also, with the availability of automated ABRs or BAEPs that can be done quickly by less skilled examiners and readers, and that are relatively inexpensive, the potential exists not to test just high-risk hearing loss newborns. Indeed using either BAEPs or otoacoustic emission tests, many centers and regions are using these techniques for universal screening of newborns and other children for hearing loss with good results. Indeed, the American Academy of Pediatrics Task Force on Newborn and Infant Hearing Loss in 1999

Table 55.6. Wave V Means and Standard Deviations (S.D.)[a] for BAEPs Performed at 40 and 25 dB nHL in Normal Hearing Newborns (Based on the Presence of a Clearly Reproducible BAEP at 25 dB nHL) of Varying Gestational Ages

Conceptional Age	Number	Mean (S.D.) (msec)	
		40 dB nHL	25 dB nHL
30–35 Weeks	29	8.47 (0.45)	9.15 (0.58)
36–38 Weeks	62	8.26 (0.47)	8.99 (0.62)
39–41 Weeks	38	8.05 (0.57)	8.76 (0.68)
42–44 Weeks	12	7.79 (0.43)	8.29 (0.81)

[a]Based on responses from either the left or right ear.

recommended that universal hearing screening of newborns and infants was advisable when screening techniques are specific enough to result in less than 4% of patients tested failing and needing to be referred for full audiological evaluations (American Academy of Pediatrics Task Force on Newborn and Infant Hearing Loss, 1999). The automated BAEP in some studies has demonstrated that degree of specificity (Norton et al., 2000; Vohr et al., 2001). Moreover, typically when patients fail one of these screening tests, they are referred for retesting, often specifically using BAEP type techniques because they are generally judged to be more reliable (Norton et al., 2000; Vohr et al., 2001).

In general, the BAEP is proving extremely useful and reliable in identifying hearing loss in newborns and other subjects difficult to test by standard behavioral methods. The problem of false positives seems surmountable, and the equipment for performing the test is readily available, decreasing in cost, and becoming easier to use. Consequently, some states in the United States have already passed legislation mandating audiometric screening of newborns at birth, and other countries have similar programs. It is expected that this will grow as the technology improves.

Another major application for BAEP testing is in assessing possible hearing loss in children after meningitis. The incidence of significant childhood hearing loss after meningitis is estimated to be between 5% and 30%, depending on numerous factors, including the type of organism responsible for the disease (Dodge et al., 1984). In young children, this hearing loss can be particularly difficult to diagnose because of the limitations of behavioral audiometry. Evoked potential audiometry has proven particularly helpful for evaluating such patients for hearing loss after meningitis. The specific nature of the loss can be assessed with evoked potential audiometry by using a latency intensity curve standardized to normal age-matched controls. Sensorineural losses tend to be considerably more severe, bilateral, and persistent. The BAEP has now been demonstrated as highly reliable and useful in evaluating and monitoring hearing loss in infants with meningitis (Dodge et al., 1984; Ozdamar et al., 1983).

Indeed, BAEP studies have proven to be useful adjuncts to standard behavioral audiometric testing in children of all ages, particularly when communication or other problems limit the reliability of behavioral audiometric studies. Numerous investigators have helped define age-specific normal ranges for BAEP studies in infants and children (Gorga et al., 1987, 1989; Krumholz et al., 1985; Thivierge and Côté, 1990).

Structural Lesions

A major clinical application of the BAEP is in diagnosing structural disorders of the brainstem or auditory nerve in children and infants as well as adults (Hecox et al., 1981). The BAEP is abnormal in cases of severe neonatal brainstem damage; BAEP abnormalities have also been described in children with hydrocephalus or posterior fossa anomalies, probably due to pressure on the brainstem (Kraus et al., 1984; Stone et al., 1983). These BAEP abnormalities can be useful for monitoring the effects of therapeutic interventions such as shunting (Kraus et al., 1984). Furthermore, brainstem

tumors such as gliomas can be identified early, and therapy monitored, using BAEPs (Hecox et al., 1981). Other tumors, such as acoustic neuromas or neoplasms that secondarily compress the brainstem, may also produce BAEP abnormalities (Chiappa, 1997). In addition, the BAEP has been used to monitor brainstem or auditory nerve function during posterior fossa surgery (Allen et al., 1981; Tucker et al., 2001).

The reproducibility of the BAEP in measuring and monitoring brainstem function has several potential applications (Chiappa, 1997). For example, it has been reported to be useful in predicting outcome after head trauma (Tsubokawa et al., 1980). Furthermore, because the BAEP is not influenced by barbiturate sedation (Sutton et al., 1982), it may be useful in monitoring brainstem function in patients with drug-induced coma. In particular, for patients treated with barbiturate coma, a popular treatment for refractory increased intracranial pressure as well as other conditions, serial BAEP measurements may help to compensate for the lack of other objective neurodiagnostic or clinical measures of neurological and brainstem function.

Systemic Disorders

Auditory evoked potentials have also been demonstrated to be useful in assessing various systemic disorders including asphyxia (Hecox and Cone, 1981), hyperbilirubinemia (Perlman et al., 1983), leukodystrophy, and some degenerative neurological diseases (Satya-Murti et al., 1980) in infants and children. In some disorders, abnormalities may be diagnostic of a specific disease or predictive of the clinical course.

Asphyxia is the most common perinatal disorder to result in serious neurological impairment and dysfunction, and specific BAEP abnormalities predictive of neurological outcome have been reported (Hecox and Cone, 1981). Hecox and others reported that, after neonatal asphyxia, some infants displayed abnormalities in the wave V/I amplitude ratio correlating with subsequent serious neurological sequelae (Hecox and Cone, 1981; Kaga et al., 1990). Other investigators, however, have failed to demonstrate as clear a predictive value in similar cases (Stockard et al., 1983; Streletz et al., 1986). In fact, there are reports of severe abnormalities and even complete BAEP loss in infants with subsequent recovery of both the BAEP and the infant (Taylor et al., 1983). Still, BAEP abnormalities, particularly abnormally low-amplitude or absent late components that are persistent and present after term, may be reliably predictive of neurological outcome in asphyxiated infants or children (Hecox and Cone, 1981; Krumholz et al., 1985).

Although the BAEP is often abnormal in individuals meeting the criteria for brain death, it has not been proposed as a standard means of determining cerebral death (Goldie et al., 1981; Starr, 1976). The BAEP abnormalities that have been described in brain death include the presence of only waves I or II and no other waves or even the absence of all waveforms (Goldie et al., 1981; Starr, 1976). However, the complete absence of any BAEP response may also occur in deafness. Although this is an unlikely error because an individual suspected to be brain dead would still be required to meet all other standard criteria for cerebral death, the fact that this could occur has tempered enthusiasm for using

BAEPs to confirm cerebral death. Under such circumstances, SEPs may be the preferable tool because a persistent initial wave can be recorded from peripheral nerves even in brain-dead individuals who have lost all brainstem activity (Goldie et al., 1981). Still, the BAEP may be useful in specific situations, for instance possible drug overdose, when some objective measure of brainstem function is needed. The preservation of the BAEP in such a situation would cause one to reconsider a clinical diagnosis of cerebral death.

Numerous authors have investigated the effects of hyperbilirubinemia on the neonatal BAEP, but the findings and their significance are still controversial (Stockard et al., 1983; Streletz et al., 1986). Many authors report some hyperbilirubinemic influence on BAEP, but this effect may be transient and often improves as the bilirubin levels fall. This finding has led to speculation that the BAEP may be useful for following the effects of hyperbilirubinemia on the developing nervous system (Perlman et al., 1983; Stockard et al., 1983). Hyperbilirubinemia may also be an important factor in neonatal hearing loss (Shannon et al., 1984; Shapiro, 2002).

Other systemic factors, such as drug effects and metabolic disorders, have been reported to influence the BAEP, but their effects are generally slight, and there have been few studies of the influence of such factors on BAEP maturation or development. Most drugs do not significantly affect the BAEP, although some, such as phenytoin, have been reported to cause BAEP delays (Chiappa, 1997; Green et al., 1982). However, most drug-related evoked potential delays are not severe; indeed, analysis of group differences is usually necessary to demonstrate significant changes (Green et al., 1982). Other drug-related changes may involve primarily BAEP amplitude rather than latency (Chiappa, 1997). Although most metabolic or toxic influences do not significantly alter BAEPs, hypothermia may produce significant delays (Stockard et al., 1978).

A particularly controversial issue is the benefit of evoked potential studies for identifying children with sudden infant death syndrome (SIDS). Several investigators have suggested that infants at risk for SIDS have a high incidence of BAEP abnormalities (Nodar et al., 1980). However, other studies have not demonstrated significant abnormalities in such children (Gupta et al., 1986; Kileny et al., 1982). In part, the difficulty in resolving this issue stems from the fact that SIDS infants are difficult to identify prior to their deaths, whereas infants with other types of apnea, such as infantile apnea and so-called near-miss SIDS, are a very heterogeneous group that cannot be fairly equated with actual SIDS victims. Furthermore, infants may incur damage to brainstem auditory centers as a direct consequence of apnea and hypoxia. This would account for some reported BAEP abnormalities but would also suggest that BAEP abnormalities in these individuals are a consequence of apnea rather than its cause, making them less valuable in terms of their predictive value (Stockard, 1981). Still, the use of the BAEP for identifying potential SIDS victims is worthy of further study because SIDS is such a serious and common health problem and there are as yet no objective neurodiagnostic means to identify at risk infants.

The BAEP has also proven useful in diagnosing systemic degenerative and demyelinating diseases. Such disorders as Friedreich's ataxia and various forms of olivopontocerebellar degeneration have been documented to have brainstem auditory evoked potential abnormalities that may prove useful in diagnosis and classification (Satya-Murti et al., 1980). BAEP abnormalities are also described in Charcot-Marie-Tooth disease or hereditary sensory motor neuropathy (Satya-Murti and Cacace, 1982). In leukodystrophies, evoked potential abnormalities appear early and may even help identify affected individuals who are still asymptomatic or even carriers of some of the disorders. Among the leukodystrophies in which abnormal BAEP potentials have been described are Pelizaeus-Merzbacher disease, metachromatic leukodystrophy, and adrenoleukodystrophy (Markand et al., 1982).

Visual Evoked Potentials

Description

Although visual evoked potentials (VEPs) were the first evoked potentials to be of practical clinical use in adults, applications in children and infants have developed slowly. The VEP has been proposed and used as an objective measure of childhood visual function and acuity (Sokol, 1978; Sokol and Moskowitz, 1985; Tyler, 1982). Furthermore, the VEP is used for establishing the presence of diseases of myelin (Markand et al., 1982), for determining the presence of compressive or infiltrating optic nerve tumors (Halliday et al., 1976; Kupersmith et al., 1981), and for documenting the adverse effects of various systemic disorders on the nervous system (Krumholz et al., 1980; Ladenson et al., 1984). Because the VEP is a cortical rather than a subcortical evoked potential, it has advantages for the study of cognitive functions and cerebral degenerative disorders. The types of visual stimuli that have been used are either flash or pattern stimuli, and the VEP components that have proven most clinically useful have been the middle to late cortical components of the response that appear 50 to 200 msec after a stimulus.

Technique

In infants and children, both pattern and flash stimuli have been used. Although pattern stimuli yield more stable and consistent responses, they depend on proper visual fixation and attention. Because these are difficult to ensure in infants, there has been greater reliance on the flash evoked potential in the very young. However, even in these very young patients one can obtain an evoked potential to pattern; as the child grows older, the response becomes more reliable (Sokol, 1978; Tyler, 1982). The standard flash stimulus used consists of either a fixed intensity strobe light or a light-emitting diode (LED). More data are available on the strobe light response, but LED systems may be easier to use, particularly outside of a controlled laboratory environment (Mushin et al., 1984). Checkerboards have been the most widely used type of pattern stimulus, but other pattern stimuli, such as sinusoidal bar gratings, may have advantages over checkerboard patterns and correlate better with psychophysiological data. The optimal size of the checks or bars used varies depending on the purpose of the test, but in general checks of from 60 to 20 minutes of arc are the most widely used. The stimulating screen should subtend a visual angle of at least 10 degrees; an even larger stimulus is desirable, particularly when there are attention or fixation problems.

Responses are recorded with electrodes placed in standard positions to allow optimal recording of clinically important potentials. The potential that is usually of greatest clinical interest is the P-100, which is maximal near the inion. Recording several channels simultaneously is preferred because it allows better visualization of the scalp distribution of the response. It can be particularly useful when interpreting atypical potentials. In addition, multiple channel recording is necessary to determine scalp distributions in assessment of the results of partial field (such as hemifield) stimulation. Standard montages for VEP recording resemble those suggested for adults (American Electroencephalographic Society, 1994; Celesia, 1984). Regardless of the techniques with which one begins recording, clarification of atypical or difficult to interpret responses may require other recording derivations or stimulating parameters.

The response to both pattern and flash stimuli is rather similar and is shown in Fig. 55.2. This response has been of principal clinical interest. It occurs maximally over the occipital regions and consists of waves with the following relative latencies (in adults): an initial negative component at about 75 msec, a major positive component at about 100 msec, and a later negative component at about 145 msec. These initial components are followed by a more variable, complex positive waveform. The P-100, the major positive peak occurring in older children and adults at about 100 msec, is the one that has been most widely studied and has proved most clinically useful.

Although attempts have been made to relate individual VEP components to specific neural generators or perceptual or cognitive processes, correlation has been difficult to substantiate. The early components, however, do seem to correlate with cortical reception of primary visual information, whereas the later components (beyond approximately 200 msec) may reflect higher cognitive processing of visual information. Still, like other forms of evoked potentials, these waveforms probably represent the sum of multiple cerebral generators, and simple anatomical or psychophysiological correlations may not be possible.

Maturation

VEPs have been successfully recorded in children and infants of all ages and have been shown to mature (Allison et al., 1984; Ellingson, 1964). A primitive evoked potential to flash can be recorded in infants prior to 30 weeks of conceptional age. The earliest recordable component is a surface negative potential of fairly long latency (in the range of 250 msec) (Hrbek et al., 1973; Mushin et al., 1984). The major occipital positive component comparable to the P-100 is less stable in the very premature infant before 30 weeks of conceptional age, but becomes more constant after about 32 weeks of conceptional age and reaches a latency of 150 to 200 msec near term (Hrbek et al., 1973). The latencies of the various VEP components shorten most quickly from 25 to 30 weeks of conceptional age at a rate of approximately 20

msec/week (Hrbek et al., 1973). Although VEP amplitude is greatest in premature infants prior to 30 weeks of conceptional age, individual wave components become better defined as infants approach term (Tsuneishi et al., 1995).

The VEP to pattern stimuli has not been studied in prematures, but has been evaluated in infants. The response can be recorded in infants before 6 months of age. A major problem in recording from such young infants is the difficulty getting infants to fixate on a screen or target. Nevertheless, VEPs to pattern stimuli have been used to assess and quantify infant visual function. The latencies of the major VEP components shorten progressively from birth to about 5 years of age and then stabilize (Levy, 1997b); after 60 years, VEP latency reportedly increases (Allison et al., 1984; Celesia, 1984). The VEP, unlike the BAEP and the short-latency SEP components, is a cortical response dependent on conscious state at the time of recording, and may be readily influenced by drugs or systemic factors. The sensitivity of the cortical evoked potential to these types of external influences make the responses more variable and less predictable in some ways, but also potentially allows monitoring of subtle influences on neuronal or cortical functions.

Visual Acuity

Because the amplitude of the VEP to pattern stimuli is maximal when refraction is optimal, the VEP can be used to assess visual acuity. Studies have demonstrated that amplitude of the VEP to pattern stimuli is attenuated as the edges of a pattern stimulus are blurred by lenses of various dioptic powers (Sokol and Moskowitz, 1985). Furthermore, it can be demonstrated that, in subjects with known refractive errors, correction of these refractive errors results in higher amplitude VEPs. These observations support the use of the VEP to pattern for the assessment of visual acuity (Rentschler and Spinelli, 1978).

The VEP is particularly promising for assessing visual acuity in subjects such as infants, who cannot be tested by behavioral methods. Using VEPs to pattern stimuli, it has been demonstrated that infants probably have considerably better visual acuity than was once thought. For example, VEP data have indicated that the 1-month-old infant has a visual acuity corresponding to 20/400 and that by 6 months of age visual acuity reaches near-adult levels of 20/20 (Sokol, 1978). These results have been confirmed by several investigators and differ from earlier reports of infant visual acuity based on preferential looking techniques and suggesting that adult levels of acuity are not reached until 2 years of age. This VEP-derived acuity estimate, however, is not a behavioral measure and may not correspond directly with visual function. Although the VEP measures the visual system's ability to transmit information to the cortex, it does not determine whether that information is being properly processed by higher centers.

The maximal VEP to pattern stimuli of varying spatial frequencies does correspond and has been directly correlated with visual acuity in adults. A maximal P-100 response correlates approximately with the check angle or size of the stimulus used (Chiappa, 1997). Although, as previously mentioned, it is difficult to get infants to attend to the stimulus, older children's attention can be held by providing them with an interesting background, such as a cartoon, that can be interrupted with the target pattern, or by simply being extremely patient and recording only when the child is fixated on the stimulus. The problem of assuring that the infant is fixating on the target is serious but probably technically solvable (Gottlob et al., 1990). For example, it may be possible to adapt currently available systems for monitoring eye position and use them to assure that individuals fixate on the stimulus (Sokol and Moskowitz, 1985). Pattern VEP is already being used in many centers to assess infant visual acuity (Derick et al., 1990; Gottlob et al., 1990; Sokol, 1978).

In newborns, VEPs to patterns stimuli are difficult to record and correlate to clinical function. Flash-evoked responses have been analyzed in children and the results broadly correlated with visual function; the absence of a VEP to flash has correlated with a poor prognosis for later vision development (Barnet et al., 1970; Duchowny et al., 1974), but the significance of less severe abnormalities such as latency delays have been correlated less consistently with clinical outcome.

VEP in Systemic Disorders

Various systemic pediatric neurological disorders are accompanied by characteristic VEP abnormalities. Disorders affecting myelin have been strongly associated with VEP abnormalities; VEP delays have been demonstrated in children with various leukodystrophies, such as metachromatic and adrenoleukodystrophy (Garg, 1983; Markand et al., 1982), as well as in older children with multiple sclerosis or optic neuritis. Other systemic disorders have also been associated with abnormal VEP latencies or amplitudes, including Huntington's chorea (Ellenberg et al., 1978; Oepen et al., 1981), Friedreich's ataxia (Carroll et al., 1980), spinocerebellar degeneration (Hammond and Wilder, 1983), and myotonic dystrophy (Gott et al., 1983). Metabolic disorders, particularly if associated with encephalopathy, have also shown VEP delays. These include renal disease (Cohen et al., 1983), thyroid deficiency (Ladenson et al., 1984), such nutritional disorders as vitamin E (Messenheimer et al., 1984) and B_{12} deficiencies (Krumholz et al., 1980), and disorders or influences that may affect CNS transmitters (Bodis-Wollner et al., 1982). Some of these abnormalities have been reversed with appropriate therapy (Krumholz et al., 1980; Ladenson et al., 1984; Messenheimer et al., 1984). However, it is worth noting that despite the numerous conditions in which VEP abnormalities or deviations have been described, the response has not proven generally useful in large screening studies as a predictor of individual neurological development (Engel and Henderson, 1973). In specific disorders such as neonatal asphyxia, however, persistent, severe VEP abnormalities may be related to outcome (Hrbek et al., 1977).

Visual Pathway Lesions

Delays in the VEP can be used to confirm visual pathway lesions in children, just as they can in adults. Compressive tumors or other structural lesions produce such delays; VEP delay can be used to diagnose and follow such problems as optic nerve gliomas, suprasellar or optic menin-

giomas, and other tumors in the region of the optic nerves (Halliday et al., 1976; Kupersmith et al., 1981; Ng and North, 2001). Other disorders that may compromise the visual pathway, for instance hydrocephalus, have also been associated with transient VEP delays that improve with treatment (Guthkelch et al., 1984).

Somatosensory Evoked Potentials
Description

Somatosensory evoked potentials are recorded from the peripheral and central nervous system in response to peripheral nerve stimulation. Both short- and long-latency evoked potentials have been used clinically in children and infants. Indeed, SEP utility relates in part to the fact that the same waveform may include components of a peripheral nerve potential, a subcortical evoked potential, and a cortical evoked potential. Short latency subcortical evoked potentials are recorded from the upper extremities, using principally the median nerve (Fig. 55.3A), and it is possible to record similar short latency responses from the lower extremities using either the posterior tibial or the peroneal nerve and to demonstrate subcortical spinal cord potentials using multiple channel recordings with electrodes over the spinal cord and over the lumbosacral plexus or cauda equina (Fig. 55.3B).

Latencies, waveforms, and wave polarities of such SEPs depend on the nerve stimulated, recording parameters, and electrode positions. In general, a wave or wave peak is characterized by its polarity, approximate average normal latency, and relation to associated waves. Abnormalities are largely determined by delays in interpeak intervals or the absence of specific waves (American Electroencephalographic Society, 1994).

Over the past decade a new type of evoked potential has been developed, the motor evoked potential. This potential is obtained by magnetic or electrical stimulation of CNS motor pathways, and the response is then recorded from peripheral muscles. The initial applications of this new form of evoked potential have been in adults (Chiappa, 1997), but the techniques used also could be applied to children (Maegaki et al., 1994).

Technique

SEP recording procedures in infants do not vary substantially from those used with adults; the nerves stimulated and recording sites are similar. In small infants, however, it is more difficult to place complex arrays of electrodes, and infants and children tend to be less tolerant than adults of long and uncomfortable recording sessions. Sedation or sleep during recording does not influence peripheral or subcortical SEPs, but later cortical evoked potential components may be affected. Remember that the young infant's peripheral nervous system conduction velocity is slower than that of adults, and matures similarly to central conduction, so age can influence both peripheral and central aspects of the SEP.

Maturation

In premature infants before 30 weeks of conceptional age, the SEP appears as a large, slow, negative deflection that, in the case of the median nerve SEP, has a contralateral rolandic maximum (Hrbek et al., 1973; Taylor et al., 1996). Later, the waveform becomes more complex and the latencies of individual components shorten; in addition, as the infants approach term, the amplitude of the response ipsilateral to stimulation also increases dramatically. SEP latency continues to shorten as the newborn ages, with peripheral latencies reaching near adult values by 3 years of age; central conduction velocity matures more slowly and does not approach adult latencies until 5 years of age (Allison et al., 1984; Cracco et al., 1979; Gilmore, 1988; Laureau and Marlot, 1990; Levy, 1997c; Smit et al., 2000).

Sensory and Motor Function

The SEP is used to monitor intraoperative sensory and motor function during surgical manipulation of the spine; it does seem to measure sensory and motor function closely enough to predict intraoperative spinal cord injury (Lueders et al., 1982; Luk et al., 2001; Macon et al., 1982; Wiedemayer et al., 2002). SEPs have also been proposed as objective measures of sensory function in situations where conversion disorders or psychogenic sensory disturbances are suspected. In general, SEP abnormality suggests organic sensory loss, but, because the SEP may be preserved in the presence of significant sensory dysfunction, normal SEP values do not completely exclude the possibility of an organic disorder.

SEP in Systemic Disorders

SEP abnormalities, primarily interpeak interval delays, have been demonstrated in numerous systemic disorders, including both degenerative and toxic or metabolic disorders. Delays and other abnormalities have been described in Friedreich's ataxia (Jones et al., 1980) and other spinocerebellar or degenerative disorders associated with ataxia (Pedersen and Trojaborg, 1981). Myelin disorders have been associated with SEP delays, as they have with BAEP or VEP abnormalities, and SEP recordings may be useful in confirming the presence of those conditions (Markand et al., 1982). Such metabolic disturbances as vitamin E and B_{12} deficiencies have also been associated with SEP abnormalities (Krumholz et al., 1980; Messenheimer et al., 1984). In addition, other metabolic disorders, for example renal failure (Vasiri et al., 1981) and diabetes (Cracco et al., 1980), have been associated with SEP abnormalities. Some of these disorders are associated with peripheral as well as central conduction disturbances.

Amplitude abnormalities or loss of specific waveforms have also been reported in childhood coma and may be good predictors of functional neurological recovery (Frank et al., 1985; Mandel et al., 2002; Pike and Marlow, 2000; Robinson et al., 2003; Tomita et al., 2003). Because of the preservation of early peripheral nerve components of the short latency SEP even in severe brainstem injury, the SEP is particularly helpful in confirming lost brainstem function in suspected cerebral death when standard diagnostic criteria provide insufficient proof (Goldie et al., 1981). In some conditions, SEPs may be abnormally enlarged; this type of abnormality has been described in epileptiform myoclonus and myoclonic epilepsy (Kelly et al., 1981; Shibasaki et al., 1978).

SEP in Somatosensory Pathway Lesions

Specific lesions along the somatosensory pathway produce SEP abnormalities; tumors, hemorrhages, and somatosensory pathway infarctions have been associated with evoked potential abnormalities and have been correlated with the clinical course (Chiappa, 1997). Intraoperative monitoring of neurological function during spinal surgery, such as major scoliosis surgery (Lueders et al., 1982; Macon et al., 1982), is now common. In addition, evidence suggests that patients with spinal cord compression or compromise related to bony abnormalities at the base of the brain, as can occur with achondroplasia, may display SEP abnormalities useful for predicting the clinical course and monitoring therapy (Nelson et al., 1984).

Cognitive Evoked Potentials

Evoked potentials may have great value in the study of cognitive processes, and these types of analyses could be particularly valuable and informative in children. The late components of the evoked potential, the P-300 and similar components, seem to have the greatest promise in this regard (Finley et al., 1985). Studies using complex statistical methods to estimate the expected distribution of electrical activity over the cortex both during steady-state studies and with various types of specific sensory stimulation have demonstrated abnormalities in such disorders as learning disabilities and attentional deficit disorder; although these types of studies hold promise, further confirmation of the techniques and their clinical value is necessary (American Academy of Neurology Therapeutics and Technology Assessment Subcommittee, 1989; Duffy et al., 1979, 1980; Nuwer, 1997).

The objective use of evoked potentials to analyze cognitive processes and discern the electrophysiological correlates of cognition and perception as they relate to intellectual development may be the next frontier in electrophysiological testing in the nervous system, but one should be careful not to draw premature conclusions on the clinical value of such studies, particularly for individual assessment and long-term prediction.

References

Allen, A.R., Starr, A., and Nudleman, K. 1981. Assessment of sensory conduction in the operating room utilizing cerebral evoked potentials: a study of fifty-six surgically anesthetized patients. Clin. Neurosurg. 28:457–481.

Allison, T., Hume, A.L., Wood, C.C., et al. 1984. Developmental and aging changes in somatosensory, auditory and visual evoked potentials. Electroencephalogr. Clin. Neurophysiol. 58:14–24.

American Academy of Neurology Therapeutics and Technology Assessment Subcommittee. 1989. Assessment: EEG brain mapping. Neurology 39:1100–1101.

American Academy of Pediatrics Joint Committee on Infant Hearing. 1995. Joint Committee on Infant Hearing 1994 position statement. Pediatrics 95:152–156.

American Academy of Pediatrics Task Force on Newborn and Infant Hearing Loss. 1999. Newborn and infant hearing loss: detection and intervention. Pediatrics 103:527–530.

American Electroencephalographic Society. 1994. Guidelines on evoked potentials and guidelines of writing clinical evoked potential reports. Clin. Neurophysiol. 11:40–76.

American Speech-Language-Hearing Association, Committee on Infant Hearing. 1989. Audiologic screening of newborn infants who are at risk for hearing impairment. American Speech-Language-Hearing Association 31:89–92.

Barnet, A.B., Manson, J.I., and Wilner, E. 1970. Acute cerebral blindness in childhood. Six cases studied clinically and electrophysiologically. Neurology 20:1147–1156.

Bodis-Wollner, I., Yahr, M.D., Mylin, L., et al. 1982. Dopaminergic deficiency and delayed visual evoked potentials in humans. Ann. Neurol. 11: 478–483.

Brazier, M.A.B. 1984. Pioneers in the discovery of evoked potentials. Electroencephalogr. Clin. Neurophysiol. 59:2–8.

Brivio, L., Grasso, R., Salvaggio, A., et al. 1993. Brain-stem auditory evoked potentials (BAEPs): maturation of interpeak latency I–V (IPL I–V) in the first years of life. Electroencephalogr. Clin. Neurophysiol. 88:28–31.

Buchwald, J.S., and Huang, C.M. 1975. Far-field acoustic response: Origins in the cat. Science 189:383–384.

Carroll, W.M., Kriss, A., Baraitser, M., et al. 1980. The incidence and nature of visual pathway involvement in Friedreich's ataxia. Brain 103: 413–435.

Celesia, G.G. 1984. Evoked potentials techniques in the evaluation of visual function. J. Clin. Neurophysiol. 1:55–76.

Chiappa, K.H. 1997. *Evoked Potentials in Clinical Medicine*, 3rd ed. Philadelphia: Lippincott-Raven.

Cohen, S.N., Syndulko, K., Rever, B., et al. 1983. Visual evoked potentials and long latency evoked potentials in chronic renal failure. Neurology 33:1219–1222.

Committee on Hearing, Bioacoustics, Biomechanics, Commission on Behavioral and Social Sciences Education, National Research Council. 1987. Brainstem audiometry of infants. American Speech-Language-Hearing Association 29:47–55.

Cox, C., Hack, M., Aram, D., et al. 1992. Neonatal auditory brainstem response failure of very low birth weight infants: 8-Year Outcome. Pediatr. Res. 31:68–72.

Cracco, J.B., Cracco, R.Q., and Stolove, R. 1979. Spinal evoked potential in man: a maturational study. Electroencephalogr. Clin. Neurophysiol. 46:58–64.

Cracco, J., Castells, S., and Mark, E. 1980. Conduction velocity in the peripheral nerve and spinal afferent pathway of juvenile diabetics. Neurology 30:370–371.

Dennis, J.M., Sheldon, R., Toubas, P., et al. 1984. Identification of hearing loss in the neonatal intensive care unit population. Am. J. Otol. 5:257–263.

Derick, R.J., Leguire, L.E., Rogers, G.L., et al. 1990. The predictability of infant visual-evoked response testing on future visual acuity. Ann. Ophthalmol. 22:432–438.

Dodge, P.R., Davis, H., Feigin, R.D., et al. 1984. Prospective evaluation of hearing impairment as a sequela of acute bacterial meningitis. N. Engl. J. Med. 311:869–874.

Duchowny, M.S., Weiss, I.P., Majlessi, H., et al. 1974. Visual evoked responses in cortical blindness after head trauma and meningitis. Neurology 24:933–940.

Duffy, F.H., Burcifiel, J.L., and Lombroso, C.T. 1979. Brain electrical activity mapping (BEAM): a method for extending the clinical utility of EEG and evoked potential data. Ann. Neurol. 5:309–321.

Duffy, F.H., Denckla, M.B., Bartels, P.H., et al. 1980. Dyslexia: Regional differences in brain electrical activity by topographic mapping. Ann. Neurol. 7:412–420.

Eggermont, J.J. 1988. On the rate of maturation of sensory evoked potentials. Electroencephalogr. Clin. Neurophysiol. 70:293–305.

Ellenberg, C., Petro, D.J., and Ziegler, S.B. 1978. The visually evoked potential in Huntington's disease. Neurology 28:95–97.

Ellingson, R.J. 1964. Cerebral electrical responses to auditory and visual stimuli in the infant (human and subhuman studies). In *Neurological and Electroencephalographic Correlative Studies in Infancy*, Eds. P. Kellaway and I. Petersén, pp. 78–116. New York: Grune and Stratton.

Engel, R., and Henderson, N.B. 1973. Visual evoked responses and IQ scores at school age. Dev. Med. Child. Neurol. 15:136–145.

Finley, W.W., Faux, S.F., Hutcheson, J., et al. 1985. Long-latency event related potentials in the evaluation of cognitive function in children. Neurology 35:323–327.

Frank, L.M., Furgiuele, T.L., and Etheridge, J.E. 1985. Prediction of chronic vegetative state in children using evoked potentials. Neurology 35:931–934.

Galambos, R., Hicks, G., and Wilson, M.J. 1984. The brainstem auditory evoked potential reliably predicts hearing loss in graduates of a tertiary intensive care nursery. Ear Hear. 5:254–260.

Galambos, R., Wilson, M.J., and Silva, P.D. 1994. Identifying hearing loss in the intensive care nursery: a 20-year study. J. Am. Acad. Audiol. 5: 151–162.

Garg, B.P. 1983. Evoked response studies in patients with adrenoleukodystrophy and heterozygous relatives. Arch. Neurol. 40:356–359.

Gilmore, R. 1988. Use of somatosensory evoked potentials in infants and children. In *Neurology Clinics*, vol. 6, No. 4, Ed. R. Gilmore, pp. 839–859. Philadelphia: W.B. Saunders, Harcourt Brace Jovanovich.

Goldie, W.D., Chiappa, K.H., Young, R.R., et al. 1981. Brain-stem auditory and short latency somatosensory evoked responses in brain death. Neurology 13:248–256.

Goldstein, P.J., Krumholz, A., Felix, J.K., et al. 1979. Brain-stem evoked response in neonates. Am. J. Obstet. Gynecol. 127:181–187.

Gorga, M.P., Reiland, J.K., Beauchaine, K.A., et al. 1987. Auditory brainstem responses from the graduates of an intensive care nursery: normal patterns of response. J. Speech Hear. Res. 30:311–318.

Gorga, M.P., Kaminski, J.R., Beauchaine, K.L., et al. 1989. Auditory brainstem responses from children three months to three years of age: normal patterns of response. II. J. Speech Hear. Res. 32:281–288.

Gott, P.S., Karnaze, D.S., and Keane, J.R. 1983. Abnormal visual evoked potentials in myotonic dystrophy. Neurology 33:1622–1625.

Gottlob, I., Fendick, M.G., Guo, S., et al. 1990. Visual acuity measurements by swept spatial frequency visual-evoked-cortical potentials (VECPs): clinical application in children with various visual disorders. J. Pediatr. Ophthalmol. Strabismus 27:40–47.

Green, J.B., Walcoff, M., and Lucke, J.F. 1982. Phenytoin prolongs far field somatosensory and auditory evoked potential interpeak latencies. Neurology 32:85–88.

Gupta, P.R., Guilleminault, C., and Dorfman, L.J. 1986. Brain stem auditory evoked potentials in "near-miss" sudden infant death syndrome. J. Pediatr. 98:791–794.

Guthkelch, A.N., Sclabassi, R.J., Hirsh, R.P., et al. 1984. Visual evoked potentials in hydrocephalus: relationship to head size, shunting, and mental development. Neurosurgery 14:283–286.

Halliday, A.M., McDonald, W.I., and Mushin, J. 1973. Visual evoked responses in the diagnosis of multiple sclerosis. Br. Med. J. 4:661–664.

Halliday, A.M., Halliday, E., Kriss, A., et al. 1976. The pattern-evoked potential in compression of the anterior visual pathways. Brain 99:357–374.

Hammond, E.J., and Wilder, B.J. 1983. Evoked potentials in olivopontocerebellar atrophy. Arch. Neurol. 40:366–369.

Hecox, K.E., and Cone, B. 1981. Prognostic importance of brainstem auditory evoked responses after asphyxia. Neurology 31:1429–1433.

Hecox, K.E., Cone, B., and Blaw, M.E. 1981. Brainstem auditory evoked responses in the diagnosis of pediatric neurologic diseases. Neurology 31:832–840.

Henderson-Smart, D.J., Petigrew, A.G., and Campbell, D.J. 1983. Clinical apnea and brain-stem neural function in preterm infants. N. Engl. J. Med. 308:353–357.

Hrbek, A., Karlberg, P., and Olsson, T. 1973. Development of visual and somatosensory evoked potentials in pre-term newborn infants. Electroencephalogr. Clin. Neurophysiol. 34:225–232.

Hrbek, A., Karlberg, P., Kjellmer, I., et al. 1977. Clinical application of evoked electroencephalographic responses in newborn infants. I. Perinatal asphyxia. Dev. Med. Child Neurol. 19:34–44.

Jacobson, J.T., and Morehouse, C.R. 1984. A comparison of auditory brain stem response and behavioral screening in high risk and normal newborn infants. Ear Hear. 5:247–253.

Jewett, D.L. 1970. Volume-conducted potentials in response to auditory stimuli as detected by averaging in the cat. Electroencephalogr. Clin. Neurophysiol. 28:609–618.

Jones, S.J., Baraitser, M., and Halliday, A.M. 1980. Peripheral and central somatosensory nerve conduction defects in Friedreich's ataxia. J. Neurol. Neurosurg. Psychiatr. 43:495–503.

Kaga, M., Murakami, T., Haruka, N., et al. 1990. Studies on pediatric patients with absent auditory brainstem response (ABR) later components. Brain Dev. 12:380–384.

Kelly, J.K., Sharbrough, F.W., and Daube, J.R. 1981. A clinical and electrophysiological evaluation of myoclonus. Neurology 31:581–589.

Kennedy, C.R., Kim, L., Cafarelli, et al. 1991. Otoacoustic emissions and auditory brainstem responses in the newborn. Arch. Dis. Child. 66:1124–1129.

Kennedy, C., Kimm, L., Thornton, R., et al. 2000. False positives in the universal neonatal screening for permanent hearing impairment. Lancet 356:1903–1902.

Kileny, P., Finer, N., Sussman, P., et al. 1982. Auditory brainstem responses in sudden infant death syndrome: comparison of siblings, near-miss, and normal infants. J. Pediatr. 101:225–227.

Kimura, J., Kimura, A., Ishida, T., et al. 1986. What determines the latency and amplitude of stationary peaks in far-field recordings? Ann. Neurol. 19:479–486.

Kraus, N., Ozdamar, O., Heydemann, P.T., et al. 1984. Auditory brainstem evoked responses in hydrocephalic patients. Electroencephalogr. Clin. Neurophysiol. 59:310–317.

Krumholz, A., Weiss, H.D., Goldstein, P.J., et al. 1980. Evoked potentials in vitamin B$_{12}$ deficiency. Ann. Neurol. 9:407–409.

Krumholz, A., Felix, J.K., Goldstein, P.J., et al. 1985. Maturation of the brain-stem auditory evoked potential in premature infants. Electroencephalogr. Clin. Neurophysiol. 62:124–134.

Kupersmith, M.J., Seigel, I.M., Carr, R.E., et al. 1981. Visual evoked potentials in chiasmal gliomas in four adults. Arch. Neurol. 38:362–365.

Ladenson, P.W., Stakes, J.W., and Ridgeway, E.C. 1984. Reversible alteration of the visual evoked potential in hypothyroidism. Am. J. Med. 77:1010–1014.

Laureau, E., and Marlot, D. 1990. Somatosensory evoked potentials after median and tibial nerve stimulation in healthy newborns. Electroencephalogr. Clin. Neurophysiol. 76:453–458.

Levy, S.R. 1997a. Brainstem auditory evoked potentials in pediatrics. In *Evoked Potentials in Clinical Medicine*, 3rd ed., Ed. K.H. Chiappa, pp. 269–282. Philadelphia: Lippincott-Raven.

Levy, S.R. 1997b. Visual evoked potentials in pediatrics. In *Evoked Potentials in Clinical Medicine*, 3rd ed., Ed. K.H. Chiappa, pp. 147–156. Philadelphia: Lippincott-Raven.

Levy, S.R. 1997c. Somatosensory evoked potentials in pediatrics. In *Evoked Potentials in Clinical Medicine*, 3rd ed., Ed. K.H. Chiappa, pp. 453–470. Philadelphia: Lippincott-Raven.

Lombroso, C.T. 1987. Neonatal electroencephalography. In *Electroencephalography*, 2nd ed., Eds. E. Niedermeyer and F. Lopes da Silva, pp. 725–772. Baltimore: Urban and Schwarzenberg.

Lueders, H., Gurd, A., Huhn J., et al. 1982. A new technique for intraoperative monitoring of spinal cord function. Multichannel recording of spinal cord and subcortical evoked potentials. Spine 7:110–115.

Luk, K.D., Hu, Y., Wong, Y.W., et al. 2001. Evaluation of various evoked potential techniques for spinal cord monitoring during scoliosis surgery. Spine 26:1772–1777.

Macon, J.B., Poletti, C.E., Sweet, W.H., et al. 1982. Conducted somatosensory evoked potential during spinal surgery. Part 1: clinical applications. J. Neurosurg. 57:349–353.

Maegaki, Y., Inagaki, M., and Takeshita, K. 1994. Cervical magnetic stimulation in children and adolescents: normal values and the evaluation of the proximal lesion of the peripheral motor nerve in the cases with polyradiculopathy. Electroencephalogr. Clin. Neurophysiol. 93:318–323.

Mandel, R., Martinot, A., Delepoulle, F., et al. 2002. Prediction of outcome after hypoxic-ischemic encephalopathy: a prospective clinical and electroencephalographic study. J. Pediatr. 141:45–50.

Markand, O.N., Garg, B.P., DeMeyer, W.M., et al. 1982. Brainstem auditory, visual and somatosensory evoked potentials in the leukodystrophies. Electroencephalogr. Clin. Neurophysiol. 54:39–48.

Messenheimer, J.A., Greenwood, R.S., Tennison, M.B., et al. 1984. Reversible visual evoked potential abnormalities in vitamin E deficiency. Ann. Neurol. 15:499–501.

Mewasingh, L.D., Christophe, C., Fonteyne, C., et al. 2003. Predictive value of electrophysiology in children with hypoxic encephalopathy. Pediatr. Neurol. 28:178–183.

Murray, A.N., Javel, E., and Watson, C.S. 1985. Prognostic validity of auditory evoked response screening in newborn infants. Am. J. Otolaryngol. 6:120–131.

Mushin, J., Hogg, C.R., Dubowitz, L.M.S., et al. 1984. Visual evoked responses to light emitting diode (LED) photostimulation in newborn infants. Electroencephalogr. Clin. Neurophysiol. 58:317–320.

Nelson, F.W., Goldie, W.D., Hecht, J.T., et al. 1984. Short-latency somatosensory evoked potentials in the management of patients with achondroplasia. Neurology 34:1053–1058.

Ng, Y.T., and North, K.N. 2001. Visual evoked potentials in assessment of optic gliomas. Pediatr. Neurol. 24:44–48.

Nodar, R., Lansdale, D., and Orlowski, J. 1980. Abnormal brainstem auditory evoked potentials in infants with threatened sudden infant death syndrome. Otolaryngol. Head Neck Surg. 88:619–621.

Norton, S.J., Gorga, M.P., Widen, J.E., et al. 2000. Identification of neonatal hearing impairment: summary and recommendations. Ear Hear. 21:529–535.

Nuwer, M. 1997. Assessment of digital EEG, quantitative EEG, and EEG brain mapping: report of the American Academy of Neurology and the American Clinical Neurophysiology Society. Neurology 49:277–292.

Oepen, G., Doerr, M., and Thoden, U. 1981. Visual (VEP) and somatosensory evoked potentials in Huntington's chorea. Electroencephalogr. Clin. Neurophysiol. 51:666–670.

Ozdamar, O., Kraus, N., and Stein, L. 1983. Auditory brainstem responses in infants recovering from bacterial meningitis. Arch. Otolaryngol. 109:13–18.

Pedersen, L., and Trojaborg, W. 1981. Visual, auditory and somatosensory involvement in hereditary cerebellar ataxia, Friedreich's ataxia and familial spastic paraplegia. Electroencephalogr. Clin. Neurophysiol. 52:283–297.

Perlman, M., Fainmesser, P., Sohmer, H., et al. 1983. Auditory nerve-brainstem evoked responses in hyperbilirubinemic neonates. Pediatrics 72:658–664.

Pike, A.A., and Marlow, N. 2000. The role of cortical evoked responses in predicting neuromotor outcome in very preterm infants. Early Hum. Dev. 57:123–135.

Prentschler, I., and Spinelli, D. 1978. Accuracy of evoked potential refractometry using bar gratings. Acta Ophthalmol. 56:67–74.

Roberts, J.L., Davis, H., Phon, G.L., et al. 1982. Auditory brainstem responses in preterm neonates: maturation and follow-up. J. Pediatr. 101:257–263.

Robinson, L.R., Micklesen, P.J., Tirshwell, D.L., et al. 2003. Predictive value of somatosensory evoked potentials for awakening from coma. Crit. Care Med. 31:960–967.

Salamy, A. 1984. Maturation of the auditory brainstem response from birth to early childhood. J. Clin. Neurophysiol. 1:293–329.

Salamy, A., Eldredge, L., and Tooley, W.H. 1989. Neonatal status and hearing loss in high-risk infants. J. Pediatr. 114:847–852.

Sasma, F. 1990. Hearing thresholds in infants and children. Audiology 29:76–84.

Satya-Murti, S., and Cacace, A. 1982. Brainstem auditory evoked potentials in disorders of the primary sensory ganglion. In *Clinical Applications of Evoked Potentials in Neurology*, Eds. J. Courjon, F. Mauguière, and M. Revol, pp. 219–225. New York: Raven Press.

Satya-Murti, S., Cacace, A., and Hanson, P. 1980. Auditory dysfunction in Friedreich's ataxia: result of spiral ganglion degeneration. Neurology 30:1047–1053.

Schulman-Galambos, C., and Galambos, R. 1979. Brain stem evoked response audiometry in newborn hearing screening. Arch. Otolaryngol. 105:86–89.

Shannon, D.A., Felix, J.K., Krumholz, A., et al. 1984. Hearing screening of high risk newborns using brainstem auditory evoked potentials: A follow-up study. Pediatrics 73:22–26.

Shapiro, S.M. 2002. Somatosensory and brainstem evoked potentials in the Gunn rat model of acute bilirubin neurotoxicity. Pediatr. Res. 52:844–849.

Shibasaki, H., Yamashita, Y., and Kuroiwa, Y. 1978. Electroencephalographic studies of myoclonus: Myoclonus-related cortical spikes and high amplitude somatosensory evoked potentials. Brain 101:447–460.

Smit, B.J., Ongerboer de Visser, B.W., de Vries, L.S., et al. 2000. Somatosensory evoked potentials in very preterm infants. Clin. Neurophysiol. 111:901–908.

Sokol, S. 1978. Measurement of infant visual acuity from pattern reversal evoked potentials. Vis. Res. 18:33–39.

Sokol, S., and Moskowitz, A. 1985. Comparison of pattern VEPs and preferential-looking behavior in 3-month-old infants. Invest. Ophthalmol. Vis. Sci. 26:359–365.

Starr, A. 1976. Auditory brainstem responses in brain death. Brain 99:543–554.

Starr, A. 1984. Auditory brainstem evoked potentials: Comments on their use during infant development. J. Clin. Neurosphysiol. 1:331–334.

Starr, A., Amile, R.N., Martin, W.H., et al. 1977. Development of auditory function in newborn infants revealed by auditory brainstem potentials. Pediatrics 60:831–839.

Stern, B.J., Krumholz, A., Weiss, H.D., et al. 1982. Evaluation of brainstem stroke using brainstem auditory evoked responses. Stroke 13:705–711.

Stockard, J.E., and Stockard, J.J. 1986. Clinical application of brainstem auditory evoked potentials in infants. In *Evoked Potentials. Frontiers of Neuroscience*, vol. 3, Eds. R.Q. Cracco and I. Bodis-Wollner, pp. 455–462. New York: Alan R. Liss.

Stockard, J.E., Stockard, J.J., Kleinberg, F., et al. 1983. Prognostic value of brainstem auditory evoked potentials in neonates. Arch. Neurol. 40:360–365.

Stockard, J.J. 1981. Brainstem auditory evoked potentials in adult and infant sleep apnea syndromes, including sudden infant death syndrome and near-miss for sudden infant death. Ann. N.Y. Acad. Sci. 388:443–465.

Stockard, J.J., Sharbrough, F.W., and Tinker, J. 1978. Effects of hypothermia on the human brainstem auditory-evoked response. Ann. Neurol. 3:368–370.

Stone, J.L., Bouffard, A., Morris, M., et al. 1983. Clinical and electrophysiological recovery in Arnold-Chiari malformation. Surg. Neurol. 20:313–317.

Streletz, L.J., Graziani, L.J., Branca, P.A., et al. 1986. Brainstem auditory evoked potentials in fullterm and preterm newborns with hyperbilirubinemia and hypoxia. Neuropediatrics 17:66–71.

Sutton, L.N., Frewen, T., Marsh, R., et al. 1982. The effects of deep barbiturate coma on multimodality evoked potentials. J. Neurosurg. 57:178–185.

Swigart, E.T. 1986. *Neonatal Hearing Screening*. San Diego: College-Hill Press.

Taylor, M.J., Houston, B.D., and Lowry, N.J. 1983. Recovery of auditory brain-stem responses after a severe hypoxic ischemic insult. N. Engl. J. Med. 309:1169–1170.

Taylor, M.J., Boor, R., and Ekert, P.G. 1996. Preterm maturation of the somatosensory evoked potential. Electroencephalogr. Clin. Neurophysiol. 100:448–452.

Thivierge, J., and Côté, R. 1990. Brain-stem auditory evoked response: normative values in children. Electroencephalogr. Clin. Neurophysiol. 77: 309–313.

Tomita, Y., Fukuda, C., Maegaki, Y., et al. Re-evaluation of short latency somatosensory evoked potentials (P_{13}, P_{14} and N_{18}) for brainstem function in children who once suffered from deep coma. Brain Dev. 25: 352–356.

Tsubokawa, T., Nishimoto, H., Yamamoto, T., et al. 1980. Assessment of brainstem damage to the auditory responses in acute severe head injury. J. Neurol. Neurosurg. Psychiatry 43:1005–1011.

Tsuneishi, S., Casaer, P., Fock, J.M., et al. 1995. Establishment of normal values for the flash evoked potentials (VEPs) in preterm infants: a longitudinal study with special reference to components of the N1 wave. Electroencephalogr. Clin. Neurophysiol. 96:291–299.

Tucker, A., Slattery, W.H., Solcyk, L., et al. 2001 Intraoperative auditory assessments as predictors or hearing preservation after vestibular schwannoma surgery. J. Am. Acad. Audiol. 12:471–477.

Tyler, C.W. 1982. Assessment of visual function in infants by evoked potentials. Dev. Med. Child Neurol. 24:853–856.

Van der Drift, J.F.C., Brocaar, M.P., and Van Zaten, G.A. 1988. Brainstem response audiometry. I. Its use in distinguishing between conductive and cochlear hearing loss. Audiology 27:260–270.

Vasiri, D., Pratt, H., Saiti, J.K., et al. 1981. Evaluation of somatosensory pathway by short latency evoked potentials in patients with end-stage renal disease maintained on hemodialysis. Int. J. Artif. Organs 4:17–22.

Vohr, B.R., Oh, W., Stewart, E.J., et al. 2001. Comparison of costs and referral rates of 3 universal newborn hearing screening protocols. J. Pediatr. 139:238–244.

Wiedemayer, H., Fauser, B., Sandalciouglu, I.E., et al. 2002. The impact of neurophysiological intraoperative monitoring on surgical decisions: a critical analysis of 423 cases. J. Neurosurg. 96:255–262.

Yamada, O., Ashikawa, H., Kokera K., et al. Frequency-selective auditory brainstem responses in newborns and infants. Arch Otolaryngol. 109: 79–82.

56. EEG and Evoked Potentials in Neuroanesthesia, Intraoperative Neurological Monitoring, and Neurointensive Care

Hans-Christian Hansen* and Jan Claassen*

Assessment of the neurological status of patients with impaired consciousness is often limited. Electrophysiological studies such as electroencephalography (EEG) or evoked potentials (EPs) have the potential to assess brain function even in the nonawake and heavily sedated patient. In the operating room (OR) these monitoring techniques are widely used to evaluate intraoperative neurological changes, e.g., during neurosurgery, and cardiovascular and spinal surgery. With the advent of interventions for neurological complications in the neurological intensive care unit (NICU), such as angioplasty for vasospasm, continuous IV infusion antiepileptic drugs for status epilepticus, total parenteral alimentation (TPA) for acute stroke, or hypothermia for ischemic brain injury, timely diagnosis becomes increasingly important for patient management. The ultimate goal of monitoring techniques in the ICU, as well as the OR, is to enable the clinician to detect impending central nervous system (CNS) injury at a time when interventions may still prevent permanent brain damage. Most established techniques such as the clinical examination, Doppler sonography, or even modern imaging tools [magnetic resonance imaging (MRI) or computed tomography (CT)] are at best serial with large time gaps in between studies. Continuous, noninvasive monitoring is needed in the ICU to facilitate early interventions in these critically ill patients.

Neurophysiological techniques may theoretically be both noninvasive and continuous. The primary tools include EEG and EPs. They may supplement the clinical examination and provide specific diagnostic information related to brain wave patterns (e.g., burst-suppression, spindles, abnormal alpha, attenuation, seizures) or anatomic function (e.g., evidence of brainstem damage on EP studies). Single or even repeated electrophysiological investigations may be as limited as other noncontinuous techniques, such as the neurological examination, represent only a discrete, brief sample of data that may not reflect the patient's overall condition. When one considers the frequent fluctuations in the clinical status of comatose patients, the cycling patterns of the background EEG (diurnal patterns), and, albeit brief, the subclinical seizures, these snapshot electrophysiological studies may not adequately reflect the patient's clinical state. If at all possible, intraoperative and ICU monitoring should be performed in a continuous fashion.

Main applications of electrophysiological monitoring in the ICU setting include (1) management of status epilepticus; (2) detection of subclinical seizures in patients with an unexplained decline of consciousness; (3) detection of ischemia particularly due to vasospasm after subarachnoid hemorrhage (SAH); (4) prognostication, particularly with EPs after traumatic brain injury (TBI); (5) assessment of neurological status, such as the presence of any electrical brain activity on EEG or the functional intactness of neurophysiological pathways after structural brain injury with EPs; and (6) evaluation of the effects of sedation and therapeutic interventions such as pentobarbital therapy for raised intracranial pressure (ICP). In the OR, these techniques may (1) define clinically important ischemic thresholds during carotid endarterectomy, (2) determine adequacy and depth of sedation possibly aided by quantitative EEG analysis (e.g., bispectral index, BIS), (3) record intraoperative seizures, and (4) guide neurosurgical operations (e.g., spinal surgery).

Technical Aspects
Critical Care Single EEG

In intensive care medicine, abnormal EEG findings are an important noninvasive diagnostic tool with many applications. This holds especially true in disorders which are not easily depicted by neuroimaging or other tests (e.g., epileptic syndromes, encephalopathies, and brain death). Brain death diagnostic protocols in some countries require an isoelectric EEG as a confirmatory test for certain subgroups of patients, e.g., in Germany for patients with infratentorial lesions (Haupt and Rudolf, 1999). Interestingly, prior to the advent of modern intensive care medicine "burst-suppression EEG" did not receive any attention. The underlying clinical phenomenon ("respirator brain") was previously unknown and signifies a comatose patient on respiratory support suffering from severe postanoxic cerebral injury (Niedermeyer et al., 1999). In contrast to evoked potential studies, EEG registrations may pick up more widespread pathology outside specific afferent or efferent systems. The EEG depicts the functional integrity of diffuse thalamocortical projections, which are modulated by parts of the ascending reticular activating system. Thus, the EEG depends on how these interacting systems modulate synaptic activity in layers 3 and 5 of the cortex and serves as a more global parameter of cerebral integrity.

Single EEG Recordings

From a single conventional EEG recording, information may be gathered about (1) reactivity to external stimuli un-

---

*Both authors contributed in equal parts to this chapter.

recognized by neurological examination; (2) separation of focal from bilateral hemispheral or subhemispheral involvement, sometimes with findings typical for certain pathologies (e.g., in Jacob-Creutzfeldt disease); (3) EEG patterns typical for coma, which may help in prognostication; and (4) epileptic patterns and their response to therapy. Nonconvulsive status epilepticus is an example of an EEG pattern that may lead to immediate therapeutic consequences.

Electrophysiological *reactivity* may appear in at least three different general categories (Evans, 1976). Acceleration of a slow EEG background can be seen in a normal arousal response (also known as desynchronization). Induction of more or less generalized delta activity by external stimuli has been termed paradoxical arousal (Evans, 1976). These series of delta waves may represent variants of abnormal K complexes (Chatrian et al., 1963). Finally, a brief period of EEG suppression may also represent EEG reactivity, which is often observed in patients undergoing sedation (Rae-Grant et al., 1991). Zschocke (2002) reported that using longer time constants may reveal the induction of sub-delta activity, which under standard recording conditions (time constant 0.3 sec) is attenuated.

The presence of any kind of reactivity suggests that the ascending reticular system receives afferent input and actively modulates cortical regions, thereby indicating some integrity of the involved pathways. Desynchronization in the EEG following external stimuli is a relatively good prognostic sign and may be preserved in deeply comatose patients [Glascow Coma Scale (GCS) 3 or 4]. Bioelectrical reactivity may further be investigated using multimodal stimuli including somatosensory, auditory, and visual input. For tactile stimulation, the face should be targeted to avoid stimulating areas with a sensory deficit (e.g., in the setting of a possibly unknown spinal level in a polytrauma patient). Adequate auditory input can be delivered by calling the patient's first name or using loud hand claps, but acquired deafness can at times play a role and lead to misleading results (e.g., inner ear trauma, or post-ototoxic antibiotic use).

Focal EEG findings are sometimes helpful suggesting specific pathological processes, such as periodic lateralized epileptiform discharges (PLEDs; see Table 56.1 for definitions) in herpes encephalitis. While injury to the hemispheres results in diffuse slowing (e.g., toxic encephalopathy), bilateral synchronous patterns can point to subhemispheric disturbance of function. Frontal intermittent rhythmic delta activity (FIRDA), although being encountered in a number of conditions and nonspecific (see Chapter 12), is often seen with dilations of the third ventricle as in aqueductal stenosis and in ICP dysregulation. In patients with SAH the appearance of FIRDA often parallels the development of hydrocephalus, suggesting the need for additional CSF drainage (Riemer et al., 1998).

EEG Patterns in Coma and Unresponsiveness

An abnormal EEG is obligatory in the comatose patient, irrespective of the underlying pathology. In unconscious patients with an unknown history of the present illness, drug-induced EEG changes may be the first hint to suspect intoxication and a suicide attempt. Typical EEG patterns include excessive beta activity (e.g., with barbiturates and benzodiazepines) and epileptiform patterns (e.g., with lithium or clozapine). Typical EEG patterns to be recorded in patients with impaired consciousness related to brain injury include diffuse slowing, FIRDA, burst suppression, triphasic waves, rhythmic delta activity, epileptic discharges, sleep patterns, alpha coma, alpha-theta coma, isoelectricity, nonconvulsive status epilepticus-like activity, and marked voltage reduction.

A normal EEG in a patient seemingly unresponsive should always raise suspicion for psychogenic unrespon-

Table 56.1. Definitions of EEG Patterns Frequently Encountered during EEG Monitoring

Name	Acronym	Definition
Electrographic seizures		Rhythmic discharge or spike and wave pattern with definite evolution in frequency, location, or morphology; evolution in amplitude alone did not qualify
Potentially epileptiform patterns		
Periodic epileptiform discharges	PEDs	Repetitive sharp waves, spikes, or sharply contoured waves at regular or nearly regular intervals and without clear evolution in frequency or location (includes PLEDs, GPEDs, BiPLEDs, triphasic waves)
Periodic lateralized epileptiform discharges	PLEDs	Consistently lateralized PEDs
Generalized PEDs	GPEDs	Bilateral and synchronous PEDs with no consistent lateralization
Bilateral PLEDs	BiPLEDs	PLEDs occurring bilaterally, but independently and asynchronously
Suppression-burst	SB	Bursts of irregular/rhythmic slow waves ± fast components, location: widespread (bisynchronous, or more focal), duration: 1–3 sec, separated by low-amplitude delta/no activity, lasting usually 2–10 sec (may be much longer)
Likely not epileptiform patterns		
Triphasic waves		Generalized periodic sharp waves or sharply contoured delta waves with triphasic morphology (typically negative–positive–negative polarity, each phase longer than the prior), at 1–3 Hz, with/without anterior–posterior or posterior–anterior lag
Frontal intermittent rhythmic delta activity	FIRDA	Moderate to high-voltage monorhythmic and sinusoidal 1–3 Hz activity seen bilaterally, maximal in anterior leads, no evolution
Uncertain if epileptiform or not		
Stimulus-induced rhythmic, periodic, or ictal discharges	SIRPIDs	Periodic, rhythmic, or ictal appearing discharges that were consistently induced by alerting stimuli, such as auditory stimuli, sternal rub, examination, suctioning, turning, and other patient care activities

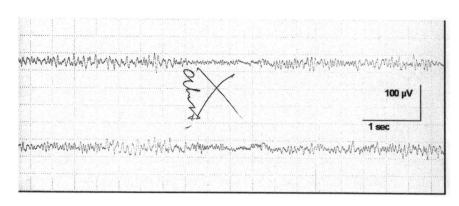

Figure 56.1. "Pseudocoma." A 19-year-old woman was admitted unconscious, after being found in the street. Eyes spontaneously closed, intact pupillary responses, Glasgow Coma Scale (GCS) score of 3, ventilation normal, computed tomography (CT) scan, and lab screens were without pathological findings. The EEG (frontoparietal leads, upper trace left, lower trace right centro-parietal leads) discloses a 11/sec alpha activity reactive to calls (*cross marks signify* auditory stimulation responded to by normal arousal). Diagnosis: dissociative state and underlying borderline personality disorder.

siveness, pseudocoma, or locked-in syndrome. Testing reactivity by passive eye opening often elicits some (volitional) eye or eyelid movement. A reactive alpha-EEG trace in a stuporous patient suggests that the patient is in a noncomatose dissociative state or locked-in syndrome. This EEG finding can be obtained by a simple two-channel bedside recording (Fig. 56.1) and allows the clinician to explore underlying psychiatric disorders such as posttraumatic stress or conversion disorders.

Certain EEG findings in coma are typical for a grave prognosis such as severe suppression in the absence of sedation and isoelectricity; others are indeterminate. In a study stratifying different EEG patterns in 80 patients suffering from hypoxic brain damage, we found that diffuse slowing with preserved reactivity in the EEG is compatible with a favorable clinical course (Fig. 56.2). This also holds true for fast frontal spindle activities resembling sleep patterns but not for slower variants of spindles in the theta domain (Kaplan et al., 2000). Interpretation of spindle patterns should include knowledge about centrally acting drugs.

Differences in definitions for EEG patterns may explain discrepancies regarding the reported prognosis for "alpha coma" (Berkhoff et al., 2000; Kaplan et al., 1999). These findings typical for coma are discussed in more detail in Chapter 24. Still today, a universally accepted EEG grading system to determine prognosis in coma does not exist. EEG prognostication of coma may be difficult in patients receiving high doses of sedatives, making the clinical applicability limited.

Besides sleep patterns, some spontaneous variability that may resemble sleep/wake cycles may be present and signal better prognosis (Bergamasco et al., 1968). Reactivity more than other factors may suggest a better prognosis in the comatose patient. Bricolo et al. (1973) found a poor outcome in only 35% when the EEG changed after stimulus application in contrast to 90% when the EEG was unreactive to external stimuli. Unlike the poor outcome being closely associated with lost EEG reactivity in coma, the relation regarding good outcome is rather loose and merely a trend. Part of this is explained by extracerebral factors interfering with the outcome in these severely ill patients. Furthermore, early EEGs may not always be able to predict complications later in the clinical course with severe impact on the outcome (such as herniation or at times status epilepticus; see below). However, Gütling et al. (1995) showed that the evaluation of EEG reactivity improves outcome prediction when assessed within the first 3 days after injury.

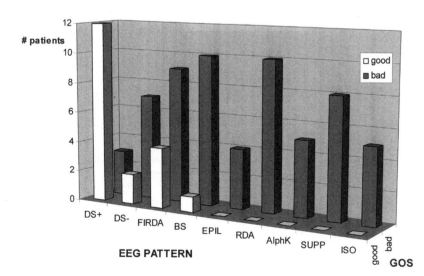

Figure 56.2. EEG patterns recorded during the first 5 days in 80 patients suffering from brain hypoxia stratified by outcome. Patients with good outcome (no or moderate disability, GOS 4 and 5, n = 19) are represented by *white columns,* and those with bad outcome (dead, vegetative state, severe disability, Glasgow Outcome Score (GOS) 1–3, n = 61) by *black columns.* EEG patterns plotted on the right. ISO, SUPP, AlphC, RA, and EPI were never observed in patients with good outcome. For the remaining EEG categories, both good and poor outcomes were observed (DS+, DS−, FIRDA, BS). Most good outcome patients showed diffuse slowing with preserved reactivity. ISO, isoelectricity; SUPP, suppression; BS, burst-suppression, AlphC, alpha coma; RDA, rhythmic delta activity; EPI, epileptic patterns; DS+, diffuse slowing with reactivity, DS−, diffuse slowing without reactivity, FIRDA, frontal intermittent rhythmic delta activity.

Few studies have analyzed EEG findings in concert with other potential predictors of poor outcome. Therefore, the independent predictive power of EEG findings remains largely unknown. A scale including etiology, age, neurological examination, and EEG findings was shown to correlate highly with mortality and functional outcome in neurological ICU patients (Hirsch et al., 2001). However, EEG findings were the weakest contributor to this score and the score requires prospective validation.

Serial EEGs

Evolving EEG patterns over time may better reflect the clinical course. Changes of EEG reactivity during the clinical course may supplement clinical and radiological data with information relevant to determining prognosis. Thus recording EEGs repeatedly may help to demonstrate stability, deterioration, or recovery in the clinical course. However, a general physiological temporal pattern for restitution, i.e., a time window in which EEG improvements must take place to achieve meaningful outcome is not known. Clearly, the longer an unreactive EEG persists, the less likely a favorable outcome will be. In experimental hypoxic-ischemic encephalopathy (in rats), the EEG following resuscitation from cardiac arrest responds with isoelectricity often followed by burst-suppression patterns that may then evolve depending on the severity of hypoxia and the degree of neurological recovery (Geocadin et al., 2002; Hansen et al., in preparation). In humans, the clinical evolution within the first 24 hours suggests a correlation with outcome: complete recovery and normalization of the EEG may occur if isoelectricity resolves within 60 minutes after onset. Full recovery has even been observed after over 3 hours of a burst-suppression EEG (Bassetti and Scollo-Lavizzari, 1987).

Continuous EEG (cEEG)

Only 10 years ago, EEG monitoring in most ICUs was performed intermittently with paper recordings. Continuous EEG (cEEG) monitoring used to be primarily limited to EEG monitoring units for the presurgical evaluation of candidates for epilepsy surgery, and seizure or spell classification (Legatt and Ebersole, 1997). Technical developments have made digital EEG monitoring, post-hoc filtering, online quantitative EEG analysis, re-montaging, sensitivity adjustments, and World Wide Web-based remote EEG interpretation possible (Scheuer, 2001). More powerful computer technology has made the collection, storage, analysis, and transmission of large amounts of continuous EEG data a reality (Scheuer, 2002). These developments have helped con-

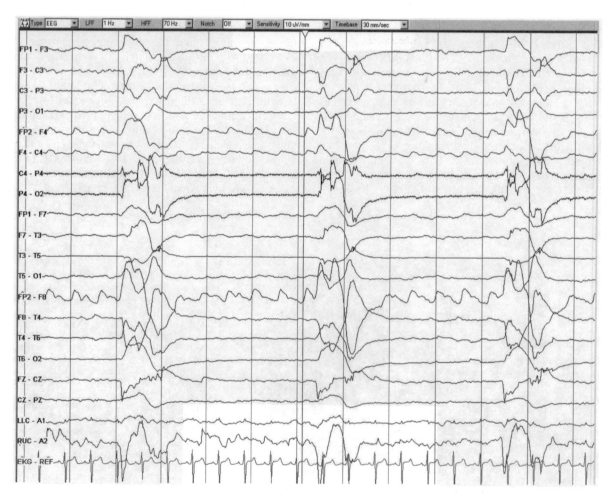

Figure 56.3. Combination of cyclic respirator artifact and right frontal pulse artifact.

tinuous EEG monitoring to be accepted as a diagnostic tool with applications in clinical management of severely sick patients rather than only as a research instrument. In this rapidly evolving field, computer technology is being developed that allows neurophysiological monitoring to be fully integrated with other data collected in the OR or the NICU, such as blood pressure, oxygen saturation, temperature, cerebral perfusion pressure (CPP), ICP, and brain tissue oxygen tension. Multimodal monitoring of this type allows optimization of physiological variables directly under our control, such as CPP and pCO_2, and provides insights into how different physiological derangements affect neurological function.

The OR and the neuro-ICU environment create substantial challenges for the recording of high-quality cEEG data that accurately reflects the patient's brain activity. In the ICU, prolonged EEG monitoring over many days may be necessary. One of the greatest difficulties is to maintain EEG electrodes for prolonged time periods on the patient's head and to provide a low-impedance, high-quality connection between patient and machine. This requires a dedicated team of well-trained EEG technicians and nursing staff, but still often results in an artifact-contaminated EEG record. Electrical noise can usually be easily filtered out of the EEG by applying a post-hoc 60- or 50-Hz filter. Other, more noncontinuous sources of artifact may be more perplexing (Hirsch and Claassen, 2002; Young and Campbell, 1999). Ventilators produce both mechanical and electric rhythmic artifact (Fig. 56.3). Nursing procedures such as chest physical therapy are other sources of activity that may at times be in the frequency range of normal or pathological brain electrical activity (Hirsch and Claassen, 2002). Completely disconnected electrodes may occasionally record activity that looks similar to that from a comatose patient with moderate to severe diffuse slowing and attenuation. Periodic or ictal-appearing EEG patterns elicited by alerting stimuli have been seen in as many as 22% of critically ill ICU patients. These were called stimulus-induced rhythmic, periodic, or ictal discharges (SIRPIDs) (Hirsch et al., 2004). Recording video during cEEG, documenting patient stimulation on the EEG by text entry, or repetitively examining patients during cEEG is necessary to recognize these patterns, avoid misinterpretation, and differentiate SIRPIDs from spontaneous seizures. For these reasons, the technologist, clinical neurophysiologist, ICU nurse, and neurointensivists must work closely together to ensure that the EEG accurately reflects cerebral activity. Team training and continuing education for clinicians are crucial to the success of any neuro-ICU cEEG monitoring program (Procaccio et al., 2001). Digital video has been shown to be particularly helpful for identifying subtle ictal phenomena (e.g., facial twitching or rhythmic eye movements), and for identifying EEG abnormalities related to artifact (Cascino, 2002).

Quantitative EEG (qEEG) Analysis

A major hurdle to overcome is the labor-intensiveness of interpreting cEEG data. Digital EEG data can be transformed into power spectra by fast Fourier transformation (FFT), creating a large number of possible quantitative EEG (qEEG) parameters. These can be displayed as numbers, or

graphically as compressed spectral arrays (CSAs), histograms, or as staggered arrays (Fig. 56.4).

These qEEG graphs may reveal subtle changes over long periods of time that may not be evident when reviewing the raw EEG. Most often CSA is used to accomplish this (Bricolo et al., 1987b). CSA based on an FFT of the EEG signal can be plotted as total power or overall amplitude, frequency activity totals (e.g., total or percent alpha power), spectral edge frequencies (e.g., the frequency below which 75% of the EEG record resides), and frequency ratios (e.g., alpha over delta ratio) (Agarwal et al., 1998; Bricolo et al., 1987a,b; Chiappa and Ropper, 1984; Suzuki et al., 1988). Other EEG data reduction display formats include the cerebral function analyzing monitor (CFAM), EEG density modulation, automated analysis of segmented EEG (AAS-EEG), and the bispectral index (BIS) monitor (Flemming and Smith, 1979; Maynard and Jenkinson, 1984; Newton, 1999).

These techniques may be used to detect delayed ischemia from vasospasm after SAH and may alert the clinician to obtain more definitive proof of vasospasm (e.g., angiography) (Claassen et al., submitted; Labar et al., 1991; Vespa et al., 1997). With the advent of powerful microprocessors, data processing of this type can now be performed in real time at the patient's bedside. qEEG analysis is readily available since most manufacturers have integrated it to some extent into their software packages.

Importantly, qEEG should never be interpreted in isolation but should always be seen in the context of the underlying raw EEG. Substantial changes of a qEEG parameter may be caused by underlying artifact alone or by noncerebral factors such as scalp swelling. Similar to raw EEG reading, interpretation of qEEG parameters should not be attempted without proper training in electroencephalography. Unfortunately, it is unrealistic to expect 24-hour coverage by an electroencephalographer in all neuro-ICUs. Possibly, well-trained ICU staff could obtain qEEG parameters and have them interpreted through a Web-based link from a remotely stationed electroencephalographer who should have access to at least an excerpt of the correlating raw EEG (Scheuer, 2001).

Automated Seizure Detection

Another approach to make EEG interpretation more time efficient is the development and improvement of seizure detection programs. This specialized EEG signal processing software can be used for screening large cEEG data sets and marking sections containing suspicious brain activity. These programs may be based on a simple FFT-based frequency analysis, may recognize specific waveform patterns, or incorporate a complex learning algorithm that recognizes more combinations and sequential developments of typical waveforms.

Based on an FFT analysis of the EEG, CSA graphs can be generated to determine the occurrence of subclincial seizures once the "CSA signature" of a seizure in an individual patient has been determined (Claassen et al., 2000). This can be used to quickly screen a 24-hour recording and quantify the frequency of seizures. Specific patterns related to the rhythmicity of electrographic seizure activity (Talwar and Torres, 1988) or accompanying muscle artifact (Prior,

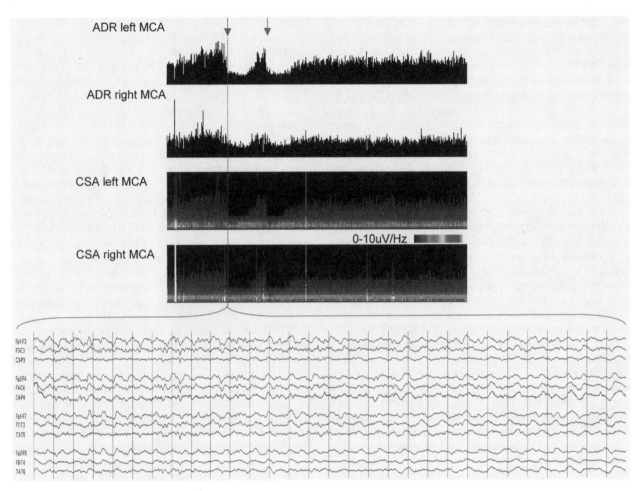

Figure 56.4. Effect of sedatives on quantitative EEG parameters. A 58-year-old woman with Hunt Hess grade four subarachnoid hemorrhage on day 5 after the bleed. Displayed are alpha delta ratio (ADR; **upper two panels**) and the compressed spectral array (CSA; **middle two panels**; color coded for intensity of the signal, with darker colors representing lower and brighter colors representing higher amplitudes) for the left and right middle cerebral artery (MCA) distribution, respectively, and an example of the raw EEG. Notice the sharp decrease of the ADR shortly after administration of a propofol bolus *(red arrow)*, which is mostly due to a loss of fast frequencies as seen in the CSA (**middle two panels:** left and right MCA) and the raw EEG (**lower panel**). (See Color Figure 56.4.)

1981) may be helpful indicators. Paroxysmal events may at times be identified using CFAM, though the sensitivity of this system for detecting partial seizures is limited (Tasker et al., 1990). Another approach to solving the problem of seizure detection has been developed by Gotman (1990), who published an algorithm for selecting parameters extracted from the digital EEG to identify ictal activity. Although the false-positive rate was quite high, the sensitivity was good, and few real ictal events are missed. Vespa et al. (1999) have developed automated seizure detection software based on multichannel, digitized real-time FFT (2 seconds per epoch, 2 minutes averaging) and trends of total EEG power, whereby some success was achieved.

Today, existing programs are far from perfect and still generate a large false-positive rate, which makes them less efficient. Even more disturbing for their ICU application is a significant false-negative rate particularly for ICU type seizures. Seizures in this setting are rarely classical, and borderline-type seizures are frequently encountered, which has led to the term *ictal-interictal continuum* (Hirsch and Claassen, 2002; Pohlmann-Eden et al., 1996). Existing automated seizure detection software that has been developed for use in epilepsy monitoring units has largely been "trained" on seizures obtained from healthy, neurologically intact patients with seizure disorders. However, these seizures differ from those of comatose, brain-injured patients, in whom ictal activity is often less organized, slower in maximum frequency, of longer duration, and without a clear on- and offset. To utilize seizure detection programs in the neuro-ICU, new software needs to be developed that can more accurately identify potentially ictal patterns in patients with brain injury.

Applications

Subclinical Seizures and Status Epilepticus

Scope of the Problem

Acute seizures and status epilepticus (SE) are common in all types of acute brain injury and are not restricted to patients with epilepsy or patients admitted with seizures or SE.

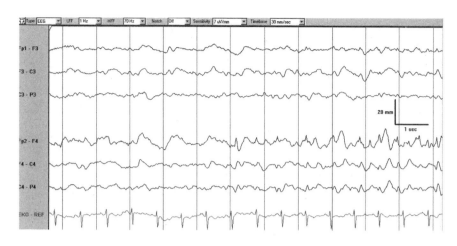

Figure 56.5. A 46-year-old man admitted with complex partial and secondary generalized tonic-clonic seizures due to underlying recurrence of a right temporal oligodendroglioma. First diagnosed 10 years prior to admission, status post-surgical resection and brain radiation, now on valproic acid. Subclinical seizures on continuous EEG (cEEG) monitoring evolving in the right hemisphere (**top and bottom panels**).

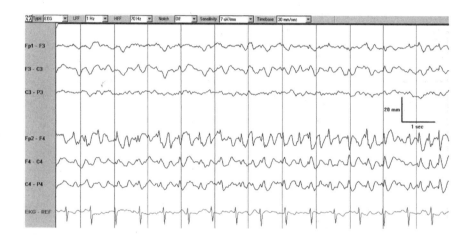

In NICU patients up to 34% have nonconvulsive seizures, and 76% of them have nonconvulsive status epilepticus (NCSE) (Jordan, 1992). Even after excluding all patients with any clinical suspicion of seizures, still 8% of comatose patients have electrographic seizures (Towne et al., 2000). Subclinical seizures (Fig. 56.5) were recorded in 18% of a cohort of 570 consecutive patients who underwent continuous EEG monitoring over a 6½-year period for the detection of subclinical seizures or unexplained impairment of consciousness (Claassen et al., submitted). In this study, seizures were more frequently recorded in (a) younger patients, (b) those with a history of epilepsy, (c) patients who had convulsive seizures prior to the start of cEEG monitoring, and (d) those who were comatose at the time cEEG monitoring was started (Claassen et al., submitted). Electrographic seizures have been described in 27% of NICU patients with altered consciousness (Privitera et al., 1994), 18% to 28% of those with severe head trauma (Claassen et al., submitted; Jordan, 1993; Vespa et al., 1999), 6% to 26% of those with ischemic stroke (Claassen et al., submitted; Jordan, 1993; Vespa et al., 2003), 29% to 33% of those with CNS infection (Claassen et al., submitted; DeLorenzo et al., 1998; Jordan, 1993), 13% to 28% of those with ICH (Claassen et al., submitted; Jordan, 1993; Vespa et al., 2003), 23% to 54% of those with brain tumor (Claassen et al., submitted; Jordan, 1993); and 18% to 60% of those with toxic-metabolic encephalopathy (Claassen et al., submitted; Jordan, 1993). These numbers tend to be higher in cohorts derived from the NICU, where monitored patients typically suffer from acute brain injury.

EEG monitoring is crucial in all SE patients who do not wake up quickly after convulsions have stopped since electrographic seizures have been documented in 48% and NCSE in 14% after control of convulsive SE (DeLorenzo et al., 1998) (Fig. 56.6). Patients on continuous IV antiepileptic drugs (cIV AEDs) for the treatment of refractory SE should always be monitored with cEEG, since subclinical seizures may occur in more than half of patients during treatment, and the majority of these patients will also have subclinical seizures after discontinuation of therapy (Claassen et al., 2001).

Impact on Outcome

It is important to diagnose these patients since the excessive metabolic demand and increased blood flow associated with ictal activity may further compromise at-risk brain tissue following acute brain insults. Most authors agree that prolonged nonconvulsive seizures can sometimes directly injure the brain and cause permanent neurological impairment (Hosford, 1999; Young and Jordan, 1998). NCSE-like conditions may also be associated with increased brain edema and midline shift after intracerebral hemorrhage

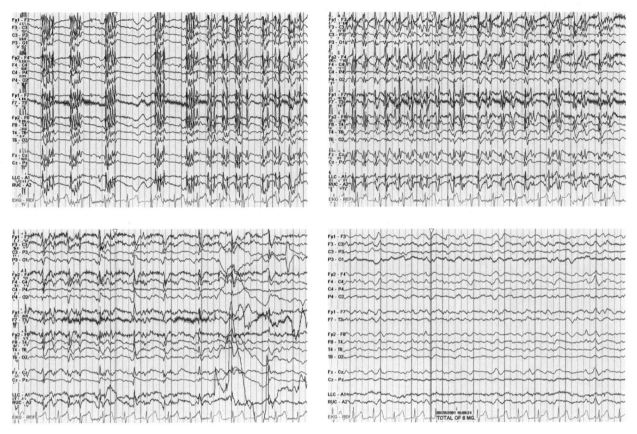

Figure 56.6. Nonconvulsive status epilepticus. An 87-year-old woman with Alzheimer's disease, possible anoxic episode, worsening confusion. EEG shows bursts of high-voltage generalized polyspikes evolving into a continuous irregular generalized spike and wave pattern at 2 to 5 Hz (**upper two panels**). Continuous generalized polyspike pattern breaks apart minutes after 6 mg of lorazepam (**bottom two panels**). Clinical condition did not improve. (See Color Figure 56.6.)

(ICH), even after controlling for other factors (Vespa et al., 2003). Although the outcome of NCSE in the setting of acute brain injury is often poor, termination of ongoing electrographic seizure activity can result in recovery of consciousness and clinical improvement (Claassen et al., 2002a). In the absence of EEG monitoring, appropriate treatment for patients with SE without overt clinical symptoms of seizures is often delayed. This may have an impact on outcome since delayed anticonvulsant therapy has been associated with poor outcome (Waterhouse et al., 1999; Young et al., 1996) and increased frequency of refractory SE (Claassen et al., 2002a; Lowenstein and Alldredge, 1993). Mortality for SE ranges between 17% and 23% (Claassen et al., 2002b; Logroscino et al., 1997; Towne et al., 1994; Waterhouse et al., 1999), and exceeds 50% in patients refractory to both first and second line therapy (Claassen et al., 2002a,c; Prasad et al., 2001; Stecker et al., 1998). The prognosis of NCSE-like conditions in the ICU setting is poor, with an overall mortality between 30% and 100% (Dennis et al., 2002; Krumholz et al., 1995; Litt et al., 1998; Young et al., 1996)—numbers that emphasize the differentiation from true NCSE, which is of benign character (Niedermeyer and Ribeiro, 2000). In NCSE-like states after TBI or SAH re-

fractory to antiepileptic medications mortality approaches 100% (Fig. 56.7) (Dennis et al., 2002; Privitera et al., 1994).

Duration of Monitoring

No general recommendation can be given for the duration of cEEG monitoring in individual patients. However, some recommendations can be given for monitoring ordered to detect subclinical seizures or to determine the cause of decreased consciousness. For a noncomatose patient with 24 hours of cEEG monitoring without evidence of ictal activity, the yield of further monitoring becomes low unless clinical changes warrant further monitoring (Claassen et al., submitted). Comatose patients may require more prolonged monitoring, as 20% do not have their first seizure until after the first 24 hours of monitoring, and 13% do not have it until more than 48 hours of monitoring (Claassen et al., submitted). Duration of cEEG monitoring should always be adjusted according to diagnostic utility in each individual patient, such as prolonged monitoring for patients on cIV-AEDs.

EEG Findings

Interpretation of cEEG in the aftermath of SE is often difficult and to some extent controversial. Seizures often pres-

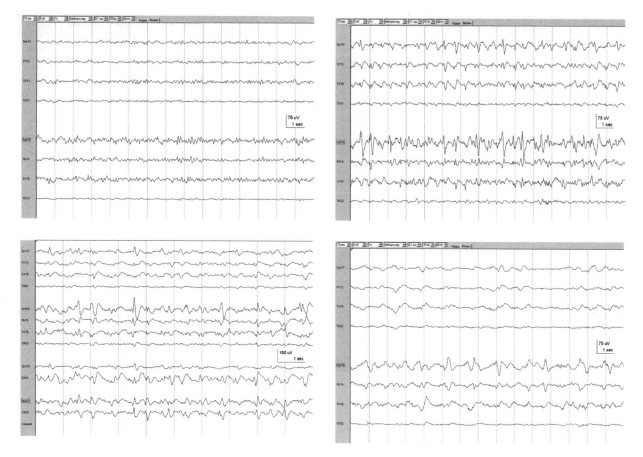

Figure 56.7. A 55-year-old woman admitted with subarachnoid hemorrhage (SAH) Hunt Hess grade III from anterior communicating cerebral artery (ACOM) aneurysm with intraventricular hemorrhage (IVH). On cEEG monitoring initially no ictal activity recorded (**upper left panel**). Later cycling between ictal activity at times evolving in frequency and location, qualifying for the diagnosis of nonconvulsive status epilepticus (**upper right panel**), more periodic epileptiform patterns without definite evolution (**lower left panel**), and recording dominated by diffuse background slowing with more isolated epileptiform discharges (**lower right panel**).

ent as paroxysmal waxing-and-waning focal slow-wave activity or PLEDs; for definitions of EEG patterns, see Table 56.1. A wide range of epileptiform discharges has been described following SE (Garzon et al., 2001; Treiman, 1995). Controversy exists regarding the interpretation and therapeutic implications of periodic epileptiform discharges that do not meet formal seizure criteria (Husain et al., 1999; Pohlmann-Eden et al., 1996). Serial EEG data (Garzon et al., 2001; Treiman et al., 1990), focal hyperperfusion single-photon emission computed tomography (Assal et al., 2001), and increased metabolism on fluorodeoxyglucose positron emission tomography (Handforth et al., 1994) have been used to argue that PLEDs following SE are often ictal. Others regard PLEDs as postictal or purely a marker of encephalopathy (Kaplan et al., 1999; Niedermeyer and Ribeiro, 2000). Periodic epileptiform discharges may represent ictal activity in the comatose patient if they are associated with some type of evolution in frequency, amplitude, and space. However, classic ictal patterns seen in epilepsy patients with otherwise normal brain function are rarely encountered in the patient with diffuse brain injury and profound EEG background suppression. Lacking a better term,

these patterns not meeting formal seizure criteria may also at times be considered part of an ictal/interictal continuum (Hirsch and Claassen, 2002; Pohlman-Eden et al., 1996). The significance of these patterns is poorly understood.

Ischemia Detection

Cerebral ischemia results in EEG changes even in the absence of infarction. Cortical layers 3 and 5, which are particularly sensitive to oxygen deficits, contribute most to the generation of electrical dipoles detected by EEG (Jordan, 1999). It has long been known that infarction may result in polymorphic delta, loss of fast activity and sleep spindles, and focal attenuation (Cohn et al., 1948). These EEG findings have been shown to reflect abnormal cerebral blood flow (CBF) and cerebral metabolic rate of oxygen as demonstrated by positron emission tomography and xenon-CT-CBF imaging (Nagata et al., 1989; Tolonen and Sulg, 1981). EEG is very sensitive for ischemia, and usually demonstrates changes at the time of reversible neuronal dysfunction (CBF 25–30 mL/100 g/min) (Astrup et al., 1981). EEG is also very sensitive for recovery and may demonstrate recovery of brain function from reperfusion earlier than the clinical examination (Jordan, 1999). The relationship between evoked potentials and ischemia is more complex since ischemia can be very focal and evoked potentials sample only a small part of the brain. Therefore, they may miss quite substantial cerebral ischemia. However, evoked potentials reliably detect changes if ischemia affects any part of the neural pathway that is studied by the particular test: somatosensory, visual, or brainstem auditory evoked potentials (BAEPs). In brainstem stroke (pontomesencephalic infarction), abnormal BAEPs correlate with an unstable clinical course and a poor prognosis (Stern et al., 1982). Central conduction time of the somatosensory evoked potential (SEP) correlates with CBF values but not closely with prognosis in comatose SAH patients (Symon et al., 1979). One study correlated serially assessed SEPs in ICU patients with cerebrovascular disease and functional outcome, assessed with the Glasgow Outcome Scale (GOS) (Haupt et al., 2000). Except for early BAEP abnormalities and infratentorial disease, outcome was closely correlated with SEP and BAEP findings in all stroke types. The high sensitivity of electrophysiological studies to changes in CBF suggests these techniques might bridge the gap between serial neurological examinations in the neuro-ICU setting, especially in comatose patients. Particularly cEEG monitoring is promising in this respect.

The sensitivity of EEG to detect reversible ischemia was clinically first applied to intraoperative monitoring, specifically to monitor CBF during carotid endarterectomy (Sharbrough et al., 1973; Zampella et al., 1991). EEG patterns, such as broad, repetitive slow waves, termed *axial bursts,* are highly correlated with clinical or angiographic evidence of vasospasm (up to 97% of the time) (Rivierez et al., 1991). In the NICU setting quantitative analysis of cEEG has been used to detect delayed cerebral ischemia (DCI) due to vasospasm in SAH patients (Claassen et al., submitted; Labar et al., 1991; Vespa et al., 1997). The qEEG parameter that best correlates with clinically significant ischemia is controversial, but most authors agree that a ratio of fast over slow activity (e.g., alpha over delta activity, or relative alpha variability) is the most practical approach (Claassen et al., submitted; Vespa et al., 1997). A number of qEEG parameters have been shown to correlate with DCI or angiographic vasospasm: trend analysis of total power (1–30 Hz) (Labar et al., 1991), variability of relative alpha (6–14 Hz/1–20 Hz) (Vespa et al., 1997), and poststimulation alpha-delta ratio (PSADR, 8–13 Hz/1–4 Hz) (Claassen et al., submitted). These qEEG parameters may detect changes up to 2 days prior to clinical changes (Fig. 56.8) (Vespa et al., 1997). Importantly, all of these studies found that focal ischemia sometimes resulted in global or bilateral changes in the EEG, and EEG changes may precede clinical deterioration by several days (Vespa et al., 1997).

Severe Head Injury

EEG monitoring in traumatic brain injury (TBI) patients may be used to diagnose posttraumatic complications, such as seizures, or more generally may be used for the monitoring of the clinical course and titration of sedatives. The goal remains to individualize therapeutic approaches in order to detect secondary brain injury as early as possible and prevent

further damage such as focal ischemia (Jones et al., 1994). Specific challenges encountered in the EEG monitoring of TBI patients include the extensive need for sedatives affecting the EEG. Furthermore, craniotomy defects and scalp edema as well as subgaleal hemorrhages have to be considered in the EEG interpretation. Communication between clinicians and electroencephalographers is crucial to prevent misinterpretations of electrophysiological recordings.

To manage intracranial pressure, high-dose barbiturate, benzodiazepines, or propofol infusions are often needed. Therapeutic efficacy relies on the reduction of cerebral metabolism, which itself decreases cerebral blood volume (CBV) and thereby ICP. Doses are often titrated with the help of on-line EEG monitoring aiming at a burst-suppression EEG tracing. During this EEG pattern cerebral metabolism is minimal and further increase of dosage produces no benefit in reducing ICP (Winer et al., 1991). A simple two-channel left and right hemisphere recording suffices to (a) titrate the therapeutic dose needed to induce burst suppression; (b) monitor for steady-state conditions; and (c) avoid unnecessarily high doses, which may result in significant cardiovascular side effects.

Vespa et al. (1999) applied cEEG monitoring and reported a detection rate of nonconvulsive seizures in 20% of their patients, which exceeds the frequency of clinically recognized events (8–10%). In the ICU, frequency of seizures may be underestimated especially in patients receiving muscle relaxants. The methods applied consisted of (a) generation of power spectra that were reviewed for peaks and (b) on-line detection by neurointensivists or nurses (Vespa et al., 1999). Peaks of power spectra were reviewed off-line in the raw EEG as to differentiate between ictal events and artifacts. Six fatal cases in this cohort were found to suffer from NCSE refractory to anticonvulsant therapy unnoticed by the clinical exam.

A quantitative EEG monitoring approach to predict outcome in TBI patients used changes in the EEG variability (Vespa et al., 2002). Data reduction was achieved by focusing on the percentage of alpha-frequencies (PA) at multiple electrodes and the determination of its variability (PAV) over time. A ratio between high and low power values was obtained and plotted in 8-hour intervals for one representative location of each hemisphere. A low PAV and especially decrease in PAV over time strongly correlated with a fatal outcome, especially in patients with low GCS. PAV values obtained during the initial 3 days after injury were significantly associated with outcome independent of clinical and radiological parameters. Although the clinical interpretation of this parameter appears straightforward, its generation implies thorough EEG analysis. Importantly, this type of qEEG monitoring requires knowledge of the underlying EEG and training in neurophysiology to be properly interpreted.

Another interesting approach to predict outcome in TBI patients utilizes EEG background attenuation and low-amplitude events in the EEG (Rae-Grant et al., 1991). It involves the quantification of periods of EEG suppression to derive the EEG silence ratio (ESR) (Theilen et al., 2000). In their study of 32 TBI patients, the authors showed that outcome at 6 month (GOS and disability scales) was closely related to ESR values obtained within the first 4 days fol-

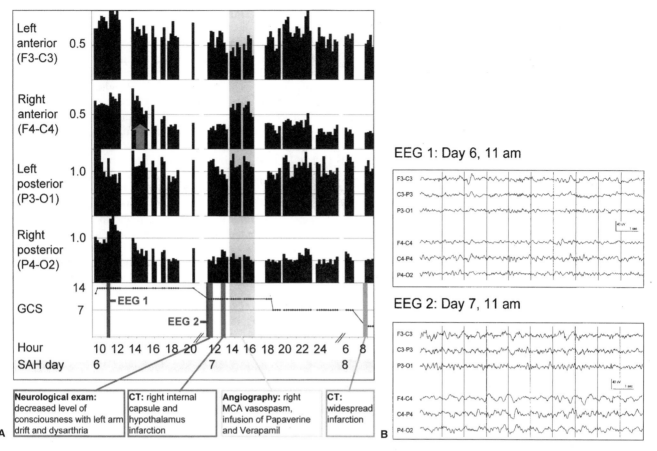

Figure 56.8. A 57-year-old woman admitted for acute SAH (admission Hunt-Hess grade 4) from a right posterior communicating aneurysm. Admission angiography did not show vasospasm. The aneurysm was clipped on SAH day 2. No infarcts were seen on postoperative CT. Postoperatively she had a GCS of 14. cEEG monitoring was performed from SAH days 3 to 8. **A:** ADR calculated every 15 minutes and GCS, shown for days 6 to 8 of cEEG monitoring. The ADR progressively decreased after day 6, particularly in the right anterior region *(orange arrow)*, to settle into a steady trough level later that night, reflecting loss of fast frequencies and slowing over the right hemisphere in the raw cEEG (**B**, EEG 2). On SAH day 6 flow velocity in the right MCA was marginally elevated (144 cm/sec), but the patient remained clinically stable with hypertensive-hypervolemic therapy (systolic blood pressure >180 mmHg). On day 7, the GCS dropped from 14 to 12 and a CT scan showed a right internal capsule and hypothalamic infarction. Angiography demonstrated severe distal right MCA and left vertebral artery spasm; however, due to the marked tortuosity of the parent vessels and the location of vasospasm, a decision was made not to perform angioplasty, but to infuse verapamil and papaverine. This resulted in a marked but transient increase of the right anterior and posterior ADRs *(yellow section)*. Later that day the patient further deteriorated clinically to a GCS of 7, with a new-onset left hemiparesis, and died on SAH day 9 from widespread infarction due to vasospasm (day 8; notice streak artifact from EEG electrodes). **B:** Sample of cEEG prior (SAH day 6) and during (SAH day 7) change in the ADR. Increase in delta and decrease in faster activity, worse on the right (bottom three channels) in EEG 2 compared to EEG 1. (See Color Figure 56.8A.)

lowing head injury. Limitations of the method include artificial increases of the ESR related to etomidate, barbiturate, and propofol use. ESR monitoring appears to be most useful in comatose TBI patients undergoing sedation with benzodiazepines and opioids.

In trauma patients the use of evoked potentials has several advantages. First, they are less susceptible to drug effects, as both SEPs and BAEPs may be recorded in barbiturate coma and even at times of an isoelectric EEG. Particularly in heavily sedated TBI patients, evoked potential studies may supplement the clinical examination. Second, serial EP studies may better monitor the physiologic integrity of afferent and efferent neuronal tracts, provided stimulus application, receptor condition (i.e., inner ear), and peripheral conduction (i.e., temperature) also remain fairly constant.

Bilaterally absent cortical SEP responses with preserved peripheral and spinal potentials are highly predictive of poor outcome after TBI (Chiappa and Hoch, 1993; Sleigh et al., 1999). In cases of bilaterally absent central somatosensory conduction the likelihood of interruption of other conduction tracts is high and therefore associated with widespread and often fatal traumatic brain damage. This strong association has been reproduced in many studies with adults and children (Chiappa and Hoch, 1993; Sleigh et al., 1999). However, circumscribed bilateral sensory tract contusions at the brainstem level may produce similar SEP loss not necessarily associated with a fatal prognosis (Pohlmann-Eden et al., 1997). Outcome is indeterminate in patients with unilaterally absent SEP potentials or conduction delays in central conduction time (Procaccio et al., 2001). Attenuation of the cortical N20-P25 may be profound, which may not be confused with complete loss of SEP potentials (Claassen and Hansen, 2001). Although normal EP studies are often seen in patients with good outcome after TBI, single EP recordings are often not able to accurately predict good outcome in the setting of neuronal damage not involving the investigated afferent or efferent tracts, and secondary injury often occurs during the hospital stay. Recovery from trauma usually is associated with recovery of SEP components (e.g., reduction of latency, normalization of amplitude). Serial SEP recordings may detect recovery after severe TBI of the diffuse axonal type earlier than the clinical exam (Claassen and Hansen, 2001).

Intracranial Pressure (ICP) Monitoring

Relatively few studies have explored the relationship between EEG patterns and ICP. EEG changes were not seen in monkeys during experimental gradual ICP rises at levels approaching mean systemic arterial pressure (Langfitt et al., 1966). In humans, no single EEG pattern has been reliably correlated with mean ICP values (Chiappa and Ropper, 1984; Munari and Calbucci, 1981). During phases without pressure waves and stable ICP, the EEG contains regular high-voltage slow waves, while an alternating EEG is seen in those patients with Lundberg B waves. It appears likely that EEG activity is not reliably influenced by increased ICP until very high levels are reached and CPP and CBF are compromised.

While visual evoked potentials (VEPs) are not sensitive to elevated ICP, BAEPs show some correlation with the ICP changes. Deterioration (Nagao et al., 1983) as well as recovery (Krieger et al., 1995) from ICP dysregulation can be monitored with BAEPs. Though the correlation between ICP and BAEPs is not strong enough to replace invasive ICP measurement in clinical practice, the BAEP trend may be used as a confirmatory test or to assess the impact of therapeutic interventions.

Monitoring of Sedation

The need for objective monitoring of the level of sedation is illustrated by the rare but dramatic occurrence of intraoperative episodes of wakefulness with intact perceptions. An objective parameter would be helpful when titrating anesthetics to minimize cardiovascular side effects while ensuring sustained surgical tolerance. Simple and user-friendly tools have been developed recently that rely on EEG monitoring requiring only a limited montage. Semiautomated analysis of single parameters extracted from a frequency analysis of the EEG (e.g., spectral edge frequency) and more complex statistical measures like the BIS can be easily derived for clinical interpretation.

Analysis of spectral EEG data using FFT reveals parameters such as spectral edge frequencies or spectral median frequencies, which show a continuous decrease following infusion of anesthetic and analgesic agents and recover to baseline during reawakening. Drummond et al. (1991) verified systematic changes of these EEG parameters in patients shortly before regaining consciousness after enflurane anesthesia. Interindividual variability of this technique, however, is high, resulting in poor sensitivity and specificity for the prediction of anesthesia depth in any individual patient. Epi-

sodes of wakefulness may not be predicted with this method (Drummond et al., 1991).

Another approach to monitoring the level of sedation is the bispectral index (BIS), which again is based on a frequency analysis and incorporates parameters that supposedly occur independently from each other. The algorithms used for the calculation of this score are controversial since the BIS is an empirically derived measurement (score between 0 and 100) based on the comparison of a patients' EEG to a database of EEGs of subjects receiving sedatives. The EEG signal input is limited to a bilateral two-channel registration at the Fp electrode locations referenced to Cz. The choice of frontopolar leads and the absence of polygraphy have been criticized given their susceptibility to artifacts. BIS values below 58 were found to be predictive of a loss of command obedience (after thiopentone bolus, Flaishon et al., 1997) and a close relation between the BIS values and the tolerance to surgical incisions has been reported (Sebel et al., 1995). However, this was not confirmed for patients undergoing isoflurane anesthesia (Sebel et al., 1995), and the cut-off values for the BIS appear to be specific for different anesthetic strategies (Vernon et al., 1995). Controversial results have been reported regarding the use of the BIS for monitoring of the sedation level in the ICU. Frenzel et al. (2002) recently reported a moderate correlation of the BIS with the level of sedation for only 60% of their ICU surgical patients. Particularly at deeper sedation levels, interindividual differences of the BIS were large.

For the electroencephalographer, the BIS is somewhat difficult to accept since "no one truly understands what physiologic phenomena the BIS measures" (Shapiro, 1999). In this context, attempts to (a) correlate the BIS with "neurologic function" as estimated by GCS and (b) look out for additive effects of "neurologic status" and pharmacologic sedation on the EEG illustrate that further experience needs to be gained and research needs to be conducted before therapeutic decisions are based on BIS values (Gilbert et al., 2001).

Other EEG processing units are also commercially available. These machines process EEG data and convert the output into changing patterns of lights or a single line representing both amplitude and frequency (e.g., cerebral function monitor; Maynard, 1979). The use of such simplistic outputs are discouraged since they give a false sense of security (ability to diagnose neurological injury) and provide limited data, increasing the possibility of false-positive diagnosis, i.e., alteration of operation based on inadequate data.

Evoked potentials are considered to be a reliable indicator of the level of sedation, especially the middle latency auditory evoked potentials (MLAEP). In contrast to BAEPs, these components originate from signal processing on a cortical level with latencies between 10 and 100 msec. Dose-dependent decreases in amplitude and increases in latency were first demonstrated by Thornton et al. (1984). Using the component Nb of the MLAEP, amnestic functions were typically preserved at latencies of <45 msec. Values above 50 msec correlated closely with amnesia (Newton et al., 1992), and latencies above 60 msec characterized a depth of sedation devoid of intraoperative arousals (Schwender et al., 1997a,b). Similar to other EEG parameters, MLAEP latency thresholds sufficiently reliable for routine applications need to be determined for various anesthetic strategies before definitive conclusions about these methods and their effectiveness in the OR can be drawn.

With increased sophistication of data presentation, the anesthesiologist assumes greater responsibility for assuring that the electrophysiological data actually reflect important physiological processes. Currently, trained neurophysiologists should always be involved in supervising the interpretation of electrophysiological data in the operating room.

Neuroanesthesia and Intraoperative EP Monitoring

Monitoring techniques during surgery or interventions (e.g., neuroradiological procedures) serve to document acute, but still reversible, changes in neurological function. Furthermore, they can be used intraoperatively to assist in identifying important neural structures (e.g., SEP-guided identification of the thalamus and the motor cortex). The motor cortex is sometimes difficult to identify (e.g., tumorous displacements) and may be located by varying intracranial electrode locations along a zone of phase shift (Fig. 56.9). Electrophysiological monitoring is also used during cardiovascular and spinal surgery and further discussed in Chapters 43 and 45.

For surgical applications, a variety of monitoring techniques may be chosen such as EEG (raw EEG; cEEG) and evoked potentials (visual, auditory, somatosensory, and motor). The choice of techniques depends on the capabilities of the surgical/monitoring team, the neural tissue at risk, and the probability of neural injury. Since the circumstances of recording are often quite different from the standard optimal conditions, it is useful to have a close working relationship between (a) an electroencephalographer with knowledge about anesthesia and familiarity with the OR and (b) an anesthesiologist specialized in both cerebral physiology and neurophysiology (i.e., neuroanesthesia).

The emphasis of interventional and intraoperative monitoring lies on the ability to detect small changes from baseline recordings in order to detect injury at the earliest and thus reversible stage (Table 56.2). The ideal technique would provide real-time detection of tissue at risk, resulting

Table 56.2. Requirements for Interventional Monitoring

- High sensitivity to neural injury
- Reasonable specificity to neural injury
- Good artifact rejection
- Low risk of monitoring procedure
- No technical interference with operating procedures
- Consequences of monitoring: option of modifying the operating procedure
- Continuous data interpretation is feasible
- Ease of data interpretation

in changes of the operating procedure. In aneurysm surgery, for example, intraoperative procedures (i.e., temporary clipping of a parent vessel) can be detected in around 10% of the patients who are monitored with SEP (see below). Although there is an obvious need to quickly correct abnormalities caused by cerebral ischemia, such abnormalities may be self-limited (Rampil et al., 1983). Rapid data generation and efficient validation should prevent unnecessary alteration of surgical procedures. Reliability must be good enough to detect most events (low rate of false negatives) without too many false positives. If false-negative diagnosis (no change in monitored parameter with neurological injury) or false-positive diagnosis (change in monitored parameter without change in neurological function) occurs, confidence in the monitoring team may be lost and an increased risk of neurological injury may result. To date, diagnostic criteria to evaluate intraoperative changes have been difficult to establish. The physician must assume that evoked potential changes in humans reflect the same neurological insults found in animals (Sohmer et al., 1983). Using conventional averaging techniques, latency changes of 7% to 15% and amplitude decreases of 45% to 50% occur without changes in postoperative neurological function in SEP (LaMont et al., 1983; Lubicky et al., 1989).

Technical Considerations

Monitoring equipment and procedures should interfere minimally with anesthetic and interventional/surgical practice. Because of surgical draping and the sterile operative

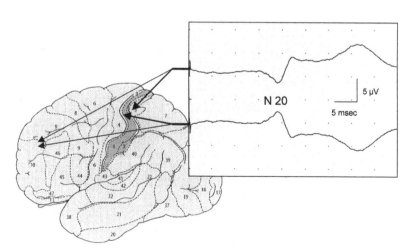

Figure 56.9. Identification of the motor cortex by intraoperative cortical SEP recording. A phase shift (especially N20 component) can be observed during displacement of the near field electrode from anterior to posterior positions across the central sulcus. (Modified after Dinkel, M., and Romstoeck, J. 1997. Neurophysiological monitoring during anesthesia. Curr. Op. Anesthesiol. 10:467–475.)

N 20

5 µV

5 msec

field, electrodes and stimulators can be difficult to apply due to the risk of dislodging cardiovascular monitors or the endotracheal tube. Careful positioning of equipment around the patient will minimize anesthetic management difficulties. To provide valuable information from intraoperative brain monitoring, fewer electrodes are necessary than in diagnostic evaluations. Rapid recognition of asymmetrical change of neural function is facilitated by comprehensive data reduction and presentation formats that provide real-time trends of one or more EEG parameters. Recent developments in computer science have facilitated this approach enormously. Irrespective of the practical considerations and extent of data reduction, raw EEG data should always be accessible for review to exclude artifacts. Electrode application techniques should provide secure attachment and prolonged, satisfactory function. Gel-filled cup electrodes attached with collodion are secure and function well (impedance less than 2 KΩ) for many hours. If the electrode location is in a sterile field, a sterile needle electrode (23 gauge) can be placed following baseline data recordings using non-sterile cup electrodes. Simultaneous monitoring of multiple electrode locations allows rapid demonstration of electrode or computer failure. Multiple-channel data acquisition and electrodes over ascending parts of the nervous system allow SEP registration to localize injury along the neural axis (McPherson and Szymanski, 1985). Sufficiently large head boxes and digital re-montage have abolished plugging and unplugging of electrodes and breaking wires.

To allow early initiation of monitoring with minimal delays in surgery, evoked potential monitoring should be undertaken prior to induction of anesthesia and surgical positioning. Equipment can be placed and electrodes applied while other operative preparations such as vascular catheter insertions are being performed. Neurological injury may be caused by surgical positioning (McPherson et al., 1984), and initiation of monitoring following positioning might lead to the incorrect assumption that evoked potential abnormalities were due solely to anesthetic agents. Suggested intraoperative monitoring time points are shown in Table 56.3.

Rapid waveform generation is necessary to assess equipment function and to effectively rule out systemic effects (drug effects). Although anesthetic agents may depress evoked potentials (especially the SEP), the signal-to-noise ratio in anesthetized patients is greatly improved because of a lack of muscle artifact (somatic muscle relaxants) and the use of high-intensity stimuli (anesthetic state). Because of the improved signal-to-noise ratio, a lower number of averages are required to produce stable waveforms. Using stimu-

lus rates of 5.9/sec for upper and 3.9/sec for lower extremity SEPs and relatively few stimuli (128–256), SEPs can be generated in less than 1 minute for the upper and lesss than 2 minutes for the lower extremity. In anesthetized subjects, stimulus frequency of 1.6, 3.1, and 5.7 Hz do not change amplitude or latencies (Delberghe et al., 1990). In patients with spinal cord injury, amplitude following posterior tibial nerve stimulation is attenuated by higher stimulus rates (>5.1 Hz), whereas good-quality waves could be obtained at lower stimulus rate (1.1 or 2.1 Hz). A majority of patients (86%) who had a decrease in amplitude with increased stimulus rate also had a discrete sensory level or bilateral lower extremity weakness or both. Of patients whose SEPs were not affected by increased stimulus rates, only 28% had similar neurological impairments (Schubert et al., 1990).

Several analysis methods for evoked potentials are available in addition to ensemble averaging. One method is the moving window average (MWA), which estimates EP components by averaging within an epoch containing the N most recent sweeps. Exponentially weighted average (EWA) estimates are obtained by weighted averaging of sweeps with the weight of older sweeps diminishing in an exponential manner. Vaz et al. (1991) compared Fourier series modeling [Fourier linear combined (FLC)] with MWA and EWA in a setting of rapid EP change after etomidate bolus. The FLC algorithm outputs a fresh estimate after each sweep and was shown to follow transient evoked potential changes much faster than EWA or MWA (Vaz et al., 1991).

Electrophysiological monitoring is periodically halted by the use of electrocautery to minimize blood loss. Although monitoring strategies should minimize disruption of surgical techniques, brain function should be assessed regularly, even if a short discontinuation of use of the electrocautery is required. Although modern equipment effectively filters high-voltage artifacts caused by the electrocautery, averaging may be automatically resumed before all components of the system have returned to baseline. A useful rule is to resume averaging only after the electrocardiogram (ECG) (which has built in delay circuits to compensate for the effect of electrocautery) has returned to normal. The BAEP is vulnerable to interruption of stimulus delivery. Transducer dislodgment, fluid in the external auditory canal, and cerumen can prevent effect stimulation.

Figure 56.10 demonstrates reversible brain dysfunction during aneurysm surgery detected by SEP monitoring. Both the time course and the characteristic changes (decreased amplitude, increased latency) are clearly shown. This case demonstrates the importance of rapid electrophysiological feedback during such procedures combined with a detailed understanding of specific operative techniques. Following aneurysm clip application, the SEP was unchanged for about 10 minutes and then changed rapidly. Since the anesthesia was not altered, the changes were correctly attributed to neurological injury. Despite rapid clip repositioning following recognition of SEP change (2–3 minutes), the patient had unilateral weakness, which resolved relatively quickly (12 hours).

The SEP is useful in demonstrating position-related neurological injury (Fig. 56.11). In this case, the rapid loss of scalp-recorded waves with preservation of waves recorded

Table 56.3.   Recommended Monitoring Time Points

- Prior to anesthesia induction
- Following anesthesia induction
- Following surgical positioning
- Before and after surgical positioning
- Before and after significant events (e.g., cardiovascular)
- Periodically or continuous during the operation
- Discontinue monitoring at end of operation or depending on the intervention continue during the postoperative phase

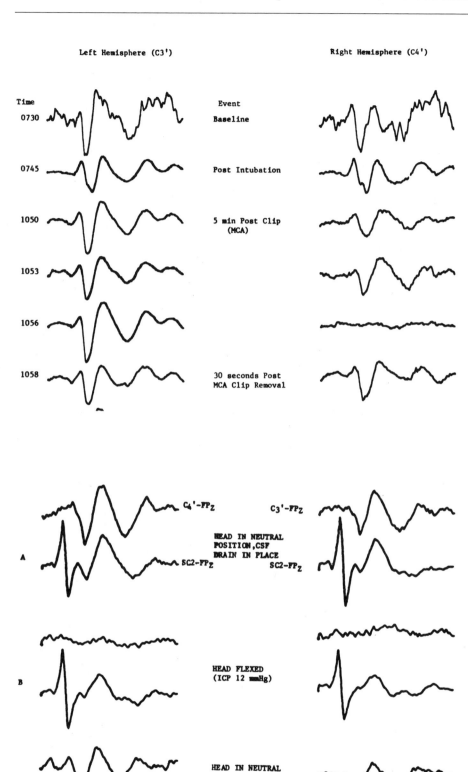

Left Hemisphere (C3')   **Right Hemisphere (C4')**

Time   Event

0730   Baseline

0745   Post Intubation

1050   5 min Post Clip (MCA)

1053

1056

1058   30 seconds Post MCA Clip Removal

Figure 56.10. Correlation of changes in median nerve SEPs and occlusion of the MCA is shown. The rapid return of the waveform following alteration of surgery (clip removal) should be noted. There was asymmetry of the SEP at the end of the operation and the patient had a transient hemiparesis that fully resolved. (From McPherson, R.W., Niedermeyer, E., Otenasek, R.J., et al. 1983. Correlation of transient neurological deficit and somatosensory evoked potentials after intracranial aneurysm surgery. J. Neurosurg. 59:146–149.)

A   C4'-FP$_Z$ C3'-FP$_Z$

HEAD IN NEUTRAL POSITION, CSF BRAIN IN PLACE

SC2-FP$_Z$ SC2-FP$_Z$

B   HEAD FLEXED (ICP 12 mmHg)

C   HEAD IN NEUTRAL POSITION

(ICP 10 mmHg)

4 u v o l t 0   ms   40

Figure 56.11. Position-related brainstem ischemia is demonstrated by SEP monitoring in a patient with a large posterior fossa tumor. Monitoring of cortical and spinal cord electrodes rapidly verified correct instrument function and localized the area of injury. (From McPherson, R.W., Szymanski, J., Rogers, M.C. 1984. Somatosensory evoked potential changes in position-related brainstem ischemia. Anesthesiology 61:88–90.)

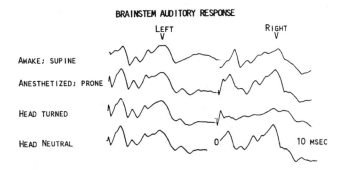

Figure 56.12. Position-related brainstem ischemia is demonstrated by brainstem auditory evoked potential (BAEP) in a young patient with right acoustic neurinoma. Prolongation of waves IV–V latency on right occurred with turning of the head and resolved quickly with return of the head to neutral position.

over the upper spinal cord localized the site of injury in the brainstem. The lack of cardiovascular changes (Cushing's response) associated with brainstem compression demonstrates that neurological monitoring is the only reliable method of recognizing such injury in patients with posterior fossa masses. The BAEP also changes (increased latency) when the surgical position causes the brainstem to be compressed (Fig. 56.12).

Patients Benefiting from Intraoperative Monitoring

Intraoperative electrophysiological monitoring is appropriate for a variety of surgical procedures. Cardiac surgery, spinal surgery, neurosurgery, major vascular surgery, and general surgery (in patients at high risk of neurological injury) are all appropriate settings for periprocedural monitoring. Within each category, these techniques can be used to identify patients who are at high risk for developing neurological deficits. Intraoperative monitoring can be initiated either by the surgeon or the anesthesiologist, depending on the institution.

Especially for neurosurgery, the benefit of monitoring is not only for prediction and identification of iatrogenic events, but also for the prevention of postoperative neurological deficits. Wiedemayer et al. (2002) reported that out of 423 operations with intraoperative monitoring, surgical decisions were successfully modified in 5.2%. Using both SEP and BAEP monitoring, the rates were: true-positive findings with intervention in 42 cases (9.9%), true-positive findings without intervention in 42 cases (9.9%), false-positive findings in nine cases (2.1%), false-negative findings in 16 cases (3.8%), and true-negative findings in 314 cases (74.2%).

Visual Evoked Potentials (VEPs)

Intraoperative monitoring of VEPs has been applied during neurosurgical interventions along the entire visual pathway, from the orbita to the optic chiasm and to the striate cortex. It is of limited use during intracranial surgery (either transsphenoidal or craniotomy approach) because of wave-

form variability possibly related to anesthetics and temperature effects (Fisher et al., 1995; Wiedemayer et al. 2003). This creates unacceptably high rates of false-positive and -negative results. Cedzich et al. (1988) assessed the use of flash VEPs in 35 patients with tumors along the visual pathway (90% symptomatic). During removal of the bone flap or during the transsphenoidal approach, a reversible loss of VEPs was observed in 11 patients, profound alteration in waveform in eight patients, and loss of single peaks in 15 patients. There was no correlation between intraoperative VEP changes and postoperative visual function. Cedzich et al. (1987) found that patients with perisellar tumors had smaller VEP amplitudes than patients with nonperisellar tumors who had similar surgery. They reported complete intraoperative VEP loss in 21 of 45 patients; however, these were not associated with postoperative neurological changes (Cedzich et al., 1987).

Brainstem Auditory Evoked Potentials (BAEP)

Kalmarchey et al. (1986) studied BAEPs during surgery for unilateral cerebellopontine angle tumors. These authors found BAEP changes with both lumbar drainage and tumor resection in their small cohort of patients, with bilateral latency prolongation in five of nine patients and ipsilateral latency increase in six of nine patients. Although the use of intraoperative monitoring was limited in these patients, post-hoc analyses suggest some additional benefit of this technique (Fisher et al., 1995). Studies have shown that intraoperative BAEP monitoring can improve outcome by reducing the rate of postoperative hearing loss from 50% to 0% (Fischer et al., 1992; Harper et al., 1992; Slavit et al., 1991). Postoperative neurological damage cannot be predicted by absolute tumor size and there are no absolute BAEP criteria available for prediction. Lam et al. (1985) reported good correlation between intraoperative BAEP and postoperative neurological function in three patients undergoing ablation of basilar artery aneurysm. Unfortunately there are currently no prospective studies to determine the benefit of this method in the operating room.

Somatosensory and Multimodal Evoked Potentials

Neurophysiological monitoring during aneurysm surgery is used to detect periods of focal cerebral ischemia, which may arise under various circumstances like brain or vessel retraction, temporary or definitive clipping, vasospasm, or induced hypotension. Various studies have shown that SEP changes may reflect critical perfusion deficits at a stage before irreversible damage occurs (Steinberg et al., 1986; Symon et al., 1988). SEP recordings may reflect critical ischemia in the distribution of the anterior cerebral artery (ACA), middle cerebral artery (MCA), and internal carotid artery (ICA) (supply of internal capsule and somatosensory cortex). BAEPs are predominantly useful for monitoring ischemia related to the branches of the posterior circulation. False-negative monitoring results are unavoidable (rates up to 4%) since ischemic events can occur outside the somatosensory and auditory afferent pathways (Friedman et al., 1987). Although the thalamic relay nuclei are fed by branches of the posterior cerebral artery (PCA), results obtained by SEP are especially disappointing with aneurysms located in the posterior circulation. Thus, bimodal monitoring with BAEP and SEP has been suggested (Lopez et al., 1999; Manninen et al., 1994). Positive monitoring results may be used to modify the operative strategy (for example, in testing vessel occlusion, clip placement), which is reported to take place in nearly 10% of the patients monitored in various studies (Emerson and Turner, 1993; Fisher et al., 1995; Friedman et al., 1991).

The temporal dynamics of SEP alterations and their recovery were investigated by Momma et al. (1987). During temporary clip application they assessed central conduction time (CCT: the time difference between the cervical spinal level and the contralateral cortex) in 40 patients with significant (25%) rates of postoperative neurological changes. In six of 40 patients, temporary arterial occlusion prolonged CCTs by up to 10 msec, and in two of those six patients postoperative neurological deficits were observed (one recovered). Loss of SEP during temporary occlusion occurred in 15 of 40 patients, and seven of 15 exhibited hemispheric deficits in the immediate postoperative period (four recovered). Permanent postoperative deficits were unlikely if the SEP disappeared slowly (over more than 3–4 minutes), and recovery was likely if the N20 component returned to baseline within 20 minutes after reperfusion. Corroborating evidence of these parameters came from Mizoi and Yoshimoto (1993), who concluded that temporary occlusion for about 10 minutes can be tolerated, provided the SEP was lost gradually.

Temporal vessel occlusion was monitored by Manninen et al. (1990), who reported persistent SEP changes despite release of occlusion in 35%. Persistent changes always predicted a postoperative neurological deficit, whereas reversible changes were followed by postoperative deficits in only five of 15 patients (false-positive rate 43%, false-negative rate 14%). When persistent SEP changes alone were considered as predictors of neurological deficits, the false-positive rate was 0%. As a predictor of neurological outcome in temporary vessel occlusion, the SEP is more useful in the carotid system than in the vertebrobasilar system. SEP changes correctly predicted a neurological deficit in only 38% of patients with vertebrobasilar artery aneurysms compared to 75% of patients with MCA or carotid artery aneurysm.

Using dual monitoring during 58 operations for intracranial aneurysmal repair, Lopez et al. (1999) detected SEP changes in 22% and BAEP alterations in 20%. Most of them were reversible after modification of the procedure (removal or adjustment of clips, adjustment of the retractor, elevating blood pressure). The mean time from the precipitating event to EP changes was 8.9 minutes and recovery time ranged from 3 to 60 minutes (mean 20 minutes). Similar to Manninen et al. (1994), they concluded that their combined use yielded lower false-negative and false-positive results and suggested the use of dual monitoring techniques, especially with posterior circulation aneurysms.

Although compared to neurosurgical clipping, endovascular aneurysm therapy has some advantages, especially for patients with aneurysms in the posterior circulation and poor-grade SAHs, it also has associated risks of ischemic complications (Groden et al., 2001; Kremer et al., 2002).

Table 56.4. Intraoperative Events Associated with Evoked Potential Changes Suggesting Neurological Injury

- Head flexion while positioning patient for surgery
- Injury to brachial plexus due to pressure or stretching
- Retraction of brainstem
- Aneurysm clip application
- Induced hypotension (in presence of vasospasm)
- Decreased arterial oxygenation
- Vertebral distraction
- Disc fragment migration

Neuromonitoring is applicable in this endovascular setting since the procedures are generally carried out under general anesthesia. In a first study (Liu et al., 2003) on 50 patients undergoing endovascular procedures (balloon test occlusion, platinum coil embolization, "coiling") and permanent vessel occlusion, neuromonitoring changes using BAEP, SEP, and EEG were seen in nine (26%) of 35 patients. The findings altered the management in five of 35 (14%) patients. In their cohort, the authors observed two false-negative monitoring results, and advocated neuromonitoring to help guide therapeutic decisions in endovascular settings.

In conclusion, intraoperative monitoring during aneurysm surgery offers the opportunity to optimize surgical strategies based on the observation of cerebral physiology in real time. Given the low rates of false-negative results, SEP findings alone can predict postoperative neurological deficits at reasonable rates and can help to guide decisions about clip placement and vessel occlusion, at least in anterior circulation aneurysm operations. Surgical and endovascular interventions in the posterior fossa seems to be better monitored by multimodal approachs including both BAEP and SEP. Table 56.4 summarizes intraoperative events in which SEP changes may indicate injury of neurological tissue. Apart from the still open question of cost-effectiveness in the standard patient, the benefit of monitoring is evident in patients considering repair of giant or multilobulated aneurysms or when occlusion therapy is discussed.

Major Contaminants for EEG and EPs
General

Limitations of electrophysiological brain monitoring in the OR or ICU setting arise from drug contamination, electrical artifact (generated by ICU equipment, e.g., ventilators), movement or manipulation of the patient (secondary to nursing procedures, agitation of the patient, or shivering). Artifacts from electrical sources and movement have been discussed in more detail above.

Anesthetic Drugs

In intensive care medicine and in the operating room, a large number of medications are routinely used that can potentially impact on electrophysiological recordings. These medications include anesthetic gases, hypnotics, opioids, sedatives, and muscle relaxants, all of which may directly alter brain electrical activity (EEG and evoked potentials), usually in a predictable dose-effect relationship. Since most

Table 56.5.   Characteristics of Commonly Used Aesthetic Drugs

	MAC[a]/iv Dose	Cerebral Blood Flow	Intracranial Pressure
Halothane	0.75%	↑	↑
Enflurane	1.7%	↑	↑
Isoflurane	1.3%	↑	↑
Nitrous oxide	105%	↑	↑
Thiopental	4 mg/kg	↑	↓
Fentanyl	25 µg/kg	↓→	↓
Etomidate	0.4 mg/kg	↓	↓
Propofol	2 mg/kg	↓	↓

[a]MAC, alveolar concentration necessary to prevent movement in 50% of subjects.

of these drugs can also affect CBF, CBV, and ICP, and hence oxygen delivery to neurons (summarized in Table 56.5), they can also indirectly exert effects on the EEG by provoking focal cerebral ischemia. The effects of reduced oxygen delivery may even overshadow the direct drug effects on brain electrical activity. Thus when neurophysiological monitoring results suggest deterioration, such indirect effects (i.e., cerebral hypoxia) must be considered first. As an example, impaired cerebrovascular and cardiovascular reflexes are common in patients with traumatic brain injury and are further blunted by vasoactive drugs like nitroglycerin. A decompensation of arterial blood pressure or increased ICP then explains deterioration of neurological function or EEG findings.

In addition to dose-related changes in the EEG, anesthetic drugs also show a typical time function in their EEG changes. Most of this temporal course can be explained by pharmacodynamic factors such as total dose, lipophilia, redistribution effects, and CBF, and may be specific to the substance. These factors determine the local drug concentration at a neuronal level, which results in alteration of both vigilance and EEG.

Most anesthetic agents produce both (a) frequency and amplitude changes of the EEG and (b) latency and amplitude changes of the EP that gradually evolve and overlap along increasing depths of anesthesia. EEG changes seen during sequential stages of anesthesia (Table 56.6) are (a) desynchronization in the excitatory phase (loss of alpha, induction of beta); (b) synchronization (higher amplitude alpha and theta components); and (c) further slowing, increasing suppression until development of burst suppression and finally general suppression. Thus, the effects on the EEG change in relation to the cerebral concentration of the anesthetic (see below). The restoration of vigilance and EEG follows a reverse course when anesthetics are washed out. Exceptions to this rule include predominant theta induction by ketamine or prominent beta activation with propofol, benzodiazepine, and barbiturate use. Certain drugs, when acting as comedication, produce EEG changes other than those known from the usual monotherapy. This is one of the challenges of monitoring the depth of sedation in balanced anesthesia during neurosurgical procedures. However, extensive experience and familiarity with the effects of anesthetic drugs on EEG and evoked potentials may enable the

neurologist or anesthesiologist to suspect neurological injury even if the anesthetic state is changing.

Epileptogenic drug side effects have to be kept in mind as nearly all anesthetics and analgesics have anti- or proconvulsive properties. Facilitation of epileptiform potentials and lowering the epileptic threshold during anesthesia may be potentially hazardous in patients with epilepsy. It has been suggested that enflurane, sevoflurane, ketamine, etomidate, and possibly also alfentanil or fentanyl be used cautiously in the epileptic patient undergoing anesthesia (Bruder and Bonnet, 2001). Under anesthesia for electrocorticography, drug-induced enhancements of the focal epileptiform activity was reported to facilitate focus localization and be helpful for the procedure (Wass et al., 2001). Others described this pharmacological activation to be counterproductive for surgical focus localization because activated areas were widely distributed (Cascino, 1998; Hisada, 2001).

Evoked potentials are generally less affected by anesthetic drugs, making them at times a good alternative to EEG monitoring. Evoked potential monitoring during anesthesia should be differentiated according to which generators are to be recorded. When inhalational anesthetics are being use, monitoring aimed at subcortical components like peripheral SEP or BAEP may be quite informative. Cortical EP monitoring is a preferential choice for combinations of intravenous agents. TIVA (propofol plus alfentanil) or alternatively an induction with etomidate plus opioids followed by anesthesia with inhalational agents are amenable to SEP recording. Regimens based on continuous drug application (steady-state conditions) are superior to bolus application because bolus injections can mimic the effects of a surgical lesion (EP amplitude depression and latency prolongation). For transcranial motor EP recording, halogenated anesthetics are inferior to opioid-based regimes (Sloan, 1998). In intraoperative monitoring, these drug-induced neurophysiological changes rarely result in levels of EEG suppression severe enough to make interpretation impossible. Importantly, recording of a baseline EEG prior to induction of the anesthesia should be available for reference, and a recording

Table 56.6.   Characteristic Pattern of EEG Changes Produced by Inhalation Anesthetics; According to Anesthesia Depth, Typical EEG Findings Can Be Expected

Clinical Situation	Characteristic EEG	Guedel Stage
Awake	Posterior alpha	I
Excitation	Activation of beta, induction of theta	II
Early anesthesia	Dominant alpha-theta, some delta	III-1
Surgical tolerance	Dominant delta, some theta	III-2
Deep surgical tolerance	Continuous, high-amplitude delta	III-3
Early overdose	Isoelectric stretches, burst-suppression EEG	III-4
Toxicity	Continuous isoelectricity	IV

Modified from Stockard, J.J., Bickford, R.G., Smith, T.N., et al. 1973. Structure-activity relationships of ether anesthetics: an electroencephalographic study of diethylether, fluroxene, isoflurane and enflurane. Electroencephalogr. Clin. Neurophysiol. 34:713(abst).

following induction of anesthesia (prior to surgical positioning) should be considered the baseline for intraoperative monitoring (Table 56.3).

Anesthetic Gases

Volatile anesthetics (desflurane, sevoflurane, halothane, enflurane, and isoflurane) are vaporized and delivered either in oxygen or in a combination of nitrous oxide and oxygen. Due to technical considerations, volatile gases are generally not used in ICU setting and are limited to the OR. The clinical measure of potency of an inhalational anesthetic agent is called minimal alveolar concentration (MAC) (Eger et al., 1965). MAC is the alveolar concentration (which equals end-expired concentration at equilibrium) at which 50% of subjects move in response to stimulation (either surgical incision or standard stimulus). MAC is decreased by increasing age (Eger et al., 1971) and by other CNS depressants such as nitrous oxide, hypnotics, and narcotics. The anesthetic concentration necessary to prevent movement is greater than that necessary to cause sedation (loss of consciousness) or amnesia (lack of memory), and muscle relaxants are frequently used to prevent nonpurposeful movement. Importantly, the inspired anesthetic gas level (indicated on the anesthesia machine) equals the alveolar concentration (which approximates brain concentration) only after a prolonged period (>30 minutes) of administration.

In general, volatile anesthetics when given in subanesthetic concentrations produce fast wave EEG activity that changes to slow components with the onset of unconsciousness (Table 56.7). Cortical evoked responses are affected by all halogenated agents and are characterized by amplitude depression (around 50% with 0.5 mol) and latency increase in a dose–effect relationship that plateaus early. Below MAC levels of 0.5 to 1.0, SEP recordings may be reliably obtained. Among volatile anesthetics, the relative order of potency is isoflurane, then enflurane, sevoflurane, and desflurane, with the least potent being halothane (Sloan, 1997). With halothane, enflurane, and isoflurane, the SEP amplitude is depressed and latency increased with coadministration of nitrous oxide (60%). Motor-evoked potentials (MEPs) are very sensitive to halogenated agents, with effects occurring at lower concentrations (Haghighi et al., 1990a,b).

Nitrous oxide (NO) has been used in anesthesia for over 100 years. Because of its low tissue solubility (rapid onset and dissipation of effect), it is frequently used to supplement intravenous agents or anesthetic gases. The NO concentration is frequently altered to maintain a stable anesthetic state and stable cardiovascular status. EEG findings change with increasing concentrations of NO. Initially, a loss of alpha frequencies may be seen at concentrations of 30% to 40%, followed by increased beta activity at NO concentrations around 50% (Yamamura et al., 1981). Gradually predominating theta components arise at concentrations of 75% to 80% (Malkin and Eisenberg, 1963). The EEG returns to baseline within 1 hour following discontinuation of NO. Used together with other anesthetic agents, its effect on the EEG varies according to the anesthetics present. It may be additive to the agent used when lower levels of NO are used and antagonistic when a higher level of anesthetic is already present, as in burst-suppression conditions (Sloan, 1998).

Under increasing levels of NO, all cortical evoked potentials undergo amplitude reductions and latency increases, whereas effects on subcortical generators are minimal. NO at 33% reduces the amplitude of both dental (tooth stimulation) and auditory (long latency) evoked potentials without alteration in latency (Fenwick et al., 1979; Harkins et al., 1982). Houston et al. (1988) found a linear decrease in BAEP amplitude with increase in NO concentration (10–40%) and also found an increase in hearing threshold that is of sufficient magnitude to explain BAEP changes due to NO. NO decreases the amplitude of pattern reversal VEP in normal subjects (Fenwick et al., 1984). The N65–N95 wave appears to be the most sensitive, being affected by concentrations as low as 10% NO. In contrast to the sensitivity of pattern reversal VEP to NO, flash-evoked VEPs are not sensitive to the effects of NO (Fenwick et al., 1979). NO depresses both magnetic MEPs (M-MEPs) and electrical MEPs (E-MEPs). In humans, the addition of NO to thiopental-fentanyl anesthesia depresses upper extremity response to 11% of baseline and lower extremity to 7% of baseline in anterior tibial muscles (Zenter et al., 1989). A similar depression is seen in human volunteers breathing 60% NO (Zenter et al., 1989).

Halothane (Fluothane) was the first of the modern anesthetic gases, providing a tremendous improvement in patient safety and comfort. Given the risk of drug-induced hepatitis (Brody and Sweet, 1963) it is infrequently used in modern anesthesia, particularly in adults. Halothane increases CBF, decreases cerebral autoregulation (Miletich et al., 1976), and may increase ICP (Fitch and McDowall, 1971). Halothane causes a progressive slowing of EEG frequencies with increasing concentrations (Gain and Paletz, 1957) and does not appear to enhance epileptiform activity (Mecarelli et al., 1981). EEG changes consisting of generalized slowing and a tendency toward posterior delta activity have been described (Burchiel et al., 1978). A significant reduction in frequency and amplitude of the posterior dominant rhythm may persist for 6 to 8 days following uncomplicated halothane anesthesia (Burchiel et al., 1978). MAC levels of 1.0 and a frequency of 11 to 16 Hz can be expected to slow to 1 Hz at MAC levels of 4.0.

Table 56.7. MAC Values of Volatile Anesthetics Necessary to Produce EEG Changes

Anesthetic Drug	MAC for Onset of	
	Epileptiform Potentials	Burst-Suppression
Diethylether	4.5	3.5
Halothane	None	3.5
Enflurane	1.0*	No suppression
Isoflurane	None	2.0
Sevoflurane	2.0	2.14
Desflurane	None	1.24

Typical MAC values of volatile anesthetics necessary to produce EEG changes under monotherapy conditions. Note that combination with nitrous oxide lowers MACs necessary to produce burst suppression. All data taken from human studies except * obtained in dogs under hypocarbia (Scheller et al., 1990).

Halothane decreases SEP amplitude in animals in a dose-dependent manner (Baines et al., 1985), and prolongs the latency of the cortical conduction time in humans (Vandesteen et al., 1991). The effect of halothane in clinically useful concentrations on BAEP is a matter of controversy ranging from no effect (Duncan et al., 1979; Sanders et al., 1979) to drug-induced increases in latency (Thornton et al., 1983). In the latter study, the increase in wave V latency at 1% end-expiratory concentration was slightly less than 1 msec. A dose-dependent effect on the VEP is characterized by an increase in latency and a decrease in amplitude (Uhl et al., 1980).

Enflurane (Ethrane) replaced halothane as the mainstay of anesthesia because of a lower incidence of liver dysfunction. Enflurane causes a dose-dependent loss of fast-wave activity (Persson et al., 1978) with periods of suppression occurring with high concentrations. Enflurane may cause generalized seizures with characteristic tonic-clonic activity and high-voltage EEG activity in humans (Niejadlik and Galindo, 1975), even at concentrations below those necessary for anesthesia. Enflurane appears to facilitate seizure activity in patients with a seizures history and possibly also in patients with a history of hyperventilation (Lebowitz et al., 1972; Oshima et al., 1981). Hypocarbia may lower the seizure threshold during enflurane anesthesia (Joas et al., 1971). The complexity of the effects of enflurane on brain electrical activity is demonstrated by a report of inhibition of seizure activity during enflurane anesthesia (Gallager et al., 1978). In this case report the addition of enflurane (40% MAC) to NO anesthesia caused rapid (<5-minute) disappearance of previously persistent seizure activity. Following discontinuation of enflurane, the seizure activity returned. Enflurane-related EEG changes [increased amplitude and groups of high-frequency, high-voltage spikes in ventroposterolateral (VPL) nucleus, nucleus centrum medianum] persist for several days in animals instrumented with chronic electrodes (Kavan et al., 1974) and may also explain postoperative seizure activity after enflurane anesthesia (Kruczer et al., 1980).

Enflurane also causes a decrease in SEP amplitude and a slight increase in latency in patients anesthetized with fentanyl and thiopental (McPherson et al., 1985). The effects of enflurane on the VEP are similar (Chi and Field, 1990). Slight increases in BAEP latency occur in a dose-dependent manner (Dubois et al., 1982; Thornton et al., 1984).

Isoflurane (Forane) is unique among the currently used anesthetic gases due to its apparent neuroprotective effects (Newberg and Michenfelder, 1983), and it is widely used to produce hypotension during intracranial aneurysm surgery. Isoflurane causes a dose-dependent increase in CBF (Cucchiara et al., 1974). Autoregulation may be preserved during isoflurane administration (Todd and Drummond, 1984). At subanesthetic concentrations (<1.2%), EEG frequency is increased and voltage slightly decreased. Isoflurane initially produces a low-amplitude EEG with a frequency of 15 to 35 Hz. With loss of consciousness, 12- to 14-Hz activity is superimposed on 2- to 5-Hz high-amplitude waves (Clark et al., 1973; Stockard et al., 1973). Anesthetic doses of isoflurane produce increasing periods of burst suppression with complete electrocortical silence appearing at an end-inspired

concentration of 2.5% (Eger et al., 1971). Isoflurane is not generally thought to cause seizure activity and has even been used to successfully treat status epilepticus (Kofke et al., 1985). However, seizure activity has been reported in a healthy patient during induction of anesthesia with isoflurane and NO (Poulton and Ellington, 1984). Increases in amplitude and periodically recurring slowing have been observed in animals up to 24 hours following isoflurane administration (Kavan et al., 1974). Although isoflurane decreases EEG frequency and increases amplitude, it does not interfere with the diagnosis of intraoperative ischemia by EEG (Campkin et al., 1985).

Isoflurane causes a decrease in SEP amplitude and an increase in latency in patients anesthetized with fentanyl and thiopental (McPherson et al., 1985). Isoflurane decreases SEP amplitude in a dose-dependent manner from 1.2 MV at 0.5 MAC (isoflurane plus NO) to 0.3 MV at 1.5% MAC (isoflurane plus NO). The effect of isoflurane on SEP may occur within a few minutes (Boston et al., 1990) and is reversible (Wolfe and Drummond, 1988). Isoflurane 1.2% end-tidal completely abolishes the VEP (Chi and Field, 1986). Isoflurane (0.5–1.5% MAC) increases latency and decreases amplitude of the E-MEP with changes occurring within 2 minutes of anesthesia induction (Haghighi et al., 1990a,b). Haghighi et al. (1990a,b) compared volatile anesthetics to basal fentanyl droperidol anesthesia on the E-MEP in rats and found dose-dependent amplitude suppression with halothane, which was more depressant than either isoflurane or enflurane.

Desflurane produces EEG alterations comparable to those seen with isoflurane or enflurane. A burst-suppression pattern can be registered around 1.24 MAC (Rampil et al., 1991) and epileptogenic effects seem to be absent (Patel and Goa, 1995). The depression of amplitude and prolongation of latency are of intermediate potency compared to other volatile anesthetics.

Sevoflurane appears to have some epileptogenic properties (Iijima et al., 2000), which may be misleading during electrocorticography (Hisada et al., 2001). Sevoflurane's epileptogenic effects are substantially reduced by coadministration of midazolam and thiopental (Nieminen et al., 2002). It produces EEG changes similar to those seen with isoflurane with a similar MAC for burst suppression (2.14 for sevoflurane, 2.17 for isoflurane). The depression of amplitude and prolongation of latency are of intermediate potency compared to other volatile anesthesia. Faster pharmacokinetics may cause EP changes to occur more rapidly in sevoflurane and desflurane.

Barbiturates are frequently used in the OR as well as in the ICU. Short-acting barbiturates are commonly used to induce anesthesia in patients at risk of neurological injury. Thiopental is the most frequently used agent for this application. In healthy individuals, 4 to 6 mg/kg thiopental produces unconsciousness lasting for 5 to 10 minutes while other agents are subsequently introduced. Thiopental directly decreases ICP (Greenbaum et al., 1975; Shapiro et al., 1973), CBF, and metabolism (Pierce et al., 1962), and may be useful in treating elevated ICP in response to surgical stimulation (Bedford et al., 1980). Furthermore, continuous pentobarbital infusions are frequently used to treat ICP elevations in the ICU and in the setting of refractory status epilepticus (for details see above).

Barbiturates cause a biphasic effect on EEG with an initial increase in fast activity with some spindles (13–30 Hz), with slowing, burst suppression, and electrocortical silence occurring with higher doses (Claassen et al., 2002c; Kiersey et al., 1950). High-amplitude delta components indicate a depth of anesthesia sufficient to tolerate surgical incision.

Early cortical SEP latencies remain nearly unaffected, even at barbiturate levels sufficient to produce an isoelectric EEG. Thiopental causes a transient dose-dependent increase in SEP latency with only moderate decreases in amplitude and only very minimal increases in BAEP latency (Drummond et al., 1985). The BAEP remains nearly unchanged at barbiturate concentrations sufficient to induce coma. Under conditions of burst suppression induced by barbiturates, component V latency can be prolonged by 0.3 msec (Drummond et al., 1987). Increasing levels of barbiturates may also increase BAEP interpeak latency (Church and Gritzke, 1987). Low doses of barbiturates appear to augment the VEP (Brazier, 1970). Transcranial M-MEPs were nearly abolished by barbiturate administration in dogs (Glassman et al., 1993).

Etomidate (Amidate) is a nonbarbiturate intravenous agent that rapidly produces unconsciousness in doses of 0.4 mg/kg. It causes less cardiovascular depression than barbiturates for induction of anesthesia and is useful when given by infusion to decrease intracranial pressure without depression of mean arterial pressure (Dearden and McDowall, 1985). However, given the possibility of adrenocortical dysfunction after prolonged infusion (Wagner et al., 1984), etomidate is now mostly used for induction of anesthesia particularly for rapid-sequence intubation.

Although myoclonus immediately following injection of etomidate is common (Ghoneim and Yamada, 1977), this is not associated with cortical seizure activity. Anesthetic induction doses of etomidate decrease CBF and cerebral metabolism (Renou et al., 1978). Etomidate increases amplitudes of theta more than alpha waves and causes a slowing of the posterior dominant rhythm with increasing doses (Doenicke et al., 1982). At increasing etomidate doses, high-amplitude theta activity may occur, followed by burst suppression (Wauquier, 1983).

Cortical, but not subcortical, EP components undergo amplitude increases with etomidate, and this appears to be a cortical effect (McPherson et al., 1986). This effect has been used clinically to augment abnormally small waves, thus allowing monitoring that would otherwise not been possible (Sloan et al., 1988). Augmentation of SEP amplitude waveform by etomidate can be on the order of 200% to 600% (Koht et al., 1988; McPherson et al., 1986). Etomidate at 0.3 mg/kg only does not change the amplitude of P100 or N70 of VEP but does slightly increase the latencies of P60, N70, P100 waves (Chi et al., 1990). During fentanyl-nitrous oxide anesthesia, a similar dose of etomidate decreases the amplitude of the P100 and increases the latencies of the P60 and N70 components. Amplitude change in E-MEP is rather small when compared to the ketamine effect (Yang et al., 1994). BAEP latencies remain unchanged or become minimally prolonged (Thornton et al., 1985).

Propofol (2.6-diisopropylphenol) is widely used in the OR and ICUs given its favorable pharmacokinetics. It is a very fast-acting agent with a half-life of 5 to 20 minutes (Sebel and Lowdon, 1989). At anesthetic doses it decreases CBF by 30% to 40% with a parallel decrease in cerebral oxygen consumption (Van-Hemelryck et al., 1990). In brain-injured patients, propofol (2 mg/kg, IV bolus plus infusion of 0.15 mg/kg/mm) decreases oxygen consumption, perfusion pressure (25%), CBF (35%), and ICP (Pinaud et al., 1990). At low doses (2 mg/kg), propofol induces an initial increase in beta activity, which is not to be confused with an excitatory effect. The evolution of EEG changes after the onset of sleep shows increases of theta and delta waves. Early reports suggested generalized convulsions with propofol (Hodkinson et al., 1987); however, the anticonvulsant actions of propofol (Dwyer et al., 1988) have recently been recognized, and this medication has been successfully used as a continuous infusion for the treatment of refractory status epilepticus (Brown and Levin, 1998; Claassen et al., 2002; Hirsch and Claassen, 2002).

Propofol produces transient decreases in amplitude and increases in latency of cortical EPs, leaving subcortical potentials nearly unchanged. The amplitudes of early SEP components (N14 and N20) are not affected, whereas amplitudes of late SEP components (more than N20) are depressed and latencies of the N20 component and central conduction time (N14–N20 latency) are prolonged (propofol dose 2.5 mg/kg) by 8% and 20%, respectively (Scheepstra et al., 1989). Propofol (bolus 2 mg/kg plus a continuous infusion) increases latencies of BAEP I, III, and V waves without changes in amplitudes, but completely suppresses middle-latency auditory waves (Chassard et al., 1989). BAEP latencies remain unaffected or very slightly prolonged by propofol (Purdie and Cullen, 1993; Savoia et al., 1988). E-MEPs and M-MEPs are both reduced in amplitude by propofol (Kalkman et al., 1992).

Ketamine typically produces a dissociative type of anesthesia (analgesia and sedation without amnesia) and has a potential to increase ICP. Furthermore, *N*-methyl-D-aspartate (NMDA)-mediated neuroprotection (via receptor antagonism) has been reported (Fitzal, 1997). Ketamine produces a characteristic EEG consisting of a high-amplitude theta activity superimposed with low-amplitude beta (20–40 Hz) components. Higher doses (above 4–5 mg/kg) are known to lower the epileptic threshold, and in patients who demonstrate ketamine-induced epileptiform changes, some may develop generalized convulsions.

Regarding evoked responses and ketamine use, the subcortical generators are nearly unchanged while cortical responses become augmented. Ketamine (2 mg/kg) increases SEP amplitudes with a maximum increase occurring within 2 to 10 minutes of initiation of an infusion (Schubert et al., 1987, 1990). Increasing doses of ketamine increase BAEP interpeak latencies (Church and Gritzke, 1987). In the monkey, incremental doses of ketamine do not decrease amplitude of M-MEP (compared to basal ketamine anesthesia at doses of <20 mg/kg). At higher doses, amplitude depression ranged from 14% to 45% with adductor pollicis brevis (APB) and 57% to 82% with adductor hallucis (AH), latency increased 12% to 18%, and stimulus threshold was increased (Ghaly et al., 1990a,b).

Droperidol, a neuroleptic drug, often combined with fentanyl, lowers the seizure threshold, but does not produce EEG excitation. At low doses, it enhances alpha activity, and at higher doses it produces high-amplitude beta and delta activities. This type of anesthesia has little effect on cortical and subcortical evoked potentials (Sloan, 1998).

Opiates are commonly used in low doses for their analgesic properties, and in larger doses during anesthesia. High doses of fentanyl produce anesthesia (Sebel et al., 1981), and it is particularly well suited for patients with cardiovascular compromise. Opioids cause a dose-dependent slowing of the EEG without initial excitation (Sebel et al., 1981). Other synthetic narcotics cause similar alterations in the EEG leading to a dominant delta activity, but without suppression intervals. This holds true in higher doses such as 20 to 30 µg/kg sufentanil, 50 µg/kg alfentanil, which compare to 0.7 µg/kg fentanyl or 3 to 10 mg/kg morphine (Smith et al., 1984). In animal models, fentanyl, alfentanil, and sufentanil can enhance spike occurrence (de Castro et al., 1979), but the opioid concentrations sufficient to elicit convulsions in this study are not used in clinical anesthesia. Epileptogenic effects, however, are visible in epilepsy patients undergoing electrocorticography on alfentanil or sufentanil (Manninen et al., 1999; Ross et al., 2001). Remifentanil, the shortest-acting opioid currently available, was reported to improve focus localization by spike activation when used in anesthesia for epilepsy surgery under electrocorticographic conditions (Wass et al., 2001). However, others have not reproduced this pharmacological activation (Herrick et al., 2002). In everyday clinical practice, synthetic narcotics rarely induce clinical or electroencephalographic seizures in patients without epilepsy (Bruder and Bonnet, 2000).

Opioids only slightly alter cortical evoked responses and leave subcortical waveforms mostly unchanged. Fentanyl causes a slight increase in SEP latency without a change in amplitude (Pathak et al., 1984). Low doses of fentanyl do not change amplitude or latency of the VEP (Loughnan et al., 1987). Even large amounts of fentanyl do not appear to alter the BAEP (Loughnan et al., 1987; Samra et al., 1984).

Benzodiazepines are commonly used in the ICU and OR setting as short- and long-term sedatives and for their anticonvulsant properties. In nonpremedicated subjects, diazepam (5 mg p.o.) reduces activity in the 4- to 7.5-Hz wave band and increases activity in the 13.5- to 26-Hz wave band (Bond et al., 1983; Fink et al., 1976). This beta activation is similar to that seen with barbiturate use and is lost in the presence of NO, opioids, or volatile anesthetics. This beta activation should not be confused with an arousal reaction. Under high-dose benzodiazepines, the EEG will often directly change to a complete suppression background and will only rarely demonstrate the burst-suppression pattern typically seen with barbiturate use. Benzodiazepines are very powerful anticonvulsant medications, with lorazepam being the most widely recommended first-line anticonvulsant medication (Claassen et al., 2003; Treiman et al., 1998). Continuous infusion of midazolam has been successfully used in refractory status epilepticus (Claassen et al., 2002).

Benzodiazepines, like opioids, mainly produce a mild decrease in the amplitude of early cortical evoked components and exert almost no effect on peripheral and subcortical generators. Diazepam depresses scalp recorded SEP waves, whereas the effect of midazolam (a shorter-acting drug of the same category) is controversial. Ebe et al. (1969) reported that diazepam reduces the amplitude of SEP components occurring within 150 msec of stimulation, whereas Koht et al. (1988) found no effect of midazolam on SEP amplitudes and a slight increase in latencies, and Sloan et al. (1990) reported mild decreases in SEP amplitudes after administration of midazolam.

Benzodiazepines do not significantly change BAEP latencies, and even in sedative doses, VEPs remain largely unchanged (Loughnan et al., 1987). Diazepam depresses the flash VEP amplitude in cats in a dose-dependent manner (Sherwin, 1971), at doses as small as 0.5 mg/kg. Differential sensitivity is noted with the later waves (>100 msec) being more depressed than the earlier waves. In patients with photosensitive epilepsy and normal subjects, diazepam (10 mg i.v.) decreases the amplitude of the flash VEP without an alteration of latency, with a return to baseline within 4 hours (Ebe et al., 1969).

Muscle relaxants seem to have no pro- or anticonvulsant properties or other effect on the EEG. However, their application may significantly improve the signal-to-noise ratio by suppression of myogenic activity, thereby somewhat enhancing the EEG and improving its analysis. Sensory evoked responses are not changed, but motor responses are abolished. Partial neuromuscular blockade, however, may improve monitoring with MEP by reduction of movement artifacts.

Hypothermia

Hypothermia-induced alterations in brain electrical activity occur due to brain metabolism decreases of approximately 55% per 10°C change (Michenfelder and Theye, 1968). Extremely low temperatures may cause brain injury and will at some point cause electrocerebral silence of the EEG (Stecker et al., 2001a). As long as the body temperature remains above 30°C, hypothermia does not significantly impact electrophysiological findings. However, with the widespread use of induced hypothermia in the intraoperative setting (Svensson et al., 1993), these effects might become clinically relevant (Stecker et al., 2001a,b). More recently, externally (e.g., cooling blankets) or internally (e.g., intravascular cooling catheter) induced hypothermia has been used in NICU patients with cerebral ischemia (Krieger et al., 2001), TBI (Clifton et al., 2001), and SAH (Badjatia et al., in press), and in mixed NICU populations (Mayer et al., 2001; Schmutzhard et al., 2002).

SEPs and EEG activity go through sequential stages during temperature shifts and have been studied during intraoperatively induced hypothermia (Stecker et al., 2001a,b). At temperatures below 29.6°C periodic complexes appear in the EEG, which become burst-suppression at around 24.4°C, and turn into electrocerebral silence at temperatures below 17.8°C (Stecker et al., 2001a). Importantly, compared to EEG signals, evoked potentials are lost at higher temperatures. During rewarming, the evoked potentials recover first, followed by EEG burst suppression, followed by a return to a continuous EEG signal (Russ et al., 1984; Stecker et al., 2001b).

The N20-P22 complex of the SEP disappears at temperatures below 21.4°C, and the N13 at 17.3°C (Stecker et al., 2001a). Hypothermia (29°C) increases the latency of long-latency SEP waves (100 msec) and is associated with a decrease in amplitude (Stejskal et al., 1980). Hypothermia increases SEP latency (Stejskal et al., 1980; Van-Rhineck-Leyssius et al., 1986) with latency changes correlating with nasopharyngeal temperature. The impact of hypothermia on amplitude is less clear with reports of no change (Van-Rhineck-Leyssius et al., 1986) or decreased amplitude with hypothermia (Stejskal et al., 1980). Hyperthermia (42°C) suppresses SEP amplitude to 15% of levels observed during normothermia (37°C) (Dubois et al., 1981).

An exponential increase in BAEP latency occurs as temperature is decreased to 19°C in both primates (Doyle and Fria, 1985) and rodents (Schorn et al., 1977). The increase in latency appears greater in the later waves. The effect of severe hypothermia (19°C) on BAEP has been studied in humans (Markand et al., 1984). As the temperature is decreased from 37° to 19°C, wave latency increases until all waves are unrecordable (at 19°C). Whereas BAEP components are easily identifiable at therapeutic levels of hypothermia (29°C), they are delayed by about 33% (Markand et al., 1984). BAEP latency is inversely related to temperature over the range of 36° to 42°C with a decrease in amplitude as temperature increases (Gold et al., 1985). It has been observed that in TBI patients, hypothermia and the combination of lidocaine and thiopental may produce BAEP changes that are similar to "preterminal" patterns (simultaneous gradual deterioration of peaks I, III, and IV). Hypothermia causes a progressive increase in VEP wave latency and a decrease in amplitude until recognizable waves disappear at about 29°C (Russ et al., 1984).

Among qEEG only the BIS has been used in patients who underwent induced hypothermia. In patients receiving cardiopulmonary bypass surgery, individuals with and without hypothermia were compared. Patients with hypothermia had lower BIS values than those with normothermia, but the authors caution that this may also be due to differences in propofol concentrations in the two groups (Schmidlin et al., 2001). To date no studies have systematically investigated the effects of induced hypothermia on electrophysiological findings in the NICU setting or in the presence of acute brain injury.

Summary

Neurophysiological monitoring in intensive care settings and during surgical or neuroradiological interventions shows promise in assisting in the noninvasive monitoring of brain function. It is, however, a complex and time consuming procedure. It is crucial that neurophysiological tools are interpreted by trained clinicians, preferably electroencephalographers, who should have access to the raw EEG data, and have knowledge of the effects that medications, temperature, and artifacts have on electrophysiological data. The aim of EEG and EP-based monitoring is to detect significant neurophysiological changes suggestive of impeding neurological injury at a time when interventions may prevent permanent neuronal damage. Issues concerning user-friendliness and cost-effectiveness should constantly be kept in mind. Given the speed of technological developments, particularly in the field of computer technology, a successful monitoring team will incorporate multidispciplnary techological advancements into their practice in order to constantly improve patient care.

Acknowledgments

The inspiration of Ernst Niedermeyer, M.D., Robert W. McPherson M.D., and Stephan Zschocke, M.D., and the assistance of the staff of the Department of Neurology of the University Hospital, Hamburg, and the Neurological Institute, New York, New York, are gratefully acknowledged. The authors are indebted to Lawrence J. Hirsch, M.D., and Kurt T. Kreiter, Ph.D., for their critical review of the manuscript.

References

Agarwal, A., Gotman, J., Flanagan, D., et al. 1988. Automated EEG analysis during long-term monitoring in the ICU. Electroencephalogr. Clin. Neurophysiol. 107:44–58.

Assal, F., Papazyan, J.P., Slosman, D.O., et al. 2001. SPECT in periodic lateralized epileptiform discharges (PLEDs): a form of partial status epilepticus? Seizure 10:260–265.

Astrup, J., Siesjo, B.K., and Symon, L. 1981. Thresholds in cerebral ischemia—the ischemic penumbra. Stroke 12:723–725.

Badjatia, N., O'Donnell, J., Baker, J.R., et al. (In press). Achieving normothermia in febrile subarachnoid hemorrhage patients: feasibility and safety of a novel intravascular cooling catheter. Neurocritical Care

Baines, D.B., Whittle, I.R., Chaseling, R.W., et al. 1985. Effects of halothane on spinal somatosensory evoked potentials in sheep. Br. J. Anaesth. 57:896–899.

Bassetti, C., and Scollo-Lavizzari, G. 1987. Der Wert des EEG zur Prognose bei postanoxischen Komata. Z. EEG EMG 18:97–100.

Bedford, R.F., Persing, J.A., Pobereskin, L., et al. 1980. Lidocaine or thiopental for rapid control of intracranial hypertension. Anesth. Analg. 59:435–437.

Bergamasco, B., Bergamini, L., and Doriguzzi, T. 1968. Clinical value of the sleep electroencephalographic patterns in post-traumatic coma. Acta Neurol. Scand. 44:495–511.

Berkhoff, M., Donait, F., and Bassetti, C. 2000. Postanoxic alpha (theta) coma: a reappraisal of its prognostic significance. Clin. Neurophysiol. 111:297–304.

Bond, A., Lader, M., and Shrotriya, R. 1983. Comparative effects of a repeated dose regimen of diazepam and buspirone on subjective ratings, psychological tests and the EEG. Eur. J. Clin. Pharmacol. 24:463–467.

Boston, J.R., Davis, P., and Brandon, B.W. 1990. Rate of change of somatosensory evoked potentials during isoflurane anesthesia in newborn piglets. Anesth. Analg. 70:275–283.

Brazier, M.A. 1970. Effect of anesthesia on visual evoked responses. Int. Anesth. Clin. 8:103–128.

Bricolo, A., Turella, G., Ore, G.D., et al. 1973. A proposal for the EEG evaluation of acute traumatic coma in neurosurgical practice. Electroencephalogr. Clin. Neurophysiol. 34:789(abst).

Bricolo, A., Faccioli, F., Grosslercher, J.C., et al. 1987a. Electrophysiological monitoring in the intensive care unit. Electroencephalogr. Clin. Neurophysiol. 39(suppl):255–263.

Bricolo, A., Turazzi S., Faccioli F., et al. 1987b. Clinical application of compressed spectral array in longterm EEG monitoring of comatose patients. Electroencephalogr. Clin. Neurophysiol. 45:211–225.

Brody, G.L., and Sweet, R.B. 1963. Halothane anesthesia as a possible cause of massive hepatic necrosis. Anesthesiology 24:29–37.

Brown, L.A., and Levin, G.M. 1998. Role of propofol in refractory status epilepticus. Ann. Pharmacotherapy 32:1053–1059.

Bruder, N., and Bonnet, M. 2001. Epileptogenic drugs in anesthesia. Ann. Fr. Anesth. Reanim. 20:171–179.

Burchiel, K.J., Stockard, J.J., Calverley, R.K., et al. 1978. Electroencephalographic abnormalities following halothane anesthesia. Anesth. Analg. 57:244–251.

Campkin, T.V., Honigsberger, L., and Smith, I.S. 1985. Isoflurane; Effect on the electroencephalogram during carotid endarterectomy. Anaesthesia 40:188–191.

Cascino. G.D. 1998. Pharmacological activation. Electroencephalogr. Clin. Neurophysiol. 48(suppl):70–76.

Cascino, G.D. 2002. Clinical indications and diagnostic yield of video-electroencephalographic monitoring in patients with seizures and spells. Mayo Clin. Proc. 77:1111–1120.

Cedzich, C., Schramm, J., and Fahbusch, R. 1987. Are flash-evoked visual potentials useful for intraoperative monitoring of visual pathway function? Neurosurgery 21:709–715.

Cedzich, C., Schramm, J., and Mengedoht, C.F. 1988. Factors that limit the use of flash visual evoked potentials for surgical monitoring. Electroencephalogr. Clin. Neurophysiol. 71:142–145.

Chassard, D., Joubaub, A., and Colson, A. 1989. Auditory evoked potentials during propofol anaesthesia in man. Br. J. Anaesth. 62:522–526.

Chatrian, G.E., White, L.E., and Daly, D. 1963. EEG patterns resembling those of sleep in certain comatose states after injuries to the head. Electroencephalogr. Clin. Neurophysiol. 15:272–280.

Chi, O.Z., and Field, C. 1986. Effect of isoflurane on visual evoked potentials in humans. Anesthesiology 65:328–330.

Chi, O.Z., and Field, C. 1990. Effects of enflurane on visual evoked potentials in humans. Br. J. Anaesth. 64:163–166.

Chi, O.Z., Subramoni, J., and Jasaitis, D. 1990. Visual evoked potential during etomidate administration in humans. Can. J. Anaesth. 37:452–456.

Chiappa, K.H., and Hoch, D.B. 1993. Electrophysiologic monitoring. In *Neurological and Neurosurgical Intensive Care,* 3rd ed., Ed. A.H. Ropper, pp. 147–183. New York: Raven Press.

Chiappa, K.H., and Ropper, A.H. 1984. Long-term electrophysiologic monitoring of patients in the neurology intensive care unit. Semin. Neurol. 4:469–479.

Church, M.W., and Gritzke, R. 1987. Effects of ketamine anesthesia on the rat brain-stem auditory evoked potential as a function of dose and stimulus intensity. Electroencephalogr. Clin. Neurophysiol. 67:570–583.

Claassen, J., and Hansen, H.C. 2001. Early recovery after closed traumatic head injury: somatosensory evoked potentials and clinical findings. Crit. Care Med. 29:494–502.

Claassen, J., Baeumer, T., and Hansen, H.C. 2000. Continuous EEG monitoring in the neurological intensive care unit: new indications and benefit for therapeutic decisions. Nervenarzt 71:813–821.

Claassen, J., Hirsch, L.J., Emerson, R.G., et al. 2001. Continuous EEG monitoring and midazolam infusion for refractory nonconvulsive status epilepticus. Neurology 57:1036–1042.

Claassen, J., Hirsch, L.J., Kreiter, K.T., et al. Quantitative continuous EEG for detecting delayed cerebral ischemia in patients with poor grade subarachnoid hemorrhage. Clin Neurophys 2004; (in press).

Claassen, J., Hirsch, L.J., and Mayer, S.A. 2002a. Critical care management of refractory status epilepticus. In *Yearbook of Intensive Care and Emergency Medicine,* Ed. J.L. Vincent, pp. 754–764. Berlin: Springer.

Claassen, J., Lokin, J., Fitzsimmons, B.F., et al. 2002b. Predictors of functional disability and mortality after status epilepticus. Neurology 58: 139–142.

Claassen, J., Hirsch, L.J., Emerson, R.G., et al. 2002c. Treatment of refractory status epilepticus with pentobarbital, propofol, or midazolam: a systematic review. Epilepsia 43:146–153.

Claassen, J., Hirsch, L.J., Mayer, S.A. 2003. Treatment of status epilepticus: a survey of neurologists. J. Neurol. Sci. 211:37–41.

Claassen, J., Mayer, S.A., Kowalski, R.G., et al. 2004. Detection of electrographic seizures with continuous EEG monitoring in critically ill patients. Neurology 2004;62:1743–1749.

Claassen, J., Hirsch, L.J., Kreiter, K.T., et al. Quantitative continuous EEG for detecting delayed cerebral ischemia in patients with poor grade subarachnoid hemorrhage. Clin. Neurophys. 2004 (in press).

Clark, D.L., Hosick, E.C., Adam, N., et al. 1973. Neural effects of isoflurane (Forane) in man. Anesthesiology 39:261–270.

Clifton, G.L., Miller, E.R., Choi, S.C., et al. 2001. Lack of effect of induction of hypothermia after acute brain injury. N. Engl. J. Med. 344:556–563.

Cohn, H.R., Raines, R.G., Mulder, D.W., et al. 1948. Cerebral vascular lesions: electroencephalographic and neuropathologic correlations. Arch. Neurol. 60:163–181.

Cucchiara, R.F., Theye, R.A., and Michenfelder, J.D. 1974. The effects of isoflurane on canine cerebral metabolism and blood flow. Anesthesiology 40:571–574.

Dearden, N.M., and McDowall, D.G. 1985. Comparison of etomidate and althesin in the reduction of increased intracranial pressure after head injury. Br. J. Anaesth. 57:361–368.

de Castro, J., Van de Water, A., Wouters, L., et al. 1979. Comparative study of cardiovascular, neurological and metabolic side effects of 8 narcotics in dogs. Pethidine, piritramide, morphine, phenoperidine, fentanyl, R 39 209, sufentanil, R 34 995. II. Comparative study on the epileptoid activity of the narcotics used in high and massive doses in curarised and mechanically ventilated dogs. Acta Anaesthesiol. Belg. 30:55–69.

Delberghe, X., Mavroudakis, N., and Zegers-de-Beyl, D. 1990. The effect of stimulus frequency on post- and pre-central short-latency somatosensory evoked potentials (SEPs). Electroencephalogr. Clin. Neurophysiol. 77:86–92.

DeLorenzo, R.J., Waterhouse, E.J., Towne, A.R., et al. 1998. Persistent nonconvulsive status epilepticus after the control of convulsive status epilepticus. Epilepsia 39:833–840.

Dennis, L.J., Claassen, J., Hirsch, L.J., et al. 2002. Nonconvulsive status epilepticus after subarachnoid hemorrhage. Neurosurgery 51:1136–1144.

Dinkel, M., and Romstoeck, J. 1997. Neurophysiological monitoring during anesthesia. Curr. Op. Anesthesiol. 10:467–475.

Doenicke, A., Loffler, B., Kugler, J., et al. 1982. Plasma concentration and EEG after various regimens of etomidate administration. Br. J. Anaesth. 54:393–400.

Doyle, W.J., and Fria, T.J. 1985. The effects of hypothermia on the latencies of the auditory brainstem response (ABR) in the rhesus monkey. Electroencephalogr. Clin. Neurophysiol. 60:258–266.

Drummond, J.C., Todd, M.M., and Hoi Sang, U. 1985. The effect of high dose sodium pentothal in brainstem auditory and median nerve evoked responses in humans. Anesthesiology 63:249–254.

Drummond J.C., Todd, M.M., Schubert, A., et al. 1987. Effect of the acute administration of high dose pentobarbital on human brain stem auditory and median nerve somatosensory evoked responses. Neurosurgery 20: 830–837.

Drummond, J.C., Brann, C.A., Perkins, D.E., et al. 1991. A comparison of median frequency, spectral edge frequency, a frequency band power ratio, total power, and dominance shift in the determination of depth of anesthesia. Acta Anaesthesiol. Scand. 35:693–699.

Dubois, M., Coppola, R., Buchsbaum, M.S., et al. 1981. Somatosensory evoked potential during whole body hyperthermia in humans. Electroencephalogr. Clin. Neurophysiol. 52:157–162.

Dubois, M.Y., Sato, S., Chassy, J., et al. 1982. Effects of enflurane on brainstem auditory evoked response in human. Anesth. Analg. 61:898–902.

Duncan, P.G., Sanders, R.A., and McCullough, D.W. 1979. Preservation of auditory-evoked brainstem responses in anesthetized children. Can. Anaesth. Soc. J. 26:492–495.

Dwyer, R., McCaughey, W., Lavery, J., et al. 1988. Comparison of propofol and methohexitone as anesthetic agents for electroconvulsive therapy. Anaesthesia 43:459–462.

Ebe, M., Meier-Ewert, K.R., and Broughton, R. 1969. Effects of intravenous diazepam (Valium) upon evoked potentials of photosensitive epileptic and normal subjects. Electroencephalogr. Clin. Neurophysiol. 27:429–435.

Eger, E.I. II, Saidman, L.J., and Brandstater, B. 1965. Minimum alveolar concentration: a standard of anesthetic potency. Anesthesiology 26:756–763.

Eger, E.I. II, Stevens, W.C., and Cromwell, T.H. 1971. The electroencephalogram in man anesthetized with Forane®. Anesthesiology 35: 504–508.

Emerson, R.G., and Turner, C.A. 1993. Monitoring during supratentorial surgery. J. Clin. Neurophysiol. 10:404–411.

Evans, B.M., 1976. Patterns of arousal in comatose patients. J. Neurol. Neurosurg. Psychiatry 39:392–402.

Fenwick, P., Bushman, J., Howard, R., et al. 1979. Contingent negative variation and evoked potential amplitude as a function of inspired nitrous oxide concentration. Electroencephalogr. Clin. Neurophysiol. 47:473–482.

Fenwick, P., Stone, S.A., Bushman, J., et al. 1984. Changes in the pattern reversal visual evoked potential as a function of inspired nitrous oxide concentration. Electroencephalogr. Clin. Neurophysiol. 57:178–183.

Fink, M., Irvin, P., Weinfeld, R.E., et al. 1976. Blood levels and electroencephalographic effects of diazepam and bromazepam. Clin. Pharmacol. Ther. 20:184–191.

Fischer, G., Fischer, C., and Remond, J. 1992. Hearing preservation in acoustic neurinoma surgery. J. Neurosurg. 76:910–917.

Fisher, R.S., Raudzens, P., Nunemacher, M. 1995. Efficacy of intraoperative neurophysiological monitoring. J Clin. Neurophysiol. 12:97–109.

Fitch, W., and McDowall, D.G. 1971. Effect of halothane on intracranial pressure gradients in the presence of intracranial space-occupying lesions. Br. J. Anaesth. 43:904–912.

Fitzal, S. 1997. *http://www.ncbi.nlm.nih.gov:80/entrez/query.fcgi?cmd= Retrieve&db=PubMed&list_uids=9163282&dopt=Abstract&itool= iconabstr.* Ketamine and neuroprotection. Clinical outlook. Anaesthesist 46(suppl 1):S65–70.

Flaishon, R., Windsor, A., Sigl, J., et al. 1997. Recovery of consciousness after thiopental or propofol. Bispectral index and isolated forearm technique. Anesthesiology 86:613–619.

Flemming, R.A., and Smith, N.T. 1979. Density modulation—a technique for display of three variable data in patient monitoring. Anesthesiology 50:543–546.

Frenzel, D., Greim, C.A., Sommer, C., et al. 2002. Is the bispectral index appropriate for monitoring the sedation level of mechanically ventilated surgical ICU patients? Intens. Care Med. 28:178–183.

Friedman, W.A., Kaplan, B.I., and Dyal, A.L. 1987. Evoked potential monitoring during aneurysm operation: Observations after fifty cases. Neurosurgery 20:678–687.

Friedman, W.A., Chadwick, G.M., and Verhoeven, F.J.S. 1991. Monitoring of somatosensory evoked potentials during surgery for middle cerebral artery aneurysms. Neurosurgery 29:83–88.

Gain, E.A., and Paletz, S.G. 1957. An attempt to correlate the clinical signs of Fluothane anaesthesia with the electroencephalographic levels. Can. Anaesth. Soc. J. 4:289–294.

Gallager, T.J., Galindo, A., and Richey, E.T. 1978. Inhibition of seizure activity during enflurane anesthesia. Anesth. Analg. 57:130–132.

Garzon, E., Fernandes, R.M., and Sakamoto, A.C. 2001. Serial EEG during human status epilepticus: evidence for PLED as an ictal pattern. Neurology 57:1175–1183.

Geocadin, R.J., Sherman, D.L., Hansen, H.C., et al. 2002. Neurological recovery by EEG after resuscitation from cardiac arrest in rats. Resuscitation 55:193–200.

Ghaly, R.F., Stone, J.L., and Aldret, A. 1990a. Effects of incremental ketamine hydrochloride doses on motor evoked potentials (MEPs) following transcranial magnetic stimulation: a primate study. J. Neurosurg. Anesthesiol. 2:79–85.

Ghaly, R.F., et al. 1990b. The effect of etomidate on transcranial magnetic-induced motor evoked potentials in primates. Anesthesiology 73:3A.

Ghoneim, M.M., and Yamada, T. 1977. Etomidate: a clinical and electroencephalographic comparison with thiopental. Anesth. Analg. 56:479–485.

Gilbert, T.T., Wagner, M.R., Halukurike, V., et al. 2001. Use of bispectral electroencephalogram monitoring to assess neurologic status in unsedated, critically ill patients. Crit. Care Med. 29:1996–2000.

Glassman, S.D., Shields, C.B., Linden, R.D., Zhang, Y.P., Nixon, A.R., Johnson, J.R. 1993. Anesthetic effects on motor evoked potentials in dogs. Spine 18:1083–1089.

Gold, S., Cahani, M., and Sohmer, H. 1985. Effects of body temperature elevation on auditory nerve brain-stem evoked responses and EEGs in rats. Electroencephalogr. Clin. Neurophysiol. 60:146–153.

Gotman, J. 1990. Automatic seizure detection: improvements and evaluation. Electroencephalogr. Clin. Neurophysiol. 76:317–324.

Greenbaum, R., Cooper, R., Hulme, A., et al. 1975. The effects of induction of anaesthesia on intracranial pressure. In *Recent Progress in Anaesthesiology and Resuscitation,* Ed. A. Arias. Amsterdam: Excerpta Medica.

Groden, C., Kremer, C., Regelsberger, J., et al. 2001. Comparison of operative and endovascular treatment of anterior circulation aneurysms in patients in poor grades. Neuroradiology 43:778–783.

Gütling, E., Gonser, A., Imhof, H.G., et al. 1995. EEG reactivity in the prognosis of severe head injury. Neurology 45:915–918.

Haghighi, S.S., Green, K.D., and Oro, J.J. 1990a. Depressive effect of isoflurane anesthesia on motor evoked potentials. Neurosurgery 26:993–997.

Haghighi, S.S., Masden, R., and Green, D.G. 1990b. Suppression of motor evoked potentials by inhalation anesthetics. J. Neurosurg. Anesth. 2:72–78.

Handforth, A., Cheng, J.T., Mandelkern, M.A., et al. 1994. Markedly increased mesiotemporal lobe metabolism in a case with PLEDs: further evidence that PLEDs are a manifestation of partial status epilepticus. Epilepsia 35:876–881.

Harkins, S.W., Benedetti, C., Colpitts, Y.H., et al. 1982. Effects of nitrous oxide inhalation on brain potentials evoked by auditory and noxious dental stimulation. Prog. Neuropsychopharmacol. Biol. Psychiatry. 6:167–174.

Harper, C.M., Harner, S.G., Slavit, D.H., et al. 1992. Effect of BAEP monitoring on hearing preservation during acoustic neuroma resection. Neurology 42:1551–1553.

Haupt, W.F., and Rudolf, J. 1999. European brain death codes: a comparison of national guidelines. J. Neurol. 246:432–437.

Haupt, W.F., Birkmann, C., and Halber, M. 2000. Serial evoked potentials and outcome in cerebrovascular critical care patients. J. Clin. Neurophysiol. 17:326–330.

Herrick, I.A., Craen, R.A., Blume, W.T., et al. 2002. Sedative doses of remifentanil have minimal effect on ECoG spike activity during awake epilepsy surgery. J. Neurosurg. Anesthesiol. 14:55–58.

Hirsch, L.J., and Claassen, J. 2002. The current state of treatment of status epilepticus. Curr. Neurol. Neurosci. Rep. 2:345–356.

Hirsch, L.J., Claassen, J., Mayer, S.A., et al. 2001. Systematic design of a prognostic scale for ICU patients with highly epileptiform EEGs. Epilepsia 42:256(abst).

Hirsch, L.J., Claassen, J., Mayer, S.A., et al. 2004. Stimulus-induced rhythmic, periodic, or ictal discharges (SIRPIDs): a common EEG phenomenon in the critically ill. Epilepsia 45:109–123.

Hisada, K., Morioka, T., Fukui, K., et al. 2001. Effects of sevoflurane and isoflurane on electrocorticographic activities in patients with temporal lobe epilepsy. J. Neurosurg. Anesthesiol. 13:333–337.

Hodkinson, B.P., Frith, R.W., and Mee, W.E. 1987. Propofol and the electroencephalogram. Lancet 2:1518.

Hosford, D.A. 1999. Animal models of nonconvulsive status epilepticus. J. Clin. Neurophysiol. 16:306–313.

Houston, H.G., McClelland, R.J., and Fenwick, P.B.C. 1988. Effects of nitrous oxide on auditory cortical evoked potentials and subjective thresholds. Br. J. Anaesth. 61:606–610.

Husain, A.M., Mebust, K.A., and Radtke, R.A. 1999. Generalized periodic epileptiform discharges: etiologies, relationship to status epilepticus, and prognosis. J. Clin. Neurophysiol. 16:51–58.

Iijima, T., Nakamura, Z., Iwao, Y., et al. 2000. The epileptogenic properties of the volatile anesthetics sevoflurane and isoflurane in patients with epilepsy. Anesth. Analg. 91:989–995.

Joas, T.A., Stevens, W.C., and Eger, E.I., II. 1971. Electroencephalographic seizure activity in dogs during anesthesia. Br. J. Anaesth. 43:739–745.

Jones, P.A., Andrews, P.J., Midgley, S., et al. 1994. Measuring the burden of secondary insults in head-injured patients during intensive care. J. Neurosurg. Anesthesiol. 6:4–14.

Jordan, K.G. 1992. Nonconvulsive seizures (NCS) and nonconvulsive status epilepticus (NCSE) detected by continuous EEG monitoring in the neuro ICU. Neurology 42:180(abst).

Jordan, K.G. 1993. Continuous EEG and evoked potential monitoring in the neuroscience intensive care unit. J. Clin. Neurophysiol. 10:445(abst).

Jordan, K.G. 1999. Continuous EEG monitoring in the neuroscience intensive care unit and emergency department. J. Clin. Neurophysiol. 16:14–39.

Kalkman, C.J., Drummond, J.C., Ribberink, A.A., et al. 1992. Effects of propofol, etomidate, midazolam, and fentanyl on motor evoked responses to transcranial electrical or magnetic stimulation in humans. Anesthesiology 76:502–509.

Kalmarchey, R., Avila, A., and Symon, L. 1986. The use of brainstem auditory evoked potentials during posterior fossa surgery as a monitor of brainstem function. Acta Neurochir. 82:128–136.

Kaplan, P.W., Genoud, D., Ho, T.W., et al. 1999. Etiology, neurologic correlations, and prognosis in alpha coma. Clin. Neurophysiol. 110:205–213.

Kaplan, P.W., Genoud D., Ho, T.W., et al. 2000. Clinical correlates and prognosis of early spindle coma. Clin. Neurophysiol. 111:584–590.

Kavan, E.M., Julien, R.M., and Lucero, J.L. 1974. Persistent electroencephalographic alteration following administration of some volatile anaesthetics. Br. J. Anaesth. 46:714–721.

Kiersey, D.K., Bickford, R.G., and Faulconer, A. 1950. Electroencephalographic patterns produced by thiopental sodium during surgical operations: description and classification. Br. J. Anaesth. 22:141–152.

Kofke, A.W., Snider, M.T., Young, R.K., et al. 1985. Prolonged low flow isoflurane anesthesia for status epilepticus. Anesthesiology 62:653–656.

Koht, A., Schutz, W., and Schmidt, G. 1988. Effects of etomidate, midazolam, and thiopental on median nerve somatosensory evoked potentials and the additive effects of fentanyl and nitrous oxide. Anesth. Analg. 67:435–441.

Kremer, C., Groden, C., Lammers, G., et al. 2002. Outcome after endovascular therapy of ruptured intracranial aneurysms: morbidity and impact of rebleeding. Neuroradiology 44:942–945.

Krieger, D.W., Jauss, M., Schwarz, S., et al. 1995. Serial somatosensory and brainstem auditory evoked responses in monitoring of acute supratentorial mass lesions. Crit. Care Med. 23:1123–1131.

Krieger, D.W., De Georgia, M.A., Abou-Chebl, A., et al. 2001. Cooling for acute ischemic brain damage (cool aid): an open pilot study of induced hypothermia in acute ischemic stroke. Stroke 32:1847–1854.

Kruczer, M., Albin, M.S., Wolf, S., et al. 1980. Postoperative seizure activity following enflurane anesthesia. Anesthesiology 53:175–176.

Krumholz A., Sung, G.Y., Fisher, R.S., et al. 1995. Complex partial status epilepticus accompanied by serious morbidity and mortality. Neurology 45:1499–1504.

Labar, D.R., Fisch, B.J., Pedley, T.A., et al. 1991. Quantitative EEG monitoring for patients with subarachnoid hemorrhage. Electroencephalogr. Clin. Neurophysiol. 78:325–32.

Lam, A.M., Keane, J.F., and Manninen, P.H. 1985. Monitoring of brainstem auditory evoked potentials during basilar artery occlusion in man. Br. J. Anaesth. 57:924–928.

LaMont, R.L., Wasson, S.L., and Green, M.A. 1983. Spinal cord monitoring during spinal surgery using somatosensory spinal evoked potentials. J. Pediatr. Orthop. 3:31–36.

Langfitt, T.W., Tannanbaum, H.M., Kassell, N.F., et al. 1966. Acute intracranial hypertension, cerebral blood flow, and the EEG. Electroencephalogr. Clin. Neurophysiol. 20:139–148.

Lebowitz, M.H., Blitt, C.D., and Dillon, J.B. 1972. Enflurane induced CNS excitation: its relationship to carbon dioxide tension. Anesth. Analg. 51:355–363.

Legatt, A.D., and Ebersole, J.S. 1997. Options for long-term monitoring. In Epilepsy: A Comprehensive Textbook, Eds. J. Engel, T.A. Pedley, pp. 1002–1010. Philadelphia: Lippincott-Raven.

Litt, B., Wityk, R.J., Hertz, S.H., et al. 1998. Nonconvulsive status epilepticus in the critically ill elderly. Epilepsia 39:1194–1202.

Liu, A.Y., Lopez, J.R., Do, H.M., et al. 2003. Neurophysiological monitoring in the endovascular therapy of aneurysms. Am. J. Neuroradiol. 24:1520–1527.

Logroscino, G., Hesdorffer, D.C., Cascino, G., et al.1997. Short-term mortality after a first episode of status epilepticus. Epilepsia 38:1344–1349.

Lopez, J.R., Chang, S.D., and Steinberg, G.K. 1999. The use of electrophysiological monitoring in the intraoperative management of intracranial aneurysms. J. Neurol. Neurosurg. Psychiatry 66:189–196.

Loughnan, B.L., Sebel, P.S., Thomas, D., et al. 1987. Evoked potentials following diazepam or fentanyl. Anesthesia 42:195–198.

Lowenstein, D.H., and Alldredge, B.K. 1993. Status epilepticus at an urban public hospital in the 1980s. Neurology 43:483–488.

Lubicky, J.P., Spadaro, J.A., Yuan, H.A., Fredrickson, B.E., Henderson, N. 1989. Variability of somatosensory cortical evoked potential monitoring during spinal surgery. Spine 14:790–798.

Malkin, M., and Eisenberg, D. 1963. Correlation between clinical and electroencephalographic findings during the first stage of nitrous oxide anesthesia. J. Oral Surg. Anesth. Hosp. Dent. Serv. 21:16–23.

Manninen, P.H., Lam, A.M., and Nantau, W.E. 1990. Monitoring of somatosensory evoked potentials during temporary arterial occlusion in cerebral aneurysm surgery. J. Neurosurg. Anesth. 2:97–104.

Manninen, P.H., Patterson, S., and Lam, A.M. 1994. Evoked potential monitoring during posterior fossa aneurysm surgery: a comparison of two modalities. Can. J. Anaesth. 41:92–97.

Manninen, P.H., Burke, S.J., Wennberg, R., et al. 1999. Intraoperative localization of an epileptogenic focus with alfentanil and fentanyl. Anesth. Analg. 88:1101–1106.

Markand, O.N., Warren, C.H., Moorthy, S.S., et al. 1984. Monitoring of multimodality evoked potentials during open heart surgery under hypothermia. Electroencephalogr. Clin. Neurophysiol. 59:432–440.

Mayer, S., Commichau, C., Scarmeas, N., et al. Clinical trial of an air-circulating cooling blanket for fever control in critically ill neurologic patients. Neurology 2001 Feb 13;56(3):292–298.

Maynard, D.E. 1979. Development of the CFM: The cerebral function analyzing monitor (CFAM). Ann. Anaesthesiol. Fr. 20:253–255.

Maynard D.E., and Jenkinson, J.L. 1984. The cerebral function analysing monitor. Anesthesia 39:678–690.

McPherson, R.W., and Szymanski, J. 1985. Intraoperative monitoring of evoked potentials. Am. J. EEG Technol. 25:175–186.

McPherson, R.W., Niedermeyer, E., Otenasek, R.J., et al. 1983. Correlation of transient neurological deficit and somatosensory evoked potentials after intracranial aneurysm surgery. J. Neurosurg. 59:146–149.

McPherson, R.W., Szymanski, J., and Rogers, M.C. 1984. Somatosensory evoked potential changes in position-related brainstem ischemia. Anesthesiology 61:88–90.

McPherson, R.W., Mahla, M., Johnson, R., et al. 1985. Effects of enflurane, isoflurane and nitrous oxide on somatosensory evoked potentials during fentanyl anesthesia. Anesthesiology 62:626–633.

McPherson, R.W., Sell, B., and Traystman, R.J. 1986. Effects of thiopental, fentanyl, and etomidate on upper extremity somatosensory evoked potentials in humans. Anesthesiology 65:584–589.

Mecarelli, O., De Feo, M.R., Romanini, L., Calvisi, V., D'Andrea, E. 1981. EEG and clinical features in epileptic children during halothane anaesthesia. Electroencephalogr. Clin. Neurophysiol. 52:486–489.

Michenfelder, J.D., and Theye, R.A. 1968. Hypothermia: effect on canine brain and whole-body metabolism. Anesthesiology 29:1107–1112.

Miletich, D.J., Ivankovich, A.D., Albrecht, R.F., et al. 1976. Absence of autoregulation of cerebral blood flow during halothane and enflurane anesthesia. Anesth. Analg. 55:100–109.

Mizoi, K., and Yoshimoto, T. 1993. Permissible temporary occlusion time in aneurysm surgery as evaluated by evoked potential monitoring. Neurosurgery 33:434–440.

Momma, F., Wang, A.D., and Symon, L. 1987. Effects of temporary arterial occlusion on somatosensory evoked responses in aneurysm surgery. Surg. Neurol. 27:343–352.

Munari, C., and Calbucci, F. 1981. Correlations between intracranial pressure and EEG during coma and sleep. Electroencephalogr. Clin. Neurophysiol. 51:170–176.

Nagao, S., Sunami, S., Tsutsui, T., et al. 1983. Serial observations of brainstem function in acute intracranial hypertension by auditory brainstem responses. In Intracranial Pressure, Eds. S. Ishii, H. Nagai, M. Brock, pp. 474–477. Berlin: Springer.

Nagata, K., Tagawa, K., Hiroi, S., et al. 1989. Electroencephalographic correlates of blood flow and oxygen metabolism provided by positron emission tomography in patients with cerebral infarction. Electroencephalogr. Clin. Neurophysiol. 72:16–30.

Newberg, L.A., and Michenfelder, J.D. 1983. Cerebral protection by isoflurane during hypoxemia or ischemia. Anesthesiology 59:29–35.

Newton, D.E., Thornton, C., Konieczko, K.M., et al. 1992. Auditory evoked response and awareness: a study in volunteers at sub-MAC concentrations of isoflurane. Br. J. Anaesth. 69:122–129.

Newton, D.E.F. 1999. Electrophysiological monitoring of general intensive care patients. Intensive Care Med. 25:350–352.

Niedermeyer, E.N., and Ribeiro, M. 2000. Considerations of nonconvulsive status epilepticus. Clin. Electroencephalogr. 31:192–195.

Niedermeyer, E.N., Sherman, D.L., Geocadin R.J., et al. 1999. The burst-suppression EEG. Clin. Electroencephalogr. 30:99–105.

Niejadlik, K., and Galindo, A. 1975. Electroencephalographic seizure activity during enflurane anesthesia. Anesth. Analg. 54:722–725.

Nieminen, K., Westeren-Punnonen, S., Kokki, H., Ypparila, H., Hyvarinen, A., Partanen, J. 2002. Sevoflurane anaesthesia in children after induction of anaesthesia with midazolam and thiopental does not cause epileptiform EEG. Br. J. Anaesth. 89:853–856.

Oshima, E., Shingu, K., and Mori, K. 1981. EEG activity during halothane anaesthesia in man. Br. J. Anaesth. 53:65–72.

Patel, S.S., and Goa, K.L. 1995. Desflurane. A review of its pharmacodynamic and pharmacokinetic properties and its efficacy in general anesthesia. Drugs 50:742–767.

Pathak, K.S., Brown, R.H., Cascorbin, H.F., et al. 1984. Effect of fentanyl and morphine on intraoperative somatosensory evoked potentials. Anesth. Analg. 63:833–837.

Persson, A., Peterson, E., and Wahlin, A. 1978. EEG changes during general anaesthesia with enflurane (Ethrane®) in comparison with ether. Acta Anaesth. Scand. 22:339–348.

Pierce, E.C., Lambertsen, C.J., and Deutsch, S. 1962. Cerebral circulation and metabolism during thiopental anesthesia and hyperventilation in man. J. Clin. Invest. 41:1664–1671.

Pinaud, M., LeLausque, J.N., Chetanneau, A., et al. 1990. Effects of propofol on cerebral hemodynamics and metabolism in patients with brain trauma. Anesthesiology. 73:404–409.

Pohlmann-Eden, B., Hoch, D.B., Cochius, J.I., et al. 1996. Periodic lateralized epileptiform discharges—a critical review. J. Clin. Neurophysiol. 13:519–530.

Pohlmann-Eden, B., Dingethal, K., Bender, H.J., et al. 1997. How reliable is the predictive value of SEP (somatosensory evoked potentials) patterns in severe brain damage with special regard to the bilateral loss of cortical responses? Intensive Care Med. 23:301–308.

Poulton, T.J., and Ellington, R.J. 1984. Seizure associated with induction of anesthesia with isoflurane. Anesthesiology 61:471–476.

Prasad, A., Worrall, B.B., Bertram, E.H., et al. 2001. Propofol and midazolam in the treatment of refractory status epilepticus. Epilepsia 42:380–386.

Prior, P. Electroencephalography in cerebral monitoring: Coma, cerebral ischemia and epilepsy. In: Stalbert, E., Young, R.R. (eds): Clinical Neurophysiology Neurology. Butterworths, 1981:347–383.

Privitera, M., Hoffman, M., Moore, J.L., et al. EEG detection of nontonic-clonic status epilepticus in patients with altered consciousness. Epilepsy Res. 1994;18:155–166.

Procaccio, F., Polo, A., Lanteri, P., et al. 2001. Electrophysiologic monitoring in neurointensive care. Curr. Opin. Crit. Care 7:74–80.

Purdie, J.A., and Cullen, P.M., 1993. Brainstem auditory evoked response during propofol anaesthesia in children. Anaesthesia 48:192–195.

Rae-Grant, A.D., Strapple, C., and Barbor, P.J. 1991. Episodic low-amplitude events: an under-recognized phenomenon in clinical EEG. J. Clin. Neurophysiol. 8:203–211.

Rampil, I.J., Correll, J.W., Rosenbaum, S.H., et al. 1983. Computerized electroencephalogram monitoring and carotid artery shunting. Neurosurgery 13:276–279.

Rampil, I.J., Lockhart, S.H., Eger, E.I. 2nd, et al. 1991. The electroencephalographic effects of desflurane in humans. Anesthesiology 74:434–439.

Renou, A.M., Veruhiet, J., Marcrez, P., et al. 1978. Cerebral blood flow and metabolism during etomidate anesthesia in man. Br. J. Anaesth. 50:1047–1050.

Riemer, G., Hansen, H.C., Theis, O., et al. 1998. Der Wert des EEG für die Hydrozephalusdiagnostik bei Subarachnoidalblutungen. Klinische Neurophysiologie 28:1–9.

Rivierez, M., Landau-Ferey, J., Grob, R., et al. 1991. Value of electroencephalogram in prediction and diagnosis of vasospasm after intracranial aneurysm rupture. Acta Neurochir. 110:17–23.

Ross, J., Kearse, L.A. Jr., Barlow, M.K., et al. 2001. Alfentanil-induced epileptiform activity: a simultaneous surface and depth electroencephalographic study in complex partial epilepsy. Epilepsia 42:220–225.

Russ, W., Kling, D., Loesevitz, A., et al. 1984. Effect of hypothermia on visual evoked potentials (VEP) in humans. Anesthesiology 61:207–210.

Samra, S.K., Lilly, D.J., Rush, N.L., et al. 1984. Fentanyl anesthesia and human brainstem auditory evoked potentials. Anesthesiology 61:261–265.

Sanders, R.A., Duncan, P.G., and McCullough, D.W. 1979. Clinical experience with brainstem audiometry performed under general anesthesia. J. Otolaryngol. 8:24–32.

Savoia, G., Esposito, C., Belfiore, F., et al. 1988. Propofol infusion and auditory evoked potentials. Anaesthesia 43(suppl):46–49.

Scheepstra, G.L., deLange, J.J., and Booij, L.H. 1989. Median nerve evoked potentials during propofol anaesthesia. Br. J. Anaesth. 62:92–94.

Scheller, M.S., Nakakimura, K., Fleischer, J.E., et al. 1990. Cerebral effects of sevoflurane in the dog: comparison with isoflurane and enflurane. Br. J. Anaesth. 65:388–392.

Scheuer, M.L. 2001. Portable remote wireless EEG review using a cellular CDMA network. Epilepsia 42:27–28(abst).

Scheuer, M.L. 2002. Continuous EEG monitoring in the intensive care unit. Epilepsia 43(suppl 3):114–127.

Schmidlin, D., Hager, P., and Schmid, E.R. 2001. Monitoring level of sedation with bispectral EEG analysis: comparison between hypothermic and normothermic cardiopulmonary bypass. Br. J. Anaesth. 86:769–776.

Schmutzhard, E., Engelhardt, K., Beer, R., et al. 2002. Safety and efficacy of a novel intravascular cooling device to control body temperature in neurologic intensive care patients: a prospective pilot study. Crit. Care Med. 30:2481–2488.

Schorn, V., Lennon, V., and Bickford, R. 1977. Temperature effects on the brainstem evoked responses (BAERS) of the rat. Proc. San Diego Biomed. Symp. 16:313–318.

Schubert, A., Drummond, J.C., and Garfin, S.R. 1987. The influence of stimulus presentation rate on the cortical amplitude and latency of intraoperative somatosensory-evoked potential recordings in patients with varying degrees of spinal cord injury. Spine 12:969–973.

Schubert, A., Licina, M.G., and Lineberry, P.J. 1990. The effect of ketamine on human somatosensory evoked potentials and its modification by nitrous oxide. Anesthesiology 72:33–39.

Schwender, D., Daunderer, M., Mulzer, S., et al. 1997a. Midlatency auditory evoked potentials predict movements during anesthesia with isoflurane or propofol. Anesth. Analg. 85:164–173.

Schwender, D., Daunderer, M., Schnatmann, N., et al. 1997b. Midlatency auditory evoked potentials and motor signs of wakefulness during anaesthesia with midazolam. Br. J. Anaesth. 79:53–58.

Sebel P.S., and Lowdon, J.D. 1989. Propofol: a new intravenous anesthetic. Anesthesiology 71:260–277.

Sebel, P.S., Bovill, J.G., Wauduler, A., et al. 1981. Effect of high dose fentanyl on the electroencephalogram. Anesthesiology 55:293–311.

Sebel, P.S., Bowles, S.M., Saini, V., et al. 1995. EEG Bispectrum predicts movement during thiopental/isoflurane anesthesia. J. Clin. Monit. 11:83–91.

Shapiro, B.A. 1999. Bispectral index: Better information for the intensive care unit? Crit. Care Med. 27:1663–1664.

Shapiro, H.M., Galindo, A., Wyte, S.R., et al. 1973. Rapid reduction of intracranial pressure with thiopentone. Br. J. Anaesth. 45:1057–1062.

Sharbrough, F.W., Messick, J.M. Jr., and Sundt, T.M. Jr. 1973. Correlation of continuous electroencephalograms with cerebral blood flow measurements during carotid endarterectomy. Stroke 4:674–683.

Sherwin, I. 1971. Differential action of diazepam on evoked cerebral responses. Electroencephalogr. Clin. Neurophysiol. 30:445–452.

Slavit, D.H., Harner, S.G., Harper, C.M. Jr., et al. 1991. Auditory monitoring during acoustic neuroma removal. Arch Otolaryngol 117:1153–1157.

Sleigh, J.W., Havill, J.H., Frith, R., et al. 1999. Somatosensory evoked potentials in severe traumatic brain injury: a blinded study. J. Neurosurg. 91:577–580.

Sloan, T.B. 1997. Evoked potentials. In *Textbook of Neuroanesthesia with Neurosurgical and Neuroscience Perspectives*, Ed. M.A. Albin, pp. 221–276. New York: McGraw-Hill.

Sloan, T.B. 1998. Anesthetic effects on electrophysiologic recordings. J. Clin. Neurophysiol. 15:217–226.

Sloan, T.B., Ronai, A.K., and Toleikis, J.R. 1988. Improvement of intraoperative somatosensory evoked potentials by etomidate. Anesth. Analg. 67:582–585.

Sloan, T.B., Fugina, M.L., and Toleikis, J.R. 1990. Effects of midazolam on median nerve somatosensory evoked potentials. Br. J. Anaesth. 64:590–593.

Smith, N.T., Dec-Silver, H., Sanford, T.J., et al. 1984. EEGs during high dose fentanyl, sufentanil or morphine-oxygen anesthesia. Anesth. Analg. 63:386–393.

Sohmer, H., Gafni, M., Goitein, K., et al. 1983. Auditory nerve brainstem evoked potentials in cats during manipulation of the cerebral perfusion pressure. Electroencephalogr. Clin. Neurophysiol. 55:198–202.

Stecker, M.M., Kramer, T.H., Raps, E.C., et al. 1998. Treatment of refractory status epilepticus with propofol: clinical and pharmacokinetic findings. Epilepsia 39:18–26.

Stecker, M.M., Cheung, A.T., Pochettino, A., et al. 2001a. Deep hypothermic circulatory arrest: I. Effects of cooling on electroencephalogram and evoked potentials. Ann. Thorac. Surg. 71:14–21.

Stecker, M.M., Cheung, A.T., Pochettino, A., et al. 2001b. Deep hypothermic circulatory arrest: II. Changes in electroencephalogram and evoked potentials during rewarming. Ann. Thorac. Surg. 71:22–28.

Steinberg, G.K., Gelb, A.W., and Lam, A.M. 1986. Correlation between somatosensory evoked potentials and neuronal ischemic changes following middle cerebral artery occlusion. Stroke 17:1193–1197.

Stern, B.J., Krumholz, A., Weiss, H., et al. 1982. Evaluation of brainstem stroke using brainstem auditory evoked responses. Stroke 13:705–711.

Stejskal, L., Travnicek, V., Sourek, K., et al. Somatosensory evoked potentials in deep hypothermia. Appl. Neurophysiol. 1980;43(1–2):1–7.

Stockard, J.J., Bickford, R.G., Smith, T.N., et al. 1973. Structure-activity relationships of ether anesthetics: an electroencephalographic study of diethylether, fluroxene, isoflurane and enflurane. Electroencephal. Clin. Neurophysiol. 34:713(abst).

Suzuki, A., Mori, N., Hadeishi, H., et al. 1988. Computerized monitoring system in neurosurgical intensive care. J. Neurosci. Meth. 26:133–139.

Svensson, L.G., Crawford, E.S., Hess, K.R., et al. 1993. Deep hypothermia with circulatory arrest. Determinants of stroke and early mortality in 656 patients. J. Thorac. Cardiovasc. Surg. 106:19–28.

Symon, L., Hargadine, J., Zawirski, M., et al. 1979. Central conduction time as an index of ischemia in subarachnoid hemorrhage. J. Neurol. Sci. 44:95–103.

Symon, L., Momma, F., Furota, T. 1988. Assessment of reversible cerebral ischemia in man: intraoperative monitoring of the somatosensory evoked potential. Acta Neurochir. (Wien) 42:3–7.

Talwar, D., and Torres, F. 1988. Continuous electrophysiologic monitoring of cerebral function in the pediatric intensive care unit. Pediatr. Neurol. 4:137–147.

Tasker, R.C., Boyd, S.G., Harden, A., et al. 1990. The cerebral function analyzing monitor in paediatric medical intensive care: applications and limitations. Intensive Care Med. 16:60–68.

Theilen, H.T., Ragaler, M., Tschoe, U., et al. 2000. Electroencephalogram silence ratio for early outcome prognosis in severe head trauma. Crit. Care Med. 28:3522–3529.

Thornton, C., Catley, D.M., Jordon, C., et al. 1983. Enflurane anaesthesia causes graded changes in the brainstem and early cortical auditory evoked response in man. Br. J. Anaesth. 55:479–486.

Thornton, C., Heneghan, H., James, F.M., et al. 1984. Effects of halothane or enflurane with controlled ventilation on auditory evoked potentials. Br. J. Anaesth. 56:315–323.

Thornton, C., Heneghan, C.P.H., Navaratnarajah, M., et al. 1985. Effects of etomidate on the auditory evoked response in man. Br. J. Anaesth 57: 554–561.

Todd, M.M., and Drummond, J.C. 1984. A comparison of cerebrovascular and metabolic effects of halothane and isoflurane in the cat. Anesthesiology 60:276–282.

Tolonen, U., and Sulg, I.A. 1981. Comparison of quantitative EEG parameters from four different analysis techniques in evaluation of relationships between EEG and CBF in brain infarction. Electroencephalogr. Clin. Neurophysiol. 51:177–185.

Towne, A.R., Pellock, J.M., Ko, D., et al. 1994. Determinants of mortality in status epilepticus. Epilepsia 35:27–34.

Towne, A.R., Waterhouse, E.J., Boggs, J.G., et al. 2000. Prevalence of nonconvulsive status epilepticus in comatose patients. Neurology 54:340–345.

Treiman, D.M. 1995. Electroclinical features of status epilepticus. J. Clin. Neurophys. 12:343–362.

Treiman, D.M., Walton, N.Y., Kendrick, C. 1990. A progressive sequence of electroencephalographic changes during generalized convulsive status epilepticus. Epilepsy Res. 15:49–60.

Treiman, D.M., Meyers, P.D., Walton, N.Y., et al. 1998. A comparison of four treatments for generalized convulsive status epilepticus. Veterans Affairs Status Epilepticus Cooperative Study Group. N. Engl. J. Med. 339:792–798.

Uhl, R.R., Squires, K.C., Bruce, D.L., et al. 1980. Effect of halothane anesthesia on the human cortical visual evoked response. Anesthesiology 53:273–276.

Vandesteen, A., Nogueira, M.C., Mavroudakis, N., et al. 1991. Synaptic effects of halogenated anesthetics on short-latency SEP. Neurology 41: 913–918.

Van Hemelrijck, J., Fitch, W., Mattheussen, M., et al. 1990. Effect of propofol on cerebral circulation and autoregulation in the baboon. Anesth. Analg. 71:49–54.

Van-Rheineck-Leyssius, A.T., Kalkman, C.J., and Bovil, J.G. 1986. Influence of moderate hypothermia on posterior tibial nerve. Anesth. Analg. 65:475–480.

Vaz, C.A., McPherson, R.W., and Thakor, N.V. 1991. Fourier series modeling of time-varying evoked potentials. III. Study of the human somatosensory evoked response to etomidate. Electroencephalogr. Clin. Neurophysiol. 80:108–118.

Vernon, J.M., Lang, E., Sebel, P.S., et al. 1995. Prediction of movement using bispectral electroencephalographic analysis during propofol/alfentanil or isoflurane/alfentanil anesthesia. Anesth. Analg. 80:780–785.

Vespa, P.M., Nuwer, M.R., Juhasz, C., et al. 1997. Early detection of vasospasm after acute subarachnoid hemorrhage using continuous EEG ICU monitoring. Electroencephalogr. Clin. Neurophysiol. 103:607–615.

Vespa, P.M., Nuwer, M.R., Nenov, V., et al. 1999. Increased incidence and impact of nonconvulsive and convulsive seizures after traumatic brain injury as detected by continuous electroencephalographic monitoring. J. Neurosurg. 91:750–760.

Vespa, P.M., Boscardin, J.W., Hovda, D.A., et al. 2002. Early and persistent impaired percent alpha variability in continuous EEG monitoring as predictive of poor outcome after traumatic brain injury. J. Neurosurg. 97:84–92.

Vespa, P.M., O'Phelan, K., Shah, M., et al. 2003. Acute seizures after intracerebral hemorrhage: a factor in progressive midline shift and outcome. Neurology 60:1441–1446.

Wagner, R.L., White, P.F., Kan, P.B., et al. 1984. Inhibition of adrenal steroidogenesis by the anesthetic etomidate. N. Engl. J. Med. 310:1415–1421.

Waterhouse, E.J., Garnett, L.K., Towne, A.R., et al. 1999. Prospective population-based study of intermittent and continuous convulsive status epilepticus in Richmond, Virginia. Epilepsia 40:752–758.

Wauquier, A. 1983. Profile of etomidate. A hypnotic, anticonvulsant and brain protective compound. Anesthesiology 38:26–33.

Wass, C.T., Grady, R.E., Fessler, A.J., et al. 2001. The effects of remifentanil on epileptiform discharges during intraoperative electrocorticography in patients undergoing epilepsy surgery. Epilepsia 42:1340–1344.

Wiedemayer, H., Fauser, B., Sandalcioglum I.E., et al. 2002. The impact of neurophysiological intraoperative monitoring on surgical decisions: a critical analysis of 423 cases. J. Neurosurg. 96:255–262.

Wiedemayer, H., Fauser, B., Armbruster, W., et al. 2003. Visual evoked potentials for intraoperative neurophysiologic monitoring using total intravenous anesthesia. J. Neurosurg. Anesthesiol. 15:19–24.

Wijdicks, E.F.M. 2002. Brain death worldwide. Neurology 58:20–25.

Winer, J.W., Rosenwasser, R.H., and Jimenez, F. 1991. Electroencephalographic activity and serum and cerebrospinal fluid pentobarbital levels in determining the therapeutic end point during barbiturate coma. Neurosurgery 29:739–741.

Wolfe, D.E., and Drummond, J.C. 1988. Differential effects of isoflurane/nitrous oxide on posterior tibial somatosensory evoked responses of cortical and subcortical origin. Anesth. Analg. 67:852–859.

Yamamura, T., Fukuda, M., Takeya, H., Goto, Y., Furukawa, K. 1981. Fast oscillatory EEG activity induced by analgesic concentrations of nitrous oxide in man. Anesth. Analg. 60:283–288.

Yang, L.H., Lin, S.M., Lee, W.Y., Liu, C.C. 1994. Intraoperative transcranial electrical motor evoked potential monitoring during spinal surgery under intravenous ketamine or etomidate anaesthesia. Acta Neurochir. (Wien) 127:191–198.

Young, G.B., and Campbell, V.C. 1999. EEG monitoring in the intensive care unit: pitfalls and caveats. J. Clin. Neurophysiol. 16:40–45.

Young, G.B., and Jordan, K.G. 1998. Do nonconvulsive seizures damage the brain? Yes. Arch. Neurol. 55:117–119.

Young, G.B., Jordan, K.G., and Doig, G.S. 1996. An assessment of nonconvulsive seizures in the intensive care unit using continuous EEG monitoring: an investigation of variables associated with mortality. Neurology 47:83–89.

Zampella, E., Morawetz, R.B., McDowell, H.A., et al. 1991. The importance of cerebral ischemia during carotid endarterectomy. Neurosurgery 29:727–730.

Zenter, J., Kiss, I., and Ebner, A. 1989. Influence of anesthetics—nitrous oxide in particular—on electromyographic response evoked by transcranial electrical stimulation of the cortex. Neurosurgery 24:253–256.

Zschocke, S. 2002. *Klinische Elektroencephalographie,* 2nd ed. Springer: Berlin.

57. Magnetoencephalography in Clinical Neurophysiological Assessment of Human Cortical Functions

Riitta Hari

Recording of weak magnetic fields outside the head by means of magnetoencephalography (MEG) emerged in the late 1960s, 40 years after the invention of the human electroencephalograph (EEG). The first instrument was an induction coil magnetometer with two million turns of wire. It was used to detect the magnetic alpha rhythm by means of signal averaging, with the electric alpha as the time reference (Cohen, 1968). The MEG method became more practical with the introduction of SQUID (superconducting quantum interference device) magnetometers in the early 1970s; since then it has been possible to record both spontaneous and evoked magnetic signals of the human brain without any electric reference. Rapid development of the technology has taken place during the last few years: sensor arrays with whole-scalp coverage are now commercially available, and signal analysis methods have progressed quickly. At present, tens of laboratories worldwide utilize MEG for exploration of normal and abnormal functions of the human brain, and MEG results continue to influence interpretation of EEG data.

This chapter reviews the basic principles of MEG, and gives examples mainly from our own laboratory. Both spontaneous and evoked activity in normal subjects and in some neurological patients are discussed. Several review articles and conference proceedings are available for consulting MEG findings directly related to basic brain research (Aine et al., 1997; Baumgartner et al., 1995; Del Gratta et al., 2001; Forss et al., 2000; Grandori et al., 1990; Hämäläinen and Hari, 2002; Hämäläinen et al., 1993; Hari and Forss, 1999; Hari and Lounasmaa, 1989; Hari and Salmelin, 1997; Hashimoto et al., 1996b; Lounasmaa et al., 1996; Lu and Kaufman, 2003; Näätänen et al., 1994; Sato, 1990). The main advantages of MEG are its good spatial resolution in locating cortical events and its selectivity to activity of the fissural cortex. The active brain areas can be located with respect to external landmarks on the head, brain structures, or functional brain regions (identified, for example, by means of sources of evoked responses).

One goal of MEG recordings is to obtain information about the neural generators of various electromagnetic signals. The EEG research has traditionally focused on temporal waveforms, and a branch of electrophenomenology has arisen around EEG "graphoelements" that have been correlated with different tasks and stimulation parameters, clinical states, and even personality factors. It is clear that a better understanding of the generators underlying the EEG signals would permit a more precise and physiological interpretation of abnormalities. This is an area where MEG has considerably contributed during the last decade, at both a conceptual and a practical level, and may have much to offer in the future.

Comparison of EEG and MEG

MEG is closely related to EEG. In spite of different sensitivities of EEG and MEG to sources of different orientations and locations, the primary currents causing the signals are the same. Similarities between the MEG and EEG waveforms, therefore, are to be expected. The advantage of MEG over EEG in source identification results mainly from the transparency of the skull and other extracerebral tissues to the magnetic field, in contrast to the substantial distortion and smearing of the electric potentials. Thus the MEG pattern outside the head is less distorted than the EEG distribution on the scalp. The magnetic recording is also reference-free, whereas the electric brain maps depend on the location of the reference electrode. As a result it is often difficult to make a reasonable guess of the source locations by visual inspection of the EEG data. Reference-free EEG presentations can be obtained by calculating the surface Laplacians (Nunez, 1989; Pernier et al., 1988). However, even then one has to proceed to neural sources for proper interpretation, and problems arise for several simultaneous sources. The Laplacians cannot be calculated for the outermost electrodes, which reduces the brain area that can be characterized.

Figure 57.1 shows a current dipole in a spherical volume conductor consisting of four layers of different conductivities that simulate the brain, the cerebrospinal fluid, the skull, and the scalp. The resulting distributions of electric potential and magnetic field are dipolar, i.e., display two extrema of opposite polarities, but are rotated by 90 degrees with respect to each other. The isocontour lines are relatively more tight in the magnetic than in the electric pattern. This is because concentric electric inhomogeneities smear only the electric potential, while the magnetic pattern is not influenced. In an ideal sphere, a single superficial tangential dipole can be found one third more accurately on the basis of magnetic than electric recordings (Cohen and Cuffin, 1983). For interpretation of MEG signals recorded from the real brain, it is sufficient to use a realistically shaped model consisting of the brain only, while accurate EEG calculations require a full multicompartment model with known conductivities and shapes for the brain, skull, cerebrospinal fluid, and scalp.

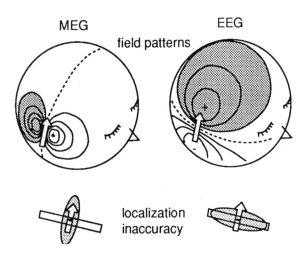

Figure 57.1. Magnetoencephalogram (MEG) and electroencephalogram (EEG) field patterns over a concentric four-layer sphere when a tangential current dipole *(arrow)* is active in an area approximating the second somatosensory cortex in the upper lip of the sylvian fissure. The shadowed areas indicate the magnetic flux out of the head (MEG) and positive potential (EEG). The lower part of the figure illustrates schematically, with shadowed ellipsoids, the inaccuracy region of the dipole location when determined "backward" from the signals on the surface. The dipole is assumed to be in a wall of a cortical fissure.

MEG's selectivity to tangential currents in the presence of several simultaneous sources is an important advantage in practical work, as is illustrated, for example, by the successful differentiation between multiple cortical areas activated by somatosensory stimuli (Forss et al., 1994a, 1996; Hari and Forss, 1999; Hari et al., 1984, 1993b; Mauguière et al., 1997). Moreover, it is often more straightforward to interpret MEG than EEG data.

Since both electric and magnetic signals are generated by the same primary currents that flow in the brain and the nearby tissues, one should pay attention to both MEG and EEG data when drawing conclusions on brain functions from either type of recordings. For example, a dipolar potential distribution could be explained equally well with two radial sources or with one tangential source. However, the existence of a clear magnetic pattern, rotated 90 degrees with respect to the electric one, would imply that the latter explanation should be favored (Hari, 1991). The minimum requirement for sound data interpretation is that the conclusions based on EEG and MEG do not contradict.

Some current sources (very deep and radial) are more reliably picked up by EEG than MEG. However, the contribution of even deep sources to the MEG signals can be probed by inserting sources to interesting brain structures (such as thalamus or hippocampus) and then calculating the best fit of this source, as a function of time, to the measured signals (Tesche, 1996, 1997). In theory, current loops are electrically silent but magnetically visible. In practice, however, ideal current loops have not been observed, and all cerebral currents that give rise to MEG signals are also expected to generate electric potentials on the scalp. For maximum information, the MEG and EEG techniques should be com-

bined, and the simultaneously recorded data should be interpreted with methods that take advantage of the complementarity of the records.

MEG Instrumentation

The magnetic field generated by cerebral currents is two orders of magnitude weaker than that produced by the heart, and only a tiny part of the steady magnetic field of the earth (Table 57.1). To avoid external magnetic artifacts caused by moving vehicles, power lines, radio transmission, etc., it is common to carry out the recordings within a magnetically shielded room, usually made of several layers of aluminum and mu-metal. Biomagnetic measurements can also be performed without magnetic shielding when special compensation techniques are available. In general, however, it is better to prevent than to compensate for artifacts. Adequate magnetically shielded rooms are commercially available.

Figure 57.2A gives a schematic illustration of the old-fashioned arrangement of a MEG recording. The subject lies in a magnetically shielded room and the neuromagnetometer, containing SQUID sensors immersed in liquid helium (at $-269°C$), is positioned close to the head. To replace the evaporating helium, the dewar container has to be refilled regularly, in modern devices about once a week. During recordings with the present-day devices that cover the whole scalp in a helmet-shaped array, such as the 306-channel neuromagnetometer in Fig. 57.3, the subject is typically sitting during the measurement.

The cerebral magnetic field is coupled into the SQUID sensors through superconducting flux transformers. The transformer configuration is important for the device's sensitivity to different source current configurations as well as to artifacts. A magnetometer, containing a single pickup loop in the flux transformer, is most sensitive to signals but also to artifacts (Fig. 57.2C). A more elaborate axial first-order gradiometer contains a compensation coil, wound in the direction opposite to the pickup coil (Fig. 57.2B,C); this configuration decreases the influence of distant disturbances that link the same magnetic flux into both coils. Therefore, the output of the axial first-order gradiometer is essentially determined by the signal of the nearby neuronal source itself. Furthermore, since the distance between the pickup and compensation coils of a first-order axial gradiometer is several centimeters, the measured signal approximates the

Table 57.1. Orders of Magnitude of Magnetic Fields (in femtotesla, fT = 10^{-15} T)

Magnetic resonance imaging	1 000 000 000 000 000 (= 1 T)
Steady magnetic field of the earth	100 000 000 000
Magnetocardiogram	100 000
Cerebral alpha rhythm	1 000
Cerebral evoked response	100
Sensitivity of magnetometers	10
Noise within a shielded room	1

Note that the sensitivity of the present-day magnetometers is below 5 fT/√Hz.

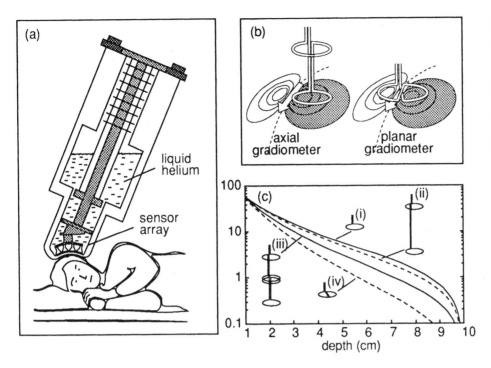

Figure 57.2. A: MEG recording. The subject is lying in a magnetically shielded room with his head supported by a vacuum cast. The dewar containing the superconducting quantum interference device (SQUID) sensors is brought as close to the head as possible, without direct contact, and the magnetic field (or its gradient) is picked up outside the head at several locations simultaneously. **B:** Two flux transformer configurations. The first-order axial gradiometer *(left)* measures essentially B_r and detects the maximum signals at both sides of the dipole. The planar gradiometer *(right)* measures the tangential derivative $\partial B_r/\partial x$ or $\partial B_r/\partial y$; the maximum signal is detected just above the dipole. **C:** Dependence of signal strength (in arbitrary units) on the depth of a current dipole when measured by *(i)* a magnetometer, *(ii)* a first-order axial gradiometer, *(iii)* a second-order axial gradiometer, and *(iv)* a planar figure-of-eight gradiometer.

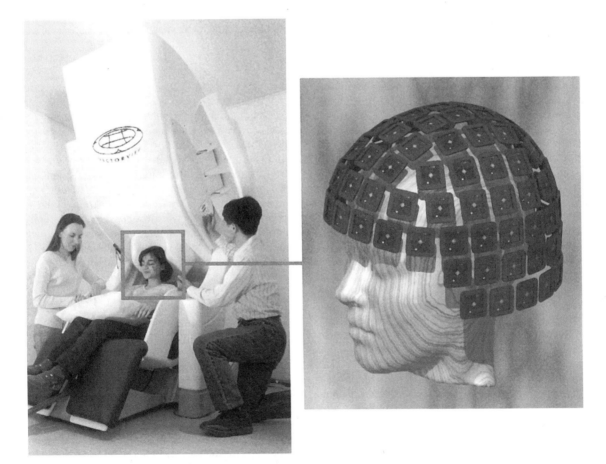

Figure 57.3. A modern 306-SQUID neuromagnetometer used in our laboratory. Each of the 102 three-channel sensor elements comprises two orthogonal planar gradiometers and one magnetometer; the helmet-shaped arrangement of the elements is shown on the right (courtesy of Mika Seppä). The planar flux transformers measure the tangential derivatives $\partial B_r/\partial x$ and $\partial B_r/\partial y$ of the radial field component B_r.

amplitude of the radial field component B_r rather than its axial derivative. Higher-order gradiometers are necessary for measurements performed without a magnetic shield; in these systems the sensitivity is reduced both to the distant artifacts and to the nearby brain currents.

The contour plots in Fig. 57.2B illustrate the pattern of B_r, the magnetic field radial to the surface, generated by a tangential current dipole in a sphere. The signal strengths measured with an axial gradiometer form a spatial pattern similar to the field itself, with extrema of opposite polarities at the two sides of the dipole. In contrast, the planar gradiometer yields the maximum signal when centered just over the dipole at the location of the steepest field gradient. The planar gradiometer is able to detect the location of the source even at the edge of the sensor array and the essential information from the field pattern can thus be obtained from a rather small measurement area. On the other hand, information about the depth of the source is more accurate with axial than planar sensors since the gradient decreases relatively more rapidly as the function of source depth than does the field itself (Fig. 57.2C). However, whole-scalp sensor coverage in part counterbalances this drawback. Although the patterns measured by both axial and planar gradiometers are easily interpreted, in practice it is often useful that the maximum signal detected by the planar gradiometers suggests the approximate source location. Methods have been developed to present data measured with different coil configurations in a standard format (Numminen et al., 1995).

An essential part of the measurement system is the head-position indicator, which gives the exact measurement sites and the orientations of the sensors with respect to the head. We obtain this information by placing three to four small wire loops on known sites on the scalp. The field pattern produced by currents led through the loops is then measured with the multichannel magnetometer. In another commonly used head-position indicator system a transmitter is connected to magnetic sensors, which are fixed on the dewar, and three receivers are placed on the subject's head. The head-position indicator devices allow the position of the magnetometer to be determined with respect to external landmarks on the head with 2- to 3-mm accuracy. The coordinate system can be either local (suitable for studies of certain sensory areas) or, preferably, global (fixed on the basis of the nasion, inion, and the preauricular points) so that it can be easily transported to, for example, the Talairach space that is commonly used in functional magnetic resonance imaging. The important landmarks on the head and the shape of the skull can be determined with a three-dimensional digitizer.

To determine the current distribution within the head, the magnetic field must be sampled at several locations, preferably simultaneously. In the early 1980s only single-channel magnetometers were in use and it sometimes took several days to complete a field map. For example, the MEG recordings of the first epileptic patients lasted for 16 hours! (Barth et al., 1982). Changes in the subject's attentive state and vigilance were thus unavoidable. With the present-day helmet-shaped magnetometers that cover the whole scalp (Fig. 57.3), the whole field pattern can be measured without moving the instrument. This progress of instruments has finally made MEG recordings feasible for comprehensive studies of integrative brain functions in health and disease.

The optimal spacing of the sensors is determined by the spatial frequency of the signal distribution, and, therefore, only marginal benefit can be obtained by reducing the sensor spacing below the distance between the source and the sensor, i.e., about 3 cm (Duret and Karp, 1984; Romani and Leoni, 1985). Thus about 150 sensors would suffice to cover the whole cortex, and the newest instruments with 200 to 300 sensors provide dense-enough spatial sampling for MEG recordings. The diameter of the sensor coil is always a matter of compromise: the larger the coil, the more sensitive it is, but also the more it averages the magnetic field, thereby leading to loss of information.

Taking into account the distance of the coils from the source, pickup coils with diameters around 2 cm are reasonably sensitive and do not lose significant information. With the present technology, the intrinsic noise of the SQUID is no longer a problem, and the main noise arises from the brain itself. Decreasing the distance to the source improves the resolution of the system. Thus it would be important to develop flux transformer arrays that can be put close to the scalp of each subject, independently of the head shape. Such systems may become feasible with the development of high-temperature$_c$ superconductors; MEG signals with an excellent signal-to-noise ratio have already been recorded with a single-channel high-temperature$_c$ neuromagnetometer (Curio et al., 1996).

Source Imaging

Since the aim of MEG studies is to obtain information about brain function, the field pattern should be interpreted in terms of cerebral currents. Yet, due to the nonuniqueness of the inverse problem—namely, that several current distributions can, in principle, produce identical magnetic field patterns outside the head—the interpretation usually requires the use of specific source and volume conductor models. Thus the situation is more complicated than in magnetic resonance imaging (MRI), functional magnetic resonance imaging (fMRI), or positron emission tomography (PET), where the inverse problem can be solved uniquely. However, physiologically meaningful solutions of MEG patterns can be found by utilizing constraints based on the known anatomy and physiology of the brain.

Current Dipole

The most commonly used source model in MEG studies is a current dipole within a sphere. The dipole can be characterized by means of five parameters, three for its three-dimensional location, one for its orientation (only the plane parallel to the surface of the sphere is relevant), and one for its strength. In the spherical model, only primary currents tangential to the surface will produce magnetic fields outside the sphere. In reality, signals may also be detected from the convexial cortex where sources are considerably closer to the detector than the currents within the wall of a fissure. Deviation of the convexial source by only 10 to 20 degrees from the radial orientation is enough to give a signal as large as that produced by a tangential dipole of the same size but 2 cm deeper in the fissural cortex. Therefore, it seems probable that under realistic conditions nearly radial sources may contribute significantly to the MEG signals. This notion is supported by simulations that took into account the real geometry of the cerebral cortex (Hillebrand and Barnes, 2002). A practical example of the possibility to detect tilted currents is the identification of magnetic counterparts of the P22 and P25 somatosensory responses, which are believed to arise in the convexial cortex (Baumgartner, 1993; Sutherling et al., 1988; Tiihonen et al., 1989a).

In dipole modeling, the location of the equivalent current dipole (ECD) is found by a least-squares fit to the data, typically at a time point of a clearly dipolar field pattern. In progressing toward a multidipole model, one may extract the field patterns produced by the already identified sources to facilitate further analysis (Lounasmaa et al., 1985; Tesche et al., 1995; Uusitalo and Ilmoniemi, 1997). The success of dipole models in MEG interpretation derives, in part, from the difficulty of discerning the details of the brain activation pattern from the typical measurement distance of at least 3 cm from the source (Fig. 57.4). Consequently, a single current dipole is a reasonably accurate description of a local active cortical area of less than 2 to 3 cm in diameter.

The adequacy of the model can be evaluated by calculating the goodness-of-fit *(g)* value (Hämäläinen et al., 1993; Kaukoranta et al., 1986b), which approximates the squared correlation coefficient between the measured signals and those predicted by the model. The *g*-value, however, depends on several factors such as the number and distribution of the measurement locations (Hari et al., 1988a). A low *g*-value means that either the brain source significantly deviates from the model or the signal-to-noise ratio is poor. It is also often useful to study the residual field, i.e., the difference between the measured field and that predicted by the model, or to compare the waveforms predicted by the model with the measured waveforms. If the residual field shows systematic features that cannot be explained by noise, a different source configuration must be considered.

The inaccuracy of MEG localization is smallest in the direction transverse to dipole orientation (cf. Fig. 57.1) and largest (about double) in the direction of depth. The locating accuracy depends drastically on the signal-to-noise ratio, which is improved by signal averaging for evoked responses but cannot be affected much—except by filtering—in the case of spontaneous activity. For comparison, note that the best localization accuracy for EEG is in the direction along the dipole (Fig. 57.1). Since the dipoles mainly reflect synchronous activation of the cortical pyramidal cells and thus are perpendicular to the cortical surface, changes in the focus of activation along the cortex are more easily seen with MEG than EEG. On the other hand, EEG may be more accurate in indicating which wall of a fissure has been activated, since here the distinction must be made along the direction of the dipole.

When a single dipole is used to model an extended cortical area consisting of a layer of dipoles, the estimates of dipole depth and, consequently, of dipole strengths may be erroneous (Fig. 57.5). Better source models are thus needed for extended areas. When multiple brain regions are simultaneously active, the relative contribution of each area to the measured signal depends on its site, strength, and synchrony. Multidipole mod-

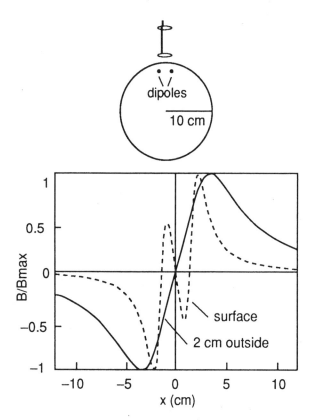

Figure 57.4. The dependence of the radial component of the magnetic field on the distance between the source and the detector. Two current dipoles are situated in a homogeneous sphere (radius 10 cm), 1 cm beneath the surface, 3 cm from each other, and symmetrically with respect to the origin. The field was calculated on an arc perpendicular to the orientation of the dipoles (x-axis). The pattern is complicated on the surface, whereas 2 cm outside the sphere the higher spatial frequencies have faded away and the dipolar term dominates. The amplitudes have been normalized according to the maximum value; the maximum field would be about seven times stronger on the surface than 2 cm above it. (Adapted from Hari, R. 1988. Interpretation of cerebral magnetic fields elicited by somatosensory stimuli. In *Springer Series of Brain Dynamics,* Ed. E. Basar, pp. 305–310. Berlin/Heidelberg: Springer-Verlag.)

els with time-varying source strengths are useful in interpreting the resulting complex field patterns (Scherg, 1990).

Neural Currents Underlying the Current Dipole

To understand the cellular events underlying the ECD, it is reasonable to divide the currents associated with postsynaptic potentials (PSPs) to transmembrane currents at the active synaptic area, intracellular currents within the neuron, and extracellular volume currents. Transmembrane currents are the driving force for both intra- and extracellular current flow. ECD calculated from the measured MEG signals reflects the direction of the net intracellular current flow. A PSP at the end of one dendrite produces an "elementary" dipole moment $Q = I \cdot \lambda \approx 10^{-14}$ nA·m, where I is the intracellular current driven by the synapse and λ is the length constant of the cell membrane (Vvedensky et al., 1985). The strength of the observed dipole moment can be strongly affected, for example, by the simultaneous calcium currents.

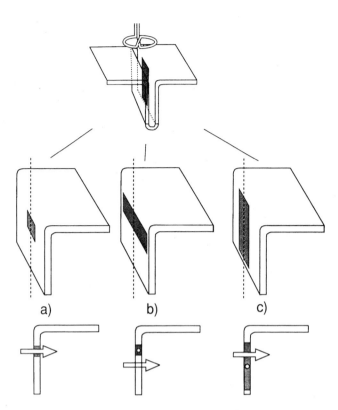

Figure 57.5. Schematic illustration of equivalent current dipole (ECD) locations when the source is (**A**) a layer of less than 2 cm in diameter, (**B**) a layer with angular extension, and (**C**) a layer extended along the radius of the sphere. The activity is assumed to occur in the wall of a cortical fissure. This behavior depends slightly on the coil configuration used. (Adapted from Hari, R. 1991. On brain's magnetic responses to sensory stimuli. J. Clin. Neurophysiol. 8:157–169.)

Since it is not known how many PSPs occur synchronously in each pyramidal cell and how much cancellation takes place within the cortex, it is not possible to derive accurate estimates for the source area of a typical evoked response on the basis of cell/synapse density and the size of the elementary dipole. Okada et al. (1996) note that many animal species across a wide phylogenetic scale (turtle, guinea pig, and swine) show an apparent invariance in the maximum current dipole moment density of 1 to 2 nA·m/mm². Considerably smaller dipole moment densities have been estimated on the basis of available information on intracortical current densities and values of cortical λ (Hari, 1990). However, intracortical current densities depend strictly on the degree of neuronal synchrony, and thus on the specimen studied, and λ may vary according to background activity (e.g., Bernander et al., 1991).

Glial cells may affect the MEG and EEG signals; they change the return paths of volume currents and have activation latencies that fit with the occurrence of long-latency evoked responses. Several important electrical events probably remain beyond the reach of both MEG and EEG measurements. For example, intracortical short-distance interactions—when viewed from the top of the cortex—are radially symmetric; only their net effect along the apical dendrites of the pyramidal cells gives rise to an MEG signal.

Minimum-Norm Estimates

An example of a different approach to the neuromagnetic inverse problem is the minimum-norm estimate (MNE) presentation of the source currents (Hämäläinen and Ilmoniemi, 1994). MNE gives the most probable current distribution, in the sense of the minimum norm, giving rise to the recorded magnetic field. Calculation of MNE does not require specific assumptions about the source configuration (one dipole, multiple dipoles, quadrupoles, etc.), which is an advantage when there is no basis for explicit models. On the other hand, the unconstrained MNE solution favors superficial currents and does not give a reliable estimate of the source depth. Therefore, MNE solutions have been limited with constraints based on the known brain anatomy and physiology (Ribary et al., 1991; Volkmann et al., 1996). Minimum-current estimates (MCEs; Uutela et al., 1999), a subclass of MNE solutions that give more local solutions, have been applied for visualization and analysis of single-subject and group-level MEG data. One example of MCE visualization is given below (see Fig. 57.14).

The distributed MNE-based source activations often look "more physiological" than the point-like current dipoles. However, a word of caution is appropriate here because the appearance of the result depends strongly on the method used; the MNE approach gives a distributed solution and the dipole approach a local solution, whatever the real current distribution is! (see Hämäläinen and Hari, 2002). In general, both dipole and MCE solutions give rather similar results, although the temporal accuracy may be better with dipole modeling and the group data may be easier to visualize with MCE (Stenbacka et al., 2002).

Combination of MEG with MRI/fMRI/PET data

A combination of structural information from MRI with functional information from MEG is routinely used. All source estimates could be improved by constraints based on the known anatomy of the brain, derived from MRI data, and forcing the dipoles/currents to the cortical tissue. In preoperative evaluation, reconstruction of the three-dimensional outer surface of the brain from MRI scans may help the surgeon to recognize the landscape after opening the skull when the brain tissue retracts and the relationship between the brain and the landmarks on the skull changes (Jack et al., 1990). Adding surface vessels to the reconstruction further facilitates the orientation during surgery (Mäkelä et al., 2001; see Fig. 57.27).

Compared with PET and fMRI (Aine, 1995), the advantage of MEG is its good temporal resolution, which allows monitoring of cortical dynamics on a millisecond scale. In combined use of multiple methods, active brain regions have been first determined with PET/fMRI and then used as source locations in the inverse solution of the MEG data to reveal their temporal behavior. However, not all changes in the synchronization of a neuronal population, reflected in the MEG/EEG signals, induce significant changes in the mean neuronal firing rates or the blood flow and metabolism, and vice versa. Therefore, MEG and fMRI results may significantly differ in certain conditions (Furey et al., 2003), and the MEG/EEG and fMRI/PET methods remain complementary in studies of human brain function. Sophisticated approaches to combine fMRI and MEG data are under development.

Volume Conductor Models

The sphere model works well in most areas of the head when the radius of the sphere is fitted to the local radius of curvature of the measurement area (Hari and Ilmoniemi, 1986), likely because the realistic noise largely masks the errors caused by the different conductor models (Tarkiainen et al., 2003). Realistic head models, however, may be beneficial for proper modeling of the temporobasal and frontobasal brain areas (Hämäläinen and Sarvas, 1989). Fortunately, it is sufficient for MEG to model the intracranial space since only a relatively small proportion of the currents flow in the poorly conducting skull. In contrast, proper modeling of the EEG signals necessitates a multicompartment model consisting of three to four concentric layers with *known* resistivities.

Some nonspherical electric inhomogeneities may also affect MEG distributions (Cuffin, 1985). For example, the falx cerebri may change volume current paths and lead to slight mislocalizations of current dipoles in the mesial wall of the hemisphere. There has been discussion about the significance of holes in the skull to the distribution of volume currents. In the intact human skull the main holes are in the base of the skull and in the orbits. The absence of electro-oculographic artifacts in intracranial recordings from the frontal lobe (Cooper et al., 1965) indicates good isolation between the outer and inner sides of the skull. Therefore, the effects of normal holes of the skull seem negligible for interpretation of MEG distributions, as is also supported by calculations showing that radial anisotropy added to a spherically symmetric conductor does not affect the external magnetic field (Ilmoniemi, 1995).

Practical Issues

Successful clinical MEG recordings need sophisticated instrumentation and close interdisciplinary collaboration. The experimental situation introduces some restrictions. Since the head has to be immobile, recordings cannot be performed during major motor seizures, and long-term monitoring is not feasible. Moreover, problems are encountered in studies of uncooperative subjects who either cannot keep still during the recording or are unwilling or unable to perform the tasks. On the other hand, multichannel MEG mappings are quick to perform, and the relative locations of the sensors, required for accurate source analysis, are exactly known without extra effort.

All magnetic materials must be avoided in the clothing of the subject. Intraoral metallic devices for orthodontics also destroy the measurement. Postoperative MEG evaluation may be impossible or limited if magnetized material is used in staples, sutures, etc. Figure 57.6 illustrates some common MEG artifacts. Since significant contamination can be caused by eye blinks and movements (Antervo et al., 1985), the electro-oculogram should be used to reject contaminated signals. Muscular artifacts may cause problems less frequently. Magnetic lung-contamination or magnetic material in clothing can cause respiration-related slow shifts. Cardiac

artifacts can be either magnetocardiographic signals (Jousmäki and Hari, 1996; Samonas et al., 1997), picked up at distance, or ballistocardiographic fluctuations, caused by the movement of magnetized material at the rhythm of the cardiac cycle. For recognition of both artifacts, simultaneously recorded electrocardiogram (ECG) is essential; the magnetocardiogram coincides with the ECG, whereas the main peak of the magnetic ballistocardiogram lags the QRS complex by several hundred milliseconds.

Special attention must also be paid to the proper design of stimulators. High-quality sounds can be produced with electroacoustic transformers placed outside the shielded room and connected through plastic tubes to the subject; the system may need sophisticated equalizing to guarantee flat frequency transfer. Excessive artifacts from electric somatosensory stimuli can be avoided by twisting the stimulator wires tightly together. Multichannel devices with balloon

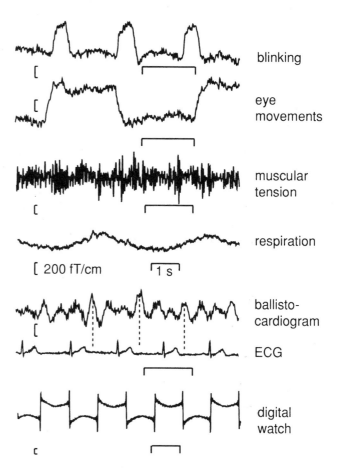

Figure 57.6. Different artifacts in MEG recordings of spontaneous brain activity over the temporal area; the measurements were made with a planar gradiometer. Blinking and vertical eye movements produce signals of about equal size; for horizontal eye movements the signals are similar in waveform but have different spatial distributions. Muscular tension refers to biting the teeth together. Respiration artifacts were due to a metallic piece over the chest of the subject. The magnetic ballistocardiogram was due to movement of magnetized metal on the bed, on which the subject was lying on his left side. Note the timing differences between the maximum signals in the ECG and the ballistocardiogram. The lowest artifact was due to a digital watch 70 cm from the dewar.

Figure 57.7. Dangers of filtering, illustrated with simulated data. A current dipole with a monophasic activation curve (*gray line* on the *left*, "no filter") and with 30 nA·m dipole moment was inserted to a site corresponding to the right auditory cortex. The field patterns above show a dipolar field pattern at peak activation at 100 msec. After high-pass filtering at 6 Hz the waveform changes (*black curve* on the *left*, "HP 6 Hz") and ghost sources appear at 60 msec and 150 msec. (See Color Figure 57.7.)

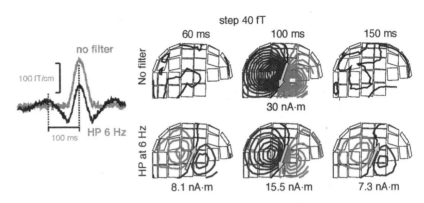

diaphragms, driven by compressed air (Mertens and Lütkenhöner, 2000), provide a nice and artifact-free method for tactile stimulation. Noxious laser heat stimuli for pain studies can be brought to the shielded room via optical cables. Visual stimuli can be transmitted through mirrors, a data projector, or a bundle of optic fibers, or the subject can view a monitor through a hole in the wall. EEG can be measured with nonmagnetic electrodes and wires without causing problems to the MEG recordings.

Figure 57.7 draws attention to dangers of filtering. A too high high-pass filter setting causes well-known distortions in the signal waveforms, but what may be less obvious is that it also transfers the dipolar field patterns, with opposite polarities, to latencies distant from the real signal and thereby leads to erroneous interpretations of brain activation.

Analysis of Spontaneous Activity

Very useful information about spontaneous activity (for a review, see Hari and Salmelin, 1997) can be obtained by calculating *frequency spectra* of the signals (Fig. 57.8) and by mapping the abundance of different frequencies at various sensor sites. The sources can then be identified either in time or in frequency domain (Lütkenhöner, 1992; Salmelin and Hämäläinen, 1995; Tesche and Kajola, 1993). In multichannel recordings, cross-spectra between channels suggest which signals arise from the same source, and time lags may indicate the sequence of activation.

We have extensively applied the temporal spectral evolution (TSE) method to quantify changes in the level of different brain rhythms (Salmelin and Hari, 1994b). The TSE method resembles the event-related desynchronization technique (Pfurtscheller and Aranibar, 1977) used to study task-dependent changes in the human scalp EEG. However, TSE preserves the original units, and the signal levels can thus be directly compared with the sizes of evoked responses. In TSE, the brain signals are first bandpass filtered, then rectified (taking absolute values of the signals), and thereafter averaged with respect to the triggering event. Thus all signals that are time-locked but not exactly phase-locked to the event will be detected. Methods have been also developed for quantification and characterization of rate-dependent stimulation effects on rhythmic activity of various cortical areas (Narici and Peresson, 1995).

Sometimes one may be interested in just seeing the signal waveform and the temporal changes in the field pattern. This type of analysis, which resembles the classical use of EEG recordings, can be helpful in screening candidates for surgical treatment; clear changes of the field pattern from one irritative phenomenon to the next discourage the assumption

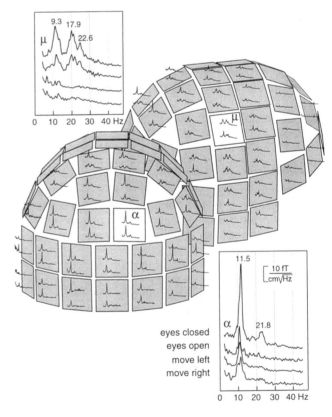

Figure 57.8. Amplitude spectra from a 1-minute period of spontaneous activity when the subject was resting with the eyes closed. Two orthogonal derivatives of the radial magnetic field were measured at each location, along the longitude and latitude. The *inserts* show reactivity of the alpha and mu rhythms to opening of the eyes and to movements of the left and right hand. (Adapted from Salmelin, R., and Hari, R. 1994a. Characterization of spontaneous MEG rhythms in healthy adults. Electroencephalogr. Clin. Neurophysiol. 91:237–248.)

of a local onset of the discharge, although they do not rule out a deeper common trigger.

Due to noise problems and the use of single-channel instruments, the first studies of epileptic MEG activity employed averaging, with the simultaneously recorded EEG signal as a trigger (Barth et al., 1982, 1984). The drawback of such a procedure is that the choice of the trigger channel largely determines the observed activity, and the method works only if well-discernible spikes or sharp waves are present. With multichannel low-noise instruments, averaging is necessary only for the detection of *pre*spikes, which might be accurate indicators of the onset area of the paroxysmal activity (Stefan et al., 1991). With template matching, signals can be automatically classified and the source locations determined separately for each class.

Spontaneous Activity of Awake Normal Subjects

Alpha Rhythm from Parieto-Occipital Areas

The typical parieto-occipital alpha rhythm, with a peak frequency around 10 Hz, is damped by opening the eyes (Fig. 57.8). In the first study of the human magnetic alpha rhythm (Cohen, 1968), a phase reversal was observed between signals measured from the right and left hemispheres, and the currents were suggested to be parallel to the longitudinal fissure.

Later, the sources of the alpha rhythm have been suggested to cluster mainly in the region of the calcarine sulcus (Chapman et al., 1984) and around the parieto-occipital sulcus (POS) (Lu et al., 1992b; Salmelin and Hari, 1994a; Vvedensky et al., 1986; Williamson et al., 1989). Figure 57.9, based on whole scalp MEG recordings, shows sources in both of these locations; typically the POS region is by far the most dominant source of the MEG alpha rhythm.

Vvedensky et al. (1986) suggested that alpha spindles often have the same generators for about 1 second, whereas the sources differ for successive spindles. Later, a multitude of MEG alpha sources was found with the help of signal-space analysis (Ilmoniemi et al., 1987). Different spindles seemed to have different sources, but the source configuration of one spindle was rather stable. Later recordings, analyzed with time-varying fixed-location dipole models, however, suggest that a typical alpha spindle cannot be explained by a single source (Salmelin and Hari, 1994a).

The parieto-occipital alpha rhythm is strongly suppressed during visual stimuli, visual memory tasks, and visual imagery (Kaufman et al., 1990; Michel et al., 1994; Portin et al., 1998; Salenius et al., 1995). When the subject has to differentiate between visually presented images of objects vs. nonobjects, the poststimulus alpha level is consistently higher after nonobjects (Vanni et al., 1997). This modulation may reflect interaction between the dorsal and ventral visual pathways during an attention-demanding task.

Early visual deprivation may lead to abolishment of parieto-occipital spontaneous rhythms; from the five *early blind* subjects in Fig. 57.10, four do not display alpha activity and

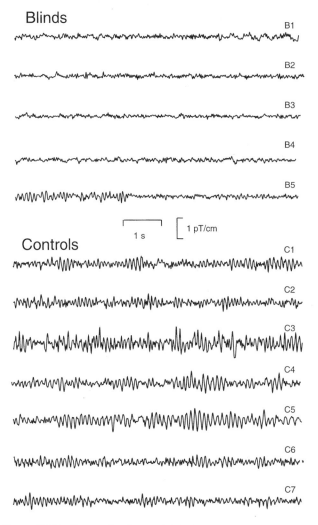

Figure 57.10. Traces of parieto-occipital alpha activity from five early blind subjects and seven control subjects. The blind subjects were 25 to 32 years in age. Subjects B2 and B3 were able to see some light; subject B5 is blind due to retinal cancer and has seen light only during her first year. (M. Huotilainen and T. Kujala participated in data collection.)

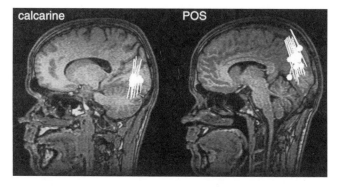

Figure 57.9. Sources of alpha oscillations superimposed on two sagittal magnetic resonance imaging (MRI) slices demonstrating a calcarine *(left)* and a parieto-occipital *(right)* source cluster. Source current orientations are also indicated. (Adapted from Hari, R., Salmelin, R., Mäkelä, J.P., et al. 1997. Magnetoencephalographic cortical rhythms. Int. J. Psychophysiol. 26:51–62.)

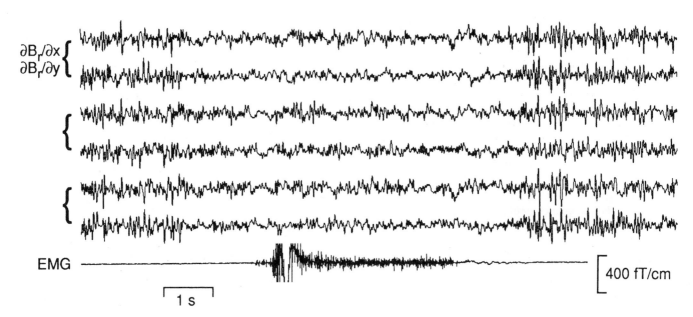

$\partial B_r/\partial x$
$\partial B_r/\partial y$

EMG

1 s

400 fT/cm

Figure 57.11. Spontaneous magnetic activity over the rolandic area, shown on six gradiometer channels, when the subject has his eyes open and clenches his contralateral fist [see the electromyogram (EMG) channel]. (Unpublished data from F. Lado and R. Hari.)

opening/closing the eyes did not have any effect on their brain rhythms. Only one subject (B5) has rhythmic alpha-like activity; she had lost her sight earlier than the other four subjects. The reason for the observed alpha absence in blinds, also known from EEG recordings (Jeavons, 1964), is unknown, but it certainly speaks against a purely idling nature of the normal alpha rhythm; otherwise one might expect strong alpha during the continuous lack of visual input.

Mu Rhythm from Sensorimotor Areas

The electroencephalographic μ-rhythm also has a magnetic counterpart. Figure 57.11 shows that the magnetic μ-rhythm dampens during a movement and that the suppression starts already 1 to 2 seconds before the HEMg. In association with unilateral movements, the suppression is bilateral, although contralaterally dominant (Salenius et al., 1997b).

The μ-rhythm consists of two main frequency components, one around 10 Hz and the other around 20 Hz (see insert in Fig. 57.8); however, these two frequencies are usually not exact harmonics and show independent temporal behaviors (Tiihonen et al., 1989b). Additional evidence for functionally separate frequency components of the μ-rhythm derives from the source locations, which center on average 5 mm more anterior for the 20 Hz than the 10 Hz frequencies (Salmelin and Hari, 1994b), suggesting the existence of separate precentral (20 Hz) and a postcentral (10 Hz) rhythms (Fig. 57.12).

In addition to movements (Nagamine et al., 1996), the magnetic μ-rhythm is modified by electric stimulation of peripheral nerves, with a clear increase, "rebound" of the 20-Hz than the 10-Hz component around 400 msec after the stimulus (Salenius et al., 1997b; Salmelin and Hari, 1994b). The poststimulus rebound is abolished when the subject moves the fingers of the same hand. Interestingly, a similar, but weaker, suppression is seen when the subject just imag-

ines making the movements, indicating involvement of the primary motor cortex in motor imagery (Schnitzler et al., 1997). Suppression of the rebound, as a sign of motor-cortex activation, also occurs when the subject views another person to make certain movements (Fig. 57.13; Hari et al., 1998).

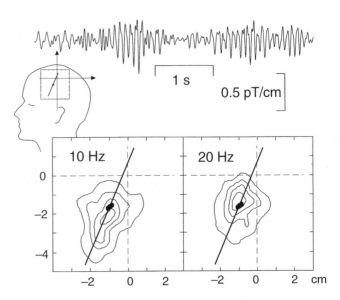

1 s

0.5 pT/cm

10 Hz   20 Hz

0

-2

-4

-2   0   2   -2   0   2   cm

Figure 57.12. *Top:* A 5-second trace of magnetic μ-rhythm from the rolandic region. *Bottom:* Isodensity clusters of sources of 10- and 20-Hz oscillations over the rolandic region of one subject, based on thousands of ECD locations. The *black ovals* show the area activated by median nerve stimulation at the wrist, and the *line* shows the estimated course of the rolandic fissure. (Adapted from Salmelin, R. and Hari, R. 1994b. Spatiotemporal characteristics of rhythmic neuromagnetic activity related to thumb movement. Neuroscience 60:537–550.)

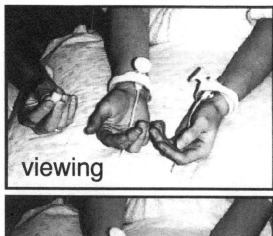

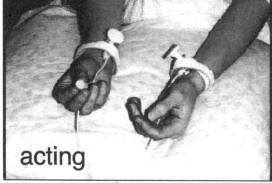

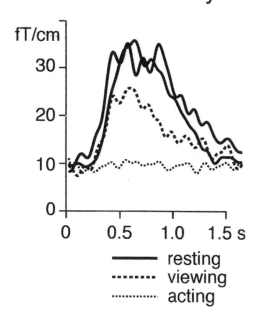

Level of motor-cortex 20-Hz activity

---- resting

········· viewing

·········· acting

Figure 57.13. Level of the 20-Hz rolandic activity after stimulation of the contralateral median nerve at when the subject either rested *(solid lines)*, viewed another person to manipulate a small object with the right hand fingers *(dashed line; "viewing")*, or manipulated the same object herself ("acting").

The sources of these 20-Hz signals were in the precentral primary motor cortex. (Adapted from Hari, R., Forss, N., Avikainen, S., et al. 1998. Activation of human primary motor cortex during action observation: a neuromagnetic study. Proc. Natl. Acad. Sci. U.S.A. 95:15061–15065.)

The 20-Hz rebounds do—whereas the 10-Hz rebounds do not—follow the moved body part in a somatotopical manner; they appear at lateral rolandic areas after mouth movements, more medially after finger movements, and close to midline after foot movements (Salmelin et al., 1995).

Recent MEG recordings after oral administration of benzodiazepine demonstrated a strong increase in the power of ~20-Hz oscillations in both hemispheres, with sources in the primary motor cortex, close to the hand area (Jensen et al., 2002, 2004; Fig. 57.14). These data suggest that the motor

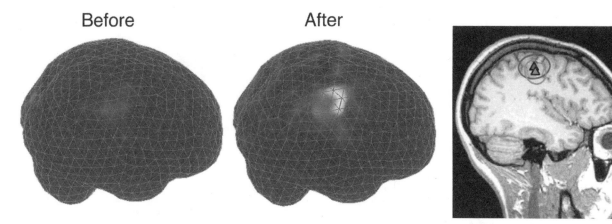

Figure 57.14. Minimum current estimates of the 20-Hz band activity projected to the brain surface of a single subject before *(left)* and after *(middle)* oral benzodiazepine administration; the brain is viewed from right. Co-registration of the sources on the subject's MRI *(right)* indicates activation of the primary motor cortex, with virtually identical source areas before

(green) and after *(red)* application of benzodiazepines. (Adapted from Jensen, O., Goel, P., Kopal, N., et al. 2003. On the human motor cortex beta rhythm: sources and modelling. Submitted.) (See Color Figure 57.14.)

cortex is an important effector site of benzodiazepine, and they also agree with the proposed generation of the rolandic 20-Hz oscillations in the motor cortex. In clinical EEG recordings benzodiazepine-related beta activity is typically seen in frontal leads, which could be explained by tangential current dipoles in the wall of the central sulcus.

Oscillatory Cortex–Muscle Coupling

The human rolandic MEG activity has been observed to have a close temporal relationship to peripheral muscular activity (Conway et al., 1995; Salenius et al., 1996, 1997a; Volkmann et al., 1996). For example, during isometric contraction of different muscles, the muscular and cortical signals are coherent at frequencies varying between 15 and 33 Hz in individual subjects (Salenius et al., 1997a). The sites of maximum coherence in the motor cortex show gross somatotopical organization, with activations during foot muscle contraction closer to the head midline than during hand muscle contractions (Fig. 57.15). The MEG signals lead the EMG signals in time, with increasing time lags with increasing brain-muscle distance. Such data strongly suggest that the 20-Hz rolandic rhythm reflects, at the population level, the common central drive to spinal motoneurons (for reviews, see Hari and Salenius, 1999 and Salenius and Hari, 2003).

Studies with different gripping tasks have led to the proposal that the cortical oscillations have a role in recalibrating the control system after a change in the cortex–muscle relationship (Kilner et al., 2000, 2003). At strong contractions, the frequency of the coherence jumps from 20 Hz to 40 Hz ("Piper rhythm"; Brown, 2000; Brown et al., 1998). The cortex–muscle coherence provides a novel tool to identify the primary motor cortex as a part of preoperative functional mapping (Mäkelä et al., 2001).

Gross et al. (2002) demonstrated, using a sophisticated dynamic imaging of coherent sources (DICS) method, developed to characterize synchronously firing neural networks in different parts of the brain, that 6- to 9-Hz velocity changes of slow finger movements are directly correlated to oscillatory activity of the primary motor cortex. Moreover, the coherence patterns suggested that the pulsatile velocity changes were sustained by a cerebellar drive through thalamus and premotor cortex.

Tau Rhythm from Auditory Areas

A third MEG rhythm, which I have started to call τ-rhythm (τ referring to *temporal lobe*), was described by Tähonen et al. (1991). This 8- to 10-Hz oscillatory activity is best seen in the planar gradiometer recordings just over the auditory cortex. Occasionally the rhythm is reduced by sound stimuli, such as bursts of noise, but it is not dampened by opening the eyes—a feature clearly different from the occipital alpha. The sources of single tau oscillations cluster to the supratemporal auditory cortex close to the generation's site of auditory evoked fields, with right-hemisphere dominance (Fig. 57.16; Lehtelä et al., 1997).

On the basis of the observed current orientations, the corresponding electric τ-rhythm should be seen mostly in the frontocentral midline where the tau sources, with dipole mo-

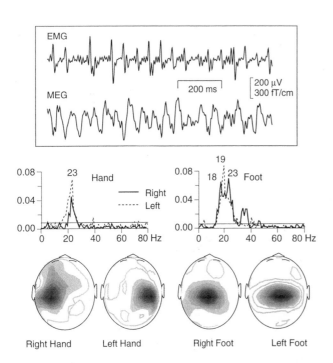

Figure 57.15. *Top:* Surface electromyogram (EMG) from isometrically contracted left hallucis brevis muscle and simultaneously recorded MEG signal over the parietal midline (3–100 Hz). *Middle:* Coherence spectra between MEG and EMG during isometric contraction of small hand and foot muscles (left- and right-sided contractions superimposed). *Bottom:* Spatial distributions of the strongest peaks of the coherence spectra. (Adapted from Salenius, S., Portin, K., Kajola, M., et al. 1997a. Cortical control of human motoneuron firing during isometric contraction. J. Neurophysiol. 77:3401–3405.)

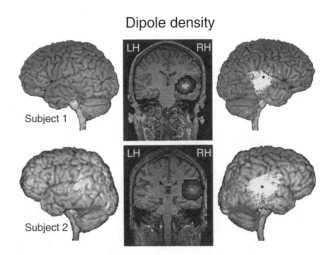

Figure 57.16. Locations of equivalent current dipoles for the tau oscillations (6.5–9.5 Hz range) in two subjects. The sources (clusters of *white dots*) are projected to the surface of the brain and shown on the subject's own MRI. The *black dot* indicates the source of the auditory N100m response. In the coronal sections *(middle),* the dipole distributions are presented as contour plots, with highest dipole densities in white and lowest in black. (Adapted from Lehtelä, L., Salmelin, R. and Hari, R. 1997. Evidence for reactive magnetic 10-Hz rhythm in the human auditory cortex. Neurosci. Lett. 222:111–114.)

ments of 40 nA·m, would lead to potentials of about 10–20 µV. In fact, such an EEG rhythm may appear during drowsiness; decreased vigilance is often considered to be associated with a spread of occipital EEG alpha toward more anterior regions, with simultaneously slightly decreasing frequency (Bente, 1964; Santamaria and Chiappa, 1987). A real spread of the alpha would be in clear contrast to the fixed, although distributed, generators of alpha, and a more plausible explanation is that the anterior alpha in fact reflects tau generated in the supratemporal auditory cortex.

The combined MEG and EEG data of Lu et al. (1992a) would agree with such a hypothesis; during the awake state (the first panel of Fig. 57.17) the occipital EEG displays rhythmic 10- to 11-Hz alpha activity, and the simultaneous MEG in the temporal region is of low amplitude, with little rhythmic activity. However, when the occipital electric alpha becomes discontinuous during light drowsiness (stage 1a) and seems to spread more anteriorly, with slightly slowed-down frequency, rhythmic activity of the same frequency appears in the MEG sensors over the temporal lobe.

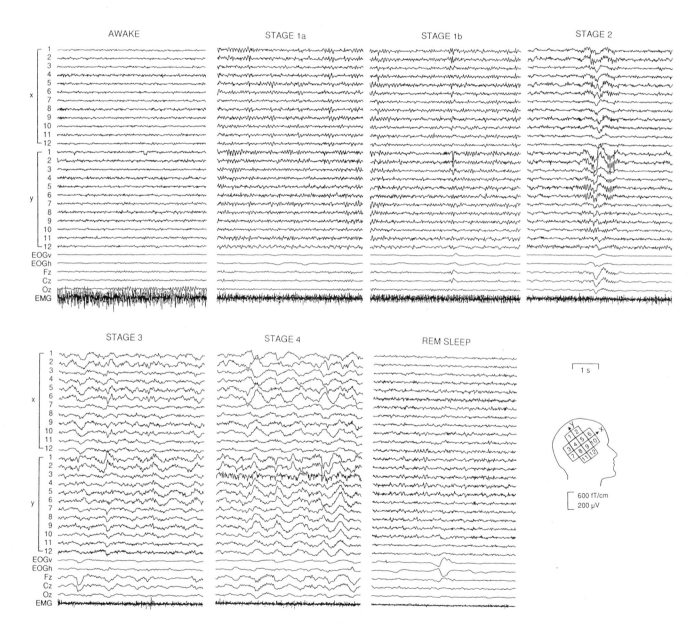

Figure 57.17. Different vigilance stages in one subject. The recording locations (24-channel planar gradiometer) are indicated on the schematic head; the x-gradients at 12 locations are plotted above and the y-gradients below. In the electric channels EOGv and EOGh refer to vertical and horizontal electro-oculograms, respectively. The electric amplitude scale refers to all other electric recordings except the EMG, for which only relative amplitudes are of importance. Note the increase of rhythmic MEG activity during stage 1a, compared with the awake stage. A typical V wave occurs during stage 1b. During stage 2, light sleep, K complexes occur both in MEG and EEG. In deep sleep, stages 3 and 4, slow activity is seen in the whole measurement area. Note the eye movements and the decreased EMG activity during the REM stage. (Adapted from Lu, S.T., Kajola, M., Joutsiniemi, S.L., et al. 1992a. Generator sites of spontaneous MEG activity during sleep. Electroencephalogr. Clin. Neurophysiol. 82:182–196.)

Therefore, the apparent spread of the EEG alpha during drowsiness might reflect changed relative contributions from the occipital alpha and from the temporal tau generators. Epidural electrode recordings (Niedermeyer, 1990, 1991) show that also the temporal-lobe 6- to 11-Hz activity arising from the convexial cortex is strikingly resilient to decreased vigilance.

A Note on Nomenclature

The existence of local cortical rhythms explains in part the confusion in the literature concerning effects of various tasks on the spontaneous EEG. Some people consider alpha to refer to the occipital "Berger rhythm," independently of its shape (i.e., frequency composition), whereas others refer to alpha as all signals falling in the 8- to 13-Hz frequency range, independently of the brain area where they are generated. To avoid confusion, it would be necessary to characterize each rhythm both by its site of origin and by its frequency range.

Other Brain Rhythms

A 7- to 9-Hz "sigma" rhythm has been demonstrated in recent MEG recordings in the second somatosensory cortex (Narici et al., 2001). Single median-nerve stimuli elicited some sigma oscillations, and the level of sigma was enhanced during rhythmic stimulation at the rhythm's dominant frequency.

Theta-range MEG activity has been scarcely studied. Sasaki et al. (1994) recorded 5- to 7-Hz MEG signals from the frontal cortex during mental calculation and intensive thinking. Tesche (1997) estimated the temporal waveforms of sources (computationally) inserted to the hippocampus and found in some subjects around 5-Hz rhythmic activity during mental calculation.

Much attention has been recently paid to the 40-Hz frequency band, often supposed to have a role in perceptual binding (Gray and Singer, 1989; Llinas, 1990). Both stimulus-related and later "induced" 40-Hz activity has been reported, with differences between visual EEG and MEG 40-Hz signals (Ribary et al., 1991; Tallon-Baudry et al., 2000). Although the 40-Hz activity, according to animal experiments, results from thalamocortical interaction, it is at present unknown how strongly the subcortical structures contribute to the MEG signals, which are strongly biased toward cortical currents.

Spontaneous Activity During Sleep

In the first MEG studies of sleep, performed with single-channel MEG devices, it was difficult to draw conclusions about the relationship between the electric and magnetic spontaneous signals (Hughes et al., 1976; Nakasato et al., 1990; Ueno and Iramina, 1990).

Figure 57.17 illustrates the first multichannel MEG recording of sleep. It was possible to classify the different stages of vigilance on the basis of both EEG and MEG (Lu et al., 1992a). The activity during awake stage and the appearance of τ-rhythm during stage 1a were discussed above. During deep drowsiness and light sleep (stages 1b and 2), vertex waves of 150- to 250-msec duration appeared in the frontocentral EEG leads and on several MEG channels. The electric and magnetic V waves did not always coincide.

Magnetic spindles of 11 to 15 Hz in frequency and 0.3 to 2 seconds in duration appeared during stage 2. The spindles were occasionally superimposed on high-amplitude transients, thereby resembling the typical electric K complexes. Often the successive magnetic V waves and K complexes differed in waveform and distribution. For example, the

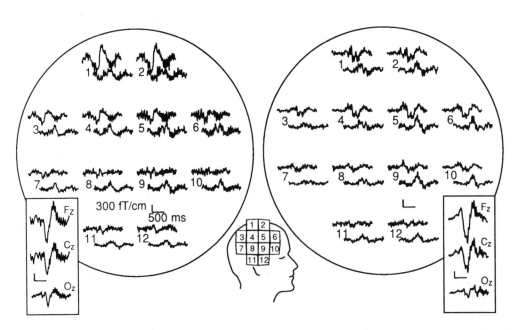

Figure 57.18. Two K complexes from the same subject, recorded from the same location. In the magnetic signals, the *upper traces* of each pair indicate the vertical gradient and the *lower trace* the horizontal gradient of the magnetic field; the recording locations are shown on the *insert head*. Si-

multaneous electric signals from the midline are shown in the *inserts;* their amplitude calibration is 100 μV. (Adapted from Lu, S.T., Kajola, M., Joutsiniemi, S.L., et al. 1992a. Generator sites of spontaneous MEG activity during sleep. Electroencephalogr. Clin. Neurophysiol. 82:182–196.)

midline distributions of two electric K complexes of Fig. 57.18 resemble each other, whereas the simultaneous magnetic distributions differ. A typical magnetic K complex lasted 0.8 to 1.2 seconds.

During slow-wave sleep (stages 3 and 4; Fig. 57.17), 0.5- to 2-Hz polymorphic MEG activity was widely spread over the measurement area. During the rapid-eye-movement (REM) stage, defined on the basis of rapid eye movements and decreased submental muscular tone, MEG activity was lower in amplitude and faster in frequency than during the other sleep stages. Sharp magnetic transients, resembling the V waves, were frequently seen.

In the first whole-scalp MEG study of sleep (Numminen et al., 1996), the sources of K complexes in the two hemispheres were active independently. Only in one subject out of six were the K-complex distributions satisfactorily explained by two current dipoles, one in each inferior parietal lobe, i.e., in line with the model suggested by Lu et al. (1992a). In the five other subjects the distributions were more complex. Therefore, the K complexes do not appear to be stereotyped responses of the cortex to external or internal stimuli, comparable to evoked responses, but rather they seem to reflect a diffuse and variable reaction involving large cortical areas.

Up to now, no focal activation spots have been detected during slow-wave sleep. The sources underlying the spindles also seem very complex. In principal component analysis, four to six separate components were often needed to explain at least 90% of the field variance during 1 second of the spindle activity (Lu et al., 1992a). Complexity of spindle generation, with a multitude of sources and frequencies, has also been suggested in animal experiments (Buser, 1987), in human depth electrode and scalp topography studies (Niedermeyer, 1982; Scheuler et al., 1990), as well as in recent MEG recordings applying synthetic aperture magnetometry (Ishii et al., 2003).

Llinas and Ribary (1993) point out that while the spontaneous activity is rather similar during awake and REM sleep stages, responses to repetitive 40-Hz stimulation are damp-

ened during REM sleep compared with wakefulness, possibly reflecting the brain's isolation from the external world during the REM stage.

Anesthesia

Burst-suppression patterns have been recorded from a dog during enflurane and propofol anesthesia (Jäntti et al., 1995). The signal pattern during the bursts was extremely complex and the signal did not show any organized structure (Fig. 57.19). A practical message from these recordings is that an essentially artifact-free MEG measurement can be obtained during respirator-assisted anesthesia when the respirator is kept outside the magnetically shielded room and when special care is taken in choosing nonmagnetic tubings and valves.

MEG in Epilepsy

The first MEG recording of an epileptic individual was reported by Cohen (1972); slow EEG and MEG activity increased during hyperventilation in a patient with psychomotor epilepsy. Starting from the early 1980s, a number of epileptic subjects have been studied in several laboratories (e.g., Barkley and Baumgartner, 2003; Barth et al., 1982, 1984; Baumgartner et al., 2000; Ebersole, 1996; Iwasaki et al., 2002; Knowlton, 2003; Lamusuo et al., 1999; Lin et al., 2003; Merlet et al., 1997; Modena et al., 1982; Nakasato et al., 1996; Paetau et al., 1990, 1992, 1994; Rose et al., 1987; Sato, 1990; Sutherling and Barth, 1989; Tiihonen et al., 1990; Van't Ent et al., 2003; Watanabe et al., 1996). In November 2003, the PubMed database already contained 400 publications with keywords of "MEG and epilepsy," and therefore it is impossible to cover here the progress in this rapidly expanding field.

The earliest MEG recordings were used to locate both single and multiple irritative brain areas (Barth et al., 1982, 1984; Modena et al., 1982). In one study, both scalp and sphenoidal EEG spikes were used as triggers for averaging the magnetic spikes. The latter had different latencies for the two triggers, consistent with propagation of the epileptic activity (Sutherling and Barth, 1989). The sources of the magnetic spikes were deeper for sphenoidal than for scalp triggers in all five subjects studied, suggesting propagation of the discharge between different parts of the temporal lobe.

Differentiation between ictal and interictal spikes is as difficult in MEG as it is in EEG. Since MEG recordings can only infrequently be performed during motor seizures, the relevance of the interictal MEG focus has been questioned. Sometimes the activity just preceding the seizure, assumed to have the best localizing value, can be detected. One possibility to reveal the significance of the observed focus is to tailor an electrode array on the basis of the interictal MEG distribution, by calculating the forward potential solution from the identified sources, and then to monitor the ictal activity during telemetric EEG recordings to ascertain whether the interictal focus is responsible for triggering the seizure.

In preoperative evaluation of epileptic patients it is important to know whether the epileptic discharges are focal, whether there are multiple foci, and whether these foci show any systematic time lags. One should also find how close the foci are to functionally irretrievable brain regions, such as

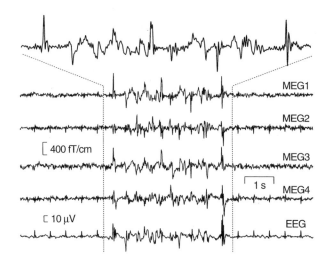

Figure 57.19. Four MEG channels and one EEG channel from a dog during burst-suppression phase induced by enflurane anaesthesia. (Adapted from Jäntti, V., Baer, G., Yli-Hankala, A., et al. 1995. MEG burst suppression in an anaesthetized dog. Acta Anaesth. Scand. 39:126–128.)

the sensorimotor and speech areas, and whether the source configuration is stable over time. MEG seems especially suitable for identifying epileptic foci in the convexial neocortex. MEG results have been also used to guide placement of intracranial electrodes and to suggest re-evaluation of structural MRI data.

Two examples of epileptic MEG discharges are presented below. Fig. 57.20 shows spikes, field patterns, and dipole moments of a 18-year-old woman who suffered from complex partial epilepsy (Hari et al., 1993a). During the night her 20- to 30-second seizures included awakening and bilateral increase of muscular tone, as well as tonic jerks in left extremities. During daytime she had epochs of paresthesia and loosening of the grip in the left hand. The abundant

spikes, recorded with a 122-channel whole-scalp magnetometer, could be adequately modeled with two current dipoles, one in each posterior parietal cortex. The peak activity occurred consistently 20 msec later in the left than the right hemisphere, suggesting callosal conduction of the signals from right to left. Such time lags are useful in differentiating the primary and the secondary (mirror) foci.

Figure 57.21 illustrates an ictal MEG recording of a man who suffered from left-sided hemifacial convulsions that were often triggered by touching the left mouth region (Forss et al., 1995a). Computed tomography and PET revealed no abnormalities. The MEG recording displays abundant epileptic spikes, which become increasingly polyphasic during the 14-second seizure. In the beginning, spikes appear only in the right hemisphere, with a source in the motor face area (defined on the basis of evoked responses and anatomical structures), whereas later during the seizure spikes also appear in the homologue area in the left hemisphere, again (as in Fig. 57.22) with about a 20-msec time lag compared with the other side.

In patients with Landau-Kleffner syndrome (LKS), stereotypic 3 cycles per second spike-and-wave complexes have been shown to be generated in the auditory cortex (Morrell et al., 1995; Paetau, 1994; Paetau et al., 1991, 1999), and the continuous epileptic discharges in the auditory cortices of LKS children likely prevent the proper analysis of sounds, including speech.

Spontaneous Activity in Other Patients

Ischemic Lesions

Ischemic hemispheric lesions are associated with slow magnetic shifts and with considerable slowing of cortical activity (Vieth et al., 1989). Gallen et al. (1992) showed that 2- to 3-Hz MEG activity was mainly concentrated in the damaged but viable tissue at the periphery of the infarcted area. It is not known, though, to which extent the changed tissue conductivities at the lesion area contributed to the measured signals.

Local unilateral lesions in the left anteromedial thalamus have been shown to cause extensive and surprisingly symmetric changes in the parieto-occipital spontaneous activity; the frequency spectra were broadened in the parieto-occipital area, but the reactivity to eye opening was preserved and the generation sites of the activity were similar as in normal subjects (Mäkelä, 1996; Mäkelä et al., 1998b).

Infantile Neuronal Ceroid Lipofuscinosis

As expected, patients with infantile neuronal ceroid lipofuscinosis (INCL) have flat MEG, pointing toward a total absence of cortical activity (R. Paetau, P. Santavuori, S.-L. Vanhanen, and R. Hari, unpublished observations, 1991). Brains of INCL patients show almost total neuronal loss and strong gliosis. Therefore, the flat MEG from these patients also indicates that glial cells have negligible contribution to the MEG signals in the absence of neuronal activity.

Migraine

Spreading depression (SD) has been suggested as the neurophysiological basis of migraine aura. In turtle cerebellum, induced SD is associated with strong magnetic fields

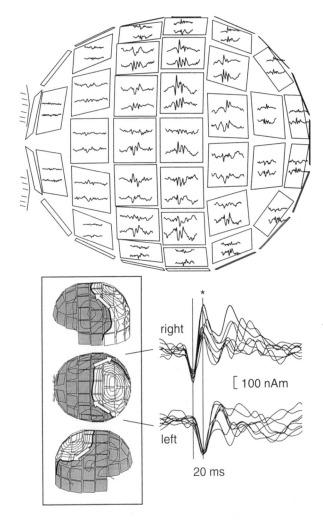

Figure 57.20. *Top:* Spatial distribution of one multispike displayed on the 122-channel sensor array viewed from top. *Bottom left:* Field pattern during the spike (*asterisk* above the curves); the sensor array is viewed from left, top, and right. The *shadowed areas* indicate magnetic flux emerging from the head; the isocontours are separated by 400 fT/cm. The *arrows* indicate the sites and orientations of the two ECDs required to account for the field pattern. *Bottom right:* Dipole moments as a function of time in both hemispheres. Each trace corresponds to one unaveraged spike, whose distribution was explained by the two-dipole model. (Adapted from Hari, R., Ahonen, A., Forss, N., et al. 1993a. Parietal epileptic mirror focus detected with a whole-head neuromagnetometer. Neuroreport 5:45–48.)

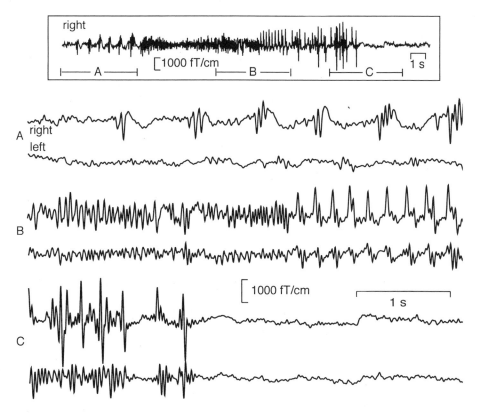

Figure 57.21. Epileptic discharges after voluntary triggering. The *top trace* illustrates MEG activity from the right hemisphere during the whole 14-second seizure. In the middle and lower parts, selected periods **(A–C)** are expanded and signals from the corresponding area in the left hemisphere are shown for comparison. (Adapted from Forss, N., Mäkelä, J.P., Keränen, T., et al. 1995b. Trigeminally triggered epileptic facial convulsions. Neuroreport 6: 918–920.)

(Okada, 1990). Consequently, it has been proposed that SD propagating in the human brain during the prodromal phase of migraine could be detected by MEG, and such shifts have been reported during the migraine aura (Barkley et al., 1991). The propagation of SD, assumed to be about 3 mm/min on the basis of changes in the scotoma in the vi-

sual field, has been elegantly demonstrated in fMRI recordings (Hadjikhani et al., 2001).

Effects of Electroconvulsive Therapy

Electroconvulsive therapy (ECT), efficient in treatment of severe depression, is known to increase slow EEG

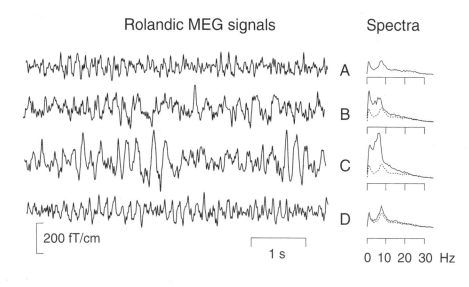

Figure 57.22. Effects of electroconvulsive therapy on rolandic MEG signals and their frequency spectra. *A,* before treatment; *B,* after four treatments; *C,* after eight treatments; and *D,* 1 month after the last treatment. On the *right,* the before-treatment *(A)* spectrum is shown for comparison in all other conditions *(dashed lines).* (Adapted from Salmelin, R., Mäkelä, J.P., Heikman, P., et al. 1996a. Human brain rhythms and electroconvulsive therapy. Soc. Neurosci. Abstr. 22(pt 1):342.)

rhythms. Salmelin et al. (1996a) and Heikman et al. (2001) tracked the temporal and spatial modulation of spontaneous oscillations in five ECT-treated depressive patients. ECT resulted in a prominent increase of frequencies below 8 Hz, which largely disappeared within 1 month after the last treatment (Fig. 57.22). In three patients, relief of depression was accompanied by an increase of the 4- to 8-Hz oscillations by at least 50% after the first four treatments and up to 500% after eight treatments, particularly in the temporal and rolandic areas.

Encephalitis

In herpes simplex encephalitis, sources of abnormal MEG waveforms have been identified in the temporal lobes (Mäkelä et al., 1998a). Further similar studies might help in the evaluation of the sites and extent of the functionally disturbed brain areas in postencephalitic patients.

Parkinsonian Tremor

Volkmann et al. (1996) found strong coherence, at the frequency of the 3- to 6-Hz resting parkinsonian tremor, between oscillatory MEG activity in premotor and somatomotor cortices and muscle activity (Volkmann et al., 1996). Previously, Mäkelä et al. (1993b) had noted that in patients with hemiparkinsonism the onset of tremor induces a similar dampening of the 10- and 20-Hz components of the μ-rhythm as do normal movements. It was thus suggested that parkinsonian tremor activates cortical mechanisms that normally produce rapid alternating movements.

Salenius et al. (2002) observed suppression of the normal 15- to 30-Hz cortex-muscle coherence in parkinsonian patients who were withdrawn from medication from the preceding evening; the coherence was, to a large part, restored with the patients' normal levodopa treatment. Abolishment of the normal 15- to 30-Hz synchronized oscillatory activity has been proposed to lead in bradykinesia (Brown et al., 2001).

In a more extensive analysis with the DICS method, Timmermann et al. (2003) demonstrated coherence between 4- and 6-Hz parkinsonian tremor and activity of several cerebral areas. Coherence was seen both at the tremor frequency and, even more strongly, at its double. The analysis of partial coherence and phase shifts was especially interesting; the interaction between M1 and EMG agreed with previous studies, indicating that cortex leads the muscle, whereas the interaction between EMG and diencephalic areas was bidirectional. Moreover, a direct afferent coupling was evident from EMG to second somatosensory cortex and to posterior parietal cortex. Cerebellum and premotor areas seemed to be connected with the periphery via other cerebral areas.

Auditory Evoked Fields

The first demonstrations of the generation of the main auditory evoked field (AEF) deflections in the superior surface of the temporal lobe (Elberling et al., 1980; Hari et al., 1980), deduced from the measured field patterns, considerably enlightened the origin of the coinciding electric evoked potentials, which had been previously believed to be non-specific due to their maximum amplitude at the vertex. Con-

sequently, various long-latency EEG and MEG responses are used nowadays widely as tools to study functions of the supratemporal auditory cortex.

Transient Responses

Figure 57.23 shows examples of middle-latency and long-latency auditory evoked magnetic fields, obtained using different stimulus repetition rates, different filter settings, different analysis periods, and different number of averaged responses. After the earliest cortical auditory responses around 19 to 20 msec, the interindividually variable but otherwise reliable middle-latency responses peak around 30 msec (Mäkelä et al., 1994; McEvoy et al., 1994; Pelizzone et al., 1987b; Yoshiura et al., 1994) and are followed by longer-latency responses around 50, 100, and 200 msec (P50m, N100m, and P200m, respectively). A sustained field is seen during long sounds. All these responses have cortical origin, and their generation sites differ slightly, indicating contribution from different cytoarchitectonic areas in the supratemporal auditory cortex. Also hippocampal activity may be seen during an auditory detection task (Nishitani et al., 1998). The clear dependence of the auditory N100m response on the interstimulus interval (ISI), with saturation at ISIs of 4 to 8 seconds (Hari et al., 1982, 1987) has been related to the duration of sensory memory (Lu et al., 1992c; Mäkelä et al., 1993a,b; Sams et al., 1993a).

Different ECD locations for N100m depending on the frequency and amplitude of the sound have been suggested to reflect tonotopic and amplitopic organization of the auditory cortex (Pantev et al., 1988, 1989a; see, however, the recent critical evaluation by Lütkenhöner et al., 2003). The auditory cortex is very sensitive to amplitude and frequency modulations (Mäkelä et al., 1987) as well as to various changes within the stimuli (Kaukoranta et al., 1987; Mäkelä et al., 1988). Direction of attention can modulate activity of at least two areas in the supratemporal cortex (Arthur et al., 1991; Hari et al., 1989b; Kuriki and Takeuchi, 1991; Rif et al., 1991). The auditory cortex also reacts to small changes in the direction of binaural stimuli, tested for example by changes in the interaural time difference of binaural click trains (McEvoy et al., 1993; Sams et al., 1993b).

The reactivity of the auditory cortex to changes in the stimulus sequence has been studied extensively (for reviews, see Alho, 1995; Hari, 1990; Näätänen, 1992, 2003; Näätänen and Picton, 1987; Näätänen et al., 1994). Infrequent deviations in a monotonous sound sequence evoke mismatch fields (MMFs) in the close vicinity of the generation site of the auditory N100m, often with right-hemisphere dominance. MMF, related to automatic sound processing, can be used in testing of auditory cortical functions, including the duration of echoic memory (Sams et al., 1993a). A total omission of a tone from a monotonous sequence activates several brain areas, including the supratemporal auditory cortex, the superior temporal sulcus, and the frontal lobe, all with right-hemisphere dominance (Raij et al., 1997).

The AEFs with known sources are good tools to study brain functions. For example, Sams et al. (1991) showed, applying the so-called McGurk illusion related to speech-sound perception, that articulation movements seen from a videotape have an effect on AEFs evoked by acoustical syl-

Middle-Latency AEFs

Long-Latency-AEFs

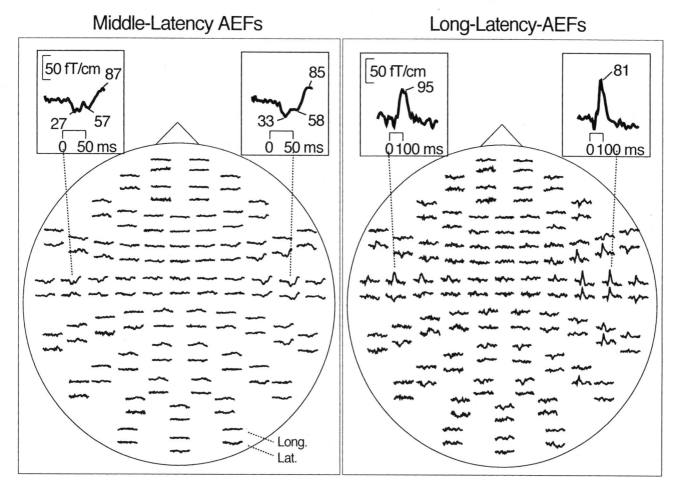

Figure 57.23. Example of middle-latency *(left)* and long-latency *(right)* auditory evoked magnetic fields recorded from one subject with a 122-channel device. (Adapted from McEvoy, L., Mäkelä, J.P., Hämäläinen, M., et al. 1994. Effect of interaural time differences on middle-latency and late auditory evoked magnetic fields. Hear. Res. 78:249–257.)

lables. It was thus demonstrated that visual information from lip movements can modify activity of the auditory cortex, a finding supported by later fMRI recordings (Calvert et al., 1997).

Steady-State Responses

Tonotopic organization of the human auditory cortex was first shown by steady-state recordings (Romani et al., 1982). The amplitude of the auditory steady-state response reaches its maximum at repetition rates around 40 Hz. This so-called 40-Hz response (Galambos et al., 1981) has a cortical origin (Mäkelä and Hari, 1987; Ross et al., 2002). (To avoid confusion, it is important to emphasize that the notion "cortical origin" refers to the major contributor to the measured signal. It does not, by any means, deny the possibility of a subcortical trigger, or simultaneous activity in some subcortical areas. However, in many cases the adequate explanation of the signal patterns by cortical sources indicates negligible contribution from subcortical areas to the measured MEG/EEG signals.)

The amplitude enhancement of the steady-state response around 40 Hz has been adequately explained by summation of subsequent single responses, each with a 40-Hz content, thereby suggesting linearity of the responses at least at stimulation rates from 10 to 40 Hz (Gutschalk et al., 1999; Hari et al., 1989a). In other words, those results do not indicate stronger reactivity or "resonance" of the auditory cortex at stimulation rates of 40 Hz. However, a recent PET study, quantifying regional cerebral blood flow during repetitive auditory stimulation, came to the conclusion that the 40-Hz response enhancement reflects increased cortical synaptic activity (Pastor et al., 2002); further studies are required because the behavior of response strengths as a function of stimulus repetition rate differed between EEG and PET recordings.

Stimulus-related 40-Hz oscillations, elicited by paired clicks, have been related to temporal binding of successive sounds (Joliot et al., 1994).

During normal binaural hearing, sounds from each ear reach the auditory cortices of both hemispheres. Therefore, the binaural cortical responses, even when recorded from one hemisphere only, are unknown mixtures of inputs from both ears. A recent solution to this problem is to "frequency-tag" the inputs from both ears (Fujiki et al., 2002; Kaneko et al., 2003); continuous tones, presented either monaurally to left or right ear, or binaurally, are amplitude modulated with different frequencies in the two ears, and the MEG signals of each hemisphere are analyzed in either time or frequency domain. Such analysis demonstrates significantly stronger suppression of the ipsilateral than contralateral input during binaural hearing.

AEFs in Patients

Ischemic lesions of the temporal lobe often cause marked defects in speech perception and production. Details of symptomatology, however, cannot be determined from the anatomical lesion alone and additional methods are welcome. In patients with different types of ischemic brain lesions, AEFs disappeared only when the lesion extended to the deep region of the temporal lobe (Leinonen and Joutsiniemi, 1989; Mäkelä et al., 1991). Figure 57.24 illustrates the extent of the lesion in one such patient (Mäkelä and Hari, 1992). The responses are normal in the healthy left hemisphere but totally abolished in the lesioned right hemisphere. The finding is of interest also from the source analysis point of view; although MEG source modeling is hampered by the nonunique inverse problem, this kind of result strongly supports the correctness of dipole modeling of normal AEFs, i.e., sources in the auditory cortices of both hemispheres.

In deaf *patients with cochlear prosthesis,* AEFs have been used to show that the auditory cortex reacts to very artificial input (Hari, 1997; Hari et al., 1988b; Hoke et al., 1989b; Pelizzone et al., 1987a). AEFs also provide a tool to study reorganization of central auditory pathways after various peripheral lesions or congenital disorders (Vasama and Mäkelä, 1995; Vasama et al., 1994a,b).

Mismatch fields are very sensitive indicators of different sensory and brain disorders at group level (for a review, see Näätänen, 2003), but, unfortunately, the specificity of the responses has not yet been rigorously addressed and thus the clinical usefulness of MMFs at single-subject level remains to be shown. For example, MMFs are altered in patients with *thalamic infarction*, but without clear relationship to the degree of memory deficit (Mäkelä et al., 1998b).

Patients with *Alzheimer's disease* have dampened cortical 40-Hz responses and delayed ipsilateral N100m responses, probably as signs of deteriorated cortical processing (Pekkonen et al., 1996; Ribary et al., 1991). The N100m responses were delayed and dampened during auditory *hallucinations* in schizophrenic patients, most likely indicating top-down activation of the sensory-specific cortices (Tiihonen et al., 1992).

Patients with *tinnitus* may have a significantly decreased amplitude ratio between P200m and N100m (Hoke et al., 1989a). In tinnitus due to acute noise trauma, the P200m/N100m amplitude ratio can normalize during the period of recovery from tinnitus (Pantev et al., 1989b). However, many contradictory findings have been presented as well (Colding-Jørgensen et al., 1992; Jacobson et al., 1991), most likely due to different types of patients studied and to variations in the experimental setups and filter settings. In support of the early tinnitus studies, Shiomi et al. (1997) showed that lidocaine in-

jection-induced tinnitus release is associated with narrowing of the N100m deflection; such a change could reflect tinnitus-related modulation of neuronal mechanisms underlying the P200m response. Tinnitus, similarly as exposure to external sounds, can be related to plastic reorganization of the auditory cortex (Muhlnickel et al., 1998).

AEFs have been frequently studied in *dyslexic* individuals, both as indicators of problems of phonological processing and as signs of a more general disorder in processing of rapidly presented auditory stimuli. For example, Nagarajan et al. (1999) observed that N100m to the second sound of a pair, at short stimulus onset asynchronies, is smaller in dyslexic than normal-reading adults. The result was interpreted to indicate an abnormal neural representation of brief and rapidly successive sensory input, and thereby to be a probable correlate of poor reading ability. Renvall and Hari (2003) noted decreased responses to acoustic frequency changes in the left auditory cortex of dyslexic adults.

Gootjes et al. (1999) developed a simple paradigm to predict language lateralization in right-handed subjects by presenting vowels, tones, and piano notes in pairs of two stimuli. Responses recorded when the subjects had to indicate when the two stimuli were the same showed, in all the

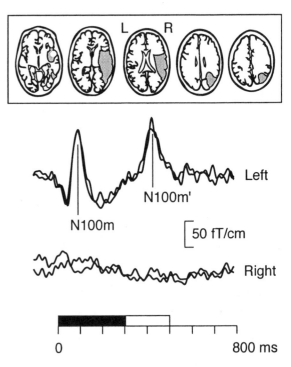

Figure 57.24. Auditory responses from a patient with an extended lesion of the right temporal lobe; the *shadowed areas* in the brain slices show the extent of the lesion. Responses are shown for a representative left- and right-hemisphere channels. The stimuli were noise/square-wave sequences (shown on the time scale) that typically elicited one onset response (N100m) and one transition-related response N100m′. (Adapted from Mäkelä, J.P., and Hari, R. 1992. Neuromagnetic auditory evoked responses after a stroke in the right temporal lobe. Neuroreport 3:94–96.)

11 subjects studied, left-hemisphere dominance for responses to vowels.

Somatosensory Evoked Fields

Responses from SI

The spatial distribution of sources of somatosensory evoked fields (SEFs) represents well the known somatotopic organization of the primary somatosensory cortex SI (Baumgartner, 1993; Brenner et al., 1978; Hari et al., 1984, 1993b; Suk et al., 1991; Yang et al., 1993). Since MEG mainly picks signals from tangential currents, the convexial cortex is either silent or poorly represented in the SEF distributions. At SI, the hand area signals, therefore, should arise mainly from cytoarchitectonic area 3b, whereas in the foot SI all cytoarchitectonic areas should produce currents tangential to the skull, and thus their changed relative contributions should be seen as rotation of the field patterns. Evoked field data to lower-limb stimulation suggest that such rotations really occur as signs of successive activation of several cytoarchitectonic areas (Fujita et al., 1995; Hari et al., 1996; Hashimoto et al., 2001; Huttunen et al., 1987; Kakigi et al., 1995b).

Figure 57.25 shows one subject's responses to left tibial nerve stimuli, with the largest signals at the top of the head (Hari et al., 1996). The field patterns rotate as a function of time, as predicted above. A two-dipole model, with one dipole in area 3b and the other in area 5, both in the mesial wall of the hemisphere, explained the data during the first 100 msec, with a consistent 3-msec time difference in their initial peak latencies. Other source models were rejected on the basis of their inconsistencies with experimental data and/or anatomical information. A slightly different two-source model for tibial-nerve SEFs was suggested by Hashimoto et al. (2001) on the basis of beam-former analysis.

SEFs from the SI cortex are typically strictly contralateral. However, tactile interference applied on the palm suppresses the median-nerve 30-msec response at the contralateral SI but enhances it in the ipsilateral SI (Schnitzler et al., 1995), implying that tactile input from one hand has access to the SI cortices of both hemispheres, probably through callosal connections. Some long-latency MEG responses from the ipsilateral SI have been reported (Korvenoja et al., 1995). However, transfer of stimulus- or movement-related vibrations to the other hand has been demonstrated as one possible cause of ipsilateral responses (Hari and Imada, 1999).

Brief bursts of about 600-Hz oscillations are superimposed on the earliest cortical deflections, the 20-msec N20m response (Curio et al., 1994; Hashimoto et al., 1996a). These high-frequency responses will be discussed in detail elsewhere in the text.

Quantification of source strengths may be very useful in some applications. For example, Elbert et al. (1995), determining source strengths for tactile finger stimulation at SI cortex, found increased cortical representations for the left hands of string players, implying practice-related cortical reorganization (see also Pantev et al., 2001).

Figure 57.26 illustrates the use of SEFs in preoperative identification of the sensorimotor strip. Superposition of

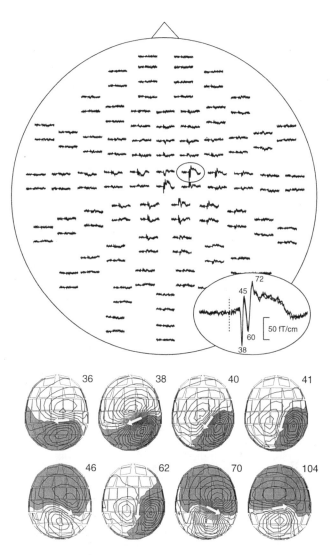

Figure 57.25. *Top*: Responses of one subject to electric stimulation of the left tibial nerve at the ankle. The traces are averages of 800 single responses. The *insert* shows enlarged two sets of 400 responses from successive experiments superimposed. The passband is 0.03 to 275 Hz. *Bottom*: Magnetic field patterns and equivalent current dipoles of the same subject as a function of time (indicated in msec). The isocontours are separated by 20 fT. (Adapted from Hari, R., Nagamine, T., Nishitani, N., et al., 1996. Time-varying activation of different cytoarchitectonic areas of the human SI cortex after tibial nerve stimulation. NeuroImage 4:111–118.)

sources for median and tibial nerve stimulation on the patient's MRI illustrates that her cavernous angioma is about 1.5 cm away from the somatomotor hand area. The angioma was later successfully operated, without causing any sensory or motor impairments.

In Figure 57.27, the preoperative evaluation includes, in addition to SEF recordings, identification of the primary motor cortex, anterior to the central sulcus, by means of cortex-muscle coherence (see Fig. 57.15 and the related text). Visualization of the somatosensory and motor landmarks on a brain rendering with veins superimposed (right) helps the

Figure 57.26. *Left*: Sources for responses to left median and tibial nerve stimulation superposed on the MRI reconstruction of the subject. The section passes through both sources to illustrate the central sulcus just anterior to them. *Right*: A parallel section slightly deeper, with the cavernous angioma indicated. The patient, a 50-year-old woman, was later successfully operated on by Prof. Herbert Silfvenius (Umeaå, Sweden). The MRI reconstructions were made by Mika Seppä.

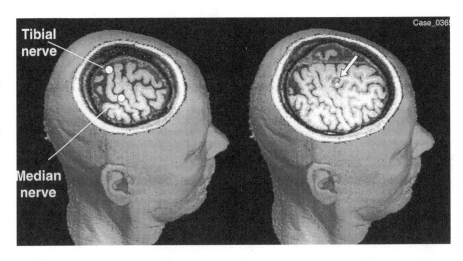

neurosurgeon to navigate during the operation (Mäkelä et al., 2001).

Responses from SII and Other Nonprimary Cortical Areas

MEG recordings have indicated that somatosensory stimuli also activate bilaterally areas close to the upper lip of the sylvian fissure, i.e., most probably at the second somatosensory area SII (Hari et al., 1983a, 1990, 1993b; Kaukoranta et al., 1986a). Although the SI/SII differentiation was possible already with small MEG sensor arrays, the more recent whole-scalp recordings have given more detailed information about the cortical somatosensory network, with spatially and temporally distinct activations also in the posterior parietal cortex, in the mesial cortex, and in the frontal lobes (Forss et al., 1994a, 1996; Hari and Forss, 1999; Mauguière et al., 1997). The field patterns of Fig. 57.28 illustrate activation of the right (contralateral) SI, left and right SII, and the posterior parietal cortex after electric stimulation of the

left thumb. Tactile stimulation activates essentially the same brain regions as does electric stimulation, but with slightly different latencies and relative amplitudes (Forss et al., 1994b). The MEG source locations in SI and SII cortices agree with fMRI data collected from the same subjects (Del Gratta et al., 2002; Tuunanen et al., 2003).

The representations of fingers of both hands overlap strongly in the bilaterally activated SII cortices, whereas the SI cortex (area 3b) has representations of fingers of one hand only, and with much weaker overlap (Simões et al., 2001). Bilateral median-nerve stimulation elicits left-hemisphere-dominant SII activation, suggesting handedness-independent functional specialization of the human SII cortices (Simões et al., 2002).

Differentiation of various source areas of SEFs has started to provide enlightening information about the functions of the cortical somatosensory network (Forss et al., 1995a; Hari and Forss, 1999; Hari et al., 1993b; Huttunen et al., 1996), and recordings of SEFs in patients with various lesions (Forss et al., 1999) and analysis, for example, of

Figure 57.27. Preoperative functional localization in a patient with a parietal-lobe tumor. The postcentral somatosensory cortex has been identified by measuring somatosensory evoked fields (SEFs) to median-nerve (hand) and tibial-nerve (foot) stimulation. In addition, cortex-muscle coherence for hand and foot small muscles has been used to identify the precentral primary motor cortex. On the right, veins are superimposed on the surface rendering. (Courtesy of CliniMEG, Brain Research Unit, Low Temperature Laboratory, Helsinki University of Technology.)

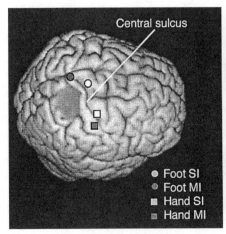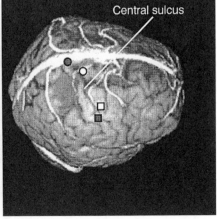

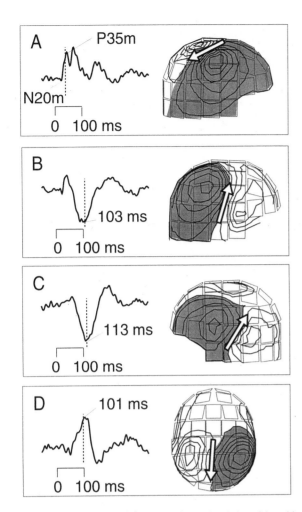

Figure 57.28. Field patterns of SEFs to electric stimulation of the subject's left thumb; interstimulus interval (ISI) 4 seconds. Illustrative responses are shown from four areas (contralateral SI, both SII regions, and the posterior parietal cortex) and the corresponding field patterns at the time of maximum response from each region. (Adapted from Forss, N., Jousmäki, V., and Hari, R. 1995a. Interaction in the human somatosensory cortex between afferent input from different fingers. Brain Res. 685:68–76.)

phase locking between areas (Simões et al., 2003) may bring new information about the debate on parallel vs. serial processing in different somatosensory cortical areas.

SEFs in Multiple Sclerosis

In patients with clinically diagnosed multiple sclerosis (Karhu et al., 1992), the N20m deflection was dampened and delayed by 2.5 to 3 msec. The 50- to 80-msec responses were often of larger amplitude than in control subjects, especially in patients who had periventricular plaques in MRI. The source locations of N20m and P60m in the somatosensory hand area did not differ between the groups.

It is probable that enhancement of the corresponding electric SEPs has remained undetected with the typical high-pass filter settings at 10 to 20 Hz and the analysis periods of 30 to 50 msec, applied in many laboratories.

SEFs in Myoclonus Epilepsy

Karhu et al. (1994) suggested that progressive myoclonus epilepsy (PME; Unverricht-Lundborg type) is associated with thalamocortical hyperreactivity in the sensorimotor but not in the auditory system. The patients were adequately medicated and their MEG did not show spikes. The amplitudes of the 30-msec SEFs were up to sixfold compared with the response of normal subjects but the source locations agreed with activation of the somatosensory hand area. Patients of juvenile neuronal ceroid lipofuscinosis and late infantile neuronal ceroid lipofuscinosis, also show enhanced SEFs (Lauronen et al., 1997, 2002).

"Giant" SEFs from SI have been recorded from a genetically homogeneous group of PME (Unverricht-Lundborg) patients (Forss et al., 2001). Figure 57.29 shows that strongly enhanced responses at the contralateral SI of a patient as a sign on hyperreactivity and responses also in the ipsilateral SI, in contrast to the healthy control subject; the latency difference of about 20 msec suggests facilitated callosal transfer to the ipsilateral side. Moreover, in spite of the enhanced SI responses, no clear SII responses are seen in the patient. Findings like this encourage the clinical neurophysiologist to assess functions of the somatosensory circuitry beyond the primary somatosensory cortex, as the dysfunctions may have direct consequences for the prognosis or rehabilitation of the patient.

Noxious Stimulation

MEG responses have also been recorded to painful stimuli, with activations around SII and/or the frontal operculum to electric stimulation of the tooth pulp, carbon dioxide stimulation of the nasal mucosa, and noxious (electric or CO_2 laser) stimulation of the skin (Forss et al., 2004; Hari et al., 1983b; Huttunen et al., 1986; Joseph et al., 1991; Kakigi et al., 1995a, 2003; Kanda et al., 2000; Ploner et al., 1999, 2002). Whole-scalp recordings indicated a clear right-hemisphere predominance to painful CO_2 stimulation of the nasal mucosa (Hari et al., 1997).

With laser heat it is possible to stimulate rather selectively Aδ- and C-fibers by applying different stimulus intensities to stimulus areas of different sizes (Bragard et al., 1996; Forss et al., 2004; Kakigi et al., 2003). Figure 57.30 shows that that the evoked responses from the contralateral SII cortex peak to Aδ-fiber stimuli at about 160 msec and to C-fiber stimuli around 800 msec, in agreement with the conduction velocities of these two fiber types (Forss et al., 2004). Interestingly, monitoring of the level of the 20-Hz motor-cortex activity strongly suggests that the painful laser stimuli automatically activate the primary motor cortex and therefore might be informative about the mechanisms underlying pathological muscle contraction in tension pain (Hari et al., 2003; Raij et al., 2003, 2004). In patients with chronic pain, enhanced activation of the motor cortex occurs after innocuous tactile stimuli (Juottonen et al., 2002).

Visual Evoked Fields

Visual evoked fields (VEFs) were reported for the first time in 1975 (Brenner et al., 1975; Teyler et al., 1975).

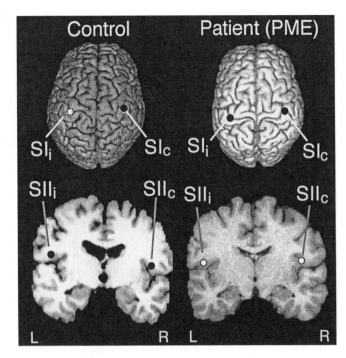

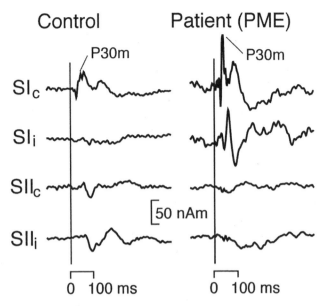

Figure 57.29.   Source locations *(left)* and source waveforms as a function of time *(right)* to electric stimulation of the left median nerve in a healthy control subject and in a patient suffering from Unverricht-Lundborg-type progressive myoclonus epilepsy. The *black circles* indicate source locations and the *white circles* indicate possible source locations that did not show any activation; c and I refer to contralateral and ipsilateral hemispheres. (Adapted from Forss, N., Silén, T., and Karjalainen, T. 2001. Lack of activation of human secondary somatosensory cortex in Unverricht-Lundborg type of progressive myoclonus epilepsy. Ann. Neurol. 49:90–97.)

Figure 57.30.   *Top left:* Averaged responses (*N* = 100) of a single subject from right SII region to selective Aδ- *(upper trace;* weak pricking pain) and C-fiber *(lower trace;* weak burning pain) thulium-laser stimuli presented to the dorsum of the left hand once every 4.5 to 5.5 seconds. *Top right and bottom:* The mean source locations of responses in the SII *(top)* and PPC *(bottom)* region to Aδ-fiber stimuli. The *ovals* indicate the mean ± standard error of the mean (SEM) locations across eight subjects superimposed on slices of a mean brain of the subjects, calculated by means of elastic transformations of their MRIs. (Modified from Forss, N., Raij, T.T., Seppä, M., et al. 2004. Common cortical network for first and second pain. Neuroimage, under revision.)

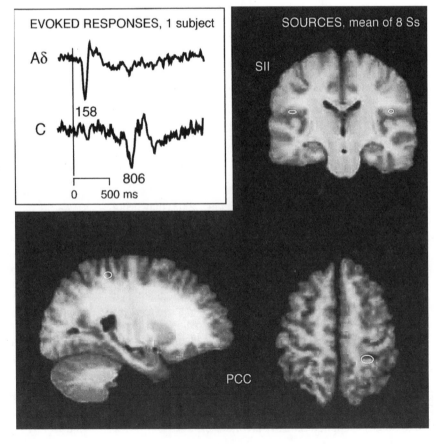

With flash stimuli, VEFs and visual evoked potentials (VEPs) did not peak simultaneously, and the responses depended on luminance in different manner, thereby suggesting separate sources for VEFs and VEPs (Teyler et al., 1975). Steady-state recordings with gratings reversing at 13 Hz (Brenner et al., 1975) allowed determination of the sources; the field patterns evoked by half-field stimuli agreed with activation of the contralateral occipital cortex and the patterns to full-field stimulation were the sums of the two half-field patterns. The retinotopic organization of the occipital visual cortex has been studied with MEG by presenting stimuli to different parts of the visual field (Ahlfors et al., 1992; Aine et al., 1996; Maclin et al., 1983; Tabuchi et al., 2002).

Outside the occipital cortex the visual field patterns are very complex and the utilization of VEFs as tools of clinical neurophysiology is still scarce. Figure 57.31 shows responses to half-field pattern and luminance stimuli. The first responses are generated in the occipital cortex but a later response is clear, especially for luminance stimuli, in the region of the parieto-occipital sulcus (POS).

The very same POS area close to the midline can be activated by various visual stimuli (Aine et al., 1996) as well as by voluntary eye blinks (Hari et al., 1994) and saccades (Jousmäki et al., 1996). Anatomically, the posterior parietal midline region, which also produces the most prominent MEG alpha activity, could well be the human homologue of

the monkey V6/V6A region, influenced, for example, by saccades and eye position, and proposed to be related to spatial coding of extrapersonal visual space and to visuomotor integration (Galletti et al., 1995). The V6/POS region is a part of the dorsal visual stream and thus of interest for both basic neuroscience and for some neurological disorders affecting visuomotor coordination.

The human homologue of the monkey MT/V5 cortex, a brain area selective to visual motion, has also been identified by MEG recordings (Anderson et al., 1996; ffytche et al., 1995; Uusitalo et al., 1997a,b). Better understanding of neural origin of different VEF components should bring invaluable information about temporal relationships in the activation of different visual areas. Interestingly, the activation order of human visual cortices can deviate from the simple serial activation pattern (Vanni et al., 2001), in agreement with both monkey recordings (Schmolesky et al., 1998) and simulation studies (Petroni et al., 2001), thereby indicating the importance of reciprocal interareal connections in a hierarchically connected network.

Responses to Faces and Language Stimuli

In agreement with both clinical and other imaging data, MEG responses to pictures of *faces* indicate activation of extrastriate visual areas, predominantly in the right posterior fusiform gyrus (Halgren et al., 2000; Linkenkaer-Hansen et al., 1998; Lu et al., 1991; Sams et al., 1997). Face-catego-

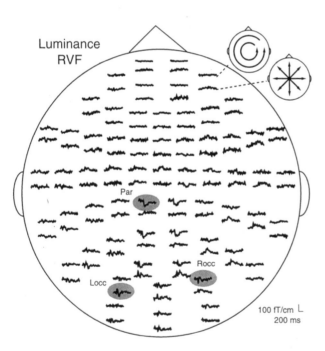

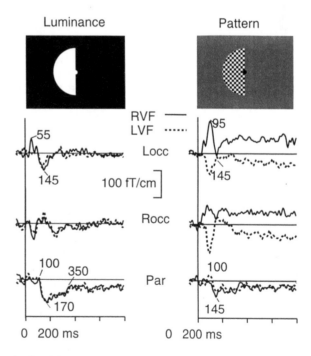

Figure 57.31. *Left*: Responses to stimulation of the right visual hemifield by luminance stimuli. *Right*: Responses of the same subject to left- and right hemifield (LVF, RVF) luminance and pattern stimuli (radius 8 degrees) from the parietal region (Par) and from left and right occipital areas (Locc, Rocc). Note the predominance of the parietal response to luminance

stimuli and the very clear LVF vs. RVF difference in the occipital channels for pattern, but not for luminance, stimuli. (Adapted from Portin, K., Salenius, S., Salmelin, R., et al. 1998. Activation of the human occipital and parietal cortex by pattern and luminance stimuli: neuromagnetic measurements. Cereb. Cortex 18:253–260.)

rization-related activity has been reported as early as 100 msec after the stimulus (Liu et al., 2002), whereas the typical face-specific response peaks at 160 to 170 msec (Furey et al., 2004), and the activation shows a systematic amplitude dependence on the degree of "faceness" of the stimulus (Halgren et al., 2000).

MEG's excellent temporal resolution is of high value in studies of *language* perception and production. Salmelin et al. (1994) were able to follow the cortical activation sequence from the posterior brain areas toward more anterior regions when the subjects named pictures of objects. Signs of considerable parallel processing were evident and both hemispheres were activated by the task. Interestingly, MEG studies of incongruities in musical syntax suggest that Broca's region and its right-hemisphere homologue area process syntactic information that is less language-specific than usually believed (Maess et al., 2001).

More recently, MEG has been increasingly applied for studies of reading and naming, both in healthy subjects (Cornelissen P. et al., 2003) and in aphasic patients (Cornelissen K. et al., 2003), stuttering subjects (Salmelin et al., 2000b), as well as dyslexic individuals (Helenius et al., 1999; Salmelin et al., 1996b, 2000a).

Saccade-Related Activity

Figure 57.32 shows saccade-related MEG signals, averaged on the basis of the saccade onsets (Jousmäki et al., 1996). The MEG channels close to the orbits recorded eyeball-related signals. Two other signal maxima were observed, one in the parietal midline and another in the lowest posterior channels. Source modeling suggested that the former response was generated in the POS region and the latter signal in cerebellar vermis. Both source activations peaked about 170 msec after the saccade onset, and the cerebellar signal started already 30 msec before the saccade. The POS signal was abolished when the lights of the experimental room were turned off, whereas the cerebellar response was only slightly delayed. The possibility to noninvasively follow the temporal behavior of human cerebellar activation

may open new windows to monitoring of neurological patients. Early cerebellar signals related to somatosensory stimulation have been observed (Tesche and Karhu, 1997), as have oscillations anticipating omissions of somatosensory stimuli (Tesche and Karhu, 2002).

Human Mirror-Neuron System

MEG recordings have been recently used for studies of the human mirror-neuron system (MNS). Mirror neurons were first described in monkey premotor cortical area F5 (Rizzolatti et al., 1996); the neurons discharged both when a monkey executed a hand action and when he observed a similar action made by another monkey or by the experimenter; the neurons assumed to match action, observation, and execution (for a review, see Rizzolatti et al., 2001). In humans, the MNS comprises at least the primary motor cortex (Fig. 57.13) and Broca's area, with contributions from superior temporal sulcus and inferior parietal lobe. These areas are activated in a specific order during viewing of other person's motor acts (Nishitani and Hari, 2000, 2002). Moreover, the primary and secondary somatosensory cortices react to observed hand movements. The human MNS may play an important role both in action imitation and in understanding the meaning of actions made by other subjects, thereby also having relevance for social interactions (for a recent review, see Hari and Nishitani, 2003).

Conclusions

MEG has established a position as a tool of basic neuroscience, and clinical applications have started to rapidly develop as neuromagnetometers with whole-scalp coverage have been installed in hospital environments. During the last few years, a combination of functional information, deduced from MEG, and structural information, obtained from MRI, has become routine, and co-registration of MEG and fMRI data has started to become popular as well. Instead of instrumental development, which already has reached a very user-friendly stage, the efforts of the neuromagnetism community

Figure 57.32. MEG signals from three locations (shown on the schematic head) during a visually guided saccade task. The signals were averaged with respect to the onset of horizontal saccades (leftward or rightward); the horizontal EOG used as the trigger is depicted above. Signals recorded during darkness and with lights on are illustrated with *dashed* and *solid lines,* respectively. (Adapted from Jousmäki, V., Hämäläinen, M., and Hari, R. 1996. Magnetic source imaging during a visually guided task. Neuroreport 7:2961–2964.)

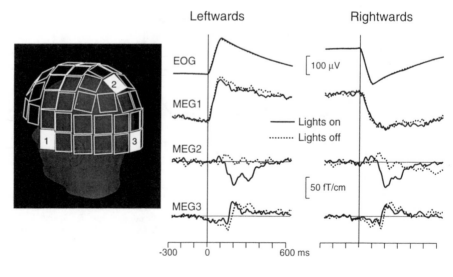

are now increasingly focusing on development of new signal analysis approaches (e.g., Baillet et al., 2001).

MEG's clinical applications in neurology, neurosurgery and audiology are expanding rapidly, and the method will probably be useful also in developmental neuroscience and in neuropsychiatry. In addition to conventional studies of the auditory, visual, and somatomotor systems, stimulation techniques are available to obtain selective MEG responses also from olfactory and gustatory systems, and reliable data have been obtained with real-life-like stimulation. With the whole-scalp neuromagnetometers, MEG can be applied in a variety of behavioral conditions, designed for assessment of neural basis of cognitive functions.

MEG allows studies of the temporal activation order of several cortical areas, thereby offering new noninvasive information of basic functions of the human brain. A clinical neurophysiologist naturally looks for practical applications, appropriate to the functional assessment of sensory pathways and the cortex. In this respect, MEG's ability to locate sources of various electric signals, which are frequently measured with scalp EEG, is very helpful. Better knowledge of cortical evoked responses and spontaneous rhythms will further widen the clinical scope of both EEG and MEG recordings. The necessity to map and interpret complex dynamical activation sequences of cortical circuitries requires future clinical neurophysiologists to obtain good understanding about modern electrophysiological and imaging methods, but also about system-level basic and cognitive neuroscience.

Acknowledgments

This study has been supported by the Academy of Finland and the Sigrid Jusélius Foundation. The skill, support, and enthusiasm of the members of the Brain Research Unit of the Low Temperature Laboratory, Helsinki University of Technology have been decisive for collecting the MEG data presented in this chapter.

References

Ahlfors, S., Ilmoniemi, R., and Hämäläinen, M. 1992. Estimates of visually evoked cortical currents. Electroencephalogr. Clin. Neurophysiol. 82: 225–236.

Aine, C.J. 1995. A conceptual overview and critique of functional neuroimaging techniques in humans: I. MRI/fMRI and PET. Crit. Rev. Neurobiol. 9:229–309.

Aine, C., Supek, S., George, J., et al. 1996. Retinotopic organization of human visual cortex: departures from the classical model. Cereb. Cortex 6:354–361.

Aine, C., Okada, Y.C., Stroink, G., et al. (Eds.) 1997. *Advances in Biomagnetism: Biomag96.* New York: Springer-Verlag.

Alho, K. 1995. Cerebral generators of mismatch negativity (MMN) and its magnetic counterpart (MMNm) elicited by sound changes. Ear Hear. 16: 38–51.

Anderson, S.J., Holliday, I.E., Singh, K.D., et al. 1996. Localization and functional analysis of human cortical area V5 using magneto-encephalography. Proc. R. Soc. Lond. B 263:423–431.

Antervo, A., Hari, R., Katila, T., et al. 1985. Magnetic fields produced by eye blinking. Electroencephalogr. Clin. Neurophysiol. 61:247–254.

Arthur, D., Lewis, P., Medwick, P., et al. 1991. A neuromagnetic study of selective auditory attention. Electroencephalogr. Clin. Neurophysiol. 78: 348–360.

Baillet, S., Mosher, J.C., and Leahy, R.M. 2001. Electromagnetic brain mapping. IEEE Signal Proc Magaz. 18:14–30.

Barkley, G.L., and Baumgartner, C. 2003. MEG and EEG in Epilepsy. J. Clin. Neurophysiol. 20:163–178.

Barkley, G., Moran, J., Takanashi, Y., et al. 1991. Techniques for DC magnetoencephalography. J. Clin. Neurophysiol. 8:189–199.

Barth, D., Sutherling, W., Engel, J.J., et al. 1982. Neuromagnetic localization of epileptiform spike activity in the human brain. Science 218: 891–894.

Barth, D.S., Sutherling, W., Engel, J., et al. 1984. Neuromagnetic evidence of spatially distributed sources underlying epileptiform spikes in the human brain. Science 223:293–296.

Baumgartner, C. 1993. *Clinical Neurophysiology of the Somatosensory Cortex.* Wien: Springer-Verlag.

Baumgartner, C., Deecke, L., Stroink, G., et al. (Eds.) 1995. *Biomagnetism: Fundamental Research and Clinical Applications.* Amsterdam: Elsevier.

Baumgartner, C., Pataraia, E., Lindinger, G. et al. 2000. Magnetoencephalography in focal epilepsy. Epilepsia 41(suppl 3):S39–47.

Bente, D. 1964. *Die Insuffizienz des Vigilitätstonus.* Habilitationsschrift. University of Erlangen-Nürnberg.

Bernander, O., Douglas, R., Martin, K., et al. 1991. Synaptic background activity influences spatiotemporal integration in single pyramidal cells. Proc. Natl. Acad. Sci. USA 88:11569–11573.

Bragard, D., Chen, A.C., and Plaghki, L. 1996. Direct isolation of ultra-late (C-fibre) evoked brain potentials by CO_2 laser stimulation of tiny cutaneous surface areas in man. Neurosci. Lett. 209:81–84.

Brenner, D., Williamson, S.J., and Kaufman, L. 1975. Visually evoked magnetic fields of the human brain. Science 190:480–481.

Brenner, D., Lipton, J., Kaufman, L., et al. 1978. Somatically evoked magnetic fields of the human brain. Science 199:81–83.

Brown, P. 2000. Cortical drives to human muscle: the Piper and related rhythms. Prog. Neurobiol. 60:97–108.

Brown, P., Salenius, S., Rothwell, J.C., et al. 1998. The cortical correlate of the Piper rhythm in man. J. Neurophysiol. 80:2911–2917.

Brown, P., Marsden, J., Defebvre, L., et al. 2001. Intermuscular coherence in Parkinson's disease: relationship to bradykinesia. Neuroreport 12: 2577–2581.

Buser, P. 1987. Thalamocortical mechanisms underlying synchronized EEG activity. In *A Textbook of Clinical Neurophysiology,* Eds. A. Halliday, S. Butler, and R. Paul, pp. 595–621. Chichester: John Wiley & Sons.

Calvert, G.A., Bullmore E.T., Brammer M.J., et al. 1997. Activation of auditory cortex during silent lipreading. Science 276:593–596.

Chapman, R.M., Ilmoniemi, R.J., Barbanera, S., et al. 1984. Selective localization of alpha brain activity with neuromagnetic measurements. Electroencephalogr. Clin. Neurophysiol. 58:569–572.

Cohen, D. 1968. Magnetoencephalography: evidence of magnetic field produced by alpha-rhythm currents. Science 161:784–786.

Cohen, D. 1972. Magnetoencephalography: detection of the brain's electrical activity with a superconducting magnetometer. Science 175:664–666.

Cohen, D., and Cuffin, B. 1983. Demonstration of useful differences between MEG and EEG. Electroencephalogr. Clin. Neurophysiol. 56: 38–51.

Colding-Jørgensen, E., Lauritzen, M., Johnsen, N.J., et al. 1992. On the evidence of auditory evoked magnetic fields as an objective measure of tinnitus. Electroencephalogr. Clin. Neurophysiol. 83:322–327.

Conway, B., Halliday, D., Farmer, S., et al. 1995. Synchronization between motor cortex and spinal motoneuronal pool during the performance of a maintained motor task in man. J. Physiol. 489:917–924.

Cooper, R., Winter, A., Crow, H., et al. 1965. Comparison of subcortical, cortical and scalp activity using chronically indwelling electrodes in man. Electroencephalogr. Clin. Neurophysiol. 18:217–228.

Cornelissen, K., Laine, M., Tarkiainen, A., et al. 2003. Adult brain plasticity elicited by anomia treatment. J. Cogn. Neurosci. 15:444–461.

Cornelissen, P., Tarkiainen, A., Helenius, P., et al. 2003. Cortical effects of shifting letter position in letter strings of varying length. J. Cogn. Neurosci. 15:731–746.

Cuffin, B. 1985. Effects of fissures in the brain on electroencephalograms and magnetoencephalograms. J. Appl. Phys. 57:146–153.

Curio, G., Mackert, B., Burghoff, M., et al. 1994. Localization of evoked neuromagnetic 600 Hz activity in the cerebral somatosensory system. Electroencephalogr. Clin. Neurophysiol. 91:483–487.

Curio, G., Drung, D., Koch, H., et al. 1996. Magnetometry of evoked fields from human peripheral nerve, brachial plexus and primary somatosensory cortex using a liquid nitrogen cooled superconducting quantum interference device. Neurosci. Lett. 206:204–206.

Del Gratta, C., Pizzella, V., Tecchio, F., et al. 2001. Magnetoencephalography—a noninvasive brain imaging method with 1 ms time resolution. Rep. Progr. Physics 64:1759–1814.

Del Gratta, C., Della Penna, S., Ferretti, A., et al. 2002. Topographic organization of the human primary and secondary somatosensory cortices: comparison of fMRI and MEG findings. NeuroImage 17:1373–1383.

Duret, D., and Karp, P. 1984. Figure of merit and spatial resolution of superconducting flux transformers. J. Appl. Phys. 56:1762–1768.

Ebersole, J.S. 1996. New applications of EEG/MEG in epilepsy evaluation. Epilepsy Res. Suppl. 11:227–237.

Elberling, C., Bak, C., Kofoed, B., et al. 1980. Magnetic auditory responses from the human brain. A preliminary report. Scand. Audiol. 9:185–190.

Elbert, T., Pantev, C., Wienbruch, C., et al. 1995. Increased cortical representation of the fingers of the left hand in string players. Science 270: 305–307.

ffytche, D.H., Guy, C.N., and Zeki, S. 1995. The parallel visual motion inputs into areas V1 and V5 of human cerebral cortex. Brain 118:1375–1394.

Forss, N., Hari, R., Salmelin, R., et al. 1994a. A novel source area in the human parietal cortex activated by median nerve stimulation. Exp. Brain. Res. 99:309–315.

Forss, N., Salmelin, R., and Hari, R. 1994b. Comparison of somatosensory evoked fields to airpuff and electric stimuli. Electroencephalogr. Clin. Neurophysiol. 92:510–517.

Forss, N., Jousmäki, V., and Hari, R. 1995a. Interaction in the human somatosensory cortex between afferent input from different fingers. Brain Res. 685:68–76.

Forss, N., Mäkelä, J.P., Keränen, T., et al. 1995b. Trigeminally triggered epileptic facial convulsions. Neuroreport 6:918–920.

Forss, N., Merlet, I., Vanni, S., et al. 1996. Activation of human mesial cortex during somatosensory attention task. Brain Res. 734:229–235.

Forss, N., Hietanen, M., and Hari, R. 1999. Modified activation of somatosensory cortical network in patients with right hemisphere stroke. Brain 122:1889–1899.

Forss, N., Nakasato, N., Ebersole, J., et al. 2000. Clinical use of magnetoencephalography. Suppl. Clin. Neurophysiol. 53:287–297.

Forss, N., Silén, T., and Karjalainen, T. 2001. Lack of activation of human secondary somatosensory cortex in Unverricht-Lundborg type of progressive myoclonus epilepsy. Ann. Neurol. 49:90–97.

Forss, N., Raij, T., Seppä, M., et al. 2004. Common cortical network for first and second pain. Neuroimage, under revision.

Fujiki, N., Jousmäki, V., and Hari, R. 2002. Neuromagnetic responses to frequency-tagged sounds: A new method to follow inputs from each ear to the human auditory cortex during binaural hearing. J. Neurosci. 22: RC205(1–4).

Fujita, S., Nakasato, N., Matani, A., et al. 1995. Short latency somatosensory evoked field for tibial nerve stimulation: rotation of dipole pattern over the whole head. In Biomagnetism: Fundamental Research and Clinical Applications, Eds. C. Baumgartner, L. Deecke, G. Stroink, et al., pp. 95–98. Amsterdam: Elsevier.

Furey, M.L., Tanskanen, T., Beauchamp, M., et al. 2004. Modulation of early and late neural responses to faces and houses by selective attention. Submitted.

Galambos, R., Makeig, S., and Talmachoff, P.J. 1981. A 40-Hz auditory potential recorded from the human scalp. Proc. NY Acad. Sci. 78:2643–2647.

Gallen, C., Schwartz, B., Pantev, C., et al. 1992. Detection and localization of delta frequency activity in human stroke. In Biomagnetism. Clinical Aspects, Eds. M. Hoke, S.N. Erné, Y.C. Okada, et al., pp. 301–305. Amsterdam: Excerpta Medica.

Galletti, C., Battaglini, P., and Fattori, P. 1995. Eye position influence on the parieto-occipital area PO (V6) of the macaque monkey. Eur. J. Neurosci. 7:2486–2501.

Gootjes, L., Raij, T., Salmelin, R., et al. 1999. Left-hemisphere dominance for processing of vowels: a whole-scalp neuromagnetic study. Neuroreport 10:2987–2991.

Grandori, F., Hoke, M., and Romani, G.-L. (Eds.) 1990. Auditory Evoked Magnetic Fields and Potentials. Advances in Audiology, Vol 6. Basel: Karger.

Gray, M., and Singer, W. 1989. Stimulus-specific neuronal oscillations in orientation columns of cat visual cortex. Proc. Natl. Acad. Sci. U.S.A. 86:1698–1702.

Gross, J., Timmermann, L., Kujala, J., et al. 2002. The neural basis of intermittent motor control in humans. Proc. Natl. Acad. Sci. U.S.A. 99: 2299–2302.

Gutschalk, A., Mase, R., Roth, R., et al. 1999. Deconvolution of 40 Hz steady-state fields reveals two overlapping source activities of the human auditory cortex. Clin. Neurophysiol. 110:856–868.

Hadjikhani, N., Sanchez del Rio, M., Wu, O., et al. 2001. Mechanisms of migraine aura revealed by functional MRI in human visual cortex. Proc. Natl. Acad. Sci. U.S.A. 98:4687–4692.

Halgren, E., Raij, T., Marinkovic, K., et al. 2000. Cognitive response profile of the human fusiform area as determined by MEG. Cereb. Cortex 10:69–81.

Hämäläinen, M., and Hari, R. 2002. Magnetoencephalographic characterization of dynamic brain activation: Basic principles, and methods of data collection and source analysis. In Brain Mapping. The Methods, Eds. A.W. Toga and J.C. Mazziotta, 2nd ed., pp. 227–253. Amsterdam: Academic Press.

Hämäläinen, M., and Ilmoniemi, R. 1994. Interpreting magnetic fields of the brain: minimum norm estimates. Med. Biol. Engn. Comp. 32: 35–42.

Hämäläinen, M.S., and Sarvas, J. 1989. Realistic conductivity geometry model of the human head for interpretation of neuromagnetic data. IEEE Trans. Biomed. Eng. BME-36:165–171.

Hämäläinen, M., Hari, R., Ilmoniemi, R., et al. 1993. Magnetoencephalography—theory, instrumentation, and applications to noninvasive studies of the working human brain. Rev. Mod. Physics 65:413–497.

Hari, R. 1990. The neuromagnetic method in the study of the human auditory cortex. In Auditory Evoked Magnetic Fields and Potentials. Advances in Audiology, vol. 6, Eds. F. Grandori, M. Hoke, and G. Romani, pp. 222–282. Basel: Karger.

Hari, R. 1991. On brain's magnetic responses to sensory stimuli. J. Clin. Neurophysiol. 8:157–169.

Hari, R. 1997. Neuromagnetic approach to human auditory cortical functions, with emphasis on subjects with cochlear implants. In Cochlear Implant and Related Sciences Update. Adv. Otorhinolaryngol., Vol. 52. Eds. I. Honjo and H. Takahashi, pp. 15–18. Basel: Karger.

Hari, R., and Forss, N. 1999, Magnetoencephalography in the study of human somatosensory cortical processing. Proc. Royal Soc. Lond. B 354:1145–1154.

Hari, R., and Ilmoniemi, R.J. 1986. Cerebral magnetic fields. CRC Crit. Rev. Biomed. Engin. 14:93–126.

Hari, R., and Imada, T. 1999. Ipsilateral movement-evoked fields (MEFs) reconsidered. NeuroImage 10:582–588.

Hari, R., and Lounasmaa, O.V. 1989. Recording and interpretation of cerebral magnetic fields. Science 244:432–436.

Hari, R., and Nishitani, N. 2004. From viewing of movement to imitation and understanding of other persons' acts: MEG studies of the human mirror-neuron system. Functional Neuroimaging of Visual Cognition. Attention and Performance XX. Eds. N. Kanwisher and J. Duncan, pp. 463–479. Oxford: Oxford University Press.

Hari, R., and Salmelin, R. 1997. Human cortical rhythms: a neuromagnetic view through the skull. Trends Neurosci. 20:44–49.

Hari, R., and Salenius, S. 1999. Rhythmical corticomuscular communication. Neuroreport 10:R1–R10.

Hari, R., Aittoniemi, K., Järvinen, M.L., et al. 1980. Auditory evoked transient and sustained magnetic fields of the human brain. Localization of neural generators. Exp. Brain Res. 40:237–240.

Hari, R., Kaila, K., Katila, T., et al. 1982. Interstimulus-interval dependence of the auditory vertex response and its magnetic counterpart: implications for their neural generation. Electroencephalogr. Clin. Neurophysiol. 54:561–569.

Hari, R., Hämäläinen, M., Kaukoranta, E., et al. 1983a. Neuromagnetic responses from the second somatosensory cortex in man. Acta Neurol. Scand. 68:207–212.

Hari, R., Kaukoranta, E., Reinikainen, K., et al. 1983b. Neuromagnetic localization of cortical activity evoked by painful dental stimulation in man. Neurosci. Lett. 42:77–82.

Hari, R., Reinikainen, K., Kaukoranta, E., et al. 1984. Somatosensory evoked cerebral magnetic fields from SI and SII in man. Electroencephalogr. Clin. Neurophysiol. 57:254–263.

Hari, R., Pelizzone, M., Mäkelä, J.P., et al. 1987. Neuromagnetic responses of the human auditory cortex to on- and offsets of noise bursts. Audiology 25:31–43.

Hari, R., Joutsiniemi, S.L., and Sarvas, J. 1988a. Spatial resolution of neuromagnetic records: theoretical calculations in a spherical model. Electroencephalogr. Clin. Neurophysiol. 71:64–72.

Hari, R., Pelizzone, M., Mäkelä, J., et al. 1988b. Neuromagnetic responses from a deaf subject to stimuli presented through a multichannel cochlear prosthesis. Ear Hear. 9:148–152.

Hari, R., Hämäläinen, M., and Joutsiniemi, S.L. 1989a. Neuromagnetic steady-state responses to auditory stimuli. J. Acoust. Soc. Am. 86:1033–1039.

Hari, R., Hämäläinen, M., Kaukoranta, E., et al. 1989b. Selective listening modifies activity of the human auditory cortex. Exp. Brain Res. 74:463–470.

Hari, R., Hämäläinen, H., Tiihonen, J., et al. 1990. Separate finger representations at the human second somatosensory cortex. Neuroscience 37:245–249.

Hari, R., Ahonen, A., Forss, N., et al. 1993a. Parietal epileptic mirror focus detected with a whole-head neuromagnetometer. Neuroreport 5:45–48.

Hari, R., Karhu, J., Hämäläinen, M., et al. 1993b. Functional organization of the human first and second somatosensory cortices: a neuromagnetic study. Eur. J. Neurosci. 5:724–734.

Hari, R., Salmelin, R., Tissari, S., et al. 1994. Visual stability during eyeblinks. Nature 367:121–122.

Hari, R., Nagamine, T., Nishitani, N., et al. 1996. Time-varying activation of different cytoarchitectonic areas of the human SI cortex after tibial nerve stimulation. NeuroImage 4:111–118.

Hari, R., Portin, K., Kettenmann, B., et al. 1997. Right-hemisphere preponderance of responses to painful CO_2 stimulation of the human nasal mucosa. Pain 72:145–151.

Hari, R., Forss, N., Avikainen, S., et al. 1998. Activation of human primary motor cortex during action observation: a neuromagnetic study. Proc. Natl. Acad. Sci. U.S.A. 95:15061–15065.

Hari, R., Forss, N., and Raij, TT. 2003. Neuromagnetic exploration of the connection between pain and the motor cortex. In *Psyche, Soma and Pain. Acta Gyllenbergiana IV,* Eds. E. Kalso, A.-M. Estlander, and M. Klockars, pp. 145–153. Helsinki: Signe and Ane Gyllenberg Foundation.

Hashimoto, I., Mashiko, T., and Imada, T. 1996a. Somatic evoked high-frequency magnetic oscillations reflect activity of inhibitory interneurons in the human somatosensory cortex. Electroencephalogr. Clin. Neurophysiol. 100:189–203.

Hashimoto, I., Okada, Y.C., and Ogawa, S. (Eds.) 1996b. *Visualization of Information Processing in the Human Brain.* Amsterdam: Elsevier.

Hashimoto, I., Sakuma, K., Kimura, T., et al. 2001. Serial activation of distinct cytoarchitectonic areas of the human SI cortex after posterior tibial nerve stimulation. Neuroreport 12:1857–1862.

Heikman, P., Salmelin, R., Mäkelä, J., et al. 2001. Relation between the frontal 3–7 Hz MEG activity and the efficacy of ECT in major depression. J. ECT 17:136–140.

Helenius, P., Salmelin, R., Service, E., et al. 1999. Semantic cortical activation in dyslexic readers. J. Cogn. Neurosci. 11:535–550.

Hillebrand, A., and Barnes, G.R. 2002. A quantitative assessment of the sensitivity of whole-head MEG to activity in the adult human cortex. NeuroImage 16:638–650.

Hoke, M., Feldman, H., Pantev, C., et al. 1989a. Objective evidence of tinnitus in auditory evoke magnetic fields. Hear. Res. 37:281–286.

Hoke, M., Pantev, C., Lütkenhöner, B., et al. 1989b. Magnetic fields from the auditory cortex of a deaf human individual occurring spontaneously or evoked by stimulation through a cochlear prosthesis. Audiol. 28:152–170.

Hughes, J.R., Hendrix, D.E., Cohen, J., et al. 1976. Relationship of the magnetoencephalogram to the electroencephalogram. Normal wake and sleep activity. Electroencephalogr. Clin. Neurophysiol. 40:261–278.

Huttunen, J., Kobal, G., Kaukoranta, E., et al. 1986. Cortical responses to painful CO_2 stimulation of the nasal mucosa. Electroencephalogr. Clin. Neurophysiol. 64:347–349.

Huttunen, J., Kaukoranta, E., and Hari, R. 1987. Cerebral magnetic responses to stimulation of tibial and sural nerves. J. Neurol. Sci. 79:43–54.

Huttunen, J., Wikström, H., Korvenoja, A., et al. 1996. Significance of the second somatosensory cortex in sensorimotor integration: enhancement of sensory responses during finger movements. Neuroreport 7:1009–1012.

Ilmoniemi, R. 1995. Radial anisotropy added to a spherically symmetric conductor does not affect the external magnetic field due to internal sources. Europhys. Lett. 30:313–316.

Ilmoniemi, R., Williamson, S., and Hostetler, W. 1987. Method for the study of spontaneous brain activity. In *Biomagnetism '87,* Eds. K. Atsumi, M. Kotani, M. Ueno, et al., pp. 182–185. Tokyo: Tokyo Denki University Press.

Ishii, R., Dziewas, R., Chau, W., Sörös, P., et al. 2003. Current source density distribution of sleep spindles in humans as found by synthetic aperture magnetometry. Neurosci. Lett. 340:25–28.

Iwasaki, M., Nakasato, N., Shamoto, H., et al. 2002. Surgical implications of neuromagnetic spike localization in temporal lobe epilepsy. Epilepsia 43:415–424.

Jack, C., Marsh, W., Hirschorn, K., et al. 1990. EEG scalp electrode projections onto three-dimensional surface rendered images of the brain. Radiology 176:413–418.

Jacobson, G., Ahmad, B., Moran, J., et al. 1991. Auditory evoked cortical magnetic field (M100/M200) measurements in tinnitus and normal groups. Hear. Res. 56:44–52.

Jäntti, V., Baer, G., Yli-Hankala, A., et al. 1995. MEG burst suppression in an anaesthesized dog. Acta Anaesth. Scand. 39:126–128.

Jeavons, P. 1964. The electro-encephalogram in blind children. Br. J. Ophthalmol. 48:83–101.

Jensen, O., Goel, P., Ermentrout, B., et al. 2003. On the benzodiazepine-induced beta rhythm in the human motor cortex: sources and modelling. Submitted.

Jensen, O., Pohja, M., Goel, P., et al. 2002. On the physiological basis of the 15–30 Hz motor-cortex rhythm. In *Proceedings of the 13th International Conference on Biomagnetism;* Eds. H. Nowak, J. Haueisen, F. Giessler and R. Huonkler, pp. 313–315 Berlin: VDE Verlag GMBH.

Joliot, M., Ribary, M., and Llinas, R. 1994. Human oscillatory brain activity near 40 Hz coexists with cognitive temporal binding. Proc. Natl. Acad. Sci. U.S.A. 91:11748–11751.

Joseph, J., Howland, E., Wakai, R., et al. 1991. Late pain-related magnetic fields and electric potentials evoked by intracutaneous electric finger stimulation. Electroencephalogr. Clin. Neurophysiol. 80:46–52.

Jousmäki, V. and Hari, R. 1996. Cardiac artifacts in magnetoencephalogram. J. Clin. Neurophysiol. 13:172–176.

Jousmäki, V., Hämäläinen, M., and Hari, R. 1996. Magnetic source imaging during a visually guided task. Neuroreport 7:2961–2964.

Juottonen, K., Gockel, M., Silén, T., et al. 2002. Altered central sensorimotor processing in patients with complex regional pain syndrome. Pain 98:315–323.

Kakigi, R., Koyama, S., Hoshiyama, M., et al. 1995a. Pain-related magnetic fields following painful CO_2 laser stimulation in man. Neurosci. Lett. 192:45–48.

Kakigi, R., Koyama, S., Hoshiyama, M., et al. 1995b. Topography of somatosensory evoked magnetic fields following posterior tibial nerve stimulation. Electroencephalogr. Clin. Neurophysiol. 95:127–134.

Kakigi, R., Tran, T.D., Qiu, Y., et al. 2003. Cerebral responses following stimulation of unmyelinated C-fibers in humans: electro- and magnetoencephalographic study. Neurosci. Res. 45:255–275.

Kanda, M., Nagamine, T., Ikeda, A., et al. 2000. Primary somatosensory cortex is actively involved in pain processing in human. Brain Res. 853:282–289.

Kaneko, K., Fujiki, N., and Hari, R. 2003. Binaural interaction in the human auditory cortex revealed by neuromagnetic frequency-tagging: No effect of stimulus intensity. Hearing Res. 183:1–6.

Karhu, J., Hari, R., Mäkelä, J., et al. 1992. Somatosensory evoked magnetic fields in multiple sclerosis. Electroencephalogr. Clin. Neurophysiol. 83:192–200.

Karhu, J., Hari, R., Paetau, R., et al. 1994. Cortical reactivity in progressive myoclonus epilepsy. Electroencephalogr. Clin. Neurophysiol. 90:93–102.

Kaufman, L., Schwarz, B., Salustri, et al. 1990. Modulation of spontaneous brain activity during mental imagery. J. Cogn. Neurosci. 2:124–132.

Kaukoranta, E., Hari, R., Hämäläinen, M., et al. 1986a. Cerebral magnetic fields evoked by peroneal nerve stimulation. Somatosens. Res. 3:309–321.

Kaukoranta, E., Hämäläinen, M., Sarvas, J. et al. 1986b. Mixed and sensory nerve stimulations activate different cytoarchitectonic areas in the human primary somatosensory cortex SI. Exp. Brain Res. 63:60–66.

Kaukoranta, E., Hari, R., and Lounasmaa, O.V. 1987. Responses of the human auditory cortex to vowel onset after fricative consonants. Exp. Brain Res. 69:19–23.

Kilner, J., Baker, S., Salenius, S., et al. 2000. Human cortical muscle coherence is directly related to specific motor parameters. J. Neurosci. 20:8838–8845.

Kilner, J.M., Salenius, S., Baker, S.N., et al. 2003. Task-dependent modulations of cortical oscillatory activity in human subjects during a bimanual precision grip task. NeuroImage 18:67–73.

Knowlton, R.C. 2003. Magnetoencephalography: clinical application in epilepsy. Curr. Neurol. Neurosci. Rep. 3:341–348.

Korvenoja, A., Wikström, H., Huttunen, J., et al. 1995. Activation of ipsilateral primary sensorimotor cortex by median nerve stimulation. Neuroreport 6:2589–2593.

Kuriki, S., and Takeuchi, F. 1991. Neuromagnetic responses elicited by auditory stimuli in dichotic listening. Electroencephalogr. Clin. Neurophysiol. 80:406–411.

Lamusuo, S., Forss, N., Ruottinen, H.-M., et al. 1999. [18F]FDG-PET and whole-scalp MEG localization of epileptogenic cortex. Epilepsia 40: 921–930.

Lauronen, L., Heikkilä, E., Autti, T., et al. 1997. Somatosensory evoked magnetic fields from primary sensorimotor cortex in juvenile neuronal ceroid lipofuscinosis. J. Child Neurol. 12:355–360.

Lauronen, L., Huttunen, J., Kirveskari, E., et al. 2002. Enlarged SI and SII somatosensory evoked responses in the CLN5 form of neuronal ceroid lipofuscinosis. Clin. Neurophysiol. 113:1491–1500.

Lehtelä, L., Salmelin, R., and Hari, R. 1997. Evidence for reactive magnetic 10-Hz rhythm in the human auditory cortex. Neurosci. Lett. 222:111–114.

Leinonen, L., and Joutsiniemi, S.L. 1989. Auditory evoked potentials and magnetic fields in patients with lesions of the auditory cortex. Acta Neurol. Scand. 79:316–325.

Lin, Y.-Y., Chang, K.-P., Hsieh, J.-C., et al. 2003. Magnetoencephalographic analysis of bilaterally synchronous discharges in benign rolandic epilepsy of childhood. Seizure 12:448–455.

Linkenkaer-Hansen, K., Palva, J.M., Sams, M., et al. 1998. Face-selective processing in human extrastriate cortex around 120 ms after stimulus onset revealed by magneto- and electroencephalography. Neurosci. Lett. 253:147–150.

Liu, J., Harris, A., and Kanwisher, N. 2002. Stages of processing in face perception: an MEG study. Nat. Neurosci. 5:910–916.

Llinas, R. 1990. Intrinsic electrical properties of mammalian neurons and CNS function. In Fidia Research Foundation Neuroscience Award Lectures, pp. 175–194. New York: Raven Press.

Llinas, R., and Ribary, U. 1993. Coherent 40-Hz oscillation characterizes dream state in humans. Proc. Natl. Acad. Sci. USA 90:2078–2081.

Lounasmaa, O.V., Williamson, S.J., Kaufman, L., et al. 1985. Visually evoked responses from non-occipital areas of human cortex. In Biomagnetism: Applications and Theory, Eds. H. Weinberg, G. Stroing, and T. Katila, pp. 348–353. New York: Pergamon Press.

Lounasmaa, O.V., Hämäläinen, M., Hari, R., et al. 1996. Information processing in the human brain—magnetoencephalographic approach. Proc. Natl. Acad. Sci. USA 93:8809–8815.

Lu, Z.L., and Kaufman, L. (Eds.) 2003. Magnetic Source Imaging of the Human Brain. Mahwah, NJ: Lawrence Erlbaum.

Lu, S., Hämäläinen, M., Hari, R., et al. 1991. Seeing faces activates three brain areas outside the occipital visual cortex in man. Neuroscience 43: 287–290.

Lu, S.T., Kajola, M., Joutsiniemi, S.L., et al. 1992a. Generator sites of spontaneous MEG activity during sleep. Electroencephalogr. Clin. Neurophysiol. 82:182–196.

Lu, Z.L., Wang, J.Z., and Williamson, S. 1992b. Neuronal sources of human parieto-occipital alpha rhythm. In Biomagnetism. Clinical Aspects, Eds. M. Hoke, S. Erne, Y. Okada, et al., pp. 33–37. Amsterdam: Excerpta Medica.

Lu, Z.L., Williamson, S., and Kaufman, L. 1992c. Behavioral lifetime of human auditory sensory memory predicted by physiological measures. Science 258:1668–1670.

Lütkenhöner, B. 1992. Frequency-domain localization of intracerebral dipolar sources. Electroencephalogr. Clin. Neurophysiol. 82:112–118.

Lütkenhöner, B., Krumbholtz, K., and Seither-Preisler, A. 2003. Studies of tonotopy based on wave N100 of the auditory evoked field are problematic. NeuroImage 9:935–949.

Maclin, E., Okada, Y., Kaufman, L., et al. 1983. Retinotopic map on the visual cortex for eccentrically placed patterns: first noninvasive measurement. Nuovo Cimento 2D:410–419.

Maess, B., Koelsch, S., Gunter, T.C., et al. 2001. Musical syntax is processed in Broca's area: an MEG study. Nat. Neurosci. 4:540–545.

Mäkelä, J.P. 1996. Neurological application of MEG. In Visualization of Information Processing in the Human Brain: Recent Advances in MEG and Functional MRI (EEG Suppl. 47), Eds. I. Hashimoto, Y. Okada, and S. Ogawa, pp. 343–355. Elsevier.

Mäkelä, J., and Hari, R. 1987. Evidence for cortical origin of the 40-Hz auditory evoked response in man. Electroencephalogr. Clin. Neurophysiol. 66:539–546.

Mäkelä, J.P., and Hari, R. 1992. Neuromagnetic auditory evoked responses after a stroke in the right temporal lobe. Neuroreport 3:94–96.

Mäkelä, J.P., Hari, R., and Linnankivi, A. 1987. Different analysis of frequency and amplitude modulations of a continuous tone in the human auditory cortex: A neuromagnetic study. Hear. Res. 27:257–264.

Mäkelä, J.P., Hari, R., and Leinonen, L. 1988. Magnetic responses of the human auditory cortex to noise/tone-transitions. Electroencephalogr. Clin. Neurophysiol. 69:423–430.

Mäkelä, J.P., Hari, R., Valanne, L., and Ahonen, A. 1991. Auditory evoked magnetic fields after ischemic brain lesions. Ann. Neurol. 30:76–82.

Mäkelä, J.P., Ahonen, A., Hämäläinen, M., et al. 1993a. Functional differences between auditory cortices of the two hemispheres revealed by whole-head neuromagnetic recordings. Human Brain Mapp. 1:48–56.

Mäkelä, J.P., Hari, R., Karhu, J., et al. 1993b. Suppression of magnetic mu rhythm during Parkinsonian tremor. Brain Res. 617:189–193.

Mäkelä, J.P., Hämäläinen, M., Hari, R., et al. 1994. Whole-head mapping of middle-latency auditory evoked fields. Electroencephalogr. Clin. Neurophysiol. 92:414–421.

Mäkelä, J.P., Salmelin, R., Hokkanen, L., et al. 1998a. Neuromagnetic sequelae of herpes simplex encephalitis. Electroencephalogr. Clin. Neurophysiol. 106:251–258.

Mäkelä, J.P., Salmelin, R., Kotila, M., et al. 1998b. Modification of neuromagnetic cortical signals by thalamic infarctions. Electroencephalogr. Clin. Neurophysiol. 106:433–443.

Mäkelä, J., Kirveskari, E., Seppä, M., et al. 2001. Three-dimensional integration of brain anatomy and function to facilitate intraoperative navigation around the sensorimotor strip. Human Brain Mapp. 12:181–192.

Mauguière, F., Merlet, I., Forss, N., et al. 1997. Activation of a distributed somatosensory cortical network in the human brain. A dipole modelling study of magnetic fields evoked by median nerve stimulation. Part I: Location and activation timing of SEF sources. Electroencephalogr. Clin. Neurophysiol. 104:281–289.

McEvoy, L., Hari, R., Imada, T., et al. 1993. Human auditory cortical mechanisms of sound lateralization: II. Interaural time differences at sound onset. Hear. Res. 67:98–109.

McEvoy, L., Mäkelä, J.P., Hämäläinen, M., et al. 1994. Effect of interaural time differences on middle-latency and late auditory evoked magnetic fields. Hear. Res. 78:249–257.

Merlet, I., Paetau, R., Garcia-Larrea, L., et al. 1997. Apparent asynchrony between interictal electric and magnetic spikes. Neuroreport 8: 1971–1076.

Mertens, M., and Lütkenhöner, B. 2000. Effective neuromagnetic determination of landmarks in the somatosensory cortex. Clin. Neurophysiol. 111:1478–1487.

Michel, C.M., Kaufman, L., and Williamson, S.J. 1994. Duration of EEG and MEG-α suppression increases with angle in a mental rotation task. J. Cogn. Neurosci. 6:139–150.

Modena, I., Ricci, G.B., Barbanera, S., et al. 1982. Biomagnetic measurements of spontaneous brain activity in epileptic patients. Electroencephalogr. Clin. Neurophysiol. 54:622–628.

Morrell, F., Whisler, W.W., Smith, M.C., et al. 1995. Landau-Kleffner syndrome. Treatment with subpial intracortical transection. Brain 118:1529–1546.

Muhlnickel, W., Elbert, T., Taub, E., et al. 1998. Reorganization of auditory cortex in tinnitus. Proc. Natl. Acad. Sci. U.S.A. 95:10340–10343.

Näätänen, R. 1992. Attention and Brain Function. Hillsdale, NJ: Lawrence Erlbaum.

Näätänen, R. 2003. Mismatch negativity: clinical research and possible applications. Int. J. Psychophysiol. 48:179–188.

Näätänen, R., and Picton, T. 1987. The N1 wave of the human electric and magnetic response to sound: a review and analysis of the component structure. Psychophysiology 24:375–425.

Näätänen, R., Ilmoniemi, R., and Alho, K. 1994. Magnetoencephalography in studies of human cognitive brain function. Trends Neurosci. 17: 389–395.

Nagamine, T., Kajola, M., Salmelin, R., et al. 1996. Movement-related slow cortical magnetic fields and changes of spontaneous brain rhythms. Electroencephalogr. Clin. Neurophysiol. 99:274–296.

Nagarajan, S., Mahncke, H., Salz, T., et al. 1999. Cortical auditory signal processing in poor readers. Proc. Natl. Acad. Sci. U.S.A. 96:6483–6488.

Nakasato, N., Kado, H., Nakanishi, M., et al. 1990. Magnetic detection of sleep spindles in normal subjects. Electroencephalogr. Clin. Neurophysiol. 76:123–130.

Nakasato, N., Seki, K., Kawamura, T., et al. 1996. Cortical mapping using an MRI-linked whole head MEG system and presurgical decision making. In *Visualization of Information Processing in the Human Brain: Recent Advances in MEG and Functional MRI (EEG Suppl. 47)*, Eds. I. Hashimoto, Y. Okada, and S. Ogawa, pp. 333–341. Elsevier.

Narici, L., and Peresson, M. 1995. Discrimination and study of rhythmical brain activities in a band: a neuromagnetic frequency responsiveness test. Brain Res. 703:31–44.

Narici, L., Forss, N., Jousmäki, V., et al. 2001. Evidence for a 7- to 9-Hz 'sigma' rhythm in the human SII cortex. NeuroImage 13:662–668.

Niedermeyer, E. 1982. Depth electroencephalography. In *Electroencephalography. Basic Principles, Clinical Applications and Related Fields*, Eds. E. Niedermeyer, and F. Lopes da Silva, pp. 519–536. Baltimore–Munich: Urban & Schwarzenberg.

Niedermeyer, E. 1990. Alpha-like rhythmical activity of the temporal lobe. Clin. Electroencephalogr. 21:210–224.

Niedermeyer, E. 1991. The 'third rhythm': further observations. Clin. Electroencephalogr. 22:83–96.

Nishitani, N., and Hari, R. 2000. Temporal dynamics of cortical representation for action. Proc. Natl. Acad. Sci. U.S.A. 97:913–918.

Nishitani, N., and Hari, R. 2002. Viewing lip forms: Cortical dynamics. Neuron 36:1211–1220.

Nishitani, N., Nagamine, T., Fujiwara, N., et al. 1998. Cortical-hippocampal auditory processing identified by magnetoencephalography. J. Cogn. Neurosci. 10:231–247.

Numminen, J., Ahlfors, S., Ilmoniemi, R., et al. 1995. Transformation of multichannel magnetoencephalographic signals to standard grid form. IEE Trans. Biomed. Engn. 42:72–77.

Numminen, J., Mäkelä, J., and Hari, R. 1996. Distribution and sources of magnetoencephalographic K-complexes. Electroencephalogr. Clin. Neurophysiol. 99:544–555.

Nunez, P.L. 1989. Estimation of large scale neocortical source activity with EEG surface Laplacians. Brain Topogr. 2:141–154.

Okada, Y. 1990. Magnetoencephalography as a noninvasive tool for electrophysiological characterization of auras in classic migraine. In *Advances in Neurology, Vol. 54, Magnetoencephalography*, Ed. S. Sato, pp. 133–140. New York: Raven Press.

Okada, Y.C., Papuashvili, N., and Xu, C. 1996. Maximum current dipole moment density as an important physiological constraint in MEG inverse solutions. Tenth International Conference on Biomagnetism, Santa Fe, NM, Volume of Abstracts, p. 149.

Paetau, R. 1994. Sounds trigger spikes in the Landau-Kleffner syndrome. J. Clin. Neurophysiol. 11:231–241.

Paetau, R., Kajola, M., and Hari, R. 1990. Magnetoencephalography in the study of epilepsy. Neurophysiol. Clinique 20:169–187.

Paetau, R., Kajola, M., Korkman, M., et al. 1991. Landau-Kleffner syndrome: epileptic activity in the auditory cortex. Neuroreport 2: 201–204.

Paetau, R., Kajola, M., Karhu, J., et al. 1992. Magnetoencephalographic localization of epileptic cortex—impact on surgical treatment. Ann. Neurol. 32:106–109.

Paetau, R., Hämäläinen, M., Hari, R., et al. 1994. Presurgical MEG evaluation of children with intractable epilepsy. Epilepsia 35:275–284.

Paetau, R., Granström, M.L., Blomstedt, G., et al. 1999. Magnetoencephalography in presurgical evaluation of children with the Landau-Kleffner syndrome. Epilepsia 40:326–335.

Pantev, C., Hoke, M., Lehnertz, K., et al. 1988. Tonotopic organization of the human auditory cortex revealed by transient auditory evoked magnetic fields. Electroencephalogr. Clin. Neurophysiol. 69:160–170.

Pantev, C., Hoke, K., Lehnertz, K., et al. 1989a. Neuromagnetic evidence of an amplitopic organization of the human auditory cortex. Electroencephalogr. Clin. Neurophysiol. 72:225–231.

Pantev, C., Hoke, M., Lütkenhöner, B., et al. 1989b. Tinnitus remission objectified by neuromagnetic measurements. Hear. Res. 40:261–264.

Pantev, C., Engelien, A., Candia, V. et al. 2001. Representational cortex in musicians. Plastic alterations in response to musical practice. Ann. N.Y. Acad. Sci. 930:300–314.

Pastor, M.A., Artieda, J., Arbizu, J., et al. 2002. Activation of human cerebral and cerebellar cortex by auditory stimulation at 40 Hz. J. Neurosci. 22:10501–10506,

Pekkonen, E., Huotilainen, M., Virtanen, J., et al. 1996. Alzheimer's disease affects parallel processing between the auditory cortices. Neuroreport 7:1365–1368.

Pelizzone, M., Hari, R., Mäkelä, J., et al. 1987a. Cortical activity evoked by a multichannel cochlear prosthesis. Acta Otolaryngol. 103:632–636.

Pelizzone, M., Hari, R., Mäkelä, J.P., et al. 1987b. Cortical origin of middle-latency auditory evoked responses in man. Neurosci. Lett. 82:303–307.

Pernier, J., Perrin, F., and Bertrand, O. 1988. Scalp current density fields: concept and properties. Electroencephalogr. Clin. Neurophysiol. 69:385–389.

Petroni, F., Panzeri, S., Hilgetag, C.C., et al. 2001. Simultaneity of responses in a hierarchical visual network. Neuroreport 12:2753–2759.

Pfurtscheller, G., and Aranibar, A. 1977. Event-related desynchronization detected by power measurements of scalp EEG. Electroencephalogr. Clin. Neurophysiol. 42:138–146.

Ploner, M., Schmitz, F., Freund, H.J., et al. 1999. Parallel activation of primary and secondary somatosensory cortices in human pain processing. J. Neurophysiol. 81:3100–3104.

Ploner, M., Gross, J., Timmermann, L., et al. 2002. Cortical representation of first and second pain sensation in humans. Proc. Natl. Acad. Sci. U.S.A. 99:12444–12448.

Portin, K., Salenius, S., Salmelin, R., et al. 1998. Activation of the human occipital and parietal cortex by pattern and luminance stimuli: neuromagnetic measurements. Cereb. Cortex 8:253–260.

Raij, T., McEvoy, L., Mäkelä, J., et al. 1997. Human auditory cortex is activated by omissions of auditory stimuli. Brain Res. 745:134–143.

Raij, T.T., Forss, N., Stancak, A., et al. 2003. Noxious input activates the human motor cortex: implications for tension-type pain? Soc. Neurosci. Ann. Meet. 2003, No. 238.3.

Raij, T.T., Forss, N., Stancak, A., et al. 2004. Modulation of motor-cortex oscillatory activity by painful A-and C-fiber stimuli. Neuroimage. in press

Renvall, H., and Hari, R. 2003. Diminished auditory mismatch fields in dyslexic adults. Ann. Neurol. 53:551–557.

Ribary, U., Ioannides, A., Singh, K., et al. 1991. Magnetic field tomography of coherent thalamocortical 40-Hz oscillation in humans. Proc. Natl. Acad. Sci. USA 88:11037–11041.

Rif, J., Hari, R., Hämäläinen, M., et al. 1991. Auditory attention affects two different areas in the human auditory cortex. Electroencephalogr. Clin. Neurophysiol. 79:464–472.

Rizzolatti, G., Fadiga, L., Gallese, V., et al. 1996. Premotor cortex and the recognition of motor actions. Brain Res. Cogn. Brain Res. 3:131–141.

Rizzolatti, G., Fogassi, L., and Gallese, V. 2001. Neurophysiological mechanisms underlying the understanding and imitation of action. Nat. Rev. Neurosci. 2:661–670.

Romani, G., and Leoni, R. 1985. Localization of cerebral sources by neuromagnetic measurements. In *Biomagnetism: Applications and Theory*, Eds. H. Weinberg, G. Stroink, and T. Katila, pp. 205–220. Oxford: Pergamon.

Romani, G.L., Williamson, S.J., and Kaufman, L. 1982. Tonotopic organization of the human auditory cortex. Science 216:1339–1340.

Rose, D.F., Smith, P.D., and Sato, S. 1987. Magnetoencephalography and epilepsy research. Science 238:329–335.

Ross, B., Picton, T.W., and Pantev, C. 2002. Temporal integration in the human auditory cortex as represented by the development of the steady-state magnetic field. Hear. Res. 165:68–84.

Salenius, S., and Hari, R. 2003. Synchronous oscillatory cortical acivity during motor action. Curr. Opin. Neurobiol. 13:678–684.

Salenius, S., Kajola, M., Thompson, W.L., et al. 1995. Reactivity of magnetic parieto-occipital alpha rhythm during visual imagery. Electroencephalogr. Clin. Neurophysiol. 95:453–462.

Salenius, S., Salmelin, R., Neuper, C., et al. 1996. Human cortical 40-Hz rhythm is closely related to EMG rhythmicity. Neurosci. Lett. 21:75–78.

Salenius, S., Portin, K., Kajola, M., et al. 1997a. Cortical control of human motoneuron firing during isometric contraction. J. Neurophysiol. 77: 3401–3405.

Salenius, S., Schnitzler, A., Salmelin, R., et al. 1997b. Modulation of human rolandic rhythms during natural sensorimotor tasks. NeuroImage 5:221–228.

Salenius, S., Avikainen, S., Kaakkola, S., et al. 2002. Defective cortical drive to muscle in Parkinson's disease and its improvement with levodopa. Brain 125:491–500.

Salmelin, R., and Hari, R. 1994a. Characterization of spontaneous MEG rhythms in healthy adults. Electroencephalogr. Clin. Neurophysiol. 91: 237–248.

Salmelin, R., and Hari, R. 1994b. Spatiotemporal characteristics of rhythmic neuromagnetic activity related to thumb movement. Neuroscience 60:537–550.

Salmelin, R., and Hämäläinen, M. 1995. Dipole modelling of MEG rhythms in time and frequency domains. Brain Topogr. 7:251–257.

Salmelin, R., Hari, R., Lounasmaa, O.V., et al. 1994. Dynamics of brain activation during picture naming. Nature 368:463–465.

Salmelin, R., Hämäläinen, M., Kajola, M., et al. 1995. Functional segregation of movement-related rhythmic activity in the human brain. NeuroImage 2:237–243.

Salmelin, R., Mäkelä, J.P., Heikman, P., et al. 1996a. Human brain rhythms and electroconvulsive therapy. Soc. Neurosci. Abstr. 22(Pt 1):342.

Salmelin, R., Service, E., Kiesilä, P., et al. 1996b. Impaired visual word processing in dyslexia revealed with magnetoencephalography. Ann. Neurol. 40:157–162.

Salmelin, R., Helenius, P., and Service, E. 2000a. Neurophysiology of fluent and impaired reading: a magnetoencephalographic approach. J. Clin. Neurophysiol. 17:163–174.

Salmelin, R., Schnitzler, A., Schmitz, F., et al. 2000b. Single word reading in developmental stutterers and fluent speakers. Brain 123:1184–1202.

Samonas, M., Petrou, M., and Ioannides, A. 1997. Identification and elimination of cardiac contribution in single-trial magnetoencephalographic signals. IEEE Trans. Biomed. Engn. 44:386–393.

Sams, M., Aulanko, R., Hämäläinen, M., et al. 1991. Seeing speech: visual information from lip movements modifies activity in the human auditory cortex. Neurosci. Lett. 127:141–145.

Sams, M., Hari, R., Rif, J., et al. 1993a. The human auditory sensory memory trace persists about 10 s: neuromagnetic evidence. J. Cogn. Neurosci. 5:363–370.

Sams, M., Hämäläinen, M., Hari, R., et al. 1993b. Human auditory cortical mechanisms of sound lateralization: I. Interaural time differences within sound. Hear. Res. 67:89–97.

Sams, M., Hietanen, J., Hari, R., et al. 1997. Face-specific responses from the human inferior occipitotemporal cortex. Neuroscience 77:49–55.

Santamaria, J., and Chiappa, K. 1987. The EEG of drowsiness in normal adults. J. Clin. Neurophysiol. 4:327–382.

Sasaki, K., Tsujimoto, T., Nambu, A., et al. 1994. Dynamic activities of the frontal association cortex in calculating and thinking. Neurosci. Res. 19: 229–233.

Sato, S. (Eds.). 1990. *Magnetoencephalography. Advances in Neurology, vol. 54.* New York: Raven Press.

Scherg, M. 1990. Fundamentals of dipole source potential analysis. In *Auditory Evoked Magnetic Fields and Potentials, Advances in Audiology, Vol. 6,* Eds. F. Grandori, M. Hoke, and G.L. Romani, pp. 40–69. Basel: Karger.

Scheuler, W., Kubicki, S., Scholz, G., et al. 1990. Two different activities in the sleep spindle frequency band–discrimination based on the topographical distribution of spectral power and coherence. In *Sleep '90,* Eds. J. Horne, pp. 13–16. Bochum: Pontenagel Press.

Schmolesky, M.T., Wang, Y., Hanes, D.P., et al. 1998. Signal timing across the macaque visual system. J. Neurophysiol. 79:3272–3278.

Schnitzler, A., Salmelin, R., Salenius, S., et al. 1995. Tactile information from the human hand reaches the ipsilateral primary somatosensory cortex. Neurosci. Lett. 200:25–28.

Schnitzler, A., Salenius, S., Salmelin, R., et al. 1997. Involvement of primary motor cortex in motor imagery: a neuromagnetic study. NeuroImage 6:201–208.

Shiomi, Y., Nagamine, T., Fujiki, N., et al. 1997. Tinnitus remission by lidocaine demonstrated by auditory-evoked magnetoencephalogram. Acta Otolaryngol. (Stockh.) 117:31–34.

Simões, C., Mertens, M., Forss, N., et al. 2001. Functional overlap of finger representations in human SI and SII cortices. J. Neurophysiol. 86:1661–1665.

Simões, C., Alary, F., Forss, N., et al. 2002. Left-hemisphere-dominant SII activation after bilateral median nerve stimulation. NeuroImage 15:686–690.

Simões, C., Jensen, O., Parkkonen, L., et al. 2003. Phase locking between human primary and secondary somatosensory cortices. Proc. Natl. Acad. Sci. U.S.A. 100:2691–2694.

Stefan, H., Schneider, S., Abraham-Fuchs, K., et al. 1991. The neocortico-to mesio-basal limbic propagation of focal epileptic activity during the spike-wave complex. Electroencephalogr. Clin. Neurophysiol. 79:1–10.

Stenbacka, L., Vanni, S., Uutela, K., et al. 2002. Comparison of minimum current estimate and dipole modeling in the analysis of simulated activity in the human visual cortices. NeuroImage 16: 936–943.

Suk, J., Ribary, U., Cappell, J., et al. 1991. Anatomical localization revealed by MEG recordings of the human somatosensory system. Electroencephalogr. Clin. Neurophysiol. 78:185–196.

Sutherling, W.W., and Barth, D.S. 1989. Neocortical propagation in temporal lobe spike foci on magnetoencephalography and electroencephalography. Ann. Neurol. 25:373–381.

Sutherling, W., Crandall, P., Darcey, T., et al. 1988. The magnetic and electric fields agree with intracranial localizations of somatosensory cortex. Neurology 38:1705–1714.

Tabuchi, H., Yokoyama, T., Shimogawara, M., et al. 2002. Study of the visual evoked magnetic field with the m-sequence technique. Invest. Ophthalmol. Vis. Sci. 43:2045–2054.

Tallon-Baudry, C., Bertrand, O., Wienbruch, C., et al. 2000. Combined EEG and MEG recordings of visual 40 Hz responses to illusory triangles in human. Prog. Neurobiol. 60:97–108.

Tarkiainen, A., Liljeström, M., Seppä, M., et al. 2003. The 3D topography of MEG source localization accuracy: effects of conductor model and noise. Clin Neurophysiol. 114:1977–1992.

Tesche, C.D. 1996. Non-invasive imaging of neuronal population dynamics in human thalamus. Brain Res. 729:253–258.

Tesche, C.D. 1997. Non-invasive detection of ongoing neuronal population activity in normal human hippocampus. Brain Res. 749:53–60.

Tesche, C., and Kajola, M. 1993. A comparison of the localization of spontaneous neuromagnetic activity in the frequency and time domains. Electroencephalogr. Clin. Neurophysiol. 87:408–416.

Tesche, C.D., and Karhu, J. 1997. Somatosensory evoked magnetic fields arising from sources in the human cerebellum. Brain Res. 744:23–31.

Tesche, C.D., and Karhu, J.Y. 2000. Anticipatory cerebellar response during somatosensory omission in man. Human Brain Mapp. 9:119–142.

Tesche, C.D., Uusitalo, M.A., Ilmoniemi, R.J., et al. 1995. Signal-space projections of MEG data characterize both distributed and well-localized neuronal sources. Electroencephalogr. Clin. Neurophysiol. 95:189–200.

Teyler, T.J., Cuffin, B.N., and Cohen, D. 1975. The visual magnetoencephalogram. Life Sci. 17:683–692.

Tiihonen, J., Hari, R., and Hämäläinen, M. 1989a. Early deflections of cerebral magnetic responses to median nerve stimulation. Electroencephalogr. Clin. Neurophysiol. 74:290–296.

Tiihonen, J., Kajola, M., and Hari, R. 1989b. Magnetic mu rhythm in man. Neuroscience 32:793–800.

Tiihonen, J., Hari, R., Kajola, M., et al. 1990. Localization of epileptic foci using a large-area magnetometer and functional brain anatomy. Ann. Neurol. 27:283–290.

Tiihonen, J., Hari, R., Kajola, M., et al. 1991. Magnetoencephalographic 10-Hz rhythm from the human auditory cortex. Neurosci. Lett. 129:303–305.

Tiihonen, J., Hari, R., Naukkarinen, H., et al. 1992. Auditory hallucinations may modify activity of the human auditory cortex. Am. J. Psychiatry 149:255–257.

Timmermann, L., Gross, J., Dirks, M., et al. 2003. The cerebral oscillatory network of parkinsonian resting tremor. Brain 126:199–212.

Tuunanen, P.I., Kavec, M., Jousmäki, V., et al. 2003. Comparison of BOLD fMRI and MEG characteristics to vibrotactile stimulation. NeuroImage 19:1778–1786.

Ueno, S., and Iramina, K. 1990. Modeling and source localization of MEG activities. Brain Topogr. 3:151–165.

Uusitalo, M., and Ilmoniemi, R. 1997. Signal-space projection method for separating MEG and EEG into components. Med. Biol. Engn. Comp. 35:135–140.

Uusitalo, M., Jousmäki, V., and Hari, R. 1997a. Activation trace lifetime of human cortical responses evoked by apparent visual motion. Neurosci. Lett. 224:45–48.

Uusitalo, M., Virsu, V., Salenius, S., et al. 1997b. Human cortical activation related to perception of visual motion and movement after-effect. NeuroImage 5:241–250.

Uutela, K., Hämäläinen, M., and Somersalo, E. 1999. Visualization of magnetoencephalographic data using minimum current estimates. NeuroImage 10:173–180.

Vanni, S., Revonsuo, A., and Hari, R. 1997. Modulation of the parieto-occipital alpha rhythm during object detection. J. Neurosci. 17: 7141–7147.

Vanni S., Tanskanen, T., Seppä, M., et al. 2001. Coinciding early activation of human primary visual cortex and anteromedial cuneus. Proc. Natl. Acad. Sci. USA 98:2776–2780.

Van't Ent, D., Manshanden, I., Ossenblok, P., et al. 2003. Spike cluster analysis in neocortical localization related epilepsy yields clinically significant equivalent source localization results in magnetoencephalogram (MEG). Clin. Neurophysiol. 114:1948–1962.

Vasama, J.P., and Mäkelä, J.P. 1995. Auditory pathway plasticity in adult humans after idiopathic sudden unilateral sensorineural hearing loss. Hear. Res. 87:132–140.

Vasama, J.P., Mäkelä, J.P., Parkkonen, L., et al. 1994a. Auditory cortical responses in humans with congential unilateral conductive hearing loss. Hear. Res. 78:91–97.

Vasama, J.P., Mäkelä, J.P., Pyykkö, I., et al. 1994b. Modification of central auditory pathways after unilateral permanent deafness due to removal of acoustic neuroma. Neuroreport 6:961–964.

Vieth, J., Sack, G., Schueler, P., et al. 1989. Ischemic and epileptic lesions measured by AC- and DC-MEG. In *Advances in Biomagnetism,* Eds. S.

Williamson, M. Hoke, G. Stroink, et al., pp. 307–310. New York: Plenum Press.

Volkmann, J., Joliot, M., Mogilner, A., et al. 1996. Central motor loop oscillations in parkinsonian resting tremor revealed by magnetoencephalography. Neurology 46:1359–1370.

Vvedensky, V., Hari, R., Ilmoniemi, R., et al. 1985. Physical basis of neuromagnetic fields. Biophys. 30:154–158.

Vvedensky, V., Ilmoniemi, R., and Kajola, M. 1986. Study of the alpha rhythm with a 4-channel SQUID magnetometer. Med. Biol. Eng. Comput. 23:11–12.

Watanabe, Y., Fukao, K., Watanabe, M., et al. 1996. Epileptic events observed by multichannel MEG. In *Visualization of Information Processing in the Human Brain: Recent Advances in MEG and Functional MRI (EEG Suppl. 47),* Eds. I. Hashimoto, Y. Okada, and S. Ogawa, pp. 283–391. Elsevier.

Williamson, S., Wang, J.-Z., and Ilmoniemi, R. 1989. Method for locating sources of human alpha activity. In *Advances in Biomagnetism,* Eds. S. Williamson, M. Hoke, G. Stroink, et al., pp. 257–260. New York: Plenum Press.

Yang, T.T., Gallen, C.C., Schwartz, B.J., et al. 1993. Noninvasive somatosensory homunculus mapping in humans by using a large-array biomagnetometer. Proc. Natl. Acad. Sci. USA 90:3098–3102.

Yoshiura, Y., Ueno, S., Iramina, K., et al. 1994. Effects of stimulation site on human middle latency auditory evoked magnetic fields. Neurosci. Lett. 172:159–162.

58. EEG Analysis: Theory and Practice

Fernando Lopes da Silva

Analysis of electroencephalography (EEG) signals always involves questions of quantification; such questions may concern the precise value of the dominant frequency and the similarity between two signals recorded from symmetric derivations at the same time or different times. In these examples, there is a question that can be solved only by taking measures with regard to the EEG signal. Without such measures, EEG appraisal remains subjective and can hardly lead to logical systematization. Classic EEG evaluation has always involved measuring frequency and/or amplitude with the help of simple rulers. The limitations of such simple methods are severe, particularly when large amounts of EEG data must be evaluated and the need for data reduction is felt strongly, as well as when rather sophisticated questions are being asked, such as whether EEG signal changes occur in relation to internal or external factors, and how synchronous are EEG phenomena occurring in different derivations.

Clear replies to these questions require some form of EEG analysis. However, such analysis is not only a problem of quantification; it also involves elements of pattern recognition. Every electroencephalographer knows that it is sometimes extremely difficult to cite exact measures for such EEG phenomena as spikes, sharp waves, or other abnormal patterns; the experienced specialist is able to detect them only by "eyeballing." These types of problems may be solved using pattern recognition analysis techniques, based on the principle that features characteristic of the EEG phenomena have to be measured. This phase of *feature extraction* is followed by *classification* of the phenomena into different groups. EEG analysis thus implies not only simple quantification but also feature extraction and classification.

The primary aim of EEG analysis is to support electroencephalographers' evaluations with objective data in numerical or graphic form. EEG analysis, however, can go further, actually extending electroencephalographers' capabilities by giving them new tools with which they can perform such difficult tasks as quantitative analysis of long-duration EEG in epileptic patients and sleep and psychopharmacological studies.

The choice of analytic method should be determined mainly by the goal of the application, although budget limitations must also be taken into consideration. The development of an appropriate strategy rests on such practical facts as whether analysis results must be available in real time and online or may be presented offline. In the past, the former requirement would pose considerable problems, solvable only by adopting a rather simple form of analysis; the development of new computer technology has provided more acceptable solutions. Another practical consideration is the number of derivations to be analyzed and whether the corresponding topographic relations have to be determined or the analysis of one or two derivations is enough; the latter may suffice during anesthesia monitoring or in sleep research. Whether the analysis of a relatively short EEG epoch is sufficient or must involve very long records, for instance up to 24 hours, is another important factor.

In short, the *method* of analysis must be suited to the *purpose* of the analysis. Among the different purposes are the following: (a) determining whether a relatively short EEG record taken in a routine laboratory is normal or abnormal; (b) classifying an EEG as abnormal, for example as epileptiform or hypofunctional; (c) evaluating changes occurring in serial electroencephalography; and (d) evaluating trends during many hours of EEG monitoring, such as under intensive care conditions for heart surgery or in long-term recordings in epileptic patients.

General Characteristics

The EEG is a complex signal, the statistical properties of which depend on both time and space. Regarding the temporal characteristics, it is essential to note that EEG signals are ever-changing. However, they can be analytically subdivided into representative epochs (i.e., with more or less constant statistical properties).

Estimates of the length of such epochs vary considerably because of dependence on the subject's behavioral state. When the latter is kept almost constant, Isaksson and Wennberg (1976) found that, over relatively short time intervals, epochs can be defined that can be considered representative of the subject's state; in this study, some 90% of the EEG signals investigated had time-invariant properties after 20 seconds, whereas less than 75% remained time invariable after 60 seconds. Empirical observations indicate that EEG records obtained under equivalent behavioral conditions show highly stable characteristics; for example, Dumermuth et al. (1976) showed that variations in mean peak (beta activity) of only 0.8 Hz were obtained in a series of 11 EEGs over 29 weeks. In this respect it is interesting to consider the studies of Jansen (1979) and Grosveld et al. (1976); these authors investigated the possibility of correctly assigning EEG epochs (duration 10.24 seconds) to the corresponding subject by means of multivariate analysis, using half of the EEG epochs recorded from 16 subjects as a training set for the classification algorithm. Using 4 to 10 EEG features, it was found that in 80% to 90% of the cases of EEG epochs were assigned correctly to the corresponding subject. McEwen and Anderson (1975) introduced the concept of wide-sense stationarity in EEG analysis; they proposed a procedure for determining whether a set of signal samples (e.g., an EEG signal) can be considered to belong to a wide-sense stationarity process. Their procedure consisted of calculating the amplitude distributions and power spectra of sample subsets and showing that they do not differ significantly using the Kolmogorov-Smirnov statistic. From this study it was concluded that, for EEG epochs (awake condition or during anesthesia) of less than 32 seconds, the assumption of wide-sense stationarity was valid more than 50% of the time.

On the basis of this type of empirical observation, it can be assumed that relatively short EEG epochs (~10 sec) recorded under constant behavioral conditions are quasi-stationary. Elul (1972) remarked that the EEG is related to intermittent changes in the synchrony of cortical neurons; thus he characterized the EEG as a series of short epochs rather than a continuous process.

The fact that EEG signals have different characteristics depending on the place over the head where they are recorded is essential to all EEG recordings. Therefore, in any method of EEG analysis, topographic characteristics have to be taken into account. This means that one should choose EEG montages carefully, in view of the objectives of the analysis. The topographic aspects appear most clearly in the simple case of comparing EEG records from symmetrical derivations; indeed, the use of the subject as his or her own control through right-left comparisons is a cornerstone of the neurological examination. Therefore, right-left comparisons are also paramount in any practical clinical system of EEG analysis.

Basic Statistical Properties

Some of the underlying assumptions of the most common methods of EEG analysis will be discussed briefly. Gasser (1977) has provided a more fundamental discussion of this topic; here, general concepts will suffice.

The exact characteristics of EEG signals are, in general terms, unpredictable. This means that one cannot foresee precisely the amplitude of an EEG graphoelement or the duration of an EEG wave. Therefore, it is said that an EEG signal is a realization of a *random* or *stochastic* process. Indeed, it is possible to determine some statistical measures of EEG signals that show considerable regularity, such as an average amplitude or an average frequency. This is a general characteristic of random processes, which are characterized by probability distributions and their moments (e.g., mean, variance, skewness, and kurtosis) or by frequency spectra or correlation functions. Such a description of an EEG signal as a realization of a random process implies a mathematical, but not a biophysical, model.

It should be stressed (Siebert, 1959) that the biophysical process underlying EEG generation is not necessarily random in nature, but it may have such a high degree of complexity that only a description in statistical terms is justified. Gasser (1977) has also emphasized this point; even in the case of signals that are deterministic (e.g., sinusoids) but very complex (e.g., made of many components), a stochastic approach may be the most adequate.

EEG signals are, of course, time series; they are characterized by a set of values as a function of time. An important problem, however, is whether the general methods for analyzing time series can be applied without restrictions to EEG signals.

In Chapter 4, which discusses EEG dynamics, it was mentioned that modern mathematical tools are being used to analyze EEG signals, assuming that signal generation can be described using sets of nonlinear differential equations. These techniques have been developed within the active field of mathematical research called "deterministic chaos." In essence, nonlinear dynamic systems such as the neuronal networks generating EEG signals can display chaotic behavior; that is, their behavior can become unpredictable for relatively long periods, and EEG signals may be an expression of chaotic behavior. Since new mathematical tools, based on the analysis of complex nonlinear systems such as the correlation dimension were introduced in electroencephalography, it became clear that EEG signals may be high-dimensional so that in many cases it is difficult, or even impossible, to distinguish whether these signals are generated by random or by high-dimensional nonlinear deterministic processes (Pijn et al., 1991).

Sampling, Probability Distributions, Correlation Functions, and Spectra

EEG signals are continuous variations of potential as a function of time. However, in most practical cases where quantitative analysis is applied, signals must be digitized so they can be processed by digital computer. This means that the EEG signal must be processed in such a way that the random variable, potential as a function of time, will have only one set of discrete values at a set of discrete time instances. In technical terms, the process of analog-to-digital (AD) conversion involves *sampling* combined with the operation of *quantizing*. According to definitions commonly used (Jay, 1977), sampling is the "process of obtaining a sequence of instantaneous values of a wave at regular or intermittent intervals" and quantization is the "process in which the continuous range of values of an input signal is divided into non-overlapping sub-ranges and to each sub-range a discrete value of the output is uniquely assigned."

EEG signal sampling must be performed without changing the statistical properties of the continuous signal. Generally, one samples an EEG signal at equidistant time intervals (Δt), thus transforming the continuous signal into a set of impulses with different heights separated by intervals Δt (Fig. 58.1). An important question is the choice of the sampling frequency. This choice is based on the *sampling theorem*: assuming that a signal x(t) has a frequency spectrum X(f) such that X(f) = 0 for f_N; no information is lost by sampling x(t) at equidistant intervals Δt with $f_N = 1/(2\Delta t)$; f_N is called the folding or Nyquist frequency. The sampling frequency, therefore, must be at least equal to $2f_N$. A consequence of this theorem is that care has to be taken to ensure that the signal to be sampled has no frequency components above f_N. Therefore, before sampling, all frequency components greater than f_N should be eliminated by low-pass filtering. One should keep in mind that sampling at a frequency below $2f_N$ is not equivalent to filtering; it would produce aliasing or signal distortion due to folding of frequency components larger than f_N onto lower frequencies (Lopes da Silva et al., 1976). The analogue voltages of the signal at the sampling moments are converted

SAMPLING

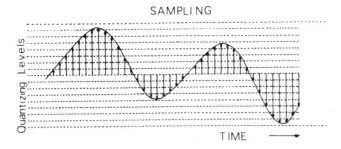

TIME ⟶

Figure 58.1. Analog-to-digital (AD) conversion of the continuous signal is performed at equidistant time intervals, digitizing its amplitude according to the corresponding quantizing levels. (Adapted from Lopes da Silva, F.H., Cooper, R., Dumermuth, G., et al. 1976. Sampling, conversion, and measurement of bioelectrical phenomena. In *Handbook of Electroencephalography and Clinical Neurophysiology,* Ed.-in-chief, A. Remond, vol. 4, Ed., M.A. Brazier, Part A. Amsterdam: Elsevier.)

to a number corresponding to the amplitude subrange or level. Most EEG analysis can be performed using 512 to 2048 amplitude levels (i.e., 9–11 bits). Technical details of AD conversion may be found in Susskind (1957) and, for the special case of EEG signals, in Lopes da Silva et al. (1976) and Steineberg and Paine (1964).

The continuous EEG signal is thus replaced by a string of numbers $x(t_i)$ representing the signal amplitude at sequential sample moments; the latter are indicated by the index i along the time axis. The signal is assumed to be a realization of a stationary random process $\underline{x}(t_i)$, which is indicated by underlining the letter ($\underline{x}$). In general, a collection of EEG signals of a certain length recorded under equivalent conditions is available for analysis. The entire collection of EEG signals is called an *ensemble*; each member of the ensemble is called a sample function or a *realization.*

Probability Distributions

The digitized EEG signal values $x(t_i)$ can be considered realizations of one stochastic variable $\underline{x}(t_i)$ and may be characterized when stationarity is assumed by a histogram; when in an interval $0 > t > T$ there are n_a sample points in the interval $a \pm 1/2\Delta$, n_a/N is called the relative frequency of occurrence of the value a, where N is the total number of samples available. One can define the relative frequencies of all other values similarly. When N becomes infinitely large and Δ infinitely small, n_a/N will tend to a limit value $p(x(t_i) = a)$, called the probability of occurrence of $x(t_i) = a$. The set of values of $p(x(t_i))$ is called the signal *probability distribution,* characterized by a mean and a number of moments. Considering that the discrete random variable x can take any of a set of values from 1 to M, the mean or *average* of the sample functions is given as follows (E is the symbol for expectation):

$$E[\underline{x}(t_i)] = \left[\sum_{a=1}^{M} a \cdot p(\underline{x}(t_i) = a) \right] = m_i \quad (58.1)$$

Also definable is a class of statistical functions characteristic of the random process: $m_n = E[\underline{x}^n(t_i)]$ with $n = 1, 2, 3, \ldots$; these functions are called the *nth moments* of the dis-

crete random variable $\underline{x}(t_i)$. The implicit assumption here and in the following discussion is that the statistical properties of the signal do not change in the interval T. Therefore, the moments are independent of time t_i.

The first moment $E[\underline{x}(t_i)]$ is called the *mean* of $\underline{x}(t_i)$. It is often preferable to consider the *central moments* (i.e., the moments around the mean); the second central moment is then:

$$E[(\underline{x}(t_i) - E(\underline{x}(t_i)))^2] = m_2 \quad (58.2)$$

or σ^2 or *variance* of $\underline{x}(t_i)$.

Similarly, the third central moment $E[(\underline{x}(t_i)(E(\underline{x}(t_i)))^3] = m_3$ can be defined; from this can be derived the *skewness* factor $\beta_1, = m_3/(m_2)^{3/2}$. The fourth central moment is $E[(\underline{x}((t_i) - (E(\underline{x}(t_i)))^4] = m_4$, from which can be derived the *kurtosis excess:* $\beta_2 = m_4/(m_2)^2$. In case of a symmetrical amplitude, distribution is $\beta_1 = 0$; all odd moments are equal to zero. For a gaussian distribution the even moments have specific values, e.g., $\beta_2 = 3$; derivatives from this value indicate the peakedness ($\beta_2 > 3$) or flatness ($\beta_2 < 3$) of the distribution (Fig. 58.2).

Correlation Functions and Spectra

In general terms, successive values of a signal, such as an EEG, which results from a stochastic process are not necessarily independent. On the contrary, it is often found that successive discrete values of an EEG signal have a certain degree of *interdependence*. To describe this interdependence, one may compute the signal *joint probability distribution.* As

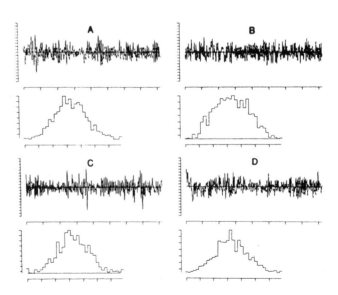

Figure 58.2. Examples of EEG signals with corresponding amplitude distributions. For the EEG signals, the time marks along the horizontal axis give the intervals in seconds; the vertical axis is in μV; for the amplitude distributions, the horizontal axis is in μV, and the vertical axis gives the number *(N)* of times a certain amplitude class has been measured in the corresponding EEG epoch. The signals were sampled at 20 Hz. The amplitude distribution of the four EEG signals has the following values of skewness (S) and kurtosis (K): **A,** S = 0.17, K = 3.09; **B,** S = 0.09, K = 2.41; **C,** S = 0.10, K = 3.37; **D,** S = 0.07, K = 2.98. The hypothesis that the amplitude distribution belongs to a normal distribution can be rejected at $p > 0.01$ whenever S > 0.464 and/or 2.45 > K > 4.13 with N = 160.

an example, consider the definition of the joint probability applied to a pair of values at two discrete moments, $\underline{x}(t_1)$ and $\underline{x}(t_2)$; assume that one disposes of N realizations of the signal; the number of times that at t_1 a value v and at t_2 a value u are encountered is equal to n_{12}. Thus, the joint probability of $\underline{x}(t_1)$ *and* $\underline{x}(t_2) = u$ may be defined as follows:

$$p(\underline{x}(t_i) = v, \underline{x}(t_2) = u) = \lim_{N \to \infty} \frac{n_{12}}{N} \quad (58.3)$$

A complete description of the properties of the signal generated by a random process can be achieved by specifying the *joint probability density function:*

$$\rho((\underline{x}(t_1), \underline{x}(t_2) \ldots \underline{x}(t_n)) \quad (58.4)$$

for every choice of the discrete time samples $t_1, t_2, \ldots t_n$ and for every finite value of n. The computation of this function, however, is rather complex. A simpler alternative to this form of description is to compute a number of *averages* characteristic of the signal, such as *covariance, correlations,* and *spectra.* These averages do not necessarily describe a stochastic signal completely, but they may be very useful for a general description of signals such as EEG.

The *covariance* between two random variables at two time samples $\underline{x}(t_1)$ and $\underline{x}(t_2)$ is given by the following expectation:

$$E[(\underline{x}(t_1) - E(\underline{x}(t_1))) \, (\underline{x}(t_2) - E(\underline{x}(t_2)))] \quad (58.5)$$

Estimating the covariance between any two variables $\underline{x}(t_1)$ and $\underline{x}(t_2)$ requires averaging over a number of realizations of an ensemble. Another way to estimate the covariance, provided that the signal is stationary and ergodic (for a discussion of these concepts see Jenkins and Watts, 1968), is by computing a time average, for one realization of the signal, of the product of the signal and a replica of itself shifted by a certain time τ_k along the time axis. This time average is called the *autocorrelation function:*

$$\Phi_{xx}(\tau_k) = \langle \underline{x}(t_i)\underline{x}(t_i + \tau_k) \rangle = \frac{1}{T} \sum_{i=1}^{N} \underline{x}(t_i)\underline{x}(t_i + \tau_k)$$
$$(58.6)$$

where $\tau_k = k \cdot \Delta t.$

The following description considers continuous random variables x(t), for the sake of simplifying the formulas. Assuming that every sample function, or realization, is representative of the whole signal being analyzed, it can be shown that for stationary and ergodic processes the time average $\Phi_{xx}(\tau)$ for one realization $\underline{x}(t)$ is an estimate of the ensemble average $R_{\underline{xx}}(\tau)$:

$$R_{\underline{xx}}(\tau) = E[x(t)\underline{x}(t + \tau)] \quad (58.7)$$

assuming that the signal $\underline{x}(t)$ has mean zero. For the value $\tau = 0,$

$$R_{\underline{xx}}(0) = E[\underline{x}^2(t)] = \lim_{T \to \infty} \frac{1}{2T} \int_{-T}^{T} \underline{x}^2(t)dt \quad (58.8)$$

which is the signal's average power or variance σ. An important property of the autocorrelation function is that its Fourier transform (FT) is:

$$S_{xx}(f) = \int_{-\infty}^{\infty} R(\tau)\exp(-j2\pi f\tau)d\tau = FT(R_{xx}(\tau)] \quad (58.9)$$

S_{xx} (f) is called the power density spectrum, or simply the *power spectrum,* a common method of EEG quantification (Fig. 58.3). The power spectrum S_{xx} (f) is a function of frequency (Hz); it gives the distribution of the squared amplitude of different frequency components. It should be noted that the word *power* does not have the meaning of dissipated power in an RC circuit but is used here in another sense. This discussion deals with a question of time series analysis. In general, a stochastic time function may be expressed in one of several ways, as a voltage, a length, a velocity, a number of occurrences of a certain event, and so forth. The power spectrum or simply the spectral density of the time function is the FT of the autocorrelation function, the dimension of which is the function's amplitude dimension squared. In case the signal dimension is in volts [V], the power spectrum is in [V²·sec] or [V²·Hz⁻¹]. Of course, if the function's amplitude is in any other dimension, the intensity of the corresponding power spectrum would be yet another dimension. It is useful to keep a clear distinction between electric power dissipated in an electric circuit (P = 1/T $\int_0^T$ V²/Rdt with units [V²·sec Ω^{-1}]) and power spectrum.

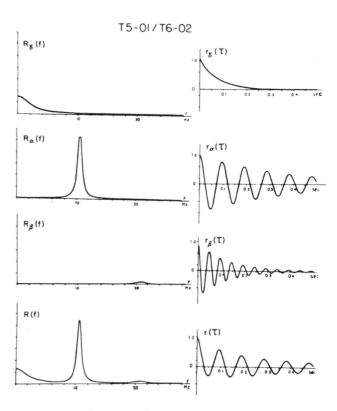

T5-0I / T6-02

Figure 58.3. The power spectrum of an EEG signal is shown in the *lower left plot;* vertical axis power indicated here as *R(f);* horizontal axis frequency, *f,* in Hz. On the lower right the corresponding autocorrelation function *r(τ)* is plotted. The power spectrum and autocorrelation functions are considered to be composed of three components (δ, α, β) corresponding to three EEG frequency bands. (Adapted from Zetterberg, L.H. 1973a. Experience with analysis and simulation of EEG signals with parametric description of spectra. In *Automation of Clinical Electroencephalography,* Eds. P. Kellaway and I. Petersen, pp. 161–201. New York: Raven.)

A function that represents the average correlation between two signals $\underline{x}(t)$ and $\underline{y}(t)$ may be defined in terms equivalent to expression 58.7:

$$R_{xy}(\tau) = E[\underline{x}(t)\underline{y}(t + \tau)] \qquad (58.10)$$

where the signals $\underline{x}(t)$ and $\underline{y}(t)$ are assumed to have means of zero. $R_{xy}(\tau)$ measures the correlation between the two signals and is called the *cross-correlation function*. Similarly, one can define the FT of R_{xy}, which is the *cross-power spectrum* between signals $\underline{x}$ and $\underline{y}$.

$$S_{xy}(f) = FT[R_{xy}(\tau)] \qquad (58.11)$$

Fundamental discussions of power spectra and related topics are found in many textbooks on signal analysis, for example Blackman and Tukey (1958), Jenkins and Watts (1968), Bendat and Piersol (1971), and Otnes and Enochson (1978). Application of the frequency analysis principle to EEG signals analysis has a long history, beginning with the pioneering work of Dietsch (1932), Grass and Gibbs (1938), Knott and Gibbs (1939), Drohocki (1938), and Walter (1943a,b). Brazier and Casby (1952) and Barlow and Brazier (1954) first computed the autocorrelation functions of EEG signals. The general principles on which this work has been based have remained essentially the same since Wiener proposed these signal analysis methods (for a review, see Wiener, 1961). An important advance in computing power spectra has been achieved with the introduction of a new algorithm for computing the *discrete Fourier transform,* known as the *fast Fourier transform* or FFT (Cooley and Tukey, 1965). In this case it is assumed that one wants to compute the power spectrum of a discrete EEG signal; the epoch $[\underline{x}(t_i)]$ is considered as a signal sampled at intervals Δt, $x(n\Delta t)$ with a total of N samples $(n = I \ldots N)$. By using the discrete FT, the so-called *periodogram* $F(f_i)$ can be computed:

$$F_{xx}(f_i) = \frac{\Delta t}{N}\left| \sum_{n=1}^{N} x(t_n)\exp(-j2\pi \cdot i\Delta f \cdot n\Delta t)\right|^2$$
$$(58.12)$$

where $f_i = i \cdot \Delta f$ with $i = 0, 1, 2 \ldots N$. The periodogram can be smoothed by means of a window $W(f_k)$ in order to obtain $P_{xx}(f_k)$, which is a better estimate of the real power spectrum $S_{xx}(f)$:

$$P_{xx}(f_i) = \sum_{k=-p}^{p} W(f_k)F_{xx}(f_{i+k}) \qquad (58.13)$$

where $W(f_k)$ is the smoothing window with a duration of $(2p + 1)$ samples or data points. Similarly, one can compute a smoothed estimate of the cross-power spectrum (S_{xy}), which might be called $(C_{xy}(f))$.

The FFT power spectral analysis and its applications are discussed in more detail below.

The close relationship between the concepts of variance σ^2, autocorrelation (equations 58.6 and 58.7), and power density spectrum (equation 58.9) has already been made apparent; in fact $R_{xx}(0) = \sigma^2$ and

$$\sigma^2 = \int_{-\infty}^{\infty} S_{xx}(f)df \qquad (58.14)$$

The autocorrelation function $R(\tau)$ and the power density spectrum $S(f)$ correspond thus to the second-order moment of the probability distribution of the random process.

In case the signals are not gaussian, higher order spectra moments must be considered. These can be derived as follows. Assuming that the signal has mean = 0, one can write (as in expression 58.7)

$$R_{xx}(\tau_1, \tau_2) = E[\underline{x}(t)\underline{x}(t + \tau_1)\underline{x}(t + \tau_2)] \qquad (58.15)$$

Similar to Expression 58.9, the two-dimensional Fourier transform FT_2 of $R_{xx}(\tau_1, \tau_2)$ can be defined as the *bispectrum* or *bispectral* density:

$$B_{xx}(f_1, f_2) = FT_2[R_{xx}(\tau_1, \tau_2)] \qquad (58.16)$$

This discussion cannot go into details about ways of estimating the bispectrum B_{xx}. For a detailed account of bispectral EEG analysis, refer to Huber et al. (1971) and to Dumermuth et al. (1971). It is, however, interesting to note that high B_{xx} values for a couple of frequencies, f_1 and f_2, indicate phase coupling within the frequency triplet f_1, f_2, and $(f_1 + f_2)$. The third moment of the probability distribution, or skewness, is related to the bispectrum. When there exists a sufficiently strong relation between two harmonically related frequency components in a signal, there will exist a significant bispectrum and skewness. The process in such a case is not gaussian; if it were gaussian with mean zero, the bispectrum would be zero. The bispectrum can be used to determine whether the system underlying the EEG generation has nonlinear properties. An example of this form of analysis is given in Fig. 58.4.

This section has demonstrated the progression from the basic principles of probability distribution and corresponding moments to the concepts of autocorrelation, power spectra, and high-order spectra. It is also of interest to examine the *moments* of the spectral density $S_{xx}(f)$, because this analysis leads to another set of concepts applicable to EEG analysis, the so-called descriptors of Hjorth (1970). Thus, one can define the nth spectral moment as follows:

$$a_n = \int_{-\infty}^{\infty} (2\pi f)^n S_{xx}(f)df \qquad (58.17)$$

The zero-order moment is then:

$$a_0 = \int_{-\infty}^{\infty} S_{xx}(f)df \qquad (58.18)$$

which is equal to the variance σ^2.

It can be shown (for derivation, see Zetterberg, 1977) that the second-order moment is defined by the following expression:

$$a_2 = \int_{-\infty}^{\infty} (2\pi f)^2 S_{xx}(f)df = -\left.\frac{d^2R_{xx}(\tau)}{d\tau^2}\right|_{\tau=0} = E\left[\frac{d\underline{x}(t)}{dt}\right]^2$$
$$(58.19)$$

and the fourth-order moment is:

$$a_4 = \int_{-\infty}^{\infty} (2\pi f)^4 S_{xx}(f)df = -\left.\frac{d^4R_{xx}(\tau)}{d\tau^4}\right|_{\tau=0} = E\left[\frac{d^2\underline{x}(t)}{dt^2}\right]^2$$
$$(58.20)$$

BICOHERENCE CONTOURMAP OF AN AVERAGE OF 4 FILES

CONTOURS AT 0.25 0.35 0.45

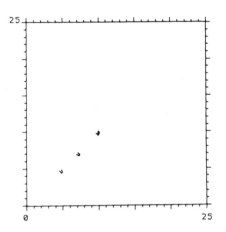

Figure 58.4.   Contour map of the normalized bispectrum (also called bicoherence) of an EEG signal recorded from a subject who presented an alpha variant (the corresponding power spectrum is shown in Fig. 58.8). The plot shows three maxima in the value of bicoherence (>0.25). One is at the intersection of approximately 5 Hz and 5 Hz (phase coupling between 5 Hz, 5 Hz, and 10 Hz); another one is at the intersection of about 7 Hz and 7 Hz (phase coupling between 7 Hz, 7 Hz, and 14 Hz). Still another is at the intersection of about 10 Hz and 10 Hz (phase coupling between 10 Hz, 10 Hz, and 20 Hz). This means that the two peaks seen in the power spectrum of Fig. 58.8 at 5 Hz and 10 Hz, respectively, are harmonically related, i.e., 5 Hz is one-half subharmonic of the dominant alpha frequency. Moreover, there is another component at 20 Hz, difficult to see in the power spectrum, of Fig. 58.8, which is also harmonically related to the alpha frequency (i.e., a second harmonic of the alpha component is also present). Another component at about 7 Hz related to 14 Hz can also be identified. (This component may be distinguished as a small notch at the flank of the 10-Hz peak in the power spectrum of Fig. 58.8.)

In this way the spectral moments relate to the derivatives of the autocorrelation function $R_{xx}(\tau)$ and of the signal $\underline{x}(t)$. The discussion below illustrates how these spectral moments a_0, a_2, and a_4 are related to the descriptors proposed by Hjorth.

Interval or Period Analysis

An alternative method of EEG signal analysis is based on measuring the distribution of intervals between either zero or other level crossings, or between maxima and minima.

A level crossing may be defined in general terms, as the time at which a signal $\underline{x}(t)$ passes a certain amplitude level b; b = 0 is a special case referred to as zero crossing (Fig. 58.5). Knowledge of the probability density function of the intervals between successive zero crossings can be useful in characterizing some statistical properties of the signal $\underline{x}(t)$ (mean value 0). $p_0(\tau)$ can be called the probability distribution density function of the intervals between any two successive zero crossings and $p_1(\tau)$, corresponding to the total time τ between successive zero crossings at which the signal changes in the same direction (i.e., from positive to negative or vice versa). In practice, these functions can be approximated by computing histograms of the interval length between two successive zero crossings or between zero

crossings at which the signal has a derivative with the same sign. The moments of the distribution function can also be computed; the simplest case is to compute the average number of zero crossings per time unit (N_0) (e.g., per second) of the signal $\underline{x}(t)$:

$$N_0^{-1} = \bar{\tau} = \int_0^\infty \tau p_0(\tau)d\tau \qquad (58.21)$$

This means that the number of zero crossings per time unit N_0 equals the reciprocal of the mean interval length τ.

In some cases it is helpful to determine the probability density function of the intervals between two adjacent zero crossings where the sign of $\underline{x}(t)$ changes from negative to positive or vice versa. In this case, it is necessary to compute additionally the zero crossing interval distribution of the first derivative of $\underline{x}(t)$, $\underline{y}(t)$ (i.e., $\underline{y}(t) = d\underline{x}(t)/dt$). If the signal $\underline{x}(t)$ to be analyzed is quasi-stationary and has a gaussian distribution, a mathematical relation between N_k, the average rate of zero crossings of the kth derivative of $\underline{x}(t)$, and the power spectrum $S_{xx}(f)$ can be shown (Cohen, 1976; Rice, 1954; Saltzberg et al., 1968):

$$N_k = 4\left[\frac{\int_0^\infty f^{2k+2}S_{xx}(f)df}{\int_0^\infty f^{2k}S_{xx}(f)df}\right]^{1/2} \qquad (58.22)$$

In interval analysis, only the values N_k for k = 0, 1, 2 are usually computed. N_0 thus represents the average rate of zero crossings of $d\underline{x}(t)/dt$ (i.e., the rate of intervals between extremes of the signal $\underline{x}(t)$); N_2 represents the average rate of

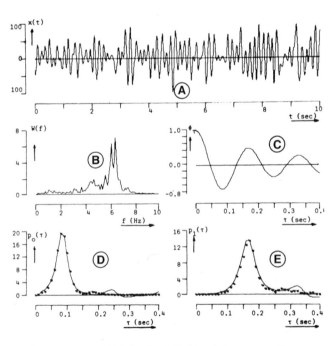

Figure 58.5.   **A:** An EEG signal $x(t)$. **B:** Plot of the corresponding power spectrum $w(f)$ as function of frequency f in Hz. **C:** Plot of the autocorrelation function (τ). **D:** Plot of $p_0(\tau)$ (i.e., the distribution density function of the intervals between any two successive zero crossing). **E:** Plot of $p_1(\tau)$ (i.e., the distribution density function of the time τ between successive zero crossings at which the signal $x(t)$ changes in the same direction, from positive to negative or vice versa). (Illustration courtesy of R.A.F. Pronk.)

zero crossings of $d^2 \underline{x}(t)/dt^2$ (i.e., the rate of intervals of the inflection points of $\underline{x}(t)$).

It can be shown (Cohen, 1976) that expression 58.22 can also be given in terms of the autocorrelation function:

$$\frac{N_0}{2} = \left[(\pi\tau)^2 \left[1 - \frac{R_{xx}(\tau)}{R_{xx}(o)} \right] \right]^{1/2} = f_g \quad (58.23)$$

where f_g is the so-called gyrating frequency (Matousek et al., 1973).

These relations between the number of zero crossings per time unit and either spectral moments or the autocorrelation function for EEG signals have been studied in detail by Saltzberg and Burch (1971), who concluded that, when the purpose is to monitor long-term changes in the statistical properties of EEG signals, it is legitimate to use average zero-crossing rates to calculate moments of the power spectral density.

Instead of measuring intervals between zero crossings, one can characterize a signal by determining intervals between successive maxima (or minima), which defines a "wave," or between a maximum and the immediately following minimum or vice versa, which defines a "half-wave." This chapter's section on mimetic analysis considers some of the variants of interval analysis as applied to EEG signals; the straightforward applications of interval analysis are described in the section on time domain analysis.

EEG Signal Processing Methods in Practice

The previous section considered the statistical properties of EEG signals as realizations of random processes, explaining how such signals can be characterized by the corresponding probability distribution and its moments, by the autocorrelation function or the power spectrum, or by distribution of intervals between level crossings. In all cases, the EEG was treated as a stochastic signal without a specific generation model. Therefore, all the previously described methods and related ones are *nonparametric methods*. *Parametric methods* may also be used to analyze EEG signals; in such cases one assumes the EEG signal to be generated by a specific model. For example, assuming that the EEG signal is the output of a linear filter given a white noise input allows characterization of the linear filter by a set of coefficients or parameters (e.g., it may correspond to an autoregressive model as explained below).

Therefore, EEG analysis methods can be divided into two basic categories, *parametric* and *nonparametric*. Such a division is conceptually more correct than the more common differentiation between frequency and time domain methods because, as has been explained, such methods as power spectra in the frequency domain and interval analysis in the time domain are closely related; indeed, they represent two different ways of describing the same phenomena. The methods of EEG analysis described here are classified as shown in Table 58.1.

Not all EEG analysis methods can be assigned to one of the two general categories just described. Those having mixed character (i.e., methods that have, as a starting point,

a nonparametric or a parametric approach that is combined with pattern recognition techniques) must be considered separately. The latter fall into the category of *pattern recognition* methods. Last, this section shall discuss *topographic analysis* methods, in which the emphasis is on topographic relations between derivations. Not included here are the evoked potentials, which are discussed elsewhere.

A thorough review of the main techniques currently in use in EEG analysis has been edited by Gevins and Remond (1987). For more details on methods of analyzing brain electric signals, the reader is referred to this authoritative handbook.

Nonparametric Methods

Amplitude Distribution

A random signal can be characterized by the distribution of amplitude and its moments. An example of an amplitude distribution is shown in Fig. 58.2. The first question that is asked regarding the amplitude distribution of an EEG epoch is whether the distribution is normal or gaussian. The most common tests of normality are the chi-square goodness-of-fit test (Otnes and Enochson, 1978), the Kolmogorov-Smirnov test, or the values of skewness and kurtosis (Gasser, 1975, 1977). It has been shown (Lilliefors, 1967) that, for the small EEG samples usually analyzed, the Kolmogorov-Smirnov test is more powerful than the chi-square test. It should be emphasized that in order to apply these tests of goodness-of-fit, two requirements must be satisfied: stationarity and independence of adjacent samples. The first requirement was considered in the previous sections. The second requirement is a well-known prerequisite for the application of the statistical tests of the type we consider here. Persson (1974) has clearly pointed out the pitfalls of applying goodness-of-fit tests to EEG amplitude distributions. The problem is that the EEG signals are usually recorded at such a sampling rate that, depending on the spectral composition of the signal, adjacent samples are more or less correlated. In this way, the

Table 58.1.   EEG Analysis Methods

Nonparametric methods
   Amplitude distributions
   Interval or period distributions
   Amplitude-interval scatter plots
   Correlation functions
   Auto- and cross-correlation
   Complex demodulation
   Power spectral analysis
   Time-varying spectra
   Cross-spectral functions (coherence and phase)
   Bispectra
   Walsh and Haar transforms
   Hjorth slope descriptors

Parametric methods
   Autoregressive and autoregressive moving average (ARMA) models
   Inverse autoregressive filtering
   Time-varying signals; Kalman filtering
   Segmentation analysis

Mimetic analysis
Matched filtering or template matching
Topographic analysis

second requirement is commonly violated. This has also been shown clearly by McEwen and Anderson's (1975) statistical study of EEG signals. The degree of correlation between adjacent samples can be deduced from the autocorrelation function. Persson found that a correlation coefficient of 0.50 or larger for adjacent samples introduces a considerable error in interpreting a goodness-of-fit test. His experience with EEG signals led to the conclusion that sampling rates in most cases should be restricted to about 20/sec in order to achieve an acceptably small degree of correlation between adjacent samples.

It is of general interest to know an EEG sample's type of amplitude distribution. Several studies have been carried out, mainly investigating whether or not EEG amplitude distributions were gaussian. Saunders (1963), using a sample rate of 60/sec, epoch lengths of 8.33 seconds, and the chi-square test, concluded that alpha activity had a gaussian distribution; this confirmed previous results from Lion and Winter (1961) and Kozhevnikov (1958), who used analogue techniques. On the contrary, Campbell et al. (1967), using a sample rate of 125/sec, epoch lengths of 52.8 seconds, and the chi-square test, concluded that most EEG signals had nongaussian distributions; however, it is likely that in this case the dual requirements of stationarity and independence were not met.

The results obtained by Elul (1969) are of special interest because he examined EEG time-varying properties using amplitude distributions for epochs of 2 seconds (200 samples/sec, chi-square goodness-of-fit test); this study most certainly failed to meet the requirement of independence. Nevertheless, Elul found that a resting EEG signal could be considered to have a gaussian distribution 66% of the time, whereas, during performance of a mental arithmetic task, this incidence decreased to 32%. Evaluating a small series of waking EEGs in twins, Dumermuth (1968, 1969) found amplitude distribution deviations from gaussianity in the majority of the subjects; he tested the normality hypothesis by way of the third- and fourth-order moments, skewness, and kurtosis. In adult sleep EEG, skewness and kurtosis also deviated significantly from the values expected for a gaussian distribution depending on sleep stage (Dumermuth et al., 1972, 1975). These observations have led to a study of higher order moments of the spectral density function using bispectral analysis.

The method recommended to test whether EEG amplitude distributions are gaussian is that proposed by Gasser (1975, 1977); it involves calculating skewness and kurtosis after correction in view of the possibility that adjacent samples may have a large (e.g., >0.50) degree of correlation. The allowed kurtosis and skewness values can be found in statistical tables. Kurtosis in most cases without paroxysmal activity or artifacts is within the limits allowed to accept the normality hypothesis; skewness different from zero is encountered particularly in those cases in which harmonic components are present in the power spectra. In such instances, the bispectrum exists (see below).

An alternative method of calculating measures of EEG amplitude was developed by Drohocki (1948) and is used mainly in psychopharmacologic and psychiatric studies (see review in Goldstein, 1975). This method involves measuring the surface of rectified EEG waves. Its usefulness for routine EEG analysis is limited.

Interval Analysis

Interval or period analysis has been used, as described above, to study the statistical properties of EEG signals in general and in relation to other analysis methods, such as autocorrelation functions and power spectra. This discussion considers a more practical aspect, the simplicity of evaluating EEG signals using interval analysis. The method, as originally applied by Saltzberg et al. (1957) and Burch et al. (1964), has been shown to be useful primarily in quantifying EEG changes induced by psychoactive drugs (Fink, 1969, 1974, 1975; Itil et al., 1979), in monitoring long-term EEG changes during anesthesia (Pronk et al., 1975, 1976), in psychiatry (Itil, 1975), and in sleep research (see review by Matousek et al., 1973).

When using interval analysis, it is good practice to compute not only the zero crossings of the original EEG signal but also those of the signal's first and second derivatives, to obtain more information about the spectral properties of the signal. One disadvantage of this method is sensitivity to high-frequency noise in the estimation of zero crossings. This problem can be avoided by introducing hysteresis, that is, by creating a dead band (e.g., between $+a\mu V$ and $-a\mu V$) so that no zero crossing can be detected when the signal has an amplitude between those limits. In this way, Pronk et al. (1975) have found that a dead band between $+3\mu V$ and $-3\mu V$ is a good practical choice. Another disadvantage is that, when examining histograms of zero-crossing counts, it is easy to underestimate the contribution of low-frequency components, of which there may be very few, and to overestimate fast frequency components. These disadvantages are particularly evident when zero-crossing histograms and power spectra of the same signal are compared as shown in Fig. 58.6. Sometimes corrections are made to enhance the number of long intervals in relation to the short ones, but this may complicate the interpretations even more.

Another approach is to compute zero-crossing intervals only within determined frequency bands; this may solve the problem of missing superimposed waves (Legewie and Probst, 1969; Schwarzer and Reets, 1966).

The main advantage of zero-crossing analysis is ease of computation, which makes this method particularly attractive for the online quantification of very long EEG records, for example, during sleep or intensive monitoring. To perform interval analysis, it is useful to combine it with prefiltering (Zetterberg, 1977) in the analysis of narrow band signals.

Interval-Amplitude Analysis

Interval-amplitude analysis is the method by which the EEG is decomposed in waves or half-waves, defined both in time, by the interval between zero crossings, and in amplitude by the peak-to-trough amplitudes. This hybrid method had been proposed repeatedly in the past by Marko and Petsche (1957), Leader et al. (1967), Legewie and Probst (1969), and Pfurtscheller and Koch (1972); it has been applied intensively in a clinical setting by Harner (1975) and Harner and Ostergren (1976). The latter called this method

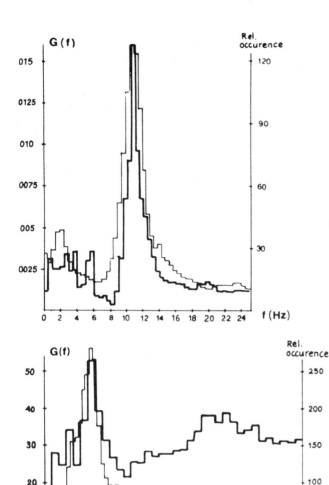

— iterative interval analysis

— power spectral analysis

Figure 58.6. Two examples for comparison of iterative interval analysis and power spectra of the same EEG signals. The intervals are plotted as inverse frequencies. The agreement is fairly good in the case presented above, a pronounced rhythmic component (peak at about 11 Hz) is present. However, in the case below, the interval analysis emphasizes in a marked way the high frequency components. (Adapted from Matejeck, M., and Schenk, G.K. 1973. Die iterative Intervall-Analyse-Ein methodischer Beitrag zur Quantitativen Beschreibung des Elektroenzephalogramms in Zeitbereich. In *Die Quantifizierung des Elektroenzephalogramms,* Ed. G.K. Schenk, pp. 293–306. Konstanz: AEG Telefunken.)

"sequential analysis" because the amplitude and interval duration of successive half-waves are analyzed, displayed, and stored in sequence in real time. The method used by these authors requires that the sampling rate be at least 250/sec, the zero level be updated continuously by estimating the running mean zero level, and, as just discussed, there be a dead band to avoid the influence of high-frequency noise. The high-frequency sampling is desirable in order to obtain

a relatively accurate estimate of the peaks and troughs. The amplitude and the interval duration of a *half-wave* are defined by the peak-trough differences in amplitude and time; the amplitude and the interval duration of a *wave* are defined by the mean amplitude and the sum of the interval durations of two consecutive half-waves. These data are displayed in a scatter diagram as illustrated in Fig. 58.7.

Correlation Analysis

In practical terms, the computation of correlation functions in the 1950s and 1960s constituted the forerunner of contemporary spectral analysis of EEG signals (Barlow and Brazier, 1954; Barlow and Brown, 1955; Brazier and Barlow, 1956) and provided an impetus to implement EEG quantification in practice. However, the computations were time consuming and therefore not widely used. A simplified form of correlator was introduced, based on the fact that auto- or cross-correlation functions can be approximated by replacing the signals $\underline{x}(t)$ and $\underline{x}(t + \tau)$ (see equation 58.4) by their signs (sign $x(t)$ and sign $x(t + \tau)$ where sign $x(t) = +1$ for $x(t) > 0$ and sign $x(t) = -1$ for $x(t) \le 0$), as demonstrated by McFadden (1956). The function thus defined is

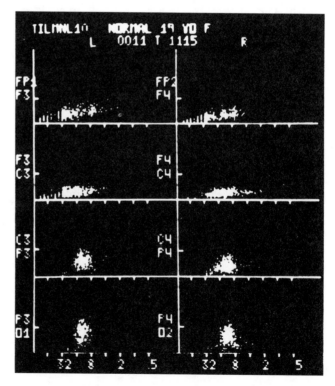

Figure 58.7. A display of sequential analysis obtained in real time. The *dots* represent individual half-waves displayed within 2 msec of their occurrence in each of eight channels. The distribution of *dots,* for example, in the 8- to 16-Hz range (frequency equivalents of wavelength are used) gives an indication in amplitude and frequency of the alpha rhythm. Side-by-side comparison of homologous areas allows assessment of symmetry. Marking in y axis indicates 50 μV. (Illustration courtesy of R.N. Harner; also in Lopes da Silva, F.H., Cooper, R., Dumermuth, G., et al. 1976. Sampling, conversion, and measurement of bioelectrical phenomena. In *Handbook of Electroencephalography and Clinical Neurophysiology,* Ed.-in-chief, A. Remond, vol. 4, Ed., M.A. Brazier, Part A. Amsterdam: Elsevier.)

called the polarity coincidence correlation function, and it has proved useful in EEG analysis (Kaiser and Angell, 1957; Lopes da Silva, 1970; Sologub, 1965; Stebel and Schwartze, 1967). Another simplified form of EEG analysis that is akin to correlation has been used by Kamp et al. (1965), Lesèvre and Remond (1967), and Remond et al. (1969). It can be called autoaveraging and consists of making pulses at a certain phase of the EEG (e.g., zero crossing, peak, or trough) that are then used to trigger a device that averages the same signal (autoaveraging) or another signal (cross-averaging). In this way, rhythmic EEG phenomena can be detected and some characteristic measures obtained.

However, correlation analysis has lost much of its attractiveness for EEG analysts since the advent of FT computation of power spectra. The latter technique is less time-consuming and therefore more economical, and, in general terms, more powerful. Above all, it is difficult to determine from an autocorrelation function EEG components when the signals contain more than one dominant rhythm, an investigation that can be done simply by using the power spectrum (Fig. 58.8). Nevertheless, it should be noted that the simplified methods of correlation analysis just described and used in the 1960s can still have practical value in simple problems, such as computing an alpha average.

The computation of autocorrelation functions has been revived due to the introduction of such parametric analysis methods as the autoregressive model, which, as described below, implies the computation of such functions. Michael and Houchin (1979) have even proposed a method of segmenting EEG signals based on the autocorrelation function.

Related to correlation functions is the method of *complex demodulation* (Walter, 1968b). With this method, a particular frequency component (e.g., ~10 Hz) can be detected and followed as a function of time. In this case a priori knowledge of the component to be analyzed is necessary. Assuming, thus, that in an EEG signal a component at about 10 Hz exists and

Figure 58.8. **Left-hand column:** Different ways of plotting the spectrum of the same EEG epoch, the bicoherence of which is shown in Fig. 58.4. First plot: y axis, power in dB, and x axis, frequency (Hz) along a linear scale; the 90% confidence band of the spectral estimate is indicated. Second plot: y axis, power in µV²/Hz, and x axis as above. Third plot: y axis, power in dB, and x axis, frequency (Hz) logarithmic scale (this way emphasizes somewhat the low-frequency components). Fourth plot: y axis, power in µV²/Hz, and x axis, frequency (Hz) along a logarithmic scale. **Right-hand column:** First plot: squared coherence (Coh or (γ²) between two symmetric EEG signals; the power of one is shown in the plots on the left side. Second plot: the same function as above; along the vertical axis the z transformed coherence is plotted z = 1/2 ln ((1 + γ)/(1 − γ)); the advantage of this form of presentation lies in the fact that, in this case, the confidence bands are the same for the whole curve and are not dependent on the value of γ². Third plot: phase spectrum corresponding to the coherence spectrum shown above.

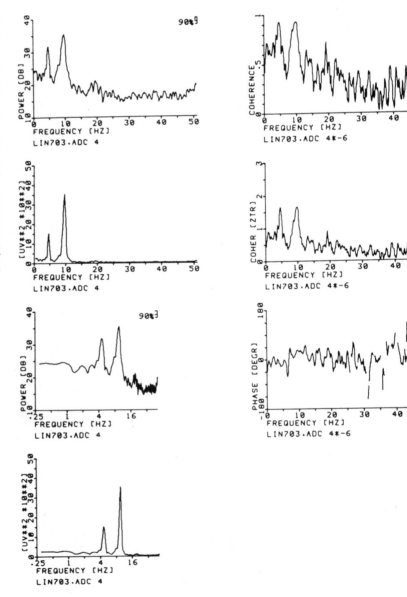

should be followed, one can set an "analysis oscillator" at 10 Hz; the oscillator output and the signal are then multiplied. The product contains components at the sum frequency (~20 Hz) and at the difference (~0 Hz). This product is smoothed so that only the difference components (at about 0 Hz) are considered. In this way, phase and amplitude of EEG frequency components can be detected and their modulation in time determined. Complex demodulation has been used to analyze rhythmic components of visual potentials (Childers and Pao, 1972) and sleep spindles (Kumar, 1975) This method is similar to a direct Fourier analysis in which an EEG signal is multiplied by sines and cosines at a particular frequency in the study of evoked potentials (Regan, 1977) and also the method of phase-locked loop analysis as used to detect sleep spindles (Broughton et al., 1978; Campbell et al., 1980).

Power Spectra Analysis

A classical way of describing an EEG signal is in terms of frequency as established by the common EEG frequency bands. It is possible to obtain information on the frequency components of EEG signals using interval or period analysis. However, the most appropriate methods in this respect are analog filtering or Fourier analysis, using either expression 58.9 (i.e., the FT of the autocorrelation function) or expressions 58.12 and 58.13 (i.e., the periodogram). Several forms of analog filtering were introduced in the early days of EEG research; that technique reached a technical level appropriate for clinical application mainly due to the work of Walter and collaborators (Walter, 1943a,b). Even in the 1960s banks of active analog filters were used to decompose EEG signals into frequency components (Kaiser et al., 1964; Matousek et al., 1975; Storm van Leeuwen, 1961, 1964). In 1975, Matousek and collaborators compared analog and digital techniques of EEG spectral analysis and demonstrated clearly the superiority of digital techniques. Digital methods are more accurate and flexible; using digital computers simplifies multichannel analysis.

The crucial landmarks in the development of EEG quantification methods have always followed technical advances: first, banks of active analog filters as just described; second, large digital computers (Walter, 1963; Walter and Adey, 1965); and third, a fast algorithm for digital computation of discrete FTs, Cooley and Tukey's (1965) so-called FFT. The latter has since been used extensively in EEG analysis (review in Dumermuth, 1977).

This chapter cannot discuss the technical aspects of applying FFT spectral analysis to EEG quantification; for these aspects, the reader is referred to Matousek et al. (1973), Dumermuth (1977), and the books of Jenkins and Watts (1968), Otnes and Enochson (1978), and Gevins and Remond (1987). It is sufficient to state here that, when planning to perform FFT spectral analysis, the electroencephalographer should consider the following basic issues.

Digitization and Prefiltering

Digitization and prefiltering were discussed in relation to the sampling process. It is necessary to define beforehand the frequency range over which the spectrum should be computed, not only to avoid aliasing, but also to minimize computation time.

Length

The length of the epoch T to be analyzed must be selected. It is important to take into account that the epoch should be short enough to avoid nonstationarity segments but long enough to obtain the desired level of frequency resolution f; the maximum Δf is, of course, $\Delta f = 1/T$. In many clinical applications one uses T = 5 or 10 seconds.

Frequency Smoothing and Ensemble Averaging

The estimate of one frequency point of a periodogram F_{xx} (f_1) of one EEG epoch has a chi-square distribution with only 2 degrees of freedom. The number of degrees of freedom must be increased and the estimate variance reduced by averaging either for a number of equivalent epochs or by smoothing over adjacent frequency components. Sometimes both ensemble averaging and frequency smoothing are used. Generally, the spectral estimate P_{xx} (f_1) (equation 58.13) should correspond to at least 60 degrees of freedom (Vos, 1975), which allows acceptable estimates of spectral values. This implies that an ensemble of at least 30 epochs should be used if only ensemble averaging is carried out. The number of degrees of freedom can also be increased, at the expense of frequency resolution Δf, by using a spectral window $W(f_k)$ (see equation 58.13). A spectral window is defined by its form and duration. The duration at the base is given by the distance between truncation points. Using a window with a large base reduces the variance but increases the bias of the estimator. An excessively large window decreases too greatly the equivalent frequency resolution Δf. In practice, therefore, a complex compromise between all the aforementioned points must be reached. Details about the technicalities of choosing the appropriate form $W(f_k)$ can be found in Jenkins and Watts (1968) and Künkel et al. (1975). A good deal of freedom in the choice of the spectral window is tolerable; the appropriate choice depends on the practical use of spectral analysis. In EEG quantification in the clinical routine, it is common to compute average spectra by making averages of ensembles of 10 epochs of 10 seconds (N = 1,024) each, using an elliptic window five sample points wide for smoothing; the equivalent bandwidth is thus 0.5 Hz. The resulting estimate corresponds, therefore, to less than 100 (more precisely, 93) degrees of freedom, owing to the fact that for each frequency component the power estimate is based on 2 degrees of freedom; this number must be multiplied by 10 (epochs), by 5 (window width), and by a factor 0.93 which corresponds to the fact that the window is elliptic.

Calibration

The dimension of power spectra in EEG analysis is intensity per bandwidth; the unit of measurement is in V^2/Hz (Walter, 1968a). Calibration can be carried out using sine waves, as proposed by Abraham et al. (1968), Clusin et al. (1970), Dumermuth and Flühler (1967), and Matousek et al. (1973); Sciarretta and Erculiani (1978) proposed a simple method, using a single rectangular pulse, that has practical advantages.

Graphic Representation

The graphic representation of power spectra merits special attention. In most instances, the EEG analyst needs a

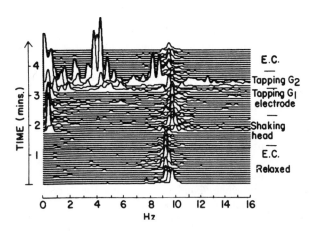

Figure 58.9. Display of a compressed spectral array showing the alpha rhythm and the effects of various artifact-inducing maneuvers on the background activity. Note the change in alpha peak frequency from the eyes-closed situation when shaking occurs. Note also the influence of artifacts in the spectra, particularly at tapping the electrodes; the large peaks at low frequencies are artifactual. (Adapted from Bickford, R.G. 1977. Computer analysis of background activity. In *EEG Informatics. A Didactic Review of Methods and Applications of EEG Data Processing,* Ed., A. Remond, pp. 215–232. Amsterdam: Elsevier.)

plot of power spectra, as shown in Fig. 58.8. In most cases, the vertical scale is simply the spectral density as computed by way of the Fourier coefficients (i.e., in $\mu V^2/Hz$). A preferred alternative is plotting the spectral intensity along a logarithmic scale. The advantage of choosing log power intensity instead of simply power intensity is that the confidence intervals of the former are independent of the values of the spectral intensity. Another technique involves computing the square root of the spectral intensity and plotting it

along the vertical axis. Frequency is usually presented along a linear scale calibrated in Hz; however, one may prefer, if the most attention is to be paid to the lower frequencies (delta and theta), to compress the frequency scale in the higher frequency range by plotting log Hz (Fig. 58.8) along the horizontal axis or a more compressed scale for frequencies higher than, for instance, 15 Hz. The presentation of a power spectrum plotting log spectral intensity vertically and frequency horizontally, and where the higher frequency components are plotted in a more compressed way than the lower ones, is useful in routine clinical situations.

Time-Varying Spectra

Time-varying spectra are often computed in order to analyze more or less slowly changing EEG records. Such spectra can be plotted simply by using the so-called compressed spectra array (Fig. 58.9) as introduced by Bickford et al. (1973). This method is particularly valuable in obtaining an overall view of EEG spectral changes for intraoperative or sleep monitoring (Johnson et al., 1976). Another form of plotting time-varying power spectra is by using contour plots (i.e., plots of frequency against time), as shown in Fig. 58.10; in such plots, points corresponding to equal values of power spectra computed from successive epochs are connected by contour lines. These plots provide useful, easily interpretable visual displays of the evolution of power spectra as a function of time.

The computation of time-varying power spectra is particularly important in those studies in which the problem is that of characterizing EEG changes in relation to specific events, such as eyes closing/opening (Kawabata, 1973), fists closing/opening (Pfurtscheller and Aranibar, 1977), word association tests (Kamp and Vliegenthart, 1977), and similar events. The problem here is to quantify time-locked changes in EEG spectra by way of ensemble averaging, using a par-

Figure 58.10. Contour plot of power spectra: note the frequency shifts and increase in power intensity occurring in the second part of the registration. (Adapted from Dumermuth, G. 1977. Fundamentals of spectral analysis in electroencephalography. In *EEG Informatics. A Didactic Review of Methods and Applications of EEG Data Processing,* Ed., A. Remond, pp. 83–105. Amsterdam: Elsevier.)

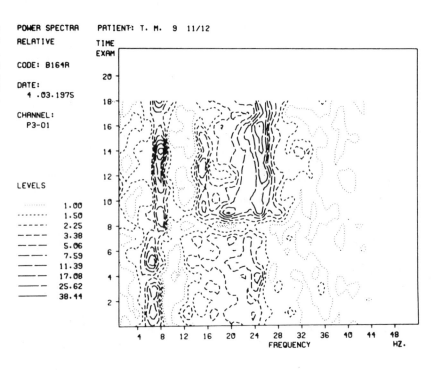

ticular event as a trigger. Kawabata (1973) considered this problem analytically and proposed a formalism to compute time-varying EEG spectra. Using this construct, he could show that initially at eye closure, power within the alpha band increases, with the greatest concentration in the center frequency; later the center frequency shifts to a lower frequency. When the eyes open, the alpha power decreases and the center frequency increases.

Pfurtscheller and Aranibar (1977) designed a method for analyzing EEG changes related to sets of stimuli such as those used to study the phenomenon of contingent negative variation (CNV). According to this method, the 6-second EEG epoch occurring before and after the event of interest is subdivided into 1-second overlapping segments. For each segment, a power spectrum is computed; in the experiment quoted above, the total power (0–32 Hz) and the power in the alpha frequency range (7–13 Hz) of each segment are averaged over a number of equivalent segments, and mean values and standard errors calculated. In this manner, these authors demonstrated phasic decreases of power in the alpha band related to sensory stimulation and to the interstimulus interval in a CNV paradigm. Pfurtscheller and Aranibar (1980) used the same method to study changes in central mu rhythms occurring in relation to opening and closing the fists in normal subjects and patients (Fig. 58.11). A large number of studies where dynamical changes of the ongoing

EEG, within different frequency components, were detected and characterized have been revised by Pfurtscheller et al. (1996).

The fact that EEG baseline values (i.e., pre-event segments) can change from trial to trial makes a statistical analysis based on ensemble averages and standard deviations particularly difficult. Kamp and Vliegenthart (1977) proposed resolving this type of difficulty by analyzing EEG epochs immediately before and immediately after the event causing the change. In this way a pre-event epoch of, for instance, 4 seconds and a postevent epoch of, for instance, 4 seconds are analyzed. A relatively large number of trials are recorded, and the degree to which the spectral value within a certain frequency band for each postevent subsegment (e.g., 1 second long) differs from the pre-event epoch evaluated using a nonparametric test (Mann-Whitney test; Siegel, 1956). The end result is given as the number of trials in which a certain frequency band changed significantly at a particular postevent segment. A similar method has been used by Arnolds et al. (1979), who compared spectral parameters of EEG segments occurring after a behavioral event with pre-event values of the same parameter simply by using the sign test (Siegel, 1956). The advantages of using this type of nonparametric method should be emphasized. Because the baseline values may vary dramatically, one runs the risk of failing to detect real EEG changes related to a particular event that exist if one compares only mean values. Directly comparing within each trial the baseline with the postevent values, particularly by means of a nonparametric statistical test, avoids the difficulty pointed out above.

Statistical Evaluation

Statistical evaluation of spectra is not done only in the analysis of time averaging EEG signals as discussed previously. Frequently, it is helpful to determine whether or not two sets of EEG power spectra differ significantly. The sets might have been obtained under two different behavioral conditions or during administration of two different treatments (e.g., a placebo or a psychotropic drug); they could have been recorded from symmetrical derivations over the scalp. The question is a simple one. Given two sets of power spectra, how can one determine whether they belong to the same population? The answer, however, is not so simple. To start with, it is necessary to emphasize that the power spectrum of a certain EEG epoch is an estimate; thus it also has a variance. A convenient way of presenting estimate variability is to present the corresponding confidence bands simultaneously with the average power spectrum as indicated previously. The question of testing whether the two sets of spectra belong to the same population has been approached using a variety of methods (for references see Dumermuth et al., 1975). Often analysis of variance (F test) and Student's *t* test are applied (Etévenon and Pidoux, 1977). The F test in principle should be the first test chosen, because power density is a quadratic function. If the number of degrees of freedom increases, the power density distribution tends to normalize so that a *t* test can be applied.

In general, it is advisable to apply to the power spectrum a logarithmic transformation, because it produces a symmetrical distribution. Confidence intervals for $\log P_{xx}$ (f)

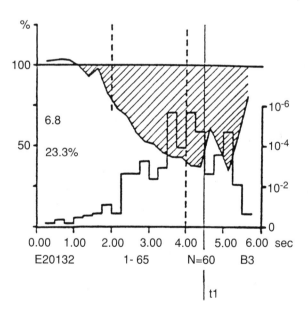

Figure 58.11. Alpha power time course over a 6-second interval calculated during voluntary hand movement (movement onset at 4 seconds). The scale on the *left* gives the percentage alpha power. Reference interval 0–2 seconds with an absolute reference power of 6.8 μV² corresponding to 100% (this reference power corresponds to 23.8% of the total power within the frequency band 0–32 Hz). The significance levels for the power decrease [event-related desynchronization (ERD)] are indicated on the right scale (10⁻² corresponds *p* < .01 etc., sign test). Note that a decrease of alpha power is indicative for ERD. (Adapted from Pfurscheller, G., and Klimesch, W. 1992. Functional topography during a visuo-verbal judgment task studied with event-related desynchronization mapping. J. Clin. Neurophysiol. 9:120–131.)

are given approximately as (Matousek et al., 1973) log P_{xx} (f) $\pm Z_{a/2}$ ($\sqrt{2/N}$) where $Z_{a/2}$ is the 100 alpha/2 percentage point of the standardized normal distribution and N is the equivalent number of degrees of freedom (Bendat and Piersol, 1971). Nevertheless, in many applications, especially if the number of degrees of freedom is small, it is preferable to apply nonparametric tests, such as the simple sign test or the more powerful Wilcoxon or Mann-Whitney tests. For a detailed analysis of the questions of statistical inference on EEG data, the reader is referred to Gasser (1977, 1979). This problem has been discussed in detail in relation to those psychopharmacologic investigations in which EEG plays a central role (Abt, 1979; Fink, 1975; Itil, 1975; Itil et al., 1979), but these aspects are too specialized to be considered here.

Cross-Spectral Analysis

Cross-spectral analysis is an important part of EEG spectral analysis because it allows quantification of the relationships between different EEG signals. The section on basic statistical properties mentioned the smoothed estimate of the *cross-power spectrum* C_{xy} (f); this quantity is the product of the smoothed discrete FT of one signal and the complex conjugate of the other (see for details Jenkins and Watts, 1968). C_{xy} (f) is a complex quantity that therefore has a magnitude and phase:

$$C_{xy}(f) = |C_{xy}(f)| \cdot \exp[j\Phi_{xy}(f)] \qquad (58.24)$$

where $j = \sqrt{-1}$. The function of frequency Φ_{xy} (f) is the *phase spectrum.* It is useful to define a normalized quantity, the *coherence function,* as follows:

$$\text{Coh}_{xy}(f) = \frac{|C_{xy}(f)|^2}{P_{xx}(f)\,P_{yy}(f)} \qquad (58.25)$$

Examples of coherence and phase functions are shown in Fig. 58.8. In EEG analysis these functions are computed after the application of cross-correlation functions, which was carried out in a way similar to the autocorrelation function as described previously (see for details Matousek et al., 1973). Coherence functions have been used in several investigations of the EEG signal generation and their relation to brain functions, including studies of hippocampal theta rhythms (Walter and Adey, 1963, 1965), on limbic structures in humans (Brazier, 1968), on thalamic and cortical alpha rhythms (Lopes da Silva et al., 1973b), on sleep stages in humans (Dumermuth et al., 1972), on EEG development in babies (Prechtl and Vos, 1973; Vos, 1975), and on the spatial and temporal structures of dynamic features of local EEG signals (Bullock et al. 1995a,b). The latter measured coherence functions between EEG signals recorded using electrodes with 5- to 10-mm spacing from epileptic patients, and found that in both the subdural surface samples and those from temporal lobe depth arrays, coherence declines with distance between electrodes of the pair, on the average quite severely in millimeters. This demonstrates that coherence fluctuations are quite local.

The recommended way to evaluate coherence functions statistically is to apply Fisher's z transformation (Jenkins and Watts, 1968) as used by Lopes da Silva et al. (1973b) to analyze EEG signals. Thus, the confidence intervals and bias are dependent of the coherence values (Fig. 58.8).

The use of coherence functions in routine clinical EEG analysis has been rather limited thus far. In one system dedicated to this type of analysis, coherence functions have been applied with good results (Storm van Leeuwen et al., 1976). The important point is to define clearly which questions one wishes to answer through coherence functions application. In this context, the most relevant points are as follows.

Is it possible to differentiate spectral components with frequencies lying close to each other? For example, alpha and mu rhythms may be difficult to differentiate in plots of power spectra but are readily separated using coherence functions computed between symmetric transversal derivations because the former show large values of transversal coherences, whereas the latter have insignificant values (Storm van Leeuwen et al., 1978).

Is it possible to detect the existence of bilateral synchronous frequency components? Such components may make relatively small contributions to power spectra, whereas they may give rise to large coherence values. Coherences also may be useful in determining the topographic relations of different EEG components.

The counterpart of coherence is the phase function (Fig. 58.8), which provides information on the time relationships between two EEG signals. An explanation of the use of the term *phase* is necessary here. *Phase* is used in the present context as a mathematical notion referring to the proportion of the period of a sine wave component of a signal as obtained through Fourier analysis. The existence of a phase difference between two EEG signals as obtained from the phase function can have different meanings. First, assume that the two signals were recorded from bipolar derivations and that some components, e.g., between 0 and 3 Hz, show an inverted polarity (phase opposition, in EEG terms); in this case the phase function computed from the cross-power spectrum between the two signals will show, for the 0- to 3-Hz components, a phase difference of 180 degrees. In the second case, assuming that some components of the signal recorded from one derivation will be transmitted to the other derivation after a certain delay time Δt (in seconds) the phase difference $\Delta\Phi$ (in degrees) between the two signals will be linear with frequency in the range Δf (in Hz) corresponding to those components; in this case, the following relationship is valid:

$$\Delta t = \frac{\Delta\Phi}{360 \cdot \Delta f} \qquad (58.26)$$

Until now, phase functions have been little used in routine clinical EEG practice, probably because phase measurements are generally difficult to interpret in terms of the two models just presented. This is because scalp EEG derivations are a complex representation of underlying cortical activity, so that the potentials recorded at a distance are not easily reduced to clearcut biophysical processes at the cortical level. Nevertheless, Gotman's (1976) system of EEG analysis included phase function computation in order to detect phase opposition between the slow frequency components of different bipolar derivations. If the phase difference between the two signals is about 180 degrees with a significant coherence between the two signals, one can conclude that a phase reversal exists. In Gotman's system, the search for phase reversals is performed only in the presence of slow activity. Computing phase functions to determine time delays between EEG signals during epileptic seizures has also been proposed (Brazier, 1972). The interpretation of these results, however, poses a problem. A time delay between two signals can be concluded with certainty only if there is a linear relationship between phase and frequency within a certain frequency band; if the coherence between the two signals is significant over only a very narrow frequency band (around a peak), it may be impossible to define a best-fit line to the phase function. In such a case, the result may be impossible to interpret definitively in terms of time delay. Instead of using the simple phase function, it may be recommended to use a weighted phase function, as proposed by Carter (1976), in the sort of problems just discussed. A fundamental problem, however, is that very often the relations between EEG signals cannot be considered linear, so that the use of coherence is not justified. Alternative methods have been developed (Mars and van Arragon, 1981) in order to overcome this limitation.

Another approach to identifying the source of EEG seizure activity is use of a generalized form of coherence analysis, the so-called *spectral regression-amount of information analysis* introduced and first applied to EEG analysis by Gersch and Goddard (1970). This method has been used not only to analyze seizures (Gersch and Tharp, 1976; Tharp and Gersch, 1975), but also to investigate the process underlying the generation of hippocampal theta rhythms (Etévenon, 1977) and thalamocortical alpha rhythms (Lopes da Silva et al., 1980a,b), the organization of infantile EEGs (Vos et al., 1977), and seizure activity in animals (Rappelsberger et al., 1978). This analytic method involves computing first the coherence between two EEG signals and then the partial coherence based on a third EEG signal. Computing partial coherences implies eliminating from each of the two EEG signals that part that can be regarded as being determined by or predictable on the basis of the third signal, which constitutes a form of regression analysis. If the initial coherence decreases significantly, one can conclude that the coherence between the two initially chosen signals is due to the effect of the third one. As indicated in the references cited earlier, it is possible to thus determine the pattern of interactions between a series of simultaneously recorded EEG signals and, eventually, to find the more likely source of a given EEG phenomenon (e.g., seizure or rhythmic activity).

Bispectra

Equation 58.16 defines the bispectrum. Although the power spectrum is sufficient to describe the statistical characteristics of signals generated by a stationary gaussian process, deviation of amplitude distribution from normality indicates the need to examine spectra of higher orders. This is particularly true for the spectrum corresponding to the second-order autocovariance function $R(\tau_1, \tau_1)$: the bispectrum $B_{xx}(f_1, f_2)$ can be estimated by smoothing the triple product $F_{xx}(f_1)F^*_{xx}(f_2)F_{xx}(f_1 + f_2)$ where $F_{xx}(f)$ represents the complex FT of the signal x(t) and $F^*_{xx}(f)$ represents the complex conjugate (see for details Dumermuth et al., 1971; Huber et al., 1971). Moreover, the bicoherence of signal x(t), which is the normalized bispectrum of x(t), can be defined. (Do not confuse with coherence, which is the normal-

ized magnitude of the cross-spectrum between two signals $\underline{x}(t)$ and $\underline{y}(t)$.) Until now, few studies have put bispectral computation to practical use. Nevertheless, the specific information yielded by bispectra about the relationship between harmonic frequency components in EEG signals can be valuable. For example, Dumermuth et al. (1975) have shown that some rhythmic EEG activities have a significant bispectrum; examples are the mu rhythm, which presents significant relations between harmonics of 10 Hz (5, 20, and 30 Hz), and the psychomotor variant, with relations between 6, 12, 18, and 24 Hz. Lopes da Silva and Storm van Leeuwen (1978) found that alpha rhythms recorded from the cortex also may have a significant bispectrum with harmonic components at 10 and 20 Hz. Moreover, alpha rhythms recorded on the human scalp may also show a significant bispectrum; in a few studied cases (Fig. 58.4), the so-called alpha variant has been characterized by a significant relation between the dominant frequency at 10 Hz and the one-half subharmonic at 5 Hz. Under such circumstances, bispectrum computation disproves the alternative hypothesis that the two components at 10 and 5 Hz are independent of each other and thus that low-frequency components would correspond to abnormal occipital activity. Furthermore, bispectral analysis of some forms of visual evoked potentials (Reits, 1975) has permitted putting in evidence some essential properties of the visual system.

Walsh and Haar Transforms

Alternative ways of computing power spectra have been proposed. These include the Walsh and Haar transforms, which can improve computational speed (Dumermuth, 1977). These alternative methods, however, have not yet proved to be of practical interest, particularly because the FFT already provides a satisfactory solution.

Hjorth Slope Descriptors

The section on basic statistical properties defined the nth spectral moment of the power spectrum a_n (equation 58.17). Hjorth (1970) and Berglund and Hjorth (1973) have developed special hardware to compute in real time the spectral moments a_0 (equation 58.18), a_2 (equation 58.19), and a_4 (equation 58.20). In this way, the spectral moments are not invariant in time as described earlier; rather, spectral moments are allowed to vary as a function of time (i.e., the statistical properties of the signal can vary in time), meaning that this form of analysis can be applied to nonstationary signals.

Based on these quantities, Hjorth derived the following parameters, also called descriptors:

$$\text{activity, A} = a_0$$

$$\text{mobility, M} = [(a_2/a_0)]^{1/2}$$

$$\text{complexity, C} = [(a_4/a_2) - (a_2/a_0)]^{1/2} \qquad (58.27)$$

Note that $a_0 = \sigma_2$ (equation 58.18), i.e., the variance of the signal; a_2 is the variance of the signal's first derivative as shown in equation 58.19; a_4 is the variance of the signal's second derivative (equation 58.20). It should be noted that Hjorth's descriptors give a valid description of an EEG signal only if the signals have a symmetric probability density function with only one maximum (Denoth, 1975). This may be true for simple EEG generation models (Hjorth, 1975; Lopes da Silva et al., 1974) but not in general practice. Nevertheless, the ease of computing Hjorth's descriptors makes them attractive in real-time EEG analysis. The required calculations involve the computation of time derivatives only.

It must be noted, however, that computing the descriptor complexity implies taking the ratio between the second and first derivatives, so that the possibility of introducing large errors is considerable. To avoid this, the signal bandwidth must be rather limited. In the author's opinion, Hjorth descriptors can be useful if the EEG patterns to be analyzed have a simple character, a probability density distribution with only one maximum, and change over time is rather gradual. It is, therefore, not surprising that Hjorth's descriptors have demonstrated value in monitoring time-varying EEG signals, for instance during sleep (Caille and Bassano, 1975). This method has also been used to quantify multichannel EEG recordings obtained under routing conditions (Lütcke et al., 1973).

Parametric Methods

It is reasonable to argue that, in general terms, EEG signals may be analyzed by any suitable method regardless of precise knowledge of their biophysical origins. It may be asked, however, whether more appropriate methods of EEG analysis might be developed if more precise models of the biophysical processes underlying the generation of EEG phenomena (e.g., alpha rhythms, delta waves, spike and wave complexes, and so on) were available. In the particular case of alpha rhythm generation, there exist biophysical models that can help in formulating a reply to such questions (Lopes da Silva et al., 1974; Zetterberg, 1973c; Zetterberg et al., 1978). These alpha rhythm models have indicated that an EEG with a dominant rhythmic component in the alpha frequency range can be described by a filter network with parameters related to physiologically acceptable variables submitted to a noise input. This filter network can be analyzed in a first approximation as a linear processor. This processor can be realized in terms of a mathematical model. A special case of this model is the mixed autoregressive model as described by Zetterberg (1969) and the autoregressive model used by Gersch (1970), Fenwick et al. (1971), and Bohlin (1971). Such methods are called parametric, because in such cases the EEG signals are described in terms of a mathematical model characterized by a set of parameters.

A link may be said to exist between this type of mathematical model and the biophysical model of alpha rhythm generation, but this link is neither specific nor essential. The use of such mathematical models in EEG analysis is yet to be justified through pragmatic argument. They provide a practically useful method for quantifying EEG signals, not only in order to compute spectra (Bohlin, 1971; Fenwick et al., 1971; Gersch, 1970; Isaksson and Wennberg, 1975; Lopes da Silva et al., 1975; Pfurtscheller and Haring, 1972; Rappelsberger and Petsche, 1975; Wennberg and Zetterberg, 1971; Zetterberg, 1973a), but also to detect EEG transient nonstationarities such as epileptiform spikes and sharp waves (Herolf, 1975; Lopes da Silva et al., 1975) and to subdivide the EEG into quasi-stationary segments (Bodenstein and Praetorius,

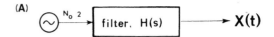

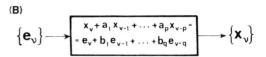

Figure 58.12. Block scheme. **A:** The filtering process on a time continuous signal. **B:** The autoregressive moving average filter model applied to a time discrete signal. (Adapted from Zetterberg, L.H. 1977. Means and methods for processing of physiological signals with emphasis on EEG analysis. In *Advances in Biology and Medical Physics,* Eds. J.H. Lawrence et al., vol. 16, pp. 41–91. New York: Academic Press.)

1977; Praetorius et al., 1977). Parametric methods allow considerable EEG data reduction. For instance, using an autoregressive model, it is possible to describe an EEG signal using a few coefficients; by following the values of these coefficients, the signal's time-varying properties can be traced. The coefficients can be used to classify EEG spectra using, for instance, cluster analysis; moreover, the model can also be used to help detect nonstationary events. The basic model can be described following the scheme of Fig. 58.12, as proposed by Zetterberg (1977). In this figure, two cases are shown: the continuous case and the discrete case. According to the continuous case, the EEG signal x(t) is assumed to result from the operation of filtering (with a filter having as transfer function H(s)) on a noise source with a flat spectrum within the frequency range of interest. In the discrete case, the EEG signal is given as a set of samples x(k) resulting from a filter operation on an input noise signal e(k) with zero mean. The filter, corresponding to the autoregressive moving average (ARMA) model, is described by a linear difference equation of the following form:

$$a_0 x(k) + a_1 x(k-1) + \ldots + a_p x(k-p) = b_0 e(k)$$
$$+ b_1 e(k-1) + \ldots b_q e(k-q) \quad (58.28)$$

where $q \leq p$. The relation between x(k) and e(k) is given by the sets of coefficients $a_1 \ldots a_p$ and $b_1 \ldots b_q$ with $a_0 = 1$. In case $b_i = 0$ for $i = 1 \ldots q$, we are left with the so-called auto-gressive (AR) model:

$$x(k) + a_1 x(k-1) + \ldots + a_p x(k-p) = e(k) \quad (58.29)$$

The computation problem, therefore, is to estimate the coefficients. An important step in this estimation is defining the minimum number of coefficients to be computed.

Fast algorithms exist to enable computation of those coefficients; they are described in detail by Zetterberg (1977), Makhoul (1975), and Eykhoff (1974) among others, and employ several criteria for estimating the order of the model. Using Durbin's algorithm, it was found in a group of EEG recordings of epileptic patients that the minimal order of the model was, in about 70% of the cases, equal to or smaller than 5 (Lopes da Silva, 1978). However, when one wishes a faithful reproduction of the power spectral density, many coefficients may be needed (Zetterberg, 1977). In most applications it is sufficient to compute the AR model of the EEG signal, so this section need not consider the special problems regarding ARMA model computation.

Computation of Power Spectra

The computation of power spectra using an AR or ARMA model presents no special difficulties. Using a special algorithm (spectral parameter analysis, SPA) developed at Zetterberg's (1977) laboratory, both an estimation of the model parameters and the best spectral representation can be obtained. In the case of the ARMA model (equation 58.28) spectral density of a signal sampled with sampling interval is given by:

$$P_{xx}(f) = \sigma^2 \left| \frac{\sum_{i=0}^{q} b_i(\exp(-j2\pi fi\Delta t))}{\sum_{i=0}^{P} a_i(\exp(-j2\pi fi\Delta t))} \right|^2 \qquad (58.30)$$

In case of the AR model, the spectral density is as follow:

$$P_{xx}(f) = \frac{\sigma^2}{\left| \sum_{i=0}^{P} a_i \exp(-j2\pi fi\Delta t) \right|^2} \qquad (58.31)$$

In both cases described, spectral density is estimated using the sets of coefficients. In Zetterberg's original computational procedure, the SPA, the EEG analysis is based on the ARMA model (1977). In this form of analysis, Zetterberg not only computes the EEG power spectrum but also decomposes the spectrum into a number of components to achieve a degree of data reduction; he usually distinguishes three spectral components so that P_{xx} (f) is written as the sum of three components (see also Fig. 58.3):

$$P_{xx}(f) = P_\delta(f) + P_\alpha(f) + P_\beta(f) \qquad (58.32)$$

The delta (δ) component is described by a first-order model; both alpha (α) and beta (β) components require second-order models. The δ component is defined by a power parameter G_δ and a frequency parameter σ_δ, which denotes the corresponding bandwidth; G_δ is defined as:

$$G_\delta = \int_{-\infty}^{\infty} P_\delta(f)df \qquad (58.33)$$

The rhythmic components (α and β) require two frequency parameters, the center or resonance frequency f_α or f_β, and two power parameters, G_α or G_β, defined as in equation 58.33. An example of the spectral decomposition of an EEG signal calculated in this way is shown in Fig. 58.13. Spectral analysis can be performed much faster with the AR than with the ARMA model. It is also easy to use this model to analyze multidimensional processes so that not only auto- but also cross-power spectra can be computed.

Inverse Autoregressive Filtering

The AR model can also be used in an inverted form, which leads to the *inverse autoregressive filtering* operation. Assuming that an EEG signal results from a stationary process, it is possible to approximate it as a filtered noise with a

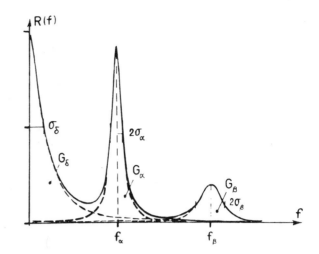

Figure 58.13. Power spectrum of an EEG signal analyzed with a fifth order model. It consists of a low-frequency component (δ) two resonance peaks (α and β); the components are described by the parameters G (power), σ (bandwidth), and f (peak frequency). *Dashed lines* denote the individual spectral components; the *solid line* indicates the total spectrum. (Adapted from Isaksson, A., and Wennberg, A. 1975. Visual evaluation and computer analysis of the EEG—A Comparison. Electroencephalogr. Clin. Neurophysiol. 38:79–86.)

normal distribution. Consequently, passing such an EEG signal through the inverse of its estimated autoregressive filter should result in a normally distributed noise N with mean zero and variance σ^2. The null hypothesis is that an EEG signal follows the assumption of stationarity and can be expressed in terms of the properties of the estimated noise, $\hat{e}(k)$, resulting from the inverse autoregressive filtering:

$$\hat{e}(k) = x_k + \sum_{i=1}^{p} a_i x(k - i) \qquad (58.34)$$

The EEG signal is said to be nonstationary for t = nT if the null hypothesis can be rejected (i.e., if $\hat{e}(k)$) deviates at a certain probability level from a noise with a normal distribution). Thus, nonstationarities in an EEG signal can be detected; this is particularly interesting in the detection of EEG transients of epileptic patients, as shown by Lopes da Silva et al. (1973a) and Lopes da Silva et al. (1975, 1977). A simple test on each sample of the estimated noise can give an indication of the stationarity of the signal at that moment. However, instead of testing $\hat{e}(k)$, a detection function d(k) is used in order to obtain a certain degree of smoothing; d(k) is defined as follows:

$$d(k) = \sum_{n=k-m}^{k+m} \left[\frac{\hat{e}(n)}{\hat{\sigma}} \right]^2 \qquad (58.35)$$

Because the square of a normally distributed variable (with unity variance) follows a chi-squared distribution, the detection function should also have a chi-squared distribution with a number of degrees of freedom (2m + 1). The null hypothesis can then be tested at a certain level, for example at $p < 10^{-3}$. An application of this process of inverse filtering for the detection of transient nonstationarities (epileptiform events) in EEG is illustrated in Fig. 58.14.

Figure 58.14. Scheme of the principle of automatic spike detection (ASD) analysis method using simulated signals. *Top,* the hypothesis is that the interictal EEG of an epileptic patient results from filtered noise to which spikes have been added. For simplification in this scheme, the spikes are not represented as being the output of a filtering process; this, however, would have been more realistic. *Bottom,* the analysis consists of computing an autoregressive filter model representing the hypothetical process, determining the corresponding inverse filter through which the EEG signal is passed, and squaring and smoothing the resulting error signal. The end result or detection signal is tested using the chi square statistic; the time samples lying above a certain level are indicated by *thin lines* under the curve. Note that in this example the ASD program detected at the correct time samples the spikes that had been added to the filtered noise. (Adapted from Lopes da Silva, F.H., van Hulten, K., Lommen, J.G., et al. 1977. Automatic detection and localization of epileptic foci. Electroencephalogr. Clin. Neurophysiol. 43:1–13.)

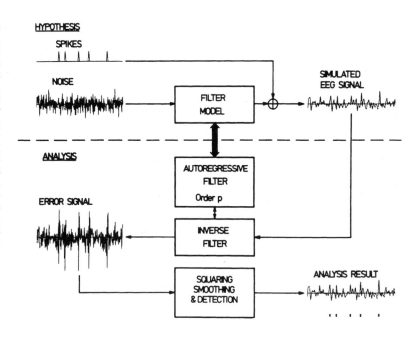

Time-Varying Signals: Kalman Filtering

Parametric models can be extended in order to analyze time-varying signals. A method of analyzing this type of EEG signal consists of applying the so-called *Kalman estimation method* of tracking the parameters describing the signals (Duquesnoy, 1976; Isaksson, 1975; Mathieu, 1976). The input signal to a hypothetical processor responsible for generating the EEG signal is assumed to be a normally distributed noise $e(k)$. A model is assumed in order to represent the observed signal; the process dynamics are represented by an autoregressive model.

The main objective of this procedure is achieved by means of a recursive algorithm called the Kalman filter to obtain estimates of the model coefficients using earlier estimated data. This involves updating based on new samples of the time series (Zetterberg, 1977). The Kalman filtering procedure is not simple to implement; for an appropriate procedure, it is necessary to choose, properly, the order of the model and the initial conditions. An application of this method in the subdivision of EEG signals (segmentation procedure) is described below. Without entering into the details of different procedures of Kalman filtering, it is of interest to note that a measure of EEG signal stationarity can be derived from the application of this method.

Isaksson (1974) has introduced for EEG analysis an algorithm called SPARK, which stands for spectral parameter analysis, based on recursive Kalman filtering. He found that an AR model of order $p* = p + q$ gave as good results as an ARMA model of order p with $q = p - 1$; a good choice appeared to be a value of $p* = 11$ or 13.

Segmentation Analysis

The original purpose of segmentation analysis as introduced by Praetorius et al. (1977) and Bodenstein and Praetorius (1977) was to find in an EEG signal those segments that could be considered to have unvarying statistical properties.

This means that those segments should be considered as being quasi-stationary, and the segments could have variable length. This necessitated the development of criteria for establishing divisions between segments. These authors based their analysis on a parametric model of the EEG, an autoregressive model as defined by equation 58.29. Consult the aforementioned references for details. Duquesnoy (1976) proposed an EEG segmentation method related to that just described. A problem in applying this analytic method is the difficulty of defining clinical-neurophysiological boundaries between segments. Therefore, judgments of whether the method produces segments acceptable on clinical-neurophysiological grounds is rather subjective and depends strongly on personal criteria. Nevertheless, this method may be useful in reducing data in analyses of long EEG records recorded under variable behavioral conditions.

Michael and Houchin (1979) proposed a similar method based simply on computing a running autocorrelation function, which ensures a quicker procedure. Barlow (1984) used the method devised by Michael and Houchin (1979) to compare the performance of automatic adaptive segmentation with those of selective analog filtering and inverse digital filtering in automatic evaluation of significant EEG changes associated with carotid clamping. Of the three methods, the former was clearly the best.

Adaptive segmentation was used to analyze a series of clinical EEGs showing a variety of normal and abnormal patterns (Creutzfeldt et al., 1985); the computer method was used based on the autocorrelation function. By means of this algorithm, EEG segments were defined; similar segments were then clustered without supervision. The study concluded that minimal supervision of the clustering process may be necessary. Nevertheless, this adaptive segmentation method is useful for obtaining significant data reduction and has practical value for the clinical neurophysiologist. A review of methods for analyzing nonstationary EEGs has appeared (Barlow, 1985).

Mimetic Analysis

This form of analysis has been developed mainly by Remond and collaborators (Baillon et al., 1976; Remond, 1975, 1978; Remond and Renault, 1972) and is based on the general concept that automatic EEG analysis should mirror the visual analysis performed by electroencephalographers in their daily practice. This is why it has been called *mimetic analysis* (Remond, 1978). However, this analytic form uses tools common to other methods, particularly those nonparametric methods based on signal features characterized in the time domain, namely interval-amplitude analysis (Harner and Ostergren, 1976). The peculiar aspect of Remond's mimetic analysis is that the whole procedure of extracting EEG features and sets of features follows a syntactic approach: half-waves and minimal descriptors correspond to linguistic characters or letters, significant waves series such as K complexes and spindles to words, segments composed of wave series such as rhythms to paragraphs, and ensembles of segments to chapters or sections.

Based on these features it is possible to construct tables or graphs that demonstrate synoptically the distribution of the different features in an EEG epoch and determine their statistical properties for several epochs and derivations. A similar type of analysis has also been proposed by Schenk (1973). These methods, which have as common background an iterative interval analysis, tend to emphasize the high-frequency components of the signal, compared directly to spectral analysis (Ahlblom and Zetterberg, 1975) (see also Fig. 58.6). The section on interval analysis stressed the rather intimate relationship between interval analysis based on the signal and its derivatives and the spectral moments (see equation 58.22). Therefore, the methodology used by Remond and collaborators does not differ essentially from spectral analysis. The main difference is that mimetic analysis combines feature extraction with segmentation and logical classification.

Matched Filtering or Template Matching

Matched filtering is a form of pattern analysis in which a certain pattern or template (i.e., a set of values in the EEG signal x(t)) is detected by using cross-correlation (equation 58.10) between x(t) and a priori defined pattern m(t). (For the sake of simplicity the underscore of the stochastic variable is omitted in the following.) As in equation 58.10, one may write:

$$s(t) = \int_0^T x(\tau - t)\, m(\tau)\, d\tau \qquad (58.36)$$

The efficiency of the estimator s(t) is defined as follows:

$$0 \le \frac{[s(t)]^2}{\left[\int_{t-T}^{t} x^2 dt\right]\left[\int_0^T m^2 dt\right]} \le 1 \qquad (58.37)$$

The estimator reaches its maximum value (= 1) when m(t) is identical to x(t) and when both signals are aligned perfectly along the time axis. In this case, the template m(t) can best be extracted from the signal x(t). Various algorithms can be used to complete this operation efficiently. Saltzberg et al. (1971), Herolf (1971), Zetterberg (1973b), Lopes da Silva et al. (1975), Barlow and Dubinsky (1976),

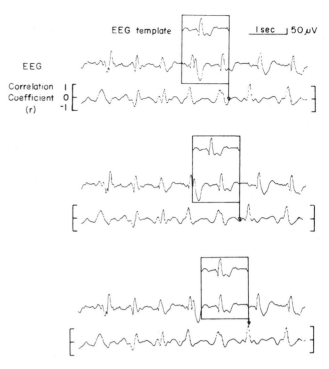

Figure 58.15. Continuous correlation coefficient write-out at three different points in time for an EEG signal and a template. In each record the *rectangle* indicates the time window for comparisons of template and EEG. In the first two instances there is no match, but in the third the template and EEG match exactly (they are identical); hence the correlation coefficient reaches a peak at 1.0. Sampling rate, 50 Hz; number of points in template, 72; duration of template, 1.24 seconds. (Adapted from Barlow, J.S., and Dubinsky, J. 1976. Some computer approaches to continuous automatic clinical EEG monitoring. In *Quantitative Analytic Methods in Epilepsy*, Eds. P. Kellaway and I. Petersén, pp. 309–327. New York: Raven.)

and Pfurtscheller and Fischer (1978) have all suggested using matched filtering to help detect epileptiform events (Fig. 58.15).

Time-Frequency Analysis

Above we have already mentioned that an important problem in EEG analysis is the fact that EEG signals, in general, can only be considered stationary during relatively short epochs. This has led to the development of several ways of analyzing such EEG signals by way of time-varying spectra, namely in the form of spectral arrays, and by applying segmentation methods. A more recent development in this respect is the introduction of methods that can combine analysis both in time and in frequency in an optimal way. Some of these methods use a special class of basis functions, the so-called wavelets. A function can be accepted as a wavelet if it satisfies the following relation:

$$\int_{-\infty}^{\infty} \psi(t)\, dt = 1 \qquad (58.38)$$

This means that wavelets have typically a waveform of a damped oscillation. The essential point of this method consists in decomposing the EEG signal in a set of wavelet functions defined as follows:

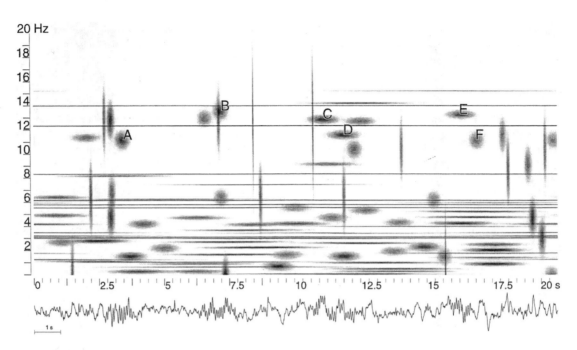

Figure 58.16. Wigner plot of the analysis of an EEG epoch of 20 seconds recorded during light sleep using a matching pursuit algorithm. Here the main objective was to detect sleep spindles automatically and to compare the results with those obtained by visual inspection by experts. The spindles automatically detected are indicated by the letters *A* to *F*. Spindles indicated by *A* and *B* were also detected by the experts. *C, D,* and *E* were classified by the experts as single spindles, but *F* was outside the section marked by the experts. (Adapted from Durka, P.J. 1996. Time frequency analyses of EEG. Ph.D. thesis, Department of Physics, University of Warsaw.)

$$\psi_{s,u}(t) = \frac{1}{\sqrt{s}}\ \psi\ \frac{(t-u)}{s} \qquad (58.39)$$

where s represents the time scale, and u is the translation variable. Based on this definition a set of orthogonal wavelets can be constructed that forms an ortho-normal basis. A given function, such as an EEG signal, may be characterized by the corresponding wavelet coefficients. For a basic theoretical treatment of this issue, the reader is referred to Mallat (1989). Wavelet analysis was applied to on-going EEG signals (Blanco et al., 1996; Schiff et al., 1994) and to evoked potentials (Bartnik and Blinowska, 1992; Geva et al., 1996) with interesting results. The set of wavelets is limited. To represent nonstationary EEG signals, a wider repertoire of basis functions is desirable. With this aim in view, the method called matching pursuit was developed by Mallat and Zhang (1993) and applied to the detection of transients in EEG signals by Durka and Blinowska (1995). A large set of basis functions can be obtained by scaling, translating and modulating a window function $g(t)$.

$$g(t) = \frac{1}{\sqrt{s}}\ g\ \frac{(t-u)}{s}\ e^{i\xi t} \qquad (58.40)$$

where in the time domain the function is concentrated around u with a width proportional to s; and in the frequency domain its energy is concentrated around ξ with a spread proportional to $1/s$.

The minimal time-frequency variance corresponds to the condition that $g(t)$ is gaussian. By means of the matching pursuit algorithm, using a dictionary of such basic functions,

a convenient expansion of a given signal can be obtained, as explained in detail by Mallat and Zhang (1993) and by Durka and Blinowska (1995). In practice, since EEG signals are available as real discrete time series the basis function has the following form:

$$g_{(\gamma,\phi)}(n) = K_{(\gamma,\phi)}g_j(n-p)\cos\left(2\pi\frac{k}{N}n + \phi\right) \qquad (58.41)$$

where the index $\gamma = (j, k, p)$ is the discrete analog of (ξ, s, u) of equation 58.40, $N = 2^L$ represents the number of samples, and the parameters p and k are sampled at intervals 2^j. The procedure is iterative and it is stopped as the set of waveforms is able to explain a given amount of the signal's variance.

The corresponding results can be visualized by means of the so-called Wigner maps, an example of which is given in Fig. 58.16 for the analysis of an epoch of sleep EEG where the detection of different types of sleep spindles is put in evidence.

An alternative way to compute the time evolution of the frequency spectrum is to apply a windowed Fourier transform that gives information about gradual changes in frequency spectra in the course of time. It was shown that this method can be useful in the analysis of ictal activity (Quian Quiroga et al., 1997).

Spatial Analysis of EEG

Typically, EEG records are obtained by sampling in space over the scalp's surface. It is of great interest to be able to infer from multiple scalp recordings obtained from different derivations the distribution within the skull of the generators responsible for different EEG phenomena. In its more specific form, the question of determining the place of intracranial sources of EEG phenomena implies solving the so-called *inverse problem* of volume conduction theory, which is to locate within a conductive medium the sources of electrical activity, given the distribution of electrical potentials at the surface enclosing the medium. In most clinical applications, only the spatial distribution of selected EEG features, i.e., their topographic displays, is made using standard brain maps that can be computed by means of commercially available software. Nevertheless, the development of more powerful algorithms is leading to an increase in the possibilities of performing more sophisticated spatial analyses than those offered by the more commonly used topographic displays. Therefore, the discussion distinguishes the three main methodological approaches: topographic displays, topologic analysis, and methods aimed at locating intracranial sources of EEG phenomena.

A general problem common to all types of spatial EEG analysis is that of sampling in space or, in simple terms, the necessary *interelectrode distance* in order to sample the EEG potential fields in an optimal way. This problem is analogous to that of sampling a time function; as discussed in that context the sampling frequency should be at least twice the highest frequency present in the signal. The question here is thus to identify the highest spatial frequency on EEG signals. This problem is difficult to solve empirically. It can be solved, however, theoretically through volume conduction models of the brain and surrounding tissues (Holman, 1979; Hosek et al., 1978; Kavanagh et al., 1978). Using such a model, it is possible to determine the spatial frequency components at the surface of the scalp model given a well-defined intracerebral source of potential. High-frequency components appear in the case of a source represented by a *radial dipole* close to the brain's surface (i.e., in the cortex). An electrode system's ability to give a good representation of the electrical potential distribution can be determined by computing the *aliasing error*, which depends on the spatial frequencies and the interelectrode distance. If the ordinary 10–20 electrode system is used with interelectrode distances of about 4.9 cm, the aliasing error for a *radial dipole* as source generator is 6%. The aliasing error can be reduced to 1% by decreasing the interelectrode distance to 3.2 cm (Holman, 1979).

Topographic Displays: A Historical Overview

In the past, several ingenious methods, including *toposcopic displays,* have been developed to depict EEG signals recorded in a compact form from different derivations, so that the spatial distribution of the most salient phenomena could be determined (see review in Petsche and Shaw, 1972). Toposcope methods essentially involve modulation of a series of light sources by the EEG signals. Thus, the signals can be visualized in a multichannel oscilloscope and filmed. The spatial information is obtained by visually scanning the oscilloscope or film display.

Walter and Shipton (1951) developed a sophisticated system allowing the display of EEG activity from 22 bipolar derivations by means of as many cathode ray tubes. Using toposcope methods, it was possible, for example, to find the distribution of time delays over the scalp of spike and wave patterns (Petsche et al., 1954). Another powerful toposcope system was developed by Livanov et al. (1964), who used their electroencephaloscope to record from 50 or 100 channels simultaneously. In another toposcope, oscilloscope output was digitized so that, in addition to a photographic display of the multichannel information, one could also have a numerical output (DeMott, 1970).

Toposcope displays, however, are difficult to interpret owing to the complexity and variability in time and space of the multichannel EEG information. Alternative methods have been developed mainly as the result of the use of digital computers. Thus, it has become feasible to map EEG potential distribution over the scalp. Two primary techniques have been used. One consists of recording EEG potentials at a specific moment, from two-dimensional arrays of electrodes, and making a contour plot of the corresponding spatial distribution using an interpolation procedure (linear or not) in order to estimate the potentials in between recording sites. In this manner, a series of spatial plots for different moments can be established. Another method consists of plotting potentials recorded using a line array of electrodes as a function of recording of place as well as time; an interpolation procedure in space may or may not be used. Remond (1968) has called these plots *chronotopograms.*

Remond (1960, 1968) and Remond and Torres (1964) conducted a particularly interesting series of studies pertaining mainly to alpha rhythms and evoked potentials using two-dimensional plots of EEG potentials (or other derived variables). In their studies of alpha rhythms, they made use of an analysis procedure to make synoptic chronotopograms; they first computed the so-called alpha average, which is obtained by triggering a computer in a particular phase of the alpha rhythm of one EEG derivation so that the activity of all derivations is averaged over a number of equivalent epochs in relation to that trigger; second, they made the two-dimensional plot of the average signals. The averaging procedure emphasizes related EEG activity in different derivations, whereas uncorrelated activity would tend to decrease. Ragot and Remond (1978) processed data from 48 EEG channels by digital computer. In constructing these plots, it is important to realize that the appearance of the topographic maps depends on the way the EEG signals have been recorded (bipolar, against a common reference electrode, or against the arithmetic mean of all electrodes). It is also necessary to consider the necessary sampling rate in space (i.e., the necessary interelectrode distance). Ragot and Remond's technique used an interelectrode distance of 4 cm; the authors contend, however, that a good representation of evoked potentials first components requires a distance of 2 cm. Lehmann (1971, 1972) and Lehmann et al. (1969) used a 48-channel recording system and computed interpolated equipotential plots that were displayed either as a series of time-specific still pictures or as a movie.

This form of spatial analysis, which is currently carried out on the basis of 64 or 128 EEG channels, yields EEG momentary maps that may represent the so-called microstates of brain activity (Lehmann, 1987). Lehmann and Michel

(1989, 1990) have extended this form of spatial analysis by computing the Fourier coefficients (sine and cosine) for a given frequency and EEG derivation. From these coefficients they estimate the dipole approximation that best fits the two-dimensional distribution of the coefficients. It should be noted that this form of FFT dipole approximation procedure gives results that are easy to interpret only if the constellation of sine and cosine values can be approximated by a straight line with a reasonably small error.

Another technique of displaying topographic information derived from a number of signals (bipolar derivations) was proposed by Harner and Ostergren (1978): *computer EEG topography*. The method consists essentially of two steps, Interval-amplitude analysis followed by use of an algorithm to display information on the time duration of individual waves occurring in different channels on a continuous two-dimensional display. These plots provide information on the spatial density of waves within a certain interval, on the corresponding amplitude, and also on the variability of wave time durations. The appearance of such displays is reminiscent of computed tomography. A similar type of display, a dot-density topogram for an EEG slow-wave pattern, has been proposed by Dubinsky and Barlow (1980).

Using color video technology, Duffy et al. (1979) introduced a topographic technique for imaging EEG power spectrum and evoked potentials, calling it BEAM, for brain electrical activity mapping. This technique has been implemented in commercially available systems and is currently used in several centers. Nagata et al. (1984) also presented a method for topographic EEG power spectrum display, called computed mapping of EEG. Such systems have been used widely to assess brain function in patients suffering from brain ischemia; numerous studies dedicated to this problem have been edited by Pfurtscheller et al. (1984a,b). Color images of sensory evoked potentials distributions have yielded results of theoretical and practical interest, especially regarding the origin of different SEP components (Desmedt and Bourguet, 1984; Desmedt and Nguyen, 1984); such images form a colored version of Remond's (1968) chronotopograms. In addition, computed EEG topography has permitted, based on a statistical evaluation of the data, brain maps displaying the regional distribution of reactivity in different frequency bands during auditory and visual stimulation (Grillon and Buschbaum, 1986).

The analysis of EEG reactivity has been extensively explored by Pfurtscheller and collaborators (1988), as indicated above (see Time-Varying Spectra). In this form of analysis both the decreases and increases in power that occur in relation to a given event, within a given frequency band, are quantified and displayed as a series of spatial maps for different time epochs. In the case of a decrease in power the authors consider that an event-related desynchronization (ERD) takes place. In the case of an increase in power they consider that an event-related synchronization (ERS) occurs. In the former case dynamic ERD mapping can be performed as shown in Fig. 58.17 (see also Color Plate 11).

Topologic Analysis: Neural Dynamics

In contrast to the previous section, in which the question of displaying EEG information was the crucial one, this discussion considers those analytic methods allowing quantitative evaluation of topologic relations. Cross-correlation and cross-spectral analysis (coherence and phase) and multivariate statistical methods are the primary approaches. Since cross-correlation, cross-spectral analysis, and spectral regression amount of information analysis have already been discussed, it is sufficient to state here that applying these methods implies a relatively large computational capacity, what nowadays is no insurmountable problem.

One of the interesting possibilities offered by the application of topologic analysis methods is the study of the electrophysiological correlates of cognitive functions as realized by Gevins (1989), Gevins and Certillo (1986), and Gevins and collaborators (1980, 1981, 1983). In these studies the interrelationship of event-related activity between different scalp derivations is quantified, using covariance or correlation analysis, in order to find the degree of functional interdependency between brain areas. It is important to note that for the study of neurocognitive relationships that may change in a fraction of a second, only methods that have a high time resolution can be used. In some cases it is possible to repeat the cognitive event a number of times, for example, the recognition of a visual pattern followed by a motor response, in order to average the results over a number of epochs.

In the last decade there was a growing interest in the field of nonlinear neural dynamics, i.e. in studying the dynamics of brain signals particularly with respect to cognitive functions. New methods have been applied and developed that allow the study of relationships not restricted to the linear domain and to measures that depend on signal's amplitudes, as is the case with covariance and cross-correlation. In essence the objective is to determine temporally correlated EEG/magnetoencephalogram (MEG) signals that may be spatially distant and not necessarily linearly related. Novel approaches explore the property that related EEG/MEG signals may show different degrees of phase synchrony. The main aim is to estimate the degree of synchronization between EEG/MEG signals as function of time, in relation to a number of events or cognitive tasks.

These mechanisms of synchronization may be analyzed through the estimation of phase synchrony. In this context the term *synchronization* means that two signals are phase-locked during a given time. Several algorithms are used in order to estimate phase synchrony. The method used by the Paris group (Le Van Quyen et al., 2001) starts by choosing EEG/MEG epochs and applying a band-pass filter to select the frequency band of interest; thereafter the instantaneous phase of the filtered signals is computed by means of the Hilbert Transform; finally the degree of phase synchrony, called phase-locking value (PLV) by these authors is estimated by averaging the phase differences on the unit circle in the complex plane:

$$PLV = \left\| 1/n \sum e^{i[\xi 1(t) - \xi 2(t)]} \right\| \qquad (58.42)$$

where n is the number of data points in each epoch. The sum is from 1 to n. PLV can vary from 1 (maximal phase grouping between a pair of signals) and 0 (independent signals, phase scattered). In this way the phase component can be obtained

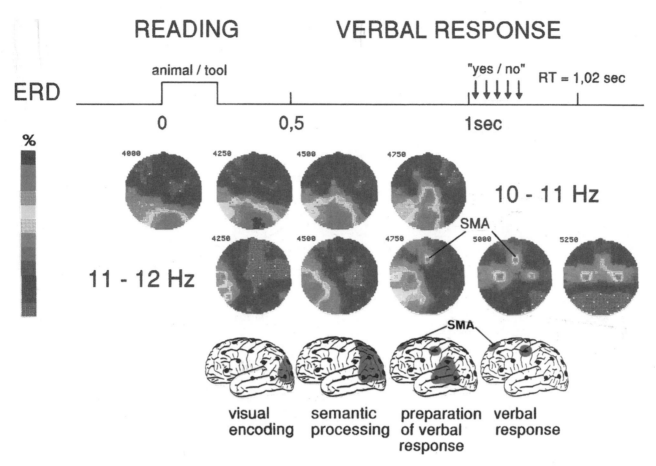

READING

animal / tool

VERBAL RESPONSE

"yes / no" RT = 1,02 sec

ERD

0   0,5   1sec

%

10 - 11 Hz

SMA

11 - 12 Hz

SMA

visual
encoding

semantic
processing

preparation
of verbal
response

verbal
response

Figure 58.17. Series of ERD maps from a normal subject computed in the 10- to 11-Hz and 11- to 12-Hz band during a visuoverbal task. The number above each map indicates the time in milliseconds when the map is computed. Color scale displays ERD% from 0% (blue) to 55% (black) for the 10- to 11-Hz band and 0% to 60% for the 11- to 12-Hz band. Red/black marks areas with decreased band power or ERD. In the lateral brain view, the approximate position of the recording electrodes and the cortical areas with high ERD magnitudes are indicated. The approximate location of the supplementary motor area (SMA) is also marked. (Adapted from Pfurtscheller G., and Klimesch, W. 1992. Functional topography during a visuoverbal judgment task studied with event-related desynchronization mapping. J. Clin. Neurophysiol. 9:120–131.) (See Color Figure 58.17.)

separately from the amplitude component for a given frequency range (Lachaux et al., 1999; Tass et al., 1998, Varela et al. 2001). Using this methodology it was shown, for example, that the scalp EEG/MEG of subjects performing the perceptive task of recognizing human faces induces a long-distance pattern of phase synchronization that represents active coupling of the underlying neural populations. This coupling appears to be necessary for the realization of this cognitive task (Rodriguez et al., 1999). An example is shown in Fig. 58.18, which illustrates how the perception of a human face induces a long-distance pattern of phase synchronization that corresponds to the moment of perception and to the subsequent motor response, while a period of desynchronization appears at the transition between these two events.

Other measures of phase synchrony have been proposed. A more generalized approach is based on the theory of nonlinear dynamical systems. Rulkov et al. (1995) introduced the concept of generalized synchronization. According to this concept synchronization between two dynamical systems X (the driver) and Y (the response) exists when the state of the response system Y is a function of the state of the driving system, X: Y = F(X). Assuming that F is continuous

and that two points on the attractor of X, x_i and x_j, are close to each other, then the corresponding points on attractor Y, y_i and y_j, will be also close to each other. The probability that embedded vectors are closer to each other than a certain small critical distance ϵ, is estimated for each discrete time pair (i,j). This is done for each signal, or channel k of a set of M channels. Thereafter, the number of channels $H_{i,j}$ for which the embedded vectors $X_{k,i}$ and $X_{k,j}$ are closer together than the critical distance can be calculated. Inspired by these theoretical concepts, Stam and van Dijk (2002) defined a synchronization likelihood $S_{k,i,j}$ for each EEG/MEG channel k and each discrete time pair (i,j) as

$$\text{If} \ |X_{k,i} - X_{k,j}| < \epsilon_{k,i}: S_{k,i,j} = (H_{i,j} - 1)/(M \, \sigma 1)$$

$$\text{If} \ |X_{k,i} - X_{k,j}| > \epsilon_{k,i}: S_{k,i} = 0 \qquad (58.43)$$

By averaging over all j, the synchronization likelihood $S_{k,i}$ can be estimated. Thus, $S_{k,i}$ is a measure that describes how strongly signal k at time i is synchronized to all other M − 1 signals. The synchronization likelihood is a measure of the dynamical interdependencies of EEG/MEG signals, both linear and nonlinear, as a function of time, and may be

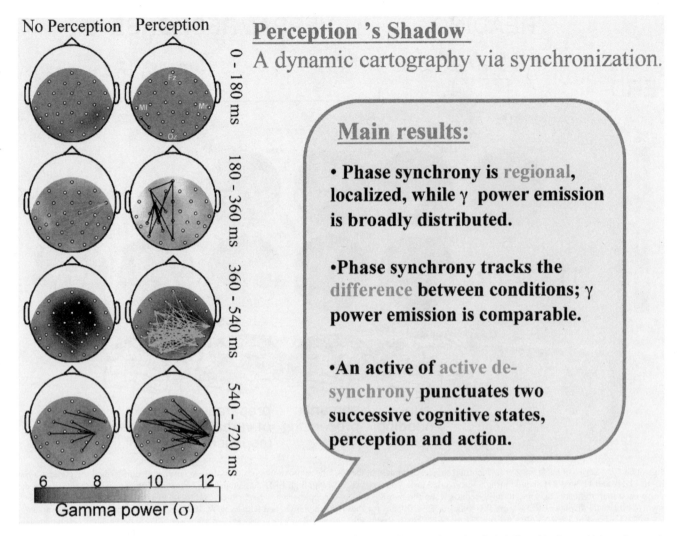

Figure 58.18. Average scalp distribution of gamma EEG activity and phase synchrony. Color coding indicates gamma power (averaged in a 34- to 40-Hz frequency range) over an electrode and during a 180-msec time window, from stimulation onset (0 msec) to motor response (720 msec). Gamma activity is spatially homogeneous and similar between conditions over time. In contrast, phase synchrony is markedly regional and differs between conditions. Synchrony between electrode pairs is indicated by *lines,* which are drawn only if the synchrony is beyond the distribution of shuffled data sets ($p < 0.01$). Black and green lines correspond to a significant increase or decrease in synchrony, respectively. (Adapted from Rodriguez, E., George, N., Lachaux, J.P., et al. 1999. Perception's shadow: long-distance synchronization of human brain activity. Nature 397(6718):430–433.) (See Color Figure 58.18.)

used to quantify phase relations of nonstationary time series. A number of applications have been published, as for example in a study of EEG changes related to the performance of a visuo-semantic task (Michelyoannis et al., 2003), and also in clinical study of EEG synchronization in mild cognitive impairment and Alzheimer's disease (Stam et al., 2003).

Another novel approach based also on a measure of phase synchronization was introduced for the analysis of visual evoked responses to intermittent light stimulation in photosensitive epileptic patients (Kalitzin et al., 2002; Parra et al., 2003). The method consists in estimating the phase dispersion of each frequency component present in the EEG/MEG. In this way a phase clustering index can be defined that differs from that used by Lachaux et al. (1999). Applying the phase clustering index it was found that the patients who develop epileptiform discharges during the light stimulation present an enhancement of the phase clustering index in the gamma frequency band in comparison to that at the driving frequency (Fig. 58.19). Thus the phase clustering index reflects the degree of excitability of the underlying neural system and it suggests the existence of nonlinear dynamics.

Multivariate Statistical Analysis Methods: Independent Component Analysis

Multivariate statistical methods can be useful in reducing data from a relatively large number of simultaneously recorded EEG signals; from the point of view of topographic analysis, they may help determine whether the variables from a number of EEG signals recorded from different der-

Distribution of Phase clustering index of Gamma frequency components over the scalp

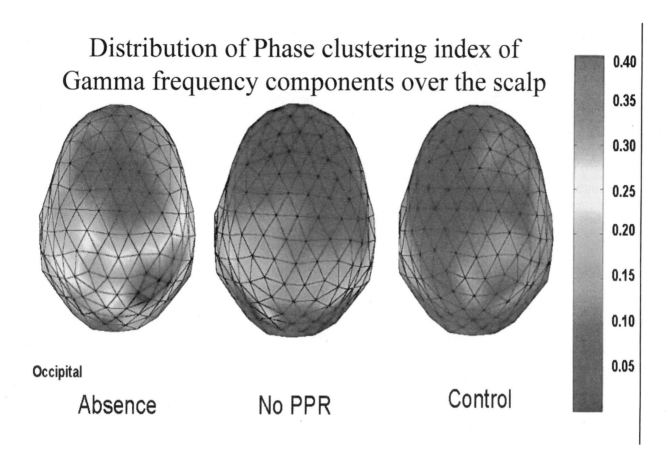

Occipital

Absence   No PPR   Control

Figure 58.19. Spatial distribution of the relative phase clustering index (rPCI) changes per magnetic sensor over the magnetoencephalography (MEG) helmet. *Left plot:* Average of the means of rPCI from four trials where intermittent light stimulation at 20 Hz was followed by a photoparoxysmal response (PPR), compared with two trials where light stimulation was not followed by PPR *(middle plot)*, and with the average of four trial in an age- and sex-matched control subject *(right plot)*. (Adapted from Parra, J., Kalitzin, S.N., Iriarte, J., et al. 2003. Gamma-band phase clustering and photosensitivity: is there an underlying mechanism common to photosensitive epilepsy and visual perception? Brain 126:1164-1172.) (See Color Figure 58.19.)

ivations and represented by, for instance, spectral values, can be described using a small number of statistically independent components. Classically this has been accomplished by factor analysis or principal component analysis. Pioneering studies of Walter et al. (1966) showed that the alpha rhythms recorded from the posterior cerebral regions cold be accounted for by way of two independent orthogonal components. It should be noted, however, that while these methods are useful in data reduction, they do not give information on the nature and location of physiological generators of EEG signals (van Rotterdam, 1970). A new approach for these kinds of analyses was developed: independent component analysis (ICA), initially proposed by Bell and Sejnowski (1995) and Makeig et al. (1996, 1997, 2002). ICA is a method that can be used to separate a number of statistically independent signals, or sources, from an equal number of linear mixtures of these sources. The basic assumption is that EEG/MEG signals recorded at a given site at the level of the scalp result from the sum of the projected activities of a number of multiple brain sources, sometimes contaminated by extracerebral (artifacts) sources. ICA

method aims at separating these sources in an optimal way. Mathematically the process of computing ICA consists of a simple transformation of one matrix (containing the sources) to another matrix (containing the mixtures or recorded signals) by multiplication with a mixing matrix. The inverse of the latter can be used to decompose the set of mixtures into the original sources. The problem is that one does not know, a priori, how the sources are combined; i.e., the coefficients of the mixing matrix are not known. To estimate these coefficients by way of the ICA method, the set of independent components are estimated by finding the minima of their mutual information. In case this process is done successfully the independent components represent the original sources. It should be realized that the sources should be nongaussian and that the number of sources should not exceed the number of mixtures. More recently, Anemüller et al. (2003) presented a generalized method that considers the EEG sources as eliciting spatiotemporal activity patterns, corresponding, for example, to trajectories of activation, propagating across the cortex. This led them to propose a model of convolutive signal superposition, in contrast to the commonly used instantaneous mixing model. In this way the sources of spatiotemporal dynamics of EEG signals recorded during a visual attention task could be identified.

The Inverse Problem in EEG and MEG

The ultimate dream of electroencephalography is to be able to find the intracranial sources of the potentials recorded at the scalp and to relate them to the activity of neural generators within the brain. This forms the *inverse problem* in electroencephalography. As stated in Chapter 5 the inverse problem has no unique solution, it is essentially ill-posed. Only approximate solutions may be estimated.

Solving the inverse problem means that first a function of three variables g(x,y,z), representing the potential at the scalp, must be estimated from measurements obtained by EEGs recorded at a number of electrode sites; this function can be obtained with an interpolation procedure. The question is then, how to find intracranial sources f(x,y,z) of the scalp potential. From the early period of EEG several researchers tried to solve this problem. In the models of Schneider (1972, 1974), Henderson et al. (1975), and Kavanagh et al. (1978), the source f is a part of a dipole. In the model of Klee and Rall (1977), the source is a part of a dipole layer. Schneider and Gerin (1973) attempted to solve this problem in practice calculating the intracerebral location of a source of epileptic discharges; Henderson et al. (1975) calculated the location of the dipole source of potentials caused by several phenomena such as eye blink artifacts, visual evoked potentials, and alpha rhythms.

To obtain a satisfactory solution of the inverse problem is not a simple task. In any case, constraints have to be introduced; namely, it is necessary to define two kinds of models: (a) of the sources, and (b) of the volume conductor. At the end we will consider the question of the relative value of the EEG and of the MEG in finding appropriate solutions to this problem.

Problems Posed by the Model of the Source

In general if the source of the potential distribution at the scalp is assumed to be described by an equivalent dipole current, the inverse problem is reduced to a six-parameter estimation problem. The estimation problem is essentially nonlinear and the parameters have to be found using an iterative procedure. The number of measurement points required to obtain an acceptable equivalent dipole estimate depends on the signal-to-noise ratio. In general, 16 to 40 measurements are enough for the main components of evoked potentials or magnetic fields (Cuffin, 1985). When multiple sources are present, ill-determined problems can arise, since the total contribution of two, or more, sources equals the sum of the contributions of each one. However, if additional information about the possible position of the sources is available, a solution may be estimated, as demonstrated by Scherg and von Cramon (1985a,b, 1986), Scherg et al. (1989), and as described in general terms in Scherg (1990). Furthermore, the signals may be described by means of a parametric model (Scherg and von Cramon, 1986), or by means of single valued decomposition, and dipoles may be fitted on the basis of the best possible linear combination of the basic functions or of the principal components, as also

proposed by Maier et al. (1987) and van Dijk and Spekreijse (1989).

However, a solution of the inverse problem can give systematical errors if a model is used that does not correspond to the physiological reality, as emphasized by Achim et al. (1988) who showed that a solution based on a single valued decomposition may not be optimal. This may occur partially because the noise may not be contained in the smallest principal values, but affect also the factor loadings corresponding to the larger principal values.

In case no extra information about the nature of the source(s) is available, a simple solution is to estimate for each time point along an EP, or evoked magnetic field, the equivalent current dipole which is allowed to change in position, orientation, and amplitude, as done by Stok (1986) and Stok and collaborators (1990).

A more general approach was proposed by de Munck (1990). This consists in splitting the model parameters into groups of linear (time functions) and nonlinear (positions and orientations) parameters. In practice it is wise to follow the proposal of Stok (1986) and of Achim et al. (1988) and start by fitting the responses with one moving dipole. In this way starting values can be obtained from which the optimal inverse procedure according to de Munck can be further applied (Lopes da Silva and Spekreijse, 1991).

Problems Posed by the Model of the Volume Conductor

In most solutions of the inverse problem in EEG or MEG, the brain and the different tissues of the head are modeled by concentric spheres. Most models, for the EEG, consist of four concentric spheres that represent, going from inside to outside, the brain, the cerebrospinal fluid (CSF), the skull, and the scalp (Cohen and Cuffin, 1983; Cuffin, 1985; Gutman and Shimoliunas, 1980; Hosek et al., 1978; Schneider, 1974; Sencaj and Aunon, 1982). The four spheres model contains eight parameters, four radii and four conductivities. Values of the radii can be obtained from magnetic resonance imaging (MRI) data, whereas the following values of the conductivities (Geddes and Baker, 1967) are generally used (in $\Omega \cdot m^{-1}$); 0.33 for the brain, 1.0 for the CSF, 0.0042 for the skull, and 0.33 for the scalp. These conductivity values have the same ratios as those used by Cohen and Cuffin (1983). As stated in Chapter 5 using an electric impedance tomography (EIT) method combined with a realistic model of the head (Ferree et al., 2000; Gonçalves et al., 2000, 2003) it was found that the ratio between the conductivities of the skull and the brain lies between 20 and 50 (for six subjects) rather than the traditionally assumed value of 80. The average values found in this investigation are the following: brain: $0.33 \text{ S} \cdot \text{m}^{-1}$; skull: $0.0081 \text{ S} \cdot \text{m}^{-1}$. It is also important to note that the variance of the estimates decreased by half when a realistic model was used, in comparison with a spherical model. However, a factor of 2.4 was found between the subject with the smallest and the largest skull conductivity, indicating that this value depends strongly on subject. Using this methodology a large number of studies have been carried out with the aim of estimating the functional localization of *equivalent dipoles* (EDs) that can account for the generation of evoked potentials and/or evoked magnetic fields (see also Chapter 5).

In Chapter 5, we have dealt with some general aspects of the numerical methods that have to be applied in this respect. Here we will consider only some more practical aspects of the problems involved in obtaining inverse solutions in EEG and MEG. We should emphasize that only in those cases where the distribution of the EEG potential or of the MEG field over the scalp is relatively simple and has a dipolar or quadrupolar character, a solution consisting of one or two, respectively, symmetrical EDs may be adequate. An increase in the number of dipoles can easily lead to rather complex and ambiguous interpretations and even to artifacts. Instead of trying to force a solution in the form of one, or more, discrete EDs, in case of more complex scalp distributions, one may attempt to describe the spatiotemporal EEG or MEG recordings in terms of sources distributed over the cortex. We refer the reader to Chapter 5 for a more fundamental description of the basic methods commonly used to estimate these cortical distributions.

In short, these methods have been developed with the objective of obtaining estimates of multiple dipoles with little a priori information, such as the MUSIC (multiple signal classification; Mosher and Leahy, 1999; Mosher et al., 1992) algorithm. A number of laboratories have pursued this issue by creating new algorithms based on the assumption that the sources are at fixed locations within the brain, using information extracted from the subject's MRI. In this way the problem is to find the linear parameters of the sources. Be that as it may, this problem is still underdetermined. This implies some form of regularization has to be introduced. To achieve this aim, several methods have been proposed (for a comprehensive review see Baillet et al., 2001): the minimum norm (MN) (Hämäläinen and Ilmoniemi, 1984, 1994), the weighted resolution optimization (WROP) method of Grave de Peralta Menendez et al. (1997), and the low-resolution brain electromagnetic tomography (LORETA), among others. The latter was proposed by Pascual-Marqui et al. (1994), and uses the discrete spatial Laplacian operator for regularization. This method yields a very smooth inverse solution (Pascual-Marqui et al., 2002). Since the latter method has an increasing scope of applications and has evolved very much in recent years, we examine here in some detail some of the specific properties of this approach. The method was originally applied to raw EEG data; later it was extended by incorporating statistical parameter mapping methodology; more recently, quantitative neuroanatomical data was added based on the digitized Talairach atlas provided by the Brain Imaging Centre, Montreal Neurological Institute. These developments have led to the wide use of LORETA and a rather extended number of publications. A new version of the basic method was introduced by Pascual-Marqui (2002) denoted as standardized low-resolution brain electromagnetic tomography (sLORETA). In general LORETA yields images that are very smoothed so that if the extent of the source is very restricted in space, for instance a small dipolar layer, the solution obtained using LORETA might be too blurred. In such cases dipole fits are to be preferred as shown for the case of epileptiform transients in Chapter 5 (Fig. 5.4).

Nonetheless, one has to emphasize that an acceptable inverse solution is very hard to achieve.

To realize the combination of EEG/MEG inverse solutions (Wood et al., 1985) with information about the dynamical properties of these signals, with the aim of determining patterns of neural dynamics and at the same time identifying which anatomical systems are involved, would be ideal. Recently, an approach was proposed with this objective by David et al. (2002). These authors use the minimum norm estimator to find source localizations; the source space can then be reduced, with the aid of surrogates, such that EEG/MEG data can be reconstructed with reduced biases both in terms of source localization and time series dynamics.

Another approach aims at estimating the distribution of EEG signals at the level of the cortical surface on the basis of the scalp distribution (reviews in Babiloni et al., 2003; He, 1999). In this way a cortical potential image may be obtained. Some approaches use the finite element method, the boundary element method, or spherical harmonics to estimate from the EEG scalp distribution that of the cortical surface (He et al., 2002; Le and Gevins, 1993; Nunez et al., 1994). Some methods estimate the equivalent dipole distribution from the EEG of the scalp, and then reconstruct the epicortical potentials by solving the forward problem (Babiloni et al., 1997; He, 1999; He et al., 1996, 2001; Sidman et al., 1990). The methods of cortical potential imaging have been applied with interesting results in a number of clinical applications, as for example in the analysis of interictal epileptiform spikes (Zhang et al., 2003).

In summary, a good deal of progress has been realized in developing methods to achieve satisfactory solutions of the inverse problem of EEG/MEG. Nevertheless, the fact that nonunique solutions, in essence, cannot be achieved makes these methods necessarily yield only approximate solutions, depending on the models and assumptions used. This should always be realized while examining the results of such methods, notwithstanding the attractiveness of the images sometimes obtained.

References

Abraham, F., Brown, D., and Gardiner, M. 1968. Calibration of EEG power spectra. Commun. Behav. Biol. Part A. 1:31.

Abt, K. 1979. Statistical problems in the analysis of comparative pharmaco-EEG trials. Pharmakopsychiatrie 12:228–236.

Achim, A., Richer, F., and Saint Hilaire, J.M. 1988. Methods for separating temporally overlapping source of neuroelectric data. Brain Topogr. 1:22–28.

Ahlblom, G., and Zetterberg, L.H. 1975. A comparative study of five methods for analysis of EEG. Technical Report No. 112, 56 pp. Stockholm: Royal Institute of Technology.

Anemuller, J., Sejnowski, T., Makeig, S. 2003. Complex independent component analysis of frequency-domain electroencephalographic data. Neural Netw. 16(9):1311–1323.

Arnolds, D.E.A.T., Lopes da Silva, F.H., et al. 1979. Hippocampal EEG and behaviour in dog. I. Hippocampal EEG correlates of gross motor behaviour. Electroencephalogr. Clin. Neurophysiol. 46:552–570.

Babiloni, F. Babiloni, C., Carducci, F., et al. 1997. High resolution EEG: a new model-dependent spatial deblurring method using a realistically shaped MR-constructed subject's head model. Electroencephalogr. Clin. Neurophysiol. 102:69–80.

Babiloni, F., Babiloni, C., Carducci, F., et al. 2003. 'The stone of madness' and the search for the cortical sources of brain diseases with non-invasive EEG techniques. Clin. Neurophysiol. 114:1775–1780.

Baillet, S., Mosher, J.C., and Leahy, R.M. 2001. Electromagnetic brain mapping. IEEE Signal Processing Magazine, November, 14–30.

Baillon, J.F., Bienenfeld, G., Findji, F., et al. 1976. Lecture, mesure et traitement automatique de l'analyse mimétique de l'EEG. Rev. Electroencéphalogr. Neurophysiol. Clin. 6:255–270.

Barlow, J.S. 1984. Analysis of EEG changes with carotid clamping by selective analog filtering, matched inverse digital filtering and automatic adaptive segmentation: a comparative study. Electroencephalogr. Clin. Neurophysiol. 58:193–204.

Barlow, J.S. 1985. Methods of analysis of nonstationary EEGs, with emphasis on segmentation techniques: a comparative review. J. Clin. Neurophysiol. 2:267–304.

Barlow, J.S., and Brazier, M.A.B. 1954. A note on a correlator system for brain potentials. Electroencephalogr. Clin. Neurophysiol. 6:321–325.

Barlow, J.S., and Brown, R.M. 1955. An analog correlator system for brain potentials. Research Lab Electronics, Technical Report No. 300. Cambridge, MA: Massachusetts Institute of Technology (MIT).

Barlow, J.S., and Dubinsky, J. 1976. Some computer approaches to continuous automatic clinical EEG monitoring. In *Quantitative Analytic Methods in Epilepsy,* Eds. P. Kellaway and I. Petersén, pp. 309–327. New York: Raven.

Bartnik, E.A., and Blinowska, K.J. 1992. Wavelets new method of evoked potential analysis. Med. Biol. Engn. Compt. 30:125–126.

Bendat, J.S., and Piersol, A.G. 1971. *Measurements and Analysis of Random Data.* New York: Wiley Interscience.

Berglund, K., and Hjorth, B. 1973. Normierte SteilheitsBeschreibungsparameter und deren physikalischer Sinn hinsichtlich der EEGDeutung. In *Quantifizierung des EEGs,* Eds. G. Schenk, pp. 249–257. Konstanz: AEGTelefunken.

Bickford, R.G. 1977. Computer analysis of background activity. In *EEG Informatics A Didactic Review of Methods and Applications of EEG Data Processing,* Ed. A. Remond, pp. 215–232. Amsterdam: Elsevier.

Bickford, R.G., Brimm, J., Berger, L., et al. 1973. Application of compressed spectral array in clinical EEG. In *Automation of Clinical Electroencephalography,* Eds. P. Kellaway and I. Petersén, pp. 55–64. New York: Raven.

Blackman, R.B., and Tukey, J.W. 1958. *The Measurement of Power Spectra.* New York: Dover Press.

Blanco, S., D'Atellis, C.A., Isaacson, S., et al. 1996. Time frequency analysis of electroencephalogram series (II): Gabor and wavelet transform. Phys. Rev. E. 54:6661–6672.

Bodenstein, G., and Praetorius, H.M. 1977. Feature extraction from the encephalogram by adaptive segmentation. Proc. IEEF 65:642–657.

Bohlin, T. 1971. Analysis of EEG signals with changing spectra. Paper TP 18.212, 118 pp. Stockholm: IBM New Lab Technology.

Brazier, M.A.B. 1968. Studies of the EEG activity of limbic structures in man. Electroencephalogr. Clin. Neurophysiol. 25:309–318.

Brazier, M.A.B. 1972. Spread of seizure discharges in epilepsy: Anatomical and electrophysiological considerations. Exp. Neurol. 36:263–272.

Brazier, M.A.B., and Barlow, J.S. 1956. Some applications of correlation analysis to clinical problems in electroencephalography. Electroencephalogr. Clin. Neurophysiol. 8:325–331.

Brazier, M.A.B., and Casby, J.U. 1952. Cross-correlation and autocorrelation of EEG potentials. Electroencephalogr. Clin. Neurophysiol. 4:201.

Broughton, R., Healey, T., Maru, J., et al. 1978. A phase locked loop device for automatic detection of sleep spindles and stage 2. Electroencephalogr. Clin. Neurophysiol. 44:677–680.

Bullock, T.H., McClune, M.C., Achimowicz, J.Z., et al. 1995a. EEG coherence has structure in the millimeter domain: subdural and hippocampal recordings from epileptic patients. Electroencephalogr. Clin. Neurophysiol. 95:161–177.

Bullock, T.H., McClune, M.C., Achimowicz, J.Z., et al. 1995b. Temporal fluctuations in coherence of brain waves. Proc. Natl. Acad. Sci. U.S.A. 92:11568–11572.

Burch, N.R., Nettleton, W.J., Sweeney, J., et al. 1964. Period analysis of the electroencephalogram on a general purpose digital computer. Ann. N.Y. Acad. Sci. 115:827–843.

Caille, E.J., and Bassano, J.L. 1975. Value and limits of sleep statistical analysis. Objective parameters and subjective evaluations. In *CEAN Computerized EEG Analysis.* Eds. G. Dolce and H. Kükel, pp. 227–235. Stuttgart: Fischer.

Campbell, J., Bower, E., Dwyer, S.J., et al. 1967. On the sufficiency of autocorrelation functions as EEG descriptors. IEEE Trans. Biomed. Eng. BME14:49–52.

Campbell, K., Kumar, A., and Hofman, W. 1980. Human and automatic validation of a phase-locked loop spindle detection system. Electroencephalogr. Clin. Neurophysiol. 48:602–605.

Carter, G.C. 1976. Time delay estimation. Rep. TR5335. New London, CT: Naval Underwater Systems Center.

Childers, D.G., and Pao, M.T. 1972. Complex demodulation for transient wavelet detection and extraction. IEEE Trans. Audio Electroacoust. AU20:295–308.

Clusin, W., Trapani, G., and Roccaforte, P.A. 1970. A numerical approach to matching amplification for the spectral analysis of recorded EEG. Electroencephalogr. Clin. Neurophysiol. 28:639–641.

Cohen, B.A. 1976. Period analysis of the electroencephalogram. Comput. Programs Biomed. 6:269–276.

Cohen, D., and Cuffin, B.N. 1983. Demonstration of useful differences between magnetoencephalogram and electroencephalogram. Electroencephalogr. Clin. Neurophysiol. 56:38–51.

Cooley, J.W., and Tukey, J.W. 1965. An algorithm for the machine calculation of complex Fourier series. Math Comput. 19:297–301.

Creutzfeldt, O.D., Bodenstein, G., and Barlow, J.S. 1985. Computerized EEG pattern classification by adaptive segmentation and probability density function classification. Clinical evaluation. Electroencephalogr. Clin. Neurophysiol. 60:373–393.

Cuffin, B.N. 1985. A comparison of moving dipole inverse solutions using EEG's and MEG's. IEEE Trans. Biomed. Eng. BME 33:854–861.

David, O., Garnero, L., Cosmelli, D., et al. 2002. Estimation of neural dynamics from MEG/EEG cortical current density maps: application to the reconstruction of large-scale cortical synchrony. IEEE Trans. Bio.-Med. Eng. 49:975–987.

DeMott, D.W. 1970. *Toposcopic Studies of Learning.* Springfield, IL: Thomas.

de Munck, J. 1990. The estimation of time-varying dipoles on the basis of evoked potentials. Electroencephalogr. Clin. Neurophysiol. 77:156–160.

Denoth, F. 1975. Some general remarks on Hjorth's parameters used in EEG analysis. In *CEAN Computerized EEG Analysis,* Eds. G. Dolce and H. Künkel, pp. 9–18. Stuttgart: Fischer.

Desmedt, J.E., and Bourguet, M. 1984. Color imaging of parietal and frontal somatosensory potential fields evoked by stimulation of median or posterior tibial nerve in man. Electroencephalogr. Clin. Neurophysiol. 62:1–17.

Desmedt, J.E., and Nguyen, T.H. 1984. Bit-mapped colour imaging of the potential fields of propagated and segmented subcortical components of somatosensory evoked potentials in man. Electroencephalogr. Clin. Neurophysiol. 58:481–497.

Dietsch, G. 1932. Fourier Analyse von Elektroenzephalogorammen des Menschen. Pflugers Arch. Ges. Physiol. 230:106–112

Drohocki, Z. 1938. L'électroencéphalographie du cerveau. C.R. Soc. Biol. 129:889–893.

Drohocki, Z. 1948. L'intégrateur de l'électroproduction cérébrale pour l'électroencéphalographie quantitative. Rev. Neurol. Paris 80:617–619.

Dubinsky, J., and Barlow, J.S. 1980. A simple dotdensity topogram for EEG. Electroencephalogr. Clin. Neurophysiol. 48:473–477.

Duffy, F.H., Burchfield, J.L., and Lombroso, C.T. 1979. Brain electrical activity mapping (BEAM): a method for extending the clinical use of EEG and evoked potential data. Ann. Neurol. 5:309–321.

Dumermuth, G. 1968. Variance spectra of electroencephalogram in twins. A contribution to the problem of quantification of EEG background activity in childhood. In *Clinical Electroencephalography in Childhood,* Eds. P. Kellaway and I. Petersén, pp. 119–154. Stockholm: Almqvist & Wiksell.

Dumermuth, G. 1969. Die Anwendung von Varianzspectra für einen quantitativen Vergleich von EEG bei Zwillingen. Helv. Paediatr. Acta 24:45–54.

Dumermuth, G. 1977. Fundamentals of spectral analysis in electroencephalography. In *EEG Informatics. A Didactic Review of Methods and Applications of EEG Data Processing,* Ed. A. Remond, pp. 83–105. Amsterdam: Elsevier.

Dumermuth, G., and Flühler, H. 1967. Some modern aspects in numerical spectrum analysis of multichannel electroencephalographic data. Med. Biol. Eng. 5:319–331.

Dumermuth, G., Huber, P.J., Kleiner, B., et al. 1971. Analysis of the interrelations between frequency bands of the EEG by means of the bispectrum. Electroencephalogr. Clin. Neurophysiol. 31:137–148.

Dumermuth, G., Walz, W., Scollo Lavizzari, G., et al. 1972. Spectral analysis of EEG activity during sleep stages in normal adults. Eur. Neurol. 7:265–296.

Dumermuth, G., Gasser, T., and Lange, B. 1975. Aspects of EEG analysis in the frequency domain. In *Computerized EEG Analysis,* Eds. G. Dolce and H. Künkel, pp. 429–457. Stuttgart: Fischer.

Dumermuth, G., Gasser, T., Hecker, A., et al. 1976. Exploration of EEG components in the beta frequency range. In *Quantitative Analytic Studies in Epilepsy,* Eds. P. Kellaway and I. Petersén, pp. 533–558. New York: Raven.

Duquesnoy, A.J. 1976. Segmentation of EEGs by means of Kalman filtering. Progress Report No. PR5, pp. 87–92. Utrecht: Institute of Medical Physics TNO.

Durka, P.J. 1996. Time frequency analyses of EEG. Ph.D. thesis, Dept. Physics, University of Warsaw.

Durka, P.J., and Blinowska, K.J. 1995. Analysis of EEG transients by means of Matching Pursuit. Ann. Biomed. Engn. 23:608–611.

Elul, R. 1969. Gaussian behaviour of the electroencephalogram: Changes during performance of mental task. Science 164:328–331.

Elul, R. 1972. The genesis of the EEG. Int. Rev. Neurobiol. 15:227–272.

Etévenon, P. 1977. Étude méthodologique de l'électroencéphalographie quantitative. Application à quelques examples. Thèse, Paris VI: Université Pierre et Marie Curie.

Etévenon, P., and Pidoux, B. 1977. From biparametric to multidimensional analysis of EEG. In *EEG Informatics. A Didactic Review of Methods and Application of EEG Data Processing,* Ed. A. Remond, pp. 193–214. Amsterdam: Elsevier.

Eykhoff, P. 1974. *System Identification. Parameter and State Estimation.* London: John Wiley & Sons.

Fenwick, P.B.C., Michie, P., Dollimore, J., et al. 1971. Mathematical simulation of the electroencephalogram using an autoregressive series. Int. J. Biomed. Comput. 2:281–307.

Ferree, T.C., Eriksen, K.J., and Tucker, D.M. 2000. Regional head tissue conductivity estimation for improved EEG analysis. IEEE Trans. Bio.-Med. Eng. 47:1584–1592.

Fink, M. 1969. EEG and human psychopharmacology. Annu. Rev. Pharmacol. 9:241–258.

Fink, M. 1974. EEG profiles and bioavailability measures of psychoactive drugs. In *Psychotropic Drugs and the Human EEG,* Ed. T.M. Itil, pp. 76–98. Basel: S. Karger.

Fink, M. 1975. Cerebral electrometry—quantitative EEG applied to human psychopharmacology. In *Computerized EEG Analysis,* Eds. G. Dolce and H. Künkel, pp. 271–288. Stuttgart: Fischer.

Gasser, T. 1975. Goodness-of-fit tests for correlated data. Biometrika 62: 563–570.

Gasser, T. 1977. General characteristics of the EEG as a signal. In *EEG Informatics. A Didactic Review of Methods and Applications of EEG Data Processing,* Ed. A. Remond, pp. 37–52. Amsterdam: Elsevier.

Gasser, T. 1979. Statistical handling of EEG data. Pharmakopsychiatrie 12:210–219.

Geddes, L.A., and Baker, L.E. 1967. The specific resistance of biological material, a compendium of data for the biomedical engineer and physiologist. Med. Biol. Eng. 5:271–293.

Gersch, W. 1970. Spectral analysis of EEGs by autoregressive decomposition of time series. Math Biosci. 7:205–222.

Gersch, W., and Goddard, G. 1970. Locating the site of epileptic focus by spectral analysis methods. Science 169:701–702.

Gersch, W., and Tharp, B.R. 1976. Spectral regression—amount of information analysis of seizures in humans. In *Quantitative Analytical Studies in Epilepsy,* Eds. P. Kellaway and I. Petersén, pp. 509–532. New York: Raven.

Geva, A., Pratt, H., and Zeevi, Y.Y. 1996. Spatiotemporal multiple source localization by wavelet-type decomposition of evoked potentials. In *Advances in Processing and Pattern Analysis of Biological Signals,* Eds. I. Gath and G.F. Inbar, pp. 103–122. New York: Plenum Press.

Gevins, A.S. 1989. Dynamic functional topography of cognitive tasks. Brain Topogr. 2:37–56.

Gevins, A.S., and Certillo, B.A. 1986. Signals of cognition. In *Clinical Applications of Computer Analysis of EEG and Other Neurophysiological Signals. Handbook of Electroencephalography and Clinical Neurophysiology* (Rev. Series, vol. 2), Eds. F.H. Lopes da Silva, W. Storm van Leeuwen, and A. Remond, pp. 335–381. Elsevier, Amsterdam.

Gevins, A., and Remond, A. (Eds.). 1987. *Methods of Analysis of Brain Electrical and Magnetic Signals. Handbook of Electroencephalography and Clinical Neurophysiology* (New Series, vol. 1), pp. 541–582. Amsterdam: Elsevier.

Gevins, A.S., Doyle, J., Yingling, C., et al. 1980. Lateralized cognitive processes and the EEG. Science 207:1105–1108.

Gevins, A.S., Doyle, J., Cutillo, B.A., et al. 1981. Electrical potentials in human brain during cognition: new method reveals dynamic patterns of correlation. Science 213:918–922.

Gevins, A.S., Schaffer, R.E., Doyle, J.C., et al. 1983. Shadows of thoughts: rapidly changing, asymmetric brain potential patterns of a brief visuomotor task. Science 220:97–99.

Goldstein, L. 1975. Time domain analysis of the EEG. The integrative method. In *CEAN—Computerized EEG Analysis*, Eds. G. Dolce and H. Künkel, pp. 251–270. Stuttgart: Fischer.

Gonçalves, S.I., de Munck, J.C., Heethaar, R.M., et al. 2000. The application of electrical impedance tomography to reduce systematic errors in the inverse EEG problem—a simulation study. Physiol. Meas. 21:379–393.

Gonçalves, S.I., de Munck, J.C., Verbunt, J.P.A., et al. 2003. In vivo measurement of the brain and skull resistivities using an EIT-based method and realistic models of the head. IEEE Trans. Bio.-Med. Engn. 50:754–767.

Gotman, J. 1976. Experiments in the automation and quantification of EEG interpretation: localized brain lesions and epilepsy. Thesis, Montreal: McGill University.

Grass, A.M., and Gibbs, F.A. 1938. A Fourier transform of the electroencephalogram. J. Neurophysiol. 1:521–526.

Grave de Peralta Menendez, R., Hauk, O., Gonzalez Andino, S., et al. 1997. Linear inverse solutions with optimal resolution kernels applied to electromagnetic tomography. Hum. Brain Map. 5:454–467.

Grillon, C., and Buschbaum, M.S. 1986. Computed EEG topography of response to visual and auditory stimuli. Electroencephalogr. Clin. Neurophysiol. 63:42–61.

Grosveld, F.M., Jansen, B.H., Hasman, A., et al. 1976. La reconnaissance des individus à l'intérieur d'un groupe de seize sujets normaux. Rev. Electroencéphalogr Neurophysiol. Clin. 9:295–297.

Gutman, A., and Shimoliunas, A. 1980. Comparison of the solutions of the direct and inverse problems of electroencephalography in models of an isolated sphere and thin membranes of the brain. Biophysics 25:715–717.

Hämäläinen, M.S., and Ilmoniemi, R.J. 1984. Interpreting measured magnetic fields of the brain: estimates of current distributions. Technical Report TKKFA559, Helsinki University of Technology.

Hämäläinen, M.S., and Ilmoniemi, R.J. 1994. Interpreting magnetic fields of the brain: minimum norm estimates. Med. Biol. Eng. Comp. 32:35–42.

Harner, R.N. 1975. Computer analysis and clinical EEG interpretation—perspective and application. In *CEAN—Computerized EEG Analysis,* Eds. G. Dolce and H. Künkel, pp. 337–343. Stuttgart: Fischer.

Harner, R.N., and Ostergren, K.A. 1976. Sequential analysis of quasistable and paroxysmal activity. In *Quantitative Analytic Studies in Epilepsy,* Eds. P. Kellaway and I Petersén, pp. 343–361. New York: Raven.

Harner, R.N., and Ostergren, K.A. 1978. Computed EEG topography. Electroencephalogr. Clin. Neurophysiol. Suppl. 34:151–161.

He, B. 1999. Brain electric source imaging: scalp Laplacian mapping and cortical imaging. Crit. Rev. Biomed. Eng. 27:149–188.

He, B., Wang, Y., Pak, S., et al. 1996. Cortical source imaging from scalp electroencephalograms. Med. Biol. Eng. Comput. 34:257–258.

He, B., Lian, J., and Li, G. 2001. High resolution EEG: a new realistic geometry spline Laplacian estimation technique. Clin. Neurophsyiol. 112:845–852.

He, B., Zhang, X., Lian, J., et al. 2002. Boundary element method-based cortical potential imaging of somatosensory evoked potentials using subject's magnetic resonance images. NeuroImage 16:564–576.

Henderson, C.J., Butler, S.R., and Glass, A. 1975. The localization of the equivalent dipoles of EEG sources by the application of electric field theory. Electroencephalogr. Clin. Neurophysiol. 39:117–130.

Herolf, M. 1971. Detection of pulse-shaped signals in EEG Telecommunication Theory, Technical Report No. 41. Stockholm: Royal Institute of Technology.

Herolf, M. 1975. A recursive detector. Telecommunication Theory, Technical Report No. 99. Stockholm: Royal Institute of Technology.

Hjorth, B. 1970. EEG analysis based on time domain properties. Electroencephalogr. Clin. Neurophysiol. 29:306–310.

Hjorth, B. 1975. Time domain descriptors and their relation to a particular model for generation of EEG activity. In *CEAN—Computerized EEG Analysis,* Eds. G. Dolce and H. Künkel, pp. 3–8. Stuttgart: Fischer.

Holman, H. 1979. Relations between depth and surface EEG. Thesis, Dept. of Electrical Engineering, Report No. 200. Twente University of Technology. Enschede, Netherlands.

Hosek, R.S., Sances, A., Jodat, R.W., et al. 1978. The contributions of intracerebral currents to the EEG and evoked potentials. IEEE Trans. Biomed. Eng. 25:405–413.

Huber, P.J., Kleiner, B., Gasser, T., et al. 1971. Statistical methods for investigating phase relations in stationary stochastic processes. IEEE Trans. Audio Electroacoust. 19:78–86.

Isaksson, A. 1974. SPARK—A sparsely updated Kalman filter with application to EEG signals. Telecommunication Theory, Technical Report No. 120. Stockholm: Royal Institute of Technology.

Isaksson, A. 1975. On time variable properties of EEG signals examined by means of a Kalman filter method. Telecommunciation Theory. Technical Report No. 95. Stockholm: Royal Institute of Technology.

Isaksson, A., and Wennberg, A. 1975. Visual evaluation and computer analysis of the EEG—a comparison. Electroencephalogr. Clin. Neurophysiol. 38:79–86.

Isaksson, A., and Wennberg, A. 1976. Spectral properties of nonstationary EEG signals, evaluated by means of Kalman filtering: application examples from a vigilance test. In *Quantitative Analytic Studies in Epilepsy,* Eds. P. Kellaway and I. Petersén, pp. 389–402. New York: Raven.

Itil, T.M. 1975. Digital computer period analyzed EEG in psychiatry and psychopharmacology. In *CEAN—Computerized EEG Analysis,* Eds. G. Dolce and H. Künkel, pp. 289–308. Stuttgart: Fischer.

Itil, T.M., Shapiro, D.M., Herrmann, W.M., et al. 1979. HZI systems for EEG parameterization and classification of psychotropic drugs. Pharmakopsychiatrie 12:4–19.

Jansen, B.H. 1979. EEG segmentation and classification. Thesis, 237 pp. Amsterdam: Free University.

Jay, F. (Ed. in Chief). 1977. *IEEE Standard Dictionary of Electrical and Electronics Terms.* The Institute of Electrical and Electronics Engineers, Inc. New York: John Wiley & Sons.

Jenkins, G.M., and Watts, D.G. 1968. *Spectral Analysis and Its Applications.* San Francisco: Holden Day.

Johnson, L.C., Hanson, K., and Bickford, R.G. 1976. Effect of flurazepam on sleep spindles and K complexes. Electroencephalogr. Clin. Neurophysiol. 40:67–77.

Kaiser, E., Petersén, I., Selldin, U., et al. 1964. EEG data representation in broadband frequency analysis. Electroencephalogr. Clin. Neurophysiol. 17:76–80.

Kaiser, J.F., and Angell, R.K. 1957. New Techniques and Equipment for Correlation Computation. Technical Memo 7668TM2, Servomechanisms Lab. Cambridge, MA: M.I.T.

Kalitzin, S.N., Parra, J., Velis, D.N., et al. 2002. Enhancement of phase clustering in the EEG/MEG gamma frequency band anticipates transitions to paroxysmal epileptiform activity in epileptic patients with known visual sensitivity. IEEE Trans. Bio.-Med. Eng. 49:1279–1286.

Kamp, A., and Vliegenthart, W. 1977. Sequential frequency analysis: a method to quantify event related EEG changes. Electroencephalogr. Clin. Neurophysiol. 42:843–846.

Kamp, A., Storm van Leeuwen, W., and Tielen, A.M. 1965. A method for auto- and cross-relation analysis of the EEG. Electroencephalogr. Clin. Neurophysiol. 19:91–95.

Kavanagh, R.N., Darcey, T.M., Lehmann, D., et al. 1978. Evaluation of methods for three-dimensional localization of electrical sources in the human brain. IEEE Trans. Bio.-Med. Eng. 25:421–429.

Kawabata, N. 1973. A nonstationary analysis of the electroencephalogram. IEEE Trans. Bio.-Med. Eng. 20:444–452.

Klee, M., and Rall, W. 1977. Computed potentials of cortically arranged populations of neurons. J. Neurophysiol. 40:647–666.

Knott, J.R., and Gibbs F.A. 1939. A Fourier transform of the EEG from one to eighteen years. Psychol. Bull. 36:512–513.

Kozhevnikov, V.A. 1958. Some methods of automatic measurement of the electroencephalogram. Electroencephalogr. Clin. Neurophysiol. 10:269–278.

Kumar, A. 1975. The complex demodulation method for detection of *a* waves and sleep spindles of the human EEG in realtime. Proc. Int. Conf. on Advanced Signal Processing Techniques, Lausanne, pp. 355–361.

Künkel, H., and EEG Project Group, 1975. Hybrid computing system for EEG analysis. In *CEAN—Computerized EEG Analysis,* Eds. G. Dolce and H. Künkel, pp. 365–385. Stuttgart: Fischer.

Lachaux, J.P., Rodriguez, E., Martinerie, J., et al. 1999. Measuring phase-synchrony in brain signal. Hum. Brain Mapping 8:194–208.

Le, J., and Gevins, A. 1993. Method to reduce blur distortion from EEG's using a realistic head model. IEEE Trans. Bio.-Med. Eng. 40:517–528.

Leader, H.S., Cohn, R., Wehrer, A.L., et al. 1967. Pattern reading of the clinical electroencephalogram with a digital computer. Electroencephalogr. Clin. Neurophysiol. 23:566–570.

Legewie, H., and Probst, W. 1969 Online analysis of EEG with a small computer. Electroencephalogr. Clin. Neurophysiol. 27:533–535.

Lehmann, D. 1971. Multichannel topography of human alpha EEG fields. Electroencephalogr. Clin. Neurophysiol. 31:439–449.

Lehmann, D. 1972. Human scalp EEG fields: evoked, alpha sleep and spike-wave patterns. In *Synchronization of EEG Activity in Epileptics,* Eds. H. Petsche and M.A.B. Brazier, pp. 307–326. New York: Springer.

Lehmann, D. 1987. Principles of spatial analysis. *Analysis of Electrical and Magnetic Signals. Handbook of Electroencephalography and Clinical Neurophysiology* (Rev. Series, vol. 1), Eds. A.S. Gevins and A. Remond, pp. 309–354. Amsterdam: Elsevier.

Lehmann, D., and Michel, C.M. 1989. Intracerebral dipole sources of EEG FFT power maps. Brain Topogr. 2:155–164.

Lehmann, D., and Michel, C.M. 1990. Intracerebral dipole source localization for FFT power maps. Electroencephalogr. Clin. Neurophysiol. 76: 271–276.

Lehmann, D., Kavanagh, R.N., and Fender, D.H. 1969. Field studies of averaged visually evoked EEG potentials in a patient with a split chiasm. Electroencephalogr. Clin. Neurophysiol. 26:193–199.

Lesèvre, N., and Remond, A. 1967. Variations in the average visual response in relation to the alpha phase "autostimulation." Electroencephalogr. Clin. Neurophysiol. 23:578–579.

Le Van Quyen, M., Foucher, J., Lachaux, J., et al. 2001. Comparison of Hilbert transform and wavelet methods for the analysis of neuronal synchrony. J. Neurosci. Methods 111(2):83–98.

Lilliefors, H.W. 1967. On the Kolmogorov-Smirnov test for normality with mean and variance unknown. J. Am. Stat. Assoc. 67:399–402.

Lion, K.S., and Winter, D.F. 1961. A method for the discrimination between signal and random noise of electrobiological potentials. Electroencephalogr. Clin. Neurophysiol. 5:109–111.

Livanov, M.N., Gavrilova, N.A., and Aslanov, A.S. 1964. Intercorrelations between different cortical regions of human brain during mental activity. Neuropsychologia 2:281–289.

Lopes da Silva, F.H. 1970. Dynamic characteristics of visual evoked potentials. Thesis, 126 pp., University of Utrecht.

Lopes da Silva, F.H. 1978. Analysis of EEG nonstationarities. Electroencephalogr. Clin. Neurophysiol. Suppl. 34:163–179.

Lopes da Silva, F.H., and Spekreijse, H. 1991. Localization of brain sources of visually evoked response: using single and multiple dipoles. An overview of different approaches. In *Event-Related Brain Research,* Eds. C.H.M. Brunia, G. Mulder, and M.N. Verbaten. EEG J. Suppl. 42:38–46. Amsterdam, Elsevier.

Lopes da Silva, F.H., and Storm van Leeuwen, W. 1978. The cortical alpha rhythm in dog: depth and surface profile of phase. In *Architectonics of the Cerebral Cortex,* Eds. M.A.B. Brazier and H. Petsche, IBRO Monograph Series, vol. 3, pp. 319–333. New York: Raven.

Lopes da Silva, F.H., Dijk, A., Smiths, H., et al. 1973a. Automatic detection and pattern recognition of epileptic spikes from surface and depth recording in man. In *Die Quantifizierung des Elektroenzephalogramms,* Ed. G.K. Schenk, pp. 425–436. Konstanz: AEG Telefunken.

Lopes da Silva, F.H., van Lierop, T.H.M.T., Schrijer, C.F., et al. 1973b. Organization of thalamic and cortical alpha rhythms Spectra and coherence. Electroencephalogr. Clin. Neurophysiol. 35:627–639.

Lopes da Silva, F.H., Hoeks, A., Smits, H., et al. 1974. Model of brain rhythmic activity, the alpha rhythm of the thalamus. Kybernetik 15:27–37.

Lopes da Silva, F.H., Dijk, A., and Smits, H. 1975. Detection of nonstationarities in EEGs using the autoregressive model. An application to EEGs of epileptics. In *CEAN—Computerized EEG Analysis,* Eds. G. Dolce and H. Künkel, pp. 180–199. Stuttgart: Fischer.

Lopes da Silva, F.H. (Ed.), Cooper, R., Dumermuth, G., et al. 1976. Sampling, conversion and measurement of bioelectrical phenomena. In *Handbook of Electroencephalography and Clinical Neurophysiology,* Ed. in Chief, A. Remond, vol. 4, Ed. M.A. Brazier, Part A. Amsterdam: Elsevier.

Lopes da Silva, F.H., van Hulten, K., Lommen, J.G., et al. 1977 Automatic detection and localization of epileptic foci. Electroencephalogr. Clin. Neurophysiol. 43:1–13.

Lopes da Silva, F.H., Vos, J.E., Mooibroek, J., et al. 1980a. Partial coherence analysis of thalamic and cortical alpha rhythms in dog. A contribution towards a general model of the cortical organization of rhythmic activity. In *EEG Activities and Cortical Functioning. Developments in*

Neuroscience, vol. 10, Eds. G. Pfurtscheller et al., pp. 33–59. Amsterdam: Elsevier.

Lopes da Silva, F.H., Vos, J.E., Mooibroek, H., et al. 1980b. Relative contributions of intracortical and thalamocortical processes in the generation of alpha rhythms revealed by partial coherence analysis. Electroencephalogr. Clin. Neurophysiol. 50:449–456.

Lütcke, A., Mertins, L., and Masuch, A. 1973. Die Darstellung von Grundaktivität, Herd, und Verlaufsbefunden sowie von paroxysmalen Ereignissen mit Hilfe der von Hjorth angegebe nen normierten Steilheitsparameter (vorläufige Mitteilungen). In *Quantitative Analysis of the EEG,* Eds. M. Matejcek and G.K. Schenk, pp. 259–280. Konstanz: AEG Telefunken.

Maier, J., Dagnelia, G., Spekreijse, H., et al. 1987. Principle component analysis for source localization of VEPs in man. Vis. Res. 27:165–177.

Makeig, S., Bell, A.J., Jung, T.P., et al. 1996. Independent component analysis of electroencephalographic data. In *Advances in Neural Information Processing Systems,* Eds. D. Touretzki, M. Mozer, and M. Hasselmo, pp. 145–151. Cambridge, MA: MIT Press.

Makeig, S., Jung, T.-P., Bell, A., et al. 1997. Blind separation of auditory event-related brain responses into independent components. Proc. Natl. Acad. Sci. U.S.A. 94(20):10979–10984.

Makeig, S., Westerfield, M., Jung, T.P., et al. 2002. Dynamic brain sources of visual evoked responses. Science 25;295(5555):690–694.

Makhoul, J. 1975. Linear prediction: a tutorial review. Proc. IEEE 63: 561–580.

Mallat, S.G. 1989. A theory of multiresolution signal decomposition: the wavelet representation. IEEE Trans. Pattern Anal. Machine Intell. 11: 674–693.

Mallat, S.G., and Zhang, Z. 1993. Matching pursuit with time frequency dictionaries. IEEE Trans. Signal Processing 41:3397–3415.

Marko, H., and Petsche, H. 1957. Ein Gerat zur gleichzettigen Frequenzund Amplitudenanalyse von EEGKurven bei frei wählbarer Zeitbasis. Arch. Psychiat. Nervenkr. 196:191–195.

Mars, N.J.I., and van Arragon, G.W. 1981. Time delay estimation in nonlinear systems using Average Mutual Amount of Information Analysis. IEEE—Trans. Acoustics, Speech and Signal Processing, vol. ASSP29, 3:619–621.

Matejcek, M., and Schenk, G.K. 1973. Die iterative IntervallAnalyse—Ein methodischer Beitrag zur Quantitativen Beschreibung des Elektroenzephalogramms in Zeitbereich. In *Die Quantifizierung des Elektroenzephalogramms,* Ed. G.K. Schenk, pp. 293–306. Konstanz: AEG Telefunken.

Mathieu, M. 1976. Analyse de l'electroencéphalogramme par prédiction linéatre. Thèse, 173 pp. Paris: Université Pierre et Marie Curie.

Matousek, M., (Ed.), Barlow, J.S., Dumermuth, G., et al. 1973. Frequency and correlation analysis. In *Evaluation of Bioelectrical Data from Brain, Nerve and Muscle,* II, Eds. M.A.B. Brazier and D.O. Walter, *Handbook of Electroencephalography and Clinical Neurophysiology,* Ed. in Chief, A. Remond, vol. 5, part A. Amsterdam: Elsevier.

Matousek, M., Petersén, I., and Friberg, S. 1975. Automatic assessment of randomly selected routine EEG records. In *CEAN—Computerized EEG Analysis,* Eds. G. Dolce and H. Künkel, pp. 421–428. Stuttgart: Fischer.

McEwen, J., and Anderson, G.B. 1975. Modelling the stationarity and Gaussianity of spontaneous electroencephalographic activity. IEEE Trans. Bio.-Med. Eng. 22:361–369.

McFadden, J.A. 1956. The correlation function of a sine-wave plus noise after extreme clipping. IRE Trans. Inform. Theory 82–83.

Michael, D., and Houchin, H. 1979. Automatic EEG analysis: a segmentation procedure based on the autocorrelation function. Electroencephalogr Clin. Neurophysiol. 46:232–235.

Micheloyannis, S., Vourkas, M., Bizas, M., et al. 2003. Changes in linear and non-linear EEG measures as a function of task complexity: evidence for local and distant signal synchronization. Brain Topogr. 15:239–247.

Mosher, J.C., Lewis, P.S., and Leahy, R.M. 1992. Multiple dipole modeling and localization from spatiotemporal MEG data. IEEE Trans. Bio.-Med. Eng. 39:541–557.

Mosher, J.C., and Leahy, R.M. 1999. Source localization using recursively and projected (RAP) MUSIC. IEEE Trans. Signal Processing 47:332–340.

Nagata, K., Yunoki, K., Araki, G., et al. 1984. Topographic electroencephalographic study of transient ischemic attacks. Electroencephalogr. Clin. Neurophysiol. 58:291–301.

Nunez, P.L., Silberstein, R.B., Cdush, P.J., et al. 1994. A theoretical and experimental study of high resolution EEG based on surface Laplacian and cortical imaging. Electroencephalogr. Clin. Neurophysiol. 90:40–57.

Otnes, R.K., and Enochson, L. 1978. *Digital Time Series Analysis.* New York: John Wiley & Sons.

Parra, J., Kalitzin, S.N., Iriarte, J., et al. 2003. Gamma-band phase clustering and photosensitivity: is there an underlying mechanism common to photosensitive epilepsy and visual perception? Brain 126:1164–1172.

Pascual-Marqui, R.D. 2002. Standardized low resolution brain electromagnetic tomography (sLORETA): technical details. Methods Findings Exp. Clin. Pharmacol. 24D:5–12.

Pascual-Marqui, R.D., Michel, C.M., and Lehmann, D. 1994. Low resolution electromagnetic tomography: a new method for localizing electrical activity in the brain. Int. J. Psychophysiol. 18:49–65.

Pascual-Marqui, R.D., Esslen, M., Kochi, K., et al. 2002. Functional imaging with low-resolution brain electromagnetic tomography (LORETA): a review. Methods Find. Exp. Clin. Pharmacol. 24(suppl C):91–95.

Persson, J. 1974. Comments on estimations and tests of EEG amplitude distributions. Electroencephalogr. Clin. Neurophysiol. 37:309–313.

Petsche, H. (Ed.), and Shaw, J.C. 1972. EEG topography. In *Evaluation of Bioelectrical Data from Brain, Nerve and Muscle,* Eds. M.A.B. Brazier and D.O. Walter, *Handbook of Electroencephalography and Clinical Neurophysiology.* Ed. in Chief A. Remond, vol. 5, part B. Amsterdam: Elsevier.

Petsche, H., Marko, A., and Kugler, H. 1954. Die Ausbreitung der "Spikes and Waves" an der Schädeloberfläche. Wien. Z. Nervenheilkd. 8:294–323.

Pfurtscheller, G., and Aranibar, A. 1977. Event-related cortical desynchronization detected by power measurements of scalp EEG. Electroencephalogr. Clin. Neurophysiol. 42:817–826.

Pfurtscheller, G., and Aranibar, A. 1980. Voluntary movement event-related desynchronization (ERD): normative studies. In *EEG Activities and Cortical Functioning,* Eds. G. Pfurtscheller, P. Buser, F.H. Lopes da Silva, et al., *Developments in Neuroscience,* vol. 10, pp. 151–177. Amsterdam: Elsevier.

Pfurtscheller, G., and Fischer, G. 1978. A new approach to spike detection using a combination of inverse and matched filter techniques. Electroencephalogr. Clin. Neurophysiol. 44:243–247.

Pfurtscheller, G., and Haring, G. 1972. The use of an EEG autoregressive model for the time saving calculation of spectral power density distribution with a digital computer. Electroencephalogr. Clin. Neurophysiol. 33:113–115.

Pfurtscheller, G. and Klimesch, W. 1992. Functional topography during a visuoverbal judgment task studied with event-related desynchronization mapping. J. Clin. Neurophysiol. 9:120–131.

Pfurtscheller, G., and Koch, W. 1972. Eine maschinelle Methode zur EEG Klassifikation. Methods Inform. Med. 11:233–237.

Pfurtscheller, G., Jonkman, E.G., and Lopes da Silva, F.H. (Eds.) 1984a. *Brain Ischemia: Quantitative EEG and Imaging Techniques. Progress in Brain Research,* vol. 62. Amsterdam: Elsevier.

Pfurtscheller, G., Ladurner, G., Maresch, H., et al. 1984b. Brain electrical activity mapping in normal and ischemic brain. In *Brain Ischemia: Quantitative EEG and Imaging Techniques,* Eds. G. Pfurtscheller, E.J. Jonkman, and F.H. Lopes da Silva. *Progress in Brain Research,* vol. 62, pp. 287–302. Amsterdam: Elsevier.

Pfurtscheller, G., Steffan, J., and Maresch, H. 1988. ERD mapping and functional topography: temporal and spatial aspects. In *Functional Brain Imaging,* Eds. G. Pfurtscheller and F.H. Lopes da Silva, pp. 117–131. Toronto: Huber.

Pfurtscheller, G., Stancak, A. Jr., and Neuper, 1996. C. Event-related synchronization (ERS) in the alpha bandan electrophysiological correlate of cortical idling: a review. Int. J. Psychophysiol. 24:39–46.

Pijn, J.P., Van Neerven, J., Noest, A., et al. Chaos or noise in EEG signals; dependence on state and brain site. Electroencephalogr. Clin. Neurophysiol. 1991 Nov;79(5):371–381.

Praetorius, H.M., Bodenstein, G., and Creutzfeldt, O. 1977. Adaptive segmentation of EEG records: a new approach to automatic EEG analysis. Electroencephalogr. Clin. Neurophysiol. 42:84–94.

Prechtl, H.F.R., and Vos, J.E. 1973. Verlaufsmuster der Frequenzspektren und Kohärenzen bei schlafenden normalen und neurologisch abnormalen Neugeborenen. In *Die Quantifizierung des Elektroenzephalogramms,* Ed. G.K. Schenk, pp. 167–188. Konstanz: AEG Telefunken.

Pronk, R.A.F., Simons, A.J.R., and de Boer, S.J. 1975. The use of the EEG for patient monitoring during open heart surgery. Proc. Comput. Cardiol. (Rotterdam) 77–81.

Pronk, R.A.F., de Boer, S.J., Cornelissen, R.C.M., et al. 1976. Computer assisted patient monitoring during open heart surgery with the aid of the

EEG. In *Progress Report No. PR6,* Eds. B. van Eijnsbergen and F.H. Lopes da Silva, pp. 224–228. Utrecht: Institute of Medical Physics TNO.

Quian Quiroga, R., Blanco, S., Rosso, O.A., et al. 1997. Searching for hidden information with Gabor Transform in generalized tonic-clonic seizures. Electroencephalogr. Clin. Neurophysiol. 103:434–439.

Ragot, R.A., and Remond, A. 1978. EEG field mapping. Electroencephalogr. Clin. Neurophysiol. 45:417–421.

Rappelsberger, P., and Petsche, H. 1975. Spectral analysis of the EEG by means of autoregression. In *CEAN—Computerized EEG Analysis,* Eds. G. Dolce and H. Künkel, pp. 27–40. Stuttgart: Fischer.

Rappelsberger, P., Petsche, H., Vollmer, R., et al. 1978. Rhythmicity in seizure patterns—intracortical aspects. In *Origin of Cerebral Field Potentials,* Eds. E.J. Speckmann and H. Caspers, pp. 80–97. Stuttgart: Thieme.

Regan, D. 1977. Evoked potentials in basic and clinical research. In *EEG Informatics Didactic Review of Methods and Applications of EEG Data Processing,* Ed. A. Remond, pp. 319–346. Amsterdam: Elsevier.

Reits, D. 1975. Cortical Potentials in Man Evoked by Noise Modulated Light. Thesis, University of Utrecht.

Remond, A. 1960. Poursuite de la signification en EEG: I—Le problème de la référence spatiale. Rev. Neurol. 102:412–415.

Remond, A. 1968. The importance of topographic data in EEG phenomena, and an electrical model to reproduce them. Electroencephalogr. Clin. Neurophysiol. Suppl. 27:27–49.

Remond, A. 1975. An EEGer's approach to automatic data processing. In *CEAN—Computerized EEG Analysis,* Eds. G. Dolce and H. Künkel, pp. 128–136. Stuttgart: Fischer.

Remond, A. 1978. From graphoelements to EEG pattern recognition. Electroencephalogr. Clin. Neurophysiol. Suppl. 34:141–145.

Remond, A., and Renault, B. 1972. La théorie des objets électroencéphalographiques. Rev. Electroencéphalogr. Clin. Neurophysiol. 2:241–256.

Remond, A., and Torres, F. 1964. A method of electrode placement with a view to topographical research. I. Basic concepts. Electroencephalogr. Clin. Neurophysiol. 17:577–578.

Remond, A., Lesèvre, N., Joseph, J.P., et al. 1969. The alpha average. I. Methodology and description. Electroencephalogr. Clin. Neurophysiol. 26:245–265.

Rice, S.O. 1954. Mathematical analysis of random noise. In *Noise and Stochastic Processes,* Ed. N. Wax, pp. 133–294. New York: Dover.

Rodriguez, E., George, N., Lachaux, J.P., et al. 1999. Perception's shadow: long-distance synchronization of human brain activity. Nature 397 (6718):430–433.

Rulkov, N.F., Sushchik, M.M., Tsimring, L.S., et al. 1995. Generalized synchronization of chaos in directionally coupled chaotic systems. Phys. Rev. E Stat. Phys. Plasmas Fluids Relat. Interdisc. Topics 51(2):980–994.

Saltzberg, B., and Burch, N.R. 1971. Period analytic estimates of moments of the power spectrum. A simplified EEG time domain procedure. Electroencephalogr. Clin. Neurophysiol. 30:568–570.

Saltzberg, B., Burch, N.R., McLennan, M.A., et al. 1957. A new approach to signal analysis in electroencephalography. IRE Trans. Med. Electron. 8:24–30.

Saltzberg, B., Edwards, R.J., Heath, R.G., et al. 1968 Synoptic analysis of EEG signals. In *Data Acquisition and Processing in Biology and Medicine,* vol. 5, Ed. K. Enslein, pp. 267–307. Oxford: Pergamon Press.

Saltzberg, B., Lustick, L.S., and Heath, R.G. 1971. Detection of focal spiking in the scalp EEG of monkeys. Electroencephalogr. Clin. Neurophysiol. 31:327–333.

Saunders, M.G. 1963. Amplitude probability density studies on alpha and alpha-like patterns. Electroencephalogr. Clin. Neurophysiol. 15:761–767.

Schenk, G.K. 1973. Die Quantifizierung des EEG mittels vektorieller Iterationstechnik, einer Simulationsmethode der visuellen Analyse. In *Die Quantifizierung des Elektroencephalogramms,* Ed. G.K. Schenk, pp. 307–343. Konstanz: AEG Telefunken.

Scherg, M. 1990. Fundamentals of dipole source potential analysis. In *Auditory Evoked Electric and Magnetic Fields, Adv. Audiol.* 6, Eds. F. Grandori, M. Hoke, and G.L. Romalni, pp. 40–69. Basel: Karger.

Scherg, M., and von Cramon, D. 1985a. Two bilateral sources of the late AEP as identified by a spatiotemporal dipole model. Electroencephalogr Clin. Neurophysiol. 62:32–44.

Scherg, M., and von Cramon, D. 1985b. A new interpretation of the generators of BAEP waves I-V; results of a spatiotemporal dipole model. Electroencephalogr. Clin. Neurophysiol. 62:290–299.

Scherg, M., and von Cramon, D. 1986. Evoked dipole source potentials of the human auditory cortex. Electroencephalogr. Clin. Neurophysiol. 65: 344–360.

Scherg, M., Vajsar, J., and Picton, T.W. 1989. A source analysis of human auditory evoked potentials. J. Cogn. Neurosci. 1:336–355.

Schiff, S.J., Aldrouby, A., Unser, M., et al. 1994. Fast wavelet transformation of EEG. Electroencephalogr. Clin. Neurophysiol. 91:442–455.

Schneider, M. 1972. A multistage process for computing virtual dipolar sources of EEG discharges from surface information. IEEE Trans Biomed. Eng. 19:1–12.

Schneider, M. 1974. Effect of inhomogeneities on surface signals coming from a cerebral dipole source. IEEE Trans. Biomed. Eng. 21:52–54.

Schneider, M., and Gerin, P. 1973. Une méthode de localisation des dipoles cérébraux. Electroencephalogr. Clin. Neurophysiol. 28:69–78.

Schwarzer, F., and Reets, H. 1966. Machines for EEG analysis. Electroencephalogr. Clin. Neurophysiol. 20:278.

Sciarretta, G., and Erculianti, P. 1978. A proposal for calibrating EFG spectrograms. Electroencephalogr. Clin. Neurophysiol. 5:674–676.

Sencaj, R.W., and Aunon, J.I. 1982. Dipole localization of average and single visual evoked potentials. IEEE Trans. Biomed. Eng. 29:26–33.

Sidman, R., Ford, M., Ramsey, G., et al. 1990. Age-related features of the resting and P300 auditory responses using the dipole localization method and cortical imaging technique. J. Neurosci. Methods 33:23–32.

Siebert, W.M. 1959. The description of random processes. In *Processing Neuroelectric Data,* Eds. Communications Biophysics Group and W.M. Siebert, pp. 66–87. Cambridge, MA: M.I.T. Press.

Siegel, S. 1956. *Nonparametric Statistics for the Behavioural Sciences.* Tokyo: McGraw-Hill.

Sologub, E.B. 1965. EEG cross correlation analysis during the formation of motor dynamic stereotype in human. Zh. Vyssh. Nerv. Deiat. 15:32–41 (in Russian).

Stam, C.J., and van Dijk, B.W. 2002. Synchronization likelihood: an unbiased measure of generalized synchronization in multivariate data series. Physica D 163:236–251.

Stam, C.J., van der Made, Y., Pijnenburg, Y.A.L., et al. 2003. EEG synchronization in mild cognitive impairment and Alzheimer's disease. Acta Neurol. Scand. 108:90–96.

Stebel, J., and Schwartze, P. 1967. Über die Verwendbarketi der Polaritätskorrelationsmethode zur Analyse von Elektroenzephalogrammen. Acta Biol. Med. Ger. 18:373–382.

Steinberg, C.A., and Paine, L.W. 1964. Methods and techniques of data conversion. Ann. N.Y. Acad. Sci. 115/2:614–626.

Stok, C.J. 1986. The inverse problem in EEG and MEG with applications to visual evoked responses. Ph.D. Thesis. Technical University of Twente, Enschede, Netherlands.

Stok, C.J., Spekreijse, H., Peters, M.J., et al. 1990. A comparative EEG/MEG equivalent dipole study of the pattern onset visual response. In *New Trends and Advanced Techniques in Clinical Neurophysiology,* Eds. P.M. Rossini and F. Mauguière. EEG J. Suppl. 41:34–50. Amsterdam, Elsevier.

Storm van Leeuwen, W. 1961. Comparison of EEG data obtained with frequency analysis and with correlation methods. Electroencephalogr. Clin. Neurophysiol. Electroencephalogr. Clin. Neurophysiol. Suppl. 20:37–40.

Storm van Leeuwen, W. 1964. Complementary of different analysis methods. Electroencephalogr. Clin. Neurophysiol. 16:136–139.

Storm van Leeuwen, W., Arntz, A., Spoelstra, P., et al. 1976. The use of computer analysis for diagnosis in routine electroencephalography. Rev. Electroencephalogr. Neurophysiol Clin. 62:318–327.

Storm van Leeuwen, W., Wieneke, G.H., Spoelstra, P., et al. 1978. Lack of bilateral coherence of mu rhythm. Electroencephalogr. Clin. Neurophysiol. 44:140–146.

Susskind, A.K. (Ed.). 1957. *Notes on Analog-Digital Conversion Techniques.* New York: John Wiley & Sons.

Tass, P., Rosenblum, M.G., Weule, J., et al. 1998. Detection of n:m phase locking from noisy data: application to magnetoencephalography. Phys. Rev. Lett. 81:3291–3294.

Tharp, B.R., and Gersch, W. 1975. Spectral analysis of seizures in humans. Comput. Biomed. Res. 8:503–521.

Thickbroom, G.W., Mastaglia, F.L., Carroll, W.M., et al. 1984. Source derivations: application to topographic mapping of visual evoked potentials. Electroencephalogr. Clin. Neurophysiol. 59:279–285.

van Dijk, W., and Spekreijse, H. 1989. Localization of the visually evoked response: the pattern appearance response. In *Topographic Brain Map-*

ping of EEG and Evoked Potentials, Ed. K. Maurer. Berlin: Springer-Verlag.

van Rotterdam, A. 1970. Limitations and difficulties in signal processing by means of the principal components analysis. IEEE Trans. Biomed. Eng. 17:268–269.

Varela, F., Lachaux, J.P., Rodriguez, E., et al. 2001. The brainweb: phase synchronization and large-scale integration. Nat. Rev. Neurosci. 2(4): 229–239.

Vos, J.E. 1975. Representation in the frequency domain of nonstationary EEGs. In *CEAN—Computerized EEG Analysis,* Eds. G. Dolce and H. Künkel, pp. 41–50. Stuttgart: Fischer.

Vos, J.E., Lammerstsma, A.A., and Van Eykeren, L.A. 1977. Ordinary and partial coherences of bipolar and quasiunipolar derivations of infant electroencephalograms. In *Random Signal Analysis,* IEE Cofn. Publ. No. 159, pp. 154–160, London.

Walter, D.O. 1963. Spectral analysis of electroencephalograms: mathematical determination of neurological relationships from records of limited duration. Exp. Neurol. 8:155–181.

Walter, D.O. 1968a. On units and dimensions for reporting spectral intensities. Electroencephalogr. Clin. Neurophysiol. 24:486–487.

Walter, D.O. 1968b. The method of complex demodulation. In *Advances in EEG Analysis,* Eds. D.O. Walter and M.A.B. Brazier. Electroencephalogr. Clin. Neurophysiol. Suppl. 27:51–57.

Walter, D.O., and Adey, W.R. 1963. Spectral analysis of electroencephalograms recorded during learning in the cat. Exp. Neurol. 8:155–181.

Walter, D.O., and Adey, W.R. 1965. Analysis of brain wave generators as multiple statistical time series. IEEE Trans. Biomed. Eng. 12:8–13.

Walter, D.O., Rhodes, J.M., Brown, D., et al. 1966. Comprehensive spectral analysis of human generators in posterior cerebral regions. Electroencephalogr. Clin. Neurophysiol. 20:224–237.

Walter, W.G. 1943a. Automatic low frequency analyzer. Electron Eng. 16:9–13.

Walter, W.G. 1943b. An improved low frequency analyzer. Electron Eng. 16:236–240.

Walter, W.G., and Shipton, H.W. 1951. A new toposcopic display system. Electroencephalogr. Clin. Neurophysiol. 3:281–292.

Wennberg, A., and Zetterberg, L.H. 1971. Application of a computer-based model for EEG analysis. Electroencephalogr. Clin. Neurophysiol. 31: 457–468.

Wiener, N. 1961. Cybernetics. Cambridge, MA: M.I.T. Press.

Wood, C.C., Cohen, D., Cuffin, B.N., et al. 1985. Electrical sources in human somatosensory cortex: identification by combined magnetic and potential recordings. Science 227:1031–1061.

Zetterberg, L.H. 1969. Estimation of parameters for a linear difference equation with application to EEG analysis. Math. Biosci. 5:227–275.

Zetterberg, L.H. 1973a. Experience with analysis and simulation of EEG signals with parametric description of spectra. In *Automation of Clinical Electroencephalography,* Eds. P. Kellaway and I. Petersén, pp. 161–201. New York: Raven.

Zetterberg, L.H. 1973b. Spike detection by computer and by analog equipment. In *Automation of Clinical Electroencephalogr. Clin. Neurophysiol.,* Eds. P. Kellaway and I. Petersén, pp. 227–234. New York: Raven.

Zetterberg, L.H. 1973c. Stochastic activity in a population of neurons. A systems analysis approach. Report No. 2.3.153/1, 23 pp. Utrecht: Institute of Medical Physics TNO.

Zetterberg, L.H. 1977. Means and methods for processing of physiological signals with emphasis on EEG analysis. In *Advances in Biology and Medical Physics,* Eds. J.H. Lawrence et al., vol. 16, pp. 41–91. New York: Academic Press.

Zetterberg, L.H., Kristiansson, L., and Mossberg, K. 1978. Performance of a model of a local neuron population. Biol. Cybern. 31:15–26.

Zhang, X., van Dronfelen, W., Hecox, K.E., et al. 2003. High resolution EEG: cortical potential imaging of interictal spikes. Clin. Neurophysiol. 114:1963–1973.

59. Computer-Assisted EEG Diagnosis: Pattern Recognition and Brain Mapping

Fernando Lopes da Silva

Pattern recognition methods form a general class of procedures. With these methods, objects characterized by a set of features such as a pattern can be assigned to a certain set. The first operation in electroencephalograph (EEG) pattern recognition is choosing a number of features that are potentially important in identifying the objects of interest. The second operation might be one of two different approaches: *classification* or *clustering*. In the former, it must be stated a priori that there exists a number of classes (e.g., clinical: normal/abnormal) to which the objects must be allocated; the latter has no predetermined number of classes. Rather, the question is which cluster can be formed given a number of objects and a certain statistical criterion. Classification uses a group of EEGs, the so-called *learning set,* to determine (for example, by way of Fisher's *linear discriminant analysis*) the set of features that gives the best possible discrimination between the classes. Thereafter, the best set of features can be used to classify any other group EEGs forming the test sets.

Clustering requires little or no specific a priori knowledge; the objects characterized by a set of features are grouped by means of a clustering algorithm. The user must determine the most useful ranging of objects relative to the result desired. Thereafter, the relevance of the clusters obtained to the specific clinical application must be evaluated.

In EEG analysis, most methods of analysis follow, explicitly or not, a pattern recognition approach. This discussion considers the most important aspects of such an approach in relation to general problems of automatic EEG diagnosis. For a thorough treatment of pattern recognition theories, the reader is referred to the books of Duda and Hart (1973), Mendel and Fu (1970), and Tou and Gonzalez (1974), and to the review of Demartini and Vincent-Carrefour (1977).

Feature Extraction: Specific Problems

The performance of any EEG analysis method depends, to a large extent, on the extraction of the relevant characteristics of the EEG signals. This section first considers the main types of features used in EEG analysis; then it examines how these features can be incorporated into EEG classification systems.

Time Domain Analysis Methods

When using EEG *amplitude analysis,* the features ordinarily chosen are mean (m), standard deviation (σ), skewness, kurtosis, and coefficient of variation [$(\sigma/m) \times 100$];

these are computed from the original signal as discussed in Chapter 58. Furthermore, one can also define similar features for the rectified signal: mean, standard deviation, and coefficient of variation.

Interval analysis of EEG signals leads to the selection of the feature's average frequency of level (zero) crossings, N0, of the original signal and also of its first derivative, N1, and second derivative, N2. Combining amplitude and interval analysis (see Chapter 58), EEG signals can be characterized by a set of features including those described above and a few others such as the signal half-wave length; and its derivatives (mean, standard deviation, and range), peak-to-peak values per wave (mean and standard deviation), and amplitude range (i.e., the difference between the largest and the smallest amplitude value within a certain time epoch). Other features that can be included in this section are Hjorth's parameters: activity, mobility, and complexity, and the results of time-frequency analyses, for example using wavelet decomposition or matching pursuit, as explained in Chapter 58.

Spectral Analysis Using Nonparametric Methods

The common features extracted from EEG power spectra include some measures of spectral intensity within the classic frequency bands, namely the mean *spectral intensity* (power and amplitude) and the average *frequency.* A fundamental question, however, is how to define the EEG frequency bands. According to the generally accepted empirical definitions, one may use the subdivision indicated in Table 59.1. Sometimes it is preferable to combine frequency bands. The question that should be asked is whether the activities in different frequency bands behave independently. This problem can be approached by applying multivariate statistical analysis to EEG spectral values. This has been investigated by Herrmann et al. (1978) using factor analysis; this study used 57 relative power values in frequency bands between 1.5 and 30 Hz with frequency resolution $\Delta f = 0.5$ Hz, as well as absolute power values. In this way, it was found that the power spectrum could be broken down into the frequency bands indicated in Table 59.1. Dymond et al. (1978) also performed factor analysis of power spectra (log transformed) of bilateral centro-occipital leads and extracted four main factors having high loadings within the following frequency bands: 0–8, 6–12, 12–20, and 20–30 Hz; they also extracted factors associated with EEG asymmetry.

It should be noted, however, that applying factor analysis to sets of power spectra is not a simple affair. The results depend on (a) whether the spectra are expressed in power or in

Table 59.1. EEG Features Obtained from Spectral Analysis

| | Frequency Bands | | | | Factor Analysis | |
| | | | Weighting Factors k | | | |
Classical Definition (Hz)	Matousek and Petersén, 1973	Gotman, 1976	Frontal Channels	Other Channels	Hermann et al., 1978	Wieneke (personal communication)
$0 \le \delta_1 \le 1.9$		0.4–1.2	1.5	2		
$2 \le \delta_2 \le 3.4$	1.5–3.5	1.6–4.0	4	4	1.5–5.5	1.5–6.0
$3.5 \le \theta_1 \le 5.4$		4.4–6.4	3	5		
$5.4 \le \theta_2 \le 7.4$	3.5–7.5	6.8–7.2	3	1	5.5–8.5	6.0–9.0
$7.4 \le \alpha_1 \le 9.9$	7.5–9.5				8.6–10.5	9.0–10.5
$9.9 \le \alpha_2 \le 12.4$	9.5–12.5	7.6–12.8	1	1.5	10.5–12.0	10.5–12.5
$12.5 \le \beta_1 \le 17.9$	12.5–17.5				12.0–18.0	12.5–15.5
$18.0 \le \beta_2 \le 23.9$		13.2–30.0	1	0.5	18.0–21.0	15.5–18.5
$24.0 \le \beta_2$	17.5–25.0				21.0–30.0	18.5–28.0
Ratios used for discrimination	$\dfrac{\theta}{\alpha + cs1}$		$\dfrac{k_1\delta_1 + k_2\delta_2 + k_3\theta_1 + k_4\theta_2}{k_5 - \alpha + k_6\beta}$			
	(θ and α in V) asymmetry Q		asymmetry ratios $\begin{cases} \delta + \theta \\ \alpha + \beta \end{cases}$			

root mean square values, (b) the way the spectra have been normalized, (c) which derivations have been used, and (d) the subject population. The results of a recent investigation at the University Hospital of Utrecht (Wieneke, personal communication), which factorized frequency bands of power spectra (logarithmic values) obtained from eight symmetric derivations in 89 patients, are shown in Table 59.1; in this case, normalization was performed using the band from 5 to 20 Hz as reference. The distribution of the most important frequency factor loadings obtained in this way for different derivations is given in Fig. 59.1. It is widely recognized that this type of analysis is sensitive to normalization and scaling. It should be noted, however, that the different frequency bands appear to form rather well-defined clusters, because the different methods presented in

Table 59.1 yield quite similar results. There is indeed considerable overlap between frequency bands calculated in this way and those used commonly in clinical electroencephalography; therefore, it may be said that a subdivision in frequency bands as used by Matousek and Petersén (1973) or Gotman et al. (1973) is acceptable for routine clinical EEG analysis. If one deals with a completely defined group of EEG (e.g., in psychopharmacological studies), factor analysis should be applied to such a specific group in order to define the optimal frequency bands that should be used.

Within the defined frequency bands, several primary spectral features, such as absolute power intensity in μV^2 or in dBs, relative power, square root of power, and average frequency within a band, can be computed. Secondary spec-

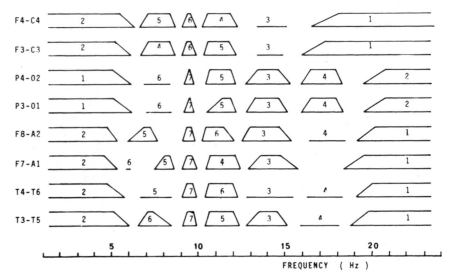

Figure 59.1. Factors found using factor analysis of EEG power spectra. Factor analysis of logarithmic power spectra for several derivations was done; power spectra were normalized in relation to the power within the frequency band between 5 and 20 Hz. Each factor is represented either by a *parallelogram* or simply by a *horizontal line*. The latter or the base of the *parallelogram* indicates the frequency interval within which the factor accounts for more than 50% of the variance; the *top line* of the *parallelogram* indicates the frequency interval within which more than 70% of the variance is accounted for by the corresponding factor. The factors are numbered in the order of decreasing eigenvalues from 1 to 6 or 7. A varimax rotation was used. The data were obtained from EEGs of 243 patients, each consisting of 100-second epochs recorded with eyes closed. (Courtesy of G. Wieneke.)

tral features can also be derived. Several types of secondary features have been proposed based on empirical criteria; clinical application has validated those proposed by Matousek and Petersén (1973) and by Gotman et al. (1973). Matousek and Petersén (1973) investigated 20 features extracted from the frequency spectrum of each EEG derivation. This study was based on the authors' claim that an increased amount of slow frequency in the EEG in abnormal cases might be considered analogous to the relatively large amount of slow activity seen in the normal but immature EEG. Initially, the EEG score chosen as the most clearly age-related was the ratio between theta band activity (3.5–7.5 Hz) and that in the alpha band (7.5–12.5 Hz) added with a constant factor.

The same group later reinvestigated this problem (Friberg et al., 1980). They used as normative data the root mean square of the spectral values computed within the frequency bands, indicated in Table 59.1, for a number of derivations (FT-T3, C3-C0, T3-T5, P3-01, and the symmetrical ones) of 562 EEG recordings from healthy individuals aged 1 through 21 years. A number of ratios between root mean square values were also computed. In total, 20 spectral features per derivation were calculated, as follows: $x(1) =$ delta activity, $x(2) =$ theta, $x(3) =$ alpha 1, $x(4) =$ alpha 2, $x(5) =$ beta 1, $x(6) =$ beta 2, $x(9) =$ alpha 1/alpha 2, $x(10) =$ beta l/(alpha 1 + alpha 2), $x(11) =$ beta 2/(alpha 1 + alpha 2), $x(12) =$ beta 1/beta 2, $x(13) =$ delta/theta, $x(14) =$ sum of delta, theta, alpha 1, alpha 2, beta 1, beta 2; features from 15 through 20 are normalized amplitudes in relation to $x(14)$ for the following bands: $x(15) =$ normalized delta, $x(16) =$ normalized theta, $x(17) =$ normalized alpha 1, $x(18) =$ normalized alpha 2, $x(19) =$ normalized beta 1, $x(20) =$ normalized beta 2.

Friberg et al.'s (1980) model is defined by the following linear equation: calculated EEG age $= a(0) + a(1) x(1) + \ldots + a(20) x(20)$. The coefficients $a(i)$, with $i = 0 \ldots 20$, have been estimated by minimizing the sum of squares of the differences between the subject's actual age and the calculated EEG age. The correlation coefficients between actual and calculated EEG age varied between 0.88 for derivations C3-C0 and C0-C4 and 0.86 for derivations F7-T3 and F8-T4. Those authors found that, according to their model, the calculated EEG age tended to be greater than zero when the line was extrapolated down to an actual age of zero. To avoid this, they introduced two new variables: the *calculated EEG maturity* and the *actual EEG maturity;* linearly related to the calculated EEG age and to the actual age, respectively. The ratio between calculated and actual EEG maturity is called the *ratio of EEG normality,* because the authors found that this ratio is closely related to the degree of EEG (ab)normality. To calculate such a ratio, the maximal actual EEG maturity of any individual is fixed to correspond to 22 years (age-related EEG changes are considered to be small beyond that age). The clinical implications of this form of feature extraction and data reduction are discussed below.

Gotman and his collaborators based their procedure for extracting spectral features on the widely accepted assumption that some kind of relation between slow and fast EEG activity should characterize the degree of EEG abnormality.

Moreover, they pointed out that a relative measure of spectral intensity is preferable to an absolute measure because the latter depends on a number of spurious factors (e.g., skull thickness). Therefore, they investigated the potential of several (delta + theta)/(alpha + beta) ratios using different weighing factors and frequency band subdivisions to discriminate the EEG of normal and abnormal (slow-wave type of abnormality) subjects. The best weighing factors for different frequency bands and areas are given in Table 59.1. The same investigators introduced still another important spectral feature, a degree of *asymmetry.* To compute this feature, the scalp was subdivided into four symmetrical regions: frontal (Fp1-F3, Fp1-F7, Fp2-F4, Fp2-F8), temporal (F7-T3, T3-T5, F8-T4, T4-T6), central (F3-C3, C3-P3, F4-C4, C4-P4), and occipital (P3-01, T5-01, P4-02, T6-02). For each region, two asymmetry coefficients were calculated, one for the slow frequencies (weighted delta and theta values as given in Table 59.1) and one for the high frequencies (weighted alpha and beta values). The value corresponding with the most active hemisphere was always placed in the numerator. Gotman et al. (1973) called the display of these ratios extracted from spectral values *canonograms (canon* is Greek for "ratio") (Fig. 59.2); the clinical validation of these features is discussed later in this chapter.

Other spectral features of interest are the spectral peak *frequencies* and corresponding *bandwidths.* There are several algorithms used to calculate peak frequencies: these involve computing a local maximum of the curve defining the spectral density. A peak is said to exist when it rises significantly above its surroundings. The bandwidth is usually calculated as the frequency interval between the -3 dB points at both sides of the peak.

A comprehensive analysis methodology that combines quantitative EEG and EP features is the approach introduced by John and collaborators and reviewed extensively in John et al. (1987, 1988) and Prichep and John (1986), under the name of *neurometrics.* This approach is based on the use of standardized data acquisition techniques, computerized feature extraction, statistical transformations in order to achieve approximately gaussian distributions, age regression equations, and multivariate statistical methods, namely discriminant and cluster analyses to achieve differential diagnosis between patients (sub)populations. In this way, neurometric test batteries have been constructed and applied to several clinical problems. A general battery consists typically of the following features: spectral composition, coherence, and symmetry indices of the spontaneous resting EEG; and brainstem auditory (BAEP) and somatosensory (BSEP) evoked potentials to unilateral stimuli, checkerboard pattern reversal or flash visual EPs, and cortical EPs to different modalities both to predictable and unpredictable stimuli. This approach is currently implemented in special-purpose personal computers.

Profiles of neurometric features that deviate from age-matched normal subjects have been obtained in several categories of patients suffering from cognitive disorders (e.g., dementias), psychiatric illnesses (e.g., different types of depressions and of schizophrenia), and neurological dysfunctions [e.g., compromised cerebral blood flow (Jonkman et al., 1985)] as discussed by John et al. (1988) and Prichep et al.

Figure 59.2. Canonogram from subject with multiple metastases in right hemisphere. The size of each *polygon* is proportional to a slow/fast EEG activity ratio, indicator of abnormality for a channel. They are arranged in a topographical pattern corresponding to the position of the derivations on the subject's head: frontal on *top*, occipital on *bottom*. *Arrows* under *horizontal lines* indicate the asymmetry in slow EEG activity; *arrows* above indicate the asymmetry in fast EEG activity. Sixteen channels, anteroposterior bipolar montage covering parasagittal and temporal regions; EEG epoch, 40-seconds. (Adapted from Gotman, J. 1978. Problems of presentation of analytical results. Electroencephalogr. Clin. Neurophysiol. Suppl. 34:191–197.)

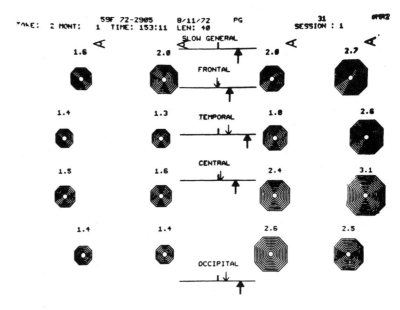

(1990). The clinical relevance of Neurometrics has been a controversial issue and has led to publications presenting opposite points of view by John (1989) and Fisch and Pedley (1989). A special effort was made by Roy John and collaborators to apply the neurometrics approach of quantitative EEG analysis to distinguish subgroups of patients with psychiatric disorders that may be potential responders to pharmacological treatments (Prichep and John, 1992). This was applied to patients suffering from obsessive-compulsive disorder (OCD) who received treatment with selective serotonin reuptake inhibitors (SSRIs) with the interesting result that the responders and nonresponders presented distinct neurometric profiles (Hansen et al., 2003; Prichep et al., 1993).

Spectral Analysis Using Parametric Methods

In Chapter 58 we discussed the general theory of spectral analysis employing ARMA or AR models. One of the main advantages of this method of computing power spectra, as proposed by Zetterberg (1973a), is precisely the fact that using spectral parameter analysis (SPA) makes it unnecessary to subdivide the spectrum in separated frequency bands. The SPA method describes the EEG as resulting from noise sources passed through a set of parallel first- or second-order filters, as illustrated in Fig. 59.3; as Isaksson and Wennberg (1975a) demonstrated, this method allows simulation of an EEG signal. The relevant spectral features can be derived simply. The first-order filter describing the low-frequency band (σ) is characterized by two features: the total power G_δ and the total bandwidth σ_δ (interval from zero to the frequency corresponding to the -3 dB point); each of the second-order filters describing theta, alpha, and beta components is characterized by the three features: G (power), σ (bandwidth), and resonance frequency (f).

Isaksson and Wennberg (1975a) have found that, for most practical applications, a SPA model of, at the highest, the fifth order is sufficient. In this case, only the first-order delta component and the second-order alpha and beta components

are described. In a few cases, it may be necessary to use a model of the seventh order to include a second-order theta component. In a study comparing the degree of visually evaluated slow activity in a large number of artifact-free EEG epochs with the features identified through SPA of the

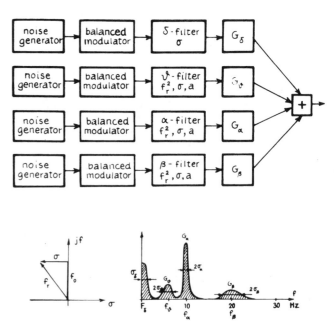

Figure 59.3. Block diagram of the EEG simulator; the δ filter represents a first-order active RC network; the δ, α, and β filters are of second order; potentiometers independently control the parameters $f(2/r)$ (which determine the resonance frequency f_0), σ (which determine the bandwidth), and α (which determine the zero of the transfer function); the power parameter is G. (Adapted from Zetterberg, L.H. 1973a. Experience with analysis and simulation of EEG signals with parametric description of spectra. In *Automation of Clinical Electroencephalography*, Eds. P. Kellaway and I. Petersen, pp. 161–201. New York: Raven Press.)

same epochs, Isaksson and Wennberg (1975b) concluded that there was, for most derivations, a significant linear correlation between the degree of slow activity encountered with visual inspection and the value of the features G_δ (positive correlation) and σ_δ (negative correlation); in a few cases there was also correlation with G_α (negative correlation) and σ_α (positive correlation).

The computation of an ARMA or AR model leads to an important degree of data reduction. The relevant information is thus condensed in the coefficients of the model; the number of coefficients corresponds to the order of the model. As shown by Mathieu (1975) and by Jansen (1979), the coefficients can be used to characterize the EEG directly. The importance of this approach for EEG pattern classification is discussed later.

The Recognition and Elimination of Artifacts: Eye Movements and Muscle Artifacts

Physiological and technical artifacts are the outstanding enemies of automatic EEG analysis. They must be eliminated if computer EEG analysis is used in practice. It is a general requirement of EEG recording in any clinical laboratory that the records have a minimum of technical artifacts, a requirement that is even more critical in automatic analysis. One way to control the quality of EEG signals while performing analog-to-digital conversion in the clinical laboratory is by simply deleting those epochs that are below acceptable standards due to technical or even physiological (e.g., ocular or muscular) artifacts. For example, the technician responsible for this operation may delete the series of digitized samples immediately preceding an identified artifact. Nevertheless, there will always be situations in which artifacts, particularly those of a physiological nature, are unavoidable. This is particularly important during long-lasting EEG monitoring in several clinical (e.g., EEG-video monitoring of epileptic patients) and experimental (e.g., sleep studies) conditions and when computer-assisted quantification is applied.

Eye movements and *muscle potentials* occur in most records of a few minutes' duration; they can distort power spectra and lead to detection of transient nonstationarities that are difficult to distinguish from epileptiform events. *Eye blinks* can be avoided by recording with eyes closed; *slow eye movements*, however, are more difficult to avoid. These are bilaterally synchronous with a maximum in frontal derivations and represent an important contribution to the power in the delta band in these derivations. In the early days of EEG quantification, Gotman (1976) discussed several methods of avoiding this type of artifact at the very first stage, e.g., by subtracting the electro-oculogram (EOG). This matter has been reviewed by Jervis et al. (1988) and by Brunia et al. (1989). However, the technique of EOG subtraction may give rise to distortion of the EEG signals, since the EOG recording also contains brain signals (Berg and Scherg, 1994) that may be partially eliminated by filtering first the EOG with a low pass of about 8 Hz. The transfer of EOG activity to the EEG can be analyzed using a frequency domain approach. Eye blinks and slow eye movements have different spectral properties and are transferred in different ways to the skull. Gain functions for transferring both types

of eye movements to the skull were computed by Gasser et al. (1985). These authors obtained average gain functions that they found to be of practical use in correcting EOG artifacts. In other studies, a frequency domain approach to correcting EOG artifacts has been proposed (Whitton et al., 1978; Woestenburg et al., 1983). Similarly, Jervis et al. (1985) found that a computerized correlation technique provides results superior to analog techniques for removing eye movement artifacts. Elbert et al. (1985) also stressed that the best correction for these types of artifact is obtained in the frequency domain, but indicated that the correction procedure should be based on more than one EOG derivation, and preferably on three. Fortgens and de Bruin (1983) also obtained good results using the method of least squares based on four EOG derivations.

Other important physiological artifacts are *muscle potentials*. Here also it is important to note that electromyographic (EMG) signals affect the EEG power spectrum not only at very high frequencies (30–60 Hz) but even down to 14 Hz (O'Donnell et al., 1974). Under normal conditions, there is very little EEG power in the 30- to 50-Hz band; if the power is significantly large, one must suspect contamination with EMG signals. Gotman (1976) proposed dealing with this problem by introducing a reduction factor with which the activity in the beta band should be multiplied; this factor depends on the spectral intensity integrated over the 30- to 50-Hz band. If this is below 1.5 μV/Hz, the reduction factor is equal to unity; if the activity is larger than 1.5 μV/Hz, the reduction factor decreased linearly to 0.1 as the spectral activity increases up to 5.0 μV/Hz.

An alternative way to deal with artifacts is that used by Gevins et al. (1977), who determine thresholds for head and body movement artifacts (under 1 Hz), high-frequency artifacts mainly caused by EMG (34–50 Hz), and eye movements (below 3 Hz in frontal derivations) based on a short segment that includes those artifacts; thereafter, EEG epochs exceeding the aforementioned thresholds are simply discarded (Barlow, 1986).

The need to avoid the contamination with artifacts of relevant EEG features is so pressing that this area of EEG signal analysis has been, for decades, in constant evolution. Here we briefly review the most relevant approaches.

Rather elaborate methods are based on decomposing a set of EEG signals into components that should represent the artifact and the EEG signals, respectively. One of these is the spatial filtering approach (Ille et al., 2003; Scherg et al., 2002). According to this method the topography of the artifact is first estimated on the basis of a specific recording where the artifact is clear evident, since this is, in general, easier to model than the EEG. Thus the artifact can be described as the product of the corresponding topography vector and time waveforms. This can be then subtracted from the EEG signals contaminated with artifact to yield the corrected signals.

Other methods have been proposed that differ in the way of separating EEG and artifact signals. With this objective Lagerlund et al. (1997) used principal component analysis (PCA), but this method has the drawback that PCA yields uncorrelated components while the EEG signals and the artifacts may be correlated. Independent component analysis

(ICA) (see Chapter 58) is very effective in separating EEG signals from artifacts as shown in a number of applications (Jung et al., 2000; Makeig et al., 1996; Vigário, 1997; Vigário et al., 1998), but it needs some form of postprocessing to identify the components corresponding to the EEG signals and the artifacts. Several strategies and combinations of approaches are compared, particularly with respect to their practical implementation, and discussed by Ille et al. (2003).

Transient Nonstationarities: Epileptiform Events

The detection of epileptiform events is a typical example of the application of a pattern recognition approach in EEG analysis. In this problem, the epileptiform events (spikes, sharp waves, and spike and waves) are considered to constitute the "signal," whereas the background activity constitutes the "noise." This necessitates the distinction of signals known to be sharp and embedded in background noise. Several methods have been used to increase the signal-to-noise ratio. Most of them are akin to the classic approach of Carrie (1972, 1976), who used as a criterion the ratio between the amplitude of the second derivative of the EEG signal and the moving average of similar measurements from a number (e.g., 128, 256) of preceding consecutive waves; a ratio of four or five was said to indicate an epileptiform event. Most other relevant studies have proposed similar types of measures (Gevins et al., 1976; Goldberg et al., 1973; Gotman and Gloor, 1976; Harner and Ostergren, 1976; Saltzberg et al., 1971). All these methods involve a preprocessing stage that constitutes a form of high-pass filtering (e.g., computing the signal's second derivative).

The method used by Lopes da Silva et al. (1973, 1975, 1976, 1977; Lopes da Silva, 1978) is based on an essentially more general form of preprocessing. In this method, an EEG epoch is described by way of an AR model, which can be viewed as providing the best fit to the background activity. The basic operation to improve the signal-to-noise ratio consists of passing the EEG signal through the inverse filter of the estimated AR model; this inverse filtering yields a new signal that ideally should have the properties of an uncorrelated white noise. The statistical properties of this new signal are then determined; deviation of the new signal resulting from inverse filtering from a normal distribution at a certain probability level is thought to identify a transient nonstationarity (see Chapter 58, Fig. 58.12). The essential feature of this method is that inverse filtering of the EEG epoch eliminates in an optimal way the background activity, allowing the transient nonstationarities to emerge clearly. The operation of inverse filtering using the AR model corresponding to the same epoch provides the best least-squares fit filter to the background activity. After this preprocessing stage the detected transient nonstationarities can be further classified, in a second stage, using a set of rules adapted from the pattern recognition algorithm introduced by Ktonas and Smith (1974). This constitutes a two-stage analysis approach (Guedes de Oliveira and Lopes da Silva, 1980).

Not all transient nonstationarities, however, are necessarily epileptiform events; some may be physiological artifacts or other forms of EEG transients (e.g., lambda waves or sharp bursts of alpha waves). After detecting transient nonstationarities using one of the above-mentioned preprocessing methods of improving the signal-to-noise ratio, one must

apply a form of pattern recognition to select those that can be accepted as being epileptiform in nature. Two main pattern recognition methods have been proposed; one is based on a matched filtering approach and the other on piece-wise characterization of the transient. Matched filtering using as template a spike-and-wave pattern has been used (Zetterberg, 1973b) to detect epileptiform transients even without preprocessing. Barlow and Dubinsky (1976) used a comparable method, computing the running correlation coefficient between the EEG signal and a template (see Chapter 58, Fig. 58.14). However, the variability of the waveforms characteristic of such transients presents a serious difficulty in dealing with this problem in practice. Pfurtscheller and Fischer (1978) combined a preprocessing stage using inverse autoregressive filtering and a template matching stage for postselection of relevant epileptiform events.

Several investigations have led to the establishment of a quantitative description of epileptiform transients in a piece-wise fashion. Smith (1972) and Ktonas and Smith (1974) categorized epileptiform spikes in terms of five features (Fig. 59.4): S_1 and S_2, the maximum slopes, respectively, before and after reaching the peak of the spike; S_3, taken by the

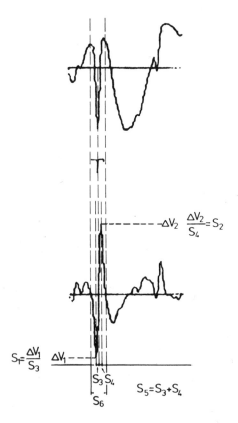

Figure 59.4. *Top,* an epileptiform spike; *bottom,* the corresponding first/derivative. The parameters proposed by Ktonas and Smith (1974) are shown: S_1 and S_2 are the maximal spike slopes, respectively, before and after reaching the peak; S_3, time taken by the spike to reach the peak after it attained maximal slope; S_4, time taken by the spike to reach maximal slope after the peak. The sum $S_3 = S_3 + S_4$ is a measure of the duration of the sharp part of the peak. The time interval between two zero crossings of the same polarity of the first derivative is S_6. The time duration of the signal shown is 1 second. (Adapted from Lopes da Silva, F.H. 1978. Analysis of EEG non-stationarities. Electroencephalogr. Clin. Neurophysiol. Suppl. 34:163–179.)

spike to reach the peak after it attains maximum slope; and S_4, time taken by the spike to reach maximum slope after the peak. The sum $(S_3 + S_4)$ of the time intervals measures the duration of the epileptiform spike (S_5). The interval between two consecutive zero crossings of the same polarity of the first derivative (S_6) is also a relevant feature.

Frost (1979) considered the problem in a simpler form, proposing the following characteristic features. Assuming that an epileptiform spike is a triangular wave with a point of origin M at the base, an apex S, and a point of termination P, Frost defined *amplitude* as the largest value of MS or SP and *duration* as the interval MP. Furthermore, he used as a measure of sharpness D, an estimate of the signal's second derivative. The initial processing step involves comparing the value of D with a threshold, so that, whenever D is larger than a certain value, a candidate spike is detected.

Extracting the features described here requires a relatively high rate of EEG sampling—at least 200/sec. The next section considers the practical implications of these methods in assessing the EEGs of epileptiform patients.

According to the method of Gotman and Gloor (1976), at the end of an analysis session the computer displays all transients detected, whether true or false. The distinction between the two types is made off-line in an interactive way. This form of analysis represents a considerable data reduction and provides a reliable account of the main types of epileptiform transients present in a given record.

The methods of analysis described in this section not only are useful in detecting the presence of epileptiform events, but also provide *quantitative information* on the morphology of such events, on their distribution over long periods of time, and on their spatial distribution. Using this methodology, Ktonas and Smith (1974), Lopes da Silva and van Hulten (1978), and Gotman (1980) observed that most epileptiform spikes, at the scalp, present a second slope that is steeper than the first, contrary to the qualitative description of Gloor (1977). However, Lemieux and Blume (1983) found that the spikes recorded directly from the cortex presented a first slope that was steeper than the first more often than the reverse.

Another interesting analysis that can be realized using these methods consists in the quantification of the distribution of epileptiform spikes in relation to the occurrence of seizures. Gotman and Marciani (1985) found that the level of spiking is not related to the probability of seizure occurrence, but they reported an increase in spiking in the days following seizures.

Very much as in the case of the detection of artifacts, the analysis of epileptiform events has attracted the interest of many researchers and new approaches are often being introduced. In most cases new methods are published without a comprehensive comparison with older methods, which makes it difficult to compare the performance of different approaches. An exception is the study of Dumpelmann and Elger (1999), which we discuss in detail below (see CADS and Epileptiform Events).

Classification and Clustering in EEG Analysis

The previous section considers different ways to find sets of features that can characterize EEG signals. This section considers very briefly the next phase in pattern recognition, *classification* and/or *clustering*. For a detailed account of this problem, the reader is referred to Duda and Hart (1973). It is necessary to consider this question here in order to be able to evaluate quantitative EEG analysis methods in the clinical laboratory. The essential problem is one of diagnosis; given a set of EEG epochs that have been analyzed and characterized by a number of features, it is necessary to determine the value of the analysis in order to classify the EEG epochs in a certain number of diagnostic categories (e.g., normal/abnormal, sleep stages) or some EEG patterns (e.g., spikes) as epileptiform.

One way to solve this problem is to use, for instance, *discriminant analysis,* which is possible only if one knows a priori that the EEG signals belong to a defined number of classes. Assume that the analysis involves classifying EEG signals into two classes, normal and abnormal, and disposing of a set of features, i.e., a feature vector, extracted from power spectra. The feature vector defines a point in n-dimensional space.

In discriminant analysis, the space where all objects (e.g., EEG epochs characterized by a vector set) are contained must be subdivided into a number of regions; the objects within a region form one class. The functions that generate the surface separating the regions are called *discriminant functions.* An object is assigned to a certain region or class by several types of *decision* rules; these are described in detail by Demartini and Vincent-Carrefour (1977), among others.

To develop and test a classifier, it is important to dispose of a sufficiently large *learning set* (i.e., a set of N objects that have been classified a priori using independent criteria); in the case of EEG analysis, the independent criteria ought to be clinically valid. This implies that the objects must be classified by raters (electroencephalographers) using their common criteria of visual inspection of the records added to other clinical information. The learning set should contain at least a number of objects $N = 5 \times n \times k$ where n is the number of features and k the number of classes (Demartini and Vincent-Carrefour, 1977). One way to develop an automatic method of EEG analysis is to divide the experimental set into two parts. The first part (learning set) is used to develop the classifier and the second to test its performance. A useful alternative if the experimental set is too small is the "hold one out" strategy, which involves removing one object from the learning set and then resynthesizing the classifier and trying to recognize the selected object. This operation should be repeated for each object. The resulting error rate is a good estimate of the classifier's performance.

The quality of the learning set is of primary importance. To start with, it is necessary to have knowledge about rater *reproducibility* (intra-rater agreement) and *validity* (inter-rater agreement) as regards evaluation of the EEG records constituting the learning set. A few studies have addressed electroencephalographers' overall characterizations of EEG records as normal or abnormal; in such cases the validity of the visual assessment is about 80% to 90%. Although most raters generally agree on the division of the EEG into two classes (normal or abnormal), classification of short segments or of epileptiform transients is much less consistent. The same applies to intra-rater agreement. For instance, Jansen (1979) reported that he presented EEGs from four subjects (two renal patients and two normal volunteers) to one electroencephalographer who was asked to mark state transitions and then lump together segments corresponding to the same state. When the records were first presented, visual segmentation resulted in 11 types of segments; on a second session, the same rater found seven types, only two of which coincided with those initially identified.

In the assessment of EEG patterns corresponding to different sleep stages, however, a good degree of interrater agreement can be expected; thus it is not surprising that methods of automatically classifying sleep stages have been those more often evaluated in a quantitative way. In assessing epileptiform events (spikes, sharp waves, spikes and waves), a large degree of interrater variability is also encountered. Gose et al. (1974) found considerable variability in the human detection of spikes; a total of 948 events were marked as spikes by one or more electroencephalographers, but only 104 events were marked by five raters. However, disagreement between raters on individual spikes is not very important; a comparison on a patient basis (30 records seen by five raters) is more important; seen from this viewpoint, the average error rate was only 4%.

For the classification of EEG records in the learning set, it is important to utilize a *structural report* such as used by Volavka et al. (1973), Rose et al. (1973), Gotman et al. (1978), Gotman and Gloor (1976), and Gevins (1979). In other words, EEG classification classes should be defined unambiguously; the abnormal EEG can be classified paroxysmal or irritative, hypofunctional (cortical or centrencephalic) or mixed; the location of the abnormality (focal: frontal, temporal, central, occipital, lateralized, or diffuse) should also be specified. Furthermore, one may use a complementary second-order classification into diagnostic types related to the global medical diagnosis: space-occupying lesions, metabolic disorders, cerebrovascular insufficiency, seizure disorders, or psychiatric disorders.

EEG Segmentation and Clustering

This chapter stresses repeatedly that EEG records are generally nonstationary. Although in the clinical laboratory it is usually possible to obtain representative EEG epochs by tightly controlling the subject's behavioral state, it is desirable to be able to quantify the EEG so different types might be separated automatically. This is even more important in the case of EEG recorded under intensive care conditions, such as during anesthesia, or in other long-duration records. Ideally, one would like to segment the EEG into epochs with different statistical properties; equivalent segments thereafter could be grouped together, thus defining a number of classes. An effort in this direction was made by Bodenstein and Praetorius (1977), who proposed a general method of EEG segmentation; they assumed that an EEG should be considered as a sequence of quasi–stationary segments of varying duration. They used an AR model as described in Chapter 51.

By setting appropriate thresholds, Bodenstein and Praetorius (1977) have been able to formulate explicit criteria for EEG segmentation. The point is that the identified segments should correspond to (patho)physiologically meaningful

states. The problem, however, is that the validity of this segmentation procedure in relation to clinically clearly defined states has not yet been demonstrated. Jansen (1979) made an interesting effort along a similar line by using an algorithm akin to that discussed above but based on a Kalman filter and following a different strategy; this method is called Kalman-Bucy (KB) clustering. Defining segments of variable length based on statistical criteria proved to be too difficult because a good learning set could not be constructed. Therefore, Jansen (1979) divided the EEG into segments with a fixed duration of 1.28 seconds and classified them using an *unsupervised learning clustering* approach. In other words, he used a clustering algorithm to group segments with similar properties into a number of classes that have not been defined a priori. Each 1.28-second segment is characterized by a feature vector consisting of the five coefficients of the corresponding AR model estimated using a Kalman filter, often complemented by a measure of amplitude, which is the largest range between a maximum and a minimum. The statistical approach used in this case is a form of clustering (see review in Anderberg, 1973).

Clustering can be partitional or hierarchical; the former is based on a priori knowledge of the place occupied by some objects, which are then used as "seed points" around which clusters grow. The latter can have two forms, agglomerative or divisive, depending on whether one starts from an assembly of as many clusters as objects or from one cluster encompassing all objects. Jansen (1979) used the agglomerative hierarchical clustering approach to group EEG segments of a number of types. This type of clustering involves an iterative process through which the two most similar clusters of the previous step are merged into a new cluster. The user can stop the process at any point, depending on the application. Using statistical criteria, it is possible to delimit the number of classes in such a way that the distance between their centroids does not fall below a certain value.

Hierarchical clustering of epileptiform spike events is being used in the analysis of interictal EEGs. Guess and Wilson (2002) presented an application by means of which spike events are separated into groups, based on topology and morphology, which provides an efficient method of performing detailed analysis of long time series. Van't Ent et al. (2003) reported a spike clustering analysis that yield meaningful results in neocortical localization-related epilepsy, in magnetoencephalogram (MEG).

This type of analysis may be criticized similarly to the segmentation method described earlier. Here also the number and types of classes are arbitrary; the advantage of the present method, however, is more flexibility; the same data may be clustered in several ways. This is feasible because all information necessary to characterize the EEG segments is stored in the form of a small number of coefficients (e.g., the five coefficients of the AR model). The presentation of the results by this clustering method is synthetic without losing clarity; one way of presenting the so-called profile of an EEG epoch obtained in this way is shown in Fig. 59.5. It is also possible to transform the parameters of the AR model characterizing the different classes into the frequency domain and thus present the result in the form of a series of power spectra. It is also possible to present the different

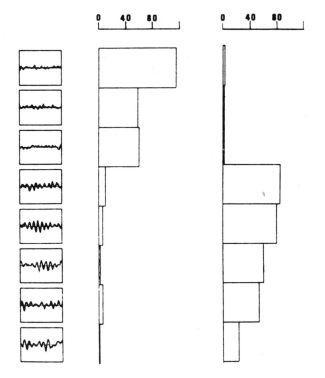

Figure 59.5. Presentation of two profiles of the elementary patterns of an EEG signal that have been submitted to cluster analysis. Two realizations were analyzed by subdividing the signal in epochs 1.28 seconds long; for each epoch, an autoregressive model using a Kalman filter was constructed. Using a cluster analysis procedure, the 1.28-second epochs were assigned to the class of elementary EEG patterns for which the distance function was the smallest; in these examples, eight classes resulted from the cluster analysis. The number of elementary patterns that belong to each class are shown in the *histograms* plotted to the side of the traces representing the different EEG patterns. The two profiles were computed from the same EEG at different times, corresponding to two states of alertness. (Adapted from Jansen, B.H. 1979. EEG segmentation and classification. Thesis, Free University, Amsterdam.)

types of segments, appropriately labeled, as functions of time, which may be relevant to relating EEG and behavioral state changes. Some applications of this method are discussed in the following section.

Neural Network-Based EEG Classification

Neural networks have been employed to classify EEG features. Several research groups have explored successfully this approach. This appears particularly interesting for the classification of single EEG epochs. Three types of neural network-based classifications of EEG data were reported: classification of single-EEG trials for selective averaging (Gevins and Morgan, 1986); classification of averaged and nonaveraged multichannel EEG data; and classification of single-trial, multichannel EEG data (Pfurtscheller et al., 1991). For these classifications, different types of neural networks were applied.

A back-propagation network was used by Gevins and Morgan (1986). Self-organizing feature maps followed by a learning vector quantizer (LVQ), both introduced by Koho-

nen (see review, 2001), were used by Pfurtscheller et al. (1991).

Pfurtscheller et al. (1991) used a neural network approach to analyze and classify nonaveraged multichannel EEG data from an experiment where the subject had to press a microswitch either with the left or right hand, whereby the side of movement was indicated by a cue stimulus. On the basis of the spatiotemporal alpha event-related desynchronization (ERD) prior to movement, this method of automatic classification was able to predict the side of the hand movement. One part of the data was used for training the neural network, the other part to test the performance of the network as classifier.

Peters et al. (1998), using autoregressive modeling of EEG time series and artificial neural nets (ANNs), developed a classifier that can tell which movement is performed from a segment of the EEG signal from a single trial. The classifier's rate of recognition of EEGs not seen before was 92% to 99% on the basis of a 1-second segment per trial. Thus the classifier was considered suitable for a so-called brain-computer interface, a system that allows one to control a computer, or another device, by means of EEG signals (see also Chapter 60A).

Segmentation and Classification in Sleep EEG Analysis

Several attempts have been made to develop an automatic sleep analyzer based on EEG records, in combination with EOG and EMG or independently (see a review of classic studies by Johnson, 1977). The development of an automatic processor has been preceded by a thorough quantitative study of the EEG characteristics during different stages of sleep. These studies have been directed mainly to quantitative analysis of EEG signals recorded from C3-A1 and C4-A2, of EOGs recorded from the outer canthus of each eye referenced to the ipsilateral mastoid, and of EMGs from the submental muscle. A somnogram (Bickford), or typical analysis of a period of sleep, is shown in Fig. 59.6. Three main characteristics of the sleep EEG have been identified by computer analysis.

1. *Sleep spindles* have been shown (Johnson et al., 1969) to range in frequency from 12.4 to 14.6 Hz in young adults. Gondeck and Smith (1974), however, found that frequency can vary about 2 Hz between different spindles; spindle duration varies between 0.5 and 0.8 seconds. Based on a model of the generation of sleep spindles, Kemp et al. (1985) have introduced an optimal detector for this type of activity.

2. *Delta activity* is the primary feature distinguishing waking and sleep stages; Johnson et al. (1969) concluded that the most consistent peak in the spectrum during different sleep stages lies between 0.8 and 1.8 Hz. The delta activity increases between stage 1 (and rapid eye movement, REM) and stages 2, 3, and 4. With age, delta activity decreases in amplitude but not in incidence (Smith et al., 1977). In addition, a very slow oscillation, at 0.5 to 1 Hz, during sleep, was described by Steriade et al. (1993) in cats, which differs from delta waves. This very slow

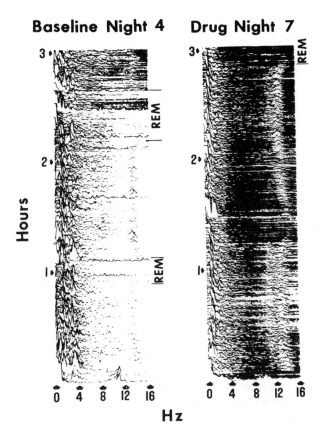

Figure 59.6. Compressed spectral arrays according to Bickford et al. (1972), obtained from sleep EEG, the somnogram. **Left:** Somnogram for the first 3 hours of sleep under control conditions (baseline night 4). **Right:** Somnogram of a corresponding period under the influence of a drug. Note the decrease in delta activity and increase in sleep spindles on drug night 7. (Adapted from Johnson, L.C. 1977. The EEG during sleep as viewed by a computer. In *EEG Informatics. A Didactic Review of Method and Applications of EEG Data Processing,* Ed. A. Remond, pp. 385–406. Amsterdam: Elsevier.)

sleep oscillation was recorded during natural sleep in the EEG (Achermann and Borbély, 1997) and MEG (Simon et al., 2000) in humans.

3. *K complexes* have been difficult to analyze automatically, probably because of their large variability. Bremer et al. (1970) were able to develop a hybrid pattern recognition method for detecting K complexes.

Rosa et al. (1991) proposed a method for the automatic detection of K complexes that yields good practical results. The method of Rosa et al. is based on a simple model of the neuronal network that is responsible for background EEG signals according to the proposal of Kemp (1987). In the model, the main pathway is represented by a frequency-selective feedback loop. The central frequency of the network depends on the time constants of the neuronal elements in the network. Rosa et al. constructed a model that represents the delta activity typical of slow-wave sleep. The K complex is represented as the impulse response of such a delta model.

This section discusses some of the attempts to analyze automatically EEG signals in relation to sleep stages. The

learning sets have been classified according to visual inspection, usually on the basis of criteria proposed by Dement and Kleitman (1957) or Rechtschaffen and Kales (1968). Künkel (1972) summarized the results obtained by several investigators who used as the first extraction procedure one or another form of spectral or hybrid frequency analysis (Larsen and Walter, 1970; Lubin et al., 1969; Smith and Karacan, 1971) or period analysis alone or combined with analog filtering (Itil et al., 1969; Rossler et al., 1970). The mean rate of correct recognition of sleep stages varied for the different studies between 60% and 79%, depending largely on the visual classification method used and on the learning set. Martin et al. (1972) and Viglione and Martin (1973) reanalyzed this problem using a comprehensive methodology; they used power spectra combined with a time-domain technique to detect delta waves (period ≥ 0.55 seconds) exceeding 75 µV amplitude and two EOGs to detect horizontal eye movements. Interval analysis of delta waves was necessary because the power in the delta frequency band (0–2 Hz) was shown not to be proportional to the number of delta waves counted by human observers. EOG recordings were considered necessary in order to help distinguish between REM and waking states. These authors validated their automatic sleep analyzer on sleep recordings of nine young subjects. Data from four subjects were used as learning sets and those of the other five as test sets. The sleep stages were classified visually by three human raters. For the five subjects, the average agreement between raters ranged from 85.8% to 91.4%; the agreement between the program and raters ranged from 77.7% to 86.2% and the agreement between the program and the consensus of raters (majority decision) ranged from 78.8% to 86.4%.

Using hybrid systems, Smith and Karacan (1971), Gaillard et al. (1972), and Gaillard and Tissot (1973) reported similar figures. Poppl (1975) used as the first feature extraction method a time-domain amplitude and interval analysis procedure, which allowed considerable data reduction; by mapping the feature space to maximize the variance ratio between classes (in relation to the variance within classes) and using linear discriminant analysis, a very good (91%) recognition rate for a test run was obtained using the hold-one-out strategy. Mathieu et al. (1975) obtained EEG features using an autoregressive model of order nine, fitted to a large number of 30-second epochs from five sleep EEG recordings of three different subjects. They found for the three subjects a recognition rate of 81% in a test run; when applied to a single patient's EEG, the recognition rate was 91%. The lower recognition rate obtained when using different subjects is a consequence of the relatively large intersubject variability. Mathieu et al. pointed out that grouping subjects by age classes might reduce variability. In any case, the most difficult operation of the automatic classifier was discriminating, on the one hand, between REM sleep and wakefulness and, on the other, between sleep stages 3 and 4. This would probably be facilitated if the AR model features had been combined with EOG data and with a supplementary method of detecting delta waves, as described above. This technique may be improved still further by incorporating a more accurate detection of EOG data during REM. Regarding the distinction between stages 3 and 4, the difficulty of the automatic methods is shared by the human raters; thus, many observations combine stages 3 and 4 into one stage called, simply, slow-wave sleep (SWS). The usefulness of computer analysis in sleep analysis is still unconfirmed; data reduction is an obvious advantage, but the purpose of the effort being carried out must be clearly defined. A possible interesting application is in psychopharmacological studies, such as those illustrated in Fig. 59.6.

Probabilistic models describing the statistical properties of the hypnogram (i.e., the transitions between stages and their duration) have been developed (Bowe and Anders, 1979; Ursin et al., 1983; Yang and Hursch, 1973; Zung et al., 1965). Kemp and Kamphuisen (1986) have introduced a model combining probabilistic and deterministic aspects of sleep. Such models, based on a Markow chain process, may offer new possibilities for computerized analysis of hypnograms. An account of several classic computerized methods of sleep analysis has been published by Hermann and Kubicki (1984).

We should note that sleep staging involves a rather fuzzy process of detection and identification, such that it is not an easy task to perform a computer-assisted analysis since the standards are not well defined. This is a caveat that should be taken into consideration. Most likely this is the reason why many ingenious algorithms developed in the past decades have not gained wide acceptance in practice. One general feature of these algorithms is that they are rule-based, and in general their performance depends very much on the learning population for which they were developed. When they are tested in other populations and other laboratories many problems arise. Agarwal and Gotman (2001, 2002) attempted to solve these limitations by developing an automatic sleep staging method using evolving schemes that can be adjusted depending on the type and quality of polysomnographical recordings. This algorithm adapts the sleep staging rules to the user preferences and the record being analyzed.

Segmentation and Classification in Intensive EEG Monitoring

Automatic intensive monitoring of the EEG is of great importance when the cerebral circulation is in acute danger, such as during open heart or carotid surgery, in states of recovery or worsening of cerebral function after brain damage, in coma, or during hemodialysis. Monitoring of cerebral function during extended anesthesia is also of interest. EEG changes during anesthesia are well known (see review of early literature in Brechner et al., 1962); in this situation, a complex of factors may affect neuronal function, cerebral circulation, and the general acid-base equilibrium in blood and tissues. Disturbances of these physiological functions are reflected in EEG changes. Some special uses of EEG computer analysis in clinical environments, with particular emphasis on continuous monitoring of EEG spectra combined with EPs, are discussed in more detail in Chapter 57.

Surgery and Anesthesia

Open-heart surgery jeopardizes cerebral function by efforts using extracorporeal circulation and cooling, and because of the chance of embolism. Carotid surgery directly menaces cerebral function due to the unavoidable disturbance of the blood flow to the brain.

Automatic EEG monitoring in the conditions described above requires on-line real-time systems and is aimed primarily at detecting and monitoring EEG changes caused by compromised cerebral blood flow and metabolism in anesthesia or other conditions. These changes are characterized mainly by a power spectrum shift in the direction of the slower frequencies, accompanied by changes in amplitude. Therefore, compressed spectral arrays (Bickford et al., 1972) have been used in monitoring these conditions. Because significant data reduction is desired in order to implement real-time EEG monitoring at reasonable cost, it is not surprising that systems have been developed based on drastic simplification of the EEG signal; for example, in the cerebral function monitor (CFM) developed by Maynard et al. (1969) and Prior et al. (1971), the EEG signal is reduced to its mean amplitude after filtering between 2 and 15 Hz. The CFM output is written on a paper chart at very low speed, achieving a form of time smoothing by monitoring only slowly occurring changes in the state of the EEG. Considering that, in this form of automatic monitoring, signal quality may be affected by several forms of technical artifacts, the CFM has a second trace indicating whether the system output may be compromised by interference caused by diathermy or movement artifacts. Thus, a record of the electrode impedance is also provided. The original CFM has been extended by using a microprocessor to provide frequency analysis by way of the proportion of activity in each of six frequency bands in the range 0 to 40 Hz. This system (Maynard, 1977) also provides outputs showing average peak, mean, and minimum EEG signal levels and allows plotting of the mean frequency. This system also reduces the amount of data, providing a simple means of giving information on EEG trends, but the pattern recognition task of evaluating those trends is left to the human observer. The CFM system has been found useful in monitoring anesthesia levels and states of hypoxia and ischemia (Prior, 1979).

A somewhat more sophisticated EEG monitoring system, particularly useful in monitoring during open-heart surgery, has been developed by Simons et al. (1977) and Pronk et al. (1977). In this system, EEG data reduction takes place by zero-crossing interval analysis of signals recorded from four EEG derivations combined with a measure of the mean signal amplitude. The histograms of the intervals and the mean amplitude computed over 60-second epochs are displayed continuously on a video screen as shown in Fig. 59.7. This system also provides a display of complementary information on other physiological variables, such as temperature and blood pressure, together with data reporting the administration of anesthetics or other drugs. All this information is stored in a permanent memory and used to document the operation. The presentation of these data on the video monitor gives easily readable information on slowly developing trends; moreover, this system makes it possible to compute indices that give information on interhemispheric asymmetry, on excessive slow frequencies, and on excessively low EEG amplitude. These indices can be used to give alarm signals so that the user may act to correct the patient's state.

Figure 59.7. Video display of the monitored parameters during an open-heart operation. On the *left* side, the real time scale. From *left* to *right,* the interval (wave duration) histogram of the EEG recorded from the left hemisphere (fronto-occipital montage), the EEG variance of the same derivation, the interval histogram of the EEG recorded from a symmetrical derivation, the curve of blood pressure (mm Hg), and the curve of temperature *(C)* markers indicating the type of anesthesia and/or other drugs administered. Note the slowing of the EEG activity during cooling between 10.40 and 10.50 hours. (Courtesy of R.A.F. Pronk and A.J.R. Simons.)

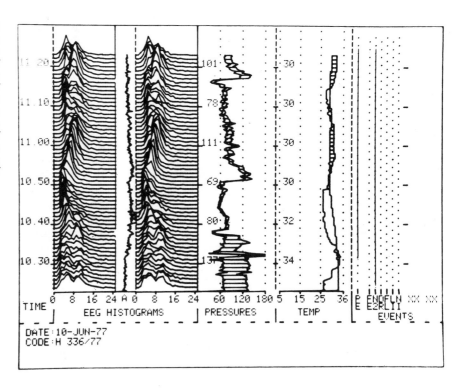

The pattern recognition technique used in this alarm system is rather simple, and it has been empirically developed.

Barlow's (1984) investigation of the performance of different analysis methods (selective bandpass filtering, matched-inverse filtering, and adaptive segmentation) to detect EEG changes associated with carotid clamping has revealed that preference should be given to automatic adaptive segmentation. Pronk (1986) has published a review of computerized methods in perioperative monitoring. More recently the digital techniques used in continuous EEG monitoring in the intensive care unit were reviewed by Scheuer (2002), including conditions such as cerebral ischemia, acute severe head injury, and coma. Since this form of monitoring generates large quantities of data it is important to perform data reduction without loss of relevant information, by way of quantitative EEG analysis and attractive display techniques. In most applications this involves the use of spectral analysis performed in real time. The analyzed information is presented in the form of color spectrograms, compressed spectral arrays, spectral edge displays. In practice it is necessary to combine these analyses with methods that allow intermittent review by specialists that can be established making use of virtual private, secure protected, networks, with Internet-based communication channels. This technology will enable specialists to review the EEG data and the corresponding analyzed data even at remote sites.

Hemodialysis

Computer-assisted EEG monitoring can also be useful during hemodialysis in renal patients. In these cases, cerebral function is disturbed by a complex of factors that can be related to accumulation in the blood of several substances of different molecular sizes (creatinine, urea, etc.) and to changes in ionic concentrations (pH, potassium, etc.) that are reflected in EEG changes.

Kiley et al. (1976a,b) have studied serial EEG recordings of renal patients with regard to frequency and amplitude, particularly using power spectra. A form of data reduction has been studied by Teschan (1974), who proposed that the ratio between the EEG power within the 3- to 7-Hz and 3- to 13-Hz bands was a good measure of EEG deterioration in renal insufficiency. This power ratio was found to be proportional to the serum creatinine and the blood urea nitrogen concentrations and thus was reported to be a useful measure of hemodialysis efficiency (Bourne et al., 1975). However, in a later study (Chotas et al., 1979), no significant statistical correlation between creatinine and the power ratio was obtained, probably because of differences in the patient population.

Formal pattern recognition techniques useful in classifying EEG patterns in renal patients have been investigated by Bowling and Bourne (1978). They used as learning sets three classes of subjects: a group of normal subjects, a low azotemic patient group (i.e., patients having less than 10 mg/100 mL creatinine in the blood), and a high azotemic group (patients with more than 10 mg/100 mL blood creatinine). A stepwise discriminant analysis was carried out using as input data the spectral values corresponding to 100 frequency bands. Two discriminant functions were used to maximize the distance between the three classes (Fig. 59.8). Considerable data reduction was achieved, because only 34 spectral values were left over as significant for the discrimination. The classifier's performance was tested in the EEGs of normal individuals and 14 patients with renal insufficiency, records that had been visually evaluated by one electroencephalographer. The validity of the method can be

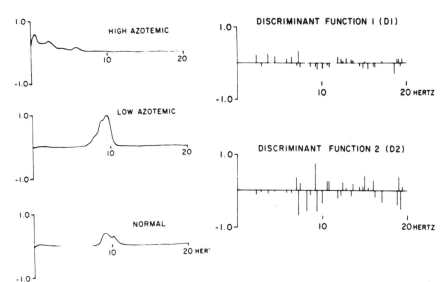

Figure 59.8. *Left side,* normalized ensemble average power spectra from each of three groups of subjects in the training set (20 power spectra from five EEGs in each group, i.e., 100 spectra). Note that the high azotemic group contains much more low-frequency activity than the two other groups, and that the low-azotemic group contains more frequency components below 8 Hz than the normal group. *Right side,* the discriminant functions D_1 and D_2 derived by stepwise discriminant analysis using EEG data from three groups. Each function is a set of weights distributed among the 34 frequency values; these 34 components insured maximum group separation. (The remaining 66 frequencies were discarded because they did not produce significant contributions.) (Adapted from Bowling, P.S., and Bourne, J.R. 1978. Discriminant analysis of electroencephalograms recorded from renal patients. IEEE Trans. Biomed. Eng. MBE-25:12–17.)

considered in two ways, in comparison with the EEG rater's visual assessment or in relation to the clinical state as defined by the creatinine concentration. According to the former criterion, only one of the 19 EEGs was classified erroneously. However, according to the latter, there was one high azotemic patient who was classified in the low azotemic group and two patients in the low azotemic group whose EEGs were classified normal. In all these cases, however, the automatic classifier agreed with the EEG rater. In the same investigation, the performance of the previously proposed power ratio index (power in 3–7 Hz/power in 3–13 Hz) was tested using the same EEG population as far as the visual assessment of the EEG rater was concerned. In this case, two normals and three patients were misclassified (error rate: 5/19); in this test, a threshold for the power ratio index was fixed as one standard deviation from the mean index of a large population of normal subjects. The discriminant functions developed in this investigation were also shown to be useful for following the trends of patients with renal failure.

The same research group (Chotas et al., 1979) studied heuristically the performance of a number of features extracted from the spectrum in order to find a simplified EEG measure useful in EEG analysis of renal failure patients. The spectral features investigated included such classic features as the average frequency, mean frequency of averaged spectrum, average maximum peak, and maximum peak of averaged spectrum as well as some new ones.

Other techniques for primary EEG processing in renal insufficiency have been proposed, namely Hjorth's descriptors (Spehr et al., 1977) and modeling with Kalman filtering and clustering (KB clustering) (Jansen, 1979). Spehr et al. (1977) showed that a combination of power spectral features (delta activity) and Hjorth's descriptors (mobility and complexity) offered a good indication of EEG improvement after hemodialysis. Jansen (1979) computed the elementary patterns found in a number of EEGs recorded before and immediately after dialysis, as well as 1 day and some weeks later; it was found that in four of the five patients investigated, the pro-

files of the elementary EEG patterns 1 day after dialysis differed significantly from those before dialysis.

Jansen (1986) described the possibilities offered by applying techniques emanating from the area of artificial intelligence (usually known as "expert systems") to the problem of classifying EEGs in renal patients. Such systems have been developed by Jagannathan et al. (1982) and Sandell et al. (1983). The expert system employed a knowledge base consisting of 37 rules for classifying EEGs as normal or abnormal. The artificial intelligence system employed a fuzzy logic. The latter system was tested on a set of 67 EEGs; its accuracy relative to that of human raters was 88%.

Computer-Assisted Diagnostic System (CADS)

It is useful for descriptive reasons to distinguish two types of computer-assisted diagnostic systems, because they are based on rather different design philosophies. One pertains to the diagnosis of what might be called *hypofunctional states* of brain function, commonly characterized by some slowing of the dominant EEG frequency components or the appearance of extra-slow components; the other pertains to the diagnosis of so-called *irritative states* or the different forms of epilepsy.

CADS and Hypofunctional States

Most systems currently used in clinical laboratories include subroutines designed to detect and evaluate hypofunctional states. In this field, two of the systems combine a high degree of sophistication with considerable clinical practicality and include comprehensive data reduction and specific displays for the clinician's use. These are the systems introduced by Matousek et al. (1975, 1978), Friberg (1980), Friberg et al. (1980), Gotman (1976, 1978), Gotman et al. (1973, 1978), Gevins et al. (1975), Künkel et al. (1975), Storm van Leeuwen et al. (1976), Mauslby et al. (1973), McGillivray and Wadbrook (1975), Binnie et al. (1978), Harner (1975), Harner and Ostergren (1978), Ebe et al.

(1973), and Bickford et al. (1973). The success of the available systems depends not so much on the exact method of EEG analysis, but rather on (a) the system's capacity to avoid and/or eliminate artifacts, (b) the degree of data reduction possible without distortion of information, (c) the graphic potential to convey adequate communication to the user, and (d) operating ease and flexibility.

In this respect, it is of paramount importance that the CADS allow interactive operation, in order to avoid an overflow of information and thus speed up the computations. At the same time, it should enable users to adopt their own strategies of selecting analytic facilities to give information on the most interesting features in a particular EEG.

Because a generally accepted CADS does not yet exist, only a few indications of the most relevant points one should take into consideration when implementing such a system in the clinical laboratory will be given here.

To evaluate the basic method of EEG analysis and the possible *degree of data reduction,* a comparative statistical study of different EEG analysis techniques in the same database has been carried out (Matousek et al., 1978). The database, however, was limited; it consisted of 57 EEG records obtained from patients with renal insufficiency (two), hepatic coma (five), brain injury (three), and patients without organic disease, but under psychotropic treatment (three); moreover, only EEGs recorded from derivation T3-T5 were analyzed. The EEG records were visually assessed by two independent raters; a structured report was used. The EEG records were sampled at 204.8 Hz. The correlation between a number of EEG features and the visually assessed degree of abnormality was computed and the following features extracted: the RMS (root mean squared) value as indicator of mean amplitude; mean frequency number of delta and theta waves calculated using zero-crossing interval analysis; power content in the delta and theta frequency bands calculated using fast Fourier transform (FFT) and the subdivision of frequency bands indicated in Table 59.1 (Matousek and Petersén, 1973); power content in the delta and theta frequency bands as percentage of total power; the ratio between power in the theta and alpha bands (theta/alpha); the ratio between power in the delta plus theta bands and that in the alpha plus beta bands (delta plus theta/alpha plus beta); and the so-called EEG age quotient (Matousek and Petersén, 1973) mentioned previously. All measures defined in terms of power were recomputed in terms of amplitude because amplitude is the unit used when employing analog frequency analysis.

A few conclusions can be drawn from this study. Time domain features give, in general terms, worse results than features obtained using spectral analysis; the two most revealing features that emerged from this study were the relative power in delta plus theta band (normalized to total power) and the EEG age quotient. Friberg continued this research line, using mainly the so-called *ratio of EEG normality* (Friberg et al., 1980) mentioned earlier in order to obtain an automatic EEG assessment in several groups of subjects. Furthermore, he used the variance of the activity in different frequency bands. The overall agreement rate between automatic and visual EEG interpretation in several groups of patients was about 80%. Two types of EEG were difficult to classify: those with an alpha activity of 7 to 8 Hz, which the program tended to classify as abnormal (contrary to the visual assessment), and those with very low amplitudes.

In terms of both informative display and interactive operation, the most attractive system proposed to date is that of Gotman and his collaborators (Gotman and Gloor, 1976; Gotman et al., 1973, 1978). A typical output of the original system is shown in Fig. 59.2. The striking advantages of this form of display are the comprehensive presentation of topographical information and the degree of information compression achieved. Furthermore, it is possible to obtain, using such a system in an interactive way, other outputs of spectral analysis, such as plots of spectra of the EEG channels, of coherence and phase functions, as well as an output indicative of the variability of the four main frequency bands (Harner, 1975; Matousek et al., 1975). These basic systems have been made more sophisticated in the course of time.

It is interesting to note that the main EEG frequency ranges that represent ischemic changes in the brain, in a clinical setting, were examined in detail by Visser et al. (2001), who determined EEG spectral changes as function of time in the course of brain ischemia caused by short periods of circulatory arrest during surgery. After onset of circulatory arrest, the log spectral changes of three-epoch moving averages were calculated relative to the baseline spectrum. Factor analysis was carried out; 17 EEG periods were selected that showed changes progressing to an isoelectrical period. This analysis revealed four factors that represented the spectral EEG changes occurring during circulatory arrest and recovery. The frequency intervals of these factors were 0 to 0.5 Hz, 1.5 to 3 Hz, 7.5 to 9.5 Hz, and 15 to 20 Hz for all channels. The sequence of events was similar for all derivations. The first EEG change after circulatory arrest was an initial increase in alpha power and a decrease in beta power. On average, after approximately 15 seconds alpha power started to decrease, beta power decreased further, delta-1 power started to increase, and delta-2 power started to decrease. After approximately 25 seconds, the delta-1 power increase appeared to plateau or to decrease. Thus to detect intraoperative cerebral ischemia, monitoring of changes in these four frequency ranges is preferable to monitoring changes in the classically defined frequency bands.

CADS and Epileptiform Events

In contrast to the systems used to analyze EEG patterns in hypofunctional states, those that have been derived for automatic recognition and display of epileptiform events have received a good deal of attention in the past decade. Most interest in these systems is in laboratories directly involved in the diagnosis and care of a large population of epileptic patients, particularly in those locations where extensive EEG investigations using intracranial electrodes are performed as a guide for neurosurgery and where routine long-term EEG recording is carried out in combination with the determination of plasma levels of antiepileptic drugs.

CADS in epilepsy may have different objectives, such as detecting *interictal epileptiform transients;* detecting *epileptic seizures,* namely petit mal absences; or *localizing an epileptogenic area* in the brain. In the last decade the development of methods that may permit the automatic *anticipation of epileptic seizures* generated wide interest.

The principal aims of developing CADS for detecting *interictal epileptiform transients* are quantifying long-term variations in transient occurrence rates, especially in relation to antiepileptic drug therapy, and determining the topographical distribution of such events. The basic methodologies used have been described in Chapter 51. One basic problem is the difficulty of defining precisely a subject population containing a large variety of events of interest. A pioneering investigation in this respect was carried out by Gose et al. (1974); this study revealed considerable intra- and interrater variability. The difficulty here lies in the definitions of transients and their lack of objectivity. In 1949, Jasper and Kershman classified these events into *spikes* (duration 10–50 msec) and *sharp waves* (duration 50–500 msec). The Terminology Committee of the International Federation of EEG Societies defined spikes as waves with a duration of $1/12$ second (83 msec) or less, and sharp waves as waves with a duration of more than $1/12$ second and less than $1/5$ second (200 msec) (Storm van Leeuwen et al., 1966). Later, this Federation committee gave somewhat different duration limits for these phenomena, with spikes having a duration from 20 to under 70 msec and sharp waves having a duration of 70 to 200 msec (Chatrian et al., 1974). A few other characteristics have been identified. Spike and sharp waves are clearly distinguished from background activity and have a pointed peak (at conventional paper speeds); their main component is generally negative relative to other scalp areas, and their amplitude is variable. A distinction between spikes and sharp waves has descriptive value only. The parameters characteristic of spikes found in the human EEG have been studied by Celesia and Chen (1976).

The criteria mentioned above are imprecise and open to subjective interpretation. Nevertheless, experience has shown that they have pragmatic value. Furthermore, it is also important to consider the problem of rejecting artifacts that may have characteristics similar to epileptiform transients, such as EMG, lambda waves, vertex waves, or K complexes in sleep, and positive occipital sharp transients.

Taking into consideration the above discussion, it seems desirable to develop CADS in which users can choose whether they want to have detected those events classified with a high probability by a consensus of electroencephalographers as epileptiform or all events that any electroencephalographer would accept as epileptiform (Guedes de Oliveira et al., 1983). The strategic choice would depend on the clinical setting in which the analysis takes place. For instance, in routine clinical EEGs, one would probably prefer a stringent criterion in order to minimize the chance of false positives, whereas the investigator monitoring long EEG and plasma levels of antiepileptic drugs in known epileptic patients might be inclined to follow less stringent criteria. The rule-based algorithms developed by Gotman (1990, 1991) and collaborators (Gotman and Wang, 1991, 1992), and implemented in software packages have practical value, especially when the objective is to detect epileptiform transients in long EEG recordings, such as during a whole night. In this respect, the fact that the performance of these algorithms takes into account the well-known influence of the

state of the ongoing EEG, namely of the sleep stages on the occurrence of epileptiform events, is particularly valuable. In general, these automatic methods yield a relatively large number of false positives, and thus it is always necessary to perform a secondary visual reevaluation of the detected events. Nevertheless, this automatic CADS achieves a very comprehensive data reduction. Other algorithms have been proposed that may yield smaller rates of false positives (Hosteler et al., 1992; Webber et al., 1993, 1994, 1996). A practical conclusion of such studies is that visually corrected (a posteriori) automatic analysis of epileptiform events is a cost-effective procedure for the presurgical evaluation of epileptic patients associated with video-EEG monitoring (Spatt et al., 1997).

No matter which detection method is chosen, it is always necessary to provide a comprehensive display of the results so that topographical interpretation may be made, particularly with regard to the existence of an epileptogenic area.

To validate the clinical relevance of CADS, it is important to compare different methods according to a comprehensive protocol. Such a study was carried out by Dumpelmann and Elger (1999), who reported the results of a comparison of the performance of two specialist reviewers and of three spike-detection approaches with respect to the detection of epileptiform spikes in intracranial recordings from subdural and intrahippocampal depth electrodes in seven patients. The systems analyzed were (a) the rule-based system of Gotman's group, (b) the two-stage system consisting of an inverse autoregressive filter and a second rule-based stage of Lopes da Silva's group (Guedes de Oliveira et al., 1983), and (c) a system using wavelet coefficients of the intracranial EEG data developed by the authors. The results are quite revealing: the agreement between the two human reviewers with respect to spike identification was less than 50%. The automatic systems achieved agreements of 24% (rule-based system), 26% (wavelet detector), and 32% (two-stage system) with the individual human reviewers. In spite of the small proportion of agreements, the same anatomical regions were identified by human and automatic EEG analysis as generators for the majority of spikes. This led the authors to conclude that the poor agreement between the human EEG reviewers suggests that the definition of spikes and spike-like episodes in intracranial electrodes is far from unequivocal, although the localizing information is highly consistent by either visual or automatic spike detection, independent of the algorithm used for automatic spike detection. These conclusions are not really surprising since in our experience (Guedes de Oliveira et al., 1983) there is considerable variability in how experienced reviewers score epileptiform transients, while the performance of the automatic methods described above does not differ appreciably from a consensus of a panel of eight reviewers provided that there is not much contamination with artifacts. Wilson et al. (1996) made a larger reliability study of the performance of human experts in detecting epileptiform spikes and concluded that the average inter-reader correlation was 0.79. These authors proposed that this database could serve as a "gold standard" for testing computer algorithms or other readers. The same group (Wilson et al., 1998) developed later a neural network approach that performed automatic grouping of spikes via hierarchical clustering (using topology and morphology), the performance of which was close to that of human experts.

Since the advent of the magnetoencephalogram, it has been assumed that this new methodology would be useful for the localization of epileptiform events (Rose et al., 1987). The early literature has been reviewed by Sutherling and Barth (1990), Ricci (1990), and Engel and Ojeman (1993). In the 1990s, the development of large arrays of sensors for MEG recordings combined with advanced realistic models of the brain and surrounding tissues based on magnetic resonance imaging (MRI) scans, has led to a number of interesting investigations with the aim of improving spike source localization (Ebersole et al., 1995; Hari et al., 1993; Kettenmann et al., 1996; Knowlton et al., 1997; Lewine and

Orrison, 1995; Merlet et al., 1996; Paetau et al., 1992, 1994; Roth et al., 1997; Smith et al., 1995; Stefan et al., 1994). A preliminary conclusion that can be derived from these and similar studies is that the localization of epileptiform sources based on MEG data, especially if combined with EEG data, using realistic models of the head based on MRI scans, can provide valuable diagnostic information of particular interest in the evaluation of candidates for epilepsy surgery. The investigation of van't Ent et al. (2003) is an example; these authors detected several types of epileptiform transients in MEG recordings of patients with neocortical localization-related epilepsy. Subsequently the selected spikes were processed by grouping events with similar field maps yielding a set of signal matrices. Thereafter, Ward's method of hierarchical clustering was applied to identify a

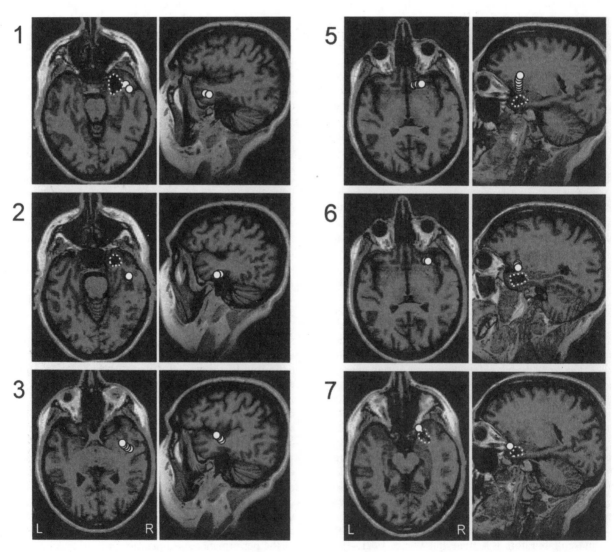

Figure 59.9. Equivalent current dipole (ECD) estimates of magnetic fields of the epileptiform spike clusters of a patient with a lesion in the right temporal pole. The locations of the ECDs are displayed on axial and sagittal magnetic resonance imaging (MRI). On the *left,* from *top* to *bottom,* the ECD positions for clusters 1, 2, and 3. On the *right* the ECDs for clusters 5, 6, and 7 (two other clusters, 4 and 8, did not yield ECDs with residual error <10%, and thus are not displayed in MRI). When present in the MRI slice, the structural lesion is delineated. Note that the ECDs of cluster 1 are positioned very close and at the lateral border of the lesion; all the others are also the right hemisphere but more distant from the lesion. (Adapted from van't Ent et al., 2003.)

number of significant clusters of spikes. After this, spike averages were computed for each cluster and the underlying sources were estimated using a single equivalent current dipole model (see Chapter 5, Fig. 5.4). A dipole was estimated at each time sample during the same time window as used in the clustering procedure. For the forward computations, a segmentation of the brain from MRI of each subject was used as volume conductor. Dipole solutions were accepted only when the residual error was less than 10%. The MEG data was transformed to the MRI coordinate system by matching fiducial markers. The estimated dipole locations are presented on MRI, as shown in Fig. 59.9). Some of these clusters are very close to the lesion visualized in the MRI.

In *clinical practice* epileptiform spike detectors are currently used in digital acquisition software applied on-line. Although these methods may differ in detail, they all derive from the results obtained in the previous studies described above (for review see Gotman, 1999). In general terms they are based on the identification of waveform parameters, such as sharpness, duration, slopes and relative amplitude. Furthermore, a measure of EEG state is very important since detection is always a process of extracting a signal (the spike) from the background, and the changes of the latter necessarily affect the performance of the detector, as used by Gotman and Wang (1992). In addition, information about the distribution in space of the detected events is commonly used (Flanagan et al., 2002; Glover et al., 1989; Gotman, 1999; Guedes de Oliveira and Lopes da Silva, 1980; van't Ent et al., 2003). As pointed out by Flanagan et al. (2002) the computation of equivalent dipole models, using appropriate detection and preprocessing methods, as indicated above, provides a spatial parameter for each detected epileptiform event, and this may constitute valuable information for the clinical assessment of a patient that can be readily combined with MRI and other relevant data. A new development in this area of endeavor is the exploration of the possibilities offered by the combination of EEG and functional MRI recordings (Ives et al., 1993) in search for ways of improving the localization of sources of epileptiform events. Al-Asmi et al. (2003) studied patients with focal epilepsy and frequent spikes who were subjected to spike-triggered or continuous functional MRI (fMRI) with simultaneous EEG. The activated regions in fMRI were concordant with EEG localization in almost all studies and confirmed by intracerebral EEG in some patients. Bursts of spikes were more likely to generate an fMRI response than were isolated spikes. The authors concluded that combining EEG and fMRI in focal epilepsy yields regions of activation that are presumably the source of spiking activity. These regions are highly linked with epileptic foci and epileptogenic lesions in a significant number of patients. This research area is most promising since the quality of simultaneously recording of EEG and fMRI is becoming practically reliable (Salek-Haddadi et al., 2003).

Automatic detection of seizures presents another kind of problems. In the initial phase of computer-assisted detection of seizures, the recognition of *petit mal absences* characterized by 3/sec spike-and-wave complexes was one main area of investigation. This is understandable considering that these seizures are relatively simple to detect in the EEG,

while they are of clinical interest in order to investigate correlations between such phenomena and behavior. The technique proposed by Ehrenburg and Penry (1976) was designed to recognize generalized spike and wave patterns whose main components, the *absence spike,* should be detected by way of a procedure based on zero-crossing analysis. The EEG records were classified visually by three raters; the consensus of all three was employed as a criterion for assigning the program's correct responses. In a test population of 12 patients, the program agreed with the consensus in 85% of the cases, and it had 1% overrecognitions. (The percentage of overrecognitions is defined here as the number of discharges detected automatically but classified by none of the raters, divided by the total number of discharges recognized by one or more of the raters.) The program's agreement with the consensus improved to 92% when all sleep sections were eliminated from the analyzed EEG. This particularly well-designed study led the authors to conclude that clinical applications of this CADS will lead to reduced costs over visual EEG assessment. Other CADS with the same main objective as the one described above have been developed (Carrie, 1972, 1976; Carrie and Frost, 1977; Frost, 1979). The advantages of this type of CADS in petit mal epilepsy are already widely appreciated by researchers interested in quantitative clinical studies.

Quite another sort of problem is the automatic recognition of other types of epileptic seizures, mainly of the *partial complex seizures* characteristic of temporal lobe epilepsy. The interest in automatic detection of this type of seizure stems from the fact that the central objective of electroencephalography in epilepsy is recording an electroclinical seizure. In the early phases of computer-assisted diagnosis in epilepsy, technical and computer facilities enabled recording EEG continuously for further off-line analysis (Ives et al., 1976; Kamp et al., 1979).

Babb et al. (1974) proposed an analog device with the objective of performing automatic seizure detection, based on the recognition of high-frequency activity occurring over several seconds. In this system, false alarms were quite frequent (30%). Currently, there is software available for the detection of seizures in clinical settings that provides reliable results, although it is not perfect.

In a few laboratories these systems are being used in combination with methods of stimulation to influence the development of seizures. Peters et al. (2001) described an integrated bedside system for real-time seizure detection and automated delivery of electrical stimulation directly to the brain of subjects undergoing invasive epilepsy surgery evaluation. These authors conclude that this network system is proof of the concept of a portable or implantable device that could serve identical functions. Viglione et al. (1970) and Viglione (1974) attempted to develop miniature automatic seizure recognition and warning systems that could be carried by patients; this system was successful in some cases but led to too many false alarms.

A related question is how to estimate the *localization of an epileptogenic area,* i.e., where within the brain epileptic seizures originate. There have been some efforts to localize possible sources of seizures on the basis of scalp recordings, and using dipole fitting methods, however, with much difficulty (Gotman, 2003). This is not surprising since it is not likely that the neuronal networks involved in the initiation of an epileptic seizure may be anatomically restricted to an area that might correspond to a discrete dipolar layer. Nevertheless, this was attempted by Kobayashi et al. (2000), who developed a noninvasive analysis to localize the source and visualize the time course of seizures, and to provide the location and orientation of the equivalent dipole generating this activity. This method was applied to scalp seizures in three patients with temporal lobe epilepsy and single-focus seizures confirmed by intracerebral recordings. A realistic head model based on MRI was used for computation of field distributions. When seizure activity was still not visually identifiable on the scalp, the method demonstrated in all scalp seizures a source in the temporal neocortex corresponding to the region of seizure activity in intracerebral recordings. More experience with this kind of methodology is needed to validate this approach.

The objective of localizing an epileptogenic area is particularly important in patients with complex partial seizures resistant to pharmacological therapy who are candidates for temporal lobectomy. On the basis of intracranial EEG recordings, useful results have been obtained by computing the time relations between EEG signals recorded from different sites. In this respect the pioneer work of Brazier (1972, 1973) was particularly influential. She computed cross-power spectra (*coherence* and *phase*) between EEG seizure records from different derivations. By determining the phase (Φ in degrees) between pairs of derivations at a frequency (f in Hz) with pronounced coherence, estimated time delay can be computed. Although interesting results have been obtained, mainly in cases of seizures studied with electrodes implanted in limbic structures, it should be noted that this method can give ambiguous results. To decide that there is a time delay depends on finding a linear relation between phase and frequency over a sufficiently wide frequency band. A difference in phase ($\Delta\Phi$) corresponding linearly to a difference in frequency (Δf) will represent a time delay computed as $\Delta t = (\Delta\Phi/\Delta f \times 360°)$. The latter method is preferred. Alternative methods were proposed by Gersch and Goddard (1970), Gersch and Tharp (1976), and Tharp and Gersch (1976). The latter were able to interpret the origin and spread of seizure activity within the brain of a patient carrying chronically indwelling electrodes, conclusions not possible on the basis of visual inspection of the records. Gotman (1981) applied the same principles to the analysis of some intracranial EEG records and was able to show that at a contralateral site the seizure activity is delayed by a few milliseconds compared with the seizures at the focal area. In the same way Gotman and Levtova (1996) were able to determine the relationships between amygdala and hippocampus in temporal lobe seizures.

From these studies, it became clear that the coherence of, and time delays between, different EEG channels during an epileptic seizure usually changes rapidly in the course of time. This implies that such seizures must be analyzed using short EEG segments. An interesting method, also aiming at determining the time relations between different EEG signals in such a way that it is possible to estimate the flow of information between different brain sites, has been proposed by Kaminski and Blinowska (1991), based on the framework of autoregressive models. This method can yield interesting results with respect to how epileptiform seizure activities may spread in the brain from a focal area (Franaszczuk et al., 1994).

To circumvent the limitations of linearity of the methods described above, new approaches were pursued. In this context Mars and van Arragon (1981) proposed to compute a measure of the average amount of mutual information (AAMI), in the sense of Gelfand and Yaglom (1959), between pairs of EEG signals as a function of the delay time introduced between both signals. It should be noted that this method is related to the cross-correlation as defined by equation 58.10 of Chapter 58, but is more general, since AAMI is not constrained by a linear relation between both signals. The AAMI method of analysis was used for focus localization in animals having a kindled epileptogenic focus (Mars and Lopes da Silva, 1983). In this way, time delays could be found for certain phases of epileptic seizures and the spread pattern of these seizures obtained. The same method was also applied to human seizures (Mars et al., 1985). The algorithms based on AAMI, however, proved to be rather cumbersome to apply in practice. This led to the creation of a new method of nonlinear regression analysis (the h^2 method of Lopes da Silva et al., 1989; Pijn, 1990; Pijn et al., 1989). This consists of computing a general coefficient of nonlinear fit between any pair of signals. The applications of this nonlinear regression coefficient to EEG signals recorded during seizures in animals (Fernandes de Lima et al., 1990) revealed that a large number of EEG signals recorded from different, but functionally related, brain areas present clear nonlinear relations. The same applies to EEG signals recorded from intracranial electrodes in patients (Pijn, 1990; Pijn and Lopes da Silva, 1993). Thus this method offers perspectives for the determination of the site of an epileptogenic focus, based on a set of simultaneously recorded EEG signals.

An exciting development is the possibility of detecting changes in the EEG that may occur before an epileptic seizure is manifest in the EEG, i.e., to be able to *anticipate a seizure*. Early attempts were not successful (Duckrow and Spencer, 1992; Rogowski et al., 1981; Viglione, 1974; Viglione et al., 1970). Recently, efforts have been made to apply mathematical tools derived from the theory of nonlinear dynamical systems in order to investigate whether it would be possible to predict the occurrence of epileptic seizures. Some of the basic notions with respect to the theory of nonlinear dynamical systems were discussed in Chapter 4. In essence, this approach, which has been called *neurodynamics,* assumes that the EEG is a signal of the activity of neuronal networks that is not purely stochastic but is governed by specific dynamical factors that are not detectable by classic linear methods. In the 1970s and 1980s, the first attempts to accomplish epileptic seizure prediction took shape, but the more convincing proof-of-principle experiments were published in the late 1980s and 1990s. At the present time this research line is an area of exciting theoretical, experimental, and clinical investigation.

The earliest attempts to use this theoretical framework in the analysis of epileptic seizures were made by Iasemidis et al. (1990, 1994), who used Lyapunov exponents to characterize dynamical changes occurring just before and during seizures. The maximum Lyapunov exponent is a measure of the maximum rate of generation, or destruction, of information as detected in EEG signals (Iasemidis et al., 1997). This group reported a preictal transition characterized by a progressive entrainment of dynamical measures, namely the maximum Lyapunov exponent, within a number of EEG signals recorded from specific sites. Shortly later a number of other studies appeared using different measures derived from the theory of nonlinear dynamics, such as the correlation dimension. These were applied to estimate EEG signal complexity, especially by the Bonn group (Elger and Lehnertz, 1998; Elger et al., 1997; Lehnertz and Elger, 1995) and the Paris group (Martinerie et al., 1998). This group introduced later another variant that was considered more robust, namely a measure of dynamic similarity (Le Van Quyen et al., 1999, 2000, 2001, 2003; Navarro, 2002). In this respect the latter methods differ from previous approaches by focusing on measures that detect changes in EEG signals properties, relative to some baseline period, and not on the nature of the change as such. A similar approach was used by Hively et al. (2000, 2003), Savit et al. (2001), and Li et al. (2003). This field is quickly evolving and new methods are appearing at a fast pace. It is noteworthy that in addition to the univariate measures initially used, also bivariate measures for phase synchronization and cross-correlation are being explored for discriminating preictal from interictal epochs (Mormann et al., 2003). Also changes in EEG signal energy were considered to have predictive value with respect to epileptic seizures (Litt et al., 2001). D'Alessandro et al. (2003) presented a method for training, testing, and validating a seizure prediction system on data from individual patients.

The application of these methods has led to the conclusion that there exists a *preseizure stage* that has dynamical properties different from both the interictal stage and the seizure. Nevertheless, the question of how one can optimally detect this preseizure state is still a controversial matter. Savit et al. (2001) summarized the problems inherent to these forms of analysis by stating that the underlying basis for the problems encountered in the validation of these analysis methods remains uncertain. Indeed, it is crucial to pay close attention to potentially confounding factors such as behavioral and other state changes, and to study and report in detail the ways in which relevant nonlinear measures behave in the presence of such changes, independent of seizure onset. Recently, a study along these lines was reported by Aschenbrenner-Scheibe et al. (2003), who searched for the identification of a preseizure state using the correlation dimension in 24-hour EEGs but with very few positive results. Most likely univariate measures may not be sensitive enough to characterize on their own the preictal state. More sophisticated multivariate measures should be further investigated in this context.

In short, a caveat of these various attempts to develop methods for the characterization of preseizure EEG features is that most of these studies have neglected to determine the specificity and the sensitivity of the observed effects in a comprehensive way.

Finally some theoretical considerations should be put forward. In our view (Lopes da Silva et al., 2003a,b), the activity of systems, such as neuronal networks, is characterized by the existence of states, or attractors in phase space, toward which the system tends to evolve as function of time. Some systems have simple attractors, like the case of a damped harmonic oscillator (point attractor) or a limit cycle (an oscillator), but the attractor may also have a complex structure called a manifold. The latter are characteristic of high-dimensional systems with so-called chaotic dynamics. These systems display sensitive dependence on initial conditions. As time evolves, small fluctuations in some parameters may drastically change the behavior of the system. These theoretical concepts are schematically illustrated in Fig. 59.10. This shows that a normal EEG pattern corresponds to an attractor that has no apparent structure, i.e., appears to be random and has a high dimension, although these values are only approximate estimates, while an EEG with abundant spikes can be represented by an attractor with both random and regular components and a slightly lower dimension; in contrast, a seizure EEG has an attractor with a complex but regular geometry and a low dimension. The transition from one to another kind of attractor in a complex nonlinear system, such as a neuronal network, may occur abruptly or not. Applying these concepts to the problem of the evolution of epileptic seizures, we may state that an abrupt transition occurs in many cases of absence seizures. Such transitions may be unpredictable because they may be caused by random fluctuations of an input or other parameters. In many instances of complex partial seizures, however, the transition may have an intermittent character, where approximately periodic behavior is intermittently interrupted, or mingled, with bursts of spikes (see Chapter 4, Fig. 4.19). Indeed, transitions from interictal EEG to seizure activity often occur in ways that are reminiscent of intermittent behavior. An epileptic seizure may take place when some critical parameters of a neuronal network change in such a way that a bifurcation to a lower dimensional attractor occurs. This change may develop gradually as shown in the model of Wendling et al. (2002), as described in Chapter 4. This is likely the case in some limbic epileptic seizures. Accordingly we may assume that in these cases changes of dynamics may *precede* the seizure and may be detectable in the preseizure EEG using appropriate methods. Furthermore, it is necessary to advance also in our understanding of which changes in dynamics of neuronal networks are relevant, combining experimental studies in animal models, more specific clinical observations in patients with intracranial electrodes, and computer modelling.

Computer System for Routine EEG Analysis

Computer technology has advanced very rapidly with the generalized use of microprocessor technology. Thus, nowa-

Characterizing the Epileptogenic Process
- State Space Reconstruction and Dimension -

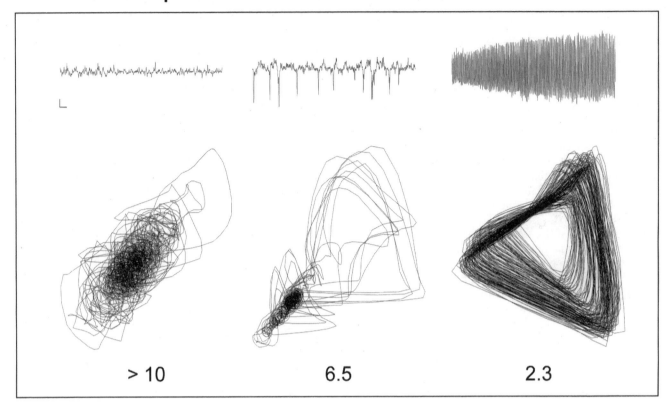

Figure 59.10. State-space representation of the attractors representing three dynamical states of neuronal networks underlying epileptic activity. On the *left* the attractor corresponding to normal EEG activity shown above, is depicted; it has a random character and a high dimension (>10); in the *middle* the attractor corresponding to an EEG with interictal spikes and with a dimension of 6.5 is displayed; on the *right* the attractor corresponding to a seizure, with a lower dimension is shown. (Adapted from Lehnertz, K., Andrzejak, R.G., Arnhold, J., et al. 2001. Nonlinear EEG analysis in epilepsy: its possible use for interictal focus localization, seizure anticipation, and prevention. J. Clin. Neurophysiol. 18:209–222.)

days, there is a wide choice of computer systems that can be used in the clinical routine EEG laboratory. These systems offer the possibility of data acquisition, editing and processing the data, artifact rejection, statistical analysis, and brain mapping.

Brain Mapping: Methodology

Brain mapping is the current term used for the methodology of representing the EEG activity, either spontaneous or evoked, in the spatial domain as a topographic map projected onto the scalp. The feature represented may be an amplitude of a given peak, a spectral variable, or a correlation measure. In essence, an EEG feature is extracted for all derivations at a given time sample, and a contour map of the distribution of the corresponding values over the scalp is constructed. A detailed discussion of questions of brain mapping methodology is given in Lopes da Silva (1990). Here only a general outline of such a discussion is presented.

Topographic EEG analysis has its roots in the toposcopic displays of Walter and Shipton (1951) and in the topograms pioneered by Remond (1968) and Remond and Torres (1964) and by Lehmann (1971), as discussed in Chapter 58. In the 1980s, brain mapping came of age with the widespread availability of fast and relatively cheap digital computers, associated with color video technology (Duffy, 1986; Duffy et al., 1979, 1981, 1984). Brain mapping is particularly attractive because it furnishes in a single image an overall view of the EEG activity of interest at a given moment. In most cases, the main interest lies in differentiating between normal and pathological activity and in following up the course of the pathological process. In this chapter, the emphasis is on brain mapping of the ongoing EEG activity; evoked potentials (EPs) are not discussed. I have chosen this focus since mapping of ongoing activity is a central issue in a clinical setting, whereas the mapping of EPs is dealt with in specialized sections.

General Factors Influencing the Construction of Brain Maps

The construction of brain maps depends on how the EEG feature being displayed has been sampled in space. Of course, the time variable is also of importance. This is discussed below. In a clinical situation, one wants to standardize the recording conditions as much as possible. However, if one is interested in obtaining interpretable brain maps, one must pay special attention to the choice of derivations and reference electrode.

Sampling in Space

From theoretical considerations, it is known that adequate sampling of a signal, whether in time or in space, requires that the sampling frequency should be at least twice the highest frequency present in the signal. In the time domain, this is usually easy to accomplish in an adequate way. However, this problem is not so easy to solve empirically in the spatial domain. Theoretically, it can be solved using models of electrical sources within a volume conductor, as discussed in the section Spatial Analysis of EEG in Chapter 58. Similarly to the time domain, it can be shown that the ability to adequately represent an electrical potential distribution in space by a certain electrode array can be given in terms of an aliasing error. This error depends on the spatial frequency content of the signal and on the interelectrode distance that corresponds to the sampling frequency in space. How can one determine the spatial frequency of a given signal? In practice, this cannot be determined in a simple way for each case. Therefore, it is necessary to define an upper limit for the spatial frequency. This upper limit is given by a source represented by a single radial dipole situated close to the brain surface, i.e., in the cortex. This may correspond, in practice, to an epileptogenic cortical focus or to some early components of EPs. In the International 10–20 System (interelectrode distance about 4.5 cm), the aliasing error for such a source is about 6%. If one wishes to reduce this error to the more adequate level of 1%, one must decrease the interelectrode distance to 3.2 cm, which means that 64 electrodes must be used. Gevins and Bressler (1988) indicate that even a system with 128 electrodes (interelectrode distances of about 2 cm) may be desirable in some cases. Therefore, we must conclude that the 21-electrode array commonly used provides a poor approximation of the spatial distribution of some features of the EEG. Indeed, the 10–20 system has been considered insufficient for some clinical applications not involving automatic topographic mapping, and this led researchers to add new electrode placements. A comprehensive extended system, called the 10% system, includes electrode sites halfway between each of the principal 10–20 placements (Chatrian et al., 1985). Its use should be encouraged (Nuwer, 1987). It should be added that it is important to use some electrode for checking artifacts.

Reference Electrode System

The choice of the reference electrode affects the appearance of any brain map. To avoid this type of problem, Lehmann and Michel (1989) have advised the use of the average reference, since all other reference sites may be close to the site of a maximum or a minimum potential. A disad-

vantage of this system is that, in the case of focal pathology, the potentials from the corresponding area may influence all recordings. Another system that is widely used is the linked earlobes reference (John et al., 1988). It is important to note that linked ears may yield distortion of a brain map (Fisch and Pedley, 1989) because of possible differences in impedance between the two ears. In these cases, it is advisable to add a high resistance between the ear electrodes to reduce such an effect. In fact, there is no ideal reference system. In general, a safe practice is to record the same data using several reference systems in order to determine how robust a particular brain map is (Rappelsberger, 1989). For example, this was done by Faux et al. (1990), who, incidentally, did not find statistically significant topographic differences between the use of a linked ears reference and a nose reference in a study of P300 brain maps.

To obtain a more precise spatial representation of the brain potentials at the scalp, one could use the more sophisticated approach of the Laplacian operator. It should be realized that electric sources within the brain cause potentials at the scalp that are spread over a relatively large area, due to the volume conductor properties of the brain and surrounding tissues. Therefore, the potentials measured between any two sites over the scalp represent the summation of signals from many cerebral, and even extracerebral, sources. The use of the Laplacian operator reduces the spatial blurring distortion at the scalp. The Laplacian operator is a mathematical procedure by means of which the potential at each electrode is converted to a quantity that represents the current density entering or leaving the scalp at that site. In this way, the need for a common reference electrode can be avoided. Of course, the computation of the Laplacian operator also poses some problems. Hjorth (1975, 1980) proposed a simplified method of performing such an operation. The use of the Laplacian combined with a large number of electrodes (e.g., 64 at least) provides the best way to collect EEG data to construct reliable brain maps (Fig. 59.11). In this context a technique that is currently being explored is the cortical potential imaging (CPI) (see Chapter 58), in which a biophysical model of the volume conductor is used to deconvolve a given scalp potential distribution into a distribution of electric potential over the epicortical surface (He, 1999; Zhang et al., 2003). The choice of the placement of the electrodes should always be guided by the question that one wants to answer. For instance, a detailed study of the topographic distribution of epileptiform spikes over the temporal region needs different coverage of the scalp than a study of sleep spindles.

What Is a Representative Brain Map?

This question cannot be answered without first clearly defining what the purpose of the investigation is. The main issue is to define whether one is interested in investigating the EEG under a steady-state condition or to study the dynamics of the spatial distribution of a given EEG feature.

Maps Representing Steady States

This is probably the most widespread application of brain maps in a clinical setting. Accordingly, it is necessary to have strict control over the conditions under which the EEG

Figure 59.11. ERD map obtained during a reading task displaying the probability of finding a change in the power spectra within the frequency range 8 to 12 Hz. The effect of different derivations can be seen: monopolar, transverse bipolar, local average or source derivations, average reference, and the Laplacian operator. Note that the ERD appears to be more widespread and to extend over frontal areas in the monopolar and common average reference but is more restricted to the occipital areas with the bipolar and Laplacian derivations. (Adapted from Pfurtscheller, G., and Lopes de Silva, FH. 1988. (Eds.). *Functional Brain Imaging*. Toronto: Hans Huber.)

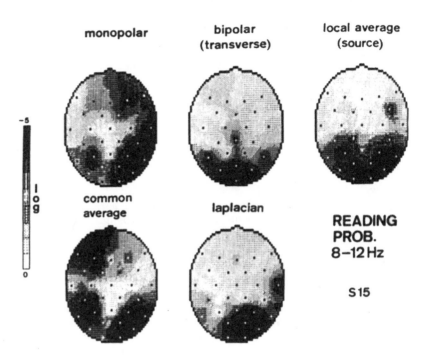

signals were recorded in such a way that the latter may be considered to be quasi-stationary. It is particularly important to discriminate between a change in the state of the subject and a pathological condition, but this is a general requirement in clinical EEG. The duration of a representative map for a given patient and condition should correspond to at least 60 to 100 seconds of artifact-free recording.

Maps Representing Dynamic States

These maps represent the change of the ongoing brain activity, within a given frequency band, induced by some event, for instance, a sensory stimulus or a movement. The name *event-related desynchronization* (ERD) has been given to this phenomenon, since in most cases such a change is characterized by a reduction of the EEG amplitude (Pfurtscheller et al., 1984). In this way, both in healthy subjects and in patients, the degree of cortical activation can be quantified, and its spatial distribution may be mapped over the scalp. Brain maps of the distribution of ERD have been shown to be useful in the assessment of patients suffering from cerebrovascular diseases (Koepruner et al., 1984). This methodology has been shown to be of interest in assessing cognitive functions in normal subjects, particularly attention and memory (Klimesch et al., 1988), and in some neurological disorders.

Use of Color

Color is not an essential element of a brain map. It is equally possible to present maps in shades of gray as in color. What is important is to have the possibility of viewing the contour lines and of changing the scale in order to focus on specific aspects of a brain map. Although the attractiveness of color to an observer cannot be underestimated, a word of caution should be put forward here. Color can be

used inadvertently in a misleading way because of the dependence on the scale used. Since a brain map is always the representation of a statistical variable, one should not only look at the colors but also take into consideration the statistical significance of the data, as discussed below.

Assessment of Brain Maps: Normality Versus Abnormality

The question of whether a map is abnormal, or not, depends on the multivariate statistics of the chosen set of topographic quantitative EEG features, independent of whether a brain map is drawn or not.

Two main approaches can be followed in order to define whether a brain map is normal or abnormal: a statistical approach and a correlational approach. The former is based on the definition of a normal distribution of healthy subjects (cf. Duffy, 1988) and on the use of statistical criteria for classifying those cases lying outside the confidence bands of the normal distribution as potentially abnormal. The latter is based on studies of the correlation between well-defined pathological cases, taking the clinical history and other examinations into consideration, and the set of features of the corresponding brain maps. These two approaches are not independent and usually they are followed jointly. In both cases, a basic requirement is that a representative normative database must be available. For clinical EEG studies it is necessary to take into consideration the age of the subjects. This aspect has been thoroughly studied by John et al. (1987, 1988) and Prichep and John (1986). The EEG features include univariate and multivariate descriptors of absolute and relative power, mean frequency, coherence, and asymmetry between homologous derivations. These researchers have constructed brain maps that depict the average deviations, for a given EEG feature, from the values predicted by the developmental equations for groups of patients with mild cognitive impairment, primary degenerative dementia, schizophrenia, alcoholism, and unipolar and bipolar depression.

In these brain maps, the scale (whether in color or not) represents the probability that the value found (e.g., percent of delta, theta, alpha, beta power) is within the normal range. For details about the statistical analysis, the reader is referred to the original publications of John et al. (1987, 1988). It is sufficient to state here that it is necessary to apply multivariate statistical analysis to sets of features in order to accomplish an automatic classification of an individual patient. However, it must be realized that different EEG derivations are often correlated. Therefore, the correlated measures of the same EEG feature occurring in brain maps must be corrected before abnormality is decided. This can be done by first calculating the covariance matrix among the set of measures. In this way, a normative covariance matrix can be defined for each particular brain map. John et al. (1988) proposed the use of a multivariate metric called Mahalanobis distance to assess deviations from the normative covariance matrix. With the same purpose, a convenient statistical method is to reduce the data set to a small number of variables using principal component or factor analysis (Skrandies and Lehmann, 1982; see also Chapter 50). In this way, an EEG data set derived from 21 derivations can be represented by five or six components that may account for 99% of the total variance. A related method, the singular value decomposition algorithm (Golub and Reinsch, 1970), has been applied to analyze multichannel topographic EEG data (Harner and Riggio, 1989), but a discussion of this problem lies outside the scope of this chapter.

In addition to statistical analyses of a given brain map obtained from a subject who may be considered abnormal, one should always resort to repetitive measurements in clinical practice. Those features that lie outside the confidence bands of the normal population in several maps, obtained on different occasions, warrant special attention and are most likely not spurious.

Phenomenology Versus Model-Based Analysis

Brain maps may be constructed simply to be used as illustrations of the EEG state of a given subject. In these cases, the map becomes by itself the phenomenon that characterizes the EEG of a subject in a given state. Following this approach, a phenomenology of brain mapping can be developed, by means of which different patterns are considered to be characteristic for certain EEG states of a given category of patients. This approach is free of any model-based assumptions. However, one can go beyond brain mapping if it is possible to assume that a given EEG spatial distribution corresponds to a definable electric source within the brain. This may be the case when sensory evoked potentials or epileptiform spike-and-wave complexes are analyzed.

It is often stated that the ultimate aim of EEG is to find the brain sources of the potential distribution recorded at the scalp. This constitutes the *inverse problem* in EEG (see Chapter 5). In these cases, one must assume a specific model of the source of a given brain map. The simplest form of an equivalent source is a simple current dipole. This should not be considered, however, as a discrete dipole somewhere in the brain, but rather as the best representation of the centroid of a dipole layer that corresponds to the activity of a patch of cortex. In those cases in which such a model proves appropriate to account for a given brain map, one can achieve an important degree of data reduction, and one can speak of real functional imaging of brain sources. Until now, this approach has not been much explored in clinical EEG, with the exception of the field of epilepsy (see also Sato and Malow, 1993), as described above and in Chapter 5.

Do Brain Maps Add Value to Multivariate Quantitative EEG Analysis?

Brain mapping implies that a set of multiple EEG signals has been quantified in some way, i.e., that one or more features were extracted and that the corresponding values were plotted in some sort of contour plot. Three types of features may be plotted: (a) a direct variable such as the amplitude value in microvolts at a given time sample, e.g., at the peak of an epileptiform spike; (b) a transformed variable such as absolute power (total or per frequency band), relative power per frequency band, mean or peak frequency (total or per frequency band); and (c) the result of a statistical test applied to a given EEG feature and represented in the form of a probabilistic map. Such a map can give, for example, the probability that the value of a given feature does not belong to the range of normative values. In addition to these features, other quantitative aspects of the EEG may be of importance, although they may not be so simple as to be represented in the form of a map, such as the interhemispheric or intrahemispheric coherence (total or per frequency band), the degree of asymmetry between homologous derivations, or the correlation and delay between different derivations as done by Gevins and Bressler (1988), as shown in Fig. 59.12 (see also Color Plate 8), and changes in power within a defined frequency band in relation to a given event (ERD), as done by Pfurtscheller et al. (1984) (Fig. 59.11). All of these features may be used for comparing clinical cases with normative EEG data using multivariate statistics. It should be emphasized that in this respect the graphic representation in the form of a brain map is neither necessary nor sufficient. In fact, it is enough to have a table with the values of the features of interest for all derivations and the corresponding normative data, in order to perform multivariate statistical analysis. Accordingly, the question may be asked whether the construction of a brain map has any added value to such a table of quantitative data.

The answer may be positive on two accounts. First, it is more attractive to the human observer to look at a map and extract out of it a characteristic pattern than it is to interpret a table of numbers. Second, a brain map can give information that may be used directly for a more extended interpretation. Indeed, a brain map may help to make direct comparisons (correlative approach of the previous section) between the topographic distribution of EEG features and an anatomical image given by MRI, positron emission tomography (PET), or similar brain scan; in addition, the topologic

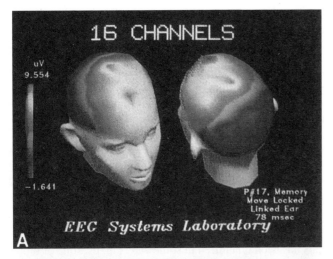

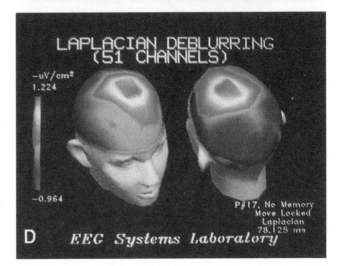

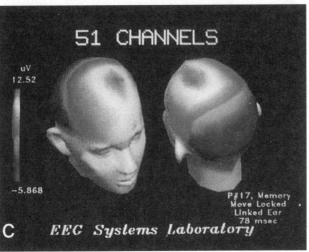

Figure 59.12. Movement-locked average event-related potentials (ERPs) at 78 msec after start of right index finger flexion, recorded against a linked ears reference with 16 channels (**A**), 27 channels (**B**), 51 channels (**C**), and after application of a Laplacian operation to the 51 channel ERPs (**D**). There is a false localization with 16 channels due to insufficient spatial sampling. The 27- and 51-channel ERP recordings show the true potential distribution with increasing resolution. Improvement in topographic localization with the Laplacian is self-evident. (Adapted from Gevins, A.S., and Bressler, S.L. 1988. Functional topography of the human brain. In *Functional Brain Imaging*, Eds. Pfurtscheller, G. and Lopes da Silva, F.H., pp. 99–116. Toronto: Hans Huber Publishers.) (See Color Figure 59.12.)

characteristics of the brain map may permit defining whether the source of the feature being mapped may be considered to correspond to a dipolar, or a more complex, electrical field (model-based approach of the previous section). If this is the case, one may go *beyond brain mapping* and test whether the map may be due to one (or more) equivalent dipole current sources within the brain. This is the essence of the process of functional localization of brain sources of activity. It is interesting to note that, in MEG, one always draws contour plots of the magnetic fields and usually tries to test whether dipolar sources are present. In this respect, MEG provides data that can be interpreted directly in a simpler way than EEG data, since the latter are more distorted by the properties of the volume conductor than the former

(cf. Chapter 5). In addition, most MEG studies have dealt with transient responses such as sensory evoked fields, which, in general, are easier to interpret in terms of equivalent source models than the ongoing activity. However, the location of discrete generators (alphons) of individual alpha spindles was derived using an array of 14 magnetic sensors (Williamson and Kaufman, 1989), and has been studied in more detail, using 151 MEG sensors in comparison with the sources of mu rhythms and sleep spindles (Manshanden et al., 2002) as shown in Fig. 59.13. With the availability of new multichannel neuromagnetic technology, it may be expected that the methodology of inverse (electro)magnetoencephalography may begin to significantly contribute to the clinic.

MEG: distribution of sources per voxel

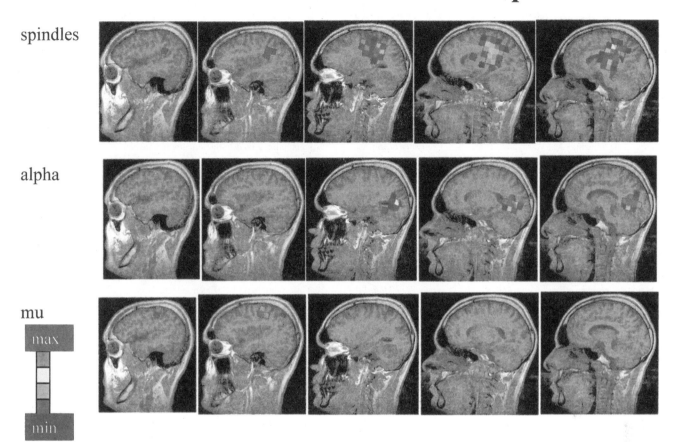

Figure 59.13. Epochs with alpha or mu rhythmic activity or sleep spindles were selected and band-pass filtered (9–16 Hz). At each sample point within the selected epochs the source was calculated using an equivalent dipole source model in a spherical model of the head (i.e., a time-varying dipole model). The optimal dipole positions and orientations were defined by using the least squares cost function that uses a global search strategy. In the model the constraint was applied that two sources, one in each hemisphere, should be symmetrical in space, whereas orientation and strength could vary between hemispheres. Only data points with a residual error lower than 10% were accepted for the displays. The dipoles were projected on the MRI of the subject using the image-fusion software package Con-Quest viewer. Additionally the MR image was divided into voxels with a size of 1 cm³. The number of dipoles the position of which fell within a given voxel, was counted. This number is displayed on the MRI slices that contain the corresponding voxel using a color code. The MEG alpha cluster was concentrated around the parieto-occipital sulcus, and the dipoles of the MEG mu rhythm were mainly restricted to the central sulcus. There was hardly any overlap between alpha and spindle dipole clusters. (Adapted from Manshanden, I., De Munck, J.C., Simon, N.R., et al. 2002. Source localization of MEG sleep spindles and the relation to sources of alpha band rhythms. Clin. Neurophysiol. 113(12):1937–1947.) (See Color Figure 59.13.)

References

Achermann, P.A., Borbély, A. 1997. Low-frequency (<1 Hz) oscillations in the human sleep. Neuroscience 81:213–222.

Agarwal, R., and Gotman, J. 2001. Computer-assisted sleep staging. IEEE Trans. BioMed Eng. 48:1412–1423.

Agarwal, R., and Gotman, J. 2002. Digital tools in polysomnography J. Clin. Neurophysiol. 19:136–143.

Al-Asmi, A., Benar, C.G., Gross, D.W., et al. 2003. fMRI activation in continuous and spike-triggered EEG-fMRI studies of epileptic spikes. Epilepsia 44(10):1328–1339.

Anderberg, M.R. 1973. *Cluster Analysis for Application.* New York: Academic Press.

Aschenbrenner-Scheibe, R., Maiwald, T., Winterhalder, M., et al. 2003. How well can epileptic seizures be predicted? An evaluation of a nonlinear method. Brain. 126(pt 12):2616–2626.

Babb, T.L., Mariani, E., and Crandall, P.H. 1974. An electronic circuit for detection of EEG seizures recorded with implanted electrodes. Electroencephalogr. Clin. Neurophysiol. 37:305–308.

Barlow, J.S. 1984. Analysis of EEG changes with carotid clamping by selective analog filtering, matched inverse digital filtering and automatic adaptive segmentation: a comparative study. Electroencephalogr. Clin. Neurophysiol. 58:193–204.

Barlow, J.S. 1986. Artifact processing in EEG data processing. In *Clinical Application of Computer Analysis of EEG and Other Neurophysiological Signals. Handbook of Electroencephalography and Clinical Neurophysiology,* New Series vol. 2, Eds. F.H. Lopes da Silva, W. Storm van Leeuwen, and A. Remond, pp. 15–64. Amsterdam: Elsevier.

Barlow, J.S., and Dubinsky, J. 1976. Some computer approaches to continuous automatic clinical EEG monitoring. In *Quantitative Analytical Methods in Epilepsy,* Eds. P. Kellaway and I. Petersen, pp. 309–327. New York: Raven Press.

Berg, P., and Scherg, M. 1994. A multiple sources approach to the correction of eye artifacts. Electroencephalgr. Clin. Neurophysiol. 90:229-241.

Bickford, R.G., Billinger, T.W., Fleming, N.I., et al. 1972. The compressed spectral array (CSA). A pictorial EEG. Proc. San Diego Biomed. Symp. 11:365–370.

Bickford, R.G., Brimm, J., Berger, L., et al. 1973. Application of compressed spectral array in clinical EEG. In *Automation of Clinical Electroencephalography,* Eds. P. Kellaway and I. Petersen, pp. 55–64. New York: Raven Press.

Binnie, C.D., Batchelor, B.G., Bawring, P.A., et al. 1978. Computer-assisted interpretation of clinical EEGs. Electroencephalogr. Clin. Neurophysiol. 44:575–585.

Bodenstein, G., and Praetorius, H.M. 1977. Feature extraction from the encephalogram by adaptive segmentation. Proc. IEEE 65:642–652.

Bourne, J.R., Miezin, F.M., Ward, J.W., et al. 1975. Computer quantification of electroencephalographic data recorded from renal patients. Comput. Biomed. Res. 8:461–473.

Bowe, T.R., and Anders, T.F. 1979. The use of the semi-Markow model in the study of the development of sleep-wake states in infants. Psychophysiology 16:41–48.

Bowling, P.S., and Bourne, J.R. 1978. Discriminant analysis of electroencephalograms recorded from renal patients. IEEE Trans. Biomed. Eng. MBE-25:12–17.

Brazier, M.A.B. 1972. Spread of seizure discharges in epilepsy: Anatomical and electrophysiological considerations. Exp. Neurol. 36:263–272.

Brazier, M.A.B. 1973. Electrical seizure discharges within the human brain: the problem of spread. In *Epilepsy, Its Phenomena in Man,* Ed. M.A.B. Brazier, pp. 155–171. New York: Academic Press.

Brechner, V.L., Walter, R.D., and Dillon, J.B. 1962. *Practical Electroencephalography for the Anesthesiologist.* Springfield, IL: Charles C Thomas.

Bremer, G., Smith, J.R., and Karacan, I. 1970. Automatic detection of the K complex in sleep electroencephalograms. IEEE Trans. Biomed. Eng. BME-17:314–323.

Brunia, C.H.M., Möcks, J., van den Berg-Lenssen, M.M.C., et al. 1989. Correcting ocular artifacts in the EEG: a comparison of several methods. J. Psychophysiol. 3:1-50.

Carrie, J.R.G. 1972. A hybrid computer technique for detecting sharp EEG transients. Electroencephalogr. Clin. Neurophysiol. 33:336–338.

Carrie, J.R.G. 1976. Computer-assisted EEG sharp transient detection and quantification during overnight recording in an epileptic patient. In *Quantitative Analytic Studies in Epilepsy,* Eds. P. Kellaway and I. Petersén, pp. 225–235. New York: Raven Press.

Carrie, J.R.G., and Frost, J.D. 1977. Clinical evaluation of a method for quantification of generalized spike-wave EEG patterns by computer during prolonged recordings. Comput. Biomed. Res. 10:449–457.

Celesia, G.G., and Chen, R. 1976. Parameters of spikes in human epilepsy. Dis. Nerv. Syst. 37:277–281.

Chatrian, G.E., Bergamini, L., Dondey, M., et al. 1974. A glossary of terms most commonly used by electroencephalographers. Electroencephalogr. Clin. Neurophysiol. 31:538–548.

Chatrian, G.E., Lettich, E., and Nelson, P.L. 1985. Ten present electrode system for topographic studies of spontaneous and evoked EEG activities. Am. J. EEG Technol. 25:83–92.

Chotas, H.G., Bourne, J.R., and Teschan, P.E. 1979. Heuristic techniques in the quantification of the electroencephalogram in renal failure. Comput. Biomed. Res. 12:299–312.

Creutzfeldt, O.D., Bodenstein, G., and Barlow, J.S. 1985. Computerized EEG pattern classification by adaptive segmentation and probability density function classification by clinical evaluation. Electroencephalogr. Clin. Neurophysiol. 60:373–393.

D'Alessandro, M., Esteller, R., Vachtsevanos, G., et al. 2003. Epileptic seizure prediction using hybrid feature selection over multiple intracranial EEG electrode contacts: a report of four patients. IEEE Trans Biomed Eng. 50(5):603–615.

Demartini, J., and Vincent-Carrefour, A. 1977. Topics on pattern recognition. In *EEG Informatics A Didactic Review of Methods and Applications of EEG Data Processing,* Ed. A. Remond, pp. 107–126. Amsterdam: Elsevier.

Dement, W., and Kleitman, N. 1957. Cyclic variations in EEG during sleep and their relation to eye movements, body motility dreaming. Electroencephalogr. Clin. Neurophysiol. 9:673–690.

Duckrow, R.B., and Spencer, S.S. 1992. Regional coherence and the transfer of ictal activity during seizure onset in the medial temporal lobe. Electroencephalogr. Clin. Neurophysiol. 82:415.

Duda, R.O., and Hart, P.E. 1973. *Pattern Classification and Scene Analysis.* New York: John Wiley & Sons.

Duffy, F.H. 1986. *Topographic Mapping of Brain Electrical Activity.* Boston: Butterworth.

Duffy, F.H. 1988. Issues facing the clinical use of brain electrical activity mapping. In *Functional Brain Imaging,* Eds. G. Pfurtscheller and F.H. Lopes da Silva, pp. 149–160. Toronto: Hans Huber Publishers.

Duffy, F.H., Burchfield, J.L., and Lombroso, C.T. 1979. Brain electrical activity mapping (BEAM): a method for extending the clinical utility of EEG and evoked potential data. Ann. Neurol. 5:309–321.

Duffy, F.H., Bartels, P.H., and Burchfield, J.L. 1981. Significance probability mapping: an aid in the topographic analysis of brain electrical activity. Electroencephalogr. Clin. Neurophysiol. 51:455–462.

Duffy, F.H., Albert, M.S., and McAnulty, G. 1984. Brain electrical activity in patients with presenile and senile dementia of the Alzheimer type. Ann. Neurol. 16:439–448.

Dumpelmann, M., Elger, C.E. 1999. Visual and automatic investigation of epileptiform spikes in intracranial EEG recordings. Epilepsia 40(3):275–285.

Dymond, A.M., Coger, R.W., and Serafetinides, E.A. 1978. Preprocessing by factor analysis of centro-occipital EEG power and asymmetry from three subject groups. Ann. Biomed. Eng. 6:108–116.

Ebe, M., Homma, I., Ishiyama, Y., et al. 1973. Automatic analysis of clinical information in EEG. Electroencephalogr. Clin. Neurophysiol. 34:706.

Ebersole, J.S., Squires, K.C., Eliashiv, S.D., et al. 1995. Applications of magnetic source imaging in evaluation of candidates for epilepsy surgery. Functional Imaging. 5:267–287.

Ehrenburg, B.L., and Penry, J.K. 1976. Computer recognition of generalized spike-wave discharges. Electroencephalogr. Clin. Neurophysiol. 41:25–36.

Elbert, T., Lutzenberger, W., Rockstroh, B., et al. 1985. Removal of ocular artifacts from the EEG—a biophysical approach to the EOG. Electroencephalogr. Clin. Neurophysiol. 60:455–463.

Elger, C.E., Lehnertz, K., Widmann, G., et al. 1997. Chaos analysis of intracerebral ECoG-data: its role in epileptic surgery. Electroencephalogr. Clin. Neurophysiol. 103:17(P).

Elger, C.E., Lehnertz, K. 1998. Seizure prediction by non-linear time series analysis of brain electrical activity. Eur. J. Neurosci. 10(2):786–789.

Engel, J., and Ojeman, G.A. 1993. The next step. In: Engel, J. (Ed.), *Surgical Treatment of the Epilepsies,* 2nd ed., New York: Raven Press.

Faux, S.F., Shenton, M.E., McCarley, R.W., et al. 1990. Preservation of P300 event-related potential topographic asymmetries in schizophrenia with use of either linked-ear or nose reference sites. Electroencephalogr. Clin. Neurophysiol. 75:378–391.

Fernandes de Lima, V.M., Pijn, J.P.M., Filipe, C.N., et al. 1990. The role of hippocampal commissures in the interhemispheric transfer of epileptiform after-discharges in the rat: A study using linear and nonlinear regression analysis. Electroencephalogr. Clin. Neurophysiol. 76:520–540.

Fisch, B.J., and Pedley, T.A. 1989. The role of quantitative topographic mapping or 'neurometrics' in the diagnosis of psychiatric and neurological disorders: the cons. Electroencephalogr. Clin. Neurophysiol. 73:5–9.

Flanagan, D., Agarwal, R., and Gotman, J. 2002. Computer-aided spatial classification of epileptic spikes. J. Clin. Neurophysiol. 19:125–135.

Fortgens, C., and de Bruin, M.P. 1983. Removal of eye movement and EOG artifacts from the non-cephalic reference EEG. Electroencephalogr. Clin. Neurophysiol. 56:90–96.

Franaszczuk, P.J., Bergey, G.K., Kaminski, M.J. 1994. Analysis of mesial temporal seizure onset and propagation using the directed transfer function method. Electroencephalogr. Clin. Neurophysiol. 91(6):413–427.

Friberg, S. 1980. A program system for the automatic evaluation of the background activity in the human electroencephalogram. Technical Report, 3:80. Research Laboratory of Medical Electronics, Chalmers University of Technology, Gothenburg, Sweden.

Friberg, S., Matousek, M., and Petersen, I. 1980. A mathematical model for the age development of the background activity in the human electroencephalogram. Technical Report, 2:80. Research Laboratory of Medical Electronics, Chalmers University of Technology, Gothenburg, Sweden.

Frost, J.D., Jr. 1979. Microprocessor-based EEG spike detection and quantification. Intl. J. Biomed. Comput. 10:357–373.

Gaillard, J.M., and Tissot, R. 1973. Principles of automatic analysis of sleep records with a hybrid system. Comput. Biomed. Res. 6:1–13.

Gaillard, J.M., Krassvievitch, M., and Tissot, R. 1972. Analyse automatique du sommeil par un systeme hybride. Electroencephalogr. Clin. Neurophysiol. 33:403–410.

Gasser, T., Sroka, L., and Mocks, J. 1985. The transfer of EOG activity into the EEG for eyes open and closed Electroencephalogr. Clin. Neurophysiol. 61:181–193.

Gelfand, I.M., and Yaglom, A.M. 1959. Calculation of the amount of information about a random function contained in another such function. Am. Math. Soc. Transact. 12:199–246.

Gersch, W., and Goddard, G. 1970. Locating the site of epileptic focus by spectral analysis methods. Science 169:701–702.

Gersch, W., and Tharp, B.R. 1976. Spectral regression—Amount of information analysis of seizures in humans. In *Quantitative Analytic Studies in Epilepsy,* Eds. P. Kellaway and I. Petersen, pp. 509–532. New York: Raven Press.

Gevins, A.S. 1979. Quantitative aspects of electroencephalography. In *Electrophysiological Approaches to Neurological Diagnosis,* Ed. M.J. Aminoff. London: Churchill Livingstone.

Gevins, A.S., and Bressler, S.L. 1988. Functional topography of the human brain. In *Functional Brain Imaging,* Eds. G. Pfurtscheller and F.H. Lopes da Silva, pp. 99–116. Toronto: Hans Huber Publishers.

Gevins, A.S., and Morgan, N.H. 1986. Classifier-directed signal processing in brain research. IEEE Trans. Biomed. Eng. BME-33(12):1054–1068.

Gevins, A.S., Yeager, C.L., Diamond, S.L., et al. 1975. Automated analysis of the electrical activity of the human brain (EEG): A progress report. Proc. IEEE 63:1382–1399.

Gevins, A.S., Yeager, C.L., Diamond, S.L., et al. 1976. Sharp-transient analysis and thresholded linear coherence spectra of paroxysmal EEGs. In *Quantitative Analytical Studies in Epilepsy,* Eds. P. Kellaway and I. Petersen, pp. 463–482. New York: Raven Press.

Gevins, A.S., Yeager, C.L., Zeitlin, G.M., et al. 1977. On-line computer rejection of EEG artifact. Electroencephalogr. Clin. Neurophysiol. 42:267–274.

Glover, J.R. Jr, Raghavan, N., Ktonas, P.Y., et al. 1989. Context-based automated detection of epileptogenic sharp transients in the EEG: elimination of false positives. IEEE Trans. Biomed. Eng. 36:519–527.

Gloor, P. 1977. The EEG and differential diagnosis of epilepsy. In *Current Concepts in Clinical Neurophysiology,* Eds. H. van Duijn, D.N. Donker, and A.C. van Huffelen, pp. 9–21. The Hague: Trio.

Goldberg, P., Samson-Dollfus, D., and Gremy, F. 1973. An approach to an automatic pattern recognition of the electroencephalogram: background rhythm and paroxysmal elements. Methods Inf. Med. 12:155–163.

Golub, G.H., and Reinsch, C. 1970. Singular value decomposition and least squares solutions. Numer. Math. 14:403–420.

Gondeck, A.R., and Smith, J.R. 1974. Dynamics of human sleep sigma spindles. Electroencephalogr. Clin. Neurophysiol. 37:293–297.

Gose, E.E., Werner, S., and Bickford, R.G. 1974. Computerized spike detection. Proc. San Diego Biomed. Symp. 13:193–198.

Gotman, J. 1976. Experiments in the automation and quantification of EEG interpretation: localized brain lesions and epilepsy. Thesis, McGill University, Montreal, Canada.

Gotman, J. 1978. Problems of presentation of analytical results. Electroencephalogr. Clin. Neurophysiol. Suppl. 34:191–197.

Gotman, J. 1980. Quantitative measurements of epileptic spike morphology in the human EEG. Electroencephalogr. Clin. Neurophysiol. 48:551–557.

Gotman, J. 1990. Automatic seizure detection: improvements and evaluation. Electroencephalogr. Clin. Neurophysiol. 76:317–324.

Gotman, J. 1981. Interhemispheric relations during bilateral spike-and-wave activity. Epilepsia 22:453–466.

Gotman, J. 1991. Automatic detection of seizures and spikes in the EEG. In: H. Lüders (Ed.), *Epilepsy Surgery,* pp. 307–316. New York: Raven Press.

Gotman, J. 1999. Automatic detection of seizures and spikes. J. Clin. Neurophysiol. 16:130–140.

Gotman, J. 2003. Noninvasive methods for evaluating the localization and propagation of epileptic activity. Epilepsia 44(suppl 12):21–29.

Gotman, J., and Gloor, P. 1976. Automatic recognition and quantification of interictal epileptic activity in the human scalp EEG. Electroencephalogr. Clin. Neurophysiol. 41:513–529.

Gotman, J., and Marciani, M.G. 1985. EEG spiking activity, drug levels and seizure occurrence in epileptic patients. Ann. Neurol. 17:597–603.

Gotman, J., and Wang, L.Y. 1991. State-dependent spike detection: concepts and preliminary results. Electroencephalogr. Clin. Neurophysiol. 79:11–19.

Gotman, J., and Wang, L.Y. 1992. State-dependent spike detection: validation. Electroencephalogr. Clin. Neurophysiol. 83:12–18.

Gotman, J., Skuce, D.R., Thompson, C.J., et al. 1973. Clinical applications of spectral analysis and extraction of features from electroencephalograms with slow waves in adult patients. Electroencephalogr. Clin. Neurophysiol. 35:225–235.

Gotman, J., Gloor, P., and Schaul, N. 1978. Comparison of traditional reading of the EEG and automatic recognition of interictal epileptic activity. Electroencephalogr. Clin. Neurophysiol. 44:48–60.

Gotman, J., and Levtova, V. 1996. Amygdala-hippocampus relationships in temporal lobe seizures: a phase-coherence study. Epilepsy Res. 25:51–57.

Guedes de Oliveira, P.H.H., and Lopes da Silva, F.H. 1980. A topographical display of epileptiform transients based on a statistical approach. Electroencephalogr. Clin. Neurophysiol. 48:710–714.

Guedes de Oliveira, Queiroz, and Lopes da Silva, F.H. 1983. Spike detection based on a pattern recognition approach using a microcomputer. Electroencephalogr. Clin. Neurophysiol. 56(1):97–103.

Guess, M.J., and Wilson, S.B. 2002. Introduction to hierarchical clustering. J. Clin. Neurophysiol. 19:144–151.

Hansen, E.S., Prichep, L.S., Bolwig, T.G., et al. 2003. Quantitative electroencephalography in OCD patients treated with paroxetine. Clin. Electroencephalogr. 34(2):70–74.

Hari, R., Ahonen, A., Forss, N., et al. 1993. Parietal epileptic mirror focus detected with a whole-head neuromagnetometer. Neuroreport 5:45–48.

Harner, R.N. 1975. Computer analysis and clinical EEG Interpretation—Perspective and application. In *CEAN-Computerized EEG Analysis,* Eds. G. Dolce and H. Kunkel, pp. 337–343. Stuttgart: Fischer.

Harner, R.N., and Ostergren, K.A. 1976. Sequential analysis of quasi-stable and paroxysmal activity. In *Quantitative Analytic Studies in Epilepsy,* Eds. P. Kellaway and I. Petersen, pp. 343–353. New York: Raven Press.

Harner, R.N., and Ostergren, K.A. 1978. Computed EEG topography. Electroencephalogr. Clin. Neurophysiol. Suppl. 34:151–161.

Harner, R.N., and Riggio, S. 1989. Application of singular value decomposition to topographic analysis of flash-evoked potentials. Brain Topogr. 2:91–98.

He, B. 1999. Brain electric source imaging: scalp Laplacian mapping and cortical imaging. Crit. Rev. Biomed. Eng. 27:149–188.

Hermann, W.M., and Kubicki, S. 1984. Various techniques of computer analysis in nocturnal sleep. In *Epilepsy, Sleep and Sleep Deprivation,* Eds. R. Degen and E. Niedermeyer, pp. 207–229. Amsterdam: Elsevier.

Hermann, W.M., Fichte, K., and Kubicki, S. 1978. Mathematische Rationale für die klinische EEG-Frequenzbander. I. Faktorenanalyse mit EEG Powerspektralschtzungen zur Definition von Frequenzbandern. EEG-EMG 9:146–154.

Hively, L.M., Protopopescu, V.A., Gailey, P.C. 2000. Timely detection of dynamical change in scalp EEG signals. Chaos 10(4):864-875.

Hively, L.M., and Protopopescu, V.A. 2003. Channel-consistent forewarning of epileptic events from scalp EEG. IEEE Trans. Biomed. Eng. 50(5): 584–593.

Hjorth, B. 1975. An on-line transformation of EEG scalp potentials into orthogonal source derivations. Electroencephalogr. Clin. Neurophysiol. 39:526–530.

Hosteler, W., Doller, H.J., and Homan, R.W. 1992. Assessment of a computer program to detect epileptiform spikes. Electroencephalogr. Clin. Neurophysiol. 83:1–11.

Iasemidis, L.D., Sackellares, J.C., Zaveri, H.P., et al. 1990. Phase space topography and the Lyapunov exponent of electroencephalograms in partial seizures. Brain Topogr. 2:187–201.

Iasemidis, L.D., Olson, L.D., Savit, R.S., et al. 1994. Time dependencies in the occurrence of epileptic seizures: a nonlinear approach. Epilepsy Res. 17:81–94.

Iasemidis, L.D., Principe, J.C., Czaplewski, J.M., et al. 1997. Spatiotemporal transition to epileptic seizures: a non-linear dynamical analysis of scalp intracranial recordings. In: *Spatiotemporal Models in Biological and Artificial Systems,* Eds. F.H. Lopes da Silva, J.C. Principe, and L.B. Almeida, pp. 81–88. Amsterdam: IOS Press.

Ille, N., Berg, P., and Scherg, M. 2003. Artifact correction of the ongoing EEG using spatial filters based on artifact and brain signal topographies. J. Clin. Neurophysiol. 19:113–124.

Isaksson, A., and Wennberg, A. 1975a. An EEG simulator—A means of objective clinical interpretation of EEG. Electroencephalogr. Clin. Neurophysiol. 39:313–320.

Isaksson, A., and Wennberg, A. 1975b. Visual evaluation and computer analysis of the EEG—a comparison. Electroencephalogr. Clin. Neurophysiol. 38:79–86.

Itil, T.M., Shapiro, D.M., Fink, M., et al. 1969. Digital computer classifications of EEG sleep stages. Electroencephalogr. Clin. Neurophysiol. 27:76–83.

Ives, J.R., Thompson, C.J., and Gloor, P. 1976. Seizure monitoring: a new tool in electroencephalography. Electroencephalogr. Clin. Neurophysiol. 41:422–427.

Ives, J.R., Warach, S., Schmitt, F., Edelman, R.R., Schomer, D.L. 1993. Monitoring the patient's EEG during echo planar MRI. Electroencephalogr. Clin. Neurophysiol. 87(6):417–420.

Jagannathan, V., Bourne, J.R., Jansen, B.H., et al. 1982. Artificial intelligence methods in quantitative electroencephalographic analysis. Comput. Progr. Biomed. 15:249–258.

Jansen, B.H. 1979. EEG segmentation and classification. Thesis, Free University, Amsterdam.

Jansen, B.H. 1986. Quantitative EEG analysis in renal disease. In Clinical Applications of Computer Analysis of EEG and Other Neurophysiological Signals. Handbook of Electroencephalography and Clinical Neurophysiology, vol. II, Eds. F.H. Lopes da Silva, W. Storm van Leeuwen, and A. Remond, pp. 239–260. Amsterdam: Elsevier.

Jasper, H., and Kershman, J. 1949. Classification of the EEG in epilepsy. Electroencephalogr. Clin. Neurophysiol. Suppl. 2:123–131.

Jervis, B.W., Nichols, M.J., Allen, E.M., et al. 1985. The assessment of two methods for removing eye movement artifact from the EEG. Electroencephalogr. Clin. Neurophysiol. 61:444–452.

Jervis, B.W., Ifeachor, E.C., Allen, E.M. 1988. The removal of ocular artefacts from the electroencephalogram: a review. Med. Biol. Eng. Comp. 26:2–12.

John, E.R. 1989. The role of quantitative EEG topographic mapping or 'neurometrics' in the diagnosis of psychiatric and neurological disorders: the pros. Electroencephalogr. Clin. Neurophysiol. 73(1):2–4.

John, E.R., Prichep, L.S., and Easton, P. 1987. Normative data banks and neurometrics: Basic concepts, methods and results of norm construction. In Handbook of Electroencephalography and Clinical Neurophysiology (Revised Series), Vol. I: Methods of Analysis of Electrical and Magnetic Signals, Eds. A.S. Gevins and A. Remond. Amsterdam: Elsevier.

John, E.R., Prichep, L.S., Fridman, J., et al. 1988. Neurometrics: computer-assisted differential diagnosis of brain dysfunctions. Science 239:162–169.

Johnson, L.C. 1977. The EEG during sleep as viewed by a computer In EEG Informatics. A Didactic Review of Methods and Applications of EEG Data Processing, Ed. A. Remond, pp. 385–406. Amsterdam: Elsevier.

Johnson, L., Lubin, A., Nautoh, P., et al. 1969. Spectral analysis of the EEG of dominant and non-dominant alpha subjects during waking and sleeping. Electroencephalogr. Clin. Neurophysiol. 26:361–370.

Jonkman, E.J., Poortvliet, D.C.J., Veering, H.M., et al. 1985. The use of neurometrics in the study of patients with cerebral ischemia. Electroencephalogr. Clin. Neurophysiol. 61:333–341.

Jung, T.P., Makeig, S., Westerfield, M., et al. 2000. Removal of eye activity artifacts from visual event-related potentials in normal and clinical subjects. Clin. Neurophysiol. 111:1745–1758.

Kaminski, M.J., Blinowska, K.J. 1991. A new method of the description of the information flow in the brain structures. Biol. Cybern. 65:203–210.

Kamp, A., Mars, N.J.I., and Wisman, T. 1979. Long term monitoring of the electroencephalogram in epileptic patients. In Handbook on Biotelemetry and Radio Tracking, Eds. C.J. Amlaner, Jr., and D.W. MacDonald, pp. 499–503. Oxford: Pergamon Press.

Kemp, B. 1987. Model-based monitoring of human sleep stage. Thesis, University of Twente, Enschede, The Netherlands.

Kemp, B., and Kamphuisen, H.A.C. 1986. Simulation of human hypnograms using a Markov chain model. Sleep 9:405–414.

Kemp, B., Jaspers, P., Franzen, J.M., et al. 1985. An optimal monitor of the electroencephalographic sigma sleep state. Biol. Cybern. 51:263–270.

Kettenmann, B., Hummel, C., Stefan, H., et al. 1996. Multichannel magnetoencephalographical recordings: separation of cortical responses to different chemical stimulation in man. Electroencephalogr. Clin. Neurophysiol. Suppl. 46:271–274.

Kiley, J.E., Pratt, K.L., Gisser, D.G., et al. 1976a. Techniques of EEG frequency analysis for evaluation of uremic encephalopathy. Clin. Nephrol. 5:279–285.

Kiley, J.E., Woodruff, M.W., and Pratt, K.L. 1976b. Evaluation of encephalopathy by EEG frequency analysis in chronic dialysis patients. Clin. Nephrol. 5:245–250.

Klimesch, W., Pfurtscheller, G., and Mohl, W. 1988. ERD mapping and long-term memory: The temporal and topographical pattern of cortical activation. In Functional Brain Imaging, Eds. G. Pfurtscheller and F.H. Lopes da Silva, pp. 131–142. Toronto: Hans Huber Publishers.

Knowlton, R.C., Laxer, K.D., Aminoff, M.J., et al. 1997. Magnetoencephalography in partial epilepsy: clinical yield and localization accuracy. Ann. Neurol. 42(4):622–631.

Kobayashi, K., James, C.J., Yoshinaga, H., et al. 2000. The electroencephalogram through a software microscope: non-invasive localization and visualization of epileptic seizure activity from inside the brain. Clin Neurophysiol. 111(1):134–149.

Koepruner, V., Pfurtscheller, G., and Auer, L.M. 1984. Quantitative EEG in normals and in patients with cerebral ischemia. In Brain Ischemia. Quantitative EEG and Imaging Techniques, Eds. G. Pfurtscheller, E.J. Jonkman, and F.H. Lopes da Silva, Progr. Brain Res. 62:29–50. Amsterdam: Elsevier.

Kohonen, T. 2001. Self-Organizing Maps. Springer Series in Information Sciences, Vol. 30, Berlin/Heidelberg/New York: Springer, Third Edition, 501 pages.

Ktonas, P.Y., and Smith, J.R. 1974. Quantification of abnormal EEG spike characteristics. Comput. Biol Med. 4:157–163.

Künkel, H. 1972. Die Spektraldarstellung des EEG. EEG-EMG 3:15–24.

Künkel, H., and EEG Project Group. 1975. Hybrid computing system for EEG analysis. In CEAN—Computerized EEG Analysis, Eds. G. Dolce and H. Kunkel, pp. 365–383. Stuttgart: Fischer.

Lagerlund, T.D., Sharbrough, F.W., Busacker, N.E. 1997. Spatial filtering of multichannel electroencephalographic recordings through principal component analysis by single value decomposition. J. Clin. Neurophysiol. 14:73–82.

Larsen, L.E., and Walter, D.O. 1970. On automatic methods of sleep staging by EEG spectra. Electroencephalogr. Clin. Neurophysiol. 28:459–467.

Lehmann, D. 1971. Multichannel topography of human alpha EEG fields. Electroencephalogr. Clin. Neurophysiol. 31:439–449.

Lehmann, D., and Michel, M.E. 1989. Intracerebral dipole sources of EEG FFT power maps. Brain Topogr. 2:155–164.

Lehnertz, K., and Elger, C.E. 1995. Spatio-temporal dynamics of the primary epileptogenic area in temporal lobe epilepsy characterized by neuronal complexity loss. Electroencephalogr. Clin. Neurophysiol. 95:108–117.

Lehnertz, K., Andrzejak, R.G., Arnhold, J., et al. 2001. Nonlinear EEG analysis in epilepsy: its possible use for interictal focus localization, seizure anticipation, and prevention. J. Clin. Neurophysiol. 18:209–222.

Lemieux, J.F., and Blume, W.T. 1983. Automated morphological analysis of spikes and sharp waves in human electrocorticograms. Electroencephalogr. Clin. Neurophysiol. 55:45–50.

Le Van Quyen, M., Martinerie, J., Baulac, M., et al. 1999. Anticipating epileptic seizures in real time by a non-linear analysis of similarity between EEG recordings. Neuroreport 21:2149–2155.

Le Van Quyen, M., Adam, C., Martinerie, J., et al. 2000. Spatio-temporal characterizations of non-linear changes in intracranial activities prior to human temporal lobe seizures. Eur. J. Neurosci. 12(6):2124–2134.

Le Van Quyen, M., Martinerie, J., Navarro, V., et al. 2001. Anticipation of epileptic seizures from standard EEG recordings. Lancet 357(9251):183–188.

Le Van Quyen, M., Navarro, V., Martinerie, J., et al. 2003. Toward a neurodynamical understanding of ictogenesis. Epilepsia. 44(suppl 12):30–43.

Lewine, J.D., and Orrison Jr., W.W. 1995. Magnetoencephalography and magnetic source imaging. In Functional Brain Mapping, pp. 369–417. St. Louis: Mosby-Year Book.

Li, D., Zhou, W., Drury, I., et al. 2003. Linear and nonlinear measures and seizure anticipation in temporal lobe epilepsy. J. Comput. Neurosci. 15(3):335–345.

Litt, B., Esteller, R., Echauz, J., et al. 2001. Epileptic seizures may begin hours in advance of clinical onset: a report of five patients. Neuron. 30(1):51–64.

Lopes da Silva, F.H. 1978. Analysis of EEG nonstationarities. Electroencephalogr. Clin. Neurophysiol. Suppl. 34:163–179.

Lopes da Silva, F.H. 1990. A critical review of clinical applications of topographic mapping of brain potentials. J. Clin. Neurophysiol. 7:535–551.

Lopes da Silva, F.H., Blanes, W., Kalitzin, S., et al. 2003a. Dynamical diseases of brain systems: different routes to epileptic seizures. IEEE Trans. Biomed. Eng. 50(5):540–548.

Lopes da Silva, F.H., Blanes, W., Kalitzin, S.N., et al. 2003b. Epilepsies as dynamical diseases of brain systems: basic models of the transition between normal and epileptic activity. Epilepsia 44(suppl 12):72–83.

Lopes da Silva, F.H., and van Hulten, K. 1978. Analyse quantitative de l'activite intercritique en EEG et SEEG dans l'epilepsie. Rev. EEG Neurophysiol. 2:198–204.

Lopes da Silva, F.H., Dijk, A., Smits, H., et al. 1973. Automatic detection and pattern recognition of epileptic spikes from surface and depth recording in man. In *Die Quantifizierung des Elektroenzephalogramms,* Ed. G.K. Schenk, pp. 425–436. Konstanz: AEG-Telefunken.

Lopes da Silva, F.H., Dijk, A., and Smits, H. 1975. Detection of nonstationarities in EEGs using the autoregressive model—An application of EEGs of epileptics. In *CEAN—Computerized EEG Analysis,* Eds. G. Dolce and H. Kunkel, pp. 180–199. Stuttgart: Fischer.

Lopes da Silva, F.H., ten Broeke, W., van Hulten, K., et al. 1976. EEG nonstationarities detected by inverse filtering in scalp and cortical recordings of epileptics: statistical analysis and spatial display. In *Quantitative Analytic Studies in Epilepsy,* Eds. P. Kellaway and I. Petersén, pp. 375–387. New York: Raven Press.

Lopes da Silva, F.H., van Hulten, K., Lommen, J.G., et al. 1977. Automatic detection and localization of epileptic foci. Electroencephalogr. Clin. Neurophysiol. 43:1–13.

Lopes da Silva, F.H., Pijn, J.P.M., and Boeijinga, P.H. 1989. Interdependence of EEG signals: Linear versus nonlinear association and the significance of time delays and phase shifts. Brain Topogr. 2:9–18.

Lubin, A., Johnson, L.C., and Austin, N.T. 1969. Discriminations among states of consciousness using EEG spectra. Psychophysiology 6:122–132.

Makeig, S., Bell, A.J., Jung, T.P., et al. 1996. Independent component analysis of electroencephalographic data. In *Advances in Neural Information Processing,* Eds. D. Touretzky, M. Mozer, M. Hasselmo, pp. 145–151. Cambridge, MA: MIT Press.

Manshanden, I., De Munck, J.C., Simon, N.R., et al. 2002. Source localization of MEG sleep spindles and the relation to sources of alpha band rhythms. Clin. Neurophysiol. 113(12):1937–1947.

Mars, N.J.I., and Lopes da Silva, F.H. 1983. Propagation of seizure activity in kindled dogs. Electroencephalogr. Clin. Neurophysiol. 56:194–209.

Mars, N.J.I., and van Arragon, G.W. 1981. Time delay estimation in nonlinear systems using Average Mutual Amount of Information Analysis. IEEE-Acoustics, Speech and Signal Processing, vol. ASSP–29, 3:619–621.

Mars, N.J.I., Thompson, P.M., and Wilkus, R.J. 1985. The spread of epileptic seizures activity in humans. Epilepsia 26:85–94.

Martin, W.B., Johnson, L.C., Viglione, S.S., et al. 1972. Pattern recognition of EEG-EOG as a technique for all-night sleep stage scoring. Electroencephalogr. Clin. Neurophysiol. 32:417–427.

Martinerie, J., Adam, C., Le Van Quyen, M., et al. 1998. Epileptic seizures can be anticipated by non-linear analysis. Nat. Med. 4(10):1173.

Mathieu, M., Tirsch, W., and Poppl, S.J. 1975. Multichannel online EEG analysis by means of an autoregressive model with applications. In *Die Quantifizierung des Elektroenzephalogramms,* Eds. M. Matejcek and G.K. Schenk, pp. 475–486. Konstanz: AEG-Telefunken.

Matousek, M., and Petersén, I. 1973. Frequency analysis of the EEG in normal children and adolescents. In *Automation of Clinical Electroencephalography,* Eds. P. Kellaway and I. Petersén, pp. 75–102. New York: Raven Press.

Matousek, M., Petersén, I., and Friberg, S. 1975. Automatic assessment of randomly selected routine EEG records. In *CEAN—Computerized EEG Analysis,* Eds. G. Dolce and H. Kunkel, pp. 421–428. Stuttgart: Fischer.

Matousek, M., Arvidsson, A., and Friberg, S. 1978. Implementation of analytical methods in daily clinical EEG routine. Electroencephalogr. Clin. Neurophysiol. Suppl. 34:199–204.

Mauslby, R.L., Saltzberg, B., and Lustick, L.S. 1973. Toward an EEG screening test: a simple system for analysis and display of clinical EEG data. In *Automation of Clinical Electroencephalography,* Eds. P Kellaway and I. Petersen, pp. 45–53. New York: Raven Press.

Maynard, D.E. 1977. The cerebral function analysis monitor (CFAM). Electroencephalogr. Clin. Neurophysiol. 43:479.

Maynard, D.E., Prior, P.F., and Scott, D.F. 1969. Device for continuous monitoring of cerebral activity in resuscitated patients. Br. Med. J. 4:545.

McGillivray, B.B., and Wadbrook, D.G. 1975. A system for extracting a diagnosis from the clinical EEG. In *CEAN—Computerized EEG Analysis,* Eds. G. Dolce and H. Kunkel, pp. 344–364. Stuttgart: Fischer.

Mendel, J.M., and Fu, K.S. (Eds.). 1970. *Adaptive Learning and Pattern Recognition Systems.* New York/London: Academic Press.

Merlet, I., Garcia-Larrea, L., Grégoire, M.C., et al. 1996. Source propagation of interictal spikes in temporal lob epilepsy. Correlation between spike dipole modelling and [^{18}F]fluorodeoxyglucose PET data. Brain 119:377–392.

Mormann, F., Kreuz, T., Andrzejak, R.G., et al. 2003. Epileptic seizures are preceded by a decrease in synchronization. Epilepsy Res. 53(3):173–185.

Navarro, V., Martinerie, J., Le Van Quyen, M., et al. 2002. Seizure anticipation in human neocortical partial epilepsy. Brain. 125(pt 3):640–655.

Nuwer, M.R. 1987. Recording electrode site nomenclature. J. Clin. Neurophysiol. 4:121–133.

Nuwer, M.R., Jordan, S.E., and Ahn, S.S. 1987. Quantitative EEG is abnormal more often than routine EEG in mild stroke. Neurology 37:369.

O'Donnell, R.D., Berkhout, J., and Adey, W.R. 1974. Contamination of scalp EEG spectrum during contraction of craniofacial muscles. Electroencephalogr. Clin. Neurophysiol. 37:145–151.

Paetau, R., Kajola, M., Karhu, J., et al. 1992. Magnetoencephalographic localization of epileptic cortex—impact on surgical treatment. Ann. Neurol. 32:106–109.

Paetau, R., Hamalainen, M., Hari, R., et al. 1994. Magnetoencephalographic evaluation of children and adolescents with intractable epilepsy. Epilepsia 35:275–284.

Peters, B.O., Pfurtscheller, G., Flyvbjerg, H. 1998. Mining multi-channel EEG for its information content: an ANN-based method for a brain-computer interface. Neural Netw. 11(7–8):1429–1433.

Peters, T.E., Bhavaraju, N.C., Frei, M.G., et al. 2001. Network system for automated seizure detection and contingent delivery of therapy. J. Clin. Neurophysiol. 18(6):545–549.

Pfurtscheller, G., and Fischer, G. 1978. A new approach to spike detection using a combination of inverse and matched filter techniques. Electroencephalogr. Clin. Neurophysiol. 44:243–247.

Pfurtscheller, G., and Lopes da Silva, F.H. (Eds.). 1988. *Functional Brain Imaging.* Toronto: Hans Huber.

Pfurtscheller, G., Ladurner, G., Maresch, H., et al. 1984. Brain electrical activity mapping in normal and ischemic brain. In *Brain Ischemia: Quantitative EEG and Imaging Techniques,* Eds. G. Pfurtscheller, E.J. Jonkman, and F.H. Lopes da Silva, Progr. Brain Res. 62:287–302. Amsterdam: Elsevier.

Pfurtscheller, G., Flozinger, G., and Mohl, W. 1991. Prediction of the side of hand movements form single-trial multi-channel EEG data using a neural network; preliminary results Institutes for Information Processing, Graz. Report 299, pp. 1–11.

Pijn, J.P.M. 1990. Quantitative evaluation of EEG signals in epilepsy. Nonlinear associations, time delays and nonlinear dynamics. Ph.D. Thesis, University of Amsterdam.

Pijn, J.P., and Lopes da Silva, F.H. 1993. Propagation of electrical activity: nonlinear associations and time delays between EEG signals. In *Basic Mechanisms of the EEG,* Eds. St. Zschocke and E.-J. Speckmann, pp. 41–61. Boston: Birkhauser.

Pijn, J.P.M., Vijn, P.C.M., Lopes da Silva, F.H., et al. 1989. The use of signal analysis for the localization of an epileptic focus: A new approach. Adv. Epileptol. 17:272–276.

Poppl, S.J. 1975. Computer allocation rules for automatic EEG classification. In *CEAN—Computerized EEG Analysis,* Eds. G. Dolce and H. Kunkel, pp. 202–215. Stuttgart: Fischer.

Prichep, L.S., and John, E.R. 1986. Neurometrics: Clinical applications. In *Clinical Applications of Computer Analysis of EEG and Other Neurophysiological Signals. Handbook of Electroencephalography and Clinical Neurophysiology,* vol. 2, Eds. F.H. Lopes da Silva, W. Storm van Leeuwen, and A. Remond, pp. 153–170. Amsterdam: Elsevier.

Prichep, L.S., John, E.R., and Mas, F. 1990. Neurometric functional imaging: 1. Subtyping of schizophrenia. In *Machinery of the Mind,* Ed. E.R. John, 460–471. Boston: Birkhauser.

Prichep, L.S., John, E.R. 1992. QEEG profiles of psychiatric disorders. Brain Topogr. 4(4):249–257.

Prichep, L.S., Mas, F., Hollander, E., et al. 1993. Quantitative electroencephalographic subtyping of obsessive-compulsive disorder. Psychiatry Res. 50(1):25–32.

Prior, P. 1979. *Monitoring Cerebral Function: Long-term Recordings of Cerebral Electrical Activity.* Amsterdam: Elsevier.

Prior, P.F., Maynard, D.E., Sheaff, P.C., et al. 1971. Monitoring cerebral function: clinical experience with new device for continuous recording of electrical activity of brain. Br. Med. J. 2:736.

Pronk, R.A.F. 1986. Peri-operative monitoring. In *Clinical Applications of Computer Analysis of EEG and Other Neurophysiological Signals Handbook of Electroencephalography and Clinical Neurophysiology,* vol. 2, Eds. F.H. Lopes da Silva, W. Storm van Leeuwen, and A. Remond, pp. 93–130. Amsterdam: Elsevier.

Pronk, R.A.F., Simons, A.J.R., and de Boer, S.J. 1977. EEG as a monitoring parameter during open heart surgery. Technical aspects. Electroencephalogr. Clin. Neurophysiol. 43:542.

Rappelsberger, P. 1989. The reference problem and mapping of coherence: a stimulation study. Brain Topogr. 2:63–72.

Rechtschaffen, A., and Kales, A. 1968. *Manual of Standardized Terminology, Techniques and Scoring System for Sleep Stages of Human Subjects.* National Institutes of Health Publication No. 204. Washington, DC: U.S. Government Printing Office.

Remond, A. 1968. The importance of topographic data in EEG phenomena, and an electrical model to reproduce them. Electroencephalogr. Clin. Neurophysiol. Suppl. 27:27–49.

Remond, A., and Torres, F. 1964. A method of electrode placement with a view to topographical research. I. Basic concepts. Electroencephalogr. Clin. Neurophysiol. 17:577–578.

Ricci, G.B. 1990. Italian contributions to magnetoencephalographic studies on the epilepsies. Magnetoencephalogr. Adv. Neurol. 54:247–260.

Rogowski, Z., Gath, I., Bental, E. 1981. On the prediction of epileptic seizures. Biol. Cybern. 42(1):9–15.

Rosa, A.C. da, Kemp, B., Paiva, T., et al. 1991. A model-based detector of vertex waves and K complexes in sleep electroencephalogram. Electroencephalogr. Clin. Neurophysiol. 78:71–79.

Rose, S.W., Penry, J.K., White, B.G., et al. 1973. Reliability and validity of visual EEG assessment in third grade children. Clin. Electroencephalogr. 4:197–205.

Rose, D.F., Smith, P.D., and Sato, S. 1987. Magnetoencephalography and epilepsy research. Science 238:329–335.

Rossler, R., Collins, R., and Rostman, A. 1970. A period analysis, classification of sleep stages. Electroencephalogr. Clin. Neurophysiol. 29:358–362.

Roth, B.J., Ko, D., von Albertini-Carletti, I.R., et al. 1997. Dipole localization in patients with epilepsy using the realistically shaped head model. Electroencephalogr. Clin. Neurophysiol. 102:159–166.

Salek-Haddadi, A., Lemieux, L., Merschhemke, M., et al. 2003. EEG quality during simultaneous functional MRI of interictal epileptiform discharges. Magn. Reson. Imaging 21(10):1159–1166.

Saltzberg, B., Lustick, L.S., and Heath, R.G. 1971. Detection of focal spiking in the scalp EEG of monkeys. Electroencephalogr. Clin. Neurophysiol. 31:327–333.

Sandell, H.S.H., Jansen, B.H., Bourne, J.R., et al. 1983. A rule-based evaluation and explanation system for EEG analysis. In *MEDINFO 83,* Eds. J.H. van Bemmel, M.J. Ball, and O. Wigertz, pp. 541–544. Amsterdam: North-Holland.

Sato, S., and Malow, B.A. 1993. Electroencephalography and magnetoencephalography in epilepsy and nonepileptic disorders. Curr. Opin. Neurol. 6:708–714.

Savit, R., Li, D., Zhou, W., and Drury, I. 2001. Understanding dynamic state changes in temporal lobe epilepsy. J. Clin. Neurophysiol. 18(3):246–258.

Scherg, M., Ille, N., Bornfleth, H., et al. 2002. Advanced tools for digital EEG review: virtual source montages, whole head mapping, correlation and phase analysis. J. Clin. Neurophysiol. 19:91–112.

Scheuer, M.L. 2002. Continuous EEG monitoring in the intensive care unit. Epilepsia 43(suppl 3):114–127.

Simon, N.R., Manshanden, I., Lopes da Silva, F.H. 2000. A MEG study of sleep. Brain Res. 860(1–2):64–76.

Simons, A.J.R., Pronk, R.A.F., and de Boer, S.J. 1977. EEG as a monitoring parameter during open heart surgery. Electroencephalogr. Clin. Neurophysiol. 43:526.

Skrandies, W., and Lehmann, D. 1982. Spatial principal components of multichannel maps evoked by lateral visual half-field stimuli. Electroencephalogr. Clin. Neurophysiol. 54:662–667.

Smith, J.R. 1972. Automatic analysis and detection of EEG spikes, IEEE Trans. Biomed. Eng. BME-21:1–7.

Smith, J.R., and Karacan, I. 1971. EEG sleep stage scoring by an automatic hybrid system. Electroencephalogr. Clin. Neurophysiol. 31:231–237.

Smith, J.R., Karacan, I., and Yang, M. 1977. Ontogeny of delta activity during human sleep. Electroencephalogr. Clin. Neurophysiol. 43:229–237.

Smith, J.R., Schwartz, B.J., Gallen, Ch., et al. 1995. Utilization of multichannel magnetoencephalography in the guidance of ablative seizure surgery. J. Epilepsy 8:119–130.

Simon, N.R., Manshanden, I., Lopes da Silva, F.H. 2000. A MEG study of sleep. Brain Res. 860:64-76.

Spatt, J., Pelzi, G., and Mamoli, B. 1997. Reliability of automatic and visual analysis of interictal spikes in lateralizing an epileptic focus during video-EEG monitoring. Electroencephalogr. Clin. Neurophysiol. 103:421–425.

Spehr, W., Sartorius, H., Berglund, K., et al. 1977. EEG and haemodialysis. A structural survey of EEG spectral analysis, Hjorth's EEG descriptors, blood variables and psychological data. Electroencephalogr. Clin. Neurophysiol. 43:787–797.

Stefan, H., Schuler, P., Abraham-Fuchs, K., et al. 1994. Magnetic source localization and morphological changes in temporal lobe epilepsy: comparison of MEG/EEG, ECoG and volumetric MRI in presurgical evaluation of operated patients. Acta. Neurol. Scand. Suppl. 152:83–88.

Steriade, M., Contreras, D., Curro Dossi, R., Nunez, A. 1993. The slow (<1 Hz) oscillation in reticular thalamic and thalamocortical neurons: scenario of sleep rhythm generation in interacting thalamic and neocortical networks. J. Neurosci. 13(8):3284–3299.

Storm van Leeuwen, W., Bickford, R., Brazier, M.A.B., et al. 1966. Proposal for an EEG terminology by the Terminology Committee of the International Federation for Electroencephalography and Clinical Neurophysiology. Electroencephalogr. Clin. Neurophysiol. 20:293–320.

Storm van Leeuwen, W., Arntz, A., Spoclstra, P., et al. 1976. The use of computer analysis for diagnosis in routine electroencephalography. Rev. EEG Neurophysiol. 6:2:318–327.

Sutherling, W.W., and Barth, D.S. 1990. Magnetoencephalography in clinical epilepsy studies: the UCLA experience. Magnetoencephalogr. Adv. Neurol. 54:231–246.

Teschan, P.E. 1974. Electroencephalographic and other neurophysiological abnormalities in uremia. In Proc. Conf. on Adequacy of Dialysis, Monterey, CA.

Tharp, B.R., and Gersch, W. 1976. Spectral analysis of seizures in humans. Comput. Biomed. Res. 8:503–521.

Tou, J.T., and Gonzalez, R.C. 1974. *Pattern Recognition Principles.* Reading, MA: Addison-Wesley.

Ursin, R., Moses, J., Naitoh, P., et al. 1983. REM-NREM cycle in the cat may be sleep-dependent. Sleep 6:1–9.

Van 't Ent, D., Manshanden, I., Ossenblok, P., et al. Spike cluster analysis in neocortical localization related epilepsy yields clinically significant equivalent source localization results in magnetoencephalogram (MEG). Clin. Neurophysiol. 114(10):1948–1962.

Vigário, R.N. 1997. Extraction of ocular artefacts from EEG using independent component analysis. Electroencephalogr. Clin. Neurophysiol. 103:395–404.

Vigário, R.N., Jousmäki, V., Hämäläinen, M., et al. 1998. Independent component analysis for the identification of artefact in magnetoencephalographic recordings. In *Advances in Neural Information Processing Systems 10,* Eds. M.I. Jordan, M.J. Kearns, and S.A. Solla, pp. 229–235. Cambridge, MA: MIT Press.

Viglione, S.S. 1974. Validation of epilepsy seizure warning system MDAC Paper APA 74133. West Huntington Beach, CA: McDonnell Douglas Astronautics Co.

Viglione, S.S., and Martin, W.B. 1973. Automatic analysis of the EEG for sleep staging. In *Automation of Clinical Electroencephalography,* Eds. P. Kellaway and I. Petersen, pp. 269–285. New York: Raven Press.

Viglione, S.S., Ordon, V.A., and Risch, F. 1970. A methodology for detecting ongoing changes in the EEG prior to clinical seizures MDAC Paper WD 1399, West Huntington Beach, CA: McDonnell Douglas Astronautics Co.

Visser, G.H., Wieneke, G.H., Van Huffelen, A.C., et al. 2001. The development of spectral EEG changes during short periods of circulatory arrest. J. Clin. Neurophysiol. 18(2):169–177.

Volavka, J., Matousek, M., Feldstein, S., et al. 1973. The reliability of EEG assessment. EEG-EMG 4:123–130.

Walter, W.G., and Shipton, H.W. 1951. A new toposcopic display system. Electroencephalogr. Clin. Neurophysiol. 3:281–292.

Webber, W.R.S., Litt, B., Lesser, R.P., et al. 1993. Automatic EEG spike detection: what should the computer imitate? Electroencephalogr. Clin. Nerurophysiol. 87:364–373.

Webber, W.R.S., Litt, B., Wilson, K., et al. 1994. Practical detection of epileptiform discharges in the EEG using an artificial neural network: a comparison of raw and parametrized EEG data. Electroencephalogr. Clin. Neurophysiol. 91:194–204.

Webber, W.R.S., Harner, R.N., Duffy, F.H., et al. 1996. Spike detection. I. Correlation and reliability of human experts. Electroencephalogr. Clin. Neurophysiol. 98:186–198.

Wendling, F., Bartolomei, F., Bellanger, J.J., et al. 2002. Epileptic fast activity can be explained by a model of impaired GABAergic dendritic inhibition. Eur. J. Neurosci. 15(9):1499–1508.

Whitton, J.L., Lue, F., and Moldofsky, H. 1978. A spectra method for removing eye movement artifacts from the EEG. Electroencephalogr. Clin. Neurophysiol. 44:735–741.

Williamson, S.J., and Kaufman, L. 1989. Advances in neuromagnetic instrumentation and studies of spontaneous brain activity. Brain Topogr. 2:129–140.

Wilson, S.B., Harner, R.N., Dufy, F.H., et al. 1996. Spike detection I. Correlation and reliability of human experts. Electroencephalogr. Clin. Neurophysiol. 98:186–198.

Wilson, S.B., Turner, C.A., Emerson, R.G., et al. 1999. Spike detection II.: automatic, perception-based detection and clustering. Clin. Neurophysiol. 110(3):404–411.

Woestenburg, J.C., Verbaten, M.N., and Slangen, J.L. 1983. The removal of the eye-movement artifact from the EEG by regression analysis in the frequency domain. Biol. Psychol. 16:127–147.

Yang, M.C.K., and Hursch, C.J. 1973. The use of a semi-Markow model for describing sleep pattern. Biometrics 29:667–676.

Zetterberg, L.H. 1973a. Experience with analysis and simulation of EEG signals with parametric description of spectra. In *Automation of Clinical Electroencephalography,* Eds. P. Kellaway and I. Petersén, pp. 161–201. New York: Raven Press.

Zetterberg, L.H. 1973b. Spike detection by computer and by analog equipment. In *Automation of Clinical Electroencephalography,* Eds. P. Kellaway and I. Petersén, pp. 227–242. New York: Raven Press.

Zhang, X., van Drongelen, W., Hecox, K.E., et al. 2003. High resolution EEG: cortical potential imaging of interictal spikes. Clin. Neurophysiol. 114:1963–1973.

Zung, W.W.K., Naylor, T.H., Gianturco, D., et al. 1965. A Markov chain model of sleep EEG pattern. Electroencephalogr. Clin. Neurophysiol. 19:105.

60. EEG-Based Brain-Computer Interfaces

Gert Pfurtscheller and Christa Neuper

Introduction and Basic Principles

A relatively recent development in applied neurophysiology is an approach called electroencephalogram (EEG)-based brain-computer interfaces (BCIs), by means of which specific features automatically extracted from EEG signals are used to operate computer-controlled devices to assist patients who have highly compromised motor functions, as is the case of tetraplegic patients. This novel approach became possible due to advances both in methods of EEG analysis and in information technology, allied to a better understanding of the psychophysiological correlates of certain EEG features. Therefore, it is interesting to take notice of the emerging field of BCI, which is a technical system that allows direct communication between brain and computer (Vidal, 1973). BCI provides a communication channel that can be used to convey messages and commands directly from the brain to the external world. For this purpose, the processing of brain signals [EEG, electrocorticogram (ECoG), multiunit activity] has to be done in real time.

The current, most important applications of a BCI include the restoration of communication for patients in a locked-in state and the control of neuroprosthesis in patients with spinal cord injuries (Pfurtscheller and Neuper, 2001; Wolpaw et al., 2002). In addition to these applications, we should also note the field of neurofeedback therapy and the upcoming field of multimedia and virtual reality applications (Ebrahimi et al., 2003).

A BCI system, in general, contains components for feature extraction and classification (detection) of EEG events (Fig. 60.1). The goal of the feature extraction component is to find a suitable representation of the EEG signal that simplifies the subsequent classification or detection of specific patterns of electrical brain activity. That is, the signal features should encode the commands sent by the user, but should not contain noise and other signal components that can impede the classification process. There are various feature extraction methods used in current BCI systems. A nonexhaustive list of these methods includes amplitude and band power measures, Hjorth parameters, autoregressive parameters, and wavelet coefficients (Graimann et al., 2003; Obermaier et al., 2001; Pfurtscheller and Neuper, 2001).

The task of the classifier is to use the signal features provided by the feature extractor to assign the recorded samples of the signal to a given category of EEG patterns. In the simplest form, detection of an EEG pattern may be made, for instance, by means of a threshold method (Birbaumer et al., 2000; Levine et al., 2000). More sophisticated classification algorithms of different EEG patterns depend on the use of linear or nonlinear classifiers (Blankertz et al., 2002; Millan et al., 2002; Pfurtscheller and Neuper, 2001).

The classifier output, which can be a simple on-off signal or a signal that encodes a number of different classes, is transformed into an appropriate signal that can then be used to control a variety of devices. For most current BCI systems, the output device is a computer screen, and the desired output consists of the selection of certain targets. Advanced applications include controlling of spelling systems or other external apparatuses such as prosthetic devices and multimedia applications.

Feedback of performance is usually obtained by visualization of the classifier output on a computer screen or by presentation of an auditory, tactile, or visual feedback signal. Feedback is an integral part of the BCI system because the users have to receive information about the behavior of the devices that they controlled, by means of the brain signals they produced.

When the user performs a mental task and, therewith, intends to transmit a message, the BCI enters into operation. In principle, two distinct modes of operation can be distinguished, the first being externally paced (cue-based, computer-driven, synchronous BCI) and the second internally paced (non-cue-based, user-driven, asynchronous BCI). In the case of a synchronous BCI, a fixed, predefined time window is used. After a visual or auditory cue stimulus, the subject has to act and produce a specific brain pattern. Nearly all known BCI systems work in such a cue-based mode (Kübler et al., 2001; Pfurtscheller and Neuper, 2001; Wolpaw et al., 2002). An asynchronous protocol requires a continuous analysis and feature extraction of the recorded brain signal. Thus, such BCIs are in general, even more demanding and more complex than BCIs operating with a fixed timing scheme. To date, only a few research groups have been working on asynchronous BCI systems (Blankertz et al., 2002; Graimann et al., 2003; Levine et al., 2000; Mason and Birch, 2000).

EEG Patterns Used As Input for a BCI

In the EEG (as well as in the ECoG) two types of phenomena can be differentiated that are relevant for a BCI system:

1. Event-related potentials (ERPs), including evoked potentials, slow cortical potential (SCP) shifts, and steady-state evoked potentials.
2. Event-related changes of ongoing EEG activity in specific frequency bands. Event-related desynchronization (ERD) defines an amplitude (power) decrease of a rhythmic component, whereas event-related synchronization (ERS) characterizes an amplitude (power) increase (Pfurtscheller and Lopes da Silva, 1999; see also Chapter 51).

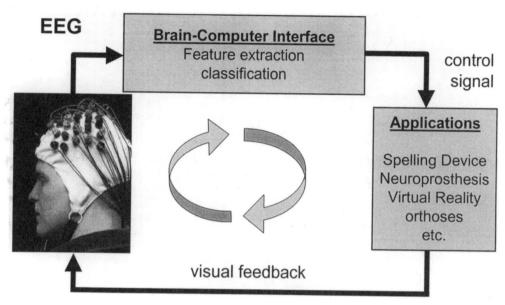

Figure 60.1. Basic principle of an EEG-based brain–computer interface (BCI) system. EEG signals from the user's brain are acquired and processed to extract specific features used for classification. The classifier output is transformed into a device command to operate the respective application, which, at the same time, provides feedback to the user.

In a simplified form it may be assumed that ERPs represent the summative responses of cortical neurons due to changes of the afferent activity, while ERD/ERS reflect changes of the activity of local interactions between main neurons and interneurons that control the frequency components of ongoing EEG/ECoG components.

Slow cortical potentials (SCPs) are slow shifts of the EEG with a duration from 300 ms to several seconds. These signals have been used by Birbaumer et al. (1999) to operate the so-called EEG-based thought–translation device, in which the subjects learn to produce negative or positive SCP shifts by means of biofeedback.

A communication system that made use of the P300 component of visual evoked potentials (VEPs) was developed by Donchin et al. (2000). This BCI is based on the presentation of a 6 × 6 letter matrix in which rows and columns are flashed at short intervals. When the user's attention focuses on a certain item, a large P300 amplitude is produced.

BCI systems based on the evaluation of steady-state visual evoked potentials (SSVEPs) were reported by Middendorf et al. (2000) and Cheng et al. (2003). The system of Cheng et al. uses 13 buttons arranged as a virtual telephone keypad and flickering at different frequencies. The subject has to direct his/her gaze to one of the flashing buttons in order to enhance the amplitude of the corresponding flicker frequency (SSVEP).

With the BCI system of Wolpaw et al. (2000, 2002) subjects with motor disabilities learn to control the amplitude of mu and beta rhythms and use these control signals to move a cursor, in one or two dimensions, to targets on a computer screen. In a similar way, the Graz-BCI system transforms the dynamics of mu and central beta rhythms (ERD, ERS) during motor imagery into a control signal that can be used to operate a virtual keyboard (Neuper et al., 2003; Ober-

maier et al., 2001), or to control the operation of a prosthetic device to restore hand grasp function (Pfurtscheller et al., 2000, 2003b) (for more details, see Applications, below).

Motor Imagery As Control Strategy

Several EEG studies indicate that primary sensorimotor areas are activated when subjects imagine the execution of a hand movement. Klass and Bickford (1957) and Chatrian et al. (1959) observed blocking or desynchronization of the central mu-rhythm with motor imagery. By means of quantification of the temporal-spatial ERD pattern, it was clearly shown that one-sided hand motor imagery can result in a lateralized activation of sensorimotor areas, similarly to that found in the preparatory phase of a self-paced hand/finger movement (Pfurtscheller and Neuper, 1997). Furthermore, measurements of slow potential shifts (Beisteiner et al., 1995) have shown that similar changes over the contralateral hand area can be observed during execution and imagination of movement. Also multichannel neuromagnetic measurements demonstrated the effect of motor imagery on brain oscillations generated in primary motor areas (Schnitzler et al., 1997).

An example is shown in Fig. 60.2 in the form of band power time courses of 11- to 13-Hz EEG activity. The ERD/ERS curves show different reactivity patterns during right and left motor imagery, displaying a significant band power decrease (ERD) over the contralateral hand area. It is of interest to note, first, that contralateral to the side of motor imagery an ERD and ipsilaterally an ERS were present and, second, that feedback enhanced the difference between both patterns and therewith the classification accuracy (see also Neuper et al., 1999).

The enhancement of oscillatory EEG activity (ERS) during motor imagery is a very important aspect in BCI

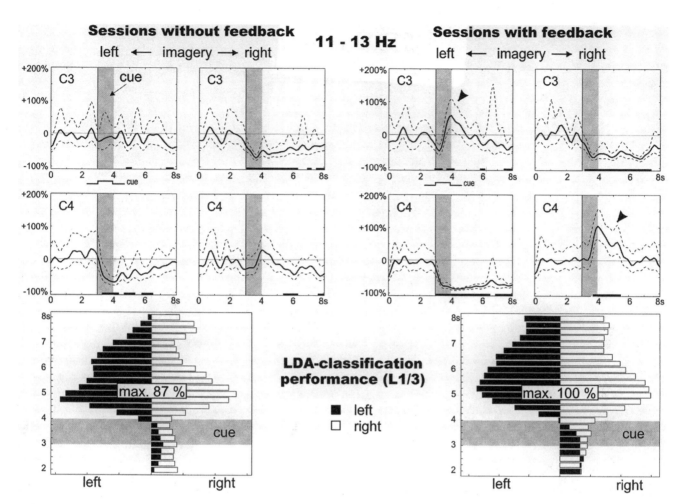

Figure 60.2. **Top:** Event-related desynchronization (ERD)/event-related synchronization (ERS) curves (11–13 Hz; 95% confidence intervals indicated) of one representative subject during imagined movements of the left versus right hand, in sessions without feedback (**left panels**) and in sessions with continuously present feedback (**right panels**). Data were recorded from the sensorimotor cortex (C3, C4). The time period of cue presentation is indicated by a *gray vertical bar.* **Bottom:** Examples of classification results of single trials (based on linear discriminant analysis, LDA) of two selected sessions, one without (**left side**) and one with feedback (**right side**), respectively. The x-axis denotes the average size of the distance function (resulting from LDA) for all left and right trials of one session (for details, see Neuper et al., 1999). In the session with feedback, the average distance corresponds to the average length of the feedback bar presented on the screen. *Black bars* indicate bar movements to the left side of the screen, *white bars* indicate bar movements to the right side. The y-axis displays the time points used for classification. The best classification accuracy for each session is indicated.

research. For example, foot motor imagery can induce beta oscillations over the foot representation area close to the vertex (Fig. 60.3), but also mu oscillations over both hand representation areas (Neuper and Pfurtscheller, 1999).

Summarizing, it can be stated that motor imagery can modify sensorimotor rhythms in a similar way to that observed in the preparatory phase of an executed movement. Since motor imagery results in somatotopically organized activation patterns, mental imagination of different movements (e.g., left vs. right hand; hand vs. foot) can be an efficient strategy to operate a BCI based on oscillatory EEG activity. The challenge is to detect the imagery-related changes in ongoing, unaveraged EEG recordings.

Training Paradigm and Information Transfer Rate

The use of the P300 component (Donchin et al., 2000) or the SSVEP (Cheng et al., 2002) for communication requires some conscious control of eye muscles and therefore is not applicable for some categories of patients, e.g., in the late stages of amyotrophic lateral sclerosis (ALS). In these cases EEG-based control by means of a motor imagery strategy may be the only way to establish a communication channel. A very important step in EEG-based communication with motor imagery is that the computer has to learn to recognize EEG patterns associated with one or more states of mental imagery. This implies that the computer has to be adapted to

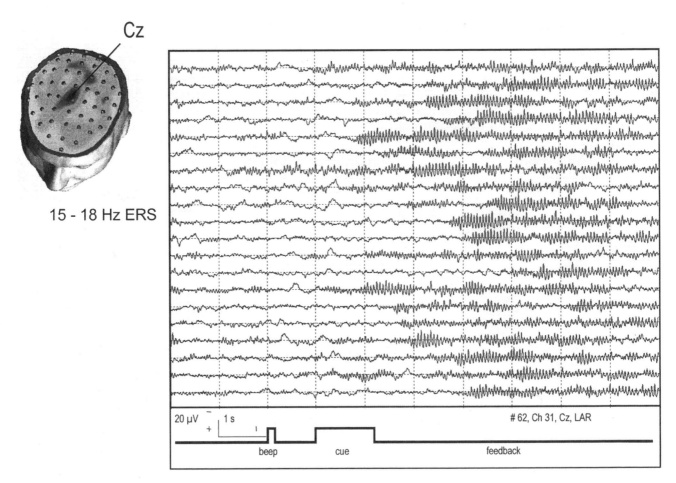

Figure 60.3. Right side: Examples of single EEG trials (tetraplegic patient T.S.) during foot motor imagery showing trains of 17-Hz beta oscilla- tions. **Left side:** Topographic map indicating the localized 17-Hz ERS close to the electrode position Cz.

the brain activity of a specific subject, a process that can last for many days or weeks. After a learning or training process, and when a classifier is available, the online classification of single EEG trials can start, and feedback can be provided. To keep the training period as short as possible, an efficient training strategy is necessary. One example of this is the so-called basket game, in which the user has to mentally move a falling ball into the correct goal ("basket") marked on the screen (Fig. 60.4, left side) (Krausz et al., 2003). The horizontal position of the ball is controlled via the BCI output signal and the falling speed can be adjusted by the investigator. Four male volunteers with spinal-cord injuries participated in a study using this paradigm. None of them had any prior experience with BCI. Two bipolar EEG signals were recorded from electrode positions close to C3 and C4, respectively. Two different types of motor imagery (either right vs. left hand motor imagery or hand vs. foot motor imagery) were used and band power within the alpha band and the beta band were classified. The patient's task was to hit the highlighted basket (which changed side randomly from trial to trial) as often as possible. The speed was increased run by run until the patient judged it as too fast. In this way it was attempted to find the optimal speed for a maximum in-

formation transfer rate. After each run users were asked to rate their performance and to suggest whether the system operated too slow or too fast. The highest information transfer rate of 17 bits/min was reached with a trial length of 2.5 seconds (Fig 60.4, right side) (Krausz et al., 2003).

The Wadsworth BCI (Wolpaw et al., 2002) is designed to improve the communication and control capacities and quality of life in patients with severe motor disabilities. This BCI has focused primarily on EEG rhythms recorded from sensorimotor cortex to control cursor movement in one or two dimensions with the goal to select characters. Well-trained users have achieved an information transfer rate (ITR) of up to 20 to 25 bits/min, by directing a horizontally moving ball in one of up to eight different targets (McFarland et al., 2000). At this time, beside brain oscillations also other signal features as ERP components were included to improve speed and accuracy (Wolpaw et al., 2003). In a different approach, an EEG-based BCI with three mental tasks, Millan and Mourino (2003) reported an average ITR of 13 bits/min in four trained subjects.

When the amplitude of brain oscillations is used to control a BCI, the ITR is limited by the time needed for EEG desynchronization and synchronization to be detected. For exam-

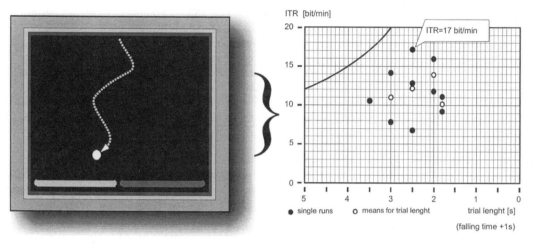

"Move the ball into the indicated basket."

falling time varied between 3 – 5 s (pause 1s)

Figure 60.4. **Left side:** Graphical display of the "basket-paradigm." The subject has to direct the ball to the indicated goal ("basket"). The trial length varies across the different runs. **Right side:** Information transfer rate (ITR) for one subject in relation to trial length. The *black line* represents the maximum possible ITR for an error-free classification. (Modified from Krausz, G., Scherer, R., Korisek, G., et al. 2003. Critical decision speed and information transfer in the Graz Brain-Computer Interface. Appl. Psychophysiol. Biofeedback, in press.)

ple, in the case of alpha rhythms at least several seconds are needed for desynchronization and resynchronization to become evident. In the case of a (de)synchronization time of 3 seconds, a maximum theoretical ITR of 20 bits/min is possible with two mental tasks. The ITR can be slightly increased when, instead of alpha, faster reacting beta rhythms are used for control. But, independent of the used frequency components, the most crucial factor for obtaining a high ITR in BCI applications is the classification accuracy. When the ITR with two mental tasks and 100% classification accuracy is 12 bits/min, the ITR drops to 4 bits/min with 80% classification accuracy (Wolpaw et al., 2002).

Also of interest is the work of the Berlin group (Blankertz et al. 2003). In a first attempt they were able to predict movement preparation (right vs. left-hand finger movement) from single trial EEG by classification of the Bereitschaftspotential (readiness potential) with nearly 100% accuracy. In four subjects they reported an ITR of 6 to 10 bits/min.

Applications

Currently, there are two important applications of a BCI. The first is to provide a new communication channel for patients severely affected by loss of all voluntary muscle control, including eye movement, and suffering, for example, from ALS or brain state stroke. The second is to restore muscle functions in patients with spinal cord injuries either to control functional electrical stimulation (FES) or to operate a neuroprosthesis or orthoses. For both applications, speed and accuracy are important.

It was demonstrated that patients suffering from advanced ALS can acquire the ability to operate a spelling device referred to as a "thought translation device" (TTD) by regulating their slow cortical potentials (Birbaumer et al., 1999). The selection of one character takes 4 seconds. During a 2-second period the user's cortical potential level is measured and compared with a 2-second baseline level. The potential difference is displayed as vertical cursor movement and used to select letters or characters. Patients with ALS were able to operate the TTD with one to two characters per minute. Over the past years more than 18 patients diagnosed with neuromuscular diseases were trained to control the TTD; in the case of a few patients the feasibility of long-term BCI use (e.g., for more than 5 years) was confirmed (Kübler et al., 2001; Neumann et al., 2003).

Moreover, it was also shown that a BCI based on oscillatory EEG changes, induced by motor imagery, can be utilized to restore communication in severely disabled people (Neuper et al., 2003). The novel aspect was that a patient, diagnosed with cerebral palsy who had lost all voluntary muscle control learned how to control, how to enhance, and how to suppress specific frequency components of the sensorimotor EEG by using a motor imagery strategy. In order for the patient to obtain control over his brain oscillations, BCI training sessions had to be conducted two times a week over a time period of several months.

In a project with a tetraplegic patient, FES resulting in hand grasp was controlled by ongoing EEG activity based on an asynchronous BCI. The patient underwent a large number of BCI training sessions with varying types of motor imagery over a period of several months (Pfurtscheller et al., 2000). At the end he was able to induce trains of 17-Hz beta oscillations focused on the electrode position near the vertex (Cz) by foot motor imagery (Fig. 60.3). These mentally induced 17-Hz oscillations were used as a simple asynchronous brain switch to generate a control signal for the operation of the FES using surface electrodes (Fig. 60.5). With this method the patient was able to grasp a glass at "will" (for a detailed description of the procedure see Pfurtscheller et al., 2003b).

Perspectives for the Future

A clear challenge for the future is to realize more effective BCI control paradigms, offering, for instance, three-dimensional (3D) control over a neuroprosthesis or the operation of a spelling device with a speed of at least five to ten characters/minute. Both applications should be realizable by either an enhancement of the classification accuracy or the discrimination between three or more brain states.

We should note that an improvement of speed and accuracy is possible when, instead of EEG records, one would use directly cortical potential changes recorded with ECoG electrode strips or grids or even to record neuronal firing patterns using intracortical semi-microelectrode recordings.

The advantage of the ECoG over the EEG is the better signal-to-noise ratio and therefore also the easier detection of gamma activity. Recently, bursts of gamma activity between 60 and 90 Hz in ECoG recordings during self-paced limb and tongue movements were reported (Crone et al., 1999; Pfurtscheller et al., 2003a). These gamma bursts are short lasting, display a high somatotopic specificity and are embedded in the alpha and beta ERD lasting for some seconds. Patient-oriented work with subdural electrodes and ECoG single trial classification has shown initial promising results (Graimann et al., 2003; Levine et al., 2000).

Studies in monkeys have shown that 3D control is possible when multiunit activity is recorded in cortical areas. Between 32 and 96 microwires were implanted in different cortical motor areas. After a training period with distinct motor tasks, the monkeys were able to achieve 3D control over the movement of a robotic device by real-time transformation of neuronal multiunit neuronal activity (Wessberg et al., 2000). The feasibility of direct cursor control for the selection of icons or letters using an implanted neurotropic cortical electrode in patients was already demonstrated by Kennedy et al. (2000).

At this time, nearly all BCI systems (for a comprehensive review see Wolpaw et al., 2002) are cue-based or computer-driven (synchronous BCI). This means that the time window

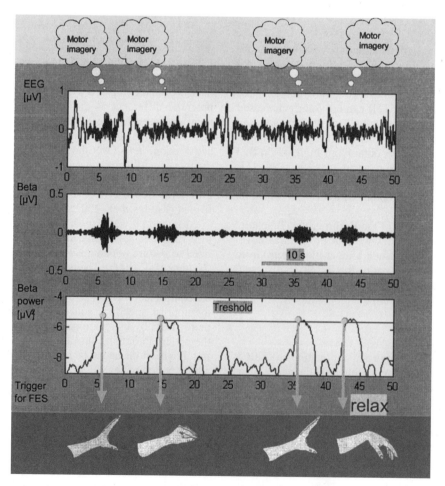

Figure 60.5. Examples of bipolar EEG recording (tetraplegic patient T.S.) from the vertex *(upper trace)*, band pass filtered (15–19 Hz) EEG signal *(middle trace)*, and band power time course *(lower trace, arbitrary units)* over a time period of about 1 minute. Each imagined foot movement induced a beta burst; depending on the threshold, a trigger pulse was initiated to control functional electrical stimulation to restore hand grasp.

where a mental task has to be recognized is predefined. An uncued or user-driven BCI (asynchronous BCI) where the EEG (ECoG) has to be analyzed and classified continuously is more complex. In this case, the major problem is to detect all true positives (hits) classification associated with predefined imagery tasks and to minimize the false-positive classification while the user is in the resting or idling state. Recently, Birch et al. (2002) reported true-positive rates of 70% and false-positive rates below 3% in subjects with high-level spinal cord injury using an asynchronous BCI and self-paced imagined movements.

One line of research has to be directed to design an application-independent, BCI-based pointing device as proposed by Mason and Birch (2003). Such a system uses a visual stimulator and is based either on P300 component (Donchin et al., 2000) or on SSVEPs (Cheng et al., 2002). The main goal of such a system is to overcome the limitation of the information transfer rate that is currently at about 20 bits/min, when a motor imagery strategy is used. Future research should also be focused on learning more about the underlying mechanisms of brain activity patterns related to motor imagery.

References

Beisteiner, R., Höllinger, P., Lindinger, G., et al. 1995. Mental representations of movements. Brain potentials associated with imagination of hand movements. Electroencephalogr. Clin. Neurophysiol. 96:183 -193.

Birbaumer, N., Ghanayim, N., Hinterberger, T., et al. H. 1999. A spelling device for the paralysed. Nature 398:297-298.

Birbaumer, N., Kubler, A., Ghanayim, N., et al. 2000. The thought translation device (TTD) for completely paralyzed patients. IEEE Trans. Rehab. Eng. 8(2):190-193.

Birch, G. E., Bozorgzadeh, Z., and Mason S.G. 2002. Initial on-line evaluations of the LF-ASD brain-computer interface with able-bodied and spinal-cord subjects using imagined voluntary motor potentials. IEEE Trans. Neural Syst. Rehab. Eng. 10:219-224.

Blankertz, B., Dornhege, G., Schäfer, C., Krepki, R., Kohlmorgen, J., Müller, K.R., Kunzmann, V., Losch, F., and Curio, G. 2003. Boosting bit rates and error detection for the classification of fast-paced motor commands based on single-trial EEG analysis. IEEE Trans. Neural Sys. Rehab. Eng. 11(2):127–131.

Chatrian, G.E., Petersen, M.C., and Lazarte, J.A. 1959. The blocking of the rolandic wicket rhythm and some central changes related to movement. Electroencephalogr. Clin. Neurophysiol. 11:497 -510.

Cheng, M., Gao, X., and Gao, S. 2002. Design and implementation of a brain-computer interface with high transfer rates. IEEE Trans. Biomed. Eng. 49:1181-1186.

Crone, N.E., Miglioretti, D.L., Gordon, B., et al. 1998. Functional mapping of human sensorimotor cortex with electrocorticographic spectral analysis. II. Event-related synchronization in the gamma band. Brain 121:2301–2315.

Donchin, E., Spencer, K.M., and Wijesinghe, R. 2000. The mental prosthesis: assessing the speed of a P300-based brain-computer interface. IEEE Trans. Rehabil. Eng. 8(2):174-179.

Ebrahimi, T., Vesin, J.-M., and Garcia, G. 2003. Brain-computer interface in multimedia communication. IEEE Signal Processing Magazine 20(1): 14-24.

Graimann, B., Huggins, J.E., Levine, S.P., et al. 2003. Detection of ERP and ERD/ERS patterns in single ECoG channels. Proc. 1st Int. IEEE EMBS Conf. Neural Eng., Capri Island, Italy, 614-617.

Kennedy, P.R, Bakay, R.A.E., Moore, M.M., et al. 2000. Direct control of a computer from the human central nervous system. IEEE Trans. Rehabil. Eng. 8(2):198-202.

Klass, S.G., Bickford, R.G., 1957. Observations on the rolandic arceau rhythm. Electroencephalogr. Clin. Neurophysiol. 9:570.

Krausz, G., Scherer, R., Korisek, G., and Pfurtscheller, G. 2003. Critical decision speed and information transfer in the Graz Brain-Computer Interface. Appl. Psychophysiol. Biofeedback 28(3):233–240.

Kübler, A., Kotchoubey, B., Kaiser, J., et al. 2001. Brain-computer communication: unlocking the locked in. Psychol. Bull. 127(3):358-375.

Levine, S.P., Huggins, J.E., BeMent, S.L., et al. 2000. A direct brain interface based on event-related potentials. IEEE Trans. Rehabil. Eng. 8(2): 180-185.

Mason, S.G., and Birch, G.E. 2000. A brain-controlled switch for asynchronous control applications. IEEE Trans. Biomed. Eng. 47(10):1297-1307.

Mason, S.G., and Birch, G.E. 2003. A general framework for describing brain-computer interface design. IEEE Trans. Neural Syst. Rehabil. Eng. 11:72-87.

McFarland, D.J., Sarnacki, W.A., Vaughan, T.M., and Wolpaw, J.R. 2000. EEG-based brain-computer interface (BCI) communication: effects of target number and trial length on information transfer rate. Soc. Neurosci. Abst. 26:128.

Middendorf, M., McMillan, G. Calhoun, G., et al. 2000. Brain-computer interfaces based on the steady-state visual-evoked response. IEEE Trans. Rehabil. Eng. 8:211-214.

Millan, J., and Mourino, J. 2003. Asynchronous BCI and local neural classifiers: an overview of the adaptive brain interface project. IEEE Trans. Neural Syst. Rehabil. Eng. 11(2):159-161.

Millan, J., Mourino, J., Franze, M., et al. 2002. A local neural classifier for the recognition of EEG patterns associated to mental tasks. IEEE Trans. Neural Networks 13:678-686.

Neumann, N., Kübler, A., Kaiser, J., et al. 2003. Consciouis perception of brain states: mental strategies for brain-computer communication. Neuropsychologia 41:1028-1036.

Neuper, C., and Pfurtscheller, G. 1999. Motor imagery and ERD. In *Event-Related Desynchronization. Handbook of Electroencephalography and Clinical Neurophysiology,* revised edition, Eds. G. Pfurtscheller and F.H. Lopes da Silva, vol. 6, pp. 303-325. Amsterdam: Elsevier.

Neuper, C., Schlögl, A., and Pfurtscheller, G. 1999. Enhancement of left-right sensorimotor EEG differences during feedback-regulated motor imagery. J. Clin. Neurophysiol. 16(4):373-382.

Neuper, C., Muller, G.R., Kübler, A., et al. 2003. Clinical application of an EEG-based brain-computer interface: a case study in a patient with severe motor impairment. Clin. Neurophysiol. 114(3):399-409.

Obermaier, B., Neuper, C., Guger, C., et al. 2001. Information transfer rate in a five-classes brain-computer interface. IEEE Trans. Neural Syst. Rehabil. Eng. 9(3):283-288.

Pfurtscheller, G., and Lopes da Silva, F.H., 1999. Event-related EEG/MEG synchronization and desynchronization: basic principles. Clin. Neurophysiol. 110:1842 -1857.

Pfurtscheller, G., and Neuper, C. 1997. Motor imagery activates primary sensorimotor area in humans. Neurosci. Lett. 239:65-68.

Pfurtscheller, G., and Neuper, C. 2001. Motor imagery and direct brain-computer communication. Proc. IEEE 89(7):1123-1134.

Pfurtscheller, G., Guger, C., Muller, G., et al. 2000. Brain oscillations control hand orthosis in a tetraplegic. Neurosci. Lett. 292(3):211-214.

Pfurtscheller, G., Graimann, B., Huggins, J.E., et al. 2003a. Spatiotemporal patterns of beta desynchronization and gamma synchronization in corticographic data during self-paced movement. Clin. Neurophysiol. 114: 1226-1236.

Pfurtscheller, G., Müller, G.R., Rupp, R., et al. 2003b. "Thought"-control of functional electrical stimulation to restore hand grasp in a tetraplegic. Neurosci. Lett. 351(1):33-36.

Schnitzler, A., Salenius, S., Salmelin, R., et al. 1997. Involvement of primary motor cortex in motor imagery: a neuromagnetic study. Neuroimage 6:201-208.

Vidal, J., 1973. Toward direct brain-computer communication. Annu. Rev. Biophys. Bioeng. 2:157–180.

Wessberg, J., Stambaugh, C.R., Kralik, J.D., et al. 2000. Real-time prediction of hand trajectory by ensembles of cortical neurons in primates. Nature 408:361-365.

Wolpaw, J.R., McFarland, D.J., and Vaughan T.M. 2000. Brain-computer interface research at the Wadsworth center. IEEE Trans. Rehabil. Eng. 8:222-226.

Wolpaw, J.R., Birbaumer, N., McFarland, D.J., et al. 2002. Brain-computer interfaces for communication and control. Clin. Neurophysiol. 113(6): 767-791.

61. Multimodal Monitoring of EEG and Evoked Potentials

Gert Pfurtscheller

General Aspects

The most comprehensive form of monitoring of cerebral functioning is obtained when electroencephalograph (EEG) and different modality evoked potentials (EPs) are recorded and analyzed continuously and simultaneously. This means that EEG spectra, brainstem auditory evoked potentials (BAEPs), and cervical and cortical somatosensory evoked potential (SEPs) are computed at intervals of seconds to minutes and displayed in a compressed form. In addition to EEG and EPs, other physiological signals, such as heart rate, ventilation, temperature, oxygen saturation, and blood pressure, may be useful, depending on the particular condition. This monitoring can be performed in the operating room, in the intensive care unit, in the sleep laboratory, or in the outpatient clinic. For extensive literature on this subject, see Nuwer (1986) and Chapters 42, 47, and 48 of this book.

Technical Aspects of Continuous Monitoring of EEG Spectra Combined with EPs

The techniques necessary for long-term monitoring of EEG and BAEPs were established in normal subjects by Maresch et al. (1983). They used two EEG channels (Cz-A1, Cz-A2) with broad-band amplifiers (1.5 Hz to 1.5 kHz); after amplification the signals were divided into low-frequency (EEG; lower cutoff frequency 30 Hz) and high-frequency (BAEP; upper cutoff frequency 250 Hz) branches. In other studies these responses were complemented with recordings of SEPs (Pfurtscheller et al., 1987; Steller et al., 1990). The main technical considerations in this type of analysis are that (a) different sampling frequencies must be used because of the rather different frequency contents of the signal, e.g., EEG and BAEP; and (b) the number of samples should be minimized to save memory storage, since the analysis must be done over long periods of time. A way to solve these technical problems is introduced in Fig. 61.1 by the sampling schema.

Measurements in the operating room or intensive care unit (ICU) may be easily affected by noise. To avoid main artifacts (50-Hz or 60-Hz), the interstimulus interval between auditory and somatosensory stimulation should be variable. More specifically, intervals should be alternatively small or large (e.g., to cancel 50 Hz: auditory stimulation 110/90 msec; somatosensory stimulation 210/190 msec). In addition, the stimuli should be applied either on the positive or negative peak of the main frequency EEG component.

With this technique, fairly good results are obtained in unshielded rooms and with electrical equipment nearby.

Long-Term Monitoring in the Intensive Care Unit

A great number of patients in the ICU are comatose or recovering from coma, since coma can be caused by many disorders including severe head injury, vascular lesions, encephalitis, posthypoxic or postischemic events, and drug intoxication, among others. The monitoring of ICU patients is important to detect critical situations as fast as possible, to facilitate therapeutic decisions, to monitor the level of impaired consciousness, and to predict the clinical outcome. Another important feature in the ICU is the determination and documentation of brain death, which is a prerequisite for most organ transplantations.

The following case report of a patient with unfavorable outcome underlines the importance of monitoring of comatose patients:

A 57-year-old woman with hypernephroma suffered hypertension for several years. She was admitted with a left hemisphere hemorrhage and was soporous. She had a right hemiplegia and responded appropriately to painful stimuli on the left side. The dominant EEG frequency was 5 to 6/sec, and there was a delta-wave focus over the left hemisphere. On the first day, a ventricular drainage of cerebrospinal fluid was performed. In the following 6 days, the patient's condition deteriorated. After 2 days, she developed anisocoria. One day later, respiration was insufficient. The patient showed extensor responses to painful stimuli. After 5 days, pupillary light reaction and ciliospinal, cornea, and oculocephalic reflexes were negative, and there was no longer any reaction to painful stimulation. The cranial computed tomography (CT) scan showed an enlargement of the hemorrhage and signs of an increased intracerebral pressure.

Figure 61.2 shows the various parameters registered from the time of admission, throughout the critical rise of intracerebral pressure (ICP), and until brain death was clinically determined. Five days after admission, at 6:20 a.m., the intracranial pressure rose to a critical level of 56 mm Hg, in spite of the ventricular drainage. Amplitudes of the cortical SEPs decreased and finally disappeared 30 minutes later. The peak of the EEG spectra shifted to lower frequencies. Pathological heart rate and heart rate variability were observed. Seven hours later, BAEP components IV/V vanished; another 30 minutes later, wave III disappeared, and 60 minutes later, all BAEP components were abolished.

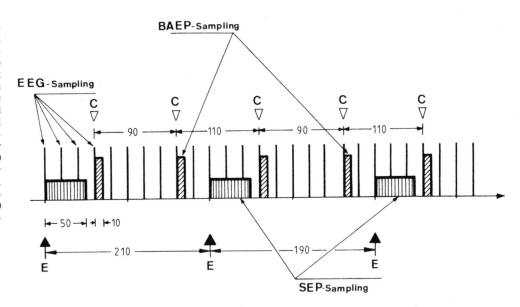

Figure 61.1. Sampling scheme of EEG, somatosensory evoked potential (SEP), and brainstem auditory evoked potential (BAEP) during computer controlled click (C) and electrical (E) median nerve stimulation as used for the data displayed in Figs. 61.2 and 60B.3; sampling and electrical and auditory stimulation are indicated. BAEP sampling lasts for 10 msec, SEP sampling for 50 msec, the SEP sampling window is variable in a range of 90 msec. Computer-controlled SEP stimulation in intervals of 210/190 msec and BAEP stimulation in intervals of 111/89 msec.

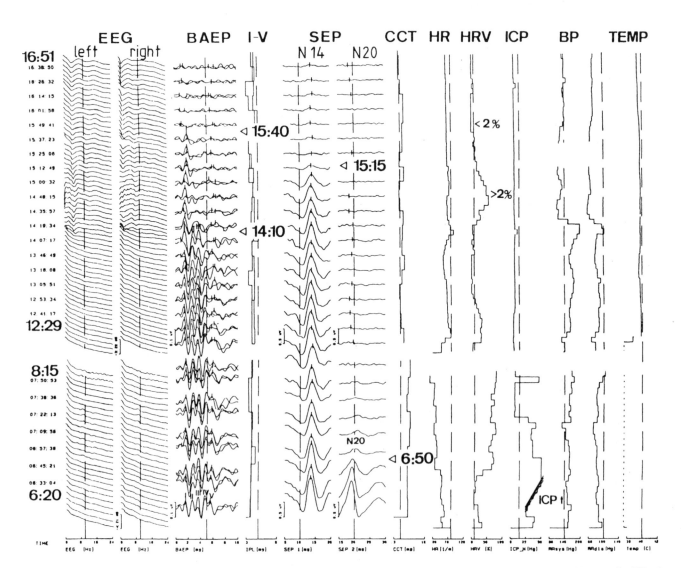

Figure 61.2. Protocol from a 57-year-old patient with a left hemispheric hemorrhage during deterioration of the comatose state and ending with brain death. From *left* to *right:* compressed EEG spectra from left and right hemispheres; brainstem auditory evoked potential (BAEP) to ipsi- and contralateral ear stimulation; BAEP interpeak latency (I–V); cervical (N14) and cortical (N20) SEPs; central conduction time (CCT); heart rate (HR); heart rate variability (HRV); intracranial pressure (ICP); systolic (BPsys) and diastolic (BPdia) blood pressure; and rectal body temperature (TEMP). Important events are indicated by *arrows.* For further explanation, see text. (Modified from Hilz, M.J., Litscher, G., Weis, M., et al. 1991. Continuous multivariable monitoring in neurological intensive care patients—preliminary reports on four cases. Intensive Care Med. 17:857–893.)

This example provides evidence that monitoring of only one signal gives incomplete information. From the SEPs alone, it can be seen that the cortical component disappeared at 6:50 a.m., whereas the cervical component remained unchanged for about 8 additional hours. The cortical component N20 is very sensitive to ischemia (Branston et al., 1984), and its disappearance signals that cortical damage occurred early in the morning. BAEPs show gradual deterioration of the waves V, IV, III, and II in the time between the disappearance of the cortical and cervical SEP components. This can be interpreted to mean that the brainstem function deteriorated during that time (starting from the midbrain level). In summary, it is clear that the most comprehensive picture of the cerebral state in comatose patients can be obtained only by monitoring different neuronal systems and signals with use of EEG, SEPs, and BAEPs.

The importance of multimodality EP measurements in patients with severe head injury was documented by Anderson et al. (1984), Greenberg et al. (1981), and others. EPs can be even more reliable than intracranial pressure measurements in predicting the clinical outcome (Anderson et al., 1984). Combined EEG and EP monitoring can also be used to differentiate comas due to structural lesions from those of metabolic origin (Guerit, 1999).

Besides EEG and EPs, the heart rate (HR) and heart rate variability (HRV) are displayed in Fig. 61.2. The HRV was initially high, dropped at 1:00 p.m., and remained depressed, with an exceptional increase during the disappearance of the cervical component of the SEP. The HRV indicates the spontaneous physiological variations in the heart rate modulated by the parasympathetic and sympathetic activity of the cardiac nerves. This activity originates mainly in the medullary circulatory center but is also influenced by higher centers (Sayers, 1973). HRV in normal subjects and in brain death was reported by Schwarz et al. (1987) and in newborns by

Mehta et al. (2002). Strong correlations exist between EEG and HRV during sleep (Ako et al., 2003). The measurement of HRV, therefore, is a sensitive parameter to monitor brainstem functions in parallel with or instead of BAEPs (BAEP measurements are not always possible in patients with severe head injury). A decrease of heart rate variability, therefore, can also indicate deterioration of brainstem function.

Monitoring in the Operating Room

In the operating room, there are two different applications for cerebral monitoring systems. One is to provide the surgeon with continuous information and warnings about potential damage to the spinal cord and other neuronal structures. Monitoring, therefore, is indicated in spinal cord operations involving risk of ischemia from compression of feeding blood vessels, aneurysm surgery, cerebrovascular procedures, and posterior fossa operations (Grundy, 1983; Nuwer, 1986). The prognostic significance of SEP, BAEP, and serum S-100B monitoring after aneurysm injury was documented by Schick et al. (2003). The second reason for cerebral monitoring is to assist the anesthetist in avoiding brain damage caused by hypoxic and/or ischemic events (Prior and Maynard, 1986), to control the depth of anesthesia, and to avoid intraoperative wakefulness (Pichlmayr et al., 1984). Further details on intraoperative monitoring are presented in Chapter 42.

Because of the different neuronal systems involved in the generation of EEG, SEPs, and BAEPs and their different sensitivity to the effect of drugs, particularly anesthetics, it is very understandable that combined monitoring of all brain signals together gives more information on neuronal signals than the monitoring of one signal alone.

An example of multiparametric monitoring of EEG spectra combined using different modality EPs under halothane anesthesia is demonstrated in Fig. 61.3. The recordings were

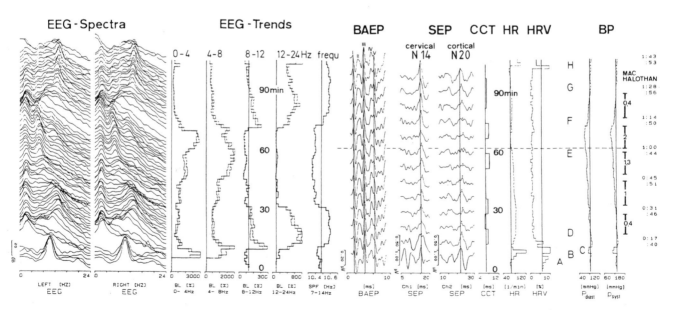

Figure 1.3. Protocol from a case under halothane anesthesia. From *left* to *right:* compressed EEG spectra, power trend curves (0–4 Hz, 4–8 Hz, 12–24 Hz), mean frequency (7–14 Hz), BAEPs, cervical and cortical SEPs, CCT, HR, HRV, and diastolic and systolic blood pressure (BP). On the *right* side, the level of anesthesia is marked. See text for further explanation.

taken from a 31-year-old patient during the initial phase of an orthopedic surgical intervention without neurological complications. Collection of the biological data started before anesthesia. Approximately 1 minute after administration of etomidate (Hypnomidate) (23 mg), the expected EEG changes occurred (Fig. 61.3; marked with *A*). The cardiovascular effects intensified after intubation *(B)* and after application of pancuronium (4 mg) *(C)*. With increasing concentration of halothane, changes in EEG spectra and cortical SEPs were accentuated *(E)*. The patient was monitored for more than 90 minutes. Despite the massive changes in the EEG as demonstrated in the band power trend curves due to the individual concentration, the BAEPs remained nearly unchanged. The cervical SEP showed an increase in latency of 1 msec, and the cortical N20 component was not identifiable with deeper levels of anesthesia. Synchronous systolic blood pressure measurements displayed a decrease from 135 to 85 mm Hg.

The protocol of Fig. 61.3 is a good example of the influence of the level of anesthesia on different neuronal systems. EEG and cortical SEPs are heavily changed, while BAEPs and cervical SEPs are only slightly modified during high levels of halothane. It is of interest to see the different behavior of power trend curves dependent on the frequency band used. Blood pressure and heart rate measurements give additional information on the cardiovascular system and should be also recorded.

Sleep Monitoring in Infants at Risk

In polysomnography, a great number of different signals must be recorded and analyzed. One goal of the sleep polygraphy in infants is to study babies at risk for sudden infant death syndrome (SIDS), that is, babies with sleep apnea and near-miss SIDS (Brass et al., 1986; Steinschneider, 1972). In this type of monitoring, in addition to the EEG, different physiological signals such as heart rate electro-oculogram (EOG), electromyogram (EMG), pO_2, and pCO_2 must be recorded and analyzed to reliably classify sleep stages and to differentiate between rapid-eye-movement (REM) (active sleep) and non-REM (NREM) (quiet sleep) state. Additional recording of BAEPs is technically possible and allows for monitoring of the brainstem at the same time. Monitoring of BAEPs during nocturnal sleep cycles was reported by Bastuji et al. (1988). They found that the latency of wave V was increased and related to physiological hypothermia during the night. This gives evidence of how sensitive BAEP measurements are and that brainstem signals are affected not only by pathophysiological but also by physiological variations.

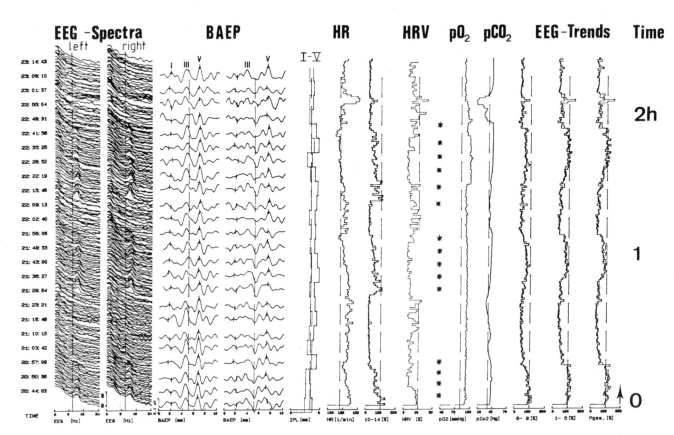

Figure 61.4. Monitoring protocol from a 4-month-old baby during active and quiet sleep. From *left* to *right:* compressed power spectra from left and right hemisphere; BAEPs ipsi- and contralateral to auditory stimulation; BAEP interpeak latency (I-V); HR; 10- to 14-Hz power trend; HRV; pO_2; pCO_2; and EEG power trend curves. For further explanation see text.

An example demonstrating the simultaneous recordings of EEG and BAEPs in a 4-month-old baby is shown in Fig. 61.4. EEG power trend curves, heart rate, po_2, and pco_2 show characteristic patterns in active sleep and quiet sleep. Slow EEG waves, spindle activity (10–12 Hz), and pco_2 increased during quiet sleep, and HR and HRV decreased. In active sleep, HR and HRV increased, and slow-wave activity and spindles decreased. A period of arousal is indicated by heart rate increase. This example again demonstrates the usefulness of simultaneous monitoring of various cardiovascular and cerebral parameters, as, for example, heart rate, oxygen saturation, EEG spectra, SEPs, and BAEPs.

References

Ako, M., Kawara, T., Uchida, S., et al. 2003. Correlation between electroencephalography and heart rate variability during sleep. Psychiatr. Clin. Neurosci. 57(1):59.

Anderson, D.C., Bundlie, S., and Rockswold, G.L. 1984. Multimodality evoked potentials in closed head trauma. Arch. Neurol. 41:369–374.

Bastuji, H., Larrea, L.G., Bertrand, O., et al. 1988. BAEP latency changes during nocturnal sleep are not correlated with sleep stages but with body temperature variations. Electroencephalogr. Clin. Neurophysiol. 70:9–15.

Branston, N.M., Ladds, A., Lindsay, S., et al. 1984. Somatosensory evoked potentials in experimental brain ischemia. In *Brain Ischemia: Quantitative EEG and Imaging Techniques, Progress in Brain Research,* vol. 62, Eds. G. Pfurtscheller, E.J. Jonkman, and F.H. Lopes da Silva, pp. 185–199. Amsterdam: Elsevier.

Brass, M., Kravath, R., and Glass, L. 1986. Death-scene investigation in sudden infant death. N. Engl. J. Med. 315:100–105.

Greenberg R.P., Newlon, P.G., Hyatt, M.S., et al. 1981. Prognostic implications of early multimodality evoked potentials in severely head-injured patients. J. Neurosurg. 55:227–236.

Grundy, B.L. 1983. Intraoperative monitoring of sensory-evoked potentials. Anesthesiology 58:72–87.

Guerit, J.M. 1999. Medical technology assessment EEG and evoked potentials in the intensive care unit. Clin. Neurophysiol. 29(4):301–317.

Hilz, M.J., Litscher, G., Weis, M., et al. 1991. Continuous multivariable monitoring in neurological intensive care patients—preliminary reports on four cases. Intensive Care Med. 17:857–893.

Maresch, H., Pfurtscheller, G., and Schuy, S. 1983. Brain function monitoring: a new method for simultaneous recording and processing of EEG-power spectrum and brainstem potentials. Biomed. Tech. 5:117–122.

Mehta, S.K., Super, D.M., Connuck, D., et al. 2002. Hear rate variability in healthy newborn infants. Am. J. Cardiol. 89:50–53.

Nuwer, M.R. 1986. *Evoked Potential Monitoring in the Operating Room.* New York: Raven Press.

Pfurtscheller, G., Schwarz, G., Schroettner, O., et al. 1987. Continuous and simultaneous monitoring of EEG-spectra and brainstem auditory and somatosensory evoked potentials in the intensive care unit and the operating room. J. Clin. Neurophysiol. 4(4):389–396.

Pichlmayr, I., Lips, K., and Künkel, H. 1984. *The Electroencephalogram in Anesthesia. Fundamentals, Practical Applications, Examples.* Berlin: Springer-Verlag.

Prior, P.F., and Maynard, D.E. 1986. *Monitoring Cerebral Function.* Amsterdam: Elsevier.

Sayers, B. 1973. Analysis of heart rate variability. Ergonomics 16:17–32.

Schick, U., Dohnert, J., Meyer, J.J., et al. 2003. Prognostic significance of SSEP, BAEP and serum S-100B monitoring after aneurysm surgery. Acta Neurol. Scand. 108(3):161–169.

Schwarz, G., Pfurtscheller, G., Litscher, G., et al. 1987. Quantification of autonomic activity in the brainstem in normal, comatose and brain dead subjects using heart rate variability. Funct. Neurol. 2:149–154.

Steinschneider, A. 1972. Prolonged apnea and the sudden infant death syndrome: clinical and laboratory observations. Pediatrics 50:646–654.

Steller, E., Litscher, G., Maresch, H., et al. 1990. Multivariables Langzeit-monitoring von zerebralen und kardiovaskulären Größen mit Hilfe eines Personal-Computers. Biomed. Tech 35:90–97.

Index

Page numbers followed by the letter "*f*" refer to figures; those followed by the letter "*t*" refer to tables.